Medical–Surgical Nursing Practice

Medical–surgical nursing practice is defined as the nursing care of adults with known or predicted physiological alteration, with trauma, or with disability. Nursing care includes the care and treatment necessary to provide comfort; to assist individuals in the promotion and maintenance of health and the prevention, detection, and treatment of illness; to promote restoration to highest possible productive capacities; and to assist with a peaceful death. Medical–surgical nursing practice encompasses patient assessment, planning, implementation, and evaluation. It takes into account the interrelatedness of biological, psychological, and social components of the patient's response or adjustment to the physiological alteration, trauma, or disability.

The field of medical–surgical nursing makes use of theories that address ethics, stress/adaptation, learning and communication, behavioral change, disease, and systems. A body of knowledge for practice is emerging from scholarly conceptualizations and research findings generated from intra- and inter-disciplinary studies.

Medical–surgical nursing encompasses the following elements:

1. Maintenance or restoration of normal patterns of functioning in areas such as sleep, rest, ventilation, activity, nutrition, elimination, sexuality, and skin integrity

2. Pain and discomfort

3. Emotional problems related to illness and treatment, such as grief, loss, anxiety, and depression

4. Knowledge for maintenance of health

5. Self-care

6. Decision making and exercise of personal choice

7. The dying process and death

From "*A Statement on the Scope of Medical–Surgical Nursing Practice*," American Nurses' Association, Division on Medical–Surgical Nursing Practice. Kansas City, MO: 1980. Reprinted with permission.

Adult
Health
Nursing

A Biopsychosocial Approach

Adult
Health
Nursing

A Biopsychosocial Approach

Carol Ren Kneisl, RN, MS
SueAnn Wooster Ames, RN, MS, RNC

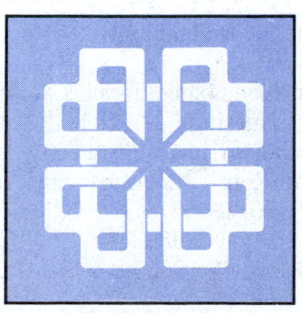

Addison-Wesley Publishing Company

Reading, Massachusetts ● Menlo Park, California ● Don Mills, Ontario ● Wokingham, England
Amsterdam ● Sydney ● Singapore ● Tokyo ● Madrid ● Bogotá ● Santiago ● San Juan

This book is dedicated to clients and the nurses who care for them

Sponsoring Editor: Nancy Evans
Production Supervisor: Glenda Epting
Production Coordinator: Anne Friedman
Art Coordinator: Helene Harrington
Permissions: Maureen Schaeffer
Developmental Editors: Mary Berry, Charles Campbell,
Shirley Hentzell, Lillian Rodberg, Robin Fox
Copyeditor: Patricia Patterson
Book Design: John R. Lanning
Cover Design: Michael Rogondino
Illustrations: Steve Beebe, Stephanie McCann,
Susan Strawn
Photographs: Unit openers, Karen Rantzman; William T.
Thompson, Unit 5
Proofreaders: Melissa Andrews, Elliot Simon,
Toni Murray
Galley Readers: Patricia Ann Brown, RN, PhD, Adelphi
University; Marilyn Murphy, RN, BSN, MS, University
of Texas, San Antonio
Indexers: Steve Sorensen, subject index; Katherine
Pitcoff, drug index
Typesetter: Graphic Typesetting Service, Los Angeles,
CA; Cathy Rundell, Project Coordinator

The authors and publishers have exerted every effort to ensure that drug selection and dosage set forth in this text are in accord with current recommendations and practice at the time of publication. However, in view of ongoing research, changes in government regulation, and the constant flow of information relating to drug therapy and drug reactions, the reader is urged to check the package insert for each drug for any change in the indications of dosage and for added warnings and precautions. This is particularly important where the recommended agent is a new and/or infrequently employed drug.

Library of Congress Cataloging-in-Publication Data

Adult health nursing.

  Includes bibliographies and index.
  1. Nursing. 2. Holistic medicine. 3. Humanistic
psychology. 4. Physiology, Pathological. I. Kneisl,
Carol Ren. II. Ames, Sue Ann. [DNLM: 1. Nursing Care.
WY 100 A2443]
RT42.A34 1986   616   86-3639
ISBN 0-201-12650-8

ABCDEFGHIJK–RN–89876

 Addison-Wesley Publishing Company
Health Sciences Division
2727 Sand Hill Road
Menlo Park, CA 94025

Contributors

SUEANN WOOSTER AMES, RN, MS, RNC
Associate Professor
School of Nursing
State University of New York at Buffalo
Buffalo, New York
Adult Nurse Practitioner
Health Care Plan
West Seneca, NY

JANIS P. BELLACK, RN, MN
Associate Professor
College of Nursing
University of Kentucky
Lexington, Kentucky

LINDA RAE BELSKY, RN, MSN
Oncology Clinical Nurse Specialist
St. Elizabeth Medical Center
Yakima, Washington

SHEILA BITTLE, RN, MS, RNC
Clinical Director, Psychiatric Nursing Practice
University of Utah Health Science Center;
Private practice in psychotherapy;
Auxiliary Assistant Professor
College of Nursing
University of Utah
Salt Lake City, Utah

JOYCE M. BLACK, RN, MSN
Assistant Professor
College of Nursing
University of Nebraska
Omaha, Nebraska
Editor-in-chief
Plastic Surgical Nursing

MARGARET A. BRADY, RN, MS, CPNP
Associate Professor, Department of Nursing
California State University
Long Beach, California

PENNY BRESNICK, RN, MS
Instructor, School of Nursing
University of Southern Maine
Orono, Maine

KAREN A. BROWN, RN, MS
Clinical Instructor
College of Nursing
University of Utah
Salt Lake City, Utah

PATRICIA ANN BROWN, RN, PhD
Associate Professor
Marion A. Buckley School of Nursing
Adelphi University
Garden City, New York

PATRICIA A. BURNS, MS, RN
Assistant Professor
School of Nursing
State University of New York at Buffalo
Buffalo, New York

JEANETTE K. CHAMBERS, RN, MS, CS
Renal Clinical Nurse Specialist
Riverside Methodist Hospital
Columbus, Ohio

RITA A. COLICCHIA, RN, MS, RNC
Adult Nurse Practitioner, Rheumatology
Kenmore Medical Group
Tonawanda, New York

JANICE LECH DUSEK, RN, MS
Assistant Director of Nursing, Critical Care
Scarborough Grace General Hospital
Scarborough, Ontario, Canada

NANCY J. EVANS, BS
Senior Editor, Health Sciences
Addison-Wesley Publishing Company
Redwood City, California

ELIZABETH SCHEIDT FARREN, RN, MSN
Assistant Professor
School of Nursing
Baylor University
Nurse Practitioner, Casa de Los Amigos
Dallas, Texas

JANICE COOKE FEIGENBAUM, RN, MS
Assistant Professor
D'Youville College
Buffalo, New York

MARY LYN FIELD, RN, MSN
Department of Primary Care
University of North Carolina
Chapel Hill, North Carolina

THERESA M. FLAHERTY, RN
Staff Nurse
Stanford University Hospital
Palo Alto, California

MARION J. FRANZ, RD, MS
  Director of Nutrition
  International Diabetes Center
  Minneapolis, Minnesota

CAROLYN GORCZYCA, RN, MS
  Professor of Nursing
  Erie Community College
  Buffalo, New York

VICKY ROSE HARTWELL-IVINS, RN, MSN
  Formerly Clinical Instructor
  School of Nursing
  State University of New York at Buffalo
  Buffalo, New York

BRENDA P. HAUGHEY, RN, PhD
  Assistant Professor of Nursing
  Social and Preventive Medicine;
  Research Associate, Program in Social Epidemiology
  State University of New York at Buffalo
  Buffalo, New York

JANE ESTHER HOKANSON HAWKS, RN, MSN
  Private Duty Supervisor
  Family Home Care
  Formerly, Assistant Professor
  College of Nursing
  University of Nebraska
  Omaha, Nebraska

PHYLLIS FOSTER HEALY, RN, MS
  Assistant Professor
  School of Nursing
  University of Southern Maine
  Portland, Maine

PATRICIA HORRIGAN-CREAHAN, RN, BS, RNC
  Nurse practioner in a nephrology practice

DOROTHY KAMINSKI, RN, CNRN, CNOR
  Clinical Supervisor
  Neurosurgical Operating Room
  Mount Sinai Hospital
  New York, New York

LESLIE S. KERN, RN, MN, CCRN
  Cardiothoracic Surgery Clinical Nurse Specialist
  University of California at Los Angeles Medical Center
  Los Angeles, California

CAROL REN KNEISL, RN, MS
  Clinical Associate Professor
  School of Nursing
  State University of New York at Buffalo
  Buffalo, New York
  President and Educational Director
  Nursing Transitions, Inc.
  Williamsville, NY

NANCY NUWER KONSTANTINIDES, RN, MS, RNC
  Metabolic Nurse Specialist
  University of Minnesota Hospitals
  Minneapolis, Minnesota

DOMINICA ANN LIMBURG, RN, MS, RNC
  Adult Nurse Practitioner
  Gerontological Nurse Practitioner
  Austin, Texas

MARTHA FIRTH MARKARIAN, RN, MS
  Clinical Instructor
  School of Nursing
  State University of New York at Buffalo
  Buffalo, New York

LYN MARSHALL, RN, MSN
  Clinical Nurse Manager
  Eating Disorders Program
  Northwestern Memorial Hospital
  Chicago, Illinois

CAROLYN FRITZ McCAIN, RN, MSN
  Assistant Professor
  School of Nursing
  University of North Carolina
  Chapel Hill, North Carolina

LINDA HEIM McCAUSLAND, RN, MS
  Clinical Assistant Professor
  School of Nursing
  State University of New York at Buffalo
  Buffalo, New York

LeANN ANDERSON McNEIL, RN, MS
  Research Director
  International Diabetes Education Center
  Minneapolis, Minnesota

MARDY NORD MEADOWS, RN, BS
  Staff Nurse, Surgical Intensive Care
  Stanford University Hospitals
  Palo Alto, California

CAROLYN CZECH MONTGOMERY, RN, MSN, RNC
  Adult Nurse Practitioner
  Health Care Plan
  Buffalo, New York

SUSAN KATHLEEN NEVINS, RN, MA
  Clinical Instructor, Neurosurgery
  Mount Sinai Hospital and Medical Center
  New York, New York

THOMAS E. OBST, MS, CRNA
  Clinical Assistant Professor
  Co-Director, Nurse Anesthesia Program
  School of Nursing
  State University of New York at Buffalo
  Veterans Administration Medical Center
  Buffalo, New York

ROSEMARY CAROL POLOMANO, RN, MSN, CS
Oncology Clinical Specialist
Hospital of the University of Pennsylvania
Clinical Lecturer, University of Pennsylvania
School of Nursing, Graduate Program
Philadelphia, Pennsylvania

YVONNE KRALL SCHERER, RN, MS
Clinical Assistant Professor
School of Nursing
State University of New York at Buffalo
Buffalo, New York

SANDRA E. SEFF, RN, PhD
Assistant Professor
University of Maryland
School of Nursing
Baltimore, Maryland

CONSTANCE A. SETTLEMYER, RN, PhD
Professor of Nursing
Nursing Department
Indiana University of Pennsylvania
Indiana, Pennsylvania

BARBARA TOBIAS SHIRK, RN, MS
Clinical Nurse Specialist
Associated Internal Medicine Physicians of Central Illinois
Peoria, Illinois
Adjunct Professor
Mennonite College of Nursing
Bloomington, Illinois

ANNE HERRSTROM SKELLY, RN, MS, RNC
Nurse Practitioner
Diabetic Clinic
Erie County Medical Center
Clinical Assistant Professor
State University of New York at Buffalo
Buffalo, New York

FRANCES L. STIER, RN, MSN, RNC
Adult Nurse Practitioner
Health Care Plan
West Seneca, New York
Critical Care Consultant
Educational Services
Hamburg, New York

DIANE WIND WARDELL, RN, MS, RNC
Assistant Professor of Nursing
Houston Baptist University
Houston, Texas

DEE WONCH, RN, MSN
Educational Nurse Administrator
Roswell Park Memorial Institute
Buffalo, New York

Contents

UNIT 8

The Client With Gastrointestinal System Dysfunction

Contemporary nursing practice requires more of nurses than ever before. The new realities facing nurses today are a turbulent health care delivery system, a dynamic society, and increasing responsibility, accountability, and autonomy.

Health and illness are not one-dimensional phenomena. They are the result of interacting physiological, cultural, psychological, sociological, developmental, economic, and lifestyle factors. These biopsychosocial factors are the antecedents of health and illness. *Adult Health Nursing: A Biopsychosocial Approach* reflects these new realities by synthesizing nursing process, pathophysiology, and clinical nursing practice in a holistic, humanistic context.

Designed for use in undergraduate courses in medical-surgical nursing, *Adult Health Nursing* seeks to fill a void in the nursing literature by providing a balanced presentation of pathophysiological and psychosocial content, emphasizing family and lifestyle implications of health and illness. Central themes in this text are: the holistic nature of humans; the importance of individuality, self-worth, and dignity; and the essentially humanitarian nature of nursing. It has an uncompromising focus on nursing care, using a nursing process format. In addition to traditional medical-surgical content, this text discusses such often-neglected topics as physiological and psychosocial implications of illness for the client, malnutrition, obesity and eating disorders, substance abuse in non-psychiatric settings, and care of the dying.

CONTEMPORARY FOCUS AND TONE

Innovative in approach and content, *Adult Health Nursing* acknowledges our beliefs about the nature of nursing, the meaning of health and illness, and the role of the health consumer. The beliefs that guided the development of this book are:

- It is essential for nurses to understand the biopsychosocial influences on health and illness.
- Adult health nursing focuses on the health needs of persons who are well, who are ill, or who are at risk.
- The nursing process provides the framework for contemporary nursing practice.
- Nurses have a major impact on health status because of broad access to clients in all age groups, in all settings, and during all phases of their lives.
- Health care consumers are clients. Clients participate in health care decision-making and self-care to the fullest extent possible, and assume primary responsibility for their own health.

- Positive health practices can reduce many of the health risks that persons face. Teaching lifestyle modification is a crucial role in nursing.

Many nurse educators have indicated through their reviews during the development of this book that they share these beliefs and that their teaching is based on these concepts.

To help students put these concepts into practice, we have used several special features throughout the text:

- Generic nursing care plans in each nursing process chapter
- Case studies that include specific nursing care plans
- Resource lists for clients, their families, and nurses describing self-help groups and other organizations, telephone hotlines, and health education material for client/family teaching and self-care
- Highlighted tables and boxes featuring health teaching guidelines
- Tables summarizing both the physiological and the psychosocial/lifestyle implications of specific surgical procedures for clients and their families
- Nursing research notes that annotate current and relevant research from the nursing literature

CONSISTENT, CLINICALLY RELEVANT ORGANIZATION

The text is organized in 13 units. Unit 1 orients the student to the shared experience of health and illness—changing health care in a changing society, basic pathophysiological concepts and processes, the experience of illness and how clients cope with it, and assessment of the adult client. Unit 2 discusses multisystem stressors affecting the client such as malnutrition, obesity and eating disorders, substance abuse, infection, cancer, trauma, surgery, burns, and dying and death. The material in these two units is fundamental to understanding the units that follow.

Units 3 through 13 focus on caring for clients with dysfunction of specific body systems. Because nursing practice uses a nursing model parallel to, rather than instead of, a medical model, each of these units in *Adult Health Nursing* presents a clear classification in the familiar language of body systems as follows:

- A review of anatomy, physiology, pathophysiology, and psychosocial/lifestyle influences and effects
- The nursing process for clients with health needs related to the body system
- The nursing care unique to clients with specific disorders of the body system

- The nursing care of clients having surgery for dysfunction in the body system

Each body system unit includes at least one case study and a nursing care plan based on that study: 23 case studies and 34 care plans in all. This consistency of organization within each unit and each chapter makes information readily accessible to students and helps them relate theory to nursing practice in the clinical setting.

INVITING FORMAT

More than 700 photographs and drawings, the majority of them commissioned expressly for this text, enliven the content and facilitate understanding. A superbly illustrated two-color format enhances the teaching value of many illustrations. Boxes and tables, screened in blue, and the liberal and consistent use of headings help locate important information. The typographical design makes the book pleasing to look at and easy to read. The clear, lively style of writing makes the subject matter interesting as well as meaningful to students and faculty.

IN-TEXT LEARNING AIDS

In addition to the special features mentioned earlier, this text includes a number of other learning aids. Student-oriented **Objectives** help students identify their learning goals. The **Chapter Highlights** at the end of each chapter review the key points covered in the chapter. Current references are in the **Bibliography**. Annotated **Suggested Readings** at the end of each chapter pinpoint other sources for students to explore. **Tables and Boxes** highlight and emphasize essential information throughout the text. **Cross-referencing** within the chapters reminds students of related discussions in other chapters and helps to avoid duplication of content. **Important terms** are set in boldface type throughout the text and defined in the **Glossary** at the end of the book. A **List of Abbreviations** used in the text and in the case studies is in the Appendix. The **International System of Units (SI)**, the most up-to-date metric system of measurement, is included on the inside back cover and used throughout the text to facilitate international use.

COMPREHENSIVE SUPPLEMENTS PACKAGE

Adult Health Nursing is the heart of a complete teaching-learning system in medical-surgical nursing. The **Instructor's Manual,** written by Irene M. Russo, includes the student study objectives referenced to pages in the text, correlates the objectives with the Student Learning Guide, provides almost 200 multiple-choice questions referenced to pages in the text and to the student study objectives, and annotates audiovisual resources (including computer programs) with complete ordering information. A **Student**

Learning Guide, written by Karen M. Falkner, suggests a variety of in-class and out-of-class activities such as group discussions; written projects; family and client interviews; role-playing; matching, essay, and review questions; and other activities designed to reinforce students' learning. A **computerized testbank** (Apple and IBM compatible), a **two-color transparency resource kit** containing 100 transparencies of both in-text illustrations and additional illustrations not in the text, and a **set of 60 slides** showing photographs from the book in full color enhance both teaching and learning. An innovative **Instructor's Resource Manual** to hold the complete teaching-learning system is available to faculty who adopt the text for their course.

HOW TO USE THIS BOOK

We believe that the biopsychosocial approach of *Adult Health Nursing* will prove uniquely effective in preparing nurses who will base their practice not only on clinical and pathophysiological knowledge, but also on an understanding of the whole person, and of the nurse's role as health teacher and client advocate.

Adult Health Nursing has been organized with readers' needs clearly in focus. Information is presented from unit to unit and from chapter to chapter in a systematic way so that readers will be able to easily find what they need.

The body system units, Units 3–13, are organized according to a specific pattern. The first chapter of each unit is divided into four sections, with general discussions covering the structural and functional interrelationships of the system in question, the pathophysiologic influences and effects, the related system influences and effects, and finally, psychosocial/lifestyle influences and effects.

The second chapter of each unit examines the nursing process. The nursing assessments required in establishing a data base are presented, including how to take a health history, medication history, and what elements are involved in subjective data gathering; physical assessment; and diagnostic studies. The nursing diagnoses are then presented and followed by means of planning and implementation. The chapter ends with a discussion of how to evaluate the nursing care.

The following chapter(s) examines specific disorders. Clinical disorders of multifactorial origin, degenerative, immunologic, infectious, neoplastic, or traumatic disorders, if relevant, are covered. Each disorder is examined in terms of the clinical manifestations, therapeutic measures, and specific nursing measures.

Each unit concludes with an overview of surgical approaches to the specific disorders, if available. Each procedure is examined by discussing the particular procedure, the implications for the client (physiologic and psychosocial/lifestyle) and the nursing implications, which include preoperative care, postoperative care, and discharge planning. The indexes, both subject and drug, are invaluable resources in using this book.

Acknowledgments

Contemporary nursing practice also requires more of nursing authors than ever before. A textbook of this size can never be the product of one or two persons' imagination or experience. Many have had a hand in shaping it and supporting and sustaining its authors, and we acknowledge them with our deepest thanks.

- Our contributors, who represent all regions in the United States and the country of Canada, shared their nursing acumen and enthusiasm for their subject.

- The talented professionals at Addison-Wesley Publishing Company provided publishing expertise and unbounded enthusiasm. Nancy Evans, our Sponsoring Editor, who knows and respects nurses and nursing, worked long and hard with us in all phases of the project. Nick Keefe, Vice President and General Manager, for his advice, support, encouragement, and commitment to this text. Glenda Epting, Production Supervisor, for her energy and personal grace under constant pressure during the production process and throughout a variety of publishing crises. Helene Harrington whose skill at organizing the 800 illustrations and photographs made working with her a delight. R. Wayne Oler, President, who sponsored this book from its very beginning in 1981 when he was general manager of the Medical-Nursing Division and continues to maintain a personal interest in it. John Connolly, Vice-President Higher Education, who gave his strong publishing support and smoothed the way.

- Our colleagues and friends, Barbara Kozier and Glen Erb, the authors of the respected Addison-Wesley nursing texts *Fundamentals of Nursing* and *Techniques in Clinical Nursing,* were part of the early planning conferences and helped to design the organization of this text.

- Mary Berry for her expertise as the developmental editor on the majority of the chapters, before she left to demonstrate her expertise as a new mother.

- Pat Patterson who copyedited the entire book and helped with developmental editing in Unit 2, coped willingly with an erratic schedule while she safeguarded the consistency of the writing style.

- Joan Schurr of the Medical Photography Department at Millard Fillmore Hospital in Buffalo, NY, who generously spent endless hours providing many of the unique photographs in the text and in the slide supplement.

- Amina Najar, MD, radiologist, and Betty Everett and her staff of the Radiology Department at Health Care Plan in West Seneca, NY are responsible for researching and providing many of the excellent x-rays used in the text. The staff in suite D in Health Care Plan, West Seneca, NY, and the staff at Health Care Plan, Sheridan Drive, were invaluable resources.

- Cathy Rundell, Elliott Derman, and the entire staff at Graphic Typesetting Service for the extra effort and superb skills demonstrated time and again during our production process.

- Sandy Sherer of Sherer Word Processing Service, Buffalo, NY for her skill, enthusiasm, energy, and willingness to work on the weekend and well into the early hours of the morning. Kathy Holst, Pat Brock-Eisenstein, Yvonne Bish, and June Santomauro all helped at crucial moments.

- The manuscript reviewers who critiqued the manuscript at various stages: Dolores Alabrodzinski; Susan Alden; Madalon Amenta; Marilyn Bayne; Peggy Birney; Barbara Bloom; Lynne Braun; Laurel Brodsley; Jo Brown; Kris Brown; Pat Brown; Barbara Bunker; Verna Carson; Mary Lou Cheatham; Virgien Clark; Jane Colley; Marcia Costello; Deanna Cross; Dorothy Crowder; Irene Cullen; Mary Cunningham; Louise Curtis; A. Jann Davis; Virginia M. Dowd; Joanne Damon; Linda Duli; Jean DuPont; Christine Farris; Paul Femea; Juanita Flint; Roxie Foster; Nancy Franke; Vivian Frantz; Nancy Fredholm; Cecilia Freeman; Elise Gardiner; Gloria Goldman; Patty Gray; Peggy Guenter; Theresa Haley; Ruth Harboe; Pat Heringa; Kay Holmes; Marguerite Jackson; Jill Jaeckle; Pam Jeffries; June Johnson; Virginia Kahn; Leslie Kern; Parry Knauss; Kristin Koehler; Elaine Larson; Marlene Loringer; Patricia Lisk; Suzanne Malloy; Janet Marvin; Esther Matassarin-Jacobs; Andrea Walsh Matz; Mary Mayers; Pat McKnight; Donna Miotke; Kathi Mooney; Patricia Moschel; Marilyn Murphy; Mary Lou Muwaswes; Holly Myers; Virginia Neelon; Mary B. Neiheisel; Martha Orr; Elizabeth Palmer; Gertrude Redmond; Sharon Reed; Gayle Reiber; Rosemary Rhodes; Linda Robertson; Dennis Ross; Vincent Rudan; Elaine Sampson; Olive Santavenere; Delores Schoen; Jane Shelby; Sandra Smith; Rita Snyder-Halpern; Denise Stevens; Elizabeth Stokes; Nancy Stotts; Charleen Strebel; Dorothy Stuppy; Elvira Szigeti; Debbie Thorpe; Ruth Taylor; Joy Ufema; Kathleen Wallace; Jean Watson; Jean Weist

- The following persons who assisted and supported the contributors in invaluable ways: Ralph Argen MD; Bonnie Bullough RN, PhD; Faith B. Davis MD; Phyllis Dion RN; Julia Eggert RN, MS; John Fath MD; Catherine Fogel; Marianna Fraser RN, MS; Patricia Greene RN, MS; Roberta Hammerschmidt RN, BSN; Mary Hynan RN; Diane Kiuhara RN, BS; Leonard I. Malis MD; Kathi Mooney RN, PhD; Rosemary Murray RN, MS; Normal Rolls RN; Elizabeth Tornquist; Andrew T. Turrisi III MD; Dana Weinkle MD; Cheryl Welch; Mary Zink; Rosario Zuppulla MD.

- And, finally, our families, who were patient and supportive through many trying moments, and learned more about coping than they ever wanted to.

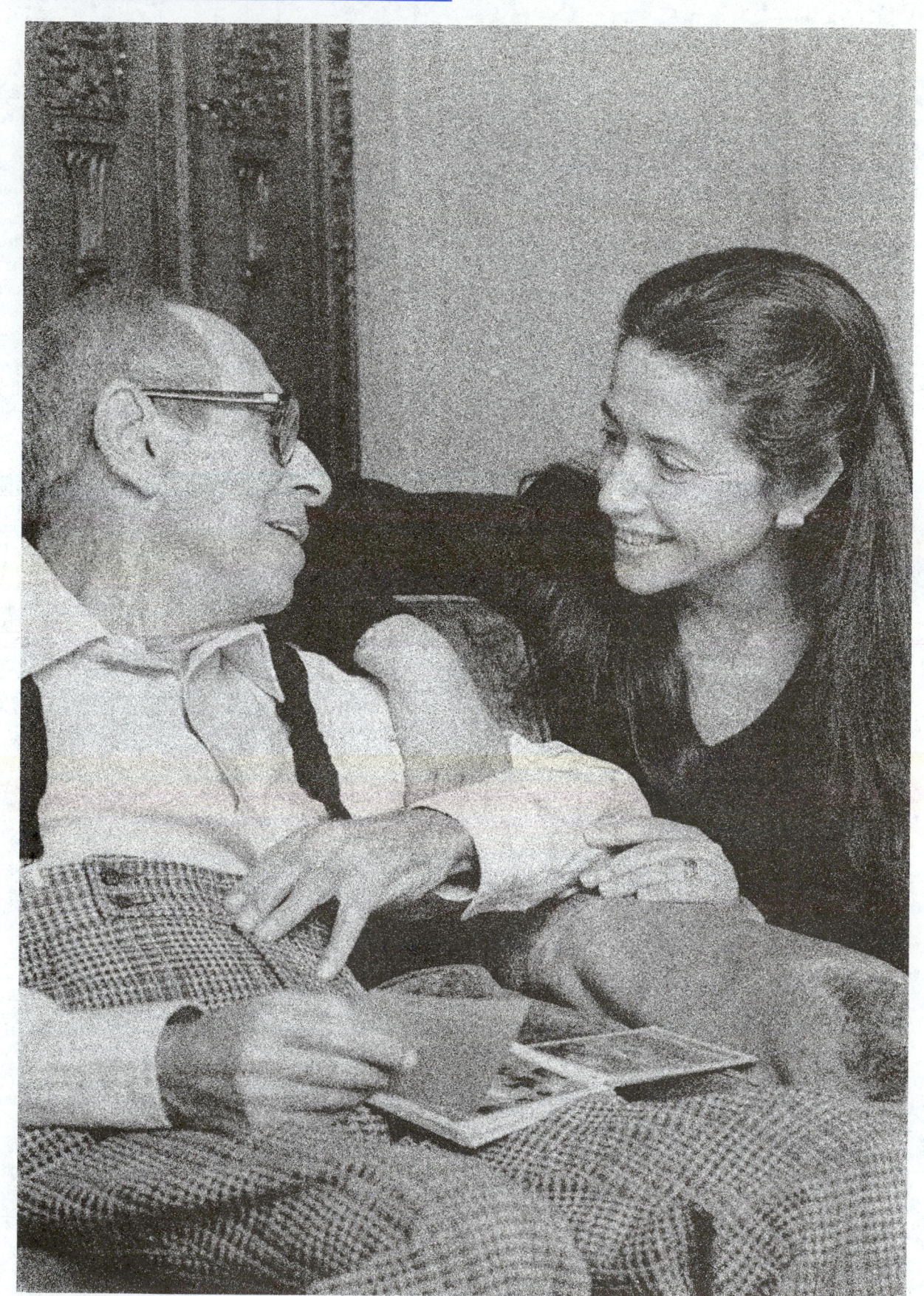

The Shared Experience of Health and Illness

Chapter 1

Changing Health Care in a Changing Society

Carol Ren Kneisl
SueAnn Wooster Ames
Nancy Evans

Objectives

When you have finished studying this chapter, you should be able to:

Describe the effects of changes in family structure, life expectancy, environment, values, cultural diversity, and health patterns on health care.

Identify the relation between poverty and health problems.

Delineate the factors responsible for spiraling health care costs.

Discuss the technologic developments affecting health care.

Explore the personal responsibility of each individual in maintaining health.

Differentiate among primary, secondary, and tertiary health care.

Discuss how changes in society, economics, and technology affect the nurse's role.

Appreciate the importance of the nursing process, nursing theory, and nursing research in clinical nursing practice.

Transplants, implants, artificial organs, laser surgery, birthing rooms, trauma centers, hospices—health care continually changes and is changed by practices of birth, life, and death. Because all change is stressful, changes in lifestyles, economics, technology, and values affect health in significant and not-so-significant ways. As the pace of change accelerates to a certain point, it becomes what Toffler (1970) termed *"future shock . . .* the shattering stress and disorientation that we induce in individuals by subjecting them to too much change in too short a time." Meeting the challenge of caring in the computer age means understanding not only sociologic, economic, and technologic changes but also how they affect the health care consumer, the health care system, and the roles and responsibilities of nurses.

Section I: Sociologic Changes

During the second half of the twentieth century, many aspects of society have undergone dramatic and rapid change. Family structure, life expectancy, environment, values, cultural diversity, and health patterns have all been affected.

FAMILY STRUCTURE

The character and mobility of the American family have changed markedly during the past three decades. For many years, the family provided care, stability, and support for its members in both health and illness. Families lived in the same geographic area for generations. Today, the tra-

ditional nuclear family no longer typifies the client population, and 17% of Americans move every year (Louis Harris, 1982). Reliance on the extended family for support and help is not always possible. In 1982, married couples were only 59% of total households, a decrease of 12% since 1970. Couples who marry may choose to remain childless or to delay first pregnancy until the wife is past 30.

Divorce and greater acceptance of children born outside marriage have led to an increase in the number of single-parent families. More than 9 million families (11% of all households) are headed by women, an increase of 72% since 1970. A serious illness and hospitalization could create major financial and logistical problems for a single mother unless she has family or friends available to help.

In many parts of North America, the number of homosexual couples is increasing. Generally, the health care system does not acknowledge these or other nontraditional relationships as legitimate, recognizing only the rights of "immediate family," even though the partner may be the most important "significant other" to the ill person.

In the midst of this affluent society, in which a higher standard of living is potentially health-promoting, homelessness is epidemic. More Americans were homeless in 1985 than at any point since the Great Depression of the 1930s. Some are welfare mothers who have been evicted from tenement rooms. Many are former mental hospital clients who, after release from the institution, have fallen through the cracks of an inadequate system of follow-up and become society's rejects. At least 20% of the homeless are over age 65. Although much media attention has been focused on the plight of the homeless, only short-term solutions to the problem have been proposed, such as food and shelter. Senator John Heinz (R-PA), chairman of the Senate Special Committee on Aging, stated in early 1985: "We can no longer view the crisis of homelessness as a short-term phenomenon. We must develop long-range policies which not only get people off the street for a couple of nights, but get them back to secure, independent living in the community."

LIFE EXPECTANCY

Butler and Lewis (1983) have called this "a century of old age—the first century in which people have a greater chance than otherwise of living out the entire cycle of human life." Nearly 80% of all babies born will live to be old. There are now more Americans over 65 than there are teenagers. This growing population of persons over 65—more than 27 million—presents one of the greatest health care challenges. Of the $1 billion America spends each day on health care, more than 30% is allocated to meet the needs of this group. Chronic rather than acute problems account for this population's need for care; more than 85% of persons over age 65 have one or more chronic conditions such as arthritis, impairments in hearing and vision, hypertension, and cardiovascular problems.

Because female life expectancy exceeds that of males, a majority of these older persons are women, often widows. Their chronic physical problems may be combined with loneliness and depression, conditions that can lead to poor nutrition or excessive use of alcohol or other drugs. Poor nutrition can also result from living on a fixed income in an age of inflation and can lead, in turn, to a myriad of other health problems.

The fastest growing segment of the population is the group over age 85, the *oldest old*, also referred to as the frail elderly. Now numbering more than 2.6 million, this group is expected to increase to 5 million by the year 2000. As their numbers increase, the oldest old will find health care a growing financial burden. Thus, an urgent need exists for more research into the health and economic condition of this population.

It is important to remember that persons over age 65 are a diverse group emotionally, physically, behaviorally, economically, socially, and politically. Only 5% are institutionalized because of health problems. Even in the oldest old, many persons work and live independently. Unfortunately, health policy and often the health care system tend to categorize and stereotype all older persons as a homogeneous group.

Life expectancy also reflects health problems and how they are dealt with. Among blacks, life expectancy is 69.3 years, 6 years less than for whites. Black infant mortality in 1983 was 22.1 deaths per 1000 live births, almost double the rate for whites. These differences reflect, at least in part, differences in income, nutrition, and health education plus limited access to health care.

ENVIRONMENT

Since the 1950s, awareness has grown of the air and water pollution that threatens life and health throughout the world. Industrial and agricultural wastes have found their way into the water supply of many communities. The Love Canal area of Niagara Falls, NY, is a deserted wasteland where an abandoned school and dozens of abandoned homes stand on foundations through which a foul-smelling green-black viscous fluid seeps. The families who once lived there experienced an unusually high number of infertility problems, spontaneous abortions, birth defects, malignancies, and neurologic disorders. Many cities, such as Los Angeles, publish a daily *air quality index* so persons with respiratory complications will know whether the outside air is safe to breathe. Every industrial city lives in the shadow of the tragic industrial chemical leak that killed 2000 people in Bhopal, India, in 1984.

On a less spectacular but equally dangerous level, the daily hazards of the work environment require further research to arrive at definitive answers about their effects. Black lung in coal miners, brown lung in textile workers, and asbestosis in construction workers have been acknowledged as occupationally related disorders. Other potential hazards in the work environment include anesthetic gases, video display terminals (VDTs), airport security machines, and other radiation-emitting devices.

VALUES

On August 6, 1985, the world paused to remember the birth of the nuclear age, the dropping of the atomic bomb on Hiroshima, Japan, in 1945. That event made clear the potential for worldwide destruction and therefore the uncertainty of the future. This uncertainty seems to have altered the emphasis in society from living carefully and planning for the future to living for the present and experiencing as much as possible in the time allotted. This emphasis on the experience-packed present, plus the stresses of modern life, have fostered escapism. Escapism is made easier by mobility and relative affluence.

More liberal attitudes about sex have led to increased promiscuity and, with it, the problems of rampant sexually transmitted diseases (STD), now second in incidence only to the common cold. The incidence of chlamydia infection, herpes genitalis, gonorrhea (see Chapters 64 and 67), and the most alarming of all because of its universally fatal outcome, acquired immune deficiency syndrome (AIDS; discussed in Chapter 29) is increasing each year. The rate of teenage pregnancy has reached new heights in the United States; more than 523,000 girls under age 18 gave birth in 1984 (Children's Defense Fund, 1985). These statistics are cause for concern, not only because of the immediate physiologic risk for mother and infant but also because of the long-term psychologic and economic problems created, not the least of which is the potential for child abuse.

Another outcome of escapism is the growing use of mood-altering drugs, including alcohol. One of the most popular recreational drugs is cocaine, second only to marijuana in its widespread use. Despite its devastating effects on health and life, cocaine continues to attract new users, as does alcohol. Estimates are that more than 40 million persons in the United States are seriously affected by excessive use of alcohol by one or more family members (ADAMHA News, 1984). Because substance abuse frequently leads to accidents or other health problems, health professionals may encounter persons experiencing withdrawal symptoms who have been admitted for a problem not clearly drug related (see Chapter 10).

CULTURAL DIVERSITY

Long considered a cultural "melting pot," the United States continues to attract immigrants from all over the world. During the 1970s, more than 450,000 immigrants were legally admitted to the United States. Illegal immigration also continues to expand the population, although accurate statistics are not available.

The 1980 census showed more than 77% of the United States population as white; the remainder is grouped as follows: blacks, 12%; Hispanics, 6%; American Indians, Eskimos, Aleuts, Asians, and Pacific Islanders, 5% (Spain, 1983). Each group has its own beliefs and values that may differ markedly from those of the dominant white culture. As Leininger (1981) indicates, "Cultural values are the blueprints for human behaviour and determine what cultural groups will do to maintain their health status and how they care for people when they become ill." Suggestions for considering cultural values are in Chapter 4.

Studies continue to show that ethnic minorities do not have equal access to health care, not only because of differences in cultural beliefs and values but also because of language barriers and inequities in income and education. The 1982 National Access Survey (Louis Harris, 1982) showed that black families were less likely than whites to obtain care when they needed it and were more dissatisfied overall with the American health care system. Hispanics also indicated greater than average dissatisfaction than whites or blacks with the system, particularly with emergency care.

Caring for clients from cultural groups different from one's own requires sensitivity to the client's beliefs and values and respect for them. Although it would be difficult, if not impossible, to be aware of the total range of possible health beliefs, values, and practices among the diverse cultural groups found in the United States, it is possible to broaden one's knowledge of transcultural nursing, the area of nursing study that examines the health and illness practices, beliefs, and values of different cultures and subcultures. Study of transcultural nursing can help in developing a more global view of health and nursing's role in improving the health of the world's people.

Recent immigrants to North America, particularly those from developing countries, experience a kind of culture shock when they are thrust into the high-tech health care system. According to Hendricks (1982), "The experience of culture shock often encompasses feelings of helplessness, irritability, and fears of being cheated, contaminated, injured or disregarded." Recognizing that clients may have these feelings can help nurses plan and implement care more appropriately.

HEALTH PATTERNS

With the reduction in infectious disease and improvement in nutrition, life expectancy has increased. Longer life, with its increased potential for chronic health problems, is sometimes a mixed blessing, however. Arthritis alone affects nearly 40 million Americans (see Chapter 59). Cataracts (discussed in Chapters 71 and 72) and other sensory losses related to aging are common problems of the elderly. More than 2.5 million Americans suffer Alzheimer's disease, the little-understood dementia; 120,000 Americans die each year from Alzheimer's (see Chapter 37). Researchers predict that by the year 2030, the incidence of Alzheimer's disease will have increased at an alarming rate (Powell & Courtice, 1983).

Improved technology and growing clinical knowledge have provided another source for chronic health problems. Persons with disorders such as cerebral palsy or cystic fibrosis who would not have lived beyond adolescence in the 1940s have received treatment sufficient for survival into adulthood. Early diagnosis and more effective treatment have meant cancer is not always a terminal diagnosis. Hundreds of thousands of persons are living reasonably normal lives despite surgery to remove a malignancy of the colon, larynx, or breast.

For more than two decades, the skilled technology of newborn intensive care units has kept alive severely compromised premature infants, many of whom survive with moderate to severe central nervous system damage and other chronic problems. The long-term sociologic and economic effects of this technology are unknown and will be difficult to measure.

Section II: Economic Changes

Economic factors are playing an increasingly important role in modern life. The growing incidence of poverty plus escalating health care costs are creating a revolution in the health care system.

POVERTY AND HEALTH

Poverty goes hand in hand with health problems, an increased need for health services, and an inability to pay for them. Persons living below the poverty level often do not have health insurance or a regular source of health care, either because of their financial problems or lack of information. An example of poverty's impact on health is the disproportionately high number of black males who die from lung cancer each year (Figure 1–1), even though they smoke at about the same rate as white males. (Lung cancer is discussed in Chapter 20.) Cooper and Simmons (1985) attribute the difference to occupational hazards and various consequences of poverty.

HEALTH CARE ECONOMICS

Health care is big business, the second largest industry in the United States, exceeded in size only by the automotive

industry. America spends $1 billion a day on health care—$365 billion annually—and the price is going up. During the two decades between 1965 and 1985, medical care costs increased more than 429%, an increase far above the general rate of economic inflation. Four fundamental factors have been responsible for this tremendous increase (Lee, Estes, & Ramsay, 1984):

1. Inflation.
2. Improved and costly techniques and technologies.
3. An increase in the number of persons who use health services.
4. The way in which physicians and hospitals have been paid.

Until recently, hospitals were reimbursed according to their costs. Physicians are paid a fee for service. Insurers have traditionally paid a large percentage of those charges, no matter how high. The average daily cost for a semi-private hospital room in America in 1985 was $213.

In an effort to stem the upward spiral of health care costs, Congress passed prospective payment legislation in 1983 to limit the amount paid to hospitals by Medicare. This legislation uses a classification system known as diagnosis-related groups (DRGs). Hospitals are paid a pre-determined amount for a client with a given medical diagnosis rather than being reimbursed for the cost of services. This system has forced hospitals to take steps to reduce the cost of client care. Savings from this new system of hospital payment are projected at $20.4 billion by 1988 (Coleman, Dayani, & Simms, 1984).

Among the effects of this prospective payment system on client care is earlier discharge of clients, reduction of services, and reduction of staff, particularly LPN/LVN staff and nurse's aides. Many hospitals are changing to all-RN staffs, nurses able to deliver the broadest range of care. Earlier discharge of clients from hospitals means greater need for nursing care at home, creating a surge in home care agencies.

The DRG system has caused concern among health professionals that the quality of care will be sacrificed for the sake of cost reduction. In addition, research indicates that DRGs are less than 30% accurate in predicting total client care costs because the medical diagnosis alone does not measure the acuteness of the person's illness, coexisting health problems, or any complications that occur. For this reason, the Health Care Financing Administration is funding research to study alternative systems for classification of severity of illness.

A study by Sovie and colleagues (1985) found that combining data from nursing on the severity of clients' illnesses with DRG data was 89% accurate in predicting total costs of care. This study also showed that professional

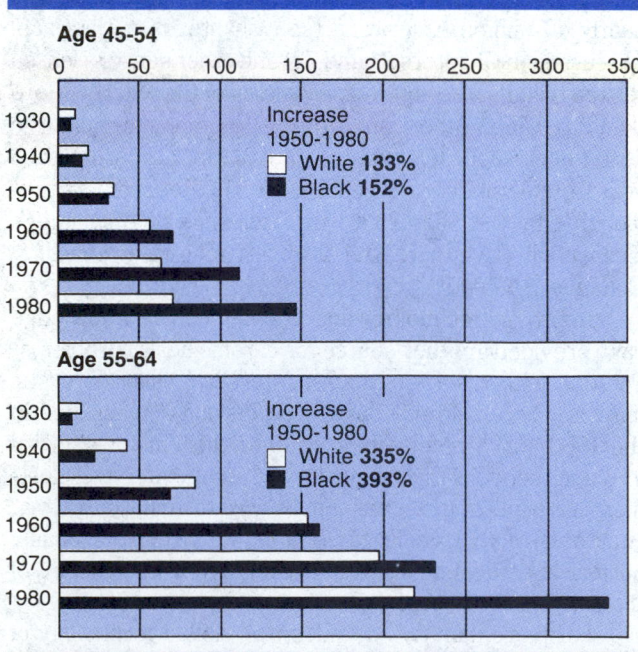

Figure 1–1

Lung cancer deaths among US men ages 45 through 54, per 100,000.
SOURCE: *NY J Med*, August 1985.

nursing care (using a staff composed of 92% RNs) is both safe and cost effective.

Many nursing leaders think that the prospective payment system is an opportunity to demonstrate the importance of nursing care and its cost effectiveness. As Diers (1985) stated:

> DRGs were invented to define the product of the human service institution called a hospital, and now it's clear that a great deal of the work of that institution is nursing. The decision to use DRGs as the basis for reimbursement suddenly made it possible to value nursing, to attach a value called dollars to it. While that has made us lose some of the mystery of the work when it cannot be defined or measured, the advantages of being able to understand, monitor, predict, control and improve nursing and see its effects valued far outweigh the disadvantages. Nursing has been treated for hospital accounting purposes as a *cost* center. When reimbursable services to patients can be identified and assigned to nursing, nursing becomes a *revenue* center. Nursing generates income, and those who make the money get to decide how to spend it.

Section III: Technologic Changes

Health care today is *high tech* and *high ticket*. Modern technology makes it possible to medicate, monitor, and maintain most body functions for extended periods with little human intervention. In this atmosphere, care can become routine and depersonalized unless it is also *high touch*. The same technology that saves lives also raises questions about the quality of lives saved. Is the individual able to live with reasonable freedom, dignity, and comfort? Questions such as this will arise more frequently as technology increases in sophistication.

COMPUTERS

In 1983, *Time* magazine chose the computer as "Man of the Year." During the past two decades, the computer has intruded in every facet of modern life. Modern health facilities are highly computerized; from accounting to intensive care, information is managed by computer. These sophisticated systems are part of the life support equipment that sustains the critically ill when they cannot sustain themselves. Computers are literally the heart of pacemakers, the commonplace devices that regulate the pulses of thousands of Americans.

TRANSPLANTS

New developments in pharmacologic and bioengineering technology have offered new hope to persons who can benefit from an organ transplant or an artificial implant. Transplant surgery is now possible to replace the pancreas, heart, lungs, veins, pituitary gland, kidneys, liver, cornea, and bone marrow. Immunosuppressant drugs such as cyclosporine reduce the risk of the body's rejection of a donated organ.

Although increasingly common, transplant surgery is still high in risk and costly; the average cost of a heart transplant in 1981 was $110,000, and the cost for a liver transplant was $200,000. Though many insurance companies do cover these costs, others consider transplant surgery to be experimental and not generally accepted.

Shortage of donor organs continues; in 1982, only 2200 donors were available to the 4500 persons waiting for a kidney. In January 1986, New York State enacted a law requiring hospitals to ask the families of all deceased clients for organ donations. The intent of the law is to provide support for physicians in requesting organ donation, so they will not be perceived by families as insensitive toward the death of their loved ones. Sponsors of this law also hope it will make more hearts, livers, and kidneys available, estimating that only 15% of the potential number of available organs is being retrieved. Oregon was the only other state with a similar law.

IMPLANTS

Far more common than transplant surgery, implant surgery to replace damaged body parts is highly sophisticated. Approximately 900,000 intraocular lens implants (see Chapter 72) are performed each year (American Intraocular Implant Society, 1985). Replacement of joints damaged by arthritis with plastic or metal prostheses (see Chapter 60) has brought increased mobility and pain relief to hundreds of thousands since the early 1960s. Pacemakers, another kind of implant (see Chapter 25), can now transmit information to physicians by home-based monitoring systems.

As hospital cost cutting pushes health care back into the home, and as individuals assume greater responsibility for their own health, home-based technology is certain to follow. Already, many homes have apnea monitors for infants at risk for sudden infant death syndrome. Persons with diabetes are using insulin pumps and performing blood glucose testing at home (see Chapter 42). Bioengineering experts are working to simplify the operation of medical instrumentation and the reading of basic laboratory results at home.

ETHICAL ISSUES

At the turn of the century, the average life expectancy for Americans was 47 years; in 1983, it was 75. Although it is now possible to live longer, controversy continues over the quality of extended life.

Chronic illness is a fact of life for many over age 65, limiting mobility and eroding independence and self-esteem.

What is the quality of a solitary, pain-filled life? In almost every life-threatening illness, some treatment procedure can delay the time of death. In human terms, what purpose is served by such a delay if the remaining life is without comfort or dignity? These questions continue; slowly, some states are developing legislation that protects the rights of the individual at the end of life.

Since the Karen Ann Quinlan case arose in 1976, efforts have been made for the terminally ill to gain the right to refuse or discontinue treatment. Gallup and Harris polls in 1985 showed that 8 out of 10 persons believe that the terminally ill have the right to have life support measures withdrawn. Nonetheless, complex legal and ethical questions surround this issue; these issues are discussed further in Chapter 16.

Section IV: Change and the Health Consumer's Responsibility

This society is health conscious, spending billions of dollars on health and fitness activities and equipment and billions more on health care. Health and health care are regarded as a right. Too few persons think of health as a personal responsibility, however, even though the leading health problems—cardiovascular disease, cancer, cerebrovascular disease, accidents, homicides, and suicides—result from how persons live and the environments they create.

The language used to discuss health care—eg, "the health care delivery system"—reflects a concept of health that has been generally accepted for many years. Health care is regarded as a product that can be "delivered" to each person if the system functions properly; in fact, the product is illness care. The most significant health care is what individuals do for themselves in the way they live, eat, exercise, manage stress, and avoid excessive use of alcohol and other drugs.

Gradually, this concept of health and health care is changing. The death rate for cardiovascular disease fell by one-third between 1950 and 1980 (Lee, Estes, & Ramsay, 1984). The death rate from peptic ulcer, strokes, and cirrhosis of the liver also fell significantly during that period. In some parts of North America and within some socioeconomic groups, there are growing applications of the abundant new knowledge about nutrition, exercise, and stress management. Nationally, however, less than 3% of the total annual expenditure on health is spent on disease prevention and control measures, and less than 1% each is spent for health education and for improving the organization and delivery of health care. Yet research indicates that increasing the expenditure for disease prevention and control measures and health education can significantly reduce health care costs. For example, a study of asthma clients conducted at Johns Hopkins University School of Hygiene and Public Health demonstrated a savings of $10 for every $1 spent on client education (Maiman et al., 1979). By increasing client compliance through education about medications and the total treatment regimen, costly complications that could require hospitalization were avoided. Since the Surgeon General's first report on the health haz-

ards of smoking, the size of the smoking population as a whole has decreased, particularly the teenage male population.

SELF-CARE, SELF-RESPONSIBILITY

A survey by the American Board of Family Practice (1985) indicated that Americans are asserting their rights in health care issues and assuming the responsibilities that accompany those rights. In this study, two groups were surveyed, members of the general public and physicians. A majority of both groups agreed that education about health maintenance and disease prevention is essential.

Self-care is not a new idea but an ancient one. As Levin (1981) described it:

> The care we provide to ourselves and to our families for common health problems constitutes about 75 percent of all health and medical care. This includes most health-promoting and disease-preventing activities, 81 percent or more of care for minor illnesses and injuries, and the vast proportion of continuing care of chronic diseases after a physician has been consulted. Tooth brushing, treating minor injuries, taking aspirin for arthritis pain, self-medicating for a cold, and self-injection for diabetes are all examples of self-care.

Without self-care practices, the health care system would be overwhelmed. Yet makers of public policy too often consider health care synonymous with professional care. In reality, increasing self-care competence is the most cost-effective means of improving health and the quality of health care. Self-care supplemented with professional care appears to be the only reasonable solution to the health care crisis. Implementing this solution, however, requires dramatic changes in public policies. Instead of trying to reform the professional care system—increasing the number of providers, improving training and distribution, and reorganizing—policies need to reflect the strength of self-care resources and emphasize that professional resources are supplementary.

THE CONSUMER MOVEMENT IN HEALTH CARE

Since the mid-1900s, a national movement has grown to protect the rights of consumers through legislation mandating such practices as truth in advertising, honest packaging, fair pricing, and improved safety standards. This movement has broadened to include health care, partly as a result of dissatisfaction with the present system. The public is aware that professional care is less than perfect. Indeed, professional care is regarded as about 10% effective overall and 10% ineffective or even dangerous (Levin, 1981). Media reports of unnecessary surgery and malpractice litigation have tarnished the image of the physician as all-knowing and infallible. Reports of incompetent treatment and lack of sensitivity have tarnished the image of all health care workers, including nurses.

Evidence of the consumer movement in health care is everywhere—in the more than 3500 health and medical self-help books; in newsletters, conferences, and workshops related to health promotion and management of acute and chronic disease; and in the more than 500 national self-help or mutual support groups. It is readily apparent that individuals want more control over their primary health care needs. In the case of chronic health problems, they recognize that an increased level of involvement in self-care is essential. At the end of each nursing process chapter in this text is a list of self-help groups and health education material that can be used in health promotion.

Mutual support groups such as Alcoholics Anonymous, Reach for Recovery, and Make Today Count, were formed by persons who felt their needs were not being met by existing institutions and health professionals. Today, more than 17 million persons have joined these groups for mutual support and education in dealing with their health problems. Alcoholics Anonymous, formed in 1935 and the model for many mutual support groups, doubled its number of chapters between 1972 and 1982 (Buch & Borman, 1982).

Today, there is a mutual support group for nearly every major health problem or life crisis. Although most are helpful, some may be less than effective or even harmful. For this reason, nurses who may wish to refer clients to these groups or perhaps participate as an advisor or group leader must be able to assess the probable effectiveness of a particular self-help group and its appropriateness for a particular client and family (Newton, 1984). The National Self-Help Clearinghouse can provide information on current support groups plus guidelines on how to start a self-help group (see Chapter 4).

Section V: Change and Health Care Delivery

A retired nurse in Arizona, weary from a day spent taking her husband to three different physicians' offices, observed: "Health care delivery? Not for us. We have to go and get it."

As health care costs continue to rise, more may question the term health care *delivery*. Is health care really being "delivered"? Ambulatory care clinics, home care, outpatient surgery—all are considered "growth industries" as health care moves out of the hospital because the price is too high. All require more initiative and responsibility by the client in seeking services than traditional health care. A study for the American College of Hospital Administrators (1984) predicted that the following trends will continue into the 1990s:

- Shift to outpatient care
- Sharing of costs between consumers and third-party payers
- Self-care
- Competition among health care providers
- Cutbacks in Medicare and Medicaid

Individually and collectively, these trends have significant implications for both consumers and providers of health care.

PRIMARY CARE

Viewing health care from the perspective of primary, secondary, and tertiary care, changes throughout the system are readily apparent. Primary care—comprising health maintenance, health promotion, and disease prevention—holds the greatest hope for reducing costs and improving health. Settings for primary care include homes, schools, community clinics, physicians' offices and increasingly, business and industry. Many corporations, alarmed by the cost of health care (20 cents for every dollar of salary paid), are initiating primary care programs to help employees lose weight, stop smoking, reduce stress, and improve their overall fitness. In addition, many offer free medical screenings. Through client education and self-care, primary care will no doubt expand remarkably during the next decades.

Health Maintenance Organizations

One of the largest, most influential types of primary care organizations, the *health maintenance organization* (HMO), offers a comprehensive range of services in exchange for a fixed periodic payment. In 1984, there were 265 HMOs in the United States, and their number continues to increase.

More than 50,000 American businesses include membership in an HMO plan as part of their employee benefits package.

By encouraging preventive care and ambulatory visits, HMOs have helped reduce the hospitalization rate of members. The total cost of premiums plus out-of-pocket expenses are less to employees covered through an HMO plan than to employees covered by traditional health insurance plans. HMO participants appear satisfied with their care, which seems to equal, and in some cases, improve on that received in the traditional fee-for-service system. Members seem satisfied despite the fact that participants' choice of health care providers is, in many HMOs, limited to those employed by the HMO. By introducing competition into the health care marketplace, HMOs have helped reduce the cost of conventional health insurance.

Preferred Provider Organizations

In response to the growing surplus of physicians and the competition offered by HMOs, another health care innovation has emerged, the *preferred provider organization* (PPO). The providers, hospitals and physicians, negotiate discounted fee-for-service rate schedules with insurers. These rates usually amount to 80% to 85% of the "usual and customary" rates (Katz, 1983) in return for quick, guaranteed claims payment. Physicians can contract with one or several PPOs, and consumers can choose among the PPO physicians or ask their own physicians to join. Consumers receive complete coverage for services rendered by the PPO and reduced coverage for services rendered elsewhere. Hospitals, physicians, and insurance companies are the principal sponsors of PPOs, usually in response to requests from companies or unions. As of June 1985, there were 334 PPOs nationwide, 96 of them in California. About 10 million persons now have the option of choosing PPOs, compared with more than 20 million in HMOs.

Because PPOs have only been in operation since 1980, it is too soon to tell whether their long-term savings will be substantial. The federal government's three-year study of several PPOs will conclude in 1988.

SECONDARY CARE

Secondary care, interventions that prevent complications of disease conditions, is no longer exclusively the province of the hospital. Ambulatory care clinics, outpatient surgical centers, and home health agencies are competing, offering clients an alternative to hospitalization.

Ambulatory Care Clinics

Ambulatory care clinics (also called freestanding emergency clinics), have proliferated since the first one opened in 1973. Designed to handle a variety of minor emergencies, these clinics number more than 2000 in the United States, and another opens each day. Clients often prefer these facilities rather than hospital emergency rooms or formal appointments with health care providers because the clinics are conveniently located, no appointment is necessary, and the average charge is about $50—less than half the cost of a hospital emergency room visit.

Outpatient Surgical Centers

New technology and the growth of freestanding surgical centers have created a boom in outpatient surgery. From tonsillectomies to the once-complex cataract extraction, clients are gaining the benefits of less expensive one-day surgery. The number of freestanding surgical centers doubled between 1980 and 1985 and is expected to reach 600 by 1988. Forced to compete with these innovative facilities, many hospitals have opened their own centers for outpatient surgery, boosting the outpatient surgery rate at hospitals by 77% between 1979 and 1983, while inpatient operations fell 7% during the same period. Initial concern that clients would develop complications that could not be handled at home have proven unfounded. Careful preoperative screening and examination of clients minimize the risk of complications.

Hospitals

Once the unchallenged controllers of secondary care, hospitals are undergoing cataclysmic changes. The trends toward outpatient care in freestanding clinics and HMOs, reduced government support, and competition among themselves have forced hospitals to adopt business methods and strategies to survive. In many areas of the United States, hospitals are operating at less than 60% of capacity. Some experts think that by 1990, 20% of the nation's hospitals will either close, merge, or sell out to large multihospital for-profit corporations. Firms such as Humana Inc, Hospital Corporation of America, American Medical International, and National Medical Enterprises now own 11.4% of hospitals in the United States.

To replace revenue formerly supplied by Medicare and Medicaid payments, hospitals are marketing innovative services to consumers. Services may include fitness and nutrition classes, day-care for the elderly, or taxi service for persons who have been drinking. Some hospital management experts question the value of these services, believing that a better way to compete is by developing low-cost products and services. In addition to cost containment of inpatient services, for example, many hospitals now have formed their own home health agencies and outpatient surgery clinics. Others have established alternative birth centers (ABCs) to attract new families who may eventually need more expensive services. In addition to providing a homelike environment for the birth experience, ABCs may include such incentives as candlelight gourmet meals or gifts and discounts on pharmaceuticals, photo sessions, and baby clothes. Although some of these services may be less than profitable, they are considered an investment in future business by building a positive image and thereby persuading clients to return when they do require hospitalization.

As economic forces are changing hospitals' methods of operation, demographic forces are changing the very nature of hospitals. Despite the trend toward ambulatory care, the chronically ill and older segments of the population are increasing the demand for acute care. All but the most seriously ill persons are treated in one or more outpatient facilities, and only the most acutely ill enter the hospital. The American Hospital Association predicts a 15% increase in the number of inpatient days between 1980 and 1990; 89% of that increase will be attributable to those over 65. With this development, former general hospitals are fast becoming large intensive care centers.

Home Health Care

Like self-care, discussed earlier, home care is not a new idea but an old one enjoying unprecedented popularity. Home care began before 1800 in Boston and became the domain of nursing in the 1880s when voluntary agencies opened in Boston, Philadelphia, and Buffalo; these agencies became the visiting nurse associations (VNAs).

Once considered strictly long-term or tertiary care, home health care today spans both secondary and tertiary care. Earlier discharge from hospitals and high-tech client support systems used in treating chronic illness have fueled an explosion in home care. In 1985, there were more than 4000 Medicare-certified home care agencies employing more than 17,000 home health care providers. Growth is so rapid that accurate statistics are difficult to obtain. In Dallas, for example, the number of home care agencies tripled between 1982 and 1983.

Many types of agencies and services exist, ranging from one- or two-service providers to large, multiservice agencies (offering both professional and nonprofessional services). Some agencies are nonprofit, either private or voluntary (such as the traditional VNAs mentioned above); some are proprietary (for profit), either extensions of hospital services or national home care corporations. These agencies may be owned by physicians, nurses, business persons, or pharmaceutical companies (Griffith, 1984).

Home care agencies are providing services for sicker persons: clients on respirators, oxygen, intravenous therapy, total parenteral nutrition (TPN), chemotherapy, and dialysis. In addition to skilled nursing care, home care clients may require a host of other services such as a homemaker, home attendant, or Meals-on-Wheels.

Home care nursing services can be grouped into three major categories: professional intermittent or part-time services; professional continuous or extended care; and paraprofessional care. Professional intermittent care might include such activities as teaching a client and family a procedure or skill, providing ongoing assessment of a client's condition, changing dressings, and administering medication. Professional extended care can range from 4 to 24 hours per day and requires experienced, highly skilled nurses to care for clients with acute health problems. These skilled professionals manage such clients as those requiring respiratory support or parenteral nutrition and teach family members how to assist in this care. Paraprofessionals, such as certified nurses' aides, home health aides, and homemakers, can be employed when skilled care is not needed. Their assistance includes such services as bathing or feeding the client and relieving family members, at least briefly, from the stress of constant care. Also known as respite care, these services can make it possible for families to care for a chronically ill or disabled family member at home (Griffin, 1985) by supplementing the family's caregiving capabilities. Home care not only offers a more humane alternative to institutionalized care and a more therapeutic environment for restoration of health but enormous cost savings as well (see Table 1–1).

TERTIARY CARE

Also called rehabilitation or long-term care, tertiary care consists of helping to restore maximum function and/or helping the client live with illness, whether chronic or terminal. Home health care, discussed earlier as secondary care because it often involves care of the acutely ill, is the largest segment of the tertiary care delivery system. Other institutions involved in tertiary care include rehabilitation centers, nursing homes and other extended care facilities, and hospices. Rehabilitation centers and nursing homes have been part of the health care delivery system for decades. With the increase in physical trauma from auto accidents and other vehicular accidents and a burgeoning population over 65, their numbers can only increase. Hospice is a concept relatively new to this country. Initiated in England largely through the efforts of Dame Cicely Saunders, hospice care offers palliative care for the dying and their families, either at home or in the hospice facility. The National Association for Home Care has begun development of a hospice service to meet the needs of persons with remittent or progressive cancer but must wait for accreditation by the National Hospice Association. Hospice care may be intermittent or extended, depending on the needs of the client and family for support services (Griffith, 1984). Hospice is also discussed in Chapter 16.

Table 1–1   The Savings From Health Care at Home

Diagnosis	Acute Care Cost per Month in Hospital	Alternate Care Cost per Month at Home	Savings per Month
Baby born with breathing and feeding problems	$60,970	$20,209	$40,761
Spinal cord injury with quadriplegia	23,862	13,931	9,931
Neurological disorder with respiratory problems	17,783	196†	17,587
Severe cerebral palsy with uncontrolled seizure disorder	8,425	4,867‡	3,558

† After initial cost of equipment
‡ In extended care unit of hospital
Data: Aetna Life and Casualty Company
SOURCE: Reprinted with permission from: Insurance companies' big push to cut medical costs. *Business Week* (May 28, 1984); 128, 130.

Section VI: Change and the Nurse's Responsibility

Cost containment, assertiveness of health care consumers, an aging population, and increasing chronic health problems are rapidly reshaping the health care system. The changes are creating new opportunities for nurses who understand their meaning for nurses and for nursing. Economic forecasters predict the demand for registered nurses will be up 49% by 1995 (*American Demographics*, 1985). Those who do not understand these changes may find their effectiveness as caregivers and their economic welfare severely compromised. Concern for the client, clinical and technical skills, and sound clinical judgment are only the beginning requirements for a successful nursing career in today's health care system. Nurses need to understand the economics and the politics of health care; they need to gain a voice in shaping health policy at every level (Mason & Talbott, 1985). They need to be computer literate and share a universal professional language based on the nursing process and nursing diagnoses.

NURSING PROCESS AND NURSING THEORY

Since the 1960s, the use of the term *nursing process* to describe nurses' overall function has gained nearly universal acceptance. First outlined in four steps, then further delineated as five in 1982, the nursing process comprises assessment, analysis (or nursing diagnosis), planning, implementation (or intervention), and evaluation.

Nursing diagnosis, the most controversial step in the nursing process, has greatly contributed to standardizing the terms that define client characteristics and actual or potential nursing care needs. In 1982, a list of nursing diagnoses approved by the North American Nursing Diagnosis Association (NANDA) was published. These nurs-

ing diagnoses are tested, discussed, periodically refined, and updated in the nursing literature (Kim, McFarland, & McLane, 1984).

Nursing diagnoses may or may not relate to the client's medical diagnosis; they do relate to the actual purpose of nursing as defined by the American Nurses' Association (ANA): "the diagnosis and treatment of human responses to actual or potential health problems" (ANA, 1980). Nursing diagnoses help nurses to describe thoughtfully the phenomena that are the human responses to illness as they apply to the special and unique characteristics of each client. Understanding and using nursing diagnoses appropriately help nurses to separate nursing care from "room and board" in hospital cost accounting and also help refine the client classification system on which prospective payment depends.

Nurses are actively engaged in scholarly inquiry into the very nature of nursing. The purpose of theory construction in nursing is to move the profession away from an intuitive base toward an intellectual base. Several conceptual models or theories of nursing have been proposed, each with its proponents and critics. Although these models of nursing are diverse, they share several themes: the holistic nature of humans; the importance of individuality, self-worth, and dignity; and the essentially humanitarian nature of nursing. These commonalites undergird the framework of this text.

CLIENT/FAMILY ADVOCACY AND EDUCATION

The traditional nursing roles of client advocate and health teacher assume new importance in today's health care climate. In the midst of monitors, tubes, and technology, nursing reaches out to the person, offering "human contact . . . human responses to fundamentally human needs. Nurses can provide the critical 'high-touch' element essential for a high-tech world. They are the fulcrum which balances high technology and human response in health care'' (Curtin, 1984). As cost containment threatens to erode the quality and even the safety of care, nursing must assert its rights to protect the rights of the client and family. To support the important self-care trend, nursing needs to reemphasize one of its central roles, that of client teacher.

None of this is possible without nursing acknowledging and exercising its power, what Benner (1984) describes as the "power of caring." One of the qualities of this power is *advocacy power*, "the kind of power that removes obstacles or stands alongside and enables" (Benner, 1984). When clients cannot understand medical jargon or negotiate the seemingly mysterious workings of the health care system, the nurse can make a positive difference. This kind of power is exemplified by the nurse who convinced the physician to delay giving medications that would take away a client's own respiratory drive, even though the client was hyperventilating and his blood gases were compromised. The nurse helped calm the young man so he could maintain control over his last remaining set of functioning muscles. The nurse described this powerful act of caring:

> It took three and a half hours before he began to relax. He needed to understand what had happened, and was presently happening to him. He needed to be reassured, and most of all to learn to trust us. He needed to know what the future might hold for him. He needed to know that we cared about *him*, as an individual not just another helpless patient. As he began to comprehend these things, he learned to trust us. That was the key. He needed to be involved, not just prescribed to. He felt so very helpless . . . . The point was made by one simple statement he mouthed to me late in the day . . . when he had a respiratory rate in the 20s, and he was no longer threatened with having the remaining functional muscles chemically paralyzed: His words were: "Thank you. You've really helped me a lot. I don't want to imagine what would have happened to me if you weren't here and hadn't cared" (Benner, 1984).

Since Nightingale, nurses have recognized the importance of teaching the client about health and illness. Today teaching is even more important because clients want and need to learn about their own health, how to maintain and improve it, and how to help restore it when accident or illness occurs. Benner (1984) has described this role, or domain, of nursing practice as the *teaching–coaching function*. Among the competencies listed in that domain are those in Box 1–1.

Within this domain, nurses have what Benner terms *integrative power*, the power that can reintegrate the individual into his or her own social world, despite prolonged or permanent disability. This kind of power is illustrated in the following nurse's description of an early experience in her career:

> When I was very young, I worked for the Visiting Nurse Association. One woman I went to see on consultation hadn't been out of her bedroom for five years and was just dying of depression. She'd had a stroke and had not had much physical therapy. She

Box 1–1 The Teaching–Coaching Domain of Nursing Practice

Timing: Capturing a patient's readiness to learn

Assisting patients to integrate the implications of illness and recovery into their lifestyles

Eliciting and understanding the patient's interpretation of his or her illness

Providing an interpretation of the patient's condition and giving a rationale for procedures

The coaching function: Making culturally avoided aspects of an illness approachable and understandable

SOURCE: Reprinted with permission from Benner P: *From Novice to Expert*. Menlo Park, CA: Addison–Wesley, 1984, p 79.

> had one completely frozen arm and very little mobility with her right leg. At the time, I knew very little about her chances for recovery. There were no orders for physical therapy. "Her heart is bad, the exercises might kill her," I was told. (Now you have to remember, that this was many years ago.) And I said, "She's dying anyway, she is dying because her whole world is just the four walls." And I wanted the opportunity to help, and I asked the doctor to give me the opportunity, by giving an order for physical therapy. And I promised to talk to the husband and to her about the fact that it is taking a big chance and that she may die. The doctor reluctantly gave me an order, and I exercised that woman, and got her out of bed. I got a book out of the library and read up on CVA physical therapy because I knew very little about physical therapy. She never regained the use of the hand and arm, of course, but she did get to the point that she could walk with help. And the first day she walked out of her bedroom, she just burst into tears. She died five and a half years later while cooking dinner. She had learned to peel potatoes with her one hand, wedging them against her paralyzed arm. She was a marvelous lady who was dying because she was being treated like an invalid, and she felt useless and hopeless (Benner, 1984).

The power of caring as Benner defines it is not a dominating, coercing, or controlling kind of power. Instead, it is a power that nurses can and do use to empower their clients. Some nurses are uncomfortable with the concept of being powerful and using power (Dumas, 1985); however, nurses need to assert their power not only to protect the rights of the clients and families they care for but also to preserve and protect the profession.

PRIMARY NURSING

One of the most vivid examples of nursing's increased autonomy and responsibility is the widespread implementation of primary nursing, the system in which one nurse is responsible for total client care around the clock, 7 days a week (Manthey, 1980). Primary nursing was introduced in the 1960s as a means of affording individualized and more consistent care and offering greater satisfaction for both nurses and clients. Studies during the past two decades have demonstrated that primary nursing does, in fact, achieve these goals. In addition, primary nursing is cost effective.

The concept of primary nursing fixes responsibility and accountability on the primary care nurse who is assigned total care of a client. When the primary nurse is off duty, care is given by associate nurses who report to the primary nurse. In addition, the primary nurse is responsible for communicating information about the client to the entire health care team, of which the client is considered a part. Also central to this concept are continuity of care through the use of nursing care plans, autonomy of the primary care nurse who makes the decisions about the care of the client, and an emphasis on client-centered and personalized, not task-oriented, nursing care.

The cost effectiveness of primary nursing is related not to salaries of the RN staff (which may be slightly higher than that of a staff of RNs plus LPNs or aides) but to the reduced incidence of complications, quicker recovery, and shortened hospital stay that results. Despite the studies that have demonstrated this cost effectiveness, however, the current cost-containment climate means that nurses will have to continue to prove to hospital managers the value of primary nursing. Fortunately, nursing's growing sophistication in the use of computers and research is making that task easier.

COMMUNITY NURSING

Nursing's roots in the community go deep. In America, the visiting nurse associations mentioned earlier were some of the first organized groups to serve the public. As the community again becomes a principal setting for care, nursing is finding new opportunities for autonomy and growth. Settings include the traditional public health areas, such as city, county, or state health departments; VNAs; community mental health centers; well-baby clinics; schools; and industry. In addition, nurses are practicing in and sometimes managing home care agencies, neighborhood health centers, and rural health centers.

Experts predict that outpatient care markets will grow more than 200% between 1984 and 1988 (Coleman et al., 1984). This dynamic and exciting situation holds great promise for nurses, particularly nurse practitioners and clinical specialists who want to practice more autonomously. Hospitals are quickly moving into this expanding market, but they need not control it. As Coleman and associates (1984) indicated, "All this work is essentially nursing work; therefore, nurses should step forward to grasp its organization. There are no reasons or justifications why they can't organize more alternative ambulatory and outpatient care delivery systems."

INDEPENDENT PRACTICE

In 1971, Lucille Kinlein "hung out her shingle," becoming the first independent practitioner of nursing in America. Since then, thousands of nurses have followed suit. Some are family care practitioners, others are health educators, still others are nurse-midwives or psychiatric nurse specialists. They practice in rural and urban settings, and in some cases, compete with other providers such as physicians.

Competition with other practitioners fosters controversy and even litigation that tests state nursing practice acts. This circumstance arose in November 1983, when Missouri's new nursing practice act was tested in the state supreme court. A lower court had ruled that two nurse practitioners were practicing unauthorized medicine when they obtained clients' histories, performed pelvic examinations, and offered information about contraceptives and other health-related issues. The supreme court reversed the decision of the lower court and ruled in favor of the two nurses, stating that Missouri's nursing practice act reflects the desire of the legislature to expand the scope of authorized nursing practice. The court held that these nurses' activities were what the legislature had envisioned when it granted nurses the "right to make assessments and nursing diagnoses."

RESEARCH IN NURSING

Just as every scientific discipline uses research as a primary tool to broaden and deepen its understanding of the world, nursing uses research to enhance its understanding of health and illness. The ANA Commission on Nursing Research (1981) defines nursing research as:

> Investigating . . . the areas of knowledge where the physical and behavioral sciences meet and influence one another, in an effort to study how health problems relate to human behavior and how behavior relates to health and illness. . . . Research in nursing addresses the human and behavioral questions that arise in the treatment of disease and the prevention of illness and maintenance of health.

Nursing research relates directly to nursing as defined in the ANA social policy statement: "the diagnosis and treatment of human responses to actual or potential health problems." For example, while the Centers for Disease Control in Atlanta study the AIDS virus, nurses in San Francisco, New York, and other major cities are studying the impact of this epidemic on clients and families, their relationships, and their abilities to cope with a potentially fatal illness.

In 1983, nursing research reached two critical milestones. First, the ANA established the Center for Research for Nursing. The functions of this center include supporting the work of policy-making bodies within ANA, administration of extramurally funded research projects, preparing grant applications to secure research funding, and coordinating external fund-raising activities.

The second milestone was the introduction in Congress of legislation to establish a National Institute of Nursing within the National Institutes of Health (NIH). This action was prompted by recommendations in a 1983 Institute of Medicine report calling for a federally funded entity to *place nursing research in the mainstream of scientific investigation*. This legislation was passed by both houses of Congress in 1984 but vetoed by President Ronald Reagan. Despite that veto, the Center for Nursing Research was established in early 1985 within the Division of Human Services, Department of Health and Human Services. Many nurses do not consider this a reasonable alternative because only a National Institute of Nursing within NIH would put nursing in the mainstream of scientific research.

Nursing research must belong to all nurses, not just the academicians and the career nurse scientists. As Wilson (1985) stated: "If nursing is to build a scientific body of knowledge and if nursing practice is to be shaped by research findings rather than tradition, intuition, or habit, then the investigative skills of all nurses, regardless of

their educational level, must be as integral to their repertoire as communication skills and sterile technique."

Priorities for future research identified by ANA focus on health care and illness prevention, development of cost-efficient systems for delivery of nursing care, and strategies for effective care of high-risk groups. Equal in importance to these priorities is making nursing research visible, both within and outside the profession. For nursing research to change the practice of nursing, it must be disseminated. More potential avenues for its publication exist today than ever before—four journals exclusively devoted to nursing research and dozens of others actively seeking articles based on research but written in a less formal style. The Nursing Research boxes throughout this text demonstrate the integral role of nursing research within nursing practice.

Chapter Highlights

Sociologic, economic, and technologic changes affect the health care consumer, the health care system, and the roles and responsibilities of nurses.

The character and mobility of the American family has changed markedly over the past three decades.

One of the greatest health care challenges is being posed by the growing population of persons over 65. Unfortunately, health policy and the health care system often categorize and stereotype older persons.

Environmental pollution and occupational hazards threaten life and health throughout the world.

The United States, a traditional cultural "melting pot," continues to attract immigrants from a variety of other cultures; their cultural blueprints affect their health care needs.

Poverty goes hand in hand with health problems, an increased need for health services, and an inability to pay for them.

The health care business is the second largest industry in the United States; health care costs have spiraled far above the general rate of economic inflation.

Implementing the DRG system for prospective payment concerns health professionals who worry that quality will be sacrificed to cost consciousness.

Highly technologic health care is expensive; it also runs the risk of becoming depersonalized care.

Increasing numbers of individuals are asserting their rights in health care and assuming the responsibilities that accompany those rights.

Primary care—health maintenance, health promotion, and disease prevention—holds the greatest hope for reducing costs and improving health.

Secondary care services have expanded outside of the hospital to ambulatory care clinics, outpatient surgical centers, and home health care.

Home health care can be either a secondary or tertiary care service.

Conceptual models or theories of nursing share several commonalities—the holistic nature of humans; the importance of individuality, self-worth, and dignity; and the essentially humanitarian nature of nursing.

The purpose of theory construction in nursing is to move the profession away from an intuitive base toward an intellectual base.

The traditional nursing roles of client advocate and health teacher assume new importance in today's health care climate. These roles help nurses balance high technology with human response.

Nurses can shape the nature of nursing practice through participating in nursing research, no matter what their educational level.

Bibliography

ADAMHA News, 1984, 10(1); 1.

American Board of Family Practice, 1985, 228 Young Drive, Lexington, KY 40505.

American College of Hospital Administrators, 1984, 840 N Lakeshore Drive, Chicago, IL 60611.

American Demographics, PO Box 68, Ithaca, NY 14851.

American Intraocular Implant Society, 3700 Pender Drive, Suite 108, Fairfax, VA 22030.

American Nurses' Association: *Nursing: A Social Policy Statement*. Kansas City, MO: ANA, 1980.

American Nurses' Association Commission on Nursing Research: *Research Priorities for the 1980s*. Kansas City, MO: ANA, 1981.

Benner P: *From Novice to Expert: Excellence and Power in Clinical Nursing Practice.* Menlo Park, CA: Addison–Wesley, 1984.

Buch R, Borman L D: *Self-Help Groups and Pastoral Care.* Care Cassettes. College of Chaplains, 1982; 9:8.

Butler R L, Lewis M: *Aging and Mental Health*, 3rd ed. St Louis: Mosby, 1983.

Children's Defense Fund: Strong national and state leadership urged to meet 1990 infant health goals. (Press release.) Washington, DC, Feb 27, 1985.

Coleman J R, Dayani E C, Simms E: Nursing careers in the emerging systems. *Nurs Management* (Jan) 1984; 15:19–27.

Cooper R, Simmons B E: Cigarette smoking and ill health among black Americans. (July) 1985; 85(7): 344–347.

Curtin L.; Nursing: High-touch in a high-tech world. *Nursing Management* (July) 1984; 15:7–7.

Diers D: Nursing intensity and DRGs. Paper presented at *National League for Nursing* convention, June 1985.

Dumas R: Two perspectives on power: Women and power. In: *Political Action Handbook for Nurses: Changing the Workplace, Government, Organizations, and Community.* Mason D, Talbott S (editors). Menlo Park, CA: Addison–Wesley, 1985.

Griffin M: Home nursing care needs more exposure. *Calif Nurse* (July-Aug) 1985.

Griffith E: Home care today. (Interview.) *Am J Nurs* 1984; 84:3 341–342.

Health, United States, 1983. Department of Health and Human Services, Washington, DC, 1984.

Heinz J: Hearing before the Special Committee on Aging, United States Senate, Philadelphia, December 12, 1984.

Hendricks B: The transitional experience for the missioner; an inward/outward journey. *Orientation.* New York: Maryknoll Sisters, 1982.

Katz C: Preferred provider organizations: New relation of the HMO. *Postgrad Med* (June) 1983; 73:143–146.

Kim M J, McFarland G K, McLane A M: *Pocket Guide to Nursing Diagnoses.* St. Louis: Mosby, 1984.

Lee P R, Estes C L, Ramsay N B: *The Nation's Health*, 2nd ed. San Francisco: Boyd & Frazer, 1984.

Leininger M: In: *International Nursing.* Masson V (editor). New York: Springer–Verlag, 1981.

Levin L S: The role of the individual in health care. In: *The Nation's Health,* 2nd ed. Lee P R, Eses C L, Ramsay N B (editors). San Francisco; Boyd & Fraser, 1984.

Living Bank, Houston, Texas.

Louis Harris L & Associates: National access survey, 1982. In *Special Report.* Princeton, NJ: Robert Wood Johnson Foundation, 1983.

Maiman L A, Green L W, Gibson G, Mackenzie E J: Education for self-treatment by adult asthmatics. JAMA 1979; 241(18): 1919–1922.

Manthey M: *The Practice of Primary Nursing.* Boston: Blackwell, 1980

Mason D J, Talbott S W: *Political Action Handbook for Nurses: Changing the Workplace, Government, Organizations, and Community.* Menlo Park, CA: Addison–Wesley, 1985.

McCormick K A: Preparing nurses for the technologic future. *Nurse Health Care* 1983; 4(7): 379–382.

Nelson J P, Carlstrom J A: A new confrontation: Nursing education and computer technology. *Image* (Summer) 1985; 17(3): 86–87.

Newton G: Self-help groups: can they help? *J Psychosoc Nurs* (July) 1984; 22:27–31.

Power L S, Courtice K: *Alzheimer's Disease: A Guide for Families.* Reading, MA: Addison–Wesley, 1983.

Sovie M D, Tarcinale M A, Vanputee A W, Stunden A E: Amalgam of nursing acuity, DRGs and costs. *Nurs Management* (March) 1985; 16:22–42.

Spain D: Country profile: The United States: Just the facts. In: *American Demographics, Inc, Special Report. Ithaca, NY: American Demographics,* June 1983.

Toffler A: *Future Shock.* New York: Random House, 1970.

Wilson H S: *Research in Nursing.* Menlo Park, CA: Addison–Wesley, 1985.

Suggested Readings

Curtin L: What we say/what we do. (Editorial.) *Nurs Management* (January) 1984; 15:7–8. This though-provoking editorial discusses the professional and economic importance of using the language of nursing process and nursing diagnosis in all communication, particularly documentation.

DeCrosta T: Megatrends in nursing: 10 new directions that are changing your profession. *Nurs Life* (May-June) 1985; 5:17–19. A director of nursing service identifies the major trends that are reshaping the entire field of health care, including nursing.

Griener PA: What has become of the traditional nurse? *Nurs Outlook* (Dec) 1981; 29:720–721. This article briefly reviews half a century of changes in health care that have altered the roles, responsibilities, and practice of the nurse.

Griffith H: Who will become the preferred providers? *Amer J Nurs* 1985; 85(5): 538–542. This article identifies how nurse-managed and nurse-serviced PPOs can provide nurses with the opportunity to be creative and innovative while providing health services for lower fees.

LaForme S: Primary nursing: Does good care cost more? *Can Nurse* (April) 1982; 78:42–49. The demonstrated cost effectiveness of primary nursing in one hospital is reported in this article.

Levenstein A: Storm clouds on the horizon. *Nurs Management* (April) 1985; 16:52–53. Written by an attorney, this column projects the implications for nursing of continuing cuts in the federal health care budget and how nurses need to respond, both individually and collectively.

Mitchell K: The next economy: Where will nurses fit? (Editorial.) *J Pediatr Nurs* (Nov-Dec) 1984; 10:381. Nursing's future in an economy in transition is the topic of this insightful editorial.

Whitman M: Toward a new psychology for nurses. *Nurs Outlook* (Jan) 1982: 30:48–52. This article describes the impact of the women's movement on nursing's increasing autonomy and power.

Chapter 2

How Illness Develops

SueAnn Wooster Ames
Carol Ren Kneisl

Objectives

When you have finished studying this chapter, you should be able to:

Interpret the multiple-causation theory of illness as a basis for nursing practice.

Describe the effects of stress on an individual.

List the sources of stress.

Identify the role of the immune system and immune response in health and illness.

Explain why the process of inflammation is a positive bodily response to tissue injury.

Enumerate the categories of genetic disorders and approaches to preventing them.

Identify the potential injurious effects of benign and malignant neoplasms.

Describe the normal physiological changes associated with aging and list possible lifestyle effects of each.

Propose strategies for assisting clients in maintaining maximum health as they age.

List the most frequent causes of traumatic injury and suggest approaches to reducing the high incidence of trauma.

What causes disease? The biomedical theory of disease focuses on cells, organs, or organ systems and explains disease on the basis of the physical and biological sciences. The social, psychological, or behavioral dimensions of health alterations are not acknowledged in the biomedical approach, which has dominated health care since René Descartes (1596–1650) formulated his theory of mind–body dualism. A holistic view of humans, as this text advocates, bridges the gulf between mind and body, between "illness" care delivery and "health" care delivery—acknowledging that disease is directly related to the sum of all factors affecting a person's life.

Section I: Disease Versus Illness (Dis-ease)

Unlike medical theory, which has traditionally emphasized *disease* at the subsystem level of the cell, the organ, or the organ system, nursing theory has its roots in holistic concepts (Figure 2–1). Nurses base their practice on the multiple-causation theory of health alterations, considering such suprasystem problems as unemployment, racism, urban congestion, pollution, and stressful living patterns as major components in explaining why persons become ill. The concept of *illness*, while recognizing that biological and genetic factors contribute to disease, is strongly related to

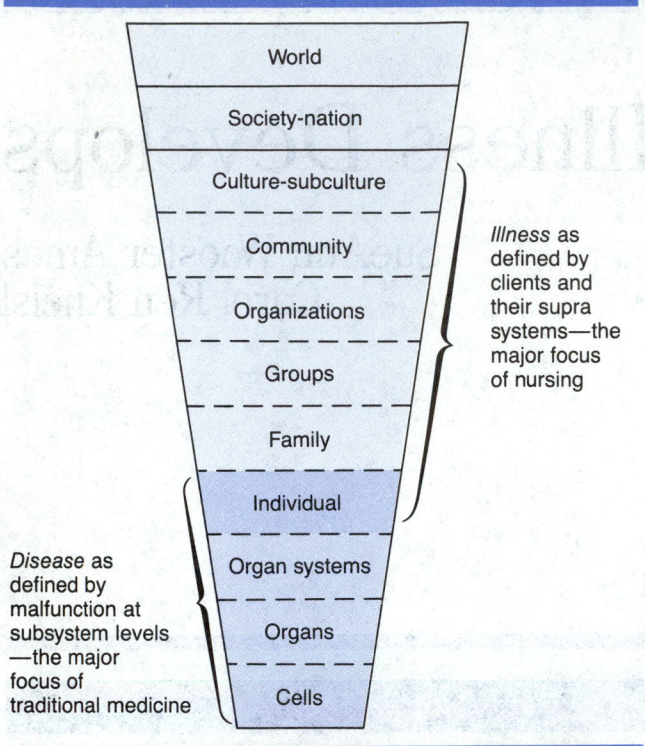

Figure 2–1

A systems hierarchy differentiating illness from disease and nursing from traditional medicine.
SOURCE: Adapted from Ames SA, Gelein J, Humphrey E, Mason-Kaufman J, Osborne JE: A systems approach to curricula in primary health care nursing. In *Approaches to Teaching Primary Health Care*, Knopke HJ, Diekelmann NL (editors). St. Louis: Mosby, 1981.

the total individual and the individual's family, social network, environment, and culture. Disease is merely one inhibitor of health. *Illness is the human experience of disease.*

For example, many factors, from neoplasia to stress, can alter the amount and frequency of a woman's menstrual flow. A cultural belief that menstruation is a process that rids the body of "dirty blood," strongly influences the woman's interpretation of the meaning of an alteration in flow for her health. If her flow decreases, she will believe something is wrong—she is ill. If her flow increases, she may view herself as cleansed of impurities and therefore in excellent health. Suppose this woman enters the American health care system. Her care provider, evaluating a history of a month or two of decreased flow with no addi-

tional problems, will probably view her as healthy. Conversely, a history of increased flow associated with a fibroid or other uterine tumor will be interpreted as disease. The client, who will probably retain the beliefs of her culture, will find herself in conflict with the health system.

Although the word *disease* derives from the prefix *dis* (without) and the French *aise* (ease)—literally meaning "without or lacking ease,"—disease is usually discussed as pathology—some abnormality in an organ or organ system that results in certain symptoms and signs. Disease may be further described by such terms as *acute* or *chronic, communicable, congenital, degenerative, functional, malignant, psychosomatic,* or *idiopathic.* The causation of a disease is called its etiology, and often a disease is discussed as if there were one specific etiology. But whenever disease exists, a *whole person* is involved—not only an organ or organ system.

Consider Mrs W, who has a urinary tract infection (UTI). The organism *Escherichia coli* is cultured, and appropriate antibiotic therapy is begun. The infectious agent may not entirely account for the illness, however. In women, *E. coli* is always present in the perineal region, yet women do not continuously have UTIs. Perhaps before the onset of the UTI, Mrs W inadvertently wiped her perineal area from back to front during toileting. Perhaps she reduced her fluid intake from her usual eight glasses of water a day, or perhaps she neglected to void after intercourse. To carry the analysis further, perhaps she was upset over losing her job, so she neglected perineal hygiene or forgot to consume enough fluids. This brief example points out the multifactorial origin of *dis-ease,* or illness. Regarding disease, the cause of this woman's urinary tract infection is the bacterium *E. coli.* But the origin or cause of the illness (dis-ease) was multifactorial.

In this text, all illness is considered multifactorial; in the fundamental sense, all disease is illness. Nevertheless, a nurse must understand certain basic internal and external mechanisms of disease or degeneration that influence the onset and duration of illness. These factors, which closely interrelate with psychosocial and environmental influences, are stress, the immune system and immune response, infection and inflammation, genetic predispositions, neoplasia, aging, and trauma. As an overview of these factors, this chapter reviews concepts discussed in earlier courses and lays the foundation for the more extensive discussions of each of these factors in the specific disorders chapters in each body systems unit.

Section II: Stress: A Cause and an Effect of Illness

Stress is a part of being alive. Standing erect stresses the musculoskeletal system (muscles and bones must work together to keep the body erect), eating stresses the

digestive system (enzymes must be produced and nutrients absorbed), and breathing stresses the respiratory system (carbon dioxide and oxygen must be exchanged). In unseen ways, the immune system is constantly engaged in a war with the bacteria in the body. The interaction and eventual balance among these various forces constitute the routine stress with which all humans contend.

THE FIGHT-FLIGHT RESPONSE TO STRESS

Beyond this routine and essential stress, humans risk encountering undesirable or excess stress that threatens well-being and may even be life threatening. They cope with such threats through either a *fight* (aggression) or *flight* (withdrawal) response. The fight-flight response was first discussed by Walter Cannon, a physician, in 1932 when he identified stress as an actual cause of disease. Consider the following situation of extreme stress: A woman is walking down a dark, deserted street when a man with a knife emerges from the shadows just in front of her. Does she try to defend herself? Does she run away? Whichever action she takes has been enabled by a variety of physiologic responses to extreme danger. According to Mason (1980), when a person faces such a situation:

- The heartbeat increases to pump blood throughout the necessary tissues with greater speed, carrying oxygen and nutrients to cells and clearing away waste products more quickly.
- As the heart rate increases, the blood pressure rises.
- Breathing becomes rapid and shallow.
- Epinephrine and other hormones are released into the blood.
- The liver releases stored sugar into the blood to meet the increased energy needs of survival.
- The pupils dilate to let in more light; all the senses are heightened.
- Muscles tense for movement, either for flight or protective actions, particularly the skeletal muscles of the thighs, hips, back, shoulders, arms, jaw, and face.
- Blood flow to the digestive organs is greatly constricted.
- Blood flow increases to the brain and major muscles.
- Blood flow to the extremities is constricted, and the hands and feet become cold. This is protection from bleeding to death quickly if the hands or feet are injured in fight or flight and allows blood to be diverted to more important areas of the body.
- The body perspires to cool itself, because increased metabolism generates more heat.

Although these physiological responses seem appropriate for the situation described, imagine the wear and tear on the body if humans responded to all stress in these ways.

THE GENERAL ADAPTATION SYNDROME

Hans Selye, a Canadian endocrinologist and the most well known and widely recognized stress researcher, developed another framework for understanding how persons respond to stress. Each person has a limited amount of energy to use in dealing with stress. How quickly it is used and, therefore, how quickly one adapts to stress depend on several factors such as heredity, mental attitude, and lifestyle, among others.

Stress can be appraised by measuring the structural and chemical changes it produces in the body. These changes are called the *general adaptation syndrome* (GAS) because when stress affects the whole person, the whole person must adjust to the changes.

While a medical student, Selye made an interesting and important observation that became the cornerstone of his stress-adaptation theory. He observed that, regardless of the diagnosis, most clients had certain symptoms in common—they lost their appetites, they lost weight, they felt and looked ill, and they had aches and pains in their joints and muscles. He introduced his observations and the general adaptation syndrome concept in 1936 in a letter to the editor of *Nature*.

A long series of experiments (1956) led to more objective evidence of actual body damage—enlargement of the adrenal glands; shrinkage of the thymus, spleen, and lymph nodes; and the appearance of bleeding gastric ulcers. These symptoms, he said, were part of the body's *alarm* reaction to disease, the first stage in the general adaptation syndrome. In the second stage, the stage of *resistance*, the body tries to return to equilibrium despite continuing disease. If the stress persists, the person becomes exhausted from the wear and tear required by constant adjustment. This third stage is appropriately named the stage of *exhaustion*. The physical and psychological manifestations in all three stages are described in Table 2–1.

LIFE CHANGES AS STRESSFUL EVENTS

Although most persons readily recognize undesirable or traumatic life experiences as stressful, fewer recognize that stress is also associated with what is normally viewed as positive—graduating from nursing school, being promoted on the job, getting along better with the boss. The cumulative effect of both positive and negative life changes may reduce a person's ability to handle stress and may even promote subsequent illness.

The research into life changes as stressful events has been continuing since the late 1960s when Holmes and Rahe (1967) began their studies. They explored life changes and developed a scale that assigned value rankings to 43 life events associated with stress. Each life event is assigned a value determined by the degree of stress involved. These rankings are called life-change units (LCU). The higher

Table 2–1 The Stress Adaptation Syndrome

Stage	Physical Change	Psychosocial Changes
Stage I: Alarm reaction (mobilization of the body's defensive forces and activation of the "fight-or-flight" mechanism)	Release of norepinephrine and epinephrine causing vasoconstriction, increased blood pressure, and increased rate and force of cardiac contraction	Increased level of alertness
		Increased level of anxiety
	Increased hormone levels	Task-oriented, defense-oriented, inefficient, or maladaptive behavior may occur
	Enlargement of adrenal cortex	
	Marked loss of body weight	
	Shrinkage of the thymus, spleen, and lymph nodes	
	Irritation of the gastric mucosa	
Stage II: Stage of resistance (optimal adaptation to stress within the person's capabilities)	Hormone levels readjust	Increased and intensified use of coping mechanisms
	Reduction in activity and size of adrenal cortex	
	Lymph glands return to normal size	Tendency to rely on defense-oriented behavior
	Weight returns to normal	
Stage III: Stage of exhaustion (loss of ability to resist stress because of depletion of body resources)	Decreased immune response with suppression of T cells and atrophy of thymus	Defense-oriented behaviors become exaggerated
	Depletion of adrenal glands and hormone production	Disorganization of thinking
		Disorganization of personality
	Weight loss	Sensory stimuli may be misperceived with appearance of illusion
	Enlargement of lymph nodes and dysfunction of lymphatic system	Reality contact may be reduced with appearance of delusions or hallucinations
	If exposure to the stressor continues, cardiac failure, renal failure, or death may occur	If exposure to the stressor continues, stupor or violence may occur

the total score of a person's life-change units, the more likely the person is to become ill within the next year. Review the life-change events in Table 2–2 and consider carefully the following example:

Mr J recently graduated from nursing school (LCU 26), where he received the award for excellence in bedside nursing at graduation (LCU 28). The following week, he married one of his classmates (LCU 50), and they went on a 2-week automobile trip across the country (LCU 13) that combined a honeymoon and a move to another state (LCU 20), where both partners obtained staff nurse positions in a large hospital. The only event marring the vacation was receiving a $20 traffic ticket for not coming to a complete stop at a stop sign (LCU 11). Mr J enjoyed his new location, his new job, and his vastly improved financial status (LCU 39) now that both he and his wife had gone from being financially strapped nursing students to full-time day-shift staff nurses. He did, however, miss the frequent visits he used to have with his parents and his brother and sister when they all had lived near one another (LCU 15). Within less than a year, Mr J received a coveted promotion to assistant head nurse (LCU 29) on the night shift. The promotion required him to

change his usual hours of sleep (LCU 16). Because he and his wife now worked different shifts, extensive changes in their social activities had to be made (LCU 18).

Although it appears on the surface that Mr J's life had changed for the better with his improved financial status and promotion to assistant head nurse, his score is 265 LCUs. According to Table 2–2, his score puts him in the 51% risk category for an illness within the next year or two. Suppose further that Mr and Mrs J are considering beginning a family soon. Gaining a new family member through birth would add 39 points to his LCU score, putting him near the 79% risk category. In Chapter 4 is a discussion of how nurses can teach and counsel clients such as Mr J about their LCU scores. Other researchers have adapted this tool to fit specific circumstances. An adaptation by two nurses measuring stress factors based on events that affect hospitalized persons is also discussed in Chapter 4.

Table 2–2 Social Readjustment Rating Scale

Item Number	Life Event (Item Value)	Item Value	Item Number	Life Event (Item Value)	Item Value
1	Death of spouse	100	27	Begin or end school	26
2	Divorce	73	28	Change in living conditions	25
3	Marital separation	65	29	Revision of personal habits	24
4	Jail term	63	30	Trouble with boss	23
5	Death of close family member	63	31	Change in work hours or conditions	20
6	Personal injury or illness	53	32	Change in residence	20
7	Marriage	50	33	Change in schools	20
8	Fired at work	47	34	Change in recreation	19
9	Marital reconciliation	45	35	Change in church activities	19
10	Retirement	45	36	Change in social activities	18
11	Change in health of a family member	44	37	Mortgage or loan less than $10,000	17
12	Pregnancy	40	38	Change in sleeping habits	16
13	Sex difficulties	39	39	Change in number of family gatherings	15
14	Gain of a new family member	39	40	Change in eating habits	15
15	Business readjustment	39	41	Vacation	13
16	Change in financial state	39	42	Christmas	12
17	Death of a close friend	37	43	Minor violations of the law	11
18	Change to a different line of work	36			
19	Change in number of arguments with spouse	35			
20	Mortgage over $10,000	31			
21	Foreclosure of mortgage or loan	30			
22	Change in responsibilities at work	29			
23	Son or daughter leaving home	29			
24	Trouble with in-laws	29			
25	Outstanding personal achievement	28			
26	Spouse begins or stops work	26			

Scoring:

150–199	Mild risk
200–299	Moderate risk
300 or more	Major risk

The higher the risk level, the more likely it is that the person will encounter illness within the year. Of the subjects Holmes and Rahe studied, 37% in the mild risk category, 51% in the moderate risk category, and 79% in the major risk category had associated health changes.

SOURCE: Reprinted with permission from Holmes TH, Rahe RH: The social adjustment rating scale. *J Psychosom Res* 1967; 11: 213–218.

Section III: The Immune System and Immune Response

The immune system is one of the body's principal defenses against disease; however, disturbances of the immune system or, in some cases, dysfunctional immune responses, can themselves cause illness. The system consists of a complex group of organs, tissues, and cells located in various parts of the body. The thymus, bone marrow, lymph nodes, spleen, tonsils, appendix, and the Peyer's patches of the small intestine constitute the organs of the immune system. Lymphocytes, plasma cells, and macrophages are its principal cells.

The function of the lymphocytes (a specific type of white blood cell or leukocyte) is the key factor in all immune responses. Lymphocyte cells migrate through tissues, circulate in blood and lymph, and accumulate in the spleen and lymph nodes. The two major types of lymphocytes are B cells and T cells. **B-lymphocytes** mature in the bone marrow. When triggered by an antigen, they differentiate into antibody-producing cells. **T-lymphocytes** are a heterogeneous group of cells that mature in the thymus gland and differentiate into a variety of **effector T cells**, namely killer cells, helpers, and suppressors. These cells are essential in regulating the intensity of the body's fight against invasive organisms and in summoning antibody production.

Macrophages, derived from monocytes (large leukocytes), are cells of the reticuloendothelial system that can engulf foreign particles. This process is called **phagocytosis**. The uptake of antigens by the macrophages is the first step in the processing of antigen leading to antibody production.

THE IMMUNE RESPONSE

The essence of an immune response is the capacity of the host to recognize and react to foreign substances. Antigens signal the host that a "nonself" invader is within.

An **antigen** is a foreign protein or protein complex capable of stimulating a specific immune response when it is present in the body. An antibody is a specialized plasma protein called an **immunoglobulin** (Ig) produced by the B-lymphocytes in response to the presence of an antigen. The five major classes of immunoglobulins are IgG, IgM, IgA, IgD, and IgE (Table 2–3).

The complement system is a group of at least 15 plasma proteins activated in an ordered sequence when an antibody couples with its antigen, producing substances that participate in inflammation and host defense. IgG and IgM can activate the complement system, which in turn enhances phagocytosis, vascular permeability, and cellular lysis (destruction of the cell).

When an antigen enters the body, the B-lymphocyte system is stimulated to begin gradual production of antibodies. This *primary response* sensitizes the immune system of the host so subsequent exposure to the antigen stimulates a rapid outpouring of antibodies (Figure 2–2). This *secondary response* depends on a specific subgroup of B cells called **memory cells**, which signal the system that previous exposure to an antibody has occurred.

MECHANISMS OF IMMUNITY
Cell-Mediated and Humoral Immunity

Immunological responses are classified as either humoral or cell-mediated. **Humoral immunity** is mediated by antibodies that circulate in the blood and are present in the body fluids. The action of those antibodies occurs at a distance from the B cells that produce them. **Cell-mediated immunity** depends on the local action of the T-lymphocyte when it becomes sensitized by contact with a specific antigen.

Natural and Artificial Immunity

Specific immunity to an antigen may be acquired naturally or through artificial introduction. **Active immunity** occurs when the host produces antibodies in response to antigenic

stimulation. **Passive immunity** is essentially "borrowed." It is acquired when antibody and complement are transferred to a person without the active participation of the body. For example, *natural active immunity* can be acquired by having a disease and recovering successfully from it or by being exposed to an antigen for a long time without actually developing the disease. *Natural passive immunity* occurs when a child receives antibodies from the mother across the placental barrier or through colostrum. *Artificial active immunity* is achieved through immunization with an antigen—as in routine childhood immunization against diphtheria, pertussis, tetanus, rubella, measles, mumps, or polio. *Artificial passive immunity* involves injection of serum that contains antibodies from a sensitized donor—as when immune globulin is given to persons exposed to viral hepatitis. Immunization is discussed further in Chapter 11.

IMMUNE REACTIONS THAT PRODUCE TISSUE DAMAGE
Autoimmunity

When the immunological system of the host attacks normal cellular components within the host, *autoimmune disease* may result. Viruses may be the initiating factor in the pathogenesis of autoimmunity. Diseases currently considered to have autoimmune involvement include lupus erythematosus, rheumatic fever, scleroderma, ankylosing spondylitis, rheumatoid arthritis, multiple sclerosis, and thyroiditis among others (Table 2–4).

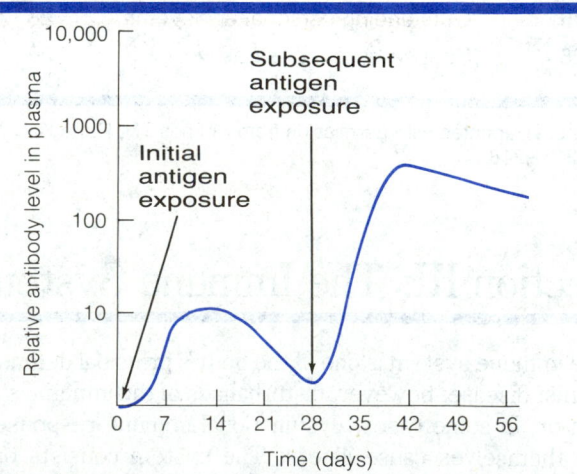

Figure 2–2

Antibody production following initial exposure to an antigen and subsequent exposure to the same antigen.

SOURCE: Spence AP, Mason EB: *Human Anatomy and Physiology*. Menlo Park, CA: Benjamin/Cummings, 1983, p. 562.

Table 2–3 Characteristics of Antibodies (Immunoglobulins = Ig)

Name	Major Area of Concentration	Pertinent Information
IgG	Principal Ig in serum	Only Ig that crosses the placental barrier; major Ig for secondary immune responses
IgM	Present in moderate amounts in serum	Major Ig for primary immune response
IgA	Present in colostrum; saliva; tears; secretions of GI, GU, and respiratory tracts	Protects mucosal surfaces of GI, GU, respiratory tracts
IgD	Present in small amounts in serum	Specific activity unknown
IgE	Present in small amounts in serum	Mediates immediate hypersensitivity reactions and anaphylaxis

Table 2–4 Diseases Believed to Have Autoimmune Involvement

Classification	Disease	Tissue or Organ Affected
Organ-specific diseases	Thyroiditis (Hashimoto's disease)	Thyroid gland
	Gastritis (in pernicious anemia)	Gastric mucosa
	Idiopathic Addison's disease	Adrenal cortex
	Myasthenia gravis	Skeletal muscle
	Multiple sclerosis	Central nervous sytem
	Ulcerative colitis	Mucosa of sigmoid colon
	Type I diabetes mellitus	Beta cells of pancreas
	Hemolytic anemia	Red blood cells
Collagen Diseases*	Rheumatoid arthritis	Synovia of joints
	Lupus erythematosus	Skin, kidney, other viscera
	Scleroderma	Skin
	Rheumatic fever	Joints, heart, kidney
	Ankylosing spondylitis	Articulations of spine
	Polyarteritis nodosa	Connective tissue of blood vessels

*Even though the pathology may be most noticeable at certain sites, these ailments involve the connective tissues throughout the body.
SOURCE: Reprinted with permission from Ramsey JM: *Basic Pathophysiology*. Menlo Park, CA: Addison–Wesley, 1982 p. 406.

HLA Complex

Recently, studies have shown that individual differences in surface antigens of human lymphocytes are related to susceptibility to certain diseases. Understanding of the role of human leukocyte antigen (HLA) complex in human immune responses is limited.

Apparently, **HLA antigens** are implicated in rejection of transplanted organs, as Figure 2–3 illustrates. HLA studies may also be of value in genetic counseling for certain rare genetic diseases. In addition, diseases such as Type I diabetes mellitus, lupus erythematosus, myasthenia gravis, and multiple sclerosis show HLA associations. A highly significant HLA association has been found with HLA antigen B27 and ankylosing spondylitis.

Hypersensitivity or Allergy

Hypersensitivity or **allergy** is an altered bodily state in which an exaggerated response occurs with exposure to an antigen. Substances capable of inducing hypersensitivity are called **allergens**. The individual's initial exposure to the allergen—called the sensitizing dose—does not cause a reaction. Subsequent exposure to the allergen does cause a hypersensitivity reaction, however.

Immediate hypersensitivity reactions such as urticaria, anaphylaxis, and allergic rhinitis (hay fever) are mediated by immunoglobulins—a humoral response. *Delayed hypersensitivity* reactions, such as a reaction to a tuberculin skin test, are mediated by the T-lymphocytes—a cell-mediated response. An example of a hypersensitivity response

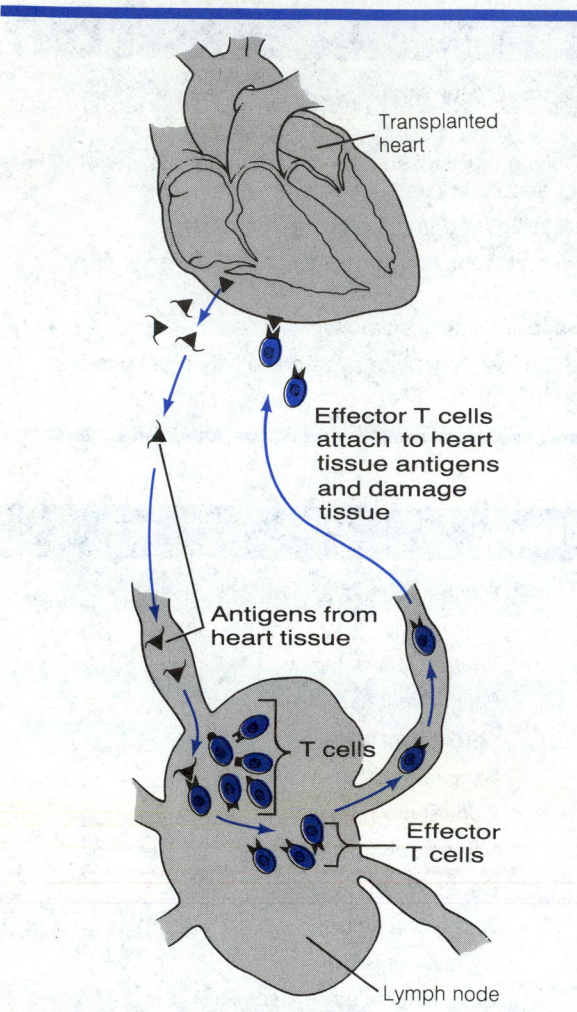

Figure 2–3

Role of cell-mediated immune responses in transplant rejection.

SOURCE: Spence AP, Mason EB: *Human Anatomy and Physiology*. Menlo Park, CA: Benjamin/Cummings, 1983, p. 565.

requiring immediate nursing action is anaphylaxis, which is discussed in Chapter 5.

FACTORS THAT AFFECT IMMUNE RESPONSE

Stress

Many studies have investigated the association of psychosocial stress with immune system dysfunction. Autoimmune, hypersensitivity, infectious, and malignant disease all may be somehow related to life stress.

Studies such as those by Riley (1981) lend credence to the idea that emotional, psychosocial, or anxiety-stimulated stress can produce an increase in plasma concentration of certain hormones associated with injury to parts of the immune system. The individual then may be vulnerable to the action of latent oncogenic (tumor-inducing) viruses (see Chapter 12), newly transformed cancer cells, or other pathological processes that would normally be checked by a heathy immune system.

Age

Developmental factors may also play a role in vulnerability to immune system dysfunction. Levels of immunoglobulin reserve—especially IgG and IgA—are highest between ages 20 and 60 (Figure 2–4). The idea that children and adults over 60 are more susceptible to health problems directly related to the immune system seems plausible considering the major health problems of the very young and the elderly. Infections (eg, otitis media and tonsillitis) and allergy are common in the young. Infections, autoimmune problems, and malignancy are common problems of the elderly. All these disorders are related to immune-system dysfunctions.

Section IV: Infection and Inflammation

Infection occurs when the body is invaded by a pathogen that multiplies and produces injurious effects. *Inflammation* is the bodily reaction to injury. Although the terms *infection* and *inflammation* are sometimes used synonymously, they are not interchangeable. Inflammation is a nonspecific response of the body to any tissue injury. Infectious agents are only one of many possible initiators of the inflammatory response.

INFECTION

Preventing foreign microorganisms from entering the body is the easiest way to avoid infection. The skin and mucous membranes, when intact, are impermeable to most infectious agents. A variety of bacteria inhabit the normal skin but are kept in check by the secretions of the sweat and sebaceous glands. The mucous membranes secrete mucus that entraps small particles, which can then be swept away by the action of cilia, expelled by coughing or sneezing, or engulfed by phagocytic cells. Many of the secreted bodily fluids contain bactericidal components (eg, lysozymes in tears and acids in gastric juice).

The washing action of tears, saliva, and urine also helps protect epithelial surfaces. The nurse who instructs a woman to void after intercourse to prevent urinary infections is applying this principle. Passing urine helps wash

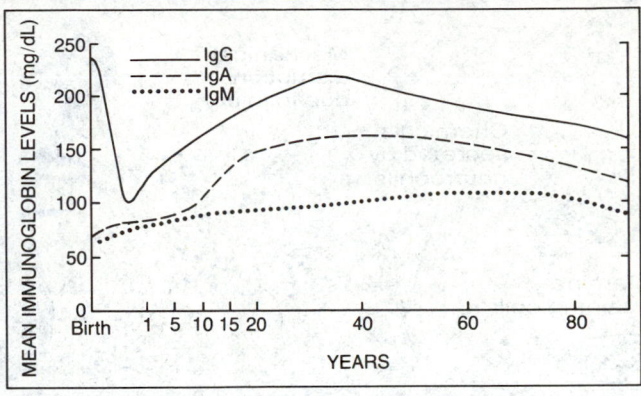

Figure 2–4

Average plasma immunoglobulin levels throughout life. Observe that the lower levels are found at the early and late periods of life, whereas the most substantial levels occur between the ages of 20 and 60, at least for IgG and IgA. (Constructed from a combination of data sources.)

SOURCE: Ramsey JB: *Basic Pathophysiology: Modern Stress and the Disease Process*. Menlo Park, CA: Addison–Wesley, 1982, p. 484.

out any organisms that have been milked into the urethra and bladder during sexual intercourse.

When host defenses against infection are impaired, the individual becomes susceptible to microbial agents; such a client is called a **compromised host**. Often, the alteration in the defense mechanisms is incompletely understood. From the nurse's standpoint, however, knowing what predisposes the alcoholic client to infection is less important than knowing that the client is a compromised host and at risk. A comprehensive history and physical assessment should always include specific attention to the possibility of infection in any client who could be considered a compromised host. The principle of the compromised host is further discussed in Chapter 11.

INFLAMMATION

The inflammatory response is the body's response to cell injury. Many factors can initiate the process of inflammation, including invasion of the body by microorganisms, mechanical trauma, chemical agents, heat, and cold. The inflammatory response is essentially the same, regardless of the damaging agent. Inflammatory reactions can be local or systemic. *Pain, heat, erythema,* and *edema* are the cardinal subjective and objective findings with local inflammation. Systemic inflammation is associated with *fever* and *leukocytosis.*

How Inflammation Occurs

The vasoconstriction immediately after injury is followed by vasodilation, increasing the blood flow to the area and

thereby delivering phagocytes and plasma proteins. Erythema and increased warmth are related to this increased localized blood volume. The permeability of capillaries and venules increases, and plasma fluid and solutes leak from the blood vessels into the inflamed tissues, producing edema. Pain is thought to be secondary to localized pressure from the swelling as well as to action of chemicals on the nerve endings.

Blood viscosity increases as fluid and solutes are lost, and clumping of the red blood cells (erythrocytes) slows the blood flow to the area. Fibrinogen moves from the blood to the tissue spaces and is converted to fibrin, creating a clot that walls off the injured area. Leukocytes enter the damaged tissue and phagocytize invading organisms and cellular debris.

Chemical Mediators of Inflammation

Many chemical substances are activated when tissue damage takes place. *Histamine,* which is present in most tissues, is released when injury occurs, leading to vasodilation and vascular permeability (Figure 2–5). The *kinins,* a group of polypeptides, also increase vascular permeability and induce pain. In addition, the complement system is involved in enhancing vasodilation, vascular permeability, and phagocytosis. Other substances thought to increase vascular permeability are the *prostaglandins* (a specialized group of fatty acids).

Interferon is a protein produced by T-lymphocytes and many other cells in response to the presence of viruses and other parasites. Interferon seems to protect the body initially against invading viruses until the slower-acting

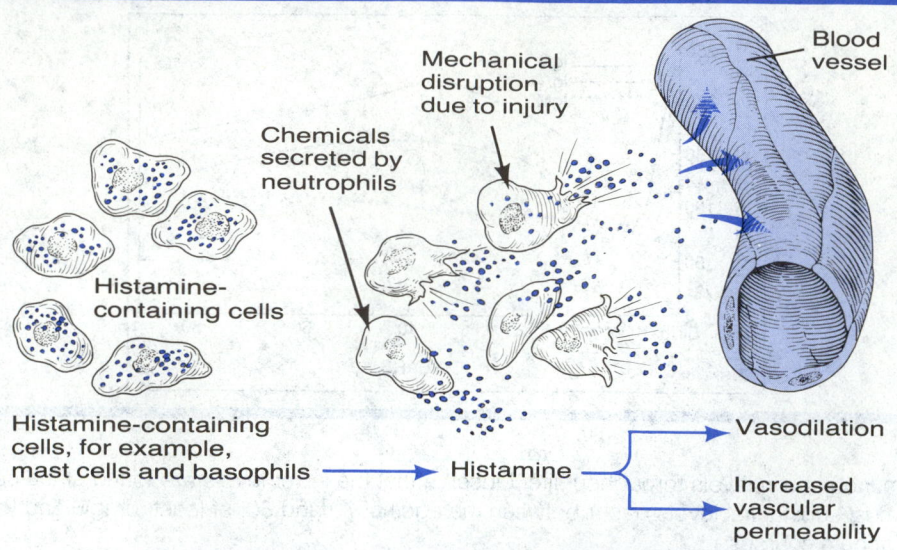

Figure 2–5

Role of histamine as a chemical mediator of the inflammatory response. Histamine can be released through injury to histamine-containing cells, or chemicals secreted by neutrophils are attracted to the site.
SOURCE: Spence AP, Mason EB: *Human Anatomy and Physiology*. Menlo Park, CA: Benjamin/Cummings, 1983, p. 557.

immune response is activated. The possible role of interferon in protecting the body against some cancers is receiving considerable research attention. Use of injected interferon as an anticancer agent has been promising in some clinical studies (see Chapter 12). Generalized stress, which can alter the immune response, may also reduce interferon production by the body.

Section V: Genetic Influences

Heredity is the transmission of certain characteristics from parent to offspring through *genes*—specific sections of molecules of deoxyribonucleic acid (DNA) carried in the chromosomes within the nucleus of each cell. Genes are arranged linearly along the chromosome, with each gene occupying a specific position, or locus, on a particular chromosome. Each human cell is estimated to contain enough genes to govern about 50,000 traits.

The nucleus of every healthy human cell contains 46 threadlike strands of genetic material (*chromosomes*) arranged in 23 pairs, one of each pair derived from each parent. Of the 23 pairs of chromosomes, one pair is sex chromosomes, and the other 22 pairs are called autosomes. In the female, the sex chromosome is made up of two X chromosomes, and in the male, the sex chromosome contains one X and one Y (Figure 2–6). The Y chromosome of the male combines with the X chromosome of the female to produce a boy. An X chromosome from each parent produces a girl.

A given gene (eg, hair color) can exist in one of several different states. Alternative forms of the same gene (blond hair versus brown hair) are called *alleles*. The **homo-**zygous individual has two identical alleles of the gene determining the characteristic under consideration. That is, the person with two identical alleles for blond hair will have blond hair. A person who is **heterozygous** has two different alleles (an allele for blond hair from one parent and an allele for brown hair from the other) at the same locus. In the heterozygous state, one gene may mask or suppress the effect of the other. The brown hair allele will mask or suppress the blond hair allele. The gene characteristic that is expressed (brown hair) is said to be *dominant*, and the one that is masked (blond hair) is called *recessive*. When both alleles of a pair are expressed in the heterozygous state, the genes are said to be *codominant*. Sickle cell anemia, sickle cell trait, and blood type AB are examples of a codominant mode of inheritance.

Genotype is a term that refers to the actual genetic constitution or make up of the individual. Phenotype refers to the way in which the genetic information is expressed as particular traits or characteristics; in other words, the individual's appearance, or what can be observed about that person. Phenotype is influenced by environment as well as by genes. For example, a child may have the genetic

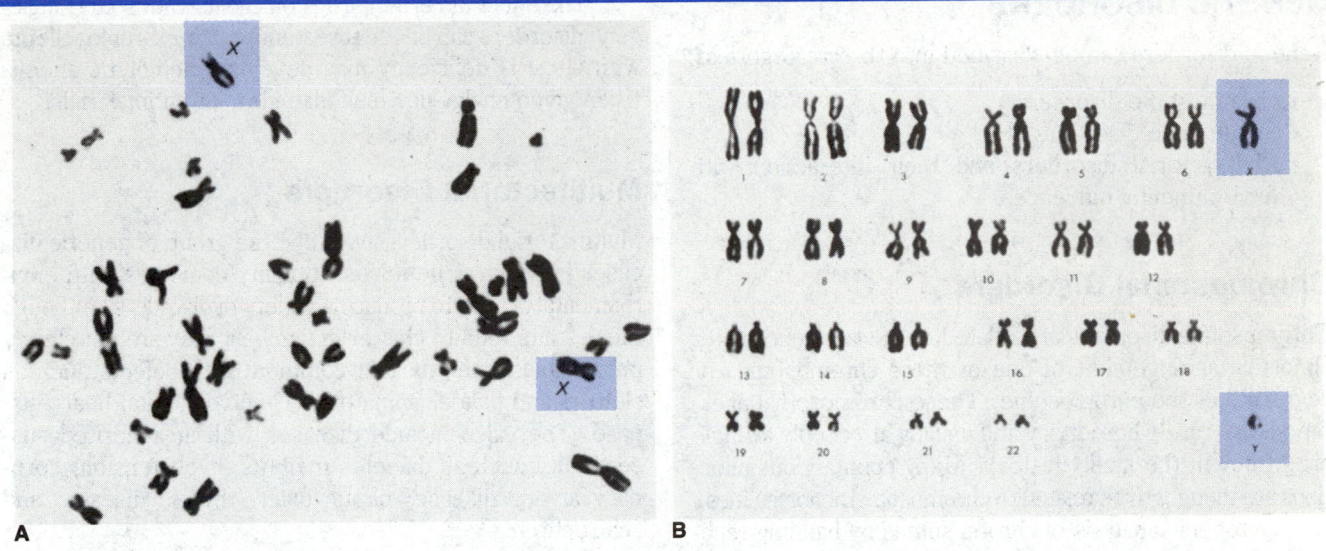

Figure 2–6

Human chromosomes. **A.** Chromosomes of a female with X sex chromosomes indicated. **B.** Chromosomes of a male with homologous chromosomes arranged in pairs. X and Y are sex chromosomes. Note X and Y chromosomes in color boxes. SOURCE: Spence AP, Mason EB: *Human Anatomy and Physiology*. Menlo Park, CA: Benjamin/Cummings, 1983, p. 74.

capacity for great intelligence but may not achieve that potential because of inadequate nutrition, lack of stimulation, residual defects from birth injury, or diseases of infancy and childhood.

INHERITANCE PATTERNS: SOME EXAMPLES

If an individual who is heterozygous for a dominant gene (Gg) conceives a child with someone who is not carrying the dominant gene, the probability is that half of their children will be affected by the dominant trait. This probability is illustrated in the pedigree pattern (a schematic method for classifying inheritance) in Figure 2–7A. If both individuals are heterozygous for the dominant gene, the probability is that one-fourth of the children will be homozygous dominant (GG), half will be heterozygous (Gg), and one-fourth will be unaffected (Figure 2–7B).

Remember that chance plays a major role in these probability levels, which are based on a large population. For example, in Figure 2–7B where both parents are heterozygous for the trait, the assumption is that if four children are born, two will be Gg, one will be GG, and one will be gg. All four could be GG, or gg, or Gg, however. The probabilities are based on the hypothesis that if these two people could manage to produce a sample size of 100 or so offspring, 50% would be Gg, 25% would be GG, and 25% would be gg.

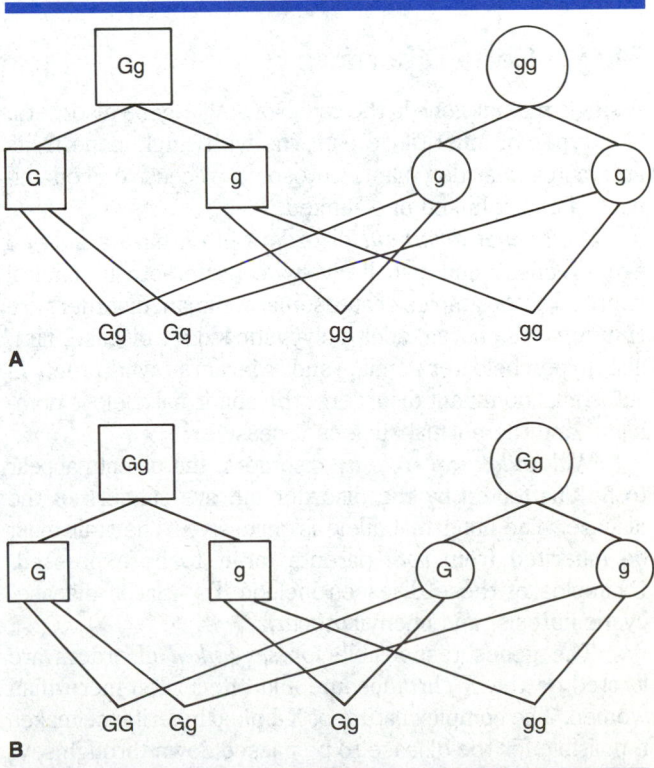

Figure 2–7

Inheritance patterns. **A.** One parent heterozygous, one parent homozygous. **B.** Both parents heterozygous.

GENETIC DISORDERS

Genetic disorders can be classified into three categories:

- Chromosome disorders
- Single-gene disorders
- Multifactorial disorders and their interaction with environmental influences

Chromosomal Disorders

Chromosomal disorders are related to the lack, excess, or abnormal arrangement of one or more chromosomes or segments of the chromosome. These chromosomal aberrations are rarely hereditary and usually affect only a single pregnancy in the family history. Many spontaneous abortions are thought to be related to chromosomal abnormalities.

Cytogenic analysis of chromosomes by banding techniques has been a major breakthrough in the study of chromosomal disorders. A small sample of heparinized blood is all that is required for analysis. Special staining techniques create alternating patterns of light and dark bands, which are highly characteristic for each chromosome, so individual chromosomes may be recognized. Photographs of an individual's banded chromosomes may then be assembled to show a picture of that person's karyotype, or chromosomal arrangement. Down's syndrome is the most common chromosomal disorder.

Single-Gene Disorders

A single mutant gene is the cause of single-gene disorders. The types of inheritance patterns with single-gene traits are: autosomal dominant, autosomal recessive, codominant, and sex linked or X-linked.

Autosomal dominant disorders often have a delayed age of onset and usually vary considerably in clinical expression. Examples of autosomal dominant disorders are Huntington's chorea, adult polycystic kidney disease, familial hypercholesterolemia, and Marfan's syndrome. In autosomal dominant disorders, the abnormal allele is dominant, and the normal allele is recessive.

With *autosomal recessive* disorders, the parents appear to be unaffected by the disorder but are carriers of the disease. The abnormal allele is recessive. The trait must be inherited from *both* parents for it to be expressed. Examples of these diseases include Tay–Sachs disease, cystic fibrosis, and phenylketonuria.

The genes responsible for *sex-linked* disorders are located on the X chromosome and affect men more than women. The complex nature of X-linked inheritance makes it possible for the disease to be passed down through several generations of a family without manifesting itself. Among the most common X-linked disorders are hemophilia A, color blindness, and glucose-6-phosphate dehydrogenase (G-6-PD) deficiency.

The effect of certain drugs on clients with some single-gene disorders can be life threatening. For example, clients with G-6-PD deficiency may develop a hemolytic anemia when given analgesics, sulfonamides, or antimalarials.

Multifactorial Disorders

Multifactorial disorders are a diverse group of genetic diseases in which genetic susceptibility combines with environmental factors to produce a variety of disorders. Although these traits tend to cluster in families, they are not clearly predictable. They include common birth defects such as cleft lip and palate, spina bifida, and congenital heart disease. They also include diseases with an inherited susceptibility such as diabetes mellitus, hypertension, coronary artery disease, peptic ulcer, thyroid disease, and schizophrenia.

GENETIC COUNSELING

The best way to combat inherited disorders is prevention. Through genetic counseling, prospective parents can learn about the relative probabilities of transmitting a genetic disorder. A thorough family history is gathered, with special attention to diseases and causes of death that have tended to run in the family, as well as for symptom complexes that may give clues to genetic problems. Ethnic origin is carefully traced, as is possible consanguinity (parents descended from a common ancestor). Pedigree patterns are constructed as in Figure 2–7 but in more detail to give an idea of susceptibility to disease.

It has been well documented that chromosomal abnormalities seem to increase with maternal age and, to a lesser degree, with paternal age, so considering pregnancy when either parent is over age 40 is accompanied by a degree of risk. Amniocentesis for prenatal diagnosis of genetic disease permits diagnosis at an early enough stage to terminate the pregnancy, if the couple wishes to do so.

Another major avenue of prevention relates to those multifactorial diseases for which a susceptibility may be inherited. Individuals with a strong positive family history of hypertension should learn from childhood to avoid foods high in sodium and to avoid adding salt to their food. Their blood pressures should be monitored semiannually, and clients who show any tendency toward hypertension should be taught to take their own blood pressures at home. The nurse who instructs these clients should have them bring in their own sphygmomanometers so they can be checked for accuracy. Clients should be aware of early symptoms and signs of health problems for which they are at risk and should learn about the possibility of preventing these problems. Nurses have a major responsibility in educating the public about practices that not only promote health but may assist in avoiding diseases for which some have a hereditary predisposition.

Section VI: Neoplasia

BENIGN VERSUS MALIGNANT NEOPLASIA

The word neoplasia means "new growth" (*neo + plasia*), and **neoplasm** is generally used synonymously with tumor. Neoplasms are classified as *benign*—meaning the dividing cells adhere to each other and the tumor remains circumscribed—or *malignant*—meaning that the tumor cells invade surrounding tissue. The cells of malignant tumors (cancers) also may enter natural channels such as the blood vessels or the lymphatics and spread from their original site to other parts of the body. There they produce secondary growths called *metastatic lesions*.

Tumor nomenclature is not entirely consistent, so it is sometimes difficult to ascertain from the name of a tumor whether it is benign or malignant. Generally, the suffix "oma" combined with the name of the affected tissue designate a benign tumor; eg, a lipoma is a benign tumor of the lipid (fat) tissue. Malignant tumors are first differentiated according to the cellular structure from which they arise. Malignant tumors arising from epithelial tissue are called carcinomas. Those arising from connective tissue are called sarcomas. These lesions are further subclassified (Table 2–5).

Benign neoplasms do not invade surrounding tissue or metastasize, but they can cause injurious local and systemic effects. For example, pressure from a benign tumor can be life threatening if the tumor is located in the brain where there is no room for expansion. A benign tumor can also cause obstruction (eg, within the intestine or in a bronchus) leading to potentially serious sequelae. Some benign tumors secrete hormones that have injurious effects; eg, an adenoma of the islets of Langerhans in the pancreas leads to an oversupply of insulin and thereby to hypoglycemia.

Because malignant neoplasms can infiltrate surrounding tissues and metastasize to distant structures, their potential for destruction is immense. Like benign tumors, cancers can cause pressure and obstructive problems as well as overproduction of hormones if a gland is involved. Among the devastating effects associated with cancer are the following: hemorrhage, anemia, ulceration, infection, pathological fractures, pain, and **cachexia** (a term denoting the progressive weakness, malnutrition, weight loss, and emaciation that sometimes occurs with advanced cancer).

Much remains to be learned about what causes cells to overproliferate, forming tumors. Research on malignant neoplasms has generated a number of theories, including genetic composition of the host, immunological factors, viruses, environmental and occupational exposures, drugs and radiation effects, diet, and stress. Because all persons

Table 2–5 Classification of Benign and Malignant Neoplasms

Origin	Benign	Malignant
Epithelial tissue:	"-oma"	"-carcinoma"
Glandular	Adenoma	Adenocarcinoma
Surface	Papilloma	Carcinoma (squamous cell, basal cell, transitional cell)
	Polyp	
Connective tissue:	"-oma"	"sarcoma"
Smooth muscle	Leiomyoma	Leiomyosarcoma
Striated muscle	Rhabdomyoma	Rhabdomyosarcoma
Cartilaginous	Chondroma	Chondrosarcoma
Bone osteoblast	Osteoma	Osteosarcoma
Blood vessels	Hemangioma	Angiosarcoma
Lymphatics	Lymphangioma	Lymphangiosarcoma
Fibrous	Fibroma	Fibrosarcoma
Nerve sheath	Neurofibroma	Neurofibrosarcoma
Adipose	Lipoma	Liposarcoma
Embryonic tissue:	"-oma"	"-blastoma"
Kidney	—	Nephroblastoma
Retina	—	Retinoblastoma
Sympathetic ganglia and adrenal medulla	Ganglioneuroma	Neuroblastoma
Germ-cell layers:	Benign Teratoma	Malignant teratoma

exposed to known carcinogens do not develop cancer, host factors are thought to play a major role in the process. Therefore, a multifactorial approach seems the most promising in finding a cancer cure. See Chapter 12 for a full discussion of cancer and care of the client with malignant neoplasia.

EARLY DETECTION AND PREVENTION OF CANCER

Cancer of the cervix, breasts, bowel, oral cavity, and testes can be detected early by relatively noninvasive techniques practiced by health care providers or in some cases, by clients themselves. Self-examination of the mouth, the breasts, and the testicles requires that the client receive careful instruction initially and understand the importance of routine self-assessment (eg, monthly). In their ability to detect disease early, the value of yearly Pap smears for women, digital rectal examinations for both men and women, and testing of stool for occult blood outweigh the possible embarrassment they may cause.

Until recently, efforts at cancer prevention have primarily included cessation of smoking, reducion of exposure to the sun, and protection of workers against known carcinogens in the workplace. Currently, there is considerable interest in evidence that high-fat diets are implicated in cancer of the colon, rectum, breast, and perhaps prostate. Cancer of the colon and rectum have also been linked to diets low in fiber. In light of current evidence on the connection between diet and cancer, it appears sensible to increase the fiber content and decrease the fat content in the average daily diet. (Diet in cancer is further discussed in Chapter 12.)

The link between stress and cancer is somewhat more nebulous. Part of the human stress response involves an increased production and release of adrenocorticotropic hormone (ACTH) from the pituitary, which in turn stimulates production of glucocorticoids in the adrenal cortex. Elevations of ACTH and glucocorticoids suppress immunocompetence by causing involution of the thymus and lymphatics and reducing the number of circulating lymphocytes. Some researchers believe that this stress-produced alteration in the immune response may be a contributing component in the development of cancer. Incorporating stress-reduction approaches in daily living may therefore be another way to reduce the risk of cancer. Stress reduction approaches are discussed in detail in Chapter 4.

Section VII: The Aging Process and Degeneration

Why do humans age? What degenerative changes are invariably associated with aging? These questions are the focus of a great deal of research. An overview of theories of aging is presented in Table 2–6. Physiologic theories of aging center on the immune system, genetic programming, metabolic changes, and a lifetime of wear and tear. Immune system research suggests that the decrease in size and function of the thymus gland and the resulting

Nursing Research Note

Chang BL, Uman GC, Linn LS, Ware JE, Kane RL: Adherence to health care regimens among elderly women. *Nurs Res* 1985; 34:27–31.

After viewing videotaped interactions between nurse practitioners (NPs) and clients, 26 older adults rated components of the NPs' care according to whether the measures would affect the client's intent to adhere to the care plan. The components—technical quality, psychosocial care, and client participation—were not found significant. Significant factors included widowhood, religion, perceived importance of the exam, social network, and pre-existing satisfaction with health care. These results reinforce the necessity of identifying a client's supportive networks and previous health experiences in determining intent to adhere to a plan of care.

decline in T cell activity with age impair the body's ability to fight off infection. An autoimmune process may also occur in which the body begins to attack its own cells. Another theory suggests that aging is caused by cumulative damage from environmental insults to the genetic information systems of the cell—DNA and RNA. Degenerative theories speculate that the body's ability to reproduce new cells or repair damaged ones decreases over time and eventually cannot keep up with the years of destruction. Other theories suggest that cellular aging is programmed to produce tissue death and that chemical substances called "free radicals" are active in the aging process.

As persons age, they are at greater risk for certain types of diseases and injuries. The degree of disability from these disorders appears to increase with age, yet many elderly persons are never afflicted with serious health problems. Of problems that do occur, many are preventable (eg, falls), most are treatable (eg, hypertension), and the majority can be compensated for in one way or another (eg, decreased auditory or visual acuity).

Being aware of the normal physiological changes associated with aging is important for nurses so they can help clients cope with the changes. Using the approach of *promoting* health and *preventing* disease, nurses can do much to offset the effects of aging. The most common changes related to aging are summarized in Table 2–7.

Table 2–6 Theories of Biological Aging

Theory	Description
Genetic theory	The cells contain a genetic clock that controls the speed of metabolic processes and the number of cell divisions possible.
Metabolic waste theory	The cells are slowly poisoned by metabolic waste products that cannot be excreted and so interfere with cellular metabolism.
Free radical theory	Unstable free radicals (pieces of molecules, often the result of oxidation of organic materials such as protein, fat, and carbohydrates) accumulate in the cells, inducing chromosome changes, accumulation of pigment, or alteration of cell membrane permeability to electrolytes so the cell cannot regenerate itself.
Random error theory	Aging is the result of accumulation of errors in the sequence of transmission of information in cells. This may be due to failure of DNA to replicate or malfunction of RNA or related enzymes.
Wear-and-tear theory Stress-adaptation theory Deprivation theory	Aging is a result of cellular loss and degeneration as a result of a lifelong attempt to maintain internal homeostasis. Cells and organs "wear out," and thus are unable to sustain life. Since organ systems are interrelated, one organ system's malfunction will cause others to malfunction. Cardiopulmonary system malfunction results in inadequate delivery of essential nutrients and oxygen to cells.
Immunological theories Slow virus theories	Older cells are less effective in synthesizing normal antibodies, so susceptibility to infection increases. Viruses that have incubated for decades may now be able to cause damage to organ systems.
Autoimmune theories	Antibodies are unable to differentiate between body cells and foreign substances so they inactivate body cells.
Cross-link theories Collagen theories	Chemical reactions create strong bonds between molecular structures that are normally separate, especially in collagen tissues, causing stiffness, chemical instability, and insolubility of connective tissue and DNA.

SOURCE: Reprinted with permission from Bellack JP, Bamford PA: *Nursing Assessment: A Multidimensional Approach*. Monterey, CA: Wadsworth, 1984, p. 128.

Muscle groups generally weakened in the elderly (pectorals, abdominal muscles, pelvic and hip extensors) can be firmed by muscle-strengthening activities. Swimming, riding a stationary bicycle, and performing regular stretching exercises make both muscles and joints more flexible. Walking, swimming, and dancing are excellent ways to improve cardiopulmonary function and to combat fatigue. Clients can learn that avoiding quick head movements or rapid change in position can help them avert falls. Yearly visual examinations with tonometry aid in detecting glaucoma early and preventing blindness.

Homes can be made safer with support rails in the bathtub and on stairways, rubber mats or nonskid strips on the tub or shower floor, smoke detectors, assistance with proper footwear, and precautions with heating pads and hot water bottles. The client can be encouraged to plan dietary changes, such as increasing fiber consumption to prevent constipation or reducing fat and sugar intake to prevent weight gain. Dietary measures can also assist in controlling or preventing Type II diabetes mellitus and hypertension. Dental problems and periodontal disease can be minimized by avoiding sugars, brushing and flossing the teeth thoroughly each day, and having them cleaned pro-

fessionally twice a year. Dentures or partial plates should be worn for proper chewing, and discomfort or sores secondary to their use should be evaluated immediately. Malignancies in the elderly can be detected early through oral self-examinations, breast self-examinations, testing stools for occult blood, mammography, and Pap smears.

The aging process is not merely a function of physiology. Social factors are crucial to how the aged view their health, and, in fact, to how healthy they actually are. The traditional, disease-oriented health care system tends to view the older person with degenerative joint disease and decreased hearing as diseased. Yet the elderly person who has adjusted well to the gradual limitations imposed by age may be content with life, may participate fully in social roles, and may feel healthy both physically and psychologically. Some research has shown that elderly persons who maintain active social contact with others are more satisfied with life and are more likely to view themselves as healthy than those who are socially isolated. Although it is clear that as aging progresses, the body gradually loses its capacity for peak performance, it is also clear that much can be done to maximize health and the quality of life as persons grow older.

Table 2–7 Physiological Changes Associated With Aging

Organ or System	Physiological Change
Skin	• Becomes thinned and dry; ↓ in subcutaneous fat; ↓ in activity of hair follicles, sweat glands, and sebaceous glands • Atrophy of melanocytes with graying of hair • Thickening of nails
Eyes	• Pupil loses its ability to dilate fully, contributing to ↓ in vision and development of glaucoma • Lens gradually loses elasticity, resulting in presbyopia • Lens gradually yellows, altering color vision • Lens may opacify causing ↓ in vision, falls • Lifetime exposure of rods and cones to light results in damage, contributing to ↓ in vision, falls
Ears	• ↓ Elasticity of tympanic membrane, impaired articulation of ossicles, resulting in ↓ hearing • Degenerative cochlear changes and loss of cells from the organ of Corti, causing ↓ hearing • Possible degeneration in vestibular function contributing to loss of balance
Respiratory system	• ↑ Rigidity of chest wall; ↓ elasticity of lungs, resulting in ↓ in vital capacity • ↓ In phagocytic activity of macrophages and ↓ in efficiency of cilia lining the respiratory tract, resulting in susceptibility to respiratory infections
Cardiovascular system	• ↓ Stroke volume, ↓ heart rate, resulting in ↓ cardiac output • Sinus node dysfunction, contributing to atrial dysrhythmia • Thickening of the intima of the arterial wall with gradually increasing rigidity of vessels, contributing to hypertension and aneurysm formation
Kidneys	• ↓ Blood flow, resulting in ↓ glomerular filtration rate and ↓ urea clearance • ↓ In renal tubule function, resulting in ↓ ability to concentrate urine
GI system	• Atrophy of taste buds and ↓ salivary flow • Enamel loss, ↑ pigmentation of teeth and recession of gums • ↓ Motility, resulting in constipation • ↓ Intestinal blood flow, which may affect drug absorption
Muscles	• ↓ Skeletal muscle mass with resultant ↓ strength and ↓ agility, ↑ in falls
Bones	• Loss of calcium from bones (more severe in postmenopausal women), resulting in osteoporosis • Bone matrix breaks down, resulting in brittleness.
Joints	• Progressive loss of cartilaginous joint surface, resulting in degenerative joint disease
Neurological system	• ↓ Velocity of nerve conduction • ↓ In memory • Alterations in circadian rhythms, sleep patterns • ↓ In brain size and weight; ↓ cerebellar function resulting in loss of balance, falls
Endocrine system	• Decline in glucose tolerance • Menopause with ↓ estrogen secretion and thermoregulation alterations in women • ↓ Testosterone, ↑ estrogen in males resulting in prostatic hyperplasia, possible gynecomastia
Immune system	• ↓ Thymus activity, ↓ T cell function • ↓ B cell response • ↑ Susceptibility to infection, autoimmune disease, and malignancy

Section VIII: Trauma

Injuries rank as the fourth leading cause of death in the United States for all age groups (*Morbidity and Mortality Weekly Report*, May 14, 1982). Considering years of life lost prematurely, injuries rank first (see Chapter 13). The risk of injury from motor vehicle accidents, falls, burns, accidental poisoning, drowning, sports activities, and occupational accidents is inherent in daily living. Certain groups are at higher risk for specific types of trauma; for example, motor vehicle collisions are a major cause of disability and death for children aged 1 to 14, whereas for the elderly, falls are the most likely to bring about permanent or fatal injury. Reducing traumatic injury depends upon efforts of heath care providers, employers, legislators, equipment designers and manufacturers, and individuals to monitor policies and practices that promote health and safety. Groups such as MADD (Mothers Against Drunk Driving) have been effective in introducing tougher legislation on drunk driving, a major factor in senseless injury and death for thousands each year.

MOTOR VEHICLE ACCIDENTS

Occupants of motor vehicles sustain the largest percentage of fatal injuries for all ages up to age 75. Risk of injury and death is highly correlated with amount of highway travel, road characteristics, speed of vehicle, vehicle size, and use of restraint systems. Alcohol use is a major contributing factor.

For a number of years, efforts have been under way to require automobile manufacturers to design systems that provide passive (automatic) crash protection, especially for those in the front seat who tend to receive the most serious injuries. Active restraint systems, such as seat belts and infant/child car seats, have been shown to reduce drastically the likelihood of serious injury and death. But these systems require individuals to participate actively in protecting themselves and others. Unfortunately, knowing about the benefits of such systems is not enough to induce people to use them. Although several states have laws mandating the use of front seat belts and infant/child seat restraints, not everyone adopts these health-protecting measures.

Passive protection, already built into the vehicle, is generally accepted as the best way to prevent serious injury and death for the general population. Tests have shown that airbags or seat belts that are automatically positioned diagonally across the torso when the car door is closed can substantially reduce occupant injury and death. Energy-absorbing steering wheels, windshields, and instrument panels, padding on projecting surfaces, and crash-resistant bumpers also make vehicles safer.

Pedestrian deaths from motor vehicles are also a major problem. Those most likely to be killed are the aged, the very young, or individuals impaired by alcohol or drugs. Children under age 5 tend to be struck when running out from between parked cars. The elderly, who often hear or see poorly and who cannot move swiftly, are most often injured at intersections. Efforts to protect pedestrians include better illumination, traffic lights timed to favor pedestrian traffic, and placing bus stops farther from intersections.

Many states have raised the legal drinking age to 21 to reduce motor vehicle accidents and have imposed severe penalties on those who are apprehended for driving while

Nursing Research Note

Valanis BG, Yeaworth R: Ratings of physical and mental health in the older bereaved. *Res Nurs Health* 1982; 5:137–146.

The subjects of this study were surviving spouses who were interviewed 3 to 4 months after their spouses' deaths. The self-ratings of mental and physical health of these bereaved elderly subjects were compared to ratings of them by nurse interviewers. A multidimensional functional assessment questionnaire from Duke University and the Zung self-rating depression scale were used.

Women in the study tended to underestimate the severity of their health problems. Older women were especially optimistic compared with nurse interviewer ratings. Mental health self-ratings were also better than nurse interviewer ratings.

The authors suggest that the elderly may identify symptoms of illness as normal problems of aging and therefore set lower standards for physical and mental health. Nurses, on the other hand, may have a broader view of optimal heath for the elderly.

intoxicated. Comprehensive driver education programs for teenagers and raising the legal driving age are other approaches to preventing vehicle-related injuries and death.

Motorcycles, mopeds, and bicycles are responsible for a significant number of head injuries each year as well as for other traumatic injuries such as fractures of the long bones of the extremities. The use of helmets has been the most effective approach to reducing severe head injury and death in motorcyclists. In states where mandatory helmet laws were repealed after they were no longer federally required, the incidence of grave head trauma dramatically increased. Helmets absorb shock, thereby reducing impact. Helmet use by all who ride on two-wheeled vehicles would markedly reduce the number of permanent injuries and deaths to cyclists yearly.

FALLS

Fatal falls occur most often in the home. Falling is also a major factor in occupational deaths, especially among construction workers. The elderly are at high risk of falling; moreover, sequelae of fractures from falls prevent many elderly victims from resuming independent lives after their injuries.

Reducing the distance a person in a high-risk situation can fall or modifying the surface on which a fall is likely to occur can effectively reduce the impact. For example, lifelines should be used by construction workers and mountain climbers. Hospital beds, diving boards, and high chairs can be lowered; floors and stairs can be carpeted or padded. Padded clothing and helmets may be worn by those at particular risk. Falls can be prevented by providing proper illumination, installing window guards and handrails, using nonslip surfaces in bathtubs, removing clutter of furniture and toys, and wearing shoes that properly support the foot and provide sufficient friction between the shoe sole and the walking surface.

BURNS

Residential fires are a leading cause of accidental death and an important source of disability and disfigurement. Injuries and deaths related to house fires can be reduced by installing smoke detectors, providing alternative exit routes, using drapes and clothing made of flame-retardant fabric, and using flame-retardant paint and construction materials. Tap water scald injuries can be prevented by keeping the water heater temperature no higher than 120° F (48.9° C). Having fire extinguishers readily accessible and in good working order, not smoking in bed, and not overloading electrical circuits are all important fire and burn prevention measures. The nursing care of the burned client is discussed in Chapter 15.

ACCIDENTAL POISONING

Nurses have many opportunities to teach clients how to avoid accidental poisoning. Unfortunately, teaching is often done only after an accident. Among the toxic substances that pose a hazard are household cleaning products, medications, pesticides, cosmetics, alcohol, poisonous indoor and outdoor plants, and lead paint. Many cities have poison control centers that can give information quickly about most toxic substances and provide protocols for treatment for clients of any age. Poisoning is specifically discussed in Chapter 13.

Nurses should be aware of folk remedies that may cause lead poisoning. Some Hispanics use fine powders for chronic diarrhea, called greta or azarcón, which have a high lead content. Children from the Hmong tribe in northern Laos now living in Minnesota, were found to have lead poisoning secondary to the use of pay-loo-ah, a red and orange powder used to treat fever or rash (*Morbidity and Mortality Weekly Report*, Oct 28, 1983). Elevated blood levels of lead secondary to inhalation and ingestion are an occupational hazard among workers involved in smelting; recovery of scrap; cutting of steel; and manufacture of batteries, lead pigment, and stained glass (*Morbidity and Mortality Weekly Report*, April 29, 1983).

DROWNING AND AQUATIC INJURIES

Spinal cord injuries from diving and sliding into the water head first permanently paralyze many teenagers and young adults each year. Surfing and water skiing are also implicated in spinal cord trauma. Drowning and serious trauma are more likely when alcohol or drug use are part of aquatic recreational activities. Drowning, near drowning, and spinal cord injuries from aquatic sports are discussed with emergency nursing interventions in Chapter 13.

SPORTS INJURIES

Athletic safety depends on the physical conditioning of the participant, proper protective equipment, and control of the sports environment. Informal sports and recreation, in which there are little physical preparation and use of protective equipment, may be an even greater threat to personal health and safety than organized sports. The rate of sports-related injury and illness can be reduced by wearing face masks and helmets; designating obstacle-free zones around playing fields; eliminating common injury-producing maneuvers from the sport; preventing heat cramps, heat stroke, hypothermia, and frostbite; and doing warming-up exercises before vigorous activity. (Heat stroke and hypothermia are discussed in Chapter 13; frostbite is in Chapter 79.)

Nurses can counsel their clients about these precautions—treatment of a minor injury can be a good occasion for health teaching. An unfortunate side effect of recently heightened public interest in fitness has been injury or illness when a previously sedentary individual plunges into a demanding exercise regimen. Cautioning the client to "start slowly" is an important part of encouraging exercise as a lifestyle change.

WORK-RELATED INJURIES

On-the-job injuries are common in construction, manufacturing, mining, and agriculture. Types of wounds include abrasions, lacerations, contusions, fractures, concussions, crushing injuries, and traumatic amputations. More work time is lost from low-back pain than any other related injury; low-back pain also is the main category of workers' compensation payments. Injury from inhaled gases, vapors, and smoke is not uncommon in firefighters and those involved in manufacturing synthetic materials such as plastics and polyurethanes.

The preemployment history and physical can be helpful in identifying persons who might be at increased risk for on-the-job injury (eg, those with impaired sight, hearing, or balance or those taking medications that produce drowsiness, such as antihistamines). The occupational health nurse can be instrumental in preventing accidents on the job by referring employees at risk—such as those with visual or hearing loss—to appropriate health care providers and recommending appropriate jobs.

The nurse in industry is also responsible for employee education programs dealing with risk reduction. Occupational trauma may be prevented, or at least reduced, by teaching workers how to bend and lift properly, how to care for the machinery they use, and how to spot potential hazards. Workers should be encouraged to use such safety equipment as earplugs, protective goggles, and respirators. Constant vigilance—assessing the work area and work practices continually for potential hazards—is crucial to preventing injury.

Chapter Highlights

Illness (dis-ease) is directly related to the sum of all factors affecting a person's life.

Nursing practice is based on holistic concepts and a multifactorial view of illness.

Stress, with its physiological and psychosocial concomitants, causes wear and tear on the whole person. Continued and unabated stress may even cause death.

Common human events, both joyous and catastrophic, are likely to cause stress when they occur in clusters.

Internal and external factors affecting physiology, such as stress, immune response, infection and inflammation, genetic predispositions, neoplasia, aging, and trauma, are closely interrelated with psychosocial and environmental influences on the individual.

Nurses have a major responsibility in educating the public in avoiding diseases for which they have a hereditary predisposition.

The immune system is one of the body's principal defenses against disease. Disturbance or dysfunction of the immune system itself can cause disease, however.

Microbial agents can produce injurious effects in the body. Inflammation is the body's response to cell injury.

Inherited disorders can result from a defect in a chromosome or chromosomal segment, a defect in a single gene, or an interaction between genetic susceptibility and environmental factors.

Neoplasms can cause both injurious local and systemic effects.

Degenerative changes, usually associated with aging or the cumulative effects of wear and tear on a body part, can cause illness.

Traumatic injuries are a leading cause of death for all age groups. The incidence of traumatic injury can be reduced through public education and legislation.

Bibliography

Allen JC: *Infection and the Compromised Host*, 2nd ed. Baltimore: Williams & Wilkins, 1981.

Ames SA, Gelein J, Humphrey E, Mason–Kaufman J, Osborne JE: A systems approach to curricula in primary health care nursing. In: *Approaches to Teaching Primary Health Care.* Knopke HJ, Diekelmann NL (editors). St Louis: Mosby, 1981.

Atchley RC: *Aging: Continuity and Change*. Belmont, CA: Wadsworth, 1983.

Beard MT: Trust, life events, and risk factors among adults. *ANS* (July) 1982; 4:26–43.

Flynn ME: Influencing repair and recovery. *Am J Nurs* 1982; 82:1550–1558.

Flynn ME, Rovee DT: Wound healing mechanisms. *Am J Nurs* 1982; 82:1543–1550.

Folk remedy-associated lead poisoning in Hmong children—Minnesota. *MMWR* (Oct 28) 1983; 32:555–556.

Gold EB: *The Changing Risk of Disease in Women: An Epidemiologic Approach*. Lexington, MA: Collamore, 1984.

Holmes TH, Rahe RH: The social readjustment rating scale. *J of Psychosom Res* 1967; 11:213–218.

Kenney RA: *Physiology of Aging: A Synopsis*. Chicago: Yearbook Publishers, 1982.

Lead poisoning from Mexican folk remedies—California. *MMWR* (Oct 28) 1983; 32:554–555.

Leiberman MA, Tobin SS: *Experience of Old Age*. New York: Basic Books, 1983.

Mason, LJ: *Guide to Stress Reduction*. Culver City, CA: Peace Press, 1980.

Pelletier KR: *Healthy People in Unhealthy Places: Stress and Fitness at Work*. New York: Doubleday, 1984.

Ramsey JM: *Basic Pathophysiology: Modern Stress and the Disease Process*. Menlo Park, CA: Addison–Wesley, 1982.

Results of blood lead determinations among workers potentially exposed to lead—United States. *MMWR* (April 29) 1983; 32:216–219.

Richter MA: *Clinical Immunology: A Physician's Guide*, 2nd ed. Baltimore: Williams & Wilkins, 1982.

Riley V: Psychoneuroendocrine influences on immunocompetence and neoplasia. *Science* 1981; 212:1100–1109.

Selye H: *The Stress of Life*. New York: McGraw–Hill, 1956.

Unintentional and intentional injuries—United States. *MMWR* (May 14) 1982; 31:240,245–248.

Walter JB: *An Introduction to the Principles of Disease*, 2nd ed. Philadelphia: Saunders, 1982.

Suggested Readings

Caplan AL, Engelhardt HT Jr, McCartney JJ: *Concepts of Health and Disease: Interdisciplinary Perspectives*. Reading, MA: Addison–Wesley, 1981. Concepts of health and disease are analyzed from both historical and contemporary perspectives. The ongoing controversies concerning the direction and significance of health care are discussed by social scientists, physicians, philosophers, nurses, and others.

Porcino J: *Growing Older, Getting Better*. Reading, MA: Addison–Wesley, 1983. This comprehensive sourcebook for women over 40 offers thorough information on the special concerns of women in their middle and later years. The second half of the book focuses on physical and mental health issues of older women and how they can become activated, knowledgeable consumers of health care. Good reading for nurses and their clients!

Reed P: Implications of the life-span developmental framework for well-being in adulthood and aging. *ANS* (October) 1983; 5:18–25. Adult development is presented as a progressive phenomenon involving a series of trade-offs from one phase to the next. The importance of interactions with others and with the environment is emphasized as a major factor in the well-being of adults and their approach to life's problems and conflicts, including health-related events.

Silverman J: On the meta-physical aspect of health care: Attitudes, values, and other thoughts we use to think. *Fam Comm Health* (Aug) 1980; 2:93–103. A thought-provoking article that encourages health workers to question the core beliefs and assumptions they hold that affect their ability to help clients take charge of their own lives. It also encourages self-care for the health worker.

The Addison–Wesley Series on Occupational Stress. This series of six softcover books on occupational stress (*Stress Management* by L. J. Warshaw, *Blue Collar Stress* by A. Shostak, *Management Stress* by L. Moss, *Preventing Work Stress* by L. Levi, *Work Stress and Social Support* by J. S. House, and *Work Stress* by A. A. McLean) treat three key concepts— stress, stressor, and stress reactions—from differing perspectives. The books are concerned with the improvement of unhealthy environments and stimuli in the world of work as well as in the other aspects of life affected by work.

Wright CC: Cost containment and health promotion. *J Occup Med* 1982; 24:965–68. This article discusses the effect of health promotion programs provided for the employees of one industry. Improvement in employee self-image, job satisfaction, company loyalty, morale, and productivity were directly attributed to the physical fitness programs. The traditional executive medical exam was found to be problematic and not cost effective.

Chapter 3

Disease Patterns and Lifestyle Factors

Brenda P. Haughey

Objectives

When you have finished studying this chapter, you should be able to:

Distinguish between morbidity and mortality

Describe the relation of time, place, and personal characteristics to disease patterns

Identify the shifting patterns in causes of death and their effects on the focus of health care

Discuss the relation between lifestyle and health risk

Compare lifestyles favorable to health with lifestyles unfavorable to health

Advocate risk-reducing lifestyle modification and increased health consciousness

Health depends on a multitude of factors: body structure and function, family history, where and how one lives, and the quality and accessibility of health care in a society at a particular time. Some factors affecting health are under an individual's control; some are not. All are interrelated; all vary from person to person, and many vary within the same person from time to time. The combination of factors is unique to each person.

Many factors that affect health will be explored in later chapters. Meanwhile, remembering that health is multidimensional will help in analyzing patterns and incidence of disease, the subject of this chapter. The knowledge from this analysis will benefit both nurse and client, regardless of age, origin, culture, or lifestyle.

Section I: Identifying Patterns of Illness

To gather data on health or illness, one must first define health. Many writers have tried to define health, and none has been wholly successful. A useful definition would be applicable to the special values and circumstances of individuals in their day-to-day lives. But such an all-encompassing definition of health is difficult to develop because concepts of health vary greatly among health care professionals as well as the general public.

One client may tell the nurse, "If I'm not in pain, I'm well." Another may say, "If I can't use my body to its maximum potential, I'm sick." A client with a long-term condition like diabetes may think of himself or herself as healthy as long as no obvious symptoms or complications appear, and the client is living in accordance with the prescribed regimen. Those caring for the client will identify him or her as being chronically ill, however.

It is much easier to establish illness than health (although this, too, presents difficulties). Thus, patterns of health have traditionally been described according to standards that actually pertain to illness: morbidity and mortality.

The term **morbidity** refers to illness; the term **mortality** refers to death. In the United States and Canada, as in most industrialized nations, mortality data are widely collected and generally accurate. Such figures reflect how many persons have died and the causes of their deaths. But they tell nothing about less-than-fatal illness and disability.

Augmenting mortality data with information about frequency and duration of illness and personal characteristics of those who are ill offers a clearer picture of the health of given populations, such as women over 40, emigrants from Japan, or elderly persons in nursing homes. But morbidity data are less clear than mortality figures because morbid episodes are less easily identified than deaths.

For example, deaths are recorded because they are reported to a central agency—usually the local government. Illness is generally not reported, except in special cases of communicable disease. Duration of illness is hard to assess because there is no precise standard for determining when an illness begins or even that it has occurred. If a person who is ill does not seek professional health care, the illness is unlikely to be entered in the data pool.

Nevertheless, knowing patterns and incidence of disease is essential to effective health care planning and disease prevention on both the micro level (for individuals) and the macro level (for whole regions and societies). It is no wonder, then, that disease statistics have been collected in some form by virtually all societies throughout their recorded histories.

In the United States, various criteria are used to estimate the frequency and effect of illness, including such obvious data as hospital admissions records and number of visits to health care facilities. The most frequent indicators are summarized in Box 3–1.

FACTORS THAT INFLUENCE HEALTH AND ILLNESS

Knowing the factors that affect disease trends helps in evaluating the extent of a public health problem and the influence of interventions on severity and spread of a disease. This information is crucial on the macro level.

Time

Important information can be gained from studying time and its relation to the secular, or long-term, patterns of disease. For instance, Figure 3–1 shows the rates of gonorrhea in the United States from 1941 through 1981. (Gonorrhea is the most frequently reported communicable disease in the United States at present). Note that the number of cases increased sharply during the 1960s and early 1970s, both in absolute numbers and as a percentage of population.

Box 3–1   Common Indicators of Illness Patterns

- Hospital admissions records
- Hospital discharge rates
- Length of hospital stay
- Restricted activity days
- Bed disability days
- Rates of acute and chronic conditions
- Immunization records
- Most common problems brought to the attention of physicians
- Leading surgical procedures performed
- Primary diagnoses of nursing home residents
- Smoking behaviors
- Perceptions of health
- Visits to physicians

Beginning in 1975, there is a downward trend. The increase has been attributed to the "sexual revolution" and to improved case detection; the decrease, to federally assisted disease control programs initiated in 1973 (US Department of Health and Human Services, 1982).

Disease patterns also vary seasonally. Before vaccines against poliomyelitis were developed, parents dreaded "polio season," which tended to occur in late summer. Reported cases of the recently discovered legionnaires' disease (legionellosis) fluctuate from month to month (Figure 3–2). More persons are hospitalized with acute symp-

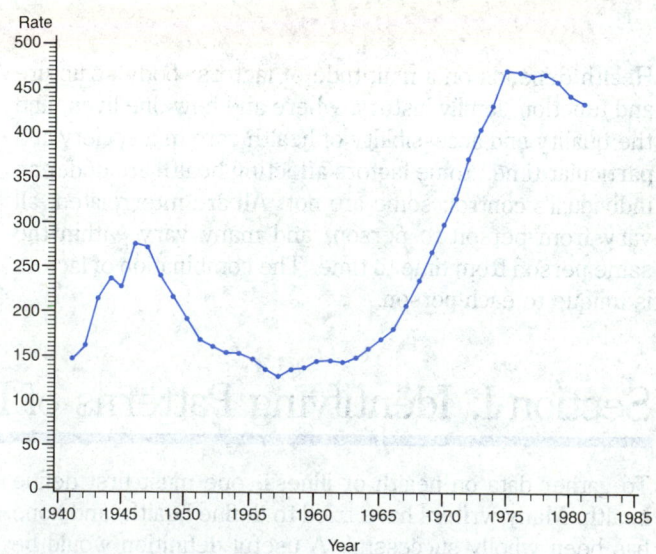

Figure 3–1

Reported civilian cases of gonorrhea per 100,000 population by year, United States, 1941–1981.

SOURCE: Reprinted from US Department of Health and Human Services. *MMWR*. HHS Publication No. (CDC) 82–8241, Oct 30, 1982, p 38.

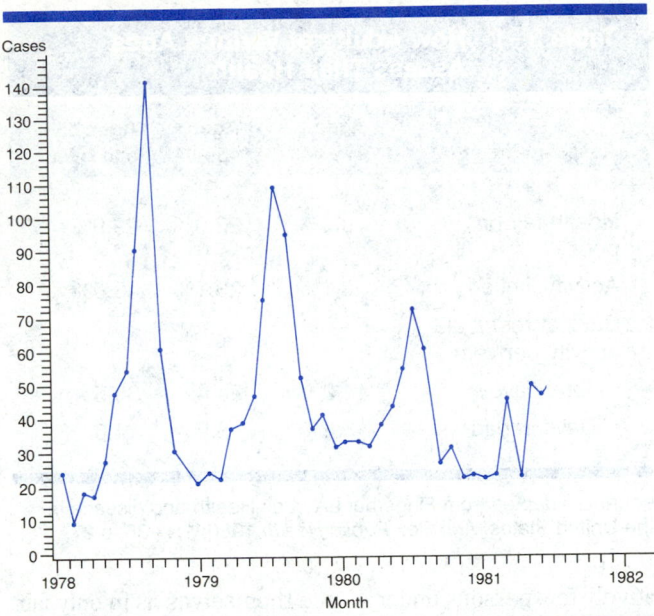

Figure 3–2

Reported sporadic cases of legionellosis by month of onset, United States, 1978–1981.

SOURCE: Reprinted from US Department of Health and Human Services. *MMWR*. HHS Publication No. (CDC) 82–8241, Oct 30, 1982, p 50.

toms of ulcers in spring and fall than in summer or winter. Food poisoning is more common in summer; suicide attempts become more frequent during the Christmas holidays in the United States and during the "dark" season in regions above the Arctic Circle such as parts of Norway and Sweden.

Knowing when a disease "peaks" is useful in allocating health care resources such as hospital beds, vaccines and other pharmaceuticals, and public health personnel. Sometimes seasonal peaks provide clues in tracing the etiology of a disease—eg, an illness related to insect vectors or seasonal activities.

Nurses can often observe seasonal patterns of client problems in hospital units, clinics, and ambulatory care facilities. Hospital admission diagnoses and absences from school or work may help in spotting a local trend. Health department records or records from the Centers for Disease Control (CDC) in Atlanta may verify trends in reportable diseases. *Morbidity and Mortality Weekly Report*, prepared by the CDC, is another resource. Any or all of these may be used in nursing research.

Place

Morbidity and mortality often show distinct patterns of geographic distribution. For example, Figure 3–3 shows comparative rates of death per 100,000 population for heart disease and stroke in countries where these diseases are among the most common causes of death. It is evident that two persons die of heart disease in Scotland for every one who dies of the disorder in France. Interestingly, although both heart disease and stroke are cardiovascular disorders, the mortality rates for these two diseases show opposite patterns in Canada and Japan: three Japanese die of stroke

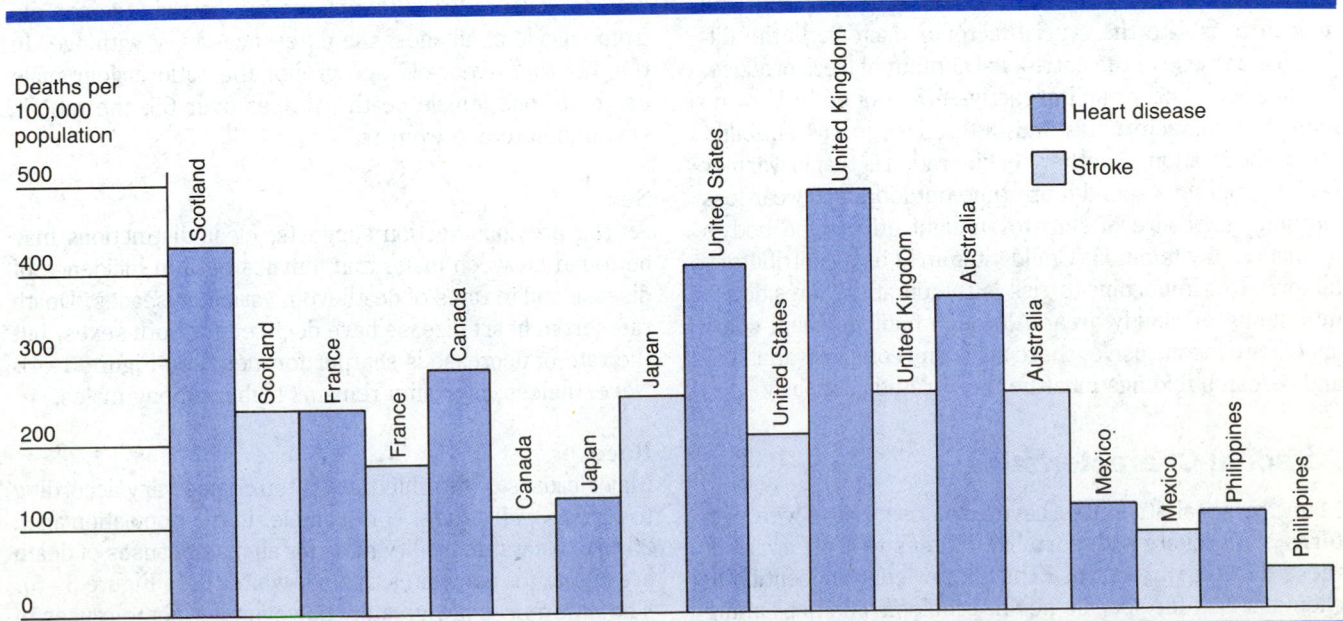

Figure 3–3

Comparison of death rates from heart disease and stroke in nine countries, all ages, 1966 (where the disease was ranked in the top ten causes of death in the country).

SOURCE: Adapted from United States Senate: *Leading Causes of Death in Selected Areas of the World*. Washington, DC: US Government Printing Office, Dec 1972.

for every Canadian who does, but more than three Canadians die of heart disease for every Japanese.

Death rates for heart disease also tend to be higher in industrialized nations. Some theorists believe this is due to higher income in these nations, and when incomes rise, lifestyles change. People eat more high-cholesterol foods (which have been linked to atherosclerosis); they are less active at work and at leisure; they often smoke and drink more. Competition and stress are generally higher in industrialized nations, which could be a factor in development of heart disease (see Chapters 2 and 22).

Rates of morbidity and mortality also vary within nations by region and in rural areas and cities. Climate varies by region, of course, and there are other environmental differences. For example, exposure to industrial chemicals in air and water is higher in urban areas. In some rural areas, water comes from private wells, and human wastes are disposed of in private septic tanks; this has implications for diseases spread by contaminated drinking water. A disease transmitted directly or indirectly by certain animals (eg, equine encephalitis) may be more common in or near farms; an illness related to overcrowded living conditions (eg, tuberculosis) may be more common in cities.

Although being aware of such patterns is useful, remember that correlation is not the same as causation. Illness is multifactorial, and determining its causes can be complex. For example, one study has shown that rates of colon cancer in various regions differ according to days of sunlight, with rates being lower where the number of "sun days" is higher. How might one interpret this association? Most areas with more sun have longer growing seasons. People who live there may eat more fresh fruits and vegetables than those in colder regions. Even so, it is still difficult to isolate the crucial factor or factors. Is the difference because of the nutritional content of fresh produce, the fiber content, or an interactive effect of both? How do individual characteristics and differences in susceptibility affect the relation? Another consideration is that in warmer regions, persons spend more time outdoors and wear less clothing; exposure of skin to sunlight affects the body's formation of vitamin D. Could vitamin D be a contributory factor? How important to risk is the duration of residence in a sunny or cloudy area? Although findings about colon cancer are inconclusive, there are many complex variables, and research findings must be interpreted cautiously.

Personal Characteristics

Many personal attributes have been associated with patterns of morbidity and mortality. Nurses who are aware of these associations can use their knowledge in identifying clients at risk for specific health problems and in planning health teaching and preventive regimens.

Age

Age affects health and mobility and influences how individuals view their health status. As Table 3–1 shows, rel-

Table 3–1   How Adults of Various Ages Assess Their Health

Assessment	Ages 17–44	Ages 45–64	Ages 65 and over
Health fair or poor	8.5%	22.0%	29.9%
Activity limited	8.1%	23.1%	43.0%
Days of restricted activity per year			
Total days	14.2	24.4	36.5
Days in bed	5.4	8.2	14.5

SOURCE: Adapted from Fingerhut LA et al: Health and disease in the United States. *Ann Rev Public Health* 1980; 1:1–36, p 27.

atively few persons under 45 see themselves as in only fair or poor health. Their activity is less apt to be restricted by health problems. But one out of five persons between ages 45 and 64 reports fair or poor health. And two out of five persons 65 and older report limitation of activity.

Causes of death—and, by implication, types of morbidity—are also related to age. Incidence of diseases of the heart, malignant neoplasms, and cerebrovascular disorders increases with age in persons of both sexes (see Table 3–2). Pneumonia, influenza, diabetes mellitus, cirrhosis of the liver, and arteriosclerosis are also more frequent causes of death in older persons. Accidental deaths, on the other hand, are most common among the elderly *and* young adults—men and women 65 or older and young men aged 15 to 24. Although more men than women die from suicide at all ages, the differences vary with age. In the 15- to 24-year-old age group, the ratio is four male deaths to one female death. At ages over 65, the ratio is seven men to one woman.

Sex

As the previous section suggests, clear distinctions may be found between males and females both in incidence of disease and in rates of death from various diseases. Death rates from heart disease have declined for both sexes, but the rate of decrease is sharper for men (see Figure 3–4). Nevertheless, mortality remains higher among males.

Race

Major causes of death in the United States vary according to race as well as age. For example, in the population aged 25 to 64 years, mortality rates for all major causes of death are higher for nonwhites than for whites (see Figure 3–5). The differences are greater, however, for some causes of death than for others. Mortality related to specific diseases also varies with race—as do rates of disease occurrence. Hypertension, for example, is more prevalent in blacks than in whites (Fingerhut et al., 1980). The lifespan of nonwhites is shorter than that of whites in the United States

Table 3–2 Mortality Rates by Sex and Age for Most Common Causes of Adult Death, 1978 (per 100,000 population)

Cause of Death	Age 15–24 M	Age 15–24 F	Age 25–44 M	Age 25–44 F	Age 45–64 M	Age 45–64 F	Age 65 and Older M	Age 65 and Older F
Heart disease	3.2	2.1	37.2	12.0	526.7	177.9	2812.6	2001.5
Malignant neoplasm	7.7	4.9	26.9	31.0	345.7	268.9	1357.0	759.0
Cerebrovascular disease	1.2	1.1	5.8	5.5	55.0	44.2	812.3	658.7
Accident	100.5	28.0	69.1	17.9	64.2	23.1	129.6	80.2
Pneumonia and/or influenza	1.6	1.1	3.9	2.4	22.4	11.2	239.8	161.2
Diabetes mellitus	.3	.4	2.9	2.2	18.3	17.2	93.4	106.7
Cirrhosis of liver	.3	.3	11.0	5.2	51.7	24.4	57.0	22.1
Arteriosclerosis	—	—	.1	—	3.7	1.9	109.6	118.7
Suicide	20.0	4.7	24.0	8.0	25.3	10.5	38.0	7.5

SOURCE: Adapted from Madden TA et al: *The Health Almanac.* New York: Raven, 1982, p 138.

(Table 3–3). (Remember that "nonwhites" does not mean only "blacks." Breaking down the "nonwhite" category might reveal further differences; for instance, between blacks and Orientals.)

Ethnicity and Religion

Different ethnic and religious groups have varying risks for particular diseases. Polish–American males have a high risk of lung and esophageal cancer; Italian–American males have a higher risk of bladder, pharyngeal, and colon cancer than other foreign-born males (Graham et al., 1963). Whether these risks are related to diet, occupation, or heredity is a matter for further study. Seventh-Day Adventists and Mormons have cancer mortality rates consider-ably lower than that of the general population, with the predominately Mormon state of Utah having the lowest rate in the United States (Phillips, 1975; Enstrom, 1975). Seventh-Day Adventists are vegetarians; Mormons neither smoke nor drink and also avoid caffeine. What relation these factors have to cancer rates—if any—has yet to be determined.

Certain genetic disorders occur primarily or exclusively in particular ethnic, religious, or racial groups. Tay-Sachs disease, for example, is found almost exclusively in Ashkenazic Jews. When disease incidence differs *within* ethnic and racial groups, nongenetic etiologic factors are likely to be responsible. Consistent variations *among* racial and ethnic groups support genetic hypotheses.

The Special Case of Emigrants

In the "melting pot" society of the United States, successive waves of emigrants from other nations have found permanent or temporary homes. Although the largest waves of immigration occurred in the late nineteenth century, immigrants from many societies continue to arrive, becoming new clients of the health care system.

Individuals who live out their lives in their country of birth may have different disease patterns than those who emigrate. Gordon (1957) reported that Japanese men aged 55 to 64 who lived in Japan died of heart disease only half as often as Japanese men of the same age who lived in the mainland United States. (The rate for Japanese men living in Hawaii was halfway between the two.)

On the other hand, the highest rates for stroke occurred among Japanese living in Japan and the lowest rates among Japanese in the continental United States. Smith (1956) reported that the pattern for gastric cancer among the same groups was similar to that for stroke: highest for

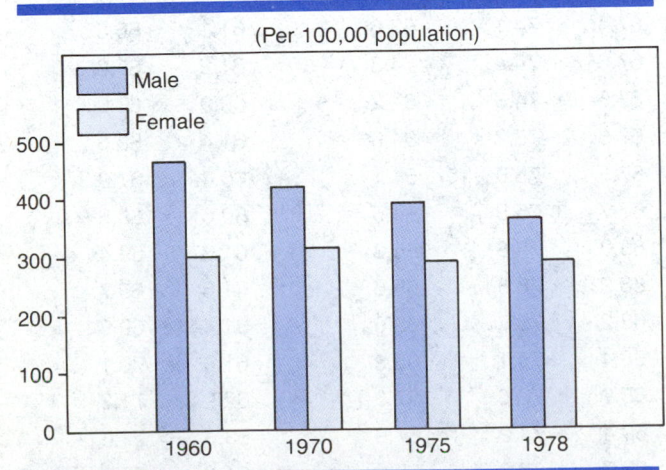

(Per 100,00 population)

Figure 3–4

Death rates from heart disease, 1960–1978.
SOURCE: Reprinted with permission from Madden TA et al: *The Health Almanac.* New York: Raven, 1982, p 123.

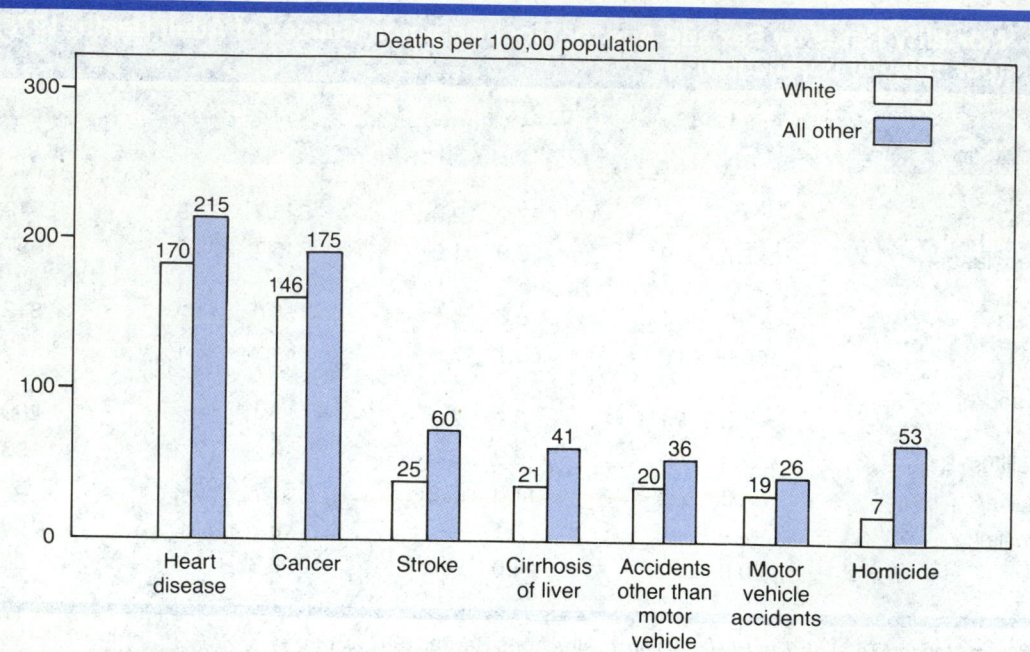

Figure 3–5

Major causes of death among persons 25 to 64 years by race, 1976.
SOURCE: Reprinted from United States Department of Health, Education and Welfare. *Health: United States 1980*. DHEW Publication No. HRA–76–1232, Figure 106.

	Total			White			All Other		
Year	Both Sexes	Male	Female	Both Sexes	Male	Female	Both Sexes	Male	Female
1950	68.2	65.6	71.1	69.1	66.5	72.2	60.8	59.1	62.9
1955	69.6	66.7	72.8	70.5	67.4	73.7	63.7	61.4	66.1
1960	69.7	66.6	73.1	70.6	67.4	74.1	63.6	61.1	66.3
1965	70.2	66.8	73.8	71.1	67.6	74.8	64.3	61.2	67.6
1966	70.2	66.7	73.9	71.1	67.5	74.8	64.2	60.9	67.6
1967	70.5	67.0	74.3	71.4	67.8	75.2	64.9	61.4	68.5
1968	70.2	66.6	74.1	71.1	67.5	75.0	64.1	60.4	67.9
1969	70.5	66.8	74.4	71.4	67.7	75.3	64.5	60.6	68.6
1970	70.8	67.1	74.7	71.7	68.0	75.6	65.3	61.3	69.4
1971	71.1	67.4	75.0	71.9	68.2	75.8	65.6	61.6	69.7
1972	71.1	67.4	75.0	72.0	68.2	75.9	65.6	61.4	69.9
1973	71.3	67.5	75.2	72.1	68.4	76.1	65.9	61.8	70.1
1974	71.9	68.1	75.8	72.7	68.9	76.6	67.0	62.9	71.3
1975	72.5	68.7	76.5	73.2	69.4	77.2	67.9	63.6	72.3
1976	72.8	69.0	76.7	73.5	69.7	77.3	68.4	64.2	72.7
1977	73.2	69.3	77.1	73.8	70.0	77.7	68.8	64.6	73.1

Table 3–3   Estimated Average Length of Life in Years, by Race and Sex, Selected Years 1950–1977

SOURCE: Reprinted from National Center for Health Statistics: Life tables. *Vital Statistics of the United States, 1977*. Vol 2. Hyattsville, MD: US Department of Health, Education and Welfare, 1979, p 16.

Japanese in Japan; lowest for Japanese on the US mainland; intermediate for Hawaii.

Do these differences reflect dietary factors, climate, lifestyle changes, or even the stress of adapting to a new culture? More research is clearly needed. Meanwhile, the nurse taking a history would be wise to ask whether a client is native or foreign born.

CHANGING PATTERNS OF HEALTH IN THE UNITED STATES

Patterns of disease and mortality change over time, as already suggested. Diseases that once decimated whole populations (eg bubonic plague) may become so rare that a modern health professional in the United States or Canada would scarcely recognize their symptoms. It is highly unlikely that the typical American health professional of today has ever seen a client with typhoid fever—a disease that regularly reached epidemic proportions only 50 years ago. Among the US population in the last few decades, mortality from all causes has declined steadily, and the relative importance of specific causes of death has shifted significantly.

Decline in Total Mortality

In the United States, age-adjusted death rates for all causes combined have declined (Table 3–4). The most significant figure is in the fifth column, which shows the 1978 death rate as a percentage of the 1900 rate.

Table 3–4 Age-Specific Mortality Rates, United States: 1900, 1970, and 1978

Age Groups (years)	Age-Specific Mortality Rates (per 1,000 population)			
	1900	1970	1978	1978 Rate as % of 1900 Rate
1–4	19.8	0.8	0.7	3.5
5–14	3.9	0.4	0.3	7.7
15–24	5.9	1.3	1.2	20.3
25–34	8.2	1.6	1.4	17.1
35–44	10.2	3.1	2.4	23.5
45–54	15.0	7.3	6.1	40.7
55–64	27.2	16.6	14.5	53.3
65–74	56.4	35.8	31.3	55.5
75–84	123.3	80.0	74.9	60.7
85 plus	260.9	163.4	147.0	56.3

SOURCE: Reprinted with permission from Madden TA et al: *The Health Almanac.* New York: Raven, 1982, p 103.

By far, the greatest improvement has been in ages 1 to 4; the 1978 rate is a mere 3.5% of the 1900 rate. This improvement is largely attributable to the control of infectious diseases through immunization and antibiotic therapy. On the other hand, the reduction in early deaths from congenital disorders means that more individuals are surviving into adolescence and adulthood and will be seen by the adult health nurse.

Note the percentages for adults over 64: the mortality rates for ages 65 and up have been cut nearly in half. As a result, more persons once considered very old are found in the general population and among the nurse's clients. As the general population ages, society must reevaluate its concept of who is "old": not long ago, a person aged 55 was considered elderly. What was old age in an earlier day is now vigorous maturity.

Shifts in Leading Causes of Death

Some diseases that were major killers in 1900 no longer ranked as fatal in 1978: gastroenteritis (once ranked third), chronic nephritis (once ranked sixth), and diphtheria (once ranked tenth) (Table 3–5). Tuberculosis, the second leading cause of disease in 1900, now ranks 19th.

Conversely, some diseases have gained in importance. The death rate for malignancies in 1978 was nearly three times that for 1900, and cardiovascular disease, once ranked fourth, now ranks first. Changing lifestyle patterns doubtless affect specific causes within the more general categories: the "all accidents" category for 1900 had virtually no automobile fatalities; the situation in 1978 was quite different.

Note also that the leading three causes of death in 1900—influenza and pneumonia, tuberculosis, and gastroenteritis—are infectious disorders. The current "top three"—cardiovascular disease, malignancies, and cerebrovascular disease—are not. These diseases primarily affect adults of middle age or older—especially persons over 65 (see Table 3–2).

Remember also that the elimination of a disease as a cause of early death may mean that people are *living* with the disease or illness. For example, trauma units and health care facilities designed to treat acute life-threatening situations may have reduced the number of deaths from accidents while increasing the number of clients in need of long-term rehabilitation. Before the development of insulin, most persons with type I (insulin-dependent) diabetes mellitus died in early adulthood; now clients with type I diabetes form a significant part of any health care professional's practice. And type II (noninsulin-dependent) diabetes is becoming a major health concern, in part because more persons are living to its age of onset. Diabetes is one example of a trend that is having major effects on health care in the United States: long-term illnesses, often related to lifestyle, are becoming the significant health problems of Americans.

Table 3–5	Leading Causes of Death in the United States: A Comparison Between 1900 and 1978			
Rate per 100,000 and Rank				
Rank Order	**1900 Rate**	**Diseases**	**1978 Rate**	**Rank Order**
	1719.1	**All causes**	883.4	
1	202.2	Influenza and pneumonia	26.7	5
2	194.4	Tuberculosis	1.3	19
3	142.7	Gastroenteritis	—	—
4	137.4	Cardiovascular disease	442.7	1
5	106.9	Cerebrovascular disease	80.5	3
6	81.0	Chronic nephritis	—	—
7	72.3	All accidents	48.4	4
8	64.0	Malignancies	181.5	2
9	62.6	Certain diseases of early infancy	10.1	10
10	40.3	Diphtheria	—	—
15	22.9	Bronchitis, emphysema and asthma	10.0	8
19	12.5	Cirrhosis of the liver	13.8	7
25	11.0	Diabetes mellitus	15.5	6
26	10.2	Suicide	12.5	9

SOURCE: Reprinted with permission from Madden TA et al: *The Health Almanac.* New York: Raven, 1982, p 111.

Long-Term Disease and Lifestyle

Early in this century, communicable acute disease was a primary concern of health professionals. More recently chronic, or long-term, disease has been the model that guides approaches to disease prevention. In the model for a communicable disease (Figure 3–6), a single agent (eg, the typhoid bacillus) acts upon the host. Within a relatively short time (days or weeks at most), the host either recovers or dies. The illness is usually a transient episode in life.

In the model of noncommunicable disease (Figure 3–7), many agents act upon the host, with an outcome that ranges from recovery to disability or death. The process takes varying amounts of time—usually a long time, and often a lifetime.

Figure 3–8 illustrates how the noncommunicable disease model applies to a specific disorder, coronary atherosclerosis, as it leads to a secondary disorder, myocardial infarction. Many factors affect the host, leading first to atherosclerosis, then to myocardial infarction, then to disability and/or death. The entire cycle occurs over a long time.

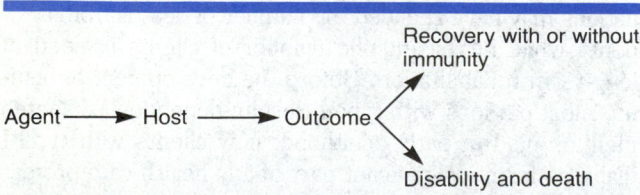

Figure 3–6

Communicable disease model.
SOURCE: Reprinted with permission from Leppink H: Health risk estimation. In: *Promoting Health Through Risk Reduction.* Faber MM, Reinhardt AM (editors). New York: Macmillan, 1982, p 38.

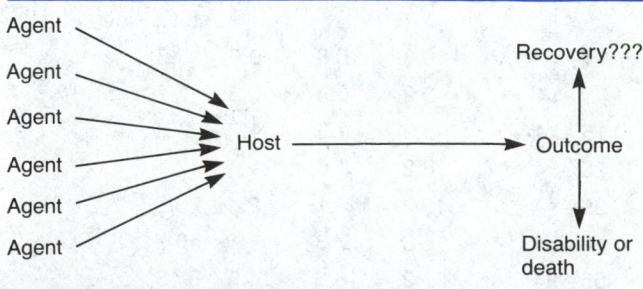

Figure 3–7

Noncommunicable disease model.
SOURCE: Reprinted with permission from Leppink H: Health risk estimation. In: *Promoting Health Through Risk Reduction.* Faber MM, Reinhardt AM (editors). New York: Macmillan, 1982, p 38.

Among the major characteristics of the long-term disorders that are now the principal causes of death in the United States are: they are relatively irreversible (ie, there is no specific "cure"), they have multiple causes, they tend to develop over long periods, and many show a strong association with the lifestyle of the host. In this regard, Dever (1976) has reported that:

- 11% of deaths are influenced by the health care organization.
- 19% are influenced by environment.
- 27% are influenced by human biology.
- 43% are influenced by lifestyle.

Moreover, studies have suggested that, for persons aged 40 to 64, current medical practices have less potential for saving lives than significant reductions in inactivity, overnutrition, alcoholism, and hypertension (Pender, 1982). No wonder, then, that lifestyle is receiving increasing attention for its potential for prevention of illness.

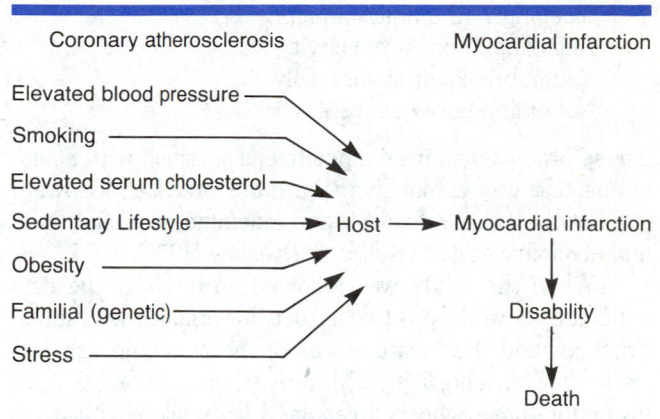

Figure 3–8

Noncommunicable disease model applied to coronary atherosclerosis and myocardial infarction.

SOURCE: Reprinted with permission from Leppink H: Health risk estimation. In: *Promoting Health Through Risk Reduction.* Faber MM, Reinhardt AM (editors). New York: Macmillan 1982, p 39.

Section II: Lifestyle and the Promotion of Health and Prevention of Illness

Of the various causes of disease mentioned at the beginning of this chapter, lifestyle is uniquely subject to each individual's control. Individual life patterns such as eating, exercise, drinking, coping with stress, and using substances such as tobacco and drugs are known to be modifiable causes of illness. Environment is sometimes, though not always, subject to societal control or modification.

An individual's lifestyle is a unique composite of thoughts, feelings, customs, and habits that often have cultural and historical roots. Just as each person's health status ranges along a continuum from optimum health through illness to death, so lifestyles range along a continuum from health enhancing to self-destructive. The issue of lifestyle in relation to health is discussed in Chapter 4. In this chapter, lifestyle is discussed as it relates to risk, to changing patterns of disease already discussed, and to changing concepts of health prevention and maintenance that significantly affect the nurse's role.

HEALTH RISKS

The identification of health risk factors is an important part of the health hazard appraisal (HHA). The concept of risk factors is crucial to understanding the multifactorial approach to illness, in contrast to simple cause and effect.

A risk factor entails probability; ie, if the risk factor is elevated, more individuals in a given group will be affected by the risk. But not everyone in a high-risk group will inevitably develop a given disorder—and not everyone in a low-risk group will escape it.

How long a person is exposed to a risk and the intensity of exposure affect the probability of that individual's developing the disorder. Moreover, in at least some cases, risk factors are synergistic; ie, if several risk factors are present, the probability that disease will develop is greater than the sum of the individual probabilities associated with the risks. Cardiovascular disease is one example of this effect. Again, remember that the connection between a risk factor and development of a disease is not absolute, even in well-studied cases. The association between lung cancer and cigarette smoking is well established—more than 80% of lung cancer among men is attributable to smoking (Gett, Cortese, & Fontana, 1983)—yet only a small proportion of heavy smokers develops cancer of the lung.

Lifestyles Favorable to Health

A major advance in establishing a connection between lifestyle, well-being, and longevity is a study of adults residing in Alameda County, Calif, begun in 1965. Many studies of morbidity and mortality are based on hospitalized populations. In this study, however, members of a general community population were studied to determine the relation, if any, among health status and seven favorable health practices:

- Never having smoked
- Limiting alcohol consumption
- Controlling weight

- Sleeping 7 to 8 hours a night
- Engaging in physical activity
- Eating breakfast almost daily
- Not eating between meals

These practices showed a positive association with health status that was cumulative (the more practices followed, the healthier the individual) and independent of age, sex, and economic status (Belloc & Breslow, 1972).

When the study was followed up in 1974, the data collected showed a positive association among the first five practices and the health status of the surviving subjects (Wiley & Comacho, 1980). Moreover, mortality rates were lower for those who had reported favorable health practices in 1965 than for those who had not (Breslow & Enstrom, 1980). A national survey conducted in 1979 and 1980 indicates that the results of the Alameda study are applicable to the general population of the United States (Wilson & Elinson, 1981).

Lifestyles Unfavorable to Health

Relations between lifestyle and disease have also been documented. For example, the following lifestyle factors have been identified as risk factors for malignant neoplasms at various sites:

- **Cigarette smoking:** cancer of the lung, oral cavity, larynx, urinary bladder, and pancreas have been linked to this practice. Cigarettes have been linked to more cancer incidence and mortality than any other carcinogenic agent (*Health: United States*, 1980).
- **Alcohol consumption:** increased risk of cancer of the mouth, pharynx, larynx, esophagus, and liver has been linked to alcohol consumption (Rothman, 1980).
- **Dietary factors:** various dietary substances have been linked to either increased or decreased risk of cancer: dietary fiber, vitamins A and C, fats, minerals (eg, selenium), nonnutritive sweeteners, and food additives and contaminants (National Research Council, 1982).
- **Sexual practices:** higher risk for cancer of the cervix has been associated with multiple sexual partners and early age at first intercourse (Graham et al, 1982). A high incidence of Kaposi's sarcoma, a relatively rare form of malignancy, has been seen among victims of AIDS (acquired immune deficiency syndrome), many of whom are homosexual men (Allen & Mellin, 1982).

Driving habits also have a significant effect on injury, disability, and death in the United States. Indeed, automobile accidents are a major cause of death for persons up to middle age. Although wearing seat belts has been shown to reduce death or injury by 30% to 50%, studies indicate that only 10% to 15% of drivers and passengers use them (Fielding, 1982b). The nurse caring for an accident victim is in a good position to discuss with the client and family the benefits of using seat belts.

The Prospective Model of Health Care

Traditionally, medical practice has concentrated on caring for clients while they are sick rather than keeping them well. With this approach, health care costs have escalated. In 1929, US per-capita expenditures on health care were $29 annually, and the total was 3.5% of the gross national product (GNP). By 1980, US health care expenditures per capita had risen to $1,067—9.4% of the GNP (Table 3–6).

Despite this vast increase in expenditure, many Americans are far from being in ideal health. One reason for this situation is that caring for an ill individual costs a great deal more than prevention and is apt to be less effective (Haggerty, 1977; Peddecord, 1980).

Traditional medicine has been practiced primarily according to the communicable disease model, emphasizing early discovery of illness rather than maintenance of health. The ill person's role has been essentially passive; and health care personnel have tended to believe the "patient" had "little need to understand the disease process, only to accept the ministrations of the healer" (Leppink, 1982).

There is evidence that this attitude is changing. The increased importance of long-term illnesses, rising costs, dissatisfaction with conventional therapies, and public demand for more involvement in health-related decision making have combined in a new perspective. The changing goals of health care stress both avoidance of illness and positive improvement of health status.

To understand this *prospective* approach, in contrast to what might be called the *retrospective* approach, consider the stages of disease:

- Stage 1. No risk is present.
- Stage 2. The individual is at risk from encounter with a causative agent.
- Stage 3. The agent is present and active, but no signs or symptoms of disease are yet apparent.
- Stage 4. Signs are present and detectable, but the individual is unaware of them.
- Stage 5. Symptoms alert the individual to the presence of a problem.
- Stage 6. Overt disease is present, and a definitive diagnosis is established (Leppink, 1982).

Stage 4 marks the passage from wellness to illness. Before this point, the progression of disease could be controlled or reversed. From this point on, behavioral changes and other interventions have less and less potential for altering the course of disease.

The traditional model has concentrated on stages 5 and 6. Prospective health care, on the other hand, focuses on stages 1, 2, and 3. That is, the focus is on well people and a principal aim is identification of persons at risk. In prospective health care, the client is an active participant, not a passive recipient of interventions by others. Responsibility rests with both client and provider.

The potential of the prospective approach for reducing

Table 3–6 US Per Capita Health Care Expenditures in Relation to GNP, Selected Years 1929–1980 (Data compiled by the Health Care Financing Administration)

Year	Gross National Product (in Billions)	National Health Expenditures		
		Amount (in Billions)	Percent of Gross National Product	Amount per Capita
1929	$ 103.4	$ 3.6	3.5	$ 29.49
1935	72.2	2.9	4.0	22.65
1940	100.0	4.0	4.0	29.62
1950	286.5	12.7	4.4	81.86
1955	400.0	17.7	4.4	105.38
1960	506.5	26.9	5.3	146.30
1965	691.0	41.7	6.0	210.89
1970	992.7	74.7	7.5	357.90
1971	1,077.6	83.3	7.7	394.23
1972	1,185.9	93.5	7.9	437.77
1973	1,326.4	103.2	7.8	478.34
1974	1,434.2	116.4	8.1	534.63
1975	1,549.2	132.7	8.6	603.57
1976	1,718.0	149.7	8.7	674.14
1977	1,918.0	169.2	8.8	754.81
1978	2,156.1	189.3	8.8	835.57
1979	2,413.9	214.6	8.9	936.92
1980	2,628.8	247.2	9.4	1,067.06

SOURCE: Reprinted from Gibson RM, Waldo DR: National health expenditures, 1980. *Health Care Financing Review.* Health Care Financing Administration. Publication No. 03123. Washington, DC: US Government Printing Office, Sept 1981.

human suffering is incalculable. The potential for reducing the cost of health care is difficult to calculate, but some estimates of cost-benefit ratios appear in Table 3–7. Note that the cost of a number of measures is virtually nothing; instead of requiring vast facilities and ever more costly technological advances, preventive measures can often be performed at home during daily living for almost nothing. Consider the cost of toothbrushes compared with the cost of ultrasonic dental drills or the cost of walking briskly for an hour a day compared with the cost of even one day in a coronary care unit.

EFFECTING LIFESTYLE CHANGE

Clearly, lifestyle modification has vast potential for raising national and individual levels of health. Nurses can identify exciting possibilities for teaching their clients about health risks and working with their clients in developing healthier lifestyles. Nevertheless, altering customary practices and attitudes is always a formidable task.

Deterrents to Lifestyle Modification

Most persons still think of health in terms of "not being sick." As long as people do not feel ill, they may be disin-

clined to change their ways—especially when change means giving up enjoyable foods, walking instead of driving, and otherwise sacrificing present pleasures for a vague promise of "better health" on some future day. Many persons say or feel that living 10 years less but doing what they want is preferable to the "penal servitude" that a life of "self-control" and "moderation" suggests to them. They are especially likely to take this view when the "10 years less" is not a clear and present danger.

Habits and attitudes are formed over many years, and these practices embrace all dimensions of life. Changing lifestyles is difficult; it takes concentration and dedication, especially when others urge "just one more" drink, piece of pie, or cigarette; when the seat belts in friends' two-year-old cars are still wrapped in plastic; when it is hot outside and sitting by the television with a cold beer seems far more appealing than taking a two-mile walk. In the absence of an overt threat to health—and even if a threat is present—motivation may be lacking.

Models for Lifestyle Change

Individual motivation to initiate change is probably the most significant factor in successful lifestyle change. The health consciousness of Americans is apparently rising, but wide-

Table 3–7 Estimated Costs of Illness and Potential Savings for Selected Preventive Interventions in the United States (1975)

Disease or Condition	Magnitude of Problem	Intervention	Estimated Preventable Cases	Estimated Cost ($ Billion)	Estimated Cost of Preventive Intervention	Potential Savings as a Result of Intervention	Benefit-to-Cost Ratio
Hypertension	Prevalence: 20+ million; largely unknown to victims	Detection, drugs	10 million	$15.9	$4–6 billion	$4–6 billion	4:1 to 2:1
Cancer of colon	Incidence: approximately 100,000/year	Diet	17,000	3.5	Unknown	1.23 billion	Unknown
Heavy cigarette smoking	22 million heavy smokers	Cessation (25% success)	5.5 million	20.3	2.75 billion	5.1 billion	1.8:1
Alcohol abuse	9 million alcoholics; 4.8 million males (target population)	Intensive program and follow-up (60% success)	60% of 4.8 million	33.6	6 billion	14 billion	2.3:1
Screening for colon cancer among all persons over 55	Incidence: approximately 3/100 over 55	Screen for stool guaiac	20% improved survival; reduced costs 50% in ⅓ of cases	0.47	80 million (screening)	670 million	8.38:1

SOURCE OF DATA: Kristein M: Economic issues in prevention. *Prev Med* 1977; 6:252–264.

spread apathy toward health remains what one writer has called "the plague of the twentieth century" (Lafferty, 1979). Once a threshold of concern has been reached, however, lifestyle modification is best approached in stages. According to Milsun (1980), these stages consist of:

- Being aware of risk and accepting that the risk applies to one personally (eg, "*I* might develop cancer if I continue to smoke").

- Integrating the knowledge; ie, making the desired modification part of the self-image. ("*I* am, or at least can be, a nonsmoker.")

- Making the effort to change (deciding how to modify behavior and then sustaining the effort).

Plunging into change without informed motivation is unlikely to bring long-term improvement.

PROMOTING HEALTH BY REDUCING RISK

Promoting health and preventing disease are responsibilities of both the society at large and of individuals. The individual, or micro, level is currently receiving the most attention, and most strategies aim at reducing individual risk. Although few data have yet been identified to support this approach, logic and experience strongly suggest it is valid.

Promoting health by reducing risk entails several steps, the first of which is screening individuals for risk factors or precursors of disease. Once this has been done, the degree of risk can be appraised, systematic reduction of risk can be planned, and health education can be directed toward permanent change in individual behavior.

Nursing Research Note

DeVon HA, Powers MJ: Health beliefs, adjustment to illness, and control of hypertension. *Res Nurs Health* 1984; 7:10–16.

In a study of 15 controlled and 15 uncontrolled hypertensive subjects, there were no significant differences in health beliefs affecting compliance, but there were significant differences in several areas related to psychosocial adjustment to illness. The uncontrolled hypertensive subjects reported difficulty in their domestic lives, more disturbances in their extended family relationships, and increased psychological stress. This finding suggests that for uncontrolled hypertensive clients, noncompliance may not be the problem. Assessing for psychosocial/lifestyle problems may assist the nurse in promoting a realistic, effective treatment outcome.

Instruments known as **health risk appraisals,** or **HRAs,** are used to gather the data on which risk reduction planning and education are based. Different techniques are used, but the basic intention of the HRA is to provide a quantitative measure of lifestyle factors and personal characteristics and thereby estimate an individual's probability of dying from a particular cause within a specified time. Computer-based statistical procedures are used to determine a "risk age" and an "achievable age." The risk age reflects how hazardous behaviors affect the individual's chronological age. The achievable age delineates the potential improvement in longevity that behavioral change might bring. Presenting these data to the client is believed to motivate the client to change.

Wagner and associates have suggested (1982) that HRAs have been favorably received because (1) they provide a rationale and focus for health counseling; (2) they can be efficiently and economically applied to large groups; (3) they fit well with American values regarding science and technology, statistics, and the computer; (4) they are congruent with a prevailing belief that lifestyles and disease are associated; and (5) HRA packages are commercially profitable.

Not all observers are optimistic, however. They suggest that users of HRAs may propose lifestyle changes that scientific evidence does not support and that conflict with cultural values and traditions. Others suggest that such programs amount to "blaming the victim" and take insufficient account of social and environmental factors that influence health.

Certainly, the validity of risk factors has not been fully explored; it may be known, for example, that obesity and hypertension are associated, but absolute, precise predictions of risk are not yet possible. Data based on group experience may not apply to specific individuals. Moreover, the statistics available may not apply to certain groups (eg, individuals of different race from those for which the most data have been compiled). There are also psychological risks in presenting clients with such apparently precise estimates of risk and longevity. Whether the HRA approach will have a significant effect on health behavior remains to be determined.

HEALTH PROMOTION, THE FUTURE, AND THE NURSE

No single strategy is likely to succeed in promoting health through risk reduction. Earlier attempts to improve health through education of individuals have been less successful than educators had hoped. Legislative constraints on hazardous behaviors have been more successful. But legislative measures that attempt to control individual lifestyles are often difficult to enforce (eg, laws mandating that individuals use seat belts) and impinge on personal choice to an extent at odds with the American tradition of individual freedom.

Haggerty (1977) has suggested a number of measures that might be helpful in gaining public acceptance of risk-reducing lifestyle changes:

- Working more closely with self-help and community groups
- Intensifying health education efforts in health care settings
- Capitalizing on the capabilities of mass media by such techniques as call-ins following health presentations, discussion groups, and personal follow-up

Haggerty also suggests what he terms "managerial prevention" that would necessarily involve government:

- Taxation of alcohol, cigarettes, candy, and soft drinks (most of which are already taxed fairly heavily)
- Using legislation to bypass hazardous behaviors; eg, requiring automatically locking seat belts
- Providing tax-funded payments to reward behavior such as seeking prenatal care during the first trimester of pregnancy
- Offering tax reductions and grants to industries and institutions that institute health-oriented environmental changes

Increased availability of reduced insurance premiums for those who maintain desirable weight, for example, has also been suggested.

These and other approaches will necessarily be a blend of micro and macro interventions. Much study will be needed to determine which measures are successful and what the costs are in money and resources as well as in individual liberty and choice.

The prospective approach to health care offers both a challenge and opportunity to professional nurses. Nursing education and research have traditionally emphasized providing care for the ill. Approaching nursing from the perspective of maintaining health will profoundly alter the nurse's role, the client's role, and the interactions between nurse and client and nurse and other health care professionals.

Chapter Highlights

Patterns of health are traditionally described in terms of illness (morbidity) and death (mortality).

Knowing the patterns and incidence of disease is essential to effective health care planning and disease prevention.

(continued)

Chapter Highlights (continued)

Important information can be gained from studying the factors that affect disease trends such as time, place, age, sex, race, ethnicity, religion, and emigration.

The leading causes of death in the United States have shifted over the past century. Long-term illnesses, often related to lifestyle, are becoming the significant health problems of Americans.

Lifestyles range along a continuum from self-enhancing to self-destructive. Many aspects are under an individual's control; some are not.

Favorable health practices—never having smoked, limiting alcohol consumption, controlling weight, sleeping 7 to 8 hours a night, engaging in physical activity, eating breakfast almost daily, and not eating between meals—are positively associated with health status independent of age, sex, and economic status.

Traditional medical practice has concentrated on caring for people while they are sick, rather than keeping them well. This approach is more costly than measures related to prevention and is likely to be less effective.

Crucial nursing goals are raising the health consciousness of the public and advocating lifestyle modification.

Health risk appraisals (HRAs), derived from a quantitative measure of lifestyle factors and personal characteristics, estimate an individual's probability of dying from a particular cause within a specified time and delineate the potential improvement in longevity from behavioral change.

Presenting HRA information to a client may provide the necessary motivation for change in health-risk behavior.

Bibliography

Allen J, Mellin G: The new epidemic: Immune deficiency, opportunistic infections, and Kaposi's sarcoma. *Am J Nurs* 1982; 82:1718–1722.

Belloc NB, Breslow L: Relationship of physical health status and health practices. *Prev Med* 1972; 1:409–421.

Breslow L, Enstrom JE: Persistence of health habits and their relationship to mortality. *Prev Med* 1980; 9:469–483.

Dever GEA: An epidemiological model for health policy analysis. *Soc Indicators Res* 1976; 2:453–466.

Enstrom JE: Cancer mortality among Mormons. *Cancer* 1975; 36:825–841.

Fielding JE: Appraising the health of health risk appraisal. *Am J Public Health* 1982a; 72:337–340.

Fielding JE: Risk reduction goals throughout life. In: *Promoting Health Through Risk Reduction*. Faber MM, Reinhardt AM (editors). New York: Macmillan, 1982b, pp 4–18.

Fingerhut LA et al: Health and disease in the United States. *Ann Rev Public Health* 1980; 1:1–36.

Gett JR, Cortese DA, Fontana RS: Lung cancer: Current concepts and prospects. *Ca* 1983; 33:74–86.

Gordon T: Mortality experiences among the Japanese in the United States, Hawaii, and Japan. *Public Health Report* 1957; 72:543–553.

Graham S et al: Ethnic derivation as related to cancer at various sites. *Cancer* 1963; 16:13–27.

Graham S et al: Sex partners and herpes simplex virus type 2 in the epidemiology of cancer of the cervix. *Am J Epidemiol* 1982; 115:729–735.

Haggerty RJ: Changing lifestyles to improve health. *Prev Med* 1977; 6:276–289.

Kannel WB: Cardiovascular risk factors: The Framingham study. In: *Proceedings of Fifteenth Annual Meeting Society for Prospective Medicine*, St Petersburg, FL, Oct 1979.

Lafferty J: A credo for wellness. *Health Ed* 1979; 10:10–11.

Leppink H: Health risk estimation. In: *Promoting Health Through Risk Reduction*. Faber MM, Reinhardt AM (editors). New York: Macmillan, 1982.

Madden TA et al: *The Health Almanac*. New York: Raven, 1982.

Milsum JH: Health, risk factor reduction and life-style change. *Fam Commun Health* 1980; 3:1–13.

National Research Council. *Diet, Nutrition, and Cancer*. Washington, DC: National Academy Press, 1982.

Peddecord KM: Competing for acute care dollars: The economics of risk reduction. *Fam Commun Health* 1980; 3:25–40.

Pender NJ: *Health Promotion in Nursing Practice*. Norwalk, CT: Appleton–Century–Crofts, 1982.

Phillips RL: Role of life-style and dietary habits in risk of cancer among Seventh-Day Adventists. *Cancer Res* 1975; 35:3513–3522.

Rothman K: The proportion of cancer attributable to alcohol. *Prev Med* 1980; 9:174–179.

Safety Belt Usage: Survey of Care in the Traffic Population. November 1977–June 1978. Opinion Research Corporation, National Highway Traffic Safety Administration, Department of Transportation, Washington, DC, 1979.

Smith RL: Recorded and expected mortality among the Japanese in the United States and Hawaii with special reference to cancer. *JNCI* 1956; 17:459–473.

US Department of Health, Education and Welfare. *Health: United States*. DHEW Publication No. HRA–76–1232, 1980.

US Department of Health and Human Services. *Health: United States*. DHHS Publication No. PHS–82–1232, 1981.

US Department of Health and Human Services. Annual summary 1981. *MMWR*. HHS Publication No. (CDC) 82–8241, Oct 30, 1982.

Vierke S: The lifestyling program: Moving toward high level wellness. *Health Values* 1980; 4:237–241.

Wagner EH et al: An assessment of health hazard health risk appraisal. *Am J Public Health* 1982; 72:347–352.

Wiley JA, Comacho TC: Life-style and future health: Evidence from the Alameda County study. *Prev Med* 1980; 9:1–21.

Wilson RW, Elinson J: National survey of personal health practices and consequences: Background, conceptual issues, and selected findings. *Public Health Report* 1981; 96:218–225.

Suggested Readings

Donabedian A, Axelrod SJ, Wyszewianski L (editors): *Medical Care Chartbook*. Washington, DC: AUPHA Press, 1980. Charts depict data in nine general categories relevant to health care: population characteristics, mortality and morbidity, use of health care services, health care costs and expenditures, health personnel, health facilities, quality of care, tax-supported programs, and medical care insurance. This is an excellent resource for students.

Faber MM, Reinhardt AM (editors): *Promoting Health Through Risk Reduction*. New York: Macmillan, 1982. This collection of readings addresses important issues relevant to health promotion, with emphasis on application of health promotion strategies. Four major parts of the book include: Overview and Definition of Health Risk Estimation and Risk Reduction, Risk Reduction Methods, Present Programs for Risk Reduction and Health Promotion, and Future Directions for Risk Reduction.

Friedman GD: *Primer of Epidemiology*. New York: McGraw–Hill, 1980. This basic text explains epidemiologic principles, concepts, and methods. The relations between epidemiology and client care and medical care and health of the community are explored. Study problems are included in each chapter.

Sobel ME: *Lifestyle and Social Structure*. New York: Academic Press, 1981. The author presents an interesting analysis of the concept of lifestyle (in the abstract and as related to American society) and discusses the sociological factors related to differences in lifestyles. Data and methods for implementing a sociological theory of lifestyle differentiation are also included.

Chapter 4

The Experience of Illness

Carol Ren Kneisl
SueAnn Wooster Ames

Objectives

When you have finished studying this chapter, you should be able to:

Demonstrate awareness of the experience of illness from the client's perspective.

Discuss the relevance of sociocultural factors in adult health nursing practice.

Apply understandings of self-concept and self-esteem in the nursing process.

Demonstrate sensitivity to the body image changes clients experience.

Recognize the importance of providing for and maintaining support systems for both clients and nurses.

Identify individuals who are at high risk for illness.

Describe the nursing role in activating clients to take steps to protect and maintain their own health.

Teach clients how to manage stress creatively.

Incorporate the principles and methods of stress reduction into your personal as well as your professional life.

Illness is common to almost all humans. The response to being ill is a deeply personal but also a universal human experience. Perceptions of illness are shaped by a number of factors, such as the subculture whose values have been internalized, health beliefs and health practices, self-concept and body image, support systems available during the crisis of illness, even the health technology encountered during illness. These factors are a central concern of this chapter.

There is no question that a client's life is richer in other roles than it is in the sick role. Although some clients come to health care settings with considerable autonomy and others have developed autonomy to a lesser extent, all give up some of the control they are accustomed to having over their lives.

Fagin and Diers (1983) have identified the dilemma nurses face when their clients are not fully in charge of their own lives:

Nurses do for others publicly what healthy persons do for themselves privately. Nurses, as trusted peers, are there to hear secrets, especially the ones born of vulnerability. Nurses are treasured when these interchanges are successful; but most often people do not wish to remember their vulnerability or loss of control, and nurses are indelibly identified with those times.

For their own well-being, as well as the well-being of their clients, nurses must encourage autonomy in clients and help them regain control over their lives. Doing so requires an understanding of the client's culture and values; self-esteem, self-concept, and body image; available or potential support systems, and methods for assisting clients to assume responsibility for their own health care.

Because clients do not exist in a vacuum but are in constant interaction with their environment, another concern of this chapter is to emphasize the meaning of the experience of illness to the client's significant others—family, friends, and nurses. The final section of this chapter is focused on helping clients take charge of their health. Activating the client to adopt health-preserving practices to prevent illness is a central nursing role.

Section I: Culture and Values

Imagine what it is like to be ill, especially to be ill in a hospital. Asked to describe a client's attributes, the admitting clerk might list age, sex, marital status, race, religion, or even the physician's name; the business officer would detail the financial status or the third-party reimburser likely to pay part or all of the hospital bills; the laboratory technician might know the client as "the stat CBC, type and crossmatch on the ninth floor." Even the nurse might describe the client as "the possible bowel obstruction in room 909" or perhaps "the alteration in the pattern of bowel elimination." Imagine also by what attributes the client knows the nurse: As a comforting, nurturing parent? As a sex object? As a rescuer? As the person who carries out the physician's orders? As an autonomous professional?

What happened to the big picture? Does anyone see the whole person, whether client or nurse?

VIEWS OF THE WORLD

Based on their experiences, individuals develop a set of assumptions to help them to make sense of the world. Assumptions such as "parents only do what is in their child's best interest," "the way to get ahead in this world is to strike the first blow," or "God takes care of those who help themselves" are used to predict how others are likely to behave and what effects behavior might have on others. These assumptions form a person's *world view* and guide the person's perceptions, behavior, and even emotional state and feeling of well-being.

One's assumptive world view is formed during the early years. Culture and values are transmitted by the family, neighbors, church, school, and workplace. In tightly knit or isolated groups, the world view is more likely to be highly shared than it is in more mobile cultures. For example, persons who live in an ethnic enclave in a large metropolitan area have more in common than condominium dwellers in a resort community.

The interactions among those who share world views are more likely to be satisfying than the interactions among those whose assumptive worlds fail to fit together. Mismatched world views are often the basis for frustration and interpersonal conflict. The client who believes nurses should behave as comforting and nurturing parents will be acutely disappointed in the nurse who is guided by the principle of "God helps those who help themselves."

Mismatched world views often account for clients' dissatisfactions with health care providers and health care providers' dissatisfactions with clients. Problems are magnified when opposing views are strongly held. World views closely related to a person's sense of self-worth or to the person's feelings of well-being are likely to be the most enduring.

For example, the intensive care unit (ICU) nurses in a hospital in a medium-sized midwestern city were engaged in an ongoing battle with a tribe of gypsies. One of the critically ill clients in intensive care was the king of the tribe. The members of the tribe had been gathering in the parking lot, the corridors outside the ICU, and in the ICU itself for days. The clan had come together, in accord with tradition, to mourn the probable passing of their king and to preside, upon his death, at the ceremony honoring the new king. Tradition demanded that respect be shown to the dying king. One way of showing respect was to mourn together at a death watch. The nurses, on the other hand, believed that the tribe interfered with their ability to give effective and safe nursing care to the gypsy king and to their other clients. In their view, the constant commotion was distracting and jeopardized the well-being of their other clients and their families and friends. When the king died, the nurses celebrated the departure of the gypsy tribe. The gypsy tribe was relieved to no longer have to argue with the nurses or cajole them into allowing them to display their respect.

HEALTH BELIEFS AND HEALING PRACTICES

Culture determines how illness and health are perceived and therefore how they are thought to exist, what causes illness, how it should be diagnosed, what symptoms of illness are, how it should be treated, and who should do the treating. This perception may be the basis for decisions about where health care will be sought, and even if health care will be sought.

For a long time, administrators at a hospital in a Texas community near the Mexico border were unable to understand why their obstetrical unit had many more empty beds than the obstetrical unit at the other local hospital. Although it had been known for some time that many more women of Mexican or Mexican–American ancestry had their babies at the competing hospital, the administrators could not identify the reason. One day, a nurse who often talked with one of the orderlies (a Mexican–American) heard from him that his wife was in the other hospital after having delivered their third child. She commented that it would have been more convenient for him if his wife was hospitalized where he was employed. The orderly revealed that his wife and her friends looked forward to the special burrito dinner prepared by the Mexican cooks at the other hospital. Providing tasty Mexican food was proof of the other hospital's personal interest in its clients.

A strong contradiction between traditional and folk health care systems is not unusual. In some ethnic groups (Chinese–Americans; Japanese–Americans; and the Indians of North, Central, and South America), herbal products are used to treat physical and emotional disorders. Figure 4–1 compares herbal dispensing practices in a Chinese–American community and in the People's Republic of China where herbal medicine is integrated with Western medicine. In these cultures, herbs are commonly used to treat hypertension. The culturally unaware health care provider may not know that herbs are being used or that they can produce both positive and negative interactions with medications. In the hypertensive client being treated

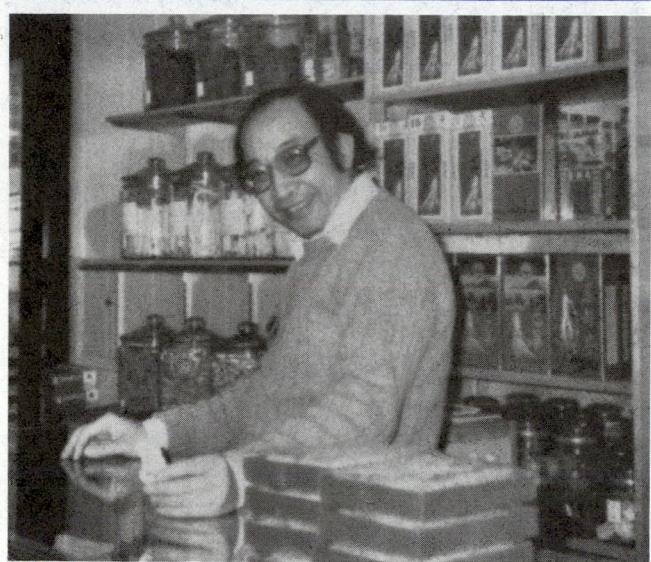

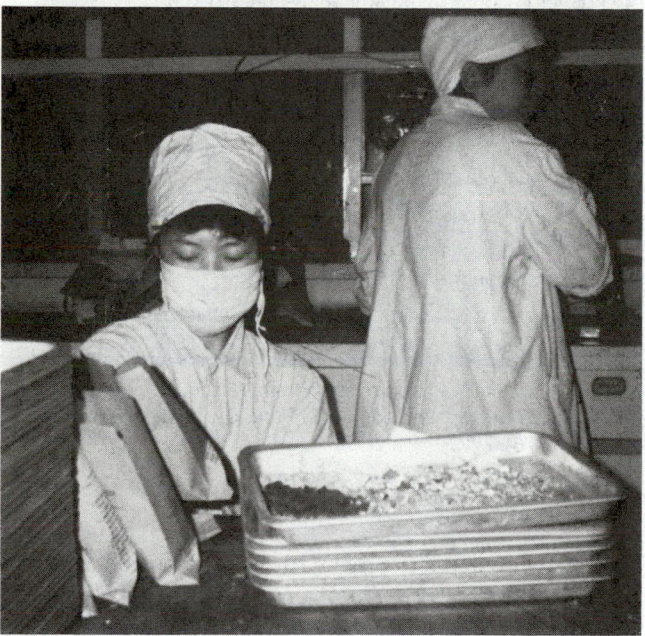

Figure 4–1

Top. Herbalist in a Chinese community in the United States.
Bottom. Herbal pharmacy in a Peking hospital.

with a beta-adrenergic blocker such as propanolol (Inderal) who is simultaneously being treated with herbs, the effects of the drug may be potentiated.

Members of some cultural groups, such as Appalachian whites and Mexican–Americans, may believe that illnesses caused by witches' spells do not respond to medications or that taking medicines may cause increased harm. The culturally unaware health care provider may label the client's failure to take prescribed medication as noncompliance.

Most health care providers in Western societies accept microbes, viruses, chemicals, or chromosomal abnormalities as causes of disease. This view is not shared by many persons in developing countries who may believe that supernatural forces cause illness and that witches, sorcerers, or medicine men can cure the sick through magic. Being aware of clients' folk health care systems will help the nurse to provide more effective and individualized health care. Becoming more culturally sensitive can help to humanize the care given to clients.

NURSING PROCESS AND SOCIOCULTURAL DIFFERENCES

If sociocultural differences are not to impede the interactions between nurse and client, the nurse's practice must be based on fundamental transcultural nursing premises (Henderson & Primeaux, 1981):

- Nurses cannot solve clients' problems, but they may be able to help clients solve their own problems.
- The easiest, least creative response to transcultural conflict is to pretend it does not exist.
- Every client behaves according to unwritten ethnic customs and traditions.
- Every successful effort by nurses to teach clients the elements of scientific medicine alienates clients from relatives and friends who do not have this knowledge.
- Previous transcultural experience is a valuable asset when used as a general guide. Such experience can be a liability, however, if the nurse believes it provides the answer to every transcultural problem.
- Nurses will make mistakes in transcultural interactions, but they should learn from mistakes and not repeat them.

These six points are reinforced in this section.

Assessment of the Client

Sociocultural assessment is an integral component of the subjective health assessment or health history. From the first contact with the client, the nurse attempts to identify the relevance of sociocultural aspects to the health history. The client's appearance and personal data such as name and address may be useful in some instances but only to form an initial impression. The initial impression must be validated by gathering additional information.

A number of opportunities to gather sociocultural information arise. During the health history, the nurse might ask about what the client believes may have caused the illness or health problem. It is also important to determine whether the client has received treatment for the condition elsewhere. Has the client attempted self-treatment or used other healers? How about herbal teas, pastes, and poultices? What ideas does the client have about how he or she could be helped? What are the health practices of the client's family, friends, and neighbors? Gathering accurate data is invaluable in the planning and intervention phases.

Assessment of the Nurse

Before nurses can truly understand and appreciate their clients' backgrounds, they must understand themselves, their own backgrounds, and the influence of their sociocultural heritage on their nursing practice. The questions in Box 4–1 are designed to help in assessing sociocultural heritage. Be honest and complete in responding to them; then apply the questions to current clients.

A second helpful step is for the nurse to explore specific sociocultural beliefs and attitudes. The statements in Box 4–2 provide direction. How might these beliefs and attitudes be the same as, or different from, the beliefs and attitudes of clients?

Planning and Implementation

Four major missteps can be made in the planning phase. The first is to stereotype the client by cultural group. Assuming all members of one ethnic or racial heritage are alike fails to allow for individualized nursing care. Essentially, stereotyping dehumanizes the client, robbing the client of personal uniqueness. Although consulting the literature or a resource person about a culture is often useful and helpful, the data obtained must be placed in the proper perspective.

The second major misstep is to assume that differences among cultural groups do not exist. Nurses must be

---

Box 4–2   Exploring Specific Sociocultural Attitudes

I accept opinions different from my own.

I respond with compassion to poverty-stricken people.

I think interracial marriage is a good thing.

I would feel uncomfortable in a group in which I am the ethnic minority.

I consider failure a bad thing.

I invite people I don't like to my home.

I believe that the Ku Klux Klan has its good points.

I set realistic life goals.

I would enjoy serving as a juror in a rape case.

I am concerned about the treatment of minorities in employment and health care.

I feel uncomfortable in low-income neighborhoods.

I prefer to conform rather than disagree in public.

I value friendship more than money.

I maintain high ethical standards as a professional.

I would not object to premarital sex for my children.

I spend a lot of time worrying about social injustices without doing much about them.

I believe that almost anyone who really wants to can get a good job.

I have a close friend of another race.

I would rather attend a concert than an athletic contest.

SOURCE: Reprinted with permission from Wilson HS, Kneisl CR: *Psychiatric Nursing,* 2nd ed. Menlo Park, CA: Addison–Wesley, 1983, pp 776–777.

Box 4–1   Questions That Acknowledge Sociocultural Heritage

What ethnic group, socioeconomic class, religion, age group, and community do you belong to?

What experiences have you had with people from ethnic groups, socioeconomic classes, religions, age groups, or communities different from your own?

What were those experiences like? How did you feel about them?

When you were growing up, what did your parents and significant others say about people who were different from your family?

What about your ethnic group, socioeconomic class, religion, age, or community do you find embarrassing or wish you could change? Why?

What sociocultural factors in your background might contribute to being rejected by members of other cultures?

What personal qualities do you have that will help you establish interpersonal relationships with persons from other cultural groups? What personal qualities may be detrimental?

What assumptions do you hold about the people who populate our world?

SOURCE: Reprinted with permission from Wilson HS, Kneisl CR: *Psychiatric Nursing,* 2nd ed. Menlo Park, CA: Addison–Wesley, 1983, p 776.

---

able to recognize differences so they can be considered in clinical practice. A third problem, trying to ignore cultural differences in the hope they will magically go away, is also ineffective.

The fourth major misstep involves making assumptions about clients based on the nurse's own value system. It is essential to interpret clients' behavior and plan their care from the context of the client's own culture, not the nurse's and to judge their behavior by their standards, not the nurse's.

Essential to the entire nursing process is the ability to communicate effectively with clients from other cultures. Language barriers often increase the sense of helplessness and alienation clients feel in their experiences with a health culture different from their own. Some strategies have been helpful in communicating with clients from different cultures. (Table 4–1).

In planning and implementing the nursing care of clients with strong folk health beliefs and healing practices, the nurse may be able to reinforce practices that will enhance the client's feeling of well-being. For example, many His-

Table 4–1 Communicating With Clients From Different Cultures

Strategy	Rationale

1. If you don't speak the language of your client try the following:
 	
  a. Enlist the aid of a family member or friend of the client.
 	
  b. Seek out a bilingual staff member in the setting.
 	
  c. Ask another client to translate.
 	
  d. Use other agencies as resources.
	Being able to help will increase the helper's self-esteem. Knowing that a concerned person is directly participating may help the client feel less anxious.
	
	Larger institutions often have bilingual employees on their staffs. Smaller agencies often employ indigenous staff.
	
	Another client can be helpful in translating cultural beliefs as well as language. Being able to help boosts self-esteem.
	
	Health and social services departments, international institutes, college language departments, neighborhood houses, or cultural centers will often know of people who are willing to volunteer as translators.

2. Select the words you use carefully, avoiding buzz words and jargon. Speak clearly, pacing yourself to be neither too fast nor too slow.	Words that are slurred, have many syllables in them, or are too technical make communication more difficult. Speaking too fast may overload the client and make it difficult for the client to follow. Speaking too slowly may lose the client's attention.
3. Select the gestures you use with care, using your nonverbal behavior to underscore your words and your actions.	The proper use of gestures can clarify a message, and drawings can sometimes be helpful. Be careful, however; not all gestures mean the same thing in all cultures.
4. Listen to your client's words and watch your client's gestures carefully. Do your best to understand and validate the meaning they have for you.	Listening carefully to the client will help you avoid focusing on what you will say or do next and will demonstrate your genuine concern for the client's distress.

SOURCE: Reprinted with permission from Wilson HS, Kneisl CR: *Psychiatric Nursing,* 2nd ed. Menlo Park, CA: Addison–Wesley, 1983, p 778.

panic–Americans believe in the *hot–cold* (caliente–frío) theory of disease causation and treatment, which originated with Hippocrates, the father of medicine. This theory stems from the belief that the four body humors (blood, phlegm, black bile, and yellow bile) must be in balance in relation to both temperature and moisture—blood is hot and wet, phlegm is cold and wet, black bile is cold and dry, and yellow bile is hot and dry. A healthy body has achieved a balance so the body is warm and somewhat wet (Murillo–Rohde, 1982).

Illness occurs when the humors are not balanced—when, for instance, the body is very hot, cold, dry, or wet. The normal balance is restored by using the proper "hot" or "cold" foods, herbs, or medicines to counteract the effects of imbalance. Cold diseases are treated by hot foods, herbs, or medicines and vice versa. Some hot and cold foods, herbs, medicines, and illnesses are listed in Table 4–2. The list is necessarily incomplete because hot and cold foods, illnesses, and treatments vary from one subcultural group to another. Within its limits, the list can be used as a general guide for clients with Hispanic–American or Asian–American backgrounds. Often, foods and medicines that support the hot–cold theory may be compatible with the client's health needs and can augment the treatment plan. The hot–cold theory may be responsible, at

least in part, for why some of the Mexican–American clients described earlier preferred one Texas hospital over another. Perhaps the burrito dinner not only signified a personal interest in the client; it also may have been seen as restoring balance to the woman's body. They might have believed that eating spicy and protein-rich foods after delivery helps to replace the heat believed to be dissipated from the body during labor and delivery.

Clients who may take comfort in continuing contact with a familiar folk healer should be allowed and even encouraged to do so. Folk healers may not only support the client but may indirectly enhance the quality of the interpersonal relationship between client and nurse when clients see that the nurse respects and supports them in their search for meaning.

Objects may be important to the client in recovery from illness. A client may believe that the medicine bundle containing charms, herbs, roots, or plants left at the bedside by the Native American's shaman after a tribal healing ceremony wards off evil and cures. The tiny bag of salt or garlic or scapulars of the saints placed around the neck or wrist of the Hispanic–American client may be believed to be protection from the evil eye (mal de ojo). Although a nurse may not believe in the evil eye or in the power of charms to ward off evil or illness, the client may.

Table 4-2 Hot–Cold Diseases or Conditions and Their Treatment					
Hot Diseases or Conditions	**Cold Diseases or Conditions**	**Hot Foods**	**Cold Foods**	**Hot Medicines and Herbs**	**Cold Medicines and Herbs**
Infections	Cancer	Chocolate	Fresh vegetables	Penicillin	Bicarbonate of soda
Kidney diseases	Earache	Cheese	Tropical fruits	Aspirin	Milk of magnesia
Diarrhea	Rheumatism	Temperate-zone fruits	Dairy products	Castor oil	Sage
Rashes and other skin eruptions	Tuberculosis	Chili peppers	Low-prestige meats (goat, fish, chicken)	Cod liver oil	Linden
Sore throat	Common cold	Cereal grains	Honey	Iron preparations	Orange flower water
Warts	Headache	Goat milk	Raisins	Vitamins	
Constipation	Paralysis	High-prestige meats (beef, water fowl, mutton)	Bottled milk	Anise	
Ulcers	Stomach cramps	Oils	Barley water	Cinnamon	
Liver complaints	Teething	Hard liquor	Cod	Garlic	
	Menstrual period	Aromatic beverages		Mint	
	Joint pain	Coffee		Ginger root	
	Malaria	Onions		Tobacco	
	Pneumonia	Peas			
		Eggs			

SOURCE: Reprinted with permission from Wilson HS, Kneisl CR: *Psychiatric Nursing*, 2nd ed. Menlo Park, CA: Addison–Wesley, 1983, p 774.

Section II: Self-Concept, Self-Esteem, and Body Image

Self-concept, self-esteem, and body image are sometimes considered three different concepts. Actually, they are so closely interrelated that separating them may be impossible.

SELF-CONCEPT

The **self-concept** is the total set of beliefs and feelings one holds about one's self. It consists of the body image or physical self—persons' perceptions of what they look like, how their body functions, and its relation to the outside world—and the personal self—the personality, attitudes, and values that identify the person and make that person unique. Problems of body image and body-image alteration are discussed later in this chapter. Problems or inconsistencies in self-concept often coincide with client behaviors that nurses may view as problematic. These behaviors are discussed in Chapter 6.

SELF-ESTEEM

The personal value placed on oneself is called **self-esteem**. It involves the extent to which one loves or values oneself.

Self-esteem is based on the reflected appraisals of significant others. That is, when significant individuals (a parent, a sibling, a lover, a nurse on whom one must depend) lets a person know he or she is valued, cherished, or respected, the person feels good about himself or herself. Self-esteem is positive and at a high level. When the feedback from significant others signals that a person is "bad," immoral, stupid, weak, or not valued, self-esteem is lowered, and the person feels inadequate, inferior, or even worthless.

Although self-esteem begins to develop in infancy in response to caretakers (most often parents), it continues to be modified and altered by interactions with others. The greater their influence and significance, the greater the effect on self-esteem. This is a crucial point for nurses to remember. Nurses frequently see clients and their families during critical life junctures or transitions when vulnerability is heightened and self-esteem can be readily altered. Wittingly or unwittingly, a nurse can be responsible for increasing a person's positive self-regard or a person's feelings of worthlessness. Problems with self-esteem often coincide with certain patterns of behavior. These patterns, their bases, and the nursing process are discussed in Chapter 6.

BODY-IMAGE ALTERATION

The **body image** is a person's concept of the size, shape, and functioning of the body and its parts. Because body image is a component of self-concept, body image also arises, in part, from the attitudes and responses of other persons to one's body. Sensations that arise within the body also influence body image.

The body image extends beyond the physical body to objects with which one is intimately connected—a wheelchair, an artificial limb, clothes, makeup, hair style, and jewelry. Other objects, such as a nurse's cap or a symphony conductor's baton, may be meaningful symbols and incorporated into the body image, not only by the person but by the public as well.

A person generally has a stable body image developed over a long time. Changes in body image are usually made with great difficulty. Threats to, or alterations in, self-concept/body image heighten anxiety.

Consider the impact on body image of receiving a transplanted heart or an artificial heart. In this culture, great meaning is attached to the heart. In discussing grave issues, one is said to be "going to the heart of the matter"; persons have "a heart of gold" or are "blackhearted"; greeting cards with hearts and heart-shaped boxes of candy are sent on Feb. 14 to demonstrate love and affection; the disloyalty of a formerly trusted friend or colleague feels like a "knife thrust to the heart"; those who are very liberal politically are derogatorily labelled "bleeding hearts"; when someone is reluctant to complete a task, it is said that his or her "heart's not in it"; and a person who fails to show sympathy is said to have "no heart at all." The heart recipient's life depends, not on his own flesh-and-blood core of being but on someone else's or on a mechanical device. Furthermore, the artificial heart client is unalterably tied to a series of machines and devices whose beeps and whirrs are constant reminders not only of the great body-image alterations he is experiencing but of his partial mechanization as well.

NURSING PROCESS AND BODY-IMAGE ALTERATION

Assessment

Assessment of the client's body image is not likely to be easily accomplished on first meeting. The nurse and client may have many discussions before the client reveals highly personal data.

The nurse's specific questions or opening statements help the client reveal body-image concerns or misconceptions. Consider asking: "What changes have you noticed in how your body looks?" "What does it feel like to have a body that . . .?" "What changes in your body do you expect as a result of this illness (surgery, treatment)?" "How have the important persons in your life reacted to the changes in your body?" "If you had to guess how the important people in your life will react to the anticipated change in your body, what would you say?"

Assess the client's body image and the effects of body-image alterations whenever the client or the client's family and friends give clues that imply concern. Clues are not always given, however. It is good practice to make these assessments whenever a client's illness or treatment is associated with body-image alterations.

Nursing Diagnoses

General nursing diagnoses for clients with body-image alteration are likely to include:

• Disturbance in body image.
• Ineffective individual (or family) coping.
• Anticipatory grieving.
• Dysfunctional grieving.
• Knowledge deficit.
• Noncompliance.
• Sexual dysfunction.

Specific nursing diagnoses show the special relation of the diagnosis to each client. Examples might be:

• Disturbance in body image, related to above-the-knee amputation of left leg.
• Sexual dysfunction, related to abdominal perineal resection.
• Noncompliance with treatment plan, related to rejection of diagnosis of terminal illness.
• Anticipatory grieving, related to forthcoming mutilating surgery.

Planning and Implementation

Helping clients with disturbances in body image requires a supportive approach by the nurse. Being supportive means accepting and facilitating the client's discussion of the changes in body image as the client begins to consider them and the meaning they have. It means being able to tolerate expressions of rage, frustration, helplessness, hopelessness, fear, and grief even though that may be difficult. Being supportive also implies the ability to help the client in more concrete ways, to look at strengths and capitalize on them and to assist the client in problem solving for the limitations or alterations caused by the body change.

When impending body image changes are known ahead of time, *anticipatory guidance* helps clients cope. This process involves discussing future body changes, anticipating the problems that may arise, and considering solutions in advance. Anticipatory guidance lays the foundation for effective grief work and helps to prevent dysfunctional grieving (Chapter 16).

Sexual dysfunction often occurs when body image has been altered. Clients may fear that their sexual partners will be repelled by their bodies after mutilating surgery or when illnesses cause unsightly or disfigured appearances. Surgery or alterations in the body may actually make it difficult or even impossible to engage in certain sexual activities. For instance, perineal prostatectomy (see Chapter 68) may cause permanent nerve damage with resulting impotence (inability to achieve or maintain an erection). Sexual dysfunction that results from surgery or other body alterations is discussed in the appropriate chapters. For example, the effect of myocardial infarction on sexuality is in Chapter 23, the effect of prostatectomy is in Chapter 68, and the effect of urinary and fecal diversion is in Chapters 34 and 50.

Evaluation

Expected outcomes for clients with body-image alteration are:

- Verbalizes feelings and thoughts related to body-image alteration.
- Engages in anticipatory grieving.
- Gives evidence of understanding limitations imposed by body-image alteration.
- Acknowledges own strengths and abilities.
- Demonstrates interest in learning about the body changes that are occurring.
- Is able to look at or touch a disfigured body part.

Section III: Support Systems for Clients and Nurses

Few individuals manage the crisis of illness without some type of support system. Most often, ill persons have health system support. If they are fortunate, health system support continues throughout the illness and remains available after recovery. In many instances, health system support occurs only during acute illnesses usually because the client is hospitalized and health care personnel are available. An exception is in health maintenance organizations, which offer support to persons along the entire health–illness continuum. Nurses are often the main support of clients during illness. More than any other health care provider, nurses spend the most time around-the-clock with sick clients. Their support, or lack of it, is significant.

Certain actions by clients make it difficult for some nurses to provide the support clients may need during illness. Most nurses hold values consistent with the health system culture in which they spend such a large part of their day. For example, clients who seem self-destructive because they do harm to their own bodies may be threatening to the views nurses hold. The following habits and behaviors may make it difficult for nurses to do their best:

- Cigarette smoking (because it causes cancer of the lung, emphysema, chronic bronchitis, and is linked with coronary artery disease)
- Alcohol abuse (because it leads to cirrhosis of the liver, malnutrition, and motor vehicle and other accidents causing severe injuries and deaths)
- Drug abuse (because it leads to addiction, drug reactions, death from overdose, accidents, and severely anxious and even violent behavior)
- Attempted suicide (because it throws nurses into ethical conflict, and it may lead to permanent body damage)
- Obesity (because it may cause damage to many body systems)
- Carelessness in sexual behavior (because it leads to sexually transmitted diseases, some of which have no cure)

Nurses often have little or no support system to help them to manage stresses incurred in caring for clients. Their supports are more likely to be social ones; many employing organizations provide little if any formal support.

TYPES OF SUPPORT SYSTEMS

There are three main types of support systems. One is the professional caregiving system of the community. For clients, the hospital, neighborhood walk-in clinic, health maintenance organization, home health care association, or social service agency provide professional services.

The professional caregiving system less frequently provides support to nurses. The reasons are probably varied. One obvious reason is budgetary—less money is available to fund continuing education programs or other forms of personal and professional help for nurses. Another reason may be that administrators fail to recognize the support needs of their nursing staff. Nurses often request discussion groups, often with a psychiatric–mental health nurse, to help them to deal with the everyday stresses of their work.

Self-help groups are a second type of support system. These groups offer support and practical guidance for dealing with problems such as weight loss, ostomy care, diabetes monitoring, or use of prostheses—strengthening self-care efforts and self-image. Whether dealing with alcoholism, unresolved grief over loss of a child, or body-image problems following radical surgery, self-help groups have been more effective than the traditional health care system in providing positive reinforcement; empathy; morale building; and opportunities for sharing, self-disclosure, and catharsis.

Clients in self-help groups often go through a problem-solving or nursing process approach without being aware of it. The group usually assists members in assessing their situation, determining priorities, planning approaches, taking action, and evaluating the action taken. Nurses should be familiar with the self-help groups in their communities, recognize their contribution to health care, and refer clients and the public to these groups. Self-help groups are included in the resources list at the end of each nursing process chapter and in many of the chapters in Units I and II.

The third type, called a natural support system, includes family and friendship groups, local informal caregivers such as nurse–friends or folk healers, and social clubs. Natural support systems have the potential to provide four different types of support (Tietjen, 1980):

- Emotional sustaining help (support and nurturance)
- Problem-solving help (information, ideas, direct intervention)
- Indirect help (accessibility, availability, willingness to help)
- Advocacy (intervention on behalf of the person)

Natural support systems are important because they offer the following possibilities—continuity over time, relationships that have depth as well as breadth, mutual choice, and the opportunity to give help to another as well as to receive help. This last aspect, of course, is not usually available in professional caregiving systems.

Natural support systems are important for both nurses and clients. They take on added importance when the person has cultural values not shared with persons in professional caregiving systems or when the person needs an advocate in dealing with professional caregiving systems.

IDENTIFYING SUPPORT NETWORKS

Persons with strong support networks are happier and live longer. What better rationale could there be for identifying support networks and helping clients to do the same for themselves? One simple way to identify support systems is to place a client's name in a circle in the center of a blank piece of paper. Add circles with the names of friends and relatives the client thinks of next as the most significant (these circles should overlap with the central circle with the client's name). The next series of circles might represent persons, social clubs, or mutual help groups that the client could incorporate in the natural support system network, and so on. A similar method can be used to identify the important persons and organizations in a professional caregiving support system.

CLIENT ACTIVISM AND CLIENT ADVOCACY

Clients who become activists and participate in their own health care help to ensure that their rights are not violated and that they receive effective and efficient health care. While it may be difficult, or even impossible, for an acutely ill client to stand up for his or her own interests, there are certain steps clients can take to protect themselves. The most obvious, and one discussed frequently in this book, is to collaborate with health care personnel in decisions and treatment and to assume as much self-care as possible and practical within the limits set by illness. Once a person becomes acutely ill, it may be necessary for another to take on this role. Suggest that clients ask a trusted family member or friend to serve as advocate and to intercede on the client's behalf when necessary. Although nurses can and do serve as client advocates, conflicts are eliminated when the role is taken on by someone from the client's own natural support system. Some hospitals have special personnel hired to serve as client advocates. Such personnel are often called ombudsmen or patient representatives. They can help safeguard the rights of clients who are without an advocate or serve as the liaison between the client and the institution or between the client's advocate and the institution. (See the resources section for a listing of paperback books for clients and advocates.)

Section IV: Helping Clients Take Charge of Their Health

Nurses are readily available to clients in industry, homes for the aged, hospitals, physician's offices, clinics, schools, community agencies, and health maintenance organizations. Their accessibility offers unlimited potential for developing health-protective behaviors. Assisting clients to understand their potential susceptibility or helping clients acknowledge that they are exposing themselves to potentially health-damaging situations (eg, by not wearing seat belts) are opportunities for developing health-promoting strategies.

Nurses are often present when clients and families are especially vulnerable. It is the nurse who establishes a relationship with the daughters of a woman who has just had a mastectomy. The nurse naturally spends the most nursing time in the postoperative care of the mother and helping the family become involved in supportive care. But the nurse also recognizes that the daughters are at increased risk for breast cancer. The nurse is in an excellent position to help them understand that risk, to teach them breast self-examination, and thus to enhance their future health and the health of all women born into that family.

The nurse in the college health center has access to a population potentially at high risk for motor vehicle accidents, alcohol and drug abuse, sexually transmitted diseases, sports injuries, and cancer of the testicle. The nurse can help these young adults, who are concerned with developing independent lifestyles, to be aware of how these risks threaten their future; to work out approaches to combat the risks; and to assist in developing alternative health-promoting lifetime patterns.

IDENTIFYING CLIENTS AT RISK

The first step in preventing illness and promoting health is identifying the client at risk. Risks to health are identified in Table 4–3. Learning to identify risks is important because of the many variables besides physiology that determine whether illness occurs. **Health risk appraisal** (HRA, also called health hazard appraisal) is a method that attempts to define an individual's risk of illness. A variety of appraisals is available (see the resources list) based on national data related to disease prevalence and mortality from specific causes. Information is gathered from a client's health history, physical examination, and laboratory data to quantify the risks to that client's health. The data are summarized so the client's chronological age can be compared with his or her "risk age." Individuals can then see clearly, on paper, what changes need to be made in their lifestyles or habits to alter their risk.

In the traditional health care system, the annual physical examination has long been the standard approach to assessing health and illness. Studies indicate, however, that the annual physical and the accompanying diagnostic studies are not cost effective and do not effectively alter the outcome of many diseases. Numerous approaches to screening have been proposed as more cost effective in promoting health and preventing disease.

The lifetime health monitoring program (Breslow & Somers, 1977) is one suggested alternative to the annual physical. The life span is divided into ten periods based on developmental changes, lifestyle alterations, health needs, and risk factors. Age-appropriate health goals and services are provided. Such a program considers reasonable preventive measures periodically and offers diagnostic studies appropriate for age and risk factors without overemphasizing examining and testing.

For example, health goals for the older middle-age group (40 to 59 years) focus on prolonging maximum physical energy and optimum mental and social activity as well as early detection of major chronic diseases. A complete history and physical examination every 5 years are recommended for this age group, including tests for hypertension, heart disease, diabetes, and cancer, as well as evaluation of vision and hearing. Updating immunizations and counseling regarding changing nutritional needs and physical activity are included. Smoking habits and use of alcohol and drugs are explored. Issues of job satisfaction and family life, including sexual activity, are discussed. Annual dental prophylaxis is recommended and, for those over 50, annual tests for hypertension, obesity, and certain cancers are advised.

Others have proposed similar periodic preventive health screening schedules with minor variations. This approach places much more responsibility on the individual for self-care and health surveillance—which is as it should be. Most persons, however, have not been adequately prepared to monitor themselves, assess their risks, and make good judgments about symptoms and signs. Nurses have a major responsibility in correcting this knowledge gap in the move toward greater self-responsibility for health.

REDUCING RISK

Assuming for the moment that individuals know what must be done to alter their risk, will they act? Many researchers have studied variables that may influence preventive health action.

Considering the Client's Health Beliefs

The health belief model developed by Rosenstock links attitudes of the individual to health actions. The health belief model assumes that consumer attitudes and beliefs are important determinants of personal efforts to prevent illness. Four variables are used:

- The individual's own view of his or her vulnerability to illness
- Beliefs about the potential severity of that illness on the person's life

Table 4–3	Risks to Health
Risk Factors	**Potential Damage to Health**
Smoking	Coronary artery disease, lung cancer, chronic obstructive pulmonary disease; additive factor in occupational lead exposures leading to toxicity
Elevated blood pressure	Coronary and hypertensive heart disease, cerebrovascular accident (CVA)
Rich diet (high in saturated fat, cholesterol, sugar, calories, salt)	Coronary artery disease, hypertension, CVA, obesity, diabetes; breast, colon, rectal, and possible prostate cancer
Diet low in fiber	Colon and rectal cancer
Alcohol	Motor vehicle accidents, cirrhosis, suicide, homicide, falls
Obesity	Diabetes; coronary artery disease with marked obesity
Diabetes	Heart and vascular disease, CVA
Sedentary lifestyle	Coronary artery disease, obesity

- Perceived benefits associated with actions to reduce the threat to health
- Evaluation of potential barriers to the proposed action (eg, pain, finances)

The first two variables are associated with the individual's subjective state of readiness to take health action. The latter two act as opposing cost-benefit forces which, in combination with the individual level of readiness to act, determine the probability and kind of health action that will be taken. Moreover, action must be triggered by an internal or external cue. Perhaps the person is experiencing pain that "won't go away" or "feels different somehow"— an internal cue. Perhaps a television commercial or program (an external cue) heightened the person's awareness of a health problem. Perhaps a health care provider furnished the necessary nudge into action. Perhaps the motivator was a similar symptom in a friend or a character in a book or movie. The cue may be a major event or as casual as seeing an advertisement on a subway car card, depending on the individual's level of readiness at the time. And readiness is particularly affected by the client's perception of vulnerability.

The results of a number of studies using the health belief model show that perceived vulnerability to illness has consistently been the most important attitude in understanding preventive health activity. The idea that individuals will not undertake health-promoting actions unless they are psychologically ready has major implications for nurses in their approach to educating clients.

Considering the Client's Locus of Control

Locus of control, a concept from social learning theory proposed by Rotter in 1962, is also relevant in considering who is most likely to take health action. Persons who have an internal locus of control *(internals)* believe they exert a major influence on their own lives and on their health states. Those with an external locus *(externals)* believe their lives are controlled by outside forces such as chance, luck, or powerful others. Internally controlled individuals tend to be more assertive and to engage in more goal-directed activity than externals.

Johnson and Sarason (1978) found significant correlations between life-change events and depression and anxiety in subjects with an external locus but not in those with an internal locus. Weight-loss programs have been more successful when structured according to each subject's locus of control. Internals did better in a self-directed program, whereas externals were more successful in a program relying on social pressure as motivation (Wallston, Wallston, Kaplan, & Maides, 1976).

Many other psychosocial considerations are undoubtedly involved in determining who will readily take positive health action and who will not. Social support networks, coping style, social class, health status, self-esteem, educational level, age, and religion may all be partial predictors of individual health behaviors.

Nursing Research Note

Lewis FM: Experienced personal control and quality of life in late-stage cancer patients. *Nurs Res* 1982; 31:113−118.

This study examined the relation between personal control and quality of life in terminal cancer clients. Four scales were used and tested—self-esteem, purpose in life, locus of control, and anxiety.

The results suggested that greater personal control over one's life is associated with higher levels of self-esteem, greater purpose in life, and decreased self-report of anxiety. There was a statistically significant relation between higher levels of personal control over health and higher levels of purpose-in-life measures. The relation between personal control over health and anxiety and self-esteem was not significant statistically. It was also found that as length of time since diagnosis increased, the subjects experienced less personal control over their health.

Fostering in clients a sense of personal control over their lives may encourage increased self-esteem and purpose in life. Because personal control in health issues did not enhance self-esteem, nurses may need to assess clients' psychological states in preparing them to take control over health issues. Nurses must determine how each client is coping and plan intervention accordingly.

THE ACTIVATED CLIENT

Whether practicing in the hospital or in the community, the nurse has as a major goal assisting clients to assume responsibility for their own health care. A client with a colostomy must be sensitively and patiently helped to look at the incisional area and stoma, encouraged to watch while the colostomy bag is changed, and assisted to begin participating in the irrigation, with the eventual goal of assuming self-care. For some reason, the importance of assisting clients to work toward independence with a laryngectomy, colostomy, or artificial limb seems more obvious and immediate than teaching health-protective behaviors. Yet developing the same level of conscientious effort in assisting clients to convert health-damaging habits into health-promoting ones offers the nurse great and lasting psychic rewards.

Self-care competencies can be identified through discussion with the client. Consider a woman who is learning breast self-examination (BSE). Does she know why BSE is important? At what point in her monthly cycle she should do it? What the technique is? How an abnormal finding looks or feels? What to do about a finding that worries her? Suppose a client with fibrocystic breast disease is immobilized with fear and unable to do BSE because her mother died of breast cancer and she is terrified of finding a lump? Besides working with the client over a long period to overcome these fears, the nurse might teach a loving friend or spouse to perform BSE on the client monthly as a short-term alternative.

Participation in self-help groups (discussed earlier in this chapter) can also be valuable in motivating clients and helping clients assume responsibility for their own health. These groups provide both emotional and informational support.

Reading material is another avenue for assisting the consumer to assume more personal autonomy for positive health practices. Bookstores are filled with books on diet, exercise, first aid, medication, self-improvement, and a host of other topics. (Health education material is included in the resources list.) Besides giving consumers valuable information about how to avoid illness and care for themselves, these books also assist in developing clients who are better informed and who know what to ask when they enter the health care system. Browsing in the self-help section of the bookstore or library can contribute to the nurses' own knowledge as well as client referral.

Setting short-term and long-term goals helps activate the client. Remember that *the goals should be the client's*. The nurse's part is making sure the client has enough information to understand fully the health risks associated with any behavior that is to be changed, knows the options available for reducing those risks, and acknowledges the personal benefits associated with the planned changes. For example, if the nurse has communicated effectively with Mrs T, an obese, hypertensive client, she will probably agree that decreasing salt intake, losing weight, and reducing blood pressure consistently to acceptable levels are desirable goals. But she may *not* agree. Further exploration may reveal barriers to communication or learning or perceived short-term disadvantages that, to the client, may outweigh the long-term benefits.

The educational, cultural, religious, personal, and philosophical barriers to incorporating new practices into one's lifestyle would fill an entire volume. By being sensitive to each client's uniqueness—including a set of beliefs and values that may be quite different from the nurse's—the nurse can gradually develop a trusting relationship with the client that will enable asking the right questions. Much effort is wasted in health education activities because unique elements of each client's lifestyle are never discovered.

Consider Mrs T again. What kinds of foods does she eat now? Does she eat at home? In a restaurant? Do time pressures necessitate her using many prepared foods? Many prepackaged, frozen, or "fast" foods are high in sodium; "fast" foods are also high in fat. Does she use canned foods, perhaps because they are inexpensive? Canned foods are usually very high in sodium. Does she cook for a family? What foods are they used to? Are ethnic foods among her or her family's favorites? Soy sauce—much used in Oriental cooking—is very high in sodium. Lox, a favorite of many Jews, has a high sodium and fat content; so does smoked fish. Lists of "foods to avoid" often include ethnic favorites; lists of "foods to eat" often ignore ethnic preferences. Neither list will help the client if it is not related to what, where, and how the client eats. Moreover, many foods—especially ethnic foods or childhood favorites—have "comfort value" that transcends their food value. Remember that asking the client to change her eating habits means

also asking for a lifestyle change that the client may perceive as unpleasant. Should the client be asked to forgo all such foods, or can compromises be arranged? In their zeal to bring clients to optimum health, professionals often forget that any change is better than no change, and a small change faithfully followed is better than a major "remake" that is soon abandoned.

How does Mrs T's husband feel about his wife's losing weight? Does he consider a stout wife a sign of his success? (Or the opposite?) Perhaps he makes statements such as, "If you were slim, some other guy would steal you away from me." "Jokes" of this kind may reveal profound feelings. The nurse may want to arrange a family counseling session so Mr T can be made aware that losing his wife to a heart attack instead of a rival is a real threat.

Lack of family support, lack of money, lack of transportation—and lack of self-esteem, feeling "unworthy to be well"—all may underlie a client's resistance to beginning or continuing a plan of care (see Chapter 6). Unrealistic goal setting may also be at fault. These problems, in turn, point to inadequate history taking at the initial stages of the client's care.

THE ACTIVATED NURSE

It is not easy to modify one's lifestyle, as those who have tried can testify. Some are successful and some are not. For those who are successful, was it because they were psychologically ready? Because they perceived themselves as vulnerable? Because they entered into a behavior modification program that fit their needs? Because they are internals? Externals? Women? Men? Young? Old? The best answer is probably that at that particular point in their lives, all factors came together, and the internal factors combined with the external factors to motivate them to act in a positive way.

Remember that lifestyle modification is often triggered by a factor external to the health care system. Clients spend the majority of their lives outside of health facilities in environments that have far greater impact on their health. A woman with mild hypertension whose sister just had a stroke might be motivated to take action after hearing a nurse speak on high blood pressure at her church women's group. Picking up a pamphlet on diet and heart attack at the YMCA could be the trigger factor for an overweight man whose business partner just suffered a coronary. Often, the well-publicized illness of a celebrity is the impetus for taking health action. For example, the practice of breast self-examination rose markedly following First Lady Betty Ford's mastectomy in 1974.

Activated nurses look beyond day-to-day responsibilities on the job. They should work individually and in groups to protest advertising destructive to health. They should write to the television networks protesting the frequent use of alcohol and cigarettes on daytime and prime-time programs. And they should make a greater effort to serve as role models for clients. A lecture on smoking from a nurse with a pack of cigarettes in a shirt pocket has little positive impact.

Although much of nursing involves caring for clients who are already ill, the future demands that nursing be instrumental in helping consumers in the area of health promotion and illness prevention. When the long-term impact of the nurse's role is considered, stressing wellness instead of illness is perhaps the most significant contribution nursing can make to improving the quality of life and decreasing the cost of health care.

MANAGING STRESS CREATIVELY

Helping clients to manage stress creatively and helping nurses to manage their own stress creatively is the subject of the final section of this chapter. Although no one can escape all the stresses of life completely, one can learn to counteract habitual counterproductive responses to them. Being able to relax decreases the alarm response to stress and returns the body to a more normal or balanced state.

The suggestions and techniques discussed will help persons to reestablish their equilibrium. It is not necessary to use every single suggestion. If a particular technique for stress reduction or relaxation doesn't seem to help, move on to another one. What is important is to give them a fair trial. Research indicates that, although exactly how stress reduction techniques work is not yet known, most persons find them helpful. Because they are better able to control their lives or to choose to relax and ease tension before it goes out of bounds, people find that the quality of their lives has been enhanced.

Anyone undertaking a stress reduction program should first discuss the program with their health care provider. Because these techniques lower the blood pressure, decrease the heart rate, and decrease pain and anxiety, persons undertaking a stress reduction program should have their medications closely monitored. Stress management is not magical; one has to work at it and enhance chances of success through regular practice. It is unrealistic to expect that reading about the techniques in this book is all that is required to be able to call upon them in times of stress or that everyone will be able to make a commitment to daily practice. Nurses can make it easier for clients to make the commitment and to follow through by:

- Recommending stress reduction strategies to clients and their families.
- Providing information about stress reduction strategies that are likely to meet the client's specific needs.
- Encouraging the client to make the decision to practice relaxation.
- Encouraging the client to take this time for himself or herself alone.
- Enlisting the family's support in meeting the client's need for uninterrupted time in a quiet setting.
- Encouraging family members to lend verbal support to the client.

- Reminding family members that because they are also under stress, they too may find relaxation techniques helpful.

The techniques described can be used by nurses in any setting. Other techniques such as autogenic training, self-hypnosis, and biofeedback require additional training or equipment and are not discussed in this chapter. To learn more about them, refer to the suggested readings at the end of this chapter.

Awareness of Sources of Stress

To manage stress, a person must have identified major sources of stress. Recall the earlier discussion of life crisis events in Chapter 2; a person is likely to ignore some sources of stress, fail to recognize others, and significantly underestimate how often events force an adjustment. Filling out the Schedule of Recent Experience (SRE) in Chapter 2 is a good start. It helps to focus attention on the amount of recent stress a person has experienced within the past year. The Hospital Stress Rating Scale in Table 4–4 is specifically related to the stresses of hospitalization. Studying the rating scale carefully will increase awareness of the many stresses hospitalized clients face that nurses and other health personnel take for granted. Some stresses are not under the nurse's control, but many are.

Identifying sources of stress helps us to anticipate them. Most persons are able to deal more effectively with stressful events when they are prepared for them. Knowing how much stress one is under is the key to preventing stress or reducing it. Like Mr J, the nurse described in Chapter 2, nurses can make lifestyle decisions according to the results of their personal SRE to avoid accumulating a high life-events score. The suggestions in Box 4–3 can help nurses and clients use the SRE to maintain health and prevent illness.

Awareness of Body Tension

Many persons fail to recognize stress when it occurs. They direct their attention to the outside world rather than to the internal world of their own experiences. Because stress and body tension are simultaneous, one of the first steps in recognizing stress is to recognize tension in the body. Recognizing body tension helps in recognizing stress and anxiety. *Body scanning* helps increase awareness of muscular tension.

Make sure that the spine is straight before beginning body scanning or any of the other exercises described in this chapter. Stand, sit, or lie on the floor—whichever is most comfortable—while maintaining good posture (Figure 4–2).

Begin by closing your eyes and turning your attention to your own internal world by focusing on your body. Focus on your toes and move up slowly. As you do this, ask yourself: Where am I tense? Become aware of all of the muscles in your body and especially of the parts of your

Table 4-4 Hospital Stress Rating Scale

Assigned rank	Stress value	Event	Assigned rank	Stress value	Event
1	13.9	Having strangers sleep in the same room with you	21	23.2	Having to eat cold or tasteless food
2	15.4	Having to eat at different times than you usually do	22	23.3	Not being able to call family or friends on the phone
3	15.9	Having to sleep in a strange bed	23	23.4	Being cared for by an unfamiliar doctor
4	16.0	Having to wear a hospital gown	24	23.6	Being put in the hospital because of an accident
5	16.8	Having strange machines around	25	24.2	Not knowing when to expect things will be done for you
6	16.9	Being awakened in the night by the nurse	26	24.5	Having the staff be in too much of a hurry
7	17.0	Having to be assisted with bathing	27	25.9	Thinking about losing income because of your illness
8	17.7	Not being able to get newspapers, radio, or TV when you want them	28	26.0	Having medications cause you discomfort
9	18.1	Having a roommate who has too many visitors	29	26.4	Having nurses or doctors talk too fast or use words you can't understand
10	19.1	Having to stay in bed or the same room all day	30	26.4	Feeling you are getting dependent on medications
11	19.4	Being aware of unusual smells around you	31	26.5	Not having family visit you
12	21.2	Having a roommate who is seriously ill or cannot talk with you	32	26.9	Knowing you have to have an operation
13	21.5	Having to be assisted with a bedpan	33	27.1	Being hospitalized far away from home
14	21.6	Having a roommate who is unfriendly	34	27.2	Having a sudden hospitalization you weren't planning to have
15	21.7	Not having friends visit you	35	27.3	Not having your call light answered
16	21.7	Being in a room that is too cold or too hot	36	27.4	Not having enough insurance to pay for your hospitalization
17	21.1	Thinking your appearance might be changed after your hospitalization	37	27.6	Not having your questions answered by the staff
18	22.3	Being in the hospital during holidays or special family occasions	38	28.4	Missing your spouse
19	22.4	Thinking you might have pain because of surgery or test procedures	39	29.2	Being fed through tubes
			40	31.2	Not getting relief from pain medications
20	22.7	Worrying about your spouse being away from you	41	31.9	Not knowing the results or reasons for your treatments

Assigned rank	Stress value	Event	Assigned rank	Stress value	Event
42	32.4	Not getting pain medication when you need it	47	35.6	Thinking you might lose a kidney or some other organ
43	34.0	Not knowing for sure what illness you have	48	39.2	Thinking you might have cancer
44	34.1	Not being told what your diagnosis is	49	40.6	Thinking you might lose your sight
45	34.5	Thinking you might lose your hearing	TOTAL		
46	34.6	Knowing you have a serious illness			

SOURCE: Reprinted with permission from Volicer BJ, Bohannon MW: A hospital stress rating scale. *Nurs Res* 1975; 24:352–359.

body that feel tense or tight. Note the location of the tenseness and talk to yourself about it, reminding yourself that muscular tension is self-produced. Perhaps you might say: "The muscles in the back of my neck feel tight. This means that I'm creating tension in my body. Tension causes me problems."

Body scanning should be a prelude to the stress-reduction techniques that follow. Use the body-scanning method to determine where tension collects in your body.

Breathing Exercises

Under most circumstances, breathing is taken for granted as an automatic body function. About the only time persons are aware of their pattern of breathing is when it has gone awry, such as when they are out of breath. Nurses notice the apneic client or the client with Cheyne–Stokes respirations because they know something has gone wrong and that breathing is essential to life. Breathing properly can,

---

Box 4–3 Suggestions for Using the Schedule of Recent Experience

Study the life events list and the amount of change the events require (their mean values) to become familiar with them.

Put the list where it can readily be seen several times throughout the day.

Identify life events as they happen.

Take time to think about the life event and its meaning for you.

Identify the feeling produced in you by the life event.

Determine the choices available to you for adjusting to the life event.

Take time in arriving at any decisions about changes in your lifestyle.

Anticipate life changes.

Plan for life changes well in advance.

Pace yourself, even when you are in a hurry.

Consider the accomplishment of a task as a part of everyday life—don't view it as an end or a time for letting down.

Remember, the higher the change score, the more likely you are to get sick.

Work hard to stay well, especially if your life change score is high.

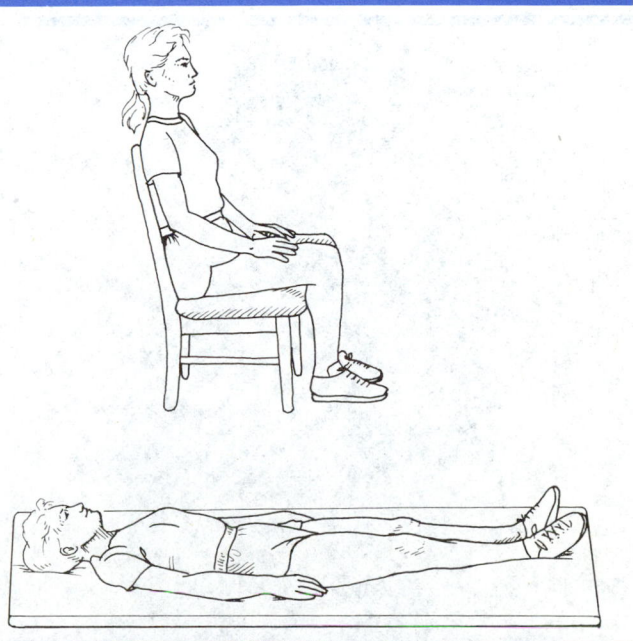

Figure 4–2

Body postures for stress-reduction exercises. **A.** Sitting. **B.** Lying.

by itself, reduce stress. How breathing can be used to reduce tension has been recognized by psychiatric nurses and by maternal health nurses who coach expectant women in breathing techniques during labor. Unfortunately, breathing techniques are virtually ignored in other clinical areas.

Breathing calmly and deeply keeps the blood well oxygenated and purified. It helps to remove waste materials from the blood and clears thinking. Poorly oxygenated blood may contribute to fatigue, mental confusion, anxiety, muscular tension, and feelings of depression. The following exercises are designed to facilitate proper breathing.

Awareness of Breathing

Do you breathe properly or does your breathing actually deprive you of oxygen? Take time to pay attention to your own breathing in the same way the person in Figure 4–3 is doing. Begin by placing one hand just below your rib cage and taking a deep breath. Note what happened when you inhaled. Did your hand move in? Did your hand move out? Did your hand move at all? If your hand moved out, you were breathing properly. But if your hand moved in or didn't move at all it was probably because you learned, as most did, to hold your stomach in and push your chest out while breathing. Although breathing this way may look good, it prevents using the full lung capacity by using only the top third or top half and failing to use the lower part.

Deep Breathing

You are breathing deeply when you move the diaphragm downward and fill the lower part of the lungs with air. The chest expands as the middle part fills with air, and the

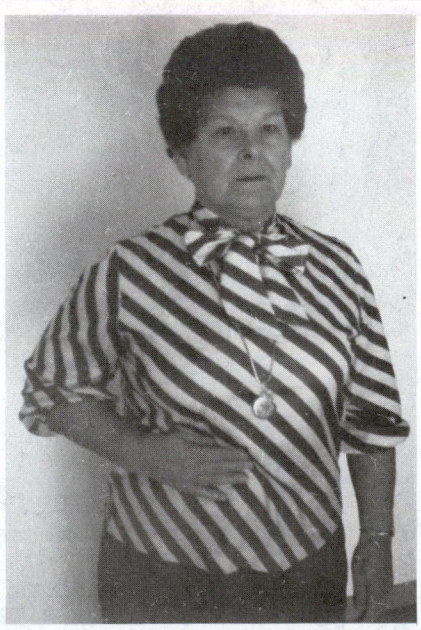

Figure 4–3

Breathing awareness.

Box 4–4   Deep-Breathing Guidelines

1. Sit, stand, or lie with your spine straight.
2. Scan for body tension.
3. Place one hand on your chest and the other on your abdomen.
4. Inhale slowly and deeply so your abdomen pushes up your hand.
5. Visualize your lungs slowly filling with air. Your chest should move only slightly as you inhale, but you should be aware of the movement of your abdomen.
6. Exhale through your mouth, making a soft, whooshing sound by blowing gently. Keep your face, mouth, and jaw relaxed.
7. Be aware of what it feels like and what you sound like when you breathe properly.
8. Continue to take long, slow, deep breaths for at least 10 minutes at a time, once or twice a day.
9. Increase the frequency if you wish once you have mastered the technique.
10. Scan your body for tension again, comparing the tension to what it was like before you began the deep-breathing exercise.

shoulders move upward as the upper part fills. To teach yourself or a client how to take deep, healthful breaths follow the directions in Box 4–4.

Deep breathing becomes easier with practice. It may become almost automatic. This is an exercise few resist—it is easy to do, it is inconspicuous, and it gives fast results.

Ten-to-One Count

This exercise is also quick and simple. Inhale, taking a deep breath, while saying the number 10 to yourself and then exhale slowly, letting out all the air in your lungs. Inhale again saying the number 9 to yourself. As you exhale, tell yourself: "I feel more relaxed than I did at number 10." With your next breath, say the number 8 to yourself, and as you exhale remind yourself: "I feel more relaxed than I did at number 9." Continue this procedure through your countdown and experience increasing calmness as you approach the number 1. Some persons use an abbreviated version and begin counting at the number 5; others require the full 10 count to feel calm.

Alternate-Nostril Breathing

This somewhat-more-difficult general relaxation exercise also helps to reduce tension and sinus headaches. First, close off your right nostril by lightly pressing it with your right thumb. Now inhale through your left nostril as slowly and quietly as possible, as the woman in Figure 4–4 is doing. Remove your thumb from the right nostril and use your forefinger to close off the left nostril. Now exhale slowly through your right nostril. Inhale through your right nostril as slowly and quietly as possible and follow the same

Progressive relaxation decreases pulse and respiratory rates, blood pressure, and perspiration. In addition, it helps to reduce anxiety. Clients with muscle spasms, lower back pain, tension headaches, insomnia, anxiety, depression, fatigue, irritable bowel, hypertension, or mild phobias are among those who can achieve positive results using this technique.

Mastering progressive relaxation may take longer than the other stress reduction techniques. With practice, one can learn to relax faster and easier.

Active Progressive Relaxation

Active progressive relaxation helps in identifying which muscles or muscle groups are chronically tense by distinguishing between sensations of tension (purposeful muscle tensing) and deep relaxation (a conscious effort to relax the muscles). Each muscle or muscle grouping is tensed for 5 to 7 seconds and then relaxed for 20 to 30 seconds and repeated. Four major muscle groups are covered— hands, forearms, and biceps; head, face, throat, and shoulders; chest, abdomen, and lower back; thighs, buttocks, calves, and feet. Use the instructions in Box 4–5 as a guide to a typical exercise. This guide was written by a nurse (Flynn, 1980) who uses these principles in her clinical practice.

Counsel clients to observe some cautions while carrying out this technique. The muscles of the neck and back should not be excessively tightened to avoid soft tissue and spinal injury. Tightening the muscles of the toes and feet too vigorously could also result in uncomfortable muscle cramps.

Progressive relaxation should be practiced while lying down or seated in a chair with a head support. Remember to check for muscle groups that are only partially relaxed and return to them to bring about deeper relaxation.

Passive Progressive Relaxation

In passive progressive relaxation, the muscles are not tensed. The focus of this form of progressive relaxation is to relax the muscles without first tightening them.

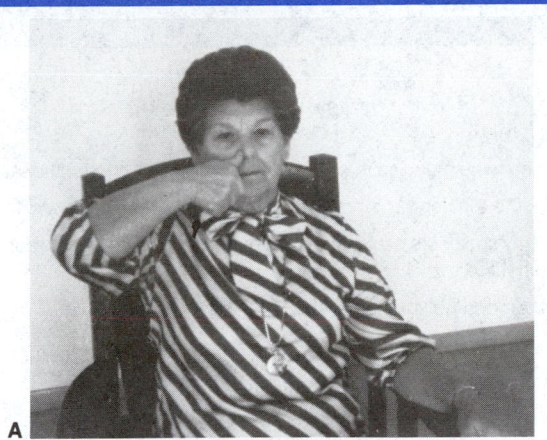

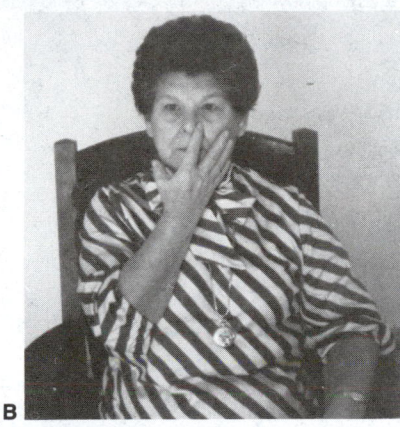

Figure 4–4

Alternate-nostril breathing. **A.** Inhale through the left nostril slowly and quietly while using the thumb to keep the right nostril tightly closed. **B.** Use the index finger to close the left nostril, and exhale through the right nostril. Then inhale through the right nostril and repeat A and B.

procedure outlined above, closing your right nostril with your right thumb while simultaneously exhaling through your left nostril.

The basic cycle for alternate-nostril breathing should begin with 10 breaths and can be increased up to 25 breaths. It may be easier to breathe through the right nostril at certain times of the day and through the left nostril at other times. The reason is that the primary breathing nostril changes approximately every 4 hours.

Progressive Relaxation

Progressive relaxation is based on the mind–body interrelatedness theory developed in 1929 by Chicago physician Edmund Jacobsen. He believed it is impossible for an anxious mind to exist in a relaxed body. The technique of progressive relaxation is based on the premise that muscle tension is the body's physiologic response to anxiety-provoking thoughts. Muscular tension increases the feeling of anxiety and reinforces it. Deep muscle relaxation, on the other hand, decreases physiological tension and blocks anxiety.

Nursing Research Note

Pender NJ: Effects of progressive muscle relaxation training on anxiety and health locus of control among hypertensive adults. *Res Nurs Health* 1985; 8:67–72.

The study investigated the effects of progressive muscle relaxation (PMR) on anxiety and perceptions of personal control over health status in a group of 22 hypertensive clients. Compared with the control group, those instructed in relaxation demonstrated lower anxiety at 4-month follow-up. Moreover, this group scored higher on beliefs of personal control of health and lower on beliefs of chance affecting health outcomes. Relaxation techniques have proven an effective nursing treatment plan in assisting clients to prevent and cope with stress.

Box 4−5   Active Progressive Relaxation Exercise

Sit or lie in a comfortable position and let your eyes close.

I take a moment to be here (allow time).

I focus my attention on my right hand, and I make a fist.

Slowly and steadily, I clench my fist and study the tension.

Now I let go and feel the difference.

I repeat that.

I clench my fist, tightly, feeling the tension.

I let go and enjoy the contrast in my feelings.

Now I tense my right forearm.

Studying the tension.

And let go and notice the difference.

Now I tense my biceps—tighten.

And let go.

I stretch my arm straight out and feel the tension in my arm and shoulder.

I let go and appreciate the difference.

Now I focus my attention on my left hand, and I make a fist.

Slowly and steadily, I clench my fist and study the tension.

Now I let go and feel the difference.

I do that again.

Clenching my fist, tightly, feeling the tension.

And let go and enjoy the contrast in my feelings.

Now I tense my left forearm.

Studying the tension.

And let go and notice the difference.

Now I tense my biceps—tighten.

And let go.

I stretch my arm straight out and feel the tension in my arm and shoulder.

I let go and appreciate the difference.

I focus my attention on my scalp.

I tighten it.

And now I smooth it out.

I pay attention to the muscles of my forehead—I frown.

And study the tension as I frown.

I let go and notice the difference.

I raise my eyebrows and hold them for a few seconds.

And let go.

Now the muscles around my eyes—I tense and tighten them.

And let go.

The muscles of my cheeks, I tighten them.

And release, acknowledging the difference.

Now I tighten my jaw muscles, tighter—

And let go.

I bring my tongue to the roof of my mouth and tighten it.

(continued next column)

And let go.

I let it relax.

And now the muscles in the back of my neck—I tighten those.

I feel the tension, and now I let it go.

I pull my shoulders back and up and tighten the muscles between my shoulders.

Tighten and notice the tension.

And let go.

Now I tighten the muscles of my upper back.

Tighten—and let go.

I focus my attention now on the muscles of my lower back.

I tighten them and notice the tension and

Let go.

Now the muscles of my buttocks.

Tighten—feel the tension.

And let go.

Breathing easily and calmly, deeply and efficiently.

I bring my attention to the muscles of the front of my neck.

I tighten them, bringing my chin up.

And let go.

Now I tighten my chest muscles—tighten.

And let go.

I let myself take in a good deep breath and hold it, feeling all my muscles expand.

And now I let go—letting all the breath out.

I repeat this and notice my feelings.

I tense the muscles of my abdomen.

I tighten them and notice the tension.

And let go and appreciate the relaxation.

And my pelvic muscles—I tighten them—tight.

And let go.

My thighs—I tighten those muscles.

And let go noticing the difference.

Now the muscles of my calves and lower legs.

I tense them tighter and note the tension.

And let go.

And the muscles of my feet—tighten them.

Letting go and appreciating the difference.

And now I take a moment to scan my body—noticing any part of my body that still needs relaxation.

And I tense that part and let go.

Any other muscles—I take a moment to tense them.

And let go.

And now feeling the pleasure of this relaxation, I take a few moments to bring my attention back to this time and this place, and filled with energy and peace I open my eyes, stretch, and get up.

SOURCE: Reprinted with permission from Flynn PAR: *Holistic Health: The Art and Science of Care.* Bowie, MD: Brady, 1980, pp 165−167.

The body-part sequence varies from that of the active progressive method, beginning with muscles easiest to relax (in the toes) and progressing to muscles most difficult to relax (in the head). The sequence is:

- Feet
- Lower legs
- Knees and upper legs
- Hips and buttocks
- Lower back
- Lower arms and hands
- Chest and diaphragm
- Abdomen
- Pelvis and genitals
- Neck
- Forehead and upper face
- Mouth and jaw

Some report feeling less alert after using this exercise. When alertness is important, one of the other exercises is probably best.

Visualization

A French pharmacist, Emil Coue, began to use the power of imagination with clients around the turn of the century. Carl Jung used it in his psychiatric practice in the early part of the century. Most recently, Carl Simonton and Stephanie Matthews Simonton have had remarkable success in treating cancer clients with visualization. Author Norman Cousins has written of his control over serious illness by using the healing power of his own imagination.

Positive visualizations use a person's own imagination and positive thinking to reduce stress or promote healing. It was Coue who asked his clients to repeat this now-famous phrase 20 times to themselves on awakening: *"Every day in every way I am getting better and better."* He believed that predicting failure or success in advance was bound to make it happen. Thus, positive visualizations anticipating success reduce stress. Visualization should be used in conjunction with the body scanning and deep-breathing exercises discussed earlier.

Not everyone finds that using the imagination in this way is easy, and the technique may not work for everyone. Constructing a detailed, effective visualization requires time, patience, and practice.

Visualization for Relaxation

Relaxing through visualizing is enhanced by constructing in one's own mind a relaxing environment. Depending on the person, that environment may take many forms. Some find the soothing sounds of a seashore calming; others prefer to imagine themselves floating above the world on a soft cloud or a magic carpet; and still others relax as they imagine themselves descending on a slow-moving escalator into a calmer and more relaxed state.

If visualization seems difficult (or if a warm bath, hot tub, or swimming pool is relaxing) try constructing a visualization while in warm water, combining the physiological effects of the warm water with the products of the imagination (see Box 4–6, next page).

Visualization for Symptom Control or Healing

Although visualization techniques for symptom control or healing are practiced in a variety of health care settings around the country, they should be part of a well-rounded health program. For example, visualization can be used with conventional medical treatment for cancer clients and with preoperative clients to control postoperative pain and enhance tissue healing. Persons with vascular problems— migraine headache, hypertension, Raynaud's syndrome— benefit from visualization. Allergies, asthma, rheumatoid arthritis, gastritis, colitis, peptic ulcer, insomnia, depression, and chronic pain all respond to visualization with a reduction in symptoms. Two sample visualizations for the reduction of pain are in Table 4–5.

Enhancing Relaxation With Music

Many persons find that listening to certain kinds of music is relaxing. Dentists have used music to help their clients relax and to mask the sounds of the drill. Several health care facilities use soothing music in conjunction with guided visualizations on audiotape or videotape to replace analgesics and tranquilizers when the client chooses. Sometimes the tapes are prescribed before or during surgery, during chemotherapy, or kidney dialysis, and during recovery from spinal injury or burns.

In fact, the therapeutic use of music has led to a new health-related career. Music therapists use a combination of visual imagery and music to teach clients to lower their blood pressure 10 to 20 points and to help those with cardiac dysrhythmias achieve a more relaxed heart rate by using music with a 60-beats-per-minute tempo.

How does music achieve its relaxing effect? One the-

Table 4–5 Visualization for Relief From Pain	
Alternative I	**Alternative II**
Imagine that your body is filled with orange and blue lights.	Concentrate on the part of your body where the pain exists.
The orange lights signify areas of pain or tension.	Attach a symbolic visual image to the pain (a knot in your stomach, a hammer pounding your head).
The blue lights signify pain-free or calm areas.	
Imagine changing the orange lights to blue lights.	Imagine the symbol being relaxed, becoming looser, getting smaller or weaker as you feel your pain becoming less and less.
Note that the pain is going away and that you're feeling more and more relaxed.	

Box 4–6   Visualization for the Bath

In a warm bath, it is difficult to worry or to sustain an anxiety attack. The body feels lighter, muscles are relaxed by the heat and movement of the water, and circulation is increased. Being in warm water for a half hour will lower the blood pressure and slow down your breathing. Though the effects will be the opposite for the first 2 minutes and you may feel stimulated, the calming properties of warm water will soon soothe you.

This visualization can be used in a bathtub, hot tub, heated swimming pool, or any warm body of water. The temperature should not be over 103°F, and you should not stay in the water for longer than 30 minutes. If you are alone, ask someone to call you on the phone after one-half hour or set a music alarm to rouse you. Turn out the lights and light a candle or use a small night light.

Get into a comfortable position, either reclining or sitting. Be sure that your back is supported and your breathing unconstricted. Take a full, deep breath and exhale fully and completely. Slowly close your eyes and feel your heart beating strongly and then begin to slow down. Let your thoughts just drift through your consciousness, as you allow them to leave with the warm air. Imagine that with each and every breath, you can breathe away tension or anxiety, as you allow yourself to relax more and more. All the day's burdens, worries, and expectations are leaving your consciousness and evaporating with the hot, moist steam. Feel your arms floating on the water, and the warm, soothing water gently lifting and caressing your body. As you continue to breathe slowly and naturally, let go of any thoughts still remaining in your mind. Watch as your thoughts flow through you and out of you, and see them disappear into the air, leaving your mind clear and calm.

Gently turn your attention to your body, and scan your body for any tension that you might still be holding. Allow it to leave with the next exhalation, as the warm water evaporates into steam. As you continue to breathe slowly and calmly, turn your awareness to your feet and to your legs. The water tenderly massages your legs and your feet, as the tension flows through you and out of you. With your next breath, breathe away any tightness still remaining in your feet. Move your attention to your abdomen and your chest, allowing the muscles to just let go, and the tension to melt away from your body. Feel your abdomen and your chest relax, as you gently loosen all the muscles and just breathe away any remaining tension. Focus on relaxing your arms and your hands, letting the muscles go completely loose and limp. Relax your fingers, and your hands, and let the feeling of deep relaxation spread up into your arms. Breathe away any tension still remaining.

Now, relax the muscles of your shoulders and your neck, and feel the heaviness gradually increase throughout your musculature, as all your muscles just let go. The muscles in your back go loose and limp, as the water gently supports your whole body. Allow the relaxation to spread to your head and your face, and the muscles around your eyes, in your jaw, your tongue, and in your forehead. Let yourself drift deeper into a dreamlike state of calm relaxation.

Imagine that the blue water becomes the sky, and the soft clouds gently support you as you drift up above the trees. You no longer feel the weight of your head upon your shoulders, and gravity no longer ties you to the earth. The warm, soft, billowy, pink clouds support you as the sun's gentle heat penetrates through any remaining tension. As you peacefully float through the warm air, the golden sun fills your body with warming heat and light. This golden light penetrates through any tension still remaining in your body. As you free-float in space, your body is becoming lighter and lighter.

When you have floated as high as you wish, you become still, and the clouds gently cradle you in the warmth of the sun's golden rays. The golden sun finds any tension still remaining in your body, and dissolves it in the warm, glowing light. Whenever you are ready, you may return. Feel the warm, pink clouds transform into water, and become aware of the water gently cradling you. Take a few, deep breaths, becoming more and more aware of your surroundings. When you are ready to become fully alert, take a full, deep breath and gently open your eyes on the exhalation. Take a few more deep breaths, and slowly get out of the water, gently drying yourself and feeling the relaxation throughout your body.

SOURCE: Reprinted with permission from Mason JL: *Guide to Stress Reduction*, pp 61–63. © 1980, 1986, Celestial Arts, Box 7327, Berkeley, CA 94707.

ory is that music produces endorphins in the brain—the same "feel-good" chemicals that running and meditation produce. These natural opiates, secreted by the hypothalamus, reduce the intensity with which pain is felt (see Chapter 5).

Because persons vary in their response to music, encourage clients to experiment with different kinds of music to discover which has positive effects and then to develop their own personal library. Tape and records specifically for stress reduction are sold in bookstores and through catalogs. They are often available through the public library. Recommend that clients pay attention to their breathing as they listen to music; if breathing is slow and deep, the music is relaxing.

Stress management is a creative and powerful tool as long as clients know the methods and how to use them. Nurses can play a significant role in bringing these methods to clients' awareness and facilitating their effective use.

Chapter Highlights

The experience of illness is both universal and unique to each person. Perceptions of illness are shaped by culture.

Persons develop a set of assumptions to help them make sense out of the world in which they live. These assumptions form a person's world view.

Mismatched world views between clients and nurses often account for the dissatisfactions they experience with one another.

It is important to understand and appreciate one's own sociocultural heritage as well as that of clients.

Folk health beliefs and healing practices that enhance the client's sense of well-being can be reinforced and incorporated into the nursing care plan.

Supporting clients means being able to accept and facilitate the client's discussion of the experience, whether positive or negative, and to tolerate expressions of fear, rage, frustration, grief, helplessness, and hopelessness among others.

Anticipatory guidance helps clients cope with impending body-image alteration, lays the foundation for effective grief work, and prevents dysfunctional grieving.

Self-help groups are important sources of support for clients and help clients assume responsibility for their own health.

Natural support systems are as crucial to clients as professional caregiving systems.

The health subculture values that nurses hold affect their relationships with clients.

It is important that nurses as well as clients identify their personal support networks.

Clients who perceive themselves as vulnerable to certain health problems are more likely to take health action than those who do not.

Clients who believe they have control over what happens in their lives are more likely to become involved in activities that reduce their risk of illness.

Stressing wellness instead of illness is perhaps the most significant contribution nursing can make to improving the quality of life and decreasing the cost of health care.

Most persons, including clients and nurses, find stress reduction techniques such as deep-breathing exercises, progressive relaxation, and visual imagery helpful in counteracting habitual counterproductive responses to the stresses of life.

Nurses can have a major impact on general health because of their broad access to clients in all age groups and in all phases of their lives. To affect health, nurses must make every individual and group encounter with clients an opportunity for teaching lifestyle modification.

Bibliography

Bonaparte B: Ego-defensiveness, open-closed mindedness and nurses' attitude toward culturally different patients. *Nurs Res* 1979; 28:166–172.

Breslow L, Somers AR: The lifetime health-monitoring program. *N Engl J Med* 1977; 296:601–608.

Delgado M: Hispanic natural support systems: Implications for mental health services. *J Psychosoc Nurs* 1983; 21(4):19–24.

Fagin C, Diers D: Nursing as metaphor. *Am J Nurs* 1983; 83:1362.

Flynn PAR: *Holistic Health: The Art and Science of Care.* Bowie, MD: Brady, 1980.

Harris DM, Guten S: Health-protective behavior: An exploratory study. *J Health Soc Beh* 1979; 20(3):17–29.

Harwood A: *Ethnicity and Medical Care.* Cambridge, MA: Harvard, 1981.

Henderson G, Primeaux M: *Transcultural Health Care.* Menlo Park, CA: Addison–Wesley, 1981.

Johnson JH, Sarason IG: Life stress, depression, and anxiety: Internal-external control as a moderator variable. *J Psychosom Res* 1978; 22:205–208.

Murillo–Rohde I: Hispanic american patient care. In: *Transcultural Health Care.* Henderson G, Primeaux M (editors). Menlo Park, CA: Addison–Wesley, 1982.

Pender NJ: *Health Promotion in Nursing Practice.* Norwalk, CT: Appleton–Century–Crofts, 1982.

Schneiderman LJ: *The Practice of Preventive Health Care.* Menlo Park, CA: Addison–Wesley, 1981.

Seeman, M, Seeman TE: Health behavior and personal autonomy: A longitudinal study of the sense of control in illness. *J Health and Social Beh* 1983; 24(6):133–160.

Simonton SM: *The Healing Family.* New York: Bantam, 1984.

Tausig M: Measuring live events. *J Health and Social Beh* 1982; 23(3):52–64.

Tietjen AM: Integrating formal and informal support systems: the Swedish experience. In: *Protecting Children from Abuse and Neglect.* Garbarino J et al (editors). San Francisco: Jossey–Bass, 1980.

Tripp–Reimer T: Cultural assessment. In: *Nursing Assessment: A Multidimensional Approach.* Bellack JP, Bamford PA (editors). Monterey, CA: Wadsworth, 1984.

Wallston B, Wallston K, Kaplan G, Maides S: Development and validation of the health locus of control scale. *J Cons Clin Psychol* 1976; 44:580–585.

Wilson HS, Kneisl CR: *Psychiatric Nursing,* 2nd ed. Menlo Park, CA: Addison–Wesley, 1983.

Volicer BJ, Bohannon MW: A hospital stress rating scale. *Nurs Res* 1975; 24:352–359.

Suggested Readings

Henderson G, Primeaux M: *Transcultural Health Care.* Menlo Park, CA: Addison–Wesley, 1981. A major theme is how the client's perceptions of health and illness are influenced by ethnic/cultural background. The subculture of poverty as well as third world and European cultures are discussed.

Jamieson M, Martinson I: Block nursing: Neighbors caring for neighbors. *Nurs Outlook* 1983: 31:270–273. An alternative health care delivery system—block nursing—is described. A unique way of providing social and health supports for clients (in this instance, for elderly clients), the block nurse program has helped some clients remain at home and avoid institutional care.

Marchewka AE: When is paternalism justifiable? *Am J Nurs* 1983; 83:1072–1073. This article discusses dilemmas that arise when the person in authority is the caregiver rather than the client. Five criteria to help nurses determine whether their actions are paternalistic are presented and analyzed.

Miller A: When is the time ripe for teaching? *Am J Nurs* 1985; 85:801–804. This practical article includes methods for assessing a client's readiness to learn, strategies to help clients remember important points, and a helpful section on selecting sound and appropriate health education materials.

Puetz BE: *Networking for Nurses.* Rockville, MD: Aspen, 1983. How to identify, maintain, and form a support system among nurse colleagues is described in this book.

Rosenberg ML: *Patients: The Experience of Illness.* Philadelphia: Saunders, 1980. This sensitively written and photographed picture–essay by a physician–photographer offers insight into the personal illness experiences of six clients and their families, based on tape-recorded interviews.

Tripp–Reimer T: Barriers to health care: Perceptual variations of Appalachian clients by Appalachian and non-Appalachian health care professionals. *Western J Nurs Res* 1982; 4:179–191. In this study, two groups of health professionals (Appalachian professionals and non-Appalachian professionals) were interviewed and asked to identify behaviors characteristic of Appalachian clients. Although both groups identified similar behaviors in their clients, they came to disparate conclusions about their meanings.

Walters J: Coping with a leg amputation. *Am J Nurs* 1981; 81:1349–1352. Although written specifically about leg amputation, this article has general application to caring for clients with body-image change. Major focus is the four phases the client undergoes in adjusting to the loss of a limb.

Resources

SELF-HELP GROUPS AND OTHER ORGANIZATIONS

InterHealth
2970 Fifth Ave
San Diego, CA 92103
Phone: (714) 291-9490

This preventive health organization was founded in 1913 by former president William Howard Taft and other leading citizens. It provides a health risk appraisal called the InterHealth Risk Profile that can be used in health care programs.

National Clearinghouse for Mental Health Information
National Institute of Mental Health
Room 11A33, Parklawn Bldg
5600 Fishers La
Rockville, MD 20857
Phone: (301) 443-4517

This division of the federal government provides information on stress control programs and resources throughout the country.

National Self-Help Clearinghouse
Graduate School University Center
City University of New York
33 W 42nd St
New York, NY 10036
Phone: (212) 840-7606

This organization monitors hundreds of self-help organizations throughout the US and Canada.

Wellness Associates
42 Miller Ave
Mill Valley, CA 94941

An organization that publishes the Wellness Inventory, a broad-based paper-and-pencil questionnaire that individuals can use to determine stress levels and to promote wellness. It does not require laboratory testing or computer analysis, as other more detailed health risk appraisals do, and its results are more general.

HOT LINES

National Health Information Clearinghouse
Phone: (800) 336-4797; in Virginia (703) 522-2590

Provides health and medical information, lists of other toll-free numbers, referrals to appropriate organizations, and researches answers to health questions. Also provides government-produced pamphlets such as *Healthstyle: A Self Test.*

Tel-Med Telephone Tape Library
Phone: Check local telephone directories

Free health information on audiotapes is available in over 200 communities in the United States. Check the local telephone directory for the number for more than 300 recorded messages on health-related topics.

HEALTH EDUCATION MATERIAL

Specific health education material is identified in appropriate chapters. Of interest might be the *Self-Care Catalog,* published and distributed free by:

Medical Self-Care Magazine
PO Box 717
Iverness, CA 94937

This catalog provides information on affordable home-based medical equipment. *Medical Self-Care Magazine* is also of interest.

The following softcover books on client advocacy and informed health care consumerism are of interest to both clients and nurses.

Berman H, Burhenne D, Rose L: *The Complete Health Care Advisor.* New York: St. Martin's, 1983. (The authors are a physician, a psychologist, and a medical writer.)

Huttman B: *The Patient's Advocate: The Complete Handbook of Patient's Rights.* New York: Penguin, 1981. (The author is a nurse committed to the concept of client advocacy.)

Nierenberg J, Janovic F: *The Hospital Experience: A Guide for Patients and Their Families,* 2nd ed. New York: Berkley, 1985. (The authors are a nurse and a medical writer.)

Chapter 5

How the Body Maintains and Protects Homeostasis

SueAnn Wooster Ames
Patricia A. Burns
Penny Bresnick

Objectives

When you have finished studying this chapter, you should be able to:

Define diffusion, osmosis, and active transport.

Explain the terms isotonic, hypertonic, and hypotonic.

Discuss the role of the lungs, kidneys, cardiovascular system, pituitary gland, adrenal glands, and parathyroid glands in maintaining homeostasis.

Specify how the body normally maintains fluid equilibrium.

Compare and contrast the major electrolyte imbalances.

Describe the major buffer systems for maintaining the pH of the extracellular fluid.

Summarize the acid–base changes that occur in both acidosis and alkalosis.

Compare and contrast hypovolemic shock, cardiogenic shock, and distributive shock.

Anticipate the common clinical manifestations of shock and identify clients at risk for shock.

Describe how gate control theory and theories about the role of endorphins and enkephalins explain the phenomenon of pain and pain control.

Distinguish between acute pain, chronic pain, referred pain, and phantom pain.

Enumerate at least five nonpharmacological approaches to pain relief.

Specify how the nurse can individualize nursing approaches to keep clients pain free.

The human body maintains its homeostatic balance through the complex interaction of all bodily systems. This chapter is concerned with the processes that normally preserve a state of equilibrium—the balance of fluids, electrolytes, acids, and bases. In addition, this chapter considers processes that protect the body from internal and external insults—the phenomena of shock and pain. Although these processes are often considered physiological, it is clear that the mind has a significant influence on these bodily responses.

Section I: Fluid and Electrolyte Balance

Proper fluid and electrolyte balance in the body is essential for good health and for life itself. This balance of fluid and electrolytes must be maintained within a normal range and is an essential component of the body's homeostatic processes. The body's physiologic processes maintain this balance in health, but almost all illnesses or states of disequilibrium threaten the balance. The young, the old, and those with chronic illness are the most susceptible to imbalances.

PROPORTIONS AND DISTRIBUTION OF BODY FLUIDS

Water is the largest single constituent of the body, composing 55% of the average healthy woman's weight and 57% of an average man's weight. This volume of body fluid remains relatively constant in health, varying less than 0.2 kg (0.5 lb) in 24 hours, regardless of the amount of fluid ingested. The percentage of total body fluid varies with a person's sex, age, and amount of total body fat. An early human embryo is 97% fluid. This percentage decreases with age; an elderly adult is composed of approximately 45% fluid. Body fat is essentially water-free, and persons with less body fat have a greater proportion of water to body weight. Women after puberty have proportionately more fat than men and, therefore, have a smaller percentage of fluid in relation to total body weight.

FLUID COMPARTMENTS

Body water is divided into two major compartments: intracellular and extracellular. Intracellular fluid (ICF), also referred to as cellular fluid, is within the cells and makes up two-thirds to three-quarters of total body fluid, or about 25 L. Extracellular fluid (ECF), fluid outside the cells, makes up the remainder of the body's fluid, about 15 L. ECF is subdivided into interstitial fluid and intravascular fluid, or plasma. Interstitial fluid surrounds the cells and contains lymph, providing the cells with the external medium for cellular metabolism. Intravascular fluid, the liquid part of the blood, is found within the vascular system. Plasma contains colloids (plasma proteins), and in conjunction with the red blood cells, maintains vascular volume.

The fluids in the ICF and ECF compartments are not static and move freely among the cells, tissue spaces, and plasma. ECF serves as the transportation system of the body via two mechanisms: the movement of blood through the circulatory system and the movement of fluid between the cells and the blood capillaries. Plasma carries nutrients, water, and electrolytes to the cells and removes the waste products of cellular metabolism from them. Additionally, plasma carries oxygen from the lungs to the capillaries and removes carbon dioxide, returning it to the lungs. The lymph component of interstitial fluid also transports wastes from the cells, ultimately entering the vascular circulation through the thoracic duct.

Transcellular fluids, or the body's secretions and excretions, are also part of the ECF volume. A *secretion* is the product of a gland, such as saliva, gastrointestinal secretions, cerebrospinal fluid, and synovial fluid. *Excretions* are waste products produced in the body, such as urine and feces. These transcellular fluids must remain in balance for effective bodily function. Excessive excretions deplete the ECF volume and then the ICF volume. Inadequate or excessive secretions may also interfere with digestion and elimination. Eventually, these imbalances alter homeostasis.

ELECTROLYTES

Extracellular and intracellular body fluids contain both electrolyte and nonelectrolyte particles. *Electrolytes* are substances, often salts or minerals, whose molecules dissociate in water. When the molecules dissociate, they disintegrate into electrically charged ions (*ionization*) that are capable of conducting a weak electrical charge, hence the term *electrolyte*. Nonelectrolyte substances, such as glucose and urea, do not dissociate in water, nor do they develop electrical charges. When a salt such as sodium chloride dissociates and ionizes, the particles develop either a positive charge, becoming *cations* or a negative charge, becoming *anions*. Sodium is always a cation with one positive charge (Na^+), and chloride is an anion with a negative charge (Cl^-). Body water contains both cations and anions, maintaining electrolyte balance. Thus, each cation is balanced chemically by an anion: eg, sodium chloride (Na^+Cl^-).

The common cations with one electrical charge (*monovalent* cations) are sodium (Na^+) and potassium (K^+); the common cations with two electrical charges (*bivalent*) are calcium (Ca^{2+}) and magnesium (Mg^{2+}). The common monovalent anions are chloride (Cl^-) and bicarbonate

(HCO_3^-), whereas the bivalent anions are sulfate (SO_4^{2-}) and hydrogen biphosphate (HPO_4^{2-}).

MEASUREMENT AND DISTRIBUTION OF BODY ELECTROLYTES

Electrolytes exist in both fluid compartments of the body in differing concentrations and compositions. They are measured according to numbers of particles, osmotic activity, or chemical activity. The number of particles per unit of volume is expressed as moles or millimoles (1/1000 of a mole). This unit of measure, expressed as grams or milligrams per 100 mL, gives no direct information as to the number of ions or to the numbers of electrical charges the particles carry. For this reason, this measurement is seldom used in referring to electrolyte concentrations.

Osmols and milliosmols (1/1000 of an osmol) are the units of measurement based on osmotic activity. They are the measures of the amount of work dissolved particles can do in drawing fluid through a semipermeable membrane. *Osmotic activity* depends on the number of actual particles in solution irrespective of any charge they may carry; even nonionizable charges such as glucose and urea exert an osmotic effect.

Electrolytes are usually measured in milliequivalents per liter of water (mEq/L). The term *milliequivalent* means 1/1000 of an equivalent, with an equivalent referring to the chemical combining power of a substance. The chemical combining power of a substance is the power of cations to unite with anions to form molecules and is measured in relation to the chemical combining power of hydrogen (H^+). Sodium and chloride ions are equivalent because they combine equally; eg, 1 mEq of Na^+ = 1 mEq of Cl^-. The milliequivalent system is used most often clinically because the reacting capacity and number of solute particles are known, and electrical imbalances and shifts are easier to evaluate and follow.

The predominant electrolytes in the ECF are sodium and chloride, whereas the major electrolytes in the cells or ICF are potassium and phosphate. The ion composition of the two major subdivisions of ECF (plasma and interstitial fluid) are similar; the main difference is that plasma has a higher concentration of protein. Electrolyte levels are measured in the intravascular portion of the ECF. The plasma is relatively easy to sample, but the electrolyte composition of cellular fluid is difficult to measure and varies somewhat from tissue to tissue. Therefore, the "normal range" of electrolyte values used clinically is a *serum measurement*, which is only an approximate measurement for the cellular fluids. The normal ranges for the four most commonly measured electrolytes are: Na^+, 136–145 mEq/L; K^+, 3.5–5.0 mEq/L; Ca^{2+}, 4.3–5.3 mEq/L; and Cl^-, 100–106 mEq/L.

The transcellular fluids such as urine, bile, and saliva each has its distinct electrolyte composition, which tends to be stable in health. Average normal values for fluids in the body compartments are shown in Figure 5–1.

MOVEMENT OF BODY FLUID AND ELECTROLYTES

Substance transport and fluid movement within the body can be described in three phases. First, nutrients and fluids are absorbed by the plasma from the lungs and gastrointestinal tract and carried within the circulatory tract. Second, the interstitial fluid and its components move between the capillaries and cells, carrying the nutrients from the plasma. Third, fluid and its solutes move from the interstitial fluid into the cells. The process then reverses itself, ending with the kidneys receiving the by-products of cellular metabolism carried by the plasma. Fluids and their carried substances move by diffusion, active transport, and osmosis.

Diffusion

Diffusion is the mixing of molecules caused by the tendency of molecules to move continuously and randomly in a solution or a gas. Particles move from an area of greater concentration to an area of lesser concentration. The greater the difference in concentration, the faster the rate of diffusion. Two other factors affect the rate of diffusion: molecule size and temperature of the solution. The larger the molecule, the slower the process because larger molecules need more energy to move. Also, higher temperatures increase the rate at which molecules move and, therefore, increase the rate of diffusion. When discussing the diffusion of electrolytes, remember that the particle's electrical charge also affects the process, because ions are pulled toward ions with opposite charges. Body electrolytes diffuse between the membrane pores in the capillaries and the interstitial fluid.

Active Transport

Active transport is the movement of small particles across cell membranes from an area of greater concentration to lesser concentration. This movement requires energy from an outside source (ie, metabolic energy provided by enzymes) and, therefore, differs from osmosis and diffusion. Other substances requiring transport combine with their specific carrier outside the cell membrane to enter the cell. Once inside the cell, they separate, releasing the substance. This active transport system is used within the body to help maintain the proper concentrations of sodium and potassium ions in their appropriate fluid compartments.

Osmosis

Osmosis is the movement of water through a semipermeable membrane, such as a cell wall, from an area where there is more water to where there is less water. An area with a greater percentage of water contains a smaller percentage of particulate matter; therefore, osmosis can also be described as the movement of water from an area of

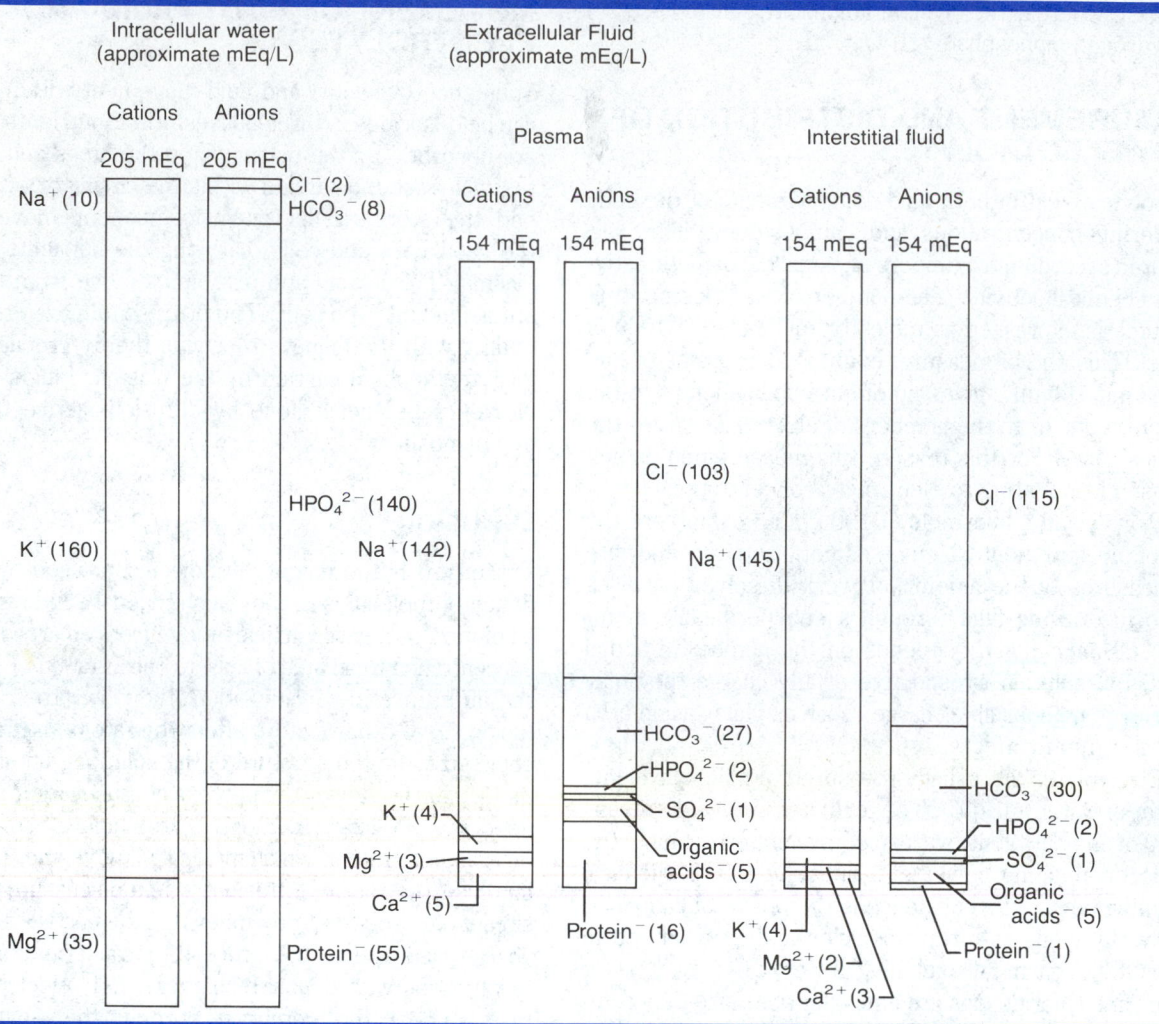

Figure 5–1

Comparison of electrolyte distribution of intracellular fluid to extracellular fluid.
Note: The anions (negative-charged electrolytes) always balance the cations (positive-charged electrolytes).

lesser concentration of particles to an area of greater concentration of particles. The osmotic process continues until an equilibrium in the concentration of particles is reached on each side of the semipermeable membrane.

Two terms are used when discussing the concentration of particles in solution—osmolality and osmolarity. **Osmolality** refers to the number of osmols (particles in solution) per liter of solvent. **Osmolarity** refers to the number of osmols per liter of solution. Osmolality is approximately equal to osmolarity when the concentration of solute is small. Therefore, the two terms are used interchangeably in this text, with a preference for the term *osmolality* because it is slightly more precise.

Osmosis occurs when two solutions have different osmolalities, and water moves from a solution of lesser osmolality to a solution of greater osmolality. **Osmotic pressure** is the force exerted by particles in the solution to stop osmosis. Osmotic pressure is exerted by molecules or ions that cannot penetrate the semipermeable membrane and is directly proportional to the concentration or degree of osmolality of the solution. The greater the degree of osmolality on one side of a semipermeable membrane, the greater the osmotic pressure and attraction for water on that side. Because of osmotic pressure, water flows toward the solution of greater concentration until the osmolality of the solutions is equalized.

CLINICAL APPLICATION

The administration of intravenous solutions is a clinical example of osmosis. Usually, intravenous solutions, such as 0.9% NaCl, are **isotonic**; they have the same osmolality as blood plasma, preventing shifts of fluids and electrolytes. This type of intravenous therapy simply replaces fluid and maintains the normal electrolyte balance in the body. A **hypertonic** solution, such as 50% glucose, has a greater osmolality than blood plasma and causes a rapid influx of water from the cells and interstitial spaces into the plasma. Glucose is sometimes used to reduce cerebral edema temporarily. **Hypotonic** solutions have a lower

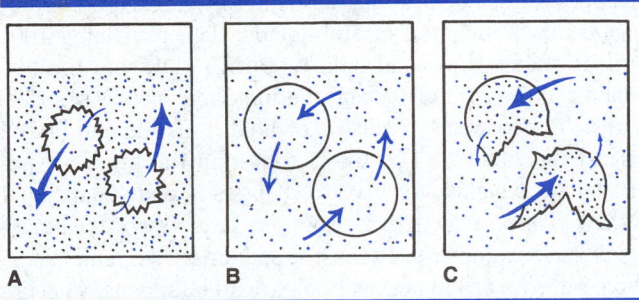

Figure 5–2

Osmosis. **A.** Hypertonic solution. Osmotic pressure is greater in the solution than in the cell, causing water to move out of the cell, with destruction or crenation of the cell. **B.** Osmotic pressure in the solution is the same as that in the cell, therefore the movement of solution is equal. **C.** Hypotonic solution. Osmotic pressure is greater in the cell than in the solution, causing water to move into the cell, with eventual rupturing or hemolysis of the cell.

osmolality than blood plasma, causing water to move from the plasma into the cells (Figure 5–2).

BODY HOMEOSTASIS

Body homeostasis is a dynamic equilibrium that maintains the body's fluid balance in a relatively constant state. This homeostasis is based on the amount of fluid taken in a normal diet and the volume of fluid excreted daily. Clinically, a healthy adult eating a normal diet satisfies the need for electrolytes and fluid and, with the help of the body's regulating mechanisms, excretes an appropriate amount of fluid to maintain this critical balance. Illness and interference with normal intake and output can seriously derange the electrolyte and fluid balance. The client can become critically ill in a matter of days and in some instances, hours.

Homeostatic regulation of the body is maintained by lungs, kidneys, cardiovascular system, pituitary gland, adrenal glands, and parathyroid glands. These organs and their regulating mechanisms control the body's fluid volume, electrolyte concentration, and the electrolyte composition of body fluids.

Lungs

The lungs maintain the composition of the blood's oxygen and carbon dioxide levels. Carbon dioxide is derived from the dissociation of carbonic acid in the blood:

$$H_2CO_3 \underset{\text{carbonic anhydrase}}{\overset{\longrightarrow}{\longleftarrow}} H_2O + CO_2$$

(carbonic acid)　(water)　(carbon dioxide)

Thus, the lungs play an important role in maintaining the balance between acid and alkali in extracellular fluid. The lungs also influence body water loss through respiration.

Kidneys

The kidneys maintain the volume and composition of the extracellular fluid, including the regulation of electrolytes and blood volume. The kidneys have an ability to reabsorb electrolytes selectively and assist in regulating acid–base balance. Reabsorption takes place mainly in the distal renal tubules, but some occurs in the proximal tubules. The kidneys also remove wastes and maintain urine volume and concentration.

Cardiovascular System

The heart and blood vessels provide the kidneys with sufficient plasma to permit regulation of water and electrolyte content of body fluids. If cardiovascular function is decreased, the blood pressure decreases, diminishing blood flow to Bowman's capsule in the kidney and decreasing the volume of urine filtered.

Pituitary Gland

The pituitary gland releases a water-conserving hormone, antidiuretic hormone (ADH), from its posterior lobe. ADH is primarily secreted by the hypothalamus and stored in the pituitary until needed. Osmoreceptors in the hypothalamus sense the need for secretion of ADH and deliver impulses to the posterior pituitary to release the stored ADH.

The normal action of ADH is to stimulate reabsorption of water from the distal renal tubule and collecting duct. If the blood becomes more diluted, the osmolality decreases and less ADH is released. Conversely, as the plasma osmolality increases, so does the release of ADH.

The anterior pituitary gland also contains a growth hormone, which helps maintain glomerular filtration, renal plasma flow, and tubular function. Additionally, the anterior pituitary produces diuretic hormone, which directly increases urine output.

Adrenal Glands

The adrenal glands secrete cortical hormones, which normally cause the reabsorption of sodium and water and the excretion of potassium in the distal renal tubule. The principal hormone is the mineralocorticoid aldosterone, which promotes the retention of sodium and the subsequent retention of water.

Constriction of either the carotid or renal arteries increases aldosterone production. Decreased arterial pressure in the carotid baroreceptors or directly in the renal arteries stimulates the renin–aldosterone mechanism. The decreased blood flow stimulates the release of the enzyme *renin* from the *juxtaglomerular* cells of the afferent arterioles of the kidney. This increased renin aids in converting the plasma protein angiotensinogen produced in the liver to angiotensin I. A converting enzyme in the lungs then

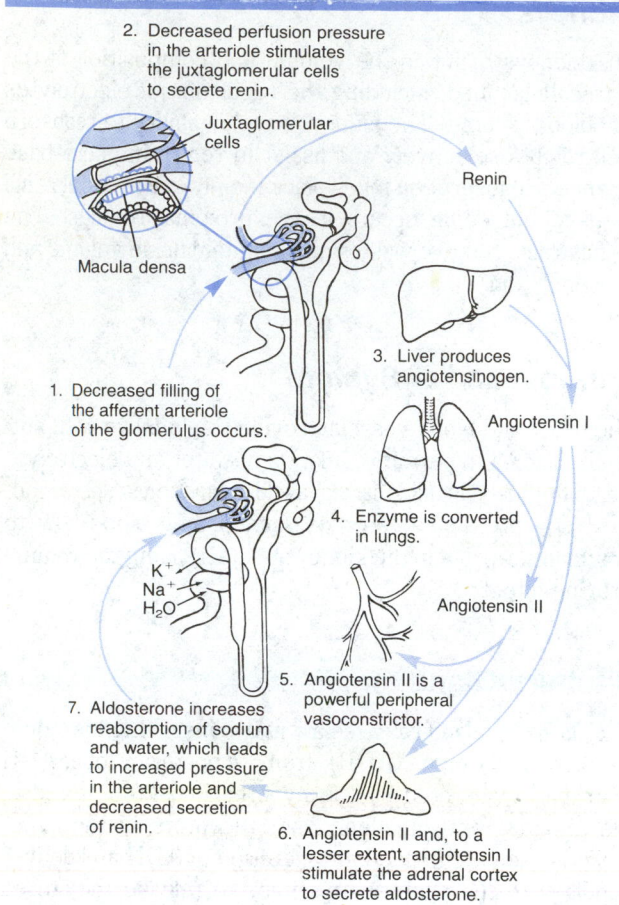

2. Decreased perfusion pressure in the arteriole stimulates the juxtaglomerular cells to secrete renin.

Juxtaglomerular cells

Renin

Macula densa

1. Decreased filling of the afferent arteriole of the glomerulus occurs.

3. Liver produces angiotensinogen.

Angiotensin I

4. Enzyme is converted in lungs.

K^+
Na^+
H_2O

Angiotensin II

7. Aldosterone increases reabsorption of sodium and water, which leads to increased presssure in the arteriole and decreased secretion of renin.

5. Angiotensin II is a powerful peripheral vasoconstrictor.

6. Angiotensin II and, to a lesser extent, angiotensin I stimulate the adrenal cortex to secrete aldosterone.

Figure 5–3

Renin aldosterone mechanism.

converts angiotensin I to angiotensin II, causing systemic vasoconstriction. This activity increases the production of aldosterone by the adrenal cortex and the subsequent retention of sodium and water, which increases the systemic blood pressure (Figure 5–3).

Parathyroid Glands

The parathyroid glands maintain the level of ionized calcium in the blood and regulate calcium and phosphorus metabolism. A low serum calcium concentration stimulates parathyroid secretion. Parathyroid hormone is also indirectly under the influence of the serum phosphate concentration. A high phosphate concentration causes a secondary lowering of serum calcium concentration, which in turn stimulates the parathyroid hormone. This phenomenon occurs in clients with severe renal disease and phosphate retention, who then develop secondary hyperparathyroidism (renal rickets).

NORMAL INTAKE AND OUTPUT

The body maintains fluid equilibrium by equalizing its intake and output in a state of health. A healthy body in moderate

temperatures needs about 2500 mL of water daily, but only 1500 mL is ingested in oral liquids. The remaining 1000 mL is acquired in solid food (700 mL) and from the oxidation of these foods during the metabolic processes (300 mL). The primary regulator of fluid intake is the body's thirst mechanism. The thirst center in the brain's hypothalamus is highly sensitive to changes in body fluid osmolality. Thirst may result from decreased water intake, excessive water loss, excessive sodium intake, and excessive infusion of a hypertonic solution. Thirst usually occurs when the water loss is equal to 2% of the body weight. These circumstances result in cellular dehydration, reduced blood volume, and hyperosmolality of the ECF. In dehydration, the increased osmolality of the serum stimulates the thirst center via neurologic impulses, and the person feels thirsty. Conversely, overhydration diminishes the drive to drink.

Fluid intake is balanced by the body's water losses. The major organs of fluid loss are the kidneys, which are responsible for approximately 1500 mL of urine produced daily. This volume approximates the daily oral fluid intake of an adult. Two other ways that the body normally excretes fluid are through insensible loss and feces. Insensible losses occur through the skin and lungs and cannot be measured accurately. The fluid is exhaled in expired air and diffused through the skin. Insensible losses account for 800 mL, and fluid in feces, for 200 mL in 24 hours (Table 5–1).

FLUID AND ELECTROLYTE IMBALANCES

Fluid and electrolyte imbalances can be categorized into two types of conditions according to causes: (1) a deficit or excess of essential body substances, such as water, sodium, hydrogen, potassium, calcium, or magnesium or (2) an abnormal shift of fluid from one compartment to another, or volume imbalances. Almost every hospitalized client is susceptible to water and electrolyte imbalances. Illness upsets the delicate state of body homeostasis, and certain conditions, diseases, and treatments make a client even more vulnerable to fluid and electrolyte imbalance.

Table 5–1 Twenty-Four-Hour Fluid Balance in a Healthy Client			
Intake	**mL**	**Output**	**mL**
Oral fluid intake	1500	Urine	1500
H_2O in food	700	Insensible loss:	
H_2O from oxidation	300	Respiration	350–400
	2500	Perspiration	350–400
		Feces	200
			2400–2500

Diseases and conditions such as kidney disease; burns; congestive heart failure (CHF); diabetes; cirrhosis of the liver; pulmonary disease; and treatments such as surgery, diuretic therapy, low-sodium diets, and intravenous therapy may all cause serious threats to body homeostasis. A client suffering from any of these conditions or therapies requires careful recording of intake and output and careful observation for symptoms and signs of imbalance.

Water–Sodium Imbalances

Osmolar imbalances involve disturbances in osmolality and, therefore, water distribution in the fluid compartments in the body. Water always moves from an *area of lesser solute concentration* to an *area of greater solute concentration* until both are equal. A clinical measure of osmolality in the body is the measurement of the solute sodium in the serum. An elevated serum sodium level or *hypernatremia* (high solute concentration), indicates hyperosmolality. A lowered serum sodium level, or *hyponatremia* (low solute concentration), indicates hypo-osmolality.

Hyperosmolar Imbalances

Hyperosmolar imbalances or water deficit syndromes result from either water depletion or extracellular solute excess. In water depletion, the amount of solute is correct, but the solute is dissolved in too little water. With solute excess, there is an excess of solute per unit of water. Either condition leads to hyperosmolality, which causes cell shrinkage and dehydration. The ECF becomes hypertonic in relation to the ICF, causing water to leave the cells and enter the ECF, causing cellular dehydration. The causes of hyperosmolar imbalances are shown in Table 5–2.

The symptoms and signs of hyperosmolar states, regardless of cause, stem from dehydration. The client may have a dry mouth; dry, furrowed tongue; and be thirsty. The eyeballs are soft and sunken in severe cases. Decreased skin turgor, especially over the forehead and chest, and elevated temperature are seen. The client becomes restless and apprehensive. Untreated, this condition can progress to delirium, convulsions, and death. As a compensatory mechanism, the kidneys concentrate the urine produced, and eventually, oliguria and anuria occur. Laboratory findings include a high urine specific gravity (> 1.030), elevated hemoglobin, and hypernatremia (> 150 mEq/L).

The treatment for hyperosmolar disturbances is to administer water. In mild dehydration, oral fluid replacement is sufficient. In severe dehydration, intravenous solutions of isotonic glucose (5% glucose) are administered in proportion to the degree of dehydration, adjusted for each client. Water should not be replaced too quickly, or water intoxication may result.

Hypo-osmolar Imbalances

Hypo-osmolar imbalances, or water-excess syndromes, result in either fluid overloads or solute deficits. Water

Table 5–2	The Causes of Hyperosmolar Imbalances
Water Deficit	**Solute Excess**

Decreased intake:
  NPO
  Water unavailable
  Coma
  Severely ill or
  immobilized
  Sense of thirst
  impaired
 	
Increased output:
  GI: Diarrhea,
     vomiting,
     suction
 	
  Renal: Inability to
       concentrate
       urine
 	
       Excessive
       urine output
       (ie, diabetes
       insipidus)
 	
  Lungs: Hyperventi-
       lation,
       tracheos-
       tomy
 	
  Skin: Excessive
     perspiration,
     burns, high
     fever
	• Infusions of hypertonic solutions
	
	• Excessive IV glucose administration
	
	• Excessive IV sodium bicarbonate administration
	
	• Uncontrolled diabetes mellitus with hyperglycemia

intoxication is an excess of water in the extracellular compartment with a normal amount of solute. Solute-deficit imbalances result when the solute concentration is normal but is diluted in too much water. Either situation results in swollen cells. The causes of hypo-osmolar imbalances are shown in Table 5–3.

The symptoms and signs of all hypo-osmolar states are due to cellular edema. The client may gain considerable weight in the presence of anorexia, nausea, and vomiting. Signs of fluid overload such as peripheral and periorbital edema, a bounding pulse, pulmonary rales, and shortness of breath without exertion may also be seen. Neurological abnormalities due to cerebral edema can be observed, especially when the hypo-osmolar state has occurred suddenly. These include headache and personality changes that progress to confusion and delirium, muscle weakness, twitching, and decreased reflexes. ADH secretion is decreased, and healthy kidneys attempt to excrete as much urine as possible; therefore, polyuria with a decreased specific gravity will be observed. Hemodilution also produces decreased hemoglobin and hematocrit values, as well as decreased Na^+ and K^+ values.

The treatment for hypo-osmolar imbalances is to restrict water until homeostasis is achieved. In moderate fluid excess,

Table 5–3	The Causes of Hypo-osmolar Imbalances
Water Excess	**Solute Deficit**
Excessive H$_2$O ingestion in a short time	Inadequate salt intake; ie, diuretics, low-salt diet
Excessive infusions of isotonic IV solutions	Replacement of Na and H$_2$O losses with only water; ie, replacing vomitus losses (which contain Na+) with plain H$_2$O
Malfunction of the homeostatic mechanisms:	
• Pituitary: ADH secretion	
• Renal: ↑ aldosterone, water retention in kidney failure	
• Adrenal: hyperaldosteronism; excessive administration of adrenal cortical hormones	

oral fluids are restricted for 24 hours, and administration of intravenous solutions is decreased or discontinued. More severe fluid excesses caused by underlying disease processes must be treated appropriately; ie, CHF may be treated with digoxin and diuretic therapy.

Volume Imbalances

Volume imbalances occur in the ECF compartment only as a result of the movement of sodium and water between the plasma and interstitial fluid. It is important to note that, in fluid shifts, both the solvent (H$_2$O) and solute (Na$^+$) move in equal proportions, creating isotonic fluid imbalances. This condition is in contrast to osmolar imbalances, in which the solute and solvent move disproportionately, as previously described.

Extracellular Volume Depletion/Hypovolemia

Extracellular volume depletion, or hypovolemia, is caused by a shift of Na$^+$ and H$_2$O from the plasma to the interstitial fluid. Any condition that results in large acute losses of salt and water can precipitate hypovolemia. Severe burns, hemorrhage, diarrhea and vomiting, fever, and kidney disease are examples. Symptoms and signs of hypovolemia are those of shock: pallor, decreased blood pressure, tachycardia, weakness, restlessness, and unconsciousness. The client's red blood cell count is increased in hypovolemia because of the concentration of the plasma. Extracellular volume depletion can be treated quickly, once recognized, by intravenous administration of isotonic solutions.

Extracellular Volume Excess/Hypervolemia

Extracellular volume excess, or hypervolemia, is caused by a shift of Na$^+$ and H$_2$O from the interstitial fluid to the plasma. Excessive increases in proportionate amounts of H$_2$O and Na$^+$ can cause hypervolemia. Causes include excessive infusions of normal saline; cortisone therapy; and disease states such as cardiac, renal, or hepatic failure. Symptoms of hypervolemia include a bounding pulse, weight gain and pitting edema, engorged peripheral veins, and pulmonary edema. The treatment of hypervolemia includes fluid restriction and diuretic therapy.

Electrolyte Imbalances

Each of the major electrolytes—sodium, potassium, calcium, and magnesium—performs specific roles in bodily function. Their normal concentrations must be maintained to sustain life.

Sodium

Sodium (Na$^+$) is the major cation of the extracellular fluid. Two important facts about sodium are: (1) the sodium ion moves rapidly between the plasma and the interstitial fluid within the ECF, and (2) sodium and water move together. Therefore, sodium is the primary regulator of ECF volume and concentration. Sodium affects not only the fluid balance in the body but also is responsible for the osmotic pressure of the ECF. Additionally, sodium establishes the electrochemical state necessary for muscle contraction and transmission of nerve impulses. Imbalances of sodium, therefore, affect fluid volume, blood volume, and the nervous system.

Hyponatremia. Hyponatremia is a sodium deficiency of the ECF, reflected in a serum sodium level of less than 135 mEq/L. This deficiency may be a result of a loss of sodium or a gain in water but is always due to proportionately greater amounts of water than sodium. It is always a hypo-osmolar state. The hypo-osmolar state causes a shift of fluid from the extracellular compartment into the intracellular compartment and results in cellular swelling. The causes of hyponatremia are summarized in Table 5–4.

The clinical symptoms and signs of hyponatremia directly depend on the cause, severity, and rapidity with which inadequate serum sodium level develops. With gradual loss of sodium, the client feels apathetic and weak. GI symptoms can occur, such as anorexia, nausea, vomiting, and abdominal cramping. As the serum sodium level becomes progressively lower, neurological signs such as confusion, muscle twitching, seizures, and coma develop, which are directly related to brain swelling. Laboratory findings include a serum sodium level of less than 135 mEq/L, sometimes as low as 100 mEq/L; a low urinary specific gravity, usually 1.002–1.004; a decreased blood volume; and increased hemoglobin and hematocrit values.

Table 5−4 Causes of Hyponatremia	
Fluid Gain	**Na⁺ Loss**
• Excessive administration of intravenous solutions (usually 5% dextrose in water) • Excessive ingestion of H_2O • Syndrome of inappropriate antidiuretic hormone (SIADH) secretion • Renal failure	• Diuretic therapy, especially thiazide diuretics • Low-salt diets • Loss of GI secretions, ie, vomiting, diarrhea, GI suction or drainage, excessive sweating • Addison's disease (decreased aldosterone causes Na^+ loss) • Extensive burns • Sequestering of Na^+ in body cavities, ie, peritonitis

Treatment of sodium loss is sodium replacement, usually by the parenteral route. If the client's fluid volume is low, an isotonic salt solution (0.9% NaCl) may be used; however, a small amount of hypertonic saline can be used if the plasma volume is normal or excessive. If excessive fluid volume is the cause for hyponatremia, fluid restriction and diuretic therapy are indicated.

Syndrome of Inappropriate Antidiuretic Hormone. Syndrome of inappropriate antidiuretic hormone (SIADH) is a type of hyponatremia associated with water excess or hypo-osmolality. The urine of SIADH clients is either hypertonic or not maximally dilute. Sodium continues to be excreted by the kidneys. Although hyponatremia is present and there is no edema, the physiologic disturbance in SIADH stems from excessive ADH activity, resulting in water retention and consequent hyponatremia. The syndrome is termed "inappropriate" because ADH production continues in spite of hypotonic plasma; hypotonic plasma normally serves as a regulatory mechanism for antidiuretic hormone secretion. Sodium continues to be lost in the urine because aldosterone does not conserve it; the normal renin–angiotensin system for stimulation of aldosterone production is not functioning in SIADH.

The causes of SIADH are either sustained secretion of ADH by the hypothalamus or aberrant ADH production from a malignancy. See Unit Seven for more information on SIADH.

The symptoms and signs of SIADH are similar to those previously described for hyponatremia. Nursing measures to monitor for SIADH include recognizing clients at high risk for the syndrome because it is potentially fatal if not recognized and treated. Other measures are careful monitoring of the client's weight, intake and output, serum sodium levels, and GI symptoms and/or neurological changes. Treatment of SIADH centers on correcting the cause of excessive ADH secretion and alleviating excessive water retention.

Hypernatremia. Hypernatremia is a sodium excess of the ECF, reflected in a serum sodium level of greater than 145 mEq/L. This excess may be a result of a gain of sodium or a loss of water but is due to a disproportionate amount of sodium to water; it is a hyperosmolar state. This hyperosmolar state causes a shift of fluid from the intracellular space to the extracellular space, causing shrinking or dehydration of the cells. The causes of hypernatremia are summarized in Table 5−5.

Table 5−5 Causes of Hypernatremia	
Fluid Loss	**Na⁺ Gain**

• Diabetes insipidus, uncompensated
• Excessive perspiration and other insensible losses
• Copious diarrhea
• Impaired renal function, ie, polyuria in nephritis
• Decreased fluid intake (common in elderly, young, confused, or comatose clients; also in clients on ventilators or with tracheostomies)
• Peritoneal dialysis with glucose solutions
	• Parenteral administration of salt solutions (hypertonic saline, sodium bicarbonate, isotonic saline)
	• Hypertonic saline abortions
	• Excessive intake of table salt
	• Partial drowning in salt water
	• Homeostatic mechanism failures:
	  - CHF, ↓ cardiac output, ↓ renal flow, ↑ Na^+ retention
	  - Nephrotic syndrome and cirrhosis:
	    ↑ Aldosterone production
	    ↑ Na^+ retention

Box 5–1 Causes of Hypokalemia

Inadequate K⁺ intake

Poor nutrition
NPO with IV fluids without K^+
Nausea, anorexia, acute alcoholism, starvation

Excessive use of K⁺ within the body

Healing phase of burns
Hyperinsulinism
Recovery from diabetic acidosis

Loss of K⁺ from the body

Medical treatments:

• Diuretics, especially thiazide and furosemide
• Low-/or no-salt diets
• High-dose corticosteroid therapy
• Prolonged administration of K^+-free IVs and hyperalimentation fluids

Parenteral administration of insulin and glucose (causes glycogen formation with a shift of K^+ into the cells)

Gastrointestinal disturbances:

• Excessive vomiting, diarrhea
• Fistula drainage
• Ulcerative colitis
• Surgical treatments such as ileostomy, colostomy

Excessive perspiration

Metabolic disease:

• Diabetes mellitus
• Hyperaldosteronism
• Adrenal tumor, cirrhosis, CHF

Renal disease:

Particularly tubular necrosis/acidosis

The clinical symptoms and signs of hypernatremia are related to the central nervous system (CNS) and are directly correlated to the degree and rapidity of the rise of serum sodium. The client may at first note a dry, red, sticky tongue and mouth and become restless and irritable. This condition progresses to delirium, twitching, seizures, and coma. Accompanying these CNS signs are increased muscle tone, hyperactive deep tendon reflexes, metabolic acidosis, and death. Laboratory findings include an elevated serum sodium level (greater than 145 mEq/L), an increased serum osmolality greater than 295 mOsm/kg (normal = 280–295 mOsm/kg), and a urine specific gravity of greater than 1.015.

The treatment of hypernatremia is to lower the serum sodium, primarily by infusing a hypotonic electrolyte solution, often 0.3% NaCl. The gradual reduction of serum sodium over 48 hours has been recommended to lower the risk of cerebral edema and brain damage.

Potassium

Although found in all the body compartments, potassium (K^+) is the major intracellular cation, with 98% of the body's potassium contained within the cells. That remaining 2% of potassium helps regulate the proper functioning of the entire body's neuromuscular system. In addition, potassium regulates intracellular osmolality and promotes cellular growth; in fact, any condition that disrupts cell wall integrity produces a potassium shift. Finally, potassium promotes proper heart muscle function and assists with acid–base balance.

Although the movement of potassium within the body is complex, it is important in understanding potassium's functions. Potassium is essential to life yet cannot be stored in the body, so a daily dietary intake of potassium is required. The average adult dietary intake ranges from 50 to 100 mEq per day, with 40 mEq essential for life. Eighty percent of the daily excretion of potassium is by way of the distal renal tubules in the urine. The remaining 20% is lost through the bowels and sweat glands. Potassium is dynamic in that it is constantly moving through the cell walls in reaction to the body's needs. The amount of potassium in a cell at a given time depends on the integrity of the cell wall, the ability of the kidney to conserve some K^+ when the cells are depleted, and the sodium–potassium pump.

The *sodium–potassium pump* is a mechanism by which Na^+ is actively excluded from the cells, allowing K^+ to be present in the cells. Glucose metabolism and alkalosis are both conditions in which potassium moves into the cells. Potassium moves out of the cells during any cellular destruction or impairment of cellular metabolism, during acidosis, or after strenuous exercise. Potassium balance is also affected by aldosterone. When the renin–angiotensin mechanism is stimulated, usually by decreased blood flow through the kidneys, aldosterone is produced by the adrenal cortex. Increased aldosterone production conserves Na^+ and, therefore, promotes K^+ excretion by the kidneys.

Hypokalemia. A potassium deficit, or hypokalemia, associated with a serum potassium level of less than 3 mEq/L, can be deadly. Hypokalemia results from decreased K^+ intake, excessive K^+ loss, and excessive use of K^+ within the body. See Box 5–1 for causes of hypokalemia.

The clinical symptoms and signs of hypokalemia include disturbances of the neuromuscular, cardiovascular, gastrointestinal, and respiratory systems as well as H^+ balance (see section on acid–base balance). Neuromuscular symptoms include general weakness, diminished or absent deep tendon reflexes, weak leg muscles, and leg cramps. Cardiovascular changes such as a weak pulse, low blood pressure, and faint heart sounds are seen. In the ECG, ST segment depression, varying degrees of heart block, and depressed T waves are common. There is an increased sensitivity to digitalis, and premature atrial and ventricular beats are frequently seen in hypokalemic clients with digitalis toxicity. The client may also have a marked decrease in blood pressure on assuming an upright position (postural hypotension). Gastrointestinal symptoms such as vomiting and decreased bowel motility often occur and can progress to an ileus (intestinal muscle paralysis). Respiratory changes include shortness of breath and shallow respirations.

Treatment of hypokalemia begins with the correction of the underlying cause of the hypokalemia. Mild hypokalemia can be corrected by oral replacement of potassium. Hypokalemia with serum levels of less than 2.0 mEq/L requires parenteral replacement. The replacement amount is usually 40 mEq of K^+ in 1000 mL of IV solution over 8 hours. Faster replacement of potassium requires constant ECG monitoring in a coronary care unit.

Hyperkalemia. Hyperkalemia is less common than hypokalemia but can be more life threatening. The condition is unusual in clients with normal kidney function and is reflected by a serum potassium level of greater than 5.5 mEq/L. See Box 5–2 for the causes of hyperkalemia.

The clinical symptoms and signs of hyperkalemia include musculoskeletal, GI, and cardiac symptoms. Muscular symptoms including weakness, paresthesia, cramps, and pain are common. Indications of gastrointestinal hyperactivity include nausea, intermittent GI colic, and diarrhea. Cardiac changes on the ECG include tented T waves, small to nonvisible P waves, widened QRS complexes, and life-threatening dysrhythmias. Supraventricular and/or ventricular tachycardias, premature ventricular beats, and ventricular fibrillation may all lead to cardiac arrest.

Treatment for hyperkalemia includes restricting both parenteral and oral K^+ intake and reducing serum K^+ by administering cation-exchange resins such as Kayexalate. Intravenous administration of glucose and insulin may be ordered to facilitate movement of K^+ into the cells. Severe hyperkalemia is an emergency and should be treated in an intensive care unit.

Calcium

Calcium (Ca^{2+}) exists in two forms in the body: ionized calcium and nonionized calcium. Nonionized calcium is in the serum and is bound to proteins, primarily albumin. Ionized serum calcium is physiologically active and plays a role in muscle contraction, neural function, and the formation of prothrombin for blood coagulation. There is a reciprocal relation between ionized and nonionized calcium, with a rise in one causing a decrease in the other. The calcium level routinely measured is the total serum calcium level; the ionized portion is estimated according to simultaneous measurement of serum protein (ie, albumin). Because serum albumin levels and serum calcium levels fall and rise together, it is important to evaluate them together. Changes in the arterial pH cause more calcium to become bound to protein ($\uparrow$ pH = alkalosis) or less calcium to be bound ($\downarrow$ pH = acidosis), whereas the total serum calcium remains unchanged.

The release of calcium into the serum is primarily controlled by the parathyroid glands. Parathyroid hormone (PTH) promotes a transfer of calcium from bones to the plasma, stimulates intestinal resorption of calcium, and

---

Box 5–2 Causes of Hyperkalemia

Retention of K^+ within the body

  Renal failure, with an inability of the kidneys to excrete potassium

  Adrenocortical insufficiency

Release of K^+ from the cells

  Burns

  Massive trauma and crushing injuries

Potassium "overdose"

  Excessive administration of intravenous infusions containing K^+

---

enhances renal reabsorption of calcium. Conversely, calcium is moved from the serum back into bones by the action of calcitonin, produced by the thyroid gland, thus lowering the serum calcium. Finally, calcium levels are influenced by phosphorus levels. As calcium levels rise, phosphorus levels decrease and vice versa.

Hypocalcemia. Hypocalcemia can be due to an acute loss of calcium from the body secondary to acute diarrhea, acute pancreatitis, hypoparathyroidism, and renal disease. Additionally, if there is an increased need for calcium, as in pregnancy and lactation, calcium deficiencies can occur unless dietary intake is increased.

Symptoms and signs of hypocalcemia include increased neuromuscular irritability, which causes tetany-type muscle spasms; fatigue; laryngospasm, sometimes with airway obstruction; and positive Trousseau's and Chvostek's signs, which are tests for tetany (Figure 5–4).

A prolonged QT interval is seen on the ECG due to decreased cardiac contractility. Laboratory findings include a serum Ca^{2+} level of less than 4.5 mEq/L and an elevated serum phosphorus level.

Treatment of hypocalcemia consists of re-establishing the normal plasma level of ionized calcium by correcting the underlying clinical problems. If the Ca^{2+} deficit is acute, 10 to 20 mL of calcium gluconate (10%) is administered intravenously over 10 to 15 minutes. In nonacute cases, oral calcium supplements (calcium lactate) and a high-calcium diet are prescribed. Vitamin D is also a part of treatment for hypocalcemia because it facilitates the absorption of calcium supplements. Dosage usually ranges from 50,000 to 250,000 units per day.

Hypercalcemia. Hypercalcemia may result from excessive calcium or vitamin D intake (increases calcium absorption in the intestines), including overuse of antacids. Hypercalcemia may also result from conditions that increase calcium absorption or prevent renal excretion of calcium. Hyperparathyroidism or a tumor of the parathyroid glands increases Ca^{2+} catabolism and increases the amount of ionized Ca^{2+} in the serum. When bone destruc-

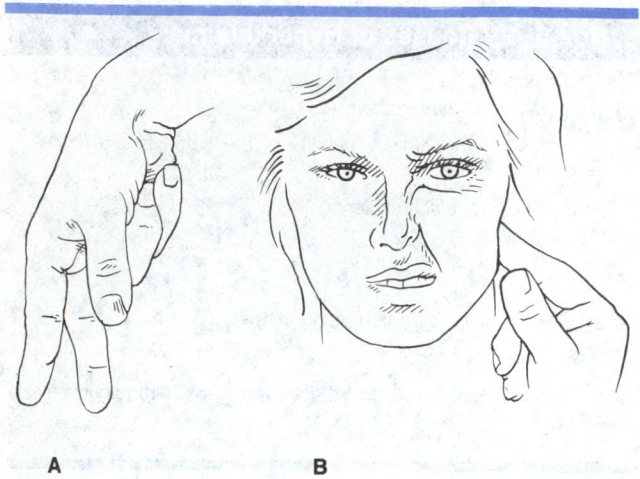

Figure 5—4

Trousseau's sign and Chvostek's sign in hypocalcemia.
A. Trousseau's sign. (1) Apply blood pressure cuff to arm and inflate above systolic pressure; leave inflated for several minutes. (2) Positive Trousseau's sign is carpopedal spasms of hands when the blood supply is decreased or the nerve is stimulated. **B.** Chvostek's sign. (1) Tap facial nerve 2 cm anterior to ear lobe, below zygomatic process. (2) Positive Chvostek's sign is muscle spasm of muscles supplied by facial nerve.

tion is greater than bone production, as in Paget's disease or osteolytic metastasis, serum calcium is elevated as well.

Symptoms and signs of hypercalcemia are opposite those of hypocalcemia, with decreased muscle tone and decreased neuromuscular irritability. Reflexes are hypoactive, and there is generalized muscle weakness and fatigue. Bone pain, osteoporosis, and eventual pathological fractures can occur. Gastrointestinal symptoms include constipation, anorexia, nausea, and vomiting. Neurological manifestations usually begin with decreased memory and attention span and can progress to psychosis, if untreated. Cardiac changes on ECG show shortened ST segments, resulting in a shorter QT segment and a widened and rounded wave. Hypercontractility of heart muscle can lead to cardiac arrest in systole if hypercalcemia is severe. Laboratory findings indicate a serum calcium level of greater than 5.8 mEq/L or 10.5 mg/dL.

Treatment of mild to moderate hypercalcemia begins with correcting the underlying cause and restricting calcium intake. If a hypercalcemic crisis occurs, the first treatment is to provide adequate hydration. Rehydration is with a normal saline infusion, usually 1000 mL every 4 to 6 hours. If diuresis does not occur, additional loop diuretics such as furosemide should be given. Oral phosphates are administered because they are successful in treating both acute and chronic hypercalcemia. Phosphate is usually given orally as sodium phosphate solution (Fleet Phospho-Soda) 5 mL three to four times daily.

Corticosteroids and mithramycin are also used to treat high serum levels of calcium. Doses of steroids range to 40 mg per day and require several days for maximal effect. Mithramycin is given by IV push for 2 days. Its use is reserved for treating hypercalcemia secondary to the side effects of cytotoxic drugs.

Magnesium

Magnesium (Mg^{2+}) is the second most abundant intracellular cation, but its importance in helping maintain proper bodily function has only recently been investigated. Consequently, its role is poorly understood, and it is still not routinely ordered when an electrolyte balance is being evaluated. The normal adult body contains approximately 20 to 25 g of magnesium, about 70% of which is stored with calcium and phosphorus in the bones. The remainder is divided intracellularly (28%) among the soft tissues of the liver, heart, skeletal muscles, and body fluids; extracellularly (2%), most of the magnesium is in the cerebrospinal fluid. The normal dietary requirements of magnesium for adults is 200 to 300 mg daily, with an increase of up to 400 mg for lactating mothers. Dietary sources of magnesium include nuts, soybeans, seafood, and whole grains.

About half the magnesium ingested is absorbed in the GI tract, and the rest is excreted in the feces. Urinary excretion of magnesium is minimal because the kidneys efficiently conserve Mg^{2+}. Calcium and magnesium are both regulated by the parathyroid glands and appear to have a mutually suppressive effect. Calcium in abundance will be absorbed over magnesium and vice versa. Additionally, if the body's magnesium level is low, the kidneys will excrete more potassium, and hypokalemia may result. Therefore, with any imbalance of calcium, phosphorus, or potassium, a parallel magnesium imbalance may also exist and warrants investigation.

Magnesium is essential for neuromuscular integration, regulation of the blood phosphorus level, and in activating multiple enzymatic reactions. Magnesium is especially important in the generation and use of adenosine triphosphate (ATP) energy produced in carbohydrate metabolism in the body because it serves as a cofactor for ATP and many other enzymes.

Hypomagnesemia. Magnesium deficiency, the most common magnesium disorder, develops when the serum concentration of Mg^{2+} is below the normal range of 1.5 to 2.5 mEq/L. Causes of magnesium depletion include conditions in which there is an inadequate magnesium intake or an excessive magnesium loss. Chronic states of malnutrition or malabsorption predisposing clients to hypomagnesemia are chronic alcoholism, intestinal bypass surgery, starvation, hyperalimentation without replacement of magnesium, and simple inadequate dietary intake. Magnesium loss occurs by several means including diarrhea, prolonged nasogastric suctioning, diuretic therapy, primary aldosteronism (causing increased urinary and fecal losses of Mg^{2+}, hypoparathyroidism, and the diuretic phase of acute renal failure.

The clinical symptoms and signs of magnesium depletion are predominantly neuromuscular and cardiac. Nervous system irritability results in coarse tremors, hyperreflexia, muscle cramps, generalized convulsions, positive Chvostek's and Trousseau's signs, and paresthesia of the hands and feet. Stimulation of the CNS causes visual and/or auditory hallucinations, intense confusion, and disorientation. Ventricular dysrhythmias (including ventricular premature contractions and ventricular fibrillation), tachycardia, and hypotension (due to decreased cardiac function) are signs of cardiac irritability. ECG findings include tall T waves and widening QRS complexes in mild magnesium deficiency to prolonged P-R intervals (first-degree block); wide QRS complexes; and/or broad, flat or inverted T waves in severe hypomagnesemia associated with hypocalcemia and hypokalemia (usually 0.2 to 0.6 mEq/L).

Magnesium deficiencies are treated by the administration of magnesium by oral, intramuscular, or intraveous routes, depending on the severity of the clinical situation. Intramuscular administration of magnesium sulfate is painful and should be given deep in the gluteal muscle. In severe hypomagnesemia, 5 g or 40 mEq of magnesium sulfate may be added to 1L of 5% dextrose in water and given as a slow infusion. A too-rapid infusion of magnesium sulfate can cause cardiac arrest. In an acute neurologic crisis such as convulsions, 1 to 2 g of magnesium sulfate can be given by direct IV push. Nurses should be alert for cardiac abnormalities during magnesium therapy and should be certain that adequate urine output (at least 100 mL every 4 hours) is maintained to allow renal elimination of magnesium.

Hypermagnesemia. Excess serum magnesium, a rare imbalance, can be caused by renal insufficiency, excessive magnesium administration during replacement therapy, excessive use of magnesium-containing antacids by clients in renal failure, and severe dehydration causing oliguria and retention of Mg^{2+}.

The main clinical symptoms and signs result from a marked decrease in neuromuscular irritability. They include a warm sensation, hyporeflexia leading to flaccid paralysis, hypotension, lethargy progressing to coma, depressed respirations, and cardiac arrest. Laboratory findings include a serum magnesium level in excess of 3 mEq/L.

Treatments of hypermagnesemia include eliminating the source of excessive magnesium intake and offsetting the toxicity of the condition. Calcium gluconate can be administered to antagonize the action of magnesium, and hemodialysis or peritoneal dialysis can be done as an emergency.

Section II: Acid–Base Balance

Acid–base balance depends on the homeostasis of the hydrogen (H^+) ion concentration in body fluids. Hydrogen ion concentration determines the acidity and alkalinity of body fluids concentration. An *increase* in hydrogen ion (H^+) makes a solution more acid, and a *decrease* makes it more alkaline. The concentration of hydrogen ions, as indicated by the symbol pH, denotes the power of the hydrogen ion. The weight of the H^+ ion is about .0000001 g/L and is expressed as 10^{-7}, or a *pH of 7*. This hydrogen ion concentration is usually expressed as the negative logarithm of the weight of ionized hydrogen in water. Because of the *negative* logarithm, *a higher H^+ ion* concentration *means a lower pH* (ie, 6.5, 6.0, 5.0), and a *lower H^+ ion* concentration indicates a *higher pH* (ie, 7.5, 8.0).

A solution having a pH of 7 is neutral because at that time, the hydrogen (acid) ions (H^+) equal of the hydroxyl (base) (OH^-) ions. Therefore, an *acidic* solution has a *pH below 7.0*, and a base or *alkaline* solution has a *pH above 7.0*. These facts are important to health care providers because *extracellular fluid* is slightly alkaline, having a *pH of 7.35 to 7.45*. For life to be maintained, the pH of the extracellular fluid must be between 6.8 and 8.0 (Figure 5–5). Slight changes in the pH or H^+ ion concentration cause marked changes in the cellular chemical reactions. If the body is in acidosis or increased H^+ ion concentration, the client can die in a coma. Conversely, if the client has a decrease in H^+ ion concentration, alkalosis and tetany or convulsions may result.

The following facts are necessary to understand and relate the chemical principles previously discussed to basic bodily physiology:

- Basic physiologic processes produce an excess of acid.
- Two major types of acids are produced: (1) carbonic acid (H_2CO_3) and (2) nonvolatile acids.

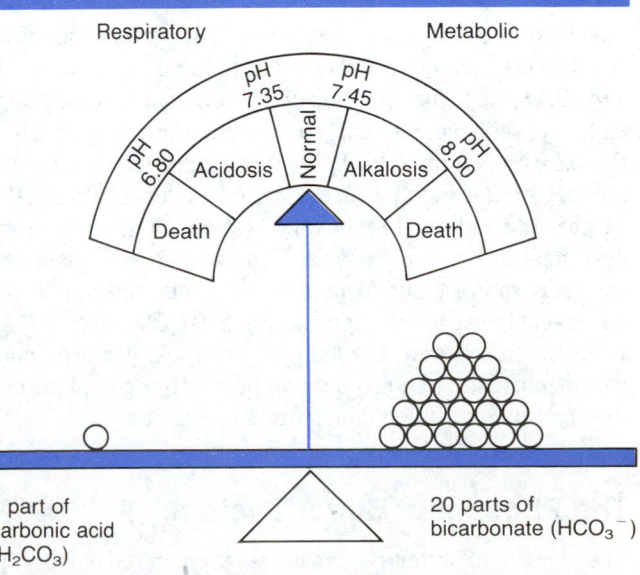

Figure 5–5

Normal acid–base balance.

• The renal, respiratory, and circulatory (blood buffer) systems act as part of the body's response as it attempts to rid itself of these acids.

Normally, the body maintains the pH between *7.35 and 7.45*. This body pH is stabilized by the buffering capacity of the body fluids. Three defense mechanisms are used to maintain the body's acid–base balance: the circulatory (blood buffer) system, respiratory system, and renal system.

DEFENSE MECHANISMS

A buffering system maintains the pH of ECF within the normal range. A *buffer* is a substance that has the ability to bind or release hydrogen H^+ in solution, keeping the pH of the solution relatively constant despite the addition of considerable quantities of acid or base. A buffer system consists of a weak acid in combination with one of the salts of that acid.

The Bicarbonate Blood Buffer System

The blood buffer system reacts within less than a second to prevent excessive changes in the H^+ ion concentration. Although the body has several blood buffer systems, the most important in the ECF is the carbonic acid (H_2CO_3)–sodium bicarbonate $(NaHCO_3)$ system. Normally, to maintain acid–base balance, the ratio of carbonic acid to sodium bicarbonate is 1:20 (see Figure 5–5). There are also small amounts of potassium bicarbonate, calcium bicarbonate, and magnesium bicarbonate. The symbol $BHCO_3$ is used to indicate any of these base bicarbonates. The bicarbonate buffer system is not an exceedingly powerful buffer for two reasons: (1) it does not operate at its fullest buffering capacity at the normal ECF pH of 7.4, and (2) there are small concentrations of bicarbonate in the blood buffer system. Yet the system is important and effective because the concentrations of the two elements (CO_2 and HCO_3^-) of the bicarbonate system can be easily regulated, carbon dioxide (CO_2) by the respiratory system and the bicarbonate ion (HCO_3^-) by the kidneys. As a result, the pH of the blood can be shifted up or down by the respiratory and renal regulatory systems. The respiratory system activates rapidly within 1 to 3 minutes to eliminate excess carbon dioxide formed from the dissociation of carbonic acid to carbon dioxide and water ($H_2CO_3 \longrightarrow H_2O + CO_2$). In contrast, the kidneys, the most powerful control mechanism, require several hours to a complete day to effect hydrogen ion concentration changes.

The Phosphate Buffer System

The phosphate buffer system is important in red blood cells and other body cells, especially in the kidney tubule cells where it enables the kidney to excrete hydrogen ions. The buffer acts similarly to the bicarbonate buffer system but is composed of the following elements: sodium dihydrogen phosphate (NaH_2PO_4) and sodium monohydrogen phosphate (Na_2HPO_4). When a strong acid is added to a mixture of these two substances, the following reaction occurs:

HCl (hydrogen chloride) + Na_2HPO_4 (sodium monohydrogen phosphate) $\longrightarrow$ NaCl (sodium chloride) + NaH_2PO_4 (sodium dihydrogen phosphate)

In other words, a strong acid is converted to a neutral salt (sodium chloride) by a phosphate buffer salt. Similarly, if a strong base such as sodium hydroxide (NaOH) is introduced into the body, the following reaction occurs:

$NaOH + NaH_2PO_4 \longrightarrow Na_2PO_4 + H_2O$

A strong base is converted into water, and the phosphate buffer salt sodium dihydrogen phosphate (NaH_2PO_4) is converted from a mild acid to a mild base, sodium monohydrogen phosphate (Na_2HPO_4).

The Protein Buffer System

Three-quarters of all the chemical buffering power of the body fluids is inside the cells and results from intracellular proteins. These proteins act as anions in the alkaline pH of the body. Existing as either acids or alkaline salts, they can operate in both acidic and basic buffering systems, binding or releasing hydrogen ions as needed.

THE RESPIRATORY SYSTEM

Carbon dioxide is constantly formed in the body by different intracellular metabolic processes. CO_2 is then transported to the lungs and exhaled. If the rate of metabolic formation of carbon dioxide increases, the concentration of carbon dioxide in ECF increases. Excretion of carbon dioxide is directly related to respiration; therefore, extracellular CO_2 *decreases* as the respiratory rate *increases*. Conversely, if the respiratory rate *decreases*, the amount of carbon dioxide in the ECF *increases*.

The respiratory center in the medulla responds when the hydrogen ion concentration increases because of the ability of carbon dioxide to combine with water to form carbonic acid:

$$H_2CO_3 \underset{\text{(carbonic anhydrase)}}{\overset{CA}{\rightleftarrows}} H_2O + CO_2$$

H_2CO_3 (carbonic acid) H_2O (water) CO_2 (carbon dioxide)

The respiratory center stimulates the respiratory system to increase the rate and depth of respiration to give off carbon dioxide. This respiratory mechanism operates *within a minute* with a 75% efficiency partially to restore the pH level.

THE RENAL SYSTEM

Normal metabolism produces an excess of acids. The kidneys compensate for this acidity by excreting acids and returning bicarbonate to the plasma and extracellular water. This process is accomplished by the following mechanisms: (1) reabsorption of bicarbonate, (2) acidification of phosphate buffer salts, and (3) secretion of ammonia.

In *acidosis*, all of these renal mechanisms are exaggerated. The excretion of acids and chloride is increased, and the absorption of bicarbonate into the plasma to correct the acidosis is increased. Conversely, in *alkalosis* these mechanisms slow or cease. Although the renal system requires more time to correct the pH than other systems (10 to 20 hours), it is more powerful, removing up to 500 mmol of acid or alkali daily.

CHANGES IN ACID–BASE BALANCE

Deficits or excesses of base bicarbonate or carbonic acid are designated as acid–base imbalances. A normal balance consists of a ratio of 1 part carbonic acid (H_2CO_3) to 20 parts bicarbonate (HCO_3^-) (1:20) (see Figure 5–5). An acid–base imbalance may occur as an increase (3:20) or a decrease (0.5:20) in carbonic acid or an increase (1:25) or decrease (1:15) in bicarbonate.

Acidosis occurs whenever a disturbance in the acid–base balance results in an increase in H^+ concentration. That is, the 1:20 ratio is altered, and the proportion of carbonic acid to bicarbonate is greater than 1:20. This can be caused by an increase in carbonic acid (ie, 2:20) or a decrease in bicarbonate (ie, 1:18) (Figure 5–6).

Alkalosis is a disturbance in acid–base balance that results in a decrease in the hydrogen ion concentration. The normal ratio of 1:20 is altered as the proportion of carbonic acid to bicarbonate changes to less than 1:20. The cause may be either a decrease in carbonic acid (ie, 0.6:20) *or* an increase in bicarbonate (ie, 1:24) (Figure 5–7). The ratio of carbonic acid to bicarbonate in the ECF determines the concentration of hydrogen ions. This balance can be altered by either a metabolic or a respiratory disorder.

Metabolic disorders affect the base bicarbonate by either adding to the base or subtracting from it. Consequently, either a *metabolic acidosis* (subtracting HCO_3^-) or *metabolic alkalosis* (adding HCO_3^-) occurs (see Figures 5–6, 5–7).

Respiratory disturbances affect carbonic acid by adding to the carbonic acid or subtracting from it. Consequently, either a *respiratory acidosis* (adding H_2CO_3) or *respiratory alkalosis* (subtracting H_2CO_3) occurs (see Figures 5–6, 5–7).

Respiratory Acidosis

Respiratory acidosis occurs whenever there is an accumulation of carbon dioxide and therefore carbonic acid due to an interference with the alveolar exchange of oxygen and carbon dioxide. This condition may develop from prolonged overbreathing of carbon dioxide; hypoventilation secondary to paralysis of the respiratory muscles—eg, poliomyelitis; upper airway obstructions due to emphysema or asthma; and depression of the medullary respiratory centers from head trauma, brain tumor, narcotic or barbiturate poisoning, or spinal cord injury.

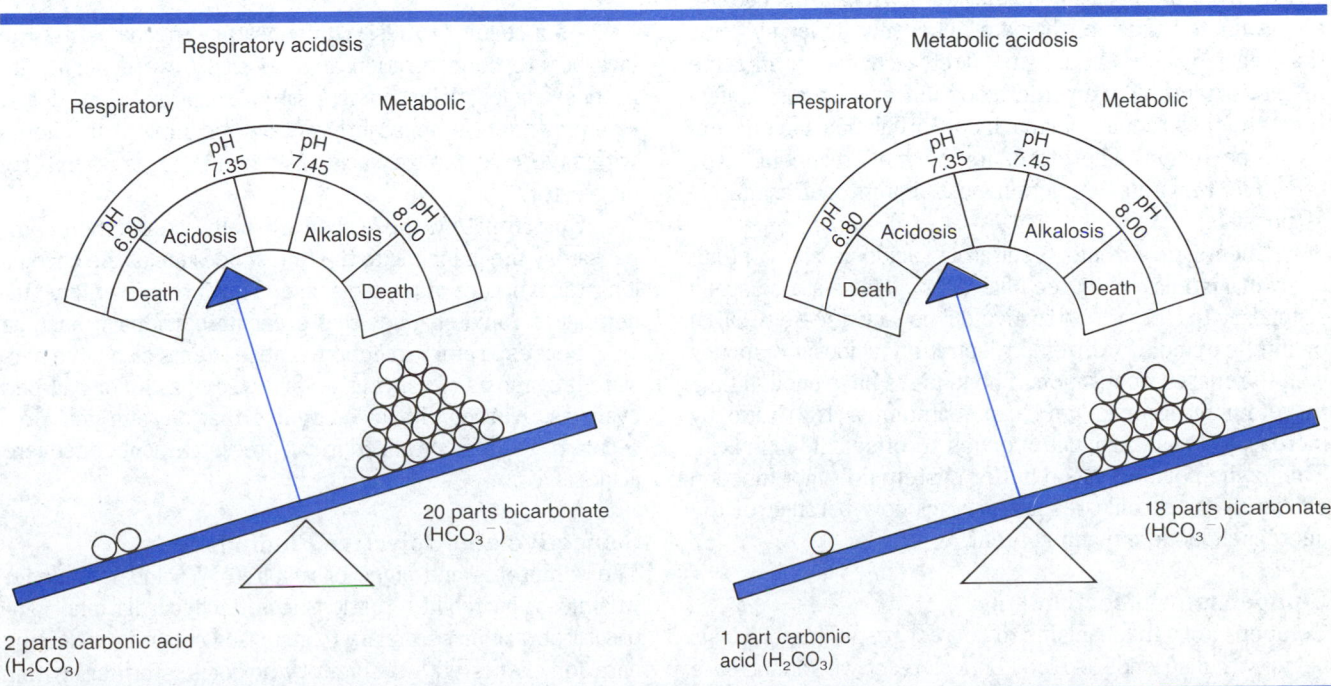

Figure 5–6

Left. Respiratory acidosis. **Right.** Metabolic acidosis.

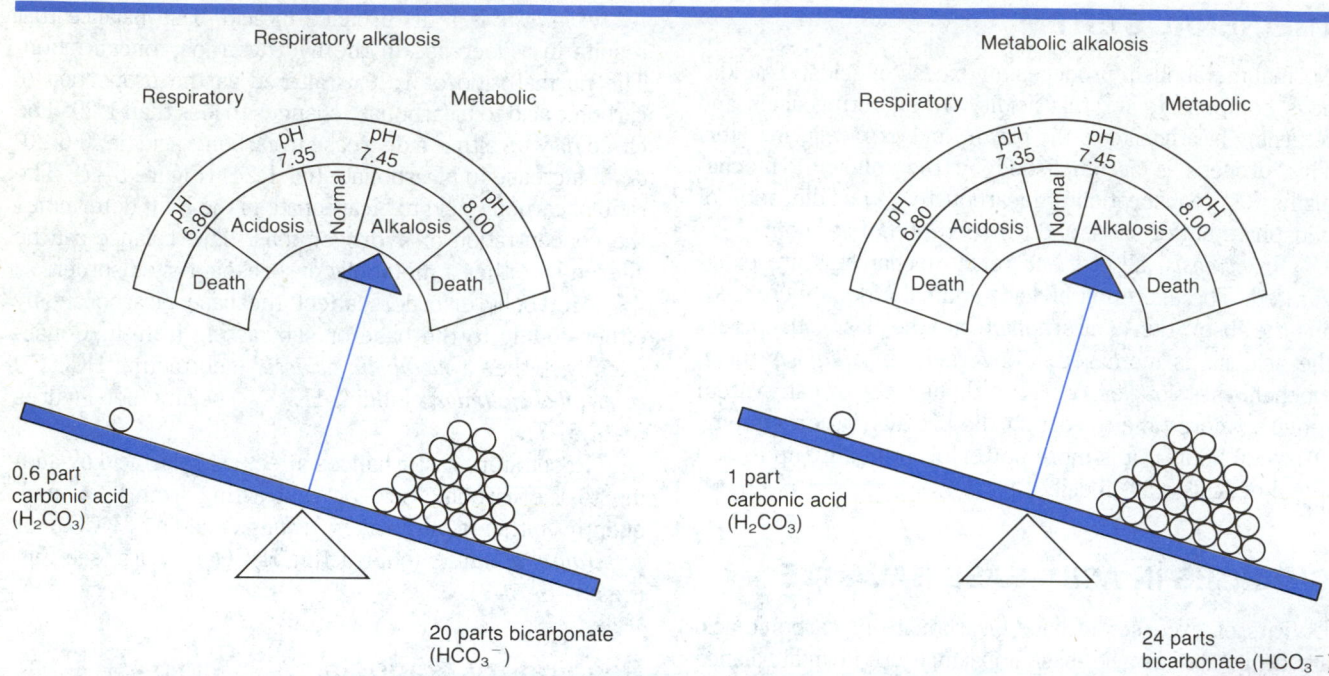

Figure 5–7

Alkalosis.

Interference with ventilation is often classified as either acute or chronic respiratory acidosis. Acute respiratory acidosis results in a severe change in an acidotic state. The most common causes include atelectasis, pneumothorax, respiratory paralysis, or drug-induced respiratory suppression.

Clients with acute respiratory acidosis do not benefit greatly from the body's compensatory mechanisms because of the limited time mechanism. The only buffer systems that react quickly enough to effect a change in an acute respiratory problem are the blood buffer systems. Unfortunately, they require normal blood circulation and efficient tissue perfusion. Therefore, for normal treatment to be effective, respiratory function must be improved as quickly as possible.

Clients in chronic respiratory acidosis are continuously in a moderate degree of acidosis. This state is usually secondary to chronic obstructive pulmonary disease (COPD) or lung carcinoma. Chronic respiratory acidosis responds well to renal compensation. The kidneys have enough time to retain bicarbonate and can maintain a 1:20 ratio by increasing the bicarbonate portion to offset the high acid. The oxyhemoglobin blood buffer system does not function efficiently in chronic respiratory acidosis because of the decreased blood oxygen content.

Compensatory Mechanisms

Compensatory mechanisms to correct respiratory acidosis begin within seconds as blood buffers react with an increase in carbon dioxide to reestablish the ratio from 2:20 to 1:20. Within hours, the kidneys attempt to excrete the hydrogen ion and compensate the acid–base imbalance through:

- Formation and excretion of the ammonium ion (NH_4)
- Retention of HCO_3^- (bicarbonate ions) and excretion of chloride (CI^-)
- A shift in electrolytes as hydrogen (H^+) and sodium ions (Na^+) move into the cells, and potassium (K^+) ions are exchanged and move from the ICF into the ECF, causing the serum potassium level to rise.

As a result of these compensatory mechanisms, the bicarbonate concentration and pH rise toward normal to produce a partially compensated respiratory acidosis. Compensation is apparently always incomplete in clients with severe respiratory acidosis when PCO_2 is 80 mm Hg or greater.

Unfortunately, these clients usually stretch their compensatory mechanisms to the fullest because of the chronic long-term nature of their disease. They are extremely vulnerable to rapid changes that precipitate acidosis, such as an upper respiratory infection. These clients also have persistent cyanosis of varying severity, seen as lip or nail-bed cyanosis. Nurses should recognize that any surgical procedure or respiratory infection can precipitate acute or severe acidosis.

Subjective and Objective Findings

The symptoms and signs of respiratory acidosis include: weakness, irritability, restlessness, tachycardia, and ventricular fibrillation secondary to increased potassium. Nursing care for clients with respiratory acidosis is critical within the first 24 to 48 hours. Providing an adequate airway and ventilation is the first priority. An endotracheal tube or tracheostomy may be needed to provide a patent airway to remove excess carbon dioxide. Suctioning is important to maintain a patent airway. Giving fluids to thin secretions, with pulmonary physiotherapy to loosen secretions, is also necessary. Postural drainage adds gravity to remove loosened mucus. Normally, increased levels of carbon dioxide stimulate the respiratory center to increase respirations and increase the inhalation of needed oxygen. In clients with chronic respiratory acidosis, sustained high levels of carbon dioxide lose their effect to stimulate the respiratory center, and an oxygen deficit is the only stimulus to breathe. The oxygen deficit is maintained by giving 1 to 2 L of oxygen per minute via cannula unless arterial blood gases and client symptoms indicate that higher levels are warranted and will be beneficial.

Respiratory Alkalosis

Respiratory alkalosis occurs when there is an excess loss of H_2CO_3 (carbonic acid) and therefore a decrease on the carbonic acid side of the carbonic acid–bicarbonate ratio. This condition is not as frequent as respiratory acidosis and is usually the result of hyperventilation secondary to hypoxia at high altitudes, encephalitis, or fever and an excessive loss of carbon dioxide. Salicylate poisoning (aspirin overdose) also causes a direct stimulus to the respiratory center and, in early stages, alkalosis. Alkalosis may also occur from rapid mechanical ventilation and hysterical hyperventilation, both of which increase the exhalation of carbon dioxide. Acute respiratory alkalosis can also be a compensatory reaction due to the sudden increase in alveolar ventilation in clients with respiratory acidosis who have a tracheostomy.

Compensatory Mechanisms

Compensatory mechanisms to restore the normal pH are carried out by the renal system. The normal excretion of acid urine by the kidneys decreases. The kidneys reduce ammonia formation (NH_4), excretion of hydrogen (H^+) and chloride (Cl^-), and no longer conserve bicarbonate (HCO_3^-). In addition, potassium moves from the extracellular water into the cells in exchange for hydrogen and sodium ions in an attempt to add acid (H^+) to the extracellular fluid. As a result of all of these changes, a compensatory metabolic acidosis develops.

Subjective and Objective Findings

The clinical picture of respiratory alkalosis includes: lightheadedness, circumoral paresthesia, numbness and tingling of the fingers and toes, tinnitus, dyspnea or air hunger, palpitations, diaphoresis, panic, muscle cramps, and/or lower abdominal pain. The signs of tetany such as carpopedal spasms also occur due to the decreased availability of calcium. As the pH rises in an alkalotic state, calcium binds to protein, and its availability for cellular functions decreases. Chvostek's and Trousseau's signs of hypocalcemia may be elicited.

Treatment is aimed at increasing the PCO_2 and

decreasing the pH. If hyperventilation is the cause, having clients breathe into a paper bag and rebreathe their own carbon dioxide may improve the symptoms.

Clients with cerebral lesions can breathe a combination of 5% carbon dioxide and 95% oxygen until the condition improves. Mechanical ventilation should be adjusted to decrease the respiratory rate and/or increase the dead space on the ventilation tubing to reduce excessive loss of CO_2.

Nursing care should center on:

- Restoring a normal respiratory breathing pattern.
- Encouraging appropriate breathing techniques.
- Providing emotional support and being alert to iatrogenic causes of respiratory alkalosis.
- Assessing for symptoms and signs of other disease processes that could be masked by respiratory alkalosis

Metabolic Acidosis

Metabolic acidosis develops because of an increased amount of acid or a decreased amount of base in the body. The normal bicarbonate-to-acid ratio of 20:1 is decreased, and the pH falls *below 7.35*.

Clients with metabolic acidosis can be divided into two categories, related to the concentration of unmeasured anions: (1) normal anion gap (delta) (*16 mEq or less*) and (2) abnormally large anion gap (*22 mEq or more*). The anion gap is determined by subtracting the values of the major anions in the ECF (HCO_3^-, Cl^-) from the values of the major cations (Na^+, K^+). Examples of a normal anion gap and an abnormal anion gap are shown in Box 5–3.

Box 5–3 Anion Gaps

Normal anion gap

$$Na^+ = 142\,mEq/L$$

$$K^+ = 4\,mEq/L$$

$$HCO_3^- = 27\,mEq/L$$

$$Cl^- = 103\,mEq/L$$

Anion gap = $(Na^+ + K^+) - (HCO_3^- + Cl^-)$

(delta) $(142 + 4) - (27 + 103)$

$146 - 130 = 16\,mEq/L$ (normal anion gap)

Abnormal anion gap

$$Na^+ = 142\,mEq/L$$

$$K^+ = 4\,mEq/L$$

$$HCO_3^- = 27\,mEq/L$$

$$Cl^- = 90\,mEq/L$$

Anion gap = $(Na^+ + K^+) - (HCO_3^- + Cl^-)$

Anion gap = $(142 + 4) - (27 + 90)$

$146 - 117 = 29\,mEq/L$ (increased anion gap)

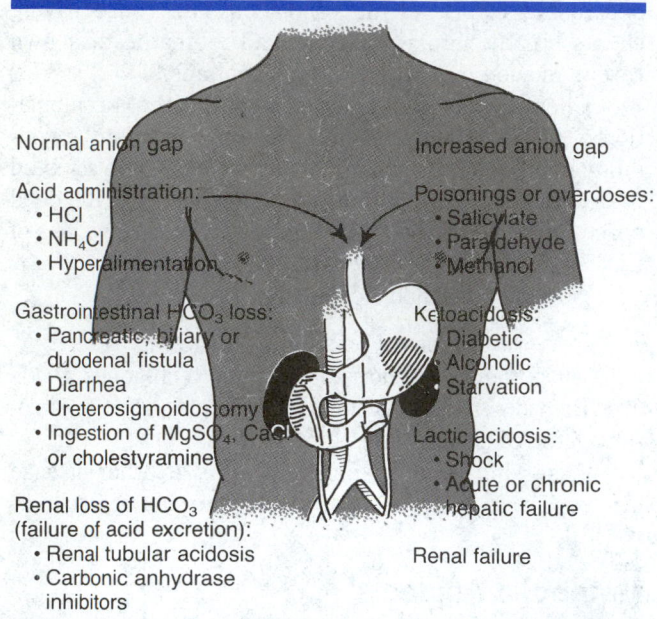

Normal anion gap

Acid administration:
• HCl
• NH₄Cl
• Hyperalimentation

Gastrointestinal HCO₃ loss:
• Pancreatic, biliary or
  duodenal fistula
• Diarrhea
• Ureterosigmoidostomy
• Ingestion of MgSO₄, CaCl₂
  or cholestyramine

Renal loss of HCO₃
(failure of acid excretion):
• Renal tubular acidosis
• Carbonic anhydrase
  inhibitors

Increased anion gap

Poisonings or overdoses:
• Salicylate
• Paraldehyde
• Methanol

Ketoacidosis:
• Diabetic
• Alcoholic
• Starvation

Lactic acidosis:
• Shock
• Acute or chronic
  hepatic failure

Renal failure

Figure 5–8

Etiologic factors in metabolic acidosis.

A metabolic acidosis in which the anion gap is normal results from inappropriate wasting of bicarbonate (as in diarrheal states) or failure of the kidney to excrete the normal endogenous acids (ie, renal tubular acidosis). In either situation, the bicarbonate concentration is reduced and replaced by an increase in the chloride (Cl^-) concentration.

In the secondary category of metabolic acidosis, the anion gap is increased or abnormal because of the circulating residual anions that are the result of the acids dissociating. These abnormal anions accumulate in lactic acidosis (lactate anions present), in diabetic ketoacidosis (unmeasured aceto-acetic acids), in salicylate poisoning (organic acid anions), and in azotemia or renal failure (phosphoric, sulfuric, and organic acid anions). See Figure 5–8 for further etiologic factors of normal and abnormal anion gap metabolic acidosis.

Compensatory Mechanisms

As the pH decreases in metabolic acidosis, the respiratory center is stimulated. Repirations increase in rate and depth in an attempt to lower carbonic acid concentration H_2CO_3 ——> $H_2O + CO_2$ (exhaled) and thereby restore the normal pH. Pulmonary compensation is usually not complete and is markedly inadequate with chronic pulmonary disease and respiratory acidosis (eg, a client with severe emphysema and in diabetic acidosis).

If the renal compensatory mechanism is operational (ie, not involved in the cause of the metabolic acidosis), the following mechanisms develop:

• Secretion and excretion of hydrogen ions increase.
• Hydrogen is excreted in the form of ammonium ions.
• The negative anion bicarbonate (HCO_3^-) is retained, and chloride (Cl^-) is excreted instead.

As a result of acidosis and the increase of hydrogen ion concentration, an electrolyte shift develops. Hydrogen and sodium move into the cells, and potassium moves into the ECF. This may cause an abnormally high potassium level in acidotic clients, leading to ventricular fibrillation and death.

The aims of treatment are to correct the metabolic disturbance and restore the electrolyte balance. In clients with diabetic acidosis, insulin is necessary to restore normal glucose metabolism and return glucose to the cells. Treatment of metabolic acidosis due to loss of intestinal fluids is aimed at restoring sodium, potassium, water, and other electrolytes through administration of intravenous fluids. As treatment progresses, potassium re-enters the cells, and hypokalemia may result. Administration of potassium chloride with monitoring of potassium levels is necessary. Correction of acidosis from renal failure requires peritoneal or hemodialysis and a low-protein, high-calorie diet.

Normally, alkalinizing solutions (sodium bicarbonate) are reserved for the seriously ill. The quickest method to overcome life-threatening acidosis is to replenish the supply of bicarbonate buffer by giving intravenous bicarbonate (1 to 3 ampules of sodium bicarbonate, with 44.6 mEq per ampule).

Subjective and Objective Findings

A mild metabolic acidosis may be asymptomatic. As the acidosis increases in severity, the client may experience weakness, malaise, or dull headache. Nausea, vomiting, and/or abdominal pain can also be present. Deep respirations (Kussmaul's breathing) are more often present in clients with acute metabolic acidosis rather than chronic metabolic acidosis. When the pH falls below 7.0, respiratory depression may occur.

The cause of the acidosis has a major effect on the client's clinical picture. Clients in diabetic acidosis may have a fruity, acetone breath odor and signs of severe water loss, eg, thirst, dry mucous membranes, and signs of sodium loss such as loss of skin turgor and shock. In addition, there are high glucose levels in the blood and urine and ketonemia (ketones in the blood and urine). Uremic clients may share these symptoms and have a fruity breath odor with signs of water or sodium loss (eg, loss of skin turgor).

Nursing care is directed toward prevention and early detection of life-threatening situations. Diabetic clients should be taught to monitor their blood glucose levels and to manage their diets and insulin correctly.

Metabolic Alkalosis

Metabolic alkalosis results from a loss of hydrogen (and chloride) ions or an excess of base bicarbonate ions.

Metabolic acidosis can occur in the following situations:

- With the excessive oral or parenteral administration of sodium bicarbonate or other alkaline salts such as sodium or potassium acetate, lactate, or citrate.

- With the excessive use of milk and antacids in ulcer treatment, producing alkalosis and severe hypercalcemia (*milk–alkali syndrome*).

- When hydrochloric acid (hydrogen ions) is lost because of vomiting and gastric suction, the bicarbonate ion passes into the bloodstream unneutralized and the pH rises, leading to alkalosis.

- Whenever excessive potassium ions are lost through diarrhea, vomiting, or diuretic therapy.

Compensatory Mechanisms

When the hydrogen ions are lost, the bicarbonate ions are retained. The bicarbonate–carbonic acid ratio increases, and the pH rises. The kidneys respond by suppressing hydrogen ion formation and ammonia formation, and they cease conservation of bicarbonate. The respiratory system responds by decreasing the rate and depth of respirations and allowing the PCO_2 to rise so a respiratory acidosis develops to compensate for the metabolic alkalosis.

The most important electrolyte shift involves the potassium and hydrogen ion exchange. With a *potassium deficit*, the hydrogen (H^+) ion, instead of the potassium (K^+) ion, is exchanged for *sodium* in the distal convoluted tubule. This exchange is an effort to preserve and increase potassium levels, thus depleting the H^+ concentration and increasing the level of bicarbonate (HCO_3^-), and promoting alkalosis. In addition, hydrogen moves into the cells so intracellular potassium (K^+) can enter the ECF to raise the potassium concentration.

Conversely, metabolic alkalosis promotes the development of potassium deficit (K^+). In alkalosis, K^+ enters the cell in exchange for H^+. In addition, K^+ rather than the hydrogen ion is exchanged for sodium in the distal tubules. Therefore, *metabolic alkalosis* causes a potassium deficit, or *hypokalemia*, and *hypokalemia* causes a reciprocal *metabolic alkalosis*.

Subjective and Objective Findings

Recognition of metabolic alkalosis strongly depends on recognition of the underlying causes of this acid–base imbalance, especially if the client also has signs of hypokalemia. Anorexia, nausea, and vomiting occur after an excessive amount of antacids has been ingested for a prolonged period. The client may have sensorium changes (eg, confusion) and be mentally unreliable. Tetany is also a common sign of metabolic and respiratory alkalosis, because tetany is caused by a lowering of the pH, which decreases the ionization of calcium.

Nursing care focuses on observation of the client's state of consciousness, restlessness, and respiratory signs. It is also important to monitor replacement of fluids in clients in alkalosis, especially potassium replacement. Because chloride is still being excreted by the kidneys and being lost in HCl through the GI tract, replacement therapy should be given using potassium chloride (KCl).

Clinical Determination of Acid–Base Balance

A client's acid–base balance can be assessed through an arterial blood gas (ABG) determination. This measurement provides specific information about the acid–base imbalance and crucial clues for early intervention. Blood gas analysis measures:

- Acidity or alkalinity, as determined by the pH.

- The partial pressure of carbon dioxide in the blood. The dissociation of H_2CO_3 (carbonic acid) forms CO_2 and H_2O. The lungs regulate CO_2 levels; therefore, an increase or decrease in CO_2 represents respiratory acid or base problems.

- The bicarbonate level in the blood, which can be plotted on a nomogram to determine levels of compensation. The bicarbonate ratio is regulated by the kidneys and is affected by metabolic acid or base disturbances.

In respiratory acidosis, the pH is low, and the PCO_2, high. Conversely, respiratory alkalosis is associated with a high pH and a low PCO_2 (Table 5–6).

Metabolic acidosis or alkalosis affects the base bicarbonate side of the 1:20 acid–base ratio. In uncompensated metabolic acidosis, the pH is low with a low base bicarbonate. Uncompensated metabolic alkalosis demonstrates an increased pH and an increased base bicarbonate (Table 5–6).

Table 5–6	Blood Gas Changes in Uncompensated Acid–Base Imbalances		
Acid–Base Imbalance	pH	HCO_3^- (Bicarbonate)	PCO_2 (Carbon Dioxide)
Respiratory acidosis	7.3 (decreased)	Normal	Increased
Respiratory alkalosis	7.5 (increased)	Normal	Decreased
Metabolic acidosis	7.3 (decreased)	Decreased	Normal
Metabolic alkalosis	7.5 (increased)	Increased	Normal

Section III: The Client in Shock

Shock is a state of widespread reduction in tissue perfusion resulting in inadequate oxygenation and nutrition of vital organs. The three major classifications of shock are shown in Box 5-4. Regardless of whether shock results from hypovolemia, myocardial damage, or altered distribution of blood volume, inadequate tissue perfusion is the common denominator in all types.

Hypovolemic Shock

Hypovolemic shock is caused by a massive loss of blood, plasma, or ECF from the intravascular compartment. Hypovolemic shock is usually caused by multiple trauma, gastrointestinal bleeding, or severe burns. The goal of care with these clients is prompt replacement of intravascular volume to reestablish perfusion of vital organs, resulting in adequate oxygenation at the cellular level.

Cardiogenic Shock

Cardiogenic shock occurs when the heart is unable to pump adequately (pump failure). The most common cause is myocardial infarction. Other etiologies include disturbances of heart rate or rhythm, trauma to the heart, rupture of the interventricular septum, pericardial tamponade, or any insult compromising the heart's ability to pump—eg, congestive heart failure. The goal of care is to maintain coronary perfusion by raising the arterial blood pressure with vasopressor drugs and adequate volume replacement.

Distributive Shock

Distributive shock is a result of abnormal distribution of blood volume due to altered vessel resistance. Neurogenic, septic, and anaphylactic shock are included in this category. In neurogenic shock, normal vasoconstrictive stimuli are lost, leading to vasodilation. Anesthesia, vasomotor center depression secondary to drug overdose, spinal cord injury, and severe pain are all possible causes. In septic and anaphylactic shock, vasodilation and increased capillary permeability occur. One goal of care in all types of distributive shock is replacement of circulating volume.

ASSESSMENT OF THE CLIENT IN SHOCK

Careful client assessment is the best way to monitor clients in shock. The common clinical manifestations of shock are in Table 5-7. Heart rate and rhythm and an estimate of arterial pressure and stroke volume are best gauged by palpation of the carotid or femoral pulses. Evaluation of skin temperature and peripheral pulses (brachial, radial, posterior tibial, and dorsalis pedis) give an estimate of cardiac output and peripheral vasoconstriction. For example, cardiac output is high if the fingers, toes, ears, and nose are warm. These structures are cold and blue with vasoconstriction and reduced cardiac output. Temperature of the great toe has been suggested as a measure of tissue perfusion. The great toe temperature is normally 82.4° F (28° C). The temperature falls to 71.6° F (22° C) with low cardiac output and raises to 96.8° F (36° C) with maximum vasodilation (Houston, Thompson, & Robertson, 1984).

Blood pressure readings are not particularly helpful in monitoring shock because of the client's markedly altered hemodynamics. True arterial pressure is usually underestimated when peripheral resistance is high. Use of vasoconstrictors in this circumstance can dangerously elevate the arterial pressure. Palpating the central arteries (carotid or femoral pulses) is a better gauge of arterial pressure, and the discrepancy between full bounding pulses and a blood pressure of 80/50 tells the nurse that the blood pressure is inaccurate.

Diminished cerebral perfusion is indicated by confusion, disorientation, restlessness, convulsions, or coma. Oliguria is evidence of reduced glomerular filtration. Mental status and urine output are extremely important parameters in evaluation of shock. Nursing diagnoses applicable to the client in shock are listed in Box 5-5.

Identifying Clients at Risk for Shock

Nurses must be fully aware of clients at risk for shock, and that risk should be emphasized in the plan of care. The health history is crucial in documenting risk factors. Has the client recently had invasive diagnostic testing of the gastrointestinal, biliary, or genitourinary tracts (eg,

---

Box 5-4   Classification of Shock

Hypovolemic shock:

- Hemorrhage secondary to trauma (accidental or surgical), GI bleeding, coagulation disorders, childbirth, carcinoma
- Plasma loss secondary to burns, dehydration, excessive diuretic use

Cardiogenic shock:

- Myocardial damage secondary to myocardial infarction, prolonged dysrhythmias, pericardial tamponade

Distributive shock (Altered distribution of blood volume):

- Neurogenic shock secondary to general or spinal anesthesia, spinal cord injury resulting in decreased peripheral resistance
- Septic shock secondary to gram-negative bacilli (and occasionally other organisms) resulting in increased capillary permeability and hypovolemia
- Anaphylactic shock secondary to antigen–antibody reaction resulting in bronchoconstriction, peripheral arteriolar dilation, and increased capillary permeability

Table 5–7 Clinical Manifestations of Shock

Organ or System	Objective Data
Skin*	Pallor, cyanosis, sweating; altered temperature of fingers, toes, ears, nose
Brain	Restlessness, disorientation, confusion, coma
Cardiovascular*	Tachycardia, ↓ BP, ↓ cardiac output, dysrhythmias, ischemic ECG changes
Pulmonary	Increased respiratory rate
Renal*	Reduced glomerular filtration, low urine output (< 30 mL/h)
Blood	Agglutination of platelets, leukocytes, and erythrocytes; sludging (red cells flowing in clumps), contributing to poor perfusion of tissues
Metabolic	Acidosis, hypoglycemia

*In septic shock, some clients go through an early phase called "warm shock" in which they have warm extremities, high or normal cardiac output, normal blood pressure, and normal urinary output; later, "cold shock" occurs with the findings in the table.

endoscopy or cystoscopy)? Has the client recently had a baby? A miscarriage? An abortion? Does the client have a known malignancy or coagulation disorder? Does the client take excessive diuretics? These clients may be at risk for hypovolemic shock.

Has the client had an MI in the past? Has the client had any previous cardiac problems such as dysrhythmias? These clients may be at risk for cardiogenic shock.

Has the client ever had an adverse reaction to drugs? To anesthesia? If the client is a menstruating woman, does she use tampons during the menses? Does she use a diaphragm or the contraceptive sponge? Is the client on immunosuppressants? These clients may be at risk for distributive shock.

Nurses caring for postoperative clients must be constantly vigilant for signs of hypovolemic shock. Nurses in coronary care units must be equally observant for signs of cardiogenic shock. Emergency room nurses should consider any client a potential candidate for shock.

Nursing Implications

Hypovolemic Shock

When the normal compensatory mechanisms following extensive fluid loss are inadequate to maintain effective tissue perfusion, hypovolemic shock occurs. Cardiac output falls, arterial blood pressure drops, and blood flow through tissues becomes inadequate to meet metabolic requirements. Tissue cells are damaged from progressive hypoxia and from the accumulation of waste products, leading to acidosis.

Shock is called reversible when the client recovers following rapid, effective treatment, such as blood transfusion. Sometimes blood pressure continues to drop in spite of vigorous efforts, the client deteriorates, and death ensues. This process is called irreversible or decompensated shock.

With multiple trauma, basic life support is the first priority. The client is placed in a horizontal position. Airway, breathing, and circulatory status are evaluated. The

client is then checked for signs of external hemorrhage. As soon as the client has a patent airway, is being ventilated with oxygen, and has a discernible pulse, attention is directed toward control of further blood loss. Intravenous lines are established, and crystalloid solutions containing electrolytes and water, such as lactated Ringer's solution, are administered until blood can be typed and cross matched. Blood transfusion is generally required when the estimated blood loss exceeds 25% of the circulating volume. Colloids containing large molecular weight molecules, such as albumin, hetastarch, or high-molecular-weight dextran, may also be used. Use of colloids in initial management of shock is somewhat controversial, although clients with burns may need them early.

Box 5–5 Nursing Diagnoses Applicable to the Client in Shock

Diagnoses directly related to shock

- *Tissue perfusion, decrease in*, related to loss of circulating volume
- *Tissue perfusion, decrease in*, related to impaired myocardial contractility
- *Tissue perfusion, decrease in*, related to altered distribution of blood volume
- *Gas exchange, impaired*, related to ventilation/perfusion imbalance
- *Urinary elimination, decrease in*, related to impaired renal perfusion
- *Thought processes, alteration in*, related to impaired cerebral perfusion

Additional potential nursing diagnoses

- *Anxiety*, related to change in health status
- *Powerlessness*, due to illness-related regimen
- *Comfort, alteration in*
- *Injury, potential for*, related to invasive treatment

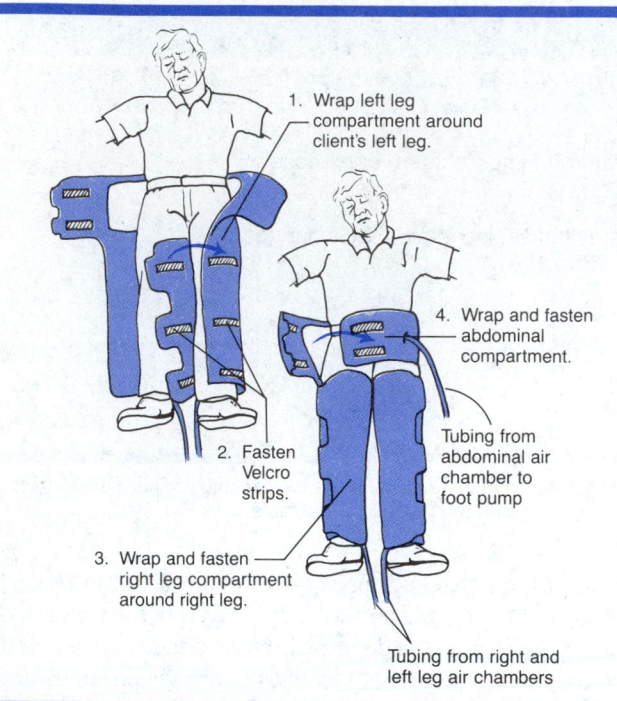

1. Wrap left leg compartment around client's left leg.

2. Fasten Velcro strips.

3. Wrap and fasten right leg compartment around right leg.

4. Wrap and fasten abdominal compartment.

Tubing from abdominal air chamber to foot pump

Tubing from right and left leg air chambers

Figure 5–9

Antishock trousers.

Volume replacement and cardiac function are monitored by central venous pressure (CVP) or pulmonary artery occlusive pressure measurement. The CVP line is placed by threading a long polyethylene catheter into the superior or inferior vena cava. The catheter tip is located at the junction of the vena cava and right atrium. The CVP reflects the pressure in the right atrium and systemic veins but does not reliably reflect left ventricular pressures.

Pulmonary artery wedge pressure approximates left ventricular pressure. A flow-directed, balloon-tipped catheter (eg, Swan–Ganz catheter) is placed similar to a CVP line but is advanced through the right heart to wedge into a branch of the pulmonary artery. This pressure reflects left atrial pressure and thus, left ventricular pressure, if there are no mitral valve problems. Using the CVP or pulmonary artery wedge pressure, a fairly accurate assessment can be made of volume depletion, volume overload, and myocardial function, helping to determine the need for additional volume replacement or cardiac support drugs.

Antishock trousers (Figure 5–9) provide for rapid treatment of hypovolemic shock in emergencies. The trousers were developed for use with military casualties and are now being used in emergency departments with some success. Sometimes called a MAST (military antishock trouser) suit, the inflatable nylon garment is applied from below the 12th rib to the ankles to compress bleeding sites in the pelvis and extremities. The feet are exposed so circulation can be monitored. Box 5–6 lists indications for use of antishock trousers.

Pulmonary edema is an absolute contraindication to use of antishock trousers. Other possible contraindications include pregnancy, increased intracranial pressure, decreased ventilation, pneumothorax, and cardiac tamponade.

When the client is stabilized, antishock trousers may be removed by gradual deflation, beginning with the abdominal compartment. Blood pressure measurement guides the rate of deflation. Shock, dysrhythmia, and death can occur with too rapid removal of the MAST suit.

Other approaches to management of hypovolemic clients include continuous ECG monitoring to alert care providers to impending dangerous dysrhythmias, insertion of an in-dwelling catheter to measure hourly urine output for assessment of renal perfusion, and arterial blood gases, especially if oxygen or ventilatory therapy is needed.

Cardiogenic Shock

Myocardial infarction is the most common cause of cardiogenic shock. With MI, the infarcted area is nonfunctional, and the surrounding area may only contract weakly. The resultant poor cardiac pump activity and decreased cardiac output are reflected by hypotension, diaphoresis, clammy skin, reduced urinary output, and altered levels of consciousness. Cardiogenic shock is the most lethal variety of shock.

Basic management is similar to care in hypovolemic shock—establishment of an airway, ventilation, oxygenation, correction of acidosis, and pain relief. Another major treatment objective in cardiogenic shock is increasing cardiac output. Output is increased by increasing the cardiac preload (the volume in the ventricle just prior to systole), improving myocardial contraction with drugs, and lowering the afterload against which the heart must pump (blood pressure and vascular system).

Volume expansion with colloids, use of antishock trousers, or leg elevation will increase the preload, which results

---

Box 5–6   Indications for Antishock Trousers

Hypovolemic shock:

- Trauma
- GI hemorrhage
- Ruptured spleen
- Leaking aortic aneurysm
- Postpartum hemorrhage
- Ruptured ectopic pregnancy
- Postoperative shock
- Hemorrhage in the lower extremities

Stabilization of fractures of the pelvis or lower extremities

May aid in venous access for IV lines in the upper extremities by increasing venous pressure

in an amplification of left ventricular stroke work. CVP or pulmonary artery wedge pressure measurement are necessary to guide fluid management to avoid the complication of pulmonary edema. Myocardial contractility can be improved with drugs such as dopamine (Intropin), dobutamine (Dobutrex), isoproterenol (Isuprel), or digitalis.

Coronary artery perfusion can be improved using the intra-aortic balloon pump, which is inserted into the descending aorta via the femoral artery. The balloon inflates during diastole and deflates during systole. Because the coronary arteries are filled during diastole, the inflated balloon increases diastolic filling and coronary blood flow while decreasing afterload and the work of the heart. Vasodilators may also be used to reduce afterload by decreasing peripheral vascular impedance.

Distributive Shock

Neurogenic Shock. Neurogenic shock occurs with a loss of vasomotor influences from the medulla, resulting in peripheral vasodilation. Circulating blood volume is sequestered in the capillary system, and blood pressure falls. Venous return to the heart is decreased, leading to reduced cardiac output that is inadequate to maintain tissue perfusion. Brain damage, spinal cord injury, severe pain, drugs, and general or spinal anesthesia may cause neurogenic shock. Fainting is considered a transient form of neurogenic shock.

Nursing care is directed toward maintaining the client in a supine position and administering IV fluids to restore normal blood pressure. Other nursing activities involve specific client care related to the cause of shock, eg, spinal cord injury or postoperative sequelae.

Septic Shock. Septic shock is usually associated with gram-negative bacteremia, although gram-positive bacilli and viruses can also be the cause. It is unclear whether the bacteria themselves or the toxins released by the bacteria are the causative factor in septic shock.

Clients most susceptible to septic shock are those with indwelling catheters, venous and arterial cannulation, postpartum infection, peritonitis, burns, or immunosuppression. Any client having instrumentation or surgery of the genitourinary, gastrointestinal, or biliary tracts is also at risk. Toxic shock syndrome (TSS) is septic shock secondary to use of tampons or the vaginal contraceptive sponge. Nasal packing can also cause TSS.

Prevention of infection is a major nursing responsibility. Clients who are to give themselves injections or change their own dressings at home must be taught good sterile technique. Women should be cautioned to avoid superabsorbent tampons and to change all tampons frequently. Vaginal contraceptive sponges and diaphragms should not be left in longer than eight hours after intercourse.

Nurses working on burn units, in the operating room, on the IV team, in the cystoscopy laboratory, in the coronary care and intensive care units, and anywhere injec-

tions are given, blood is drawn, and dressings are changed must be impeccable in their use of asepsis and vigilant about breaks in technique. Hand-washing for both client and care provider is basic to maintaining a safe environment. Overuse of antibiotics in illness care has resulted in drug-resistant bacterial strains, particularly in the hospital. As a result, hospital-acquired (nosocomial) infections are more difficult to treat.

Before beginning antibiotic treatment, obtain all needed specimens and send them for culture. Culture specimens may include blood, urine, sputum, cerebrospinal fluid, or purulent aspirates or drainage. Antibiotics are then selected and started according to the suspected microorganism, the source of the organism, the site of the infection, and the underlying disease of the client. Antibiotics are generally given intravenously because decreased perfusion makes the intramuscular and oral routes less reliable. It is difficult for antibiotics to penetrate an area that is sealed off, such as an abscess. Surgical incision and drainage of abscesses are essential to remove the septic focus.

Anaphylactic Shock. Anaphylactic shock is a life-threatening immediate hypersensitivity response of a previously sensitized person to an antigen—a foreign protein or drug. The response is caused by a damaging antigen–antibody reaction occurring on the surface of certain cells, which causes histamine, slow-reacting substance of anaphylaxis (SRS-A), and other mediators to be released. IgE antibodies predominate in the anaphylactic response.

Within seconds to minutes after introduction of the antigen, bronchospasm may occur, causing respiratory distress and hypoxemia. Urticaria, a cutaneous eruption of well-circumscribed, intensely pruritic wheals with erythematous raised borders and blanched centers, may appear. These wheals (also known as hives) can coalesce into localized or well-distributed giant wheals.

Angioedema, edema of the subcutaneous tissue and mucous membranes, may also occur, possible leading to mechanical obstruction of the epiglottis and larynx. Widespread vasodilation results in hypotension, circulatory insufficiency, lowered cardiac output, and decreased perfusion of the brain and coronary arteries. Death results from asphyxiation or circulatory failure. Table 5–8 summarizes the subjective and objective findings in anaphylaxis.

The major causes of systemic anaphylaxis are injections of therapeutic drugs, diagnostic contrast media, and insect stings. Penicillin is perhaps the most common drug implicated, although many drugs—even vitamins—are capable of eliciting a systemic anaphylactic reaction.

Early recognition of an anaphylactic reaction is essential. Urticaria and pruritus can be controlled with subcutaneous injection of 0.2 to 0.5 mL of 1:1000 epinephrine, which can be repeated at 3-minute intervals in the event of a severe reaction. If the reaction was secondary to an insect sting or drug injection, a tourniquet applied proximal to the site of injection may reduce absorption of the antigenic material. When an insect stinger remains, it should

Table 5–8	Anaphylaxis: Subjective and Objective Data	
Subjective Data	**Objective Data**	
Pruritus	Skin eruptions: Wheals, giant wheals	
Sensation of a lump in the throat	Localized skin edema of face, neck, hands	
Shortness of breath, tightness in chest	Dyspnea, wheezing, cough, laryngeal stridor, hoarseness, cyanosis	
Abdominal cramps, nausea	Diarrhea, vomiting	
Extreme apprehension	Rapid weak pulse, drop in blood pressure	

Table 5–9	Diagnostic Studies for Clients in Shock to Monitor Potential Physiological Dysfunctions	
Diagnostic Study	**Physiological Dysfunction**	
Central venous pressure (CVP) Pulmonary artery wedge pressure Intra-arterial blood pressure Hematocrit, electrolytes	Volume depletion or volume overload	
ECG, CVP, pulmonary artery wedge pressure, intra-arterial pressure	Altered cardiac function	
Creatinine, BUN, urinalysis	Altered renal function	
Arterial blood gases (ABG)	Altered acid–base balance	
Blood lactate levels	Altered cellular metabolism	
White blood cell count and differential; blood cultures	Sepsis	
Coagulation studies	Disseminated intravascular coagulation (DIC)	

be removed without compression. Epinephrine 0.2 mL is administered into the sting or injection site.

When the reaction takes place in a clinical setting, in addition to the previous treatment, an IV is started to provide a route for IV administration of epinephrine if needed as well as for volume expanders and vasopressors, if extreme hypotension occurs. Oxygen is administered, and endotracheal intubation or tracheostomy may be necessary. Additional possible therapeutic agents include diphenhydramine for urticaria and angioedema and aminophylline for bronchospasm.

Individuals with a known hypersensitivity should wear a Medic-Alert bracelet and have an emergency kit on hand for self-administration of epinephrine. Persons with allergy to insect stings should always carry epinephrine during seasons when contact with insects is possible.

Diagnostic Studies

Table 5–9 provides an overview of some diagnostic studies useful in evaluating the possible physiological alterations in shock. Many of these studies are invasive, involving inserting a venous or arterial line for client monitoring. The client's already tenuous situation may be aggravated by complications from the tests. The nurse must be alert for the possibility of thrombus formation, embolism, hemorrhage, dysrhythmia, or infection.

Complications of Prolonged Shock

Shock lung, or adult respiratory distress syndrome (ARDS), is a serious pulmonary complication that may follow shock from all causes. Initially, there seems to be an increased permeability of the alveolar capillaries to plasma proteins with development of interstitial edema. Tracheobronchial secretions, tachypnea, and cyanosis increase. As the condition progresses, arterial blood gases show a decreasing PaO_2 and an increasing $PaCO_2$. Later, atelectasis, microthrombosis, hemorrhage, and fibrosis occur.

Acute tubular necrosis (ATN) is another possible complication from any type of shock. ATN results from destruction of tubular epithelial cells secondary to impaired perfusion, which can lead to renal failure and death.

Disseminated intravascular coagulation (DIC) is a serious complication of septic shock. Stasis of blood in capillary beds leads to uncontrolled microcirculatory clotting with widespread organ ischemia and necrosis.

Section IV: Understanding and Caring for the Client in Pain

Pain is a universal experience. Everyone has known pain to some degree. Pain is often a useful protective signal because it is a warning of potential health problems, eg, the dysuria caused by a bladder infection or the earache of otitis media. Pain is also a consequence of some normal bodily functions (eg, mild dysmenorrhea or the pain of childbirth). Pain can also warn of emotional or stress-related problems (eg, the headache, gastritis, or low-back pain caused by tension, anxiety, or the stress of daily living).

Pain is a totally subjective personal experience. No one can fully appreciate the pain of another. No two persons feel the same degree of pain in the same way. Pain is a complex perceptual phenomenon. There is no direct relation between pain stimulus and individual response.

Fortunately for most, pain is transitory. Often cuts and bruises, a fleeting gas pain, discomfort following sports activity, or a few days of postoperative pain are the only identification with the pain experience. Consider what it must be like to have persistent, unrelenting, immobilizing chronic pain. Every day is disrupted, and lives are crippled, controlled by the fine balance between activity and pain exacerbation.

Despite the universality of pain, much is still unknown about what actually causes a sensation to be perceived as painful. The reappraisal of theories of pain by Melzack and Wall in 1965 stimulated great interest in pain research. The following brief review of pain physiology and pain theories provides a background for caring for the client in pain.

PATHWAYS OF PAIN

Pain signals in peripheral nerves are transmitted by small-diameter, thinly myelinated A-delta fibers and unmyelinated C fibers. The A-delta fibers are slightly larger and transmit information rapidly, whereas C fibers have a slow conducting velocity. Pain produced by A-delta fibers is a sharp, well-localized pricking pain called **epicritic** (discriminating) pain. C fiber pain is a slower, diffuse, burning or aching pain that is poorly localized. It is called **protopathic** (undiscriminating) pain.

Sensory nerve fibers enter the spinal cord via the dorsal root of a spinal nerve. They synapse in the substantia gelatinosa, a functional unit of densely packed cells that extends the length of the spinal cord. The substantia gelatinosa is located in the dorsal horns on either side of the cord (Figure 5–10). The impulses cross over and ascend

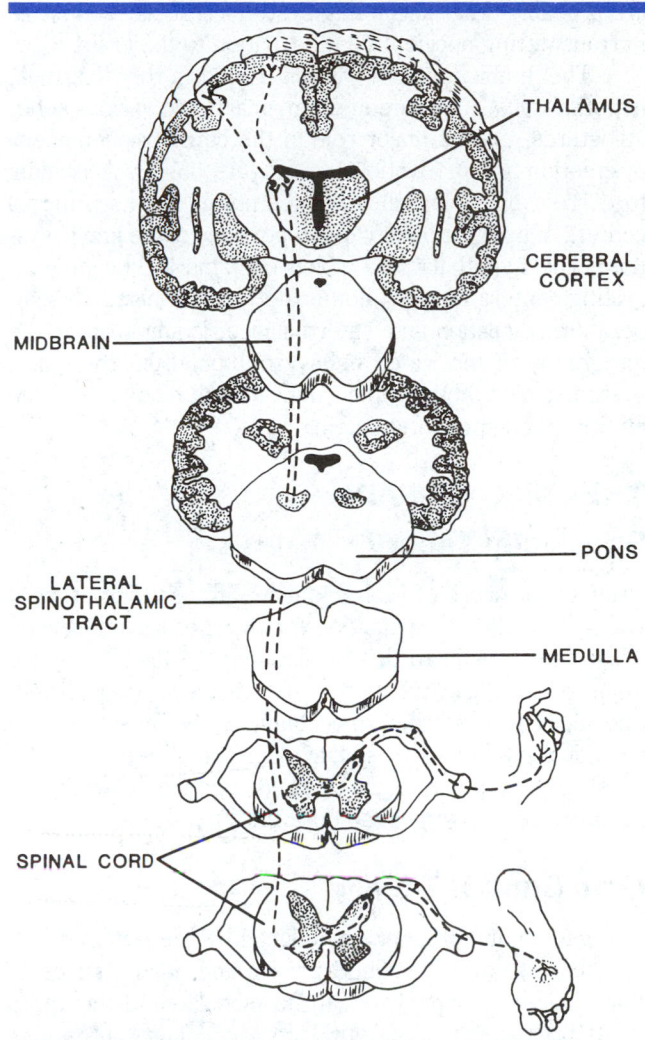

Figure 5–11

Sensory pathways for pain and temperature within the lateral spinothalamic tracts.
SOURCE: Vick RL: *Contemporary Medical Physiology*. Menlo Park, CA: Addison–Wesley, 1984, p. 75.

contralaterally in the lateral spinothalamic tracts to the thalamus and then move on to the cerebral cortex (Figure 5–11). The sensations of pain and temperature ascend the spinal cord in the same fiber tracts.

Previously, it was thought that **nociceptive impulses**, impulses giving rise to sensations of pain, were transmitted straight through to the brain without modulation. It is now known, however, that pain can be inhibited all along the course of transmission. The dorsal horn has been found to be a complex structure anatomically, physiologically, and biochemically. Its synaptic arrangements permit reception and transmission as well as local integration and selection.

Although the spinothalamic tract has been considered the specific pain and temperature tract, there is evidence that it may have other functions as well. In addition, there

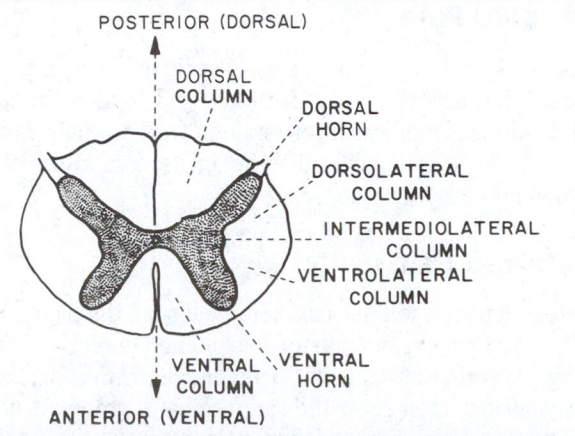

Figure 5–10

Cross-section of spinal cord showing major divisions. Shaded area represents gray matter, which contains cell bodies and unmyelinated fibers. Unshaded portions represent white matter, which consists of ascending and descending myelinated fibers.
SOURCE: Vick RL: *Contemporary Medical Physiology*. Menlo Park, CA: Addison–Wesley, 1984, p. 73.

are probably other ascending systems that play some role in transmitting nociceptive information to the brain.

The limbic system, which includes the thalamus, hypothalamus, hypocampus, amygdala, and various other structures, plays a major role in the complex phenomena of emotion and motivation (see Figure 35–3). According to current physiological theory, emotion has its principal centers of integration in various portions of the limbic system. The hypothalamus, which contains the major integrating centers for such homeostatic mechanisms as temperature regulation and water balance, is important in the integration of motivated behavior. Input from the limbic system is also thought to account for the motivational and emotional components of pain.

THEORIES OF PAIN
Specificity Theory

Prior to the work of Melzack and Wall, specificity theory was the accepted explanation for the mechanism of pain. This theory assumed that the intensity of the nociceptive impulse and the perception of pain were directly related. Specificity theory failed to account for the broad range of individual responses to similar pain stimuli (eg, why two persons undergoing uncomplicated appendectomy experience postoperative pain so differently).

Gate Control Theory

The gate control theory, introduced by Melzack and Wall and subsequently modified by them and others, suggests that nociceptive impulses can be modulated in the spinal cord, brainstem, or cerebral cortex. These authorities postulate that neural mechanisms in the substantia gelatinosa in the dorsal horns act as a gate that can increase or decrease the flow of nerve impulses from peripheral fibers to the spinal cord cells that transmit these impulses to the brain.

A few brief clinical applications of the theory may more fully explain its usefulness. The theory suggests that activity in large-diameter nerve fibers closes the gate and decreases or eliminates the pain. Transcutaneous electrical nerve stimulation (TENS), in which electrodes are applied to the skin, has been used for pain relief with some success. TENS is thought to stimulate the large rapid-velocity fibers, which effectively closes the gate. Reducing clients' anxiety also often reduces their pain. It is thought that inhibiting impulses from the cerebral cortex and thalamus closes the gate. Analgesic drugs act on the central nervous system, essentially reducing or abolishing the integration of the pain experience.

Although the gate control hypothesis may only partially explain the pain phenomenon, this theory has made major contributions to the understanding and treatment of pain. The concept of a gate mechanism is a scientific explanation for the uniqueness of each pain experience and the multidimensional influences on that experience.

Endorphins and Enkephalins

The discovery of the endorphin system in the mid-1970s added an entire new dimension to pain research. Endorphins, literally meaning the "morphine within," are opioid-like substances in the brain, spinal cord, and gastrointestinal tract. The endorphins apparently combine with specific receptors to produce analgesic activity similar to that of the drug morphine.

Enkephalins, part of the endorphin system, are central nervous system neurotransmitters that mediate the transmission of pain information. Enkephalins may inhibit the release of substance P, a peptide released in the dorsal horn with nociceptive stimulation. Substance P seems to function as a sensory neurotransmitter for relay of pain signals.

Stress and pain both activate the endorphin system. Endorphin release is also thought to accompany other pain-relief measures such as acupuncture and TENS. Naloxone, an opiate antagonist drug, has been found to reverse the analgesic effects of the endorphins.

PAIN AS DEFINED BY THE HEALTH PROFESSIONAL
Acute Pain

Acute pain is usually of rapid onset, varies in intensity from mild to severe, is self-limiting, and is of less than 6 months' duration. Common examples of acute pain are dental pain, postsurgical or postpartum pain, and pain from injury or infection. Acute pain is usually successfully treated with analgesic medications or hypnosis, or it may require no specific intervention. If tissue damage was the cause of pain, pain declines steadily as the tissue heals.

Chronic Pain

Chronic pain is an ongoing pain experience of 6 months or longer that fails to resolve naturally and does not respond to traditional medical intervention. Chronic pain is now thought to be a specific disease in its own right rather than a symptom of disease.

Referred Pain

Referred pain is felt in a part removed from the pain's point of origin. One explanation for this phenomenon is that sensory neurons that transmit pain signals from a particular body surface area enter the same spinal segment as nerve fibers from the diseased internal organ. The ascending neurons carry pain signals to the brain from both locations. Because cutaneous pain is more common than visceral pain, the brain interprets the pain as originating in the skin. Many conditions are diagnosed by the pattern of referred pain. For example, pain radiating into the left shoulder and down the left arm is associated with myocardial infarction. For common skin sites of visceral referred pain see Figure 5–12.

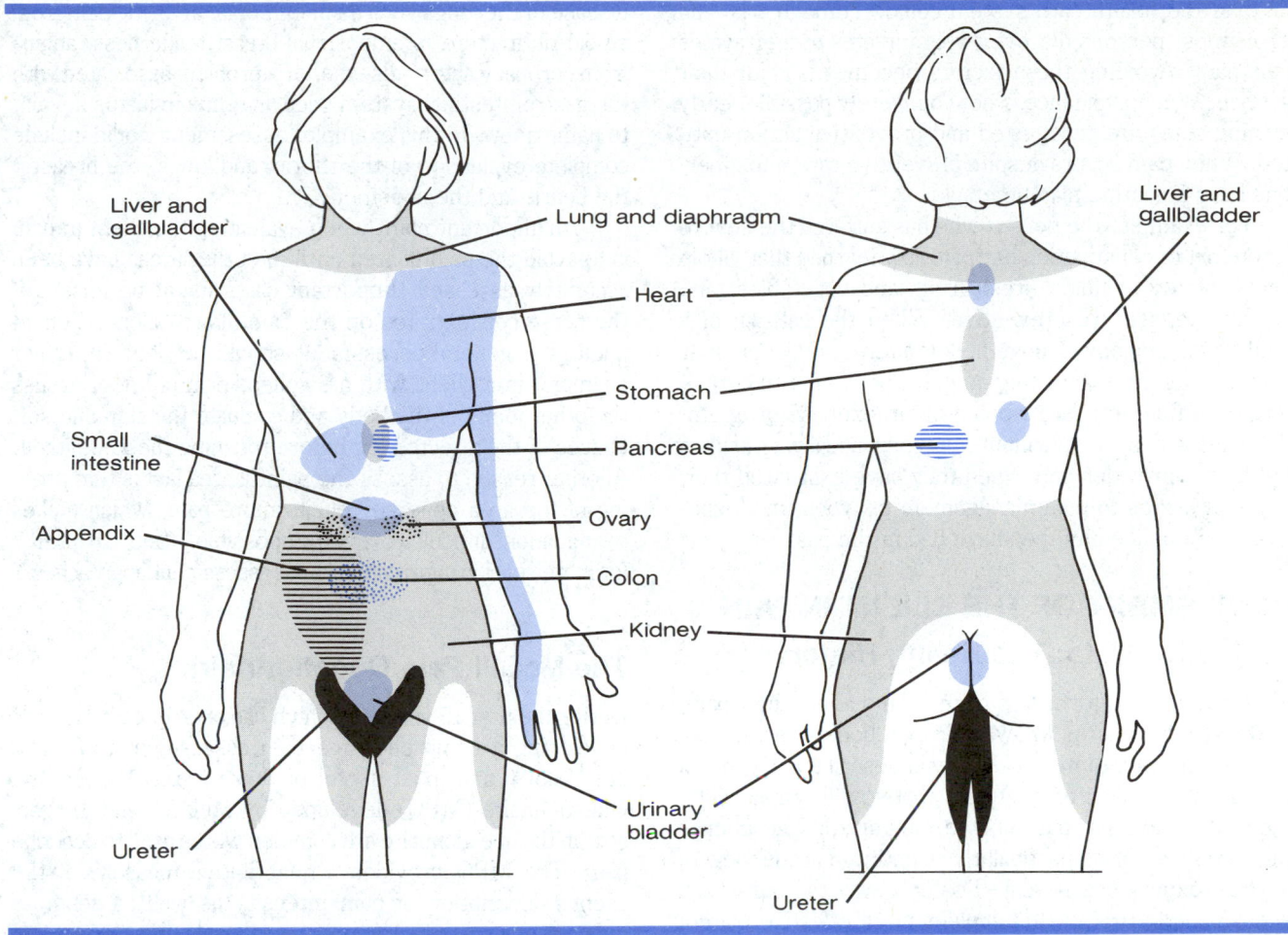

Figure 5–12

Cutaneous areas to which pain from certain viscera is referred.
SOURCE: Spence AP, Mason EB: *Human Anatomy and Physiology*, 2nd ed. Menlo Park, CA: Addison–Wesley, 1983, p. 345.

Phantom Pain

Phantom pain is a sensation in a body part that has been amputated. Even though the nerves supplying the amputated part were severed, the remaining neurons may continue to send impulses to the same area of the brain as before. Some time may elapse before the brain stops interpreting impulses from the severed neurons as if the part were still present.

PAIN AS EXPRESSED AND ACTED ON BY CLIENTS

Persons in pain react in a wide variety of ways. Some attempt to keep their pain hidden and say nothing. Others verbally express their discomfort using descriptive words and phrases. Sometimes body language tells the story. How individuals express their pain and attempt to deal with it depends on a myriad of factors including family tradition and upbringing, culture, religion, previous pain experience, bodily part involved, and beliefs about health and illness—to name a few.

Approaches to pain relief are highly individual. The use by North Americans of over-the-counter (OTC) analgesics containing acetylsalicylic acid, acetaminophen, or ibuprofen has spawned a multimillion dollar drug industry geared toward relief of common human discomforts. Think for a moment about how persons learn to deal with aches and pains when growing up. Perhaps they are told to "grin and bear it," to take two aspirin and go to bed, or to use ice or heat. Perhaps a child is given a piece of candy or distracted when complaining of a minor discomfort. More severe pain may be dealt with in the same way, or perhaps a physician is called or the person is taken immediately to the emergency room. Perhaps a knowledgeable neighbor, a grandmother, a nurse in the family, or a healer associated with the cultural or religious beliefs of the family is consulted. If the treatment suggested by the consultant is not effective, further information probably is gathered until an effective approach is found, or the pain goes away by itself.

Most adults, having developed their own approach to pain management from childhood and having lived with their unique aches and pains for some time (eg, tension headaches, tennis elbow), self-treat these discomforts better than the health care system could. Through trial and error, most persons discover what initiates or aggravates their pain. Avoiding these factors becomes part of their lifestyle. When avoidance is not completely possible, early warning signs are recognized and preventive action initiated. When pain occurs despite preventive care, most persons have a routine plan of attack.

For example, the person who has suffered the severe discomfort of constipation has probably learned that whole grains, plenty of fluids, fresh fruits and vegetables, and regular exercise are preventive. When the pattern of a regular morning bowel movement is altered, the client may initiate action such as eating an extra bowl of bran cereal, increasing fluid intake, stepping up an exercise program, or taking a dose of psyllium. Persons usually consult a health care provider only when they have exhausted their own approaches to pain management or when they experience pain unlike any they have had in the past.

ASSESSMENT OF THE CLIENT IN PAIN

Subjective Data: The Health History

When gathering information from clients about their pain, appreciate that clients know their own bodies better than anyone else. Sometimes a client will describe a pattern of pain or an approach to treatment that sounds implausible. These descriptions must not be minimized. The client's language may not be particularly scientific, but the view of the pain experience is real. The only way the nurse can assess pain accurately and implement an effective plan of care is to understand fully each client's pain experience.

The history should include questions about factors that *provoke* or *palliate* the pain, the *quality* of the pain, the *region* of the body involved, and the *severity* and *timing* of the pain—the PQRST of pain evaluation (see Chapter 7). The history should also attempt to describe any cultural, familial, or religious influences on the client's feelings and beliefs about pain. There may also be specific cultural or religious approaches to managing pain or limitations on types of treatment. Information about previous pain experiences and previous encounters with the health care system are helpful to discuss and document.

Objective Data: Physical Assessment

While taking the health history, especially observe the client's facial expression and body language. Is the client extremely restless or lying rigid in bed? Does the client clutch at or massage a particular body region? Does the client maintain a certain position or pace the floor? What is the skin color? Is diaphoresis present? Are the respirations rapid or shallow? Before beginning a physical examination, obtain as much data as possible by observing the client during history taking.

Specific physical assessment depends on the bodily system involved, although in many instances, this is not known. For example, a client with chest pain could have a

disease of the lungs such as pneumonia, arthritic pain from an old rib fracture, premenstrual breast tenderness, angina from coronary artery disease, or a problem associated with the gastrointestinal system such as reflux in hiatus hernia, to name a few. In this example, assessment would include complete evaluation of the thorax and lungs, the breasts, the heart, and the abdomen.

An important point when evaluating the client in pain is to avoid the painful area until the other areas have been accurately assessed. Important clues might be missed if the nurse concentrates on the painful area alone. Consequently, a general assessment should be done first. For example, in a client with a swollen, painful knee, assess the other joints of the body and evaluate the skin and soft tissues of the affected leg before touching the knee itself. Another reason to assess the painful area last is that probing of the area generally elicits more pain, which makes examination difficult or even impossible. (See Chapter 7 for more specific information about assessment approaches.)

The McGill Pain Questionnaire

During the past 15 years, research has been directed toward developing a comprehensive pain assessment tool. The best known and most useful of these is the McGill Pain Questionnaire (MPQ) developed by Melzack and Torgerson. In the questionnaire are common words used to describe pain. The MPQ provides a quantitative measure of the client's description of pain intensity as well as separate indexes of sensory, affective, and evaluative aspects of pain (Figure 5–13).

The MPQ has been used as a diagnostic tool as well as for assessment of pain relief. Studies using the MPQ have found that the words clients use in describing their pain, particularly the affective terms, provide an expedient approach to measurement of the subjective pain experience. The MPQ has several components:

- Pain rating index (PRI): The 20 groups of words in Figure 5–13A that describe pain quality; these words are divided into three categories of pain—sensory (S), affective (A), and evaluative (E) (Figure 5–13B).

- Present pain intensity (PPI): The client selects one word from a group of five that best describes the intensity of pain; the values range from 1 (mild) to 5 (excruciating), as shown in Figure 5–13A.

- Line drawings of the body: The client attempts to pinpoint the painful area and state whether the pain is external (E), internal (I), brief, intermittent, or constant (Figure 5–13A).

A tool such as the MPQ can assist both the nurse and the client to compare the pain experience before and after pain-relieving approaches. The tool can be used with clients who have acute pain as well as for those with long-term chronic pain.

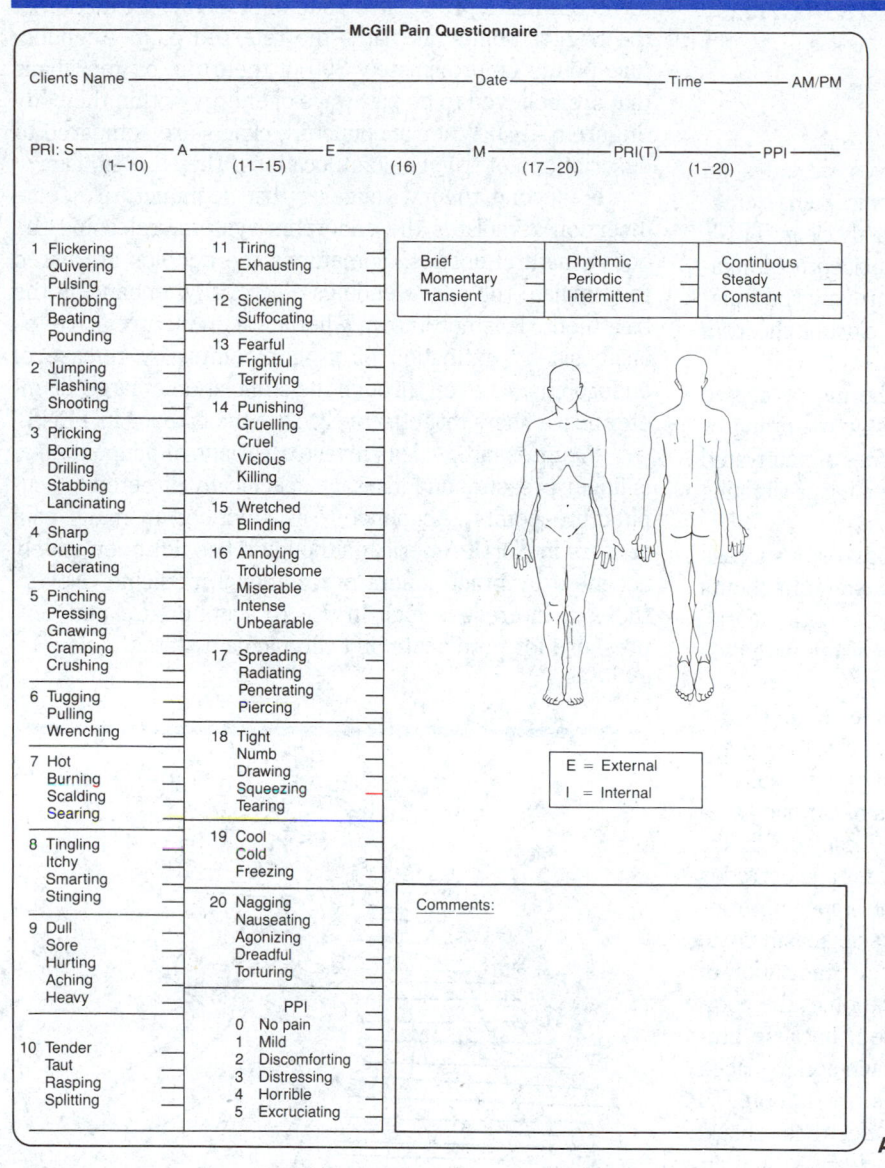

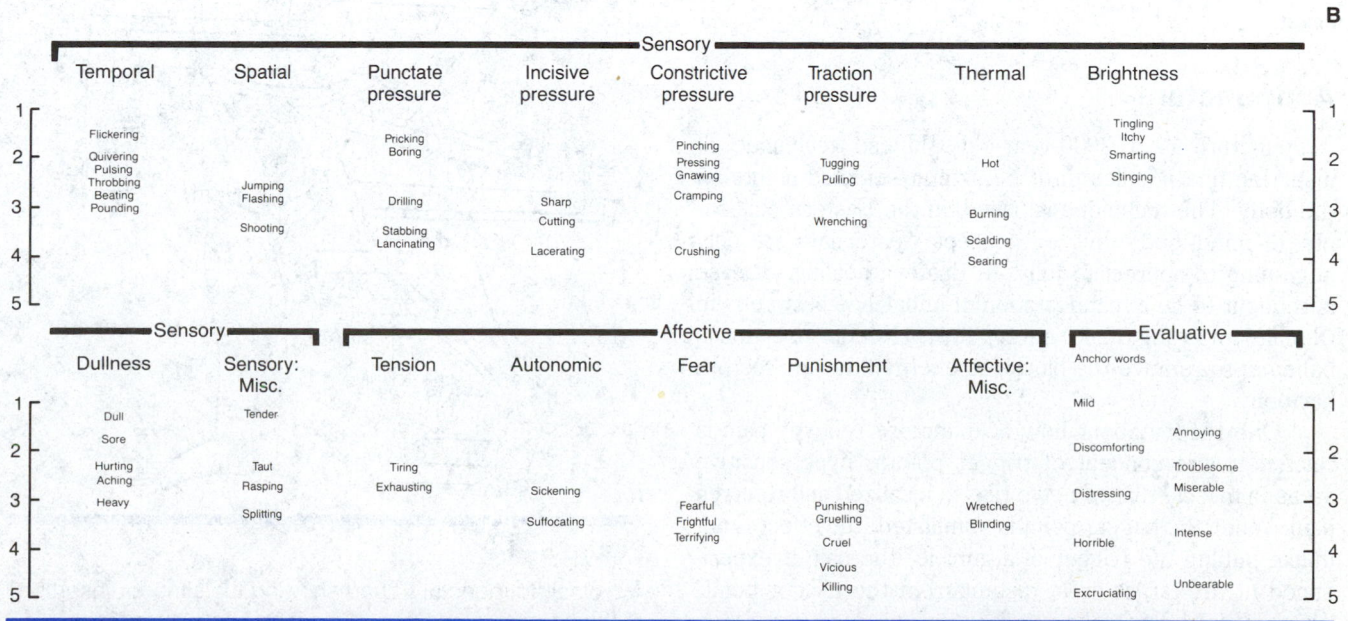

Figure 5–13

A. McGill pain questionnaire. The descriptors fall into four major groups: sensory, 1 to 10; affective, 11 to 15; evaluative, 16; and miscellaneous, 17 to 20. The rank value for each descriptor is based on its position in the word set. The sum of the rank values is the pain rating index (PRI). The present pain intensity (PPI) is based on a scale of 0 to 5. **B.** Spatial display of pain descriptors based on intensity ratings by clients. The intensity scale values range from 1 (mild) to 5 (excruciating).

SOURCE: A and B reprinted with permission from: Melzack R: *Pain Measurement and Assessment.* New York: Raven, 1983.

NONPHARMACOLOGICAL APPROACHES TO PAIN MANAGEMENT

Transcutaneous Electrical Nerve Stimulation

Electrical stimulation of peripheral nerves provides an analgesic effect in both acute and chronic pain states. Although the mechanism of action is not exactly clear, TENS is thought to modify the transmission of nociceptive impulses in the central nervous system by improving the function of the large-diameter nerve fibers, closing the pain gate.

Flexible electrodes that are self-adhering or coated with a conductive gel are applied to the skin overlying or proximal to the painful region. The electrodes are activated by a battery-operated device to produce a tingling or vibrating sensation in the painful area.

TENS has been used with varying degrees of success for pain modulation in postoperative clients and in clients with phantom limb pain, stump pain, postherpetic neuralgia, low back pain, arthritis, and pain associated with dysfunction of the temporomandibular joint.

Although TENS is noninvasive and generally safe, certain precautions are indicated. Safety of TENS in pregnancy is not documented, and the electrical stimulation with TENS can interfere with some types of cardiac pacemakers. A pacemaker may also alter the efficacy of TENS. Because TENS can stimulate muscle spasm, electrodes should not be placed in areas such as the upper anterior neck where laryngeal and pharyngeal muscle spasm could cause laryngeal spasm and airway closure. Stimulation of the carotid sinus in the neck at the bifurcation of the common carotid artery should also be avoided, because bradycardia can result. TENS electrodes should not be placed over an incision line or on an area of skin irritation. To prevent skin irritation from TENS use, the electrodes should be removed daily and the skin carefully cleansed and air dried.

Acupuncture

Acupuncture is a 2000-year-old Chinese technique of inserting fine needles into the skin at selected points on the body. The technique is based on the Eastern philosophy of mind–body unity, a concept Westerners are only beginning to appreciate fully. In Eastern healing, disease is thought to be a manifestation of imbalance between yin (female) and yang (male) energy flows. Needle insertion is believed to remove the blocks to energy flow and restore harmony.

One theory about how acupuncture relieves pain is related to the concept of trigger points, hypersensitive areas in muscle that can give rise to localized and referred pain. When the trigger point is stimulated, the effect is not unlike pulling the trigger of a gun; ie, the pain is experienced in the target area, distant from the trigger point. This referred pain does not follow usual dermatome patterns but has a predictable zone of referral. Extinction of the trigger points alleviates the referred pain. Acupuncture points (approximately 800 of them) lie on meridians that are believed to be pathways of energy within the body (Figure 5–14). When acupuncture charts are compared to descriptions of trigger-point locations, they are similar.

A second theory suggests that acupuncture needle insertion stimulates the endorphin system, releasing the body's natural opiates. Sometimes the needles are wired to stimulate the nerve endings electrically, enhancing the treatment. It is not known whether acupuncture achieves analgesia by extinction of trigger points, by release of endorphins, or even through the stimulation of large-diameter nerve fibers that effectively close the gate, as in TENS.

Acupressure, a less invasive variant of acupuncture, is finger pressure and massage specifically directed to acupuncture points. Acupuncture is practiced in many pain centers in North America, although it has not been widely accepted by practitioners of traditional medicine. Nevertheless, interest is high in use of acupuncture and acupressure for both acute and chronic pain states.

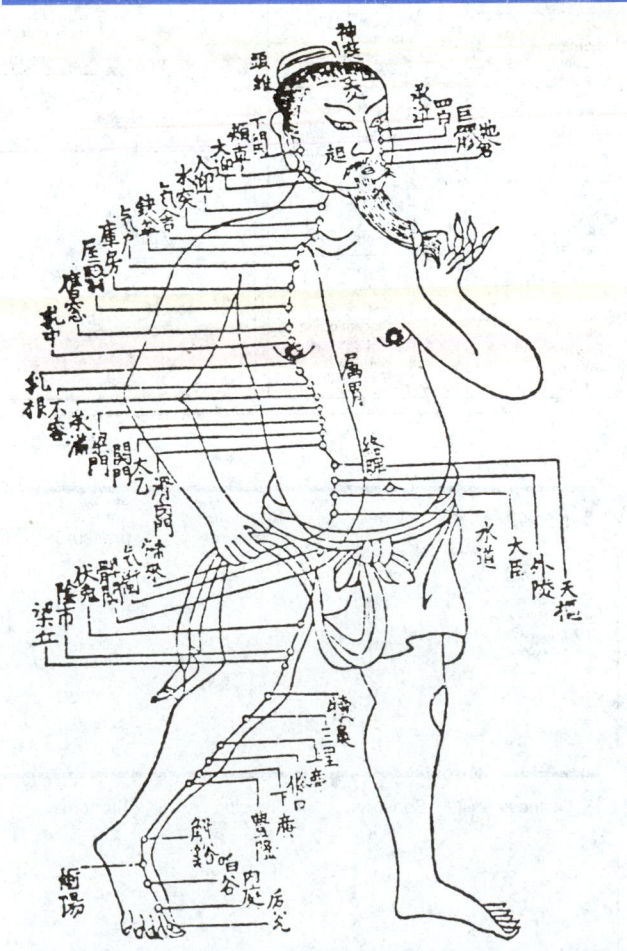

Figure 5–14

A typical acupuncture chart showing the sites for insertion of the needles along one of the major body meridians.

Nerve Blocks

Interrupting nerve function or myofascial trigger points by injecting a local anesthetic such as 1% lidocaine or 0.5% bupivacaine can provide temporary pain relief in some clients with acute or chronic pain. Nerve blocks are also done for severe muscle spasticity, such as that in clients with multiple sclerosis. Neurodestructive agents such as phenol or alcohol can be injected to achieve a longer-lasting effect, although adjacent tissue destruction can be a serious problem. Clients are carefully selected for this more permanent type of blockade.

Biofeedback

Biofeedback is a teaching method that assists clients to tune in to their bodies and eventually learn to control certain visceral responses, eg, muscle tension, hand temperature, heart rate, and blood pressure. A selected physiological activity is monitored by attaching the client by electrodes or transducers to an electronic instrument that amplifies the bodily response with lights, digital readings, graphs, or auditory signals. The client is thus able to see or hear fluctuations of physiological activity and develop an awareness of how to reproduce the desired response. Through concentration, the client can learn to shift brain wave activity patterns from the usual beta waves of daily activity to alpha waves, which characterize relaxation and tranquility. Achieving a high degree of alpha rhythm is helpful in controlling certain pain states, particularly those related to muscle tension.

The eventual goal of biofeedback training is to have clients develop skills that can be used outside the clinical setting to achieve the relaxed alpha wave state. Biofeedback is often used in conjunction with stress management techniques such as guided imagery, diaphragmatic breathing, and progressive muscle relaxation (see Chapter 4). Biofeedback as the sole modality in pain control is not as effective as biofeedback accompanied by other ancillary relaxation techniques.

Hypnosis

Hypnosis is a self-induced state of relaxation and concentration in which cognitive thinking is bypassed, allowing the client to be more susceptible to suggestion. Hypnosis has been used for pain reduction with dental procedures, in labor and delivery, and in clients with cancer. In recent years, hypnosis has increased in popularity as an approach to weight loss and smoking cessation. Although some question whether hypnosis is a sound approach to pain control, the literature reports many dramatic accounts of hypnotic analgesia in a wide variety of acute and chronic pain states (Barber & Adrian, 1982).

Placebo Effect

The relief of pain or other symptoms by a so-called "useless" medication or treatment is called the placebo effect.

In the past, clients who responded favorably to a placebo were considered malingerers. More recently, the placebo response has been explained as mind–body interaction; a heightened expectation of positive effects caused those effects to take place. In essence, the placebo worked because the person believed it would. The current thinking is that placebos relieve pain or other symptoms by causing the body to release endorphins, which have analgesic and other opioid properties.

Much is still unknown about the placebo response. Some persons do not seem to respond to placebos at all. Some consistently respond, and others respond only occasionally. Some experts suggest that the degree of placebo response depends on what medication clients believe they are receiving. Others suggest that a care provider the client perceives as honest and convincing can affect the degree of response with a statement such as, "Here is your medication. I believe it will help."

Because the prescribing of placebos seems to involve a degree of client deception, their use is controversial. Research has certainly disproved that persons who respond to a placebo have imaginary symptoms. Until more is understood about the totality of the placebo effect, however, the debate about placebo use will continue.

PHARMACOLOGICAL APPROACHES TO PAIN MANAGEMENT

Aspirin

Acetylsalicylic acid (ASA), or aspirin, is the most frequently used OTC analgesic, antipyretic, and anti-inflammatory drug in North America. Aspirin seems to produce analgesia by a peripheral action on synthesis of prostaglandins, substances generated by tissue damage. Aspirin is absorbed in the stomach and upper intestine, reaching adequate plasma concentration within 30 minutes and peak concentration in 2 hours. The usual adult dose of aspirin is 325 to 650 mg PO q. 4–6 h.

High doses of aspirin, as used in rheumatoid arthritis, or prolonged use of aspirin can cause epigastric distress and occasionally, gastrointestinal bleeding. Excessive doses can also produce tinnitus. Buffered aspirin (a combination of aspirin and antacids) and enteric-coated aspirin reduce the gastric irritation of plain aspirin. Because aspirin affects blood platelets, prolonging bleeding time, clients with peptic ulcer, on anticoagulants, or with bleeding disorders should not take aspirin. Aspirin is a common ingredient in many OTC and prescription drugs. Therefore, clients who cannot take ASA should remind their nurse, physician, and pharmacist when medications are prescribed.

Acetaminophen

Acetaminophen (Tylenol, Datril) is the second most common OTC analgesic, antipyretic drug sold. Acetaminophen does not have the anti-inflammatory properties of aspirin but neither does it interfere with clotting nor produce epigastric distress. The usual adult dose of acetaminophen is the same as aspirin—325 to 650 mg PO q. 4–6 h. Toxicity is uncommon with acetaminophen, although serious hepatic necrosis and death have occurred after large overdoses.

Nonsteroidal Anti-Inflammatory Drugs

Nonsteroidal anti-inflammatory drugs (NSAIDs) have analgesic, antipyretic and anti-inflammatory properties. The therapeutic effects of NSAIDs result from inhibition of prostaglandin synthesis. **Prostaglandins** are a group of compounds synthesized from unsaturated fatty acids that seem to have a role in both acute and chronic inflammatory reactions. There is a known variable clinical response in different clients to the NSAIDs. Therefore, a client who fails to respond to one drug may be helped considerably by another NSAIDs. Table 5–10 lists common NSAIDs and their maximum daily dosages.

Adverse effects of NSAIDs are mainly gastrointestinal. Dyspepsia, heartburn, gastritis, and gastric or duodenal ulcer have been reported. The gastrointestinal side effects seem to be less severe than those of aspirin, however. Renal function in clients with preexisting renal disease can be impaired with NSAIDs. Edema formation, blurring of vision, insomnia, and constipation are other reported adverse effects.

Narcotic Analgesics

Narcotic analgesics produce analgesia by acting directly on the central nervous system. They seem to activate an endorphin-mediated network in the CNS designed to inhibit nociceptive transmission. The central analgesic effect is often accompanied by enhanced feelings of well-being or euphoria and sometimes drowsiness and mental clouding. Respiratory depression and nausea and vomiting may also occur. Table 5–11 lists the common narcotic analgesics, the usual dose range for analgesia, and the route and frequency of administration.

Alternative approaches to administering narcotics for pain control have been used with some success. Continuous administration of morphine by IV infusion, titrated to the client's needs, has provided effective analgesia in some clients and decreased the total amount of drug needed for pain relief (Boyer, 1982). Extravascular infusion of meperidine (Demerol) or a local anesthetic such as bupivacaine via a catheter placed in the epidural space for 5 to 7 days has also been effective in some clients with chronic pain. The brachial plexus, celiac plexus, or lumbar sympathetic chain are other areas used for catheter placement and drug infusion (Alberico, 1984).

Other drugs effective for pain relief, alone or in combination with narcotics, include amphetamines and antidepressants. Amphetamines seem to reduce the amount of narcotic required to control pain. Some clients welcome the stimulant effect of amphetamines to counteract the sedative effect of many narcotic analgesics. Tricyclic anti-

Table 5–10	Nonsteroidal Anti-Inflammatory Drugs
NSAID	**Maximum Daily Dose**
Indomethacin (Indocin)	25–50 mg q.i.d.
Sulindac (Clinoril)	150–200 mg b.i.d.
Tolmetin (Tolectin)	400 mg t.i.d. or q.i.d.
Meclofenamate (Meclomen)	50–100 mg q.i.d.
Naproxen (Naprosyn)	250–500 mg b.i.d.
Fenoprofen (Nalfon)	200–600 mg q.i.d.
Ibuprofen (Motrin, Rufen, Advil*, Nuprin*)	200–600 mg q.i.d.

*Advil and Nuprin are available OTC in 200-mg tablets.

depressants (amitriptyline, imipramine) have been most successful in relieving pain associated with depression. Clients on these drugs should have urinary output monitored carefully because tricyclic antidepressants can cause urinary retention.

NURSING IMPLICATIONS

The effect of pain on the life of the client and loved ones is as variable and unique as each person. Some generalizations can be made that are important for nursing care, however. Clients often reduce their food and fluid intake, so they may be malnourished and dehydrated. Clients may be unable to sleep, resulting in chronic fatigue. Because of their decreased energy, they are unable to participate in strategies to cope with their pain (guided imagery, relaxation techniques, and distraction); consequently, the pain cycle is exacerbated. Social and sexual relationships deteriorate, reinforcing the client's isolation and feelings of frustration, helplessness, and anger in loved ones. Planning and nursing intervention for these problems are discussed in other chapters. This discussion will focus on comfort and pain relief.

Nurses have known for years that certain measures relieve pain in many clients. For example, touch, massage, breathing techniques, repositioning, explanation, and teaching have all been documented by nurses as helpful for promoting comfort and relieving pain. The physiological reasons for the effectiveness of these approaches are only beginning to be understood. For example, cutaneous stimulation, massage, and pressure may stimulate the large-diameter nerve fibers and close the pain gate. Careful explanation and teaching may decrease anxiety and reduce pain by stimulating release of endorphins. Diversion or distraction, as with relaxation approaches (music, watching TV, Lamaze breathing, guided imagery, and meditation), may also reduce muscle tension and modify pain perception through endorphin release. When the client is also receiv-

Table 5–11 Narcotic Analgesic Drugs

Analgesic	Average Dose Range	Route of Administration	Frequency of Administration
Codeine	15–60 mg	PO, SC	q.4h. p.r.n.
Hydromorphone (Dilaudid)	2 mg 3 mg	PO, SC, IM, IV Rectal suppository	q.4.–6h. p.r.n. q.6–8h. p.r.n.
Meperidine (Demerol)	50–150 mg	PO, SC, IM	q.3–4h. p.r.n.
Methadone (Dolophine)	2.5–10 mg	PO, SC, IM	q.3–4h. p.r.n.
Morphine	5–15 mg	PO, SC, IM, IV	q.3–4h. p.r.n.
Oxycodone (Percodan, Percocet)*	5 mg	PO	q.4h. p.r.n.
Propoxyphene (Darvon, Dolene)	32–65 mg	PO	q.4h. p.r.n.
Pentazocine (Talwin)	30 mg 50 mg	SC, IM, IV PO	q.3–4h. p.r.n. q.3–4h. p.r.n.

*Percodan contains 325 mg of aspirin; Percocet contains 325 mg of acetaminophen.

ing analgesic medications, nursing activities involving touch, explanation, and listening enhance the effect of the drug.

The nurse is the care provider most responsible for evaluating the clients need for analgesic medications. Medications are frequently ordered with variable dosage and variable timing, eg, Demerol 50 to 100 mg q. 3-4 h. p.r.n. The nurse decides how much of the drug will be given and how soon. Unfortunately, nurses often do not medicate the client soon enough or with a sufficient dose. Consequently, the client never achieves a level of comfort compatible with rest. Anxiety and muscle tension increase, and the pain is exacerbated.

Nurses often worry that a client will become addicted. Clients and families also frequently express the same concern. Addiction can be a problem in some instances, but when responsible health care providers are working with clients in pain, they continually evaluate the client's response, and adjust the medication schedule accordingly. The age and weight of the client, the severity of the health problem, other extenuating factors, and history of response to analgesic medication are considerations in deciding about medication management. Although it could be assumed that a small, elderly person needs less medication than a 25-year-old, 250-lb football player, health care providers should continuously evaluate the client's response to medication. The elderly client might suffer unnecessarily because of insufficient dosing for weight and age but be too stoic to ask for better pain relief. Carefully monitoring the client during the first two to three dose intervals helps the nurse to gauge the efficacy and duration of the analgesic effect as well as any adverse side effects.

Postoperative clients need analgesics for 24 to 72 hours after surgery and perhaps longer, depending on the procedure. Withholding narcotics or encouraging the client to "wait a little longer" in the first postoperative days only increases the client's level of discomfort and may cause feelings of guilt, embarrassment, or weakness in asking for pain relief.

There should be less fear of addiction in terminally ill clients in excruciating pain. It is difficult to justify an attitude that encourages living with unbearable pain while dying. Nurses often feel helpless in working with clients with relentless pain. Their discussions with physicians about more effective pain control measures may lead nowhere, often because physicians are equally frustrated when they are unable to keep a client comfortable. This helplessness and inability to control a situation may cause both physician and nurse unconsciously to withdraw from the client and family.

Nursing Research Note

Wells N: The effect of relaxation on postoperative muscle tension and pain. *Nurs Res* 1982; 31(4):236–238.

Relaxation has been used to control pain following abdominal surgery. This study examined the effect of relaxation training on muscle tension and subjective reports of pain. Of two groups of subjects who had cholecystectomies, one group received relaxation instruction and the other received standard preoperative instruction.

The results indicated that relaxation training reduced the psychological discomfort associated with pain but had no significant effect on physiologic measures. Muscle tension was not significantly altered by either technique. In applying these findings, nurses can incorporate relaxation training into preoperative teaching and encourage clients to use such techniques postoperatively.

The hospice movement and the increasing efforts to give clients more control over their lives, whether hospitalized or at home, is a promising development in pain management. Clients on oral medication can easily be given control over their own dosing schedules. Even when on parenteral medications, clients and their families can titrate the dosage and adjust the dose intervals as needed. On some days, clients in pain may feel good and only need oral aspirin and relaxation techniques. On other days, clients may be uncomfortable enough to need sufficient parenteral medication to make them completely unaware of their surroundings or their pain. Individualizing approaches to medication management in the terminally ill client in pain improves the quality of life for the client and family. Health care providers also see the wisdom in giving clients and families more control over decisions that so profoundly affect their lives.

PAIN CLINICS

Persons with chronic pain are frequently unable to find help in the traditional health care system. Many are now being helped in multidisciplinary pain clinics, of which there are a growing number in North America. Treatment at a clinic begins with a thorough health history, physical examination, and psychological evaluation. Clients dependent on narcotics are weaned from them, and methadone is substituted, if necessary. Psychological counseling, physical therapy, hypnosis, biofeedback, TENS, and acupuncture are potential approaches to treatment. The rehabilitation program is individually designed for each client.

Some clinics encourage inpatient treatment, and others favor an outpatient approach. Clients learn new patterns of moving and living that ameliorate the pain. Reduction in pain medication, resumption of more normal activities, and a positive self-image are the eventual goals.

Other centers may meet the needs of individual clients. Holistic health centers usually provide programs to promote relaxation and reduce stress. Hospice programs provide terminally ill clients in pain and their families with thoughtful, supportive, humanistic care. Organizations such as the National Committee on the Treatment of Intractable Pain are valuable resources to clients and families.

Chapter Highlights

Osmols are the measures of the amount of work dissolved particles can do in drawing fluid through a semipermeable membrane. Osmolality refers to the number of osmols per liter of solvent.

Isotonic solutions have the same osmolality as blood plasma, preventing shifts of fluids and electrolytes.

Hypertonic solutions have a greater osmolality than blood plasma, causing a rapid influx of water from the cells and interstitial spaces into the plasma.

Hypotonic solutions have a lower osmolality than blood plasma, causing water to move from the plasma into the cells.

Homeostatic regulation of the body is maintained by the lungs, kidneys, cardiovascular system, pituitary gland, adrenal glands, and parathyroid glands.

Fluid and electrolyte imbalances include water–sodium imbalance, volume imbalance, and electrolyte imbalance.

Sodium is the primary regulator of extracellular fluid volume and concentration. Potassium is the major intracellular cation.

Acid–base balance depends on the homeostasis of the hydrogen ion concentration in body fluids. An acidic solution has a pH below 7.0. A base or alkaline solution has a pH above 7.0. Extracellular fluid is slightly alkaline, having a pH from 7.35 to 7.45.

A buffer is a substance that has the ability to bind or release hydrogen in solution, maintaining the pH of the solution relatively constant despite the addition of considerable quantities of acid or base.

Acidosis occurs whenever a disturbance in the acid–base balance results in an increase in hydrogen ion concentration. Alkalosis is a disturbance in acid–base balance that results in a decrease in hydrogen ion concentration.

Respiratory acidosis occurs whenever there is an accumulation of CO_2 and, therefore, carbonic acid due to an interference with the alveolar exchange of O_2 and CO_2.

Respiratory alkalosis occurs when there is an excess loss of carbonic acid and, therefore, a decrease on the carbonic acid side of the acid–bicarbonate ratio.

Metabolic acidosis develops because of an increased amount of acid or a decrease in the amount of base.

Metabolic alkalosis results from a loss of hydrogen and chloride ions or an excess of base bicarbonate.

Shock is a state of widespread reduction in tissue perfusion resulting in inadequate oxygenation and nutrition of vital organs. The three major classifications of shock are hypovolemic shock, cardiogenic shock, and distributive shock.

Clients at risk for hypovolemic shock include those

with recent surgery, trauma, burns, invasive diagnostic testing, childbirth, miscarriage, or abortion; clients with a malignancy or coagulation disorder; and clients who take excessive diuretics.

Clients at risk for cardiogenic shock include those in the coronary care unit and those with previous cardiac problems such as myocardial infarction or dysrhythmias.

Clients at risk for distributive shock include those with known or unknown allergy to drugs or anesthesia; women using tampons, diaphragms, or contraceptive sponges; and clients on immunosuppressants.

Pain produced by A-delta fibers is a sharp, well-localized pain called epicritic pain. Pain produced by C fibers is a diffuse, poorly localized pain called protopathic pain.

Chronic pain is pain of 6 months or longer that fails to resolve and does not respond to traditional medical intervention.

Because clients understand their bodies better than anyone else, nurses should listen carefully to the ways in which clients describe their pain experience and approaches they have found helpful.

Bibliography

Fluid and Electrolyte Balance/Acid–Base Balance

Collins R, Douglas MD: *Illustrated Manual of Fluid and Electrolyte Disorders*, 2nd ed. Philadelphia: Lippincott, 1983.

Flink E: Nutritional aspects of magnesium metabolism. *West J Med* 1980; 133:304–312.

Goldberger E: *A Primer of Water, Electrolyte and Acid–Base Disorders*, 6th ed. Philadelphia: Lea & Febiger, 1980.

Lane G, Peirce AG: When persistence pays off: Resolving the mystery of an unexplained electrolyte imbalance. *Nurs 82* (Jan) 1982; 12:44–47.

Maxwell MH, Kleeman CR: *Clinical Disorders of Fluid and Electrolyte Metabolism*, 3rd ed. New York: McGraw–Hill, 1980.

Menzel LK: Clinical problems of electrolyte balance. *Nurs Clin North Am* 1980; 15(3):559–576.

Menzel LK: Clinical problems of fluid balance. *Nurs Clin North Am* 1980; 15(3):549–558.

Metheny N, Snively WD: *Nurse's Handbook of Fluid Balance*, 4th ed. Philadelphia: Lippincott, 1983.

Stroot V, Lee C, Barrett C: *Fluid and Electrolytes: A Practical Approach*, 3rd ed. Philadelphia: Davis, 1984.

Urrows ST: Physiology of body fluids. *Nurs Clin North Am* 1980; 15(3):537–547.

Weldy NJ: *Body Fluids and Electrolytes*, 2nd ed. St Louis: Mosby, 1980.

Witkowski AS: *Pulmonary Assessment: A Clinical Guide*. Philadelphia: Lippincott, 1985.

Zucker AR, Chernow B: Diabetes insipidus and the syndrome of inappropriate antidiuretic hormone release. *CCQ* (Dec) 1983; 6:63–74.

Shock

Ayres SM et al: Rescuing the patient in cardiogenic shock. *Patient Care* (July 15) 1983; 17:255–278.

Christopher KL: The use of a model for hemodynamic balance to describe burn shock. *Nurs Clin North Am* 1980; 15(3):617–627.

Gaunder BN, Winkle D: Anaphylaxis: Managing and preventing a true emergency. *Nurse Pract* (May) 1984; 9:17–20.

Houston MC, Thompson WL, Robertson D: Shock: Diagnosis and management. *Ann Intern Med* 1984; 144:1433–1439.

Lamb LS: Think you know septic shock? *Nurs 82* (Jan) 1982; 12:34–43.

Nursing care of patients in shock. (Programmed instruction) 1. Pharmacotherapy. 2. Fluids, oxygen, and the intra-aortic balloon pump. 3. Evaluating the patient. *Am J Nurs* 1982; 82:943–964; 1982; 82:1401–1422; 1982; 82:1723–1746.

Purcell JA: Shock drugs: Standardized guidelines. *Am J Nurs* 1982; 82:965–974.

Pain

Alberico JG: Breaking the chronic pain cycle. *Am J Nurs* 1984; 84:1222–1225.

Barber J, Adrian C: *Psychological Approaches to the Management of Pain*. New York: Brunner/Mazel, 1982.

Battenfield BL: Suffering: A Conceptual description and content analysis of an operational schema. *Image* (Spring) 1984; 16:34–41.

Boyer MW: Continuous drip morphine. *Am J Nurs* 1982; 82:602–604.

Clark PE, Clark MJ: Therapeutic touch: Is there a scientific basis for the practice? *Nurs Res* 1984; 33:37–41.

Ersek RA: *Pain Control With TENS: Principles and Practice*. St Louis: Green, 1981.

Escobar PL: Management of chronic pain. *Nurse Pract* (Jan) 1985; 10:24–32.

Geden E et al: Self-report and psychophysiological effects of five pain-coping strategies. *Nurs Res* 1984; 33:260–265.

Hendler NH, Long DM, Wise N: *Diagnosis and Treatment of Chronic Pain*. Boston: Wright, 1982.

Horsley JA: *Pain: Deliberative Nursing Interventions*. New York: Grune & Stratton, 1982.

Huhman M: Endogenous opiates and pain. *ANS* (July) 1982; 4:62–71.

Kane RL, Bernstein L, Wales J, Rothenberg R: Hospice effectiveness in controlling pain. *JAMA* (May 10) 1985; 253:2683–2686.

Kotarba JA: *Chronic Pain*. Beverly Hills, CA: Sage, 1983.

Levin RF: Choice of injection site, locus of control, and the perception of momentary pain. *Image* (Feb-Mar) 1982; 14:26–32.

McGuire D: The measurement of clinical pain. *Nurs Res* 1984; 33:152–156.

Meinhart NT, McCaffery M: *Pain: A Nursing Approach to Assessment and Analysis*. Norwalk, CT: Appleton–Century–Crofts, 1983.

Melzack R: *Pain Measurement and Assessment.* New York: Raven, 1983.

Moore DE, Blacker HM: How effective is TENS for chronic pain? *Am J Nurs* 1983; 83:1176–1177.

Panayotoff K: Managing pain in the elderly patient. *Nurs 82* (Aug) 1982; 12:53–57.

Randolph GL: Therapeutic and physical touch: Physiological response to stressful stimuli. *Nurs Res* 1984: 33:33–36.

Taylor AG et al: How effective is TENS for acute pain? *Am J Nurs* 1983; 83:1171–1174.

Taylor AG, Skelton JA, Butcher J: Duration of pain condition and physical pathology as determinants of nurses' assessments of patients in pain. *Nurs Res* 1984: 33:4–8.

Turk DC, Meichenbaum D, Genest M: *Pain and Behavioral Medicine.* New York: Guilford, 1983.

Suggested Readings

Copp LA: Pain coping model and typology. *Image.* Summer 1985; 17(3):69–71. The author goes beyond the descriptors in the McGill Pain Questionnaire by obtaining additional words from pain sufferers to describe their pain. Five self-image types with a corresponding pain descriptor are identified. A coping model is presented for each type.

Miller TW, Jay LL: Cognitive-behavioral and pharmaceutical approaches to sensory pain management. *Top Clin Nurs* (Jan) 1985; 6:34–43. The authors review definitions and levels of pain and discuss pain management techniques. The goal of the cognitive behavioral approach to pain management is to help clients cope with their pain by altering their interpretation of the pain sensation. An individualized approach using the client's own skills and resources is suggested as the most beneficial method in modulating pain perception.

Update on pain. *Female Patient* (Jan) 1985; 10:96–104. At the 4th World Congress on Pain, participants from more than 50 countries discussed pain concepts, including the social and psychological impact of chronic pain and the use of extradural opiates for long-term pain. This article reviews these discussions as well as the treatment of headaches and use of hypnosis with intractable pain.

Witt JR: Relieving chronic pain. *Nurse Pract* (Jan) 1984; 9:36–38. Four methods of relieving chronic pain are discussed—therapeutic touch, myotherapy, guided imagery, and relaxation combined with rhythmic breathing.

Resources

(See also resources in Chapter 36 for headaches)

SELF-HELP GROUPS AND OTHER ORGANIZATIONS

American Pain Society
340 Kingsland St.
Nutley, NJ 07110
Phone: (201) 235–0587

Biofeedback Society of America
4301 Owens St.
Wheat Ridge, CO 80033

Biogenic Institutes of America
615 S 10th St.
LaCrosse, WI 54601
This nonprofit corporation offers client training in pain control through biofeedback, autogenic training, and external electrical stimulation at facilities throughout the United States. Clients must be referred by their own physician.

Chronic Pain Outreach
8222 Wycliffe Ct.
Manassas, VA 22110

Committee on Pain Therapy
American Society of Anesthesiologists
515 Busse Hwy
Park Ridge, IL 60068
Phone: (312) 825–5586

National Committee on the Treatment of Intractable Pain
PO Box 9553 (Friendship Station)
Washington, DC 20006
Phone: (301) 983–1710
This committee of individuals was organized to promote education and research on more effective management of intractable pain. Information on the latest methods of pain management and current research can be obtained by contacting their Pain Control Information Clearinghouse. Referrals to other agencies for pain control information or treatment are available upon request.

National Hospice Organization
1311 Dolley Madison Blvd
McLean, VA 22101
Phone: (703) 356–6770

Pamphlet available:
Chronic Pain: Hope Through Research, April 1982
NIH Publication No. 82–2406
National Institutes of Health
Bethesda, MD 20205

Booklet available: *Questions and Answers About Pain Control*, 1983
American Cancer Society, Inc
777 Third Ave.
New York, NY 10017

Paperback books from local bookstores:
Benjamin BE, Borden G: *Listen to Your Pain.* New York: Penguin, 1984.

Olshan NH: *Power Over Your Pain Without Drugs.* New York: Beaufort, 1983.

Smollen B, Schulman B: *Pain Control: The Bethesda Program.* New York: Zebra Books, Kensington, 1982.

Chapter 6

Coping With Illness

Carol Ren Kneisl

Objectives

When you have finished studying this chapter, you should be able to:

Describe constructive and destructive coping strategies in response to the stress of illness.

Discuss the reasons why clients may have difficulty in following treatment plans.

Identify common defense-oriented behaviors.

Assess anxiety, anger, denial, depression, and dependence in clients.

Develop nursing diagnoses for clients who are anxious, angry, denying, depressed, or dependent.

Plan and implement the nursing care of clients experiencing anxiety, anger, denial, depression, or dependence.

Evaluate nursing interventions for clients experiencing anxiety, anger, denial, depression, or dependence.

Everyone deals with illness in his or her own way. Illness is difficult to cope with because it alters, sometimes in permanent and irreconcilable ways, both internal and external environments. Instead of feeling safe and secure, a person may feel vulnerable and threatened. A previously stable and predictable existence may become unsettled and inconstant, and a person may lose confidence that events will work out for the best. To make the situation even more complex, being ill may require clients to be more, not less, coherent, in charge, and capable. Rapid technical innovations in health care seem to have surpassed the ability to deliver care in ways that consistently protect the client's right to self-determination.

Section I: The "Noncompliant Patient" Label

Consider the following clinical situation from the perspective of the client as well as the nurse:

Mr J K was well known to the staff of 5 West; this was his third hospitalization within the past 10 months. During his first hospital visit, he was diagnosed as having Buerger's disease; his second admission was prompted by small ulcerations of the feet and ankles; this third hospitalization followed his discovery of black areas around the nails of two toes of his left foot.

Since the original diagnosis of Buerger's disease, Mr K has

had complication after complication. The health care professionals working with Mr K have advised him to stop smoking; to keep his extremities warm and reduce exposure to cold weather; to avoid either standing or sitting in one position for too long; and to continue taking a prescribed vasodilator, tolazoline hydrochloride (Priscoline).

One hour after his admission, 5 West was in turmoil. Mr K was standing at the doorway to his room loudly arguing with John Baker, his nurse, who had made another of many attempts to persuade his client to change jobs and stop smoking. Mr K's job as a chairlift handler at a ski resort requires him to stand outdoors all day regardless of temperature to assist skiers into the chairlifts on their way up the mountain. He almost always has a cigarette dangling from his lips. John Baker vented his frustration by delivering an angry lecture on the harm Mr K was doing to himself by not complying with the prescribed medical regimen. Later, at the change of shift report, John said: "If that man really wanted to get better and save his leg, he'd get his act together and do what we tell him. He's getting good advice. Why doesn't he follow it?"

Why don't some clients follow the good advice they get from well-meaning health professionals? In Mr K's case, the reason may be that the required changes seem too overwhelming, too threatening, or too anxiety provoking. His self-view may not comfortably allow for the necessary lifestyle alterations. Perhaps Mr K does not understand the reasons behind John Baker's suggestions. Possibly John Baker has not been clear enough in his attempts at health teaching. It may even be that Mr K cannot afford to change jobs because too many persons depend on the money he earns at the ski resort. On the other hand, Mr K may not really believe he is susceptible to the long-term complications his nurse has identified. It is also possible that he thinks the physical and psychosocial costs outweigh the potential benefits.

Clients like Mr K who do not follow the advice of their caregivers are often labeled resistive or "noncompliant." Sometimes such clients fail to enter a treatment program, or they drop out. Often they do not keep follow-up or referral appointments. At other times, clients do not take prescribed medication, or they do not alter their lifestyles or activities. Implicit in the "noncompliant" label is the belief that these clients are troublemakers who refuse to do what is good for them.

Labels seem to become attached to persons—almost permanently, at times. After the noncompliant label has been "earned" (ie, perceived by health care providers as accurate) it often remains attached to the client regardless of behavior or future compliance. Labels turn nurses into adversaries instead of advocates, and what should be a mutual effort toward recovery becomes a tug-of-war between client and nurse. Being an advocate, rather than an adversary, is much easier when nurses are able to acknowledge that persons face stress differently.

REASONS FOR NONCOMPLIANCE

Nurses may be able to avoid labeling clients as "resistive," "noncompliant," or "problem patients" by understanding their social, emotional, and practical needs. These factors may make it difficult if not impossible for clients to perform exactly as nurses deem proper or appropriate.

Knowledge Deficit

In some cases, a client resists treatment or fails to cooperate because of a knowledge deficit. The client may not know what is happening in his or her body or why the condition is being treated as it is.

Knowledge deficit can exist for a variety of reasons. The health care provider may not have taken the time to explain events to the client. Or perhaps the health care provider's "bedside manner" alienated the client. Misunderstandings may also arise because nurse and client come from different cultural or ethnic groups (see Chapter 4). The client's ability to understand explanations may have been impaired by a cognitive or intellectual deficit or by an emotional state.

Unfortunately, some health care providers (including nurses) mistakenly think they can change clients' behavior by using fear. Lessons from the past dispel the myth that fear encourages adherence to the medical regimen.

In 1967, Leventhal, Watts, and Pagano used a variety of techniques to encourage their cigarette-smoking subjects to stop smoking, including an anxiety-provoking color film of the surgical removal of a lung blackened by smoking and obstructed with cigarette tar. After viewing this film, the smokers feared for their health, expressed their determination to stop smoking, and actually reduced the number of cigarettes they smoked during the following week.

In addition, some smokers received instruction on how to stop smoking, and some did not. The detailed instructions from a booklet used in antismoking clinics included:

- Avoiding conditions conducive to smoking
- Preparing excuses for refusing cigarettes offered by others
- Carrying gum
- Not carrying matches or lighters
- Taking deep breaths when the urge to smoke was strong

By the end of the first week, there was little difference between the two groups—both groups had smoked much less. At one month and again at three months, the instructed group held to their gains, but the uninstructed group moved back toward the original level of smoking. In other words, *the effect of fear petered out*. Effects lasted in those who knew what to do and when to do it. The instruction they received had equipped them with the cognitive coping strategies they needed to carry out their intent to stop smoking.

When no knowledge deficit exists, one must look elsewhere for explanations of noncompliance. The rewards of compliance with medical advice simply may not be worth the cost to the individual.

The Cost of Acknowledging Ill Health or Health Risk

The reality of illness or being at health risk may provoke anxiety. Denial offers a certain amount of comfort to most. Illness happens to others, not to oneself—it can be viewed from a safe distance. Adhering to a treatment program is a constant reminder of vulnerability. (Denial is discussed further later in this chapter.)

Being at risk frequently carries duties but seldom offers payoffs. Attending to medical or nursing advice may not help a person feel better. Social and work obligations are not lessened, and one is seldom praised for maintaining a prudent diet or increasing physical exercise. Society seldom gives rewards for "being good."

The Cost of Imposed Lifestyle Burdens

Compliance with a medical regimen may impose unfavorable lifestyle burdens. Medication or treatment regimens and schedules may require a change in work schedule or even a change in jobs. Because of dietary restrictions, dining out may no longer be the simple pleasure it once was. Further, the treatment plan may contradict the values, customs, beliefs, and behaviors of the client's cultural or social group.

Duration of treatment—whether an illness is temporary or permanent—affects how drastic the lifestyle change is perceived to be. Those who place high value on independence feel threatened by the thought of assuming a sick role and becoming dependent on others.

The Cost of Painful, Disfiguring, or Hazardous Treatments

Some treatments cause clients pain and/or disfigurement, and many carry risks. Clients may question whether they will be safe from untoward side effects and disfigurement. It may not be possible to unequivocally reassure the client about the risks, or even whether the treatment will work. Some clients may be faced with risking pain, disfigurement, even death, without assurance that they will feel better or that their health status or lives will be improved. Radical head and neck surgery causes disfigurement, a heart transplant is certainly a hazardous procedure, and treatment with certain hormones may greatly increase one's risk of developing cancer. Although these examples may seem extreme, nurses encounter many clients who face these and similar concerns daily to varying degrees.

The Cost of Financial Burdens

Being ill or being at risk for illness may entail financial burdens. Some medications and treatments and home health care services carry high price tags. Although insurance plans, health maintenance organizations, and tax deductions ease the burden for many, this is not the case for everyone. Not all insurance coverage is adequate or available to everyone, and the client and the client's family may have to take up the financial slack. Even the cost of staying well may seem exorbitant; consider the ongoing cost of insulin syringes and blood sugar monitoring for a diabetic.

Indirect costs may arise because treatment schedules require clients to change to jobs that pay less but have more convenient hours. Some treatments may be so time consuming or debilitating that it is difficult, or even impossible, for an individual to maintain a job; a nonpaid leave of absence may be necessary.

The Cost of Submitting to Outside Authority

Most clients of the health care system relinquish some control over their lives. Although this loss of control may not disturb some, others may find it anxiety provoking. Clients who fail to follow a prescribed treatment plan may be trying to regain control and autonomy. Being submissive or compliant may be frightening for some persons. They may want to be partners with their nurses and physicians and to participate in health care decisions that involve them. Deprived of this opportunity, they engage in a power struggle with the staff.

The Cost of Burdening Family and Friends

Medical regimens cause changes not only in the lives of clients but also in the lives of their family and friends. Family and friends may also experience lifestyle changes related to the client's medication and treatment schedules. Moreover, the costs of health care may reduce the amount of money available for the needs of other family members.

Families and friends may also be called upon for emotional support. Depending on the quality of their own lives, they may or may not have enough energy to provide the client with emotional and pragmatic support. Knowing this, some clients may be reluctant to undertake courses of treatment that add to the problems facing an already-stressed family system. The problem may be particularly severe when there is family instability or disharmony.

PREDICTING NONCOMPLIANCE

In most health care settings, the staff tend to expect noncompliance primarily from clients who have personality problems or who are poorly educated. However, noncompliance has been found among all socioeconomic groups, among all types of persons, and in all types of health care settings. Research has indicated that, although it is difficult to predict exactly which clients will not follow a treatment plan, noncompliance is more likely for:

- Clients with unstable or disharmonious families
- Clients who live alone and lack the support of family and/or friends
- Clients with a low level of fear about their condition
- Clients with a high level of fear about their condition

One cannot assume that clients will always comply in the absence of these conditions, however. It is important to also consider the many reasons for noncompliance discussed in the preceding section.

Section II: Coping With Illness

Coping strategies are a set of behaviors persons under stress use in struggling to improve their situations. Coping strategies can be thought of simply as ways of getting along in the world.

WAYS OF COPING

A person can cope on different levels, including the physical, social, cognitive, and emotional levels. Problem solving, daydreaming, drinking or taking drugs, meditating, getting angry, praying, working out, and accepting the situation are common methods of coping.

Most often, individuals use behaviors that have worked well for them in the past. Sometimes they behave in a certain way because it is the only method they have of coping with stress or because other coping strategies failed to work. Some persons learn to turn to others for protection and nurturance; some learn to turn to chemicals or to food; some rely on self-discipline and keeping a stiff upper lip; others feel better after the intense expression of feelings; some withdraw physically and/or emotionally; still others work out or talk the problem out. Table 6–1 lists some of the common and not-so-common coping methods identified in the literature. Most are task-oriented behaviors at the cognitive or thinking level and are directed toward solving problems or reducing conflict. They are as varied as individuals. Some work; some don't.

Table 6–1 Coping Methods

Affect-Oriented Coping Methods	Problem-Oriented Coping Methods
Hope things will get better	Try to maintain some control over the situation
Eat, smoke, chew gum	Find out more about the situation so you can handle it better
Pray, trust in God	Think through different ways to handle the situation
Get nervous	Look at the problem objectively
Worry	Get an objective opinion
Seek comfort or help from family or friends	Try out different ways of solving the problem to see which works the best
Want to be alone	Draw on experience to help you handle the situation
Laugh it off, figuring things could be worse	Try to find meaning in the situation
Try to put the problem out of your mind	Seek advice
Daydream, fantasize	Set specific goals to help solve the problem
Prepare to expect the worst	Accept the situation as it is
Get mad, curse, swear, shout	Talk the problem over with someone who has been in the same type of situation
Cry, get depressed	Settle for the next best thing
Go to sleep, figuring things will look better in the morning	Do anything just to do something
Don't worry about it; everything will probably work out fine	Let someone else solve the problem
Withdraw from the situation	Read
Work off tension with physical activity	
Take out your tensions on someone or something else	
Drink alcoholic beverages	
Resign yourself to the situation because things look hopeless	
Resign yourself to the situation because it's your fate	
Deny the situation	
Do nothing in the hope that the problem will take care of itself	
Blame someone else for your problems	
Do meditation, yoga, biofeedback, self-hypnosis	
Take drugs, smoke marijuana, overeat	

SOURCE: Compiled from Jalowiec A, Powers MJ: Stress and coping in hypertensive and emergency room patients. *Nurs Res* 1981; 30:13; and Ziemer MM: Coping behavior: A response to stress. *Top Clin Nurs* 1982; 2(4):8.

COPING RESOURCES

Early classic research on coping was concerned with how individuals respond to specific stresses in a laboratory setting. More recent studies that consider the whole being in interaction with the environment have helped in viewing coping as a dynamic process that involves the demands and restrictions on a client as well as the resources available. For example, according to Antonovsky (1980), persons stay healthy or cope with stress because they possess what he calls *generalized resistance resources* (GRRs). A GRR is any factor in the person, group, or organization that helps in managing tension.

Physical and biochemical GRRs are physiological characteristics, such as genetic features and levels of immunity. These GRRs also include interaction of the nervous and endocrine systems that help in adaptation (eg, interactions involving adrenocorticotropic hormone or ACTH, thyroid-stimulating hormone or TSH, vasopressin, norepinephrine, and insulin and their influence on human behavior). Not only are individuals different in their genetic and biochemical makeup, but the physiological effects of illness and stress (see Chapter 2) may also alter the person's ability to use physical and biochemical GRRs positively.

Material goods and relative wealth constitute the *artifactual and material* GRRs; having these attributes makes it easier to cope with illness. Money helps to ensure the best health care available. Effective coping is often interrelated with one's socioeconomic status simply because the higher the socioeconomic status, the greater the resources to help the person cope. For example, household help not only relieves an ill person's worries but also reduces the practical burden.

Cognitive GRRs have to do with intelligence and knowledge. When persons know about stressors, they can avoid them. They can also predict when periods of stress are imminent and thus reduce their impact (see the discussion of life changes as stressful events in Chapter 2). Knowing what community services are available is also a cognitive GRR.

Emotional GRRs are possessed by those who are self-aware—who know their own capacities and potentials and have a well-developed sense of themselves. Emotional GRRs determine the extent of psychological hardiness. In general, they have to do with how competent and self-assured one feels.

Valuative and attitudinal GRRs are the products of a person's culture and environment. Persons are apt to respond in learned ways. The attitudinal aspect also is related to how flexible, rational, and farsighted the person is. The more rational or accurate one's appraisal of a threatening situation and the more flexible one is in approaching the situation and envisioning the consequences, the greater one's resources for coping.

Interpersonal–relational GRRs are available social support systems. The greater a person's social contacts, the greater the social resources available to augment the ability to deal with stress. Love, affection, and nurturance

Nursing Research Note

Dixon J: Group self-identification and physical handicap: Implications for patient support groups. *Nurs Health* 1981; 4:299–308.

The relation between attitudes toward self and attitudes toward general types of handicapped and nonhandicapped persons were examined. Data were collected from subjects who had no handicaps and from individuals with one of the following physical impairments: amputation, arthritis, emotional disturbances, spinal cord injuries, or stroke. The subjects were tested for willingness to associate with handicapped persons and evaluated themselves with reference to handicapped and nonhandicapped individuals.

The results indicated a strong identification between subjects and their own handicap group for amputees, clients with spinal cord injuries, and stroke subjects. Subjects with arthritis and emotional disturbances did not strongly identify with their own handicap group but identified more with the average person. The nonhandicapped had a significant identification between self and the average person and a nonsignificant level of association between self and concepts associated with the handicapped.

The study suggests that some individuals may benefit from self-help groups but not all. Nurses should assess each client individually and determine if group identification would help or hinder psychological adjustment.

are hallmarks of interpersonal–relational GRRs.

Institutional structures that facilitate coping are called *macrosociocultural* GRRs. These resources include governmental programs such as Aid to Dependent Children as well as cultural institutions such as death and funeral rites, religious rituals, and ceremonies. Both institutional and interpersonal–relational structures are discussed in Chapter 4 under social support systems.

According to this model, the ability to stay healthy or to cope with illness is determined by the extent and effectiveness of each person's generalized resistance resources. Yet the actual process of coping remains unclear. Exactly which personal resources should be mobilized and under which conditions still is not fully understood.

Little research has been performed on the preferred coping methods of "normal" subjects (those not facing a crisis). One nursing study (Ziemer, 1982) found that over 50% of the study population reported that their preferred method of coping was to talk to someone. This finding has profound implications for nursing, because nurses are the health care providers who spend the most time with clients. It also has profound implications for clients whose ability to communicate freely is restricted.

CONSCIOUS AND UNCONSCIOUS MODES OF COPING

The coping methods in Table 6–1 are largely conscious strategies used by persons in specific stressful situations (hypertensive clients and emergency room clients). What happens to the client who has no one to talk with, who can't jog 5 miles, or who can't laugh off the problem?

When a person is unable to ward off stress or reduce tension in the usual way, anxiety mounts as the client feels increasingly inadequate to cope with the situation. Under these circumstances, the person is more likely to engage in *defense-oriented behavior*. Rather than specifically attempting to solve a problem, defense-oriented behaviors, often called *defense mechanisms*, are geared toward reducing anxiety regardless of cost.

Defense mechanisms are primarily unconscious and often inflexible coping patterns that protect a person through intrapsychic distortions that are really self-deceptions. The person usually has little awareness of what is happening or even less control over events. Although these reactions may help keep the lid on anxiety, they also limit the ability to grow from and savor the experience, they interfere with rational decision making and the ability to work productively, and they impair and erode interpersonal relationships. Even adaptive devices can go wrong.

COMMON DEFENSE-ORIENTED BEHAVIORS

Several kinds of defense-oriented behaviors have been identified in the literature. The common ones are discussed in this section. The three the nurse sees most often employed by ill clients are denial, regression, and suppression.

Denial

The father is reacting with *denial* when he shouts, "No, it can't be true; there must be a mistake," when told his 8-year-old son has just died in the trauma unit of injuries incurred when his bicycle collided with an automobile. The person who denies may totally disregard the reality of the situation or may transform the situation into a less threatening one.

Denial can be constructive when it provides temporary protection from a threatening event or an unpleasant reality until an individual has shored up coping ability. Denial can also be harmful or destructive when it interferes with a person's ability to take steps to ensure health. A later section of this chapter discusses the nursing process with clients who are using denial to cope.

Regression

Regression is a means of reducing anxiety by retreating from the present to a more pleasant past. The person reverts to behavior more characteristic of an earlier developmental level. The behavior is less mature but more comforting.

Suppose a nurse who is ill with an upper respiratory infection takes to her bed, enjoys being medicated with Vick's Vaporub, and asks her spouse or children to bring her apricot nectar to drink, as her mother did when she was a girl. She is demonstrating regression—reverting from an independent health care provider to being temporarily dependent on others, a move that provides comfort while she is feeling ill. An extreme form of regression is the infantile behavior of some acutely ill schizophrenic clients. This form of regression is less temporary for the schizophrenic client (who has little control over it) than regression is for the nurse with the cold.

Like denial, temporary regression can help a person to reconstitute defenses. Remember, temporary regression is not harmful. It could be good medicine.

Repression

Repression, the basis of all defense mechanisms, is the dynamic behind much of "forgetting." When persons regress, they unconsciously exclude distressing emotions, thoughts, or experiences from awareness. In this way, they avoid the conflicts these emotions, thoughts, or experiences could bring. The rape victim in the emergency room who cannot recall the circumstances surrounding the rape or what the rapist looks like is repressing.

Suppression

A middle-aged male business executive discovers bright red rectal bleeding the day before he is to leave for a visit to his company's international offices in three European countries. His decision to put off worrying about the bleeding until he returns in 3 weeks is an example of using *suppression* to deal with the emotional discomfort of this discovery. Suppression is an intentional act that helps to keep thoughts, feelings, wishes, or actions that cause anxiety out of conscious awareness.

Rationalization

When a person substitutes "good" or plausible reasons for questionable behavior to justify it, that person is said to be *rationalizing*. Rationalizing helps to avoid social disapproval and to bolster flagging self-esteem. Rationalization appears to be operating, for example, when a nurse who is late in administering a preoperative sedative explains to the head nurse that "it'll probably work out to the good" because the operating suite is busy, and the client's surgery is likely to be delayed anyway.

Displacement

Displacement is the act of transferring unacceptable emotions associated with a threatening person, idea, or object to a less threatening person, idea, or object. For example, a preoperative client shouts at the nurse after an unsatisfying visit from the surgeon. Rather than risk threatening the relationship with the person who will perform the surgery, the client vents his hostility toward the nurse.

Identification

Acting or behaving like an admired person is called *identification*. An example is the freshman college student who after hospitalization for minor surgery decides to switch to a major in nursing.

Introjection

Introjection is a more intense form of identification in which the person actually assumes the values, beliefs, and attitudes of another and incorporates them into his or her personality. For example, while in nursing school, the college student assumes the gestures, speech mannerisms, and values of an admired nursing instructor.

Fantasy

Fantasy is a way of satisfying a wish that cannot be realized. A client with advanced multiple sclerosis who imagines herself a famous ballerina with complete control of her body is engaging in fantasy. Fantasy and imaging can also be useful tools for reducing stress and promoting health (see Chapter 4).

Compensation

A young research scientist who has severe scars from facial burns and devotes all his energies to scientific study in his laboratory is *compensating* for his perceived body defect by emphasizing his intellectual strengths. Doing so helps to relieve fears of failure in one area by emphasizing an area in which there is a greater likelihood of success. Compensation can be adaptive for clients who are limited because of the effects of their illness.

THE ROLE OF ANXIETY IN COPING

Anxiety is a state of uneasiness or discomfort experienced to varying degrees. Beyond the mild level, anxiety is often described as a feeling of terror or dread; anxiety is believed to be the most uncomfortable feeling a person can experience. In fact, anxiety is so uncomfortable that most persons try to get rid of it as soon as possible. The coping strategies and defense-oriented behaviors discussed earlier in this chapter are the results of attempts to control or reduce anxiety. Other behavior patterns to control or reduce anxiety commonly seen in clients are discussed later in this chapter.

Sources of Anxiety

Anxiety is an inevitable condition of human existence in the attempt to maintain equilibrium in a changing world.

Generally, anxiety stems from two major kinds of threats: threats to biological integrity and threats to the security of the self. It is crucial to understand that either actual *or* impending interference may cause anxiety (ie, actual interference with a biological or psychosocial need is not a necessary condition). All that is necessary for anxiety to arise is the *anticipation* of one of these major threats.

Threats to biological integrity or to the fulfillment of such basic human needs as food, drink, warmth, and shelter are a general cause of anxiety. Threats to the security of self are not as easily categorized. In some instances, they are obvious; in others, they are more obscure because each person's sense of self is unique. To one person, power and prestige may be essential; to another, independence; to a third, being of service to others.

Consider the last category—being of service to others. Suppose that Mrs C, a nurse, is convinced that a particular client would feel much better if he expressed his fears about impending surgery to her. But no matter how often she provides the opportunity, he insists, "This is not the time to talk about it," and thwarts her attempt. She is not able to help him in a way that is important to her sense of self. In addition, she believes that the unit's head nurse (whose communication skills she admires) expects her to have been successful in this endeavor. When unmet needs or expectations related to essential values (eg, being of service to the client) are coupled with the actual or anticipated disapproval of others who are important (the head nurse), anxiety is generated.

Anxiety as a Continuum

It is helpful to think of anxiety as a continuum. Anxiety is a potent force. At low levels, it may stimulate constructive action. At higher levels, it may become a problem in its own right.

Mild Anxiety
Mild anxiety helps one deal constructively with stress. A mildly anxious person has a broad perceptual field (ie, mild anxiety heightens the ability to take in sensory stimuli). Such a person is more alert to what is going on and can make better sense of what is happening with others and the environment. The senses take in more—the person hears better, sees better, and makes logical connections between events (Figure 6–1). The person feels relatively safe and comfortable. Because learning is easier when one is mildly anxious, mild anxiety helps clients learn how best to give their own insulin. Mild anxiety can also help a nursing student review the nursing care of the client with dysfunction of the endocrine system before a final examination.

Moderate Anxiety
In moderate anxiety, a person remains alert, but the perceptual field narrows (see Figure 6–1). The moderately anxious person shuts out the events on the periphery while focusing on central concerns. For example, if the nursing

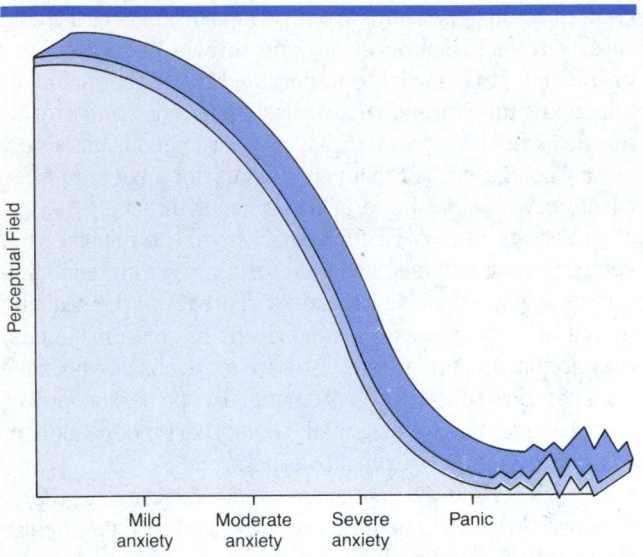

Figure 6–1

The effect of anxiety on the perceptual field.

student is moderately anxious about the final examination, he may be able to focus so intently on his studies that he is not distracted by an argument between his roommates, loud music on the stereo, and a rousing chase scene on television. He shuts out the chaos in the environment and focuses on what is of central importance to him—preparing for the exam. This process of taking in some sensory stimuli while excluding others is called *selective inattention.*

Selective inattention may also be used to cope with anxiety-provoking stimuli. This phenomenon may account for the anxious preoperative client who fails to remember what the nurse said about postoperative pain or the need to cough and deep breathe after surgery.

Although the perceptual field is narrowed and the person sees, hears, and grasps less, there is an element of voluntary control. The moderately anxious individual can, with direction, focus on what has previously been inattended.

Severe Anxiety

In severe anxiety, sensory reception is greatly reduced (see Figure 6–1). Severely anxious persons focus on small or scattered details of an experience. They have difficulty in problem solving, and their ability to organize is also reduced. They seldom have the complete picture. Selec-

tive inattention may be increased and may be less amenable to voluntary control. The person may be unable to focus on events in the environment. New stimuli may be experienced as overwhelming and may cause the anxiety level to rise even higher.

The sympathetic nervous system is activated in severe anxiety, causing an increase in pulse, blood pressure, and respiration and an increase in epinephrine secretion, vasoconstriction, and even body temperature. A multitude of physiological changes may be observed, which are described in the nursing process section that follows.

Many clients in health care settings are severely anxious. An unfavorable diagnosis or prognosis or a painful or disfiguring treatment may threaten both biological integrity and the security of the self.

Panic

The panic level of anxiety is characterized by a completely disrupted perceptual field (see Figure 6–1). Panic has been described as a disintegration of the personality that is experienced as intense terror. Details may be enlarged, scattered, or distorted. Logical thinking and effective decision making may be impossible. The person in panic is unable to initiate or maintain goal-directed action. Behavior may appear purposeless, and communication may be unintelligible.

Not all those in panic behave alike. At the scene of an auto accident in which an elderly couple lost control of the travel trailer they were towing, the husband remained immobile in the driver's seat, hands firmly fixed to the steering wheel, eyes focused on some distant spot despite the threat of explosion from the smoking car. The wife ran around in circles. Having lost her shoes in the accident, she was unaware she was running through the broken glass of the windshield in her bare feet despite numerous bleeding cuts.

Automatic Responses to Anxiety

Because anxiety is such an uncomfortable feeling, persons learn early in life to try to reduce it or diminish its effect as soon as possible. Although individuals use a variety of behaviors described in this chapter, behavior generally falls within a few categories. The most common automatic responses to anxiety are anger, withdrawal, and somatization. Automatic responses are limiting, rigid, and inflexible. Because they are automatic, these responses are called out under anxiety-provoking conditions, preventing a creative response to the threat and inhibiting learning.

Section III: The Nursing Process in Problems of Coping With Illness

Anxiety influences an individual's ability to cope as well as the individual's type of coping strategies. This section begins

with a discussion of the nursing process with anxious clients. Other behavior patterns common to anxious clients—anger, denial, depression, and dependence—follow. Keep in mind that this chapter applies to family members and friends as well as clients under direct care.

ANXIETY

Anxiety affects a person's thinking, behavior, and feeling. Anxiety may enhance a wellness/illness experience so learning and creativity result, or it may be a destructive force that interferes with the ability to keep well or to get well. For this reason, intervening effectively in clients' anxiety is crucial.

Nursing Assessment: Establishing the Data Base

Anxiety can be assessed in the physiological, cognitive, and emotional/behavioral dimensions. Objective data, particularly nursing observations, may be critical because of the nature of anxiety. Selective inattention and dissociation interfere with the client's awareness of anxiety and ability to give accurate reports. Families and friends also can contribute data useful to the assessment of anxiety.

Physiological Dimension

Observations of the client's physiological state are likely to indicate autonomic nervous system responses, particularly sympathetic effects. (The autonomic nervous system is discussed in Chapter 35.) Various organs may be affected, such as the adrenal medulla, heart, blood vessels, lungs, stomach, colon, rectum, salivary glands, liver, pupils of the eyes, and sweat glands (Figure 6–2). Anxious clients may have an increased heart rate, increased blood pressure, difficulty in breathing, sweaty palms, trembling, dry mouth, "butterflies in the stomach" or a "lump in the throat," as well as other symptoms.

Laboratory tests are not routinely done to evaluate anxiety because observation is faster and more accurate, but anxiety affects the results of laboratory tests. Blood studies may show increased adrenal function, elevated lev-

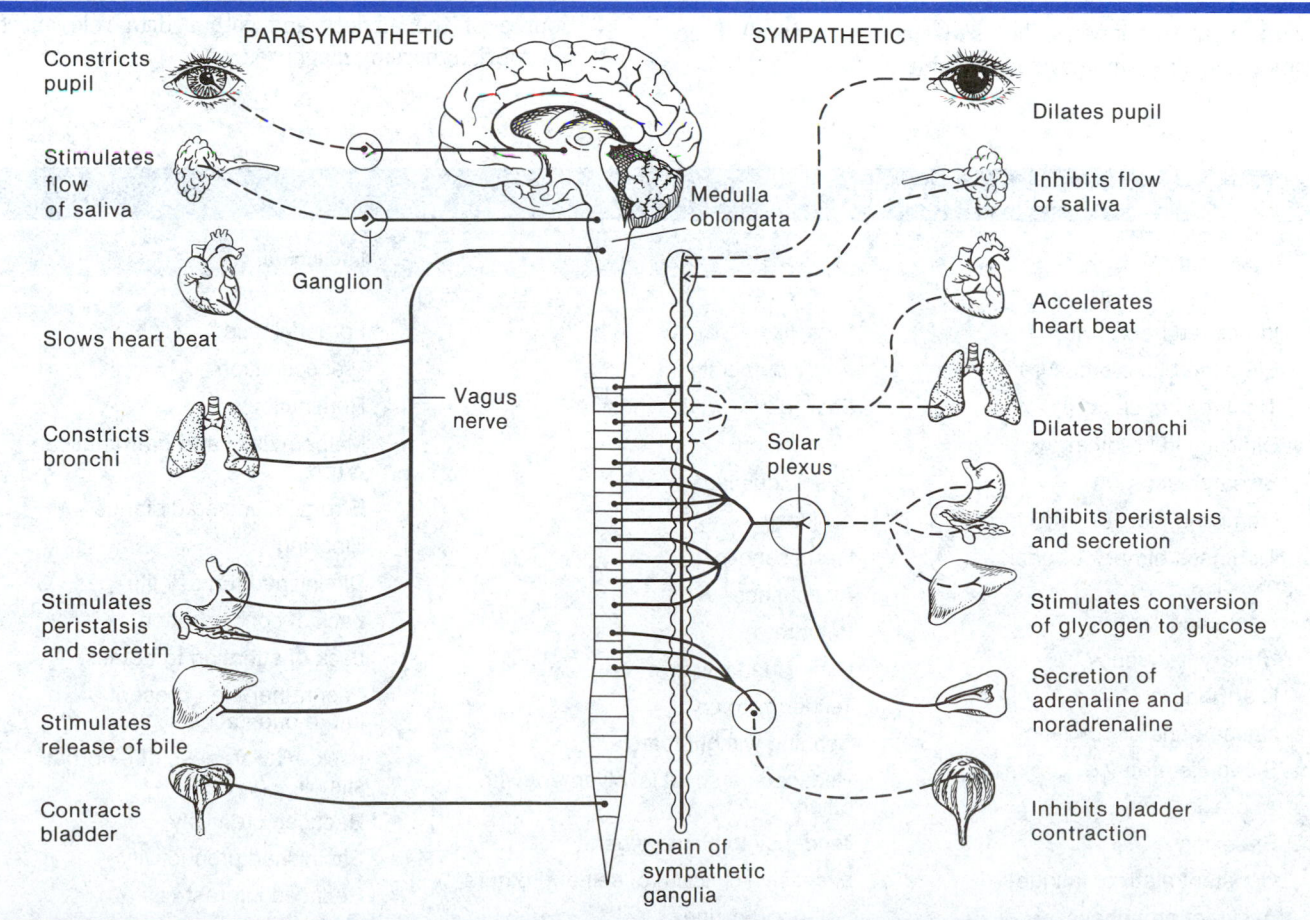

Figure 6–2

The autonomic nervous system and some of the organs it innervates. In anxiety, sympathetic nervous system responses are most common.

SOURCE: Ramsey JM: *Basic Pathophysiology: Modern Stress and the Disease Process*. Menlo Park, CA: Addison–Wesley, 1982, p. 46.

els of glucose and lactic acid, and decreased parathyroid function and oxygen and calcium levels. Urinary studies may indicate increased levels of epinephrine and norepinephrine.

Cognitive Dimension

Assessment of cognitive function may indicate difficulty in logical thinking, narrowed or distorted perceptual field, selective inattention or dissociation, lack of attention to details, difficulty in concentrating, or difficulty in focusing. The extent to which cognitive function is affected is determined by the level of anxiety. Mild, moderate, severe, or panic level of anxiety is assessed according to the descriptions earlier in this chapter.

Emotional/Behavioral Dimension

In the emotional/behavioral dimension, clients may be irritable, angry, withdrawn, restless, or they may cry. The affective response can often be assessed through the client's subjective description. Clients may describe themselves as "on edge," "uptight," "jittery," "nervous," "worried," or "tense." They may feel dizzy or faint and may experience a feeling of impending doom as if something terrible were about to happen. The assessment cues in all three dimensions are summarized in Table 6–2.

Determining the Source of Anxiety

In the assessment phase, it is essential to determine not only whether the client is anxious and, if so, how anxious, but also to attempt to determine the source of the anxiety. Knowing the source will help in planning and implementing effective care. These two steps can be useful:

1. Help the client to recognize and name the experience as anxiety. The nurse might say something like: "You're trembling. How are you feeling?" Some clients will be able immediately to connect their behavior with feeling anxious. For clients who do not, it is helpful to make the connection: "Often persons tremble because they're feeling anxious (or nervous, uncomfortable, or worried). I was wondering if you could be feeling anxious (or nervous, uncomfortable, or worried) right now."

2. Help the client to discuss the experience more fully by moving into the cognitive dimension. It would be premature to ask the client why he or she feels anxious. Encouraging clients to discuss what they are thinking about is more likely to bring their concerns out into the open. Then the nurse can determine the source of the anxiety and gather data relevant to appropriate nursing diagnoses.

Table 6–2 Assessment of Anxiety

Physiological	Emotional	Intellectual
Increased heart rate	Irritability	Forgetfulness
Elevated blood pressure	Angry outbursts	Preoccupation
Tightness of chest	Feeling of worthlessness	Rumination
Difficulty in breathing	Depression	Mathematical and grammatical errors
Sweaty palms	Suspiciousness	Errors in judging distance
Trembling, tics, or twitching	Jealousy	Blocking
Tightness of neck or back muscles	Restlessness	Diminished fantasy life
Headache	Anxiousness	Lack of concentration
Urinary frequency	Withdrawal	Lack of attention to details
Diarrhea	Diminished initiative	Past rather than present or future orientation
Nausea and/or vomiting	Tendency to cry	Lack of awareness of external stimuli
Sleep disturbance	Sobbing without tears	Reduced creativity
Anorexia	Reduced personal involvement with others	Diminished productivity
Sneezing	Tendency to blame others	Reduced interest
Constant state of fatigue	Excessive criticism of self and others	
Accident proneness	Self-deprecation	
Susceptibility to minor illness	Lack of interest	
Slumped posture		

SOURCE: Reprinted with permission from Wilson HS, Kneisl CR: *Psychiatric Nursing*, 2nd ed. Menlo Park, CA: Addison–Wesley, 1983, p 357.

The exception to this general strategy occurs when clients are in panic or are extremely anxious. In this case, formal data gathering is suspended in favor of immediate, direct action to reduce anxiety (see section on Planning and Implementation).

Nursing Diagnosis

A number of nursing diagnoses are relevant to anxiety. In addition to the nursing diagnosis of anxiety itself, the most obvious are ineffective individual coping and ineffective family coping. In considering the varying physiological, cognitive, and emotional effects of anxiety, a variety of other nursing diagnoses may be important.

Alterations in physiological functioning because of anxiety may prompt nursing diagnoses such as:

- Alteration in bowel elimination, related to constipation (or, diarrhea)
- Ineffective breathing pattern
- Alteration in nutrition: less than body requirements (or more than body requirements)
- Self-care deficit
- Sleep pattern disturbance
- Alteration in pattern of urinary elimination

Alterations in cognitive functioning because of anxiety may prompt nursing diagnoses such as:

- Knowledge deficit
- Impaired verbal communication
- Alteration in thought processes

Alterations in emotional, social, and behavioral functioning because of anxiety may prompt nursing diagnoses such as fear, noncompliance, and disturbance in self-concepts.

Planning and Implementation

The planning and implementation phases of the nursing process with anxious persons depend on a careful and accurate assessment of the level of anxiety and the determination of appropriate nursing diagnoses. It is important for planning and implementation to take place as soon as possible. Not only does anxiety often escalate, but anxiety is also communicated interpersonally. Other persons, such as the client's family and friends or other clients and staff in the health care setting, may be caught up in the tension as well.

Talking About Anxious Feelings
Many times, simply offering the client the opportunity to acknowledge and discuss feelings of anxiety helps the client to regain control. Having followed the two steps outlined in the section on assessment, the nurse may find the client's anxiety has already abated somewhat. At this point, clients are more likely to share their concerns because the nurse has already taken the first steps in demonstrating genuine interest and concern in the client's experiences.

It is important to tolerate the client's expression of feelings and concerns once their expression has been encouraged. Clients may express fear, anger, sadness, disappointment, or alienation, and it may be difficult to hear about the client's pain. Some nurses feel helpless in the face of their client's catharsis and think they should be able to provide ready answers. Instead, ready answers are more likely to interfere with and thwart the client's communication. Genuine, concerned listening without judgments is an effective intervention in itself.

Physical Activity
Simple physical activities often help to reduce anxiety to more tolerable levels. What is important is to encourage adaptive coping mechanisms that work. A client could:

- Soak in a warm bath.
- Listen to soothing music.
- Take a walk or exercise.
- Have a massage or back rub.
- Drink a warm beverage.
- Engage in whatever activity is found relaxing.
- Take slow, deep breaths to counteract the effects of hyperventilation, breathing in harmony with the nurse for support.

Stress Reduction Strategies
A nurse could also teach the client a variety of stress reduction strategies and encourage their use. Deep breathing, active progressive relaxation, and imaging techniques such as those described in Chapter 4 are helpful in reducing anxiety. Meditation and biofeedback techniques are other approaches. Teaching clients about these self-management approaches encourages self-care and provides the client with tools to use at home, at school, and on the job as well as in the health care setting.

Decreasing Knowledge Deficit
If a knowledge deficit has contributed to anxiety, providing the client with useful information helps reduce anxiety. Explanations should be simple, clear, and concise. Be careful not to overload the moderately or severely anxious person with more information than can be processed. If anxiety has contributed to knowledge deficit, the anxiety level will have to be reduced before trying to teach about health or provide information. Unless the cognitive conditions (such as narrow or disrupted perceptual field) have changed, the client will be unable to assimilate the information.

Direction and Structure in Severe Anxiety or Panic
Clients who are extremely anxious or in panic require more immediate, direct, and structured intervention. During an acute panic attack, perception and personality are disrupted to such a degree that the client cannot solve problems or discuss the source of anxiety. The first priority is

Table 6–3 Nursing Intervention Into Panic	
Strategy	**Rationale**
Stay with the client	Being left alone may further increase the anxiety
Maintain a calm, serene manner	Knowing that the nurse is calm and in control may be calming to the client
Use short, simple sentences	Because the client's perceptual field is disrupted, the client will experience difficulty in focusing
Use a firm and authoritative voice	Conveys the nurse's ability to provide external controls
Move the client to a quieter, smaller, and less stimulating environment	Prevents further disruption of the perceptual field by sensory stimuli
Focus the client's diffuse energy on a repetitive or physically tiring task	Repetitive tasks or physical exercise can help to drain off excess energy
Administer antianxiety medications if ordered	Antianxiety medications may help reduce anxiety

to reduce the anxiety to more tolerable levels (see Table 6–3). The suggested strategies can be applied wherever nurses engage with persons who are extremely anxious or in panic—the emergency room, the trauma unit, or at the scene of a crisis or disaster.

Antianxiety Medication

Antianxiety medication may be appropriate for anxious persons. The minor tranquilizers such as chlordiazepoxide (Librium) and diazepam (Valium) are commonly administered. Major tranquilizers, or antipsychotic medications, such as thioridizine (Mellaril), prochlorperazine (Compazine), or chlorpromazine (Thorazine) may be used for extreme anxiety or panic.

Use antianxiety medication cautiously and sparingly. Certain antianxiety medications (diazepam, for one) are among the most prescribed, overprescribed, and abused drugs in the United States and Canada. Valium overreliance is a serious medical problem that has prompted the formation of a self-help group, Valium Anonymous (see the resources list at the end of Chapter 10), to help addicted persons to get off the drug. Certain groups such as the elderly are particularly sensitive to the effects of central nervous system depression associated with diazepam.

Although medications may alleviate the symptoms of anxiety, they do nothing to help clients to understand its source nor to manage their own lives in more comfortable ways. At best, these drugs should be used for the short-term treatment of anxiety—meaning days or even weeks but not months or years.

Anticipating Anxiety

Anticipating anxiety and preparing clients and their families to cope with it ahead of time will often help prevent it. Illness and treatment, because they threaten biological integrity and the security of the self, precipitate anxiety. Nurses can expect clients and their families to become anxious in the face of the unknown or potentially painful, dangerous, or disfiguring events.

Evaluation

Nursing interventions related to anxiety may be considered successful when the client's anxiety has been reduced to a level that the client can more readily manage. Observations verifying this outcome include a broadening of the perceptual field and reduction in sympathetic nervous system effects.

When the client can openly discuss the experience of anxiety, consider its sources, and attempt self-management practices to reduce it, then nursing interventions have helped to attain successful outcomes.

ANGER

Anger is an intense emotion of strong displeasure usually linked with antagonism. In fact, the word derives from the Latin *angere*: to strangle. With anger, the feeling of powerlessness stemming from anxiety is converted into power. Anger is one of the learned automatic responses to anxiety.

Because many situations in health care settings can arouse anxiety, there are also many opportunities for anger. Clients may feel as if they are subject to the whims of health care personnel. Removed from familiar surroundings where they were in charge, clients are forced to deal with unknowns, to wait to have needs met, and to worry about what will happen to them and their families. Their biological needs and their sense of self-security are threatened from all sides.

Anger is the fight response to anxiety. Unfortunately, even though the angry person may feel restored to power, others who may be the objects of anger feel threatened, frightened, pushed away, or angry in turn.

Nursing Assessment: Establishing the Data Base

Most of the time, anger can be readily assessed. Angry people look tense and tight—the face may be contorted, the jaw tightened, the fists clenched, the cords and veins of the neck protruding, the posture tensed, and the nostrils flared. Angry persons may hold their breath or take deep, rapid breaths with sighing expirations. The pupils may be dilated, and the angry person appears to be glaring. The angry person's voice changes, becoming louder, harsher, and more strident. The person may curse or may be sarcastic, rude, accusatory, or hurtful. The angry person may become physical, pounding one fist into the other palm, pounding on an object, slamming a door, breaking or throwing something, hitting, shoving, pushing, or otherwise striking out. Occasionally, an angry person looks rigid.

Physiological changes from the autonomic nervous system response to increased secretion of epinephrine may include increased blood pressure and heart rate, decreased gastrointestinal peristalsis and increased hydrochloric acid secretion, increased salivation, and increased urination. Angry persons also become hyperalert and have difficulty relaxing or falling asleep.

As with anxiety, it is essential in the assessment phase to determine not only whether the client is angry but also the source of the anger or the anxiety that preceded it. Knowing the source will help in planning and determining effective care. The following two steps can be useful:

1. Help the client to recognize and name the experience as anger. The nurse might say: "You're shouting. You seem angry." This often helps the client make the connection.
2. Help the client to discuss the experience more fully by moving into the cognitive dimension. Asking the client what the anger is about will encourage open discussion and facilitate the gathering of data relevant to appropriate nursing diagnoses.

Sometimes, anger may be harder to assess. Those who value controlling their angry feelings may have learned to disguise these expressions or to deny their anger. In these instances, cues may be more subtle. Look for mixed messages, in which verbalization and behavior are not consistently matched. Suppose a client says he is "a little upset (or annoyed, or irritated)" because he had to wait 50 minutes before his request for medication to relieve postoperative pain was fulfilled. Do his tone of voice and body actions indicate a more profound anger? If so, adapt step 1. Because the client may not recognize his anger, try to make the client's mixed message evident. Say something such as "You say it doesn't matter, but you look angry."

Nursing Diagnosis

Anger is considered an automatic response to anxiety. Therefore, the nursing diagnoses relevant to anxious clients are also relevant to angry clients.

Planning and Implementation

The first and most obvious action is to reduce the sources of anxiety. This action will indirectly reduce the angry responses resulting from anxiety.

It is essential that nurses recognize anger as a response to anxiety and not as an aggressive act specifically directed toward them. Keeping in mind that the client is responding to a real or anticipated threat to biological well-being or self-esteem is a reminder of the need for a professional instead of a social relationship between client and nurse.

Respecting the Client as a Person
Respecting a client's privacy, territory, autonomy, and need for information may help prevent clients from becoming angry with health care providers. In one study (Maagdenberg, 1983), when clients were asked what made them angry with the nursing staff, they identified the following conditions:

- When nursing staff failed to ask permission before touching
- When nurses and physicians inspected incisions or body parts without providing privacy
- When nurses failed to explain beforehand what they planned to do to the client
- When nurses failed to ask permission before performing a nursing task

The study also found that few staff members knew why clients became angry. Being aware of these needs and providing for them in planning and administering nursing care may avoid problems.

Providing for the Nonharmful Expression of Anger
When anger is situational—ie, a response to the stress and anxiety generated by illness—the nurse can more directly intervene by acknowledging the client's anger and encouraging discussion of the events preceding it. Interventions depend on the source of the anger. Corrective steps can be taken by nursing and medical staff to place clients back in charge and respect their privacy and dignity. The nurse and client can explore alternatives together—eg, discussing the anger rather than throwing the bedpan, working out in the gym, or taking up carpentry or leather working. Occupational therapists will have ideas on how to help angry persons channel their energy in more constructive directions. The objective is to allow the expression of anger in more acceptable and less harmful ways. Review the suggested verbal interventions in the section on anxiety because they also apply in the nursing care of angry clients.

Setting Rational and Reasonable Limits
Of course, limits must be set on the behavior of angry clients if it endangers the client or others. Limits should be set in a nonjudgmental way. While acknowledging the

client's angry feelings, also let the client know that hurting oneself or others or destroying property is not allowed. Although nurses in psychiatric settings may sometimes see violent or assaultive clients, this behavior is not common in most other health settings. Assaultiveness or violence may result from alcohol, drugs, certain medications, and head injury. Nurses in emergency or trauma settings and on neurologic units may encounter such clients.

Under these circumstances, it is wise to seek assistance from other staff to help monitor the client's behavior and enforce limits. Precautions should be taken against physically overwhelming the client and endangering the client's well-being. Some clients have died as the result of the staff's overeagerness to control disruptive behavior. In one explosive situation, a violent client who had assaulted staff and other clients was subdued in a neck hold by a male nursing supervisor. During the melee, the client suffered laryngeal damage and died of suffocation. Training programs in nonviolent management of disruptive, assaultive, or out-of-control behavior (see resource list at the end of this chapter) are useful for staff who are likely to encounter such clients.

Referring to Other Resources
For some persons, anger, hostility, and even rage are a way of dealing with the world. In addition to the interventions discussed, the nurse might also consider other resources. The assistance of a mental health–psychiatric nurse would be beneficial to the client, family, friends, and the staff.

Understanding One's Own Feelings
Of crucial importance is that nurses not retaliate or allow themselves to be alienated from angry clients. Remember that anxiety came before anger in the client's experience. Although the nurse may feel angry at the client or frightened, these feelings can interfere with developing realistic goals and effective interventions.

Supporting Family and Friends
Families and friends of angry clients may need the nurse's help as well. They may be embarrassed about the behavior of their family member or friend. They may need help in understanding the behavior and its source and help in dealing with the problems it may bring them. Explain that the client has the need to express both positive and negative feelings about health, illness, and/or hospitalization. Help them to understand when the anger is displaced and when it is not personally directed. Encourage family and friends to accept the angry verbalizations without being judgmental—and acknowledge their efforts.

If their loved one is assaultive or violent, family and friends may also be frightened, confused, or angry. Helping them to understand the client's responses as part of the client's traumatic or toxic condition will also support them in their efforts to manage the situation. They may also need help in setting limits and strategies for reducing the anger.

Evaluation
In evaluating the potential client outcomes, determine whether:

- The client is able to recognize the anger.
- The client is able to discuss the anger and consider the possible sources.
- The client is able to convert the expression of anger to behavior that is not dangerous to the self or to others, preferably in words.
- The client is able to use other more constructive outlets for the expression of anger.
- The client is able to exert greater self-control over the expression of anger.
- The client is able to be increasingly self-directed in managing situations that provoke anger.

In evaluating potential outcomes in relation to family and friends, consider whether:

- Family or friends are able to spend time in the client's company and do not withdraw their presence or their support.
- Family or friends do not personalize the anger and respond defensively.
- Family or friends allow the client to express both positive and negative feelings about what is happening.
- Family or friends are able to accept the client's verbal expressions of anger.
- Family and friends are able to set limits if necessary.
- Family and friends are able to implement strategies for anger reduction.

Do not set overly optimistic expectations. Clients for whom anger has been a lifestyle may have passed an important milestone by simply being able to acknowledge previously unrecognized anger.

DENIAL
Earlier in this chapter, denial was described as a self-protective measure. Denial helps reduce the anxiety associated with illness, trauma, loss (see Chapter 16), and other major life changes. A diagnosis of a life-threatening illness or an illness that requires unwanted major life changes may bring intolerable anxiety. Clients or family members may use denial essentially to "buy time" so they will not feel overwhelmed before the associated anxiety abates. Denial is usually limited in time. Persistent denial hinders well-being when it interferes with steps that can be taken to regain health or to prevent further deterioration of health. Persistent denial also drains psychic energy. Denial may also be a factor in noncompliance.

Nursing Assessment: Establishing the Data Base
Clients may be using denial when they give mixed messages to questions about symptoms or how they are feeling

(ie, the verbal and nonverbal communications do not match). The grimacing client who denies pain is an example. Denial may also be operating when clients or their families disbelieve the diagnosis, prognosis, or information they are given. This does not mean clients and their families must always unquestioningly accept what the health care provider says or does. In fact, if they did, fewer second opinions would be sought, which would not be in the best interests of health care consumers. Sometimes, however, persons distort information so they can maintain denial without being aware they are doing so. Denial should be suspected when a client refuses to discuss a condition or upcoming surgery; fails to carry out recommended procedures or self-care such as colostomy care; refuses to look at a mastectomy incision or the stump of an amputated limb; or refuses medication, treatment, or diagnostic studies.

Nursing Diagnosis

Nursing diagnoses relevant in the care of clients who are denying are:

- Anxiety
- Ineffective individual coping
- Ineffective family coping
- Dysfunctional grieving
- Noncompliance

Also consider the diagnoses of self-care deficit, disturbance in self-concepts, and alteration in thought processes.

Planning and Implementation

In planning and implementation, it is important to understand that the client uses denial because of its protective function. The client needs to deal with the stressful situation at the pace that can be tolerated. Interfering with the protective function of denial before the client is ready is usually not helpful and may be harmful. The exception is when the denial is actually causing the client damage.

To ensure denial is not causing harm, monitor the client with this in mind. By spending time with the client and providing opportunities for verbalization, the nurse can begin to create a climate in which the client may feel freer to relax and begin to cope with the anxiety brought on by the threatening situation.

Without pressuring the client, begin introducing reality-based observations and/or health instructions. A comment on how the incision is healing or on what prostheses are available provides an opening for further discussion. Do not support the denial by agreeing with it or by giving false reassurance. Instead, acknowledge that accepting unpleasant or frightening realities can be difficult. Support any progress the client has made in overcoming or reducing the denial. Encourage the client's continuing efforts in this direction.

If family or significant others are denying, the same interventions can be useful in helping them. Remember that the stability of a family system can be threatened by the illness of one of its members. Family and friends can help the client cope with the denial if they understand what is happening and how they can help. Meeting with family and friends to provide health teaching and to enlist their cooperation will help them as well as the client.

As the client begins to accept reality, the anxiety level may again increase. When anxiety rises, consider implementing the strategies discussed earlier in the section on anxiety.

Evaluation

Expected potential outcomes are that the client and/or family and friends will be able to accept reality and give up denial. They will be able to discuss the previously denied prognosis, diagnosis, or body alteration. The client may begin to implement self-care activities. An additional potential outcome might be a temporary increase in anxiety immediately after the denial has been discarded.

DEPRESSION

Depression is an alteration of affect or mood to sadness or even despair. The condition has been called "the common cold" of mental health because almost everyone is subject to it at one time or another. Depression is also the next most common condition after cardiovascular and musculoskeletal problems.

An estimated one out of every six Americans is likely to be depressed at some point in life. The condition is most prevalent among women and the elderly (American Psychiatric Association, 1980), but the reasons are unclear. Recent research indicates that heredity, environment, and changes in body chemistry may contribute to depression.

Depression may follow real or perceived loss. Clients who have experienced biological or self-esteem losses may respond with depression. Nurses are likely to encounter many persons depressed by the stress of illness, surgery, lifestyle changes, and body image alterations common to health care clients.

Nursing Assessment: Establishing the Data Base

Look for the following emotional and behavioral manifestations of depression:

- Looking and feeling sad, despairing, hopeless, or tired
- Loss of interest in work, hobbies, self, and environment
- Inability to experience pleasure or joy
- Lowered self-esteem
- Thoughts of death or suicide

Physiological manifestations include:

- Loss of appetite usually accompanied by weight loss or, because some people eat more when feeling depressed, weight gain

- Sleep disturbances such as insomnia, early morning awakening, or being unable to get up to face the new day
- Decreased activity level evidenced in slowed-speech and movement
- Constipation
- Decrease in sexual activity

Cognitive manifestations include: difficulty in concentrating, slowed thinking, and difficulty in decision making.

History taking should include family and friends. They may be able to share important information about the type and severity of losses the client has recently experienced, the events that led to the client's feeling depressed, and the client's responses to these situations.

Although there are no laboratory tests to diagnose depression, the dexamethasone suppression test (DST) helps determine whether the client's depression is amenable to somatic treatment, such as antidepressant medications.

Nursing Diagnosis

A number of nursing diagnoses are appropriate in caring for persons who are depressed. The primary diagnoses are ineffective individual coping and dysfunctional grieving. Other relevant nursing diagnoses are:

- Alteration in bowel elimination: constipation
- Impaired verbal communication
- Deficit in diversional activity
- Impaired physical mobility
- Alteration in nutrition: less than body requirements (or more than body requirements)
- Self-care deficit
- Sexual dysfunction
- Sleep pattern disturbance
- Distress of the human spirit
- Alteration in thought processes

This list demonstrates the interrelation among the physiological and psychosocial concerns of depressed persons.

Planning and Implementation

Physiological needs of depressed clients require special attention to hydration, nutrition, and bowel elimination. A depressed client may not be able to tend to these needs. Because the whole body slows down, the client may be prone to constipation. The client may need more assistance than usual in carrying out personal hygiene and activities of daily living. Comfort measures such as back rubs, a warm drink, a warm bath, or soothing music may promote relaxation and sleep.

Because depressed persons are withdrawn and quiet, they are sometimes forgotten. Be sure to spend time with the client, offering opportunities to express feelings related to the losses the client has experienced. When the client is unable or unwilling to talk, simply being there can demonstrate genuine interest in the client's welfare. Touching the client—a pat on the hand, a touch on the shoulder, or a hug if the client seems open to it and it seems appropriate—is often comforting.

Be careful not to offer empty reassurance to the client. In the client's view, life may look bleak. Attempting to make light of these feelings only demonstrates lack of understanding. Instead, help the client to understand the relation between the client's feelings and recent events that may have provoked the depression. Acknowledge that the client has had a bad time and is going through a period of mourning.

Remember that depressed persons are slowed not only in their motor skills but in their thinking. Allow more time than usual to carry out direct client care activities. The client should be encouraged to undertake self-care activities as able, and allow more time than usual for these activities. The client's activity level can be gradually increased.

Clients who continue to be severely depressed may benefit from mental health intervention by a psychiatric-mental health nurse or other professional. Interventions may include counseling or somatic treatments such as antidepressant medication.

Evaluation

Expected outcomes are that the client's depression will lessen and the client will be able to assume self-care activities. Sleep pattern disturbances should diminish, and the client should feel less fatigued and apathetic. With counseling, the client should be able to identify the events and losses that led to the depression and be able to express the feelings associated with them.

DEPENDENCE

Everyone relies on someone or something else at some time for support and to have needs met. As infants, persons learn to rely on parents or other caregivers. As adolescents, they struggle with becoming independent. By the time they reach adulthood, most have learned interdependence—a balance between dependent and independent behavior.

At various times, adults may find that, no matter how independent or how interdependent they usually are, circumstances may require dependence on others. Illness and hospitalization are two of these circumstances. Consider the client whose femur is fractured in an automobile accident. In the early stages, this person will probably have to depend on others to meet physical needs and emotional needs for support and caring. As healing progresses, however, the client begins to meet more of his or her own needs, relying on others to a lesser degree. The behavior is considered *adaptive dependent behavior* because the client was able to be as dependent as necessary to regain health.

In another situation, the client might continue to be dependent for physical needs even though healing has progressed, and the condition no longer warrants it. This is an example of *maladaptive dependent behavior*. As a method of coping, it is unrealistic and inappropriate. The behavior may come about because the client has not had early needs for dependence met in a satisfying way. These clients fear being left alone and find it difficult to trust that others will take care of them when necessary. Or perhaps the client has learned that anxiety can be reduced by depending on others. Regardless of the reason, the results are problems in the interpersonal relationship between client and nurse that cause obstacles to health care.

Although overly dependent persons may appear helpless, their behavior actually controls others as it becomes demanding. Health care personnel often respond with anger to the client's unrealistic and inappropriate demands. Their anger may only increase the client's anxiety and dependence.

It is important that nurses recognize how their own needs for dependence and independence influence their expectations of clients. Nurses who feel rewarded and fulfilled when clients are overly dependent on them do not assist clients to function at their optimum health level. Nurses who cannot tolerate a client's dependence will not deal effectively with a client's realistic dependence and interfere with the client's return to health. A nurse can help dependent clients most by facilitating adaptive dependent behavior, setting limits on maladaptive dependent behavior, and encouraging eventual independence or interdependence.

Nursing Assessment: Establishing the Data Base

Adaptive dependent behavior is assessed by observing the circumstances under which the dependent behavior occurs. Adaptive dependent behavior is a flexible response to a change in the health situation. Evidence of maladaptive dependent behavior may include:

- The client refuses to participate in self-care.
- The client asks the nurse or other health care personnel to perform tasks that are within the client's capabilities.
- The client frequently uses the call light or calls for nursing personnel.
- The client frequently expresses a lack of confidence, helplessness, and feelings of isolation and alienation.
- The client is reluctant to discontinue treatment or, if hospitalized, to be transferred to a unit, such as an intermediate or ambulatory care unit, that requires greater independence.
- The client refuses to learn to carry out tasks associated with a body change or claims inability to learn.

Also assess how long the maladaptive behavior has been used. Is dependence an ongoing method of coping with life? Or is dependence situational (ie, a method of coping with anxiety brought on by illness [or threat of illness] or hospitalization)? Data relevant to these questions can be obtained from the client as well as from family and friends. Be sure also to identify other coping methods the client has employed.

Nursing Diagnosis

Several nursing diagnoses apply to dependent behavior. Among them are ineffective individual coping, self-care deficit, disturbance in self-concepts, and noncompliance.

Planning and Implementation

The first priority is to initiate frequent contacts with the client. It is essential to demonstrate interest in the client and willingness to spend time with the client other than time the client requests or demands. At the same time, it is important to identify when the client can next expect to see the nurse or another health care worker. Telling the client when a nurse or someone else will return and then doing so helps the client develop trust and may reduce anxiety.

Next, encourage the client to begin self-care activities one step at a time. The intent is to assist the client toward greater independence and not to be punitive. As the client begins to take on self-care activities, provide encouragement and acknowledge the client's efforts. Collaborating with the client in developing a step-by-step plan is likely to result in a more effective plan than one determined solely by the nurse. In some cases, verbal or written contracts between client and nurse assist in establishing common goals and clarify the rights and responsibilities of each party. It goes without saying that adaptive dependence needs are met until the client is physiologically able to participate in self-care.

If dependence has been a lifelong coping strategy for the client, it is probably unrealistic for the nurse to expect to be able to change the behavior. The nurse may not be able to meet the unrealistic and perhaps insatiable demands of such clients. Efforts to encourage self-care activities may not be successful. If that is the case, rational limits may have to be set on the extent to which the client's dependence needs will be met.

Let clients know why their increasing independence is being encouraged. Express interest in helping the client be as self-sufficient as possible and explain that doing everything for the client diminishes autonomy. Criticizing dependent behavior is more likely to increase anxiety than to encourage behavior change.

Family and friends should also participate in the planning and implementation. They often have useful suggestions because they know the client well. They will be in a position to reinforce the client's moves toward greater independence. Family and friends may be helped by explanations that account for the client's dependent behavior.

The nurse can help them to learn when to perform activities for the client and when they should encourage independent functioning.

Evaluation

In a successful plan, the client demonstrates an increased ability for self-care. Client requests for help or attention should decrease in frequency. As the client gains greater self-confidence and trusts the nurse to help when necessary, the client will be more interested in greater independence, be pleased with the changes in activity, and be less reluctant to rely more on self than on others. The client's objections to transferring to an intermediate care unit or ambulatory care unit will decrease or cease.

Chapter Highlights

Being ill not only makes clients vulnerable; they also must be more (not less) coherent, in charge, and capable in the face of an unsettled existence.

The social, emotional, and practical needs of clients may make it difficult, if not impossible, for them to perform or behave as the nurse thinks appropriate. Labeling such clients "resistive," "noncompliant," or "a problem patient" obstructs effective use of the nursing process.

Clients who fail to follow a treatment program may do so because of knowledge deficit. Assess for this possibility to correct it.

Complying with a treatment regimen may have costs to the client, such as the anxiety of acknowledging the reality of illness or health risk; imposed lifestyle burdens; being subjected to painful, disfiguring, or risky treatments; financial burdens; the need to submit to the authority of health care personnel; and the possibility of burdening family and friends.

Persons cope with stress in a variety of ways that seem to have worked in the past. Some talk it over with others; some jog; others pray or laugh off the problem.

When someone is unable to ward off stress or reduce anxiety in the usual way, tension mounts. Persons may have to rely on largely unconscious and inflexible coping patterns that are self-deceptive. The three most common patterns are denial, regression, and suppression.

Anxiety is the reason why persons use coping strategies. Anxiety is an uncomfortable feeling that stems from threats to biological integrity and the security of the self.

Quick and accurate assessment and interventions for anxiety are important, because at higher levels, anxiety interferes with a client's ability to get well or to keep well.

Nurses can expect clients and their families to become anxious in the face of unknown or potentially painful, dangerous, or disfiguring events.

Anger is the fight response to anxiety that reduces the powerlessness the anxious client feels. In planning an intervention for anger, the nurse should understand that anger was preceded by anxiety.

Denial helps clients and their families "buy time" as a self-protective measure to reduce the anxiety associated with illness, trauma, loss, and major life changes.

Depression is not uncommon in clients and families under stress. The condition often follows real or perceived biological or self-esteem losses. Depression interferes with a person's ability to carry out self-care activities.

Maladaptive dependent behavior exists when a client continues to depend on the nurse to meet physical needs when the client's condition no longer warrants. The behavior creates obstacles to effective health care.

Bibliography

American Psychiatric Association: *Diagnostic and Statistical Manual of Mental Disorders*, 3rd ed. Washington, DC: American Psychiatric Association, 1980.

Antonovsky A: *Health, Stress, and Coping.* San Francisco, CA: Jossey–Bass, 1980.

Barry PD: *Psychosocial Nursing Assessment and Intervention.* Philadelphia: Lippincott, 1984.

Brigman C, Dickey C, Zegeer LJ: The agitated aggressive patient. *Am J Nurs* 1983; 83:1409–1412.

Garber J, Seligman MEP: *Human Helplessness: Theory and Applications.* New York: Academic Press, 1980.

Hoff LA: *People in Crisis: Understanding and Helping.* 2nd ed. Menlo Park, CA: Addison–Wesley, 1984.

Jalowiec A, Powers MJ: Stress and coping in hypertensive and emergency room patients. *Nurs Res* 1981; 30:10–14.

Kneisl CR, Wilson HS: *Handbook of Psychosocial Nursing Care.* Menlo Park, CA: Addison–Wesley, 1984.

Leventhal H, Watts JC, Pagano F: Effects of fear and instructions on how to cope with danger. *J Personal Soc Psychol* 1967; 6:313–321.

Maagdenberg AM: The "violent" patient. *Am J Nurs* 1983; 83:402–403.

Vogel CH: Anxiety and depression among the elderly. *J Gerontol Nurs* 1982; 8:213–216.

Wilson HS, Kneisl CR: *Psychiatric Nursing*, 2nd ed. Menlo Park, CA: Addison–Wesley, 1983.

Yoos L: Compliance: Philosophical and ethical considerations. *Nurse Pract* 1981; 6(5):27 + .

Ziemer MM: Coping behavior: A response to stress. *Top Clin Nurs* 1982; 2(4):4–12.

Suggested Readings

Barash DA: Defusing the violent patient before he explodes. *RN* (March) 1984; 47:34–37. This practical article describes the early warning signs of mounting tension that could escalate into violence. Various approaches to handling conflict are discussed. Especially useful is "do's and don'ts" of dealing with violence.

Brigman C, Dickey C, Zegeer LJ: 1983. The agitated aggressive patient. *Am J Nurs* 1983; 83:1409–1412. Although written for nurses who work with head injury clients, this article is useful for any nurse who cares for agitated or aggressive clients. Promoting client safety, protecting oneself, reducing stimulation, minimizing confusion, and dealing with inappropriate behavior are discussed. There is a small section on reducing the family's anxiety.

Davis AJ: *Listening and Responding*. St Louis: Mosby, 1984. This book focuses on the skills of listening and responding to clients with concern, sensitivity, and compassion throughout the life cycle.

Miller JM: Inspiring hope. *Am J Nurs* 1985; 85(1):22–25. Based on the belief that hope positively influences the healing response and is necessary to prevent the physical and mental deterioration brought on by despair, this author presents practical hope-inspiring nursing strategies, based on an existential framework, that can be incorporated into the care of seriously ill clients.

Scarf M: *Unfinished Business*. New York: Simon & Schuster, 1981. Written by noted feminist author Maggie Scarf, this book on depression is warm, caring, and interesting. It makes the pain of depression real to the reader.

Tavris C: *Anger: The Misunderstood Emotion*. New York: Simon & Schuster, 1983. This book challenges the assumption that ventilation of anger is basically healthy and suppressed hostility, medically dangerous. The author takes the view that expressing anger makes one angrier, solidifies an angry attitude, and establishes a hostile habit.

Zangari M, Duffy P: Contracting with patients in day-to-day practice. *Am J Nurs* 1980; 80:451–455. The philosophical base of this article is that nurses and clients are equal partners in health care with certain responsibilities toward established common goals. The authors present the theoretical basis for contracting, explain how contracting can be used with hospitalized clients, and provide case examples.

Resources

Crisis Prevention Institute
Lakewood Building
3575 N Oakland Ave
Milwaukee, WI 53211
Phone: (414) 332–4663
Toll-free number: (800) 558–8976

This organization has offered nonviolent physical crisis intervention programs in health, education, social welfare, security, and correctional facilities since 1972. Staff are trained in the prevention and management of disruptive, assaultive, or out-of-control behavior. The group also offers a quarterly publication, the *CPI National Report*, focusing on current facts and techniques in managing aggressive behavior.

Chapter 7

Comprehensive Health Assessment of the Adult

SueAnn Wooster Ames

Objectives

When you have finished studying this chapter, you should be able to:

Identify approaches to facilitating nurse–client communication.

Elicit and record a comprehensive health history.

Explain the need for a thorough psychosocial/lifestyle history.

Become comfortable obtaining a sexual health history.

Recognize the importance of a review of the family health history and its implications for the long-term health of the client.

Maintain client dignity and comfort throughout the health assessment process.

Demonstrate techniques of physical assessment and explain appropriate alterations in their sequence depending on the body system being examined and the condition of the client.

Specify areas to be assessed in each bodily system.

Describe common assessment findings that may appear abnormal but are within the wide range of normal.

Anticipate some of the age-related changes often observed during the health assessment process.

Discuss the difference between invasive and noninvasive diagnostic tests.

Demonstrate the role of the nurse as client advocate by presenting an actual or simulated nurse–client interaction involving informed consent with an invasive diagnostic study.

To assess the health of adults comprehensively, the nurse must be able to communicate effectively with clients and families, assemble a complete data base, and synthesize the information gathered to form an accurate picture of the client's health. Use of the nursing process is fundamental to the accomplishment of this goal.

The nursing process is a problem-solving approach to the care of clients. The essential steps of the nursing process are:

- Assessment (gathering the subjective and objective client data base).
- Establishing a nursing diagnosis.
- Developing a plan of care with the client.
- Implementing the plan.
- Evaluating the plan and revising it as needed.

The crucial step is the data-gathering phase. If important aspects of the client's life are overlooked or given only cursory attention during the health history, the nursing diagnoses and plan of care will be deficient.

Section I: Communicating With Clients

Each client and each nurse bring to the client–nurse interaction a unique set of variables that influences the relationship in a variety of ways. Age and sex, background, culture and life experience, religion or belief system, attitudes and values, expectations, hopes and fears all affect the relationship. Some of these factors enhance communication; others may create barriers.

No matter what their status in the outside world, clients enter the health care system with a perceived loss of status, power, and most of all, control. These losses are often intensified by a system that subtly rewards "good patients" who passively comply with a plan of care devised and directed by health professionals who barely know them. The assertive client who asks pointed questions and demands input into decisions about care is labeled "difficult."

Of the members of the team of health professionals concerned with the client's care, the nurse knows the client and family best. Thus, the nurse often assumes the position of client advocate; reinforcing to the physician the concerns of the client and family; getting answers to unanswered questions; and in general, presenting the case for the client. The nurse also assumes the role of interpreter, restating and explaining the physician's statements to the client in terms appropriate to the client's level of understanding and current emotional state.

Besides functioning as advocate and interpreter, the nurse is responsible for identifying clients' strengths and social resources; evaluating their knowledge of health and illness; becoming acutely aware of sociocultural and religious influences that may affect their responses; and detecting subtle cues of pain, anxiety, emotion, or deteriorating condition. Fulfillment of these numerous respon-

sibilities depends in large part on the nurse's ability to assess a client, blending communication strengths with a systematic approach to history taking and skill in physical assessment.

During the assessment process, nurses integrate their own natural communication style into the communication approaches learned in nursing fundamentals courses. Listening, body language, touch, and silence—as well as verbal approaches like open-ended questions, clarifying, and paraphrasing—are techniques basic to nursing. These must become more than mere techniques; they must be purposefully cultivated so they become "second nature."

When clients come from cultures other than the care provider's, their views of their illness and its cause will be quite unlike the views of the caregivers. Often the client's questions will not be answered satisfactorily because the significance of the query is not clear to the health professional. To provide effective care to clients from different sociocultural backgrounds, the nurse must understand their health beliefs and practices. For example, many Hispanic clients classify illnesses, drugs, and foods according to their belief in the "hot–cold" theory, which may have significant bearing on how the client responds to diagnosis and treatment. If a different belief system is interfering with the client's care, it is the nurse's responsibility to investigate these beliefs by asking the client about them in a nonjudgmental manner.

Section II: Subjective Health Assessment: The Health History

Health assessment should be the area in which the nurse is most expert. Whether in an acute care or primary care setting, the nurse, rather than the physician, spends the most time in direct contact with the client. Each interchange, no matter how brief, should strengthen the base on which a nursing diagnosis is made as well as strengthen the nurse–client relationship. The nurse's observation and communication skills can be the key to proper diagnosis and treatment, not only nursing diagnosis but medical diagnosis as well.

In the medical diagnostic approach to gathering subjective data, the client's history is taken in an organized sequence, beginning with the chief concern (CC) and ending with a review of systems (ROS). This organized approach to data gathering is a strength of the medical model. The overall focus of the medical model is a search for symptoms—a disease approach. Nurses have long recognized that health and illness are influenced by the totality of one's life and have redesigned the health history format to reflect this fact. Consider the following example:

Mrs JS enters the health care system obviously ill with vertigo, malaise, and muscle weakness of sudden onset. She has a number of noninvasive and invasive diagnostic studies. All test results are within normal limits. In talking with the client, the

nurse asks her about her life, her habits, how she usually spends her day, and how happy she is in her marriage. At this point, the client bursts into tears and blurts out the story of her husband's extramarital affair. Her symptoms developed shortly after learning of his infidelity. The nurse consults with the physician and arranges for the mental health clinical nurse specialist to see Mrs S. As individual counseling and marital counseling continue, her symptoms gradually resolve.

This example is not meant to suggest that physicians do not obtain psychosocial/lifestyle information about clients. Rather, it suggests that nurses, who are educated in a holistic mode, find this information essential to a comprehensive picture of the client. Only with such a picture is it possible to make an accurate nursing diagnosis, to consider fully the goals of care, and to develop with the client a mutual plan to achieve these goals.

APPROACH TO THE HEALTH HISTORY

To depict the health history as an organized whole, history taking will be discussed as though the nurse is taking an initial complete history. Actually, in a clinical situation, history taking continues throughout the nurse–client relationship. A complete history is taken when the client is admitted to an inpatient unit or when the client comes into

Nursing Research Note

Bramwell L: Use of the life history in pattern identification and health promotion. *ANS* (Oct) 1984; 6:37–44.

This qualitative research pilot study was conducted with a selected sample of eight adults over age 60. The life history process incorporated aspects of reminiscence and life review with a comprehensive view of the past from earliest recollections to current circumstances.

In phase 1 of the study, participants jotted on 5 × 7 cards events as they came to mind, one card for each decade of life. The cards were organized chronologically in preparation for phase 2, tape-recorded, 45-minute interviews. Phase 2 took place in the participant's home with only the participant and interviewer present. Two or three sessions were required to complete the data gathering. Field notes were also recorded on each participant from the time of consent to the final interview.

A number of unifying themes emerged from the analysis of each life history. Examples of themes included "wide and varied interests," "satisfying social relationships," and "altruism." Combinations of themes also occurred.

Putting life events in context provided an opportunity for participants to obtain perspective of themselves. Comments by study participants supported this process as a vehicle for expanding consciousness and thus promoting health.

an ambulatory facility for a complete physical examination or for a health problem. Even so, the history-taking process continues for as long as the nurse and the client are in contact. If the history is viewed as a task to be completed and not thought of again, important data may be missed.

In the initial encounter with the care provider, clients are often anxious, worried, or embarrassed about their health problem. They may simply forget important information or perhaps consciously withhold it. One advantage of an ongoing nurse–client relationship, as in inpatient settings, is that clients can easily share previously withheld information later when they remember it or become more comfortable with the nurse.

FORMAT FOR THE HEALTH HISTORY

Some portions of the health history are almost self-explanatory; eg, personal data includes such information as name, address, and age. Source of history and reliability of informant refer to circumstances in which the client may not be able to give a clear history, eg, because of a language barrier, aphasia, facial or oral injury, or coma. Identify the person who gave the history (client, parent, spouse, friend) and record a judgment of the overall reliability of the informant. A complete health history appears later in this chapter in Box 7–3.

Chief Concern

The chief concern (CC) is the main reason the client sought health care. Usually, the CC is recorded in the client's own

words; eg, "[I have had this] severe pounding headache over both eyes for 2 days."

To make the CC more concise, the nurse might translate the client's words into a brief statement. Suppose the client says, "I came to the clinic today because I was in an auto accident a week ago. Since then, I have had aching in both my lower legs and pain in my left arm. My lower back hurts since the accident. I've had low back pain on and off for 10 years, but the accident made it much worse." The CC in this instance might be translated:

CC: Numerous aches and pains both legs, left arm 2° to auto accident 1 week ago.
Low-back pain × 10 years, aggravated by accident.

History of the Present Illness

The history of the present illness (HPI) is the heart of the health history. It is a chronological review of the client's health problem in narrative form. Various approaches to tracking down a symptom have been developed to be certain important historical information is not overlooked (see Boxes 7–1 and 7–2).

For example, when taking the HPI on the client with a CC of severe pounding headache over both eyes for 2

Box 7–1   Seven Guidelines to Evaluate a Symptom

1. Bodily location
2. Quality
3. Quantity: intensity, volume, number, size or extent
4. Chronology or timing: onset, duration, frequency, course
5. Setting
6. Aggravating and alleviating factors
7. Associated manifestations

SOURCE: Reprinted with permission from Morgan WL Jr, Engel GL: *The Clinical Approach to the Patient.* Philadelphia: Saunders, 1969, p. 35.

Box 7–2   Mnemonic to Evaluate the Symptom of Pain

P: provocative/palliative factors

Q: quality

R: region

S: severity

T: timing

days, the interviewer would initially use the seven guidelines (Box 7–1), or the PQRST mnemonic (Box 7–2) if that is easier to remember. For *bodily location* the nurse might say, "Point to the places on your head where you feel the pain." *Quality* can be evaluated by asking what the pain is like. If the client cannot give an example the nurse might ask, "Does it feel like someone pounding on your head or like a tight band around your head?" To assess *quantity* of the pain, ask the client to describe its severity: "Is it mildly annoying, moderate, severe? Or is it unbearable?"

Chronology begins with the onset of the symptom; eg, "When did these headaches first begin?" Duration, frequency, and course are then reconstructed. "How long do they usually last?" "How often do they tend to recur?" "Have you noticed any pattern to them? For example, are your headaches often associated with your menstrual cycle, or do you seem to develop a headache when you are under stress?"

The *setting* where a symptom is experienced often gives a clue to the diagnosis. Does the client experience headaches only on weekends? Only at work? Only on vacation? Only during allergy season? Or does the setting seem to have no relation at all to the headache?

Conditions that *aggravate* or *provoke* the headache are assessed. "When you have a headache, what seems to make it worse? For example, is the headache made worse by bright lights, potent smells, loud noises, bending over? Factors that *alleviate* or *palliate* the headache are also addressed. "Have you found anything that helps your headache once you have one? For example, is the headache made better by lying down in a dark room? An ice bag? A hot towel? A specific medication?" Any other *symptoms associated* with the headache are also considered. For example, does the client also experience nausea and/or vomiting, photophobia, or vertigo?

Information gathered during the evaluation of the symptom guides the examiner to the next phase of the HPI. For example, if the client associates eating patterns with the headache, the next step is a dietary history. Substances associated with headache are tracked down carefully. Examples are foods containing tyramine (cheese, beer, red wine) or monosodium glutamate (MSG), frequently found in Chinese food and in many "fast-food" preparations. Perhaps the headache occurs when the client misses a meal or is secondary to caffeine withdrawal. Any association the client notes should be followed up in the HPI.

With experience and an increasing knowledge base, the nurse also begins to associate symptom complexes and to develop ability to identify information that directly contributes to the client's chief concern. When completed, the HPI should provide a clear picture of the client's problem from onset to the present and should convey an appreciation for how the client's lifestyle has contributed to and been affected by the health problem.

Past Health History

The client's past health is reviewed and recorded as concisely as possible. Childhood illnesses are listed, and specific questions are asked about rheumatic fever, scarlet fever, or any major health problems the client recalls from childhood. An immunization history is obtained. Many adults are unaware that they should have a tetanus–diphtheria (Td) booster every 10 years. Because a booster is given with dog bites or with injuries in which the skin is broken in an unclean manner, the client may be able to associate the most recent Td with such an event.

A review of medical problems and surgical procedures follows. Major diagnostic studies with dates (eg, an intravenous pyelogram) are listed, as are blood transfusions. For the female client, a pregnancy history is obtained, and weight of infants if over 9 lb is noted. A client who has given birth to a large infant may be prediabetic.

Both physical and psychological trauma are evaluated. A history of fractures or concussions as well as major life stress events that may be unresolved are important to note. Any psychiatric hospitalizations or other hospitalizations not covered under the previous categories are also listed.

An allergy history is obtained, including allergy to pollens, foods, clothing, insects, animals, drugs, diagnostic test contrast media, and anesthetic agents. The client's reaction to the allergen is recorded. Does the client state a penicillin allergy is present because of diarrhea 6 days after beginning the drug, or because of becoming extremely short of breath and cyanotic shortly after taking it? This information may make a major difference in future treatment.

The client's history of medication use is of prime importance. Many clients think of "medicine" as prescription drugs and do not consider over-the-counter (OTC) drugs significant. Yet an OTC medication that the client forgot to mention may interfere with the action of a prescribed drug. For example, antacids inhibit the absorption of tetracycline. OTC drugs may also cause serious side effects if not used carefully. For example, phenylpropanolamine, found in many nasal decongestants and in diet pills, has been reported to cause headaches, seizures, and psychic disturbance in previously healthy persons. Few clients think of vitamins and oral contraceptives as drugs, so the nurse should ask specifically about them.

Family History

Because many health problems tend to run in families, either through genetic transfer or environmental influence (eg, diet), the nurse gathers a thorough family history (FH). If the client has been adopted, the genetic aspect will not apply, but a discussion of the general health of the entire family is still helpful in obtaining an impression of the client and family relationships. The family history may be recorded in outline format or in the form of a **genogram,** a diagram

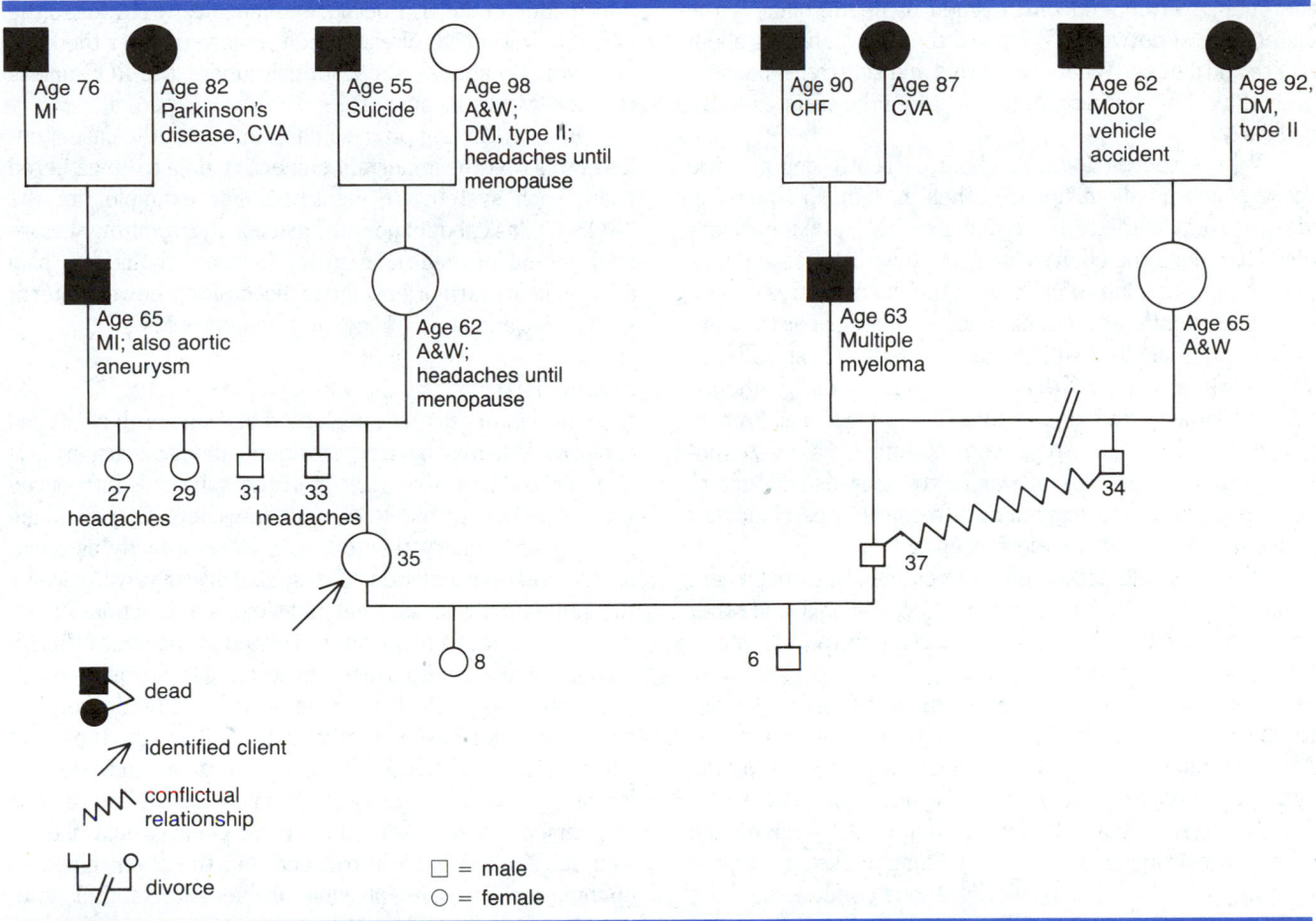

Figure 7–1
Example of a genogram. In this genogram, the identified female client, age 35, is the oldest of five children. Her mother and grandmother are both living. She is married to a 37-year-old man who has some conflict with his younger brother. His parents were divorced. The client and her husband have a daughter and a son. Her family history is positive ⊕ for cardiovascular disease, diabetes mellitus type II, Parkinson's disease, aortic aneurysm, suicide, and headache until menopause. Her husband's family history is ⊕ for cardiovascular disease, diabetes mellitus type II, and multiple myeloma.

of the family tree. Interactional as well as genetic information can be noted on the genogram (Figure 7–1).

The age, health, and cause of death of blood relatives is recorded. Maternal and paternal grandparents, parents, siblings, and children all are included in this history. In addition, ask whether any blood relatives have a history of elevated blood pressure, cerebrovascular accident (CVA), myocardial infarction (MI), hypercholesterolemia, tuberculosis (TBC), alcoholism, cancer of any organ, or diabetes mellitus (DM). It is helpful to follow up with a question such as, "Are there any diseases your family thinks tend to run in the family?" The answer may reveal problems such as migraine headache, cystic fibrosis, or familial polyposis that may not have surfaced during the discussion. Another useful follow-up question is, "Does anyone else in the family have a problem similar to yours?" The response is often revealing and helps put the client's symptoms in perspective. In the client with the headaches, consider what approach to use if the client said, "My best friend

who was just my age died last week of a brain tumor. Her symptoms started out just like mine."

The racial and ethnic origins of the family are of great importance when gathering a history. Blacks should be asked about a family history of sickle cell disease or sickle cell trait. Jews should be questioned about Tay–Sachs disease in the family. Uncovering these facts early provides an opportunity to direct the unmarried and/or not-yet-pregnant client to a genetic counselor for counseling and education.

Personal/Social History

The personal/social portion of the health history helps the nurse develop a feeling for what clients' lives are like; how they spend an average day; and their interests, beliefs, and habits. Does the client have strong religious beliefs that are a source of hope and spiritual strength? Who are the significant persons in the client's life? Are there persons the client can depend on in times of need? What is the client's social network? What are the client's beliefs about health and illness? What preventive and self-care measures does the client routinely practice? Does the client exercise regularly?

What stresses does the client currently identify? Are there concerns about finances, health, family responsibilities, or social life? Are there multiple changes in the client's life? How does the client usually cope with stress and how does he or she plan to cope with the current stressors?

The client's educational and occupational history are discussed, including future goals. Is the client satisfied with work or school? What occupational or environmental hazards is the client exposed to? Military service and recent travel experiences are reviewed, not only to assess exposure to toxic chemicals of war or to diseases endemic to certain geographic areas but also to consider psychological consequences of such experiences.

The client should be questioned about practices contributing to poor health such as tobacco, alcohol, and other drug use. Smoking is quantified according to pack years. (One package of cigarettes per day for 1 year equals 1 pack year.) Thus, a client who has smoked 2½ packs per day (PPD) for 20 years has a 50-pack-year smoking history. Alcohol intake should also be quantified, if possible, by the number of ounces of beer, wine, or liquor per day.

A careful dietary history is obtained by asking the client to describe in detail food and fluid intake for a typical 24-hour period. Ask specifically about caffeine, sodium, and fat intake. Does the client make an attempt to incorporate foods from the basic four food groups, or is the eating pattern haphazard? Does the client prepare meals at home or eat out? Are there mobility or transportation problems that prevent the client from shopping for food? What type of restaurants does the client frequent? Are there any restrictions on the client's diet because of finances, religious beliefs, cultural preferences, food intolerance, or health status? Is the client on a weight-reduction diet and, if so, what kind? Is the client a vegetarian? Does the client take vitamin or mineral supplements? (See Chapters 8 and 9 for information on malnutrition, obesity, and eating disorders.)

Review of Systems

The review of systems (ROS) is a verbal rundown from head to toe of the client's overall state of health and the health of each bodily system. The review serves as a memory prod for both the nurse and the client in obtaining missing data. For example if, in questioning the client with headaches, vision was omitted during the HPI, ask under "ROS-Eyes" when the last vision exam was done. The client might respond that it was 3 years ago when glasses were prescribed for reading, but she never wears them. She then talks about how tired her eyes feel at times and states that this probably doesn't help the headaches. In this instance, when recording the history, place the eye

information in the HPI because it specifically relates to the CC. If a system has already been reviewed under the HPI, however, do not ask about it again under the ROS unless the review was incomplete.

In each nursing process chapter and in the case studies in this text the important subjective data to be gathered about each system are identified. For example, for the "ROS-GI" ask about appetite, nausea and vomiting, nature and amount of emesis, food intolerance, flatulence, pain such as heartburn or epigastric discomfort, bowel pattern, stool color and consistency, and hemorrhoids.

Sexual History

A sexual history is often neglected because both client and care provider may have reservations about discussing this intimate and sensitive subject. If the subject is introduced with ease during the ROS, and the client is questioned about genitourinary function as matter-of-factly as about gastrointestinal function, the sexual history will receive the same emphasis as other physiological functions.

After a series of questions related to the overall health of the client's genitourinary system, ask an open-ended question about sexual functioning, eg, "How do you feel about the sexual aspects of your life?" Perhaps the client will not answer. Perhaps nonverbal messages indicate hesitation or discomfort. Suggest that it would be fine to raise the subject some other time, if the client would like to. The subject has been introduced and the client given an opening for discussing possible problems at another time.

If the client has a health problem that may cause concurrent alterations in sexual function, pursue the questioning further. For example, in taking a history from a woman who has a cystocele and rectocele and a concern about stress incontinence, the nurse might say, "Many women who lose urine with coughing or sneezing, as you do, find that the fear of losing urine interferes with their sexual relationship. Has this been true for you?" To a man who is taking an antihypertensive drug that may cause impotence, the nurse might say, "Some men have a problem getting an erection when they are taking certain blood pressure medicines. Has this ever happened to you?" Such approaches also let clients know they are not alone with their problems. That knowledge may encourage them to explore the subject further with the nurse or with their physician.

At the completion of the health history, the nurse should ask, "Do you have any other concerns about your health you would like to discuss?" Perhaps an issue important to the client has not been mentioned or pursued. By now enough rapport has usually been established to make the client comfortable in discussing other matters with the nurse. The concerns shared at this point may be the most significant and should not be taken lightly. The client's deepest worry may be signaled by an off-hand question such as, "By the way, do you think this little lump under my arm means anything?" A sample health history write-up is shown in Box 7–3.

Box 7-3   Sample Health History

Personal data:

Date and time: 3-2-85 1 PM

Full Name: Sarah Harris

ID number (Social Security, insurance number): 000-11-1111

Address: 19 Elmwood, Cassadaga, NY

Telephone: Home: 000-0000; Work: 000-0000

Sex: Female

Age: 35

Birthdate: 1-3-50

Marital status: Married

Race/culture: Caucasian

Religion: Protestant

Occupation: Nurse

Usual health care providers: R. Collins, MD; S. Montgomery, RN, NP

Informant: History given by client, who seems credible

CC: Severe, pounding headache over both eyes for 2 days

HPI: Yesterday, Ms Harris awoke with a pounding headache over both eyes, for which she took two OTC sinus pills with no relief. Later, she tried an ice bag, which had helped headaches she'd had in the past, and ASA, with no relief. The pain, which she described as an annoying pounding gradually increasing to severe pain, remained steady all day. It was made worse by bending over and by bright lights. She continued to work but was unable to eat because the pain made her nauseated. She went to bed early and slept all night but still had the headache on awakening this AM. Her menstrual period began today.

Ms Harris has had similar headaches since she was a sophomore in college. She always got one once a month premenstrually and occasionally at other times, "usually after a stressful experience or when I am overtired." She had no headaches during her two pregnancies. Her mother and grandmother had "sick headaches" similar to hers. Their headaches resolved at menopause.

Ms Harris's headaches are always accompanied by nausea and sometimes vomiting. She feels that at times they may be triggered by foods such as cold cuts or chocolate. Red wine also seems to bring them on. She now avoids these substances. She is a heavy coffee drinker at work and sometimes gets a dull headache at home from "caffeine withdrawal."

Ms Harris states she is a "headachy person" and also tends to get other types of headache that are different from her current symptoms and associated with tension, sinus congestion, or eyestrain. She admits to needing glasses for reading but rarely wearing them.

Ms Harris is not a smoker, is not on oral contraceptives, has no known hx of high BP or hx of head trauma.

She suspects her headaches may be migraines because her younger sister, who has similar headaches, was recently diagnosed as having migraines.

Past Health Hx:

Childhood: Chickenpox; denies rheumatic fever, scarlet fever

Immunization: All childhood immunizations; last Td 1982, stitches for cut on hand while working in the garden

Medical problems: None

Surgeries: Tonsils, age 4, Deaconess Hospital, Buffalo NY

Pregnancies: $P_2 G_2$

Trauma: Physical, fx rt clavicle, age 9; psychological, father's death, 1981

Other hospitalizations: None

Blood transfusions: None

Allergies: To tomatoes; reaction—hives

Medications: Prescription, none; OTC, sinus medication spring and fall; occasional ASA or acetaminophen for headaches; multi-vitamin $\bar{\top}$ q.d.

Family Hx (see Figure 7–1 for more genogram format for FHx):

Father: Died age 65, MI; also had aortic aneurysm, benign polyps of colon

Mother: Age 62, A&W; had headaches until menopause

Sisters ×2: Ages 29, 27; A&W; youngest $\bar{c}$ headache

Brothers × 2: Ages 33, 31; A&W; oldest $\bar{c}$ headache

Husband: Age 37, A&W

Daughter: Age 8, A&W

Son: Age 6, A&W

PGF: MI

PGM: CVA, Parkinson's

MGF: Suicide

MGM: DM, type II; headaches until menopause
No ⊕ FHx of Ca, HTN, TBC

Personal/Social Hx: Client received a BS in nursing and is currently working toward an MS degree. She works part-time 3 to 11 PM on a surgical unit of a small hospital. Now that both children are in school all day, she is considering taking a full-time 8 to 4 PM job in an HMO close to her home.

She is happily married × 10 years; the family enjoys many activities together, such as bike riding and swimming.

She never smoked and has an occasional glass of white wine on the weekend; she denies ever having used drugs. A typical diet for a 24-hour period includes orange juice, bran muffin, and coffee for breakfast; yogurt for lunch; and a salad and meat such as broiled chicken or fish and roll for dinner. She rarely eats desserts and watches her fat intake because of her father's CV disease.

Reading, biking, sewing, and playing board games or video games with the children are her major leisure activities.

They are financially stable; her spouse owns a small appliance store, which is doing well.

She copes with stress by talking things over with her sisters, with whom she is very close, or by weeding her garden or cleaning a messy closet.

She feels she has many strengths, good support systems, and a positive attitude toward her future.

ROS:

General state of health: States she is in excellent health with no lack of energy; weight is stable

(continued)

Box 7–3 Sample Health History (continued)

Skin/hair/nails: Occasional facial pimple premenstrually

Eyes: Last eye exam, 1982; no probs c̄ eye pain, blurring of vision, or rings around lights; see HPI

Ears: States hearing is excellent; no ear pain or discharge; no dizziness or tinnitus

Nose and sinuses: Occasional sinus headache spring and fall relieved by OTC medicines; no known seasonal allergies; no nasal trauma or epistaxis

Mouth and teeth: Yearly dental exam, no dentures; no problems with gums, tongue, or change in taste

Throat and neck: Rare sore throat; no difficulty swallowing, hoarseness, or neck stiffness

Breasts and axillae: Does monthly BSE; no nipple discharge, no known lumps or lesions

Respiratory: No cough or wheezing; last chest x-ray 15 years ago, wnl; always has ⊕ TB skin test as was given BCG vaccine in nursing school

Cardiovascular: No DOE, PND, orthopnea; no known heart murmur; no ankle edema; has varicose veins since last pregnancy, wears support stockings; no phlebitis hx

Gastrointestinal: No anorexia, n & v except c̄ CC; no food intolerance, flatulence, change in bowel habits; states stools are brown in color; has BM q.d.; no abdominal pain or abdominal surgery; no hx of jaundice or hemorrhoids

Gynecological: Menarche age 14; q. 28–30-day cycle, 5-day

flow; currently menstruating; no longer uses tampons since TSS scare; no prob c̄ dysmenorrhea, dyspareunia, or vaginal discharge; no birth control—husband had vasectomy; has intercourse approximately once a week; states sexual aspect of her marriage has "always been good"; see HPI for headaches associated c̄ menses

Urinary: No problems of urgency, frequency, dysuria, nocturia, or hematuria; no hx of stress incontinence, UTI, or renal calculi

Musculoskeletal: No problems c̄ low back pain, muscle weakness, leg cramps, joint pain or stiffness; no foot problems

Neurologic: Headaches—see HPI; no problems c̄ vertigo, tremor, sleep disturbances, memory; no paralysis, numbness and tingling, or decreased sensation to any bodily part

Psychological: No problems c̄ mood swings, paranoid feelings, periods of depression or indecision; no hx of suicidal thoughts or attacks of severe anxiety; saw a nurse mental health counselor monthly for about 8 months after her father's death to sort out her feelings about God and life after death; she found the counseling experience helpful and would return if she felt the need to do so

Endocrine: No polyuria, polydipsia, polyphagia; no changes in skin or hair; no intolerance to heat or cold

Lymphatic: No known enlarged nodes in neck, axillae, or groin

Hematopoietic: No hx of anemia or abnormal bleeding or bruising

---

Section III: Objective Health Assessment: The Physical Examination

Using sight, hearing, touch, and smell to examine the client is the objective aspect of the health assessment process. Physical examination of the client will be combined with the client's subjective account of health to arrive at a nursing diagnosis.

The nurse has already made numerous observations about the client throughout the history-taking process. A general impression has been formed; ie, this client is the picture of health or is acutely or chronically ill. Personal hygiene; general intelligence; degree of cooperation; and orientation to time, place, and person have been noted. Body size and shape, body symmetry, posture and gait, and overall speech patterns have already been assessed to some extent. In addition, the skin, the largest organ of the human body, has been observed and was probably touched during the initial handshake. The integument is the window to the human body. Thorough assessment of the skin can reveal a great deal about health and illness.

General observations of the client during the history are translated into a brief description, recorded at the beginning of the physical exam; for example:

Chronically ill, very thin 55-yr-old black male, appears older than stated age, oriented × 3, with scleral icterus, who scratches continuously throughout the history.

General guidelines for approaching the physical examination include:

- Good lighting is essential.
- If the examiner is right handed, examine from the client's right side.
- If the client is an inpatient, position the bed to a proper height.
- The environment should be private and as quiet as possible.
- Explain to the client as the examination proceeds.
- Adequately expose areas being examined.

Subjective data gathering continues throughout the physical assessment as each area is examined in sequence (eg, "Tell me about this small scar on your right breast," or "How long have you had this dark mole on your neck?")

TECHNIQUES OF PHYSICAL ASSESSMENT

In the usual sequence of physically assessing body organs, inspection always comes first and is followed by palpation, percussion, and auscultation. In assessing the abdomen, this sequence changes slightly. Auscultation is performed after inspection because the intestine is sensitive to touch, and palpation and percussion of the abdomen may alter peristaltic sounds.

Inspection

Careful inspection of the area is the most important part of physical assessment. Placing a stethoscope on the chest before looking at the chest is a common error. Each anatomical region should be inspected carefully *before* it is touched with the examiner's hands or instruments, because valuable information can be obtained by thorough observation.

Palpation

Palpation uses the sense of touch to examine all accessible body parts. Using palpation, the following evaluations are made:

- Size and shape (organs, masses)
- Pulsatility
- Mobility
- Consistency
- Tenderness or pain
- Swelling
- Surface temperature
- Muscle rigidity or spasm
- Presence or absence of masses

Keeping the client comfortable and relaxed facilitates thorough palpation. Muscle tension during examination not only interferes with adequate palpation but may also make the client uncomfortable and reluctant to continue with the examination.

Tender areas should always be palpated last. Suppose the client has pain in the left upper quadrant (LUQ) of the abdomen. Examining the involved area first can create considerable discomfort. The client will guard the abdomen, making it impossible to perform an adequate assessment. Many examiners tend to focus in too quickly on the problem area without thoroughly examining surrounding areas where the problem might actually originate.

The nurse should also be comfortable while palpating, and the hands should be warm. Parts of the hand used during palpation are:

- Fingertips for fine tactile discrimination, lymph nodes, skin texture.
- Dorsa of hands for temperature (because dorsal skin is thinner).

- Palmar and ulnar surfaces for vibratory sensation.
- Grasping position of fingers for tissue consistency.

Light palpation helps to relax and reassure the client. It aids in identifying regions of tenderness and muscle resistance. The pads of the fingertips with the fingers together are used in a gentle dipping motion.

Deep palpation is essentially the same as light palpation except that the examiner is pressing much deeper. The approach can be single handed, or the palpating hand (the dominant hand) can be reinforced with fingers of the other hand (Figure 7–2). In this instance, the underlying hand receives the tactile sensations while the upper hand exerts the pressure.

Rebound is a palpatory technique often used for assessment of peritoneal inflammation with appendicitis. Only experienced examiners should palpate for rebound tenderness. Great caution is necessary. The fingertips are pressed deeply into the abdominal wall and quickly withdrawn. Pain felt after withdrawal of pressure is called **rebound tenderness** and is a reliable sign of peritoneal inflammation.

Bimanual palpation is the use of two hands in assessing an organ or mass. One hand may be placed at either side of the mass, grasping it, or one hand may support an organ to move it upward or more forward to make it more accessible to the examining hand. Bimanual palpation is routinely done in examining the kidneys, liver, spleen, and uterus.

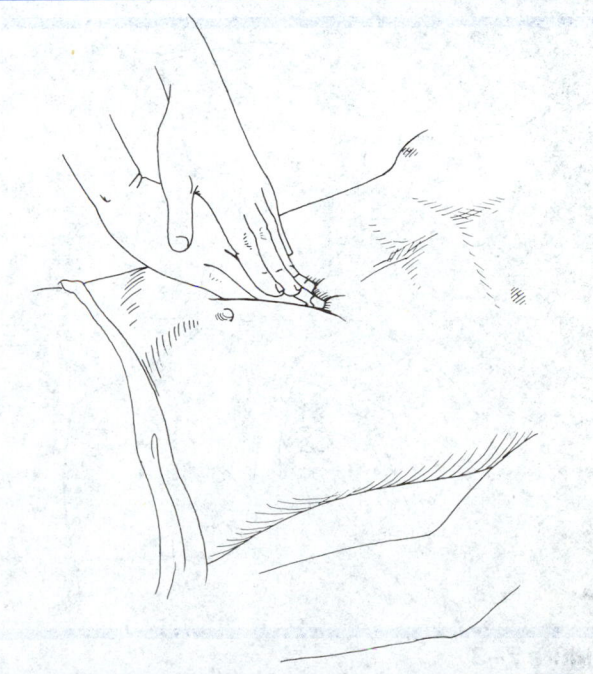

Figure 7–2

Deep palpation. The examiner uses two hands to press deeper into the client's abdomen.

Ballottement is used when fluid is suspected. The fingers are thrust into the area of a suspected mass so a freely movable mass may bound upward, touching the examiner's fingertips. Ballottement should also be done cautiously.

Percussion

Percussion is the technique of striking a body surface lightly but sharply to produce sounds. The sounds enable the examiner to determine position, size, and density of an underlying organ.

In *indirect percussion,* the middle finger of the non-dominant hand (the **pleximeter**) is placed against the body surface with palms and other fingers raised off the skin. The tip of the middle finger of the dominant hand (the **plexor**) strikes the base of the distal phalanx of the pleximeter in a quick, sharp stroke. A series of two to three quick blows is struck. The pleximeter is then moved to a new site, and percussion continues in symmetrical regions, comparing the sounds from side to side (Figure 7–3). Percussion notes are:

- Resonance: A loud, low note heard over normal lung tissue.
- Hyperresonance: A louder, lower, longer note heard over an emphysematous lung.
- Tympany: A loud musical note with a drumlike quality, heard over air-filled viscera such as the stomach or bowel.

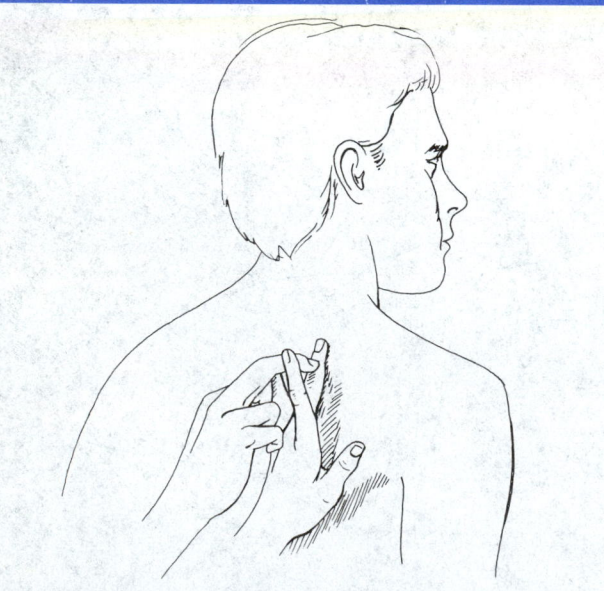

Figure 7–3

Indirect percussion technique to assess the lung sounds. A right-handed examiner uses the middle finger of the left hand as the pleximeter and the middle finger of the right hand as the plexor.

- Dullness: Medium sound heard in areas of increased density, eg, over the liver.
- Flatness: A short, high-pitched sound produced over solid tissue such as the muscles of the thigh.

Direct percussion is a gentle direct striking of the body with one or more fingers or with the ulnar surface of the clenched fist. This technique is useful in assessing tenderness in an underlying organ such as a sinus, a kidney, or the liver.

Auscultation

Auscultation is accomplished by use of a stethoscope to evaluate sounds arising from the lungs, the abdomen, and the cardiovascular system. Basic to proper auscultation is a good stethoscope with both a bell and a diaphragm. The stethoscope should be warmed before being applied to the client's bare skin. The bell of the stethoscope is used for low-pitched sounds such as murmurs and bruits and is applied lightly to the skin surface. The diaphragm is firmly applied and is used for detecting high-pitched sounds. The bell is also useful on male chests whose hair may scratch against the diaphragm or on a thin client where the diaphragm will not lie flat between the ribs.

Smell

The odor of the breath, sputum, ear drainage, vomitus, urine, feces, vaginal discharge, or pus may be diagnostic. The nurse is exposed repeatedly to these smells, and observations about them may offer important diagnostic clues. For example, foul-smelling sputum may be indicative of a lung abscess or bronchiectasis.

THE PHYSICAL EXAMINATION
The Normal Sequence of the Physical Examination

An examination may be a regional examination (eg, a neurologic assessment), a combined regional examination (eg, respiratory, cardiac, and abdominal assessment), or a complete physical assessment from head to toe. An organized, sequential approach to the physical examination is important because it saves unnecessary position change for the client and assists the examiner in remembering all parts of the assessment. The approach also saves time. The sequence in Table 7–1 is suggested for clients who are not limited in the positions they can assume. Remember that the skin of every bodily part is carefully inspected during each phase of the examination.

A review of previous client records, if available, and the results of diagnostic studies complete the data base. A section on general diagnostic testing at the end of this chapter is presented as preparation for the more specific tests in each nursing process chapter. A sample physical examination write-up is shown in Box 7–4, p. 142.

Table 7–1 Sequence of the Physical Examination

Client Position	Areas Assessed
Supine, seated, and standing	Blood pressure and other vital signs
Seated	Hands and arms (skin, nails, pulses, ROM); head and face; eyes; ears; nose and sinuses; mouth and pharynx; neck; (all cranial nerves have now been evaluated); posterior thorax (includes CVA tenderness); anterior thorax; breasts/axillae
Supine	Breasts; heart; abdomen/inguinal region; anus and rectum; female genitourinary system (lithotomy position); hips, knees, ankles, feet (joints, ROM, muscle strength, pulses, vascular findings); sensory function (light touch, pinprick); Babinski's sign
Seated	Reflexes; hands, arms, shoulders (muscle strength); cerebellum (rapid alternating movements); sensory function (stereognosis)
Standing	Spine, ROM; varicose veins; cerebellum, gait; male genitourinary system

Vital Signs

Body temperature, pulse, respirations, and blood pressure, along with measurement of height and weight are the first assessments taken. Specifics of each procedure are taught in nursing fundamentals courses. The additional important aspects of blood pressure and pulse in total assessment will be mentioned in this section.

Blood pressure should be measured in three positions—supine, seated, and standing—to evaluate the effect of position change. To obtain a baseline supine reading, have the client remain flat for about 10 minutes. Allow 2 to 3 minutes with each position change to assess seated and standing pressures. In orthostatic hypotension, dizziness or even syncope (fainting) occurs when the client stands, associated with a sudden drop in arterial blood pressure. Common causes of *orthostasis* include prolonged immobility, peripheral venous stasis, and use of antihypertensive drugs. In a specific assessment for orthostasis, the standing blood pressure is taken immediately and again after the client has been standing for 3 minutes to note the early drop followed by return to normal.

Blood pressure should also be measured in both arms. Blood pressure normally varies somewhat from arm to arm but should not vary widely. A rudimentary cervical rib or a tight scalene muscle may compress the brachial plexus

or subclavian artery on one side. In this circumstance, the blood pressure may not be auscultated or palpated on the affected side. To confirm a suspicion of this problem, which is called *thoracic outlet syndrome,* ask the client to turn the head to the affected side, extend the neck, and take a deep breath. Obstruction of the brachial pulse constitutes a positive *Adson's test* for thoracic outlet syndrome.

Normally, leg blood pressures are somewhat higher than blood pressures in the arm because the muscle mass of the thigh offers resistance to arterial compression. Hypertension in the arm pressures of a young client should alert the nurse to the possibility of coarctation of the aorta. To evaluate a client for aortic coarctation:

- Ask the client to assume the prone position.
- Apply a large blood pressure cuff appropriate to the size of the thigh.
- Place a stethoscope over the popliteal artery.

In aortic coarctation, the arm pressures are hypertensive and the leg pressures markedly lower. A comparison of the pulses finds weak femoral pulses with full, bounding brachial and radial pulses.

Assessment of the Skin

The skin is the largest organ of the human body and one of the most visible. Following evaluation of vital signs, begin the physical assessment with inspection of the visible skin. Through inspection and palpation of the skin, the nurse can easily identify cyanosis, icterus (jaundice), fever, dehydration, and edema. Subtle skin lesions may be an incidental finding during a health assessment. Skin lesions are classified as primary or secondary. A *primary lesion* is an original skin lesion from which a *secondary lesion* may result

Nursing Research Note

Tachovsky B: Indirect auscultatory blood pressure measurement at two sites in the arm. *Res Nurs Health* 1985; 8:125–129.

Indirect auscultatory blood pressure measurements at the upper arm (brachial) site and the forearm (radial) site were compared. The forearm site is often recommended for measuring blood pressure on obese clients. For the brachial site, a pressure cuff was applied at the right arm 2.5 cm above the antecubital fossa. For the radial site, a cuff was applied between the middle and distal third of the forearm.

The results, obtained from a sample of 98 female nursing students, indicated a statistically significant systolic difference. The brachial site readings averaged 7.35 mm Hg higher than at the forearm site. There was also a statistically significant difference in diastolic readings. The forearm site had a mean diastolic reading of 14.1 mm Hg higher than the brachial site.

One might ask how clinically significant these findings are. The brachial site remains the site of choice, and pressure should be measured with the appropriate-sized cuff.

Box 7–4 Sample Physical Examination Write-Up

Height: 5 ft 4 in

Weight: 125 lb (56.8 kg)

Temperature: 97.8°F (36.6°C)

Pulse: 76

Respiration: 14

BP: Lying, 100/60 right arm, 96/62 left arm; seated, 106/70 right arm, 102/68 left arm; standing, 110/70 right arm, 108/70 left arm

WD/WN pleasant, articulate white female who appears younger than her stated age, wearing sunglasses to protect her eyes from the light

Skin, hair, nails: Pink; good skin turgor, no lesions or changes in pigmentation; hair glossy with appropriate distribution; nails s̄ brittleness, good capillary refill

Head and face: Normocephalic, symmetrical scalp s̄ lesions or areas of tenderness

Eyes: Vision 20/30 OD, OS OU, Snellen's chart; lashes and brows present; conjunctivae clear, sclerae white; PERRLA; EOMs nl, no nystagmus, no lid lag or ptosis; VFs intact; fundi benign

Ears: Hearing intact to whisper test bilat; Weber s̄ lateralization, Rinne AC > BC bilateral; auricles s̄ lesions; ear canals c̄ small amount cerumen; TMs pearly gray and mobile, landmarks visible

Nose and sinuses: Nose symmetrical, both nostrils patent; nasal mucosa slightly edematous and erythematous; watery discharge; frontal and maxillary sinuses s̄ tenderness

Mouth and pharynx: Lips s̄ lesions; teeth in good repair, no dentures or partial plates; buccal mucosa pink s̄ lesions; tongue mobile, s̄ lesions and protrudes midline; uvula rises midline on phonation; gag reflex present; tonsils absent; pharynx not injected; TMJ c̄ full ROM s̄ crepitation

Neck: Symmetrical; no obvious masses or pulsations; thyroid not palpable, trachea midline; one pea-sized freely movable, nontender posterior cervical node on left; full ROM; JVP not elevated; ō carotid bruits

Breasts and axillae: Symmetrical, ō dimpling, ō retraction, ō discharge, ō masses; ō axillary adenopathy

Chest: Expansion = bilat; AP diameter not ↑; tactile fremitus = bilat; resonant to percussion; diaphragmatic excursion = bilat; clear to auscultation; no rales, rhonchi, or wheezes

Heart: PMI visible 5th LICS just medial to the MCL; PMI also palpable; no precordial thrills or lifts; apical rate 66, NSR; S_1S_2 nl, split S_2 at pulmonic area; no murmur, no gallop

Abdomen: Flat, s̄ scars or skin lesions; ō bruits; bowel sounds normoactive; ō tenderness or masses; liver, spleen, kidneys not palpable; liver 8 cm at rt MCL; ō CVA tenderness, ō inguinal adenopathy

Pelvic: External genitalia s̄ lesions; vaginal vault c̄ small amount menstrual blood; cervix pink, s̄ lesions. Bimanual: uterus retroverted, mobile, firm, smooth, not enlarged; adnexae s̄ tenderness; rectal: no external lesions, good sphincter tone; no masses; stool heme ⊖

Extremities: Joints s̄ swelling; full ROM joints and spine; muscle strength intact; no pedal edema; varicose veins bilat, more severe on rt leg

Pulses: (on a 4-point scale)	Radial	Ulnar	Brachial	Carotid	Femoral	Popliteal	Posterior tibial	Dorsalis pedis
Right:	4+	3+	4+	4+	4+	3+	3+	3+
Left:	4+	3+	4+	4+	4+	3+	3+	3+

Neurologic: Oriented ×3; recent and remote memory intact; speech clear; CN II–XII intact; CN I not tested; sensory intact; gait nl; Romberg negative, rapid alternating movements nl

Reflexes: (graded on a 4-point scale)

(eg, from scratching or infection). Common primary and secondary skin lesions are discussed in Chapter 78.

The fingernails and skin of the hands and arms are inspected carefully and any visible lesions palpated. The head, scalp, and hair are inspected. The examiner parts the hair with the fingers to examine the underlying skin carefully. Then with each phase of the physical assessment that follows, the exposed skin areas are examined during the inspection and palpatory phases.

Specific skin lesions must be observed systematically, or important information will be overlooked. Description of each lesion and group of lesions includes:

- Type of lesion:
  Flat (eg, macule)

  Elevated (eg, papule)
  Depressed (eg, ulcer)
- Shape of the individual lesion.
- Color of the lesion (include dominant hue and color pattern).
- Configuration of groups of lesions:
  Linear
  Annular (circular)
  Serpiginous (snakelike or creeping)
  Iris (bull's eye pattern)
  Zosteriform (in the area of a nerve distribution)
- Surface characteristics of the lesions:
  Scaly
  Dry

Wet

Greasy

- Anatomical distribution of lesions.

Skin turgor, the normal fullness and elasticity of the skin, is assessed by picking up and releasing a small area of skin. This assessment is best done on the forearm, the dorsum of the hand, or over the sternum. Healthy skin springs back into position immediately. Dehydrated skin remains elevated for some time. Skin loses some elasticity in the course of normal aging.

In addition to common primary and secondary skin lesions, the examiner may observe:

- Alopecia areata: A patchy loss of hair involving the scalp and sometimes the beard.
- Comedones: Whiteheads and blackheads commonly seen on the face, chest, and back of clients with acne.
- Dandruff: Noninflammatory diffuse scaling on the scalp.
- Ecchymosis: Extravasation of blood into the skin or mucous membrane; "bruising"; larger than petechiae.
- Folliculitis: A staphylococcal infection that begins around the hair follicles.
- Furuncles: "Boils," which usually develop from a superficial staphylococcal folliculitis.
- Hirsutism: Having darker, thicker body hair than the average client.
- Intertrigo: Superficial dermatitis involving the skin folds, commonly seen in obese clients in hot weather; principally found under the breasts and in the axillary and inguinal folds.
- Keloids: Hypertrophic scars more common in blacks, although caucasians can also develop them.
- Petechiae: Small hemorrhagic areas on the skin.
- Tinea cruris: "Jock itch" or ringworm of the groin, frequently seen in obese men in the summer; also seen in joggers.
- Urticaria: "Hives" or intensely pruritic circumscribed wheals commonly seen in allergic reactions.
- Vitiligo: Absence of pigmentation in areas of the skin.
- Xanthelasma: Slightly raised, yellowish, well-circumscribed plaque frequently seen in the elderly; appears most often on the nasal aspect of one or both eyelids.

Assessment of the Head and Face

Inspect the head and face for asymmetry, obvious deformities, and areas of erythema. Observe color, character, and distribution of hair. Palpate the head and scalp for lumps, lesions, or areas of tenderness and feel hair for flexibility, brittleness, or dryness.

Two cranial nerves are evaluated during assessment of the face. The trigeminal nerve, or fifth cranial nerve (CN V), is involved with facial sensation and chewing. A mixed nerve with both sensory and motor components, CN V is tested by evaluating the client's ability to open and close the mouth. The sensory portion is checked by touching the client, whose eyes are closed, with a sharp and a dull object in symmetrical areas on the face and by having the client say whether the sensation is sharp or dull. The corneal reflex, blinking when the cornea is touched with a wisp of cotton, also evaluates CN V. This test should be done with care, and a clean piece of cotton should be used for each eye. Corneal sensation may be decreased in clients who have worn contact lenses for many years.

The facial nerve, or seventh cranial nerve (CN VII), is involved with facial movement, tasting, salivation, and crying. Also a mixed nerve with both sensory and motor components, CN VII is tested by asking the client to wrinkle the forehead, raise the eyebrows, frown, smile, puff out the cheeks, and close the eyes so tightly the examiner is unable to open them forcibly. Observe for any asymmetry, especially in the nasolabial folds.

Assessment of the Eyes

Visual Acuity

Evaluation of visual acuity is an important aspect of health assessment. Snellen's chart is commonly used (see Chapter 70). Clients stand (or sit) 20 ft from the chart and cover one eye at a time, reading the letters on the chart from the top down. The last row in which the client can read all but one or two of the letters is recorded as the visual acuity for that eye. After the right eye (OD) and the left eye (OS) have been tested individually, both eyes (OU) should be tested together. If the client wears corrective lenses, these should be worn during the exam. In Snellen's chart, the upper number refers to the distance at which the normal eye would see the letter; eg, a notation of 20/50 vision OD indicates that the right eye sees at only 20 ft what a normal eye could see at 50 feet.

Other means to evaluate visual acuity include having clients read from a hand-held card developed for use at the bedside or reading from a newspaper or any printed matter; having them count fingers or, in the case of severe visual problems, checking for perception of light and dark. Assessment of visual acuity is one measure of the function of the optic nerve, or the second cranial nerve (CN II).

Alignment, Lids, Conjunctivae, Lacrimal Apparatus

The internal and accessory structures of the eye are shown in Figures 69–1 and 69–2. The eyes are inspected for symmetry and width of palpebral fissures. The lids are inspected for edema, exudate, scaling, or ptosis. The conjunctivae are evaluated for pallor, vascular injection, edema, and **pinguecula** (yellow raised fatty plaques usually seen nasally). If a foreign body (FB) is present, the upper lid can be everted, exposing the upper palpebral conjunctiva and perhaps the foreign body (Figure 70–2B).

The lacrimal gland is located in the superior lateral region of the upper eyelid. When swollen, the gland may be visible between the upper lid and eyeball when the lateral upper lid is elevated. The puncta of the lacrimal ducts lie in the medial corner of each upper and lower lid. Excess tears are drained via these ducts into the lacrimal sac and the nasolacrimal duct, which empties into the nasal cavity. When the lacrimal sac is inflamed, erythema and edema may be present between the medial canthus and the nose. Pressure on this area may cause backward flow of purulent matter through the puncta. Inflammation of the lacrimal sac is called *dacryocystitis.*

Cornea

Shine a light obliquely on the cornea and note any scars, abrasions, elevations, or ulcers. **Arcus senilis,** a peripheral corneal opacity, is common in clients over age 60. It does not interfere with vision.

Pupils

Evaluate the pupils for shape, size, equality, and position. A pupil size chart is available on neurologic units; a millimeter ruler may also be used. Darken the room and test the pupillary reaction to light by having the client fix on an object in the distance. Then shine a penlight into the client's eye from the side. The pupil should constrict, and consensual constriction should occur in the unexposed eye. Test the other eye in the same manner. The pupils are also tested for **accommodation,** the process by which the eye adjusts for distance, maintaining a clear visual image with a shift in gaze. To assess accommodation, ask the client to look into the distance and then at the nurse's finger, which is held about 12 in from the client's nose. The eyes should converge (move inward), and both pupils should constrict. These pupillary assessments evaluate the oculomotor nerve, or the third cranial nerve (CN III). A normal pupil examination is recorded as PERRLA—pupils equal, round, reactive to light and accommodation.

Extraocular Muscles

Six pairs of extraocular muscles control the motions of the eyeball (globe): the superior, lateral, inferior, and medial rectus muscles and the superior and inferior oblique muscles. Three cranial nerves innervate these muscles: the oculomotor nerve (CN III); the troclear nerve, or fourth cranial nerve (CN IV); and the abducens nerve, or sixth cranial nerve (CN VI). To remember which nerve innervates which muscles, use the mnemonic LR_6SO_4. Translated, it means the lateral rectus is innervated by CN VI and the superior oblique, by CN IV. This leaves CN III to innervate the other muscles.

To test extraocular movements (EOMs), have the client follow the nurse's finger with the eyes in the six cardinal positions of gaze (Figure 69–6). Both eyes should move in unison. At the extremes of lateral gaze, some clients demonstrate an involuntary rhythmic oscillating motion of the eyes called **nystagmus.** A few beats of nystagmus in these extreme positions is considered normal. In disease states, the pattern of nystagmus is helpful in differentiating labyrinthine and brain stem disorders.

Lid Lag

During evaluation of the EOMs, lid lag is also evaluated. Normally, no portion of the sclera is visible above the iris when the client is gazing straight ahead. With lid lag, the upper lid does not follow the movement of the eyeball when the eyes move from an upward position downward, and rims of sclerae remain visible above the irises. Lid lag is sometimes seen in clients with hyperthyroidism.

Visual Fields

A gross estimate of the visual fields (VFs) is done by confrontation testing, a method of examination in which the VFs of the client are compared to those of the examiner.

- The nurse and the client are at the same eye level, about 3 ft apart.
- Have the client cover the left eye while the nurse covers the right. The client's uncovered eye should be fixed on the nurse's uncovered eye.
- The nurse holds a pencil in the hand midway between nurse and client; the nurse's arm is extended beyond the limits of the field of vision.
- Advance the pencil inward from the periphery toward the center, and ask the client to indicate when the pencil tip appears in the client's field of vision.

The testing should proceed from eight equally spaced directions. The entire procedure should then be repeated with the other eye.

When lesions occur in the optic chiasm, optic tract, or brain, the visual fields are affected, resulting in a variety of possible defects, depending on the specific location of the lesion. Glaucoma may also cause visual-field defects. More specific mapping of visual fields, using a perimeter, is indicated whenever a visual-field defect is suspected on confrontation testing. This mapping is usually done by an ophthalmologist or neurologist.

Ophthalmoscopic Examination

The **fundus** of the eye (the retinal area) is accessible to examination with the ophthalmoscope (Figure 7–4A). Initial attempts to use the ophthalmoscope can be frustrating, but practice yields exciting results. Because viewing the retina by ophthalmoscopic exam is the only way to see blood vessels directly (except in the operating room), the skill is well worth developing.

Within the ophthalmoscope is a series of lenses, identified by red and black numerals that range from 1 to 25 on the red side and 1 to 40 on the black side, depending on the age and make of the scope. The lenses are adjusted to compensate for the myopia or hyperopia of both the client and examiner. The red numerals are used when the client and examiner are myopic, and the black are used for a hyperopic pair. The zero lens is used when no correction is needed. When one person is myopic and the other hyper-

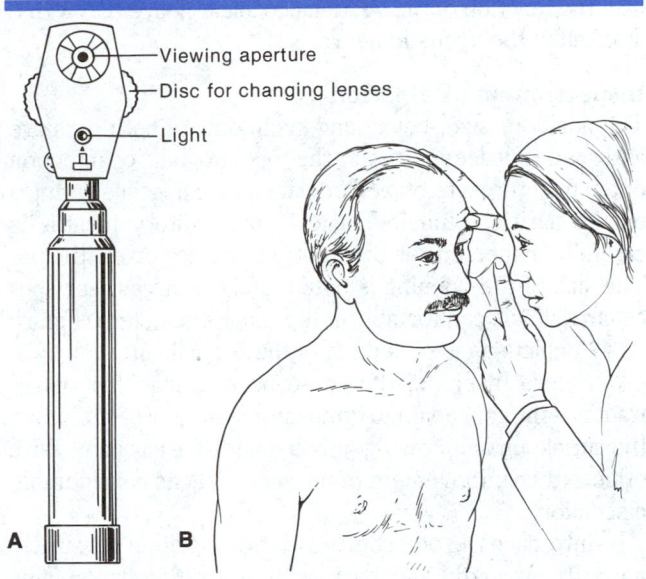

Figure 7–4

Ophthalmoscopic examination. **A.** An ophthalmoscope for viewing the retina of the eye. **B.** Position of client and examiner for ophthalmoscopic examination.

opic, the lens adjustment could be zero or anywhere on the wheel, depending on the severity of each person's refractive error. The ophthalmoscope also contains several apertures and light filters. The small or large white beam of light is best for most examinations.

If the client wears eyeglasses, these should be removed. Contact lenses may remain in unless the client prefers to take them out. The examiner may examine with or without eyeglasses.

The right eye of the examiner is used for examining the client's right eye, and the ophthalmoscope is held in the examiner's right hand. The reverse procedure is used for the left eye. The room is darkened so the pupil is dilated as much as possible. To examine the right eye, the examiner gently retracts the client's right upper lid with the left hand. The client is asked to stare straight ahead (Figure 7–4B).

- Stand lateral to the client, 12 to 15 in away, and focus the light beam on the client's pupil. A uniform red glow (the red reflex) should be seen.

- Keeping the red reflex in view, the examiner gradually moves in closer to the client's eye until the forehead touches the examiner's other hand, which is supporting the client's upper lid.

- Whatever detail is seen through the ophthalmoscope should be brought into focus by rotating the lens wheel.

In a systematic way, the optic disk, the retinal vessels, the retinal background, and the macular area are evaluated (Figure 7–5). The disk is examined for size, shape, color, clarity of its margins, and the size of the physiological cup, if present. The arterioles and veins are evaluated for color and size. The ratio of arteriole size to venous size (A:V

ratio) is noted. The ratio should be 2:3 or 3:4, the arterioles being smaller than the veins. The blood column in the vessels and the areas of arteriovenous crossings are assessed.

The periphery of the retina is examined for hemorrhages or exudates (HorE) or any unusual coloration. The normal retinal background varies in color. A fair-skinned person has a pinkish yellow fundus, whereas a black person has a fundus that looks brownish purple. The macula is more temporal in location than the disk, which is more nasal. The macula is evaluated last because of its extreme sensitivity to light. The macula is avascular and may be found by asking the client to look at the light, which moves the macula into the examiner's field of vision.

Palpation for Increased Intraocular Pressure

For a rough evaluation of intraocular pressure, ask the client to close the eyes. The examiner places the tips of both index fingers on the closed upper lid in the area of the center of the globe. The fingers are moved back and forth alternately, gently indenting the globe. The normal globe indents slightly with pressure and rebounds against the withdrawing finger. The client with glaucoma has increased intraocular pressure. The globes will be hard and will not rebound, but this is often a subtle distinction. Measurement of intraocular tension with an instrument called a tonometer is a much more accurate method of detecting glaucoma (Chapter 70).

Auscultation for Bruits

Listening for bruits over the globe, with the eyelids closed, should be part of the total assessment of clients with cer-

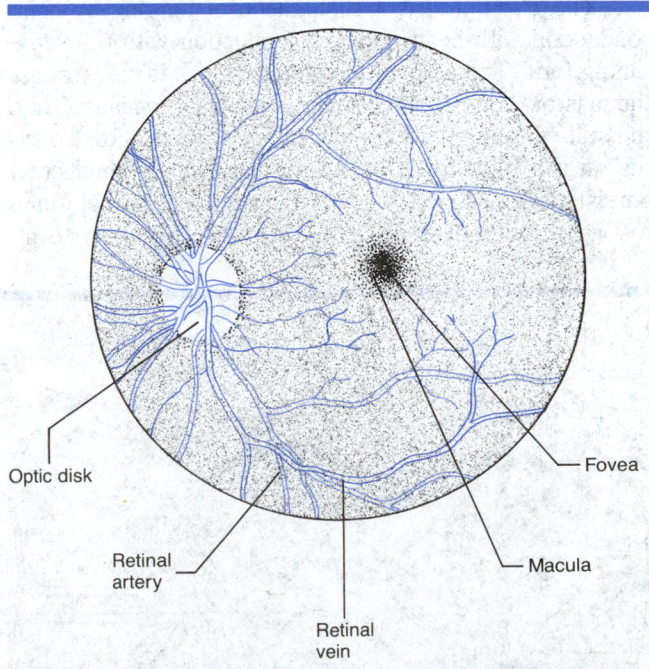

Figure 7–5

The fundus of the left eye. Note the optic disk, retinal arteries and veins, and macula.

ebrovascular disease. The bell of the stethoscope is gently placed on the closed upper lid. A **bruit,** an audible murmur in a blood vessel secondary to turbulent blood flow, may be indicative of arteriovenous malformation (AVM), a tangle of atypical vessels creating abnormal channels between the arterial and venous systems. A bruit may also be a sign of carotid occlusion. The bruit is heard over the globe on the side opposite the occlusion. This is thought to reflect the increased blood flow through the remaining patent vessel (Petersdorf et al., 1983).

Assessment of the Ears

Auditory Acuity
When evaluating hearing, only one ear is tested at a time. The other ear must be occluded with a finger, either the examiner's or the client's. Whispered and spoken voice tests are common ways of evaluating hearing. Stand 1 to 2 ft from the client's unoccluded ear and whisper in a quiet, medium, and loud tone. Have the client repeat what was heard. Next, check the hearing while speaking in a quiet, medium, and loud voice. Be sure the client is not lip reading. Repeat the tests with the other ear.

Tuning Fork Tests
Conductive or nerve deafness can be evaluated by use of Weber's and the Rinne tests (Figure 7–6). In a person with normal hearing, when the stem of a vibrating tuning fork is pressed against the midline of the scalp, the sound will be heard equally in both ears. In a person with conductive loss, the test will lateralize to the affected ear. This is *Weber's test*.

The *Rinne test* is a comparison of hearing by bone conduction with hearing by air conduction with the same tuning fork. The stem of the vibrating fork is held against the mastoid bone until the sound is no longer audible. Then the still-vibrating tines are held opposite the auditory meatus on the same side. In the normal ear, air conduction persists twice as long as bone conduction. A normal Rinne test is recorded AC > BC. The various hearing tests eval-

uate the function of the vestibulocochlear nerve (CN VIII), also called the acoustic nerve.

Inspection and Palpation
The position, size, color, and symmetry of both ears are assessed. Sebaceous cysts, the tophi of gout, or infection of the puncture site of pierced ears all are possible findings on the auricle (pinna). The external auditory meatus is carefully inspected for discharge, swelling, or erythema. The size of the opening is noted, and the largest ear speculum that will comfortably fit the canal is selected. (Figure 73–2 depicts a cross section of the normal ear.)

Before inserting the otoscope speculum for visualization of the ear canal and tympanic membrane (TM), move the auricle up and down gently to check for ear pain. With otitis externa, movement of the auricle elicits considerable discomfort.

Introduce the otoscope slowly while pulling the auricle upward, outward, and back with the other hand. This straightens the curve of the external auditory canal, facilitating otoscope insertion. Observe the ear canal as the scope is passed, noting any swelling, erythema, or lesions of the canal. Note any cerumen, discharge, or foreign bodies. Identify the landmarks of the tympanic membrane (Figure 7–7). The normal TM is shiny, translucent, and pearly gray. The TM should also be mobile, which is easily tested with an insufflator attached to the otoscope.

Notice the odor of any ear discharge on the ear speculum tip, because certain organisms causing external otitis produce a distinctive bad odor. For example, the odor of ear discharge from a Pseudomonas infection is pungent and sweet, whereas the odor from a staphylococcal infection is like overripe cheese.

Assessment of the Nose and Sinuses

The Nose
The contour of the external nose is examined for symmetry and palpated for areas of tenderness. Patency of each nostril is tested by occluding one while the client inhales through the other. The olfactory nerve, or first

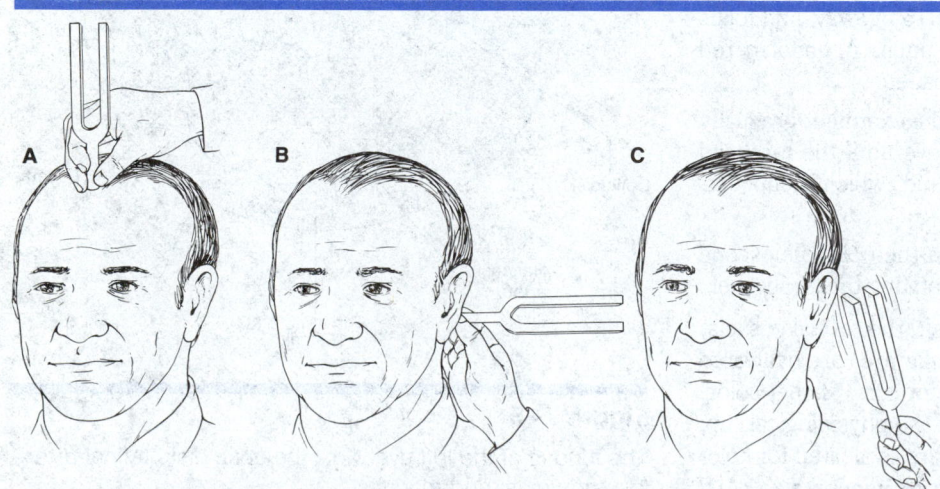

Figure 7–6

Tuning fork tests. **A.** The Weber test to evaluate whether the sound remains centralized or lateralizes to one side or the other. **B & C.** The Rinne test to compare bone conduction and air conduction.

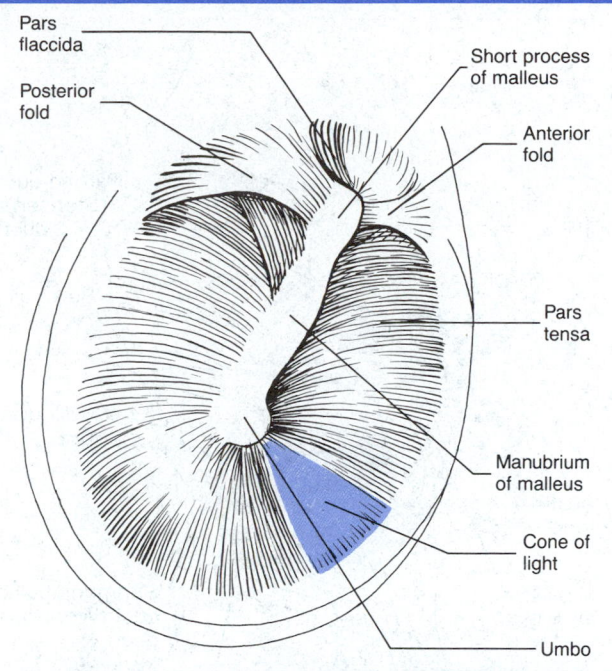

Figure 7–7

The right tympanic membrane. Note the cone of light pointing to 5 o'clock.

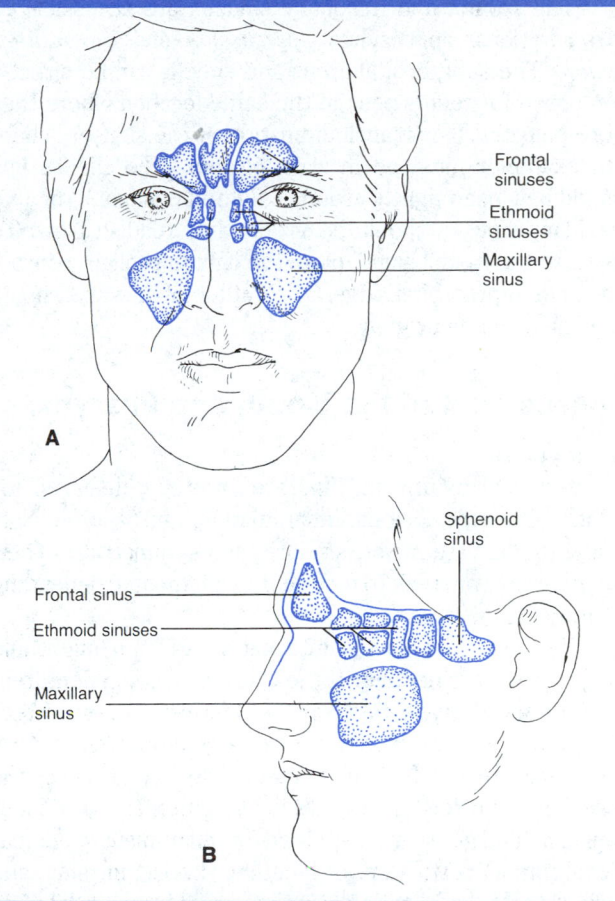

Figure 7–8

The paranasal sinuses. **A.** Frontal view. **B.** Lateral view.

cranial nerve (CN I), is tested by having the client identify specific odors, eg, soap, tobacco, alcohol, or coffee. Each nostril is tested separately while the client's eyes are closed.

The short nasal speculum is attached to the otoscope head and inserted into the nostril, avoiding any contact with the sensitive nasal septum. The nasal mucosa, normally pink, may be bright red secondary to inflammation or blue gray in allergic rhinitis. A nasal mucosa that is edematous and moist is often described as *boggy*. The nasal septum is assessed for bleeding points, ulcers, deviation, or perforation.

The Sinuses

There are four pairs of paranasal sinuses: the frontal, maxillary, sphenoid, and ethmoid (Figure 7–8). Only the fron-

tal and maxillary sinuses are accessible to evaluation by physical assessment techniques. The ethmoid and sphenoid sinuses must be studied radiographically.

The frontal sinuses are evaluated by palpation of the supraorbital ridge. The maxillary sinuses are assessed by palpation of the maxillary portions of the cheek (Figure 7–9). Firm steady pressure is used during palpation. Tenderness to palpation indicates sinus inflammation.

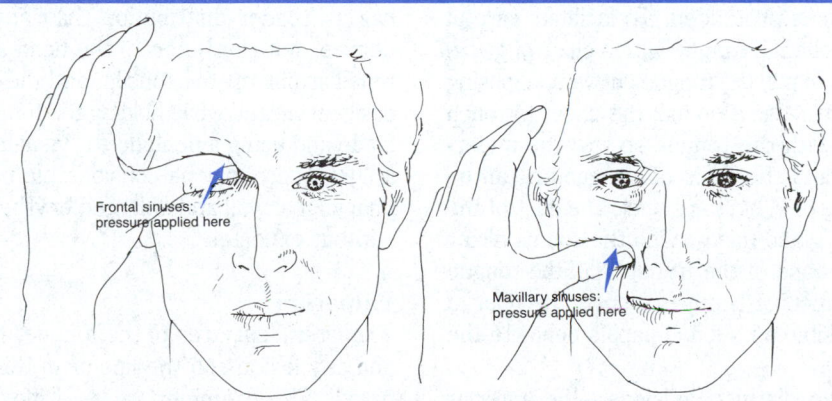

Figure 7–9

Palpation of the frontal and maxillary sinuses.

The frontal and maxillary sinuses are accessible to two additional approaches—*percussion* and *transillumination*. The supraorbital areas and cheeks can be directly percussed for tenderness in the same location where they were palpated. For transillumination of the sinuses, client and examiner must be in a dark room. The client's lips should be closed tightly around a lighted penlight. The two maxillary sinuses should be visible as a reddish glow. To visualize the frontal sinus, place the lighted penlight beneath the inner supraorbital ridge. The outline of the sinus should be visible as a faint glow.

Assessment of the Mouth and Pharynx

Inspection
The external mouth and lips are carefully observed for color, symmetry, lesions, inflammation, and fissures. Normally, the lips are moist, smooth, and symmetrical. Their color varies from pink to more darkly pigmented depending on the client's race.

For inspection of the internal mouth, a penlight and tongue blade are needed. If the client is wearing dentures, the bite and the general fit of the dentures are evaluated. The dentures are then removed so that the entire oral cavity can be carefully inspected. The buccal mucosa is assessed for color, ulcers, areas of pigmentation, and leukoplakia. The gums are inspected for inflammation, edema, pigmentation, retraction, or bleeding. Loose, missing, and carious teeth are noted. Normally, adults have a total of 32 permanent teeth. The color of the teeth may vary. Coloration may indicate conditions such as chronic smoking (yellow brown). Brownish pigmentation may indicate exposure to tetracycline in utero or having received tetracycline before age 7.

The tongue is carefully inspected for size, color, lesions, mobility, and symmetry. The client is asked to stick out the tongue, which should appear symmetrical, should protrude midline rather than deviate laterally, and should be movable from side to side. **Fasciculations** (fine twitchings) should not be present. These observations evaluate the hypoglossal nerve, or twelfth cranial nerve (CN XII). The lateral surfaces of the tongue are carefully inspected while the client's tongue is protruded. To facilitate careful observation, grasp the client's tongue with a piece of gauze and apply gentle traction to pull the tongue outward, exposing the posterior lateral surfaces. Also ask the client to touch the roof of the mouth with the tongue so that the undersurface of the tongue and the floor of the mouth can be inspected. The opening of Wharton's duct, the duct of the submandibular salivary gland (also called the submaxillary gland), is visible at the base of the frenulum of the tongue (Figure 7–10). The orifice of Stensen's duct, the duct of the parotid gland, is visible as a small papilla opposite the second upper molar.

The palate has two distinct divisions—the anterior two-thirds, or hard palate, and the posterior third, the soft palate, to which the uvula is attached. An unusual-appear-

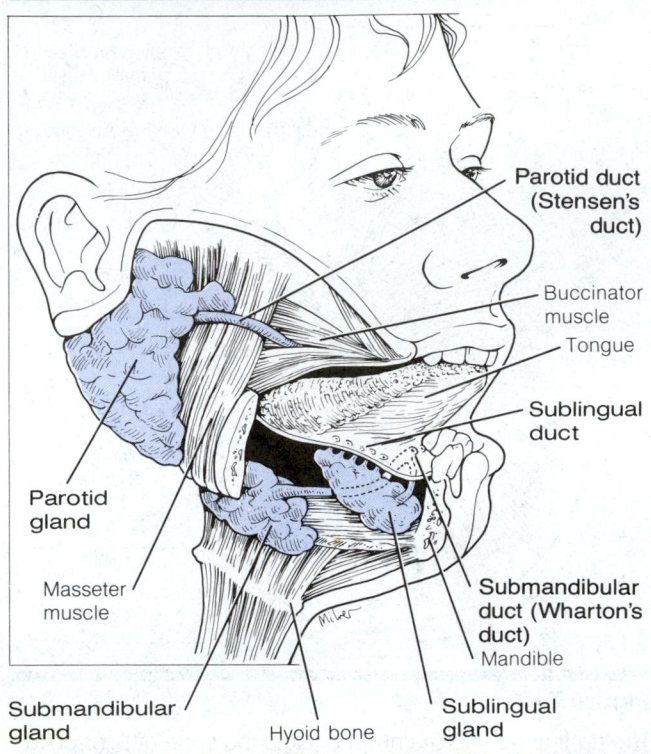

Figure 7–10

The salivary glands. Note the location of Stensen's and Wharton's ducts.
SOURCE: Spence AP, Mason EB: *Human Anatomy and Physiology,* 2nd ed. Menlo Park, CA: Benjamin/Cummings, 1983.

ing but relatively common finding on the hard palate is a midline bony outgrowth called **torus palatinus.** The uvula varies in width and length, occasionally becoming edematous with upper respiratory infections (URI), causing greater irritation in the throat. The glossopharyngeal nerve (CN IX), and the vagus nerve (CN X), are partially tested by inspecting for midline position of the uvula and rise of the soft palate when the client says "ahhh." Stimulation of the gag reflex by touching the pharyngeal wall with a tongue blade is also a test of CN IX and CN X. The vagus nerve has a broader distribution than any of the other cranial nerves, not restricted to the head and neck regions. The tonsillar pillars, the tonsils, and the posterior pharynx are easily evaluated while holding the tongue down with a tongue blade and using a penlight for visualization. In a client with a URI, there may be considerable mucus on the posterior pharyngeal wall and enlarged erythematous tonsils with or without exudates.

Palpation
The lateral surfaces of the tongue, the floor of the mouth, and any lesions on the lips or in the mouth should be palpated. The examiner wears a glove for this part of the assessment. Lesions should be described according to their size, shape, consistency, location, and tenderness.

The temporomandibular joint (TMJ) (Figure 7–11), which is moved when the jaw is opened and closed, is one of the most active joints in the body. Whenever a person talks, chews, yawns, or swallows, the TMJ is exercised. Estimates are that the TMJ opens and closes 1500 to 2000 times a day. The TMJ must not be neglected when the mouth is assessed, because malocclusion or arthritic problems may damage the joint.

The TMJ is best palpated by placing the index fingers in the external auditory meatus and pressing anteriorly while the client slowly opens and closes the mouth. The joint is assessed for crepitation, clicking, pain, and range of motion (ROM).

Assessment of the Neck

The sternocleidomastoid muscles divide the neck into one anterior and two posterior triangles. Structures within the anterior triangle include the larynx, trachea, and thyroid. The internal jugular veins and carotid arteries lie partially beneath the sternocleidomastoid muscle. Their pulsations are often visible in the anterior triangle (Figure 7–12).

Trachea and Thyroid
The anterior neck is carefully inspected for asymmetry, masses, abnormal pulsation, limitation in ROM, and tracheal deviation. The lower half of the anterior triangle is observed for enlargement of the thyroid gland. To inspect the thyroid, offer the client a glass of water and watch the

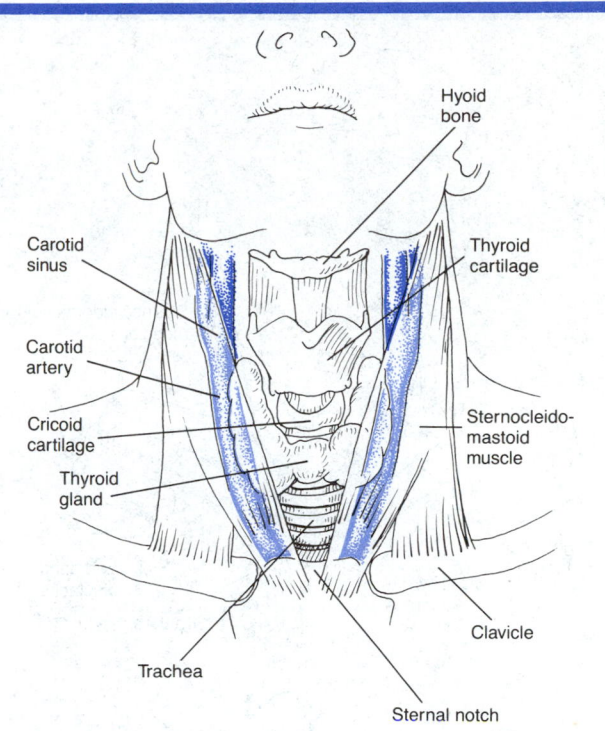

Figure 7–12

Anterior triangle of the neck, showing proximity of structures to carotid artery.

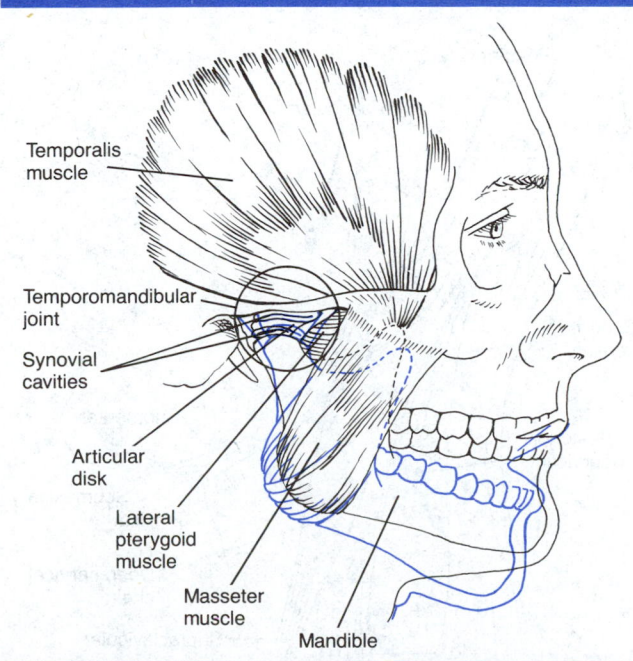

Figure 7–11

The temporomandibular joint (TMJ) is moved by the muscles of mastication (masseter, temporalis, and pterygoid muscles), which are innervated by CN V.

neck during swallowing, looking for any ascending mass in the midline or arising from behind either sternocleidomastoid muscle. Thyroid tissue ascends during swallowing.

The trachea is normally seen in the midline and should be palpable at the suprasternal notch. Localized disease or disease within the cardiopulmonary system may cause tracheal deviation.

The thyroid may be palpated from either a posterior or an anterior approach (Figure 7–13). With the posterior approach, the examiner stands behind the client, with the client's neck extended slightly. The client may be most relaxed and comfortable with the head resting against the examiner. The fingertips of both hands of the examiner lie gently over the thyroid area. The client is asked to swallow, and the thyroid isthmus is located as it elevates under the fingertips. The client then is asked to tilt the head slightly forward and to the right for examination of the right lobe. The thyroid cartilage is displaced with the left hand, and the right lobe is palpated with the right hand. The procedure is reversed to examine the left lobe.

With frontal palpation of the thyroid (Figure 7–13B), the client's neck is slightly extended, and the thyroid isthmus is located by having the client swallow. The same palpatory procedure described for posterior palpation is repeated, although the examiner's right hand will now be evaluating the client's left lobe. Presence of any nodules is noted, as well as the size, shape, and consistency of each lobe.

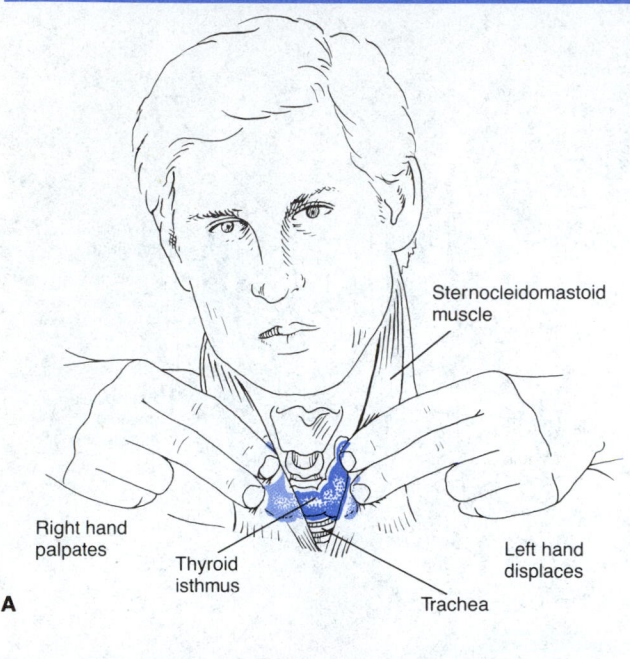

A

Right hand palpates

Sternocleidomastoid muscle

Thyroid isthmus

Left hand displaces

Trachea

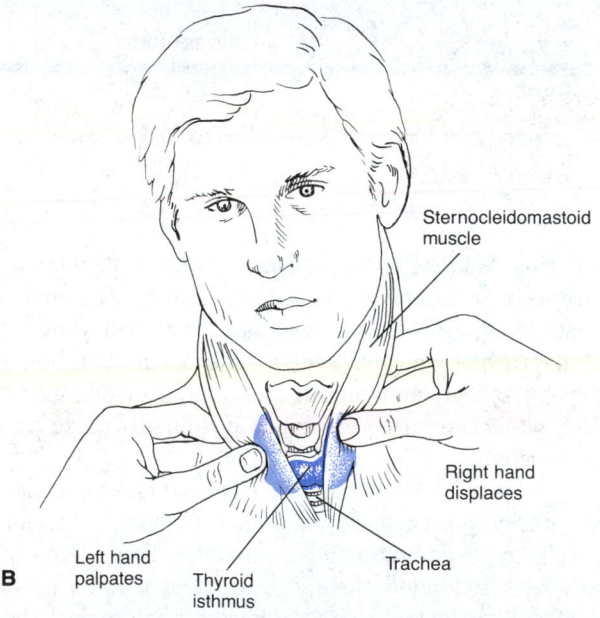

B

Left hand palpates

Sternocleidomastoid muscle

Right hand displaces

Thyroid isthmus

Trachea

Figure 7–13

Palpation of the thyroid gland. **A.** Posterior palpation of the thyroid. The examiner stands behind the seated client, displacing the thyroid gland with one hand while palpating with the other. **B.** Anterior palpation of the thyroid. Facing the client, the examiner displaces the thyroid with one hand while palpating with the other.

The Lymph Nodes

Lymph nodes of the head and neck are shown in Figure 7–14. Normally, these lymph nodes are not palpable. They enlarge secondary to a variety of disease processes, the most common being a URI. Most persons have had these so-called "swollen glands" at one point or another in their lives. Occasionally, an individual will have an isolated persistently enlarged lymph node in the neck. One isolated

node that does not change in size or consistency is not abnormal. In fact, instructors often look for these in their students so others can learn what an enlarged lymph node feels like. They are called "teaching nodes."

The fingertips are used to evaluate the cervical lymph nodes. The neck is palpated sequentially in the areas of the various lymph node groups, beginning with the preauricular node slightly anterior to the tragus. The posterior auricular, occipital, tonsillar, submaxillary, submental, superficial cervical, posterior cervical chain, deep cervical chain, and supraclavicular nodes are examined in sequence. Any palpable nodes should be described in terms of their location, size, shape, consistency, mobility, tenderness, and whether they are discrete or clumped.

An isolated node in the supraclavicular region may be an ominous sign. The *sentinal node* or *Virchow's node,* usually seen in the left supraclavicular group, indicates metastasis from a carcinoma in the upper abdomen (DeGowin & DeGowin, 1981).

Neck Range of Motion and the Eleventh Cranial Nerve

To check ROM of the neck, have the client touch chin to chest (anteflexion), tilt the head backwards (dorsiflexion),

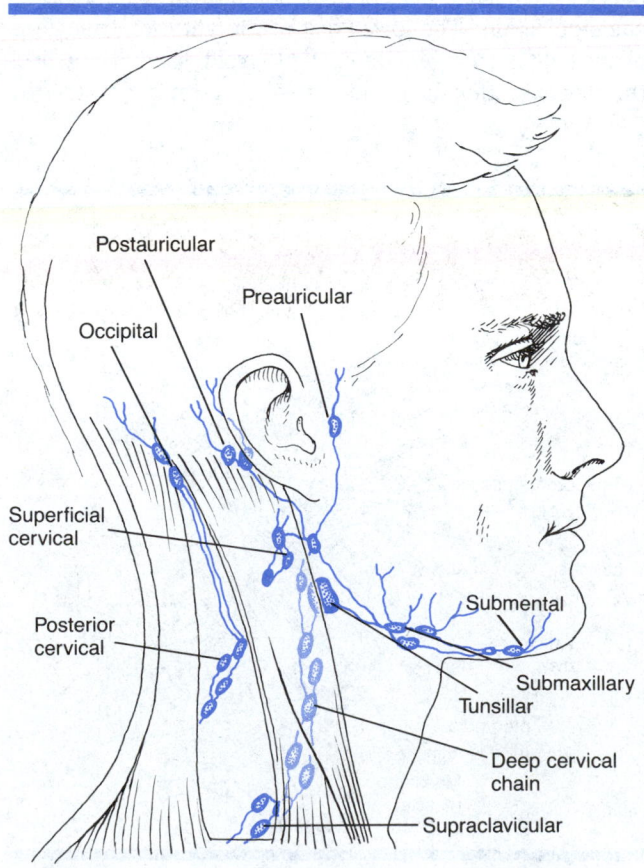

Postauricular

Preauricular

Occipital

Superficial cervical

Posterior cervical

Submental

Submaxillary

Tunsillar

Deep cervical chain

Supraclavicular

Figure 7–14

Lymph nodes of the head and neck. Palpate for each lymph node group with the fingertips.

Table 7–2	Differentiating the Internal Jugular Venous Pulsation From the Carotid Arterial Pulsation	
Internal Jugular Venous Pulsation	**Carotid Arterial Pulsation**
Easily compressed with gentle pressure	Requires firm pressure for obliteration
Has two or three undulations with each heart beat	Has one brisk wave with each heart beat
With inspiration, the pulse wave in the neck descends, and rises on expiration	Not affected by respiration
With the client supine, pulsations in the neck veins become more prominent	Not affected by change in position
Pressure over the liver in the RUQ of the abdomen under the costal margin may cause a rise in the jugular venous pulsation, called hepatojugular reflux (HJR)	Abdominal pressure does not alter the carotid pulsation

touch the chin to each shoulder (rotation), and touch the ear to each shoulder (lateral flexion). The accessory nerve (CN XI) is a motor nerve that supplies the trapezius and sternocleidomastoid muscles. (CN XI was formerly called the spinal accessory nerve.) To test its function, ask the client to shrug the shoulders against resistance. Note the strength of the trapezius muscles. Then have the client turn the head to each side while the examiner resists with pressure against the client's chin. Observe the prominence of the opposite sternocleidomastoid muscle and the strength of the client's movement against resistance.

The Carotid Arteries and Jugular Veins

Inspect the neck carefully for any pulsations. The carotid pulsations may be visualized just medial to the sternocleidomastoid muscles. Palpate the carotid pulses individually, comparing one side with the other. Take care to avoid the carotid sinus, located below the upper level of the thyroid cartilage; pressure on the carotid sinus may slow the heart (Figure 7–12).

The carotids are auscultated for bruits with the bell of the stethoscope. Auscultate along each carotid in low, middle, and high positions on the neck, because bruits may be fairly localized. Because the client's normal breath sounds interfere with auscultation, ask the client to hold his or her breath. If the examiner will be listening for an extended period, give the client plenty of opportunity to breathe normally between assessments. Carotid bruits may be heard in clients with atherosclerosis. Auscultation should continue over the thyroid if any thyroid abnormalities were found on inspection and palpation.

Observation of the jugular veins in the neck provides an estimate of venous pressure, the pressure exerted in the venous system by the blood. The neck veins are generally distended when clients are supine and collapsed when clients are upright. Venous pulse waves of both the internal and external jugular veins may be visible in the right neck when the client is positioned at a 45° angle. The internal jugular vein is more reliable for determining venous pressure, but its pulsation must be carefully differentiated from

the carotid pulsation because both vessels lie deep along the sternocleidomastoid muscle. See Table 7–2 for approaches to differentiation of these pulsations.

To measure the jugular venous pressure (JVP), assist the client to a supine position with the head and shoulders elevated to a 45° angle. Direct a lighted penlight at the right neck to look for the pulsations of the right internal jugular vein underlying the sternocleidomastoid muscle. When the pulsation has been identified, measure the distance of the upper level of distention in the internal jugular vein from the sternal angle (Figure 7–15). Pressures greater than 4 cm above the sternal angle (angle of Louis) are considered elevated. Because the sternal angle is approximately 5 cm above the right atrium, the measurement obtained may be added to 5 cm to estimate central venous pressure.

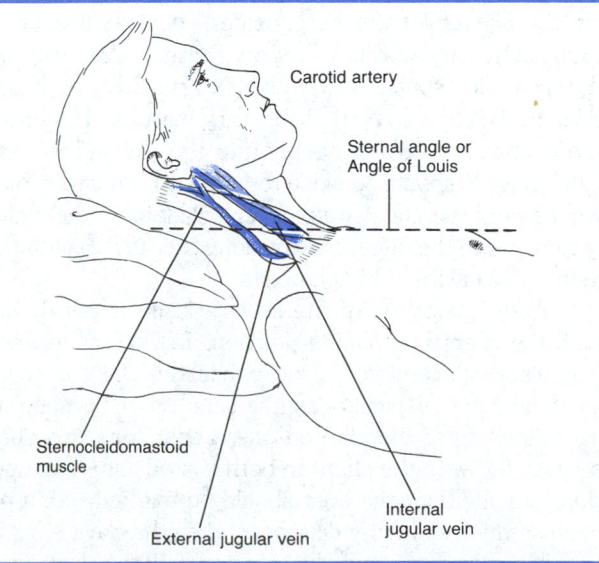

Figure 7–15

Measurement of jugular venous pressure using the internal jugular vein.

Assessment of the Breasts

Although this discussion of breast assessment focuses on the female breasts, men also develop breast problems, including malignancy. Consequently, the male breast and axilla should be examined routinely in physical assessment. The approach to examination is identical for both sexes.

Inspection

The client is seated and exposed from the waist up for adequate visualization. The breasts are inspected for symmetry, skin dimpling, nipple retraction, nipple inversion, lesions, or masses. One breast may be slightly larger than the other, and sometimes there is a marked difference between the size of the breasts. Asymmetry is a normal finding if it has existed since breast development and abnormal if it is recent.

The breasts are then inspected while the client places hands on hips and tenses the chest muscles and while raising the arms over the head. The breasts are assessed again for size and shape, skin alterations, and changes in nipples and areolae. Also note whether both breasts elevate symmetrically when the arms are raised. If the breasts are extremely pendulous have the client assume alternative positions to visualize adequately sections of the breast tissue. Having the client lean forward with hands on the back of a chair for support will demonstrate whether the breasts fall away from the thorax as they should. The axillary, supraclavicular, and infraclavicular regions should also be inspected for evidence of bulging, retraction, edema, or asymmetry.

Palpation

Initial palpation of the breast and surrounding areas is done with the client seated. The supraclavicular and infraclavicular regions are assessed for enlarged lymph nodes. Having the client elevate the shoulders permits deeper palpation in the supraclavicular region. During axillary palpation, the examiner supports the client's arm, keeping it quite close to the chest to relax the axillary muscles. This enables the examiner to reach deeply into the axilla. The examiner's fingers should be close together with the palm of the hand facing the chest wall. After palpation of the axillary region, move the fingers down along the surface of the ribs feeling for enlarged lymph nodes.

Actual palpation of the breast tissue is usually done with the client in a supine position. In several instances, it is also important to palpate while the client is seated. Certainly, if a suspicious sign is seen on inspection, such as a dimpling of the skin on one breast, this area should be palpated with the client in both seated and supine positions. In addition, the area should be marked with a pen, because the finding may disappear when the client is supine. Very large breasts should be palpated with the client seated as well as supine, because positive findings may be concealed, and palpation in various positions offers the best chance of locating early lesions.

Begin systematic palpation with the client supine and the arm on the side to be examined raised over the head to flatten the breast tissue. The pads of the fingertips of the middle three fingers are used for palpation. Peripheral breast tissue is composed of adipose tissue held in place by connective tissue. Centrally, the breast contains approximately 20 lobes of glandular tissue, each of which is drained by a single duct that opens onto the nipple (see Figure 61–6 in Chapter 61). There is a wide variation in how normal breast tissue feels. Age, stage of menstrual cycle, weight, pregnancy, and diet all affect the consistency of the tissue. During palpation, keep in mind the normal structures of the breast and the information gathered about the client when the history was obtained.

The breasts are palpated in a rotary motion with the pads of the fingers, compressing the breast tissue against the chest wall. Systematic palpation is imperative so a section of tissue will not be overlooked. Four approaches have been recommended (Figure 7–16):

- A quadrant-by-quadrant approach
- A concentric-circle approach beginning at the nipple and working outward or beginning at the clavicular region and working inward
- From the sternum to the anterior axillary line
- From the anterior axillary line to midline; from sternum to midline

Regardless of the sequence, the objective is a complete assessment of the breasts. The axillary tail, a section of breast tissue extending into the axilla, must not be overlooked. Throughout the assessment, teach the client the importance and proper technique of breast self-examination (Figure 7–17). In most instances, the examination sequence should be consistent with what is taught and with

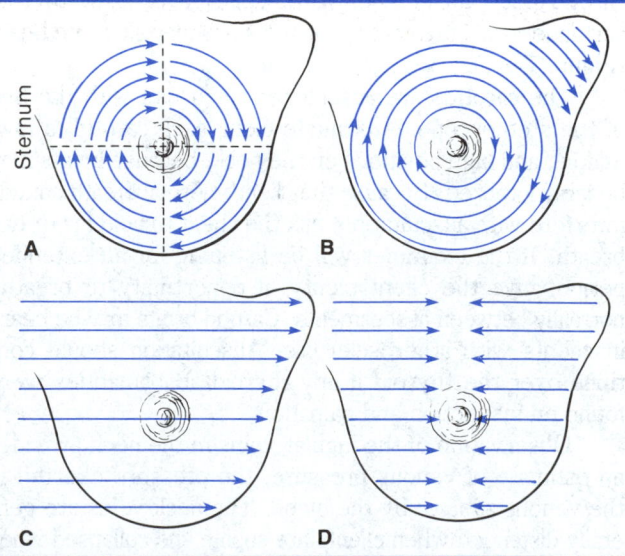

Figure 7–16

Four approaches to breast palpation. **A.** Quadrant-by-quadrant approach. **B.** Concentric-circle approach. **C.** From sternum to AAL. **D.** From AAL to midline; from sternum to midline.

Step 1

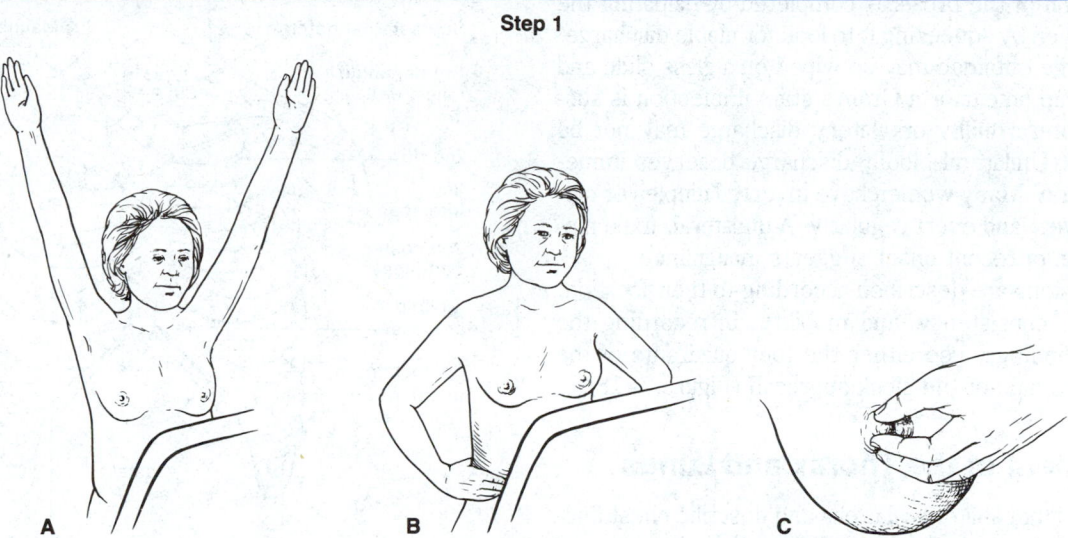

A. *In Front of a Mirror:* Look for any change in the size or shape of the breast, puckering or dimpling of the skin, or changes in the nipple. **B.** *Inspect in Three Positions:* With arms relaxed at sides; with arms held overhead; with hands on hips, pressing in to contract the chest muscles. Turn from side to side to view all areas. **C.** *Nipple Examination:* Gently squeeze the nipple of each breast between your thumb and index finger, looking for any nipple discharge.

Step 2

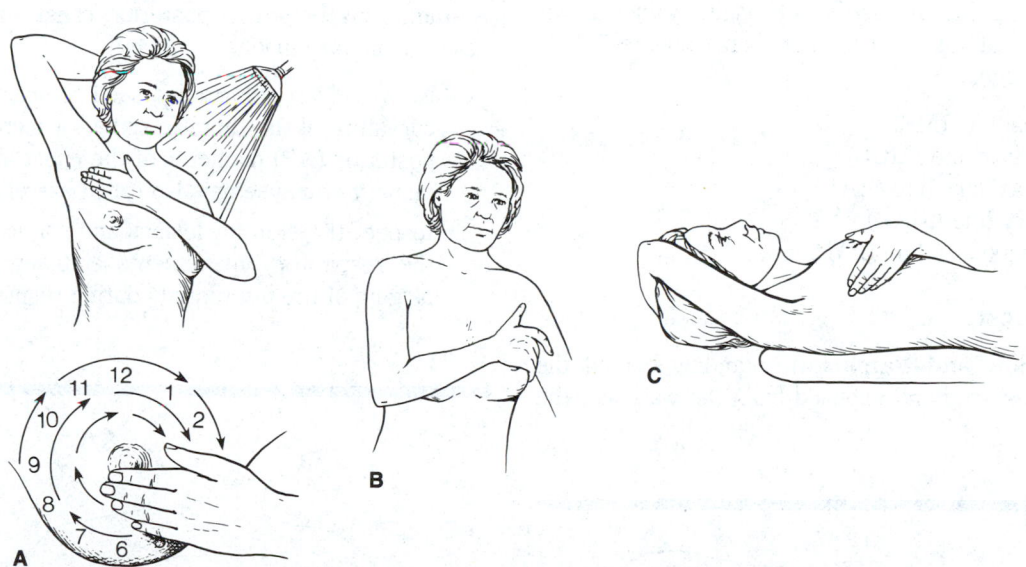

A. *In Shower or Bath:* Fingers will glide over wet soapy skin, making it easier to feel any changes in the breasts. Check the breast for a lump, knot, tenderness or for any change in the consistency of normal breast tissue. To examine your right breast, put your right hand behind your head, with the pads of your fingers of your left hand held flat and together, gently press on the breast tissue using small circular motions. Imagine the breast as the face of a clock. Begin at the top, 12 o'clock and so on, making a circle around the outer area of the breast. Move in one finger width, continue in smaller and smaller circles until you have reached the nipple. Cover all areas including the breast tissue leading to the arm pit. Reverse the procedure for the left breast. At the lower border of each breast, a ridge of firm tissue may be felt. This is normal. **B.** *Underarm Examination:* Examine the left underarm with your arm held loosely at your side. Cup the fingers of the opposite hand and insert them high into the underarm area. Drop fingers down slowly, pressing in a circular pattern, covering all areas. Reverse the procedure for the right underarm. **C.** *Lying Down:* While lying flat, place a small pillow or folded towel under the right shoulder. Examine the right breast using the same circular motion as was used in the shower. Cover all areas. Repeat this procedure for the left breast. Press firmly but gently while examining your breasts, rolling the tissue between your fingers and the chest wall.

Figure 7–17

Breast self-examination. **Step 1.** Inspection. **Step 2.** Palpation or feeling. (Courtesy of Department of Cancer Control and Epidemiology, Roswell Park Memorial Institute, Buffalo, NY)

any printed information given to the client. If it is not, explain why the examination was conducted in one way, but the printed pamphlet suggests another. For example, say, "The pamphlet I gave you shows a woman examining her breasts in concentric circles. Because you are a large-breasted woman, I can feel your breast tissue better by starting at your breast bone, moving to your nipple, and then repositioning your breast and examining from under your arm across to the nipple. Let's see which approach works best when you examine yourself."

Palpation of the breast is completed by palpating the nipple and then by squeezing it to look for nipple discharge. Any discharge obtained may be wiped on a glass slide and sent for a Pap smear or a Gram's stain if infection is suspected. Bilateral milky or watery discharge may not be problematic. Unilateral bloody discharge deserves immediate attention. Many women have inverted nipples or nipples that invert and evert regularly. A unilateral, fixed nipple inversion of recent onset suggests malignancy.

Any lesions are described according to their location, size, shape, consistency, and mobility. In recording the location of findings, use either the four quadrants of the breast or the face-of-the-clock approach (Figure 7–18).

Assessment of the Thorax and Lungs

To locate certain anatomical areas and describe chest findings adequately, the nurse must be familiar with common reference points on the chest. The manubrium of the sternum, the sternal angle or angle of Louis, the intercostal spaces, the costochondral junctions, and the xiphoid process all are important anterior landmarks (Figure 7–19). Additional reference points are a series of imaginary lines drawn on the anterior, lateral, and posterior thorax (Figure 7–20). These include the:

- Midsternal line (MSL)
- Midclavicular line (MCL)
- Anterior axillary line (AAL)
- Midaxillary line (MAL)
- Posterior axillary line (PAL)

Posterior Chest

Inspection and Palpation. Standing behind the client, who is seated and exposed from the waist up, the

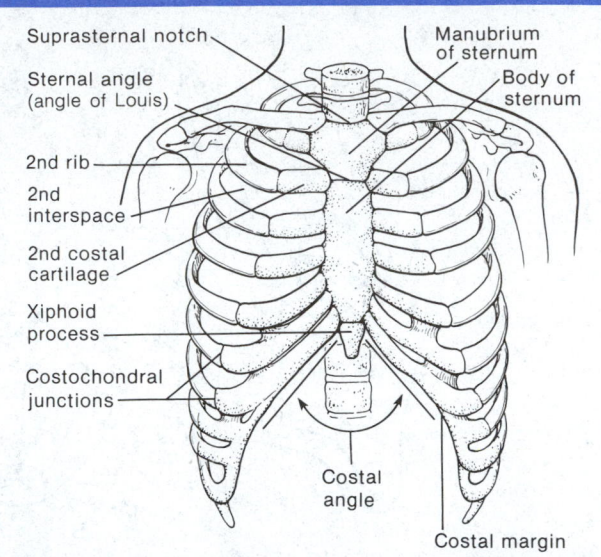

Figure 7–19

Anatomic landmarks on the anterior chest.

examiner inspects the posterior chest. The following assessments are made:

- Note skeletal deformities such as scoliosis, a lateral curvature of the thoracic spine, or increased anteroposterior (AP) diameter of the chest as seen in pulmonary emphysema (also called barrel chest).
- Inspect the skin for lesions and surgical scars. Note the respiratory movements and any retraction or bulging of the interspaces during respiration.

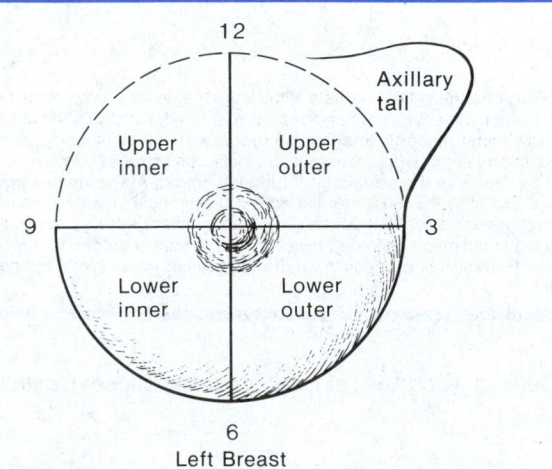

Figure 7–18

Quadrant and face-of-clock method of recording breast findings.

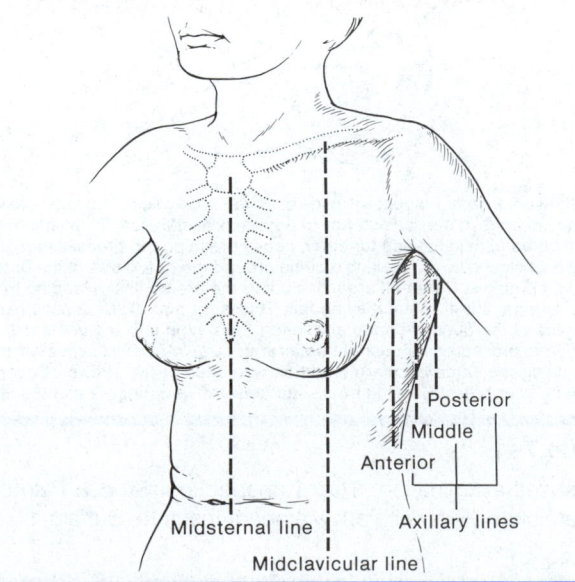

Figure 7–20

Reference points on the chest for describing the location of physical findings.

- Position the hands on the lateral lower rib cage with thumbs close to the spine, with a loose fold of skin between them. With normal respiratory excursion, the entire thorax should move as a unit. Therefore, as the client inhales, the examiner's hands should move in synchrony and the thumbs should diverge equally from the midline.

The posterior chest is palpated for tenderness and areas of crepitation. **Crepitation,** a coarse crackling sensation, is caused by escape of air from the lungs into the subcutaneous tissue, usually as a result of thoracic trauma or surgery. This condition is called *subcutaneous emphysema.*

Assess the chest for **tactile fremitus,** a palpable vibration of air through the airways as a person speaks. Have the client say "99" repeatedly while the examiner places the palmar bases of the fingers of the dominant hand on the interspaces. Some examiners find the ulnar surface of the hand more sensitive for assessing vibratory palpation. The examining hand is moved in sequence while symmetrical chest areas are compared side to side. If fremitus is faint, ask the client to lower the pitch of the voice. Increased fremitus is normally found anteriorly over the parasternal regions and posteriorly in the interscapular areas because these areas lie closest to the main-stem bronchi. Increased lung density transmits air vibrations better than the healthy air-filled structures of the lungs. Therefore, any condition that increases lung density (eg, the consolidation that occurs in pneumonia) increases the vibration and thus palpatory fremitus. With pleural thickening, fluid in the pleural space, or bronchial obstruction, tactile fremitus is decreased or absent.

The level of the diaphragm on each side may also be estimated by vibratory palpation. The ulnar surface of the hand is placed on the interspaces, parallel to the diaphragm, beginning in the midlung fields and working downward to the costovertebral angle. The diaphragmatic level is approximated in the area where fremitus is no longer palpable.

Percussion. Areas of the posterior chest for percussion and auscultation are shown in Figure 7–21. Posterior chest percussion is done while the client is seated. The percussion note heard over healthy lung tissue is described as *resonant.* Begin percussion along the top of each shoulder at the lung apices and work down the chest wall in the interspaces to the lower lung field. Percussion is impaired over the scapular muscles and bones, so avoid these areas. As in palpatory fremitus, symmetrical regions are compared, and the symmetry of sound is evaluated.

Various pathological conditions can alter the percussion note. *Hyperresonance* is heard when the amount of air in the lungs is increased, as in pulmonary emphysema. *Dullness* or impaired resonance is heard when there is considerable solid or liquid matter in the underlying lung tissue. Therefore, dullness to percussion would be expected in pleural effusion or over areas of consolidation.

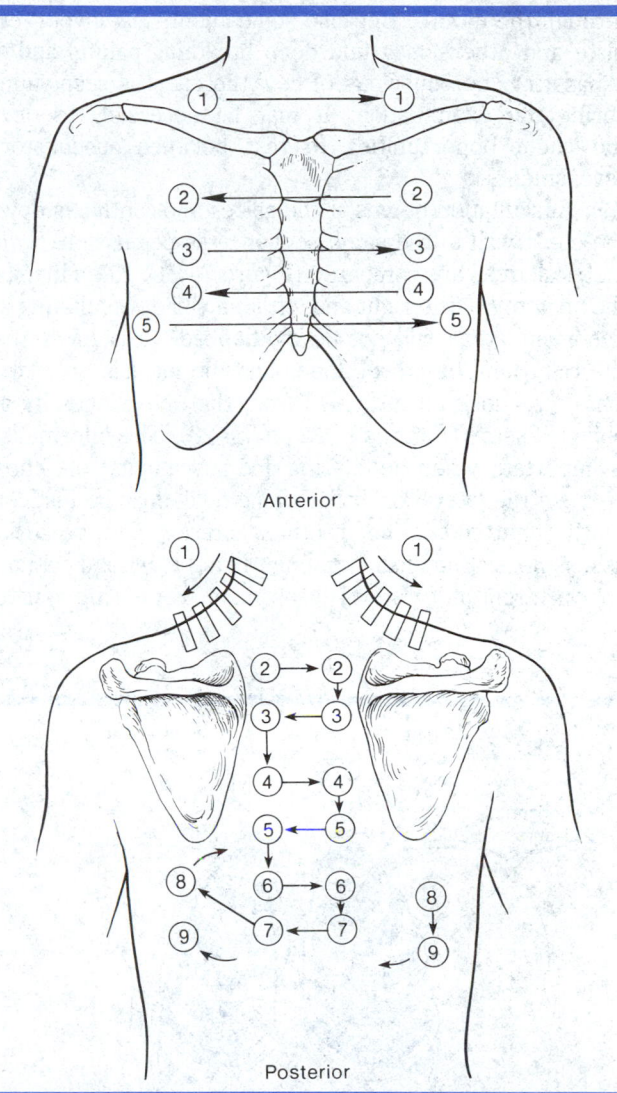

Anterior

Posterior

Figure 7–21

Areas on the anterior and posterior chest for percussion and auscultation.

The amount of diaphragmatic excursion on each side is also obtained by percussion. The client is asked to take a deep breath and hold it. The level of the diaphragm is obtained by noting the change in percussion note from resonance to dullness. This level is marked with a pen. The client is then asked to exhale completely and hold it. The percussion note again changes from resonance to dullness but at a higher level. This level is also marked, and the distance between the two markings is measured to estimate diaphragmatic movement. The same assessment is repeated on the other side to note the symmetry between left and right posterior chest. A low diaphragm with reduced diaphragmatic excursion is often seen in pulmonary emphysema.

Auscultation. The lungs are auscultated with the diaphragm of the stethoscope placed firmly on the interspaces. The client is asked to breathe slowly and deeply through the mouth. Because some clients may hyperventilate and others may find deep breathing painful and/or exhausting, be conscious of how the client is responding during the examination. It may be necessary to offer the client opportunities to rest between auscultatory assessments.

Auscultation begins at the apices and continues down the chest wall in the same sequence as percussion. Symmetrical areas are compared (Figure 7–21). Keep in mind the anatomy of the right and left lung while auscultating so important areas will not be overlooked. Remember that the right lung has three lobes and the left has only two. The lower lobes are divided from the upper lobes by an oblique fissure (Figures 7–22 and 7–23). This information is important when percussing and auscultating the chest because the lateral or axillary lung fields may be inadvertently omitted during routine anterior and posterior assessment. Significant findings may be missed without special attention to lateral assessment. For example, path-

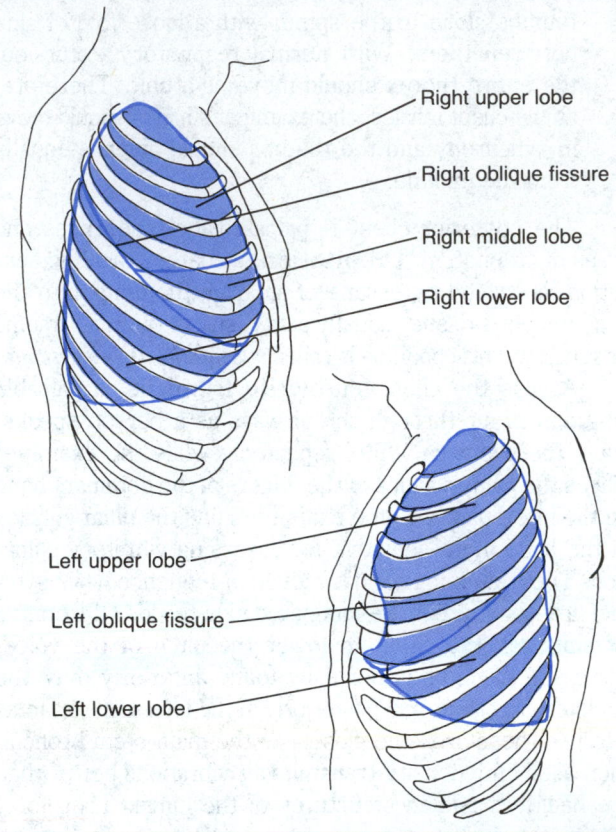

Figure 7–23

Major lung fissures and lobes projected on the lateral surfaces of the chest. **A.** Right. **B.** Left.

ologic conditions in the right middle lobe can be detected only in the right axilla and anterior thorax.

Normal breath sounds are of three types: vesicular, bronchovesicular, and bronchial (see Table 7–3). Abnormal breath sounds *(adventitious sounds)* often auscultated with pulmonary disease include:

- **Rales** (pronounced "rahls")—sounds heard over the smaller bronchi or alveoli. Rales are produced by passage of air through bronchi that contain fluid or exudates or are constricted by spasm or thickening.
- **Rhonchi**—gurgling sounds originating in the larger air passages; these are also called *coarse rales*.
- **Wheezes**—whistling sounds resulting from the narrowing of respiratory passages.
- **Pleural friction rub**—leathery, grating sound produced when inflamed or roughened pleural surfaces rub together.

Two additional auscultatory techniques may be used for further evaluation of suspected pathology. In **whispered pectoriloquy,** the client is asked to whisper. Normally, a whisper is barely audible through the stethoscope; pulmonary consolidation will transmit a whisper clearly. In **egophony,** the client is asked to say "ee." Normally, an "ee" sound is transmitted unchanged through the stethoscope; a long "a" sound is transmitted with consolidation.

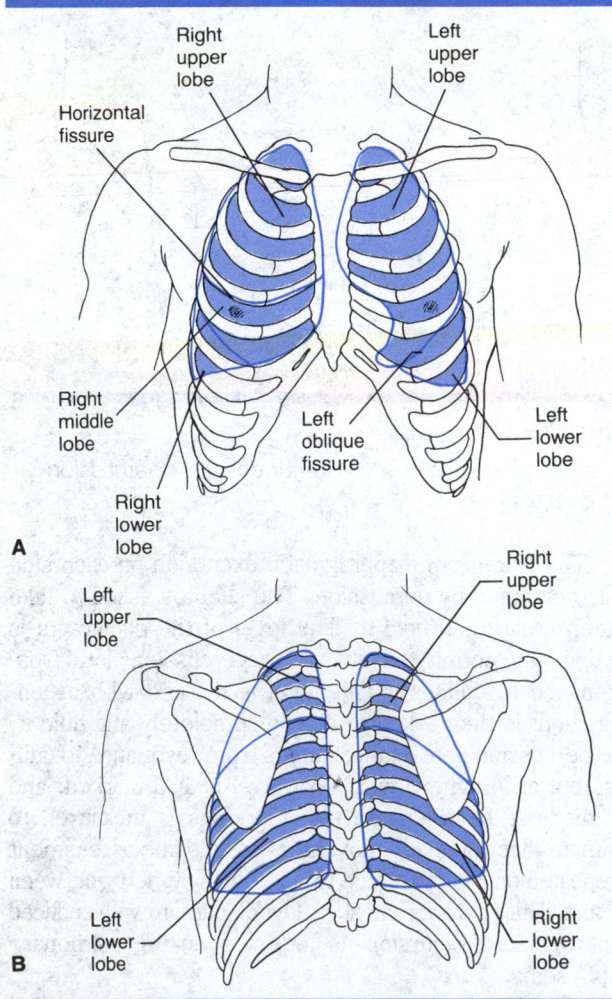

Figure 7–22

Major lung fissures and lobes projected on the anterior and posterior surfaces of the chest. **A.** Anterior. **B.** Posterior.

Table 7–3   Normal Breath Sounds and Their Characteristic Patterns

Description of Normal Breath Sounds	Characteristic Pattern		
Vesicular: Have a long inspiratory phase and short expiratory phase and are heard over most of the lung surface.	Inspiration	Vesicular	Expiration
Bronchovesicular: Have equal inspiratory and expiratory phases and are heard over the main-stem bronchi.	Inspiration	Bronchovesicular	Expiration
Bronchial or tubular: Have a short inspiratory phase and long expiratory phase; bronchial sounds are not normally heard over the lung but are the normal sounds heard when listening over the trachea.	Inspiration	Bronchial	Expiration

Anterior Chest

Assessment of the anterior chest proceeds in the same sequence: inspection, palpation, percussion, auscultation. Anterior assessment may be done with the client seated or supine. In the female client, the breast tissue is flattened or displaced during percussion and auscultation. In percussion of the anterior chest, normal resonance is altered to dullness on the right by the liver and on the left by the cardiac border. Tympany is also noted on the left in the region of the *gastric air bubble,* an air bubble of varying size normally found in the stomach. More will be said about these findings in the sections on cardiac and abdominal assessment that follow.

Assessment of the Heart

Inspection and Palpation

With the client supine, the **precordium,** the area of the anterior chest overlying the heart (Figure 7–24) is inspected

for visible pulsations and areas of retraction. Tangential lighting is helpful. The **point of maximal impulse** (PMI) is specifically sought. The PMI represents the systolic thrust of the cardiac apex, which is sometimes visible in the fifth left intercostal space (LICS) at or just medial to the left MCL. Left ventricular hypertrophy displaces the PMI downward and to the left, lateral to the left MCL.

Palpate for the PMI in the fifth LICS at the MCL whether or not it is visible. Then palpate over the entire precordium, using the palmar bases of the fingers, which are most sensitive to vibration. Evaluate the precordium for **thrills** (palpable vibrations similar to those felt on the throat of a purring cat), thrusts, or lifts. A lifting motion of the lower left parasternal area during systole is indicative of right ventricular hypertrophy.

Percussion

The left border of cardiac dullness (LBCD) can be percussed, indicating cardiac position and size. Because the

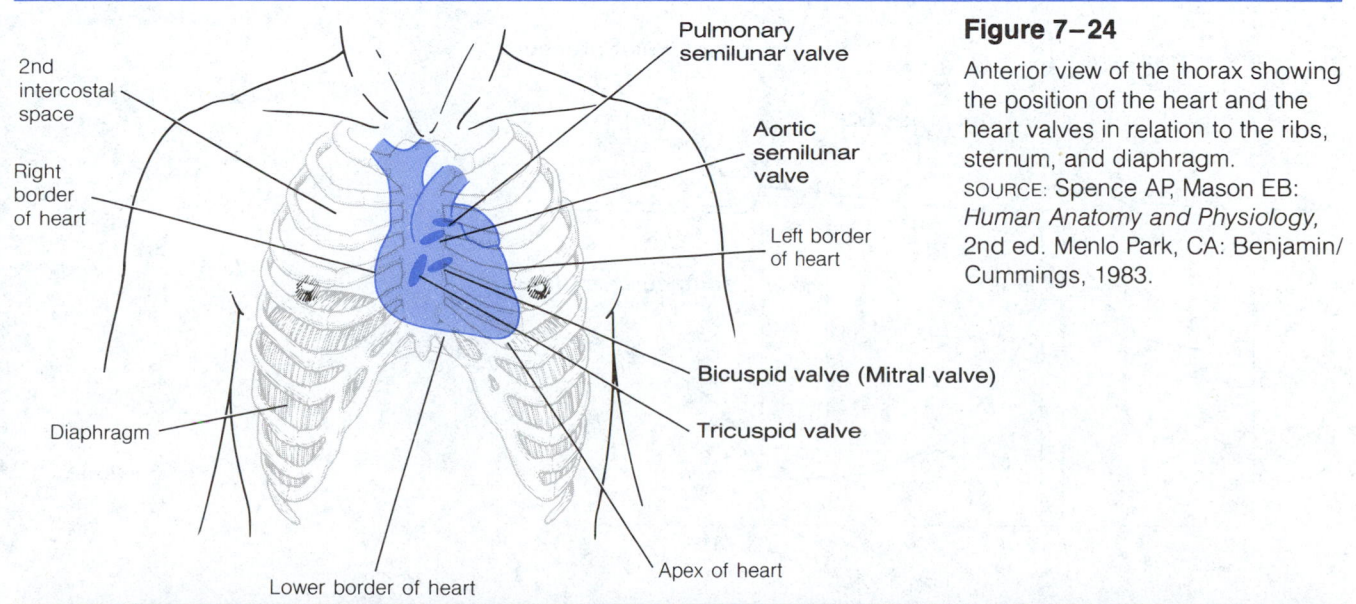

Figure 7–24

Anterior view of the thorax showing the position of the heart and the heart valves in relation to the ribs, sternum, and diaphragm.
SOURCE: Spence AP, Mason EB: *Human Anatomy and Physiology,* 2nd ed. Menlo Park, CA: Benjamin/Cummings, 1983.

2nd intercostal space

Right border of heart

Diaphragm

Lower border of heart

Pulmonary semilunar valve

Aortic semilunar valve

Left border of heart

Bicuspid valve (Mitral valve)

Tricuspid valve

Apex of heart

chest x-ray is more precise in delineating the size and contour of the heart, percussion is not often done. Percussion is helpful in determining cardiac enlargement, however, and it can be a useful assessment tool when a chest x-ray is not available. Begin at the left AAL in the fourth, fifth, and sixth interspaces and percuss across from resonance to dullness. Mark the point of change in percussion note at each interspace. This locates the LBCD.

The Cardiac Cycle and Related Heart Sounds

A review of the normal events in the cardiac cycle may help in understanding the heart sounds and what they mean. During diastole, pressure in the left atrium, which has been filled by blood returning through the pulmonary veins, slightly exceeds pressure in the left ventricle; therefore, blood flows across the open mitral valve from left atrium into the left ventricle. Just before the onset of ventricular systole, the atrium contracts (the *atrial kick*), forcing more blood into the ventricle. As the ventricle begins to contract, the pressure within it rises rapidly, exceeding the pressure in the atrium, forcing the mitral valve closed. The rising ventricular pressure soon exceeds the pressure in the aorta, causing the aortic valve to open. As the blood

is ejected, ventricular pressure continues to rise and then drops off when most of the blood has been emptied. The aortic valve closes when left ventricular pressure drops below aortic pressure. As left ventricular pressure continues to drop, it falls below left atrial pressure; the mitral valve opens and ventricular filling begins anew. The same events also occur on the right side of the heart, almost simultaneously, but events on the left side occur a little sooner.

Pressure changes, volume changes, and valve actions in the left heart are shown in Figure 7–25. Although these events occur similarly on the right side, right ventricular peak pressure is considerably lower. The pressure curve in Figure 7–25 demonstrates a systolic pressure of 120 mm Hg during left ventricular systole. A pressure curve of the right heart depicting right ventricular systolic pressure would show a pressure of about 30 mm Hg. Pressure is lower on the right side because the right ventricle has to pump blood only into the pulmonary circulation, whereas the left ventricle is responsible for the entire systemic circulation.

In Figure 7–25, curve a is the pressure curve of the left atrium. Line 1 shows the closing of the mitral valve

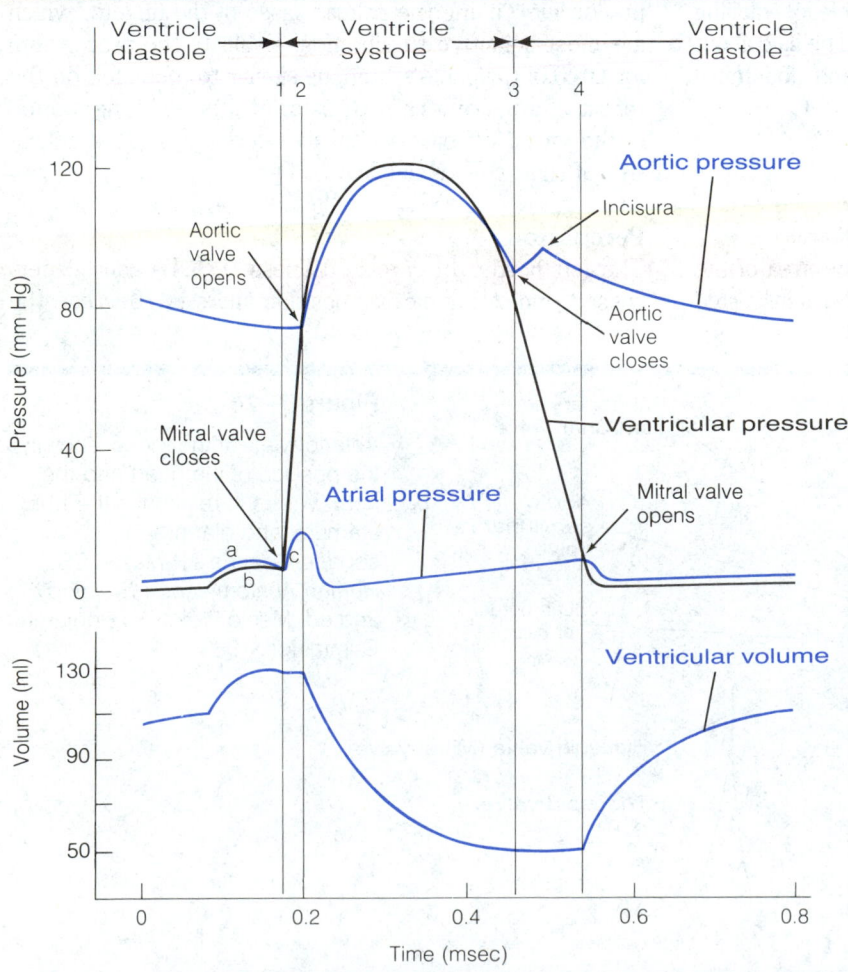

Figure 7–25

The cardiac cycle. Comparisons of pressure changes, volume changes, and valve actions within the left chambers of the heart during a single cardiac cycle. Note that the duration of a complete cycle is 0.8 sec.
SOURCE: Spence AP, Mason EB: *Human Anatomy and Physiology*, 2nd ed. Menlo Park, CA: Benjamin/Cummings, 1983.

when left ventricular pressure exceeds left atrial pressure. With the sudden increase in left ventricular pressure the mitral valve bulges slightly into the left atrium, increasing left atrial pressure, which is depicted by curve c. This increased left atrial pressure continues until the aortic valve opens, depicted by line 2. The pressure within the left atrium drops to almost 0 mm Hg. Pressure in the left atrium gradually increases as it is filled by the pulmonary veins. When left atrial pressure exceeds left ventricular pressure, the mitral valve opens (line 4).

In Figure 7–25, curve b is the ventricular pressure curve. The pressure within the left ventricle rises rapidly during systole, as clearly seen between lines 1 and 2. At the end of ventricular systole, left ventricular pressure drops below aortic pressure, causing blood from the aorta to flow backward, closing the aortic valve (line 3).

Left ventricular pressure continues to drop until it is lower than left atrial pressure, allowing blood in the left atrium to push open the mitral valve (line 4). Left ventricular blood volume is at its lowest point, as shown by the ventricular volume change curve at the bottom of Figure 7–25.

The aortic pressure curve shows well the ability of the aorta to expand and recoil, which helps to maintain pressure on the blood. As seen on the curve, aortic blood pressure does not drop below 80 mm Hg. Line 3 shows a brief rise in aortic pressure when the aortic valve closes, indicated by the incisura (notch) on the diagram.

Heart Sounds. Closure of the valves causes normal heart sounds. The most important sounds are the *first heart sound* (S_1) and the *second heart sound* (S_2) because they divide the cardiac cycle into systole and diastole. The first heart sound (S_1) is synchronous with the apical impulse (PMI) and corresponds to the onset of ventricular systole. Closure of the mitral and tricuspid valves produces S_1, which sounds like the syllable "lub."

The second heart sound (S_2) occurs at the termination of systole and corresponds with the onset of ventricular

diastole. Closure of the aortic and pulmonic valves produces S_2, which sounds like the syllable "dup." Both S_1 and S_2 are clearly audible over all valve areas in healthy persons and together sound like "lub dup."

The third heart sound (S_3), if present, occurs in early diastole during the phase of rapid ventricular filling, as blood flows from left atrium to left ventricle. It is considered normal when heard in children and young adults. The fourth heart sound (S_4), if present, occurs late in diastole or just prior to S_1 and is caused by atrial contraction (atrial kick). The sound is often heard in healthy persons. An S_3 may indicate ventricular failure in older adults. An S_4 may suggest cardiac disease such as aortic stenosis or hypertension.

Relation of Heart Sounds to the Chest Wall. The precordial areas where the heart sounds are most audible do not correspond to the anatomical valve locations as seen in Figure 7–24 but to the following auscultatory areas (Figure 7–26):

- Mitral (or apical or bicuspid) area—fifth LICS at, or just medial to, the MCL
- Tricuspid area—fifth LICS at the LSB
- Pulmonic area—second LICS at the LSB ⎫ base of
- Aortic area—second RICS at the RSB ⎭ the heart

The first heart sound (S_1) is louder than S_2 at the cardiac apex and fainter than S_2 at the pulmonic and aortic areas. Because S_1 has two valvular components, mitral and tricuspid closure, and because events in the left heart occur slightly before events on the right, the sound of S_1 is occasionally split. The split of S_1 may be heard better in the tricuspid area, whereas a single component of S_1 is usual in the mitral area.

The second heart sound (S_2) also has two valvular components, the pulmonic and the aortic. S_2 is louder than S_1 at the base of the heart. The aortic component of S_2 is audible in all auscultatory areas, but the pulmonic component, which is weaker, is usually heard only in the second

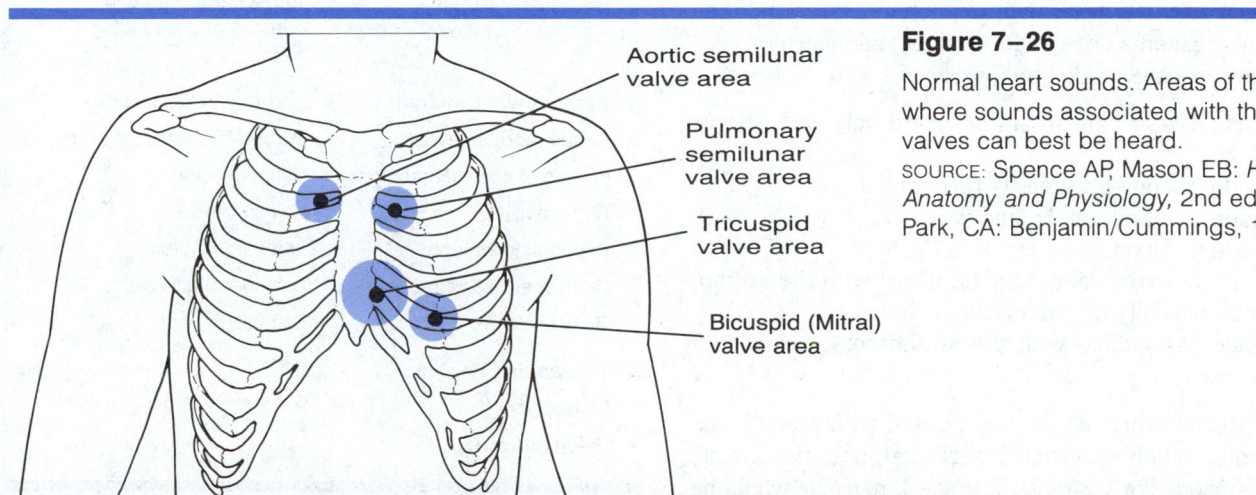

Aortic semilunar valve area

Pulmonary semilunar valve area

Tricuspid valve area

Bicuspid (Mitral) valve area

Figure 7–26

Normal heart sounds. Areas of the chest where sounds associated with the heart valves can best be heard.
SOURCE: Spence AP, Mason EB: *Human Anatomy and Physiology*, 2nd ed. Menlo Park, CA: Benjamin/Cummings, 1983.

LICS at the LSB. Splitting of S_2 is considered normal only in the pulmonic area (DeGowin & DeGowin, 1981).

If audible, S_3 and S_4 are both heard best at the apex (mitral area). Because they are both low-pitched sounds, they are best heard with the bell of the stethoscope. The term **gallop rhythm** refers to auscultation of an S_3 or S_4 or both, along with S_1 and S_2, which altogether resemble the canter of a horse.

Heart Murmurs. Heart **murmurs** are sounds resulting from vibrations produced by turbulence of blood flow in the heart or great vessels. Mechanisms of murmur production include increased velocity of blood flow; constriction or dilation of a cardiac valve, cardiac chamber, or great vessel; or shunting of blood through an abnormal opening. Murmurs are described according to their:

- Location (where best heard on the precordium)
- Radiation
- Timing (systolic or diastolic; early, middle, or late)
- Quality
- Intensity (grade 1 to 6)

The location on the precordium where a cardiac murmur is heard best and the areas to which it radiates are helpful in identifying the origin of the murmur. For example, the murmur of aortic valve stenosis is usually loudest in the second RICS at the RSB and often radiates into the neck.

Whether a murmur occurs in systole or diastole is also important in diagnosis. Systolic murmurs are much more common than diastolic murmurs, and many are benign. Diastolic murmurs are almost always pathological. Holosystolic or pansystolic murmurs are heard throughout systole. If the murmur occurs during a certain phase of systole, it is recorded as early systolic, midsystolic, or late systolic.

The quality of a murmur describes whether it is harsh, blowing, or musical; its pitch (high or low); and its configuration. If the pitch increases, the pattern is crescendo. If the pitch decreases, the pattern is decrescendo. A diamond pattern is a murmur whose pitch increases and then decreases, called a crescendo–decrescendo murmur.

Murmurs are graded on a scale of 1 to 6:

- Grade 1—so faint it can be heard only with special effort
- Grade 2—quiet but easily recognized
- Grade 3—moderately loud
- Grade 4—loud
- Grade 5—very loud; may be heard with the stethoscope partially off the chest
- Grade 6—audible with the stethoscope entirely off the chest

A palpable thrill is often associated with grade 5 and 6 murmurs. When a murmur is recorded, note that a scale of 6 was used. For example, a grade 2 murmur would be recorded as "grade 2/6."

Pericardial Friction Rub. A pericardial friction rub arises from the rubbing together of the pericardial surfaces secondary to inflammation of the pericardial sac. The rub may be heard over the entire precordial region. The sound is usually described as scratchy, grating, or squeaky and may be heard through both systole and diastole. The rub may disappear and reappear. Having the client change position may alter the audibility of the rub.

Auscultation

When the first three steps of cardiac assessment—inspection, palpation, and percussion—have been completed, begin auscultation by placing the diaphragm of the stethoscope on the mitral area (apex) and identifying the sounds of S_1 and S_2. Count the apical rate for 1 minute. *Pulse deficit* is the difference between the apical rate and the peripheral pulse rate. Listen carefully for any rhythm irregularity. **Normal sinus rhythm** (NSR) is the orderly rhythm of the healthy heart, whose rate at rest is between 60 and 100 beats per minute.

Then move the stethoscope sequentially to the tricuspid, pulmonic, and aortic areas, listening for S_1, S_2, and any extra sounds in systole or diastole. Turn to the bell of

---

Box 7–5   Abdominal Organs Located in the Four Abdominal Quadrants and the Suprapubic Region

Right Upper Quadrant	Left Upper Quadrant
Liver and gallbladder	Left lobe of liver
Pylorus	Spleen
Duodenum	Stomach
Head of pancreas	Body of pancreas
Right adrenal gland	Left adrenal gland
Right kidney	Left kidney
Hepatic flexure of colon	Splenic flexure of colon
Ascending colon and portions of transverse colon	Transverse colon and portions of descending colon

Right Lower Quadrant	Left Lower Quadrant
Cecum and appendix	Portion of descending colon
Portion of ascending colon	Sigmoid colon
Right ovary ♀	Left ovary ♀
Right fallopian tube ♀	Left fallopian tube ♀
Right spermatic cord ♂	Left spermatic cord ♂
Right ureter	Left ureter

Suprapubic Region

Bladder

Pregnant uterus ♀

NOTE: Portions of the small intestine are located in all quadrants.

the stethoscope and repeat the listening sequence in all auscultatory areas.

Ask the client to turn onto the left side while auscultating at the apex with the bell of the stethoscope. Murmurs and other sounds may be accentuated in this position, called the left lateral decubitus (LLD) position. Cardiac sounds can be further evaluated by having the client sit up and lean forward. The squatting position may intensify some heart murmurs.

Assessment of the Abdomen

Within the abdomen lie numerous organs and blood vessels, all of which must be considered during the assessment process. In description of examination findings, two topographic divisions of the abdomen are used. Figure 7–27 depicts the abdomen divided into four quadrants, probably the most common divisions. Figure 7–28 shows the abdomen sectioned into nine regions. This system is useful because of its three central areas—the epigastric, umbilical, and suprapubic. For example, it is clearer to describe the bladder as being in the suprapubic region than as being split between the right and left lower quadrants. Many clinicians use the four quadrant descriptions except for centrally located findings. During abdominal assessment, remember the organs found in each quadrant (see Box 7–5).

Inspection

With the client supine and the entire abdomen exposed, look carefully at sequential areas of the abdomen and note:

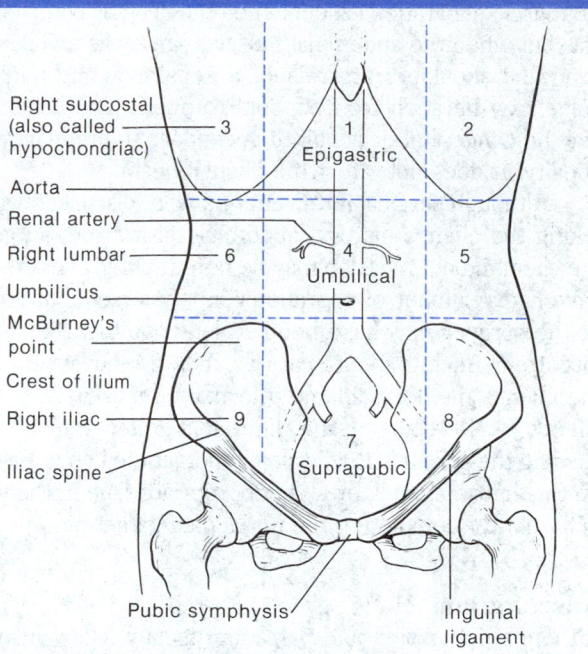

Figure 7–28

The nine abdominal regions: **1.** Epigastric region. **2** and **3.** Right and left subcostal or hypochondriac regions. **4.** Umbilical region. **5** and **6.** Right and left lumbar regions. **7.** Suprapubic or hypogastric region. **8** and **9.** Right and left inguinal or iliac regions.

- Skin color and lesions
- Striae (stretch marks)
- Scars
- Engorged veins
- Visible pulsations
- Visible peristalsis
- Umbilical position
- Herniation
- Abdominal profile

Abdominal distention is frequently seen when observing the abdominal profile. A mnemonic, the 6 Fs, aids in remembering the six common causes of a distended abdomen:

- Fat
- Fluid
- Feces
- Flatus
- Fetus
- Fatal mass

Another common finding on visual inspection is an abdominal hernia. Incisional hernias (herniations adjacent to old surgical scars) and umbilical hernias are the most usual. **Diastasis recti,** a separation of the two rectus abdominis muscles, is sometimes mistaken for a hernia.

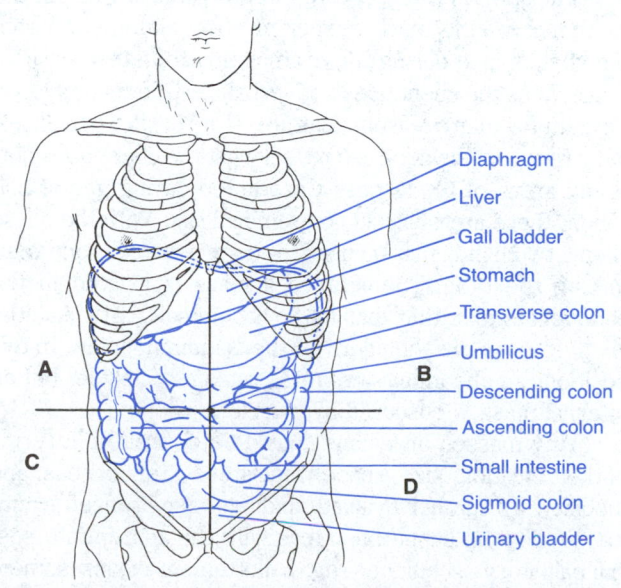

Figure 7–27

The four abdominal quadrants. **A.** Right upper quadrant (RUQ). **B.** Left upper quadrant (LUQ). **C.** Right lower quadrant (RLQ). **D.** Left lower quadrant (LLQ).

No muscle separation is seen when the client is completely flat, but when the abdominal muscles are tensed while the head and shoulders are raised, a separation and midline bulge may be seen from xiphoid to pubis. The condition may be congenital or acquired secondary to pregnancy or obesity. It does not affect the client's health.

Although surgical interventions were discussed when taking the client's history, abdominal scars from surgery the client did not mention may be noted. Often clients who have had a number of operations simply forget about one, or the surgery may have been so long ago that they have forgotten. Asking about scars as they are observed jogs the client's memory, adding information important to the client's health record. If the client deliberately avoided discussing the surgery, that is also important to know. Follow up this information later at an appropriate time in the plan of care after completing the initial data gathering.

Auscultation

Although percussion and palpation usually follow inspection, auscultatory findings may be altered by these techniques. Thus, auscultation precedes them in abdominal assessment.

Listen for the normal peristaltic sounds (gurgles) below and to the right of the umbilicus. High-pitched sounds may be indicative of early intestinal obstruction or severe diarrhea. The complete absence of peristaltic sounds is seen in paralytic ileus. To establish that the abdomen is silent, however, the examiner must listen for 5 minutes.

Another auscultatory sound is the peritoneal friction rub indicative of peritonitis. The rub sounds much like the leathery pleural friction rub in the chest and often emanates from the splenic or hepatic region.

Bruits are best heard with the bell of the stethoscope. An abdominal aortic aneurysm, renal artery stenosis, or partial occlusion of any major blood vessel can cause a bruit. In young, thin, healthy clients, a bruit over the abdominal aorta is sometimes heard; this is not considered pathological. See Figure 7–29 for the areas where abdominal sounds are best heard.

Palpation

Most abdominal structures cannot be felt in the healthy abdomen. Structures that may normally be palpable include the:

- Abdominal aorta
- Lower pole of the right kidney
- Liver edge as it descends on inspiration
- Ascending colon ——————————— when they
- Descending colon and sigmoid   contain stool
- Distended bladder
- Pregnant uterus

The abdomen is palpated using a gentle dipping motion of the fingertips, keeping the fingers together. All four quadrants are examined. In the ticklish client, placing the

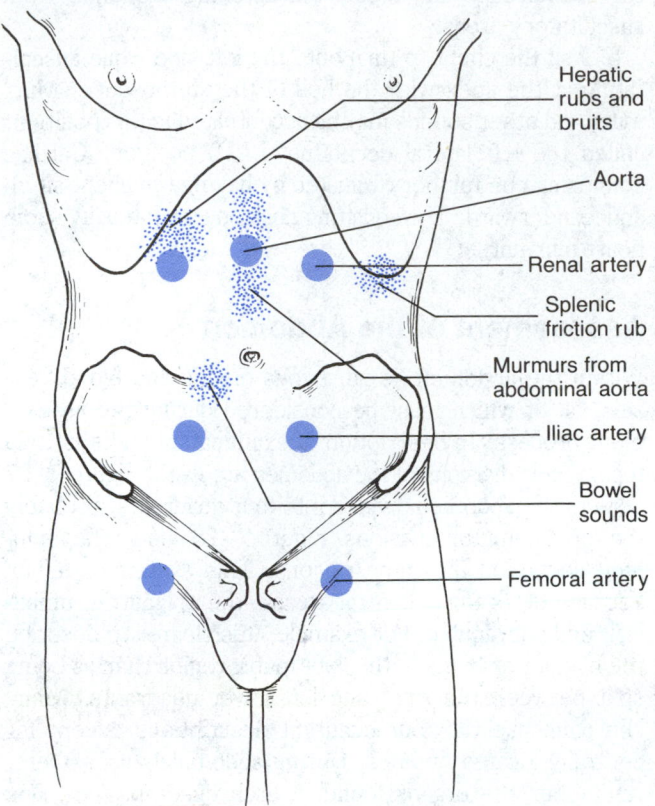

Figure 7–29

Areas for listening to sounds in the abdomen.

client's hand on top of the examiner's during palpation will help in desensitizing the client.

Palpation is then repeated in the same way, with the examiner feeling much deeper into the abdomen. Watch the client's face during the examination to detect areas of tenderness the client does not verbalize. Clients deny having pain for many reasons (culture, fear, past experience), but careful observation can reveal what the client does not. If any areas of tenderness were noted during gentle palpation, these areas should be examined last. With the obese client, two hands may be used for deep palpation, one reinforcing the other. Sometimes a mass is located in the abdominal wall rather than in the abdominal cavity. Ask the client to raise the shoulders off the examining table. In this position, an abdominal wall mass remains palpable, but an internal mass is obscured by muscle tension.

Any masses or lesions should be described in terms of their location, size, shape, consistency, tenderness, and mobility. To further evaluate findings, experienced examiners follow up suspicious areas with the appropriate special palpatory technique—eg, ballottement or assessment for rebound tenderness.

Specific organs are palpated in sequence. To palpate the liver, the left hand is placed under the client's right flank, parallel to and supporting the 11th and 12th rib areas. This bimanual technique is used to bring the liver more forward. The examiner's right hand is placed on the right midabdomen in the area of the right MCL with fingers pointing toward the costal margin (Figure 7–30). Ask the client to inhale deeply, which may bring the liver edge down toward the palpating fingers.

In palpating the kidneys, remember that the right kidney is generally slightly lower than the left because of the location of the liver. To palpate the right kidney, use the same bimanual technique as liver palpation, but position the right hand below the right costal margin with the fingers pointing toward the umbilicus. As the client takes a deep breath, press the two hands together, and try to feel the lower pole of the right kidney slipping between the fingers. The same technique is used for the left kidney, but the examiner should move to the client's other side.

To palpate the spleen, have the client turn onto the right side, toward the examiner. Support the client's left side with the left hand. With the right hand low in the abdomen, fingertips pointed toward the left costal margin, press in toward the spleen as the client takes a deep breath. The spleen must be enlarged significantly to be palpable.

The aortic pulsation is often visible slightly to the left of the midline, above the umbilicus. To palpate the aortic pulsation, press into the middle of the upper abdomen. The normal aortic pulsation is in an AP direction. An examiner who palpates a pulsatile mass with lateral as well as AP movement should suspect an abdominal aortic aneurysm.

The inguinal region of the lower abdomen must not be overlooked. The femoral pulses are palpated, graded, and compared side to side. Palpation is also useful in detecting enlarged inguinal lymph nodes. Enlarged nodes may be

secondary to regional infections such as vaginitis or urinary tract infections (UTI).

Percussion

Light percussion in all quadrants assesses the general distribution of tympany and dullness. Tympany is heard over the air-filled regions in the bowel and stomach and is the predominant sound in the abdomen.

Liver size is percussed by beginning below the umbilicus in the right MCL in an area of tympany and percussing upward toward the costal margin. When the percussion note changes to dull, the lower liver edge has been located. Mark this spot with a pen. To find the upper liver border, begin high in the right thorax at the MCL and percuss in the interspaces until lung resonance changes to dullness. Mark the upper border and measure between the two marks to obtain the liver span. The normal liver span is 6 to 12 cm at the MCL.

Blunt percussion is sometimes done over the liver to assess for tenderness when acute hepatitis or acute cholecystitis is suspected. The left palm is placed over the right ribs just above the costal margin. The back of the left hand is struck lightly by the ulnar side of the examiner's right fist. The impact causes pain in acute hepatitis and acute cholecystitis (DeGowin & DeGowin, 1981).

The gastric air bubble of the stomach is percussed in the left upper quadrant in the area of the sixth or seventh left intercostal space. Sometimes it is located in the epigastric region.

The spleen may be located by percussing for splenic dullness near the tenth rib in the left MAL. To assess for splenic enlargement, percuss the lowest interspace in the AAL. The percussion note here should be tympanic. Ask the client to take a deep breath and hold it. Repercuss the area. If dullness replaces tympany, the spleen may be enlarged.

Percussion for renal tenderness is usually done during assessment of the posterior chest while the client is seated. The technique is discussed in this section because the kidneys are abdominal organs. The kidneys are situated on the posterior wall of the abdominal cavity on each side of the vertebral column in front of the 12th rib. This anatomical area is called the *costovertebral angle* (CVA), and the procedure is thus called assessing for CVA tenderness. The examiner's left hand is placed over each CVA and struck very gently with the ulnar side of the right fist. Tenderness in the area indicates inflammation of the kidney.

Examination of the Rectum

Assessment of the rectum is an important aspect of evaluation of the gastrointestinal tract. The rectal examination also is helpful in assessing for disorders of the genitourinary tract (eg, prostatic hypertrophy in men).

The position of the client for the exam varies. If the rectal examination is done during the pelvic exam, the woman is in the lithotomy position. If it is combined with exami-

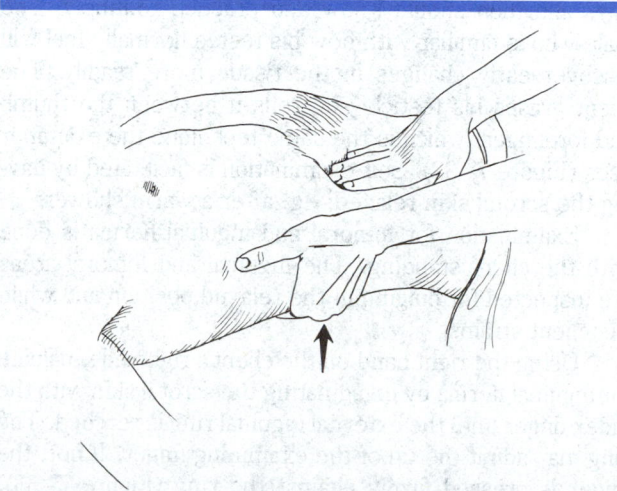

Figure 7–30

Bimanual palpation of the liver. In bimanual palpation of the liver, the posterior rib cage is lifted with the examiner's left hand as the palmar surface of the fingers of the right hand are pressed gently into the abdominal wall. The client inspires slowly and deeply to cause the liver edge to descend and meet the tips of the palpating fingers.

nation of the male genitalia, the client may be standing, leaning over the examining table. If examination of the rectum follows the abdominal evaluation and a pelvic or male genital examination will not be done, the client may be positioned on the left side with the knees up close to the chest.

The buttocks are spread apart, and the sacrococcygeal and perianal areas are inspected for inflammation, rashes, lesions, hemorrhoids, fissures, or evidence of scratching. The client is asked to strain as if to defecate, and the anus is observed for internal hemorrhoids, which may prolapse into view.

To palpate the anus, use a gloved index finger to explore any external lesions that were observed. Assess the area for tenderness. Lubricate the gloved index finger with a water-soluble lubricant and place the pad of the fingertip against the external anal sphincter to relax the sphincter. Having the client breathe through the mouth also aids in relaxation. Insert the finger gently into the anal canal as far as possible. The anal canal slants downward and backward, so the finger should be pointing toward the umbilicus as it is inserted. The rectal wall is palpated in sequence: right lateral, posterior, left lateral, and anterior surfaces. Areas of tenderness or masses are identified. Often hard stool is found in the rectum.

In the male client, the prostate gland is evaluated (Figure 7–31). The prostate, a gland the size of a chestnut, surrounds the male urethra and is located just anterior to the rectum. With the examining finger on the anterior wall, identify the lateral lobes of the prostate and the median sulcus between them. The normal prostate feels firm and

slightly compressible. The size, shape, consistency, nodularity, or tenderness of the prostate are noted.

With the female client, the uterine cervix or the retroverted uterine fundus is frequently palpable through the anterior rectal wall. With both male and female clients, asking them to strain may bring a mass beyond the examiner's fingertip downward, enabling it to be located and examined. Any fecal matter on the gloved finger should be inspected and tested for occult blood.

Assessment of the Male Genitalia

Although a complete examination of the male genitalia may not be part of a routine nursing assessment, nurses should be familiar with the components of the exam. Teaching of testicular self-examination is a nursing responsibility.

The skin of the penis is inspected, and the foreskin, if present, is retracted either by the client or the examiner. The glans penis and the urethral meatus are assessed for lesions and discharge. If lesions are present, gloves are applied before penile palpation. The shaft of the penis is palpated for nodules. Note any areas of tenderness.

The skin of the scrotum is inspected carefully, lifting it to view the posterior surface. In clients who are confined to bed, the scrotum often becomes edematous, excoriated, and inflamed. The scrotum is palpated, and areas of tenderness or swelling are noted. To determine whether a scrotal swelling is serous or more solid, transilluminate the scrotum in a darkened room. Serous fluid transmits a red glow; blood or masses do not.

Both testes in the scrotal sac are gently palpated. Their size, shape, and consistency are compared. Areas of tenderness are noted. Testicular self-examination is an important health maintenance technique that adolescent boys and men should know and practice routinely. The male who is familiar with how his testes normally feel will discover early changes in the tissue more readily. The client grasps his testicle and rolls it between the thumb and forefinger, which is the same technique the examiner uses (Figure 7–32). Self-examination is facilitated by having the scrotal skin relaxed; eg, after a warm shower.

Examination for femoral and inguinal hernia is done with the client standing. The inguinal and femoral areas are inspected for bulging in the relaxed position and while the client strains.

Using the right hand on the client's right side, palpate for inguinal hernia by invaginating the scrotal skin with the index finger until the external inguinal ring is reached. The ring may admit the tip of the examining finger. If not, the finger is pressed firmly against the ring (Figure 7–33). Ask the client to cough, feeling for a bulge against the fingertip. The left inguinal region is then checked with the left hand.

Assessment of the Female Genitalia

The pelvic examination is one that many women dread. The nurse has an important role in assisting women to

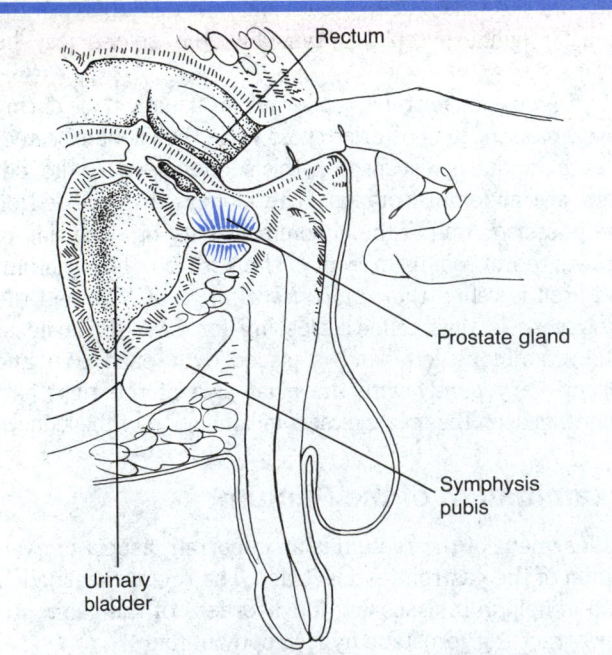

Figure 7–31

Palpation of the male prostate gland.

How to do TSE: Testicular self-examination is a simple procedure that all young men should learn to do. Palpation, or feeling, of the testicles is best done using two hands as illustrated in the figure. Explore each testicle individually. Using both hands, gently roll the testicle between the thumbs and fingers. If pain is experienced, too much pressure is being applied.

The examination should be done at least once each month, preferably after a warm bath or shower when the scrotal skin is most relaxed.

What to look for: A normal testicle is egg-shaped, somewhat firm to touch, and should be smooth and free of lumps. When doing TSE, you should be looking for any changes in the size or consistency of the testicle. If you do find something abnormal, most likely it will be an area of firmness or small lump on the front or on the side of the testicle. Do not confuse the epididymis (the soft tubelike structure at the back of the testis) with a tumor. If you do find something abnormal, you should have the condition checked immediately by a physician.

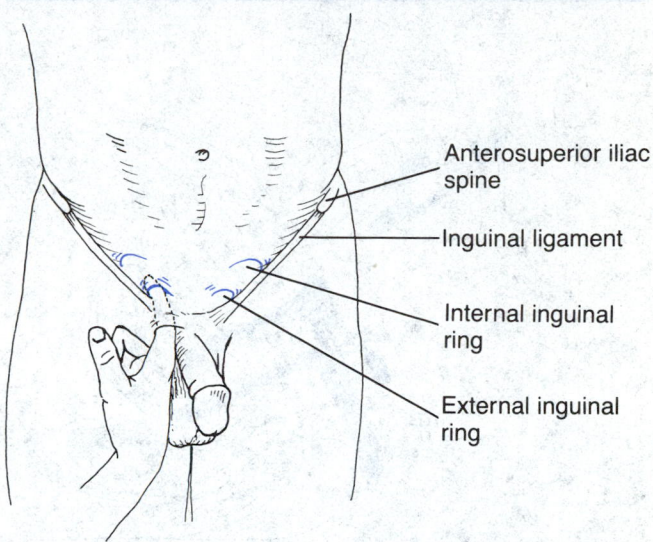

Anterosuperior iliac spine

Inguinal ligament

Internal inguinal ring

External inguinal ring

Figure 7–33

Examination for right inguinal hernia.

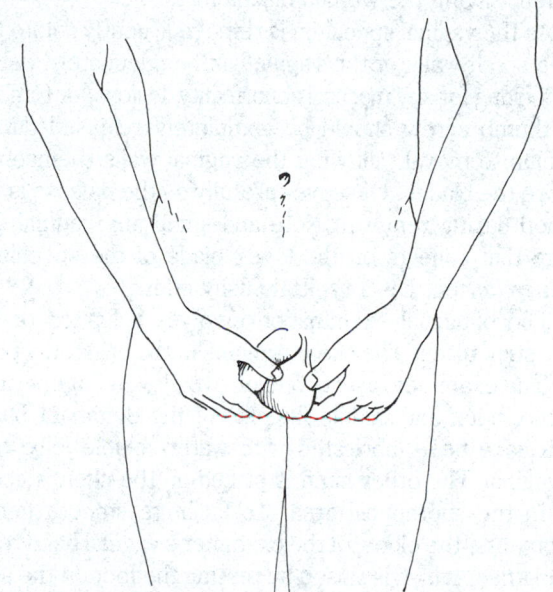

What happens if cancer is found? When detected early enough, testicular cancer is one of the most curable types of cancer. Most early tumors are confined to one testicle. Surgical removal of one testicle does not leave a person impotent; the remaining testicle is capable of maintaining sexual fertility, erection, and orgasm.

Figure 7–32

Teaching the client about testicular self-examination (TSE). (Courtesy of Department of Cancer Control and Epidemiology, Roswell Park Memorial Institute, Buffalo, NY)

understand why the embarrassing lithotomy position is needed for an adequate pelvic exam and to appreciate the complete evaluation of the genitourinary and gastrointestinal system the pelvic exam affords. Positioning the client in a semiseated position and providing a properly placed mirror allows the client to see what is being visualized. Although some women prefer not to look, many women are pleased to see their own cervix so clearly. This experience greatly enhances their appreciation of the importance of the exam.

The woman is in the lithotomy position with her buttocks partially hanging over the edge of the examining table to facilitate distensibility of the inferior vaginal wall. The external genitalia (see Figure 61–1) are carefully inspected. Note any ulceration, discharge, swelling, inflammation, nodules, or lesions. Ask the client to bear down while the labia are separated by the examiner's fin-

gers. Note any bulging of the vaginal walls. An anterior bulging indicates a cystocele (bladder relaxation into the vagina), and a posterior bulging indicates a rectocele (rectal prolapse into the vagina). These problems of pelvic support are secondary to childbearing. Note any loss of urine (stress incontinence), which is also related to loss of adequate muscular supporting mechanisms, rarely seen in nulliparas and commonly seen in multiparas. See Figure 61–2 to see the relation of the bladder, vagina, and rectum.

With gloves on, palpate any suspicious areas. If inflammation of Skene's glands (paraurethral glands) is suspected, insert the index finger into the vagina and gently massage the urethra from inside out. Any discharge obtained is cultured. If labial swelling is noted, insert the index finger into the vagina at the inferior end of the introitus and position the thumb opposite on the labia majora. Palpate this area of Bartholin's gland between the two fingers, noting tenderness and swelling. Normally, these glands cannot be visualized or palpated.

A speculum of the appropriate size is selected and warmed with warm water. Specula with narrow blades are used for women who are not sexually active and often for elderly women who have atrophic vaginal changes. Take great care to use the proper sized speculum, or the exam will be extremely uncomfortable for the client.

The examiner inserts one or two fingers into the introitus and, holding the closed speculum vertically with the other hand, inserts the blades gently into the vagina (Figure 7–34A). The speculum is rotated into a horizontal position. Downward pressure is maintained on the vagina during the speculum exam, because the inferior vaginal wall is more distensible and less sensitive than the superior vaginal wall. The blades of the speculum are gradually opened after full insertion, and the speculum is maneuvered until

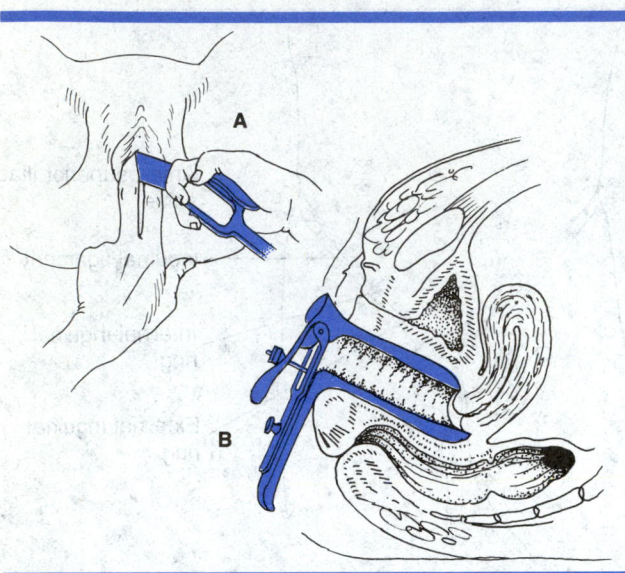

Figure 7–34

The speculum examination. **A.** Insertion of vaginal speculum for inspection. **B.** The vaginal speculum in place with the cervix in view.

the cervix comes into view. When the entire cervix and cervical os are well visualized, the screws on the speculum are tightened (Figure 7–34B).

The cervix and its os are carefully inspected. The os can be small, round, or oval. The os of a parous cervix has a slitlike appearance (Figure 7–35). Note the color of the cervix and any lesions, ulcerations, inflammation, cysts, nodules, bleeding, erosion, or discharge. If the client has an intrauterine contraceptive device (IUD), the IUD string should be seen exiting from the cervical os. Chadwick's sign, cyanosis of the vaginal and cervical mucosa secondary to pregnancy, is seen near the end of the second month of pregnancy as a bluish hue of the cervix and vagina.

The Papanicolaou (Pap) smear is obtained during the speculum exam. The Pap smear is a cytologic smear of the cervix for early detection of cervical cell changes predisposing to cancer of the cervix. A woman should begin having Pap smears at the age of 20 or earlier if she is

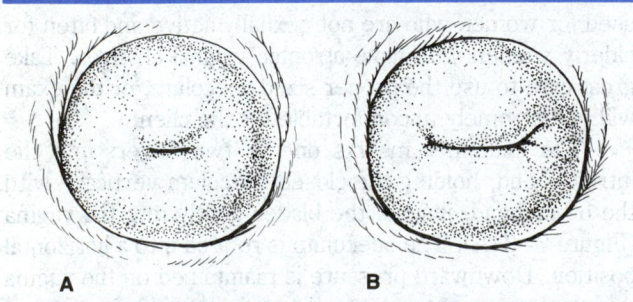

Figure 7–35

The female cervix and its os. **A.** Nulliparous cervix. **B.** Parous cervix.

sexually active or at increased risk for malignancy in the genital tract (eg, as in daughters of women who took diethylstilbestrol [DES] during their pregnancy). Specimens for culture can also be taken at this time if infection is suspected.

Some common organisms causing vaginitis can be readily seen under the microscope. If the examiner suspects monilial vaginitis (yeast), trichomonal vaginitis, or vaginitis caused by *Hemophilus* (now more commonly called Gardnerella vaginitis), a wet smear can be obtained during the exam and examined immediately under the microscope. The diagnosis can be made at once and treatment initiated, saving the woman discomfort.

As the vaginal speculum is removed, gently rotate the blades so all walls of the vagina can be adequately visualized, looking for any mucosal abnormality, lesions, or tumors. The thumb screw should be completely released during speculum removal, allowing the vaginal walls themselves to close the blades. Observe carefully so the mucosa is not pinched during removal. Note and smell any vaginal discharge that collects on the lower blade of the speculum. *Gardnerella*, eg, has a typically fishy odor.

The bimanual examination involves palpation of the pelvic structures. The client remains in the lithotomy position. The examiner inserts one or two gloved fingers (usually the index and middle fingers) of the dominant hand, which have been lubricated with water-soluble jelly, into the vagina. The other hand is placed on the client's abdomen in the suprapubic area. To facilitate smooth gentle movements, the elbow of the examiner's vaginal hand rests on the knee, which is raised by resting the foot on the step at the base of the examining table.

The size, shape, consistency, mobility, and configuration of the cervix are noted. If an IUD string was not visible (eg, because of a large amount of vaginal discharge), the string may still be palpable in the os, reassuring the client of the presence of the IUD. Next, the uterus is palpated by pushing upward on the cervix and downward with the abdominal hand, entrapping the uterine fundus between the two hands (Figure 7–36). A mnemonic (MCSTPS) helps in remembering the important aspects of uterine evaluation:

- Mobility
- Consistency
- Size
- Tenderness
- Position
- Shape

The ovaries are evaluated by moving the internal fingers into each right and left lateral fornix while pushing downward with the abdominal hand in the corresponding right and left abdomen, about 5 cm medial to the anterior superior iliac spines. The abdominal fingers are pushed in deeply to approach the vaginal fingers. The vaginal hand should feel the ovary, which is normally palpable in thin clients or if it is enlarged. The normal fallopian tube is usually not palpable.

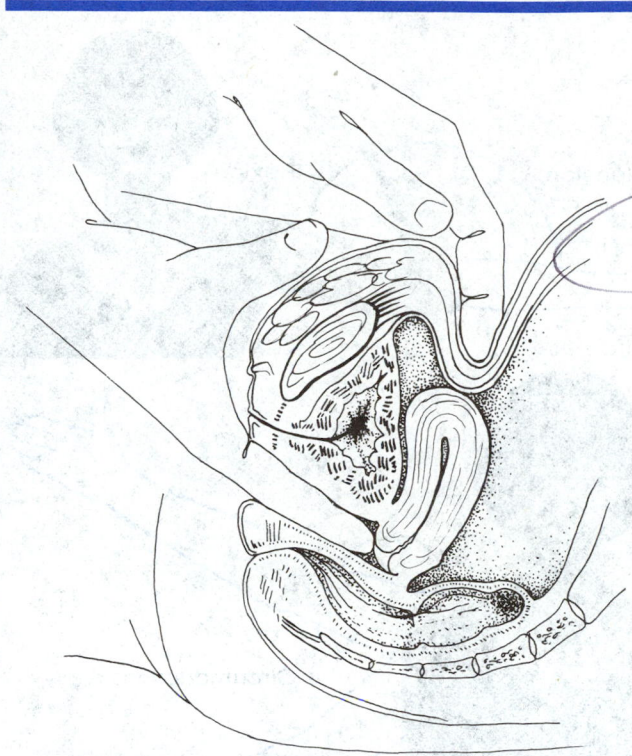

Figure 7–36

Bimanual palpation of the uterus, entrapping the uterine fundus between the two examining hands.

In addition, a rectovaginal exam is often done. For this exam the index finger is placed in the vagina, and the middle finger, which is well lubricated, is inserted into the rectum. The maneuvers of the previous bimanual exam are repeated, with particular attention to the rectovaginal septum and the area behind the cervix. The examiner then proceeds to the rectal exam. If bleeding occurred during any part of the previous exam, the examiner should change the glove before the rectal exam to prevent obtaining a false-positive result from test of the stool for occult blood. Another rationale for changing gloves between the vaginal and rectal exams is to prevent the spread of gonorrhea from vagina to rectum.

Assessment of the Musculoskeletal System

The Synovial Joints

Range of motion (ROM) of many of the joints has already been observed and tentatively assessed to some extent. For example, shoulder motion was noted when the client raised the arms in the air during assessment of the breasts. Mobility of the knees and hips of the woman was partially evaluated when she was assisted into the lithotomy position. All joints are now inspected for swelling, erythema, deformity, symmetry, ROM, and condition of surrounding skin. General joint palpation includes assessment for increased warmth, tenderness, crepitation (a palpable grating

sensation produced by joint movement), or bogginess caused by a thickened synovium.

The Hands, Fingers, and Wrists

Note the number of digits on each hand. Inspect the distal and proximal interphalangeal joints (DIP, PIP) (Figure 7–37). Heberden's nodes, a bony enlargement of the DIP joint, and Bouchard's nodes, a bony enlargement of the PIP joint, are often seen in degenerative joint disease (DJD). Clubbing of the fingers, a bullous enlargement of the distal segment of a digit, should alert the examiner to the possibility of cardiac or pulmonary disease, although the condition may be hereditary (Petersdorf et al., 1983). Ask the client to make a fist and then to extend and spread the fingers of the hand. Have the client flex, extend, hyperextend, abduct, and adduct both wrists. Palpate the metacarpals, the metacarpophalangeal joints, and the PIP and DIP joints. Palpate the wrist.

The Elbows and Shoulders

Ask the client to flex, extend, supinate, and pronate both elbows (Figure 7–38). Palpate the elbow, noting any pain or tenderness over the lateral epicondyle of the humerus, which is suggestive of tendinitis or "tennis elbow." Palpate the ulnar nerve in the groove in the posterior aspect of the medial epicondyle of the humerus. Tenderness in this area indicates nerve irritation, often secondary to direct

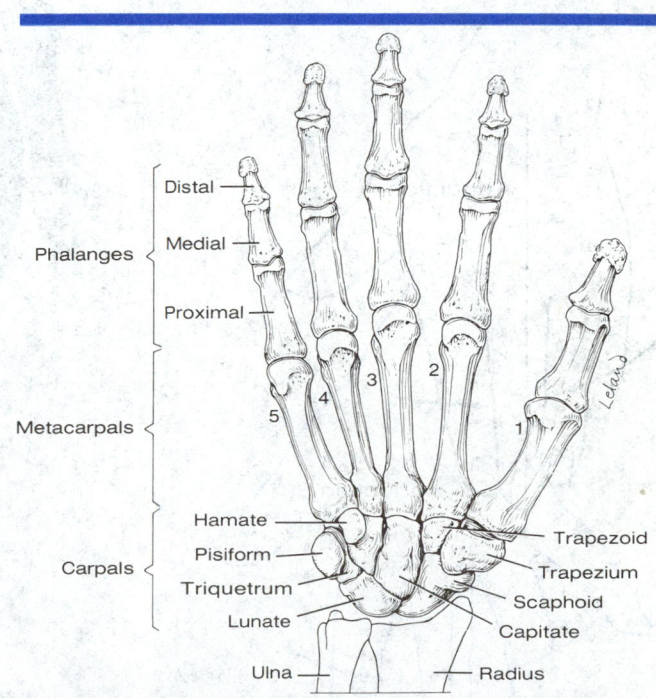

Figure 7–37

Palmar view of the joints and bones of the right hand and wrist.

SOURCE: Spence AP, Mason EB: *Human Anatomy and Physiology*, 2nd ed. Menlo Park, CA: Benjamin/Cummings, 1983.

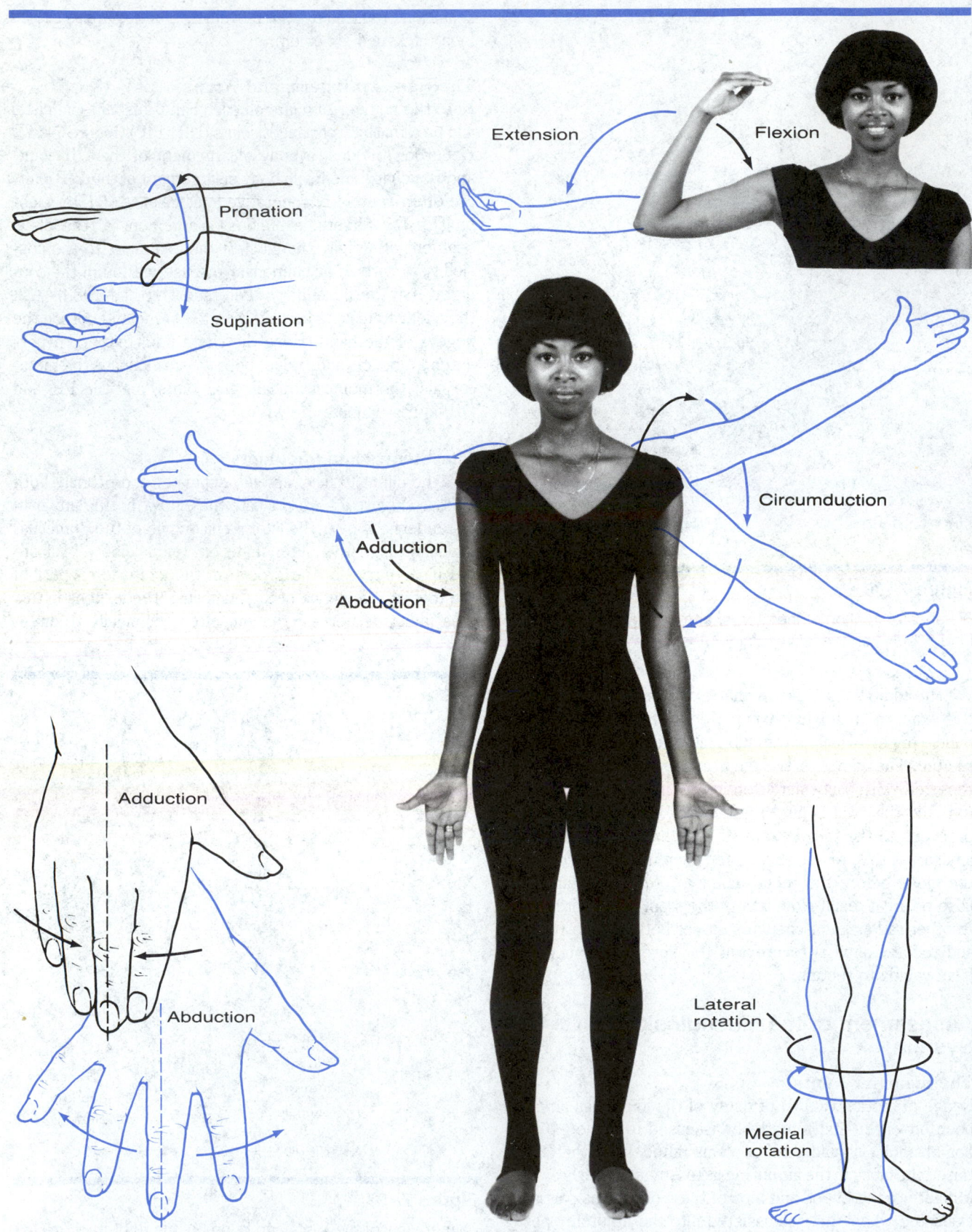

Figure 7–38

Angular and circular movements of diarthrodial joints.
SOURCE: Spence AP, Mason EB: *Human Anatomy and Physiology,* 2nd ed. Menlo Park, CA: Benjamin/Cummings, 1983.

trauma or to fracture of the elbow. This nerve is commonly called the "funny bone" because of the pain and tingling that occurs when it is struck.

To assess ROM of the shoulder, ask the client:

- To raise both arms to a vertical position at the sides of the head (flexion).
- To place the hands behind the neck with the elbows out to the side (external rotation).
- To place the hands behind the small of the back (internal rotation).

In addition, assess abduction, adduction, extension, and circumduction (Figure 7–38). Place a hand on the joint to note any crepitation with motion. Palpate the sternoclavic-

ular joint, the acromioclavicular joint, and the greater tubercle of the humerus. The rotator cuff, which is composed of four muscles, inserts into the greater tuberosity of the humerus and is a common site of abduction problems.

The Hips

Observe the client's gait carefully, because many problems in the hip are readily seen during ambulation. ROM of the hip includes flexion and extension, abduction, adduction, circumduction, and internal and external rotation (Figure 7–39). Have the client bring the knee to the chest while supine (hip flexion). The thigh of the other leg should remain flat on the table. If flexion contracture of the hip is present on the unflexed side, the thigh does not remain flat but

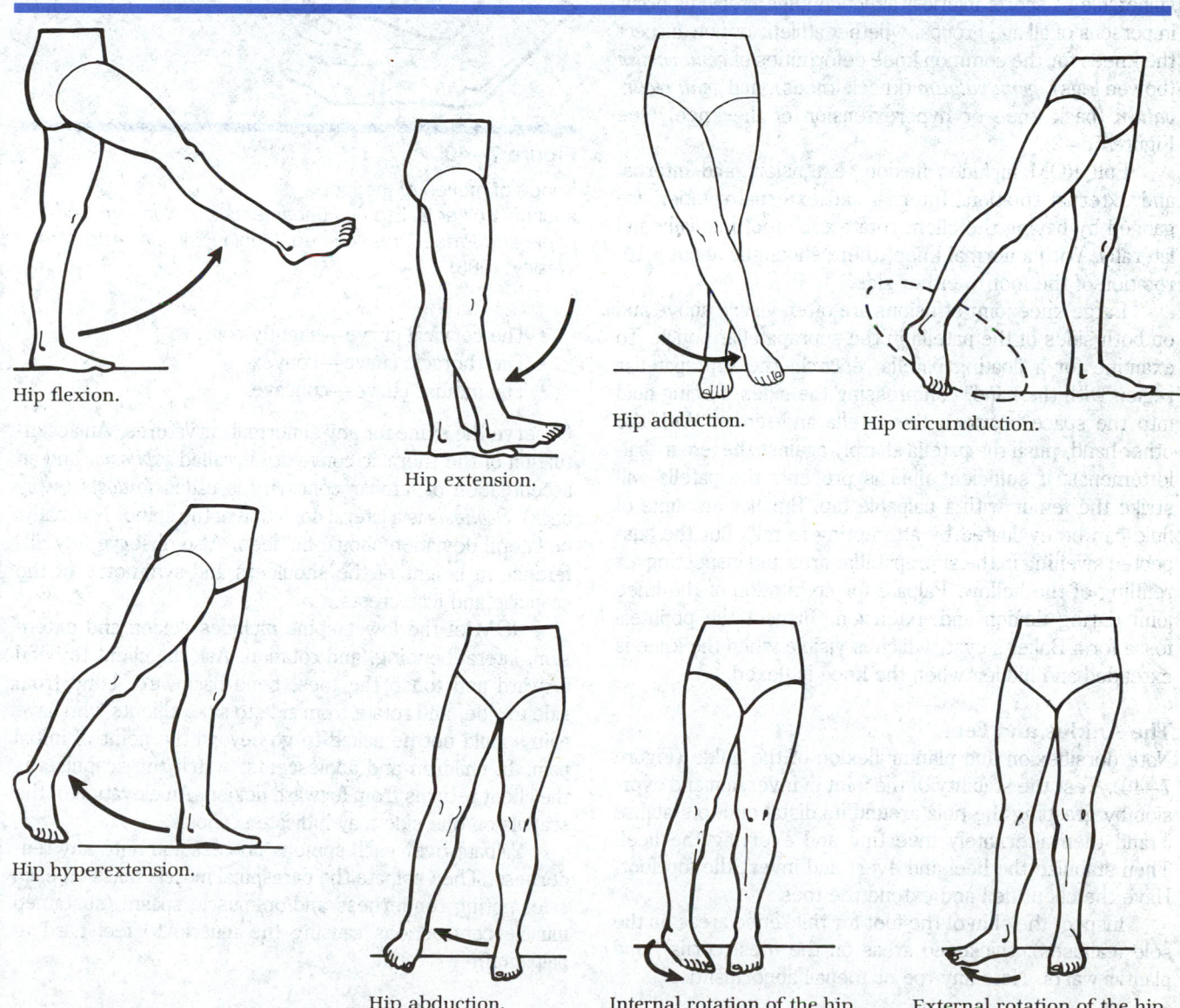

Hip flexion.

Hip extension.

Hip adduction.

Hip circumduction.

Hip hyperextension.

Hip abduction.

Internal rotation of the hip.

External rotation of the hip.

Figure 7–39

Range of motion of the hip.

SOURCE: Kozier B, Erb G: *Fundamentals of Nursing: Concepts and Procedures,* 2nd ed. Menlo Park, CA: Addison–Wesley, 1983.

pulls up into flexion when the opposite knee and hip are fully flexed. This is called the *Thomas test* for flexion contracture of the hip.

Shortening of one leg can be caused by a number of problems including disorders of the hip. With the client supine, measure leg length with a flexible tape measure from the anterosuperior iliac spine to the medial malleolus (see Figure 56–1). The leg measurements are compared. A leg-length discrepancy of as little as ¼ in can cause low back pain or greater trochanteric bursitis on the side of the longer leg.

The Knees

The knee joint is the largest joint in the body and is poorly protected by fat or muscle mass. The joint is especially vulnerable to sports injuries, although knee problems occur in persons of all age groups, whether athletic or not. Inspect the knees for the common knee deformities of *genu varum* (bowed legs), *genu valgum* (knock knees), and *genu recurvatum* (back knee or hyperextension of the knee) (see Figure 56–2).

Full ROM includes flexion, extension, and internal and external rotation. Internal and external rotation are gauged by having the client rotate each foot medially and laterally. With a normal knee, there should be about a 10° rotation of the foot to either side.

Large knee joint effusions are often visible above and on both sides of the patella in the suprapatellar pouch. To examine for a floating patella, encircle the suprapatellar region with the hand, compressing the sides, forcing fluid into the space between the patella and femur. With the other hand, push the patella sharply against the femur (ballottement). If sufficient fluid is present, the patella will strike the femur with a palpable tap. Smaller amounts of fluid can be evaluated by attempting to milk out the suspected swelling in the suprapatellar area and inspecting for refilling of the hollow. Palpate for crepitation of the knee joint during flexion and extension. Inspect the popliteal fossa for a Baker's cyst, which is visible when the knee is extended and hidden when the knee is flexed.

The Ankles and Feet

Note dorsiflexion and plantar flexion of the ankle (Figure 7–40). Test the stability of the joint in inversion and eversion by grasping the tibia around its distal end to stabilize it and then alternately inverting and everting the heel. Then stabilize the heel and evert and invert the forefoot. Have the client flex and extend the toes.

Inspect the skin of the foot for thickened areas on the sole (calluses), thickened areas on the toes (corns), and plantar warts. Note any toe or toenail abnormalities.

The Back and Spine

There are 33 vertebrae in the vertebral column and 31 pairs of spinal nerves exiting above or below the corresponding vertebrae. Viewed laterally, three curves are normally noted in the vertebral column (Figure 7–41):

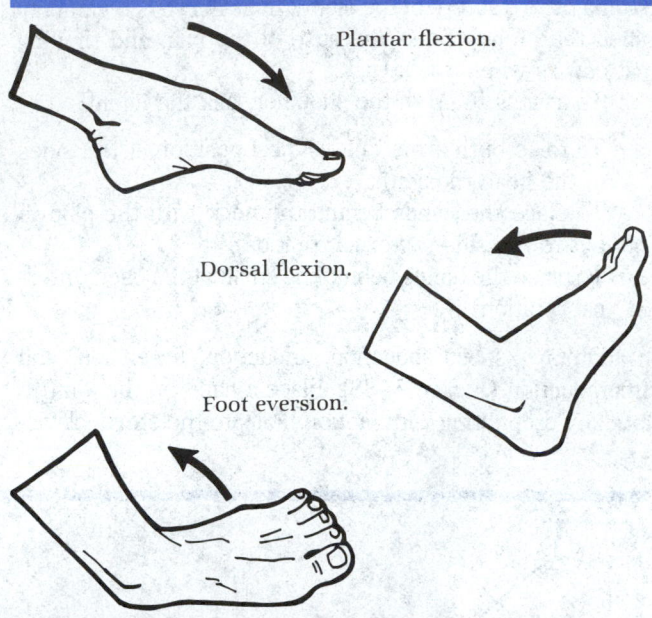

Figure 7–40

Range of motion of the foot.
SOURCE: Kozier B, Erb G: *Fundamentals of Nursing: Concepts and Procedures,* 2nd ed. Menlo Park, CA: Addison–Wesley, 1983.

- The cervical curve—slightly concave
- The thoracic curve—convex
- The lumbar curve—concave

Observe the spine for any abnormal curvatures. An accentuation of the thoracic convexity is called *kyphosis,* and an accentuation of lumbar concavity is called *lordosis* (sway back). *Scoliosis* is a lateral deviation of the spine. Normally, no lateral deviation should be seen. Also observe any difference in height of the shoulders and symmetry of the scapulae and iliac crests.

ROM of the lower spine includes flexion and extension, lateral bending, and rotation. Ask the client to bend forward and touch the toes, bend backward, bend from side to side, and rotate from side to side. Clients who have pain should not be asked to go beyond the point of initial pain. In children and adolescents, watch the scapulae as the client returns from forward flexion. An elevation of the scapula on one side may indicate scoliosis.

Palpate over each spinous process and note any tenderness. Then palpate the paraspinal muscle mass on each side, noting tenderness and/or muscle spasm (sustained muscle contractions causing the muscle to feel hard to palpation).

Assessment of the Neurologic System

Evaluation of the neurologic system includes:

- The mental status exam as a test of general cerebral function.

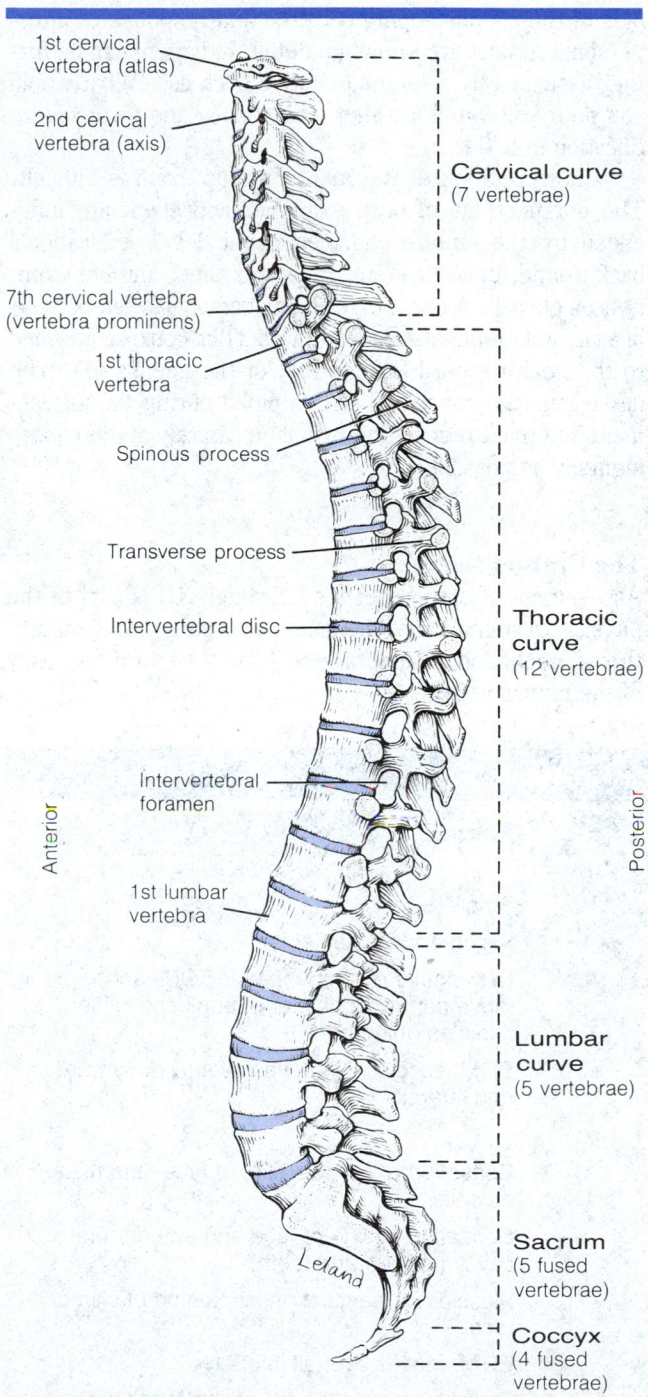

1st cervical vertebra (atlas)

2nd cervical vertebra (axis)

Cervical curve (7 vertebrae)

7th cervical vertebra (vertebra prominens)

1st thoracic vertebra

Spinous process

Transverse process

Intervertebral disc

Thoracic curve (12 vertebrae)

Intervertebral foramen

Anterior

Posterior

1st lumbar vertebra

Lumbar curve (5 vertebrae)

Leland

Sacrum (5 fused vertebrae)

Coccyx (4 fused vertebrae)

Figure 7–41

Lateral view of the vertebral column.
SOURCE: Spence AP, Mason EB: *Human Anatomy and Physiology*, 2nd ed. Menlo Park, CA: Benjamin/Cummings, 1983.

- Assessment of cranial nerves I through XII.
- Assessment of the sensory system.
- Assessment of the motor system.
- Assessment of the reflexes.
- Tests for cerebellar function.

The Mental Status Exam

The mental status exam begins during history taking when the examiner is noting general appearance and grooming, language use, thought processes, emotional state, attention span, and memory. A problem suspected in any area is followed up carefully during the neurologic assessment. If the client's ability to understand and communicate in words is impaired, the sequence of examination is reordered. Vision and hearing are evaluated first. Then a specific assessment of language deficits is begun.

Language. The examiner points to common objects and asks the client to name them. The client is asked to read some words and to match the printed and written words with pictures. Simple commands such as "point to your toes" can be written out for the client to perform, and simple verbal commands can be offered such as "raise your right arm."

As the client speaks, note the loudness, flow, speed, quantity, and logic of the words. For example, clients with hypothyroidism, Parkinson's disease, and depression often have slow, monotonous speech. Various types of aphasia have characteristic speech patterns. Clients with motor aphasia (Broca's aphasia) have painfully slow speech, poor articulation, and a tendency to delete prepositions and pronouns. Clients with auditory receptive aphasia (Wernicke's aphasia) have abundant speech with appropriate expressiveness and many incorrect words (paraphasia). *Perseveration*, a pattern of repeating the same response as different questions are asked, is common in all forms of aphasia.

Orientation and Memory. Assess whether the client seems relatively trusting, granting the normal suspiciousness many clients have about health professionals. Note excessive evasion and suspicion. Evaluate the client's orientation to time, place, and person, which can be done naturally with questions during the history about specific dates, places, and persons. Ask the client about any difficulty with memory. Question specifically about the day of the week, date of the month, and the year.

Immediate recall and concentration can be tested by giving the client a series of three digits to repeat. The number of digits is gradually increased until the client fails to repeat the series correctly. Start again with a series of three digits, gradually increasing the number. This time ask the client to repeat them backwards. The average person can repeat a series of seven digits in order and four digits in reverse order.

Recent memory is assessed by assigning the client three facts to remember such as an address, a color, and an object. Have the client repeat all three and request that he or she remember them. Later in the interview, ask the client to recall all the items. Remote memory is evaluated by asking the client to describe an event several years in the past. An example might be the Watergate cover-up.

Intellect. Much of the assessment of intelligence is derived from the detail and subtleties of clients' accounts of themselves and their health problems. In addition, a number of testing techniques are helpful in evaluating higher intellectual functions. Some approaches include asking the client to count backwards from 100 by subtracting 7s, naming the last four presidents and their political affiliations, or calculating the cost of three eggs if a dozen costs 92 cents.

Evaluate abstract reasoning by giving the client a proverb to interpret. Examples would be "a stitch in time saves nine" or "people who live in glass houses shouldn't throw stones." Concrete interpretations may indicate a problem or may simply indicate level of education. Normally, an abstract or semiabstract interpretation is expected. Asking the client to explain how two things are alike such as "an orange and an apple" or how two things are different such as "climate and season" also assists in evaluating abstract thinking.

The client's judgment has already been assessed to some degree during the personal/social part of the health history. If that portion of the history was done well, exam-

ples of the client's coping patterns and response to interpersonal conflict are known in detail. Judgment can be further assessed by asking a question such as, "What would you do if you found a wallet with money and owner identification in it?"

Interpretation of the mental status exam is difficult. The perspectives of both examiner and client are influenced by the culture, socioeconomic level, educational background, belief system, race, sex, age, and life experiences of each. A client may be unfavorably labeled because of a cultural misunderstanding—a label that could be attached to the health record for the rest of the client's life. The nurse must be conscious of this pitfall during the assessment and must record findings as accurately and nonjudgmentally as possible.

The Cranial Nerves

Assessment of cranial nerves I through XII is part of the physical examination of the face, eyes, ears, nose, mouth, throat, neck, and shoulders. See Table 7–4 for a summary of the cranial nerves.

Table 7–4   Summary of the Cranial Nerves and Their Functions

Nerve	Name	Type of Nerve	Function
I	Olfactory	Sensory	Smell
II	Optic	Sensory	Vision and visual fields
III	Oculomotor	Motor	Extraocular eye movement (EOM) and movement of sphincter of pupil and ciliary muscles of lens
IV	Trochlear	Motor	EOM, specifically moves eyeball downward and laterally
V	Trigeminal	Motor and sensory	
	Ophthalmic branch	Sensory	Sensation of cornea, skin of face, and nasal mucosa
	Maxillary branch	Sensory	Sensation of skin of face and anterior oral cavity (tongue and teeth)
	Mandibular branch	Motor and sensory	Muscles of mastication; sensation of skin of face
VI	Abducens	Motor	EOM, moves eyeball laterally
VII	Facial	Motor and sensory	Facial expression; taste (anterior tongue)
VIII	Vestibulocochlear (acoustic)		
	Vestibular branch	Sensory	Equilibrium
	Cochlear branch	Sensory	Hearing
IX	Glossopharyngeal	Motor and sensory	Gag reflex, tongue movement, taste (posterior tongue)
X	Vagus	Motor and sensory	Sensation of pharynx and larynx; swallowing and phonation
XI	Accessory	Motor	Head movement; shrugging of shoulders
XII	Hypoglossal	Motor	Protrusion of tongue

SOURCE: Reprinted with permission from Kozier B, Erb G: *Fundamentals of Nursing: Concepts and Procedures,* 2nd ed. Menlo Park, CA: Addison–Wesley, 1983, p. 351.

Assessment of Sensory Function

Loss or change in somatic sensation is an important manifestation of neurologic disease. Assessment of the sensory system is difficult, however, because the tests are somewhat crude, and interpreting them is quite subjective. Knowledge of segmental and peripheral nerve distribution in the skin is important for understanding the process (see Figure 36–1).

Testing of *superficial sensation* involves light touch, pain, and temperature. *Deep sensation* testing includes position and vibratory sense. Evaluation of higher integrative functions includes testing for two-point discrimination, stereognosis, and graphesthesia.

Response to light touch is assessed by lightly touching the client's skin with a wisp of cotton while the client's eyes are closed; ask the client to say "yes" when the cotton is felt. Start from the toes and move up the body symmetrically, comparing the client's response from side to side.

Because pain and temperature fibers run together in the spinal cord, testing of pain sensation alone is satisfactory for general assessment. If pain sensation is altered, temperature sensation is then evaluated. A pin is used to assess pain. Clients close their eyes and say "yes" whenever they feel the pinprick. Symmetrical areas are evaluated.

Position (proprioceptive) sense is tested by passive movement of the client's fingers and toes. With the client's eyes closed, the examiner grasps a finger or toe and flexes or extends it. The client must state what position the digit is in ("down" or "up"). Several digits are checked on each hand and foot.

Vibratory sense is evaluated by placing the end of a vibrating tuning fork on the bony prominences. The distal phalanx, lateral malleolus, tibial tuberosity, iliac crest, costal margin, clavicle, elbow, wrist, and distal phalanx on the hand all are tested. The tuning fork should be struck in the same way and applied to the bone with the same pressure. The client's appreciation of vibration is evaluated and compared symmetrically. Vibratory sense is diminished in pernicious anemia, diabetic neuropathy, and alcoholic polyneuritis.

Two-point discrimination involves the ability to distinguish the separation of two simultaneous pinpricks to the skin. The objective is to determine the smallest distance at which the two points are still distinct.

Testing of *stereognosis* involves the client's ability to identify objects by palpation alone. One hand is tested at a time with the client's eyes closed. The examiner places an object in the client's hand (eg, a key, a coin, or cloth) for identification. To test for *graphesthesia*, assess the client's ability to recognize a number traced in the palm of the hand.

Assessment of Motor Function

Evaluation of the motor system includes careful attention to muscle atrophy, muscle tone, muscle strength, and involuntary muscular movements. For inspection of muscles for atrophy or hypertrophy, the client must be exposed well enough for good visualization of major muscles. Corresponding muscle areas in the extremities are measured and compared side to side. The client's occupation must be considered. For example, professional tennis players would be expected to have disproportionate muscle hypertrophy in the dominant arm.

Muscle tone is the tension in the resting muscle—the slight resistance felt when the relaxed limb is passively moved. In a client with upper motor neuron disease, the tone of the passively moved muscle is increased (spasticity). In lower motor neuron disease, the tone of the passively moved muscle is decreased (flaccidity). Muscle strength is tested as shown in Table 7–5; a grading scale is found in Box 56–2.

Involuntary muscle movements may be normal in some instances. Many healthy persons have an exaggeration of normal physiological tremor secondary to caffeine intake or situational anxiety. A few types of tremor are recognized as related to certain disease processes. For example, a coarse, rhythmic tremor reduced or eliminated by voluntary movement (intention tremor) is characteristic of Parkinson's disease. A combined rest and intention tremor is often seen in multiple sclerosis.

Clonus, a series of involuntary muscle contractions precipitated by a sudden passive stretch of muscle, is most often elicited at the knee and ankle joints. This sign of disease in the central nervous system may be elicited by dorsiflexion of the foot with the knee flexed or may be seen during assessment for the deep reflexes.

Deep and Superficial Reflexes

Assessment of reflex arcs at specific levels of the brain stem and spinal cord is an important aspect of neurologic assessment. A normal reflex indicates that every element in the reflex arc is intact and that the motor tracts descending from levels above the reflex center are healthy (DeGowin & DeGowin, 1981).

The deep tendon reflexes (DTRs) are tested by striking the tendon with a reflex hammer. The client should be relaxed, not anticipating the strikes. The examiner holds the hammer loosely between the thumb and index finger, swinging it from the wrist. The reflexes most commonly tested include the:

- Biceps
- Triceps
- Brachioradialis
- Patellar
- Achilles tendon (ankle)

To elicit the biceps reflex (C-5 to C-6), support the client's elbow with the arm at a 90° angle and the examiner's thumb over the tendon. Strike the thumb with the reflex hammer. The normal response is elbow flexion (Figure 7–42A).

The triceps reflex (C-7 to C-8) is elicited by striking the triceps tendon above the elbow while the client's arm

Table 7–5   Testing Muscle Strength

Muscle	Client/Examiner Activity
Deltoid	Client holds arm up and resists while examiner tries to push it down.
Biceps	Client fully extends each arm and then tries to flex it while examiner attempts to hold arm in extension.
Triceps	Client flexes each arm and then tries to extend it against the examiner's attempt to keep arm in flexion.
Wrist and finger muscles	Client spreads the fingers and then resists as examiner attempts to push the fingers together.
Grip strength	Client grasps the index and middle fingers of the examiner while the examiner tries to pull the fingers out.
Hip muscles	Client is supine, both legs extended; client raises one leg at a time while the examiner attempts to hold it down.
Hip abduction	Client is supine, both legs extended. Examiner's hands are on the lateral surface of each knee; client is asked to spread the legs apart against the examiner's resistance.
Hip adduction	Client is in same position as for hip abduction; the examiner's hands are now placed between the knees; client is asked to bring the legs together against the examiner's resistance.
Hamstrings	Client is supine with both knees bent. Client resists while examiner attempts to straighten them.
Quadriceps	Client is supine with knee partially extended; client resists while examiner attempts to flex the knee.
Muscles of the ankles and feet	Client resists while examiner attempts to dorsiflex the foot back and again resists while examiner attempts to flex the foot.

is folded across the chest (Figure 7–42B). The normal response is elbow extension. To test the brachioradialis reflex (C-5 to C-6), strike the distal radius an inch or so (2.5 cm) above the wrist. The normal response is elbow flexion and supination of the forearm.

The patellar reflex (L-2 to L-4), also called the quadriceps reflex or knee jerk, is elicited by having the client seated with legs hanging freely over the edge of the examining table. The patellar tendon is tapped directly, normally resulting in quadriceps contraction with extension at the knee (Figure 7–42C).

The ankle jerk or Achilles reflex (L-5 to S-2) is assessed by having the examiner dorsiflex the client's foot with one

hand while striking the Achilles tendon with the hammer (Figure 7–42D). Plantar flexion of the ankle is the normal response. Also note the speed of relaxation. In hypothyroidism, delayed return of ankle reflexes is seen.

Superficial reflexes include the upper and lower abdominal reflexes (T-8 to T-12) and the cremasteric reflex (L-1 to L-2). The abdominal reflexes are tested by stroking the skin lightly in all four quadrants with a brisk stroke toward the umbilicus. The wooden end of a cotton applicator or tongue blade broken in two longitudinally can be used. The normal response is movement of the umbilicus toward the quadrant stimulated.

To test the cremasteric reflex in males, lightly stroke

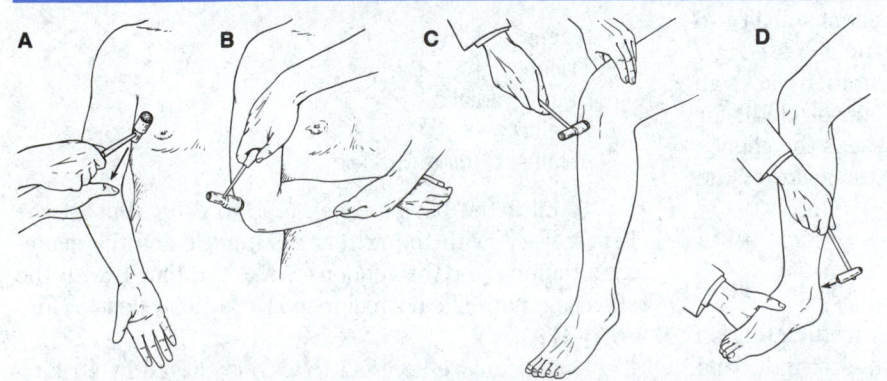

Figure 7–42

Assessing reflexes. **A.** Testing the biceps reflex. **B.** Testing the triceps reflex. **C.** Testing the patellar reflex. **D.** Testing the Achilles reflex.

the skin of the inner surface of the upper thigh downward. The normal response is prompt elevation of the testis on the ipsilateral (same) side.

Babinski's Sign
Babinski's sign is a test for pyramidal tract disease. With the client supine, stroke the lateral sole of the foot with a moderately sharp object such as a key. The stroke moves from the heel laterally to the toes and then curves toward the great toe. The normal response is toe flexion. The classic Babinski's sign is slow dorsiflexion of the great toe and fanning of the other four toes (Figure 7–43).

Recording of Reflexes
All reflexes are recorded on a stick figure to depict clearly the symmetry or asymmetry of the response (refer back to Box 7–4). Reflexes are graded on a scale from 0 to 4:

Grade	Description
0	Absent
1+	Hypoactive
2+	Normal
3+	Hyperactive
4+	Hyperactive with clonus

Some authorities use a scale of 0 to 5. Note whether a four-point or five-point scale is being used when recording the assessment.

Assessment of Cerebellar Function
The cerebellum modulates and coordinates skeletal muscle activity and maintains body posture and muscle tone. A person with cerebellar damage experiences muscle weakness, a loss of muscle tone, and difficulty standing erect and walking. Testing for cerebellar function involves evaluating coordination and the ability to perform rapid alternating movements in both upper and lower extremities.

The upper extremities are tested by having the client alternately supinate and pronate the hand as rapidly as possible and pat the leg with the hand as fast as possible. Then the client is asked to touch the tips of the fingers to the thumb in rapid sequence. Each hand is tested and compared with the other. Instruct the client to touch the index finger of the extended arm to the nose and then return the arm to the extended position. This is done repeatedly, first with the eyes open and then with them closed (finger-to-nose test). With eyes open, the client touches a finger to the nose and then to the examiner's finger while the examiner changes the position of that finger. This activity is repeated with increasing speed. These tests are performed bilaterally.

The lower extremities are tested by having the client tap a foot against the floor or against the examiner's hand as rapidly as possible. While supine, the client places the heel of one foot on the opposite knee and slides the heel slowly down the shin (heel-to-knee test). Both legs are tested. Abnormal findings in these tests include tremor; slow, jerky movements; and breaks in rhythm.

Equilibrium is assessed by asking the client to stand erect with feet together and eyes open. Then assess the

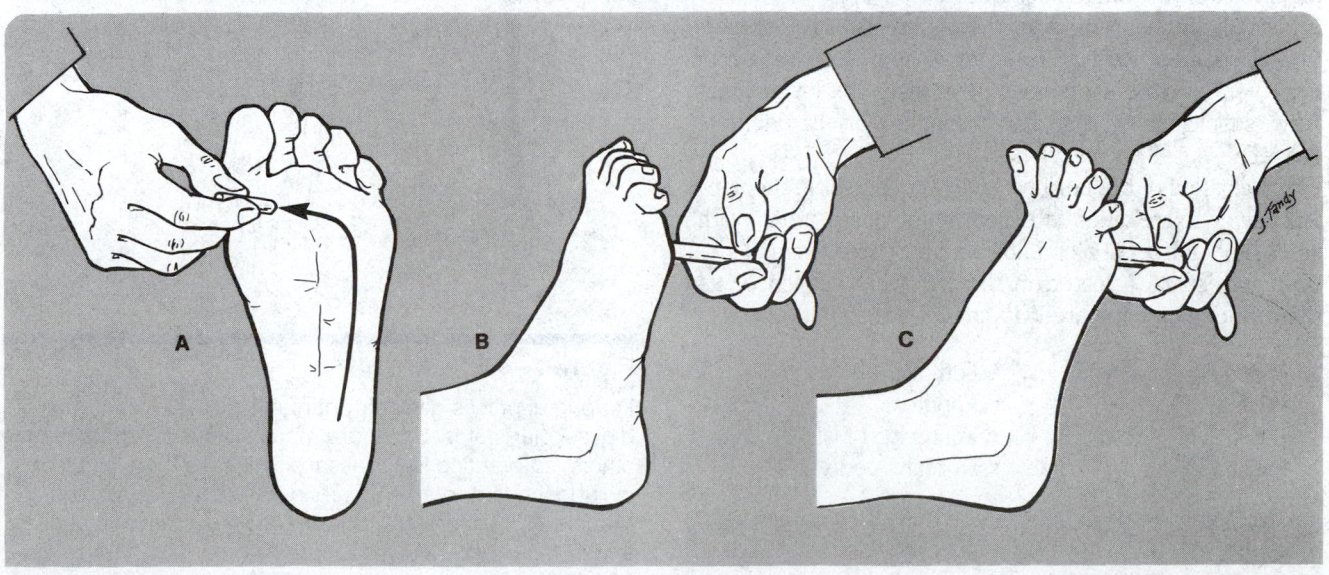

Figure 7–43
Testing for Babinski's sign. **A.** The line of stroking. **B.** Negative Babinski's sign (normal). **C.** Positive Babinski's sign (abnormal).
SOURCE: Kozier B, Erb G: *Fundamentals of Nursing: Concepts and Procedures,* 2nd ed. Menlo Park, CA: Addison–Wesley, 1983.

client's ability to maintain an upright position with the eyes closed. A loss of balance with the eyes closed is called a positive Romberg's sign. Obviously, the examiner should remain close to support the client who begins to sway or fall. Ask the client to walk across the room to assess the normal gait. Then have the client walk as if walking a tightrope (heel to toe) in a straight line. Clients with cerebellar disease will lose their balance after two or three steps and will place one foot to the side to avoid falling.

Assessment of the Peripheral Vascular System

The examiner inspects the legs for obvious swelling and checks for pitting edema by applying thumb pressure over the bony prominences in the lower-leg and ankle regions. Pitting edema in an adult indicates at least 10 lb (4.5 kg) of fluid accumulation (DeGowin & DeGowin, 1981). In pitting edema, a depression occurs where thumb pressure against the bone has been applied, and the depression persists for a short time. The depth of the pit is estimated and recorded. The distribution of edema is noted. Bilateral edema indicates a systemic problem, whereas unilateral edema indicates local disease.

Inspect the legs for signs of venous thrombosis, looking for swelling and duskiness of the calf and pitting edema on the ankle of the affected side. The calf is often warmer to the touch and may be tender to gentle palpation. The calf should be measured and its circumference compared with the other leg. *Homans' sign,* pain in the calf or popliteal region when the foot is sharply dorsiflexed with the knee slightly flexed, is a nonspecific but well-known test for deep vein thrombophlebitis.

With the client standing, the legs are carefully inspected for varicosities. *Varicose veins* are dilated, tortuous superficial veins in the saphenous system of the lower limbs. Any suspicious veins are palpated for hardness or tenderness.

Palpation of the peripheral arterial pulses in the upper and lower extremities is essential for assessment of the adequacy of arterial blood flow to the systemic circulation. The pulses are palpated in the following sequence, and their volume is compared (Figure 7–44):

- Radial
- Ulnar
- Brachial
- Carotid
- Femoral
- Popliteal
- Posterior tibial
- Dorsalis pedis

Pulses are classified on a scale of 0 to 4, with 4 being normal:

- 0 = completely absent
- 1+ = barely palpable
- 2+ = moderately impaired
- 3+ = slightly impaired
- 4+ = normal; full and bounding

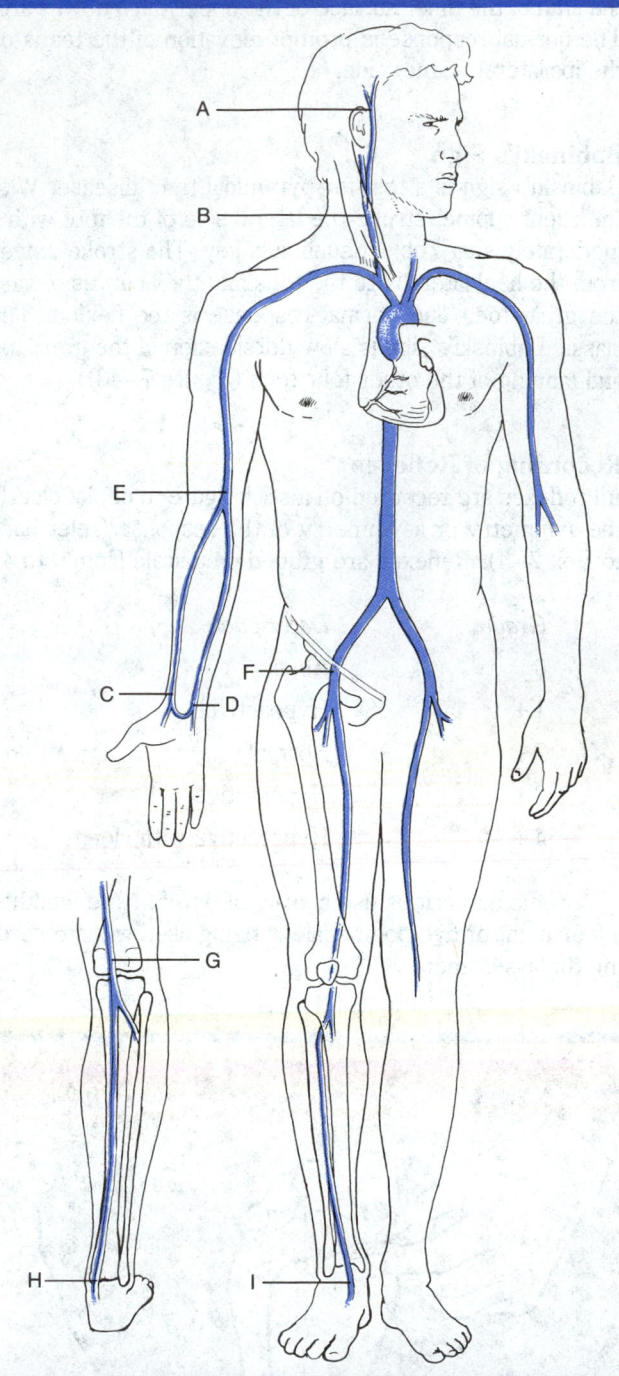

Figure 7–44

Peripheral pulses give important clues to the client's cardiovascular status. Some are more difficult to locate than others, so practice is necessary. Pulses to be evaluated include the temporal (A), carotid (B), radial (C), ulnar (D), brachial (E), femoral (F), popliteal (G), posterior tibial (H), and dorsalis pedis (I).

The popliteal pulses are often difficult to palpate. To facilitate assessment, flex the knee to relax the popliteal fossa and palpate deeply, lateral to the midline.

Section IV: Diagnostic Testing

Diagnostic tests are generally classified as invasive or noninvasive. Noninvasive tests, those performed on the exterior of the body, include:

- Examination of bodily fluids such as blood, urine, sputum, sperm, or vaginal discharge
- Recording of sounds (eg, ultrasound) and currents (eg, ECG)

In invasive tests, an instrument such as a scope, a catheter, or a scalpel is used for observation of internal body parts. Examples of invasive testing include:

- Endoscopy (eg, sigmoidoscopy)
- Arteriography (eg, coronary arteriography)
- Biopsy (eg, biopsy of the liver or kidney)

Invasive diagnostic procedures usually require more preparation, last longer, are often uncomfortable or painful, and involve greater risk for the client than noninvasive tests. The nurse is usually the person responsible for preparing clients, both physically and psychologically, for tests they will undergo. Client preparation for "routine" studies is often overlooked. Remember that a client who has never had an ECG or a client who requires a blood test but had a large, painful hematoma with a previous venipuncture needs information and reassurance.

For any invasive procedure involving some risk to the client, the client signs a written consent for the procedure, and the signature is witnessed. Before signing the form, the client must be fully informed. The process of informed consent is intended to ensure that the client knows what the test involves, the potential risk(s), and the possible negative side effects. The client should also understand what the test results will show, what the potential benefits are, and what alternatives exist if he or she does *not* consent to the test. Informing the client about proposed tests is the physician's responsibility, but a nurse usually helps the client resolve apprehension and ambivalence about the testing.

The most important point to keep in mind regarding consent is that clients have choices. They are responsible for their own bodies and have the right—indeed the responsibility—to make the best decision for themselves. What they need is information. If the information the client has is inaccurate or incomplete, the nurse has the responsibility to make certain the client has sufficient information to make an informed decision. A nurse who is knowledgeable about the procedure may provide the information or call the physician, explaining the client's concerns and ask the physician to return to discuss the procedure now that the client has had more time to think about it.

ROENTGENOGRAPHY (X-RAY)

X-rays are high frequency electromagnetic rays of short wave length capable of penetrating solid material, destroy-ing living tissue, and affecting a photographic plate. Wilhelm Roentgen, a German physicist, discovered x-rays in 1895. X-ray procedures are among the most frequently used noninvasive diagnostic approaches in health care. X-ray procedures are considered invasive when they involve contrast media such as radiopaque dyes administered by intravenous or retrograde injection. Clients need to be well prepared for procedures using contrast material because these studies often involve considerable discomfort during and after the procedure (eg, barium enema). Clients should also know that they will be alone in the room when the actual x-rays are taken. However, they should be told a technician can see and hear them if they require assistance. Fluoroscopy is an x-ray with an image of an organ projected on a screen much like a television screen so movement of contrast media can be evaluated.

Clients and health personnel must be protected from unnecessary exposure to radiation, which can damage body tissue. Protective approaches include increasing distance from the source, reducing exposure time, and shielding with a dense material such as lead. Film badges are worn by all personnel exposed to radiation to monitor the amount of exposure over time. Clients in their childbearing years should ask whether a proposed x-ray procedure will potentially damage their reproductive organs. Pregnant women should avoid x-ray exposure.

The major therapeutic use of radiation is in the treatment of cancer. Because malignant cells are more sensitive to radiation than normal cells, radiotherapy is carefully calculated to destroy malignant cells without damaging healthy nearby tissue. Radiation therapy may be delivered internally or externally. Internal therapy includes the use of ^{131}I for thyroid cancer and radium implants for cancer of the uterus, cervix, or nasopharynx. External radiation, in which a small amount of tissue is irradiated at high doses for short intervals, is the treatment of choice in some malignancies. Radiation is also used for palliation.

RADIOACTIVE ISOTOPE EXAMINATION

Many radiocompounds can be used for diagnosis and treatment. Among the most common are technetium 99m, ^{131}I, thallium-201, and gallium-67. Radiocompounds are selected according to their ability to localize in a particular organ or type of tissue. The compounds can be administered by mouth, intrathecally, or by intravenous injection. The emissions from the radioactive substance are picked up by a scintillation detector (scanner) and converted to an image. Clients are asked to lie still during the scanning procedure. Organs most frequently evaluated by radionuclide scanning include the brain, thyroid, liver, pancreas, spleen, lung, myocardium, kidneys, and bone.

Clients are often concerned about the radiation hazards of radioactive isotopes and sometimes believe that the scanning device is actually emitting radiation rather than receiving it. Clients should be helped to understand that the actual radiation dose is small in most scanning procedures and that the scanner is a recording device and not a machine that emits radiation.

COMPUTERIZED TOMOGRAPHY SCANNING

A variety of contemporary technologies, including the ability of the computer to detect subtle differences in tissue, has made computerized tomography (CT) scanning possible. Other terms for the technique are computed transverse tomography, CTT, and computed axial tomography, CAT. It uses computer-assisted radiology to produce a reconstructed image of a cross section of the body, which closely resembles an anatomic section. CT scanning is often used in combination with intravenous contrast material to enhance the image. CT scanning is considered a noninvasive procedure, although the client is often apprehensive because of the size of the equipment and the need to lie completely still throughout the scanning process. CT scanning is used in diagnosing intracranial, intrathoracic, mediastinal, and intra-abdominal abnormalities. This technology has virtually eliminated the need for many invasive and relatively uncomfortable diagnostic studies.

ULTRASONOGRAPHY

Ultrasonography uses ultrasonic pulse-echo techniques to detect differences in tissue density in various areas of the body. A transducer is moved over the body part to be studied. The transducer emits an ultrasonic wave, which is reflected back and converted into radio frequency impulses that can be recorded. The recorded image results from the passage of the sound wave through the junction of two tissues of differing densities. The client is asked to lie completely still during the test, which is noninvasive and does not use IV contrast material.

Ultrasonography is useful in detecting fluid-filled areas (eg, cysts and abscesses) and pulsating structures. It is used to evaluate thyroid nodules and pancreatic, gallbladder, renal, hepatic, and splenic cysts; tumors; and abscesses. In gynecology and obstetrics, ultrasonography has numerous uses including detecting ovarian and pelvic lesions, estimating fetal growth, and determining multiple pregnancies and fetal abnormalities. Pregnant clients are asked to drink several glasses of water before the examination because a full bladder pushes the uterus out of the pelvis, aiding visualization of uterine contents. A full bladder also enhances transmission of sound waves. Other common clinical applications of ultrasound include echocardiography, echoencephalography, and the Doppler shift technique, which evaluates the motion of blood in the arterial and venous systems.

ENDOSCOPY

Direct visualization of hollow organs of body cavities can be accomplished with an *endoscope,* a lighted tube containing an optical system. Some endoscopes are rigid (eg, cystoscopes) and others are flexible (fiberoptic endoscopes). The scope is equipped with channels for biopsy and air insufflation, snares for foreign body removal, and attachments for suction and irrigation. Endoscopy is an invasive procedure requiring a considerable amount of client preparation. Clients are on NPO status before most procedures. Enemas are given before lower GI endoscopy. Whether local or general anesthesia is used depends on the type of procedure and the condition of the client. The most common endoscopic procedures are listed in Table 7–6.

STUDIES OF ELECTRICAL ACTIVITY OF BODY TISSUE

Electrical activity of certain body tissues can be recorded and analyzed by means of electrodes. The following are studies of electrical potentials of tissue:

- Electrocardiography (ECG)—a recording of the electrical activity of the heart by surface electrodes.
- Electromyography (EMG)—a recording of electrical activity associated with skeletal muscles by insertion of small needle electrodes into the muscle.
- Electroencephalography (EEG)—recording of the electrical activity of the brain by scalp electrodes.
- Electronystagmography (ENG)—a recording of nystagmus by detecting the electrical activity of the extraocular muscles.
- Electroretinography (ERG)—a recording of the alterations in the electrical potential of the retina following light stimulation; the cornea is anesthetized and a contact lens electrode used.
- Electroneurography—a recording of the action potentials of the larger peripheral sensory and motor nerve fibers by surface electrodes.

Client preparation varies depending on the invasiveness of the electrodes.

LABORATORY TESTS

Laboratory evaluation of tissues, body fluids, and excreta is part of the objective data base. Laboratory testing generally involves:

- Hematology—the study of blood, the cellular constituents of blood, and the metabolic processes by which blood components are formed.
- Urinalysis—the study of the organic and inorganic substances in the urine.
- Chemistry—the chemical analysis of blood, urine, and

Table 7–6 Common Endoscopic Procedures

Procedure	Instrument	Nursing Implications
Esophagoscopy Gastroscopy Duodenoscopy	Fiberoptic endoscope	Inserted via mouth; local anesthesia
Laryngoscopy	Rigid scope	Inserted via mouth; the fiberoptic scope can be inserted through the nose; local or general anesthesia
Bronchoscopy	Rigid or fiberoptic scope	
Anoscopy Proctoscopy (rectum) Sigmoidoscopy	Rigid scope	Inserted via rectum
Colonoscopy	Fiberoptic scope	Inserted via rectum
Cystoscopy (bladder)	Rigid scope	Inserted via urethra
Colposcopy (cervix)	Binocular microscope used to visualize cervix	Vaginal speculum is in place; similar to pelvic exam
Culdoscopy (pelvic viscera)	Rigid scope	Inserted via vagina, through posterior fornix into peritoneal cavity
Peritoneoscopy (laparoscopy)	Rigid scope	Inserted via a small abdominal incision to visualize abdominal structures; local anesthesia
Arthroscopy (joint—most often the knee)	Rigid scope	Inserted into joint; usually done in OR with local or general anesthesia

cerebrospinal fluid for electrolytes, enzymes, proteins, glucose, and other constituents.

- Microbiology (bacteriology)—examination of specimens from various sites for identification of specific bacterial pathogens. Bacteriology specimens may be obtained from blood; urine; feces; sputum; pleural and cerebrospinal fluid; vaginal discharge; pus from abscesses or other draining wounds; and throat, nasal, and eye cultures.

- Serology—the study of serum for evaluation of antigen–antibody reactions in diagnosing bacterial, fungal, parasitic, or viral disorders; also for identification and measurement of immunoglobulins.

- Toxicology—the study of body fluids for evidence of poisons or toxins.

Laboratory tests should be interpreted cautiously, relating results closely to the history and physical examination of the client. Laboratory values are affected by the method of specimen collection, drugs the client is taking, dietary factors, the position of the client, and recent exercise. For example, clients who have been ambulating or who have been jogging may demonstrate proteinuria, yet a follow-up early morning urine specimen will be negative for protein.

INTERNATIONAL SYSTEM OF UNITS

Many nations record laboratory data with an international system of units (SI), the most current metric system of measurement. SI is founded on seven units called "base units" (Table 7–7). All traditional units of measurement from calorie counts to radiation doses are converted to a new language and new system with SI. Canada is currently converting to this system. A listing of SI units applicable to health is found on the inside back cover. In the future, laboratory tests will probably be listed with both traditional values and SI equivalents.

Table 7–7 International System (SI) Base Units

Physical Quantity	Base Unit	Symbol
Length	Meter	m
Mass	Kilogram	kg
Time	Second	s
Amount of substance	Mole	mol
Thermodynamic temperature	Kelvin	K
Electric current	Ampere	A
Luminous intensity	Candela	cd

SOURCE: Reprinted with permission from *SI Manual in Health Care,* 2nd ed. Ottawa, Canada: Metric Commission, 1982.

Chapter Highlights

Nurses play a key role in helping clients to understand their rights and the need for them to exercise their rights.

Clients from various sociocultural backgrounds may not understand questions and often find it difficult to cooperate with examinations and procedures that contradict their belief systems.

Nurses must be aware of the universal potential for cultural, religious, age, socioeconomic, racial, sexual, and lifestyle differences and develop communication skills that facilitate an understanding of these differences to improve client care.

An organized, sequential approach to health assessment is important in gathering a complete data base.

Obtaining a comprehensive data base is the most important phase of the nursing process because all subsequent client care depends on this information.

The most significant step in physical assessment is careful visual inspection.

Nurses should understand the complete physical assessment process so they can adequately prepare clients for examination, even though they may not be doing some components of the assessment themselves.

Invasive diagnostic tests may involve potential health risks to clients of which they may be unaware.

An international system of measurement, called SI, will probably become the universal standard for all traditional units of measurement in health care.

Bibliography

Bates B: *A Guide to Physical Examination*, 3rd ed. Philadelphia: Lippincott, 1983.

Bramwell L: Use of the life history in pattern identification and health promotion. *ANS* 1984; 6:37–44.

Davis AJ: Informed consent: How much information is enough? *Nurs Outlook* 1985; 33(1):40–42.

DeGowin EL, DeGowin RL: *Bedside Diagnostic Examination*, 4th ed. New York: Macmillan, 1981.

Delp MH, Manning RT: *Major's Physical Diagnosis,* 9th ed. Philadelphia: Saunders, 1981.

Konikow NS: Alterations in movement: Nursing assessment and implications. *J Neurosurg Nurs* (Feb) 1985; 17:61–65.

Kreps GL, Thornton BC: *Health Communication*. New York: Longman, 1984.

Lindberg SC: Periodic preventive health screening schedule for adult men and women. *Nurse Pract* (Sept–Oct) 1980; 5:9–13, 21.

Malasanos L et al: *Health Assessment,* 3rd ed. St. Louis: Mosby, 1985.

Meyer LS: Untangling communication lines to connect consumers and providers. *Nurs Health Care* (Sept) 1985; 6:367–368.

Ozuna J: Alterations in mentation: Nursing assessment and intervention. *J Neurosurg Nurs* (Feb) 1985; 17:66–70.

Pagana KD, Pagana TJ: *Diagnostic Testing and Nursing Implications.* St. Louis: Mosby, 1982.

Petersdorf RG et al: *Harrison's Principles of Internal Medicine,* 10th ed. New York: McGraw–Hill, 1983.

Primrose RB: Taking the tension out of pelvic exams. *Am J Nurs* 1984; 84:72–74.

Prior JA, Silberstein JS: *Physical Diagnosis: The History and Examination of the Patient,* 6th ed. St. Louis: Mosby, 1981.

Tietz NW: *Clinical Guide to Laboratory Tests.* Philadelphia: Saunders, 1983.

Widmann FK: *Clinical Interpretation of Laboratory Tests,* 9th ed. Philadelphia: Davis, 1983.

Suggested Readings

Delancy VL, North C: Skin assessment. *Top Clin Nurs* (July) 1983; 5:5–10. The significance of skin problems throughout history are emphasized. There is a brief but excellent section on psychosocial assessment.

Ginnetti J, Greig AE: The occupational health history. *Nurse Pract* (Nov–Dec) 1981; 6:12–13. The authors discuss important aspects of an occupational health history that can be incorporated into a general health history. Nurses must be aware of the hazards to health in the workplace, and this article offers guidelines for gathering pertinent information from clients.

Pickwell S: Health screening for Indo-Chinese refugees. *Nurse Pract* (April) 1983; 8:20–25, 35. Many Indo-Chinese persons are currently living in the United States. The author discusses the health problems these refugees may have and the important adaptations to be made in the health history and physical assessment to assess their health properly.

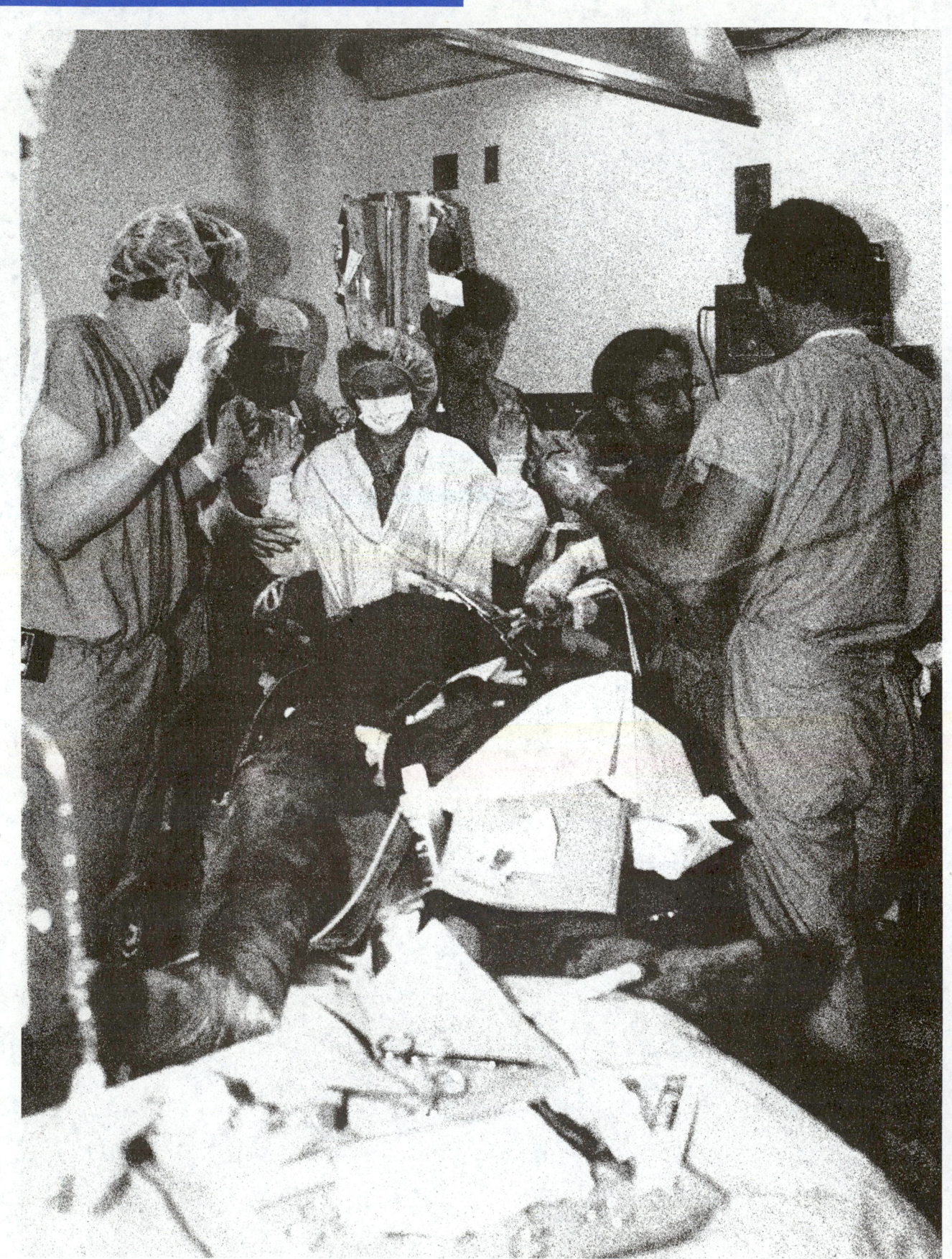

UNIT 2

Multisystem Stressors

Chapter 8

Malnutrition

Nancy Nuwer Konstantinides

Objectives

When you have finished studying this chapter, you should be able to:

Define malnutrition.

Identify the incidence of and reasons for malnutrition in hospitalized clients.

Discuss the physiological and psychosocial causes of malnutrition.

Describe the multisystem effects of malnutrition.

Identify clients at high risk for developing malnutrition.

Discuss subjective and objective data collection in nutritional assessment.

Develop a plan of care for the client with malnutrition.

State nursing responsibilities in administering and monitoring tube feedings and total parenteral nutrition (TPN).

Good health and good nutrition go hand in hand. Although more people are making informed choices about what they eat, malnutrition remains a worldwide problem. Chronic malnutrition has tragic consequences. It depletes energy and capacity for work; decreases resistance to infectious disease; and adversely affects concentration, motivation, and learning ability.

That malnutrition is prevalent in third-world countries is well known. But malnutrition is also a serious problem in industrialized nations, especially for the poor, the elderly,

and certain groups such as migrant workers and Native Americans (Hui, 1983). The affluent may not be aware of the principles of good nutrition or may ignore them. A person may enter the hospital well nourished only to leave malnourished. Clients with devastating illnesses and inherited disease also suffer from malnutrition. Even health professionals do not always have an adequate background in nutrition. This chapter discusses the health problem of malnutrition and the role of the nurse in its prevention and treatment.

Section I: The Problem of Malnutrition

Nutrition is the process of taking in and utilizing necessary nutrients. These nutrients must be consumed (ingested), digested (broken down to basic particles), absorbed (transported into cells or the bloodstream), and used by the body. Good nutrition is the daily ingestion of adequate amounts of essential nutrients including protein, carbohydrates, fats, vitamins, minerals, and water. Each of these

nutrients is important in either providing energy for body processes, structural material for tissues, or regulation of biochemical processes (Box 8–1). The overall role of good nutrition is to promote growth and development, maintain health, prevent illness, and treat disease.

Malnutrition is a serious consequence of continued poor nutrition. Growth, development, and cognition may

Protein—Structural element of cells, enzymes, glandular secretions, and hormones; necessary for growth and structural maintenance; made of amino acids, 16% of which is nitrogen. Some amino acids cannot be synthesized by the body, so intake is essential. There are 4 calories per gram of protein.

Carbohydrates—The major source of food energy; easiest nutrient to digest; adequate amounts can spare protein used for energy; primary energy source for lung, brain, and nerve tissue; source of fiber, an undigested plant product that provides bulk in the stool. There are 4 calories per gram of carbohydrate.

Fats—High-energy nutrients that provide more than twice the calories per gram as carbohydrates; necessary for utilization of fat-soluble vitamins; some fats cannot be synthesized by the body, so intake is essential; contribute to cell wall structure; necessary for the production of some hormones. There are 9 calories per gram of fat.

Vitamins—Most cannot be synthesized, so intake is essential; play a role in many vital functions in cells and tissues. Some vitamins function like hormones; some contribute to formation of red blood cells and clotting factors. Some are fat soluble (A, D, E, and K), and some are water soluble (thiamine, riboflavin, B_6, B_{12}, C, folic acid, niacin, biotin, and pantothenic acid).

Minerals—Inorganic compounds necessary for chemical processes throughout the body. Some contribute to acid–base balance; calcium and phosphorus contribute to bone formation. Some regulate osmosis. Some are constituents of body secretions.

Water—Approximately 55% to 60% of adult weight is from water, which is essential to the function of every organ. Structural component of cells, tissues, and secretions; medium for chemical reactions; regulator of body temperature.

be impaired and disease can develop. Malnutrition can prolong disease and complicate treatment, perhaps extending hospitalization.

The term **malnutrition** most commonly describes a condition of reduced intake or utilization of nutrients, particularly protein and calories, in relation to requirements. Calories, or heat energy, are supplied primarily by carbohydrates and fats. (A calorie is the unit of energy necessary to raise the temperature of 1 kg of water by 1°C.) Malnutrition has been defined as an inappropriate reduction in the lean body mass, which consists of skeletal muscle made up primarily of protein (Cerra, 1984). The term **nutrient deficiency** generally refers to specific vitamin and mineral deficiency states.

INCIDENCE IN HOSPITALIZED CLIENTS

Even with recent advances in nutritional support, malnutrition among hospitalized clients continues to be a serious problem. In a study of 134 medical clients, researchers found that the 48% who were malnourished when admitted had prolonged hospitalizations and a high mortality rate. In 75% of those admitted with normal nutritional values, nutritional parameters worsened during their hospitalizations (Weinsier & Butterworth, 1981). Another expert reports that 25% to 50% of clients are malnourished upon admission (Cerra, 1984). Of those well nourished when entering the hospital, 25% to 30% will develop malnutrition. Cerra estimates that 69% of all hospitalized clients will demonstrate declining nutritional status, whether they are admitted well nourished or malnourished. With malnutrition, there are increases in mortality and morbidity, including surgical complications and prolonged hospitalization.

Malnutrition induced by treatment in the hospital is referred to as *iatrogenic malnutrition*. Factors contributing to iatrogenic malnutrition are discussed later in this chapter.

TYPES OF MALNUTRITION

There are several types of malnutrition. A client may be deficient in a specific nutrient such as vitamin A or have severe protein or calorie deficiency requiring several months of treatment before repletion takes place. By determining the type, the nurse will find it easier to identify causal factors, assess the physiological and psychosocial impact, and determine the appropriate nutritional approach.

Nutrient Deficiencies

Specific nutrient deficiencies are considered types of malnutrition. Gaps in nutrient intake cause related physical changes. For example, a diet with few fruits and vegetables may lead to a vitamin C deficiency, causing bleeding gums. (Objective and subjective data related to nutrient deficiencies are discussed later in this chapter in Table 8–3.) Often several simultaneous deficiencies are found. The diet lacking in fruits and vegetables will also result in deficiencies of a number of other vitamins, such as A and B. Most nutrient deficiency states are easily reversed by providing the necessary nutrient.

Marasmus

Marasmus, or simple starvation, refers to protein and calorie malnutrition, generally occurring as the result of a chronic reduction of protein and calorie intake. It is associated with severe depletion of fat stores and muscle wasting. The World Health Organization (WHO) describes the client with marasmus as emaciated "skin and bones." Those with marasmus will require adequate protein and calories over several months to replace muscle loss.

Kwashiorkor

Kwashiorkor is protein malnutrition resulting from a protein-poor diet or from protein loss due to physiological stress. The client may not appear malnourished because although fat stores may be depleted, edema maintains the weight level. Malnutrition occurring with obesity is of this type. WHO describes the person with kwashiorkor as edematous and apathetic. Persons with kwashiorkor are given protein with adequate calories to improve the protein status.

A mixed form of marasmus–kwashiorkor can occur. This is most often observed in chronically malnourished persons who develop acute stress from disease, which alters their metabolism.

CAUSES OF MALNUTRITION

Clients may be malnourished because they have not ingested enough calories (starvation) or because a disease state has altered their metabolism. The hospitalized client may develop iatrogenic malnutrition, which results from aspects of treatment during hospitalization.

Starvation

Starvation is a state of insufficient intake of necessary calories to supply the body's energy needs. Insufficient intake can occur because of physiological, psychological, or socio-economic factors.

Physiological Causes

Physiological causes of starvation include disease factors, drug-nutrient interactions, or dietary restrictions. Disease-induced starvation results from disorders that impair nutrient intake, prevent nutrient absorption, or promote nutrient losses. Nutrient intake may be impaired because of difficulty in chewing, such as with poorly fitted dentures, or disease-induced generalized weakness. With oral lesions or inflammation of the throat or esophagus, chewing and swallowing can be painful, difficult, or impossible. Constriction of the throat and esophagus may cause difficulty in swallowing. Some disorders, such as hiatal hernia with reflux esophagitis, result in pain upon swallowing from lower esophageal inflammation. Cancer in the upper gastrointestinal tract may also make eating difficult because of pain or obstruction.

Disease states may prevent nutrient absorption. Malabsorption, the defective absorption of ingested nutrients, can result from various causes (see Unit Eight). Diarrhea may speed the passage of nutrients through the intestines, decreasing the time for nutrient absorption. Any gastrointestinal surgery in which the small intestine is removed or bypassed will cause some degree of reduced nutrient absorption.

Several conditions promote nutrient losses. Among these are open draining wounds, fistulas, abscesses; renal dialysis; severe burns; and major blood loss. With prolonged, unreplaced nutrient depletion, starvation may develop. Some gastrointestinal diseases, such as celiac sprue, scleroderma, and regional enteritis cause protein excretion into the stool.

Drug therapy may be associated with starvation or

Nursing Research Note

Heitkemper M, Marotta S: Role of diets in modifying gastrointestinal neurotransmitter enzyme activity. *Nurs Res* 1985; 34(1):19–23.

This study examined the effects of fasting on the synthesis and degradation of acetylcholine and norepinephrine, neurotransmitters in the gastrointestinal tract. The study also examined the effects of choline-deficient diets on neurotransmitter enzyme activity. Dietary deficiencies in choline intake occur with total parenteral nutrition (TPN), self-imposed food restriction, inadequate oral intake, starvation, and anorexia.

Starvation decreased adrenergic enzyme activity and increased cholingeric activity. The stress of starvation also resulted in increased plasma and adrenal cortisol levels. Choline-deficient diets decreased adrenergic enzyme activity but did not alter cholingeric enzyme activity.

Nurses might apply these findings in nursing assessment of dietary alterations and the effects on the GI tract. Because the adrenergic and cholingeric neurotransmitters affect the entire central nervous system, behavior as well as physiology can be altered. Fasting clients, clients on TPN, and clients receiving medications such as lecithin or choline are likely to exhibit disequilibrium in parasympathetic/sympathetic activity and experience GI symptomatology. These symptoms must be evaluated and interventions planned to reduce discomfort.

nutrient deficiencies. Drugs that cause a decreased hunger drive (eg, amphetamines), decreased nutrient absorption (eg, antibiotics), or decreased metabolism (eg, barbiturates), can contribute to malnutrition or nutrient deficiency states. Table 8–1 outlines examples of common drugs and their effect on nutritional status. Many drugs such as caffeine, amphetamines, and chemotherapeutic drugs, can reduce the appetite and induce nausea. Drugs causing malabsorption of some nutrients include antacids containing aluminum hydroxide (Maalox, Gelusil, Mygel, Gaviscon); antigout preparations such as colchicine, antibiotics such as neomycin, and some laxatives such as mineral oil. Drugs that alter metabolism of nutrients by affecting biochemical processes include some anticonvulsants and steroids.

The elderly are particularly prone to poor dietary intake. The physiological changes of aging and the presence of disorders significantly affect appetite and ability to ingest and absorb nutrients. Taste perception is impaired, making food less appetizing. Salivation decreases with aging, so eating and swallowing are more difficult. Age-related dental changes, such as osteoarthritis and dentures that fit poorly, impair chewing. Gastrointestinal changes of aging, such as decreased secretions and decreased absorption, alter nutrition status. Constipation, common to the elderly, may diminish appetite. Altered cardiac and respiratory functions may contribute to fatigue or shortness of breath during eating. Some elderly persons are unable to prepare meals because of poor vision, strength, balance, and coordination, and reduced mobility can make food shopping difficult.

Table 8–1 The Effects of Common Drugs on Nutritional Status

Drug	Clinical Usage	Possible Direct and Indirect Effects on Nutritional Status
Alcohol	A minor ingredient in medications	Thiamine and magnesium deficiencies most common; deficiencies of folic acid, niacin, and pyridoxine may also occur. May decrease absorption and utilization and increase excretion of affected nutrients
Alkylating agents	Cancer chemotherapy	
Cyclophosphamide (Cytoxan)		Anorexia, vomiting, nausea, hemorrhagic cystitis and colitis, ulceration of intestinal mucosa
Nitrogen mustard (Mustargen)		Anorexia, vomiting, nausea, diarrhea, and metallic taste
Analgesics	Multiple uses	
Aspirin		May fluctuate blood glucose, deplete body folic acid and vitamin C. Stomach bleeding may result in iron-deficiency anemia. Potential hypernatremia, especially undesirable for heart or kidney patients
Cocaine		Decreases sensitivity of taste, especially of bitterness and sweetness
Phenylbutazone		May ulcerate stomach walls, decrease intestinal mucus secretion
Antacids	Buffering stomach acids	
Aluminum hydroxide		Chronic ingestion results in hypophosphatemia, especially low phosphate intake. Also causes constipation and potential vitamin malabsorption
Calcium carbonate or too much milk		Milk-alkali syndrome; hypercalcemia, which can be serious
Sodium bicarbonate		Hypernatremia, especially undesirable for kidney and heart patients
Antibiotics	Destruction of pathogenic organisms	Most drugs can irritate intestinal walls, causing diarrhea, thus fluid and electrolyte imbalance. Causes malabsorption of various nutrients to different extents; decreases nutrient contribution by intestinal flora (eg, vitamins such as K, folic acid, biotin, and B_{12} and amino acids)
Bleomycin (Blenoxane)	Cancer chemotherapy	May cause stomatitis, anorexia, nausea, vomiting, fever, oral ulceration
Cycloserine	Antituberculosis; treatment of urinary tract infection	Folic acid and pyridoxine deficiencies
Dactinomycin (actinomycin D. Cosmegen)	Cancer chemotherapy	May cause stomatitis, anorexia, nausea, vomiting, diarrhea, oral ulceration
Griseofulvin	Controlling growth of some dematophytes	May cause loss of taste sensitivity; nausea
Isoniazid	Antituberculosis	Niacin and pyridoxine deficiencies
Neomycin (and kanamycin)	Nonabsorbable; gut sterilization and prevention of coma from liver failure	May damage small intestine walls; malabsorption of various nutrients usually not significant because of short-term usage
Para-aminosalicylic acid (PAS)	Antituberculosis	Decreases absorption of fat and vitamin B_{12}, especially if given at high dosage
Tetracycline	Multiple uses (systemic effect)	May specifically affect bone growth, malabsorption of various nutrients. Usually not significant because of short-term usage
Anticholinergics	Treatment for peptic ulcer	May cause dry mouth, constipation, and urinary retention
Belladonna		
Propantheline bromide		
Anticoagulants	Preventing blood clotting	
Coumarin		Works by counteracting the function of vitamin K (ie, synthesis of prothrombin)
Phenindione		Steatorrhea. May bring about loss of fat-soluble vitamins and essential fatty acids in the stool

Drug	Clinical Usage	Possible Direct and Indirect Effects on Nutritional Status

Anticonvulsants (including sedatives)
  Barbiturates
  Dilantin
  Diphenylhydantoin
  Others
	Sedation, tranquilizing, control of epilepsy	Folic acid and vitamin D deficiencies; sometimes vitamin K deficiency

Antihistamines
  Chlorpheniramine
  Promethazine
	Multiple uses (eg, antiallergy)	Dry mouth, increased appetite, intestinal problems may cause malabsorption of nutrients

Antihyperglycemic drugs (oral)
  Biguanides
  Metformin
  Phenformin
  Sulfonylureas
	Lowering blood glucose; optional treatment for diabetes	May interfere with vitamin B_{12} absorption
		
		May increase appetite

Antihyperlipidemic drugs
  Cholestyramine
  Clofibrate
 	
  Niacin
	Lowering blood cholesterol	Both may interfere with the absorption of fat-soluble vitamins A, D, and K, fat, iron, and vitamin B_{12}. Clofibrate may also induce nausea and abnormal muscle metabolism
		May interfere with glucose metabolism

Antihypertensives
  Hydralazine
 	
  Propranolol
	Lowering blood pressure	Vitamin B_2 deficiency by binding with B_2 and increasing its excretion
		Hypoglycemia

Anti-inflammatory drugs Colchicine	Treatment for gout	Maldigestion and malabsorption. Diarrhea and steatorrhea. Sodium, potassium, B_{12}, lipid, nitrogen, fat-soluble vitamins may be lost in stool. Decreases disaccharidases in intestine. Lowers blood carotene concentration. Damages the intestinal walls
Antimanic depression agents Lithium carbonate	Treatment for mental disorders	Blocks release of thyroid hormone, which can cause hypothyroidism with possible goiter. Strange, unpleasant taste sensation. May affect renal function and fluid and electrolyte balance

Antimetabolites
  Cytarabine (Cytosar)
 	
  5-Fluorouracil
  6-Mercaptopurine
 	
  Methotrexate
	Cancer chemotherapy	Most produce nausea, vomiting, and diarrhea
		Also anorexia, megaloblastic anemia. Antagonist to pyrimidine
		Also stomatitis, gastrointestinal ulceration, and bleeding
		Also stomatitis, fever. Antagonist to purine and pantothenic acid
		Also stomatitis, anorexia, abnormal liver function, and gastrointestinal ulceration

Antipsychotic drugs
  Butyrophenone
  Phenothiazines
  Thioxanthenes
	Treatment of psychiatric problems	Weight gain, hyperglycemia, lactation, temperature irregularities, and paralytic ileus

Appetite depressants
  Amphetamine
  Fenfluramine
	For losing weight	Decreased food intake results both in decreased caloric and essential nutrient intake

Bulking agents
  Guar gum
  Methylcellulose
	For losing weight	These substances take up fluid and swell in the intestine; there may be decreased caloric and essential nutrient intake

Cardiovascular drugs
  Digitalis and its glycosides
 	
  Quinidine
  Procainamide
	Treatment of heart problems Increasing the force and velocity of cardiac contraction
	Treatment of dysrhythmias
		Most can produce anorexia, nausea, and vomiting

(continued)

Table 8–1   The Effects of Common Drugs on Nutritional Status (continued)

Drug	Clinical Usage	Possible Direct and Indirect Effects on Nutritional Status

Chelating agents
    Deferoxamine
    Penicillamine
	Treatment of poisoning with heavy metals; sometimes used for other diseases such as arthritis and Wilson's disease	May also chelate essential minerals such as calcium and iodine

Diuretics	Removing excess water from body	
Benzothiadiazine Thiazide Diazoxide		Diabetogenic; increased urinary excretion of potassium, hypokalemia
Furosemide Ethacrynic acid Spironolactone		Increased urinary potassium, hypokalemia Increased urinary calcium, hypocalcemia Hyperkalemia, decreased urinary excretion of potassium
Triamterene		Hyperkalemia, hypocalcemia, possible folic acid deficiency
Chlorothiazide Hydrochlorothiazide Thiazides		Increased urinary potassium, hypokalemia Decreased urinary calcium, hypercalcemia
Chlorthalidone Furosemide		Increased urinary excretion of zinc
Herbal medicines	Multiple uses in some countries	Diarrhea may cause loss of fluid and electrolyte. Presence of oxalic acid in plant parts may cause some essential mineral elements to precipitate. Some plant parts, when ingested, may cause hypoglycemia

Hormones
    Insulin
    Oral contraceptive pills (mestranol, conjugated estrogens, ethinyl estradiol)
	Lowering blood glucose
	Contraception
		Increases appetite
		Multiple and profound effects on the nutritional status of a woman. May produce vitamin B_6, B_{12}, and folic acid deficiencies. Affects the body metabolism of protein, fat, carbohydrate, calcium, phosphorus, magnesium, and zinc. Effects of the new "low-dose" contraceptive pills are unknown

Steroids (corticosteroids such as cortisone and prednisone)	Multiple uses	Diabetogenic; growth retardation; muscle protein catabolism, adipose tissue deposition; electrolyte imbalances, hypernatremia, hypokalemia, hypocalcemia, fluid retention; potential osteoporosis; increased excretion of zinc and iodine; peptic ulcer

Purgatives
    Mineral oil
    Phenolphthalein
	Laxatives (cathartics)	May result in loss of fat-soluble nutrients in the stool
		May interfere with the absorption of calcium and vitamins

Miscellaneous Marijuana (either smoked or ingested)		May increase appetite

SOURCE: Hui YH: *Human Nutrition and Diet Therapy.* Monterey, CA: Wadsworth, 1983, pp. 390–393.

Psychosocial Causes

Dietary habits greatly affect nutritional status. Some poor dietary habits contribute to starvation and the development of malnutrition or nutrient deficiencies. It is best to ask the client to record intake over several days to determine if deficiencies exist. Fad diets and religious or cultural limitations may provide insufficient amounts of nutrients. Dieters often attempt to lose weight by fasting or eliminating foods that contain important nutrients. Those who avoid these foods must learn to balance food intake so protein needs are met. Vegetarians who consume milk, milk products, and eggs usually meet their nutritional needs. Bad eating habits may provide sufficient caloric intake but insufficient nutrients, such as in a diet consisting solely of high sugar starchy foods (cakes, breads, etc). Other diets may have enough protein but not enough vitamins. Alcohol intake may be a substitute for food for some people, resulting in malnutrition. Teenagers often prefer to skip mealtimes, choosing instead to satisfy hunger with snack foods such as chips, french fries, soda pop, candy, or ice cream.

Nursing Research Note

Mallick MJ: Health problems associated with dieting activities of a group of adolescent females. *West J Nurs Res* 1982; 4(2):167–177.

This study examined the characteristics of adolescent dieters, types of diets followed, and the incidence of health problems associated with these diets. Diet types were classified as informal (dieter's own dietary restrictions) and formal diets (those found in books, magazines, etc) Data were collected from a group of 144 women who were high school juniors and seniors.

In this sample, 23% were below weight and height norms for their age, 33% were at norms for age, and 44% were above weight and height norms for their age. Of the 144 respondents, 120 had symptoms associated with dieting. The average number of symptoms was 2.79 for informal dieters and 3.21 for formal dieters. Underweight and above-weight respondents had the greatest number of symptoms.

As would be expected, hunger was the most frequently reported symptom for both formal and informal diet types. Weakness, preoccupation with food, nausea, nervousness, dizziness, and susceptibility to infection were most frequently reported by those following informal diets. Headache, fatigue, poor concentration, and changes in menstrual patterns were cited as symptoms of formal diets. The researcher concluded that diets with the most drastic changes in nutrient intake resulted in the most symptoms.

In dealing with overweight adolescents, nurses must encourage proper dieting techniques and moderation. They must also stimulate interest in physical activity. Because growth is still occurring during these years, nutritional status must be closely assessed in this population. Including a nutritional history in an adolescent's health assessment allows for early and appropriate intervention.

Such a diet may result in overnutrition yet be deficient in vital nutrients. A teenager's intake may need to be recorded to evaluate diet.

The nurse should also be familiar with psychological conditions that may result in starvation from inadequate intake of nutrients or from induced vomiting following eating. Anorexia nervosa and bulimia, extreme conditions occurring primarily in adolescent females, are discussed in Chapter 9. Psychosis may precipitate psychogenic malnutrition. The psychotic person may have delusions of food poisoning and fear eating foods purchased or prepared by others. Severe depression or apathy may reduce the hunger drive. These persons need to be encouraged to eat frequent, small, nutritious meals.

Psychological stress precipitated by an anxiety-provoking event such as a speaking engagement or an athletic competition may cause transient difficulty in swallowing or loss of appetite. Stress from work or family pressures may reduce appetite and interfere with mealtimes. The psychological stress of loss through death, divorce, or separation often reduces appetite to a point where rapid weight loss jeopardizes health.

Socioeconomic factors may contribute to poor nutritional status. Persons in lower socioeconomic groups may not be able to afford an adequate diet. The poorly educated may not know what constitutes a proper diet, although lack of nutritional knowledge occurs at every socioeconomic level. Poor refrigeration or cooking facilities may affect nutritional intake or contribute to food contamination. Environmental sanitation and water supply will affect the quality of nutrient intake. A water supply deficient in minerals such as iodine or fluoride may contribute to nutrient deficiencies or dental problems. At any socioeconomic level, drug and alcohol abuse interfere with good nutrition.

Altered Metabolism

Certain disease states contribute to the development of malnutrition because of altered metabolism, which affects how nutrients are used. Conditions that cause physiological stress, such as fever, infection, trauma, hyperthyroidism, and burns, increase metabolism and alter the ways in which the body can use nutrients. This increased metabolism, or hypermetabolism, increases the demand for nutrients. At the same time, many of these conditions diminish appetite. A paradox results: increased demand and decreased supply. Malnutrition may develop if the stress state is severe and prolonged and the person does not receive nutritional support.

Chronic disease states may also contribute to poor nutritional status. Diabetes alters the metabolism of carbohydrates, fats, and protein while decreasing circulation to areas where some nutrients are metabolized. Diseases that alter oxygenation of tissues, such as hypertension, coronary artery disease, and chronic obstructive lung disease, reduce the supply of oxygen to cells that need it to metabolize nutrients.

Cancer and cirrhosis are chronic diseases that have a particularly serious effect on metabolism, often leading to malnutrition. The altered metabolism of cancer increases the need for calories and protein while depressing the appetite and altering taste perception. The wasting process is accelerated because the body's fat and protein are broken down to meet metabolic demands. Cancer treatment can cause nausea, vomiting, oral lesions, and intestinal absorption problems, worsening nutritional status.

Cirrhosis—progressive liver failure—alters metabolism of fat, protein, and carbohydrates, in part because the liver is a major center of nutrient metabolism. The liver's ability to produce protein from amino acids and to store glucose as glycogen is impaired. Increasing amounts of protein in the diet may contribute to mental confusion because the liver cannot properly metabolize the dietary protein.

Iatrogenic Malnutrition

Treatment-induced malnutrition is a serious problem for hospitalized clients. Nurses should be alert for medical and nursing practices such as diffusion of responsibility for client care and rotation of staff that may inadvertently contribute to a client's malnourished state. The problem may begin at admission. Failure to assess nutritional status at that point allows altered nutritional status to go unnoticed. For example, if baseline height and weight are not recorded, there will be no means for comparing weight changes.

Nutritional assessment must continue throughout hospitalization. Failure to observe and record food intake means poor nutritional intake will not be identified. Withholding meals for diagnostic tests further lowers nutritional intake for clients who may already be at risk for malnutrition. Providing low glucose and saline intravenous solutions as the sole nutrient intake over several days also promotes development of malnutrition. Nutritional needs may be unmet if there is inappropriate use of nutrient products through ignorance or carelessness. Similarly, failure to recognize increased nutritional requirements from injury and illness and failure to determine whether nutritional status is satisfactory before performing surgery may also result in unmet needs. Delays in initiating appropriate nutritional support until clients are seriously malnourished exposes them to its results until treatment can take effect.

MULTISYSTEM EFFECTS OF MALNUTRITION

Malnutrition affects all body systems. Early identification and prevention of malnutrition will prevent a multitude of physical, emotional, social, and economic problems. When malnutrition progresses without early identification and treatment, many physiological problems can be observed. Among malnourished clients, the nurse will notice poor resistance to illness, poor response to illness and stress, poor response to therapy including surgery, prolonged hospitalization, and increased mortality.

Identifying those at risk for malnutrition and those with malnutrition is an important nursing responsibility. When identified, these clients require special nutritional management. Until renourished, they will present special problems for nursing and medical management.

The nurse should be familiar with the physiological changes that occur with progressive malnutrition. With starvation, the body will use reserves of carbohydrates and fats to meet energy demands. There are no true reserves of protein; therefore, in starvation, functional protein tissue is broken down to meet protein demands. Eventually, the metabolic rate decreases, along with body temperature. Weight loss and a wasted appearance ensue.

With malnutrition, illness and response to therapy are worsened. In a malnourished client, resistance to infection is poor because of lowered body temperature and decreased ability to produce antibodies, which require protein. Higher morbidity and mortality rates are especially evident in malnourished clients undergoing surgery. When preoperative nutritional repletion is overlooked, the risks of surgery and anesthesia multiply. Following abdominal surgery, the incidence of wound infection, pneumonia, major complications, and mortality is increased in malnourished clients, espe-

cially if nutritional support continues to be poor (Muller et al. 1982). Surgical recovery may be prolonged.

In acute starvation, organ efficiency is reduced with no change in organ mass. With progressive malnutrition, organs are reduced in size (mass) and in function (effi-

Table 8–2 Multisystem Effects of Malnutrition

System	Effect
Neurological	
Temperature regulation	Decreased metabolism causes decreased baseline temperature
Mental changes	Apathy, depression, irritability, depressed cognitive function, impaired reasoning and judgment
Immune	
White blood cell (WBC) production	Very sensitive to protein status resulting in decreased antibody formation; increased risk of developing infection also enhanced because of decreased temperature
Musculoskeletal	Decreased muscle mass, agility, and coordination
Cardiovascular	
Heart	Decreased muscle mass and decreased pumping efficiency; increased dysrhythmias
Red blood cells	Decreased synthesis of red blood cells
WBCs	Decreased production of WBCs
Respiratory	Muscle atrophy; increased pneumonias
Gastrointestinal	Decreased mass; decreased enzymes for digestion; decreased absorption; impaired motility; shortened transit time; increased bacterial overgrowth; diarrhea
Hepatic–biliary	Altered metabolism; reduced ability to store glucose; reduced ability to produce glucose from amino acids; reduced protein synthesis; reduced clotting factors
Integumentary	Easy breakdown of skin
Urinary	Kidney atrophy; altered efficiency in filtration, fluid and electrolyte balance, and acid–base balance

ciency). The nurse should be familiar with the response to malnutrition of the major organs or organ systems (Table 8–2). Prolonged malnutrition can cause atrophy of the heart muscle and reduced cardiac efficiency, which may result in heart failure and easy fatigue. Decreased respiratory efficiency from malnutrition of the respiratory muscles causes poor oxygenation of the blood and shortness of breath with minimal exertion. Depressed gastrointestinal function because of atrophy from poor nutrition may inhibit intestinal absorption of nutrients and drugs and cause diarrhea. Because advanced malnutrition affects the liver, metabolism of carbohydrates, fats, and protein may be altered. Depressed white blood cell function contributes to poor wound healing and increased infections. Malnutrition can cause anemia because production of hemoglobin is altered.

Malnutrition compounded by illness or stress can lead to apathy, depression, irritability, poor appetite, fatigue, low energy levels, and skin breakdown. In clients with chronic malnutrition, body temperatures are below normal because metabolism is reduced.

Pharmacologic therapy will be altered with malnutrition. Drug absorption is impaired because of the gastrointestinal effects. Drug metabolism will be altered when malnutrition affects the organs involved in metabolizing drugs. Some drugs depend on blood proteins to prevent toxic effects. When a person is malnourished, blood proteins are reduced, increasing the chance of toxicity with normal doses. Drug doses must be altered according to the degree of malnutrition. Pharmacists know which drugs are likely to be toxic in such cases.

The physiological signs and symptoms of malnutrition generally occur with prolonged malnutrition. Nutritional repletion should be instituted as soon as symptoms are noted; months of continued nutritional support may be needed before the problems are corrected.

Section II: Nursing Process in Malnutrition

ASSESSMENT: ESTABLISHING THE DATA BASE

Malnutrition is a prevalent problem, which the nurse may encounter in any setting. The nursing approach to malnutrition includes an assessment of nutritional status to provide information essential for devising an appropriate plan of care. This assessment should identify clients with overt malnutrition or subclinical nutritional deficiencies. The nutritional assessment should identify contributing factors, especially high-risk factors, indicating a potential for nutritional problems. The nutritional assessment includes gathering subjective and objective data from a detailed dietary history, a complete physical examination, and diagnostic studies. No single physical finding, measure, or index indicates a definitive diagnosis of malnutrition. It is essential to examine these numerous variables simultaneously.

Subjective Data

The subjective data obtained from nutritional assessment should reflect the potential physiological and psychosocial causes of malnutrition with special attention to identifying the high-risk client (Box 8–2). Ask the client about any disorder that would decrease food ingestion or absorption, increase nutrient losses, or alter nutrient metabolism. A decrease in food ingestion can result from difficulty in chewing or swallowing or nausea and vomiting. A decrease in food absorption accompanies digestion problems, diarrhea, pancreatic disease, gastrointestinal disorders, or surgery. An increase in nutrient losses can occur with draining wounds, burns, blood loss, or renal dialysis. Altered metabolism occurs with fever, infection, burns, hyperthyroidism, trauma, or surgery. Chronic diseases contributing to malnutrition are: diabetes, cancer, heart disease, hypertension, liver disease, kidney disease, and psychosis.

Obtain information on recent and current drug therapy. Drugs contributing to malnutrition are those that decrease the appetite or alter nutrient absorption or metabolism. Appetite suppressants include caffeine, amphetamines, and cancer chemotherapy drugs. Medications that alter absorption of nutrients include antacids,

---

Box 8–2 Identifying the High-Risk Client

Grossly underweight: Weight-for-height below 80% of standard

Grossly overweight: Weight-for-height above 120% of standard (risk due to tendency to overlook protein and calorie requirements in the acutely obese patient)

Experiencing recent weight loss: 10% or more of usual body weight

Alcoholic

Taking nothing by mouth: More than 10 days while being given simple IV solutions

Experiencing protracted nutrient losses: Malabsorption syndromes; short-gut syndromes/fistulas; renal dialysis; draining abscesses, wounds

Experiencing increased metabolic needs: Extensive burns, infection, trauma; protracted fever

Taking drugs with antinutrient or catabolic properties: Steroids, immunosuppressants, antitumor agents

SOURCE: Morgan J: Nutritional assessment of critically ill patients. *Focus on Critical Care* 1984; 11(3):30. (Adapted from Weinsier RL, Butterworth CE: *Handbook of Clinical Nutrition.* St. Louis: Mosby, 1981, pp. 7–8.)

antigout preparations, antibiotics, and laxatives. Altered nutrient metabolism occurs with steroids or some anticonvulsants. (Table 8–1 includes examples of common drugs that affect nutrition.)

Information on usual and current nutrient intake is essential. When gathering subjective data for nutritional assessment, determine the client's dietary history as outlined in Box 8–3. A thorough diet history will reveal eating habits including recent changes. It is preferable to request a 3-day record or a 24-hour recall from the client or client's family, if appropriate. The client or family should record time, food, and amount ingested using household measures. For the hospitalized client, the nurse should observe what is eaten at meals and what is brought in by family members. Also obtain a history of weight gain or loss.

Ask about any gross inadequacies or excesses in intake from the major food groups: milk, meat, vegetables, fruits, breads, and cereals. Intake of fiber foods should be noted. Ask about seasonings used with cooking or on food. Determine intake of fatty foods (such as butter, oils, nuts, gravy, sauces), simple carbohydrates (such as jelly, jams, sugar, cakes, pies, cookies, candy), and snack foods (such as pretzels and potato chips). Inquire about food preparation, such as frying or broiling, and frequency of meals. It is helpful to ask if the client usually eats at home or at a restaurant. Information about food intolerance should be requested, along with data on specific nutrients (Table 8–3) and cultural and religious diet limitations.

Fad diets may be deficient in some nutrients. Ask if the client is following a fad diet, such as a liquid protein diet or diets that consist only of "nutritious" pills. A vegetarian diet may be deficient in protein, especially when milk and eggs are omitted. Review diet information with a nutritionist to determine nutritional content and any gross inadequacies.

Some alcoholics substitute excess alcohol intake for food. The elderly client may indicate problems with eating,

such as constipation, disinterest in food, decreased taste, or ill-fitting dentures. A poor appetite, especially with loss of taste acuity, may be associated with illnesses, especially cancer. Poor intake or no intake for 10 days or more is of concern. The time span is even less for extremely malnourished individuals.

Explore any psychological causes for decreased intake. The client should be asked why food intake is decreased to determine if the reason is delusions, depression, psychological stress, or a recent loss. Pressure of school or work may leave little time for preparing and eating food. If the client is reluctant to provide information, use communication techniques such as reflecting, clarifying, or paraphrasing.

Socioeconomic factors may contribute to malnutrition. Ask the client if obtaining food is a financial burden or a serious inconvenience. If appropriate, ask about refrigeration and cooking facilities. The interview should also provide an opportunity for the client to ask about nutrition practices.

Objective Data

Physical Examination

In the physical examination, look particularly for signs that support or rule out the suspected nutritional disorders. The physical signs of malnutrition and nutrient deficiencies may not always be obvious. Many signs do not appear until the deficiency is advanced. Multiple deficiencies may exist, making the determination of a specific deficiency difficult. Some physical signs of malnutrition such as dry, flaking skin have nonnutritional causes. Obesity may mask protein malnutrition because wasting is not apparent. Since no single sign is diagnostic, the best approach to physical assessment is also to consider the subjective data and laboratory results when drawing conclusions.

The clinical findings of malnutrition and nutrient deficiencies are outlined in Table 8–4. When examining the hair, ask the client if hair collects on the client's pillow, brush, or comb. If any skin lesion is observed, note the body distribution. When examining the mouth, note the status of the teeth. Poor dentition will contribute to poor intake. Muscle mass is assessed by feeling the calves and/or the upper arms. In severe muscle wasting, a decrease in mass is noted throughout the body so the outline of bones is visible. Decreased muscle mass of the hands and the upper chest is seen in advanced protein malnutrition.

In clients where malnutrition has progressed, signs of multisystem effects, as described earlier in Table 8–2, can be observed. Baseline temperature in chronic malnutrition can be as low as 96°F (35.5°C). Record the baseline because elevations may indicate a fever even when below the usual normal of 98.6°F (37°C). Mental changes such as apathy or depression may be detected in advanced malnutrition. Shortness of breath, fatigue, pallor, peripheral edema, and heart rhythm abnormalities may be observed.

Box 8–3 Elements of a Dietary History

Frequency of intake of each food group: milk, meat, fruit, vegetable, and grains

Current nutritional intake versus usual nutritional intake (if it varies)

Meal and snacking patterns

Nutritional supplements

Nutritional preferences and intolerances

Weight history

Food acquisition and preparation habits

Special diet as monitored by health care provider or by client

Cultural or religious dietary considerations

Smoking, caffeine, and alcohol intake

Physical activity

Table 8-3   Selected Nutrient Deficiencies

Nutrient Deficiency	Subjective Data	Objective Data	Primary Food Sources
Vitamin A deficiency	Inadequate dietary intake; night blindness; disorder of fat malabsorption	Dry, scaling, rough skin; shrinking mucous membranes; swelling and redness of eyelids; clouded cornea; Bitot's spots	Leafy green and yellow—orange vegetables and fruits
Thiamine (B_1) deficiency (beriberi)	Inadequate dietary intake; malabsorption; chronic alcohol abuse; apathy; confusion; recent memory loss; nausea, vomiting, anorexia	Cardiomegaly, dyspnea; increase or absence of deep tendon reflexes; peripheral edema; muscle cramps; muscle wasting; pallor; ophthalmoplegia; nystagmus; paresthesia; neuropathy; ataxia	Whole or enriched breads or cereals, pork, beans, nuts, ham, liver, peas, asparagus
Riboflavin (B_2) deficiency	Inadequate dietary intake; chronic alcoholism; taking oral contraceptives	Cheilosis, stomatitis; conjunctivitis; edema; neuropathy; seborrheic dermatitis in nasolabial folds; generalized dermatitis; dimness of vision; purplish-red tongue; glossitis	Milk, meat, fish, leafy green and yellow vegetables, enriched breads
Niacin deficiency (pellagra)	Inadequate dietary intake; carcinoid syndrome; chronic alcohol abuse; headache; confusion; muscle weakness; diarrhea	Reddened mouth, tongue, and lips; dermatitis, especially in sun-exposed area(s); glossitis; loss of memory	Liver, halibut, tuna, chicken, turkey, veal, peanuts, and peanut butter
Pyridoxine (B_6) deficiency	Alcohol abuse; inadequate dietary intake; taking oral contraceptives	Dermatitis; neuritis; convulsions	Pork, lamb, veal, legumes, potatoes, wheat germ, bananas
Cobalamin (B_{12}) deficiency	Strict vegetarian diet; malabsorption from gastrectomy or ileal resection; history of pernicious anemia; hand and feet paresthesia	Lemon-yellow pallor; bright red tongue; congestive heart failure; pale conjunctivas; glossitis; peripheral neuropathy	Seafood, meats, eggs, dairy products
Vitamin C deficiency (scurvy)	Inadequate dietary intake; pain and swelling of limbs and joints; easily fatigued	Swollen, bleeding gums; loosening teeth; delayed wound healing; anemia; petechiae; ecchymosis; depression; weakness; easily bruised	Fresh fruits and vegetables, citrus fruits and juices, strawberries, canteloupe, spinach, broccoli
Vitamin D deficiency (adult rickets; osteomalacia)	Inadequate dietary intake; malabsorption; inadequate sunlight exposure	Bone malformations; low serum calcium levels	Fortified milk
Vitamin K deficiency	Prolonged use of anticoagulants or antibiotics; malabsorption; biliary obstruction	Bleeding tendencies, especially into gastrointestinal tract, muscles, and joints; petechiae and ecchymoses	50% from intestinal bacterial synthesis; cauliflower, broccoli, cabbage, spinach, beef liver
Iron deficiency	Inadequate dietary intake; iron malabsorption such as with diarrhea or gastrectomy; blood loss; anorexia, flatulence, constipation; paresthesias in extremities; pregnancy; fatigue	Brittle spoon-shaped nails; cracked corners of the mouth, smooth tongue; tachycardia; dyspnea; listlessness; irritability; pallor; pale conjunctivas; decreased serum iron	Liver, beef, lamb, pork, veal, baked beans, molasses, prunes, enriched breads and cereals, green leafy vegetables
Iodine deficiency	Inadequate dietary intake; poor memory; chills; amenorrhea; anorexia	Hoarseness; thick tongue; hearing loss; decreased blood pressure; enlarged thyroid gland	Table salt, seafood, plant food from soil high in iodine

(continued)

Table 8–3	Selected Nutrient Deficiencies (continued)		
Nutrient Deficiency	**Subjective Data**	**Objective Data**	**Primary Food Sources**
Folic acid deficiency	Inadequate dietary intake; chronic alcohol abuse; malabsorption; diarrhea; pregnancy	Severe pallor; glossitis; anemia; cardiac enlargement; pale conjunctivas	Leafy vegetables, organ meats, beef, wheat, fish, legumes
Zinc deficiency	Gastrointestinal losses	Altered taste; flaky dermatitis; impaired healing; loss of hair	Seafood (especially oysters), meat, liver, eggs, milk, whole grain products

As the nurse progresses through the physical exam, signs of preexisting disorders should also be observed, especially if possibly related to malnutrition. For example, an enlarged thyroid gland may occur with hyperthyroidism, which is associated with increased metabolism.

Diagnostic Tests

Information from diagnostic tests sensitive to nutritional intake is another aspect of objective data. For the purposes of this chapter, diagnostic tests include body measurements, skin testing, and laboratory tests. The information gathered from these diagnostic tests will further support the evidence from the subjective data and the physical examination in determining the presence of malnutrition or nutrient deficiencies.

Laboratory tests are used primarily to assess protein status because protein is sensitive to nutritional status. Other than protein status indicators, blood levels of minerals and vitamins can be determined when nutrient deficiencies are suspected.

Anthropometric Measurements. Body measurements, or *anthropometric measurements*, are useful for nutritional assessment because they are altered by states of nutrition. The measurement of body weight, skinfold thickness, and certain body circumferences are the most useful in assessing malnutrition.

Body weight and height should be obtained with the initial nutritional assessment, as a basis for comparison, and at regular intervals thereafter. Ideally, repeated weights should be taken on the same scale. Some clients need a chair or litter scale if their medical condition limits their ability to stand. The present weight should be compared to the reported usual weight and the history of weight gains and/or losses. The present weight should also be compared to the ideal or desired weight. The Metropolitan Life Insurance Company periodically publishes standard weight-to-height tables that are widely used (Table 8–5). This is only one standard that can be used for comparison.

Skinfold measurements (measurements of a fold of skin and subcutaneous fat) are used to estimate body sub-

cutaneous fat to determine total body fat (or calorie) stores. These measurements can be obtained in the triceps, biceps, subscapular, suprailiac, and thigh areas. The triceps skinfold is the most easily obtained. It is measured on the back of the nondominant upper arm at a midpoint between the olecranon process of the elbow and the acromial process of the shoulder. (When determining the upper arm midpoint, the arm should hang loosely at the person's side.) Using a device called a caliper, a lengthwise fold of skin and fat is measured in millimeters (Figure 8–1). This measurement is then compared to a table of standards, such as the one in Table 8–6. Other standards are available in most clinical nutrition texts. The result indicates the degree of increased or decreased body fat stores. For accurate triceps skinfold measurement, one individual should take an average of three readings and avoid the following common errors:

- Using the wrong arm
- Measuring the midarm point incorrectly
- Identifying the posterior plane incorrectly
- Measuring an arm that does not hang freely
- Having an unequal level between client and examiner
- Applying the caliper too deeply or too superficially
- Placing the caliper jaws at the wrong site
- Reading the measurement too early or too late
- Releasing the skinfold before the measurement is obtained
- Failing to take an average of three readings
- Failing to release the caliper handle fully between repeat measurements

The midarm circumference is measured at the same point on the arm as the triceps skinfold. The circumference is measured in centimeters using a 7- to 12-mm-wide tape made of a nonstretchable but compliant material. The tape is positioned snugly at the upper arm midpoint, but not tightly enough to cause skin contour indentation. This measurement, along with the triceps skinfold, is used in calculating the arm muscle circumference, also an indication of protein stores. Subtract the triceps skinfold measurement from the midarm circumference to arrive at a mea-

Table 8–4   Clinical Nutrition Exam

Clinical Findings	Consider Deficiency of:	Clinical Findings	Consider Deficiency of:
Hair, nails		**Glands**	
Flag sign (transverse depigmentation of hair)	Protein, copper	Parotid enlargement	Protein
Hair easily pluckable	Protein	Sicca syndrome	Ascorbic acid
Hair thin, sparse	Protein, biotin, zinc	Thyroid enlargement	Iodine
Nails spoon-shaped	Iron	**Heart**	
Nails lackluster, transverse ridging	Protein-calorie	Enlargement, tachycardia, high-output failure	Thiamine ("wet" beriberi)
Skin		Small heart, decreased output	Calories
Dry, scaling	Vitamin A, zinc, essential fatty acids	Sudden failure, death	Ascorbic acid
Flaky paint dermatosis	Protein	**Abdomen**	
Follicular hyperkeratosis	Vitamins A, C; essential fatty acids	Hepatomegaly	Protein
Nasolabial seborrhea	Niacin, pyridoxine, riboflavin	**Muscles, extremities**	
Petechiae, purpura	Ascorbic acid, vitamin K	Calf tenderness	Thiamine, ascorbic acid (hemorrhage into muscle)
Pigmentation, desquamation (sun-exposed area)	Niacin (pellagra)	Edema	Protein, thiamine
Subcutaneous fat loss	Calorie	Muscle wastage (especially temporal area, dorsum of hand, spine)	Calories
Eyes		**Bones, joints**	
Angular blepharitis	Riboflavin	Beading of ribs (child)	Vitamins C, D
Corneal vascularization	Riboflavin	Bone and joint tenderness (child)	Ascorbic acid (subperiosteal hemorrhage)
Dull, dry conjunctiva	Vitamin A	Bone tenderness (adult)	Vitamin D, calcium, phosphorus (osteomalacia)
Fundal capillary microaneurysms	Ascorbic acid		
Scleral icterus, mild	Pyridoxine	**Neurological**	
Perioral		Confabulation, disorientation	Thiamine (Korsakoff's psychosis)
Angular stomatitis	Riboflavin	Decreased position and vibratory senses, ataxia	Vitamin B_{12}, thiamine
Cheilosis	Riboflavin	Decreased tendon reflexes, slowed relaxation phase	Thiamine
Oral cavity		Ophthalmoplegia	Thiamine, phosphorus
Atrophic lingual papillae	Niacin, iron, riboflavin, folate vitamin B_{12}	Weakness, paresthesias, decreased fine tactile sensation	Vitamin B_{12}, pyridoxine, thiamine
Glossitis (scarlet, raw)	Niacin, pyridoxine, riboflavin, vitamin B_{12}, folate	**Other**	
Hypogeusesthesia (also hyposmia)	Zinc, vitamin A	Delayed healing and tissue repair (eg, wound, infarct, abscess)	Ascorbic acid, zinc, protein
Magenta tongue	Riboflavin		
Swollen, bleeding gums (if teeth present)	Ascorbic acid		
Tongue fissuring, edema	Niacin		

SOURCE: Morgan J: Nutritional assessment of critically ill patients. *Focus on Critical Care* 1984; 11(3):32–33. (Adapted from Weinsier RL, Butterworth CE: *Handbook of Clinical Nutrition.* St. Louis: Mosby, 1981, pp. 30–31.)

Table 8–5   1983 Metropolitan Height and Weight Tables*

MEN					WOMEN				
Height		Small Frame	Medium Frame	Large Frame	Height		Small Frame	Medium Frame	Large Frame
Feet	Inches				Feet	Inches			
5	2	128–134	131–141	138–150	4	10	102–111	109–121	118–131
5	3	130–136	133–143	140–153	4	11	103–113	111–123	120–134
5	4	132–138	135–145	142–156	5	0	104–115	113–126	122–137
5	5	134–140	137–148	144–160	5	1	106–118	115–129	125–140
5	6	136–142	139–151	146–164	5	2	108–121	118–132	128–143
5	7	138–145	142–154	149–168	5	3	111–124	121–135	131–147
5	8	140–148	145–157	152–172	5	4	114–127	124–138	134–151
5	9	142–151	148–160	155–176	5	5	117–130	127–141	137–155
5	10	144–154	151–163	158–180	5	6	120–133	130–144	140–159
5	11	146–157	154–166	161–184	5	7	123–136	133–147	143–163
6	0	149–160	157–170	164–188	5	8	126–139	136–150	146–167
6	1	152–164	160–174	168–192	5	9	129–142	139–153	149–170
6	2	155–168	164–178	172–197	5	10	132–145	142–156	152–173
6	3	158–172	167–182	176–202	5	11	135–148	145–159	155–176
6	4	162–176	171–187	181–207	6	0	138–151	148–162	158–179

*Weights at ages 25–59 based on lowest mortality. Weight in pounds according to frame (in indoor clothing weighing 5 lb for men and 3 lb for women; shoes with 1 in heels).

Source of basic data 1979 Build Study Society of Actuaries and Association of Life Insurance Medical Directors of America 1980. Copyright 1983 Metropolitan Life Insurance Company.

sure of arm muscle circumference (Figure 8–2). To obtain an accurate midarm circumference measurement, avoid the following common errors:

- Using the wrong arm
- Measuring the midarm point incorrectly
- Measuring an arm that does not hang freely

- Having an unequal level between client and examiner
- Using a tape that is too thick, creased, stretched, or too rigid
- Placing the tape at the wrong site
- Pulling the tape too taut or leaving it too loose

The value of anthropometric measurements is ques-

Table 8–6   Standards for Triceps Skinfold and Arm Circumference

Anthropometric Norms	Men		Women	
	Jelliffe Standard	U.S. Population Ages 25–34 Years*	Jelliffe Standard	U.S. Population Ages 25–34 Years*
Weight (kg)†	70.1	79.1	58.3	64.5
Triceps skinfold (mm)	12.5	11.0	16.5	19.0
Arm circumference (mm)	293	310	285	275
Arm muscle circumference (mm)	253	270	232	213

*Population data from Ten-State Nutrition Survey and Health and Nutrition Examination Survey

†Weight for 175-cm man or 163-cm woman

SOURCE: Gray GE, Gray LK: Anthropometric measurements and their interpretation: Principles, practices, and problems. *J Am Diet Assoc* 1980; 77:534–538.

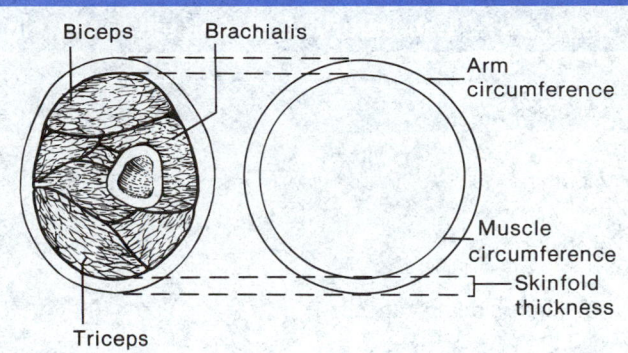

Figure 8–2

Arm muscle circumference. Given arm circumference and double thickness of the skinfold layer, the inner circumference, or arm muscle circumference, may be derived as follows (convert all measurements to centimeters): Arm muscle circumference = (arm circumference) − π (triceps skinfold). This index of body muscle mass does not take into account the bone, fascia, and other nonmuscle tissues below the skinfold; nor does it take into account the ellipsoid shape of most arms. However, as a comparative measurement, for which standards have been developed, it correlates well with other more elaborate methods of measuring muscle mass. (See Table 8–6 for population standards.)

SOURCE: Willard MD: *Nutrition for the Practicing Physician.* Baltimore, MD: Williams & Wilkins, 1982.

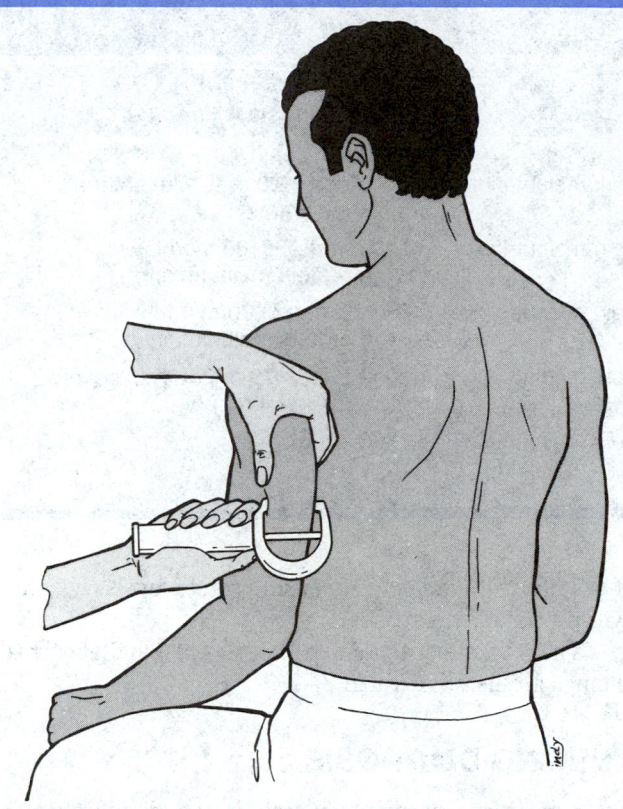

Figure 8–1

Measuring the triceps skinfold. Using the thumb and forefinger, pick up a double thickness of skinfold and gently pull it away from the underlying muscle. Use the posterior part of the arm and vertical pinch. Practice is required to isolate the skinfold for accurate measurement. To measure triceps skinfold thickness, maintain the skinfold isolation, and apply the caliper jaws at the arm midpoint. Read in 2 or 3 seconds. Reapply the calipers two more times for a total of three readings. Do not release the isolation of the skinfold until the thickness is determined by the calipers (the calipers exert mild pressure but will not maintain skinfold isolation). (See Table 8–6 for population standards.)

SOURCE: Kozier B, Erb G: *Fundamentals of Nursing: Concepts and Procedures,* 2nd ed. Menlo Park, CA: Addison–Wesley, 1983.

tioned in some situations, such as: acute starvation because anthropometric changes may lag behind the immediate changes; altered hydrational status from dehydration or overhydration because they also alter the measurement, yielding false high or false low measures; and in the elderly because standard tables were determined on younger people. The results are most useful when observing trends in serial measurements. The trend may indicate an improvement or a decline in nutritional status.

Skin Testing for Delayed Cutaneous Hypersensitivity. Another diagnostic test useful in nutritional status is skin testing for delayed cutaneous hypersensitivity. Skin testing with various substances (recall antigens) can provide gross information on immune response to those substances. Immune function is particularly sensitive to nutritional status because lymphocytes and antibodies are produced from proteins. Poor protein and/or calorie intake alter the body's ability to produce lymphocytes and antibodies needed to fight infections. In essence, skin tests create a localized infection by introducing antigens that the immune system should recognize and respond to. Malnutrition impairs this response.

Skin testing, often the nurse's responsibility, involves the application (usually by injection) and interpretation of skin test antigens. Common antigens used for this purpose include *Candida*, mumps, and tuberculin purified protein derivative (PPD). Each antigen (0.1 cc) is injected, usually on the inner aspect of the forearm. Because these antigens exert a delayed hypersensitivity response, the sites are observed at 24 and 48 hours. A positive response occurs when the site is indurated with a raised swelling 5 mm in diameter (Jensen et al., 1983). Erythema (redness) alone does not constitute a positive response. Skin tests are most useful as one aspect of a nutritional assessment because many variables—recent surgery, trauma, radiation therapy, immunosuppressive drug therapy, and cancer—can cause false negative responses. It is important to observe trends in serial assessments to determine improving or potentially worsening nutritional status.

Nitrogen Balance Determination. One assay of protein and nutrition status is nitrogen balance, since pro-

Table 8–7   Laboratory Tests Related to Protein Malnutrition

Laboratory Test	Normal Expected Value	Disease State	Expected Abnormal Findings
Albumin	3.5–5.5 g/dL	Protein malnutrition	<3.5 g/dL; <2.0 g/dL with severe protein malnutrition
Transferrin	200–400 mg/dL	Protein malnutrition	<200 mg/dL; <100 mg/dL with severe protein malnutrition
Total iron-binding capacity	250–420 µg/dL	Protein malnutrition	<250 µg/dL; <180 mg/dL with severe protein malnutrition
Prealbumin	20–50 mg/dL	Protein malnutrition	<20 mg/dL; <15 mg/dL with severe protein malnutrition
Lymphocyte count	1500–4500 cells/µL	Protein malnutrition	<1500 µL

tein is made of nitrogen. Nitrogen balance is determined by subtracting the nitrogen intake from the nitrogen output during the same 24-hour period. Nitrogen intake is determined by recording the protein intake, from which the nitrogen intake is derived. (There is approximately 1 g of nitrogen in 6 g of protein.) Nitrogen output is determined by analyzing a 24-hour urine collection, with allowances for estimated stool and insensible nitrogen losses. A negative nitrogen balance is an indication of protein breakdown exceeding protein intake, which occurs more in acute malnutrition or in acute stress with chronic malnutrition. With chronic malnutrition, muscle mass is minimal, minimizing the amount of protein available to break down into nitrogen. A nitrogen balance near zero or greater reflects good use of ingested protein. Nitrogen balance studies are usually done in hospital settings and involve both nursing and dietary personnel.

Serum Albumin, Transferrin, and Prealbumin. Protein status is also assessed by evaluating the liver's production of transport proteins including albumin, transferrin, and prealbumin. Albumin, a serum protein, has a long half-life of about 20 days. Albumin is not a sensitive indicator of nutrition status because it takes about 20 days to respond to nutritional depletion or repletion. Therefore, it is not reliable in acute starvation, but it is a useful and inexpensive screening measure. Transferrin has a half-life of 8 to 10 days, making this test more sensitive to changes in nutrition status (Cerra, 1984). Some laboratories do not measure transferrin levels. In those cases, an estimate can be made from total iron-binding capacity (TIBC) using the following equation:

$$\text{Transferrin} = 0.8 \times \text{TIBC} - 43$$

Prealbumin, another transport protein, with a half-life of 2 to 3 days, is highly sensitive to nutritional status.

Lymphocyte Count. Lymphocyte production is sensitive to protein availability because lymphocytes are made of protein; with depressed serum protein levels, lymphocyte production decreases.

The laboratory tests and their normal and abnormal findings are listed in Table 8–7.

NURSING DIAGNOSIS

The nurse plays an important role in the identification of malnutrition. The suspected cause of malnutrition should be recognized so appropriate nutrition therapy can be implemented. By thorough collection of subjective and objective data, the nurse should be able to identify specific client problems and determine nursing diagnoses related to malnutrition. The nursing diagnoses commonly related to malnutrition are listed in Box 8–4 and discussed below.

Box 8–4   Nursing Diagnoses Commonly Related to Malnutrition

Nutrition, alteration in: less than body requirements

Bowel elimination, alteration in: diarrhea, related to reduced bowel surface area

Fluid volume deficit, potential, related to fluid loss or fluid displacement

Injury, potential for, related to accentuated risk for tissue injury

Knowledge deficit, related to diet

Impaired physical mobility, related to fatigue and loss of strength

Self-care deficit, related to impaired mobility

Self-concept, disturbance in: body image

Self-concept, disturbance in: self-esteem

Self-concept, disturbance in: role performance

Sexual dysfunction, related to altered body structure

Skin integrity, impairment of

Alterations in Nutrition

Malnutrition has many detrimental effects, described earlier in this chapter. As the severity increases, the body's overall health declines. The nurse should note situations where iatrogenic malnutrition can develop, such as prolonged periods when food is withheld for tests or prolonged intravenous glucose and saline infusions when the client is not eating.

Alterations in Bowel Elimination

Malnutrition affects all body systems, including the gastrointestinal tract. Bowel surface area is reduced because of atrophy of the intestinal lining. With a reduced surface area, nutrients and fluids are absorbed less efficiently, causing diarrhea. Also, excess fluids and electrolytes may be lost, leading to a fluid deficit.

Potential for Fluid Volume Deficit

Since many foods contain fluid or water, a reduction in food intake may result in reduced fluid intake. Fluids can also be displaced, causing a deficit. Fluid lost in diarrhea is a good example. Reduced plasma protein from malnutrition alters the vascular compartment osmotic gradient. Edema may result because of the reduced gradient to maintain the fluids in the circulatory system. Edema can develop, especially in dependent areas such as the extremities, buttocks, or in the abdomen. This fluid imbalance will result, in part, in poor skin turgor.

Potential for Injury and Impaired Physical Mobility

Malnourished clients experience fatigue and loss of strength. The easy fatigue and loss of strength affect the client's ability to move quickly to avoid danger or trauma. Tasks requiring physical strength may become difficult if not impossible to carry out. Decrease in tissue nourishment also places the client at risk for tissue injury and prolongs healing.

Knowledge Deficit

Some clients may be malnourished because they do not realize that their diets may be lacking in nutrients, that malabsorption may also cause malnutrition, or that medications they are taking may adversely affect their nutritional status. Fad diets used for weight control and "fast food" diets also contribute to inadequate dietary intake.

Disturbances in Self-Concept

Malnutrition can result in disturbances in self-concept related to body image, self-esteem, and role performance. Those with severe wasting may see themselves as deformed and

helpless. The easy fatigue and loss of strength alter the ability to continue with usual activities. Time away from work or the inability to carry on a usual line of work may further intensify feelings of helplessness. The client's role in the family may change because of physical limitations, placing a strain on established relationships. Other family members may need, as a result, to take on additional responsibilities and burdens.

Alterations in Sexual Functioning

As malnutrition progresses, sexual functioning may become impaired because of fatigue and decreased strength and muscle mass. Body changes from malnutrition lessen feelings of sexual attractiveness. This will result in guilt feelings for the malnourished person and potential frustration for the partner. Libido may be decreased and, in the woman, decreased vaginal lubrication may cause dyspareunia (painful intercourse).

Alterations in Skin Integrity

Skin integrity is sensitive to the state of nutrition. Malnutrition predisposes the client to alterations in skin integrity because the skin relies heavily on good nutrition. Pressure areas on the skin, especially the buttocks, will be prone to skin breakdown. Infection occurs easily in broken-down skin because malnutrition impairs the infection-fighting ability of the body. Skin excoriation around the anus may be caused by diarrhea.

PLANNING AND IMPLEMENTATION

The plan of nursing care for clients with malnutrition should be directed toward correction of the poor nutritional state as described in the sample nursing care plan in Table 8–8. Along with proper nutritional repletion, therapy should be implemented to correct the cause of the malnutrition. The specific therapies will be based on the established data base and the client assessment and are carried out in collaboration with the dietitian and the nutrition support team. The nurse has an important role in facilitating the correction of some causes of malnutrition. For example, the nurse can request correctly fitting dentures, identify drug therapy that worsens nutrition, recommend counseling for alcohol abuse or poor dietary habits, and identify socioeconomic causes.

Improving Nutritional Intake

Reinforcing instructions from the dietitian regarding good eating habits contributes to dietary counseling. Determining food preferences and taking measures to obtain these foods encourage eating. Removing foul odors from drainage and bedpans will provide a pleasant environment at mealtime. Encouraging or providing oral care before and after meals helps to make food more appetizing. The nurse

Table 8–8   Sample Nursing Care Plan for Clients With Malnutrition

Nursing Diagnoses	Client Care Goal	Plan/Nursing Implementation	Expected Outcomes
Nutrition, alteration in: less than body requirements	Return to healthy state of nutrition; understanding of importance of good nutrition and elements of adequate dietary intake	Correct reversible problems leading to malnutrition such as: poorly fitting dentures, diarrhea, draining wounds, drug therapy, poor dietary habits, alcohol abuse, and socioeconomic causes; modify nutritional approach in the presence of relatively irreversible causes of malnutrition such as cancer, cirrhosis, chronic disease, difficulty swallowing, malabsorption, and age-related changes in the elderly; counsel clients on good dietary intake; determine and provide food preferences; provide a relaxed atmosphere free of foul odors and secretions; provide antiemetics in the presence of nausea; provide for oral care before and after meals; monitor tube feeding or total parenteral nutrition for safety	Malnutrition and/or nutrient deficiency will be corrected; signs and symptoms of deficiency will normalize; adequate nutritional intake will be maintained
Bowel elimination, alteration in: diarrhea	Return of normal bowel movements; reversal of excoriation from diarrhea; reversal of fluid loss from diarrhea	Encourage adequate nutritional intake; provide antidiarrheals as ordered; promote good hygiene following bowel movements to prevent skin excoriation; provide fluids to replace fluid loss; record frequency and amount of diarrhea	Bowel movements will solidify and become less frequent
Fluid volume deficit, potential	Fluid status balance	Administer fluids to replace fluid loss; monitor daily weights; note skin turgor; record intake and output; note presence of edema in extremities, buttocks, and abdomen	Client will have good skin turgor; balanced intake and output; absence of edema
Self-concept, disturbance in: body image	Acceptance of body image	Help client to understand reason for body image change; inform client that nutritional repletion should improve body image; allow client and family to ventilate feelings	Client's body image will improve when malnutrition is reversed
Skin integrity, impairment of: actual	Maintenance of skin integrity	Provide health teaching on relationship of poor nutrition and skin integrity; prevent prolonged pressure on pressure points by regular change in position; prevent skin breakdown and infection	Client has healthy skin free of breakdown and infection; client has improved skin integrity with reversal of malnutrition

may involve family members in mealtime activities when their involvement improves nutrient intake. If oral supplements are ordered, provide them as the client prefers, eg, on ice, served cold, flavored, or mixed with foods. Encourage good nutritional intake especially prior to surgery and during infections. It is also important to be knowledgeable about nutrient contents of tube feedings, nutrition supplements, and multivitamins. Some elderly persons with limited physical abilities and income require support systems such as communal dining or Meals on Wheels to maintain good nutritional intake.

Principles of Nutritional Management

Some clients require sophisticated nutritional therapy to supply calories, protein, and other nutrients specific to their needs. Nutritional support refers to the administration of oral supplements and enteral and parenteral feedings. Many institutions have nutrition support teams consisting of a multidisciplinary group (physician, dietitian, pharmacist, and nurse specialist) with the responsibility of assuring the appropriate use of and monitoring for nutritional support regimens. Nursing participation in the team is essential to assure proper identification of client candidates and optimal administration and monitoring of those receiving nutritional support. Some factors that influence the selection of a nutritional therapy route are listed in Figure 8–3.

The nutrition support team can help the nurse in recognizing clients who may suffer from metabolic problems associated with rapid refeeding. In the presence of chronic malnutrition, the body adapts to the state of poor nutrition. If the body is suddenly overwhelmed by nutrients, they are handled poorly (Heymsfield, 1982). Blood sugar is poorly controlled because of chronic low insulin production. The malnourished heart will be stressed with refeeding because of the high demand for oxygen in the tissues where nutrients are metabolized. Electrolyte imbalances occur because of increased cellular activities related to nutrient metabolism (see Chapter 5). In nutritional therapy for chronic malnutrition, measures must be taken to replete nutrients slowly.

Tube Feedings

Tube feedings may be necessary for those suffering from malnutrition or those at high risk for developing malnutrition who cannot obtain an adequate oral intake. Tube feedings are given directly into the gastrointestinal tract when the client is unable to eat by mouth, such as after massive head and neck surgery or when swallowing is impaired. Tube feedings are administered through soft, flexible tubes that may be passed through the nose into the stomach or small intestine or inserted directly into the gastrointestinal tract during surgery (esophagostomy, gastrostomy, and jejunostomy). These surgically inserted feeding tubes have special nursing considerations, described in Chapters 47 and 50.

The nurse is responsible for administering the tube feeding. With malnutrition, diarrhea will develop if feedings are given too rapidly. When feedings are first initiated, the nutrients should be diluted in water and administered very slowly over 1 hour or continuously by a feeding pump. It may take 4 to 7 days before the client can tolerate the full amount of tube feeding necessary to meet nutritional requirements.

The nurse is also responsible for preventing complications of tube feeding. Plugging of the tube is prevented by flushing the tube with water periodically and after the administration of medications. Formula contamination is prevented by handling the formula and the administration setup carefully. Aspiration of formula into the lungs may be prevented by elevating the head of the bed, checking for tube placement, checking the amount of residual feeding remaining several hours after administration, and by responding to complaints of fullness. The nurse should ask the client whether any nausea, bloating, cramping, or sweating occurs in relation to the feeding. These and other

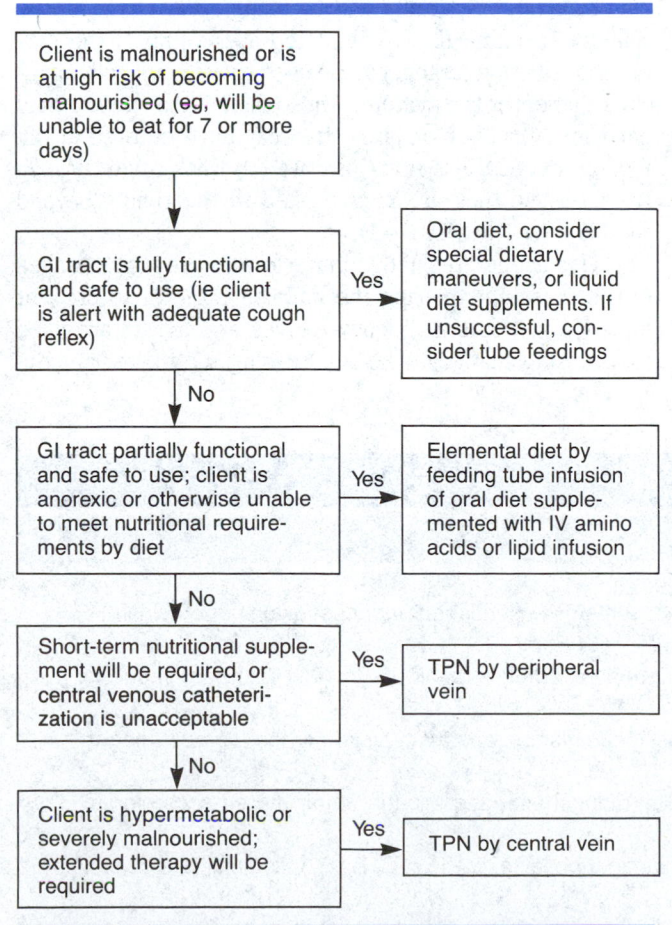

Figure 8–3

Factors in selection of nutritional therapy route.
SOURCE: Willard MD: *Nutrition for the Practicing Physician.* Baltimore, MD: Williams & Wilkins, 1982.

nursing responsibilities of tube feedings are described in detail in Chapter 47.

Total Parenteral Nutrition

When the gastrointestinal tract cannot be used to maintain good nutritional status, nutrients must be delivered intravenously. Gastrointestinal conditions such as major surgery, obstruction, or inflammation may impair the ability to digest and absorb nutrients adequately. When this occurs, nutrients can be administered directly into the vein on a short-term or long-term basis.

Total parenteral nutrition (TPN), also referred to as *hyperalimentation,* consists of the intravenous infusion of all necessary nutrients. The components of parenteral nutrition are outlined in Table 8–9. Carbohydrates in the form of dextrose, protein in the form of crystalline (synthetic) amino acids, electrolytes, vitamins, and minerals are mixed in a container. Intravenous fat emulsions, containing primarily essential fatty acids, are administered from a separate container because of problems with stability when mixed with the other components of the parenteral nutrition solution. The amount of parenteral nutrition and fat delivered varies with the individual nutritional needs. Nutritional status can be maintained indefinitely by the intravenous route.

The nurse plays an important role in the safe and effective administration of parenteral nutrition. Parenteral nutrition is administered by the nurse into peripheral or central (major) veins. Figure 8–4 illustrates a client receiving TPN through a central venous catheter inserted into the external jugular vein. Because the peripheral veins are easily irritated by high concentrations of dextrose, the amount of dextrose (or carbohydrate calories) that can be infused in the parenteral nutrition solution is limited. The peripheral veins can only tolerate up to a 10% dextrose solution (10 g dextrose per 100 mL of solution). Central veins tolerate dextrose better because of the high volume of blood flow. Usually, central parenteral nutrition solution contains 15% to 25% dextrose, allowing for a greater carbohydrate caloric intake.

Because of the dextrose concentration, parenteral nutrition is administered by an infusion pump (see Figure 8–4). The pump precisely regulates the rate of infusion, controlling the rate of dextrose administration. The proper rate of intravenous dextrose infusion will help regulate glucose homeostasis and cause an appropriate insulin response. Monitor blood and urine glucose to assess for blood glucose imbalances.

The nurse should also monitor fluid and electrolyte balance when administering parenteral nutrition. Initial weight gain is common because of the fluid intake. Weight should be monitored daily and daily records kept of fluid intake and output. Electrolyte balance is best assessed by monitoring serum levels.

Take measures to prevent contamination of the parenteral nutrition solution and the infusion catheter. Fungi grow readily in the parenteral solution and bacteria in the fat emulsion. Solutions and infusion tubing should be handled carefully, especially when setting up or changing the tubing. An inline filter, connected at the end of the parenteral nutrition tubing, can be used to collect small organisms that enter the system. These filters also collect small particles of rubber or glass that may have entered in the mixing process. Fat emulsions are too thick to go through the filter, so they are piggybacked to the tubing beyond the filter (see Figure 8–4).

Use aseptic technique in performing regular changes of the dressing covering the infusion catheter to prevent infection at this site. Ideally, gloves and masks are used for dressing changes. The old dressing is removed and the

Table 8–9 Components of Parenteral Nutrition	
Component	**Description**
Protein	Supplied as crystalline synthetic amino acids; contains essential and nonessential amino acids (4 calories/gram of protein; 1 gram nitrogen/6 grams protein)
Carbohydrate	Supplied as dextrose at 3.4 calories/gram. Peripheral administration 0% to 10% dextrose; central administration up to 50%, although usual is 20% to 25%
Electrolytes	Added to formula; can include sodium, potassium, chloride, acetate, calcium, phosphorous, magnesium; administered according to need
Minerals	Added to formula; can include zinc, chromium, manganese, and copper; administered according to need
Vitamins	Recommended allowances of vitamins A, thiamin, riboflavin, B_6, B_{12}, C, D, E, folic acid, niacin, biotin, and pantothenic acid*
Fat	Contains primarily essential fatty acids; requires separate container due to stability problems

*10 mL of MVI-12 (USV Labs) provides 100 mg ascorbic acid, 3300 IU vitamin A, 200 IU vitamin D, 10 IU vitamin E, 3 mg vitamin B_1, 3.6 mg vitamin B_2, 4 mg vitamin B_6, 40 mg niacinamide, 15 mg pantothenic acid, 60 mg biotin, 400 mg folic acid, and 5 mg vitamin B_{12}.

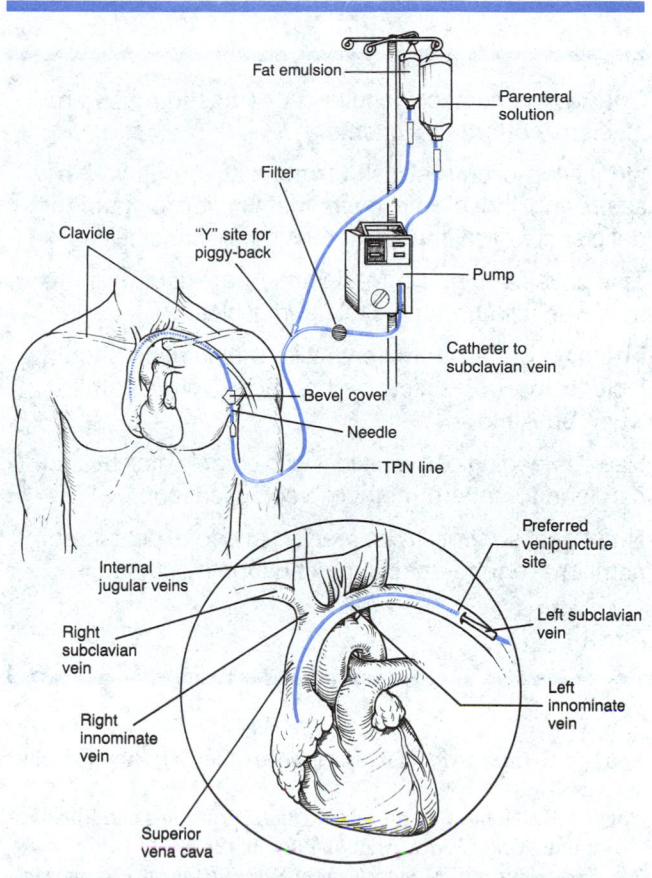

Fat emulsion

Parenteral solution

Filter

"Y" site for piggy-back

Clavicle

Pump

Catheter to subclavian vein

Bevel cover

Needle

TPN line

Preferred venipuncture site

Internal jugular veins

Left subclavian vein

Right subclavian vein

Left innominate vein

Right innominate vein

Superior vena cava

Figure 8–4

Total parenteral nutrition (TPN) through a central vein. The left subclavian vein is most commonly used because of its gentle arch.

site observed for redness or purulent drainage. An antiseptic solution such as povidone-iodine (Betadine) is used to cleanse the skin around the site, and an antiseptic ointment is applied at the site to prevent infection. A sterile dressing should be applied to cover and protect the infusion catheter site.

The client receiving TPN is at risk for a variety of complications. Some complications resulting from the procedure itself are air embolism, catheter misplacement, circulatory overload, pneumothorax, and hemothorax. Infection (both systemic and at the infusion site) is possible. Metabolic complications are possible, such as acidosis; hyperkalemia; hyperglycemia or hypoglycemia; HHND (hyperosmotic, hyperglycemic, nonketotic dehydration); hypermagnesemia, and deficiencies of sodium, magnesium, calcium, and phosphate; as well as prerenal azotemia.

Improving Bowel Elimination

Bowel elimination can be improved by an adequate dietary intake. Foods high in fiber content, such as bran cereals and muffins, whole grain breads and cereals, fruits, and vegetables add bulk to stool. Antidiarrheals, such as diphenoxylate hydrochloride (Lomotil) or kaolin–pectin mixture, may relieve diarrhea, especially during tube feedings. Fluids should be given to replace excess fluid loss from diarrhea, preventing dehydration.

Improving Volume Deficit

With potential dehydration, fluids should be administered to maintain fluid balance. Fluids are given orally or intravenously, depending on tolerance. Daily weights and fluid intake-and-output records will help to assess the client's fluid needs and response to fluid replacement.

Improving Self-Concept

The nurse can help the client's self-concept by facilitating an understanding of the physical changes of malnutrition. If the nurse emphasizes the positive effects of good nutrition, the client may be motivated to improve nutritional intake. The client should be allowed to ventilate feelings related to body image change.

Improving Skin Integrity

Improved nutritional status will improve skin integrity. Frequent position changes will prevent undue pressure at points where skin breakdown can occur. Measures should be taken to prevent infection at any skin breakdown sites. If skin excoriation develops from diarrhea, good hygiene should be encouraged following each loose stool.

EVALUATION

Malnutrition and/or nutrient deficiency have been corrected when laboratory results normalize and physical signs improve. Malnutrition, especially severe malnutrition, may take months to reverse. Along with reversing malnutrition, another expected outcome is maintaining adequate nutritional intake, whether by oral feeding, tube feeding, or intravenous feeding.

The frequency of bowel movements should diminish, and stools should approach a semisolid state. Bowel movements should assume a regular pattern. This problem may take time to reverse as nutritional status is improved.

Balanced fluid intake and output with good skin turgor and absence of edema are an expected outcome. The client should express knowledge of fluid balance and necessary intake.

Self-concept should improve in response to positive body changes as nutritional status improves.

Skin integrity should improve as the nutritional intake improves. Skin should be healthier and free of breakdown or infection.

Chapter Highlights

Malnutrition is a condition that results from a prolonged reduction of the supply of nutrients or improper utilization of nutrients in relation to demand. It affects all body systems.

Malnutrition is present in 25% to 50% of clients upon admission to the hospital; of those admitted well nourished, 25% to 30% will develop malnutrition during the hospitalization.

Malnutrition significantly contributes to the incidence of morbidity, mortality, and prolonged hospitalizations.

Malnutrition can result from physiological and psychosocial causes.

Disease states that alter the metabolism of nutrients can lead to malnutrition.

The incidence of infection greatly increases with malnutrition.

Chronic malnutrition results in decreased mass and efficiency of organ systems.

Identifying clients at risk for malnutrition as well as assessing those with overt malnutrition or nutrient deficiencies are important nursing responsibilities.

The physical signs of malnutrition are found in the hair, skin, mouth, and skeletal muscles.

The plan of care for clients with malnutrition should include the correction of the cause of malnutrition when possible.

Rapid refeeding of the patient with chronic malnutrition can lead to severe metabolic complications.

Nutritional support (tube feeding and total parenteral nutrition) require special precautions by nurses.

Bibliography

Anderson MA, Aker SN, Hickman RO: The double-lumen Hickman catheter. *Am J Nurs* 1982; 82:272–274.

Anderson L et al: *Nutrition in Health and Disease*. Philadelphia: Lippincott, 1982.

Baker DJ: Ten years of TPN at home. *Am J Nurs* 1984; 84:1248–1249.

Butterworth CE, Weinsier RL: Malnutrition in hospital patients: Assessment and treatment. Pages 667–684 in: *Modern Nutrition in Health and Disease*. Goodhart RS, Shils ME (editors). Philadelphia: Lea & Febiger, 1980.

Cerra FB: *Pocket Manual of Surgical Nutrition*. St. Louis: Mosby, 1984.

Friedman JD, Cerra FB: Impact of nutritional derangement on organ function. *Infections in Surgery* 1984; 217–221.

Gray GE, Gray LK: Anthropometric measurements and their interpretation: Principles, practices, and problems. *J Diet Assoc* 1980; 77:534–538.

Hennessy K: HHNK dehydration. *Am J Nurs* 1983; 83:1425–1426.

Herrmann CS: Performing intradermal skin tests the right way. *Nurs 83* 1983; 13:50–53.

Heymsfield SB: Metabolic changes associated with refeeding. *Aspen Update* 1982; 4(3):1–2.

Hui YH: *Human Nutrition and Diet Therapy*. Monterey, CA: Wadsworth, 1983.

Hutchison M McG: Administration of fat emulsions. *Am J Nurs* 1982; 82:275–277.

Jensen TG et al: Delayed hypersensitivity skin testing: Response rates in a surgical population. *J Am Diet Assoc* 1983; 82:17–23.

Morgan J: Nutritional assessment of critically ill patients. *Focus on Critical Care* 1984; 11(3):28–34.

Muller JM et al: Preoperative parenteral feeding in patients with gastrointestinal carcinoma. *Lancet* 1982; 63:68–71.

Nurses quick guide to nutritional disorders. *Nurs 83* 1983; 13:56–57.

Roe DA: *Geriatric Nutrition*. Englewood Cliffs, NJ: Prentice-Hall, 1983.

Rogers BL: Home Parenteral Nutrition: Principles and Management. *Nurse Pract* (March) 1984; 9:42–52.

The Treatment and Management of Severe Protein–Energy Malnutrition. Geneva: World Health Organization, 1981.

Weinsier RL, Butterworth CE: *Handbook of Clinical Nutrition*. St. Louis: Mosby, 1981.

Suggested Readings

Forlaw L, Bayer LM (editors): Nutrition. *Nurs Clin North Am* 1983; 18:1–128. This series of articles addresses nutrient metabolism and nutrition in specific disease states.

Forlaw L, Bayer L, Grant J: *Introduction to Nutritional and Physical Assessment of the Adult Patient for the Nurse*. (Monograph.) Washington, D.C.: American Society of Parenteral and Enteral Nutrition, 1983. A good basic overview of nutritional assessment.

Konstantinides NN: Home parenteral nutrition: A viable alternative for patients with cancer. *Oncology Nursing Forum* 1985; 12:23–29. Excellent source for helping clients and families prepare to administer parenteral nutrition at home.

Munro-Black J: The ABC's of total parenteral nutrition. *Nurs 84* 1984; 14:50–56. Specific nursing measures in administration and monitoring of parenteral nutrition, showing catheter insertion, setup of solution, and dressing change.

Strotts NA, Friesen L: Understanding starvation in the critically ill patient. *Heart Lung* 1982; 11:469–478. How the physiological stress from critical illness causes malnutrition.

Teitelman R: Skeletons in the closet. *Forbes* (April 9) 1983; 133:156–157. An economic examination of the problem of hospital malnutrition.

Chapter 9

Obesity and Eating Disorders

Barbara Tobias Shirk
Lyn Marshall
Carol Ren Kneisl

Objectives

When you have finished studying this chapter, you should be able to:

Differentiate between obesity and overweight.

Define anorexia nervosa and bulimia.

Explain how environment, biology, and psychological aspects interact in the development of obesity.

Identify three theories of development related to eating disorders.

Cite the major health problems caused by obesity.

State the physical effects and psychological disturbances of anorexia and bulimia.

Collect appropriate subjective and objective data for nursing assessment.

Select appropriate nursing diagnoses.

Outline a comprehensive treatment program.

Use the problem-solving method to guide the client through the implementation and evaluation processes.

Eating is the focus of our physical, emotional, and social lives. Food means more than sustenance. It is an expression of love and comfort and a means of reward and punishment. Nourishment is an important part of bonding between mother and infant. In child-rearing, food may be used as a tool to modify behavior, and parent–child relationships take shape during mealtime. Social rituals, such as holidays, weddings, and funerals, are marked by lavish meals in which food may take on a symbolic meaning.

The emphasis on food is strong, but the value placed on physical appearance is equally strong, particularly for women. Although the ideal form for men has changed little since the ancient Greeks, the ideal female form has shifted with fashion. Slim and ample figures have been in and out of vogue. The full, fecund female form was immortalized by the 16th century painter Rubens and the Victorian Gibson Girl. In contemporary Western society, thin is the ideal, particularly for the middle and upper classes. The attitude "never too thin or too rich" is heavily reinforced by advertising and entertainment. There is a cultlike devotion to achieving the appropriate shape through diet and exercise.

Considering the emotional and psychological investment in eating and physical appearance, it is not surprising that obesity and eating disorders are serious health problems. Until recently, obesity received only perfunctory attention from health professionals. Now this pervasive problem is known to be a high risk factor for a variety of disorders such as diabetes and coronary artery disease. Considerable attention has also been focused on two unusual eating disorders—anorexia nervosa and bulimia. Affecting primarily young women, both anorexia nervosa and bulimia seem to be on the increase. This chapter provides an overview of obesity and eating disorders and the appropriate nursing care.

Section I: Obesity

A problem for all age groups, obesity is not limited by social, economic, or ethnic boundaries. The terms *obesity* and *overweight* are not synonymous. **Obesity** is an excess of relative body fat; **overweight** is an excess in body weight. *Morbid obesity* is the maintenance of 100 lb over ideal body weight for 1 year.

Obesity is common. In the United States, an estimated 7 million men (13%) and 14 million women (22%) between the ages of 20 and 74 are obese and overweight. More women are classified as obese across all age groups. The incidence of obesity rises for women between the ages of 34 and 44 years and for men between the ages of 20 and 34 years (Abraham, Carroll, Najjar, & Fulwood, 1983). Demographic studies have shown obesity to be correlated with lower social economic groups, particularly for women. However, the prevalence of obesity is not correlated with either race or culture in the United States or in western Europe.

CLASSIFICATION

Obesity is classified according to adipose tissue morphology (structure and form); age of onset; and definition. The terms describing tissue morphology are **hypertrophy**, an increase in the size of a fat cell, and **hyperplasia**, an increase in the number of fat cells. Hyperplasia–hypertrophy is an increase in both the size and number of fat cells. The terms *juvenile* and *adult* refer to the age at onset. Juvenile onset obesity begins between the ages of 32 weeks' gestation and 15 years. Adult onset obesity begins after age 15. There is a correlation between age of onset and tissue morphology. Juvenile onset obesity is also known as hypertrophy–hyperplasia; adult onset obesity is denoted as hypertrophy. By definition, individuals are classified as overweight–not obese, obese–overweight, obese–not overweight, and other combinations suitable to specific conditions. For example, a well-conditioned athlete may weigh far more than the norm for his ideal body weight but have less body fat content than normal. He would be termed overweight–not obese. A young mother's weight may be near her ideal body weight, but her body may contain a larger percentage of fat. She would be classified as obese–not overweight.

FAT FORMATION

The overconsumption of fats, proteins, and carbohydrates, in any combination, promotes the development of adipose tissue. Since fat is the primary substrate in the formation of adipose tissue, fat digestion, fat assimilation, and fat storage are important to understand.

Fat is digested primarily in the small intestine through the interaction of bile and pancreatic lipase upon the fat molecule, resulting in degradation to monoglycerides, glycerol, and free fatty acids. Other lipases in the saliva and stomach have only a small effect on fat digestion. However, when the pancreas fails to secrete pancreatic lipase into the small intestine, the client experiences **steatorrhea** (bulky, clay-colored, fatty stools; see also Unit Eight). About 97% of the fat is absorbed. During the absorption through the villi in the intestinal wall, monoglycerides, glycerol, and free fatty acids are resynthesized into triglycerides. Cholesterol follows a similar digestive and absorption process. Then the triglycerides combine with cholesterol and phospholipids to form chylomicrons. The chylomicrons, carried in the lymph system, enter the venous circulation at the juncture of the jugular and the subclavian veins. The circulating chylomicrons are quickly taken up by the adipocytes with the aid of lipoprotein lipase (LPL). LPL is an enzyme that hydrolizes (splits) the chylomicrons into free fatty acids and glycerol and facilitates their absorption into the cells and their conversion to triglycerides within the cell for storage. In a similar fashion, insu-

Nursing Research Note

Salter E, Golden M: Obesity in lower and middle socioeconomic status mothers and their children. *Res Nurs Health* 1985; 8(2):147–153.

The relation between child and maternal obesity, socioeconomic status, maternal nutritional knowledge, and locus of control were studied. Two socioeconomic groups, middle and lower status, were compared by examining maternal obesity, child obesity, maternal locus of control, and maternal nutritional knowledge.

The results demonstrated that mothers of lower socioeconomic status on the average were significantly heavier than middle-class mothers. Children from lower socioeconomic levels were not significantly more overweight than the middle-class group; however, there was a trend toward obesity in the lower-status sample. The amount of adiposity in mothers and children from the lower socioeconomic group was significantly correlated. This was not the case for the middle-class sample. Mothers of lower socioeconomic status scored lower on nutritional knowldge tests and were found to be more external in their locus of control.

This study suggests that in lower-status families, there is a greater trend toward obesity. Nursing intervention for clients of lower socioeconomic status may need to center on nutritional education, developing clients' beliefs that they can control their own body weight, and guidance for nutritional planning for the entire family.

lin acts upon glucose, providing the necessary substrate to complete triglyceride formation within the cell.

When the fat is needed for energy, lipases in the adipocyte convert the stored triglycerides into free fatty acids and aid in their extrusion across the cell membrane for assimilation into the blood serum. Fatty acids, reformed as triglycerides, are transported to the liver, where hydrolization again takes place, providing fatty acids and glycerol for cellular energy. Excess serum glucose and excess serum protein, not needed for energy, are also converted by the liver into triglycerides and subsequently stored as fat (Guyton, 1981).

CAUSES OF OBESITY

Obesity is a complex, multidimensional problem. Vigorous investigation of the obesity problem in the past 20 years has generated considerable controversy. The etiology of obesity is central to this debate because effective classification and treatment depend on its determination. The possible physiological and psychosocial causes of obesity are discussed below and outlined in Box 9–1.

Physiological Causes

Genetics

Heredity and environment are so closely intertwined in the developmental process that it is difficult to discern which component is dominant. In rare instances, single gene defects and other genetic deficiencies cause obesity. More prevalent causes are lineage (family genes) and somatotype (body configuration). Succeeding generations within a family follow similar patterns of weight gain and body fat accumulation. Studies show that three-fourths of the children of two obese parents will be obese, but only one-tenth of the children of two lean parents will be obese. Studies of fraternal twins reared together showed significant weight differences. Identical twins reared together had minimal weight differences when compared to identical twins reared apart, who showed marked differences in weight. The weight of adopted children does not correlate with that of adoptive parents or siblings. Inconsistent results of these and similar studies indicate the difficulty of separating the effects of environment and heredity (Greenwood & Turhenkopf, 1983).

Differences in somatotype are genetic and sex specific. Males generally have a larger muscle mass and larger bones than females. In the android body configuration, characteristic of males, fat is deposited in the arms, chest, and abdomen. Excessive fat deposits usually accumulate in the abdomen, surround the viscera, and cover the abdominal surface. In the gynoid configuration of females, the fatty deposits are found in the breasts, hips, upper thighs, and gluteal regions. Although somatotypes are useful

Box 9–1 Possible Causes of Obesity
Physiological
Familial predisposition
Inherited body configuration
Defect in hypothalamus
Imbalance between energy intake and output
Defect in metabolism
Individual setpoint for body weight
Psychosocial
Excess caloric intake
Inappropriate eating behaviors
Stimulation by advertising and availability of fast foods
Learned family eating patterns and food preferences
Sedentary lifestyles
Response to emotional experiences
Life stresses

descriptors of body shapes, the actual assessment of body fat content is best accomplished by other methods, such as skinfold measurements described in Chapter 8.

Hunger and Satiety

Hunger is defined as a physiological response to the lack of food, characterized by distressful sensations in the epigastric area coinciding with contractions of the stomach. *Appetite* is more cerebral and can be present without hunger sensations. The thought of food results in a pleasant sensation. *Satiety* is a sense of physiological fullness.

Until recently, hunger and satiety centers were thought to be located solely in a specific area of the hypothalamus (the hunger center in the lateral hypothalamus and the satiety center in the ventromedial nuclei) and that stimulation of the hunger center initiated food-seeking behaviors, whereas stimulation of the satiety center inhibited feeding. The hypothalamus is presently viewed as an integrating and control center for the autonomic nervous system and the neurohormones. (See Unit 6 for a complete discussion of the neurologic system.)

Other areas of the brain such as the brainstem are now known to be involved. The mechanical aspects of feeding, chewing, salivation, and swallowing are controlled by the brainstem. These movements also occur when the limbic area, contiguous with the hypothalamus, is stimulated. Stimulation of the cortical area of the limbic system perpetuates food-seeking behaviors, without regard to either hunger or satiety. Stimulation of the amygdaloid body induces autonomic nervous system responses of gastrointestinal motility and both inhibition and excitation of gastric secretions.

Other biological factors are involved in regulating hunger and satiety. They are stimulated and inhibited by fluctuations in blood serum levels of glucose, amino acids, free fatty acids, blood temperature, insulin, and gastrointestinal secretions. The level of free fatty acids in the serum is thought to be the most influential long-term regulator. Chewing, swallowing, and tasting also influence the satiety center.

Current neuroendocrine research proposes that the hunger and satiety areas serve only as integrating sites for neurological and hormonal input. The neuroreceptors, neurotransmitters, and neuromodulators affect food-seeking behaviors. Of the neurotransmitters, some monamines (dopamine, alpha-agonists) and the peptides (enkephalins, endorphins, and dynorphin) increase food-seeking behaviors. Other monoamines and peptides (serotonin, beta-agonists, cholecystokinin, bombesin, and calcitonin) inhibit food-seeking. Six neuropeptides are also classified as food-seeking inhibitors: thyrotropin releasing hormone, histidylproline diketopiperazine, pancreatic polypeptide, glucagon, somatostatin, and insulin (Morley & Levine, 1982). These substances and their effects are summarized in Table 9–1. The complex interaction between the neurotransmitters themselves, the neuromodulators, and the other substrates (choline, tryptephan, acetylcholine, and many more) is currently being studied. Experiments with rats have demonstrated changes in food-seeking behaviors when the autonomic nerve fibers are severed, when endogenous opiates are introduced directly into the rats' brains, and when rats were subjected to psychic stress. In humans, brain tumors and trauma have induced changes in food-related behavior. Although the physiology of hunger and satiety are not clearly understood, evidence suggests that these endogenous components have a major role.

Energy Balance

In the energy equation, energy intake equal to energy output yields a stable body weight. Any change in caloric intake or caloric expenditure will affect body weight. Weight is gained when caloric intake is increased, energy expenditure is decreased, or both. Conversely, weight is lost when caloric intake is decreased, caloric expenditure is increased, or both. Energy balance is sensitive to small changes. A pound of body fat contains 3500 calories. Elimination of 250 calories from the daily caloric intake while holding the energy expenditure constant will result in a weight loss of 1 lb in 14 days ($3500 \div 250 = 14$).

Thermogenesis

Food-seeking behaviors are inhibited by the thermal effect of eating. All metabolic processes produce heat (thermogenesis). The exact mechanism for heat production after eating a meal is not completely understood. Two mechanisms thought to contribute to the thermal effect are the mechanical activity of the stomach during digestion and the oxidation of food substrate in the gut. Heat is also produced in the liver as an outcome of metabolism of amino acids and fats. The consumption of a high-carbohydrate diet produces more heat than a diet high in fat.

The brown fat theory offers an explanation of why some individuals are able to ingest large numbers of calories without appreciable weight gain while others who eat fewer calories in proportion to body mass gain weight. Brown fat is a type of adipose tissue found in rodents, hibernating animals, and various other mammals including human embryos and newborns. The theory is based on rat experiments, and its application to humans is controversial.

Table 9–1 Endogenous Substances Thought to Be Involved in Appetite Regulation

	↑ Feeding	↓ Feeding
Monoamines	Dopamine Alpha-agonists	Serotonin Beta-agonists
Peptides	Enkephalins Endorphins Dynorphin	Cholecystokinin Bombesin Calcitonin Thyrotropin releasing hormone Histidylproline diketopiperazine Pancreatic polypeptide Glucagon Somatostatin Insulin (central)
Miscellaneous	Gamma-amino butyric acid (Muscimol)	Glucose Fatty acids Amino acids

In rats, stimulation of brown fat by the sympathetic nervous system increases the metabolic rate of the brown fat cells, increasing the production and dissipation of heat. Thus, the excess energy is expended and not stored as fat. This physiological response is activated by exposure to cold and by overeating. Prolonged activation of the brown fat mass causes hyperplasia of the tissue, promoting greater energy loss.

The thermogenesis induced by overeating is inactivated by a defect in any part of the hypothalamus, the sympathetic nervous system, or the brown fat tissue mass. Rats unable to induce thermogenesis eat ravenously and become obese. Moreover, genetically obese rats, which are incapable of diet-induced thermogenesis, become even more obese with overfeeding.

From these observations in rats, experts have theorized that obesity in humans may be the result of similar defects. Applying the theory to humans is difficult, however, because techniques for determining brown fat content are not adequately developed. In addition, humans lose the bulk of their brown fat before adolescence, and it is not known if a sufficient amount remains to expend enough energy to prevent obesity in adults (Himms-Hagen, 1983).

Setpoint Theory
Also known as the lipostat theory, ponderstat theory, or apostat theory, this theory proposes that the body has an internal control mechanism, called a *setpoint,* located in some yet-to-be-determined portion of the brain. Exactly how the setpoint is established is unknown. The essential element of the theory is that each person has a set amount of body fat mass determined by genetic and biological factors. Whenever the body fat mass changes above or below the setpoint, the body adjusts its metabolic rate to keep the percentage of fatty tissue the same. The setpoint may be altered, or reset permanently, if the changed body mass is maintained over an extended period of time.

This anatomy-is-destiny theory is controversial. Proponents argue that other physiological processes, such as blood glucose and body temperature, are regulated by similar mechanisms. Additional support for the theory comes from studies in which one group increased weight 15% to 25% by overfeeding, whereas another group reduced theirs by 25% by restricting food intake. When all subjects ate as they wished, all returned to their original weights. Two other studies showed that morbidly obese persons who lost weight regained it within 2 to 5 years (Keesey, 1980).

On the other hand, flaws in the theory are cited. Some people who lose weight maintain the reduced weight. Also, the average weight of the Western population has increased over the past 30 years, as shown by changes in the standard weights in the Metropolitan Life Insurance Company tables (see Chapter 8). Furthermore, studies have found that although disruptions of the hypothalamus cause hyperphagia, eating patterns return almost to normal within several weeks. Obesity caused by hyperphagia continued only

if the food was highly palatable; with a nonpalatable diet, weight returned to normal.

Psychosocial Causes

Psychological Causes
The psychological causes of obesity have not been delineated. No specific personality pattern or personality disorder seems to characterize the obese. Well-controlled studies have failed to find evidence that individual characteristics of the obese differ from those of the nonobese either in psychological or psychiatric examinations. On the other hand, one psychiatrist (Bruch, 1973), in a now classic work, considers juvenile onset obesity to be developmental, a response to flawed family relationships. Bruch sees adult onset obesity as a response to a crisis or trauma.

Many obese people have low self-esteem and a poor self-concept, reflecting societal opinion and family and peer pressure. They may be socially isolated, unable and unwilling to subject themselves to society's ridicule. They may participate minimally in life and have low-paying jobs. They may feel ashamed. They may believe they have a disease. Some find self-destruction the answer. In contrast, other

---

Nursing Research Note

Wineman NM: Obesity: Locus of control, body image, weight loss and age-at-onset. *Nurs Res* 1980; 29(4):231–237.

Psychological characteristics of the obese individual were studied to ascertain whether there are subgroups within the obese population. Age-at-onset subgroups were defined as childhood onset, adolescent onset, and adulthood onset. Locus of control, body image, and weight loss were studied in subjects with these subgroup age onsets.

The results indicated that age at onset was not significantly related to sex, percentage of overweight, length of time in a weight-loss group, or social status. There was no significant relation among weight-loss success, time of joining a weight-loss program, and age at onset. Age at onset and time of joining the weight-loss group were not significantly affected by locus of control. Statistically significant results were isolated for body image and age at onset by time joined. That is, the older members of weight-loss groups with adolescent onset had a greater degree of satisfaction with their bodies. Adolescent-onset subjects with recent membership in a weight-loss group had the least satisfaction with their body image. Older members with adult onset had lower satisfaction, whereas new members with adult onset had higher satisfaction. In addition, there was no relation between locus of control and weight loss in all the subgroups. Men exhibited a greater degree of satisfaction with their bodies than women. Men also exhibited a greater weight loss.

This research addresses some factors that may lead to obesity. If a developmental link exists between obesity in childhood and adolescence and if life events in adulthood can lead to obesity, nursing intervention must be directed at these links to be effective. A developmental age-at-onset assessment might provide clues for treatment.

obese persons have a positive attitude, viewing themselves as powerful, important, sensuous, attractive, intelligent, and affectionate. The National Association to Aid Fat Americans has as its motto, "Fat is beautiful."

Overeating is categorized as an addictive behavior similar to alcoholism and drug addiction. The discovery that food metabolism causes release of natural opiates supports this contention. The intake of alcohol, drugs, and food elicits the same set of physiological responses. The person feels warm, relaxed, and euphoric. These pleasant feelings are easily replicable. Such pleasure is difficult to deny one's self, particularly when society approves and promotes excessive food intake. In addition, obesity may be a means of maintaining emotional equilibrium. Obese people report eating because of feelings of loneliness, frustration, boredom, guilt, depression, anxiety, insecurity, and changes in their personal relationships. They eat to cope with life's stresses. They also eat to celebrate the positive aspects of life (Cozens, 1982). Some think the obese may use their corpulence as a shield from others, a protective device. Therefore, they suggest that moderately obese people who are emotionally stable and happy should not be urged to lose weight unless they are at risk for a life-threatening disease.

Environmental Causes

The diet consumed by many overweight people is higher than recommended in fats, proteins, and simple carbohydrates and lower than recommended in complex starches. Although they may have decreased the actual amount of food consumed, they have increased the caloric content. This excessive caloric intake coupled with a sedentary lifestyle promote obesity.

Cues for eating are the availability, the sight, the smell, and the taste of food. Inability to resist these stimuli results in inappropriate eating behaviors. Research has shown that food intake is excessive when foods are eaten fast, not chewed thoroughly, eaten in large bites, and not savored.

Highly palatable, high calorie foods are available everywhere in supermarkets, fast food restaurants, gas stations, and laundromats. Examples are chocolate, chips, candy, and soft drinks. More people eat away from home than ever before. The proliferation of fast food and specialty restaurants reflects this trend. In the home, appliances to store and prepare food promote consumption. Advertising in magazines, newspapers, and particularly television commercials, emphasizes the desirability of preparing and eating foods. Cookbooks are often among the ten best sellers.

Cultural Causes

Behaviors, beliefs, and attitudes are influenced by social, cultural, and family mores. Eating is a central social activity throughout society and across cultures. Religious and national holidays are celebrated with feasts. In some cultures, a fat wife confers social status on the husband, and obesity is an acceptable condition. These ethnic standards

are usually acculturated into the American's norms within one generation (Friemer, Echenberg, & Kretchmer, 1983). Beliefs promote overfeeding. Examples are the belief that a fat baby is a healthy baby and that carbohydrates give energy. Adults who require children to clean their plates and offer food as a comfort or reward teach children to eat when they are not hungry. They learn to respond to life situations by eating. Children also learn family eating patterns, food preferences, and food preparation. These learned behaviors are retained in adulthood and passed to the next generation. It is not unusual for most members of a nuclear family and many members of their extended families to be obese.

Sedentary lifestyles have developed over the past 30 years with automation. Labor-saving devices in the home and workplace as well as passive entertainment have reduced energy expenditure. Spectator sports have replaced active participation for many. The fitness revolution seems to have attracted those persons who tend to be active participants regardless; it has not significantly increased the overall number of active people.

OBESITY AS A MULTISYSTEM STRESSOR

Obesity is a stressor to all body systems. An obese person is at greater risk for health-related problems than a person of normal weight. Obesity is identified as a major risk factor for gallstones and Type II diabetes. It contributes to coronary artery disease; congestive heart failure; hypertension; and cancers of the breast, uterus, prostate, and colon. Obesity also aggravates arthritis, low back pain, stress incontinence, varicosities, and thrombophlebitis. In addition, obesity impairs pulmonary function and wound healing, and promotes wound dehiscence. The major health problems associated with obesity are discussed here. These and other health-related problems are listed in Box 9–2.

Cardiovascular System

Atherosclerosis

Obesity is well documented as a risk factor for atherosclerosis, the major cause of coronary artery disease. Atherosclerosis is characterized by narrowing of the lumen of a coronary artery or by total obstruction (see Chapter 24). Degenerative changes in the intima are followed by deposits of fibrous materials and fat, composed primarily of cholesterol. Over time the plaque formation accumulates, decreasing the diameter of the lumen, increasing peripheral resistance, and reducing blood flow (Guyton, 1981).

In the obese state, high density lipoprotein (HDL) serum levels are reduced. The primary role of HDL is to transport cholesterol from the peripheral tissue to the liver. A deficiency of HDL promotes high serum levels of cholesterol, providing substrate for plaque formation. Low HDL serum levels are thought to occur in the following way. The enlarged fat mass and increased number of hypertrophied fat cells—which are highly active metabolically—rapidly break down the HDL. Concurrently, the liver produces less HDL. The HDL is also redistributed in the vascular spaces. In addition, ingestion of a high-carbohydrate, high-fat diet promotes low-density lipoprotein (LDL) production in the liver. Because LDL serves as the transport system for cholesterol from the liver to the peripheral tissues, additional cholesterol is provided for plaque formation. Excessive caloric intake also causes overproduction of very low-density lipoproteins (VLDL) from the breakdown of excessive triglycerides. Large quantities of circulating VLDL also contribute to plaque deposits (Morlin, 1984).

Serum cholesterol levels in the obese are often elevated. Contrary to common belief that excessive ingestion of exogenous cholesterol causes this problem, diets high in saturated fats are more of a contributing factor. Saturated fats stimulate the liver to produce cholesterol. Cholesterol is also produced in the small intestine. Although extremes in cholesterol ingestion can affect blood serum levels, the liver maintains balance by regulating the ratio of endogenous cholesterol to the exogenous amount ingested. Therefore, many authorities dispute the use of a low cholesterol diet as treatment for high cholesterol levels. This remains a controversial issue.

Hypertension

There is no direct correlation between obesity and high blood pressure; as many obese persons have hypertension as those who do not. In the massively obese, the heart and the kidneys enlarge. This compensatory enlargement facilitates normotension. Often the diagnosis of hypertension is based on inaccurate measurements made by using an inappropriately sized cuff and by placing the cuff incorrectly on the upper arm. Elevated blood pressure indicates increased peripheral resistance. It is unclear if the increased peripheral resistance is in response to the expanded intravascular volume accompanying the enlarged body mass or if it is secondary to increased cardiac output and other autoregulatory mechanisms. Some studies are finding that a decrease in body weight results in a decrease in blood pressure.

Congestive Heart Failure

In the obese, the highly vascular fat mass, with the increased metabolic activity of the hypertrophied fat cells, increases demand for cardiac output. As the stroke volume increases, the left ventricle dilates, causing the myocardium of the posterior walls and septum to thicken. Eventually, left ventricle function is impaired, progressing to congestive heart failure.

Respiratory System

Obese persons often experience respiratory difficulties upon exertion. The extra fat and concomitant decrease in mobility hinder ventilation, making the obese more susceptible to postoperative complications such as atelectasis and

Box 9–2 Health-Related Problems in Obesity

Atherosclerosis

Cardiac enlargement

Kidney enlargement

Congestive heart failure

Diabetes mellitus, Type II

Impaired pulmonary function

Hypertension

Hiatus hernia

Cholecystitis and cholelithiasis

Prolonged labor and delivery

Pregnancy-induced hypertension

Arthritis

Chronic renal failure

Arteriosclerosis

Higher incidence of postoperative complications such as pneumonia, atelectasis, wound dehiscence or evisceration, thrombosis, embolism

Cancers of the breast, uterus, prostate, and colon

Low back pain

Muscle sprains and strains

Stress incontinence

Varicosities

Thrombophlebitis

pneumonia. In addition, obese persons with pickwickian syndrome are subject to a number of severe and uncomfortable respiratory problems such as hypoventilation and periodic respirations. The syndrome is also characterized by somnolence, twitching, cyanosis, polycythemia, right ventricular hypertrophy, and heart failure. Marked improvements occur with diuresis and weight loss.

Endocrine System

Truncal obesity (obesity of the trunk of the body), hypertrophied fat cells, genetic predisposition, and the lack of exercise are factors in the development of adult onset noninsulin-dependent (Type II) diabetes. Two physiological mechanisms contribute to the insulin resistance of fat, liver, and skeletal muscle cells:

1. The cells become less sensitive to glucose as a result of diminished receptor sites on the cell surface.

2. There is a defect in glucose metabolism within the cell.

These conditions, combined with a high-fat, high-carbohydrate intake, create higher than normal serum plasma levels of triglycerides, glucose, and insulin. This produces overt symptoms of glucose intolerance.

Thyroid hormone, cortisol, and growth hormone are also factors in obesity. Both cortisol and growth hormone are decreased during the weight-gaining phase and during maintenance of massive obesity. Less growth hormone promotes fat storage by inhibiting lipolysis. In addition, evidence suggests that low cortisol levels cause an increase in gluconeogenesis, lipogenesis, and fat storage while depressing fat utilization.

Overeating a high-carbohydrate diet causes an increase in triiodothyronine (T_3) and a decrease in reverse-triiodothyronine (rT_3) with no change in thyroxine (T_4). Thyroid hormones do not respond to high fat meals. Changes do occur, however, when food is restricted: T_3 values decrease and rT_3 values increase. There is no concurrent increase in thermogenesis. During weight loss, adaptation to lower levels of T_3 slows the basic metabolic rate, and energy requirements decrease. Therefore, lipolysis is slowed, and weight loss slows or reaches a plateau. The body uses calories far more efficiently; fewer need to be taken in to maintain weight, and more must be cut back to achieve weight loss.

TREATMENT OF OBESITY

The treatment of the obese person is rewarding when the client successfully loses weight and frustrating when the client is unable to do so. Throughout their lives, many persons gain and lose weight on a regular cycle (the yo-yo syndrome). The problem often seems insurmountable. A variety of treatments have been used with minimal success. Presently, bariatric specialists (health professionals who focus on the problems of obesity) recommend a lifestyle that incorporates changes in food intake and physical activity. A comprehensive program includes an eating plan for weight loss and long-term maintenance, physical exercise, behavioral change, social support, and cognitive restructuring. Surgical interventions and drug therapies are other possibilities.

Motivation is a stimulus to change actions or behavior. Each individual is spurred by unique, specific needs and perceptions that are often subconscious. Many persons cite health problems as reasons for losing weight, such as diabetes, hypertension, angina, or arthritis. Others are motivated by psychological or emotional problems (eg, feelings of embarrassment, social isolation, shame, and guilt). Still others find motivation in the wish to purchase fashionable clothing, wear bathing suits, or attract the opposite sex. These motives are usually effective only until the problems or feelings have been resolved. During the weight loss process, additional motivators must be found to meet the long-term goals of achieving ideal body weight and weight maintenance. Assisting clients to develop awareness of their needs is helpful. At the beginning of their weight loss program, ask them to list reasons for losing weight and to add to this list as they proceed through the program. Motives should be reviewed daily, particularly when tempted and when making difficult choices.

Regulation of Food Intake

The regulation of food intake is the cornerstone of a weight-loss program. Weight is lost when energy intake is less than energy expenditure. In this text, the term *dieting* is avoided because it connotes short-term behaviors that usually have little success. In fact, it may be that repeated dieting causing the yo-yo effect causes the greatest health risk.

The variety of weight-loss plans is almost unlimited. Restricted food plans proliferate in popular magazines and books. Most of these fad diets lack nutrients and, therefore, are detrimental when followed for more than a few weeks. In the 1970s, a liquid protein diet consisting of hydrolized gelatin and collagen but deficient in essential amino acids, caused more than 50 deaths (almost all of which were linked to cardiac dysrhythmias). Usually, these plans are found to be boring and unsatisfying and are not continued more than a few weeks. This perpetuates the yo-yo syndrome and reinforces feelings of failure and inadequacy. Nutritional instruction focused on long-term weight maintenance assists a client to view changes in behavior as permanent. Patience and persistence are required for long-term adherence to an eating plan. A brief discussion of the more popular eating plans is presented below and summarized in Table 9–2.

Fasting

Short-term fasting that omits solid foods for several days or weeks is one treatment approach. It is essential to provide nutrient supplements for fasting clients and to encourage adequate fluid intake to avoid dehydration. Fasting is usually prescribed for the massively obese (50% to 100% above ideal body weight) and is conducted in a supervised inpatient setting.

Protein-Sparing Modified Fast

The protein-sparing modified fast uses high biological protein in the form of fish, fowl, and lean meat as the only energy source. The protein is supplemented with multivitamins with iron, calcium, potassium, and large quantities of fluids. The stored body carbohydrates in the liver and muscle are depleted and, finally, fat is used for energy. Ketosis develops, promoting anorexia so the client does not experience hunger. Weight loss that occurs during the first two weeks is from diuresis; loss then tapers to an average of 3 to 4 lb per week. Electrolyte imbalance, hyperuricemia, kidney stones, and cardiac arrhythmias are potential problems. Adherence to the plan is recommended for approximately 3 months under the careful supervision of a health professional, so that electrolytes and electrocardiogram results can be closely monitored.

Low-Carbohydrate Plans

In the most popular versions of the low carbohydrate diets, carbohydrate intake is limited to 60 g or less and combined with either unlimited fat or unlimited protein food sources.

Table 9–2   Types of Restricted Diets Used for Weight Reduction (*Note that most of the diets are not safe or effective*)

Diet Type	Description	Possible Health Effects
Balanced diets of 1200 kcal or more	Usually consist of ordinary, readily available, high-nutrient-density foods in limited amounts; often moderate in protein and carbohydrate and most restricted in fat	Can meet the RDA if carefully chosen; weight loss is usually 1–2 lb per week; can be liberalized to stabilize weight for safe lifetime use
Diets of fewer than 1200 kcal	Usually composed of ordinary, readily available, high-nutrient-density foods in very limited amounts; often moderate in protein and very restricted in fat and carbohydrate	Diet often fails to meet the RDA for many nutrients; ketosis may occur; weight loss is often 3 or more pounds per week, much due to water loss; regain is more likely than with slower weight loss
High-carbohydrate, high-fiber diets	Emphasize whole grain breads, cereals, raw fruits and vegetables, moderate amounts of animal proteins, dairy products, avoidance of highly processed foods; supplemental fiber is sometimes recommended	Calculated nutrient intake is nearly adequate, but fiber (especially if supplemented) may reduce availability of minerals
Formula low-kcal diets	Powders, liquids, or wafers constitute diet of 1000 kcal with supplemented vitamins and minerals; provide 20% protein, 30% fat, and 50% carbohydrate	Adequate in vitamins and minerals; may be constipating; ketosis may occur; requires no food choice decisions or contact with food; often discontinued due to monotony or unpalatability; weight regain is likely because old eating habits remain; more acceptable as one meal per day within a low-kcal diet plan
Low-carbohydrate, high-protein, high- or moderate-fat diets	Emphasize high-protein foods, severely limit carbohydrate to 50 g; usually low in kcal because allowed foods become unappealing	Diet may meet RDA if chosen carefully; ketosis occurs, causing fluid loss; can cause increase in blood fat and cholesterol levels; may cause menstrual dysfunction, dehydration, osteoporosis, aggravation of gout, kidney failure or stones; much of lost weight due to water loss
One-food diets	Emphasize one food or food type, such as fruit, rice, or ice cream, as mainstay of the diet	Inevitably deficient in some nutrients, excessive in others; discarded quickly because of monotony; lost weight regained
Fasting	Water and no-kcal beverages allowed; vitamin and mineral supplements given; person usually hospitalized for monitoring	May result in nutrient deficiencies, low blood pressure, ketosis, emotional disturbances; death may result if prolonged; causes weight loss of 3–5 lb per week; regain begins when person begins eating again but has not learned new eating behaviors; former weight usually regained in time
Protein-supplemented fasting	Like fast, but with protein supplement of up to 1.5 g/kg of ideal body weight; protein in form of lean animal products, liquid protein isolates, or amino acids	May result in ketosis, nausea and vomiting, diarrhea or constipation, weakness, muscle cramps, mineral imbalance, irritability; former weight usually regained in time; over 50 deaths attributed to use of over-the-counter liquid protein products

SOURCE: Christian JL, Greger JL: *Nutrition for Living.* Menlo Park, CA: Benjamin-Cummings, 1985, pp. 248–249.

Advocates of these low-carbohydrate diets believe that the development of ketosis and anorexia will limit the protein and fat intake.

The protein diet provides essential amino acids for tissue maintenance and energy. Excessive protein calories above energy needs will be stored as fat, however. Fat intake in the form of large amounts of unsaturated oils is unpalatable and calorically dense. With both plans, the caloric deficits are small, producing minimal weight loss. The adverse effects of these plans are similar to those of the protein-sparing modified fast.

Very Low Carbohydrate Plans

Very low carbohydrate plans comprise 30 to 45 g of carbohydrate daily with either high biological protein or a formula diet (eg, Cambridge and Optifast, which also contain essential amino acids). These plans avoid adverse side effects and facilitate weight loss in the massively obese. The formula plans are supplemented by one 600-calorie meal per day. Supporters of these programs point out that they preserve anorexia and nitrogen balance while preventing electrolyte imbalance, refeeding edema, and muscle weakness. The Cambridge diet is usually sold by untrained "counselors" and has been linked by the Food and Drug Administration to six deaths. Optifast is used as part of a strictly supervised medical program.

Calorie Counting

Calorie counting is the simplest and most frequently used method of restricting calories. Clients follow books or printed lists with the calorie content of food. Clients are instructed to record the number of calories eaten and to restrict the total food intake to the designated calorie limitations. Among the disadvantages are that nutritional guidelines are not used, clients usually forget to record the calories, and they tire quickly of the process.

Balanced Deficit Plan

The food exchange system developed jointly by the American Diabetes Association and the American Dietetic Association outlines a balanced nutritional food plan using household measurements that can be used as a weight reduction regimen. Divided into six food groups, designating food quantities of equal equivalence, this plan permits unlimited variations. Cookbooks and exchange lists for fast food restaurants, frozen food, and other commercially prepared foods are available. Instructional material, food models, and booklets are also available. The balanced deficit diet is the eating plan of choice for most authorities. Nutritional eating behaviors learned during the weight loss period are used for life-long maintenance.

Exercise

Many authorities believe obesity is related more to inactivity than overeating (Bjorntorp, 1983). Studies show the obese move less and expend less energy than lean persons. A conditioned muscle requires more energy for movement than an unconditioned muscle. In most activities, only low-level energy is expended (eg, a 150-lb male walking for approximately 10 minutes expends only about 25 calories). The expenditure of energy is cumulative over time, so it does contribute to weight loss. The rate of loss is accelerated with calorie restriction. Elevating the resting heart rate between 40% and 60% of maximum will use stored fat for energy.

An exercise program is designed in progressive steps with a goal of 20 to 30 minutes of continuous activity three to four times per week. The basic exercise program includes flexibility exercises (bending and stretching), muscular strengthening, muscular endurance, and cardiovascular conditioning (Figure 9–1). Each session consists of a warm-up, the activity, and a cool-down period. Calisthenics and flexibility exercises are done in the warm-up and the cool-down portions. Calisthenics using 3- to 5-lb weights, aerobic dancing, running, rowing, bicycling, and cross country skiing are activities that produce muscle strengthening and muscle endurance along with cardiovascular conditioning. For an exercise program to be effective, it must be practical, pleasurable, and an activity the client will perform. It should also fit into the person's daily schedule.

For the morbidly obese, a low-level walking program or merely an increase in the activities of daily living will facilitate weight loss. A walking program consists of flexibility exercises and walking 10 to 15 minutes per day, 7

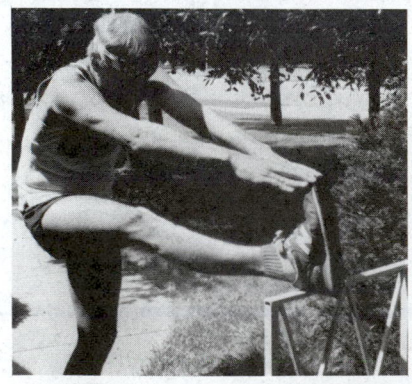
A

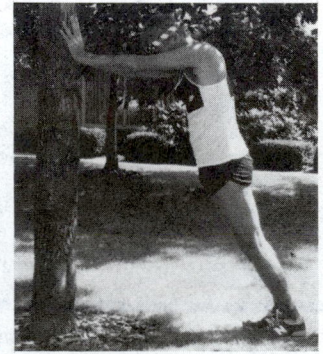
B

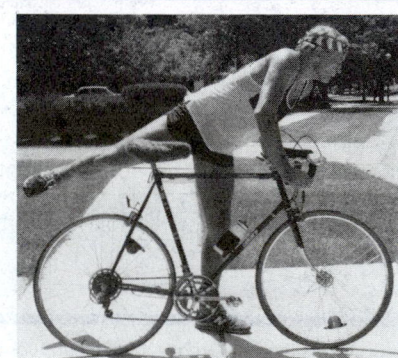
C

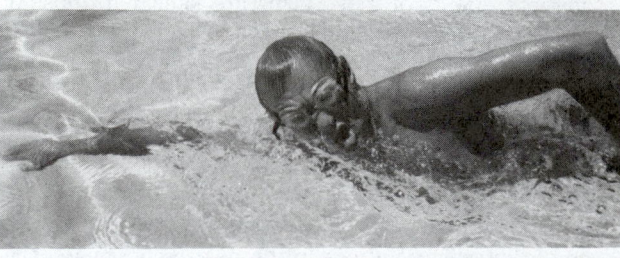
D

Figure 9–1

Exercise program. Flexibility exercises such as those in **A** and **B** are an important part of an exercise program. They provide a warm-up to the more strenuous activities shown in **C** and **D** that include muscular strengthening and endurance and cardiovascular conditioning.

days a week, progressing to 1 hour per day. All persons should be encouraged to increase routine activities by using the stairs instead of the elevator, parking further from store entrances, and increasing bending and stretching during household chores.

Exercise has added physiological benefits. With conditioning, changes occur in the cardiovascular system—the pulse rate is lowered, the stroke volume increases, and peripheral vascular resistance is lessened. Muscle work promotes increased cellular metabolism, suppresses hunger, and increases lipid utilization. Psychologically, individuals develop self-confidence, improve their perceptions of themselves, develop a more positive attitude toward their bodies, feel more in control, and recognize the body as a source of pleasure. These new attitudes foster improved interpersonal relationships and social interactions.

Behavioral Change

In the healthy person, most behavior related to food seeking and food intake are the result of habits learned throughout life. Learned behaviors can be changed or modified by experience during any stage of the life cycle. According to behavioral therapists, the "cure" for obesity lies not solely in dieting, but rather in behavioral change. Behavior modification, a process characterized by the conscious alteration of responses to stimuli, combined with the action-oriented problem-solving approach, assists with this process. First, the client's specific problems and goals are defined. Then the client's life history is obtained and analyzed. Identification of the "triggers" or stimuli for inappropriate food seeking and food intake is the next step in the process. Appropriate alternate behaviors are then identified. The individual selects the most suitable alternate behavior and plans ways for implementation. After the plan is implemented, progress is monitored and the outcomes are evaluated. If results are satisfactory, the behavior is repeated. When unsatisfactory results occur, an alternative strategy is selected, and the process begins again until a solution is found. Each success contributes to feelings of control and progress. Gaining control encourages the setting of short-term and long-term goals, which structure the arduous process of weight loss. Thus encouraged, the individual develops patience and persistence.

Due to the complexity of food-seeking behaviors, changes in responses to the environment and physiological and psychosocial stimuli are required. The examples of behavioral strategies listed in Box 9–3 are not inclusive. Additional suggestions are found in the literature and are only limited by the creativity of the individuals involved.

Social Support

Social support from family, friends, peers, coworkers, and professionals may help or hinder the weight-loss program.

Box 9–3 Strategies for Behavioral Change

Methods for controlling the environment are:

1. Purchase low-calorie food.
2. Shop from a prepared list and on a full stomach.
3. Keep all foods in the kitchen.
4. Store all foods in the refrigerator or in cabinets in opaque containers.
5. Prepare exact portions of food to eliminate leftovers.
6. Become an expert on preparing low-calorie foods.
7. Eat all foods in the same place, avoiding the kitchen.
8. Avoid eating when watching television or reading a book.
9. Reduce the frequency of eating out at restaurants, parties, picnics, etc.

Methods for controlling physiological responses to food are:

1. Eat slowly in small bites, allowing 20 minutes for a meal.
2. Eat a salad or drink a hot beverage before a meal.
3. Chew each bite thoroughly and slowly.
4. Put eating utensils or food down between bites.
5. Concentrate on the eating process; savor the food.
6. Lengthen the time between courses.
7. Stop eating with the first feelings of fullness.

Methods of controlling psychological responses to food are:

1. Appreciate the aesthetic experience of eating.
2. Use attractive dinnerware and prepare a formal setting for eating.
3. Use small plates and cups to make servings of food look larger.
4. Concentrate on conversations and socialization during the meal.
5. Use nonfood rewards for meeting a goal.
6. Acknowledge small successes and improvements in all behavior.
7. Substitute other activities for eating (eg, reading, exercise, hobbies).
8. Problem-solve.
9. Identify feelings.
10. Use assertive behavior.

The direct involvement of selected family members in the program will often foster understanding and cooperation. Group programs may also produce positive effects as members learn from one another, identify with each other, and develop feelings of belonging. A variety of self-help and mutual support groups are described in the resources list at the end of this chapter. These groups are available in most cities. Clients can often, with help, start their own groups.

Cognitive Restructuring

Cognitive restructuring means to change beliefs, attitudes, and thoughts by interpreting reality in new and different ways. The origins of beliefs and attitudes are embedded in life-long psychological development. Therefore, change requires conscious, sustained effort. Focusing on changes in eating behaviors and on implementing an exercise program helps identify areas for change. Introspection and discussion with a therapist, in groups, and with family or friends will facilitate the process.

Language changes are also required because thinking is the use of language. Perceptions of self and the world depend on words used. Self-esteem is a reflection of how a person believes the world views him or her. Low self-esteem and feelings of guilt, anxiety, and depression are common among the obese. Many obese people use negative words and phrases when speaking of themselves, reinforcing negative feelings. They need to change these word choices and thought patterns. For example, compare these phrases for feeling: "I am bad," "I have no will power," "I cheated," with "I did not meet my goal," "I choose to," "I ate an apple." The positive statements reflect an objective, in-control attitude that is conducive to building self-esteem.

Surgery

Surgery can be used to treat obesity in difficult cases. Criteria for surgical candidates include morbid obesity, a stable personality, failure to lose weight by conventional methods, age between 25 and 50 years, and no previous or existing medical problems. Surgery is effective only if the client also changes lifestyles and adheres to a diet. Ingestion of high-calorie foods and fluids will cancel the benefits of surgery.

Not considered effective in controlling weight are jaw-wiring and ear-stapling. The once-popular ileojejunal bypass loop is no longer widely used. The technique involved bypassing most of the jejunum and diverting food into the ileum. Serious complications, including death, result from nutrient malabsorption and adverse effects on liver, kidneys, and bones.

Currently, the most widely accepted procedures involve compartmentalizing the stomach. One technique is gastroplasty, similar to the Billroth II operation for stomach ulcers. The stomach is stapled across the cardiac portion to create a 50 cc to 65 cc pouch. A small opening in the pouch is connected to the duodenum, making a 1-cm to 2-cm lumen for passage of food. The newest procedure is gastric banding. A broad band is placed on the exterior surface of the stomach. The stomach is constricted to create an internal lumen about 9 to 10 mm in diameter. The duodenum is not involved. Risks are considered low and complications minimal (Bo & Modalski, 1983). These surgical procedures and the associated nursing care are illustrated and described in Chapter 50.

Drug Therapy

Because of the many causes of obesity, no single drug modality is effective. Research is focused on drugs that intervene at critical points in the food-intake and food-processing systems in the brain, the gastrointestinal tract (stomach, small intestine), and the adipose tissue. Many pharmacological approaches have been tried. Diuretics have numerous side effects and are essentially not effective since the weight lost through diuresis is body water, not fat. Drugs containing cellulose produce a feeling of fullness by absorbing water and expanding the stomach; their effectiveness is unknown. Thyroid hormones have also been administered in attempts to increase body metabolism. However, they must be used in high doses that cause hazardous cardiovascular symptoms, and the effect is transitory.

In the past, the primary anorectic drugs (hunger suppressants) were amphetamines. Amphetamines affect the catecholomines, neurotransmittors of the sympathetic nervous system, causing loss of appetite, hyperactivity, and euphoria. These addictive drugs have a number of serious side effects such as hypertension, allergy, blood disorders, and paranoid reactions (see Chapter 10). A newer drug, fenfluramine (Pondimin), derived from amphetamines, may act peripherally by mediating adipocyte cellular metabolism. The basic action of fenfluramine is believed to be on the brain neuroregulators, but the exact mechanisms for its actions are unknown.

For weight loss, appetite-suppressing drugs are usually prescribed only for the first few weeks and are used in conjunction with a low-calorie eating plan. Research shows these drugs promote quick weight loss, which is enhanced by behavioral change. Unfortunately, study results also showed the weight was regained over the long term. It was thought that some of the weight gain was in response to the drugs (Sullivan, Nauss-Karol, & Cheng, 1983).

NURSING PROCESS WITH OBESE CLIENTS

To be effective in assisting obese clients, nurses must examine their own beliefs, attitudes, and feelings about obese persons. Preconceived notions and prejudices will affect the total therapeutic plan. Health professionals may have negative perceptions of the obese, viewing them as lazy, undisciplined, neurotic, and lacking in character. The physical difficulties in providing care reinforce these negative feelings. Obtaining reliable data from the physical examination is difficult and often requires special skills and equipment. The thickened subcutaneous fat interferes with auscultatory techniques and percussion, obscures abnormalities detectable by inspection, and inhibits palpation. Attempts to give physical care, such as bathing, repositioning, ambulating, and venipuncture, are impeded. A clear understanding of this problem is required to circumvent the negative views of the obese and promote a positive therapeutic milieu.

Nursing Assessment: Establishing the Data Base

Recall the earlier discussion of the health risks to obese people. An accurate and thorough assessment is important for several reasons. Obese persons have more health-related problems than persons of normal weight and require a comprehensive treatment plan that includes attention to them as well as attention to the obesity. Relevant data must be collected and analyzed to determine the most effective approach to a plan for healthful living.

Subjective Data

The weight history elicits data about:

- Chronological development of obesity
- Familial attitudes, beliefs, and lifestyle, including ethnic and cultural influences
- The individual's self-perceptions: self-esteem, self-concept, and body image
- Motivation
- Participation in other weight-loss programs
- Food intake and physical activity

More accurate than the weight history is an evaluation of food intake and activity from a recorded analysis. A recorded analysis is a more accurate method of evaluating exercise and food intake because people tend to overestimate their activity levels and underestimate their food intake. Record forms are available or may be developed for individual situations. These records integrate the biopsychosocial areas associated with food intake behavior. The self-analysis includes recording the time of eating; length of time required to eat; eating site (kitchen, bedroom, den); physical position (sitting, standing); companion; mood (happy, sad, bored); hunger level; amount and types of food intake; and types of meal (meal, snack). Also recorded are the type, amount (repetitions), and time spent in physical activity. A typical recorded analysis is illustrated in Figure 9–2.

Objective Data

Determining the degree of obesity or overweight is accomplished both by gross and precise methods. The gross methods include the simple inspection of the individual body, preferably in the nude, for marked fat deposits. The *pinch test* is performed by grasping the skin between the forefinger and thumb. If the skinfold is greater than an inch, the area contains excessive fat deposits. Overweight and obesity can be estimated by comparing a person's height and weight with the tables developed by the Metropolitan Life Insurance Company (see Chapter 8). Compared with 1959 tables, 1983 tables reflect an increase in ideal body

Time	Minutes spent eating	M or S*	H**	Activity while eating	Place of eating	Food and quantity	Others present	Feeling while eating
8:10 a.m.	17	M	1	standing, fixing lunch	kitchen	1 c O.J. 1 c corn flakes ½ c whole milk 2 t. sugar black coffee	—	sleepy
10:30 a.m.	10	S	1	sitting, taking notes	classroom	12 oz cola	class	busy
11:45 a.m.	2	M	2	sitting, talking	union	1 sandwich 1 apple 2 cookies black coffee	friends	good
2:30 p.m.	15	S	1	sitting, studying	library	12 oz cola	friend	bored
5:30 p.m.	15	M	3	sitting, talking	kitchen	1 chicken leg 1 baked potato 2 T. butter lettuce 1 oz dressing 1 c whole milk 4 cookies	roommate	good
8:15 p.m.	10	S	0	sitting, studying	living room	12 oz cola	—	tired

* M or S: Meal or snack
** H: Degree of hunger (0 = none; 3 = maximum)

Figure 9–2

Food record form.
SOURCE: Christian JL, Greger JL: *Nutrition for Living*. Menlo Park, CA: Benjamin/Cummings. 1985, p. 252.

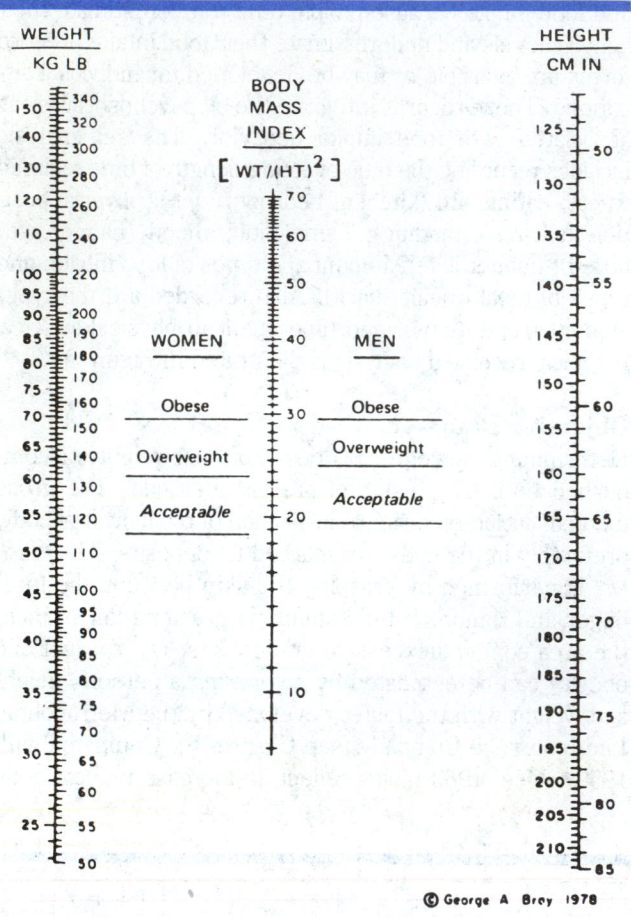

Figure 9–3

Nomogram for body mass index (BMI). To determine your BMI, use a straightedge between your weight in Column A and your height in Column B. The point where the line crosses Column C is your BMI. Note the obese, overweight, and acceptable ranges.
SOURCE: Adapted from Department of Health, Education, and Welfare. Obesity in America: An overview. In: *Obesity in America.* Bray GA (editor). Washington, DC: Government Printing Office, 1980.

weight. The tables do not indicate the amount of body fat, nor do they consider age factors (many people over 40 are overweight); therefore, these weights should be used only as guidelines and not as standards (Abraham, Carroll, Najjar, & Fulwood, 1983). Another method, the Hamwi method, calculates the ideal body weight for women of medium frame as 100 lb for the first 5 ft and 5 lb for every inch over 5 ft. Weights for men of medium frame are calculated at 106 lb for the first 5 ft and 6 lb for every inch over 5 ft. Although adjustments for large and small frames are made, this method is subject to the same drawbacks as the standard tables.

More precise methods for determining obesity and overweight are skinfold measurements and calculating the body mass index (BMI). Skinfold measurements using skin calipers yield relative body fat values. The normal body fat content is approximately 15% for men and 18% to 25% for women. The number of millimeters obtained from the measurements of the skinfolds of the triceps, biceps, subscapular area, suprailiac crest, thigh, lower chest wall, abdomen, and buttocks are totaled, and the sum is compared to age-differentiated standard charts (see Table 8–6). The triceps and the subscapular measurements are also used to predict body fat percentages mathematically, although some expertise is required to obtain accurate measurements. Expensive LED calipers are a popular item in catalogs that cater to persons interested in physical fitness. Skinfold measurements are discussed and illustrated in Chapter 8.

The BMI is thought by many experts in obesity research to be a more reliable indicator of obesity than the height–weight table ranges. It can be calculated by dividing a person's body weight (in kilograms) by the person's height (in meters) squared. Calculation can be avoided by using a nomogram (Figure 9–3) that converts height and weight to BMI and lists the acceptable, overweight, and obese ranges.

Also useful in assessment are laboratory values for serum plasma levels of glucose, triglycerides, cholesterol, cortisol, T_3 and T_4 (see Chapter 8), as well as skull x-rays and an ECG.

More sophisticated assessment methods used by researchers are underwater weighing, also known as water displacement; ultrasound; computerized tomography (CT) scanning; and measurement of total body electrical conductivity.

Nursing Diagnosis

Nursing diagnoses related to the obese and overweight client are listed in Box 9–4. The complexity of this disorder may require development of additional diagnosis or alteration of standard diagnoses.

Planning and Implementation

In some instances, the identified problems are outside the scope of the nurse's practice and are referred to an appropriate resource; examples are counseling for marital problems or severe psychological dysfunction and the medical treatment of physical problems. The plan depends on the care setting: inpatient, clinic, or private practice. Depending on available resources and the client's needs, the nurse might recommend group sessions or individual counseling. Also influencing the plan is the availability of ancillary support from dietitians and activity assistants and physical facilities. Time constraints for both the nurse and the client must also be considered. Since there will be frequent appointments over a long period, they must be scheduled to avoid conflicts with employment. The cost of the program and reimbursement must also be considered. Some insurance policies cover weight loss associated with high-risk health problems. Prepaid health plans, such as health maintenance organizations (HMOs), emphasize health promotion and therefore are more liberal in benefits.

Generally, a treatment plan prescribes a change in lifestyle through goal setting, problem solving, and information exchange. Specific techniques are recommended for food intake, exercise, behavior, and cognitive restructuring. These techniques are discussed in the section on treatment.

The implementation of the plan may be negotiated by the nurse or other health care provider and the client during counseling sessions. The nurse is responsible for providing information and guiding problem solving and goal setting. The client and his or her support systems are responsible for implementation and evaluation.

Evaluation

Although the treatment plan will be individualized, evaluation can be based on several common outcomes. The client can be expected to:

- Maintain normal weight for height, age, sex, and body structure as determined by the assessment tool
- Modify food-intake behaviors
- Participate in an exercise program
- Demonstrate positive cognitive restructuring
- Maintain optimal nutritional status
- Apply principles of nutrition to food choices and food preparation
- Demonstrate an improvement in health problems and develop no additional problems

---

Box 9–4 Nursing Diagnoses Commonly Related to Obesity

Diagnoses Directly Related to Obesity

Self-concepts, disturbance in

Activity intolerance

Coping, ineffective individual

Knowledge, deficit, related to nutrition, exercise

Mobility, impaired physical

Breathing pattern, ineffective

Nutrition, alterations in: more than body requirements

Additional Potential Diagnoses

Social isolation

Powerlessness

Coping, ineffective family

Cardiac output, alteration in: decreased

Gas exchange, impaired

Self-care deficit

Skin integrity, impairment of

Section II: Eating Disorders

Within the past several years, anorexia nervosa and bulimia have captured the attention of both scientists and the general public. There seem to be several reasons for the interest and concern. First, incidence seems to be increasing among the group that is primarily affected—women in adolescence and young adulthood. Also, the etiology is not fully understood even though anorexia nervosa was first described in the clinical literature nearly 300 years ago. Until recently, bulimia was included with anorexia, and researchers are only starting to define and explain its specific aspects. Finally, there is a fascination with the symptomatology. The willpower and denial exercised by emaciated anorexia clients can be astounding even to experts. The numbers of calories ingested by the bulimic client and the vomiting and laxative abuse seem horrifying.

The symptoms are more than just bizarre phenomena. Prolonged starvation, repeated vomiting, and laxative abuse may lead to a life-threatening situation. The body is simply not equipped to withstand starvation and the complications of the extreme weight-loss methods. The mortality rate has been variously estimated in the range of 5% to 21%, with the higher percentage having relevance for anorexia. Worse yet, both disorders have proven difficult to treat. Follow-up studies on clients with anorexia indicate that eating symptoms and other problems are persistent (Garner & Garfinkel, 1982). Although follow-up studies on bulimia are rare, an ominous sign is that these clients often do not seek treatment for many years after the onset of symptoms. The nurse who encounters these clients faces a serious and challenging task that will require understanding both the physiology and psychopathology of the two disorders.

Anorexia nervosa is a complicated disorder involving self-inflicted starvation that may be accompanied by vomiting, laxative abuse, and hyperactivity. The term *anorexia* is misleading because the individual does not initially experience a loss of appetite. Rather, intake is purposefully reduced to achieve and maintain goal weight well below the minimum norm for body size. In most cases, the target weight continues to drop until weight loss reaches life-threatening proportions. The drive to be thin is propelled by a distorted belief that one's body is "too fat" despite extreme emaciation. Although the disorder may begin as simply a conscious effort to lose weight, weight loss eventually becomes the primary focus in the individual's life. Not eating can be viewed as an attempt to cope.

Anorexia nervosa may be distinguished from bulimia, sometimes called bulimarexia or bulimia nervosa. The word *bulimia* comes from the Greek word meaning "ox hunger." It is characterized by episodic and frenzied binging on large quantities of usually soft-textured, easily eaten, highly caloric food, consumed in a brief period of time, followed by purging with vomiting, laxatives, or diuretics. In some cases, people with bulimia will follow binging behavior with a period of restricted intake and/or rigorous exercising. Binge–purge cycles are usually followed by self-deprecation, a depressed mood, and the realization that the eating pattern is abnormal. Clients with bulimia are usually striving to maintain weight and do not have the distortions in body image common to anorexics. They may in fact be at or above normal weight for their body size, varying from about 10 to 15 lb in either direction at any given time. For the bulimic, eating becomes an uncontrolled, embarrassing, and frightening impulse.

DIAGNOSTIC CRITERIA

Currently, the DSM III (Diagnostic and Statistical Manual, 1980) diagnostic criteria for anorexia nervosa and bulimia are the most widely used (Table 9–3). There is a continuing effort to refine diagnostic criteria for both eating disorders. Controversies about symptomatology and etiology may create confusion for nurses who encounter these clients. There are similarities between features present in eating disorders and other psychiatric diagnoses such as depression, schizophrenia, and obsessive-compulsive behavior. For example, symptoms such as depressed affect, sleep disturbances, decreased ability to concentrate, and low self-esteem may occur in both eating disorders and depression. Sometimes clients qualify for more than one diagnosis concurrently (Garner & Garfinkel, 1982). In addition, symptoms of anorexia nervosa and bulimia tend to overlap. There are individuals who alternate between extended periods of restricted intake and periods of bulimia and who reach extremely low body weights. These clients are sometimes referred to as "bulimic-anorexics" or "bulimic-restrictors." Hilde Bruch, the renowned authority on eating disorders, is unconvinced that bulimia is truly a separate clinical entity but sees it as a symptomatic feature of other conditions, including anorexia nervosa (Bruch, 1984). Other experts defend the validity of a separate diagnostic category for bulimia but see the criteria for diagnosis as limiting, given the wide range of underlying psychopathology seen clinically.

In her classic work on eating disorders, Bruch (1973) described the psychopathology of anorexia nervosa and identified three cardinal symptoms that experts agree are central to the diagnosis of eating disorders:

1. Body image distortion, which was described in the definition.
2. A disturbance in the perception of internal states, in which the client is unable to recognize and label sensations such as hunger, fatigue, and cold, as well as emotional states.
3. A "paralyzing sense of ineffectiveness," the overwhelming lack of feeling competent in any arena aside from weight control. Clients feel worthless and empty

Table 9–3 Diagnostic Criteria for Anorexia Nervosa and Bulimia	
Anorexia Nervosa	**Bulimia**
Intense fear of becoming obese, which does not diminish as weight loss progresses	Recurrent episodes of binge eating (rapid consumption of a large amount of food in discrete period of time, usually less than 2 hours)
Disturbance of body image (eg, claiming to "feel fat" even when emaciated)	1. Consumption of high-calorie, easily ingested food during a binge
Weight loss of at least 25% of original body weight (if under 18 years of age, weight loss from original body weight plus projected weight gain expected from growth charts may be combined to make the 25%)	2. Inconspicuous eating during a binge
Refusal to maintain body weight over a minimal normal weight for age and height	3. Termination of such eating episodes by abdominal pain, sleep, social interruption, or self-induced vomiting
No known physical illness that would account for the weight loss	4. Repeated attempts to lose weight by severely restrictive diets, self-induced vomiting, or use of cathartics or diuretics
	5. Frequent weight fluctuations greater than 10 lb due to alternating binges and fasts
	Awareness that the eating pattern is abnormal and fear of not being able to stop eating voluntarily
	Depressed mood and self-deprecating thoughts following eating binges
	Bulimic episodes not due to anorexia nervosa or any known physical disorder

inside and see themselves as incapable of meeting the demands of adolescent and young adult life.

Treatment of the client with an eating disorder is often more successful when initiated in the early stages of symptom development. Be alert for individuals who may be vulnerable to eating disorders or who are already symptomatic. Susceptibility is difficult to recognize because of their apparent good health and the secrecy involved with the symptoms. Frequently, the onset of symptoms occurs during adolescence, but early detection is difficult because many adolescent girls engage in some form of dieting behavior. Sometimes the symptoms begin following a separation from friends or family. Beginning high school or college and moving to a new city or school are life changes that are potential triggers to the development of symptoms.

In attempting to identify the client at risk, pay careful attention to preoccupation with dieting and weight. Although many dieters share similar beliefs, clients with eating disorders carry them to an extreme. Evaluate the degree to which dissatisfaction with body size is incongruent with the individual's actual size, weight, and appearance. Individuals with eating disorders have characteristic belief systems. For example, the client may feel that a 1- or 2-lb weight gain will result in appearing "too fat." Often three-digit numbers are a source of extreme anxiety: The client may tolerate 99 lb but be terrified at 100 lb. Certain foods may be regarded as "dangerous," and the client will avoid them completely. Snack foods that are easy to eat, or foods with sauces, like spaghetti, may stimulate binging behavior in bulimic clients. Anorexic clients may find these foods too difficult to monitor for specific caloric content.

At times, family members may offer warning signs for an individual at risk. Family members may be concerned about problem behaviors but not recognize the severity of the eating disorder. Sometimes, the family struggles to coax the individual to eat more but watches in frustration as the person simply pushes food around the plate. In cases of bulimia, parents may see food disappearing and grocery bills mounting before they realize the implications. The nurse can help families to face these indicators and encourage them to seek treatment for the individual.

ETIOLOGY

A variety of theories have been used to explain the etiology of eating disorders. Most experts agree that anorexia and bulimia develop from an interaction of biological, psychological, and sociocultural factors. Theories relating to the early psychological development of these clients pertain primarily to anorexia nervosa, since bulimia has only recently been considered as a separate phenomenon. Even the earliest descriptions of anorexia stressed a psychological component. Recent trends, however, explore the influence of hereditary and physiological factors. Few would deny that society's current norms for thinness play a role in the increasing incidence of eating disorders, but a complete understanding of the interplay of all these factors has not yet been achieved.

Developmental Theory

Hilde Bruch thinks that eating disorders result in part from faulty learning beginning at infancy. That is, the parents of these individuals did not respond appropriately or at least consistently to their infant's cues for physical and emotional needs. A pattern of erratic reinforcement laid the groundwork for the child's inability to identify and satisfy his or her own bodily needs. Faulty communication between parent and infant was the precursor to the development of a sense of ineffectiveness. Instead of developing a sense of ownership of their own bodies and feelings of competence in communicating and satisfying their needs, these children learned instead to respond to the parent's needs and emotions. Bruch believes that this background leads to the compliant behavior characteristic of these clients during their latency years (Bruch, 1973).

Psychoanalytic Theory

Traditional psychoanalytic theorists believe, like Bruch, that problems in early childhood contribute to personality development that predisposes the individual to eating disorders. The belief is that during the toddler years, the child fails to develop a sense of an independent, complete self separate from the caretaking parent. The parent rewards the child with affection for clinging, dependent behavior but withdraws emotional support when the child demonstrates assertive, autonomous behavior (Masterson, 1978). This theory is complex but in essence describes a child who fears emotional displays that may drive away the parent and other important figures. This leads to a quality of relating to others characterized by the desire to please. Problems arise later during adolescence when there is a pull toward increasing autonomy and independence from the family. The child may experience this as a threat of loss of emotional support. Rather than risk the loss of emotional support that could result from increased autonomy and independence, these adolescents remain overly compliant and pleasing. A sense of control and autonomy is achieved through the eating disorder by restricting food intake or engaging in vigorous exercise, for example.

Family Systems Theory

Systems theorists view the client within the context of the whole family. The family is viewed as a hierarchy with the parents as the executive subsystem and the children as the sibling subsystem. Ideally, there is a clearly defined boundary between the two levels that maintains the leadership role of the parents. The boundary is supported by a mutually satisfying parental relationship that allows the parents to work as a team to foster the growth and development of the children. Conflict between the parents is addressed and resolved from within the parental subsystem.

In 1974, Minuchin identified several interaction patterns that are still considered characteristic in families of anorexic children. *Enmeshment* refers to a lack of clear boundaries between the generations as well as between individual members. Members become overly sensitive to one another. Emotions and needs of one individual are shared by the other members of the system, and the members feel endangered by conflict. There is a tendency to avoid conflict, become overprotective of one another, and maintain a facade of harmony. Since every marital system or family has conflict, problems are in effect deflected onto the child, who becomes symptomatic. The family becomes focused on the child with anorexia, freeing the parents and the other family members from addressing their own problems. This system becomes self-perpetuating, and the families become locked into a rigid, unchanging pattern.

EATING DISORDERS AS MULTISYSTEM STRESSORS

Eating disorders have adverse physiological effects on many different body systems. They are discussed briefly below and listed in Table 9–4.

Physiological Effects of Starvation

Prolonged restriction of intake will lead not only to weight loss but also to a general state of malnutrition affecting all systems of the body (see Chapter 8). Many symptoms of anorexia nervosa are actually a direct result of the starvation process. Features such as obsessive thinking about food, mixing unusual combinations of foods, hoarding food-related items, and depressed affect have been observed in victims of starvation. The physical effects of anorexia nervosa are often a result of both poor dietary intake and fluid depletion secondary to vomiting or inadequate intake. Typically, the client is dehydrated with poor circulation. Muscle breakdown and lack of padding of the bones and nerves contribute to fatigue and pain when sitting and lying down. A common yet serious complication of starvation is amenorrhea. Researchers have found that in some cases amenorrhea may precede weight loss; however, it is generally thought that cessation of menstruation accompanies loss of body fat (Garner & Garfinkel, 1982). Numerous hormonal changes may occur secondary to changes in the hypothalamic–pituitary axis.

Physiological Effects of Binging and Purging

The most severe medical complications may occur in clients who engage in repeated vomiting and laxative abuse. Loss of fluid and electrolytes, especially potassium, along with the already compromised nutritional status may lead to renal dysfunction and cardiac dysrhythmia. A less serious though

Table 9–4	Health Consequences of Eating Disorders	
Anorexia Nervosa	**Bulimia**
Amenorrhea	Dehydration
Hormonal imbalances	Lightheadedness
Hypokalemia resulting in fatigue, seizures, cardiac dysrhythmias, nephropathy related to chronically low levels of potassium	Hypokalemia
	Esophageal irritation, erosion, or bleeding
Constipation	Dysphagia
Edema	Swelling, pain, and tenderness in the salivary glands
Abdominal bloating	
Vitamin and mineral deficiencies	Excessive tooth decay and erosion of tooth enamel
Bradycardia	Gum disorders
Muscle wasting	Menstrual irregularity
Gastrointestinal intolerance to food	Hemorrhage of blood vessels in the eyes
Susceptibility to infection	Hormone imbalances
Loss of hair	Erosion of stomach lining
Infertility	Difficulty in retaining food even in small amounts (spontaneous regurgitation)
	Constipation because of bowel atony

more common complication of vomiting is dental caries and inflammation and erosion of the gums caused by the hydrochloric acid from the stomach. Mild to severe cases of constipation may occur, either because the client's food intake is below the level necessary to provide intestinal bulk or because of bowel atony resulting from prolonged laxative abuse. Esophageal and gastric problems may potentially become severe. Clients may even experience spontaneous regurgitation—difficulty in retaining food when they want to.

EATING DISORDERS AS PSYCHOSOCIAL STRESSORS

Not only do eating disorders result from psychosocial stress; they may be psychosocial stressors as well.

Body Image, Self-Esteem, and Self-Confidence

The body image and self-image are closely intertwined concepts. For the individual with an eating disorder, the two become centered around the achievement of thinness. The person believes that in becoming thin, all problems will be solved and happiness found. This notion is supported by both internal and external feedback. The process of dieting is inherently rewarding in its measurable successes. Beyond this, friends and family members often congratulate early successes in dieting. Certainly, society equates thinness with success and happiness. The potential anorexic is vulnerable to all these influences because of an already poor sense of self-worth and a belief that she or he has little to offer as a unique individual. Many clients will say they are "nothing" if they are not thin.

In view of their low self-worth and of social influences, it is not surprising that clients with eating disorders persist in a self-destructive pattern. The harmful aspects of starvation elude them. Instead, they are boosted by the self-discipline involved in restricting intake and in long hours of study, work, and exercise. Discipline and success in weight loss become the core of the individual's self-esteem and self-confidence.

In many ways, the anorexic individual fears developing the primary symptom of bulimia—uncontrolled binging. These clients fight the loss of control involved in a binge. Persons with bulimic symptoms may have tried to accomplish the self-discipline of anorexia and in succumbing to the binge, feel deeply humiliated. They share the anorexic's desire to be thin and the low feelings of self-worth, but they lack the pride associated with the symptoms of the restriction. Instead, they harbor their symptoms in secrecy from friends and family. At the same time, the binging behavior itself may become a source of pleasure because it is often used to soothe tension or to create a sense of euphoria, similar to that of drug or alcohol abuse. Consequently, these individuals find their symptoms to be a complicated blend of pleasure and pain, and thus difficult to relinquish.

Autonomy, Independence, and Isolation

Often, individuals who develop eating disorders appear to be healthy and functioning well, aside from their symptoms. This facade may have been long-standing. These clients have frequently assumed the role in their families of the "least needy" child (Levinkron, 1982). That is, they have been problem-free and have won the love of their parents through a kind of pseudoindependence. They appear to take care of themselves and often assume the role of caring for others. An internal dilemma arises, however, because they deny their own needs for nurturance and support. The symptoms serve as a kind of symbolic representation of their own neediness. In developing a thin body, they take on a childlike quality and receive the care and attention they are often ill-equipped to ask for directly.

The style of relating begun with the family is continued in relationships with others. These clients become kind, supportive friends and are good "listeners," but they seldom identify problems for themselves. They feel guilty asking others to support them. On the surface, clients with bulimia may appear more outgoing and engaging than clients with anorexia, who may appear more reserved and aloof. Beneath the external appearance, however, both types are focused more on other's needs and wants than on their own. The symptoms become a means of coping with the resulting frustrations. The client with anorexia denies neediness and withdraws from others. The bulimic client may remain superficially engaged with others but uses the symptoms to soothe inner tensions from unexpressed anger.

TREATMENT OF EATING DISORDERS

Treatment of eating disorders usually combines behavior modification and psychotherapy in an interdisciplinary approach. In many settings, the physician, nurse, dietitian, psychotherapist, social worker, and occupational therapist, among others, work as a team in development of a treatment plan. Each professional assumes a different role in relating to the client and family, but all members of the team cooperate in the development and implementation of the treatment plan. Communication among members is essential in this system, and often the primary nurse will coordinate among team members.

Behavior Modification

In most cases, some principles of behavior modification will be incorporated into treatment for clients with eating disorders. Although specific interventions may vary, clients will usually be reinforced for weight gain. Reinforcements might include increased time for diversional activities, less time under direct supervision of staff, visiting privileges, increased exercise, or passes to leave the unit. Outpatients might be told they must gain weight to avoid hospitalization. Inpatients often will be given liquid protein supplements to drink or receive tube feedings for uneaten portions of meals. These interventions should not be presented as punishment but rather as life-saving measures.

The behavioral principles of desensitization and response prevention are frequently used. The inpatient may be desensitized to eating by beginning a low-calorie diet using stated food preferences. Gradually, calories are increased, and foods are introduced that the client fears (such as spaghetti). Staff supervision after meals to prevent vomiting or laxative abuse allows the client gradually to tolerate the feeling of fullness. It is important to include the opportunity to talk about feelings generated by eating, such as fear, anger, or guilt.

Behavioral techniques such as cognitive restructuring may be particularly helpful. The nurse can provide didactic information on the harmful effects of binging and purging and remind the client that vomiting and laxative abuse are not effective means of weight control. Alternatives to binging may be suggested, such as taking a walk or calling a friend. Helping the patient to plan a daily mealtime regimen can provide a structure for the client's intake and may help relieve anxiety concerning control of eating. This is an important element in treatment because many clients will not eat all day, adding hunger to the precipitating factors of a binge. All of these techniques work to help change the client's thinking about the usefulness of the symptoms.

Psychotherapy

Most behavioral programs are used in conjunction with individual psychotherapy, family therapy, or both. The goal of individual therapy is to increase the client's understanding of the reasons for the symptomatic behavior and to increase self-esteem. Family therapy can assist the family members to cope with the feelings generated by the client with the eating disorder. It may also be helpful in sorting out other problems in family relationships that may affect the family group as a whole.

NURSING PROCESS FOR THE CLIENT WITH AN EATING DISORDER

Caring for clients with anorexia nervosa and bulimia is challenging. Not only do they have complex physiological and emotional problems, but they may resist treatment. For the anorexic, the disorder may be life threatening. Extended therapy with repeated hospitalizations is not unusual. Many bulimics also require long-term treatment. The nurse sets the tone for treatment by conducting a thorough assessment and establishing a supportive therapeutic relationship.

Nursing Assessment: Establishing the Data Base

Identifying clients at risk for developing an eating disorder has been discussed in the earlier section on diagnostic criteria. The following discussion is more directly related to the hospitalized client.

Subjective Data

When the client is admitted to a hospital unit for severe malnutrition or serious electrolyte abnormalities, it may be difficult to gather subjective data from the client. The client's condition may preclude accurate reporting, and family members may need to supply additional information. The nurse should determine the circumstances of the admission, such as whether the client entered treatment voluntarily. If not, the client may deny the severity of the condition and give incomplete data regarding the history of symptoms.

The nurse may need to alter the approach to data gathering depending on the client's age and previous experience with hospitalization. A young client in an initial hospitalization may be frightened and need reassurance before feeling comfortable offering a history. The initial interaction with the client can be extremely important in setting the tone for the course of the hospitalization.

The initial history should include a detailed description of the previous dieting behavior. The goal will be to assess

the chronology, nature, and severity of symptoms as well as the client's investment in them. In particular, the nurse will need to know the client's previous high and low weights, the ideal or goal weight, the age of onset of dieting and/or binging, the frequency of use of vomiting or purgatives, the amount of time spent exercising, and percentage of time spent thinking about food and weight control. In addition, ask about the reasons for initiating a diet, such as having been teased about increasing weight or pubertal development. If the client has binging episodes, assess the client's ability to identify what factors trigger a binge.

The interview should illuminate the extent to which the eating disorder interferes with other areas of functioning. Open-ended questions are often helpful. For example, the nurse might ask the client to describe a typical day, detailing all activities including eating. Many clients will spend hours working, studying, or exercising to avoid thinking about food. It is important to elicit information about time spent with friends or family members and the client's response to that time. Individuals may avoid activities with friends that might include a meal and eventually withdraw from relationships altogether.

Objective Data

Physical assessment of the malnourished client has been discussed in Chapter 8. The nurse monitors electrolyte values both initially and regularly thereafter to determine if the client is continuing with vomiting or laxative abuse. It is also important to observe the client's affective state. Although the client may be unable to identify depressed feelings, facial expression, posture, eye contact, and tone of voice provide information about internal states.

Nursing Diagnosis

Identification of client problems relating to the effects of malnutrition is outlined in Chapter 8. Specific nursing diagnoses for clients with anorexia nervosa or bulimia are listed in Box 9–5. For clients with eating disorders, there is the added dimension of refusal to eat or the lack of impulse control related to binging, vomiting, exercising, and laxative abuse. The nurse will be instrumental in establishing goals and interventions to help the client eliminate destructive behavior and establish healthy eating patterns. At the same time, the nurse can assist the client in developing alternative coping mechanisms that will promote better physical and mental health.

Although detrimental eating behaviors are the most apparent problems with these clients, they are closely linked to disturbances in body image and self-esteem. Disturbances in self-concept are usually long-standing and difficult to change.

Planning and Implementation

The nurse working closely with the client will want to establish reasonable short-term goals that will ultimately lead to an improvement in self-regard. Sometimes a first step will be the client's ability to express anger at the nurse. It is important not to feel insulted and to view this as a gain. Often being able to work out a conflict with the nurse and develop open communication are the highlights of the client's treatment experience.

The treatment of eating disorders is a long, complicated process, and the nurse will need to reevaluate and update goals and interventions. The steps toward improvement may be small and subtle. The goal will be gradually to increase the client's ability to manage independently yet to be able to recognize the need to seek assistance and support when necessary. Many anorexic persons require inpatient treatment, while outpatient treatment is usually manageable in bulimia.

Planning and implementation involve both clients and their families. Although dysfunctional family interactions might contribute to the development of eating disorders, it is important that the nurse not make judgments about the client's family. Remain sensitive to the fact that the family members of anorexic clients may have been struggling for many months to force the client to eat. The distress of watching a family member willfully starve may be enough to cause chaos in a household. Parents, siblings, friends, and spouses will likely feel guilty, ineffective, and depressed about the situation and will need support from the nurse with regard to these feelings. At the same time, be aware that family and friends may inadvertently collude in obstructing the client's treatment. For example, clients may complain that the nurse is cruel and punitive, leading families into taking them home before it is medically safe. Forewarn them about this phenomenon and encourage them to discuss this with the nurse. Instruct them also not to discuss eating and weight with the client but to let the staff handle this aspect of care.

Inpatient Care: Strategies for Client and Family

Nursing interventions are aimed at the goal of restoring weight and adequate nutrition within a supportive emotional context. In the treatment of severe emaciation, the client's condition may necessitate intravenous infusions to correct electrolyte imbalance, nasogastric tube feedings (see Chapters 5 and 47), and in some cases, total parenteral nutrition (see Chapter 8). It is crucial not to overload the client's circulatory system, risking congestive heart failure from the body's inability to handle fluid overload. Too rapid administration of food and the calories the client has been attempting to avoid may result in a sudden and severe escalation of the client's anxiety level to the extent of panic. The process of weight restoration should be initiated slowly, preferably with a balanced diet of 1200 calories with no added salt, incorporating the client's food preferences. Ideally, the client should be monitored closely for at least 1 hour during and after meals. Clients with anorexia may experience anxiety, guilt, and panic after eating because of the distorted belief that all food is "bad" and will lead to excessive weight gain. This belief leads to desperate

---

Box 9–5 Nursing Diagnoses Commonly Related to Eating Disorders

Diagnoses Directly Related to Eating Disorders

Bowel elimination, alteration in: constipation, related to insufficient intake of food or laxative abuse

Coping, ineffective individual

Fluid volume deficit, actual or potential, related to diuretic abuse

Injury, potential for

Nutrition, alterations in, less than body requirements

Self-concepts, disturbance in, body image, self-esteem

Tissue perfusion, alteration in

Mucous membrane, alteration in, related to induced vomiting

Additional Potential Nursing Diagnoses

Cardiac output, alteration in: decreased, related to arrhythmia from electrolyte imbalance

Coping, ineffective family

Sexual dysfunction

Skin integrity, impairment of

Social isolation

Nutrition, alterations in: potential for more than body requirements, related to binging

Injury, potential for, related to dehydration and lightheadedness

---

behavior, such as hiding food during meals or postmeal vomiting. If the patient refuses food, liquid protein supplements may be given in caloric amounts equivalent to uneaten food portions.

Eating after prolonged periods of starvation or chronic laxative abuse can lead to edema, abdominal distention, and constipation. The nurse will need to monitor such potential problems, keeping in mind that clients with anorexia frequently complain of feeling "bloated" after meals because of their psychological discomfort with eating.

Weights are usually taken daily at the same time with the client wearing the same clothing. Clients should void before weigh-ins because they may attempt to increase their weights by drinking large quantities of water. To promote weight gain, activity should be restricted to a minimum. In some cases, bed rest may be necessary initially.

In most cases, clients will resist treatment despite an initial sense of relief that the treatment team has assumed responsibility for their decisions. Although anorexic clients usually are not attempting to commit suicide, they are overwhelmed with fear at the idea of gaining weight. The difficulties that arise during eating may surprise staff because of the client's generally pleasing, compliant facade. It is not unusual for some nurses to feel angry and avoid the client because of the apparent refusal to accept treatment. Remember during this stressful time that clients are not maliciously attempting to sabotage efforts of the staff, but rather need to maintain some sense of control.

It is good practice to consult with a psychiatric nurse specialist when caring for clients with eating disorders. Staff members often need assistance in implementing a consistent, firm approach to eating. Clients will need encouragement to explore their feelings after eating, without being given false reassurances. Avoid power struggles with the client about particular food items or portions. Make an effort to see that one nurse is not identified as more strict or more lenient than another. In general, firm limits combined with genuine emotional sensitivity and support will be most helpful to the anorexic client.

Outpatient Care: Strategies for Client and Family

If the client's condition is not severely compromised medically, it may be preferable to attempt outpatient treatment. The nurse may play a key role in establishing a relationship with the client. Often the nurse will be required to make highly skilled judgments in responding to the client. At times, firm limits may need to be set on the symptomatic behavior. At other times, empathy and supportive statements can motivate the client to continue treatment.

The nurse will probably work closely with a physician and perhaps a dietitian in establishing weight goals with the client. Usually, the nurse weighs the client weekly. Some clients who have not achieved their goal weight attempt to hide this fact to avoid hospitalization. Others may actually hide objects on their bodies to increase weight. The nurse who discovers such techniques should avoid acting punitive, angry, or shocked. It is preferable to use a matter-of-fact approach in reweighing the client and later trying to elicit feelings about the difficulty of giving up the symptoms.

Techniques for reducing symptoms of bulimia were discussed earlier in this chapter. It may be helpful to have clients with either anorexia or bulimia complete weekly food diaries as well. The bulimic individual may discover patterns or trends to the binging behavior. The anorexic client may be able gradually to introduce additional food items with encouragement from the nurse. The nurse can provide nutritional teaching and include information about the harmful effects of inadequate nutrition.

A number of organizations offer mutual support groups for individuals with anorexia and bulimia. Some clients may be interested in using a peer group as an adjunct to other treatment. They may benefit from the relationships that develop with other group members who share similar problems. Group members may trade ideas on helpful steps to controlling symptoms. Most individuals will need to continue medical follow-up, however, to monitor side effects of the symptoms.

EVALUATION

The nurse will play an important role in determining the client's response to treatment interventions. For the client in the hospital, physical stability and weight gain are two critical variables. Many clients will return to the symptoms and begin to lose weight upon discharge. Recovery from anorexia and bulimia can be a long, complicated process, and some persons will require multiple hospitalizations. Most individuals will need some form of follow-up treatment to include ongoing therapy as well as routine monitoring of weight and electrolytes.

The nurse can be helpful in determining the psychological readiness to manage diet and weight. Decisions might be based on the client's ability to plan menus and tolerate eating without direct supervision. The nurse will want to consider the client's level of insight with regard to the relationship between emotional state and symptomatic behavior. Eating disorders involve a complicated blend of physiological and psychosocial processes. With the support of all treatment team members, the nurse can intervene successfully in restoring the health and well-being of these individuals.

Chapter Highlights

Obesity is an excess of relative body fat; overweight is an excess in body weight.

Anorexia nervosa is a disorder of self-inflicted starvation often resulting in extreme emaciation.

Bulimia is a disorder involving episodes of binging on food, usually followed by purging by vomiting or laxatives.

In obesity, both sides of the energy equation—intake and expenditure—are of equal importance.

Obesity is a stressor to all body systems.

Eating disorders result from a blend of biological, psychological, and sociocultural forces.

Prolonged starvation and purging can result in general malnutrition, dehydration and electrolyte imbalances, hormonal changes, and multiple effects on all systems.

Understanding the causes of obesity is central to development of an effective, individualized treatment plan.

Weight loss and long-term weight maintenance are accomplished only with a permanent lifestyle change.

Effective treatment of obesity is based on long-term motivation, a nutritious eating plan, and a practical activity program.

Clients with eating disorders base their self-esteem on ability to lose weight.

Treatment of eating disorders can be a long, complicated process because it involves both weight restoration and psychological changes.

Nursing goals for eating disorders promote weight gain and adequate nutrition in a supportive emotional context.

In the initial phase of inpatient treatment, the client may need close monitoring to ensure adequate intake.

Bibliography

Abraham S et al: Obese and overweight adults in the United States. *Vital Health Statistics* 1983; 230:1–93.

Bjorntorp P: Physiological and clinical aspects of exercise in obese persons. *Exercise and Sports-Science Reviews,* 1983; 11:159–180.

Bo O, Modalski O: Gastric banding: A surgical method of treating morbid obesity: Preliminary report. *Int J Obes* 1983; 7:493–499.

Brownell K: The psychology and physiology of obesity: Implications for screening and treatment. *J Diet Assoc* 1984; 84(4):406–413.

Bruch H: *Eating Disorders: Obesity, Anorexia Nervosa and the Person Within.* New York: Basic Books, 1973.

Bruch H: Four decades of eating disorders. In: *Handbook of Psychotherapy for Anorexia Nervosa and Bulimia,* pp. 7–18. Garner D, Garfinkel P (editors). New York: Guilford, 1984.

Cozens RE: Obesity in the aged: Not just a case of overeating. *Nurs Clin North Am* 1982; 17(2):227–232.

Diagnostic and Statistical Manual of Mental Disorders, 3rd ed. (DSM-III). Washington, DC: American Psychiatric Association, 1980.

Friemer N, Echenberg D, Krutchmer N: Cultural variation—nutritional and clinical implications. *West J Med* 1983; 139(6):928–933.

Garner D, Garfinkel P: *Anorexia Nervosa: A Multidimensional Perspective.* New York: Brunner/Mazel, 1982.

Goodsett A: Self psychology and the treatment of anorexia nervosa. In: *Handbook of Psychotherapy for Anorexia Nervosa and Bulimia,* pp. 55–82. Garner D, Garfinkel P (editors). New York: Guilford, 1984.

Greenwood MRC, Turhenkopf IJ: Genetics and metabolic aspects. In: *Obesity,* pp. 193–208. Greenwood MRC (editor). New York: Churchill Livingstone, 1983.

Guyton AC: *Textbook of Medical Physiology.* Philadelphia: Saunders, 1981.

Harris MB: Eating habits, restraint, knowledge and attitudes toward obesity. *Int J Obes* 1983; 7:271–286.

Himms-Hagen J: Brown adipose tissue thermogenesis in obese animals. *Nutr Rev* 1983; 40(9):261–267.

Keesey RE: A set point analysis of the regulation of body weight. In: *Obesity,* pp. 144–165. Stunkard AJ (editor). Philadelphia: Saunders, 1980.

Levinkron S: The nurturant authoritative approach. *Psychotherapeutic Approaches to the Treatment of Anorexia and Bulimia.* Symposium presented at the Conference of the Center for the Study of Anorexia and Bulimia. New York, November 1982.

Masterson J: The borderline adolescent: An object relations view. In: *Adolescent Psychiatry,* pp. 344–359. Feinstein S, Giovacchini P (editors). Chicago: University of Chicago, 1978.

Minuchin S: *Families and Family Therapy.* Cambridge, MA: Harvard University Press, 1974.

Morley JE, Levine AS: The role of the endogenous opiates as regulators of appetite. *Am J Clin Nutr* 1982; 35(4):757–761.

Morlin RJ: Atherosclerosis: Advances in prevention and treatment. *Geriatric Consultant* 1984; (Nov–Dec):11–17, 31.

Sullivan A, Nauss-Karol C, Cheng L: Pharmalogical treatment, II. Pages 139–158 in: *Obesity.* Greenwood MRC (editor). New York: Churchill Livingstone, 1983.

Wagner PL, Kirsch ER: Obesity complications in critical care. *Dimensions Crit Care Nurs* 1985; 4(2):81–91.

Suggested Readings

Boskind-White M, White WC: *Bulimarexia: The Binge/Purge Cycle.* New York: Norton, 1983. This book is based on the Whites' work with over 2000 bulimarexic women. It describes their therapy and their clients' experiences.

Bruch H: *The Golden Cage: The Enigma of Anorexia Nervosa.* Cambridge, MA: Harvard University Press, 1978. A book of case examples by a leading authority on anorexia nervosa, summarizing and updating her earlier classic work.

Cozens RD: Obesity in the aged: Not just a case of overeating. *Nurs Clin North Am* 1982; 17(2):227–232. The problems of aging and obesity are briefly presented. The nursing process is used as a framework for a case study of an elderly obese female. The psychological, physiological, social, cultural, and developmental aspects are considered in the formulation of the nursing care plan.

McBride AB: Obesity of women during the childbearing years: Psychosocial and physiologic aspects. *Nurs Clin North Am* 1982; 17(2):217–225. The impact of traditional social expectations on the psychological development of women and the conflicts that arise when the hopes and desires of women are not congruent with these values are emphasized.

Orbach S: *Fat is a Feminist Issue II.* New York: Berkley, 1982. A best-selling soft cover book with a feminist perspective that focuses on compulsive eating. The author provides strategies to break the addiction to compulsive eating.

Popkess-Vawter S: Reducing cardiac risk factors in the obese patient. *Nurs Clin North Am* 1982; 17(2):233–244. A case study of a yo-yo diet incorporates an outline for nursing interventions that promotes holistic self-care. An update of atherosclerosis and a cardiac risk profile and questionnaire are featured.

Sanger E, Cassino T: Eating disorders: Avoiding the power struggle. *Am J Nurs* (Jan) 1984; 84:31–33. Article provides helpful strategies for avoiding power struggles with clients hospitalized for treatment of anorexia nervosa.

White JH: An overview of obesity: Its significance to nursing. Definition, prevalence, etiologic concerns and treatment strategies. *Nurs Clin North Am* 1982; 17(2):191–198. A clear, succinct overview of obesity is presented. The psychological problems are highlighted.

Resources

SELF-HELP GROUPS AND OTHER ORGANIZATIONS

American Anorexia Nervosa Association, Inc (AANA)
133 Cedar La.
Teaneck, NJ 07666
Phone: (201) 836-1800 weekdays, 10 AM to 2 PM EST
   A self-help group that provides information and help.

Anorexia Nervosa and Related Eating Disorders, Inc
   (ANRED)
PO Box 5102
Eugene, OR 97401
Phone: (503) 344-1144
   A nonprofit organization that responds to requests for information and referrals.

Drs Marlene Boskind-White and William C. White
67 W. Malloryville Rd.
Freeville, NY 13068
   The authors of *Bulimarexia: The Binge/Purge Cycle* will help to locate a knowledgeable and reputable therapist, send a reading list about bulimarexia, and answer all inquiries. Send a stamped, self-addressed envelope.

National Association to Aid Fat Americans, Inc (NAAFA)
PO Box 43
Bellerose, NY 11426
   In existence since 1969, the group fights prejudice and discrimination against obese people and promotes self-acceptance and societal acceptance.

National Association of Anorexia Nervosa and Associated
   Disorders (ANAD)
Box 271
Highland Park, IL 60035
Phone: (312) 831-3438
   This mutual support association was founded by Vivian Meehan, a nurse recognized for her achieve-

ment by the American Nurses' Association. It will provide advice on joining a self-help group or forming one.

Overeaters Anonymous (OA)
2190 190th St.
Torrance, CA 90504
Phone: (213) 320-7941

In Canada:
Overeaters Anonymous
Box 224, Postal Station Z
Toronto, Ontario, Canada M5N 2Z4
Phone: (416) 783-9445
   Patterned after the philosophy of Alcoholics Anonymous, this self-help organization views compulsive eating as a disease that can be arrested but not cured. No dues or fees. Literature available upon request. Over 100,000 members.

UNIVERSITY- AND HOSPITAL-AFFILIATED EATING DISORDERS PROGRAMS

Behavioral Health Clinic
University of Minnesota Hospital
420 Delaware St., SE
Box 301 Mayo
Minneapolis, MN 55455
Director: Dr. Richard Pyle

Eating Disorders Program
New York Hospital-Cornell University
   Medical Center
Westchester Division
21 Bloomingdale Rd.
White Plains, NY 10605
Director: Dr. Katherine Halmi

Eating Disorders Program
Northwestern Memorial Hospital
Superior Street and Fairbanks Court
Chicago, IL 60611
Directors: Dr. Steven Stern, Dr. Craig Johnson
Clinical Nursing Manager: Lyn Marshall, RN, MSN

Eating Disorders Program
UCLA Neuropsychiatric Institute
760 Westwood Plaza
Los Angeles, CA 90024
Director: Karen Lee-Benner, RN, MSN

Eating and Weight Disorder Clinic
Henry Phipps Psychiatric Clinic
Johns Hopkins Hospital
600 N. Wolfe St.
Baltimore, MD 21205
Director: Dr. Arnold E. Anderson
   These sources will supply information and may be able to recommend local specialists.

Chapter 10

Substance Abuse

Sheila Bittle
Janice Cooke Feigenbaum
Carol Ren Kneisl

Objectives

When you have finished studying this chapter, you should be able to:

Identify the scope of substance abuse problems.

Discuss general theories related to etiology of substance abuse problems.

Define psychological and physical dependence and tolerance.

Compare and contrast the effects of major drugs of abuse.

Use the nursing process with clients who have problems related to substance abuse.

The use and abuse of prescription, over-the-counter (OTC), and illicit drugs is a problem of staggering proportions in America. Many people use a variety of substances to relax, induce sleep, alleviate pain, relieve depression, increase energy and alertness, alter mood, and heighten fun. Alcohol, sedative-hypnotics, stimulants, and antianxiety drugs are being consumed more often and by more people than ever before.

The history of using mind-altering drugs to excess, or in a manner disapproved by society, is as old as the human race. Fermented beverages were probably used by prehistoric humans, who depicted their effects on cave walls. The Bible and the writings of the ancient Egyptians described their effects. Opium and marijuana have been in worldwide use for centuries, and the Indians of South America recognized the stimulant properties of the coca plant long before the Spanish conquest.

Each society develops rules and guidelines for the use of drugs. Although the Bible frequently mentions wine in approving terms, it warns against drunkenness. In some cultures, men may drink fermented beverages to intoxication; women and children who do so may be punished. Alcohol use is widely accepted in Western society, but its use is prohibited and condemned in Moslem cultures that often tolerate marijuana. In the Eastern world, opium was once a widely accepted recreational drug. In the United States and England, it was available on grocery store shelves until the late nineteenth century. Cocaine, the ingredient that was responsible 75 years ago for making Coca-Cola "the pause that refreshes," is now an illegal drug in the United States.

Section I: The Problem of Substance Abuse

Drugs are being produced in increasing numbers, making them more readily available through both legal and illicit channels. A drug culture lifestyle with its own jargon sup-

ports and maintains its members in their drug-seeking behavior and helps to make the illicit market profitable.

Substance abuse is a major social and public health

problem. The abuse of one drug—alcohol—currently is the third major cause of death in the United States, ranking only behind coronary diseases and cancer. Substance abuse costs the American economy billions of dollars a year in lost productivity, health care and treatment costs, and crime.

Nurses have frequent contact with individuals who abuse drugs—clients, friends, neighbors, and colleagues. It has been estimated that 25% of all hospitalized clients experience problems related to substance abuse. Each person who is a substance abuser will have an adverse effect on the health and well-being of family members, friends, and work associates. They, in turn, become clients in the broadest sense, needing assistance in learning how to cope with their substance-abusing relative, friend, or colleague. Nurses have a high rate of substance abuse within their own ranks.

WHAT CONSTITUTES SUBSTANCE ABUSE

A wide variety of chemical agents, illegal as well as legal, is commonly ingested in this society. Consider this frequently heard comment: "A substance abuser is someone who uses more of it (alcohol, cocaine, caffeine) than I do." Substance abuse or misuse is not easily defined, and the parameters are not clear-cut. The definition also depends on one's perspective.

Substance use is a general term applied to the occasional use of a chemical substance. It includes a wide range of behaviors—trying the drug out of curiosity or because of peer pressure, using the drug in religious or cultural rituals, using modest amounts for their pleasurable or recreational effects, or using a stimulant to stay awake to study for an exam or while driving. Occasional use, however, may lead to using more of the drug more often.

Substance abuse can be defined as the continued use of chemical agents despite the emotional, social, legal, and health problems their use creates. One of the hazards of using mind- and mood-altering drugs is dependence. **Drug dependence** develops with the repeated use of certain chemical agents; a person requires the effects of a specific drug to function. Two forms of dependence—psychological and physical—may develop. Some substances cause one form of dependence, whereas others generate both types.

Psychological dependence occurs when a person has a compulsion to continue using the substance, craving its effects to experience a sense of self-esteem and well-being. In **physical dependence,** an individual experiences physiological symptoms of withdrawal when the drug is discontinued. The time from the last ingestion of the substance to withdrawal, as well as the withdrawal symptoms, are drug-specific and depend on the type and amount of drug taken. Diazepam (Valium) causes both psychological and physical dependence. Besides severe physical symptoms accompanying withdrawal (Table 10–1), the diazepam user has a craving to resume using the drug.

Imipramine hydrochloride (Tofranil), used to treat depression, is a good example of a drug causing physical dependence but not psychological dependence. When Tofranil is discontinued after prolonged administration, the client may experience nausea, vomiting, muscle aches, anxiety, and difficulty in sleeping but does not feel compelled to resume its use.

Tolerance is the result of the body's attempts to adapt to repeated exposure to specific chemical agents. Tolerance means that, with repeated use of the drug, the user requires increasingly larger amounts to produce the same effects previously attained with smaller amounts. Another dangerous aspect is that tolerance does not develop uniformly to all of a drug's effects. For example, users of alcohol and barbiturates develop tolerance to the intoxicating effect of the drug, but the potentially lethal dose does not change appreciably. The amount the user then needs to feel good may be nearly enough to cause death.

A concurrent state of **cross-tolerance** may also develop. This condition occurs when the person has developed a tolerance to one agent and then requires larger doses of pharmacologically similar drugs to achieve the desired effect. For example, an alcoholic client admitted for an appendectomy will probably require larger dosages of meperidine (Demerol) to experience relief from postoperative pain than another client who is not dependent on alcohol. An individual tolerant to methaqualone (Quaalude) will also be tolerant to sodium pentobarbital (Nembutal).

Addiction is another term often applied to substance abuse. Although it has been deleted from the diagnostic classifications of the American Psychiatric Association and the World Health Organization (WHO), the term continues to be used by professionals and clients to describe psychological dependence, physical dependence, and both. To avoid confusion, this chapter will use the term *dependence.*

At any given time, some chemicals may be more popular among substance users than others. Preferences change, and some substances become either more or less available. A current trend is toward polydrug use, using many different drugs at the same time. Many drinkers combine alcohol with marijuana, cocaine, and amphetamines. Clients taking prescribed antipsychotic agents, antianxiety agents, and antidepressants often use them concomitantly with alcohol.

Polydrug use may result in the following interactions, depending on which drugs are used simultaneously:

- Additive effect. When two or more drugs that produce the same effects by the same physiologic mechanism are used together, the effects are greater than would be expected from one drug alone. Effects do not exceed what would be expected from simple addition of the drug effects, however.

- Potentiation effect. When one drug enhances the effects of another drug taken in combination with it by intensifying or prolonging its effect, it is said to have a potentiative (synergistic, supraadditive) effect. The drug actions may be much greater than with simple addition. Central nervous system depressants, such as barbiturates, benzodiazepines, and opioids, are examples of drugs that have a synergistic effect with alcohol.

• Antagonistic effect. When drugs are combined, one drug may inhibit (lessen or block) the effects of the other. Caffeine, a weak antagonist, is often added to antihistamine drugs to counter the drowsiness they cause. Alcohol and barbiturates are often taken by amphetamine abusers to "take the edge off" their anxiety and agitation. Naloxone (Narcan) is an opioid antagonist used in emergency treatment to counteract respiratory depression caused by opioids.

Polydrug use is a hazardous practice leading to serious medical emergencies and physiologic crises. Be aware that some health problems of clients could be related to drug interactions from polydrug use. The ultimate effects of ingesting many different drugs together remain unknown.

ETIOLOGY OF SUBSTANCE ABUSE

Despite the hundreds of studies focused on the problem of substance abuse, the cause (or causes) remains unknown. No one physical, social, developmental, psychological, cultural, or genetic factor can be singled out.

No matter why a person becomes a substance abuser, once dependent on a chemical agent, the person will be motivated to continue its use to experience a sense of self-esteem and worth, to prevent or relieve withdrawal symptoms, or both. In effect, once dependent, the person comes to view the substance as a "best friend." Although the question of why one person becomes dependent on a drug while another does not remains unanswered, several explanations have been offered.

Availability and Encouragement

Sedatives and antianxiety agents are not only produced in massive numbers, but they are also excessively prescribed. One of them, diazepam (Valium), is the best-selling drug of all time. Others are easily available on the street through illegal sources. Vigorous advertising campaigns make many chemical substances seem appealing and socially acceptable. The combination of availability and mass media influence is thought to contribute to substance use and abuse. Peer pressure is another strong motivator.

Adverse Social Conditions

Poverty, unemployment, racial discrimination, and lack of social and educational opportunities have been correlated with high rates of substance abuse. Some people may abuse substances as a means of coping with these adverse social conditions. The social conditions themselves may also result from substance abuse: substance abusers who are unable to function on the job or to keep up with the demands of an educational program may find themselves without employment (and without money).

Developmental Factors

Developmental theorists propose a link between substance abuse and parental loss (either through death, abandonment, or divorce) or the inability of parents to form satisfying emotional relationships with their children. Parents are important role models for their children's behavioral and emotional development; thus, children of substance-abusing parents are at greater risk for developing substance abuse problems.

Psychological Factors

Psychoanalytic theory links substance abuse with fixation at the oral stage of development. Substance abuse is viewed as self-destructive behavior that stems from lack of adequate self-love and aggression that is turned inward. Other psychological causes are thought to be unfulfilled dependence needs, depression, low self-esteem, and hostility; thus, substance abusers depend on chemicals to fill emotional needs.

Genetic Predisposition

Recent research has suggested that substance abusers (particularly alcoholics) have a genetic predisposition to dependence. Researchers suspect that alcoholism is caused by a genetically transmitted biochemical defect, resulting in a lack of production of certain enzymes or hormones. This creates a particular kind of homeostatic balance that can only be maintained by ingestion and metabolism of alcohol. Although conclusive evidence is yet to be found, it is anticipated that identification of biological causes will enhance the treatment and rehabilitation of alcoholics and other substance abusers.

Neurotransmitter Defects

An exciting aspect of current neurochemical and physiological research is the study of neurotransmitters and their relationship to substance abuse. Neurotransmitters are chemicals in the nerve endings (axons) that are important in the transmission of nerve impulses to the next cell by way of the synapse, the microscopic space between the axon and the receptor of the next nerve cell (dendrite).

Depressant drugs (such as alcohol and antianxiety agents) appear to depress the nerve cell action by inhibiting or interfering with neurotransmitters. Stimulants increase the synthesis and release of neurotransmitters by mimicking the neurotransmitter or inhibiting its reuptake. Chapter 35 discusses neurotransmitters in greater detail.

(continued on page 238)

Table 10—1 Commonly Abused Substances

Name of Drug	Street Names	Onset of Action	Duration of Action	Desired Effect	Dependence Potential: Psychological/ Physical
Depressants					
Alcohol	Booze, juice, sauce	30 min	5—6 h up to 72 h	Reduction of anxiety; "high" feeling	High/High
Barbiturates:	Sleepers, downers	30—60 min	1—16 h	Relaxation and euphoria	High/High
Amobarbital (Amytal)	Blues				
Butabarbital (Butisol)	Yellows, yellow jackets				
Pentobarbital (Nembutal)					
Phenobarbital	Purple Hearts				
Secobarbital (Seconal)	Redbirds, red devils				
Secobarbital and amobarbital (Tuinal)	Heavens, tooies, rainbows				
Chloral hydrate (Noctec)		30 min	Half-life is 7—11 h	Sleep promotion, relaxation, and euphoria	Moderate/ Moderate
Chlordiazepox-ide hydrochloride (Librium)		15 min—4 h	Half-life PO is 5—30 h	(See chloral hydrate)	High/High
Diazepam (Valium)		15—60 min	3 h up to 3—4 d	(See chloral hydrate)	High/High
Glutethimide (Doriden)		30 min	Half-life is 5—22 h	(See chloral hydrate)	High/High
Meprobamate (Equanil, Miltown)		1 h	Half-life is 6—17 h	(See chloral hydrate)	High/High
Methaqualone (Quaalude, Sopor)	Quads, sopors, ludes	30 min	Half-life is 10—42 h	(See chloral hydrate)	High/High
Narcotics	Dope				
Opium/paregoric	Op, poppy	Minutes	4—6 h	Pain relief, sensation of pleasure (same for all narcotics)	High/High
Morphine sulfate	M, white stuff	Minutes	8—12		High/High
Methylmorphine, codeine	Schoolboy	Minutes	4—6 h		Moderate/ Moderate
Diacetylmor-phine (heroin)	H, horse, smack, junk, stuff, scag, brown sugar	Minutes	4—6 h		High/High

Tolerance	Usual Mode of Administration	Potential Reactions	Cues to Overdose	Symptoms of Withdrawal
Yes	Oral	Slurred speech, disorientation (same for all depressants)	Intoxication	Increased pulse, BP, temperature; diaphoresis; tremors; inner shakiness; hallucinations; delirium; convulsions; death (same for all depressants)
Yes	Oral, IM, IV		Cold, clammy skin; shallow breathing; weak, rapid pulse; dilated pupils; coma; death (same for all other depressants except alcohol)	
Yes	Oral			
Yes	Oral, IM, IV			
Yes	Oral, IM, IV			
Yes	Oral			
Yes	Oral			
Yes	Oral			
Yes	Oral, smoked	Drowsiness, euphoria, respiratory depression, constricted pupils, nausea (same for all narcotics)	Clammy skin; slow, shallow respirations; convulsions, coma, possible death (same for all narcotics)	Yawning, anorexia, insomnia, irritability, tremors, running nose, chills, panic, diaphoresis, cramps, nausea
Yes	IV, IM, smoked			
Yes	Oral, IV, IM			Milder than morphine but may last several weeks
Yes	IV, sniffed			(Same as methylmorphine)

(continued)

Table 10-1 Commonly Abused Substances (continued)

Name of Drug	Street Names	Onset of Action	Duration of Action	Desired Effect	Dependence Potential: Psychological/ Physical
Narcotics					
Meperidine hydrochloride (Demerol)	Cube	20–30 min	3 h		High/High
Methadone hydrochloride (Adanon, Dolophine)	Dolly	20–30 min	4–6 h	Heroin substitute	High/High
Stimulants					
Amphetamine sulfate (Benzedrine)	Speed, wake-ups, pep pills, bennies, lid poppers	Minutes	4–6 h	Alertness, increased feeling of energy, euphoria	High/Possible
Dextroamphe-tamine sulfate (Dexedrine)	Dexies, oranges, hearts	Minutes	4–6 h	(Same as amphetamine sulfate)	High/Possible
Cocaine hydrochloride*	Coke, C, snow, star dust, flake, gold dust, leaf, speed, lady	Minutes	4–6 h	Euphoria, excitation	Yes/Yes
Hallucinogens					
Lysergic acid diethylamide (LSD)	Acid, sugar cubes, big D, sunshine, blue dragon	Few minutes	10–12 h	Insight, exhilara-tion, increased energy (same for all halluci-nogens)	Unknown/None
Mescaline	Mesc, cactus, chief, peyote, white light, pink wedge	Few minutes	12–24 h		Unknown/None
Phenyclidine (PCP)	Angel dust, peace pill, hog, horse	Few minutes	12–24 h		Unknown/None
Psilocybin	God's flesh, exotic mush-room, silly putty	Few minutes	12–24 h		Unknown/None
Central Nervous System Toxins					
Cannabis sativa: marijuana	Pot, grass, joint, reefer, tea, Mary Jane, weed	Few minutes	Great range: 2–12 h	Relaxation, euphoria, increased per-ceptual abilities, sense of escape	Moderate/ Unknown
Hashish	Hash, Acapulco gold, ace, butter, black hash (con-tains opium), black Russian (contains very potent hashish)	Few minutes	Great range: 2–12 h	(Same as for marijuana)	Moderate/ Unknown
Nicotinia tabacum, nicotene	Fag, coffin nail	1–2 min	15 min–2 h	Relaxation	High/Possible

*Designated a narcotic under the Controlled Substances Act

Tolerance	Usual Mode of Administration	Potential Reactions	Cues to Overdose	Symptoms of Withdrawal
Yes	Oral, IM, IV			Shorter than morphine; begins 3 h after last dose; peaks at 8–12 h
Yes	Oral, IM, IV			Slower to develop than morphine; acute symptoms may last up to 6 wk; vague physical complaints for up to 6 mo
Yes	Oral, IM	Dilated pupils, increased pulse and blood pressure, anorexia, insomnia (same for all stimulants)	Agitation, fever, hallucinations, convulsions, death (same for all stimulants)	Apathy, fatigue and sleepiness, depression, disorientation (same for all stimulants)
Yes	Oral, IM			
Yes	Sniffed, IV			
Yes	Oral, IV	Illusions, hallucinations, decreased perception of time and distance (same for all hallucinogens)	Psychosis, flashbacks, brain damage, death (same for all hallucinogens)	None reported
Yes	Oral, IV			None reported
Yes	Oral, IV			None reported
Yes	Oral, IV			None reported
Yes	Smoked, oral	Relaxed inhibition, increased appetite, disorientation	Fatigue, paranoia, psychosis	Unclear; possible syndrome of anorexia, insomnia, hyperactivity
Yes	Smoked, oral	(Same as for marijuana)	(Same as for marijuana)	(Same as for marijuana)
Yes	Smoked, chewed, sniffed	Anorexia		Agitation, insomnia, nausea, headache, impaired concentration

Section II: Substances of Abuse

Abused drugs are categorized based on their effects on the central nervous system. The five primary classifications are: depressants (including alcohol and anxiolytic agents), narcotics, stimulants, hallucinogens, and central nervous system toxins.

All of the drugs in these five groups have one point in common: each drug can produce a pleasurable state by either elevating the mood and creating a "high" feeling or decreasing anxiety or tension. With frequent or repeated use, many of these drugs result in psychological and/or physical dependence. Recall that dependence motivates future substance use. The potential for psychological and physical dependence is identified in Table 10–1.

DEPRESSANTS (ALCOHOL AND ANXIOLYTIC AGENTS)

The drugs in this category have a depressant effect on the central nervous system; they include alcohol and the prescription medications known as anxiolytic agents because they reduce anxiety. In addition to decreasing anxiety, anxiolytic drugs also have sedative (promoting relaxation) or hypnotic (producing sleep) effects. Anxiolytic agents include, among others, the barbiturates such as phenobarbital, sodium pentobarbital, and secobarbital (Seconal) and non-barbiturate drugs such as chlordiazepoxide (Librium) and diazepam. Many people, including nurses, use these agents rather than problem-solving methods to help them cope with the pressures of life. Worldwide, the anxiolytic agents are the most frequently prescribed group of medicines for symptoms of sleeplessness and anxiety (Gilman, Goodman & Gilman, 1984).

Alcohol

Alcohol is one of the most easily available and frequently abused drugs in America. Of the adult population 18 years and older who report drinking behavior, the average daily consumption is about three drinks per day. Of course, a smaller proportion of people drinks more than average, and a larger proportion drinks much less. Of those who drink, 1 in 10 will become alcoholic (alcohol-dependent). Alcoholism is also a serious problem in the Soviet Union, France, and Sweden.

Alcohol is related to about half of all fatal automobile accidents and is cited in a high percentage of other accidental deaths such as drownings, fires, suicides, and homicides. Public concern with drunk driving has increased. The educational and lobbying efforts of such groups as MADD (Mothers Against Drunk Driving; see resources listing in Chapter 13) have resulted in tougher laws at both local and national levels. Some states have raised the legal drinking age to 21 and imposed strict fines and penalties for driving under the influence of alcohol.

Alcoholism costs the economy an estimated $50 billion annually because of lost productivity, property damage, medical expenses, rehabilitation programs, family disruptions, alcohol-related illnesses, alcohol-related violence, and neglect and abuse of children. The estimated 13 million Americans who are believed to be alcoholics or problem drinkers are associated with an annual toll of 50,000 traffic fatalities (Chiras, 1985), 15,000 suicides and homicides, most of the family violence, and half of the 5 million arrests each year (Wilson & Kneisl, 1983).

Although some may have a hereditary predisposition to alcoholism, for others, environmental stresses are important. Cultural factors also play a role. In some countries where drinking wine is a regular practice among youth and adults at family gatherings, incidence of alcoholism is lower. Certain other cultural groups are at high risk for alcoholism. Persons at risk according to the criteria developed by Seixas (1982) are identified in Box 10–1.

Alcohol use can impair health; its abuse leads to many life-threatening, chronic physical, and emotional illnesses. Alcohol abuse is, in reality, a potentially fatal illness. Jellinek's (1952) classic model with an insightful description of the phases of alcoholism, is outlined in Table 10–2. Although widely accepted, Jellinek's model does not hold true in every circumstance. Not all symptoms are present in alcoholics, and the sequence may vary. Women may also progress through the phases more rapidly than men.

Effects and Absorption

Alcohol is a central nervous system depressant that is rapidly absorbed from the stomach and small intestine and becomes evenly distributed throughout the body. Absorption from the stomach can be slowed by ingesting food or milk. Absorption rate and blood alcohol level are affected by the amount and concentration of alcohol ingested, the rate of drinking, and body weight. For example, a large

---

Box 10–1   Persons at High Risk for Developing Alcoholism

The potential for alcoholism is high when the following factors exist:

A family history of alcoholism

A family history of abstinence or strong moral controls

A family history with a high incidence of depression among female relatives

A history of divorce or parental disorder in the family of origin

Being a member of certain cultural groups (Irish, Scandinavian, Native American)

Being a heavy smoker

Table 10–2 Jellinek's Phases of Progressive Alcoholism

Phase	Description
Phase I Prealcoholic phase	Use of alcohol for relaxation and relief of tension and anxieties. Results in gradual increase in physiological tolerance.
Phase II Early alcoholic phase	Ushered in by first "blackout" (brief period of amnesia during or directly after drinking). Followed by further blackouts, sneaking of drinks, growing preoccupation with drinking situations, defensiveness about drinking, rationalizations and excuses, guilt about drinking, and increased denial of the problem.
Phase III Crucial phase	Frank addiction occurs, and physiological dependence is evident, with loss of control over drinking. Social and interpersonal difficulties result in job loss, marital disruption, and increased aggressive behavior. Life goals are replaced by goal to continue drinking.
Phase IV Chronic phase	Alcoholic goes on "benders," has decrease in tolerance, develops physiological deterioration and illnesses. With abrupt cessation, may experience alcohol withdrawal. Severe depression and other psychological and emotional symptoms become pronounced.

SOURCE: Adapted from Jellinek EM: Phases of alcohol addiction. Reprinted by permission from *Quarterly Journal of Studies in Alcohol*, 1952; 13:673–684. Copyright Journal of Studies on Alcohol, Inc., Rutgers Center of Alcohol Studies, New Brunswick, NJ 08903.

man can usually tolerate more alcohol than a small woman, provided the large man's size is not from excess fat.

The level of concentration of alcohol in the blood (the blood alcohol level, or BAL) determines the extent of the psychophysiological effects. A person who weighs 160 lb would have a BAL of 0.1% (the legal criterion for alcohol intoxication in almost all states) after drinking, in a 2-hour period, the amount of alcohol illustrated in Figure 10–1. Although caloric content varies, a "drink" of each type of beverage contains about the same total amount of alcohol. As tolerance to alcohol develops, these figures are no longer accurate; persons addicted to alcohol may reach higher blood alcohol levels without significant changes in their ability to control motor and CNS functions.

Menstrual cycle is sometimes said to affect the absorption rate of alcohol, although the actual mechanism has not yet been scientifically established. In a recent study of premenstrual syndrome (PMS), many women described

alcohol cravings and feeling intoxicated after drinking even small amounts (one or two beers or one or two drinks of hard liquor) during peak PMS symptoms (Norris, 1983).

The body metabolizes 90% to 98% of the ingested alcohol, mostly in the liver. The rest is excreted by the kidneys through the urine, by the lungs through exhalation, and by the skin through perspiration. Alcohol metabolism differs from that of most substances. Its rate of metabolism is constant with time; it is not increased by a rise in alcohol blood concentration. Thus, metabolism is not affected by the amount of alcohol ingested at one time, and the elimination of progressively higher concentrations of alcohol requires progressively longer periods of time. For example, in a person of average size, the average rate of alcohol metabolism is about 10 mL/h. Thus, it requires 5 to 6 hours to metabolize the amount of alcohol contained in 120 mL (4 oz) of whiskey or 1.2 L of beer.

This relatively slow and constant metabolic rate is

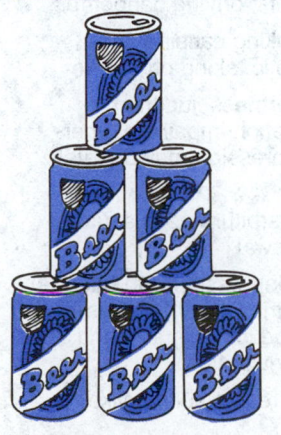
6 beers (12 oz)

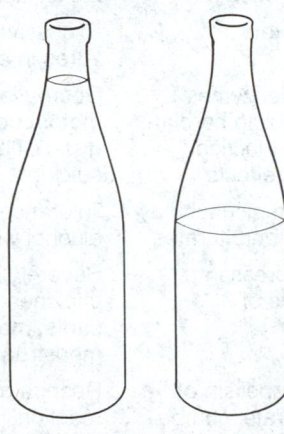
24 ounces of table wine   15 ounces of fortified wine

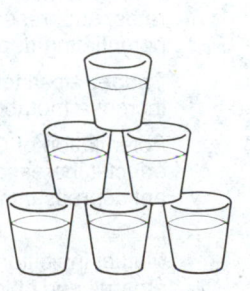
6 glasses of liquor (1.3 oz 80 proof)

Figure 10–1

Legally drunk. These amounts of alcoholic beverages, when consumed within a 2-hour period, will make a 160-pound person legally drunk in most states (BAL of 0.10 percent).
SOURCE: Combs BJ, Hales DR, Williams BK: *An Invitation to Health*, 2nd ed. Menlo Park, CA: Benjamin/Cummings, 1983.

responsible for the limits on the amount of alcohol that can be consumed over a period of time before a person becomes intoxicated. *Intoxication* occurs when more alcohol is consumed than can be metabolized. Various other factors, such as diet, hormones, and medications, may alter the metabolism of alcohol. For example, severe malnutrition lowers the rate of alcohol metabolism, but insulin raises it. Because such effects are slight, they probably have minimal significance in the treatment of acute alcohol intoxication. Drug interactions that alter the metabolism of alcohol are discussed in Table 10–3.

Multisystem Effects

The immediate effects of alcohol on all systems are relatively minor. Difficulties develop with prolonged use of large amounts of alcohol and the development of tolerance. Excessive consumption of alcohol often results in a reaction popularly known as the *hangover,* with headache, nausea and vomiting, dizziness, tremor, diaphoresis, thirst, and gastritis. Other disturbances associated with hangover are alterations in liver function, acid-base balance, and electrolyte homeostasis.

Even though the symptoms and signs of hangover are

Table 10–3 Drug Interactions With Alcohol (Ethanol)

Type of Drug	Physiologic Mechanism	Complications
Additive effect		
Analgesics, such as the salicylates (aspirin)	Ethanol damages gastric and intestinal mucosa; aspirin combined with hydrochloric acid can produce further damage and bleeding; inhibits ADP-induced blood platelet aggregation	Gastrointestinal bleeding and hemorrhage
Antianginals, such as the nitrates (amyl nitrate)	Side effects accentuated by ethanol	Postural hypotension
Antihypertensives, such as reserpine (Serpasil), methyldopa (Aldomet), hydralazine (Apresoline), guanethidine (Esimil, Ismelin), ganglionic blockers, propranolol (Inderal)	Additive hypotensive effect	Hypotension or syncope
	Propanolol may produce hypoglycemia by inhibiting transformation of glycogen in hepatic and skeletal muscle	Propanolol may mask symptoms and signs of alcohol-induced hypoglycemia (rapid heart beat, profuse sweating)
Diuretics, such as the thiazides (Esidrix, Oretic), furosemide (Lasix), chlorthalidone (Hygroton)	Alcohol inhibits release of antidiuretic hormone	Hypotension, isosmotic over-hydration
Marijuana	Enhanced euphoria with ethanol	Poor judgment, poor motor coordination, driving dangerous
Potentiating effect		
Antihistamines	Block histamine receptors; can both stimulate and depress CNS; alcohol potentiation of sedative effects	Most common side effect sedation with slow reflex activity and potential for accidents; driving dangerous
Anticonvulsants, such as phenytoin (Dilantin)	Metabolized at a faster rate	Excessive drinking causing seizures in epileptic taking phenytoin
Sedative-hypnotics, such as the barbiturates	Alcohol inhibits hepatic enzymes responsible for metabolizing barbiturates; suppresses CNS function, potentiating depressant effects	Decreased alertness, judgment; motor coordination impaired; synergistic CNS depression may be fatal; suicide
	Sudden abstinence from alcohol may increase metabolism of barbiturates	Tolerance to barbiturates in acute alcohol withdrawal
Methaqualone (Quaalude, Sopor)	Potentiation of CNS depressant effects; increases effects of antidepressants	Severe CNS depression with phenothiazines and tricyclic antidepressants; may produce epistaxis and menstrual irregularities
Chloral hydrate	Mutual inhibition of metabolism of ethanol and chloral hydrate; combination called "Mickey Finn"; increased CNS depressant effects	Respiratory arrest; disulfiramlike reaction

Type of Drug	Physiologic Mechanism	Complications
Benzodiazepines such as diazepam (Valium), chlordiazepoxide (Librium), flurazepam (Dalmane)	Ethanol increases absorption of benzodiazepines and increases CNS depressant effects	Some cross-tolerance, respiratory depression, impaired motor coordination and judgment
Meprobamate (Equanil, Miltown)		High potential for drug abuse
Phenothiazines	Metabolism of phenothiazines enhanced	Hypotension; lowered seizure threshold during alcohol withdrawal (should be used with caution); impaired psychomotor function and death; obstructive jaundice
Chlorpromazine (Thorazine)	May block uptake of guanethidine into sympathetic nerves, blocking antihypertensive effects	
Fluphenazine (Prolixin)		
Thioridazine (Mellaril), perphenazine (Trilafon)	Cardiac depressant effects with strong anticholinergic action, causing tachycardia	
Antidepressants (MAO inhibitors) Isocarboxazid (Marplan), nialamide (Niamid)	Metabolism of ethanol slowed; potentiated depressant effect	Disulfiramlike reaction
Phenelzine (Nardil)	Interaction with tyramine contained in many alcoholic beverages (especially beer and wine)	May cause hypertensive crisis
Tricyclic antidepressants such as: Amitriptyline (Elavil), imipramine (Tofranil), desipramine (Norpramin, Pertofrane), nortriptyline (Aventyl), doxepin (Sinequan)	Metabolism in liver may be interrupted by damaged liver; produce quinidine-like effect on heart, prolonging atrioventricular conduction time	Lowered seizure threshold; psychomotor skills severely affected; dangerous to drive or operate machinery; orthostatic hypotension
Narcotics, such as opioids (morphine), hydromorphone (Dilaudid), meperidine (Demerol), propoxyphene (Darvon)	Ethanol may increase metabolism of narcotics, potentiating CNS depressant effects	Respiratory depression, hypotension, death
Anesthetics, such as ether, chloroform	Ethanol and ether interaction is addictive; tolerance to ethanol may induce cross-tolerance to anesthetics	May require increased dosage; prolonged postoperative recovery; respiratory complications
Nicotine	See discussion of tobacco abuse	Secondary complications from smoking; respiratory complications
Antagonistic effect		
Anticoagulants, such as coumarin	Metabolism is increased; action may be enhanced because of diminished formation of prothrombin in alcohol-liver disease	May require increased dose; danger of hemorrhage; decreased anticoagulant effects
Antibiotics: nitrofurans such as chloramphenicol (Chloromycetin), metronidazole (Flagyl), furazolidine (Furoxone), quinacrine (Atabrine)	Enzyme inhibition by antibiotics, preventing oxidation of acetaldehyde	May provoke disulfiramlike reaction (flushing, headache, nausea, vomiting); possibly seizures
Hypoglycemics: sulfonylureas such as tolbutamide (Orinase), tolazamide (Tolinase), chlorpropamide (Diabinese), acetohexamide (Dymelor)	Ethanol produces hypoglycemia, may increase the rate of metabolism of hypoglycemics; unpredictable fluctuations of plasma concentrations in chronic ethanol consumption; decreases half-life of tolbutamide	Hypoglycemic reactions; disulfiramlike reactions
Disulfiram (Antabuse)	Markedly alters the intermediary metabolism of alcohol; blood acetaldehyde concentration rises 5–10 times higher	Disulfiram or acetaldehyde syndrome; may produce hypotension and shock
Stimulants, such as caffeine (coffee, tea, cola); amphetamines, such as methylphenidate (Ritalin)	Antagonize CNS depressant effects of alcohol (may be synergistic)	Untoward effects on cardiovascular system; hypertension and excessively rapid heartbeat; serious in client with decreased cardiac function secondary to alcoholism; can promote seizure disorders

well recognized, their possible biochemical background is not well understood. The pathogenesis of hangover has been associated with the accumulation of lactic acid and acetaldehyde in the blood and with hypoglycemia. Experimental evidence is varied and contradictory, however. Ordinarily, alcoholic drinks rich in congeners (such as gin) induce a more severe hangover than those that are nearly pure alcohol (such as vodka). It is probable, however, that alcohol alone in large doses is capable of inducing severe hangovers.

The effects of excessive alcohol use on the hepatic, nervous, cardiovascular, musculoskeletal, gastrointestinal, and reproductive systems are discussed below. Some of the medical problems attributed to chronic excessive use of alcohol are listed in Box 10–2.

Hepatic System. Although nearly every body system is eventually affected by prolonged use of alcohol, the system most often affected is the hepatic system, specifically the liver (Figure 10–2). A major effect of ethanol includes the development of fatty liver, which leads to Laennec's cirrhosis if the individual continues to ingest alcohol. If alcohol ingestion is stopped before the onset of cirrhosis, the fatty liver can return to normal, and cirrhosis is avoided. It may take from 5 to 20 years of chronic alcohol ingestion for Laennec's cirrhosis to result (see Chapter 53).

Neurologic System. Alcohol has significant effects on the nervous system. It has an immediate central nervous system depressant effect, causing less efficient func-

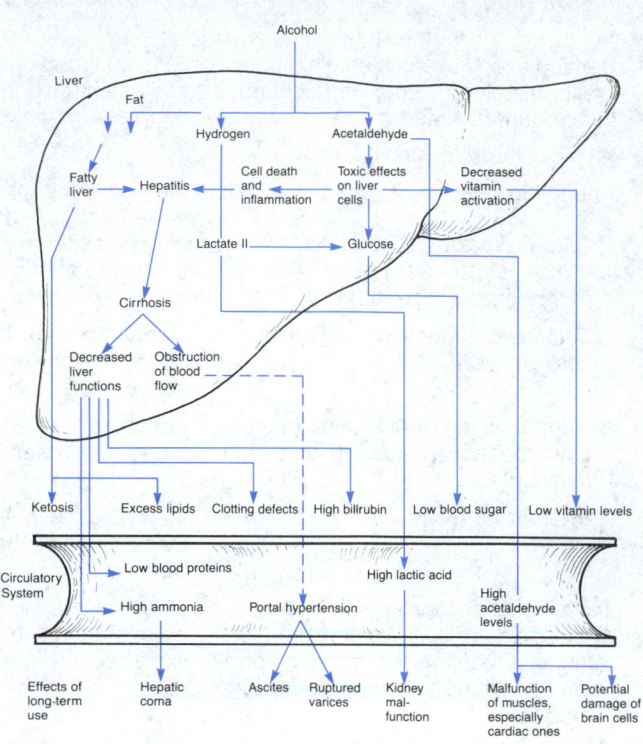

Figure 10–2

Long-term effects of alcohol abuse on liver function.

tioning. Although people often refer to alcoholic beverages as stimulating, the apparent stimulation results from the depression of the brain's inhibitory control mechanisms. The effects are increased compulsive behavior and unrestrained activity that often occur early in progressive intoxication. Alcohol simply eliminates the usual ability to repress such behavior.

Chronic excessive use of alcohol is directly associated with serious neurologic consequences. Although this is partially because of the toxic effects of alcohol itself, it is also a by-product of the nutritional problems of most heavy drinkers, who prefer alcohol to food. The serious nutritional deficiencies may lead to anemias, beriberi, heart disease, and cheilosis (scaling and lesions around the lips and mouth), Wernicke–Korsakoff syndrome (associated with thiamine deficiency), and peripheral neuropathy (associated with vitamin B deficiency). Marchiafava–Bignami disease, central pontine myelinosis, cerebellar degeneration, and alcoholic amblyopia may also occur (Estes, Smith-DiJulio, & Heinemann, 1980). The last four conditions are rare and incompletely understood.

Alcoholic peripheral neuropathy is slow, insidious, and progressive. It is the most common form of peripheral neuropathy and results from multiple nerve degeneration because of nutritional deficiency, principally of the B vitamins. Although thiamine is important for its role in the

Box 10–2	Medical Problems Attributed to Chronic Excessive Use of Alcohol
Anemia	Hepatitis
Atherosclerosis	Hypokalemia
Atrial fibrillation	Hypomagnesemia
Beriberi	Impotence
Cancers of gastrointestinal system	Leukopenia
Cardiomyopathy	Megaloblastic hematopoiesis
Cheilosis	Myopathy
Cirrhosis	Pancreatitis
Diabetes	Peptic ulcers
Duodenal ulcers	Peripheral neuropathy
Esophagitis	Sterility in males
Fatty liver	Testicular atrophy
Fetal alcohol syndrome	Thrombocytopenia
Gastritis	Wernicke–Korsakoff syndrome
Gynecomastia	

conversion of glucose (needed for nerve cell function), deficiencies of niacin, pantothenic acid, and pyridoxine may also be present.

In some persons, the syndrome may occur rapidly over a few days, but in others, symptoms may go unnoticed. The person may first experience pain or tenderness in the calf muscles or feet or tingling, burning, prickling, or numbness in the lower extremities. Varying degrees of sensory, motor, and reflex loss typically occur in the feet before they do in the hands and arms. As the degenerative process continues, muscle weakness, wasting, and diminished sensation characterized by an ataxic, wide-based gait may occur.

Recovery, which depends on the degree of nerve degeneration, may be rapid for those whose condition was diagnosed early but longer for those requiring extensive nerve regeneration. Treatment includes abstinence from alcohol, correction of nutritional deficiencies, and high doses of supplemental B vitamins.

The *Wernicke–Korsakoff syndrome* is an extreme on the continuum of cognitive impairment resulting from alcohol-induced brain damage. Because this syndrome was originally described as two separate entities, it may be helpful to distinguish Wernicke's encephalopathy from Korsakoff's psychosis. However, since their etiology is the same, they occur together, and their treatment is the same, they are now recognized as one syndrome. Wernicke's encephalopathy is a degenerative brain condition involving lesions in several areas of the brain. Symptoms are a global confusional state, somnolence and disinterest, ataxia (lack of muscular coordination), ophthalmoplegia (ocular muscle paralysis), and nystagmus (rhythmic jerking motion on horizontal gaze). In addition, polyneuropathies may be present (pain, loss of sensation, and weakness of legs and arms).

A typical person with these symptoms is likely to be a chronic alcoholic between 40 and 60 years of age in a confused and excited state. Within a few days, this person develops diplopia (double vision) from palsy of the abducens nerve (CN VI). Diplopia is a critical diagnostic criterion of Wernicke's encephalopathy because many alcoholics may appear confused, excited, or delirious without actually having Wernicke's. Once diplopia develops, the client's mental state may progress from quietness to stupor. Treatment must be initiated immediately to prevent fatal midbrain hemorrhage (Estes & Heinemann, 1982).

Korsakoff's psychosis is characterized by degenerative changes in the thalamus caused by a deficiency of B complex vitamins, particularly thiamine and vitamin B_{12}. The most striking and common symptoms of Korsakoff's psychosis are severe amnesia, confabulation, and remarkable personality changes. Memory disorder involves two forms of amnesia: anterograde (difficulty in remembering new information since the onset of the illness) and retrograde (difficulty in recalling events prior to the brain damage).

Treatment with high doses of thiamine and other vitamin supplements should be started as soon as possible and abstinence from alcohol encouraged. After 2 or 3 weeks of IV thiamine therapy (usually an initial dose of 100 mg by IV push, followed by daily doses of 50 to 100 mg until the client is taking a balanced diet daily), the ocular symptoms, ataxia, and global confusion disappear or improve greatly (Budassi, 1982). Recovery from Wernicke–Korsakoff's syndrome varies depending on the stage of the disease process but is usually slow and incomplete. Unfortunately, clients who suffer severe neurologic alterations have the poorest and most incomplete recovery; they may require supervisory care (usually in an institution) for the remainder of their lives.

Cardiovascular System. Alcohol has both direct and indirect effects on the cardiovascular system. In low doses, alcohol increases heart rate and cardiac output. With increased consumption, however, heart rate and cardiac output are decreased. Eventually, with prolonged excessive use of alcohol, the efficiency of the cardiac muscle, valves, conduction system, blood supply, and neural mechanisms is reduced. Impairment of the heart's pumping function eventually results in alcoholic cardiomyopathy.

Alcoholic cardiomyopathy is a syndrome of cardiac dysfunction primarily involving the heart muscle, with relatively little effect on the rest of the cardiovascular system. Clinical symptoms have a slow, insidious onset and are similar to those in congestive heart failure and cardiac dysrhythmias. Treatment includes absolute, continuous absti-

Nursing Research Note

Lenehan–Pisarcik G, Gastfriend D, Stetler C: Use of haloperidol with alcohol-intoxicated ED patients. *JEN* (March-April) 1985; 11:72–79.

This study examined the effectiveness and safety of haloperidol in calming and treating acutely intoxicated, agitated, and aggressive clients. Emergency room clients who met the criteria for the study were monitored for changes in heart rate and blood pressure as well as changes in behavioral states. These observations were collected at timed intervals. The results suggest that haloperidol causes a decrease in blood pressure and heart rate. This drop was not associated with clinical evidence of shock or physiological decompensation. The drug did cause somnolence in 67% of the sample. There was no evidence of dystonic reactions. Haloperidol resulted in a trend toward calmness, positive verbal and nonverbal behaviors, and cooperative behavior.

This study indicates that use of haloperidol for agitated alcohol-intoxicated clients needs further investigation. The results suggest the drug has a positive effect when used to calm agitated clients. Nurses should evaluate haloperidol use with alcohol-induced agitation and assess for changes in behavior, side effects, and alterations in physiological parameters.

nence from alcohol and management of congestive heart failure symptoms: tachycardia, palpitations, dyspnea, orthopnea, decreased tolerance for exercise, and nonproductive cough. Mild diuresis and rest are effective interventions in the early stage. Additional treatment measures—oxygen, digitalization, sodium restriction—are instituted for severe symptoms (refer to Chapter 24).

Other indirect effects of excessive alcohol ingestion on the cardiovascular system are: hypokalemia (from low potassium levels), hypomagnesemia (from increased magnesium secretion in urine), hyperlipidemia (causing atherosclerosis), and altered fluid balance (from decreased circulating levels of antidiuretic hormone or diuresis). Beriberi heart disease (from marked thiamine deficiency) is another complication. In contrast to alcoholic cardiomyopathy, beriberi heart disease is characterized by increased cardiac output and decreased circulation time due to marked reduction in peripheral vascular resistance. Peripheral neuropathies are also present. Treatment includes vigorous thiamine replacement, general nutritional improvement, and abstinence from alcohol.

Hematopoeitic System. A variety of hematological abnormalities occur with alcohol ingestion. Inhibition of folate metabolism induces megaloblastic hematopoiesis, ineffective cell production, anemia, leukopenia, and thrombocytopenia. These conditions, discussed in detail in Chapter 29, can be corrected by improving the client's nutritional status or administering folate as a dietary supplement.

Musculoskeletal System. Excessive alcohol use has a damaging effect on the skeletal muscles in three clinical forms: acute alcoholic myopathy, subclinical alcoholic myopathy, and chronic alcoholic myopathy. The exact mechanism by which alcohol induces muscle damage has not been completely established. Muscle damage seems to be related to the direct toxic effects of alcohol; these toxic effects cause alterations in muscle cell permeability and interfere with the normal electrochemical and metabolic functions of the cell.

In acute alcoholic myopathy, clients have muscle pain, tenderness, and edema following an episode of excessive alcohol intake. These symptoms are most common in the proximal muscles of the arms and legs, the pelvic and shoulder girdle, and the thoracic cage. In subclinical alcoholic myopathy, clients actually have acute alcoholic myopathy, but the symptoms are masked by the symptoms of concurrent acute intoxication or withdrawal. With appropriate treatment, including alcohol abstinence, balanced nutrition, and vitamin supplementation, symptoms gradually become less severe and abate within a few weeks. Symptoms may return, however, with a future episode of excessive drinking. In chronic alcoholic myopathy, clients have slow, insidious muscle wasting and weakness in the same muscles affected in acute alcoholic myopathy but without pain and tenderness. Treatment is the same as for acute alcoholic myopathy.

Gastrointestinal System. Alcohol stimulates the secretion of gastric acid, irritates the gastric mucosa, and causes gastritis. It aggravates preexisting peptic disorders or may even cause them. Alcoholics are prone to esophagitis because of increased gastric secretions and frequent vomiting. Severe vomiting may also lead to the development of Mallory–Weiss syndrome (lacerations of the mucosa at the gastroesophageal juncture) or the more serious Boerhaave's syndrome (rupture of the lower portion of the esophagus). Excessive alcohol intake may lead to acute and chronic pancreatitis. Insufficient food and bulk intake and malabsorption of fat, xylose, folic acid, B vitamins, and minerals in the digestive tract lead to nutritional deficiency diseases. Alcoholics also suffer from nausea, abdominal pain, erratic bowel function (constipation and diarrhea), gastrointestinal hemorrhage, and jaundice.

Although the exact reason is unknown, alcoholics have a high incidence of digestive tract cancers. This may be because of carcinogenic substances in alcoholic beverages and the possibility that ethanol itself acts as a carcinogen. That many alcoholics are also chronic smokers is also related to their susceptibility to cancer. Because cigarette smoking alone is known to increase the risk of cancer in some of the same body areas, separating the two factors is difficult. One theory is that alcohol increases the metabolizing enzymes in the liver, thereby speeding the conversion of noncarcinogens to carcinogens. In clients with cirrhosis of the liver, the liver may not be able to detoxify carcinogens such as tobacco.

Reproductive System. Sexual problems result from the ineffective and deteriorating relationships common in alcoholism. Early use of alcohol may lessen inhibitions on sexual behavior, and some users may experience a psychological sexual arousal. Excessive alcohol use generally reduces performance ability, however. In fact, in men, chronic use of alcohol may lead to impotence, sterility, and gynecomastia (excessive development of the mammary glands). Women also become anorgasmic. Recovery from alcoholism is usually paralleled by recovery from sexual dysfunction.

Fetal alcohol syndrome (FAS), one of the three leading causes of birth defects, occurs in infants born to mothers who chronically ingest large amounts of alcohol. Because alcohol rapidly crosses the placenta and affects the developing fetus, FAS babies have growth deficiencies, characteristic clusters of facial deformities, a variety of minor and major abnormalities, intellectual impairments, and psychomotor retardation. At birth, the infant may need to be gradually withdrawn from alcohol just as the infant born to a heroin addict must be withdrawn from heroin. It is not known exactly how much alcohol consumption causes FAS or during which stage of pregnancy the fetus is most likely to be affected. Although light social drinking does not appear to produce FAS, it is wise to advise pregnant women to refrain completely from drinking alcohol.

Anxiolytic Agents

The initial anxiolytic agents were the barbiturates. Because of their ability to reduce anxiety and tension, their use, misuse, and abuse became extensive. Other dangers soon became apparent. The barbiturates create tolerance and cross-tolerance to other depressant drugs, dependence, severe life-threatening withdrawal symptoms, and death from overdose. These problems stimulated the search for a replacement. The drugs that emerged to replace the barbiturates for daytime sedation and treatment of anxiety symptoms were the benzodiazepines. Unfortunately, these drugs possess dangers similar to the barbiturates: tolerance, dependence, and overdose.

Effects and Absorption

The benzodiazepines, first prescribed in the 1950s, are currently used in the treatment of neurotic reactions. They are also used to reduce anxiety, induce sleep, promote relaxation of the skeletal muscles, and to produce an anticonvulsant effect. These agents are thus prescribed for clients experiencing withdrawal symptoms.

The precise mechanisms of action of the benzodiazepines have not been clearly delineated. All the benzodiazepines are absorbed and metabolized similarly. They are rapidly absorbed when administered orally. Then, metabolism proceeds according to two phases. Initially, a portion of the drug is quickly eliminated within a few hours. The rest is converted to active metabolites. Since these drugs are lipid-soluble, they are then widely dispersed throughout the body's fat tissues. The accumulation of these metabolites may produce a cumulative effect resulting in oversedation and/or ataxia.

Since the benzodiazepines tend to precipitate in muscle, they are poorly absorbed when administered intramuscularly. If it is necessary to administer a benzodiazepine intramuscularly, however, the injection should be given slowly and deeply into the gluteus muscle.

The barbiturates are basically salts or derivatives of barbituric acid. They produce sedative effects with low dosages or hypnotic effects with high dosages. Since they are derived from the same source, all of the barbiturates possess the same mechanisms of action, problems, and side effects. Very high doses of the barbiturates will produce a feeling of euphoria or a "high" similar to alcohol-induced states.

Barbiturates produce all degrees of depression of the central nervous system, ranging from mild sedation to general anesthesia. When barbiturates are given in sedative or hypnotic doses, there is little effect on skeletal, cardiac, or smooth muscle. If depression is severe, however, as in acute barbiturate intoxication, serious deficits in cardiovascular and peripheral functions occur. The barbiturates alter the stages of sleep and depress respiration. In hypnotic doses, depressant effects on respiration are minor; however, when clients have pulmonary insufficiency or overdose, severe respiratory depression may occur. In small doses, barbiturates have a hyperanalgesic effect and may increase the client's reaction to pain. Thus, in the presence of pain, barbiturates may produce a paradoxical effect: overexcitement rather than the usual sedation (Gilman et al., 1984).

The barbiturates are readily absorbed and metabolized in the liver. A dangerous side effect of barbiturates is their capacity to increase the synthesis of porphyrins (nitrogen-containing compounds necessary for heme biosynthesis in hemoglobin); thus, they should not be given to clients with acute intermittent porphyria. Since cirrhosis increases both the half-life of some barbiturates and the client's sensitivity to the drug, barbiturates should also not be administered to clients with cirrhosis. Clients receiving anticoagulant therapy should also be monitored carefully since barbiturates decrease the action of anticoagulant drugs.

The barbiturates continue to be used for analgesia and anesthesia and for the treatment of some gastrointestinal disorders, hypertension, asthma, cardiovascular disease, insomnia, and epilepsy. Therefore, they continue to be available for illicit drug use and are often used by amphetamine ("speed") abusers to counter the agitated effects of "overamping" (overuse). Infants born to women who are physically dependent on depressants have symptoms similar to those in infants born to women addicted to heroin. Postnatal withdrawal syndromes vary in severity (see section on narcotics).

Patterns of Abuse With Anxiolytic Agents

Three patterns of abuse with anxiolytic agents have been identified:

- An individual, usually a middle-class woman between the ages of 30 and 60, gradually begins to increase the prescribed dose without consulting her physician. She may begin to "shop" around, procuring a number of prescriptions from various other physicians for sleep disturbance or anxiety. Several months may pass before a pronounced dependence occurs, bringing the consequences of withdrawal and other complications of high-dose maintenance.

- In periodic recreational intoxication, usually by teenagers or young adults, the pattern is becoming "high" at concerts, social functions, or any event that provides the motivation for use. Risks associated with this pattern include obtaining drugs on the black market that may be "mixed" or have unreliable content, accidents occurring during an intoxicated or out-of-control state, overdose danger because of the trend to mix drugs with alcohol or other depressants, and the potential for addiction.

- A third pattern is specific to the intravenous use of barbiturates. The "barb freak" is characteristically a young adult who has experimented or abused many and various drugs and chooses barbiturates for the "rush" experienced with intravenous injection. Serious health risks include overdose, infections, allergic reactions from contaminants, and accidental injection into an artery.

Physiological and psychological dependence and tolerance develop quickly with these drugs. If untreated, withdrawal usually produces serious medical consequences resulting in coma, respiratory depression, and death. When tolerance develops, accidental overdose can easily occur because the upper limit of tolerance is close to the lethal dose. Overdose occurs when the client accidentally takes more medication than is therapeutically indicated or actually attempts suicide.

NARCOTICS

Throughout history, the narcotics have been used for medicine or pleasure. They continue to be used as analgesics in treating both acute and chronic pain. Because of their rapid action and propensity for physical dependence, however, the abuse of these drugs poses a major problem for society. This class of drugs refers to the natural derivatives from the oriental poppy *(Papaver somniferum)*—opium, morphine, codeine—as well as synthetic chemicals that have morphinelike action such as heroin, meperidine (Demerol), and methadone (Dolophine). Narcotics cause mood changes, mental clouding, pain reduction, and drowsiness. Addicts describe a state of euphoria with the use of narcotics similar to that experienced during orgasm.

Codeine is more commonly abused than heroin because it is less expensive and more readily available in cough elixers and syrups or analgesic tablets. Codeine withdrawal is similar to morphine withdrawal though less severe. For differences in withdrawal patterns for codeine, meperidine, and methadone, see Table 10–1.

All narcotics create psychological and physical dependence and tolerance and have similar properties, mechanisms of action, and withdrawal syndromes (refer to Table 10–1). Dependence occurs in individuals who take drugs as a way of life rather than in those who use drugs during a specific traumatic time in their lives or for a short-term medical reason.

When heroin was first introduced at the end of the nineteenth century, it was as a cough suppressant and a cure for opium and morphine dependence. By various estimates and depending on the availability of heroin on the illicit market, there are between 400,000 and 750,000 heroin addicts in the United States at any time. Heroin abuse is not confined to large metropolitan areas. It can be found in medium-sized communities and small cities, and the drug is abused by persons from all socioeconomic and ethnic segments of the population.

In addition to having a high annual mortality rate, approximately 10 per 1000 heroin-addicted persons are subject to multiple health and personal hazards (American Psychiatric Association, 1980). The heroin user is at high risk for hepatitis and other infections from contaminated equipment. Heroin addicts are also one of the high-risk groups for contracting acquired immune deficiency syndrome (AIDS) (see Chapter 29). The drug often contains impurities because of carelessness in manufacture or the purposeful addition of impurities to "cut" the heroin or extend it, increasing bulk and profit for the seller. These impurities also put the addict at high risk for poisoning, inflammation, and a variety of other disorders. The heroin user is also at risk for overdose and death and for chronic undernutrition. In addition, social, work, and family relationships are often disrupted.

Because heroin is rapidly converted to morphine in the bloodstream, the actions as well as the withdrawal pattern are essentially the same, except withdrawal symptoms may occur earlier with heroin than morphine. The severity of withdrawal is determined by two factors: (1) the amount of the dose and (2) the method of administration. Symptoms are more severe in persons who take high doses or administer the drug intravenously (Bennett et al., 1983).

Abrupt morphine abstinence produces the pattern of withdrawal signs and symptoms shown in Figure 10–3. Earliest signs of withdrawal are:

- Coryza
- Extreme yawning
- Diaphoresis
- Gooseflesh
- Dilated pupils

Following the last dose, withdrawal generally begins within 8 to 12 hours becoming most intense by 36 to 48 hours. After the onset of early symptoms, there is a period of "yen," or fretful sleep. Upon wakening, symptoms worsen. The acute phase lasts 10 to 14 days. Prolonged irritability, anxiety, inability to cope with minor problems, and physical complaints are symptoms of chronic withdrawal and are associated with the compulsion to obtain more drugs.

Pregnant women who have been taking opioids regularly will deliver infants who are physically dependent. Signs of withdrawal in these infants include (in varying degrees of severity), irritability, excessive high-pitched crying, tremors, frantic sucking of fists, hyperactive reflexes, increased respiratory rate, increased stools, sneezing, yawning, vomiting, and fever. Signs of heroin withdrawal commonly appear within the first 24 hours of birth, but may not appear for several days when the mother has been taking methadone. The dose the mother takes, or how long she has taken it, does not always correlate with the intensity of the syndrome. Although there is no consensus on the best method of treating physically dependent infants, the use of paregoric (0.2 mL orally 3 to 4 h, increased as needed) seems to be one effective approach as long as simultaneous dependence on alcohol or other sedatives is not present (Gilman et al., 1984).

STIMULANTS

Stimulants are most popular with the student population (ages 18 to 25) but are used and abused by many people

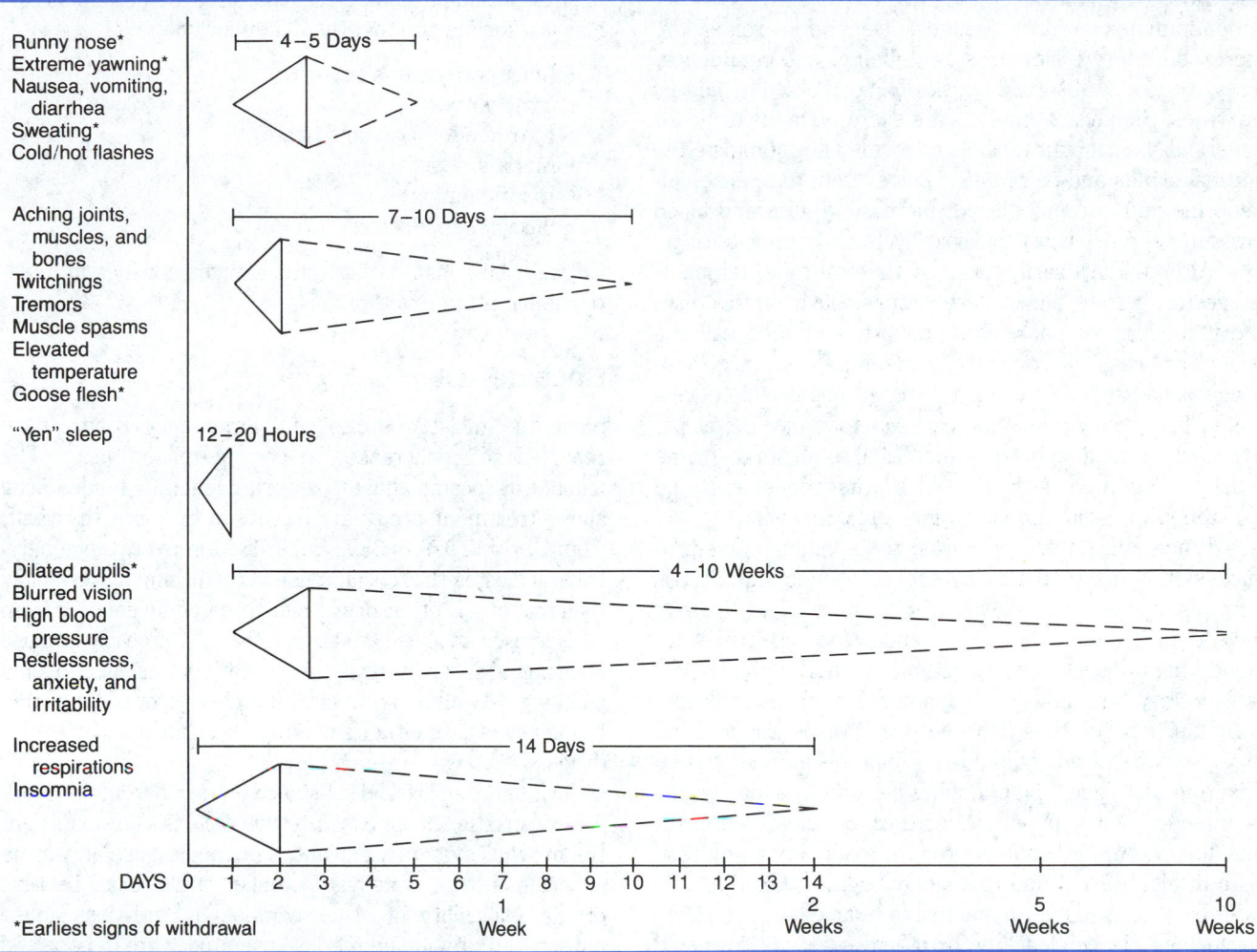

Runny nose*
Extreme yawning*
Nausea, vomiting, diarrhea
Sweating*
Cold/hot flashes
|— 4–5 Days —|

Aching joints, muscles, and bones
Twitchings
Tremors
Muscle spasms
Elevated temperature
Goose flesh*
|— 7–10 Days —|

"Yen" sleep
12–20 Hours

Dilated pupils*
Blurred vision
High blood pressure
Restlessness, anxiety, and irritability
|— 4–10 Weeks —|

Increased respirations
Insomnia
|— 14 Days —|

DAYS 0 1 2 3 4 5 6 7 8 9 10 11 12 13 14

1 Week   2 Weeks   5 Weeks   10 Weeks

*Earliest signs of withdrawal

Figure 10–3

Signs and symptoms of morphine withdrawal.
SOURCE: Woolf D: Opioids. In: Bennett G, Vourakis C, Woolf DS (editors), *Substance Abuse: Pharmacologic, Developmental, and Clinical Perspectives*. New York: Wiley, 1983.

to combat fatigue, elevate mood, increase alertness, and suppress appetite. Stimulants include two major categories—amphetamines and cocaine—as well as other substances such as caffeine and nicotine contained in some antihistamines and cold preparations. Stimulants are sympathomimetic amines that act on the cerebral cortex and the reticular activating system, elevating mood and decreasing fatigue and appetite. In general, stimulant drugs do not produce physical dependence in the same sense as the depressants and narcotics. All seem capable, however, of producing a psychological dependence, which may range from weak to extremely strong.

Millions of legal prescriptions are written each year for these drugs despite their high propensity for psychological dependence and abuse. Stimulants are used to treat the common cold (Benzedrine inhalers), narcolepsy, hyperactivity in children, and mild depression. Because of their recognized potential for abuse and the speed with which tolerance develops (8 to 12 weeks), current accepted medical use is generally limited to treating hyperkinesis in children and narcolepsy.

Amphetamines

Athletes and entertainers have long been known to abuse stimulants to increase performance and endurance. The stimulant effects falsely signal to athletes that they are "up" and ready to compete. A danger is that the effects of amphetamines mask signs of fatigue and alter judgment. Thus, athletes who use them may perform beyond the safety level in endurance events such as bicycle marathons and risk cardiovascular collapse and death.

Amphetamines as "diet pills" were once popular for weight control. Although they do suppress appetite, they lose their anorexic effects within about 4 to 8 weeks. Beyond this point, the dieter is in danger of developing tolerance and using amphetamines to elevate mood and ward off depression.

Physiologic Effects

Amphetamines produce feelings of euphoria, relaxation, increased energy, alertness, well-being, and confidence. They are readily absorbed but slowly metabolized by hepatic enzymes. Significant amounts are excreted in the urine for several days in an unmetabolized form. They stimulate the adrenal glands and central nervous system to release epinephrine and norepinephrine, increasing pulse and blood pressure, serum glucose and lipid levels, and muscle tension.

Although ordinarily taken by the oral route, amphetamines can also be administered intravenously. In this case, the immediate response is a euphoric sensation called a "flash" or "rush," accompanied by feelings of extreme adequacy, self-confidence, unlimited energy, and complete well-being. Frequency of use increases as tolerance develops; eventually, the dose must be increased to obtain the same results. The time between "runs" (injections) must be shortened to avoid intense fatigue and depression.

When abused in high doses, the amphetamines produce symptoms mediated by the autonomic and central nervous system. Cardiovascular symptoms of toxicity include tachycardia, headache, and when taken in sufficiently high doses, life-threatening dysrhythmias. Hypertension may be followed by hypotension when cardiovascular function becomes impaired. Cerebrovascular accident may also occur. Gastrointestinal symptoms include nausea, vomiting, diarrhea, and cramping. Diaphoresis may occur, or in some cases, hyperthermia may develop, and death may follow. Amphetamines produce irritability and jitteriness in high doses, and users may begin to take barbiturates or other sedative-hypnotics to reduce these unpleasant feelings. Dependence on both "uppers" and "downers" results.

Toxic Psychosis

A toxic psychosis from amphetamine abuse may occur in chronic abusers. Amphetamine psychosis closely resembles the clinical picture of paranoid schizophrenia with the following symptoms:

- Paranoid ideation with well-formed delusions
- Stereotyped compulsive behaviors such as agitated pacing
- Visual, auditory, tactile, and olfactory hallucinations
- Increased libido
- Severe to panic levels of anxiety with potential for violent behavior

It is important to note that although the two psychoses appear similar, the client with an amphetamine psychosis does not experience the thought disorders common in schizophrenia. Also, the schizophrenic client seldom has tactile and olfactory hallucinations but is more likely to have visual or auditory hallucinations. Rather than the flat, bland affect common in schizophrenia, the client with an amphetamine psychosis appears highly anxious.

Although no physical withdrawal syndrome follows the abrupt discontinuation of amphetamine use, a combination of physical and psychological symptoms are prominent and may last for several months. They include:

- Long periods of sleep
- Irritability
- Extreme lethargy and apathy
- Marked depression
- Disorientation
- Suicidal tendencies

Clients who abuse barbiturates simultaneously will experience barbiturate withdrawal.

Cocaine

Since the mid-1970s, hospital emergency rooms have reported sharp increases in cocaine-related visits. The number of cocaine abusers entering federally funded drug abuse treatment programs increased by more than half, from 1961 in 1979 to 3393 in 1981. Moreover, the general trend indicates that cocaine use is increasing more rapidly than that of any other drug. Life-threatening dangers from cocaine use and abuse are also on the rise, probably because of changing patterns of administration such as injecting and smoking as well as an overall increase in prevalence and frequency of use, either alone or in combination with other drugs.

Cocaine, an alkaloid substance extracted from the South American coca shrub, *Erythroxylon coca,* is a powerful central nervous system stimulant. The medical use of cocaine is limited because of its high potential for abuse and because of the availability of other compounds with less abuse potential. Its two main medical uses today are in nose and throat surgery as an effective local anesthetic that also constricts blood vessels and reduces bleeding at the operative site and as an ingredient in Brompton's cocktail given to clients with terminal cancer (see Chapter 16).

Because of its ability to produce intense euphoria and a profound sense of well-being, cocaine is a favorite drug for social and recreational use among the middle and upper socioeconomic classes. Users believe it enhances sociability and talkativeness, elevates mood, and reduces fatigue without clouding the sensorium or causing disorientation. Although the biological mechanisms responsible for cocaine's ability to produce mood elevation or euphoria have not been clearly identified, the drug is thought to have a direct effect on cortical cells or the ascending reticular activating system and to alter catecholamine levels.

The question of whether cocaine causes physical dependence requires further study. Cocaine does have a strong potential for psychological dependence, however. Among those who develop a pattern of chronic, high-dose use, the abrupt cessation of cocaine use produces an abstinence syndrome with symptoms of craving for the drug, prolonged sleep, fatigue, hunger, and depression.

The usual or preferred method of administration is "snorting" or inhalation for absorption through the nasal mucosa. Prolonged use of cocaine by this method can damage and erode the nasal mucosa, with eventual perforation of the nasal septum. "Freebasing" is a method of making cocaine more palatable for smoking by removing water-soluble adulterants from street-grade cocaine to obtain a white talclike powder. Overdosing can occur when cocaine is smoked or injected subcutaneously or intravenously, and death can occur from respiratory paralysis and cardiovascular collapse.

Cocaine psychosis may result from high doses of the drug or prolonged use. The psychosis is characterized by symptoms similar to those of schizophrenia or paranoia. A specific type of tactile hallucination known as *formication*— the sensation of insects or bugs crawling on the skin or burrowing under the skin ("cocaine bugs")—may lead to scratching, gouging, and excoriation of skin. Nurses may see the cocaine abuser in the withdrawal state, which is similar to amphetamine psychosis except that symptoms are less severe, of shorter duration, and transient.

Caffeine

Caffeine—a methylxanthine derivative from coffee beans, tea leaves, cocoa, and cola nuts—is the most popular central nervous system stimulant in America. Caffeine is found in a variety of beverages such as coffee, tea, cocoa, and cola drinks; approximately 90% of American youth and adults use coffee and other caffeine-containing beverages. It is also found in a number of OTC preparations—analgesics such as Anacin, Bromo Seltzer, and Midol; stimulants such as NoDoz and Vivarin; cold preparations such as Dristan; and weight-control aids such as Dexatrim. The approximate caffeine content of selected beverages and OTC drugs according to various sources is listed in Table 10–4. Caffeine is misused and abused when taken excessively for its stimulating effects or when it continues to be used in the face of uncomfortable symptoms or health hazards. These are identified later.

Caffeine is classified as a mild CNS stimulant. In addition to its CNS stimulant effects, caffeine has diuretic properties. It is rapidly absorbed in the gastrointestinal tract, reaching maximum plasma concentrations within 1 hour of ingestion. Stimulant effects are noticeable within 30 minutes after ingestion and last for 3 to 5 hours.

The degree to which caffeine stimulates an individual varies with the amount taken and the development of tolerance. Although some people claim caffeine does not interfere with their sleep after five to six evening cups of coffee, an individual sensitive to its effects may become restless, agitated, and unable to sleep after only one cup. Other effects that vary among users are increased respirations, tachycardia, relaxed smooth visceral muscles, decreased peristalsis, nervousness, gastrointestinal upset, and fine tremors. Toxicity causes insomnia, restlessness, excitement, muscle twitching, increased respirations, tachycardia, and extrasystoles. Mild sensory disturbances such as ringing in the ears and flashes of light (at higher doses) are known to occur.

Table 10–4	Caffeine Content of Certain Beverages and Drugs	
Source	**Approximate Caffeine Content per 1 Cup (5 oz) or Tablet or Capsule**
Beverages	
Drip coffee	56–176 mg (average 112)
Percolated coffee	39–168 mg (average 74)
Instant coffee	29–117 mg (average 66)
Decaffeinated coffee	1–8 mg (average 3)
Tea (bag or leaf)	30–91 mg (average 27)
Cocoa	2–7 mg (average 4)
Cola drinks (12 oz)	30–46 mg
OTC drugs	
Analgesics	
Aspirin (plain)	0 mg
Anacin, Bromo Seltzer, Cope, Empirin Compound, Midol	32 mg
Excedrin	65 mg
Vanquish	33 mg
Stimulants	
NoDoz	100 mg
Vivarin	200 mg
Caffedrine	250 mg
Cold preparations	
Coryban-D, Triaminicin	30 mg
Dristan	16 mg
Diuretics	
Aqua-Ban	100 mg
Weight control aids	
Dexatrim, Dietac	200 mg
Prolamine	140 mg

Caffeine produces acid indigestion, and because it stimulates gastric acid and pepsin, it may cause or aggravate peptic ulcers. In clients with unregulated glaucoma, caffeine can produce increased intraocular pressure. Cardiac clients are advised against using substances containing caffeine because it increases myocardial contractions, causes tachycardia, and increases plasma glucose and lipid levels. The relationship between caffeine and myocardial infarction is currently being investigated. An abstinence syndrome occurs when a person who regularly ingests more than five cups of coffee (or equivalent) per day ceases regular use. The main signs of the abstinence syndrome are nausea, lethargy, and headache.

HALLUCINOGENS

Hallucinogens, also called psychedelics, are the "mind expanders" that gained notoriety in the United States in the 1960s and continue to be used but to a lesser extent. Hallucinogens are capable of altering time and space perception; changing feelings of self-awareness, body image, and emotions; increasing sensitivity to textures, shapes, sounds, and taste; and bringing on visions of luminescence, flashes of light, kaleidoscopic patterns, and landscapes. They can also induce hallucinations and feelings of having had a religious experience.

Many natural and synthetic hallucinogens are in use today. Naturally occurring hallucinogens include mescaline (which can be found in buttons of the peyote cactus and can also be produced synthetically), psilocybin (known as "God's flesh," from the "divine" mushroom; actually found in about 100 mushroom species), morning glory seeds, nutmeg, jimsonweed, and a great many more. The most commonly used hallucinogenics—lysergic acid diethylamide (LSD) and phencyclidine (PCP)—are both synthetics. PCP is included in this discussion because it causes hallucinations; however, it has a number of other effects not shared by hallucinogenics such as LSD. LSD is the most potent by weight, and also the best researched, of all the hallucinogenics. Other synthetic hallucinogenics include 5-methoxy-3,4 methylenedioxyamphetamine (MMDA), dimethyltryptamine (DMT), paramethoxyamphetamine (PMP), and trimethoxyamphetamine (TMA).

LSD

LSD, first developed in the late 1930s, was used in research to investigate its mystical and creative potential as well as the biochemical etiology of schizophrenia. Its illicit use overshadowed its clinical experimental use in the early 1960s. LSD use reached its peak in the late 1960s and has since declined, stabilizing at a low level.

The usual method of taking LSD is orally; the clear liquid is placed on sugar cubes or other materials and ingested. With rapid absorption in the stomach, it appears to concentrate in the visual cortex, limbic system, and reticular formation. The mechanism by which LSD produces its hallucinogenic effect—called a *"trip"*—remains largely unknown. Autonomic nervous system effects include dizziness, hot and cold flashes, dry mouth, dilated pupils, elevated body temperature, and increased blood pressure. Sometimes excessive salivation occurs. Central nervous system effects include labile mood; synesthesia (stimulation of one sense is perceived as another sense; eg, a sound produces a sensation of color); visual hallucinations; and abnormal color, time, and space perception. Feelings of possessing unusual power or having the ability to perform impossible feats or acts may lead the individual into impulsive actions such as jumping off a building to fly.

Although the hallucinogens do not create physical or psychological dependence, tolerance develops rapidly. Cross-tolerance also occurs between LSD, mescaline, and psilocybin but not between these and other hallucinogens. Adverse reactions are the panic reaction, aggressive outbursts, overt psychosis, the "bad trip," and the "flash-back." Panic reactions are acute anxiety attacks, usually brought on because the person fears not being able to regain control and return from the "trip." Overt psychosis occurs as the person loses touch with reality; it is more likely in individuals who are vulnerable to personality disorganization. A person having a "bad trip" experiences anxiety, panic, and paranoid feelings magnified by the distortion of time perception. Because time seems to have no end, terror sets in, and the individual may be subject to aggressive, violent, or unpredictable self-destructive or grandiose behavior. Flashbacks are frightening recurrences of the LSD "trip" weeks or months after ingesting the drug. They are unpredictable, but may be more pronounced when a person is under stress or lacking sleep. They vary with frequency and eventually decrease when hallucinogen use is discontinued.

PCP

Also known as "angel dust," "rocket fuel," and "horse tranquilizer," PCP is rapidly increasing in popularity in America. It is relatively inexpensive and is readily manufactured in small basement or garage laboratories, making it easily available to persons with limited funds. It was developed in 1959 as the first in a class of new dissociative anesthetics (and in fact, is related to the anesthetic ketamine) but was quickly abandoned for human use because it caused agitation, delusions, and irrational behavior. Approved only for veterinary use, PCP is still used for immobilizing animals.

In its pure form, PCP is a water-soluble crystalline powder. It is sold on the street in a variety of colors and forms. PCP can be taken as a pill; snorted as a powder; or sprayed as a liquid on parsley, mint, or other leafy substances to be smoked. Because it has so many street names and has often been misrepresented as another drug (mescaline, psilocybin, methaqualone, or cocaine), some users may not even know they have used PCP. Because the dose sold on the street varies widely, the effect is difficult to predict.

The effects of PCP are experienced quickly—usually within 5 minutes of smoking it. Initially, users tend to experience an active fantasy life and focus inward while appearing oblivious to others. Feelings of euphoria, peace, floating, warmth, and tingling are experienced. Users may also experience depersonalization; hallucinations; and distortions of time, space, and body image. Anxiety and labile affect (alternating moods) have also been reported (Kaplan & Sadock, 1985). The "high," which lasts for 4 to 6 hours, may be followed by a mild depression.

Adverse effects and overdoses may be treated in emergency departments, usually because in addition to the above, the client also demonstrates suicidal or aggressive behavior. In some instances, the symptoms abate as the PCP is absorbed. At other times, the symptoms worsen and may require hospitalization. Clients with PCP intoxication may have hypertension, nystagmus, hyperthermia, ataxia, seizures, and other symptoms of neurological involvement. Respiratory arrest is also possible. The most dramatic of PCP's effects is its ability to mimic acute schizophrenia. In fact, some unusually long, severe, and treatment-resistant initial episodes of what was thought to be schizophrenia have turned out to be responses to PCP. The user may experience delusions and hallucinations (usually auditory, sometimes visual), irrational behavior, blocked speech, body image alteration, and violent behavior. Because PCP also has anesthetic effects, the user's sensations of touch and pain are dulled, making the user unusually resistant to outside control.

CENTRAL NERVOUS SYSTEM TOXINS (NICOTINE AND CANNABIS)

Included in this category are two chemical agents that have mixed effects on the central nervous system and, thus, are difficult to categorize elsewhere. The substances are nicotine and cannabis, both of which tend to have a toxic effect on the central nervous system.

Nicotine

Europeans and Asians discovered tobacco after it was brought back to Spain from the Caribbean islands by one of the early Spanish explorers. By the early 1600s, tobacco was smoked in pipes and cigars, chewed, and sniffed by men, women, and children and used as a medicinal herb. Not until 250 years later in the mid-nineteenth century did tobacco appear in cigarettes, its most widely used form today.

Nicotine is one of the few natural liquid alkaloids. It is isolated from leaves of tobacco, *Nicotiana tabacum,* and has no therapeutic application. Nicotine is a colorless, volatile base that turns brown and acquires the odor of tobacco when exposed to air. Nicotine use usually begins in adolescence or early adulthood.

Nicotine dependence is recognized by the American Psychiatric Association's *Diagnostic and Statistical Manual* (DSM III) as a substance use disorder. An individual is considered tobacco dependent who has used tobacco continuously for at least 1 month, has unsuccessfully attempted to quit or significantly reduce the amount of use, has developed nicotine withdrawal, or continues to smoke in the presence of a serious physical disorder that is directly linked to smoking (American Psychiatric Association, 1980).

Effects and Absorption

Although many people begin tobacco use for psychosocial reasons (identification with peers and response to stress and tension), nicotine appears to have specific stimulant properties. It increases alertness, relaxes muscles, and decreases appetite and irritability. Nicotine is quickly absorbed from the lungs, usually bypasses the liver, and reaches the brain within 8 seconds after inhalation—more rapidly than an intravenous dose of heroin. Chewing tobacco

Nursing Research Note

Kneeshaw MF: Smoking cessation in nurses: A report on a self-selected population at the Presbyterian Hospital in New York City. *Occup Health Nurs* 1985; 33:338–342.

The number of nurses who smoke is greater than the average in the female population and greater than the number of physicians smoking. Cigarette breaks at this hospital were considered a good reason for a rest period, contributing to increased tobacco use among nurses.

A survey of nursing employees assessed the prevalence of smoking among nurses and determined the number of nurses who would be interested in a program that encouraged smoking cessation. Of the 32 nurses who stated they would be interested in a cessation program, only 3 actually attended.

As health care professionals, nurses should be role models for the general population and encourage cessation of tobacco use. Lung cancer has markedly increased in women. More research should be conducted to find ways to assist nurses with smoking cessation.

is absorbed through the buccal mucosa and snuff, through the nasal mucosa. Pipe and cigar tobacco is usually puffed and not inhaled, so it, too, is absorbed through the buccal mucosa.

Cessation of use may lead to the tobacco withdrawal syndrome, which varies in intensity, duration, and signs and symptoms. The onset of symptoms may begin within hours of the last cigarette or may be delayed for several days. Symptoms last from a few days to several months. The symptoms of tobacco withdrawal syndrome are:

- Craving for tobacco
- Restlessness
- Irritability
- Anxiety
- Sleep disturbance
- Drowsiness
- Headache
- Impaired concentration
- Gastrointestinal disturbances

Although this syndrome alone is not life-threatening, the added stress and anxiety associated with the symptoms may place the medical or surgical client at a higher risk for complications.

Multisystem Effects

Cigarette smoke contains some 4000 chemical substances, including at least 15 different types of known carcinogens and a number of toxic hydrocarbons or solvents (Bennett et al., 1983). Nicotine, carbon monoxide, and tar are the three toxic components in tobacco most likely to contribute to health hazards of smoking. Each year approximately 320,000 deaths occur from lung and other cancers, chronic pulmonary disease, and cardiovascular diseases directly linked to smoking. Smoking is considered the major etiologic factor in emphysema and bronchitis. Smokers who live or work in areas where dust and other pollutants are prevalent are more likely than nonsmokers to develop lung cancer and other associated respiratory illness. Since pipe and cigar smokers do not ordinarily inhale, they are considered at lower risk than cigarette smokers for developing serious health complications. They are also less likely to develop dependence on nicotine and find it easier to quit when advised to do so.

Although campaigns recognizing the hazards of smoking have resulted in a decline in smoking among all adults (more than 30 million have quit), women's smoking has declined at a slower rate than men's. Despite these campaigns and warning labels, 39% to 40% of the adult population continue to smoke. The potential for developing health problems linked to smoking increases with exposure, but cessation of smoking reduces this potential. For example, 5 to 10 years after quitting, former smokers are at only slightly higher risk than nonsmokers (Surgeon General, 1981). The federal government has targeted three issues for study in the 1980s: the health consequences to women smokers, the implications of the growing promotion of "low-tar" cigarettes in decreasing hazards of smoking, and the long-term effects of side-stream smoking (the effects of smoking on nonsmokers).

Smoking has been directly correlated with prematurity and low-birth-weight infants. Offspring of smoking mothers have a higher incidence of upper respiratory problems and pneumonia in the first 2 years of life. Nicotine is excreted in the milk of lactating mothers, which may contain 0.5 mg/L.

In addition to smokers' high mortality rate from diseases cited earlier in this section, smokers are at higher risk for peptic ulcers and cirrhosis. In addition, women smokers over 35 who take birth control pills are at risk of hemorrhage, especially cerebral hemorrhage. Accidental deaths from fires started by people who smoke in bed or fall asleep while smoking are a major hazard. The incidence is higher with alcoholism.

Physiological changes from smoking cessation include electroencephalographic changes such as decreased high-frequency activity (characteristic of arousal) and increased low-frequency activity (characteristic of drowsiness and hypoarousal), lowered heart rate and blood pressure, and increased peripheral blood flow. The appetite increases, and weight gain is common over time. Coughing and other respiratory symptoms improve. It is not completely known how many people successfully quit smoking on their own. Of those who seek formal help, about 66% actually quit for a few days, but only 10% to 40% remain abstinent for 1 year (Bennett et al., 1984). Programs to help smokers give up the habit are in the resources list at the end of Chapter 18.

Cannabis

Cannabis sativa, the Indian hemp plant, produces a strong fibrous material that has been used to make clothing and rope. Its origin is the plains of Central Asia, from where it spread to the Middle East, North Africa, and Europe. It is used as a mind-altering drug by large numbers of persons in North America, Great Britain, Australia, Sweden, the Netherlands, and West Germany. Its use is increasing among young people in India, Egypt, and Jamaica. Its use is not limited to any specific age, social, economic, or educational group.

The primary psychoactive agent is delta^6-3,4-tetrahydrocannabinol (THC), which is concentrated in the resin secreted from the flowering tops and leaves of the cannabis plant and acts as a central nervous system depressant. The potency of any cannabis preparation is determined by the amount and potency of the resin. The three most common forms of cannabis in street use are:

- Marijuana, the most prevalent, which is the dried leaves, stems, and flowers of the cannabis plant and has a THC content of 5% to 6%
- Hashish, or hash, which is more potent because it has a higher THC concentration (up to 10%), from the flowering tops of the plant
- Hashish oil, which has the most concentrated THC (may reach 63%) and is produced by boiling hashish in a solvent to filter out the solid material

Effects of Marijuana

Marijuana is usually smoked but can be eaten or taken in pill form, and the effects last for a few hours. Blood levels of THC in chronic users have been detected for up to 6 days following the last inhalation. Chronic marijuana smokers are at risk for developing asthma, chronic bronchitis, and adverse pulmonary effects. The "tar" produced by marijuana is considered more carcinogenic than the tar produced by tobacco (1 marijuana cigarette, or joint = 5.0 mg tar; 1 tobacco cigarette = 1.2 mg tar); thus, chronic users are considered at high risk. The harmful effects of one joint a day on the lungs has been compared to the effect of smoking 20 tobacco cigarettes per day because marijuana smokers usually inhale more deeply and hold the smoke in the lungs longer to obtain a heightened effect.

The effects of marijuana that account for its popularity as a recreational drug include:

- The "high"—euphoria, relaxation, reduced anxiety, feelings of well-being
- A sense of hilarity and excitement
- Increased clarity and sensitivity
- Heightened sense of awareness
- Feeling pleasantly detached, floating
- Having ideas that flow freely

Other less pleasurable effects may cause problems in thinking, motor performance, and interpersonal relationships. They are:

- Impaired logical thinking, irrelevant thoughts, and gaps in thoughts or memory

- Rapid, slurred, or otherwise impaired speech and loose associations
- Difficulty in concentrating or making decisions
- Impaired reality testing (auditory and visual hallucinations are possible) that make operating machinery or driving a car dangerous
- Altered sense of time and space
- Increased suggestibility
- Alteration in libido and sexual performance (either increased or decreased)
- Altered body image and self-identity
- Increased anxiety and panic
- Apathy with prolonged use

In addition, cannabis overdose may cause fear, anxiety, panic, suspiciousness, agitation, ataxia, tremors, acute depression, disorientation, and distorted perceptions.

An amotivational syndrome may also occur in the chronic user characterized by apathy; a lack of concern for the future; decreased effectiveness at school or work; and difficulty in completing complex tasks, performing routines, or mastering new experiences. Whether this syndrome can be isolated as a consequence of chronic marijuana use or is a manifestation of personality disorganization that occurred before its use is difficult to study and continues to be somewhat controversial.

Marijuana may also have medically therapeutic effects. It is being used in selected health centers, on a limited experimental basis, to help alleviate the nausea associated with cancer chemotherapy and to help reduce the intraocular pressure in clients with open-angle glaucoma.

Multisystem Effects

While the illegal status and the harmful effects continue to be debated, national concern is growing over the large number of young people who regularly use and abuse marijuana. Long-term use and cannabis accumulation in the body cause chromosomal mutations and the development of micronucleic white blood cells. Findings indicate that abuse of cannabis may result in a high incidence of birth defects in offspring and a high risk of disease due to lowered resistance to infection. Other hazards of cannabis use are associated with the unpredictability of other chemicals (such as PCP) found in cannabis preparations and the health hazards associated with cigarette smoking. The incidence of cigarette smoking among marijuana users is high and therefore poses all the health hazards described for nicotine dependence.

Withdrawal

Although infrequent, tolerance and physical dependence have been reported in the chronic marijuana user. Tolerance depends on the dose and duration of use, but as tolerance develops, mild physical dependence also occurs. Mild withdrawal symptoms, which may occur within hours of the last dose, include restlessness, anxiety, insomnia, excitability or irritability, nausea, vomiting, anorexia, and diarrhea. Acute psychotic episodes may occur in certain vulnerable individuals. Mild to moderate adverse symptoms ameliorate within a few hours in a quiet supportive environment. Psychotic episodes may last from 1 to 6 weeks or longer.

Section III: The Nursing Process for Clients Who Abuse Substances

Be aware of the possibility that many clients, regardless of diagnosis, have problems related to the abuse of chemical agents either because they themselves abuse substances or because significant others do. Nurses in general hospitals, ambulatory care facilities, schools, industry, and community environments are often unaware that clients they are seeing for one reason—to have a broken leg set, an emergency appendectomy, a nose and throat culture, a scoliosis check, a preemployment physical, or a home visit after hospital discharge—may also be substance abusers. If frequent contact continues, the nurse will eventually notice symptoms.

Some of the most dangerous situations occur when misdiagnoses are made: the client in a diabetic coma is mistakenly thought to be drunk and is left to "sleep it off" rather than given insulin; an intoxicated client is mistakenly thought to be a diabetic and receives insulin that further reduces an already extremely low blood sugar level not uncommon in clients in alcoholic coma; a client with a heroin overdose fails to receive naloxone (Narcan) to coun-

teract the respiratory depression. In these situations, immediate appropriate action is imperative. Being alert to possible misdiagnosis facilitates early intervention and helps to prevent complications arising from substance abuse.

Historically, nurses' reactions to substance abusers have followed two patterns. Both reactions appear to stem from nurses' own anxieties about substance abuse and their fear of it. These feelings come about, in part, because many nurses feel helpless in the face of substance abuse.

The first reaction pattern is one of disgust and revulsion. This stems from the nurse's belief that substance abuse is irreversible and the substance abuser is helpless and hopeless. Some nurses who react this way tend to withdraw from the client, feeling less responsible for the client's care. Other nurses try to inspire the client to give up the drug, preaching to them about willpower or providing information designed to frighten clients into abstinence. These behaviors only increase the client's feelings of low self-esteem and futility.

The second reaction pattern is one of enabling. Ena-

Box 10–3   Guide to Analyzing Personal Responses Toward Substance Abusers

Analyze your responses to the following questions:

1. What thoughts and feelings does the term alcoholic evoke in me?

2. What thoughts and feelings does the term addict evoke in me?

3. Do I believe that substance dependence occurs out of moral weakness?

4. Do I believe that substance dependence is an illness that can be treated?

5. Is the person who abuses substances deliberately destroying his or her life and the lives of significant others?

6. Who in my personal life has abused drugs, alcohol, or other chemicals?

7. How does my experience with relatives, friends, colleagues, or clients who have abused substances affect my attitude toward caring for a substance-abusing client?

8. Is substance abuse a social problem, an emotional-psychological problem, or a physical abnormality?

9. How do I view the family, spouse, or friends of the substance abuser? Do they encourage the abuse, or otherwise "enable" the person to continue their abuse? Or are they victims?

10. How does my own personal use of nicotine, caffeine, drugs, or alcohol affect my attitude toward clients?

bling is defined as supporting condoning, or covering up an individual's continued use of the substance or protecting the person from the ultimate consequences of substance abuse. In effect, the nurse, family member, or friend assumes responsibility for the client's actions. The nurse who enables:

- Encourages the substance abuser's use of denial by concurring that the client is only an infrequent "social drinker" or that the client only uses drugs when a "little nervous"

- Apologizes for asking questions about the person's drug use habits

- Ignores cues to possible substance abuse, choosing instead to explore cues to anxiety or depression

- Emphasizes repeatedly that the problem can be overcome if the client will only use "willpower"

- Counsels the person to seek psychiatric help for anxiety or depression, yet overlooks the underlying problem of substance abuse

- Sympathizes with the client's reasons (work, financial, and family problems) for using the substance, denying the reality that the difficulties are often the result, and not the cause, of substance abuse

The result of both reaction patterns is that the client fails to receive the needed help; the ultimate result with some drugs, such as alcohol, is death. Nurses need to increase their knowledge of substance abuse and their skill in implementing the nursing process with chemically dependent people. The ability to analyze one's own feelings and reactions to substance abusers regularly helps avoid withdrawing from, preaching to, or enabling the substance abuser. The questions in Box 10–3 will help in analyzing feelings, beliefs, and attitudes toward substance abuse.

NURSING ASSESSMENT: ESTABLISHING THE DATA BASE

Assessing for substance abuse requires a cautious, objective, holistic approach. No one sign or symptom definitely and exclusively pinpoints substance abuse. Consider all cues carefully to be able to intervene effectively, but avoid jumping to hasty and stigmatizing conclusions that erroneously brand clients and may negatively affect the quality of health care clients receive.

Subjective Data

In beginning to assess each client by completing the health history, the nurse simultaneously observes for cues of substance abuse. It is imperative to observe the client's nonverbal cues and to listen carefully to how questions are answered. These cues may give a more accurate picture than actual words of whether a problem with substance use exists.

Begin by collecting data about ingestion of alcohol. To determine the frequency, ask the client: "How often do you drink alcoholic beverages?" The magnitude can be determined by asking: "When you do drink, how much do you drink?" Remember to ask about the conditions under which the client drinks. Asking: "When do you tend to drink alcohol?" and "Under what circumstances?" and "With whom?" will help to gather specific facts. Remember also to ask, "When was your last drink?" to be able to anticipate the onset of symptoms of withdrawal in an alcoholic. Other behavioral clues are listed in Table 10–5.

The history also explores the client's current and past use of drugs, including prescription and nonprescription medications. At this point, the aim is to assess the client's pattern of drug use. Ask the client what drugs are being taken. It may be useful to tell the client: "I need to know all the drugs/medications that you are taking because it may be dangerous to abruptly stop taking some of them," or "I need to know all the drugs/medications that you have been taking because it is important not to mix certain chemicals, and some stay in the body for a long time." Since it is not unusual for the client to know only the drug's street name, be prepared to correlate street names with pharmacologic names (no easy task, since the street names frequently change). Some street names included in Table 10–1 may be helpful.

Determine how much is being taken, how often, and

Table 10–5 Clues in the Appraisal of Alcohol-Related Problems

Physical Clues	Behavioral Clues
An illness, under treatment, not responding as it should because the person may be drinking and not taking medicine as prescribed	Rapid response to questions
"Hash marks" of various ages, particularly in women, on forearms from oven burns	Very slow, prolonged responses to questions about alcohol as though person is being extremely careful about what to say
Multiple small cigarette burns on hands or chest, the latter from smoking while drinking in a reclining position	Preoccupation with alcohol in conversation, with frequent references to being "bombed" or "stoned"
Bruises, old and new, particularly at coffee and kitchen table height, caused by psychomotor incoordination during intoxication	Expressing undue concern about welfare of health care provider: "I don't want to bother you; you're busy; just phone in my prescription to the drug store"
Periorbital and pretibial edema caused by retention of fluid following a drunk	"Doctor shopping" to get what is wanted, particularly sedative drug prescriptions
Healed or unhealed slash marks across wrists, reflecting suicide attempt	Coming to scheduled appointment with alcohol on breath
Flushed face due to vasodilation effects of alcohol	Failure to report for health care after an injury for a period of time, as result of not wanting to be seen intoxicated or from fact that pain is masked by anesthetic property of alcohol
Numerous scars on hands and face from falling when drunk or from fights	
Appearing older than stated age from debilitating effects of excessive alcohol use	Frequent Monday morning absences from work because of "flu"
Aseptic necrosis of head of femur without trauma	Pattern of taking maximal sick leave during year
Skin stigmata of cirrhosis	Frequent calls to health care personnel seeking justification for sick leave
Cardiac dysrhythmias	Not performing as well as usual on job
Palpably enlarged liver	Poor self-image
	Dropping out of nondrinking relationships
	Giving up old pastimes and hobbies to spend time drinking
	Employment choices that facilitate drinking, such as those in which a person can function without direct supervision or those that allow business conducted over lunch

SOURCE: Estes N, Smith–DiJulio K, Heinemann M: *Nursing Diagnosis of the Alcoholic Person.* St. Louis: Mosby, 1980, p. 104.

for low long. Ask how it has affected the client's social, work, and sexual relationships. Carefully observe the nonverbal cues, acknowledging that the topic of substance abuse will be difficult for both nurse and client to discuss. Anticipate that if the person is abusing chemical agents, particularly illicit ones, this information is not likely to be offered voluntarily. Sometimes family members verbalize their concerns about the client's substance abuse; others tend to conceal this data.

Objective Data

Observation of Physical and Behavioral Symptoms
Objective data can be gathered during the physical examination or more indirectly when interacting with the client for other reasons. The client may have dilated or constricted pupils, needle tracks from intravenous administration, or ulcerations in the nares. Note whether the client appears intoxicated, agitated, stuporous, assaultive, severely

anxious, or panicky. Any one, or a combination, of these physiological or behavioral cues may indicate substance use or abuse, untoward reactions, or drug overdose (see Table 10–1 for specifics).

In monitoring vital signs, observe for respiratory depression. Fluctuations in pulse and blood pressure for no seemingly plausible reason can indicate that the client is in the process of withdrawal from a depressant, narcotic, or stimulant. Signs of withdrawal for specific substances have been discussed earlier. Withdrawal from alcohol is discussed in the section on planning and implementation.

Response to Anesthetics and Medications
Does the client demonstrate the anticipated physiological response to analgesics, anesthetics, or sedative–hypnotics? If the response is "less than expected," this may be a cue to cross-tolerance. The client may require larger than usual doses of the medication to achieve the desired response. If the response is greater than expected, the client may be unknowingly or surreptitiously taking

Nursing Research Note

Forchuk C: cognitive dissonance: Denial, self-concepts and the alcoholic stereotype. *Nurs Papers* 1984; 16(3):57–67.

This study examined denial, negative self-concept, and the acceptance of the alcoholic stereotype within the theorectical framework of cognitive dissonance. According to the author, the alcoholic stereotype assumes the alcoholic is not worthwhile and is "weak" and "bad." The theory of cognitive dissonance holds that if a person's knowledge, opinions, or beliefs (cognitions) are inconsistent with those of important others, the individual will be motivated to change and hold similar beliefs and opinions. Alcoholics can avoid dissonance by either denying their drinking problem or accepting this negative self-concept. This attitude presents a problem in treating alcoholics.

Using a sample of 116 men and women in an alcoholic treatment program, the author measured acceptance of the alcoholic stereotype, denial, and self-concept. The results indicated that 61% accepted their alcoholism, 28% felt they had a drinking problem but denied alcoholism, 6% denied alcoholism, and the remaining 5% did not answer the denial questions. There was a positive relation between improving self-concept and self-esteem and denial. As denial increased so did self-esteem. The subjects consistently rated alcoholics as more negative than themselves. Similarly, for those denying their alcoholism, there was a greater distance between self-rating and ratings for alcoholics. Problem drinkers and those accepting their alcoholism rated themselves more closely to alcoholics in their traits. On the average in this study, alcoholics accepted the alcoholic stereotype and rated other alcoholics more negatively than themselves, supporting the cognitive dissonance theory.

Health teaching and counseling are necesary to encourage alcoholic clients to reject the alcoholic stereotype. The client must accept the problem but not accept the social stigma attached to the disease. In addition, when treating the alcoholic, nurses must focus on the client's positive qualities and enhance the self-image.

Nurses must also become aware of their own feelings regarding alcoholics and alcoholic stereotyping. Alcohol problems are not limited to the psychiatric setting but are present in all health care settings. Therefore, all nurses must become familiar with alcoholism, treatment modalities, and nursing interventions.

medications similar to those administered by the nurse. The case of Mrs. J. is an example of such a situation.

Mrs. J. is a 67-year-old widow with chronic generalized rheumatoid arthritis, diagnosed 20 years ago. She was admitted to an orthopedic unit for her third total joint arthroplasty of the left knee. She had had previous right total knee and bilateral total hip arthroplasty procedures. She was stylishly dressed and presented an attractive and meticulous physical appearance. The nurse who carried out the preoperative assessment noted that Mrs. J. had a sound understanding of her illness. This was her first admission to this metropolitan hospital since she moved to the city 2 years ago to be near her children after her husband's death. She was gracious, friendly, and cooperative with the nursing and medical staff. When asked what medications she took for her arthritis, she responded, "Well, dear, I take one or two extra-strength Anacin about twice a day when my joints ache. That's about it."

Following her surgery, Mrs. J. was returned to the orthopedic floor with an order for meperidine (Demerol) 50–75 mg IM q. 3–4 h for pain for 3 days. Because of her age and small stature (105 lb), she was given 25 mg of meperidine. Within an hour, she was complaining of severe pain, asked the nurse for more pain relief, and was given another 25 mg of meperidine. After receiving little relief after another hour, her family requested additional assistance from the nurse. The physician was called to request an order for hydroxyzine (Vistaril) 25 mg IM q. 3–4 h. The pain continued to be severe, and the analgesic orders were changed to hydroxyzine 50 mg and morphine 10 mg. The following day, diazepam (Valium) 5 mg PO q. 6 h was administered to reduce discomfort from muscle spasms.

On the third postoperative day, Mrs. J.'s medications were changed to acetaminophen with codeine 32 mg (Tylenol-3), one to two tablets q. 3 h. Because of Mrs. J.'s continued discomfort, the nurse administered two tablets of acetaminophen with codeine q. 3 h. On the evening of the third day, Mrs. J.'s nurse observed her to be sleepy and lethargic. Diagnostic tests were ordered to rule out cerebral vascular accident, pulmonary embolism, and postoperative anemia. Although the results were negative, the nurse continued to be concerned about Mrs. J.'s lethargic and mildly disoriented state. She told Mrs. J. of her concern and asked whether Mrs. J. was taking any other medications. Mrs. J. smiled weakly and said, "Why, no, dear, nothing but my Anacin," and motioned to her bedside table. The nurse looked in the drawer and found an Anacin bottle in Mrs. J.'s cosmetic bag. Inside the bottle were numerous pills of many varieties: Valium, Librium, Percocet, Talwin, and her usual arthritis medications—Motrin, Darvocet, and Anacin.

The nurse sat down beside Mrs. J., told her she had found Mrs. J.'s medications, and said it was important that Mrs. J. no longer take her own medications while she was in the hospital. The nurse explained that one of the reasons Mrs. J. continued to feel so uncomfortable was that she had become dependent on a variety of medications so the normal doses of her pain medications were not effective. She asked Mrs. J.'s permission to discuss the problem with her son on one of his frequent visits so arrangements could be made for Mrs. J. to be seen in the hospital's pain clinic. With Mrs. J.'s permission, the son was consulted and informed that because his mother had probably been taking a variety of medications over the years to relieve arthritic pain and discomfort, she would need some special assistance and support to reduce her reliance on multiple drugs.

A pain consultation was requested and a follow-up appointment made for the outpatient clinic. The son and his family were informed that Mrs. J. would require special care and consideration during her recovery from surgery and during longer term management of her arthritis pain. She was successfully maintained on morphine 10 mg q. 3–4 h during the remainder of her postoperative hospital period.

Diagnostic Studies

Routine laboratory studies may provide indirect cues to undiagnosed substance abuse. For example, unexplained abnormal liver function studies may suggest the need to evaluate a client for possible alcohol or heroin abuse. On the whole, routine studies point to complications of long-term abuse. Once a client is identified as a substance user, laboratory and diagnostic studies such as complete blood count (CBC), serologic studies, chest x-ray, ECG, EEG, and others suggested by the history or physical examination help to uncover related health problems and complications.

Blood and urine specimens, and sometimes gastric specimens, may be collected for forensic or legal purposes, especially in the investigation of drug or alcohol abuse, suicide, and intentional poisoning. It is crucial that in medicolegal investigations, the chain of possession remains unbroken from the time the specimen is collected until courtroom testimony is completed. Each person obtaining or handling such specimens should be sure that each step in the collection, processing, and handling of a medicolegal specimen is witnessed and properly documented. Certain precautions will help to ensure the legal credibility of laboratory test results. The nursing responsibilities in relation to these precautions are outlined in Box 10–4.

Drug Screening. A toxicologic screen of 100 mL of urine and 20 mL of blood may indicate the presence of a variety of drugs of abuse. Although a toxicologic screen can identify use, it cannot identify abuse (how long and how often the individual uses the drug). Negative results may mean either that the individual does not use drugs or that the drug is no longer detectable. For example, cocaine traces last for only a relatively brief time, but heroin can often be detected in the urine as long as 48 hours after use. Sometimes a toxicology screen gives negative results except for the presence of quinine (frequently used as a diluent with many drugs of abuse), which can be detected

as long as 5 to 6 days after use. The presence of quinine is not definitive for drug abuse, however, since quinine is also found in some cold remedies and soft drinks.

While the results of a toxicologic screen are often useful in guiding long-term treatment, they may not always be available soon enough to aid in the management of emergency situations such as coma or respiratory depression. In these emergencies, health care providers will need to rely on subjective data and the specific physical findings discussed earlier in this chapter when giving immediate treatment. Specific toxicological tests for barbiturate levels and blood alcohol levels are discussed below.

Barbiturate Levels. The measurement of barbiturate levels requires the collection of a venous blood specimen. Since each barbiturate varies in its duration of action and rate of absorption, different barbiturates produce coma at different blood levels. Short-acting barbiturates such as pentobarbital and secobarbital are more toxic and produce coma at low concentrations. Long-acting barbiturates such as phenobarbital (Luminal) are absorbed more slowly and do not produce coma until higher concentrations are reached. Table 10–6 correlates barbiturate blood levels with clinical findings.

High concentrations of several drugs can falsely elevate barbiturate levels:

- Glutethimide (Doriden)
- Phenytoin sodium (Dilantin) and other hydantoins used to treat epilepsy
- Meperidine
- Methyprylon (Noludar)
- Nitrazepam
- Salicylamide
- Theophylline and its derivatives

An accurate medication history will help to avoid treatment based on falsely elevated toxicology reports.

Blood Alcohol Levels. Laboratory analysis of blood alcohol level (BAL) is used to identify the presence of alcohol intoxication, to establish its degree, and to help determine appropriate treatment. It is essential to differentiate between alcohol intoxication and other conditions such as diabetic coma, cerebral trauma, and drug overdose. For example, the fruity breath odor of a person in diabetic coma, caused by the excretion of accumulated ketones by the lungs, can be mistaken for the breath odor of alcohol intoxication caused by congeners, the various substances such as methanol, esters, and aldehydes in alcoholic beverages. An error in diagnosis can have serious consequences for the client. The concentration of alcohol in the blood or urine is the major reliable indicator of alcohol intoxication and is essential to the differential diagnosis.

Because blood alcohol concentration levels may be used for medicolegal purposes, strict requirements for specimen collection must be followed. For example, alcohol should not be used for cleansing the client's arm, and the exact

---

Box 10–4 Nursing Responsibilities in Ensuring the Legal Credibility of Toxicology Reports

1. Obtain a signed consent form before collecting the specimen.

2. Collect the specimen in the presence of a witness, using appropriate collection containers and equipment.

3. Have the witness sign the laboratory request slip, noting the time the specimen was collected.

4. Seal the collection container with tape to prevent tampering.

5. Label the container with the date, contents, and subject's name. Be sure to sign the label.

6. Complete the laboratory request slip, including the type, source, and weight or volume of the specimen, data obtained, and test requested. Sign the laboratory request slip.

7. Maintain a continuous record of the chain of possession for the specimen. Each person who receives the specimen must sign the laboratory request slip, recording the exact time and date the exchange took place. Keep the number of people who handle each specimen to a minimum.

8. Seal the specimen and laboratory request slip in a package and label it "Medicolegal Case" on all sides.

9. Deliver the specimen to the laboratory immediately. If transportation is delayed, lock the specimen in a container and refrigerate the entire container and its contents.

SOURCE: Byrne JC, Saxton DF, Pelikan PK, Nugent PM: *Laboratory Tests: Implications for Nursing Care,* 2nd ed. Menlo Park, CA: Addison–Wesley, 1986, pp. 357–358.

Table 10–6 Barbiturate Blood Levels and Clinical Findings

Classification	Clinical Findings
Short-acting (secobarbital)	
1–5 µg/mL	Therapeutic range
10–20 µg/mL	Mild toxicity; marked sedation
20–30 µg/mL	Moderate toxicity; comatose; reflexes present
30–40 µg/mL	Marked toxicity; comatose; reflexes absent; respiratory depression
>40 µg/mL	Acute toxicity; deep coma; cardiovascular collapse
Intermediate-acting (amobarbital)	
5–15 µg/mL	Therapeutic range
15–30 µg/mL	Mild toxicity; marked sedation
30–50 µg/mL	Moderate toxicity; comatose; reflexes present
50–70 µg/mL	Marked toxicity; comatose; reflexes absent; respiratory depression
>70 µg/mL	Acute toxicity; deep coma; cardiovascular collapse
Long-acting (phenobarbital)	
10–40 µg/mL	Therapeutic range
40–50 µg/mL	Mild toxicity; marked sedation
50–80 µg/mL	Moderate toxicity; comatose; reflexes present
80–110 µg/mL	Marked toxicity; comatose; reflexes absent; respiratory depression
>110 µg/mL	Acute toxicity; deep coma; cardiovascular collapse

SOURCE: Adapted from Byrne CJ, Saxton DF, Pelikan PK, Nugent PM: *Laboratory Tests: Implications for Nursing Care,* 2nd ed. Menlo Park, CA: Addison–Wesley, 1986, p. 381.

Box 10–5 Nursing Procedure for Obtaining a Valid BAL Specimen

1. Cleanse the client's arm for the venipuncture with an aqueous germicidal solution rather than the usual alcohol swab or antiseptic. For example, a solution of benzalkonium chloride may be used to clean the skin, but a tincture should not be used because it contains alcohol and may contaminate the test specimen. Note the substance used on the laboratory slip.

2. Collect 5 mL of venous blood in a tube containing EDTA or oxalate anticoagulant (vacuum tube with a lavender or black stopper); a serum specimen tube (red stoppered tube) may also be used.

3. Label the tube carefully, recording the exact time the specimen was drawn and the time it was sent to the laboratory. Each step of specimen collection may eventually become part of the legal evidence.

SOURCE: Byrne CJ, Saxton DF, Pelikan PK, Nugent PM: *Laboratory Tests: Implications for Nursing Care,* 2nd ed. Menlo Park, CA: Addison–Wesley, 1986, p. 363.

Planning and Implementation

Nurses become involved in planning and implementation for the substance-abusing client at a variety of different levels. The case of Tom W. is an example of the several different roles nurses may fill in the planning and implementation phases.

Tom W., age 21, arrived in the emergency room by ambulance, following a motorcycle accident in which he sustained a compound fracture of the tibia. The paramedics noted they "smelled liquor on his breath." His condition was stabilized, and he was taken to surgery where an open reduction was performed; then he was transferred to the orthopedic unit. His vital signs upon admission to the orthopedic unit were: temperature 100.2°F (37.9°C), pulse 92, respirations 24, and blood pressure 132/86.

Postoperative medication orders included morphine 10–12 mg IM q. 3–4 h for pain, with hydroxyzine (Vistaril) 50 mg IM q. 3–4 h p.r.n. to augment the effectiveness of the narcotic.

At this point, the nurse completed the health history. Tom W. indicated that he had not been taking any medications, either prescribed or OTC. In response to the nurse's inquiry about alcohol use, Tom W. responded by saying in a defensive tone, "Well, if you really must know, I drink about a beer a day." He further stated that he liked to "smoke a joint with my friends after work."

Three hours after Tom W. arrived on the unit, he was given morphine 12 mg IM and hydroxyzine 50 mg IM for pain. When the nurse inquired 30 minutes later, he said that he still had "much pain." Later during the shift, the results of his laboratory tests became available. In checking the results, the nurse noted that Tom W.'s admission BAL was 0.11%. Meanwhile, Tom W. continued to state that he was experiencing "real severe pain" and asked for more "pain medication." Recognizing that the particular operative procedure Tom W. had can result in severe pain, the nurse became increasingly concerned. The nurse carefully and frequently assessed Tom for cues of compartment syndrome, which would account for severe pain, or fatty embolus syndrome, which would be marked by disorientation (see Chapter 60).

Approximately 24 hours after his admission, Tom became

times when the specimen was collected and sent to the laboratory should be noted. The nursing procedure for obtaining a valid BAL specimen is described in Box 10–5. Be sure to also follow the guidelines outlined in Box 10–4.

Nursing Diagnoses

As has become evident in this chapter, the abuse of chemical substances has complex physiological and psychosocial ramifications. Diagnoses may be relevant to the usual physical or behavioral effects of the substance, alterations due to overdose, alterations due to withdrawal, or alterations due to health complications. Nursing diagnoses relevant to the plan of care for substance-abusing clients span this wide range. The list of nursing diagnoses in Box 10–6 is by no means all-inclusive and needs to be individualized for each client.

diaphoretic, restless, and began to have hand tremors. His vital signs were: temperature 101.4°F (38.6°C), pulse 104, respirations 28, and blood pressure 152/94. Based on an analysis of the data the nurse had gathered—the BAL, changes in vital signs, physical symptoms, and Tom W.'s failure to receive pain relief from the analgesics—the nurse tentatively determined that Tom was experiencing symptoms of withdrawal from alcohol. In consultation with Tom W.'s physician, the decision was made to encourage Tom to drink a cup of weak tea with 2 tablespoons of sugar. When the nurse assessed his vital signs 30 minutes later, they were: temperature 101.2°F (38.0°C), pulse 90, respirations 22, and blood pressure 140/86.

The nurse shared these findings with Tom W., explaining that the data appeared to indicate that he might be dependent on a chemical substance, and expressed concern regarding his recovery. The nurse did not tell Tom W. that he was an alcoholic. When the nurse requestioned Tom W. on his use of chemical substances, he seemed embarrassed when he admitted that he drinks "one to two six-packs of beer a day along with smoking a couple of joints." Next, the nurse directed the conversation toward discussing a plan to facilitate Tom W.'s withdrawal from alcohol and referral to a drug-alcohol counselor.

Intoxication

Clients in intoxication or overdose need prompt emergency treatment. The nursing care plan focuses on alleviating the effects of the substance. Later, the nurse helps the client decide whether to learn to live without the substance by guiding the problem-solving process.

Drug and alcohol intoxication is usually self-limiting. In a physiological emergency, hospitalization is needed. Attending to any secondary complications, such as those related to falls, infections, and physical injuries is a priority once the emergency is under control.

Intoxication occurs when an individual has consumed a drug in excess of the body's ability to metabolize it (Table 10–7). For example, most people become intoxicated when their blood level is between 100 and 200 mg/dL (BAL = 0.10% to 0.20%). Maladaptive behaviors resulting from intoxication may include aggressiveness; altered judgment; and other social, personal, or work-related impairment. Psychological characteristics include euphoria, irritability, impaired attention or concentration, loquacity, and emotional lability. Physiologic characteristics include flushed face, slurred speech, lack of coordination, unsteady gait, and nystagmus. Intoxicated persons must be supervised to make sure they do not mistakenly assume that they can drive safely.

Intoxication may alter or accentuate the individual's usual behavior. Shy or inhibited persons may become outgoing and gregarious, whereas a person who tends to be mistrustful may become extremely suspicious. In the early stage of intoxication, individuals may experience an increased sense of well-being and confidence. They may talk as if they are experts who can solve the problems of the world, or they may become overbearing and opinionated, demanding that those around them agree with their point of view. The early behavioral manifestations of intoxication may appear uninhibited. In later stages, however, persons may become depressed, speech and thoughts are slowed down,

and they may become withdrawn and even lose consciousness, or "pass out."

The duration of intoxication depends on the amount of the drug ingested over what period of time and whether food was taken at the same time. Weight, height, age, and sex also affect the rate of alcohol metabolism. The individual's tolerance for alcohol also affects the length of intoxication, as do individual variations and susceptibility.

The usual manifestations of alcohol intoxication require no specific nursing intervention or medical treatment. There are no proven methods to speed up the metabolism of a drug. Such time-honored remedies used for alcohol intoxication as a warm shower followed by a cold one, strong coffee, forced activity, or induced vomiting may provide some comfort but should not be suggested as a means for increasing the rate of dissipation of alcohol from the blood. Pathological intoxication, characterized by increased excitement and combativeness, may require restraints and administration of sedatives such as sodium luminal 100 mg subcutaneously, or amobarbital sodium (Amytal) 500 mg IM, repeated once in 30 or 40 minutes.

Intoxicated persons in an emergency room may cause a critical nursing situation. Some medical and nursing personnel may see them as a nuisance and may refuse them entry to the ER or call the police department. Instead, the astute nurse evaluates the person for level of intoxication, determines the drug history, and evaluates the potential

---

Box 10–6 Nursing Diagnoses Commonly Related to Substance Abuse

Anxiety

Breathing patterns, ineffective, related to respiratory depression

Coping, ineffective individual

Coping, ineffective or disabled family

Gas exchange, impaired

Injury, potential for, related to substance abuse

Knowledge deficit, related to polydrug abuse

Mobility, impaired physical, related to perceptual or neuromuscular impairment

Nutrition, alteration in: less than body requirements, related to lack of interest in food

Powerlessness

Self-concepts, disturbance in: body image, self-esteem, role performance, personal identity

Sensory-perceptual alterations: visual, auditory, kinesthetic, tactile, related to chemical alterations from alcohol or drugs

Sexual dysfunction

Skin integrity, impairment of, related to parenteral administration of drugs

Thought processes, alteration in

Tissue perfusion, alteration in: cerebral

Violence, potential for

Table 10–7   Effects of Blood Alcohol Concentration

Ounces of Whiskey	Concentration	Effects
1–2	10–50 mg/dL (0.01%–0.05%)	Subclinical, with no intoxication; mild euphoria; sedation; tranquility
3–4	50–100 mg/dL (0.05%–0.1%)	Sociability; talkativeness; mild influence on stereoscopic vision and dark adaptation; lack of coordination; slurred speech
	100 mg/dL (0.1%)	Decreased attention; diminished control; slow mental response; legal intoxication
5	100–150 mg/dL (0.1%–0.15%)	Emotional instability; euphoria; disappearance of inhibition; loss of critical judgment; prolonged reaction time; driving ability significantly reduced; some incoordination
6–7	150–200 mg/dL (0.15%–0.2%)	Decreased sensory response; obvious intoxication; slightly disturbed equilibrium and coordination; poor color perception; loss of inhibition; reaction time greatly prolonged; moderately severe poisoning
8–9	200–250 mg/dL (0.2%–0.25%)	Disorientation; decreased sense of pain; disturbances of equilibrium and coordination; exaggerated emotional states; retardation of thought processes; clouding of consciousness
10–14	250–350 mg/dL (0.25%–0.35%)	Apathy; inability to stand; unconsciousness; tremors; sweating; incontinence; vomiting; beginning stupor; confusion; marked intoxication; severe degree of poisoning
15–20	350–500 mg/dL (0.35%–0.5%)	Anesthesia; unconsciousness; decreased reflexes; deep, possibly irreversible or fatal coma; incontinence; circulatory and respiratory collapse
20–30	500–800 mg/dL (0.5%–0.8%)	Fatal concentration

SOURCE: Reprinted from Byrne JC, Saxton DF, Pelikan PK, Nugent PM: *Laboratory Tests: Implications for Nursing Care,* 2nd ed. Menlo Park, CA: Addison–Wesley, 1986, p. 362.

for physiological complications and medical emergency (pathological intoxication, alcoholic coma, or potential for alcohol withdrawal) to determine the need for treatment.

Coma

Coma from a drug overdose is a medical emergency requiring an immediate assessment of the physical state and depth of coma. Important information frequently can be obtained from those accompanying the client. When the coma is profound, the immediate danger is death from respiratory depression. For respiratory depression from a narcotic overdose, a narcotic antagonist agent such as naloxone hydrochloride counteracts the respiratory depression. The response to naloxone is dramatic: the client's respiratory rate increases, pupils dilate, and level of consciousness improves.

Once emergency measures are established and the client is stable, assess the client for the common acute complications of heroin addiction and overdose such as cardiac dysrhythmias, sepsis, and pulmonary edema. The following measures must also be taken:

- Maintain a clear airway by insertion of an endotracheal tube.
- Prevent aspiration of secretions and vomitus. (If no injury to head or neck is obvious, place the client in a semiprone position.)

- If the client is in shock, treat immediately with fluids, vasopressor drugs, and steroids.
- Empty the bladder and institute drainage if urinary retention occurs.
- Measure vital signs frequently.
- Remove accumulated mucus by suction; turn the client to the side.
- Provide mechanical ventilation in case of respiratory paralysis.

If the client is in an alcoholic coma, begin intravenous infusion of 5% glucose to reduce hypoglycemia. Assess for and treat other injuries and complications such as subdural hematoma, pneumonia, meningitis, hepatic failure, and gastrointestinal bleeding. Gastric lavage is unnecessary because alcohol is rapidly absorbed in the stomach and because there is a danger of aspiration of gastric contents. Gastric lavage or hemodialysis may be undertaken if a large number of pills has been swallowed.

Withdrawal

Whether withdrawal is gradual or "cold turkey" (all at once) depends on the specific substance being abused. Regardless of whether withdrawal is gradual or abrupt, the goals of nursing are:

- Preventing death
- Preventing serious complications related to withdrawal

- Keeping the use of other chemical agents to a minimum
- Helping the client understand the withdrawal experience as the result of substance abuse

The care plan for individuals withdrawing from a depressant, narcotic, or stimulant incorporates similar principles. The specific withdrawal symptoms and the anticipated time of their onset differ depending on the category of drug, however. With some drugs, especially narcotics, the dosage is gradually decreased to avoid dangerous withdrawal states. The care plan should follow the principles outlined below for the client withdrawing from the effects of alcohol.

Withdrawal from alcohol progresses through a series of increasingly dangerous physiological and behavioral states as outlined in Table 10–8. Skilled nursing intervention prevents the final three stages (auditory hallucinosis, delirium tremens, and "rum fits"). Since the client withdraws from alcohol "cold turkey," the nurse provides psychosocial as well as physiological support.

Beginning with admission and continuing until vital signs are stable, the nurse monitors the client's pulse, respiration, blood pressure, and temperature every 2 hours while awake. Vital signs are the most reliable objective evidence of withdrawal symptoms that require medication. Once the vital signs are stable, encourage the client to tolerate the tremors and feelings of inner shakiness without resorting to diazepam, chlordiazepoxide, or paraldehyde. Acknowledging how difficult it is to tolerate these

experiences helps clients to cope with them. Pointing out that these symptoms result from the effects of alcohol on the body helps the client to connect the uncomfortable experiences with alcohol abuse.

The vital signs increase prior to the occurrence of hallucinations or convulsions. As the vital signs begin to rise, some clinical settings give liquids or foods with a high glucose content; 8 oz of Kool-Aid with 1 to 2 tbsp of Karo syrup is recommended. If this is unavailable, 8 oz of apple juice with 1 tbsp of sugar may be given if the client's gastrointestinal system is able to tolerate it. Recheck vital signs in 30 minutes. If they have not decreased, administer medications to promote relaxation and increase the seizure threshold. Diazepam or chlordiazepoxide are commonly prescribed for this purpose. Since the intent is to produce a state of calm wakefulness, administering diazepam or chlordiazepoxide should not be delayed too long. Waiting until hallucinations or convulsions occur is too late. Administering these drugs may be necessary to stabilize the client's vital signs or control escalating withdrawal symptoms.

In other clinical settings, diazepam or chlordiazepoxide is administered during the detoxification period. This essentially requires replacing alcohol with diazepam or chlordiazepoxide and then withdrawing the client from this drug in a controlled way. For example, a client taking the equivalent of 12 oz of alcohol daily would receive approximately 300 mg of diazepam on day 1. The dose is decreased by one-half on successive days—150 mg on day 2, 75 mg on day 3, 35 mg on day 4—until day 5 when the client is

Table 10–8   Stages of Withdrawal From Alcohol

State	Peak Time of Onset After Last Drink	Symptoms	Potential Duration of Symptoms
Tremulousness	24 h	At rest: slight tremors; during activities: gross and irregular tremors	1 wk
		Diaphoresis	3–4 d
		Anorexia, nausea, and vomiting	3–4 d
		Increased vital signs	3–4 d
		Sense of agitation and inner shakiness	2 wk
		Insomnia with nightmares of seemingly real events	2 wk or longer
Tremors and transitory hallucinosis	24 h	Above cues plus visual hallucinations of events (eg, having an accident while driving drunk)	3 d
Auditory hallucinosis	24 h	Cues of tremulousness state plus vivid persecutory and auditory hallucinations, agitation, increased suicide and preassaultive potential	3 d–2 wk
Delirium tremens	24–48 h	Cues of tremulousness state plus delirium, grand mal seizures, disorientation for time and place, visual hallucinations, agitation, panic level of anxiety	3–5 d
Rum fits	24–48 h	2–6 grand mal seizures; cues of delirium tremens	3–5 d

withdrawn from the drug. The dose is not decreased by more than half in any 24-hour period. The belief in these centers is that controlled detoxification allows for maximum client comfort and safety. Monitor the client's intake and output and weigh the client daily. Encourage, but do not force, the client to drink fluids since overhydration (which promotes cerebral edema, restlessness, and agitation) must be avoided.

Keeping a night light on helps to reduce disorientation. Intervene into hallucinations by acknowledging that, while the experience seems real to the client, the nurse does not have the same experience. For example, saying, "I understand the voice seems real to you, but I don't hear it," presents the real situation without arguing with the client. Empathizing with the client about how frightening these experiences are helps to reduce the client's anxiety and keep it within bounds. Letting the client know that these experiences are the result of alcohol withdrawal and that they will abate will help reduce anxiety.

Reactions to Hallucinogens

Hallucinogens often cause high levels of anxiety and panic. The goals of intervention should be to reduce anxiety to a mild to moderate level and to prevent suicide or violence. Environmental stimuli must be reduced. Helpful measures include lowering the volume of televisions and radios and turning off bright lights. Do not leave the client alone. Speak slowly and calmly in sentences limited to five to six words so the client can follow them. Monitor vital signs every 2 hours while the client is awake.

Watching a client experiencing panic from a hallucinogen may be frightening. It is important to recognize and attempt to control these feelings so as not to increase the client's anxiety. Have another staff member stand close by but not near enough to overwhelm or threaten the client. Once the client's level of anxiety has decreased, carefully assess suicide potential. Implement the approach to hallucinations discussed in the section on withdrawal.

Promoting More Healthful Coping

After the withdrawal symptoms have decreased, or the panic level of anxiety has been reduced, focus on promoting more healthful methods of coping. The client will have to decide whether to learn to live without the chemical agent.

Recognize that the drug has become like a best friend to the client and empathize with how difficult it will be to live without its effects. The client who is serious about wanting to refrain from drug use may experience grief over the loss of the valued drug. Anticipate, however, that many clients will continue to minimize and deny the gravity of the situation. Instead, they will focus energy on reasons for using the drug. Avoid being caught up in this topic. Focus instead on how the client will avoid using chemical agents from this point on.

Inpatient Treatment Programs. Community agencies that provide intensive 2- to 4-week inpatient treatment programs following withdrawal are often useful referrals. Encouraging the client to investigate and use such a program stresses the seriousness of the problem. These programs usually involve a number of treatment modalities, including individual, group, and family psychotherapy; psychodrama; recreational therapy; lectures on substance abuse; and support groups. These programs seem to be successful in helping individuals cope with all forms of substance abuse, including polydrug abuse.

Self-Help Groups. The importance of self-help groups should also be emphasized. Most, but not all, support groups are modeled after the Alcoholics Anonymous program. Encourage clients to investigate and attend a number of different groups to identify which ones will best suit their needs. Some, such as Women for Sobriety, are particularly suited to women. Others more directly focus on adolescents or young adults, on polydrug users, or on cocaine abusers. These and other resources are briefly described in the resources section at the end of this chapter. Emphasize that, for the initial year of recovery, the client should attend as many meetings as possible. Alcoholics Anonymous advises recovering alcoholics to attend five to ten meetings each week. A supportive network, particularly during the initial year of recovery, is especially important.

Methadone Maintenance Programs. Methadone maintenance programs were developed in the 1960s in response to heroin addiction, which had grown to epidemic proportions, particularly in inner cities. Methadone (Dolophine) is a synthetic compound, which in moderate or high doses, blocks the effects of heroin.

Although methadone is the most frequent treatment for heroin addiction in the United States, controversy surrounding its use has both physiological and psychosocial implications. Those who support methadone maintenance programs say that methadone:

- Effectively reduces the craving for heroin
- Has long-lasting effects
- Has few known side effects
- Can be administered orally
- Is cost effective compared to other forms of treatment
- Reduces criminal heroin-seeking behaviors
- Allows clients to return to their jobs, decreasing the number of heroin addicts receiving governmental assistance

Those who argue against this form of treatment make the following claims:

- Dependence on methadone is merely substituted for dependence on heroin.
- Methadone treatment is simply a chemical solution; it

fails to encourage finding solutions to the complex problems that led to drug abuse in the first place.
- The majority of heroin addicts are not attracted to methadone maintenance programs.
- Many clients who enter methadone programs leave before treatment is completed.
- A significant proportion of clients either begin to abuse or continue to abuse a wide spectrum of other drugs, including alcohol, tranquilizers, and barbiturates.

One hazard of prolonged methadone maintenance is, in fact, dependence. Methadone withdrawal is similar to morphine withdrawal except the symptoms develop more slowly and are prolonged. Acute symptoms last for 2 to 3 weeks but may continue until 4 to 6 weeks after abstinence. Other symptoms, such as irritability, fatigue, lethargy, and a variety of physical discomforts, may last up to 6 months (Bennett et al., 1983). Although it is clear that methadone is not the best or final answer to heroin dependence, it is recognized as one approach to a complex socioeconomic, psychological, and physical problem.

Disulfiram (Antabuse) Treatment. Disulfiram is used in the treatment of alcoholism as a deterrent to drinking. The usual dose is 250 mg/day. By inhibiting the action of acetaldehyde dehydrogenase, disulfiram causes an accumulation of toxic acetaldehyde when alcohol is ingested. If an individual drinks even a small amount of alcohol within a 2-week period after taking disulfiram, a reaction occurs: nausea, vomiting, flushing, dizziness, and tachycardia. Cardiovascular collapse and potential death are possible, depending on how much alcohol is ingested.

While disulfiram can be a powerful deterrent to drinking, the risks must be carefully and individually assessed before prescribing it. Disulfiram is contraindicated in clients with myocardial disease because of the cardiovascular effects that occur in a disulfiram reaction and in those who are taking metronidazole (Flagyl) because it can cause a disulfiram reaction. Clients should be clearly instructed, verbally and in writing, against using alcoholic beverages or paraldehyde and to avoid preparations such as cough and cold medicines or mouthwashes that contain alcohol. Some OTC cough and cold preparations and the percentage of alcohol they contain are listed in Table 10–9. As little as 1 tablespoon of some of these preparations is enough to cause a disulfiram reaction.

Evaluation

Initially, identifying whether the physiological and behavioral effects of abused substances have abated helps the nurse determine the effectiveness of the intervention. Cues that indicate successful withdrawal include:

- Stable vital signs
- Orientation to the "here and now"
- Improved appetite

Table 10–9 Alcohol Content of Selected OTC Cough and Cold Mixtures and Mouthwashes

Preparation	Amount of Alcohol (%)
Cough and cold mixtures	
Benylin Cough Syrup	5
Consotuss Antitussive Syrup	10
Halls Mentho-Lyptus Decongestant Cough Syrup	22
Novahistine DMX Decongestant Cough Formula	10
Nyquil Nighttime Colds Medicine	25
Quiet-Nite Liquid	25
Robitussin Night Relief Colds Formula	25
Romilar III	20
Sudafed Cough Syrup	2.4
Vicks Formula 44 Cough Mixture	10
Mouthwashes	
ACT Fluoride	7
Cepacol	14
Fluorigard	6
Listerine	26.9
SCOPE	18.5
Signal	14.5

These cues will usually be observed within 1 week of the last dose of the substance. Alcohol withdrawal is usually complete within 3 to 5 days. Even after the vital signs have been stabilized, continue to monitor them at least once per shift. Be alert to the development of other behavioral and physical cues; polydrug abusers may be beginning to withdraw from another chemical agent.

Long-term evaluation of whether the individual has achieved the goal of living life without the drug (if the client has chosen to) is difficult. The nurse may never again see the client who successfully achieves this goal. On the other hand, the person who does not achieve this goal or who chooses not to give up drugs, may return to the health care setting frequently. Nurses may feel discouraged, helpless, angry or frustrated, and hopeless when clients return to the health care setting; they may feel they have somehow failed the client. It is important to acknowledge these feelings and examine how they affect the nursing care of clients who are substance abusers.

Nurses need to assume the attitude that drug abuse is a long-term, chronic problem that can be altered. When an individual has a relapse, focus on the present and future instead of on the past. Also take the view that the current episode is possibly the right time and situation to motivate the person to be successful in recovering from the drug problem. In effect, focus on one day at a time when caring for clients with substance abuse problems.

Section IV: Chemical Dependence Among Health Care Professionals

Health professionals live and work in an environment that puts them at high risk (15% to 20%) for developing substance abuse problems. Nurses, physicians, and other health care professionals are at risk because of:

- Easy access to substances that might be abused
- Knowledge of the health care system, which makes it easier to obtain drugs for personal use
- Stressful and tiring work
- Professional, ethical, and personal conflicts inherent in the care provider role

Alcohol, meperidine, and morphine are the substances most commonly abused by health providers. Fentanyl (Sublimaze) is fast approaching similar levels of abuse among anesthesiologists and nurse anesthetists (Bissell & Haberman, 1984).

Although professionals and the general public have increased knowledge and awareness about alcohol and drug abuse problems, many professionals continue to deny the existence of an obvious problem in their ranks. Covering for a substance-abusing colleague, avoiding confrontation, and ignoring negligent performance result in situations often dangerous for both clients and the abusing professional. Terminating the employment of a nurse or other health care provider without a referral for treatment not only allows the nurse to seek other employment and continue potentially hazardous nursing practice but also perpetuates the nurse's substance abuse problem. Each nurse should be prepared to intervene effectively with a substance abusing coworker.

Consider the following situation:

Ann, a 35-year-old registered nurse, worked in the operating room of a large hospital and was also on the trauma triage team in the emergency room. She was suspected of using narcotics while working in the operating room but was never detected taking drugs by the other staff. Her colleagues and supervisor failed to discuss their suspicions with her, and she was eventually fired from her job in the OR for "chronic absenteeism."

She continued to work on the triage team and was considered an effective trauma nurse. Again, her peers began to suspect drug use, but were unable to detect that she was abusing narcotics. Soon, both clients and staff reported a number of valuables missing. Rather than confront her directly, the staff informed the administration of their suspicions. The narcotic drawer was dusted by security personnel, and she was apprehended when the dye was revealed on her hands under ultraviolet light. She admitted to having had a narcotic drawer key made and to taking morphine and replacing it with saline.

Ann was fired and informed that she should admit herself to a drug rehabilitation program. No formal charges were filed, however, and she was not reported to the licensing board. Like many of her chemically dependent colleagues in similar circumstances, Ann did not seek treatment on her own. Instead, she found employment in another hospital and continued to abuse morphine, placing herself and her clients in jeopardy.

To avoid control by the government and other authorities over professional practice, nursing and other professions have assumed responsibility for governing professional practice, protecting the public, and providing active assistance to the abusing professional. The American Nurses' Association has issued a policy statement regarding responsibility of the nursing profession to promote education, early identification, and recovery for chemically dependent nurses. Many state nurses' associations have adopted model programs to address the problem and offer support. These programs include telephone hot lines, or crisis information and treatment referral; volunteer peer assistance to aid the nurse in receiving help; and self-help peer support groups to assist in the recovery process. In some states, boards of nursing and state nurses' associations have collaborated on methods for taking disciplinary action and encouraging treatment. The aim of intervention is to protect the client and keep the nurse in active practice, perhaps with certain limitations. If suspension of pro-

Nursing Research Note

Bissell L, Jones RW: The alcoholic nurse. *Nurs Outlook* 1981; 29(2):96–101.

A survey of 100 nurses recovering from alcoholism showed that their pattern is like that of other women in the general population. It is believed that 5% of 1.5 million nurses are alcoholic. In addition, high-risk factors contribute to alcoholism in nurses, including demanding, stressful work; lack of recognition; changing shifts; and unpredictable sleep patterns. The recovered alcoholic nurses were found to be high academic achievers in professional school, had a higher incidence of suicide attempts, and were more likely to be addicted to other drugs.

Alcoholism among nurses is a significant problem. Knowing about alcohol and other drugs does not make nurses invulnerable to their effects. Denial by peers and nurses themselves suggests that more education programs and support groups should be organized to help nurses deal with alcoholism and other drug-related problems. Rehabilitation programs and helping addicted nurses return to productive, satisfying employment while safe-guarding client care are crucial.

fessional practice is indicated, the aim is to return the nurse to full practice as soon as feasible.

In a state where a peer assistance program is operating, or where legislation allows for alternatives to the customary revocation of a chemically dependent nurse's license, the outcome of Ann's case might have been quite different. Her colleagues could have requested intervention by a peer assistance team usually comprised of two nurses, one of whom is a chemically dependent recovering nurse. Ann's coworkers' observations would have been presented in a manner intended to assist Ann in seeking treatment. Alternatives to being fired would be negotiated, a leave of absence or sick leave arranged, and revocation of licensure avoided. Peer support groups provide the opportunity for discussion and consideration of re-entry into practice and alternatives to working in settings with ready access to controlled substances. The recovering nurse is encouraged to continue after-care treatment or psychotherapy as well as involvement in other support groups such as those in the resource list.

Chapter Highlights

Substance abuse is a problem of major proportions. The abuse of only one drug—alcohol—is the third major cause of death in the United States and is a major health problem in many other countries.

Substance abuse has far-reaching effects on individuals, families, friends, work associates, and neighbors.

One in four hospitalized clients is estimated to have problems related to substance abuse.

Dependence—requiring the effects of a specified drug to function—can be physiological, psychological, or both.

Tolerance to drugs develops with repeated use and requires increasingly higher, and potentially lethal, doses.

A nursing care problem develops in clients who develop a cross-tolerance to drugs that are pharmacologically similar.

No one physical, social, developmental, cultural, or genetic factor is the cause of substance abuse.

Substance abuse affects all the systems of the body, and with chronic abuse, results in debilitating physical and emotional illness.

Nurses may not always know that a client is a substance abuser; being alert to this possibility helps to prevent complications and promotes opportunities for appropriate treatment referral.

Analyzing their own feelings, beliefs, and attitudes toward substance abuse will help nurses to implement the nursing process effectively.

States of intoxication, coma, and overdose require immediate and accurate assessment and emergency measures.

Nurses and other health professionals are at high risk for developing substance abuse problems. The professions are assuming active responsibility and promoting programs of prevention, education, intervention, and peer assistance.

Bibliography

American Psychiatric Association. *Diagnostic and Statistical Manual of Mental Disorders,* 3rd ed. Washington, DC: American Psychiatric Association, 1980.

Bennett G, Vourakis C, Woolf E: *Substance abuse: Pharmacologic, Developmental, and Clinical Perspectives.* New York: Wiley, 1983.

Betemps E: Management of the withdrawal syndrome of barbiturates and other central nervous system depressants. *J Psychiatr Nurs Mental Health Serv* 1981; 19(9):31–34.

Bissell L, Haberman P: *Alcoholism in the Professions.* New York: Oxford, 1984.

Bry B: Substance abuse in women: etiology and prevention. *Issues Mental Health Nurs* 1983; 5(1-4):253–272.

Budassi S: Wernicke's encephalopathy and Korsakoff's psychosis. *Am J Nurs* 1982; 82:295–297.

Byrne CJ et al: *Laboratory Tests: Implications for Nursing Care.* 2nd ed. Menlo Park, CA: Addison–Wesley, 1986.

Chiras DC: *Environmental Science: A Framework for Decision Making.* Menlo Park, CA: Benjamin/Cummings, 1985.

Cohen S: The substance abuse problem. New York: Haworth, 1981.

Dennison D, Prevet T, Affleck M: *Alcohol and Behavior: An Activated Education Approach.* St. Louis: Mosby, 1980.

Estes NJ, Heinemann ME (editors): *Alcoholism: Development, Consequences, and Interventions,* 2nd ed. St. Louis: Mosby, 1982.

Estes N, Smith–DiJulio K, Heinemann M: *Nursing Diagnosis of the Alcoholic Person.* St. Louis: Mosby, 1980.

Gilman AG, Goodman LS, Gilman A: The Pharmacological Basis of Therapeutics, 7th ed. New York: Macmillan, 1984.

Jellinek EM: Phases of alcohol addiction. *Quarterly J Studies Alcohol* 1952; 13:673–684.

Kaplan HI, Sadock BJ: *Comprehensive Textbook of Psychiatry,* 4th ed. Baltimore: Williams & Wilkins, 1985.

Malin H et al: An epidemiologic perspective in alcohol use and abuse in the United States. In: *Alcohol Consumption with Related Problems*. Alcohol and Health Monograph No. 1. National Institute on Alcohol Abuse and Alcoholism, 1984.

Mauge CE, Dragan DK: Heroin maintenance: the second time around. In: *Drug Abuse and Alcoholism: Current Critical Issues*. Cohen S (editor). New York: Haworth, 1981.

McCoy S, Rice M, McFadden K: PCP intoxication: psychiatric issues of nursing care. *J Psychiatr Nurs Mental Health Serv* 1981; 19(7):17–23.

Naegle M: The nurse and the alcoholic: Redefining a historically ambivalent relationship. *J Psychosoc Nurs Mental Health Serv* 1983; 21(6):17–23.

Norris R: *PMS: Premenstrual Syndrome*. New York: Rawson, 1983.

Pierce RO, Pierce GW: The effect of alcohol on the skeletal system. *Ortho Rev* 1985; 14(1):45–49.

Pilette W: Caffeine: Psychiatric grounds for concern. *J Psychosoc Nurs Mental Health Serv* 1983; 21(8):19–24.

Solomon J: *Alcoholism and Clinical Psychiatry*. New York: Plenum, 1982.

Surgeon General: *The Health Consequences of Smoking: The Changing Cigarette*. DHHS Publication No. PHS 81-50156. US Government Printing Office, 1981.

US Department of Health and Human Services: *Fourth Special Report to the Congress on Alcohol and Health*. DHHS Publication No. ADM 81-1080. US Government Printing Office, 1981.

Wilson HS, Kneisl CR: *Psychiatric Nursing,* 2nd ed. Menlo Park, CA: Addison–Wesley, 1983.

Suggested Readings

Alcoholism and the family: Putting the pieces together. A special focus section. *Alcoholism* (Jan–Feb) 1981; 19–47. Entire issue reports on alcoholism as the top concern of the 1980 White House Conference on Families. Among family-related issues covered are: the children of alcoholics, spouses of alcoholics as victims or villains, family violence, recovery, rebuilding the family, family dynamics, and family treatment programs.

Folkers BL: Recognition and management of the alcohol dependent trauma patient. *Ortho Nurs* 1985; 4(2):34–36. A brief but practical article for recognition of alcohol dependence in the trauma client. Includes guidelines for nursing management.

Ford B: *The Times of My Life*. New York: Ballantine, 1978. This is the former first lady's autobiographical description of her own struggle with alcoholism and her recovery process. Mrs. Ford poignantly describes her family's influence and insistence that she receive professional help and the feelings and emotions of a woman in political life suffering from alcoholism. A major outcome of her recovery is the establishment of the Betty Ford Center, a $5 million 60-bed chemical dependence hospital in California.

Gold M: *800–Cocaine*. New York: Bantam Books, 1984. This paperback is a straightforward, up-to-date, prescriptive manual that addresses the cocaine problem. It has a no-nonsense, sensitive approach well worth the $2.95 it costs. Helpful for clients, families, and health care professionals.

Help for the helper: *Am J Nurs* 1982; 82:572–587. This series of articles describes how nursing is reaching out to help colleagues impaired by drugs or alcohol. It includes articles on confronting and helping a chemically impaired colleague, an employee assistance program in a hospital, and activities of state nurses' associations directed toward helping substance-abusing nurses.

The hospitalized alcoholic: *Am J Nurs* 1982; 1861–1879. This series of articles on alcoholism covers diagnosis, crisis assessment, communication interventions, and treatment planning.

Johnson V: *I'll Quit Tomorrow*. New York: Harper & Row, 1980. The Johnson technique described in this book includes gathering the family in what is described as "loving confrontation." Success is said to be more likely when the whole family is in treatment, and this technique is a way of breaking through the denial that accompanies alcoholism.

Mitchell R: Breakdown: Commonsense psychiatry for nurses. 1. Alcoholism. *Nurs Times* (Oct 13) 1982; 1704–1706. This first part in a monthly series deals with descriptions and case studies of common psychiatric disorders. This article discusses alcoholism as a major public health problem; presents two case studies; and describes causes, effects, and treatment of alcoholism.

Resources

SELF-HELP GROUPS AND OTHER ORGANIZATIONS

Alcoholics Anonymous World Services, Inc.
PO Box 459
Grand Central Station
New York, NY 10017

> The organization is composed of people who share experiences with alcoholism and provide support for each other in overcoming alcoholism. Pamphlets useful for health professionals are *If You Are a Professional, Alcoholics Anonymous Wants to Work with You* and *Alcoholics Anonymous and the Medical Profession*.

In Canada write to:
Intergroup Office, AA
272 Eglinton Ave., West
Toronto, Ontario, Canada M4R 1B2

Al-Anon Family Group Headquarters
PO Box 182
Madison Square Station
New York, NY 10010
Phone: (212) 475-6110

> This organization for relatives and friends of alcoholics includes Alateen for children of alcoholics. The organization functions separately from Alcoholics Anonymous and publishes several pamphlets, books (catalog available), and a monthly newsletter *Forum*. Write for a catalog of pamphlets. No dues or fees; donations at meetings.

Nar-Anon Family Group
PO Box 2562
Palos Verdes Peninsula, CA 90274
Phone: (213) 547-5800

An organization for the partners and families of persons who abuse narcotics. No dues or fees; donations appreciated. There are groups in both the United States and Canada (check local telephone book).

Narcotics Anonymous
PO Box 622
Sun Valley, CA 91352
Phone: (213) 764-4880

A worldwide fellowship of recovered narcotics addicts who meet regularly to help one another stay off drugs, this organization is based on the Alcoholics Anonymous philosophy. Membership is open to all; no dues or fees. Local chapters publish the *Narcotics Anonymous Newsletter*.

National Association of Recovered Alcoholics
PO Box 95
Staten Island, NY 10305
Phone: (213) 448-6094

Members are recovered alcoholics who help one another deal with economic, legal, social, and vocational problems. Sponsors a job-placement service and a job opportunities newsletter.

National Clearinghouse on Alcohol Information
PO Box 2345
Rockville, MD 20852
Phone: (301) 468-2600

This branch of the National Institute on Alcohol Abuse and Alcoholism makes available current information on alcohol use and abuse. They will conduct computerized searches for specific materials, provide bibliographies, provide referrals to local alcohol abuse programs, and give notification of newly published research results. Several pamphlets and books on alcohol are available at no charge or minimal charge.

National Clearinghouse on Drug Abuse Information
Room 10A53, Parklawn Building
5600 Fishers La.
Rockville, MD 20857
Phone: (301) 443-6500

This branch of the National Institute on Drug Abuse provides educational materials and referrals to drug abuse treatment programs.

National Council on Alcoholism, Inc.
733 Third Ave.
New York, NY 10017
Phone: (212) 968-4433

This national voluntary health agency consists of state and local affiliates as well as the American Medical Society on Alcoholism and National Nurses Society on Alcoholism (see listing under Nursing Organization). It cooperates with, and supports, self-help groups. The NCA Library Information Service invites questions by telephone or letter.

Pills Anonymous
443 W. 50th St.

New York, NY 10019
Phone: (212) 247-1700

Modeled after AA, this organization has the goal of helping people live a drug-free life. Most members have or had dependence problems with tranquilizers, sedatives, or analgesics. No dues or fees; contributions at meetings.

Salvation Army
National Information Service
50 W. 23rd St.
New York, NY 10010
Phone: (212) 620-4900

Sponsors both alcohol and drug rehabilitation programs, halfway houses, drop-in centers, and family service bureaus.

Therapeutic Communities of America, Intl.
54 W. 40th St.
New York, NY 10018
Phone: (212) 354-6000

This organization monitors the activities of drug-free therapeutic communities throughout the United States and will make referrals to those that meet its standards. Referral resources do not include methadone maintenance programs.

Valium Anonymous
Box 404
Altoona, IA 50009

This self-help group for persons "hooked" on Valium was founded in 1978 and now has chapters around the country. It provides support and helpful strategies for persons who wish to discontinue their dependence on Valium.

Women for Sobriety, Inc.
Box 618
Quakertown, PA 18951
Phone: (215) 536-8026

This is a network of over 200 self-help groups for women alcoholics only. It is supported by contributions and donations at group meetings. Monthly newsletter.

HOT LINES

Alcoholics Anonymous

Local phone books in the United States and Canada list the number of the closest 24-hour answering service.

Federal Drug Administration
Bureau of Drugs
Phone: (301) 443-1016

Offers information on drug interactions and side effects (weekdays 7 AM to 4:30 PM EST).

National Cocaine Helpline
Phone: 800-COCAINE

This 24-hour nationwide referral and information service is a resource for cocaine users, nonuser victims, and health care professionals, who can request information on cocaine research. It is based at Fair Oaks Hospital in Summit, NJ. Its founder, Dr. Mark S. Gold, is the author of *800-Cocaine*, described in the Suggested Readings.

NURSING ORGANIZATIONS

National Nurses Society on Addictions (NNSA)
2506 Gross Point Rd
Evanston, IL 60201
Phone: (312) 475-7300

This organization for nurses working in the addiction field publishes a newsletter four times a year. It also provides information on treatment and research in addiction, certification for nurses working in the field, and a chemically dependent nurse network.

National Nurses Society on Alcoholism
733 Third Ave.
New York, NY 10017
Phone: (212) 968-4433

An affiliate of the National Council on Alcoholism, this is an organization for nurses interested in alcoholism programs or the care and treatment of alcoholics. Publishes a newsletter four times a year.

Chapter 11

Infection

Carol Ren Kneisl
Joyce Black

Objectives

When you have finished studying this chapter, you should be able to:

Identify the sequence of events necessary for transmission of infection.

Describe susceptibility to infection.

Discuss the physiological and psychosocial/lifestyle factors that can compromise the immune system.

Describe the assessment of the potentially infected client.

Implement isolation precautions.

Employ direct measures to prevent or limit nosocomial infection.

Educate clients regarding immunization, hygiene and sanitation, and food handling.

Discuss principles of infection prevention and control in the nursing care of all clients.

Infectious diseases have aroused fear from the time of the ancient Greeks and Chinese to the present. During the Middle Ages, an estimated three-fourths of the population of Europe contracted smallpox. Many died or were left with disfiguring scars. At about the same time, the black death, or bubonic plague, destroyed about one-fourth of the total population of Europe. Yellow fever endangered the successful completion of the Panama Canal. Poliomyelitis terrorized the United States in the late 1940s and early 1950s; many children and adults were left to cope with its paralyzing effects. More recently, legionellosis, or legionnaires' disease, a pneumonialike illness, frightened the citizens of Philadelphia in 1976 when 182 American Legion conventioneers became ill, and 29 of them died. Women who used superabsorbent tampons in the early 1980s feared toxic shock syndrome; and homosexuals, bisexuals, and entire populations fear contracting what is proving to be an exceptionally insidious and lethal disease, acquired immune deficiency syndrome (AIDS).

An infection occurs when potentially pathogenic (disease-producing) organisms invade or colonize the body, or host. Not all contact with these microorganisms is harmful,

and therefore, not all infections cause disease. In fact, people live in constant contact with infectious agents throughout their lives. Corynebacteria normally inhibit the surface of the eye; mycobacteria, the external ear; and lactobacilli, the vagina and the stomach epithelium. Usually, a balance between the host's immune system and the virulence of the organism keeps the host healthy. But when the balance is tipped, such as when the immune system is penetrated or when the organism is particularly pathogenic, infectious disease occurs. All body systems are vulnerable to infectious disease; therefore, infection is a multisystem stressor.

This chapter provides a general overview of infection, its prevention and control, and nursing measures relevant to infectious disease. Selected diseases such as botulism, tetanus, and rabies, among others, are also discussed here. Other infectious diseases and related nursing measures are discussed in each of the specific disorders chapters in the units on body system dysfunction. For example, influenza, legionnaires' disease, pneumonia, and mononucleosis are described in Chapters 19 and 20 with disorders of the respiratory tract. Acquired immune deficiency syndrome is discussed in Chapter 29 with specific disorders of the blood and blood-forming organs. Infectious gastroenteritis is discussed in Chapter 49 with disorders of the stomach, intestines, and pancreas. Hepatitis is discussed with disorders of the hepatic-biliary system in Chapter 53. Infectious arthritis is included with other joint disorders in Chapter 59. Syphilis, gonorrhea, and herpes genitalis appear in Chapters 64 and 67 with reproductive system disorders, whereas herpes simplex and herpes zoster can be found in Chapter 79 with disorders of the integumentary system.

Infectious disease affects health care and human behavior at many different levels. It can influence or be influenced by culture, economics, religion, environment, and various lifestyle factors. Because all body systems are vulnerable to infectious disease, the thread of infection is woven throughout the fabric of this text.

Section I: The Problem of Infection

Despite the development of antimicrobials and methods of infection prevention and control, infectious diseases remain a major cause of illness and death, especially in third world countries. It has been estimated that pathogenic microorganisms cause at least half of all human diseases.

HOST AND MICROBE

The relationship between host and microbe varies from mutually beneficial to seriously harmful, depending on the condition of the host and the virulence of the microbe. The relationship between a healthy person and that person's *normal flora* (the microorganisms that normally inhabit the inside as well as the outside of the human body) is called *symbiosis*. The normal flora usually found in healthy individuals are identified in Table 11–1.

When a human and a microorganism mutually benefit from their symbiotic relationship, the term is *mutualism.* Normal intestinal microbes such as *Escherichia coli* live on ingested food; in return, they aid in synthesis of vitamin K, vitamin B_{12}, thiamine, and riboflavin.

In *commensalism,* one organism is benefitted and the other is unaffected. The corynebacteria that live on sloughed-off cells and secretions on the surface of the eye apparently neither benefit nor harm their human host. On the other hand, lactobacilli in the vagina help maintain a vaginal pH of 4.0 to 4.5, inhibiting yeast infection from *Candida albicans.*

The relationship is known as *parasitism* when one organism benefits at the expense of the other; eg, in a serious infection, microbes benefit at the expense of a human. Many microorganisms causing disease are parasites.

Under certain circumstances, a relationship of peaceful coexistence can change, and organisms such as *E. coli* may become harmful. If the client is ill for another reason, or if the integrity of the skin or mucous membranes has been compromised (accidentally or purposefully through an invasive procedure such as surgery or diagnostic testing), allowing the organism access to a body site in which it is not normally found, a normally harmless organism can become pathogenic. For example, when *E. coli* invades the urinary bladder or a surgical wound, it can cause infections or abscesses. Even hygienic measures or drug therapy sometimes disrupts peaceful coexistence. When lactobacilli in the vagina are eliminated through douching, vaginal deodorants, or treatment with wide-spectrum antibiotics or immunosuppressive drugs, *C. albicans* flourishes, causing infectious vaginitis (see Chapter 64). These potentially pathogenic organisms are called **opportunists.**

It is important to keep this concept in mind when delivering hands-on nursing care or teaching clients and their families. Alert clients and health care providers can reduce the risk of opportunistic organisms becoming harmful ones. Specific nursing measures are discussed in Section III.

In addition to the normal flora, other microorganisms usually regarded as pathogenic may be present on or in the body without causing disease. For example, the varicella-zoster virus, a member of the herpesvirus group that causes chickenpox, can remain latent in nerve cells after recovery. Serious illness, trauma, or psychological stress are factors thought to reactivate the virus, causing a related disease known as herpes zoster, or shingles. The poliovirus has been found to remain latent in the anterior horn cells of the upper spinal cord where it can be reactivated decades later. Some adults who had polio as children are discovering new paralytic symptoms similar to those of the original poliomyelitis 30 and 40 years after having had the disease.

THE SPREAD OF INFECTIOUS DISEASE

Until scientists established that specific organisms caused specific diseases, infections were thought to be caused by foul odors from sewage, poisonous swamp vapors, the night air, or by the gods who brought illness down upon a person, family, or community as a punishment for misdeeds. The germ theory of disease was first proven a little over a century ago in 1876 when Robert Koch, a young German physician, first proved that bacteria caused the cattle disease, anthrax.

Now it is known that a sequence of events is necessary for infection to spread (Figure 11–1). First is a *disease-producing agent*—a bacterium, virus, fungus, rickettsia, protozoan, or helminth (worm). Second, the organisms must have a source, called a *reservoir,* in which the organism survives but may or may not multiply. Although the human body is the most common reservoir for the microorganisms that cause human disease, a reservoir can also be animal or inanimate. Amazingly, about 150 diseases can be transmitted to humans by animals, birds, or insects. Inanimate reservoirs include soil and water as well as other

Table 11–1   Normal Flora in Commonly Cultured Sites of Healthy Individuals

Location	Organism	
Anterior nares	*Staphylococcus epidermidis* *Streptococcus pneumoniae* (pneumococcus, diplococcus) *Neisseria* species including *meningitidis* (except gonococci)	Nonhemolytic *Streptococcus* Diphtheroids *Staphylococcus aureus*
Mouth, nasopharynx	*Neisseria catarrhalis (Branhamella catarrhalis)* *Streptococcus viridans* (alpha-hemolytic *Streptococcus*) *Staphylococcus epidermidis* or *aureus* *Streptococcus,* nonhemolytic and anaerobic; various fungi, viruses, and mycoplasma	*Fusobacterium* *Bacteroides* species *Borrelia* species Diphtheroids *Hemophilus* species
Trachea, bronchi and lungs, sinuses, inner or middle ear	Often sterile, these structures may often become contaminated with many nasooropharyngeal organisms	
Stomach	Often sterile but varies with digestive activity	
Small bowel	Few aerobic organisms	
Large bowel	*Bacteroides* and *Fusobacterium* (bifidobacteria in breast-fed infants) *Clostridium* (*perfringens* and *tetanus,* among others) Enterococcus (group D *Streptococcus*) viruses, fungi, and protozoa	*Lactobacillus* *Escherichia coli* *Klebsiella-Enterobacter* group *Proteus* species *Pseudomonas* species *Serratia* species
Vagina: premenopausal	*Lactobacillus* (small numbers of nasooropharyngeal flora) Anaerobes including species of *Bacteroides, Clostridium, Peptostreptococcus, Propionibacterium, Selenomonas*	
prepubertal and postmenopausal	Enterobacteriaceae family Streptococci, yeasts	
Skin	Diphtheroids (*Propionibacterium* and aerobic *Corynebacterium*) *Staphylococcus epidermidis* (coagulase-negative) *Staphylococcus aureus* (coagulase-positive) *Acinetobacter* (*Herellea*), yeasts Anaerobic streptococci	
Urinary bladder	Usually sterile or contaminated with low numbers of organisms in distal urethra	
Blood, spinal fluid	Sterile	

SOURCE: Reprinted with permission from Hargiss CO, Larson E: How to collect specimens and evaluate results. *Am J Nurs* 81; 1981:2168.

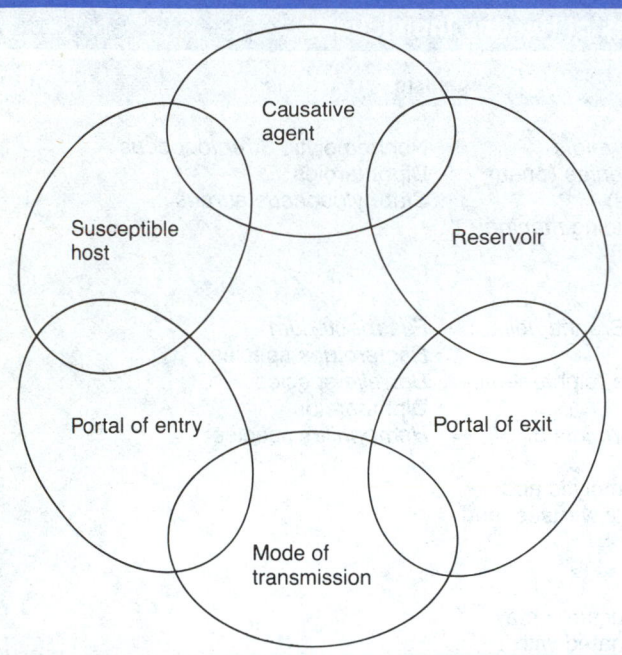

Figure 11–1

The chain of infection. Components of the infectious disease process.
SOURCE: Soule BM: *The APIC Curriculum for Infection Control Practice.* Vol 1. Dubuque, IA: Kendall/Hunt, 1983.

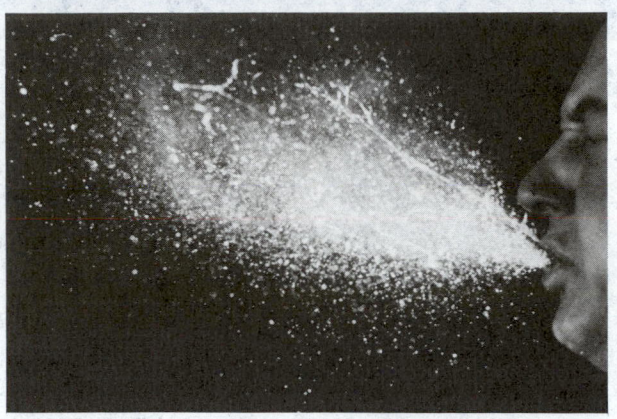

Figure 11–2

This high-speed photograph shows the spray of small droplets that comes from the mouth during a sneeze.
SOURCE: Tortora GJ, Funke BR, Case CL: *Microbiology;* 2nd ed. Menlo Park, CA: Benjamin/Cummings, 1986.

substances or objects not normally considered reservoirs of infection; eg, *Salmonella* organisms can multiply in contaminated turkey at a family gathering, and *Pseudomonas* organisms can multiply in nebulizers, eye drops, and cosmetics. Although most microorganisms multiply in the reservoir, viruses are unable to multiply in nonliving reservoirs. A *portal of exit* is the organism's escape route from the reservoir. Common portals of exit from human reservoirs are the gastrointestinal system (through saliva or feces), the respiratory system (through coughing, sneezing, and even laughing or talking), the urinary system (through the urine), the reproductive system (through the semen or secretions from the penis or vagina), and skin or wound infections (through wound drainage).

Next is a *mode of transmission* from the reservoir to the host. Organisms are transmitted by direct contact, indirect contact, and arthropod vectors. Infection might spread by direct body contact when a nurse accidentally sticks herself with a needle from a hepatitis B client or handles a contaminated wound dressing and forgets to wash her hands before rubbing her eyes. The common cold and venereal diseases are also spread directly from one person to another through such close associations as handshaking, kissing, and sexual intercourse. Droplet spread from talking, coughing, and sneezing, usually limited to 3 ft or less, is another form of direct contact (Figure 11–2).

Food or objects provide for indirect contact. A contaminated suction catheter used for endotracheal suctioning is an example of an object that provides for indirect contact; another is the contaminated turkey at the family gathering. Because many more steps are involved in indirect transmission, it is a less likely mode of transmitting infectious agents than direct contact. Consider this scene in a dialysis unit: (1) A hemodialysis nurse gets blood on her hands from a client with hepatitis B. (2) The nurse handles the dialysis machine knobs, transferring the hepatitis B virus to them. (3) A second nurse also handles the knobs, picking up the hepatitis B virus. (4) The second nurse starts an intravenous infusion on a second client. (5) On palpating the second client's vein, the nurse transfers the virus to the access route. Airborne transmission, an indirect method that spreads diseases such as tuberculosis, covers greater distances than droplet spread. Some organisms that live in dry desert soil are transmitted by the wind or in dust storms.

Arthropod vectors include the insects that carry disease and transmit it either mechanically or biologically. Houseflies carry infectious organisms on their feet and transfer them mechanically to food that is later swallowed. In malaria and yellow fever, pathogens reproduce in mosquitoes, which transmit them biologically by injecting them through the skin.

A pathogen gains access to the body by a *portal of entry*. Common portals are the respiratory and gastrointestinal tracts. Pathogens can also enter the body through broken skin, mucous membranes, or by the parenteral route—injections, blood transfusions, wounds, surgery, punctures, cuts, and bites. Table 11–2 lists some common causative organisms by portal of entry. Finally, to cause an infection, the pathogen must find a *susceptible host,* one whose body defenses are ineffective against the pathogen. The susceptible host is discussed in greater detail later in this chapter.

Table 11–2   Causative Agents for Some Common Diseases by Portal of Entry

Portal of Entry	Causative Agent*	Disease	Incubation Period
Mucous membrane Respiratory tract	*Corynebacterium diphtheriae*	Diphtheria	2–5 days
	Neisseria meningitidis	Bacterial meningitis	1–7 days
	Streptococcus pneumoniae	Pneumococcal pneumonia	Variable
	*Mycobacterium tuberculosis***	Tuberculosis	Variable
	Bordetella pertussis	Whooping cough (pertussis)	12–20 days
	Myxovirus	Influenza	18–36 hours
	Paramyxovirus	Measles (rubeola)	11–14 days
	Togavirus	German measles (rubella)	2–3 weeks
	Epstein–Barr virus (herpesvirus)	Infectious mononucleosis	2–6 weeks
	Varicella-zoster (herpesvirus)	Chickenpox (varicella)	14–16 days
	Poxvirus	Smallpox (variola)	12 days
	Coccidioides immitis (fungus)	Coccidioidomycosis (primary infection)	1–3 weeks
	Histoplasma capsulatum (fungus)	Histoplasmosis	5–18 days
Gastrointestinal tract	*Shigella* species	Bacillary dysentery (shigellosis)	1–2 days
	Brucella melitensis	Brucellosis (undulant fever)	6–14 days
	Vibrio cholerae	Cholera	1–3 days
	Salmonella enteritidis, Salmonella typhimurium, Salmonella cholerae-suis	Salmonellosis	7–22 hours
	Salmonella paratyphi	Paratyphoid fever	7–24 days
	Salmonella typhi	Typhoid fever	5–14 days
	Hepatitis A virus (picornavirus)	Infectious hepatitis	15–50 days
	Paramyxovirus	Mumps	2–3 weeks
	Picornavirus	Poliomyelitis	4–7 days
	Trichinella spiralis (helminth)	Trichinosis	2–28 days
Skin, or parenteral route	*Clostridium perfringens*	Gas gangrene	1–5 days
	Clostridium tetani	Tetanus	3–21 days
	Neisseria gonorrhoeae	Gonorrhea	3–8 days
	Leptospira interrogans	Leptospirosis	2–20 days
	Yersinia pestis	Plague	2–6 days
	Rickettsia rickettsii	Rocky Mountain spotted fever	3–12 days
	Treponema pallidum	Syphilis	9–90 days
	Hepatitis B virus** (picornavirus)	Serum hepatitis	6 weeks–6 months
	Rhabdovirus	Rabies	10 days–1 year
	Togavirus	Yellow fever	3–6 days
	Plasmodium species (protozoan)	Malaria	2 weeks

*All causative agents are bacteria, unless indicated otherwise. For viruses, only the viral group is given, except where the virus has a name different from the disease it causes.

**These pathogens can also cause disease after entering the body via the gastrointestinal tract.

SOURCE: From Tortora GJ, Funke BR, Case CL: *Microbiology*, 2nd ed. Menlo Park, CA: Benjamin/Cummings, 1986.

THE NATURE AND SCOPE OF INFECTIOUS DISEASE

Infectious diseases are classified and understood according to their nature and scope. A disease that can be transmitted from one person to another is a *communicable disease*. Tuberculosis and typhoid fever are communicable diseases. A *noncommunicable disease* is one that is not transmitted from one person to another. Noncommunicable diseases are caused by organisms normally inhabiting the body that only occasionally cause disease or by organisms that reside outside the body causing disease when introduced into it. Tetanus is an example of a noncommunicable disease. Diseases, such as measles and chickenpox, that can be easily spread from one person to another are termed *contagious diseases*. The initial infectious disease is called a *primary infection*. When an opportunist organism causes a different infection in a body already weakened by a primary infection, the condition is called a *secondary infection*.

Of great concern recently has been the frequent occurrence of pneumocystis pneumonia caused by *Pneumocystis carinii* as a secondary infection in persons whose immune systems have been disrupted by the virus that causes AIDS. A person can also have a *subclinical infection* in which there are no apparent symptoms.

Knowing about the incidence, prevalence, and frequency of occurrence also helps in understanding infectious diseases. (Incidence and prevalence have previously been discussed and defined in Chapter 3.) A variety of terms describes the frequency of infectious diseases. An *endemic* disease is usually present within a certain population or within a geographic area. For example, yellow fever is endemic in Africa and Central and South America, and coccidioidomycosis is endemic in the American Southwest (especially the San Joaquin Valley of California) and northern Mexico (Figure 11–3). Whenever there is an excess incidence of a disease over that expected within an area in a relatively short time, a disease is said to be *epi-*

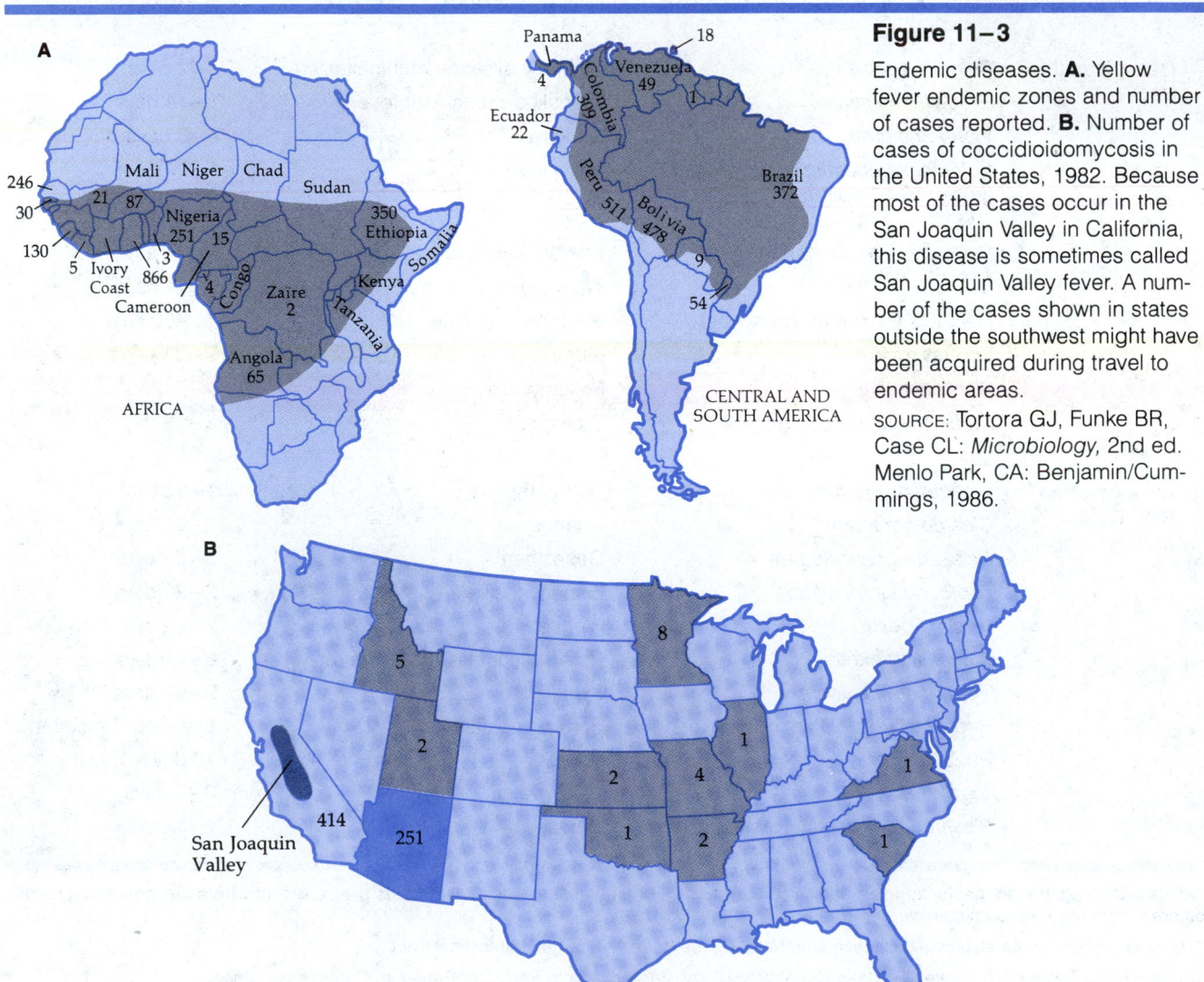

Figure 11–3

Endemic diseases. **A.** Yellow fever endemic zones and number of cases reported. **B.** Number of cases of coccidioidomycosis in the United States, 1982. Because most of the cases occur in the San Joaquin Valley in California, this disease is sometimes called San Joaquin Valley fever. A number of the cases shown in states outside the southwest might have been acquired during travel to endemic areas.

SOURCE: Tortora GJ, Funke BR, Case CL: *Microbiology,* 2nd ed. Menlo Park, CA: Benjamin/Cummings, 1986.

demic. Measles, smallpox, and poliomyelitis historically have occurred in epidemics. Some sexually transmitted diseases are thought to have reached epidemic proportions. A *pandemic* is an epidemic disease that affects several countries or occurs worldwide. Influenza and bubonic plague have been pandemic.

Infectious diseases may also be classified according to the extent to which the body is affected. For example, in a pimple or an abscess, the infection is confined to a limited area of the body. This is called a *local infection.* A *systemic infection* is generalized rather than limited. The disease is spread throughout the body by the blood and the lymphatics. Typhus and typhoid fever are examples of systemic diseases. A *focal infection* is one that had its beginnings as a local infection but spread to another part of the body. Infections in the teeth and sinuses may spread to the brain via the lymphatics and blood supply.

SUSCEPTIBILITY TO INFECTION

Although everyone has frequent contact with potentially infectious organisms, most persons do not often become ill. They remain well either because the organism's *virulence* (ability to produce disease) is low or because the host's resistance to disease is high. Resistance to disease depends on an equilibrium among these factors. When there is an imbalance, infection is more likely.

The *virulence* of an organism, or its ability to produce disease, is influenced by a variety of factors. The first factor is the number of organisms involved; the likelihood of disease increases with the number of pathogens. Recall the earlier example of *C. albicans;* normally present in the vagina, this organism does not usually cause disease unless it proliferates.

A second influencing factor is an organism's *invasiveness,* its ability to colonize and multiply in a host and interfere with body function. A third factor is the organism's ability to produce poisonous substances called **toxins.** A fourth factor is the organism's ability to cause changes in cells themselves that result in cell death. These factors are discussed in the later sections on selected diseases.

In the past, organisms were considered the dominant factor in infection. Now the role of the host figures as prominently. From experience with chemotherapeutic agents, immunosuppressants, and antimicrobials, it is known that any organism can cause an infection if the host's resistance is sufficiently suppressed. A person with impaired resistance is referred to as a **compromised host.** A person may be a compromised host for a number of reasons such as age or general health, malnutrition, defects in the immune system, chronic disease, injury to the integumentary or respiratory systems, or psychosocial/lifestyle factors. Other causes of a weakened immune response are splenectomy and administration of potent antimicrobials, immunosuppressants, and chemotherapeutic agents. Factors compromising the host's ability to resist infectious

Table 11–3 The Compromised Host

Conditions Placing Clients at Risk for Infection	Altered Defense Mechanism
Severe burns, extensive trauma	Skin and mucous membranes
Malnutrition	Cell-mediated immunity
Diabetes mellitus	Microcirculation, inflammatory response
Leukemia, lymphoma, multiple myeloma, sarcoidosis	Immune system
Immunosuppressive drugs	Immune system
Broad-spectrum antibiotics	Normal bacterial flora
Glucocorticosteroids	Cell-mediated immunity
Anatomic defects, eg, scoliosis	Respiratory function
Chronic heavy alcohol use	Normal cough and glottal closure; humoral and cell-mediated immunity
Heavy tobacco smoking	Normal ciliary function, oxygen level, platelet responses
Stress	Immune system

disease are discussed in the following sections and listed in Table 11–3.

Age and General Health

Infants are born with passive immunity from their mothers that protects them from illness for a short time. After the first few weeks of life, infants must be protected from unnecessary exposure to contagious illness and immunized on schedule because they have not developed their own immunity. The infant's immunity can be extended by breast feeding because the mother passes antibodies to her infant in the breast milk.

As children grow older, their immune systems mature. Although young children are easily infected, they recover from most infections without problems. They build immunity against many diseases through exposure and immunization. Young adults are less easily infected than children and normally recover readily from local infections. For middle-aged adults in good health, minor contagious diseases are the primary infection problem. By the later years, however, susceptibility to infection increases because of a variety of factors. Chronic diseases, such as diabetes and pulmonary and cardiovascular diseases, which are most common in the elderly, reduce the ability to fight infectious disease. During the winter many elderly persons die from influenza, in part because of their debilitated state.

Nutritional Status

Poor nutritional status increases the risk of infection. Insufficient protein in the diet reduces the numbers of antibodies formed because antibodies are a protein substance. This reduces host resistance. Because caloric and protein needs increase during illness, the malnourished person with an infection may become trapped in a cyclical disease state. Malnutrition exacerbates infection and vice versa, so a minor infection may have serious consequences. A person without normal serum protein levels can sometimes even acquire a disease from the small dose of antigens given in an immunization.

Nurses caring for malnourished clients should be aware of the effect of nutritional status on the immune system. Hospitalized clients are at particular risk for malnutrition and consequently for infection. Certain hospital practices, such as withholding food before tests, can contribute to this iatrogenic malnutrition (see Chapter 8).

Immune System Defects

The immune system is a complex group of organs, tissues, and cells that is mobilized to identify, resist, and destroy foreign substances. A complete discussion of the immune system and immune response is in Chapter 2.

Conditions affecting the production, lifespan, or function of white blood cells reduce the host's ability to fight infection. When the blood neutrophil count drops below 1000 μL, particularly if the count falls below 100 μL, the risk of infection is greatly increased. Low neutrophil counts (neutropenia) occur with leukemia, agranulocytosis, and aplastic anemia, discussed in Chapter 29.

Other acquired diseases specifically affecting the immune system are multiple myeloma, Hodgkin's disease, Crohn's disease, and sarcoidosis. Of growing concern is AIDS, an infectious disease that involves a defect in cell-mediated immunity and for which there is, as yet, no known cure. AIDS is fully discussed in Chapter 29.

Persons can also be born with a variety of congenital immune abnormalities that affect the production of antibodies, complement, or cellular immunity. A few children with severe congenital combined immune deficiencies have been placed in clear plastic "bubbles" to protect them from pathogens, but such precautions are extremely expensive.

Chronic Disease

Among chronic diseases suppressing the immune system are uremia and diabetes. Studies have shown that persons with uremia from chronic renal failure have a decrease in the number of circulating lymphocytes as well as malnutrition and other factors that impair the body's defenses. Diabetics have an increased incidence of infection, although research has not demonstrated that their immune response is reduced. The increased risk of infection probably results from vascular damage and neurovascular changes. Deficits in sensation place the client at risk of injury, and impaired

circulation to the injured area delays healing, increasing the risk of infection. It is also possible that elevated levels of blood glucose and ketones impair the inflammatory response.

Injury to Integumentary and Respiratory Systems

The skin and mucous membranes provide the first barrier to invading organisms. The body is protected by the skin's tough outer layer, the stratum corneum, and by antimicrobial substances produced by the sweat and oil glands.

In the respiratory tract, mucus and other substances prevent organisms from colonizing or invading. Cilia lining the respiratory tract sweep mucus upward on a so-called "ciliary escalator," taking bacteria along so they can be expelled (Figure 11–4). The sneeze and cough reflexes also expel foreign matter from the airway. Urine, tears, and saliva wash infectious organisms away from body orifices.

Injuries to these protective mechanisms increase a person's infection risk. Burns, decubitus ulcers, and extensive trauma are examples of injuries that leave the skin raw and vulnerable to infectious organisms. These wounds often become infected. Persons with diabetes or atherosclerosis can develop ulcers on the legs and feet that are prone to infection.

Damage to the respiratory tract from inhalation burns, mechanical ventilation, or infection can alter the normal resistance of lung epithelium, increasing the risk of pneumonitis and pneumonia. Intubation and tracheostomy with or without mechanical ventilation also increase the risk of pulmonary infection because the normal protective barriers are interrupted or bypassed. These procedures provide direct communication between the environment and underlying tissues.

Psychosocial/Lifestyle Factors

Host resistance is also influenced by psychosocial and lifestyle factors such as finances, environment, occupation, avocation, recreation, and stress. When finances are limited, a common tendency is to delay purchasing health services such as immunizations for preventable diseases. Tuberculosis is a good example of how psychosocial and lifestyle factors influence the development of disease. In the United States, tuberculosis is most prevalent among the poor where overcrowding facilitates the airborne transmission of the causative organism, and malnutrition and stress are likely. Yet, large numbers of the population have a positive reaction to tuberculosis skin testing, indicating previous exposure to the causative organism, without developing active disease.

Where one lives can also make a person more susceptible to certain infectious diseases. Histoplasmosis, a fungal disease of the respiratory system, is essentially limited in the United States to states surrounding the Ohio and Mississippi Rivers, where the moisture and pH provide ideal growing conditions for the fungus (Figure 11–5). Recall

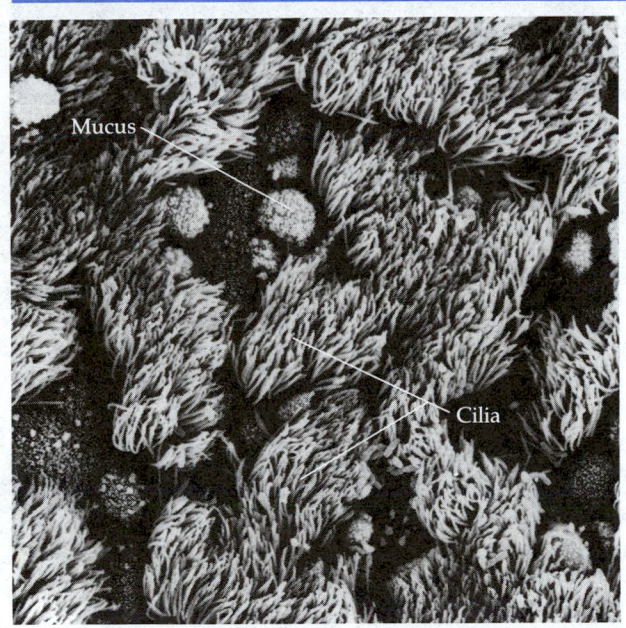

A

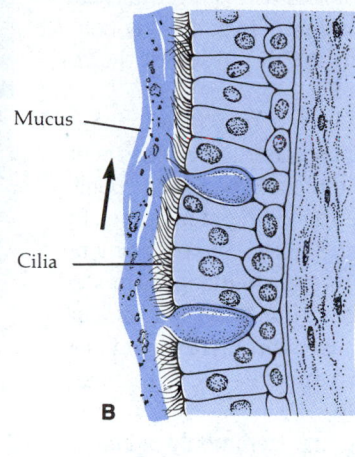

Figure 11–4

Mucous membrane of the trachea. **A.** Micrograph of cilia and mucus-secreting goblet cells, from which blobs of mucus are emerging (×1500).
B. Action of the ciliary escalator.
SOURCE: Tortora GJ, Funke BR, Case CL: *Microbiology*, 2nd ed. Menlo Park, CA: Benjamin/Cummings, 1986.

also that coccidioidomycosis is more likely to be found in the San Joaquin Valley of California and the desert regions of Arizona where the dry, highly alkaline soils favor the growth of the fungus that causes it.

Travel exposes persons to infectious diseases that, although rare in one part of the world, are common in another. Travelers have contracted Asiatic cholera in India, schistosomiasis (infestation by a flatworm parasite in contaminated water) in Africa and the Caribbean, and yellow fever in Brazil.

Occupation and avocation may place people at risk for infection. For example, farmers are susceptible to organisms that tend to use animals, the earth, and water as

reservoirs. Lifestyle is yet another influencing factor. A person who values health and fitness is more likely to stay away from situations of risk. A person with multiple sex partners is at greater risk for contracting a sexually transmitted disease. A street person who lives on a park bench or seeks shelter in an abandoned building is more likely to become undernourished and exposed to a wide variety of organisms.

Splenectomy

Persons who have their spleens removed, usually because of traumatic injury, seem to have a greater incidence of bacterial infections. Pneumococcal infections are the most common. The increased infection risk after splenectomy is related to a defective production of immunoglobulins and delayed mobilization of macrophages.

Clients receiving organ transplants in the past may also have had their spleens removed to reduce the risk of rejection of the transplanted organ. Regardless of the reason for splenectomy, these clients have increased susceptibility to infectious diseases.

Drug Therapy

Antibiotics, glucocorticoids, and immunosuppressants can alter normal resistance to infection. Antibiotics change the normal balance of flora, especially when broad-spectrum agents are given in combination with other antibiotics. With alteration in normal flora, a **superinfection** (secondary infection resulting from overgrowth of normal flora during antibiotic treatment) can occur. An organism responsible for many superinfections is *Pseudomonas aeruginosa*. This organism is resistant to many antibiotics and becomes a dominant commensal when other more susceptible bac-

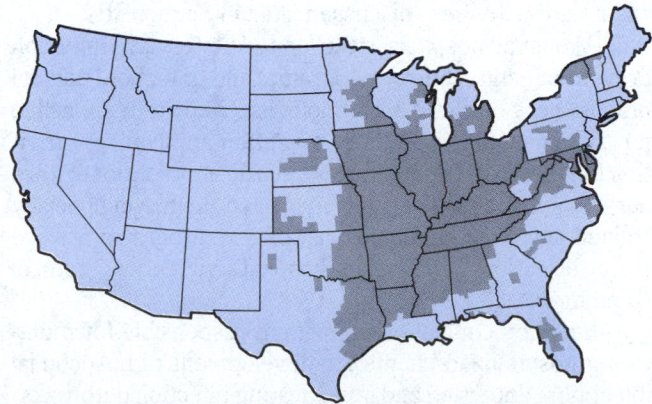

Figure 11–5

The dark area indicates the geographical distribution of histoplasmosis in the United States.
SOURCE: Tortora GJ, Funke BR, Case CL: *Microbiology*, 2nd ed. Menlo Park, CA: Benjamin/Cummings, 1986.

teria are suppressed by an antibiotic. It is often the cause of hospital-acquired respiratory infections in already compromised clients. Superinfections are discussed further in Section III.

Glucocorticoids reduce the body's response to infection by reducing inflammation. In the laboratory, it has been observed that steroids decrease mobilization of neutrophils to the site of infection, decrease the killing of microbes by monocytes, and interfere with cell-mediated immune response. Clients with a disease requiring long-term steroid therapy have a high incidence of infection. It is difficult to diagnose these infections because steroid treatment may inhibit the signs of inflammatory response—heat, redness, pain, and swelling.

Immunosuppressive drugs are commonly administered to clients with cancer and those who have had organ transplants. These agents produce side effects of neutropenia, lymphocytopenia, and monocytopenia because they reduce the ability to produce white blood cells. Immunosuppressants also impair the growth of new cells in other body sites. One result is damage to the mucous membrane epithelium, which is normally repaired rapidly. Clients may develop stomatitis, affecting their ability to eat, drink, or talk. Breakdown of mucous membranes also provides entry for microorganisms.

NOSOCOMIAL INFECTIONS

According to the Centers for Disease Control (CDC), 5% to 10% of all clients admitted to acute care hospitals in the United States develop a nosocomial (hospital-acquired) infection. With certain operations such as surgery of the large intestine and amputations, the infection rate approaches 30% (Tortora, Funke, & Case, 1982). It is estimated that fully one-third of all infections in hospitalized clients are nosocomial (Kochar, 1983).

Hospitalized clients are more vulnerable to infectious diseases than outpatients or healthy persons. Catheters, intravenous lines and devices, and endotracheal tubes are some of the invasive objects used in hospitals that disturb the normal barriers to infections. In some instances, reusable devices are not properly cleaned and disinfected or sterilized between use in one client and the next. In addition, many clients have coexisting conditions that alter the body's ability to combat organisms that have entered the bloodstream or tissues. (See discussion of the compromised host.)

The majority of nosocomial infections are caused when an organism normally present in a client overwhelms an impaired immune system. (These normal flora have been listed in Table 11–1.) Common examples are *E. coli* causing urinary tract infections and *Klebsiella* causing pneumonia. These and other bacteria that account for the majority of nosocomial infections are listed in Table 11–4.

The remainder of nosocomial infections is acquired from organisms within the hospital environment. Inhalation therapy and hemodialysis equipment are reported to have been sources of infection from gram-negative organisms.

Table 11–4	Six Bacteria That Account for Over 60% of All Nosocomial Infections	

Bacterium	% of Infections
Escherichia coli	18.6
Staphylococcus aureus	10.3
Enteroocci	10.7
Pseudomonas species (79% *P. aeruginosa*)	10.6
Klebsiella species	7.4
Coagulase-negative *Staphylococci*	6.1

SOURCE: From Tortora GJ, Funke BR, Case CL: *Microbiology*, 2nd ed. Menlo Park, CA: Benjamin/Cummings, 1986.

The source of most nosocomial infections caused by *Streptococcus* and *Staphylococcus aureus* is usually the client. These infections can also be acquired from other clients or hospital personnel and sometimes from contaminated equipment or inanimate objects. Nurses are also at risk for hospital-acquired infections. A nurse who is not wearing gloves, but has a fresh cut on a finger, can be at risk when suctioning a client. For example, if the client harbors the herpesvirus in oral secretions, the nurse could develop herpetic whitlow from the transfer of the virus from the client's oral secretions to the cut even though there are no obvious lesions on the client's lips.

Because many nosocomial infections are caused by organisms from the client's normal flora, nosocomial infections cannot be completely eliminated. An active infection control program, however, can be effective in identifying interventions that can reduce nosocomial infection risk and in teaching personnel to use these interventions in their client care activities (discussed later in Section III).

Almost all hospitals in the United States have infection prevention and control programs and infection control practitioners or nurse epidemiologists who are responsible for the day-to-day infection prevention and control activities for the hospital. About 85% of these practitioners are nurses; some large hospitals may have their own specially trained physician epidemiologist. These programs receive their direction from the hospital's infection control committee.

Infection control personnel are responsible for monitoring hospitalized clients for development of nosocomial infections, detecting and investigating infection outbreaks, monitoring isolation precautions for clients admitted with infection and clients who develop infection while hospitalized, educating hospital personnel about infection control risks and prevention strategies, and developing hospital infection control policies and procedures consistent with the latest information. Infection control practitioners can be a valuable resource to the nursing staff.

Section II: Epidemiology and Disease Control

Epidemiology is the study of the occurrence, distribution, and determinants of disease and other health conditions in populations. When an outbreak of disease occurs, such as salmonellosis, or when a new disease appears, such as toxic shock syndrome, epidemiologists go to work analyzing the incidence and transmission patterns. Some large medical centers employ epidemiologists to identify, investigate, and recommend strategies to reduce the incidence of nosocomial infection and to solve related problems. Epidemiology is also an important function of government at all levels. By gathering information and sharing resources, state, federal, and international agencies can spot trends and recommend disease control measures.

State law specifies which communicable diseases must be reported to the state health department. Listed in Box 11–1 are the diseases that typically must be reported. The lists may vary slightly from state to state. State health departments, in turn, report outbreaks to the federal government. Infection control personnel often provide the link between the hospital and the local or state health department. Nurses who work in other types of health care settings such as a community clinic or a physician's office may be responsible for reporting these diseases.

The CDC in Atlanta is the federal agency charged with disease prevention and control. The CDC administers national programs for the prevention and control of communicable and vector-borne diseases as well as other preventable conditions, such as lead-based paint poisoning and urban rat infestations. The CDC also participates with other national and international agencies in this endeavor. Occupational safety and health research and other activities are carried out by the CDC agency, the National Institute for Occupational Safety and Health.

The World Health Organization (WHO), a division of the United Nations, assists with international cooperation for improved health conditions. WHO has been directed to promote attainment of the highest possible level of health for all people. For infectious disease, WHO sponsors measures for disease prevention and control by promoting vaccinations, sanitation, and use of antibiotics and insecticides. The agency has also standardized quarantine measures.

This section discusses selected infectious diseases not discussed elsewhere in this text. A comprehensive summary of the epidemiology and prevention of infectious diseases is in Table 11–5.

(continued on p. 288)

Box 11–1   Reportable Communicable Diseases

Acquired immune deficiency syndrome (AIDS)

Amebiasis (amebic dysentery)

Anthrax

Botulism

Brucellosis (undulant fever)

Cholera, Asiatic

Conjunctivitis, acute infectious (of the newborn, not including trachoma)

Diarrhea of the newborn, epidemic

Diphtheria

Encephalitis (Eastern, Western, equine, St Louis, other)

Food poisoning (Staphylococcus enterotoxin)

Glanders

Hepatitis (A, B, non-A/non-B)

Legionellosis

Leprosy (Hansen's disease)

Leptospirosis (Weil's disease, hemorrhagic jaundice)

Malaria

Measles (rubeola and rubella)

Meningococcal infections (meningococcal meningitis, meningococcemia)

Paratyphoid fever

Pertussis (whooping cough)

Plague

Poliomyelitis, paralytic or nonparalytic

Psittacosis

Q fever

Rabies

Salmonellosis (food infections)

Shigellosis (bacillary dysentery)

Smallpox (Variola)

Tetanus

Trachoma

Trichinosis

Tuberculosis

Tularemia

Typhoid fever, cases and carriers

Typhus fever, endemic (flea borne)

Typhus fever, epidemic (louse borne)

Venereal diseases (syphilis, gonorrhea, lymphogranuloma venereum, chancroid, granuloma inguinale)

Yellow fever

Table 11-5   Summary of Epidemiology and Prevention of Selected Infectious Diseases

Disease	Causative Agent	Mode of Transmission	Incubation Period	Communicable Period	Isolation Precautions	Prevention
Acquired immune deficiency syndrome (AIDS)	Human T-cell lymphoma virus, type III (HTLV-III)	Sexual contact; blood and blood product transfusion; contaminated needles; possible transplacental transfer	Believed to be a few months to 5 yr or more	Unknown; carrier state possible	Blood/body fluid precautions	Public education about risk factors; caution in handling blood and needles; testing of donor blood for HTLV-III antibody
Amebiasis (amebic dysentery)	Protozoa: *Entamoeba histolytica*	Water or food contaminated with *E. histolytica* cysts	Variable, but may be 2–4 wk	As long as individual has cysts in stools (may be years)	Enteric precautions	Hand-washing after defecating and before eating or handling food; sanitary disposal of human feces; thorough cooking of foods; treating water with 8 gtt of tincture of iodine per quart when camping or whenever contamination is suspected or possible; removal of carriers from food handling
Anthrax	Bacteria: *Bacillus anthracis*	Contact inhalation or ingestion of heavy spore concentrations from infected animals (cattle, goats, sheep, etc) or infected materials such as hides, wool, and animal hair (especially in imported handicrafts); cutaneous infection from contaminated tissues of animals	1–7 d	Contaminated articles and soil can remain infective for years; not transmitted person to person	Drainage/secretion precautions during illness for cutaneous or inhalation anthrax	Immunization of high-risk persons; early detection and control of disease in animals; importation restrictions on possibly contaminated animal products
Botulism	Bacteria: *Clostridium botulinum*	Ingestion or contact with infected food or soil	12–72 h	Not applicable	Enteric precautions	Public education on home canning, food preservation; avoiding foods suspected of spoilage; proper industrial canning techniques; avoid giving honey to infants under 1 yr of age

Disease	Causative Agent	Mode of Transmission	Incubation Period	Communicable Period	Isolation Precautions	Prevention
Brucellosis (undulant fever)	Bacilli of Brucella genus: *B. abortus, B. canis, B. melitensis, B. suis*	Ingestion of or contact with unpasteurized dairy products, meat, blood, or aborted fetuses and placentas of infected animals (cattle, goats, pigs, dogs)	5–30 d; may be several mo	Not transmitted person to person	None	Pasteurization of milk and milk products; early detection of disease in animals; education of animal and meat handlers
Cat-scratch fever	Not yet established; may be a gram-negative bacteria	Cat scratch or bite	3–14 d	Unknown; not transmitted person to person	None	Declawing of domestic cats; teaching cats not to claw or bite; thorough cleansing of scratches or bites
Chancroid	Bacteria: *Hemophilus ducreyi*	Direct contact, especially sexual contact	2–5 d; up to 14 d	While lesions are present; usually weeks	None	Treatment of infection; prophylactic treatment of contacts; avoid sexual contact with infected person
Chickenpox (varicella)	Herpesvirus (herpes zoster virus, also known as varicella-zoster virus)	Airborne droplets and direct or indirect contact with contaminated secretions from mucous membranes or vesicles on skin	7–21 d	1 d before skin lesions appear to 6 d after they appear, or when first crop of vesicles has crusted	Strict isolation (in hospitals); isolation impractical in the community	Human varicella-zoster immune globulin for immunodeficient clients upon exposure; a live attenuated varicella-zoster vaccine is under investigation
Cholera	Bacteria: *Vibrio cholerae*	Fecal–oral route; contaminated water and food	1–5 d (usually less than 3 d)	While organism is present; carrier state may persist for several months	Enteric precautions	Protection of water and food from fecal contamination; vaccination for travelers to endemic areas not required in US but is required in a few countries
Cytomegalovirus infection	Cytomegalovirus (CMV) (Herpesvirus family)	Placental transfer, blood transfusion, skin or mucus membrane contact with infectious tissues, secretions, or excretions, and possibly passage through infected birth canal	Unknown	Unknown but may be several years	None; secretion precautions for hospitalized clients excreting the virus	Isolation of infected persons from pregnant women and newborns
Diphtheria	Bacteria: *Corynebacterium diphtheriae*	Droplet; airborne; respiratory secretions of healthy carriers	2–5 d; may be longer	As long as organism is present (usually 2 wk); chronic carriers are rare	Strict isolation	Immunization

(continued)

Table 11–5   Summary of Epidemiology and Prevention of Selected Infectious Diseases (continued)

Disease	Causative Agent	Mode of Transmission	Incubation Period	Communicable Period	Isolation Precautions	Prevention
Encephalitis	Arbovirus: St. Louis, western equine, eastern equine, Californian, Venezuelan, Japanese Enterovirus: Coxsackievirus, echovirus, poliovirus Herpesvirus: Herpes simplex Myxovirus: Mumps Rabies virus	Mosquito bite; tick bite or ingestion of infected milk or food	2–21 d, depending on specific organism	Not transmitted person to person; mosquitoes and ticks remain infective for life	Enteric precautions (unless known not to be caused by enteroviruses)	Mosquito and tick control; other measures depend on organism
Food poisoning, bacterial	*Clostridium perfringens*	Contaminated food and drink	8–24 h	Not applicable	Enteric precautions	Proper refrigeration and cooking of food; infected persons should not prepare food; proper sanitation and hand-washing during food preparation
	Salmonella	Inadequate cooking of food; infected food handlers; ingestion of contaminated food and drink; pet turtles, chicks, and ducklings	6–72 h	Throughout the course of infection; temporary carrier state may exist for months	Enteric precautions	As above
	Staphylococcus	Contamination of food by infected food handlers; improperly refrigerated food	30 min–7 h (usually 2–4 h)	Not applicable	None	As above
Giardiasis	Protozoan: *Giardia lamblia*	Ingestion of contaminated water; asymptomatic carriers	4–10 d (may be as long as 25 d)	As long as individual has cysts in stools	Enteric precautions	Avoid drinking tap water or using ice made from tap water in areas with high incidence of giardiasis; avoid drinking untreated wilderness water
Gonorrhea	Bacteria: *Neisseria gonorrhoeae*	Mucous membranes of genitourinary tract and conjunctiva through sexual transmission or direct contact during vaginal delivery	2–5 d (symptoms may not appear for 3 mo)	As long as organism is present; usually until 4 d after onset of antibiotic therapy	None	Treatment of infection; prophylactic treatment of contacts; prophylaxis in eyes of newborns

Disease	Causative Agent	Mode of Transmission	Incubation Period	Communicable Period	Isolation Precautions	Prevention
Granuloma inguinale	Bacteria: *Calymmatobacterium granulomatis*	Probably sexual contact	Unknown; may be from 1 wk to almost 3 mo	Unknown; probably while lesions are open	None	Treatment of infection; prophylactic treatment of contacts
Hepatitis Type A	Hepatitis A virus	Direct or indirect contact with feces of infected individual; ingestion of contaminated water or food, particularly shellfish, meat, and milk; blood transfusion possible but rare	2–4 wk but may be as long as 7 wk	1–2 wk before onset of symptoms to a few days up to a week after onset of jaundice	Enteric precautions	Proper hand-washing; enteric precautions; passive immunization with immune globulin possible if instituted before anticipated contact (eg, travel to highly endemic areas) or soon after but before disease has developed
Type B	Hepatitis B virus	Parenteral route: transfusion of whole blood or plasma; contaminated equipment that pierces the skin (needles, dental, or medical instruments); sexual contact	45–180 d (usual 60–90 d)	From weeks before the onset of symptoms through chronic carrier state (may last for years)	Blood/body fluid precautions	Avoid unnecessary needle piercing or blood transfusion; careful screening of potential blood donors; hepatitis B vaccine for individuals at risk; hepatitis B immune globulin for prophylaxis after exposure
Non-A, Non-B	Specific viruses unknown	Contaminated water; fecal–oral route possible	14–64 d	Probably similar to hepatitis A	Blood/body fluid precautions	Same as hepatitis A
Herpes simplex	Herpesvirus (herpes simplex virus): Type I ("cold sores"), Type II (genital herpes)	Direct contact (Type I), sexual intercourse (Type II)	2–12 d	Up to 7 wk (Type I), 4–7 d (Type II)	Contact isolation	Avoid contact with infected person; cesarean section delivery of Type II infected pregnant woman
Histoplasmosis	Fungus: *Histoplasma capsulatum*	Inhalation of spores in caves inhabited by bats and in soil nourished by dried bird droppings	5–18 d	Not transmitted person to person	None	Minimize exposure to dust or dried soil in contaminated environments
Hookworm	Helminth: *Ancylostoma duodenale* (hookworm: Old-World type); *Necator americanus* (hookworm: tropical type)	Skin, usually feet; possibly mouth (larva)	Unknown; could be a few weeks to many months	Not transmitted person to person; untreated infected person could contaminate soil	None	Wear shoes while walking in soil; use sanitary disposal systems
Infectious mononucleosis	Epstein–Barr virus (herpesvirus)	Oral–pharyngeal direct contact via saliva; possibly parenteral (transfusions, syringes, etc)	4–6 wk	Unknown; may persist for a year as a latent infection	None	None known

(continued)

Table 11–5   Summary of Epidemiology and Prevention of Selected Infectious Diseases (continued)

Disease	Causative Agent	Mode of Transmission	Incubation Period	Communicable Period	Isolation Precautions	Prevention
Influenza	Myxovirus: Myxovirus influenzae hominis types A, B, and C; types A and B include variants or subgroups; type A subgroups cause the following influenzas: Asian, Hong Kong, Russian, swine, Texas, Victoria, among others	Direct or indirect contact with contaminated respiratory droplets	Variable: 18–36 h the most common	Probably 3 d from onset of symptoms	Contact isolation	Limit smoking and provide environmental humidity for susceptible persons during flu season; specific vaccines available
Legionnaires' disease (legionellosis)	Bacteria: Legionella pneumophila	Aerosols from contaminated air-conditioning cooling tower water; contaminated hot and cold water systems; soil and water from creeks and ponds	2–10 d	Not transmitted person to person	None	Disinfection of environmental air system
Leprosy (Hansen's disease)	Bacteria: Mycobacterium leprae	Transfer of exudates from lesions through breaks in skin or mucous membranes	Variable but usually 3–5 yr; may be 1½–10 yr	Unknown; infectiousness usually lost with regular treatment	Contact isolation	Early detection of infectious cases; protection of contacts not necessary
Lymphogranuloma venereum	Chlamydia: Chlamydia trachomatis	Direct contact, especially sexual contact	3–12 d; may be as long as 30 d	While lesions are active (from weeks to years)	None	Use of condoms; treatment of infected person; prophylactic treatment of contacts
Malaria	Protozoa: Plasmodium vivax, P. falciparum, P. ovale, P. malariae	Bite of infected female Anopheles mosquito; infected blood transfusions; contaminated needles and syringes	12–30 d, depending on specific organism; P. vivax, P. falciparum, and P. ovale 12–14 d and P. malariae 30 d	3–14 d after symptoms appear; may last for years, depending on organism and treatment; mosquito remains infective for life	Blood/body fluid precautions	Prophylactic therapy for travelers to endemic areas; mosquito control; screening of blood donors; prompt and effective treatment of cases
Measles (rubeola)	Paramyxovirus	Direct or indirect contact with respiratory secretions of infected person; droplet spread	7–14 d	4–5 d before appearance of rash and throughout catarrhal inflammation, which usually lasts 4–5 d	Contact isolation (in hospitals); isolation impractical in the community	Vaccination; immune globulin for high-risk contacts
Meningococcal meningitis	Bacteria: Neisseria meningitidis	Contact with a healthy carrier or infected person via respiratory tract; droplet	2–10 d (usually 3–4 d)	As long as organism present in discharges from nose and mouth	Respiratory isolation	Vaccine for population at high risk
Mumps (infectious parotitis)	Myxovirus parotidis	Direct contact with infected human salivary secretions; droplet	14–21 d	1–6 d before symptoms appear until about 9 d after	Respiratory isolation	Immunization

Disease	Causative Agent	Mode of Transmission	Incubation Period	Communicable Period	Isolation Precautions	Prevention
Pertussis (whooping cough)	Bacteria: *Bordetella pertussis*	Respiratory secretions; droplet	7–20 d (usually within 10 d)	High communicability in early catarrhal stage and decreases over 3 wk; 5–7 d after onset of therapy	Respiratory isolation	Immunization
Plague	Bacteria: *Yersinia pestis*	Bite of infected flea from rats and other rodents; airborne droplets of persons with pneumonic form of the disease (bacteria carried by blood to lungs)	2–6 d	As long as organism present; fleas remain infective for months	Strict isolation	Flea and rat control; vaccination for high-risk persons and travelers to endemic areas
Pneumococcal pneumonia	Bacteria: *Streptococcus pneumoniae*	Healthy carriers; droplet spread; direct oral contact; indirect contact with respiratory discharges; primarily a disease following viral respiratory infection or other stress	Variable; believed to be 1–3 d	As long as organism present	None; if organisms are antibiotic resistant, then contact isolation	Vaccine available for those at high risk
Poliomyelitis	Poliovirus, an enterovirus; serotypes include 1, 2, and 3	Direct contact; contaminated saliva, vomitus, and feces	3–35 d but usually 7–14 d	Uncertain; virus persists in pharynx for at least 1 wk and in feces for a minimum of 3–6 wk or more	Enteric precautions	Immunization
Rabies	Rabies virus (a rhabdovirus)	Bite of a rabid animal; sometimes virus is transmitted by saliva or a break in the skin	10 d to 1 yr (usually 2–8 wk)	Not usually transmitted person to person	Contact isolation	Vaccination of domestic animals; vaccine for persons at risk or those who have been exposed
Rocky Mountain spotted fever	Rickettsia: *Rickettsia rickettsii*	Bite of infected wood or dog tick (4–6 h of attachment required)	3–12 d	Not transmitted person to person; tick remains infective for life	None	Wear protective clothing in tick-infested areas; check body and clothing for ticks; remove ticks carefully and promptly; inspect dogs for ticks
Rubella (German measles)	Togavirus	Direct or indirect contact with respiratory secretions, blood, urine, or feces of infected individual; transplacental	2–3 wk	7 d before rash to approximately 5 d after rash	Contact isolation (in hospitals)	Vaccine; immune globulin for high-risk contacts
Scarlet fever	Bacteria: erythrogenic toxin-producing strains of *Streptococcus pyogenes*	Inhalation of infected droplets or contaminated dust	1–3 d	As long as organism is present	Drainage/secretion precautions	Prophylactic antimicrobial therapy for contacts

(continued)

Table 11–5 Summary of Epidemiology and Prevention of Selected Infectious Diseases (continued)

Disease	Causative Agent	Mode of Transmission	Incubation Period	Communicable Period	Isolation Precautions	Prevention
Shigellosis (bacillary dysentery)	Bacteria: Shigella genus: S. dysenteriae, S. flexneri, S. boydii, S. sonnei	Direct or indirect contact with feces of infected individual; ingestion of contaminated water, milk, and food	24–48 h but may be as long as 7 d	Until stool cultures are negative; usually 1–4 wk but may be as long as 1 yr	Enteric precautions	Proper hand-washing and personal hygiene; treatment of water supply; infected persons should not be food handlers
Smallpox* (variola)	Variola virus	Direct contact with infected person, crustations of lesions, or contaminated articles; may be airborne	7–14 d	1–2 d before rash until shedding of crusts (usually 3–4 wk); most communicable during first week	Strict isolation until all scabs have separated	Vaccination may be required for international travel or exposure to infected person; routine vaccination no longer justified
Syphilis	Bacteria: Treponema pallidum	Sexually, parenterally, transplacentally (after fifth month); by direct contact with body fluids, chancre, or secretions of individuals during the infectious primary and secondary stages	10–90 d (usually 3–4 wk)	Variable; extremely infectious during primary and secondary stages; usually not infectious about 2 yr after start of latent stage; noncontagious during tertiary stage	Blood/body fluid precautions in primary and secondary stages (in hospitals)	Avoid sexual contact with infected person; use condom; treatment of infected person; prophylactic treatment of contacts
Tetanus	Bacteria: Clostridium tetani	Skin penetration (usually via puncture) of clostridium endospores, usually from soil contaminated with animal fecal wastes	3–21 d	Not transmitted person to person	None	Thorough wound cleansing and debridement; immunization; immune globulin to exposed nonimmunized persons
Toxoplasmosis	Protozoa: Toxoplasma gondii	Ingestion of oocysts of the organism, which are found in contaminated meat and feces of many birds and animals, especially cats; inhalation; transfusions; transplacental	Usually 10–23 d but may be months	Not transmitted person to person except in utero	None	Avoid eating undercooked foods; avoid inhaling dried feces of cats while cleaning litter box; pregnant women should not clean litter box
Trichinosis	Helminth: Trichinella spiralis	Ingesting cysts in insufficiently cooked contaminated pork	10–14 d; can be as long as 45 d	Not transmitted person to person	None	Cook all pork and pork products thoroughly; garbage for hogs should be cooked; eat only inspected meat

Disease	Causative Agent	Mode of Transmission	Incubation Period	Communicable Period	Isolation Precautions	Prevention
Tuberculosis	Bacteria: *Mycobacterium tuberculosis* (acid-fast baccillus)	Droplet or sputum of infected human; infected unpasteurized dairy products; dust containing organism; reinfection can occur endogenously years after the primary infection by release of viable bacilli from old tuberculous Ghon's lesions	4–12 wk	While sputum, secretions, and urine contain causative organism	AFB isolation	BCG immunization in endemic areas; avoid unpasteurized dairy products; prophylactic treatment for close contacts
Tularemia	Bacteria: *Francisella tularensis*	Handling infected animals (ground squirrels, rabbits); bites of infected deer flies, ticks, or lice; ingestion of contaminated water or undercooked meats; droplet spread has occurred in laboratory workers	2–7 d	Not directly transmitted person to person	Drainage/secretion precautions for open lesions	Avoid contact with infected animals; cook meats thoroughly; vaccine available for high-risk laboratory workers
Typhoid fever	Bacteria: *Salmonella typhi*	Water or food, usually raw fruits and vegetables, shellfish, and milk contaminated by urine and feces of infected individuals or carriers	Usually 5–14 d; may be as long as 3 mo or for life if the individual becomes a chronic carrier	Until three consecutive negative cultures of feces taken at least 24 h apart; may be as long as 3 mo or for life if the individual becomes a chronic carrier	Enteric precautions	Vaccination for travelers to endemic areas and those with intimate exposure to the infected person; good personal hygiene; thorough washing and cooking of foods; proper sewage disposal; decontamination of water sources; infected person or carrier should not handle food; pasteurization of milk
Typhus	Rickettsia: epidemic typhus: *Rickettsia prowazekii*; murine typhus: *Rickettsia typhi*	Bites of infected fleas or lice	1–2 wk	While infested	Not required after delousing	Sanitary living conditions; rat control; vaccine for travelers to endemic areas

*Although smallpox has been eradicated from the world, the occurrence of even a single case in a non-immune population, could result in a major disaster. Therefore, all health professionals should be familiar with it.

BACTERIAL DISEASES

Of the multitudes of bacteria species, relatively few cause human disease. These diseases are a major health problem, however, especially in developing countries. In industrialized countries, bacterial infections are the most common fatal infectious diseases.

Pathogenic bacteria cause disease in two basic ways: by invasion and by producing toxins. Invading bacteria establish residence in the host and, through metabolism and multiplication, interfere with phagocytosis, damage cells, and interfere with metabolism. There are two types of toxins: exotoxins and endotoxins. **Exotoxins** are particularly lethal substances, usually produced by gram-positive bacteria, that are released by the bacteria. When transported by the blood or the lymph, exotoxins can cause cellular damage far from the site of infection. They are disease specific and are responsible for producing the signs and symptoms of that particular infectious disease. Exotoxins are produced in gas gangrene, tetanus, botulism, diphtheria, and scarlet fever. **Endotoxins,** although toxic, are not as lethal as exotoxins in the same amount; that is, their lethal dose is considerably larger. Endotoxins are actually part of the outer cell wall, usually of gram-negative bacteria, and are released only upon destruction of the cell wall. They are not disease specific; rather, they produce generalized symptoms such as fever, weakness, generalized aches, and shock, regardless of which bacterium is involved. Endotoxins are produced in shigellosis (bacillary dysentary), tularemia, and epidemic meningitis.

Selected bacterial diseases such as bacteremia, septicemia, staphylococcal and streptococcal infection, bacterial food poisoning, botulism, tetanus, and gas gangrene

are discussed here. Specific antimicrobial treatment is in Table 11–6.

Bacteremia

Asymptomatic bacteremia (the presence of bacteria in the blood) often occurs following tooth extraction and in up to 10% of clients who have barium enema, sigmoidoscopy, cystoscopy, and tracheal suctioning (Kochar, 1983). The organisms involved are not usually virulent enough to cause problems, and the client's own defenses can usually combat the organisms. On the other hand, bacteremia in hospitalized clients can be a serious problem. The organisms are often more virulent, and the client's defenses to combat the invasion are often reduced. The nurse should be alert for symptoms such as fever, tachycardia, hypotension, tachypnea, and confusion. Specific diagnosis is by positive blood cultures. Cultures are also collected from possible sites of infection, such as the urinary tract, lungs, abdomen, or skin. Antibiotics and antipyretics may be prescribed.

Nursing actions include monitoring the client for response to the bacteremia. Vital signs should be checked frequently. Antibiotics should be administered only after blood cultures are collected, because they can disguise or destroy the organism. Urine output and mental status should also be monitored.

Septic Shock

Approximately 40% of clients with bacteremia develop septic shock or septicemia (Kochar, 1983), sometimes called "blood poisoning" by the public. In septicemia, the organisms in the blood multiply rapidly. Although many organisms can cause septic shock, gram-negative bacilli are the most common cause. The endotoxin these bacteria produce increases capillary permeability. Circulation of endotoxin stimulates complement activation and may cause disseminated intravascular coagulation (DIC), a derangement in the clotting mechanism. Initially, DIC is marked by accelerated clotting, causing occlusion of the small blood vessels and organ necrosis. The accelerated clotting starts a chain reaction that may eventually lead to consumption of platelet and clotting factors. Bleeding, and eventually massive hemorrhage, can occur because of these coagulation defects. DIC is discussed in Chapter 29.

Symptoms of gram-negative septic shock are fever, hypotension, and oliguria. Peripheral vascular resistance is usually decreased, so the extremities are warm. Clients are confused because of reduced blood flow to the brain, and acid–base imbalances often occur.

A specific diagnosis is made from cultures collected from blood, urine, and possible infected sites. Clients are generally cared for in an intensive care unit because they are physiologically unstable. These clients often require respiratory assistance, parenteral antibiotics, blood prod-

---

Nursing Research Note

Baker N, Cerone SB, Gaze N, Knapp T: The effect of type of thermometer and length of time inserted on oral temperature measures of afebrile subjects. *Nurs Res* 1984; 33(2):109–111.

Accuracy of readings of electronic thermometers and mercury in glass thermometers was compared. The effect of oral insertion time on temperature readings in both thermometers was also studied.

The results suggest there is no significant difference between the readings given by electronic thermometers and/or mercury in glass thermometers. Insertion times had a statistically significant effect on readings, however. Both thermometers when inserted for extended periods (the mercury thermometer for 4 minutes and the electronic thermometer for 4 minutes after the buzzer) gave readings 0.12°C higher than for nonextended insertion times of 2 minutes for the mercury and until the buzzer sounds in the electronic. The researchers concluded that 0.12°C may be statistically significant but its clinical significance is questionable in terms of convenience and expense for both nurse and client.

Table 11–6 Summary of Common Antimicrobial Drugs (continued)

Antimicrobial Drug	Effect on Microorganisms	Mode of Action	Clinical Use/Toxicity
Synthetic drugs:			
Sulfonamides	Bacteriostatic	Competitive inhibition	*Neisseria meningitidis* meningitis and some urinary tract infections
Isoniazid (INH)	Bacteriostatic	Competitive inhibition	With streptomycin and rifampin to treat tuberculosis
Ethambutol	Bacteriostatic	Competitive inhibition	With INH to treat tuberculosis
Antibiotics:			
Penicillin, natural (penicillins G, V)	Bactericidal	Inhibition of cell wall synthesis	Gram-positive bacteria
Penicillin, semisynthetic (ampicillin, methicillin, oxacillin, and others)	Bactericidal	Inhibition of cell wall synthesis	Broad spectrum; resistant to penicillinase and stomach acid
Aminoglycosides	Bactericidal	Inhibition of protein synthesis	
Streptomycin			Gram-negative bacteria
Neomycin			Topical ointment
Gentamicin			Gram-negative bacteria
Cephalosporins	Bactericidal	Inhibition of cell wall synthesis	Penicillin-resistant *Staphylococci*
Tetracyclines	Bacteriostatic	Inhibition of protein synthesis	Very broad spectrum; some toxic side effects include tooth discoloration and liver and kidney damage
Chloramphenicol	Bacteriostatic	Inhibition of protein synthesis	*Salmonella;* aplastic anemia occasional side effect
Macrolides (erythromycin)	Bacteriostatic	Inhibition of protein synthesis	Diphtheria; Legionnaires' disease; various infections in individuals allergic to penicillin
Polypeptides Bacitracin	Bactericidal	Inhibition of cell wall synthesis	Gram-positive bacteria primarily; toxic to kidneys; usually used as topical ointment
Polymyxin B	Bactericidal	Injury to plasma membranes	Gram-negative bacteria, including *Pseudomonas;* toxic to brain and kidneys
Rifamycins (rifampin)	Bactericidal	Inhibition of RNA synthesis	Gram-positive bacteria, some gram-negatives, chlamydias, and poxviruses; often used with INH and ethambutol to minimize drug resistance
Polyenes (nystatin, amphotericin B, and others)	Fungicidal	Injury to plasma membranes	*Candida* infections of skin and vagina (nystatin); histoplasmosis, coccidioidomycosis, and blastomycosis (amphotericin B)
Imidazoles (Ketoconazole, miconazole)	Fungicidal	Injury to plasma membranes	Topical use for fungal infections (miconazole); systematic fungal infections (ketoconazole).

(continued)

Table 11–6 Summary of Common Antimicrobial Drugs (continued)

Antimicrobial Drug	Effect on Microorganisms	Mode of Action	Clinical Use/Toxicity
Griseofulvin	Fungistatic	Inhibition of mitotic spindle function	Fungal infections of skin, primarily ringworm
Antiviral drugs:			
Idoxuridine	Antiviral	Inhibition of DNA synthesis	Herpes eye infections
Adenine arabinoside	Antiviral	Inhibition of viral multiplication	Herpes eye infections, chickenpox, viral encephalitis
Amantadine	Antiviral	Inhibition of nucleic acid release from viruses into host cells	Influenza A prophylaxis and treatment
Antiprotozoan and antihelminthic drugs:			
Quinine and chloroquine	Antiprotozoan	Inhibition of DNA and RNA synthesis	Malaria
Emetine	Antiprotozoan	Blocks protein synthesis	Amebic infections
Metronidazole	Antiprotozoan	Inhibition of certain oxidases	*Trichomonas* infections
Niclosamide	Antihelminthic	Inhibition of oxidative phosphorylation	Tapeworm infections
Piperazine	Antihelminthic	Causes paralysis of helminth	Pinworm infections
Antimony compounds	Antihelminthic	Inhibition of glycolysis	Schistosomiasis and other helminthic infections

SOURCE: Reprinted with permission from Tortora GJ, Funke BR, Case CL: *Microbiology*, 2nd ed. Menlo Park, CA: Benjamin/Cummings, 1986.

ucts, vasoactive drugs, and acid–base imbalance correction. Nurses monitor the client's response to therapy by frequently checking vital signs and urinary output. Cardiac, respiratory, and mental status must be closely observed. Even with appropriate therapy, the mortality for septic shock is 50% (Kochar, 1983).

Staphylococcal Infection

Of the several *Staphylococcus* organisms, *S. aureus* is the most common cause of infections, ranging from mild to severe. *Staphylococcus epidermidis,* a normal resident of the skin, is usually not pathogenic, but it may cause disease under certain circumstances. The organisms are spread by direct contact. Many persons, including hospital personnel and clients, carry *S. aureus* in the nares, axilla, and rectum.

Frequent sites of staphylococcal infections are furuncles, carbuncles, chalazia, cellulitis, and wounds. Staphylococcal pneumonia is most common in clients with influenza or chronic bronchopulmonary disease and in newborns; it often ends in abscess formation or empyema. *S. aureus* may cause osteomyelitis and septic arthritis, particularly

in children. Toxin or proteases from certain strains of *S. aureus* and *S. epidermidis* are leading causes of bacterial endocarditis. Intravenous drug users and persons with prosthetic heart valves are at highest risk for staphylococcal endocarditis. Narcotic users have an increased incidence of *S. aureus* colonization on the skin; prosthetic valve clients are vulnerable to staphylococcal contamination of the implant site.

Staphylococcal food poisoning is caused, not by the organism itself, but by protein toxins produced during the growth of *S. aureus* in food. Food poisoning is discussed later.

Staphylococcal infections are usually treated with penicillinase-resistant penicillins. Many strains are resistant to penicillin G, ampicillin, carbenicillin, streptomycin, and the tetracyclines. Seriously ill clients may require parenteral treatment. Food poisoning usually does not require antibiotic treatment.

Clients with staphylococcal infections are often placed in contact isolation. Hospital personnel with staphylococcal infections such as boils should not be allowed to care for clients until personnel have begun antibiotic treatment.

Streptococcal Infection

Among the *Streptococcus* organisms, group A *Streptococcus* is responsible for many diseases, including pharyngitis, scarlet fever, nephritis, rheumatic fever, impetigo, and puerperal infection. Streptococci are a major cause of subacute bacterial endocarditis, urinary tract infections, neonatal sepsis, and meningitis.

Infections by group A streptococci and *S. viridans* are treated with penicillin. Enterococcal species, which may be resistant to penicillin, are also treated with an aminoglycoside. Symptomatic treatments are also prescribed.

Because streptococcal infections are spread by personal contact, infected clients should be placed in contact isolation until they have received antibiotic treatment and are deemed noninfectious. Assess for complications such as otitis media, nephritis, abscesses, arthritis, pneumonia, and septicemia.

With respiratory infections, the client's room should have good ventilation and high humidity to prevent drying of the mucous membranes of the upper respiratory tract. The nose and throat should be kept clean to ease breathing and reduce the risk of sinus infections. Vital signs and urinary output should be assessed frequently.

Bacterial Food Poisoning

Food poisoning may be caused by *Staphylococcus, Salmonella, Shigella,* and many other less common agents. Some organisms, such as *Staphylococcus,* cause illness by producing **enterotoxins,** exotoxins that impair intestinal absorption and provoke secretion of electrolytes and water. In contrast, some *Salmonella* and *Shigella* species invade the mucosa of the small bowel or colon, producing microscopic ulceration, bleeding, and secretion of electrolytes and water.

Staphylococcal food poisoning often begins with a food preparer who is a carrier; the organism is transferred to the food, where the enterotoxin is produced. Animals are the reservoir for *Salmonella,* and the organisms are transmitted through animal-derived food and feces. Common food reservoirs are meat, poultry, eggs and egg products, and unpasteurized milk and dairy products. Outbreaks have also been associated with household pets such as turtles. *Shigella* organisms are found in infected human feces. The organism is spread from person to person by the fecal–oral route or indirectly through food, such as shrimp, milk, eggs, and cheese.

Staphylococcal food poisoning is an acute gastroenteritis typically occurring suddenly in a group of people who have eaten in the same place, such as at a picnic or wedding reception. The incubation period is from 1 to 6 hours, with diarrhea lasting from 8 to 24 hours. Symptoms include nausea with explosive vomiting, abdominal cramps, diarrhea, and sweating and chills; usually, there is no fever.

With salmonella gastroenteritis, there are chills and fever, nausea and vomiting, abdominal pain, and diarrhea, which may be bloody. The incubation period is 8 to 72 hours, with diarrhea for 5 to 7 days.

Symptoms of shigellosis are similar to those for other types of food poisoning: fever, abdominal cramps, nausea and vomiting, and watery diarrhea, which may contain blood and mucus. Symptoms appear in 1 to 3 days, with diarrhea lasting for 3 to 7 days. Some cases of "tourist diarrhea" may actually be milder forms of shigellosis.

Usually, gastroenteritis from food poisoning resolves by itself, and treatment is symptomatic. Most persons recover without complications, although the fluid loss from vomiting and diarrhea may be dangerous for infants and children, the elderly, and debilitated clients.

Strict hand-washing procedures and proper handling of food (see the food handling section later in this chapter) are the keys to reducing transmission. Nurses can contribute to disease control by educating their clients about handwashing and the proper preparation and handling of foods. For specific nursing measures for clients with infectious gastroenteritis, see Chapter 49.

Botulism

Botulism is a particularly severe type of food poisoning that may lead to death. The disease is usually contracted from home-canned foods with a high pH (low-acid foods such as beans and corn), which have been inadequately sterilized. These foods provide an anaerobic condition for the growth of the spore-forming organism, *Clostridium botulinum.* The toxin produced by this bacteria is highly lethal; 1 mg is enough to kill 1 million guinea pigs. Death can occur from simply tasting, not swallowing, a contaminated food. Cases involving commercially prepared foods are rare.

Wound and infant botulism are other forms of the disease. In wound botulism, the organism grows in infected tissue. Infant botulism occurs when ingested spores colonize in the gastrointestinal tract. One possible cause is honey, which may contain *C. botulinum* spores; honey should not be given to infants under 1 year. Adults do not acquire botulism from honey (Wehrle & Top, 1981).

Food-borne botulism usually occurs 18 to 36 hours after ingesting the contaminated food, although onset varies from 4 hours to 8 days. Initial symptoms are nausea, vomiting, dry mouth, dilated pupils, diplopia, and dysphagia. Neurological symptoms appear later, with a bilateral symmetrical descending paralysis. With wound botulism, there are no GI symptoms, but neurological symptoms are the same as with the food-borne variety. Infant botulism is marked by constipation and neuromuscular paralysis.

In management, respiratory failure is the first priority. The disease progresses rapidly, so those who are suspected to have botulism should be hospitalized in case a tracheotomy and mechanical ventilation are required. Antitoxin should be given as soon as botulism has been diagnosed before neurologic impairment occurs because it cannot reverse neurologic impairment. Antitoxin is available through the CDC.

Because foods and materials contaminated with *C. botulinum* are highly toxic, they require special handling. Specimen-handling instructions are available from the CDC.

Public education is the major preventive measure. For more information on prevention, see the discussion of food handling in the section on prevention.

Tetanus

Tetanus is caused by *Clostridium tetani,* an anaerobic spore-forming organism with reservoirs in the soil and animal feces. The spores of the bacteria usually enter the body through deep wounds or foreign bodies. A puncture wound from an object lying in the dirt provides a perfect avenue for infection. However, *C. tetani* may also enter the body through what appear to be relatively minor wounds such as abrasions or insect stings or through dental surgery. Intravenous drug users are also vulnerable, as are those with surgical and burn wounds. The organism produces a neurotoxin, which causes generalized muscle spasms followed by contraction of the muscles of the jaw. This explains the popular term, "lockjaw." Eventually, opisthotonos, abdominal rigidity, and other symptoms of increased sympathetic nervous system activity occur. Tetanus is usually severe and is difficult to treat, even for experts. The mortality rate is 50%, but when recovery occurs, it is complete (Kochar, 1983).

Wounds should be cleaned and debrided as soon as possible because dirt and necrotic tissue provide a medium for growth of *C. tetani.* Depending on the immunization status and the nature of the wound, prophylaxis may be administered. Most persons receive tetanus toxoid immunization during the DPT (diphtheria, pertussis, tetanus) series of immunizations given in childhood; boosters are given every 5 to 10 years. With a serious wound, immunity should be renewed with a booster dose of tetanus toxoid (Table 11–7). Tetanus toxoid is not effective after an injury, however, if the person has not been immunized.

When immunization is inadequate or uncertain, tetanus immune globulin is an alternative that provides temporary immunity lasting for about 1 month. Use of human tetanus immune globulin (HTIG) is preferred. If HTIG is unavailable, the client must be tested for sensitivity to horse serum immune globulin before that type of antitoxin is given because of the risk of *serum sickness,* an immune complex disorder in which antibodies are produced against the horse serum. The symptoms of serum sickness include fever, rash, joint lesions, and kidney dysfunction.

Clients with tetanus are usually treated in intensive care units. Treatment includes supportive care as well as antitoxins and sedative-relaxant drugs for seizures or convulsions. Mechanical ventilation may be needed. Aseptic technique should be used when disposing of drainage and respiratory fluids.

Although tetanus is difficult to treat, it can be prevented effectively with tetanus toxoid. Immunization is more effective than prophylaxis at the time of injury.

Gas Gangrene

Gas gangrene can be caused by several species of *Clostridium,* but *Clostridium perfringens* is the most common. The organisms are introduced into traumatic and surgical wounds from the soil or from the person's own intestinal or vaginal flora. Devitalized or necrotic tissues that have lost their blood supply provide the perfect conditions for the growth of the anaerobic organisms.

As the organisms multiply, they ferment carbohydrates in the tissues and actually produce gases (carbon dioxide and hydrogen) that cause the tissue to swell. Combined with the exotoxins and enzymes produced by these microorganisms, these conditions cause further necrosis and spread of the infection. Severe toxemia and death result without immediate and aggressive treatment.

Treatment includes penicillin and aggressive surgery, such as debridement and amputation. Hyperbaric oxygen therapy is sometimes used, especially for gas gangrene in the abdominal cavity, although experts disagree about its effectiveness. Therapy is administered in a hyperbaric chamber that provides an oxygen-rich atmosphere under pressure. Immediate and thorough cleansing of all serious wounds along with prophylactic antibiotic therapy are the best preventive measures.

VIRAL DISEASES

Unlike living cells that contain both nucleic acids DNA and RNA, viruses contain a core of only one (never both) surrounded by a protein coat and sometimes by an additional lipid membrane, called an envelope. Because viruses contain only one nucleic acid, they are unable to carry out chemical reactions or to reproduce unless within living cells. In other words, viruses are inert when outside living cells. For this reason, it is unclear whether viruses are living microorganisms whose essential characteristics differ fundamentally from other living microorganisms or whether viruses are exceptionally complex nonliving chemicals.

When viruses invade the body, they attach to receptor sites on a host cell surface. The virus and host cell fuse, allowing the virus to penetrate the host cell. Viruses can also be taken into host cells by phagocytosis. Once inside the cell, viruses replicate either in the cytoplasm or the nucleus; mature viruses escape through the cell wall and invade other cells.

Among the wide variety of infections caused by viruses are rubella, rubeola, varicella, mumps, herpes simplex and zoster, hepatitis, influenza, mononucleosis, and rabies. Only

(continued on p. 296)

Table 11–7 Immunologic Agents

Official Nonproprietary and Trade Names	Dosage and Administration	Comments
Agents for active immunization:		
BCG vaccine USP (from bacillus Calmette–Guérin)	0.1 mL by intradermal injection; 0.05 mL for infants less than 28 d old	Preparation of an attenuated live strain of BCG bacillus for preventing tuberculosis in clients with negative tuberculin skin tests who are exposed to active cases of pulmonary tuberculosis
Cholera vaccine USP	0.2 mL given intradermally in two doses 1 wk to 1 mo apart for people 5 yr of age and above. Also SQ or IM in doses of 0.2–1 mL at intervals of 1 wk to 1 mo or more	Suspension of killed *Vibrio cholerae* for prevention of cholera in travelers to areas where the disease is endemic, with boosters required every 6 mo for continued protection
Diphtheria toxoid USP and diphtheria toxoid, adsorbed USP	0.5 mL IM in three doses at 2, 4, and 6 mo of age; or two doses at intervals of 6–8 wk; booster 1 yr later at about 18 mo	Regular and precipitated adsorbed preparations for pediatric use, preferably combined with tetanus toxoid
Diphtheria and tetanus toxoids USP and diphtheria and tetanus toxoids, adsorbed USP	0.5 mL IM as above; further booster doses recommended every 10 yr and at lesser intervals with traumatic wounds that are severe or contaminated	Toxins inactivated by treatment with formaldehyde or adsorbed with aluminum phosphate for routine immunization of children
Diphtheria and tetanus toxoids and pertussis vaccine USP and the same in an adsorbed USP preparation	0.5 mL IM at 4- to 8-wk intervals, followed by a fourth dose about 1 yr after the third primary dose	Combination of three antigens for use in children up to 7 yr of age
Hepatitis B vaccine (Heptavax-B)	Three IM injections, initially and at 1 and 6 mo; 0.5 mL each for children under 10 yr of age; 1 mL each for older children and most adults; 2 mL each for dialysis patients and immunocompromised patients in two 1-mL doses injected at different sites	Indicated for immunization of clients at increased risk of infection with all subtypes of hepatitis B virus but not other hepatitis viruses
Influenza virus vaccine USP (Fluax, Fluogen, Fluzone)	See manufacturer's literature for the current year for dosage volume and administration instructions	Inactivated viruses of strains prevalent in a particular year for use in the prevention of disease in clients in high-risk categories
Measles virus vaccine, live, USP (Attenuvax; others)	0.5 mL SQ; no booster needed	Attenuated live rubeola virus for immunizations of children 15 mo or older
Measles and rubella virus vaccine, live USP (M-R-Vax II)	Inject the total volume of a vial SQ into the outer aspect of the upper arm	Mixture of two attenuated live viruses for simultaneous immunization against measles and German measles in children 15 mo or older and adults
Measles and mumps virus vaccine, live USP	Inject the total volume of a vial SQ into the outer aspect of the upper arm	Mixture of two live vaccines for immunization of children and adults
Measles, mumps and rubella virus vaccine, live USP (M-M-R$_{II}$)	Inject the total volume of the reconstituted vaccine into the outer aspect of the upper arm	Triple antigen live virus vaccine for simultaneous immunization against rubeola, rubella, and mumps in children 15 mo of age or older and in adults
Meningococcal polysaccharide vaccine (group A, group C, and groups A & C combined) (Menomune-A, -C, -A/C; Meningovax A/C)	0.5 mL injected SQ in a single immunizing dose	Not for routine immunization but for special situations to protect against *Neisseria meningitidis* infections in populations at high risk

(continued)

Table 11–7   Immunologic Agents (continued)

Official Nonproprietary and Trade Names	Dosage and Administration	Comments
Mixed respiratory vaccine (MRV)	0.05 mL SQ initially, followed by doses of up to a total of 0.5 to 1 mL	Contains antigens from strains of several types of bacteria considered responsible for producing allergic symptoms, including asthma and rhinitis
Mumps virus vaccine, live USP (Mumpsvax)	Inject total volume SQ into outer aspect of upper arm	Used to induce protective antibodies against mumps in children 12 mo or older and in adults
Pertussis vaccine USP and pertussis vaccine, adsorbed USP	IM 0.5 mL in three doses in 4- to 8-wk intervals and with boosters about 1 yr later and upon starting school	Mainly for immunization of infants, starting at 2 mo of age; should not be used after 6 yr
Plague vaccine USP	Adults and children over age 10 receive a series of three IM injections: two doses of 0.5 mL each administered 1 mo or more apart and third dose of 0.2 mL given 4 to 12 wk later; fractional doses for children under 10	Used mainly to immunize travelers to countries where plague is endemic and persons in US who come in contact with wild rodents during their work
Pneumococcal vaccines, polyvalent (Pneumovax 23)	0.5 mL SQ or IM in the deltoid muscle or in lateral area of midthigh	For prevention of pneumococcal pneumonia and bacteremia caused by 23 of the most prevalent types of organisms, especially in high-risk populations
Poliovirus vaccine, inactivated USP (Salk vaccine)	Three doses of 1.0 mL given SQ at 4- to 6-wk intervals, followed by a fourth dose 6 to 12 mo later	Formalin-treated virus is nonparalytic; it is preferred for clients whose immune systems are deficient and for prevention of poliomyelitis in adult travelers to areas where they may be exposed
Poliovirus vaccine, live, oral USP (Sabin vaccine, TOPV)	0.5 mL contents of a single dose container are taken orally by infants at 2 and 4 mo and sometimes at 6 mo, with booster given at 18 mo and at 4 to 6 yr	Orally administered attenuated live virus vaccine is convenient, safe, and effective for protecting against infections by the three types of virus that cause the natural disease. Rarely, paralytic polio occurs in those who receive this vaccine or in people in close contact with them
Rabies vaccine, human diploid cell strain (HDCV: Imovax; Wyvac)	*Preexposure immunization:* 1 mL IM (eg, in deltoid area) on days 0, 7, and 21 or 28	Preexposure immunization is indicated for medical and laboratory personnel and others at high risk of exposure to rabies virus
	Postexposure immunization: 1 mL IM (eg, in deltoid area) as soon as possible after exposure and on each of days 3, 7, 14, and 28 after the first dose, plus a sixth dose recommended 90 d after the first dose	Postexposure treatment is employed after individual evaluation of each exposure; local treatment of wounds and combined use of the vaccine with passive antirabies treatment are recommended in most cases
Rabies vaccine USP (duck embryo vaccine, DEV)	*Preexposure:* 1 mL SQ in a series of 4 injections, first 3 a wk and final one, 5 or 6 mo later	Caution in patients with a history of allergy to chicken or duck eggs; local reactions are common; minor neurological reactions include headache and photophobia; major neurological reactions such as those seen with previously available rabbit brain vaccine are rare. Use together with passive antirabies treatment
	Postexposure: 1 mL SQ in 21 daily doses, or 2 doses a day for 14 days and 7 more daily doses	

Official Nonproprietary and Trade Names	Dosage and Administration	Comments
Rubella virus vaccine, live USP (Meruvax II)	Inject total volume of vial SQ into outer aspect of the upper arm	For immunization against German measles in children from 12 mo to puberty; also for adolescent and adult males and for *nonpregnant* adolescent and adult females
Rubella and mumps virus vaccine, live USP (Biavax II)	Inject total volume of vial SQ into outer aspect of the upper arm	For simultaneous protection against infection by both viruses in children 12 mo or older and in adults
Smallpox vaccine USP (Dryvax)	Deposit vaccine on site and administer by multiple pressure technique	No longer employed routinely in US; administered only to laboratory personnel working with variola virus and to travelers to and from certain countries
Tetanus toxoid USP and tetanus toxoid, adsorbed USP	0.5 mL IM three injections with second given 4 to 6 wk after the first and third 6 to 12 mo later; booster dose every 10 yr	Adsorbed form is preferred to fluid for protection against *Clostridium tetani* infections
Tetanus and diphtheria toxoids, adsorbed for adult use USP	0.5 mL IM two injections at intervals of at least 4 wk an additional dose 6 to 12 mo later and booster doses every 10 yr	For simultaneous primary and booster immunization against both bacterial infections in children over 7 yr of age and in adults
Typhoid vaccine USP	0.5 mL SQ in two doses at intervals of 4 wk or more for adults and children over 10 yr; 0.25 mL for children under 10 yr	For immunization of travelers to areas where typhoid is endemic and of individuals exposed to a carrier
Typhus vaccine USP	Two SQ doses in recommended amounts at intervals of 4 wk, followed by a single SQ booster dose after 6 to 12 mo	Protection against louse-borne infections by *Rickettsia prowazekii* for travelers to areas where the disease is endemic
Yellow fever vaccine USP	0.5 mL SQ for children over 6 mo and adults; revaccinate after 10 yr	Live, attenuated virus vaccine for long-lasting immunity in persons traveling to or living in countries where the disease is endemic

Agents for passive immunization:

Botulism antitoxin USP	Inject 10,000 units IV q. 4 h	Neutralizes toxin in clients with botulism. Test for hypersensitivity to avoid immediate and delayed reactions in sensitive clients
Diphtheria antitoxin USP	Inject 20,000 to 80,000 units or more IV at one time, depending on the seriousness of the illness; or for prophylaxis 1000 to 10,000 units IM	Administer immediately upon diagnosis, together with the appropriate antibiotic therapy
Hepatitis B immune globulin USP (HBIG; Hep-B-Gammagee; HyperHep)	IM 0.06 mL/kg, or 3 to 5 mL as soon as possible after exposure	For prophylaxis following accidental exposure to blood and other materials positive for hepatitis B surface antigen
Immune globulin USP (gamma globulin)	IM 0.02 to 0.04 mL/kg for prevention of hepatitis A; IM 0.25 mL/kg for prevention of measles; IM 0.05 mL/kg (up to 15 mL) for modification of measles	For hepatitis A, give before expected exposure or soon after but not for treatment after disease has developed; for measles, give within 6 d after exposure
Immune globulin, intravenous (Gamimune)	100 mL/kg IV of a 5% solution (ie, 2 mL/kg body weight) once a month by infusion	Indicated for maintenance prophylaxis in clients with immune system deficiency syndromes such as congenital agammaglobulinemia

(continued)

Table 11–7 Immunologic Agents (continued)		
Official Nonproprietary and Trade Names	**Dosage and Administration**	**Comments**
Mumps immune globulin (Hyparotin)	IM 2 to 10 mL for prevention following exposure; IM 1.5 to 4.5 mL for modification or treatment	Provides protection for 6 to 12 wk; serum sickness reaction has occasionally developed
Pertussis immune globulin USP (Hypertussis)	IM 2.5 mL for prophylaxis; IM or IV 1.25 mL daily for treatment	Prepared from blood of humans hyperimmunized with pertussis vaccine; effectiveness is uncertain
Rabies immune globulin USP (HRIG; Hyperab)	IM 20 IU/kg as soon as possible after exposure, together with the first dose of rabies vaccine; half the dose may be used to infiltrate the wound site	Advantage; does not cause serum sickness, as may occur with the equine antirabies vaccine
Antirabies serum USP	IM 40 IU/kg, half of which is infiltrated in the area of the wound	Test patient for sensitivity to this hyperimmune horse serum to avoid allergic reactions in sensitive patients
Tetanus antitoxin USP	IM 3000 to 5000 units for prophylaxis within 24 h after treatment; 10,000 to 20,000 units after 48 h; for treatment, IV 40,000 to 100,000 units	Use only when tetanus immune globulin is not available because of the risk of hypersensitivity reactions to this equine blood product
Tetanus immune globulin USP (Homo-Tet; Hu-Tet; Hyper-Tet)	IM 250 units for prophylaxis; for treatment, 3000 to 6000 units is the usual dose, but larger amounts have been administered	This product, obtained from the plasma of hyperimmunized humans, is preferred because of its relative freedom of hypersensitivity reaction risk
Vaccinia immune globulin USP	IM 0.6 mL/kg	Used to counteract adverse effects of smallpox vaccination and to modify the disease itself, this substance obtained from human plasma rarely causes hypersensitivity reactions
Varicella-zoster immune globulin (human)	IM (deep gluteal) injection of the entire contents of a 2.5 mL vial containing 125 units	Used to reduce the severity of chickenpox in immunodeficient children, in whom pneumonia and encephalitis are possible complications

SOURCE: From Rodman MJ, Smith DW: *Clinical Pharmacology in Nursing,* 3rd ed. Philadelphia: Lippincott, 1984, pp. 603–606.

influenza and rabies will be discussed in this chapter. Complete information about the other viral diseases that affect adults is found in other chapters. For information on viral infections during childhood, consult a pediatric nursing textbook. Specific antimicrobial treatment is in Table 11–6. Effective vaccines are available against a number of viral diseases (Table 11–7).

Influenza

Influenza, or "the flu," is a viral infection as well known as the common cold. Epidemics of influenza spread rapidly through large geographic areas almost annually and have been pandemic at various times. The pandemic of 1918–1919 caused 20 million deaths, many of them from secondary bacterial infections rather than the viral disease itself. One of these bacteria was mistakenly determined to cause influenza and named *Hemophilus influenzae* to link it with the

disease. It is now known that *H. influenzae* was one of several secondary invaders responsible for many of the deaths but was not a cause of the disease. (*H. influenzae* causes bacterial meningitis and acute epiglottitis.)

The symptoms of influenza include fever, chills, headache, and general muscular aches, followed by coldlike symptoms after the fever subsides. If not complicated by a secondary bacterial infection, influenza runs its course in a few days. Treating the symptoms will help clients feel more comfortable. For secondary bacterial infections, antibiotic treatment is appropriate. Because of the availability of antibiotic treatment today, a pandemic such as the one of 1918–1919 is unlikely to have such a high mortality rate. Amantadine (Symmetrel), an antiviral drug (see Table 11–6), can reduce the severity of the symptoms of influenza caused by the Influenza A virus if treatment is begun immediately. Amantadine has also been used as a prophylactic measure to reduce the rate of Influenza A infection and illness. It is not effective against the Influenza B virus.

Vaccines consisting of killed viruses are available against influenza. Vaccinations are administered in the fall before the winter flu season and are used primarily for the elderly and other high-risk individuals. Immunity is effective in about 10 days and lasts 3 to 6 months; thus, yearly immunization is required. Influenza vaccines are not completely effective for several reasons. First, in years when a new strain or subtype appears, vaccine cannot be produced fast enough to be available. Minor antigen changes occur every 2 to 4 years, and there is a major shift about every 10 years. Different strains of the Influenza A and B virus (and the less common C virus) are often named for the location in which they are first identified (eg, Hong Kong flu, Russian flu). Also, not everyone develops immunity after vaccination, and some persons will not seek out or accept immunization.

Local skin reactions can occur with vaccination. Persons allergic to egg or egg products may develop anaphylactic reactions. A rare complication of the swine influenza vaccine administered during the swine influenza vaccine program in 1976 was Guillain-Barré syndrome, an acute, rapidly progressive form of polyneuropathy. Subsequent influenza vaccines have not been associated with increased risk of this disorder.

Rabies

Rabies (sometimes called hydrophobia), a viral disease transmitted through saliva, is virtually 100% fatal if untreated. The few who do survive experience severe neurological damage. Fortunately, human rabies is rare in the United States with only one to four cases per year (Tortora et al., 1986). The disease is usually transmitted through an animal bite. The most common animal reservoirs in this country are wild animals including skunks, bats, foxes, and raccoons. Domestic dogs are less often sources of the disease because of canine rabies vaccination. Rabbits and rodents are rarely infected with rabies.

Infection occurs when the rabies virus comes in contact with mucous membranes or the dermal layer of the skin, almost always through a penetrating bite. The virus can also enter through minute abrasions in the skin. Cave explorers have also contracted rabies by inhaling aerosols of the virus in bat caves, as have laboratory workers exposed to these aerosols during laboratory accidents.

Rabies symptoms usually appear 18 to 60 days after exposure although there have been instances up to a year or more before the onset of symptoms. Among the early symptoms are fever, headaches, anorexia, nausea, and paresthesias in the area of the bite. Over the next 2 weeks, neurologic symptoms progress to coma. One characteristic symptom is painful pharyngeal spasms when attempting to swallow liquid or sometimes merely at the sight or thought of water (the basis for the term *hydrophobia*, fear of water). Finally, flaccid paralysis develops, and death follows.

As soon as possible after the bite, the wound should be cleaned thoroughly with soap and water. This is a highly effective first aid measure. Vaccinated domestic animals should be observed for rabies symptoms for 10 days; this may be a legal requirement. If an unvaccinated domestic animal develops rabies symptoms, it should be killed immediately and examined for rabies virus in brain smears. Wild animals should be killed at once and examined. If the laboratory test is negative for rabies virus, the client does not require prophylaxis.

The client is given rabies prophylaxis if the animal is rabid, suspected to be rabid, or has escaped before rabidity has been determined. Postexposure treatment begins with passive immunization with human rabies immune globulin (HRIG). Active immunization with five doses of human diploid cell vaccine (HDCV) over a 4-week period and a sixth dose 2 months later follows the passive immunization. Reactions with HDCV are less frequent than with the former duck embryo vaccine, which required a series of 23 subcutaneous injections. Local reactions, occurring in about 25% of cases, consist of swelling, itching, pain, and induration. Less common are the systemic symptoms of nausea, fever, myalgia, and abdominal pain. Because the series of immunizations must continue, any reactions are treated symptomatically. Active immunization with HDCV before exposure to the rabies virus is given to veterinarians and laboratory personnel.

Animal vaccination is the best method of rabies control. Nurses can assist in educating the community about the importance of having pets vaccinated. A rigid quarantine program has kept islands such as Australia, New Zealand, and the Hawaiian chain free of the disease.

RICKETTSIAL DISEASES

Rickettsia organisms are smaller than bacteria but larger than viruses. Like viruses, they can reproduce only within a living cell. However, they more closely resemble bacteria in their structure and biochemistry. They are nonmotile and often parasites of insects. The microbes usually invade by an insect bite, producing a rash and a generalized inflammatory and antibody response. Examples of rickettsial diseases are Rocky Mountain spotted fever, Q fever, and typhus. *Chlamydia* organisms are also categorized as rickettsias. Unlike most rickettsias, however, they are transmitted by direct contact or airborne routes and do not require insects for transmission. There are only two known species of chlamydias. *Chlamydia trachomatis* causes trachoma (discussed in Chapter 71). It also causes lymphogranuloma venereum and nongonococcal urethritis, the most common sexually transmitted disease in the United States (discussed in Chapter 67). *Chlamydia psittaci* causes psittacosis, a form of pneumonia spread by contact with bird droppings. Specific antimicrobial treatment is in Table 11–6.

Rocky Mountain Spotted Fever

Despite its name, Rocky Mountain spotted fever is most common in the southeastern United States and Appalachia. Its name is derived from the fact that it was first identified in the Rocky Mountain area. The disease is caused by *Rickettsia rickettsii,* a parasite of ticks, and usually spreads to humans by tick bites. Most cases occur in children, and the disease is most common in spring and summer.

The symptoms appear suddenly about 7 days after the bite by a dog tick or wood tick. Initial symptoms are severe headache, high fever, chills, prostration, and muscular pain. About 4 days after exposure, a rash appears on the palms and soles, spreading to the face and neck, buttocks, and trunk. DIC may occur. The mortality rate is 5% to 10%.

Antibiotic therapy with tetracycline and chloramphenicol is effective in the early stages of the disease. Supportive care is required for vasculitis, the distinguishing pathological characteristic of Rocky Mountain spotted fever. The client needs management for inadequate blood volume, circulatory collapse, fluid and electrolyte imbalance, and renal insufficiency. Hematologic values must be monitored for signs of DIC.

No vaccine is commercially available, but research is continuing. The best preventive measure is to prevent ticks from attaching to the skin or removing them promptly. Persons frequenting tick-infested areas should use repellent, dress in clothes that inhibit tick attachment (eg, boots and coveralls), and inspect their bodies (and the bodies of domestic animals) daily, especially hairy areas, for ticks. Ticks usually do not transmit infection until they have been feeding for at least several hours.

An attached tick can be removed with gentle traction of a forceps on the mouth parts; if possible, wear a gown and gloves for protection. Try not to crush the tick, because this can contaminate the bite. Wash the bite thoroughly with soap and water. Take care when removing an engorged tick from an animal by hand, because the infection can be transmitted into small abrasions on the skin.

PROTOZOAL DISEASES

Protozoa are single-celled animals that can move about independently. They are equipped with structures enabling them to feed, breathe, excrete waste, and attach themselves to other objects. Protozoal infections are not limited to third-world countries; they also occur in the United States. Persons who have traveled to other countries and those who have emigrated from countries with endemic protozoal infections may bring the diseases to the United States.

Common examples of protozoal diseases are malaria, amebiasis, and toxoplasmosis, which are discussed in this section. Some other examples are kala-azar and African sleeping sickness (trypanosomiasis). *P. carinii,* which causes an often fatal pneumonia in compromised hosts and may be endemic in hospitals and institutions (Benenson, 1985), is a protozoan. Specific antimicrobial treatment is in Table 11–6.

Malaria

Caused by four protozoans classified as *Plasmodium,* malaria causes more disability and economic strain worldwide than

any other parasitic disease. Carried by mosquitoes, malaria occurs mainly in the tropics, although it has been transmitted by blood transfusions and unsterilized syringes. The disease affects 200 million people throughout the world. In Africa, it is estimated that one-fourth of adults have malaria at one time or another. Carriers of the sickle-cell gene are resistant to malaria because of the special characteristics of their red blood cells that lower the potassium needed for the protozoan's survival. Malaria is rare in the United States, but occasional small epidemics have been caused by returning military personnel; travelers and emigrants may also bring the disease into the country (Figure 11–6). Malaria remains a serious problem in tropical Asia, Africa, and Central and South America.

Four types of the *Plasmodium* organism *(P. vivax, P. falciparum, P. malariae,* and *P. ovale)* cause malaria, with varying patterns. Most cases (95%) are caused by *P. falciparum* and *P. vivax.*

Depending on the type of malaria, there may be an abrupt onset or a prodromal phase with symptoms including intermittent fever, malaise, headache, myalgia, and chills. The disease is characterized by episodes of shaking chills with fever. Untreated vivax malaria subsides spontaneously in 10 to 30 days but may recur; untreated fulciparum malaria has a high mortality rate.

Treatment depends on diagnosis of the *Plasmodium* species. Acute attacks for all except drug-resistant *P. falciparum* are treated with chloroquine. The resistant strains of *P. falciparum* are treated with a combination of quinine, pyrimethamine, and a sulfonamide. For *P. falciparum,* treatment must be prompt and immediate, because the disease progresses rapidly and may lead to coma and death.

Drug treatment for the acute attack will cure the dis-

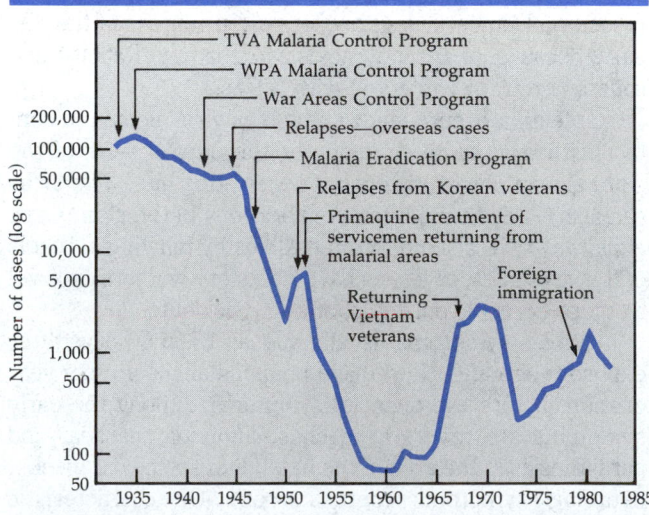

Figure 11–6

Reported cases of malaria in the United States, 1933–1983.

SOURCE: Tortora GJ, Funke BR, Case CL: *Microbiology,* 2nd ed. Menlo Park, CA: Benjamin/Cummings, 1986.

ease. Some strains, particularly those in Southeast Asia and Latin America, are also resistant to pyrimethamine and sulfonamides. In this case, treatment is with quinine sulfate and a tetracycline.

Clients may require oxygen if anemia and tissue hypoxia are present. Fluid status should be monitored. Other nursing care centers on control of fever, myalgia, and headache. Precautions should be used in disposing of blood and body fluids (see Box 11–4 later in this chapter).

The best prevention in high-risk areas is destroying mosquito breeding places and avoiding exposure to mosquito bites with repellent, screens, and mosquito nets. Drug prophylaxis is used but may be unreliable in areas of Southeast Asia and Latin America because of resistant strains. For nonresistant strains, prophylaxis is with chloroquine phosphate. For resistant strains, pyrimethamine and sulfadoxine are also taken; there is no reliable protection against strains also resistant to these drugs. The drugs are taken 2 weeks before arrival in the area and for 6 weeks after leaving.

Amebiasis

Amebiasis, or amebic dysentary, is spread by ingestion of cysts of *Entamoeba histolytica* in food or water contaminated by human feces, flies, or hands of infected food handlers. It is common in the tropics but uncommon in temperate climates. Infected persons are often asymptomatic cyst passers. Symptoms of the disease range from mild diarrhea to colitis with fever and profuse bloody diarrhea. Complications include hemorrhage, intestinal perforation, and liver abscess.

Treatment is with metronidazole (Flagyl), diiodohydroxyquin (Diodoquin), or diloxanide furoate (Furamide). Supportive care includes symptomatic relief and rehydration.

Toxoplasmosis

Toxoplasmosis is an insidious disease because infected adults are often asymptomatic. A pregnant woman can transmit the disease through the placenta to the fetus. The result may be abortion, stillbirth, or the birth of a child with congenital disease, which can be severe.

Toxoplasma gondii, the protozoan responsible for the disease, is a parasite of warm-blooded animals. Adults usually acquire the infection by eating raw or undercooked meat containing cysts or by being exposed to cat feces with cysts, often while cleaning a litter box. A large number of cats in urban areas have been shown to be infected with the organism, although they apparently are not ill.

Adults with symptoms usually have lymphadenopathy, fever, and malaise. Congenitally infected newborns may be asymptomatic or have severe, fulminating disease. Most symptoms appear months or years later, including chronic chorioretinitis, severe jaundice, hepatosplenomegaly, rash, purpura, central nervous system symptoms, and hydrocephaly or microcephaly. There may be blindness and mental retardation.

Adults with mild infections usually do not require treatment. Newborns, pregnant women, and immunosuppressed clients receive drug therapy with pyrimethamine in combination with trisulfapyrimidines or sulfadiazine.

Nurses can assist in educating the public, particularly pregnant women and immunocompromised clients, about the dangers of toxoplasmosis. These persons should:

- Avoid contact with any area that might have cat feces, such as litter boxes and sand boxes.
- Wash all fruits and vegetables before eating.
- Cook meat to at least 150°F (66°C) and not eat raw meat.
- Wash hands after handling raw meat.

HELMINTHIC DISEASES

Three major types of helminths (worms) invade the human intestines: nematodes (roundworms), cestodes (tapeworms), and trematodes (flukes). The life cycle of parasitic helminths is complex and often involves a succession of hosts such as humans, domestic animals, fish, and snails. Enterobiasis, or infestation by pinworms *(Enterobius vermicularis),* which causes perianal itching, is the most common worm infection in the United States. It occurs principally in children. Consult a pediatric nursing textbook for more information on this condition. A disease caused by nematodes—trichinosis—will be discussed in this chapter. Specific antihelminthic drug treatment is in Table 11–6.

Trichinosis

Trichinosis (trichinellosis) is caused by ingesting encysted larvae of the nematode *Trichinella spiralis,* usually in pork. The larval cysts are imbedded in pork muscle; if pork is undercooked, the cysts may remain intact. When the meat is eaten, gastric juices digest the cyst wall, and the larvae burrow into the intestinal mucosa, where they multiply. The new larvae are carried into the bloodstream and disseminated throughout the body, but only those imbedding skeletal muscle survive. There they mature, encyst, and eventually calcify; the organisms may live for several years.

Many of those infected are asymptomatic. There may be initial symptoms of gastrointestinal distress and fever, or the disease may first appear as edema of the upper eyelids on about the 11th day after infection. Other ocular symptoms including hemorrhage, pain, and photophobia may follow. Shortly thereafter, systemic symptoms appear, including muscle pain, chills, fever, weakness, sweating, urticaria, and eosinophilia. Most likely to be involved are muscles of the diaphragm and tongue as well as the pectoral, eye, and intercostal muscles. The inflammatory reaction to the disseminated larvae may produce a variety of other systemic symptoms. Within about 3 months, most symptoms subside, although the client may feel weak for months.

Symptomatic and supportive care focuses on relief of pain and fever as well as nutrition and fluid replacement.

Corticosteroids may be given. Thiabendazole is effective in destroying organisms, but its use is controversial because of possible hypersensitivity response.

Public education is important in prevention. Pork and pork products should always be thoroughly cooked until no longer pink in the center. Less obviously, ground beef may be contaminated by a meat grinder that was not cleaned after grinding pork. Thus, eating raw hamburger meat is to be avoided.

Section III: Nursing Measures in Infectious Disease

Since Florence Nightingale outlined her principles and practices of "fever nursing" in 1863, nursing interventions in infection have traditionally been directed toward the care of the already infected client. Since Nightingale's day, scientific discoveries have radically changed the principles and practices of caring for the already infected client. These principles and practices are discussed in this section. Contemporary health care often involves exposing uninfected clients to potentially infective agents or altering the normal flora. Thus, prevention of infection and protection of the immunocompromised client are also significant nursing responsibilities. Keep these important principles in mind when planning care for *all clients:*

- Health care personnel and the health care environment harbor many organisms—normal flora and potentially pathogenic organisms.
- All secretions and tissues (of clients, their families, and health care personnel) contain organisms that are potentially harmful to others.
- Many clients are compromised hosts and are therefore at greater risk from these organisms.
- The single most important preventive strategy is adequate hand-washing.
- Knowledge of the methods of transmission of microorganisms is the basis for developing strategies to protect clients from infection.

This section discusses nursing measures for the prevention of infection as well as the treatment of infection. The nursing measures for specific infectious diseases can be found in the specific disorders chapters in the units on body systems.

PUBLIC EDUCATION AND PREVENTION

Whether they work in health care facilities, physician's offices, or the community, nurses can educate people about disease prevention and promote immunization. In addition, nurses are often the first to see signs of infections. By recognizing infection, nurses can refer clients for medical care leading to early arrest of the disease; they can also take measures to prevent its spread. Nurses should be well informed about these subjects so they can counsel clients as well as friends and neighbors about preventive measures.

Immunization

Immunization with a vaccine induces a state of immunity in a host. Most vaccines consist of attenuated (living but weakened) organisms or killed organisms. Many diseases, such as poliomyelitis, tetanus, diphtheria, pertussis, measles, and rubella, can be prevented by immunization. The immunologic agents currently available for the prevention and treatment of infectious disease are listed in Table 11–7. Current research is studying the use of **recombinant DNA** techniques (the artificial introduction of DNA into a cell to alter it; the new DNA is replicated along with the natural DNA) to make genetically engineered vaccines that are safer, or to make new vaccines not now available. The possibility of producing a new "supervaccine" using genetic engineering is another new concept in immunization. Researchers are experimenting with genetic manipulation of vaccinia, the large cowpox virus used in smallpox vaccine, so that it will also provide immunity against infections such as herpes, hepatitis, and influenza in addition to providing immunity against smallpox. These studies indicate that it may be possible in the future to produce a single, multipurpose vaccine to provide protection against as many as a dozen infections. The use of such a vaccine would have to be weighed against the serious side effects—including brain damage—that sometimes result from smallpox vaccine. The third area in immunology research investigates the prospect of producing synthesized vaccines. These are entirely man-made vaccines produced by stringing together short chains of synthetic protein. New delivery methods, such as administering flu vaccine through nose drops rather than injections, are also being investigated. To date, no immunologic agents are effective against protozoal or helminthic infections.

Nurses are in a position to teach the public about the advantages of immunization and to encourage participation in immunization programs. The nurse should explain:

- What disease the immunization is for
- Why immunization is recommended
- When booster doses are needed
- The relative safety and advantages of immunization

Clients should be instructed to keep up-to-date vaccination records, which may be required when entering school or applying for a passport. Public health clinics often provide immunizations at little or no cost. For example, public health nurses may provide influenza immunization at senior citizen clinics.

International travel may also require immunization. The Bureau of Epidemiology of the CDC distributes a weekly "blue sheet" to health departments, physicians, and public and private health agencies that lists countries infected with diseases requiring quarantine. A toll-free hot line is available to provide the traveler with immediate health information. (Both are listed in the resources section at the end of this chapter.) Travelers arriving from these countries may be required to provide evidence of vaccination. If immunizations are necessary, travelers should allow enough time for a full course of treatment and for discomfort or reactions to subside.

Assess clients before immunization because there are contraindications to vaccination as well as contraindications to the use of certain substances. Before using any immunologic product, read the package insert carefully for indications, precautions, and side effects. Vaccines prepared in chicken or duck embryos may cause an allergic reaction in clients allergic to eggs. Recall that hypersensitivity to horse serum can cause serum sickness. Testing for hypersensitivity should precede immunization whenever possible.

Attenuated virus vaccines should not be given to clients with altered immune status because viral replication after administration might be unchecked. Because trivalent oral poliovirus vaccine (TOPV) viruses are excreted by an immunized person, clients living with an immunocompromised person should not receive TOPV. Attenuated virus vaccines also should not be given to a client who has a cold or other infection because the inflammatory reaction may be greater than usual. Use of these vaccines is also avoided in pregnant women because of the theoretical risk to the fetus. Attenuated virus vaccines should not be given at the same time as passive immunization because passively acquired antibodies can interfere with the response to the live vaccine. All vaccines should be withheld from clients with acute severe febrile illness until the illness is over.

Before leaving the clinic, the client or family members should be instructed about the expected effects of the inoculation. They should be told to contact the physician or go to an emergency room if unexpected symptoms develop. These might include severe headache, palpitations, paresthesias, pruritus, difficulty breathing, nausea and vomiting, urticaria, and joint pain. When antitoxins, antisera, and antivenoms are given, the client is observed for 20 to 30 minutes because symptoms of severe allergic response, as described earlier, usually appear within that time.

Some persons refuse immunization because of religious beliefs. Others hesitate to be immunized or to have their children immunized because of fear about potential side effects. An example is Guillian–Barré syndrome, an acute polyneuritis that is a rare complication of rabies and swine influenza vaccination. There has also been concern about pertussis immunization in children because of potential neurotoxicity. The nurse might explain when the benefits of immunization far outweigh risk of side effects. In the United Kingdom, for instance, the incidence of pertussis and pertussis-related deaths significantly increased after immunization was suspended from 1974 to 1978. On the other hand, a national campaign in the United States of preventive inoculations for swine influenza in the 1976–1977 flu season caused an incidence of

Guillian–Barré syndrome five to six times higher in vaccinated than unvaccinated persons. In retrospect, this campaign seems to have been ill advised because the anticipated outbreak of swine influenza did not materialize. This situation points out a serious problem with large-scale inoculation programs against a new strain of flu virus—the immunization program must begin as soon as possible to be effective, often before the new vaccine has been thoroughly tested and before it is known whether the epidemic would actually occur.

Adult clients need to be reminded to complete an immunization series, such as for polio, and to keep tetanus immunization up to date. Those employed in health care should maintain immunity against poliomyelitis, diphtheria, and tetanus. Personnel are often given a tuberculin test on employment, especially if the incidence of tuberculosis in the area warrants it. Policies on follow-up testing and chest x-rays vary by location. In Europe, those in high-risk groups may be immunized against tuberculosis with BCG (bacillus Calmette–Guérin) vaccine, although this vaccine is rarely used for this purpose in the United States today. According to the CDC (Williams, 1983), adequate surveillance and control measures, rather than BCG vaccination, are all that is necessary to protect clients and personnel in the United States.

Immune globulins can prevent or modify the severity of hepatitis. Immune serum globulin (ISG) is used against the three types of viral hepatitis. ISG is not usually given to those, including hospital personnel, who have had only casual contact with clients with hepatitis A. Persons who receive needle-stick injuries or are otherwise exposed while caring for those with hepatitis B, however, should receive hepatitis B immune globulin (HBIG) as soon as possible after exposure, or ISG if HBIG is not available. Vaccine against hepatitis B, Heptavax-B, is also available and is recommended for persons such as surgeons, dentists, nurses, and laboratory workers who are at high risk for hepatitis B because they frequently come into contact with blood and for clients at increased risk for hepatitis B. More information can be obtained from the Public Health Service Advisory Committee on Immunization Practices listed with the resources at the end of this chapter.

Hygiene and Sanitation

Public health depends on adequate community sanitation. A clean water supply, sewage treatment, and garbage disposal are the fundamental means of controlling disease in a society. In general, communities in the United States do an adequate job in these areas. On the other hand, precautions must be taken in areas where sewage disposal might not be adequate. An example is rural areas where residents have their own wells and septic tanks. Contamination of drinking water is possible if proper measures are not taken.

With the renewed interest in outdoor recreation, persons may also be vulnerable to infectious organisms.

Campers may drink water from streams or lakes without adequate attention to sanitation. Nurses can encourage outdoor enthusiasts to seek the latest information from local authorities before drinking from these water supplies. They can also instruct campers and hikers to boil their water or carry effective water purification tablets.

Personal hygiene is also a factor in preventing disease. Thorough and frequent hand-washing by hospital personnel is an important means of preventing the spread of nosocomial infections. Food handlers in the home, restaurants, and institutions must also be conscientious about hand-washing and personal care. Specific measures to limit the spread of infectious diseases in health care settings or in the home are discussed later in this chapter.

Food Handling

Proper food handling is an important means of preventing food poisoning and infection spread. Foods that are improperly prepared, preserved, or stored provide an ideal growth medium for microorganisms. Nurses can help raise public awareness of appropriate food handling regardless of the setting where they practice. General principles for food handling are:

- Wash hands before preparing food.
- Keep hot foods hot and cold foods cold.
- Cook all meat thoroughly.

If there is any question about spoilage, the food should be discarded without tasting. Commercial food preservation is highly sophisticated, and commercial products are rarely contaminated. Home canning, on the other hand,

can cause food poisoning, especially in low-acid foods. Figure 11–7 illustrates temperatures associated with microorganisms and food spoilage. Home canners should be instructed to purchase jars and lids intended specifically for home canning and follow the manufacturer's directions exactly.

Travelers to foreign countries often have their trips interrupted by gastroenteritis characterized by diarrhea, abdominal cramps, nausea and vomiting, and occasional headache and fever. Known by various colorful names such as "Montezuma's revenge," "Rangoon runs," "Casablanca crud," and "Delhi belly," this condition was thought to be due to changes in diet or the use of cooking oils with a laxative effect. Evidence now shows that an enterotoxin produced by *E. coli* is the most common cause (Rodman & Smith, 1984). Although the use of prophylactic antimicrobial drugs such as doxycycline (Vibramycin) for travelers is controversial, nurses can advise travelers about food and water precautions. For example, fresh fruits and vegetables should be peeled before they are eaten. It is generally not safe to eat lettuce or green salads unless they have been washed in a chlorinated solution. Another good piece of advice is to recommend drinking bottled beverages. Using ice cubes in bottled beverages defeats the purpose. Drinking water and milk should be boiled before drinking. Using antidiarrheal agents once diarrhea has begun is also controversial; it may be best to let the diarrhea run its course and rid the body of the offending organisms. Clients should be sure to seek health care if symptoms are severe or if they persist, if they become dehydrated, or if they are very young or old or have a chronic illness, or if they are a compromised host. See the

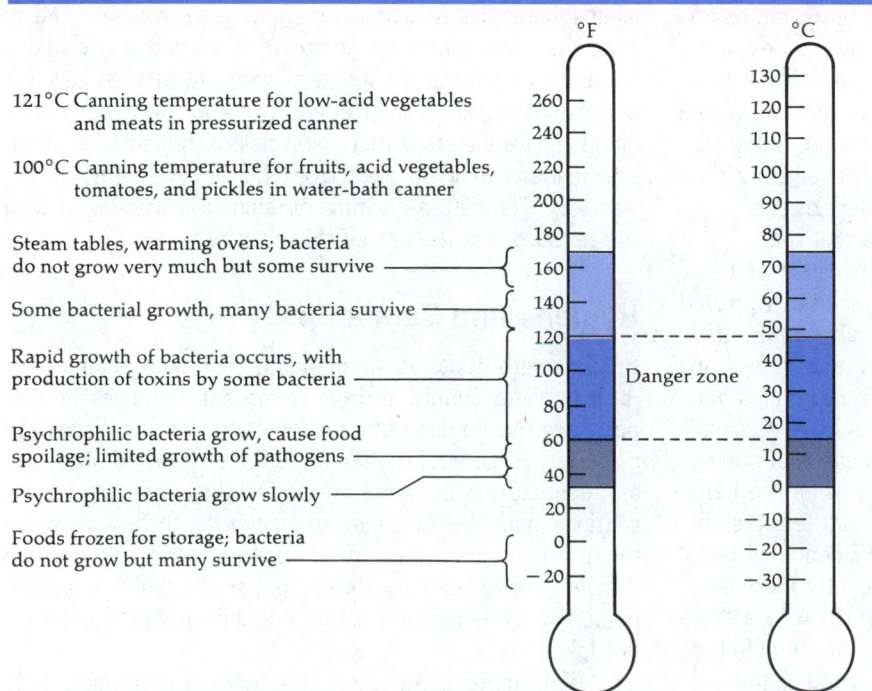

Figure 11–7

Some important temperatures associated with microorganisms and food spoilage.
SOURCE: Tortora GJ, Funke BR, Case CL: *Microbiology*, 2nd ed. Menlo Park, CA: Benjamin/Cummings, 1986.

resources listing at the end of this chapter for organizations that provide health services to travelers.

ASSESSMENT OF THE POTENTIALLY INFECTED PERSON

A comprehensive assessment is essential in planning the care for a potentially infected person. A comprehensive assessment will help determine:

- Whether infection exists
- The most probable primary source of infection
- Which organisms are most likely to be responsible
- Which antimicrobials are indicated
- Whether special procedures such as isolation measures or measures for controlling the spread of the suspected disease should be instituted
- What information and health teaching are needed for client and family

The health history, physical assessment, and diagnostic studies are all part of the assessment phase.

Subjective Data

Collection of a detailed history is essential to the diagnosis of infectious disease. Most infectious diseases begin with nonspecific symptoms such as headache, anorexia, fatigue, and joint and muscle pain. A thorough history may help in pinpointing the diagnosis. Asking where and what a client has eaten in the last few days might aid in reaching a diagnosis of food poisoning. For example, has the client attended a banquet or a company picnic? Are others attending also ill? Has the client eaten pork or raw meat? Some questions to ask during history taking are in Table 11–8. It is as important to record what is absent as well as what is present. For example, a pertinent negative finding is the absence of back pain with a urinary tract infection. This usually indicates that the infection has not ascended to the kidney.

The client with an infectious disease may harbor feelings of inadequacy or inferiority. Some infectious diseases are stigmatized, especially sexually transmitted diseases, tuberculosis, and AIDS. Clients may feel "dirty" and blame themselves for acquiring the disease. They may shun social contact. Depending on the severity of the disease, they may also fear long-term disability or death. If the disease carries a social stigma, the nurse must be particularly perceptive in assessing the client's attitude toward the illness, and eliciting the client's concerns. Inquire about the attitudes of family members and friends to determine the client's social support and to help develop a plan of care that considers the psychosocial needs of clients, family members, and friends.

Objective Data

After a history is obtained, a physical assessment should be performed. Particular findings that might indicate an infectious process are:

- Dehydration
- Neck rigidity
- Open or draining lesions

Table 11–8 Questions to Ask When Infectious Disease is Suspected	
Questions	**Rationale**
1. What are the symptoms? When did they begin?	Provides data about duration of illness and specific information to assist with diagnosis
2. Is there fever? With or without chills? What is the pattern: intermittent, recurrent, or constant?	Fever patterns vary with the organism; pattern may help in identifying microbe
3. Is there a stiff neck? Pain when knee and hip are flexed and knee is straightened?	May indicate meningitis
4. Is there back pain?	May indicate kidney infection
5. Is there dysuria?	May indicate bladder infection
6. Is there diarrhea?	May indicate gastrointestinal infection
7. Are there draining wounds?	May indicate wound infection
8. Is there use of prescription, over-the-counter, or illegal drugs?	Identifies client's routine drug use as well as potential problems with self-medication or blood-transmitted infections (eg, hepatitis)
9. Does the client have a chronic disease (eg, diabetes)? Is the client taking an immunosuppressant?	Identifies increased risk for infection through impaired immune response
10. Has the client traveled recently, especially outside the country?	Identifies exposure to foreign diseases
11. Has the client been bitten by an animal, insect, or human? Has the client been in contact with animals?	Identifies exposure to diseases transmitted by bites

- Inflamed throat
- Enlarged lymph nodes
- Rashes
- Elevated temperature

As with the history, the absence of a finding may also be important. The absence of a fever might indicate a particular kind of infection, or it might indicate that the infection is improving. For example, there is usually no fever with staphylococcal food poisoning, but there may be with other types. Clinical signs highly specific for selected infections have been identified in Section II of this chapter and in the specific disorders chapters in each body systems unit.

A variety of diagnostic studies is useful in determining the causative organism and identifying the appropriate antimicrobial drug therapy (Table 11–9). The nurse's role includes teaching the client about the planned procedure, obtaining cultures and specimens, assisting with diagnostic

Table 11–9 Diagnostic Studies Common in Infectious Disease

Laboratory Test	Normal Expected Value	Expected Abnormal Findings
Total white blood cell count (WBC)	4000–12,000 µL (up to 35,000 in newborns and 15,000 in 1-yr-olds	↑ In most systemic infections
Differential WBC count:		
• Lymphocytes	25%–33%	↑ In many viral infections
• Segmented and banded neutrophils (left shift)*	Up to 60%	↑ In many bacterial infections
• Monocytes	Up to 7%	↑ In mononucleosis
• Eosinophils	Up to 600 µL	↑ In many parasitic infestations
Erythrocyte sedimentation rate	Men: 0–8 mm/h Women: 0–15 mm/h Children: 4–13 mm/h	↑ In many bacterial infections
Peripheral blood smear		Parasites
Urine (clean, void, unspun):		
• WBCs	0–4 WBCs/high power field	↑ In most urinary tract infections (UTIs)
• Gram's stain	None	↑ In most UTIs
Stool examination:		
• Mucus (or white cells on smear)	None or minimal	↑ In invasive processes (eg, bacillary dysentery) rather than toxin reactions (eg, staphylococcal food poisoning)
• Blood	None	↑ In bacillary dysentery
Cerebral spinal fluid:		
• Glucose	40%–80 mg/dL (at least one-half blood glucose level)	Usually low in bacterial meningitis and fungal infections
• Protein	5%–40 mg/dL	Usually high in bacterial meningitis, tuberculous meningitis, poliomyelitis
• WBC count	0–7 cells	↑ In viral infections (poliomyelitis and aseptic meningitis), CNS syphilis, bacterial meningitis
• Gram's stain	No organisms	Differentiates between gram-positive and gram-negative bacteria
X-rays, scans, thermography, ultrasonography	Normal anatomy	Abscesses or cyst (eg, liver, lung); infiltrates (eg, pneumonia); bony abnormalities (eg, osteomyelitis)
Cultures:		
• Urine	0–10⁴ bacteria/mL	>10⁵ organisms of single species
• Blood, CSF, synovial fluid	No organisms	Pathogens
• Sputum, stool, etc	Normal flora	Pathogens
Skin tests (for tuberculosis, diphtheria, scarlet fever, brucellosis, tularemia, toxoplasmosis, trichinosis, mumps, blastomycosis, lymphogranuloma venereum, coccidioidomycosis, histoplasmosis)	Test-specific and variable	May indicate an immunity to the disease or the presence of either an active or inactive case (of little value in confirming ongoing infection)

Laboratory Test	Normal Expected Value	Expected Abnormal Findings
Immunologic tests: • Immunofluorescence tests (for syphilis, toxoplasmosis, and Epstein–Barr virus) • Precipitation tests (for coccidioidomycosis and schistosomiasis) • Agglutination tests (for atypical pneumonia, malaria, influenza A and B, mycoplasma pneumonia, determination of immunity to rubella, staphylococcemia, African trypanosomiasis) • Complement fixation tests (for histoplasmosis, rickettsial diseases, blastomycosis, trichinosis, schistosomiasis) • Enzyme-linked immunosorbent assay (ELISA) (for detecting rubella and hepatitis)	Test-specific and variable	Results specific and variable

*See the discussion of left shift in Chapter 22.

procedures, and providing emotional support to the client. Gram's stain and culture and sensitivity tests are briefly described because they are the principal means of diagnosis in infection.

Gram's stain, a laboratory procedure performed on a specimen, is one of the most useful and most important procedures for identifying bacteria. If the test is negative, no organisms were identified, indicating the specimen was not infected with bacteria. If the test is positive, signifying a bacterial infection, the Gram's stain indicates whether the bacteria are gram-positive or gram-negative. The Gram's stain reaction provides important information for treatment. Because it requires no incubation of the organism, results can be obtained faster than by a laboratory culture, meaning antimicrobial treatment can begin sooner.

Laboratory cultures of specimens may also be done to identify organisms. Urine, spinal fluid, and blood are normally sterile, and a culture will not reveal organisms in the absence of infection. In contrast, stool has a normal population of bacteria. Interpretation of culture results must consider whether the material is normally sterile. Cultures may be done on all of the specimens discussed in Box 11–2, next page. Results may take 3 or more days. The specimen for culture should be obtained before antimicrobial therapy is begun for more accurate results. The laboratory also can determine the sensitivity and resistance of an organism to antimicrobials. This information is used in selecting an antimicrobial to which the organism is sensitive (Figure 11–8).

An exception is the emergency treatment of septicemia. In this situation, a combination of an aminoglycoside-type antibiotic such as gentamicin and a penicillin-type drug such as ampicillin or carbenicillin may be administered without delay because of the seriousness of septic shock

(Rodman & Smith, 1984). The organisms primarily responsible for septic shock are usually sensitive to one or both of these classes of drugs.

PREVENTING NOSOCOMIAL INFECTION

Precautions to prevent nosocomial infections and to avoid becoming infected oneself begin with the recognition that

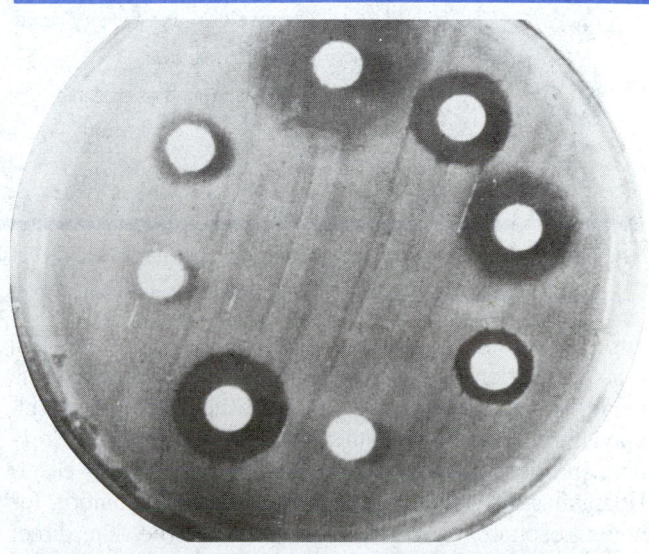

Figure 11–8

Culture plate with filter paper disks impregnated with various antibiotics. The clear areas indicate where bacterial growth has been inhibited; these agents are effective to varying degrees against the microorganism being tested.

Box 11–2 Guidelines for Obtaining Specimens for Cultures

Blood

Requires venipuncture

Aseptic technique must be rigorously followed

Obtain two 10-mL samples from separate sites

One sample is for aerobic bacteria; the other is for anaerobic bacteria

Cerebrospinal fluid

Iliac crest landmark

Sterile-prepped area 1 2 3

Requires lumbar puncture

Aseptic technique must be rigorously followed

Obtain three samples for smear, culture, and chemistries

Transport to laboratory within 30 minutes

Cervical–Vaginal

Rotate sterile swab*

Obtain as much as possible

Ear

Cleanse skin and auditory canal

Rotate sterile swab*

Obtain as much as possible

Eye

Use sterile swab*

Gently obtain specimen from lower conjunctiva

Massage lacrimal duct to obtain specimen if dacryocystitis is suspected

Feces

Use a rectal swab* or obtain a small amount of feces (about the size of a walnut)

Samples of feces are preferred for most purposes and required for ova and parasites; rectal swab may be adequate for *Shigella*

Transport to laboratory within 60 minutes

Do not refrigerate

Nasal or nasopharyngeal

Use sterile swab* or small wire-loop swab

Client's head must be held firmly; procedure may cause sneezing

For nasal culture: moisten swab with sterile normal saline and gently rotate swab in both external nares and deeper recesses of the nose

For nasopharyngeal culture: moisten swab with sterile normal saline; insert small wire-loop swab gently and quickly through nares into nasopharyngeal area; gently rotate swab

*Chemicals on cotton swabs are bactericidal and may affect the culture; use specially prepared swabs for cultures.

unrecognized or subclinical infections are prevalent and that prevention begins before a diagnosis of infection is made. (Recall the earlier example of the nurse who developed herpetic whitlow.) Nurses should incorporate the recommendations in Box 11–3 (p. 308) in caring for any client. Hospital staff should seek prompt medical attention for upper respiratory problems and breaks in the skin; direct client care should be avoided if these conditions exist. Be especially cautious when caring for clients whose immune systems are suppressed. Additional environmental protection such as protective isolation or the use of patient-isolator units, although recommended by some, does not appear warranted for most compromised clients. Instead,

routine techniques such as hand-washing should be emphasized and enforced, and these clients should be in private rooms whenever possible and away from other clients who may make infection transmission likely (Garner & Simmons, 1983).

Urinary tract instrumentation is the most common cause of urinary tract infections, and the urinary tract is the most common site of nosocomial infections. According to Hargiss and Larson (1981), the nurse can use several strategies to minimize the risk to clients of contracting a nosocomial urinary tract infection. The most important is to avoid catheterization whenever possible. If this is not possible, using condom catheters or intermittent cathet-

Skin lesion

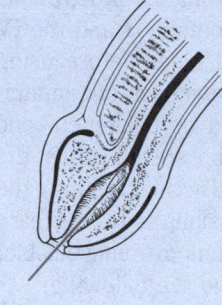

Cleanse area with normal saline

Use either sterile swab* or syringe to aspirate fluid (disinfect the area first if aspirating)

Obtain as much as possible

Sputum

Morning samples preferred

Client should rinse mouth thoroughly before raising sputum from deep within the bronchi and expectorating into sterile container

Use sterile suction catheter and aseptic technique for tracheal aspiration

Obtain 2 to 3 mL of sputum (not saliva)

Transport to laboratory within 60 minutes

Do not refrigerate

Throat

Use sterile swab*

Stand to the side of the client (most clients cough or gag)

Depress client's tongue with tongue depressor

Avoid touching the lips or tongue

Rotate swab firmly and gently over both tonsils, back of the throat, and any areas of inflammation, ulceration, or exudation

Obtain as much as possible

Urethra

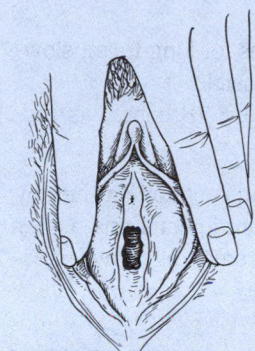

Use small urethral wire-loop swab

In males, prior massage of prostate may increase yield

Obtain as much as possible

Urine

Early morning specimens are best because bacterial counts are highest then

Females: cleanse vulvar area; client collects midstream specimen while holding labia apart

Males: cleanse glans penis; obtain midstream specimen

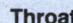

Use aseptic technique when aspirating specimens from in-dwelling catheter with sterile needle and syringe

Obtain at least 1 mL for culture (5 mL for urinalysis)

Use sterile container

Transport to laboratory immediately; refrigerate if not cultured immediately but transport within 2 hours

Wound

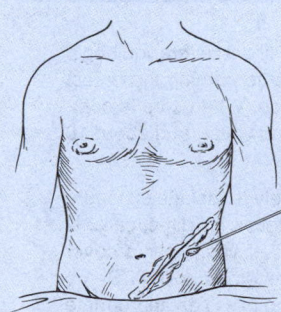

Cleanse wound with sterile saline to remove skin flora

Use sterile swab* or syringe

Obtain as much as possible

Take care not to contaminate surrounding tissue

Transport within 60 minutes

---

erization rather than an in-dwelling catheter reduces the risk. If an in-dwelling catheter is unavoidable, preventive measures include:

- Using aseptic technique when inserting in-dwelling catheters or when obtaining specimens
- Keeping the entire collection system closed
- Avoiding obtaining specimens from connecting tubing (which may not be self-sealing) if the system does not have an inline port; using a sterile needle and syringe to aspirate through the catheter
- Preventing reflux of urine by keeping the drainage bag below the bladder at all times
- Separating clients with urinary tract infections from

clients with in-dwelling catheters; also separating clients with in-dwelling catheters from one another

- Removing catheters as soon as possible
- Changing catheters whenever crusting develops at the catheter-meatal junction or in the catheter itself or if it becomes necessary to manipulate the catheter to maintain the flow of urine
- Irrigating catheters only when necessary; if irrigations are necessary to maintain patency, use a closed three-way system

Incorporating these suggestions into the nursing care of every client with an in-dwelling catheter will do much to limit the incidence of catheter-related infections.

Bacteremias that occur in hospitalized clients with no underlying site of infection are likely to have resulted from contaminated intravenous fluids or from the intravenous delivery system. Check all IV fluid containers and the IV infusion system itself for cracks and holes before using them and inspect the fluid for visual evidence of contamination. Do not use any suspect fluid or equipment and notify infection control personnel who should notify the appropriate agencies and take remedial action. Limiting the need for and use of intravenous infusions is the primary preventive strategy. When IV infusions are unavoidable, Hargiss and Larson (1981) recommend the following:

- Maintain scrupulous aseptic technique.
- Use steel needles whenever possible.
- Change the site of a peripheral IV infusion if inflammation or phlebitis develops.
- Avoid the use of glucose solutions for long-term, slow-running infusions whenever possible.
- Change IV fluid and tubing every 48 hours, as recommended by the CDC.

Respiratory instrumentation and respiratory therapy are major risk factors in hospital-acquired pneumonia. Other risk factors are ineffective coughing, smoking, other infec-

Nursing Research Note

Nichols E, Barstow R, Cooper D: Relationship between incidence of phlebitis and frequency of changing IV tubing and percutaneous site. *Nurs Res* 1983; 32(4): 247–251.

This study examined the development of phlebitis related to IV tubing change and changing IV sites percutaneously. No statistically significant difference was found in phlebitis development when tubing was changed at 24 hours and 48 hours. There was not a statistically significant difference in phlebitis development when tubing was changed at 48 hours and 72 hours. Subjects who had tubing changed every 24 hours had less clinical evidence of phlebitis, however.

When IV sites were rotated, there was no statistical significance between site rotation at 48 hours and 72 hours. Clinically, however, 48-hour site rotation coupled with 24-hour tubing change resulted in a trend toward less phlebitis development.

Nurses are responsible for maintaining IV therapy and assessing clients' IV sites for infection. Monitoring sites and regular tubing changes may result in lower incidence of phlebitis formation. More research is needed to determine scientifically what nursing approaches are most effective.

Box 11–3 Recommended Nursing Measures When Infection is Unrecognized or Subclinical

Assess what you are going to do for the client *before* you begin an episode of care. When you anticipate coming in contact with body substances, glove your hands. When care is completed, *wash your hands*. Soap, running water, and about 10 seconds of friction are usually enough.

Is the client bleeding or is your care likely to include exposure to blood? If the answer is yes, wear gloves for direct care. Is bleeding enough to soil your uniform? If yes, wear a cover gown and change your uniform if it becomes soiled. (Scrub clothes are available in all hospitals, and this is an appropriate use for them.)

Is the wound draining? If yes, wear gloves for direct care. Is drainage copious? If yes, wear a cover gown.

Is the client incontinent? If yes, wear gloves for contact with urine or stool and a cover gown if you are changing the client's bed linen or if a great deal of soilage is likely.

Will you be suctioning the client? If yes, glove both hands to avoid skin contact with sputum or oral secretions.

It is not always possible to anticipate contact with body substances. When such episodes of care are completed, it is essential to wash hands well before continuing with client care.

The same logic applies to handling linen and trash soiled with body substances. If linen or trash from any client is likely to expose personnel to direct contact with body substances, it should be securely bagged and marked for careful handling.

SOURCE: Adapted from Jackson MM, Lynch P: Infection control: Too much or too little? *Am J Nurs* 1984; 84:208–210.

tion, and tracheal suctioning. Adequate sterilization and disinfection of all respiratory equipment and frequent changes of respiratory therapy equipment is an important preventive measure. Nurses should focus on encouraging deep breathing and effective coughing (as discussed and illustrated in Chapter 14) in postoperative clients as well as in any clients at risk. Aseptic technique should be used for laryngotracheal suctioning (see Chapter 18).

Preventing surgical wound infection requires concerted effort during the entire perioperative period because many factors can cause infection. Examples of client risk factors are:

- Less-than-optimal surgical technique
- Presence of organisms at the operative site
- Duration of surgical procedure
- Severe underlying disease
- Presence of infection at other sites
- Length of hospitalization before surgery
- Break in aseptic technique in the operating room
- Inappropriate use of antibiotics
- Extremes of age
- Obesity
- Malnutrition

All surgical clients should be closely monitored. Violating the integrity of the skin during preoperative shaving and exposing the client to infected staff or clients after the operation also contribute to the development of wound infection.

During the preoperative period, nurses can ensure that the client's skin is kept intact and that preoperative preparation such as enemas and antibiotic administration before bowel surgery is carried out. The circulating nurse acts as the client's advocate during surgery by monitoring the surgical team and the operating room environment for adherence to standards of surgical asepsis. Aseptic postoperative care of wounds is another important measure. Preventing postoperative wound infection is discussed further in Chapter 14; preoperative bowel preparation is described in Chapter 50.

PROVIDING PHYSIOLOGIC SUPPORT

Clients with infectious disease should have vital signs assessed at least every 4 hours. Even afebrile clients should have their temperature documented to establish any fever pattern. Arterial blood pressure monitoring may be required for clients in septic shock.

Tepid water baths may be used to reduce high fever. Be careful not to cause shivering, which only increases temperature. In some situations, alcohol baths bring temperatures down more quickly; however, they are more likely to cause shivering and dry the skin. In critical situations, hypothermia blankets may be used. Antipyretic drugs are usually given.

The profuse diaphoresis, vomiting, and diarrhea that accompany many infectious diseases may cause dehydration and fluid and electrolyte imbalance. Monitor the client's state of hydration, encourage oral fluids, and administer intravenous fluids as indicated. Measure and record intake and output and weigh the client at regular intervals.

PROMOTING COMFORT

Weakness and generalized aches often accompany infectious diseases. Physical activity should be reduced to avoid further fatigue and weakness. Pillows, pads, frequent position changes, and back rubs often help to reduce the discomfort associated with aching. Analgesics may also be useful.

Bathing and frequent linen changes reduce the discomforts associated with diaphoresis. For clients with skin rashes, bathing with sodium bicarbonate, applying antipruritic lotions, or administering antipruritic medications can help reduce the itching associated with skin rashes.

Dehydration, fever, and coughing adversely affect the mucous membranes. Frequent oral hygiene is important. Warm gargles are often comforting, as is providing warm, humidified air.

MONITORING ANTIMICROBIAL THERAPY

Antimicrobial drugs are available to control most microbes and parasites, but as yet, few are effective against viruses (Table 11–6). Most infections can be quickly controlled. If an organism is resistant to the drug, the drug may have to be discontinued, and an alternative drug or combination of drugs may be tried. If the client is immunosuppressed, antimicrobial therapy alone may not be enough to control or treat the infection. In other situations, clients may even be made worse by drug-induced adverse effects such as direct tissue toxicity, hypersensitivity reactions, and superinfections.

Direct-tissue toxicity takes a number of forms. Some oral antimicrobials irritate the mucosa of the gastrointestinal tract, causing nausea, vomiting, and diarrhea. Others cause local pain when administered intramuscularly, and some cause phlebitis when administered intravenously. The most severe effects result in nephrotoxicity (kidney damage) and neurotoxicity (damage to cranial nerve VIII, the vestibulocochlear nerve). Aminoglycosides and polymyxins are more likely to cause nephrotoxic effects. Monitor the results of laboratory reports of kidney function for signs of drug-related renal impairment. Aminoglycosides can also cause neurologic impairment; monitor the client for dizziness, vertigo, and impaired hearing.

Hypersensitivity reactions, common with penicillin-type antibiotics, can occur immediately after administration of an antimicrobial, or they can be delayed. Hypersensitivity is more likely in persons having other allergies and in those who have been treated with these agents frequently. This is a good reason for not using antibiotics to treat minor upper respiratory tract infections, because most are caused by viruses not sensitive to these drugs. Health care providers have reportedly developed hypersensitivity reactions because of careless handling of antibiotics (eg, spilling a liquid preparation on the hands; handling tablets; or inadvertent injection of parenteral antibiotics during preparation, administration, or disposal of equipment).

Superinfections result from the overgrowth of the client's own normal flora. The antimicrobial eliminates susceptible organisms, permitting the growth of pathogens normally kept under control. Superinfections are often more serious than the original infection being treated. Superinfections are often associated with various procedures and equipment such as intravenous catheters, parenteral nutrition, heparin locks, arterial catheters and angiographic procedures, hemodialysis and peritoneal dialysis, cerebrospinal fluid shunts, pressure transducers, nebulizers, endotracheal intubation or tracheostomy, and transtracheal aspiration of local neck infections (Sen et al., 1982). Clients who have undergone these invasive procedures should be carefully monitored for infection. Prosthetic valves, cardiac pacemakers, total hip and knee prostheses, vascular grafts, intraocular lens implantation, and breast implants are devices that are associated with superinfection. With some devices such as cerebrospinal fluid shunts, 50% of the infections occur within the first week. With total hip and knee protheses, it may take as long as 2 years before infection occurs (Sen et al., 1982). Clients with prostheses must not only be monitored by nurses during the postoperative period in the hospital, but must also be instructed to observe for superinfection on discharge.

Nurses must be able to administer antimicrobials properly as well as to advise clients and their families on how to administer them and how to avoid their misuse. The proper administration of antimicrobials will be facilitated by following these guidelines:

- Determine whether the client is allergic to any drugs, especially penicillin or other antimicrobials, before administering them; if so, do not administer the drug.

- Monitor the client closely for adverse effects, such as drug-induced toxicity or hypersensitivity, and report them immediately.

- Maintain therapeutic blood levels of antibiotics by administering them at the appropriate intervals.

- Administer oral antibiotics with food to diminish any unpleasant gastrointestinal symptoms, but check first to be sure food will not interfere with the absorption of the antibiotic.

- Report nausea and vomiting immediately so oral administration can be changed to parenteral administration if necessary.

- Observe the client closely to determine the effect of the drug; report signs of continuing or worsening infection.

- Handle needles and syringes with extreme care to protect oneself from inadvertent infection with contaminated equipment.

- Avoid careless handling of antibiotics.

Advising clients and their families on how to administer antimicrobials safely and avoid misuse will help to ensure that clients are not deprived of the use of a valuable drug when needed. The following guidelines will help to achieve these goals:

- Inform clients that using antimicrobials to treat trivial infections may not only be useless, but it may also render the drug ineffective in a future illness.

- Advise clients to continue taking the drug for the recommended length of time, even if symptoms seem to have abated. (This prevents relapses.)

- Instruct clients to take the drug in the recommended dose. (This prevents chronic infection because of undertreatment as well as the later emergence of resistant strains because of less-than-optimal doses.)

- Caution clients about any special adjunctive measures such as taking sulfonamides with large amounts of fluid; avoiding alcohol when taking moxalactam disodium (Moxam) and other cephalosporin-related drugs; and avoiding dairy products, antacids, and iron salt preparations with tetracyclines.

- Remind clients not to treat themselves with antimicrobials left over from another illness.

These guidelines apply to clinical situations that nurses commonly encounter. Keep in mind there are many different types of antimicrobials, all with different effects and precautions. Consult a pharmacology textbook for detailed information on specific antimicrobials.

IMPLEMENTING ISOLATION PRECAUTIONS

Health care institutions have isolation procedures to prevent transmission of infectious organisms to clients, visitors, and personnel. In 1983, the CDC issued new recommendations for isolation precautions (Box 11–4). The previous five categories of isolation have been expanded to seven. Clients with infections are assigned to the appropriate category. For example, clients with a wound infection are placed in contact isolation because wound infections are spread by contact. The seven isolation categories are:

- Strict isolation
- Respiratory isolation
- Tuberculosis (AFB) isolation
- Enteric precautions
- Contact isolation
- Drainage/secretion precautions
- Blood/body fluid precautions

Refer to the CDC guidelines to determine appropriate isolation precautions for specific infectious diseases. Each category includes specific information, such as whether a private room is indicated, whether protective clothing must be worn, and the proper handling of contaminated articles. Refer also to a nursing fundamentals text for a discussion of the principles of protective asepsis. The CDC also offers the option of disease-specific isolation precautions as well as the option for hospitals to develop their own system. Health care facilities may differ from one another in this regard. The infection control practitioner should be consulted regarding specific institutional procedures.

Clients assigned to isolation precautions have a variety of psychosocial needs that require sensitive handling. First, client and family need thorough explanations about the disease, the planned treatment, and the rationale for isolation. Although the initial explanation is probably given by the physician, the nurse reinforces, clarifies, and provides additional information as needed.

Depending on the isolation category, the client may be in a private room, perhaps with the door closed. Isolation may lead to withdrawal and possibly even sensory deprivation because the normal sources of stimulation are removed. Assess the client's need for stimulation regularly. Spending time with the client when not providing physical care is one way to provide stimulation. See that the client has means of diversion, such as television, a telephone, books and magazines, craft projects, and other forms of entertainment. Try to provide as much variety in activities as the isolation requirements allow. Friendly conversation that provides opportunities for the client to talk and demonstrates the nurse's interest is perhaps the most important stimulation measure. These measures also help in reducing withdrawal.

Box 11–4 CDC Guidelines for Isolation Precautions

Strict isolation

Strict isolation is an isolation category designed to prevent transmission of highly contagious or virulent infections that may be spread by both air and contact.

Specifications for strict isolation:

1. Private room is indicated; door should be kept closed. In general, clients infected with the same organism may share a room.

2. Masks are indicated for all persons entering the room.

3. Gowns are indicated for all persons entering the room.

4. Gloves are indicated for all persons entering the room.

5. Hands must be washed after touching the client or potentially contaminated articles and before taking care of another client.

6. Articles contaminated with infective material should be discarded or bagged and labeled before being sent for decontamination and reprocessing.

Diseases requiring strict isolation:

Diphtheria, pharyngeal

Lassa fever and other viral hemorrhagic fevers, such as Marburg virus disease*

Plague, pneumonic

Smallpox*

Varicella (chickenpox)

Zoster, localized in immunocompromised patient or disseminated

Contact isolation

Contact isolation is designed to prevent transmission of highly transmissible or epidemiologically important infections (or colonization) that do not warrant strict isolation.

All diseases or conditions included in this category are spread primarily by close or direct contact. Thus, masks, gowns, and gloves are recommended for anyone in close or direct contact with any client who has an infection (or colonization) that is included in this category. For individual diseases or conditions, however, one or more of these three barriers may not be indicated. For example, masks and gloves are not generally indicated for care of infants and young children with acute viral respiratory infections, gowns are not generally indicated for gonococcal conjunctivitis in newborns, and masks are not generally indicated for care of clients infected with multiple-resistant microorganisms, except those with pneumonia. Therefore, some degree of "overisolation" may occur in this category.

Specifications for contact isolation:

1. Private room is indicated. In general, clients infected with the same organism may share a room. During outbreaks, infants and young children with the same respiratory clinical syndrome may share a room.

2. Masks are indicated for those who come close to the client.

3. Gowns are indicated if soiling is likely.

4. Gloves are indicated for touching infective material.

5. Hands must be washed after touching the client or potentially contaminated articles and before taking care of another client.

6. Articles contaminated with infective material should be discarded or bagged and labeled before being sent for decontamination and reprocessing.

Diseases or conditions requiring contact isolation:

Acute respiratory infections in infants and young children, including croup, colds, bronchitis, and bronchiolitis caused by respiratory syncytial virus, adenovirus, coronavirus, influenza viruses, parainfluenza viruses, and rhinovirus.

Conjunctivitis, gonococcal, in newborns

Diphtheria, cutaneous

Endometritis, group A *Streptococcus*

Furunculosis, staphylococcal, in newborns

Herpes simplex, disseminated, severe primary or neonatal

Impetigo

Influenza, in infants and young children

Multiple-resistant bacteria, infection or colonization (any site) with any of the following:

1. Gram-negative bacilli resistant to all aminoglycosides that are tested. (In general, such organisms should be resistant to gentamicin, tobramycin, and amikacin for these special precautions to be indicated.)

2. *Staphylococcus aureus* resistant to methicillin (or nafcillin or oxacillin if they are used instead of methicillin for testing).

3. *Pneumococcus* resistant to penicillin.

4. *Hemophilus influenzae* resistant to ampicillin (beta-lactamase positive) and chloramphenicol.

5. Other resistant bacteria may be included if they are judged by the infection control team to be of special clinical and epidemiologic significance.

Pediculosis

Pharyngitis, infectious, in infants and young children

Pneumonia, viral, in infants and young children

Pneumonia, *Staphylococcus aureus* or group A *Streptococcus*

Rabies

Rubella, congenital and other

Scabies

Scalded skin syndrome, staphylococcal (Ritter's disease)

Skin, wound, or burn infection, major (draining and not covered by dressing or dressing does not adequately contain the purulent material) including those infected with *Staphylococcus aureus* or group A *Streptococcus*

Vaccinia (generalized and progressive eczema vaccination)

(continued)

Box 11–4   CDC Guidelines for Isolation Precautions (continued)

Respiratory isolation

Respiratory isolation is designed to prevent transmission of infectious diseases primarily over short distances through the air (droplet transmission). Direct and indirect contact transmission occurs with some infections in this isolation category but is infrequent.

Specifications for respiratory isolation:

1. Private room is indicated. In general, clients infected with the same organism may share a room.

2. Masks are indicated for those who come close to the client.

3. Gowns are not indicated.

4. Gloves are not indicated.

5. Hands must be washed after touching the client or potentially contaminated articles and before taking care of another client.

6. Articles contaminated with infected material should be discarded or bagged and labeled before being sent for decontamination and reprocessing.

Diseases requiring respiratory isolation:

Epiglottitis, *Hemophilus influenzae*

Erythema infectiosum

Measles

Meningitis

Hemophilus influenzae, known or suspected
Meningococcal, known or suspected

Meningococcal pneumonia

Meningococcemia

Mumps

Pertussis (whooping cough)

Pneumonia, *Hemophilus influenzae,* in children (any age)

Tuberculosis isolation (AFB isolation)

Tuberculosis isolation (AFB isolation) is an isolation category for clients with pulmonary TB who have a positive sputum smear or a chest x-ray that strongly suggests current (active) TB. Laryngeal TB is also included in this isolation category. In general, infants and young children with pulmonary TB do not require isolation precautions because they rarely cough and their bronchial secretions contain few acid-fast bacilli (AFB) compared with adults with pulmonary TB. On the instruction card, this category is called AFB isolation to protect the client's privacy.

Specifications for tuberculosis isolation (AFB isolation):

1. Private room with special ventilation is indicated; door should be kept closed. In general, clients infected with the same organism may share a room.

2. Masks are indicated only if the client is coughing and does not reliably cover mouth.

3. Gowns are indicated only if needed to prevent gross contamination of clothing.

4. Gloves are not indicated.

5. Hands must be washed after touching the client or potentially contaminated articles and before taking care of another client.

6. Articles are rarely involved in transmission of TB. However, articles should be thoroughly cleaned and disinfected, or discarded.

Enteric precautions

Enteric precautions are designed to prevent infections that are transmitted by direct or indirect contact with feces. Hepatitis A is included in this category because it is spread through feces, although the disease is much less likely to be transmitted after the onset of jaundice. Most infections in this category primarily cause gastrointestinal symptoms, but some do not. For example, feces from clients infected with poliovirus and coxsackieviruses are infective, but these infections do not usually cause prominent gastrointestinal symptoms.

Specifications for enteric precautions:

1. Private room is indicated if client hygiene is poor. A client with poor hygiene does not wash hands after touching infective material, contaminates the environment with infective material, or shares contaminated articles with other clients. In general, clients infected with the same organism may share a room.

2. Masks are not included.

3. Gowns are indicated if soiling is likely.

4. Gloves are indicated if touching infective material.

5. Hands must be washed after touching the client or potentially contaminated articles and before taking care of another client.

6. Articles contaminated with infective material should be discarded or bagged and labeled before being sent for decontamination and reprocessing.

Diseases requiring enteric precautions:

Amebic dysentery

Cholera

Coxsackievirus disease

Diarrhea, acute illness and suspected infectious etiology

Echovirus disease

Encephalitis (unless known not to be caused by enteroviruses)

Enterocolitis caused by *Clostridium difficile* or *Staphylococcus aureus*

Enteroviral infection

Gastroenteritis caused by:
　　Campylobacter species
　　Cryptosporidium species
　　Dientamoeba fragilis
　　Escherichia coli (enterotoxic, enteropathogenic, or enteroinvasive)
　　Giardia lamblia
　　Salmonella species
　　Shigella species
　　Vibro parahaemolyticus
　　Viruses, including Norwalk agent and rotavirus

Enteric precautions (continued)

> *Yersinia enterocolitica*
> Unknown etiology but presumed to be an infectious agent

Hand, foot, and mouth disease

Hepatitis, viral, type A

Herpangina

Meningitis, viral (unless known not to be caused by enteroviruses)

Necrotizing enterocolitis

Pleurodynia

Poliomyelitis

Typhoid fever *(Salmonella typhi)*

Viral pericarditis, myocarditis, or meningitis (unless known not to be caused by enteroviruses)

Drainage/secretion precautions

Drainage/secretion precautions are designed to prevent infections that are transmitted by direct or indirect contact with purulent material or drainage from an infected body site. This newly created isolation category includes many infections formerly included in wound and skin precautions, discharge (lesion), and secretion (oral) precautions, which have been discontinued. Infectious diseases included in this category are those that result in the production of infective purulent material, drainage, or secretions, unless the disease is included in another isolation category that requires more rigorous precautions. For example, minor or limited skin, wound, or burn infections are included in this category, but major skin, wound or burn infections are included in contact isolation.

Specifications for drainage/secretion precautions:

1. Private room is not indicated.

2. Masks are not indicated.

3. Gowns are indicated if soiling is likely.

4. Gloves are indicated for touching infective material.

5. Hands must be washed after touching the client or potentially contaminated articles and before taking care of another client.

6. Articles contaminated with infective material should be discarded or bagged and labeled before being sent for decontamination and reprocessing.

Diseases requiring drainage/secretion precautions:

The following infections are examples of those included in this category provided they are not (a) caused by multiple-resistant microorganisms, (b) major (draining and not covered by a dressing or dressing does not adequately contain the drainage) skin, wound, or burn infections, including those caused by *Staphylococcus aureus* or group A *Streptococcus,* or (c) gonococcal eye infections in newborns. See contact isolation if the infection is one of these three.

Abscess, minor or limited

Burn infection, minor or limited

Conjunctivitis

Decubitus ulcer, infected, minor or limited

Skin infection, minor or limited

Wound infection, minor or limited

Blood/body fluid precautions

Blood/body fluid precautions are designed to prevent infections that are transmitted by direct or indirect contact with infective blood or body fluids. Infectious diseases included in this category are those that result in the production of infective blood or body fluids, unless the disease is included in another isolation category that requires more rigorous precaution, eg, strict isolation. For some diseases included in this category, such as malaria, only blood is infective; for other diseases, such as hepatitis B (including antigen carriers), blood and body fluids (saliva, semen, etc) are infective.

Specifications for blood/body fluid precautions:

1. Private room is indicated if client hygiene is poor. A client with poor hygiene does not wash hands after touching infective material, contaminates the environment with infective material, or shares contaminated articles with other clients. In general, clients infected with the same organism may share a room.

2. Masks are not indicated.

3. Gowns are indicated if soiling of clothing with blood or body fluids is likely.

4. Gloves are indicated for touching blood or body fluids.

5. Hands must be washed immediately if they are potentially contaminated with blood or body fluids and before taking care of another client.

6. Articles contaminated with blood or body fluids should be discarded or bagged and labeled before being sent for decontamination and reprocessing.

7. Care should be taken to avoid needle-stick injuries. Used needles should not be recapped or bent; they should be placed in a prominently labeled, puncture-resistant container designed specifically for such disposal.

8. Blood spills should be cleaned up promptly with a solution of 5.25% sodium hypochlorite diluted 1:10 with water.

Diseases requiring blood/body fluid precautions:

Acquired immune deficiency syndrome (AIDS)

Arthropod-borne viral fevers (for example, dengue, yellow fever, and Colorado tick fever)

Babesiasis

Creutzfeldt–Jakob disease

Hepatitis B (including HBsAg antigen carrier)

Hepatitis, non-A, non-B

Leptospirosis

Malaria

Rat-bite fever

Relapsing fever

Syphilis, primary and secondary with skin and mucous membrane lesions

*A private room with special ventilation is indicated.

SOURCE: Adapted from CDC Guidelines for Isolation Precautions in Hospitals. *Infection Control* 1983; 4:245–290.

Chapter Highlights

The relation between host and organism varies from mutually beneficial to seriously harmful, depending on the host's condition and the type of organism.

A series of events is necessary for an infection to occur: a disease-producing agent, a reservoir, a portal of exit, a mode of transmission, a portal of entry, and a susceptible host.

Although susceptibility is not entirely understood, it depends on several factors, including virulence and number of organisms, age and general health, nutritional status, and the immune system's ability to destroy the invading organisms.

Susceptibility to disease is also influenced by psychosocial/lifestyle factors such as finances, environment, occupation, avocation, recreation, and stress.

A person with an impaired immune system is referred to as a compromised host.

The majority of nosocomial (hospital-acquired) infections occur when an organism normally present in a client overwhelms an impaired immune system; the remainder is acquired from organisms in the hospital environment.

Nurses have a major role in disease control through promoting prevention and public education.

Nurses should assess clients before immunization and instruct them about possible side effects.

Because most infections begin with nonspecific symptoms, a thorough history and physical assess-ment can help in arriving at a diagnosis. The absence of findings is often clinically significant.

Assessing the client's and family's attitudes toward the infectious disease is essential in determining psychosocial needs.

Clients with infectious disease often feel inadequate or inferior and shun social contact. Because of the stigma attached to infectious disease, clients may be shunned by others.

Gram's stain and laboratory cultures of specimens are two common diagnostic studies. Sensitivity determinations are often made to select an appropriate antimicrobial.

Nurses should employ direct measures to prevent or limit nosocomial infections in all clients.

In addition to providing physiological support and promoting comfort, monitoring antimicrobial therapy is an important nursing responsibility.

Advising clients and their families on how to administer antimicrobials safely and avoid misuse helps to ensure that clients are not deprived of the use of a valuable drug when needed.

The CDC recommendations for the isolation of infected clients should be followed to reduce the risk of cross-transmission of organisms between clients and personnel or via personnel to other clients.

Because isolation may lead to withdrawal and sensory deprivation, the nurse must meet the client's need for stimulation.

Bibliography

Arking LM, McArthur BJ (editors): Symposium on infection control. *Nurs Clin North Am* 1980; 15(4):651–908.

Benenson AS (editor): *Control of Communicable Diseases in Man,* 14th ed. Washington, DC: American Public Health Association, 1985.

Brooks PM et al: Problems of antibiotic therapy in the elderly. *J Am Geriatr Society* (March) 1984; 32:36–41.

Carroll M: Infection control in long-term care. *Geriatr Nurs* (March) 1984; 5:100–103.

Centers for Disease Control: *Guidelines for the Prevention and Control of Nosocomial Infections.* Atlanta: US Department of Health and Human Services, Public Health Service, 1984.

Corman LC: The relationship between nutrition, infection, and immunity. *Med Clin North Am* 1985; 69(3):519–531.

Derore W, Jackson V, Piening S: TORCH infections. *Am J Nurs* 1983; 83:1660–1665.

Garner J, Simmons B: CDC guidelines for isolation precautions in hospitals. *Infect Control* 1983; 4:245–325.

Hargiss CO, Larson E: Guidelines for prevention of hospital-acquired infection. *Am J Nurs* 1981; 81:2175–2183.

Jackson MM, Lynch P: Isolation practices: A historical perspective. *Am J Infect Control* (Feb) 1985; 13:21–31.

Keithley J: Infection and the malnourished patient. *Heart Lung* 1983; 12:23–27.

Kochar M: *Textbook of General Medicine.* New York: Wiley Medical, 1983.

Kottra C: Infection in the compromised host: An overview. *Heart Lung* 1983; 12:10–14.

Pfaff SJ, Terry BA: Discharge planning: Infection prevention and control in the home. *Nurs Clin North Am* 1980; 15(4)896–903.

Quinn T: Precautions for patients hospitalized with acquired immunodeficiency syndrome. *Infect Control* 1983; 4:79–80.

Rodman MJ, Smith DW: *Clinical Pharmacology in Nursing,* 3rd ed. Philadelphia: Lippincott, 1984.

Sen P, Kapila R, Chmel H, Armstrong DA, Louria DB: Superinfection: Another look. *Am J Med* 1982; 73:706–717.

Soule B (editor): *The ADIC Curriculum for Infection Control Practice*. Dubuque, IA: Kendall/Hunt, 1983.

Tortora GJ, Funke BR, Case CL: *Microbiology*, 2nd ed. Menlo Park, CA: Benjamin/Cummings, 1986.

Wehrle P, Top F: *Communicable and Infectious Diseases*. St. Louis: Mosby, 1981.

Williams WW: Guidelines for infection control in hospital personnel. *Infect Control* 1983; 4:326–349.

Suggested Readings

Alexander J et al: The influence of hair removal methods on wound infections. *JAMA* 1983; 118:347–352. The influence of shaving versus clipping preoperative wounds was studied in 1013 patients. Clipping hair the morning of surgery was found to have the lowest infection rate.

Cunha B: Nosocomial urinary tract infections. *Heart Lung* 1983; 11:545–551. A comprehensive review of nosocomial urinary tract infection. The pathogenesis, indications for catheterization, and methods to reduce infection rates are reviewed.

Dobson J: IV tube changing: 24 or 48 hours? *NITA* 1981; 4:349–350. Discussion of the CDC recommendations on intravenous tubing changes. Also reviewed are studies challenging the CDC's recommendations and protocol for a 48-hour tubing change.

Eron C: *The Virus That Ate Cannibals: Six Great Medical Detective Stories*. New York: Macmillan, 1981. These six nonfiction stories chart the adventures of scientific virologist sleuths and their attempts to understand and combat yellow fever, polio, RNA viruses that cause cancer in laboratory animals, herpes, the common cold, and the slow-virus disease called kuru (the title story).

Hotter A: Physiologic aspects and clinical implications of wound healing. *Heart Lung* 1982; 11:522–531. A thorough review of wound healing with emphasis on client disease states that alter normal physiological events.

Nichols R: Techniques known to prevent postoperative wound infection. *Infect Control* 1982; 3:34–37. A discussion of factors relating to wound infection: antibiotics, preoperative stay, preoperative shower and scrub, surgical gloves, shaves, instruments, drapes, length of surgery, and environment.

Roderick M (editor): Infection control in critical care. *CCQ* 1980; 2:1–108. A collection of nine articles on infection in critical care.

Roueche B: *The Medical Detectives*. New York: Times Books, 1980. Often fascinating nonfiction stories describe how epidemiologists from the CDC and local health departments track down sources of infection.

Resources

(Resources for AIDS are in Chapter 28 and resources for sexually transmitted diseases are in Chapters 63 and 66.)

ORGANIZATIONS

Bureau of Epidemiology
Centers for Disease Control

US Public Health Service
Atlanta, GA 30333
> This arm of the CDC distributes weekly "blue sheets," updates on quarantinable diseases worldwide. It also publishes *Morbidity and Mortality Weekly Report* (MMWR), which contains data on the incidence of specific notifiable diseases and the deaths from these diseases (usually organized by state).

International Association for Medical
Assistance to Travelers (IAMAT)
Empire State Building
350 Fifth Ave., Suite 5620
New York, NY 10001
Phone: (212) 279-6465

In Canada:
1268 St Clair Ave., West
Toronto, Ontario, Canada M6E 1B9
Phone: (416) 654-8291
> This organization provides medical assistance to travelers, provides a directory of English-speaking physicians worldwide who can be reached 24 hours a day, and offers information on local sanitation and required immunizations. No fee, but donations are accepted.

Pan American World Health Organization
525 23rd St., NW
Washington, DC 20037
> This is the World Health Organization Regional Office for the Americas. It coordinates international health efforts in North, Central, and South America.

Public Health Service Advisory Committee
on Immunization Practices (ACIP)
Centers for Disease Control
US Public Health Service
Atlanta, GA 30333
> A resource for the latest information on immunization, available vaccines, and ongoing research. Will provide current recommendations regarding specific infectious diseases.

World Health Organization (WHO)
Palais de la Santé
Geneva, Switzerland
> The organization responsible for coordinating international health efforts according to international health regulations.

HOT LINE

Worldwide Health Forecast
Phone: (800) 368-3531 (24-hr toll-free number)
> This travelers' information service is provided by Health Care Abroad, a Washington, DC, company that is the USA's major supplier of travelers' health insurance. A 2½ minute recording, changed weekly, provides medical alerts as well as weather and political news about more than 100 countries. Information is obtained from the CDC, the WHO, and the Department of State. Consultants are also available to answer questions about specific countries.

HEALTH EDUCATION INFORMATION

Copies of the two-volume *The ADIC Curriculum for Infection Control Practice* (1983) can be obtained from the Association for Practitioners in Infection Control (see Professional Organization). The cost is $55 for members and $65 for nonmembers, with the association paying for postage if a check is enclosed with the order.

Copies of *CDC Guideline for Isolation Precautions in Hospitals* (1983), can be obtained for $5.50 from:
Superintendent of Documents
US Government Printing Office
Washington, DC 20402
In ordering, ask for GPO #017-023-00148-5.

Copies of *Control of Communicable Diseases in Man* by A. S. Benenson (14th ed., 1985) can be obtained for about $10 from:
American Public Health Association
1015 15th St., NW
Washington, DC 20005

From: Channing L. Bete, Inc.
45 Federal St.
Greenfield, MA 01301
Phone: (413) 774-2301

Isolation, a booklet explaining why isolation is sometimes necessary, including common rules and procedures in isolation. To help further understanding of clients, their families, and friends.

SPECIALTY ORGANIZATION

Association for Practitioners in
Infection Control
505 E. Hawley St.
Mundelein, IL 60060
Phone: (312) 949-6050

APIC is open to physicians, nurses, and others concerned with infection control problems. APIC holds an annual meeting in the spring.

Chapter 12

Cancer

Rosemary Polomano
Dee Wonch

Objectives

When you have finished studying this chapter, you should be able to:

Summarize the impact of recent trends in cancer care on survival rates.

Differentiate between characteristics of benign and malignant neoplasia.

Compare various theories of cancer causation.

Discuss the nurse's role in primary and secondary prevention.

Relate the importance of nutrition to cancer prevention and causation.

Describe the basic principles of each major treatment modality: surgery, chemotherapy, radiation therapy, and immunotherapy.

Analyze the biological and psychosocial responses to cancer in the early and late phases of illness.

Identify the common side effects of chemotherapy and radiation therapy, appropriate nursing interventions, and expected client outcomes.

Explain the assessment parameters and associated nursing implications of oncologic emergencies.

Discuss the nurse's role in the psychosocial aspects of cancer care.

In 1986, an estimated 930,000 Americans faced a diagnosis of cancer. Of these, about 350,000 or three out of eight could expect to still be alive 5 years after the diagnosis (American Cancer Society, 1986). Although these statistics may seem discouraging, great strides continue to be made in cancer treatment and research. In the past, some forms of leukemia, testicular cancer, and lymphomas were almost always fatal. Today, with effective combination chemotherapy regimens and advancements in radiotherapy techniques, the potential for long-term cure of these cancers has improved. Fifteen years ago, many clients with breast cancer not cured by surgery alone could expect a short survival of less than 5 years. Currently, many women with breast cancer (even with spread of the disease) live significantly longer as a result of chemotherapy and hormonal manipulation. With these advancements, metastatic breast cancer can now in many cases be considered a chronic illness.

Nevertheless, pessimistic perceptions about cancer remain. Many clients still perceive a cancer diagnosis to be a sentence to a painful, lingering death—a series of mutilating surgeries accompanied by therapies "worse than the disease." A newly diagnosed cancer client is likely to be plagued with fear, well founded in society's attitudes and beliefs toward cancer and reinforced by personal experiences with others having cancer. Almost everyone knows someone who has had terminal cancer. Clients tend to relate the cancer experience of others to themselves, particularly when those experiences involved loved ones.

When caring for a newly diagnosed client, be sensitive to their fears and concerns while stressing the individual nature of this disease and its response to therapy. This approach may discourage clients from interpreting the experiences of others as their own. Public and professional education are necessary to dispel the strong associations of cancer with pain, suffering, and death. Helping clients to understand their disease, maximize their potential for living, cope with the effects of therapy, live with the fear of recurrence, and face imminent death with dignity and comfort makes oncology nursing a special challenge.

Oncology nursing is a specialty. Yet every nurse encounters and cares for clients with cancer in all phases from diagnosis to the end stage of the disease. Nurses see the woman in the surgeon's waiting room who has just been instructed to arrange for a biopsy for the lump she found in her breast, the client on a medical unit receiving chemotherapy or radiation therapy in hopes of controlling or arresting the disease, and the client at home in the terminal phase of illness.

By becoming thoroughly familiar with the neoplastic process, its physiologic and psychosocial effects, its forms and their prognoses, its treatments and their side effects, the nurse can help clients participate actively in the management of their disease and avoid the despair that so often accompanies it. Comprehensive care of the client with neoplastic disease meets the needs of the body while offering solace and encouragement to the human spirit. As this chapter demonstrates, cancer is a multisystem stressor. The care of clients with specific forms of cancer is discussed in Units Three through Thirteen.

Section I: Incidence and Trends

The poor survival rate at least partially explains the extreme apprehension a diagnosis of cancer evokes. Yet survival has improved over the long prevailing rate of one in three. The improvement in percentages may not seem significant (37.5% compared to 33.3%, a difference of only 4.2%). Yet, for 1985 alone, the improved survival rate means that 50,000 more persons will survive beyond the fifth year.

It is important to remember that 5-year survival is not synonymous with cure. Moreover, cancer, the second leading cause of death in the United States, is not one disease but many. Some forms of cancer are far more common than others (Figure 12–1), and survival rates vary widely, from far better than the overall average to far worse. For example, the 5-year survival rate for cancer of the breast, the most common cancer among women, is 65%; breast cancer accounts for 26% of cases of cancer in women

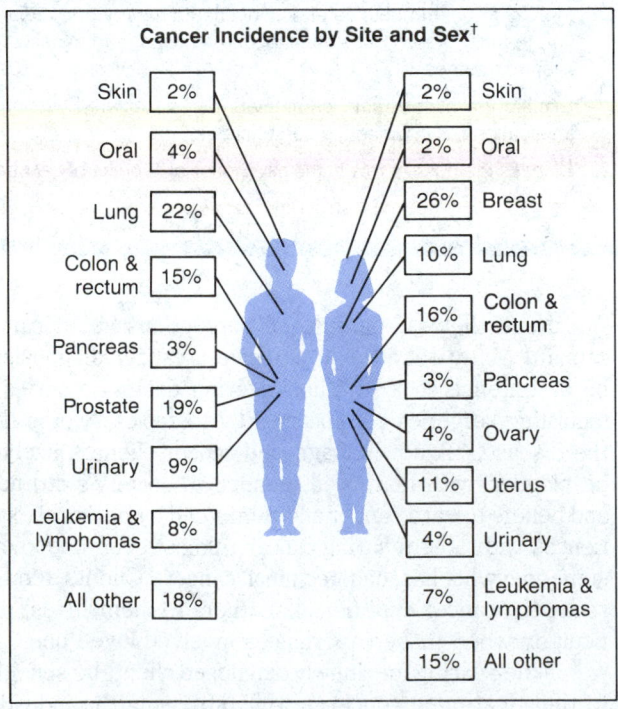
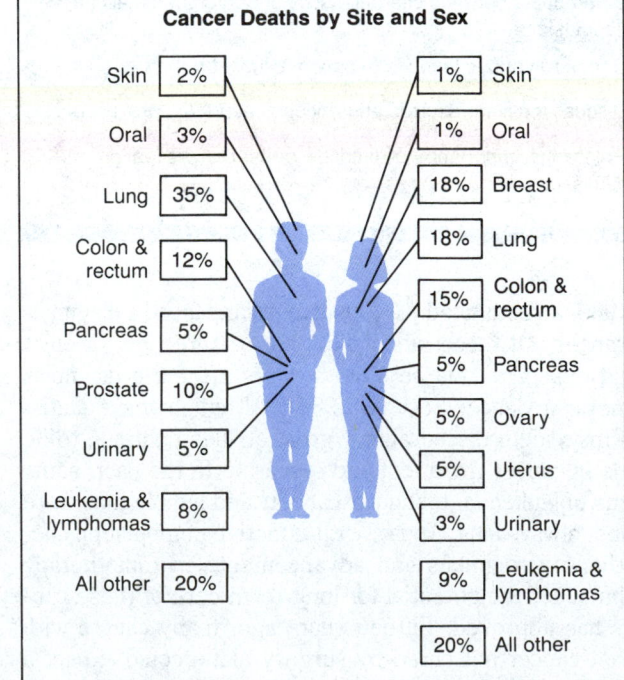

†Excluding nonmelanoma skin cancer and carcinoma in situ.

Figure 12–1

Estimates of cancer incidence and deaths by site and sex, 1985.

SOURCE: American Cancer Society: *Cancer Facts and Figures*. New York: American Cancer Society, 1985.

and 18% of female cancer deaths. The 5-year survival rate for cancer of the lung, the most common cancer affecting men, is only 10%. And for cancer of the pancreas, a relatively rare disease accounting for only 3% of male and female cancers, the 5-year survival rate is only 1%. Table 12–1 shows estimates of cancer incidence and cancer deaths for 1985. Figure 12–2 shows 5-year survival rates for various malignant neoplasia.

These differences reflect many factors, including the etiology and course of the various forms of neoplasia, the effectiveness of screening techniques in early detection of particular forms of cancer, and the efficacy of treatment modes. The general psychological and physical health of the individual client are also factors affecting survival. These issues will be discussed later in this chapter.

Cancer accounts for nearly 21% of all deaths in the United States. Although the probability of a 5-year survival after a diagnosis of cancer is better than in the past, the national rate of deaths from cancer has gradually but steadily risen since 1930. The number of cancer deaths per 100,000 population was 143 in 1930; in 1981, it had increased to 167 per 100,000 population. In 1985 it was estimated that about 462,000 persons would die of cancer, compared to an estimated 452,000 persons in 1984. Although the mortality rates for some cancers have been declining (eg, gastric and uterine cancers), the mortality rate for lung cancer has increased. In fact, it has risen so steeply that

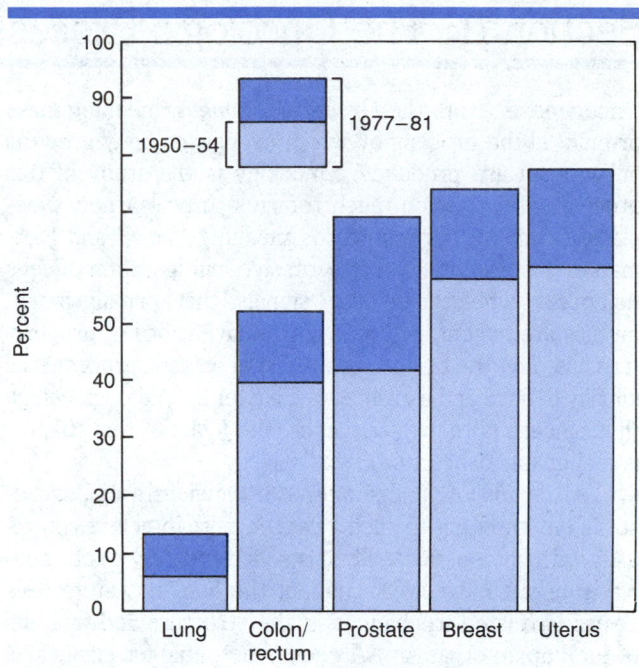

Figure 12–2

Five-year cancer survival rates: trends for selected sites (1950–54 to 1977–81).
SOURCE: American Cancer Society. *Cancer Facts and Figures.* New York: American Cancer Society, 1985.

Table 12–1	Estimated New Cases and Deaths for Major Sites of Cancer, 1985*	
Site	Number of Cases	Deaths
Lung	144,000	126,000
Colon-rectum	138,000	60,000
Breast (female)	119,000	38,000
Prostate	86,000	26,000
Urinary	60,000	20,000
Uterus	52,000**	10,000
Oral	29,000	10,000
Pancreas	25,000	24,000
Leukemia	25,000	17,000
Skin	22,000***	7,000
Ovary	19,000	12,000

*Figures rounded to nearest 1000.

**If carcinoma in situ is included, cases total over 100,000.

***Estimated new cases of nonmelanoma over 400,000.

SOURCE: American Cancer Society. *Cancer Facts and Figures.* New York: American Cancer Society, 1985, p 15.

the overall increase in mortality for the entire category of cancer may be attributed to lung cancer alone (American Cancer Society, 1985).

The incidence of cancer is higher in men than in women. Moreover, both incidence and mortality rates for men are increasing, and those for women—except for lung cancer—are decreasing. When age is considered, however, the picture is altered. The incidence of cancer in women aged 20 to 40 is three times that for men in the same age group.

Both incidence and mortality are higher for black Americans than for whites. Cancers of the lung, colon, rectum, prostate, and esophagus have increased slightly in the black population. Studies attribute this higher rate to socioeconomic and environmental factors rather than biological factors.

The relation of age, sex, and cultural groups to both the incidence and mortality statistics are useful indicators for identifying high-risk populations, monitoring the success of prevention and detection programs, and evaluating the effectiveness of educational efforts and cancer treatment modalities. These statistics are also helpful in suggesting the future direction of oncology nursing. Understanding the process by which neoplasms develop is also essential to any approach to prevention, diagnosis, or treatment.

Section II: The Oncologic Process

Oncogenesis (from the Greek word *onkos,* meaning mass or bulk) is the process by which neoplasms (new growths or tumors) are produced. Oncology is the study of this process, about which much remains to be learned. Neoplasia (from the Greek words meaning "new" and "formation") is essentially a progressive multiplication of cells that occurs when the cellular "signals" that normally inhibit mitosis are absent, altered, not received, or not properly translated by the target cells. (The neoplastic process was initially defined and explained in Chapter 2.) Although benign (noncancerous) neoplasia occur, the focus of this chapter is malignant (cancerous) neoplasia.

All forms of cancer alter the individual's biopsychosocial environment to such a degree as to interfere continually with homeostasis. The presence and growth of a neoplasm creates stress throughout the human system; this stress is related to changes in the structure and function of the human organism. A client's potential for survival is clearly related to how effectively the bodily defenses of the individual respond to this multisystem assault. This response may vary in the same individual according to both internal and external influences (see Chapter 2).

Early diagnosis is the most important single factor affecting a favorable prognosis or cure. The method of treatment as well as its timing also clearly affects the prognosis. In 1985, an estimated 160,000 persons could have been saved if their cancers had been diagnosed and treated earlier. The importance of both diagnosis and treatment is related to the unique characteristics of the cancer cell.

THE CANCER CELL

The cell is the basic unit of life—an entity so complex that hundreds of researchers have not discovered all of its secrets. Although much remains to be learned, it is known that neoplasia, an abnormal growth process, is related to disturbances in normal cell growth, replication, and migration. Understanding the similarities and differences between normal and neoplastic cells is essential to comprehend the overall effects of neoplastic disease on the body.

The life cycle of both normal and neoplastic cells is referred to as the *cell cycle.* It comprises five phases described below and illustrated in Figure 12–3:

- The G_0 (gap 0), or resting phase.
- The G_1 (gap 1) phase, in which RNA and protein are synthesized in preparation for DNA synthesis.
- The S (synthesis) phase, during which DNA is synthesized.
- The G_2 (gap 2) phase, poorly understood, in which preparation for mitosis (splitting) continues, RNA is synthesized, and chromosomes condense.
- The M (mitosis) phase, during which two new cells are formed by the splitting of the original cell. Mitosis

occurs in four major stages: prophase, metaphase, anaphase, and telophase.

Knowledge of cellular growth is important, because these phases and their durations are critical to the treatment of cancer by chemotherapy. Some chemotherapeutic agents are only effective in a specific phase or phases of the cell cycle.

Malignant cells behave much differently than normal cells because of their selective growth advantages and abilities to invade and spread. These distinguishing features are unique and characteristic of the cancer process and are summarized in Table 12–2.

The growth control mechanisms of normal cells are not clearly understood. It is believed, however, that cells stop growing because of cell-to-cell surface contact or "contact inhibition" and because certain locally active substances (not yet identified) act as signals to regulate cell division or replication. Somehow, probably because of quantitative cell-surface changes, malignant cells either do not appropriately receive these messages or are unable to respond to them, allowing progressive growth. Keep in mind that both cancer and normal cells divide at comparable rates (not all cells dividing with equal frequency), meaning that cell cycle growth time is somewhat similar. The loss of effective regulatory control mechanisms is primarily what permits growth in excess of body demands.

Normally, body tissues have a balanced ratio of differentiated cells, capable of differentiation into mature cells, to stem cells or precursor cells. Stem or precursor cells usually remain undifferentiated until injury or aging eliminates cells in normal tissues. The stem cells then produce differentiated daughter cells for regeneration and repair. Neoplastic tumor cells are mutated stem cells that do not

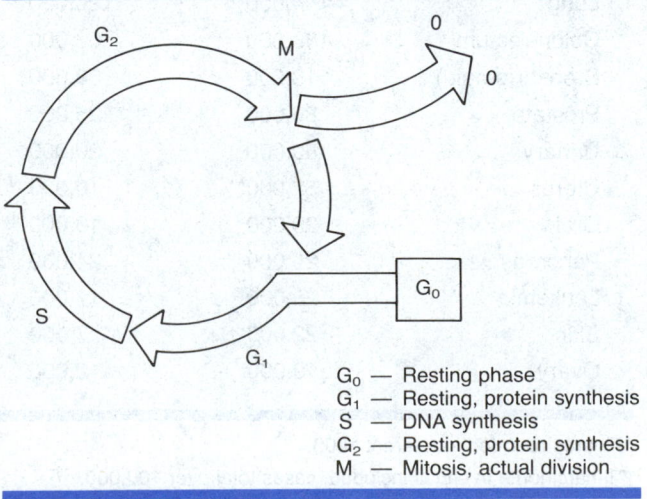

Figure 12–3

The cell cycle.

Table 12–2 Characteristics of Benign and Malignant Neoplasms

Benign Neoplasms	Malignant Neoplasms
Grow slowly	Grow rapidly or very rapidly
Usually are encapsulated	Rarely are encapsulated
Grow by expansion causing minor tissue damage	Grow by expansion as well as infiltration of surrounding tissue, causing marked changes, inflammation, ulceration, and necrosis
Show little or no tendency to recur when surgically removed	Show a strong tendency to recur when surgically removed if residual tumor remains
Do not spread, remain localized	Spread or metastasize to adjacent and distant structures by direct extension, lymphatics, blood, and implantation
Microscopically resemble tissue of origin	Usually differ in appearance from tissue of origin in varying degrees
Produce little or no generalized symptoms unless affecting the endocrine glands	Produce generalized symptoms such as cachexia and weight loss
Generally do not cause death unless pressure or obstruction of vital structures occurs	Usually cause death from spread to vital organs

respond to the structural and chemical signals that normally regulate the replication of cells (Figure 12–4). The degree of undifferentiation varies, and the most undifferentiated-appearing cells are also called "anaplastic cells."

The aggressive growth patterns of some tumors compared with others may be related to the ratio of stem cells to differentiated ones, as well as to cell death rate. For example, when malignant neoplasms have a large number of stem cells in comparison to differentiated cells, coupled with a low cell death rate, then overall tumor growth may be rapid. Conversely, if there are small differences in numbers of stem cells to differentiated cells and increased cell death, the tumor mass may grow more slowly. At best, this explanation may account for varying tumor growth rates. In summary, a major factor in the rate of tumor growth is the percentage of actively dividing stem cells in the tumor at any given time—the higher the percentage, the faster the tumor grows.

In general, once the neoplastic tumor cells outgrow the available blood supply, malignant cells tend to revert to the resting phase (G_0) or die. The overall tumor growth slows. Moreover, inactive cells are less responsive to some forms of treatment, strongly supporting the concept that the tumor response to chemotherapy is invariably poorer with large tumor masses than with smaller ones.

Another unique feature, the highly invasive property of malignant cells, results from the production of proteolytic enzymes, one of which may be hyaluronidase, released at the margin of the tumor and normal tissue (Nowell, 1982). These enzymes literally digest surrounding tissue—a phenomenon reflected in the popular phrase, "eaten up by cancer." A benign tumor is usually clearly delineated from normal tissue, whereas a malignant tumor has no boundaries (Figure 12–5).

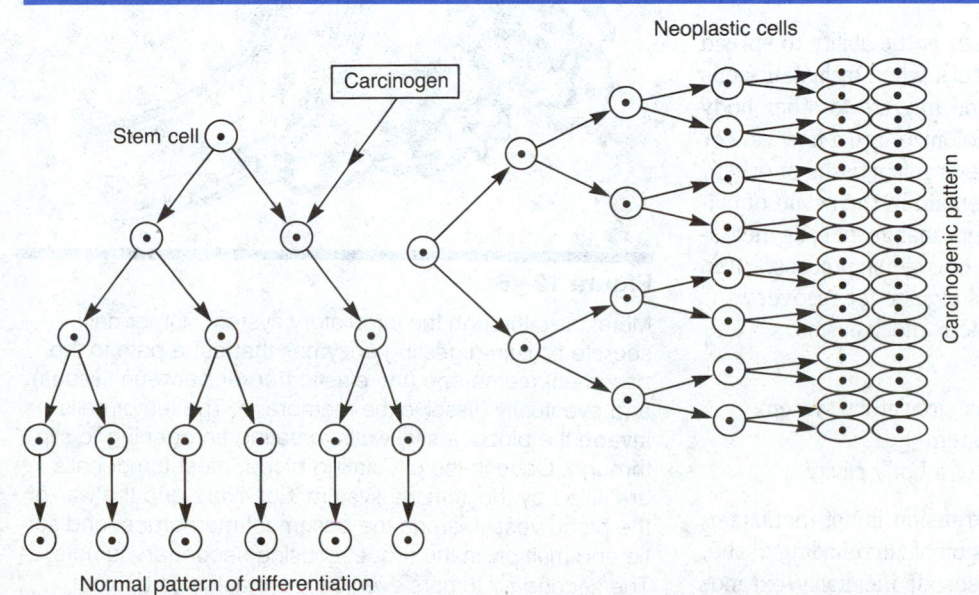

Figure 12–4

Carcinogenesis. The carcinogen causes a stem cell to mutate. The mutated stem cell produces neoplastic tumor cells with an aggressive growth pattern.

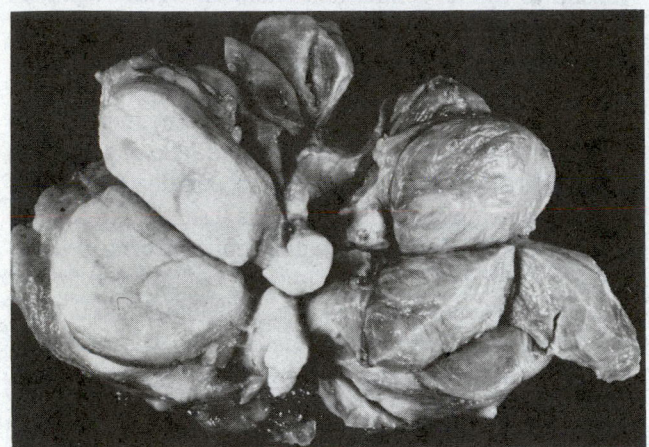

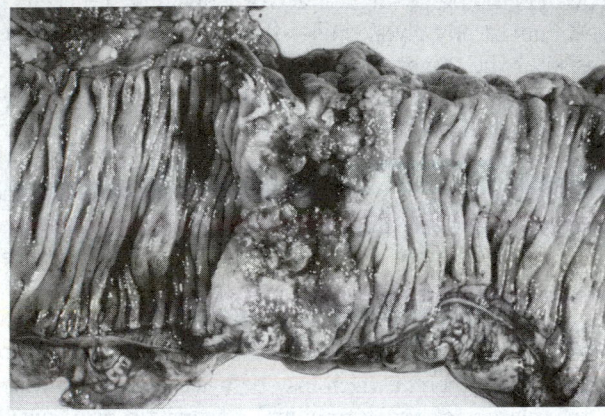

Figure 12–5

Benign and malignant neoplasms. **Top.** Multiple benign leiomyomas of the uterus. These are encapsulated. **Bottom.** Infiltrating adenocarcinoma of the colon (center). Surrounding it is normal lumen of the colon. (Courtesy of Surgical Pathology Department, Hospital of the University of Pennsylvania)

A final characteristic of cancer is the ability to spread or metastasize. **Metastasis** occurs when malignant cells detach from the parent tissue and migrate to other body tissues. These malignant cells colonize into a new cancer cell mass that grossly reflects the primary tissue of origin. Usually, normal daughter cells remain in the tissue of origin. Benign cells do not spread, but malignant cells metastasize and can do so early in the oncogenic process, often negatively influencing the client's chance for recovery.

Metastasis occurs through four mechanisms:

- By direct extension
- By way of the arteriovenous circulatory system
- By way of the lymphatic system
- By implantation or seeding of a body cavity

Strictly speaking, direct extension is not metastasis to a distant site; rather, it is invasion of surrounding tissue. As the mass of a tumor increases, it inevitably extends into adjacent areas. Muscle tissue and connective tissue

initially act as barriers to extension, but in time, these, too, are invaded by the neoplasm.

A convenient route for migration of malignant cells is the arteriovenous circulatory system (Figure 12–6). Neoplastic microemboli migrate to the small capillary beds, where growth of a new mass begins. Research has shown that a subpopulation of malignant cells is shed into the bloodstream when a tumor reaches a critical size.

The process of embolization is also the mechanism by which cancer spreads through the lymphatic system. Although lymphatic metastasis is slower than vascular metastasis, it is noteworthy especially because metastasis is often first detected by nodal enlargement.

Cavitary seeding may occur inadvertently during surgery; the surgeon's hand or a surgical implement may transfer tumor cells to a new site. Malignant cells may also

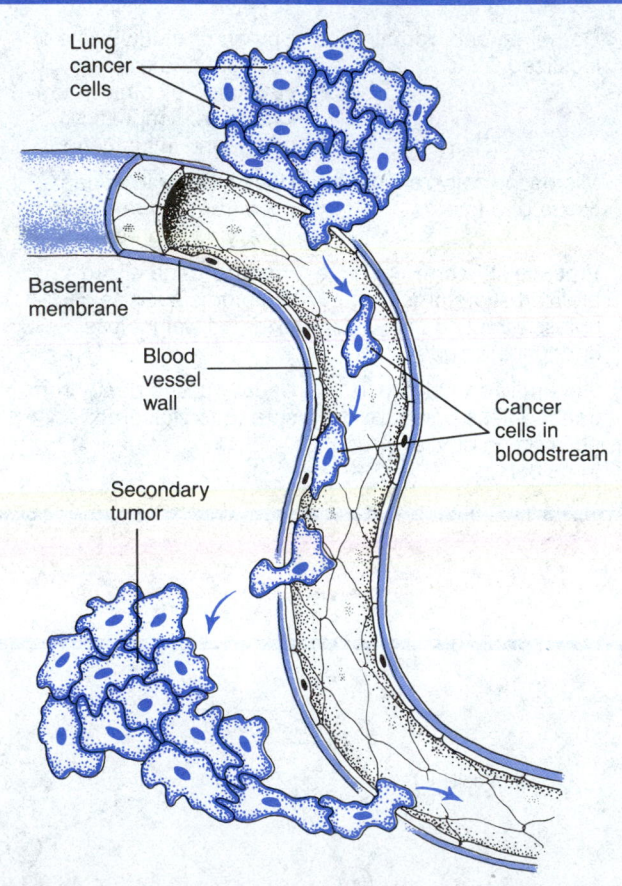

Figure 12–6

Metastasis through the circulatory system. Tumor cells secrete protein-digesting enzymes that cut a path to the basement membrane (the elastic barrier between tissues) and eventually dissolve the membrane. The tumor cells invade the blood vessel walls, creating an opening to slip through. Once in the circulating blood, most tumor cells are killed by the immune system. Survivors grip the wall of the blood vessel, erode the basement membrane, and settle and multiply in the tissue, causing secondary tumors. The secondary tumors eventually metastasize to other locations.

be implanted as a tumor enlarges and extends. In either event, new colonies of malignant cells begin to multiply in cavities of the body, eg, in the peritoneal cavity. Before intracavitary seeding was discovered, surgical procedures could initiate the metastatic process. Today precautions are taken to prevent microembolic seeding and intracavitary spread.

Different forms of cancer have a predilection for metastasis to different sites, depending on such factors as proximity to lymph nodes or blood vessels.

THEORIES OF CAUSATION

Many hypotheses have attempted to explain the origin of cancer. No single theory is universally accepted as the primary explanation for cancer; rather, the current trend in oncologic research supports the likelihood of multiple etiologies. Among the etiologic factors believed to be related to the development of cancer are:

- Viruses
- Oncogenes
- Genetic predisposition, heredity
- Cellular (somatic) mutations
- Environmental carcinogens (cancer-producing agents) such as chemicals, radiation, and dietary substances
- Immunologic factors
- Psychological factors such as stress, lifestyle, and geographic location
- Nutrition

Various forms of cancer have been linked to or attributed to one or more of these factors.

Viral Theory

The viral theory of cancer causation was given new impetus by investigators pursuing an earlier theory that cancer might be hereditary. Because viruses have been shown to cause tumors in exposed animals (eg, the feline leukemia virus in cats), it is possible that tumor viruses also influence the development of cancer in humans. The human T-cell leukemia virus (HTLV-I) has been linked to leukemia, and the Epstein–Barr virus, to Burkitt's lymphoma. In the past, DNA-type viruses were believed to be associated with cancer. Today, evidence suggests RNA-type viruses, or oncoviruses, induce tumorigenesis. This type of virus, also called a retrovirus, incorporates viral RNA into DNA through a process called reverse transcription (Morgan, 1983).

Oncogenes

By the early 1970s, researchers were working toward a unifying theory of cancer causation that hypothesized the existence of **oncogenes**—genetic material that can bring about malignant transformation and is thought to be latent in the chromosomes of some individuals. Oncogene precursors, called proto-oncogenes have been found in normal cells. The term *proto-oncogene* implies the ability of a nor-

mal gene to become oncogenic when altered, either directly or indirectly, by carcinogens such as radiation or chemicals. More recently, viruses have also been implicated in malignant changes caused by oncogenes (see the preceding viral theory section). Oncogenes may be present in the entire population, lying dormant in those who never acquire cancer or becoming activated in the one in four persons who does develop cancer.

Genetics and Heredity

The tendency of specific tumor types to demonstrate patterns of inheritance (eg, breast and colon cancers, and melanoma) led researchers to analyze closely the familial patterns of cancer. The question is whether these patterns are caused by inherited genetic material or by shared environmental exposures among family members. Researchers have already linked chromosomal aberrations to certain cancers; eg, trisomy 21 or Down's syndrome has been linked to leukemia, and the Philadelphia chromosome has been linked to chronic myelogenous leukemia. In addition, oncogenes or virogenes latent in the DNA of host cells can be passed on to subsequent generations, eventually becoming activated and expressing oncogenic characteristics.

Somatic Mutation Theory

The somatic mutation theory rests on the premise that cancer is characterized by qualitative or mutational changes in cellular DNA. These changes are thought to be directly or indirectly related to repeated exposure to carcinogens; ie, a single mutational insult is not sufficient to cause cancer. Rather, successive changes from several mutational insults over the life span create conditions for oncogenesis.

Environmental Theories

It is agreed that 85% of all human cancers are related to environmental carcinogens such as chemicals, radiation, viruses, hormones, and irritants (Groer & Shekleton, 1983). Many substances or agents in the human environment can cause cancer or contribute to its development. These include exogenous chemicals such as polycyclic hydrocarbons, dyes, alkylating agents, urethane, nitrosamines, and polymers; endogenous chemicals such as hormones and cholesterol; ionizing and ultraviolet radiation; irritations from burns and wounds; and substances ingested in foods. Individuals are exposed to these agents through their work in medical treatments and in ordinary pursuits. Some types of exposures are avoidable (cigarette smoking being a notable example); others are not.

Immunologic Factors

The immune system (specifically the T-cell lymphocyte responses) is responsible for eradicating cancerous cells as they arise within the body. Failure of the immune system to respond to these tumor cells, either from an inherent defect or intentional suppression from immunosuppressive treatment, may result in cancer. For example, clients receiving immunosuppressive therapy, such as renal transplant clients, have a higher incidence of cancer than the general population, particularly tumors of suspected viral origin.

Psychological Factors

The association among psychosocial influences, stress, and cancer is unknown. Studies attempting to detect such a relation have been hampered by difficulties in establishing reliable and valid measurement tools, controlling variables, and interpreting apparent biases. Research reports are thus far inconclusive, and there is little information relating cancer to psychological attributes in the literature. Despite the limiting and conflicting data, there is general agreement that psychological determinants affect cancer incidence and survival. Several factors believed to be associated with cancer have been identified. These include unresolved conflicts; personality characteristics; lifestyle changes; loss of a significant other; feelings of hopelessness, helplessness, powerlessness and frustration; psychosomatic disturbances, anxiety, and depression; and sexual disturbances.

The relation of stress to cancer is of growing concern. Immunologic theories of cancer causation have attempted to link stress with changes in the immune mechanisms likely to permit expressions of malignant mutations. Early reports cited by Oppenheimer (1982) propose that stress may damage or alter the immune response, creating a favorable environment for the development of cancer. Because of the complexity of stress-related neurologic and immunologic responses, specific stress-induced effects are difficult to ascertain, however.

Recently, investigators have tried to confirm a common observation—cancer clients with a strong will to live and a positive attitude survive longer than those who passively accept and submit to their illnesses. The so-called "fighting spirit," or strong desire to live, has been associated with improved survival rates among clients with breast cancer (Derogatis, Abeloff, & Melisaratos, 1979; Greer, Morris, & Pettingale, 1979).

Although psychological factors are believed to play a role in cancer, the extent to which these influence cancer etiology and prognosis remains in question. Future research will perhaps uncover the mystifying effects of psychic attributes on health and illness.

Nutrition and Cancer

The role of nutrition in neoplastic disease has been of growing public concern. Widespread geographic epidemiologic evidence supports the notion that dietary habits play an important role in preventing and causing cancer. For example,

the American diet, high in dietary fat, may be linked to the high incidence of breast and colon cancer, which occur at much lower rates in Asian countries, where dietary fat intake is low. However, in Asian countries including Japan, where the consumption of salted and pickled foods is high, gastric cancer is much commoner than in the United States. It is very difficult to confirm a direct cause-and-effect relation between nutrition and cancer because so many preexisting environmental carcinogens are responsible for cancer.

In search of more information, a Committee on Diet, Nutrition, and Cancer was formed under the direction of the National Cancer Institute to review the scientific data and formulate recommendations. The committee concluded that certain dietary factors are possibly linked to cancer:

- Obese persons tend to be at greater risk for cancer.
- A high-fat diet may increase the risk for cancer of the colon, prostate gland, and breast.
- Dietary fiber may protect against colon cancer. This association is a difficult one to assume because high-fiber diets are generally low in fat.
- High caloric intake may increase the risk for cancer in general because obesity and high fat intake are more likely.
- Carbohydrates show no demonstrable effects on carcinogenesis.

In addition, the American Cancer Society advocates avoiding obesity; cutting down on total fat intake; eating more high-fiber foods; consuming foods rich in vitamins A and C; eating cruciferous vegetables (named for their cross-shaped flowers) such as cabbage, cauliflower, broccoli, brussels sprouts, and kohlrabi; eating less salt-cured, smoked, and nitrite-cured foods; and drinking alcohol in moderation (no more than two drinks a day) if one drinks (American Cancer Society, 1984). A variety of other nutrients and their roles in cancer prevention and causation are outlined in Table 12–3.

PHYSIOLOGIC EFFECTS OF THE ONCOGENIC PROCESS

As a malignant neoplasm develops and grows, many physiologic effects ensue, although millions of cancer cells may form before physical symptoms become apparent. Initially, effects may be localized. Eventually, as the tumor grows, becomes established, and metastasizes, systemic symptoms occur. Although the effects of tumor development vary according to the type of lesion and its location, certain effects are generally characteristic of all malignant neoplasms.

Local Effects

The three major local effects of increase in tumor mass are pressure, erosion of adjacent tissue, and obstruction.

Table 12–3   Common Foods and Their Role in Cancer

	Role in Cancer	Sources	Recommendations	Hazards of Megadoses
Vitamin C	Probably minor. Deficiencies increase risk of stomach and esophageal cancer. Seems to block the conversion of nitrites in smoked and cured meats to carcinogenic nitrosamines	Citrus fruit, tomatoes, strawberries, broccoli, kale, potatoes, cabbage, green peppers, cantaloupe	At least 60 mg daily—the amount in 4 oz of orange juice—especially if eating preserved meats like bacon and ham	More than 1000 mg a day can cause diarrhea, kidney and bladder stones, and problems metabolizing some prescription drugs
Vitamin A	Deficiencies seem to increase the risk of cancer of the lung, cervix, skin, bladder, and colon	Animal foods such as eggs, cheese, and liver. Yellow, orange, and green vegetables contain beta-carotene, which converts to vitamin A	Two or three servings daily of foods rich in vitamin A and beta-carotene	More than 50,000 IU a day for adults can cause dizziness, headache, vomiting, and liver, bone, and brain damage
Vitamin E	Still unknown. Prevents genetic mutations in certain bacteria: these mutations cause cancer in animals. Impedes the formation of nitrosamines in animals	Vegetable oils, margarine, wheat germ, whole grain cereals, bread, liver, dried beans, and leafy green vegetables	At least 10 mg a day (about 1 tablespoon of margarine). Supplements should be used only with medical supervision	May cause high blood pressure, headaches, blurred vision, fatigue, and muscle weakness, and aggravate diabetes and thyroid problems
Selenium	Still uncertain. Animal studies show that it protects against cancers like those of the breast, liver, and colon—but only at levels 25 times higher than people can safely consume	Wheat germ, seafood, egg yolks, chicken, whole grain cereals, milk, and meat	Most people get enough (between 0.05 and 0.20 mg daily) from grains and cereals. Supplements require medical supervision	Very toxic. In humans it can cause nausea and loss of hair, fingernails, and toenails. In animals it can cause death
Zinc	Uncertain. Animal studies suggest that zinc can either enhance or retard the growth of certain cancers	Seafood, meat, poultry, eggs, milk, and whole grains	At least 15 mg daily for adults, the amount found in about half a pound of beef liver, or three 8-oz glasses of milk	Can cause nausea, anemia, stomach pain, premature birth, and stillbirth
Fiber	High-fiber diets may protect against colon cancer because of the fiber itself or because such diets are usually low in fat	Fresh vegetables and fruit, whole grain cereals and bread, beans, nuts, and peas	30 to 40 g a day (at least four slices of whole wheat bread). Substitute high-fiber foods for fatty foods	Intestinal gas, bloating, and diarrhea; can interfere with the body's absorption of important vitamins and minerals
Fat	Increases the risk of breast, colon, and prostate cancer. Studies in both animals and people suggest that polyunsaturated fats seem to pose as great a risk as saturated fats	Saturated fats: fatty meats and lard, butter, cream, cheese, and vegetable shortening. Unsaturated fats: most vegetable oils, fish, nuts	Reduce fat intake. Fats should make up no more than 30% of the calories consumed daily	Excessive weight gain, atherosclerosis and heart disease, and cancer
Protein	Still uncertain, but protein-rich foods are often high in fat, which appears to be carcinogenic	Meat, fish, poultry, eggs, cheese, milk, dried beans and peas, and peanut butter	A third of a gram daily for every pound of body weight; about 6 oz of meat, fish, or poultry for a 150 lb adult, more for children	Extreme thirst, frequent urination, kidney failure. May cause the body to lose calcium

(continued)

Table 12–3	Common Foods and Their Role in Cancer (continued)			
	Role in Cancer	**Sources**	**Recommendations**	**Hazards of Megadoses**
Nitrates and Nitrites	Probably pose a risk only if vitamin C intake is low. Both convert to nitrosamines and cause stomach and esophageal cancer in laboratory animals. Vitamin C prevents this conversion	Nitrites: cured foods like bacon, sausages, and ham. Nitrates: vegetables like spinach and beets	Fewer nitrite-preserved foods, and more foods rich in vitamin C. Nitrate-containing vegetables probably pose no risk in sensible amounts	Stomach and esophageal cancer
Salted and pickled foods	Probably minor in the United States. In Asia, where consumption is high, stomach cancer is common, but that may be due to low vitamin C intake and excess nitrites	Pickled vegetables and meats	For general good health, less salted food. No more than 2000 mg of salt (roughly 1 teaspoon) a day	Excessive thirst. Too much salt raises blood pressure and can cause hypertension
Cholesterol	No known risk at present, but cholesterol-rich foods are often also high in fat, which does cause cancer	Beef liver and kidneys, eggs, shrimp, butter, and mayonnaise	No more than 300 mg a day, roughly the amount in one medium-sized egg	Atherosclerosis, heart attacks, or stroke
Alcohol	Heavy drinking, especially combined with smoking, increases the risk of cancers of the mouth, esophagus, throat, and liver. More than two beers a day is linked with rectal cancer	Wine, beer, and liquor	No more than two drinks a day	High blood pressure, abnormal heart rhythms, damage to heart and muscle cells, liver disease, birth defects
Caffeine	Questionable. Some studies blame a high intake of coffee for bladder and pancreas cancer, although more recent ones fail to confirm the association	Coffee, tea, cola drinks, cocoa, and chocolate	None are possible at present because the evidence is inconclusive	Jitteriness, headaches, upset stomach, heartburn, and general anxiety
Cruciferous vegetables	Seem to reduce the risk of colon, lung, and esophageal cancers, possibly because they block the activity of certain cancer-causing chemicals in laboratory animals	Cabbage, brussels sprouts, kohlrabi, cauliflower, and other members of the mustard (Brassicaceae) family	At least two or three servings a week	Unknown
Artificial sweeteners	Large doses of saccharin cause bladder cancer in animals. At present there is no evidence that aspartame causes cancer in animals or humans	Saccharin, aspartame (found in diet foods and soft drinks)	Moderate saccharin consumption, though researchers have yet to establish danger level. Avoid during pregnancy and early childhood	Unknown
Browned foods	Charring creates chemical substances called mutagens that produce cancer-causing changes in the genes of laboratory animals	Meat, fish, poultry, or other high-protein foods, fried, broiled, or grilled at high temperatures (500° to 600°F)	Avoid charring foods. Bake, stew, simmer, sauté, or poach foods at 200° to 300°F instead	Unknown

SOURCE: Reprinted with permission from: Grady D, Siwolop S: An anti-cancer diet? *Discover* 1984; 5(6):24–25.

As the uncontrolled replication of the cancer cells causes the tumor to grow continually, the enlarging mass causes pressure atrophy in surrounding tissue. Necrosis of normal cells ensues, and tumor cells may also become necrotic as the mass enlarges. These effects are related to the sheer bulk of the tumor mass but also result from the invasive properties of cancer previously discussed. To supply the ever-increasing amounts of nutrients, particularly nitrogen, required by the enlarging tumor, an intricate system of collateral circulation develops. This enhanced vascularity is often a significant factor in diagnosis; eg, vascularity distinguishes a renal neoplasm from a renal cyst, which has no vascular supply. As this circulatory network grows, the risk of hemorrhage increases. The tumor mass may also exert pressure on adjacent organs or may obstruct an organ or the flow of blood or lymph.

Generalized Systemic Effects

The spectrum of local and systemic effects from cancer is manifested in conditions as diverse as the kinds of tumors and their sites. It is important to remember that during the course of the disease, a client may encounter one, many, or all such common physiologic problems as anemia, hemorrhage, infection, cachexia, and pain. The client may experience psychosocial responses ranging from anxiety or depression to profound changes in body image and lifestyle. Keep in mind that the degree of these problems depends on the type and extent of the tumor as well as treatment implications. Neoplastic disease as it affects specific organ systems is discussed in each specific disorders chapter in the body systems units.

Effects originally manifested locally may have systemic sequelae; eg, pressure of a tumor on the optic nerve can cause blindness; pressure on the spinal cord may cause paralysis; and obstruction of the bronchus interferes with respiration. A tumor may cause hypersecretion or hyposecretion of glandular hormones, leading to life-threatening systemic complications; eg, hypersecretion by the parathyroid glands may lead to hypercalcemia.

Probably the most universal systemic effect is cancer's ability to alter immunologic responses. Early in the development of malignant neoplasia, the immune system attempts to defend the host by attacking and destroying antigens on the surface of tumor cells. Eventually, in advanced malignant disease, the immune response is impaired. It is speculated that billions of tumor cells may deplete or overwhelm the immune system, reducing or destroying its capacity to defend the body from other insults such as trauma or infection.

Anemia

Anemia, a common problem for clients with cancer, may be related to the neoplastic process itself or to cancer therapies. Recurrent hemorrhage, malnutrition, or infection may be contributing factors.

Several theories have been proposed to account for the anemia associated with cancer; a mild reduction in the survival capacity of erythrocytes, a level of erythropoietin lower than the existing degree of anemia would explain, and poor responsiveness of apparently normal bone marrow are among the mechanisms proposed. This type of anemia is usually mild, and specific treatment may not be indicated unless the client is symptomatic from the anemia or a correctable contributing cause such as hemorrhage or malnutrition can be identified. Anemia in a client with cancer has diagnostic significance because it indicates extensive disease progression.

Another type of anemia in clients with cancer is associated with tumor invasion of the bone marrow, either as a primary or metastatic site of involvement. Erythrocyte precursor stem cells may be impaired in leukemias, or erythrocyte development may be limited because marrow has been replaced with tumor cells (eg, metastasis from breast tumors and lymphomas). This type of anemia may be severe, necessitating blood replacement therapy.

Tumor-associated autoimmune hemolytic anemia is related to the body's immune defense against red blood cell antigens that have been stimulated by the tumor. The exact cause of this tumor-mediated response remains unknown. Autoimmune hemolytic anemia more often develops in clients with non-Hodgkin's lymphoma and chronic lymphocytic leukemia than in clients with other types of malignancies.

Anemia associated with blood loss is common in clients with gastrointestinal, head and neck, urinary, and uterine malignancies. As the tumor invades vascular structures and erodes tissues, bleeding results. Blood loss may be overt, an early symptom of cancer. The client may seek professional health care advice after noticing blood in the urine or stool or because of irregular vaginal bleeding.

Anemia is associated with many conditions other than cancer; however, because of its frequent association with malignant neoplasia, any anemic condition should be thoroughly investigated. When anemia occurs in a client in whom cancer has already been diagnosed, treatment is necessary to provide the optimal state of health consistent with the client's condition.

Hemorrhage

Spontaneous hemorrhage may occur when a tumor obstructs an organ or blood vessel, impinges on or erodes a blood vessel during growth, or is surgically disrupted or manipulated. Severe bleeding, secondary to thrombocytopenia, may be an initial symptom of some malignancies of blood cells or blood-forming tissues (eg, leukemias, lymphomas, and multiple myeloma). Hemorrhage may be profound and visible or slow and occult. Detection of occult blood in the stool during a routine nursing assessment may signal a previously undetected malignancy.

When hemorrhage occurs, it must be diagnosed promptly. The site of hemorrhage must be quickly determined because emergency measures involve local control of bleeding along with replacement of necessary blood constituents (eg, red blood cells and platelets). Regardless of severity, location, or cause, hemorrhage is a potentially life-threatening condition that must be recognized and treated immediately.

Infection

Any condition that impairs the body's immunologic defenses creates a favorable environment for infection. In clients with cancer, the immune system may be compromised by the disease process, the treatment modality, or both. Infections may be bacterial, fungal, viral, or protozoal. These infections are usually opportunistic, resulting from overgrowth of normal flora (eg, oral candidiasis) or because flora that normally reside in one location gain access elsewhere (eg, *E. coli* septicemia). About 50% of infections in neutropenic clients are caused by gram-negative bacteria, most commonly *E. coli* and *Klebsiella pneumoniae*, normally found in the intestines, and *Pseudomonas aeruginosa*, a common hospital pathogen (the EORTC International Antimicrobial Therapy Project Group, 1978).

No single agent of infection has been found to have a predilection for cancer clients; therefore, it is assumed that predisposing factors related to the client's physiologic status or surroundings govern infection. Common sites of infection in cancer clients are the lungs, gastrointestinal tract, anorectal area, skin, mouth, pharynx, urinary tract, and bloodstream. Although uncommon, the site of infection may be associated with the site of neoplastic lesion.

Infection related to neutropenia and immunosuppressive therapy is a major cause of mortality in clients with cancer. Because immunosuppression depresses or eliminates some of the usual signs of infection, diagnosis may be delayed. Therefore, the client must be observed carefully to detect signs of local infections such as erythema, induration, swelling (remember pus formation may be absent in severely leukopenic clients), pain, cough, and signs of systemic infections including elevated temperature and chills. Prompt therapy for immunologically suppressed clients with infections is essential to prevent life-threatening consequences such as septic shock. Because most infections are bacterial, antibiotic therapy may be instituted at the first sign of infection, even before identification of the causative organism. When anti-infective therapy is not effective in controlling the infection, granulocyte transfusions may be administered to clients who are neutropenic. See Chapter 11 for a complete discussion of infection and related nursing care.

Cachexia

Weight loss, related primarily to decreased caloric intake and in part to the increased metabolic requirements of the multiplying neoplastic cells, is a common initial symptom of cancer. On the other hand, cachexia related to anorexia is a life-threatening complication that usually develops late in the course of the disease. **Cachexia** is a syndrome characterized by anorexia, weakness, and emaciation—the "wasting away" associated with cancer. Cachexia is known to be related to decreased food intake, impaired absorption of nutrients, and alterations in metabolism, but the pathogenesis of the anorexia has not been clearly determined.

Researchers suspect that anorexia is caused from a combination of factors predominantly related to the tumor, therapy, and psychosocial effects. For example, lipid mobilizing factor, believed to be released from tumors, breaks down body fats, resulting in hyperlipidemia, which in turn suppresses the hypothalamic appetite center. Additionally, the tumor itself may directly release noxious substances leading to nausea and anorexia. Among the factors believed to be associated with anorexia in clients with cancer are:

- Pain, fever, nausea, and other nonspecific manifestations
- Intestinal obstruction
- Alterations in metabolism
- Toxins produced by neoplastic tumors
- Lipid mobilizing factor
- Ketosis (see Chapter 5)
- Reactions related to treatments such as chemotherapy and radiation therapy
- Alterations in olfactory perceptions
- Psychological factors (fear, anxiety, depression)

The anorexic client is trapped in a deadly cycle: caloric (energy) requirements continually increase as the neoplasm grows; nutritional intake continually declines as factors related to the disease and therapy exacerbate the client's anorexia.

The nurse is a crucial participant in the client's struggle to halt or at least slow the life-threatening cycle. Providing small, palatable meals (blenderized if necessary), relieving pain and nausea, offering comfort measures, and removing offensive food odors are part of a multifaceted approach to cancer-related cachexia. At some point in the course of the disease, total parenteral nutrition may become necessary (see Chapter 8).

Pain

Of all the psychological manifestations of cancer, pain is undoubtedly the best known and most feared. It has been estimated that each year 450,000 to 600,000 cancer clients experience pain to some degree (Silverberg, 1982). Ironically, fear and anxiety can potentiate the pain and interfere with therapies offered to relieve or mitigate it. Although pain is almost inevitable with the oncologic processes of invasion, pressure, and tissue erosion, the degree of pain varies greatly among individuals—even among those with similar diseases. As with many other cancer problems, factors such as tumor type, extent of disease, and site of involvement greatly influence the amount of pain.

The psychophysiologic mechanisms of pain are discussed in Chapter 5. In addition, specific physiologic as well as psychological components of the cancer pain experience must be considered. The physical mechanisms include:

- Tumor destruction of bone
- Venous engorgement
- Arterial ischemia
- Pressure on nerves
- Inflammation, infection, ulceration, and necrosis

Bone pain from cancer is particularly devastating. A possible reason for the pain is that tumor invasion of bone causes the release of *prostaglandins,* hyperalgesic substances that sensitize nerve fibers, making them more vulnerable to painful stimuli (Twycross & Lack, 1983). Nonsteroidal anti-inflammatory agents (eg, Motrin, Indocin), which inhibit prostaglandins, are widely accepted in the treatment of tumor-induced bone pain.

The psychosocial aspects of a cancer diagnosis greatly influence the perceptions and response to pain. Common fears and concerns often expressed by clients with cancer include:

- Fear of death
- Fear of pain
- Changes in lifestyle
- Alterations in body image
- Social isolation

Along with others, these fears can intensify the pain experienced.

In caring for the client with cancer, as with any client whose illness is accompanied by chronic pain, the nurse must continually explore the individual's perception of the pain and response to it. The site, intensity, and characteristics of pain should be assessed. Because the painful stimuli from cancer generally originate in body tissues that are not well innervated (eg, bone, blood vessels, and organs), the pain may be perceived as diffuse, vague, and poorly localized. The characteristics of the pain, often changing over time, may be difficult to express. The nurse can best help the client describe the pain sensation by asking the client to relate it to a situation or event that may illustrate the feeling. A client with severe abdominal pain who could not find one word to describe how awful it was said, "It's like a little soldier is walking around in my belly with no set path or destination, stepping on mines!" The client was experiencing an unpredictable, exploding type of pain. Remember that clients with cancer need structure in the pain assessment process. Simply asking a client with cancer pain, "How is your pain?" may be too broad an inquiry. Ask simple and specific questions to elicit information. Examples of words to describe pain are in Figure 5–13, the McGill Pain Questionnaire, in Chapter 5.

For many clients with cancer pain, a cycle of pain, anxiety, and depression leads to frustration, relentless suffering, and mental anguish. The primary goal of managing cancer pain is to prevent the recurrence or worsening of the pain—to interrupt the cycle. Consistent pain relief is usually accomplished through around-the-clock, not p.r.n., medication schedules; usually, a narcotic analgesic is given in accordance with its relief duration. Unfortunately, medication is sometimes withheld because of an unfounded fear that it will lead to drug addiction. In clients experiencing cancer pain, drug addiction is not a serious problem. In fact, very few cancer clients actually become addicted. It seems unnecessary to worry about an uncommon problem.

Pharmacologic agents as well as other pain-relieving measures must be a part of a holistic approach. Mild diversion and distraction, relaxation therapy, hypnosis, cutaneous stimulation techniques (eg, transcutaneous electrical nerve stimulation, or TENS), and application of heat and cold may be helpful. These techniques are discussed in Chapters 4 and 5.

Section III: The Diagnosis of Cancer

Diagnosis of cancer has become a specialty in itself. Not only is early detection of malignant neoplasia crucial to the favorable outcome of treatment, but choice of treatment depends on correct identification of the tumor and evaluation of its stage of development. Improper diagnosis and delayed or inappropriate treatment can have fatal consequences.

Symptoms suggesting cancer should be investigated without delay. If the results of initial diagnostic evaluations are even slightly ambiguous, or if precancerous lesions are discovered, the client's progress must be monitored closely and frequently.

Initial assessment of the client consists of a physical examination including visual inspection and palpation of the skin, lymph nodes, and organs as well as percussion of underlying body tissues. Often, such an examination is part of a routine physical examination (see Chapter 7) with no prior suspicion of cancer. For female clients, a periodic Papanicolaou (Pap) smear is part of routine health maintenance; a Pap smear may also be ordered if a client reports such symptoms as dysmenorrhea or spotting. Hematologic studies and studies of the urine and stool are also part of the preliminary evaluation. Suspicious findings may be further investigated by x-ray, computerized tomography (CT) scan, ultrasonography, or thermography. These techniques are described in Chapter 7. Skin tests for immunologic response may also be employed.

Among new diagnostic techniques are tests for *circulating tumor markers,* blood-borne substances that are diagnostic of some forms of cancer. Although a number of tumor-associated substances are known, not all meet the criteria for a tumor marker. For example, not all are measurable by widely available methods; some are not associated exclusively with cancer; and the levels of some do not rise and fall in relation to the progress of the disease or the success of therapy.

Carcinoembryonic antigen (CEA) is being employed as a tumor marker with some success. CEA is one of several glycoproteins produced by fetal cells that either do not occur in normal mature tissue or occur only in trace amounts. Human chorionic gonadotropin (HCG) and alpha-fetoprotein are glycoproteins useful in the diagnosis of germ cell tumors such as testicular cancer. When epithelial cells, especially those in the digestive tract, multiply rapidly, CEA secretion is increased. This is especially true in clients with colorectal adenocarcinoma. Because CEA is generally not detectable in the early stages of cancer, however, it is not used to diagnose malignancy. On the other hand, high levels of CEA have been correlated with large tumors or with metastasis. Thus, serial determinations of CEA are a means of monitoring the response of colorectal cancer to surgical removal of the tumor. CEA levels also may be elevated in carcinoma of the breast, prostate gland, lung, and pancreas; in hypothyroidism, liver disease, inflammatory bowel disease, neuroblastoma; and in smokers (Byrne et al., 1986).

As diagnostic techniques become more precise, earlier detection and timelier treatment may improve the rate of cure. Meanwhile, histologic examination of tissue or body secretions (ie, biopsy and cytologic examination) remains the cornerstone of diagnosis.

HISTOLOGIC EXAMINATION

Cancer can be diagnosed by microscopic evaluation because the morphology of cancer cells differs significantly from that of normal tissue (Figure 12–7). *Biopsy* refers to the removal and examination of a sample of tissue; *cytologic diagnosis* is microscopic evaluation of body secretions or body tissues to determine whether abnormal cells are present.

A biopsy may be performed as a separate procedure or during surgery. The specimen may be examined in a laboratory by embedding the tissue in paraffin and sectioning it for diagnosis, although this is time consuming. A faster method is the *frozen section* technique. Within minutes, a pathologist can ascertain whether a lesion is benign or malignant or whether malignancy has spread to lymph nodes or distant parts of the body. A portion of tumor tissue or adjacent tissue is frozen solid at subzero temperature. A microtome slices off a thin section, which is prepared, stained, and microscopically examined. A frozen section can be performed during an operation so results are available immediately.

Techniques for obtaining a biopsy specimen include excisional biopsy, incisional biopsy, and needle (aspiration) biopsy. *Excisional biopsy* removes the entire tumor with a wide margin of normal tissue. Depending on the findings, further surgery may be performed. If the tumor is large, an *incisional biopsy* may be performed to remove a small section of the tumor. Incisional biopsy may be done during endoscopic surgery (eg, transurethral resection of the prostate). The amount of tumor and marginal tissue removed must be sufficient to permit a reliable diagnosis. One danger of incisional biopsy is seeding of tumor cells.

Needle or *aspiration biopsy*, a less definitive procedure, does not involve surgery. A hollow needle is inserted into the lesion, twisted, and withdrawn, bringing a core of tissue with it. One drawback of this technique is that, in the case of negative findings, one cannot be certain the appropriate site (the lesion) was sampled. Tumors with increased vascularity (eg, tumors of the thyroid gland) may hemor-

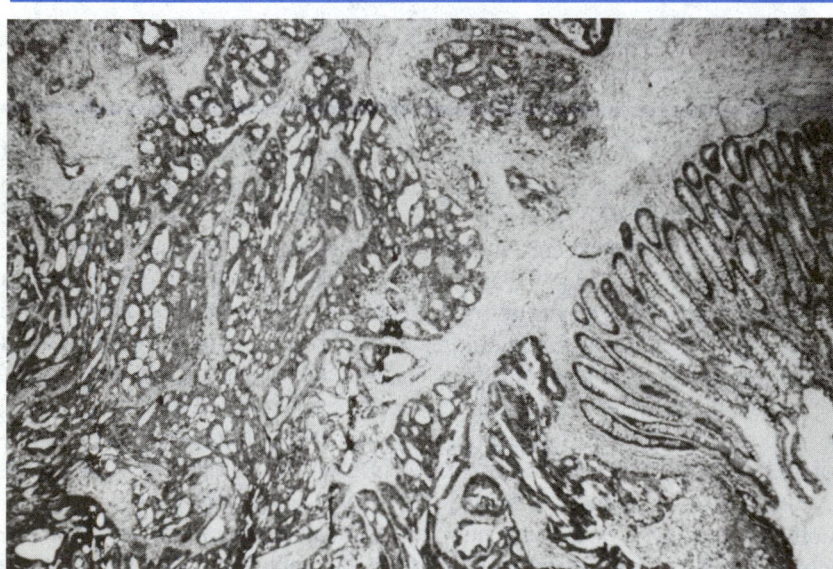

Figure 12–7

The morphologic appearance of normal cells of the colon (right) and malignant adenocarcinoma cells (left). (Courtesy of Hospital of the University of Pennsylvania)

rhage insidiously after the procedure. The possibility of tumor cell seeding along the needle track is controversial. Needle biopsy has been used, however, in tumors involving the breast, lungs, and lymph nodes. Excisional, incisional, and aspiration biopsy are discussed further in Chapter 65. *Punch biopsy,* a method to obtain a superficial sample of skin, is discussed in Chapter 78.

CYTOLOGIC EXAMINATION

Tumors shed abnormal cells; these cells may be detected in body fluids and secretions that come into contact with the tumor. Sometimes cytologic examination can detect a tumor when it is still microscopic, long before symptoms develop. One well-known cytologic technique is the Pap smear developed by Dr George Papanicolaou. The Pap smear involves analysis of cervical cells and vaginal secretions to detect cancer of the uterine cervix (see Chapter 63). Its widespread use has played an important role in reducing mortality associated with this disease.

CLASSIFICATION AND STAGING

Once the existence of a neoplasm has been established, it must be classified and staged before appropriate treatment can be initiated. *Classification* identifies the neoplasm according to type and tissue of origin. *Staging* describes the extent of the disease.

Classification

Benign tumors may be classified as *polyps* if they arise from mucous membrane or *papillomas* if they arise from surface epithelium. Other benign tumors are identified by the suffix *oma* combined with a prefix denoting the cell of origin; eg, a benign tumor arising in neural tissue is called a *neuroma.* The term *lymphoma* is the exception to this classification since it is used to denote a malignant process.

Malignant neoplasms are generally classified as carcinomas, sarcomas, leukemias, or lymphomas. A cancerous tumor is generally categorized according to the tissue of origin. A carcinoma is a malignant tumor that arises from surface, glandular, or parenchymal epithelium, eg, the outer layer of the skin, the lining of the thyroid gland, the glandular area of the breast, or the parenchyma of the kidney. Malignant tumors arising from surface epithelium are called *squamous cell carcinomas,* and those from glandular or parenchymal tissues are referred to as *adenocarcinomas.* Typically, carcinomas spread first through the lymph system and later through blood.

A *sarcoma* is a malignant tumor originating primarily in connective tissue such as bone, blood vessels, cartilage, muscle, adipose tissue, and neural tissue. In contrast to carcinomas, sarcomas usually spread initially through the blood, with less frequent metastases through the lymphatics.

Although the leukemias, some types of lymphomas, and multiple myeloma constitute their own separate categories, they share a common feature. Unlike carcinomas and sarcomas that generally are solid masses, these tumors proliferate diffusely throughout the blood and blood-forming organs. Because cells are scattered throughout the blood, these tumors are sometimes called *liquid tumors.* Classifications of neoplasms are listed in Table 2–5 in Chapter 2.

Staging

The American Joint Committee for Cancer Staging has developed a universal system of staging classification, the so-called TNM system. Stages of tumor growth are designated by a combination of letters and subscripts; eg, T designates a primary tumor; N designates lymph node involvement; and M designates metastasis. Numbers from 0 (no evidence) to 4 designate degree of involvement. TIS designates **carcinoma in situ,** or noninfiltrating carcinoma.

Not all tumors can be staged by this system, and other systems have been developed. Staging systems for specific types of malignant neoplasms are presented in the appropriate specific disorders chapters.

NURSING IMPLICATIONS DURING THE DIAGNOSTIC PROCESS

The nurse's role in prevention, education, and early screening procedures is discussed in a later section of this chapter. This section considers care of the client undergoing diagnostic studies after a symptom or sign has suggested the presence of cancer. These clients and their significant others will have many questions, voiced and unvoiced. Underlying all those questions is a fundamental one: What is going to happen to me—right now, in the hospital or outpatient area? How will it affect my life?

The Prediagnostic Phase

Waiting for a definitive diagnosis has been described as "the longest wait in the world." Nurses can best assist clients through this tense and anxious time by first assessing the client's knowledge base, attitudes, and possible misconceptions. Has someone the client knows well died of cancer? What type? What treatments were employed? How did the client view them? As effective? Painful? Palliative? Futile?

Does the client have current information about the suspected type of cancer? Is the information reliable? Or is it a compendium of TV "horror stories" and popular myths? Has the client understood the physician's explanation? (Teaching does not always mean that learning has taken place.) Does the client have at least a general understanding of the tests to be performed? If the tests are painful or uncomfortable, is the client prepared for this?

Are the client's significant others a source of support or of additional concern? Might friends or a spiritual counselor help the client through the waiting period? Or does the client truly prefer solitude? (Some individuals do.)

The prediagnostic phase is a good time to initiate client education about possible outcomes. Once a definite diagnosis of malignancy has been made, the nurse can assist the client in understanding and adjusting to the cancer experience.

The Postdiagnostic Phase

Characteristics of neoplastic disease account for some of the dread and despair the cancer diagnosis frequently evokes in clients and their significant others:

- The onset of cancer is often insidious and difficult to diagnose.
- Cancer metastasizes.
- If not discovered early and promptly controlled, cancer may be incurable; yet even early diagnosis does not necessarily guarantee cure.
- The etiology of the disease is not yet understood; treatment techniques have not been perfected.
- The treatments may be painful or disfiguring.
- No matter how willingly the client cooperates, the treatment regimen may fail, and the client may die.

Each individual confronts the diagnosis of cancer with a unique world view developed over a life span. A young, unmarried man with carcinoma of the testis will have one outlook and set of problems; the mother of three children who has cancer of the breast will have another. The child-

less widow whose relatives have all died before her will have an entirely different set of questions.

At the beginning of the cancer experience, the client may feel physically strong, yet the prospect of eventual disability must be faced. "Who will take care of me?" asks the client who lives alone. "Who will take care of them?" asks the parent of small children. "Who will support the family and pay my medical bills?" "Will it hurt? How much? For how long?" "Can I work? Garden? Take one last trip to the places I've always wanted to see?" "Will I live? Will I die? Will I live maimed?" A surprising number of persons may ask—or hesitate to ask—"Is it catching?"

Often the nurse is best qualified to address these spoken and unspoken concerns. The client's history and the nursing assessment provide clues on how to begin. Does the client understand the diagnosis and prognosis? If the client's mind is churning with anxieties and concerns, the physician's explanation may not have been absorbed. Was the information given in terms the client can understand? "The probability of metastasis is minimal" may need translation into "the cancer is not likely to have spread." The client's intelligence may be unaffected by the disease process, but the client's level of comprehension is almost certainly diminished by anxiety, pain, debilitation, or the side effects of medication.

Clients often hesitate to question their physicians; the nurse who has established trust and rapport during routine care may seem more approachable. Listening to the client is essential, and listening means attending to the client in several senses. Nonverbal signals may say more than words: the hesitant gesture that heralds a stifled impulse to speak, the slight frown that greets an unfamiliar phrase, the tensed facial muscles that reflect unvoiced pain. The nurse alert to these signals can encourage the client to ask questions about diagnostic studies, treatment options, and lifestyle changes and can encourage both client and family to voice their concerns. In responding, the nurse must be open and honest, engendering neither false hope nor unwarranted despair.

When the client's concerns have been identified, the nurse may consult other members of the health care team or the community. The dietitian may offer recipes for blenderized meals that can be easily prepared at home; a local church or charitable organization may provide a hospital bed or other equipment for home care. A self-help organization may offer counsel from a member whose cancer has been cured or arrested; the psychiatric nurse specialist may suggest how the client can cope with fears. Simple interventions may do much to alleviate anxiety and offer the client hope. Examples are providing a catalog of wigs for the client undergoing chemotherapy or describing speech aids to the client awaiting a laryngectomy.

To provide this kind of assistance to the client, whether in the hospital, in a physician's office or outpatient facility, or in the client's home, the nurse must be familiar with the therapeutic options available to the client with cancer and those involved in his or her care.

Nursing Research Note

Oleske D: Questions about cancer: Indicators for patient education. *Top Clin Nurs* (Jan) 1981; 2:1–8.

Inquiries about cancer received at a phone-in information center were analyzed. Most of the callers were women with ratios of 3 to 1 and 2 to 1 over male callers; 92% of the callers were white. The majority of inquiries were regarding breast cancer. Other sites frequently discussed were the lung, colon, cervix, and uterus. Prostatic cancer was ranked in the least-requested category. Most questions dealt with treatment and follow-up. Most of the callers were family members of a cancer client. Often callers were angry and hostile about not finding a cure through conventional therapies. Questions about unproven cancer therapies were frequent. Nurses can take an active role in educating all consumers of health care services about cancer. Important information for clients with cancer and their families may include treatment, plans for care, follow-up, anticipatory guidance, and emotional support systems. Oral information must be supplemented with written material and instructions to reinforce learning.

Section IV: Primary and Secondary Prevention

Prevention is a concept not formerly associated with cancer; even a decade ago, the word was rarely heard in this connection. Today, cancer prevention offers exciting opportunities for nurses, especially in outpatient and ambulatory care. Nursing assessment and education can make a life-saving difference.

Primary prevention of cancer (ie, prevention of its occurrence) presents difficulties because knowledge of the etiology of many forms of cancer is incomplete. Even with known carcinogens, a simple cause-and-effect relation may not have been demonstrated. For example, although cigarette smoking has been clearly associated with lung and laryngeal cancer, not all smokers contract the disease.

Primary prevention is presently directed at eliminating occupational and environmental carcinogens, identifying high-risk populations, and protecting individuals who have been exposed to carcinogenic agents, eg, asbestos. Major risk factors and symptoms and signs of common cancers are in Table 12–4. A painstaking nursing assessment, particularly the health history, can contribute a great deal to identifying individuals at risk and providing follow-up investigation and lifestyle education.

Cancer does not have the infectious properties of other diseases for which prevention programs have been successful. Measures such as isolation of affected individuals or mass inoculation are not applicable to cancer. For this reason, *secondary prevention* (early detection) is significant in reducing cancer-related morbidity and mortality.

For many years, community education has stressed regular checkups and awareness of cancer's seven warning signals (Box 12–1). More recently, self-administered screening such as self-examination of the breasts and testing for blood in the stool and noninvasive cytologic testing such as the Pap smear have been emphasized. Comprehensive programs of public education directed at both primary and secondary prevention of cancer include:

- Informing the community that some cancers are preventable and explaining preventive measures.
- Enhancing public awareness of risk factors, including those related to lifestyle.
- Teaching techniques all persons can use to detect early evidence of neoplasia, eg, breast, testicular, and oral self-examination.

Table 12–4	Major Risk Factors and Common Symptoms and Signs for Common Cancers
Type of Cancer	**Risk Factors, Signs, and Symptoms**
Colon-rectum	History of rectal polyps; rectal polyps run in family; history of ulcerative colitis; blood in stool; over age 40
Lung	Heavy cigarette smoker over age 50; started cigarette smoking at age 15 or before; smoker working with or near asbestos
Uterine-endometrial	Unusual bleeding or discharge; late menopause (after age 55); diabetes, high blood pressure, and overweight; aged 50 +
Uterine-cervical	Unusual bleeding or discharge; frequent sex in early teens or with many partners; low socioeconomic background; poor care during or following pregnancy
Breast	Lump or nipple discharge; history of breast cancer; close relatives with history of breast cancer; over age 35, especially over age 50; never had children; first child after age 30
Skin	Excessive exposure to sun; fair complexion; work with coal tar, pitch, or creosote
Oral	Heavy smoker and drinker; poor oral hygiene
Ovarian	History of ovarian cancer among close relatives; aged 50 + ; never had children
Prostate	Aged 60 + ; difficulty in urinating
Stomach	History of stomach cancer among close relatives; diet heavy in smoked, pickled, or salted foods

SOURCE: Reprinted with permission from *Cancer Facts and Figures 1980.* New York: American Cancer Society, 1980.

Box 12–1	Cancer's Seven Warning Signals

1. Change in bowel or bladder habits
2. A sore that does not heal
3. Unusual bleeding or discharge
4. Thickening or lump in breast or elsewhere
5. Indigestion or difficulty in swallowing
6. Obvious change in wart or mole
7. Nagging cough or hoarseness

SOURCE: Reprinted with permission from American Cancer Society.

- Informing the public of the advantages of early detection, eg, publishing comparative mortality and morbidity data.
- Explaining diagnostic techniques used for early detection of cancer, including information on where to obtain these services.

Guidelines for the early detection of cancer are in Box 12–2.

SCREENING TECHNIQUES

Most screening techniques are not designed for diagnosis of specific malignancies. Rather, screening evaluates the well population and detects signs that might indicate neoplasia. Individuals with positive signs are referred for more precise evaluation. Health teaching, including personal hygiene, lifestyle risk factors, and self-examination techniques, may also be part of a screening program.

Noninvasive diagnostic techniques in early detection of cancer include:

- Examination of stool for occult blood (Hemoccult test) as a routine part of assessment.
- Ultrasonography, mammography, and thermography for mammary or prostatic cancer.
- Injection of radiopharmaceuticals to detect hypervascularization or irregular vascularization of masses (ie, radioisotope scan).
- Cytological study of serum or body fluids (eg, Pap smear of nipple discharge).

By explaining these techniques, which are painless and relatively simple outpatient procedures, the nurse can encourage clients and the public to seek prompt evaluation of any suspicious symptoms.

Box 12–2   Guidelines for the Early Detection of Cancer in Persons Without Symptoms

Age 20–40

Cancer-Related Checkup Every 3 Years
Should include the procedures listed below plus health counseling (such as tips on quitting cigarettes) and examinations for cancers of the thyroid, testes, prostate, mouth, ovaries, skin, and lymph nodes. *Some persons are at higher risk for certain cancers and may need to have tests more frequently.*

Breast
- Exam by health care provider every 3 years
- Self-exam every month
- One baseline mammogram between ages 35 and 40

Higher risk for breast cancer: personal or family history of breast cancer, never had children, first child after 30

Uterus
- Pelvic exam every 3 years

Cervix
- Pap test—after two initial negative tests 1 year apart—*at least* every 3 years, includes women under 20 if sexually active

Higher risk for cervical cancer: early age at first intercourse, multiple sex partners

Age 40 and Over

Cancer-Related Checkup Every Year
Should include the procedures listed below plus health counseling (such as tips on quitting cigarettes) and examinations for cancers of the thyroid, testes, prostate, mouth, ovaries, skin, and lymph nodes. *Some persons are at higher risk for certain cancers and may need to have tests more frequently.*

Breast
- Exam by doctor every year
- Self-exam every month
- Mammogram every year after 50 (between ages 40 and 50, ask your doctor)

Higher risk for breast cancer: personal or family history of breast cancer, never had children, first child after 30

Uterus
- Pelvic exam every year

Cervix
- Pap test—after two initial negative tests 1 year apart—*at least* every 3 years

Higher risk for cervical cancer: early age at first intercourse, multiple sex partners

Endometrium
- Endometrial tissue sample at menopause if at risk

Higher risk for endometrial cancer: infertility, obesity, failure of ovulation, abnormal uterine bleeding, estrogen therapy

Colon and Rectum
- Digital rectal exam every year
- Guaiac slide test every year after 50
- Proctological exam—after two initial negative tests 1 year apart—every 3 to 5 years after 50

Higher risk for colorectal cancer: personal or family history of colon or rectal cancer, personal or family history of polyps in the colon or rectum, ulcerative colitis

---

SOURCE: Reprinted with permission from American Cancer Society.

SELF-EXAMINATION TECHNIQUES

Self-examination of the breasts and testes is described in Chapter 7, and oral cavity self-examination is described in Chapter 47. Although breast examination has been widely publicized, many women still do not practice it. The nurse can encourage more widespread use of this lifesaving technique by stressing the value of early diagnosis in possibly avoiding the radical dissection that women fear.

Testicular self-examination has been less widely publicized than examination of the breasts. Yet carcinoma of the testis is the third most common tumor in males between ages 20 and 35 – the prime reproductive years (Nixon, 1982). Tragically, the usual time between onset of this disease and diagnosis is 6 months; if not detected early, testicular cancer can spread rapidly. Obviously, greater public awareness is needed.

Oral self-examination also has not received as much emphasis as breast self-examination. Yet, because minor lesions in the mouth are common, an early sign of oral cancer may easily be missed. Counsel clients to consult a health professional promptly if a sore in the mouth fails to heal within a few weeks. Regular dental checkups should include a meticulous oral examination; more frequent teaching of oral examination by dentists is encouraging.

NURSING IMPLICATIONS OF CANCER PREVENTION

In recent years, nurses have become more involved in early detection and screening. Community prevention activities are often managed by nurses. Urban and rural cancer detection clinics are gaining wider acceptance. Nurses working in these settings, in physician's offices, and in health maintenance organizations are finding that inspection, palpation, auscultation and percussion, as well as a careful health history, are valuable in cancer detection.

Section V: Treatment of Neoplastic Disease

The basic treatment modalities for cancer have changed little in the past decade; surgery, chemotherapy, and radiation therapy remain the mainstays of therapy. What has changed are the precision of these techniques and the skill with which they are combined.

SURGERY

Surgery, alone or in combination with other therapies, continues to be the preferred treatment for many forms of malignancy. Surgery may be performed for diagnostic purposes (eg, biopsy), for staging (ie, to determine the extent of the tumor), to control effects of the tumor (eg, pressure, obstruction, or hemorrhage), or for palliation (eg, to alleviate pain). In some cases (eg, carcinoma in situ), surgery alone may be curative.

Principles of Surgical Treatment

Curative or definitive surgery was performed more frequently before the concept of micrometastasis was fully understood. It was thought that the more extensive the surgery, the better the chance for cure. Traditionally, large masses were excised with a considerable amount of normal marginal tissue, often at great physical and emotional cost to the client. The classic example is the radical Halsted mastectomy, which included extensive surgical removal of chest wall muscles and axillary lymphatics and resulted in severe image changes (eg, concave chest wall and lymphedema of the affected arm). Recently, studies have shown no significant difference in survival between the Halsted procedure and less radical procedures such as the modified radical or simple mastectomy (see Chapter 65). The benefits of wide local resections of tumor and normal tissue are questionable now that it is known that tumor cells may spread to distant areas even at an early stage. Radical surgery is still performed, but the trend is toward supplementing less extensive surgical procedures with chemotherapy, radiation therapy, or immunotherapy.

Palliative surgery has the goal of client comfort rather than cure. For example, a tumor may be surgically reduced to relieve invasion of adjacent tissue or remove obstruction, improving the client's condition and allowing time for systemic treatments to take effect. *Ablative* surgery, which involves surgical alteration of the endocrine system, may be employed in clients who have hormone-dependent tumors. Examples of ablative surgery, which is considered palliative, are hypophysectomy, adrenalectomy, oophorectomy, and orchiectomy (discussed in Units Seven and Eleven).

A controversial procedure known as "second-look surgery" is sometimes a part of treatment, usually for gastrointestinal or ovarian cancer. An exploratory laparotomy is performed at the site of a resection to determine whether chemotherapy or radiation treatment has been successful.

Regardless of whether surgery is for curative or noncurative purposes, certain principles apply (Patterson, 1983):

- Some normal tissue surrounding the malignant neoplasm must be removed.
- The initial surgical treatment of a tumor is more likely to be successful than subsequent operations to remove recurrent malignancy.
- Some tumors, especially carcinomas and less frequently sarcomas, readily metastasize to adjacent lymph nodes. Therefore, removal of adjacent lymph nodes is recommended.
- Some cancers do not metastasize readily and may be cured by extensive resection.

- Surgical intervention is most effective in treating neoplasms that grow slowly.
- Combination therapy may be an effective alternative to some extensive resections.
- The status of the client's immune system is an important consideration in planning surgery.
- Precise identification and staging of the neoplasm must precede curative surgery.

Surgical approaches to specific forms of cancer are discussed in Units Three through Thirteen.

Nursing Implications of Surgical Treatment

General principles of perioperative care are discussed in Chapter 14. Nursing implications of specific surgical procedures are described in the surgical approaches chapters in Units Three through Thirteen. Underlying all nursing care of the client with cancer must be an awareness of the psychic and physiologic stress imposed by neoplastic disease. The client recovering from first-time surgery asks first, "Will my cancer recur?" After subsequent procedures, the question may be, "Did they get it all this time?" All clients wonder, "What will happen now?"

Surgical treatments for cancer produce changes in body image and lifestyle, some of them profound. No matter how well prepared a client may have been for these changes, the immediate postoperative period may hold surprises, even shocks.

Clients who have had mutilating surgery may fear they are repulsive to others. Habits of a lifetime must be changed; actions taken for granted must be relearned. Significant others, too, must adapt to a changed status. For these reasons, the nurse's continuing assessments, care planning, and evaluation of outcomes must encompass psychosocial as well as physiologic status. As much as possible, the client and the family must be involved in decision making and encouraged to participate in care. (A plan for nursing care related to psychosocial aspects is in Section VI. Rehabilitation is discussed in Section VII.)

CHEMOTHERAPY

Antineoplastic drug therapy is an outgrowth of an incidental discovery during World War I. Military personnel who had been exposed to mustard gas were found to have depressed leukocyte counts. It was postulated that a derivative of this gas would be beneficial in treating certain types of leukemia. Thus, the first chemotherapeutic agent, mechlorethamine (Mustargen), was developed, which was effective in the treatment of Hodgkin's disease. This discovery provided the foundation for a new mode of cancer therapy.

Today a wide range of chemotherapeutic agents is available for treating neoplastic disease. All act in some fashion to destroy cancer cells or inhibit their function. Unfortunately, these agents do not affect cancer cells exclusively; normal cells may be damaged or destroyed as well.

Principles of Chemotherapy

No single drug has been found capable of destroying tumor cells during all stages of the cell cycle. Some kill proliferating cells more effectively than resting cells. These agents are labeled *cell cycle specific* (CCS). *Phase-specific* agents kill or arrest dividing cells during a specific phase of the cell cycle. Others that kill both dividing and resting cells are called *cell cycle nonspecific* (CCNS).

Agents used in treating human cancers generally can be assigned to one of seven categories:

- Alkylating agents
- Nitrosoureas
- Antimetabolites
- Antibiotics
- Plant alkaloids
- Hormones and steroids
- Miscellaneous agents

Specific chemotherapeutic agents are listed in Box 12–3.

Alkylating agents all have an alkyl group, a highly reactive and unstable group that binds and braces the double-helix DNA strands, preventing the strands from separating (a necessary step for replication). Nucleic base pairs between DNA and RNA may also be affected. Although alkylating agents, *nitrosoureas* are classified in a separate category based on their lipid solubility and unique ability to cross the blood-brain barrier.

The chemical structure of *antimetabolites* closely resembles that of normally occurring compounds needed by the tumor cell for functional processes or mitosis. Once the tumor cell has incorporated the "imitation," its function is inhibited or destroyed.

Antibiotics are generally considered anti-infectious agents. Many antibiotics are important in antineoplastic therapy, however. Like antimetabolites, they prevent the tumor cell from synthesizing DNA and RNA by interfering with synthesis of nucleic acids.

Plant alkaloids, such as vincristine and vinblastine found in the periwinkle plant *(Vinca rosea),* and etoposide (VP-16-213) derived from podophyllotoxin, are all strong mitotic inhibitors. It is believed these agents interfere with microtubule protein synthesis of the mitotic spindles, the apparatus necessary for mitosis.

Hormones and steroids are used in the treatment of hormonally dependent tumors such as some breast and prostate cancers. Hormonal therapy disrupts the hormonal environment, making it unfavorable for the tumor to survive. Hormonal therapy has two principle modes of action: (1) synthetic hormones replace naturally occurring ones by competitive inhibition on tumor receptor sites, and (2) some hormones block the production of certain endogenous hormones. Steroids such as prednisone and dexamethasone (Decadron) are included in this category.

Miscellaneous agents share little or no common prop-

Box 12–3   Classification of Antineoplastic Agents

Alkylating agents
Bis (chloroethyl) amines:
*Mechlorethamine, nitrogen mustard (Mustargen)
Cyclophosphamide (Cytoxan, Neosar)
L-phenylalanine mustard, melphalan (Alkeran)
Chlorambucil (Leukeran)

Ethylenimine derivatives:
Thiotepa (Triethylenethiophosphoramide)

Alkyl sulfonates:
Busulfan (Myleran)

Triatenes:
*Dacarbazine, DTIC (DTIC-Dome)

Nitrosoureas
BCNU, carmustine
CCNU, lomustine (CeeNU)
Methyl-CCNU
Streptozocin (Zanosar)

Antimetabolites (inhibitors of nucleic acid biosynthesis)
Folic acid antagonists:
Methotrexate, MTX, amethopterin

Purine antagonists:
6-mercaptopurine, 6-MP (Purinethol)
6-thioguanine, 6-TG

Pyrimidine synthesis inhibitors:
+5-azacytidine
5-fluorouracil, 5FU, fluorouracil (Adrucil)
Cytosine arabinoside, ARA-C (Cytosar)

Antibiotics
*Doxorubicin hydrochloride (Adriamycin)
Bleomycin (Blenoxane)
*Dactinomycin, actinomycin D (Cosmegen)
*Daunorubicin, daunomycin (Cerubidine)
*Mithramycin (Mithracin)
*Mitomycin, mitomycin-C (Mutamycin)
+Mitoxantrone (Novantrone)

Plant alkaloids
++*Vindesine (Eldesine)
++*Teniposide, VM-26
*Vinblastine, VLB (Velban)
*Vincristine, VCR (Oncovin)
Etoposide, VP-16-213 (VePesid)

Hormones
Steroids:
Prednisone
Dexamethasone (Decadron)

Sex hormones:
Diethylstilbestrol (DES)
Conjugated estrogens
Androgens
Progesterones
Antiestrogens:
Tamoxifen

Miscellaneous
++*Amsacrine, M-AMSA
Cisplatin (Platinol)
L-Asparaginase (Elspar)
Procarbazine (Matulane)
Hydroxyurea (Hydrea)

*Vesicant/sclerosing agents
+ Investigational (not yet commercially available)

erties or mechanisms of action with previously classified drugs. Although cisplatin is thought to inhibit DNA and RNA synthesis in a manner similar to that of alkylating agents, it is generally classified in the miscellaneous group.

Chemotherapeutic agents may be administered alone or in combination. *Single-agent therapy* is usually reserved for the treatment of tumors showing little or no response to other agents. 5-Fluorouracil alone is commonly employed for colon cancer, because this tumor type rarely responds to other drugs. Because of increased drug toxicity, high-dosage chemotherapy (dosages exceeding the normal range of a particular drug) is usually administered as single-agent therapy to avoid added toxicities of other drugs. High-dosage therapy may be used for tumors refractory to lower therapeutic dosages.

Combination chemotherapy is preferred to single-agent therapy. The major intent is to optimize "cell kill" and minimize additive side effects or toxicities by combining drugs with varied tumoricidal actions and different side effects. Usually, a drug regimen includes cycle-specific agents or phase-specific agents along with cell cycle non-specific agents. The administration of chemotherapy is designed to produce maximum "cell kill" using alternating or intermittent cycle-specific and phase-specific agents. For example, a phase-specific agent of the vinca alkaloid category causing metaphase arrest may be followed by another phase-specific agent from the antimetabolite category causing cell kill at the S-phase (see Figure 12–3). Combination drug regimens are discussed in the specific disorders chapters in the body systems units.

Clinical Trials of Chemotherapeutic Agents

Investigation of new chemotherapeutic agents and methods of administration continues. Extensive research projects, commonly referred to as protocols, or clinical trials, are underway. A protocol is a formal research document with all information necessary to conduct clinical trials, including an informed consent form. A client participating in any investigative protocol should be aware of the risks and benefits of treatment as well as the conventional treatment available. Before being approved by the Food and Drug Administration (FDA), a drug must be subjected to research trials. To ensure valid and reliable findings, the National Cancer Institute has developed strict standards

Nursing Research Note

Farrel S, Bubela N, Hall–Burlein S: High-volume chemodialysis: A new outpatient program. *Can Nurse* (Feb) 1985; 81:44–47.

This ongoing research is attempting to determine the effectiveness of high-volume intraperitoneal chemotherapy for the treatment of cancer. Chemotherapy is instilled via a Tenckhoff catheter, currently the most widely used catheter for peritoneal dialysis.

Although the efficacy of this procedure for cancer treatment is unknown, the researchers have found many psychosocial benefits. Because the dressing procedure itself is lengthy, it allows for nurse–client interaction. This treatment also has been found to provide additional hope for a response to treatment. The treatment form has reduced hospitalization time and is less disruptive to the client's daily life. It also promotes client participation and reduces feelings of dependence, loss of control, and helplessness. Clients have also taken pride in participating in experimentation for cancer cure.

for clinical trials. After a new agent or treatment has proved effective in laboratory tests, clinical trials in human subjects are begun. A clinical trial comprises four phases:

- Phase 1: The maximal tolerated dosage in humans is established, and the safety of the drug(s) in humans is evaluated. In this phase, the only clients enrolled are those with advanced malignant neoplasms that conventional therapies have failed to control.

- Phase 2: Clinical measurements (eg, x-rays) are used to determine whether the drug or method has antitumor activity in humans. In this phase also, experimental treatment is offered to clients with measurable neoplasia whom standard therapies have failed to help.

- Phase 3: This phase is initiated after the drug or method has been proven (1) safe in humans and (2) capable of producing antitumor activity in humans. In this phase, the new drug or treatment protocol is systematically compared with the established modality known to have the maximal effect in a given type of malignancy. A large random selection of clients is enrolled. To pass this phase, the new method must prove at least as effective as standard methods.

- Phase 4: Upon approval by the FDA, limited marketing of the drug or limited clinical use of the method begins. More data are gathered before wide-scale commercial distribution by using the drug in combination chemotherapy regimens.

Clients undergoing clinical trials should be encouraged to raise questions and discuss concerns about the options at hand. For these clients, the National Cancer Institute's *What Are Clinical Trials All About?* is a helpful client information booklet (see the resources listing at the end of this chapter).

Administration of Chemotherapy

Many nurses care for clients receiving chemotherapy, but only those who are specially trained should administer these drugs intravenously. Chemotherapeutic agents can be irritating to the veins. Some agents, referred to as irritants (eg, BCNU, etoposide), may cause phlebitis. Therefore, good vein care is essential. Measures include changing IV sites every 48 to 72 hours, flushing the drug through the vein adequately, and applying warm soaks to phlebitic sites.

Other drugs classified as sclerosing agents or vesicants (see Box 12–3) cause severe tissue inflammation and necrosis if **extravasation** (leakage of a drug into the surrounding tissues) occurs. It is generally agreed that only skilled phlebotomists should administer these drugs. Management of extravasation depends on the individual drug and is highly controversial. The Oncology Nursing Society (1984) has developed recommendations for chemotherapy drug extravasations. If extravasation is suspected with drugs *other* than the plant alkaloids, immediate care includes these measures:

- The intravenous needle should remain in place, and ice is applied to the area.

- Steroids or anti-inflammatory agents may be injected through the needle or into the surrounding tissues.

- For extravasation of plant alkaloids, heat is applied to the area, and hyaluronidase injections are given via the IV needle and subcutaneously into the extravasation site.

Many antineoplastic drugs are mutagenic, and some are carcinogenic, posing hazards for health professionals handling them. Mutagenic changes have been found in the urine of nurses preparing and administering these agents (Falck, et al., 1979). Because these drugs can be absorbed through skin and mucous membranes by inhalation and direct skin contact in an unprotected environment, any person mixing or giving chemotherapeutic agents should take precautions. The Public Health Service (US Department of Health and Human Services, 1983), the National Study Commission on Cytotoxic Exposure (1984), and the Oncology Nursing Society (1984) have developed guidelines for safe handling of parenteral cytotoxic agents:

- All parenteral chemotherapeutic agents should be prepared by skilled personnel under a vertical laminar flow unit or biological safety cabinet.

- Personnel mixing should wear a long-sleeved protective garment, surgical latex gloves, and face mask and goggles if a protective glass shield is not available.

- Surgical latex gloves should be worn for all chemotherapy-related preparation, handling, and disposal. (Polyvinyl chloride gloves are permeable and should *not* be worn.)

- All materials used in preparation and administration of antineoplastic drugs should be disposed of as toxic waste.

Institutional policies should be developed to protect those handling these agents from hazards. The National Institute for Occupational Safety and Health (NIOSH) and the Occupational Safety and Health Administration (OSHA) are developing guidelines for chemotherapeutic (cytotoxic) agents.

Toxic Effects of Chemotherapy

Because chemotherapy affects both normal and malignant cells, some normal cellular function is sacrificed. Many of the effects on normal cells are reversible; however, the repair or recovery time of normal cells often determines or limits the dosage, frequency, and total duration of antineoplastic therapy. Each neoplastic drug has a maximum tolerated therapeutic range beyond which certain toxicities may occur, some irreversible. Constant monitoring is necessary to ensure toxicity does not exceed predetermined limits.

Myelosuppression (suppressive alteration in the function of the bone marrow), a side effect of most antineoplastic agents, is reflected by leukopenia (neutropenia), thrombocytopenia, and less frequently anemia. Usually leukopenia and thrombocytopenia are more pronounced than anemia because the life span of erythrocytes is approximately 120 days, whereas the life span of leukocytes and thrombocytes is much shorter. Because erythrocytes are less affected, anemia associated with chemotherapy is generally mild. The peak suppressor effect on the marrow (called the *nadir*) is the point at which the leukocyte, thrombocyte, and erythrocyte counts are at their lowest. The nadir is usually a delayed effect that differs among the chemotherapeutic agents and is useful in determining drug schedules. For example, the nadir for cyclophosphamide occurs 7 to 14 days after therapy, with recovery of the marrow cells around day 21; therefore, cyclophosphamide doses are usually repeated every 21 days. In some instances, the dangers of myelosuppression may be lessened by blood component therapy. Life-threatening complications can ensue if these conditions are not treated.

Hemorrhage may be a life-threatening consequence of thrombocytopenia associated with bone marrow suppression. Clients should be cautioned to report immediately to a health care professional if blood is found in the stool or urine or any signs of obvious bleeding are noted. Clients should also be alerted to watch for signs such as ecchymoses or petechiae and to be careful in handling sharp objects or tools. Because straining at stool or passing hard feces can induce hemorrhage, clients should avoid constipation by using stool softeners or increasing fluid intake and dietary fiber, if tolerated.

Cytotoxicity is especially likely to affect cells that proliferate rapidly. For example, some cells of the gastrointestinal tract are replaced every 3 days. Drugs that kill cells during the S phase of the cell cycle (eg, antimetabolite drugs) generally cause toxic side effects in the gastrointestinal tract. Diarrhea, mucositis, or stomatitis as well as nausea and vomiting may result from cell damage. Nausea and vomiting probably are caused by central nervous system irritation or excitation, which triggers the vomiting center of the brain.

Integumentary side effects of chemotherapy include alopecia (hair loss), rashes, hyperpigmentation, and altered nail growth. Although these conditions may not be life threatening, they are disturbing to clients, who may already be dealing with severe alterations in body image related to surgical treatment.

Long-term administration of certain antineoplastic agents may produce cumulative effects on the tissue of the lungs, liver, heart, kidney, and nerves. Examples include doxorubicin and daunorubicin cardiotoxicity and bleomycin lung toxicity. Physiologic testing is often used regularly to monitor the status of each organ system. Long-term influences of antineoplastic chemotherapy on the reproductive system are under study. Use of these agents is associated with abnormal sperm production and possibly sterility in males. The ova may be less affected than the sperm, although women may also have temporary or permanent sterility. The drug, dosage, and duration of administration are important variables determining the effects on fertility in any client.

Nursing Implications of Chemotherapy

In addition to their underlying disease, clients receiving chemotherapy experience unpleasant, worrisome, and sometimes life-threatening side effects related to the therapy. Offering emotional support and information on which the client can base decisions is essential.

Nursing diagnoses related to the client receiving chemotherapy are included in Table 12–5. The nursing care plan in Table 12–5 outlines the goals, interventions, and evaluations related to these diagnoses. Diagnoses related to anxiety, knowledge deficit, and body image changes experienced by clients on chemotherapy are addressed in the psychosocial care plan presented later in this chapter in Table 12–7.

Clients undergoing chemotherapy are at serious risk of developing infections because of the suppressed immune response. The nurse should review general infection control guidelines with clients. For example, clients should be instructed to avoid crowds and contact with individuals having colds or infections and to observe for signs and symptoms of infection, such as coughs or redness, swelling or tenderness of any body part, burning on urination, and fever. Clients should also be instructed to report immediately a temperature at or higher than 100°F. Stress the importance of recognizing and reporting symptoms of infection because prompt treatment is necessary to control infections in the leukopenic client. Review oral and body hygiene measures (eg, operation of a WaterPic, use of sitz baths to cleanse the perineal area, and cleansing the perineal area from front to back in women).

(continued on p. 345)

Table 12–5 Nursing Care Plan for the Client Receiving Chemotherapy

Nursing Diagnoses	Client Care Goal	Plan/Nursing Implementation	Expected Outcome
Alteration in nutrition, less than body requirements related to: nausea and vomiting; anorexia; mucositis/stomatitis; diarrhea; constipation	Prevent or minimize nausea and vomiting; increase nutritional intake during and after treatment; minimize weight loss	Monitor intake and output. Encourage fluids >2 L/d; administer antiemetics as premedication ½–1 h before chemotherapy treatment (eg, Decadron, Compazine, Reglan) and continue posttreatment; monitor weights at least weekly; encourage good oral hygiene (see alterations in mucous membranes); encourage high-protein foods such as cheeses, meats, yogurt, milkshakes (be aware lactose intolerance resulting in diarrhea may occur in adults who seldom drink milk); suggest cold foods without strong odors (eg, cottage cheese, cold fruits, cold cuts); consult a dietitian if necessary; institute calorie counts; ask clients at home to keep a diet history; assess for peripheral edema and sacral edema from decreased serum protein	Client will state causes of nausea and vomiting; identify methods of controlling nausea and vomiting; modify diet to enhance food and fluid intake; maintain a stable weight during treatment
Alteration in nutrition, more than body requirements related to: adjuvant chemotherapy for breast cancer; steroid therapy; hormonal therapy: estrogens, antiestrogens, androgens	Prevent or minimize weight gain; assist the client in coping with side effects of therapy	Monitor daily weights; provide dietary counseling for caloric intake control; warn client of potential side effects of steroids (weight gain; increased blood glucose; gastrointestinal upset; acne of face, neck, and chest areas; fluid retention; fat deposition on cheeks, shoulders, and abdomen; emotional changes); warn female clients of potential side effects of androgens (masculinization; fluid retention; weight gain); warn female clients of potential effects of antiestrogens (amenorrhea; hot flashes; weight gain); warn client of potential side effects of estrogens (gynecomastia; fluid retention); instruct client to avoid food high in sodium; assess for edema of hands and ankles and for pedal edema from fluid retention; administer diuretics as ordered; monitor blood and urine glucose for clients on steroid therapy; instruct client in signs and symptoms of hyperglycemia if taking steroids	Client will manifest minimal weight gain (<5 lb) and fluid retention; modify diet appropriately; cope with changes in physical appearance; state signs and symptoms of hyperglycemia if on steroids
Fluid and electrolyte imbalance related to: nausea and vomiting; anorexia; diarrhea; constipation; dehydration; hypokalemia as a result of steroid therapy; hypomagnesemia as a result of cisplatin	Maintain optimal fluid and electrolyte balance	Encourage fluid intake of greater than 2 L/day; monitor intake and output; assess skin turgor; monitor urine specific gravity if necessary; check blood chemistry studies for Na^+, K^+, Cl^-, Mg^{++}; institute measures to control: nausea and vomiting, diarrhea, and constipation to prevent fluid and electrolyte loss and promote fluid intake; administer K^+ and Mg^{++} supplements as ordered	Client will consume more than 2 L/day of fluids with output comparisons ⅔ of intake; laboratory studies will remain within normal limits
Alterations in bowel elimination: diarrhea, as a result of cytotoxic effects on intestinal mucosa	Maintain integrity of the GI mucosa	Assess number and consistency of stools; administer antidiarrhea medications as ordered (Lomotil, Imodium), higher doses of Metamucil (2 Tbsp in water or juice q.i.d.) to add bulk to stool; encourage fluids (no fruit juices); instruct client to avoid raw fruit, vegetables, and bran-containing foods high in fiber and to eat a low-residue diet; encour-	Client will state the importance of recording number and consistency of stools; modify diet appropriately; experience none or few problems with diarrhea

Nursing Diagnoses	Client Care Goal	Plan/Nursing Implementation	Expected Outcome
		age foods high in potassium; test all stools for occult blood; assess for abdominal pain or distention; observe for signs and symptoms of GI bleeding, (black tarry stools, decreased Hct and Hb, hypotension, tachycardia)	and/or intestinal ulceration
Alteration in elimination: constipation, related to: neurotoxicity from vinblastine and vincristine administration; immobilization and decreased fluid intake	Prevent or minimize constipation	Administer stool softeners as ordered and laxatives if no bowel movement q. 48 h; force fluids and high-fiber diet; encourage ambulation; place client on daily bowel check; instruct client to report frequency of stool	Client will experience no problem with constipation; modify diet and fluid intake appropriately
Alteration in tissue perfusion related to direct cytotoxic effects on bone marrow reserves (iliac crests and sternum): leukopenia; thrombocytopenia; anemia	Leukopenia; prevent and minimize potential risk for infection	Monitor temperature and other vital signs q. 4 h; assess areas of body for signs and symptoms of infection: mouth: lesions, changes in color (pallor vs erythema), soreness, swelling; rectum: tenderness, induration, discoloration, hemorrhoids; GI: constipation/diarrhea daily bowel checks, institute measures to avoid constipation; skin: redness, swelling, induration, lesions, pain; urinary: pain, burning on urination, frequency/urgency, odor; respiratory: pain, cough, secretions (note color and amount). Control environmental factors: strict handwashing, no fresh flowers, no fresh fruits or vegetables, screen visitors for colds, viruses (eg, nausea and vomiting, diarrhea, etc), exposure to infectious diseases (eg, chickenpox); avoid invasive procedures: no IM injections; no rectal temperatures, enemas, or suppositories; no urinary catheters; intermittent straight catheter preferred to indwelling when necessary; provide client education: instruct client to avoid trauma, use electric razor, wear shoes when out of bed, avoid straining at BM; teach client signs and symptoms of infection to observe for and report; teach client to take own temperature when at home and report elevations >100.5°F or shaky chills immediately	Leukopenia: client will manifest minimal signs and symptoms of infection; identify signs and symptoms of infection to observe and report; practice appropriate health behaviors to prevent infection
	Thrombocytopenia: prevent and minimize potential risk for bleeding	Check platelet counts daily: normal count 150,000–300,000 μL; instruct clients with platelet count <100,000 μL to: use electric razor (no straight-edge blades); use soft toothbrush; report any bruising or bleeding from rectal area, vagina (menstruation), gums, nose; assess daily for signs and symptoms of bleeding; check oral mucosa and dependent parts for petechiae; test all excreta: urine, stool, emesis, sputum; assess neurologic status (headache, blurred vision) for clients with platelet counts <20,000 μL; check skin for ecchymosis, purpura, petechiae; do a pad count for menstruating women; avoid invasive procedures if platelet count <75,000 μL; no IM injections, rectal temperatures; no urinary catheters, espe-	Thrombocytopenia: client will be free from active bleeding; recognize factors that increase risk for bleeding; observe and report early signs of actual or potential bleeding; practice appropriate behaviors to prevent or minimize bleeding

(continued)

Table 12–5	Nursing Care Plan for the Client Receiving Chemotherapy (continued)		
Nursing Diagnoses	**Client Care Goal**	**Plan/Nursing Implementation**	**Expected Outcome**
		cially if platelet count <50,000 µL; avoid prolonged BP cuff use, or tourniquet application if platelet count <50,000 µL; apply pressure to venipuncture sites 3–5 min; place clients with active bleeding on bed rest; clients with platelet count <20,000 µL should have activity modifications (bed rest, ambulation with assistance); avoid administration of any aspirin-containing compounds; administer platelet transfusions if necessary; assess for fever >101°F, and report to physician because circulating platelet survival time is decreased with fevers	
	Anemia: adequate tissue perfusion will be maintained	Observe for signs and symptoms of anemia: SOB, H/A, pallor, dizziness, hypotension, tachycardia, palpitations; instruct client to report these symptoms if present; check Hb and Hct; administer blood transfusions as ordered	Anemia: client will state the signs and symptoms of anemia
Alterations in oral mucous membranes, related to: direct cytotoxic action causing inflammation of buccal and gingival membranes, decrease in saliva, changes in normal flora (usually seen with antimetabolite chemotherapeutic agents); myelosuppression; poor oral hygiene	Maintain integrity of oral mucosa; foster compliance with good oral hygiene practices	Institute preventive measures; instruct client to: brush teeth in AM and PM with soft brush or oral swabs and mild nonabrasive toothpaste (preferably Crest, Sensodyne); rinse with saline q.i.d. (P.C. and H.S.); avoid commercial mouthwashes; remove ill-fitting dentures between meals; assess for signs and symptoms of early mucositis and alert client to these: swollen, thick mucous membranes; erythematous or pale membranes; increased sensitivity to hot and cold foods; oral discomfort; burning sensation in mouth. Inspect oral mucous membranes daily for ulcerations or lesions, color changes (erythema/pallor), swelling, candidiasis (white opaque lesions), and mouth ulcers. Administer mycostatin mouth rinses or lozenges to prevent or treat oral candidiasis. Institute measures to manage mucositis if present: reinforce preventive measures; soft diet if tolerated; warm, frequent saline rinses or lavage; determine appropriate solution(s) for oral irrigations or rinses with physician (¼–½ strength hydrogen peroxide, modified Dakin's ¼ strength, sodium bicarbonate or other solutions); keep mucous membranes clean and moist (frequent rinses, artificial saliva); teach client to avoid alcoholic beverages, cigarette, pipe, and cigar smoking. Institute comfort measures: administer: local anesthetics if ordered (2% viscous lidocaine, 0.5% dyclonine, and 0.5% dyphenhydramine); milk of magnesia or kaolin mouth rinses to coat oral membranes; systemic pain medication if prescribed by physician. Instruct client with dry mouth to drink fluids frequently, suck on ice chips, and use gravies and sauces on foods	Client will experience minimal or no oral mucous membrane problems as a result of disease or therapy; recognize and report early signs of mucositis; practice appropriate preventive and management measures

Nursing Diagnoses	Client Care Goal	Plan/Nursing Implementation	Expected Outcome
Impairment of skin integrity related to: alopecia; local effects of intravenous administration of chemotherapy: phlebitis, tissue sclerosis from extravasation or infiltration of vesicant/sclerosing agents (see Box 12–3 for list); photosensitivity, especially from 5-fluorouracil; rashes, urticaria, and pruritus from hypersensitivity reactions; erythema or skin reactions in previously irradiated areas, from chemotherapy-induced "radiation recall"; striae and skin fragility from high doses of steroids	Prevent or minimize integument toxicities; maintain skin integrity	Teach client that alopecia may occur with certain chemotherapy agents; instruct client that hair loss is temporary and hair will regrow, possibly with a different color or texture; instruct client to keep scalp clean with mild shampoo; encourage client to wear wigs or scarves; be informed about scalp tourniquet and scalp hypothermia, which is only effective in minimizing hair loss with certain IV-push, low-dose medications such as doxorubicin and is not effective with PO or infusion-method chemotherapy; institute measures to prevent phlebitis and preserve veins (eg, change IV sites q. 48–72 h, warm soaks to phlebitic areas, avoid high concentrations of K^+ in IV fluids); be aware that all sclerosing agents should be administered by skilled phlebotomists via a free-flowing IV; instruct clients susceptible to photosensitivity to avoid prolonged exposure to the sun and to use sunscreens; observe for rashes and other skin reactions; be aware that some clients who have had previous radiation may have erythema in the irradiated area after the administration of certain chemotherapy agents (called "radiation recall"); instruct client that striae and skin fragility may occur with long-term high doses of steroids; poor wound healing may also occur with steroids	Client will know alopecia is temporary; care for scalp appropriately; experience little or no skin or vein problems
Alteration in elimination: urinary, related to: hemorrhagic cystitis from cytoxan administration; oliguria or renal toxicity from cisplatin administration; dysuria secondary to cystitis; renal calculi from hyperurecemia	Prevent renal and/or bladder toxicities	Force fluids >2 L/day while taking cyclophosphamide (Cytoxan); encourage client to void frequently; dipstick urine for blood for 24 h after PO or IV cyclophosphamide dose; prehydrate with >150–200 mL of fluid/h and ensure urine output is >100 mL/h prior to cisplatin dose; monitor strict input and output post cisplatin administration, urine output should remain >100 mL/h during and at least 4 h post cisplatin; notify physician immediately if urine output decreases below 100 mL/h; check renal function studies; assess for pain in urination, odor of urine, cloudy urine, and frequency and urgency; collect urine for culture and sensitivity if urinary infection suspected; be aware that clients with leukemias and lymphomas may produce increased levels of uric acid from tumor lysis; maintain urine pH at 7.5, force fluids, and administer allopurinal to prevent uric acid formation or sodium bicarbonate or acetazolamide (Diamox) to alkalinize urine	Clients receiving cyclophosphamide will manifest no signs of hemorrhagic cystitis Clients receiving cisplatin will excrete >100 mL/h prior and post cisplatin 4–12 h; manifest renal function studies within normal limits Clients receiving any chemotherapeutic agent will manifest no signs and symptoms of cystitis or increased renal toxicity; maintain a blood uric acid level within normal limits and a urine pH of 7.5 during therapy

(continued)

Table 12-5   Nursing Care Plan for the Client Receiving Chemotherapy (continued)

Nursing Diagnoses	Client Care Goal	Plan/Nursing Implementation	Expected Outcome
Alteration in sensory perception: auditory, kinesthetic, tactile, olfactory, related to: cytoxicity from cisplatin; neurotoxicity from vinblastine, vincristine, etopiside, and cisplatin administration; taste and smell changes	Prevent or minimize alterations in sensory perception	Instruct client to report tinnitus or decreased hearing if receiving cisplatin; baseline audiogram should be done prior to drug; assess for signs and symptoms of neurotoxicity such as numbness and tingling in extremities, decreased sensation, constipation, paralytic ileus, decreased deep tendon reflexes, foot drop, ataxia; place client on daily bowel check; administer stool softener daily and laxatives if no BM in 48 h (for clients on vincristine and vinblastine); monitor BP prior to and q. 15 min during infusion of etopiside, over 30 min to 1 h; instruct clients to avoid foods with strong odors and to eat cold foods such as poultry, cottage cheese, yogurt, milkshakes, cold cuts and cold fruits; be aware that clients may have an aversion to red meats and sweets	Client will experience no hearing loss; state signs and symptoms of neurotoxicity and report if these occur; experience no problems with constipation; experience no hypotension from etopiside; modify diet appropriately
Impaired gas exchange, related to: pulmonary fibrosis from bleomycin therapy; atelectasis; pneumonia from myelosuppression	Maintain adequate respiratory function	Assess for signs and symptoms of respiratory distress: dyspnea, SOB, pallor, cyanosis; auscultate lungs for rales, decreased breath sounds, and stridor; observe for cough, increased sputum production (note amount, color, and consistency) and hemoptysis; monitor temperatures q. 4 h; assess respiratory patterns (eg, rate, depth, and regularity of respirations and use of accessory muscles); check chest x-ray reports, pulmonary function studies, ABGs and blood chemistry; encourage turning, coughing, and deep breathing exercises (diaphragmatic breathing); monitor fluid status input and output; instruct client to avoid strenuous exercise, smoking, and contact with individuals with URIs; encourage frequent rest	Client will experience no respiratory problems during therapy; demonstrate effective breathing exercises; maintain respiratory parameters within normal limits
Injury: trauma, related to effects of chemotherapeutic agents on body tissue: cardiotoxicity, usually from dose-related effects of daunorubicin and doxorubicin; phlebitis from chemical irritants: 5-fluorouracil and etopiside; tissue sclerosis from extravasation of sclerosing agents: doxorubicin, daunorubicin, mechlorethamine, mithramycin, mitomycin, vinblastine, vincristine, dacarbazine; hepatotoxicity from cyclophosphamide, methotrexate	Prevent or minimize potential toxicities	Assess for cardiac toxicity: dysrhythmias, increased cardiac enzymes, signs and symptoms of CHF, chest pain; prevent phlebitis by floating all chemotherapeutic agents through the vein, change IV sites q. 48-72 h; apply warm soaks to phlebitic areas; know that sclerosing agents should only be administered by skilled phlebotomists via a newly started, free-flowing IV; if extravasation is suspected, stop infusion; apply ice to area and notify physician or nurse skilled in management of extravasations; observe for hepatotoxicity, enlarged liver, elevated liver function tests, jaundice, and pruritus	Client will manifest no signs of tissue injury as a result of cardiotoxicity, phlebitis, tissue sclerosis, and hepatotoxicity

Nursing Diagnoses	Client Care Goal	Plan/Nursing Implementation	Expected Outcome
Sexual dysfunction, related to: altered body image; fatigue and other distressing symptoms; changes in hormone levels	Assist client and sexual partner to understand reasons for sexual changes; promote adaptation to altered body image changes and sexual dysfunction	Discuss with the client sexual concerns; explain changes in sexual desire, responsiveness, and function may occur from fatigue, hormonal changes, and other distressing symptoms (eg, nausea, vomiting, pain, diarrhea); teach female clients who are still menstruating that amenorrhea, irregular menses, hot flashes, and decreased vaginal lubrication may occur; a vaginal lubricant can be suggested; contraception methods should be reviewed because genetic mutation can occur; conception during and shortly after chemotherapy is not recommended; the effects of drug related infertility may be temporary or permanent and will vary according to the drug, dosage, and therapy; instruct female clients receiving chemotherapy who have decreased WBC counts to check with their physician about sexual intercourse; inform male clients that decreased hormone production and decreased spermatogenesis may occur; contraceptive methods should be reviewed; impotence and decreased libido or lack of interest may result from fatigue and/or other discomforts; suggest alternate expressions of physical and sexual contact; refer client for sexual counseling, if necessary; stress the importance of open and honest communication with significant others	Client will express sexual concerns if present; explain reasons for sexual changes; take appropriate actions to cope with sexual changes

Although many of the side effects of chemotherapy are unpleasant, clients may be less frightened if they have been prepared for the side effects and given an idea of their possible severity and duration. For example, the client may purchase wigs and scarves before initiating therapy that may cause alopecia. Nausea and vomiting may be alleviated by diversional therapy or relaxation techniques, hypnosis, and touch or music therapy as well as by adjustment of meal times and antiemetic therapy. Some of these techniques can be taught to the client in advance.

Many clients have concerns about the effect of the therapeutic regimen and the disease on sexual activity. Although few clients raise questions about sex, the nurse who has established rapport with the client may introduce the subject casually, perhaps during hygienic care or when explaining the effects of chemotherapy. It is important for clients to understand that decreased sexual desire and responsiveness may be secondary to fatigue, anxiety, and other distressing symptoms associated with the cancer or therapy (eg, nausea, diarrhea, or pain). Female clients may experience decreased vaginal lubrication as a result of hormonal changes; a water-soluble lubricant can be recommended to them. Good precoital and postcoital hygiene should be stressed (eg, cleansing the perineal area) because of the danger of infection. Female clients with severely depressed leukocyte and thrombocyte counts should check with their physician about sexual intercourse. The nurse

can also help to reassure the client and partner by addressing the unspoken question, "Is it catching?"

RADIATION THERAPY

Radiation therapy plays an important role in the treatment of localized malignancies, whether alone or in combination with surgery or chemotherapy. Approximately 60% of clients with cancer receive some form of radiotherapy (Phillips, 1982). This treatment modality has been used since the early 1900s. Earlier in the century radiotherapy usually affected only superficial lesions (generally at the cost of severe skin reactions) and did little for deep-seated tumors. With advancements in radiobiology, tumoricidal effects were enhanced without increasing toxicity to normal tissues.

Principles of Radiation Therapy

In radiation therapy, ionizing radiation is delivered in cancericidal doses to destroy tumor cells. The radiation may be given externally or internally. Ionizing radiation includes both particulate radiation (alpha and beta particles) and electromagnetic or gamma radiation (x-ray or gamma rays). Alpha radiation has poor penetration ability and is rarely used in therapeutic radiation therapy. Beta radiation, with more penetration potential than alpha radiation, is generally emitted from radioactive isotopes (^{32}P, ^{131}I) and used for internal source radiation. Electromagnetic or gamma radiation penetrates deeper areas of the body. In the most common form of radiotherapy, x-rays or external photon radiation is administered by an electrical machine capable of transferring energy from electrons as they interact with a heavy metal. Internal source radiation usually employs gamma rays emitted from radioactive isotopes as they decay.

External x-rays may be delivered in either high- or low-energy beams; the higher the energy, the deeper the penetration potential. Gamma rays have a wide range of energy yield and can penetrate the body at any depth. Both types of radiation pose hazards for clients and those who administer the treatment; gamma rays from internal sources may also present a risk to caregivers and visitors. Precautions are discussed later in this section.

Ionizing radiation damages both normal and malignant cells. Damage may be directly related to the disruption of DNA strands or indirectly as free radicals and ions produced in the intracellular water affect the DNA. Chromosomes may be damaged as parts break off and rejoin other chromosomes; these deletions and translocations lead to chromosomal aberrations that may lead to cell death or mutations if not correctly repaired.

The dual objectives of radiation therapy are to maximize tumor cell destruction ("cell kill") and minimize destruction of neighboring normal cells. Achievement of these goals primarily depends on the differences in radioresponsiveness between normal and malignant cells, whether the tolerance of normal cells has been exceeded, and the capacity of normal cells to repair themselves when damaged. Some tumors are more radioresponsive (a term used to describe tumor regression following radiotherapy) than others. Many lymphomas are exquisitely responsive to radiation; breast, prostate, and lung cancers are responsive to a lesser extent; melanomas and hypernephromas are highly radioresistant.

Normal cells also have some degree of radiosensitivity (cell sensitivity to the effects of radiation) and radioresistance. Radiation has a predilection for rapidly dividing cells such as blood cells (leukocytes, thrombocytes, and to a lesser extent, erythrocytes), cells lining the gastrointestinal tract, and hair follicles. The more radioresistant normal cells include muscle, nerve, and some organ (visceral) cells. Although total dose limitations for certain body tissues have been established, toxicity to normal tissues may still occur. Dose fractionation (ie, dividing the total dose over a period of time) often allows for more efficient normal cell repair.

Selection of the type of x-ray beam is critical in maximizing tumor cell destruction. High-energy or deeper penetrating beams are used for tumors deep within the body; low-energy beams are used for surface lesions. The x-ray beam must be carefully focused to deliver the radiation dose to the tumor. In a process called simulation, a diagnostic quality film of the malignant tumor and surrounding structures taken by a simulator or diagnostic x-ray machine may be visualized with the client in the treatment position. The exact treatment area is localized, the external skin surface over the treatment area is marked, and blocks are fashioned to shield or protect adjacent structures from full dose radiation.

Methods of Delivery

Radiation is measured in the following units:

- The *curie* (Ci), the unit of activity
- The *roentgen* (R), the unit of exposure
- The *radiation absorbed dose* (rad), the unit of absorbed dosages. (The term *gray*, abbreviated as Gy, may also be used; 1 gray = 100 rads.)
- The *roentgen equivalents man* (rem), the dosage equivalent commonly used in radiation safety to quantify radiation exposure

External beam radiotherapy or teletherapy is the delivery of radiation to a tumor by means of an external machine at a predetermined distance. A linear accelerator machine (Figure 12–8) or Cobalt 60 machine may be used.

Internal radiation therapy or brachytherapy may be delivered by systemic, interstitial, or intracavitary means. *Systemic radiotherapy* may be administered intravenously or by oral ingestion of radioisotopes. *Interstitial radiotherapy* involves implantation of radioactive needles, wires, or seeds (tiny radioactive particles) into the tissues. Implants may be placed in body cavities to administer *intracavitary*

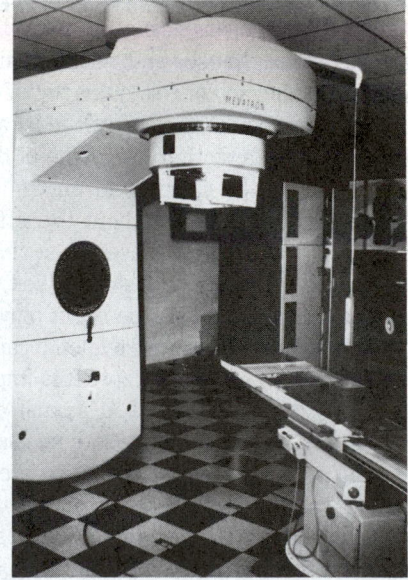

Figure 12–8

Linear accelerator machine (LA-3) emits proton and electron beams. (Courtesy of Hospital of the University of Pennsylvania Radiation Therapy Department)

radiation. A surgical procedure may be necessary to place the radioactive material.

Time, Distance, and Shielding Factors

Factors to consider in evaluating the client's exposure to radiation are:

- The radioactive source
- Duration of exposure
- Distance from the source
- Shielding (protecting untreated areas)

These factors are especially important in evaluating exposure hazards from internal radiation sources for those administering the therapy, caregivers, and others such as visitors and family.

Clients receiving external radiotherapy are not radioactive; they pose no risk for caregivers. Personnel in radiation therapy departments (especially those administering treatment) should wear monitoring devices (eg, a film badge) to measure cumulative radiation exposure.

With internal source radiation, the amount of radiation received is directly related to the duration of exposure. Distance is the most effective reducer of radiation, because the amount of exposure is inversely proportional to the distance between the source and receiver. The source must also be considered. For example, a radioisotope such as ^{32}P (phosphorus) emits poorly penetrating beta particles and presents minimal risks to caregivers; whereas ^{137}Cs (cesium) and ^{192}Ir (iridium) emit both beta and gamma rays (higher penetrating rays), which pose greater risks for radiation exposure. Care of the client must not be compromised because of fear. Risk can be substantially lowered with specific information and guidelines for exposure for the individual client; there is no one overall standard guideline. For specific information on radioisotopes, guidelines for time and distance exposure, and methods of collecting and isolating body secretions, consult a radiation safety officer or radiation therapy department personnel.

Shielding or preventing unnecessary exposure is an important factor in handling displaced radiation sources and bodily wastes contaminated by radiation. If dislodged from the body, the radiation source should never be directly handled without forceps. Radioactive wastes should be placed in closed, marked, shielded containers (usually made of lead). The lead aprons usually worn for protection against low-level radiation (eg, dental x-rays) do not provide sufficient protection from high-level radiation from implanted sources.

Goals of Therapy

Response to radiation therapy depends on the type of tumor. Radiation alone may be curative. For example, tumors arising in the hematopoietic system respond favorably to radiation therapy. Radiation is often combined with surgery and/or chemotherapy to effect a cure.

Palliative radiotherapy may also be employed for symptomatic relief when there is no hope of cure. Local radiation to bone metastases may relieve pain. Reduction of tumor size by radiation may also relieve pain, and radiotherapy may reduce distress from obstruction, effusion, spinal cord compression, and superior vena cava syndrome (see section on oncologic emergencies).

Side Effects of Radiation Therapy

Radiation therapy invariably destroys or damages both normal and malignant cells. Some cells recover, some die. Certain cells cannot reproduce; others die in the attempt.

Localized effects are generally related to the field of treatment. For example, alopecia from cranial radiation, localized skin reactions, and dysphagia from radiation to the esophagus may occur. Generalized symptoms include fatigue and sometimes nausea and vomiting, both related to cellular breakdown products. The client may experience debilitating fatigue and lassitude. Bone marrow depression can result from radiation to bone marrow reserves (ie, iliac crests, sternum), which may be more pronounced in clients concurrently receiving chemotherapy and may be severe enough to warrant stopping treatment.

Although newer methods of treatment have reduced them, localized skin reactions still may occur. The three stages of skin reaction are:

1. Erythema (usually the only reaction)
2. Dry desquamation with flaking
3. Moist desquamation with shedding of surface epithelium (preventable)

Alopecia caused by epilation occurs at the radiation site and possibly at the site where the radiation exits. Effects at the exit site are usually minimal, however, because as the radiation enters the body, it diverges, and some is absorbed by the underlying body tissues.

Intermediate reactions occur when radiation has been delivered to slowly reproducing cells. Pneumonitis and pericarditis may occur 2 or 3 months after radiotherapy. Late side effects may occur years after treatment. Tissue necroses, fistulas, and pulmonary fibroses are long-term problems. Secondary cancers, such as leukemia, may also arise following radiotherapy.

Nursing Implications of Radiation Therapy

Nursing diagnoses related to radiotherapy are similar to those for chemotherapy. A nursing care plan for the client undergoing radiotherapy is in Table 12–6. Psychosocial aspects are addressed in Table 12–7.

(continued on p. 351)

Table 12–6 Nursing Care Plan for the Client Receiving Radiation Therapy

Nursing Diagnoses	Client Care Goal	Plan/Nursing Implementation	Expected Outcome
Alteration in nutrition: less than body requirements, related to nausea and vomiting, anorexia as result of: release of cellular waste products; intestinal mucosal alterations from abdominal radiation; direct cranial radiation; delayed smell and taste changes, dry mouth, mucositis from local head and neck radiation; psychological factors; poor nutritional status	Prevent or minimize vomiting and nausea; increase nutritional intake during treatment; minimize weight loss	Monitor intake and output; encourage fluids 2 L/day; administer antiemetics ½–1 h before treatment for clients receiving abdominal and cranial radiation if nausea and vomiting after treatment is a problem; clients should be instructed to take antiemetics regularly for nausea and vomiting; encourage good oral care, especially for clients receiving head and neck radiation (see alteration in oral mucosa membranes); monitor weights at least weekly; encourage high-protein foods such as cheeses, meats, nutritional supplements, milkshakes (be aware lactose intolerance may occur in adults who seldom drink milk); suggest cold foods for individuals with taste and smell changes; consult a dietitian if necessary; institute calorie counts if client is hospitalized or if the client is at home; encourage client to keep diet history; assess for peripheral and sacral edema from decreased serum protein; recommend a soft diet with full liquids for clients experiencing esophagitis; thicker fluids are easier to swallow than water or juices; avoid drinking fluids with meals; these can cause bloating, and feelings of fullness; fluids should be encouraged between meals	Client will state causes of nausea and vomiting, identify methods of controlling nausea and vomiting; modify diet to enhance food and fluid intake; maintain a stable weight during treatment
Alterations in bowel elimination: diarrhea, related to the effects of radiation on the intestinal mucosa	Refer to Table 12–5	Refer to Table 12–5	Refer to Table 12–5
Fluid and electrolyte imbalance related to: nausea and vomiting; anorexia; diarrhea; constipation; dehydration	Maintain optimal fluid and electrolyte balance	Encourage fluid intake of 2 L/day; monitor intake and output; assess skin turgor; monitor urine specific gravity if necessary; check blood chemistry studies Na^+, K^+, Cl^-; institute measures to control diarrhea and constipation to prevent fluid and electrolyte loss and promote fluid intake	Client will consume 2 L/day of fluid with output comprising approximately ⅔ of intake; laboratory studies will remain within normal limits
Alteration in tissue perfusion, related to the direct cytotoxic effects on bone marrow reserves (iliac crests and sternum): leukopenia; thrombocytopenia; anemia	Refer to Table 12–5	Refer to Table 12–5	Refer to Table 12–5
Alterations in oral mucous membranes related to: direct result of mucosal damage from head and neck radiation, causing inflammation of buccal and gingival membranes, decrease in saliva, changes in normal flora	Refer to Table 12–5	Refer to Table 12–5	Refer to Table 12–5

Nursing Diagnoses	Client Care Goal	Plan/Nursing Implementation	Expected Outcome
Impairment of skin integrity, related to the local effects of radiation on the skin	Maintain skin integrity; institute measures to prevent skin discomfort during and after treatment	Instruct client to avoid the use of soaps, ointments, creams, cosmetics, powder, and deodorants on treated skin area during treatment unless prescribed by physician: avoid washing off markings; keep skin area dry; use Ivory soap for bathing, and do not wash or wet the treated area; check skin area for increased erythema, dryness, burning, discomfort, dry or wet desquamation; instruct client to: report changes in skin; avoid tight-fitting clothing against treated area (100% cotton clothing is recommended); avoid using applications of heat (hot water bottle, heating pads, heat lamp) to treated area during or after treatment; protect skin from sunlight during a few months after treatment; institute comfort measures if skin discomfort is present: use cool air to affected area by fan or blow dryer; administer pain medication; avoid pressure to the area; apply cold Vigilon (C.P. Bard, Inc.) dressing during and after treatment if allowed by physician; encourage the use of wigs and scarves for alopecia from cranial radiation; reassure client that hair will regrow after therapy, usually slowly (3–4 months)	Client will experience minimal skin changes or problems during and after treatment; state appropriate skin care measures necessary to prevent skin problems on the treated areas
Impaired gas exchange, related to the effects of radiation to lung fields, potentially resulting in: pulmonary fibrosis; interstitial pneumonitis; atelectasis	Refer to Table 12–5	Refer to Table 12–5	Refer to Table 12–5
Sexual dysfunction, related to: altered body image; fatigue and other distressing symptoms; changes in hormone levels	Refer to Table 12–5	Refer to Table 12–5 Also, instruct female clients who are receiving radiation in the pelvic and genital organs to check with their physician about sexual intercourse	Refer to Table 12–5

Table 12–7   Psychosocial Nursing Care Plan for the Client and Family

Nursing Diagnoses	Client Care Goal	Plan/Nursing Implementation	Expected Outcome
Anxiety related to: fear of death; fear of body mutilation and pain; prevailing attitudes and beliefs about cancer and cancer therapies; fear of social isolation/role alteration; financial concerns	Minimize or alleviate anxieties associated with diagnosis, treatment, and long-term effects of cancer; provide emotional support to promote effective coping strategies	Acknowledge that anxiety associated with a diagnosis of cancer is normal; assist client and family in expressing concerns; explore attitudes and beliefs about cancer, dispel misconceptions; stress that responses to the effects of cancer and cancer therapies are individual; implement an organized teaching plan with consumer education materials; emphasize the client and family participation; instruct client regarding relaxation exercises; encourage client and family participation in support groups and educational	Client will express concerns related to cancer; maintain optimal level of self-care, independence, and family and social interactions; use effective coping strategies to deal with effects of cancer

(continued)

Table 12–7   Psychosocial Nursing Care Plan for the Client and Family (continued)

Nursing Diagnoses	Client Care Goal	Plan/Nursing Implementation	Expected Outcome
		programs, if available; assist client in formulating realistic goals for self-care, participation in therapy, and family and social interactions; allow client to maintain independence to the extent possible; use an open, honest approach for communication; recommend individual and family counseling, if necessary; offer hospice or palliative care, if available, for clients in the terminal phase of illness	
Disturbance in self-concept, body image, related to: effects of cancer: weight loss, cachexia, and visible changes (eg, skin lesions, ascites, or lymphedema); effects of cancer therapies such as surgery (physical alterations) and radiation and chemotherapy (alopecia, weight loss or gain)	Promote a positive body image	Develop an honest and trusting relationship with client; explore with the client the perceived body-image changes; assist the client in coping with body-image changes: allow verbalization of feelings, encourage client to discuss feelings with significant others, allow client to focus on body parts that may not be affected, encourage client to look at physical alterations while the nurse or significant other is present to lend support; explore ways of minimizing altered body image (wigs, scarves, prosthesis); encourage adequate nutrition if possible to minimize weight loss	Client will express concerns regarding altered body image; exhibit ways of promoting a more positive body image (eg, taking interest in appearance)
Ineffective client/family coping, related to: role performance expectations; financial concerns; altered communication patterns	Establish or maintain effective communication patterns between client and family; provide client- and family-centered care	Assess the family system (eg, communication patterns, role expectations, coping patterns); assess previous client and family losses and ways of dealing with these in the past; encourage open, honest communication; include the family in educational activities and encourage participation in client-centered activities; assist client to set realistic expectations for role as part of a family unit; refer client and family for counseling, if necessary; encourage the client to seek financial advice, if necessary	Client will discuss concerns related to illness with family
Disturbance in self-concept: role performance, related to inability to maintain personal and social responsibilities	Assist the client in establishing realistic goals for personal and social role performance; encourage optimal participation in activities of daily living	Assist the client to identify strengths and weaknesses and to set realistic goals; allow the client to verbalize feelings of loss or grief over inability to maintain previous role function; assist the client to identify realistic role expectations that can be achieved and maintained; offer the client means of maintaining control and providing input into the plan of care; positively reinforce goal-oriented behaviors	Client will formulate realistic goals; manifest optimal interactions with family and environment; maintain optimal level of self-care and independence
Knowledge deficit, related to impaired learning ability, secondary to: denial; anxiety; learning disabilities; pain and other discomforts	Motivate clients and families to learn; encourage optimal client and family participation in care	Assess readiness to learn (usually can be determined by client and family expressing concerns and questions); remember clients who seem disinterested, preoccupied with other thoughts, denying effects of disease or therapy, or extremely anxious may not benefit from teaching plan until motivated and able to concentrate; identify information regarding the disease and effects of therapy that is essential for clients and families for optimal participation in care; prioritize necessary information and formulate a structured	Client will be able to repeat or know where to seek information essential to the plan of care; demonstrate behaviors indicative of learning

Nursing Diagnoses	Client Care Goal	Plan/Nursing Implementation	Expected Outcome
		teaching plan to coincide with expected effects from disease or therapy; use various teaching methods, such as consumer publications (see Resources list); remember teaching does not ensure learning; remember the elderly may need more time to learn; repeat teaching activities as necessary; evaluate the effectiveness of teaching plan; observe behaviors or desired outcomes as a result of teaching; encourage the client and family to write down their questions; for clients whose learning capacities are impaired, be sure to include family members in all teaching activities	

IMMUNOTHERAPY

Still under investigation, immunotherapy seeks to stimulate specific immune responses or to boost overall nonspecific responses against tumor growth. Conventional treatments (surgery, chemotherapy, and radiation) along with the oncogenic process suppress the body's natural immunologic defenses. (The immune response is discussed in Chapter 2.) Combining immunotherapy with conventional treatments may improve the client's prognosis.

Principles of Immunotherapy

Four basic principles govern selection of clients for participation in immunotherapy protocols.

1. The type of tumor and the extent of involvement is critical. Clients with limited disease whose immune systems have not been severely compromised by conventional treatments may benefit from immunotherapy in cases of skin cancer, malignant melanoma, leukemias, bronchogenic carcinoma, colon cancer, tumors of the head and neck, osteogenic sarcomas, ovarian carcinomas, and Hodgkin's disease.

2. Removal of the tumor or reduction of tumor bulk by surgery or radiation in preparation for immunotherapy enhances the client's immune responses.

3. Skin testing before therapy may be used to indicate a certain degree of immune response. The test entails intradermal injection of antigens (substances capable of eliciting an immune response). If no reaction is noted, usually within 48 hours, the client is considered anergic, or not able to demonstrate allergic responses. An anergic response can indicate some degree of immune suppression.

4. Therapy must be planned to stimulate the immune response at the most critical times when conventional therapies have limited the numbers of proliferating cells.

Types of Immunotherapy

In *active immunotherapy,* the client's immune responses are directly stimulated through the use of tumor antigens. In *specific active immunotherapy,* the source of antigenic materials is vaccines. These vaccines contain tumor cell antigens either collected from the client's own tumor or from individuals with the same type of tumor. The antigenicity of these cells may be enhanced by chemicals. To prevent formation of new tumor growths, cells may be irradiated before administration. The vaccine is injected into the client with the hope of stimulating antibody production against the tumor.

Nonspecific active immunotherapy, the most common method, uses antigens and agents that do not originate from tumor cell sources. No attempt is made to stimulate immunity against a specific tumor. Among the common agents are the bacillus Calmette–Guerin (BCG); MER (methanol extraction residue), an extract of BCG; *Corynebacterium parvum;* and levamisole.

Passive immunotherapy uses lymphocytes or serum factors from a healthy person or from a cured client with a similar tumor. These substances are injected into the cancer client to produce an immune response. *Specific passive* or *adoptive immunotherapy* transfers an immune response from a donor to the client. Currently the least used method, passive immunotherapy has the fewest consistent reports of success, perhaps because of its short-lived effect.

Side Effects of Immunotherapy

Generally, the side effects of immunotherapy are much less severe than those of chemotherapy or radiotherapy. Localized erythema or pruritus may occur at the injection site. More severe localized reactions may include pustule formation, necrosis, weeping patches, inflammation at previous injection sites, or regional lymph node involvement. Systemic reactions may include flulike symptoms such as fever, shaking chills, fatigue, arthralgia, or headache. The nurse can reassure the client that these side effects are generally of short duration. Scarring of the injection site persists in some cases.

Allergic responses may also occur. Depending on the individual client's response to a specific immunologic agent, these responses may range from localized urticaria to severe, possible life-threatening anaphylaxis characterized by dyspnea, cyanosis, and convulsions. Treatment of anaphylactic reactions is discussed in Chapter 20.

Monoclonal Antibodies

One of the most promising leads in immunotherapy is the use of **monoclonal antibodies.** Monoclonal antibodies are specially produced antibodies directed toward the antigens or foreign substances on the cell surface of cancer cells. This antigen–antibody mediated response offers a moderate level of specificity against tumor cells, unlike the generalized normal and malignant cell destruction of chemotherapy and radiation therapy. Although not yet perfected, monoclonal antibody treatment is based on the principle that antigenic cell surface changes occur as a cell undergoes malignant transformation. These cell surface antigens are expressed on cancer cells but are absent from normal cells. Some researchers are also studying the possibility of developing a vaccine for cancer from monoclonal antibodies.

The manufacture of monoclonal antibodies begins when malignant tumor cells processing a variety of tumor-associated antigens are injected into an animal (usually a mouse). The tumor-associated antigenic materials stimulate antibody production in the animal's spleen. The spleen is removed from the animal, and B-lymphocytes are procured. Because B-lymphocytes cannot survive for long outside the body, they are fused with rapidly proliferating cancer cells such as myeloma cells to produce an "immortal" cell line, enhancing survival and indefinite production of antibodies relatively specific to the cancer cell antigens. The resulting fused cell, a hybrid, is called *hybridoma* (from the combination of *hybrid* and *myeloma*). This single cell, the hybridoma, can be cloned (reproduced exactly) to produce an endless supply of a single antibody (hence the name monoclonal antibody). This process is illustrated in Figure 12–9.

Monoclonal antibody treatment for cancer is under investigation. The approach has been studied in a variety of cancers such as colon and breast cancer, melanoma, leukemias, and lymphoma. A potential advantage of monoclonal antibodies is their usefulness in diagnosing specific tumors (Morton & Giuliano, 1985).

Monoclonal antibodies are collected and processed for intravenous administration. Allergic-type reactions such as anaphylactic shock or serum sickness are rare. Close monitoring of the client receiving monoclonal antibodies is warranted, including frequent vital signs and observation for anaphylaxis. Fevers and myalgias a few days after therapy may be early signs of serum sickness.

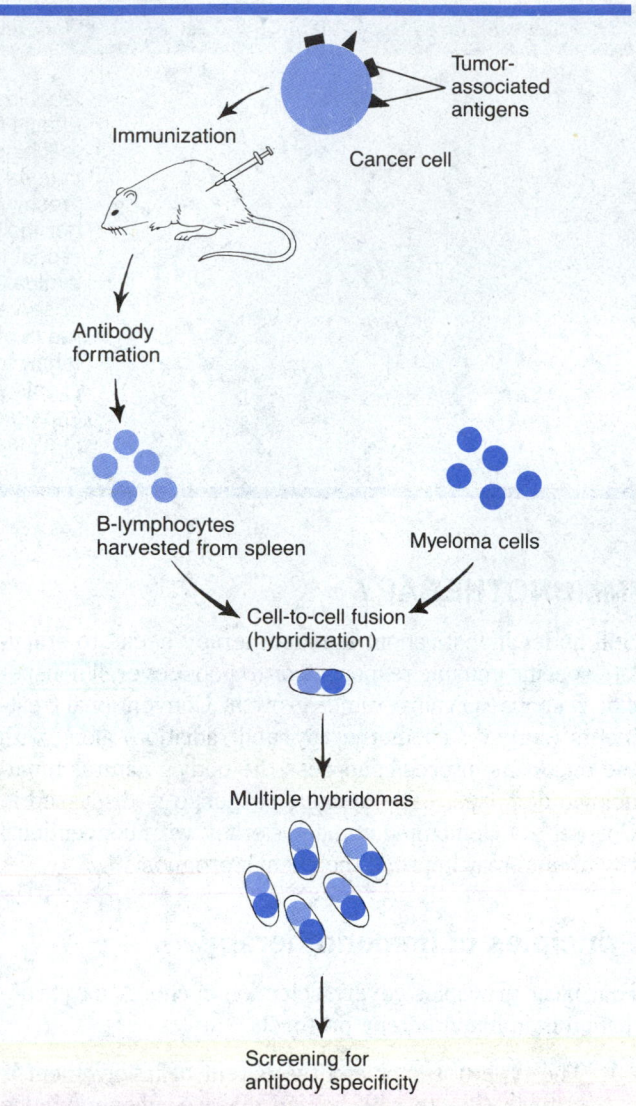

Figure 12–9

Monoclonal antibody production.

Nursing Implications of Immunotherapy

By conscientious application of assessment skills and close observation, nurses can make a significant contribution to progress in this promising new field of cancer therapy. Caring for clients during testing of treatment protocols may yield opportunities for nursing research. Thorough familiarity with immunologic agents, treatment techniques, and their side effects is necessary for prompt intervention if complications develop as well as for client education.

COMBINED THERAPIES

All treatments have strengths and limitations. In *combination therapy* two or more treatment modalities are used simultaneously or alternately for optimal effect. The idea is not that "more is better"; rather, combined therapy attempts to employ the advantages of each type of treatment. For example, the use of chemotherapy in addition to surgical resection may make it possible to avoid radical and disfiguring surgery. Surgical removal of a portion of a tumor may alleviate pain or obstruction while allowing time for chemotherapeutic measures to take effect, or surgery may enhance the effectiveness of immunotherapy.

Adjuvant therapy (auxiliary therapy), combined with surgery, is intended to eradicate any microscopic spread of tumor, prolonging a disease-free state. This type of therapy is of little or no benefit for certain tumors (eg, colon cancers). Adjuvant therapy has improved overall survival for breast, testicular, and head and neck cancers, however. Adjuvant therapy may involve chemotherapeutic, radiologic, or immunologic approaches.

NUTRITION AND TREATMENT

The role of nutrition in cancer therapy is controversial. It is generally agreed that enteral or parenteral nutritional support has no demonstrable effects on stimulating tumor growth in humans, although it has in animals. On the other hand, there is agreement that nutritional repletion may increase tumor responsiveness to chemotherapy and radiation therapy, while minimizing side effects such as nausea and vomiting, mucositis, and diarrhea. Adequate nutrition is also necessary for promoting healing after surgery and enhancing effective immunologic responses.

The client with cancer often experiences anorexia from causes previously discussed. The net result of decreased food intake is malnutrition and cachexia. Enteral hyperalimentation via oral, nasogastric, gastrostomy, and jejunostomy feedings (see Chapter 47) as well as intravenous hyperalimentation (see Chapter 8) may be indicated to restore adequate nutrition and prevent the progressive cachexia associated with cancer. Box 12–4 has helpful eating tips for cancer clients that can be incorporated into the nursing care plan as well as shared with the client and family.

ONCOLOGIC EMERGENCIES

The oncologic emergencies are potentially life-threatening disorders occurring either as a direct effect of malignant tumors or as a consequence of therapy. Included are conditions such as septic shock, disseminated intravascular coagulation (DIC), spinal cord compression, superior vena cava syndrome (SVCS), malignant pericardial and pleural effusions, and hypercalcemia. Depending on its nature, etiology, and severity, the problem, if untreated, might lead to cardiovascular shock, hemorrhage, severe vital organ impairment, neurologic deficits, metabolic alterations, and even death. Therefore, early detection and prompt treatment are necessary if these conditions are to be reversed or controlled.

All nurses caring for clients with cancer should be familiar with these oncologic emergencies, know who is at risk, and be able to recognize and assess the signs and symptoms. Although each condition requires a specialized approach, emotional support and comfort are an essential part of any nursing plan of care. The conspicuous physical alterations, coupled with immediate initiation of therapy, can be alarming to clients and families. Their overwhelming fear can be alleviated to some degree by client education. Explanations of procedures and treatments must be directed toward the client's and the family's levels of comprehension.

Septic Shock

Septic shock associated with a malignancy is often a result of an overwhelming infection in an immunologically compromised host. Because the normal immunologic controls are impaired, individuals at risk include clients with neoplastic invasion of the bone marrow from leukemias, lymphomas, or solid tumors; bone marrow suppression from chemotherapy or radiation therapy; or advanced malignant disease. The infective agent, usually gram-negative bacteria, uncontrollably proliferates, releasing an endotoxin. The endotoxin affects the cardiovascular system, causing a sequence of events leading to decreased cellular oxygenation, hypoxia, metabolic acidosis, and eventually death. The clinical manifestations and nursing implications are discussed in Chapter 11.

Disseminated Intravascular Coagulation

Acute *disseminated intravascular coagulation* is a pathologic state of abnormal coagulation secondary to another underlying process. DIC is characterized by abnormal release and utilization of clotting factors, which is precipitated either by a malignant tumor or infectious process. Thromboplastin, the stimulus for the clotting cascade, is abnormally released from malignant tumors—certain carcinomas, acute promyelocytic leukemia, and neuroblastomas—either as a result of cellular proliferation or lysis, without regard for clotting necessity. In turn, the widespread coagulation stimulates fibrin degradation by the fibrinolytic pathway, breaking down clots as fast as they are formed. The lack of available clotting constituents leads to generalized bleeding. The nurse's role in caring for clients with DIC is discussed in Chapter 29.

Spinal Cord Compression

Spinal cord compression usually results from extradural involvement (outside the cord) as a result of a tumor impinging on the dura mater or from vertebral collapse. This condition can be caused by lymphomas, multiple myeloma, and solid tumors. A less common cause is intramedullary lesions from within the cord itself. Compression may occur at the thoracic, lumbar, or sacral levels. Most clients initially experience either localized or radiating pain (a band or girdle of tightness radiating from the back to the chest or abdomen). Neurologic assessment may find

Box 12–4   Helpful Eating Tips for Cancer Clients

Eat smaller meals more frequently throughout the day. Chew food slowly. Eat whenever you feel hungry.

Keep snacks handy for nibbling. People tend to eat more when food is easily available.

Try eating a snack before you go to bed in addition to your other meals.

If morning is your best mealtime, try to eat as much as you can then without overstuffing yourself.

Rely on food you really love, especially during your not-so-hungry periods. But remember what sounds unappealing today may sound good tomorrow.

Vary the color of foods served on the plate. Make the meal eye appealing. Serve it on a small plate, adding garnishes—an orange or tomato slice or a sprig of parsley.

Make your mealtime a relaxing experience with attractive table settings, bright surroundings, music, and good company.

Stay away from high-fat and greasy foods.

Try resting before a meal. Stop and pause while eating.

Make sure your liquids are nutritious. Do not take a beverage with your meal. Take your beverage between meals to reduce the volume of material in your stomach at eating time.

If protein foods, such as red meat, don't taste right, try eating protein foods cold or at room temperature. Try chicken.

Extra salt may improve the taste of food if you are not on a salt-restricted diet. Try cold cuts.

To enhance taste, meats may be marinated in wine, teriyaki sauce, soy sauce, or Italian dressing.

Tart foods may enhance flavors. Orange juice, pickles, lemonade, vinegar, and lemon juice may be used as seasonings.

Sweeter protein foods may not taste bitter, eg, ice cream, milkshakes, puddings.

Consider using different seasonings, eg, mint, basil, curry, oregano.

When foods taste sweet, use unsweetened (water-packed) fruits and more bland-tasting foods, or rinse canned fruits with water.

If you have an aversion to sweet-tasting foods, try adding a lot of cream to your milkshakes.

Stimulate your appetite with light exercise, such as walking. Check with your doctor about trying wine, dry sherry, or beer before a meal.

Experiment with a diet low in meat but high in other protein foods.

Good odors, such as freshly baked bread or cakes baking, can take your mind off a slumping appetite. If food odors are a problem, don't eat in the room where the food is prepared. And if you feel up to it, try going to a restaurant. Avoid foods that have a strong smell, such as fish.

You can sometimes take away that strange taste in your mouth by eating foods that leave their own tastes in the mouth, such as fresh fruit or hard candies.

In addition to your regular diet, a nutritional supplement containing the needed vitamins, minerals, and nutrients may be used. Ask your doctor about such supplements.

If you wear dentures, make sure they fit properly. Have your dentist rule out dental problems causing bad taste.

Practice good mouth care. Brush teeth gently with a soft toothbrush.

If your mouth is sore, avoid hot spicy foods and eat warm or cool soft, bland foods, eg, cold cuts, cottage cheese, fruits.

If your mouth feels dry, try brushing your teeth before meals or rinsing your mouth with water. Both will stimulate saliva. Also try drinking small sips of fluid with your food.

Consult the American Cancer Society cookbook *Nutrition* and the National Cancer Institute's *Eating Hints: Recipes and Tips for Better Nutrition During Cancer Treatment* (see the resources list at the end of this chapter).

Adapted with permission from American Cancer Society, Philadelphia Division, Cheltenham Unit. Developed in consultation with Rosemary C. Polomano, RN.

muscle weakness, ataxia, urinary or fecal incontinence, and sensory impairment. Severe or prolonged cord compression can cause progressive paralysis with loss of sphincter control.

Immediate radiotherapy is usually instituted for local control along with high doses of corticosteroids to reduce swelling and inflammation. In some circumstances, a decompression laminectomy is required. Both systemic and intrathecal chemotherapy may be used, depending on the type of tumor and its symptoms. The important nursing considerations include frequent neurologic assessment below the level of the lesion, effective pain control, and physical and emotional support in coping with neurologic deficits and proposed therapies. A primary nursing responsibility is astute observation and follow-up of clients' pain or neurologic deficits to detect spinal cord compression before it

progresses to the point where the client is unlikely to become ambulatory again.

Superior Vena Cava Syndrome

Superior vena cava syndrome, characterized by compression of the superior vena cava or intracaval thrombosis of this vessel, obstructs venous blood flow from the head, neck, and upper extremities. Approximately 90% of individuals with this condition are found to have a malignancy. SVCS is most common with bronchogenic carcinomas and, to a lesser degree, with lymphomas and carcinomas of the head and neck, breast, thymus, and testes.

The clinical manifestations of SVCS are those of impaired venous circulation causing fullness in the head and chest, headache, visual changes, dyspnea, cough, wheezing, dysphasia, and syncope. Progression may lead to mental changes; lethargy; and eventually, severe respiratory distress. Obvious signs include distended neck, chest, and arm veins along with facial, neck, and possibly arm edema. Because of this congestion, clients prefer an upright position for effective breathing.

Treatment usually begins with a tissue diagnosis by bronchoscopy or mediastinoscopy to confirm SVCS, because other conditions, such as aortic aneurysm, can cause the same symptoms. For clients requiring a biopsy, be aware of the risk of hemorrhage because of vessel engorgement and the risk of respiratory distress from compression of the trachea. Careful assessment of respiratory and cardiovascular status is essential. Radiotherapy is usually used to achieve a quick response in tumor reduction because death can ensue if the obstruction is not relieved. Capable of effecting a response in drug-sensitive tumors, chemotherapy is used although effects may be somewhat slower. Nursing goals are aimed at promoting comfort by positioning the client in a high Fowler's position and supporting edematous upper extremities, modifying activity, and managing the effects of therapy.

Malignant Pericardial Effusion

Malignant pericardial effusion is an accumulation of fluid between the visceral layer of the pericardium (the lining directly over the heart) and the parietal pericardium (the lining of the pericardial sac) as a result of malignant cell infiltration. As it accumulates, the fluid restricts the heart's expansion capacity during the diastolic or ventricular filling phase. As the heart is compressed, effective cardiac output cannot be maintained; consequently, dyspnea, anxiety, restlessness, chest discomfort, and eventually circulatory collapse may occur. This condition, called *cardiac tamponade*, is described in Chapter 24. Physical assessment parameters include jugular vein distention, tachycardia, rapid respiratory rate, decreased blood pressure secondary to decreased cardiac output, and mental status changes.

The condition can be caused by spread of tumor cells from lung and breast cancers, lymphomas, leukemias, and malignant melanoma as well as by high doses of radiation therapy to the heart. Treatment includes the creation of a pericardial window to allow fluid to escape into surrounding lymphatics and pericardial stripping, removing the fluid-producing membrane layer. Chemotherapy is used if the condition is caused by breast cancers, leukemias, and lymphomas. Radiotherapy may have a general role for all tumor types but not for conditions precipitated by radiation toxicity. Knowledge of the signs and symptoms along with skill in cardiovascular system assessment are important nursing considerations.

Malignant Pleural Effusion

A *pleural effusion* is an accumulation of fluid between the visceral layer (outer lining) of the lung and the parietal layer (lining of the pleural cavity). When caused by a malignancy, the condition is generally secondary to tumor cells in the lung (either primary lung cancer or metastatic disease from other tumor types), seeding or implanting on the parietal lining, or from spread of tumor cells through the blood to the parietal pleura. As the fluid builds up, the area for lung expansion decreases. The severity of symptoms depends on whether there is unilateral or bilateral involvement and on the amount of fluid in the pleural space. Symptoms such as shortness of breath, dyspnea, chest pain, and cough may be present. Usually, a chest tube is inserted to drain the fluid. A sclerosing agent (a drug that causes widespread tissue irritation) may be instilled through the chest tube to initiate a widespread inflammation resulting in fibrosis and scarring and decreasing fluid secretion. Care of the client with a chest tube is discussed in Chapter 18. Chemotherapy is most frequently used for tumors that are drug sensitive. Local radiation therapy is reserved for drug-resistant tumors.

Hypercalcemia

Hypercalcemia, the most common oncologic emergency, is a rise in the blood calcium level beyond what can be incorporated into the bone or excreted by the kidneys. Tumors generally cause calcium elevations by: metastatic tumor invasion of bone (usually from breast cancers), prostaglandin release from tumors, or release of an activating substance associated with multiple myeloma. These mechanisms act on the target osteoclast cells of the bone, causing release of calcium. Uncontrolled excess blood calcium levels may lead to mental status changes (lethargy and confusion), muscle weakness, coma, and eventual cardiac arrest.

The preferred treatment is to eradicate the stimulus for calcium release, usually the tumor. In addition, attempts are made to control the rise in the calcium concentration by increasing renal excretion through fluid diuresis and medications. Hypercalcemia is discussed further in Chapter 5.

ALTERNATIVE THERAPIES

Alternative therapies are therapeutic approaches other than the conventional modalities of surgery, chemotherapy, and radiotherapy. (Immunotherapy might be considered a frontier.)

Some alternative techniques supplement conventional therapy, often to improve client comfort, eg, self-hypnosis, psychological counseling, or relaxation techniques. Some researchers are exploring the possibility that nutritional factors underlie the oncogenic process. At present, however, nutritional therapy, including total parenteral nutrition, is used to potentiate conventional therapy.

New drugs or treatment protocols not yet commercially available may be available to selected clients in oncology centers. New drugs or combinations of drugs as well as various forms of high-dose chemotherapy are continually being tested. Other promising techniques that require further study include bone marrow transplantation, interferon, red light (hematoporphyrin) therapy, hyperthermia, visual imagery, and limb salvage surgery techniques.

Bone Marrow Transplantation

Bone marrow transplantation (BMT) is essentially an auxiliary technique that facilitates use of higher doses of chemotherapeutic agents and radiation. In some cases, the dose sufficient to produce tumoricidal effects may suppress bone marrow activity to a life-threatening extent. If transplanted bone marrow can generate the production of new bone marrow to replace what was destroyed, higher doses can be given before the transplant. Either *autologous marrow* (from the client's own body) or *allogeneic marrow* (from a donor) may be used. Bone marrow transplantation has been used with some success in clients with leukemia, anaplastic anemia, and severe immunodeficiency. The BMT procedure is described in Chapter 30.

Interferon

Interferon has received much publicity as a new hope for cancer clients. Essentially, **interferon** is a form of protein produced by the body as a by-product of the physiologic response to a viral infection. When stimulated by interferon, certain body cells produce substances that inhibit the reproduction of viruses. Interferon was initially tested in clients with cancer in the hope it might stimulate body cells to inhibit cancer cell mitosis. It has been found that, in addition to any antitumor activity, interferon may enhance the activity of the client's immune defense system. Any improvement of immune defenses would greatly benefit clients with cancer. Interferon therapy is still being studied. Side effects include extreme malaise, fever, myalgias, depressed bone marrow production, and excessive or insufficient production of antibodies.

Photodynamic Therapy

Photodynamic therapy, or red light therapy, uses a light-sensitive drug called hematoporphyrin derivative. When administered intravenously, this drug is quickly washed out by normal cells but is stored by cancer cells. When a fiberoptic beam of red light, usually from a laser, is directed at the hematoporphyrin-containing cancer cells, the drug produces a form of oxygen that is lethal to the cancer cells. Researchers are beginning to report disease regressions with certain kinds of cancers such as lung and esophageal cancer. The treatment has little effect on slow-growing cancers with a poor blood supply and is only effective on tumors that can be visualized. Clients have photosensitivity for about a month after treatment and must avoid sun

and bright light. Strictly experimental, phototherapy is available in only a few research centers and has not yet been approved by the FDA.

Hyperthermia

Hyperthermia is based on the premise that certain types of neoplastic cells are more responsive to antineoplastic drugs if they have been exposed to high temperatures. In 1984, the FDA approved a device that uses controlled microwave energy to treat melanoma, squamous cell carcinoma, adenocarcinoma, and sarcoma in clients who have recurrent or regressive cancers of those types despite conventional therapy (Thompson, 1984). A palliative treatment, hyperthermia suppresses cancer growth by heat, or thermal energy. The hyperthermia device radiates energy, much like a microwave oven. A hornlike applicator on the microwave machine directs a beam of energy to the tumor, heating the cancer cells to 108° to 113°F (42° to 45°C) causing the tumor cells to die. In normal tissue, heat is carried away by the blood that flows through it. Because solid malignant tumors are much less vascular, the heat is not carried away as quickly, and the tumors reach a relatively higher temperature than surrounding normal tissue. The temperature of the tumor and the surrounding tissue is constantly monitored during the treatment by needlelike thermometers inserted into the tissues that automatically adjust the power to maintain the desired temperature. Hyperthermia is an experimental technique available only in a few cancer centers.

Visual Imagery

Visual imagery, a technique developed by the Simontons (Simonton, Matthews-Simonton, Creighton, 1978), stems from the theory that the mind can stimulate the body's natural defenses to withstand neoplastic disease. The theory is not one of "mind over matter"; rather, it is based on advances in understanding of the interrelation of mind and body. The Simonton regimen includes counseling, relaxation, and exercises in visual imagery; eg, clients are encouraged to visualize leukocytes devouring bacteria within the bloodstream or to visualize themselves pursuing a cherished activity. The Simontons advise that this technique be used in conjunction with standard acceptable medical practices. Later work by Stephanie Matthews-Simonton focused on involving the cancer client's family in the creation of a healing environment (1984).

Limb Salvage Surgery

New *limb salvage surgery* techniques allow clients to avoid amputation, eg, in cases of bone cancer. Transplants of bone from cadavers and grafts made of space-age synthetics are being studied (see the section on bone grafting in Chapter 60).

UNORTHODOX THERAPIES

Given the poor prognosis associated with many forms of cancer and the painful and debilitating side effects of some conventional therapies, it is not surprising that cancer victims and their families may be susceptible to unorthodox practitioners who hold out hope—however faint—of cure. To take a recent and well-known example, an estimated 70,000 Americans have tried *laetrile (amygdalin) therapy,* despite the lack of reliable evidence that this compound has an antineoplastic effect (Nixon, 1982).

The principle danger of unorthodox therapies is that conventional treatment may be delayed until it is too late, or treatment may be foregone entirely. Another danger is that clients who have tried unorthodox therapies may be reluctant to inform health care providers of this fact, for fear of scorn and disapproval. Side effects of unorthodox therapy—eg, cyanide poisoning in users of laetrile—may thus go unrecognized and untreated (Nixon, 1982).

By establishing rapport with the client and responding empathically to expressions of fear and despair, the nurse can caution client and family to be alert for fraudulent claims. Several characteristics suggest unscrupulous practice:

- The treatment regimen is secret.
- Histologic verification of cancer is not required.
- Conventional treatments are denigrated.
- Record keeping is scanty or nonexistent.
- The care provider may have unusual degrees from unfamiliar institutions.
- Treatment is extremely costly compared with conventional therapies.

Proponents of unorthodox therapies may not have mercenary motives and be sincere in their beliefs. The rationale for some therapies may seem plausible; eg, it seems reasonable to believe that nutrition may play a greater role in cellular structure and function than has heretofore been attributed to it. Indeed, the American Cancer Society has recently conducted studies of the relation between cancer and nutrition and made several recommendations listed earlier in this chapter.

Another unorthodox approach to cancer therapy is the macrobiotic diet, introduced into the United States by the Japanese in the 1960s. This diet largely comprises whole grain cereals, vegetables, and supplementary foods, with occasional consumption of white-meat fish and dried and fresh fruits. The predominantly vegetarian diet forbids the ingestion of red meats and dairy products. Proponents of the macrobiotic diet believe that the Western diet including red meats, poultry, milk, eggs and other dairy products promotes carcinogenesis. They believe cancer evolves from an imbalance of yin and yang forces; certain food classifi-cations consumed in excess are believed to have the tendency to cause cancer in the lower or upper part of the body. Besides imposing restrictions on food intake, the diet is not very palatable, and preparation is inconvenient. Because the diet lacks essential nutrients, severe malnutrition may occur. Health-care providers do not advocate this diet because scientific evidence shows no benefits in cancer prevention, cure, or control.

Clients must be cautioned to evaluate *all* treatment modalities carefully in the light of the best current thinking about the nature of the neoplastic process and in the light of their personal experience, values, and goals.

SUPPORTIVE CARE

For some clients with cancer, the time comes when nothing further can be done to cure the disease or arrest its course. All treatment options may have been exhausted, or the client may choose not to submit to treatments that might prolong life by sacrificing its quality. Some members of the health care team or the family may find such a decision difficult to accept. In such cases, the nurse may assume the role of client advocate, affirming the client's fundamental right to determine the conditions under which he or she chooses to live.

Supportive care is the palliative treatment of the symptoms and effects of an advancing, incurable, terminal disease process. The underlying premise of supportive care is not based on curative or disease control measures; rather, it is a shift from the focus on arresting disease and prolonging life to providing the maximum possible quality of life while encouraging the client to cope with and prepare for death.

Cassileth and Cassileth (1982) have outlined general assumptions underlying supportive care for clients with cancer:

- The oncologic process is not curable.
- The neoplasm is the cause of the client's symptoms.
- Treatment goals must be set realistically in light of these facts.
- Effective communication with client and family must be established.
- Care and treatment should be planned to avoid debilitating side effects.

Control of pain (see Chapters 5 and 16) becomes the first priority in supportive care. Nutritional support with emphasis on palatability, control of infection, and comfort measures including emotional support are other important goals. The client may choose to spend the final stage of life at home receiving hospice care, or a hospice facility may seem the best alternative. The dying process and nursing principles applicable to terminal illness are discussed in Chapter 16.

Section VI: Psychosocial Dimensions of the Cancer Experience

The neoplastic process adds an extra dimension to the experience of illness (see Chapter 4). The client with cancer must cope with a multitude of internal and external stressors, and the client's significant others have their own problems to face.

A pertinent question during initial assessment is, "What problems and coping resources did the client have *before* the cancer was diagnosed?" For example, does the client have a history of depressive illness? How might this affect response to the current diagnosis? To stresses imposed by treatment? To necessary adjustments of lifestyle? What social or environmental stressors might be affecting client or family in addition to those associated with neoplastic disease? Financial problems? Divorce or widowhood? Ill health of a spouse or child? What about attitudes toward cancer in the client's family? Social or cultural group? Work environment?

There is a "cancer mythology" in Western society— beliefs that influence societal attitudes toward persons with cancer and persons' attitudes toward themselves. These myths include:

- The *contagious myth*—the belief that cancer is "catching."

- The *pain myth*—the belief that the pain of cancer is inevitable, immediate, excruciating, unending, and uncontrollable.

- The *treatment myth*—the belief that all cancer treatments are lengthy and painful.

- The *mutilation myth*—the belief that all cancers cause mutilation and disfigurement and that all treatments cause extensive, permanent disfigurement.

The myth of contagion is without foundation. Others carry sufficient truth to account for their longevity—cancer *may* be painful, and treatments *may* be debilitating and temporarily or permanently disfiguring. But myths that make the client's situation seem worse than it is impose unneeded burdens on both the client and society. For example, fear of contagion can isolate clients when they need maximum support from family and friends. Fear of contagion or a partner's unfounded concerns about damaging the client's health can unnecessarily curtail the client's sexual activity. Fear and misunderstanding can underlie societal discrimination against the individual with cancer; clients whose cancer is cured or in remission may lose their jobs or be unable to find employment. Those who have been treated for cancer at any time in their lives find insurance almost impossible to obtain.

Cancer imposes a large financial burden on client, family, and society. Individuals have expended their life savings on treatment; billions have been spent on research aimed at eradicating neoplastic disease. This burden is increased when individuals with cancer are restrained from leading productive lives because of cancer mythology.

Individuals respond to a diagnosis of cancer in themselves or a loved one in individual ways: fear ("Will I die?" "What will happen?"); guilt ("Am I too much of a burden?"); anger ("Why must this happen to *me*?"); despair ("It's no use; I know I'm doomed."). Families have similar reactions, whether directed inward or at the client. Hostility or fear, for example, may engender oversolicitude. Either client or significant others may relieve stress by lashing out angrily at others, including the nurse. Although the cost in time and patience may seem high, the gift of listening may be the greatest the nurse can offer the client. A psychosocial nursing care plan for the client with cancer is in Table 12–7.

Section VII: Rehabilitation

For too long, public attitudes and sometimes those of health professionals, have focused on supportive care of the client dying with cancer. Because survival among cancer clients has significantly improved, rehabilitation is assuming a new role in oncology as a necessary and integral aspect of cancer care. In recent years, publicity about the cancer experiences of well-known figures such as former First Lady Betty Ford and television personality Betty Rollins has provided a more optimistic view of cancer.

Rehabilitation is a dynamic, holistic process in which the individual with cancer is assisted in achieving optimal function in all areas of life. Rehabilitation for clients with cancer should be similar to that for disabilities and handicaps secondary to other health problems. The rehabilitative process is directed toward maximizing function and fostering psychosocial adaption to lifestyle changes imposed by cancer. Rehabilitation should provide opportunities for the client and family to set new priorities and reformulate realistic goals, all for the purpose of making life more meaningful. Rehabilitation involves clients, significant others, and community support groups, as well as the health care team. Physical rehabilitation includes physical and occupational therapy, nutritional support, and enterostomal therapy as well as reconstructive surgery. Vocational rehabilitation, financial planning, and spiritual and psychological support care are also essential components of the rehabilitative process.

The type and extent of cancer, the magnitude of physical and emotional impairments, and the available treatment options and response to therapies are important in constructing a rehabilitative program. The clients' and families' motivational levels, availability of social resources, and financial support play equally important roles.

Rehabilitation does not begin with client discharge. Rehabilitative efforts should start with admission to the hospital and continue throughout the hospitalization as the client's life is actually or potentially affected by cancer. The process begins with an assessment. Factors to be considered are:

- The pathologic state. (Is it progressive or stable?)
- The physical or functional impairments. (Are these reversible or irreversible?)
- The client's strengths (motivational, physical, and emotional).
- The family system and supports.
- The availability of financial and community resources.

The trend toward greater client involvement in health care planning and treatment regimens (see Chapter 2) is reflected in the growing number of community resources available to clients with cancer and to their families. Some groups offer financial assistance; some offer counseling; some offer mutual support with sharing of the cancer experience. The American Cancer Society offers many kinds of assistance, including homemaker services, blood donors, transportation, equipment, and supplies. Self-help groups such as Reach for Recovery (breast cancer), the International Association of Laryngectomees, and the United Ostomy Association offer the invaluable counsel of those who "have been there." And groups such as Make Today Count offer both practical and emotional support. (A list of support groups is at the end of this chapter.) By informing the client about these services and encouraging the client to use them, the nurse performs the dual service of offering the client practical assistance and reassuring the client that the cancer experience need not be endured alone.

Chapter Highlights

Cancer alters the biopsychosocial environment to such a degree that it continually interrupts the body's state of equilibrium.

Oncology nursing is a specialty. Because cancer is a widespread health problem, however, nurses from every practice area have the opportunity to care for cancer clients.

The fundamental differences between a benign and malignant cell are the malignant cell's abilities to infiltrate surrounding tissue and metastasize.

Basic knowledge of the oncologic process is necessary for implementing the nursing process during all phases of the client's cancer experience.

The evolution of cancer probably results from a combination of factors. No one theory of causation is universally accepted.

Generalized systemic effects from cancer may include fatigue, anemia, infection, cachexia, organ impairment, hormonal imbalance, and pain. The degree to which these occur depends on the type and extent of the malignant tumor as well as the body area involved.

Prime objectives of community prevention and detection programs have been to increase awareness of cancer's seven warning signals and to promote compliance with self-examination and cancer check-ups.

Self-examination at recommended intervals may lead to early detection of cancers, optimizing chances for cure.

Surgery remains the primary treatment of choice for many types of cancer. With more effective chemotherapy regimens and advancements in radiotherapy, these treatments are more widely used in combination or alone.

Adjuvant chemotherapy and radiation therapy are aimed at eradicating microscopic spread of the disease in combination with another form of primary therapy.

Common side effects of chemotherapy include alopecia, bone marrow suppression (leukopenia and thrombocytopenia), and gastrointestinal side effects (mucositis and diarrhea).

Sexual desires and responses may be altered as a result of body image changes and generalized effects from cancer and cancer therapy.

Systemic generalized effects of radiotherapy may include fatigue, weakness, anorexia, and perhaps mild nausea. More severe nausea and vomiting may occur from cranial and abdominal irradiation. Local effects are hair loss in the irradiated area and possibly skin toxicity.

Primary objectives of immunotherapy are to stimulate specific immune responses and potentiate overall immunity. This type of therapy is not generally effective in advanced disease.

Early assessment and recognition and prompt treatment of oncologic emergencies are important factors in reversing or controlling these conditions.

(continued)

Chapter Highlights (continued)

Unproven methods of cancer treatment may cause clients to delay acceptable conventional therapies or may deter them from seeking conventional therapies.

Clients with cancer and their families should be informed and educated about their disease and treatment to enhance participation in care.

Rehabilitation of the client with cancer requires an interdisciplinary approach.

Clients who are dying are also living. Supportive care for the dying should include adequate pain and symptom control, emotional and social support, and spiritual care.

Bibliography

American Cancer Society: *Cancer Facts and Figures*. New York: American Cancer Society, 1985.

American Cancer Society: *Nutrition Common Sense and Cancer*. ACS Publication 84-IMM-No. 2096-LE. New York: American Cancer Society, 1984.

American Joint Committee on Cancer: *Manual for Staging of Cancer*, 2nd ed. Philadelphia: Lippincott, 1983.

Bersani G, Carl W: Oral care for cancer patients. *Am J Nurs* 1983; 83:533–536.

Byrne CJ et al: *Laboratory Tests: Implications for Nursing Care*, 2nd ed. Menlo Park, CA: Addison–Wesley, 1986.

Cassileth BR, Cassileth PA (editors): *Clinical Care of the Terminal Cancer Patient*. Philadelphia: Lea & Febiger, 1982.

Chernecky CC, Ramsey PW: *Critical Nursing Care of the Client with Cancer*. Norwalk, CT: Appleton–Century–Crofts, 1984.

Cline BW: Prevention of chemotherapy-induced alopecia: A review of the literature. *Cancer Nurs* 1984; 7:221–228.

Copeland EM et al: Nutritional changes in neoplasia. In: *Surgical Nutrition*. Fischer, JE (editor). Boston: Little, Brown, 1983.

Derogatis LR, Abeloff MD, Melisaratos N: Psychological coping mechanisms and survival time in metastatic breast cancer. *JAMA* 1979; 242:1504–1508.

Devita V, Hellman S, Rosenburg S (editors): *Cancer: Principles and Practices of Oncology*, 2nd ed. Philadelphia: Lippincott, 1985.

Donaghue M, Nunnally C, Yasko JM: *Nutritional Aspects of Cancer Cure: A Self-Learning Module*. Reston, VA: Reston, 1985.

Donovan MI, Girton SE: *Cancer Care Nursing*. Norwalk, CT: Appleton–Century–Crofts, 1984.

EORTC International Antimicrobial Therapy Project Group: Three antibiotic regimens in treatment of infection in febrile granulocytopenic patients with cancer. *J Infect Dis* 1978; 137:14–29.

Falck K et al: Mutagenicity in urine of nurses handling cytotoxic drugs. *Lancet* (June 9) 1979; 1:1250–1251.

Frank–Stromberg M et al: Psychological impact of the "cancer" diagnosis. *Oncol Nurs Forum* 1984; 11(3):16–22.

Greer S, Morris T, Pettingale KW: Psychological response to breast cancer. *Lancet* 1979; 2:785–787.

Groer ME, Shekleton E: *Basic Pathophysiology: A Conceptual Approach*, 2nd ed. St. Louis: Mosby, 1983.

Gunn AE: *Cancer Rehabilitation*. New York: Raven, 1984.

Higby DJ: *The Cancer Patient and Supportive Care*, 2nd ed. Boston: Martinus Nijhoff, 1985.

Howard–Ruben J, Miller NJ: Unproven methods of cancer management. Part 2: Current trends and implications. *Oncol Nurs Forum* 1984; 11(1):67–73.

Klatersky J: *Infections in Cancer Patients*. New York: Raven, 1982.

Knopf MK, Fischer DS, Welch-McCaffrey D: *Cancer Chemotherapy: Treatment and Care*. Boston: Hall, 1984.

Matje SD: Stress and cancer: A review of the literature. *Cancer Nurs* 1984; 7:399–404.

Maxwell MB: When the cancer patient becomes anemic. *Cancer Nurs* 1984; 7:321–326.

McNally JC, Stair JC, Somerville ET (editors): *Guidelines for Cancer Nursing Practice*. New York: Grune & Stratton, 1985.

Morgan HR: Virology: Relationship of viruses to malignant disease in animals and man. In: *Clinical Oncology for Medical Students and Physicians: A Multidisciplinary Approach*. Rubin P (editor). New York: American Cancer Society, 1983.

Morton PL, Giuliano AE: Cancer immunology and immunotherapy. In: *Cancer Treatment*, 2nd ed. Haskel, CM (editor). Philadelphia: Saunders, 1985.

National Study Commission on Cytotoxic Exposures: *Recommendations for Handling Cytotoxic Agents*. Syracuse, NY: Bristol Laboratories, March 1984.

Nixon D: *Diagnosis and Management of Cancer*. Menlo Park, CA: Addison–Wesley, 1982.

Nowell PC: Tumor biology: Evolution toward terminal illness. In: *Clinical Care of the Terminal Cancer Patient*. Cassileth BR, Cassileth PA (editors). Philadelphia: Lea & Febiger, 1982.

Oncology Nursing Society: *Cancer Chemotherapy: Guidelines and Recommendations for Nursing Education and Practice*. Pittsburgh, PA: Oncology Nursing Society, 1984.

Oppenheimer S: *Cancer: A Biological and Clinical Introduction*. Boston: Allyn and Bacon, 1982.

Patterson WB: Principles of surgical oncology. In: *Clinical Oncology for Medical Students and Physicians: A Multidisciplinary Approach*. Rubin P (editor). New York: American Cancer Society, 1983.

Phillips TL: Principles of radiobiology and radiation therapy. In: *Principles of Cancer Treatment*. Carter SK, Glatstein E, Livingston RB (editors). New York: McGraw–Hill, 1982.

Silverberg E: Cancer statistics, 1982. *CA* 1982; 32:15–31.

Simmons CC: The relationship between life change losses and stress levels for females with breast cancer. *Oncol Nurs Forum* 1984; 11(2):37–41.

Simonton OC, Matthews-Simonton S, Creighton JL: *Getting Well Again: A Step by Step, Self-Healing Guide to Overcoming Cancer for Patients and Their Families*. New York: Bantam, 1978.

Thompson RC: Heat used to fight some cancers. *FDA Consumer* 1984; 18(3):26–27.

Twycross RG, Lack SA: *Symptom Control in Far Advanced Cancer: Pain Relief.* London: Pitman, 1983.

US Department of Health and Human Services, Public Health Service and National Institutes of Health: *Recommendations for the Safe Handling of Parenteral Antineoplastic Drugs.* Publication No. 83-2621, 1983.

Valentine AS, Stewart JA: Oncologic emergencies. *Am J Nurs* 1983; 83:1282–1285.

Yasko JM: *Care of the Client Receiving External Radiation Therapy: A Self-Learning Module.* Reston, VA: Reston, 1982.

Yasko JM: *Guidelines for Cancer Cure: Symptom Management: A Self-Learning Module.* Reston, VA: Reston, 1983.

Suggested Readings

Baxley KO et al: Alopecia: Effect on cancer patients' body image. *Cancer Nurs* 1984; 7:499–503. A research study demonstrated the impact of hair loss on the client's total body image.

Hassey K: Demystifying care of patients with radioactive implants. *Am J Nurs* 1985; 85:788–792. Accompanied by photographs, this article discusses the hospital and home care of clients with radioactive vaginal, breast, head-and-neck, and prostatic implants. General as well as specific guidelines are provided for both temporary and permanent implants.

Kaempfer SH, Hoffman DJ, Wiley FM: Spermbanking: A reproductive option in cancer therapy. *Cancer Nurs* 1983; 6:31–38. This article describes the use of sperm banking for male clients before radiation therapy or chemotherapy. The authors conclude that sperm banking is a comfort to many clients because the integrity of their reproductive functioning is kept intact.

Maxwell MB: Dyspnea in advanced cancer. *Am J Nurs* 1985; 85:673–677. This article focuses on reducing the dyspnea experienced by many ambulatory cancer clients and identifying the difference between acute breathlessness and slowly developing dyspnea. Useful illustrations on pursed-lip breathing and work simplification are included.

Nealon E, Blumberg B, Brown B: What do patients know about clinical trials? *Am J Nurs* 1985; 85:807–810. A pilot study by the National Cancer Institute to investigate the education needs of cancer clients considering clinical trials is described. The study's outcome, a booklet with basic information about clinical trials, is also described. (See the resources list at the end of this chapter for directions on how to obtain a copy of *What Are Clinical Trials All About?*)

Pageau MG, Mroz WT, Coombs DW: New analgesic therapy relieves cancer pain without oversedation. *Nurs 85* (April) 1985; 15:46–49. The article describes continuous intraspinal morphine infusion. Morphine is infused through an infusion pump implanted in the abdomen and a catheter inserted in the intraspinal space to relieve intractable pain in cancer clients.

Simonton SM, Shook RL: *The Healing Family.* New York: Bantam, 1984. Based on the classic earlier work by the Simontons (*Getting Well Again: A Step By Step, Self-Healing Guide to Overcoming Cancer for Patients and Their Families.* New York: Bantam, 1978), this book helps individual cancer clients and their families learn how to mobilize the client's immune system through visual imagery. Included are strategies for

clients without a traditional family—whether single, widowed, or elderly and alone—to create their own healing family through intimates and friends.

Resources

In addition to these resources, see the listings in other chapters throughout this text for information about cancer in specific body systems. For example, resources for the client with leukemia are listed in Chapter 28; for the client with a laryngectomy, in Chapter 18; and for the client with a mastectomy, in Chapter 63.

SELF-HELP GROUPS AND OTHER ORGANIZATIONS

American Cancer Society
National Headquarters
777 Third Ave.
New York, NY 10017
Phone: (212) 371-2900

> This voluntary organization has about 3000 chapters, staffed largely by volunteers, to provide services to cancer clients, educational programs, and research. Sponsors the "I Can Cope" program to address the educational and psychological needs of clients and families through lecture and group discussion. Also sponsors a number of cancer prevention programs through local units.

Corporate Angel Network (CAN)
Hangar F
Westchester County Airport
White Plains, NY 10604

> A group of 310 firms will provide free transportation on corporate flights to cancer clients in need of treatment. This is an especially useful service because most insurance plans do not cover medical travel costs. To qualify, clients must be able to walk, have proof they are being treated, and be fit to fly. Organized by Priscilla Blum, a pilot and former cancer client.

Make Today Count
PO Box 303
Burlington, IA 52601
Phone: (319) 754-7266

> A mutual support group for persons with cancer and other life-threatening illnesses, this group also provides support to clients' families and assists members of the professional community to meet these needs.

United Cancer Council, Inc.
1803 N. Meridian St.
Indianapolis, IN 46202
Phone: (317) 923-6490

> This federation of voluntary cancer agencies provides a cancer control program through service, education, and research.

HOT LINES

Cancer Information Services
Phone: (800) 4-CANCER (in Hawaii, Oahu (808) 524-1234, neighboring islands call collect; in Washington, DC, and sub-

urbs in Maryland and Virginia (202) 636-5700; in Alaska (800) 638-6070

This service, sponsored by the National Institutes of Health, provides the latest facts on all types of cancers, educational materials available for consumer education, and information on coping with the disease. Spanish-speaking staff members are available to callers from the following areas (daytime hours only); California (area codes 213, 619, 714, 805), Florida, Georgia, Illinois, northern New Jersey, New York City, and Texas.

NURSING ORGANIZATIONS

American Radiological Nurses Association
Johns Hopkins Hospital
Radiology Division, Dept N83
600 N. Wolfe St.
Baltimore, MD 21205
Phone: (301) 955-5784

An organization of nurses working in radiology, this group has educational and clinical practice goals. In addition to representing the radiology nurse, it serves as a resource to persons in nursing education and acts as client advocate with families, nurses, physicians, and radiology personnel. Dues $25 for RNs; $15 for associate membership for LVNs and LPNs.

Oncology Nursing Society
3111 Banksville Rd.
Pittsburgh, PA 15216
Phone: (412) 344-3899

A professional organization for RNs interested in oncology or practicing oncology nursing to promote high standards in oncology nursing, provide peer support and networking, encourage specialization by nurses in oncology, develop educational programs, and encourage nursing research. Dues $38.

HEALTH EDUCATION MATERIAL

From: American Cancer Society (the booklets below as well as many others are available from local units)

Cancer Facts and Figures (a booklet of annually updated statistics for health professionals)

I Have a Secret Cure for Cancer! (a booklet on quackery)

Nutrition (a cookbook)

From: National Cancer Institute
Office of Cancer Communications
Building 31, Room 10A18
Bethesda, MD 20205

Cancer Treatment: An Annotated Bibliography of Patient Education Materials

Chemotherapy and You: A Guide to Self-Help During Treatment

Eating Hints: Recipes and Tips for Better Nutrition During Cancer Treatment

Radiation Therapy and You: A Guide to Self-Help During Treatment

Taking Time: Support for People With Cancer and the People Who Care About Them

What are Clinical Trials All About?

What Black Americans Should Know About Cancer

Trauma and Other Emergencies

Janis P. Bellack

Daily news accounts of traumatic injuries and deaths are an inescapable part of contemporary life. Consider the following news headlines:

- 32-year-old woman electrocuted when hair dryer falls into bathtub
- 25-year-old man drowns in rough waters while canoeing
- 1 teenager dead, 3 critically injured in single-car accident
- 50-year-old construction worker sustains severe 2nd and 3rd degree burns
- Farm tractor overturns, 46-year-old driver paralyzed
- 70-year-old woman robbed, beaten, and sexually assaulted
- Street-gang fight erupts. Multiple stabbings and gunshot wounds, 2 dead, 4 seriously wounded

Industrialization, technology, increasing population, high crime rates, and lifestyle practices and behaviors have increased the risk of serious injury or death. Everyone is a potential victim. Trauma is a mushrooming health and social problem. Because of the potential physiological and psychological consequences, trauma victims and their families pose a special challenge to nurses.

Clients suffering from a medical emergency or traumatic injury face numerous stressors. Physiologically, the client's illness or injury may be life threatening, calling on all the body's systems to battle for survival. Psychologically, the suddenness and seriousness of the client's illness or injury may precipitate an emotional crisis for the client and family. Although physiological stabilization of the client must take precedence over emotional well-being, psychological support is an essential part of optimal nursing care in an emergency. This chapter discusses trauma and emergency care. Trauma is also discussed in all body systems units in the specific disorders chapters.

Section I: Trauma and Emergency Nursing: An Overview

Trauma generally refers to a physical injury or wound resulting from accidental or intentional impact to the body. Traumatic injuries include such conditions as head and spinal injuries, electrical shock, chest and abdominal wounds, limb injuries or amputations, or a combination of these *(multiple trauma)*. Forcible rape is also considered trauma, even in the absence of physical wounds.

Medical emergencies, on the other hand, are acute physiological threats to the body and its systems that are potential threats to life. Acute myocardial infarction (MI), stroke (cerebrovascular accident, or CVA), drowning, sudden obstructed airway, drug overdoses, poisonings, and hypothermia are examples of medical emergencies.

A *disaster* refers to a sudden, destructive event that results in major damage to or loss of property and life. Disasters such as floods, fires, earthquakes, and tornadoes usually cause distress and suffering for a large number of persons or even an entire community.

Emergency nursing is a specialty role in clinical nursing practice, the focus of which is providing professional nursing care for clients who are suffering from a medical emergency, trauma, or a disaster. The various roles in emergency nursing will be discussed later in this chapter.

SCOPE AND COSTS OF TRAUMA

In the United States and Canada, the incidence of death and disability caused by physical trauma is staggering. In the United States, for example:

- Trauma is the leading cause of death in individuals from birth to age 40. Because trauma affects the most productive and healthy segment of the population, its cost to society is even greater than the following numbers indicate.

- In 1982, there were approximately 165,000 deaths from trauma.

- The trauma death rate for individuals ages 15 to 24 has increased 56% since 1976.

- For every trauma death, two persons are left permanently disabled.

- Trauma cases account for one-third of all hospital admissions.

- The annual cost of trauma to society, including trauma care expenses, lost productivity, and permanent disability, is estimated to be $50 billion (over $135 million a day).

- Traumatic injuries account for more years of life lost than heart disease and cancer combined.

In Canada, the incidence of accidental death (from all causes) is significantly less. In 1981, the number of Canadians who lost their lives from trauma was less than one-third the US incidence (2 per 10,000 in Canada compared to 7 per 10,000 in the United States).

Trauma has been called a "neglected epidemic." It is certainly a major health and social problem. Because trauma is potentially preventable, public education and legislation aimed at reducing the incidence of trauma by increasing public awareness of the problem is imperative. For example, stiffer penalties for drunk drivers, laws requiring safety helmets for motorcyclists, maintaining and enforcing the current 55 mph speed limit, enforcing occupational safety standards, and taking normal safety precautions in the home could significantly reduce the high incidence of traumatic injuries and deaths.

Despite the epidemic proportions of trauma, funds for research are scarce. Few research dollars are spent on trauma research compared with research for cancer and heart disease. On the other hand, trauma care has received increased attention in recent years, especially the organization and delivery of trauma care services.

TRENDS IN TRAUMA AND EMERGENCY CARE

Today's emergency health care services range from community "urgent treatment" centers providing round-the-clock, immediate, noncritical health care services to complex, fully equipped trauma centers that specialize in the care of the multisystem trauma victim. Emergency health care specialties in nursing and medicine have evolved as increasingly aware consumers have recognized the need for professionals trained explicitly to care for trauma and acute medical emergency victims. Advances in health care technology have, in turn, increased demand for emergency services. In most communities, the public now expects swift and competent care be given to trauma victims or persons suffering from serious acute illness. As with other health care services, the public has followed the lead of the medical profession in adopting a crisis-oriented, treatment–cure approach to trauma and serious life-threatening illness rather than a prevention-oriented approach. The organization and proliferation of trauma care services has, albeit unintentionally, perpetuated and reinforced this crisis-oriented attitude.

Nonemergency use of emergency facilities has increased in the past decade. Approximately 85% of visits to emergency departments are for conditions that are not life threatening. Reasons include:

- Increasing mobility of the population, so fewer persons have a regular family physician.

- Increased perception by the public that emergency facilities provide nonacute backup care when other sources of care are not available (eg, evenings, nights, and weekends).

- Differences between what the public and the health professional perceives as an emergency.
- Changes in emergency department staffing patterns; many emergency departments in medium-sized and large communities have qualified emergency physicians 24 hours a day.
- Referral of clients to emergency facilities by their regular physicians (for the convenience of the referring physician).

Respiratory illnesses are the most frequent cause for nonemergency visits to emergency departments. Nonwhite persons under age 44 whose family income is less than $10,000 are most likely to use emergency facilities for nonemergency reasons.

As use of emergency departments for nonlife-threatening conditions has increased, the number of free-standing urgent treatment centers has grown. These centers are designed and staffed to provide immediate care to persons with noncritical health problems, helping to meet the public's need for extended availability of health care services. Most centers are open at least 16 hours a day, 7 days a week. Some provide 24-hour service. Nonemergency health care in these facilities can be provided at a much lower cost to the consumer and, ideally, decreases nonemergency use of emergency and trauma facilities.

Emergency Medical Services Systems

The concept of an emergency medical services system (EMSS) originated with military field experiences in caring for war casualties. In fact, the model for a regional EMSS was tested in the Korean War with its MASH (Mobile Army Surgical Hospital) units and was improved during the Vietnam conflict. The EMSS was officially established in 1973 by public law to provide a comprehensive, integrated, nationally coordinated system for delivering quality emergency care.

An EMSS generally includes such elements as prehospital emergency care, emergency transport, and 24-hour emergency department availability as well as professional and public emergency care education programs. The United States currently has over 300 EMSS regions. The Canadian provinces offer similar emergency services through their Emergency Health Services Commissions.

Regionalization of Trauma Care

Regional trauma centers, an outgrowth of the EMSS, have been developed to improve the quality of emergency services, to save lives, and to reduce cost by avoiding duplication of services. The American College of Surgeons Committee on Trauma has established criteria for effective trauma care that focus on three "rights": getting the *right client* to the *right facility* at the *right time*. The "right facil-

Nursing Research Note

Lauck BW, Bigelow D: Why patients follow through on referrals from the emergency room and why they don't. *Nurs Res* 1983; 32(3): 186–187.

Thirty-one clients who had been referred for further treatment after an emergency room visit were interviewed to determine if they had followed through with the referral.

The result indicated that clients were more likely to come to the referral office if they had an appointment. Follow-up was improved when the client understood why the referral was made and agreed that it was necessary. Follow-up was also more likely if the client and care provider both understood what the clients' needs were and if the clinician understood the clients' feelings. Clinicians' understanding of the problem did not enhance follow-up.

In treating emergency room clients, examine their expectations of care to gain insight into the motivation behind seeking care and follow-up. Clients without previous treatment history need special attention, and referrals must be specific. Appointments should be confirmed and the client should be told about them in detail.

ity" *may not mean the nearest hospital;* rather, it may mean the hospital best equipped to handle a particular victim's emergency. The three levels of trauma care designated by the committee are listed in Box 13–1. (The major difference between Level I and II facilities is that Level I facilities must be engaged in providing education and conducting research related to trauma.)

It has been estimated that, with the exception of burn victims and those with spinal cord injuries, 85% of trauma victims can be cared for in Level III facilities; 10%, in Level II; and 5% (those most critically injured), in Level I. For those with spinal cord injuries and burns, these percentages are reversed; ie, 85% of these victims require care at a Level I facility. Studies show that as many as 85% of neurologically injured clients who died could have been saved had they been treated initially in a trauma care center.

Box 13–1 Designated Levels of Trauma Care

Level I facility: Regional; optimal; resuscitation, initial care, surgical intervention, critical care management, specialized care; education of qualified personnel in the region; trauma research

Level II facility: Limited geographic area; intermediate; resuscitation, initial care, standard surgical intervention, and critical care management

Level III facility: Local; minimal; resuscitation, stabilization of victim within the facility's capabilities

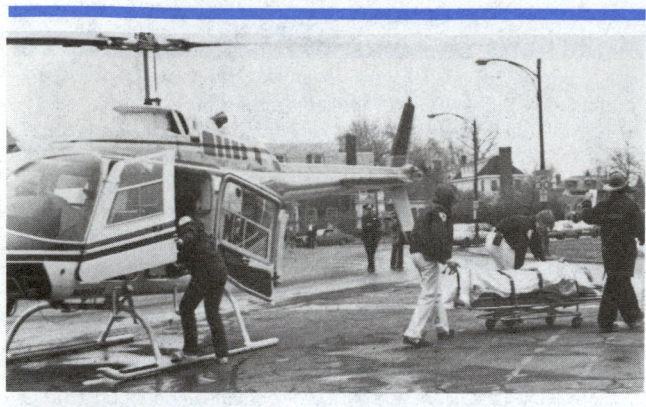

Figure 13–1

Trauma service helicopter with client. (Courtesy of Millard Fillmore Hospital, Buffalo, NY)

The Trend Toward Prehospital Care

With the trend toward regionalization of emergency health care, there has been a concomitant trend toward prehospital care delivered by specially trained staff, such as emergency medical technicians (EMTs) and emergency nurses. Basic or advanced life-support mobile rescue units are equipped so the rescue team can quickly render care to individuals who are suffering from trauma or sudden life-threatening illness. Many of these units offer sophisticated monitoring and life-support equipment as well as direct communication with the service's hospital base, usually the emergency department. Under the supervision of the physician at the base station, the prehospital management team is trained to assess and manage potentially life-threatening conditions at the scene. It has been estimated that prehospital care has saved 18% of victims who otherwise would have died.

Access to such services remains a concern for many small or rural communities. Rural communities, especially, may lack the funds to equip, staff, and support a mobile rescue unit. Moreover, the nearest appropriate emergency facility may be so distant that ill or injured clients' lives are in jeopardy. In some rural communities, air transport units (eg, helicopters or small airplanes) are available to transport critically ill victims as quickly and safely as possible to the nearest appropriate facility (Figure 13–1).

The Trend Toward Operating Room Management

Another recent trend is to shift management of the major (multiple) trauma victim from the emergency department to the operating room. Upon admission to the hospital or trauma center, the victim is immediately transferred to the operating room, where the controlled aseptic environment and specialized equipment enhance the victim's chance for immediate and long-term recovery. Early surgical inter-

vention has dramatically increased the trauma victim's chances of survival.

Multidisciplinary Care of the Trauma Victim

Many members of the health team are involved in early and ongoing care of the trauma victim. The professional nurse plays a unique and valuable role in working with and coordinating the services of the various disciplines involved. Because the priority for care usually involves medical and surgical intervention, the physician retains primary responsibility for directing the trauma victim's care during the initial critical stages following the injury. The nurse serves as the necessary link between the client and other professionals involved in emergency care, such as laboratory and radiology personnel, the respiratory therapist, and social services personnel. The nurse is also the critical link between the client and the family and between the health team and the family, keeping the family informed and offering them emotional support during a time of intense anxiety.

LEGAL CONSIDERATIONS IN EMERGENCY CARE

An emergency is legally defined as any illness or injury that is likely to result in death or disability if not rapidly attended to. State laws govern the obligations of health providers and hospitals to render emergency treatment to persons in potentially life-threatening situations. Generally, emergency care is considered an individual's right. Tax-exempt hospitals with emergency departments can be held legally liable for refusing to treat clients suffering from serious illness or injury, regardless of the client's ability to pay for care rendered.

Deciding what constitutes an emergency or who is in need of emergency care is the responsibility of the individual in charge. In many instances, this person is the nurse. The emergency room nurse is often the professional who screens clients and decides who should be treated first. From a legal standpoint, the nurse is expected to make decisions consistent with the accepted standard of reasonable practice for someone with similar education and experience.

Although health professionals who are passersby at the scene of an emergency are not legally required to render emergency aid, all 50 states in the United States have enacted Good Samaritan laws to encourage such assistance. Some state laws protect physicians from civil liability in giving care at the scene of an emergency, and some states extend this immunity to nurses. Immunity usually applies only to persons who do not receive remuneration for rendering emergency aid. Health professionals may be judged by what might be expected of a similar professional under the same circumstances. Some states provide immunity for all persons who give emergency aid at the scene.

Good Samaritan laws protect persons covered by the statute from being sued for negligence so long as the care was rendered "in good faith." Nurses should be familiar with the protection provided by Good Samaritan laws in their own state or province.

Certainly, nurses have an ethical if not a legal obligation to give whatever assistance they can to persons in potentially life-threatening situations, as long as their own lives are not in danger. No health professional has ever been successfully sued for providing such aid.

Informed Versus Implied Consent

At the prehospital site, clients may be treated under a doctrine of *implied consent*. The client's need for emergency intervention takes precedence over obtaining written consent to treatment, and it is assumed that the client would grant such consent if able to do so. Once the client's condition is stabilized or the client has been transported to a health care facility, then written, informed consent to treatment must be obtained. If the client's condition makes written consent impossible to obtain (eg, in the case of brain injury or continuing severe bleeding) treatment may continue under implied consent, or consent may be obtained from the next of kin. Implied consent, of course, is restricted to interventions within the accepted standards of current medical and nursing practice.

Legal Guidelines

Guidelines for notifying a client's family, releasing information, and transferring or discharging clients from the emergency facility vary among institutions. The professional emergency nurse has an obligation to be familiar with specific state laws and institutional policies and to act in accordance with these measures.

Generally, the nurse or physician is responsible for notifying immediate family members when a client is admitted for emergency treatment. If able, the client should designate who is to be notified. Otherwise, immediate family members (spouse, parent, son or daughter, guardian, partner, companion) should be contacted.

Information concerning the client's condition should be released *only* to appropriate family members. The nurse should realize that, in some instances, the most appropriate "family" member may be a live-in partner or close friend. In cases of criminal injury or death, the nurse is also obligated to release information to the appropriate legal authorities.

Clients should not be transferred to another hospital until medically able to tolerate a transfer. This means the client's condition has been stabilized to the extent that moving the client will not cause additional harm.

Discharge of clients from an emergency facility is usually prescribed by a physician or by a nurse practicing under medical protocol. As long as acceptable standards of practice concerning client discharge are followed, there is minimal legal risk to the hospital and its personnel.

Documentation of Emergency Care and Preservation of Evidence

Professionally and legally, the nurse has an obligation to document emergency care rendered a client. Specifically, pertinent assessment data, nursing and other professional interventions, and the client's responses should be carefully recorded clearly, systematically, and chronologically. Information should be entered in the client's record as close to the time of occurrence as possible. The written health record may become a crucial source of information later, especially in cases of civil or criminal legal action. In addition, a carefully documented record ensures that gaps and overlaps in care will be avoided. Flow sheets or other systematic records facilitate recording of information in emergencies.

In cases of traumatic injuries or sexual assault, an important part of the nurse's role is to assist in the preservation of evidence that may later become part of legal action. Hospitals generally have policies that govern how potential evidence such as clothing and specimens (eg, blood, urine, nail scrapings, bullet fragments) is to be handled. These policies should be strictly followed. In addition, the client's pertinent statements should be immediately recorded verbatim because they may later be admissible as court evidence.

THE PROFESSIONAL NURSE'S ROLE IN TRAUMA AND EMERGENCY CARE

Because of the many advances in the care of emergency victims, emergency nursing has become highly specialized. The professional nurse may assume a variety of roles. As mentioned earlier, the nurse may function as a member of the prehospital management team. In this role, the nurse may be involved in ground or air transport of victims to appropriate facilities as well as on-site management of the emergency victim. More often, however, the professional emergency nurse is a staff member of a hospital emergency or trauma department.

Nurses who work in this capacity must have skills that prepare them to deliver high-quality care to emergency victims. At the very least, preparation for emergency nursing requires education and licensure that qualifies the nurse to practice as a registered nurse. The Emergency Department Nurses' Association (EDNA) (1983), the professional specialty organization of emergency nurses in the United States and Canada, specifies that emergency staff nurses should also have "advanced knowledge of physiologic and psychosocial concepts and the application of therapeutic interventions" that enables them to provide comprehensive, safe nursing care to emergency clients. This knowledge includes the ability to provide basic life support (cardiopulmonary resuscitation, CPR) to clients. The emergency nurse may also achieve professional certification through EDNA as a Certified Emergency Nurse (CEN) for excellence in the specialty. In addition, emergency nurses have a professional obligation and, in a number of states a legal mandate, to maintain and improve their skills through continuing education.

More advanced preparation for emergency nurses is available through several programs. These are primarily intense, short-term certificate programs that prepare nurses to function in an expanded role in an emergency facility or trauma center. Several major medical centers in the United States offer emergency nurse training programs or trauma nurse specialist programs. A major component of these programs is emergency medical or nursing procedures, including advanced cardiac life support (American Heart Association standards), with emphasis on preparing nurses to assess, establish priorities, and effectively intervene with clients who have life-threatening conditions.

Standards and Guidelines for Emergency Nursing Care

Standards of Emergency Nursing Practice
An important part of developing specialized roles in emergency nursing has been criteria for assuring high-quality emergency nursing care in a variety of emergency settings. The *Standards of Emergency Nursing Practice,* written, adopted, and published by EDNA, "delineate safe nursing practice and excellence in emergency nursing." These standards have four components: practice, professionalism, research, and education. These standards communicate to other professionals and the public what emergency nurses are capable of doing (the scope of emergency nursing practice) and increase accountability for the delivery of emergency nursing care. Each standard specifies the expected level of practice and includes a rationale, component standards, and measurable outcome criteria for evaluating emergency nursing care.

Emergency Care Guidelines
In 1982, a joint committee of EDNA and the American College of Emergency Physicians developed "Emergency Care Guidelines" for ensuring the delivery of safe, effective emergency care for persons with life-threatening conditions. The guidelines are based on the philosophy that all critically ill or injured persons have a right to receive prompt, appropriate health care. They are intended to assist emergency health care providers in planning for and offering appropriate emergency health services to the public. Guidelines concerning professional responsibility and public expectations, principles of emergency care (administration, staffing, physical facilities, and equipment), and continuity of care for victims of critical illness or injury assure the public of safe, accessible, and acceptable emergency health care services.

JCAH Emergency Services
In addition to these standards and guidelines, the Joint Commission on Accreditation of Hospitals (JCAH) provides for the evaluation of hospital emergency services as part of its accreditation process (JCAH, 1983). Eight standards

and specific interpretations are spelled out under the general principle, "Any individual who comes to the hospital for emergency medical evaluation or initial treatment shall be properly assessed by qualified individuals, and appropriate services shall be rendered within the defined capability of the hospital."

Prevention and Public Education

An important responsibility of the professional nurse is education of clients and the public concerning appropriate measures that can lessen the incidence of accidental injury and death. Teaching persons how to modify their lifestyles and educating them concerning proper assistance for emergency victims could significantly lessen the tragic toll of trauma on individuals; their families; and in some instances, entire communities.

Nurses have numerous informal and formal opportunities for educating the public about prevention and early intervention. First, nurses can teach family members and friends ways to lessen the risk of accidental injury. Nurses, of course, should be role models for others by observing safety precautions such as use of seat belts and demonstrating optimal health behaviors, such as weight control, not smoking, consuming alcohol only in moderation, and so forth. More formal opportunities for educating others include participation in community education events such as first aid classes, health fairs, and radio and television messages aimed at risk reduction.

Specific areas for public education include:

- Drug and alcohol use and abuse (see Chapter 10).
- Safe driving practices (staying within the speed limit, wearing seat belts, maintaining vehicles in safe working condition).
- Occupational safety practices.
- Accident-proofing the home (such as keeping poisons out of reach, having treads on stairs and slip-free rugs, storing solvents and paints properly, not smoking in bed, installing smoke detectors, taking care in do-it-yourself projects (especially those involving electrical and chemical hazards), storing food safely, and safely using home equipment such as power saws and lawn mowers).
- Knowing how to swim.
- Safe camping, hiking, and boating practices.
- Sports safety.
- Personal protection (avoiding dark or isolated areas, especially at night; knowledge of self-defense techniques).
- Proper disposal of hazardous wastes.
- Basic life support (CPR) techniques.
- Use of Medic-Alert identification.
- First aid and emergency assistance measures.

Public education also involves educating people about the availability and appropriate use of emergency health care facilities. Consumers should be urged to familiarize themselves with the locations of the nearest emergency facilities. Emergency telephone numbers, such as emergency rescue, police, and fire protection and poison control centers, should be readily accessible to family members, guests, and babysitters.

Nurses should be familiar with concepts and principles of treating trauma and life-threatening illness. The emergency client must cope with numerous physiological multisystem stressors. In addition, the client who is alert or semiconscious may also face psychological stressors, as may the client's family and friends.

THE ABCs OF EMERGENCY CARE

In any emergency, it is crucial for the rescuer to assess the client's:

- **A**—airway
- **B**—breathing
- **C**—circulation

The rescuer must first stabilize the head and neck if a possibility of spinal cord injury exists before rapidly assessing the patency of the victim's airway, the presence and character of breathing, and the victim's circulatory status (see also Box 13–2 later in this chapter). Of course, establishing an airway is the primary consideration in any emergency. The airway should be cleared, and oxygen should be administered, if available. If the client is not breathing, initiate artificial mouth-to-mouth respiration. If pulses are absent or severely weakened and bradycardic, begin cardiac compression (closed chest massage).

Cardiac Arrest

The emergency victim may go into cardiac arrest from a variety of causes, including MI, trauma, drowning, electrical shock, drug overdose, or hypersensitivity reactions. These conditions usually lead to cardiac dysrhythmias, such as ventricular tachycardia or fibrillation, which if untreated, will cause the heart to stop beating. Treatment of the monitored client in cardiac arrest is discussed in Chapter 24. With cardiac arrest, irreversible brain damage from tissue anoxia follows within 4 to 6 minutes.

Clinical manifestations of cardiorespiratory arrest include:

- Unresponsiveness
- Absence of breathing
- Absence of carotid pulses
- Cyanosis, especially of lips and nail beds
- Dilated pupils that become fully dilated and fixed approximately 2 minutes after the heart stops beating

Cardiopulmonary Resuscitation

Cardiopulmonary resuscitation (CPR) must begin as soon as unresponsiveness and the absence of breathing and carotid pulses are noted. CPR provides for oxygenation of vital tissues (ie, brain and myocardium) until cardiac functioning can be restored, preventing irreversible cerebral or cardiac damage. The rescuer should open the individual's airway using a head-tilt maneuver (Figure 13–2A) and then listen and feel for the victim's breath on the rescuer's cheek (Figure 13–2B). If the victim is not breathing, the rescuer should:

- Pinch the victim's nostrils to prevent an air leak.
- Take a deep breath.
- Seal the victim's mouth with his or her mouth and breathe forcefully **four times** in rapid succession, while watching for the victim's chest to rise (Figure 13–2C). **The elapsed time should be no more than 3 to 5 seconds.**

If the victim's pulses are absent, cardiac compression must be instituted, using the following steps:

- Move the victim to a firm surface, such as the floor or a resuscitation board.
- Kneel on one side of the victim, keeping elbows straight and shoulders parallel, directly over the victim's sternum.
- Locate the correct anatomic landmark: 2 to 3 fingers above the xiphoid process (Figure 13–3A).
- Place the heel of the working hand on the landmark with the heel of the second hand directly on top, interlacing the fingers (Figure 13–3B). Only the heel of the working hand should be in contact with the victim's chest.
- Apply sufficient downward pressure to depress the sternum 3.8 to 5.0 cm (1.5 to 2 in). Release pressure to allow the heart to refill.
- Deliver 15 compressions at a rate of 80 per minute (or 60 per minute if two people are performing the procedure), pacing the compressions by counting, "one, and two, and three. . . ." Compressing on "one" and releasing on "and" will keep the pressure and release times even.
- Continue this cycle at a rate of *two breaths to 15 cardiac compressions at a rate of 80 compressions per minute (one breath to 5 cardiac compressions at a rate of 60 compressions per minute when two people are performing the procedure).*
- Pause after 1 minute to check the victim's carotid pulse and breathing. Thereafter, pause to check every 4 to 5 minutes.

If the victim is wearing secure-fitting dentures, they can be left in place to help the rescuer maintain an airtight seal. If dentures are loose, they should be removed. If the victim

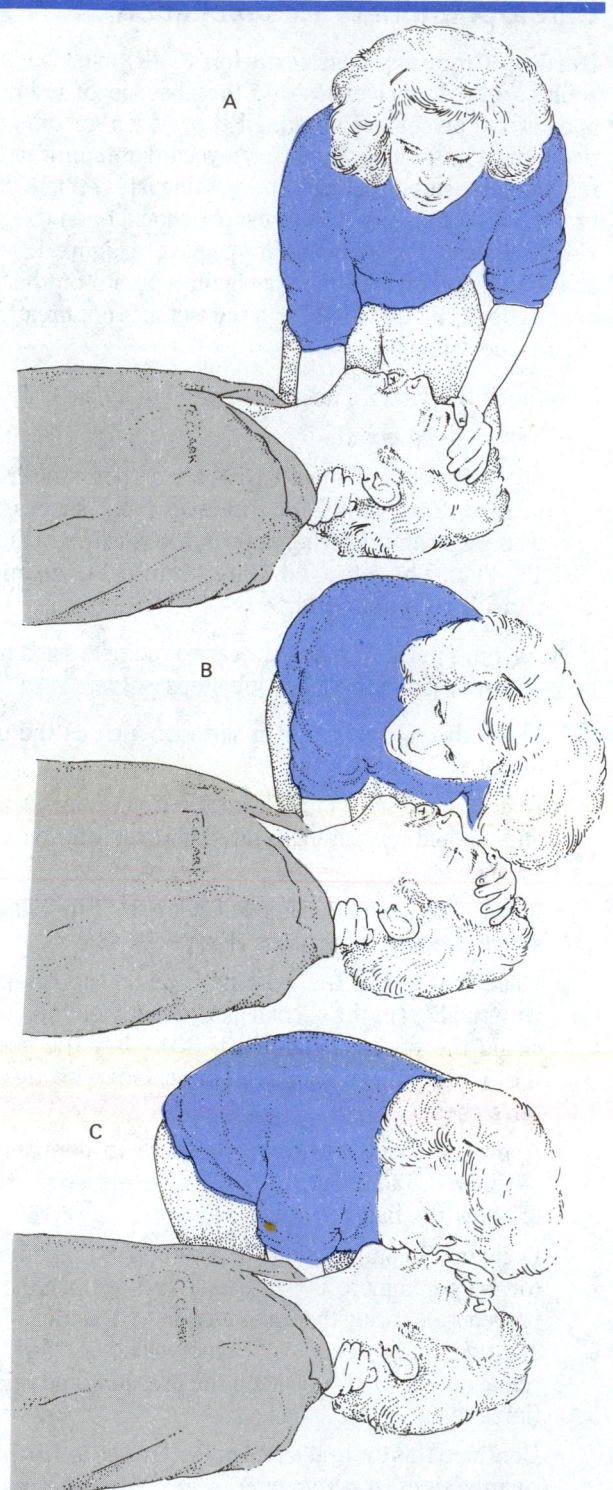

Figure 13–2

Cardiopulmonary resuscitation. **A.** Open the victim's airway using head-tilt maneuver. **B.** Listen and feel for breath on cheek. **C.** If victim is not breathing, pinch the victim's nostrils, take a deep breath, seal victim's mouth with your mouth, and breathe forcefully four times in rapid succession, watching for the victim's chest to rise.

SOURCE: Saxton DF et al.: *Addison–Wesley Manual of Nursing Practice.* Menlo Park, CA: Addison–Wesley, 1983.

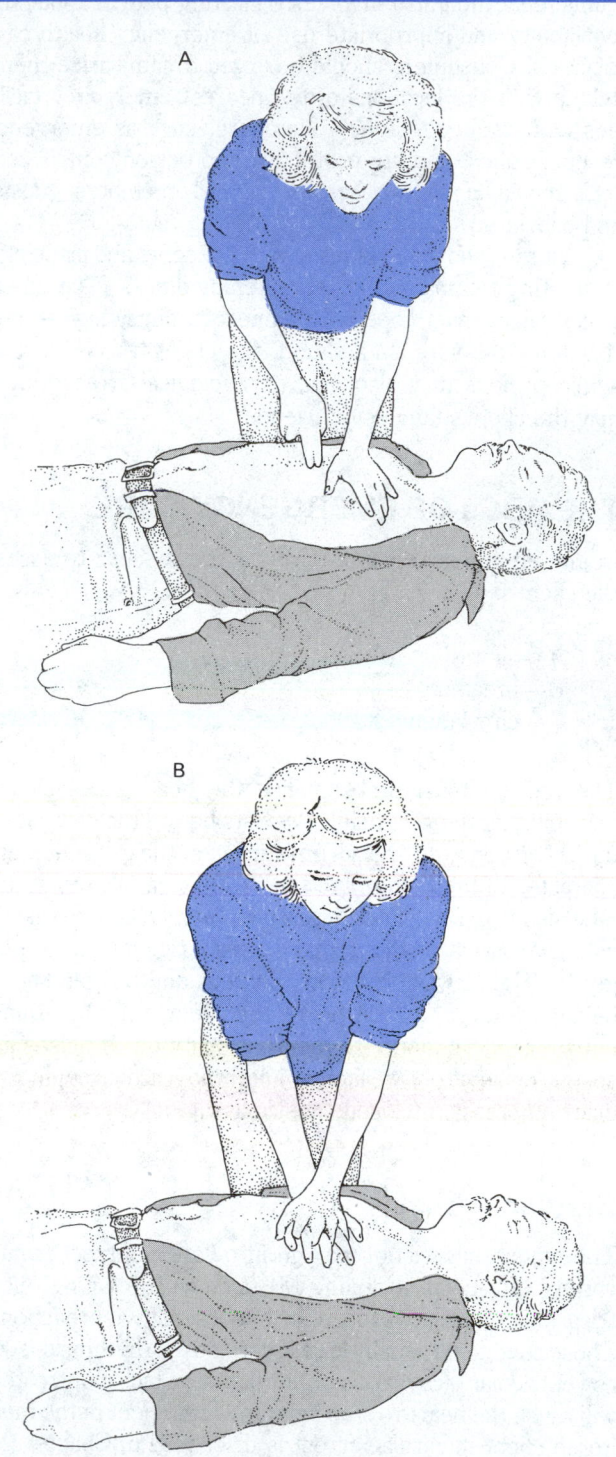

Figure 13–3

External cardiac compression. **A.** Locate the xiphoid process. **B.** Position hands on landmark (heel of working hand on landmark, covered by heel of second hand with fingers interlaced).

SOURCE: Saxton DF et al.: *Addison–Wesley Manual of Nursing Practice.* Menlo Park, CA: Addison–Wesley, 1983.

has a laryngectomy or tracheostomy, direct mouth-to-stoma ventilation should be used. If gastric distention occurs during CPR, reposition the airway to be sure it is patent.

Once CPR is initiated, it should be continued until the client's breathing and heartbeat are restored, the client can be turned over to an experienced resuscitation team, or the client is pronounced dead by a physician or coroner.

Every nurse, especially a nurse who works in an acute or critical care setting such as an emergency facility, has a professional and ethical obligation to be certified in basic life support. Such certification is available through the American Heart Association and the American Red Cross in hundreds of communities around the country.

Section II: Trauma and Other Emergencies as Multisystem Stressors

Shock, metabolic imbalance, neurologic insult, and even cardiac arrest are potential responses of the body to the stress of trauma or sudden, life-threatening illness. These responses, in turn, place the client's life in jeopardy. Rapid assessment and intervention are imperative if the client is to have an optimal chance for recovery.

SHOCK SYNDROME

Shock syndrome is a defect in cell and tissue perfusion resulting from a decrease in cardiac output. This circulatory failure can rapidly lead to tissue hypoxia or anoxia. Shock syndrome is a medical and nursing emergency related to a variety of conditions: blood loss (hemorrhage), spinal cord trauma, burns, hypersensitivity reactions, MI, or severe psychological distress. Classification of shock, clinical manifestations of shock, assessment of the client in shock, and nursing implications related to the management of shock are discussed in Chapter 5.

The nurse who suspects a client is in shock should act quickly to prevent its worsening. Emergency nursing care of the client in shock includes the following measures:

- Place the client in a supine position with legs elevated at a 45° angle (12 to 16 in). Do *not* place the client in a Trendelenburg position, because this can impair cerebral blood flow and interfere with lung ventilation.
- If the client has a head or chest injury, elevate the head slightly.
- Control external bleeding by applying direct pressure to the wound or indirect pressure to the nearest proximal pressure point (Figure 13–4).
- Loosen restrictive clothing.
- Keep the client warm but do not overheat.
- Provide calm reassurance to the client and anxious others.
- Transport the client to an appropriate facility; if already in the hospital, obtain medical attention immediately.

Ongoing nursing care of the shock victim involves carefully and frequently assessing the client's vital signs and responses to treatment and carrying out the nursing interventions described in Chapter 5.

METABOLIC RESPONSES TO TRAUMA

Trauma poses a major insult to the body's metabolic functions. Metabolic responses to trauma occur in three phases: ebb, stress, and recovery.

Ebb Phase

The first phase is the *ebb phase,* which is the shortest, lasting approximately 24 hours. Body heat production drops during this early phase. This drop in heat decreases the need for oxygen, allowing the body to meet the increased metabolic demands imposed by the stress of traumatic injury. With certain types of trauma, such as burns or wounds resulting in severe blood loss, fluid loss may be great. At this point, however, changes in hormonal levels and body metabolites are not observable.

Stress Phase

The *stress phase* follows the ebb phase. Its duration varies in accordance with the nature and severity of the client's injury. During the stress phase, numerous metabolic changes occur in relation to stimulation of the sympathetic nervous system (caused by the stress of trauma). Release of hormones by the hypothalamus, pituitary gland, adrenal glands, pancreas, and thyroid glands is triggered by sympathetic stimulation. Specifically:

1. The hypothalamus secretes corticotropin-releasing factor, which in turn stimulates the anterior pituitary gland.
2. The anterior pituitary then releases adrenocorticotropic hormone (ACTH), which acts on the adrenal cortex to stimulate the release of cortisol and cortisone.
3. These glucocorticoids speed up the process of gluconeogenesis (breakdown of protein into carbohydrate), increasing the level of glucose in the blood and urine ("diabetes of injury") and the level of nitrogen in the blood in the form of urea.
4. Increased glucose production raises the basal metabolic rate, leading to a "hypermetabolic" state.
5. Aldosterone secretion is also greatly increased (especially when blood loss is significant), leading to sodium retention and potassium loss.

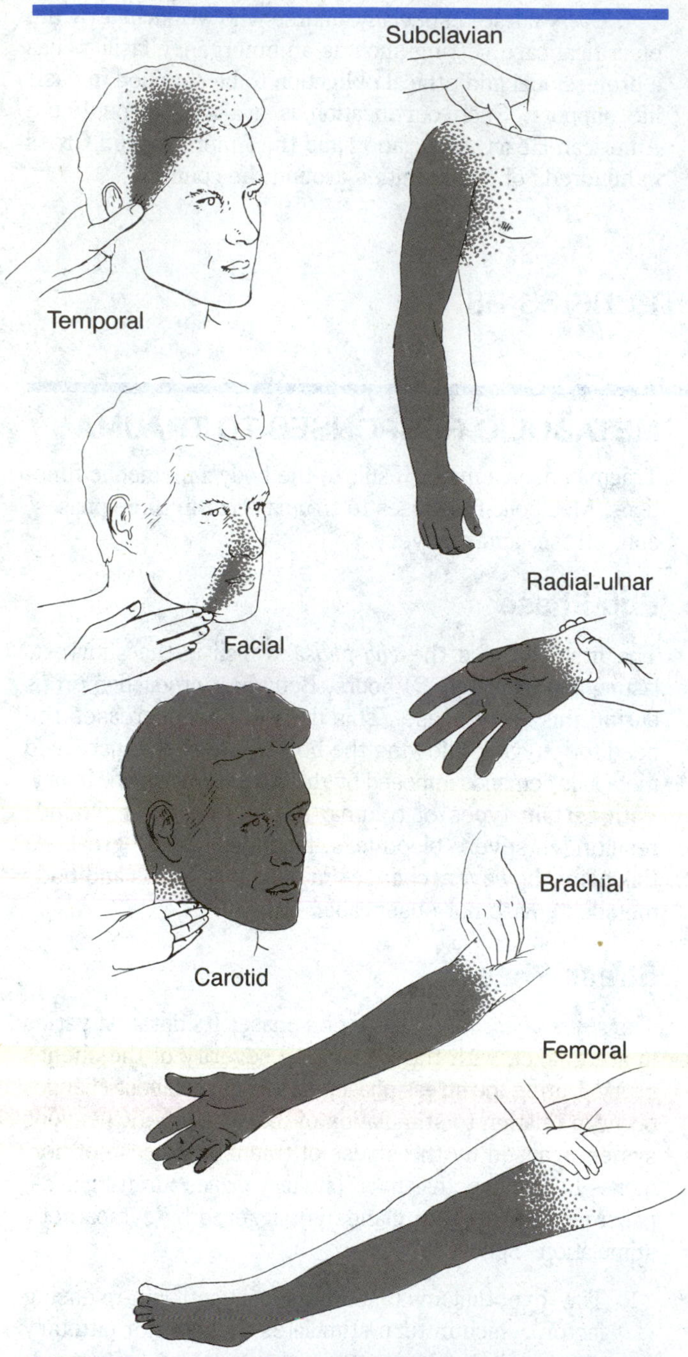

Subclavian

Temporal

Radial-ulnar

Facial

Brachial

Carotid

Femoral

Figure 13–4

Location of pressure points.

6. Catecholamines are released from the adrenal medulla, stimulating the breakdown of skeletal muscle protein. (This muscle breakdown occurs because the body needs additional energy in the form of glucose as well as blood protein and enzymes to deal with the stress of trauma.) Breakdown of muscle protein (catabolism) places the client in negative nitrogen balance. Body temperature may increase, and the client begins to lose weight.

Recovery Phase

The final phase is termed *recovery*, or the *anabolic phase*. The length of this phase is highly variable and, according to Hui (1983), depends on the nature and severity of the injury, the amount of body weight the client loses during the stress phase, and the extent of nutrient depletion. During this phase, normal sympathetic nervous system function resumes, stimulating increased production of insulin and growth hormone. These hormones aid in tissue repair and the restoration of muscle mass. The phases of metabolic response to trauma are summarized in Table 13–1.

Intervention is aimed at restoring fluid and electrolyte balance, correcting any acid–base imbalance, and providing nutritional support. Nutritional therapy is discussed later in this chapter.

NEUROLOGIC INSULT

Trauma may precipitate a direct or indirect insult to the brain. Head injury, severe shock, drowning, cardiorespiratory arrest, strangulation, suffocation, smoke inhalation, certain poisonings, or severe hypersensitivity reactions may cause anoxia and resulting ischemia of cerebral tissues. This damage causes cerebral edema and may lead to increased intracranial pressure.

Medical measures are aimed at minimizing cerebral edema to prevent permanent neurologic damage. Certain medications such as steroids (usually dexamethasone), diuretics, or hypertonic glucose (50% glucose) may be prescribed. Fluid intake is usually restricted to prevent further increases in intracranial pressure. The client is hyperventilated, usually with a mechanical ventilator, to reduce the $PaCO_2$, promoting vasoconstriction of cerebral blood vessels, which lowers the intracranial pressure. Barbiturate coma and hypothermia may be induced to further decrease the oxygen demands of the brain. Surgical intervention may be indicated when cerebral damage is severe, eg, with depressed skull fractures or subarachnoid hemorrhage (see Chapter 39).

Nursing care for the trauma client who has suffered neurologic insult involves careful and frequent assessment of the client's neurologic status (eg, vital signs, pupil reaction, and reflexes), maintenance of artificial ventilation, monitoring of fluid status and fluid replacement therapy, and administration of prescribed drugs. The client's responses to interventions must also be carefully evaluated. If the client has not suffered a spinal injury, the head is usually elevated approximately 30° to promote venous drainage and thus decrease intracranial pressure.

NUTRITIONAL SUPPORT OF THE TRAUMA VICTIM

Clients with traumatic injuries have increased nutritional needs that must be met to promote recovery and prevent complications. The client who is hospitalized following a major injury is at great risk of malnutrition.

Table 13–1 Metabolic Responses to Trauma

Stage	Medical Term	Duration (days)	Hormonal Changes	Variations in Body Metabolites	Body Composition and Temperature Changes
1	Ebb phase, early phase	1	Not definitive	Not definitive	Decreased heat production; decreased oxygen consumption
2	Stress phase, catabolic phase, acute phase, flow phase, hypermetabolic phase	2–10	Increased blood catecholamines, glucagon, corticosteroids, thyroid hormones; decreased blood insulin	Increased blood and urine glucose and nitrogen (in the form of urea)	Muscle protein and fat breakdown, weight loss; possible body water and electrolyte loss; possible increase in body temperature and heat production; possible skin loss; loss of potassium and retention of sodium
3	Recovery phase; anabolic phase, adaptive phase	3–10	Increased blood insulin and growth hormone; decreased blood catecholamines	Increased blood ketone bodies; decreased blood glucose; slightly elevated to normal blood and urine nitrogen (in the form of urea)	Nutrient deposition; building up of body muscle

SOURCE: Reprinted with permission from Hui YH: *Human Nutrition and Diet Therapy.* Monterey, CA: Wadsworth, 1983, p 745.

Tissue injury, surgery, shock, and prolonged hospitalization often associated with major trauma place great demands on the trauma victim's body stores. Even previously healthy clients are at risk, and those whose nutritional status was less than optimal are especially vulnerable. (Malnutrition and its effects are discussed in Chapter 8.)

The trauma victim's needs are great for increased caloric intake and adequate amounts of vitamin A, B complex, C, and K. Nitrogen loss following trauma is related to breakdown of skeletal muscle. The average trauma victim loses approximately 50 g of nitrogen in the first 5 days following injury. Nitrogen is excreted in the urine in the form of urea, creatinine, and creatine, leading to a negative nitrogen balance. Potassium loss accompanies protein depletion, and hypokalemia may result. Carbohydrate stores are rapidly depleted after traumatic injury, usually within the first 8 to 24 hours postinjury. In addition, the physiological and psychological stress of trauma may increase energy demands on the body by so much as 50% to 60% (Sheldon, Harper, & Way, 1981).

Factors that influence an individual client's nutritional needs include:

- The client's pretrauma nutritional status
- The type and severity of the injury
- The client's metabolic responses to the injury (Hui, 1983)

Following major trauma, clients generally require as much as 6.25 g/kg of protein daily to restore and maintain a positive nitrogen balance. Caloric needs for the average adult trauma victim are 45 to 60 kcal/kg/day. In addition, the client needs sufficient potassium to restore potassium balance and aid in the synthesis of muscle protein during recovery. The trauma victim also requires more than the recommended daily allowance of vitamin B complex (to meet increased metabolic demands), vitamins A and C (to facilitate wound healing), and vitamin K (for prothrombin production).

To compound the situation, traumatic injury often interferes with normal dietary intake. After trauma, the client may be unable to tolerate food and fluids and may be NPO for days, even weeks. Clearly, nutritional needs are great during the stress and recovery phases following injury, especially if the client has suffered severe burns, abdominal trauma, or spinal cord injury, which are associated with prolonged recovery. (Nutritional needs of burn victims are discussed in Chapter 15.) In such instances, the client may be placed on total parenteral nutrition to decrease the risk of nutritional deficiencies and other complications, such as infection.

Careful assessment of the trauma client's nutritional status is an important nursing function. The nurse should collaborate with the physician and clinical nutritionist to assure that the client's nutritional needs are recognized and met to ensure optimal recovery.

PHARMACOLOGIC INTERVENTION

A variety of pharmacologic agents must be readily available in emergency care settings. The emergency nurse is often called on to anticipate which drugs may be needed. Knowledge of commonly used emergency drugs is necessary for safe administration and evaluation of a client's responses. Drugs used in cardiorespiratory emergencies are discussed in Chapters 20 and 24. Immunologic agents are discussed in Chapter 11. Pharmacologic treatment of common poisonings is summarized later in this chapter.

Section III: Trauma as a Psychosocial Crisis

Anyone who has been through a trauma experience knows that a sudden life-threatening illness or injury can be intensely stressful and frightening for all involved. The importance of attending to the victim's and family's emotional needs in an emergency cannot be overemphasized. Sudden, acute illness or injury is an unexpected event that places victims and their loved ones in a state of extreme emotional vulnerability.

Needless to say, the victim's physiological needs must be the priority in an emergency. Indeed, family members and friends *want* to be reassured that everything medically and humanly possible is being done to save the victim's life and promote the victim's potential for a full recovery. In the process, however, the client's and family's emotional needs are often ignored, and the experience leaves them feeling depersonalized and devalued. It is not enough to care for the victim's physiological needs if the victim and family are left with long-term unresolved psychological sequelae.

PSYCHOLOGICAL IMPACT ON THE VICTIM

Trauma victims must deal with a number of potential threats. The body's stress response (see Chapter 2) is called into action to maintain or restore homeostasis. Psychological stress may intensify or aggravate the client's physical injuries or illness. If the client's fears and anxieties can be calmed, treatment measures are more easily carried out and are more likely to be effective. It is imperative that emergency health care providers recognize the importance of assessing and intervening to minimize the psychological impact of trauma.

If conscious, the victim must grapple with immediate fears of death or disability. Will medical help arrive in time? Will I live? Will I be disabled as a result of this? Are others injured? In the hospital setting, these fears continue as the client is faced with many unknowns. The outcome of the illness or injury may be unpredictable. People and equipment are unfamiliar and often frightening. Fears of procedures, pain, anesthesia, and surgery may all heighten the victim's initial anxiety.

Behavioral Threats to the Client's Well-Being

Other immediate threats to the client's psychological stability include loss of control, threats to autonomy and independence, changes in body image resulting from damage to body structure or function, and threats to self-esteem (see Chapter 4). Upon admission to the hospital, emergency clients are usually unable to do things for themselves or are prevented from doing so. Clothing and other personal belongings are removed. The client is attached to tubes and wires and becomes totally dependent on others for basic needs and even for survival. The client may feel helpless and out of control. In one sense, clients may feel comforted and secure knowing that competent, knowledgeable professionals are caring for their immediate needs. This total dependence, however, is also likely to cause feelings of helplessness and frustration (see Chapter 6).

The nature of an emergency also impairs the client's feelings of autonomy and independence. Invading the client's body space—a necessary part of treatment—may be distressing, especially if the victim is a modest and private person. This invasion can lead to feelings of shame and loss of dignity.

Injuries may cause structural or functional damage to the client's body. For example, a gunshot wound to the face that results in disfigurement and blindness, accidental limb amputation, a severe cerebral vascular accident (CVA), burns, or a spinal cord injury is likely to interfere significantly with the client's body image.

The loss of a body part or a permanent change in body functioning requires long-term adaptation to the change. Of course, the client must begin almost immediately to incorporate potential body image alterations into conscious awareness.

Emergency victims may even be embarrassed or apologetic about their injuries or illness. Victims of sudden obstructed airway (eg, choking on a piece of food in a busy restaurant) often later report their intense embarrassment in the situation. A young man who suffered a traumatic amputation of the ends of three of his fingers from a riding power mower exclaimed, "How could I be so dumb!"

Body image alterations may also damage the client's self-esteem (feelings of self-worth). Long-term hospitalization or permanent impairment of body functioning may wreak emotional havoc on clients and their families. The victim may lose employment and suffer permanent disability. Role status and role relationships may be severely impaired. The emotional and financial stressors of serious injury may disrupt family functioning. Unresolved feelings of anger and grief can surface long after the client's physical recovery.

Legal matters may further complicate the victim's full emotional recovery. Obtaining worker's compensation benefits, Social Security disability payments, or insurance reimbursement may involve legal complications, or there may be lawsuits by or against the victim to recover actual or punitive damages. Legal matters may take years to resolve and may be expensive. In some cases, victims may face criminal prosecution once they recover from their physical injuries (eg, an injured driver who was drunk and also seriously injured other persons).

Nursing Interventions Related to Psychosocial Effects on the Client

Emergency nursing interventions should be aimed at allaying the victim's anxiety and fear, promoting a sense of control, and minimizing threats to esteem and autonomy. The following nursing interventions can be easily performed while stabilizing the client:

- Remember that a real person is connected to the tubings, wires, ventilator, and other devices.
- Address the victim by name, in a clear, reassuring tone of voice. Don't shout at the client.
- Provide clear, brief explanations of procedures while preparing to institute them. Use terms the client can understand (avoiding medical jargon) and briefly describe how the client will feel. For example, say, "Mr Cavanaugh, I am going to insert a needle into your left arm. This may hurt some, but please try to lie still" or "Mr Cavanaugh, you are having trouble breathing because your chest was injured in the accident. We're giving you oxygen through the tube in your nose. Please try to relax."
- Keep the client covered to the extent possible to minimize exposure and embarrassment. This is especially important for sensitive areas such as breasts and genitals.
- Provide realistic reassurance. For example, a client with a spinal cord injury, severity unknown, asks, "I can't feel my legs and feet. Will I be able to walk again?" The nurse responds, "You have injured your back, but at this point the doctors haven't determined how badly. We will tell you more as soon as we know more about your injury. How can I make you more comfortable?"
- Even when a client is comatose, the nurse should briefly explain what is being done ("We're going to turn you on your side, Mrs Carlos.").

These sensitive nursing interventions will help the victim begin to cope with the psychological stresses of sudden acute illness or traumatic injury. If the victim dies, the nurse has the satisfaction of knowing the client's last moments or hours of life were more comfortable and less frightening. If the client lives and recovers, supportive nursing intervention will have helped the client's recovery.

At the very least, the client will have been helped to cope with the potential psychological consequences of sudden life-threatening illness or injury.

PSYCHOLOGICAL IMPACT ON THE FAMILY OR SIGNIFICANT OTHERS

The family of the emergency client may experience the same emotional responses as the client, perhaps more intensely because they need not simultaneously deal with physiological stressors. Anxiety and fear for the victim's well-being are paramount concerns. Separated from their loved one and given no time to prepare for this sudden, unexpected event, they are thrown into an emotional whirlwind.

The immediate shock and disbelief are accompanied by anxious worry, gnawing fear, and sometimes anger and guilt. Anger may be directed toward known or unknown persons who are believed to be responsible for the illness or injury, toward the emergency staff, and even toward the victim "for not being more careful." Guilt may be expressed, especially if family members perceive they are in some way responsible for the victim's injury ("I shouldn't have let him install that TV antenna on the roof") or if unpleasant words or emotions were exchanged the last time they were with the client.

Family and friends may sit helplessly in the waiting room, passively waiting and "accepting" what has befallen them. Or they may become verbally aggressive or abusive, or even physically violent. Reactions are highly individual from family to family and even among individual family members. How they respond depends a great deal on their usual patterns of coping with stressful situations. The client's roles in the family, the emotional attachments among family members, and the circumstances and nature of the client's illness or injury all influence the family's unique responses and coping behaviors.

Unfortunately, too often the emotional needs of the family are overlooked. The family may be seen as "getting in the way," "overreacting," "demanding," or "harrassing." In a study by Yoder and Jones (1982), 47% of emergency nurses said it was unrealistic to expect them to care for the emotional needs of emergency clients' families. However, 84% believed they had a responsibility to inform family members of the client's care, treatment, and responses. Surely, this information can be imparted in a way that is supportive and responsive to the family's emotional distress.

Some families overreact, making the nurse's task of handling their responses more difficult. This is especially the case when family members become verbally abusive to the nurse or try to strike a staff member. Although firm, restraining intervention may be necessary, it should be done in a calm, authoritative (not punitive) manner. The staff should try to remember it is the family's intense distress, or even panic, that is causing this unacceptable behavior.

Cultural Considerations

The family's cultural beliefs and values play a major role in their responses to emergencies. The family and the victim may believe they are being "tested" or punished by God, or they may simply accept the situation as "God's will."

The family's religious or spiritual beliefs often are a major source of strength and hope during the crisis. Sometimes, though, the family's beliefs may interfere with treatment. For example, a trauma victim who is a Jehovah's Witness may refuse permission for needed blood transfusions, without which the client may die. Health professionals who have dedicated themselves to aggressive treatment of emergency victims often have a difficult time dealing with this ethical dilemma and may react with hostility or anger toward the family.

Families whose cultural backgrounds are vastly different from those of the health professionals caring for their loved one may experience feelings of isolation and alienation. If there is a language barrier, the situation is even more difficult and frustrating for all involved. If the client and family speak a different language, an interpreter (if available) may be helpful. Nevertheless, in the crisis, there may be misinterpretations and misunderstandings about what is happening with the victim and what the family's role is. Helpful strategies for communicating with clients from different cultural backgrounds are given in Table 4–1 of Chapter 4.

Some cultural groups value close attendance of ill family members. Numerous relatives may arrive at the emergency department, each anxiously inquiring about the victim and requesting to see him or her. A large number of relatives and friends may be overwhelming to emergency staff and may interfere with maintaining a calm atmosphere.

Another frequent problem in today's "high-tech" emergency environment is the *technological gap* the family feels when faced with complex, unfamiliar, and confusing treatment measures and equipment. Even family members familiar with health care advances (such as computed tomography [CT] scans or cardiac monitors) may be intimidated and frightened by the complex environment surrounding their loved one. The technology becomes even more of a problem if the family has had little or no experience with a modern hospital. The family may be so frightened that they become anxious, agitated, or even angry about treatment measures. This technological gap and the family's anxiety intensify when staff use medical jargon to explain the client's condition and treatment.

Nursing Interventions Related to Psychological Effects on the Family

The family's needs for information and support can be met in a variety of ways during their often agonizing wait in the emergency department:

- As soon as possible, the family's presence should be acknowledged, with reassurance that they will be kept informed of the client's condition and progress.

- Explanations (in terms family members can understand) and reports of the client's status should be provided as frequently as possible, at least every 15 minutes.

- A pleasant waiting environment should be provided, with chairs or couches, restrooms, telephones, and vending machines.

- Admitting clerks should be trained to be sensitive when obtaining necessary information, such as insurance data.

- The immediate family should be allowed to see the client as soon as possible, if only for a few moments. Family members often imagine the worst. Seeing their loved one, even comatose or attached to equipment, can be reassuring. This measure is especially important if the client is going to surgery and death is a possibility.

- In Level I and II facilities that handle large emergency caseloads, a specifically trained professional should be available as a liaison between the family and emergency department staff. This person can be an experienced, sensitive emergency department staff nurse, clinical nurse specialist, or social worker. This liaison can help close the cultural and technological gaps by providing appropriate explanations and ongoing emotional support.

- An interpreter should be available in facilities where there is a large non-English speaking population in the community (or staff members should be able to speak the language).

- When numerous family members are present, a family spokesperson should be identified. All information may then be channeled through this person.

- If the hospital facility cannot physically accommodate large numbers of family members, the family can be asked to gather somewhere nearby, leaving one or two family members in the emergency department as liaisons.

- Perhaps most important, family members should be treated with respect, patience, and sensitivity. Avoiding family members may only compound their distress and grief and may result in feelings of anger and hostility toward the staff and hospital. Such feelings may linger for months and may interfere with the family's resolution of their grief.

When the family's worst fears are realized and the victim dies, their needs for supportive nursing intervention are even greater. (Refer also to Chapter 16.) The victim may have been pronounced dead on arrival at the hospital or may die sometime after admission. In either case, the survivors have special nursing needs. The nurse can help the family to begin to deal with their grief and the responsibilities associated with their loved one's death, such as arranging for the funeral or taking care of personal belongings. Interventions might include:

- Informing the family as soon as possible. A study by Jones and Buttery (1981) found that survivors would rather have been informed of their loved one's death by a compassionate nurse than by a physician who was knowledgeable but not as caring.

- Informing the survivors in a quiet room or area separate from the general emergency waiting area, where they can express their grief privately.

- Conveying the news in clear and specific words. Saying, "I'm sorry, Mr Michaels, but your wife is gone," may leave the survivor confused. Saying instead, "Mr Michaels, your wife suffered a severe head injury. We did everything we could to save her, but she died a few moments ago. I'm terribly sorry," is clear yet sensitive.

- Explaining what measures were instituted to try to save the victim. Families need reassurance that everything possible was done.

- Giving the survivors an opportunity to ask questions or to talk about the deceased.

- Making sure family members understand what they have been told. Often, in their shock and acute grief, family members hear only part of what they are told. They need time to think about what has happened and to clarify any misunderstandings.

- Providing the family an opportunity to have some time alone with the deceased. Unnecessary equipment (eg, IV tubing, endotracheal tubes, and monitor leads) should be disconnected and the body cleaned and covered. On the other hand, the presence of monitors and other equipment in the area may help reassure the survivors that all possible measures were employed to save the victim's life. Changes in the body, such as visible injuries or discoloration, should be explained. Family members should be gently reassured that it is all right to touch, kiss, and hold their loved one if they wish. This process can help make the death more real and facilitate the family's coping. The family should be left alone with their loved one for a few minutes if they desire.

- Assisting the survivors with completing the required paperwork and making the necessary contacts (eg, minister, priest, or rabbi; funeral director; other family members).

- Handling the victim's personal belongings with sensitivity and care. Clothing, jewelry, and other personal effects should be neatly assembled and given to the family in a compassionate manner, preferably not in an impersonal "brown bag." The victim's personal belongings often provide family members with a final link to their loved one.

- Informing the family when it is all right for them to leave the emergency department. In their research, Jones and Buttery (1981) found that survivors stated that a "concluding process" would have been helpful. By this, they meant being told, "You have done all you can here. It's okay for you to leave now." Providing a follow-up contact in the emergency department is also helpful if the family thinks of additional questions later.

PSYCHOLOGICAL IMPACT ON THE EMERGENCY NURSE

The emergency nurse is not immune to the psychological stressors of working with victims of life-threatening injuries or illness. Having to deal on a regular basis with death and critical illness or injury and with grief-stricken families places great demands on a nurse's physical and emotional stamina. These demands can be emotionally draining. Over time, the nurse risks becoming desensitized to the emotional needs of victims and their families as a self-protective mechanism. On the other hand, a nurse who becomes too emotionally involved with clients and families and overidentifies with their reactions may be unable to meet their needs for support because of concern with his or her own emotional responses. Finding a balance between these extremes is not easy, but the emergency nurse can learn to convey empathy, caring, and compassion through a conscious conviction that these qualities are an essential part of emergency nursing.

Section IV: The Nursing Process in Trauma and Other Emergencies

Application of the nursing process in emergencies involves the same steps as in any health care situation. The difference in applying the nursing process in emergency settings is the speed with which the nurse proceeds through these phases. In emergencies, the nurse may seem to be assessing, analyzing, planning, implementing, and evaluating all at once. The reason is that the nurse is drawing on knowledge and experience to focus on the significant aspects of the situation quickly. For example, the nurse may be administering oxygen (implementing), asking questions about events that led up to the illness or injury (assessing),

deciding on the next priority for care (planning), and determining the client's response to the oxygen (evaluating) simultaneously.

NURSING ASSESSMENT

Assessment is perhaps the most important phase of caring for an emergency client. If an inaccurate assessment is made, the nurse or other health professionals may implement measures that are ineffective or even harmful to the client. The nursing assessment of the emergency client

Nursing Research Note

Jones S, Ring S, Jones P, Katz J: ED use in relation to health care experiences and behavior. *JEN* 1985; 11(3):145–148.

Emergency department (ED) users were examined for two variables: early socialization to emergency department utilization and preventive health care behavior. Early socialization to ED use was found to be a factor in emergency room utilization in adulthood. ED users had been taken to the ED as children and had learned to use the ED as a health care facility. Men and women used the ED services equally. However, men used the ED for accident-related injuries, whereas women used it for illnesses. Both ED users and nonusers practiced preventive health care and did not use the services for primary care.

This research indicates that early socialization to ED services is a factor in frequent ED use by adults. Nurses can teach parents and the general public about proper emergency department utilization. Education may help to reduce this early socialization process and help to reduce unnecessary use of emergency care resources.

should be conducted rapidly yet systematically so important parameters are not missed. The assessment includes interviews with the client or significant others and a thorough head-to-toe clinical appraisal.

ABC Assessment

In the initial contact with the emergency client, a rapid yet thorough assessment is necessary to determine if any life-threatening condition is present. The client should quickly be appraised to determine whether a possibility of a spinal cord injury exists. If such an injury is suspected, the client's head and neck should be stabilized as the rescuer begins

Box 13–2   The ABCs of Emergency Assessment

Step 1: Is there a possibility of spinal cord injury (because of the circumstances of the accident)? If so, stabilize head and neck and proceed with rapid ABC assessment.

Step 2: A = Airway

1. Is the airway patent?
2. Is there a partial or complete obstruction of the airway?

Step 3: B = Breathing

1. Is the client breathing (inhaling and exhaling)?
2. Is chest movement with each breath symmetrical?
3. Are audible breath sounds present bilaterally?

Step 4: C = Circulation

1. Is skin color pale or cyanotic?
2. Are pulses (carotid and femoral) present? If so, are they regular or irregular? Are they full, weak, or bounding?
3. Does the client's skin feel clammy or cold?
4. Is there any external bleeding? Is it arterial or venous?

to conduct an assessment of the client's airway, breathing, and circulation (ABCs). The client's ABCs should be assessed within the first 60 seconds (Box 13–2). If any life-threatening condition is present (eg, airway obstruction, respiratory or cardiac cessation, or severe external bleeding), the nurse must intervene at once to correct the situation. Once the threat to life has been averted, a more thorough emergency assessment can be done.

Emergency History (Subjective Data)

The emergency history is usually obtained during or immediately following the initial ABC assessment. The victim should be queried if conscious. Immediate family, friends, bystanders, or police and rescue workers may have to be questioned if the client is unable to provide complete information, or they may help validate the client's description of the problem. Obtain the following information:

• The nature of the emergency. (What is the client's chief concern?)

• The circumstances surrounding the emergency, including time and place of occurrence, precipitating and alleviating factors, the client's and others' responses, and any measures already instituted.

• The client's subjective complaints or concerns, including pain and other subjective symptoms such as nausea or chills.

• The client's health history (allergies; current medications; and history of illness such as diabetes, heart disease, or hypertension).

Be alert for inconsistencies in the history given by the client or others. For instance, a 62-year-old man brought to the emergency department with complaints of chest pain says, "This is just like the pains I always get." His wife tells the nurse, "I can tell this is much worse. He's never had nausea and sweating before, and he took four nitroglycerin tablets. He usually only needs one or two to get relief." Such information helps guide further questioning and pinpointing of the actual problem.

Clinical Appraisal of the Emergency Victim (Objective Data)

The clinical appraisal usually takes place while the nurse is gathering subjective information from the client, especially if there is concern or evidence that the client's life is in immediate danger. Following initial appraisal of the client's ABCs, a head-to-toe clinical assessment should be conducted. The nurse should use the senses to gather pertinent data: *observe, inspect, listen, touch,* and *smell* to determine or validate the nature of the emergency. The clinical appraisal is outlined in Box 13–3. The objective data obtained should be compared with the client's subjective reports for consistency and cross-validation.

Box 13-3 Clinical Appraisal of the Emergency Client

Oxygenation status (see Box 13-2)

- Are there signs of respiratory distress or shock?
- Is the trachea in the midline?
- Is the chest wall symmetrical?
- Is there evidence of external or internal injury (eg, contusions, lacerations, opening in chest wall)?
- Is there evidence of pain on inhalation or exhalation (wincing, shallow respirations, holding chest)?
- Are there any changes in vital signs (pulse, respiration, blood pressure)?

Neurologic status

- Is the client responsive to verbal and other stimuli?
- Is the client oriented to time, place, and person?
- What is the pupillary response of both eyes?
- Is blood or clear fluid leaking from ears or nose?
- Does the client's breath smell of alcohol or acetone?
- Is there evidence of lacerations, depressions, or contusions of the skull?
- Is the client stuporous, convulsing, or comatose?

Abdomen/pelvis

- Are femoral pulses present?
- Is there any femoral swelling or hematoma formation?
- Is the abdominal wall distended, rigid, or asymmetrical (abdominal girth should be measured if intra-abdominal injury is suspected)?

- Are there external signs of injury (lacerations, pelvic fracture, penetrating wounds, contusions)?
- Is there localized pain or rebound tenderness?
- Are bowel sounds present, and what is their quality?
- Is the urinary bladder distended?
- Is there evidence of trauma to external genitalia?
- Are there lacerations or hematomas of the perineum (including urethral meatus, vagina, or anal sphincter)?

Extremities

- Is the client able to move all four extremities?
- Is the client able to distinguish sensations (eg, sharp, dull) in extremities?
- Is there evidence of fractures or dislocations (swelling, lacerations, asymmetry of extremities or joints, projecting bone fragments, pain on movement)?
- Are peripheral pulses present? What is the quality of the peripheral pulses (brachial, radial, popliteal, pedal)?
- Are there any muscle tremors or contractions?
- Do fingers and toes blanch easily? Do nail beds refill quickly? Are fingers and toes pink and warm to the touch?

Behavioral manifestations

- What are the client's verbal responses (eg, questioning, cursing, verbal abuse, expressions of fear or anger)?
- Are there signs of severe anxiety or hypoxia (restlessness, distress, muscle tensing, twitching or tremors, disorientation)?
- Is the client calm and cooperative or combative and uncooperative?

It is especially important that subtle manifestations of injury or illness not be overlooked because of obvious or dramatic signs and symptoms. Oversights are more likely when the emergency team is attending to more than one victim simultaneously. For instance, a middle-aged couple was admitted to the hospital following an auto accident. The husband was comatose and bleeding from an obvious head injury. His wife was alert and oriented, and on admission, her vital signs were stable. As the team attended to her husband, she developed hypovolemic shock from internal bleeding and died. *Frequent and ongoing assessment of the emergency client is imperative.*

Diagnostic Profile

Certain diagnostic tests may be indicated to help confirm or rule out a particular medical diagnosis in the emergency client. The specific diagnostic tests that are ordered for an emergency victim depend on the information gathered during the history and clinical appraisal and the client's known or suspected injury or illness. For example, a client admitted with abdominal pain suggestive of appendicitis would

likely have a complete blood count (CBC) with white cell differential and a urinalysis. A client with suspected intra-abdominal bleeding may have a hematocrit, serum amylase, abdominal x-rays, and a paracentesis to aid in the diagnosis. Angiography or CT scan may be used to diagnose intracranial trauma, such as a ruptured cerebral aneurysm or other intracranial hemorrhage.

The emergency nurse must be familiar with common laboratory tests and their normal values. A typical diagnostic profile for a trauma victim includes:

- CBC with white cell differential (hematocrit, hemoglobin, red blood cell [RBC] count, leukocyte count, and differential white cell count).
- Coagulation profile (this may include bleeding and clotting times, clot retraction, platelet count, partial thromboplastin time, prothrombin time, and fibrinogen assay).
- Arterial blood gases (pH, PCO_2, PO_2, and oxygen saturation).
- Serum electrolytes (sodium, potassium, CO_2, chloride, and magnesium concentrations).

- Serum amylase (elevated in intra-abdominal trauma).
- Blood type and crossmatch (emergency crossmatch should be performed only when the urgent need for blood volume replacement is greater than the risk of a blood transfusion reaction) (Byrne et al., 1986).
- Urinalysis (especially for blood cells).

Other laboratory tests may be ordered for specific conditions such as toxicology tests for clients with suspected poisonings; lactate dehydrogenase (LDH) and SGOT (serum glutamic-oxaloacetic transaminase) levels in clients with MI; cerebrospinal fluid analysis in clients with suspected meningitis or intracranial hemorrhage; and selected tests for victims of sexual assault, including aspiration and analysis of vaginal contents for motile sperm and acid phosphatase levels.

NURSING DIAGNOSIS

After the data have been gathered, they must be analyzed to arrive at appropriate and valid nursing diagnoses. Certain nursing diagnoses, such as *impaired gas exchange, ineffective airway clearance,* and *altered cardiac output,* must be determined rapidly so appropriate actions can be initiated. Other nursing diagnoses must also be attended to after the client's physiological functioning has been stabilized, eg, *fear* or *anxiety* related to potentially life-threatening illness or injury; *impaired physical mobility* related to fracture or spinal cord injury; and *alteration in comfort* related to pain from intra-abdominal trauma or rib fractures.

Typical nursing diagnoses for clients experiencing trauma or sudden, life-threatening illness are listed in Table 13–2. Some possible etiologic factors for each diagnosis are also included.

PLANNING

Planning care for the emergency client is especially concerned with establishing priorities for medical and nursing intervention. Of course, the client's needs for a patent airway, breathing, and adequate circulation vital to basic life processes must be attended to first. Other priorities include protecting the client from further injury (eg, stabilizing the head and neck of a client with a possible spinal cord injury), restoring fluid and electrolyte balance, thermal regulation, and pain control. While attending to the emergency client's basic physiological needs, the nurse can begin planning to meet less pressing but nevertheless important needs, such as those involving emotional support and client and family teaching.

Triage

In emergencies in which several or many ill or injured persons must be cared for simultaneously, clients must be **triaged** (sorted) according to the severity of their injuries and the potential outcomes of treatment. Triage decisions are based on the findings of the initial assessment. Generally, there are three triage categories:

Category 1: Clients who will probably die unless treatment is begun immediately. Examples: Sudden obstructed airway, cardiac arrest, severe chest injuries, major burns, severe or profound shock, severe hemorrhage.

Category 2: Clients with serious but not life-threatening injuries whose treatment may be delayed up to 1 hour without risk of death. Examples: Compound fractures, head and neck injuries, abdominal wounds.

Category 3: Clients with minor injuries who can be treated after clients in the first two categories have been attended to. Examples: Simple fractures, minor burns, lacerations or other minor soft tissue injuries.

An additional category in major disasters includes victims who will probably die even if treatment is instituted (those with severe cardiac or crushing chest injuries or massive burns). Clients with the least chance of survival are assigned the lowest priority for care because resources and personnel must be used to save the greatest number of victims possible.

Nursing Care Plans for the Emergency Client

Every emergency client should have a nursing care plan. In cases of minor, easily treated injuries the nursing care plan may be recorded as part of the nursing interventions; eg, "tetanus toxoid, 0.5 mL given in deltoid; dry sterile dressing applied to abrasions; client instructed in home care of abrasions." In more serious illness or injury, the emergency nursing care plan should be documented as part of the client's health record. Standardized nursing care plans should be available for clients with common illnesses or injuries, such as acute MI, near-drowning, burns, abdominal injury, and so forth. EDNA has delineated the emergency nurse's responsibility with regard to nursing care planning: "Emergency nurses shall develop and utilize standardized care plans as a systematic, uniform, and consistent method to provide safe, effective [client] care" (EDNA, 1983). When using standardized nursing care plans, the emergency nurse must individualize the plan to fit each client's situation, taking into account the client's age, past history, current responses, and cultural background.

A sample nursing care plan for a trauma client is in Table 13–3. This plan includes priorities for care, independent nursing interventions, related medical interventions carried out by the nurse, and the desired client outcomes.

Emergency Supplies and Equipment

An important part of the nurse's role is to ensure that emergency supplies and equipment are readily available and in working order. In most emergency settings, the

Table 13–2   Possible Nursing Diagnoses of Trauma or Emergency Victims

Nursing Diagnosis	Possible Etiology	Nursing Diagnosis	Possible Etiology
Airway clearance, ineffective	Foreign body in trachea; laryngeal edema from smoke inhalation; client comatose or convulsing		body integrity (eg, spinal cord injury, burns, traumatic amputation, chronic disability)
Anxiety	Life-threatening illness or injury; emergency hospitalization or surgery	*Injury, potential for***	Unsafe conditions at home or work; risk-taking behaviors (driving while intoxicated, use of illegal drugs, street violence, not wearing seat belts); suicidal or homicidal behavior
Breathing patterns, ineffective	Chest injuries; pulmonary embolus; diabetic ketoacidosis; status asthmaticus; near-drowning; anaphylaxis; poisoning (drug overdose, carbon monoxide, corrosive ingestion)	*Mobility, impaired physical*	Head and spinal cord injuries; fractures; cerebral vascular accident; prolonged bed rest because of major trauma or illness
Cardiac output: alteration in (decreased)*	Internal or external hemorrhage; shock syndrome; acute myocardial infarction or congestive heart failure; cardiac arrest; chest injuries	*Powerlessness*	Dependence and loss of control caused by sudden, life-threatening situations
Comfort, alteration in: pain	Acute myocardial infarction; burns; corrosive ingestion; traumatic injuries	*Rape trauma syndrome*	Sexual assault
Communication, impaired verbal	Cerebral vascular accident (stroke); intubation or tracheostomy	*Self-concept: disturbance in*	Burns; trauma to body parts resulting in loss, disfigurement, or altered functioning; alcoholism or drug abuse
Coping, ineffective (individual or family)	Sudden life-threatening illness or injury	*Sensory-perceptual alteration*	Head, spinal cord, and eye injuries; toxic ingestions; sensory overload or deprivation in "high-tech" environment; anxiety; hypoxia
Fear	Life-threatening illness or injury; emergency hospitalization or surgery; loss of control (dependence)		
Fluid volume deficit: actual or potential	Internal or external hemorrhage; shock syndrome; heat exhaustion or heat stroke; burns	*Skin integrity, impairment of*	Burns; penetrating trauma; lacerations
Fluid volume excess	Near-drowning; congestive heart failure; pulmonary edema	*Distress of the human spirit*	Life-threatening illness or injury that causes the client/family to doubt their religious beliefs or causes conflicts with spiritual values
Gas exchange: impaired	Shock syndrome; hypoxia; carbon monoxide poisoning; near-drowning; pulmonary embolus; sudden airway obstruction; hyperventilation or hypoventilation; chest injuries; diabetic ketoacidosis; anaphylaxis; status asthmaticus	*Thought process, impaired*	Head injury; shock syndrome; sensory deprivation or overload
		Tissue perfusion, alteration in	Shock syndrome; hemorrhage; trauma to body part
Grieving, anticipatory	Expected loss (eg, of loved one); threats to	**Violence, potential for**	Reactions of rage to trauma or death of loved one; suicidal or homicidal behavior; some drug overdoses

*Diagnoses shown in boldface require immediate referral for medical evaluation and treatment.

**This nursing diagnosis applies to the preventive role of the nurse in trauma.

Table 13–3 Sample Nursing Care Plan

Emergency Nursing Assessment

Mr JC is a 41-year-old white male admitted to the emergency department at 9:10 PM following a two-vehicle collision. He has an IV of 5% dextrose in water infusing into his left forearm and a nasal O_2 cannula in place. His left leg is in a full leg splint. Mr C is complaining of chest and leg pain. His chest pain is aggravated on inhalation. He is guarding his abdomen and says he feels like vomiting.

Mr C says he has minimal recall of the accident. He says he was coming home from a practice football game and was proceeding through an intersection at approximately 30 mph through a green light when he felt a sudden impact "from nowhere!" against the driver's side of the car. He says he was dazed and barely remembers being transported to the emergency department. Mr C reports no current illnesses or medications and says he has no allergies.

Clinical Appraisal

Oxygenation status: Airway patent; R—32, shallow; wincing on inhalation; chest wall movement symmetrical; bilateral breath sounds; obvious contusions of left chest wall.

P—92, regular, slightly weak; BP—110/60; skin slightly pale, cool, and moist to touch; no external bleeding.

Neurologic status: Responsive to verbal commands; oriented × 3; PERRLA; no alcohol odor on breath; no external injuries of skull or back evident; apprehensive.

Abdomen/pelvis: Femoral pulses present bilaterally but weak; no hematomas or edema; abdominal wall slightly distended with extreme tenderness on palpation; no external wounds; bowel sounds all four quadrants; no apparent injury of bladder, genitalia, or perineum.

Extremities: Left leg splinted. Contusions and swelling of left anterolateral thigh; able to wiggle toes; toes pink and warm to touch, blanch easily; able to distinguish sharp/dull in all extremities; pedal pulses present but weak; full ROM in other extremities.

Behavioral: Asking for family. Apprehensive but cooperative. Asked, "Are you taking me to surgery?"

Probable Medical Diagnoses

Fractured ribs, left rib cage; intra-abdominal bleeding with potential for hypovolemic shock; fractured left femur

Nursing Diagnosis*	Client Care Goal	Plan/Nursing Implementation	Expected Outcome
Ineffective breathing pattern, related to chest injuries	Promote ventilation and prevent further respiratory compromise	Elevate head of bed 10–20° to decrease pressure on diaphragm and increase lung expansion; monitor respiratory status for change; administer O_2 as prescribed; splint left chest with pillow to decrease pain and facilitate breathing	Respiratory status remains stable or improves; client breathes more comfortably; documentation of frequent respiratory assessment entered in record
Potential fluid volume deficit, related to intra-abdominal injuries	Prevent hypovolemic shock; restore fluid balance	Place in supine position with legs elevated 12–16 in; continue to monitor fluid/electrolyte and circulatory status for change; administer IV fluids and blood products as prescribed and monitor response; administer prescribed antiemetic rectal suppository; prepare client for emergency exploratory laparotomy (eg, lab studies, informed consent—see Chapter 14)	Vital signs remain WNL; signs of fluid balance WNL; no vomiting; correctly prepared for surgery; documentation of fluid therapy and client response entered in record
Alteration in comfort: pain, related to injuries	Relieve pain and promote physical comfort	Splint chest wall with pillow; elevate legs to decrease pressure on abdomen; encourage client to relax; administer prescribed analgesics; move client as little as possible before surgery	Client verbalizes fewer complaints of pain; says he feels more comfortable; clinical manifestations of pain (wincing) decrease; documentation of client's response to interventions entered in record

Nursing Diagnosis*	Client Care Goal	Plan/Nursing Implementation	Expected Outcome
Fear, related to injuries and anticipated surgery and hospitalization	Decrease fear and apprehension; promote psychological comfort	Explain procedures and provide preop teaching in clear, concise, understandable terms; provide honest answers to client's questions; explain expected outcomes of medical and surgical interventions; allow family members to visit with client before surgery; provide for family members' comfort during waiting	Increased evidence of calm; decreased apprehension; cooperation with treatments; family members visit with client; family members kept informed of client's treatment and progress; family members' comfort needs met during wait
Self-concept, potential disturbance in, related to intrusive procedures, loss of control, lack of privacy, leg injury, anticipated surgery, abdominal incision, hospitalization, and separation from loved ones	Promote increased sense of control; promote self-esteem; provide privacy to extent possible	Use client's name; speak to (not about) client; explain to client why personal belongings have been removed and reassure him he can have them back postop; minimize number of different persons caring for client to the extent possible; keep body parts covered (especially genital area) to extent possible; keep curtain drawn around bed or door to room closed (if possible); encourage client to participate in decision making whenever possible	Client is treated with dignity and respect; personal belongings are safely stored and transported to postop room; privacy is provided to extent possible; client participates in decision making concerning his care and treatment whenever possible (eg, informed consent, acceptance of analgesics)

*Nursing diagnoses have been prioritized.

nursing staff is responsible for frequent, periodic checks of emergency equipment to ensure it is ready for use. Supplies and equipment used during an emergency should be replaced as quickly as possible thereafter. The American College of Emergency Physicians publishes a recommended equipment list for emergency facilities.

IMPLEMENTATION

The implementation phase of the nursing process in an emergency setting involves both independent nursing actions and actions that may be carried out according to preestablished medical protocols (eg, oxygen administration, starting IV fluids, administering emergency drugs, and ordering lab tests). Nursing actions should be carried out effectively, efficiently, and with utmost consideration for the client's safety. The nurse should implement nursing measures calmly and confidently to reassure and comfort the emergency client (and family, if present).

Because victims are often in pain and are highly anxious or frightened, the emergency nurse is in a key position to modify the emergency environment to promote the client's physical and psychological comfort. Some general nursing

interventions that promote client comfort in an emergency setting are:

- Explain procedures to the client before carrying them out or as they are being implemented.

- Use terminology familiar to the client. Help interpret for the client explanations given by others that appear to be confusing or are only partially understood.

- Reduce noxious stimuli in the environment to the extent possible (eg, minimize the number of persons in the immediate environment, remove unnecessary equipment, and talk in normal tones).

- Be alert to verbal and nonverbal behaviors that indicate the client is having pain.

- Encourage relaxation if the client is tense and anxious (eg, use of conscious, slow deep-breathing and thinking of something pleasant). (Refer to Chapter 4.)

- Position the client for maximum comfort (if not contraindicated by health conditions).

- Administer prescribed analgesics, sedatives, or tranquilizers as needed and monitor the client's response.

- Provide emotional support and realistic reassurance

to the client and family (keep them informed; make appropriate use of listening, reflection, and touch to convey compassion and caring; elicit client's and family's concerns and questions). Support the client's and family's attempts to cope with the stress and crisis.

- Identify and utilize appropriate resources, such as a chaplain or social worker, to assist the client and family to cope.

EVALUATION

Evaluation of the client's responses according to observable behavioral outcomes is the last step of the nursing process. The desired client outcomes defined during the planning phase should be used to evaluate whether client goals have been achieved and whether any revisions or modifications in the nursing care plan are needed (see Table 13–3 for examples).

In addition to evaluating outcomes of care for individual clients, use the Standards of Emergency Nursing Practice (EDNA, 1983) to evaluate the quality of emergency nursing care in a particular emergency facility. Periodic evaluation of whether the standards are being met and to what extent can identify problems or deficiencies in the level of emergency nursing practice so they may be corrected.

Section V: Specific Emergencies

Common medical and traumatic emergencies such as sudden airway obstruction, drowning and near-drowning, allergic reactions and anaphylaxis, thermal emergencies, and poisonings, along with related emergency nursing and medical management, are reviewed in this section. Traumatic injuries are also described in general. Specific emergency care of the client with acute MI, aneurysm, CVA, pulmonary embolus, acute respiratory failure, and status asthmaticus is discussed in Units Three, Four, and Six and will not be repeated here. Specific traumatic injuries are discussed in the appropriate body systems chapter—injuries to the head and spine are discussed in Chapters 37 and 38; injuries to the bony structures of the face in Chapter 19; eye injuries in Chapter 71; flail chest and pneumothorax in Chapter 20; cardiac tamponade in Chapter 24; abdominal injuries in Chapters 33, 49, 53, 64, and 67; fractures or traumatic amputation of the extremities in Chapter 57; and injuries from sexual assault in Chapter 64.

SUDDEN AIRWAY OBSTRUCTION

Sudden occlusion of the airway is most common when a large or whole piece of food, such as a chunk of meat, a peanut, an ice cube, or a marshmallow, becomes lodged in the trachea. The passage of air is obstructed, and respiration ceases. Symptoms mimic those of an MI. This condition has been called the "café coronary" because it frequently occurs while dining in a restaurant. The food may have been chewed insufficiently, or the individual's gag reflex may be diminished because of alcohol intake. Airway obstruction is also common in persons with poorly fitting dentures that interfere with food chewing.

The nurse is more likely to encounter this emergency in a public place than in the emergency department. If the obstruction is not attended to immediately, death from a blocked airway will ensue in 4 to 6 minutes from cardiorespiratory arrest.

Symptoms of an obstructed airway are those of acute respiratory distress. They may be further delineated according to partial or total obstruction (Saxton et al., 1983):

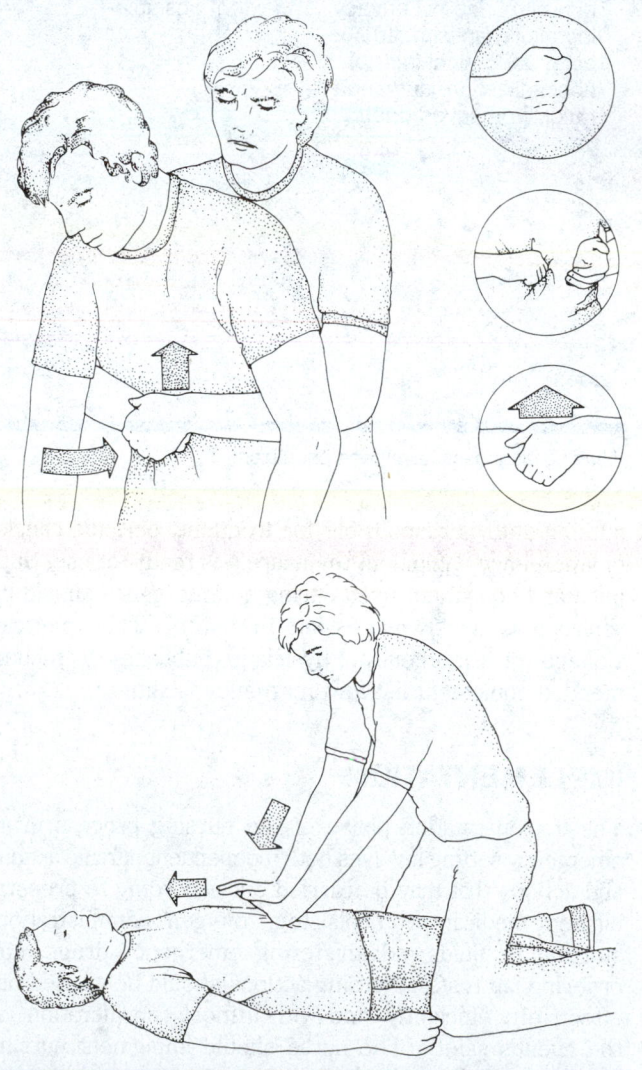

Figure 13–5

Heimlich maneuver. **Top.** Individual in upright position. **Bottom.** Individual in recumbant position.
SOURCE: Saxton DF et al. *Addison–Wesley Manual of Nursing Practice.* Menlo Park, CA: Addison–Wesley, 1983.

Partial obstruction:

• Noisy respiration
• Dyspnea, gasping
• Lightheadedness
• Dizziness
• Flushing of face
• Bulging of eyes
• Restless and fearful behavior
• Repeated coughing

Total obstruction:

• Cessation of breathing; lack of air flow in or out of the nose or mouth
• Inability to speak or cough; may make strident noises
• Exaggerated movements when attempting to inhale; head may be extended; suprasternal and supraclavicular notches may be indented
• Facial pallor or cyanosis
• Bulging of the eyes
• Behavior that is fearful or panicky; victim may clutch at the throat
• Unconsciousness

Appropriate intervention for sudden airway obstruction has been delineated by the American Heart Association and is included as a part of basic life support instruction. If the victim is conscious, the rescuer should:

1. Validate with the victim that the airway is obstructed. (Ask the victim, "Can you breathe?")
2. Use an abdominal thrust (Heimlich maneuver) to clear the airway (Figure 13–5).
3. Continue using abdominal thrusts until the airway is cleared or the victim becomes comatose.

If the victim becomes unconscious, turn the victim's head to the side and "sweep" the mouth using a cross-finger technique (Figure 13–6) to remove any loosened material. Mouth-to-mouth resuscitation should then be attempted, and the victim should be transported as quickly as possible to the nearest emergency facility.

Sometimes a cricothyroidotomy may be indicated if the previous attempts do not clear the airway and the victim is comatose. A cricothyroidotomy involves cutting an opening in the trachea below the cricoid cartilage (see Chapter 21).

The nurse has a responsibility to educate the public concerning prevention of airway obstruction, using the following guidelines:

• Avoid laughing or talking with food in the mouth.
• Take small bites.
• Have dentures fitted properly and use them when eating.
• Be familiar with the universal choking signal (Figure 13–7).
• If alone when the obstruction occurs, use a table edge, countertop, or chair to thrust against just below the rib cage in the middle of the upper abdomen.

DROWNING AND NEAR-DROWNING

Drowning is the fourth leading cause of accidental death in adults. Boating and swimming accidents account for the largest number of drownings, and many are alcohol related. Drowning is defined as death from asphyxia while the victim is submerged in water (or other type of fluid). Near-

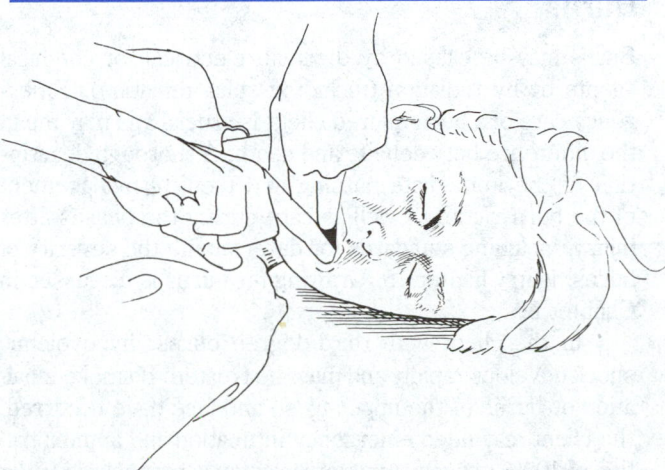

Figure 13–6

Sweeping the mouth with the cross-finger technique.

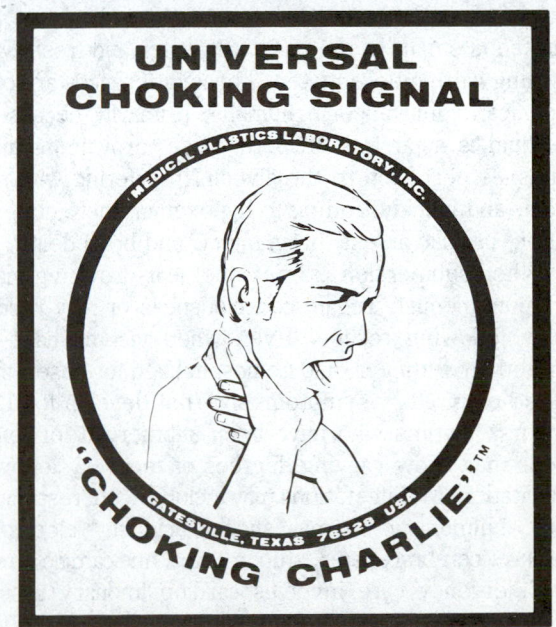

Figure 13–7

Universal choking signal.
SOURCE: Medical Plastics Laboratory, Inc., P.O. Box 38, Gatesville, Texas 76528.

drowning applies to victims who survive for at least 24 hours after rescue from submersion. Victims of near-drowning, if rescued and resuscitated quickly enough, may fully recover. In many instances, however, near-drowning victims are left with mild to severe neurologic sequelae. Even if the victim has been submerged in water for some time (as much as 1 hour or more), vigorous attempts at resuscitation are indicated because of documented recovery following such incidents.

Factors that influence the extent of damage in near-drowning include the length of time submerged, the temperature of the water, and the victim's resistance to asphyxia and anoxia. Recovery may be more successful if the victim drowns in cold water, because the induced hypothermia lowers the body's metabolic demands and, therefore, oxygen needs. On the other hand, extremely cold water may decrease the victim's core body temperature so rapidly that death from hypothermia may actually occur before drowning.

Generally, there is an inverse relation between the victim's age and the victim's resistance to asphyxia and anoxia; ie, the younger the victim, the greater the resistance. This resistance is especially strong in very young victims (usually under 2 or 3 years of age) because of the diving reflex triggered in young children when the face is immersed in very cold water. Blood is shunted to the vital organs, especially the brain and the heart. Although the victim suffers severe bradycardia, the remaining oxygen supply is concentrated in the heart and the brain. The diving reflex is generally not a factor in adult drownings.

Approximately 10% of drowning victims develop laryngospasm concurrently with the first gulp of water and, thus, do not aspirate fluid ("dry drowning"). Even in the majority of victims who do aspirate, the amount of fluid aspirated is small. In the past, salt-water and fresh-water drowning were differentiated. These differences are of little clinical significance in humans, primarily because so little fluid is aspirated. In both cases, drowning quickly diminishes perfusion to the alveoli, interfering with ventilation, and quickly leading to hypoxemia, ineffective circulation, cardiac arrest, brain injury, and brain death.

When submersion is brief, the near-drowning victim may spontaneously regain consciousness or may recover quickly following rescue. Even when victims have not aspirated fluid, they should be hospitalized for observation because respiratory symptoms may not develop for 12 to 24 hours. Victims who have been submerged for longer periods may show varying degrees of recovery following resuscitation. Manifestations may include acute respiratory failure, pulmonary edema, shock, acidosis, electrolyte imbalance, cerebral edema, stupor, coma, and cardiac arrest.

Emergency care involves cardiopulmonary resuscitation, intubation, and mechanical ventilation with 100% oxygen. Positive end-expiratory pressure (PEEP) may be needed to achieve adequate ventilation (see Chapter 18).

Metabolic acidosis results from the severe hypoxia. Arterial blood gases should be monitored frequently. Sodium bicarbonate is usually administered to correct the acidosis.

Barbiturate coma (with pentobarbital or thiopental) may be induced and a state of hypothermia maintained for several days following the near-drowning. These interventions reduce the metabolic and oxygen demands of the brain. Diuretics are prescribed to treat pulmonary and cerebral edema.

Fluid therapy must be monitored carefully to prevent fluid overload and promote adequate renal function. The nurse should frequently evaluate and document the client's responses to therapy.

ALLERGIC REACTIONS AND ANAPHYLAXIS

A number of substances can precipitate severe allergic (hypersensitivity) reactions: certain foods (when eaten in large amounts); food additives and chemicals (such as monosodium glutamate); medications such as penicillin, aspirin, horse-serum based antitoxins, or iodinated contrast media; insect bites or stings; and snake bites. The body's immune response to ingested or injected toxins, including anaphylactic shock, and emergency management are fully described in Chapter 5.

Symptoms of specific types of bites and stings and emergency nursing prescriptions are in Table 13–4. For localized allergic responses from spider bites or insect stings, antihistamines, such as diphenhydramine (Benadryl) injection, capsule, or elixir, may be administered every 4 to 6 hours until the edema and other symptoms subside.

THERMAL EMERGENCIES

Thermal emergencies include exposure to extremes of heat (burns, heat exhaustion, heat stroke) or cold (hypothermia, frostbite). These conditions may be life threatening or limb threatening and require immediate intervention.

Burns

Burns may be caused by thermal, electrical, or chemical agents or by radiation (including solar radiation). Emergency care of a burn-injured client is crucial and may mean the difference between life and death. A thorough description of the immediate nursing and medical management of the burn victim as well as care during the phases after injury, including standards for determining the severity of burns, is in Chapter 15. Grafting for burns is discussed in Chapter 80.

In the client with third-degree burns, hypovolemic shock develops rapidly and must be treated. If smoke inhalation or burns of the upper torso and face have occurred, the client may need emergency intubation and administration of 100% oxygen. Appropriate tetanus prophylaxis (refer to Table 11–7) should be administered. Tetanus immunizations are generally painful, and the nurse should instruct clients who receive them that localized redness, swelling,

Table 13–4 Bites and Stings: Symptomatology and Nursing Prescriptions

Type of Bite or Sting	Symptomatology	Nursing Prescriptions
Animal bites	Laceration, puncture, or abrasion; bleeding; swelling; erythema, ecchymosis; loss of function if nerves or bone involved; pain may vary considerably depending on damage done; if the nerve supply has been interrupted, pain may be absent in spite of extensive damage; anxiety and fear	Flush bite with water; cleanse with soap or antiseptic solution; control hemorrhage; apply pressure to pressure points or wound to stop bleeding; apply dry sterile dressing; transport to emergency room for tetanus inoculation, antibiotics, surgical repair, and Pasteur or hyperimmune serum if animal cannot be located or is known to have rabies; report to local authorities, such as police or health department, to assist in location, capture, and testing of animal
Bee, wasp, or ant stings	Presence of bite, with or without stinger imbedded in skin; local swelling, redness, and pain *Generalized allergic reaction:* nausea, vomiting, diarrhea; uticaria, pruritus; anaphylactic shock, collapse; hypotension; shortness of breath, wheezing; tightness of chest; anxiety; unconsciousness *Delayed reaction (serum sickness):* fever; malaise; lymphadenopathy; joint pain; skin eruptions	Remove stinger, if present, by scraping skin with sharp object; do not squeeze to prevent further injection of venom; apply tourniquet 2 in above bite on extremity to obstruct lymphatic but not arterial flow; release every 5 min briefly and reapply; neutralize with alkaline solutions, such as ammonia water, alcohol, bicarbonate of soda, soap and water, or a paste of baking soda applied as a compress; apply ice packs to localize poison and limit pain and edema; watch for anaphylactic reaction; if multiple stings, treat for shock; keep flat and warm and transport to emergency room immediately; advise individuals with hypersensitivity reactions to see allergist
Snake bites Coral	Presence of bite without fang marks; severe, burning pain; stupor and collapse; nausea and vomiting; incontinence; shortness of breath and dyspnea; signs of shock and vascular collapse; respiratory arrest; symptoms develop rapidly	Immobilize the part, keeping lower than the rest of body; keep individual flat and quiet; reassure to allay anxiety; loosen restrictive clothing; apply tourniquet lightly several inches above the bitten extremity to impede circulation of venom; do not occlude arterial pulse; release for 2 min out of every 10 min; apply ice or cold pack, if possible, to limit circulation of venom, pain, and edema; transport to nearest aid station for antivenin, tetanus toxoid, and other treatment as soon as possible; if transport is delayed for 30–60 min, incise skin ⅛ to ¼ in deep through fang marks; suck wound by mouth or suction cup for 1 h (do not swallow venom or suck wound if rescuer has open wounds in mouth); cleanse and bandage wound; monitor vital signs; treat for shock if present
Pit vipers (rattlesnakes, copperheads, and water moccasins)	Presence of bite with one or more puncture marks; intense, localized pain radiating eventually; edema and erythema; weakness, tingling, and numbness of extremities or around the mouth; feeling of suffocation with dyspnea; nausea and vomiting; generalized urticaria; usually occurs about an hour after the bite; diaphoresis; diarrhea with melena; signs of shock and vascular collapse	See above.

(continued)

Table 13–4 Bites and Stings: Symptomatology and Nursing Prescriptions (continued)

Type of Bite or Sting	Symptomatology	Nursing Prescriptions
Spider bites		
Black widow	Local erythema; small, red puncture wounds; localized pain; severe cramping and pain in muscles; rigidity of the abdomen; begins within 60 min, usually subsides after 48 h; dyspnea; diaphoresis; nausea and vomiting; paresthesias; increased temperature; tachycardia; constipation; urinary retention; convulsions; respiratory arrest	Keep victim quiet; apply ice to site to limit venom absorption; apply alcohol or hydrogen peroxide to site to prevent infection; transport to medical facility for medical attention; antivenin *(Latrodectus mactans),* muscle relaxants, antibiotics, antihistamines, steroids, and tetanus immunization may be ordered; monitor vital signs; administer oxygen when available if respiratory distress occurs
Brown recluse	Local reactions within 2–8 h; pain; edema; formation of blisters; ulceration and bleeding at site; occurs 7–10 days after bite; rash; nausea and vomiting; fever and chills; weakness and malaise; joint pain; petechiae; healing of site begins in about 3 wk and may take 6–8 wk	See above.

SOURCE: Saxton D et al: *Addison–Wesley Manual of Nursing Practice.* Menlo Park, CA: Addison–Wesley, 1983, pp. 1052–1053.

and soreness of the injection site are common side effects. A warm, moist compress may help relieve the discomfort. If the client is in pain or very anxious, analgesics or sedatives may be given. Because burns are frightening, devastating, and painful injuries, do not overlook the client's needs for emotional support.

Heat Exhaustion and Heat Stroke

Heat exhaustion and heat stroke are most common during hot weather. A comparison of heat exhaustion and heat stroke and nursing and medical management appear in Table 13–5.

Hypothermia

Hypothermia is a sudden decrease in body temperature that results when the body is exposed to cold, and heat is lost through the skin (especially of the head and chest) and lungs. Body heat loss causes constriction of peripheral blood vessels as the body tries to conserve heat.

Persons most susceptible to hypothermia are those who participate in winter sports, especially hiking, cross-country skiing, and climbing; persons lost in isolated areas; the elderly, who may be unable to pay their heating bills or who may keep their environmental temperature extremely low to reduce costs; alcoholics (alcohol causes vasodilation and thus increases susceptibility to cold); and "street people" who lack adequate clothing and shelter. Elderly persons have decreased physiological resistance to temperature extremes. Extremely cold temperatures accompanied by wind can increase the risk of hypothermia during normal outdoor activities such as construction work, jogging, or snow shoveling.

In cold weather, the body's heat requirements increase. If the individual is not adequately protected by clothing and shelter, hypothermia may result. An increase in caloric intake or activity during very cold weather helps counteract susceptibility to hypothermia. Symptoms of hypothermia include:

- Severe shivering
- Decrease in body temperature
- Drowsiness
- Lack of muscle coordination
- Difficulty speaking
- Disorientation
- Coma (when body temperature reaches 20°C (84°F)

Emergency management of the hypothermic client focuses on warming the body by covering with blankets (wet clothing should first be removed), giving warm liquids to drink (or warmed IV fluids), and using a hypothermia blanket set on "warm." The client's body temperature and vital signs should be monitored frequently until body temperature returns to normal.

Frostbite

Frostbite is a more localized body response to extremely cold temperatures. Frostbite causes vasoconstriction and thrombosis of the affected part; without treatment, tissue necrosis occurs, and surgical amputation may be necessary. The clinical manifestations, therapeutic measures, and specific nursing measures related to frostbite are discussed in Chapter 79. In general, priority nursing management includes slowly rewarming the affected part. Rapid rewarming and massage are contraindicated because they may further damage tissue and increase pain.

Table 13–5	**Comparison of Heat Exhaustion and Heat Stroke**	
	Heat Exhaustion	**Heat Stroke**
Pathophysiology	Dehydration and salt depletion result from prolonged or severe sweating (as much as 3–4 L of perspiration and 60–200 mEq of Na^+ can be lost in 1 h); accumulation of blood in peripheral circulation (due to decreased blood volume) causes circulatory insufficiency and decreased cerebral perfusion.	Especially likely when environmental temperature and humidity are high; thermal regulatory mechanisms of body fail; decreased perspiration and increased body temperature (above 40.6°C (105°F) lead to increased oxygen and cardiac demands; high temperature can cause pulmonary edema, tubular necrosis of kidney, convulsions, and heart failure.
Commonly affected persons	Individuals engaged in strenuous exercise; women; elderly; obese persons; alcoholic individuals; clients with circulatory impairments	Men; elderly persons; obese persons; alcoholic individuals; individuals taking medications that affect thermal regulation (thyroid extracts, antihistamines, phenothiazines, anticholinergics)
Symptoms*	Fatigue, dizziness, syncope; pale, damp, diaphoretic skin; headache; anorexia, nausea, vomiting; muscle cramps; weak, rapid pulse; normal or subnormal temperature; possible dilatation of the pupils	Weakness, dizziness, nausea; headache; visual disturbances; mental confusion, irrational behavior, feeling of euphoria or impending doom, diminished level of consciousness, loss of consciousness that may be abrupt; hot, flushed, dry skin (ashen, gray color may indicate impending cardiovascular collapse); rectal temperature above 40.6°C (105°F); cessation of diaphoresis; strong, rapid pulse progressing to weak, rapid pulse; slow, deep respirations; muscle cramps; convulsions (may occur early or late); signs of shock

Management*	1. Place the afflicted individual in a recumbent position in a cool, shaded environment; loosen all tight clothing; avoid exposure to heat.
	2. Encourage the liberal intake of cool fluids.
	3. Replace lost sodium (1 tsp of table salt diluted in 200 mL water).
	4. Monitor vital signs.
	5. Elevate the legs and lightly rub the muscles to help relieve cramps.
	6. Refer to a primary health care provider or transport to a medical facility for medical follow-up; serum levels of sodium and chloride and urine specific gravity may be determined.
	7. Stress the importance of avoiding excessive physical activity and the need for adequate intake of fluids and salt in warm environments to prevent future episodes of heat exhaustion; salt tablets prevent heat exhaustion but are too slow acting to be useful in any heat-related emergency.
		1. Place the afflicted individual in a cool, shaded environment; remove as much clothing as possible.
		2. Reduce the body temperature to 39°C (102°F) as rapidly as possible; avoid a rapid reduction of temperature to below 39°C, because this will induce shivering, which raises body temperature and increases the cardiac workload.
		  a. Sponge the body with tepid water.
		  b. Place the individual in a tub of cool water.
		  c. Place ice packs on the head, axillae, and groin.
		  d. Allow a fan to blow across the body to increase evaporation.
		  e. Chilled saline enemas or a hypothermia blanket may be administered at a medical facility.
		3. Monitor vital signs and the level of consciousness.
		4. Ensure an adequate airway; administer oxygen if available.
		5. Encourage the intake of cool fluids and a salt solution (1 tsp per 200 mL of water) if conscious.
		6. Protect the individual from injury during convulsions; note the type and duration of convulsions.
		7. Monitor intake and output; save urine for urinalysis.

(continued)

Table 13–5 Comparison of Heat Exhaustion and Heat Stroke (continued)	
Heat Exhaustion	**Heat Stroke**
	8. Transport the individual immediately to a medical facility for temperature stabilization and prevention or treatment of complications.
	9. Advise the individual to avoid immediate reexposure to heat because hypersensitivity may be lifelong, necessitating a move to a cooler climate.

*Symptoms and management adapted from Saxton D et al.: *The Addison–Wesley Manual of Nursing Practice.* Menlo Park, CA: Addison–Wesley, 1983, pp. 1048–1049.

POISONINGS

Numerous substances are accidentally or intentionally ingested or inhaled by adults each year. Poisonous substances are present in many household and gardening products and in the general environment (eg, auto exhaust and by-products of manufacturing). Therapeutic and illegal (street) drugs as well as alcohol may also be ingested in toxic amounts. (Emergency care for drug or alcohol overdose is given in Chapter 10.)

Glue sniffing or inhalation of toxic substances such as carbon monoxide, oxide of nitrogen, or lead fumes from auto exhaust may result in death or permanent neurologic or pulmonary impairment. Other substances cause injury by direct contact with the skin. Benzene poisoning may cause serious or fatal blood dyscrasias, and carbon tetrachloride can severely damage liver tissue. Other caustic substances, such as lye or acids, may cause moderate or extensive burns of the skin and mucosa.

Prompt recognition and management of poisoning are essential to prevent death or permanent disability. Depending on the substance ingested or inhaled, manifestations may include:

- Abrupt onset of nausea and vomiting; abdominal pain; diarrhea
- Dizziness; headache
- Thirst; fever
- Salivation; lacrimation
- Tinnitus
- Visual disturbances; dilated or constricted pupils
- Fear and anxiety
- Confusion; disorientation; stupor
- Agitation, tremors, twitching; convulsions
- Myalgia
- Hemorrhage; purpura, hematemesis, hemoptysis
- Alterations in skin color; pallor, cyanosis, pink or cherry-red skin
- Reddened, irritated, inflamed, edematous skin; burns around the mouth; burning pain
- Irregular or altered respirations
- Odor of ingested material on the breath (eg, alcohol or petroleum products)
- Kussmaul's respirations
- Diaphoresis
- Circulatory collapse
- Paralysis
- Delirium and coma (Saxton et al., 1983)

Emergency nursing management is concerned with identifying the substance and eliminating it from the body or neutralizing its effects. The first action should be to identify the poisonous substance and the amount ingested, either from the container or physical evidence such as burns about the mouth or breath odor. Any vomitus or urine should be saved and brought to the hospital for laboratory analysis.

Once the poison has been identified, the priority is to eliminate the poison from the body, usually by inducing vomiting or using gastric lavage, or to neutralize its effects. The local poison control center should be called immediately for advice concerning the best action. The victim should be kept calm to decrease the rate of absorption. Generally, vomiting should be induced to rid the body of the substance by stimulating the gag reflex or administering syrup of ipecac (30 mL followed by 3 to 4 glasses of water). *Do not induce vomiting if the victim is comatose or convulsing or the poison is a corrosive or caustic substance or a petroleum distillate,* such as turpentine, gasoline, or kerosene. If vomiting if contraindicated and the victim is conscious, an appropriate antidote should be administered.

If the poison is an inhalant, the victim should be removed from its source as quickly as possible and placed in a well-ventilated environment. Artificial respiration should be administered if breathing has stopped. Cardiopulmonary resuscitation should be administered if the victim is breathless and pulseless. The victim should be transported to the nearest appropriate emergency facility as soon as possible. Emergency management of poisonous ingestion or inhalation may also require laboratory tests and correction of fluid and electrolyte imbalances.

Topical poisons should be neutralized by flushing the

skin with liberal amounts of water. Toxic oils can be removed by washing the skin with warm soapy water. Clothing should be removed to prevent further contact with the poisonous substance, and the victim should be taken to an emergency facility for appropriate treatment.

Food poisoning may occur following ingestion of contaminated foods. Causes of food poisoning include bacterial toxins (eg, *Clostridium botulinum*, *Salmonella*, *Staphylococcus*); chemical agents from acid foods stored in containers lined with antimony, cadmium, lead, or zinc; and from unwashed foods sprayed with insecticides. Food poisoning from bacterial toxins is discussed in Chapter 11.

TRAUMATIC EMERGENCIES

Traumatic injuries result from direct impact to the body by a stationary or moving object, such as a steering wheel, pavement, a bullet, or a knife. Traumatic injuries may affect a single body part, as in an eye injury or soft tissue lac-eration of a limb, or may involve several body parts (multiple trauma).

Trauma may be categorized as blunt, penetrating, contrecoup, or crushing. *Blunt trauma* occurs when a blunt object forcibly hits the body, such as a steering wheel, fist, or the ground in a fall. *Penetrating injuries* involve actual penetration of the body by a foreign object, such as a knife or bullet. When the velocity of impact against a blunt object causes internal organs to bounce forcefully against the internal body wall or bony structures surrounding the organs, a *contrecoup injury* results. Severe head and chest injuries often involve this "shifting" type of trauma. *Crushing trauma* results when body parts are literally crushed or smashed. This type of injury may occur in falls from high places or motor vehicle accidents where the force of impact collapses or crushes body structures. Accidents involving equipment such as farm tractors or industrial machinery often cause crushing injuries. Traumatic injuries are discussed in the specific disorders chapters in each body systems unit.

Chapter Highlights

The professional nurse has a responsibility to educate the public about preventive measures to lessen the incidence of trauma.

The regionalization of trauma services and the development of the Emergency Medical Services System (EMSS) have improved the quality of emergency health care services and decreased the incidence of death and disability from trauma and sudden, life-threatening illness.

Nursing care of emergency clients should conform with the Standards of Emergency Nursing Practice developed by the Emergency Department Nurses' Association.

The emergency nurse must be able to communicate and collaborate effectively with all members of the emergency team.

The three priorities for managing the emergency client are: A—airway, B—breathing, and C—circulation.

The emergency client must cope with numerous multisystem stressors, including shock, metabolic imbalance, neurologic insult, and psychological stress. The emergency nurse has a responsibility to intervene with emergency clients to assist them in coping with these stressors.

The emergency nurse should be familiar with specific pharmacologic and nutritional measures to promote stabilization and ultimate recovery of the emergency client and should be able to implement these measures rapidly.

Trauma or life-threatening illness precipitates a psychological crisis for victims and their loved ones. The emergency nurse has a major responsibility to implement nursing measures to help clients and their loved ones cope with the psychological impact of trauma or life-threatening illness.

The emergency nurse must be knowledgeable about the recognition and emergency management of victims with specific life-threatening illnesses or injuries.

Bibliography

American College of Emergency Physicians: Emergency care guidelines (position paper). *Ann Emerg Med* 1982; 11:222–226.

American Heart Association: *Cardiopulmonary Resuscitation*. New York: American Heart Association, 1978.

Boyd DR: Comprehensive regional trauma and emergency medical services delivery systems: A goal of the 1980s. *CCQ* (Dec) 1982; 5:1–21.

Brown AJ: Your "heat of the moment" guide to emergency drugs. *RN* (June) 1982; 9:27–31.

Byrne CJ et al: *Laboratory Tests: Implications for Nursing Care,* 2nd ed. Menlo Park, CA: Addison–Wesley, 1986.

Emergency Department Nurses' Association. *Standards of Emergency Nursing Practice.* St. Louis: Mosby, 1983.

Fanslow J: Needs of grieving spouses in sudden death situations: A pilot study. *JEN* (July–Aug) 1983; 9:213–216.

Hui YH: *Human Nutrition and Diet Therapy.* Monterey, CA: Wadsworth, 1983.

Joint Commission on Accreditation of Hospitals. *Accreditation Manual for Hospitals.* Chicago: JCAH, 1983.

Jones WH, Buttery M: Sudden death: Survivors' perceptions of the emergency department experience. *JEN* (Jan–Feb) 1981; 7:14–17.

Rodman MJ, Smith DW: *Clinical Pharmacology in Nursing,* 2nd ed. Philadelphia: Lippincott, 1984.

Saxton D et al: *Addison–Wesley Manual of Nursing Practice.* Menlo Park, CA: Addison–Wesley, 1983.

Sheldon GF, Harper HA, Way LW: Surgical metabolism and nutrition. In: *Current Surgical Diagnosis and Treatment,* 6th ed. Way LW (editor). Los Altos, CA: Lange, 1985.

Trunkey DD: Trauma. *Sci Am* (Aug) 1983; 249:28–35.

Yoder L, Jones SL: The family of the emergency room patient as seen through the eyes of the nurse. *Int J Nurs Studies* 1982; 19:29–36.

Suggested Readings

Braulin JLD, Rook J, Sills GM: Families in crisis: The impact of trauma. *CCQ* (Dec) 1982; 5:38–46. A review of the family's response to traumatic injury with a case presentation to illustrate the use of a crisis intervention model in trauma.

Cardona VD: Trauma postop: The real nursing challenge. *RN* (March) 1982; 9:23–27. A discussion of immediate postoperative nursing care of the multiple trauma victim. Includes a body systems assessment checklist.

Holloway N: *Nursing the Critically Ill Adult: Applying Nursing Diagnosis.* Menlo Park, CA: Addison–Wesley, 1984. This is an excellent comprehensive nursing reference of the problems and complications of the critically ill patient. The author logically organizes the material with a nursing diagnosis framework, stressing appropriate nursing interventions.

Jones WH, Buttery M: Sudden death: Survivors' perceptions of the emergency department experience. *JEN* (Jan–Feb) 1981; 7:14–17. Discussion of the findings of a study of immediate survivors of victims of unexpected death. Recommendations for nursing interventions are included.

Pisarcik G: On compassion. (Editorial). *JEN* (Nov–Dec) 1981; 7:237–239. The dehumanization of clients in emergency departments is discussed. A plea is made for more compassion for ill or injured clients and their families in emergency settings.

Zwicke DL, Bobzien WF, Wagner EH: Triage nurse decisions: A prospective study. *JEN* (May–June) 1982; 8:132–138. An evaluation of the appropriateness of triage decisions made by the emergency nurse compared with the emergency department attending physician or resident. The authors conclude that an experienced emergency nurse can function in a safe, efficient, and cost-effective manner as a triage officer.

Resources

SELF-HELP GROUPS AND OTHER ORGANIZATIONS

American Red Cross
National Headquarters
17th and D St., NW
Washington, DC 20006
Phone: (202) 737-8300

> Provides assistance in disasters and offers classes in safety, first aid, and cardiopulmonary resuscitation. Contact the local unit.

American Trauma Society
857 N. Michigan Ave.
Chicago, IL 60611
Phone: (312) 649-1810

> The society's mission is to reduce needless death and disability by increasing public and professional support for improved systems of prehospital and inhospital emergency and trauma care. It also promotes research and educational programs related to trauma, with emphasis on prevention of injury and death. *Trauma Center Newsletter* and *Traumagram Newsletter* are published by the Society.

Medic-Alert Foundation International
1000 N. Palm
Turlock, CA 95380
Phone: (209) 632-2371

> For a $15 lifetime membership, this organization will provide a bracelet or necklace with medallion stating the wearer's medical problem, a wallet-sized card with personal information about allergies and medicines being taken, a computer information file containing the wearer's complete medical history, and a 24-hour answering service with operators available to relay the medical history to emergency personnel (the phone number is engraved on the medallion). The computer file can be updated for $4. This organization has over 700,000 members in the United States and Canada; the emblem is registered in over 40 other countries.

Mothers Against Drunk Driving (MADD)
5330 Primrose, Suite 146
Fair Oaks, CA 95628
Phone: (916) 966-6233

> A relatively new organization that acts as a voice for victims of drunk driving accidents and their families. The group is active in supporting highway patrol programs and lobbying for state and federal legislation for reform of drunk driving laws. MADD also provides counseling services for victims and families and publishes brochures and a newsletter aimed at widespread public education.

National Clearinghouse for Poison Control Centers
US Department of Health and Human Services
Public Health Service
5401 Westbard Ave.
Bethesda, MD 20016

> Provides a list of Poison Control Centers in the United States. Publishes a news bulletin and distributes poison information cards (Poison Control Cards).

National Drivers Association for the
Prevention of Traffic Accidents
PO Box 604
Bakersfield, CA 93302

This association conducts educational programs, including dissemination of information to government officials, and publishes monographs dealing with causes of traffic accidents. The group is active in recommending proposals to prevent and reduce the incidence of traffic accidents.

National Institute for Occupational Safety
and Health (NIOSH)
Centers for Disease Control
Robert A. Taft Laboratory
4676 Columbia Pkwy.
Cincinnati, OH 45226
Phone: (513) 684-8326

This arm of the Centers for Disease Control serves as a clearinghouse for information and research on occupational safety and health.

National Safety Council
425 N. Michigan Ave.
Chicago, IL 60611
Phone: (312) 527-4800

This organization gathers and distributes information to the public and to professionals concerning the causes of accidental death and disability with a focus on methods of prevention. The goal is to reduce the number and severity of all types of accidents and occupational illnesses.

Occupational Safety and Health Administration (OSHA)
Office of Public and Consumer Affairs
US Department of Labor (Room N3637)
200 Constitution Ave., NW
Washington, DC 20210
Phone: (202) 523-8151

This federal agency is responsible for overseeing and enforcing safety practices and regulations in occupational and industrial work settings.

HOT LINES

Poisoning Information Hotline
Phone: (412) 681-6669 (24 hours)

Provides information to aid victims of accidental poisoning, supplies the address of the nearest poison treatment center, and calls the center while the victim is en route to ensure prompt attention. Sponsored by the National Poison Center Network at Pittsburgh Children's Hospital.

HEALTH EDUCATION MATERIAL

From: Poisondex
Washington, DC 20201

A computer retrieval service that outlines the management of poisonous ingestions (available on computer printout or microfiche).

NURSING ORGANIZATION

Emergency Department Nurses' Association (EDNA)
666 N. Lake Shore Dr.
Chicago, IL 60611
Phone: (312) 649-0297

This professional association for nurses who work in emergency nursing or are interested in the field is concerned with establishing standards for optimum emergency care. Provides public education and continuing education in emergency nursing and conducts a certification program. Also publishes the *Journal of Emergency Nursing*.

Chapter 14

Surgery

Patricia Brown
Carol Ren Kneisl
Thomas E. Obst

Objectives

When you have finished studying this chapter, you should be able to:

Discuss the roles and responsibilities of the members of the surgical team.

Anticipate the physiological and psychosocial factors that influence surgical risk.

Describe the wound-healing process, the factors that influence it, and nursing interventions that foster it.

Formulate nursing interventions aimed at decreasing surgical risk.

Integrate legal aspects, ethical codes, advocacy, and clients' rights into the care of surgical clients.

Apply the nursing process throughout perioperative care.

Identify the components of a comprehensive plan for preoperative care that includes physiological and psychosocial preparation of the client for surgery.

Discuss the role of the nurse in maintaining the client's safety during surgery and recovery from anesthesia.

Discuss nursing responsibilities in preventing postoperative complications.

Formulate a comprehensive plan for the postoperative recovery and discharge of the surgical client.

The art and science of surgery have been practiced since antiquity. Early practitioners were primarily concerned with repair of wounds caused by trauma. They also attempted to control the spread of infection by means such as amputation, even though the mechanism of infection was not understood. Modern techniques of anesthesia, asepsis, and control of hemorrhage have enabled surgical teams to perform virtual miracles, as sophisticated procedures such as organ transplants and open heart surgery have gradually become commonplace. The early unsterile, crudely equipped operating "theater" has evolved into the technology-dominated operating suite of today in which nurses play major roles.

Although most surgery continues to be performed in hospital operating rooms, this is changing. Ambulatory or outpatient surgery (sometimes called same-day surgery) is becoming increasingly prevalent. The client may enter an outpatient facility, undergo surgery, and return home the same day. The cost of hospitalization and the stresses associated with it are thus reduced. An estimated 20–40% of surgical procedures performed annually in the US could be safely performed in an outpatient setting. The trend toward outpatient surgery affects the role of the nurse, especially in educating clients about postoperative self-care.

As techniques advance and as circumstances surrounding surgery change, the nursing knowledge base continues to expand. Cryosurgery, laser surgery, the use of intraoperative hypothermia, and the introduction of client-controlled analgesia are among the innovations that challenge the nurse who provides perioperative care, whether in the operating room, the intensive care unit, or the client's home.

This chapter discusses the nursing process as it relates to perioperative care in general. Nursing care for specific surgical procedures is discussed in the units about specific body systems.

Section I: General Principles of Surgical Treatment

Although surgical procedures vary greatly, both in technique and in the demands they impose on the body, certain fundamental principles are common to all. With a comprehensive understanding of these principles and an empathic attitude, the nurse can assist the client and family in coping with the physiological and psychosocial stresses of surgery to promote an optimum recovery.

CLASSIFICATION OF SURGICAL PROCEDURES

Surgical procedures may be classified in several ways, according to the purpose, the extent of trauma, or whether the procedure is elective or an emergency (Table 14–1). *Diagnostic* and *exploratory* procedures determine the origin of a client's symptoms or the extent of a lesion or disease. *Curative* surgery attempts to remove a lesion or to reconstruct or replace diseased, defective, or injured tissues or organs. *Palliative* procedures are used to alleviate symptoms. Any of these types of surgery may be classed as *major* or *minor* according to their traumatic effect. Most surgical procedures are *elective* in the sense that competent clients of legal age determine whether to undergo them; the exception is an *emergency* in which an imminent threat to life or limb exists.

Knowledge of the type of surgery a client is to undergo as well as the rationale for the procedure are prerequisites for planning nursing care. The client's motivation affects recovery and so does emotional status. For example, a client scheduled for diagnostic or exploratory surgery may be intensely apprehensive about the findings, especially if a diagnosis of malignancy is involved. The client undergoing palliative surgery may feel an overwhelming sense of hopelessness. Conversely, the client anticipating cosmetic surgery may feel joyful expectation of an improved appearance. By knowing the individual client's situation, the nurse can be prepared to offer appropriate psychosocial as well as physical support.

SURGERY AS A MULTISYSTEM STRESSOR

Surgery imposes stress on all body systems. It imposes psychological stresses as well, both on the client and on significant others. Physiological stresses accompanying surgery are related not only to the surgical wound but to the effects of anesthesia and other adjunctive measures and to immobility, which has profound effects on homeostasis. These stresses are superimposed on those related to any existing disease.

The nurse's responsibility includes recognition of these stresses, accurate assessment of their extent, and anticipation and prevention of their consequences to the extent possible. By keeping the client informed of what to expect, reinforcing the physician's explanations in understandable terms, and frankly addressing spoken and unspoken concerns about pain and disability, the nurse can make a major contribution to the client's effort to recover. The specific effects of surgery and anesthesia are discussed later in this chapter. The present discussion is concerned with generalized responses.

Physiological Stresses

In response to the surgical invasion, the body mobilizes defenses to maintain homeostasis. Most of these mechanisms, which are summarized in Table 14–2, are generally favorable to survival and healing; if uncontrolled or prolonged, however, they may promote the development of complications. Systemic responses to stress are explained in Chapter 2, and strategies for coping with them are explained in Chapter 4. In addition to systemic responses, local stress reactions also occur in response to tissue injury.

Table 14–1	Classification of Surgical Procedures
Classification	**Purpose or Definition**
Purpose	
Diagnostic	To determine etiology of client's disorder
Exploratory	To determine a diagnosis and/or to evaluate the extent of a lesion
Curative	
Ablative	To remove diseased tissue or organ(s)
Constructive	To build tissues and/or organs that are absent, anomalous, or have been destroyed or altered by trauma or disease
Reconstructive	To repair or replace tissues or organs (see above)
Palliative	To alleviate symptoms of disease without necessarily altering the disease process
Extent of Trauma	
Major	Imposes extensive trauma and/or is associated with serious risk
Minor	Imposes minimal trauma and is associated with minimal risk
Urgency	
Elective	Recommended, but delay imposes no additional risk on the client
Emergency	Immediately necessary for preservation of life

Table 14–2 Consequences of Selected Systemic Responses to Surgical Stress

Specific Systemic Responses	Protective Consequences	Negative Consequences
Increase in blood coagulation; peripheral vasoconstriction	Prevention of excessive blood and fluid loss	May increase tendency for postoperative thrombus formation
Increase in the rate and force of the heartbeat, which increases cardiac output and blood pressure; dilatation of coronary arteries	Maintenance of cardiac perfusion and oxygenation when the work load of the heart is increased	Prolonged or repeated effect can promote hypertension and increase work load of the heart, resulting in failure
Increased reabsorption of Na$^+$ from the kidney, causing retention of Na$^+$ and water	Maintenance of blood volume, blood pressure, and cardiac output	
Decreased GI peristalsis; increased gastric acidity	Other body functions favored	Paralytic ileus, constipation, stress ulcer
Smooth muscle relaxation promotes dilatation of bronchioles	Improvement of gas exchange and tissue oxygenation	
Increased protein breakdown	Availability of amino acids for tissue repair	If prolonged and uncontrolled, promotes negative nitrogen balance and catabolic effect
Connective tissue proliferation	Promotion of wound healing	
Over a long period, anti-inflammatory effect occurs, with shrinkage of lymphoid tissue		Decreases ability to fight infection
Increase in circulating glucose and mobilization of fat from reserve stores	Provision of needed energy	Chronic increase in glucose and fat stores can promote development of diabetes and atherosclerosis
Increase in basal metabolic rate	Provision of needed energy and tissue nourishment	Sweating in response can be uncomfortable and render the client susceptible to fluid imbalance and decubitus ulcers

These localized effects promote wound healing, which is discussed later in this chapter.

Inactivity related to the surgery also takes its toll on the individual. Although rest aids healing, it may also have detrimental effects on body systems. Hazards associated with immobility are discussed later in this chapter with postoperative care (see also Unit Ten).

Psychosocial Stresses

Although physiological and psychosocial stresses are discussed separately, they are inseparable. The holistic view of health care recognizes that mind and body are inseparable and that mental and emotional states such as fear, anxiety, and uncertainty affect physical as well as psychological recovery. By minimizing negative responses and encouraging positive ones, the nurse can assist the client in summoning inherent coping strengths. Coping with the experience of illness is discussed in Chapter 6.

ASEPSIS AND THE CARE OF THE SURGICAL CLIENT

Scrupulous adherence to the principles of infection control is especially important in caring for the surgical client.

Once the protective barrier of the integument has been breached, the individual becomes highly susceptible to invasion by pathogenic organisms that may cause local or systemic infections. Moreover, the many invasive procedures associated with surgery create ideal conditions for nosocomial infection. Endotracheal tubes, suctioning apparatus, urinary and drainage catheters, and instruments used for blood sampling and intravenous administrations may serve as reservoirs for infectious organisms or as agents of transmission.

Nurses have a major responsibility in preventing infections in surgical clients. The principles of asepsis, which are emphasized throughout this chapter, should be conscientiously followed. The general infection control recommendations of the Centers for Disease Control, which are discussed in Chapter 11, should be understood and followed. Specific guidelines for preventing surgical wound infections are reviewed later in this chapter.

WOUND HEALING

A consequence of surgical manipulation and incision is a localized stress response—the inflammatory process—which contains the tissue injury and promotes wound healing. This process, which is essentially an aggressive response to injury, is discussed in Chapter 2.

The wound-healing process, an outcome of the inflammatory process, involves three phases of repair:

- The proliferation of epithelial cells to provide a surface covering for incised tissue
- The formation of pinkish-red granulation tissue, an outgrowth of new tissue and capillaries, to draw wound edges together
- The synthesis of collagen, which facilitates connective tissue repair and draws wound edges together (scar tissue formation)

Barring complications, the time for normal wound healing depends on a number of factors:

- The extent of tissue damage from the surgery
- The amount of stress and tension placed at the incision
- The extent to which wound edges have been approximated
- The client's overall health status

Wound healing generally takes place within 7 to 10 days, although scar tissue contraction continues for some time. More extensive wounds, those prone to tension and stress, those left open to facilitate drainage, and those on a client who is malnourished, take longer to heal. Eventually, scar tissue shrinks, but occasionally keloids form. Keloidal tissue is an excessive overgrowth of scar tissue to which dark-skinned persons appear especially susceptible. Keloids can be disfiguring, and although they can be surgically removed, they frequently grow back (see Unit Thirteen).

Surgical wounds approximated and closed with clips, staples, sutures, or skin strips heal by **primary intention,** with minimal formation of granulation tissue or scar tissue and minimal loss of function in the affected area. With an infected incision or one that is purposely left open, healing involves greater formation of granulation tissue and contraction from scar tissue **(secondary intention).** Healing by **tertiary intention** involves debridement of large infected or contaminated wounds followed by mechanical skin closure.

A number of factors adversely affect wound healing. Advanced age and nutritional deficiencies are associated with poor healing. Infection also complicates the process, inhibiting tissue repair and perhaps promoting systemic infection or abscess formation. High fever; purulent drainage; and excessive erythema, edema, and tenderness at the incision site may indicate infection. Excessive strain on the incision, from overactivity, for example, can delay union of wound edges. The obese client may have special difficulties with wound healing because adipose tissue has a poor blood supply. The obese client is also prone to dehiscence or evisceration. **Dehiscence** is disruption of the superficial layers of the surgical wound. **Evisceration** is the complete disruption of the wound, with protrusion of the viscera. Often, early signs of these conditions can be detected and measures taken to prevent them. Dehiscence and evisceration are discussed in the section on the later postoperative period.

Section II: The Scope of Perioperative Nursing Care

During the early days of surgery, the nurse's role was primarily that of assistant to the surgeon. Nursing responsibilities included maintaining asepsis and passing instruments; nurses had little direct responsibility for the client, and there was little continuity of preoperative and postoperative care. Today the model of care is perioperative nursing, which encompasses care of the client before surgery (preoperative care), during surgery (intraoperative care), and after surgery (postoperative care). The safety and welfare of the client is the nurse's primary concern during all phases of the perioperative period. The Association of Operating Room Nurses (AORN), the professional association for registered nurses in operating room nursing, promotes quality care for the surgical client (see resources list at the end of this chapter).

Although health care facilities vary, the surgical client is generally cared for by four types of nurses: staff nurses, operating room nurses, nurse anesthetists, and recovery room nurses. All share responsibility for the client's well-being throughout the perioperative period, but each has a different focus. *Staff nurses* are responsible for preoperative and postoperative care on the surgical unit, although their responsibility overlaps into the intraoperative period.

The staff nurse generally is responsible for a number of surgical clients. Staff nurses need a sound knowledge of medical-surgical nursing. *Operating room nurses* care for the client primarily during the intraoperative period. Recently, however, the role of operating room nurses has expanded to include preoperative visits to prepare clients for the surgical experience as well as counseling during the postoperative phase. *Nurse anesthetists* (or physician anesthesiologists) develop a plan of anesthesia for the client during the preoperative period, administer the anesthesia during surgery, and evaluate the client's postanesthesia progress. The nurse anesthetist has responsibilities for client care throughout the perioperative period.

Postanesthesia recovery room nurses care for the client during the immediate postoperative period, carefully monitoring the client's recovery from anesthesia. Usually, their responsibility for the client is eventually passed back to the staff nurse on the surgical unit. Some clients who require specialized care are taken to the intensive care unit and do not return to the general surgical unit until later, sometimes by way of an intermediate care facility. Recovery room nurses have also become involved with preoperative consultation and postoperative follow-up.

Nurses who work primarily in the operating room or recovery area require specialized preparation, which may be acquired through inservice education programs or continuing education courses offered through educational institutions and professional organizations. Advanced preparation for surgical nurse practitioners and nurse anesthetists is moving into degree-granting programs at the master's level (Metz, 1984).

Throughout the surgical experience, the client's care should be based on the nursing process, employing the principles of assessment, diagnosis, planning, implementation, and evaluation as appropriate to the client and the procedure. In addition to the basic Standards of Nursing Practice formulated by the American Nurses' Association (ANA), specialized standards pertaining to clients undergoing surgery have been developed. ANA has developed Standards of Medical–Surgical Nursing Practice, and ANA and AORN have jointly issued Standards of Perioperative Nursing Practice. AORN also publishes other recommended practices for operating room nursing and aseptic practice. The American Association of Nurse Anesthetists (AANA) has developed standards of practice for the nurse anesthetist. (See Nursing Organizations in the resource list.)

Section III: The Nursing Process in Preoperative Care

The preoperative phase of the perioperative period begins when surgery is first considered and ends with the admission of the client to the operating suite. This phase may be long or short, depending on whether surgery is planned or is an emergency. Whatever the time frame, the client's needs must be met.

NURSING ASSESSMENT

Before surgery, the nurse participates in assessing the surgical risk, informed consent, and the client's readiness for surgery. These assessments contribute to the formulation of an individualized nursing diagnosis and to preoperative planning, implementation, and evaluation. This section discusses the general nursing role in preoperative care. The role of the nurse anesthetist is discussed in the section on physical examination.

Surgical Risk

As part of the surgical team, the nurse is involved in determining the client's risk, or potential for complications, associated with the proposed surgery. Assessing risk is important for a number of reasons:

- The client has a legal right to be apprised of all risks before consenting to surgery.
- Identified risks alert health team members to possible complications so they may be considered in planning future care.
- Identified risks can, in some cases, be rectified.

The nurse collects data regarding surgical risk from a number of sources—the health history, the physical examination, and laboratory tests and diagnostic studies. These are discussed later.

By consulting with the surgeon, the nurse can ascertain how extensive the proposed surgery will be. The more extensive the procedure, the greater the surgical risk and the more intensive the nursing care. The nurse can also use the acquired information to clarify the surgeon's instructions to the client and to prepare for postoperative care.

Through ongoing communication with the client, the nurse can encourage expression of feelings about the operation. The client may need more than one explanation, especially if intense anxiety has impeded comprehension. The client's attitude will greatly influence coping and ultimate recovery, and understanding is likely to improve cooperation with inconvenient or uncomfortable procedures such as NPO status or bowel preparation. All nurses responsible for the client's care throughout the perioperative period should be familiar with the client's risks. Preoperative interviews by the nurse anesthetist and the operating room and recovery room nurses familiarize them with the risks.

Health History

The health history provides data about the client's general health and past experiences with surgery. For example, has the client undergone major surgery before? Were there any complications? Hemorrhage? Infection? What type of anesthesia was employed? How rapid or slow was the client's return to normal function? The anesthetist will be particularly interested in the client's prior experience with anesthesia, especially if there were any adverse effects that could influence future anesthesia. In a preoperative visit, the anesthetist will gather these data as well as data about potential intraoperative and postoperative complications (Box 14–1).

A thorough history of the client's current and recent but discontinued medication use should be obtained. If the client is taking antihypertensive or antiarrhythmic agents, have they been successful? What drugs could the client be taking that might interact with anesthetic agents? These data help the anesthetist plan for preoperative medications and the specific anesthesia best suited to the client's needs.

Physical Examination

In the preoperative physical examination, the anesthetist pays special attention to the integrity of the cardiovascular

Box 14–1 Preanesthesia History

Cardiovascular system

Angina pectoris

Exercise tolerance

Myocardial infarction

Rheumatic fever

Paroxysmal nocturnal dyspnea

Dependent edema

Palpitations, tachydysrhythmias

Claudication

Respiratory system

Exercise tolerance

Dyspnea

Orthopnea

Cough

Sputum production

Asthma, bronchitis

Pneumonia

Recent upper respiratory infection

Cigarette, tobacco use

Nervous system

Injuries

Cerebral vascular accident

Transient ischemic attacks

Areas of peripheral anesthesia, parasthesias, motor weakness

Hepatic–biliary system

Hepatitis

Alcohol use

Prior exposure to halothane

Urinary system

Nocturia

Pyuria

Polyuria

Endocrine system

Diabetes mellitus

Thyroid dysfunction

Adrenal gland dysfunction

Musculoskeletal system

Arthritis

Osteoporosis

Weakness

Coagulation

Bleeding tendency

Bruising tendency

Hereditary coagulopathies

Dentition

Loose teeth

Dentures

Damaged teeth

Caps or bridges

Mouth/neck

Range of motion of neck and jaw

Prior anesthesia experience

Allergic reactions

Adverse reactions to anesthesia among family

Jaundice

Delayed awakening

Headache after spinal anesthesia

Postanesthesia nausea and vomiting

Prolonged paralysis after muscle relaxants

Hoarseness

Muscle pain

Malignant hyperthermia

and respiratory systems. Evaluation of the upper airway is critical; if the integrity of the upper airway is compromised, special consideration and planning may be required during the intraoperative period. A problematic upper airway may inhibit the maintenance of adequate ventilation during anesthesia. Upper airway problems may be caused by limited range of motion of the neck or jaw; loose oral appli-

ances; poor dentition; or a short, stocky neck. Such anatomic problems may inhibit a proper mask fit or may make standard laryngoscopic visualization of the glottis (for placement of an endotracheal tube) difficult or impossible.

The anesthetist examines the musculoskeletal system for anatomic deformities that may interfere with respiratory or cardiac function (eg, pectus excavatum or severe scoliosis) or indicate the presence of chronic obstructive pulmonary disease (eg, barrel chest). Wheezes, rhonchi, rales, and decreased or absent breath sounds may indicate the need for more extensive respiratory evaluation or therapy. Exercise tolerance can be evaluated by asking the client to walk a short distance or climb a flight of stairs.

Other musculoskeletal deformities may limit a client's ability to assume various positions during surgery. Hip dysplasia is an example of a musculoskeletal limitation that affects positioning during surgery. Clients with this hip problem will be unable to assume the dorsal lithotomy position. For example, a woman with hip dysplasia may need to have an abdominal hysterectomy rather than a vaginal hysterectomy; a man with hip dysplasia may need to have a suprapubic prostatectomy rather than a perineal prostatectomy. Clients with severe arthritis may be unable to assume even the most routine surgical positions. This information is crucial in planning anesthesia and surgery around the client's limitations, avoiding postoperative complications and unnecessary client discomfort.

The anesthetist will assess blood pressure in both arms to gather data concerning possible peripheral vascular disease. The collateral arterial blood supply to each hand should be assessed by Allen's test (occluding the radial artery to determine the blood supply to the hand provided by the ulnar artery). If the ulnar flow fails to perfuse the hand adequately in the absence of radial flow, vascular supply to the hand may be totally blocked if the radial artery is occluded during surgery because of percutaneous puncture or cannulation.

Assessment of peripheral pulses should include auscultation for carotid bruits, which indicate impaired cerebral circulation. Any history or physical findings of carotid artery disease indicate that hyperextension of the neck may occlude cerebral blood flow. This is an important finding because the neck is often hyperextended to facilitate various aspects of airway management during endotracheal intubation or when ventilating a client under general anesthesia. These determinations should be assessed in the awake state to prevent impairing cerebral perfusion during anesthesia. Aortic stenosis (discussed in Chapter 24) is another condition that has important implications for the type of anesthesia the client receives.

In the routine preoperative physical examination, the anesthetist will also evaluate potential sites for peripheral or central venous cannulation. If a regional anesthetic is planned, the site of injection should be assessed for the presence of infection; infection at the site contraindicates the use of regional anesthesia.

Laboratory Tests and Diagnostic Studies

Laboratory tests and diagnostic studies help pinpoint possible problems with respiration, circulation, and urinary excretion, as well as other risk factors (eg, previously undiagnosed diabetes or hypertension). Until recently, the client was usually admitted to the hospital for such tests some time—even days—before surgery. The current trend is to perform most tests on an outpatient basis within a week of the scheduled operation. Research has found that the threat of infection is less with shorter preoperative hospital stays (Cruse & Foord, 1980).

Which laboratory tests and diagnostic studies from the list below are carried out depends on the findings of the history and physical examination and the nature of the surgery.

- Arterial blood gas and pH: evaluates acid–base regulation and status.
- Blood type and crossmatch: identifies client's blood type and matches donor blood in case blood replacement is required.
- Blood urea nitrogen: screens for kidney disease.
- Chest x-ray: determines lung pathology and cardiac size.
- Complete blood count including hemoglobin concentration and hematocrit value: determines presence or absence of anemia and infection.
- Electrocardiogram: determines cardiac pathology; often routine for clients over 40.
- Fasting blood sugar: screens for diabetes; evaluates clients with diabetes.
- Liver function studies such as serum glutamic-oxaloacetic transaminase (SGOT), serum glutamic-pyruvic transaminase (SGPT), and lactic dehydrogenase (LDH): screen for hepatitis or liver damage.
- Prothrombin time and/or plasma thromboplastin time: screen for possible coagulating deficiencies and hemorrhagic disorders.
- Pulmonary function studies such as forced expiratory volume, vital capacity, and maximum breathing capacity: determine lung pathology such as early chronic obstructive pulmonary disease.
- Serum electrolytes such as Ca^{++}, Cl^-, H^+, K^+, Mg^{++}, Na^+: determine the electrolyte composition of the extracellular fluid.
- Urinalysis: detects infections of the urinary system as well as the presence of glucose in the urine; see Chapter 32.

Factors Contributing to Risk

During the preoperative assessment, the client is assigned a physical status category, usually by the anesthetist. This classification, developed by the American Society of Anes-

thesiologists, attempts to correlate the client's physical status with the approximate degree of risk associated with anesthesia (Box 14–2). Although an imprecise method, this classification system alerts the surgical team to the degree of risk and has been used to correlate preoperative status with anesthesia outcomes. Among the factors that have been found to contribute to surgical morbidity and mortality are advanced age, poor nutritional status, specific disease states and/or therapies, unhealthy lifestyle, and poor outlook regarding the surgery itself.

Advanced Age

Elderly or aged clients are generally considered poorer surgical risks than younger clients. Cardiac reserve diminishes with advanced age, the heart rate slows, and the individual is less able to adapt successfully to stressful situations such as surgery. Gastrointestinal responsiveness diminishes with age, making the client susceptible to constipation or fecal impaction when surgery also predisposes the client to these problems. The malnutrition common in elderly clients lowers vitality and may interfere with healing. Renal and hepatic function become depressed with advanced age, making it difficult to predict accurately the

Box 14–2 American Society of Anesthesiologists Classification of Physical Status

Class 1: Healthy clients without organic, physiologic, biochemical, or psychiatric disturbances. Surgical intervention is for a specific, limited process or disorder.
Example: A healthy client who requires inguinal hernia repair.

Class 2: Client with mild to moderate systemic disturbance caused either by the condition requiring surgical intervention or another pathophysiologic process.
Example: Client with heart disease that slightly limits or does not limit activity or clients with diabetes mellitus, hypertension, or anemia.

Class 3: Client with severe systemic disease from any cause.
Example: Clients with severely limiting heart disease, healed myocardial infarction, moderate pulmonary insufficiency.

Class 4: Client with systemic disorders of a life-threatening nature.
Example: Clients with severe heart disease with myocardial insufficiency or persistent angina or clients with advanced pulmonary, renal, hepatic, or endocrine pathology.

Class 5: Moribund client with little chance of survival even with surgical intervention.
Example: Client with ruptured aortic aneurysm and shock; client with increasing intracranial pressure associated with cerebral trauma.

Emergency (E): Client in any category 1 to 5 who requires emergency surgery is so designated by placing "E" next to the numeric class identifier.

SOURCE: Adapted from American Society of Anesthesiologists: New classification of physical status. *Anesthesiology* 1963; 246:111.

Nursing Research Note

Faherty B, Grier M: Analgesic medication for elderly people post-surgery. *Nurs Res* 1984; 33(6):369–372.

Analgesic medication prescription and administration to elderly postoperative clients were studied. Elderly clients were compared with younger postoperative clients. The results indicate that less analgesic medication was ordered for postoperative clients aged 54 years and above. Less analgesic medication was administered to clients age 44 years and over. The results also indicate that age more than weight influenced the amount of pain medication administered.

This study demonstrates a need for more research into analgesic use in the elderly population. Nursing assessment must objectively assess the true need for pain medication.

client's response to medications and anesthetics. One or more degenerative diseases may be present, compromising homeostasis in various ways. Finally, many aged clients—particularly those who are widowed—have lost the psychosocial support system that contributes to coping with illness.

Nutritional Status

The success of surgery and the eventual recovery of the client are adversely affected by malnutrition. Malnutrition alters host resistance through depression of the immune response and predisposes the client to wound infection (see Chapter 8). Laboratory studies have demonstrated a relation between nutritional status and wound repair; deficiencies of protein, vitamins, trace elements, fatty acids, and glucose all have been identified as interfering with the healing process (Flynn & Rovee, 1982). If there is a fluid and electrolyte imbalance before surgery, the client is in serious jeopardy because fluid and electrolyte loss during surgery will compound the problem.

The obese client is at particular risk, because adipose tissue is poorly supplied with blood, is prone to infection, and does not heal well (Flynn & Rovee, 1982). Not only is physiological risk increased if the client is obese, but so is the technical difficulty of surgery and anesthesia. The surgical team may find it harder to position the client appropriately. The surgeon may have greater difficulty in identifying anatomic landmarks during the operation. The anesthetist may have problems inserting and securing peripheral or central intravenous infusion lines, identifying landmarks for regional anesthesia, and securing the airway during surgery.

Finally, surgery itself has a negative effect on nutritional status. Tissue repair and wound healing require energy in excess of that needed for homeostasis; if dietary sources of energy are insufficient, a catabolic effect will occur. Visceral protein depletion (negative nitrogen balance) can significantly increase surgical morbidity and mortality.

Underlying Disorders

Disorders that alter circulation, such as peripheral vascular disease and atherosclerosis, and those that promote peripheral vascular alteration, such as diabetes, affect tissue perfusion and can inhibit tissue repair. Preexisting anemia can develop into a life-threatening condition when exacerbated by surgical blood loss. Preexisting infections may be spread by surgery and may seriously compromise the ability of the client to fight additional trauma. Unless the purpose of surgery is to treat the infection (ie, by incision and drainage), infection generally contraindicates surgery, at least temporarily. The client with an acute or chronic respiratory disorder may be at greater risk in surgery, because the stress of anesthesia and the surgery can complicate respiratory problems. The cardiovascular system may be particularly taxed during surgery, and the increased work load may overtax the heart of the client with preexisting cardiovascular disease. The client with inadequate renal or hepatic function may be at considerable risk, because the kidneys and liver play a role in wound healing, detoxification and elimination of drugs and anesthetics, and maintenance of fluid and electrolyte balance. If a client has preexisting disorders, a specialist is usually consulted regarding the risks and benefits associated with the intended surgery. Often, measures to reduce risk before surgery are recommended.

Medications and Therapies

Certain pharmacologic agents and therapeutic regimens increase surgical risk. Examples are chemotherapeutic agents, steroids, anticoagulants, depressants, and radiation therapy. The client receiving chemotherapy, radiotherapy, or steroid treatments is at increased risk of infection and poor tissue healing. Anticoagulants increase the risk of hemorrhage. Central nervous system depressants may cause hypotension or diminished responsiveness. When possible, medications that increase surgical risk are discontinued prior to surgery, but in many cases discontinuing medication may present hazards. This issue is discussed further under planning and implementation.

Lifestyle

Unhealthy practices such as cigarette smoking or abuse of drugs or alcohol can adversely affect operative risk. The client who smokes has reduced hemoglobin levels and therefore less oxygen available for tissue repair (Flynn & Rovee, 1982). Moreover, increased platelet aggregation in smokers may predispose the client to thrombus formation related to hypercoagulability—a risk superimposed on the risk of thrombosis associated with inactivity.

Clients dependent on alcohol or drugs may experience withdrawal reactions during hospitalization, further complicating recovery. The client who abuses alcohol may have impaired hepatic function (see Chapter 52) as well as nutritional deficiencies. The client who abuses drugs may have untoward reactions to anesthesia and analgesia. In some instances, abused drugs may potentiate the effects, causing dangerous levels of respiratory depression. In other instances, clients may have developed a cross-tolerance to an anesthetic or analgesic agent, increasing the amount of drug needed to achieve the desired effect. These interactions are more fully discussed in Chapter 10.

Clients who live a sedentary lifestyle may have poor exercise tolerance and reduced cardiac–respiratory reserve. They may find it difficult to adjust to the physical stresses associated with surgery and recovery.

Attitudinal Factors

The client who has a high level of anxiety or who lacks confidence in the surgeon or the therapy may also be at greater than normal risk. The highly anxious client experiences greater physiological and psychological stress, depleting energy reserves that may be needed in the intraoperative and postoperative periods. Hyperventilation accompanying anxiety may promote a respiratory alkalosis. The client who has lost hope or is depressed may suffer from fatigue, anorexia, and sleep loss, compromising the ability to cope with the stress of surgery and jeopardizing successful recovery.

Informed Consent

The doctrine of informed consent is based on the concept that clients have a right to self-determination. If the client is to make decisions about care, he or she requires complete information from the physician. Physicians must not proceed with treatment until they have *informed* the client about the facts and risks of the treatment in understandable terms and received the client's *consent*. A physician who fails to inform a client fully about treatment risks being sued for negligence or charged with assault and battery. Lack of informed consent is a common reason for malpractice lawsuits.

To give a valid consent, the client must be competent, must understand the information, and must accede voluntarily. A competent adult—a person over age 18 who is conscious, oriented, and not confused or under sedation—may sign the consent form. An emancipated minor—a person under 18 who is married or self-supporting—may also sign. In general, a family member or legal guardian must authorize treatment for minors or incompetent adults. In emergencies, treatment may be given without formal consent.

The client usually is requested to sign a form documenting consent. Most hospitals provide standard forms for this purpose. There is a tendency to confuse the mere signing of the form with informed consent. Informed consent is an exchange between the physician and client; the form is a record of the exchange. Informing the client and obtaining consent are the responsibility of the physician. These responsibilities cannot be delegated. The common practice of having nurses obtain consent—or even witness the client's signature—is highly questionable. The nurse who witnesses only the client's signature on the consent

form—and who was not present when the physician discussed the treatment or surgery and explained the benefits, risks, or alternatives, to a legally competent individual—should write on the form, "witnessing signature only" (Northrop, 1984).

As a client advocate, the nurse has an important role in assessing whether the client's consent was truly informed. The nurse can determine how well the client understands by discussing information received from the physician. Many clients are in awe of physicians and assent without completely understanding the treatment; others misunderstand what the physician tells them; some have not been adequately informed; still others are so anxious that they are temporarily unable to assimilate information. Such clients may have signed consent forms, but whether they are truly informed is questionable. A checklist for information consent, such as the one in Box 14–3, helps the nurse fulfill obligations for informed consent.

If finding that the client does not have adequate information or does not fully understand the procedure, the nurse has a responsibility to refer the problem to the physician. A client has the right to withdraw consent at any time before surgery, and the client should be informed of this right. If the client refuses surgery or withdraws consent, the nurse and physician can cooperate in determining the reason. Often the cause is misinformation or lack of information. Clients who refuse treatment have the right to be fully informed about the consequences of refusal; clients are ultimately responsible for their own bodies, however. Explanations of possible consequences should be given nonjudgmentally.

When surgery is not an emergency, clients should be informed of their right to a second opinion. Information about second opinions might be provided in a printed handout, as shown in Box 14–3. Most insurance carriers, including private insurers, Medicare, and Medicaid, encourage second opinions and will pay for them. Mandatory second opinions are becoming more common.

Client Readiness

Other factors the nurse should consider in preoperative assessment of the client relate to the client's physiological and psychological readiness for the experience. Does the client know what to expect during the perioperative period? Is the client familiar with procedures in which he or she must take part—eg, coughing and deep breathing? Previous experience with surgery does not guarantee that clients are knowledgeable, and the nurse should not neglect to assess their readiness for surgery and to give them preoperative instruction.

Research has indicated that clients who know what will happen to them during a stressful experience are less angry and anxious during the procedure (Hartfield & Cason, 1981). Does the client know what tests will be performed? What skin preparation consists of? Whether preoperative medication will be given? Why NPO status is necessary?

Box 14–3   Client Checklist for Informed Consent

To the Client:

Before agreeing to surgical treatment, you have both the right and the responsibility to be sure you understand:

- What your diagnosis is; that is, what is making you ill.
- Why surgical treatment is recommended.
- What the operation will consist of.
- What risks are involved.
- What the probable outcome will be.
- What risks are involved in *not* having surgery.
- What medical (nonsurgical) alternatives there are.

You may want to discuss your operation with your personal physician as well as the surgeon or other specialist who recommended the operation. Here are some questions to ask:

- What is the nature of my illness, in medical terms and in ordinary language?
- What tests have been (will be) done to confirm the diagnosis?
- What risks are associated with the tests?
- What are the test results and what do they mean?

What do the surgery and any additional treatments consist of?

- What will happen during the operation? (Ask for as much detail as *you* need to make a decision.)
- Are there alternative methods of surgery? What are they?
- What additional treatments, if any, will I need after surgery?
- Who will perform the operation? Who will be assisting?
- What are the reasonable risks of the operation?
- Are there any frequent complications of this operation?
- Is this operation experimental or new?

What is the probable outcome of this operation?

- What is the success rate of the operation? (That is, what proportion of the time does it cure my condition?)

- How much pain is involved under normal circumstances?
- Is any long-lasting disfigurement involved? Can it be corrected?
- How long will I be in the hospital?
- How long will I have to stay inactive at home?

What are the alternatives?

- Are there alternative medical (nonsurgical) treatments for my condition? What are they? What are their risks and/or success rates?
- What risks are involved in delaying my decision? How long?
- What is the probable outcome of *not* having surgery?

You are also entitled to obtain a second opinion from a qualified physician. Medicare, Medicaid, and most private insurers will pay for this—check with your insurer. Do not hesitate to seek a second opinion. To find another surgeon or specialist, you may:

- Ask your own doctor.
- Ask a nurse or other health care professional.
- Ask your local medical society or medical school for names of physicians specializing in your condition.
- Call the government's toll-free number to find out how to locate a specialist near you: (800) 638-6833 (in Maryland, 800-492-6603).
- If you are covered by Medicare, call your local Social Security office (listed in your telephone directory under US Government, Department of Health and Human Services).
- If you are eligible for Medicaid, call your local welfare office.
- Select a physician who is likely to be most objective and least likely to have a personal relationship with your physician.

When the trip to the operating room will take place? What sensory perceptions may be felt during the surgery while under local anesthesia, or upon awakening in the recovery room?

Early classic psychological research demonstrated that a person who knows what to expect is usually better able to tolerate the experience (Pervin, 1963; Vernon & Bigelow, 1974). Most clients fear pain associated with surgery. If the nurse says, "You will have a fair amount of pain during the first 24 hours; then it will abate," the client may be better able to cope because of knowing the pain will soon dissipate. Studies have demonstrated that giving sensory information to clients before a stressful event reduces stress and may even shorten the hospital stay (Johnson et al., 1978a; Johnson et al., 1978b). Other studies have shown that preoperative teaching is associated with less use of pain medication and a lower incidence of vomiting and complications, as well as a shorter stay. An extensive review of such studies documented the potential effectiveness of systematic preoperative teaching; further research is needed to discover the most effective components of such a teaching plan (Devine & Cook, 1983). Techniques for preop-

erative teaching are discussed under planning and implementation.

NURSING DIAGNOSIS

The assessment phase of the nursing process culminates in the formulation of nursing diagnoses. The nurse analyzes the data obtained to determine diagnoses that will provide guidance in formulating a plan of care for the individual client. Some common nursing diagnoses related to the preoperative client are in Box 14–4.

PLANNING AND IMPLEMENTATION

The preoperative plan of care is based on fundamental principles of preoperative care as they relate to the nursing diagnoses determined for the individual client. Interventions common to all surgical procedures include general physiological and psychological preparation, preoperative teaching, and immediate preparation before the surgical procedure.

Box 14–4 Common Nursing Diagnoses Related to Preoperative Care

Anxiety, related to threat to health status

Fear, related to impending diagnostic surgery

Grieving, anticipatory, related to expected loss of body part

Knowledge deficit, related to surgical procedure and associated risks

Self-concepts, disturbance in: body image, related to anticipated change in body function

Self-concepts, disturbance in: role performance, related to inability to meet usual responsibilities

Physiological Preparation

Minimization of Risk

Nursing care before surgery includes assisting with measures to eliminate or minimize identified risks. For example, the condition of the client with cardiac, hepatic, or renal dysfunction or diabetes may be stabilized. A client who smokes may reduce his or her risk by giving up smoking 2 weeks before surgery. A client with respiratory difficulties may participate in active respiratory therapy; measures may include coughing and deep breathing, incentive spirometry, and elimination of secretions by postural drainage or intermittent positive pressure breathing (IPPB) therapy. The nurse can encourage the client while assisting in carrying out these measures.

The client with poor nutritional status may be hospitalized for some time before surgery so nutritional deficiencies may be corrected by a well-balanced diet, supplementary feedings, vitamins or minerals, or, in some cases, hyperalimentation (see Chapter 8). Electrolyte imbalances are also corrected. Nursing measures to maintain and increase the client's appetite may include determining food preferences and providing for them—usually in consultation with the dietitian—by providing small, frequent feedings and by making mealtime pleasant.

The client with potential for infection may be given prophylactic antibiotics before surgery. Preoperative antimicrobial therapy is generally instituted if the wound is dirty or contaminated (eg, a ruptured appendix), with intestinal surgery, or if prosthetic devices are to be inserted. If prophylaxis is to be effective, therapeutic levels of the antibiotic in the tissues must be obtained before surgery. One study suggested that parenteral antibiotics should be administered within 1 hour of surgery and continued for 24 to 72 hours (Nichols, 1982); however, therapy is often begun earlier. Continuation of parenteral antibiotic therapy beyond the 24- to 72-hour period is considered unnecessary and may make the client susceptible to superinfection.

Preparation of Gastrointestinal Tract

Stress, sedation, general anesthesia, and the inactivity associated with surgery tend to depress gastrointestinal activity, predisposing the client to retention of food and fluids and thereby to abdominal distention and/or vomiting. Besides increasing the client's discomfort, vomiting and distention (often called "gas" by clients) place unnecessary tension on thoracic and abdominal incisions.

Depression of the gastrointestinal tract also predisposes the client to postoperative constipation or fecal impaction. Bowel cleansing by laxative or enema is frequently ordered to help prevent these problems. These measures may be ordered for the evening before surgery or for the day of surgery. For intestinal surgery, however, the bowel may be cleansed days in advance to minimize the bacterial count in the intestine so contamination of sterile areas is less likely. Cleansing the bowel is especially important in abdominal surgery, because a bowel distended with fecal material may interfere with surgical manipulation of the abdominal organs.

Maintaining NPO status is intended to prevent and alleviate gastrointestinal problems. Allowing ample time for gastric emptying decreases the risk of subsequent pulmonary aspiration of gastric contents, a serious perianesthesia concern discussed later in this chapter. However, preoperative restriction of food and fluids may lead to fluid and electrolyte imbalances in clients who are scheduled for surgery late in the day. When surgery is scheduled in the early afternoon hours, some early morning fluids may be given orally but not within 6 hours of surgery. Minor surgical procedures performed under local anesthesia outside the operating room, as well as those performed in the operating room that do not require the presence of anesthesia personnel, are often performed without dietary restrictions. Many institutions, however, require the presence of the anesthetist to closely monitor, sedate, and support the client even during local anesthesia. In such instances, either client status or the need to anticipate potential problems require the restriction of food and fluids for at least 6 to 8 hours preoperatively in the event that the need for general anesthesia should arise.

Medication Status

For the client who must be NPO, oral medications are either withheld or administered with a sip of water before surgery; however, the client's physician should be consulted before medications are withheld. Omitting even one dose of certain medications, eg, digoxin (Lanoxin), phenytoin (Dilantin), or various antihypertensives may place the client in jeopardy. An alternative route of administration such as intramuscular injection may be ordered. The physician may not remember that the client receives routine medication, so be alert to this possibility and be aware of the properties of such medications and the hazards associated with even brief discontinuance.

Also be aware of potential problems associated with routine medications. Clients who receive daily doses of intermediate or long-acting insulins, for example, require a diet that will meet carbohydrate levels to which their insulin dosage has been adjusted. On the day of surgery, when the client is NPO and the principal source of nourishment will be intravenous fluids, carbohydrate levels and insulin requirements are unpredictable. Stress associated with surgery may cause an increase in the client's blood levels of glucose, further complicating the picture. To allow for maximum flexibility, the physician will usually prescribe short-acting insulin coverage according to urinary and blood glucose tests. Sometimes a fractional dose of NPH insulin is administered once an IV of 5% D/W has been started. The client is then closely monitored in case additional insulin is required (see Chapter 42).

Preparation of the Skin

The area to be incised is usually cleansed before surgery with an antiseptic such as povidone–iodine (Betadine) or tincture of chlorhexidine to minimize the number of microorganisms on the skin (Centers for Disease Control, 1982). Hexachlorophene is no longer recommended for use as a single agent (Kneedler & Dodge, 1983). Such cleansing reduces the risk of contamination and infection of the wound. The client may be instructed to bathe or shower with antiseptic solutions the night before and/or the morning of surgery.

In the past, the area of the incision was also shaved, because hair was believed to be a potential source of microbial contamination. Recent studies, however, have brought this assumption into question. Several investigators have found that not removing hair at all, clipping hair, or using electric shavers or depilatory agents are associated with lower infection rates than traditional shaving (Cruse & Foord, 1980; Alexander et al., 1983). Fewer infections occurred when hair was removed close to the time of incision (Alexander et al., 1983). The Centers for Disease Control (1982) recommends that hair be removed, if necessary, shortly before surgery. The trend, therefore, is to remove hair immediately before surgery, often in the operating suite. The nurse responsible for hair removal should pay careful attention to preventing skin abrasion or laceration, because skin wounds may harbor microorganisms or provide an entry route for them. See a nursing fundamentals text for further discussion of hair removal before surgery.

Rest and Hygiene

A well-rested client is more relaxed and less anxious. Often a sedative is ordered to provide a good night's sleep for the hospitalized client the night before surgery. Although clients may protest that the sedative is unnecessary, they should be reminded that this medication is available. A bath or shower may also aid relaxation, ensure that the client is clean and comfortable, and reduce the number of microorganisms.

Psychological Preparation of Client and Family

Health care professionals, who may see many surgical cases every day, may forget how frightening the prospect of "being cut" is to the client. A procedure that seems minor to the nurse—eg, a dilatation and curettage—may not seem minor to the client. Some clients voice their fears openly; others become withdrawn; still others seem stoic. The prospect of surgery raises many questions, spoken or unspoken, about body image alteration, loss of control, and fear of pain or death. The client may be thinking: "What will 'they' do to me while I'm unconscious?" "Will I always have a scar?" "How quickly will the wound heal?" "When can I go back to work?" "When can I care for my kids?" And always, "How much will it hurt?" In encouraging the client to discuss fears and in helping to clarify expectations, be careful not to minimize the amount of discomfort the client can expect. Reassure the client that analgesics will be available when needed and that family and friends will be able to visit.

Often, significant others are permitted to visit on the morning that surgery is scheduled, regardless of visiting hours. The presence of a supportive person may greatly aid coping. A visit by a member of the clergy or a spiritual advisor may also be helpful, and the client should be informed that such counsel is available. By insisting on such a visit, however, the nurse might suggest to some clients that their condition is more serious than they have been told. "When they talked about calling a priest, I was sure I was a goner" is a common reaction.

Prepare the family for the experiences they are likely to encounter on the day of surgery and in the postoperative period. Family members and friends may be feeling stressed and anxious, especially in instances where the diagnosis is questionable or the outcome of the surgery is difficult to predict. Be sure to let them know what time to come to the hospital to see the client before surgery and before preoperative sedation is given. Family members and friends should know where to wait while the client is in surgery. Some hospitals permit a family member or friend to accompany the client to the operating room holding area. However, most hospitals require visitors to wait in the client's room or in a waiting area adjacent to the operating room. When surgical procedures are expected to be lengthy, family and friends will probably be more comfortable in an environment other than the hospital and may choose to return home to wait if distance permits.

Family and friends often ask the nurse how long the surgery is expected to take. Predictions about the length of surgery should be made with caution, taking into account the numerous factors (such as the extent of a lesion or even scheduling complications in the operating room itself) that could prolong the amount of time the client spends in the operating room but not necessarily the length of time of the surgery itself. Make sure that predictions are general enough so that visitors do not become unduly concerned if the client does not return to the hospital room exactly when expected.

If a waiting area is provided in the operating suite itself, the operating room nurse or other personnel may give the family and friends periodic updates. If visitors are waiting in the client's hospital room, operating room personnel can inform the staff nurse who can, in turn, relay the messages. Inform the family about the communication system before the client's surgery. Knowing how to go about obtaining information on the progress of the client's surgery is comforting to them.

Preoperative Teaching

As already noted, preoperative teaching can contribute to reducing anxiety and stress, reducing the incidence of complications, and shortening the hospital stay. Teaching can take many forms. Informal teaching occurs during routine nursing care, perhaps while the nurse is giving a bed bath or feeding the client. Often the client will be more responsive at such times. Formal teaching may involve reserving a special time. Formal group sessions in which clients can share concerns with others having similar conditions can be effective. The family should also be involved in preoperative instruction.

Each type of nurse contributes special knowledge to preoperative teaching. The surgical staff nurse provides general orientation to the entire perioperative period. The operating room nurse can explain what occurs during the actual surgery. The nurse anesthetist discusses the anesthesia experience. The recovery room nurse concentrates on immediate postsurgical recovery. It may be possible to have the client tour some areas of the operating rooms and recovery rooms and to meet personnel who will be involved in intraoperative and postoperative care. Remember that the client who has same-day surgery also needs comprehensive preparation, with additional teaching about home recovery.

General Orientation

Preoperative teaching generally includes a general orientation to the surgical experience and instruction in specific activities in which the client will participate postoperatively to avoid complications and speed recovery. Explain specific preoperative preparation such as restriction of food and fluids, including the rationale for these measures. Clients who understand the reason for procedures are more likely to remember them and to comply with the regimen. If nasogastric intubation, insertion of an intravenous line, or urinary catheterization has been ordered, prepare the client for these events. "Surprises" of this kind increase the client's apprehension and intensify concerns about control. Also reassure the client that the nurse will be available for support and will be concerned for the client's safety throughout the surgical experience.

Postoperative Moving, Turning, Coughing, and Deep Breathing

Clients should be instructed about the importance of moving and turning, coughing, and deep breathing. Explain that inactivity imposed by surgery makes blood flow sluggish and can predispose the client to thrombosis. Moving and turning help prevent this complication. Inform clients that

Nursing Research Note

Rettig F, Southby J: Using different body positions to reduce discomfort from dorsogluteal injection. *Nurs Res* 1982; 31(4):219–221.

This study analyzed body positioning related to discomfort during intramuscular injections into the greatest gluteal muscle. Four positions were compared; prone with toes pointed inward (internally rotating the femur), prone with toes pointed outward (externally rotating the femur), side lying with toes pointed in (internal rotation of femur), and side lying with toes pointed out (external rotation of femur). All subjects received the same injection, using a 22-gauge needle with a 1- to 1½-inch needle length. Medication was injected for no less than 5 seconds, and the site was massaged for 5 seconds after the injection.

Less discomfort was associated with internal rotation of the femur in both the side-lying and prone positions.

These findings demonstrate a link between research and clinical practice. Appropriate positioning can reduce the pain of IM injections.

they will be encouraged to move and turn as soon as possible after surgery. Clients who are able to move without help should be prepared to move their extremities and to turn from side to side within the limits that may be imposed by the surgeon. Tell the client who will be unable to move or turn that the nurse will assist with these activities.

Inactivity, sedation, anesthesia, and pain can cause hypoventilation. The surgical client is susceptible to atelectasis, a condition in which the alveoli collapse and adequate gas exchange cannot occur (see Chapter 19). Accumulation of mucous secretions can lead to bronchitis and pneumonia. Explain these possible complications and encourage the client to practice deep breathing and controlled coughing, so these procedures will be familiar when they are required after surgery. Recommend the sitting position or Fowler's position because they allow for maximum lung expansion and aeration. Several deep breaths (such as those described in diaphragmatic breathing below) should be followed by a short breath and cough. Or teach the client the *cascade* cough: taking a deep breath, holding it for 3 seconds, and coughing several times while exhaling. These subsequent coughs upon exhalation at successively lower lung volumes prevent small airway collapse (a potential complication of forceful coughing for clients with chronic obstructive pulmonary disease).

Clients should be told that coughing may be painful, especially if a thoracic, lumbar flank, or abdominal incision is involved. Splinting the incision—providing external support—reduces movement of the involved tissues, reduces pain, and thus facilitates coughing and deep breathing. Either the nurse or client can splint the incision by supporting it with a pillow or interlocked hands. Both methods are illustrated in Figure 14–1. The support that splinting provides often helps to alleviate clients' fear of "splitting the stitches." Reassure clients that sutures are strong and able to withstand coughing and deep breathing. Remind the client that analgesics will be available. Coughing and deep breathing, although generally a routine postoperative activity, may be contraindicated in some surgeries, such as eye surgeries, because increased pressure can damage the operative site. These contraindications are discussed in the chapters about surgical approaches to specific disorders.

Deep breathing, or diaphragmatic breathing, uses the

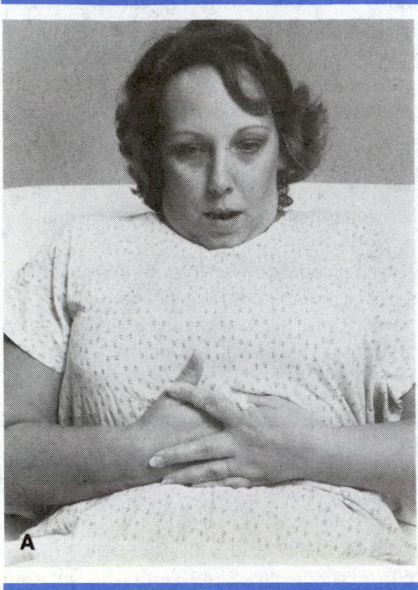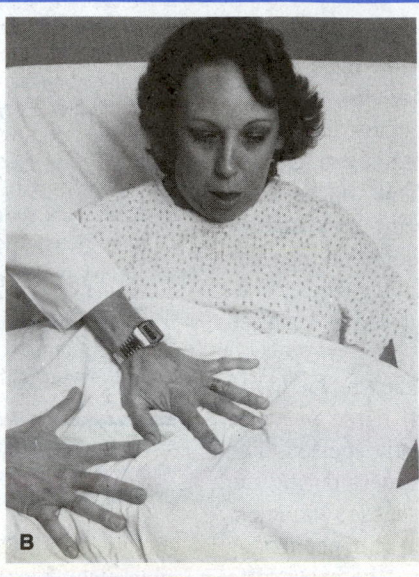

Figure 14–1

Splinting the incision for coughing. **A.** Splinting the incision during coughing by supporting it with interlocked hands. An alternative method is to press the arm and hand of the unaffected side against the operative area. **B.** A pillow, pressed against the operative area, can also provide support. Both methods can be done by the client, family member, or nurse.
SOURCE: Swearingen PL: *The Addison–Wesley Photo-Atlas of Nursing Procedures.* Menlo Park, CA: Addison–Wesley, 1984.

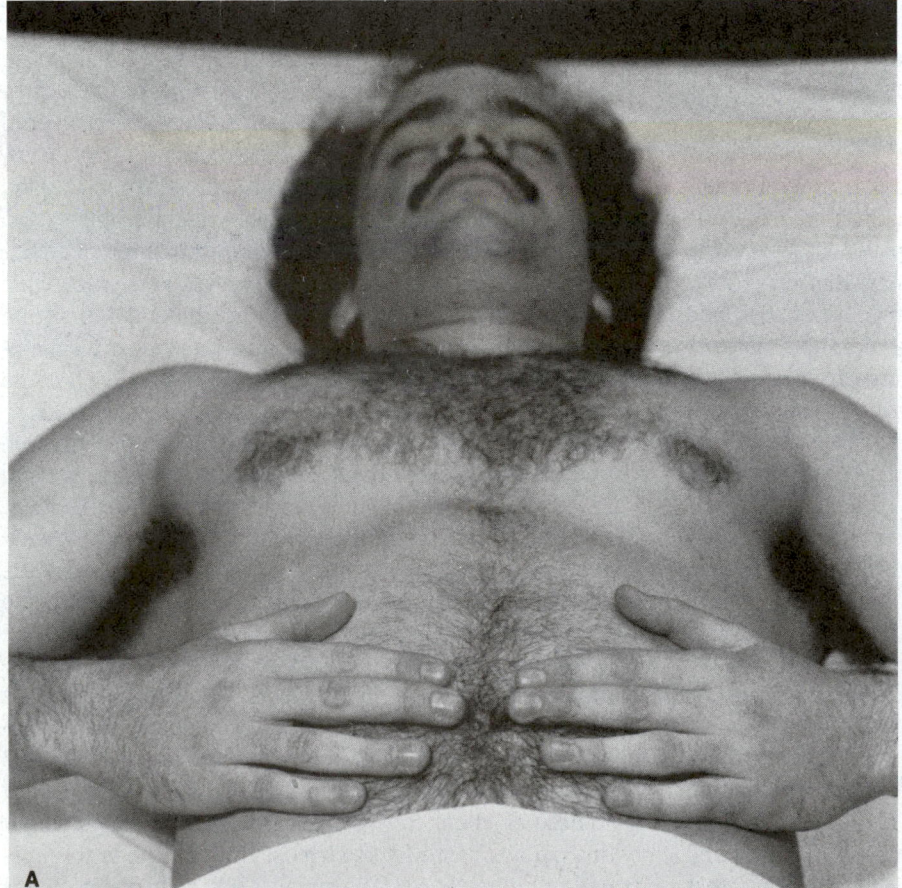

Figure 14–2

Deep-breathing exercises. **A.** Diaphragmatic breathing. The abdomen rises during inspiration and falls during expiration.

diaphragm and abdominal muscles to fully aerate the lungs. The client should relax the abdominal wall by flexing the knees and breathe in deeply and slowly through the nose while pushing the abdomen out (Figure 14–2A). The client can tell if he or she is breathing correctly by practicing with one hand on the chest and the other hand on the abdomen. The hand on the abdomen should rise with inspiration and fall with expiration. The hand on the chest should remain still. Clients with chronic obstructive pulmonary disease should exhale slowly through pursed lips.

Teach clients who are restricting or limiting upper chest movement because of pain (common with clients having chest or kidney surgery or mastectomy) the apical expansion exercises illustrated in Figure 14–2B. Basal

expansion exercises, discussed and illustrated in Figure 14–2C, promote and maintain mobility of the lower thorax. They are often helpful for clients after chest surgery when pain on the affected side inhibits bilateral chest movement.

Immediate Presurgical Preparation

In the immediate presurgical period, the nurse on the unit is responsible for ensuring that the client is physically prepared for transport to the operating room and that the appropriate records will accompany the client. Institutional policies regarding these procedures vary, but general considerations include the following measures.

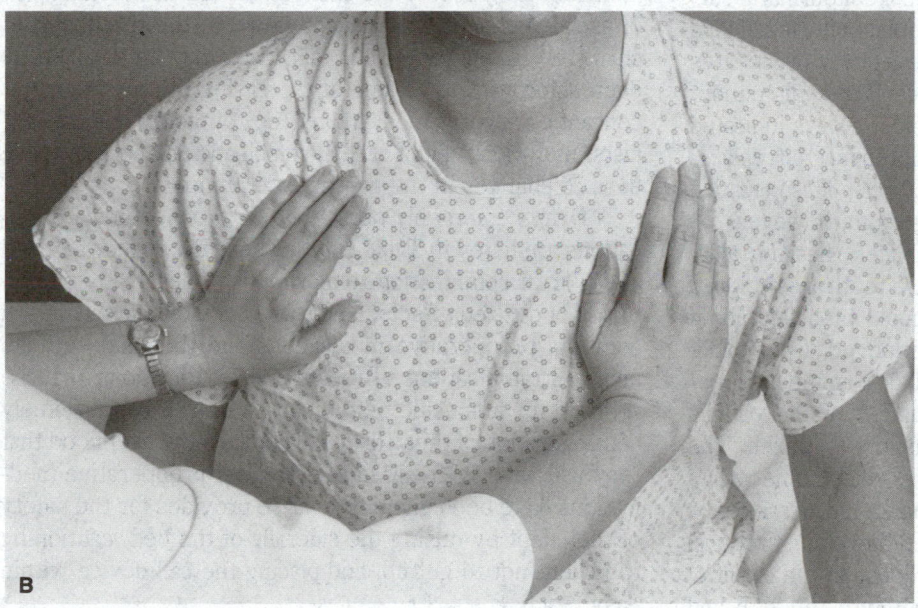

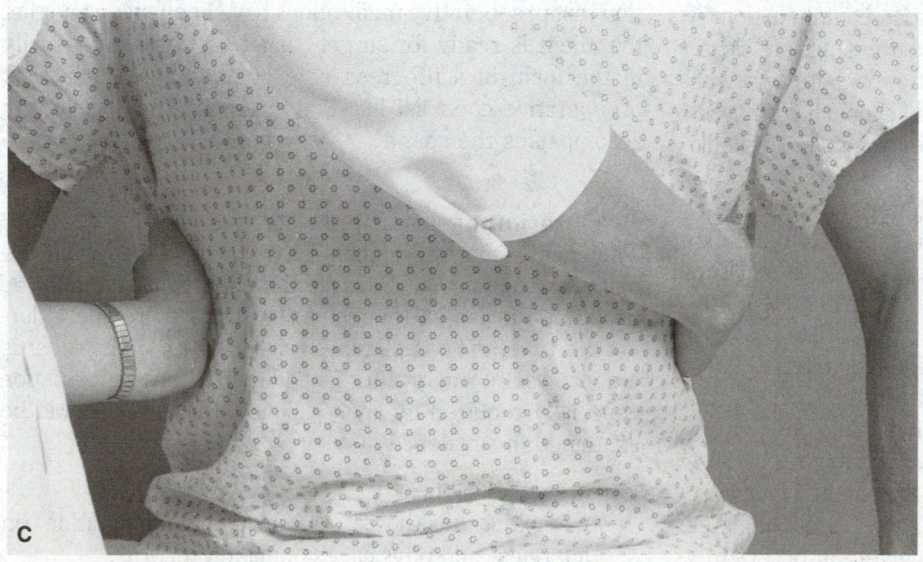

Figure 14–2 (continued)

B. Apical expansion. The client inhales, pushing the chest upward and outward, against the moderate pressure applied by the nurse. Encourage the client to retain the expansion for a few moments before exhaling quietly. **C.** Basal expansion. The client inhales, attempting to expand the lower ribs to move the nurse's hands outward. The client may use his or her own hands for both B and C, performing the exercises independently. Encourage the client to retain maximum inhalation for 1 or 2 seconds before exhaling quietly.
SOURCE: Swearingen PL: *The Addison–Wesley Photo-Atlas of Nursing Procedures.* Menlo Park, CA: Addison–Wesley, 1984.

Preparation of the Client

A checklist for preoperative preparation is shown in Figure 14–3. The checklist serves as a reminder, helping to ensure comprehensive preoperative preparation.

The importance of appropriate identification cannot be overemphasized. Asking the client's name is insufficient; check the client's identification bracelet before proceeding with the final preparation and administration of preoperative medications. Any abnormalities in vital signs should be reported. Vital signs should be monitored immediately before the administration of preoperative medications and transfer to the operating suite. Abnormalities or findings inconsistent with the client's usual values should be reported to the surgeon in case a delay of surgery is appropriate.

Preoperative nasogastric intubation is often ordered for clients having abdominal surgery and those in whom depressed gastrointestinal function may be expected. Foley catheters are usually inserted before genitourinary surgery, before major surgery when careful monitoring of fluid balance will be necessary, and before lengthy procedures that may cause urinary retention and bladder distention. Insertion of an intravenous line is almost always indicated to provide a route for anesthesia, maintenance or replacement fluids, and/or emergency medications. This insertion is usually performed in the operating room, however.

Jewelry, hairpins, prosthetic devices, hearing aids, eyeglasses and contact lenses, and false teeth are removed for the client's safety. The client should be asked about dental caps or bridges that might be dislodged during endotracheal intubation. Agency policy will determine how jewelry is secured; generally, a careful list of the client's belongings is made and security measures are taken. The client should be encouraged to send jewelry home with a relative for safekeeping. A wedding band may occasionally be left on with tape to secure it, depending on institutional policy, but this practice can be hazardous. In the event of postoperative edema, jewelry can cut into the skin and obstruct circulation. Generally, any current wound dressings are left in place to prevent cross-contamination of wounds. The nurse should ensure that dressings are clean. Nail polish, lipstick, and other cosmetics can interfere with observations for pallor and cyanosis and should be removed. Instructions to the client about not wearing makeup should include an explanation of the reason.

Clients who have not been catheterized should void before receiving preoperative medications to prevent distention of the bladder during surgery. In abdominal surgery, bladder distention may interfere with the identification of operative landmarks and appropriate surgical technique and may predispose the bladder to trauma. Postoperative bladder distention also contributes to client discomfort. After preoperative medications have been given, the client should not be permitted out of bed to void, because the sedative effects may predispose the client to injury.

Only when these preparations have been completed should preoperative medications be given as ordered by the surgeon or anesthetist. Pharmacologic preparation of the client has both physiological and psychological objectives. Perhaps the most common objective is to control anxiety and promote a state of calmness. Sedatives are usually ordered the night before surgery to help the client sleep well and may also be given the morning of surgery. Other reasons for preoperative medications are to reduce oral secretions, interrupt vagal nerve impulses that slow the heart, decrease gastric fluid volume, increase gastric fluid pH, and prevent postoperative nausea and vomiting. Clients with preexisting injuries may require narcotics to be able to tolerate movement during transfer to the operating room. Anticholinergics such as atropine or glycopyrrolate may be given to facilitate endotracheal intubation or prevent the accumulation of secretions in a client receiving general anesthesia by a mask technique.

General anesthesia, especially for the client with a full stomach, predisposes the client to the life-threatening risk of aspirating acidic gastric contents into the tracheobronchial tree (see Chapter 17). This risk may be reduced by decreasing gastric volume or increasing the pH of gastric contents. Several medications (eg, antacids, H_2-antagonists, metoclopramide) used in combination may effect these desired changes in the gastric environment.

Drugs commonly prescribed as preanesthesia medications are listed in Table 14–3. These drugs may be used alone or in combination to accomplish one or any combination of desired effects. The nurse should be familiar with common preoperative medications and their side effects and contraindications. Preoperative medications may be ordered for a specific time or on an on-call basis. Timely administration of these drugs maximizes the likelihood that they will have the desired effect. After preoperative medications have been given, the nurse provides for the safety of the client by raising the siderails of the bed, cautioning the client not to get up, and placing the call device within easy reach.

The client is taken to surgery by stretcher. Verification that preoperative medications have been given and that the client is ready for surgery must be provided, usually in the form of a progress note on the client's chart. A preoperative checklist like that in Figure 14–3 generally accompanies the client.

Preparation of the Client's Record

The client's chart accompanies him or her throughout the perioperative period. Because the client will generally be unable to furnish information to health care providers during this time, the completeness and accuracy of the records are especially important. In addition to any information especially required by agency policy, the chart should be examined for evidence of:

- Signed consent.
- Complete health history, including information on allergies, and physical examination records.

MILLARD FILLMORE HOSPITAL

☑ GATES   ☐ SUBURBAN

Ms. Sonya Green
Room 104

PRE-OP CHECK LIST

DIRECTIONS: Complete all sections of the checklist. Indicate the item was completed by writing your initials in the space in front of the item. Do not leave blank spaces. If the item is not relevant to the patient, draw a line through the item.

PATIENT INFORMATION: (include ALLERGIES, HANDICAPS, etc.)

Allergic to penicillin, meperidine. Right shoulder easily dislocated since childhood.

TO BE COMPLETED PREVIOUS TO THE DAY OF SURGERY DATE *12/1/86*

CR	H&P
CR	Medical Clearance obtained
CR	Consent signed, Witnessed and Dated
CR	Urine report in chart
CR	Bloodwork reports in chart
CR	T&X match Number of units available *2*
~~	~~Chest x-ray~~
~~	~~EKG~~
CR	Weight *131* lbs.

Area of surgical prep: _____

_____

Prep done by *Ethel O'Rourke, LPN*

Checked by *Christine Reardon, RN*

TO BE COMPLETED DAY OF SURGERY DATE *12/2/86*

The following items have been removed (Where appropriate, give short description of item and state what was done with it):

~~	~~Dentures, please circle, (upper, lower, partial) disposition~~
CR	Permanent Crown or Fixed Bridge __✓__ yes _____ no *Two fixed bridges; one upper and one lower; left jaw*
~~	~~Contact lens/glasses~~
CR	Jewelry *Gold wedding band, neck chain, wristwatch given to husband*
~~	~~Prothesis~~
CR	Make up, nail polish, hair pins, etc. *Makeup and nailpolish removed*

VITAL SIGNS: (TPR & BP) *98F, 72, 18, 126/82*

CR	Identaband in place
CR	Pre-Op hypo given: *Atropine 0.4mg IM* *Diazepam 5mg IM* } Time: *7³⁰ Am*
CR	Med sheet in chart

Sent to O.R. by: *Christine Reardon, RN*
(Nurse's Signature)

Figure 14–3

An example of preoperative checklist. (Courtesy of Millard Fillmore Hospital, Buffalo, NY)

Table 14–3 Common Preoperative Medications

Class of Drug	Drug	Typical Adult Dose (mg)	Route
Narcotics	Meperidine (Demerol)	25–100	IM, IV
	Morphine	5–15	IM, IV
Barbiturates	Sodium pentobarbital (Nembutal)	50–150	Oral, IM
	Secobarbital (Seconal)	50–150	Oral, IM
Antihistamines	Diphenhydramine (Benadryl)	25–75	Oral, IM
	Hydroxyzine (Atarax, Vistaril)	50–100	IM
Benzodiazepines	Diazepam (Valium)	5–15	Oral, IM, IV
	Lorazepam (Ativan)	1–4	Oral, IM
Anticholinergics	Atropine	0.4–0.6	IM
	Glycopryrrolate (Robinul)	0.2–0.3	IM
H_2-antagonists	Cimetidine (Tagamet)	350	Oral, IM, IV
	Ranitidine (Zantac)	150	Oral
Antacids	Particulate	15–30 mL	Oral
	Nonparticulate	15–30 mL	Oral
Gastric motility stimulant	Metoclopramide (Reglan)	10–20	Oral, IM, IV

- Completed consultation report(s), if ordered.
- Reports of diagnostic work-up, including laboratory tests and x-rays.
- Availability of any blood ordered in preparation for surgery and proof of type and crossmatch.
- Identification plate, in case additional chart forms are required.

The nurse is responsible for notifying the physician of any abnormal laboratory or diagnostic findings. Results of any ordered consultations should be obtained and reviewed by the physician before surgery.

EVALUATION

Evaluation of interventions during the presurgical period is a continual process. Goals related to the client's understanding of the surgical experience and postoperative activities may be evaluated by asking the client to repeat the information provided and to demonstrate deep breathing and coughing. Goals related to decreasing surgical risk should be met with evidence of improvement observed through physical assessment and results of laboratory tests and diagnostic studies. The preoperative checklist provides an instrument for evaluating goals of immediate presurgical care.

Section IV: The Nursing Process in Intraoperative Care

The intraoperative phase of the perioperative period begins when the client enters the operating room suite and ends with the completion of surgery and transfer of the client to the recovery room. During this period, the operating room nurse, as part of the surgical team, cares for the client. Because many of the routine procedures during this phase compromise the client's safety, comfort, and privacy, nursing care focuses on meeting these needs. Although some specific procedures vary among health care facilities, certain principles and procedures are common to all.

GENERAL INTRAOPERATIVE PROCEDURES

During the intraoperative phase, care of the client is the responsibility of the surgical team. The team is generally composed of the surgeon, one or more surgical assistants, an individual who administers anesthesia (nurse anesthetist or physician anesthesiologist), a scrub nurse or operating room technician, and a circulating nurse. For highly complex operations such as organ transplants or open heart surgery, the team is of course greatly expanded.

Functions of the Surgical Team

The surgeon performs the actual surgery; surgical assistants (generally physicians learning the surgical specialty) retract tissue and suction blood and debris from the surgical site to afford the surgeon clear visualization of the operative field. The physician anesthesiologist or nurse anesthetist maintains the client in a state of adequate surgical anesthesia while monitoring vital functions and providing for physiologic homeostasis. The scrub nurse or operating room technician assists the surgeon by providing instruments and other materials (eg, sponges or sutures) as needed. Finally, the circulating nurse serves the needs of the other team members and the client; the circulator sets up the room, maintains the necessary supply of instruments and materials, and ensures that all equipment is safe and functional. Any required blood, medications, and intravenous solutions are also obtained through the circulating nurse, who also oversees maintenance of sterile technique and alerts team members of any breaks in technique. All members of the surgical team work together to ensure the safety and welfare of the client.

In no other setting is the role of the nurse as client advocate more challenging. During surgery, the client relies entirely on the surgical team to meet physiological as well as psychosocial needs. The nurse must ensure that the informed consent the client has given is not violated.

The Operating Room Environment

The layout of the operating suite and the procedures performed there are designed to provide for efficiency, safety, and infection control. A typical suite houses operating rooms and scrub areas, clean and dirty linen supply areas, a personnel lounge and dressing room, and a client holding area. A small hospital may have two or three operating rooms, whereas a large surgical suite may have 12 to 15 rooms in a hospital of 500 to 600 beds. Some operating rooms are designed for minor procedures; others, with more sophisticated equipment, are used for major procedures. Regardless of complexity, all operating rooms should contain supplies for emergency care of the client.

Safety and infection control are primary concerns in operating room design. Gruendemann and Meeker (1983) recommend that temperature be maintained between 20°C and 24°C (68°F to 75°F) and humidity at a minimum of 50% to help control bacterial growth and prevent static electricity. The potential for bacterial contamination of the operating room is further reduced by such devices as air filters, positive pressure, and high-flow unidirectional ventilation systems. The operating room is a potentially hazardous environment containing electrical equipment and many materials, such as oxygen, that support combustion.

Operating rooms are generally adjacent to a clean supply area from which sterile supplies can be conveniently obtained. A generous supply of instruments and materials is kept on hand in case of emergency. Soiled and contaminated supplies are removed to a dirty supply area for processing, cleaning, and sterilization.

Scrub Attire

Scrub attire is worn to decrease transport of microorganisms that personnel may harbor on their skin, shoes, and clothing and in their respiratory passages. Attire includes a hat, a pantsuit or dress, shoe coverings, and a face mask.

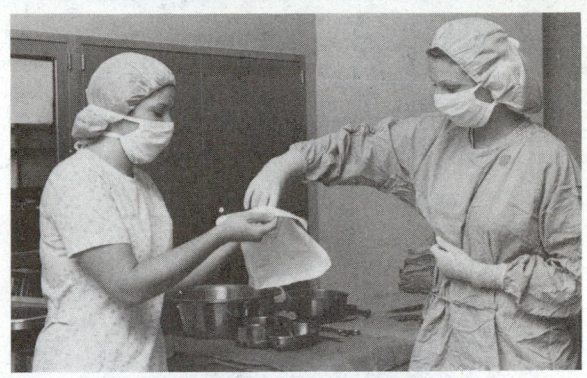

Figure 14–4

Circulating nurse (left) and scrub nurse. (Courtesy of Millard Fillmore Hospital)

Scrub clothing may be disposable or reusable, and it is clean, not sterile. Individuals who scrub for surgery (the surgeon, assistants, and scrub nurse or OR technician) also wear sterile gowns and gloves that are put on after the surgical scrub and after entering the operating room (Figure 14–4). All scrub apparel should be flame resistant, lint free, cool, and comfortable. Caps are put on first so other attire will not be contaminated by hair. Shoe covers and masks as well as any sterile garb must be changed between procedures and when leaving and reentering the operating room. Other garb may also require changing.

The Surgical Scrub

Before entering the operating room, scrub personnel perform a surgical scrub in the area provided for that purpose. The purpose of the surgical scrub is to make the hands and forearms as clean as possible, reducing the number of microorganisms that might contaminate the surgical incision. The procedure takes about 5 minutes. As with routine hand-washing, the scrub's effectiveness depends on the application of light friction and the action of an antimicrobial soap or detergent. Hands and forearms are scrubbed with a brush well above the elbows, and the nails are cleaned. The hands are held higher than the elbows for scrubbing and rinsing. (Figure 14–5) Hands and forearms are dried with a sterile towel in the operating room, and a sterile gown and sterile gloves are then donned, using aseptic technique.

ANESTHESIA

Anesthesia is administered to make the client more receptive to surgery and less susceptible to trauma by promoting narcosis (drug-induced unconsciousness), analgesia (pain relief), amnesia (loss of recall), muscle relaxation, and protection from detrimental autonomic reflex responses to surgical stimuli. The anesthetist will have visited the client before the operation to perform a preanesthesia history

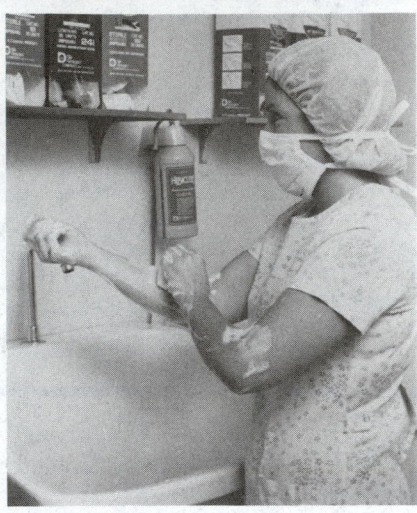

Figure 14–5

The surgical scrub. (Courtesy of Millard Fillmore Hospital)

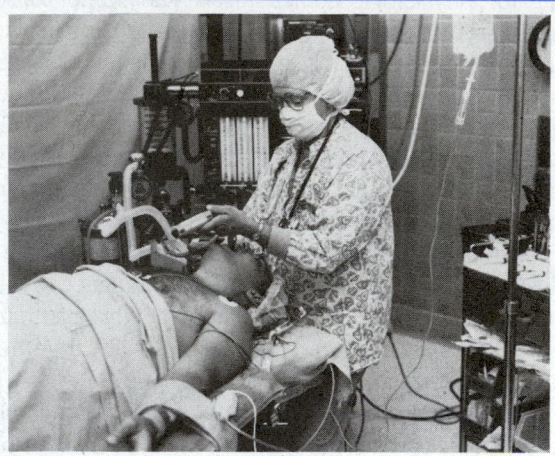

Figure 14–6

A nurse anesthetist performing a laryngoscopy during endotracheal intubation after a state of anesthesia has been induced in the client. (Courtesy of Carol Payne Zagon, RBP, VA Medical Center, Buffalo, NY)

and physical examination; to help reduce the client's anxiety; participate in preoperative teaching; and obtain information about any previous experience with surgery, associated risks, and contraindications for specific anesthetic agents. Client preferences will have been ascertained, but these are superseded by requirements imposed by the client's health history and the type of surgery to be performed. Anticipated departures from the client's preference will have been explained. Although anesthesia affords freedom from pain, its price is loss of control. Clients feel more comfortable in relegating control after having met and consulted with the anesthetist. The preanesthesia visit can help to establish lines of communication and trust between client and anesthetist.

The person in charge of administering anesthesia also is responsible for preparing necessary equipment and supplies before the operation. Throughout the surgical procedure, this surgical team member monitors all the client's vital functions (temperature, pulse, respirations, blood pressure, and ECG data) and keeps the surgeon continually informed of the client's status (Figure 14–6). Measures are taken as needed to maintain adequate blood volume, cardiac output, and blood pressure.

The Development of Modern Anesthesia

Ether vapor was first administered for surgical anesthesia in the 1840s. Although chloroform had been used for obstetrical analgesia in England during this same period, not until it was administered to Queen Victoria in 1853 during the birth of Prince Leopold was the practice accepted. Another anesthetic agent, nitrous oxide, fell into disrepute as a show-stopper for itinerant showmen who capitalized on the gas's exhilarating effects. Soon, medical students and others began using ether for recreational purposes, and "ether frolics" became a popular pastime. Later in the

nineteenth century and early in the twentieth century aseptic technique, sterilization, and anesthesia became accepted milestones in surgical practice.

After ether was first demonstrated, nearly 60 years passed before nurses and physicians began full-time professional practice in anesthesia. The first comprehensive anesthesia training program for nurses was established in 1883, the AANA was founded in 1931, and certification by examination in the specialty began in 1945. Today, approximately 50% of anesthesia in the United States is administered by nurse anesthetists (Stoelting & Miller, 1984).

General Anesthesia

General anesthetics depress cerebral function and interfere with consciousness, perception of sensations, voluntary motor function, and involuntary reflex action. They are administered by various routes, usually by intravenous administration or inhalation.

Anesthetic Agents and Adjuncts

Inhalation anesthesia requires a mask and/or an endotracheal (ET) tube. The ET tube is frequently employed because it helps maintain a patent airway, provides a route for removal of secretions, and allows for ventilatory assistance if necessary.

Only qualified personnel should insert an ET tube because expert appreciation of airway anatomy and placement technique are required to prevent serious complications such as intubation of the esophagus, soft tissue obstruction, and laryngospasm, all of which can interfere with proper oxygenation. Intubation of the esophagus is perhaps the most common problem associated with ET tube placement. This situation, lethal in its consequences, must be detected immediately and an airway rapidly made available. In addition, qualified personnel will be able to manage both soft tissue obstruction and laryngospasm, both of which are also potentially lethal.

The ET tube is usually inserted after the client is anesthetized and paralyzed with a short-acting muscle relaxant such as succinylcholine. Within this controlled environment, and with the assistance of the circulating nurse, conditions for tracheal intubation are nearly ideal, and the chances for soft tissue trauma minimized. For a typical adult female, a 7.0 mm or 8.0 mm (internal diameter) ET tube is recommended; an 8.0 mm or 9.0 mm (internal diameter) ET tube is appropriate for an adult male. During placement of the ET tube, the glottic opening is exposed by the laryngoscope whose lighted blade is passed through the mouth and over the tongue. A stylet (stiff wire) may be inserted within the ET tube to allow it to assume a rigid shape during passage through the mouth and glottic opening. The stylet is removed as soon as the tube enters the glottic opening. The tube is passed until its balloon disappears through the vocal cords. At this time, the cuff is inflated to allow for an airway with a tight seal. The tube's placement is secured by taping at the mouth or applying any of a number of appropriate ET tube securing devices. Figure 14-7A illustrates an ET tube in place in an anesthetized client. An endotracheal tube, a laryngoscope, and an oral airway are pictured in Figure 14-7B. (See also Chapter 18 which discusses the use of ET tubes in other than perioperative care.)

Inhalation anesthetics in current use are listed in Table 14-4. These agents are taken up in the lungs where molecules of the anesthetic vapor cross the alveolocapillary membrane. Once in the blood, the agents induce general anesthesia by affecting the central nervous system (CNS). They also exert many effects (usually depressant) on the cardiovascular, respiratory, urinary, hepatic–biliary, and endocrine systems.

Various intravenous drugs are in common use as anesthetic agents and as adjuncts to anesthesia (Table 14-5). Barbiturates such as thiopental sodium (Pentothal) are used most frequently to produce rapid, smooth induction of anesthesia before the use of an inhalation agent. Benzodiazepines such as diazepam (Valium), useful because of their sedative qualities, are employed during induction or as preoperative sedation. Narcotics are used during the entire perioperative period. In the intraoperative period, narcotics are usually used in conjunction with nitrous oxide and other inhalation agents. In some circumstances, narcotics may be used to induce anesthesia, and high doses may be used as the sole anesthetic agent throughout the surgical procedure. Ketamine (Ketalar) is a dissociative anesthetic that produces a trancelike state. It may be used as a sole agent to produce anesthesia or as an induction agent. Etomidate (Amidate) is a new drug useful in producing rapid, smooth induction.

Neuromuscular blocking agents, administered intravenously, are also adjuncts to anesthesia (Box 14-5). They create optimal conditions for endotracheal intubation and

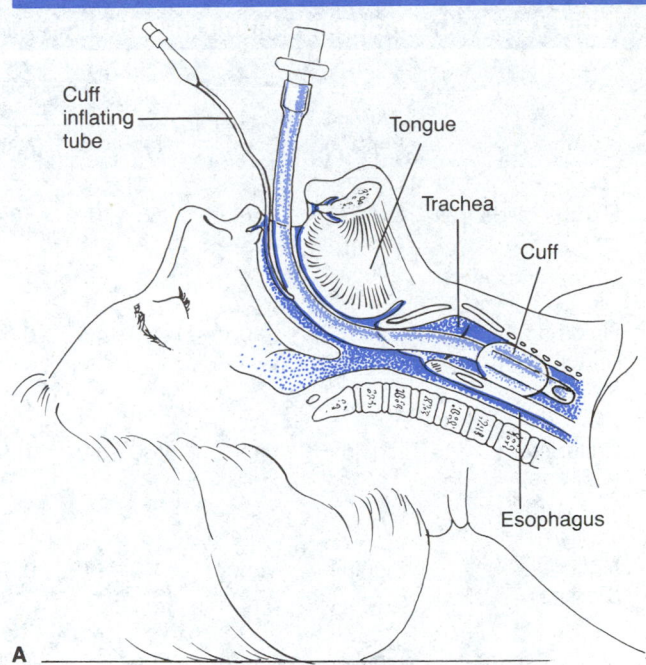

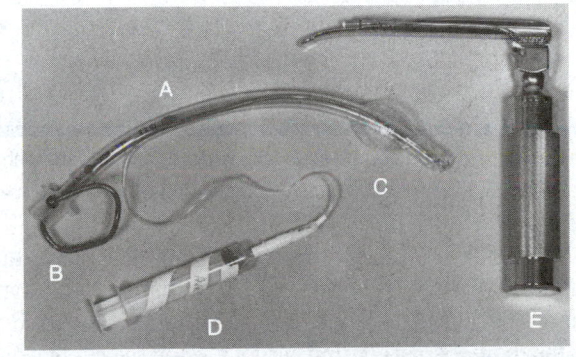

Figure 14-7

A. Endotracheal tube in position in an anesthetized client. **B.** The endotracheal tube (A) can be placed through either the oral or nasal route. The stylet (B), used only during oral placement, facilitates passage through the glottic opening. The balloon (C), at the distal end of the tracheal tube, is inflated with the air syringe (D) and allows positive pressure ventilation by sealing the space between the tracheal wall and the tracheal tube. The inflated balloon also prevents regurgitation of gastric contents into the airway. The lighted laryngoscope (E) illuminates the glottis during tracheal intubation. (Courtesy of Carol Payne Zagon, RBP, VA Medical Center, Buffalo, NY)

relax skeletal muscles. Relaxation of skeletal muscles serves several important purposes during surgery: facilitating the surgeon's access to the operative area, minimizing retraction trauma against otherwise tense muscles, and preventing client movement while surgery is being performed. Clients receiving neuromuscular blocking agents are closely monitored by the anesthetist because of possible dangerous side effects such as respiratory embarrassment, prolonged apnea, and cardiovascular complications such as hypotension and cardiac dysrhythmias. A

Table 14–4 Common Inhalation Anesthetics

Agent	Storage Form	Delivery Form	Typical Inspired Concentration (%)		Clinical Comments
			Induction	Maintenance	
Nitrous oxide*	Liquid/gas (tank)	Gas	50–70	50–70	Rapid, potent anesthesia with rapid recovery; must be mixed with oxygen; high concentrations required to achieve anesthesia may also cause hypoxia
Halothane (Fluothane)	Liquid	Vapor	1.0–4.0	0.5–2.0	Rapid anesthesia and recovery; must be supplemented by other drugs; rarely associated with postanesthetic hepatitis; may cause cardiac dysrhythmias
Enflurane (Ethrane)	Liquid	Vapor	2.0–5.0	1.5–3.0	Rapid anesthesia and recovery; nonflammable and nonexplosive; limited analgesia; may cause respiratory depression, cardiac dysrhythmias, EEG abnormalities
Isoflurane (Forane)	Liquid	Vapor	1.0–4.0	0.8–2.0	Little or no CNS excitement or cardiac dysrhythmias; client usually requires assisted ventilation because of deep respiratory depression
Methoxyflurane** (Penthrane)	Liquid	Vapor	3.0	0.25–1.0	Potent anesthetic with prolonged anesthesia; nonflammable and nonexplosive; prolonged recovery from anesthesia; deep respiratory depression and hypotension; causes direct damage to renal tubules and liver damage

*Often administered in combination with another agent (either inhalation or intravenous)

**Available but rarely used clinically because of renal toxicity

number of adjuvant drugs (eg, catecholamines, sympathomimetics, antihypertensives, antiarrhythmics, and sympathetic blockers), although not anesthetics, are used to maintain homeostasis during surgery when the client's own physiologic mechanisms cannot.

During anesthesia, the anesthetist continually monitors and adjusts the client's level of anesthesia. Traditional descriptions of the stages of anesthesia have been based on the signs elicited during ether anesthesia. Today, ether is no longer in use. It has been replaced by inhalation and intravenous agents whose actions vary from those of ether. In addition, the actions tend to be agent-specific; the stages of anesthesia tend to vary with the agent and technique used. Discussion of these stages as they occur with individual anesthetic agents is beyond the scope of this chapter and can be found in textbooks on anesthesia.

Table 14–5 Common Intravenous Anesthetics

Class of Drug	Specific Drug
Barbiturates	Thiopental sodium (Pentothal) Thiamylal sodium (Surital) Methohexital sodium (Brevital)
Benzodiazepines	Diazepam (Valium) Lorazepam (Ativan) Milazolam
Narcotics	Morphine Fentanyl (Sublimaze) Alfentonil Meperidine (Demerol) Sufentanil
Dissociative	Ketamine hydrochloride (Ketalar, Ketaject)
Imidazole derivative	Etomidate

Box 14–5 Neuromuscular Blocking Agents

Ultra short-acting agent

Succinylcholine chloride (Anectine, Quelicin, Sucostrin)

Short-acting agents

Atracurium (Tracrium)

Vecuronium

Long-acting agents

Gallamine triethiodide (Flaxedil)

Metocurine iodide (Metubine)

Pancuronium bromide (Pavulon)

Tubocurarine chloride (Tubarine)

Complications of Anesthesia

The client who has undergone general anesthesia has incurred a neurologic deficit by virtue of the general depression of the CNS by these agents. Many of the complications of general anesthesia are a direct outgrowth of these CNS effects that result in diminution or loss of protective reflexes such as the gag reflex, the corneal reflex, and sympathetic nervous system reflexes. However, the risk of complications is not determined solely by the client's responses, but may also depend on the skill level of the anesthesia care provider.

The physical status category assigned to clients undergoing anesthesia has been used as a general indicator of the anesthesia risk facing a client. An analysis of several studies of anesthesia mortality demonstrated not only the wide variation in available mortality data, but also the general usefulness of the categories in Box 14–2 for determining client risk (Dripps, Eckenhoff, & Vandam, 1982). Specific complications associated with anesthesia and the risks they present to clients are multifactorial in origin. They range from the competency of the anesthesia provider, to the integrity of sophisticated equipment, to the pharmacologic reactions to specific client pathophysiology. A list of usual and unusual complications associated with anesthesia (Orkin & Cooperman, 1983) is given in Box 14–6.

Risks to Operating Room Personnel

The operating room environment combines sophisticated technology with the potential for error in its use. Although the hazards of combustion associated with the use of flammable anesthetics has disappeared since the advent of newer nonexplosive agents, dangers such as electrical shock or electrocution have increased. Various measures have been incorporated into the operating room environment to lessen the risk of electrical shock. Isolation transformers decrease the chance of undesired faulty flow of electrical current, and line isolation monitors sound alarms when excessive leakage of current occurs from a piece of electrical equipment. Laser technology also has certain risks, which are discussed later in this chapter.

Personnel in the operating room are chronically exposed to trace levels of anesthetic gases. Available data suggest that a health hazard may exist in this chronic exposure (Lecky, 1983). Based on the association of trace gas exposure with such phenomena as increased rates of congenital malformations and spontaneous abortion among female personnel and decrements in performance on psychological tests, steps have been taken to minimize trace gas exposure. Adequate ventilation of operating rooms, closed scavenging of excess gases directly from the anesthesia machine out of the room through the ventilation exhaust or suction, and trace gas monitoring programs may be instituted. The National Institute for Occupational Safety and Health has established target levels of trace gases well below those levels at which impaired psychomotor testing is known to occur. In addition to exposure to trace gases,

---

Box 14–6 Complications Associated With Anesthesia

Pharmacologic considerations

Unusual reactions to drugs

Prior drug therapy

Clinical judgment of the person administering the drug

Respiratory system

Airway obstruction

Difficult tracheal intubation and hazards of intubation

Pulmonary aspiration of gastric contents

Hypoxemia/hypercapnia

Pneumothorax

Cardiovascular system

Dysrhythmias

Failure of peripheral circulation

Pump failure

Myocardial infarction

Air embolism

Nervous system

Altered temperature regulation
  • Unintentional hypothermia
  • Malignant hyperthermia

Increased intracranial pressure

Cerebral hypoxia

Awareness during anesthesia

Prolonged emergence from effects of anesthesia

Cranial nerve injury

Renal system

Fluid and electrolyte imbalance

Oliguria

Polyuria

Urinary retention

Gastrointestinal and hepatic–biliary systems

Nausea and vomiting

Hepatic injury

Dental complications

Hematopoetic system

Transfusion reactions

Sickling of red blood cells

Obstetrics, gynecology, neonatology

Compromise of uteroplacental blood flow

Fetal depression

Uterine atony

Hypoventilation and apnea in newborn

operating room (and especially anesthesia) personnel are at risk for substance abuse, a hazard for health care personnel that has been linked to drug availability (see Chapter 10).

Regional Anesthesia

Regional anesthetics block the conduction of nerve impulses to specific sites in the body. The anesthetics, listed in Table 14–6, act by blocking nerve pathways, preventing transmission of pain and other sensations, and inhibiting motor function. Because the client remains conscious, psychological support is necessary throughout.

Spinal anesthesia involves the injection of a local anesthetic agent into the subarachnoid space at the L-3 or L-4 interspace (Figure 14–8A), where it blocks impulse conduction in the spinal nerve roots and the dorsal root ganglia (refer to Chapter 35). In *epidural anesthesia,* a local anesthetic agent is injected into the extradural space, which lies between the dura mater and the body and ligamentous structures of the spinal canal (Figure 14–8B). Epidural anesthesia is usually given in the lumbar region but may also be given in the thoracic epidural space. A *caudal block* is a form of epidural anesthesia that involves injecting the local anesthetic agent in the sacral canal. Although the amount of the anesthetic agent required for spinal anesthesia is small, the amount required in epidural anesthesia

and caudal block can be large, meeting or even exceeding toxic levels unless the dose and concentration are carefully monitored.

Peripheral nerve block anesthesia blocks peripheral nerves at specific sites. Brachial, radial, medial, and ulnar nerve blocks are used for the upper extremity. Blocks of the sciatic, femoral, obturator, and lateral cutaneous femoral nerves and nerves of the ankle are used for the lower extremity. Peripheral nerve blocks may also be used for diagnostic purposes and to relieve pain. A *Bier block* is a form of intravenous regional anesthesia to an extremity occluded by a pneumatic tourniquet. *Infiltration anesthesia* is the intracutaneous or subcutaneous injection of local anesthetics directly into tissues that are to be surgically cut or sutured, blocking the sensory nerve pathways. This may require a single injection or multiple injections in a ring surrounding the operative area. *Topical,* or *surface, anesthesia* involves the direct external application of a local anesthetic in a cream, ointment, drops, spray, or other form. Some forms are used to anesthetize traumatized skin; others are used for mucous membranes.

Regional anesthesia has several disadvantages. Protective motor and sensory functions are lost in the body area of regional anesthesia with consequences similar to general anesthesia. Clients having spinal anesthesia may experience a spinal headache (discussed under immediate postoperative care). In both spinal and epidural anesthesia,

Table 14–6 Local Anesthetic Agents

Agent	Common Use	Maximum Single Dose (mg)
Lidocaine (Xylocaine)	Infiltration; topical; peripheral nerve block; spinal; epidural; caudal	300–500*
Prilocaine (Citanest)	Infiltration; peripheral nerve block; epidural; caudal	400–600*
Mepivacaine (Carbocaine)	Infiltration; peripheral nerve block; epidural; caudal	300–500*
Etidocaine (Duranest)	Infiltration; peripheral nerve block; epidural; caudal	300–400*
Bupivacaine (Marcaine, Sensorcaine)	Infiltration; peripheral nerve block; epidural; caudal	175–250*
Dibucaine (Nupercainal, Nupercaine)	Spinal; topical	50
Procaine (Novocain)	Infiltration; epidural; caudal	500–600*
Chloroprocaine (Nesacaine)	Infiltration; epidural; caudal	600–650*
Tetracaine (Pontocaine)	Topical; infiltration; peripheral nerve block; spinal	100
Cocaine	Topical	150
Benzocaine	Topical	Unknown

*Maximum safe dose when used with epinephrine

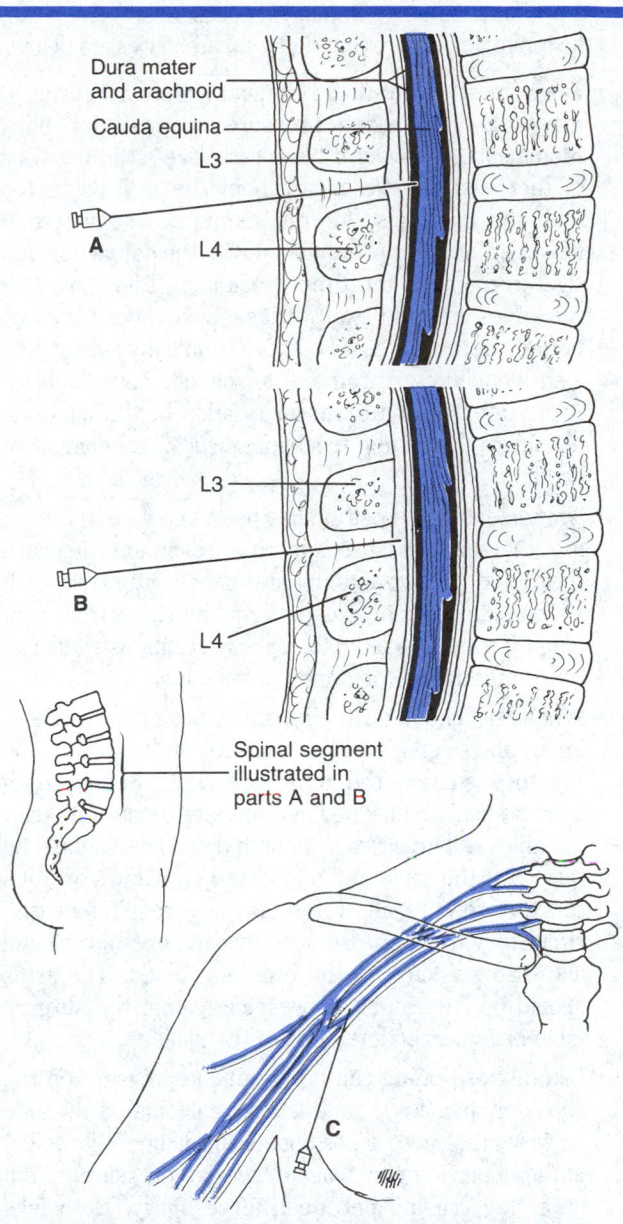

Figure 14–8

Regional anesthesia. **A.** Spinal anesthesia. The anesthetic is injected into the subarachnoid space between L-3 and L-4. **B.** Epidural anesthesia. The anesthetic is injected into the extradural space between L-3 and L-4. **C.** Peripheral nerve block. The anesthetic is injected into the brachial plexus in preparation for surgery on the client's right arm.

hypotension may occur in response to vasodilatation. With topical anesthesia of the mucous membranes of the throat (eg, for bronchoscopy), the gag reflex may be suppressed and swallowing affected for about 1 hour after the application of the anesthetic. Compromised cardiopulmonary function may require rapid resuscitation or the administration of supportive medications. The care of a client having a regional anesthetic should be as meticulous as for the client having a general anesthetic.

Other Types of Anesthesia

Other more controversial but potentially less traumatic types of anesthesia are not commonly employed in the United States. *Acupuncture* is an ancient Oriental medical practice that involves the insertion of metal needles at particular body points. The technique is used in the prevention, diagnosis, and treatment of disease as well as the control of acute and chronic pain. Why the technique is effective has not been clearly explained, but it is effective in increasing a client's pain threshold and enables most minor surgical and dental procedures to be performed without the use of other anesthetics. Acupuncture is more fully discussed in Chapter 5. *Hypnosis,* another form of anesthesia not fully understood, uses the power of suggestion to control pain. These anesthetic alternatives have advantages because vital functions are not adversely affected, postoperative respiratory and circulatory complications do not occur, and the client's food and fluid intake need not be interrupted.

SURGICAL POSITIONING

The dorsal recumbent (supine), prone, and lateral positions are the major ones used for surgery with modification for particular operations. The surgical positions are illustrated in Figure 14–9.

Poor positioning can adversely affect the musculoskeletal, neurologic, circulatory, and respiratory systems. Excessive or prolonged pressure on skin, bones, or muscles and/or poor alignment can lead to abrasions, decubitus ulcers, and postoperative pain. Pressure on superficial nerves can cause temporary or permanent paresthesia, paralysis, or loss of sensation. Excessive pressure on blood vessels can obstruct the flow of blood, depriving tissues of oxygenation and nourishment. Pressure may also contribute to pooling of blood and formation of thrombi. It is important that all nurses, not only those who work in the operating room, be aware of the inherent potentials for client injury. Damage incurred in the operating room often does not become apparent until the postoperative period.

Although clients should be securely strapped into position on the operating table, check to be sure that the client is not strapped too tightly, that bony prominences are padded, and that supporting pillows, pads, or bolsters do not cause undue pressure on a nerve or a blood vessel, thus risking nerve damage or venous thrombosis. Be sure that the extremity used for the intravenous line is properly supported and positioned to avoid excessive abduction. In the arm, excessive abduction may damage the brachial plexus causing paralysis and loss of sensation in the arm and shoulder. Radial nerve damage can cause wrist drop; damage to the medial or ulnar nerves causes hand deformities; peroneal nerve damage causes foot drop; and damage to the tibial nerve causes loss of sensation on the plantar surface of the foot. It is possible that the muscle relaxants administered to the client may contribute to the problem by reducing muscle resistance, allowing muscles to become overstretched.

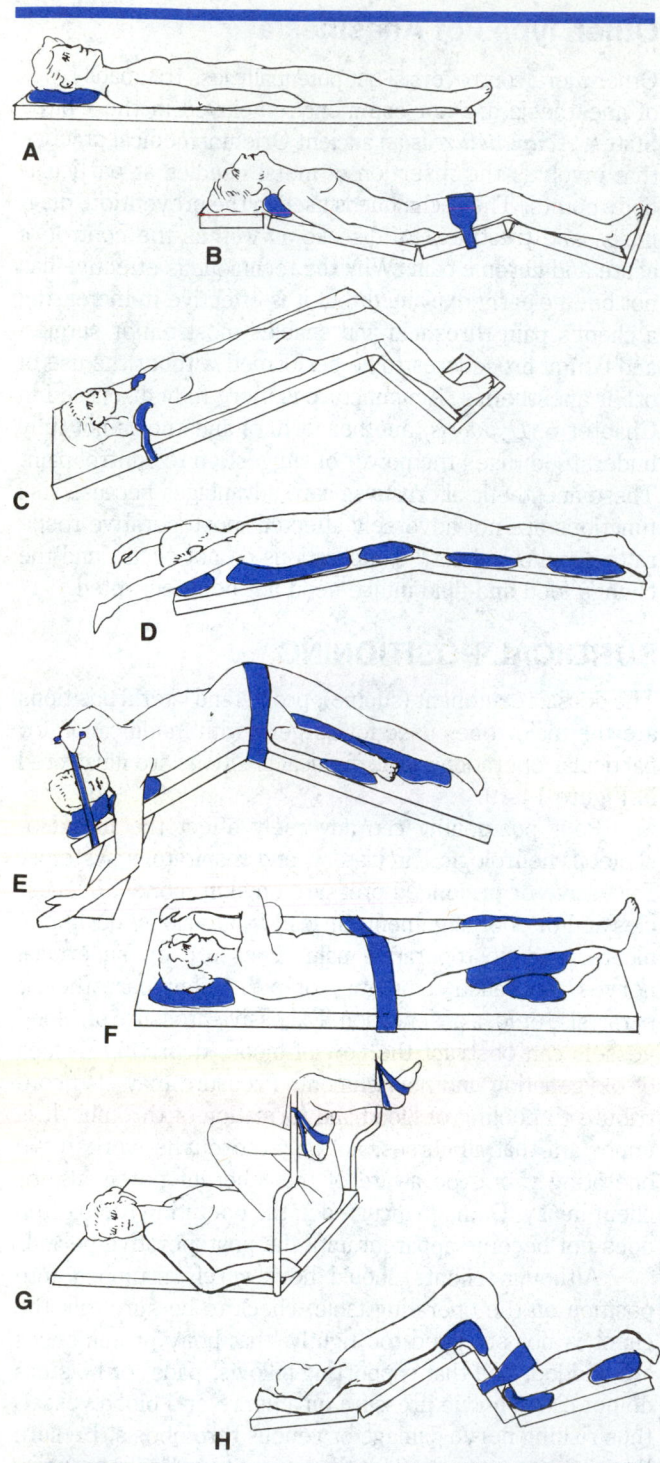

Figure 14-9

Client positions during surgery. **A.** Dorsal recumbent (supine) position for abdominal and thoracic surgery, and for surgery on the extremities. **B.** Variation of the dorsal recumbent position for operations on thyroid and neck area. **C.** Trendelenburg's position for pelvic surgery. **D.** Prone position for spinal fusion. **E.** Lateral position for kidney surgery and operations on the upper ureters. **F.** Lateral position for thoracic surgery. **G.** Lithotomy position for vaginal, perineal, or rectal surgery. **H.** Jackknife position for proctologic surgery.

Each surgical position has particular risks. The risks, and the strategies for preventing them, are discussed below.

- Dorsal positioning (used in most abdominal surgery) may cause excessive pressure on posterior bony prominences—sacrum, heels, scapulae—and the back of the head. These areas should be well protected with soft materials. Alterations in circulatory status, however, are less pronounced with the dorsal position than in many of the other positions. Take care that the knees are not flexed with supports even for short periods because vessel compression can lead to sluggish blood flow, thrombus formation, and phlebitis. Avoid internal and external rotation of the hips and shoulders by using trochanter rolls, sandbags, or padding.

- Trendelenberg's position has been known to increase intrathoracic pressure and alter respiration because the weight of the abdominal organs is redistributed. Padded shoulder braces prevent the client from slipping off the surgical table. Take precautions similar to those mentioned for dorsal positioning.

- When the client is in the prone position, the face, knees and thighs, anterior surfaces of the ankles, and the toes sustain the most pressure. Bony prominences should be padded and the feet supported under the ankles. The client's chest and abdomen should be raised off the table and supported on pillows or bolsters in order to allow for effective respiratory and circulatory function. Be sure that the eyes are closed and that pressure on the eyes is avoided. The arms should be free and not pressed against the surgical table or hyperabducted out to the sides.

- Lateral positioning can create undue pressure on the shoulder, hip, knee, and lateral malleolus on the side on which the client is positioned. In addition, the weight of the upper leg may place excessive pressure on the lower leg causing peroneal nerve injury. Both legs must be padded. Damage to the brachial plexus, medial, radial and ulnar nerves can be prevented by supporting the shoulder and preventing overextension of the arm. Using an axillary roll (a firm, cushioned pad) prevents undue pressure on the dependent axilla.

- The lithotomy position may compromise respiratory status. Improper padding or positioning in the stirrups can cause peroneal nerve damage, or damage to peripheral blood vessels. To avoid joint damage, both legs should be simultaneously manipulated into the stirrups. Be especially careful when putting elderly clients into this position.

- The jackknife position requires attention to the respiratory and circulatory status of the client, making sure that the chest and abdomen are free and unrestricted. The greatest pressure is exerted at the bends in the table. The client therefore should be supported by pads at both the groin and the knee areas and under the ankles. Precautions must be taken to avoid pressure on the nerves of the upper arm and on the lower ear and eye, to be sure that the pinna is not folded in on itself, and to avoid kinking of the neck veins.

All of these positions impede maximal inspiration and expiration. Clients having lengthy surgeries are also at risk for pressure sores and venous stasis. The client's eyes must be protected with all positions. Clients under general anesthesia will have lost the corneal reflex, and the cornea can be damaged by the movement or pressure of the surgical drape if adequate eyelid closure is not ensured. Pressure on the eyeball during surgery has been known to cause blindness resulting from thrombosis of the retinal artery.

SURGICAL TECHNIQUE

Surgery necessarily involves a break in the body tissue, compromising the host defenses of the client. As a result of surgical incising, body fluids (blood and serum) are lost. Efforts are made to minimize these consequences, but they occur nevertheless. The more extensive the surgery, the greater the consequences. Various skin closures, dressings, and drainage techniques are used by the surgeon to close the surgical incision, minimize trauma, and encourage wound healing. Nurses who are familiar with these techniques will be better able to provide intraoperative and postoperative care.

Suturing

When surgery is completed, the wound may be closed or left open. Generally, a wound or part of a wound is left open if the probability of infection is high, as with a contaminated wound. An open wound facilitates release of pus and tissue debris and allows for thorough wound cleansing.

In most cases, however, the surgical wound is closed in layers with sutures, clips, staples, skin closure strips, and even zipperlike devices. When closing the skin, the surgeon approximates the wound edges as closely as possible, manipulating the tissue as little as possible. Proper technique promotes healing with minimal scar tissue formation and loss of function.

Essentially, suturing is "sewing" tissues together; the popular term for sutures is "stitches" even though alternative closure methods such as staples may be used. Sometimes a single line of sutures is sufficient for external closure. Frequently, however, retention sutures are necessary for closure, especially in abdominal surgery or obese clients. These overlapping sutures, padded with soft material, provide additional support for the wound. Metal clips and staples bind tissue together; the mechanical methods used to apply these sutures reduce manipulation of tissue and generally cause less external scarring than suturing. Finally, skin closure strips, similar to the butterfly type of adhesive bandage, can be applied with tissues closely approximated. These strips also minimize tissue manipulation and scar tissue formation and allow for infectious drainage. When

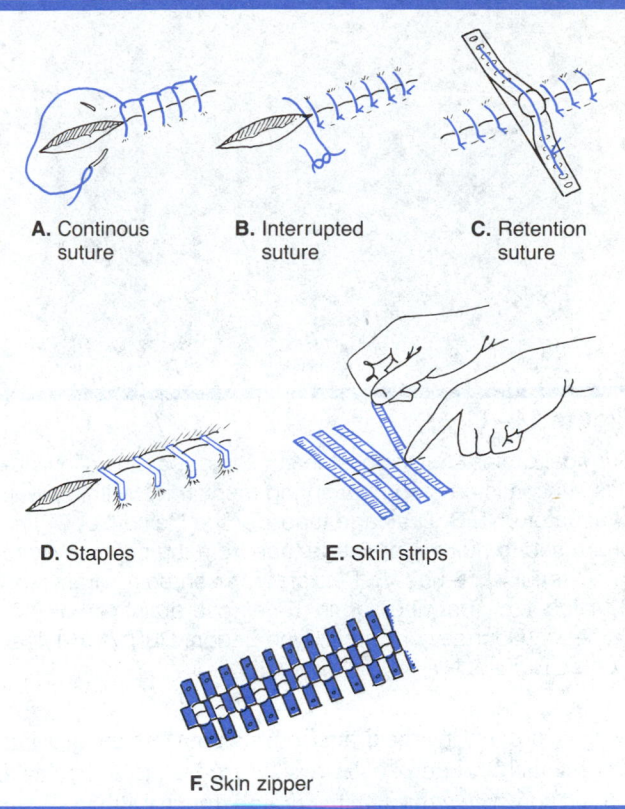

A. Continous suture B. Interrupted suture C. Retention suture D. Staples E. Skin strips F. Skin zipper

Figure 14–10

Skin closure techniques. **A.** Continuous suture **B.** Interrupted sutures. **C.** Retention suture. **D.** Staples. **E.** Skin strips. **F.** Skin zippers.

healing has progressed well, sutures, clips, and staples are usually removed within 7 to 10 days. Skin strips usually dry up and fall off as tissue heals. Types of skin closure are illustrated in Figure 14–10.

Drains and Dressings

The surgeon may place a *drain* in the incision line or may insert a drain through a separate incision near the principal wound. A drain provides an exit route for blood, serum, and debris that might otherwise accumulate in the postoperative period, causing tissue edema and pain, interfering with wound healing, and promoting infection. A drain also provides for removal of any infectious debris. The type of drain chosen depends on the depth and breadth of the wound and the need to have a drain held in place by an inflatable device (eg, a Foley catheter balloon). Drains are generally removed when a decrease in secretions indicates they are no longer needed. Types of drains are depicted in Figure 14–11.

Drains may be freestanding or attached to gravity drainage, intermittent suction (eg, Gomco suction), or to a self-contained disposable drainage system that supplies its own suction (eg, Hemovac). A common freestanding rubber drain is the Penrose drain. A sterile safety pin is generally attached to the top of the drain to provide some

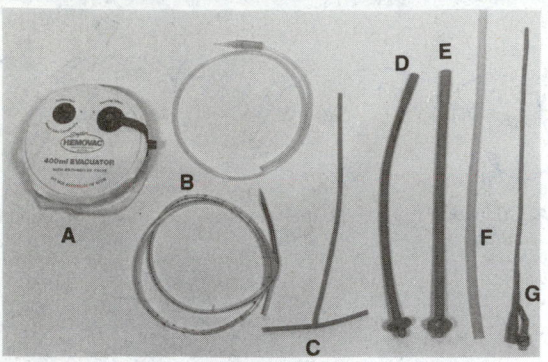

Figure 14–11

Surgical drains. **A.** Disposable suction apparatus. Continuous suction is created by a spring mechanism within the evacuator unit. **B.** Drainage tubes for the Hemovac. **C.** Trochar used to pull the drainage tube from the body cavity to the exterior. **D.** T-tube. **E.** Pezzar, or "mushroom," drain. **F.** Malecot, or "batwing," drain. **F.** Penrose drain. **G.** Foley catheter. (Courtesy of Carol Payne Zagon, RBP, VA Medical Center, Buffalo, NY)

weight, preventing the drain from slipping into the incision. Occasionally, a Penrose drain is sutured in place. Drainage should flow freely through the drain's internal lumen. When a small to moderate amount of drainage is expected, a well-padded dressing is generally sufficient for drainage absorption. When larger amounts of drainage are anticipated, bags may be applied to the skin around the drain for drainage collection. Collection bags prevent skin trauma from caustic wound drainage and facilitate the measurement of drainage as fluid output. Other types of drains, also depicted in Figure 14–11, include the T-tube, Foley catheter, mushroom drain, and Malecot drain.

A typical wound dressing is sterile gauze pads placed over the incision. The purposes of a dressing are to:

- Protect the wound from physical trauma and potential contaminants in the environment
- Absorb drainage that might otherwise accumulate, have an odor, excoriate the skin, and provide a medium for bacterial growth
- Deliver medication, either applied to the gauze (eg, povidone–iodine ointment) or imbedded in the gauze (eg, nitrofurazone or petrolatum)
- Prevent dehydration of exposed wound tissue. Wound dehydration inhibits normal wound healing by promoting unnecessary wound inflammation, discouraging epithelialization, and increasing incisional pain (Flynn & Rovee, 1982)
- Shield the wound from the client's view, especially when an incision may be perceived as a threat to body image

Recent developments in dressings include foams, gels, and transparent plastic film. The use of a transparent film

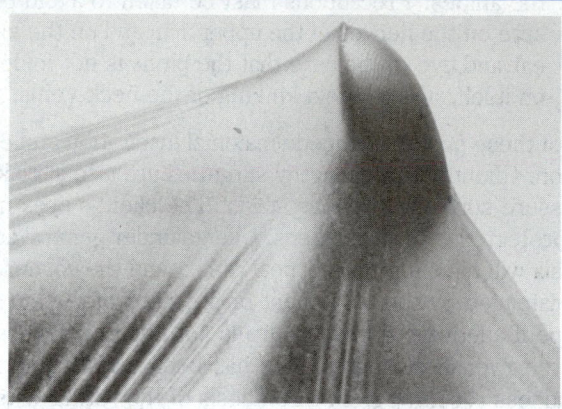

Figure 14–12

Transparent plastic surgical dressing (Tegaderm™). (Courtesy Medical Products Division, 3M, St. Paul, MN)

dressing is depicted in Figure 14–12. The transparency of these dressings allows for wound observation, protection, and aeration. Some surgeons prefer to leave a surgical wound completely undressed, avoiding potential irritation from dressings and frequent dressing changes.

Innovative Techniques

Several innovations in biomedical engineering have altered the traditional practice of surgery. The development of instruments such as the binocular operating microscope, the laser, and the cryoprobe have made possible what would once have been impossible surgery, improved the prognosis for surgical clients, decreased the extent of disfigurement the client experiences, and reduced the number of necessary postoperative lifestyle changes.

Binocular Operating Microscope

The binocular operating microscope permits the surgeon to have a brightly illuminated, enlarged three-dimensional view of the operating field. This instrument makes it possible to operate with greater precision on small structures and to visualize structures that are not visible to the naked eye without it. The subsequent development of microinstruments, microsutures, and microsurgical techniques has made it possible to perform surgeries unheard of a short time ago and to minimize damage to delicate structures. These features are extremely important in eye and ear surgery (see Chapters 72 and 76 respectively), in neurosurgery (see Chapter 39), and in surgery that requires the repair of small blood vessels or the microvascular reattachment of minute blood vessels such as occurs in free tissue transfer (see Chapter 80).

Laser

The **laser** is a device that transforms light of various frequencies into a finely focused, intense beam of light capable of mobilizing great heat and power at close range. As the beam comes into contact with tissue, the light energy is absorbed in the tissue and converted to heat. The heat causes a burn (photocoagulation) that results in a scar. The extent of tissue destruction and the depth of an incision created by the laser depends on how long the laser beam is focused on any given spot. The surgeon must be careful not to cause damage to normal tissue. The main advantage of laser surgery is that incisional surgery can be avoided in many instances. Depending on the type of operation, laser surgery can be performed without anesthesia on an ambulatory basis.

There are several different kinds of lasers in current use. They vary in which portion of the light spectrum is used to create the energy. Some wavelengths are thought to be more appropriate for specific types of surgeries, which explains why several laser types are available. The *argon laser* (blue-green) is primarily absorbed by melanin and hemoglobin and is especially effective on vascular lesions such as the port-wine stain (see Chapter 80), in removing tattoos (see Chapter 80), and in ophthalmic surgery to treat proliferative retinopathy and glaucoma (see Chapter 72). It does not remove or destroy overlying tissue. The *carbon dioxide laser* (red) produces energy which is absorbed by the fluid in cells. As the water heats and vaporizes, it causes cells to burst, destroying them. The carbon dioxide laser acts much like a surgical knife. Some of the uses of carbon dioxide lasers are in microlaryngeal and oral surgery to eradicate both benign and malignant lesions (see Chapter 21), in dermatologic surgery to treat skin lesions such as warts, neoplasms, and actinic keratosis (see Chapter 80), and in ophthalmic surgery to treat retinal lesions. The *neodymium-yttrium aluminum garnet (Nd-YAG) laser*, known more simply as the YAG laser, is a pulsed laser that is being used to treat complications of certain cataract surgeries (see Chapter 72). Unlike the other lasers, the YAG laser, called a cool laser, does not heat or burn. The newest laser, the *excimer laser*, is also a cool laser. Excimer lasers are being used for precise corneal surgery and for coronary angioplasty on an experimental basis (see Chapter 25).

The introduction of optical lasers has produced the need for operating room personnel to wear appropriate eye protection to protect themselves from stray or reflected beams of laser light. The energy from these lasers can cause eye damage, burns, or ignition of endotracheal tubes during microlaryngeal surgery for example.

An adaptation of laser therapy in which a hematoporphyrin-derivative dye is combined with a laser to treat malignant tumors has been described in Chapter 12. Other applications of laser surgery are described in the surgical approaches chapters in the units on body systems.

Cryosurgery

Cryosurgery involves the freezing and destruction of tissues through a variety of techniques. Liquid nitrogen, Freon 114, or solid carbon dioxide may be applied to tissue by a spray, with a swab, or by a super-cooled cryoprobe. Cryosurgery is most commonly used for dermatologic lesions

and cataract removal, and its specific applications are discussed in Chapters 80 and 72, respectively.

ASSESSMENT AND NURSING DIAGNOSIS

Assessment has been discussed earlier in this section. Client assessment during the intraoperative period, an ongoing process that begins with the client's admission to the operating suite, forms the basis for the general nursing diagnoses listed in Box 14–7.

PLANNING AND IMPLEMENTATION

Planning and implementation during the intraoperative period include measures to ensure emotional well-being, physical safety, and privacy. These measures are discussed in this section.

Promoting Emotional Well-Being

When entering the surgical suite, the client may experience a heightened anxiety. Anxiety may be caused by apprehension about the surgical procedure, concern about safety, and perhaps uncertainty about the diagnosis. The anxiety may bring physiological, emotional, and intellectual changes. Tachycardia with palpitations and peripheral vasodilation with flushing may occur. With mild and moderate anxiety, the client will be attentive and alert to the surroundings, although the depressive effects of preanesthesia sedation may dull cognitive and problem-solving abilities. With severe anxiety, the client's perception is less acute, tending to focus on details. With panic, the client's perception is completely disrupted; the client has lost control and is unable to understand or communicate intelligibly.

Operating room nurses can alleviate clients' anxiety in a number of ways. Nurses should introduce themselves

---

Box 14–7   Common Nursing Diagnoses Related to Intraoperative Care

Anxiety, related to awareness of surroundings during operative procedure in client having regional anesthesia

Fluid volume deficit, potential for, related to altered intake and loss of body fluids during surgery

Gas exchange, impaired, related to inability to move secretions independently

Infection, potential for, related to destruction of skin barrier by surgical incision

Injury, potential for, related to insertion of surgical instruments and supplies, loss of sensation and reflexes while anesthetized, and positioning and use of restraints

Powerlessness, related to anesthesia

Urinary elimination, alteration in, related to depressant effects of general anesthetic

to the client and explain procedures and activities before and as they are being performed. Reassure the client that the surgical team carefully monitors physiological status during surgery and that privacy will be maintained. Besides providing verbal reassurance, use touch as a means of communication. Holding the client's hand may be an especially supportive gesture. (See also Table 14–8 later in this chapter.)

If the client is to receive a general anesthetic, physical activity and talking in the operating room must be kept to a minimum until the client is unconscious. Although many activities must be performed at this time, the client should not be ignored. Once the client is unconscious, the surgical team must continue to discuss only matters relevant to the procedure. The client's sense of hearing may be especially acute during this time, and there have been reports of clients recalling conversations and their surgery even while anesthetized. In fact, there is speculation that unconscious learning may occur during anesthesia and that what is learned (eg, a grave prognosis) may influence the postoperative course. On the other hand, listening to relaxing music through headphones is thought to enhance clients' relaxation under general anesthesia.

With a regional anesthetic, the client will remain awake, although usually sedated, during the surgery. As the surgery is performed, keep the client informed of the progress. Touching and talking with the client during the procedure both distracts and supports the client.

Promoting Physical Safety and Privacy

The person accompanying the client to the operating suite (generally a staff nurse) reports to the operating room nurse (generally a circulating nurse), who admits the client to the operating suite. At this time, the preoperative preparation and medical record are again reviewed for completeness and accuracy. In particular, establish that consent has been obtained, that preoperative medication has been given if ordered, that the client has been properly identified, that blood is available as ordered, and that risks related to surgery have been identified and corrected if possible.

If the client has been sedated, accident potential is high. While the client remains on the stretcher, ensure that safety straps are secure and that the client's extremities are kept on the stretcher. Also ensure that the client is transferred from the stretcher to the operating table safely. The client should be safely secured to the table and should remain secured throughout the surgical procedure. Restraint straps should be snug but not too tight, and padding should be provided between the restraint and the client's body unless the restraint itself is padded.

As the client is positioned on the operating table, the circulating nurse should ensure that privacy and warmth are maintained as much as possible, that the body is aligned properly, and that body areas are not subjected to excessive pressure. Only necessary body areas need be exposed;

other body areas should be covered to prevent unnecessary heat loss. Reasons for heat loss include a cool temperature in the operating room, the effects of some inhalation anesthetics, and the depressant effects of general anesthesia on heat-regulating mechanisms (Kneedler & Dodge, 1983). Measures to be taken to ensure the client's safety in specific surgical positions have been discussed in the section on surgical positions.

The client's physical safety must be maintained throughout anesthetic administration. The operating room nurse shares responsibility for maintaining the client's safety, although the anesthetist carries the major responsibility. When the intended stage of anesthesia has been reached, the nurse concentrates on monitoring the client's safety and privacy. Be sure there is no excessive pressure on the client's skin, and take corrective measures as necessary. Because of the absent gag reflex and the client's inability to clear accumulated respiratory secretions, the anesthetist will suction the client if necessary. Suctioning is aided by the ET tube, if present, or an oral and/or nasal airway. The anesthetist makes sure these tubes do not place excessive pressure on the mouth or nose and protects the eyes in the absence of the corneal reflex as discussed earlier. If the client has not been catheterized, assess the client for suprapubic distention, which indicates urinary retention and, perhaps, the need for catheterization.

During the procedure, the scrub nurse helps ensure the client's safety by being efficient in anticipating the needs of the surgeon and assistants and providing instruments. Efficiency is increased if the circulating nurse has adequately prepared the room with the appropriate supplies and equipment. The circulating nurse is also responsible for ensuring the sterility of supplies and checking equipment to determine it is in safe working order. All guidelines for the maintenance and use of electrical equipment should be followed. The trend away from flammable anesthetics has reduced the chance of fire in the operating room. Nevertheless, the operating room is a hazardous environment with a great deal of electrical equipment and many substances, such as oxygen, that can support combustion.

Although all members of the surgical team use sterile technique, the circulating nurse is responsible for enforcing use of sterile technique throughout surgery. As client advocate, the circulating nurse alerts the surgical team if a break in technique is suspected. If a suspected break or actual break occurs, suspected contaminated clothing or instruments are discarded and replaced with sterile ones. The nurse also helps to protect the client from infection by appropriately disposing of contaminated materials, ensuring that instruments or supplies are cleaned and/or sterilized after surgery, and preparing the room for the next client according to agency policy.

An important aspect of protecting the client's safety is verifying that no surgical instruments, needles, or sponges (gauze pads) remain inside the client's body after suturing. Agency policies vary; most hospitals require sponge counts;

needle and instrument counts are more controversial. AORN recommends counting all three. Generally, one scrub person and one circulating person count the items both before surgery and before the surgical incision is closed. Any discrepancy must be accounted for before the incision is closed.

The client's safety is also maintained by administering appropriate fluids, as ordered, to replace body losses and prevent dehydration. Electrolyte solutions (eg, Ringer's lactate) are frequently administered during the operative period, and blood loss is replaced. When blood is administered, carefully verify that the blood has been typed and crossmatched for the particular client and that the expiration date has not been passed. Agency policy usually requires that two persons make this assessment. The nurse is also responsible for ascertaining that enough blood is on hand for the client's anticipated needs and for ordering more, if needed. In conjunction with fluid replacement, keep an accurate intake and output record, recording all administered intravenous fluids, urinary output (if the client is catheterized), blood loss, emesis (if any), and any other drainage. The intraoperative monitoring and maintenance of homeostasis and vital functions (both traditional nursing functions) are done by the anesthetist.

EVALUATION

In evaluating the effectiveness of nursing care throughout the intraoperative period, consider the following:

- Is the client less anxious as a result of the nurse's reassurance?
- Does the client remain free from tissue injury (eg, no reddened areas on the skin) from careful positioning?
- Is the client's privacy maintained by draping?
- Does the client remain free of signs of decreased circulating fluid volume (eg, hypotension) as a result of administered blood and intravenous solutions?

Section V: The Nursing Process in Postoperative Care

The central goal of postoperative nursing care is the return of the client to an optimal level of functioning. To accomplish this goal, the nurse must understand factors that affect postsurgical recovery—the expected consequences and potential complications of anesthesia and surgery in the immediate and later postoperative periods. These two periods are discussed separately in the next section, although much of the nursing care is similar.

NURSING CARE IN THE IMMEDIATE POSTOPERATIVE PERIOD

Immediately after surgery, the client is generally cared for in a postanesthesia recovery area close to the operating room. There members of the surgical team can conveniently monitor the client's progress periodically and quickly return the client to the operating room in the event of an emergency. The client is kept there under the care of a recovery room nurse until having recovered from the effects of anesthesia (motor and sensory functions begin to return), vital signs are stable, and the wound dressing remains intact with no signs of hemorrhage.

To ensure continuity of care, the surgical team reports to the recovery room nurse about the client's status upon admission to the recovery area. This report includes information about the kind of surgery performed, the presence and status of drains and dressings, the length of time the client remained in the operating room and under anesthesia, the kind of anesthesia given, the status of the client's vital functions throughout the intraoperative period, the need for oxygen and/or ventilation, the need for monitoring (central venous pressure, arterial pressure), the status of fluid and electrolyte balance and the intraoperative intake and output record, the need for blood transfusions, and the presence and patency of any other tubes (eg, a Foley catheter). Any complications during the intraoperative period (eg, bradycardia, cardiac arrest) should also be communicated, along with appropriate therapies to be instituted if they recur.

Nursing Assessment

Nursing diagnoses must be determined to plan appropriate nursing care for the client in the immediate postoperative period. Diagnoses are based on thorough understanding of the recovery of persons from anesthesia and surgery and an assessment of each client.

Recovery From Anesthesia and Residual Effects

In the immediate postoperative period, the effects of anesthesia can be expected to wear off gradually. Until motor and sensory functions return, however, the client remains at risk for injury (as discussed in the intraoperative section). The client may have an altered response to various noxious stimuli that may circumvent normal protective responses.

As the depressive effects of the anesthetic subside, motor and sensory functions gradually return. The client may begin to feel pain and react to it by moaning or moving around, potentially causing harm to himself or herself and to the incision site. The client with an ET tube or oral airway may fight it as anesthesia wears off and coughing and swallowing reflexes return. Artifical airways are removed once protective airway reflexes return, and once the client's ability to support adequate ventilation and oxygenation has been assessed to be adequate. Afterward, the client should be closely assessed for ability to breathe normally and clear secretions, and suctioning should be continued as necessary. An ET tube should not be removed until it is certain that the client has muscular control and can maintain the airway. Often, arterial blood gas determinations and tidal volume assessments are made before removal of the tube; the anesthetist, in conjunction with the recovery room nurse, determines the appropriateness of removing the tube. Premature removal of an ET tube or oral airway can result in obstruction of respiratory passages by the tongue or secretions. On the other hand, if it is determined that a postoperative ET tube is required, but the client is not tolerating the tube, measures to control ''bucking'' or ''fighting'' of the tube may be taken to ensure respiratory integrity.

The time it takes an anesthetic to wear off depends on the length of the procedure (longer procedures produce greater saturation of body tissues with anesthetics, resulting in longer recovery periods); the kind and amount of anesthetic; and the individual client's reaction to the anesthetic. With inhalation anesthetics, recovery is usually rapid; the client may be conscious and able to move when admitted to the recovery area. Nevertheless, the depressive effects of the anesthetic may still affect the client's respiratory function, cognitive and problem-solving abilities, and motor and sensory function for some time, even up to 24 hours. Recovery from intravenous anesthetics, such as ketamine, is also fairly rapid (within 3 hours), although the client may experience similar prolonged effects. Hyperactivity, delusions, and/or hallucinations may occur as the client emerges from the effects of ketamine.

Nausea and vomiting are a consequence of some anesthetics, as well as some surgical procedures, making the client uncomfortable and increasing the risk of aspiration. The client may feel chilled because the body temperature may be low, as discussed earlier. The client may shiver in an effort to create body heat, at the same time increasing oxygen needs. Oxygen needs may be greatly increased, compounded by the residual depressive effects of general anesthesia on respiratory function resulting in hypoventilation.

Recovery from regional anesthesia is also gradual. As the client's sensory functions return, pain is perceived, and nursing interventions to promote comfort will be necessary. As motor function returns to the anesthetized area, the client may move inappropriately, causing damage to a surgical area or to an unprotected body part.

The return of consciousness and the return of motor and sensory functions, occur in phases. The client who has received a general anesthetic shows signs of arousal when reflex actions, such as the corneal and swallowing reflexes, return. Initially, the client advances from stupor to lethargy and then to drowsiness before becoming fully alert and conscious. The stuporous client responds poorly to verbal and painful stimuli and is still well under the effects of anesthesia. The lethargic, drowsy client demonstrates dull behavior and may fall asleep intermittently. This client may respond to painful stimuli but still be experiencing some effects of anesthesia. The conscious client

is alert, awake, fully responsive to verbal stimuli, and has recovered from the effects of anesthesia. As motor functions return, the client may first feel a heaviness in the body, particularly in the extremities, and movements are difficult and uncoordinated. Gradually, the client's sense of self and ability to move become more definite.

Assess level of consciousness by observing the client's behavior and orientation. Does the client respond to pain? Does the client respond to name? Is the client able to carry on a conversation? Does the client know where he or she is? Generally, the client will first respond to pain; then to verbal stimuli; then to the surroundings; and eventually, the client will be able to communicate. At first, the client will be disoriented, but gradually orientation to person, place, and time return. Assess motor ability by asking the client to squeeze the nurse's hand. Motor and sensory function of the affected area can be assessed in the same manner when the client has had a regional anesthetic.

The rate, rhythm, and quality of respirations should be closely monitored, generally upon admission to the recovery room and every 5 minutes for 15 minutes and then every 15 minutes. Abnormal rate, irregular rhythm, and noisy respirations may indicate an underlying problem and require intervention. As a result of the depressive effects of a general anesthetic, bradypnea (respirations less than 10 per minute) may be noted. Generally, the client will remain in the recovery room until the respiratory rate normalizes (between 10 and 20 breaths/minute). Breath sounds should be assessed for signs of accumulated secretions in respiratory passages and/or for diminution of sounds associated with atelectasis, pneumonia, or pneumothorax. Cyanosis of the nail beds and/or lips should also be observed. Cyanosis may signal a need for the administration of oxygen, although restlessness is an earlier sign of hypoxia. Restlessness may also result from anxiety, pain, or bleeding.

Respiratory obstruction is a serious occurrence in the immediate postoperative period and may occur anywhere along the respiratory tract. The most common cause is soft tissue obstruction of the upper airway. Laryngospasm, a potentially life-threatening event, also must be recognized and treated quickly. While soft tissue obstruction is usually caused by posterior relaxation of the tongue, laryngospasm may be caused by the stimulation of the vocal cords by oral secretions, blood, or vomitus.

Residual Physiological and Psychosocial Effects of Surgery

As already noted, systemic stress responses from the surgical experience affect the entire person physically and psychologically. Although the body's stress responses generally enhance physiological and psychological coping, they may have negative consequences if unchecked. Nursing care is directed at alleviating or minimizing stress to foster a quick recovery.

Being aware of common physiological sequelae of stress helps the nurse assess an individual client's responses and plan nursing care. Blood pressure, pulse, and respiration commonly increase in the client under stress. These responses may not be apparent, however, until the client emerges from the effects of anesthesia. Hormonal regulation of renal function conserves water and sodium, maintaining circulating fluid volume and blood pressure (see Units Five and Seven). To maintain this defensive body action, fluid and electrolyte balance is carefully assessed and fluids are administered in the immediate postoperative period, with attention to preventing fluid overload. Peripheral vasoconstriction accompanying stress may contribute to the pallor commonly observed in the postoperative period. An increase in circulating glucose, as a result of physiological adaptation to provide for needed energy, can precipitate transient hyperglycemia (elevated blood sugar) and glycosuria (abnormal presence of sugar in the urine).

Aside from these generalized stress responses, specific local responses, such as inflammation and bleeding, result from the tissue trauma of surgery. Although blood loss should not be excessive postoperatively, the potential for it requires periodic assessment, especially in the immediate postoperative period.

Finally, the postsurgical client may have other more specific physiological, psychosocial, and environmental stresses. Hypoxia, metabolic changes, and fluid and electrolyte imbalances precipitated by surgery and/or anesthesia may occur. The effects of pain, drugs (including the anesthetic), and the extent of the surgical trauma all contribute as well. Psychosocial stresses include fears associated with pain, death, mutilation, and the effects of anesthesia. Furthermore, the powerlessness, depersonalization, and physical exposure of the surgical experience are stressful. Finally, overwhelming environmental stresses may contribute to sensory alteration (deprivation and/or overload). Physiological, psychosocial, and environmental sources of stress in the postoperative period are summarized in Table 14–7. These stresses all contribute to anxiety, which may be severe in the immediate postoperative period.

Nursing Diagnosis

An understanding and analysis of these factors enable the nurse to determine nursing diagnoses specific to the care of a client in the immediate postoperative period. Nursing diagnoses common to the client in this period listed in Box 14–8 can be used as general guidelines.

Planning and Implementation

Care during the postanesthesia period is planned according to the nursing diagnoses. The plan of care is aimed at ensuring a safe recovery of the client from the immediate effects of anesthesia and surgery.

Promoting Safe Recovery From Anesthesia

The primary goal of immediate postoperative nursing care is the safe recovery and arousal of the client from the effects of anesthesia. The nurse is responsible for initiating communication with the client, attempting to stir the client from the effects of anesthesia, and providing orienting cues. As the client gradually becomes oriented, alert, and able to move, the recovery room nurse can promote postanesthesia recovery by encouraging the client to breathe deeply and move the arms and legs. These actions encourage elimination from the body of inhalation anesthetics (through exhalation) and other anesthetics (through increased circulation and kidney perfusion and elimination).

Table 14–7 Sources of Stress in the Postanesthesia Recovery Period

Physiological	Psychosocial	Environmental
Hypoxia	Fear of mutilation caused by surgery	Sensory overload because of constant noise, lights, unfamiliar treatments
Metabolic changes	Fear of death	Sensory deprivation because of immobility, restraints, casts, dressings
Electrolyte imbalance	Fear of revealing too much while recovering from effects of anesthesia	Lack of familiar orienting cues given by clocks, calendars, radio or television, meals, windows, visiting hours
Drugs	Fear of complications from anesthesia	Proximity to other clients who may be confused, crying, distressed, or in pain
Pain	Separation from family and friends	Constant attendance by physicians, nurses, and other health team members
Length of time spent under anesthesia	Depersonalization	Separation from familiar environment
Extent of surgical trauma	Powerlessness	
	Pain	
	Inability to reduce tension in usual way	
	Physical exposure	

Box 14–8 Common Nursing Diagnoses Related to Immediate Postoperative Care

Comfort, alteration in, related to pressure on nerve endings caused by surgical incision and recovery from anesthetic

Communication, impaired verbal, related to depressive effects of general anesthetic and/or sedation

Fluid volume deficit, potential for, related to surgical and postsurgical fluid losses

Gas exchange, impaired, potential for, related to respiratory depression associated with general anesthesia, inability to move secretions independently associated with depressed gag reflex, and horizontal positioning for surgery

Impairment of skin integrity, potential for, related to immobility associated with anesthesia and surgery, surgical positioning, and use of restraints

Injury, potential for, related to residual effects of anesthetics and operative sedation

Sensory perceptual alteration, potential for, related to depressive effects of anesthetic, excessive and inappropriate environmental stimuli, separation from significant others and usual surroundings, or effects of ketamine anesthesia

Urinary elimination, alteration in, related to depressive effects of general anesthetics (and regional anesthetics affecting the bladder)

If the client has received spinal anesthesia, spinal headache, a potential complication of spinal anesthesia, must be prevented. Although the cause of spinal headaches is unclear, a decrease in cerebrospinal fluid (through leakage at the injection site) may be a contributing factor. These headaches are most likely to occur in clients under 60 years of age, and they are more prevalent in pregnant clients. Their incidence is less than 1% when a 25-gauge spinal needle is used. When a 25-gauge (or smaller) needle is used, there may be no reason to limit the client's activity after the return of sensory motor function. If the client experiences a headache upon elevating the head, the client should return to the supine position and increase fluid intake. In some institutions, clients are encouraged to remain supine for 6 to 24 hours after a spinal anesthetic, especially when the spinal needle used is larger than 25-gauge.

Whether the client has received a general or a regional anesthetic, safety precautions must be instituted in the immediate postoperative period. Although the client may feel alert and capable of moving, movements may be uncoordinated, and residual drowsiness and sedation probably persist. Therefore, the client should remain restrained on the stretcher throughout this period. If the client is recovering from ketamine, excessive restlessness, delusions, and hallucinations can be prevented by maintaining a quiet environment and disturbing the client as little as possible. An aspect of safety is protecting the client from the effects of hypothermia. The client's temperature is generally monitored every 15 minutes. Measures to maintain body warmth, such as covering the client, should be instituted.

Promoting Adequate Respiratory Function

Especially when the client has received a general anesthetic, nursing measures for ensuring adequate respiratory function go hand in hand with measures related to the client's recovery from anesthesia. The first concern is maintaining an adequate airway. If the client arrives in the recovery room with an endotracheal tube, it should be well secured. These devices provide a means for suctioning secretions. Often, the client with an endotracheal tube may require continued ventilatory assistance with a respirator. The nurse confers with the anesthetist about ventilatory care for the individual client.

The client must be positioned so that a patent airway is maintained, secretions can be suctioned, and oxygen can be administered, if required. Immediately after surgery, the client is usually positioned laterally to discourage pooling of secretions and vomitus. The lateral position also helps prevent the tongue from occluding the pharynx. Remember that the client will not be able to cough or swallow until the gag reflex returns, and any mucous secretions and vomitus must be suctioned by the nurse as required. Take special care in suctioning clients with head or neck surgery, because they are especially susceptible to injury from suctioning. Use proper aseptic technique when suctioning, and assess breath sounds afterward to determine whether suctioning was effective. Likewise, administer oxygen safely and appropriately, when it is ordered.

To reverse the depressant effects of anesthetics on respiratory function (hypoxia and hypoventilation with atelectasis), encourage deep breathing to expand the lungs fully and coughing to remove accumulated secretions. Clients are often surprised at the amount of secretions they expectorate postoperatively; secretions accumulate as a result of maintaining one position during surgery and the hypoventilation associated with anesthesia.

Promoting Adequate Circulatory Function

Throughout the immediate postoperative period, circulatory function may continue to be compromised by the effects of anesthesia, surgical positioning, fluid and blood losses, and general immobility. Therefore, the nurse generally monitors the client's pulse and blood pressure every 15 minutes for adequate function. An abnormally low blood pressure and increased pulse rate may signify shock and should be reported. Peripheral circulation must also be monitored to ensure adequate perfusion of peripheral tissues and prevent excessive pressure on peripheral vessels. The nurse also monitors the client's fluid balance. Adequate fluid balance is necessary to maintain blood pressure and body tissue perfusion. Fluids and blood should be administered safely and as ordered.

Remember that surgery may impose a great deal of stress on the client's heart. With preexisting cardiac disease (or even without preexisting disease), the heart may be unable to cope with the increased work load; heart failure or myocardial infarction, may occur (see Chapter 24), indicated by changes in pulse, blood pressure, and respiration.

Promoting Comfort

As the client recovers from the effects of the anesthetic, he or she will begin to feel incisional pain. Make a thorough pain assessment (including both subjective and objective observations; refer to Chapter 5) ascertaining the quality, severity, and location of the client's pain. Do not assume that "pain" necessarily means only "incisional pain." General muscular aches and pains may also occur as a consequence of prolonged surgical immobility and positioning. The client may also describe a sore throat, a residual effect of endotracheal intubation and the drying effects of anticholinergics. Also be alert for unexpected pain, which might indicate a problem such as myocardial infarction.

Nursing comfort measures to alleviate pain, such as turning, positioning, and distraction, may be useful, but pain medication will also be necessary and should not be withheld. Because general anesthetics have residual depressive effects on blood pressure, respiratory status, and circulation, the client usually receives an attenuated dose (usually one-half dose) of an analgesic. (Guidelines for modifying analgesia in the early postoperative period are given later in this chapter.) Before administering a narcotic, especially morphine, carefully assess the client's respiratory status and determine that further respiratory depression will not seriously compromise the client's status. Because these drugs may cause hypotension, blood pressure should also be assessed to ensure that further lowering of the blood pressure will not be dangerous.

Monitor the effectiveness of pain-relief techniques and drugs in relieving the client's pain. Does the client appear more comfortable? Less restless? Does the client state that the pain is less troublesome? In some cases, the nurse may need to confer with the surgeon or anesthetist, advising them that the pain medication dosage needs to be increased to bring relief.

Providing Wound Care

In the immediate postoperative period, observing for hemorrhage is a major responsibility of the nurse caring for a surgical client. A dressing is generally left in place, and the nurse should carefully monitor wound drainage by circling any drainage and reevaluating drainage spots continually for major increases in bleeding. Check both the dressing and the linen underneath the client. On first inspection, a dressing may look dry because blood is draining to a dependent location by gravity. Dressings are not generally changed but are reinforced as necessary. Unexpected severe bleeding is immediately reported to the surgeon. The client may need to be returned to the operating room for further ligation of bleeding vessels if heavy bleeding persists.

Excessive bleeding from drains may also be noted and may also signal a need for further surgery.

Drains or other equipment that may be inserted in the surgical wound should be cared for as necessary. A drain might need to be connected to suction or to gravity drainage, or a wound might need to be irrigated as ordered. Depending on the surgery, specific assessments and interventions may be called for. For example, after vascular surgery (eg, repair of an abdominal aortic aneurysm), circulation distal to the surgical area will need to be monitored. (See the chapters about surgical approaches to disorders of specific body systems.)

Reducing Anxiety and Promoting Normal Sensory Status

As discussed earlier, the postoperative client who is recovering from the immediate effects of anesthesia and surgery may experience severe anxiety. Nursing measures should be directed at reducing the client's anxiety level. Orienting the client to the environment as soon as the client is responsive and explaining procedures and equipment are especially helpful. Other nursing actions are suggested in Table 14–8.

Providing Pychosocial Support

The emotional needs of the client, family members, and friends must also be considered in the immediate postoperative period. As soon as possible after surgery, contact the client's family members or significant others and advise them that the surgery is completed and that the client is recovering as anticipated. This action can allay fears and may help to relax the client, who may be concerned that family members are worried.

Although family members generally are not permitted to visit the client in the recovery room they should be advised of the anticipated time when the client will be transferred to the surgical unit. When the client returns to the surgical unit, visiting is usually permitted, depending on the client's condition.

Providing Continuity of Care

A postoperative client is generally transferred to the surgical unit when:

- The client has fully recovered from the depressive effects of the anesthetic.
- The surgical wound is intact and without excessive unexpected bleeding or drainage.
- The client is considered stable, with respirations in the normal range, adequate palpable pulses, adequate blood pressure, and temperature approaching normal limits.

With transfer of the client, nurses provide for continuity of care by accurate and thorough written documentation of care and the client's status. The recovery room nurse should also give the surgical unit nurse a thorough

Table 14 – 8 Strategies to Reduce Severe Anxiety and Panic in Postanesthesia Clients	
Nursing Action	**Rationale**
Conduct thorough assessment	Determine whether there is a physiological basis (eg, hypoxia) for restlessness
Stay with client	Leaving client alone may further increase anxiety
Use short, simple sentences	With high anxiety, there is decreased ability to make sense of sensory input
Use firm and authoritative but kind voice	With high anxiety, internal control is lacking; it is important to convey ability to provide external controls
Minimize environmental stimuli	The client is already overwhelmed by stimuli
Focus the client's diffuse energy on a task such as deep breathing, exercising legs or feet, counting, or other simple activities	Diffuse energy may be drained off until anxiety is more manageable
Consider the need for a sedative or pain medication	Sedatives and narcotic analgesics should be given when warranted, but pronounced depression of the circulatory, respiratory, or central nervous systems may follow. The dose in the recovery room is usually about *one-half* that given after full recovery from anesthesia

oral report; this oral report facilitates the transfer and further promotes continuity of care.

Documentation in the immediate postoperative period may involve the use of flow sheets, progress records, nursing progress notes, and care plans. Whatever the form for documentation, the content is similar, including:

- Vital signs
- Respiratory and circulatory status assessment
- Client's level of consciousness and motor and sensory abilities
- Presence of pain or discomfort
- Condition of dressing and wound
- Presence and patency of tubes
- Urinary output
- Medications, intravenous fluids, and blood ordered and administered
- Nursing interventions and client responses to nursing interventions

Evaluation

During the immediate postoperative period, the nurse continually monitors the effectiveness of nursing interventions. Is the client breathing easier as a result of lying on a side? Is the client more oriented to time, place, and person as a result of the nurse's providing sensory clues? Does the client remain free from injury? Are respirations, blood pressure, pulse, and temperature within the anticipated range? Ongoing evaluation helps the nurse to decide whether particular interventions should continue or whether the nursing care plan should be revised.

NURSING CARE IN THE LATER POSTOPERATIVE PERIOD

In the later postoperative period, the client recovers from the residual effects of the surgical experience, usually on a surgical unit or in an intensive care unit, if necessary. In the final stage of recovery the client is usually at home.

Nursing Assessment

In caring for the postoperative client during recovery, the nurse must be aware of potential complications. Especially important to assess are respiratory and circulatory needs.

Assessing Respiratory Needs
A number of respiratory complications may occur in the later postoperative period. Those associated with anesthesia have been discussed in the previous section. Ventilation of the lungs is inhibited by the horizontal position during surgery and by bed rest after surgery. Mucous secretions may accumulate, leading to pneumonia, bronchitis, respiratory obstruction, or atelectasis.

After the client has been transferred back to the unit from the postanesthesia recovery room, monitoring of respiratory status is generally reduced to every half hour and then to every hour, every 2 hours, and eventually every 4 hours if the client's status is satisfactory. Auscultate and percuss the lungs periodically to be sure secretions are not building up. (Auscultation and percussion are described in Chapter 7.) Careful assessment of breath sounds; skin color; and rate, rhythm, and quality of respirations help ensure prompt detection of any complications. Assessment should be continued throughout the postoperative recovery period.

Pulmonary embolism is a serious potential complication of surgery secondary to thrombus formation. Sudden onset of dyspnea and severe chest pain may indicate this life-threatening condition and should be reported immediately. Pay special attention to clients identified as high risk in the preoperative period—those whose breathing ability has been compromised by cigarette smoking, lung disease, age, or obesity.

Assessing Circulatory Needs

During postoperative recovery, the client is at risk for pooling of blood, thrombophlebitis, and phlebothrombosis. Ongoing assessment is required for prevention and early detection of these conditions.

Venous stasis, a consequence of postoperative bed rest, increases the coagulability of the blood and the client's susceptibility to **phlebothrombosis,** the formation of a blood clot in a vein, usually in the legs. Thrombi that break free from the wall of the vein become emboli, which may be carried to other areas by the bloodstream and cause organ dysfunction. Emboli involving the heart, lungs, or brain can have fatal consequences. Inflammation of the veins **(thrombophlebitis)** may begin in the preoperative or intraoperative periods because of trauma to the veins. Careless transfer of the sedated or anesthetized client to or from the operating table, stretchers, or the client's bed can cause trauma to veins. Prolonged pressure on veins, particularly those on the calf of the leg, may also cause thrombophlebitis and embolus formation. Early signs of thrombophlebitis include calf tenderness, pain with standing, or a positive Homans' sign (pain in the leg when the foot is dorsiflexed).

Assessing Nutritional and Fluid and Electrolyte Needs

If the client remains NPO during the later postoperative period, fluid and electrolyte balance is maintained by intravenous administration. Intake and output must be carefully monitored, and the nurse must be alert for signs of fluid overload or deficit. Careful monitoring and charting of skin turgor, urinary output, and intravenous setups are imperative. Fluid and electrolyte balance is discussed in detail in Chapter 5, and total parenteral nutrition is discussed in Chapter 8.

When prolonged fasting is required, detailed nutritional assessment should be ongoing, and the client should be weighed daily. This is particularly important, because malnutrition or nutrient deficiencies (see Chapter 8) prolong wound healing. Fluid balance must be continually assessed for all such clients, and intake and output records should be scrupulously maintained and carefully analyzed. Wound drainage, nasogastric tube drainage, and vomitus must be included in intake and output charting because these may contribute to fluid imbalance. If the threat of fluid imbalance is grave or when imbalance has been identified, an in-dwelling catheter may be inserted to facilitate accurate assessment. The nurse should also observe the client for signs of dehydration: thirst, dry skin, or poor skin turgor. The nurse should also be familiar with signs and symptoms of electrolyte imbalance and should observe for them as well.

Assessing Elimination Needs

Surgery may hamper elimination of body wastes (urine and feces). Adequate activity is one of many factors influencing gastrointestinal function; a depressed activity level slows it. The acute stress of surgery itself and the general depressive effects of anesthesia and intraoperative medications also can be expected to alter gastrointestinal and urinary function for some time in the later postoperative period.

Gastrointestinal peristalsis will be depressed, possibly leading to constipation or *paralytic ileus,* a condition in which the intestinal wall is distended and aperistalsis occurs. Paralytic ileus is more likely in the client who has had a general anesthetic and/or abdominal or pelvic surgery with manipulation of organs. Until peristalsis resumes, foods will not pass normally through the gastrointestinal tract. The client will be required to follow a restricted diet which, compounded by fluid losses, may promote constipation and dehydration. Accurate assessment for return of normal peristalsis is an important aspect of postoperative nursing care. Among the signs to observe are diminished or absent bowel sounds, abdominal distention, and failure to pass flatus or stool. Periodic auscultation for bowel sounds continues until their return is evident.

Similar physiological effects on the bladder and micturition may result in oliguria (reduced amount of urine) or urinary retention with bladder distention. Although not necessarily a cause for concern, oliguria because of fluid loss and the stress of surgery should be reported. If fluids are being replaced, the amount of urine being excreted should increase. The micturition reflex may be depressed by anesthesia, however, and urinary retention may occur in the client who has had general or spinal anesthesia. If retention occurs, the client will experience suprapubic discomfort, and the nurse may observe evidence of suprapubic distention.

Assessing Comfort and Safety Needs

Surgery may compromise both comfort and safety. The nurse should continually assess the client's environment for hazardous conditions.

General comfort should also be considered. Poor hygiene, dry mouth, confinement to a single position, and abdominal or suprapubic distention can cause discomfort. Generalized muscular aches and pains may be felt in the later postoperative period as a consequence of intraoperative positioning and the use of restraints. Sore throat may also continue through this period from endotracheal intubation and/or the use of anticholinergics. The surgical incision and the actual cutting or retraction of fascia and muscles may contribute to postoperative discomfort.

Some clients may discuss the comfort problem, but

others may not, depending on their cultural orientation or physical condition. Clients having surgery of the chest, anorectum, joints, back, and upper abdomen generally experience the greatest postoperative pain. Observe the client's behavior and inquire about the client's comfort.

The client with postoperative pain appears anxious and restless. To provide medications for pain relief, obtain an accurate description of the pain if the client is able to provide it. What precipitates the pain? What relieves it? What is its quality? Sharp? Dull? Throbbing? Burning? How severe is it? How long does it last? Is it steady or intermittent? Where is it felt? In the incisional area? All over? (Tools for pain assessment are in Chapter 5.) To avoid oversedating or undersedating the client, determine what intraoperative drugs the client has received. Clients who received a tranquilizer, narcotic, or both, may be pain-free when they first arrive in their room. Those who receive only inhalant anesthesia may have received a parenteral analgesic in the recovery room. If not, they may need relief from pain upon arriving in their room. General guidelines for analgesia are:

- The client may receive a postoperative narcotic analgesic approximately 1 to 1½ hours after the intraoperative administration of meperidine (Demerol) or morphine.

- The client who has received naloxone (Narcan) to relieve respiratory depression may have severe pain in the recovery room or upon return to the unit. The client will need a postoperative narcotic analgesic because naloxone is a quick-acting narcotic antagonist.

- The client who has received intravenous droperidol (Inapsine) during surgery should have the standard dose of a narcotic analgesic reduced by one-third to one-half during the first 8 to 12 hours postoperatively because of the drug's potentiating effects on narcotics.

- The client who has received intravenous diazepam (Valium) or lorazepam (Ativan) during surgery should have the standard dose of a narcotic analgesic reduced by one-third to one-half during the first 2 to 4 hours postoperatively because these drugs also have a potentiating effect on narcotics.

Assessing Motor and Sensory Needs

As already noted, assessment during the immediate postoperative period focuses on restoration of normal motor and sensory function. During the later postoperative course, the nurse continues to assess vital signs and verbal and nonverbal communication. Is the client oriented to time, place, and person? Is the client grunting, grimacing, or otherwise responding to questions or other stimuli? Is the client showing signs of sensory overload or sensory deprivation (see Chapter 4). The client is necessarily immobilized during surgery and for some time thereafter. The longer the immobilization during and after surgery, the greater the potential for complications from immobility.

Assessing Wound Care Needs

Throughout the postoperative period, assess the wound for evidence of normal healing; expected inflammation; and unexpected complications such as infection, dehiscence, or evisceration. Check to make sure that drainage tubes are patent. A low-grade fever (below 37.8°C or 101°F), associated with the inflammatory process, is generally expected postoperatively and may persist for 2 to 3 days with uncomplicated wound healing. Thereafter, a fever generally signifies an infection.

The wound should be assessed at least daily in the later postoperative period and more frequently if problems are identified. Signs and symptoms of wound-healing problems are often subtle. For example, serous drainage, no matter how small the amount, between the 5th and 12th postoperative day should alert the nurse to the potential for dehiscence. Reporting the potential for dehiscence before it occurs saves the client pain. Observing for and reporting signs of redness, induration, or purulent drainage help to prevent or decrease the severity of infection. An infected surgical wound adds about 5 to 7 days to the hospital stay (Curtin, 1984). Sometimes clients alert the nurse to impending dehiscence or evisceration by describing a "giving" sensation in the operative area.

Assessing Psychosocial Needs

Faced with body image changes to accept, altered lifestyle patterns to adjust to, and temporary or permanent role change, clients usually continue to be anxious during the later postoperative period. The nurse is responsible for assessing the psychosocial impact of surgery on each client.

Nursing Diagnosis

From a thorough analysis of the assessment factors for the postoperative period, with other factors discussed earlier in this chapter, the nurse formulates nursing diagnoses for the later postoperative period. Some nursing diagnoses common to this period are listed in Box 14–9.

Planning and Implementation

Nursing plans and interventions for the later postoperative period are aimed primarily at meeting needs related to respiration, circulation, nutritional and fluid and electrolyte status, elimination, comfort and safety, motor and sensory status, wound care, and psychosocial status. Continuity of care is provided by adequately preparing the client for discharge. Nursing care for clients having particular surgical procedures is discussed in the units about body systems.

Meeting Respiratory Needs

Once fully recovered from anesthesia, the client must be properly positioned to facilitate adequate ventilation of the lungs. The client confined to bed should be kept in the high- or semi-Fowler's position as much as possible if the client's condition permits. The client is turned from

Box 14–9 Common Nursing Diagnoses Related to Later Postoperative Care

Airway clearance, ineffective, related to ineffective coughing

Bowel elimination, alteration in: constipation, related to decreased activity level

Breathing pattern, ineffective, related to incisional pain

Comfort, alteration in: pain, related to tissue manipulation during surgery

Fluid volume deficit, related to nasogastric and wound drainage

Gas exchange, impaired, related to failure to breathe deeply

Injury: potential for infection, related to incisional disruption of the integument

Nutrition, alteration in: less than body requirements, related to postoperative NPO status

Self-concepts, disturbance in: body image, related to loss of body part

Skin integrity, impairment of, related to surgical incision and excessive wound drainage

side to side regularly. Coughing and deep breathing should be encouraged at least every hour in the early postoperative period and periodically thereafter.

The client may be reluctant to cough and deep breathe, because this will be painful. Offer empathic support while reinforcing preoperative explanations of the rationale for coughing and deep breathing. Providing analgesics before deep breathing and coughing will make the client less uncomfortable. Splinting of the incision (as illustrated and discussed earlier in this chapter) will provide the client who has an abdominal or thoracic incision with extra support. Incentive spirometry, if ordered, should be encouraged as often as prescribed, and the nurse should assist the client as necessary (see Chapter 18).

Modify coughing and deep breathing as necessary to meet individual client needs. Elderly, weak, drowsy, or depressed clients may need frequent reminders and assistance with coughing or deep breathing and positioning. Obese clients are also likely to need help with positioning. Smokers are prone to coughing spasms, laryngospasm, and bronchospasm after surgery. In these clients, excessive coughing, as well as insufficient coughing, can cause harm by collapsing alveoli. Teach these clients the cascade cough described earlier in this chapter. Clients with chronic obstructive lung disease should also do pursed-lip breathing exercises to help rid the lungs of high levels of carbon dioxide.

Meeting Circulatory Needs

The nurse should advise the client to avoid undue pressure on blood vessels and to watch for factors that promote venous stasis, such as immobility and crossing the legs. Turning and moving in bed at least every hour or two

should be encouraged, especially while activity is restricted. The nurse should also encourage early ambulation, when permitted, and should assist the client as necessary. Elastic stockings or elastic bandages from toe to midthigh promote venous return to the heart, preventing pooling of blood in the extremities. These supports should be removed at least once daily, skin condition should be checked, and skin care provided. Clean stockings should be provided as necessary.

Bed rest, warm compresses, and anticoagulant therapy are commonly prescribed for clients who develop thrombophlebitis. Massage should be avoided because it might dislodge thrombi.

Meeting Nutritional and Fluid and Electolyte Needs

Because of the effects of stress and general anesthesia on the gastrointestinal tract, the postoperative client may be unable to tolerate food or fluids given by mouth. Nausea and vomiting are common sequelae of anesthesia, and antiemetics are often prescribed to relieve these effects. Food and fluids are generally withheld until normal gastrointestinal functioning has returned. In the meantime, the client is nourished by intravenous fluids. Dextrose, saline, and electrolyte solutions are often given, and vitamins are usually added. (Fluid and electrolyte balance is discussed in Chapter 5.) Routine IV fluids cannot meet long-term nutritional needs, however. Weight loss and nutritional deficiencies may occur.

After minor surgical procedures, intravenous administration may be discontinued soon after surgery and oral feedings may be started. After major procedures normal feeding may be postponed for up to a week. In such cases, hyperalimentation may be indicated (see Chapter 8). When oral ingestion resumes, the client will generally advance from a clear fluid diet to full fluids and, eventually, to regular foods. Once the client is permitted food and fluids by mouth, nursing measures to promote appetite can be employed (see Chapter 47).

Meeting Elimination Needs

The client should be instructed to inform the nurse when flatus or stool is passed. Generally, fluids and foods are withheld until normal intestinal peristalsis resumes. The client should be encouraged to ambulate as soon as permitted, and the diet should be adequate in fluids and fiber (roughage) to maintain normal bowel function.

If the client is uncomfortable from the inability to pass flatus, inserting a rectal tube when needed may be helpful. Abdominal distention may indicate that the client is unable to pass stool or flatus (paralytic ileus). Distention may be painful for the client, and a colonic irrigation (or Harris flush) may be prescribed. In this technique, water is instilled into the intestinal tract, as with an enema, and removed by gravity drainage, which remains in place. (Refer to a nursing fundamentals text for a full description of the colonic irrigation technique.)

Nursing measures to promote micturition include rinsing the perineum with warm water, encouraging fluids and ambulation if permitted, and stroking the abdomen. Bedpans and urinals should be kept within easy reach. Many clients find it difficult to void on a bedpan. Providing privacy is essential. A fracture pan may be more comfortable for the client than a regular bedpan. The client should notify the nurse when the first voiding is accomplished, and the specimen should be measured to ensure that the bladder has emptied adequately. Urinary retention with overflow or inadequate emptying may occur. In some cases, the client does not void, and catheterization may be ordered. A one-time catheterization with a straight catheter may be performed, or in-dwelling catheterization may be necessary. Catheterization is usually carried out if the client does not void within 8 hours of surgery.

Meeting Comfort and Safety Needs

Plan and implement measures to promote and maintain hygiene to increase the client's comfort. When the client returns to the surgical unit, removal of secretions such as blood and vomitus helps the client relax and rest. Once the client is responsive and receptive, a complete bath may be given. The perineum should be cleansed after urination and defecation. The recovering client can assume increasing responsibility for hygiene, but the nurse must assume this responsibility until the client is able.

Mouth care should be offered frequently. NPO status makes the mouth uncomfortable and can promote cracking of the lips and tongue, xerostomia (excessive dryness of the mouth), and parotitis. The lips and mouth should be lubricated frequently, and ice chips should be offered if permitted.

Nursing measures should be directed at the postoperative pain the client perceives—not the pain the nurse thinks is perceived. Individuals vary greatly in their sensitivity to pain and in pain tolerance. Distraction, relaxation techniques, changes of position, or massage may be employed, and prescribed analgesics should be given as needed. The nurse should not withhold pain medication out of fear of addiction. Pain relief is the first consideration for the surgical client, because pain and fear of pain can induce additional stress, interfering with recovery. The assurance that analgesics have been prescribed and may be requested when needed often relieves anxiety and pain. (Pain is discussed in Chapter 5.)

A relatively recent technique that gives the client some control over postoperative pain is transcutaneous electrical nerve stimulation (TENS). In the operating room, external electrodes are applied near the incision and connected to a control mechanism; the client uses the mechanism to inhibit transmission of pain impulses, inhibiting perception of pain. The TENS device may be kept on continually right after surgery; eventually, the client uses it as necessary. TENS is also discussed in Chapter 5.

Bedpans or urinals, call devices, and any supplies the client may need should be kept where the client can easily reach them. Supplies and equipment that are not needed should be removed; a bed table touching the feet of a client who cannot remove it can be extremely uncomfortable. Siderails should be raised while the client is confined to bed or under the effects of anesthesia or narcotics. When the client begins to ambulate, remove obstructing furniture from the path.

Meeting Motor and Sensory Needs

Activity will gradually increase as tolerated. As recovery progresses, the client should gradually become capable of a wider range of activity. Clients getting out of bed for the first time may feel dizzy or weak. **Postural hypotension** (a drop in blood pressure when moving from a lying or sitting to a standing position) is often associated with the dizziness or weakness. Having the client dangle the legs off the bed and assisting in a slow, relaxed transfer can minimize these symptoms. If the client appears disoriented, visits by the family may be helpful. The client should be reminded of his or her identity and kept aware of the time, day, and similar facts. Diversion and a change in environment may be helpful. If sensory overload is a problem, try to reduce stimuli.

Meeting Wound Care Needs

When drainage is excessive, either in the recovery room or on the surgical unit, the first postoperative dressing is generally reinforced rather than changed. The amount of drainage or blood loss should be noted. Drainage can sometimes be estimated by drawing a circle around the area; to estimate blood loss, note the number of soiled pads or the size of a blood spot.

The first dressing change is usually performed by the surgeon. Subsequently, the nurse may assume responsibility for dressing changes, depending on agency policy. Sterile technique must be maintained during dressing changes. The incisional area and the area around any drains should be meticulously cleansed. Unless ordered to leave the wound open, protect it from further trauma by applying a clean dressing.

When the client is allowed out of bed, an abdominal binder may be ordered to provide extra support. Clients often describe a feeling that the viscera are dropping or falling out when they first ambulate after abdominal surgery, and a binder provides a sense of security. Binders may also help prevent complications such as dehiscence and evisceration in obese clients.

Should the wound become infected, precautions must be taken to prevent transfer of infection. Drainage and secretion precautions are recommended for minor infections; for major wound infections, contact isolation should be instituted (Centers for Disease Control, 1982) (see Chapter 11). Wound irrigation is often performed.

If there are indications of dehiscence or evisceration, notify the surgeon immediately. Meanwhile, apply heavily padded pressure dressings soaked with saline. Check vital signs because hypotension and tachycardia may occur, and shock may accompany evisceration.

Meeting Psychosocial Needs

In general, assisting the client to return to customary functioning helps psychologically. Encourage independence by allowing the client to perform self-care activities, ambulate as soon as possible, and otherwise assume responsibility without endangering recovery. Visits from family members should be permitted and encouraged soon after surgery. Be available so that the client can express concerns about the prognosis, body image changes, and changes in lifestyles. Concerns about specific operations are discussed in other chapters. The client may need to assume new roles, and the nurse can assist in the transition. Strategies for assisting the client with coping are discussed in Chapter 6.

Meeting Discharge Needs

Throughout the perioperative period, keep in mind the client's eventual return home. What home care needs will the client have? Will the client have drains in place? Catheters? Do the client's significant others understand care of these devices? Will the client's diet or activity be restricted? How will the client get home? Should other agencies be consulted in anticipation of these needs?

Although instructions for postrelease care are often prescribed by the physician, the nurse does the actual teaching, explaining, and clarifying. When possible, ask the client and family to demonstrate any techniques they have been taught, such as dressing changes, and to explain why the procedure must be done in a certain way. Reassurance may also be necessary, because the client may be apprehensive about leaving the protective environment of the hospital. Written instructions will aid the client's memory. Generally, written instructions include:

- Wound care
- Diet
- Activity and/or special exercises
- Medication, including dosages, anticipated effects, and signs of overdose or side effects
- Date for follow-up visit

If necessary, contact a home care agency to provide for continuity of care. The client may also be furnished with names and addresses of self-help groups. Self-help groups and other resources are listed at the end of each nursing process chapter.

Evaluation

The client who has had surgery may leave the hospital hopeful and eager for rehabilitation, or the client may be apprehensive, angry, or regretful. The quality of nursing care can help make the difference. In all phases of the perioperative period, evaluation provides the data necessary for making decisions about the appropriateness and effectiveness of interventions so they can be continued or modified or so new needs can be addressed.

Chapter Highlights

Nursing care for clients throughout the perioperative period should conform with the Standards for Medical-Surgical Nursing Practice and the Standards for Perioperative Nursing Practice.

The role of the nurse as client advocate is especially important for surgical clients, who may be unable to take action on their own.

The prevention of nosocomial infection in surgical clients is a major nursing responsibility throughout the perioperative period.

Surgery has a profound impact on body systems as well as on lifestyle and psychosocial well-being.

Consequences and potential complications of surgery may affect the status of respiration, circulation, nutrition, fluid and electrolyte balance, elimination, safety and comfort, and motor and sensory function.

A preoperative teaching plan should include a general orientation to the surgical experience and instruction in anticipated postoperative activities.

Surgical clients who receive preoperative and postoperative teaching are less anxious, more willing to participate in their own care and to comply with prescribed medical regimens, and have fewer complications.

Excessive and/or prolonged pressure on body tissues, a potential consequence of surgical positioning, can contribute to the development of pressure sores, postoperative muscle discomfort, and neurovascular damage.

In caring for the client under anesthesia, the nurse acts as client advocate when ensuring that the client is positioned to protect privacy and with proper body alignment, and that surgical asepsis is maintained.

Clients who have had surgery may have difficulty in coping with body image alterations that may be a consequence of the surgery.

Pain relief and promotion of comfort, which require

(continued)

Chapter Highlights (continued)

a variety of medical and nursing measures, deserve high priority in the care of the postsurgical client.

Nursing interventions to promote wound healing include ensuring optimal nutritional and fluid intake, providing aseptic wound care, and avoiding unnecessary stress on the operative area.

Discharge planning for the surgical client should begin at admission. In providing discharge instructions, the nurse should consider the client's acceptance of any surgical alteration of body structure or function, the impact of any imposed limitations on usual lifestyle, the ability for self-care, and the availability of support systems.

Bibliography

Alexander J et al: The influence of hair removal methods on wound infections. *Arch Surg* 1983; 118:347–352.

American Nurses' Association: *Standards of Perioperative Nursing Practice.* Kansas City: ANA, 1981.

Andrews DR, Taylor C: Documenting post-anesthesia recovery. *Am J Nurs* 1985; 85(3):290–291.

Centers for Disease Control: *Guideline for Prevention of Surgical Wound Infection.* US Government Printing Office, March 1982.

Cruse PJE, Foord R: The epidemiology of wound infection. *Surg Clin North Am* 1980; 69(1):17–40.

Curtin L: Wound management: Care and cost—an overview. *Nurs Mgmt* (Feb) 1984; 15:22–25.

Devine EC, Cook TD: A meta-analytic analysis of effects of psychoeducational interventions on length of post-surgical hospital stay. *Nurs Res* 1983; 32:267–274.

Dripps RD, Eckenhoff JE, Vandam LK: *Introduction to Anesthesia: The Principles of Safe Practice.* Philadelphia: Saunders, 1982.

Flynn ME, Rovee DT: Promoting wound healing: Influencing repair and recovery. *Am J Nurs* 1982; 82:1550–1556.

Gruendemann BJ, Meeker MH: *Alexander's Care of the Patient in Surgery.* St. Louis: Mosby, 1983.

Hartfield M, Cason C: Effect of information on emotional response during a barium enema. *Nurs Res* 1981; 30:151–155.

Johnson JE et al: Altering patients' responses to surgery: An extension and replication. *Res Nurs Health* 1978a; 1(3):111–121.

Johnson JE et al: Sensory information, instruction in coping strategy, and recovery from surgery. *Res Nurs Health* 1978b; 1(0):4–17.

Kneedler JA, Dodge GH: *Perioperative Patient Care.* Boston: Blackwell, 1983.

Lecky JH: Problems of trace anesthetic levels. In: Orkin FK, Cooperman LH: *Complications in Anesthesiology.* Philadelphia: Lippincott, 1983, pp. 715–732.

Mattia MA: Hazards in the hospital environment: Anesthesia gases and methylmethacrylate. *Am J Nurs* 1983; 83:73–77.

Metz C: A survey of nurse anesthesia programs: A look at the trend toward graduate education. *JAANA* 1984; 52:520–529.

Nichols RL: Techniques known to prevent postoperative wound infection. *Infect Control* 1982; 3(1):34–37.

Northrop C: Legal aspects of nursing. In: Flynn J-B, Heffron PB: *Nursing: From Concept to Practice.* Bowie, MD: Brady, 1984, pp. 205–236.

Orkin FK, Cooperman LH: *Complications in Anesthesiology.* Philadelphia: Lippincott, 1983.

Pervin L: The need to predict and control under conditions of threat. *J Pers* 1963; 31:570–587.

Rosenberg H: Malignant hyperpyrexia. *Am J Nurs* 1981; 81:1484–1486.

Stoelting RK, Miller RD: *Basics of Anesthesia.* New York: Churchill Livingstone, 1984.

Vandam LD (editor): *To Make the Patient Ready for Anesthesia: Medical Care of the Surgical Patient.* Menlo Park, CA: Addison–Wesley, 1980.

Vernon D, Bigelow D: Effects of information about a potentially stressful situation on response to stress impact. *J Pers Soc Psychol* 1974; 29:50–59.

Ziemer M: Effects of information on postsurgical coping. *Nurs Res* 1983; 32(5):282–287.

Suggested Readings

Burns LA: Ambulatory surgery growing at a rapid rate. *AORN J* 1982; 35(2):260–270. An informative description of ambulatory surgery, including its definition, growth, and advantages, in the specialty journal published by AORN.

Fraulini KE, Gorski DW: Don't let perioperative medications put you in a spin. *Nurs 83* (Dec) 1983; 13:26–30. This article discusses common operative medications, their usual dosage, and desired and adverse effects.

Gruendemann BJ, Meeker MR: *Alexander's Care of the Patient in Surgery,* 7th ed. St. Louis: Mosby, 1983. This revision of a classic is a comprehensive review of the care of the client during the intraoperative period.

Hewitt D: Don't forget your preop patient's fears. *RN* (Oct) 1984; 10:63–68. This article is an assessment guide to preoperative ability to cope with stress and offers suggestions for reducing preoperative anxiety.

MacDonald JA: *Facing the Scalpel.* Englewood Cliffs, NJ: Prentice–Hall, 1981. This consumer-oriented book offers guidelines on preparing for surgery and protecting one's rights throughout the surgical experience.

Vandam LD (editor): *To Make the Patient Ready for Anesthesia: Medical Care of the Surgical Patient.* Menlo Park, CA: Addison–Wesley, 1980. Using a systems approach, this book discusses numerous medical problems. Their implications for pre- and post-anesthesia care are detailed in this book.

Resources

HOT LINE

Second Surgical Opinion Hotline
(Monday through Friday, 8 AM to 12 noon)
Phone: Nationwide: (800) 638-6833
       Maryland: (800) 492-6603

Provides the names of local surgeons who will act as consultants and give a second opinion on nonemergency operations. These surgeons will not treat persons who consult them and thus have no financial interest in whether the client has the operation. Printed information is also available.

HEALTH EDUCATION MATERIAL

From: American Medical Association
535 N. Dearborn St.
Chicago, IL 60610

"Surgery," a booklet explaining what the client will experience before, during, and after surgery.

From: American Society of Anesthesiologists
515 Busse Hwy.
Park Ridge, IL 60068

"Anesthesia and You," a booklet explaining anesthesia, the role of the anesthesiologist, and the experiences the client will undergo.

From: Consumer Information Center
Pueblo, CO 81009

"Facing Surgery? Why Not Get a Second Opinion?," a booklet describing why a second opinion is important.

NURSING ORGANIZATIONS

American Association of Nurse Anesthetists
216 Higgins Rd.
Park Ridge, IL 60068
Phone: (312) 692-7050

The membership of this organization comprises certified registered nurse anesthetists. The goals are to promote high-quality anesthesia care, to advance the science and art of anesthesiology, and to promote educational standards in the field. Annual dues are $125 for active members.

American Society of Post Anesthesia Nurses
Box 11083
Richmond, VA 23230
Phone: (804) 359-3557

Composed of RNs and LPNs who are interested in or working in postanesthesia care, this organization encourages research, education, and specialization in the care of clients during the immediate postoperative period.

Association of Operating Room Nurses
10170 E. Mississippi Ave.
Denver, CO 80321
Phone: (303) 755-6300

An organization for RNs engaged in supervisory, teaching, or staff positions in operating room nursing. Goals are to improve nursing care, provide educational programs, and encourage study and certification. Annual dues are $35.

Chapter 15

Burns

Joyce Black

Objectives

When you have finished studying this chapter, you should be able to:

Describe how burns are classified.

Describe the effects of burns on the major body systems, including the cardiovascular, respiratory, renal, gastrointestinal, hepatic–biliary, and integumentary systems.

List priorities in immediate care of burn clients.

State applications of major burn treatments, including debridement, temporary wound coverage, skin grafting, and topical antibiotics.

Identify nursing diagnoses commonly associated with care of burn clients in the emergent, acute, and rehabilitative periods.

Discuss psychosocial adjustment of clients with major burns during the three periods of care.

Burns are among the most devastating injuries a person can sustain. Not only do burns injure the body and leave the skin permanently scarred, but burns also damage the psyche by severe pain and altered body image. A client's lifestyle may also be affected by lengthy hospitalization, which may alter work patterns and finances. Recovery is likely to be long and grueling, both physically and psychologically. Physical care and emotional support for the burned client and his family require highly developed nursing skills and great sensitivity.

Section I: The Problem of Burns

CLASSIFICATION

Burns can be classified according to their causes and according to the depth of injury. Causes of burns are described as thermal, chemical, electrical, and radiation. Thermal burns include injuries caused by fire, steam, scalding water, and other hot liquids. Children often sustain thermal injuries when they play with matches or pour hot fluids on themselves. Adults are often burned while cooking, trying to ignite a fire with gas, or smoking in bed. Burns also occur when people intentionally ignite themselves or others.

Chemical burns occur most often when caustic chemicals are used in chemistry laboratories and in some industrial settings. Because of this increased risk, eye irrigating fountains and showers are installed for emergency use. Caustic home-cleaning chemicals, such as oven cleaners and toilet bowl cleaners, are also potentially dangerous.

Electrical burns are possible anywhere there is electrical current. Electrical burns in the home occur most often to children biting on electrical cords or playing with wall sockets. Adults sometimes sustain electrical burns at home while trying to repair outlets or appliances. In the work setting, linemen may sustain electrical burns when electricity in power lines has not been turned off properly.

Radiation burns are caused by overexposure to the

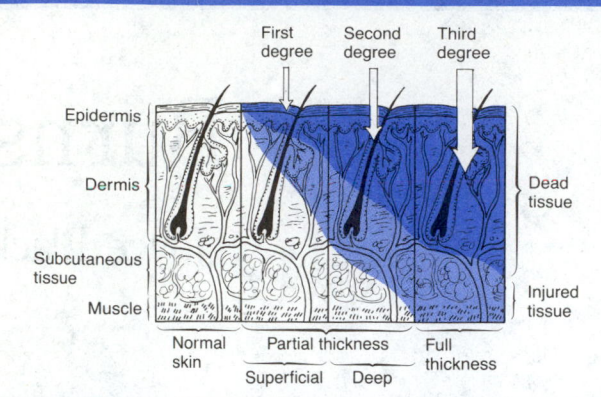

Figure 15–1

Depth of burn. The arrows represent degrees of heat or intensity of burning agent and the duration of contact with skin. The darker shaded area represents dead tissue. The lighter shaded area indicates damaged or injured tissues that will heal with good care.

sun, x-rays, and nuclear energy. Radiation burns are also seen in clients who have had radiation therapy for cancer.

Two methods are used for classifying the depth of a burn. Burns can be described as first, second, or third degree or as partial thickness or full thickness. The term **partial-thickness burn** encompasses first- and second-degree burns; **full-thickness burns** are equivalent to third-degree burns (Figure 15–1). A **first-degree burn** damages only the epidermal layer of skin; **second-degree burns** damage the epidermis and part of the dermis; and **third-degree burns** damage both the epidermal and dermal layers. Assessment of burn depth is discussed in the section on nursing process for the emergent period.

INCIDENCE OF BURN INJURY

An estimated two million people are treated for burns yearly by physicians, and approximately 70,000 are hospitalized. Burn injuries account for approximately 12,000 deaths per year. Accidents, which include burns, are the major cause of death in children aged 1 to 4.

Chances of surviving after a burn are influenced by five physical factors:

1. The amount of body surface area (BSA) burned
2. The depth of burn injury
3. The victim's age
4. Medical history
5. The part of the body burned

Assessment of these factors is discussed further in the section on nursing process for the emergent period.

Figure 15–2 depicts the average chances of survival for burned clients, based on their age and percent of body burned. Persons from ages 5 to 34 have the best chance for survival. The figure does not include other aspects of

determining burn severity, such as medical history and body part burned. It is known, however, that those with concurrent illnesses and those with burns on the head, neck, chest, or perineum have poorer prognoses than persons without those problems. Also, the more extensive the burn size, the greater the risk of mortality.

PREVENTION OF BURNS

Nurses can help prevent burns by participating in health education programs that stress fire prevention, such as "Learn Not to Burn." Legislation is another avenue in burn prevention, and nurses can work for measures that promote safety in work and home environments. Community health nurses are especially likely to see fire hazards in the home and should assist families to make their homes safe. Occupational health nurses need to be aware of hazards in the work setting and emergency care of burns. Nurses in any setting should also encourage and participate in drills and fire safety inspections. Finally, nurses should set good examples by keeping their homes and work settings free of fire hazards.

Approximately 80% of accidental burns occur in the home. Ignorance and carelessness are contributing factors. Many burns of adults occur while they are cooking, smoking, or using matches in some way. Burns are common when a person is distracted while cooking or falls asleep smoking. In the elderly, 75% of flame burns happen when they accidentally set their clothing on fire. Bathing is another burn hazard for the elderly because they have decreased sensitivity to temperature and slowed response time. One out of ten burned elderly persons were injured from bath water being too hot. Diabetics are also prone to burn injury from hot water. In the winter, malfunctioning kerosene heaters have caused home fires. Much of the suffering and financial burden caused by burn accidents is avoidable. Extensive education about risks and precautions is the long-term solution.

BURNS AS A MULTISYSTEM STRESSOR

Following a severe burn, all body systems are involved in an attempt to maintain homeostasis. Clients with severe burns generally progress through three stages of treatment. The emergent period begins at the time of injury and ends when fluid resuscitation is complete, usually within 48 hours. Massive fluid shift and shock are the immediate reactions to the severe insult. The acute period begins with complete fluid resuscitation and ends when the client has less than 20% of the body to be healed. The acute period may last from a few days to many months in major burn clients. The final period, the rehabilitative phase, begins when there is less than 20% of the body to be healed and ends with total rehabilitation. This period may last for years after the injury.

Complications are the rule, not the exception, after burn injury. A client with major burns can be expected to

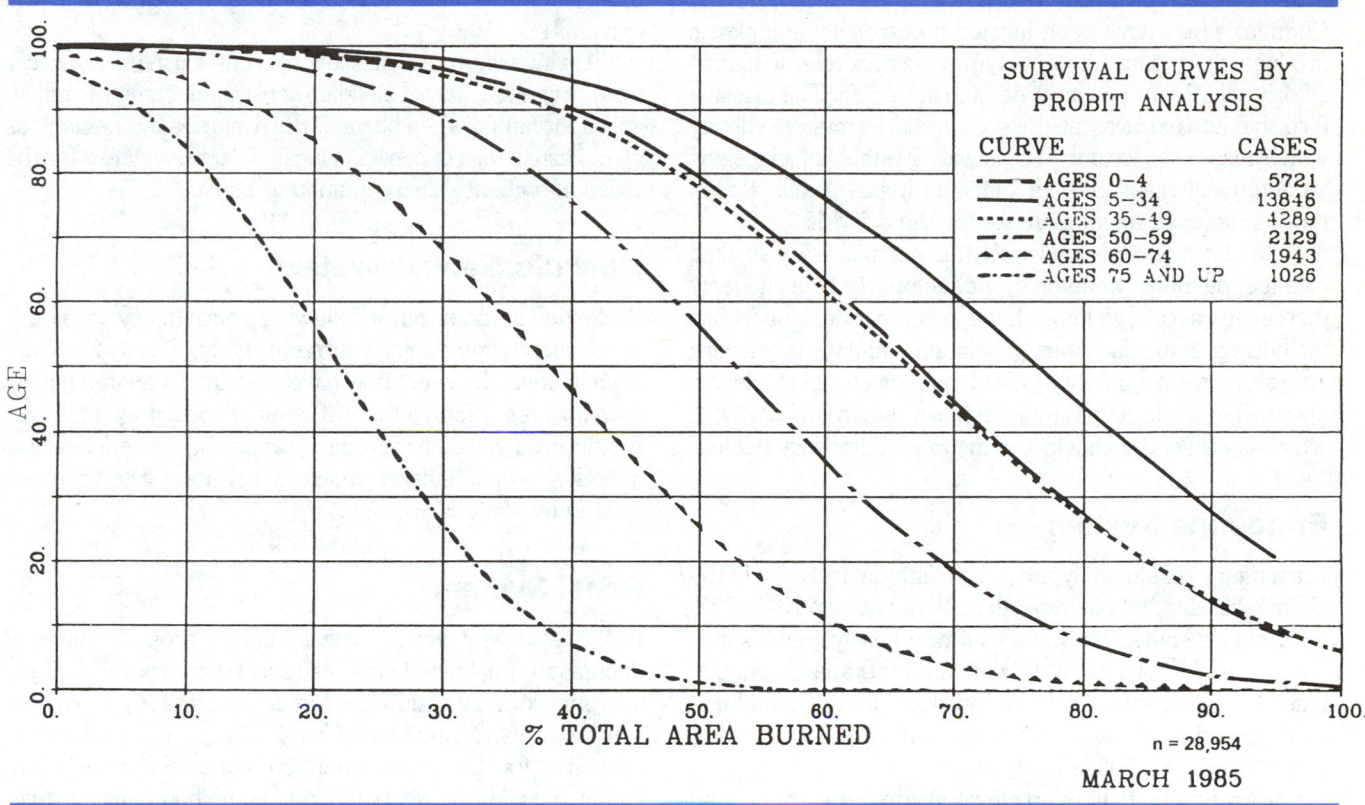

SURVIVAL CURVES BY
PROBIT ANALYSIS

CURVE	CASES
AGES 0-4	5721
AGES 5-34	13846
AGES 35-49	4289
AGES 50-59	2129
AGES 60-74	1943
AGES 75 AND UP	1026

% TOTAL AREA BURNED

n = 28,954

MARCH 1985

Figure 15-2

Burned patient survival by age, 1979 to 1984.
SOURCE: Taken with permission from Irving Feller, MD, University of Michigan Burn Center, National Burn Information Exchange, Ann Arbor, Michigan.

develop four to six major complications in addition to the burn. Complications can involve any body system because all systems are stressed during the injury and healing.

Cardiovascular System

Immediately following the burn, the body releases massive amounts of vasoactive substances, such as serotonin and histamine. These substances increase capillary permeability, allowing serum (which contains water), proteins, and electrolytes to escape into both damaged and normal tissues. This loss of serum into the tissues causes hypovolemia, which may lead to massive shock if the injury is severe enough.

Unlike hypovolemia from blood loss, there is no actual fluid loss; instead the fluid is sequestered (isolated) in the tissues where it cannot be utilized. As a result of hypovolemia, cardiac output falls, renal blood flow decreases, blood viscosity increases, and total peripheral vascular resistance increases because of peripheral vasoconstriction. Blood pressure falls because of the fluid shift and local vasodilatation from histamine. The heart rate increases from the low blood pressure and beta-receptor stimulation by epinephrine. Acute renal failure and death may follow unless appropriate measures are taken promptly.

With the fluid shift, blood values change. Hematocrit and hemoglobin values are elevated because of the escape of fluid from the blood. There may be hypernatremia because of dehydration and hyperkalemia because of release of intracellular potassium during the injury. Heat also destroys red blood cells, releasing free hemoglobin into the bloodstream. The client may be disoriented as a result of the decreased cerebral circulation and hypoxia caused by hypotension, dehydration, electrolyte shifts, pain, and shock.

Within 36 to 48 hours of a major burn, capillary permeability returns to normal, and fluids sequestered in body tissues reenter vascular spaces, increasing blood volume. Hemoglobin and hematocrit values will return to normal or below-normal levels. In this phase, clients will exhibit profound diuresis and elevated blood pressure unless fluids were titrated closely to urine output in the emergent phase. They may also develop circulatory overload because of strain on the heart. Cardiovascular complications include congestive heart failure from fluid overload, stroke, disseminated intravascular coagulation (DIC), and suppurative thrombophlebitis from coagulated blood in vessels.

Respiratory System

Pulmonary damage from smoke, super-heated gases, chemical inhalation, and carbon monoxide intoxication, is the leading cause of death in fire victims. It is essential to assess burn victims at once for primary damage from inhalation injury and upper airway obstruction. If the fire occurred in an enclosed space, the victim will have breathed smoke. Chemicals may have been inhaled if petroleum and plastic products were burned; eg, polymer plastics release hydrochloric acid, hydrogen cyanide, and ammonia. The massive fluid shift into extravascular tissues produces massive edema, which may also occlude the airway. Metabolic acidosis is an additional result of fluid shift and hypovolemia. Respirations increase to compensate for the acidosis.

In the acute period, with the normalization of fluid balance, pulmonary edema may develop from the suddenly increased vascular volume. Later pulmonary complications include pneumonia from inhalation injury; pulmonary embolism from immobility; and pulmonary insufficiency, also called adult respiratory distress syndrome (ARDS), which is caused by shock, trauma, and pulmonary edema.

Endocrine System

Burn injury results in hypermetabolism, an increase in the client's basal metabolic rate. In a client with a 40% to 50% body surface burn, the metabolic rate nearly doubles during the first 5 days after the burn and then reaches a plateau. Increased catecholamine production and an endogenous resetting of the body's metabolic rate are the cause of the hypermetabolism.

Burned clients have an elevated core temperature and an elevated skin temperature as part of their hypermetabolism. Their core temperatures average at 38.3°C (101°F). Burned clients feel most comfortable in warmer-than-average rooms at temperatures around 30.6°C (87.0°F), in contrast to the usual room setting temperature of 21.1°C (70°F).

Endocrine system complications following burn injury are adrenal hemorrhage, adrenal insufficiency, diabetes insipidus, and inappropriate antidiuretic hormone (ADH) secretion. Adrenal hemorrhage results from increased demands on the adrenal glands to secrete steroids and catecholamines. Symptoms of adrenal hemorrhage are vague; they include upper abdominal pain, cyanotic mottling of unburned skin with cardiovascular collapse, and increased losses of sodium in the urine (over 100 mEq/day). Systemic steroids administered to clients with diagnosed adrenal hemorrhage seem to result in only temporary improvement before death. Adrenal insufficiency, diabetes insipidus, and inappropriate ADH secretion are discussed in Unit Seven.

Nervous System

Damage to peripheral nerves occurs when tissue is destroyed by any burn. Electrical burns can damage the central or peripheral nerves. If high voltage electrical current comes in contact with the skull, transmitting heat into the brain tissues, brain damage can occur. The spinal cord and peripheral nerves can also be injured by electrical current. Injuries can range from limited areas of weakness to complete paralysis. These neurologic problems sometimes reverse completely, and vigorous therapy must be insti-

tuted to maintain full range-of-motion (ROM) in these extremities.

Changes in the client's level of consciousness can occur from hypoxia, hypovolemia, sepsis, electrolyte imbalances, or falling when burned. Burn injuries by themselves do not cause loss of consciousness. Look elsewhere for the cause of a client's disorientation or coma.

Musculoskeletal System

Prolonged immobilization following a burn injury can result in muscle atrophy, joint contractures, and loss of calcium from bones. The client may have sustained a related injury, such as a leg fracture that will require special wound care. A fractured burned extremity cannot be casted because infection would quickly result. Therefore fractures are treated by skeletal traction.

Renal System

In the emergent phase, urinary output drops because of decreased renal blood flow resulting from hypotension and secretion of ADH and aldosterone. Poor tissue perfusion can progress to renal shutdown if prompt and appropriate measures for fluid replacement are not taken. Free hemoglobin released by destruction of red blood cells or myoglobin released by damaged muscle may pass into the urine through the kidney; if free hemoglobin or myoglobin block the nephrons, renal failure may develop.

In the acute period, urine output increases with the restoration of intravascular fluid balance, leading to profound diuresis. When diuresis begins, do not assume that fluids are no longer needed, however, because evaporative water loss from the wound can reach 3 to 5 L in 24 hours.

Serum electrolyte values may fall during this period because of the excess body fluids. Most electrolyte changes are from dilution. The only exception is hyperkalemia, which is caused by intracellular potassium leaking into the bloodstream. Potassium leaves the damaged cells after a burn and can reach lethal levels quickly. Serum sodium levels can assist in determining fluid needs. Other indicators of fluid status besides urinary output are the condition of the oral mucosa, skin turgor, body weight, and hemoglobin and hematocrit levels.

Gastrointestinal and Hepatic–Biliary Systems

With the initial insult, ileus often occurs because the stress of the injury shunts blood away from the gastrointestinal tract. The injury also triggers an endogenous reset of metabolism, greatly increasing metabolism over preburn levels. Sympathetic nervous system stimulation mobilizes steroids. Glycogen stores are converted to glucose for energy. The glucose stores are quickly depleted, forcing the body to use fats and proteins for energy.

With catabolism, weight loss following a burn injury can be severe and is directly proportional to the size of the burn. A client with a 40% burn can lose 20% of body weight without nutritional support. A burned client can survive only 3 to 4 weeks without food, compared with a normal, healthy adult who can survive 2 months.

Malnutrition following a major burn is still a serious problem, increasing the client's risk of complications. The increased metabolism continues until clients have less than 20% of the body unhealed. Obviously, closure of the burn wound, which resets metabolism to near normal, is essential in severe cases. Curling's ulcer, or stress ulcer, a potential complication with any major trauma, can be prevented by high doses of acid-secretion-blocking drugs such as cimetidine (Tagamet). Another complication is hepatic failure caused by sepsis.

Integumentary System

With full-thickness burns, skin loses its elasticity and does not expand to accommodate edema. Therefore, the edema caused by the shift of fluids into interstitial spaces puts pressure on underlying structures such as blood vessels and the airway. In clients with chest burns, **eschar** (thick burned skin) prevents normal chest expansion with breathing. In clients with circumferential burns of the arms and legs, nonexpanding eschar may impair circulation to the distal extremities.

As previously discussed, extensive evaporative water loss from a burn wound contributes to the body's overall fluid imbalance. Condition of the oral mucosa and skin turgor in unburned skin are two clues to fluid status. Burned clients may also lose 30 g of nitrogen per day through the wound, quickly placing them in negative nitrogen balance.

Throughout the healing period, wound care and skin integrity are major foci of care. Burn wounds can develop four major problems as they heal: contractures, keloids and hypertrophic scars, color changes, and infection. Infection is the most common complication for burn clients, accounting for 45% of all deaths. Burn wounds can become infected with bacteria, fungi, and/or viruses. Left untreated, wound infections can lead to septicemia.

Initially, burn wounds are usually sterile because heat sterilizes the burn surface. After 5 days, all burn wounds are considered contaminated, however. The eschar provides an excellent growth medium for microorganisms because eschar is dark, warm, moist, has the proper pH, and provides ample food. If the microorganisms are limited to the eschar (wound colonization), clients usually are minimally affected by their presence. When pathogens invade deeper structures of the skin, however, clients develop wound infections. When the infection enters normal tissue, sepsis can develop.

Wound contracture is not the same as wound contraction. Contraction, a normal healing process, can be defined as the drawing together of the edges of the wound by forces within the wound. All wounds undergo some contraction during healing. In contrast, contracture is an abnormal process from excessive wound contraction that causes a fixed deformity (Figure 15–3). Burn wound con-

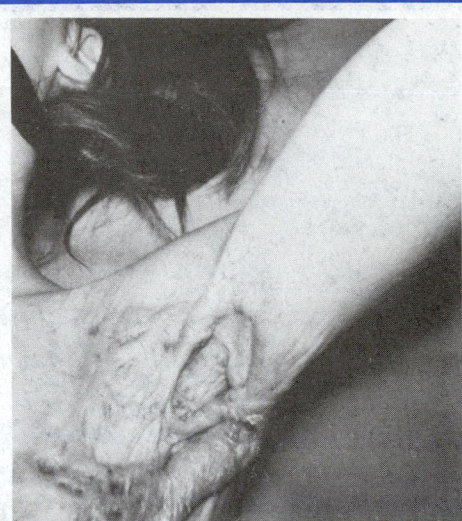

Figure 15–3

Burn wound contracture.

tracture over joints can become so severe that clients cannot move their extremities. Neck burns can contract, actually pulling the chin down onto the sternum. Mouth burns can contract to the point that clients have only a small hole the size of a dime to eat through.

A keloid is an excessive amount of tumorlike scar tissue that extends far beyond the scar line of the original wound (Figure 15–4). Hypertrophic scars, on the other hand, are raised scars that do not extend beyond the wound. The cause of keloid formation and hypertrophic scars is unknown. Although excessive scarring tends to occur more often in persons with dark or olive-toned skin, it can occur in fair-skinned people also. Keloids and hypertrophic scars are also more frequent in young people than in adults. In addition to obvious problems with appearance, keloids itch, bleed, and may be painful.

Clients may sustain burns through the melanin layer of skin. During healing, this pigment-forming layer may not be replaced by the body, and the healed areas are paler than the normal pigmentation.

After the wound is healed and grafts are completed, the burn wound scar usually matures over 1 year, changing from angry red to off-white. During this time, aggressive efforts must be taken to minimize scarring and prevent contractures. Contractures continue to be a problem over healing joints, so ROM exercises and splints must be continued until the scar matures.

TREATMENT OF BURNS

The following discussion covers emergency care of the burn victim before transfer to the hospital, as well as outpatient treatment for minor burns. Also discussed are special burn care procedures such as debridement, temporary wound coverage, skin grafting, and topical antimicrobial agents.

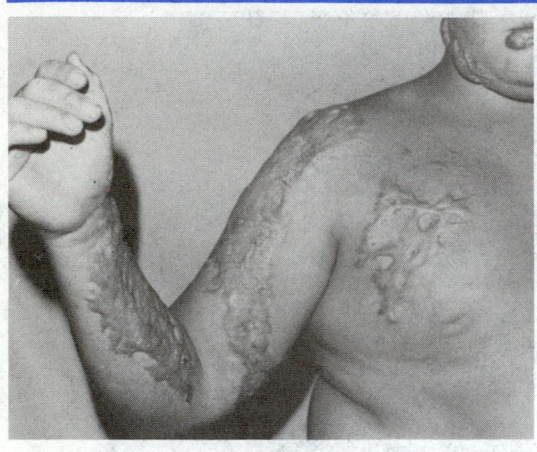
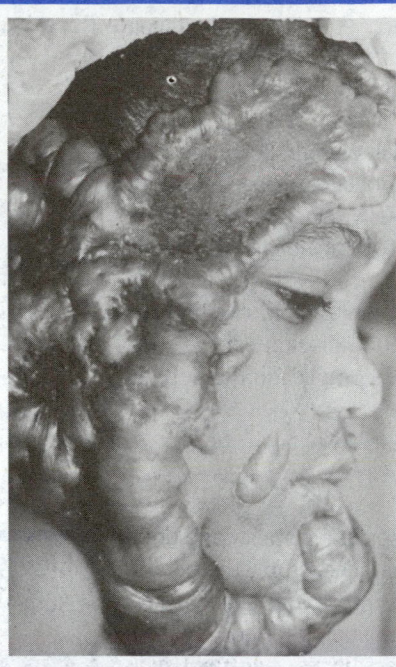

Figure 15–4
Examples of burn wound keloid.

Immediate Care of Burns

The initial care of the burned client focuses on one principle: Stop the burning process (see Box 15–1). The damage from a burn is directly related to the length of exposure and intensity of the burning agent. The same damage to

Box 15–1   Immediate Care of Burn Clients

1. Stop the burning process.

   Thermal burns:

   • Extinguish flames by rolling victim on ground or wrapping in blanket; get victim down on floor or ground.
   • If burn is less than 20% of body surface area, apply cool water (not cold; no ice). (Do not use ointment, butter, or grease.)

   Chemical burns:

   • Stop burning by flushing with large amounts of water.
   • Do not attempt to neutralize.
   • Carefully remove any clothing containing chemical.

   Electrical burns:

   • Shut off power source or disconnect client from live current without endangering self.

   Radiation burns:

   • Remove victim from source of heat if possible, avoiding exposure to radiation.

2. Assess airway, breathing, and circulation. Establish airway. Perform cardiopulmonary resuscitation if needed.

3. Cover wound with clean, lint-free, noncotton dressing.

4. Assess for other injuries such as fractures or injuries from a fall.

skin will occur in 6 hours at 111°F (43.9°C) as occurs in 1 second at 140°F (60°C).

The rescuer of the burn victim must thoroughly know the immediate plan of care. Burn clients will not always be rational and cooperative because they are frightened and in pain. The rescuer must also be able to execute the plan of care without becoming a second burn victim. It is critical that the rescuer think and remain calm before rushing into a potentially dangerous situation.

Thermal Burns

For the person who is actually on fire, the flames must be extinguished immediately by rolling the victim on the ground or wrapping him or her in a blanket. Flames travel upward toward the face; therefore, it is crucial to get the victim down on the floor or ground to reduce facial burns and airway injury. After the fire is out, evaluate the airway, breathing, and circulation (ABCs). (The ABCs are discussed in Chapter 13.) Initiate care as needed to save the victim's life.

Cool, not cold, water can be applied to the burned part if it is less than 20% of body surface (see Figure 15–7 later in the chapter). Initial cooling of burns relieves pain, speeds healing, and reduces the need for grafting because the cool temperature stops the injury. Cold water or ice can cause further injury (similar to frostbite) and can cause shock from temperature extremes. No medications should be given to the client. Ointments, butter, or grease should not be applied to the wound because ointment keeps the wound warm, potentially increasing the depth of the injury. The wound should be covered in clean noncotton-filled dressings. In the home, bed sheets work well because they are clean and do not have lint. Lint adheres to open wounds and is painful to remove.

Burns caused by tar or asphalt are difficult to treat. The tar must be removed without damaging underlying tissues. Some burn specialists feel that if it is not completely removed, the client has an increased risk of infection. Tar burns are usually very deep burns. Most tar burns result from contact with molten tar heated to 140°C to 232°C (284°F to 450°F) for roofing and road paving. Although molten tar cools rapidly when it splatters, prolonged contact can produce a serious burn. Initial treatment involves applying cold water to cool and solidify the molten tar. De-Solv-it® (Medasol) has been shown to be effective in removing tar without causing systemic side effects. Organic solvents such as mineral oil and gasoline should not be used; they are generally ineffective, can cause further injury, and have the potential to cause systemic toxicity. Follow the other steps outlined previously.

Chemical Burns

For chemical burns, initially stop the burning process by flushing the burned area with large amounts of water. Do not attempt to neutralize the chemical. Precious time will be lost searching for a neutralizing chemical. In addition, chemical reactions produce heat, which will further damage the skin. The only exceptions to irrigating chemical burns are when burns result from phenol or dry chemicals such as lime or phosphorus. Phenol burns should be irrigated with alcohol and not with water; water dilutes the phenol allowing it to penetrate to deeper layers of skin. Dry chemicals should be brushed off the client's skin or clothing; adding water would create a liquid that can penetrate the skin. After the burning sensation has lessened, carefully remove any clothing containing the chemical, being careful not to injure other tissue or self. Evaluate the client's airway, breathing, and circulation. Finally, dress the wound with a wet dressing as explained in the section on thermal burns.

Electrical Burns

In an electrical burn, shut off the power source to stop the burning process. Be cautious when moving power lines to avoid becoming a second victim. After the client is disconnected from live current, assess the airway, breathing, and circulation. Cardiopulmonary resuscitation may be required because the electricity exiting the body can disrupt the cardiac cycle. The client must also be assessed for other injuries, such as extremity fractures, because electricity can cause massive muscle contraction that can fracture bones. Wound care for electrical burn wounds is the same as described in care of thermal burns.

The damage to the body from electrical injury cannot be judged from the size of the skin wound. Severe damage occurs beneath the skin from the electrical current (Figure 15–5). As the electricity travels through the body to an electrical ground, the current causes damage to the structure through which it passes. Blood in the vessels coagulates from the heat causing necrosis of the tissues those blood vessels formerly supplied. Nerves may be destroyed; muscles may spasm severely enough to fracture bones.

The renal damage that follows electrical burns has been described earlier. In addition, tissue disruption can occur along the active path of the current. These burns are called "exit burns." Exit burns generally appear as quarter-sized red areas that open to expose deeper tissues. Exit burns may appear initially or after many days.

Radiation Burns

The victim should be removed from the source of heat if possible. The rescuer must be cautious to avoid exposure to any active source of radiation such as radium or nuclear waste during the rescue. The client should be assessed for skin damage and heat stroke if burned by the sun (see Chapter 13 for discussion of heat stroke).

Minor Burns

About 95% of burns are minor. Minor burns are superficial wounds (first and second degree), generally not exceeding 10% of the body surface. Minor burns never include electrical burns of any size or burns of the face, feet, perineum, or entire hand. Even though these are small body surface areas, the potential for complication is increased. Burns in these areas must be evaluated and usually cared for in a hospital.

Stop the the burning process by submerging the burned part in cool water or covering it with a cool wet cloth. For example, for a finger burned on the stove, place the finger in cool water until the burning sensation stops. While the burn feels warm and painful, tissue is still being injured. Thirty minutes may pass before the pain stops. No dressings need be used on the wound if skin integrity is intact. Blisters should not be broken except by a health care provider because blisters provide a sterile dressing for the wound. Blistered burns should be wrapped in loose sterile gauze. The gauze will provide a sterile environment and absorptive material when the blister breaks. Do not apply ice. Ice will cause vasoconstriction and further ischemia, damaging the wound. Irrigate chemical wounds with large amounts of water for a sustained period of time. Do not attempt to neutralize.

Assess the need for analgesia before beginning any wound care. The pain from a burn need not be described to anyone who has been burned by an oven rack. Oral narcotics may be required to control pain. Wash all debris from the wound. Running tap water on the burn or washing it in povidone–iodine solution while cleansing with a gauze pad works well to remove dead skin, dirt, or parts of clothing. Small blisters should be left intact, because the skin provides a "biologic dressing," protecting the wound. Large blisters should be covered with a bulky dressing to absorb the fluid if the blister breaks.

Systemic antibiotics are seldom indicated for minor burns because they encourage superinfection from resistant organisms. Tetanus prophylaxis should be renewed because burn wounds provide an excellent medium for growth of anaerobic organisms. Use of topical antimicrobials should be considered for burns over 15 × 30 cm. Silver sulfadiazine (Silvadene) has become the drug of choice

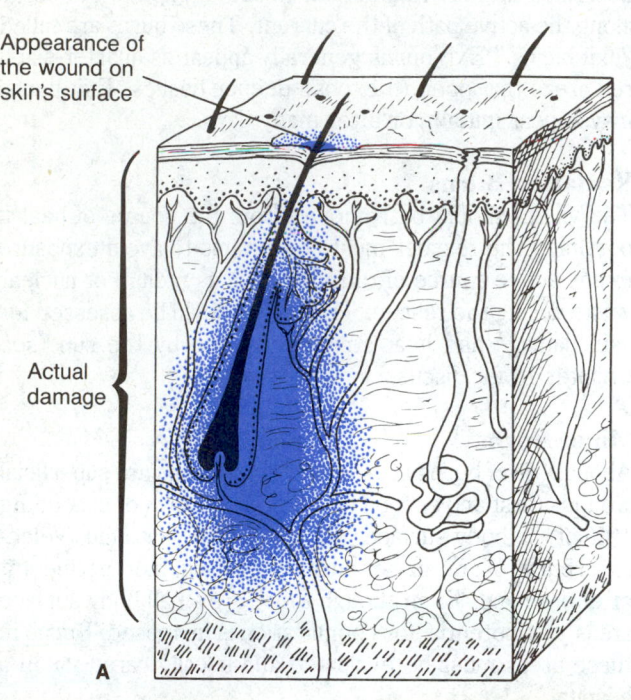

Appearance of the wound on skin's surface

Actual damage

A

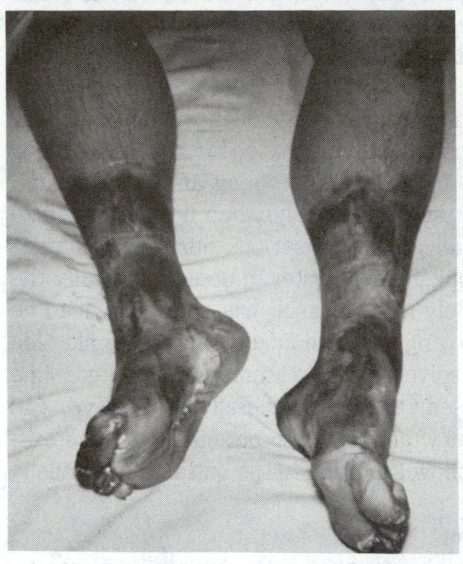

B

C

Figure 15–5

Damage to skin from an electrical current. **A.** The damage to the body from an electrical burn cannot be judged by the skin wound. There is extensive damage under the surface of the skin. **B.** Client who sustained electrical burns in an industrial accident. This photograph was taken on admission to the ICU. Note the dark eschar indicating full-thickness injury. **C.** One week after admission the client required bilateral amputation of the legs because of necrosis. Note the exit burns behind the knee; initially, they appeared as blisters.

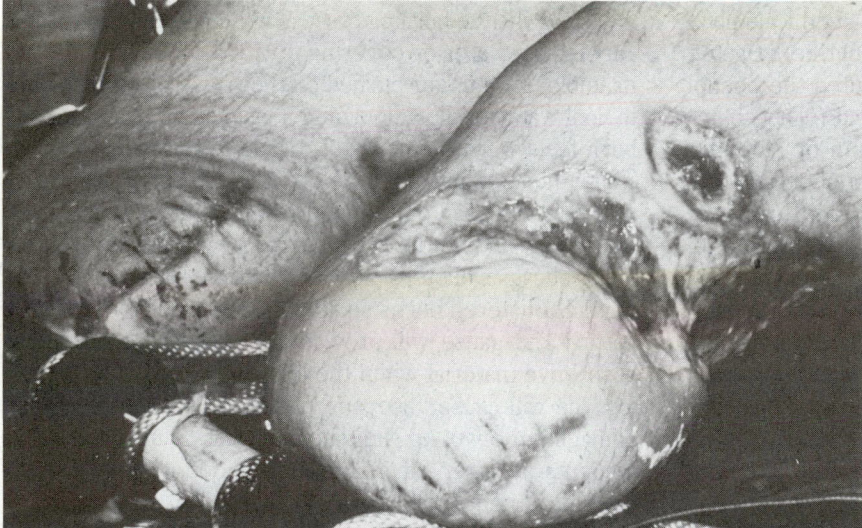

because of client comfort, antibacterial effect, and the ease of application. The cream should be applied to the wound ¼ in thick with a sterile glove or sterile tongue blade. The ointment can also be "buttered" on the dressing first and then applied to the wound. Small wounds can be cared for with ointment or grease-impregnated gauze (Xeroform, Adaptic) applied to the wound. These dressings should be held in place with a gauze wrapping.

The soiled dressing should be removed daily while dry to facilitate debridement of the wound (removal of necrotic tissue). If this is too painful, the dressings can be soaked off. Holding the burn under the shower for 10 to 15 minutes is one effective method. The wound should be examined for signs of infection, which include a foul odor, increased

redness at the edges of the wound, increased pain, a lack of healing, or regression of the burn to deeper layers of tissue. Fever need not be present with an infection. When silver sulfadiazine dressings are removed, a greenish yellow drainage does not indicate infection.

Debridement

Prior to healing or any skin-grafting procedure, the necrotic burned skin, or eschar, must be removed. There are three types of debridement: natural, mechanical, and enzymatic.

Natural debridement occurs by the body's own processes of phagocytosis. This form of debridement is slow and is not effective to clean and heal a burn over the size of a half-dollar.

Mechanical debridement uses instruments or water to speed wound cleaning. Hydrotherapy is one form of mechanical debridement. Mechanical debridement can also be performed by peeling or cutting away eschar with a scalpel or dermatome (the instrument used in skin grafting). This form of debridement is temporarily painful and may cause bleeding. Pain is caused by stimulation of cutaneous nerves, and excess bleeding is from the loss of engorged blood in the injured area.

Enzymatic debridement involves the application of proteolytic enzymes such as sutilains (Travase) to second- and third-degree burns to digest the eschar and dissolve and remove necrotic tissue. This form of debridement causes a burning sensation in the wound and should be limited to 15% of the body surface area at one time. Enzymatic debridement should not be used on pregnant women or when the burn connects with a body cavity.

The enzyme action may be inactivated if sutilains ointment is used in conjunction with iodine, nitrofurazone (Furacin), or hexachlorophene. Neomycin, mafenide acetate, streptomycin, and penicillin do not affect the enzyme activity.

The ointment is applied in a thin layer over the wound with a sterile gloved hand or a cotton applicator, overlapping onto the unburned skin by about ¼ in. A moist saline dressing is then applied over the enzyme. This dressing must be kept moist at all times.

Debridement is painful, and clients should be prepared for the experience, either with analgesics, relaxation techniques such as those discussed in Chapter 4, or self-hypnosis. General anesthesia may be used when large areas of the wound are debrided in the operating room, but it is not safe for daily wound care. Daily debridement is wearing for clients because they know they will experience pain. Clients quickly fall into a pain-anxiety cycle because of anticipation of pain. Debridement also causes anxiety because the client sees the extent of the burn as wounds are uncovered and sees whether the wound is healing.

Debridement is usually done twice daily in the physical therapy unit in large whirlpool tanks filled with warm saline. Clients are submerged in the tanks after dressings are removed (Figure 15–6). Dressings should be removed while dry to increase wound debridement. While the client is in the tank, the bubbling water softens and loosens the eschar, allowing it to be clipped off by the physical therapist. No more than a 3-sq-in area is removed at one time. Removing more eschar increases pain and potential for septicemia. The client is also assisted by the physical therapist to perform ROM while in the water. The hydrotherapy tank does not eliminate the need for personal care. Face, oral, hair, and perineal care must also be completed.

Some burn centers use flat tubs to cleanse burn clients. Clients are cleansed with sprayers instead of being submerged. The rationale for this form of therapy is that spraying can reduce the risk of septicemia because all body parts

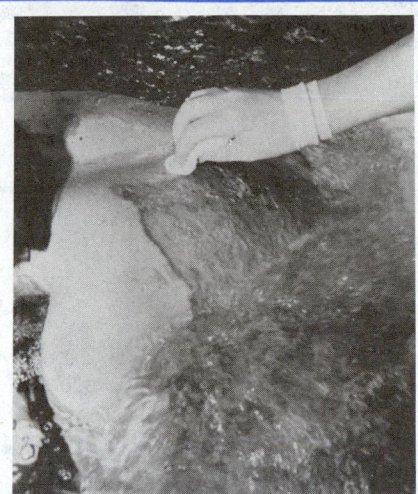

Figure 15–6
Debridement in a whirlpool tank.

are not exposed to the contaminated bath water. In either method, the client should be rinsed with clean water after hydrotherapy to reduce residual skin bacteria.

If the client is too physiologically unstable to be transported to the hydrotherapy unit, wound care can be done in the client's room using a sterile basin and sterile saline to wash the wound. The client should be assisted in performing ROM and the wound redressed according to routine.

Once the wound is cleaned and requires minimal debridement, bathtubs can be used for wound care. The tube should first be completely filled with hot water and ½ cup of bleach added. The tub should remain filled with this solution for 30 minutes before use. Then the tub should be drained, rinsed, and filled with water and table salt to make normal saline (2 tsp salt per liter of water) for the client's use.

Tangential excision is surgical removal of eschar down to bleeding tissues followed by immediate grafting or application of dressings. Tangential excision is completed during the first week after the burn and is used instead of hydrotherapy debridement for more rapid healing of the burn. Compared with more conventional therapy, tangential excision shortens hospitalization, reduces fluid losses and some complications such as sepsis, wound infection, and scarring. The major risk of tangential excision is hemorrhage. Tangential excision is limited by the amount of available skin for grafting and the client's overall condition. Bleeding is often controlled with thrombin solutions.

Temporary Wound Coverage

Burn wounds can be covered temporarily with homografts (allografts), heterografts (xenografts), or synthetic skin to reduce heat and evaporative water losses. Homografts are skin from other humans, such as cadavers and placental membranes. Heterografts are skin from animals, such as

Table 15–1 Temporary Wound Coverage

Preparation	Advantages	Disadvantages
Pigskin	Relief of pain; reduction of water and heat loss; available in several forms; can be meshed	Costly; can provoke rejection
Cadaver skin	Relief of pain; reduction of water and heat loss; can be meshed	Expensive; scarce
Amniotic membrane	Biologic dressing; relief of pain; reduction of water and heat loss; free	Difficult to apply at times
OpSite (transparent polyurethane membrane dressing)	Permeable to air; not permeable to fluid or bacteria; promotes wound healing in moist environment; no scab formation; no debridement necessary; immediate pain reduction; nonpainful removal; transparent; significantly shortens healing time	Time-consuming application; self-adhesive, can be difficult to apply; not suitable for full-thickness burns
Biobrane™ (silicone rubber and nylon with collagen)	Suitable for partial- and full-thickness wounds; semi-transparent; flexible, stretchable	Expensive

pigskin. Artificial skin includes OpSite and similar products. The only permanent wound coverage is an autograft from the burned person. Advantages and disadvantages of temporary wound covers are described in Table 15–1.

Skin Grafting

Burn wounds can reepithelialize and heal without skin grafting in 10 days to several weeks if they are not deep dermal burns. Allowing large deep burns to heal is a lengthy process and increases risk of infection and scarring, so these burns are often grafted.

Permanent skin grafting is the movement of skin from an unburned area on the client to a burned area. The burn wound must be clean and granulation tissue present before it is ready to accept a skin graft. Granulation tissue, seen in all clean wounds, is the initial step in healing. It is shiny and pale pink; on close examination, small bumps will be seen. (A detailed discussion of skin grafting is in Chapter 80.)

Burns not requiring skin grafting heal through epidermal cell replication. Hair follicles, which extend into the dermis, are lined with epidermal cells. These epidermal cells grow up into the wound and form "buds" of epidermis. The buds grow together and cover the wound. This is a long process, and problems with wound infection may mandate that a burn wound be grafted to speed healing. Burn wounds also heal by scarring. Production of scar tissue is normal in the healing of any wound but can cause special problems for the burned client.

Recently, sections of clients' unburned skin have been grown in the laboratory and then used to skin graft burned areas. Laboratory techniques can alter normal skin growth, so the skin grows 150 times faster than normal. This technique permits severely burned clients (90% of body surface area and more) to receive permanent grafts within a shorter time rather than waiting for weeks or months while their burns and donor sites healed and could be used for more grafting. All-cultured skin is still in the experimental stage, and long-term effectiveness has not yet been determined.

Topical Antimicrobial Agents

Many antimicrobial agents are used for burn care, with advantages and disadvantages. The ideal burn agent would control bacteria beneath the eschar, be painless in application, have no metabolic side effects, be easy to apply, be cost effective, and speed up the separation of eschar from the wound. Such an agent does not exist.

Topical antimicrobials do not sterilize the burn wound. They simply reduce the number of bacteria so that the client's host defense mechanisms can control bacterial replication. Controlling wound flora merely "buys time" while vigorous efforts are made to change an open, dirty wound to a closed, clean one. If this cannot be accomplished within a reasonable time (approximately 28 days), the bacterial population will grow out of control, and burn wound sepsis will follow.

Silver Sulfadiazine

Silver sulfadiazine (Silvadene), is a white water-soluble cream made from the reaction of silver nitrate and sulfadiazine. Silver sulfadiazine does not cause pain on application. It spreads easily over a burn or dressing with a gloved hand and is easily removed with water. The ointment is effective against a wide range of gram-negative and gram-positive bacteria, as well as yeast. Silver sulfadiazine acts only on the cell wall and membrane.

Mafenide Acetate

Mafenide acetate (Sulfamylon) is a topical sulfonamide drug. With intact subcutaneous blood vessels, peak concentrations occur 2 hours after application, or up to 4 hours in avascular areas. The drug is effective against *Pseudomonas aeruginosa, Staphylococcus aureus,* and *Aerobacter aerogenes.*

Mafenide acetate is applied in cream form once or twice daily with a gloved hand. It has the consistency of soft butter and burns and stings for 15 minutes to 1 hour following application because it is hydroscopic and draws water out of the tissues.

Silver Nitrate

Silver nitrate ($AgNO_3$) has been used as a burn treatment for many years. When used properly, it controls the wound's bacterial population and reduces water evaporation. Therapeutic effects are limited to the superficial tissues. Biochemical abnormalities are the major problem in the use of silver nitrate. Because of the hypotonicity of the distilled water used to carry the silver nitrate, large amounts of distilled water are absorbed into the body, and large quantities of minerals (sodium, potassium, chloride, magnesium, and calcium) are drawn out of the tissues. If clients are burned on more than 20% of their body surface area, they are likely to have a mineral deficiency unless there is regular electrolyte replacement. Daily monitoring of serum and urinary electrolytes may be necessary. Experience indicates that if the urinary sodium concentration falls below 40 mEq/L, the serum sodium concentration will fall within 24 hours. In infants and children and in some adults, these deficiencies can occur within 6 to 8 hours of beginning therapy, so careful monitoring is essential.

Povidone–Iodine

Povidone–iodine (Betadine), also used to help prevent burn wound sepsis, is effective against gram-negative and gram-positive organisms. Povidone–iodine is available in solution, foam, and ointment. It is easily applied to the burn wound with a sterile gloved hand. Gauze dressings are applied over the agent and are kept moist with povidone–iodine solution every 6 hours or as necessary. Because the agent tends to build up a crust, specific care must be given in hydrotherapy to clean the wound thoroughly.

Subeschar Clysis

With this technique, which is a valuable adjunct to topical therapy, appropriate antibiotics are infused directly into the subeschar space. A physician determines the area to be infused, as well as the antibiotic and the amount and type of carrier fluid to be used.

With a 21-gauge needle inserted into the subeschar space at a 45° angle, 25 mL of fluid are infused into a 7.5 cm^2 area (roughly the size of a softball). A new needle is used for each insertion site. This technique is often used for burns of greater than 40% of body surface area.

Section II: Nursing Process in Emergent Period

With the devastation of a burn injury, the client faces a massive insult that may be life threatening. Immediate care emphasizes the fundamental ABCs: airway, breathing, and circulation. (For discussion of the immediate care of the burn client at the scene, see Box 15–1 and the section on treatment.)

Once the client has been hospitalized and stabilized, both client and nursing staff face the prospect of a long healing process. The nurse will need to assist the client not only with serious physical needs but also with the gradual process of adjusting emotionally to what may be permanently altered appearance and functioning. Nursing care will be discussed according to the three phases of burn care: emergent, acute, and rehabilitative. Although the client may be stabilized before arriving at the hospital, initial care is strongly focused on the priorities of maintaining life.

ASSESSMENT: ESTABLISHING THE DATA BASE

Depending on the severity of the injury, initial assessment may only consist of a rapid check for a patent airway, respirations, and shock, with a more detailed assessment to be carried out later when the client's condition is stabilized.

Subjective Data

Client's History

Data about the cause of injury and the time of injury should be recorded. If the client cannot provide this information, ask the family or emergency medical technicians who brought the client to the hospital. Allergies, routine medication, and date of last tetanus immunization should be noted on the medical record.

Take special note of clients who have had chronic illnesses before a burn injury because they have an increased mortality rate. The stress of the burn may exacerbate the disease, making burn management more complex. Examples of such diseases are diabetes mellitus and chronic obstructive pulmonary disease. The stress of injury will cause gluconeogenesis from corticosteroid production. This increased need for glucose will cause irregularities in blood glucose values. Clients with lung disease will be susceptible to pneumonia because they have an ineffective cough reflex for respiratory clearance.

Psychosocial Assessment

The client's immediate adjustment to injury should be assessed. Some clients will be extremely frightened and think they are still burning. Others will be so overwhelmed by the events, they will be irrational. Burned clients will have pain. The pain level and client's coping with pain should be assessed according to the verbal and nonverbal cues and documented.

If possible, learn about the client's pretraumatic coping style from the family members. Clients who normally handle crises by crying, talking, or becoming depressed will continue to use the same methods after their burn. Knowing pretraumatic coping styles allows the nurse to prepare the nursing staff and client's family for these probable behaviors.

One of the most challenging aspects of nursing burn clients is supporting clients' coping as they adjust to their injury and its sequelae. Clients may feel angry at themselves or others for causing or contributing to the accident, guilty for not "being more careful," resentful if the injury was a punishment, and victimized if the injury was intentional. They may also be grieving for loss of home, family members who may have died in the fire, appearance changes, or inability to cope with pain. There are also potential losses, such as employment and financial security. All of these feelings are added to feelings of pain and anxiety about the final scarring and altered appearance.

The nurse should be aware that these feelings may also arise in family members as they grieve. The client's family must also be assessed for ability to cope with the crisis. While talking with the family, assess for rational and irrational thoughts, stages of grieving, behavior, and general reaction to the client and the injury.

Objective Data

Photographs should be taken of the burn wounds on admission and throughout hospitalization. Pictures can assist in documenting healing and can prove useful for insurance or legal claims.

Assessment of Size of Burn
The size of the burn is expressed as a percent of the total body surface. There are two methods to calculate burn size. The *rule of nines* divides the adult body into sections: The head is 9% of the total body; the anterior and posterior trunk are each 18%; each leg is 18%; each arm is 9%; and the perineum is 1%, equalling 100%. The rule of nines is a rapid way to estimate burn size in adults (Figure 15–7). The rule of nines is not accurate for children because their body proportions are not the same as in adults. Refer to a pediatric nursing text for a modified rule of nines for children.

Other more accurate methods are available to calculate the extent of burn injury. These methods use charts that allow for changes in body proportion with age. One such method, the *Lund–Browder method,* is illustrated in Figure 15–8. To use the Lund–Browder chart to determine burn size, shade in the area of the burn wound on the diagram for full thickness burns and use slash marks

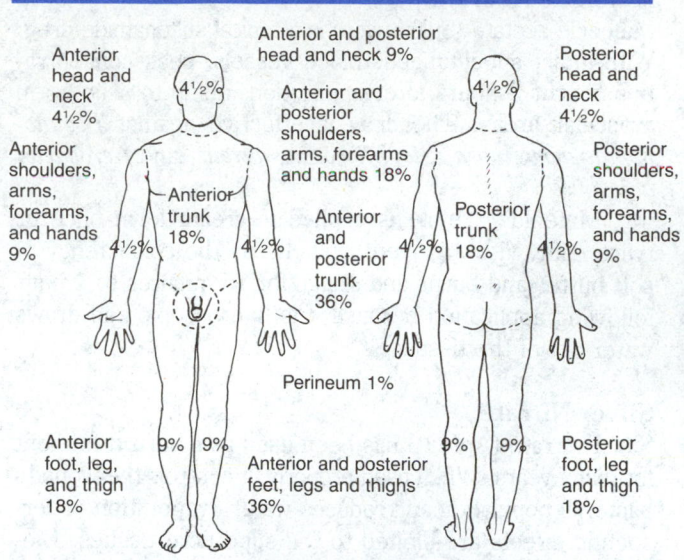

Figure 15–7

Estimating the extent of burns on the body surface area using the rule of nines.

to indicate partial thickness wounds. The numbers on each body portion indicate the percentage of body surface area for that part. For example, the anterior upper arm is 2% of BSA. Body areas that change in percentage with growth are marked with letters A, B, C. (Recall that a child's head is large in comparison to his body.) These areas are calculated by age, using the chart at the bottom of the form. For example, the anterior aspect of the newborn's head (age 0) is calculated at 9½%, the 5 year old at 6½%, and the adult at 3½%. These charts allow a rapid and yet accurate means of determining burn size.

Assessment of Depth of Burn
As previously discussed, burn wounds can be classified as first, second, or third degree or as partial or full thickness. Both sets of terms describe the depth of injury to the skin. The term *partial-thickness* includes first- and second-degree burns; *full-thickness* burns are equivalent to third-degree burns (refer to Figure 15–1).

A first-degree burn damages only the epidermal layer of the skin. Sunburn is a common first-degree burn. These wounds appear red and dry and blanche with fingertip pressure. First-degree burns are painful because cutaneous nerve endings are injured. These injuries will heal on their own within 1 week if there are no complications.

Second-degree burns, which damage the epidermis and part of the dermis, appear red and blistered. If blisters have broken, the wound will appear wet or crusted. Second-degree burns are painful because cutaneous nerves are exposed to air. Shallow second-degree burns can heal on their own over a few weeks. Deeper second-degree burns can heal on their own but are often skin grafted to speed recovery, reducing the risk of wound infection and

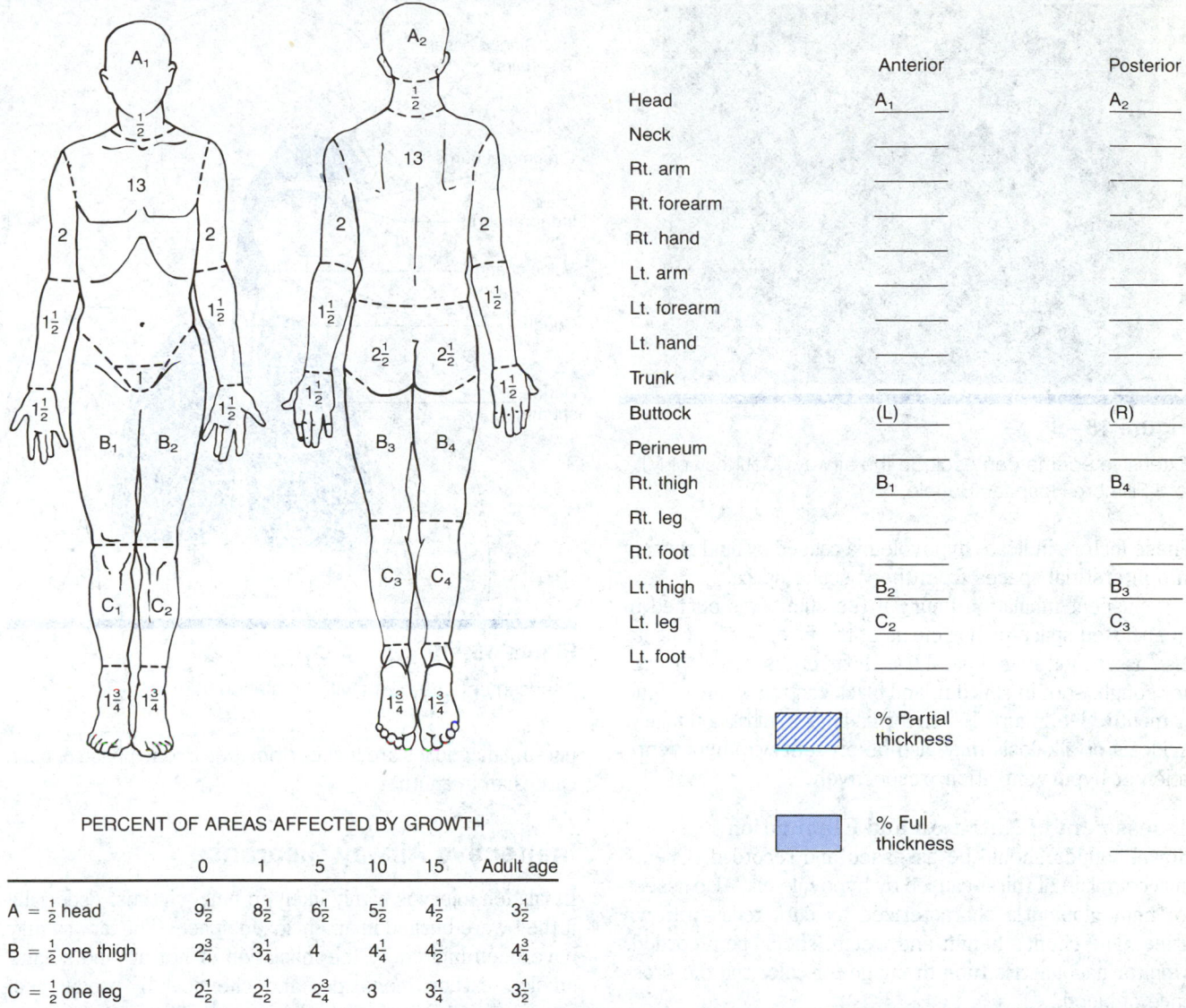

	Anterior	Posterior
Head	A₁ _____	A₂ _____
Neck	_____	_____
Rt. arm	_____	_____
Rt. forearm	_____	_____
Rt. hand	_____	_____
Lt. arm	_____	_____
Lt. forearm	_____	_____
Lt. hand	_____	_____
Trunk	_____	_____
Buttock	(L) _____	(R) _____
Perineum	_____	_____
Rt. thigh	B₁ _____	B₄ _____
Rt. leg	_____	_____
Rt. foot	_____	_____
Lt. thigh	B₂ _____	B₃ _____
Lt. leg	C₂ _____	C₃ _____
Lt. foot	_____	_____

% Partial thickness

% Full thickness

PERCENT OF AREAS AFFECTED BY GROWTH

	0	1	5	10	15	Adult age
A = ½ head	$9\frac{1}{2}$	$8\frac{1}{2}$	$6\frac{1}{2}$	$5\frac{1}{2}$	$4\frac{1}{2}$	$3\frac{1}{2}$
B = ½ one thigh	$2\frac{3}{4}$	$3\frac{1}{4}$	4	$4\frac{1}{4}$	$4\frac{1}{2}$	$4\frac{3}{4}$
C = ½ one leg	$2\frac{1}{2}$	$2\frac{1}{2}$	$2\frac{3}{4}$	3	$3\frac{1}{4}$	$3\frac{1}{2}$

Figure 15–8

Estimation of size of burn by Lund–Browder chart.

minimizing scarring. Second-degree burns will blanche and refill with fingertip pressure.

Third-degree burns, or full-thickness burns, damage both epidermal and dermal layers of skin. Subcutaneous tissue, muscle, and bone may also be injured. These wounds appear leathery and may be white, brown, red, or black. The wound will be painless because cutaneous nerve endings have been destroyed and will not blanche with fingertip pressure. Third-degree burns do not heal without skin grafting unless they are small. The deeper the burn wound, the more severe the injury because of pathophysiological changes (see previous discussion of multisystem stressors).

Assessment of Oxygenation

Nursing assessments of airway patency and vascular flow to extremities are critical. Edema of the head and neck can become so extensive that the airway swells closed (Figure 15–9). Blood flow to the foot or hand may be lost because of swelling of a circumferential burn of the arm or leg. Respiratory rate and depth, lung sounds, air hunger, peripheral pulses, and color should be assessed hourly.

Inadequately treated fluid shifts may lead to hypovolemia and shock. Assessments of blood pressure, pulse, skin temperature, urine output, and mental status must be collected frequently—every 15 minutes initially. In the assessment, be alert for:

- Low blood pressure
- Rapid pulse rate
- Absent or weak peripheral pulses
- Elevated hematocrit level
- Cool unburned skin
- Low urine output
- Confusion

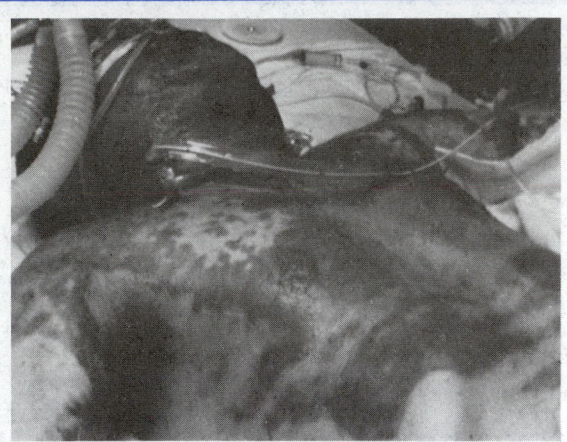

Figure 15–9

Extensive edema can occlude the airway. (Courtesy of Millard Fillmore Hospital, Buffalo, NY)

These factors indicate hypovolemia caused by fluid shifting into interstitial spaces from the vascular space.

Suspect inhalation injury if the client was burned in an enclosed space or has burns of the face, head, or neck. Also assess for singed nasal hair, hoarseness, voice change, dry cough, soot in sputum, and black coating on the tongue or mouth. See Figure 15–10 for findings in inhalation injury. Acidosis or alkalosis may also be present with hypoventilation or hyperventilation, respectively.

Assessment of Nutrition and Elimination

Bowel sounds should be assessed and recorded. Clients may complain of thirst caused by hypovolemia. Also assess for hemoglobinuria characterized by dark reddish-brown urine. The client's height and weight should be recorded. Monitor nasogastric tube drainage for color and the presence of blood.

Basic hematologic studies, complete blood count, serum electrolytes, and BUN level should be performed as a baseline for determining hydration status. Hyperkalemia should be noted and reported to the physician.

Assessment of Other Injuries or Health Problems

The health team must suspect internal organ damage, fractures, or head injuries in clients who were victims of explosions or who fell or jumped from a burning building. Existing illness will often be exacerbated by the stress of the burn. For example, diabetics will often have uncontrollable blood glucose levels caused by gluconeogenesis from stress.

NURSING DIAGNOSES

Nursing diagnoses in the emergent period reflect the priorities of caring for a person with critical and possibly life-threatening injuries. Nursing diagnoses directly and indirectly related to immediate care of the burn client are listed in Box 15–2. Diagnoses directly related to emergent care are discussed in this section. The diagnoses for the three phases of care have been prioritized for each phase. Some

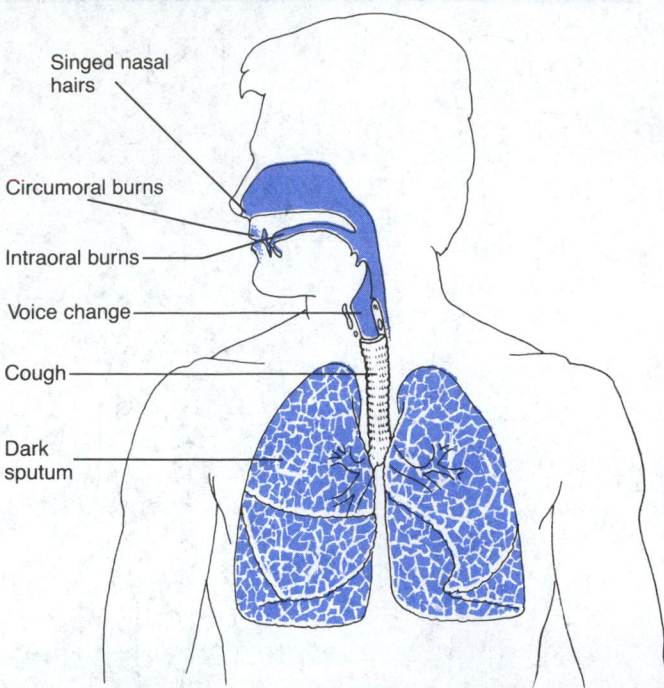

Figure 15–10

Assessment of a client with inhalation injury.

nursing diagnoses are higher priorities in one phase of burn care than in another.

Ineffective Airway Clearance

Inhalation injury is highly likely in burn victims, especially if they were burned in an enclosed space. The airway may have been injured by the inhalation of hot air and steam, smoke, carbon monoxide, and chemical by-products of combustion. Soon after the injury, the inflammatory response produces edema of the head and neck, which may be so extensive that the airway is blocked. Adding to the problem of edema is the massive fluid shift, which is the body's immediate response to a severe burn. Edema resulting from the fluid shift may also block the airway.

Impaired Gas Exchange

Burns produce a variety of problems that impair oxygenation, as previously described. First, inhalation injuries may damage the airway and lung parenchyma; edema may block the airway. The combined effects of fluid shift and hypovolemia also produce pulmonary dysfunction. The problem of decreased oxygenation is exacerbated by reactions to pain and fear.

Actual or Potential Fluid Volume Deficit

Fluid volume changes are the most significant immediate physiological response to a burn. Fluid volume replacement is a priority for the health care team. With thermal injury, capillary permeability increases, and fluid leaks into the extravascular spaces. With hypovolemia, cardiac output falls, renal blood flow decreases, blood viscosity increases, and total peripheral vascular resistance increases because of peripheral vasoconstriction. The process may result in renal failure and death without rapid treatment (see discussion of multisystem stressors).

Impairment of Skin Integrity

Skin is destroyed by burns, and the degree of injury is classified according to the depth of destruction. The depth of skin injury influences the systemic effects of the burn, how long the wound will take to heal, and the potential for complications. With loss of skin comes heat loss, and the client is subject to hypothermia.

Alteration in Tissue Perfusion

Poor tissue perfusion, a result of fluid loss and hypovolemia, has implications for all organ systems (see multisystem stressors). The body's first reaction to the insult is primary or neurogenic shock, probably from pain and fear, causing sudden collapse from generalized vasodilatation. With the massive fluid shift into tissues, cardiac output falls, and hypovolemic shock, or secondary shock, may ensue. Without immediate adequate resuscitative measures, acute renal failure and death may follow.

Alteration in Comfort

Burns cause intense pain. Immediately after the burn, the degree of pain depends on the extent of the burn. First- and second-degree burns are painful because of damage to nerve endings. The third-degree burn victim may not feel pain because cutaneous nerve endings have been destroyed. The client's response to pain varies with the pain threshold and perhaps cultural values.

Alteration in Pattern of Urinary Elimination

During hypovolemia, renal blood flow is reduced and clients can have decreased urinary output. Hemoglobinuria and myoglobinuria may also develop following severe burn injury.

Ineffective Coping

A client who has been severely burned has been through a traumatic event. In addition to the pain and anxiety caused by the burn itself, the client may also be overwhelmed by the traumatic circumstances of the fire or accident. The family is also likely to be overwhelmed by the client's injury and the events surrounding it.

Alteration in Bowel Elimination

Ileus may result from the stress of the burn injury. With fluid shift and hypovolemia, there is a drop in plasma vol-

---

Box 15–2 Nursing Diagnoses Commonly Related to Burns in the Emergent Period

Diagnoses Directly Related to Burns in Emergent Period

Airway clearance, ineffective

Gas exchange, impaired

Fluid volume deficit, actual or potential

Skin integrity, impairment of, actual and potential

Tissue perfusion, alteration in

Comfort, alteration in, related to pain

Urinary elimination, alteration in pattern of

Coping, ineffective individual and/or family

Bowel elimination, alteration in, related to ileus

Infection, potential for

Mobility, impaired physical

Additional Potential Nursing Diagnoses

Communication, impaired verbal

Fear

Grieving, anticipatory

Injury, potential for, related to trauma

Self-concepts, disturbance in, related to body image

Thought processes, alteration in

---

ume, blood volume, and cardiac output; the result is poor tissue perfusion, which impairs bowel function.

Potential for Infection

Although a burn wound is usually sterile initially, burn eschar later provides a medium for growth of microorganisms. Wound infection is the most common complication for burn victims.

Impaired Physical Mobility

Burn clients are susceptible to movement problems both because of burn wound contractures and because of immobility. Burned hands may present an especially difficult mobility problem.

PLANNING AND IMPLEMENTATION

Immediate care of burn clients is discussed in the section on treatment. This discussion focuses on nursing activities performed after the client has been stabilized and admitted to the hospital. A sample nursing care plan for the emergent period is presented in Table 15–2.

Table 15−2   Sample Nursing Care Plan for the Emergent Period

Nursing Diagnosis	Client Care Goals	Plan/Implementation	Expected Outcome
Airway clearance, ineffective	Patent airway; adequate oxygen-carbon dioxide exchange	Maintain patent airway through proper positioning, removal of secretions; establish airway if needed	Patent airway and adequate respiration maintained
Gas exchange, impaired	Adequate oxygen-carbon dioxide exchange	Provide oxygen as appropriate; assess breath sounds and respiration; monitor client on ventilator; observe for signs of respiratory distress or carbon dioxide poisoning	No signs of respiratory distress or inadequate oxygenation
Fluid volume deficit	Restoration of fluid balance	Observe vital signs, urine output, CVP, and sensorium for signs of hypovolemia or fluid overload; maintain IV lines and regulate fluids; observe electrolyte levels and report abnormal values to physician; document input and output (I and O); weigh client daily	No signs of hypovolemia or fluid imbalance
Skin integrity, impairment of	Progress in wound healing; freedom from infection	(See nursing activities for preventing infection)	Progress in wound healing; no signs of infection
Tissue perfusion, alteration in	Correction of hypovolemia with increase in cardiac output	Observe vital signs, urine output, CVP, and sensorium for signs of hypovolemia; maintain IV lines and regulate fluids; assess for dysrhythmias	No signs of hypovolemia; cardiac output adequate
	Adequate tissue perfusion	Assess peripheral pulses hourly on extremities with circumferential burns; report signs of decreased peripheral circulation or nerve or muscle ischemia to physician; elevate extremities and head of bed (see also nursing activities for fluid volume deficit, cardiac output, and urinary elimination)	No signs of inadequate tissue perfusion
Comfort, alteration in, related to pain	Control of pain	Assess pain; differentiate from hypoxia; administer IV narcotics; introduce relaxation techniques, nitrous oxide, and other adjuncts to pain relief; provide emotional support	Adequate control of pain
Urinary elimination, alteration in pattern of	Adequate urinary elimination	Monitor electrolyte levels; document I and O; weigh client daily; observe urine output for hemoglobinuria (see also nursing activities for fluid volume deficit)	
Coping, ineffective	Adequate coping skills	Maintain calm, confident manner; provide adequate pain control for painful procedures; prepare family for first visit; provide honest information as client and family seem ready	Demonstration of realistic coping skills
Bowel elimination, alteration in	Adequate bowel function	Maintain NG tube on low intermittent suction until bowel sounds return; auscultate for bowel sounds q. 4 h	Adequate bowel function returns

Nursing Diagnosis	Client Care Goals	Plan/Implementation	Expected Outcome
Infection, potential for	Freedom from infection	Use aseptic technique in client care; support immune response by prevention of shock; maintain isolation; clean client's perineum; administer antimicrobial drugs as ordered; administer tetanus prophylaxis	No signs of sepsis or wound infection
Mobility, impaired physical	Maintenance of adequate mobility	Prevent client susceptible to neck contracture from sleeping on pillow; assist in ROM exercises; encourage exercise for client with burned hand	Client performs exercises regularly; client describes reason for exercise; ROM is adequate

Maintaining Airway Clearance

Two immediate goals of treatment are maintenance of the airway and normal blood oxygen levels. Arterial blood gas values are assessed frequently to evaluate oxygenation. The head of the bed is elevated if blood pressure permits. Oxygen can be provided through the appropriate mode. If the airway or normal oxygenation cannot be maintained, tracheotomy or intubation may be performed. Clients may require mechanical ventilation. In this case, nursing responsibilities are the same as for any respirator-dependent client (see Chapter 18).

Improving Gas Exchange

Impaired gas exchange will be improved by maintaining the airway and respiration and by treating hypovolemia and fluid loss. Nursing interventions for these problems are discussed in the appropriate sections.

Restoring Fluid Volume Deficit

Massive volumes of intravascular fluids are lost to edema after a burn (see discussion of multisystem stressors). Untreated, hypovolemia will cause death; therefore, rapid replacement of fluid losses is critical for the burned client.

A large-bore intravenous line should be inserted. Major burn clients often have central venous lines (discussed and illustrated in Chapter 8). The needle should be placed through unburned skin and proximal to any burns on the extremities.

Ringer's lactate solution is the fluid of choice for resuscitation because it is physiologically similar to blood serum. If Ringer's lactate is not available, use of any other intravenous fluid is preferable to no fluid administration at all. Solutions with glucose should be administered carefully because osmotic diuresis can occur. (Osmotic diuresis is the loss of body water through the urine as the glucose is excreted.) Colloids may be administered after cell membranes have stabilized. Giving colloids too early after the burn can increase edema because the protein leaks through the altered membranes, drawing body water with it.

The volume of fluid replacement is calculated using a formula (Box 15–3). Assessing the client's response to fluid therapy is essential. Fluid resuscitation formulas are only guidelines to fluid therapy; the best indicator of fluid balance is the client. Measure vital signs every 15 to 30 minutes and urine output every hour. Signs of continuing hypovolemia should also be noted. When urine output begins to increase, intravenous fluids can be reduced. Physicians may order fluids titrated to maintain a urine output of 30 mL/h. Administer fluids to achieve this urine output, calculating and adjusting the fluid rate every 30 minutes. The client should be weighed daily to determine fluid status. Body weight is more accurate for determining fluid status than intake and output.

Hyperkalemia can be treated with potassium-binding enemas and/or with intravenous glucose and insulin solutions. Glucose and insulin solutions allow potassium to reenter the cells, temporarily reducing the serum levels of the electrolytes.

Promoting Skin Integrity

Immediate goals for skin integrity for the burned client are preventing infection and promoting wound healing with minimal scarring. Recall that hypothermia can result from

---

Box 15–3 Baxter's Formula for Calculating Fluid Requirements

4 mL × % BSA burned × kilograms = fluid to be administered in the first 24 hours post-burn

Administer one-half of total fluids in 8 hours and one-half in next 16 hours. (Calculate the first 8 hours from the time of injury.) For example, in the first 24 hours, fluid requirements for a 70 kg man with a 50% burn would be calculated as follows:

$4 \times 50 \times 70 = 14{,}000$ mL fluid in 24 hours
(7000 mL in first 8 hours; 7000 mL in next 16 hours)

loss of skin. Warm the client's room to 90°F and use heat shields, lamps, or blankets to maintain normothermia. Work quickly to redress burn wounds when exposed to room air. Monitor body temperature rectally every 2 hours.

Burn wounds should be cleaned before applying ointments or dressings. The burn wound may require soaking in a basin of water or with wet dressings to loosen burned-on debris. Loose shreds of skin should be removed with forceps. Intact blisters should not be opened. Blistered areas should be dressed loosely so the dressing will absorb the fluid and keep the wound clean when the blister breaks.

After the wound is clean, prescribed antimicrobial ointments and dressings are applied (see discussion of treatment). The ointment should be applied to the dressing to avoid touching the wound directly. This technique reduces pain and potential for contamination. The antimicrobial dressing should be secured with a gauze bandage, wrapping body parts distal to proximal.

Burn wounds covered with ointment but not dressed should be kept clean and moist. Normal saline on sterile gauze can be used to clean the wound. Crusts on the wound should also be removed. Crusts harbor bacteria, creating potential for infection and scarring.

Prophylactic antibiotics are seldom given to burn clients; they cannot penetrate the avascular eschar. The only exception is the administration of penicillin for the first 72 hours to reduce the risk of streptococcal infections. Tetanus prophylaxis is provided or renewed for burn clients. As the eschar separates from the body, an anaerobic environment is left, providing an environment for tetanus organisms to grow. If the client was rolled on the ground to extinguish the flames, risk of tetanus is higher.

Some areas of the body require special precautions. Ear tissue is primarily cartilage, which has poor circulation. Ear burns heal slowly and become infected easily. Dressings should pad the entire ear well, including the back of the ear, so the ear is not pressed onto the skull. Hands may be dressed in a variety of ways—each finger wrapped separately, the hand placed in a bag with ointment, or the hand placed in a medicated glove. Perineal burns are especially susceptible to infection. Perineal burn wound dressings must be checked after each voiding and bowel movement and changed as needed. For further discussion, see the section on immediate burn treatment.

Improving Tissue Perfusion

Tissue perfusion is improved by resuscitative measures to treat fluid loss and hypovolemia. Effects of poor tissue perfusion on the major organ systems are monitored.

Deficits in cardiac output are corrected by providing for oxygenation and fluid replacement, as discussed under airway clearance, ineffective breathing patterns, and correcting fluid volume deficit. The client should have an ECG monitor; electrodes can be placed on burned skin if necessary.

Promoting Comfort

Burn injury is extremely painful. Clients with severe burns (more than 25% of body surface area) should receive intravenous narcotics. Intravenous administration is used because circulation to the extremities is diminished and therefore, medication given intramuscularly would not be absorbed, pain relief would not be achieved, and the client would require more medication. Then when circulation was restored, all medication pooled in the extremities because of intramuscular administration would flood the body, causing an overdose.

Self-administered nitrous oxide has been effective in controlling pain and anxiety. The client holds the mask to the face until relaxation occurs and pain diminishes. If the client falls asleep, the mask is dropped, so overmedication usually is not a concern.

Improving Urinary Elimination

A drop in urinary output is the result of decreased renal blood flow from hypotension and the secretion of ADH and aldosterone. Measures to improve fluid balance will improve urinary elimination (see previous discussion of fluid volume).

An in-dwelling catheter should be inserted in all clients with major burns and in those with burns of the perineum. Urine should be sent for urinalysis, noting the amount and color. If hemoglobinuria is noted, serial urine samples should be collected until the urine is clear. A sample of 15 to 30 mL should be collected each hour and labeled clearly; the samples are lined up in sequence to monitor the change in color. Notify the physician if hemoglobinuria is noted because unpassed hemoglobin may lodge in the kidney, potentially causing renal damage. Diuretics may be required to open the nephron cell walls, allowing the large hemoglobin molecules to pass through.

Supporting Effective Coping

Effective coping can be supported by a variety of interventions. A calm, confident attitude in caring for the client will earn the client's trust. When the client screams or pulls away from a painful procedure, assess the need for safe use of additional analgesia. If no more of the analgesic can be safely administered, the client may need to be restrained to allow a necessary procedure to be completed. Keep in mind the intended outcome and need for the procedure, trying not to be distracted by the client's reaction because this will extend the time needed to complete the task.

Prepare the family for the initial visit with the client. Seeing the client swollen, in pain, covered with dressings, and surrounded by machines may be distressing for them. Before the visit, describe how the client will look, what is temporary (such as swelling), and the reason for unusual behavior, such as confusion or combativeness, especially if the client has been placed in restraints. Often the family will be more concerned initially about the client's future appearance than will the client. A discussion about scarring is best left to the physician because healing is unpredictable.

The health team should be honest with the client and family about expected outcomes. News about unfavorable outcomes should be given gradually, allowing the client and family time for effective coping. Be aware that information may need repeating because stress, fear, pain, and anxiety block clear understanding of information.

Improving Bowel Function

If a nasogastric tube has been placed for ileus, the tube should be attached to low intermittent suction. Bowel sounds should be auscultated every 4 hours.

Preventing Infection

Physiologically stable clients may have their wounds cared for in the emergency room. For unstable clients, wound care is deferred until they are stabilized. Once transferred to the burn unit, the client will require isolation precautions to reduce the risk of wound infection. In some burn units, each client has a private room; in others, the entire burn unit is isolated from the rest of the hospital.

Aseptic technique must be used for all client care. The client's own intestinal flora is the primary source of infections. For this reason, the nurse must clean the perineal area well, especially after bowel movements. Sterile linens are used if the hospital policy so specifies. The second major source of infection is the environment. The nurse is also responsible for monitoring compliance with isolation precautions by all members of the health care team.

Maintaining Mobility

Some body areas require special attention. With neck burns, the client is susceptible to contractures. Clients with neck burns should not use pillows under the head; this avoids neck flexion. ROM exercises should be performed routinely. Burned hands may also develop contractures with loss of function. Hourly exercises of hands and fingers and elevation to reduce edema are critical. Exercising hands is painful, so clients may be reluctant to do exercises. Encourage the client because hand function is important for long-term recovery. Static splints may be used to maintain a client's hands in a functional position during rest times. They are also helpful when hands are too edematous to exercise.

EVALUATION

The nursing process is completed through evaluation of the client's response to planned interventions. Expected outcomes during the emergent period are:

- Patent airway and maintenance of adequate oxygenation
- Improvement in gas exchange
- Restoration of fluid and electrolyte balance
- No further degradation of skin integrity
- Maintenance of normothermia
- Improvement in tissue perfusion
- Control of pain
- Improvement in urinary elimination
- Demonstration of adequate coping mechanisms
- Restoration of bowel function
- Freedom from wound infection
- Maintenance or improvement in mobility

Section III: Nursing Process in Acute Period

The client enters the acute period when fluid resuscitation is complete. In this phase of care, the focus is on wound care and promotion of healing. This period, which may last from a few days to many months, ends when less than 20% of the body surface is yet to be healed.

ASSESSMENT: ESTABLISHING THE DATA BASE

As the client's physiological condition stabilizes, the client faces new physical and emotional challenges. Vigilant monitoring continues for oxygenation and fluid and electrolyte balance. Because of the multisystem impact of burns, complications are a continuing threat. The nurse's assessment is the first line of defense against such potential complications as sepsis, wound infection, stress ulcer, and deteriorating nutritional status. During this period, the client

begins psychological adjustment by first confronting the extent of the injury and then beginning to come to terms with the possibility of disfigurement. The client may also need to cope with a long series of painful treatments, including debridement and perhaps surgery.

Subjective Data

Pain continues to be a serious problem in the acute period. Physical pain will be increased by anxiety, creating a pain-anxiety cycle that must be broken by controlling pain. Since pain is subjective, the nurse should not judge whether clients are in pain. Rather, assess the client's reaction to pain and other concurrent factors increasing pain or decreasing pain threshold. Pain may seem exaggerated because of loneliness, and the complaint may be a call for attention. Anxiety over anticipated procedures that may or may not be painful

Nursing Research Note

Garts K, Garland S: Marital satisfaction of the post-rehabilitation burned patient. *Occupat Health Nurs* 1983; 31(7):35–37.

A comparative study was conducted of 50 burn clients and 52 general surgical clients to determine marital satisfaction. A highly valid and reliable tool, the Locke–Wallace Marital Adjustment Test, was used to differentiate well-adjusted and maladjusted persons in marriage. Results showed that both groups were equal in marital satisfaction in all areas except for sexual relations, which showed a significant difference. Burn clients' comments about sex related to altered body image and concern for physical well-being or discomfort. Knowledge that burn clients may have sexual adjustment problems enables nurses to focus interventions on this area and offer alternatives to help the client and spouse cope effectively with their concerns.

increases pain. Muscle tension from fear lowers the pain threshold. Sleep deprivation also lowers the client's ability to cope with pain.

Clients may fear disfigurement during this period of burn care. After the emergent phase when clients feared for their lives, they begin to integrate their changed body appearance into their self-concept. The psychological assimilation of the burn event and subsequent changes is a long process requiring strong coping mechanisms. Many coping mechanisms may be used throughout hospitalization. Assess clients' behavior to determine not only the coping behavior—withdrawal, denial, anger, dependence, compliance, "a stiff upper lip," or any other of a wide variety of possible responses—but also the psychosocial needs it serves. For example, after seeing the disfigured body, a client may express a desire to abandon it through dying. On the other hand, denial of the injury and its seriousness may be assessed from statements such as, "I'll be home by next weekend," when the nurse is aware the client will be in the hospital many weeks.

Regression, the return to earlier stages of life when less mature needs were met, allows for childlike expressions of anger, frustration, and pain, conserving psychic energy when the client is overwhelmed by stress. Mild regression with any major illness is normal and can be identified in most hospitalized clients. Clients may control mild regression because they are aware that bursts of anger may have negative effects on the health care team. Severely regressed clients cannot contain anger, and their combativeness and verbal abuse may alienate the health care team. Other cues of regression are loss of bladder or bowel control, thumb sucking, whining, and pouting.

Clients often struggle against being dependent on others for basic human needs. Not only are they often kept naked for observation of the burn wounds, but severely burned clients require help eating, toileting, and ambulating. Although dependence may be difficult to accept at first,

some clients may begin to enjoy it and regress to maintain it.

Anger following a disfiguring burn can be directed inward or outward. Inwardly directed anger is often manifested as withdrawal; left untreated, it can lead to depression. Outwardly directed anger may be expressed through sarcasm, rudeness, or uncooperativeness. Clients may be angry at themselves or others for causing the accident, killing or maiming other friends or family, or not preventing the accident. Because it is essential that clients and family come to terms with the accident, be observant for cues suggesting a need to work out such feelings.

The repeated debridement, skin grafting, and plastic surgery needed to heal a burn injury may be overwhelming to clients even though they are aware surgery is essential for their survival, function, and appearance. Each operation has inherent risks: anesthesia, postoperative pain and immobility, loss of self-control while anesthetized, and possible death. Healing following a burn is a long, slow process. Daily progress may be measured only by centimeters of wound healing or joint movement. Burn care has an unknown outcome, and the health care team cannot offer empty promises that "you'll be all right."

Burn clients may view their disfigurement as a roadblock to a loving relationship with another person. Clients may feel their scarred appearance makes them untouchable and unlovable. Clients watch others for nonverbal messages about their feelings and are quick to recognize incongruent verbal statements and nonverbal signs.

During the extensive hospital stay, clients are unable to predict future activities and plans realistically. Clients are intensely aware that someone else has had to carry out their roles at home or work. This loss of fulfillment creates anxieties about their capacity to return to previous employment, or whether they are even needed.

Objective Data

Because of the changing condition of all burn clients in the acute stage, thorough head-to-toe assessments must be completed on every shift.

Assessment of Oxygenation

Oxygenation status is assessed by observing skin color and capillary refill. Lung sounds should be auscultated, listening closely for rales. The ability to cough as well as sputum consistency and color should be noted. Vital signs should be measured at least every 4 hours if the client is stable. Early changes in oxygenation status may be assessed by a change in sensorium because the nervous system is extremely sensitive to small decreases in oxygen levels. Oxygenation assessment assists in early diagnosis of cardiovascular and pulmonary complications from both the burn and immobility.

Assessment of Nutrition and Elimination

Clients should be assessed for nutritional status and signs

of weight loss. Calorie counts should be included with daily weight readings. Weight loss may be from poor intake or other problems such as infection. Daily weights should be graphed for ease in evaluation of weight changes. Laboratory values for electrolytes, blood counts, and serum protein should be assessed. Clients may require 5000 or more calories per day to meet their metabolic needs.

Assessment of Fluid Balance

The client should be assessed for signs of fluid overload during the first few days following fluid resuscitation. Include auscultation of lung and heart sounds, palpation for dependent edema, measuring intake and output, and determining whether weight gain, dyspnea, or orthopnea occur. The massive volumes of fluid administered to the client during fluid resuscitation will reenter the bloodstream once membranes have regained their integrity. Symptoms of congestive heart failure may develop if the client cannot excrete the fluid, or if the client receives too much fluid.

Assessment of Sensory–Motor Function

Clients can quickly develop flexion contractures of healing burns over both burned and nonburned joints. Burns of the hands are especially prone to contractures. Flexion and extension of all joints should be assessed, recording the actual degrees of motion. Recording ROM allows for close evaluation of progress or lack of progress. Muscle atrophy can also occur with long-term bed rest and limited activity.

Assessment of Burn Area

Integrity of burned and unburned skin must be evaluated daily. Skin over bony prominences may break down from pressure and limited movement. Burned skin must be inspected daily by the same person to evaluate the progress of healing and to recognize infection early. The best time to assess the burn wound is when clients are in the hydrotherapy tub because dressings and ointments are off. Symptoms of burn wound infections are subtle: a change in color of the wound, increased pain, conversion of a partial-thickness wound to full thickness, fever, and signs of sepsis.

The medical diagnosis of a wound infection may be made through a quantitative culture or biopsy. Quantitative culture differs from other cultures in that the tissue is evaluated for the presence of invasive infection by determining the number of bacteria per gram of tissue. A small clipping or section of burned tissue is excised from the wound. The laboratory liquefies the tissue and cultures it, determining the number and type of each bacteria present. Wound biopsy can show actual organisms invading healthy tissue, indicating invasive infection. Because burn wounds are often infected below the surface of the wound, quantitative cultures and biopsies are a more accurate method for diagnosis of infection than cultures of the wound surface.

Assessment of Complications

In burned clients, complications can involve any body system. Complete assessment of all body systems is critical.

Box 15–4 Nursing Diagnoses Commonly Related to Burns in the Acute Period

Gas exchange, impaired

Fluid volume overload, actual or potential

Infection, actual or potential

Comfort, alteration in, related to pain

Skin integrity, impairment of, actual or potential

Nutrition, alteration in, less than body requirements

Mobility, impaired physical

Coping, ineffective, individual and/or family

Self-care deficit, related to feeding, bathing/hygiene, dressing/grooming, toileting

Self-concepts, disturbance in, related to body image

Knowledge deficit, related to surgery

Sepsis is the leading cause of death in the acute period of burn care. Sepsis is caused by bacteria entering the bloodstream from infected wounds and overpowering normal defense mechanisms. Early signs of sepsis include: fever over 101°F (38°C) or below 98°F (37°C), tachycardia, tachypnea, insidious hypotension, insidious oliguria, confusion, and chills. Blood cultures verify sepsis.

The risk of stress ulcers increases with the size of the burn; ulceration begins immediately following the injury. Drugs that prevent acid secretion (cimetidine) and prompt use of antacids have reduced the incidence of stress ulcer. In assessing clients for this potential complication, look for: occult blood in stool, blood flecks in nasogastric drainage, gastric distension, pallor, and lowered hemoglobin values. Later symptoms include hematemesis, black tarry stools, nausea, vomiting, and abdominal pain.

NURSING DIAGNOSES

Nursing diagnoses in the acute period shift toward the healing process and the prevention of complications. Nursing diagnoses related to the acute period are listed in Box 15–4. Diagnoses related to the acute period are discussed in this section.

Impaired Gas Exchange

The need for close monitoring of oxygenation continues, with particular attention to potential development of pulmonary and cardiovascular complications.

Fluid Volume Overload

Fluid and electrolyte balance continues to be a concern in the acute period. In the early acute period, fluid volume stabilizes as capillary permeability is restored. During this process, the client will evidence profound diuresis and elevated blood pressure. The client may develop circulatory volume overload and pulmonary edema as well as electrolyte imbalances. Evaporative water loss from the burn wound may contribute to fluid loss.

Potential for Infection

Infection is one of the most serious threats to the client during the early recovery period. Constant vigilance is required to prevent infection from developing and to spot the early signs of sepsis. Promotion of wound healing is a primary focus of the acute period.

Alteration in Comfort

Pain is a constant companion for burn clients. Anxiety and fear may exacerbate the physical discomfort, setting up a pain–anxiety cycle. Other contributing factors may be muscle tension, sleep deprivation, and psychological needs.

Impaired Skin Integrity

During the long healing process, the skin is vulnerable to a variety of problems. The serious threat of infection has already been discussed. Other potential skin problems for healing burn wounds are contractures, keloids, and color changes. In addition, an immobilized client is susceptible to skin breakdown from pressure over bony prominences.

Alteration in Nutrition

With the metabolic changes in the postburn period, the body rapidly depletes glycogen. Severely burned clients are highly susceptible to malnutrition and often need nutritional support to offset great weight loss.

Impaired Mobility

Clients with severe burns may be immobilized for long periods. In addition, contractures may develop in the acute period if the client has been burned over joints or nonburned joints are not put through ROM. Clients who have skin grafting may also have limited mobility postoperatively. An appropriate plan for increasing ROM and ambulation is important during this period.

Ineffective Coping

In the acute period, the client must cope with a variety of stressors, such as the long time needed for healing; possible disfigurement; the continuing series of painful treatments, which may involve repeated surgeries; constant pain; and concern about reaction to his or her appearance. The family confronts similar stressors as they share the experience with the client. Clients may need assistance in developing or reinforcing coping mechanisms.

Self-Care Deficit

Immobilized clients are dependent on others for everyday tasks and personal care. They may become angry and impatient about their dependence, or they may regress to the point that they become more dependent.

Disturbance in Self-Concept

Severe burns have serious implications for self-concept because the client may face permanent disfigurement and disability. In the acute period, the client begins to assimilate changes in body image and needs support to accomplish this successfully.

Knowledge Deficit

Clients requiring skin grafting and plastic surgery will need to be educated about the procedures and their risks. They and their families will also need careful counseling about the expected outcomes.

PLANNING AND IMPLEMENTATION

Nursing interventions are designed to promote the healing process and prevent complications. A sample nursing care plan for the acute period is in Table 15–3.

Promoting Adequate Gas Exchange

In the acute period, the client's respiration will have been stabilized, although continued respiratory support may be necessary. During this period, promoting adequate gas exchange is largely a matter of monitoring. Also important is continuing assessment for pulmonary complications, which may include pulmonary insufficiency (adult respiratory distress syndrome), pneumonia, and pulmonary embolism. The immobile client should be turned every 2 hours and deep breathing and extremity exercises encouraged.

Avoiding Fluid Volume Overload

Approximately 48 to 72 hours after burn injury, the tissue membranes regain their integrity and fluid is no longer lost into the tissues. When diuresis is noted, intravenous fluid volumes should be lowered to avoid fluid overload. The potential for fluid overload still exists as fluid returns to the bloodstream. Assessing for fluid volume excess is important. Clients with circulatory overload receive similar nursing care as clients in congestive heart failure (see Chapter 24).

Preventing and Treating Infection

Infection is the most frequent cause of complications and death in burn clients. Wound infections occur because the microbial population in the wound exceeds the impaired

Table 15–3 Sample Nursing Care Plan for the Acute Period

Nursing Diagnosis	Client Care Goals	Plan/Implementation	Expected Outcome
Gas exchange, impaired	Adequate oxygen-carbon dioxide exchange	Monitor respiratory function; be alert for signs of pulmonary complications	No signs of respiratory distress or inadequate oxygenation
Fluid volume overload, potential for	No signs of fluid overload	Monitor lung and heart sounds; palpate for edema; monitor intake and output and daily weight	Diuresis with stable body weight, clear lung sounds, eupnea
Infection, actual or potential	Freedom from infection	Wash hands before client contact; cleanse client wound and body daily; apply topical antimicrobials as ordered; prevent cross-contamination; remove possible reservoirs of infection; provide donor site care; monitor graft take	No signs of wound infection or sepsis
Comfort, alteration in, related to pain	Control of pain	Assess pain; offer analgesics plus relaxation breathing, transcutaneous electrical nerve stimulation, self-administered nitrous oxide; assess and document response; assist with appropriate means of expressing pain	Adequate control of pain
Skin integrity, impairment of	Progress in wound healing; no further impairment in skin integrity	Maintain appropriate wound care, depending on severity of burn; maintain adequate room temperature and humidity; change dressings as indicated; prevent and/or control infection; take measures to minimize contractures, hypertrophic scarring, and keloids	Client shows progress in wound healing; is free of infection; wound-healing problems are prevented to extent possible
Nutrition, alteration in	Adequate caloric intake and tolerance of diet	Consult with dietitian to plan adequate intake; monitor intake and report if inadequate; monitor hyperalimentation, if given; monitor client for input and output (I and O), bowel elimination, abdominal distension	Client eats prescribed number of calories; demonstrates tolerance of diet
Mobility, impaired physical	Improved ROM and ambulation	Assist with ROM daily; document ROM; position client in open position; assist with ambulation as tolerated	Progress in ROM and ambulation; client cooperates in ROM exercises and ambulation
Coping, ineffective	Adequate coping skills	Assess client's readiness to express feelings about alteration in body image or lifestyle; provide opportunity to express feelings; maintain positive but honest approach; use other resources, such as counselors, to support coping; employ preventive psychosocial care	Client verbalizes realistic outlook on injury, treatment, and progress
Self-care deficit	Increased participation in personal care as able	Provide opportunities to participate in self-care; encourage participation; provide opportunity for client to express feelings of anger and frustration; support appropriate coping skills	Client shows willingness to participate in self-care; expresses feelings; shows improvement in coping skills
Self-concept, disturbance in	Realistic reaction to changes in body	Assess client's readiness to view burns and express feelings about altered body image; provide	Client expresses readiness to view burns; discusses feelings about

(continued)

Table 15–3	Sample Nursing Care Plan for the Acute Period (continued)		
Nursing Diagnosis	**Client Care Goals**	**Plan/Implementation**	**Expected Outcome**
		opportunity to discuss feelings; tolerate anger and regression that may aid in strengthening coping skills; reinforce feelings of self-worth; encourage family to express positive feelings toward client; refer for psychological help if appropriate	body image; family demonstrates positive attitude toward client; referral made if appropriate
Knowledge deficit, related to surgery	Accurately describe purpose of treatments, including surgery	Teach client and family about treatment procedures, even if client has had previous procedures	Client accurately describes treatment procedure; asks appropriate questions

client's immunologic ability to fend off infection. The prevention of burn wound infection includes proper handwashing prior to all client contact; use of topical antimicrobials; prevention of cross-contamination; removing possible reservoirs of infections; and wearing gowns, gloves, masks, and caps when in direct contact with the wound. Because the most frequent source of wound contamination is the client's own body flora, elimination of infection reservoirs, such as body hair and fecal material, is essential. The early detection of burn wound infection is critical and best accomplished by having the same person evaluate the wound each day.

Sepsis is treated by antibiotics, eliminating the source of infection, and by fluid replacement, steroids, and vasoactive drugs. Clients with sepsis quickly go into shock and are often cared for in intensive care units.

Promoting Comfort

After the client's pain is assessed, narcotic analgesics are used to control pain. Many clients will say, "Put me out and get this over with," because the pain seems unbearable. Be honest in explaining the physiological hazards of excessive narcotics. Antianxiety drugs are not indicated until there is adequate control of pain. Pain should be treated without a fear that the client will become addicted to the drug. Research indicates addiction does not occur when drugs are taken to control pain but when drugs are used to produce euphoria (see Chapter 10). In contrast, antianxiety drugs can produce dependence, and withdrawal from these agents is difficult. In addition to narcotics, other pain control methods have been used in burn care. They include relaxation breathing, self-administered nitrous oxide, and transcutaneous electrical nerve stimulation (TENS). Relaxation breathing and TENS are discussed in Chapter 2.

Restoring and Maintaining Skin Integrity

Promoting adequate wound healing is a major goal during this phase of recovery. The client's room temperature should

be kept at 94°F + 4 (34°C + 2) to prevent heat loss. If the client complains of chilling or body temperature drops, additional heat lamps should be used. The humidity of the room should be between 40% and 50%. If the room is drier, the eschar will crack open and bleed. If the room is too moist, the eschar will soften and separate prematurely. Portable humidifiers or dehumidifiers are effective in maintaining humidity.

Many methods of burn wound care are in use. The method used depends on the size, location, depth, and facilities available for treating the wound. Two or more methods may be used simultaneously, and methods for the same client may change during the course of healing.

Open Method

The open method of burn wound care is the application of antimicrobial ointments without dressings. This technique is used on the face, neck, upper chest, hands, and perineum because these body areas are difficult to dress. Ointments are applied with a sterile gloved hand. The heat of the room and client's skin melts the ointment, so it must be reapplied frequently. The advantages of the open method are that no dressings are required, and antimicrobials hasten eschar separation and reduce infection. The disadvantage of the open method is that frequent reapplication of ointment is necessary.

Semiclosed Method

In the semiclosed method, topical antimicrobials are applied with dressings and changed once or twice daily. This technique can be used on almost any body part (see discussion of dressing changes for technique). Advantages of the semiclosed method are:

- Wounds are inspected at least daily.
- Infection is reduced by antimicrobials.
- Eschar separation is enhanced through debridement when dressings are removed.
- Body heat loss is reduced.
- Pain is manageable except for dressing changes.

- Body parts are protected because they are not exposed.
- Clients do not continually look at their wounds.

Disadvantages are:

- Dressing changes are required.
- Painful debridement is necessary.
- Dressings can be applied incorrectly, either too tight so they restrict circulation or too loose so they fall off.

Closed Method

The closed method is the occlusive wrapping of a burn with antimicrobials and dressings that are not changed for up to 72 hours. This technique can be used on any body part according to the physician's preference. Precautions must be taken to wrap the body part in functional body alignment and not to wrap two burned body areas together, such as a burned ear on to a burned head, because they can heal fused. Outer dressings should be wrapped distal to proximal. Peripheral circulation and neurological status are assessed every 4 hours. Advantages of this method are:

- Fewer painful dressing changes.
- Body heat loss is minimized.
- Burned body parts are protected because they are not exposed.

Disadvantages are:

- Wounds cannot be inspected.
- Dressings can be applied incorrectly, either too loose, too tight, or pinning burned parts together.

Dressing Changes

Dressings should be removed after the administration of an analgesic. The nurse should don a mask, gown, and gloves before beginning the dressing change. Dressings should be removed while dry to speed debridement because the dried dressing adheres to the wound. Outer dressings should be cut and the dressing spread open and removed. Dressings should be discarded in dressing bags.

After dressings are removed, the wounds should be cleansed either in a hydrotherapy tank or bathtub, or from a basin of sterile water. Once the wound is free of ointment, loose eschar can be clipped off using sterile forceps and scissors. Eschar can be removed to the point of bleeding. If bleeding starts, direct pressure on the area will usually control it. Occasionally, topical hemostatic agents, such as thrombin, or ligation may be required to control large amounts of bleeding.

The wound should be redressed as rapidly as possible following wound care to prevent hypothermia. Dressings should be prepared before or during hydrotherapy. The exact number of dressings for wound care should be a part of each burned client's plan of care. Clients should not be left undressed and alone while nurses are searching for more dressings.

To minimize pain and save time, apply the ointment to the dressing rather than the client. Dressings can be "buttered" with the ointment like a piece of toast and stacked with ointment sides together on a sterile field while waiting for the client. Dressings with ointment should be placed on the wound and held in place by outer wrappings of gauze or netting. On extremities, outer wrappings of gauze must be applied distal to proximal to aid circulation.

To apply silver nitrate dressing, fill a plastic wash basin with warmed 0.5% silver nitrate solution. (Silver nitrate turns everything it touches black. Use caution not to touch the solution to linens or uniforms because the stain is permanent.) Soak precut and rolled dressings in the solution and then apply to all burned areas. The dressings are held in place with a bias-cut stockinette and secured with safety pins; clients are covered with dry sheets and at least one dry cotton blanket. Dry covers are important and must be changed when they become wet. The dressings must be kept soaking wet. If dressings are kept wet, reepithelialization will take place between the 15th and 40th days postburn.

During the first 7 to 14 days, the dressings need to be changed only once daily. After the eschar begins to liquefy and separate, three or four daily dressings may be necessary. As soon as treated parts are exposed to sunlight, the eschar darkens and turns brown, black, or blue, depending on the depth of the burn and the amount of sunlight. Hard blue–black eschar on wounds indicates a probable subdermal burn. Eschars of intradermal burns are brown and begin to separate after 7 to 10 days.

If infection is controlled, eschar will remain in place for weeks until finally separating from the granulating adipose tissue. If the adipose tissue is burned, eschar will begin to separate a few days after the injury. If this occurs, it must be removed promptly because liquefied eschar is an excellent medium for bacterial growth.

Burned Hands

With some first-degree burns or superficial second-degree burns, hand bags are used to reduce the pain, allow early mobility, and make it possible for clients to use their hands for daily care. A variety of such hand bags have been used including rubber surgical gloves, specially designed bags of semipermeable transparent plastic such as OpSite, and bags filled with liquid silicone. Hand bags are commonly used with topical medications, which are applied to the wound prior to covering the hands with the bags. These bags are easier to change than conventional dressings and are generally well accepted by clients.

Hand bags require several precautions. It is critical that the hand bag be loose enough not to constrict any part of the hand, particularly as the hand becomes edematous. Surgical gloves are often too tight. Precautions must be taken so normal skin does not become macerated from the increased humidity. Bacteria flourish in the moist environment. On the other hand, the bag may adhere to the burn wound if it becomes too dry. Therefore, clients with hand bags require frequent assessment.

Proper positioning of the hand is essential to reduce edema and deformities. The hand should be elevated above

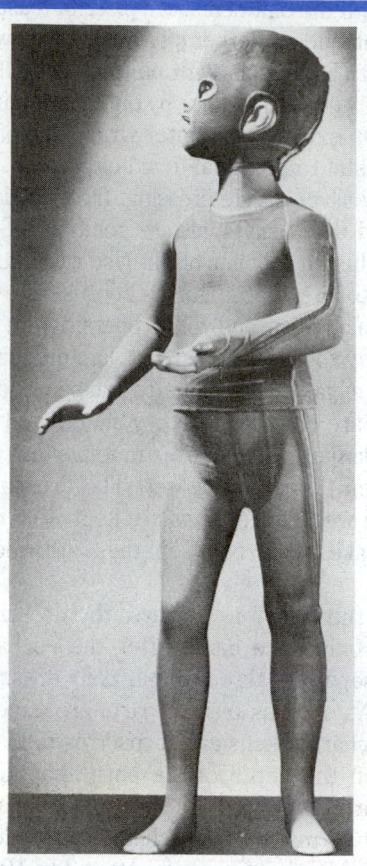

Figure 15–11

Custom-made elastic supports for prevention and correction of postburn hypertrophic scarring. (Courtesy of Jobst Co.)

the level of the heart, preferably on two pillows. This allows more freedom of movement, and cooperative clients appreciate not being tethered to an IV pole.

Problems in Burn Wound Healing

Wound contractures can be reduced in severity through excellent nursing care and client compliance. Contractures can be surgically treated by a technique known as Z-plasty, which involves rearranging and lengthening the scar tissue. Another surgical treatment is to remove the scar tissue and apply a skin graft in its place to open up the contracture. The best treatment, however, is prevention through nursing care. Applying pressure over healing wounds has been successful in reducing keloid formation. Keloids have recently been prevented by the use of lathrogen, a drug that interferes with collagen synthesis. (Scar tissue is chiefly collagen fibers.) The drug is still investigational. Steroids have also been injected into keloids but with minimal results in shrinking them. Excision of keloids usually is not successful because clients tend to be "keloid formers" and heal with keloids again. Because the etiology of keloids is unknown, the treatment varies from one physician to another. Constant pressure placed on the wound

throughout scar maturation seems to retard growth of scars. Custom-made elastic garments can be measured to fit exactly any burned body part (Figure 15–11). In most hospitals, measurements for these garments are taken by physical therapists.

As skin grafts heal, pruritus and dry skin become a problem because the sweat and oil glands are not carried along to the recipient site of skin grafts. The client should return to a normal diet if all wounds are healed and normal weight has been achieved. The client's eating should be tapered off to allow physical and psychological adjustments.

Providing Adequate Nutritional Support

Hypermetabolism following the burn quickly removes body stores of energy. Clients must be given adequate carbohydrates, fats, protein, vitamins, minerals, and fluids to support metabolism, heal the wound, and prevent catabolism and a negative nitrogen balance. Caloric needs are determined for the adult client by the following equation:

$$25 \text{ kcal} \times \text{kg body weight} + 40 \text{ kcal} \times \% \text{ burn} = \text{number of calories}$$

This caloric total may be over 5000 calories a day for major burn clients, and eating that amount of food becomes difficult. In most hospitals, dietitians work with nurses and clients to ensure adequate intake. It is critical that nurses record all that is eaten, so caloric intake can be calculated.

There are many methods to achieve the intake desired. Powdered milk or instant breakfast powder can be added to whole milk, and corn syrup can be added to orange juice; protein supplements can be given in six feedings a day. If oral intake cannot support metabolic needs, and the client loses weight, hyperalimentation or gastrostomy or nasogastric tube feedings may be used. Clients with hyperalimentation lines must be assessed closely for sepsis because the contaminated water from wound care may seep under the dressing at the needle insertion site. Concentrated tube feedings may cause osmotic diuresis and/or diarrhea. Clients should be assessed for their tolerance to their diet. Accurate intake and output, bowel movements, and abdominal distention will be clues to nutrition–elimination tolerance.

As burn wounds heal, clients' caloric needs are reduced. When burns are grafted, however, the donor sites become a new wound, and caloric requirements may need adjustment.

Improving Physical Mobility

Promoting activity tolerance is an important goal in the acute period. Joints with healing burns as well as other joints should have a ROM performed daily. The degrees of motion should be recorded to document progress or lack of progress. If contractures are forming in healing burns, frequency of ROM should be increased. Splints can be used to support joints in their functional anatomical position while in bed. Clients should be positioned in an open position to decrease flexion in joints.

Assist the client to ambulate as tolerated. After skin grafting to legs, clients will have to increase ambulation slowly. Increasing ambulation time with the grafts in dependent positions decreases potential venous engorgement and edema, which will destroy new grafts. Elastic wraps rather than support stockings should be used to support the legs because grafts can be sheared off as stockings are put on.

For a burned hand, physical therapy to maintain ROM should be initiated the first day and continued frequently throughout the healing process, which may take more than a year. ROM exercises for all hand joints will often be performed while the client is in a whirlpool twice daily. Hourly ROM exercises are also essential, however. Exercises can be done actively or passively. Increased motion can be achieved when dressings are changed. If the client has progressed to the point where hand bags can be used, the client can perform active ROM exercises with the hand bags in place. Splints are often necessary, especially during sleep.

Promoting Effective Coping

The health care team faces a great challenge in helping the client and family cope with the suffering caused by burns. Coping varies with each client and family, the support provided by the family, and the social and economic status of the client and family. How the family unit is treated throughout the healing will help determine how well they adjust physically and psychosocially.

Preventive psychosocial care will establish a trusting relationship and reduce problems throughout hospitalization. The health care team should be assured that clients and their families understand the burn injury, treatment, and prognosis. In all bedside discussions, speak directly to clients rather than talking about them to others. Allow the client as much control as possible in treatment. Finally, provide adequate analgesia.

For clients who fear disfigurement, assist the client and family to maintain hope and allow the client to adapt gradually to the body changes. Support the client's coping methods, such as denial or anger, as long as needed. Help the family understand that the client is attempting to deal with the situation. Clients will offer cues when they wish to see burned body parts or know more about their condition. They will generally ask someone they trust to help support them during their immediate reactions. Clients should not be forced to view their burns. When clients view their burns, especially facial burns, for the first time, be prepared to be supportive because the radical changes may be shocking.

Clients who deny the seriousness of their injury should be assisted to see the reality of their injury and treatment. In some cases, the need for denial may be so extreme that clients will not comprehend what is said. Some degree of

Nursing Research Note

Simmons D: Family adjustment when the breadwinner is burned. *Occupat Health Nurs* (1983); 13(7):38–40.

Four case studies of burned clients are presented to examine the financial, legal and social implications when the breadwinner is unable to be employed. Because of advances in technology and well-trained burn treatment teams, more burn clients are surviving their initial trauma. Families and clients must face a variety of stresses that must be overcome for full recovery and rehabilitation to occur. These stresses are different for each individual and must be identified early for appropriate intervention.

Anxiety management for all members of the family is essential to help them focus on problem solving and decision making. Support groups and legal aid counseling are also important. Early assessment of the social, economic, and mental health concerns of burn clients and their families is essential. Once these are identified, appropriate intervention will help facilitate rehabilitation that can foster individual growth and change.

denial is acceptable if the client does not cause harm. Families should be repeatedly informed about the true situation so they do not become confused. A firm, kind, nonrejecting approach is needed for clients coping by regression. Embarrassed and worried family members should be informed that regression is a temporary coping method and will resolve as the physical state improves.

For angry clients, the nurse must absorb the brunt of the aggression, realizing that verbal and physical abuses are not personal. The anger is directed at events surrounding the injury and its sequelae. Chemical and physical restraints are punitive; use rational methods instead for dealing with angry clients (refer to Chapter 6).

Clients and their families need support and examples of specific improvements to maintain their hope. Sincere, constant praise is needed from family members and the health care team. Clients in later stages of healing can offer much support to others. They offer positive proof that it is possible to be burned and live, boosting morale for other clients.

Convey a sense of the client's self-worth despite appearance. Recognize each client as a unique person. Clients may reject help from the health care team if they sense they are not valued. The family also needs help to develop positive feelings toward the client, even though they may feel repelled. Teach the family to touch the client without causing pain and encourage them to do so. This will help restore a sense of closeness between the family and client.

Improving Self-Care Deficit

Supporting the client in developing effective coping mechanisms will assist the client in adjusting to inabilities to provide personal care. As coping mechanisms are strengthened and the self-concept assimilates the changed body image, clients may recover from some of their anger and frustration toward their dependence.

Improving Self-Concept

It is usually during the acute period that severely injured clients first see the burns and recognize their extent. As mentioned under the discussion of coping, follow clients' cues for when they wish to view the burns for the first time. Recognize that the shock may be great and that integration of the burn into the person's self-concept may be a long and gradual process. Anger, denial, and regression may be part of the natural process of adjusting to the trauma. The nurse will need to be sensitive to the client's reaction and perceptive enough to judge when a coping mechanism has become counterproductive.

Preparing the Client for Possible Skin Grafting

For each skin-grafting procedure, clients and families should be taught about the planned procedure and preoperative and postoperative care. (These procedures are discussed and illustrated in Chapter 80.) Even if a burned client has undergone multiple skin graftings, the nurse should not assume the client and family do not have questions and anxiety about the planned surgery. The nurse can adjust the teaching to the client's needs and anxiety level.

Burn clients should have wound care completed the morning of surgery, with the wounds dressed in clear antibiotic solution or saline dressings. This eliminates the need to clean the wounds of ointment in the operating room. Burn clients are considered contaminated cases and will be the last scheduled for the operating room on the day of surgery. Some institutions use one operating room for the burn surgeries scheduled on that particular day.

EVALUATION

Expected outcomes during the acute period are:

- Adequate oxygenation
- Achievement of fluid balance
- Majority of wounds closed and absence of infection in remaining open wounds
- Adequate pain control
- Reasonable control of wound contractures and keloid formation
- Adequate nutritional status
- Demonstration of range of joint motion approaching preburn range
- Demonstration of effective coping mechanisms by both client and family
- Increased participation in self-care
- Realistic concept of changes in body image and alterations in daily activities from burn injury
- Verbalization of understanding of treatments and surgical procedures, with appropriate participation in care

Section IV: Nursing Process in Rehabilitative Period

The major focus of the rehabilitative period is preparing the client for discharge from the hospital. In the aftermath of what may have been a life-threatening injury, the client and family begin to focus more on the impact of the burn on their lifestyles.

ASSESSMENT: ESTABLISHING THE DATA BASE

Nursing assessment during the rehabilitative phase centers on the final stages of wound healing, psychological adjustment, and preparations for discharge.

Subjective Data

Clients begin to think about their functional disabilities and appearance during this phase. They begin to internalize their changed body image and often test new behaviors in the safety of the hospital. Clients become interested in other recovered burn victims and self-help groups. As clients begin to visualize reassuming responsibilities for self-care in their jobs and lives, anxiety will again rise.

Progressive desensitization—the eventual feeling that

the injury is not repulsive—occurs in this stage. The injured body is integrated into the client's self-image with less awareness of the injury. The clients will say, "Yes, I was burned once, but I'm OK now." This change allows the burned client to master body changes and again be in control.

On the other hand, maladaptive adjustments of depression, withdrawal, isolation, and regression may go on for a lifetime. Some clients feel their injury has left them so deformed that they isolate themselves from society. These clients need long-term psychological counseling and when appropriate, referral to a plastic surgeon for possible future plastic surgery. It is important that psychological problems be addressed because plastic surgery is not a panacea.

If the burn involved the face or hands, the self-concept may be seriously damaged. Burns or grafts to the face obviously alter the appearance. Furthermore, skin grafts and healed scarred wounds do not allow normal movements. Grafted facial skin does not stretch with expressions, giving a masklike appearance.

Burned clients will frequently express frustration that no one except the health care team knows what they have been through. Clients may need to discuss these feelings.

They may need assistance in planning how to react to questions that are meant to be sincere but may sound cold.

Families are primarily concerned about "doing the right thing" for the client once dismissed to home. Discharge instructions should always include the family because they become the primary caregivers. Instructions should be given in writing because the family may be as anxious as the client and may not absorb oral instructions. Having the family perform a demonstration of wound care is especially helpful in reinforcing teaching. Not only do families need to be taught what to do for clients; they need to be taught what clients can do for themselves. At times, in their zealousness to do everything possible, the family loses sight of the client's need to regain independence. Finally, the family should be reassured that they can call the burn team if questions arise.

Objective Data

Burn wounds should be assessed for development of contractures and keloids. Healed burns should be assessed for tightness, dryness, and pruritus. Unhealed wounds must be assessed for continued evidence of healing or lack of healing.

Clients will still have pain during this phase, but it should be less intense. All complaints of pain should be completely assessed before administering medications. Activity tolerance should be assessed to determine the need for ROM exercises and perhaps occupational therapy to accomplish activities of daily living.

NURSING DIAGNOSES

Nursing diagnoses in the rehabilitative period primarily involve preparing the client for hospital discharge and independent functioning. Deficits are noted in both physiological and psychosocial areas so they can be improved before the client leaves the hospital. Especially important during this period is the involvement of family because they will be central to the client's continued rehabilitation at home. Nursing diagnoses related to the rehabilitative period are listed in Box 15–5.

Disturbance in Self-Concept

Progressive desensitization to the injury is the principal sign that the client's self-concept is adjusting appropriately to the altered body image. If desensitization has not been achieved, the client may exhibit signs of ineffective coping skills, as previously discussed.

Alteration in Nutrition

During the healing period, the client may have become accustomed to a high-calorie, high-protein diet. With the change in metabolism after healing is complete, the client

---

> **Box 15–5　Nursing Diagnoses Commonly Related to Burns in the Rehabilitative Period**
>
> *Self-concept, disturbance in*, related to body image
>
> *Nutrition, alteration in, potential for more than body requirements*
>
> *Comfort, alteration in*, related to pain and pruritus
>
> *Coping skills, ineffective individual and/or family*
>
> *Knowledge deficit*, related to self-care
>
> *Mobility, impaired physical*
>
> *Skin integrity, impairment of, actual or potential*

may gain unnecessary weight if the diet and eating habits are not modified.

Alteration in Comfort

Although the client may continue to have pain, it should be diminished. By this time, pain will probably be controlled by oral agents. As the burned skin heals and becomes dry, the client is likely to experience discomfort from pruritus.

Ineffective Coping Skills

Coping skills continue to need reinforcement as the client prepares to face the world beyond the hospital. Burned clients may adapt positively or negatively to the injury and the reaction of others. Adaptive adjustments include progressive desensitization, mastery, and control. Maladaptive adjustments are depression, withdrawal, isolation, and regression.

Knowledge Deficit

In their preparation for discharge, clients and their families continue to need education about their care outside the hospital. Among the subjects on which they may need instruction are skin care, wound care, joint mobility, exposure to sunlight, nutrition, and pain management.

Impaired Mobility

In the rehabilitation period, wound contractures and ROM are the principal mobility problems. Clients need to be taught appropriate exercises and to understand their importance in restoring optimal function.

Impairment of Skin Integrity

Although healing should be largely completed by the time the client is ready for discharge, the client may still have unhealed areas. Instruction about self-care will assist the client in managing wound care and promoting wound healing at home.

PLANNING AND IMPLEMENTATION

Nursing activities, consistent with the nursing diagnoses, are focused on preparing the client to go home. A sample nursing care plan for the rehabilitative period is in Table 15–4.

Improving Self-Concept

Assisting clients to cope with permanent changes in physical appearance is not easy. In the early stages of burn care, the primary concern was for life, then wound coverage and complications. When the wounds are healed, clients and nursing staff have to come to terms with the permanence of the changed body. In many respects, clients look better than when first burned, but this is the best they probably will look. With serious signs of maladaptation—depression, withdrawal, isolation, or regression—a referral for psychological counseling may be appropriate.

Promoting Nutrition

The diet should remain high in protein until all wounds have healed. As healing takes place, the diet should be tapered off to normal caloric intake. Burn clients become used to eating a great deal of food and may develop a habit of eating frequently. After healing is complete, metabolism decreases, and the calories are deposited as fat. Clients can gain unneeded weight if the diet is not adjusted.

Promoting Comfort

Pain management may include mild analgesics and oral narcotics. Pain is generally manageable with oral agents, and the majority of pain occurs with stretching and ROM exercises. Clients should receive medication before physical therapy treatments.

The pruritus and skin drying from wound and graft healing can be relieved with the application of heavy lotion and cocoa butter. The environment should be cool and dry. The client may find cotton underwear comfortable, even in bed. Mild soap should be used in bathing to reduce irritation and prevent further drying.

Supporting and Improving Coping Skills

The client should be given an opportunity to discuss fears or ask questions. Arrange for a time when not doing treatments to have such a discussion. Give honest answers to questions, even if the answer is, "We don't know." To assist the client for going home, activities of daily living can be tried in the hospital. Alternate methods to perform activities can be discussed and tried.

Clients who fear the reaction of others should be reminded that they need not discuss every detail of their tragedy with everyone. Clients should be encouraged to be assertive and learn to say they do not care to discuss all aspects of their situation.

Psychiatric nurse clinicians, psychiatrists, or social workers are excellent resources for clients with unresolved problems. The nursing staff in the burn treatment unit does not always have time or preparation to intervene effectively in all aspects of client care. Appropriate referrals for complete and improved client care should be made without hesitation.

Improving Knowledge Deficit

Client teaching is perhaps the most important activity in preparing the client for discharge. Specific teaching activities are discussed under appropriate nursing interventions.

Improving Physical Mobility

Wound contractures can be minimized with the use of splints to hold joints in extension. ROM exercises are essential, and clients should be encouraged to begin to do their own exercises. Wound contractures cannot be completely prevented because scar contraction is a normal part of healing, but exercising will reduce their severity.

If contractures become so severe that clients cannot move a limb, their necks, or open their mouths, plastic surgery can be performed. Plastic surgical procedures include releasing the scarred tissue and sometimes skin grafting to open up the joint. These procedures are performed throughout the client's life when contractures become unmanageable.

If needed, the client should wear a custom-made elastic garment, such as a Jobst garment (Figure 15–11), 23 hours a day (1 hour to launder) to prevent keloid formation and hypertrophic scars. The garment is worn until scar maturation is complete, usually 1 year from the time of injury. After the scar has matured, contractures occur more slowly. Jobst garments should be hand washed in a mild soap and air dried.

Promoting Skin Integrity

The healed burned and grafted skin is tender and will break down more easily than normal skin because it has not formed protective calluses. Clients and family who will continue wound care at home should be taught how to do the care, including dressing removal, tubbing, debridement, application of medications, and dressings. A shower works well for debridement on small burns because the moving water rather than the client loosens and removes necrotic skin. A return demonstration is critical to evaluate learning.

Clients should be taught to avoid sunlight on burned areas for a full year because burned and grafted skin tans unevenly and unpredictably. One spot may become dark tan, and another may burn. Skin cancers are more frequent in burned skin, especially many years after a burn. There-

Table 15–4 Sample Nursing Care Plan for the Rehabilitative Period

Nursing Diagnosis	Client Care Goals	Plan/Implementation	Expected Outcome
Self-concept, disturbance in	Integration of changed body image	Assess body image and anxiety about returning to home and job; provide information about self-help resources; note signs of maladaptation (see coping skills) and refer for counseling if appropriate	Client expresses realistic self-image; does not seem unduly anxious about hospital discharge; does not show undue signs of maladaptation; accepts referral if made
Nutrition, alteration in, potential for more than body requirements	Appropriate adjustment in caloric intake; no unnecessary weight gain	Plan adjustment in calories in consultation with dietitian; explain rationale for adjusting intake; monitor intake and weight	Client explains rationale for adjusted intake; complies with diet; does not gain unneeded weight
Comfort, alteration in, related to pain and pruritis	Control of pain and pruritus	Assess pain and document; plan pain management for exercise periods; for pruritus, maintain cool, dry environment; apply lotion and cocoa butter as needed; recommend cotton underwear; use mild soap for bathing	Adequate control of pain; client does not complain of pain while exercising; client does not complain of pruritus; no signs of skin breakdown from scratching
Coping skills, ineffective	Adequate coping skills for hospital discharge	Assess coping skills; provide teaching about home care; provide information about self-help resources; note signs of maladaptation (depression, withdrawal, isolation, regression) and refer for counseling if appropriate	Client exhibits mastery of self-care skills; discusses feelings about adjustment to return to home and work; expresses interest in self-help resources; does not show undue signs of maladaptation; accepts referral if made
Knowledge deficit, related to self-care	Demonstrates understanding and mastery of self-care activities needed at home	Teach client about self-care activities to be performed at home: wound care, exercise, and nutrition	Client describes self-care activities accurately and demonstrates them correctly; states understanding of rationale for each activity
Mobility, impaired physical	Return of ROM and ambulation to near preburn levels	Assess joint mobility and ambulation; instruct client in exercises to perform at home; prescribe splints and elastic garments as needed	Client demonstrates exercises and explains rationale
Skin integrity, impairment of	Progress in wound healing; no further impairment in skin integrity	Continue to assess and monitor skin integrity; instruct client and family in wound care to be done at home; teach about susceptibility to skin breakdown, sunburn, and skin cancer	Client continues to show progress in wound healing; demonstrates wound care activities; explains rationale for wound care and skin care

fore, clients should have frequent physical examinations for the remainder of their lives. Chapter 80 discusses nursing care for clients with skin grafts.

EVALUATION

Expected outcomes during the rehabilitative phase are:

- Appropriate integration of burn into body image with less awareness of the injury.
- Successful modification of eating habits after wound healing is complete.
- Control of pain and pruritus.
- Development of adequate coping skills by client and family.
- Demonstration of necessary knowledge to perform self-care at home.
- Improved mobility.
- Demonstration of understanding of proper wound care measures and of factors that jeopardize skin integrity.

When a burn client leaves the hospital, the health care team feels a sense of accomplishment and joy at the successful recovery; they may also feel sad about the separation, regardless of the problems they faced. Some sadness may be from apprehension about the quality of life for a severely deformed client. Some health team members may be angry to see clients go home to a less-than-ideal environment or to a family that was not supportive during hospitalization. Some of these feelings may be mitigated if the client later returns for a visit, and the staff sees that he or she is functioning and adapting well.

Chapter Highlights

Burns can be classified according to their causes and depth of injury.

Clients with severe burns generally progress through three stages of treatment: emergent period, acute period, and rehabilitative period.

A client with major burns can be expected to develop four to six major complications in addition to the burn.

Massive fluid shift, which is the body's immediate response to a burn, has multisystem effects; correction of the fluid deficit is an immediate priority in burn care.

The first step in caring for a burn client is to stop the burning process. After the fire is out, the next step is to evaluate the airway, breathing, and circulation. Then initiate care to save the victim's life.

Minor burns never include electrical burns of any size or burns of the face, feet, perineum, or entire hand.

In the emergent period, initial care is strongly centered on maintaining life and on fluid resuscitation.

In the acute period, emphasis is on continued monitoring for oxygenation and fluid deficit, assessing for development of complications, preventing wound infection, and promoting wound healing.

In the rehabilitative period as the client prepares for hospital discharge, a major focus is self-care instruction for such topics as wound care and nutrition, with continuing assessment of psychosocial adjustment and appropriate referrals as necessary.

Bibliography

Boswick J (editor): Burns. *Surg Clin North Am* 1979; 58(6). [Entire issue.]

Burns among older Americans aged 70 and over. *National Burn Information Exchange Newsletter* (Aug) 1983; 2.

Demling R: Fluid resuscitation after major burns. *JAMA* 1983; 250:1438–1440.

Hill M, Achaver B, Martinez S: Tar and asphalt burns. *J Burn Care Rehab* (July–Aug) 1984; 5:271–274.

Johnson CL, Cain VJ: Burn care: The rehab guide. *Am J Nurs* 1985; 85(1):48–50.

Johnson CL, Cain VJ: Team approach to effective range of motion in burn patients. *J Burn Care Rehab* (Nov–Dec) 1981; 4:218–220.

Kibbee E: Public health nurses: A liaison between home and hospital for burned patients. *J Burn Care Rehab* (Nov–Dec) 1983; 4:427–429.

Martyn JA, Greenblatt D, Abernathy D: Increase cimetidine clearance in burn patients. *JAMA* 1985; 253:1288–1291.

Perry S, Heidrich G, Ramos E: Assessment of pain by burn patients. *J Burn Care Rehab* (Nov–Dec) 1981; 2:322–326.

Richard R et al: Autocontamination of the burn patient by hydrotherapy. *Bull Clin Rev Burn Injuries* 1984; 2:40.

Richard R et al: The effect of hydrotherapy on burn wound bacteria. *Bull Clin Rev Burn Injuries* 1984; 2:39.

Robertson K, Cross PJ, Terry JC: Burn care: The crucial first days. *Am J Nurs* 1985; 85(1):29–45.

Rosequist CC, Shepp PH: Burn care: The nutrition factor. *Am J Nurs* 1985; 85(1):45–47.

Tegtmeier R: Nursing care of patients with burned hands. *Plast Surg Nurs* 1983; 3:3–5.

Walkenstein M: Comparison of burned patients' perception of pain with nurses' perception of patients' pain. *J Burn Care Rehab* 1983; 3:233–236.

Zimmerman T, Krizek T: Thermally induced dermal injury: A review of pathophysiologic events and therapeutic intervention. *J Burn Care Rehab* (May–June) 1984; 5:193–201.

Suggested Readings

Bernstein N: *Emotional Care of the Facially Burned and Disfigured*. Boston: Little, Brown, 1976. Everyone involved in the care of injured or disfigured people should read this book. Filled with case studies, the book dissolves the fears and biases of those caring for the injured. The book shows that real people exist behind scarred faces.

Burn care. *Am J Nurs* 1985; 85(1):29–50. This collection of three articles provides a comprehensive review of burn care and includes excellent color photographs and illustrations of mobility exercises for burns of the neck, shoulder, hand, and knee.

DeCrosta T: What burn centers want you to know. *Nurs Life* (Jan–Feb) 1984; 4:45–49. Burn centers ask that emergency nurses sharpen their skills to assess accurately size and depth of burn, treat other injuries first, and know when to transfer the burn client to a burn center. Nurses caring for the burned client must devote comprehensive attention to pain relief, infection control, and fluid and electrolyte replacement.

Hurt R: More than skin deep. *Nurs 85* (June) 1985; 15:52–57. A case study of a 25-year-old man with an electrical burn.

Leeder C: Focus on burn prevention: A community education program. *Plast Surg Nurs* (Fall) 1983; 3:66–69. A series of photographs demonstrates a burn education program for the public. Various types of burn injuries are illustrated with photographs.

Surveyer J, Clougherty D: Burn scars: Fighting the effects. *Am J Nurs* 1983; 83(5):746–751. Article focuses on scar formation and abnormal scar development after burns. A series of 12 photographs illustrates positioning to prevent contractures and preserve function.

Resources

SELF-HELP GROUPS AND OTHER ORGANIZATIONS

American Burn Association
New York Hospital–Cornell Medical Center
525 E. 68th St., Rm. F0758
New York, NY 10021
Phone: (212) 371-2900

This is a clearinghouse for information on the causes, prevention, and treatment of burns that also provides referrals to medical centers that specialize in the treatment of burns. Information is also available on cosmetic surgery and rehabilitation for burn victims.

National Burn Federation
California Heritage Bank Bldg.
3737 Fifth Ave., Suite 206
San Diego, CA 92103
Phone: (714) 291-4764

This organization, founded in 1975, promotes fire safety and burn prevention programs. Membership is composed of community organizations, public interest groups, fire fighters, health personnel, and interested citizens. It also publishes educational material.

National Institute for Burn Medicine
900 E. Ann St.
Ann Arbor, MI 48104
Phone: (313) 769-9000

National statistics are tabulated here on burn injury. Also provides a burn nurse specialist program.

The Phoenix Society, Inc.
11 Rust Hill Rd.
Levittstown, PA 19056
Phone: (215) 946-4788

This national self-help organization for burned clients and their families has as its major goal easing the psychological adjustment of severely disfigured burn victims. Staff and members are usually recovered burn clients who offer one-to-one counseling services. It publishes a descriptive brochure and a quarterly publication, "The Icarus File."

Society for the Rehabilitation of the
Facially Disfigured
See resources listing in Chapter 78.

HEALTH EDUCATION MATERIAL

From: American Red Cross
(See local listing in telephone directory.) "Red Cross First Aid Module: First Aid for Burns," an 80-page programmed learning manual. Cost: 60¢.

From: The Phoenix Society
"Publications List," a 1-page flyer lists books, films, and audiocassettes on burns, disfigurement, and related topics.

PROFESSIONAL ORGANIZATIONS

American Burn Association
% Dr. Thomas Wachtel
1130 E. McDowell Rd., Suite B2
Phoenix, AZ 85006

This is a professional organization for the entire burn team. It sponsors many projects to improve burn care.

American Society of Plastic and
Reconstructive Surgical Nurses
See resources listing in Chapter 78.

International Society for Burn Injuries
% Dr. John Boswick
2005 Franklin St., Bldg. 2, Suite 600
Denver, CO 80205

The Client With Burns

I. Descriptive Data

Mr Michael Smith, age 29, was brought to the emergency room by ambulance after being rescued from his burning home. His children were playing with matches in the garage while Mr Smith was in the office above the garage. Once the fire ignited gasoline in the garage, the fire became extensive and spread rapidly. The children ran from the fire and suffered only minor burns. Mr Smith had to escape from the burning, smoke-filled house.

Mr Smith was wheeled into the emergency room on a stretcher. Some singed blond hair and a smoke-streaked face were visible at one end of the blanket, and track shoes (the right one half melted away) at the other end. His hands and arms were red and blistered with some patchy areas of full-thickness burn. His abdomen and right thigh had both partial- and full-thickness burns. He was alert and screaming in pain. According to the emergency medical technician, Mr Smith had not lost consciousness. The burn occurred at approximately 2 PM. An IV of lactated Ringer's solution had been started at the scene. Vital signs were stable.

On admission to the emergency room, Mr Smith's airway was patent. The IV fluid needs were calculated to be 7200 mL for 24 hours according to Mr Smith's reported weight of 72 kg and burn size of 35% of body area. The IV rate was adjusted accordingly. A urinary catheter was inserted, and 300 mL of dark amber urine was obtained. Mr Smith had singed nasal hairs, and because he had been trapped in a smoke-filled enclosed space, inhalation injury was suspected. The burn wounds were debrided of burned-on clothing, bathed in saline, and dressed with 1% silver sulfadiazine dressings. A nasogastric tube was inserted and connected to low suction; gastric juice returned. A tetanus booster was administered. Urine was sent for urinalysis; blood was drawn for a CBC and electrolyte values. Mr Smith was admitted to the burn unit where the following information was collected.

II. Personal Data

Date and Time:	June 14, 1986, 2:45 PM
Full Name:	Michael Smith
Social Security, Insurance Number:	000-00-0000
Address:	123 Main St.
Telephone:	Home: 000-0000
	Work: 000-0000
Sex:	Male
Age:	29
Birthdate:	6-4-57
Marital Status:	Married
Race/Culture:	White
Religion:	Lutheran
Occupation:	Accountant

Case Study written by Joyce Black.

Usual Health Care
Provider: John Jones, MD

III. Health History

Source of Information: Mrs Smith (client's wife)

Reliability of Informant: Reliable but very anxious

Chief Concern: Second- and third-degree burns of hands, arms, R thigh, chest, and neck equalling 35% BSA

History of Present
Illness: Burn occurred at 2 PM today (see descriptive data from emergency room note)

Past Health History:

Childhood: Usual childhood diseases—measles, mumps, chickenpox

Immunizations: DPT as a child, last tetanus booster 1971

Medical Problems: None

Surgeries: None

Transfusions: None

Special Diagnostic
Procedures: None

Trauma: None

Allergies: None

Medications: Occasional aspirin for headache

Family History: Father: age 55, A&W, ↑ BP

Mother: age 54, A&W

Brother: age 24, A&W, DM Type I

Sisters × 2: age 26 (twins), both A&W

No ⊕ FHx of MI, CVA, Ca, TBC

PGF, paternal uncle both with ↑ BP

Personal/Social History: Mr Smith works full time as an accountant. He is married and has two children, ages 6 and 4. His wife works part-time as a secretary. Has private medical insurance. Nonsmoker; drinks two to three beers per week. Can problem solve, deals with problems openly. Has always coped well in crisis situations.

Review of Systems:

General: Overall health has been excellent until now

Skin: No history or problems

Eyes: Wears glasses for reading

Respiratory: No DOE, cough; no hx of asthma, pneumonia, TBC

Cardiovascular: No history of ⓜ, no chest pain, no hx of elevated cholesterol or lipid levels, no family hx of MI

Gastrointestinal: Occasional "heartburn," relieved with antacids

Musculoskeletal: Rt knee pain with heavy exertion and running

IV. Physical Assessment

Height: 6 ft 1 in

Weight: 72 kg

Vital Signs: Temperature 99.9°F, pulse 116, respirations 28, BP 142/90

WD/WN: White male in acute distress from pain

Skin: Red, wet, blistered skin over arms, hands, chest to umbilicus, and neck. Remainder of the skin pale, cool, dry, and intact

Eyes: Lashes and eyebrows present, no evidence of burns; conjunctival, scleral nl; PERRLA, EOMs full; fundi, benign

Nose: Nasal hairs singed, soot evident in nose

Chest: Lung sounds clear throughout

(continued)

The Client With Burns

Cardiovascular: Heart rate rapid and regular at 116; no murmurs, rubs, S_3 or S_4
Gastrointestinal: Bowel sounds infrequent, abdomen flat
Neurological: Drowsy but arousable; complains of severe pain when awake; asks about his children; oriented × 3

V. Laboratory Studies

Chest x-ray: Normal
Urinalysis: Specific gravity 1.030; glucose negative; ketones 2+; pH 4.5; occasional hyaline cast
CBC: Hgb 17.5; Hct 49; WBC 14000; RBC 5.4
ABGs: pH 7.54; paO 80; pCO 27; HCO 26

VI. Emergency Care

Airway patent, O_2 via mask at 4 L/min. Subclavian line inserted, 2 L RL infused. Urinary catheter inserted. Wound debrided and dressed in Silvadene dressing. Chest x-ray taken. Laryngoscopy performed.

VII. Estimation of Burn Size by Lund–Browder Chart

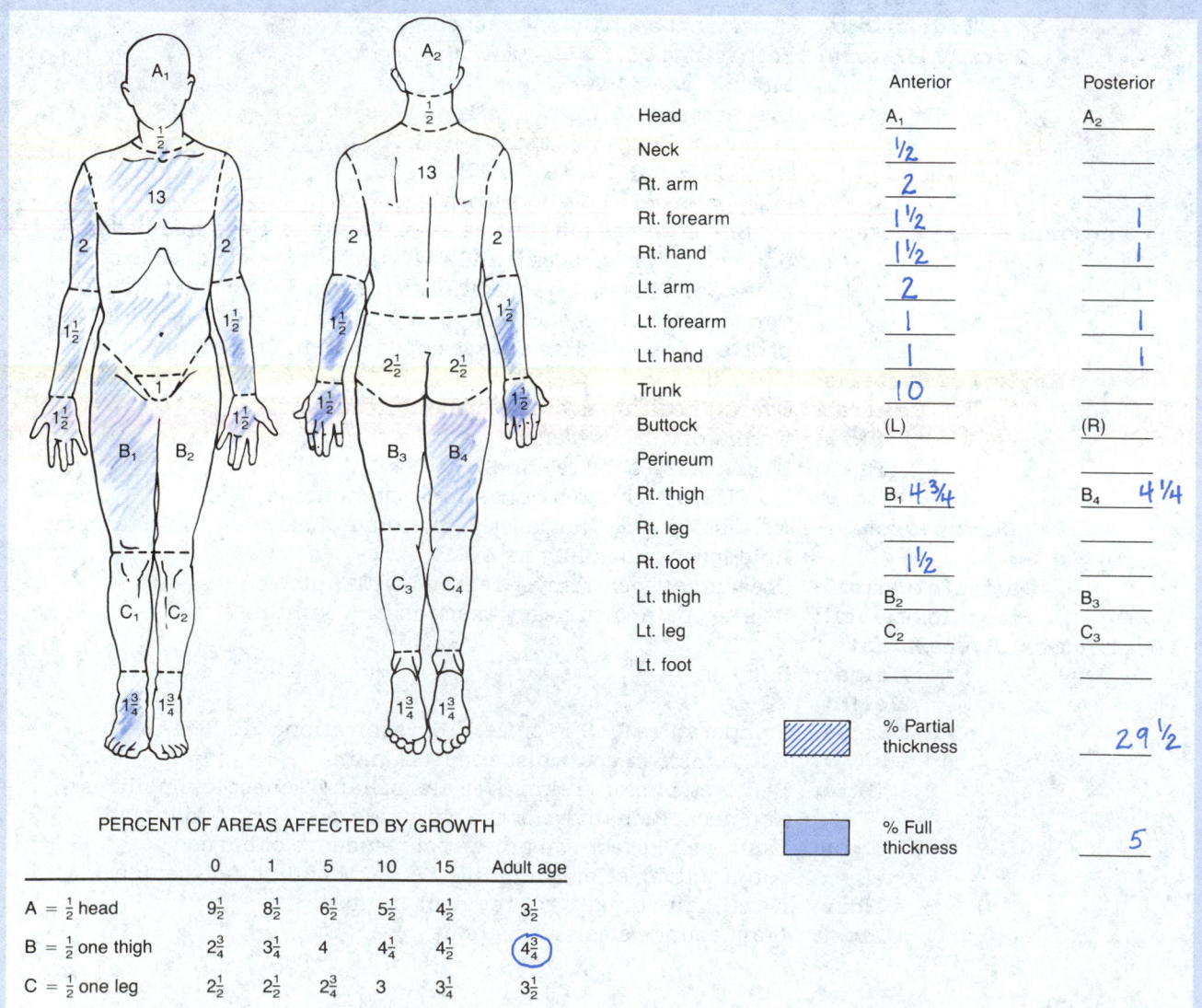

	Anterior	Posterior
Head	A_1	A_2
Neck	½	
Rt. arm	2	
Rt. forearm	1½	1
Rt. hand	1½	1
Lt. arm	2	
Lt. forearm	1	1
Lt. hand	1	1
Trunk	10	
Buttock	(L)	(R)
Perineum		
Rt. thigh	B_1 4¾	B_4 4¼
Rt. leg		
Rt. foot	1½	
Lt. thigh	B_2	B_3
Lt. leg	C_2	C_3
Lt. foot		

% Partial thickness   29½

% Full thickness   5

PERCENT OF AREAS AFFECTED BY GROWTH

	0	1	5	10	15	Adult age
A = ½ head	9½	8½	6½	5½	4½	3½
B = ½ one thigh	2¾	3¼	4	4¼	4½	(4¾)
C = ½ one leg	2½	2½	2¾	3	3¼	3½

VIII. Medical Regimen

Lactated Ringer's IV: 10,200 mL over 24 h; 5100 mL in next 8 h; 5100 mL in following 16 h
Hourly vital signs, urine output
Hct/Hb q. 8 h
Morphine 5 mg IV q. 1–2 h p.r.n. pain
NPO
Chest x-ray in AM
Wound care: 1% silver sulfadiazine dressing change b.i.d.; begin hydrotherapy in AM, if stable
Burn isolation
O_2 via nasal cannula at 2 L/min
Cimetidine 300 mg IV q.i.d.

IX. Nursing Care Plan

Nursing Diagnosis	Client Care Goals	Plan/Nursing Implementation	Expected Outcome
Comfort, alteration in: pain due to burns	Comfort increases	Morphine IV p.r.n.; observe response and respiratory rate; room temperature 90°F; keep burn wounds dressed	Severe pain reduced, requiring less analgesia
Fluid volume deficit, actual	Vital signs remain stable; urine output adequate	Infuse IV at 500 mL/h; monitor vital signs, Hb, Hct, and urine output q. 1 h; observe for respiratory distress; assess lung sounds; check pulses in arms q. 1 h; assess ABGs	Stable vital signs; urine output of 30 mL +/h; Hb and Hct in normal range; airway remains patent; pulses remain strong in extremities
Injury: potential for, inhalation	Adequate ventilation	Assess lung sounds, dyspnea, sputum color, ABGs	ABGs reveal adequate oxygenation, eupnea
Skin integrity, impairment of: actual	Normal body temperature maintained	Keep room at 90°F; keep wounds covered; use additional heat lamps during dressing changes	No hypothermia; body temperature above 98°F
	Wound healing without infection	Isolation; sterile technique for dressing changes; observe burn wound for signs of infection; monitor temperature, amount of pain, WBC count	Healed burn wound without infection
Anxiety	Client to sleep without waking up with dreams of injury	Reorient client p.r.n.; adequate analgesia; help client understand reaction is common and he will not always have such dreams	Comfortable periods of sleep increasing with time
Body image, disturbance in: related to burns of hands, arms, chest, and neck	Client to express fears about future appearance and limitation in possible use of hands	Discuss wound healing process, scar formation, and prevention of contractures with client and significant others	Client and significant others can look at burn wounds and discuss client progress openly and honestly

Chapter 16

Dying, Death, and Bereavement

Karen A. Brown
Nancy Evans

Objectives

When you have finished studying this chapter, you should be able to:

Summarize general historical trends influencing customs and rituals surrounding death and dying in Western culture.

Describe the attitudes that influence a person's perceptions of and feelings toward death and dying.

Trace how a person's concept of death develops and changes throughout life.

Identify the influences that religion, philosophy, and technology have on the understanding of death.

Delineate the criteria for determining brain death and how these criteria affect nursing practice.

Identify rights of the dying client.

Explore the importance of psychological and spiritual care to the dying person.

List the signs of impending and imminent death.

Discuss the ethical issues surrounding treatment of the dying person.

State current trends in caring for dying persons and their families.

Death, like birth, is a universal yet uniquely personal experience that each of us faces alone. In many cultures, birth is heralded with rituals expressing joy and hope; death, however, is surrounded by rituals designed to reassure and comfort. We fear death, even as we acknowledge its universality. Aware that the ultimate question about our own death is not "whether" but "when," most of us shun the subject. When confronted by impending or actual death—our own or that of a loved one—we are rarely prepared.

Nurses, in the course of their profession, may face death every day:

- The death of an accident victim, unconscious and unaware of his own dying
- The death of a client on the oncology unit after a long, painful struggle

- The death of an aged widower in his home, surrounded by children and grandchildren and mementos of a life fully lived
- The death of a young businesswoman whose life had scarcely begun

Each death evokes different emotions and behaviors from the survivors, including the nurse. Each family has different needs to which nurses can offer important responses. Nurses attend the last needs of the dying and offer solace and support to those left behind. In so doing, they must strike a delicate balance—maintaining their professional objectivity and psychological well-being without sacrificing the empathy on which their clients so often rely.

Nurses can fulfill a central role in helping clients and families work through fear, grief, guilt, and anger while helping them care for dying loved ones. Fulfilling this role requires a clear understanding of the many factors that influence everyone's responses to death, including one's own: culture, religion, family structure, and individual life experiences. Nurses must be familiar with measures com- monly used in caring for the dying, as well as ethical issues involved in such care. By exploring these and other topics of this chapter, nurses can help prepare themselves to meet the needs of the dying and those who must go on living without them.

Section I: The Problem of Dying and Death

In every culture, philosophers, religious leaders, and ordi- nary persons have pondered the meaning of life and death, wondering why humans are on earth for so short a time. All cultures associate certain rituals with death and offer some explanation of what happens to the person, soul, or spirit thereafter. The dying may themselves be held responsible for the fulfillment of certain rituals; for exam- ple, Jewish people, when dying, must acknowledge their God as the only God. If the dying are unable to perform these rituals, those close to them are responsible for such acts as summoning a priest, baptizing a dying child, or repeating special words or phrases. Individual rituals give the dying a sense of controlling their own fate; family and community rituals make them feel less alone.

DYING AND DEATH IN WESTERN CULTURE

In earlier eras of Western culture, death was part of every- day life. The dying person's family and friends attended the deathbed, and children were included in the ceremonies of death and burial. Death was not a solitary, mysterious occurrence but an everyday event with which everyone was familiar. Nor was it restricted to the old nor even the adult, because before the major infectious diseases were controlled, the death of a brother, sister, or playmate was a common childhood experience.

The present approach to death may be traced to the evolution of modern hygienic practice beginning in the late eighteenth century. "Superfluous" bystanders were ban- ished from the bedsides of the dying—especially those dying of contagious disease—as the principles of contagion became known. Hospitalization of the dying became rou- tine practice in the early twentieth century. As medical treatments became more sophisticated, control of the death experience was delegated to a cast of health care profes- sionals. Clients became, in effect, onlookers at their own deaths, and the trend toward "sparing" clients the knowl- edge that they were dying further removed the individual from participation in decisions affecting care.

Modern life-support systems have evolved to the point where "life" by some definition can sometimes be sus- tained almost indefinitely. Death has become a technical event; not a cessation of breath and heartbeat but the with- drawal of a machine or the cold determination that death has actually occurred, hedged by legalities and all too often lacking in dignity and humanity. Gonda and Ruark (1984) describe this modern way of dying as *graceless death*, char- acterized by feelings of desperation, abandonment, humil- iation, rage, and dehumanization. They indicate that grace- less death often is the result of poorly managed terminal care and carries profound consequences, both immediate and long term.

In recent years, the trend toward "technifying'" death has been reversed. Health professionals are becoming more aware of the psychosocial as well as the physiological needs of the dying and are taking an interest in *thanatology*, the study of death. **Hospices,** facilities that specialize in car- ing for the terminally ill and their families, now exist in each state of the United States and in Canada. Families who express an interest in taking their loved ones home to die are encouraged to do so if feasible. Often, the hos- pice offers ongoing support throughout the dying process and follow-up care of the survivors after the death.

Hospital care is changing, too. It is no longer custom- ary to withhold the truth from the dying and their families. In more institutions, practitioners are respecting the right of the dying to understand their proposed treatment and to accept or reject it (Box 16–1). Hospitals are allowing families to help care for their dying member, and they are trying to meet the needs of family members both before and after death. Death is again becoming the family event it has been throughout most of history.

Views of Death

Although each death is unique, depending on who is dying and the relationship, death generally can be viewed in three ways: impersonally, interpersonally, and intrapersonally (Kastenbaum & Aisenberg, 1972).

An *impersonal* view of death does not involve a sense of personal loss but rather a sense of distance from the event and the person or persons involved. The death of a stranger, multiple deaths from war or other disasters such as plane crashes, hurricanes, fires, tornadoes—usually, none of these deaths is a reminder of one's own mortality. Nurses and other health professionals are sometimes accused of having an impersonal attitude toward death. In fact, this may be a mechanism for coping with the daily stress of death. This view of death, however, can inhibit the ability to provide the empathic care and support required by the dying and their families.

An *interpersonal* view of death means there is an emotional connection to the dying person so that the death has a personal impact. Most people have many persons threaded through the fabric of their lives, and the loss of any one means not only the loss of that person but the loss of part of themselves. The intensity of reaction to a particular death depends on the importance of that relationship.

Many health care professionals whose practice is focused on care of the dying believe that an interpersonal view of death is appropriate and directly related to meeting the needs of clients and families effectively. It is difficult to imagine caring for someone throughout a terminal illness without becoming humanly involved with that person and his or her family. Remembering that every death is probably viewed interpersonally by someone can help increase awareness of the need for sensitive, respectful care of the dying and their families.

The third and most difficult view of death is *intrapersonal* because it involves the thought of one's own death and the ultimate loss, the loss of self. Confronting one's own mortality, one's nonexistence, is almost unthinkable. Writer William Saroyan's last words elucidate this concept: "I have always heard that death spares no one. However, I thought in my case they would make an exception."

Gonda and Ruark (1984) point out that health professionals can learn from the "little deaths" encountered in daily living, such as losses of self-esteem over failed expectations; loss of precious objects, health, body image, jobs or homes; and particularly, loss of loved ones. How persons cope with these losses offers important clues about how personal death will be managed.

Common Fears Associated With Dying and Death

No life event holds greater, more complex fears than dying. Choron (1964) described three primary foci for these fears: the process of dying, nonexistence, and what follows death.

Considering the pain and indignity so often associated with death in this culture, it is rational to fear dying. Many studies have shown, however, that fear of pain and indignity are secondary to fear of abandonment. Most dying persons find it more important to be with someone during the process of dying, particularly during the last moments of life.

The fear of nonexistence relates to the difficulty of imagining the world without the consciousness through which it has been perceived. Fear of the unknown has always been common in humans, and there is no more profound unknown than death and nonexistence of self.

Fears about what happens after death include those related to anticipated judgment and punishment for thoughts and behavior based on feelings of guilt and anticipation of rejection. These are not universal fears but are real and terrifying for those who have them.

Survivors also have fears about what follows the death

Box 16–1   The Dying Person's Bill of Rights

I have the right to be treated as a living human being until I die.

I have the right to maintain a sense of hopefulness, however changing its focus may be.

I have the right to be cared for by those who can maintain a sense of hopefulness, however changing this might be.

I have the right to express my feelings and emotions about my approaching death in my own way.

I have the right to participate in decisions concerning my care.

I have the right to expect continuing medical and nursing attention even though "cure" goals must be changed to "comfort" goals.

I have the right not to die alone.

I have the right to be free from pain.

I have the right to have my questions answered honestly.

I have the right to not be deceived.

I have the right to have help from and for my family in accepting my death.

I have the right to die in peace and dignity.

I have the right to retain my individuality and not be judged for my decisions, which may be contrary to beliefs of others.

I have the right to discuss and enlarge my religious and/or spiritual experiences, whatever these may mean to others.

I have the right to expect that the sanctity of the human body will be respected after death.

I have the right to be cared for by caring, sensitive, knowledgeable people who will attempt to understand my needs and will be able to gain some satisfaction in helping me face my death.

SOURCE: Barbus AJ: A dying person's bill of rights. *Am J Nurs* 1975; 75:79.

---

of another person. Guilt and a sense of unfulfilled expectations may engender a fear of retaliation for past behaviors toward the deceased. This fear may underlie the widespread fascination with ghost stories (Gonda & Ruark, 1984). A second fear of survivors is the loss of the relationship. Trying to imagine life without a valued person and a valued relationship is a realistic and painful fear. Knowing that nurses or other professionals will continue to offer support during bereavement can help relieve the intensity of that fear.

Being human, nurses often fear the complexity and intensity of caring for persons who are dying. They may fear getting too involved, not having easy answers to questions from clients and families, or feeling that they have failed when the client dies. Unless these and other common, understandable fears are acknowledged and dealt with, they can severely impede nurses' abilities to give the kind of care they would like to give and to receive. Help in dealing with the fears associated with care of the dying can come from other nurses, social workers, clergy, and other members of the health team. Venting feelings, fears, and doubts, and listening sympathetically to other caregivers can reduce the emotional burden and help create a mutual support network.

Trajectories of Death

Death can take many courses. Glaser and Strauss (1968) have grouped these courses into six types and identified them as trajectories (or courses) of death. These trajectories are:

- Abrupt surprise
- Expected swift
- Expected lingering
- Short-term reprieve
- Suspended sentence
- Entry–reentry

These forms of death affect the dying person's experience and the reactions of the family and health professionals to that experience.

A fatal heart attack, stroke, and automobile accident are examples of the *abrupt surprise* trajectory. This trajectory holds the greatest potential for shock, guilt, and unfinished business among survivors. These persons are most likely to need supportive care and counseling from the nurse or other health professional.

The *expected swift death* trajectory is most common in hospital units such as the emergency department and the critical care unit. This type of death involves a sudden severe illness or accident that is not instantly fatal.

Expected lingering is most frequently the result of chronic illness such as cancer or emphysema. This trajectory allows time for the client and the family to at least begin coming to terms with the impending death.

The *short-term reprieve* trajectory may overlap with the expected lingering death, as when a client with leukemia has a temporary remission. Short-term reprieve often reflects medical science's ability to delay but not alter the inevitable. Helping the client and family accept the temporary nature of the remission while maintaining any prescribed medical regimen is the nurse's challenge. The nurse must find a delicate balance between supporting this necessary reality orientation and simultaneously supporting hope.

The *suspended sentence* trajectory occurs when the life-threatening disease is unexpectedly cured. This situation can be difficult for families to handle, despite their joy at having their loved one spared, because they may have begun the grieving process.

The *entry–reentry* trajectory is actually a series of short-term reprieves, in which the person is in and out of the hospital. Effective nursing care depends on knowing the probable time outside the hospital, measures that will best support the client's health, individualized and updated discharge planning with interdisciplinary collaboration, and support for home care.

Critical Junctures

Glaser and Strauss (1968) also hypothesized that each death trajectory has three critical junctures:

- When the person is defined as dying
- When the hospital staff and/or the family and perhaps the client make preparations for death
- When curative treatment is withdrawn or considerably curtailed

The final phase ends only with the client's death. Nursing support at each of these junctures involves providing the client and family as much information as possible about the dying person's condition and what to expect and helping them work through their feelings when the dying process does not follow the expected course.

Time and Certainty

Because death holds many unknowns for dying persons and their families, the definition of time and certainty are important when possible. For example, if the expected time of death can be defined, the family might want to have this information. Often, however, the time of death cannot be predicted accurately. There is also a point at which uncertainty about the dying process is resolved; the questions about remissions, improvements, and death have all been answered.

In examining the relationship between certainty and time four types of death expectations can be identified:

- Certain death at a predictable time
- Certain death at an unknown time
- Uncertain death but a known time when certainty will be established
- Uncertain death and an unknown time for certainty to be established

Certain death at a predictable time means, for example, that the person will die within the hour. Certain death at an unknown time could mean knowing that the client's cancer will cause death, perhaps in hours, perhaps in months. An uncertain death but a known time to establish certainty could mean waiting for laboratory results to be analyzed. An uncertain death and an unknown time for certainty to be established may mean laboratory and diagnostic studies have been inconclusive. These factors of certainty and uncertainty can have a powerful effect on the nurse as well as the family and can make it difficult to offer essential support. In some cases, the nurse may find it helpful to consult a colleague such as another nurse, a chaplain, or a social worker.

GRIEF AND MOURNING

Grief is the subjective response to loss. Anyone faced with a serious loss begins to grieve before the loss actually occurs. A person with a diagnosis of terminal illness begins to grieve for the ultimate loss—the loss of self. Mourning is a long-range process through which grief and loss are eventually resolved. Because mourning is a painful process, some persons avoid working through it, particularly if family, friends, or others do not support and encourage expression of feelings.

In a classic book in thanatology, Kübler–Ross (1968) analyzed the grieving process of the dying person as five stages: denial and isolation, anger, bargaining, depression, and acceptance of death. Other researchers have proposed somewhat different sequences. Weisman (1980) identified four phases of dying: existential plight, mitigation and accommodation, decline and deterioration, preterminality and terminality.

Although the work of Kübler–Ross, Weisman, and other thanatologists has contributed to a better understanding of the dying, it is essential to remember that *each death is unique.* Therefore, these stages may not correspond with a particular person's experience. Individuals may move back and forth through these stages during a final illness. Moreover, one or more of the stages may be absent completely without the reaction being abnormal. Thus, nurses should not try to identify or predict a client's psychological state by mechanical application of a theory of stages. The concept of stages can be useful to help nurses recognize and deal with these reactions in whatever sequence they occur.

Anticipatory Grief

The family and friends of the dying person also experience grief from the time they learn of the impending death until after the death has occurred. Grieving for the dying person before death, termed *anticipatory grief,* is a process of letting go. The pace of this process varies among individuals. Occasionally, the process proceeds rapidly, and the course of the illness is marked by dramatic reversals. This can cause problems for the dying person who may feel that loved ones have already "let go" and that he or she is therefore alone.

Acute Grief

The classic study of acute grief, the reaction that begins at the time of death, was conducted by Lindemann (1944) with survivors of the Coconut Grove disaster in Boston where hundreds died in a fire. He described a specific symptom complex associated with the grief syndrome: somatic distress, preoccupation with the image of the deceased, guilt, hostility, and the loss of habitual patterns of conduct (see Table 16–5 later in this chapter). The length of the process varies with each individual; however, Lindemann believed that in optimal circumstances and with understanding support, acute grief might be resolved within 4 to 6 weeks. Then follows the longer process of mourning. Bowlby (1961) and Parkes (1964) have each described mourning as a three-phase process following acute grief:

Table 16–1	Phases of Mourning
Phase	**Behaviors of Bereaved**
Protest	Clings to thoughts or images of the deceased; may despair and rage at deceased or others, particularly those who encourage letting go of the deceased and returning to normal life patterns
Despair	Accepts that deceased is gone forever; exhibits disorganized behavior with anxiety and depression, a kind of disintegration
Detachment	Reintegration of personality; reorients behaviors and emotions previously centered around deceased toward other persons or activities

protest, despair, and detachment. Characteristic behaviors of these phases are shown in Table 16–1.

The total experience of grief and mourning are referred to as *grief work.* Completion of grief work is usually a slow and gradual process unique to the bereaved person that is based on the relationship with the deceased. Strongly ambivalent feelings toward the deceased can prolong the time needed for grief work, as can repression or inhibition of feelings associated with grief and mourning. Loneliness, sadness, despair, and reactive depression are natural and appropriate responses to a serious loss. To ignore or refuse to experience these emotions, however painful, can have potentially devastating effects such as the patterns of "abnormal" or "pathologic" grief described next.

Extended Grief

The uniqueness of each death and its meaning to the survivors make it difficult to establish what is "normal" and "abnormal" grief. Periods of mourning vary widely. One year is considered by many to be the minimum time for resolving grief and returning to normal life function, with the average being 1 to 2 years. Patterns of "abnormal" or "pathologic" grief have been defined by several authorities (see Table 16–6 later in this chapter). Two of these patterns relate to time: absence of grief (or massive denial) and abnormal prolongation of grief. Other variations include manic escape, dysfunctional hostility, and clinical depression.

Successful completion of mourning is essential to good mental health and a return to life satisfaction. Persons who deny their grief and resist expressing their painful feelings related to loss can experience the serious consequences described above. Repressed feelings are often stronger and more difficult to deal with when they do emerge. It is not wise to assume, however, that because persons are not expressing grief in the presence of professionals, they are not grieving.

Nursing Research Note

Wujcik D: Grief response of the primary caregiver receiving bereavement follow-up care at home. *Am J Hospice Care* 1984; 1(4):15–21.

Using a descriptive correlational survey design, this study evaluated the effect of hospice bereavement care on bereavement outcome of the primary caregiver. The results implied that follow-up may lessen the grief response to some degree at 13 months. Men were found to have more guilt and sleep disturbances than either wives or daughters. It was also determined that increased age may be a risk factor in a greater response.

Follow-up support for families who have lost loved ones is important, especially for men and older persons. Education and research are needed to identify risk factors that lead to extreme grief reactions.

ALTERNATIVES TO DEATH IN HOSPITALS

Since the mid-1970s, considerable progress and innovation have occurred in care of the dying and their families. Health professionals and families are learning to feel more comfortable caring for terminally ill clients and families, making possible more comprehensive care that allows the dying person to live more fully. With the taboo lifted from discussing death and dying, more families are discussing their wishes and concerns about these topics.

Workshops and seminars in death awareness are relatively recent. Death and dying workshops are being provided for health care professionals working with dying clients and their families. Universities and other educational centers are offering seminars to help people outside the health care community discuss and understand their feelings about death.

Through the consciousness-raising associated with death awareness comes the inverse, life awareness. By talking about and facing the issue of death, health professionals become more attuned to living. In this sense, working with dying persons provides a great benefit.

Hospice

A hospice is a specialized facility caring only for clients with terminal diagnoses. The goal of hospice care is to assist the person to live fully every day of his remaining life. Hospice care is less costly than conventional medical care, and Medicare coverage for hospice care began in 1983. With the focus on treatment of symptomatology associated with dying, clients are allowed to interact with family and friends without interruptions.

The hospice movement has grown primarily from the work of Dame Cicely Saunders, an English nurse and physician, who founded St Christopher's Hospice of London. Until the founding of St Christopher's in 1968, no facilities were available to care for only dying patients. Since then, many hospices have opened in the United States, Canada,

and around the world. Public response has been positive as more persons have experience with hospice care and its philosophy.

The National Hospice Organization (1982) has outlined the hospice philosophy: "Hospice affirms life. Hospice exists to provide support and care for persons in the last phases of incurable disease so that they might live as fully and comfortably as possible. Hospice recognizes dying

---

Box 16–2   Standards of a Hospice Program of Care

1. The hospice program complies with applicable local, state, and federal law and regulation governing the organization and delivery of health care to clients and families.

2. The hospice program provides a continuum of inpatient and home care services through an integrated administrative structure.

3. The home care services are available 24 hours a day, 7 days a week.

4. The client/family is the unit of care.

5. The hospice program has admission criteria and procedures that reflect:
   a. The client/family's desire and need for service
   b. Physician participation
   c. Diagnosis and prognosis

6. The hospice program seeks to identify, teach, coordinate, and supervise persons to give care to clients who do not have a family member available.

7. The hospice program acknowledges that each client/family has its own beliefs and/or value system and is respectful of them.

8. Hospice care consists of a blending of professional and nonprofessional services, provided by an interdisciplinary team, including a medical director.

9. Staff support is an integral part of the hospice program.

10. Inservice training and continuing education are offered on a regular basis.

11. The goal of hospice care is to provide symptom control through appropriate palliative therapies.

12. Symptom control includes assessing and responding to the physical, emotional, social, and spiritual needs of the client/family.

13. The hospice program provides bereavement services to survivors for a period of at least 1 year.

14. There will be a quality assurance program that includes:
    a. Evaluation of services
    b. Regular chart audits
    c. Organizational review

15. The hospice program maintains accurate and current integrated records on all clients/families.

17. The hospice inpatient unit provides space for:
    a. Client/family privacy
    b. Visitation and viewing
    c. Food preparation by the family

SOURCE: National Hospice Organization. Standards of a Hospice Program of Care, 1982. In: *The Hospice Alternative.* Munley A. New York: Basic Books, 1983. Reprinted with permission.

as a normal process whether or not resulting from disease. Hospice neither hastens nor postpones death. Hospice exists in the hope and belief that, through appropriate care and the promotion of a caring community sensitive to their needs, patients and families may be free to attain a degree of mental and spiritual preparation for death that is satisfactory to them."

The hospice philosophy may be applied in a number of settings. Five modes of hospice care are presently available (Munley, 1983):

- Home care services
- Hospice teams in hospitals
- Palliative care units in hospitals
- Hospices with hospital affiliations
- Autonomous or free-standing hospices

Hospice services may be offered through the visiting nurse association or the public health department. Hospice teams in hospitals generally offer their services Monday through Friday from 8 AM to 5 PM. Palliative care units in hospitals have beds for use by terminally ill clients. Hospital-affiliated hospices may be supported by the larger facility and staffed by their own staff and/or the hospital's staff. The free-standing or autonomous hospice is independent. The National Hospice Organization (see the resources listing) maintains a current directory of hospices in the United States. The Standards of a Hospice Program of Care are outlined in Box 16–2. These may be implemented in any hospital unit where terminally ill clients are found.

Home Care

The home was once the place to die. Some families are again choosing home care for dying clients. The family needs a great deal of support to make and continue with this course of action. Suggestions for the nurse counseling the family considering taking a family member home to die are in Box 16–3.

The decision to take the client home should include the following considerations (Hine, 1979):

- Sources of moral support to assist the family in taking on the responsibility
- Types of professional aid available part-time
- Kinds of special equipment necessary for adequate care
- Ease with which the family members may learn the needed nursing skills

---

Box 16–3   Death at Home: The Setting

The room chosen for the client should have:

1. Plenty of fresh air and sunshine.
2. Easy access to a bathroom.
3. Enough room to accommodate a hospital bed, if needed.
4. Access to the dining room, if the client joins the family for some meals.
5. Some of the client's favorite paintings, photos, or religious objects arranged so they can be seen from the bed.
6. Music available if the client enjoys it.
7. A tidy, well-kept appearance, with colorful linens and flowers.
8. No "sickroom" items in sight (such as medical supplies and commodes) unless actually in use.
9. Visitors as the client desires, including children and pets.

SOURCE: Dolan MB: If your patient wants to die at home. *Nurs 83* (April) 1983; 13:52. Reprinted with permission.

- Basic information concerning the death event and what to do with the body after death

Although most persons surveyed by Hine said they would prefer to die at home, the majority of the population dies in institutions.

If the family is unwilling or unable to take the dying person home or if the family admits the client to the hospital for the final days, the nurse must acknowledge the stress on the family and be supportive of their decision. Not all families can handle the burden of caring for a dying relative at home. Many families taking the client into the home readmit the client to the hospital for the actual death. They express fear at the thought of the family member actually dying in the house, or they may be exhausted by the demands care places on them. The family may have guilt feelings that the client's last wish, to die at home, is not being fulfilled through their inability to continue care. The nurse can help relieve some of this guilt by helping them to acknowledge what excellent care they gave and empathizing with how difficult it must have been for them. Also point out that the family did the best they could for as long as they could and that the client appreciates all the family did. In this way, the family may be helped to feel better about their difficult decision to readmit the client for respite care or the actual death.

Section II: The Nursing Process and Care of the Dying

The nurse has more contact with the dying person and family than any other member of the health care team. Thus, the nurse is the caregiver best able to assess, diagnose, and plan interventions to meet the needs of these clients and their families. Implementing the nursing process involves continual reevaluations and appropriate adjustments in care throughout the process of dying. Nurses also serve as the client's advocate to assure that other members of the health care team are aware of special needs and maintain continuity of care.

Box 16-4 Examining Feelings About Death and Dying

Box 16-4 Examining Feelings About Death and Dying

How comfortable do you expect to feel when talking to a dying person?

What do you anticipate you would say to a dying person?

How would you feel if you had to tell someone he or she was dying?

Do you agree with the statement, "At the point when there's nothing more medical science can do for a client, then the responsibility of the medical team is only to make the client as comfortable as possible physically"?

Do you think you could help persons adjust to the fact of their death?

Are you concerned that you may become too fond of a dying client and will therefore risk becoming "unprofessional"?

Do you imagine it is possible to overcome a fear of dying?

Do you think persons should be told they are dying, or do you think this would only add to their suffering?

Do you think death should be discussed in front of children?

Do you anticipate that being around a dying person would make you feel ill?

Have you avoided thinking about your own death?

Do you think you will ever feel comfortable with dying clients in the hospital or at home?

How would you feel if you were caring for a person who had requested not to be resuscitated?

How would you respond to someone who requested something to "stop the pain and help me die"?

Many nurses find it difficult to talk with a client or family member about death. Even those experienced in care of these clients do not find the process easy. Measures that can help the nurse to feel more comfortable in talking about death include examining feelings and life experiences, reading the literature on the topic, discussing death with nurse colleagues, and attending classes and/or seminars. By overcoming discomfort with the subject, the nurse can communicate in a more therapeutic manner with patients and families. For help in examining feelings about death, consider the questions in Box 16-4.

Care of the dying is also one of nursing's most challenging tasks. While striving to meet the client's and family's special needs, nurses must remember to meet their own needs; otherwise, the continuing emotional stress can lead to burnout. It is important for nurses to be willing to share their feelings about working with the dying, how these deaths affect them, and how they deal with the experience. Peer support groups can be valuable in lightening the emotional burden implicit in this area of nursing. In addition, members of other health professions—social workers, clergy, and psychiatrists—can be part of the support network. By caring for themselves and each other, nurses will be better able to care for dying clients and

families. Nurses who are uncomfortable with the dying should avoid working in a clinical setting where death is common. Through careful self-assessment, nurses can often determine whether they would be successful in this challenging aspect of nursing practice.

ASSESSMENT

How a person approaches death depends on what the person has been in life. Because everyone has a unique set of life experiences, each person will have differing perceptions and feelings about death and dying. It is important to understand the general characteristics and life experiences that influence perceptions of death. Many persons, including nurses, do not wish to examine their own feelings about death. This is a right. No one should be forced to examine their feelings about death. Nurses who maintain this position, however, will find it difficult to care for the dying effectively.

Nurses can play an important role in helping clients or family members explore their feelings about death and experiences with it. Verbal and nonverbal communication usually indicate when the person is ready to talk. Open-ended questions, use of silence as a communication technique, and sensitivity to the individual's needs to talk about an impending death are key skills for the nurse to develop.

Social and Cultural Values

Cultural beliefs and attitudes about death influence many aspects of care of dying persons. These beliefs and attitudes may (Ross, 1981):

- Affect assessment of comfort needs of the dying and the kind of care provided
- Influence selection, perception, and evaluation of health care givers and their methods
- Shape beliefs about the causes of death
- Determine the disposition of the body and funeral and burial rituals
- Pattern grief responses and bereavement roles

For example, in some cultures, men are expected to remain stoic, quietly accepting fate. Other cultures expect this behavior from both sexes during illness. Conversely, some cultures may expect demonstrative behavior from all members; crying, moaning, and active solicitation of care may be the norm.

The family's expectations of the ill member will influence how that member acts; each cultural group has a specific set of behaviors associated with the "patient" role. Some cultural groups or subgroups, for example, are known for their reserved reactions to crises. The mood at a relative's deathbed may be subdued, with little open crying or mourning. In contrast, those of a different cultural group may openly demonstrate their grief by wailing at the bedside.

It is crucial that nurses be aware of a family's cultural expectations surrounding death and dying and of their own cultural influences, being careful not to impose their values on the client and family. A nonjudgmental attitude and supportive approaches in working with these families will facilitate their grieving process and preserve their trust in the nurse.

Familial Roles

As a family develops and grows through time, the relationships and expectations of the family members change. Assessment of the family experiencing the terminal illness of a member requires understanding the roles of the family members.

The role a terminally ill person holds within the family constellation will influence the behavior of the client and family. For example, an unmarried man will have different concerns than a married father; an older widow will have different concerns than a young woman newly married. These differences primarily reflect the amount of responsibility placed on the person holding a certain role within the family. The terminally ill person with great family responsibility may feel guilty or angry about being ill and unable to meet the family's needs. The single person may also feel guilty and angry, perhaps more because of the loss of independence. Assessing the cause of behaviors will help the nurse organize the plan of care.

Various familial roles carry certain functions and expectations. The importance of these functions within the family determines how the family responds to the illness and death of the person in the role. A traditional family is headed by a couple in a heterosexual, monogamous relationship. When families adhere to traditional roles for husband and wife, the loss of a member can be disruptive over a long time, not only because of the loss of the individual but also because of the loss of the role. The remaining member may know little about functions previously performed by the dying person. After the husband dies, the widow is frequently bewildered by financial matters formerly handled by the deceased. Conversely, a widower may be unsure of how to prepare his own meals. The survivor may express resentment and anger toward the deceased: "How dare he die and leave me to carry on alone?" and then feel guilty about the thought.

In today's society, family roles are less concrete and more easily exchanged. Many persons choose to remain single and live alone. In young couples, men are learning to cook, and women are learning about car repair. Flexibility of roles in these families can help ease adaptation in the event of loss; a person will have been lost but not the ability to fulfill a specific role.

When a single parent dies, there may not be a counterpart to help fill this role. If there are children who will need care and guidance, the dead parent's relatives or the separated spouse may claim the children unless the parent has made other legal arrangements for their care.

Homosexual couples can share the same relationships found in traditional families. Should one of the partners be terminally ill, the other will experience the same feelings of loss and grief. If children are involved, the couple needs to consider legal provision for their guardianship. Hospital rules and regulations often reflect little sensitivity even for the rights of persons in traditional families. Persons in nontraditional relationships often have their grief compounded by frustration because health care professionals do not acknowledge them to have valid family relationships.

Communal and polygamous families consist of any number of men and women and their offspring. Because of their number and the sharing of tasks among members, they often have a substantial support system. If a member of a well-functioning system is terminally ill, many will share in the support of that person. If the dying member is a figurehead or leader of the group, another leader will need to be identified to ensure continuity and integrity of the group. Again, the amount of responsibility invested in the dying member will determine how the rest of the family reacts to the illness.

Nurses need to be aware of their own feelings and biases as they relate to family roles and duties. An independent female nurse may find it difficult to understand why a man threatened with losing his wife expresses concern about who will cook his dinner rather than about his wife's dying. It is essential for nurses to acknowledge their own expectations of familial roles and understand the concerns and needs of families with differing structures and role expectations.

Developmental Level

Attitudes and perceptions of death change with age and experience. By knowing what developmental stage the dying person is in, the nurse can better assess the person's condition and plan care. As a human being, the nurse is also experiencing a developmental stage that affects the reaction to dying and death. Recognizing this fact is important in assisting clients and families. (For information about children's perception of death, consult a pediatric nursing text.)

The Client's Level

12 to 18 Years. Persons in this age group have a mature concept of death. Because the primary developmental task at this age is to discover a unique identity, however, the teenager finds it extremely difficult to acknowledge the ultimate giving up of identity—death. Therefore, adolescents' attitudes about their own death may swing from mature one minute to childlike the next.

18 to 45 Years. Adults are fully aware of the finality of death. But during this stage of their lives, they are involved with childbearing and career development; they do not think about death often. They may take the erroneous view that only old persons die and that it couldn't happen to them. When faced with their own death, adults in this age group

Nursing Research Note

Valanis BG, Yeaworth R: Ratings of physical and mental health in the older bereaved. *Res Nurs Health* 1982; 5:137–146.

The subjects of this study were surviving spouses who were interviewed 3 to 4 months after their spouses' deaths. The self-ratings of mental and physical health of these bereaved elderly subjects were compared to ratings of them by nurse interviewers. A multidimensional functional assessment questionnaire from Duke University and the Zung self-rating depression scale were used.

Women in the study tended to underestimate the severity of their health problems. Older women were especially optimistic compared with nurse interviewer ratings. Mental health self-ratings were also better than nurse interviewer ratings.

The authors suggest that the elderly may identify symptoms of illness as normal problems of aging and therefore set lower standards for physical and mental health. Nurses, on the other hand, may have a broader view of optimal health for the elderly.

will be influenced by religious and cultural norms, discussed elsewhere in this chapter.

45 to 65 Years. Adults at this stage have accepted their own mortality. They probably have experienced the death of their parents and perhaps some peers; episodes of death anxiety may occur occasionally. When facing a terminal illness, adults of this age draw upon experience and belief systems to guide behavior.

65 Years and Older. Death for an older adult may have many meanings. Those who have lived a full life may look upon death as a reunion with deceased family members. Many adults in this age group have lost a spouse to death. Their families may be grown and self-sufficient, not requiring their guidance. Many older adults fear becoming a burden to children or relatives or suffering through a prolonged painful death. Sensitivity to life experiences of older adults will assist the nurse in assessing their needs.

The Family's Level

The family of the dying person has special needs. Each member will react to the death differently, depending on his or her age. Understanding the developmental levels of death perception will assist the nurse in assessing the needs of families.

Infancy to 5 Years. Young children experiencing a death in the family do not fully understand what is happening. This may further be compounded by adults who are uncomfortable explaining death to them. Children should have death explained realistically and consistently to them by an adult they trust. Telling the child the loved one has "gone to heaven," "gone to sleep," or "God took them away" may cause the child to fear heaven and hate God or

to be afraid to fall asleep for fear of also being "taken away." Children this age should be included in visiting the hospitalized relative and attending the funeral and other rituals surrounding the death.

Because of their egocentricity, children this age believe they have the power to make people ill or dead. This "magical thinking" may convince children they caused the relative's death. The child does not feel he or she can share this with anyone for fear of punishment. By knowing that children may think they caused an illness or death, the nurse can assist the child and family in exploring this idea.

5 to 9 Years. Although children in this age group understand the finality of death, they may still use "magical thinking." The school-age child's love for logic and knowledge will manifest itself in uncomfortable questions about the deceased. Adults need to realize the child is coping with a devastating event in the most familiar way, through the acquisition of knowledge about the deceased. Honest and consistent answers to difficult questions are important to help the child cope. Including children in visitation and funeral rituals is important when possible. Children, not adults, should determine if they want to go to the funeral, and their wishes should be honored.

9 to 12 Years. These children understand that death is inevitable, and honesty and consistency are as important for them as for younger age groups. Their wish to participate or not participate in activities surrounding the dying relative and the funeral should be respected and followed. Because children this age are learning to exert control over surroundings and events, the total loss of control that death represents may make them unable to cope with the death event. If this occurs, the nurse can help the family understand the reasons for this behavior.

12 to 18 Years. Because the adolescent's primary developmental task is to establish an identity, the total loss of identity that death signifies may be too much to handle. Responses may range from mature expressions of grief to a childlike denial of the death. Adolescents require the support of friends and family while grieving; however, their fierce drive for independence may inhibit their openly expressing this need. The family can meet these needs while allowing the adolescent to retain control over the situation by being sensitive to the adolescent's verbal and nonverbal communication. Open-ended questions such as, "How are you feeling about all this?" or "Do you have any questions or thoughts you'd like to share?" may help the adolescent express grief in a nonthreatening manner.

18 to 45 Years. Adults also may express their grief in a mature manner or deny it like children. Because adults usually have different roles than adolescents, considerations other than self-centered ones will affect their reaction to a terminally ill relative. But because they are concerned with the business of living, they may have a difficult time accepting a relative's death. To assist in assessment of the family member, the nurse might state, "This must be very difficult for you," or ask, "How are *you* doing?" with an arm around the person's shoulders.

45 to 60 Years. In this age group, adults have undoubtedly experienced the deaths of friends or relatives near their own age. Most have accepted the fact that they will die some day. During these years, many adults experience the loss of one or both parents. The loss of parents indicates to these adults that they are logically the next "in line" to die. This concept of chronological ordering of deaths will be explored later in this chapter.

65 Years and Older. Older adults will have encountered many deaths of friends and relatives. The older adult may hear of the loss of friends frequently. This can be depressing, not only because of losing relatives and friends but also because of the constant reminder that life is ending. An older adult experiencing the death of a younger adult, perhaps a daughter or son, may express anger that one so young with much to live for is dying.

Experience With Death

Clients' responses to their own death are influenced by other deaths experienced interpersonally. They will relive past deaths, comparing their experience with the experiences of others. Clients who have not been personally acquainted with someone who died in a similar manner may have no idea what to expect. Conversely, those who have witnessed a frightening or prolonged death from similar causes may expect the worst. The media can also have a powerful impact on thinking about death. Death of persons both real and imaginary has been presented vividly in television, movies, books, and magazines. For example, a young mother diagnosed with cancer might relate strongly to the role played by Debra Winger in the 1984 movie, *Terms of Endearment.*

Family members also relive past deaths, comparing experiences among themselves and perhaps with the dying person, helping each other to adapt to this new death experience. Reliving past deaths is a continuation of the grieving process discussed earlier in this chapter.

Although nurses see death more often than the general public, the deaths nurses witness cannot compare with the loss of a loved family member or friend. Drawing on experiences with death in the roles of nurse, family member, or friend, can help in better assessing and empathizing with grieving family members and clients. Because each death is uniquely painful to each of the bereaved, one person can never understand what others are experiencing; yet often, a nurse tries to comfort by saying, "I know how you must feel." Dying persons and their families will sense greater understanding and empathy in someone who says, "I can't possibly know or understand what you're going through, but if talking about it will help, I'd like to listen."

Living-Dying Interval

Pattison (1977) used the phrase "living-dying interval" to describe the time between being informed of the possibility of death and the actual death. Theoretically, the longer the living-dying interval, the more time the client and family have had to become accustomed to the death. The shorter the interval, such as in accidents, suicides, or sudden illness, the less prepared the family will be for the news of death. Assessment of the client and family should consider the living-dying interval and also the factors of death trajectory, critical junctures, and time and certainty. With this information, the nurse may better assess the client's and family's possible reaction to the death event and plan interventions accordingly.

A lengthy living-dying interval usually allows the client to initiate and progress through stages of dying discussed earlier. If the living-dying interval is short, the client may be in a state of denial up to the point of death. If there is no living-dying interval, as when sudden death occurs from an accident, the nurse focuses efforts more on the family than on the deceased.

The duration of the living-dying interval affects the family's response to the client's death through the initiation of the grief work by the family. Sanders (1982) stated that short-term chronic illness (6 months) had the most favorable adjustment to bereavement at 18 months. In comparison, sudden death and long-term chronic illness (longer than 6 months) resulting in death appeared to result in more intense bereavement at 18 months after the death. Families experiencing sudden death had an internalized emotional response resulting in prolonged physical stress. Families who experienced long-term chronic illness had an externalized bereavement resulting in dejection, frustration, and loneliness.

Occasionally, a client who has been diagnosed with a terminal disease or has been close to death is cured. Sudden recovery or remission is an extremely disruptive, although welcome, occurrence. The person must once again plan for living rather than dying. The family, although thankful, is experiencing anticipatory grief and may not be able to talk with the person about the close brush with death. In this case, the nurse may wish to explore with the client and family their feelings about the sudden remission or recovery and how this will affect their future plans. Referral to a family counselor may be necessary to help them adjust to this special circumstance.

Cause of Death

The person dying from acquired immune deficiency syndrome (AIDS), which is associated primarily with male homosexual and bisexual populations, may feel differently about the illness and impending death than a person dying from bone cancer. Some diseases in our society have values placed upon them, which may or may not be based on fact. The client's perception of the acceptability and etiology of the disease will affect the reaction to the disease and the sense of self-worth.

Families also are affected by the social values placed on various diseases. A family member dying from cirrhosis of the liver may be an embarrassment because this disorder usually is associated with chronic alcoholism. Assessment of the family's understanding of the disease, its cause, and the family's values and attitudes concerning the disease is critically important because it can have a major effect on the family's ability to support the client.

Family survivors of suicide victims often have tremendous guilt to deal with as well as their grief and, perhaps, questions that can never be answered. Those families who survive a member's murder or other type of violent death must cope with feelings of grief compounded by rage and the endless questions about why such tragedy struck their family. Special support groups formed by these families are listed with the resources at the end of this chapter.

Nurses, who see many clients with many diseases unfortunately tend to equate diseases with certain causative factors. They may make value judgments about the disease and the person who has it. The nurse who disdainfully cares for the cirrhotic client assumes the client was an alcoholic, when the condition might actually have resulted from years of work with toxic chemicals. Regardless of the cause of a disease, the nurse needs to acknowledge the dying person's humanity and offer unjudging, supportive care.

Nonchronological Deaths

There is a certain expected "order" of death. Grandparents are expected to die before parents, and parents before their children. The client's order in the family may affect the ability to cope with the thought of terminal illness. Younger people especially may become angry that they will die before those who are older.

For the family, the unexpected loss of a family member is potentially more disturbing than the loss of a member who is expected to die. For example, the death of a child through accident or disease leaves parents and grandparents to mourn the loss. No matter what the age of the child who dies, parents do not expect to outlive the child; thus, they find this the most painful death to cope with.

Nurses aware of the chronological expectations of death and the associated psychological barriers can better assess the needs of the dying person and the family. This awareness can help nurses understand the middle-aged person's potential reaction to the death of a parent or the difficulties an elderly parent experiences when a middle-aged child dies. Both the dying person and the family may have a great deal of anger that needs to be expressed.

Religious Values

Religion plays an important part in the lives of many people, especially as they face death. The beliefs of selected religious groups surrounding death, afterlife, reincarna-

tion, and funeral rituals are presented in Table 16–2. Some persons may have no religious beliefs in a supreme being or any kind of an afterlife. They may have definite ideas about how and where they wish to die, however. Their feelings and values should be respected despite any differences from those of the nurse or other caregiver.

A spiritual assessment should be included with a general assessment; however, the assessment needs to be done on the client's terms so as not to intrude on his or her privacy. The client's religious preference, recorded on admission, should be available to all who care for that person. If the dying person has no religious preference, this also needs to be communicated and respected. Religion may be a source of solace for some persons but a source of irritation for others. Assessment of religious beliefs includes noting what the person reads, watches on television, and whether he or she requests a visit from a member of the clergy. Persons without a religious preference still may wish to talk with some type of counselor.

Family members sometimes differ in their religious affiliations and beliefs. This may be a source of debate throughout the client's illness, upsetting all concerned. The family's religious preference should be assessed and recorded for its congruency or lack of congruency with the client's beliefs. The family may have specific funeral rituals they expect to carry out after the person's death that are in conflict with the client's wishes. Such differences can divide a family when their mutual support is needed and expected.

The nurse's religious beliefs will affect the care given to dying persons and their families. Effective care depends on understanding and accepting the client's and family's religious affiliation and belief system. On occasion, the nurse may be placed in the middle of a religious argument between client and family. By open acceptance of other's religious beliefs while retaining one's own beliefs, the nurse can demonstrate behaviors and attitudes that could be conducive to family unity.

Personal Philosophy

More than any other single factor, a personal philosophy about death and its meaning influences one's attitude toward death. This philosophy is shaped over time by cultural and religious background and life experience. Freud noted that to each person, death is unimaginable. In the unconscious, everyone is convinced of his or her own immortality. Death is outside the realm of experience and therefore cannot exist. Although intellectually, all persons know they will die, deep in the unconscious, they are convinced they will not.

Persons strive to give life and death meaning through measures aimed at achieving a sense of immortality. Among these are having children to carry on and remember them, doing good works that will be remembered, or creating objects of permanence that will remain after death. Those with strong religious convictions count on an afterlife or a resurrection to assure their immortality. Many persons will not have thought out or discussed their feelings on this

Table 16-2   Death-Related Beliefs and Practices of Selected Religious Groups

Group	Afterlife	Rituals/ Funerals	Autopsy	Organ Donation	Cremation	Prolonging Life
American Indian	Beliefs vary	Practices vary; most want family present	Prohibited		Practices vary	
Black Muslim		Special procedures for washing and shrouding the dead; special funeral rites				
Buddhist in America	Reincarnation; after reaching state of enlightenment, may attain nirvana	Last rite chanting at bedside	No restriction		No restriction	Permit euthanasia in hopeless illness
Church of Christ Scientist	Yes	No last rites	Only in sudden death	No	Individual decision	
Church of Jesus Christ or Latter Day Saints (Mormon)	Yes	Baptism essential; preaching gospel to dead also practiced	No restriction	No restriction	Discouraged	
Eastern Orthodox (Greek and Russian Orthodox)	Yes	Last rites (administration of Holy Communion obligatory)	Discouraged		Discouraged	Encouraged
Episcopal (Anglican)	Yes	Last rites not mandatory	No restriction	No restriction	No restriction	
Hindu	Reincarnation; after leading a perfect life, may join Brahma	Priest pours water into mouth of corpse and ties string around wrist or neck as sign of blessing; string must not be removed; family washes body	No restriction	No restriction	Preferred; ashes cast in holy river	
Islam (Moslem, Muslim)	May join Allah by being a good Moslem and observing rituals daily	Dying person must confess sins and ask forgiveness in presence of family; family washes and prepares body (female body cannot be washed by male) and turns body toward Mecca	Prohibited unless required by law	Prohibited	Prohibited	Encouraged

(continued)

Table 16–2 Death-Related Beliefs and Practices of Selected Religious Groups (continued)						
Group	**Afterlife**	**Rituals/ Funerals**	**Autopsy**	**Organ Donation**	**Cremation**	**Prolonging Life**
Jehovah's Witness			Prohibited unless required by law. No body parts may be removed	Prohibited	No restriction	
Judaism	Dead will be resurrected with coming of Messiah; man lives on through survival of memory	Body ritually washed by members of Ritual Burial Society; burial as soon as possible after death; dead not left unattended; five stages of mourning extending over a year; no embalming; no flowers at funeral because flowers are a symbol of life	Orthodox prohibit; some liberals permit; no body parts removed	Beliefs vary	Largely prohibited; beliefs vary	
Lutheran	Yes	Last rites optional	No restriction	No restriction	No restriction	
Roman Catholicism	Yes; resurrection with second coming of Christ	Rites for anointing the sick not mandatory; receiving Holy Communion mandatory	Permitted, but all body parts must be given appropriate burial	No restriction	No restriction	Discouraged
Seventh Day Adventist	Dead are asleep until return of Christ, when final rewards and punishments will be given					
Unitarian	Beliefs vary		No	No	Encouraged	Preferred

SOURCES: Ross HM: Societal/cultural views regarding death and dying. *Top Clin Nurs* 1981; 3(3):1–16; *Nurs 77* (Dec) 1977; 7:64–70.

personal matter before being faced with death. They may wish to explore these feelings with the nurse's assistance.

Each family member is also an individual; collectively, the family members may represent varied personal philosophies. As with religious values, the nurse may assist the client and family by demonstrating an attitude of acceptance of varying philosophical viewpoints.

If the nurse's personal philosophy differs from that of a client and/or family, the nurse must make every attempt to understand their philosophy. Acknowledging that everyone has a personal philosophy about meanings of life and death will help the nurse work with individuals and families facing this life event.

NURSING DIAGNOSIS

Careful assessment of the dying person may lead to several nursing diagnoses related to physical needs. There are also a variety of possible nursing diagnoses related to psychosocial needs of the individual and the family (Box 16–5). Naturally, the diagnoses will vary with each individual and family.

PLANNING AND IMPLEMENTATION

A team approach to care of the dying is extremely important. Continuous communication between members of the health care team is essential to ensure consistent care of the client and family. Care conferences should be arranged regularly to update all caregivers on new issues and evaluate the successes of past planned care. The client's chart and the nursing care plan should be updated at these conferences to maintain continuity and consistency of care.

Members of the health care team customarily involved in the team approach include nurses, physicians, social workers, appropriate members of the clergy, pharmacists, physical and occupational therapists, and respiratory therapists. Others may include psychologists and/or psychiatrists and hypnotherapists. Members of the family are occasionally asked to participate in care conferences because they know the client's private concerns. When families are a source of concern for the health care team, however, they may not be asked to attend a care conference.

Physical Care

The client's disease process will largely determine the specific needs for physical care; other chapters in this text provide information about specific diseases and disorders. There are similarities in caring for all dying patients, however. In addition to pain, which is discussed here, other distressing symptoms are common in dying clients. These include respiratory difficulty and problems of mobility, nutrition, hydration, elimination, and sensory changes. Table 16–3 summarizes these problems with suggested nursing interventions.

Health care professionals often have great concern about administering large doses of narcotics or barbiturates for fear of the client's becoming addicted. In the case of terminally ill persons, however, this is not a concern because they usually will not live long enough to become addicted. If addiction occurs, it may become secondary to the goal of keeping the person pain-free to enjoy the limited time remaining. Saunders (1982) suggests various treatments for the different kinds of pain in terminal illness, summarized in Table 16–4. For a general approach to pain management, see Chapter 5.

One of the unfortunate side effects of most narcotic analgesics and barbiturates is stupor and oversedation. The doses that relieve pain in terminally ill clients often result in their being unresponsive. Brompton's cocktail is an oral mixture of morphine sulphate (or heroin), cocaine, ethyl alcohol, and flavorings for palatability. It has proven effective in controlling pain when given on a schedule. Palliative care specialists assert that p.r.n. orders are inappropriate for pain control and only serve to increase the client's

| Box 16–5 | Nursing Diagnoses Commonly Related to Death and Dying |

Diagnoses Related to Physiological Needs

Airway clearance, ineffective

Mobility, impaired physical

Nutrition, alteration in, less than body requirements

Fluid volume deficit, actual or potential

Bowel elimination, alteration in

Urinary elimination, alteration in

Sensory perceptual alteration, visual, tactile

Diagnoses Related to Psychological Needs

Coping, ineffective individual and family, related to impending death

Coping, family, potential for growth

Grieving, anticipatory, related to expected death

Grieving, dysfunctional, related to death

Fear, related to known and unknown factors

Self-concepts, disturbance in, related to role performance, personal identity, expected death

psychological dependence (Munley, 1983). Brompton's cocktail allows the client to be pain-free without the stupor and oversedation experienced with the high doses of narcotic analgesics or barbiturates necessary to control severe chronic pain. At St Christopher's Hospice in London, morphine sulfate solution and water alone are being found to be as effective (Twycross, 1984).

Policies and procedures vary among hospitals for the continuous intravenous administration of some drugs to relieve pain. Often these policies have little justification other than the hospital's fear of being sued for overdosing a person and possibly causing death. Intravenous morphine sulfate has been successful in reducing the pain for persons with cancer. It is recommended that hospitals and units caring for large numbers of terminally ill persons seriously consider this intervention, enabling persons to live out their last days free from pain. The administration of intraspinal narcotics is a newer method of pain control (see Chapter 12).

Psychological Care

Care of the Client and Family
Care of the dying is an ongoing learning experience for the nurse; much of the learning is done by observing the persons for whom they care. After nearly 30 years of studying dying persons and grieving families, Lindemann (1972) confronted his own impending death from cancer. He summarized three key aspects of caring for the dying: open,

Table 16–3	Physiological Needs of Dying Persons
Problem	**Nursing Intervention**
Airway clearance, ineffective	• Fowler's position: conscious patients • Throat suctioning: conscious patients • Low Fowler's position: unconscious patients • Oxygen therapy as needed
Mobility, impaired physical	• Assisted out of bed periodically, if able • Regular changing of position for bedridden patients • Support in position with rolls of blankets or towels as needed • Lateral positioning in bed to decrease aspiration of saliva • Elevate legs when sitting up to prevent pooling of blood
Nutrition, alteration in, less than body requirements	• Antiemetics or alcoholic beverages to stimulate appetite • High-calorie and high-vitamin diets • Semisolid, soft, or liquid foods because of decreased gag reflex
Fluid volume deficit, actual or potential	• Continued assessment of gag reflex
Bowel elimination, alteration in	• Laxatives as needed to prevent constipation • Skin care because of incontinence of urine or feces
Urinary elimination, alteration in	• Bedpan, urinal, or commode chair within easy reach of patient • Call light within reach for assistance onto bedpan or commode • Absorbent pads placed under incontinent patient, linen changed as often as needed • Catheterization may be needed in some cases • Keep room as clean and odor-free as possible
Sensory perceptual alteration, visual, tactile	• Patients prefer a light to a dark room • Hearing is not diminished; speak clearly and do not whisper • Touch is diminished, but will feel pressure of touch

empathic communication; honesty; and tolerance of emotional expression. He offered this advice:

Rely on open communication. Don't fib. The family or the patient always will know if you do, just as children always know. That's number one, and for me it is the basis of helping.

The second important skill is to be able to take the patient's position. Even if what is said seems silly to you, take enough time to hear the patient out, because he may have a very good reason for an attitude which sounds very nonsensical to you at first. So don't brush him aside.

The third skill is not to assume that for the patient to be sad and miserable and crying for a while is bad for him. Don't assume that you have to keep a smooth surface and that the patient must smile. He may smile just to keep you happy.

Talking with a person about his or her impending death is never easy, nor is discussing that death with a family, partly because society has considered death a forbidden topic. Many dying persons have an acute need to voice their thoughts and feelings on this most personal of all topics, and often the nurse is the most convenient (and sometimes the only) person who can and will listen. These persons may need permission to discuss their dying, and if they are unable to ask for it, the nurse, through both words and actions, can either explicitly or implicitly grant that permission. Some guidelines for communicating are summarized in Box 16–6.

Organized support groups for dying persons and their families can also assist in meeting the psychological needs of these persons. Among them are the I Can Cope and Make Today Count groups (see the resources listing in Chapter 12). These groups help the terminally ill and their families confront and work through fears and feelings concerning the illness and death. Because they are sharing a common experience, the members provide empathic understanding that seems to be highly therapeutic.

On occasion, clients refuse to talk about their impending death. They may deny they are dying, deny any religious affiliation, and deny a need to talk to anyone. Denial is their way of coping. It is also their right—a right to be respected by nurses as much as they would respect another client's wish to talk about death.

Often clients who are dying are in the process of finalizing their wills or assisting in the preparation of trusts and powers of attorney. These legal documents usually require signatures from witnesses. Nurses may be asked to be witnesses to the client's signature. The general rule is that if the client is competent, there is no problem for the nurse to sign as a witness. (These wills should be distinguished from living wills, described later. In most states, witnesses to a living will should not be employees of the care-taking institution.)

Sexuality

Sexual needs of the dying person are often overlooked by nurses. Uncomfortable with discussing sexuality in any client situation, nurses may see these needs as irrelevant to persons who are dying. Sexuality refers to the "constellation of physical and psychological traits that make us male or female" (Taylor, 1983). In this sense, part of one's sexual consciousness is the life and sex roles one fills.

Taylor identifies three methods in which the nurse may assist the clients in remaining sexual beings and fulfilling their sexual needs until death: (1) attention to appearance and grooming, (2) supporting fulfillment of life roles, and (3) helping to meet the need for physical contact. Appearance and grooming reflect an individual's sexuality. Part of routine care should include helping the client look his or her best. This will reinforce sexual identity and reinforce feelings of well-being. Life roles, ascribed or assumed, are a part of the client's sexual identity. Both nurse and family can reinforce and encourage continuation of functions and duties of life roles. The need for physical contact must not be underestimated. Dying persons are often reassured by the nurse holding their hand or by other kinds of gentle, caring touch. Understandably, the same simple act from a loved one will be more meaningful for both persons. Family members often fear hurting their loved one and refrain from any physical contact. If the client is unable to ask for physical comfort and contact, the nurse might suggest that someone sit and hold the person's hand. If the person wishes to be held, rocked, or hugged, the nurse should make every effort to grant this wish because it fulfills a real need for client and family.

Privacy is essential for intimate encounters between clients and loved ones. Despite hospitals' notorious lack of privacy, nursing staff can arrange to provide privacy for a realistic time. A special sign on a completely closed door signifies a private time for the client and visitor. Thirty

Table 16–4 Treatment of Pain in Terminal Care

Cause of Pain	Primary Treatment	Secondary Treatment	To Consider
Visceral from involvement of abdominal or pelvic organs	Analgesics	Low-dose steroids may help	Celiac axis block for abdominal pain; intrathecal block for pelvic pain
Bone pain	• Palliative radiotherapy • Nonsteroidal anti-inflammatory drugs • Immobilization, eg, cervical collar or pinning	Analgesics	Nerve block; low-dose steroids may help
Soft tissue infiltration	Analgesics	Low-dose steroids and nonsteroidal anti-inflammatory drugs may help	Nerve block
Nerve compression	Analgesics	High-dose steroids	Nerve block
Secondary infection • Deep	• Systemic antibiotics including metronidazole if possibility of anaerobes; local surgery	Analgesics	Nerve block
• Superficial	• Systemic antibiotics; local applications, eg, povidone-iodine		
Pleural pain	Antibiotics if appropriate	Analgesics	Intercostal block
Colic due to bowel obstruction	Fecal softeners; antispasmodics, eg, loperamide (Imodium)	Analgesics	—
Lymphedema	Analgesics; intermittent positive pressure	High-dose steroids may help	Diuretics rarely of use
Headaches from increased intracranial pressure	High-dose steroids; raise head of bed	Avoid opiate analgesics if possible	Diuretics may help
Pain in paralyzed limb(s)	Physiotherapy and regular movement of limb(s) by nurses	Nonsteroidal anti-inflammatory drugs	Muscle relaxants

SOURCE: Saunders C: Principles of symptom control in terminal care. *Med Clin North Am* 1982; 66(5):1173. Reprinted with permission.

Box 16—6 **Guidelines for Communicating With Terminally Ill Patients and Their Families**

1. Remember that each person is unique. Rote responses will distance you from the dying patient or family member.

2. Talk with the dying person as you would a friend. Your goal is to relate person to person. Don't be afraid to show your humorous as well as your serious side.

3. Hear not only what the dying patient is saying but also what he is not saying. Use your mind, eyes, and ears to listen.

4. Recognize that people have long-standing patterns of communication and means of coping with stress. Attempting to interrupt or change their usual patterns will just increase the stress.

5. Respond to concerns with compassionate honesty. If you don't know the answer, say so. Patients often just want to know what you think.

6. Maintain a calm tone of voice—and your composure—during interactions. Your control will improve the patient's sense of control.

7. Appreciate the patient's need for privacy. Never force communication. Don't talk about a sensitive topic just because you have time. You must develop the ability to know when the patient is ready to talk.

8. Talk about the here and now at first. Let the patient direct conversations about the future of his personal life. Don't share your personal problems spontaneously.

9. Be willing to expose some of your own insecurities, fears, and vulnerabilities. You'll gain insight into your own feelings and probably learn how to be more comfortable with these personal areas.

SOURCE: Kellar MH: What is it like to be dying? *Nurs 83* (Sept) 1983; 13:66—67. Reprinted with permission.

minutes of uninterrupted privacy could make possible sharing personal thoughts and intimate pleasures. At first, the client and loved ones may not feel comfortable with private time; the nurse can explain, however, that this time is theirs to use however they wish. Consistently available private time can allow initiation of activities or conversations previously suppressed. This helps meet the sexual needs of the client and helps the nurse offer complete care to client and family.

Permission to Die

Ufema (1980) and Moody (1976) have described the occasional client who needs "permission" to die. This permission usually comes from family members or significant others whose prayers or wishes for the person to live on indefinitely seem to inhibit completion of the dying process. Moody and Ufema recount instances in which the person's family and congregation prayed daily for a cure. Living a pain-filled, useless life, the person wished to die and expressed that sincere wish to the family. After the family altered the petition in their prayers from keeping the loved one alive to assisting the person through a painless death, the person was able to die peacefully.

Although the client and family must resolve this issue, the nurse should be sensitive to unrealistic family goals for the client. The nurse may wish to assist the client and family in discussing the situation. Helping to alleviate misunderstanding can enable the family to offer support to their loved one through the dying process.

Persons sometimes resist death in order to witness or experience a meaningful life event such as the wedding of a grandchild or a holiday with special significance. After the event, the client may die within days or weeks. This power of the mind over the body is only beginning to be understood. The ability to "will" oneself to resist or accept death is an example of this power. Family members may be shocked that the person doing well before Christmas deteriorates rapidly after the new year. The nurse can help the family understand that once the client's private goal has been attained, the process of dying may be accelerated.

Self-Care for the Nurse

Caring for dying persons and their families demands great personal and emotional investment from the nurse and other caregivers. How the nurse reacts to each experience depends on many factors mentioned earlier such as culture and personal philosophy. Adams (1984) suggests six variables that affect how nurses react to a dying person:

- Length of hospitalization
- Frequency of admissions
- Role of the family
- Condition of the client when admitted
- Client's coping style
- Role of the nurse's subconscious

Because any of these factors can influence the nurse's feelings about the client and family, it is important to con-

Nursing Research Note

Korte PD: Registered nurses' anxiety about the process of dying and death. *Am J Hospice Care* 1985; 2(4):27–29.

This study investigated in a survey the level of nurses' death anxiety by using Templer's Death Anxiety Scale and the relation between certain characteristics of nurses and their level of death anxiety. The older a nurse and the more years of practie he or she had, the lower the level of death anxiety. More research was recommended because the sample was skewed toward the younger age group.

Nurses must examine their own personal beliefs and anxieties about death. How they deal with these anxieties may affect their responses to dying clients and their families. Nursing education, both in formal classes and inservice programs, might help nurses cope more effectively with their anxieties. Being open and expressing feelings at staff conferences with supportive peers may be other ways of coping with death anxiety.

sider each carefully, particularly when effective communication seems difficult. When the nurse is experiencing difficulty in working with the dying and their families, it is useful to recognize that many nurses probably share these concerns. Mandel (1981) has identified three common concerns expressed by nurses caring for the terminally ill: being overwhelmed, overidentification, and avoidance.

Being Overwhelmed. Death on a daily basis seems unendurable. In care units where life-threatening illness and death are part of the normal pattern, such as intensive care, oncology, and emergency units, nurses can become victims of burnout or emotional depletion. When great human and technologic efforts are directed at keeping the client alive, nurses may view the client's death as a professional defeat as well as a personal loss. Some nurses not comfortable with their own feelings about death might change specialties or perhaps leave nursing all together. Others who stay might find themselves dissatisfied with their careers. Some nurses believe that shorter shifts in these units might relieve the pressures on caregivers and help prevent burnout.

Overidentification. Confronted with the client's pain and the family's grief, some nurses may attempt to do more than offer understanding palliative care and try to assume some of the client's and family's burden of grief. This reaction is called the *surrogate sufferer syndrome.* Rooted in helplessness, this behavior includes attempts to shield clients and their families from difficult experiences. Although stemming from what are "good intentions," a caregiver cannot do the grief work for another or assume the pain for another. Doing so is inconsistent with self-care goals for client and family and further diminishes their already minimal autonomy. Clients and families can best be helped by assisting them to function for themselves. Being a surrogate sufferer only helps to reduce the nurse's own sense of helplessness; it does nothing to address the feelings of helplessness experienced by clients and their families.

Avoidance. A common response to dealing with death is trying to block personal feelings and reactions. Some nurses hide behind technology and avoid becoming involved. This reaction can also block the sensitivity required for effective care of the dying, and clients become objects rather than persons (Box 16–7). Although letting persons know nurses care about them as well as for them involves great emotional risk, it can be the most critical element in meeting the needs of clients and families. The nurse needs to achieve a delicate balance between objectivity and involvement to offer the kind of care needed by these families in crisis. Nurses also tend to avoid their nursing colleagues who may be grieving for a dying person. Supporting each other can do much to prevent loneliness and emotional depletion among the nursing staff.

Box 16–7   The Nurse's Reaction to Dying and Death

I am a student nurse. I am dying. I write this to you who are, and will become, nurses in the hope that by my sharing my feelings with you, you may someday be better able to help those who share my experience. . . . You slip in and out of my room, give me medications and check my blood pressure. Is it because I am a student nurse, myself, or just a human being, that I sense your fright? And your fears enhance mine. Why are you afraid? I am the one who is dying!

I know you feel insecure, don't know what to say, don't know what to do. But please believe me, if you care, you can't go wrong. Just admit you care. . . . Don't run away—wait—all I want to know is that there will be someone to hold my hand when I need it. . . . If only we could be honest, both admit of our fears, touch one another. If you really care, would you lose so much of your valuable professionalism if you even cried with me? Just person to person? Then it might not be so hard to die—in a hospital—with friends close by.

SOURCE: *Am J Nurs* 1970; 70(2). Reprinted with permission.

Spiritual Care

Frequently, persons close to death will request a visit from the clergy, and the nurse must act quickly to meet this need. Most hospitals have members of the clergy available, and they will respond promptly when their counsel is sought. Many teaching hospitals have a pastoral counseling department staffed by graduate theology students who are on call at all times. It is important to let clients know that counsel is available but not to force or coerce the client into talking with clergy.

Some clients will be unable or unwilling to talk to clergy or their families about death. If this seems to be the case, ask the client if there is anything he or she would like to talk about. Ask this question *only* when there is time to spend with the client. Closing the door to the client's room makes other staff aware that privacy is needed.

INTERVENTION AT THE TIME OF DEATH
Physiological Death

Although death may result from one or more disease processes, the actual death event is precipitated by failure of one or all of the three major organ systems: the central nervous system, the respiratory system, or the cardiovascular system (Wass, 1979). In earlier times, all three systems failed in rapid succession; however, technology can enhance the function of respiratory and cardiovascular systems, enabling them to function long beyond their normal failure following CNS shutdown. Clinical signs of impending and imminent death are described in Box 16–8.

Physiological changes at death include rigor mortis, algor mortis, and livor mortis. *Rigor mortis* occurs approximately 2 to 4 hours after death and is due to the lack of adenosine triphosphate (ATP) required for muscle relaxation. The process begins with involuntary muscle groups and then proceeds to the trunk and extremities. The body *must* be arranged for viewing by the family before rigor

---

Box 16–8   Clinical Signs of Death

Clinical signs of impending death

1. Loss of muscle tone, which results in:
   - Relaxation of the facial muscles.
   - Difficulty speaking.
   - Difficulty swallowing with decreased gag reflex.
   - Decreased activity of the gastrointestinal tract, with subsequent nausea, accumulation of flatus, abdominal distention and retention of feces, especially if narcotics or tranquilizers are being administered.
   - Possible urinary and rectal incontinence due to decreased sphincter control.
   - Diminished body movement.

2. Slowing of the circulation, which results in:
   - Diminished sensation.
   - Mottling and cyanosis of the extremities.
   - Cold skin, first in the feet and later in the hands, ears, and nose.

3. Changes in vital signs:
   - Decelerated and weaker pulse.
   - Decreased blood pressure.
   - Rapid, shallow, irregular, or abnormally slow respirations; mouth breathing, which leads to dry oral mucous membranes.

4. Sensory impairment:
   - Blurred vision.
   - Impaired taste and smell senses.

Clinical signs of imminent death

1. Dilated, fixed pupils.
2. Inability to move.
3. Loss of reflexes.
4. Faster, weaker pulse.
5. Cheyne–Stokes respirations.
6. Noisy breathing or death rattle from mucus in throat.
7. Lowered blood pressure.

Clinical signs of death

1. Total lack of response to external stimuli.
2. No muscle movement, especially breathing.
3. No reflexes.
4. Flat electroencephalogram (EEG).

SOURCE: Kozier B, Erb G: *Fundamentals of Nursing: Concepts and Procedures,* 2nd ed. Menlo Park, CA: Addison–Wesley, 1983. Reprinted with permission.

---

mortis occurs. *Algor mortis* is the process of body cooling, which takes place at approximately 1°C per hour until the body reaches room temperature. *Livor mortis,* discoloration of skin related to the pooling of red blood cells, is more apparent in dependent areas, such as the back and buttocks.

Decomposition of the body is more rapid in warm temperatures, so the body is stored in a cool place. Cool temperatures prevent growth of bacteria that initiate decomposition. Embalming destroys bacteria through the injection of chemicals into the body, retarding the process.

Care of the Body After Death

When the client dies, the nurse prepares the body and then invites the family in to view the deceased. Some families may not want to view the body, and this should be respected and accepted. They may not be ready at that time. If the family wishes to see the body, prepare them for the appearance of their loved one. For example, say, "Your father will look different than he did when you last saw him. The resuscitation efforts left some bruising on his arms and his throat where we tried to insert an IV. These procedures were necessary and we were concerned about saving him. If you wish, I'll be available to answer any questions you may have." The nurse should be sensitive to the family's grief and quietly leave the room after informing the family he or she will be available if needed. The body should be washed in areas requiring cleansing. Pads should be placed under the buttocks to absorb drainage of feces or urine released through relaxing sphincter muscles. Depending on the policy of the institution, tubes may be removed or cut 1 in from the skin and secured with tape. A clean gown, brushed hair, and removal of all soiled linen and equipment will help the family focus on the deceased rather than on a cluttered room. Before bringing in the family, turn off the harsh overhead lights and leave on the softer lights. Soft lighting will lessen the obvious discoloration from livor mortis.

After the family has viewed the deceased, shroud the body in a linen or plastic sheet, unless the family has made specific arrangements for a mortician to remove the body from the hospital room. Policies vary for shrouding and identifying the deceased. The standard procedure is to leave the wristband on, to place an additional identifying card on a great toe, and after the shroud is secured, to place an additional identifying card on the chest on top of the shroud. The body will then be transported to the hospital's morgue for cooling.

Autopsy

An autopsy (postmortem examination) may be performed on the body. Autopsies are performed for various reasons, including determination of the cause of death or as a final follow-up on the client's disease process. Occasionally, it is the nurse's responsibility to gain permission from the family for an autopsy.

Be sensitive to the family's wishes when obtaining permission for an autopsy. They may understandably have an aversion to the postmortem disfigurement of a loved one. The family is vulnerable at this time, and they may later regret their decision to allow an autopsy. Autopsies may violate the teachings of certain religious groups such as the Jewish faith. Explain to the family that, in most cases, the autopsy will contribute to knowledge about the disease from which their family member died and explain that the autopsy will not alter the appearance of the body. Their feelings about this personal matter must be respected and their refusal empathically accepted, however.

When the cause of death is in question, the law usually requires that the county medical examiner or coroner conduct the autopsy. These experts have advanced knowledge in forensic medicine and/or pathology. Special procedures must be followed in preparing the body for removal by legal officials. Customarily, no tubes are to be removed from the body, although this policy varies. After the postmortem examination, a report is filed with the district attorney's office.

Follow-Up Care for the Bereaved

If the family requests a visit from a member of the clergy, arrange a visit as soon as possible. In hospitals not having clergy on call, be aware of community religious resources. Clergy will usually visit on short notice if they are aware of the circumstances.

The support groups mentioned earlier for clients also accept family members if they wish to attend. Some family members may want this kind of support system, and others will seek the support of friends and family. Mention the availability of support groups to the family and supply them with further information if they want it.

EVALUATION

Evaluation of care continues throughout the process of dying; however, because cure is not possible, the outcome criteria for a dying person are different than those for one who is expected to recover. Constantly evaluate the person's comfort and psychological well-being.

Evaluation of the plan for the family of a dying person is also continuous. Evaluate their ability to support and empathize with the client. Also be aware that it is normal in some families not to exhibit this behavior; therefore, this is not a reflection on the nursing efforts with them. Because the family remains after the client dies, continue to evaluate care of the family after the death. Depending on the setting, responsibility to the family continues, and they may need the nurse even more after the death event.

Follow-up with the family after a death is often forgotten on busy hospital units. If anyone is in touch with the family after the funeral, it may be the primary nurse or someone who developed a special relationship with the client or family. Many hospices now have specific follow-

---

Box 16–9   Guidelines for Helping Persons Experiencing Grief

Do

1. Remember that grief resulting from the loss of a beloved person often lasts several years.

2. Listen as they "retell it" over and over again. This is part of grief work.

3. Accept what may seem to be inappropriate anger and guilt. They have to get it out through sharing.

4. Make every effort to put a family back in touch with the religious traditions of their childhood.

5. Discourage bereaved persons from making major decisions and changes in their lives during the first year.

Don't

1. Don't tell them not to cry. Cry with them. What most people are saying is that "you make me uncomfortable when you cry." That puts a burden on the people least able to carry a burden.

2. Don't be frightened when people act a "little bit crazy" soon after a death—comfort and protect them.

3. Don't shut children out of grief; share it with them.

Courtesy Grief Education Institute, 2422 South Downing Street, Denver, Colorado 80210.

---

up policies that are initiated after the death as the responsibility of the primary nurse. Measures include phone calls or home visits 1 month, 6 months, and 1 year after the death, with additional family–nurse contacts as warranted. Nurses may feel uncomfortable about calling a family, feeling the family would not wish to hear from them or fearing the evoking of unpleasant memories. On the contrary, families usually are gratified that the nursing staff remembers them. Follow-up care allows family members to speak about the deceased if other family and friends feel they should not speak of the death any longer. Family-centered nursing includes follow-up contacts with families to assess and facilitate their progress through the grieving process.

Every family and family member resolves grief in a different way. The range of normal for a grieving family is still being defined through research. Guidelines to helping those who grieve are shown in Box 16–9. One nurse described an extended grief reaction: "A mother continued to set the table for the deceased child a year after that child had died. When the family moved to a new home, the dead child's room was moved intact, as if he were expected home any minute." This is considered an abnormal bereavement response. Common grief responses are outlined in Table 16–5. If there is concern that the family's behaviors are abnormal, compare them to these responses and to those of other families cared for. Psychiatric nurses, social workers, psychiatrists, and psychologists are also valuable resources for evaluating a family's grieving

Table 16–5	Common Grief Responses
Symptom Classification	**Characteristics**
Somatic distress	Occurs in waves lasting from 20 min to 1 h; deep sighing respirations, most common when discussing grief; lack of strength; loss of appetite and sense of taste; tightness in throat; choking sensation accompanied by shortness of breath
Preoccupation with image of deceased	Similar to daydreaming; may mistake others for deceased person; may be oblivious to surroundings; slight feeling of unreality; fear of becoming "insane"
Feelings of guilt	Accuses self of negligence; exaggerates existence and importance of negative thoughts and feelings and actions toward deceased; views self as having failed deceased saying, "If I had only. . . ."
Feelings of hostility	Irritability, anger, and loss of warmth toward others; may attempt to handle feelings of hostility in formalized and stiff manner in social interaction
Loss of patterns of conduct	Inability to initiate or maintain organized patterns of activity; restlessness, with aimless movements; loss of zest; tasks and activities are carried on as though with great effort; activities formerly carried on in company of deceased have lost their significance; may become strongly dependent on whoever stimulates mourner to activity

SOURCE: Wilson HS, Kneisl CR: *Psychiatric Nursing,* 2nd ed. Menlo Park, CA: Addison–Wesley, 1983. Reprinted with permission.

Table 16–6	Extended or Unusual Grief Reactions
Symptom Classification	**Characteristics**
Delayed reaction	Most common and most dramatic reaction; postponement may be brief or prolonged for years; usually occurs when bereaved is confronted with necessity of carrying out important tasks or maintaining morale of others
Distorted reaction	Excessive activity with no sense of loss; development of physical symptoms similar to those experienced by deceased just before death; medical illness of psychophysiological nature, developed close in time to loss of important person; continued and progressive social isolation with alteration in relationships with friends and relatives; extreme hostility against specific persons somehow connected with death event; "schizophreniclike" wooden and formal conduct, masking hostile feelings; lasting change in patterns of social interaction; activities detrimental to own social and economic existence; agitated depression

SOURCE: Wilson HS, Kneisl CR: *Psychiatric Nursing,* 2nd ed. Menlo Park, CA: Addison–Wesley, 1983. Reprinted with permission.

response. Examples of extended or unusual grief reactions are summarized in Table 16–6.

Helping a dying person to live fully as a whole person until the time of death is a challenge that brings special rewards when successful. Caring for the dying and their families can enhance the value of all personal relationships.

It can develop more fully the nurse's ability to communicate sensitively and honestly. For each person, death is a journey into the unknown. Nurses who can make that journey less lonely and frightening for the persons for whom they care may find their lives enriched rather than depleted by the process.

Section III: Ethical Issues in Caring for the Dying

Ethical considerations in caring for the dying client are not new. Ethics has taken on new dimensions in light of advancing technology, however. Technology has created unprecedented ethical dilemmas, some of which will be discussed in this section.

QUALITY OR QUANTITY OF LIFE?

In caring for the terminally ill, the issue of quality or quantity of life often surfaces. Facing the possibility of sending a client home to be with the family while terminating treatment that could prolong life is difficult. Some health care professionals are reluctant to follow the client's wishes for what he or she sees as better quality of life. They hesitate when dying clients indicate they would be happier for a shorter period of time at home without treatment. All clients and families should be allowed ultimately to decide what they wish to do, and the options should be presented completely and honestly to facilitate the decision. In this way, the client will regain some of the control given up through advances in medical technology.

THE CLIENT'S RIGHT TO KNOW

There is a basic human right to know the truth about one's own health status. A sometimes paternalistic attitude often surfaces in discussions about whether to tell a client about the terminal diagnosis. Veatch (1976) attributes this unwillingness to be the bearer of bad news to the Hippocratic oath, which in part says the physician will "never do harm to anyone." The current trend is to inform the client fully about the diagnosis and allow the client to participate in decisions about care.

On occasion, a physician might tell the family the client's diagnosis but not the client. This is a breach of confidentiality in the physician–client relationship. Unless the client authorizes the disclosure of information to others, the physician may not do so. By withholding this information, the physician not only abrogates the client's rights, but prevents the dying person from initiating the grieving and mourning process described earlier. In addition, time to resolve past grievances, say good-bye to family and friends, or accomplish some final task known only to the dying person is being wasted. Avoidance of the issue hides nothing from the client, who usually knows he is dying. The dying person feels isolated and unable to talk with those who mean the most about the important impending event.

The question has been raised whether a client who knows he or she is dying is competent to grant an informed consent for medical procedures. It may be reasoned that the person is being unduly pressured, not by the medical team, but by the impending death. The issue is still under debate.

TREATMENT DILEMMAS

The question sometimes arises whether to initiate or terminate treatment of a dying person. The reasons for this question vary from situation to situation, and each situation must be judged individually. The situation can be more clearly decided if the client has signed a living will, discussed later in this section.

Decisions About Treatment

The decision not to provide treatment is always difficult, no matter who makes it. Numerous factors presented by the client, family, and health care team may influence this decision. A few of the considerations are discussed here.

The health care team is legally obligated to comply with the family and client's wishes to initiate treatment. If the client and family want treatment in spite of the opinions and recommendations of the health care team, treatment customarily is given. Treatment may not only satisfy the client and family that something is being done but also prevents legal action against the medical staff and hospital.

On occasion, families or clients will request that no treatment be initiated against the health care team's recommendations. This request may be based on several reasons, some personal and others from religious teachings. Depending on the client's age and his or her determined sanity and rationality, the court sometimes will assume custody of the client for the duration of the illness. This occurs most often in the cases of minors whose parents refuse treatment. For older persons, each case must be considered to determine the sincerity of the client and family and their convictions about not initiating treatment.

Resuscitation

One of the most common issues in care of the terminally ill is the request from the family or client that no resuscitation be attempted in the event of cardiac or respiratory arrest. Many practitioners feel uncomfortable about these "no-code" orders. Some have the conviction that life should be prolonged, no matter what the quality of life.

Because the nurse is often the first professional on the scene of a cardiopulmonary arrest, the nurse must know if the person is to be resuscitated and if an order has been written to that effect. If the physician has communicated a spoken order to the nursing staff but has not written the order on the chart, the nurse *must initiate cardiopulmonary resuscitation (CPR)*. If the order was not signed by the physician, legally it has not been written. Only the physician's signature legally validates the order.

A number of hospitals require that "no-code" orders be rewritten periodically to keep abreast of the family's wishes. It cannot be overemphasized that the nurse has a responsibility to inform the physician if the client or family (if the client is incompetent) has changed their decision about a code or no-code order. If a nurse forgets or neglects to communicate this wish, the nurse may be held legally responsible for the person's death if CPR is not initiated. All nurses working with terminally ill persons should be aware of each person's code status and of the wishes of client and family.

The ethical and emotional issues surrounding "no-code" orders are difficult to resolve. Health professionals are taught to save lives at all costs. The decision not to issue a code for a person may make the nurse feel that caring for that person is a lost cause. In reality, many persons die every year without the option of being "coded"; they may die in a setting where no one knows CPR, such as at the scene of an accident or alone on a camping trip. Being aware of a person's code status should not in any way affect the nursing care given.

Termination of Treatment

Termination of treatment that is no longer beneficial and may in fact be harmful is a serious issue. Many therapies intended to cure are unpleasant and cause severe side effects, which in some cases may be life threatening. The termination of treatment must be evaluated individually.

If the client and family want to continue treatment and the health care team decides it is no longer of benefit, the health care team usually honors the wishes of the family or client. Guilt may be a factor in the decision to continue useless treatment. The family may feel guilty they did not give the person more attention while healthy, or the person may feel guilty to be ill and dying.

On occasion, for various reasons, the client and family will decide to terminate treatment against the recommendations of the health care team. Some clients may simply be tired of the treatment regimen and feel death would be a more pleasant alternative. Occasionally, a client and family will opt for an unproven method of treatment in place of the regimen prescribed for them. It is important for the health care team to understand the rationale for the decision to leave the prescribed protocol and to support the client and family in their decision.

Euthanasia

Euthanasia, a term that literally means "good death," is more commonly used to describe "mercy killing," an illegal act. If a family member assists a person in euthanasia, that family member could be charged with murder. Euthanasia societies mentioned later publish literature describing how to end life painlessly.

Davis (1984) identifies four types of euthanasia: passive, active, voluntary, and involuntary. *Passive euthanasia* is allowing someone to die by passive means, or by doing nothing. An example would be the terminally ill cancer client who develops renal failure; the decision not to dialyze this client would passively result in the client's death. *Active euthanasia* is actively causing a death. Animals are "put to sleep," a form of active euthanasia. *Voluntary euthanasia* involves the clients' acquiescence with the decision; they decide when and how to end life. *Involuntary euthanasia* occurs when the individual is incompetent to make this decision and others make it for him or her, as in the case of infants or comatose clients.

Euthanasia continues to incite controversy. It is an emotional issue, with no clear black-and-white definitions. For example, discontinuing life-support systems for a comatose client could be considered either active euthanasia (the person is being killed) or passive euthanasia (a dying person is being allowed to continue the process of dying).

Suicide and euthanasia have the same result—death of the participant. Some contend that suicide is a basic human right. Western society's aversion to suicide is based on Judeo-Christian beliefs that only God may determine when life should end. Other cultures, notably the Japanese, consider suicide an honorable death. Various organizations in 23 countries advocate what they term "self-deliverance." Concern for Dying and the Society for the Right to Die believe that persons have the right to have life-support measures withdrawn when there is no hope for recovery. Some groups go beyond that belief, however. The Hemlock Society in the United States has published a controversial book, *Let Me Die Before I Wake*, that includes information on fatal doses of a variety of common drugs and poisons. Sometimes called a "suicide manual," it is available in most bookstores. The British Voluntary Euthanasia Society and the Scottish group, Exit, also publish how-to literature for "self-deliverance." These societies have large memberships, an indication of the need for careful evaluation of health care practices surrounding death.

Near-Death Experiences

Research begun by Moody (1976) describes an interesting phenomenon referred to as "near-death" experiences, "out-of-body" experiences, or the "Lazarus syndrome." Other researchers have verified and expanded on Moody's findings and have added to the growing body of research on this intriguing subject (Ring & Franklin, 1982; Salladay, 1982). When interviewing persons who had been pronounced dead and were subsequently resuscitated, these researchers found remarkable similarities in their stories of the experiences. This prompted further research and interviewing of persons with "near-death" experiences. These persons reported hearing themselves pronounced dead, feeling as if they were rapidly moving through a tunnel; being aware of other "beings" present to assist them (usually people they recognize as being dead); experiencing intense feelings of joy, love, and peace; seeing their life passing before them for purposes of evaluation; and approaching a barrier, sensing the barrier is not to be crossed, and returning to the physical world. Afterward, many of these persons are reluctant to discuss these events for fear of being considered "crazy." As more people are successfully resuscitated, more of these experiences can be assessed for their commonalities and differences.

It is significant that persons assumed to be comatose or dead may be aware. The nursing implications are clear for persons being resuscitated and who are newly resuscitated or newly dead. During resuscitation, someone should be at the head of the bed, if possible, telling the client what is happening. Persons frequently can repeat conversations held while they were clinically dead and being resuscitated. A person newly resuscitated, in addition to being very ill, may be angry or withdrawn because of being wrenched back into the world of the living. An understanding nurse will recognize this as an appropriate response and explore the person's experience if he or she is willing and able to discuss it.

Many physicians and nurses talk to the clinically dead person because there is a possibility the client may still be aware. A nurse who is uncomfortable talking to a dead person in front of others may request to perform post-mortem care alone to talk freely. The nurse might say to the deceased what a good battle they fought, that they are undoubtedly more comfortable and pain-free now, and that those left behind will remember them lovingly. This aspect of nursing care should not be ignored because it is the nurse's final act of caring.

Determination of Death

Determination of death has become a problem with the advent of modern technology. Health professionals find it necessary to consider not only medical issues, but legal issues surrounding the pronouncement of death.

The American Bar Association, the American Medical Association, the National Conference of Commissioners on Uniform State Laws, and the President's Commission for the Study of Ethical Problems in Medicine and Biomedical and Behavioral Research have proposed a model statute for defining **clinical death** intended for adoption in all the states (Joynt, 1984). It states, "An individual who has sustained either (1) irreversible cessation of circulatory and respiratory functions, or (2) irreversible cessation of all functions of the entire brain, including the brain stem, is dead. A determination of death must be made in accordance with accepted medical standards." Complicating this definition and therefore the determination of death are drug and metabolic intoxications and cases of shock or hypothermia where cerebral circulation is decreased. Children in particular have been found to have an increased resistance to brain damage under such conditions.

The legal determination of death is of special significance in cases of neurological damage where other organ systems are not involved or damaged. In these cases, if the client has previously given consent for organ donation, death should be pronounced before any life-sustaining equipment is removed. Cases of prolonged hypoxia resulting in brain death are the most frequent instances when the definition and testing criteria become critical. In the treatment of increased intracranial pressure, the use of high-dose barbiturates and hypothermia to decrease intracranial pressure further confuses EEG readings. Frequently, the client is maintained fully on life-support systems for many days until an accurate determination of death can be made.

Living Wills, Natural Death Acts, and Right-to-Die Acts

Living wills are documents stating a person's desires about care if he or she becomes unable to communicate. These documents usually express a desire to die a natural death without intervention to artificially prolong life. By 1985, 23 states and the District of Columbia had passed "living will" legislation. In January 1984, California enacted pioneering legislation on a durable power of attorney. This law allows persons to designate someone—a spouse, other family member, or friend—to make decisions about treatment and life-support when they cannot speak for themselves. This same law protects health professionals against litigation if they obey the instructions of an authorized person and permit an individual to die.

Such documents should be kept available in a wallet or handbag in the event they are needed. Copies should be made and distributed to persons likely to be involved with the individual's care, such as the person's physician and family members. These documents must be updated and initialed yearly to indicate that the individual has not changed intent. These documents are legal if completed appropriately according to the statute's provisions. As with any document, however, the mental competence of the signer at the time of signing may be questioned if the document is brought to court. A living will used in California under the Natural Death Act is in Figure 16–1.

Organ Donation

In organ donation, still-functioning organs are removed from a newly dead person for implant in an individual needing a new organ. An individual who wishes to donate organs may obtain a special card from various organizations which, when completed and signed by the donor and witnesses, gives permission to health personnel to use the organs for donation in the event of death.

Some religions prohibit the donation of organs or the implantation of donated organs. Some persons feel uncomfortable about donating organs, fearing they will be declared dead prematurely so their organs may be used for others. In most instances, such fears are unfounded because the process of organ donation is carefully monitored, and both applicants and recipients are screened for an appropriate match. The nurse should always be alert for such fears, however, as well as for unreasonable efforts to procure an organ to give to someone younger or more prestigious. Suspicious cases should be reported.

Families of newly deceased persons may wish to donate their family member's organs or body. Widespread metastatic cancers may also make one's organs inappropriate for donation. If the client's family wishes to donate the deceased person's organs, the nurse should follow through and help them determine feasibility. These decisions must be made immediately after death because highly vascularized organs deteriorate rapidly without deliberate continued perfusion by artificial means.

Many lives are lengthened each year by legally donated organs. The success rate of transplantation is improving as technology and pharmacology to combat rejection improve.

In 1984, Congress passed the Organ Procurement and Transplantation Act. The primary purpose of the act is to increase the supply of human organs. The act also provides for the establishment of a communications network for matching of donor organs with recipients. A Task Force on Organ Procurement was created to examine legal,

A LIVING WILL
A directive to withhold treatment and
for the administration of pain-killing drugs

To my family, my relatives, my friends, my physicians, my employers, and all others whom it may concern:
Directive made this _____ day of _____ 198 _ I, _____ (name),
being of sound mind, willfully, and voluntarily make known my desire that my life shall not be prolonged artificially under the circumstances set forth below, do hereby declare:

   1. If at any time I should have an incurable injury, disease, illness or condition certified to be terminal by two
medical doctors who have examined me, and where the application of life-sustaining procedures of any kind would
serve only to prolong artificially the moment of my death, and where a medical doctor determines that my death
is imminent, whether or not life-sustaining procedures are utilized, I direct that such procedures be withheld or
withdrawn and that I be permitted to die naturally, and that I receive whatever quantity of whatever drugs may
be required to keep me free of pain or distress even if the moment of death is hastened.

   2. In the absence of my ability to give directions regarding the use of life-sustaining procedures, I hereby appoint
_____ (name) currently residing at _____ ,
as my attorney-in-fact/proxy for the making of decisions relating to my health care in my place; and it is my
intention that this appointment shall be honored by him/her, by my family, relatives, friends, physicians and law-
yer as the final expression of my legal right to refuse medical or surgical treatment; and I accept the consequences
of such a decision. I have duly executed a Durable Power of Attorney for health care decisions on this date.[1]

   3. In the absence of my ability to give further directions regarding my treatment, including life-sustaining procedures, it is my intention that this directive shall be honoured by my family and physicians as the final expression of my legal right to refuse or accept medical and surgical treatment, and I accept the consequences of such
refusal.

   4. If I have been diagnosed as pregnant and that diagnosis is known to any interested person, this directive
shall have no force during the course of my pregnancy.[2]

   5. I have been diagnosed, and notified at least 14 days ago, as being in a terminal condition by
_____ , M.D., whose address is _____
and whose telephone number is _____ . I understand that if I have not filled in the physician's name and
address, it shall be presumed that I did not have a terminal condition when I made out this directive.[3]

   6. This directive shall have no force and effect after five years from the date (above) of its execution, nor, if
sooner, after revocation by me, either orally or in writing.[4]

   7. I understand the full importance of this directive and am emotionally and mentally competent to make this
directive. No participant in the making of this directive or in its being carried into effect, whether it be a medical
doctor, my spouse, a relative, friend or any other person shall be held responsible in any way, legally, professionally or socially, for complying with my directions.

Signed _____

City, county and state of residence _____

   The declarant has been known to me personally and I believe her/him to be of sound mind.

Witness _____   Witness _____

address _____   address _____

_____   _____

Figure 16–1
Living will conforming with the California Natural Death Act.

SOURCE: Reproduced by permission of the Hemlock Society, from which additional copies can be obtained free of charge
by sending a self-addressed, stamped business envelope to: Hemlock Society, PO Box 66218, Los Angeles, CA 90066.

ethical, and economic issues of organ procurement and transplantation.

RESEARCH

Many questions remain unanswered concerning care of the dying. Only continued research at many levels can answer these questions. Because nursing has a central role in this area of care, nurses need to help pose questions for nurse researchers and other researchers to answer. The issues range from providing appropriate pain and symptom control, to assessing the family's most important needs and priorities, to helping survivors complete their grief work. There are also questions about the caregiver and economics. What qualities does it take to be a hospice nurse? Is hospice care more cost effective than care in a hospital? What can be learned from the ethical dilemmas that spring from high-tech health care?

Many such studies are underway. For example, one study by Amenta (1984) compared 36 hospice nurses with 35 nurses working in traditional settings. Hospice nurses were found to be significantly more assertive, imaginative, forthright, freethinking, and independent than those working in traditional settings. The nurses working in traditional settings were more conventional and comfortable with structure. The results of this study suggest a useful basis for selection of hospice staff. They also suggest the need for further study of hospices as an environment where autonomous professional nursing practice can flourish.

During the past two decades, health professionals have made great strides toward the goal of giving competent, compassionate, humane care to those who are dying. This progress is in large part because hospice care has become more than a collection of services and facilities; it is a social movement (Amenta, 1984) that has changed not only attitudes toward care of the dying but care of the living as well. Hospice care has served as a model for holistic care

Nursing Research Note

Caty S, Tamlyn D: Positive effects of education on nursing students' attitudes toward death and dying. *Nurs Papers* 1984; 16(4):41–53.

The authors describe the effects of an educational seminar about death and dying on attitudes of nursing students. Using a longitudinal quasi-experimental design, the researchers compared the nursing students (the experimental group) to a control group of physiotherapy students. The nursing students attended a 2-day death education seminar, and the control group received no specific educational program. Both groups were tested for attitudes about death 2 weeks before the seminar and 3 months and 14 months after the seminar.

The nursing students had a more open and flexible attitude toward death and dying compared to the control group at the first and third testings. These findings were statistically significant. At the second testing 3 months after the seminar, there were no statistically significant differences in scores between the experimental and control groups. The experimental group showed a statistically significant difference between the first testing and the third testing at 14 months. There was no difference in scores from the first testing and the second testing. The control group had no difference between mean scores at the first, second, or third testing.

The researchers state that educational seminars on death and dying may influence attitudes. They also cite professional socialization and educational experience as factors that lead to attitude changes among nursing students over time.

that meets psychosocial and spiritual needs as well as physical needs, both of the individual and the family. This model is changing the nature of care, particularly in chronic illness such as Alzheimer's disease. Nurses have been an integral part of the hospice movement because nursing's goals and philosophy are in agreement with those of hospice—holistic care of individuals and families, both the dying and those who must prepare to live without them.

Chapter Highlights

Death is both a universal and a unique experience.

Nurses have a central role in care of dying persons and their families, throughout the dying process and during grief and bereavement.

Death is often characterized by feelings of abandonment, desperation, humiliation, rage, and dehumanization.

An individual's attitude toward death and dying will be determined by his or her social and cultural values, developmental level, family role, religious and philosophical beliefs, and total life experiences. The

nurse needs to assess attitudes toward death to care for the dying effectively.

Principal fears of dying persons include abandonment, nonexistence, and what follows death.

The hospice movement offers a humane alternative to death in hospitals, enabling families to remain together while a member is dying.

The length of the living-dying interval will have a major effect on how the dying person and the family respond to the death.

(continued)

Chapter Highlights (continued)

Psychosocial and spiritual support and care are as important as physical care of the dying person and family.

Successful completion of grief and mourning ("grief work") is unique to each bereaved person; thus, it is difficult to establish what is "normal" and "abnormal."

Modern medicine and technology have added

complexity to the issues involved in care of the dying, including termination of life-support, brain death, and organ donation.

Research is needed on how to best meet the needs of dying persons and their families and how caregivers can support each other to meet their own needs as well.

Bibliography

Adams FE: Six very good reasons why we react differently to various dying patients. *Nurs 84* (June) 1984; 14:41–43.

Amenta M: Hospice USA 1984: Steady and holding. *Oncol Nurs Forum* (Sept–Oct) 1984; 11(5):68–72.

Amenta M: Traits of hospice nurses compared with those who work in traditional settings. *J Clin Psych* 1984; 40:414–420.

Bowlby J: Process of mourning. *Int J Psychoanal* 1961; 42:317–340.

Choron J: *Modern Man and Mortality.* New York: Macmillan, 1964.

Davis AJ: *Listening and Responding.* St. Louis: Mosby, 1984.

Dolan MB: If your patient wants to die at home. *Nurs 83* (April) 1983; 13:52.

Engel GL: Grief and grieving. *Am J Nurs* 1964; 64:93–98.

Geltman RL, Paige RL: Symptom management in hospice care. *Am J Nurs* 1983; 83:78–85.

Glaser BG, Strauss AL: *Time for Dying.* Hawthorne, NY: Aldine, 1968.

Gonda T, Ruark J: *Dying Dignified: The Health Professional's Guide to Care.* Menlo Park, CA: Addison–Wesley, 1984.

Hine VH: Dying at home: Can families cope? *Omega* 1979; 10(2):175–187.

Joynt RJ: A new look at death. *JAMA* 1984; 252:680–682.

Kalish RA, Reynolds DK: *Death and Ethnicity.* Los Angeles: University of California Press, 1976.

Kastenbaum R, Aisenberg R: *The Psychology of Death.* New York: Springer–Verlag, 1972.

Kübler–Ross E: *On Death and Dying.* New York: Macmillan, 1968.

Lindemann E: Symptomatology and management of acute grief. *Am J Psych* 1944; 101:141–148.

Lindemann E: Homotransplantation and death. Edited transcript of a tape recording. Feb 17, 1972. From Gonda T, Ruark J: *Dying Dignified: The Health Professional's Guide to Care.* Menlo Park, CA: Addison–Wesley, 1984.

Mandel HR: Nurses' feelings about working with the dying. *Am J Nurs* 1981; 81:1194–1197.

Moody RA Jr: *Life After Life.* New York: Bantam, 1976.

Munley A: *The Hospice Alternative: A New Context for Death and Dying.* New York: Basic Books, 1983.

Parkes C: Effects of bereavement on physical and mental health. *Brit Med J* 1964; 2:274–279.

Pattison EM: *The Experience of Dying.* Englewood Cliffs, NJ: Prentice–Hall, 1977.

Ring K, Franklin S: Do suicide survivors report near-death experiences? *Omega* 1982; 12:191–208.

Ross HM: Societal/cultural views regarding death and dying. *Top Clin Nurs* 1981; 3(3):1–16.

Salladay SA: In the event of death. *Omega* 1982; 13(1):1–11.

Sanders CM: Effects of sudden vs chronic illness death on bereavement outcome. *Omega* 1982; 13(3):227–241.

Saunders C: Principles of symptom control in terminal care. *Med Clin North Am* 1982; 66(5):1169–1183.

Taylor PB: Understanding sexuality in the dying patient. *Nurs 83* (April) 1983; 13:54–55.

Twycross RG: personal communication, August 1984.

Ufema JK: The dying patient. In: *Family-Centered Community Nursing: A Sociocultural Framework.* Vol. 2. Reinhardt AM, Quinn M (editors). St. Louis: Mosby, 1980.

Veatch RM: *Death, Dying and the Biological Revolution: Our Last Quest for Responsibility.* New Haven: Yale University Press, 1976.

Wass H: *Dying: Facing the Facts.* New York: McGraw–Hill, 1979.

Weisman AD: Thanatology. In: *Comprehensive Textbook of Psychiatry IV,* 4th ed. Kaplan HI et al (editors). Baltimore: Williams & Wilkins, 1985.

Woods JR: Death on a daily basis. *Focus on Critical Care* 1984; 11(3):50–51.

Suggested Readings

Buckingham RW, Lupu E: A comparative study of hospice services in the United States. *Am J Pub Health* 1982; 72:455–463. Examination of various services offered by hospices and comparison of hospice settings.

Comartin MA: Dealing with the dying patient in the hospital. New directions in care, part 2. *Can Nurse* 1983; 79(2):45–46. A sensitive look at how nurses can help establish a new order of care for dying persons and their families during hospitalization.

Dobihal SV: Hospice: Enabling a patient to die at home. *Am J Nurs* 1980; 80:1448–1451. Shows how a team of hospice professionals can enable the family of a dying person to be the unit of care and caregiving and to work through grief and bereavement.

Kübler–Ross E: *Death: The Final Stage of Growth.* Englewood Cliffs, NJ: Prentice–Hall, 1975. Further expounds on the original book, *On Death and Dying,* and elaborates on the concept that dying is a growth process.

Kübler–Ross E: *Questions and Answers on Death and Dying.* New York: Macmillan, 1974. Annotated text answering numerous letters generated by *On Death and Dying.*

MacElveen–Hoehn P, McIntosh EG: The hospice movement: Growing pains and promises. *Top Clin Nurs* 1981; 3(3):29–38. Reviews the history and concept of hospice and the problems encountered in implementing the concept in North America.

Putnam ST et al: Home as a place to die. *Am J Nurs* 1980; 80:1451–1453. Report of a study of 44 patients and their families concerning where they wanted to be cared for during the terminal stages of their illnesses, where they wanted to die, factors influencing their preferences, and services they needed.

Smurl JF: Did I do the right thing? Ethical decision making for everyday nursing problems. *Nurs Life* (May–June) 1983; 49–52. Practical guide to ethical problem solving using common situations. Discusses various philosophical schools of thought.

Stowers SJ: Nurses cry, too. *Nurs Management* 1983; 14(4):63–64. Emphasizes the importance of nurses' acknowledging and sharing with each other their feelings and reactions to the death of patients.

Vago MD: Remember the roommate. *Nurs 84* (May); 14:51. Offers insight into meeting the needs of the person who shares a room with a dying person.

Resources

SELF-HELP GROUPS AND OTHER ORGANIZATIONS

Compassionate Friends
PO Box 3247
Hialeah, FL 33013
Phone: (305) 741-8866

> Founded in the United States in 1972 (originally begun in Great Britain in 1969), this is a fellowship of parents who have experienced the death of a child. Over 100 local chapters in the United States and Canada offer mutual support through self-help groups, distributed literature, and through offers of counseling and friendship to bereaved parents. This group has no religious ties, is nonprofit, and charges no membership fees or dues.

Concern for Dying
250 W. 57th St.
New York, NY 10019
Phone: (212) 246-6962

> Formerly called the Euthanasia Educational Council, this organization of physicians, lawyers, educators, religious leaders, and other interested individuals distributes literature, promotes research on death and dying, and works toward promoting the right of dying individuals to refuse extraordinary life-prolonging measures. They publish a quarterly newsletter and a "living will."

The Hemlock Society
PO Box 66218
Los Angeles, CA 90066
Phone: (213) 391-1871

> This organization, founded in 1980, supports the option of active voluntary euthanasia for the terminally ill. Its goal is to promote tolerance of the right of terminally ill persons to end their lives in a planned manner. Publishes the "Hemlock Quarterly" newsletter, various legal declarations and documents such as a "living will" and a durable power of attorney for health care, and the only guide to self-deliverance ("Let Me Die Before I Wake") for the dying in the United States. Membership fee of $20 for an individual or a couple ($15 for senior citizens) includes the newsletter.

Make Today Count

> This self-help group is sponsored by the American Cancer Society and is described in the resources section of Chapter 12.

National Hospice Organization
1910 N. Fort Myer Dr., Suite 902
Arlington, VA 22209
Phone: (703) 243-5900

> This is an organization of hospices and individuals that encourages public and professional education on caring for the terminally ill, monitors legislation affecting the hospice movement, and publishes a quarterly newsletter, "National Hospice Organization Newsletter."

HEALTH EDUCATION MATERIAL

American Association of Retired Persons
National Retired Teachers Association
1909 K St., NW
Washington, DC 20049
Phone: (202) 872-4700

> A special magazine offering advice for the elderly on coping with bereavement and death is published and distributed by this organization. Included is a bibliography on this subject.

Information Clearinghouse on Grief, Bereavement, Death, and Dying
Center for Death Education and Research
1167 Social Science Bldg.
University of Minnesota
267 19th Ave., S.
Minneapolis, MN 55455
Phone: (612) 376-3641

> This research institution disseminates research on death and dying to the public and professional communities. Request the brochure entitled "Center for Death Education and Research" for more information and "Publications List" for a list of more than 1000 titles on the topic.

From: American Cancer Society, Inc.
> 777 Third Ave.
> New York, NY 10017
> "Questions and Answers About Pain Control," a free booklet.

From: Concern for Dying
"Dilemmas of Euthanasia," a summary of the proceedings of the Fourth Euthanasia Conference.
"A Living Will" includes a sample document and the procedures for making a living will legally binding.
"Questions and Answers About the Living Will," a brochure.

From: National Hospice Organization
"Facts About Hospice," a brochure
"Philosophy and Organization of a Hospice Program," a booklet, cost: $.75.

From: National Institutes of Health
Besthesda, MD 20205
"Chronic Pain—Hope Through Research," NIH Publication No. 82-2406.

From: Public Affairs Committee
381 Park Ave. S
New York, NY 10016
"Acupuncture: Myths or Medical Treatment?," a booklet on acupuncture with guidelines for selecting an acupuncturist; cost is $.50.

The following paperback books are also available at local bookstores:
Benjamin BE, Borden G: *Listen to Your Pain.* New York: Penguin Books, 1984.
Olshan NH: *Power Over Your Pain Without Drugs.* New York: Beaufort Books, 1983.
Smollen B, Schulman B: *Pain Control: The Bethesda Program.* New York: Zebra Books, 1982.

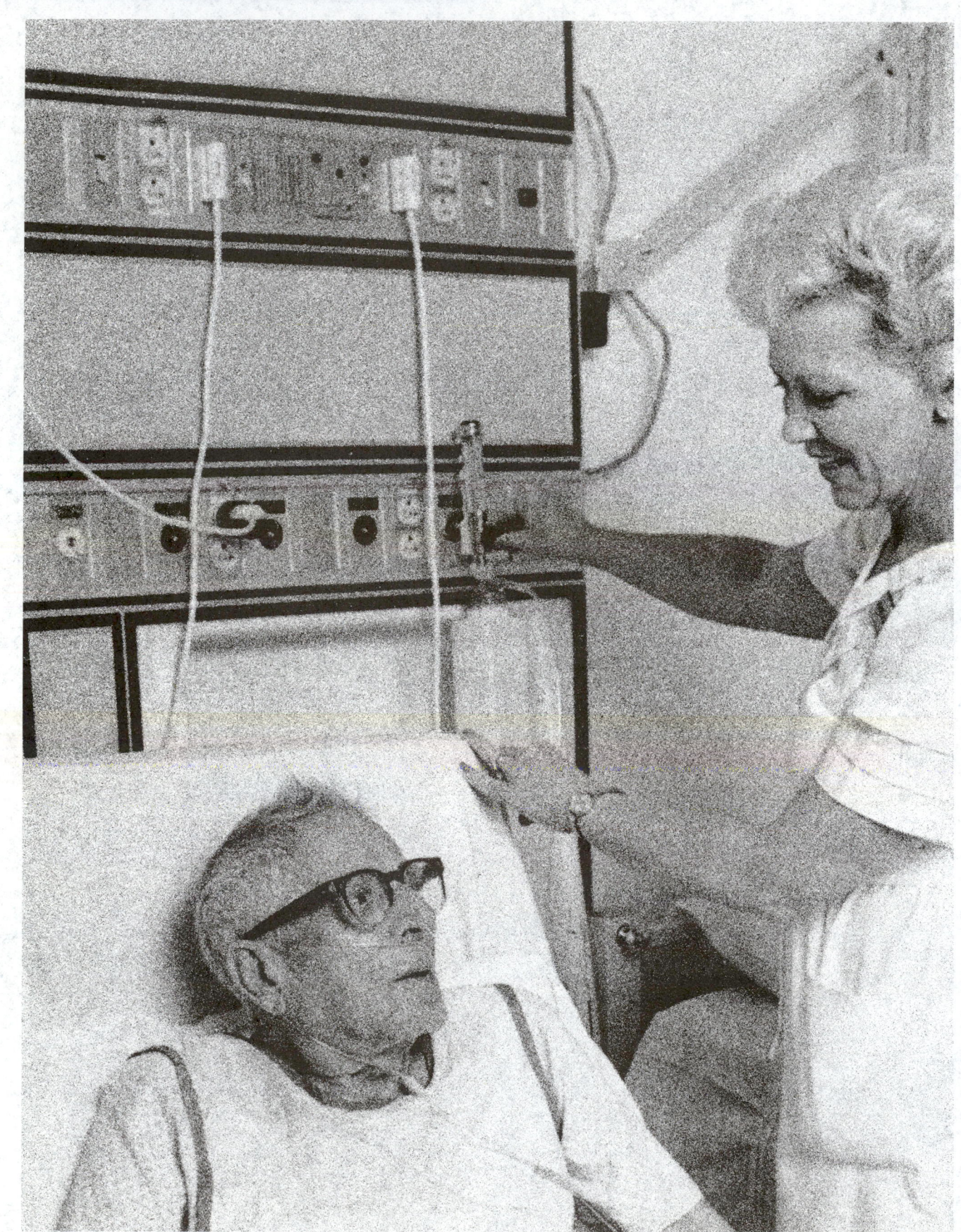

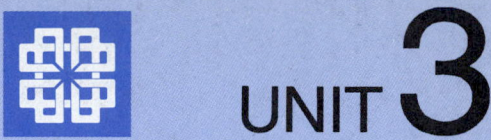

UNIT 3

The Client With Respiratory System Dysfunction

Chapter 17

The Respiratory System in Health and Illness

Yvonne Krall Scherer

Every cell in the body needs oxygen to carry out its metabolic functions, that is, to live. Likewise, every cell in the body must rid itself of carbon dioxide, a waste product of cellular metabolism. The process of transporting oxygen to the cells and removing carbon dioxide is called respiration. Any disease or trauma that interferes with respiration injures body cells. The body can survive without food for weeks and without water for a few days; without oxygen it dies in a few minutes.

Respiration involves two major body systems, the cardiovascular system and the respiratory system, under regulation of the nervous system. Oxygen and carbon dioxide, which are gases, are conveyed to and from tissues and organs by the cardiovascular system. The respiratory system delivers oxygen from the atmosphere to the bloodstream and delivers carbon dioxide from the blood to the atmosphere. The exchange of oxygen and carbon dioxide, called gas exchange, takes place in specialized structures of the lungs.

Section I: Structural and Functional Interrelationships

Although the respiratory airways and the anatomic structures where gas exchange takes place are continuous, their components are classified anatomically and functionally as belonging to either (1) the upper respiratory tract or (2) the lower respiratory tract. The muscles of the chest wall and diaphragm also participate in respiration.

THE UPPER RESPIRATORY TRACT

The upper respiratory tract is primarily an air delivery system: it warms, moistens, and filters inspired atmospheric air on its way to the lungs. Structures of the upper respiratory tract also expel foreign matter and excess secretions from the system. The principal structures of the upper respiratory tract are the nose, the paranasal sinuses, the pharynx, and the larynx (Figure 17–1).

The Nose

Air enters the system first through the nares, or nostrils—the openings of the two cavities of the nose (nasal fossae). The nasal septum separates the two fossae. The nose is composed of both bone and cartilage, and its interior surface has ridges called turbinates. The ridged configuration increases the effective surface of the nasal mucosa. An extensive bed of capillaries transfers body heat to the inspired air. Because of this rich vascularity, bleeding from injured nasal tissue can be profuse.

Mucus secreted by the membrane that lines the nose helps humidify inspired air, which attains a relative humidity of over 90% as it passes through the nares. Hairs that line the nose filter out large foreign particles, and a sticky mucus secreted by the serous glands in the mucosa traps finer dirt, dust, and microorganisms. Hairlike structures of the mucous membrane called cilia constantly propel trapped particles toward the pharynx, from which they can be expelled by sneezing or coughing.

In addition to its respiratory functions, the nose is the organ of olfaction. Sensory receptors sensitive to various odors are concentrated in the roof of the nasal fossae.

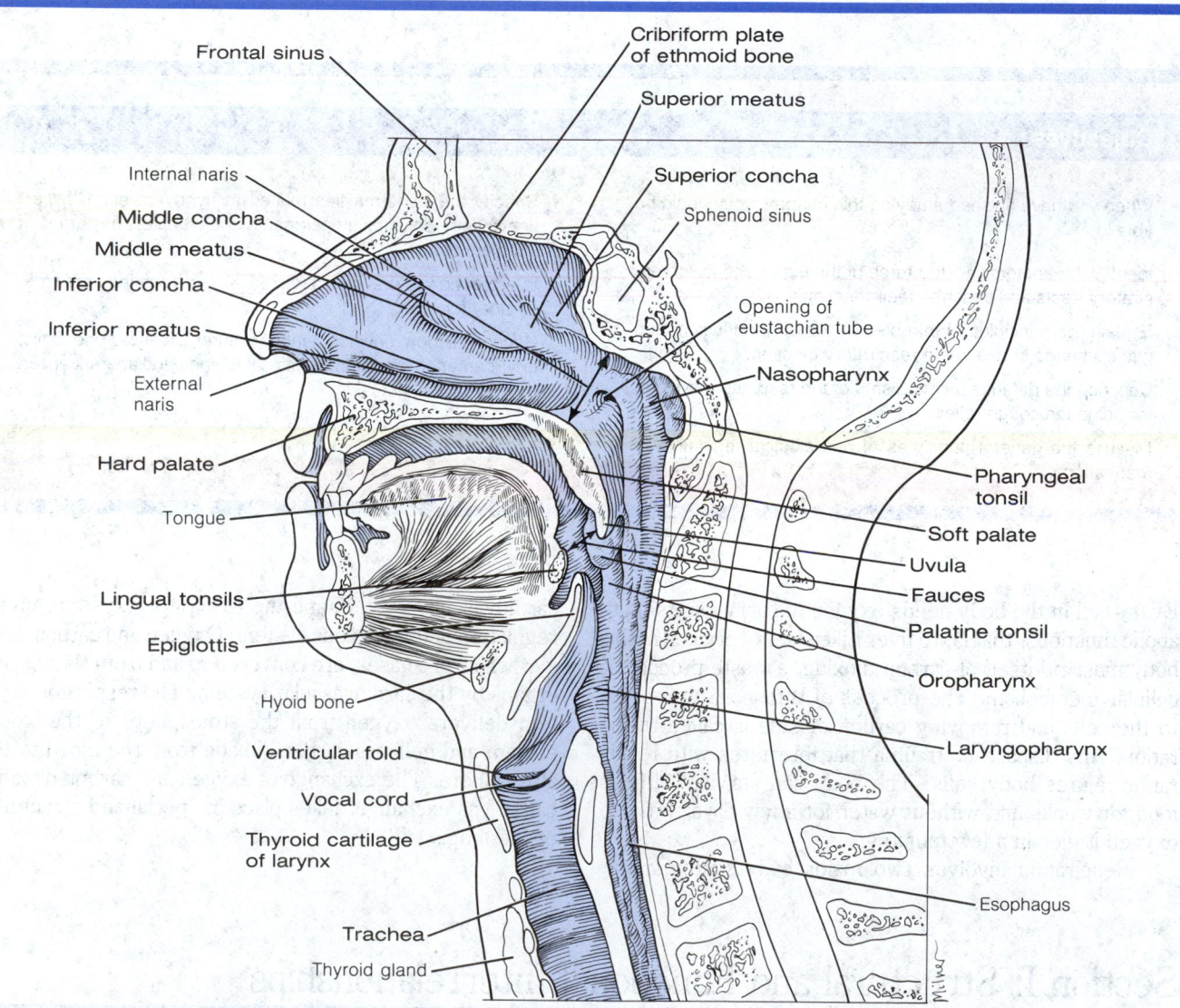

Figure 17–1

Structures of the upper respiratory tract.

SOURCE: Spence AP, Mason EB: *Human Anatomy and Physiology*, 2nd ed. Menlo Park, CA: Benjamin/Cummings, 1983.

Along with the paranasal sinuses, the nose functions as a resonance chamber for phonation; if the mucosa of these structures becomes edematous or clogged with secretions, the flat, nonresonant sound associated with "stuffy nose" occurs.

The Paranasal Sinuses

The paranasal sinuses are air-filled cavities within bony structures adjacent to the nasal cavity. These sinuses—called the ethmoid, frontal, sphenoid, and maxillary sinuses—drain through the nasal cavity. All are lined with ciliated columnar epithelium that is continuous with the lining of the nose. Because the mucosa is continuous, infection in the nasal passages can readily spread to the sinuses.

Although their function is not yet completely understood, the paranasal sinuses are thought to help insulate the delicate structures inside the skull from extremes of temperature and to make the skull lighter. Like all structures of the upper respiratory tract, the sinuses can trap foreign matter and, by ciliary movement, expel it—the respiratory system's first line of defense.

The Pharynx

The pharynx begins at the base of the skull and ends opposite the lowest cartilaginous rings of the larynx. Its three sections, from superior to inferior, are the nasopharynx, the oropharynx, and the laryngopharynx. The nasopharynx contains the adenoids—paired lymphatic structures—and the eustachian tubes, which maintain appropriate air pressure within the middle ear. Functional eustachian tubes are essential for hearing and crucial to the mechanism by which the body maintains balance. Air and food both enter the body through the oropharynx. The palatine tonsils, which, like the adenoids, are composed of lymphatic tissue, are located there. The laryngopharynx contains the lingual tonsils and the epiglottis, a small flap of tissue that covers the larynx during swallowing to prevent food or liquid from being aspirated into the lower airway.

The lining of the pharynx, like the lining of the structures that precede it, consists of mucous membrane that traps foreign particles and humidifies and warms the inspired air. The lymphatic tissue of the tonsils also traps microorganisms and disposes of them by phagocytosis before they can enter the remainder of the respiratory tract, another line of defense.

The Larynx

The larynx, often called the voice box, connects the upper and lower airways. The opening of the larynx, called the glottis, closes during swallowing to prevent aspiration. The vocal cords of the larynx, in addition to producing sound, are involved in the cough reflex, which clears the respiratory tract of foreign substances or objects and of accumulated secretions (Figure 17–2).

The Cough Reflex

The cough reflex is initiated when a foreign substance—(eg, a dust particle)—irritates specialized nerve endings within the larynx, trachea, or major bronchi. Nerve im-

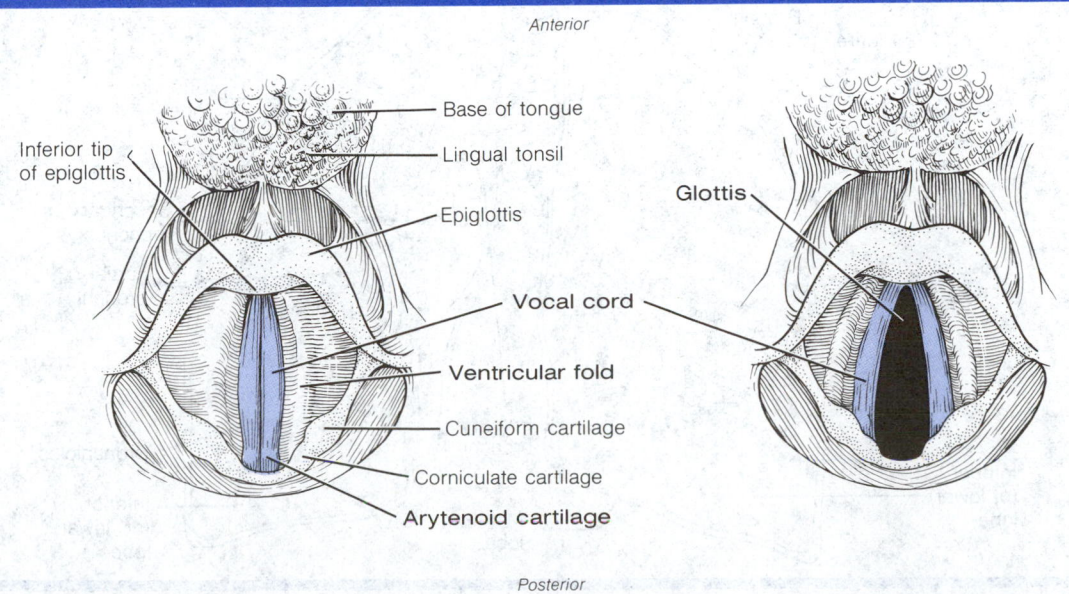

Anterior

Inferior tip of epiglottis

Base of tongue

Lingual tonsil

Epiglottis

Glottis

Vocal cord

Ventricular fold

Cuneiform cartilage

Corniculate cartilage

Arytenoid cartilage

Posterior

Figure 17–2

Superior view of the larynx showing **(left)** the glottis closed and **(right)** the glottis open.

SOURCE: Spence AP, Mason EB: *Human Anatomy and Physiology*, 2nd ed. Menlo Park, CA: Benjamin/Cummings, 1983.

pulses are sent to contract muscles that close the vocal cords and simultaneously contract abdominal muscles and muscle fibers within the respiratory tract itself. Air pressure builds up within the lower airways, and when the vocal cords reopen, a sudden rush of air carries mucus and foreign matter up to be expectorated. Because the vocal cords are crucial to the cough reflex, persons whose larynxes have been removed cannot cough and thus are deprived of an important defense against airway obstruction.

THE LOWER RESPIRATORY TRACT

The lower respiratory tract consists of the trachea, the bronchi and their branches, and the various structures of the lungs, which are protected by the chest wall. The structures of the trachea and bronchi are best visualized as an upside-down tree (Figure 17–3). The tracheobronchial tree is composed of a main "trunk" (the trachea) that bifurcates into two major branches (the right and left primary bronchi). These divide in turn into secondary and then tertiary bronchi, which branch again and again into "twigs" (the bronchioles). At the tiny outermost tips of the twigs, the terminal bronchioles, are the respiratory bronchioles, from which air passes through alveolar ducts into the alveoli, the "leaves" where gas exchange actually takes place.

The Trachea

The air passage of the trachea, or windpipe, is kept open by C-shaped cartilaginous rings in the tracheal wall, much as the flexible hose of a vacuum cleaner or hair dryer is

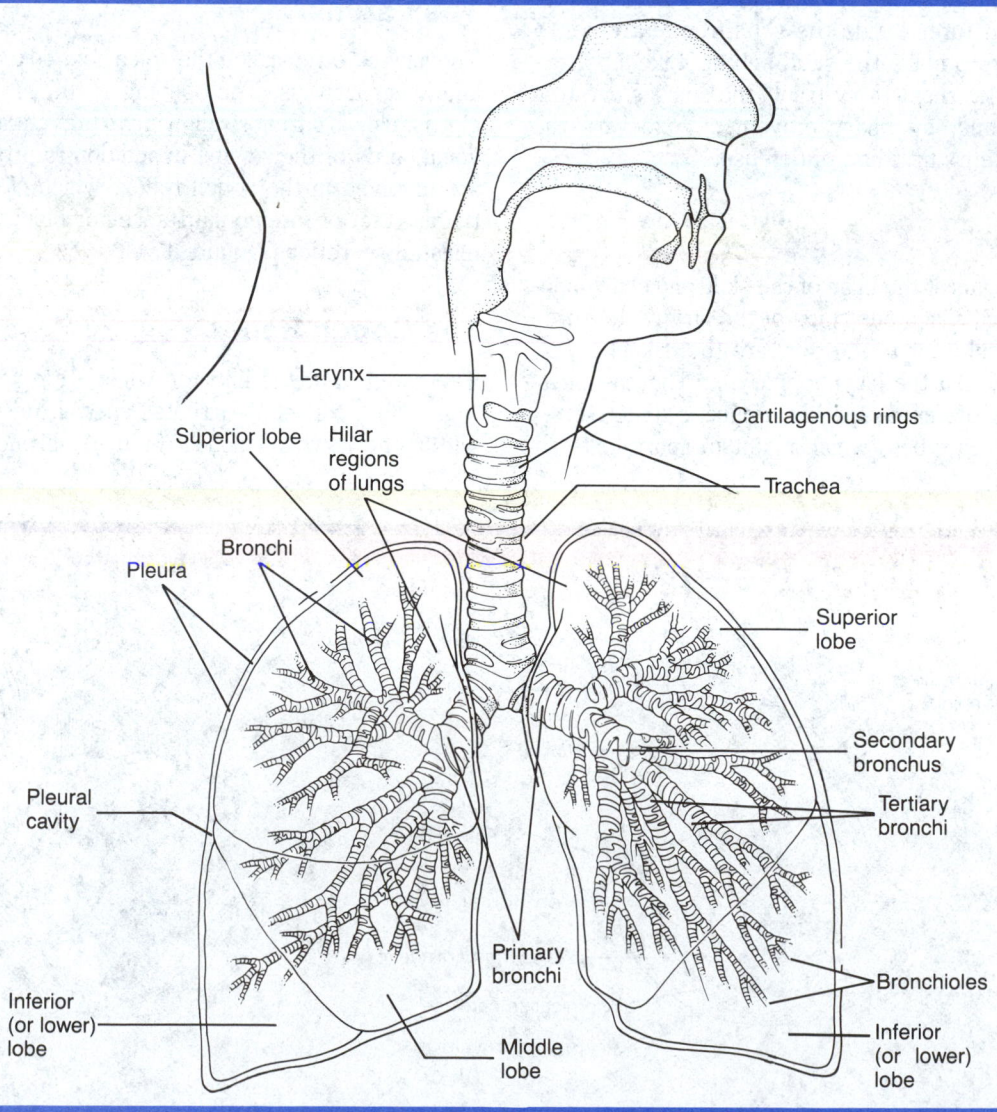

Figure 17–3

The tracheobronchial tree.
SOURCE: Tortora GJ, Funke BR, Case CL: *Microbiology: An Introduction,* 2nd ed. Menlo Park, CA: Benjamin/Cummings, 1986.

kept open by rings of plastic or metal (see Figure 17–3). The mucus-bathed ciliary epithelium that lines the trachea sweeps foreign material up into the pharynx, where the cough reflex expels it. The trachea, like the upper respiratory passages, warms and humidifies inspired air.

The Bronchi and Bronchioles

In Figure 17–3, note that the left primary bronchus exits from the trachea at a more acute angle than the right bronchus. The right bronchus might almost be considered an extension of the trachea itself. Because of the obtuse angle, foreign material is more often aspirated into the right lung than the left. The cellular structure of the bronchial lining at this point is similar to that of the trachea.

The bronchi contain sensory receptors of the parasympathetic and sympathetic nervous systems. If these nerve endings are stimulated—(eg, by an allergen)—impulses transmitted to the respiratory centers of the brain by cranial nerve X (the vagus nerve) initiate constriction of the bronchi, secretion of mucus, or the cough reflex. Thus, the lungs are protected against foreign particles.

The right primary bronchus divides into three secondary bronchi that supply the three lobes (superior, middle, and inferior) of the right lung. The left bronchus bifurcates, each segment going to one of the two lobes of the left lung. Within the lung, the bronchi branch off into smaller and smaller airways and then into tiny bronchioles.

The primary bronchi, like the trachea, are supported by partial rings of cartilage. As the airways become narrower and narrower, the proportion of smooth muscle to cartilage increases, and the number of serous glands lining the bronchiolar walls decreases. At approximately the point where a bronchiole narrows to 1 mm in diameter, the walls are entirely surrounded by smooth muscle. Thus, when the muscles of the bronchioles undergo spasm—as in an asthma attack—the lack of cartilaginous support causes air passages to collapse, and breathing becomes extremely difficult (Spence & Mason, 1983).

The terminal bronchioles mark the end of the air conduction system and open into the respiratory bronchioles. Each of these in turn branches into several alveolar ducts, which open into grapelike clusters of air-filled sacs called alveoli. The respiratory bronchioles, alveolar ducts, and alveoli form the terminal respiratory units of the lungs, called **acini** (Figure 17–4).

The Lungs

The lungs are paired, somewhat cone-shaped structures that lie in the thoracic cavity on either side of the mediastinum, which contains the heart, aorta, venae cavae, and other vital structures (Figure 17–5). The bases of the lungs rest on the diaphragm. The right lung has three lobes, the left two, and the lobes are further subdivided into smaller bronchopulmonary segments. This segmental

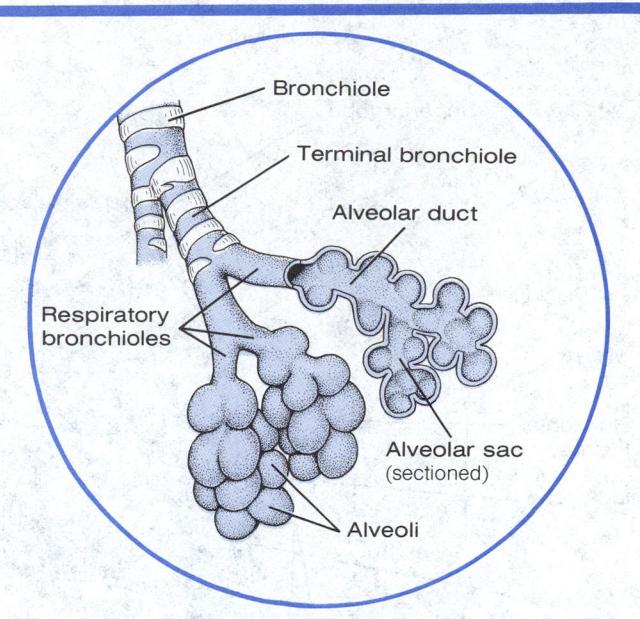

Figure 17–4

An acinus, the terminal respiratory unit of the lung.
SOURCE: Spence AP, Mason EB: *Human Anatomy and Physiology,* 2nd ed. Menlo Park, CA: Benjamin/Cummings, 1983.

structure makes it possible to remove a relatively small portion of the lung if surgical resection is necessary.

The lungs lie free within the pleural cavities of the thorax, except at the hilus, or root, on the medial surface. The bronchi and blood vessels enter and exit through the hilus. The sternum forms the anterior border of the thorax. The lateral boundaries of the thorax are composed of the twelve ribs, or costae, which are attached to the sternum by the costal cartilages anteriorly and the vertebral column posteriorly. This bony thoracic cage protects the vital structures within the mediastinum and the fragile, spongy tissue of the lungs.

The diaphragm, which lies below the lungs, is an important muscle of respiration and separates the thorax from the abdominal cavity. Each half of the diaphragm is innervated by a phrenic nerve. The phrenic nerves originate from the fourth cervical nerve. An injury to one of the phrenic nerves results in a unilateral diaphragmatic paralysis with elevation of half of the diaphragm.

The Pleura

The visceral pleura covering the lungs is continuous with the parietal pleura, which lines the thoracic cavity. Both pleurae are formed of serous membrane that secretes pleural fluid into the extremely narrow pleural cavity between the two layers. This fluid lubricates the two layers, reducing friction as the lungs and thorax move during respiration. The pleural fluid also couples the parietal and visceral pleurae and the structures to which they are attached—much

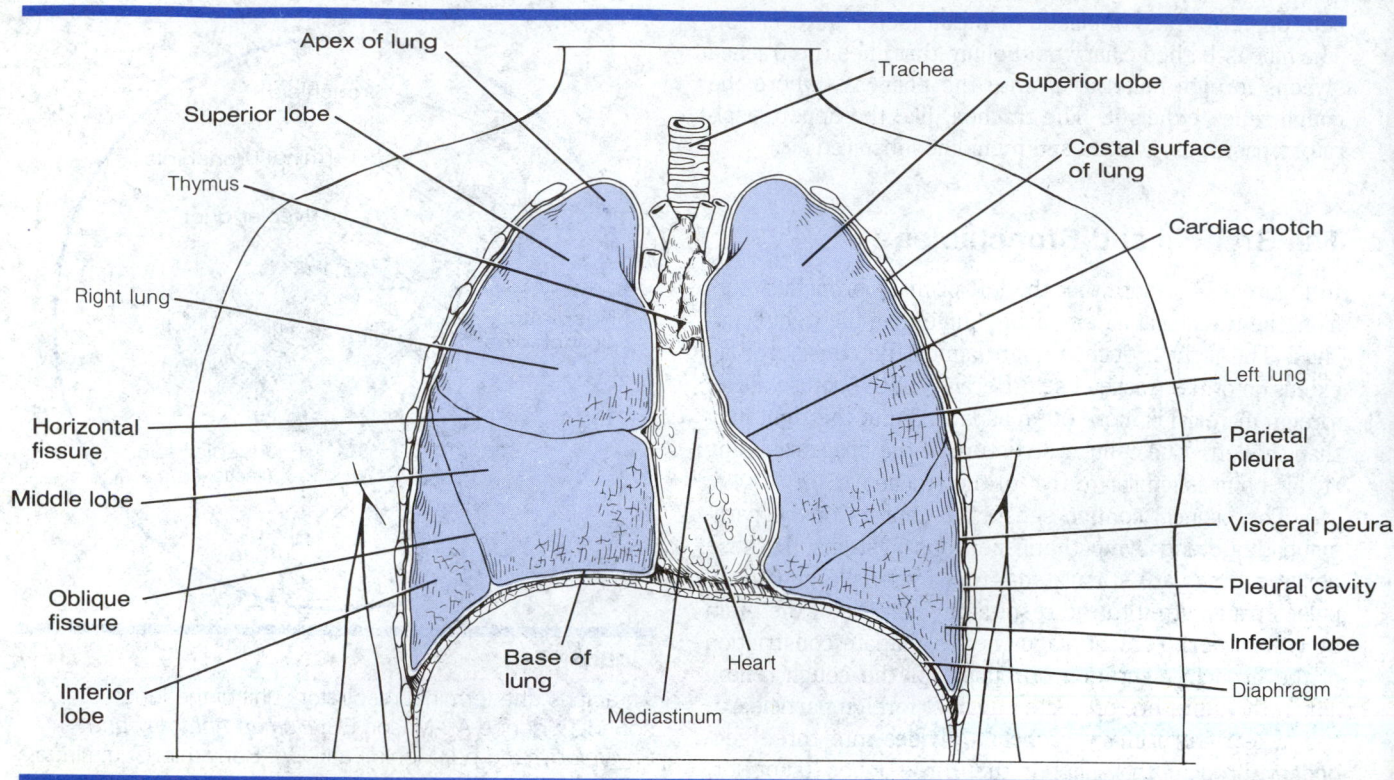

Figure 17–5

The lungs and thoracic cavity, showing the structures within the mediastinum.
SOURCE: Spence AP, Mason EB: *Human Anatomy and Physiology,* 2nd ed. Menlo Park, CA: Benjamin/Cummings, 1983.

as a drop of water between a laboratory slide and a cover plate will cause the two to adhere.

Inflammation of the pleural membrane (pleurisy)—(eg, during a bacterial infection)—causes the membrane to become dry and fibrous. The ensuing friction makes breathing painful (Spence & Mason, 1983).

Intrapleural Pressure

Because of changes that occur when breathing begins after birth, air pressure within the pleural cavity (intrapleural pressure) is lower than air pressure within the lungs (intrapulmonary pressure). This lower pressure keeps the lung expanded because of its tendency to be drawn toward the area of subatmospheric pressure. If the lung or chest wall is punctured, air rushes into the area of lower pressure, the pleural space, destroying the vacuum that keeps the lung expanded. In severe injury, the amount of air entering the intrapleural space may be sufficient to cause equalization of intrapleural pressure and atmospheric pressure. The result is collapse of the lung on the affected side.

The Pulmonary Circulation

The lungs have a dual blood supply: the tracheal and bronchial circulation, and the pulmonary circulation. The right and left bronchial arteries branch from the descending aorta and supply blood to the trachea and bronchi to the level of

the respiratory bronchioles. The terminal respiratory units of the lungs where gas exchange takes place are nourished via the pulmonary circulation.

The pulmonary circulation is where oxygenation of blood occurs. The entire output of the right ventricle leaves the heart via the pulmonary artery, which divides into the right and left pulmonary arteries. This poorly oxygenated blood circulates through the capillaries of the alveoli where gas exchange takes place. Oxygenated blood is then returned to the left atrium via the pulmonary veins. Figure 17–6 shows the pulmonary circulation.

The Alveoli and Gas Exchange

Each terminal bronchiole supplies its own unit of several alveoli, called the acinus. Exchange of gases takes place here. Essentially, each alveolus is a tiny air space enclosed by a thin wall—the alveolar septum—that consists of a network of pulmonary capillaries held together by connective-tissue fibers and lined with squamous epithelium that contains secretory cells. To appreciate how small alveoli are, consider that the tissue of an adult lung contains over 300 million alveoli (Harper, 1981). Figure 17–7 depicts an alveolus surrounded by capillaries showing the respiratory membrane that separates the air in the alveolus from the blood in the capillaries.

The secretory glands of the alveolar wall produce a

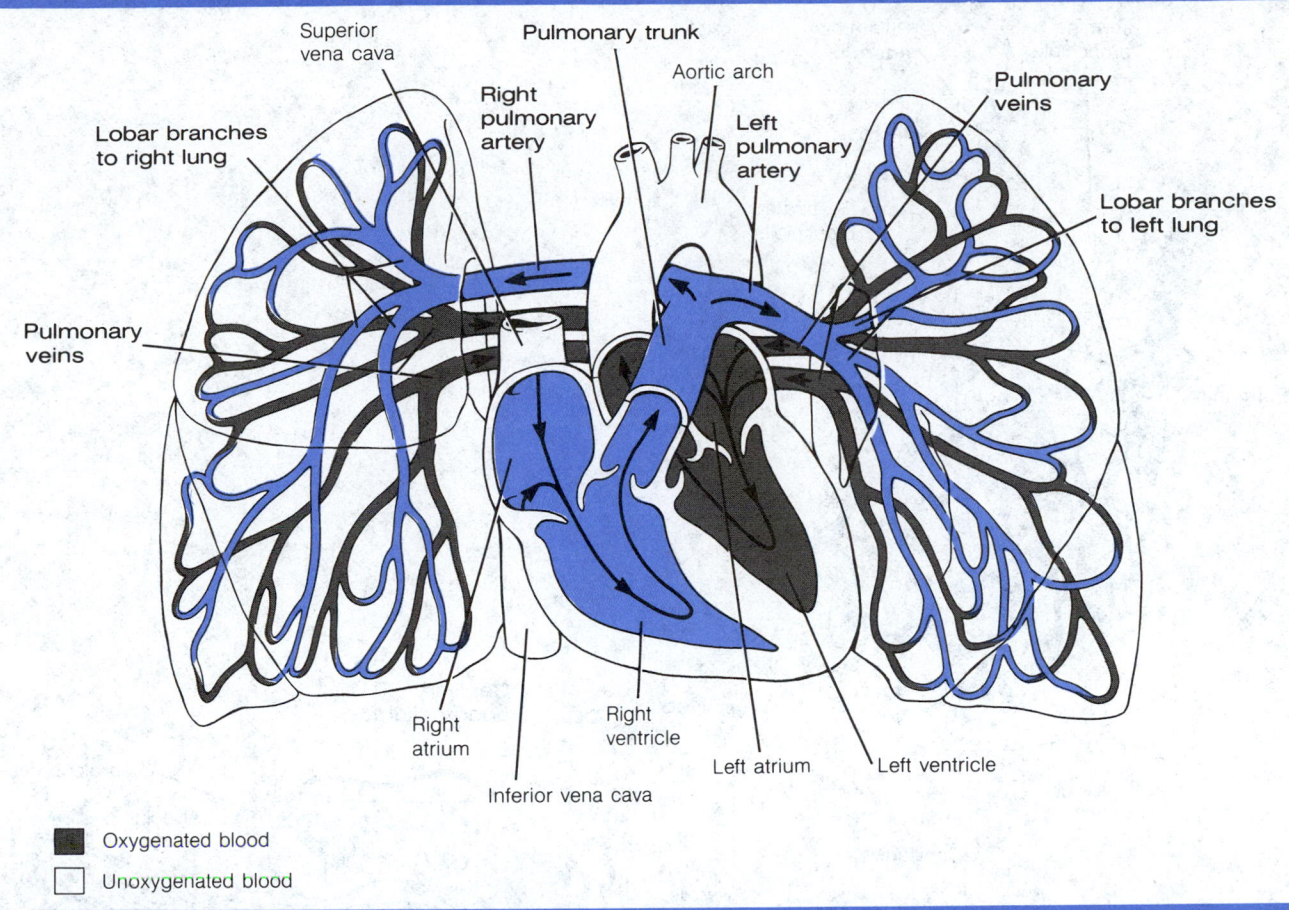

Figure 17–6

Pulmonary circulation showing the pulmonary trunk dividing into right and left pulmonary arteries, which then divide into lobar branches. Blood from the lungs returns to the left atrium through the pulmonary veins. Arrows indicate direction of blood flow.
SOURCE: Spence AP, Mason EB: *Human Anatomy and Physiology,* 2nd ed. Menlo Park, CA: Benjamin/Cummings, 1983.

fluid called **pulmonary surfactant.** (A surfactant is a substance that reduces the *surface tension* of a liquid—the attraction between molecules that causes them to form droplets instead of spreading. Dishwashing detergents contain surfactants so water will spread easily along the surface of dishes. If surface tension were to pull alveolar walls together, expansion of the lungs during inspiration would be hindered, and the alveoli would tend to collapse during expiration as the molecules of fluid cohered. Pulmonary surfactant also contains macrophages that destroy foreign material that has passed through the upper-airway defenses.

Within the alveoli, air is separated from blood by the respiratory membrane, which is formed by the basement membrane of the alveolar and capillary epithelia. This membrane is less than 1 μm thick, and gases move across it in accordance with the principle of diffusion; that is, a gas moves across a membrane from an area of greater partial pressure to one of lesser partial pressure. Partial pressure, denoted by P, refers to the proportionate pressure exerted by a gas in relation to total atmospheric pressure at sea level.

The venous blood returning from the tissues is high in carbon dioxide and low in oxygen; the air in the alveolar space is higher in oxygen and lower in carbon dioxide than the blood. Under normal conditions, the approximate partial pressures of oxygen and carbon dioxide in the alveoli and the capillaries are (Spence & Mason, 1983):

	Capillaries	**Alveoli**
Oxygen	PO_2 40 mm Hg	PO_2 105 mm Hg
Carbon dioxide	PCO_2 45 mm Hg	PCO_2 35 mm Hg

Among the prerequisites for efficient gas exchange are:

- *A large number of capillaries must be in contact with the inspired air.* The many-sectioned structure of lung tissue normally provides maximum capillary surface. If alveolar septa are destroyed by a disease process, however, and alveoli coalesce, the surface available for diffusion is reduced.

- *Diffusion of gases must be unimpaired.* If the alveolar membrane becomes fibrous and thickened by scarring, diffusion will be impeded.

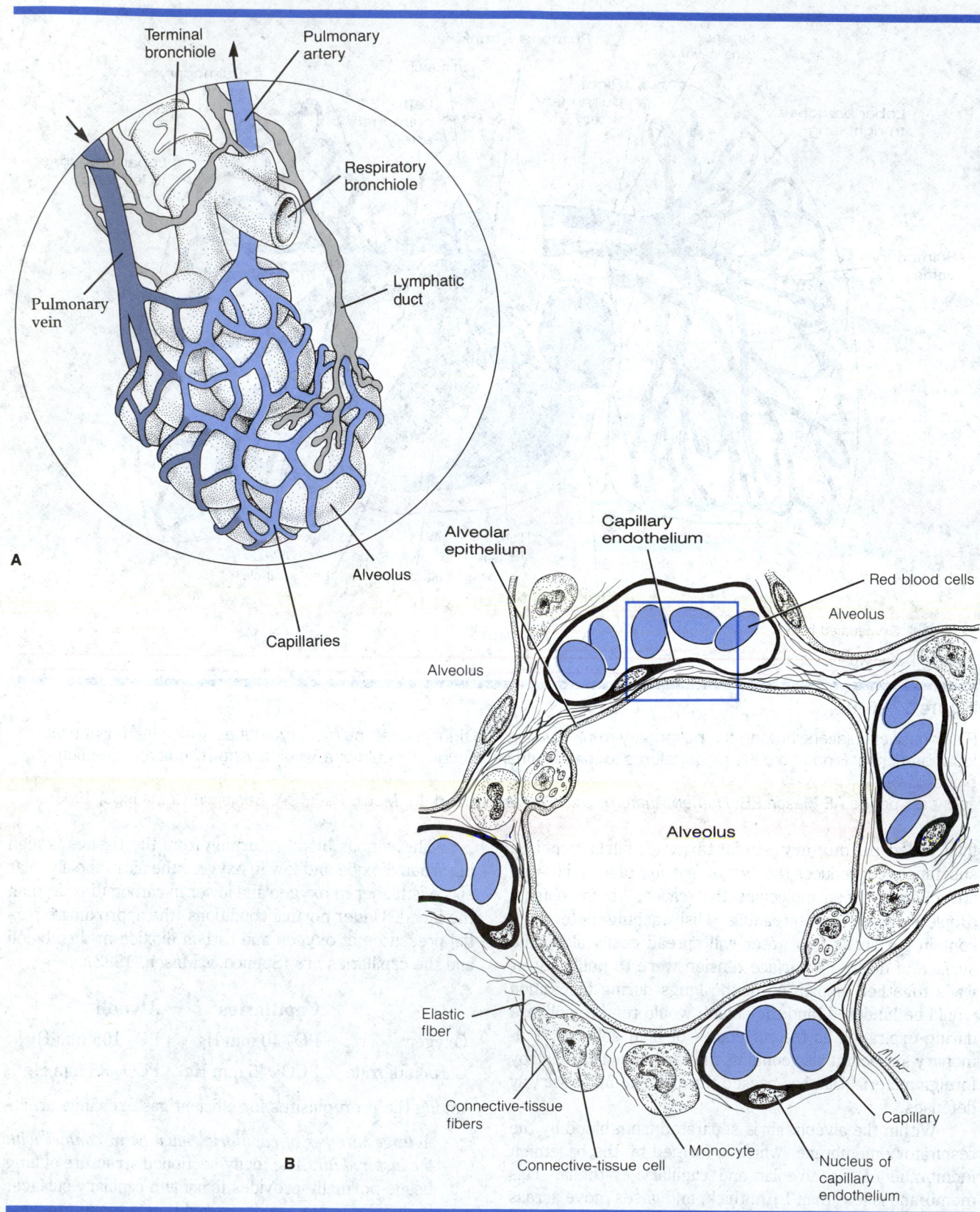

Figure 17–7

A. An alveolus surrounded by capillaries. **B.** An alveolus surrounded by capillaries, showing the respiratory membrane that separates the air in the alveolus from the blood in the capillaries.
SOURCE: Tortora GJ, Funke BR, Case CL: *Microbiology: An Introduction,* 2nd ed. Menlo Park, CA: Benjamin/Cummings, 1986.

- *Pulmonary blood flow must be normal.* If an embolus obstructs blood flow to a portion of the lung, gas exchange will be impaired.
- *Alveoli must be in normal condition.* If alveoli are filled with inflammatory exudate from infection, air cannot reach the respiratory membrane.

In other words, gas exchange, the object of the process of respiration, depends on adequate flow of blood (perfusion) and adequate flow of air (ventilation) to and from alveoli.

THE PROCESS OF VENTILATION

Ventilation is the exchange of air between the atmosphere and the alveoli. At rest, intrapulmonary pressure and atmospheric pressure are equal—760 mm Hg at sea level (Figure 17–8). During inspiration, the muscles of the diaphragm and the intercostal muscles contract, lowering the diaphragm and raising the rib cage. The volume of the intrathoracic space expands, intrapleural and intrapulmonary pressures decrease, until the intrapulmonary pressure is lower than atmospheric pressure. Air moves along the concentration gradient (from higher concentration to lower) into the upper respiratory tract, through the tracheobronchial tree, and into the alveolar tissue of the lungs. Air moves into the lungs until intrapulmonary pressure and atmospheric pressure are equal.

Neuronal receptors sensitive to stretch respond to the expansion of the thoracic cage, stimulating a rebound action of the muscles and connective-tissue fibers of the lungs.

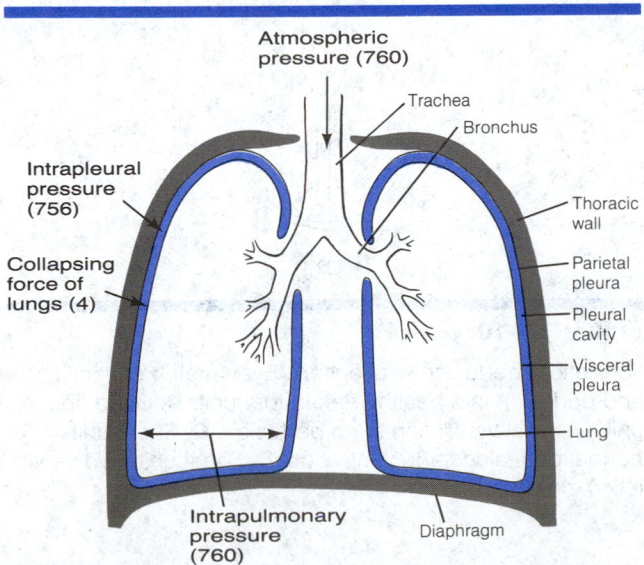

Figure 17–8

Intrapulmonary and intrapleural pressures in resting position (in mm Hg).
SOURCE: Spence AP, Mason EB: *Human Anatomy and Physiology,* 2nd ed. Menlo Park, CA: Benjamin/Cummings, 1983.

The ribs become more vertical and the diaphragm rises, causing intrapulmonary pressure to rise above atmospheric pressure. Air moves passively out of the lungs along the reversed concentration gradient, carrying out carbon dioxide (and other wastes) that have been exchanged for oxygen from the inspired air. This expiration continues until the intrapulmonary pressure is again lower than atmospheric pressure, and the cycle begins again.

During normal inspiration, most of the work is accomplished by the diaphragm, with some participation by the intercostal muscles. Movement of the rib cage may be barely perceptible during quiet respiration, as during sleep. As exertion increases, oxygen demand increases proportionately, and the intercostal muscles are called upon to an increasing extent. During forced or labored respiration, additional chest muscles and even abdominal muscles are employed in moving the thoracic cage.

MECHANISMS OF RESPIRATORY CONTROL

The rate and extent of inspiration and expiration are governed by nervous pathways that respond to various stimuli that signal increased or diminished oxygen requirements or carbon dioxide levels. Requirements are greater during exertion and least during sleep. Like other mechanisms vital to survival—(ie, heart action and digestion)—respiration proceeds without conscious control.

Cerebral control of the respiratory mechanisms is believed to be centered in the pons and the medulla oblongata, both located in the brain stem. The apneustic and pneumotaxic centers of the pons apparently control and modify the activities of the medullary center through stimulation and inhibition, respectively. Figure 17–9 is a schematic representation of the pontine and medullary pathways. The cerebral centers receive impulses from a wide array of nerve endings (dendrites and axons), some sensitive to chemical stimuli and some to mechanical stimuli. For example, as already mentioned, nerve endings sensitive to stretch (mechanical sensors) initiate the impulse sequence that ultimately stimulates expiration. Certain chemicals that build up in muscle tissue during exertion initiate impulse sequences that increase the respiration rate. If circulating carbon dioxide increases, hydrogen ions increase and pH decreases; these chemical changes stimulate neurologic pathways that ultimately effect increases in both rate and depth of ventilation. Fear or anxiety initiate response mechanisms that increase both heart rate and respirations to prepare the body for "fight or flight." Chemoreceptors in the aortic arch and the bifurcation of the internal and external carotid arteries detect changes in oxygen content of the blood and send impulses via neuronal networks to the respiratory centers to increase the ventilation rate as required. These are merely some examples of the extremely complex mechanism governing respiration.

Clearly, then, there are many prerequisites for normal

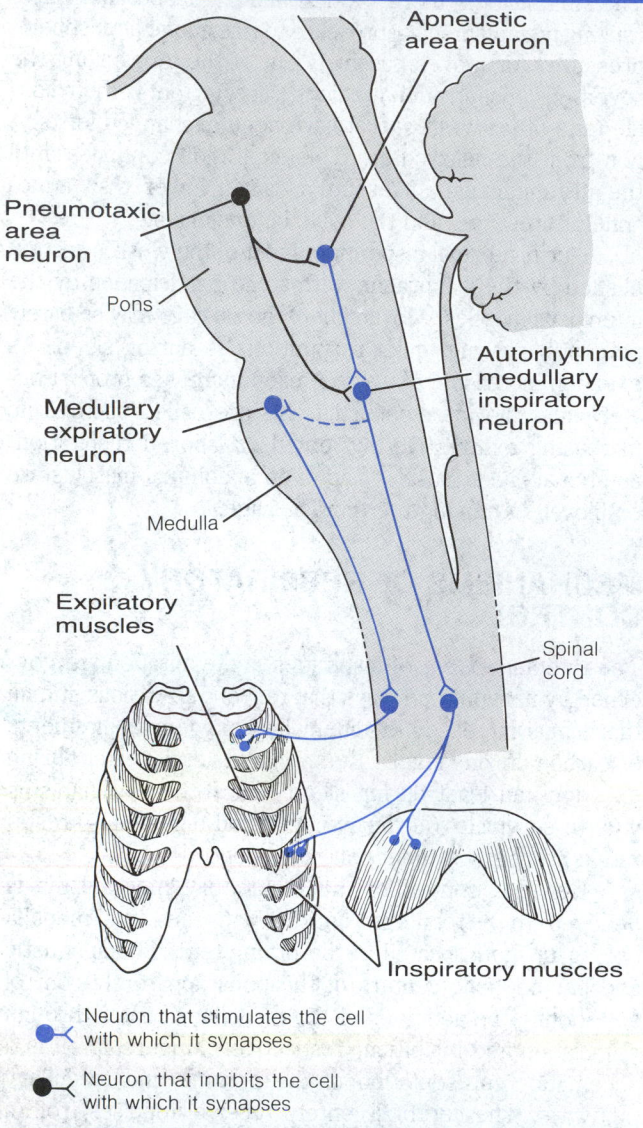

Figure 17–9

Diagrammatic representation of pontine and medullary pathways involved in control of respiration.
SOURCE: Spence AP, Mason EB: *Human Anatomy and Physiology*, 2nd ed. Menlo Park, CA: Benjamin/Cummings, 1983.

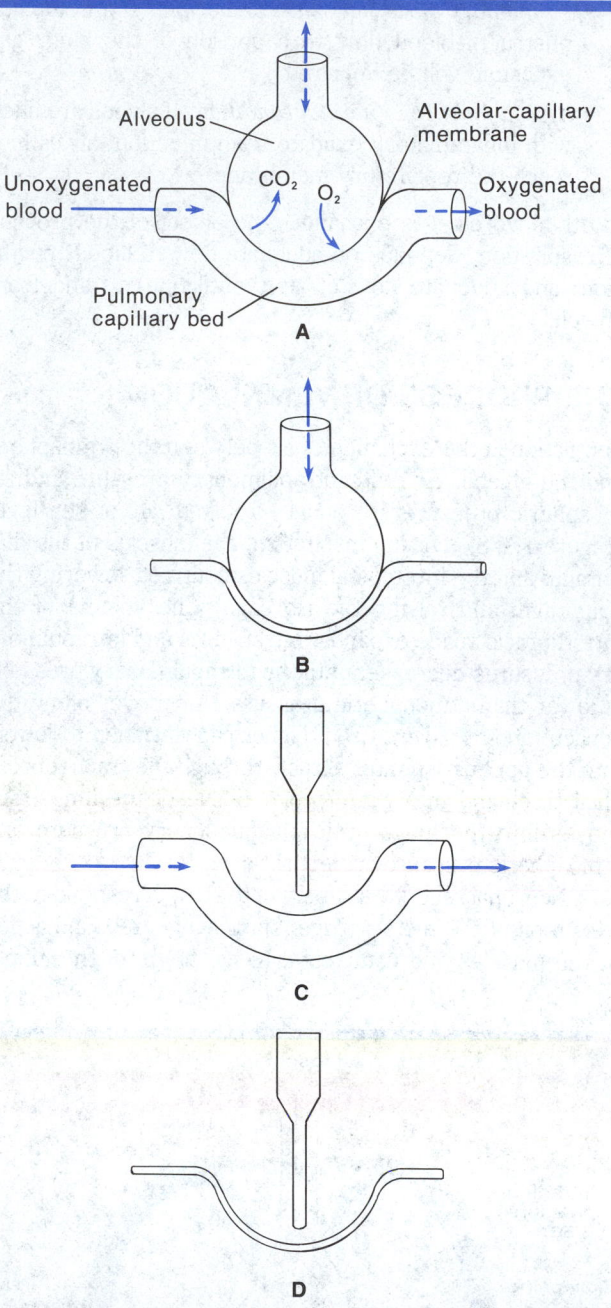

Figure 17–10

Ventilation–perfusion relations: **A.** Even match of ventilation and perfusion in a healthy respiratory unit. **B.** Dead space unit—normal ventilation to no perfusion. **C.** Shunt unit—normal perfusion to no ventilation. **D.** Silent unit—no ventilation, no perfusion.

respiration. The muscles of respiration must be capable of normal movement, the neurological pathways and centers affecting respiration must be intact and functional, and the chest wall must be mobile. Any number of alterations in the internal or external environment may adversely affect respiratory function.

Section II: Pathophysiological Influences and Effects

The basic abnormalities of oxygen–carbon dioxide exchange are hypoventilation, diffusion impairment, and ventilation–perfusion inequality, including shunt.

HYPOVENTILATION

Ventilation below the level needed to maintain normal arterial carbon dioxide tension (PCO_2) is called hypoventilation. If a client is hypoventilating, arterial blood levels of carbon dioxide (CO_2) will be above normal (**hypercapnia,** sometimes called *hypercarbia*), because alveolar ventilation is not keeping pace with body metabolism. As arterial CO_2 rises, arterial oxygen (PO_2) falls; this condition is called **hypoxemia.** Although hypercapnia can be caused only by hypoventilation, hypoxemia may be caused by several other conditions as well (Broughton, 1982).

Hypoventilation is related to many conditions; airway obstruction is one of the most common. The upper airway, especially the pharynx and larynx, may be obstructed by inflamed, edematous mucosal linings or by hypertrophic tonsils or adenoids. Polyps, tumors, or foreign bodies may partially block the airway. Impairment of the lower respiratory tract or the alveoli can have even more serious effects. Retained secretions, mucosal edema, and bronchospasm can narrow or even collapse some or all of the airways. Obstructive diseases such as emphysema cause hypoventilation because they impair air flow.

Functional alterations in the central nervous system, as well as neuromuscular or skeletal abnormalities, can also play a part in hypoventilation. Hypoventilation often occurs as a consequence of immobility or inappropriate positioning for extended periods. These effects are discussed in the section on related-system alterations.

DIFFUSION IMPAIRMENT

Remember that oxygen and carbon dioxide molecules are transported between the alveolar air spaces and the capillary beds of the alveolar septum by diffusion. The effectiveness of the diffusion process is influenced by the condition of the alveolar and capillary epithelia, the interstitial fluid, and the erythrocytic membrane, as well as by the secretion of pulmonary surfactant. There is a wide margin of safety, however. Since blood in the alveolar capillaries normally can reach the gas tension levels prevalent in the alveolar space in approximately one-third of the time it remains there, diffusion can be reduced for some time before abnormalities become apparent.

Significant diffusion abnormalities can interfere with the passage of inspired oxygen from the alveoli into the blood. Because carbon dioxide diffuses readily, the partial pressure of carbon dioxide is generally unaffected by diffusion impairment. Hypoxemia may lead to hyperventilation, however, and this, rather than diffusion impairment itself, may lower PCO_2.

Any condition that thickens the alveolar septum—(eg, interstitial fibrosis)—can impair diffusion. Metastatic carcinoma may invade the interstitial spaces. Pulmonary edema also hampers oxygen diffusion because of the increased amount of fluid in the alveoli and the interstitial spaces. If the amount of functioning lung tissue is reduced because of emphysema, pneumonectomy, or tumor growth, diffusion will also be impaired.

In the early stages of diffusion impairment, hypoxemia may occur only during exertion. As the condition pro-

gresses, hypoxemia and related symptoms (dyspnea, restlessness, tachycardia) may occur even when the client is resting.

VENTILATION–PERFUSION ABNORMALITIES

Efficient exchange of carbon dioxide for oxygen requires equality of alveolar ventilation (V) and perfusion (Q). That is, ventilation–perfusion inequality (or V/Q mismatching) is defined as an imbalance of pulmonary ventilation and perfusion. (Figure 17–10A depicts a normal V/Q.) Slight imbalances occur in healthy individuals, but excessive ventilation–perfusion imbalances are the most common cause of hypoxemia. Such abnormalities may be classified as:

- Normal ventilation to no perfusion (Figure 17–10B)
- No ventilation and normal perfusion (Figure 17–10C)
- No ventilation and no perfusion (Figure 17–10D)

Normal Ventilation to No Perfusion (Dead Space Unit)

Without perfusion, gas exchange cannot take place. This condition is called *wasted ventilation,* since ventilation of the alveoli brings about no exchange of carbon dioxide for oxygen. Conditions related to wasted ventilation include a decrease in total blood volume (eg, in hemorrhage or dehydration), pulmonary embolism, and chronic obstructive pulmonary disease (COPD) such as emphysema. Emphysema may also destroy both alveoli and capillaries within portions of the lungs, so neither ventilation nor perfusion can take place. If large areas of the lungs are affected by wasted ventilation, hypoxemia and hypercapnia with related respiratory acidosis can occur.

No Ventilation to Normal Perfusion (Shunt Unit)

In shunting, the alveolus is perfused but not ventilated (wasted perfusion). Any pathological condition that obstructs the alveoli can lead to a low ventilation-to-perfusion ratio. For example, a client who is in pain from upper abdominal surgery may take shallow breaths, resulting in atelectasis. Then unoxygenated blood from the collapsed area mixes with oxygenated blood from the unaffected areas, lowering the level of oxygen in the arterial blood. This venous admixture represents the shunting phenomenon. In addition, insufficient carbon dioxide is eliminated. Arterial hypoxemia occurs, but hypercapnia may not occur unless the lungs are severely compromised, because of the compensating effect of hyperventilation.

No Ventilation to No Perfusion (Silent Unit)

Conditions leading to diminished or absent ventilation of some alveolar units include pneumonia, atelectasis, pulmonary edema, and COPD. Conditions leading to diminished or absent perfusion of some alveolar units include compression of intrathoracic blood vessels by a neoplasm; occlusion of blood vessels by emboli or thrombi; and collapse of blood vessels because of decreased perfusion pressure, shock, or hypotension. The severity of client symptoms depends on the extent of alveolar units involved.

Section III: Related System Influences and Effects

In addition to abnormalities of the lungs and upper respiratory structures, pathophysiological processes involving other body systems can adversely affect respiratory function. Conversely, since oxygen is a primary need of every body cell, dysfunction of the respiratory system can have extensive repercussions in any body system.

Two body systems closely related to respiratory function are the neurologic and cardiovascular systems. Influences and effects ultimately felt in other systems—eg, musculoskeletal, gastrointestinal, or urinary—are often secondary to neurologic or cardiovascular disturbances.

NEUROLOGIC SYSTEM

Neurologic regulation of normal ventilation was depicted in Figure 17–9 and discussed in the accompanying text. From these descriptions, it is evident that drugs or disease processes affecting the nervous system will inevitably affect respiration to some extent. Anesthetic agents are a major example of drugs having respiratory side effects. Infections, tumors, diseases of the peripheral nervous system (ie, Guillain-Barré syndrome), neuromuscular diseases (ie, myasthenia gravis) and others, will affect respiration in various ways. The respiratory system may respond to these influences by hyperventilation, hypoventilation, a combination of the two (eg, Cheyne–Stokes respiration), or apnea. If the brain or spinal cord is damaged (eg, by trauma or subarachnoid hemorrhage) respiratory function may be greatly impaired or even totally destroyed, depending on the location and severity of the damage. So closely are the neurologic and respiratory systems interrelated that abnormalities in either can have major consequences for both.

CARDIOVASCULAR SYSTEM

The heart must not only move blood to the pulmonary arteries for exchange of oxygen and carbon dioxide but must supply oxygenated blood to the lung tissue itself. Consequently, functional alterations in the cardiovascular system affect respiratory function as well.

If severe hemorrhage depletes the volume of circulating blood, the supply of oxygen and nutrients for the airways and terminal respiratory units will also be diminished. The oxygen and nutrient deficit will be greater in pulmonary tissue because even under normal conditions, pressure in the pulmonary circulation is lower than pressure in the systemic circulation. Because the lungs are adjacent to the heart, little pressure is normally required for pumping blood to them (Harper, 1981).

Failure of the right side of the heart related to certain disease states may affect the volume of pulmonary blood circulation. Conversely, certain disorders of the respiratory system are closely related to right-sided heart failure. Left-sided heart failure also affects pulmonary function because of backup of blood in the pulmonary vasculature and related pulmonary edema (Harper, 1981). If the volume of blood circulating either to or from the lungs is compromised for any reason, oxygen, carbon dioxide, and acid–base abnormalities may occur.

Oxygen obtained during gas exchange in the pulmonary circulation must combine with hemoglobin to be transported to the tissues. Normally, the circulation contains approximately 15 g of hemoglobin to carry about 20 mL of oxygen at any given time. If the hemoglobin concentration is below normal (eg, from anemia) the capacity of the blood to transport oxygen will be reduced.

OTHER RELATED SYSTEMS

Diseases and deformities of the skeletal system can also alter respiratory functioning, generally by restricting movement of the thoracic cage (eg, scoliosis). Problems in the gastrointestinal tract such as hiatal hernia can interfere with lung expansion. Extreme obesity can restrict movement of the thoracic cage and places an abnormal load on the respiratory system by increasing the exertion required for ordinary activities.

Surgery of the gastrointestinal tract, especially procedures such as cholecystectomy that have a high abdominal incision, can be associated with pulmonary complications in the postoperative period. Pain in the surgical site inhibits adequate deep breathing and coughing, resulting in inadequate expansion of the lungs. Atelectasis or pneumonia can be the consequence.

Section IV: Psychosocial/Lifestyle Influences and Effects

Long-term impairment of respiratory function has serious effects on both clients and their families. An acute respiratory infection or chest injury can severely incapacitate an individual. But once the infection is controlled and the injury healed, the client can usually resume daily activities. Cancer of the respiratory system, on the other hand, is a progressive disease with a poor prognosis. Chronic disabling respiratory disorders of long duration, such as COPD, also have far-reaching psychosocial effects. These long-term disabilities, many of which are diseases of middle and old age, have assumed importance in recent years, as advances in epidemiology and medicine have reduced the significance of acute infectious diseases that once took a high toll of lives. Similarly, attention to environmental hazards is focusing on such matters as chemical pollution of water and air, which is often related to long-term pathologic change.

DEVELOPMENTAL INFLUENCES

Aging, although not a disease, usually diminishes respiratory capacity as it does cardiovascular function. Cerebral neurons have one of the highest metabolic rates of all body cells, and brain cells are thus the first to be affected by any reduction in respiratory efficiency. Moreover, since neurons (alone among body cells) do not reproduce once mature, destruction of neurons permanently affects cerebral function. The vagueness and forgetfulness often seen in older people can be related to oxygen deficit. These symptoms interfere with personal autonomy and are upsetting to client and family.

Regardless of age, clients react differently when breathing problems develop. A client with supportive friends and family—a support network—will find it easier to cope

Nursing Research Note

Sexton D, Munro B: Impact of a husband's chronic illness (COPD) on the spouse's life. *Res Nurs Health* 1985; 8:83–90.

When a husband has chronic obstructive pulmonary disease (COPD), the wife assumes new roles and responsibilities and faces new stresses. This research examined the effect of COPD on the life of wives.

The wives of COPD husbands reported new roles and responsibilities, poorer sleeping patterns, less frequent sexual relations, greater financial strain and reported their health status as low. The COPD wives also reported paying greater attention to their husband's health and environment than in the past and giving up social activities because of their husband. The COPD wives said their biggest problems were the husband's condition and symptoms, his attitude and irritability, and the loss of their personal freedom. These women said they live with considerable fear and worry about their husbands and the situation.

Nurses must attend to the care of both husband and wife. Nurses can provide guidance for these women. Support networks and respite care can allow the woman time for herself. Counseling and group meetings can offer the opportunity to talk and share feelings. These women need to have regular physical examinations and follow the advice of their care provider. The woman must be helped to learn to manage her daily activities in less stressful ways to attain some life satisfaction.

with disability than a client who is socially isolated. Like many vital body functions, breathing is generally taken for granted. "As natural as breathing" is a common simile for an act that takes virtually no thought or effort. When such an ordinary process becomes a matter of extraordinary concern, many areas of life are inevitably affected.

CULTURAL INFLUENCES

For many people, breathing is intimately related to deep fears about death, and even a slight interference with breathing can mobilize the primitive fear of suffocation. For example, nurses may find that clients have torn off oxygen lines while semiconscious because of a sensation of being smothered.

Masculinity in many cultures is equated with physical performance. When respiratory insufficiency impedes physical activity, self-esteem suffers. American society is work oriented, and inability to do work can have profound effects on self-esteem. Cultural expectations of self-reliance and independence can make the mere admission of illness a threat to the client's sense of self-worth.

In North American culture, the chest is a focal point of sexual identity. The "manly chest" and female breasts are symbols of masculinity and femininity. Disorders that affect the chest area thus threaten not only life but the individual's sexuality.

LIFESTYLE FACTORS

Studies have shown that positive lifestyle changes have more potential for improving health than any treatment of an illness once developed. By encouraging lifestyle modification and by setting an example, nurses offer their clients an opportunity for better long-term health. This is especially true in preventing or alleviating respiratory disorders, since smoking has clearly been implicated in cancer of the lung and a multitude of other disorders.

Smoking

More than 340,000 Americans die prematurely each year from disorders related to smoking; millions of others lead restricted lives because of pulmonary damage and cardiovascular impairment. The chemical agents in tobacco smoke reduce and eventually destroy ciliary movement in the bronchial mucosa, making the lungs more susceptible to infection. The hot smoke dries out and inflames the delicate tissues of the mouth, larynx, trachea, and lungs. Carbon monoxide in cigarette smoke combines with hemoglobin more readily than does oxygen; this competition reduces the amount of oxygen available to body tissues. Nicotine is a vasoconstrictor, and vasoconstriction also reduces oxygen supply. Sensors in the blood and the tissues thus signal the heart to beat faster to make up the deficit. Tars in cigarette smoke have produced cancerous lesions in the lungs of test animals.

Unfortunately, cigarette smoking starts as early as grade school. Nearly a million teenagers start smoking each year, and the proportion of teenage girls who smoke is higher than the proportion of boys. Smoking by teenagers is often related to peer pressure, but most teenagers who smoke also have parents who do.

Smoking not only endangers the health of the smoker but pollutes the air breathed by nonsmokers. Public awareness of the hazards of smoking has led to requests for "no smoking" areas in restaurants and other public places. Nurses, as health professionals, are well qualified to help publicize the need for such facilities.

Nutrition and Exercise

Nutritional intake has little direct bearing on respiratory disorders, but overall health related to nutrition does affect susceptibility to infection. Individuals who are poorly nourished have a higher incidence of respiratory infections; moreover, they have less capacity to withstand disease or trauma. Nutritional status affects healing in the respiratory system as elsewhere in the body.

Some allergens in food may affect respiratory function, and some clients may have to curtail their intake of dairy products because these foods apparently overstimulate mucus production.

Overweight individuals may suffer from dyspnea because the excess tissue increases oxygen requirements. Movement of the chest wall and diaphragm may be restricted, particularly in clients who are extremely obese.

Clients with dyspnea may become anorectic. The mere act of eating may require more energy than they can summon, and the presence of large quantities of food in the stomach impedes the descent of the diaphragm during inspiration. Foods that stimulate flatus formation—beans, cabbage, cucumbers—may have to be curtailed to avoid excess pressure on the diaphragm. Clients may have to eat smaller meals at more frequent intervals.

Various studies have demonstrated that moderate exercise such as walking, if done regularly, can have beneficial effects on cardiovascular and respiratory capacity, another example of the value of incorporating healthy habits into one's lifestyle.

ENVIRONMENTAL FACTORS

Airborne allergens can cause or aggravate respiratory disease. The most common respiratory disease associated with allergens is extrinsic asthma, which usually affects children but is sometimes seen in adults. Such well-known and widespread environmental allergens as ragweed pollen and animal dander are related to allergic rhinitis and the uncomfortable symptoms associated with "hay fever."

Pollution of air by industrial and agricultural chemicals can increase the severity of numerous respiratory conditions, including long-term obstructive disorders. Individuals who have such conditions as chronic bronchitis may have to change their residence or stay indoors when pollution levels are high. Although increasing public awareness of pollution hazards has stimulated efforts by government and industry to reduce the quantity of pollutants released into the air, new technology is needed and much remains to be done. Nurses experienced in caring for victims of respiratory illness can alert their clients and the general public to the ill effects of air pollution.

ECONOMIC AND OCCUPATIONAL FACTORS

Crowded living conditions often associated with low income, particularly in urban areas, increase the risk of respiratory disorders. The classic example is tuberculosis. Inadequate knowledge about risk factors and healthful lifestyles increases the likelihood of illness and decreases the likelihood that professional health care will be sought promptly.

Once long-term respiratory disease occurs, treatment can be costly, yet the earning capacity of the client is usually curtailed by disease symptoms such as dyspnea and pain. Frequent hospitalization may be necessary, disrupting employment still further, and home care equipment such as oxygen units or mechanical ventilators may have to be rented or purchased.

Occupation is a significant factor in the development of some respiratory disorders. "Black lung disease," which affects coal miners, is a well-publicized example; asbestosis is another. Solvents in paints and varnishes have also been implicated in respiratory disorders, not only among factory workers and professional painters but among hobbyists. A timely question about recent craft or hobby projects can yield a valuable diagnostic clue about a respiratory ailment. Clerks in dry cleaning establishments and beauticians exposed to permanent wave solutions (ammonia) and hair dyes may also develop respiratory abnormalities.

Existing respiratory problems can be made worse by exposure to chemical pollutants at work. The trend toward tightly insulated buildings brought about by the energy crisis has raised concerns about chemical pollution—eg, photocopying materials—in office environments that formerly were relatively hazard free. By being alert to occupational information in the client's history, the nurse can help identify individuals at risk and can counsel clients with respiratory disorders about possible hazards in their working environments.

Long-term respiratory illness will affect the client's capacity to work, often progressively. The client may have to find part-time work or a new occupation, depending on the kind of work the client does. A bank teller may be able to continue working almost indefinitely; a pneumatic drill operator will not. Loss of occupation will affect not only the client's income but the client's psychological well-being as well. Thus, occupation, income, and respiratory status are interrelated, and any plan of care for the client must consider them all.

SOCIAL FACTORS

A disease that affects so fundamental an activity as breathing necessarily influences all aspects of the client's life, from intimate relationships to casual social contacts. Fear, anxiety, and anger related to symptoms and restrictions of activity place added burdens on an already compromised respiratory system and on personal relationships. Tensions rise, and depression is common.

As work activities are restricted, people see their position and value in their family and community as being threatened or destroyed. Another family member may have to step in as breadwinner; household chores and gardening must be taken over by others; the client feels displaced and disoriented. When sports or hobbies are abandoned because they require more energy than the damaged respiratory system can supply, the social relationships accompanying these activities are also lost.

Clients with breathing difficulties may avoid sexual contact or their mates may avoid them, fearing to worsen the illness. The depression that so often accompanies long-term illness diminishes sex drive, and some medications can cause or contribute to loss of libido and impotence. Lowered self-esteem, low energy, reduced strength, and easy fatigability also contribute to sexual difficulties. Clients who are unable to bring themselves to discuss these problems with their mates often find the nurse a nonthreatening confidante. Consultation with the psychiatric nurse on the health care team may provide the client sympathetic and helpful advice.

Chapter Highlights

Transport of oxygen from the atmosphere to the cells and transport of carbon dioxide from the cells back to the atmosphere is called respiration.

The upper respiratory tract warms, filters, and humidifies inspired air. It consists of the nose, paranasal sinuses, pharynx, and larynx.

The trachea, bronchi, and bronchioles of the lower respiratory tract conduct air to and from the functional lobules of the lungs, where gas exchange takes place. The lobules are composed of respiratory bronchioles, alveolar ducts, and grapelike clusters of alveoli.

The defense mechanisms of the respiratory system include filtration, ciliary movement, mucus secretion, phagocytic action, and the cough reflex.

Respiration is regulated by apneustic and pneumotaxic centers in the brain stem in response to chemical and mechanical stimulation of sensors in the bloodstream, tissues, and organs.

The lungs are kept inflated by subatmospheric pressure in the intrapleural space. Loss of normal intrapleural pressure from leakage of air into the intrapleural space can cause the lung on the affected side to collapse.

Excess levels of carbon dioxide in the blood (hypercapnia) stimulate the respiratory centers to increase rate and depth of ventilation.

Insufficient levels of oxygen in the blood (hypoxemia) stimulate chemoreceptors in the aortic arch and carotid arteries, sending impulses to the respiratory centers to increase ventilation.

The basic abnormalities of oxygen/carbon dioxide exchange are hypoventilation, diffusion impairment, and ventilation–perfusion inequality.

Abnormalities in other systems, especially the nervous and cardiovascular systems, can adversely affect the respiratory system.

Respiratory abnormalities affect all other body systems to some degree.

Neuronal cells are especially sensitive to oxygen deprivation because of their high metabolic rate.

Oxygen is transported to the tissues by hemoglobin; therefore, a decrease in hemoglobin levels will diminish the amount of available oxygen.

Cultural factors such as the importance assigned to the chest and breasts as symbols of sexuality affect the client's response to respiratory impairment.

Cigarette smoking is a major cause of emphysema, chronic bronchitis, and lung cancer and impairs the respiratory system's defenses against disease.

Air pollution by industrial and agricultural contaminants is related to a number of respiratory disorders.

Impairment of respiratory status has profound and far-reaching effects on the individual's psychosocial status, including occupation, social and family relationships, emotional state, and self-image.

Bibliography

American Lung Association: *Cigarette Smoking—The Facts About Your Lungs*. New York: American Lung Assn, 1982.

Anderson M: *Occupational Lung Diseases: An Introduction*. New York: American Lung Assn, 1983.

Broughton JO: Pathophysiology of the respiratory system. In: *Critical Care Nursing*. Hudak C, Lohr T, Gallo B (editors). Philadelphia: Lippincott, 1982.

Crofton J, Douglas A: *Respiratory Diseases*. Boston: Blackwell, 1981.

Crowley LV: *Introduction to Human Disease*. Belmont, CA: Wadsworth, 1983.

D'Alonzo GE, Dantzker DR: Respiratory failure: Mechanisms of abnormal gas exchange and oxygen delivery. *Med Clin North Am* 1983; 67:557–571.

George RB, Light RW, Matthay RA: *Chest Medicine*. New York: Churchill Livingstone, 1983.

Harper R: *A Guide to Respiratory Care Physiology and Clinical Applications*. Philadelphia: Lippincott, 1981.

Hinshaw HC, Murray JF: *Diseases of the Chest*. Philadelphia: Saunders, 1980.

Kent DC, Smith JK: Psychological implications of pulmonary disease. *Clin Notes Resp Disease* 1977; Winter 3–11.

Petty TL: *Intensive and Rehabilitative Respiratory Care*. Philadelphia: Lea & Febiger, 1982.

Ross JS, Wilson KJW: *Foundations of Anatomy and Physiology*. New York: Churchill Livingstone, 1981.

Spence AP, Mason ER: *Human Anatomy and Physiology*, 2nd ed. Menlo Park, CA: Addison-Wesley, 1983.

Subcommittee of the Research Committee of the British Thoracic Society: Smoking withdrawal in hospital patients: factors associated with outcome. *Thorax* Sept 1984; 39(9):651–656.

Traver GA: *Respiratory Nursing: The Science and the Art*. New York: Wiley, 1982.

Suggested Readings

Callahan M: COPD makes a bad first impression, but you'll find wonderful people underneath. *Nurs 82* (May) 1982; 12:68–72. This article discusses how breathing difficulties affect emotional status. The role of the nurse in working with clients with COPD is explored.

Dudley DL et al: Psychosocial concomitants to rehabilitation in chronic obstructive pulmonary disease. *Chest* 1980; 77:413–420. Coping patterns of COPD clients and integration of psychosocial, psychological, and medical approaches are emphasized.

Chapter 18

The Nursing Process for Clients With Respiratory Dysfunction

Yvonne Krall Scherer
Vicky Hartwell-Ivins

Objectives

When you have finished studying this chapter you should be able to:

Identify subjective and objective data related to the nursing diagnoses of ineffective airway clearance, ineffective breathing patterns, and impaired gas exchange.

Describe the diagnostic studies used to assess the upper and lower respiratory tract.

Discuss the normal and abnormal findings of these diagnostic studies.

Explain the nursing implications in caring for clients undergoing diagnostic studies of the respiratory system.

Describe the different types of artificial airways and the nursing implications involved in the care of a client with an artificial airway.

Demonstrate correct technique when performing nasotracheal suctioning or suctioning via an artificial airway.

Demonstrate correct technique when performing tracheostomy care for a client who has undergone a tracheotomy or laryngectomy.

Describe the different types of mechanical ventilators.

Discuss nursing care of clients who are being mechanically ventilated.

Enumerate the nursing considerations for a client who is being weaned from mechanical ventilation.

Define the different types of closed chest drainage systems.

Explain the nursing management of the client with a chest tube.

Instruct the client, family members, or significant others in the skills necessary for the proper management of the respiratory problem.

Recognize the impact of the physiological alterations caused by respiratory dysfunction and their impact on client lifestyle.

Anticipate the psychosocial implications of respiratory dysfunction for client and family.

Specify effective coping mechanisms clients can use in dealing with the psychosocial stresses caused by respiratory disorders.

Disorders of the respiratory system produce symptoms that range in severity from an inconvenience (such as a decrease in the ability to detect odors) to life-threatening (such as inability to breathe).

Alterations in the function of the respiratory system not only have localized effects but can alter the client's systemic physiological function. For example, certain disorders may prevent the client from maintaining a clear airway or alter the mechanics of breathing. This can slowly or rapidly lead to impairment of carbon dioxide and oxygen exchange in the lungs. Nursing diagnoses used frequently when caring for clients with respiratory disorders include: airway clearance, ineffective; breathing pattern, ineffective; and gas exchange, impaired.

Clients who experience dysfunction of the respiratory system often undergo a change in body image and consequently the way in which they interact socially. The laryngectomee is confronted with a permanently altered route for breathing and permanent loss of voice. The client with chronic obstructive pulmonary disease (COPD) must cope with a limited energy reserve and dependence on medication, oxygen, and other therapy.

The nutritional status of clients may be affected by certain alterations of the respiratory system. Changes in sensations of smell and taste can make food seem less appetizing. Structural alterations from tumor or trauma can make swallowing difficult or block the oropharynx. Infectious and neoplastic disorders of the respiratory system can place increased stress on the client, increasing caloric requirements.

Nursing interventions, whether in teaching the client, using technical skills, or providing emotional support, can be essential to clients with disorders of the upper and lower respiratory system. Many clients can deal effectively with minor disorders at home when given adequate instruction. The important technical nursing skills include suctioning and cleaning of artificial airways. Emotional support for clients and family members includes clear explanations and instructions, credible reassurance, and reinforcement of information. Clients, family members, and significant others may be extremely frightened and anxious. Some disorders that interfere with breathing, speaking, and eating may seem worse than they are; others may be more severe than they seem. Clients who are terminally ill often need support and assistance through the process of dying.

Section I: Nursing Assessment: Establishing the Data Base

SUBJECTIVE DATA

Clients with disorders of the upper and lower airway may describe a variety of symptoms. These symptoms vary primarily with the location and severity of the disorder.

Airway Problems

When the nasal airway is involved, clients often report a "stuffy nose" or decreased ability to breathe through the nose and sometimes a voice with a nasal quality. Other concerns may be a "runny nose" and a headache or feeling of fullness over the paranasal sinuses. People often say they have a "sinus headache." If nasal discharge is present, the client may report soreness around the nostrils. In some instances, clients may state they have nasal stuffiness but cannot remove secretions when blowing their noses. Reports of postnasal drip are not uncommon. These symptoms may be produced by an infection such as sinusitis or rhinitis. A decrease in the size of the nasal airway may be related to disorders such as nasal polyps, a deviated nasal septum, or a tumor.

The client should be questioned about the use of nose drops and nose sprays and the frequency and amount of use. Also note if the client has obtained relief from this medication. Remember that overuse of intranasal medication can result in rhinitis medicamentosa.

Rhinitis medicamentosa results from frequent and prolonged use of local vasoconstrictor nose drops and sprays. Application of these nasal preparations results in an immediate vasoconstriction of the mucosal arterioles, which leads to temporary improvement in the airway. This is followed by vasodilation and nasal obstruction.

A common symptom in clients with respiratory disorders is difficult breathing (**dyspnea**). Dyspnea is more often caused by disorders of the lower respiratory tract, such as COPD and carcinoma of the lung. Disorders of the upper airway that may cause dyspnea include obstruction of the airway by inflammation or obstruction by a foreign body or tumor. Clients should be asked whether they are short of breath during rest or exertion and, if so, what factors aggravate and alleviate the symptom.

Another common symptom of respiratory disorders is a cough. A cough can result from irritation or from retained secretions that obstruct some part of the airway. Causative disorders in the upper airway may include sinusitis (leading to postnasal drip) and infections of the pharynx. Causative disorders in the lower respiratory tract include bronchitis, bronchiectasis, and pneumonia. The client should be asked whether the cough is productive or nonproductive. If the cough is productive, ask about the color, amount, odor, and consistency of the sputum. Ask about precipitating factors and the frequency of the cough.

Bronchospasm, retained secretions, edema, and obstruction by foreign objects can result in complaints of wheezing. This may be the chief concern of clients with asthma or allergic rhinitis. The client should be questioned about the frequency of wheezing and precipitating factors.

Chest Pain

Clients with respiratory dysfunction often describe sensations of pain and tenderness. Discomfort of the upper airway can be from an infection such as rhinitis, sinusitis, or pharyngitis. Trauma to the head and neck area can also cause pain in the upper respiratory tract.

Although chest pain is not uncommon for clients with respiratory system dysfunction, chest pain can also result from cardiovascular, gastrointestinal, hepatic–biliary, genitourinary, and musculoskeletal disorders. Difficulty with managing life stresses can also contribute to chest pain.

Use the seven dimensions or PQRST discussed in Chapter 7 as a guide to gathering a complete history of the pain. A careful history and physical examination are necessary to determine the origin of the pain so proper intervention can be carried out. Some disorders that cause chest pain, such as myocardial infarction or a punctured lung, can be fatal if not treated appropriately.

Voice Change and Dysphagia

Having determined that chest pain does not stem from a disorder demanding immediate intervention, ask whether the client has experienced any voice change. Infections of the pharynx, vocal nodules, laryngeal paralysis, and laryngeal tumors can cause a voice change. Laryngeal paralysis results from damage to the recurrent or superior laryngeal nerve or the vagus nerve. For example, pressure on the recurrent laryngeal nerve from bronchogenic carcinoma or an aortic aneurysm can lead to paralysis of the vocal cord. Ask the client how long ago the voice change occurred and whether it is associated with pain when speaking or swallowing.

Dysphagia, a decrease in the client's ability to swallow, drink, and eat may result from disorders such as pharyngitis, infectious mononucleosis, peritonsillar abscess, and tumors of the oropharynx and laryngopharynx. Ask clients how long they have experienced the difficulty, if they experience pain when attempting to swallow, and if a sensation of choking or gagging occurs. Whether any difficulty has significantly affected nutritional intake should also be assessed. Ask what and how much the client has been able to eat and drink since the problem was noticed.

Fatigue and Weight Change

Clients may also complain of generalized feelings of malaise and fatigue. This may result from respiratory infections or other conditions that alter the normal levels of oxygen and carbon dioxide in the body. Neoplastic disorders also cause fatigue because of increased metabolic demands.

Determine whether the client has had a weight change. A weight loss may be deliberate or may result from a neoplastic process or COPD. A weight gain may indicate fluid retention secondary to pulmonary edema or congestive heart failure. Ask how much weight was lost or gained, over how long, and whether the client's appetite increased or decreased during the change.

Many disorders of the respiratory tract may lead to an alteration in carbon dioxide and oxygen levels in the blood. This imbalance may manifest itself as respiratory acidosis or respiratory alkalosis. Respiratory acidosis and alkalosis are discussed in Section II of this chapter and also in Chapter 5. Clients in an acidotic state may complain of headache, double vision, weakness, drowsiness, and difficulty in breathing. These symptoms may result from hypoxia and/or hypercapnia. Clients who are in an alkalotic state may report they are dizzy and have a tingling sensation in the fingers and toes. These subjective complaints are the result of hypocapnia (Harper, 1981).

Habit History

Obtain a detailed smoking history from the client. Cigars, pipes, and chewing tobacco should be included along with cigarettes. Smoking has been implicated as a risk factor in the development of lung cancer, cancer of the head and neck, and COPD. Smoking also aggravates upper respiratory symptoms such as rhinorrhea, sinusitis, and pharyngitis because of damage to the cilia and mucous membranes. The longer the person has smoked and the greater the number of cigarettes, the greater the risk of developing respiratory disorders. Clients who smoke should be asked how many cigarettes they smoke each day? What brand? Filtered or nonfiltered? How many years have they smoked? Do they inhale? Clients who have stopped smoking should be asked the date they quit smoking in addition to the previous questions. The client's smoking history is recorded in pack years (number of packs per day $\times$ the number of years they have smoked). For example, the client who has smoked 2 packs per day for 10 years, has a 20 pack-year smoking history.

Clients should also be asked if they use chewing tobacco, since this has been implicated as a factor in the development of cancers of the mouth, larynx, throat, and esophagus (American Cancer Society, 1985). The nurse should determine how long the client has chewed tobacco and how frequently it is used.

An excessive use of alcohol has been implicated as a predisposing factor in the development of tuberculosis, pneumonia, and cancers of the mouth, larynx, throat, esophagus, and liver (American Cancer Society, 1985). Clients should be questioned specifically about what they drink, how much per day, and how long they have been drinking. Clients may tend to minimize their drinking. Therefore, a careful, sensitive, nonjudgmental approach is needed when asking questions related to alcohol intake.

Past Health History

Obtain a thorough history of past respiratory, face, neck, and thoracic problems. Has the client ever had maxillofacial trauma or rib fractures? Is there any history of scoliosis or thoracic deformity? Has the client ever had a positive tuberculosis skin test or abnormal chest x-ray? Has the client ever had respiratory complications following general anesthesia or surgery? A history of any of these could contribute to the current health problem of the client.

Allergy and Medication History

Find out whether the client has any history of allergies. Allergies can cause sinusitis, allergic rhinitis, and asthma. If the client has a history of allergies, ask how long the allergic symptoms have been present, what the symptoms are (severe difficulty breathing? a runny nose? watery eyes?), has allergy testing has been done, have specific allergens been identified, whether the client is receiving allergy shots, and what specific medications relieve the symptoms.

Ask clients about all medications they are taking and why. Also ask if clients are using medications as prescribed and if they seem to provide the desired effects.

Occupational and Travel History

Exposure to certain chemical agents and other irritants can result in respiratory disorders. Therefore, a thorough occupational history is obtained. Two common occupational diseases are asbestosis and silicosis. Clients should be asked if they work or have ever worked in a job that exposed them to chemical fumes, dust, smoke, or asbestos.

Does the client work in an environment with people who smoke? Do the windows open to allow fresh air to enter or is the air recirculated?

The client's recent travel history is important because some infectious disorders affecting the lungs are endemic to certain geographical regions.

Family History

Information should be gathered on respiratory problems in blood relatives. Any family history of allergies, asthma, chronic bronchitis, emphysema, tuberculosis, or malignancy should be documented. Did the client grow up in a family of smokers? Does the client live with a smoker? Does anyone in the home or in the family have symptoms like the client's?

OBJECTIVE DATA

Physical Assesssment

When performing a physical assessment of clients suspected of having a respiratory disorder, the nurse uses the skills of inspection, palpation, percussion, and auscultation.

Inspection

Inspection of the nose may reveal polyps, tumors, enlarged turbinates, a foreign body, secretions, or combinations of these. The size and shape of the nose should be noted. An alteration in its shape may be the result of trauma or a tumor in or near the nose. Characteristics of the nasal mucosa and the appearance of the nasal septum are important. The mucosa may be swollen and reddened in an infectious process, and in some instances may be covered with secretions. The client with allergic rhinitis often has pale nasal mucosa rather than the normal pink. Most adults have some degree of nasal septal deviation, but note any deviation that narrows or blocks the nasal airway.

Assess the characteristics of the nasal secretions. They may be watery, mucoid, mucopurulent, purulent, or bloody. Watery discharge is usually of viral origin. Secretions that are mucoid or mucopurulent may result from inflammation, as in acute rhinitis or allergic rhinitis. Mucopurulent secretions often result from infectious processes, as when acute rhinitis progresses. Purulent discharge is usually of bacterial origin. Blood may drain from the nares because of irritation or trauma.

The appearance of the inferior and middle turbinates should be assessed. Tissues overlying the turbinates may become hypertrophied in conditions such as chronic allergic rhinitis.

Sinusitis may result in a decrease in transillumination of the frontal and maxillary sinuses. Skin over these areas may also appear reddened in the presence of an infection.

Structures of the oropharynx may be enlarged, reddened, and covered with secretions. The color of the oral mucosa should be noted. White patches or spots on the mucous membrane of the cheek or tongue (leukoplakia) may indicate a premalignant lesion. Observe for inflammation, swelling, bleeding, retraction, or distortion. Inflammation and secretions are often present with infections such as pharyngitis. Bleeding, retraction, or distortion of the area may be from a neoplasm of the oropharynx or an infectious process. Inspect the uvula, fauces, and pharyngeal tonsils as part of the examination. These areas may be distorted in disorders such as peritonsillar abscess, infectious mononucleosis, and tumors of the pharynx.

Examine the neck for enlarged lymph nodes. Enlargement may be the result of common upper respiratory infections, mononucleosis, lymphoma, or metastatic cancer.

Inspection of the chest may reveal thoracic deformities such as kyphoscoliosis or an increased anteroposterior (AP) diameter (barrel chest). Kyphoscoliosis reduces thoracic movement and limits lung expansion. "Barrel chest" is a common finding in clients with COPD (Figure 18–1). Asymmetrical chest expansion can result from trauma (pneumothorax, hemothorax, flail chest).

General overall appearance such as facial expression, posture, and ease of movement should be assessed. Clients with COPD may have to sit up to breathe or lean forward in a chair resting their arms on tables for support.

Examination of sputum may reveal thick tenacious secretions; mucus plugs; or purulent, bloody, or blood-tinged sputum (**hemoptysis**). Secretions that are yellow–green or foul smelling may indicate an infectious process.

Sputum that is pink or rust-colored may indicate bleeding, which can result from irritation, infection, or neoplasia.

The pattern and character of respirations should be observed. This includes rate and depth of breathing and the presence of labored breathing. Labored breathing may be marked by nasal flaring, the use of neck and accessory chest muscles, asymmetry of chest expansion, and increase in respiratory rate. This occurs in conditions such as airway obstruction by a foreign body, COPD, and mediastinal shift. Pursed-lip breathing, a slow, relaxed expiration against pursed lips, prevents collapse of small bronchioles and reduces the amount of trapped air. It is characteristic of clients with emphysema. Chest trauma may result in sub-cutaneous emphysema (air under the skin), which can compromise the airway.

When inspecting clients with respiratory disorders, also observe for signs of respiratory acidosis, respiratory alkalosis, and hypoxemia. Disorders that can lead to acidosis are COPD, pneumonia, or respiratory depression due to trauma or drugs. Clinical manifestations of respiratory acidosis or hypercapnia include: confusion, drowsiness, dizziness, tetany, and asterixis. Tachycardia and dysrhythmias may be present. Late signs of hypercapnia are convulsions and coma (Harper, 1981).

Respiratory alkalosis occurs in conditions resulting in hyperventilation. Disorders that may lead to hyperventilation include brain injury or tumors, gram-negative sepsis, acute asthmatic attacks, and extreme anxiety. Manifestations of respiratory alkalosis are related to stimulation of the nervous system. The nurse may observe muscle spasms, which can be in the form of carpopedal spasm—contractions of the hands and feet. The client's thumb is flexed, wrist and metacarpophalangeal joints are flexed, the interphalangeal joints are hyperextended, and fingers are adducted in the form of a cone. Severe spasms can progress to tetany or continuous muscle contractions. Diaphoresis and cardiac dysrhythmias may occur. The client will be tachypneic and may lose consciousness (Harper, 1981).

When the respiratory system is affected by disease, the ability to deliver oxygen to the tissues may become impaired, resulting in hypoxia (inadequate tissue oxygen) or hypoxemia (inadequate blood oxygen levels). Conditions that limit the volume of air entering the lungs result in inadequate amounts of available oxygen at the alveolar level. Disorders leading to hypoxia or hypoxemia include restrictive lung diseases (such as pulmonary fibrosis, occupational lung diseases, and sarcoidosis), obstructive lung diseases (such as asthma, chronic bronchitis, and emphysema), and occasionally, morbid obesity. Any disorder that lowers the oxygen-carrying capacity of the hemoglobin in the blood will also produce tissue hypoxia.

The symptoms manifested by acute hypoxia are reflected in the neurological, cardiovascular, and respiratory systems. Deprivation of oxygen to the brain causes signs of restlessness, irritability, and mental confusion. Effects on the cardiovascular system include tachycardia,

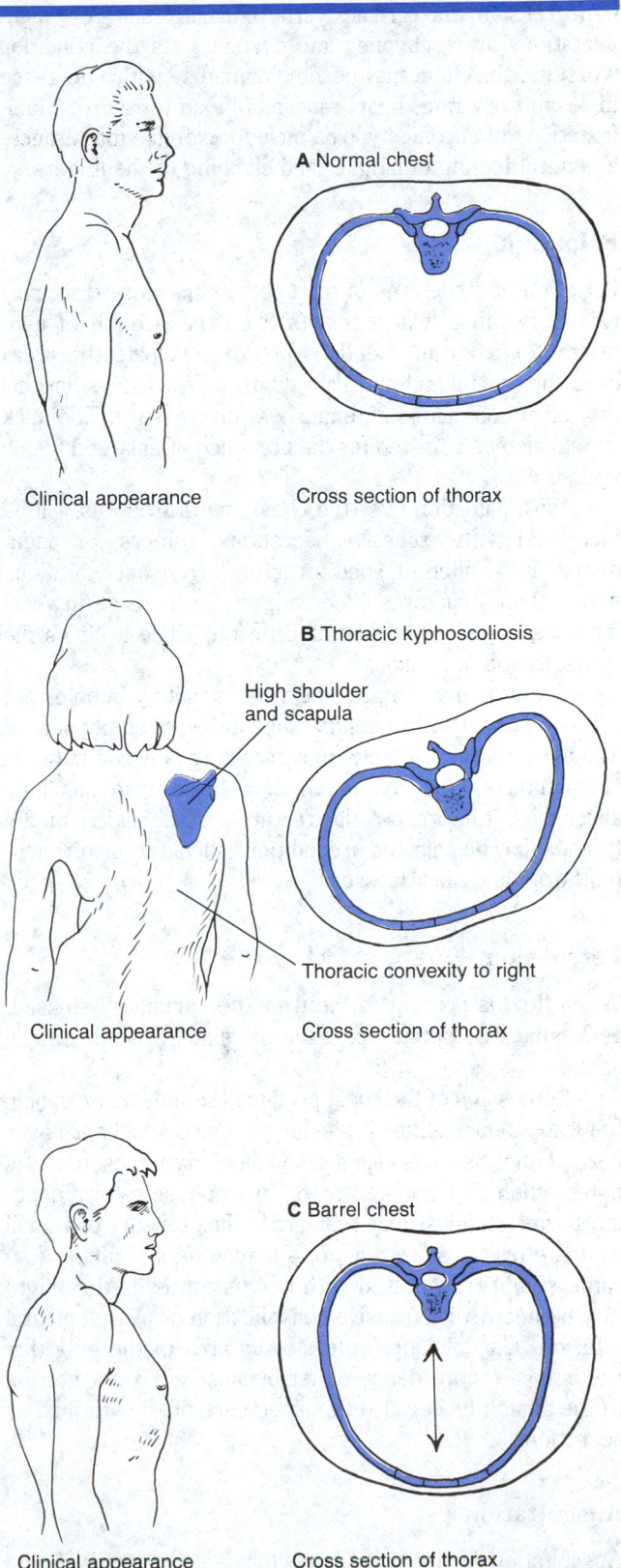

Figure 18–1

Cross section of thorax.
A. Normal. **B.** Thoracic kyphoscoliosis. **C.** Barrel chest in COPD.

hypertension, and cardiac dysrhythmias. Respiratory manifestations are tachypnea and dyspnea. As the condition worsens, the client may become comatose with a decrease in respiratory rate, heart rate, and blood pressure. Manifestations of chronic hypoxia include exercise intolerance, a general feeling of fatigue, and clubbing of the fingers.

Palpation

Palpation of structures of the upper respiratory tract may reveal swelling, which results from the growth of neoplasms or from an infectious process. Palpate the areas over the frontal and maxillary sinuses. With sinusitis, this may elicit complaints of tenderness or pressure. The neck should also be palpated for the presence of enlarged lymph nodes.

With palpation over the chest, vocal fremitus will be increased with excessive secretions, tumors, or pneumonia. Fluid-filled or solid structures transmit vibrations better than structures filled with air. A decrease in vocal fremitus is present in pleural effusion, since it slows the transmission of sound.

Crepitus may be palpated when small air bubbles are present underneath the skin (subcutaneous emphysema). Touching the area results in a crackling sensation. Intercostal bulging may be noted in a client who has lung abscesses, tumors, or rib fractures. A deviation of the trachea may be palpated in conditions such as tension pneumothorax and neck masses.

Percussion

When fluid is present in the frontal or maxillary sinuses, as in sinusitis, percussion over the sinus produces a dull sound.

Percussion of the chest produces sounds that can help to locate abnormalities in the lungs. The sound heard over normal lung tissue is called resonance. Hyperresonance is noted when air trapping occurs, in emphysema or a pneumothorax. Dullness may be heard in the presence of a small pleural effusion, atelectasis, or a hemothorax. Flatness (the same sound transmitted with percussion over the thigh) may be heard with massive consolidation or a large pleural effusion. Consolidation refers to an area of the lung that has become more dense either because air is not getting to the alveoli or because the alveoli are filled with fluid or secretions.

Auscultation

Auscultation of the lungs is performed to determine the presence or absence of abnormal breath sounds. Bronchial or tracheal, bronchovesicular, and vesicular breath sounds are normal respiratory sounds in certain areas of the lungs. However, auscultation of these sounds in areas where they are not normally heard may indicate pathology. The presence of bronchial or tracheal sounds over the periphery of

the lung may be an indication of atelectasis or consolidation. The presence of bronchovesicular sounds over the peripheral lung tissue may also indicate consolidation. Decreased vesicular sounds in the peripheral lung may be present in early pneumonia or emphysema.

Adventitious or abnormal breath sounds may also be heard during auscultation. These can include: fine to medium rales, medium to coarse rales, rhonchi, wheezing, and friction rubs. Fine to medium rales may indicate pneumonia. Medium to coarse rales are heard in bronchitis, pneumonia, bronchiectasis, emphysema, and pleural effusion. Wheezing may be noted in clients with asthma and COPD. Rhonchi indicate an obstructive mass or secretions in the larger airways. A friction rub may be heard in clients with pneumonia, lung cancer, pleurisy, or tuberculosis.

Diagnostic Studies

Diagnostic studies used when caring for clients who have respiratory dysfunction are discussed in order of increasing invasiveness.

Pulmonary Function Tests

Pulmonary function tests measure the functional ability of the lungs. More specifically, they:

- Provide objective evidence of the presence, type, and degree of lung abnormality
- Monitor the course of a disease process over time
- Evaluate the effectiveness of various medications on breathing function
- Determine the risk of respiratory complications of surgical procedures

In routine pulmonary function studies, the client's lung size and breathing ability are compared with values for normal individuals who are similar to the client in age, sex, height, and race. The spirometer is the primary instrument used in this test. Spirometry provides an easy and inexpensive method to measure lung volume with relatively little risk to the client. Several different types of spirometers are used to measure lung volumes; the most common are electronic computerized units and the kymograph.

Normal findings for pulmonary function tests are discussed under lung volumes and capacities. Table 18–1 shows abnormal findings related to specific disease states.

Pulmonary function study results can show either a restriction or an obstruction to airflow or a combination. Disease conditions that commonly result in a restriction to airflow include certain neuromuscular disorders such as myasthenia gravis, thoracic deformities such as kyphoscoliosis, restriction to lung expansion as occurs in pneumothorax and fibrosis, or infiltrative diseases such as

(continued on p. 11)

Table 18–1   Diagnostic Tests Common to the Respiratory System

Diagnostic Test	Normal Expected Value*	Disease State	Expected Abnormal Findings
Pulmonary function test			
Tidal volume (TV)	500 mL	Guillain-Barré syndrome Myasthenia gravis Thoracic deformity Kyphoscoliosis Pneumothorax Pulmonary fibrosis Tuberculosis COPD Asthma Bronchiectasis	Decreased
Inspiratory reserve volume (IRV)	3000 mL	Guillain-Barré syndrome Myasthenia gravis Thoracic deformity Kyphoscoliosis Pneumothorax Pulmonary fibrosis Tuberculosis COPD Asthma Bronchiectasis	Decreased
Expiratory reserve volume (ERV)	1100 mL	COPD Asthma Bronchiectasis	Decreased
Residual volume (RV)	1200 mL	COPD Asthma Bronchiectasis	Increased
Inspiratory capacity (IC)	3500 mL	Guillain-Barré syndrome Myasthenia gravis Thoracic deformity Kyphoscoliosis Pneumothorax Pulmonary fibrosis Tuberculosis COPD Asthma Bronchiectasis	Decreased
Functional residual capacity (FRC)	2300 mL	Guillain-Barré syndrome Myasthenia gravis Thoracic deformity Kyphoscoliosis Pneumothorax Pulmonary fibrosis Tuberculosis	Decreased
		COPD Asthma Bronchiectasis	Increased
Vital capacity (VC)	4600 mL	Guillain-Barré syndrome Myasthenia gravis Thoracic deformity Kyphoscoliosis Pneumothorax Pulmonary fibrosis Tuberculosis COPD Asthma Bronchiectasis	Decreased

(continued)

Table 18−1   Diagnostic Tests Common to the Respiratory System (continued)

Diagnostic Test	Normal Expected Value*	Disease State	Expected Abnormal Findings
Total lung capacity (TLC)	5800 mL	Guillain-Barré syndrome Myasthenia gravis Thoracic deformity Kyphoscoliosis Pneumothorax Pulmonary fibrosis Tuberculosis	Decreased
		COPD Asthma Bronchiectasis	Increased
Forced vital capacity FEV_1, FEV_2, FEV_3	Able to exhale 75% of vital capacity in 1 sec and almost all in 3 sec	COPD Asthma Bronchiectasis	Decreased
		Guillain-Barré syndrome Myasthenia gravis Thoracic deformity Kyphoscoliosis Pneumothorax Pulmonary fibrosis Tuberculosis	May be decreased in severe cases
Maximal voluntary ventilation (MVV)	Can breathe about ½ of vital capacity with each breath and can take 40−70 breaths/min	COPD Asthma Bronchiectasis	Decreased
Minute respiratory volume (MV)	6 L/min	Guillain-Barré syndrome Asthma Bronchiectasis Myasthenia gravis Thoracic deformity Kyphoscoliosis Pneumothorax Pulmonary fibrosis Tuberculosis	Decreased
Chest x-rays	Normal chest film	Pulmonary infections	Infiltration and consolidation
		Obstructive disorders such as benign or malignant neoplasms, nodules	Density
		Emphysema	Hyperaeration
		Trauma; pneumothorax, hemothorax	Air or blood in the intrapleural space and collapsed lung
		Flail chest	Fractured ribs or sternum
Sinus films	Absence of air fluid levels	Sinusitis, foreign body, stone, cyst, polyp, osteoma	Air fluid level or clouding
Facial films	Absence of edema and fractures	Hemorrhage secondary to trauma Maxillofacial trauma	Fluid Breaks or fractures of bones and/or edema of tissues
Lung scan	Normal ventilation/perfusion	Pulmonary embolism Lung cancer COPD Pulmonary edema Pulmonary infections	Abnormal ventilation/perfusion

Diagnostic Test	Normal Expected Value*	Disease State	Expected Abnormal Findings
Blood gases	ph 7.35–7.45	Respiratory acidosis	Below 7.35
		Respiratory alkalosis	Above 7.45
	PCO_2 34–45 mm Hg	Respiratory acidosis	Above 45 mm Hg
		Respiratory alkalosis	Below 35 mm Hg
	PO_2 80–100 mm Hg	Prolonged administration of high liter flows of oxygen	Above 100 mm Hg
		Any disease state resulting in hypoxemia	Below 80 mm Hg
Oxygen hemoglobin saturation (SO_2)	95%–98%	Disorders that result in a shift to the right (acidosis, hypercapnia, chronic hypoxemia, elevated temperature)	Release of oxygen made more readily to the tissues, drop in SO_2
		Disorders that result in a shift to the left (alkalosis, hypocapnia, lowered temperature)	Stronger binding of oxygen to hemoglobin, rise in SO_2
Bicarbonate (HCO_3)	22–26 mEq/L	Metabolic acidosis	Below 22 mEq/L
		Metabolic alkalosis	Above 26 mEq/L
Base excess	−2–+2 mEq/L	Metabolic alkalosis	Above +2 mEq/L
		Metabolic acidosis	Below −2 mEq/L
Culture	No growth from specimens obtained from normally sterile sites	Infections	Presence of organisms
	Presence of mixed flora in areas of the body that normally harbor microorganisms	Infections	Presence of and/or elevation of pathogenic organisms
Gram's stain	Absence of microorganisms when the specimen is taken from a normally sterile site; identification of normal flora when the specimen is obtained from areas that normally harbor microorganisms	Infections	Identification of presence and/or elevation of pathogenic organisms
Acid-fast stain	Absence of acid-fast bacilli	Tuberculosis	Presence of tubercle bacilli and other mycobacteria
Cytology	Appearance of normal cells	Carcinoma	Presence of cellular changes indicative of neoplastic activity
Mantoux intradermal skin test	0–4 mm of induration	Tuberculosis	Induration measuring 10 mm or more within 72 h; induration of between 5 and 9 mm is doubtful unless there is known exposure to the organism
Skin test for coccidioidomycosis	Less than 0.5 mm of induration	Coccidioidomycosis	0.5 mm or more of induration
Immunoglobulins	IgG 650–1600 mg/dL IgA 50–400 mg/dL IgM 18–280 mg/dL IgD 0.5–3.0 mg/dL IgE 0.01–0.04 mg/dL	Pneumonia Tuberculosis Fungal infections of the lung	Changes in the levels of one or more of the immunoglobulins

(continued)

Table 18–1   Diagnostic Tests Common to the Respiratory System (continued)

Diagnostic Test	Normal Expected Value*	Disease State	Expected Abnormal Findings
Laryngoscopy (indirect or direct)	Normal-appearing larynx	Laryngeal cancer	Neoplasm (ulceration may be seen)
		Laryngeal polyps	Polyps
		Vocal cord nodules	Nodules
		Foreign body	Foreign body
		Laryngitis	Inflammation
Bronchoscopy	Normal-appearing tracheobronchial tree	Bronchogenic carcinoma	Neoplasm, bleeding
		Tuberculosis	Nodule or lesion, bleeding
		Lung abscess	Purulent material
		Bronchiectasis	Excessive secretions
		Foreign body	Foreign body
Mediastinoscopy	Normal-appearing thoracic structure	Bronchogenic carcinoma	Neoplasm
		Sarcoidosis	
Bronchography	(Done only in the presence of a known disease)	Bronchiectasis	Evidence of bronchial dilation
Thoracentesis	No fluid present	Chylothorax	Milky white fluid
		Blood	Red-tinged fluid
		Empyema	Purulent fluid
		Anaerobic microorganisms	Foul odor
Percutaneous needle biopsy	Normal lung tissue	Malignancy	Abnormal cells in specimen

*Values given are the average for a normal young male adult.

tuberculosis and lung cancer. These restrictive conditions cause a reduction in lung compliance, which decreases chest expansion and therefore decreases the volume of air inspired and expired (Wade, 1982). Disorders that result in pathologic changes of the airways or alveoli obstruct airflow into and out of the lungs. These include chronic bronchitis, emphysema, asthma, and bronchiectasis.

Nursing Implications. To allay anxieties, clients should be told how the test will be conducted and what will be expected of them. It is important to explain that the test is not painful or harmful in any way. Some clients may need to be reassured that the degree of exertion necessary to complete the test will not cause injury to their lungs. Others may fear their lungs will burst or that they will be unable to catch their breath. Explain the technique and equipment to clients in terms they can understand. This will aid in lowering client anxiety and increasing cooperation. Clients should be told their noses will be clamped intermittently and they will be asked to breathe in and out through a mouthpiece connected to a machine. The client should understand that accurate results can be obtained only by following instructions carefully. Since gastric distention may impair ability to expand the lungs, tests should be performed before meals. Medications that may alter

respiratory function, such as bronchodilators, should be withheld unless otherwise indicated by the physician (Harper, 1981; Wade, 1982).

Before the test, the client is asked to loosen any constricting clothing that might interfere with chest expansion. The client may be either sitting or standing. The client should be told to seal both lips around the mouthpiece and keep the nose clip on because air leakage would make the test results inaccurate. The client is then asked to breathe as normally as possible through the spirometer and does not begin the next step until comfortable with breathing normally on the machine. At the completion of four or five normal breaths, the client is told to breathe in as much air as possible, to fill the lungs far more than usual, and then to blow out all the air from the lungs. The volume breathed in and that breathed out are the measures, along with the time needed for expiration.

Lung Volumes and Capacities. Lung volumes and capacities as measured by spirometry are shown in Figure 18–2. There are two lung volumes that cannot be measured by routine spirometry. These include the residual volume and the functional residual capacity. These measurements are discussed under gas dilution methods. The values given for pulmonary function tests are average values

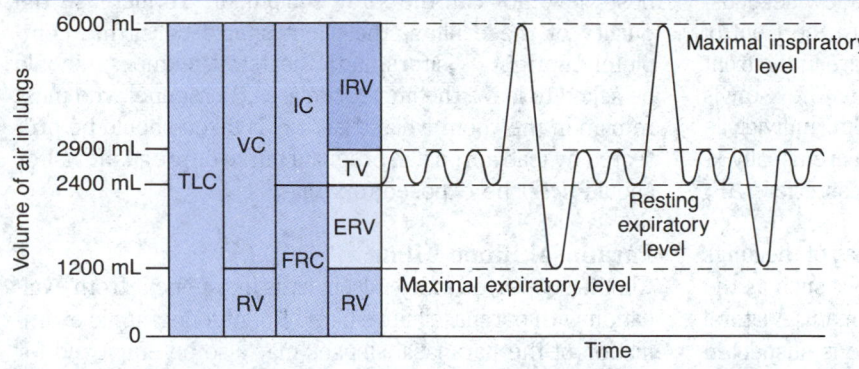

Figure 18–2

Measurement of lung volumes and capacities by spirometry.

for a young adult male. Values for women are approximately 10% to 25% less. (Some women, of course, will show higher values than some men.)

- Lung volumes
  - Tidal volume (TV) is the amount of air inspired and expired with each normal breath. The normal is approximately 500 mL.
  - Inspiratory reserve volume (IRV) is the additional volume of air that can be inspired beyond the normal tidal volume. It amounts to approximately 3000 mL.
  - Expiratory reserve volume (ERV) is the volume of air that can be forcefully expired at the end of the normal tidal expiration. This is about 1100 mL.
  - Residual volume (RV) consists of the amount of air that remains in the lungs after a forceful expiration. This equals about 1200 mL.

- Lung capacities. When discussing the pulmonary cycle, it is often helpful to consider two or more of the pulmonary volumes together. These combinations are referred to as pulmonary capacities. The four capacities include:
  - Inspiratory capacity (IC) is the volume of air that a person can inspire from a resting level. This equals the tidal volume plus the inspiratory reserve volume, and amounts to about 3500 mL.
  - Functional residual capacity (FRC) is the volume of air remaining in the lungs after a normal expiration. It equals the expiratory reserve volume plus the residual volume, and is about 2300 mL.
  - Vital capacity (VC) is the maximum volume of air that can be exhaled forcefully from the lungs following a maximal inspiration. This equals the inspiratory reserve volume plus the tidal volume plus the expiratory reserve volume; it totals about 4600 mL.
  - Total lung capacity (TLC) refers to the maximum volume to which the lungs can be expanded with the greatest possible inspiratory effort. It equals the vital capacity plus the residual volume and is approximately 5900 mL.

- Pulmonary volumes measured in time intervals
  - Forced vital capacity (FVC) is the maximal pulmo-

nary volume the client has for ventilation. The client inhales the maximum amount of air and then forcefully exhales as fast as possible. The amount of air the client can forcefully exhale within specific time periods is calculated. The usual time periods are 1, 2, and 3 seconds. Forced vital capacity is also referred to as the forced expiratory volume in 1, 2, or 3 seconds (FEV 1.0, FEV 2.0, FEV 3.0). A healthy individual can usually exhale approximately 75% of vital capacity in 1 second and all of it by 3 seconds (Harper, 1981).
  - Minute respiratory volume (MRV) is the amount of air moved into the respiratory passages each minute. This consists of the tidal volume times the respiratory rate. The normal finding is approximately 6 L/min.

Gas Dilution Method. The functional residual capacity (FRC) cannot be calculated using simple spirometry. A method of gas dilution is used to obtain this value. Once this value is obtained, the residual volume can be calculated.

One gas dilution method is the nitrogen washout technique. After a normal expiration, the person changes from breathing normal air to breathing 100% oxygen for several minutes. This serves to remove (wash out) all of the nitrogen into the expired air (atmospheric air contains approximately 79% nitrogen and 21% oxygen). By knowing how much nitrogen was in the expired air, the amount of air in the lungs at the beginning of the test can be calculated. This value is the functional residual capacity. Then the residual volume is obtained by subtracting the expiratory reserve volume from the functional residual capacity (as shown in Figure 18–2).

Chest X-ray

Chest x-ray, one of the most common procedures used to evaluate the lungs, is part of the evaluation of most clients suspected of having pulmonary disease, except during pregnancy. The evaluation should include a posteroanterior (PA) view and at least one lateral film.

In PA views, the upright position is used because the diaphragm is lower and the lungs are larger. The client is asked to take a deep breath and hold it for a few seconds. An x-ray beam is projected from the back to the front of the client. Since the heart and mediastinum are in the front of the thorax, in this position magnification on the x-ray is much less than in an anteroposterior (AP) film. Individuals who are very ill, infants, and young children are usually x-rayed lying down in the supine or anteroposterior (AP) position (George, Light, & Matthay, 1983).

Lateral views add information about areas of the lungs that cannot be viewed well in the PA position, such as the anterior part of the lung close to the mediastinum. A lateral film is always taken whenever chest disease is suspected or clients are over 40 years of age (Matthay & Sostman, 1983).

Oblique views are beneficial in delineating pulmonary or mediastinal masses or lesions, and pleural effusion that may not be well demonstrated on PA or lateral views. Oblique positions consist of the right anterior oblique (RAO), in which the right front of the client is against the film holder or *cassette* (George, Light, & Matthay, 1983).

The lateral decubitus view is used to detect a small amount of free pleural fluid, pneumothorax, cavitation, or lung abscess. This view is taken with the client in the side-lying position. The x-ray beam is aimed parallel to the floor and the area of concern is positioned closest to the film. Lordotic views are also taken to better evaluate the apical portions of the lungs, to assist in recognizing collapse of the middle lobe, and to determine if a lesion is anterior or posterior (George, Light, & Matthay, 1983).

General abnormal findings that may be evident on chest x-ray include areas of density (may be related to atelectasis, pneumonia, or a pneumothorax), hypersecretion, presence of masses, and increased vascular markings.

Nursing Implications. The procedure should be explained in terms that the client can understand. In a chest x-ray, an x-ray beam passes through the body to a film. The films obtained will provide the radiologist with information about the structure and function of the lungs. Clients may have misconceptions about the physiologic effects of exposure to diagnostic x-rays (eg, fears of cancer). Allow the client to verbalize these fears and then provide correct information. If the client is pregnant, x-rays are avoided unless absolutely necessary. If critical illness of a pregnant woman necessitates a chest x-ray, the abdomen is protected with a lead shield.

For a chest x-ray, clients are asked to remove clothing down to the waist and don an open-backed gown. They will be asked to inhale and hold their breath for a few seconds. If the client is connected to equipment such as a ventilator, the tubing should be placed above the level of the chest. Tubing and jewelry may appear as shadows on the film.

When clients are acutely ill, portable chest x-rays may be necessary. The quality of a chest film taken with a portable x-ray is not as good as the film taken in the x-ray department because the client cannot be positioned for the best view, nor can the x-ray equipment. To increase the quality of these films, the client should be sitting completely upright. Visitors and other staff members should be asked to leave the immediate area. Personnel who must remain in the room while the x-ray is taken should be protected by lead aprons. A pregnant nurse or pregnant visitor should *never* be exposed to x-rays.

Paranasal Sinus Films

Clients suspected of having sinusitis may benefit from evaluation with paranasal sinus films. Roentgenographic examination of the paranasal sinuses may also be employed for clients with head trauma and those suspected of having sinus neoplasms.

Traditional x-ray assessment of the paranasal sinuses often necessitates a series of different views. Five basic views are common for visualization of the sinuses: Caldwell's view, Water's view, lateral view, submentovertical view, and right and left oblique orbital views.

In Caldwell's view, the client's nose and forehead are positioned against the film cassette. The ethmoids are well visualized, and the frontal sinuses are best seen in this view. This view is of primary value in looking for disease of the frontal and ethmoid sinuses, orbits, and nasal cavities. This view may also contribute to the diagnosis of disease in the maxillary sinuses.

The Water's view, the most frequently used, is obtained by placing the client's nose and chin on the film cassette. It allows for excellent exposure of the maxillary sinuses. The anterior ethmoids and frontal sinuses are also visualized well. If the client's mouth is open, the sphenoid sinus may be seen. This view is helpful in diagnosis of pathology within the maxillary sinuses and fractures of the orbits.

The lateral view, as the name implies, should be obtained from the side view of the skull. The sphenoid sinus is well outlined in this view. All of the paranasal sinuses can be seen, but the right and left sinuses are superimposed. This view gives information about the frontal, sphenoid, and maxillary sinuses and the sella turcica.

The submentovertical view, obtained with the head fully extended, allows good visualization of the base of the skull and the paranasal sinuses, particularly the walls of the maxillary and sphenoid sinuses.

The right and left orbital oblique views offer views of the superior ethmoid cells, frontal sinus, and optic foramen. This view is often helpful in the diagnosis of frontal and ethmoid mucoceles, which may not be evident in Water's or Caldwell's views (Paparella & Shumrick, 1980).

An area of density on x-ray film may indicate a foreign body, stone, cyst, polyp, or osteoma in the paranasal sinuses. Osteolysis (abnormal resorption or absorption of bone) or osteoblastosis (abnormal production of bone) may be evident. In the absence of disease, the mucosal lining of the sinuses does not show up on x-ray films. An infection of the sinus may be evident on x-ray if it causes edema of the mucosal lining. Clouding of the sinus may indicate edema or accumulated fluid in the sinus. When fluid is present but does not fill the entire cavity, an air-fluid level may be seen. Fluid may be present as the result of sinusitis or hemorrhage secondary to trauma.

Nursing Implications. The nurse should explain the procedure in terms the client can understand. Clients should be told that x-ray films will be taken of their sinuses from different views, and that the process will not cause them much if any discomfort. Clients will be asked to hold the head in certain positions against the x-ray plate. The nurse might find it helpful to compare the process to a chest x-ray since most clients have had these.

Facial Films
The traditional x-ray examination to detect injury after maxillofacial trauma consists of the four views discussed under sinus films with the addition of the Panorex view of the mandible. This shows the entire mandible fairly well in one view so that breaks in the bones and edema of tissues may be seen.

Nursing Implications. If the client has severe maxillofacial trauma, the nurse will need to provide emotional support in addition to technical skill, such as maintaining a patent airway and closely monitoring vital signs.

Tomograms
Tomograms are views of the area in horizontal, sagittal, and coronal planes. This method is employed when conventional x-rays cannot detect the extent of the pathologic process or when the area is obscured by other structures. Tomograms allow visualization of minute structures. The major application of tomography of the nose and paranasal sinuses is in determining the presence of fractures or bone destruction due to a tumor. Tomography of the thorax is indicated when more precise knowledge of the morphologic characteristics of lesions is needed (Paparella & Shumrick, 1980).

Nursing Implications. Tell the client that films will be taken of the areas that allow the physician to see different sections of tissue from several angles, to identify changes that traditional x-ray films cannot show. Clients should be told that the procedure will not cause them any discomfort. Some of the equipment may be rather large and noisy, however.

Lung Scan
A lung scan may be classified as either a perfusion scan or a ventilation scan. To obtain a *perfusion* scan, radioactive dye is administered intravenously. When the dye is injected, the client should be supine and breathing normally to produce a uniform distribution of radioactive particles that are trapped in the pulmonary capillary bed. The scan may begin immediately after injection of the dye. Anterior, posterior,

both lateral views, and both posterior oblique views are obtained. An x-ray of the lung should be obtained at the same time so comparisons can be made.

Ventilation scans are usually performed using inert gases. The client should be sitting or supine. Clients will usually wear a tightly fitting facial mask that allows them to breathe radioactive gas for a few minutes. Depending on the type of gas, clients may need only to breathe through a nasal cannula.

Ventilation and perfusion scanning are used to diagnose pulmonary embolism, lung cancer, COPD, pulmonary edema, and pulmonary infections. Unlike most pulmonary function tests, the lung scan can measure regional lung function. This makes possible the diagnosis of pulmonary diseases at an earlier stage, before other parameters of respiratory function become abnormal (Wagner & Buchanan, 1980).

Nursing Implications. Explain that the purpose of the test is to determine if all of the client's lung tissue has adequate circulation and if air is reaching areas as it should.

Clients should know they will receive radioactive dye IV for a perfusion scan. Any history of an allergic reaction to dye used in diagnostic tests must be documented beforehand and brought to the attention of the physician. The nurse should stress that clients should try to relax and breathe normally during the test. Clients should be told that a machine will move over the chest to obtain different views of the lungs. A conventional chest x-ray will also be taken at that time.

Clients should be informed that during a ventilation scan they will be asked to breathe a mixture of gases through a mask or nasal cannula so that the air flowing in and out of their lungs can be traced. Inhalation of this gaseous mixture should not cause them discomfort. A machine will move over their chest to obtain different views.

Arterial Blood Gas Analysis
Arterial blood is collected for analysis of the pH, PCO_2, PO_2, oxygen saturation, bicarbonate level, and base excess. These values show how well the client's lungs are delivering oxygen to the bloodstream and eliminating the waste product of cellular metabolism, carbon dioxide. Individual values are discussed below.

pH. The normal pH of arterial blood is 7.35 to 7.45. Values below 7.35 indicate acidemia, while those above 7.45 are indicative of alkalemia. The normal pH range is maintained primarily by two buffers—carbonic acid (H_2CO_3) and bicarbonate (HCO_3).

The normal ratio of carbonic acid to bicarbonate (1:20) must be maintained; otherwise, the pH will not be within the normal range. The lungs control the carbonic acid by selectively retaining or ventilating the carbon dioxide (CO_2) that combines with water to form the carbonic acid's hydrogen ion. The bicarbonate portion of the balance is controlled by the kidneys, which excrete either alkaline or acidic urine. Chapter 5 gives a detailed explanation of acid–base balance.

The normal range of PCO_2 in the arterial blood is 35 to 45 mm Hg. An elevation of PCO_2 above 45 mm Hg may be indicative of hypoventilation, which results in respiratory acidosis, or it may result from compensated metabolic alkalosis. A PCO_2 below 35 mm Hg may arise from hyperventilation, which can result in respiratory alkalosis or from compensatory metabolic acidosis.

The normal value of PO_2 in arterial blood is 80 to 100 mm Hg. This value has no direct bearing on the pH but is an important indication of whether adequate oxygen is available for cellular metabolism. A PO_2 elevation may be seen in clients who are receiving a high-liter flow of oxygen. Prolonged elevation in PO_2 levels can result in damage to the pulmonary tissue.

Oxygen Saturation. The extent of oxygen saturation, the amount of hemoglobin combined with oxygen, is expressed as a percentage of the blood's capacity for full saturation. The normal value is 95% to 98% in arterial blood. Figure 18–3 represents the oxyhemoglobin dissociation curve—the binding capacity that hemoglobin has for oxygen. The flat part of the curve represents strong hemoglobin binding capacity for oxygen; reduction in the amount of arterial oxygen (PO_2) does not significantly reduce the percentage of saturation of hemoglobin with oxygen. The steep part of the curve represents the situation where oxygen is dissociated or released from the hemoglobin.

A shift of the curve to the *right* means oxygen is released to the tissues more readily. Factors that can cause a shift to the right include acidosis, chronic hypoxemia, hypercapnia, and an elevated temperature. A shift of the curve to the *left* can result from alkalosis, hypocapnia, and a decrease in temperature. These conditions result in increased binding of oxygen to hemoglobin.

Bicarbonate Ion. Bicarbonate is a negative ion whose normal value in arterial blood is 22 to 26 mEq/L. A lower value is indicative of metabolic acidosis or compensation for respiratory alkalosis. A value above 26 mEq/L is indicative of metabolic alkalosis or compensated respiratory acidosis.

Base Excess. The base excess represents an increase or a decrease in the total amount of buffer bases available. The normal range is −2 to +2 mEq/L in arterial blood. This value is considered a more reliable indication of the true metabolic makeup of an acid–base disturbance than the bicarbonate value. An increase indicates metabolic alkalosis or compensated respiratory acidosis. A decrease indicates metabolic acidosis or compensated respiratory alkalosis.

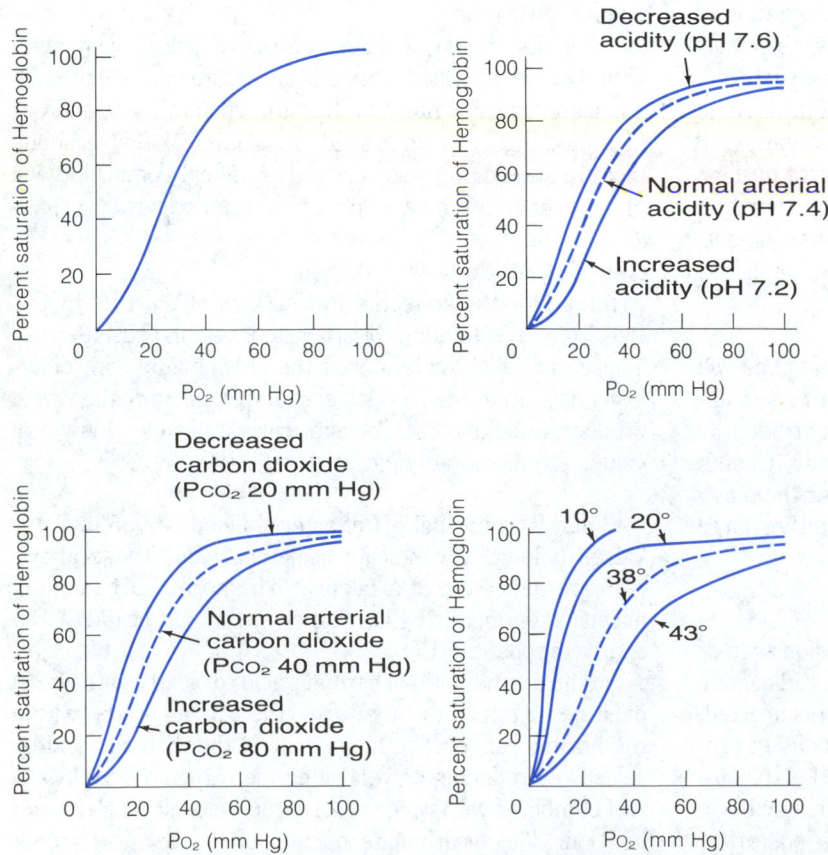

Figure 18–3

Oxyhemoglobin dissociation curves.
SOURCE: Spence AP, Mason EB: *Human Anatomy and Physiology*, 2nd ed. Menlo Park, CA: Benjamin/Cummings, 1983.

Nursing Implications. For arterial blood gas tests, tell the client that a small amount of blood needs to be obtained from an artery to determine how well the lungs are functioning in the transport of oxygen and carbon dioxide. In settings such as intensive care units or cardiac care units, nurses may be responsible for collecting this blood sample. Equipment necessary includes a heparinized syringe, alcohol swab, a basin with ice, and a piece of gauze. Heparinization is achieved by drawing up 0.5 mL of heparin (1:1000) into the syringe and wetting the entire barrel by moving the plunger up and down. Excess heparin is ejected, leaving the syringe free of air bubbles, and the needle filled with heparin. This will prevent clotting of the blood sample.

Common sites for obtaining an arterial blood gas sample are the radial, brachial, and femoral arteries. The puncture site should be thoroughly cleansed with alcohol or an antiseptic solution. The location of the artery is ascertained by palpation of the pulse. The fingers used to palpate the artery must be clean. A sterile 5 mL heparinized syringe fitted with a wide bore needle (20 to 21 gauge) will allow the easy flow of blood into the syringe. However, a smaller gauge needle results in less trauma to the artery.

A variety of techniques are used when inserting the needle into the lumen of the artery. The blood should enter the syringe with a fairly rapid, pulsatile flow. Once 3 to 5 mL of blood have been obtained, pressure should be applied above the puncture site with a piece of sterile gauze and the needle removed. Pressure must be applied for at least 5 *minutes* or longer, particularly if the client is receiving anticoagulants. This should be followed by application of a dressing, preferably a pressure dressing.

The arterial blood sample must be protected from atmospheric oxygen by removing the needle and capping the tip of the syringe. The syringe is then rotated so the blood and heparin are mixed together to prevent clotting. The sample is then immediately placed in ice (to slow down oxygen metabolism) and taken to the lab for analysis. Clients in an intensive care unit may have an arterial line from which the specimen can be directly removed (Wade, 1982).

Cultures

A culture is the growing of bacteria or other microorganisms from a specimen of material obtained in an aseptic manner or using sterile technique. Sterile technique is necessary whenever cultures are needed from areas normally free of microorganisms, such as the lungs. Sterile technique is also required when specimens are taken from areas that normally harbor microorganisms, such as the throat, because of the possibility of growing, identifying, and treating organisms introduced when the culture was taken.

The specimen is placed in an environment where organisms can grow. When the microorganisms increase, laboratory personnel can isolate and identify the pathogen. Sensitivity studies are then done to determine which antimicrobial drug is effective against the organism. The organism can be described as sensitive or resistant to spe-

cific antibiotics. This helps the physician select the most effective agent for drug therapy (Treseler, 1982).

Specimens are examined in direct smears, stained and unstained. The most frequent staining test is Gram's stain, which distinguishes among bacteria with similar morphology by classifying them as gram-negative or gram-positive. Certain organisms such as the tubercle bacilli and other mycobacteria cannot be stained using this method and require acid-fast staining techniques.

Nursing Implications. Obtaining a nose or throat culture rarely causes the client discomfort, but tell the client that a cotton swab will be inserted into the nose or throat to obtain a specimen. Explain the purpose for the specimen—that is, to identify organisms present and which antibiotic will suppress them. Nose and throat cultures are obtained by the following methods:

- For cultures from the nares, introduce the swab as far back as possible without bending it and rotate it gently.
- For cultures from the pharynx (throat), avoid touching the tongue or teeth, which would result in contamination. Depress the tongue with a tongue blade. Swab the posterior wall of the pharynx below the level of the uvula. The swab should be rotated over any involved or inflamed areas. The specimen collected on the swab should be placed in the appropriate container and taken to the laboratory as soon as possible to prevent drying of the organisms.

Sputum cultures are often indicated in problems of the respiratory system. Obtaining sputum specimens is discussed in the next section. Other culture specimens (eg, from abscesses in the lungs) are obtained during bronchoscopy.

Sputum Cytology

Sputum cytology involves the detailed examination of the cellular structures of sputum under a microscope. This is primarily done to assist in the identification of malignant cells in individuals suspected of having lung cancer.

Nursing Implications. When obtaining a sputum specimen, keep in mind:

- The optimal time for obtaining a specimen is early in the morning. The first sputum expectorated will contain secretions that have pooled in the client's lungs during the night, giving a more productive sample.
- To decrease contamination of the sputum, the client should rinse out the mouth without swallowing, brush the teeth, or both.
- For a true sputum sample (not saliva), the client should take several deep breaths and then cough forcefully.

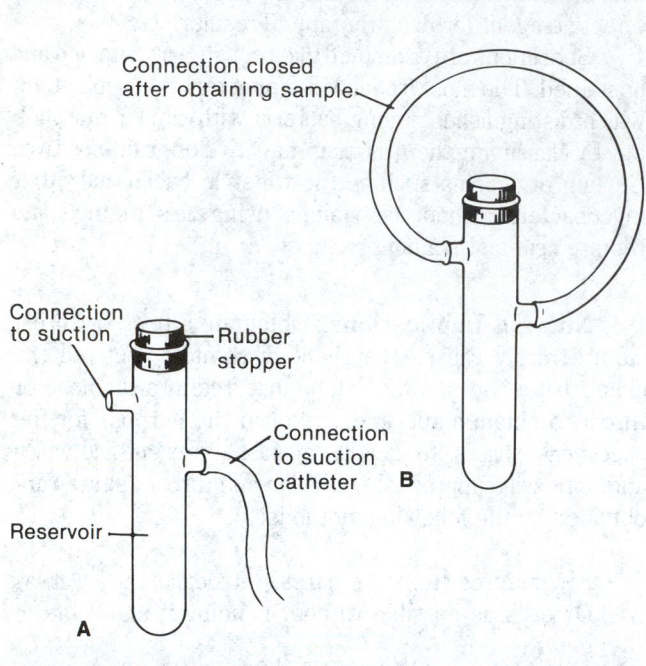

Figure 18–4

A. Sputum trap (Lukin's tube) used when suctioning is necessary to collect a sterile sputum specimen. **B.** Tubing is disconnected from suction catheter and connected to suction orifice to maintain asepsis.

- If the client cannot cough up a sputum sample, three different techniques can be used to obtain the specimen: postural drainage, inhalation of cold steam or nebulized vapor, and suctioning. If suctioning is used, a sputum collection trap is used to obtain a sterile sample (Figure 18–4).

- When cultures are being obtained, the specimens should be collected in sterile containers using sterile technique.

Skin Tests

Mantoux Intradermal Skin Test. This test is used in the detection of tuberculosis (TBC). Anyone infected with the tubercle bacillus develops hypersensitivity to certain products of the organism. These byproduct antigens are extracted and refined into a product called purified protein derivative (PPD). The PPD is then stabilized. A concentration of 5 tuberculin units of Tween-stabilized PPD-tuberculin is the strength most commonly used. The method of administering the test is to inject 0.1 mL of this solution just beneath the surface of the skin on the inner aspect of the forearm, with the bevel of the needle upward. If the fluid is injected properly, a raised area 6 to 10 mm in diameter will appear on the surface of the skin. Anyone who has been previously sensitized will show an induration and

erythema at the injection site as T-lymphocytes collect there over 48 to 72 hours. It usually requires 2 to 10 weeks after the initial infection with the bacilli for a positive tuberculin test. An induration measuring 10 mm or more within 72 hours is considered indicative of infection with *Mycobacterium tuberculosis* (Figure 18–5). A reading of between 5 and 9 mm of induration is considered doubtful unless there is known exposure to the organism. With 0 to 4 mm of induration, the result is considered negative.

The tuberculin test is not 100% accurate. In addition, a positive test merely indicates that tuberculosis exposure occurred at some point in the past. It does not mean active disease is present. Also, a negative reaction does not necessarily rule out TBC. Incorrect results may occur because of errors in the administration and reading of the test, the nature of the test material, or factors related to the test subjects. Clients with certain illnesses, those who are poorly nourished, or those on immunosuppressive drugs can have false negative reactions to the Mantoux skin test. False positive reactions can occur because *Mycobacterium tuberculosis* shares numerous antigens with many other Mycobacteria that can also produce a positive skin test.

The booster phenomenon can also occur with tuberculin skin tests. Skin test reactivity declines over time. Those who are tested after several years will show a small reaction or no reaction at all. The introduction of the tuberculin test antigen can boost this waned sensitivity. Thus, if the tuberculin test is readministered within a relatively short time, the new skin reaction may be considerably larger, leading the interpreter of the test to believe a new infection has developed. The booster effect can be controlled for by administering a second tuberculin test about 1 week after the initial reaction if that reaction was smaller than 10 mm in diameter. Since 1 week does not allow for a true conversion to take place, clients who have a reaction of 10 mm

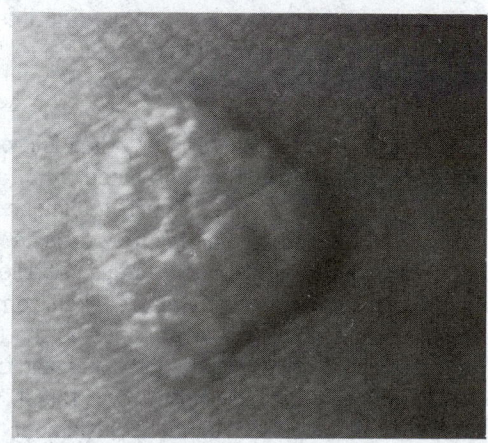

Figure 18–5

Positive Mantoux test. (Courtesy of Millard Fillmore Hospital, Buffalo, NY)

or more on the second test are classified as infected but are considered to have boosted rather than converted from negative to positive (Glassroth, 1981).

False positive results may also be due to previous administration of the BCG vaccine. Bacillus Calmette-Guerin (BCG) contains live, attenuated bovine tubercle bacilli. The substance is incapable of producing active disease. In the past, many health care providers received BCG to increase their resistance to TBC. These people will always have a positive tuberculin skin test.

Multiple puncture devices such as the tine test are not recommended for individual screening because they are not as reliable as the Mantoux test. The amount of concentrated tuberculin is not standardized in the multiple puncture technique, which is recommended only in the screening of large groups. Any positive tests should be followed with the Mantoux test.

Nursing implications for the Mantoux intradermal skin test include the following measures. Explain the procedure carefully because client cooperation is essential; the elderly may have great anxiety about TBC, as may newcomers from third-world countries; and young clients may never have heard of TBC. Reassure the client that the test is relatively painless and that the solution is injected into the superficial layers of the skin only. Question the client about whether they have had a positive tuberculin skin test in the past, have recently been exposed to anyone with TBC, or have ever received a tuberculosis vaccine (BCG). Remind the client to report back to have the skin test read after 48 hours. The nurse must communicate the importance of returning, since results of this test will indicate whether the client may require further testing and/or treatment for tuberculosis. A chest x-ray is necessary for any client with a positive Mantoux skin test.

Skin Test for Coccidioidomycosis. Skin tests for coccidioidomycosis, a respiratory fungal disease, can be performed with mycelium-derived antigen coccidioidin or the newer, more sensitive spherulin (produced from the parasitic spherule). The procedure for administering the test is similar to that for the Mantoux tuberculin test; the test is read in 24 to 48 hours. A positive reaction (0.5 mm or more of induration) indicates past infection. This test becomes diagnostic only when conversion to positive occurs during the course of the clinical illness. A positive skin test indicates intact cell-mediated immunity. This immunity is frequently lost during the course of dissemination of the disease and means a poor prognosis (Einstein, 1981).

Immunoglobulins

These serum proteins, produced by lymphocytes and plasma cells, function as antibodies in the body's immune defense system. Immunoglobulins can be separated for study by electrophoresis. The five main immunoglobulin serum proteins are IgG, IgA, IgM, IgD, and IgE. The levels of one or more immunoglobulin fractions may change in pneu-

monia, tuberculosis, and pulmonary fungal infections such as coccidioidomycosis (Byrne et al., 1986). For this test, the nurse need only prepare for the withdrawal of a venous blood sample.

Indirect Laryngoscopy

This standard diagnostic examination allows the examiner to view the vocal cords and other laryngeal structures by inserting a mirror into the oropharynx. Clients are usually positioned so they are sitting all the way back in the chair with the head and shoulders forward (Figure 18–6). Mirrors of different sizes can be used, depending on the amount of space between the tonsils. The examiner dips the mirror in warm or hot water and dries it with gauze to prevent fogging when the mirror is placed in the client's mouth. The client is asked to stick out the tongue. The examiner grasps the tongue with gauze, pulls it away from the back wall of the pharynx, and places the mirror near (but not touching) the back wall. Touching the tonsils or back of the tongue will cause the client to gag. The desired position is that from which the laryngeal orifice and the epiglottis can be seen (Figure 18–7). The examiner can inspect the area when the client is quiet and when the client says "ah."

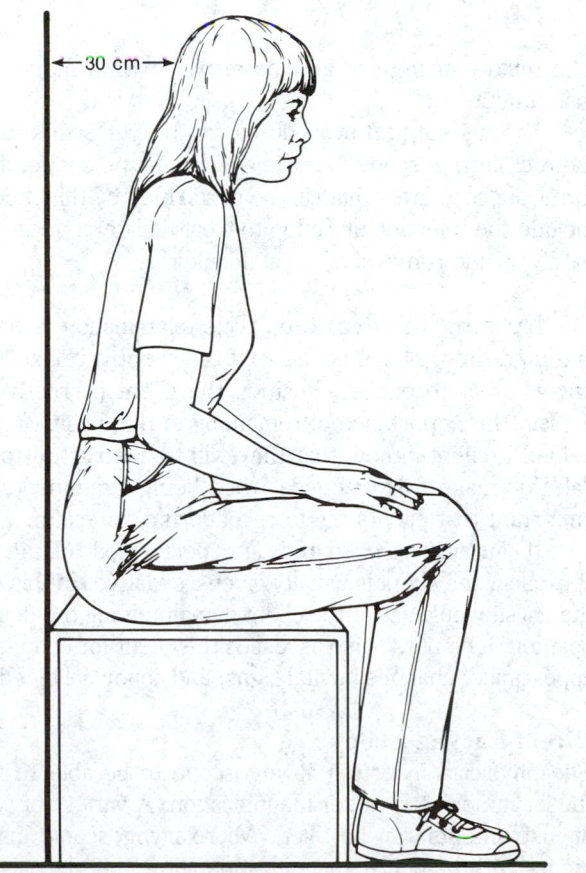

Figure 18–6

Proper client position for indirect laryngoscopy.

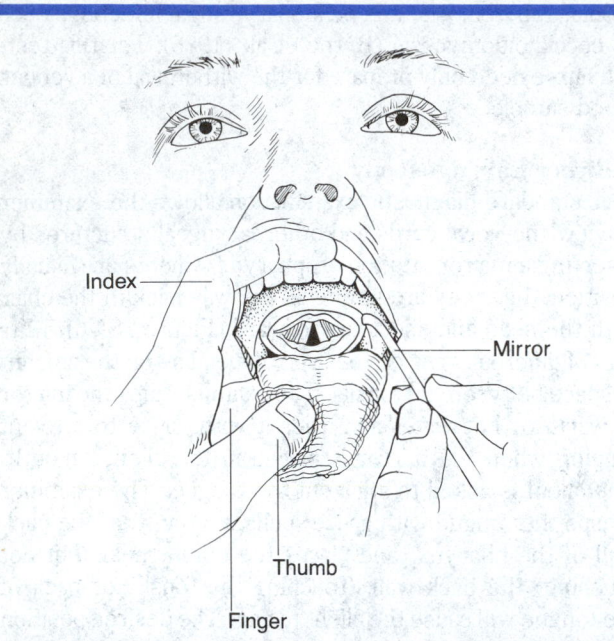

Index

Mirror

Thumb

Finger

Figure 18–7

The mirror image of the vocal cords in indirect laryngoscopy. The index finger holds up upper lip; client's tongue is
grasped with a fold of gauze.

The mirror image can also be viewed with a magnifying
instrument.

Various surgical procedures can be performed using
indirect laryngoscopy, but the client must be cooperative.
Surgical procedures that can be performed by this method
include the injection of Teflon to treat unilateral vocal cord
paralysis and removal of vocal nodules.

Nursing Implications. This examination is easier
and more information is gained if the client is relaxed and
knows what to expect. Position the client correctly and
explain the importance of remaining in that position. It is
helpful if clients know that they will be instructed to say
"ah" or make other sounds while being examined. It is
important that clients try to relax during the exam.

If surgical procedures are performed using this
approach, the client is usually given a sedative. In this case
the nurse would assist the client in maintaining the desired
position. The nurse also assesses the client for changes in
appearance, changes in vital signs, and abnormal bleeding.

Direct Laryngoscopy

The physician inserts a laryngoscope to be able to view
the larynx directly under magnification. A variety of types
of instruments can be used. Microlaryngoscopic instruments with binocular magnification allow the physician to
view changes that cannot be seen with a mirror (Paparella
& Shumrick, 1980).

Direct laryngoscopy is used to investigate signs and
symptoms associated with the larynx, such as when a client
complains of hoarseness for more than 2 weeks, but indirect laryngoscopy shows no abnormality. Direct laryngoscopy is frequently used for such surgical procedures as
biopsy of a growth on the larynx. This procedure is usually
preferred for the removal of laryngeal polyps and vocal
cord nodules and is also used for the removal of foreign
bodies from the larynx. Trauma victims may require direct
laryngoscopy to assess the extent and severity of the injury.

Nursing Implications. Direct laryngoscopy can be
performed using either local or general anesthesia. Assure
clients that they should not experience pain during the
procedure and that the airway will be maintained throughout. Preoperative medications may be administered to help
the client relax if local anesthesia is employed. The client
should not drink or eat for several hours before the procedure, and any dentures must be removed.

After the procedure, the client will be allowed to drink
soon after waking up. If a local anesthetic is used, the nurse
must ensure that clients' gag reflex has returned and that
they can swallow. A sore or irritated throat is not uncommon from passage of the laryngoscope. The client should
be observed for signs and symptoms of respiratory distress from laryngeal edema or spasm.

After the removal of laryngeal polyps or vocal cord
nodules, the client should rest the voice for several days.
Clearing the throat and coughing should be avoided if
possible.

Bronchoscopy

Bronchoscopy is the direct viewing of the trachea and
tracheobronchial tree by means of a standard metal bronchoscope or a fiberoptic bronchoscope (Figure 18–8). The
fiberoptic bronchoscope is a slender flexible tube with mirrors and a light at the distal end. A brush, biopsy forceps,
or catheter may be passed through the bronchoscope to
obtain samples for cytologic examination (Hollen, Toomey,
& Given, 1982).

The fiberoptic bronchoscope is more common today
than the rigid bronchoscope; because it is small and flexible, it allows better visualization of the segmental and
subsegmental bronchi. There is also less risk of trauma
from intubation when the fiberoptic bronchoscope is used
(Hollen et al., 1982).

Bronchoscopy is used in the diagnosis of such conditions as hemoptysis, lesions, masses, and abnormalities
seen on chest x-ray. Bronchoscopy may also be used to
treat lung abscesses, pneumonia, aspiration, to debride
mucosal eschar resulting from burns and other inhalation
injuries, and to remove foreign bodies. Bronchoscopy can
aid in removal of excessive tenacious secretions when
nasotracheal suctioning is ineffective (Cameron, 1981).

Bronchoscopy is performed with the client sitting or
supine. The fiberoptic bronchoscope is inserted either
through the client's nose or mouth, whereas the rigid bronchoscope is inserted through the mouth. The bronchoscopy tube is made up of four channels—two channels to

provide a light source; one visualizing channel to see through; and one open channel in which biopsy forceps, cytology brush, suctioning, anesthetic gas, or oxygen can be passed (Hollen, Toomey, & Given, 1982).

Nursing Implications. Bronchoscopy entails a certain amount of physical discomfort. The client is likely to be anxious not only about pain but also about the findings, especially if the procedure is being performed to confirm the presence of a tumor. Take time not only to explain the procedure but to answer any questions the client may have and allay any anxieties based on misconceptions. Clients should be told that they will receive an intravenous sedative to help them relax, and that a local anesthetic will be sprayed into the nose and mouth to suppress the gag reflex. This will produce the sensation of a dry mouth, swollen tongue, and swollen throat, and will make the client unable to swallow. Clients should be reassured that they will be able to breathe during the procedure. The client takes nothing by mouth 6 to 12 hours prior to the procedure, and any dentures are removed. Occasionally, clients will require a general anesthetic. A signed consent form is necessary.

Following bronchoscopy vital signs are monitored. The conscious client is placed in a semi-Fowler's position, and the unconscious client is positioned on one side with the head of the bed slightly elevated. An emesis basin should be provided and the client instructed to expectorate secretions into the basin rather than swallow them so the nurse can observe them. Clients should be advised that clearing the throat or coughing could dislodge a clot and possibly cause hemorrhage. Watch for subcutaneous emphysema, which may indicate tracheal or bronchial perforation. Foods and fluids are restricted until the gag reflex returns. Hoarseness and a sore throat can be relieved by gargles and throat lozenges. Watch for any breathing difficulty (from laryngeal edema or laryngospasm), hemoptysis, symptoms of a pneumothorax, and bronchospasm (Hollen et al., 1982).

Mediastinoscopy

In this procedure, the surgeon makes an incision over the mediastinum and inserts a scope to explore the area. The mediastinum is the area in which the esophagus, trachea, great vessels, and heart are located. Mediastinoscopy is also used to obtain biopsies of lymph nodes or other masses, to determine the presence of lymph node metastases due to bronchogenic carcinoma, and to diagnose intrathoracic sarcoidosis (Paparella & Shumrick, 1980). A common approach is through an incision in the suprasternal notch, which allows for endoscopic examination of the upper half of the mediastinum, including the proximal part of the major bronchi.

Nursing Implications. Mediastinoscopy can be performed under either local or general anesthesia. Tell clients that the procedure will leave a small incision with a dressing covering it postoperatively and that the incision site might be somewhat sore for a few days. The client should not eat or drink anything for several hours prior to the procedure. Clients are given a full explanation of the procedure and its purpose in terms they can understand. A signed consent is necessary.

Postoperative nursing care includes monitoring vital signs, observing for bleeding from the incision site, and alleviating discomfort by comfort measures or administering prescribed pain medication as appropriate. The nurse should also observe the wound for signs and symptoms of infection. Possible complications, in addition to hemorrhage and wound infection, include right recurrent laryngeal nerve paralysis and esophageal perforation.

Bronchography

On a chest x-ray, a small portion of the bronchial tree beyond the first two major divisions is visible. To diagnose abnormalities of the smaller sections of the bronchial tree, bronchography may be performed. The diagnostic test begins with instillation of radiopaque contrast medium through a catheter into the lumen of the trachea and bronchial tree. Chest x-rays are then taken.

Bronchography is primarily indicated for diagnosing bronchiectasis and ascertaining its location before surgical

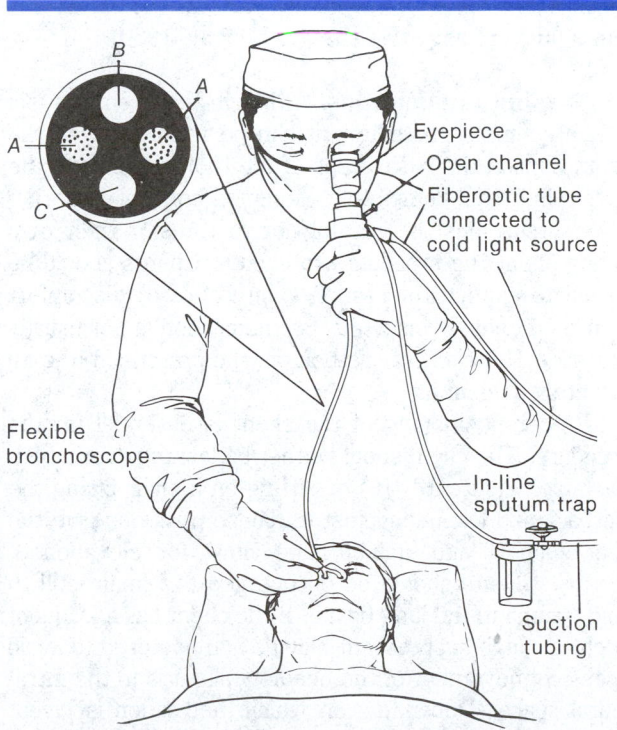

Figure 18–8

Bronchoscopy. The bronchoscopic tube, inserted through the nostril into the bronchi, has four channels (see inset). Two light channels provide a light source: one visualizing channel to see through and one open channel that accommodates biopsy forceps, cytology brush, suctioning, lavage, anesthetic, or oxygen.

resection. Bronchography may also aid in diagnosing compression, obstruction, presence of a foreign body, or a lesion in the trachea or larger bronchi. Figure 18–9 illustrates a bronchogram.

Nursing Implications. Explain the procedure and make sure that the client understands the explanation. This includes informing clients that they will be placed in various positions to aid in distribution of the dye. Question the client and also check the chart for known hypersensitivity to the dye used for the procedure.

Proper visualization requires that the airways be as free of secretions as possible. To achieve this, the nurse may have to carry out bronchial drainage, nasotracheal suctioning, or both. The client should have nothing by mouth for several hours prior to the procedure. A signed consent is necessary.

After completion of the procedure, monitor the client's vital signs. To facilitate removal of the contrast medium, deep breathing and sighing, postural drainage, and nasotracheal suctioning are usually necessary. Before allowing the client to drink, check for return of the gag reflex by stimulating the posterior pharynx with a swab or tongue blade. If the reflex is not yet present, the client will not gag and is vulnerable to aspiration.

Thoracentesis

Thoracentesis has been employed for years to aid in the identification of disease involving the pleura. The physician inserts a needle into the intrapleural space to obtain a fluid specimen for diagnostic purposes. Thoracentesis may also be performed to remove fluid from the client with a pleural effusion. After the selected area is cleansed, a local anesthetic is injected into the skin. The needle is then inserted and fluid aspirated.

The presence of fluid in the intrapleural space is abnormal. The amount, color, odor, and character of the fluid should be noted in the chart. The fluid may be described as serous, serosanguineous, or turbid. Serous fluid may be obtained from clients who have disorders of nontraumatic origin, including congestive heart failure, pleural effusion due to a malignancy, granulomatous disease, and disorders resulting in inflammation. Blood in the fluid is usually due to trauma to the lungs, but it may be seen in clients with an advanced malignancy. Turbid fluid in the intrapleural space is most commonly from an infectious process.

Rarely, hyperalimentation solution may be present in the fluid. This occurs when a central venous line is placed into the intrapleural space instead of the vena cava, and the hyperalimentation solution is infused via this intravenous line.

No more than 1000 to 1500 mL of fluid should be removed at any one time because of the danger of hypotension. The specimen is sent to the laboratory where the following tests are usually performed: red cell count, white cell count with differential, protein, sugar, lactic acid dehydrogenase, amylase, pH, cultures, bacteriologic stains, and pleural fluid cytology (Hinshaw & Murray, 1980).

Nursing Implications. Although thoracentesis is a relatively simple procedure, it can be frightening to the client. Explain the basic steps of the thoracentesis to the client calmly and completely. A signed consent is necessary. Nurses must be careful not to transfer their own anxiety about the procedure to clients. Clients should be warned to expect a sensation of pressure or discomfort when the needle is inserted. Premedication is not usually necessary. However, medication may be prescribed to calm a frightened client.

Proper positioning of the client is essential for the procedure. The client should either be leaning over a bedside table (Figure 18–10) or sitting on a chair facing the chairback and leaning against it. These positions give the client support and stability and allow for elevation of the ribs. Clients should be encouraged to remain still to avoid trauma to the lung tissue. If the client has a frequent cough, a cough suppressant may be administered to avoid excessive movement of the needle while it is in the intrapleural space. Depending on which medication is given, the timing is important for maximum effectiveness. Remain with the client throughout the procedure to provide support and monitor vital signs.

Complications of thoracentesis are relatively rare. They include hemorrhage, pain, and pneumothorax. After the procedure, monitor the client's vital signs and respiratory status to detect any adverse reactions. The insertion site

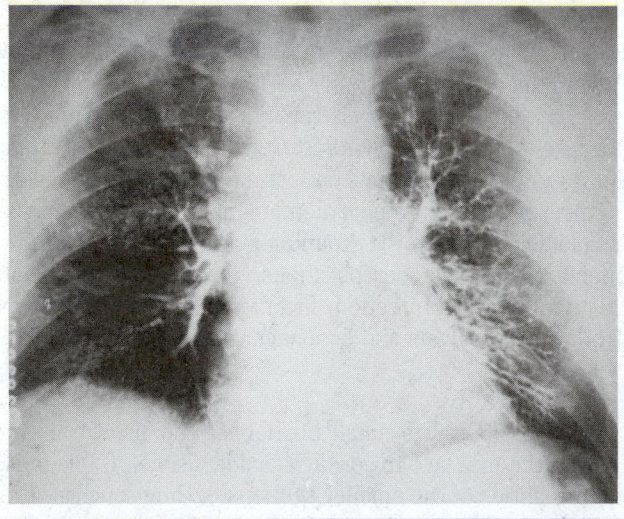

Figure 18–9

Bronchography.

SOURCE: Petty T: *Intensive and Rehabilitative Respiratory Care*, 3rd ed. Philadelphia: Lea & Febiger, 1982.

should be observed for swelling that could result from bleeding into the area.

Lung Biopsy

Both open and closed approaches are used to obtain lung tissue for cytologic analysis and culture. Closed approaches include fine needle aspiration, biopsy via a percutaneous cutting needle, and biopsy via fiberoptic bronchoscope. All closed procedures are done under local anesthesia with fluoroscopic guidance. Open lung biopsy requires a thoracotomy. This approach provides the largest volume of tissue, but general anesthesia is needed. Lung biopsy is indicated when the client's diagnosis remains unclear despite a complete work-up.

   Nursing Implications. Explain the basic procedure. If only local anesthetic is used, clients should be told that the area will be numbed, but they will probably still feel some pressure or discomfort when the biopsy is taken. Clients may be asked not to eat or drink anything for a few hours prior to the procedure. A signed consent is necessary.

   When the biopsy is completed, observe the site for swelling or bleeding, and watch the client for approxi-

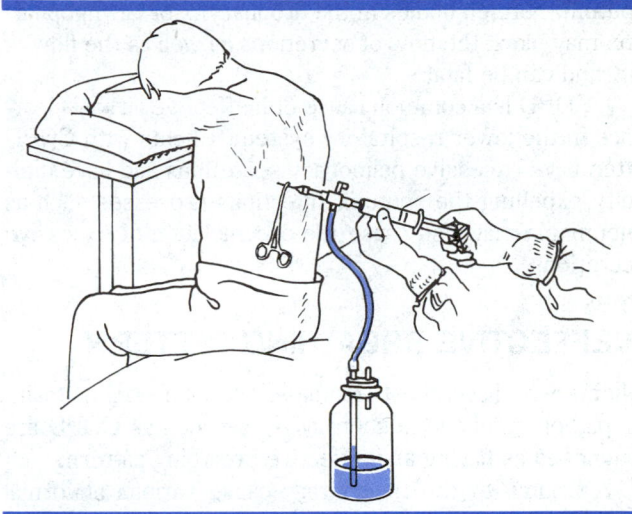

Figure 18–10

Client position for thoracentesis.

mately 24 hours for any signs and symptoms of pneumothorax, air embolism, or hemorrhage.

Section II: Nursing Diagnosis

Assessment of clients with respiratory dysfunction involves obtaining the history, a physical examination, and reviewing the results of diagnostic studies. A list of nursing diagnoses commonly related to respiratory dysfunction is shown in Box 18–1. The three major nursing diagnoses—airway clearance, ineffective; breathing pattern, ineffective; and gas exchange, impaired—are discussed in the following sections.

INEFFECTIVE AIRWAY CLEARANCE

The nursing diagnosis of ineffective airway clearance is frequent. The degree may range from mild to severe and may be related specifically to either the upper or lower respiratory system, or both. The client may experience difficulty maintaining normal airflow into and out of the lungs because of structural obstruction, foreign bodies, or the presence of excessive tenacious nasal or bronchial secretions.

   For example, the client with acute rhinitis or sinusitis may have nasal and sinus secretions that make it difficult or impossible to breathe through the nose. The presence of nasal polyps or turbinates enlarged as a result of an allergic response will also decrease the airflow through the nasal passage. Inadequate drainage of the paranasal sinuses can result in a chronic infectious sinusitis that may necessitate surgical intervention. Secretions may be present in the oropharynx from postnasal drip or an infectious

process such as pharyngitis or tonsillitis and may impair the client's ability to swallow, speak, or breathe. These symptoms can also be caused by a tumor in the oropharynx or laryngopharynx that blocks the flow of sputum when the client coughs. Enlargement of structures in the oropharynx such as the tonsils may also block attempts to expel

---

Box 18–1   Nursing Diagnoses Commonly Related to Respiratory Dysfunction

Diagnoses Directly Related to Respiratory Dysfunction

Airway clearance, ineffective
Breathing pattern, ineffective
Gas exchange, impaired

Additional Potential Nursing Diagnoses

Communication, impaired verbal
Mobility, impaired physical
Nutrition, alterations in: less than body requirements
Tissue perfusion, alteration in: cardiopulmonary
Activity intolerance
Oral mucous membrane, alterations in
Social isolation

sputum. Foreign bodies in the oropharynx or laryngopharynx may block the flow of secretions as well as the flow of air, and can be fatal.

COPD is a common cause of ineffective airway clearance in the lower respiratory system. Clients with COPD often have excessive pulmonary secretions and have difficulty expelling the sputum. Infectious processes such as pneumonia may also cause the accumulation of excessive secretions.

INEFFECTIVE BREATHING PATTERN

Clients who have chest trauma, chest or abdominal pain, or pathology of the pulmonary tissue such as COPD are diagnosed as having an ineffective breathing pattern.

Trauma to the thorax may cause various abnormal breathing patterns leading to ineffective ventilation. These may occur as a result of pneumothorax, hemothorax, flail chest, tension pneumothorax, and mediastinal shift. When these conditions prevent air from moving in and out of the lungs effectively, various signs of respiratory distress may be observed, such as dyspnea, cyanosis, or use of accessory muscles, depending on the injury.

Clients experiencing pain in the chest or abdomen often tend to "guard" by breathing as little as possible to avoid increasing the pain. This hypoventilation in turn leads to impaired gas exchange over a few days.

Clients with pathology of the pulmonary tissue often show signs that they are having difficulty moving air in and out of their lungs. For example, clients with emphysema experience "air trapping" in the alveoli and have difficulty exhaling fully. These clients often lean forward and purse their lips to facilitate movement of air. Clients with asthma or allergic reactions may experience bronchospasm and have difficulty ventilating. Wheezing can often be heard when the lungs of these clients are auscultated.

IMPAIRED GAS EXCHANGE

Any disorder of the respiratory system may result in a nursing diagnosis of impaired gas exchange, depending on the degree to which it interferes with ventilation and perfusion of the pulmonary system. This state, although abnormal, is "normal" for certain clients with respiratory disorders. For example, some clients with COPD have a higher PCO_2 and lower PO_2 than clients without a respiratory disorder.

The diagnosis of impaired gas exchange may refer to three different abnormalities: respiratory acidosis, respiratory alkalosis, and hypoxia.

Respiratory Acidosis (Hypercapnia)

Hypercapnia occurs when a disorder results in interference with gas exchange or decreases the amount of effective alveolar ventilation. The underlying cause of this abnormal state is always related to hypoventilation. Respiratory acidosis is observed in certain clients with COPD, with pneumonia, or with decreased respiratory function as a result of drugs or trauma. Clients in respiratory acidosis may exhibit the following signs and symptoms: confusion, drowsiness, headache, dizziness, tetany, asterixis, tachycardia, dysrhythmias, convulsions, and coma.

Respiratory Alkalosis (Hypocapnia)

As opposed to respiratory acidosis, respiratory alkalosis occurs in disorders resulting in hyperventilation. This impairment in gas exchange is observed in certain clients who have experienced brain injury or have intracranial tumors. It is also seen in clients with gram-negative sepsis, those experiencing an acute asthma attack, and those who are extremely anxious. Signs and symptoms of respiratory alkalosis include diaphoresis, tetany, cardiac dysrhythmias, tachypnea, and loss of consciousness.

Hypoxia

Certain disorders affect the body's ability to deliver oxygen to the tissues, resulting in hypoxia. Disorders that limit the volume of air entering the lungs and produce hypoventilation result in inadequate amounts of available oxygen at the alveolar level. Conditions that can lead to hypoxia include restrictive lung diseases such as pulmonary fibrosis, occupational lung diseases, and sarcoidosis. Hypoxia can also result from obstructive lung diseases such as asthma, chronic bronchitis, and emphysema. Signs and symptoms of hypoxia include: headache, restlessness, irritability, fatigue, tachycardia, hypertension, cardiac dysrhythmias, tachypnea, dyspnea, exercise intolerance, clubbing of the fingers, mental confusion, and coma.

Section III: Planning and Implementation

A sample nursing care plan for the client with dysfunction of the respiratory system is presented in Table 18–2 and discussed in this and the following section on evaluation.

PROMOTING AIRWAY CLEARANCE

A variety of nursing interventions may be employed when the nursing diagnosis is ineffective airway clearance. The most useful, which are included in the nursing care plan in Table 18–2, include pursed-lip breathing, diaphragmatic breathing, postural drainage, and nasotracheal suctioning. In severe disorders, the client may require intubation and placement on a mechanical ventilator.

(continued on page 28)

Table 18–2 Sample Nursing Care Plan for Clients With Respiratory Dysfunction

Nursing Diagnosis	Client Care Goals	Plan/Nursing Implementation	Expected Outcomes
Airway clearance, ineffective, related to: excessive, tenacious secretions from inflammation of the upper airway	Decrease in or absence of secretions of the upper respiratory tract	Assess for redness and swelling of the upper airway; note amount and characteristics of drainage; assess for discomfort of the nose, paranasal sinuses, and pharynx; monitor vital signs at regular intervals; administer prescribed humidified air or oxygen as appropriate; administer prescribed decongestants/antihistamines as needed; suction nasal or oropharyngeal area using aseptic technique if necessary	• Absence of nasal obstruction • Absence of nasal discharge • Absence of nasal stuffiness • Sinus films normal • Absence of inflammation, redness, and tenderness over paranasal sinuses • Absence of headache • Absence of inflammation, redness, and drainage in pharynx • Voice return to normal • Absence of sore throat • Absence of dysphagia • Normal vital signs • Intake of 2000 to 3000 mL of fluid per day
	Maintain adequate fluid intake	Encourage fluids, at least 1000 mL/shift	
	Understand measures necessary to avoid spread of infection to others	Instruct in measures to prevent spread of infectious organisms such as decreased personal contact with others, hand-washing, proper tissue disposal, and covering mouth and nose when coughing and sneezing	Acts to prevent spread of infection
	Describe the benefits of humidification and adequate hydration	Instruct that humidification and adequate hydration will facilitate removal of secretions; include cold mist or steam humidifier, pans of water around room, fluid intake	Acts to obtain the benefits of adequate hydration and humidification and implements it in the home
	Describe how to blow nose and cough to remove secretions effectively	Instruct the client how to blow the nose and cough to remove nasal and pharyngeal secretions effectively	Uses correct method of blowing nose and coughing
	Describe how to administer decongestants/antihistamines properly	Instruct client in use of decongestants/antihistamines; include family members when carrying out teaching measures	Follows proper administration of decongestants/antihistamines
Airway clearance, ineffective, related to: excessive, tenacious secretions from inflammation of the lower airway	Remove secretions from the lower respiratory tract effectively	Assess the pulmonary status of the client: monitor and record amount, consistency, and color of sputum; auscultate lungs for abnormal breath sounds (rales, rhonchi, wheezing); monitor vital signs at regular intervals; monitor for signs and symptoms of arterial blood gas abnormalities	• Absence of purulent, tenacious sputum • Sputum C&S negative • Lungs clear to auscultation • Chest x-ray normal • Vital signs are within normal limits • Arterial blood gas values within normal limits for the client
	Maintain adequate oxygen to tissues	Measures to remove excessive secretions from the lower respiratory tract may include: turning a bedridden client every 2 h; having a client cough and deep breathe at least every 2 h; if appropriate, getting client out of bed three times each shift; pursed-lip breathing, diaphragmatic breathing, and/or postural	Absence of adventitious breath sounds; absence of signs and symptoms of hypoxemia

(continued)

Table 18–2   Sample Nursing Care Plan for Clients With Respiratory Dysfunction (continued)

Nursing Diagnosis	Client Care Goals	Plan/Nursing Implementation	Expected Outcomes
		drainage as prescribed; suctioning using sterile technique; administering IPPB treatments as prescribed; administering prescribed expectorants, bronchodilators, steroids, as appropriate; administering prescribed oxygen as needed	
	Maintain acceptable intake and output	Ensure fluid intake of 2 to 3 L/day (fluid requirement will vary with weight and physical condition; fluid restrictions may be necessary in disease states such as congestive heart failure and renal failure); careful monitoring of intake and output; inspect skin turgor daily; monitor vital signs at regular intervals	• Drinks 2000 to 3000 mL fluid per day • Good skin turgor • Absence of tenacious secretions • Intake and output within acceptable limits
	Describe how to cough and perform breathing exercises	Instruct on proper technique used in coughing and breathing exercises	Performs coughing and breathing exercises correctly
	Describe how to make use of oxygen and breathing equipment	Instruct client in use and proper placement of oxygen delivery equipment; instruct in correct use of breathing equipment such as incentive spirometer	Uses oxygen and breathing equipment correctly
	Discuss proper administration of prescribed medications	Instruct in the actions, side effects, and proper administration of medications	Complies with instructions as to administration of medications, reports side effects, understands actions and reports any ineffective medication
	Identify measures to avoid development of a respiratory tract infection	Reinforce measures to prevent spread of infection; instruct in measures to prevent development of a respiratory infection such as avoiding contact with an infected individual, hand washing, and taking precautions to maintain optimal health; include family members when teaching	• Acts to prevent spread of infection • Acts to prevent development of respiratory tract infections • Actions of family members show they understand information
Breathing pattern, ineffective, related to: inadequate chest expansion from pain or trauma	Maintain normal respiratory rate and pattern	Assess client for: respiratory rate and depth; symmetrical chest expansion; abnormal breath sounds; fractured ribs; tracheal deviation; fluctuation of vital signs; pain upon inspiration and upon movement, as with a fractured rib	• Adequate aeration of lungs as evidenced by: normal breath sounds; normal chest x-ray; normal arterial blood gas values • Vital signs within normal limits • Symmetrical chest expansion (These outcomes hold for all nursing interventions under this problem)
	Remain free of complications that can result from trauma	Note signs that may indicate inadequate ventilation: stridor, use of accessory muscles, flaring of nares, dyspnea, asymmetric chest movement, paradoxical breathing, open chest wound, hemoptysis, subcutaneous emphysema, tracheal devia-	

Nursing Diagnosis	Client Care Goals	Plan/Nursing Implementation	Expected Outcomes
		tion, hyperresonance on percussion, dullness on percussion, diminished or absent breath sounds	
	Tolerate pain on breathing within limits	Assess client for location, type, and intensity of pain; provide comfort measures: positioning; splinting when coughing and deep breathing; administer prescribed analgesics as appropriate; assess respiratory rate after administration of narcotic analgesic to identify any respiratory depression; assess respiratory rate, depth, and chest expansion; monitor vital signs at regular intervals	• Pain sensation remains within tolerable limits as reported by client • Vital signs within normal limits
	Understand reasons for procedures and what to expect during them	Carefully prepare client and family members for procedures: explain reason procedure is performed, length of procedure; discuss steps involved in procedure; inform client about likely sensations during the procedure and that pain medication is available	• Expresses feelings and anxiety about conditions and situation
		Maintain a patent airway: suction as necessary; prepare to assist with intubation or tracheotomy; place in a semi-Fowler's position unless contraindicated	• Adequate ventilation and oxygenation as evidence by: normal lung sounds; normal pulmonary function studies; normal chest x-ray; normal arterial blood gas values
		Maintain optimal pulmonary ventilation: prepare for insertion of chest tube if necessary; monitor for adequate function of the closed chest tube system; encourage client to perform pulmonary hygiene measures such as coughing and deep breathing exercises on a set schedule. Administer humidified oxygen as necessary; administer IPPB treatments as necessary; monitor vital signs at regular intervals as indicated; prepare client for placement on a mechanical ventilator; monitor client who requires mechanical ventilation	• Chest tube system functioning normally • Normal function of the ventilator
Breathing pattern, ineffective, related to: pathophysiological conditions (eg, COPD, pulmonary fibrosis, infection, neuromuscular disorders, musculoskeletal disorders, and carcinoma)	Maintain optimal pulmonary ventilation	Assess for signs of inadequate ventilation: dyspnea, increased respiratory rate, shallow respiration, use of accessory muscles, nasal flaring, pursed-lip breathing, increased anterior-posterior diameter, diminished or absent breath sounds, signs of hypoxia and hypercapnia/hypocapnia; encourage measures to promote pulmonary hygiene such as coughing and deep breathing, chest physical therapy, breathing exercises, and suctioning; administer humidified oxygen as prescribed; administer IPPB treatment as prescribed; administer medications as pre-	• Improved ventilatory status as evidenced by: improved lung sounds upon auscultation; return to baseline levels for arterial blood gas values, chest x-ray, and pulmonary function studies • Decreased production of sputum

(continued)

Table 18–2   Sample Nursing Care Plan for Clients With Respiratory Dysfunction (continued)

Nursing Diagnosis	Client Care Goals	Plan/Nursing Implementation	Expected Outcomes
		scribed: antibiotics, bronchodilators, expectorants, steroids; prepare for intubation and mechanical ventilation when indicated	
	Explain reasons for procedures and pulmonary hygiene measures	Carefully prepare client and family members for necessary procedures: explain reason procedure is performed; discuss steps involved in procedure; inform client what sensations to expect during the procedure and explain that pain medication is available; explain and demonstrate breathing exercises	• Expresses feelings and anxiety about condition and situation; can demonstrate breathing exercises
	Understand and able to perform care measures needed for long-term management	Teaching intervention for long-term management should include: avoiding individuals and situations where respiratory tract infections are likely; notifying a care provider at the first sign of development of a respiratory tract infection; avoiding exposure to irritants such as smoking and other air pollutants; performing bronchial hygiene measures such as effective coughing technique, breathing exercises, and bronchial drainage; using respiratory equipment if necessary, such as nebulizers, IPPB machines, and oxygen delivery systems; reporting symptoms indicative of hypercapnia and hypoxia; maintaining adequate hydration and nutrition; following an organized pulmonary rehabilitation program	• Client and family members carry out measures for long-term management
	Maintain a positive self-concept	Consultation with social service if change in occupation is required; encourage client to express feelings related to curtailment in social interaction because of disease process	• Copes effectively with physical and psychosocial limitations imposed by disease process
Gas exchange, impaired, related to: hypoxia from problems of diffusion, ventilation, and ventilation-perfusion	Maintain adequate oxygenation for cellular metabolism	Observe for signs and symptoms of hypoxia: restlessness, irritability, impaired judgment, central cyanosis, diaphoresis, labored breathing, tachypnea, tachycardia, fluctuation in blood pressure, alteration in level of consciousness, clubbing of the fingers; perform pulmonary hygiene measures: deep breathing and coughing, breathing exercises; administration of humidified oxygen; IPPB treatments as prescribed; chest physical therapy as indicated; perform suctioning as necessary; administer appropriate medication (bronchodilators, expectorants, antibiotics, steroids); prepare to assist with intubation and mechanical ventilation when indicated; monitor client receiving PEEP for effectiveness of therapy	• Decrease in signs and symptoms of cerebral, cardiovascular, and respiratory hypoxemia • Return to baseline normal PO_2 as reflected in arterial blood gas values • Hemoglobin values come to within normal limits • O_2 saturation returns to baseline normal values

Nursing Diagnosis	Client Care Goals	Plan/Nursing Implementation	Expected Outcomes
	Maintain orientation to self and surrounding environment	Assess client's degree of orientation; if confused, attempt to reorient to time, place, and person; perform measures to prevent client from self-harm; explain to family members and significant others that confusion may be due to a lowered oxygen level; administer oxygen as prescribed	• Client responds correctly with name, date, time, place • Family members show an understanding of the cause of confusion and how to care for the client • Copes effectively with the limitations of a lowered oxygen level
	Understand the physical limitations of hypoxia	Inform client and family members about signs and symptoms of hypoxia such as shortness of breath, fatigue, and confusion	
	Understand therapy necessary to correct hypoxia	Instruct in correct use and administration of oxygen in the hospital and at home	• Client and family members respond in ways that show correct knowledge of oxygen therapy
Gas exchange, impaired, related to: hypercapnia from hypoventilation	Maintain a PCO_2 level compatible with a normal pH	Observe for signs and symptoms of hypercapnia: confusion, drowsiness, headache, dizziness, tetany, asterixis, tachycardia, dysrhythmias, convulsion, and coma; perform pulmonary hygiene measures: deep breathing and coughing, breathing exercises; administer humidified oxygen; administer IPPB treatments as prescribed; provide chest physical therapy as indicated; perform suctioning as necessary; administer appropriate medication (bronchodilators, expectorants, antibiotics, steroids); prepare to assist with intubation and mechanical ventilation when indicated	• Decrease in signs and symptoms of cerebral, cardiovascular, and respiratory hypercapnia • Return to normal blood pH of 7.35–7.45
	Understand reasons for procedures and what to expect during them	Carefully prepare client and significant others for procedures: explain reason procedure is performed; discuss steps involved in procedure; inform client what may be felt during the procedure	• Expresses feelings and anxiety about condition and situation
Gas exchange, impaired, related to: hypocapnia from hyperventilation	Maintain PCO_2 level compatible with a normal pH	Observe for signs and symptoms of hypocapnia: muscle spasm, carpopedal spasm, tetany, diaphoresis, cardiac dysrhythmia, tachypnea, alteration in level of consciousness; carry out measures to decrease client anxiety and to slow the respiratory rate: calm approach to client, reassurance and explanation, administer antianxiety medications as prescribed, administer bronchodilators and expectorants as prescribed, assist client to breathe effectively via breathing exercises Use equipment to increase PCO_2 level as prescribed, such as rebreathing mask (or paper bag), adjustment of ventilator settings	• Decrease in signs and symptoms of cerebral, cardiovascular, and respiratory hypocapnia • Return to normal blood pH of 7.35–7.45 as reflected by arterial blood gas analysis

Pursed-Lip Breathing

Pursed-lip breathing, a slow, even expiration against pursed lips, prevents collapse of small bronchioles and reduces the amount of trapped air in the lungs. The client should be sitting up. To assume the proper lip position for pursed-lip breathing, have the client pretend to blow out a candle. Clients with emphysema can use pursed-lip breathing to maximize expiration.

Diaphragmatic Breathing

Diaphragmatic breathing (abdominal breathing) facilitates maximum use of the diaphragm in breathing. This is particularly helpful for clients who have had thoracic surgery and those with COPD.

Ask the client in the sitting position to take a deep, slow breath through the nose, concentrating on maximum expansion of the abdomen. Place the client's hand on the abdomen to feel it rise. Then have the client exhale slowly through pursed lips while contracting the abdominal muscles. The client should place manual pressure on the abdomen during expiration. Use of this breathing pattern should be encouraged during daily activities so it can become an automatic approach to breathing during periods of respiratory difficulty.

Postural Drainage

Postural drainage combines the force of gravity with normal ciliary action to move secretions from smaller to larger airways, where they can be removed by coughing or suctioning. Auscultate the client's lungs prior to postural drainage to determine which segments require drainage. Auscultate afterward to determine effectiveness of the therapy. Postural drainage can be directed to any segment of the lung. Figure 18–11 shows client positions for specific pulmonary segments.

Percussion and vibrating techniques are often used with postural drainage. Percussion with a cupped hand (Figure 18–12) helps loosen secretions and stimulate coughing. The client should use diaphragmatic breathing during percussion.

Vibration involves manual pressure on the chest using a vibrating movement of the hand during expiration. The loosening and mobilizing of mucus secretions are increased with vibration. The client should cough after the procedure.

Percussion and vibration are directed to the specific lung segments involved. For example, using Figure 18–11, to loosen secretions in the right middle lobe (position f), percuss over the anterior and lateral right chest from the midaxillary line to the sternum for about 2 minutes. Then perform three to five vibrations over the same area during expiration only.

Extremely ill or elderly clients may not be able to tolerate some of the positions for postural drainage, par-

ticularly those with the head lower than the feet. Individual modifications of position will be necessary, based on the client's condition.

Schedule postural drainage exercises before meals because sputum will be minimal and vomiting and aspiration will be prevented. Postural drainage is generally done two to four times a day.

Nasotracheal Suctioning

Clients who are not intubated may require suctioning of the tracheobronchial tree. It is important to explain the procedure to the client to allay anxiety and gain as much cooperation as possible. An explanation is important even if clients are unresponsive, since they may still be aware of activities. The client is positioned at a 45° angle unless contraindicated. Clients should be hyperoxygenated before suctioning; if they are receiving oxygen, the flow rate is increased during the procedure. Box 18–2 describes the procedure for insertion of a nasotracheal suction catheter. The procedure and basic principles of suctioning are discussed later in Table 18–4 in relation to suctioning tracheostomy and endotracheal tubes. The principles essentially remain the same, however, except that oral suctioning is a clean procedure, whereas nasotracheal, tracheostomy, and endotracheal tube suctioning are sterile procedures.

The Client With Nasal Packing

Clients with epistaxis may have a nursing diagnosis of ineffective airway clearance. Some will have difficulty breathing because of the drainage of blood through the nasopharynx into the oropharynx. They may also have difficulty expectorating the blood and may swallow a significant amount, causing them to become nauseated and to vomit. Nasal packing is inserted by the physician in an effort to control the bleeding.

As described in Chapter 19, nasal packing may be either anterior, posterior, or both. When bleeding from the anterior portion of the nose cannot be controlled by either local application of vasoconstrictor drugs or cauterization, anterior packing is inserted. Bleeding from the posterior portion of the nose is often more severe, and a posterior pack is inserted to control the bleeding.

Clients with anterior nasal packing are often sent home; however, clients who require posterior packing are usually admitted to the hospital because of risk of respiratory obstruction.

Nursing Care of the Client With Anterior Packing
Prior to discharge, tell the client to:

- Observe for bloody drainage. If bleeding begins and the gauze becomes blood-soaked, the client should

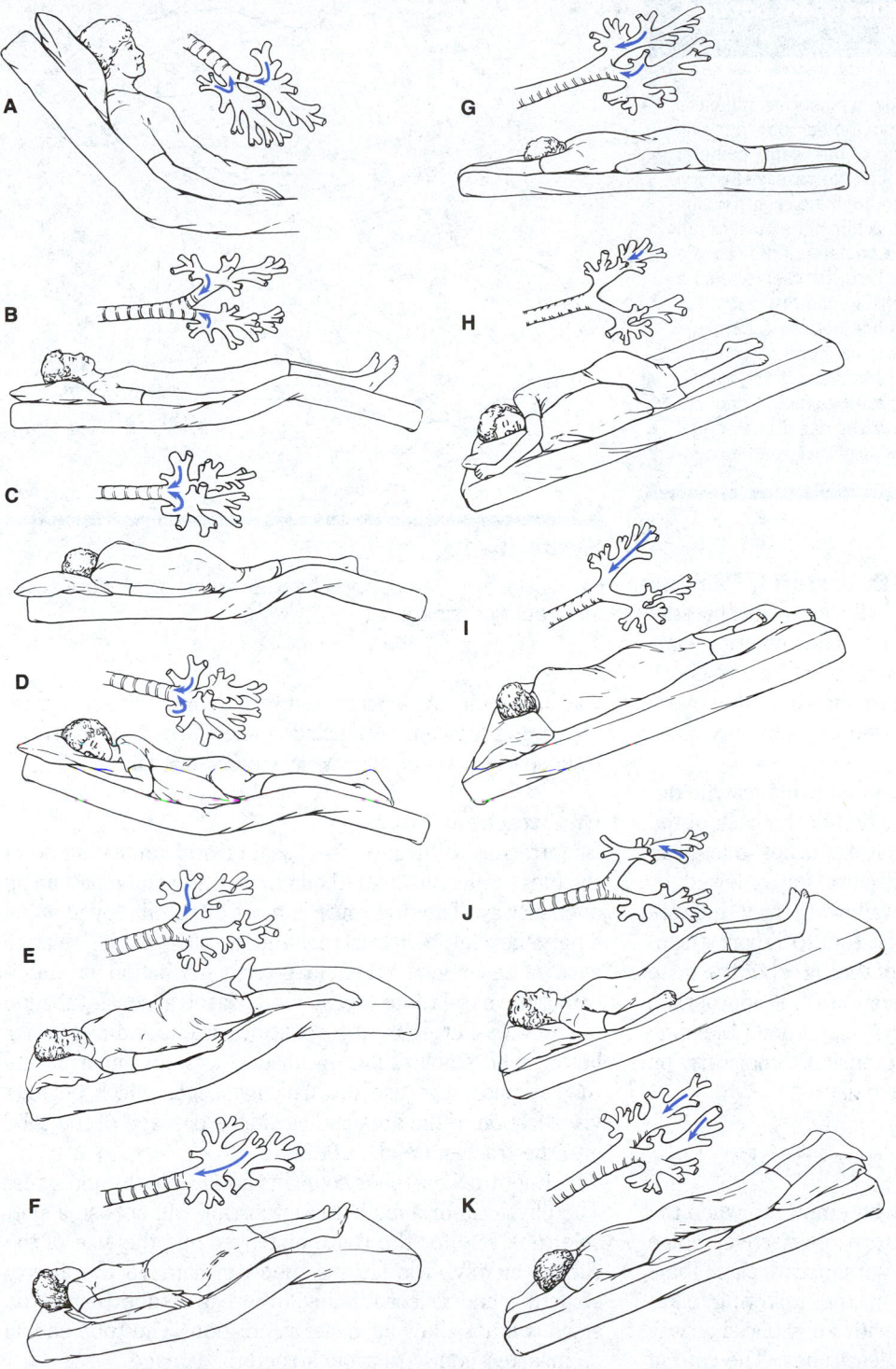

Figure 18–11

Postural drainage positions for specific pulmonary segments. **A.** Left and right upper lobes (apical segment). **B.** Left and right upper lobes (anterior segments). **C.** Right upper lobe (posterior segment). **D.** Left upper lobe (posterior segment). **E.** Left upper lobe (lingular segment). **F.** Middle lobe of right lung. **G.** Lower lobe (superior segment), client lying prone with one pillow under abdomen. **H.** Left lower lobe (lateral basal segment). **I.** Left and right lower lobes (anterior basal segments). **J.** Left and right lower lobes (anterior basal segments). **K.** Left and right lower lobes (posterior basal segments).

call the physician immediately. When bleeding recurs, the client is usually instructed to return to the office or hospital. If unable to contact a health care provider by phone, the client should go for assistance.

- Avoid picking or unnecessary touching of the packing or nose.

- Apply a lubricant around the nares to prevent drying and crusting of secretions and skin.

- Since mouth breathing is necessary, frequent oral hygiene should be given every 2 hours to prevent drying of the oral mucosa. Lubricants should be applied to the lips to prevent drying or cracking.

To find out how far the catheter should be inserted, measure off the amount of catheter needed from the ear lobe to the tip of the client's nose. Lubricate the tip of the sterile catheter using sterile water-soluble lubricant to facilitate passage through the nose. Insert the catheter gently through the client's nostril *without suction.* If the client is alert, ask him or her to stick out the tongue to prevent swallowing the catheter. If the client is not alert, hyperextend the neck and hold the client's tongue forward with a piece of gauze to facilitate catheter entry into the trachea. Entry into the trachea rather than the esophagus is indicated by coughing. If the catheter is in the esophagus, the client may gag or vomit. Avoid frequent suctioning via the same nostril to prevent traumatizing the mucosa. If frequent suctioning is necessary, a flexible rubber nasal pharyngeal airway may be inserted to prevent trauma of the nasal mucosa.

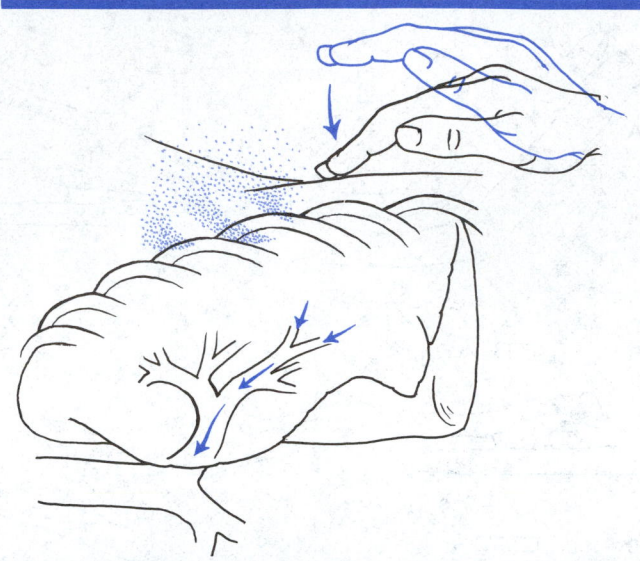

Figure 18–12

Percussion with the cupped hand over the pulmonary segment being drained.

Nursing Care of the Client With Posterior Packing

The client with posterior packing will also mouth breathe and therefore will need good oral care. The posterior pharynx should be inspected often with good lighting, to check for bleeding and to ensure that the packing has not moved. Misplacement of the packing into the oral pharynx could obstruct the upper airway.

The client should be told that swallowing may be difficult and will bring a sucking sensation in the back of the throat. Because of this, a liquid or soft diet is best tolerated.

Nurse and client should be alert for renewed or increased bleeding. Frequent swallowing may indicate bleeding. Also, the client should be told to report a sensation of fluid draining in the back of the throat or the taste of blood. Vital signs should be monitored at appropriate intervals, depending on the client's condition. Bleeding may result in tachycardia and hypotension. Stools may be tarry if bleeding has lasted for a few days.

IMPROVING BREATHING PATTERN

Several nursing interventions may be employed when the nursing diagnosis is breathing pattern, ineffective. Some of these actions are included in the nursing care plan (Table 18–2). Interventions discussed in the following paragraphs include care of the client with an artificial airway and management of clients with chest tubes. The care of clients who also require mechanical ventilation is discussed under "Improvement in Gas Exchange." These clients may also require deep breathing, coughing and breathing exercises, postural drainage, and nasotracheal suctioning (if they are not intubated).

The Client With an Artificial Airway

The indications for placement of an artificial airway are to relieve obstruction, facilitate suctioning of the lower air-

way, allow for mechanical ventilation, and to prevent aspiration. Artificial airways include the endotracheal tube, the tracheostomy tube, and the laryngectomy tube.

Endotracheal Tubes

Endotracheal intubation (by nasal or oral route) is one of the most widely used methods to institute and maintain an open airway. The oral route is most often employed when emergency intubation is required because of the relative ease of insertion. When long-term intubation is anticipated, the nasal route is preferred. Nasotracheal intubation is tolerated better by the conscious client and allows for better tube stabilization. Intubation with an endotracheal tube requires the use of a laryngoscope, which permits visualization of the area and facilitates passage of the tube into the trachea (Wade, 1982).

Endotracheal tubes come in various lengths and sizes. The physician or anesthetist intubating will choose a suitable tube size for the route employed and the size of the client's airway. Too large a tube can damage the airway structure and mucosal lining, whereas a tube that is too small will not allow adequate ventilation. The tube should be inserted gently to avoid structural damage.

Most tubes used today are disposable and are made of polyvinylchloride or silicone rubber. Nondisposable tubes are used less frequently. Most endotracheal tubes have inflatable cuffs (Figure 18–13). The cuff is inflated by injecting air into the pilot balloon. The amount of air required varies with the type of tube. The specific amount necessary is included in the package directions and may be printed on the tube. The cuff provides a seal so air does not leak around the tube when the client is ventilated. The cuff also prevents aspiration of material into the lungs. The

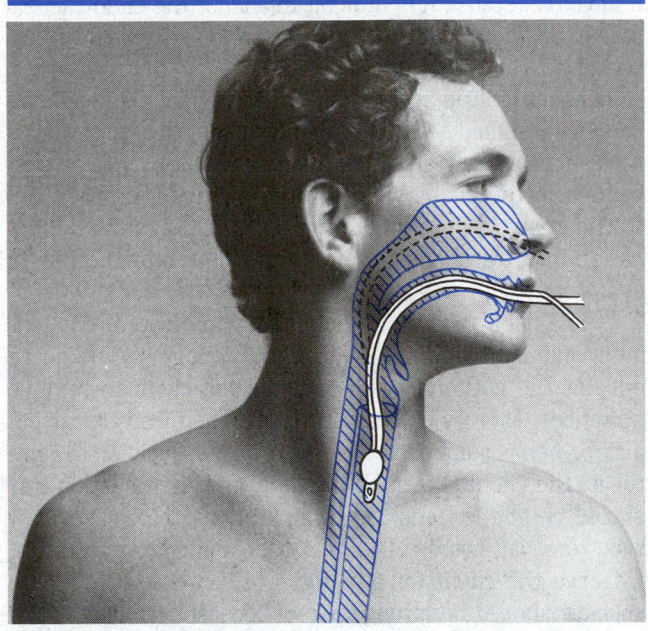

Figure 18–13

A polyvinyl chloride cuffed endotracheal tube that extends from the mouth to just above the bifurcation of the trachea. SOURCE: Swearingen PL: *The Addison–Wesley Photo Atlas of Nursing Procedures.* Menlo Park, CA: Addison–Wesley, 1984, p. 316.

newer endotracheal tubes have a low-pressure cuff that is more compliant and less likely to cause injury to the tracheal mucosa (Petty, 1982). Nursing considerations for the client with a cuffed tube are presented in Box 18–3.

Nursing Care of the Client With an Endotracheal Tube. Immediately after intubation, auscultate the lung fields to determine if the tube is placed properly. Since the right bronchus is straighter than the left, the tube is sometimes inserted into the right mainstem bronchus. This permits aeration of the right lung only. If the end of the endotracheal tube rests on the carina, partial or complete obstruction results. (The carina is the area where the trachea bifurcates into the left bronchus and right bronchus.) Inadvertent entry of the tube into the esophagus will result in gastric dilation. A chest x-ray should be obtained to ascertain the position of the tube.

Endotracheal tubes provide a means of suctioning secretions from the lower respiratory tract (Figure 18–14). Sterile technique is used.

The tube must be stabilized to prevent inadvertent removal (extubation) or change in placement. This is most often accomplished by taping the tube. When the client is intubated nasally, tape is applied at the insertion site. Stabilizing the oral endotracheal tube involves placement of an oral airway to prevent the client from biting down and obstructing the tube. Avoid applying excessive tape at the mouth, which would make inspection of the oral cavity difficult.

Box 18–3 Nursing Considerations for the Client With a Cuffed Endotracheal Tube

Effective and safe nursing care of clients with a cuffed endotracheal tube depends on an adequate understanding of the characteristics of the cuff being used. The two basic types of cuffs are air-filled and foam-filled. The newer tubes on the market (such as the Lanz or the Shiley) have a built-in control mechanism to prevent excessive pressure on the tracheal wall.

When using air-filled tubes, realize that once the syringe is removed from the one-way inflation valve, the cuff loses its ability to regulate or readjust for correct cuff pressure. For example, some cuffs are constructed to vent air when the pressure within the cuff exceeds 15 mm Hg on inflation. Once the syringe is removed from the one-way inflation valve, there is no route for escape of excess air. Therefore, an increase in tracheal and intracuff pressure will not be vented, and intracuff pressures may go above 15 mm Hg (Harper, 1981).

With the modern soft-cuff tracheostomy and endotracheal tubes, deflation of the cuffs is not necessary. However, the intracuff pressure must be checked at regular intervals. This reading can be obtained using an aneroid manometer or the Portex pressure gauge, designed specifically for this purpose (Harper, 1981).

Foam-filled cuffs work on a different principle than the air-filled type. The inflation line is left open to the atmosphere to allow the foam inside the cuff to reexpand. Air should never be injected into these cuffs since the pressure would greatly increase (Harper, 1981).

Occasionally, the nurse may care for a client who is intubated with a tube that does not have a soft cuff. To prevent damage, the "minimal leak" technique allows a small amount of air to escape around the cuff. To accomplish this, place a stethoscope on the client's neck over the trachea. During inspiration, inject air into the pilot balloon until the gurgling or hissing of air around the tube is no longer present. Then slowly remove 0.2 to 0.3 mL of air from the pilot balloon. The pressure should then be checked. Cuff pressures should never exceed 15 mm Hg, or 25 cm water.

Regardless of the type of cuff, check and record the pressures at least once each shift. Some clinicians recommend that inflatable cuffs be deflated for a few minutes every hour to relieve pressure on the tracheal lining. The benefit of periodic deflation has not been documented by research. If the cuff is deflated, however, the area above the cuff should be suctioned to prevent aspiration of secretions.

One method of securing an oral endotracheal tube is illustrated in Figure 18–15. Plastic devices may be used rather than tape to secure the tube. Meticulous oral hygiene is important for these clients. The position of the orotracheal tube should be changed daily and the tape replaced at the same time. Care must be taken to avoid skin breakdown, which can result from irritation by the tape.

The client's skin should be assessed daily when tape is changed. A rash may indicate an allergic reaction to the tape. The use of nonallergenic tape or plastic devices may then be indicated, particularly for clients, such as diabetics, who are likely to have skin breakdown and poor wound healing.

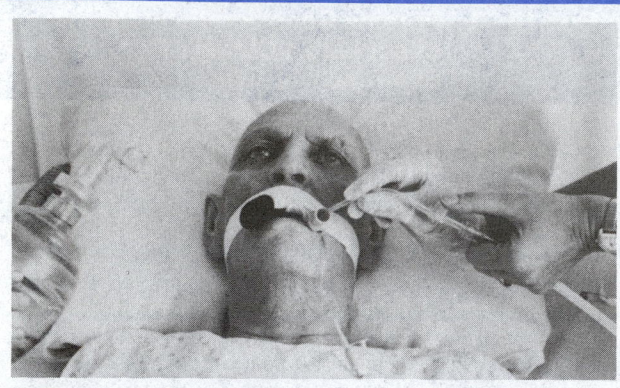

Figure 18–14

Sterile suctioning of an oral endotracheal tube.
SOURCE: Petty T: *Intensive and Rehabilitative Respiratory Care,* 3rd ed. Philadelphia: Lea & Febiger, 1982. Reprinted with permission.

Clients with endotracheal tubes should be assessed daily for complications involving the nose, mouth, pharynx, sinuses, and ears. A nasotracheal tube could obstruct the eustachian tube, causing otitis. Damage to the nasal mucosa may occur from pressure or irritation from the tube.

Other possible complications include damage to the vocal cords, laryngeal edema, and laryngeal ulcers. These complications are caused by traumatic insertion of a tube, improper stabilization of the tube once it is in place, and unnecessary manipulation of the tube. Laryngeal ulcers occur more frequently with oral intubation than with nasal

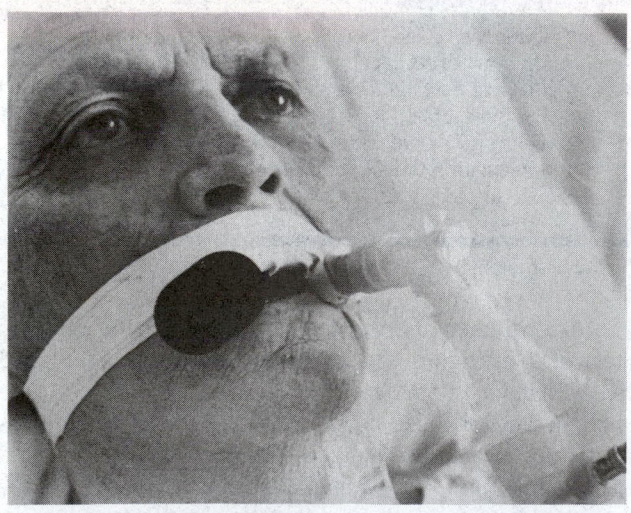

Figure 18–15

Securing an oral endotracheal tube.
SOURCE: Petty T: *Intensive and Rehabilitative Respiratory Care,* 3rd ed. Philadelphia: Lea & Febiger, 1982. Reprinted with permission.

intubation because it is difficult to anchor the endotracheal tube in the mouth, and an unanchored tube exerts pressure on the posterior rim of the glottis.

There is little agreement about how long an endotracheal tube should be left in place. The length of time varies with agency policy and the physician. If the physician suspects that the client will require prolonged intubation, a tracheotomy is performed because the longer the client has an endotracheal tube in place, the greater the risk of complications.

The client should be adequately ventilated, oxygenated, and suctioned before extubation begins. The nurse deflates the cuff and again suctions the client to remove secretions that may have accumulated. The tube is removed, and oxygen is administered. An individual qualified to reintubate the client should be present, and an intubation tray should be at the bedside. Complications that may follow tube removal include laryngeal edema and laryngospasm. Observe the client for any signs of these complications, such as labored breathing, use of accessory muscles, and stridor. Laryngospasm and laryngeal edema can result in upper airway obstruction. If these complications occur, the administration of parenteral corticosteroids and reintubation are necessary (Petty, 1982).

Tracheostomy Tubes

Other methods of establishing an artificial airway include tracheotomy and cricothyroidotomy. (Chapter 21 describes these procedures and indications for their use.) Tracheostomy tubes are placed during these procedures. These are short curved tubes and have a flange that assists in stabilization of the tube on the neck. A variety of types are available, including metal tubes or disposable tubes of polyvinylchloride or silicone. Tubes come in several sizes. Most tubes today have an inner cannula to facilitate cleansing of the inside of the tube. All tubes are packaged with an obturator, which is used to minimize trauma when the tube is inserted (Figure 18–16).

Fenestrated tracheostomy tubes are sometimes used prior to extubation of the client (Figure 18–17). This tube has an opening, or fenestration, in the outer cannula; it may or may not have a cuff. If the fenestrated tube is cuffed, the cuff should be deflated to allow the client to breathe around, as well as through, the tube. This allows the client to adjust gradually to removal of the tracheostomy tube. It also allows nursing staff to determine how the client will tolerate removal. Covering the tracheostomy tube enables the client to talk, to breathe normally through the upper airway, and to cough up secretions (Harper, 1981).

Another way of preparing the client for permanent removal of the tracheostomy tube is by applying a tracheostomy button (Figure 18–18). The button extends from the tracheostomy opening to just inside the tracheal wall. If the tracheostomy tube has a cuff, the cuff is deflated before the tracheostomy button is placed to allow the client

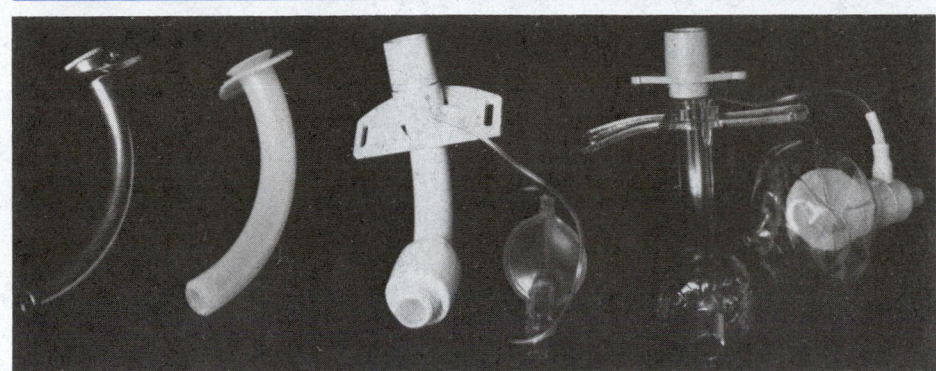

Figure 18–16
Comparison of different types of tracheostomy tubes.

to breathe around the tube. To determine readiness for decannulation, a tracheostomy button is most effective with a fenestrated tube. Placement of this button facilitates talking, coughing, and normal breathing through the upper airway. If the client has difficulty breathing or expelling secretions, the button is removed, and the client breathes through the tracheostomy tube (Harper, 1981).

Tracheostomy Care. Tracheostomy care is performed to minimize bacterial contamination and to decrease the possibility of obstruction by secretions. Routine tracheostomy care consists of cleansing of the inner cannula and the area around the stoma. The frequency of cleaning the inner cannula may vary depending on the amount of secretions present. Cleaning may be necessary as frequently as every half hour or only once a shift. There are two schools of thought regarding care of the inner cannula. Some advocate cleaning the inner cannula as often as necessary. Others believe that proper humidification and suctioning negate the need for cleansing of the inner cannula because frequent cleansing may increase the chance of infection. Table 18–3 presents the steps for routine tracheostomy care (Brown, 1982).

When caring for clients with a tracheostomy or laryngectomy tube, it is wise to have another sterile tube at the bedside in case of accidental decannulation or obstruction of the tube. A clearly labeled obturator for the tube should be in the room because it would be needed to reinsert the tube. Some nurses prefer to keep sterile forceps at the bedside since, in the early period after tube insertion, decannulation may result in closure of the stoma. The forceps would be employed to reopen the stoma. Scissors should also be at the bedside to cut the tracheostomy tube ties in case they become too tight or the tube is partially dislodged by coughing.

Prior to removal of the tube, the client is ventilated, oxygenated, and suctioned to remove tracheal and pharyngeal secretions. The cuff is deflated, and the client is again suctioned. The tube is removed, and a moist gauze dressing is placed over the stoma. Normally, the opening closes within 5 days (Petty, 1982).

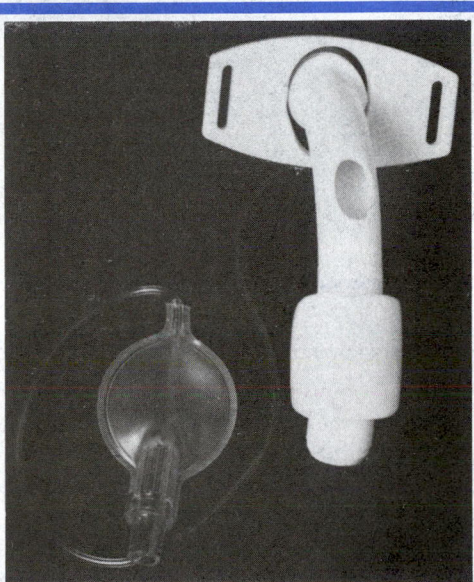

Figure 18–17
Fenestrated tracheostomy tube.

Nursing Research Note

Harris RB, Hyman RB: Clean vs. sterile tracheostomy care and level of pulmonary infection. *Nurs Res* 1984; 33:80–84.

The researchers set out to determine if clean tracheostomy care was more effective than sterile technique in preventing postoperative pulmonary infections. Based on laboratory data, they found that clean tracheostomy care was associated with fewer infections. Sterile technique and a mixed technique of clean and sterile procedures resulted in higher infection rates.

The study also found that nurses did not consistently follow written procedures and poor technique was a recurrent problem. This study reinforces the need for additional clinical experimentation in comparing tracheostomy procedures. It also substantiates the need for nurses to follow written policy to provide consistency in care and accurate assessment of the efficacy of the procedure.

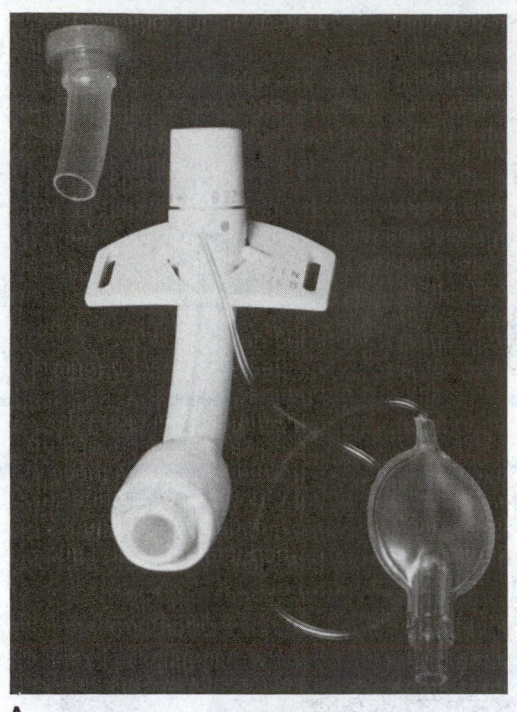
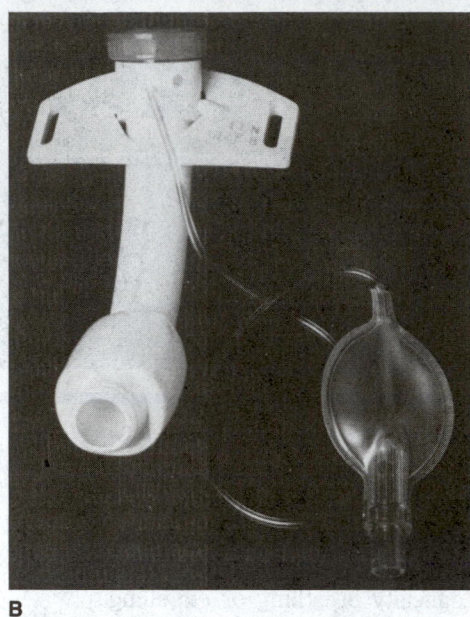

Figure 18–18

A. Shiley tracheostomy tube and tracheostomy button. **B.** Tracheostomy button in place.

Laryngectomy Tubes

The terms *tracheostomy tube* and *laryngectomy tube* are often used interchangeably. Actually, the laryngectomy tube is shorter. Metal tubes are commonly used, such as the one shown in Figure 18–19. These consist of an obturator, inner cannula, and outer cannula. These tubes are usually placed following a total laryngectomy to provide a route for removal of secretions and to maintain a patent airway.

Complications of Artificial Airways

The insertion of artificial airways can result in a variety of complications. Since inspired air bypasses the nose, air must be humidified to prevent drying of the mucosa of the lower respiratory tract. These clients are more vulnerable to the development of an infection because of altered ciliary function, trauma to the mucosa caused by suctioning and intubation, and colonization of the airway with bacteria.

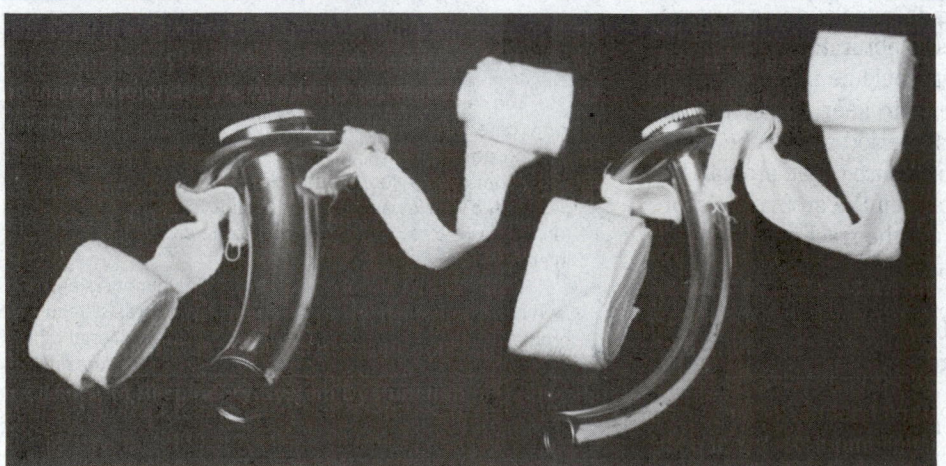

Figure 18–19

Comparison of shorter laryngectomy tube (on left) with tracheostomy tube.

Table 18–3 Tracheostomy Care—A Sterile Procedure

Nursing Implementation	Rationale
1. Assemble the following equipment: sterile drape; sterile pipe cleaners, brush, swabs, scissors, forceps, gloves; sterile gauze squares; trach ties and trach bib; two sterile basins; sterile normal saline; sterile hydrogen peroxide; paper bag.	With all the equipment at hand, it is easier to carry out the steps in an organized sequence.
2. Wash hands using soap and water.	This removes bacteria from the hands, decreasing the chance of contaminating the client's airway.
3. Explain procedure to the client and provide reassurance, even if the client is unresponsive.	Explanations help to allay the client's anxiety. Explaining the reasons for the procedure and the steps helps to involve alert clients in their own care. Later, clients can be encouraged to help with the procedure. If the tracheostomy will be permanent, it is important that clients learn the procedure and participate actively in their own care.
4. Suction the client as necessary using sterile technique.	Suctioning using strict asepsis prevents airway contamination.
5. Open the sterile drape and place on the bedside stand.	This will serve as a sterile field on which sterile equipment should be placed.
6. Open all equipment using sterile technique.	Since the lung is normally a sterile environment, trach care must be performed using sterile technique.
7. Fill one basin with hydrogen peroxide and one with sterile normal saline.	Pouring the solution before putting on the sterile gloves prevents contamination.
8. Remove the soiled tracheostomy dressing and dispose of it in the paper bag.	Proper disposal prevents contamination of the environment.
9. Loosen the inner cannula.	This facilitates removal.
10. Put on sterile gloves. One hand should be kept sterile and the other clean.	Wearing sterile gloves minimizes contamination of the respiratory tract.
11. Remove inner cannula and place it in the hydrogen peroxide solution. Allow the cannula to soak for a few minutes, then clean with the sterile brush and pipe cleaners.	This facilitates removal of secretions.
12. Rinse inner cannula with sterile saline. Cannula should then be gently shaken and reinserted.	The inner cannula should not remain out longer than 5 to 10 min to prevent the formation of crusts in the outer cannula (Brown, 1982).
13. Maintaining sterile technique, cleanse the skin around the stoma and phlanges of the tube using gauze soaked in a hydrogen peroxide solution. Care must be taken to prevent hydrogen peroxide and lint from entering the stoma.	Hydrogen peroxide facilitates the removal of secretions and crusts, which are a source of bacteria. Cotton applicators should not be used around the stoma since lint from the cotton may be aspirated into the lungs.
14. Rinse area around the stoma with sterile normal saline and dry with sterile gauze.	Hydrogen peroxide is irritating to tissue and should be removed. Drying is important because moisture provides an environment conducive to the growth of bacteria and eventual skin breakdown.
15. Inspect the surrounding area and the stoma site for inflammation, skin breakdown, and presence of secretions. Any abnormalities should be documented and reported.	Signs of impaired wound healing and infection require immediate attention.
16. Make a new tracheostomy dressing by cutting a sterile gauze square (without cotton filler) halfway up the center and place it over the incision under the faceplate of the tracheostomy tube.	Pieces of cotton could inadvertently enter the tracheostomy tube. The dressing will absorb any drainage from the incisional area.

(continued)

Table 18–3 Tracheostomy Care—A Sterile Procedure (continued)	
Nursing Implementation	**Rationale**
17. Apply a new tracheostomy bib and ties. The ties should be tight enough to prevent the tube from being dislodged yet not result in skin irritation. If the ties are fastened appropriately, the nurse should be able to insert one finger underneath the string. Secure with a square knot.	The bib prevents contamination of the airway, and the ties secure the tube.
18. Whenever possible, two people should be present when changing the trach ties. One person can then hold the trach tube securely in place while the other changes the ties. Often clients are able to assist in this way.	This prevents accidental dislodgment of the trach tube.

Organisms commonly isolated from the respiratory tract in these clients include *Staphylococcus aureus* and *Pseudomonas*.

Excessive pressure on the trachea from the cuff of endotracheal tubes will decrease blood supply to the area and cause tissue necrosis. This may lead to tracheal stenosis or a tracheoesophageal fistula.

Another complication from cuffed tubes is herniation of the cuff over the end of the tube, resulting in partial or complete airway obstruction. Signs include a significant air leak through the stoma, mouth, or nose; the sounding of the high-pressure alarm on the ventilator; and obstruction when attempting to suction the client. An underinflated cuff may be caused by instillation of an insufficient amount of air or a ruptured cuff. An air leak is detected around the stoma, nose, or mouth, and the ventilator indicates a decrease in the expired volume of air with sounding of the low pressure alarm.

Obstruction of artificial airways may occur because of accumulation of secretions or a kink in the endotracheal tube. Obstruction will result in the sounding of a high pressure alarm. It must be corrected immediately or the client will asphyxiate.

Nursing Care of the Client With an Artificial Airway

Placement of an artificial airway can be a source of anxiety and apprehension for the client and family members. A major source of anxiety is the client's impaired ability to communicate. This problem is only temporary, except for clients who have undergone a total laryngectomy. To allay the client's anxiety and fear, provide an alternative means of communication. A "magic slate" or a pad of paper and a pencil should be available. The call light should be within reach of the client at all times and should be answered promptly. The intercom at the nurses' station should be marked to indicate that the individual cannot speak. Some clients who cannot communicate by writing might use gesturing as an alternative method. The client who has had a total laryngectomy must adjust to permanent changes. Information on communication after a laryngectomy is presented in Chapter 21.

The ability of the client to remove secretions effectively is also impaired. The artificial airway prevents the client from closing the glottis and generating intrathoracic pressure to dislodge secretions. Thus, the cough is less effective. Also, the artificial airway impairs the effectiveness of the mucociliary mechanism. Secretions that accumulate in the airway may cause the client to fear suffocation. When the client is unable to cough and expel secretions, the uncomfortable and frightening procedure of suctioning must be performed. Table 18–4 describes the procedure for tracheostomy or endotracheal tube suctioning. During this procedure, the client will experience discomfort as well as a feeling of breathlessness. Attempt to allay the client's anxiety by providing an explanation of the artificial airway and the suctioning procedure.

Obviously, the placement of an artificial airway will result in a change in the client's body image. This not only affects the way in which clients view themselves but the way in which they are viewed by family members and significant others. Family members should always be included when providing information and reassurance. Hospitalization, by its very nature, puts the client in a dependent role, and having an artificial airway compounds the feeling of dependency. Clients should be encouraged to participate actively in their own care as much as possible.

For most clients, an artificial airway is temporary. They should be informed that the airway will be removed after they are able to ventilate adequately.

The Client With Chest Tubes

Inspiration and expiration depend partly on the presence of normal intrapleural pressure. Even though this pressure varies with breathing, it remains lower than atmospheric

Table 18–4   Tracheostomy or Endotracheal Tube Suctioning—A Sterile Procedure

Nursing Implementation	Rationale
1. Assemble the following equipment: oxygen source, flowmeter, Ambu bag, connecting tubing; suction source and connecting tubing; sterile suction catheter about half the diameter of the tracheostomy or endotracheal tube; sterile glove; sterile normal saline; 5 mL sterile syringe; sterile container to pour saline in; disposable bag.	Because intubated clients may require immediate suctioning, this equipment should be at the bedside at all times. A small catheter will not occlude the tracheostomy or endotracheal tube. Having all needed equipment readily available also helps the nurse to carry out the procedure in a more organized manner. This helps to allay client anxiety.
2. Wash hands using soap and water.	Bacteria on the hands could contaminate the client's airway. Hand-washing removes bacteria.
3. Explain procedure to client and provide reassurance even if client is unresponsive.	Explaining helps allay client anxieties.
4. If possible, have the client cough and deep breathe. Postural drainage may be helpful.	Measures that loosen pulmonary secretions or move them toward the major bronchi or trachea facilitate their removal.
5. Hyperoxygenate the client by using an Ambu bag connected to a high liter flow of oxygen. This procedure is more easily performed with two people, one to ventilate the client and another to suction.	Hypoxemia can occur during suctioning and could result in the development of cardiac dysrhythmias.
6. Open all equipment using sterile technique.	The lung is normally a sterile environment.
7. Put on the sterile glove.	
8. Attach the catheter to the connecting tubing. Suction of 80–120 mm Hg should be applied.	Pressure above 120 mm Hg may damage the tracheal mucosa.
9. Insert the sterile catheter carefully into the endotracheal or tracheostomy tube with the suction *off,* taking care not to contaminate the catheter. The catheter is inserted only until resistance is met.	This prevents the introduction of bacteria into the lower respiratory tract. Forcing the catheter can cause trauma to the lower airways.
10. Apply suction intermittently for no longer than 10 sec at a time. Rotate the catheter gently between gloved fingers when withdrawing the catheter.	Short-term suctioning limits the amount of oxygen removed. Suctioning for longer than 10 sec can result in hypoxemia. Continuous suctioning may damage the tracheal mucosa.
11. Turning the client's head from side to side may facilitate suctioning.	The anatomic position of the left main bronchus makes it difficult to enter with the suction catheter. Alteration in client position can facilitate positioning of the catheter.
12. The nurse again hyperoxygenates the client using an Ambu bag and evaluates respiratory status to determine if further suctioning is necessary.	Hyperoxygenation prior to, between, and after suctioning prevents hypoxemia.
13. The catheter should be inserted in the container of sterile saline and flushed after use in suctioning.	Flushing removes bacteria from the catheter so they are not reintroduced into the respiratory tract.
14. Characteristics of the sputum should be recorded, including amount, color, consistency, and odor. Removal of tenacious secretions may require the instillation of 1–3 mL of sterile normal saline prior to introducing the suction catheter into the airway.	Changes in the sputum indicate alterations in the physiological status of the client.
15. When suctioning is completed, the catheter is disposed of.	A sterile catheter must be used each time the client is suctioned.
16. The client's tolerance of the procedure is recorded.	This information is important in overall assessment of the client's physiological and psychosocial status.
17. A fresh container of sterile saline should be obtained every 24 h. When the container is first opened, the date and time should be written on the label. When not in use, the bottle should be tightly capped.	Always assume that if bacteria can grow in the solution, they will. Every effort must be made to prevent introduction of bacteria into the lungs.

pressure. Disruption of intrapleural pressure by trauma, disease, or surgery will decrease the effectiveness of ventilation. Information on normal physiology of breathing is addressed in Chapter 17. To reestablish normal intrapleural pressure, the insertion of chest tubes may be required. This procedure is described below and also in Section VII of Chapter 21.

Nursing Considerations During Chest Tube Insertion

The insertion of a chest tube is painful. If the procedure is not an emergency, analgesics or pain medications should be given about 30 minutes prior to tube insertion. The nurse may need to request the medication order from the physician. It is of utmost importance that the nurse explain the procedure and equipment used. Clients should be told that the tube (or tubes) will be placed through the chest wall to drain air, fluid, or both, so their lungs can function normally. These tubes will be secured by a dressing and connected to a drainage apparatus.

When chest tubes are inserted at the bedside, the nurse will be responsible for obtaining equipment. The equipment may vary among institutions, but basically the following will be required (Erickson, 1981):

• Local anesthetic, usually 1% lidocaine
• Antiseptic, such as povidone-iodine
• Sterile gloves
• Suture materials
• Collection receptacle
• Chest tube(s)
• Tape and petrolatum gauze for an occlusive dressing

Unless contraindicated, the client is placed in a recumbent position for insertion of the chest tube. If the tube is being inserted to remove air (pneumothorax) the client should be supine. Because air rises, the chest tube is inserted anteriorly in the midclavicular line in the second to fifth intercostal space. If the tube is being placed to remove fluid (hemothorax), the client should be placed in a semi-Fowler's position. Since fluid collects in the dependent area, the tube is inserted in the sixth to eighth intercostal space in the midaxillary line (Figure 18–20). The client who cannot tolerate a semi-Fowler's position should lie on one side with the affected side up.

Drainage Systems for Chest Tubes

The chest tube will be connected to approximately 6 ft of tubing that leads to the collection system, which is placed on the floor, considerably below the client's chest. The tubing should be long enough that it allows the client to move and turn without pulling. A long tube also decreases the chance that a deep breath would cause fluid to be sucked back into the chest.

The collection receptacle is placed below the level of the client's chest to take advantage of gravity flow, facilitating removal of air and fluid from the intrapleural space.

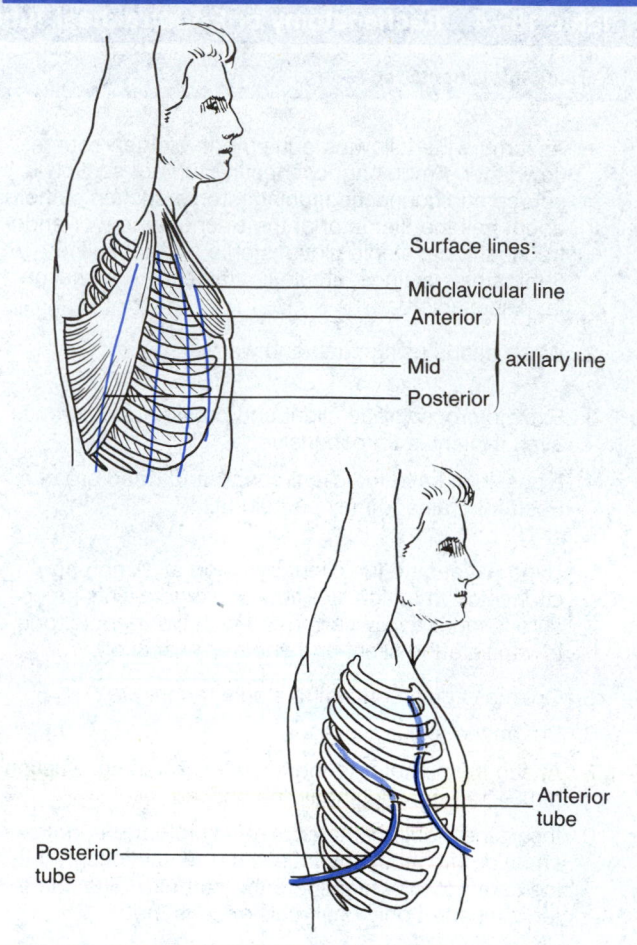

Figure 18–20

Insertion of an anterior or posterior chest tube.

This dependent position also prevents the backflow of fluid into the intrapleural space.

To prevent the reentry of air into the intrapleural space, the distal end of the tube must be submerged under water. This water seal is a necessary part of any chest drainage unit. During exhalation, the pressure in the lungs forces air out of the pleural space into the tubing, which is submerged under water (as shown by bubbling) (Erickson, 1981).

The One-Bottle System. The one-bottle system may be employed when a small portion of the lung has collapsed. Fluid or air is drained from the intrapleural space by gravity into the bottle (Figure 18–21A). The end of the connecting tube is attached to a rigid tube, which is placed into the bottle. The end of the rigid tube is submerged in about 1 in or 2 cm of sterile saline or water, creating the water seal that prevents reentry of air. As indicated in Figure 18–21A, an open vent releases air into the atmosphere and prevents excessive buildup of air inside the bottle. Water-seal drainage using one bottle is not recommended if the chest drainage is expected to be significant, because any rise in the fluid level increases the pressure the client must exert to expel air and fluid from the chest cavity. If a moderate to a large amount of drainage is expected, a second bottle is added to the system.

The Two-Bottle System. In the two-bottle system, the drainage and water-seal bottles are separate, and fluid drains only into the collection bottle (Figure 18–21B). This system allows the water-seal bottle to remain at a fixed level so chest drainage can be more accurately measured. As with the one-bottle system, gravity drives the drainage system. When gravity drainage is not sufficient to remove air or fluid from the lungs, suction may be added.

The Three-Bottle System. The three-bottle system is usually employed when suction is necessary (Figure 18–21C). The first two bottles are as explained above. The third bottle is added to control the amount of suction

applied to the intrapleural space. The bottle has three tubes: one tube is connected to a suction source (a wall suction inlet or a portable suction unit); another is connected to the water-seal bottle; the long tube is the suction control manometer and is open to the atmosphere (Figure 18–21C). Suction not only pulls air from the drainage bottles but also pulls air in from the atmosphere through the manometer. If the manometer is submerged in 15 cm of water, the amount of suction necessary to pull atmospheric air to the bottom of the manometer is −15 cm of water pressure. When this amount of suction is obtained, bubbling will occur in the suction control bottle. Increasing the amount of suction applied to the system will result in more bubbling but will not increase the amount of negative pressure applied to the intrapleural space. The depth to which the manometer tube is submerged determines the amount of suction applied to the intrapleural space. Thus, the suction control bottle acts as a breaker system to prevent excessive pressure from being exerted on the intrapleural space (Erickson, 1981).

Commercial Water-Seal Units. There are a number of variations of chest drainage units available. One of the most popular is the disposable Pleur-Evac. The advantages of the Pleur-Evac are: it is lightweight, it takes up a small amount of space, it can be placed on the floor on a stand or hung on the side of the bed to facilitate transporting the client, and it is not breakable. The Pleur-Evac functions like a three-bottle system; it can be used as a water-seal gravity drainage system, or it may be connected to suction (Harper, 1981).

Other drainage systems include the Argyle and the Emerson. The Argyle is a plastic disposable unit with a fourth chamber, whose purpose is to prevent a possible pressure buildup in the system. The Emerson unit uses two glass bottles: the first is a combined water seal and collection container; the second is a trap bottle to prevent fluid from entering the pump. There is no control bottle in the Emerson system, and pressure of up to −60 cm of water can be achieved (Erickson, 1981; Harper, 1981).

Nursing Care of the Client With Chest Tubes

The major objective of nursing care is to facilitate drainage of fluid and air, fostering lung reexpansion. After insertion of the chest tube, it is often the nurse's responsibility to apply the dressing. Sterile technique is necessary. Petrolatum gauze is wrapped around the insertion site, and wide tape is applied to provide an occlusive dressing. This prevents air from entering the intrapleural space. Even though the chest tube is sutured in place, great care must be taken to secure the tube when applying the tape. If drainage is present on the dressing, the physician should be notified.

Characteristics of the chest tube drainage should be recorded, including amount, color, consistency, and odor. Initially, the drainage characteristics should be noted every

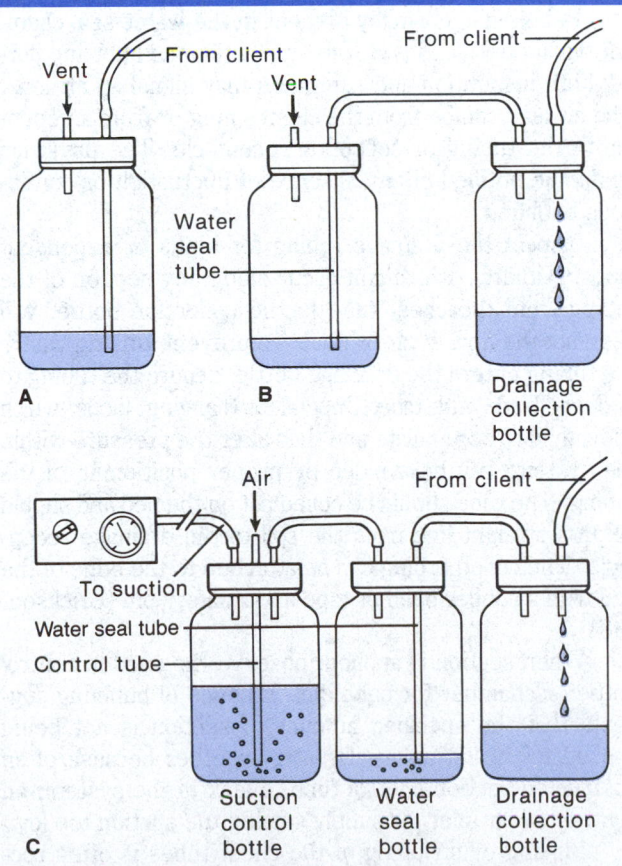

Figure 18–21

Drainage systems for chest tubes. **A.** One-bottle system. **B.** Two-bottle system. **C.** Three-bottle system.

15 to 20 minutes. If the container does not have calibrated markings, apply tape vertically and mark the level of drainage on the tape every hour. Persistent drainage of more than 100 mL per hour should be reported to the physician.

An important aspect of care for the client with chest tubes is assessment of the client's respiratory status. Clients should be questioned about their level of discomfort and any difficulty in breathing. Lung fields should be auscultated to determine if all areas of the lungs are being aerated. Watch for symmetrical expansion of the chest when the client breathes, and listen for any adventitious breath sounds. The rate, depth, and quality of respirations should be noted. To facilitate lung reexpansion and prevent complications, the client should be encouraged to cough and deep-breathe every hour.

Maintaining the Water Seal. It is essential that the water seal be maintained to prevent reentry of air into the pleural space. At least 2 to 2.5 cm of sterile water or normal saline should be placed in the water-seal bottle. Check the fluid level frequently and add sterile water or saline to replace whatever evaporates. It is important that the drainage unit be kept well below the chest level. If any part of the system is lifted above chest level, fluid may reenter the pleural space. When transporting the client, use a stretcher with a bottom shelf and place the collection unit on the stretcher shelf, keeping all of the system below the level of the client's chest. It is recommended that someone familiar with the water-seal system accompany the client.

The water seal can be lost by accidentally disconnecting the tubing or breaking the water-seal bottle. If this happens, air will enter the pleural space. Air may also enter the pleural space if the chest tube is dislodged. Disconnection should be suspected if the nurse notices an absence of fluctuation in the water-seal bottle or chamber. In the event that it becomes disconnected, the end of the disconnected tubing should be cleansed with an alcohol swab and reconnected. The nurse should then ask the client to cough deeply to remove any excessive air that may have accumulated in the intrapleural space.

If the bottle breaks, there is controversy about the actions to take. Some clinicians recommend clamping the tube for a minute or two (no longer). Check with the physician about whether chest tubes may be clamped, and record this on the care plan and in the chart. The authors believe a chest tube should never be clamped because a tension pneumothorax can develop if a continuous air leak is present. For example, when an air leak is present in the lung or bronchi, air will move into the pleural space. When the chest tube is clamped, there is no avenue of exit for the air. Thus, as the air leak continues, pressure in the pleural space increases, and a tension pneumothorax develops.

If the chest tube is pulled out or falls out of the intrapleural space, the client should be asked to exhale forcefully, and the opening should be immediately covered. Ideally, the wound should be covered with petrolatum gauze and pressure applied until the tube can be inserted. If petrolatum gauze is not available, a gauze 4 × 4 or the palm of the hand or a sheet can be used. (Tissue should not be used because lint may enter the chest cavity.) If the client develops signs and symptoms of a tension pneumothorax, the pressure should be momentarily relieved to allow air to escape (Harper, 1981). (Tension pneumothorax is discussed in Chapter 20.)

Maintaining Patency of the Drainage System. The patency of the drainage system must be maintained to facilitate expansion of the lung. Make frequent, systematic observations to determine that the system is patent. The system should be checked for loose connections and the dressing reinforced as needed. All connections should be taped to prevent disconnection of tubes.

Observe for fluctuation in the water-seal bottle or chamber. The water rises and falls with changes in intrapleural pressure. As the client inhales, fluid should be pulled up the water-seal tube or the chest tube, and the level should fall back as the client exhales. Absence of fluctuation may be caused by an obstructed tube, by a disconnected tube, or by reexpansion of the lung.

Bubbling is normally present in the water-seal chamber during exhalation. However, continuous bubbling during both inspiration and expiration may signal an air leak. The air leak can be from the client's lung or from an opening in the tubing or collection receptacle. The physician should be notified of any absence of fluctuation or continuous bubbling.

Inspect the drainage tubing for kinks or dependent loops. Kinking, which can occur along any section of the tubing from the chest tube to the collection bottle, will obstruct the flow of air or fluid. To prevent kinking where the tubing enters the drainage bottle, secure the tubing to a tongue blade with tape. Dependent (hanging) loops, which allow fluid to accumulate and thus alter the pressure within the system, can be avoided by proper positioning of the tubing. The tube should be coiled flat on the bed and should fall in a straight line from the coil to the drainage receptacle. The coiled tubing can be attached to the edge of the bed with a rubber band or tape and a safety pin (Erickson, 1981).

When suction is applied, observe the suction control bottle or chamber for bubbling. Absence of bubbling suggests that the specified amount of suction is not being applied to the intrapleural space, whether because of an obstructed suction control tube, a leak in the system, an obstructed air inlet, or simply setting the suction too low.

Milking or stripping of the chest tubes is often recommended to prevent the formation of clots or remove clots from the tubing. Grip and stabilize the tubing with the thumb and forefinger of one hand. Compress a section of the tubing by sliding the other hand from that point toward the drainage unit (away from the client to the collection receptacle). Release the first hand, and repeat the procedure along the rest of the tubing. This is facilitated by the use of lotion or lubricant. Some nurses prefer to use a special chest tube roller (Erickson, 1981).

Psychosocial Considerations for the Client With Chest Tubes

The insertion of a chest tube is a painful, invasive procedure. Explanations and reassurance should be provided for the client, family members, and significant others. During the insertion, remain with the client to provide emotional support.

Clients may restrict their breathing and movement not only to minimize pain but because they fear they may dislodge the tube. They should be informed that the tube is secured with sutures and tape. Movement such as turning, coughing, and deep breathing must be encouraged by the nurse, since this will facilitate reexpansion of the lung. The client should be told that pain medication can be given to decrease discomfort during breathing exercises. Narcotics, however, should be administered judiciously since they can depress the respiratory rate.

The collection receptacle should be explained to the client. If suction is necessary, clients should be aware that bubbling and some noise is expected. Clients, family members, and significant others should be given the opportunity to verbalize fears and ask questions regarding the procedure and equipment. Be aware that chest tubes may seem far more frightening to visitors than other sorts of tubes, and be prepared to reassure clients that it is the visitor's lack of knowledge and not the client's situation that has caused the reaction.

IMPROVING GAS EXCHANGE

The nursing diagnosis of impaired gas exchange can refer to clients with mild disorders as well as those with severe disorders. Numerous nursing measures can be employed in an effort to improve the exchange of carbon dioxide and oxygen (see the nursing care plan in Table 18–2). These clients often require highly skilled nursing care since they may require the assistance of mechanical ventilators. Other nursing measures that may be employed when caring for these clients include: deep breathing and coughing exercises, administration of oxygen, postural drainage, and suctioning.

The Client Requiring Mechanical Ventilation

Mechanical ventilation may be necessary for any client in whom the process of ventilation has been significantly altered. A significant alteration would be caused by a condition that prevents the client from maintaining normal oxygen and carbon dioxide levels in the blood.

Types of Mechanical Ventilators

There are basically three types of positive-pressure ventilators (Nielsen, 1980): time-cycled, pressure-cycled, and volume-cycled machines. Each is discussed below.

In the time-cycled ventilator, inspiration is terminated after a set time. The volume of air delivered is regulated by the length of the inspiratory cycle and the rate of flow of the pressurized gas. A disadvantage of this type is that the pressure required to deliver the gas and the tidal volume vary with each breath, depending on the compliance of the client's airway. (Compliance refers to the ability of the lungs to distend with each breath on ventilation.) The Engstrom ventilator is an example of this type.

With the pressure-cycled ventilator, the gas is delivered to the lungs until a predetermined pressure is reached; then inspiration is terminated. The disadvantage of this type is that the tidal volume delivered to the client can vary with each inspiration, depending on the condition of the client's airway. The Bennett PR-1 and PR-2 ventilators are pressure-cycled.

In volume-cycled ventilators, a set amount of air (tidal volume) is delivered for each inspiration. The advantage of this form of ventilation is that the tidal volume remains consistent and the pressure necessary to deliver the volume varies, depending on the client's lung compliance. Because of this feature, the volume-cycled type is the most frequently used with adult clients.

To understand volume ventilator settings and functions, the nurse must be familiar with certain terms. These are defined and discussed in Table 18–5.

Patterns of Mechanical Ventilation

There are four common ventilation patterns: assist control, IMV, SIMV, and PEEP. Each is discussed here.

In assist control ventilation, the inspiratory phase is initiated by the client. Modern ventilators have a built-in safety feature so that if the client becomes apneic, the machine will deliver the preset volume at the ordered rate. In controlled ventilation, the machine has complete control of the client's rate and depth of ventilation.

IMV, or intermittent mandatory ventilation, delivers a preset tidal volume at a specific rate while also providing a continuous flow of air for spontaneous breaths (Luce, Pierson, & Hudson, 1981). IMV was introduced for the purpose of gradually weaning individuals from ventilators. The use of this type of ventilation has expanded. It is now used with clients who require mechanical ventilation but are able to initiate some inspiratory effort on their own, such as a client with COPD. IMV cannot be used for someone who is apneic, such as one who has suffered damage to the brain stem. An advantage of IMV ventilation is that it allows the client to use the respiratory muscles and prevents their atrophy. Muscle atrophy may occur when a client is totally dependent on the machine for inspiratory volume.

SIMV refers to synchronized intermittent mandatory

Table 18–5 Terms Related to Ventilator Settings

Term	Explanation
Tidal volume	The amount of air moved in and out with each breath. For individuals of average build, the tidal volume can range between 500 and 1000 mL.
Respiratory rate	Averages 10–14 breaths per minute. Higher or lower rates may be necessary in some clients, depending on their specific condition.
Inspiratory/expiratory ratio	In normal breathing, the expiratory phase lasts as long as the inspiratory phase to allow for emptying of the lungs. This ratio is usually set at 2:1 (expiration, inspiration) to approximate normal physiological function.
Oxygen concentration	The fraction of inspired oxygen (FiO_2). This percentage can vary from room air (21%) to 100%. The administration of higher percentages of oxygen (beyond 50%) for prolonged periods may result in alveolar damage from oxygen toxicity.
Pressure setting	The amount of force required to deliver a specific volume of air into the lungs. Damage to the lungs may result from the use of high pressure to deliver the tidal volume. Therefore, a maximum pressure limit is set on the ventilator to avoid damage to the lungs.
Sighs	Normally, an individual sighs or takes a deep breath periodically. A mechanism for sighing is provided by the ventilator. Sighing prevents atelectasis by causing hyperinflation of the lungs.
Spirometer	The large bellowslike container on the ventilator that measures the volume of air the client expires. This amount should be equal to the tidal volume set on the ventilator. It is important to note this amount, since a decrease may indicate that the client is not receiving the set tidal volume.
Low-pressure alarm	The sounding of this alarm indicates an air leak within the client or inside the ventilator. An air leak within the client may be from leakage of air around the cuff of an endotracheal or tracheostomy tube, or to a persistent air leak after thoracic surgery. Machine air leaks can be from disconnection of the ventilator tubing.
High-pressure alarm	This alarm will sound whenever the pressure volume is reached, but the full delivery of tidal volume did not occur. This can be caused by a variety of factors: obstruction of the inspiratory tubing by kinks, condensation of water, and the body weight of the client lying on the tubing. The airway can be obstructed by herniation of the cuff over the end of the endotracheal or tracheostomy tube. The client may bite the endotracheal tube or pinch the tubing and prevent the inflow of air. Accumulation of bronchial secretions can also cause this alarm to sound, indicating that the client needs to be suctioned. (Coughing during the inspiratory cycle of ventilation will also trigger the alarm but does not indicate any problem.) Other causative factors include pneumothorax, decreased lung compliance, bronchospasm, and incorrect placement of the artificial airway.
Spirometer alarm	This alarm sounds when the volume of air exhaled is less than the amount set on the spirometer. Occasionally, the bellows may stick, causing the alarm to sound. The underlying reason can be identified by noting whether the problem is related to the high-pressure or low-pressure alarm (deToledo, 1980).

ventilation. With this method, air is delivered by the ventilator in synchronization with the client's own ventilatory efforts. For example, if the SIMV is set at a rate of 10, the client is assisted 10 times per minute.

PEEP, or positive end expiratory pressure, prevents the collapse of the airways and alveoli at the end of expiration, facilitating the diffusion of more oxygen from the alveoli into the pulmonary capillaries. PEEP allows for a reduction in inspired oxygen concentrations because oxygen can diffuse during both inspiration and expiration (Wade, 1982). The setting for PEEP is usually within the range of 1 to 15 cm of water. However, levels of over 40 cm have been used when treating clients with severe hypoxemia, as in those with adult respiratory distress syndrome.

Physiologic changes occur with the administration of PEEP. PEEP causes an increase in intrathoracic pressure, which decreases the venous return of blood to the heart. The baroreceptors in the thoracic aorta interpret the decreased venous return as hypovolemia and stimulate an increase in production of antidiuretic hormone (ADH). Increased ADH can lead to the development of hypervolemia, which results in decreased cardiac output. Another potential problem encountered is the development of a pneumothorax.

Nursing Care of the Client Who Is Mechanically Ventilated

Accidental disconnection of the client from the ventilator must be prevented. A warning should be placed on all ventilators and on the nursing care plan reminding health care personnel to leave the ventilator alarm on at all times, even during client suctioning (Box 18–4). The sound of the alarm is a minor nuisance compared to the brain damage that may occur if someone fails to remember to turn the alarm on and the client is accidentally disconnected from the ventilator.

An Ambu bag should be kept at the client's bedside to be used in the event of a power failure or ventilator malfunction. If the ventilator is not working properly, do not waste time trying to identify the mechanical difficulty. Instead, use the Ambu bag to ventilate the client, and have someone call the maintenance technician.

Clients who are ventilated mechanically often require monitoring of central venous pressure or pulmonary capillary wedge pressure. The positive pressure exerted by the ventilator will alter these readings. It is important that they be taken one way consistently, either with the client connected to or disconnected from the ventilator.

As a rule, respiratory therapists are responsible for checking the function of the ventilator at regular intervals. However, the nurse should also be familiar with the machine and how it functions. There are certain observations that the nurse should make at regular intervals.

The pressure indicator shows the amount of force required to ventilate the client's lungs. If the amount of pressure required increases or decreases significantly, assess the situation. Whenever any alarm sounds on the ventilator, respond immediately. (See Table 18–5 for what may cause the alarm to sound.) If the reason for the alarm cannot be readily ascertained and rectified, the client should be disconnected from the ventilator and ventilated manually with an Ambu bag until the ventilator can be replaced or fixed. Since the alarms can be frightening to clients and any others in the room, reassure them that the client can be adequately oxygenated.

Check the settings on the ventilator hourly. This includes making sure that the tidal volume, respiratory rate, FiO_2 (fraction of inspired oxygen), and other parameters are set as ordered. Also check the ventilator tubing for water condensation. When any is found, the tubing should be disconnected and the water emptied. This will prevent accidental aspiration of water into the trachea or impairment in ventilation.

In addition to checking the ventilator, carefully assess the client. Observe the client for overt clinical signs of hypoxia, hypercapnia, or hypocapnia. In addition, arterial blood gas values are obtained at regular intervals. Blood gas values are particularly important when ventilator settings are changed, as when the FiO_2, IMV, or PEEP settings are decreased. Assess the client to ensure that both

Box 18–4 Ventilator Warning—To Maintain Client Safety

The ventilator alarm should remain on at all times, so the staff is immediately notified if the client is accidentally disconnected or there is a problem with ventilator function. It is safe practice to leave the alarm on, even when suctioning the client.

lungs are aerated. This involves auscultating lung sounds and observing for symmetrical expansion of the chest.

A major responsibility is careful monitoring of the client's vital signs. Because the application of PEEP can result in a decrease in cardiac output, particular attention should be paid to blood pressure, pulse, and urine output. Any time the setting for PEEP is altered, the client must be reevaluated. Increasing the amount of PEEP can further compromise venous return, whereas decreasing it could result in cardiac overload and pulmonary edema. Often clients on PEEP have a central venous pressure line or a Swan–Ganz catheter, which allows for more accurate assessment of physiologic parameters. Because of the increased positive pressure exerted with PEEP, the client should be observed for signs and symptoms of pneumothorax.

Nursing care of the client who is mechanically ventilated also includes position change and skin assessment every hour, putting joints through active or passive ROM every 8 hours, and frequent mouth care. Clients who are comatose will need eye care, including use of artificial tears to keep the eyes moist, removal of crusts on lashes and lids with sterile saline or sterile water-soluble lubricant, and protection from corneal drying, irritation, or trauma by taping the eyelids closed.

Nursing Research Note

Dressler D, Smejkal C, Ruffolo M: A comparison of oral and rectal temperature measurement on patients receiving oxygen by mask. *Nurs Res* 1983; 32:373–375.

These researchers investigated the differences in temperature readings from oral and rectal sites in clients receiving oxygen mask therapy. An IVAC 2000 electronic thermometer was used. The results suggest that both oral and rectal temperatures are stable measures. Rectal temperatures were more stable than oral ones, however. The mean difference between oral and rectal readings was 1.46°F.

The implications for nursing practice are related to clinical judgment. Should a 1.46°F difference in temperature change nursing intervention to a significant degree? Is the difference worth disturbing the client for rectal temperature taking? This study indicates a need for more investigation into temperature measurement and site selection.

A client will occasionally fight the ventilator. (This is also referred to as "bucking the ventilator" or "being out of phase with the ventilator.") The client attempts to exhale actively while the ventilator is still delivering the inspired volume. This conflict must be corrected because it results in decreased volume delivery and excessively high airway pressures. Measures to alleviate the problem include manual ventilation using an Ambu bag to increase volume delivery gradually and decrease the respiratory rate. Altered inspiratory flow rates may be ordered for the ventilator to correct the situation, or medication may be prescribed to sedate the client and allow the ventilator to function more efficiently (Traver, 1982).

A complication of prolonged mechanical ventilation is the development of a stress ulcer. The mechanism of the formation of stress ulcers is not entirely understood. It is related to a combination of hypersecretion of hydrochloric acid and decreased resistance of the gastric mucosal lining. The gastric irritation may lead to bleeding. Therefore, the nurse should assess stool and nasogastric drainage for fresh and occult blood. Gastric dilation may also occur from introduction of air into the esophagus. This may necessitate the insertion of a nasogastric tube.

Psychosocial Considerations for the Client Who Is Mechanically Ventilated

Mechanical ventilation is frightening for both the client and family. Staff members are so familiar with the routines and equipment that they may forget the impact on clients and their families. It is important to take the time to explain the equipment, the alarms, the blinking lights, and the like. The client and significant others should be assured that a nurse is always close by and will respond promptly to the client's call light and alarms. Clients should not be left alone in the room until they appear relatively comfortable with the situation. Be careful not to become so involved with monitoring the equipment and performing the procedures that the client is forgotten. Allow time for the client, family members, and significant others to verbalize fears and concerns. These clients are acutely ill and may have realistic fears about being dependent on the machine and the possibility of dying (Traver, 1982).

Mechanical ventilation obviously limits client mobility. Clients confined to their rooms have limited contact with the larger world, which may lead to disorientation. Make a point to interact with the client frequently. Orientation to date, time, and place helps to minimize confusion and prevent anxiety. Lighting can be controlled to create a day–night change. Sometimes it is helpful to keep a large calendar in the room where the client can see it and cross off days. Suggest that family members bring a few pictures or other articles to the hospital to personalize the environment. Clients should be encouraged to become actively involved in their care to maintain a sense of control over their lives.

These clients require frequent attention and care, in an environment with a lot of activity and a high noise level. Clients may suffer from sensory overload, so it is important that nursing care be organized to give the client periods of uninterrupted rest.

When clients require indefinite use of mechanical ventilation even after discharge, the client and family members or significant others need instruction. Ancillary health care providers may also be needed in the home. The nurse can facilitate proper care by coordinating activities among different departments such as respiratory therapy, social service, public health nurses, and any other health team members involved.

Weaning the Client From the Ventilator

Weaning the client involves reducing both physiological and psychological dependence on the ventilator. Criteria that should be met before weaning include acceptable arterial blood gas values on a liter flow of oxygen no greater than 40% to 50%. If the client is receiving PEEP, it should be no higher than 5 cm of water; otherwise, this would interfere with the client's inspiratory efforts. Vital capacity should be greater than 15 mL/kg of body weight because this indicates that the client is able to move enough air. This measurement can be obtained using a respirometer attached to the end of the client's endotracheal or tracheostomy tube. Maximum inspiratory effort should also be assessed to determine whether the client's chest expansion is sufficient to produce a negative alveolar pressure and stimulate a deep inspiration. The greater the client's ability to inhale, the more negative the inspiratory pressure will be. This is assessed by attaching the pressure gauge from an anesthesia machine to the end of the endotracheal or tracheostomy tube and instructing the client to take in a deep breath. The client is considered to be ready for weaning when a pressure of -25 to -30 cm of water is obtained. Respiratory rate and minute volume may be taken to determine the number of breaths per minute and the tidal volume. The respiratory rate must be at least 12, but no greater than 20 per minute.

Additional criteria for weaning include: a stable chest wall, an acceptable chest x-ray, adequate cardiac output, normal temperature, adequate nutritional status, and a generally well rested condition.

Two methods used to wean clients are the T-piece and intermittent mandatory ventilation (IMV). Regardless of the weaning method employed, the cuff on the endotracheal or tracheostomy tube is usually deflated. Before beginning, the weaning process should be explained to the client. In T-piece weaning, the client is taken off the ventilator and a T-tube carrying humidified oxygen is attached to the airway (Figure 18–22). Clients should be encouraged to use the breathing exercises taught to them while they were on the ventilator. Weaning is started during the day, scheduled around medications and activities so that the client is not uncomfortable and is not interrupted. The client should be suctioned prior to disconnection from the ventilator. A semi-Fowler's position will facilitate the weaning process by preventing abdominal contents from pressing on the diaphragm.

Weaning is usually started with 15 minutes off the ventilator and then gradually increased if the client's respiratory status remains stable. The client's vital signs should be checked frequently. Indications that the weaning is being poorly tolerated are: increased respiratory rate and dyspnea, increased pulse rate, cardiac dysrhythmias, change in mentation, increase in fatigue, and decrease in pulmonary volumes. Arterial blood gas measurements are obtained for objective evidence of how well the client is ventilating.

The other method of weaning, IMV, was discussed earlier. The number of IMV breaths per minute is gradually decreased (without exceeding the client's tolerance) until the client is breathing wholly spontaneously. The same nursing implications apply as in T-piece weaning.

Psychological Considerations When Weaning Clients From the Ventilator. Clients who are mechanically ventilated for extended periods may develop a psychological dependence on the ventilator that makes weaning difficult. Mendel and Khan (1980) identified factors that impair the weaning process: fear of sudden death, anger from being asked to give up dependence on the ventilator, secondary depression when the illness is chronic, and interpersonal problems such as a resentful or impatient spouse.

Counseling may be necessary for clients, family members, or significant others when attempts to wean the client

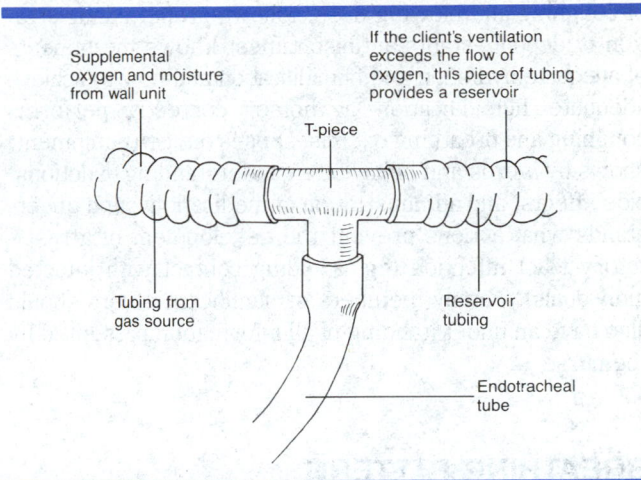

Figure 18–22

T-piece setup for weaning a client from a ventilator.

from the ventilator are resisted. This is particularly true where physiological parameters clearly indicate that weaning is feasible but difficulties are encountered.

Along with counseling, psychotropic drugs may be necessary. Antianxiety medications administered to clients who are near panic prior to weaning have been found helpful in selected clients. If depression is a problem, the physician may prescribe antidepressants. Regardless of whether medications are used, recognize that weaning difficulty can be associated with emotional factors as well as physiological deficits.

Section IV: Evaluation

The evaluation process encompasses physiological status, psychosocial function, and information and/or skills obtained through teaching. This evaluation process should include family members or significant others. Expected outcomes for the client with respiratory dysfunction, summarized in Table 18–2, are reviewed below. If data collected concerning the client's responses and those of the family or significant others do not substantiate expected outcomes, the nursing care plan requires revisions.

AIRWAY CLEARANCE

Nursing interventions related to excessive secretions in the respiratory system are successful when the client can move air in and out of the upper and lower respiratory tracts without difficulty. Subjective and objective findings verifying these outcomes include: a normal appearance of structures in the nose, oropharynx, and hypopharynx, or at least a decrease in inflammation and swelling in these structures; absence of inflammation, redness, and tenderness over the paranasal sinuses; return of the client's

voice to normal; absence of purulent, tenacious discharge or sputum; normal breath sounds on auscultation; absence of adventitious breath sounds; client verbalizations that dysphagia, cough, headache, or sore throat have disappeared; good skin turgor, with intake and output within acceptable limits. In addition, the client's vital signs, chest x-ray, and arterial blood gas analysis would be within normal limits.

These expected outcomes may never be reached by some clients with respiratory disorders. For example, a client with COPD will probably always have abnormal arterial blood gas values and most likely will have a productive cough.

Clients with infections of the upper and lower respiratory tract and their families (or significant others) may need teaching so they may take actions to facilitate resolution of the infection. Also, they must be aware of measures to prevent spread of infection. Signs that the instruction was effective include observations that the client takes action to prevent spread of infection (eg, covering mouth and nose when coughing and sneezing); uses correct method of coughing and blowing nose; follows proper administration of decongestants/antihistamines; knows the benefits of adequate hydration and humidification and how to achieve adequate humidification at home; correctly performs coughing and breathing exercises; uses oxygen equipment; shows by words and behavior an understanding of actions, side effects, and administration of medications; and understands what actions prevent the development of a respiratory tract infection (eg, avoiding contact with infected individuals). Family members or significant others should also have an understanding of all information presented by the nurse.

BREATHING PATTERN

Nursing interventions employed to improve the client's breathing pattern are successful when the lungs are aerated adequately. Findings verifying this outcome in the client who has experienced chest pain or trauma include: normal breath sounds, normal chest x-ray, normal arterial blood gas values, vital signs within normal limits, symmetrical chest expansion, and normal pulmonary function studies. When evaluating clients with chest tubes, note that the chest tube is in place, secured, and covered by a sterile dressing. The chest drainage collection receptacle should also be observed to see that it is functioning properly. If the client is on a ventilator, the function of the ventilator must be monitored as well as the condition of the client.

Findings indicating that the nursing intervention for clients with pathophysiology of lung tissue has been successful include a return to baseline values for the arterial blood gas analysis, normal chest x-ray, and pulmonary function studies. Improved lung sounds should be audible upon auscultation, and sputum production should decrease.

Respiratory disorders can significantly alter the client's ability to perform activities of daily living, as can be seen in many clients with COPD. The physiological changes can result in stress and emotional turmoil for clients and significant others. With knowledgeable and caring nursing intervention, both clients and family members should be able to cope more effectively with limitations imposed by the respiratory disorder. Examples of effective coping behavior would include active participation in developing the plan of care and performing activities of daily living. Expression of fears and anxieties related to the illness and its effects is an integral part of the coping process. Successful adaptation to the limitations imposed by the illness is manifested when the client maintains an interest in functioning at an optimal level. For some, this may mean adjusting to a change in occupation and/or a decrease in social activities.

Clients who require long-term management of their illness need to learn new techniques and skills. Instruction is successful if the client and family members or significant others are able to incorporate learned health behaviors into their everyday life.

GAS EXCHANGE

Three major abnormalities are noted when gas exchange is impaired: hypoxia, hypercapnia, and hypocapnia. Nursing interventions for clients with these abnormalities are directed toward adequate oxygenation for cellular metabolism and arterial CO_2 levels within the normal range.

When caring for the client with hypoxia, nursing interventions are successful when there is a decrease in signs and symptoms of cerebral, cardiovascular, and respiratory hypoxemia. This is evidenced by an absence of (or decrease in) restlessness, irritability, impaired judgment, central cyanosis, diaphoresis, labored breathing, tachypnea, and tachycardia. Blood pressure and level of consciousness should return to normal for that particular client (providing brain injury did not occur). Interpretation of arterial blood gas values will reveal a return to baseline normal PO_2 and oxygen saturation. A complete blood count will also show hemoglobin values within normal limits.

If the hypoxic state is a chronic condition, both clients and significant others must learn to cope effectively with the lowered oxygen level. For example, the client and significant others will plan daily activities to leave adequate time for rest periods.

Nursing measures employed with the client who is hypercapnic are successful if signs and symptoms of cerebral, cardiovascular, and respiratory hypercapnia decrease. This involves an absence of (or decrease in) confusion, drowsiness, headache, dizziness, tetany, asterixis, tachycardia, and cardiac dysrhythmias. The client will no longer experience convulsions, and the level of consciousness will improve or return to normal. Analysis of an arterial blood gas sample will show a pH of 7.35 to 7.45.

Nursing measures to correct hypocapnia are successful if signs and symptoms of cerebral, cardiovascular, and respiratory hypocapnia decrease. There would be an absence of (or decrease in) muscle spasm, tetany, diaphoresis, cardiac dysrhythmias, and tachypnea. The client would also return to a normal level of consciousness. Interpretation of arterial blood gas analysis reveals a normal pH of 7.35 to 7.45.

Clients with impaired gas exchange will experience changes in their mentation and level of consciousness. Nursing measures are directed toward orienting the client and assisting significant others in coping with the change. Measures are successful if clients know their names, the date, the time, and the place. Also, the family and significant others must understand the cause of the confusion and measures they must take to prevent the client from self-injury.

Chapter Highlights

Disorders of the upper and lower respiratory tract can result in ineffective airway clearance, ineffective breathing patterns, and impaired gas exchange.

Pulmonary function tests are used in the diagnosis of lung volume abnormalities, to monitor the course of disease, and to evaluate the effectiveness of treatment.

Roentgenologic examination such as chest x-rays and sinus films are used to diagnose abnormalities of the respiratory tract.

Arterial blood gas analysis provides an objective measurement of oxygenation, carbon dioxide elimination, and blood pH.

Oxygen is primarily transported in the blood in combination with hemoglobin. The oxygen saturation and the oxygen-hemoglobin dissociation curve are measurements of the amount of hemoglobin combined with the oxygen.

Sputum cultures are used to identify an invading organism and its sensitivity to antibiotics.

Thoracentesis involves the insertion of a needle into the intrapleural space for the purposes of removing fluid that impairs breathing and to obtain a specimen for laboratory evaluation.

Endoscopic procedures are used to assess, diagnose, or correct disorders of the upper and lower respiratory tract.

Pulmonary hygiene measures employed by the nurse to improve ventilation and enhance the removal of secretions include deep breathing and coughing, breathing exercises, and postural drainage.

Artificial airways consist of endotracheal tubes, tracheostomy tubes, and laryngectomy tubes.

Indications for placement of an artificial airway are to relieve obstruction, facilitate suctioning, allow for mechanical ventilation, and prevent aspiration.

Nursing management of the client with an artificial airway involves providing humidification, maintaining airway patency, and observing for complications.

Since the lower respiratory tract is normally a sterile environment, the nurse must use sterile technique when suctioning or performing tracheostomy care.

Mechanical ventilation is employed for clients who can no longer maintain adequate oxygenation and carbon dioxide elimination on their own.

Weaning the client from a ventilator involves reducing and eventually eliminating physical and psychological dependence on the ventilator.

The major objective of water-seal drainage is to facilitate drainage of fluid and air from the intrapleural space, fostering reexpansion of the lung.

Nursing management of the client with a chest tube consists of: assessment of respiratory status, ensuring proper function of the closed chest drainage system, assessing level of fluid drainage, and maintaining patency of the chest tube.

Evaluation of the client with a respiratory disorder includes assessment of: physiological parameters; effectiveness of teaching; and ability of the client, family members, or significant others to cope with the illness.

Bibliography

American Cancer Society: *1985 Cancer Facts and Figures.* New York: American Cancer Society, 1985.

Brown I: Trach care? Take care: Infection's on the prowl. *Nurs 82* (May) 1982; 12(5):44–49.

Burton GG, Hodgkin JE (editors): *Respiratory Care: A Guide to Clinical Practice,* 2nd ed. Philadelphia: Lippincott, 1984.

Byrne CJ, Saxton DF, Pelikan PK, Nugent PM: *Laboratory Tests: Implications for Nursing Care.* Menlo Park, CA: Addison-Wesley, 1986.

Cameron T: Fiberoptic bronchoscopy. *Am J Nurs* 1981; 81:1462–1464.

Chalikian J, Weaver TE: Mechanical ventilation—Where it's at, where it's going. *Am J Nurs* 1984; 84(11):1372–1379.

de Toledo L: Caring for the patient instead of the ventilator. *RN* 1980; 43(12):21–23.

Edlund BJ, Wheeler EC: Adaptation to breathlessness. *Top Clin Nurs* 1980; 2(3):11–25.

Einstein H: Coccidioidomycosis. *Resp Care* 1981; 26:563–569.

Erickson R: Chest tubes: They're really not that complicated. *Nurs 81* (May) 1981; 11(5):34–43.

George RB, Light RW, Matthay RA (editors): *Chest Medicine.* New York: Churchill Livingstone, 1983.

Glassroth J: Tuberculosis: A review for clinicians. *Clin Notes Resp Dis* Fall 1981; 20:5–13.

Grossbach-Landis I: Successful weaning of ventilator-dependent patients. *Top Clin Nurs* 1980; 2(3):45–68.

Guyton AG: *Textbook of Medical Physiology,* 6th ed. Philadelphia: Saunders, 1981.

Harper R: *A Guide to Respiratory Care: Physiology and Clinical*

Applications. Philadelphia: Lippincott, 1981.

Hinshaw H, Murray J: *Diseases of the Chest.* Philadelphia: Saunders, 1980.

Hollen E, Toomey I, Given S: Bronchoscopy. *Nurs 82* (June) 1982; 12(6):120–122.

Irwin MM, Openbrier DR: A delicate balance: Strategies for feeding ventilated COPD patients. *Am J Nurs* 1985; 85(3):274–280.

Irwin MM, Openbrier DR: Feeding ventilated patients safely. *Am J Nurs* 1985; 85(5):544–546.

Janowski MJ: Accidental disconnections from breathing systems. *Am J Nurs* 1984; 84(2):241–244.

Lake J: Prolonged nasotracheal intubation. *Heart Lung* 1980; 9:93–97.

Langner SR, Innes C: Breathing, holism, and health. *Top Clin Nurs* 1980; 2(3):1–10.

Luce JM, Pierson DJ, Hudson LD: Intermittent mandatory ventilation. *Chest* (June) 1981; 79(6):678–685.

Mendel JG, Khan FA: Psychological aspects of weaning from mechanical ventilation. *Psychosomatics* (June) 1980; 21(6):465–471.

Natanson C, Shelhamer JH, Parrillo JE: Intubation of the trachea in the critical care setting. *JAMA* Feb 22, 1985, 253(8):1160–1165.

Nielsen L: Ventilators and how they work. *Am J Nurs* 1980; 80:2202–2205.

Paparella M, Shumrick D (editors): *Otolaryngology.* Vol 3. Philadelphia: Saunders, 1980.

Petty T (editor): *Intensive and Rehabilitative Respiratory Care.* Philadelphia: Lea & Febiger, 1982.

Pfister S, Bullas JB: Caring for a patient with a chest tube connected to the Emerson pump. *Crit Care Nurs* 1985; 5(2):26–32.

Saum M: Taking the mystery out of chest tubes. *AORNJ* 1980; 32:86–100.

Sumner S: Refining your technique for drawing arterial blood gases. *Nurs 80* (April) 1980; 10(4):65–69.

Traver G: *Respiratory Nursing: The Science and the Art.* New York: Wiley, 1982.

Treseler K: *Clinical Laboratory Tests: Significance and Implications for Nursing.* Englewood Cliffs, NJ: Prentice-Hall, 1982.

Wade JF: *Comprehensive Respiratory Care: Physiology and Technique.* St. Louis: Mosby, 1982.

Wagner H, Buchanan J: Radioactive tracer studies in pulmonary disease. In: *Diagnostic Techniques in Pulmonary Disease.* Sacker M (editor). New York: Marcel-Dekker, 1980.

Weaver T: Bronchoscopy, laryngography, and their potential complications. *RN* (Dec) 1982; 45:64–65.

White HA, Briggs AM: Home care of persons with respiratory problems: Optimization of breathing and life potential. *Top Clin Nurs* 1980; 2(3):69–77.

Suggested Readings

D'Agostino J: Set your mind at ease on oxygen toxicity. *Nurs 83* (July) 1983; 13(7):55–56. The author provides a brief explanation of the complication of oxygen toxicity. Signs and symptoms and preventive measures are discussed.

Dunlap C, Marchionno P: Help your COPD patient take a better breath, with inhalers. *Nurs 83* (May) 1983; 13(5):42–43. The authors explain how inhaled medications (bronchodilators, corticosteroids, mast-cell inhibitors) work when used by clients with chronic lung disease. Specific guidelines and helpful hints are presented for clients who use an inhaler.

Ellmyer P, Thomas N: A guide to your patient's safe home use of oxygen. *Nurs 82* (Jan) 1982; 12(1):55–57. The author presents important ground rules for the use of home oxygen, reasons behind the rules, and specific suggestions for the client and family. The information would be useful when performing discharge teaching for clients who require oxygen therapy at home. Public health nurses who make home visits should also find this information useful.

Fuchs P: Before and after surgery, stay right on respiratory care. *Nurs 83* (May) 1983; 13(5):47–50. The author briefly reviews the effects of surgery on the pulmonary system and the importance of preparing a client physiologically and psychologically in the preoperative phase. Explanations of coughing, the use of mechanical devices to stimulate deep breathing, chest physiotherapy, and the use of small-volume nebulizers are discussed.

Resources

SELF-HELP GROUPS AND OTHER ORGANIZATIONS

American Association for Respiratory Therapy
7411 Hines Pl., Suite 101
Dallas, TX 75235
Phone: (212) 245–8000

Chapters of this health and education organization are staffed primarily with volunteers who raise funds to support research, and provide information and referral services for lung disease. Sponsor "Easy Breathers", a training program of breathing exercises for persons with emphysema, chronic bronchitis, asthma, and other lung diseases; a smoking cessation program; and a nonsmokers' rights program including assertiveness techniques.

Asthma and Allergy Foundation of America
801 Second Ave.
New York, NY 10017
Phone: (212) 867–8875

A national, voluntary health agency that sponsors research, training of asthma and allergy specialists, and information for the public. Also maintains a directory of physicians who specialize in the treatment of these disorders and provides referrals to inpatient and outpatient asthma and allergy treatment facilities.

Black Lung Association
906 W. Neville St. Box 1065
Beckley, WV 25801

This advocacy organization promotes safer mining conditions and supports legislation for increased government benefits for miners affected by pneumoconiosis. Membership consists of coal miners, their families, and other interested persons.

Cystic Fibrosis Foundation
6000 Executive Blvd., Suite 309
Rockville, MD 20852
Phone: (301) 881-9130

In addition to supporting research, educational and training programs for professionals and the public, and providing referral services, clinical care and counseling for children with cystic fibrosis, this organization provides information on asthma, emphysema, bronchiectasis, bronchitis, recurrent pneumonia, and developmental lung disorders.

Emphysema Anonymous, Inc.
PO Box 66
Ft. Myers, FL 33902
Phone: (813) 334-4266

Members of this all-volunteer, nonprofit organization have established a mutual support network of self-help groups throughout the US, Canada, and Mexico.

International Association of Laryngectomees
% American Cancer Society, Inc.
777 Third Ave.
New York, NY 10017
Phone: (212) 371-2900, ext. 246

This organization is composed of over 250 clubs known as "Lost Chord," "New Voice," or "Anamilo" (depending on geographical area). Members are persons who have undergone laryngectomies and wish to help others who have had this surgery. Local clubs sponsor counseling for clients and their families, self help meetings, voice rehabilitation services, workshops on esophageal speech and the use of other voice appliances and seminars for health educators on first aid and artificial resuscitation for laryngectomees.

In Canada
Canadian Tuberculosis and Respiratory
Disease Association
345 O'Connor St.
Ottawa, Ontario, Canada K2P 1V9

An organization, with associations in all Canadian provinces, to promote research, education, diagnosis, treatment, and client care for persons with respiratory diseases. (Check phone book for local chapters.)

Lost Chord Club
% Princess Margaret's Lodge
545 Jarvis St.
Toronto, Ontario, Canada M4Y 2H8
Phone: (416) 924-0671, ext. 405

Organization for clients who have had laryngectomies, and their families. Provides self-help and mutual support with monthly meetings of group.

STOP SMOKING PROGRAMS

American Cancer Society
777 Third Ave.
New York, NY 10017
Phone: (212) 736-3030

American Health Foundation Stop
Smoking System
320 E. 43rd St.
New York, NY 10017
Phone: (212) 953-1900

5-Day Plan to Stop Smoking
Seventh Day Adventist Church
Narcotics Education Division
6840 Eastern Ave., NW
Washington, DC 20012
Phone: (202) 722-6000

SmokEnders
50 Washington St.
Norwalk, CT 06854
Phone: (203) 846-4371

St. Helena Hospital Program
Deer Park, CA 94576
Phone: (707) 963-3611
(5-day live-in plan)

HOT LINES

Asthma Hotline
National Jewish Hospital/National
Asthma Center
Phone: (800) 222-LUNG

Questions about asthma, emphysema, chronic bronchitis, tuberculosis, juvenile rheumatoid arthritis, occupational and environmental lung diseases and other respiratory and immune system disorders are answered by a specially trained nurse.

Asthma-Allergy Hotline
American Academy of Allergy and Immunology
Phone: (800) 558-1035
in Wisconsin (414) 272-1004, collect

Twelve recorded messages by experts in the field are available through this number. A list of local specialists and research centers can be requested.

HEALTH EDUCATION MATERIAL

American Lung Association
"Cocci", a booklet on coccidioidomycosis (especially for those who live in California, Arizona, New Mexico, and Texas).
"Emphysema: Answers to Your Questions", a booklet.
"Facts About Your Lungs: Tuberculosis", a booklet.
"Health Hazards in the Arts", a booklet describing the hazards of crafts such as photography, rock tumbling, pottery, and metal working.
"Health Hazards in the Science Classroom", a booklet on some dangerous chemicals used in school science laboratories.
"Histo", a booklet (especially for those who live in the Mississippi, Ohio, and Missouri river valleys.
"Nonsmokers' Rights: What You Can Do", a brochure on how to assert nonsmoking rights.

Asthma and Allergy Foundation of America
"Asthma, Climate, and Weather", a booklet.

"Handbook for the Asthmatic", a booklet explaining treatment approaches and offering advice on how to eliminate household allergens.

Emphysema Anonymous
"Our Daily Breath", a booklet describing breathing exercises

National Interagency Council on Smoking and Health
419 Park Ave. South
New York, NY 10016
Phone: (212) 532-6035
"Smoking and Health Newsletter", a regular newsletter by subscription on research into cigarette smoking and the progress being made by antismoking organizations.

The President's Committee on Employment of the Handicapped
111 Twentieth St., N. W.
Washington, DC 20210
Phone: (202) 653-3044

"Respond to: Workers With Cystic Fibrosis", a booklet for employers and those who work with cystic fibrosis clients.

NURSING ORGANIZATION

Otorhinolaryngology Head/Neck Nurses
% Warren Otologic Group
3893 E. Market St.
Warren, OH 44484
Phone: (216) 856-4000
This organization promotes the recognition of ENT and head and neck nursing as a distinct subspecialty. Members are RNs. Annual dues are $40.

Chapter 19

Specific Disorders of the Upper Respiratory Tract

Vicky Hartwell-Ivins

Objectives

When you have finished studying this chapter, you should be able to:

Identify and discuss the etiology and clinical manifestations associated with disorders of the upper respiratory tract.

List the therapeutic measures used for clients with problems of the upper respiratory tract.

Describe the recommended nursing care for clients with upper respiratory disorders.

Specify the role of the nurse in prevention of the spread of upper respiratory tract infections.

Anticipate the psychosocial/lifestyle implications of disorders of the upper respiratory tract on clients and significant others.

Educate the general public about etiological factors associated with the development of disorders of the upper respiratory tract.

Specific disorders of the upper respiratory system cover a wide spectrum. Some may be considered minor annoyances of short duration. Other upper respiratory disorders may be related to extensive morbidity that may threaten the client's life or may seriously affect the client's lifestyle.

Section I: Disorders of Multifactorial Origin

Disorders of multifactorial origin cannot be ascribed to any single class of etiologic factors. They may be related to anatomic or physiological changes within the body, to environmental conditions, to the psychosocial status of the individual, or to any combination of these factors.

The symptoms of multifactorial disorders range from minor, easily tolerated discomforts such as the "common cold" to the life-threatening emergency of angioneurotic edema. The sensations of taste and smell may be diminished or obliterated; these alterations may in turn affect nutritional status by diminishing the client's appetite. Voice quality may be altered, in some cases to the point where alternative means of communication must be found. And the airway may be compromised in some disorders to the point at which death will occur if the appropriate interventions are not promptly undertaken.

Nurses can educate their clients and the general public about preventive measures such as cessation of smoking and avoidance of habits that abuse the vocal cords. Clients with minor disorders of the respiratory system may seek treatment as outpatients or may elect to care for themselves at home, so nurses are often consulted both formally and informally about therapeutic measures. Clients seeking professional health care for other disorders may have symptoms of upper respiratory disorders of which they are unaware. The nurse who is alert to findings that signal respiratory problems can refer these clients for more thorough evaluation that in some cases—notably early detection of malignancy—can be life-saving.

EPISTAXIS

Bleeding from the nose is a common problem that occurs in people of all ages. **Epistaxis** is not a disease; rather, it is an indication of underlying trauma or physiological abnormality. Some individuals with epistaxis can treat them-

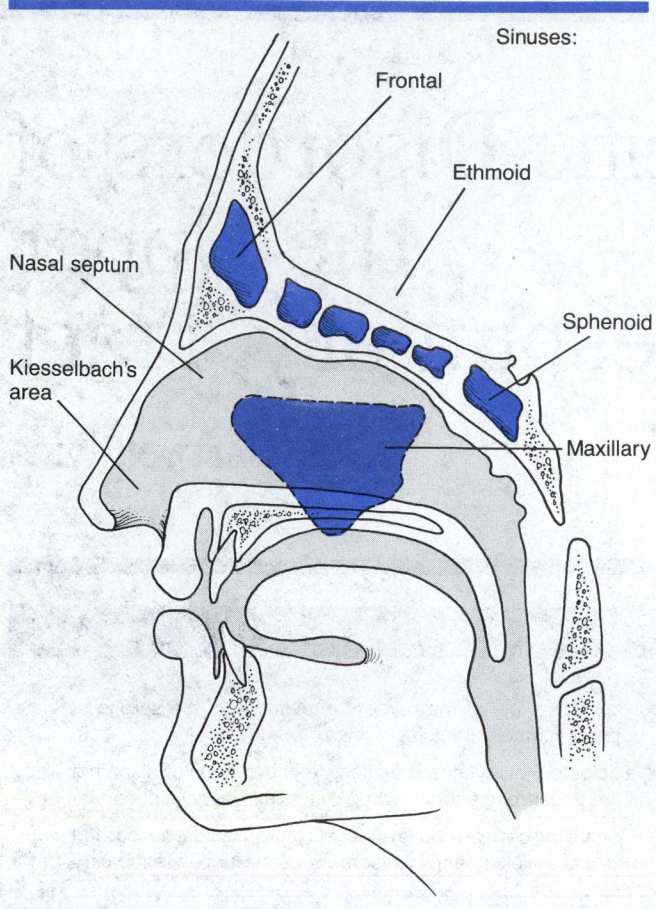

Sinuses:
Frontal
Ethmoid
Sphenoid
Nasal septum
Kiesselbach's area
Maxillary

Figure 19–1
Location of Kiesselbach's area and the paranasal sinuses.

selves at home; for others, professional intervention is required. The severity of epistaxis and the appropriate treatment depend on the specific site of the hemorrhage.

In most cases, epistaxis is related to hemorrhage from the anterior portion of the nose. The most common site of bleeding is the vascular area of the anterior nasal septum known as Little's or Kiesselbach's area (Figure 19–1). Epistaxis originating in this area is commonly observed in young and middle-aged adults. Epistaxis originating from the posterior area of the nasal septum is often quite severe and is observed more commonly in elderly people.

The most frequent cause of epistaxis is trauma. Trauma may be related to an external cause such as a blow to the nose or maxillofacial area, or minor injury such as after picking of the nose or noseblowing. Epistaxis may be related to lack of humidification, local nasal infections, or tumors of the nose or paranasal sinuses. Some systemic disorders are associated with an increased incidence of nosebleeds (eg, hypertension and arteriosclerosis). Epistaxis may be a manifestation of an underlying blood dyscrasia such as leukemia, pancytopenia, or thrombocytopenia, or it may be related to treatment with anticoagulants such as warfarin (Coumadin), heparin, or aspirin. Hereditary hemorrhagic telangiectasia, a multisystemic vascular disorder charac-

terized by hemorrhage due to localized capillary lesions, is related to severe, recurrent epistaxis.

Clinical Manifestations

Epistaxis is usually unilateral. Sometimes drainage from the posterior portion of the nose may flow behind the septum and out both nares; the nosebleed appears bilateral but is actually unilateral. Bilateral epistaxis may occur after nasal fractures. Clients who have blood dyscrasias may hemorrhage bilaterally from the nasal mucosa; generally, these clients will hemorrhage at other body sites as well.

Clients frequently swallow some of the blood and may report nausea or vomiting. If the swallowed blood passes through the gastrointestinal (GI) tract, the stools will be black, and stool guaiac testing will be positive for blood. Hypertensive clients may report headaches. If a large amount of blood is lost, the client may exhibit symptoms and signs of hypovolemia.

Therapeutic Measures

Vasoconstrictive agents may be applied locally for initial control of hemorrhage from the anterior portion of the nose. A suction catheter is used to remove clots from the nasal cavity, and a sterile cotton ball moistened with a topical vasoconstrictor, such as aqueous epinephrine 1:1000, is inserted into the nostril. Pressure is then applied to the nose for several minutes.

If epistaxis is related to a systemic disorder, measures for correcting the underlying abnormality should be undertaken. For example, antihypertensives may be prescribed, or coagulation abnormalities may be corrected. Blood transfusion and fluid replacement may also be required.

Cauterization using a silver nitrate stick, trichloroacetic acid, or an electric cautery device may be used to promote hemostasis by sealing the vessels with denatured protein. If cauterization does not control the hemorrhage, an anterior nasal pack is placed (Figure 19–2). The material commonly used for this is a long, continuous strip of half-inch petrolatum gauze. Antibiotic ointment may be applied to prevent odor.

Hemorrhage from the posterior area of the nose is often more severe than anterior hemorrhage, and the site is more difficult to treat. A posterior nasal pack is inserted to apply pressure to the site of hemorrhage (Figures 19–3A and B). A sedative or analgesic may be prescribed to help calm the client and to reduce the discomfort caused by insertion of the pack. Two methods of posterior packing are used. The first employs 4 × 4 gauze rolled up and tied with sutures as a pack. A catheter is inserted through the nostril into the nasopharynx, down into the oral cavity, and out through the mouth. The catheter is clamped, the pack is tied to it by the sutures, and the catheter is then pulled through the nose until the pack is in the appropriate position. Once the pack is in the nasopharynx, an anterior pack may be applied also. The alternative method employs a

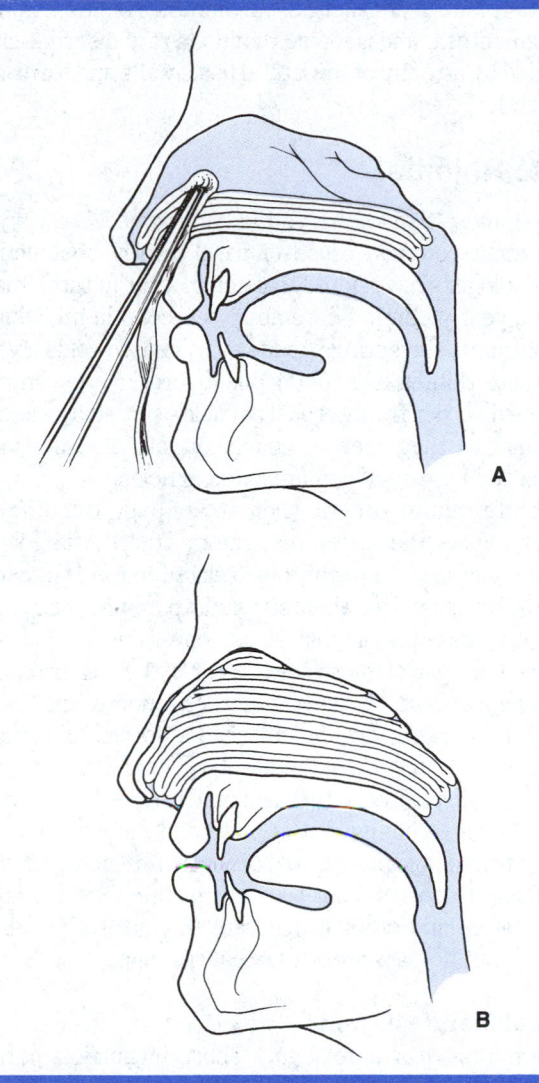

Figure 19-2

Anterior nasal pack. **A.** Gauze is layed in switch-back fashion. **B.** Both nostrils are completely packed with gauze in all crevices.

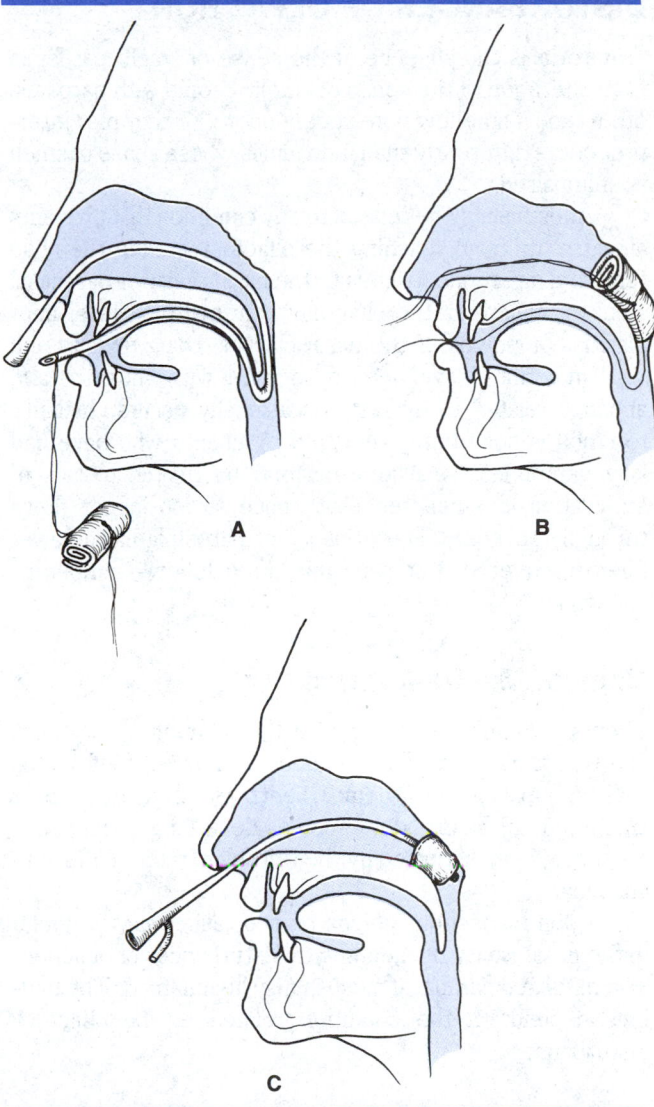

Figure 19-3

Posterior nasal pack with gauze. **A.** Catheter inserted via one nostril, passed into oral pharynx and out through the mouth; a rolled gauze sponge is attached to it. **B.** The sponge is drawn into the nasopharynx. **C.** Foley catheter method of packing the posterior portion of the nose.

Foley catheter (Figure 19-3C). The balloon is inflated with water once it is in the nasopharynx; the anterior portion of the nose is packed, and the catheter is secured. The pack is left in place for 3 to 7 days.

If a serious nosebleed cannot be controlled by packing, the internal maxillary or anterior ethmoidal artery or even the external carotid artery may have to be ligated. Usually, ligation of the internal maxillary artery accomplishes hemostasis.

Specific Nursing Measures

Seeing large quantities of blood is often frightening to the client. The nurse can offer reassurance to alleviate the client's anxiety. Clients who are not hypotensive should be seated in an upright position with the head slightly flexed forward to prevent blood from dripping into the pharynx.

Clients who cannot tolerate the upright position should be placed on their sides or supported with pillows to prevent aspiration. Blowing the nose is contraindicated. Since the client has lost blood, blood pressure and pulse must be monitored. Elevated blood pressure may be related to underlying hypertension or to agitation and anxiety. Clients who have lost a significant amount of blood may be hypotensive and are usually tachycardic.

Clients with anterior packing are usually sent home. Hospitalization is mandatory for clients with posterior nasal packing because of the risk of airway obstruction. Nursing care of the client with nasal packing is discussed in Chapter 18.

DISTURBANCES OF OLFACTION

Anosmia is the absence of the sense of smell; parosmia is an alteration of the sense of smell. People with parosmia often report smelling nonexistent odors, or they may interpret odors differently than individuals whose sense of smell is unimpaired.

Anosmia may be related to any condition that prevents air currents from reaching the olfactory area in the nose (eg, viral infections, trauma to the nasal cavity or paranasal sinuses, lesions of the olfactory neuronal pathways, neoplasms, or polyps of the nasal cavity). Drug toxicity and viral infections have been associated with anosmia, and anosmia related to hysteria occasionally occurs. Inability to smell is sometimes reported by clients who have had laryngectomies; such anosmia may be related to lack of stimulation of smell receptors once air no longer flows through the nose. The etiology of parosmia has not yet been discovered, but parosmia often follows temporary anosmia.

Clinical Manifestations

Clients with anosmia report that they cannot detect odors and that their taste discrimination is altered; food tastes flat and unpalatable to them. Clients with parosmia report smelling unpleasant odors such as decayed garbage; they are more often disturbed by their problem than clients with anosmia.

Upon inspection, polyps or neoplasms may be found in the nasal cavity of clients with disturbances of olfaction. The nasal and paranasal mucosa may be inflamed. The findings depend on the condition related to the olfactory disturbance.

Therapeutic Measures

Treatment of olfactory disturbances is directed at alleviating the underlying pathologic condition if it can be identified. For example, if an infection is present, measures should be taken to eradicate it. Nasal polyps, neoplasms, or other obstructions may be removed surgically. Administration of vitamin A, orally or by injection, has achieved limited success in the treatment of anosmia (DeWeese & Saunders, 1982).

Specific Nursing Measures

Encouraging the client to eat when the sense of taste is altered is an important nursing activity. Other interventions depend on the underlying disorder.

RHINITIS

Inflammation of the nasal mucosa, or rhinitis, has many causes. It is often accompanied by inflammation of the throat and sinuses. Among the different types are acute rhinitis, allergic rhinitis, nonallergic vasomotor rhinitis, rhinitis medicamentosa, and atrophic rhinitis (a rare disorder characterized by atrophy of the lateral nasal walls and formation of crusts).

Acute Rhinitis

Acute rhinitis, also known as the common cold or coryza, is the most common cause of nasal airway obstruction. Epidemiologists have noted that colds occur in three major waves a year—one in September, a second in midwinter, and another in the spring. Adults average two colds a year.

Acute rhinitis is a contagious disorder; one can contract the disorder from aerosol particles spread by infected individuals as they sneeze, cough, or talk. It can also be transmitted by way of contaminated articles.

Acute rhinitis occurs when any of over 100 different viruses infects the upper respiratory tract. A large percentage of cases is thought to be related to the rhinovirus, but other responsible agents include parainfluenza, influenza, respiratory syncytial virus, enterovirus, and adenovirus. One reason more colds occur in the colder months is that people tend to crowd together indoors, facilitating spread of infection; dry, heated indoor air also diminishes the protective function of the nasal mucosa. Evidence concerning predisposing factors is conflicting. Although most people believe chilling of the body and fatigue favor the development of symptoms, well controlled laboratory studies have failed to corroborate this supposition. Stress, nutritional status, and other factors are thought to be related to colds, but no data presently confirm this.

Clinical Manifestations

Acute rhinitis has a relatively short incubation period. Symptoms begin to appear within 18 to 48 hours after an individual contracts the virus. Initial symptoms include irritation or a burning sensation in the nasopharynx, nasal stuffiness, dry scratchy throat, and headache. A persistent sore throat usually does not accompany the uncomplicated common cold. On examination of the nares with a nasal speculum, the nasal turbinates will be swollen, and a mucoid nasal discharge will be visualized that may become purulent as the infection progresses. Frequent bouts of sneezing are common, and a dry, hacking cough may be present. The client may be febrile and may report malaise. The uncomplicated cold usually resolves in 5 to 6 days. Significant pain or persistent temperature elevation should make one suspect a secondary bacterial infection. Possible complications of acute rhinitis include sinusitis, otitis media, bronchitis, or pneumonia.

Therapeutic Measures

Aspirin may provide some relief from the feeling of malaise. Initially, decongestants such as pseudoephedrine may provide symptomatic relief; if not, an antihistamine–decongestant combination may be tried. Although vasoconstrictor nose drops may provide relief from nasal congestion, they should be used infrequently to prevent rhinitis medicamentosa, which is discussed later in this section. Bed rest is recommended, and adequate fluid intake should be maintained to mobilize secretions and prevent dehydration. If secondary bacterial infection occurs, antibiotics will be prescribed.

Specific Nursing Measures

Clients who develop acute rhinitis may request antibiotic therapy. The nurse should stress that antibiotics are not indicated, since acute rhinitis is caused by a virus, and antibiotics are not effective against viruses. Remind the client that aspirin, fluids, humidified air, and rest are a proven regimen. Aspirin will relieve some of the discomfort and will lower the temperature. Liquids will replace fluid lost through diaphoresis and will loosen secretions. Humidified air, especially in the bedroom during sleep, will maintain moist mucous membranes. Rest will help alleviate fatigue. The nurse should warn clients that antihistamines have side effects such as drowsiness and dry mouth. The nurse might also suggest that the client limit contact with others during the first 2 or 3 days of the infection to reduce spread of the cold. Clients can be taught hygienic measures such as good hand-washing technique and covering the nose and mouth when sneezing or coughing. Clients should also be cautioned not to blow their noses too vigorously. They should not close their mouths completely or occlude their nostrils while blowing the nose, since doing so can force nasal discharge into the eustachian tubes.

Allergic Rhinitis

Allergic rhinitis can be classified as an acute (seasonal) or chronic (perennial) allergy. Seasonal rhinitis is often referred to as hay fever. The symptoms last several weeks and recur each year. A person who has perennial allergic rhinitis may experience symptoms throughout all or most of the year.

Seasonal allergic rhinitis is related to sensitivity to pollens from flowers, grasses, or trees. Perennial allergic rhinitis is usually related to sensitivity to such substances as animal danders, wool, feathers, household dust and molds, foods, tobacco, drugs such as aspirin, and a host of other agents present in the environment.

Clinical Manifestations

Both types of allergic rhinitis are manifested by the same symptoms, although the acute form is usually related to more severe symptoms. Clients will often have nasal obstruction, sneezing, recurrent thin nasal discharge, itching of the eyes and nose, increased lacrimation, and frontal headache. If the reaction is severe, the individual may experience dyspnea related to bronchospasm. The nasal mucosa appears pale blue-gray and boggy. Microscopic examination of the nasal discharge usually reveals the presence of large numbers of eosinophils. Clients who suffer from allergic rhinitis often develop nasal polyps.

Therapeutic Measures

Antihistamines may relieve symptoms. Short-term administration of systemic steroids may benefit a client with severe allergic rhinitis, but prolonged use of steroids should be avoided because of their side effects. Ideally, the allergen would be identified and removed from the client's environment, but this is not always feasible. Desensitization may be attempted; this involves injecting gradually increasing quantities of the allergen weekly until a specific level is achieved. The process of desensitization stimulates antibody production against the specific allergen. Sometimes clients are given a series of injections prior to hay fever season to desensitize them.

Some clients will benefit from a submucous resection or a polypectomy to remove excess mucosa or nasal polyps. These procedures are explained in Chapter 21.

Specific Nursing Measures

Clients who are undergoing desensitization can benefit from explanations of the purpose and technique of the procedure; the nurse can reinforce the physician's explanation. Clients should be warned about the side effects of antihistamines and cautioned about driving or operating machinery while taking these medications. They should also be cautioned about drinking alcoholic beverages, since antihistamines can potentiate the effects of alcohol.

If the cause of allergic rhinitis is not known, the client can try the following measures to alleviate symptoms:

- Using hypoallergenic cosmetics
- Avoiding wool clothing and blankets
- Limiting chocolate, milk, and eggs in the diet
- Removing domestic animals from the home
- Installing air conditioning or air filtration equipment in the home
- Covering mattresses and pillows with plastic

Clients should be cautioned not to use vasoconstrictor nose drops or sprays frequently.

Nonallergic Vasomotor Rhinitis

Oversensitivity of the normal nasal reflexes can be related to nonallergic vasomotor rhinitis. Normally, the sympathetic and parasympathetic pathways of the autonomic nervous system interact to regulate certain nasal reflexes; sympathetic stimulation tends to shrink the nasal mucosa; parasympathetic stimulation is related to nasal congestion, increased nasal discharge, and sneezing. Nonallergic vasomotor rhinitis apparently occurs because the vasomotor system is oversensitive to certain stimuli (Paparella & Shumrick, 1980).

Emotional stress appears to be one of the factors related to this disorder. Anxiety or frustration, particularly after illness or surgery, can precipitate symptoms, as may a change of climate. Hormonal changes related to pregnancy or the use of oral contraceptives have been related to this disorder; symptoms have also been observed in clients with hypothyroidism. Several chemical substances that affect the autonomic nervous system may be indirectly related to alterations in the nasal mucosa, including aspirin, reserpine, neostigmine, chlorpromazine, ergot alkaloids, alcohol, and tobacco. Pollutants in water or air may precipitate symptoms in some clients (Paparella & Shumrick, 1980).

Clinical Manifestations

The afflicted person may experience nasal obstruction or stuffiness, watery nasal discharge, and repeated sneezing. Nasal turbinates will be swollen, and the nasal mucosa will vary in color from dark red to blue. In long-standing cases of the disorder, irreversible hypertrophy of the mucosa may occur. Symptoms are intermittent and may last for several hours. Some clients with nonallergic vasomotor rhinitis suffer atypical facial neuralgias and migraine headaches.

Therapeutic Measures

Because of the varied etiology, nonallergic vasomotor rhinitis may be difficult to treat successfully. Nose drops and other medication are usually ineffective; nose drops should be avoided because of their side effects. Clients may benefit from counseling by a psychiatric nurse clinician or other mental health professional who can help them deal with underlying stress or anxiety that may be related to the condition. In some cases, surgical treatment such as cauterization of the turbinates or even, in severe cases, turbinectomy, may have to be performed. Vidian neurectomy (severing of the vidian nerve to interrupt cholinergic stimulation to the area) may be performed if the client has excessive nasal discharge. These procedures are discussed in Chapter 21.

Specific Nursing Measures

The client may benefit from an explanation of nasal physiology leading to better understanding of why symptoms occur. Emotional support is important for these clients, who are uncomfortable with symptoms for which the cause and the care are elusive.

Rhinitis Medicamentosa

Rhinitis medicamentosa involves a so-called rebound phenomenon related to excessive use of nose drops or sprays. Short-term use of these agents may decrease engorgement of the nasal turbinates, but continued use causes reengorgement and an actual increase in nasal stuffiness. Individuals who use these products initially obtain 1 or 2 hours of relief before nasal stuffiness recurs. Most people apply the medication repeatedly, and the cycle repeats itself, with the severity of the nasal congestion increasing and the duration of relief decreasing as more and more medication is applied more and more often. Eventually, the client becomes a "nose drop addict." Inspection reveals congested, shiny red nasal mucosa. Any client with nasal obstruction that has no apparent cause should be questioned about use of nose drops or nasal sprays.

Therapeutic and Specific Nursing Measures

The client is instructed to discontinue use of all intranasal medications. Recovery usually follows in 2 to 3 weeks, but the client may be uncomfortable during this period because of the mucosal engorgement. An oral antihistamine or decongestant and humidified air may relieve some symptoms.

The nurse should explain the rebound phenomenon to reinforce the client's understanding of why intranasal medication should be discontinued.

NASAL POLYPS

Nasal polyps are not neoplasms; they are masses of hypertrophied mucosa that may contain fluid. The majority develop as an outpouching of the mucosa covering the maxillary or ethmoid sinuses. They extend from the sinuses into the nasal cavity through the ostium. A polyp that develops in a maxillary sinus and protrudes into the nasopharynx is called an antrochoanal polyp. Polyps are often multiple and may occur bilaterally. Obstruction of the nasal passages develops gradually as the polyps multiply and enlarge.

Polyps form in response to recurrent swelling of the mucosa of the nose or sinuses, but their precise etiology may be indeterminate. They may be related to long-term nasal allergy or to an infectious condition such as rhinitis or sinusitis. Nasal polyps are often observed in clients with allergic rhinitis. They are also found in clients who have aspirin-intolerant asthma, a condition characterized by aspirin sensitivity, nasal polyposis, and asthma.

Clinical Manifestations

Clients with nasal polyps may find that breathing through the nose is impeded. Disturbances of olfaction may be noted, and the voice may have a nasal quality (**rhinolalia**). Upon inspection, nasal polyps appear as smooth gray or gray-blue masses that can be readily manipulated. Their appearance has been described as that of "skinned white grapes." Infection or irritation causes the polyps to become reddened. Radiologic examination of the sinuses may show changes in the mucosa, since many nasal polyps originate in the sinuses.

Therapeutic Measures

Although systemically or locally administered steroids may effect regression of nasal polyps, steroid therapy is contraindicated by the known side effects of steroids and by the fact that regression is frequently only temporary (DeWeese & Saunders, 1982). Polypectomy—surgical removal by one of a number of procedures—is recommended for most clients. Intranasal polypectomy or more extensive surgery involving the paranasal sinuses, such as intranasal ethmoidectomy or the Caldwell-Luc procedure, may be performed. These procedures are discussed in Chapter 21.

Specific Nursing Measures

Inspection of the internal nares with a nasal speculum in any client with upper respiratory symptoms or problems with smell is an important nursing responsibility. Nasal polyps are often missed because this aspect of physical assessment is omitted. Other nursing measures are related to postoperative care.

HYPERTROPHY OF THE NASAL TURBINATES

Three nasal turbinates are seen in most clients: the inferior, middle, and superior (Figure 19–4). In a few instances, a fourth turbinate may be seen. Hypertrophy of the turbinates, which is related to nasal obstruction, generally involves the inferior turbinate and occasionally the middle turbinate. The turbinates are covered with semierectile, richly vascularized mucosa that helps warm and humidify inspired air. Under normal conditions, a congestion–decongestion reflex alternately increases and decreases congestion of opposite sides of the nose every 3 to 4 hours, so airway resistance remains constant overall. Hypertrophied turbinates do not shrink and expand normally, and consequently, the airway is obstructed.

Permanent hypertrophy of the nasal turbinates is related to long-standing inflammation (eg, in chronic rhinitis). Redundant hyperplastic mucosa is seen in the turbinates.

Clinical Manifestations and Therapeutic Measures

Clients experience continual nasal obstruction that is not relieved by nasal drops or sprays, antihistamines, or allergic desensitization. In the past, sclerosing agents were sometimes injected to shrink the turbinates, but there have been reports of blindness related to this treatment, and it is no longer generally performed (Saunders, 1982). Electrocautery may be used to reduce the size of the turbinate, or turbinectomy may be performed to remove the mucosa or a portion of the bone.

DEVIATED NASAL SEPTUM

The nasal septum, which is composed of cartilage and bone overlaid with ciliated mucosa, is normally thin and straight. A variation from this ideal is called a deviated nasal septum; variations range from a single bulge to S-shaped deviations, sharply angulated deformities, or excessive spurring of the maxillary crest. Most adults have some degree of nasal septal deviation.

In adults, deviation of the septum may be due to either congenital or traumatic factors. Deviation may be related to a single, severe trauma to the area or to a number of insignificant blows to the nose that pass unnoticed over the years.

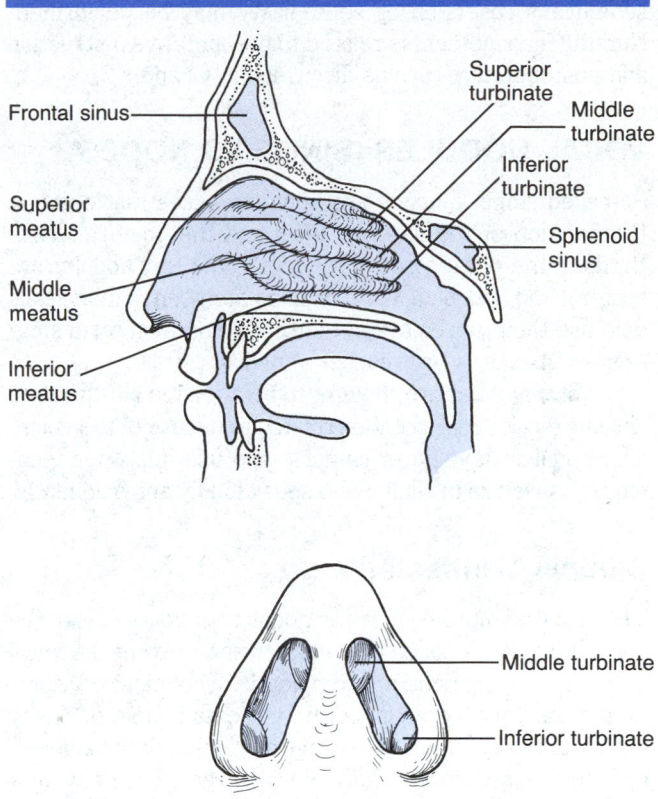

Figure 19–4

The nasal turbinates.

Clinical Manifestations

Septal deviations may produce no symptoms at all. When symptoms do occur, the most common is nasal obstruction, which may be unilateral or bilateral, intermittent or continuous. Other symptoms are nebulous. Headache is sometimes associated with a septal defect, but no etiologic relationship has been established. Deviation sufficient to cause pressure on other structures may cause pain in the nares, cheeks, or orbit. Hemorrhage can also occur. Inspiration may be obstructed, and continual exposure of the nasal mucosa to unhumidified air may lead to drying and cracking of the mucosa and to epistaxis. Clients who breathe through their mouths may experience dryness and irritation of the throat. The client may be predisposed to sinusitis because drainage from the sinuses is obstructed.

Deviation of the nasal septum is generally apparent upon inspection. If the condition has developed over a period of years, the inferior turbinate on the contralateral side may be hypertrophied. The degree of deviation does not always correspond to the degree of nasal obstruction.

Therapeutic and Specific Nursing Measures

Many individuals require no treatment. If nasal obstruction is present or if drainage from the sinuses is impeded, a submucous resection or septoplasty may be performed. Nursing management is related to preoperative instruction and postoperative care as discussed in Chapter 21.

VOCAL NODULES (SINGER'S NODES)

So-called singer's nodes are benign nodules that occur at the junction of the anterior third and the posterior two-thirds of the vocal cords. Frequently, the tiny nodules are bilateral and apposed. Vocal nodules are seen in individuals who use their voices often; hence the common term singer's (or speaker's or preacher's) nodes.

Vocal nodules are thought to be a reaction of tissue to chronic mechanical irritation related to misuse of the voice. The nodules develop in singers who use improper technique, as well as in adults who speak loudly and frequently.

Clinical Manifestations

The usual symptom of vocal nodules is hoarseness; the apposing nodules touch one another and prevent the vocal cords from approximating completely. The impaired vibration of the vocal cords gives the voice its hoarse or husky quality. Initially, the nodules appear red; as fibrosis develops, they appear white. Vocal nodules can be seen by indirect mirror laryngoscopy.

Therapeutic Measures

If the client is not disturbed by the change in voice quality, no treatment may be necessary. Speech therapy and rest may improve hoarseness. Nodules may be surgically removed by direct or indirect laryngoscopy under local or general anesthesia.

Specific Nursing Measures

A client whose vocal nodules have been surgically removed should not use the voice at all for 2 to 4 days to avoid approximation of the cords, which might cause trauma to healing structures. The nurse can help the client maintain silence by providing alternative means of communication such as a writing tablet or "magic slate." Clients who will not maintain complete silence should be advised to whisper. Remind the client that further misuse of the voice may cause recurrence of nodules.

LARYNGEAL POLYPS

A laryngeal polyp is a growth that arises from the mucous membrane of the vocal cord. Such polyps are usually benign but may become malignant or may be related to other complications. Polyps may have a thin stalk (pedunculated polyp) or they may have a broad base (sessile polyp) (Figure 19–5).

The precise etiology of laryngeal polyps is not clear. Polyps have been known to develop in relation to vocal abuse and other irritative factors such as smoking.

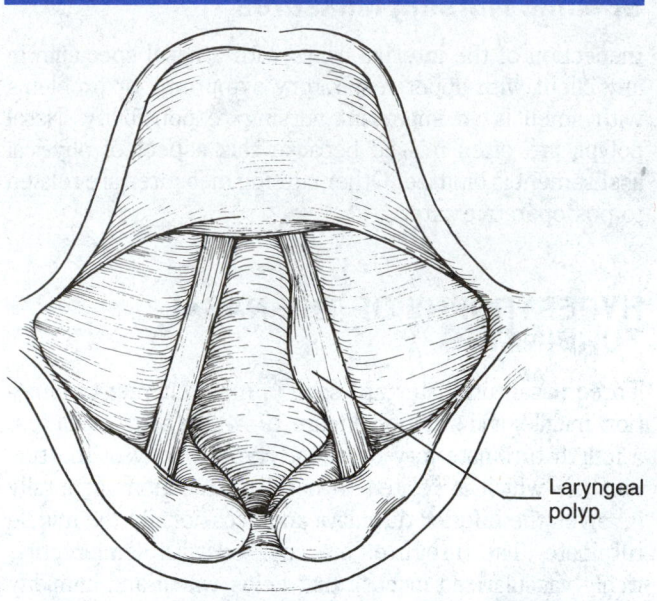

Laryngeal polyp

Figure 19–5
Large polyp of left vocal cord.

Clinical Manifestations

The principal symptom of laryngeal polyps is hoarseness. The voice assumes a deep quality because the tissue of the larynx cannot resonate properly during phonation. If the polyp is pedunculated, it may drop below the level of the vocal cords occasionally, and hoarseness may be intermittent. Sessile polyps are related to continuous hoarseness. In rare instances, a large polyp may be associated with respiratory distress.

Therapeutic Measures

Laryngeal polyps should be removed for tissue biopsy to rule out the possibility of malignancy. Polyps are generally removed by endoscopy under local anesthesia combined with sedation, but general anesthesia may also be employed. Very small polyps may be resected by microlaryngoscopy. Use of a carbon dioxide laser has reportedly been successful in eradicating laryngeal polyps.

Specific Nursing Measures

Following removal of a laryngeal polyp, the client should talk as little as possible for 7 to 10 days. The nurse can provide alternative means for communication and encourage the client to use them. Coughing and clearing of the throat should be avoided for the first few days after the procedure. If the condition has been related to abuse of the voice, the client may benefit from referral to a speech therapist.

LARYNGEAL EDEMA

Edema of the laryngeal tissue is seen in both acute and chronic forms. Rapidity of onset varies, depending on etiology and the response of the individual.

Infectious processes that involve the larynx will be related to some degree of edema. Edema may also be related to irradiation of the neck, neoplastic disease involving the region of the neck, or infections that alter the lymphatic drainage of the area. Laryngeal edema may also be secondary to iatrogenic injury in connection with intubation or surgical procedures. In some instances, edema occurs in systemic diseases that alter capillary permeability or disturb the oncotic pressure of the plasma. **Angioneurotic edema** involves an allergic response of the tissue of the larynx. Angioneurotic edema occurs rapidly with an allergic reaction to inhalants, injected substances (including contrast media), transfusions, insect bites, food, or medications.

Clinical Manifestations

The initial symptom of laryngeal edema is hoarseness. As the condition progresses, the person may be barely able to speak. When inspected by indirect mirror laryngoscopy, the laryngeal structures and vocal cords may appear swollen. As obstruction becomes more severe, dyspnea, stridor, tachypnea, and cyanosis may occur. Onset of the edema is usually gradual, involving structures other than the larynx. Onset of angioneurotic edema, however, is usually acute. Symptoms and signs of laryngeal obstruction develop rapidly, and the condition can progress to total obstruction and death.

Therapeutic Measures

Angioneurotic edema is a medical emergency. Intravenous administration of epinephrine usually brings about rapid decrease in inflammation. Corticosteroids are also sometimes used. Tracheotomy or intubation may be required to maintain a patent airway, particularly in cases of acute onset.

Laryngeal edema related to systemic disorders responds to treatments directed at the underlying condition. Serum protein and electrolyte levels may have to be monitored and corrected.

Specific Nursing Measures

Nursing responsibilities involve obtaining a history from the client of known allergies and documenting them well on the nursing care plan and in the client's chart. Clients who have been intubated should be monitored for evidence of laryngeal edema. Emergency drugs and a tracheotomy setup should be at the bedside of clients at risk and generally accessible on the unit for acute laryngeal obstruction.

LARYNGEAL PARALYSIS

Paralysis of the larynx may be unilateral or bilateral. The nature of the presenting symptoms will depend on whether one or both cords are affected and on the position of the vocal cords.

Laryngeal paralysis may be related to disease or injury to the recurrent or superior laryngeal nerves (branches of the vagus nerve) or to the vagus nerve itself. Although the underlying cause may be a disorder of the central nervous system, peripheral nerve disorders are more frequently responsible. Since the recurrent laryngeal nerve passes under the aortic arch on the left side, the nerve may be stretched and paralyzed if the client has an aortic aneurysm. Enlargement of the left atrium related to mitral stenosis may damage the nerve. Neoplasms in the chest or neck may stretch or invade the nerve. Laryngeal paralysis may also be related to trauma or to neuritis caused by metallic poisons (eg, lead) or infectious diseases (eg, diphtheria). Iatrogenic injury to the recurrent nerve or one of its branches during a thyroidectomy is a common cause of laryngeal paralysis.

Clinical Manifestations

Hoarseness may be present if vocal cord paralysis is unilateral, but the client's voice may also remain unaffected. Dyspnea does not occur with unilateral paralysis, because the functioning cord abducts to allow for a normal airway. If paralysis is bilateral, the cords are usually adducted. The client's voice will be adequate but weak. The major problem is the compromised airway; the client usually breathes normally during bed rest or minimal activity, but stridor is present upon exertion.

Therapeutic Measures

Treatment of unilateral paralysis of the vocal cords is not mandatory. Some clients are disturbed by the change in voice quality, however. In such cases, injections of Teflon into the paralyzed cord may cause it to swell sufficiently to allow the normally functioning cord to approximate it (Passy, 1982).

Bilateral paralysis of the vocal cords compromises the client's airway, sometimes so severely that a tracheotomy is required to prevent asphyxiation. Arytenoidectomy is the most frequent surgical approach for bilateral paralysis; one or both of the arytenoid cartilages are removed and one of the vocal cords is retracted laterally and sutured, enlarging the glottic opening and improving the airway.

FOREIGN BODY IN THE NASAL CAVITY

Foreign bodies found in the nasal cavity are usually objects small enough to be inserted through the nostril. Occasionally, an insect may be sucked into the nasal cavity during inspiration. Objects inserted into the nares voluntarily—

usually by a child but occasionally by a mentally ill or mentally retarded adult—make up a nearly endless list, including stones, dried peas or beans, nuts, beads, and buttons.

Clinical Manifestations

A complex of symptoms and signs including nasal obstruction, edema of the nose or the nasal mucosa, seropurulent nasal discharge, and foul odor are typically associated with a foreign body in the nose. The classic sign is lasting, unilateral foul-smelling discharge. Upon inspection, the foreign body may be visualized; the nasal mucosa is swollen, and pus may be present. Stasis of nasal discharge may be related to formation of a **rhinolith,** or nasal calculus, when the inorganic salts in nasal secretions collect around the foreign body.

Therapeutic Measures

Usually, the foreign body can be removed with forceps; curved hemostatic forceps may be used if the object is hard and smooth. To increase client comfort and exposure of the object, a topical anesthetic and vasoconstrictor, such as 2% tetracaine and 0.5% phenylephrine hydrochloride, can be used. Soft material may be removed by suction or with a blunt, right-angled hook. An anterior nasal pack may be inserted if hemorrhage occurs after removal.

Specific Nursing Measures

It is dangerous to attempt removal of a foreign body from the nose without proper instrumentation. The object could be accidentally forced into the nasopharynx or could fall into the larynx or trachea, causing airway obstruction. The client should be reassured that it is normal for some bleeding to occur when the object is removed. Nursing measures related to use of nasal packs and to epistaxis are discussed earlier in this chapter and also in Chapter 18.

FOREIGN BODY IN THE LARYNX

Foreign substances lodged in the throat may have been put into the mouth and accidentally displaced backward into the throat, or they may consist of food or substances contained in food—bones, for example. The substance becomes lodged in the oropharynx or larynx, causing partial or total obstruction of the airway. If total obstruction occurs, the person will asphyxiate in minutes unless the object is dislodged.

Foreign bodies may be aspirated in a number of ways. Many people carelessly hold objects in their mouths while working—pins, tacks, nails, and the like—and swallow or aspirate them when they are distracted. Intoxicated individuals, or those taking sedative drugs, may aspirate because their protective reflexes are impaired. Persons may aspirate a bone or other unexpected object contained in their food, or a portion of the food itself, such as a large bite of meat, may be drawn into the larynx because of difficulty in swallowing it. Individuals who talk while eating or eat hurriedly without chewing their food sufficiently are at increased risk, as are elderly people who may have poor dentition and cannot masticate effectively.

Clinical Manifestations

Any foreign body that becomes lodged in the larynx will impair respiration to some extent. If complete obstruction occurs, the victim will be unable to talk and may indicate choking by clutching the neck between the thumb and open palm. The symptoms of choking mimic those of a heart attack; hence the popular term "cafe coronary." If the airway is incompletely obstructed, the victim will exhibit signs of respiratory distress; coughing, choking, or gagging indicates that some air is moving through the respiratory tract.

Therapeutic Measures

Total obstruction of the airway is of course an emergency; the victim can die in minutes if a patent airway is not restored. The Heimlich maneuver is recommended in this situation (see Chapter 13). If the maneuver is unsuccessful, a cricothyroidotomy should be performed. If the obstruction is not total, the individual may seek medical care. No attempt should be made to remove the object, since it might be dislocated in such a way as to obstruct the airway completely. The victim should be accompanied to a health care facility, since the obstruction might shift position at any time. Endoscopic removal of the obstruction should be performed by direct laryngoscopy (see Chapter 18).

Specific Nursing Measures

A person whose airway is partially obstructed will be anxious. The nurse should remain calm and reassure the client. Nurses should be skilled in the Heimlich maneuver and take every opportunity to teach it to the public. The laryngoscopy procedure should be explained to the client and significant others. Nursing care related to cricothyroidotomy is discussed in Chapter 21.

Section II: Infectious Disorders

The term *upper respiratory infection* (URI) refers to infections of the nose and paranasal sinuses, nasopharynx, middle ear and eustachian tube, pharynx, and larynx.

Infections of the ear and eustachian tube are discussed in Chapter 75.

Infections of the upper respiratory tract are related to

invasion of the body by microorganisms that are capable of destroying tissue, either in themselves or by producing toxins (as in diphtheria). The microorganisms may be either viruses or bacteria.

Upper respiratory infections are among the most common infections found in the adult population; they are responsible for 80% of all school days missed and 40% of all workdays lost (Cluff & Johnson, 1982). Most of these infections are minor and self-limiting; if unattended, however, they may lead to more serious infections. Upper respiratory infections sometimes accompany more severe disorders, and sometimes they are manifestations of an underlying systemic disease. On occasion, an upper respiratory infection may spread to the lower respiratory tract. Thus it is possible for the infection to be related to a fatal outcome, but this is rare.

General Nursing Implications

Nurses are frequently consulted about respiratory infections, especially nurses working in outpatient facilities, health maintenance organizations, and industrial and institutional settings. Nurses are also involved in preventing the spread of infection in both the hospital and community. Thus, it is important that nurses recognize the symptoms of respiratory infection and possible complications, and that they know how symptoms can best be alleviated.

In working with clients with upper respiratory infections, preventing spread of the infection is a paramount concern. The client should be encouraged to practice proper oral and nasal hygiene: to cover the mouth when coughing or sneezing and to use disposable tissues. Contact with others should be limited, and any direct contact such as kissing should be avoided entirely. Clients' eating and drinking utensils should not be used by others. It is imperative that individuals undergoing immunosuppressive therapies—(eg, clients receiving chemotherapy or transplant recipients)—be isolated from anyone with an upper respiratory infection. Persons whose immune system has been compromised can die from an infection that would be mild in a healthy adult.

General nursing measures include encouraging bed rest, adequate hydration, and nutrition. Bed rest helps alleviate fatigue and gives the client a respite from day-to-day pressures. Hydration assists in thinning and removing secretions; dried secretions cannot be removed as readily by mucociliary and cough mechanisms and thus can lead to obstruction of the eustachian tube, sinuses, or tracheobronchial tree. Clients should be cautioned against drinking beverages containing caffeine (including tea, hot chocolate, and cola drinks as well as coffee). Caffeine acts as a mild diuretic and thus interferes with hydration (Cluff & Johnson, 1982). Gargling may provide some relief from throat irritation. Humidification aids in thinning secretions and relieves symptoms; clients should be cautioned against using steam, however. Cold-water humidification offers relief without the hazards associated with boiling water.

SINUSITIS

Sinusitis is an inflammatory change in the mucosa of the paranasal sinuses. Inflamed, edematous mucous membranes partially or totally occlude the ostia leading from each sinus into the nasal passages. Mucus accumulates in the obstructed passage and exerts pressure against the walls of the sinus. One or all sinuses may be affected.

In strict otolaryngologic terms, sinusitis refers to a suppurative infection involving bacterial invasion of the mucosa. This condition, which may be acute or long term, is relatively common. Clients may report they are suffering from "sinus trouble," however, when the actual condition is allergic rhinitis, postnasal drip, headache related to unidentified causes, or various infections of the upper respiratory tract. Of every 100 persons who consult an otolaryngologist about sinus trouble, fewer than 10 have sinusitis (DeWeese & Saunders, 1982).

Acute suppurative sinusitis often accompanies or follows acute rhinitis. So-called swimmer's sinusitis is related to contaminated water being forced into the nose during swimming or diving. Maxillary sinusitis may be related to dental infection. Certain predisposing factors contribute to development of sinusitis (eg, conditions that impede drainage, such as nasal polyps or a deviated septum). Inflammation related to allergy can also obstruct drainage. Dryness of the mucosa, which may occur in overheated rooms in winter or in chronic smokers, can interfere with mucociliary defenses. Lower resistance related to any of a number of conditions can also contribute to development of sinusitis. Bacteria most often involved in sinus infection are pneumococci, streptococci, and staphylococci.

In chronic suppurative sinusitis, the mucosal lining of one or more of the paranasal sinuses has been irreversibly damaged. Failure to treat acute sinusitis, or repeated episodes of the acute form of the disorder, can lead to chronic suppurative sinusitis.

Clinical Manifestations

Acute Suppurative Sinusitis

Onset of symptoms is gradual, except in the case of swimmer's sinusitis. The initial symptom is nasal stuffiness followed by a sensation of pressure over the infected sinus. The client will experience general malaise and may have a headache. In uncomplicated cases, temperature is only slightly elevated (99°F to 99.5°F, or 37°C to 37.5°C). The leukocyte count is usually normal. During the 48 to 72 hours after onset, the client experiences localized pain and tenderness over the affected sinus. Palpation over the involved area elicits tenderness. Severe, constant headache frequently develops. Maxillary sinusitis will cause pain in the cheek. Pain in the nasal bridge or around the eyes is related to ethmoid sinusitis, whereas clients with sphenoid sinusitis report deep pain behind the eyes and in the occipital area. Those with frontal sinusitis typically report a frontal headache. Most clients report nasal and postnasal discharge. Nasal discharge may be blood tinged initially, soon becoming copious and purulent. Postnasal drip may be accompanied by sore throat related to irritation. The client may be anorexic and nauseated.

The nasal mucosa on the involved side appears red and edematous. Purulent secretions may be observed in the nares. The face may appear swollen and red in the area over the involved sinuses, and periorbital edema may be noted. Upon radiologic examination, the involved sinus appears clouded; a fluid level may be visible (Figure 19–6). The affected frontal or maxillary sinus appears dark when examined by transillumination. The ethmoid and sphenoid sinuses cannot be examined in this manner because of their anatomic location.

Chronic Suppurative Sinusitis

Symptoms of chronic suppurative sinusitis vary in intensity. Nasal discharge is a common sign; it may be mucoid, purulent, or mucopurulent. Postnasal drip is frequently present and may be the only problem reported by the client. Related to postnasal drip may be an unpleasant taste in the mouth, frequent cough, and constant need to clear the throat. Some nasal obstruction may occur, particularly if nasal polyps are present. Unlike acute sinusitis, chronic suppurative sinusitis is not related to significant pain. Some clients may report headaches, but most do not, and pain in other areas does not generally occur unless a complication develops.

Inspection of the nasal mucosa reveals redness and edema. As in acute sinusitis, an involved maxillary or frontal sinus appears dark with transillumination. Mucosal thickening or fluid in the area may appear on x-ray.

Complications of sinusitis have become relatively uncommon since the development of antibiotic therapy. Possible complications include development of a mucocele (dilation of a cavity with mucus), osteomyelitis, orbital cellulitis, meningitis, and cavernous sinus thrombosis (infection of a cavernous sinus) (Paparella & Shumrick, 1980).

Therapeutic Measures

Acute suppurative sinusitis is usually treated medically; surgical intervention is often necessary in cases of chronic sinusitis. Analgesics, including codeine, meperidine, and morphine, may be prescribed. Vasoconstrictor nose drops or sprays may have short-term usefulness in maintaining an open nasal passage; the disadvantages of these agents have been discussed in a previous section. Commonly used decongestants include ephedrine sulfate and phenylephrine HCl (Neo-Synephrine) administered as nasal drops or as inhalants. Antibiotic therapy is prescribed on the basis of culture and sensitivity tests and the duration and extent of the infection.

If the infected sinuses become totally occluded, and conservative measures fail to bring about improvement, surgical drainage and irrigation may be indicated. Generally, surgical intervention is contraindicated during the acute

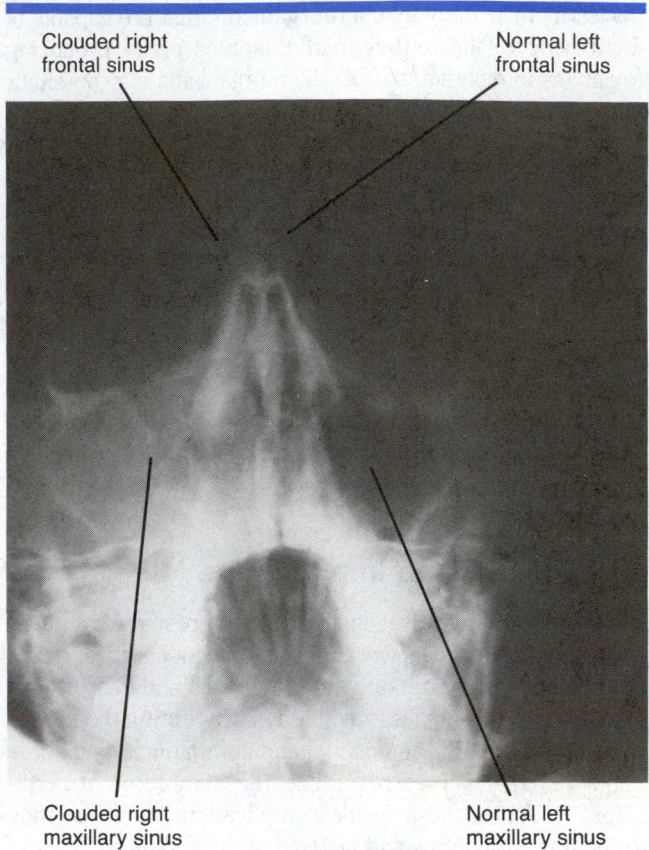

Clouded right frontal sinus

Normal left frontal sinus

Clouded right maxillary sinus

Normal left maxillary sinus

Figure 19–6

X-ray of a client with acute right frontal and maxillary sinusitis; the left frontal and maxillary sinuses are normal. (Courtesy of Health Care Plan, Buffalo, NY)

stage because of the risk of spreading the infection. Surgical treatments employed include the Caldwell-Luc approach combined with antral irrigation of the maxillary sinuses; ethmoidectomy for ethmoid and sphenoid sinuses; and frontoethmoidectomy, osteoplastic flap, and frontal trephination for the frontal sinus. Refer to Chapter 21 for description of these procedures and related nursing care.

Specific Nursing Measures

Hot wet packs applied continuously or for 1 to 2 hours four times each day may reduce inflammation. A hot water bottle may also be used for this purpose. Steam inhalation may relieve symptoms. Clients should be instructed to avoid sudden changes in temperature, which may aggravate the condition (eg, entering an air-conditioned room when it is hot outside). Smoking should be avoided, since it causes further irritation of the mucous membranes.

PHARYNGITIS

Inflammation of the mucous membranes of the pharynx, or pharyngitis, is a common, troublesome disorder causing considerable loss of time from work and school. The three major classifications of this disorder are acute pharyngitis (the most common throat inflammation), acute follicular pharyngitis, and chronic pharyngitis.

Acute pharyngitis is usually related to a viral infection but sometimes to a bacterial infection. Acute follicular pharyngitis is a bacterial infection, most commonly caused by group A beta-hemolytic streptococci. Epidemiologists have found that streptococcal pharyngitis is most prevalent during February, March, and April. The incubation period is 3 days. Staphylococci may also cause pharyngitis, most commonly in debilitated clients. Pharyngitis related to infection with *Neisseria gonorrhoeae* has been reported; the condition appears to occur most often in homosexual males (Sloane, 1982).

Chronic pharyngitis has no clearly defined etiology; one or more factors may be involved. Acute pharyngitis may become chronic if not adequately treated. Irritation of the mucous membranes by postnasal drip associated with chronic infectious disorders or allergies affecting the nose or sinuses can cause pharyngitis. Administration of anti-microbial or antiseptic agents may suppress the normal bacterial flora of the oral cavity, leading to fungal infection and related inflammation. Lack of humidification of inspired air (eg, due to mouth breathing) or impaired production of saliva can lead to dryness of the pharyngeal mucosa, which predisposes it to infection. Xerostomia (dry mouth) is often associated with irradiation and the use of anticholinergic medication. Alcohol and tobacco irritate the pharynx, and environmental pollutants may also be related to pharyngitis. The incidence of chronic pharyngitis is higher among individuals whose tonsils have been removed.

Clinical Manifestations

Acute Pharyngitis

A common cold may be preceded by acute pharyngitis. A mild sore throat, slight difficulty in swallowing, and low-grade fever may be accompanied by cough, **rhinorrhea,** and headache. Symptoms remain mild unless complications occur, and the inflammation usually resolves within 4 to 6 days. Edema and redness of the pharyngeal and nasal mucosa can be observed, with visible rhinorrhea. Enlarged lymph nodes in the neck may be palpable.

Acute Follicular Pharyngitis

Onset of inflammation is usually abrupt. Temperature elevation to 103°F (39°C) or higher may occur, accompanied by chills. The client may report headache, myalgia, and joint pain. Inspection of the throat reveals severe inflammation of the mucosa and edema of the uvula. (Structures of the pharynx are shown in Figure 19–7.) White or yellow follicles may be observed on the lymphoid areas of the throat. Tonsils (if present) are enlarged and studded with follicles.

Chronic Pharyngitis

Persistent sore throat and a constant desire to clear the throat characterize chronic pharyngitis. This disorder is

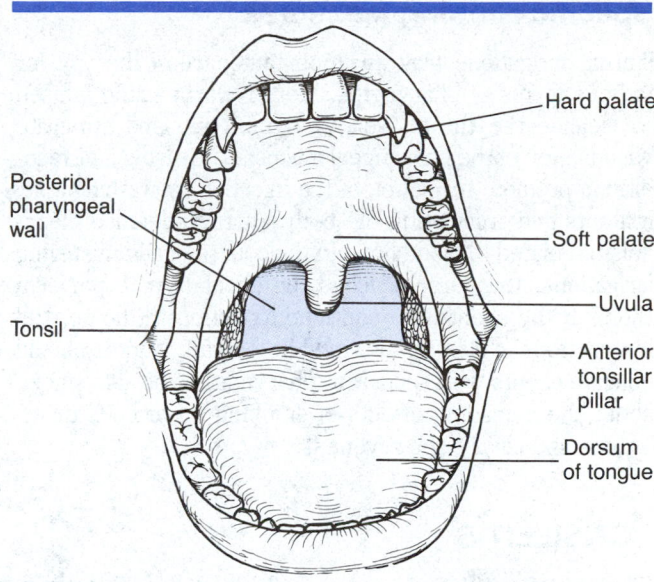

Figure 19–7

View of pharyngeal structures.

often referred to as granular pharyngitis because of the presence of prominent granules on the posterior pharyngeal walls. The mucosa appears red and dry.

Therapeutic Measures

Acute pharyngitis is usually treated at home with a combination of rest, oral fluids, warm gargles or throat irrigations, throat lozenges, and aspirin or acetaminophen. The recommended therapy for acute follicular pharyngitis consists of bed rest, throat irrigations, and the administration of antibiotics and analgesics. The majority of clients can be cared for at home. If the throat becomes so painful and swollen that fluids cannot be swallowed, the client must be hospitalized. Intravenous fluid administration may be required for 24 to 72 hours, until inflammation subsides.

Penicillin is generally the drug of choice for acute follicular pharyngitis since streptococci are the usual causative organisms. Erythromycin may be used if the client is allergic to penicillin. The client should be carefully questioned about any history of penicillin sensitivity before it is administered. To prevent recurrence of the infection, antibiotic therapy is continued for a full 10 days even though symptoms and signs of infection usually subside in 5 to 7 days.

Chronic pharyngitis that is allergy related is managed by removal of the allergen from the client's environment, if possible; if not, desensitization treatments are given. If the disorder is not allergy related, silver nitrate 10% may be applied locally by a physician. Throat irrigations are beneficial in treatment of chronic pharyngitis; irrigations are preferable to gargling because the warm fluid reaches the oropharynx.

Specific Nursing Measures

Throat irrigations play an important part in therapy for various forms of pharyngitis. Hot or warm saline is used to cleanse the throat, relieve symptoms, and stimulate vasodilation of the pharyngeal mucosa. Cleansing and vasodilation promote resolution of the infection by washing away irritants and stimulating the body's natural defense mechanisms related to blood flow. In the course of administering irrigations, the nurse teaches the client how to perform them. If the client is to continue irrigations at home, the instructions in Box 19–1 would be helpful. Nurses should educate clients with recurrent pharyngitis who also smoke about the damaging effects of smoking on mucous membranes and ciliary effectiveness.

TONSILLITIS

The term *tonsillitis* describes inflammation and enlargement of tonsillar tissue with accumulation of leukocytes, dead cells, and bacteria in the crypts. Although the condition may affect either the palatine or the lingual tonsils, only palatine tonsillitis is discussed here. Infection of the lingual tonsils is a much rarer condition.

Although the tonsils are believed to provide defensive barriers against microorganisms invading the upper respiratory system, these defenses can be overcome by invading organisms. Acute or chronic tonsillitis then develops, either as a localized infection involving only the tonsils, or as part of a generalized pharyngitis.

Acute tonsillitis may begin as a bacterial infection of the tonsils, or it may be secondary to a viral infection of the upper respiratory system. Group A beta-hemolytic streptococci are the usual etiologic agents. Droplet contamination is the primary mode of transmission. Chronic tonsillitis may follow an acute episode in which the infection lingers. The lymph follicles may harbor small residual abscesses that can trigger future episodes of acute tonsillitis.

Clinical Manifestations

The initial symptom of acute tonsillitis is a severe sore throat, often accompanied by fever, chills, headache, and muscular discomfort. The sensations of discomfort and malaise may slowly subside after the first 24 to 72 hours.

Typically, palpation will reveal swollen cervical lymph nodes, and the client will report tenderness during palpation. Inspection of the throat reveals enlarged, inflamed tonsils, and inflammation of the pharynx. The uvula and palate are red and edematous. Uncomplicated tonsillitis will usually subside in 7 to 10 days in response to bed rest, throat irrigations, and adequate fluid intake.

If tonsillitis is caused by a streptococcal infection, the tonsils are studded with yellow follicles. This condition may be referred to as acute follicular tonsillitis or "strep throat"

Box 19–1 Client Instructions for Throat Irrigation

Use hot or warm saline (110°F to 115°F or 43°C to 46°C) unless it causes discomfort (2 tsp salt to 1 qt water).

Fill an irrigation container with saline and hang it 2 to 3 ft above your head. (A 1-qt douche bag works well.)

Hold a basin under your mouth or stand over a sink to catch fluid as you irrigate.

Direct the tip of the tubing toward the back of your throat.

Hold your breath and allow the saline solution to run into the back of your throat. Stop the flow when you need to breathe or rest. Be careful not to inhale or swallow as fluid comes in contact with mucosa.

Repeat the process several times a day. Frequency of irrigation will vary from every 2 to 3 hours while you are awake, to two or three times a day, depending on how severe your sore throat is.

SOURCE: DeWeese DD, Saunders WH: *Textbook of Otolaryngology*, 6th ed. St. Louis: Mosby, 1982.

(see Figure 19–8). Streptococcal tonsillitis is marked by abrupt onset of fever, often as high as 104°F (40°C). Other symptoms include a sore throat of increasing severity, pain on swallowing, a sensation of fullness in the throat, chills, and joint and muscle pain. The client may experience referred ear pain (otalgia). The breath may smell foul. Leukocyte count and erythrocyte sedimentation rate are elevated. A throat culture is positive for group A beta-hemolytic streptococci. Also, an ASO (antistreptolysin O) titer greater than 125 in adults indicates recent streptococcal infection. Possible complications of acute tonsillitis include peritonsillar abscess, chronic tonsillitis, rheumatic fever, acute glomerulonephritis, cervical adenitis, and otitis media.

The most common initial symptom of chronic tonsillitis is recurrent sore throat. The client may report dryness of the throat and an associated unpleasant taste in the mouth. Malaise or lassitude may occur, but the client is not usually febrile. Analysis of the blood may reveal hypochromic anemia. Typically, the tonsils will be enlarged. The presence of purulent material in the tonsillar crypts is a reliable sign of chronic tonsillitis. If pus is present, it will be expressed when a wooden tongue depressor is pressed against the anterior tonsillar pillar.

Therapeutic Measures

Penicillin is the treatment of choice for "strep throat." Erythromycin may be used if the client has a penicillin allergy. The usual dose for both penicillin and erythromycin is 250 mg q.i.d. for 10 days. Analgesics and antipyretics may improve comfort and reduce temperature. Throat irrigations are helpful. Tonsillectomy may be indicated for chronic tonsillitis.

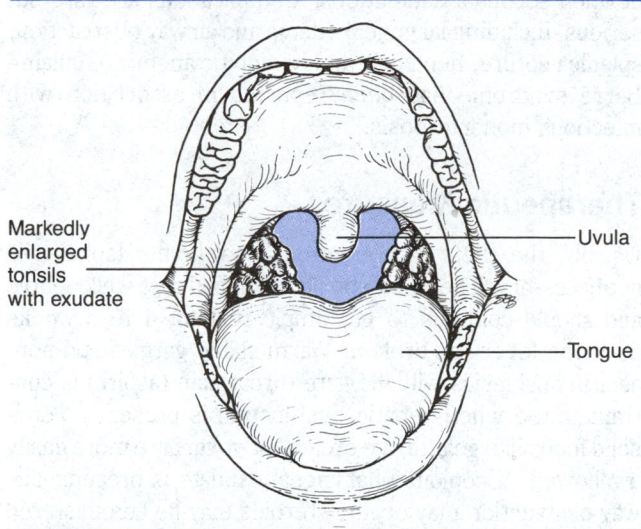

Figure 19–8
"Strep" throat.

Specific Nursing Measures

The client should be instructed regarding the need for increased oral fluids, rest, and continuation of medication therapy for the full 10 days. Throat irrigations as described in the section on pharyngitis are helpful. Refer also to general nursing implications applicable to infectious disorders of the upper respiratory tract. A soft, bland diet will help the client maintain nutritional intake.

PERITONSILLAR ABSCESS (QUINSY)

Peritonsillar abscess is an abscess, or collection of pus, between the tonsillar capsule and the superior constrictor muscle of the pharynx (Figure 19–9). Peritonsillar abscess, or quinsy, occurs as a complication of untreated or improperly treated acute bacterial tonsillitis, usually related to streptococcal or staphylococcal infection. The abscess forms when infection extends through the capsule and invades surrounding tissue. Cultures taken from the abscess may reveal *Streptococcus pyogenes, Staphylococcus aureus,* gram-negative organisms, or anaerobic organisms.

Clinical Manifestations

The client has a sore throat that persists for several days. An apparent improvement may be followed by unilateral increase in severity. Increasing dysphagia is accompanied by pain and spasm of the muscles of the jaw (trismus); inability to swallow saliva may result in drooling. Referred otalgia is not uncommon, and the client is febrile. The client's voice is muffled ("hot potato" voice).

Inspection of the oral cavity reveals edema of the soft palate on the involved side. This area is often reddened,

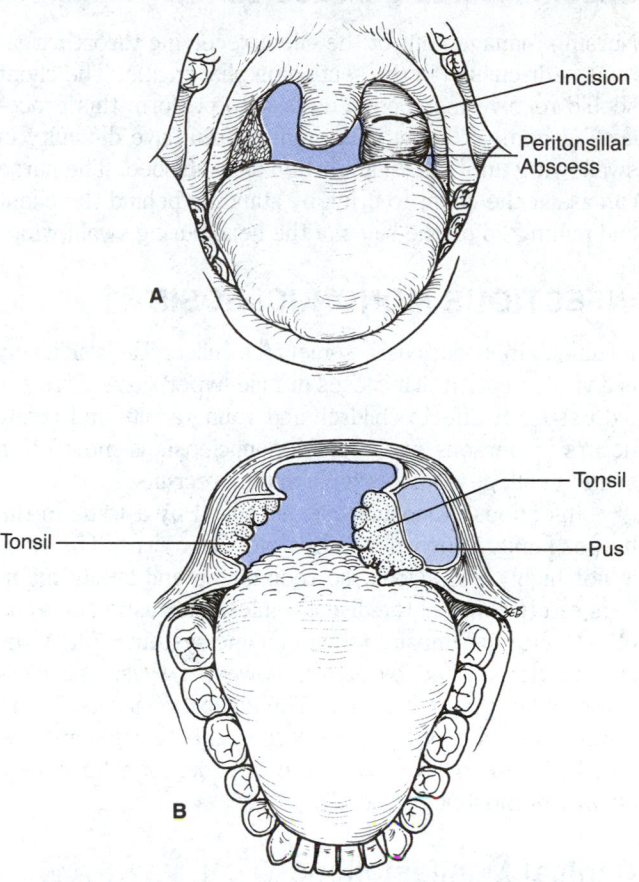

Figure 19–9
Peritonsillar abscess. **A.** A large red mass is seen in the pharynx displacing the uvula to the opposite side. Tonsil tissue on that side cannot be visualized, only red mucous membrane swelling. **B.** A collection of pus is noted between the superior constrictor muscle and the tonsil capsule. The abscess is incised halfway between the base of the anterior pillar and uvula.
SOURCE: Reprinted with permission from Schaefer WC, Fletcher MM: Diseases of the pharynx. *Surgical Rounds* (June) 1979; 2(6):17.

and palpation may reveal fluctuation. The edema causes the uvula to deviate toward the uninvolved side, and the involved tonsil is displaced toward the midline.

Therapeutic Measures

Frequently, the client must be hospitalized so that fluids and antibiotics can be administered intravenously. The abscess is incised and drained under local or topical anesthesia. Analgesics are given to relieve pain, and hot saline irrigations are administered. Once the infection has subsided, or in about 1 month, a tonsillectomy is performed to prevent recurrence.

Specific Nursing Measures

Nursing management of the client receiving throat irrigations is discussed in the section on pharyngitis. The client should receive instruction on how to perform this procedure at home. Clients with quinsy often have difficulty in swallowing until the inflammation has subsided. The nurse can assist the client to drink by standing behind the client and pulling up on the sides of the head during swallowing.

INFECTIOUS MONONUCLEOSIS

Infectious mononucleosis, sometimes called glandular fever, is a viral infection that causes diffuse hyperplasia of lymphoid tissue. It affects children and young adults and rarely occurs in persons over 30. Mononucleosis is most often seen in college students and military recruits.

Infectious mononucleosis is caused by a virus in the herpes family known as the Epstein–Barr virus. The virus is not highly contagious, so roommates and family members rarely contract the disease unless exhaustion or some other factor has impaired their immune systems. The virus can be transmitted by saliva, however; thus, the nickname, "the kissing disease." The incubation period is 2 to 7 weeks. Levels of Epstein–Barr viral antibodies are elevated in persons who have the disorder or who have a history of mononucleosis.

Clinical Manifestations

An episode of infectious mononucleosis may be mild and transient, or the client may be severely ill. Symptoms include fever, sore throat, malaise, generalized weakness, and headache. Common clinical findings include marked cervical lymphadenopathy, especially of the posterior cervical nodes, pharyngitis, splenomegaly, and elevated temperature. Mononucleosis may be suspected in clients with pharyngitis when enlargement of the cervical lymph nodes is disproportionate to the severity of the pharyngitis. The nodes are firm, discrete, and tender on palpation. Lymph glands in the groin and axilla may also be enlarged. The nasal and pharyngeal mucosa appears red and edematous, the tonsils are enlarged, and a gray membrane may cover the tonsillar tissue. Exudate in the pharynx is indicative of secondary infection.

Fever ranges from 100°F to 103°F (38°C to 39°C) and may persist for 7 to 10 days. In more severe cases, the temperature may reach 105°F (41°C). An enlarged spleen can be palpated in 75% of infected individuals. Approximately 10% of clients will have hepatic dysfunction accompanied by jaundice and hepatomegaly. Some clients will have a skin rash, petechiae, and icterus.

Laboratory studies will reveal a leukocyte count of 12,000 to 25,000, with an elevated number of atypical lymphocytes. Heterophil antibody tests and Monospot tests will be positive. Liver function studies are often abnormal.

Mononucleosis generally persists for 2 to 4 weeks, and it is not uncommon for clients with this disorder to develop secondary infections. Complications are rare but serious, including laryngeal edema and airway obstruction, splenic rupture, hepatitis, and hemolytic anemia. Guillain–Barré syndrome has been reported in association with infectious mononucleosis.

Therapeutic Measures

Usually, the client can be cared for at home. Isolation is not necessary. The client should be on bed rest while febrile and should continue to get ample rest for 4 to 6 weeks after the fever has broken. Warm saline gargles and non-aspirin analgesics will alleviate throat pain (aspirin is contraindicated when hepatic dysfunction is present). Semisolid foods like gelatin, ice cream, or yogurt are more easily swallowed. If copious pharyngeal exudate is present, airway obstruction may occur; steroids may be administered to reduce inflammation but will have no effect on the virus. Antibiotics are given only if secondary bacterial infection develops. Ampicillin should be avoided, since this drug is related to development of a rash or hypersensitivity reaction in a high percentage of clients with mononucleosis.

Hospitalization may be required if the client is severely ill with anorexia, airway obstruction, or severe splenomegaly. The abdomen of a person with an enlarged spleen should not be palpated, because splenic rupture could occur. Sudden abdominal pain in a client with splenomegaly may indicate splenic rupture; nursing interventions for hypovolemic shock should be instituted immediately if rupture occurs.

Hospitalization may sometimes be required for a client who cannot get adequate rest at home. Hepatic failure or hemolytic anemia may develop if the client does not rest sufficiently to allow the liver to regenerate.

Specific Nursing Measures

Nursing care includes careful assessment for signs of splenomegaly, administration of comfort measures and prescribed medications, and emphasizing to the client the necessity for adequate rest. Intimate contact (eg, kissing) should be avoided until laboratory results are normal.

Young people often are able to continue their routine activities, such as school attendance and homework, after the acute stage has passed. In addition to the need for increased rest, clients should know that avoiding trauma to the abdomen is important during the recovery process to prevent splenic rupture. Contact sports and playful roughhousing are to be avoided. A stool softener may be prescribed to prevent constipation and straining.

VINCENT'S ANGINA

Vincent's angina is an acute ulcerative infection of the pharynx that initially involves a tonsil—usually only one, although the infection may spread to the contralateral tonsil, the pharynx, and the gingiva. The disease occurs most often in young adults aged 15 to 35 and rarely occurs in persons who have had a tonsillectomy. Vincent's angina is not uncommon and may occur in epidemic form (Paparella & Shumrick, 1980).

Vincent's angina is related to proliferation of gram-negative organisms, spirochetes *(Borrelia vincentii)*, and fusiform bacilli, small numbers of which are normally present in the mouth. Predisposing factors include irritative oral lesions such as decayed teeth, poor oral and dental hygiene, low blood levels of vitamin C, and debilitation.

Clinical Manifestations

The client reports unilateral pharyngitis that increases in severity over several days. Additional symptoms may include referred otalgia on the involved side, an unpleasant taste in the mouth, and a fetid odor. These symptoms are usually accompanied by a generalized malaise and a mildly elevated temperature (99°F to 100°F or 37°C to 38°C). Typical findings include an ulcerated area in one tonsil that does not involve the tonsillar pillar and a gray pseudomembrane covering the affected tonsil. The membrane can be easily rubbed off, and hemorrhage of the ulcerated area usually occurs when the membrane has been removed. Gingivostomatitis (trench mouth) may accompany Vincent's angina; gingival hemorrhage may then be the principal symptom. Cervical lymphadenopathy may be noted, usually unilaterally. Diagnosis is confirmed by a Gram's stain of a specimen from the ulcerated area.

Therapeutic Measures

Penicillin is administered parenterally for approximately 1 week; sodium borate or hydrogen peroxide is applied to the ulcerated area. The therapeutic value of these agents is related to their release of oxygen; the microorganisms involved in Vincent's angina are anaerobic. Vincent's angina generally responds rapidly to treatment; complications are rare.

Specific Nursing Measures

Meticulous oral hygiene is of primary importance. The nurse should instruct the client in the use of mouthwashes and gargles (half-strength hydrogen peroxide has been recommended) and in precautionary measures to prevent spread of the infection. This disorder is transmitted by close contact or by contact with contaminated objects used by the infected person (fomites).

DIPHTHERIA

Diphtheria is a serious infectious disease that primarily affects the upper respiratory system. It is now uncommon in the United States because of widespread immunization; however, the number of cases reported annually has been increasing since 1965. The probable cause of the increase is parental reluctance about infant immunization because of greater public knowledge of rare but serious side effects, mainly associated with the pertussis (whooping cough) component of the DPT (diphtheria-pertussis-tetanus) vaccine. Diphtheria is seen most often in children over age 6, but adults are also affected. It is still common in some parts of the world.

Diphtheria is caused by the gram-positive organism *Corynebacterium diphtheriae,* which produces a protein exotoxin that has an affinity for the myocardium and neuromuscular junction. Diphtheria is usually transmitted by droplet and fomites and can occur in mild form in immunized individuals.

Clinical Manifestations

The onset of diphtheria is insidious. The affected person has a sore throat and malaise, which may be accompanied by a low-grade fever. Mild tachycardia may occur. Inspection of the pharynx reveals the blue-white or gray false membrane typical of the disease (the name diphtheria comes from the Latin word for leather, which refers to the toughness of the false membrane). The membrane may extend over the oropharynx, nasopharynx, and laryngopharynx. When the firmly attached membrane is removed, the underlying tissue hemorrhages. Involvement of the larynx is first signaled by hoarseness, followed by cough, stridor, and signs of progressive respiratory obstruction. Cervical lymphadenitis may be so severe that the client has a "bull-necked" appearance. Overall, the client appears quite ill. *Corynebacterium diphtheriae* can usually be identified by microscopic examination of the membrane; the diagnosis is confirmed by cultures. Complications of diphtheria include myocarditis and peripheral neuritis.

Therapeutic Measures

Prophylaxis is far more effective than treatment. Children should be immunized in infancy and should receive booster immunizations until age 10. Antitoxin is administered if the disease is present or strongly suspected; a single dose of 20,000 to 100,000 units is given, half intramuscularly and half intravenously. Penicillin is administered to prevent the client from becoming a carrier; it destroys the causative organisms but does not affect the course of the disease. Tracheotomy may be necessary if respiratory obstruction progresses; it may be preceded by bronchoscopy to remove membrane that has invaded the trachea and bronchi.

Specific Nursing Measures

Measures should be taken to prevent spread of the infection; these measures are discussed in Chapter 18 and at the beginning of this section. Meticulous oral and nasal hygiene is required. Emphasize the importance of following immunization timetables when talking with parents of infants and children. Parents should be encouraged to discuss their feelings about immunization with their pediatrician. Parents should also be vigilant regarding their child's response to any immunization given because an occasional child will have an untoward reaction and should not receive the remaining injections in the series.

LARYNGITIS

Laryngitis is an inflammation of the laryngeal mucosa that affects phonation and sometimes respiratory function. It occurs in both acute and chronic forms. The term *chronic laryngitis* describes long-standing inflammatory changes in the laryngeal mucosa.

Upper respiratory infections are frequently accompanied by acute laryngitis, and isolated laryngeal infections may also occur. Acute laryngitis may also be related to misuse of the voice, inhalation of hot gases, or aspiration of hot or corrosive substances.

No single etiologic factor is related to chronic laryngitis. In some instances, the disorder is related to recurrent episodes of acute laryngitis, continued vocal abuse, smoking, purulent drainage from chronic sinusitis or bronchitis, or allergies. It is sometimes related to hypometabolic states (eg, hypothyroidism). Alcohol abuse may contribute to laryngitis, since an intoxicated person may misuse or abuse the voice. Rare causes include syphilis and laryngeal tuberculosis.

Clinical Manifestations

Acute Laryngitis
The typical symptom is hoarseness or loss of the voice. The client may report roughness or a tickling sensation in the throat. A dry cough may occur, and there may be discomfort in the laryngeal area that increases during swallowing. Talking tends to aggravate the condition. General symptoms of upper respiratory tract infection will be present; if the inflammation progresses, respiratory obstruction may occur. The client may have no fever, or temperature may be as high as 104°F (40°C) depending on related factors.

When inspected by indirect mirror laryngoscopy, the vocal cords appear red and edematous. The entire larynx may be inflamed, and secretions may be present. A false membrane is not generally associated with simple laryngitis; its presence suggests the possibility of diphtheria, although a membrane may form in response to trauma caused by hot gases or steam.

Chronic Laryngitis
Hoarseness is the principal symptom of chronic laryngitis. The client may be unable to speak for a period of hours. Aching of the throat may be reported; otherwise, there is generally no pain. A dry cough is usually present, unless

there are secretions related to an associated infection such as bronchitis. The vocal cords may appear polypoid and edematous or red and thickened. If the false cords are affected, they appear red and thickened.

Therapeutic Measures

Acute laryngitis generally subsides once the accompanying upper respiratory infection is resolved. Antibiotics, steam or aerosol therapy, and voice rest may be prescribed for clients with fever, persistent cough, or stridor. They should be cautioned not to smoke. Throat lozenges containing a topical anesthetic such as benzocaine may provide some relief from hoarseness. Hospitalization and tracheotomy may be required in severe cases.

Chronic laryngitis is best treated by removing the cause, if known (eg, by ceasing to smoke). Total rest of the voice is helpful. A biopsy may be ordered to rule out the possibility of cancer of the larynx.

Specific Nursing Measures

The client should be taught to use humidification to relieve symptoms and prevent aggravation of the condition. Room humidifiers may be used, or the client can inhale steam from a shower or teakettle. Precautions against burns should be emphasized. If purulent sputum is being produced, the client should be encouraged to cough; if the cough is dry and nonproductive, coughing should be avoided. Coughing occasionally becomes a habit after a respiratory infection; such coughing should be discouraged. The nurse can encourage the client to maintain total voice rest by providing alternative means of communicating such as a tablet or a "magic slate," and by stressing the importance of voice rest to significant others. Family members can be shown how to help the client by asking questions that can be answered by nodding or shaking the head. Clients who smoke should be urged to discontinue smoking or at least to reduce the number of cigarettes smoked. *It is important that clients with hoarseness lasting more than 2 weeks be further examined to rule out malignancy.*

EPIGLOTTITIS

Inflammation of the epiglottis is considered an emergency because it can rapidly lead to total obstruction of the airway. This serious infection, sometimes called supraglottitis, is now being reported more frequently in adults, possibly because of better recognition of the disorder (Ossoff, 1981). Epiglottitis appears most commonly in young children.

Hemophilus influenzae type B is the organism most frequently implicated in cases of epiglottitis, but the disorder has also been associated with *Staphylococcus aureus,* group A beta-hemolytic streptococcus, *Neisseria catarrhalis,* and *Streptococcus pneumoniae.*

Clinical Manifestations

Typically, epiglottitis is manifested by sore throat of short duration (less than 12 hours) and rapidly increasing severity, pain in the area of the hyoid at the base of the tongue, significant dysphagia, and elevation of temperature that may reach 103°F (39°C). Secretions may be so copious that the client drools. Hoarseness, if any, is minimal, but the client's voice may have a muffled, "hot potato" quality. Respiratory obstruction becomes evident as the inflammation progresses.

The pharyngeal and tonsillar mucosa appears normal, but pooled secretions may be seen in the lower pharynx (hypopharynx). Although the enlarged, cherry red epiglottis may be seen by means of indirect (mirror) laryngoscopy, lateral x-rays of the neck taken with the client in an upright position are a less hazardous means of diagnosis;

manipulation can aggravate edema, leading to sudden total occlusion of the airway. Cultures of blood and secretions may be used to isolate the causative organism. A leukocyte count of 18,000 to 24,000 is common. The epiglottis and related structures are shown in Figure 19–10.

Therapeutic Measures

The client should be hospitalized, since respiratory obstruction can rapidly occur. The client must be closely monitored for signs of progressive respiratory obstruction. Restlessness, stridor, cyanosis, and retraction of the supraclavicular and intercostal spaces indicate a need for immediate tracheotomy. Endotracheal intubation may be an alternative to tracheotomy; if this alternative is used, precautions must be taken to prevent the client from

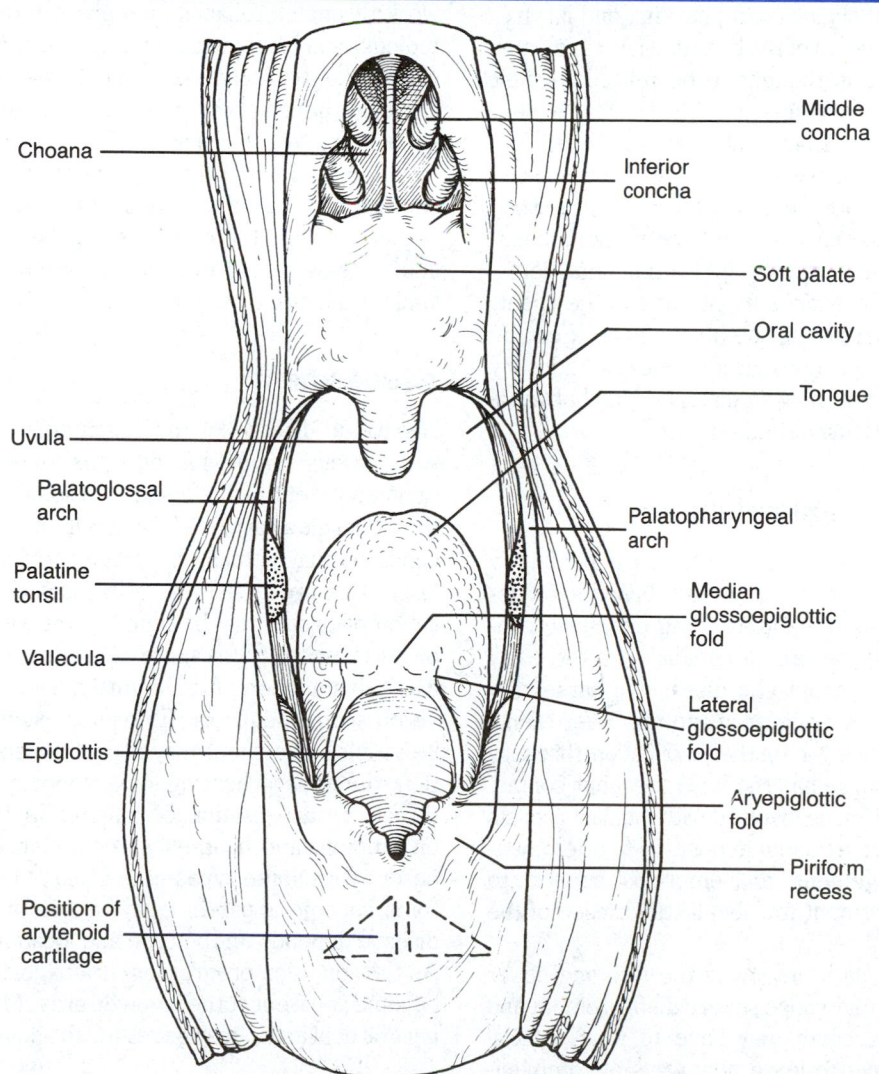

Choana — Middle concha — Inferior concha — Soft palate — Oral cavity — Tongue — Uvula — Palatoglossal arch — Palatine tonsil — Vallecula — Epiglottis — Position of arytenoid cartilage — Palatopharyngeal arch — Median glossoepiglottic fold — Lateral glossoepiglottic fold — Aryepiglottic fold — Piriform recess

Figure 19–10

The epiglottis and related structures (posterior wall of pharynx has been removed).

removing the endotracheal tube. Antibiotic therapy appropriate to the organism identified by culture studies is generally prescribed. Recovery usually follows 24 to 48 hours after treatment is initiated. Failure to recognize the seriousness of the disorder can lead to death in up to 20% of clients with epiglottitis (DeWeese & Saunders, 1982).

Specific Nursing Measures

The importance of continuous monitoring for signs of respiratory obstruction cannot be overemphasized. Onset of obstruction can be extremely rapid. A tracheotomy tray should be kept in the client's room, and the nurse should be prepared to assist in this procedure (see Chapter 21). If endotracheal intubation is used, the tube should be taped securely in place so the client cannot remove it. Confused clients may require soft wrist restraints. Both client and family are extremely frightened when symptoms of respiratory obstruction occur and the measures to relieve it initiated. Explanation, reassurance, and a caring, confident approach by the nurse are extremely important.

Section III: Neoplastic Disorders

Benign and malignant disease is defined and explained in Chapter 12. The discussion in this chapter is limited to specific benign and malignant growths affecting the nose, nasopharynx, paranasal sinuses, oropharynx, and larynx.

The incidence of cancers of the head and neck in women has recently risen; this is thought to be related to their increased use of tobacco (McGuirt, 1983). These neoplasms appear to be of multifactorial origin, however.

Neoplasia of the upper respiratory tract can cause disfigurement and death. Benign tumors can have serious consequences related to expansion and obstruction; malignant neoplasms damage tissue by infiltration and metastasis. Any diagnosis of cancer is frightening to the client, but neoplastic disease affecting the head and neck can be especially devastating psychologically because sensory functions (olfaction, vision) may be disturbed, and physical appearance may be seriously affected.

General Nursing Implications

Nurses play an important role in educating the public, by example and precept, about the health benefits of not smoking or chewing tobacco and avoiding excessive consumption of alcohol. By becoming familiar with the early symptoms and signs of neoplastic disease, a nurse may facilitate early diagnosis of malignancy and may refer clients who are especially at risk for further evaluation that may save their lives. The nurse has the most frequent contact with hospitalized clients and is involved with intimate aspects of their care. Nurses are in a unique position to offer counsel, comfort, encouragement, and emotional support to clients undergoing treatment for neoplastic disease of the head and neck.

Treatment of neoplasia involving the face and upper respiratory structures may cause severe disfigurement and loss of the voice. The client may have to wear a facial prosthesis and may have to learn new ways of communicating through artificial devices or esophageal speech. Full knowledge is necessary for decision making. Be careful, however, to avoid imposing values on the client, even if the client asks, "What would you do?" It is the client who

must make major adjustments in lifestyle and who may have to cope with a drastically altered appearance or with learning to speak all over again. It is the client who must work through a rehabilitation process that may be painful, tedious, and often discouraging. Thus, it is the client who must make the final decision about treatment. But the nurse can offer information, physical assistance, and emotional support for that decision.

Some clients will refuse therapy altogether, and this decision may be difficult to accept. Yet providing supportive care during the remainder of the client's hospital stay and, in some cases, after the return home, can be a worthwhile challenge to empathy and professional skills.

Assessment

Neoplastic disease of the respiratory tract is associated with various symptoms and signs, depending on the location and extent of the lesion. Although the client may initially consult a caregiver about a lump felt in the neck, this condition may actually be related to metastasis of a neoplasm that arose elsewhere in the body. Edema or dislocation of tissue may be found at the site of the neoplasm or adjacent to it. Pressure related to tumor growth may cause dysfunction of the cranial nerves or disturbances in vision such as diplopia. Epiphora (excessive tearing) may be visible. The client may report anosmia, nasal obstruction, tinnitus, or hearing loss. Reports of dysphagia, sore throat, or a sensation of fullness in the throat are not uncommon, and hoarseness or a change in voice quality occurs with some types of lesions. Whether these symptoms become apparent early or late in the course of the disease depends on the type and location of the neoplasm. As the condition progresses, drainage and a foul odor may become apparent at the involved area. Malnourishment and general debilitation may be related to anorexia and dysphagia.

Nursing Intervention

In general, the objectives of nursing care are related to providing adequate nutrition and fluid intake and encouraging involvement in self-care. Clients who have advanced lesions may find it difficult or impossible to swallow and may require supplementary alimentation such as enteral feeding. Some will require a tracheotomy to facilitate breathing or removal of secretions; if secretions are copious, tracheal suctioning may be necessary. Meticulous oral hygiene must be maintained, and strict aseptic technique must be employed during suctioning because of the danger of infection.

Emotional support is a major component of care. After the initial diagnosis, the client may welcome the opportunity to confide in the nurse as a knowledgeable professional who is able to combine empathy with objectivity. The importance of teaching and preparing the client intellectually and emotionally for treatment has already been discussed. The nurse's own reaction to the client is crucial; physical disfigurement and foul-smelling secretions are often associated with neoplasia of the upper respiratory tract. Cheerful words and kind gestures can be negated by body language or facial expression; a sensitive client can read the message inherent in averted glance, pursed lips, and concentration on detailed mechanics of care.

Clients who are not obviously disfigured may still have difficulty accepting the diagnosis and outcomes of treatment such as loss of vocal expression. By encouraging self-care, the nurse can help the client regain a sense of control over his or her life. For example, the client may be taught how to perform oral suctioning or administer enteral feedings.

Many clients continue to smoke and to drink alcoholic beverages even after diagnosis and treatment. Explain the irritative properties of these substances and encourage the client to discontinue or at least reduce consumption. Nevertheless, some clients find these habits to be so important to their sense of well-being that they persist despite all warnings. In such instances, there is little the nurse can do after an honest effort at teaching but recognize that the client's body is ultimately his or her own responsibility. A case study of a client with cancer of the larynx is presented at the end of this chapter.

NEOPLASMS OF THE NOSE, PARANASAL SINUSES, AND NASOPHARYNX

Malignancies of the nose, paranasal sinuses, and nasopharynx are relatively rare, accounting for approximately 0.2% of all reported cancers (Paparella & Shumrick, 1980). Because these structures are anatomically adjacent, a neoplasm that arises in one will often infiltrate or impinge upon another.

The more common benign neoplasms affecting the nose, sinuses, and nasopharynx include papillomas, angiomas, osteomas, and fibromas. Although the adenoids may become extremely hypertrophic, this disorder is rarely seen in adults.

Squamous cell carcinoma is the most common malig-

nant lesion of the nose and paranasal sinuses. Other types of malignancies affecting this region include basal cell carcinoma, adenocarcinoma, cystic sarcoma of the adenoids, fibrosarcoma, lymphosarcoma, osteosarcoma, chondrosarcoma, mixed tumors, malignant melanoma, and pituitary malignancies. Cancer of the paranasal sinuses affects the maxillary sinuses most often (in 60% of cases).

Not all neoplastic disorders affecting the nose and adjacent regions have clearly defined etiologies. A **rhinophyma** is a benign tumor of the external nares related to overgrowth of the sebaceous glands. Factors that have been associated with this lesion include long-standing fistulas related to dental extractions, chronic sinusitis, and a history of multiple nasal polypectomies. Carcinoma of the sinuses has been associated with such factors as inhalation of dust particles and chemicals used in cabinetmaking. Smoking and ingestion of alcohol have also been implicated in cancer of the sinuses. The incidence of nasopharyngeal carcinoma is higher in persons of Southern Chinese descent than in the general population, regardless of country of residence (Paparella & Shumrick, 1980).

Clinical Manifestations

Neoplastic disease of the nose, paranasal sinuses, and nasopharynx may be associated with a variety of symptoms. Because the symptoms are nonspecific and may be mistaken for those of less serious disorders, neoplasms in this area may be overlooked, especially in the earlier stage of the disease when they are most amenable to treatment. Some affected individuals will be asymptomatic. The client may report hearing loss, a feeling of fullness, or tinnitus related to extension of the tumor into the nasopharynx. Unilateral or bilateral nasal obstruction and epistaxis may be present. The voice may have a nasal quality (rhinolalia). The client may notice trismus, distortion of the soft palate (a late sign), toothache, or maladjustment of previously fitting dentures. Because these symptoms are related to dentition, a dentist may be the first health professional consulted. If nasal discharge is present, it may be serous, serosanguineous, or purulent and may have a foul odor.

If pain accompanies the disorder, it may be referred to various areas of the head and may be aggravated when the client assumes a recumbent position. Cranial nerve dysfunction may manifest as paralysis or alteration in sensory function. Proptosis, diplopia, or epiphora may be apparent, and edema and distortion of facial structures may also occur. Nodal metastasis is relatively common; in one study, 50% of clients with nasopharyngeal cancer initially sought medical attention because of a swelling in the neck (Paparella & Shumrick, 1980).

A neoplasm in the nasopharynx may be visualized by indirect mirror laryngoscopy, or a fiberoptic nasopharyngoscope may be used by a specialist in combination with careful palpation. Anatomic changes in the frontal and maxillary sinuses may be seen by transillumination. Cervical nodes are palpated. Roentgenographic studies are usually performed, and tissue biopsy may be conducted to confirm the diagnosis.

Therapeutic Measures

Treatment depends on the type of neoplasm, its location, and its extent. Rates of cure for cancer of the nasopharynx and paranasal sinuses are low, because the disease is not usually discovered until late in its course. Benign neoplasms are usually removed by surgical excision. Malignant neoplasms are treated by surgery, irradiation, or chemotherapy, alone or in combination. Surgical excision may be extensive and disfiguring [eg, successful eradication of carcinoma of the maxillary sinuses requires surgical excision of the maxilla and, occasionally, enucleation (removal of the eye) on the affected side]. Irradiation may be used in conjunction with the surgical excision. The client may require a facial prosthesis after surgery. Malignant neoplasia of the nasopharynx is treated by irradiation; malignant neoplasia of the paranasal sinuses is usually treated by irradiation, surgery, or a combination of these methods. Surgical approaches to the paranasal sinuses and related nursing care are discussed in Chapter 21.

NEOPLASMS OF THE OROPHARYNX

Neoplasia of the oropharynx may involve the tonsils and pharyngeal walls, the base of the tongue, and the soft palate. One of the most commonly detected benign tumors of this area is squamous papilloma of the tonsillar fossa. Fibromas, lymphangiomas, hemangiomas, and osteomas may also be seen, although rarely. Small pigmented nevi are not uncommon on the tonsillar pillars of adult men. Malignant neoplasms of the oropharynx, particularly the tonsil and the pharyngeal wall, tend to be less well differentiated and more aggressive than malignancies in other areas of the oral cavity (Paparella & Shumrick, 1980).

Clinical Manifestations

Because the initial symptoms of oropharyngeal neoplasia—persistent irritation or soreness of the throat—are nonspecific and common to many minor disorders, a client may experience symptoms for weeks or even months before seeking professional evaluation. The client may feel a sensation of a mass in the throat; referred otalgia, trismus, or a lump in the neck may also be present.

Clients who have *a malignancy at the base of the tongue* may have a decreased tolerance for rough or hot foods in addition to the foregoing symptoms. Fixation of the tongue may cause difficulty in swallowing, and the voice may be muffled. Unfortunately, these symptoms occur late in the course of the disease.

The first symptom of *tumor of the soft palate* is dysphagia, which is often felt in the midline. The client may also detect enlargement of a cervical lymph node.

Examination of a person with *cancer of the tonsil* will reveal a mass on the tonsil. The extent of involvement can be detected by palpation and confirmed by soft-tissue roentgenography. Tissue biopsy is used to confirm malignancy. Enlargement of cervical lymph nodes indicates metastasis.

In persons with *cancer of the base of the tongue,* inspection generally reveals fullness of the affected area. Because early symptoms are nonspecific, the tumor is often large by the time the client seeks professional care. Ability to protrude the tongue may be limited. The diagnosis is confirmed by soft-tissue studies and biopsy. Chest films should be obtained to confirm or rule out pulmonary metastasis.

Examination of an individual with *carcinoma of the soft palate* may reveal ulceration or localized erythema or edema. Diagnosis is confirmed by digital examination, inspection of the nasopharynx, roentgenography, and biopsy.

Therapeutic Measures

Therapy is often multimodal, combining surgery, irradiation, and chemotherapy. Radium implants have been effective in treating cancer at the base of the tongue, although surgical resection is also employed. Extensive lesions may be treated with dissection of the tongue and neck, sometimes in combination with laryngectomy. Glossectomy (total removal of the tongue) is sometimes required. Irradiation may be employed to treat less extensive primary lesions of the tonsil and pharyngeal wall; surgical intervention is indicated if the client cannot tolerate radiotherapy, if the lesion has recurred after radiation, if cervical metastasis occurs, or if the lesion is resistant to irradiation. Exceptionally large neoplasms also are resected. Cancer of the soft palate is treated by surgical excision, irradiation, or both.

NEOPLASMS OF THE LARYNX

Although benign neoplasms of the larynx do occur—usually small, easily removed papillomas—the following discussion centers on malignant neoplasia. Laryngeal cancers may be classified according to locus of origin; the four major types are (Figure 19–11):

- Glottic (arising from the vocal cords)
- Supraglottic (arising above the vocal cords)
- Subglottic (arising below the vocal cords)
- Transglottic

Glottic carcinoma is the most common and has the most favorable prognosis. Supraglottic lesions are more often associated with lymphatic metastasis and thus have a poorer prognosis. Subglottic lesions, the rarest of the four types, are less aggressive than supraglottic lesions but more so than glottic cancers. Transglottic cancer is highly invasive and metastasizes extensively.

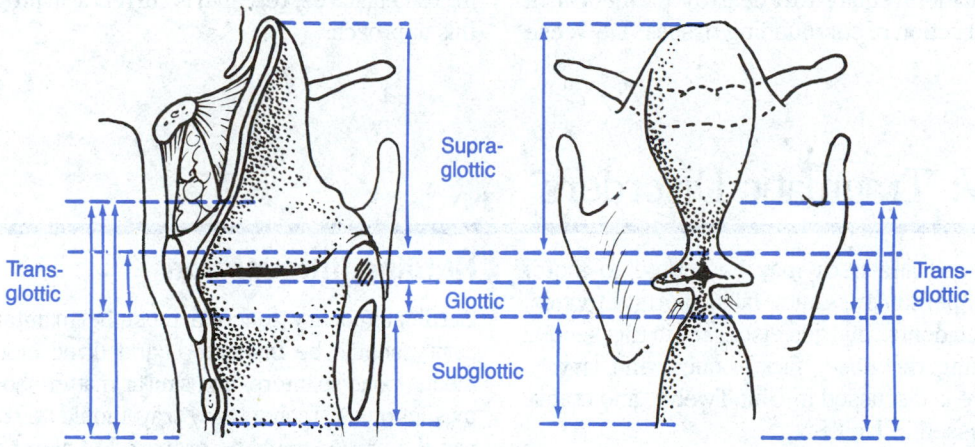

Figure 19–11

Classification of cancer of the larynx.
SOURCE: Adapted from Ballenger TJ: *Diseases of the Nose, Throat, and Ear*, 12th ed. Philadelphia: Lea & Febiger, 1977.

Laryngeal cancer has a high rate of cure *when detected early*. But the average client has consulted three physicians about persistent hoarseness over a period of 8 months by the time the condition is diagnosed (DeWeese & Saunders, 1982). The estimated morbidity and mortality for laryngeal cancer in 1985, according to the American Cancer Society, was 11,500 new cases and 3750 deaths.

Heavy cigarette smoking and ingestion of alcohol are believed to be major factors in the development of laryngeal cancer. Environmental pollution, particularly air pollution, occupational exposure to radiation, and chronic pharyngeal infection have also been related to this disorder. Although laryngeal carcinoma has predominantly affected males aged 50 to 70, incidence in women has been rising (McGuirt, 1983).

Clinical Manifestations

The most common symptom of benign laryngeal neoplasms is hoarseness, sometimes accompanied by dysphagia if the lesion is large. Symptoms of laryngeal carcinoma vary according to the type of lesion.

Glottic Carcinoma

Hoarseness occurs early in the course of the disorder. Pain may be felt in the latter stages. Dyspnea and inability to speak (aphonia) are also late signs.

Supraglottic Carcinoma

Hoarseness is uncommon. The client may report a sensation of "something in the throat" or a change in voice quality. The throat may burn when hot or acidic liquid is ingested. The client may notice a lump in the neck, which

may be the reason for consulting a professional caregiver. Pain unrelated to ulceration may occur, as may referred otalgia. Later symptoms include pain, hoarseness, and dyspnea related to obstruction of the airway.

Subglottic and Transglottic Carcinomas

In subglottic carcinoma, dyspnea may be the initial reported symptom. Hoarseness is rare. Transglottic carcinoma refers to tumors that have invaded various sections of the larynx; thus, a variety of the previously described symptoms may occur.

Lesions involving one or both vocal cords may be seen by indirect mirror laryngoscopy, as may supraglottic lesions. The latter are more likely to ulcerate than are glottic lesions. Visualization of the subglottic area requires direct laryngoscopy by a physician. Cervical nodes may be palpable if the lesion has metastasized. Roentgenographic examinations will aid in determining the extent of the disease, and biopsy specimens may be removed under local or general anesthesia.

Therapeutic Measures

Among the surgical procedures employed for laryngeal carcinoma are excision via suspension laryngoscopy, laryngofissure with partial laryngectomy, total laryngectomy, and supraglottic laryngectomy. A radical neck dissection may be performed in conjunction with total or supraglottic laryngectomy. Partial laryngectomy has the most favorable prognosis. Surgical approaches and related nursing care are discussed in Chapter 21.

In cases of localized carcinomas involving only one vocal cord, radiation may be efficacious and will have less effect on voice quality than will surgical excision. Radiotherapy is least effective with advanced lesions because the level of irradiation required to destroy the neoplasm would cause destruction of surrounding tissues (DeWeese & Saunders, 1982). Sometimes adjuvant chemotherapy is employed in an attempt to shrink the tumor and eradicate micrometastases; research is currently in progress to explore this approach.

Section IV: Traumatic Disorders

Trauma of the head and neck may be related to motor vehicle accidents, personal assaults, falls, sports activities, or occupational accidents. Injuries discussed in this section are those involving the nose, facial bones, and larynx. Trauma to the eye is discussed in Unit Twelve, and cranial injuries are discussed in Unit Six.

Trauma to the head and neck is a leading cause of morbidity and mortality in the United States (Bailey, 1982). Such trauma is serious, as it is often related to sensory impairment, permanent disability, disfigurement, and death.

General Nursing Implications

Nurses working in the community should encourage the public to take advantage of such safety features as automobile seat belts and to wear helmets when riding motorcycles. In the hospital, surgical intervention consists of reduction, stabilization, and immobilization of the injured part. Proper nursing care can greatly facilitate healing and help avoid complications. Many head and neck injuries have psychologically devastating consequences related to changed appearance and sometimes to inability to carry out normal activities. Clients with such injuries can benefit from instruction and support during recovery and rehabilitation.

Assessment

The client must be assessed for possible damage to the cervical spine prior to any manipulation except emergency life-saving measures (eg, maintaining the airway). If the cervical spine is injured, moving the client could lead to additional neurologic damage. Assessment of cranial nerves II through X should be performed. Visual disturbances such as diplopia or decreased acuity may occur. Alteration in sensation may range from pain to hypoesthesia.

Inspection for hemorrhage and drainage should be routine; edema and ecchymosis may occur in relation to profuse bleeding. Drainage from the nares should be evaluated for the presence of cerebrospinal fluid (CSF rhinorrhea), which is transparent. The presence of glucose in the fluid confirms CSF rhinorrhea. Cerebrospinal fluid dries as a yellow halolike ring and does not crust as do other types of secretions (Black & Arnold, 1982). Lacerations may be noted, with foreign debris in the wound or surrounding area. The client may experience difficulty in swallowing or speaking.

Nursing Intervention

Cardiopulmonary function must be maintained. The oral cavity should be inspected, and dried blood, tooth fragments, bone splinters, and similar matter should be removed by suction. A tracheotomy tray should be readily available, and the nurse should be prepared to assist with intubation or tracheotomy.

The client should be positioned to reduce edema and avoid asphyxiation. Elevating the head of the bed, if not otherwise contraindicated, helps decrease edema of the head and neck; application of ice is helpful during the first 24 hours after injury, with warm applications used thereafter to promote vasodilation. Blood transfusions and intravenous fluids may be given.

Wound care must be meticulous. This may involve cleansing and application of antimicrobial ointments. Dressings may be necessary, depending on the nature of the injury. The nurse must continually observe for signs of infection, and oral hygiene must be maintained.

Adequate nutritional intake is crucial to healing. Depending on the client's ability to eat, a liquid diet or intravenous fluids may be used initially. If the nature of the injury permits, nasogastric feedings may be administered. Obtain a baseline weight upon admission so nutritional status can be monitored by subsequent weighings. Clients should be encouraged to take part in self-care to the maximum extent possible; doing so helps them reestablish a sense of control over their lives. Emotional support is of utmost importance for these clients, who may face long and painful rehabilitation and major changes in appearance and lifestyle. Clients who have been disfigured may appreciate receiving information about plastic surgery.

MAXILLOFACIAL TRAUMA

Trauma to the face may cause extensive damage to soft tissue as well as damage to bone and cartilage. Facial fractures discussed in this section include injury to the nasal bone and septum, the zygomatic bone (malar bone), the maxilla, and the mandible. Because the nose is located in the center of the face and because it protrudes, it is injured more frequently than other areas of the body.

Maxillofacial trauma is related to some kind of direct blow. Nasal fractures are a common aftermath of fistfights; a blow to the cheek may fracture the zygomatic bone.

Zygomatic fractures frequently accompany maxillary fractures but may occur alone. Maxillary and mandibular fractures may be related to a variety of causes already discussed; fractures of the mandible occur most often in young adult males (Bailey, 1982).

Clinical Manifestations

Nasal Fractures

Nasal fractures are accompanied by the classic signs of nasal pain, edema, nasal obstruction, and epistaxis. They are diagnosed most easily 1 or 2 hours after the injury, before maximum edema occurs. Because nasal tissue is richly vascularized, trauma to the nose usually causes extravasation of blood that is manifested as edema and the appearance of a black eye (Paparella & Shumrick, 1980). The nasal bones may appear asymmetrical, the skin may be lacerated, and crepitation may be noted on palpation. The interior of the nose must be examined for additional damage; this can be painful for the client.

Zygomatic Fractures

Symptoms depend on the location of the fracture, which can be classified according to the LeFort system (Figure 19-12). A LeFort III fracture is the most serious. Profuse hemorrhage, edema, and hypoesthesia of the middle third of the face are common symptoms of zygomatic fractures. Malocclusion may also occur.

Mandibular Fractures

Common findings include pain on movement, malocclusion, and abnormal mobility. The dental arch will be irregular. Fractures of specific sections are often diagnosed by palpation.

Roentgenograms are usually obtained in all cases of maxillofacial trauma, although nasal fracture is often diagnosed by physical examination alone. If the client has been unconscious or has suffered a significant blow to the head, skull films may be obtained to rule out the possibility of cranial fracture.

Therapeutic Measures

If there is evidence of significant wound contamination, antibiotics are administered to clients with open fractures to avert infection. Tetanus toxoid may be given, depending on the degree of wound contamination and the client's history of tetanus immunization.

Intubation or tracheotomy may be required, hemorrhage must be controlled, and blood replacement may be necessary. Skin lesions are treated by cleansing, debridement, and suturing as indicated, and fractures must be reduced. Open reduction may be necessary for complicated fractures.

In the case of maxillary and mandibular fractures, interdental wiring may be necessary to restore correct alignment of the jaws and teeth. Dental arch bars are placed against the mandibular and the maxillary teeth, and wires or rubber bands attached to hooks on the bars are used to draw the dental structures into proper alignment (Figure 19-13). Maxillomandibular fixation must remain in place for approximately 6 weeks in adults and sometimes longer in elderly people.

Specific Nursing Measures

Clients with nasal fractures must be given the following instructions:

- Avoid blowing the nose, which could push nasal flora into tissues of the face and orbit, promoting infection.
- Try to sneeze through the mouth instead of the nose.
- Do not use decongestant nasal sprays or drops, as these medications reduce blood supply to the area and impede healing.

The following precautions should be employed in caring for clients who require interdental fixation. Maintenance of a patent airway is the predominant concern.

- A wire cutter and suction equipment should be at the bedside at all times; taping the cutter to the head of the bed may be a wise precaution. If secretions cannot be removed by suctioning or if the client shows signs of respiratory distress, the rubber bands or wires should be cut.
- If the client vomits, either tip the head forward or turn it to the side (if the client is supine) and use suction to remove the secretions. (The client may be taught how to suction secretions through a space between the teeth.)
- Mark the intercom at the nurses' station to indicate that the client cannot articulate clearly.
- Maintain meticulous oral hygiene by irrigating the oral cavity with saline or an alkaline solution. Lubricate the lips to prevent drying and cracking.
- Provide a high-calorie diet. Clients usually begin with clear liquids and may progress to blenderized soft foods.
- Provide an alternative means of communication such as a writing tablet or "magic slate."

The nurse is responsible for home care instruction because of the length of time the fixation must remain in place. A sample set of instructions that may be reproduced and given to the client appears in Box 19-2. The nurse may consult with the dietitian, who can provide the client with suggestions for palatable and nutritious meals and instructions for preparation.

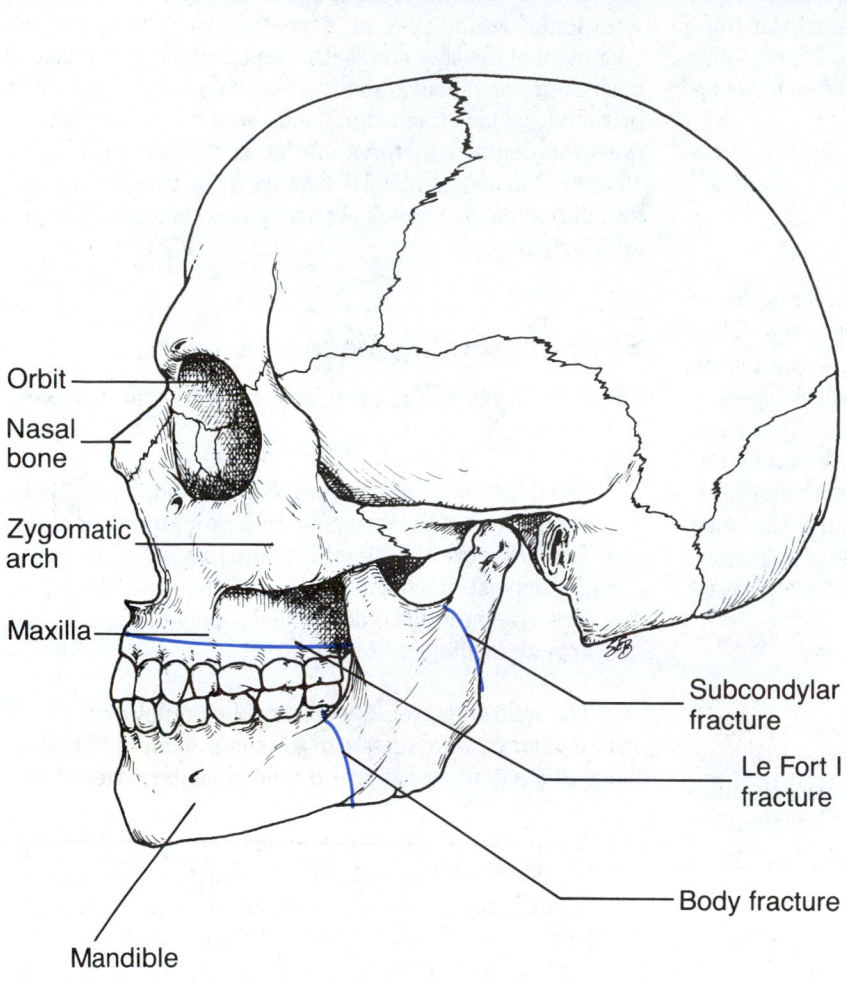

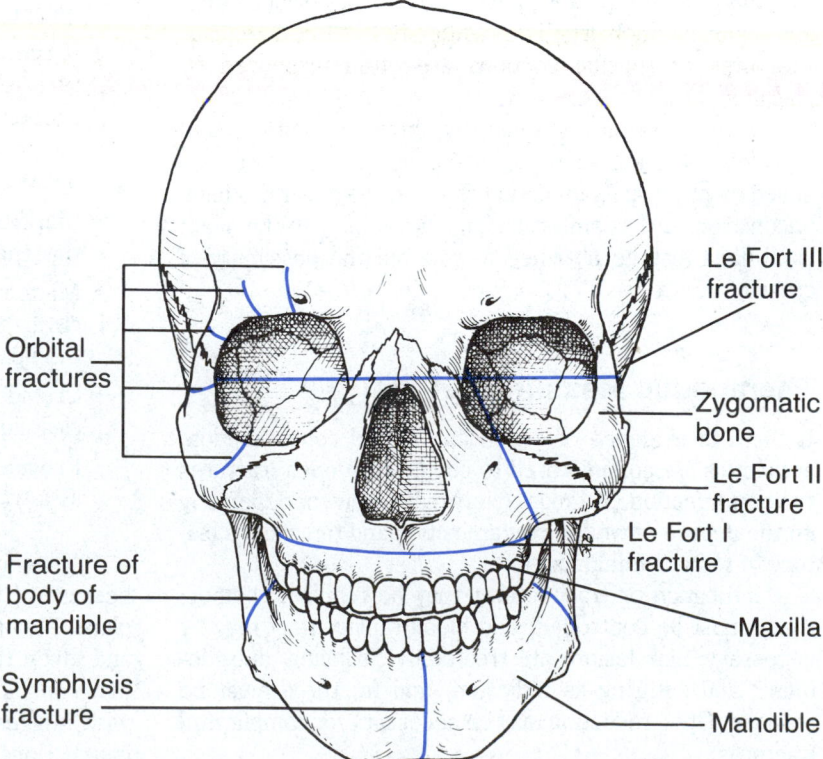

Orbit

Nasal bone

Zygomatic arch

Maxilla

Mandible

Subcondylar fracture

Le Fort I fracture

Body fracture

Orbital fractures

Fracture of body of mandible

Symphysis fracture

Le Fort III fracture

Zygomatic bone

Le Fort II fracture

Le Fort I fracture

Maxilla

Mandible

Figure 19–12

Zygomatic fractures: Le Fort I fracture—a transverse fracture through the maxilla; Le Fort II fracture—the fracture line crosses the nasal and maxillary bones, and the floor of the orbit; Le Fort III fracture—involves the zygoma, maxilla, and nasal, orbital, ethmoid, and sphenoid bones.

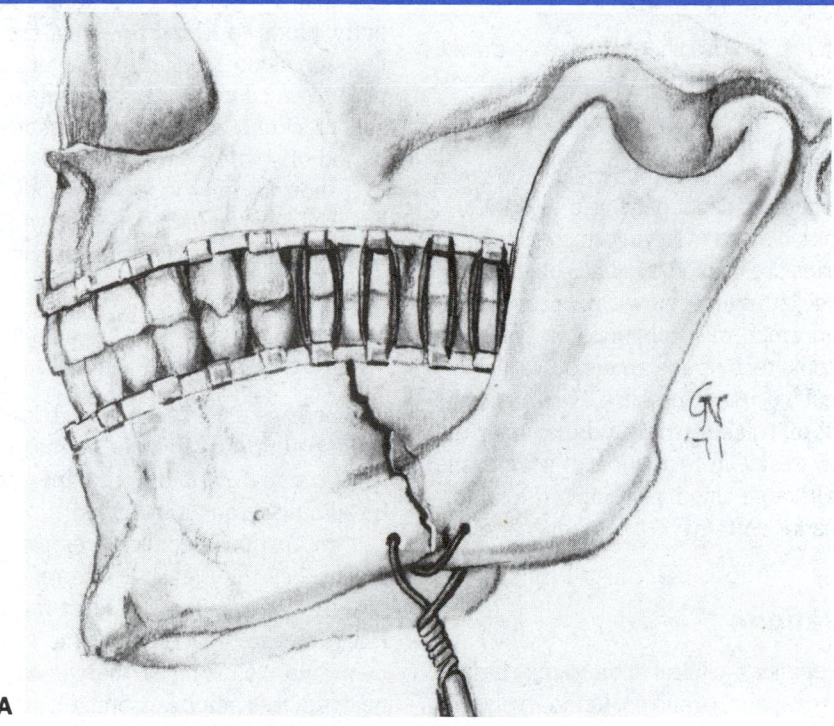

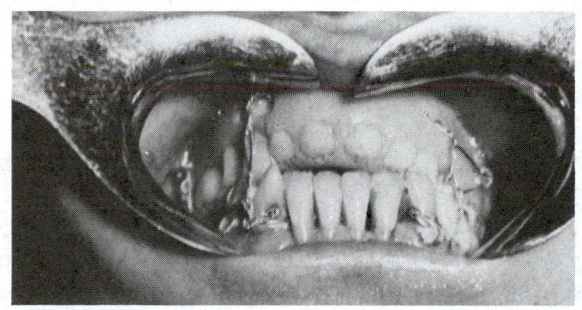

Figure 19–13

A. Wiring of mandibular fracture fragments. **B.** Photograph of a client with wiring in place. (Photo courtesy of Millard Fillmore Hospital, Buffalo, NY)

Box 19–2   Instructions for Clients With Maxillomandibular Fixation

Carry wire cutters with you at all times in case of respiratory obstruction. You and your significant others will be shown how to cut the wires before you leave the hospital. Notify your physician immediately if the wires have been cut.

Blenderize your food and maintain a high-calorie diet according to the instructions given you by the dietitian. Losing 10 to 20 pounds while your jaws are wired is not uncommon.

Maintain good oral hygiene. A Water-Pik may be helpful, but do not use too forcible a spray, and do not direct the stream of water over the lacerated area at first. You may use plain water, a mouthwash, or salt water for rinsing the mouth.

Brush your teeth regularly. Rinse your mouth after meals and at bedtime.

Apply paraffin to the ends of the wires, which will help prevent irritation of the inside of your mouth.

Refrain from swimming, because it will be hard for you to clear your throat of water.

Avoid alcoholic and carbonated beverages. Alcohol impairs the reflexes you need to clear your throat. Carbonated beverages produce foam that may make it hard for you to clear your throat.

Notify your physician of any sudden swelling or atypical pain.

SOURCE: Adapted from Black JM, Arnold PG: Facial fractures. *Am J Nurs* (July) 1982; 82(7):1086–1088.

LARYNGOTRACHEAL TRAUMA

Laryngotracheal trauma may be classified as open or closed. It may be accompanied by neural and vascular trauma of the head and neck, and fracture of the cervical spine commonly occurs with this kind of injury.

Automobile accidents in which an individual is thrown against the steering wheel or dashboard at a high rate of speed are the most common cause of laryngotracheal trauma. Some penetrating injuries are caused by sharp objects (eg, stab wounds). Iatrogenic laryngeal injury can occur in relation to endoscopy, endotracheal intubation, or tracheotomy; improper endoscopic technique can dislocate the larynx or tear the laryngeal mucosa. Pressure exerted by the cuff of an endotracheal or tracheostomy tube against the arytenoid cartilage may result in formation of scar tissue (arytenoid stenosis), although this has occurred less frequently since low-pressure cuffs have been employed.

Clinical Manifestations

Depending on the type of injury, clinical findings may include hoarseness, dysphagia, dyspnea, cyanosis, hemoptysis, and edema of the larynx and pharynx. Laryngeal fracture is generally associated with pain on swallowing and speaking and protrusion of the tongue.

An open or closed wound may be apparent on inspection. Edema may occur in the region of the larynx, and the normal prominence of the thyroid cartilage may be absent because of fracture. Subcutaneous emphysema, signs of respiratory distress, and hemoptysis accompany severe injuries. Subcutaneous emphysema is related to any disruption of the integrity of the respiratory tract that allows air to escape into the subcutaneous tissue. The client will feel pain in the affected area, and the skin may appear puffy. Upon touching the area, the nurse will feel a crackling sensation similar to that of touching wrinkled cellophane. Once the underlying disorder has been treated, subcutaneous air is usually absorbed by the body over a period of several days.

Indirect mirror laryngoscopy may reveal edema and mucosal lacerations of the pharynx and larynx. Direct laryngoscopy and x-ray studies may be ordered for further diagnosis.

Therapeutic Measures

Hemorrhage must be controlled, lost blood must be replaced, and a patent airway must be maintained. As with maxillofacial trauma, antibiotic therapy and tetanus toxoid should be administered as indicated.

Intubation is generally employed, not only to maintain respiratory function but also to stent the fractured laryngeal fragments. Tracheotomy may be necessary if severe facial fractures accompany the laryngeal injury. Debridement and cleansing of the wound is followed by repair of mucosal lacerations. Complex fractures may necessitate wiring of cartilaginous fragments.

Specific Nursing Measures

Routine nursing measures are discussed under general nursing implications in upper respiratory trauma. Clients with laryngeal trauma must be assessed for signs of damage to the carotid artery and jugular vein. This includes observing for signs of hemorrhage such as formation of a hematoma and diminution of pulses in the upper extremities. The carotid arteries should be auscultated for bruits.

Chapter Highlights

Disorders of the upper respiratory tract produce symptoms ranging from discomfort that is easily tolerated to life-threatening emergencies.

Nurses are frequently consulted about disorders of the upper respiratory tract since clients will manage many of these disorders at home.

Clients with a posterior nasal pack require hospitalization because of the risk of respiratory obstruction.

Frequent and prolonged use of vasoconstrictive nose drops or sprays will result in the development of a rebound phenomenon, which results in nasal obstruction.

In certain disorders, inflammation of the upper respiratory tract can progress to the point of airway obstruction.

Humidification and hydration of the client aid in the thinning and removal of secretions from the upper respiratory tract.

Many people say they have "sinus trouble" when, in fact, they are suffering from allergic rhinitis, postnasal drip, or other upper respiratory tract infections.

If complete airway obstruction occurs from aspiration of a foreign body into the larynx, the individual will not be able to speak or cough.

If incomplete airway obstruction results from aspiration of a foreign body, the person will be able to produce some sound such as coughing or gagging.

Disorders that prevent normal approximation of the vocal cords will result in hoarseness or a change in the quality of the voice.

Clients with hoarseness lasting more than 2 weeks should be examined to rule out a malignancy.

Malignant neoplasms of the upper respiratory tract are observed more frequently in individuals who smoke and consume large quantities of alcohol.

Neoplasms of the upper respiratory tract are frequently overlooked because of the nonspecific symptomatology.

Malignant neoplasms of the larynx have a high cure rate if diagnosed early.

Neoplastic and traumatic disorders of the upper respiratory tract can be devastating because of physical disfigurement and altered function.

Clients with traumatic disorders of the upper respiratory tract must be assessed for multisystem damage, particularly the neurological and cardiovascular systems.

Bibliography

A step-by-step workup for neck masses. *Patient Care* (April 30) 1984; 100–131.

Bailey BJ: Management of maxillofacial trauma. *Resident Staff Physician* (Dec) 1982; 28:57–68.

Bertz JE: Maxillofacial injuries. *Clin Symp* 1981; 33(4):2–32.

Black JM, Arnold PG: Facial fractures. *Am J Nurs* (July) 1982; 82(7):1086–1088.

Bumsted RM: Evaluation and therapy of nasal obstruction. *Primary Care* (June) 1982; 9(2):385–400.

Cluff L, Johnson J (editors): *Clinical Concepts of Infectious Disease,* 3rd ed. Baltimore: Williams & Wilkins, 1982.

Cummings CW, Trevye EL: Common mouth and throat infections. *Hosp Med* (Jan) 1981; 17:87–96.

Dayal VS: *Clinical Otolaryngology.* Philadelphia: Lippincott, 1981.

DeWeese DD, Saunders WH: *Textbook of Otolaryngology,* 6th ed. St. Louis: Mosby, 1982.

Donlon WC, Jacobson AL: Maxillofacial Pain. *Am Fam Physician* 1984; 30(1):151–163.

Gates G (editor): *Current Therapy in Otolaryngology: Head and Neck Surgery.* Trenton, NJ: Decker, 1982.

McGuirt WF: Head and neck cancer in women: A changing profile. *Laryngoscope* (Jan) 1983; 93(1):106.

Ossoff RH: Epiglottitis: Also deadly in adults. *Emerg Med* (Feb 28) 1981; 13(4):48–50.

Paparella M, Shumrick D (editors): *Otolaryngology.* Vol. 3. Philadelphia: Saunders, 1980.

Passy V: Hoarseness: Evaluation and treatment. *Primary Care* 1982; 9:337–354.

Saunders WH: Surgery of the inferior nasal turbinates. *Ann Otol Rhinol Laryngol* 1982; 91:445–447.

Saxton D, Pelikan PK, Nugent PM, Hyland PA: *The Addison-Wesley Manual of Nursing Practice.* Menlo Park, CA: Addison-Wesley, 1983.

Silverberg E: Cancer. *Statistics 1983* 1983; 33:9–25.

Sloane PD: Sore throats: They're common but full of surprises. *Consultant* 1982; 22:110–117.

Templer J: Removal of foreign body from the nose. *Hosp Med* (March) 1981; 17:77–84.

Suggested Readings

Denning DC: Head and neck cancer: Our reactions. *Cancer Nurs* 1982; 5:269–273. Focuses on personal reactions of nurses who care for clients who experience alteration in body image related to cancer of the head and neck.

Lee BC, Hansen EF, Poppell MR: Facial fractures take a special kind of nursing care. *Nurs 80* (Aug) 1980; 10(8):43–46. Follows hospital course of client with multiple lacerations and fractures of the head and neck, discussing nursing care from admission to emergency room until discharge.

Sumner SM, Eaton P: Emergency! First aid for choking. *Nurs 82* (July) 1982; 12(7):40–49. Reviews major causes of choking. Includes pictorial guide for assisting adult, child, and infant; also summarizes information for public education about preventive measures.

The Client With Cancer of the Larynx

I. Descriptive Data	James Curtis, age 56, has come to the medical clinic of the county hospital with a concern about hoarseness × 6 mo and recent dysphagia. He is accompanied by his wife.
II. Personal Data	
Date and Time:	October 7, 1986, 9 AM
Full Name:	James Scott Curtis
Social Security Number:	000-00-0000
Address:	1613 S. Market St., Buffalo, NY
Telephone:	Home: 000-0000
	Work: 000-0000
Sex:	Male
Age:	56
Birthdate:	10-2-30
Marital Status:	Married
Race/Culture:	Black
Religion:	Baptist
Occupation:	Truck driver
Usual Health Care Provider:	Company physician
III. Health History	
Source of Information:	Client and wife
Reliability of Informant:	Mr Curtis is moderately reliable. Has difficulty remembering time of onset of symptoms. Mrs Curtis provides detailed information regarding history, symptoms, and time of onset.
Chief Concern:	Hoarseness of approximately 6 mo duration, becoming progressively worse; slight difficulty swallowing during the past month.
History of Present Illness:	The client's wife noticed an alteration (deepening) in the quality of Mr Curtis's voice approximately 6 mo ago. He attributed this change to the aftermath of a cold and refused to seek evaluation until this time. According to Mrs Curtis, the hoarseness has progressively worsened. He has not had prolonged upper respiratory problems, postnasal drip, or sinusitis. He has no known allergies. He does not overuse his voice; does not sing—except in the shower.
	The client has lost 25 lb during the last 6 mo, going from 200 to 175 lb. He did not experience anorexia and continued to eat his regular diet. He states he has experienced slight difficulty swallowing during the past month. Mr Curtis has noticed feeling more tired than usual during work.
	He smokes 2 packs of cigarettes/day × 20 yr (40 pack yr); has a nonproductive cough, mild DOE; no history of TBC or other respiratory problems. Usual alcohol intake includes 2 beers after work and 2 to 4 beers on the weekend. He has had mild hypertension × 12 yr, controlled on hydrochlorothiazide 50 mg q.d. He takes no other medications.
Past Health History:	
Childhood:	Usual childhood diseases—chickenpox, mumps, and measles
Immunizations:	Received immunization during elementary school and in the army
Medical Problems:	Mild essential hypertension for 12 yr, which is controlled with medication
Surgeries:	1973—left inguinal herniorrhaphy
	1976—hemorrhoidectomy

Case Study written by Vicky Hartwell-Ivins.

Transfusions:	None
Special Diagnostic Procedures:	None
Trauma:	None
Allergies:	None known
Medications:	Hydrochlorothiazide, 50 mg PO q.d. for hypertension
Family History:	

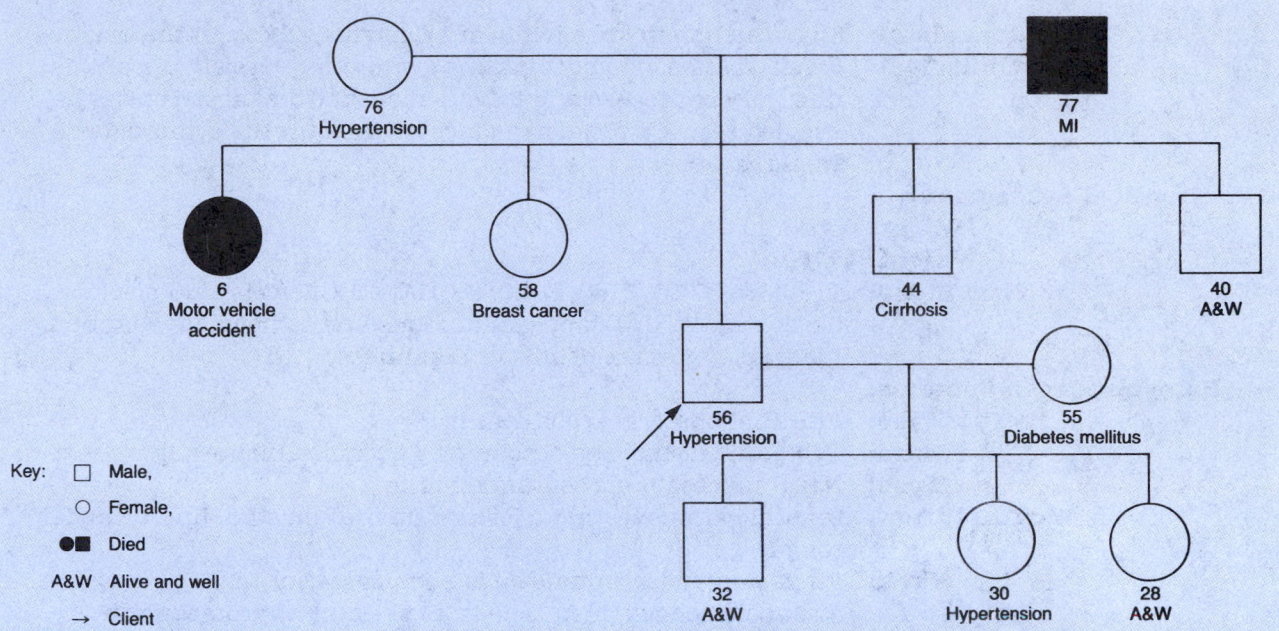

Key:
- □ Male,
- ○ Female,
- ●■ Died
- A&W Alive and well
- → Client

Personal/Social History: The client is married and lives with his wife in their suburban home, which they own. Their three children have their own homes in the surrounding community. His wife works as a school teacher. The client spends 10 to 12 hr a day driving a truck; has worked for the same company for 22 yr; plans to retire in 9 yr; total yearly combined income is $38,000. After work, he stops at the local tavern and visits with his friends. Enjoys working in his garden on weekends. Also enjoys football and horse races. Sleeps approximately 7 hr each night without difficulty. Mr Curtis completed high school. He was a private in the army; remained in the United States through his tour of duty.

Diet: Mr Curtis's physician has instructed him to follow a low-sodium diet. The client states that he eats what he wants. His regular diet is high in fats and carbohydrates. He eats a large proportion of fried foods. He does not add salt at the table, and his wife does not cook with salt.

Review of Systems: Generally feels more tired than usual; 25 lb weight loss over past 6 mo

Throat/Neck/Chest: See history of present illness

Cardiovascular: Experiences headaches when blood pressure is elevated; no chest pain, epistaxis, ankle edema, or claudication; wife takes BP at home. Ranges from high of 160/100 to low of 130/90; average BP 140/92.

(continued)

The Client With Cancer of the Larynx

Gastrointestinal: No change in appetite or bowel habits; no melena, hematemesis, diarrhea, constipation, or ulcer hx; slight dysphagia during the past month

Genitourinary: Denies dysuria, UTI, impotence; sexually active without difficulty

Musculoskeletal: Slight aching in knee joints after driving all day in the truck

Psychological: States that he did not think his symptoms were significant; is now very concerned and fearful about the diagnosis; states he avoided seeing a physician since he thought the symptoms would disappear

IV. Physical Assessment

Height: 6 ft 1 in

Weight: 175 lb

Vital Signs: T. $98^8°$F ($37°$C), P. 88, R. 20, BP 150/90. Client is a 56-yr-old black male in NAD; appears anxious and somewhat reliant on his wife to give the details of his illness.

Relevant Organ Systems:

Eyes: PERRLA, bilateral arcus senilis

Ears: Tympanic membrane obscured by cerumen bilaterally

Nose: Nasal mucosa pink, septum midline

Mouth/Throat: Several carious teeth; no lesions on oral mucosa, lips, or under tongue

Neck: Firm, nontender, nonmovable node posterior to sternocleidomastoid muscle in rt neck; no thyromegaly; no bruits

Chest: Breath sounds equal bilaterally c̄ basilar rhonchi; bilaterally resonant to percussion; no axillary adenopathy

Cardiovascular: S_1, S_2 nl; regular rate and rhythm s̄ murmurs or gallops; pedal pulses 2+ and symmetrical

Abdomen: Muscular and flat; well-healed left inguinal herniorrhaphy scar; active bowel sounds; abd. nontender s̄ masses; liver palpable 1 cm below rt costal margin; liver span at MCL, 10 cm by percussion

Genitourinary: Normal uncircumcised male; testes s̄ masses

Rectal: Normal prostate s̄ nodules; no hemorrhoids or masses; stool occult blood test negative

Extremities: No cyanosis, clubbing, or edema; full ROM

Neurological: Cranial nerves II–XII grossly intact; DTRs 2+ and symmetrical; normal motor and vibratory sense

Psychological: Appears anxious; has difficulty sitting still; constantly tapping fingers and feet; relies on wife to answer some questions; does not offer information without being questioned specifically

V. Diagnostic Data

Indirect laryngoscopy: mass present on rt vocal cord. Laboratory tests: moderately elevated liver enzymes; mild anemia

VI. Summary

Mr Curtis underwent a direct laryngoscopy with biopsy.

Findings: Mass on right true vocal cord and beneath it, 1 mm subglottic extension; pyriform sinuses clear

Diagnosis: Well-differentiated squamous cell carcinoma of the larynx

Medical Plan: Mr Curtis was scheduled for a total laryngectomy with right radical neck dissection on 10-14-86

Nursing Diagnosis	Client Care Goals	Plan/Nursing Implementation	Expected Outcomes
Nutrition, alterations in: less than body requirements, related to increased metabolism of malignant cells	• Remain well hydrated • Understand importance of adequate intake of food and fluids	Encourage client to eat low Na diet including adequate amounts of calories, protein, carbohydrates and fats: 2500 calories daily, 160 g protein; encourage fluids, at least 3000 mL/24 h; initiate a nutritional consult so client receives food he likes and is familiar with, in accordance with his low Na diet; provide environment conducive to eating; administer dietary supplements and vitamins prescribed by physician; stress importance of maintaining present weight by good nutritional intake; explain that cancer increases body's need for intake of adequate calories	• Takes in well-balanced low-sodium diet of at least 2500 calories with 160 g of protein • Takes in 2000 to 3000 mL of fluid per day • Good skin turgor • BP, heart rate wnl • Describes what constitutes adequate nutritional and fluid intake
Airway clearance, ineffective, potential for, related to dysphagia	• Remain free of foreign objects such as food or liquids in airway • Understand importance of taking small bites, chewing food well, and eating in unhurried manner	Encourage client to eat and drink in an unhurried manner, taking small bites and chewing food well; observe for signs and symptoms of choking—grasping throat, difficulty or inability to speak, dyspnea/stridor, use of accessory muscles, nasal flaring, skin color changes; keep suction machine and suction catheter in the room in case he should choke and oral suction becomes necessary	• Discusses importance of eating in an unhurried manner, taking small bites, and chewing food well • Demonstrates proper eating as described and does not choke
Anxiety, related to the diagnosis of cancer and impending surgery	• Cope effectively with the diagnosis and impending surgery • Understand basic information regarding laryngeal cancer and his symptoms	Approach client and significant others in calm, unhurried manner; assess level of understanding of client and family regarding laryngeal cancer and impending surgery; provide atmosphere in which the client and significant others will verbalize fears and anxieties related to the illness and management; explain in basic terms the disease of laryngeal cancer and the relationship of the client's symptoms to the disease; clarify misconceptions	• Client will exhibit signs and symptoms of decreased anxiety level (eg, blood pressure, respiratory rate, and pulse wnl) • Client and family will express their feelings and anxieties about the diagnosis and impending surgery • They willl be able to say "cancer" when discussing the diagnosis
	• Understand in basic terms the procedure of a total laryngectomy and radical neck dissection	Provide preoperative teaching and counseling related to a total laryngectomy and a radical neck	• Describes total laryngectomy and radical neck dissection • Discusses his situa-

(continued)

The Client With Cancer of the Larynx

VII. Nursing Care Plan (continued)

Nursing Diagnosis	Client Care Goals	Plan/Nursing Implementation	Expected Outcomes
		dissection; administer antianxiety medications when appropriate as prescribed by physician; initiate consultation with speech therapist and psychologist in the preoperative phase; introduce client to a well-adjusted client who has undergone a total laryngectomy; share information about self-help groups and other resources for laryngectomy clients	tion and expected outcome of surgery with speech therapist and psychologist • Interacts with a well-adjusted laryngectomee • Describes available support groups and resources
Knowledge deficit, related to planned surgery	• Understand the surgical procedure and what to expect postoperatively	Explain the procedure of a total laryngectomy and radical neck dissection to the client and significant others in terms they can understand; inform client and significant others that his route for breathing will be permanently altered; include the following information: • He will breathe through a stoma (opening) in his lower neck • Initially, humidified oxygen will be administered to compensate for loss of humidification by the nose • Suctioning through the stoma will be necessary to remove excessive secretions • Drains inserted under the skin are connected to a suction source to promote drainage of fluid • Suture lines will be inspected frequently to assess the healing process • Suture lines will be cleansed, and an antibiotic ointment may be applied • Edema (swelling) may be present in the face • VS will be monitored at frequent intervals, initially every 15 min, then q.1h, 2 h, and 4 h	• Explains the surgical procedure in general terms • Discusses the postoperative events related to the altered airway

Nursing Diagnosis	Client Care Goals	Plan/Nursing Implementation	Expected Outcomes
	• Recognize the parts of a laryngectomy tube • Demonstrate interest in becoming involved in his own care	Show client a laryngectomy tube; explain that the tube will remain in the stoma for a period of time (often 2–3 weeks after surgery); explain that the tube is removed every day (after 2 or 3 postoperative days) and a sterile tube reinserted; the inner cannula is removed and cleansed as often as necessary, depending on the amount of secretions that accumulate on inner cannula; initially, this will be done by a nurse; however, soon he will be expected to learn the procedure	• Able to identify the three parts of a laryngectomy tube • Recognizes that he will be encouraged to participate actively in his care in the early postoperative period (ie, cleansing the laryngectomy tube and stoma)
	• Know physical limitations that result from the procedure of a total laryngectomy • Understand that after surgery he will no longer be able to communicate as he does at the present time	Explain that the client will no longer be able to perform certain actions (eg, swimming, drinking through a straw, blowing his nose, Valsalva's maneuver); also his sense of smell will be diminished or absent, and taste sensation may be altered; inform client and significant others that his ability to communicate will be permanently altered	• Verbally describes or lists required alterations in current lifestyle after surgery • Will discuss altered communication status and its significance to him
	• Know that several options are available as methods of communication	If client is receptive, discuss alaryngeal methods of speech he may choose from (ie, esophageal speech and artificial aids such as electrolarynx or Cooper–Rand device); explain that immediately after surgery he can communicate by writing and gesturing; reassure him that he will have a call bell to alert staff; explain that many laryngectomees develop excellent communication skills and return to their previous jobs and activities	• Verbalizes feelings and emotions regarding loss of ability to produce a natural voice • Gives some thought to communication options available following laryngectomy and discusses them with staff and family • Expresses interest in communicating with a well-adjusted laryngectomee • Copes with impending loss of "natural" voice
	• Know method by which he will receive nutrition in the postoperative period	Inform client and significant others that an NG tube will be placed in surgery as a route for providing nutrition in the postoperative period; soon after surgery, he will receive liquid feedings through the tube every 2–3 h; initially, this will be done by a nurse. Then client will be	• Verbalizes an understanding of the liquid diet he will receive via NG tube in the postoperative period

(continued)

The Client With Cancer of the Larynx

VII. Nursing Care Plan *(continued)*

Nursing Diagnosis	Client Care Goals	Plan/Nursing Implementation	Expected Outcomes
		expected to learn the procedure; the NG tube will remain in place approximately 1 to 2 weeks; explain that he will receive fluids through an intravenous infusion for a short time after surgery	
		The client will need to rinse his mouth frequently with a solution that will be provided	• Discusses importance of good oral hygiene after surgery
	• Recognize need for close monitoring postoperatively	Explain that he will be in an intensive care unit for a few days after surgery so he can be monitored closely; take client and significant others through intensive care unit (depending on individual and family)	• Expresses feelings and anxiety about the postoperative period; asks questions
	• Explain necessity of performing ROM exercises to his rt shoulder and arm	Explain that client will experience some discomfort and limited movement of his rt shoulder because of the surgery; teach ROM exercises client will be instructed to perform postoperatively; determine the effectiveness of preoperative instruction; ask client and significant others to repeat information provided	• Demonstrates ROM exercises to rt shoulder and arm • Client and significant others discuss information presented demonstrating an understanding of the preoperative instruction
Comfort, alteration in, pain	• Maintain a relatively pain-free state during his postoperative course	Explain that during the first postoperative days, the nursing staff will medicate him for pain q. 3–4 h; after the first few days, he will be medicated for pain as he feels he needs it; inform the client and family that they should not hesitate to request medication when the client feels pain	• Client and family both express satisfaction with client's level of comfort in the postoperative period • Verbalizes he will not hesitate to ask for pain medication if he feels significant discomfort

Chapter 20

Specific Disorders of the Lower Respiratory System

Yvonne Krall Scherer

Objectives

When you have finished studying this chapter, you should be able to:

Identify the major respiratory diseases categorized under multifactorial, infectious, neoplastic, obstructive, and traumatic causation.

Describe the appropriate therapeutic measures involved in the medical management of clients with specific respiratory diseases.

Explain appropriate nursing interventions based on the nursing diagnoses of clients with specific respiratory diseases.

Specify the appropriate health teaching for clients with specific respiratory diseases.

Anticipate the psychosocial/lifestyle impact that specific respiratory disorders can have on the lives of clients, their families, and significant others.

Demonstrate the role of the nurse in health education by not smoking and by actively teaching others the health dangers of cigarette smoking and exposure to respiratory irritants.

Discuss the significance of rehabilitation and the measures employed in rehabilitation of clients with chronic respiratory disorders.

Problems of the lower respiratory tract constitute a major concern in health care. These disorders can range from a minor bout of acute bronchitis to major life-threatening conditions such as acute respiratory failure. Many of the disorders are chronic and debilitating, making it necessary for clients and their families (or significant others) to make long-term adjustments in lifestyle. Clients admitted to a hospital with other debilitating conditions frequently develop respiratory difficulties in the form of atelectasis, retained respiratory tract secretions, and pneumonia. A majority of these are preventable with good nursing care. Interpersonal nursing intervention skills are also required. Dysfunction of the respiratory system can arouse many disturbing feelings and concerns, including anxiety, helplessness, fear, despair, and depression. Air hunger is a primal drive—stronger even than hunger and thirst. The nurse must be equipped to deal with the problems these feelings produce and assist clients and their families to cope.

Section I: Disorders of Multifactorial Origin

Some of the respiratory disorders addressed in this section are referred to as occupational lung diseases. Sarcoidosis and adult respiratory distress syndrome are also discussed here. Occupational lung diseases result from exposure to offending respiratory agents in the workplace. The pathogenic agents can be classified (Table 20–1) as mineral (inorganic) fibers or dusts, organic fibers and dusts, and irritant gases and chemicals (Weill, 1981).

Table 20–1 Occupational Lung Diseases

Inhalant	Disease	Exposure
Mineral (inorganic) dusts		
	Fibrosis and malignancy	
Free silica	Silicosis	Hard-rock or metal mining, foundry work, sandblasting, pottery industry, slate industry.
Asbestos	Asbestosis, lung cancer, mesothelioma	Mining and milling; manufacture of asbestos products; installation or removal of asbestos insulation
Coal dust	Progressive massive fibrosis	Coal mining
Diatomaceous earth, kaolin, talc, mica, tungsten carbide	Varying degrees of fibrosis	Mining, manufacturing
	Maculae	
Coal dust	Simple coal workers' pneumoconiosis	Coal mining
Iron oxide	Siderosis	Welding
Barium sulfate	Baritosis	Mining
Tin oxide	Stannosis	Mining
Organic dusts		
	Diffuse hypersensitivity pneumonia (extrinsic allergic alveolitis)	
Moldy hay	Farmer's lung	Farming
Bagasse (sugar cane waste)	Bagassosis	Manufacture of wallboard, paper
Avian droppings or serum	Bird breeder's lung	Bird handling
Mushroom spores	Mushroom worker's lung	Mushroom farming
	Variable airways obstruction (occupational asthma)	
Grain	Asthma	Grain-elevator work
Castor or coffee beans	Asthma	Castor oil or coffee manufacturing
Proteolytic enzyme detergents	Asthma	Detergent manufacturing
Western red cedar dust	Asthma	Lumbering, woodworking
Cotton, flax, hemp	Byssinosis	Textile industry
Irritant gases and chemicals		
Acute heavy exposure	*Diverse pathology*	
Chlorine, phosgene, nitrogen oxide, ammonia	Tracheobronchitis, bronchiolitis, pulmonary edema	Transportation accidents, manufacturing accidents or malfunction
Chronic low level exposure (continuous or intermittent)		
Toluene diisocyanate (TDI), phthalic anhydride, trimellitic anhydride	Occupational asthma	Plastics industry
Wide variety of irritants	Industrial bronchitis	Chemical industry
Chemical carcinogens:	Lung cancer	
Chlormethyl ethers		Chemical industry
Uranium		Mining
Coke-oven emission		Steel industry
Metals (arsinic, chromates, nickel)		Mining or manufacturing

SOURCE: Weill H: Occupational lung diseases. *Hosp Pract* (April) 1981; 16(4):68.

According to estimates by the National Institute for Occupational Safety and Health, approximately 2 million Americans are partially or severely disabled by occupational diseases. The Department of Labor estimates that approximately 65,000 US workers develop a respiratory disease related to their jobs, and 25,000 persons die from these diseases (American Lung Association, 1983).

Since occupational lung diseases are for the most part considered preventable, nurses need to encourage and support measures directed toward reducing polluted air at the workplace. Nurses need to support legislation aimed at ensuring safe and healthy working conditions.

It is also important to educate the public about occupational hazards and resulting diseases so employees are aware of the dangers and how to combat or minimize their effects. Many employees may know of no alternative but to accept the risk and hope for a better life for their children.

OCCUPATIONAL LUNG DISEASE (THE PNEUMOCONIOSES)

The pneumoconioses are lung diseases resulting from inhalation of inorganic dusts. Silicosis, asbestosis, and coal workers' pneumoconiosis fall in this category.

Clinical Manifestations

The clinical manifestations of the pneumoconioses are similar in that these disorders can lead to pulmonary fibrosis. This condition causes the lungs to become stiff and nonelastic, reducing lung volume. Also, the development of a thickened pulmonary membrane can interfere with gas exchange.

Silicosis may occur in various forms. The most common is chronic or classic silicosis, which occurs in individuals who have inhaled relatively low concentrations of dust for 10 to 20 years. Initially, the accumulated dust and tissue reaction result in the development of scattered nodules throughout the lungs and shortness of breath upon exertion. Chronic silicosis may become more serious, resulting in increased shortness of breath, cough, and sputum production. In complicated silicosis, fibrosis of the lung occurs, leading to restriction in lung function and right-sided heart failure. Respiratory impairment is severe. Those with silicosis may also develop tuberculosis. Caplan's syndrome, the development of rheumatoid arthritis and concomitant fibrotic lesions, may occur (Cohen, 1981). Acute silicosis, most commonly due to exposure to high concentrations of silica dust (as in sandblasting), is a rapidly progressive disease leading to severe disability and death within 5 years of diagnosis.

Asbestosis is a diffuse interstitial fibrosis of the lungs resulting from repeated trauma caused by the impact and deposition of asbestos fibers on the alveolar walls. As the

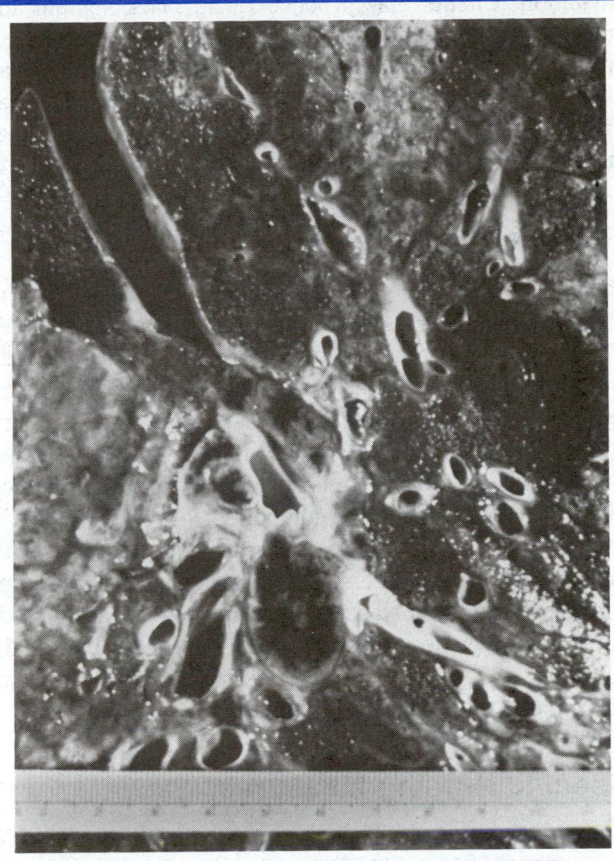

Figure 20–1

Asbestosis of the lung. (Courtesy of Millard Fillmore Hospital, Buffalo, NY)

fibrosis becomes widespread, the elasticity and compliance of the lung are reduced (Figure 20–1). Fibrosis results in a thickening of the alveolar walls and interstitial space, which in turn reduces the oxygen diffusion to the pulmonary capillary bed. Pulmonary function studies show a reduced forced vital capacity. X-rays reveal linear opacities, especially in the lower lung fields. Unfortunately, physical findings are few until the disease is relatively advanced (Cohen, 1981). Individuals may see their care provider for symptoms of a productive cough, shortness of breath, and weight loss. Asbestosis has no cure and usually results in death after a period of years. Lung cancer is associated with all types of asbestos inhalation. Mesothelioma, a cancer of the pleura, accounts for 7% to 10% of the deaths of asbestos workers.

Coal workers' pneumoconiosis results from the accumulation of coal dust in the lungs, which accounts for its common name, black lung disease. Simple coal workers' pneumoconiosis, not complicated by other lung conditions, causes no symptoms or respiratory difficulty. A small percentage develop progressive massive fibrosis with large lesions consisting of fibrous tissue, coal dust, and central cavitation. Clients may produce thick, black sputum and suffer from shortness of breath and dyspnea. X-rays reveal large opacities, and pulmonary function studies indicate an obstructive deficit. The large-mass lesions produced may eventually lead to pulmonary hypertension, cor pulmonale, and death from congestive heart failure (Cohen, 1981).

Therapeutic Measures

Pulmonary function studies and chest x-ray assist in the diagnosis and in assessing the degree of lung impairment. Therapeutic measures are not curative but only supportive.

Superimposed respiratory tract infections are treated with antibiotics. Antituberculosis medications are administered if tuberculosis develops in clients with silicosis. Bronchodilators may be beneficial when there is evidence of a reversible obstructive component.

Oxygen therapy may be necessary for individuals with low arterial oxygen levels. Cardiotonic drugs may be prescribed if the cardiovascular system has been affected. Bronchial hygiene measures such as deep breathing, coughing, and postural drainage are often indicated. Clients are advised to discontinue exposure.

Specific Nursing Measures

Nursing management is supportive. Stress the importance of avoiding further exposure to the harmful agent. Smoking will aggravate the symptoms. Answering client questions, explaining the disease process, and explaining treatments, will give clients more knowledge about how to cope effectively with their illness.

Be aware that many people will be afraid to leave a job they know how to do. Others, unable to leave a geographical area and with responsibility for a family, will feel their options are limited. They may choose to stay on the job even though it interferes with their health. If nurses acknowledge the reality of the client's situation, their health teaching efforts may be more readily accepted.

SARCOIDOSIS

Sarcoidosis is a multisystem disorder characterized by non-caseating granulomas in many organs. It is most common in young adults and more prevalent among blacks. Objective findings include bilateral hilar lymphadenopathy, pulmonary infiltration, and skin or eye lesions. Other areas affected can include the liver, spleen, heart, muscles, peripheral lymph nodes, mucous membranes, parotid glands, phalangeal bones, and nervous system.

The etiology of sarcoidosis is unknown, but immune system involvement is suspected. The tubercle bacillus and genetic susceptibility are also under investigation. The illness can vary from self-limiting with spontaneous remission to a progressive widespread granulomatous inflam-

mation and fibrosis. Death is usually from advanced pulmonary disease.

Clinical Manifestations

Intrathoracic lesions are the most common manifestation of sarcoidosis and the most frequent indication for treatment. There is usually dyspnea and a cough that may be severe, incapacitating, and occasionally occurring in paroxysms that lead to vomiting. There is scanty sputum, which occasionally can be blood streaked from straining. Wheezing and pulmonary obstruction also can occur. Physical examination reveals crackling rales that are diffuse or only at the bases of the lungs. Restricted pulmonary excursion and an accentuated or split-second heart sound in the pulmonic area can be heard if pulmonary hypertension is present. Hemoptysis and spontaneous pneumothorax are also possible. Systemic features of sarcoidosis include fever, weight loss, fatigue, and night sweats. Tuberculosis must be ruled out by careful examination. Mediastinal and hilar lymph nodes are most commonly involved. There also may be peripheral lymphadenopathy that is generalized or localized to axillary or femoral areas. The nodes found are discrete, firm, nontender, and usually symmetrical. Epitrochlear nodes are often palpable.

Other extrathoracic lesions may produce symptoms and signs in any organ system. Skin lesions may range from maculopapular eruptions, plaques, and raised nodules to erythema nodosum (Figure 20–2). The most common specific lesions are reddish purple, soft, asymptomatic nodules observed most often on the nares (Figure 20–3), eyelid margins, and back of the neck. Ocular involvement is possible, including conjunctivitis, retinal lesions, and lacrimal gland enlargement. Acute granulomatous inflammation of the iris, ciliary body, and choroid (uveitis) may occur, producing pain and clouding of vision that can progress to severe visual impairment and blindness. A careful slit-lamp examination is important for all clients with sarcoidosis.

There may be asymptomatic enlargement of the parotid, sublingual, and submaxillary glands. A syndrome of fever, uveitis, and lacrimal and salivary gland enlargement is known as Heerfordt's syndrome.

Sarcoidosis may involve the liver and spleen, causing abnormalities in laboratory tests (eg, elevation in serum alkaline phosphatase levels, leukopenia, and anemia). The kidneys also can be affected because of unexplained hypercalcemia in sarcoidosis. The heart is often affected because of lung involvement. Pulmonary hypertension and cor pulmonale can develop, or there may be sudden death from conduction disturbances or paroxysmal dysrhythmias. Occasionally, a pacemaker is needed.

Granulomas can also form in muscles. Although they do not always produce pain, severe weakness and incapacitation can result. Arthralgias may occur, along with erythema nodosum and fever. Arthritis, most often involving the ankles, also may be seen. Bone lesions in the phalanges of the hands and feet are often visualized on x-ray examination. Various neurological manifestations occur, such as facial nerve (CN VII) palsies, swallowing disorders, pituitary involvement, and peripheral neuropathies.

Abnormal laboratory test results include signs of anemia, eosinophilia, and elevated serum globulins and serum calcium. X-rays of the chest show hilar lymphadenopathy bilaterally and translucent lesions in bones.

The Kveim test may be done; an intradermal injection of sterilized sarcoidal or lymph node material is followed by biopsy of the area in 2 to 3 weeks. A positive test will show a noncaseating granuloma. This test has questionable value because of the lack of standardization of the test material and false-positive responses.

Pulmonary function studies demonstrate decreased lung compliance and loss of diffusing surface. Vital capacity and carbon monoxide diffusing capacity also are decreased. These two indexes are indicators of progression of the illness and the client's response to treatment. Significant pulmonary function impairment can remain even after the x-ray is clear. The vital capacity will always be slightly decreased, even after treatment or spontaneous remission of the disease.

Diagnosis is made by clinical features, along with histological evidence of granulomas composed of epithelioid cells from tissue biopsy. Most biopsied tissue should come from superficial or palpable lesions in the skin or lymph nodes. When the predominant lesions are in the lung, lung biopsy via fiberoptic bronchoscopy or mediastinoscopy with lymph node biopsy can be performed, but these are much more invasive procedures.

Therapeutic Measures

No treatment is required if the client is asymptomatic. Most asymptomatic clients will have spontaneous resolution of the disease within 1 to 2 years. Corticosteroids have a dramatic impact on the symptomatic client by suppressing the active inflammatory reaction. Indications for corticosteroid therapy include:

- Active ocular disease
- Persistent, progressive pulmonary involvement
- Hypercalcemia or hypercalciuria
- Central nervous system involvement with functional impairment
- Significant evidence of myocardial problems
- Persistent constitutional symptoms, such as fever and weight loss
- Any progressive deterioration of a vital organ

Sarcoidosis can remain in remission after corticosteroid treatment but can recur in some clients when treatment is reduced. X-rays and pulmonary function tests are

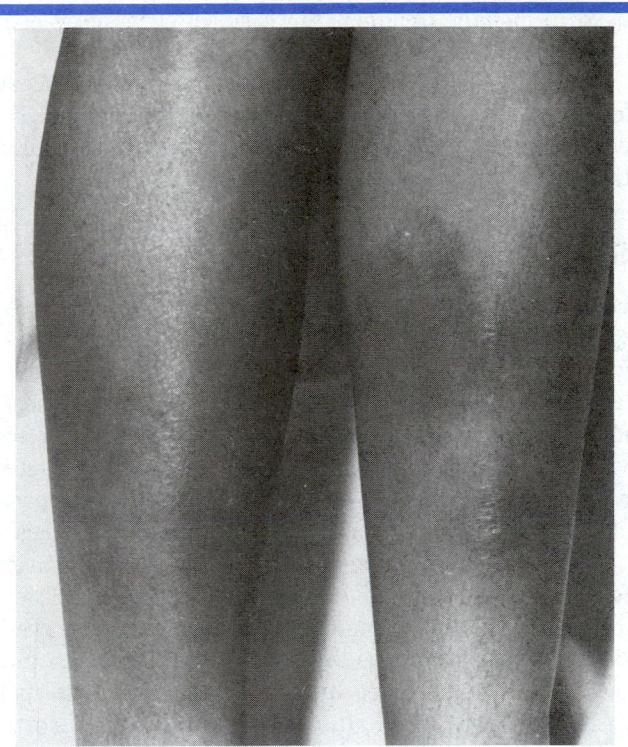

Figure 20–2

Erythema nodosum in a client with sarcoidosis.
SOURCE: Binnick SA: *Skin Diseases: Diagnosis and Management in Clinical Practice.* Baltimore: Williams & Wilkins, 1982, p. 258.

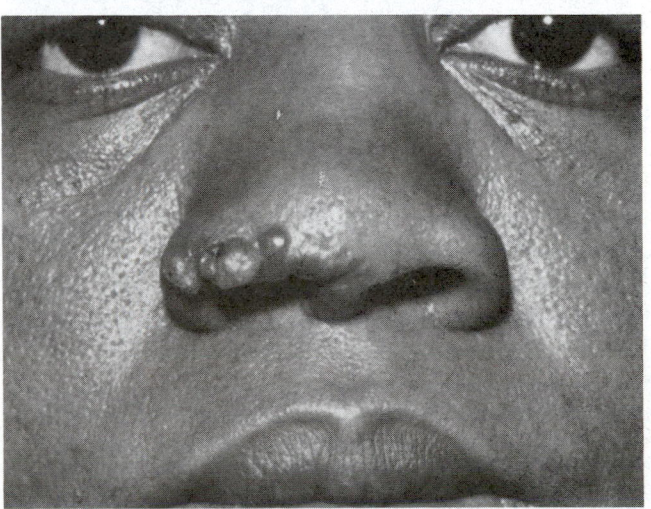

Figure 20–3

Nodules on the nose of a client with sarcoidosis.
SOURCE: Binnick SA: *Skin Diseases: Diagnosis and Management in Clinical Practice.* Baltimore: Williams & Wilkins, 1982, p. 291.

used to monitor treatment. Occasional clients may need lifelong treatment.

Chloroquine (Aralen) improves skin and mucosal lesions, but they return when the drug is discontinued. For clients receiving this medication, it is important to monitor the retina for damage.

Specific Nursing Measures

Because sarcoidosis can affect any body system, the nurse must continuously assess the client for new system involvement. For example, the nurse observes the skin for lesions and auscultates the lungs for rales and the heart for dysrhythmias and an abnormal S_2. Record weight and vital signs frequently, and provide comfort measures according to the client's symptoms. Follow laboratory reports closely, especially pulmonary function and x-ray studies.

If the client is taking corticosteroids, check the urine for glucose and acetone, and carefully evaluate the client for other signs and symptoms of side effects. The client taking corticosteroids is vulnerable to infection, so protection may be provided by use of the reverse isolation technique. During and after withdrawal from corticosteroids (which must be gradual), watch for vomiting, orthostatic hypotension, hypoglycemia, restlessness, anorexia, malaise, and fatigue.

Discharge planning includes encouraging clients to avoid working in an environment subject to dust or chemicals because of the continuing pulmonary involvement. Clients should not smoke for the same reason. Clients taking chloroquine should have ophthalmologic examinations every 6 months, and more often if visual symptoms develop. Those with hypercalcemia may benefit from a diet with low calcium levels and decreased vitamin D.

ADULT RESPIRATORY DISTRESS SYNDROME

Adult respiratory distress syndrome (ARDS) is a pathophysiological state best recognized in clients with no previous underlying lung disease who have suffered a sudden catastrophic, often multisystem insult, which has led to the development of severe dyspnea, hypoxemia, loss of pulmonary compliance, and noncardiogenic pulmonary edema (Petty, 1982). ARDS is not a clearly defined disease but a name given to a group of conditions of different etiology but having similar manifestations (Burrell & Burrell, 1982). ARDS has also been called shock lung, white lung, DaNang lung, adult hyaline membrane disease, stiff lung syndrome, wet lung, and many other names (Petty, 1982). Petty and his colleagues first described ARDS as a clinical syndrome in 1967. Approximately 150,000 cases of ARDS are reported each year in the United States.

Many factors can lead to the development of ARDS, including major insults such as shock from any cause, mul-

---

Box 20–1 Clinical States Associated With ARDS

Related to Primary Disorder

Shock of any etiology

Trauma
  Fat embolism
  Lung contusion
  Massive soft tissue injury
  Head injury
  Burns

Aspiration
  Gastric contents
  Near drowning

Infections
  Sepsis
  Pneumonia
  Severe pneumonitis

Hematologic disorders
  Disseminated intravascular coagulation
  Massive transfusions
  Prolonged cardiopulmonary bypass
  Transfusion reactions

Chemical lung injury
  Smoke inhalation
  Inhaled chemicals

Drug ingestion and overdose

Miscellaneous
  Pancreatitis
  Uremia
  Eclampsia
  Anaphylaxis
  Radiation pneumonitis
  Amniotic fluid embolism

Related to Treatment

Oxygen toxicity

Excessive fluid administration

Microatelectasis

SOURCE: Holloway NM: *Nursing the Critically Ill Adult*, 2nd ed. Menlo Park, CA: Addison-Wesley, 1984, p 404.

---

tisystem trauma, aspiration, overwhelming infections, overdoses of drugs, and inhaled toxic substances (Petty, 1982). See Box 20–1 for the clinical states most commonly associated with ARDS.

Clinical Manifestations

There is often a latent period of 12 to 48 hours between the initial injury or insult and the development of ARDS. The pathophysiology in ARDS is caused by diffuse damage to either side of the alveolar–capillary membrane (Figure 20–4). Whether the damage is alveolar or capillary, the result is an increase in vascular permeability with edema and hemorrhage. Fluid and red blood cells leak into the interstitial space and into the alveoli. The resulting pulmonary edema leads to decreased lung volume and impaired oxygenation. The presence of fluid in the alveoli results in a decrease in surfactant activity, causing an increased tendency of the alveoli to collapse. In alveoli that are collapsed or filled with edema fluid, little or no ventilation can take place. Since oxygen-poor blood is still perfused to these nonventilated alveoli, the result is an abnormally low ventilation-to-perfusion ratio with an increased right to left intrapulmonary shunt. This is responsible for the severe hypoxemia that is refractory to increases in inspired oxygen concentrations (Traver, 1982).

The fluid accumulation in the interstitial space and alveoli causes the lungs to become less compliant, or stiff. The functional residual capacity also decreases because of alveolar instability and collapse (Petty, 1982). These destructive factors will increase the work of breathing, causing clients to hyperventilate in an effort to correct the hypoxemia. Initially, the hyperventilation may result in a lower than normal arterial carbon dioxide tension. As the condition worsens, dyspnea will become more severe. Grunting respirations along with intercostal and suprasternal retractions may be present. Cyanosis is present along with tachycardia, diaphoresis, and confusion (Cline & Fisher, 1982). The client may have rales and rhonchi. Chest x-rays usually reveal pulmonary edema without evidence of heart failure. Arterial blood gases reveal hypoxemia, the cardinal feature of ARDS despite the initiation of high liter flows of oxygen. Hypocapnia may be present initially. Unless treatment is begun, the client will eventually no longer be able to hyperventilate, and this may result in CO_2 retention and respiratory acidosis.

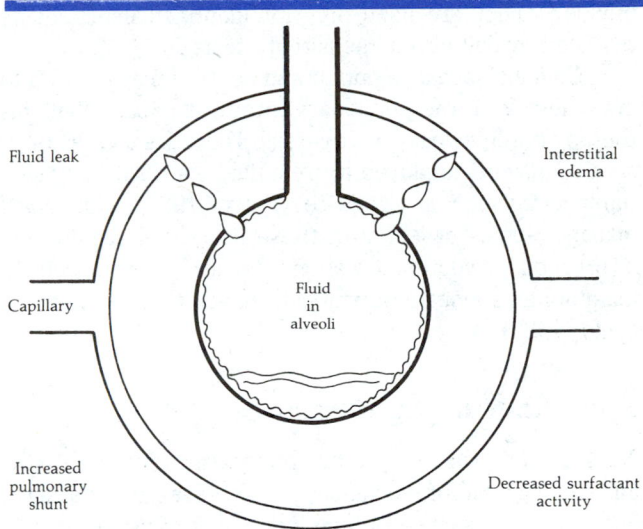

Pathophysiologic sequence

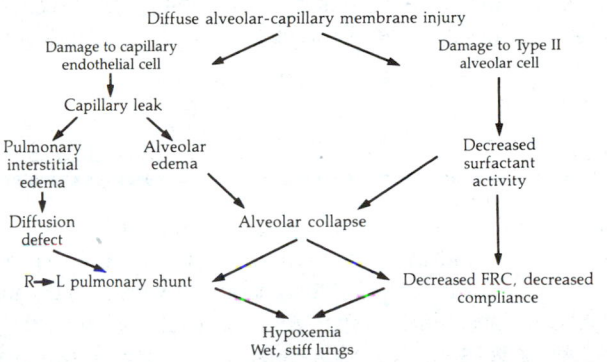

Figure 20–4

Pathophysiological sequence in ARDS.
SOURCE: Holloway NM: *Nursing the Critically Ill Adult,* 2nd ed. Menlo Park, CA: Addison–Wesley, 1984, p. 405.

Therapeutic Measures

Therapeutic measures begin with anticipating which clients are candidates for ARDS. These clients should be closely monitored for early signs of abnormal lung functioning so preventive measures can be instituted.

Treatment of ARDS requires that the client's ventilation be supported and adequate inspired oxygen be delivered to correct the life-threatening hypoxemia. The client must be intubated and placed on a mechanical ventilator with supplemental oxygen to maintain an arterial PO_2 between 60 and 70 mm Hg. A volume ventilator is most often used, and large tidal volumes are given along with supplemental oxygen. Positive end expiratory pressure (PEEP) is frequently instituted to prevent or minimize alveolar collapse at the end of expiration. This improves oxygenation, enabling a reduction in oxygen concentra-

tions. (High inspired oxygen concentrations can lead to oxygen toxicity.)

Careful monitoring of fluid administration is critical because of the increased pulmonary capillary permeability. Overhydration could increase the existing pulmonary edema, shunting, and compliance abnormalities; underhydration could result in inadequate pulmonary and systemic perfusion. A pulmonary artery catheter is frequently used to aid in determining fluid status and left ventricular functioning.

The use of corticosteroid drugs in the treatment of ARDS remains controversial. Corticosteroids may improve surfactant elaboration in ARDS but their potentially harmful effect on the function of lung macrophages can result in a decrease in the lung's defense against bacterial infection. A recommended steroid is methyprednisolone sodium succinate 30 mg/kg body weight for 24 to 48 hours (Petty, 1982). The use of prophylactic antibiotics is not recommended. They are used only for identified infections as revealed by culture and sensitivity tests.

Colloids such as albumin and dextran may be used to draw fluid from the pulmonary interstitial space, but this therapy is somewhat controversial. Diuretics such as furosemide may be employed to treat fluid overload when systemic circulation is adequate (Petty, 1982). Nutritional management is essential in these acutely ill clients, and intravenous hyperalimentation should be employed to maintain an adequate nutritional balance (Hudak, Lohr, & Gallo, 1982).

Specific Nursing Measures

Nurses need to be alert to the precipitating causes of ARDS and closely monitor individuals at risk, assessing vital signs and any abnormalities of lung function such as atelectasis, rales, shortness of breath, and symptoms of hypoxia.

Once ARDS has been diagnosed, nursing care becomes complex. Nursing care of the client's airway requires suc-

tioning, postural drainage, and proper management of the endotracheal or tracheostomy tube. The nurse must be alert to the possible complications of PEEP and mechanical ventilation (see Chapter 18).

Close attention must be paid to arterial blood gases. The level of arterial oxygen needs to be monitored closely to guard against both hypoxemia and oxygen toxicity. Careful monitoring of fluid balance is imperative. Daily weights along with accurate intake and output records are important. Also be alert to the possibility of electrolyte imbalances.

The cardiovascular system may be affected by the various therapeutic interventions. Measurement of central venous pressure, pulmonary artery pressure, and pulmonary capillary wedge pressure are frequently made by the nurse in the intensive care setting.

Since these clients are acutely ill, they and their families require emotional support. The equipment used and the procedures performed on the client can be frightening, and the nurse must take time to explain what is being done and why.

Section II: Infectious Disorders

Infectious disorders of the lower respiratory tract occur when microorganisms invade this normally sterile area and grow unchecked, causing inflammation. A variety of organisms can cause infections: viruses, bacteria, and fungi (including yeasts). Infectious disorders vary in severity and can be acute or chronic.

Of all infectious diseases, lung infections are the most common life-threatening diseases, accounting for significant morbidity and mortality in North America (Putnam, 1980). In the hospital setting, nursing assessment and intervention can be instrumental in preventing the development of pulmonary infections in clients.

ACUTE BRONCHITIS

Acute bronchitis is primarily an infection of the larger bronchi in clients whose airways are otherwise normal. This infection is most commonly viral, and usually starts as an extension of an upper respiratory infection.

Clinical Manifestations

The major symptoms include coughing, a burning substernal sensation (often aggravated by a deep breath), and sputum production. The amount of sputum may be slight initially, but as the infection progresses, the sputum becomes mucoid or purulent. The client may or may not have an elevated temperature. Malaise, muscle aches, and headache are common. Chest auscultation reveals rales, rhonchi, and wheezes. The disease is self-limiting, and the

duration depends on the underlying causative organism. Smoking tends to prolong and aggravate the condition.

Therapeutic Measures

Treatment is aimed at relieving the symptoms. Bed rest may be ordered initially. Debilitated clients sometimes require hospitalization. Hot or cold steam inhalation or intermittent positive pressure breathing (IPPB) will liquefy and loosen secretions so they can be more easily expectorated. Antipyretics such as aspirin may be ordered if temperature is elevated; expectorants may be ordered to loosen secretions or antitussives to quiet a chronic nonproductive cough. Lozenges may be used to soothe an irritated throat. Antibiotics are not routinely given unless sputum cultures identify a superinfection with a bacterial agent.

Specific Nursing Measures

Since acute bronchitis is contagious, clients should learn to guard against spreading the infection by properly disposing of tissues, using good hand-washing technique, covering the nose and mouth when coughing or sneezing, and not sharing drinking glasses or towels. Clients may need instruction on proper deep breathing and coughing techniques. Bronchial drainage may be required in situations where secretions are numerous and the client has difficulty in expectorating them. In more debilitated clients who have a poor cough reflex, suctioning may be necessary. Increased fluid intake of at least 2 to 3 L/day should be encouraged unless contraindicated to help prevent dehydration and to keep respiratory tract secretions liquid so they can be more easily expectorated.

Nutritional management should include an adequate intake of fluids such as soft drinks and fruit juices. Light meals consisting of toast, gelatin, puddings, and cereals should be encouraged. This type of diet is easily tolerated and digested while helping to meet caloric needs.

The environment should be kept warm and dry and free of drafts to prevent chilling. Clients should be encouraged to rest and to avoid becoming overly fatigued. A period of convalescence is usually necessary after the infection, and clients should be cautioned to avoid further exposure to infection, to dress warmly, eat properly, get enough rest, avoid people with colds, and avoid environmental irritants such as cigarette smoke and other pollutants.

THE PNEUMONIAS

Pneumonia is an inflammation of the alveolar spaces caused by infection. Many different organisms can cause pneumonia with a resultant variation in symptomatology. Microorganisms can enter the alveolar spaces when infected airborne droplets are inhaled, when food or fluid is aspirated, or when an infection is spread to the lungs by the bloodstream (George, Light, & Matthay, 1983).

Pneumonia is most common in the elderly, but it can occur at any age. Although relatively healthy adults can contract pneumonia, certain predisposing conditions make individuals more susceptible. One predisposing condition is impaired upper airway defense mechanisms such as can occur with cigarette smoking, trauma, or decreased levels of consciousness (eg, impaired gag reflex). Abnormalities of the lungs or thorax, such as those in chronic obstructive pulmonary diseases, are another predisposing factor, as is general debility from heart disease, diabetes mellitus, or chronic alcoholism. Diseases known to impair immunity, such as leukemia or aplastic anemia, can also lower resistance to pneumonia-causing organisms (Mitchell & Petty, 1982). Hospitalized clients may develop pneumonia, especially those who are debilitated and bedridden, those with artificial airways such as tracheostomies, and certain high-risk postoperative surgical clients.

Overall, pneumonia accounts for more than 10% of all hospital admissions and occurs in about 5% of the clients admitted for other reasons (nosocomial pneumonia). During one recent year, over 2 million cases of pneumonia were reported, and pneumonia is listed as the fifth leading cause of death in the United States. As shown in Table 20–2, the pneumonias and their causative organisms can be divided into those commonly acquired in the community and those that are more frequently hospital acquired (Ryan, 1982).

Table 20–2 Common Types of Pneumonia	
Types of Pneumonia	**Etiological Agent**
Community-acquired pneumonias	
Pneumococcal pneumonia	*Streptococcus pneumoniae*
Mycoplasmal pneumonia	*Mycoplasma pneumoniae*
Legionnaires' pneumonia	*Legionella pneumophila*
Viral pneumonia	Influenza virus (Type A or Type B)
Hospital-acquired pneumonias	
Staphylococcal pneumonia	*Staphylococcus aureus*
Klebsiella pneumonia	*Klebsiella pneumoniae* (Friedländer's bacillus)
Pseudomonal pneumonia	*Pseudomonas aeruginosa*
Aspiration pneumonia	Aspiration of a foreign body, gastric contents, or bacteria from the upper respiratory tract

Clinical Manifestations

Pneumococcal Pneumonia

Pneumococcal pneumonia, caused by *Streptococcus pneumoniae,* is the most common community-acquired bacterial pneumonia. This pneumonia, which may be preceded by an upper respiratory tract infection, is usually lobar or segmental, involving one or two lobes of the lung. The rest of the lung may remain free of infection. The onset is abrupt beginning with shaking chills, severe pleural pain, rapidly rising fever (as high as 106°F or 41°C), and a hacking cough. A cough productive of purulent sputum that is greenish, bloody, or rusty is common. Generalized symptoms such as malaise, weakness, headache, nausea, and vomiting occur frequently. Clients are diaphoretic and generally uncomfortable but usually remain alert.

These clients are acutely ill. Respirations are rapid and shallow, and hypoxemia (usually not severe) can result. Nasal flaring and grunting in response to hypoxemia can occur. There may be splinting of the lung on the affected side. Percussion will reveal dullness over the affected area. Rales, rhonchi, pleural friction rub, and egophony may also be present. The elevated temperature increases the client's metabolic rate, and tachycardia occurs.

Lobar consolidation is shown on x-ray (Figure 20–5). Laboratory studies usually reveal leukocytosis, respiratory alkalosis, mild hypoxemia, and an elevated erythrocyte

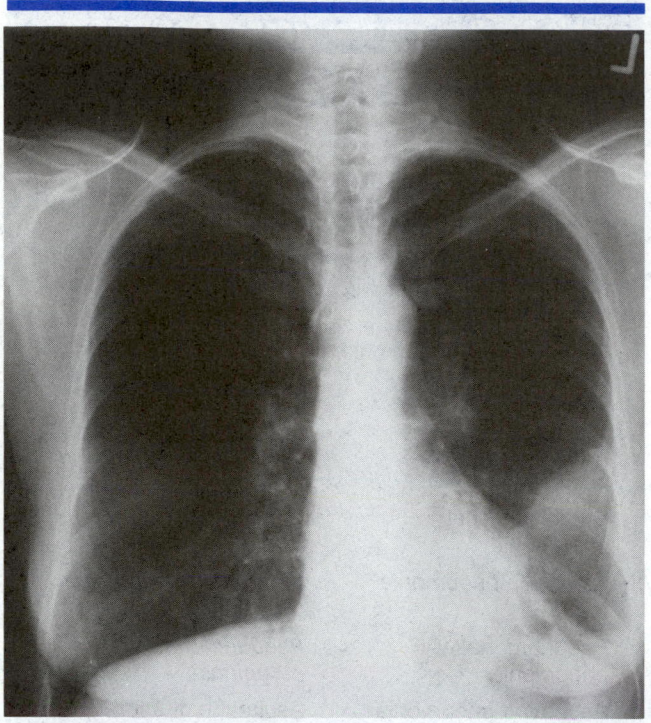

Figure 20–5

A female client with pneumonia. Chest x-ray shows large areas of consolidation in the left lower lobe. (Courtesy of Health Care Plan, Buffalo, NY)

sedimentation rate. Fewer than half may have a positive blood culture. If the medical management and treatment with antibiotics are unsuccessful, the organism can spread to other areas of the body causing meningitis, endocarditis, and joint inflammation. Complications within the lungs themselves can result in pleural effusions (fluid in the pleural space), atelectasis, lung abscess, and empyema.

In those who improve without antibiotic treatment, recovery usually begins between the seventh and fourteenth day (George, Light, & Matthay, 1983). With antibiotic treatment, uncomplicated pneumococcal pneumonia usually responds within 24 hours (Tuazon, 1980). The ultimate prognosis depends on the extent of involvement and the client's underlying condition. Older clients who have underlying debilitating conditions and involvement of more than one lobe have a high mortality rate because of the development of septicemia and septic shock.

Mycoplasmal Pneumonia

Mycoplasmal pneumonia, caused by *Mycoplasma pneumoniae,* is referred to as an "atypical" pneumonia, primarily to distinguish it from the more common bacterial pneumonias. The atypical pneumonias more closely resemble viral infections, but they usually respond to antibiotic therapy.

Mycoplasma pneumoniae is a common cause of pneumonia in children and young adults, but this pathogen is now recognized to be an important cause of pneumonia in all age groups (Murray & Tuazon, 1980). The organism is not highly contagious, and significant outbreaks usually stem from close interpersonal contact, as in schools or families.

The onset is gradual. The most common symptoms, developing over 3 to 4 days, are a low-grade fever, malaise, headache, sore throat, and a cough with minimum sputum production, which is often mucoid. As the illness progresses, earache, tracheal irritation, and chest pain commonly accompany the cough. Clients appear mildly to moderately ill. Tachypnea and tachycardia are not pronounced. Chest x-rays reveal areas of bronchopneumonia. The white blood count may or may not be elevated, depending on the severity of the infection. In most instances, this pneumonia is self-limiting, with recovery beginning in 10 to 14 days. Deaths are extremely rare.

Legionnaires' Disease

Legionnaires' disease is another type of pneumonia that conforms most closely to the atypical syndrome. The disease received national attention when an outbreak of severe respiratory illness was traced to the 1976 American Legion Convention in Philadelphia. The causative organism was later named *Legionella pneumophila,* a gram-negative bacterium (Mitchell & Petty, 1982).

Although all age groups can be affected, those over 50 are more susceptible. Males are more vulnerable than females, as are those who smoke, are on immunosuppressive therapy, or have an underlying chronic debilitating condition. The exact source of contamination with this organism is unknown, but large outbreaks have been traced to contaminated water and air conditioning systems and to soil at contaminated excavation sites (Devereux & Goldstein, 1980).

This organism can cause a range of symptoms, from a flulike illness to an overwhelming pneumonia. Initially, the general symptoms are weakness, malaise, nausea and vomiting, diarrhea, and headache. The cough is nonproductive but later can become productive of minimally purulent or nonpurulent sputum. As the illness progresses, fever rises to about 104°F (40°C), but is accompanied by bradycardia rather than tachycardia. Pulmonary symptoms and signs include dyspnea, rales, bronchial breath sounds, and dullness to percussion. The chest x-ray may show various forms of involvement. Pulmonary consolidation and pleural effusion can occur. Confusion marked by subtle changes in affect is common, as are involvement of the kidneys and liver (Devereux & Goldstein, 1980). The general course and prognosis depend on the underlying risk factors of clients and appropriate management of care. With the administration of the appropriate antibiotics, the death rate is between 5% and 10%, primarily from shock or respiratory failure (Cordes & Fraser, 1980).

Viral Pneumonia

The cause of viral pneumonia in adults is primarily the influenza virus, either Type A or Type B (Reichman & Dolin, 1980). Influenza pneumonia is more common in elderly clients who have underlying chronic debilitating disease. Clients appear acutely ill with a sudden onset of chills, malaise, anorexia, headache, and tearing, burning eyes. The cough produces bloody sputum. Belated bronchial involvement occurs, along with dyspnea and cyanosis. Individuals have a high fever accompanied by tachycardia. Again, the duration and outcome of this pneumonia depend on the underlying condition of the client and control of secondary bacterial infections.

Staphylococcal Pneumonia

Staphylococcal pneumonia is primarily a disease of hospitalized clients or clients with altered defense mechanisms. Because of new antibiotics, staphylococcal pneumonia is not as prevalent in hospitals as it once was. *Staphylococcus aureus* is normally present in the nose and skin of healthy individuals and can be spread by aerosol or direct contact. Debilitated adults whose resistance to infection is hampered are targets for the development of infections from this organism. The organism can also be spread hematogenously (via the bloodstream) from infected areas to the lungs in those with bacteremia, such as in endocarditis and infections from in-dwelling catheters. Intravenous drug abusers are also susceptible to developing staphylococcal pneumonia via the blood.

Staphylococcal infections of the lungs leading to pneumonia usually begin suddenly. The client is very ill, with chills, diaphoresis, and spiking temperatures. Dyspnea, pleural pain, hypoxemia, and a cough that produces yellow, blood-tinged sputum are present. Chest x-rays most commonly show patchy, rapidly spreading areas of bronchopneumonia. Tissue necrosis and abscess formation can occur. There is a moderately elevated white blood count, and positive blood cultures can occur. The destructive nature of this organism may lead to permanent lung damage in the form of fibrosis or bronchiectasis. Empyema and lung abscesses are other complications. The prognosis varies with the age and general condition of those affected (Hinshaw & Murray, 1980).

Klebsiella Pneumonia

Klebsiella pneumonia (also known as Friedländer's bacillus) produces an especially lethal form of pneumonia with a predilection for older men who are debilitated by some form of chronic illness, especially alcoholism. The onset is abrupt. Symptoms include marked respiratory distress, high fever, violent chills, pleuritic chest pain, and a cough producing copious amounts of thick grey–green or reddish brown sputum (often described as resembling currant jelly). Rales and rhonchi are present. Chest x-rays show dense lobar consolidation with infiltration. A high mortality is associated with this pneumonia (often called "the old man's friend") because of the overall debilitated condition of those most likely to contract it and because of the virulence of the organism (Hinshaw & Murray, 1980).

Pseudomonal Pneumonia

Pseudomonas aeruginosa is an important cause of hospital-acquired infections. Pneumonias caused by this organism usually result from aspiration of organisms indigenous to the upper respiratory tract or inhalation of the organism from contaminated nebulizers. Susceptible clients are debilitated and suffer from underlying chronic lung or heart disease or burns, are on steroids or antibiotics, or are intubated and on nebulizer breathing devices. Initial symptoms include an elevated temperature, chills, dyspnea, cyanosis, and a cough productive of copious amounts of foul smelling yellow or green sputum. Apprehension and confusion are also present. Chest x-rays reveal diffuse bronchopneumonia, which is often bilateral, involving several lobes. Abscesses and pleural effusions can develop. Leukocytosis, azotemia, and abnormal liver function tests are likely (Reyes, 1980). The treatment is long and the prognosis poor because of underlying debilitating disease and the lack of responsiveness of the organism to antibiotics (Hinshaw & Murray, 1980).

Aspiration Pneumonia

Aspiration pneumonia usually occurs in clients with impaired gag or swallowing reflexes. Several processes are associated with aspiration. A foreign substance may be aspirated that is large enough to obstruct the airway and cause asphyxiation. A chemical pneumonia can occur secondary to aspiration of gastric contents. Whenever the level of consciousness is depressed, the reflex response preventing aspiration diminishes (eg, postsurgical clients have a depressed cough and gag reflex). Others at risk are those with tracheostomies, elderly and chronically ill bedridden clients, those with nasogastric feeding tubes, and those on antidepressant drugs or under the influence of alcohol. The pH of the aspirated liquid determines the severity of the resulting damage to the lungs. If the pH is above 2.4, the effects are comparable to the aspiration of the same amount of saline. A pH below 2.4 will cause an intense inflammatory response (Fishman, 1980). The presence or absence of food or bacteria also plays a part in the pathophysiology of aspiration pneumonia. Plain aspirated hydrochloric acid spreads rapidly throughout the lungs. Damage to pulmonary tissues occurs quickly, resulting in diffuse hemorrhage and pulmonary edema (Johanson & Harris, 1980). Massive inhalation of gastric contents can lead to respiratory failure. Infection may complicate either type of aspiration pneumonia.

Aspiration pneumonia can be caused by the aspiration of bacteria from the upper respiratory tract. The organ-

Table 20–3	Pharmacological Management of Pneumonia
Types of Pneumonia	**Usual Antibiotic(s) of Choice**
Pneumococcal pneumonia	Penicillin G or erythromycin
Mycoplasmal pneumonia	Erythromycin or tetracycline
Legionnaires' disease	Erythromycin
Viral pneumonia	Amantadine for prophylaxis (antibiotics useless for a virus)
Staphylococcal pneumonia	Nafcillin, oxacillin, cephalothin, amikacin
Klebsiella pneumonia	Gentamicin or tobramycin with or without cephalothin
Pseudomonal pneumonia	Tobramycin, gentamicin, or amikacin
Aspiration pneumonia	Penicillin G, or nafcillin if client acquires staphylococci while in the hospital

isms most frequently involved are *Bacteroides melaninogenicus,* streptococci, and fusobacteria, which are all anaerobic pathogens. In hospitalized clients, *Pseudomonas aeruginosa, Escherichia coli,* and *Enterobacter cloacae* are common pathogens (Gracey, 1981). The same factors that predispose persons to the aspiration of gastric contents can lead to the aspiration of bacteria.

Anaerobic pulmonary infections usually begin as a pneumonitis characterized by alveolar filling with edema and inflammatory cells. The right upper lobe and the apical segments of the lower lobes are most commonly involved because when the client is supine, the organism has easiest access to these areas. Simple uncomplicated pneumonitis is rather mild. Foul-smelling sputum is absent. Acute disease responds well to treatment with antibiotics. If untreated, pneumonitis may progress to a necrotizing pneumonia or lung abscess consisting of consolidation and cavitation of the lung tissue (Johanson & Harris, 1980).

Therapeutic Measures

The treatment of the bacterial pneumonias centers around selecting the antibiotic or antibiotics to which the infecting organism is most sensitive. Table 20–3 lists the usual antibiotics of choice for the various pneumonias. Most viral pneumonias have no specific therapy. Amantadine has had limited success in the treatment of one specific influenza strain. Polyvalent pneumococcal vaccine can be used to prevent the development of pneumococcal pneumonia, providing protection for at least 3 years against 14 serotypes causing 75% of this type of pneumonia (Mitchell & Petty, 1982).

Antipyretics and analgesics such as acetylsalicylic acid (aspirin) or acetaminophen may be given. Narcotics may be required if chest pain is severe. Codeine is most frequently given. Expectorants are given to reduce the viscosity of pulmonary secretions; examples are terpin hydrate orally or acetylcysteine (Mucomyst) by nebulization. Antitussives may be ordered to treat nonproductive coughs.

Clients are frequently placed on bed rest because of the debilitating nature of pneumonia. Hospitalization may also be required. IPPB along with other pulmonary hygiene measures such as postural drainage may be ordered. Supplemental oxygen may be required if arterial oxygen levels become too low. Hospitalized clients may receive intravenous fluids as well as oral fluids to replace fluid loss caused by an elevated temperature, increased cellular metabolism, tachypnea, and diaphoresis. Electrolytes may also need to be replaced. Between 3 and 4 L of fluid per day are required unless contraindicated. A high-calorie, high-protein diet is ordered to help the body fight the infection. If the client is unable to eat, nasogastric feedings or hyperalimentation may be ordered. If respiratory failure occurs, intubation and placement on a mechanical ventilator are required. Depending on the infectious agent, clients may have to be placed in respiratory isolation. If a pleural effusion develops, a thoracentesis may be performed.

Specific Nursing Measures

Although the symptomatology of pneumonias varies, the overall nursing care is similar. Since bed rest is frequently needed during the acute phase of pneumonia, nursing care for hospitalized clients should be organized to allow periods of uninterrupted rest combined with turning, coughing, and deep breathing at least every 2 hours. Postural drainage measures may also be needed. If clients are not able to cough up secretions effectively, tracheal suctioning may be required.

Careful monitoring and assessment of respirations identifies any improvement or deterioration in the client's condition. Remain alert to the complications pneumonia can cause in the lungs such as pleurisy, pleural effusion, empyema, lung abscess, and pulmonary edema (which may lead to respiratory failure). Monitoring for systemic complications (septicemia, septic shock, meningitis, endocarditis, and renal and liver involvement) is also important so they can be recognized and treated early (Burrell & Burrell, 1982).

Since sputum specimens play such an important part in identifying the causative organism, efforts should be made to collect an adequate sputum sample and not saliva (see Chapter 18). Tracheal suctioning may be required for clients who cannot cough effectively. If the client has an elevated temperature and is diaphoretic, tepid baths along with frequent changes of bed linen are needed as comfort measures and to prevent chilling.

Keeping the client hydrated is important to loosen secretions so they can be more easily expectorated and to prevent dehydration. Fluid intake should be closely monitored, and set amounts should be given for each shift. Urinary output is a good indicator of hydration. If clients can eat, good mouth care may help to improve the appetite.

Preventing cross-infection is important. Clients should cover the nose and mouth when they cough and dispose of tissues in a paper bag. Strict hand-washing by staff, clients, and families will help to reduce the spread of bacteria.

Clients who are acutely ill with pneumonia may suffer from fears or anxiety related to respiratory impairment caused by the infection. This is especially true if the pneumonia is superimposed on another illness such as chronic lung disorders. Symptoms such as shortness of breath, expectoration of blood-streaked sputum, and chest pain can arouse undue anxiety for both client and family. Take time to answer questions and explain procedures. If clients are bothered by chest pain, analgesics may be needed. If narcotic analgesics are ordered however, it is important to observe the client for signs of respiratory depression. Splinting the chest during coughing and deep breathing exercises will help to reduce chest pain (Figure 20–6). Family members should be taught to do this, keeping the fingers together to apply firm support.

Discharge planning involves reviewing medications, their actions, and side effects with client and family. Clients should understand how to avoid overfatigue by increasing activities gradually. Clients with an underlying chronic debilitating condition should be made aware of their increased susceptibility to respiratory tract infections and should know the techniques of avoiding infections that may lead to further pneumonia (eg, sufficient rest, well-balanced diet, avoiding people with colds, and not getting chilled). Clients should be told to contact their physician if they develop a cough, notice a change in the color or amount of sputum they normally produce, or suffer any shortness of breath. Cigarette smokers should be made aware of their higher risk and told that the American Lung Association or the American Cancer Society has information on how they can stop smoking. Alcohol abusers should also know their risks and should be told about Alcoholics Anonymous or other treatment programs for alcoholism. Offering to get them information about these organizations is important. If these measures are not at least attempted, the chances of the recurrence of pneumonia are greater (Ryan, 1982).

Specific nursing measures should be employed to prevent aspiration and hence, aspiration pneumonia. Semicomatose or comatose clients should be placed on their side with the foot of the bed elevated 6 to 9 in unless contraindicated. Support the client with pillows behind the back, between the knees, and in front of the chest. The client should be turned q. 2h. to prevent formation of decu-

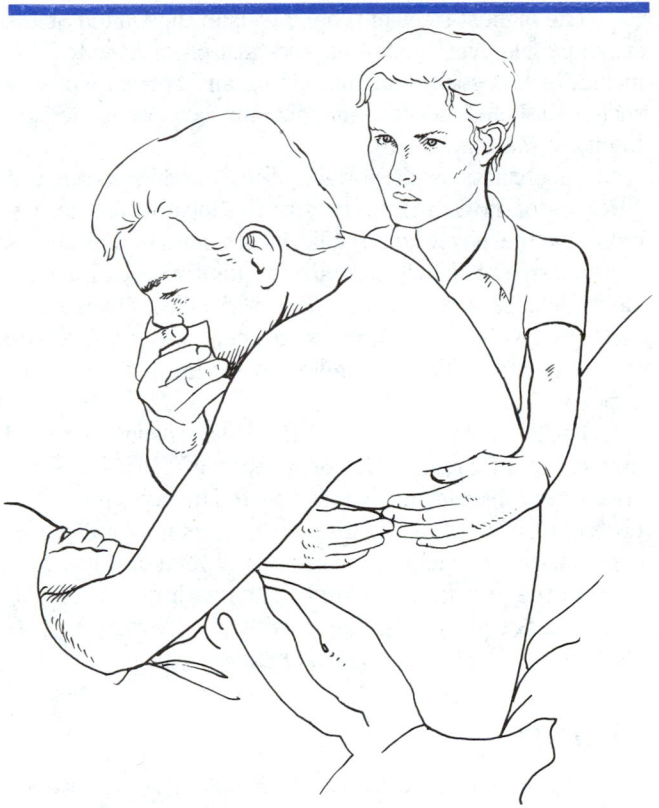

Figure 20–6

Splinting a painful area of the chest during coughing.

biti. The head of the bed should be elevated at least 30° during feeding and for 1 hour after completion of the feeding. Gag and cough reflexes should be checked before feeding. Before administering a nasogastric feeding, check for proper placement of the tube in the stomach. Aspirate for stomach contents, and if 100 mL or more is withdrawn, hold the feeding and consult with the physician. Administer the tube feeding slowly over 20 minutes and remain with the client. If the tube feeding is continuous, keep the head of the bed elevated. Frequent mouth care and the removal of secretions that accumulate in the back of the throat will help to prevent the aspiration of organisms into the lower respiratory tract (Ryan, 1982).

TUBERCULOSIS

Tuberculosis (TBC), an infectious disease caused by *Mycobacterium tuberculosis,* is not the dreaded disease it once was. The improvements in public health and sanitation and the development of effective antituberculosis drugs starting during the 1950s resulted in a progressive decline in the incidence of tuberculosis in the United States until 1979. The influx of Indochinese refugees into North America in recent years has contributed to a small increase in new cases of TBC (Petersdorf, 1983). Worldwide, tuberculosis remains the most prevalent infectious disease.

The highest rates of tuberculosis in the United States are in people over age 50. Factors that predispose to TBC include a low socioeconomic status and certain illnesses such as diabetes mellitus, silicosis, and alcoholism (George, Light, & Matthay, 1983).

Tuberculosis is a reportable disease, which means that all cases of TBC are reported to the local health department by the physician. Public health nurses and nurses working in ambulatory care are frequently responsible for identifying contacts of the client with TBC. These contacts receive skin testing and a chest x-ray if the skin test is positive. They are followed for up to a year after exposure.

Bacillus Calmette–Guerin (BCG) vaccinations are used in many other countries for prevention of TBC. BCG vaccination involves giving live, attenuated mycobacteria. The protection from BCG is neither permanent nor predictable; wide variations in efficacy have been reported. It has been used in the past in the United States with groups continuously exposed to TBC (eg, health care workers). BCG has also been used in cancer immunotherapy.

Etiology

Mycobacterium tuberculosis is a nonmotile, acid-fast, weakly gram-positive, aerobic bacillus. The organism is transmitted by inhaling invisible infective particles (droplet nuclei) produced when an infected person speaks, coughs, laughs, or sneezes. Only droplet nuclei 1 to 5 μm (.001 to .005 mm) can be inhaled into the terminal bronchioles and alveoli to cause infection (Glassroth, 1981). Larger infected inhaled particles are removed by the mucociliary action of the respiratory airways. Bacteria that land on furniture or other surfaces are not contagious, since they can no longer be inhaled and are usually quickly killed by the ultraviolet rays of sunlight or by drying. Tuberculosis is not highly contagious; transmission generally requires close, frequent, or prolonged contact with the infected individual. Infected cattle have been eliminated as a source of contagion by pasteurizing milk and slaughtering infected animals.

When infected droplet nuclei are inhaled into the alveoli of a susceptible adult, tubercle bacilli begin to multiply slowly. A small area of bronchopneumonia develops at the site, known as the primary focus (or primary disease). In spite of the body's reaction to phagocytize the invading organism, there is little or no resistance to the multiplication of the bacilli. As a result, bacilli are disseminated from the primary site, primarily by the lymphatics with extensive involvement of the regional (hilar) lymph nodes (Figure 20–7). The primary peripheral lesion in the lung and the associated enlarged draining lymph nodes form what is called the Ghon complex. From the lymphatics, the organism drains into the systemic circulation, potentially spreading the bacilli to all the organs and tissues of the body. Other portions of the lung tissue may also be reseeded.

The infected individual is, in most cases, asympto-

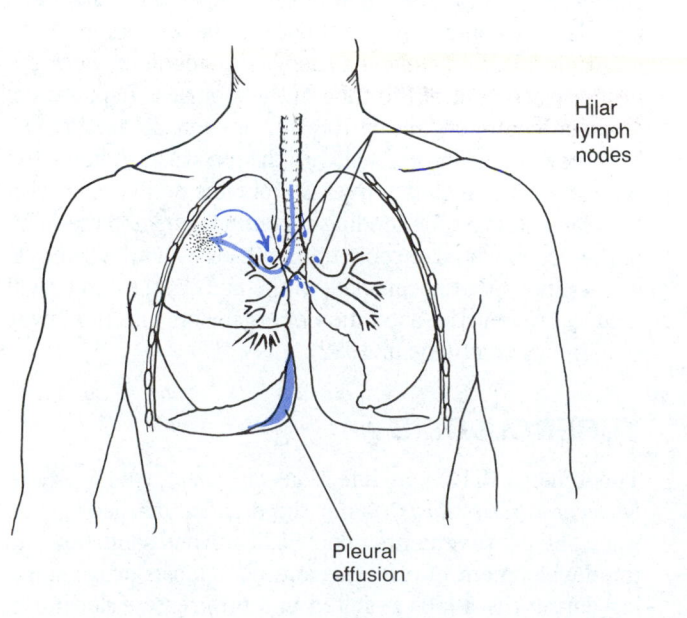

A

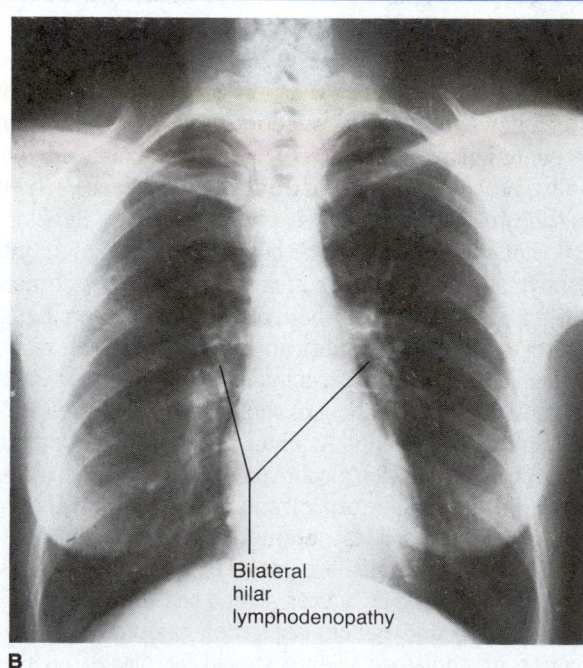

B

Figure 20–7

Hilar lymph node involvement in TBC. **A.** Anatomic relationship of the hilar lymph nodes to the pulmonary structures. **B.** Chest x-ray of a female client with bilateral hilar lymphadenopathy. (X-ray courtesy of Health Care Plan, Buffalo, NY)

Box 20–2   Diagnostic Standards and Classification of Tuberculosis

0. No tuberculosis exposure: Not infected (no history of exposure, reaction to tuberculin skin test not significant).

1. Tuberculosis exposure: No evidence of infection (history of exposure, reaction to tuberculin skin test not significant).

2. Tuberculous infection: No disease (significant reaction to tuberculin skin test, negative bacteriologic studies [if done], no clinical and/or roentgenographic evidence of tuberculosis).
   Chemotherapy status (preventive)
     None
     On chemotherapy since (date)
     Chemotherapy terminated (date)
       Complete (prescribed course of therapy)
       Incomplete

3. Tuberculosis: Current disease (*M Tuberculosis* cultured [if done], otherwise *both* a significant reaction to tuberculin skin test *and* clinical and/or roentgenographic evidence of current disease).
   Location of disease
     Pulmonary
     Pleural
     Lymphatic
     Bone and/or joint
     Genitourinary
     Disseminated (miliary)
     Meningeal
     Peritoneal
     Other
   The predominant site shall be listed. Other sites may also be listed. Anatomic sites may be specified more precisely.
   Bacteriologic status
     Positive by
       Microscopy only (date)

       Culture only (date)
       Microscopy and culture (date)
     Negative (date)
     Not done
   Chemotherapy status
     On chemotherapy since (date)
     Chemotherapy terminated, incomplete (date)
   The following data are necessary in certain circumstances:
     Roentgenogram findings
       Normal
       Abnormal
         Cavitary or noncavitary
         Stable or worsening or improving
     Tuberculin skin test reaction
       Significant
       Not significant

4. Tuberculosis: No current disease (history of previous episode(s) of tuberculosis, or abnormal stable roentgenographic findings in a person with a significant reaction to tuberculin skin test, negative bacteriologic studies [if done], no clinical and/or roentgenographic evidence of current disease).
   Chemotherapy status
     None
     On chemotherapy since (date)
     Chemotherapy terminated (date)
       Complete
       Incomplete

5. Tuberculosis suspect (diagnosis pending)
   Chemotherapy status
     None
     On chemotherapy since (date)

SOURCE: Penn R, George RB: Respiratory infections. In: *Chest Medicine.* George RB, Light RW, Matthay RA (editors). New York: Churchill Livingstone, 1983, p 447.

Adapted with permission from American Thoracic Society: Diagnostic standards and classification of tuberculosis and other mycobacterial diseases. *Am Rev Respir Dis* 123(3):357–358, 1981.

matic at this time. Infection with *Mycobacterium tuberculosis* does not necessarily mean developing active TBC. (See Box 20–2 for the diagnostic standards and classification of TBC and other mycobacterial diseases.) Rarely, hematogenous spread of the organism results in meningitis or acute miliary tuberculosis (massive dissemination of tubercle bacilli throughout the body via the bloodstream). In most cases, after a few days or weeks the multiplication of the virulent tubercle bacilli markedly decreases, the pneumonic process resolves, and there is no further spread of the bacilli by the lymphatics or blood.

This pattern is the same in any other organs infected with tubercle bacilli. The body's defenses can effectively contain the organisms. Macrophages engulf the bacilli, forming clusters of cells that give rise to the granuloma, the characteristic lesion of TBC. This reaction usually occurs over 4 to 10 weeks and results in reactivity to the tuberculin skin test. A relative immunity to exogenous reinfec-

tion (reinfection from another active case) by the tubercle bacilli also appears to develop.

In most adults, the healed granulomas remain stable and may calcify. While some of the bacilli are destroyed as the lesions heal, a significant number of bacilli become dormant. Thus, a person infected with the bacilli but not treated with antimicrobial drugs may develop tuberculosis in the future.

The full-blown disease may never develop; if it does, it may develop weeks or many years after the initial infection. For the first 1 or 2 years after infection, the risk of developing TBC for the newly infected individual is about 4% (Glassroth, 1981). The likelihood of developing the disease diminishes as the time from infection lengthens.

In approximately 5% to 15% of individuals infected with TBC, one of the granulomas in the lung or elsewhere breaks down, the tubercle bacilli multiply, and the individual becomes ill with tuberculosis (Glassroth, 1981). The adult can also become reinfected through contact with a host who has active TBC. Because the organism requires oxygen to grow, the apices of the lungs where the concentrations of oxygen are highest, are favored. The initial lesion of reinfection or reactivation is characterized by a localized necrosis. The necrosis is due to the destructive nature of the inflammatory reaction in an adult previously sensitized to the organism. The lesion is localized because acquired cellular immunity is operating in adjacent tissue and the lymphatic system. Dissemination of the tubercle bacilli by the lymphatics to other organs and tissues does not occur as readily with reinfection as with the initial infection. Caseation necrosis (resembling cheese) can spread to adjacent tissue with progression of the inflammatory process. The infection may spread when a bronchus or a blood vessel is eroded by infectious material. This caseous material may be expectorated, leaving a cavity or hole in the lung tissue. Large numbers of bacilli are contained in this material, and it is highly infectious.

The reasons why a person develops active TBC are not clearly understood. Certain factors such as aging, degenerative diseases, malnutrition, diabetes mellitus, silicosis, chronic obstructive pulmonary disease (COPD), and immunosuppressive therapy, all of which lower resistance to infection, promote the development of TBC.

Clinical Manifestations

Tuberculosis of the lung most often develops as a chronic illness, and symptoms appear over weeks or months. Symptoms can include anorexia, weight loss, fatigue, a low-grade fever that usually occurs in the afternoon, irregular menses in women, and night sweats. A cough occurs, which progressively becomes productive of mucoid or sometimes mucopurulent sputum. There may be chest pain or a feeling of tightness in the chest. Caseous material may erode into the pleural space, causing a pleural effusion, which is painful (see Figure 20–6). Hemoptysis occurs and is often the reason the client seeks health care.

A history of possible exposure to TBC is important, but the exposure could have occurred years before, and the client may not even have been aware of it. Making the diagnosis is crucial not only for treatment of the infected individual but also to reduce spread of the disease. Contacts must be screened because they may have become infected with the bacilli and may require treatment to prevent TBC.

A positive Mantoux intradermal skin test (Chapter 18) or a positive tine test may confirm the diagnosis of infection with *Mycobacterium tuberculosis,* but false positive (and false negative) tests occur. The chest x-ray can show active or calcified lesions. The Ghon complex and characteristic cavity in the lung tissue can be seen on x-ray. The problem with making a definitive diagnosis with a chest x-ray is that other diseases of the lungs (pneumonia or malignant tumors) can look like TBC.

A definitive diagnosis of TBC can only be made when *M tuberculosis* is cultured from secretions or tissues. In TBC of the lung, sputum samples are obtained for smear and culture. In the sputum smear, specimens are stained by the Ziehl–Neelsen technique for acid-fast organisms. Smears can also be quickly screened by low-power microscopy using the fluorochrome technique. The smear will be positive only if the bacilli are numerous. A positive smear is therefore important in identifying highly infectious cases.

A culture and sensitivity report takes more time because of the slow growth of the bacilli. A culture and sensitivity report may take over 8 weeks. A culture can detect smaller numbers of bacilli and permit a positive identification of tuberculosis. Sensitivity to antibiotics can be determined at the same time.

Therapeutic Measures

Ten drugs currently available in the United States have been approved for the treatment of tuberculosis. These drugs are divided into three categories: primary, secondary, and tertiary (Table 20–4). The primary drugs, isoniazid and rifampin, are highly effective, especially if used together, and the frequency of toxicity is relatively low.

The secondary drugs are not as effective and have more toxic side effects. They are usually used in combination with one or both of the primary drugs. Since the organism can develop resistance to any single drug, combining two or three drugs helps to maintain drug effectiveness. Recent studies have shown that combining isoniazid with rifampin has a more rapid effect in the treatment of tuberculosis than the usual standardized treatment of combining isoniazid, ethambutol, and streptomycin (Traver, 1982).

The tertiary medications are not as effective as the primary or secondary drugs and have greater toxic side effects. They are introduced when drug resistance develops to a medication in the other two groups.

In individuals who are being treated for TBC for a second time, different drugs should be used than were used for the previous treatment. Response to medication therapy is fairly rapid, and individuals become noninfectious within a period of weeks. To prevent the recurrence of active disease, drug therapy is continued for 18 months to 2 years. The drug regimen of isoniazid with rifampin may take only about 9 months. (Ethambutol may be combined with these two drugs for the first 2 months.) This short-course therapy is usually used in the treatment of initial cases of TBC and is not used in retreatment protocols or in clients with other medical problems.

Another drug treatment regimen found effective is intermittent therapy. The treatment consists of daily drug therapy for the first 1 to 4 months, followed by twice weekly therapy with larger doses of the drug for an additional 8 to 24 months. This form of treatment has been beneficial for clients who find it difficult to comply with the more standard

Table 20–4 Pharmacological Management of Tuberculosis

Drug	Dosage	Adverse Side Effects
Primary (highly effective, rarely toxic)		
Isoniazid (INH)	5 mg/kg/day (300–400 mg)	Hepatotoxic; inhibits phenytoin metabolism leading to ↑ blood levels and toxicity; peripheral neuropathy
Rifampin	450–600 mg q.d.	Hepatotoxic; when used with INH, ↑ incidence of liver damage; accelerates catabolism of quinidine, warfarin, corticosteroids, and oral contraceptives
Secondary (less effective, may have more toxic side effects, usually used in combination with one or both primary drugs)		
Ethambutol	15 mg/kg	Optic neuritis
Para-aminosalicylic acid (PAS)	8–12 g/day	GI disturbance
Streptomycin	1 g/day IM for 60 days	Ototoxic (CN VIII); paresthesia; rash; fever; nephrotoxic
Pyrazinamide	20–35 mg/kg (but no more than 3 g/day)	Hepatotoxic; urate retention leading to gout
Tertiary (usually used only when resistance develops to previous drugs)		
Capreomycin	1 g/day IM	Nephrotoxic; ototoxic
Cycloserine	500 mg to 1 g/day in divided doses	Personality changes; convulsions; rash
Ethionamide	500 mg to 1 g/day in divided doses	GI disturbance; peripheral neuritis; hepatotoxic
Kanamycin	15 mg/kg/day IM in two equally divided doses 12 h apart	Ototoxic; nephrotoxic

daily dose therapy. Increased side effects are more common with this therapy because of the increased dosages of the drugs administered.

Isoniazid has also been used alone for 12 months to prevent clinical symptoms in certain individuals with dormant TBC who show a positive skin test, such as household contacts.

Monitoring of clients is required during the course of drug therapy. This monitoring involves sputum smears and cultures, which usually will be negative after 2 months of therapy. If the smears remain positive, a new treatment regimen must be started. Change in the client's symptoms and chest x-rays will also show how well the client is progressing with treatment. Once an adequate course of therapy has been completed, clients can be discharged from further supervision.

Since the advent of effective chemotherapy against TBC, surgical intervention such as thoracoplasty or resection is rare.

Specific Nursing Measures

Although TBC can be cured, many clients are fearful when the diagnosis is made. Feelings of shame may also be present because of the association of the illness with poverty and overcrowding. It is therefore important that the nurse explain what TBC is, how it is transmitted, and that it can be cured. Nursing staff may also react with fear toward the client with tuberculosis, leaving the client isolated and often ignored. All staff need a proper understanding of the disease.

If clients require hospitalization, they are routinely placed in isolation. The only isolation measures necessary are careful handling and disposal of secretions and the avoidance of direct face-to-face contact. Tissues contaminated with sputum should be discarded in a paper bag and burned. The client's room should be properly ventilated with nonrecirculating air. Laminar flow or ultraviolet lighting will accomplish the same purpose as nonrecirculating ventilation. Masks are not routinely required for persons who come in contact with the client or for clients themselves. Clients should cover the nose and mouth when they cough or sneeze. Clients who are very ill and unable to cover their mouths when they cough should be masked when direct care is given. The mask must be capable of filtering out the small droplet nuclei. No other isolation measures, such as gowning or wearing gloves, are necessary. Within 2 weeks after chemotherapy is begun, the possibility of transmitting the disease is markedly reduced.

Since strict adherence to the medication schedule is required if tuberculosis is to be cured, make certain that clients understand and accept the importance of following the medication schedule. Both clients and family members must give this aspect of care precedence over other needs. The family and significant others can assist in the therapeutic regimen by checking on and supporting client compliance with the medication schedule (Spires, 1980). Even after the client is discharged from the hospital, many more months of medication therapy are required. The medications are provided by the county health department, and clients must not let their medications run out.

The importance of follow-up must be stressed, not only so progress can be monitored but also to check for possible side effects from the antituberculosis medications and to make sure drug resistance has not developed. Clients should be instructed to see a physician immediately if symptoms of TBC recur or if they develop any side effects from the medication they are taking. Side effects of the common TBC drugs are listed in Table 20–4. The responsibility for client care and education falls not only on hospital nurses but on public health nurses who must continue to monitor both clients with tuberculosis and their contacts (Traver, 1982).

NONTUBERCULOUS MYCOBACTERIAL DISEASE

Since the discovery of the tubercle bacillus, many other strains of mycobacteria have been identified. Not all of these organisms cause disease in humans. The two other most common species of mycobacteria affecting humans are *M avium intracellulare,* and *M kansasii.*

Clinical Manifestations

The pathophysiology of diseases caused by these organisms is similar to illnesses caused by *M tuberculosis.* As in TBC, any organ of the body can be affected; the most common is the lung. Because these organisms are less virulent however, the disease progresses slower, and the symptoms are not as readily manifested.

The disease caused by *M kansasii* is more common in males than females. Individuals of any age can be affected; however, some underlying lung disease (such as fibrosis or COPD) is common. Beginning symptoms are mild, consisting of a productive cough, dyspnea, fever, chills, and sometimes hemoptysis. X-rays commonly show bilateral lung involvement. Without treatment, the condition will progress, sometimes destroying an entire lung.

The disease caused by *M avium intracellulare* is most common in rural areas at low altitude with high humidity and soil with a high organic content. The predisposing conditions mentioned under *M kansasii* hold true for this organism as well. The disease course can be benign or it can be progressive, destroying an entire lung.

These diseases do not have to be reported to the health department because direct transmission from person to person has not been documented.

Therapeutic Measures

A combination of rifampin, isoniazid, and ethambutol is administered to treat *M kansasii* infection until sputum cultures have been negative for 1 year. A two-drug combination is continued for an additional year.

Strains of *M avium intracellulare* are usually highly resistant to antituberculosis medications. If the client is clinically ill, as many as six antituberculosis medications may be administered at one time until the sputum cultures are negative for at least 1 year. Three or four drugs are given for an additional year. A major drawback in this type of therapy is the development of drug toxicity or failure of the treatment to have any appreciable effect on the organism.

The benefits and risks of drug treatment for *M avium intracellulare* infections must be carefully weighed because of the high incidence of drug toxicity. If the disease does not seem to be worsening, drug therapy may be omitted or delayed. If drug therapy is indicated, hospitalization is initially required so clients can be closely monitored for side effects.

In clients with *M avium intracellulare,* surgical resection of the lung is sometimes the treatment of choice for those judged able to tolerate the procedure. This choice is made because of the side effects and questionable sensitivity of the organism to medication therapy.

Specific Nursing Measures

Client education is the primary concern of nursing management. Clients and families need to understand the illness and the treatment. Follow-up care is stressed so sputum cultures, progression of the disease, and signs and symptoms of drug toxicity can be monitored.

LUNG ABSCESS

A *lung abscess* is a circumscribed suppurative area of inflamed and infected lung parenchyma associated with central tissue necrosis. Communication with the bronchial tree results in the eventual expectoration of purulent material (Burrell & Burrell, 1982). Lung abscesses are not as common today as they once were because of the effective treatment of pneumonia with antibiotics. Also, improved management of clients during and after surgery has reduced the incidence of aspiration pneumonia (Hinshaw & Murray, 1980).

Etiology

Single lung abscesses usually result from an inflammatory response to a bronchial obstruction or aspiration. The aspiration of foreign material such as food, gastric contents, or blood can lead to obstruction. Benign or malignant tumors or large amounts of thick, sticky secretions can obstruct an airway. Pneumonia, although not as common a cause of lung abscess formation, still may be a causative factor in some cases.

The organisms most frequently responsible for lung abscess formation are *Staphylococcus aureus, Klebsiella pneumoniae,* some strains of mycobacteria, the bacteroides, certain funguses, and parasites such as the lung fluke. Multiple lung abscesses can result from the hematogenous spread of organisms to the lungs or from septic emboli. Immunosuppressive therapy is a predisposing factor in the development of lung abscesses (Mitchell & Petty, 1982).

Clinical Manifestations

The symptomatology of a lung abscess depends on the etiology. The most common symptoms include fever, chills, malaise, anorexia, cough, and pleuritic chest pain. When the abscess ruptures into a bronchus, the cough is productive of copious amounts of purulent sputum, which may be foul smelling and bloody. Leukocytosis is frequently present. Cavitary lesions (holes) that result from abscess formation are visible on chest x-rays. The prognosis of lung abscess, if not complicated by an underlying malignancy or other progressive lung disease, is generally good if the organisms responsible are treated with antibiotic therapy.

Therapeutic Measures

Specific antibiotics to treat a lung abscess or abscesses depend on the causative organism identified. Some of the more frequently used medications are penicillin G, 2 to 6 million units IV daily, or penicillin G procaine IM for milder cases. For those clients who are allergic to penicillin, clindamycin, lincomycin, or erythromycin may be used. Sometimes streptomycin or tetracycline may be added (Mitchell & Petty, 1982). Antibiotics are usually given for at least 6 weeks.

Bronchoscopy is indicated for removal of foreign matter that may be blocking a bronchus or to obtain a specimen for diagnostic purposes. Pulmonary hygiene measures such as postural drainage and suctioning may be ordered. Surgical drainage of an abscess by means of a thoracotomy is rarely performed today but may be done if the abscess will not clear using antibiotic therapy.

Specific Nursing Measures

Nursing measures for clients with lung abscess include coughing and deep breathing exercises, tracheal suctioning, and postural drainage. Client and family teaching cen-

ters around explaining the disease process and the treatment modalities.

Preventing semiconscious (postsurgical, sedated, or semicomatose) clients from aspirating has markedly decreased the incidence of lung abscess. Good oral hygiene in clients semiconscious for more than a few hours is important because bacterial growth in the oral cavity can, through aspiration, lead to lung abscess formation.

EMPYEMA

Empyema is the accumulation of pus in the pleural space or a purulent pleural effusion. The use of antibiotics in the treatment of lung infections has greatly reduced the occurrence of empyema.

The most common cause of empyema is extension of a pulmonary infection from the lung. Less often, empyema is a complication of a penetrating chest wound or thoracic surgery. Anaerobic bacteria are the most common organisms isolated from empyema fluid. Aerobic organisms most frequently involved are *Staphylococcus aureus* and enteric gram-negative rods. Infections can be from a mixture of anaerobic and aerobic organisms (George, Light, & Matthay, 1983).

Clinical Manifestations

Empyema may involve the whole pleural space, or it can be localized. Fibrinous adhesions between the lung and the chest wall can develop as part of the inflammatory process. Common symptoms include fever, pleuritic chest pain, dyspnea, and anorexia. Breath sounds are absent over the affected area, and there is dullness to percussion. There may be a productive cough; blood-stained sputum can result from the development of a bronchopleural fistula. If not treated, pleural fibrosis can cause chest wall deformity. The movement of the chest on the affected side becomes restricted, and the ribs become flattened and crowded. A fibrothorax or trapped lung can result, in which the lung adheres to the chest wall. Chest x-rays show a dense opacity over the affected area, which may or may not be localized by adhesions. The prognosis for individuals with empyema is good if it is properly and promptly treated with antibiotics and/or surgery.

Therapeutic Measures

Antibiotics are selected on the basis of Gram's stain and culture and sensitivity reports. Surgery is also usually required. A thoracentesis is usually performed to make a definitive diagnosis. A chest tube is then inserted to drain the infection from the pleural space. Repeated needle aspirations may be performed in lieu of chest tube insertion.

If treatment is started too late or chest tube drainage is not able to remove thick purulent drainage, an open thoracotomy with rib resection may be required. A fibrothorax or trapped lung may necessitate removal of the thickened pleura by decortication. Although rare, a thoracoplasty may be required to close a persistent empyema space.

Specific Nursing Measures

The nursing management of clients with empyema is the same as the preoperative and postoperative nursing care of clients undergoing chest surgery and the care of clients with chest tubes (Chapters 18 and 21).

FUNGAL INFECTIONS

Fungal infections of the lungs generally are the result of infectious spores that are inhaled into the distal air spaces, multiply, and cause an inflammatory response. The fungi that cause diseases in humans are nonmotile yeasts or molds. The infection can spread from the lungs to other organs, including the skin, bones, and the central nervous system. Many fungi can cause respiratory diseases, all of which have similar pathological findings, symptomatology, and treatment. Coccidioidomycosis, histoplasmosis, and blastomycosis are three of the most common fungal infections.

Coccidioidomycosis

Coccidioidomycosis, caused by *Coccidioides immitis,* is a common deep mycosis in the United States, with more than 100,000 new cases reported each year (Bayer, 1981). The disease is also known as San Joaquin Valley fever, desert rheumatism, and "the bumps" (Einstein, 1981). Although coccidioidomycosis has been reported worldwide, it is endemic only in the Americas, especially the southwestern United States, including parts of New Mexico, Utah, California, Texas, and Arizona. The growth of the organism is supported by a semiarid hot climate with a short, intense rainy season. *Coccidioides* is called a dimorphic fungus because it occurs in two forms. In the soil, it takes the form of arthrospores and is infectious to humans; once in the tissues (and under special in vitro conditions), it assumes the form of endosporulating spherules (Bayer, 1981). The arthrospores are inhaled from spore-laden dust. Person-to-person transmission has not been documented because the organism does not grow in the lungs as arthrospores but as spherules.

Clinical Manifestations

Once the arthrospores are deposited in the lungs, they enter a vegetative cycle producing spherules and endospores. A granulomatous host reaction follows similar to that in TBC. This cell-mediated response in most cases limits the extent of the illness and gives lifelong immunity. Approximately 50% to 60% of those infected with coccidioidomycosis in this primary form are only subclinically

affected. The rest develop influenzalike symptoms 1 to 3 weeks after infection, including cough, fever, chest pain, headache, and fatigue. Symptoms of infection other than in the lungs include arthralgia, conjunctivitis, and erythema nodosum, a skin rash seen primarily on the lower legs of young women. Chest x-rays can show infiltrates that may occur in any part of the lungs, hilar adenopathy, pneumonia, and pleural effusions. Leukocytosis is present because of the inflammatory response. In most cases, the disease process is self-limiting, and complete clinical and x-ray resolution will occur within 6 to 8 weeks (Bayer, 1981).

Some clients develop a chronic progressive coccidioidal pneumonitis. These individuals often remain very ill, exhibiting symptoms such as persistent fever, prostration, productive cough, hemoptysis, and chest pain. The course is unpredictable but tends to depend on the underlying condition of the host and/or the use of immunosuppressive drugs. Chest x-ray lesions generally worsen, showing destruction of lung tissue, cavity formation, and fibronodular lesions (Bayer, 1981).

Dissemination of the disease to other parts of the body accounts for most of the morbidity and the mortality; however, dissemination occurs in only about 1% of clients. Dissemination is more common in nonwhites, diabetics, pregnant women, and individuals who are immunosuppressed by disease or drugs. The sites involved in order of frequency are the skin, bones and joints, meninges, lymph nodes, genitourinary tract, liver, and adrenal glands (Einstein, 1981). On chest x-ray, the lung may have a miliary appearance because of hematogenous spread. Symptomatology depends on the organs involved. The most serious complications are osteomyelitis and meningitis.

Therapeutic Measures

In the simple primary infection, no antibiotic is required, only symptomatic care. In progressive coccidioidal pulmonary disease and in disseminated coccidioidomycosis, the antibiotic amphotericin B, 0.5 to 0.7 mg/kg IV daily, is the treatment of choice. In osteomyelitis and meningitis, intravenous and local or intrathecal administration are advocated.

Miconazole, a less toxic antifungal agent, can also be given intravenously and intrathecally, but it is not the first agent of choice. Ketoconazole, a relatively new drug reported to have low toxicity, has shown promise for long-term oral treatment of nonmeningeal coccidioidomycosis.

Skin tests with either coccidioidin or spherulin will convert from negative to positive in 24 to 48 hours in primary pulmonary coccidioidomycosis. False positives and false negatives do occur.

Serologic tests are helpful in confirming the diagnosis. IgM antibodies are detected early; later IgG antibodies appear. Rising titers signify dissemination of the disease. Presence of IgG antibodies in cerebrospinal fluid is diagnostic of coccidioidal meningitis. Cultures of sputum, body fluids, pus, and tissue biopsy may demonstrate the fungus. Surgical resection may be required for cavities that cause severe and frequent hemorrhage or may spread the infection to the pleura (Mitchell & Petty, 1982).

Histoplasmosis

Histoplasmosis is caused by the dimorphic fungus *Histoplasma capsulatum.* Histoplasmosis is a worldwide infection. In the United States, it is more prevalent in the Mississippi and Ohio River valleys. The organism likes a temperate climate, and its growth is enhanced in soil that contains chicken, starling, or blackbird droppings, or bat guano. The fungi become airborne when the soil is disturbed and can be inhaled, leading to infection. Transmission from person to person does not occur.

Clinical Manifestations

Once the spores are implanted in the lungs, they mature and rupture, releasing yeast forms of the organism. These yeast forms are surrounded and engulfed by macrophages. The pathogenesis of this disease is similar to that of tuberculosis. Caseating granulomas form, and delayed hypersensitivity develops. Invariably, the organism invades the bloodstream, spreading to various organs, especially the liver and spleen. In most cases, the disease is brought under control by the body's defense mechanisms (Hinshaw & Murray, 1980). Histoplasmosis can be asymptomatic, acute, or chronic. Acute histoplasmosis is most common in infants and small children. Acute histoplasmosis in adults is most often a reinfection with a large number of fungi. Symptoms include fever, chills, malaise, dry cough, and muscle aches. Pulmonary infiltrates plus hilar and mediastinal lymphadenopathy are visible on x-ray. This form of histoplasmosis is usually self-limiting, with symptoms persisting for about a week. Lesions on the lung eventually calcify, leaving a so-called "buck shot" appearance (George et al., 1983). In some cases, a severe pneumonia results that is sometimes fatal.

Chronic histoplasmosis is most common in middle-aged or older white males who have a history of smoking and COPD. Symptoms that usually persist over several months include a low-grade fever, chronic cough, and weight loss. There is a progressive loss of lung tissue. X-rays reveal cavitary lesions and fibrosis along with obstructive airway disease.

Acute disseminated histoplasmosis is rare. Clients who are immunosuppressed and young children are more likely to develop this form of histoplasmosis.

Therapeutic Measures

No antifungal medication is required for the primary infection under most circumstances. Amphotericin B is indicated for chronic progressive pulmonary disease and for acute disseminated disease.

A histoplasmin skin test antigen is available to test for infection. Skin testing is of limited use because of the high rate of false positive and false negative results. Serologic tests can be done, but because they are often made positive by the histoplasmin skin test, blood should be drawn prior to the skin test. The organism can be better identified from cultures of sputum, blood, urine, and tissue biopsy. Surgery is rarely performed but may be done to resect compressing nodes (Mitchell & Petty, 1982).

Blastomycosis

Blastomycosis, caused by the fungus *Blastomyces dermatitidis,* is most common in the southeastern United States and in the Mississippi and Ohio River valleys. It also occurs in Canada, Mexico, and parts of South America and Africa. *Blastomyces* has been found in the soil and is acquired by inhaling the spores into the lungs.

Clinical Manifestations

Once spores are deposited in the lung, the inflammatory response occurs as with coccidioidomycosis and histoplasmosis. Subclinical and mild infections can occur with this disease, but more frequently clients present with a progressive pulmonary disorder often associated with dissemination. Symptoms include a cough, which is productive of purulent material and sometimes contains blood, a low-grade fever, weakness, and weight loss. Chest x-rays may show diffuse fibronodular infiltration, cavitations, bronchopneumonia, or miliary lesions. The pleura may be affected. The disease may be limited to one lobe or may involve all parts of both lungs. The most common area to be affected by dissemination is the skin, where lesions consist of granulomas surrounding small abscesses. The other two most common sites of spread are the bone and the male genitourinary system. The mortality rate for untreated progressive blastomycosis is high (Hinshaw & Murray, 1980).

Therapeutic Measures

Amphotericin B, IV is used in the treatment of progressive and disseminated disease. A drug that can be used for isolated cutaneous lesions is hydroxystilbamidine.

Skin tests and serologic studies are considered of little value because they can be negative even when the disease is present. A definitive diagnosis must be made by culturing the organism from sputum, tissues, or body fluids.

Surgical intervention is not indicated in the treatment of this disease but may be used to assist in the diagnosis by needle aspiration or open biopsy of a pulmonary lesion.

Specific Nursing Measures

Nursing care for clients with fungal diseases of the lungs centers around explaining the disease and treatment and monitoring potential side effects of drugs. Clients and their families may be apprehensive that the disease is contagious, so it is important to explain that person-to-person spread does not occur.

Since the primary drug used in the treatment of fungal infections, amphotericin B, can cause kidney damage and other serious side effects such as liver damage, severe chilling, and malaise, monitor the administration of this IV medication closely. Inquire about any effects experienced by the client, and note results of laboratory tests indicating impaired liver and renal function. The color and consistency of urine should also be observed and urinary output measured. The client's skin should be inspected in natural light to detect any jaundice.

Section III: Obstructive Disorders

Obstructive disorders of the respiratory system are lung diseases that cause a persistent obstruction of bronchial air flow. Different names have been applied to this group of diseases. The most common are chronic obstructive pulmonary disease (COPD) and chronic airway obstruction (CAO). Chronic bronchitis and emphysema are the most common diseases associated with COPD, but asthma, bronchiectasis, and cystic fibrosis are also included (Traver, 1982).

The prevalence of COPD and its death rate have increased to epidemic proportions in recent years. In 1976, 43,907 deaths were attributed to COPD. COPD affects males more frequently than females. Statistics on worker disability allowances under the Social Security Administration ranked COPD sixth among the most frequent disabilities for males and ninth for females (American Lung Association, 1983).

Besides losses in productivity, the cost of medical care for those with COPD is significant. A National Institutes of Health Task Force Report on Respiratory Disease estimated the direct costs of treatment for COPD are approximately $1 billion annually (American Lung Association, 1983).

Since these diseases are chronic and debilitating, nurses play a significant role in the long-term management and rehabilitation of clients with obstructive lung diseases. Nurses can also provide valuable support for clients and their families or significant others, who frequently become discouraged and depressed.

BRONCHIECTASIS

Bronchiectasis is a permanent abnormal dilatation of one or more large bronchi because of the destruction of the elastic and muscular components of the bronchial wall (Hinshaw & Murray, 1980). In the past, bronchiectasis was considered a disease of children, and few individuals lived beyond their third or fourth decade. Before antibiotics, children developed the disease after bacterial pneumonia, which followed such diseases as measles and pertussis. While the number of people developing bronchiectasis as a complication of severe pulmonary infections is decreas-

ing, there are more clients in whom bronchiectasis is a complication of an underlying systemic disorder, particularly cystic fibrosis (Hinshaw & Murray, 1980).

Etiology

The basic disturbance in bronchiectasis is a weakness of the bronchial wall that may be congenital, acquired, or both (Hinshaw & Murray, 1980). Developmental anomalies of the bronchial system can lead to bronchiectasis by promoting infection in the involved airways. Immotile cilia syndrome, a genetic disorder causing immotility of cilia in the respiratory tract, leads to recurrent sinus and bronchial infections, which eventually result in bronchiectasis. Certain hereditary immune-deficiency diseases are frequently complicated by bronchiectasis because affected clients are predisposed to development of infections of the upper and lower airways.

Most forms of bronchiectasis are associated with prolonged respiratory tract infections and prolonged bronchial obstruction. At times, it is difficult to determine whether the infection caused the bronchiectasis or whether the infection is superimposed on an underlying congenital, hereditary, or local obstruction that causes the development of bronchiectasis. Occasionally, bronchiectasis may follow the aspiration of corrosive chemicals or the aspiration of gastric fluid.

Some clients likely to have recurrent lower respiratory tract infections may develop bronchiectasis even with the use of antibiotics. Those most likely to develop such bronchiectasis have disorders with diffuse airway involvement such as cystic fibrosis, bronchial asthma, chronic bronchitis, and ciliary immotility disorders (Hinshaw & Murray, 1980).

Partial obstruction of an airway or airways favors the development of bronchiectasis by impairing the clearance mechanisms. Bacteria, rather than being cleared out by the cilia, are free to grow. Tumors, foreign bodies, and bronchostenosis caused by inflammation can lead to bronchiectasis. Because of antibiotics and corrective surgery, bronchiectasis secondary to obstruction is rare today (Hinshaw & Murray, 1980).

Clinical Manifestations

The signs and symptoms of bronchiectasis vary depending on its extent, severity, location, and complications. If only one bronchopulmonary segment is involved, the symptoms may be mild; however, if the bronchiectasis is diffused throughout the lungs, the disease may be incapacitating (Sexton, 1981).

The infectious process involved in bronchiectasis destroys parts of the bronchial mucosa. These areas are then replaced by fibrous tissue. Since this scar tissue has no resilience, the dynamics of breathing cause the affected airways to become permanently deformed and dilated. The involved airways can dilate up to four times their normal size and take on cylindrical, fusiform (varicose), or saccular shapes. The cylindrical bronchi are dilated with regular outlines; the dilatation may have a square end because of obstruction by mucus. Fusiform bronchi are irregular in form and size with irregular areas of constriction; the ends of the bronchial tree are bulbous and distorted. In the saccular form, the bronchi increase in diameter progressively and end in large blind sacs (Figure 20–8). These structural changes may be located in one or both lungs. The lower lobes, particularly the left lower lobe, are most frequently affected. The right middle lobe is also frequently affected. The most severe involvement tends to occur in the smaller bronchi and bronchioles (Sexton, 1981).

The impaired bronchial wall movement and loss of cilia, coupled with nonaerated alveoli distal to the bronchiectatic area, cause secretions to pool, stagnate, and become infected. The retained secretions, along with obliteration of the bronchioles distal to the affected areas, also cause diffuse bronchial obstruction and ventilation–perfusion abnormalities.

The primary clinical feature of bronchiectasis is a chronic, loose cough that is usually productive of large amounts of mucopurulent, often foul-smelling sputum. In advanced cases, the sputum will settle out into three layers: cloudy mucus on top, clear saliva in the middle, and cloudy purulent material on the bottom (Mitchell & Petty, 1982). Hemoptysis is a frequent occurrence, and recurrent bronchopulmonary infections are common. Clients can suffer from dyspnea, chronic malnutrition, fatigue, and anemia as the disease progresses (Sexton, 1981). Chronic paranasal sinusitis is frequently associated with bronchiectasis. Advanced bronchiectasis is often associated with anastomosis between the bronchial and pulmonary vessels, resulting in right-to-left shunts, which in turn lead to hypoxemia, pulmonary hypertension, cor pulmonale, and clubbing of fingers (Mitchell & Petty, 1982).

Auscultation of the chest usually reveals rales. Chest x-rays may show chronic inflammatory changes, at times including recognizable dilatations. Pulmonary function studies may be normal if involvement is minimal; however, in diffuse disease, findings similar to those of the other

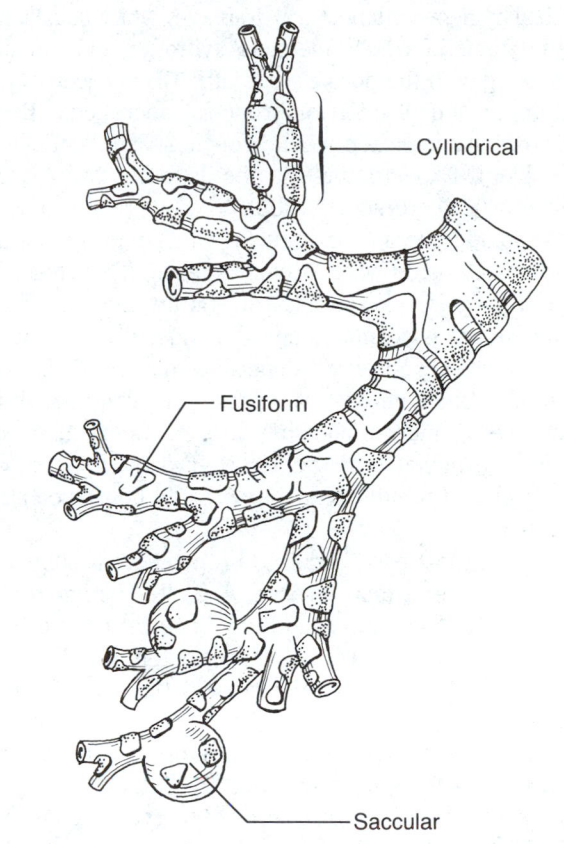

Figure 20–8

Bronchiectasis. Examples of cylindrical, fusiform, and saccular bronchi.

chronic obstructive pulmonary disorders are usually evident. Arterial blood gas values reveal a reduced PO_2 because of perfusion of poorly ventilated alveoli; PCO_2 is often normal (Sexton, 1981).

The prognosis of severe untreated bronchiectasis is generally poor, with a survival rate of 10 to 15 years. The use of antibiotics has greatly improved the outlook for this disease, however.

Therapeutic Measures

Bronchiectasis can often be diagnosed from the history alone and sometimes by a routine chest x-ray showing dilated sacs with fluid levels. Often the chest x-ray is normal. Bronchography can confirm the disease by demonstrating the permanent bronchial dilatation. Because of the possible untoward effects of this procedure, it is recommended only for clients with known or suspected bronchiectasis who are being considered for resection of one or more lobes of the lung.

The cornerstone of treatment in bronchiectasis is daily bronchial hygiene with postural drainage, which usually has to be continued for life. Adequate hydration and humidification along with the possible use of IPPB is necessary to assist in the liquefaction of bronchial secretions. Bronchodilators are indicated when bronchospasm compounds the problem. Expectorants may be used but are of questionable value (Petersdorf, 1983).

Antibiotic therapy is used in the treatment of the infection associated with bronchiectasis. The choice of antibiotic is guided by results of sputum culture. If the sputum culture is normal, ampicillin is usually prescribed. Prolonged use of antibiotics, especially multiple antibiotics, should be avoided because it tends to eliminate the drug-susceptible organisms, allowing drug-resistant organisms to multiply (Mitchell & Petty, 1982). Treatment of accompanying sinusitus with decongestants and humidified air is also important.

For the most part, acquired bronchiectasis should be considered a preventable disease. Aspirated foreign bodies should be removed immediately by bronchoscopy or surgery. Pneumonia should be appropriately treated with antibiotics to prevent complications that can lead to bronchiectasis.

Surgery and resection of the lung are rarely used today as a treatment for bronchiectasis. Successful resection depends on the demonstration of irreversible involvement of localized areas with freedom from involvement of all other areas of both lungs. Palliative surgery is seldom beneficial except in cases where there is a severe symptom, such as recurrent hemoptysis, limited to one portion of the lung. It is important that surgery be deferred until all efforts at medical management, such as antibiotic therapy, bronchoscopy, and pulmonary physical therapy, have failed.

Specific Nursing Measures

Since bronchiectasis is a chronic condition, clients and their families need to learn how to perform deep breathing and coughing exercises as well as bronchial drainage. These measures aid in mobilizing and removing bronchial secretions, controlling problems of accumulation and stagnation, preventing the development of pneumonia. Adequate fluid intake and humidified air may also help to liquefy secretions.

Clients must avoid exposure to infections and other situations, such as smoke or heavy smog, that could aggravate their condition. All persons living in the home should know that smoking cigarettes, cigars, or pipes will exacerbate the client's condition. Visitors to the home should be forewarned that smoking of any kind is not allowed. Obviously, the client must not smoke.

Nutritional management should be stressed, because clients with bronchiectasis are anorexic due to coughing and sputum production which leaves a foul taste in the mouth. A nutritious diet is necessary to keep resistance up, so clients are better able to ward off respiratory tract infections (Sexton, 1981).

Clients will be more likely to eat a nutritious diet if they have good oral hygiene before meals and get as much rest as possible. Bronchial hygiene measures before eating may help reduce coughing and expectoration during eating. Clients and families should be aware that any exacerbation in the bronchiectasis warrants immediate attention by the physician so prompt antibiotic therapy can be started. Clients should be encouraged to receive the influenza vaccine yearly and the pneumococcal vaccine every 3 years.

Because of the productive cough and frequent need to expectorate sputum, clients often markedly curtail their social lives, rarely eat out, and many times feel rejected by friends and family. Emotional support is important for both client and significant others as they cope with a disease that does not necessarily alter life expectancy but may interfere with the client's work, sexual relationships, and other important aspects of life.

ASTHMA

Millions of Americans suffer from asthma. The American Lung Association estimates that 66% of the 6 million asthmatics are over 17 years of age. Asthma can begin at any age, with about one-half of the cases developing in childhood and another third before age 40. The number of hospital admissions is in the hundreds of thousands, and at least 2000 people die of asthma each year in the United States (Raffin & Roberts, 1982).

The American Thoracic Society defines asthma as a disease characterized by increased responsiveness of the trachea and bronchi to various stimuli, manifested by a difficulty in breathing caused by generalized narrowing of the airways. This narrowing of the airways changes in degree, either spontaneously or because of therapy. Asthma differs from the other obstructive disorders in that it is a reversible process, and individuals may be asymptomatic for extended periods. When asthma and bronchitis occur together, airway obstruction persists. The condition is then called chronic asthmatic bronchitis.

Etiology

No single specific factor is recognized as the causative agent of asthma. Asthma is routinely classified according to the type of precipitating factor: extrinsic (exogenous, immunologic, or noninfectious); intrinsic (endogenous, nonallergic, nonimmunologic, or infectious); and mixed (a combination of intrinsic and extrinsic).

Extrinsic asthma develops before the age of 35 with the onset frequently in childhood. Those who develop this type of asthma often have a history of accompanying allergies, such as hay fever or eczema. Individuals with extrinsic asthma are atopic, that is, they are susceptible to hypersensitization from common environmental allergens. An inhaled, ingested, or parenterally introduced allergen results in the formation of sensitizing antibodies (immunoglobulins, particularly IgE). This type of sensitization develops rapidly in response to exposure to allergens occurring in the environment. In extrinsic atopic asthma, IgE is elevated.

The interaction of the antigen and antibody sensitizes the individual, and skin tests to purified antigens are usually positive. When the allergen enters the tissues of a sensitive person, chemical substances referred to as mediators are released. These substances include histamine, slow reacting substance of anaphylaxis (SRS-A), eosinophil chemotactic factor of anaphylaxis (ECF-A), bradykinin, and prostaglandins (Sexton, 1981). The release of these mediators in the lung tissue affects the smooth muscle and glands of the respiratory tract, causing bronchospasm, mucous membrane swelling, and excessive mucus production (Figure 20–9). (These chemical mediators are involved in the clinical manifestations of asthma regardless of whether the cause is intrinsic or extrinsic.) A wide variety of environmental substances may precipitate an asthmatic attack, including pollens, animal dander, molds, certain foods, and drugs such as aspirin.

Intrinsic asthma occurs in adults. In this form of asthma, no immunologic reaction or reactivity to injected antigens has been demonstrated. Asthmatic symptoms frequently occur with a respiratory tract infection. IgE levels are normal, and skin tests are nonreactive. This type of nonallergic asthma can be precipitated by various factors, including respiratory tract infections, exercise, cold air, tobacco smoke, polluted air, and emotionally stressful situations (Sexton, 1981). In intrinsic asthma, exposure to certain respiratory irritants such as smoke can stimulate airway nerve endings, causing the release of an increased amount of acetylcholine, which can directly cause bronchoconstriction as well as stimulate the production of the chemical mediators discussed above.

Clinical Manifestations

Sporadic paroxysmal attacks characterize bronchial asthma. In extrinsic asthma, symptoms are provoked by seasonal and environmental changes, and response to therapy is generally good. Intrinsic asthma is usually less responsive to pharmaceutical therapy, is more difficult to treat, and requires long-term rather than intermittent therapy (George et al., 1983).

Individuals having an asthma attack experience chest tightness, shortness of breath, wheezing, difficulty getting air in and out of their lungs, and a cough. The cough is productive of thick mucoid or white tenacious mucus. Asthmatics also experience marked anxiety, profuse diaphoresis, tachycardia, and an elevated blood pressure. Accessory muscles may be used in breathing as they struggle to

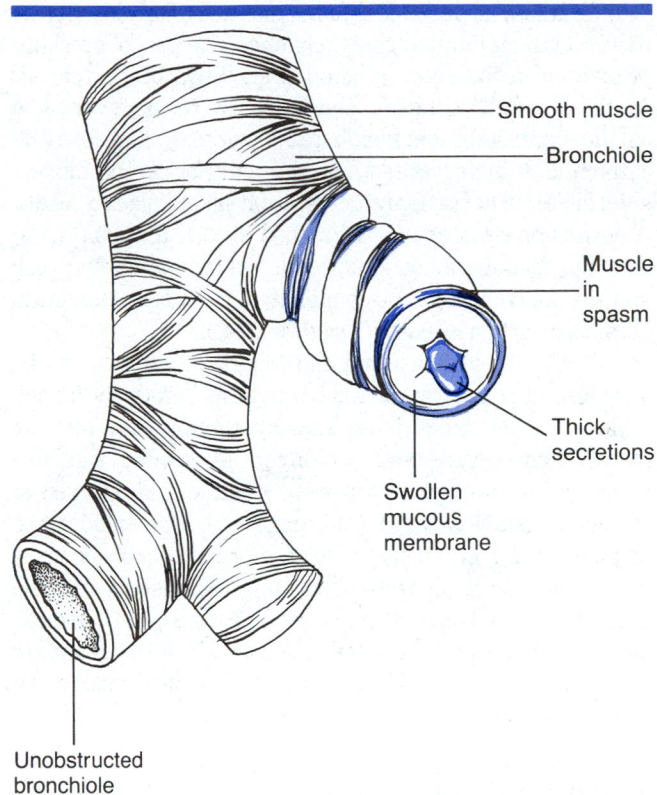

Figure 20–9

Bronchiole obstruction in asthma.

maintain adequate ventilation. This increased work of breathing, along with the anxiety, can cause marked fatigue (Sexton, 1981).

The pathophysiology behind the symptoms is primarily related to a decrease in the size of the airways because of bronchial constriction, inflammation and edema of the bronchial mucosa and an increase in mucus secretion (Sexton, 1981). The decrease in airway size is responsible for the primary symptom of asthma—wheezing. Also, the thick, tenacious mucus produced during an asthma attack tends to adhere to the bronchial walls, further obstructing the flow of air. The primary obstruction to airflow occurs during expiration, because the airways normally narrow during this phase of breathing. This physiological process, along with added bronchial constriction, edema, and mucus plugs, can severely impede or totally obstruct the expiratory flow of air. This can cause alveolar hyperinflation and collapse (Traver, 1982).

Obstruction of the expiratory airflow is reflected in pulmonary function studies, which show an increase in residual volume, an increase in the functional residual capacity (FRC), and a decrease in the vital capacity (VC). Chest x-rays may reveal hyperinflation and atelectasis of the lungs. Rales and rhonchi may be heard throughout the lungs, along with inspiratory and expiratory wheezes.

Ventilation–perfusion abnormalities can also occur, resulting in ineffective gas exchange. The partial pressure of oxygen in the arterial blood (PaO_2) will be decreased. As the attack progresses, the PaO_2 can become very low as the ventilation–perfusion ratio worsens. Because the asthmatic is hyperventilating, the arterial carbon dioxide level is below normal, and respiratory alkalemia can result. A normal or elevated arterial carbon dioxide tension (PCO_2) is a sign that airway obstruction is becoming more severe and the individual can no longer hyperventilate enough to eliminate carbon dioxide (Traver, 1982).

Both the severity and the length of asthma attacks vary greatly. Treatment may bring the asthmatic attack under control rapidly, or the symptoms can become increasingly severe and prolonged. A severe and prolonged asthma attack that resists treatment is referred to as *status asthmaticus*. In this instance, more and more alveoli become either hyperinflated or collapsed; the arterial oxygen level decreases, causing hypoxemia; and the arterial carbon dioxide level rises. This rise in carbon dioxide can lead to respiratory acidosis. Unless treatment reverses the condition, the client will go into respiratory failure and die.

Therapeutic Measures

Medications to dilate the bronchioles are used in both the prevention and treatment of asthmatic attacks. Examples include aminophylline-theophylline compounds and beta-adrenergic stimulators, which relax smooth muscle, and oral and parenteral corticosteroids, which moderate the inflammatory response. Cromolyn sodium, an inhaled medication that is not a bronchodilator but prevents the release of chemical mediators of anaphylaxis, is also used to prevent attacks.

In an acute asthma attack, the beta-adrenergic drugs (epinephrine, isoproterenol, metaproterenol, and terbutaline) and the theophyllines are used. Epinephrine may be given initially subcutaneously (0.3 to 0.5 mL of a 1:1000 solution) and repeated in 15 to 30 minutes if bronchospasm is not relieved. If the condition continues to worsen, intravenous aminophylline is started. The beta-adrenergic drugs are given either subcutaneously or by inhalation, along with aminophylline (Mitchell & Petty, 1982).

Status asthmaticus is refractory to the theophyllines and beta-adrenergic medications. Administration of intravenous corticosteroids is required (Mitchell & Petty, 1982).

In individuals with chronic persistent asthma or frequent attacks, continuous therapy is required. Theophylline administered orally is often accompanied by an oral or inhaled beta-adrenergic such as terbutaline and metaproterenol. If this is not effective, oral steroids such as prednisone may have to be given (Mitchell & Petty, 1982).

Sedatives or tranquilizers may be administered to calm the anxious client who is not threatened with ventilatory failure. Antibiotics may be prescribed if an infection is pres-

ent. Clients whose asthma is triggered by common allergens may undergo treatment to reduce their sensitivity to the substances.

Since the client ill enough to visit the physician or emergency room is almost always suffering from hypoxemia, the administration of humidified oxygen is required and is guided by the monitoring of arterial blood gas values. The administration of fluids is also important; asthmatics are frequently dehydrated by diaphoresis, hyperventilation, and the inability to drink.

Breathing exercises along with bronchial drainage are ordered to assist in removing retained secretions. Because of the reported risk of sudden death, the use of IPPB is not advocated for acute asthma attacks (Mitchell & Petty, 1982). Aerosol therapy to loosen secretions may be ordered.

Careful monitoring of chest x-rays, arterial blood gas reports, pulmonary function studies, and sputum cultures is a necessary part of medical management, since these tests will reflect the client's response to treatment. If the client's condition worsens to the point of impending respiratory failure, the client will be intubated and placed on a mechanical ventilator.

Specific Nursing Measures

During an acute asthmatic attack, clients are frequently frightened, anxious, and exhausted because of labored breathing. It is important from the start to give clients all needed emotional support and assurance that the nurse will remain with them. Nothing is as terrifying as not being able to breathe and, even though the client and family may have been through the experience many times, each attack generates the fear of dying. To be effective, the nurse must overcome personal anxieties about acute asthmatic attacks by gaining a good understanding of asthma and its treatment.

Interact with the client and family in a calm and caring manner. Clients frequently prefer to sit up, bending forward. They can be made more comfortable if the bedside table is set so they rest their arms on it. To help allay the feeling of suffocation, clients may prefer not to be closed in (eg, by bedside curtains). A quiet environment with as few interruptions as possible should be maintained. Clients should be protected from drafts and chills; wet linen from diaphoresis should be changed quickly.

Because shortness of breath interferes with ability to talk, do not tire the client further by trying to take an admission history or asking nonessential questions. Needed information can be obtained more easily from family members.

Any instructions given to asthmatics during an acute attack, such as instructions for breathing exercises, should be given slowly and repeated as necessary, since anxiety may interfere with the ability to comprehend what is being said (Traver, 1982). Clients should avoid any unnecessary exertion since they will need all their energy to breathe. As the condition warrants, activity levels can be increased, but initially, asthmatic clients require assistance in carrying out activities of daily living.

Fluid intake and output must be monitored; unless contraindicated, clients should receive 3000 to 4000 mL per day. The nutritional intake of asthmatics can be severely hampered if shortness of breath makes them unable to eat. Monitor their intake of food as well as fluids. High-nutrient liquid supplemental feedings are sometimes needed.

Attention to good bronchopulmonary toilet is essential. Breathing exercises along with bronchial drainage are important aspects of care. Suctioning may be required if secretions cannot be expectorated. The sputum expectorated should be observed and charted for amount, consistency, and color.

Respiratory and cardiac assessment is an ongoing responsibility of the nurse, as is careful monitoring of blood gas values and pulmonary function studies. Cardiac dysrhythmias, tachycardia, tremors, nervousness, nausea, and headache are possible adverse effects from the beta-adrenergic stimulators as well as from aminophylline or theophylline. As the health professional with continuous client contact, the nurse is in the best position to synthesize the client's subjective reports and objective findings to evaluate client response to treatment.

Since asthma is a chronic condition, clients, their families, and significant others require instruction in its cause, care, and treatment. If possible, help clients to identify precipitating factors in the development of their attacks and take measures to avoid them. This is especially important if specific allergens such as pollen, animal dander, or dust are involved. Other environmental irritants should be avoided, such as cigarette smoke, aerosol sprays, overly dry air, and extremes in temperatures. Since these irritants may precipitate an attack, clients should be encouraged to seek medical care at the first sign of a respiratory tract infection, tonsillitis, or sinusitis (Sexton, 1981). Clients should also avoid people with respiratory tract infections.

If emotional stress seems to be a precipitating factor, encourage the client to identify stressful factors and how they might manage stress more effectively. Stress management intervention should be aimed at identifying ways to prevent a stressor from disrupting the client's life or to lessen the degree of reaction. Stress management techniques such as relaxation training can be beneficial in assisting individuals to deal with stressful situations more positively.

Asthmatics should be encouraged to maintain as active and as normal a life as possible, avoiding only activities that may precipitate an attack. An individualized medication program may help to control exercise-induced asthma. Sufficient rest is important, since fatigue may make it more difficult for asthmatic clients to handle daily stresses. Breathing exercises will help reduce the amount of residual volume of air in the lungs during an attack, and bronchial drainage will help to prevent the buildup of secretions.

Clients must be aware of the nature, proper admin-

istration, and side effects of the medications they are taking. Clients need to understand why they should not discontinue, start, or increase medication without consulting with the physician or care provider. For example, abrupt discontinuation of corticosteroids such as prednisone is likely to cause a serious "steroid rebound" effect (withdrawal syndrome). Propranolol (Inderal) should not be given to clients with asthma because of its potential to cause bronchoconstriction. Antihistamines and decongestants should be avoided because of their tendency to dry airway secretions, making expectoration difficult.

CHRONIC BRONCHITIS

The American Thoracic Society defines chronic bronchitis as a clinical disorder characterized by excessive mucus secretion in the bronchi, manifested by chronic or recurrent productive cough. The cough is present for a minimum of 3 months per year for at least 2 successive years, and other causes of productive cough, such as specific pulmonary infections, have been excluded. Chronic bronchitis may precede and accompany pulmonary emphysema. Chronic bronchitis is a disabling disease. It has been estimated that at least 14 million Americans have chronic bronchitis or emphysema.

Etiology

There is conclusive evidence that cigarette smoking is the most consistently important factor in the development of chronic bronchitis. Atmospheric pollution from industry and automotive pollutants, such as sulfur oxides, nitrogen oxides, carbon monoxide, and many hydrocarbons, also irritates the respiratory structures, causing nonspecific inflammatory reactions in the lungs (Wade, 1982). Air pollution raises both the morbidity and mortality of chronic bronchitis sufferers. Occupational pollutants are also important predisposing factors in this disease. Some high-risk occupations are sandstone workers, copper miners, cotton strippers, and grinders (Fishman, 1980).

Respiratory tract infections are associated with chronic bronchitis because recurrent infections damage the structures of the respiratory system. Conversely, the increased secretions of chronic bronchitis make individuals more susceptible to recurrent respiratory tract infections.

Genetic factors are believed to play a part in the development of the chronic obstructive pulmonary diseases, including chronic bronchitis. Relatives of bronchitic subjects have a higher prevalence of bronchitis than do relatives of controls. There is also the possibility of increased susceptibility to respiratory irritants among those heterozygous for a certain gene (Fishman, 1980). This would explain why people exposed to the same amount of a respiratory irritant such as cigarette smoke do not show the same damage.

Chronic bronchitis is more common in men than women,

occurs more frequently in whites than nonwhites, and is more common in city dwellers than those who live in the country. City dwellers may experience more air pollution and occupational exposure. Those who live in a poor socioeconomic environment are also more frequently affected (Fishman, 1980).

Clinical Manifestations

In simple chronic bronchitis, the client experiences only a cough with intermittent wheezing. In the more severe forms, there are constant wheezing, sputum production, dyspnea, and episodes of acute respiratory failure (George, Light, & Matthay, 1983). The changes in the airways usually occur gradually, over 25 to 40 years (Traver, 1982).

The peripheral conducting airways are the primary site of pathological changes. The chronic inflammatory response stimulates the bronchial mucous glands, causing hypertrophy and hyperplasia. This is accompanied by chronic inflammatory cell infiltration and edema of the bronchial mucosa. These factors combine with the hypersecretion of mucus to cause a narrowing of the bronchial airways, with increasing resistance to airflow. The narrowing increases the effort needed for breathing.

Cilia activity is either diminished or destroyed by the inflammation, which results in retained secretions. This mucus becomes an excellent medium for the growth of bacteria, subjecting individuals to recurrent respiratory tract infections, which in turn contribute to an increase in inflammation and mucus production (Traver, 1982). The inflammatory responses and retained secretions do not occur uniformly throughout the lungs, which results in ventilation–perfusion mismatching. Repeated infections along with inflammation and persistent obstruction can lead to necrotizing, scarring, and sometimes destruction of the small bronchioles.

Individuals with chronic bronchitis tend to be overweight and dusky. The disease usually affects individuals between 40 and 55 years of age and has a gradual onset. The first symptom is an early morning cough, frequently described as a "cigarette cough" (Sexton, 1981). As the condition progresses, the cough, which is productive of copious secretions, becomes continual. The client experiences acute exacerbations from respiratory tract infections. Dyspnea becomes more and more severe, and the client becomes more inactive and debilitated. Table 20–5 compares characteristics of clients with predominant chronic bronchitis to those with predominant emphysema.

Those with chronic bronchitis are frequently referred to as "blue bloaters" because of their bloated, cyanotic appearance. The cyanosis is from the hypoxemia of chronic bronchitis, which is caused by alveolar hypoventilation. Why individuals with chronic bronchitis tend to hypoventilate is not clearly understood, but it appears to be a type of compensatory mechanism (Wade, 1982). The hypoventilation results not only in a low arterial oxygen level (hypoxemia) but also in an elevation of carbon dioxide (hypercapnia). The combination of hypoxemia, hypercapnia, and possible respiratory acidosis can lead to vasoconstriction, resulting in increased vascular resistance. This causes an increase in pulmonary artery pressure and an increase in the work required by the right ventricle of the heart. This, in turn, can lead to right-sided heart failure, or cor pulmonale (Wade, 1982). Compensatory polycythemia may occur as a result

Table 20–5	Characteristics of Clients With Predominant Chronic Bronchitis or Predominant Emphysema	
Characteristic	**Predominant Bronchitis**	**Predominant Emphysema**
History	Recurrent pulmonary infections	Insidious dyspnea
Smoking history	Usual	Usual
General appearance	"Blue bloater," cyanotic	"Pink puffer," pursed lip breathing, use of accessory muscles
Weight loss	Absent or slight	Often marked
Dyspnea	Moderate	Severe, often disabling
Cough	Before onset of dyspnea	After onset of dyspnea
Sputum	Copious, purulent	Scanty, mucoid
Chest x-ray	Normal diaphragm position; cardiomegaly; increased bronchovascular markings at bases	Bilateral low, flat diaphragm; long, narrow cardiac silhouette; bullae; absence of bronchovascular markings in lung periphery
Cor pulmonale	Common	Uncommon, except terminally

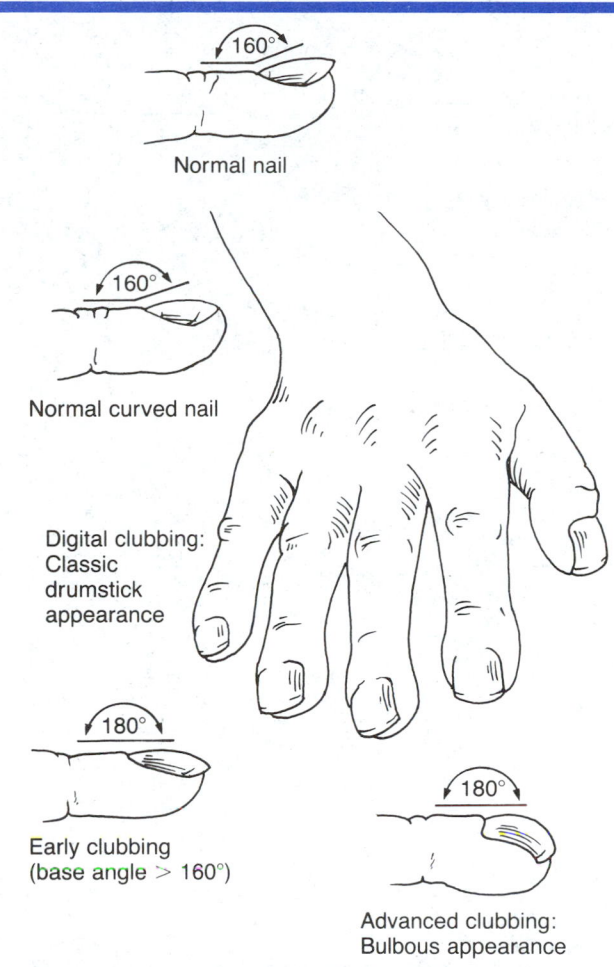

Figure 20–10

Clubbing of the fingers in chronic bronchitis.

of the chronic hypoxemia (George, Light, & Matthay, 1983). Clubbing of the fingers because of the development of secondary polycythemia may also be present (Figure 20–10).

Therapeutic Measures and Specific Nursing Measures

The therapeutic management of chronic bronchitis and specific nursing measures in the care of clients with chronic bronchitis are covered under pulmonary emphysema because they are so closely related.

PULMONARY EMPHYSEMA

Pulmonary emphysema is a chronically progressive pulmonary disease in which there is an enlargement of the air spaces distal to the terminal nonrespiratory bronchioles with destruction of the alveolar walls. Emphysema ranks

high among the diagnostic categories awarded disability allowances. Of the three chronic obstructive pulmonary diseases (emphysema, chronic bronchitis, and asthma), approximately 84% of the disability allowances were awarded to men with emphysema. Emphysema has been estimated to be three times more prevalent in men than in women (Oregon Thoracic Society, 1981). Although chronic bronchitis and emphysema can occur separately, they frequently coexist.

Etiology

The etiology of emphysema is essentially unknown. The predisposing factors discussed under chronic bronchitis are applicable to emphysema. Cigarette smoking is again the major culprit.

Theories attempt to explain why certain people are more likely to develop emphysema. Research has shown an apparent failure of the connective tissue of the lungs to protect against protein digestion from enzymes released from the alveolar macrophages and leukocytes (Mitchell & Petty, 1982). Human serum, lung tissue, peripheral airways, and bronchial mucus have been shown to contain inhibitors of these enzymes. It is postulated that tissue damage to the lungs occurs when there is not enough of these enzyme inhibitors to control the enzymes released from the macrophages and the leukocytes (Traver, 1982). It has been demonstrated that a hereditary deficiency of alpha$_1$-antitrypsin, one of the main agents inhibiting the action of these enzymes, results in the development of emphysema at an early age (usually during the fourth decade of life). This deficiency is found in less than 2% of all cases of severe emphysema, however (Fishman, 1980). Recent studies indicate that cigarette smoke contributes to alveolar wall damage by interfering with the enzyme-inhibitor balance (Mitchell & Petty, 1982).

Clinical Manifestations

The development of emphysema is insidious and progressive. The obstruction in emphysema typically begins in the small, peripheral bronchioles, due to inflammation, infection, retained secretions, and edema. The narrowing of the airways traps air in the alveoli. As the disease progresses, alveolar walls become disrupted by hyperinflation, and some alveolar tissue septa are destroyed. The alveolar walls degenerate into a lacy pattern made up of thin strands of collagen fibers. There is an accompanying destruction of the pulmonary capillaries of the involved alveoli and the development of air spaces (Wade, 1982). Because of the loss of elasticity of the lung tissue, the minute respiratory and terminal bronchioles tend to collapse prematurely during exhalation. This causes increased airway resistance and a slowing of expiratory airflow, making exhalation of air from the lungs more difficult. Ventilation–perfusion abnormalities occur, since the alveolar and vascular changes are not uniform throughout the lungs. Some alveoli will be ventilated and not perfused, and others will be perfused but underventilated (Sexton, 1981).

Emphysema is classified into two principal types: centrilobular and panlobular emphysema. These types may occur together or separately.

Centrilobular Emphysema

Centrilobular emphysema (CLE), or centriacinar emphysema, affects the central portion of the lung lobule close to the respiratory bronchiole (Figure 20–11). As the disease progresses, the destruction of the lobule occurs from the center outward (Wade, 1982). Upper portions of the lung are usually more severely affected, and the disease tends to be distributed unevenly. Centrilobular emphysema is more common than panlobular and is much more prevalent in males than in females. This type of emphysema is usually associated with chronic bronchitis and is seldom found in non-smokers (Wade, 1982).

Panlobular Emphysema

Panlobular emphysema (PLE), or panacinar emphysema, results in the destruction of the acinus or terminal respiratory unit, which includes the respiratory bronchiole and the alveolar ducts and sacs (see Figure 20–11). There is a concomitant destruction of the pulmonary capillary bed (Wade, 1982). PLE tends to be diffuse but is more severe in the lower lung areas. This type of emphysema is often found to some degree in older people who do not have chronic bronchitis or clinical impairment of lung function and is as common in women as in men. PLE is a characteristic finding in those deficient in alpha$_1$-antitrypsin.

Individuals with emphysema are generally older. Because emphysema has an insidious onset, symptoms may not appear until 20% to 30% of the lung tissue is destroyed unless an individual is active (Wade, 1982). Dyspnea on exertion is the first recognized symptom. As the disease progresses, the client must work harder and harder at breathing, especially exhalation. Individuals will often exhale through pursed lips to prolong expiration and reduce the tendency of airways to collapse, thus removing more air from the lungs. As the emphysema becomes more severe, clients use all their accessory muscles to breathe and usually sit with their hands firmly supported. The anterior–posterior diameter of the chest usually increases due to expansion of the chest wall and loss of lung elasticity, giving the chest a barrel-shaped appearance. Anorexia and weight loss are common, causing an emaciated appearance and concomitant muscle wasting (Figure 20–12). Cough and sputum production are not common, unless the client develops a respiratory tract infection—a frequent occurrence during the winter months (Sexton, 1981).

Auscultation of the chest may reveal rhonchi, prolonged expiration, and diminished breath sounds. Hyperresonance is noted on percussion. Tactile and auditory

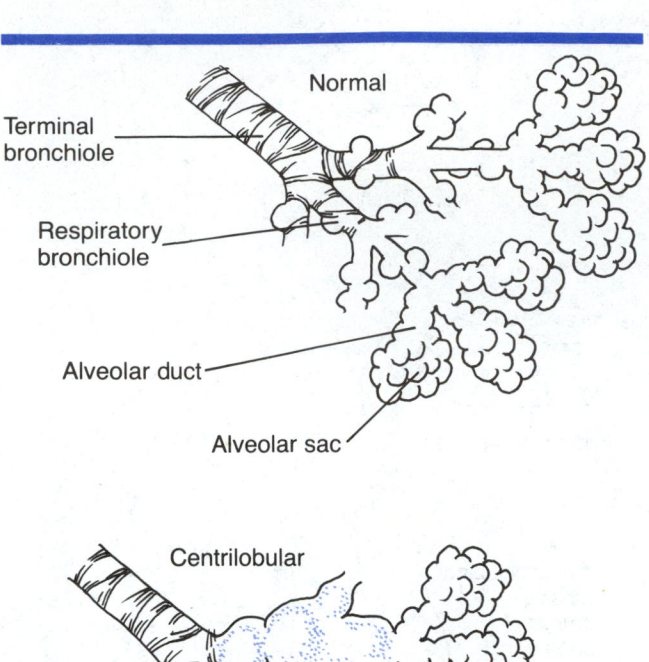

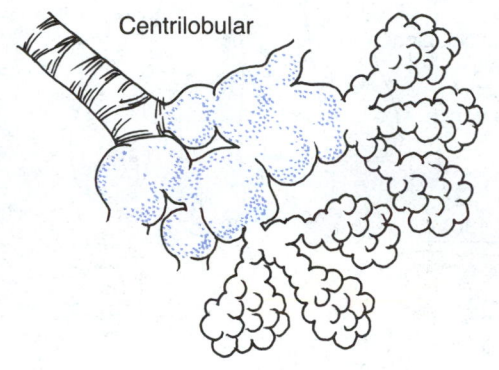

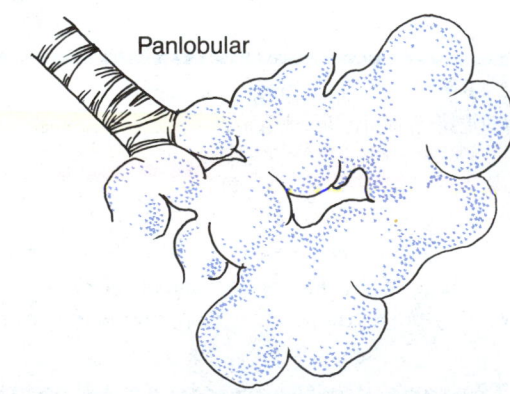

Figure 20–11

Alterations in alveolar structure in centrilobular and panlobular emphysema.

fremitus is reduced. Chest x-ray may show a low, flattened diaphragm and hyperaeration of the lungs (Figure 20–13). Bullae—bubblelike structures containing air that project from the lung surface—can occur from progressive trapping of air and may be seen on chest x-ray. The cardiac silhouette is often lengthened and narrowed although hypertrophy of the right ventricle can occur if cor pulmonale is developing (Mitchell & Petty, 1982). Pulmonary function tests usually show decrease in vital capacity and

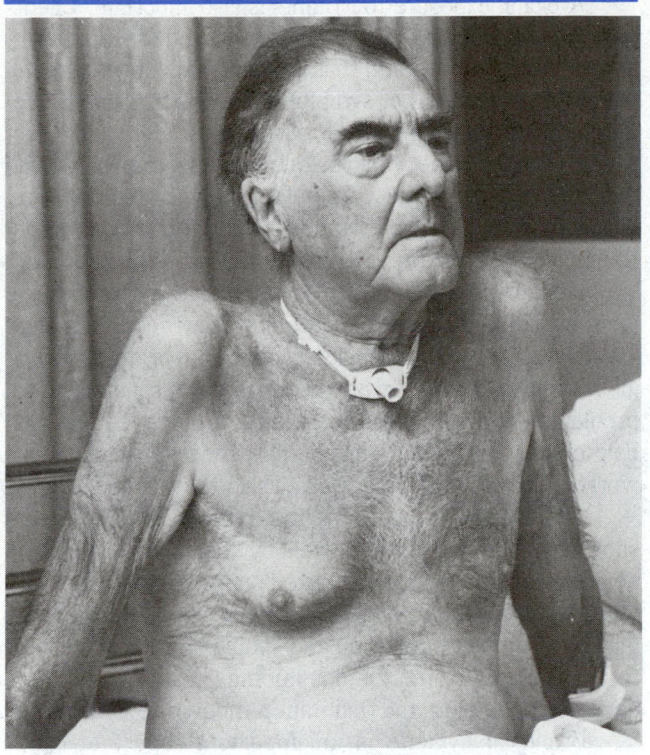

Figure 20–12

Typical appearance of a client with advanced pulmonary emphysema. Photograph by Carol Payne-Zagon.

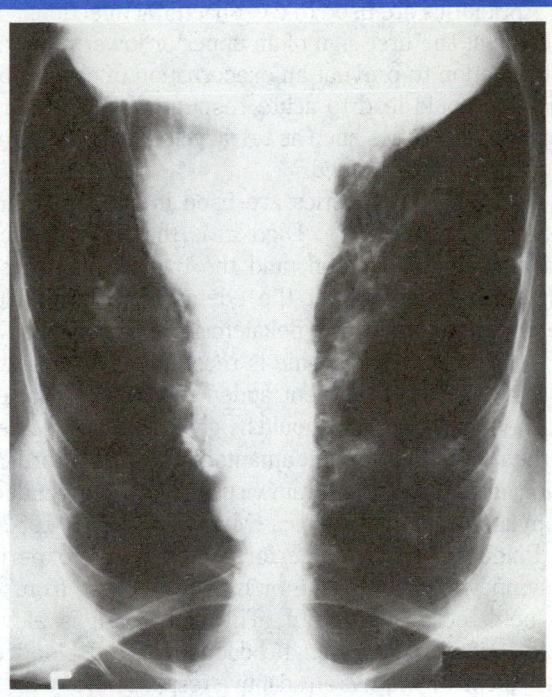

Figure 20–13

Chest x-ray of a male client with advanced pulmonary emphysema. Note the bilateral lowering and flattening of the diaphragm, the lengthened and narrowed cardiac silhouette, and the absence of bronchovascular patterns in the lung periphery. (Courtesy of Health Care Plan, Buffalo, NY)

an increased resistance to expiratory airflow, with a decrease in forced expiratory volume and in maximal voluntary ventilation.

Arterial blood gas values may show normal or slightly reduced arterial oxygen at rest. Even in the presence of severe disease, clients can maintain relatively normal blood gas levels. This happens because alveolar destruction is accompanied by pulmonary capillary destruction and, although this is not always uniform, the ventilation-to-perfusion ratio is close enough to maintain relatively normal blood gas values. In contrast, those with chronic bronchitis have a ventilation–perfusion mismatch that is more abnormal (Sexton, 1981).

Those with COPD, especially emphysema, may show elevated arterial carbon dioxide levels. If elevation has developed gradually, the kidneys will have attempted to compensate for rising CO_2 levels by conserving bicarbonate, maintaining a normal pH. Therefore, clients whose arterial blood gas values show an elevated CO_2 and a normal pH are considered to have compensated for respiratory acidosis.

The hematocrit is frequently elevated because of the development of polycythemia, giving clients a "pink puffer" appearance. With progression or exacerbation of the disease because of a superimposed respiratory tract infection, alveolar ventilation may be inadequate to maintain normal blood gas values. A low oxygen and an elevated carbon dioxide level with a low pH indicate respiratory acidosis that may lead to respiratory failure.

As with chronic bronchitis, finger clubbing may occur. Distended neck veins may be present along with cor pulmonale because of the loss of pulmonary vasculature, with a resulting increase in pulmonary vascular resistance.

Clients with emphysema can become totally disabled, unable to do anything for themselves except fight for every breath of air. They are frequently drained emotionally by anxiety, fear, and depression over their disease state.

Therapeutic Measures

Since bronchitis and emphysema are chronic conditions that will last a lifetime, treatment centers around controlling the symptoms, retarding further deterioration of function, rehabilitation, and client education (Sexton, 1981).

Bronchodilators are used in the treatment of reversible bronchospasm, if present. Pulmonary function studies may be done before and after the administration of the medication to see if the medication has any effect on reducing the bronchospasm. Frequently used bronchodilators include theophylline and epinephrine or terbutaline.

Antibiotics are used to treat bacterial infections. They are given at the first sign of an upper or lower respiratory tract infection to prevent an exacerbation of chronic bronchitis that could lead to acute respiratory failure. Broad-spectrum antibiotics such as tetracycline or erythromycin are commonly prescribed.

Digitalis and diuretics are used in the treatment of right-sided heart failure. Digoxin is the most commonly used digitalis preparation, and the thiazide diuretics are most often used to treat the edema. Clients should be carefully monitored for hypokalemia and hypoxemia.

Yearly influenza vaccine is recommended for individuals with COPD to prevent added respiratory problems. The pneumonia vaccine should be given every 3 to 4 years, and the new antiviral agent amantadine, which affords protection against many A-strain viruses, is recommended for prophylaxis during epidemics (Mitchell & Petty, 1982).

Phlebotomy may be performed for clients experiencing symptoms of headache or mental clouding from very high hematocrits (over 60). The hematocrit is elevated because of the increased production of red blood cells (polycythemia), which is an adaptive response to hypoxemia.

In the treatment of chronic bronchitis and emphysema, surgery is limited to treatment of a spontaneous pneumothorax caused by rupture of an emphysematous bleb, which requires the insertion of chest tubes.

Specific Nursing Measures

The nurse must work with health team members in the care of clients with COPD. Frequently, physical and respiratory therapists are involved in client rehabilitation.

As stated in the discussion of psychosocial aspects of respiratory diseases in Chapter 17, clients with chronic lung conditions frequently feel angry, depressed, and anxious over their condition. It is important to know this, acknowledge their feelings, and answer their questions honestly. It is even more important that clients learn which aspects of their condition are reversible, such as accumulation of secretions and bronchospasm, and which are not. The potential for reversibility is greatest in treating chronic bronchitis and least in treating emphysema. Clients should understand that if they conscientiously carry out the treatment plan, they can expect improvement. By understanding their condition and how to manage their symptoms, they will be better able to cope with chronic respiratory disease.

Since infection is a threat, clients should be instructed to avoid persons who have colds or other respiratory tract infections. At the first sign of a cold, or of any change in the color, amount, or consistency of sputum, they should notify the physician. Sometimes clients have antibiotics on hand, which the physician has instructed them to take at the first sign of a cold. Stress that if the antibiotics do not begin to relieve the symptoms within 24 to 48 hours, clients should consult the physician.

Avoiding exposure to irritants is also important. Clients who are still smoking should be encouraged to stop. It may help if clients understand that stopping smoking will result in some improvement of symptoms and will markedly retard further deterioration. Direct smokers to a smoking cessation clinic, to the American Lung Association, or the American Cancer Society for help on how to stop smoking. Nicorette gum, available by prescription, has been effective in aiding smokers to give up their smoking habit.

If clients are exposed to irritants on the job and there is no way of avoiding exposure, they may need to change jobs to avoid becoming completely disabled. Having to change jobs or stop working can be upsetting and result in financial problems. Nurses need to be aware of these feelings and help clients and their families work through them. Social workers can offer useful advice on how to manage finances.

Air pollution can aggravate respiratory disorders; clients should avoid high pollution levels by staying indoors. Daily pollution levels are often reported on television, especially when levels are high. Dusts, powders, and aerosol sprays may be a source of irritation and should be avoided or kept to a minimum. Home air conditioning may be helpful to decrease pollutants and maintain temperature control.

Bronchial hygiene is an important aspect of client instruction. Topics should include how to cough effectively, do breathing exercises, and aid bronchial drainage. To facilitate the expectoration of secretions and reduce bronchospasm, an IPPB machine may be ordered for use at home. Medications such as isoetharine (Bronkosol) and saline can be added to the nebulizer of the machine to loosen secretions and reduce bronchospasm. Steam inhalation may also loosen secretions. The nurse may have to teach clients and families how to procure and use the equipment.

Continuous home oxygen therapy may be required if the client's arterial oxygen level is low. Reservoir tanks can be placed in the home, and portable oxygen units can be filled from the reservoir. Because those with chronic bronchitis and emphysema may have a hypoxic drive to breathe, continuous low flow oxygen therapy must be carefully monitored with regular arterial blood gas levels. Clients and their families must know why it is essential to use only the flow of oxygen ordered by the physician and not to increase the flow. As with the IPPB machines, clients may require assistance in how to procure, use, and pay for oxygen equipment.

The most frequent symptoms of hypoxia and hypercapnia should be reviewed with the client and especially family members, since these symptoms may signify impending respiratory failure. Symptoms include increased shortness of breath, restlessness, lethargy, headache, and confusion.

Clients should learn to weigh themselves daily, because a weight gain of 2½ kg (5½ lb) could indicate fluid retention from right-sided heart failure. Hydration is an important aspect of care because water helps to liquefy secretions in the lung. Unless contraindicated, clients should be instructed to drink 8 to 10 glasses of fluid a day. Coffee and tea have a diuretic effect and should not be counted as fluid intake.

Nutrition is another important aspect of care. High-calorie meals are necessary for clients with emphysema who are underweight and undernourished. Small, frequent meals may be more easily tolerated by those who are short of breath; eating large meals may require more energy than the client can afford. Also, large meals can interfere with the downward descent of the diaphragm during inspiration, adding to the breathing difficulty. (Gas-forming foods should be avoided for the same reason.) Salt-restricted diets may be necessary for those with right-sided heart failure. Foods high in potassium are important for clients taking diuretics.

The positive effects of physical reconditioning exercises have been well established in the literature. Those with chronic bronchitis and emphysema frequently fear exercise because of the dyspnea that may result. Exercise training and instruction are usually begun in the hospital and continued at home. Once breathing exercises are mastered, the client's tolerance to exercise is gradually increased by walking on a treadmill and/or riding a stationary bicycle. Stair climbing is also included. Clients continue to increase exercise until they reach their tolerance level. Blood gases, pulmonary function tests, and cardiac status are monitored.

Since walking and controlled breathing are the main components of the program, clients are encouraged to carry out these activities daily at home. If the weather is cold and rainy, clients can do their walking in a shopping mall.

Pulmonary rehabilitation programs have helped clients return to more active and productive lives. This author has seen clients, once bedridden, who have completed a rehabilitation program to the point that they are able to drive a car again, go to the grocery store, and engage in social activities they previously could not tolerate. Besides increasing their exercise tolerance, the program usually improves their sense of well-being.

Many pamphlets and teaching materials are available through the American Lung Association. These can be given to clients and their families to help them learn more about their respiratory disease and its care.

ACUTE RESPIRATORY FAILURE

Acute respiratory failure is the sudden inability of the respiratory system and the heart to maintain adequate arterial oxygenation and adequate carbon dioxide elimination. The arterial blood gas level arbitrarily used to define acute respiratory failure is an arterial oxygen tension of less than 55 mm Hg, with or without carbon dioxide retention. An acute elevation of carbon dioxide to more than 50 mm Hg is referred to as acute ventilatory failure. Acute ventilatory failure can result in acute respiratory failure if the level of ventilation decreases enough that hypoxemia occurs. Acute respiratory failure is encountered frequently; it can be caused by a variety of conditions.

Etiology

Arterial oxygen and carbon dioxide levels are maintained by the normal dynamics of ventilation, diffusion, and circulation (Chapter 17). Should problems arise that alter any of these mechanisms, gas exchange can be impaired, resulting in respiratory failure. Of the diseases of the lungs, the chronic obstructive pulmonary diseases such as emphysema and chronic bronchitis are the most frequent causes of respiratory failure (Mitchell & Petty, 1982). Disturbances of the chest wall, such as kyphoscoliosis or neuromuscular diseases such as Guillain-Barré syndrome, can impair ventilation, leading to respiratory failure. Overdoses of certain drugs, such as narcotics, barbiturates, and tranquilizers, can depress or damage the respiratory center. Cerebral infarction or brain trauma can suppress the respiratory drive leading to respiratory failure (Mitchell & Petty, 1982).

Clinical Manifestations

The signs and symptoms of acute respiratory failure combine those of the underlying disease with the signs of hypoxemia, hypercapnia, or both. The onset of respiratory failure may be gradual and subtle, or it may be dramatic.

Clinical manifestations of hypoxemia affect the nervous system first because the brain is the organ most sensitive to oxygen deprivation. Neurological symptoms include headache, mental confusion, anxiety and agitation, restlessness, impaired judgment, euphoria or depression, double vision, weakness, drowsiness, and coma. Effects on the cardiovascular system include tachycardia, hypertension, and dysrhythmias. Respiratory effects include tachypnea and dyspnea (Harper, 1981). Central cyanosis may be present, but the hemoglobin saturation must be as low as 78% before cyanosis becomes apparent (Wade, 1982).

The marked increases in carbon dioxide levels depress the central nervous system, leading to symptoms of drowsiness or lethargy, inability to concentrate, headache, dizziness, muscle twitching, a gradual loss of consciousness, and coma. A rise in arterial carbon dioxide will decrease arterial oxygen because of hypoventilation. If the carbon dioxide level increases rapidly, the kidney will not have enough time to compensate by conserving bicarbonate, and respiratory acidosis will result. The four most common signs of acute respiratory failure are restlessness, headache, confusion, and tachycardia (Mitchell & Petty, 1982).

Therapeutic Measures

Bronchodilators may be used to decrease edema of the airways and bronchospasm. Aminophylline may be administered as a bolus followed by intravenous drip. Corticosteroids may be administered to reduce bronchial inflammation and bronchospasm. Antibiotics may be necessary if an underlying infection is present. Cardiac drugs are

Nursing Research Abstract

Woodburne C, Powaser M: Mechanisms responsible for the sustained fall in arterial oxygen tension after endotracheal suctioning in dogs. *Nurs Res* 1980; 29:312–316.

Endotracheal suctioning can decrease arterial oxygen tension below presuction levels for up to 5 minutes. This study examined the decline in PaO_2 in anesthetized dogs. The researchers examined ventilated dogs and spontaneously breathing dogs for changes in PaO_2 after various manipulations before and after suctioning.

In spontaneously breathing dogs, arterial oxygen tension fell after catheter insertion with or without application of suction pressure. The decrease in oxygen tension persisted through 15 minutes. At 30 minutes after suctioning, oxygen tension had partially or completely returned to presuction levels. Hyperinflation and pretreatment with isoproterenol mist did not prevent the sustained drop in PaO_2.

The sustained PaO_2 drop was also seen in mechanically ventilated dogs both before and after suctioning or catheter insertion without suction. Again, hyperinflation and isoproterenol did not prevent the decline in PaO_2 after suctioning.

The researchers concluded that mechanical stimulation of the airway by a suction catheter causes the sustained PaO_2 drop. The nurse must carry out suctioning efficiently and effectively as well as assess client tolerance and need for suctioning.

given if cardiac failure or dysrhythmias occur. Sodium bicarbonate is administered in respiratory acidosis.

Acute respiratory failure can be a medical emergency requiring such life-saving measures as intubation and a mechanical ventilator. When the client's breathing is not as severely compromised as in COPD, respiratory failure can be treated by more conservative measures. These clients may be treated judiciously with the medications mentioned previously, closely monitored oxygen therapy, and chest physiotherapy. IPPB has not proven highly effective in the treatment of acute respiratory failure, since inhaled drugs can be administered as effectively with nonpressurized nebulizers. Also IPPB therapy can tire a client, lead to pneumothorax, and result in gastric distention from air swallowing (Mitchell & Petty, 1982).

Whether endotracheal intubation and mechanical ventilation will be required depends on the clinical evaluation of the client and on arterial blood gas abnormalities. If the client's arterial oxygen level cannot be maintained at 60 to 70 mm Hg, or if the rise in arterial carbon dioxide level results in respiratory acidosis, intubation and mechanical ventilation are required. Three general indications for endotracheal intubation and mechanical ventilation are unconsciousness, copious secretions that cannot be cleared by coughing, and severe hypoxemia or respiratory acidosis that does not respond promptly to lesser measures (Mitchell & Petty, 1982). Along with maintaining adequate ventilation, the underlying cause of the acute respiratory failure must be identified and treated.

Specific Nursing Measures

If the conservative approach to management is used in the treatment of respiratory failure, monitor the client carefully for signs and symptoms of hypoxia and hypercapnia. The COPD client who is difficult to arouse from sleep or is irritable may be exhibiting the symptoms of hypercapnia (Wade, 1982). Close monitoring of arterial blood gas values can also indicate any deterioration in the client's condition.

Besides monitoring the respiratory status, assess the client's cardiac status. Hypoxia, hypercapnia, and acidosis can lead to cardiac dysrhythmias and depressed myocardial contractility. Serum electrolyte values also require close monitoring (Sexton, 1982).

Be alert to the possibility of carbon dioxide narcosis, especially in those with COPD. CO_2 narcosis occurs when the level of carbon dioxide in the arterial blood becomes so high that it no longer is a stimulus to breathe. The stimulus to breathe then comes from low arterial levels of oxygen. Oxygen should be administered continuously, since any interruption in the flow can result in a drastic drop in the arterial oxygen level. On the other hand, administering a high flow of oxygen raises the arterial oxygen levels, so the client no longer has any hypoxemic stimulus to breathe. Respiratory arrest can occur.

Some clients may find it difficult to keep an oxygen mask on or may be aggravated by a nasal cannula. They may find the oxygen irritating to the mucous membranes of the nose or mouth, experience a feeling of suffocation, or simply be confused. It is important to use the proper comfort measures when these oxygen delivery devices are used. Explaining to the client why the mask or cannula must be worn may help elicit more cooperation.

Provide bronchial hygiene instruction. If clients cannot raise secretions effectively, tracheobronchial suctioning may be necessary (Sexton, 1982). If intubation and mechanical ventilation are required, the nurse's responsibilities expand to proper management of the endotracheal tube and care for clients who are mechanically ventilated (Chapter 18).

Psychological support for both clients and their families is important. Clients with acute respiratory failure are very ill, and many of the life-saving measures employed in their treatment are frightening.

Section IV: Neoplastic Disorders

Lung cancer, like other cancers, is the uncontrolled growth of abnormal cells. The origin and clinical characteristics of these malignant cell types differ, depending on where they originate. The World Health Organization (WHO) has classified pleuropulmonary neoplasms into 13 categories (Box 20–3). More than 90% of lung cancers belong to the group

Box 20–3 WHO Classification of Malignant Pleuropulmonary Neoplasms

I. Epidermoid carcinoma (squamous cell)

II. Small cell carcinoma (oat cell)

III. Adenocarcinoma
   - Bronchogenic
   - Bronchioloalveolar

IV. Large cell carcinoma

V. Combined epidermoid carcinoma and adenocarcinoma

VI. Carcinoid tumors

VII. Bronchial gland tumors
   - Cylindromas
   - Mucoepidermoid tumors

VIII. Papillary tumors of the surface epithelium

IX. "Mixed" tumors and carcinosarcomas

X. Sarcomas

XI. Unclassified

XII. Mesotheliomas

XIII. Melanomas

called bronchogenic carcinoma, meaning that the cancer originates in the bronchi or bronchioles.

According to the American Cancer Society, more than 25% of American cancer deaths are from cancer of the lung, which accounts for 5% of all deaths in this country (Jett, Cortese, & Fontana, 1983). Lung cancer is the leading cause of cancer death in men and women. The average age at onset is around 60 years. The incidence of lung cancer has increased in women because of increased smoking rates in women. Among cancers, the survival rate for lung cancer is one of the poorest because this disease is seldom detected early and tends to metastasize quickly.

Since lung cancer is among the most preventable of all diseases, nurses can do much to alert the public to avoid the primary cause of lung cancer, which is cigarette smoking. Also, nurses can encourage people who are at risk for lung cancer (those with a history of smoking for 20 or more years or with exposure to industrial substances such as asbestos), to have routine chest x-rays and sputum cytology studies. For those clients diagnosed as having lung cancer, the nurse can function as an important source of support both for the client and family.

A recent study in Minnesota (1985) reported that drinking more than five cups of coffee a day increased the risk of lung cancer. Smoking magnified the risk. Nurses should be alert to these possible health risks and watch the literature for conclusive studies.

BRONCHOGENIC CARCINOMA

Bronchogenic carcinoma, which accounts for 90% of all lung cancers, can be divided into four cytologic types: epidermoid carcinoma, small-cell carcinoma, adenocarcinoma, and large-cell carcinoma. Epidermoid carcinoma is the most common type, accounting for about 40%. Epidermoid carcinoma most often appears as a centrally located lesion and usually does not metastasize early. This type of carcinoma tends to grow into the lumen of the bronchi, causing obstruction leading to obstructive pneumonitis.

Small-cell carcinomas account for approximately 25% of the bronchogenic carcinomas. Of the four cell types, the small-cell carcinoma has the poorest prognosis because of its rapid growth rate and its tendency to metastasize early. It is also most often associated with ectopic hormone production, paraneoplastic syndromes, and metastasis to the central nervous system (Jett et al., 1983).

The adenocarcinomas account for approximately 25% of the lung cancers (Greco & Hande, 1982). This cell type tends to arise peripherally and is not associated with the major bronchi. The tumor may be quite large when discovered and appear as a pleural effusion. This cell type also has a tendency to spread to the central nervous system (Jett et al., 1983).

Large-cell cancers account for about 10% of lung cancer. This category includes lung neoplasms that do not exhibit the better defined patterns of the other cell types. These tumors tend to appear as large peripheral masses (Jett et al., 1983). It is important to note that any of the bronchogenic carcinomas may have features typical of the four common types.

Etiology

The increased incidence of lung cancer in this country is related to several factors, the most important being the inhalation of cigarette smoke. According to the American Lung Association, 1 in 10 heavy smokers will eventually get lung cancer. Other factors are related to the development of lung cancer, including atmospheric pollution and occupational exposures. Occupational factors, including exposure to coal tars and asbestos; mining of radioactive ores; and exposure to arsenic, nickel, iron-oxide, or chromium, have been documented as contributing to the development of lung cancer (Greco & Hande, 1982). Since everyone exposed to respiratory carcinogens does not develop lung cancer, certain host factors are believed to play a part in susceptibility (Carr, 1981). Lung cancer is more common in scarred and chronically diseased lungs.

Clinical Manifestations

Lung cancers are usually far along in their development before physical manifestations appear. The tumors have usually been present for a long time and may have metastasized. In general, signs and symptoms depend on the location and size of the primary tumor and whether metastasis is present (Greco & Hande, 1982). Localized symptoms of bronchogenic carcinoma can include cough or a change in a smoker's cough, dyspnea, hemoptysis, stridor

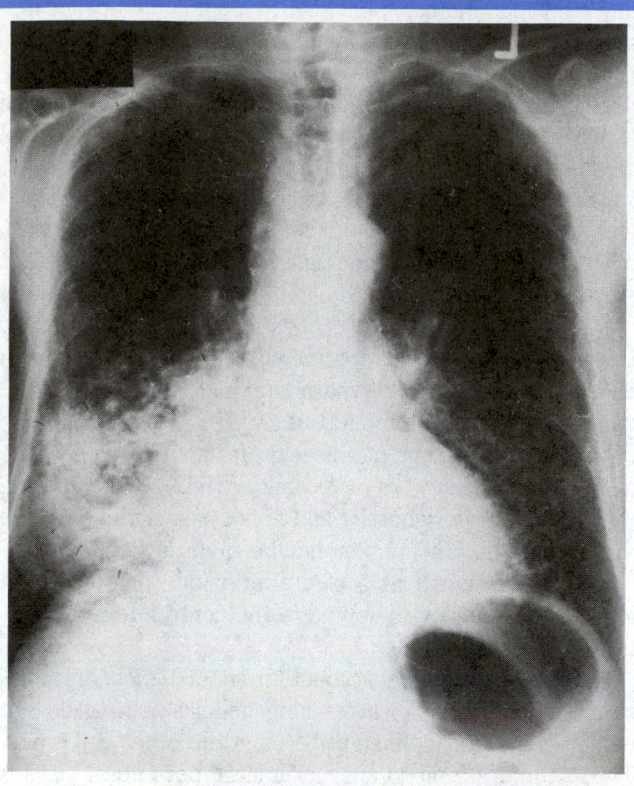

Figure 20–14

Chest x-ray of a male client with bronchogenic carcinoma of the right middle lobe. A normal gastric air bubble is evident on the lower left. (Courtesy of Health Care Plan, Buffalo, NY)

or wheeze, and signs of obstructive pneumonitis. Figure 20–14 shows a chest x-ray of a male client with bronchogenic carcinoma of the right middle lobe.

The effects of spread to adjacent thoracic structures may cause the client's initial symptoms. Clients may experience pain in the chest where the tumor impinges on nerves or where it is invading the chest wall or mediastinum. Left vocal-cord paralysis can result from involvement of the left recurrent laryngeal nerve. The spread of the tumor to the outside surface of the lung may cause accumulation of fluid, resulting in a pleural effusion (Figure 20–15), which can cause chest pain and difficulty in breathing. Invasion of the mediastinum may cause obstruction of the superior vena cava or the esophagus. Pericardial effusion with tamponade may also result from invasion of the cancer to the mediastinum or chest wall. Sometimes the initial symptoms may be associated with organs that are the primary sites of metastasis: the liver, brain, bones, kidneys, and adrenals (Carr, 1981).

Therapeutic Measures

A careful history and physical examination are important in establishing the diagnosis of lung cancer. The history and physical are followed by a chest x-ray. When neces-

sary, fluoroscopy, tomography, bronchoscopy, and angiography may be required to further define the nature and extent of involvement. The diagnosis of lung cancer requires histologic confirmation. Bronchoscopy may be carried out to locate the tumor, to obtain bronchial washings for sputum examination, or to take a biopsy specimen. Sputum cytology studies are done to test for the presence of cancer cells and identify the type. Bronchial brush biopsies, percutaneous needle biopsies, scalene lymph node biopsy, and mediastinoscopy may be carried out to diagnose or rule out metastasis. Bone marrow biopsy may also be performed to check for metastasis. An exploratory thoracotomy may be performed as a diagnostic test when the previous measures have failed to locate a suspected tumor or show the extent of a known one. This procedure is performed only when physicians are reasonably sure there is a possibility for a cure. Usually sputum cytology, bronchoscopy, mediastinoscopy, and percutaneous biopsy are effective in the histologic confirmation of lung cancer. Complete blood counts and routine blood chemistries should also be performed (Greco & Hande, 1982).

The treatment of lung cancer depends on the cell type, the stage of the cancer, and the client's general condition. Basically, lung cancer can be treated in three ways: surgery, radiation therapy, and chemotherapy. One or a combination of these methods may be used.

Surgery is used primarily to treat individuals for whom all diagnostic evidence suggests that the entire tumor can be removed surgically. The presence of distant or extrathoracic metastasis is a contraindication for surgery. Palliative resections are not advocated since symptoms can usually be alleviated by other treatment. A thoracentesis may be performed to relieve pain or shortness of breath caused by a collection of fluid in the pleural space due to metastasis of the tumor.

Many clients receive radiotherapy at some time during their illness. It may be used as definitive treatment for localized intrathoracic lung cancers, in combination with chemotherapy, postoperatively in combination with surgery, or as a palliative treatment.

Chemotherapy is frequently used in treating lung cancer either because metastasis is present on diagnosis or because it is expected. (Metastasis occurs in 90% of clients with lung cancer.) The small-cell cancers have been shown to be the most responsive to chemotherapy, and partial and complete remissions have been reported. The chemotherapeutic regimen usually involves administration of cyclophosphamide, methotrexate, vincristine, doxorubicin, and procarbazine in varying three or four drug combinations concurrently (Petersdorf, 1983).

Immunotherapy has been used in the past to see if it could help individuals by stimulating their natural immune system. Usually, bacillus Calmette-Guerin (BCG) or *Corynebacterium parvum* was used in clinical trials. The value of immunotherapy has not been confirmed, however, and it is currently recommended only as a part of carefully controlled research studies and not as a routine therapy.

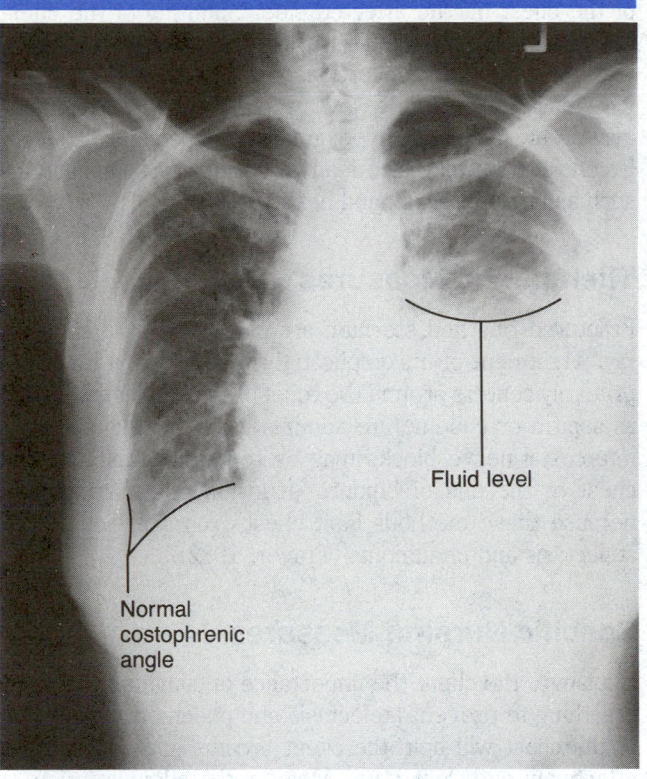

Figure 20–15

Chest x-ray of a female client with a left pleural effusion. Note the normal costophrenic angle (angle between the diaphragm and rib cage) on the right and the obliteration of the angle on the left. Also note the upward concavity of the fluid (effusion) level on the left. (Courtesy of Health Care Plan, Buffalo, NY)

Specific Nursing Measures

Clients and their families may react in many ways to the diagnosis of lung cancer. There may be feelings of shock and disbelief, anger, depression, and anxiety. The nurse can assist clients and their significant others to work out their feelings, giving support and guidance as needed. Clients and their families need to be educated about lung cancer. They need to understand the various diagnostic procedures and therapeutic interventions. The side effects associated with radiation and chemotherapy need to be explained.

Many of these clients will not survive. Clients need to know the reality of their situation so they can organize their affairs and plan for the time they have remaining. Nurses often need to encourage physicians to be honest and direct with clients and families about the prognosis, because false hope may prevent them from coping realistically with the situation. There is a fine line between hope and realism; health care professionals do not want to destroy the client's desire to live or motivation to fight. On the other hand, when only a miracle will help, the client and family need to know that, although miracles do happen, the situation is ominous.

Pain is a great concern of both clients and families. Whether the client is hospitalized or cared for in the home, pain management approaches need to be planned so clients are comfortable but not overly sedated when they prefer to be alert. At other times, heavy sedation will be a great relief. The nurse may have to take the initiative in developing the pain management approaches, based on observations of the client.

Good nutrition is important to help clients maintain their strength and prevent tissue breakdown. Adequate vitamins, minerals, protein, and calories are necessary, even though clients undergoing treatment often do not feel like eating. Families can help clients by learning new food selection and preparation ideas.

Medications may need to be ordered to relieve nausea. Good oral hygiene can help to improve the taste of food. Small and more frequent feedings are more readily tolerated. Supplemental vitamins and feedings may be necessary if the client's food intake is poor.

Section V: Traumatic Disorders

Chest trauma is an injury resulting from penetrating or blunt trauma to the chest. Penetrating chest injuries, also referred to as "open chest" trauma, result from penetration through the chest wall. Open chest trauma is caused by gunshot wounds, stab wounds, and wounds from other penetrating objects. Blunt chest trauma—nonpenetrating injury to the chest—is primarily caused by traffic accidents. Other causes include falls, blasts, explosions, and airplane crashes. Blunt chest trauma is by far the most common type of injury to the chest (Traver, 1982). Chest injuries may involve the bony framework of the chest, the heart, the great vessels, the lungs, or a combination of these. Damage to the liver and spleen are frequently associated with chest trauma.

Chest injuries are particularly hazardous because damage to the many vital structures contained in this area can be life threatening. In the United States, trauma is the third leading cause of death. Of the deaths resulting from trauma, approximately 75% involve chest injury (Traver, 1982).

General Nursing Implications

Chest trauma victims are frequently brought in with multiple injuries that present a serious challenge to nurses. Trauma victims are most often encountered first in the emergency room, where careful assessment skills are required to ascertain the extent of the injuries and the effects of these injuries on vital life structures. Trauma victims require close monitoring since the full extent of their injuries may not always be evident. When assessing a client with chest trauma, remember the ABCs ($+$C$+$C)—airway, breathing, circulation, cervical spine, and consciousness (Hoyt, 1983).

The airway may be obstructed by the tongue, secretions, blood, or injury to airway structures. Breathing in clients with chest trauma may be accompanied by pain, dyspnea, asymmetrical chest movement, paradoxical chest movement, a sucking sound, poor tidal volume, and symptoms of hypoxia or hypercapnia. (Cyanosis may be a later manifestation.) Circulation may be affected, detected by such signs as jugular venous distention, tachycardia, dysrhythmias, hypovolemic shock, and cardiogenic shock. Auscultation may reveal diminished or absent breath sounds on the affected side, respiratory stridor, crepitation, rales, muffled heart sounds, paradoxical pulse, and a narrow pulse pressure. Palpation may demonstrate subcutaneous emphysema, tenderness, or tracheal deviation. Percussion may detect dullness on the affected side, hyperresonance, or tympany (Hoyt, 1983). Expectorated secretions may be present. Always assume that a chest trauma victim has suffered a spinal cord injury until x-rays prove otherwise. Clients with chest trauma may be alert and oriented, comatose, or somewhere in between; if alert, they may be very apprehensive.

If the client has a penetrating chest wound and the instrument (eg, knife) is still in place, it should not be removed. In most situations, the instrument serves as a mechanical tampon for the lacerated vessels, and removing the instrument may result in hemorrhage (Kenner, Guzzetta, & Dossey, 1981). The control of pain is important. Analgesics may be ordered, and the nurse must evaluate for depressive respiratory side effects.

RIB OR STERNAL FRACTURES

Fractured ribs may pose few or many problems, depending on how many ribs are affected and whether there has been damage to the underlying tissue. A fractured sternum is usually not considered hazardous but, because of the amount of bone marrow in the sternum, there is some danger that the client may develop a fat embolism (Burrell & Burrell, 1982). Fractured ribs puncturing the wall of the trachea or bronchi, the aorta or other major blood vessels, or the heart can be a life-threatening emergency.

Fractured ribs and sternum are almost always caused by blunt chest injuries. Because the first and second ribs are relatively well protected, fractures of these ribs are usually associated with severe crushing injuries (Traver, 1982). Fractures of the fourth through eighth ribs are the most common.

Clinical Manifestations

With simple uncomplicated rib fractures, the client's only complaint may be pain, tenderness at the site, and splinting

of the chest on the affected side. Splinting of the chest because of pain can result in shallow breathing, leading to atelectasis, retained secretions, and pneumonia. In clients who minimize breathing, low ventilation-to-perfusion ratios may occur, leading to hypoxemia and hypercapnia as well. Fractured ribs may also lead to secondary complications such as pneumothorax and hemothorax.

Therapeutic Measures

Fractured ribs and sternum are diagnosed by a chest x-ray. Treatment of uncomplicated rib and sternal fractures primarily centers around the relief of pain. Analgesics such as aspirin or codeine are administered. In severe cases, intercostal nerve blocks may be required. Taping of the chest or the use of binders is no longer recommended because these methods limit chest excursion, leading to atelectasis and pneumonia (Traver, 1982).

Specific Nursing Measures

Explain to the client the importance of coughing and deep breathing to prevent atelectasis and pneumonia. Splinting of the chest will help the client breathe and cough more effectively with less pain. Monitor the administration of analgesics and watch for side effects, particularly respiratory depression. Also be alert for the possible complications of rib and sternal fractures.

FLAIL CHEST

A flail chest occurs when multiple adjacent rib fractures and/or costosternal separations result in "floating" of a segment of the rib cage (Kenner et al., 1981). Flail chest is the result of blunt trauma in which there is a crushing injury to the chest. The flail segment may occur anteriorly, laterally, or posteriorly. Posterior injuries occur less frequently because of the musculature and the protection afforded by the scapula (Traver, 1982).

Clinical Manifestations

A primary symptom of flail chest is the paradoxical motion of the chest wall during inspiration and expiration (Figure 20–16). The flail segment is pulled into the chest on inspiration because of the effect of the negative pleural pressure on the unstable segment. As the person exhales, the pleural pressure becomes more positive, and the flail segment moves outward. This can impair ventilation and lead to hypoxia, hypercapnia, and respiratory failure. A sternal flail, in which the sternum itself becomes free floating, can result in myocardial injury leading to heart failure (Kenner et al., 1981). The degree of dysfunction is now thought to depend more on underlying damage than the flail injury itself. Flail chest may also be accompanied by a pneumothorax, a hemothorax, or both.

Mediastinal structures may shift toward the uninjured

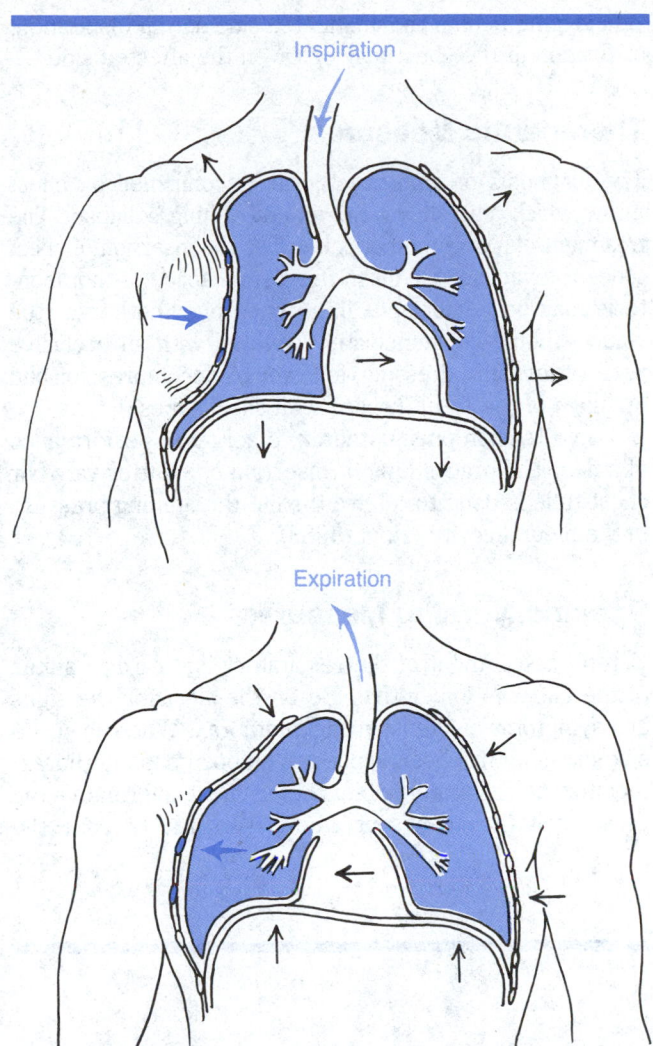

Figure 20-16

Flail chest. The blue large arrows indicate movement of the flail segment on inspiration and expiration after multiple rib fracture.

lung, compressing it and reducing the amount of ventilation the unaffected lung can provide. This mediastinal shift may also cause kinking and obstruction of major vessels.

Victims complain of pain, which tends to be severe, resulting in limited respiratory effort and an ineffective cough. Other manifestations include dyspnea, tachycardia, restlessness, and cyanosis (Burrell & Burrell, 1982).

Therapeutic Measures

As a first-aid measure, the flail segment can initially be stabilized by exerting firm but gentle pressure on the segment with the palm of the hand. Sandbags, a pressure dressing, or positioning the client on the affected side may be used as temporary measures or to treat milder injuries.

Supplemental oxygen and nerve blocks to decrease pain may also be employed.

If the client's ventilation becomes more severely compromised as reflected by hypoxemia and hypercapnia, however, the treatment of choice is intubation and mechanical ventilation. The positive pressure exerted by the ventilator causes internal stabilization of the flail segment and supports ventilation. Mechanical ventilation is usually continued only until the client can maintain adequate spontaneous ventilation and not until the flail segment has stabilized (Traver, 1982). The use of PEEP along with intermittent mandatory ventilation (IMV) has been shown to be advantageous in treating flail chest (Kenner et al., 1981).

Surgical intervention to stabilize the flail through fixation of the broken rib fragments is seldom used. Closed chest drainage may be necessary if a pneumothorax or hemothorax is present.

Specific Nursing Measures

Coughing and deep breathing are imperative to prevent atelectasis and pneumonia. Suctioning may be required. The client's level of pain needs to be assessed and the effect of analgesics monitored. Close observation of vital signs and level of consciousness as well as for additional respiratory or cardiac complications is necessary. Nursing care of the client who is intubated and on a ventilator is discussed in Chapter 18.

PNEUMOTHORAX

A pneumothorax occurs when there is a communication between the atmosphere and the pleural space, with resultant loss of the negative intrapleural pressure, causing partial or total collapse of the lung.

A pneumothorax can be open or closed. In an open pneumothorax, the injury creates an opening in the chest wall, allowing air to flow into the pleural cavity (Figure 20–17). The increased intrapleural pressure causes a partial or total collapse of the lung.

In closed pneumothorax, also called spontaneous pneumothorax, the chest wall remains intact, and air enters the pleural space from the lung surface (Figure 20–18). A closed pneumothorax may be caused by blunt chest trauma, in which a fractured rib pierces the lung, or from sudden compression of the thoracic cavity at the height of inspiration, with the glottis closed, causing rupture of the alveoli from excessive pressure (Hoyt, 1983). Pneumothorax can also be a complication of thoracentesis or CVP line insertion.

A spontaneous pneumothorax can also be caused by rupture of a bleb (a small vesicle) or a bulla (a large vesicle) on the lung surface, allowing air to leak from the lung into the pleural space. A bleb or a bulla may form from an infection or from congenital weakness in the lung tissue. Stress or strain, such as coughing or mechanical ventilation, can rupture the bleb or bulla (Woodin, 1982).

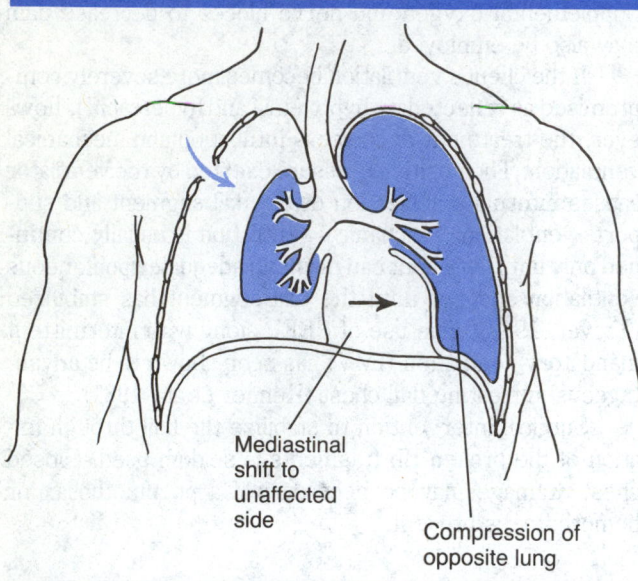

Figure 20–17

Open pneumothorax. An opening in the chest wall causes air to enter the pleural space, causing lung collapse and mediastinal shift to unaffected side.

Mediastinal shift to unaffected side

Compression of opposite lung

Clinical Manifestations

A client with a pneumothorax may complain of pain with breathing. Clients may also exhibit dyspnea, tachypnea, and unilateral diminished breath sounds. The respiratory movement on the affected side may be diminished or absent. In an open pneumothorax, a sucking sound may be heard near the wound. There may be hyperresonance on the affected side. Tachycardia and hypoxemia may be present along with cyanosis. There may be subcutaneous emphysema in the neck and upper chest.

A tension pneumothorax is a complication of either a closed or open pneumothorax. Air enters the pleural cavity during inspiration but is unable to escape during expiration because the wound creates a one-way valve. With each inspiratory cycle, the amount of air increases, causing progressive compression of the lung. The high intrathoracic pressure on the affected side causes pressure on the mediastinum, resulting in a shift of the mediastinum (along with the heart, trachea, esophagus, and great vessels) to the unaffected side. This *mediastinal shift* compresses the unaffected lung, decreasing ventilation. Distortion of the vena cava impairs venous return to the heart with a resultant decrease in cardiac output. These abnormalities can lead to hypoxia, hypercapnia, and acidosis. Symptoms include marked dyspnea, severe chest pain, restlessness, agitation, cyanosis, intercostal retraction, nasal flaring, and tachycardia. Jugular vein distention may be present. Subcutaneous emphysema may occur (Traver, 1982). There may be asymmetrical chest movement, with the affected

side lagging behind the unaffected side during inspiration, or fixation of the chest may occur on the affected side.

Therapeutic Measures

The diagnosis of a pneumothorax is confirmed by chest x-ray, which also shows the extent of lung collapse. The treatment of a pneumothorax involves the insertion of chest tubes to evacuate the air in the pleural space; a thoracentesis may be performed. In an open pneumothorax, the wound should be immediately covered with an occlusive petrolatum gauze dressing, followed by decompression and drainage of the pleural space with chest tubes.

In a tension pneumothorax, emergency performance of a needle thoracostomy or insertion of a flutter valve or chest tube is done to relieve the life-threatening pressure in the pleural cavity (Hoyt, 1983).

Specific Nursing Measures

Careful assessment of the respiratory and cardiac status of the client is imperative. Be on the alert for the signs and symptoms of a tension pneumothorax. When an occlusive dressing has been applied to an open pneumothorax, monitor the respiratory status of the client and remove the dressing if the client's breathing worsens, because the

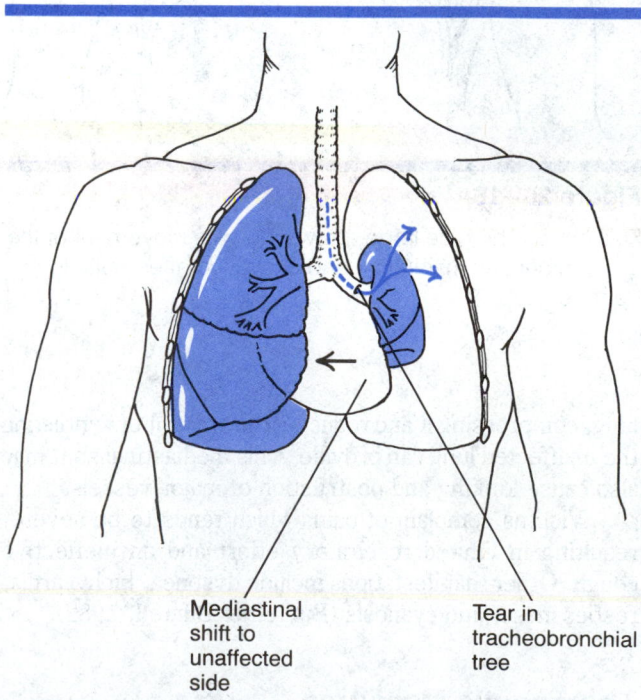

Mediastinal shift to unaffected side

Tear in tracheobronchial tree

Figure 20–18

Closed pneumothorax. Tear in tracheobronchial tree allows air to enter pleural space, causing lung collapse and mediastinal shift to unaffected side.

dressing may be creating a tension pneumothorax. Positioning the client in a semi-Fowler's position may facilitate breathing. Deep breathing and coughing must be encouraged. In penetrating injuries, be alert to the possibility of infection introduced by the penetrating object. Be prepared to assist the physician in a thoracostomy and insertion of chest tubes. Nursing care of a client with chest tubes is discussed in Chapter 18.

Teach clients with a history of spontaneous pneumothorax to avoid scuba diving and flying in unpressurized aircraft at high altitudes. A case study of a client with pneumothorax is presented at the end of this chapter.

HEMOTHORAX

A hemothorax is the accumulation of blood in the pleural space. The usual sources of bleeding in a hemothorax are the pulmonary parenchyma and vessels, the intercostal and internal mammary arteries, the heart, the aorta and great vessels, and the liver and spleen (Kenner et al., 1981).

A hemothorax may result from either blunt or penetrating trauma to the chest, but it is more common in penetrating trauma. A hemothorax should be considered in severe blunt or decelerating accidents (such as car crashes), which can result in ruptured intrathoracic vessels and cause aortic tears (Kenner et al., 1981). Fractured ribs caused by blunt trauma are commonly responsible for lacerations leading to a hemothorax.

Clinical Manifestations

Signs and symptoms depend on the source and the amount of accumulated blood loss. A hemothorax may result not only in respiratory and cardiac impairments but also in hypovolemic shock if large amounts of blood are lost. The total accumulation of blood can range from less than 300 mL in a small hemothorax to over 1500 mL in a severe hemothorax. In a small hemothorax, the client may be asymptomatic. In more severe bleeding, partial or total lung collapse may occur as blood accumulates in the pleural cavity. There may be increasing dyspnea, asymmetric chest movement, chest tightness, ecchymosis over the affected lung, and hemoptysis (Hoyt, 1983). Dullness and decreased breath sounds can be present, and there may be a mediastinal shift to the unaffected side. Tachycardia, restlessness, hypotension, and hypovolemic shock may occur.

Therapeutic and Specific Nursing Measures

A chest x-ray will confirm the diagnosis, showing accumulation of fluid in dependent areas and the amount of lung collapse. Clients with a small hemothorax may require no treatment because of the absorptive power of the pleura (Traver, 1982). In symptomatic cases, a thoracentesis may be performed initially. Chest tube drainage is the most

effective means of treating a hemothorax. Replacement of lost blood volume is indicated. A thoracotomy may be necessary in cases where there is a large amount of recurrent bleeding.

The nursing measures are comparable to those for pneumothorax. The emphasis is on monitoring for hypovolemic shock and carrying out fluid and blood replacement therapy.

TRACHEOBRONCHIAL INJURIES

Tracheobronchial injuries are small lacerations, tears, or ruptures of the trachea and bronchi caused by trauma. These types of injuries are rare, but when they do occur, mortality is approximately 30% (Traver, 1982).

Tracheobronchial injuries can result from blunt or penetrating chest trauma. In blunt trauma, the damage occurs when the anteroposterior diameter of the chest narrows suddenly while the transverse diameter simultaneously expands, exerting a shearing force on the trachea, bronchi, or both (Hoyt, 1983). This may occur during a crash when a driver hits the steering wheel. Penetrating chest trauma, such as that caused by a bullet or knife, can also damage the trachea and bronchi.

Clinical Manifestations

This type of injury should be suspected when a persistent air leak is not controlled by chest tubes and there are deep cervical emphysema or extensive mediastinal emphysema, massive dyspnea, hemoptysis, and stridor due to an obstructed airway from blood or secretions. Fractures of the upper thoracic ribs may be another indication of a ruptured bronchus. A pneumothorax or mediastinal emphysema may be the only indication of a ruptured airway. Tracheal rupture frequently results in death before the victim reaches the hospital (Kenner et al., 1981).

Therapeutic Measures

If a ruptured airway is suspected, an endoscopic examination with a fiberoptic bronchoscope is indicated to locate the injury and make a positive diagnosis. A chest x-ray may also show air surrounding a bronchus.

Endotracheal intubation or a tracheostomy may have to be performed, depending on the degree of impairment in ventilation. Surgery is then required to repair the rupture.

Specific Nursing Measures

If possible, the client should be placed in a high Fowler's position to facilitate breathing. Monitor the client's ventilation and other vital signs closely. Be prepared for the possibility of emergency intubation. Once the airway has been established, prepare the client for chest surgery (Hoyt, 1983).

PULMONARY CONTUSION

Crushing and bruising of the lung parenchyma are referred to as contusion. This injury can occur with or without rib or sternal fractures.

A sudden blow to the chest causing compression of the thoracic cavity and lung followed by an equally sudden decompression can result in pulmonary contusion (Hoyt, 1983). This type of parenchymal injury most frequently occurs as a result of blunt chest trauma. It can occur as a result of penetrating trauma, but this is not as common.

Clinical Manifestations

The injury results in extravasation of blood into the lung parenchyma. Depending on the extent of the injury, there may be intra-alveolar destruction, hemorrhage, and interstitial edema. With an increased accumulation of fluid and cellular debris, there are a progression of atelectasis and a decrease in lung compliance. A low ventilation-to-perfusion ratio can occur, leading to hypoxemia. With extensive lung contusion, hypoventilation may develop. The client may exhibit such external symptoms as dyspnea, cough, hemoptysis, increasing hyperpnea, tachypnea, and restlessness. Breath sounds may be decreased, and rales

may be present. In a mild pulmonary contusion, few or no symptoms develop (Traver, 1982).

Therapeutic Measures

The specific treatment for a lung contusion depends on the extent of the damage. In mild contusions, clients are treated with supplemental oxygen and closely monitored. Because lung contusions can result in the development of septicemia, broad-spectrum antibiotic coverage is initiated. Fluid must be restricted because there is damage to the pulmonary capillaries, and administration of large amounts of fluids can cause pulmonary fluid overload. In more severe contusions, where hypoxemia cannot be corrected or there is hypoventilation, and client may have to be intubated and placed on a ventilator.

Specific Nursing Measures

When possible, the client should be placed in a high Fowler's position to facilitate breathing. Careful monitoring of respiratory status and vital signs is necessary. Clients should be instructed to cough and deep breathe. Tracheal suctioning may be required.

Chapter Highlights

Occupational lung diseases are preventable; nevertheless, they continue to affect a great many people, causing physical disability, lost earnings, suffering, and death.

Adult respiratory distress syndrome is associated with increased fluid in the lung. It can be caused by acute pulmonary infections, aspiration, inhalation of toxins and irritants, overdoses of drugs, and trauma, to name a few.

Pneumonias, which can be community or hospital acquired, are the fifth leading cause of death in the United States.

Nurses play a significant part in the prevention of nosocomial or hospital-acquired pneumonias.

Tuberculosis, although not the dreaded disease it once was, still can evoke feelings of fear in those affected and their families.

Client teaching regarding tuberculosis should stress that strict adherence to a prolonged treatment with antituberculosis drugs is necessary to cure the disease.

Fungal infections of the lungs result from inhalation of nonmotile yeasts or molds; these infections do not spread from person to person.

The prevalence and death rate from chronic obstructive pulmonary disease (COPD) has increased markedly in recent years.

The most common diseases associated with COPD are chronic bronchitis and emphysema. Asthma, bronchiectasis, and cystic fibrosis are also included under this category.

Pulmonary rehabilitation programs, which encompass client teaching, respiratory hygiene measures, and conditioning exercises, form the cornerstone of intervention for COPD clients.

Lung cancer in this country is increasing at a greater rate in women.

Nursing interventions for clients with lung cancer center around helping them to cope with their diagnosis and treatment and to live as productive and fulfilling lives as their condition allows.

Acute respiratory failure is a life-threatening condition that occurs because of the lungs' inability to maintain adequate oxygenation of the blood.

Nursing intervention for victims of chest trauma centers around assessment of the airway, breathing, circulation, cervical spine, and level of consciousness.

Clients with elevated arterial carbon dioxide levels and low arterial oxygen levels are stimulated to breathe by the hypoxemia. Administration of high liter flows of oxygen can eliminate this hypoxemic drive to breathe, resulting in respiratory arrest.

In penetrating chest wounds when the instrument is still in place, it should remain in place until surgery; hemorrhage may result if it is removed.

Bibliography

American Cancer Society: *Cancer Facts and Figures*. New York: American Cancer Society, 1985.

American Lung Association: *Occupational Disease: An Introduction*. New York: American Lung Association, 1983.

Bayer A: Fungal pneumonias: Pulmonary coccidioidal syndromes. Part 1. *Chest* 1981; 79:575–583.

Burrell LO, Burrell Z Jr: *Critical Care*. St. Louis: Mosby, 1982.

Cancer facts and figures. *Occup Health Nurs* (July) 1982; 30:42–43.

Catanzaro A: Pulmonary coccidioidomycosis. *Med Clin North Am* (May) 1980; 64:461–473.

Cline B, Fisher M: A.R.D.S. means emergency. *Nurs 82* (Feb) 1982; 12:62–67.

Cohen R: Occupational lung disease: Pneumoconiosis. *Occup Health Nurs* (April) 1981; 29:10–13.

Cordes L, Fraser D: Legionellosis: Legionnaires' disease, Pontiac fever. *Med Clin North Am* (May) 1980; 64:395–416.

D'Agostino J: Teaching tips for living with COPD at home. *Nurs 84* (Feb) 1984; 14:57.

D'Agostino J: You can breath new life into your COPD patients. *Nurs 83* (Sept) 1983; 13:72–77.

Daniele R: Sarcoidosis: Diagnosis and management. *Hosp Pract* (June) 1983; 18:113–122.

Devereux P, Goldstein E: Legionnaires' disease: Finding answers to the riddle. *Am J Nurs* 1980; 80:81–85.

Diethorn M: Prevention of sensory deprivation for the COPD victim's spouse. *Top Clin Nurs* 1985; 6(4):64–71.

Einstein H: Coccidioidomycosis. *Respiratory Care* (June) 1981; 26:563–569.

Fishman A: *Pulmonary Diseases and Disorders*. New York: McGraw-Hill, 1980.

Gentry L: Pneumonia and bronchitis: Causes, diagnosis, and treatment. *Consultant* (March) 1980; 20:161–165.

George R, Light R, Matthay R (editors): *Chest Medicine*. New York: Churchill Livingstone, 1983.

Gibbs CJ, Coutts II, Rock R, Finnigan OC, White RJ: Premenstrual exacerbation of asthma. *Thorax* (Nov) 1984; 39(11): 833–836.

Glassroth J: Tuberculosis: A review for clinicians. *Clinical Notes on Respiratory Diseases* (Fall) 1981; 20:5–13.

Gracey D: *Pulmonary Disease in the Adult*. Chicago: Year Book Medical Publishers, 1981.

Greco FA, Hande K: *Lung Cancer Management: Progress and Prospects*. Wayne, NJ: Lederle Laboratories, 1982.

Griffin F: Rational antibiotic selection for pneumonia. *Consultant* (Jan) 1981; 21:47–57.

Harper R: *A Guide to Respiratory Care: Physiology and Clinical Applications*. Philadelphia: Lippincott, 1981.

Hinshaw H, Murray J: *Diseases of the Chest*. Philadelphia: Saunders, 1980.

Hoyt S: Chest trauma: When the patient looks bad, act fast. When he looks good, act fast. *Nurs 83* (May) 1983; 13:34–41.

Hudak C, Lohr T, Gallo B (editors): *Critical Care Nursing*. Philadelphia: Lippincott, 1982.

Jett J, Cortese D, Fontana R: Lung cancer: Current concepts and prospects. *CA* 1983; 33:74–85.

Johanson WG Jr, Harris G: Aspiration pneumonia, anaerobic infections and lung abscess. *Med Clin North Am* (May) 1980; 64:385–394.

Keller C, Solomon J, Reyes V: *Respiratory Nursing Care*. Englewood Cliffs, NJ: Prentice-Hall, 1984.

Kenner C, Guzzetta C, Dossey B: *Critical Care Nursing: Body-Mind-Spirit*. Boston: Little, Brown, 1981.

Macher A: Histoplasmosis and blastomycosis. *Med Clin North Am* (May) 1980; 64:459–477.

Mitchell R, Petty T (editors): *Synopsis of Clinical Pulmonary Disease*. St. Louis: Mosby, 1982.

Murray H, Tuazon C: Atypical pneumonias. *Med Clin North Am* (May) 1980; 64:507–527.

Oregon Thoracic Society. *Chronic Obstructive Pulmonary Disease*. New York: American Lung Association, 1981.

Petersdorf RG et al: *Harrison's Principles of Internal Medicine*, 19th ed. New York: McGraw-Hill, 1983.

Petty TL: *Intensive and Rehabilitative Respiratory Care*. Philadelphia: Lea & Febiger, 1982.

Putnam J, Tuazon C: Forward. *Med Clin North Am* (May) 1980; 64:317.

Raffin T, Roberts P: The prevention and treatment of status asthmaticus. *Hosp Pract* (Feb) 1982; 17:80A–80Z-6.

Reichman R, Dolin R: Viral pneumonias. *Med Clin North Am* (May) 1980; 64:491–506.

Reyes M: The aerobic gram-negative bacillary pneumonias. *Med Clin North Am* (May) 1980; 64:363–383.

Ryan MA: Pneumonia: Aggressive treatment is the key. *RN* (Aug) 1982; 45:44–50.

Sbarbaro J: Tuberculosis. *Med Clin North Am* (May) 1980; 64:417–431.

Sexton D: *Chronic Obstructive Pulmonary Disease: Care of the Child and Adult*. St. Louis: Mosby, 1981.

Sexton DL, Munro BH: Impact of a husband's chronic illness

(COPD) on the spouse's life. *Res Nurs Health* (March) 1985; 8(1):83–90.

Spires R: Tuberculosis today: The siege isn't over yet. *RN* (Aug) 1980; 43:43–47.

Stockdale-Wooley R: Sexual dysfunction and COPD: Problems and management. *Nurse Pract* (Feb) 1983; 8:16–18.

Tellis C, Putnam J: Pulmonary disease caused by nontuberculosis mycobacteria. *Med Clin North Am* (May) 1980; 64:433–446.

Traver G: *Respiratory Nursing: The Science and the Art.* New York: Wiley, 1982.

Tuazon C: Gram-positive pneumonias. *Med Clin North Am* (May) 1980; 64:343–361.

Wade J: *Comprehensive Respiratory Care: Physiology and Technique.* St. Louis: Mosby, 1982.

Weill H: Occupational lung disease. *Hosp Pract* (April) 1981; 16:65–80.

Wiley L: Adult respiratory distress syndrome: A true test of nursing skills. *Nurs 80* (May) 1980; 10:51–56.

Woodin L: Your patient with a pneumothorax: A patient in distress. *Nurs 82* (Nov) 1982; 12:50–56.

Suggested Readings

Anderson SJ: Sarcoidosis: A multisystem disease. *Am J Nurs* (Oct) 1982; 82:1566–1569. Comprehensive, up-to-date description of the pathophysiology of sarcoidosis and the appropriate nursing interventions.

Cohen R: Occupational lung disease: Pneumoconiosis. *Occup Health Nurs* (April) 1981; 29:10–13. Concise presentation of the diseases of the lung caused by inorganic dust. Causes, symptomatology, and treatment are addressed.

Hoyt S: Chest trauma—When the patient looks bad, act fast, when he looks good act fast. *Nurs 83* (May) 1983; 13:34–41. Very comprehensive article on the various types of injuries that can occur due to chest trauma, their clinical manifestations, and nursing interventions. Case studies are presented.

Krokosky NJ: Black lung and silicosis. *Am J Nurs* 1985; 85(8):883–886. The author reviews the diagnosis, prevention, and treatment of black lung disease. Worker's compensation and sources of help for dust-related breathing problems are discussed.

The Client With a Pneumothorax

I. Descriptive Data

John Armstrong, age 21, is brought to the College Health Service directly from a soccer practice. While playing, he was accidentally kicked in the left chest. Shortly thereafter, he developed pain in the left chest and became short of breath.

II. Personal Data

Date and Time:	April 4, 1986, 2:30 PM
Full Name:	John David Armstrong
ID Number:	000-00-0000
Local Address:	Kimball Hall 916
Home Address:	50 Cherry St., Long Island, NY
Telephone:	Local: 000-0000
	Parents: 000-000-0000
Sex:	Male
Age:	21
Birthdate:	2-26-65
Marital Status:	Single
Race/Culture:	Caucasian/American
Religion:	Roman Catholic
Occupation:	College student
Usual Health Care Provider:	Harvey Stone, MD, New York City

III. Health History

Source of Information:	Client and soccer coach
Reliability of Informants:	Reliable
Chief Concern:	Stabbing pains in the left side of his chest and shortness of breath
History of Present Illness:	Today during a routine soccer practice, John was accidentally kicked in the left lower chest area by a teammate; he experienced pain in the area and began to have difficulty breathing almost immediately, which has become progressively worse. He has had no prior breathing difficulties, doesn't smoke, has not had a recent URI, takes no medications. He has been in good health all his life; was hospitalized once for an appendectomy at age 14; is allergic to penicillin—reacts with hives.

Past Health History:

Childhood:	Chickenpox; bronchitis, age 4
Immunizations:	Last Td 1983; had all childhood immunizations
Medical Problems:	None
Surgeries:	Appendectomy, age 14
Special Diagnostic Procedures:	None
Trauma:	None
Allergies:	Penicillin (hives)
Medications:	None

(continued)

Case Study written by Yvonne Krall Scherer.

The Client With a Pneumothorax

Family History:

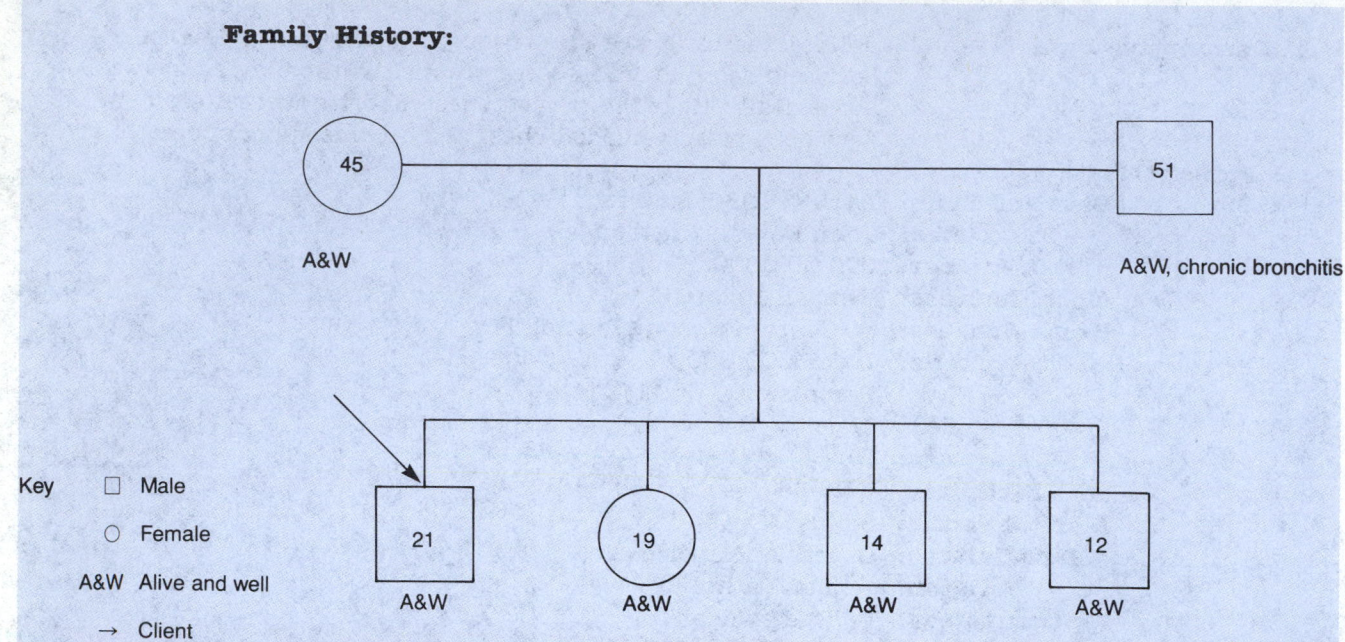

Key
☐ Male
○ Female
A&W Alive and well
→ Client

Personal/Social History: No ⊕ FHx of DM, MI, ↑ BP, CVA, TBC, or cancer
John is a full-time student majoring in business administration; currently a junior, maintains a B+ average; his tuition is paid by his parents; he has a student loan and works two part-time jobs at a hardware store and a gas station to help pay for his college expenses; he enjoys school and has many friends including a special girlfriend; he maintains good relationships with his parents and siblings; he sees them on holidays and returns home each summer.

Habits: Appetite is good, mainly eats in college cafeteria; likes sub sandwiches, hamburgers, pizza; eats fruits but a minimal amount of vegetables; drinks beer mainly on weekends (5 to 6 bottles); does not use any drugs; tried cigarettes as a teenager but decided not to smoke because of enjoyment of sports and the advice of his father who is a heavy cigarette smoker and has chronic bronchitis; gets approximately 6 h of sleep per night; not bothered by insomnia; frequent exercise (jogging, swimming, tennis, soccer).

Sexually active with girlfriend whom he says he will probably marry; uses condoms for birth control; is Catholic but does not go to church on a routine basis; girlfriend is Jewish; copes with stresses of college life by actively engaging in sports and talking with his male friends and girlfriend.

Review of Systems: States general health is excellent
Skin: No problems with acne
EENT: Vision and hearing excellent; infrequent URIs
Chest: See HPI

Heart:	No hx of (m) , no DOE, no ankle edema, no chest pain except for current injury
Gastrointestinal:	No n & v, no food intolerance, daily BM without problems, stool brown in color
Genitourinary:	No hx of hernia, no dysuria, no pain with intercourse
Musculoskeletal:	No hx of fractures, no trauma except for current injury
Psychosocial:	Feels good about his life and his potential; no suicidal thoughts

IV. Physical Assessment

Height:	6 ft 1 in
Weight:	165 lb
Vital Signs:	Temp. 99.8°F (37°C), P. 120 (regular), R. 40 (labored), BP 120/60 (RA) seated
Skin:	Erythematous, ecchymotic golf-ball size lesion in left anterior lower chest
Eyes:	PERRLA
Ears:	Both TMs obscured by cerumen
Mouth/Throat:	Teeth in good repair; no lesions
Neck:	Full ROM; no lymphadenopathy; thyroid not enlarged; no bruits
Chest:	Labored breathing with retraction of the intercostal spaces, neck, and chest muscles; asymmetrical chest movement with poor expansion left chest; no evidence of subcutaneous emphysema; trachea slightly deviated to the right; pain and tenderness felt at level of left fifth and sixth rib anteriorly; hyperresonant on the left; decrease in tactile fremitus; no evidence of crepitus; absent breath sounds in the left lower lobe region; diminished breath sounds heard in the upper lobe of the left lung
Cardiovascular:	Apical rate 120; regular s̄ (m) or gallop; S_1, S_2 nl; pedal pulses 3+ and symmetrical; no jugular venous distention
Abdominal:	Flat, muscular; RLQ appendectomy scar; normoactive bowel sounds; ō bruits; nontender s̄ masses; liver palpable 1 cm below rt. CM - 9 cm by percussion
Genitourinary:	Normal, circumcised male; testes without masses
Rectal:	Normal prostate without nodules; no hemorrhoids; stool occult blood test negative
Musculoskeletal:	Joints nl; full ROM; no cyanosis, clubbing or edema
Neurological:	Cranial nerves II through XII grossly intact; DTRs 2+ and symmetrical; normal motor and vibratory sense
Psychological:	Somewhat anxious and restless due to pain and shortness of breath

V. Diagnostic Data

	Chest x-ray revealed single fractures of the fifth and sixth ribs, left anterior chest; a lowering of the diaphragm on the left; air in the left pleural space; and an 85% collapse of the lung on the left.
Diagnosis:	Closed pneumothorax secondary to punctured left lung from fractured ribs

VI. Medical Regimen

- Insertion of chest tube between the second and third anterior intercostal space
- Oxygen at 28% via nasal cannula
- Codeine 60 mg q.4h. p.r.n. for chest pain
- Repeat chest x-ray
- Arterial blood gases
- CBC

(continued)

The Client With a Pneumothorax

VII. Nursing Care Plan

Nursing Diagnosis	Client Care Goals	Plan/Nursing Implementation	Expected Outcome
Breathing pattern, ineffective: related to inadequate chest expansion secondary to pneumothorax	Maintain ventilation of normal depth with symmetrical chest expansion	Prepare client for chest tube insertion: inform client of the reason for chest tube insertion; answer questions client may have; administer pain medication as ordered; request it if not ordered. Gather equipment for chest tube insertion: • Local anesthetic • Antiseptic solution • Sterile gloves • Suture material • Collection setup • Chest tube • Tape and petrolatum gauze • Thoracotomy tray	Client is prepared for chest tube insertion as evidenced by decrease in anxiety level; understanding and verbalization of reason for chest tube insertion; cooperation during chest tube insertion; decrease in pain
	Reduction of anxiety level	Assist MD with insertion of the chest tube. Monitor for correct functioning of chest tube drainage system: fluctuation in the water seal chamber; inspect drainage tubing for dependent loops or kinks; observe suction control chamber for bubbling and correct suction pressure; assess and record chest tube drainage q.h. (amount, color); milk or strip chest tube as ordered; assess respiratory status including rate, depth, quality of respirations; observe for symmetrical chest expansion and use of accessory muscles; auscultate lung fields	Chest tube functions correctly as evidenced by improvement in client condition such as: improvement in breathing; chest expansion symmetrical; increased aeration of affected lung; decrease in anxiety; chest x-ray shows reexpansion of lung; vital signs normal; blood gases return to normal
	Remain free of complications that can result from pneumothorax	Note signs and symptoms that may indicate respiratory complications, especially a tension pneumothorax, hemothorax, and infection. Observe for: severe pain with breathing; dyspnea; stridor; use of accessory muscles; asymmetric chest movement; jugular vein distention; tracheal deviation; paradoxical breathing; hyperresonance or dullness to	Absence of complications as evidenced by: normal breath sounds, normal chest x-ray, normal arterial blood gas values; vital signs within normal limits

Nursing Diagnosis	Client Care Goals	Plan/Nursing Implementation	Expected Outcome
		percussion; continued absence of breath sounds on the affected side; adventitious breath sounds (rales, rhonchi, friction rub); chest tube drainage that is straw-colored or purulent; signs and symptoms of hypoxemia or hypercapnia; abnormal vital signs (increased pulse, respiratory rate, and elevated temperature); increased anxiety or other behavior changes	
	Tolerate pain upon breathing within reasonable limits	Assess client for location, type, and intensity of pain: provide comfort measures—positioning (semi-Fowler's), splinting when coughing and deep breathing; administer analgesics as prescribed; assess respiratory rate after administration of narcotic analgesic	Pain sensation remains within tolerable limits as indicated by client's verbalization or vital signs
	Understand and be able to perform measures to improve respiratory status and prevent complications	Explain importance of deep breathing and coughing exercises q. 1–2 hr: demonstrate deep breathing and coughing exercises; assist client in carrying out these pulmonary hygiene measures; when acute symptoms have been relieved, assist client to sit in a chair and to ambulate	Client and significant others will verbalize reasons for and correctly carry out measures to improve respiratory status
Gas exchange, impaired: related to hypoxemia from impairment in ventilation and diffusion caused by the pneumothorax	Maintain adequate oxygenation for cellular metabolism	Observe for signs and symptoms of hypoxemia: restlessness; irritability; impaired judgment; central cyanosis; labored breathing; tachypnea; tachycardia; fluctuation in blood pressure; alteration in level of consciousness	Absence of signs and symptoms of cerebral, respiratory, and cardiovascular hypoxemia Arterial PO_2 normal
		Administration of supplemental oxygen as ordered (28% FIO_2 via nasal cannula); explain reason for oxygen administration to client and significant others; answer questions client and significant others have about oxygen administration	Client and significant others verbalize an understanding of and comply with supplemental oxygen delivery No evidence of nasal irritation or skin breakdown caused by nasal prongs
	Sustain client comfort during O_2 administration	Employ comfort measures necessary with oxygen administration such as:	No evidence of irritation behind ears Client verbalizes that

The Client With a Pneumothorax

VII. Nursing Care Plan *(continued)*

Nursing Diagnosis	Client Care Goals	Plan/Nursing Implementation	Expected Outcome
		humidify oxygen delivered to client, observe for irritation of nasal mucosa caused by nasal prongs, water-soluble lubricant to nasal opening, check for irritation behind ears, provide padding (4 × 3 gauze) behind ears if client is bothered by elastic straps used to anchor nasal cannula, carry out nursing measures involved with chest tubes and pulmonary hygiene measures as outlined under ineffective breathing pattern	oxygen delivery is comfortable
Gas exchange, impaired: related to respiratory alkalosis from hypocapnia caused by hyperventilation	Maintain PCO_2 level compatible with a normal pH	Observe for signs and symptoms of hypocapnia: muscle spasm, carpopedal spasm, tetany, diaphoresis, tachypnea, alteration in level of consciousness	
		Employ measures to slow client's respiratory rate: assist with insertion of chest tube, reassure and explain, administer pain medication as ordered, assist client to breathe more efficiently via breathing exercises	Absence of signs and symptoms of cerebral, respiratory, and cardiovascular hypocapnia; return of arterial blood gases to normal
Anxiety, related to inability to breathe effectively	Reduction of client's anxiety level to within tolerable limits	Carefully prepare client and significant others for procedures; maintain a calm, relaxed manner when interacting with client or significant others; offer reassurance; allow client and significant others to verbalize questions and concerns; carry out measures to alleviate respiratory distress: monitor functioning of chest tube, administer O_2 as ordered, position client in semi-Fowler's, carry out pulmonary hygiene measures, administer analgesics for pain	Anxiety remains within tolerable limits as evidenced by: client's verbalization, stable vital signs, nursing observation

Nursing Diagnosis	Client Care Goals	Plan/Nursing Implementation	Expected Outcome
Powerlessness	Regain independence and full control over his life	Encourage client when condition permits to become an active participant in own care; encourage client to participate in goal setting; encourage verbalization of concerns over disruption of studies, athletics, etc; begin plans for discharge as soon as condition warrants: when client can return to school, when client can resume sports, when client can return to work	Client becomes an active participant in own care Client verbalizes concerns over temporary loss of independence

Chapter 21

Surgical Approaches to Respiratory Dysfunction

Vicky Hartwell-Ivins

Objectives

When you have finished studying this chapter, you should be able to:

Define and describe the surgical procedures presented involving the nose, paranasal sinuses, pharynx, trachea, larynx, neck, and lungs.

Discuss the physiological and psychosocial/lifestyle implications of each surgical procedure for the client.

Specify the nursing implications for each procedure, including preoperative care, postoperative care, and discharge teaching.

Explain the complications of head and neck surgery and the related nursing interventions.

Explain the complications of thoracic surgery and the related nursing interventions.

Educate clients and their significant others about the specific surgical procedures presented in this chapter.

Clients who undergo surgery of the respiratory system are often very ill and very frightened. Their breathing may be compromised, they may be in pain, and they may be anxious. They, and their families and friends, often require a great deal of teaching, support, and encouragement to cope with the enormous alterations in lifestyle faced by some. To be effective, the nurse who cares for these clients must blend technical competence and human sensitivity.

Section I: Surgical Approaches to Disorders Affecting the Nose

Client and nursing implications are similar for most types of nasal surgery and are discussed in detail under the first procedure. Complications of head and neck surgery are specified with each surgical procedure. In addition, Table 21–3 later in this chapter describes complications common to all head and neck surgeries. Surgery of the nose can be performed under local or general anesthesia, depending on the preference of the surgeon and client. Local anesthesia consists of topical or injectable medication, or both.

This is often accompanied by the administration of a sedative and an analgesic.

SUBMUCOUS RESECTION OF THE NASAL SEPTUM

A submucous resection (SMR) is a procedure to correct a deviated nasal septum. An incision is made through the mucosa of the nose to remove cartilage or bone in an effort to correct the abnormality.

A deviated nasal septum is common among the general population; relatively few require surgical correction. The five major indications for a submucous resection are:

- Nasal obstruction by a deviated septum (the most common indication).
- Obstruction of the drainage of one of the paranasal sinuses.
- To allow better access to the site of bleeding during epistaxis from the posterior area of the nose.
- To allow better access to the nose and sinuses when inspecting or treating polyps, enlarged turbinates, or tumors or removing a rhinolith.
- Correction of the nasal septum for cosmetic reasons (perhaps in conjunction with a rhinoplasty).

Surgical Procedure

This procedure may be done with the client in a sitting or reclining position. Local anesthesia is accompanied by less bleeding than general anesthesia because local anesthetic also has a vasoconstricting property. The face, nose, and nasal vestibules are cleansed. Then cotton pledgets on applicators and gauze strips in a topical anesthetic solution (such as 10% cocaine) are placed in the nose. The topical anesthetic takes full effect in 10 to 15 minutes. In addition, an injectable local anesthetic such as lidocaine (Xylocaine) 1% or 2% with epinephrine 1:80,000 is administered in different sections of the septum and nose.

Different surgical approaches depend on the character and location of the deviation. Usually, the surgeon makes a vertical incision through the mucosa and perichondrium at the anterior end of the septum and separates the mucosa on both sides from the bone or cartilage, removing the deviated area with special forceps (or, if necessary, with a hammer and gouge). Once the cartilage is removed, the nasal cavities are separated only by the adjacent layers of mucoperichondrium. The surgeon then places bilateral nasal packing to prevent postoperative bleeding and to hold the mucoperichondrial flaps together. The gauze packing may be impregnated with an antibiotic ointment to prevent infection and odor. The packing is left in place approximately 24 to 36 hours (Saunders et al., 1979).

Implications for the Client

Physiological Implications
The nasal packing may give the client a sensation of suction in the throat when swallowing. This occurs because the packing prevents air from entering the nose, and a partial vacuum forms in the throat during swallowing. The nasal packing may also interfere with sleep. The client is likely to experience pain for the first few hours postoperatively.

Complications that can follow submucosal resection of the nasal septum include: septal hematoma, septal abscess,

Table 21–1 Nasal Surgery: Implications for the Client	
Physiological Implications	**Psychosocial/Lifestyle Implications**
Presence of nasal packing; discomfort; localized edema and ecchymosis with submucous resection of nasal septum, septoplasty, turbinectomy, and rhinoplasty	Temporary alteration in appearance from ecchymosis and swelling
Minimal discomfort is experienced with a nasal polypectomy	Rhinoplasty clients may fear that cosmetic effects will not be as expected or that significant others may not approve of their new appearance

perforation of the septum, postoperative nasal deformities, and adhesions between the nasal septum and turbinates (synechia). A septal hematoma is characterized by bulging of the mucous membrane of the septum on one or both sides, which results in some degree of nasal airway obstruction. It is a result of bleeding into the mucous membrane of the septum. Septal hematomas readily become infected and can progress to a septal abscess, which requires incision and drainage of the area.

Accidental septal perforation during the surgery is usually discovered by the surgeon and closed in the operating room. Postoperative nasal deformities can result from removal of too much of the nasal septum, the supportive structure of the nose.

Adhesions between the nasal septum and inferior turbinate may result in a sensation of a foreign body in the nose and obstruction of the airway on the affected side. Treatment consists of separation of the adhesions followed by the application of a sheet of dental wax for 2 or 3 weeks to prevent recurrence (Paparella & Shumrick, 1980).

Psychosocial/Lifestyle Implications
This surgery usually does not cause dramatic changes in the person's life. According to Gates (1982), these clients can usually return to a desk job in several days. Those who perform vigorous physical labor may miss 1 week of work. Clients may be anxious about their appearance because of ecchymosis (especially around the eyes), and edema. Once the bruising and swelling decrease, clients look positively on their changed physical appearance. Alteration in the sound of the voice also decreases after edema subsides. Client implications are summarized in Table 21–1.

Nursing Implications

Preoperative Care
The client should be informed about the events that will precede the operation. The client must not eat or drink within 6 to 8 hours of surgery, to prevent aspiration of

stomach contents. Preoperative medication is usually given about an hour prior to surgery—usually a sedative and/or analgesic.

It is important that the client understand the purpose of a submucous resection, which is usually to improve a nasal airway narrowed by a deviated septum. Some clients expect that the surgery will reduce postnasal drip or relieve headaches. They should be told the expected results so they do not consider the surgery a failure if postnasal drip or headaches do not disappear.

Explain the procedure and why it is performed under local anesthesia. (Bleeding is less, the operative area is free of equipment necessary in general anesthesia, and the client has some awareness of what is happening.) Tell the client to expect a sensation of pressure during the surgery when local anesthesia is used, to expect the nasal pack to be in place for 24 to 36 hours, and to breathe through the mouth during that period. It is sometimes helpful for the client to practice mouth breathing prior to surgery. Gauze will be folded and taped under the client's nose to catch drainage in the postoperative period. This is referred to as a mustache dressing or a gauze snuffer. Some degree of ecchymosis and edema will be present because of manipulation of the nose during surgery. In fact, the client may appear to have black eyes.

Postoperative Care

The major goal of nursing care in the postoperative period is to maintain safety and comfort. Hemorrhage is a potential problem because of the rich vascular supply of the nose. Bleeding is usually controlled by the nasal packing. Observe the gauze *under the nose* frequently and change it as it becomes blood-soaked. Remember to be gentle with dressing changes since the area may be tender. As a rule, the amount of bleeding is small, only enough to color the gauze two or three times a day in the first 24 to 36 hours. The client can be taught to change the gauze. The physician should be notified if frank bleeding is present or additional packing needs to be inserted.

After the operation, the client's vital signs should be monitored every 15 minutes until stable and then every 4 hours during the first day. The temperature should be taken rectally. The client should be instructed to avoid sneezing and, if that is impossible, to keep the mouth open while sneezing. Frequent swallowing may be an indication of blood dripping into the pharynx. The client should be instructed to expectorate postnasal drainage instead of swallowing it. Inspect the back of the throat at regular intervals for bleeding. If the client has swallowed blood, stools may appear tarry for a day or two. Because the client mouth-breathes while the packing is in place, frequent use of a mouthwash and lubrication of the lips are indicated. Because the nasal packing may interfere with sleep, a sedative may be helpful at night.

Edema of the nasal tissues is caused by manipulation of the nose during any nasal surgery. The edema may cause varying degrees of obstruction. Obstruction of the sinus ostia may result in a headache in addition to the general discomfort caused by the swelling. When the client returns from the operating room, placement in a semi-Fowler's position will increase venous return from the head. (An unconscious client should be turned to the side.) Ice packs can be applied during the first 24 hours to minimize the swelling and discoloration around the eyes.

Some physicians recommend after the nasal packing is removed that clients irrigate the nose with normal saline at regular intervals. Steam inhalations or decongestant tablets such as ephedrine or an antihistamine may help to alleviate the edema. Like nasal packing, edema that obstructs the nasal airway makes swallowing more difficult. The client may benefit from a soft diet and drinking through a straw. Regular diet can be introduced as tolerated.

Postoperative tenderness and pain are generally experienced. Initially, the client may require analgesics such as meperidine, 50 to 100 mg or morphine, 10 mg for one or two doses. Later the discomfort can be relieved by medication such as acetaminophen.

The surgical procedure irritates the nasal lining. More mucus is produced than normal, and the client has a bothersome nasal discharge. Decongestant tablets assist in decreasing the discharge.

Infections rarely develop after a submucous resection because of the rich vascular supply of the nose. Nevertheless, any temperature elevation should be reported, as should any unusual redness or tenderness of the nasal tissues, which may indicate an infection. Antibiotics may be prescribed.

Discharge Teaching

Clients should be instructed not to blow the nose vigorously for the first 2 weeks and to avoid other sources of trauma to the nose. They also should be informed that the tip of the nose may be numb for weeks or months either because of the swelling or because nerve endings were severed, or both. The sense of smell may also be altered by the swelling.

SEPTOPLASTY

Septoplasty, reconstruction of the nasal septum, is used to conserve the nasal septum as much as possible. When too much of the cartilaginous septum is removed during a submucous resection, the tip of the nose can collapse because of lack of support. Septoplasty is an effort to avoid this by straightening rather than removing the deviated piece of septum. The surgeon removes any section of bone that prevents the straightening. The septum is held in place by a suture or nasal packing. The physiological and psychosocial implications for the client (see Table 21–1) and nursing implications are the same as for a submucous resection.

TURBINECTOMY

Turbinectomy refers to a partial or total resection of a nasal turbinate. The surgery may consist of a submucous resection of the turbinate bone, excision of hyperplastic tissue over the turbinate, or a combination of the two. The procedure is most often performed to correct nasal airway obstruction by the inferior turbinate, but may be applied to the middle turbinate as well.

A partial or radical turbinectomy may be indicated in the following situations:

- Chronic rhinitis, which can cause permanent hypertrophy of the mucosa of the turbinate, resulting in some degree of nasal airway obstruction.
- Nasal septal deviations present over a long period of time, which may be accompanied by hypertrophy of the inferior turbinate on the side opposite the septal deviation.
- To facilitate drainage of a frontal sinus, a resection of the anterior end of the middle turbinate may be necessary.
- The presence of a neoplasm that involves a turbinate.

Surgical Procedure

If the prominence of the bony structure of the turbinate causes obstruction, a submucous resection of all or part of the turbinate bone is performed. The surgeon makes an incision down to the bone of the turbinate and elevates the soft tissue. The surgeon may use a chisel to fracture the bone. After the skeletal tissue is removed, the mucous membrane is repositioned. Gauze packing impregnated with antibiotic ointment is inserted to prevent postoperative bleeding.

Sometimes the inferior turbinate is crushed laterally to alleviate the nasal obstruction. This procedure is not usually totally effective because the turbinate tends to return to its original position. If the client has hypertrophy of the mucosa covering the turbinate, the treatment consists of removing the redundant tissue with scissors or with a snare for tissue at the posterior end of the turbinate.

Other surgical methods include electrocautery, cryosurgery, and the injection of sclerosing agents. Electrocautery is performed by either stripping the surface of the turbinate with the blade of a cautery instrument or inserting an electrode under the mucosa. Either method causes tissue destruction and subsequent scarring, which reduces the size of the turbinate. Cryosurgery involves the use of the cryoprobe to freeze the nasal turbinate. The advantages include more controlled tissue destruction, lack of bleeding problems, and the lack of pain since the nerve endings are frozen. In the past, some physicians injected sclerosing agents and steroids into the turbinate. Because of reports of blindness resulting from injections with steroids, these injections are no longer performed by most physicians (Saunders, 1982).

Implications for the Client and Nurse

Depending on the technique, the client may or may not develop ecchymosis of the area. The nasal pack must be

left in place at least 48 hours. Most surgeons recommend that it be left in for 3 or 4 days and removed on an outpatient basis. The main complication of this procedure is hemorrhage caused by removing the nasal packing too soon.

According to Saunders (1982), half of the soft tissue of the turbinate can be removed without causing dryness and crusting of the nasal mucosa. Since one function of the turbinate is to warm and humidify inspired air, some clients may find this capacity reduced after turbinectomy.

The implications for the client are the same as those mentioned for the submucous resection in Table 21–1. Nursing implications are also the same as those described for a submucous resection.

RHINOPLASTY

Rhinoplasty, reconstruction of the nose, is used to reconstitute and shape the anatomic features of the nose into a more pleasing form without impairing physiologic function. Rhinoplasty may also be performed to improve respiratory function when posttraumatic or developmental deformities result in nasal obstruction. This surgery is often done in conjunction with reconstruction of the nasal septum.

Surgical Procedure

This procedure can vary from minor corrections to complete reconstruction of the nose. Basically, the operation involves rearranging and remodeling the nasal bones and cartilage. The classic rhinoplasty consists of the following interrelated steps: (1) remodeling the tip of the nose, (2) removing the nasal hump (cartilage and bone), (3) narrowing the nose, and (4) reconstructing the nasal septum. After the surgery is completed, packing is inserted, the nasal tip is strapped into position with tape, and an external splint is applied. The purpose of the dressing is to control the swelling and secure the nose in the desired shape (Conlee, 1981).

Implications for the Client

Physiological Implications
The packing and splint are removed on the fifth to seventh day after surgery. At that time, more tape may be applied to hold the nose in position for 5 or 6 days. Potential complications of a rhinoplasty consist of hemorrhage and infection. If a septoplasty is performed, complications associated with that procedure can occur. Refer also to the implications described under submucous resection.

Psychosocial/Lifestyle Implications
The nose is especially significant since it is one of the most visible features of the body. It has secondary sex characteristics and is often referred to as feminine or masculine. Facial appearance is obviously related to the client's body image; an alteration of the nose may have either a positive or negative effect.

Clients who have elective cosmetic surgery sometimes become emotionally upset, particularly around the third postoperative day. The disturbance may be caused by their temporary physical appearance (swelling and ecchymosis), discomfort from the operation, a fear that the results will not be as expected, or all of these. The client may also be anxious about the change in physical identity and how significant others will react to the altered appearance.

It is important to tell the client that appearance does not stabilize at once. Appearance a few weeks after surgery may change further over a year, because of the healing process. The final result of the surgery may not be seen until 18 to 24 months afterward. Physiological and psychosocial/lifestyle implications are briefly discussed in Table 21–1.

Nursing Implications

Preoperative Care
Most clients admitted to the hospital for elective cosmetic surgery are motivated, healthy individuals. Because of this, nurses may think these clients do not need much attention; however, this is not the case. They will be anxious about the procedure and the anticipated alteration in appearance. Some may even feel guilty that they are in the hospital but are not "ill."

Postoperative Care
Nursing care is the same as described for the submucous resection, with a few additions. After surgery, the client's nose will be covered by a layered dressing of tape and a splint. Nasal packing will be in place with pieces of gauze folded and taped under the nose. Caution the client not to pick at the dressing and to limit talking and facial movement as much as possible. As with other types of nasal surgery, the client is likely to show edema and ecchymosis. After a rhinoplasty, the eyes may be swollen shut. The nurse may need to reassure the client that this will pass in a matter of hours. The nasal packing is removed the first or second postoperative day. Warn the client against sniffing, blowing, picking, or feeling the nose—actions that could produce bleeding. Make sure the client also understands that the inside of the nose should *not* be cleaned until the surgeon indicates it is appropriate.

Discharge Teaching
Following rhinoplasty, clients usually go home on the first or second postoperative day. Instruct the client to seek assistance immediately if frank bleeding begins, since hemorrhage can occur up to 1 week after surgery. The nasal splint remains in place for 5 to 10 days. About 10 days after surgery, the client is allowed to clean the inside of the nose with cotton-tipped swabs soaked in 3% hydrogen peroxide. Clients with rhinoplasty can usually resume normal activity within 1 week, but should avoid contact sports for 5 to 6 months to prevent damage to the nose. Clients who must wear eyeglasses should tape them to the forehead for 3 to 6 weeks instead of letting them rest on the nose (Conlee, 1981).

NASAL POLYPECTOMY

A nasal polypectomy, the removal of nasal polyps, is done when polyps result in some degree of nasal airway obstruction. The procedure is not used to remove an antrochoanal polyp or long-standing polyps with secondary infection.

Surgical Procedure

This procedure is often performed in an outpatient setting with the use of topical anesthesia and premedication. A wire snare is looped around the stalk of the polyp, closing the snare so the polyp is evulsed in one piece. The polyp is removed via suction or forceps and sent to the laboratory for examination.

Implications for the Client

Physiological Implications
Nasal polypectomy is often followed by some bleeding. If bleeding is significant, the client will probably be admitted to the hospital for observation.

Psychosocial/Lifestyle Implications
This minor surgical procedure does not usually affect lifestyle, body image, or require psychosocial adjustments. Refer also to Table 21–1.

Nursing Implications

The nurse should make sure the client understands that nasal polyps tend to recur and that decreasing the intensity of any allergy (or avoiding the allergen) may slow polyp recurrence. Chapter 19 describes nursing management of clients with allergic rhinitis.

Section II: Surgical Approaches to Disorders of the Paranasal Sinuses

Surgical procedures performed on the maxillary, frontal, ethmoid, and sphenoid sinuses—the paranasal sinuses—are often used to treat chronic sinusitis but may be done for a variety of reasons.

ANTRAL IRRIGATION

Antral irrigation (lavage) is one of the most common surgical procedures performed on the maxillary sinus. The maxillary sinus may be lavaged either as a diagnostic procedure to confirm chronic sinusitis, or as treatment for subacute sinusitis, to remove purulent secretions.

Surgical Procedure

This procedure is often carried out in the outpatient clinic under local anesthesia. In certain adults and children, it has been performed using a general anesthetic. The client should be in a sitting position. The physician either punctures the wall below the inferior meatus with a trocar or inserts a cannula into the ostium of the middle meatus. Sterile normal saline, heated to body temperature (about 98.6°F, or 37°C), is then run through connecting tubing to the cannula. The fluid washes purulent material through the natural ostium, out of the nose, into a receptacle held by the client or nurse. The irrigation is continued until returning fluid is clear.

Implications for the Client

Physiological Implications
The client should not feel pain but may experience a cracking sound and a sense of pressure as the instrument passes through the sinus wall. Complications of the procedure include bleeding and puncture of the lateral wall or roof of the sinus. Swelling of the cheek or area around the eye as the fluid is introduced means an accidental puncture has occurred.

Psychosocial/Lifestyle Implications
This procedure does not usually disrupt the client's lifestyle to a significant degree. Table 21–2 lists the client implications of surgery on the sinuses.

Nursing Implications

Postoperative Care
Observe the client for at least 30 minutes after completion of the procedure. Most clients will have a slight nosebleed lasting approximately 15 minutes. If epistaxis continues, the client will be admitted to the hospital for observation. Some clients may faint.

CALDWELL–LUC PROCEDURE

This radical antrum operation, named after two surgeons, is commonly used to gain access to the maxillary sinus to manipulate or remove the contents of the antrum.

The Caldwell–Luc procedure is used primarily for treatment of chronic sinusitis by removal of a part or the entire lining of the maxillary sinus. The Caldwell–Luc approach to the maxillary sinus is used in carrying out the following procedures:

- Removal of an antrochoanal polyp
- Examination and biopsy of a suspected sinus-cavity neoplasm
- Removal of a foreign body from the sinus cavity, such as the root of a molar tooth
- Repair of a fistula between the oral cavity and the sinus
- Surgery on a dental cyst that involves the sinus
- Reducing a blowout fracture of the eye

Surgical Procedure

The procedure may be performed under either local or general anesthesia with the client in a semisitting position.

Table 21–2	Surgery of the Sinuses: Implications for the Client	
Surgery	**Physiological Implications**	**Psychosocial/Lifestyle Implications**
Antral irrigation	No residual effects	Does not significantly alter lifestyle
Caldwell–Luc procedure	May experience numbness of upper lip, gum, and cheek temporarily or permanently; edema of lip, cheek, and/or eye; ecchymosis may be present	Anxiety from temporary alteration in appearance
Total maxillectomy	Discomfort; impaired ability to swallow; impaired ability to speak; if accompanied by orbital exenteration, loss of sight in one eye	Alteration in body image because of change in appearance and function; adjustment to the use of a dental prosthesis if used; may require reconstructive surgery if extensive resection accompanies maxillectomy
Ethmoidectomy	Discomfort; presence of packing	Anxiety from swelling and ecchymosis
Frontal trephination	Discomfort; catheter may be left in place for a short time	No significant alteration; may experience anxiety because of presence of catheter
Osteoplastic flap	Discomfort; presence of dressings and drain	Temporary alteration of body image because of shaved head if scalp incision is employed
Sphenoidotomy	Same as for ethmoidectomy	

An incision is made under the upper lip (Figure 21–1). A section of the anterior wall of the antrum is removed. The surgeon then removes the infected lining of the sinus, leaving a large nasoantral window through the bone that separates the maxillary sinus from the nose. This window is left open to heal to promote drainage from the antrum. The sinus may be packed with gauze in an effort to control bleeding. Bleeding from the bone may be minimal however; in that case, packing is not necessary.

Implications for the Client

Physiological and Psychosocial/Lifestyle Implications

The client may experience temporary (for months) or permanent numbness of the upper lip, gum, and cheek as a result of damage to the infraorbital nerve. Other complications include heavy bleeding and osteomyelitis of the maxilla (DeWeese & Saunders, 1982). Even when no complications occur, edema and a black eye may be present for 1 or 2 weeks after surgery, and the client will experience some postoperative discomfort.

Clients may be anxious about their appearance because of the swelling and ecchymosis. Client implications are listed in Table 21–2.

Nursing Implications

Postoperative Care

Ice packs may be applied to minimize the edema. Ensure that the client has adequate oral hygiene. The upper lip may be quite swollen for several days, making it difficult for the client to brush the teeth. The nurse can assist by providing soft toothbrushes or sponges and mouthwash. Explain the danger of irritating the incision above the teeth, since if the area is numb, the client may not be aware of abrading the surface. Check for unusual bleeding. When the packing is removed 24 to 48 hours after surgery, blood may drip from the nose for approximately 20 minutes. Analgesics such as acetaminophen or codeine may be required during the first week after surgery (Saunders et al., 1979).

Discharge Teaching

The client is usually discharged the second or third postoperative day. Make sure the client understands the importance of not blowing the nose for 2 weeks. (The pressure could force air from the nose into the maxillary sinus and out the incision.) The client should also be instructed to avoid chewing on the operative side and should not wear an upper denture plate for 2 weeks after surgery. Clients tolerate a liquid diet best for several days before advancing to a soft diet.

MAXILLECTOMY

Maxillectomy, the surgical removal of part or all of the maxilla, is primarily performed to remove malignant lesions

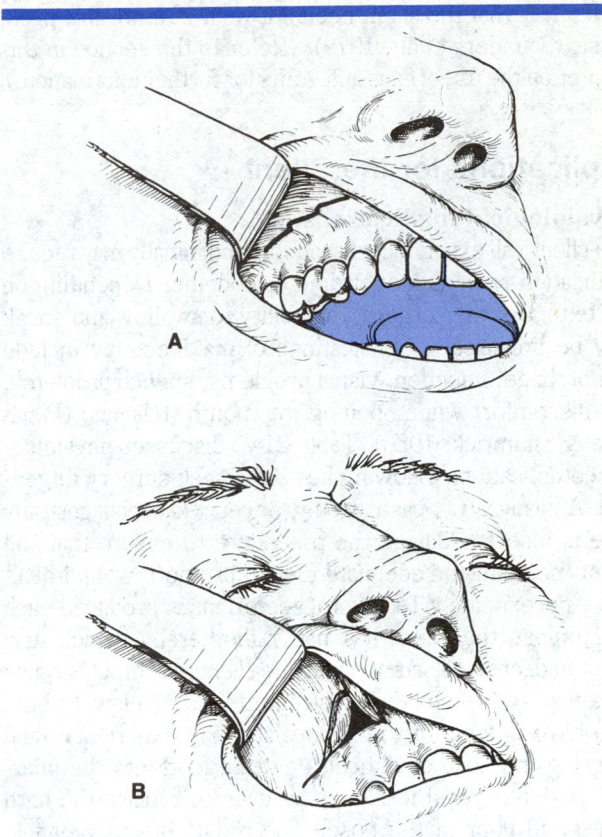

Figure 21–1

Caldwell-Luc radical antrum surgery. **A.** A horizontal incision is made in the canine fossa, the soft tissue is elevated, the sinus is entered through its anterior wall, and enough of the wall is removed to provide adequate exposure. **B.** The diseased membrane in the sinus is removed and a large window is made under the inferior turbinate. The incision in the canine fossa is then sutured.

from the maxillary or maxilloethmoidal sinuses. Benign lesions are occasionally removed via partial or complete maxillectomy.

Surgical Procedure

Maxillectomy is performed under general anesthesia. A partial maxillectomy is an individualized operation to remove a specific lesion. The surgeon may remove a part of the palate, a portion of the anterior maxilla, or other areas. A total maxillectomy involves the removal of the entire upper jaw and may be accompanied by removal of the orbit (eye) and resection of the cheek. After surgical excision, a split-thickness skin graft is removed from the thigh and used to line the cavity, which is then packed with gauze containing antibiotic ointment. Ideally, a previously manufactured prosthesis is available. The packing remains in place for approximately 5 days. Some surgeons prefer to use muscle flaps to reconstruct this area. This can be done in such a way that the client need not wear a removable prosthesis (Saunders et al., 1979). (Refer to the section in this chapter on the use of flaps and grafts for further information.)

Implications for the Client

Physiological Implications
The client will experience discomfort and initially may require medication such as meperidine or codeine. Depending on the extent of the surgery, the ability to swallow and speak may be impaired. Complications of maxillectomy include hemorrhage, infection, visual problems, speech problems, and discomfort when opening the mouth (trismus) (Paparella & Shumrick, 1980). Table 21–3 discusses physiological complications following head and neck surgery in general. A nasogastric, gastrostomy, or cervical esophagostomy tube is inserted during the procedure to ensure that the client maintains an adequate diet to promote wound healing. Approximately 1 L of oral secretions is produced each day (unless the client has had radiotherapy, which may result in decreased secretions). The client may drool because of pain and discomfort when attempting to swallow. Clients who have defects of the soft palate may experience fluid entering the nose or difficulty getting food into the pharynx. A dental prosthesis may be used to replace the hard palate and floor of the nose. The prosthesis may enable the client to swallow and speak. If the orbit is removed, the client will have to adjust to the loss of sight in one eye.

Psychosocial/Lifestyle Implications
The client may face the diagnosis of cancer and fear recurrence or death. After surgery, the client will have to deal with altered appearance, which may entail significant physical disfigurement if a large amount of tissue was resected in addition to the maxilla. (A maxillectomy performed without resection of other areas will not cause severe external deformity.) The client who is unable to perform previously routine acts such as swallowing and speaking will feel helpless and will mourn the loss of these abilities and the change in physical appearance. Table 21–4 discusses the psychosocial difficulties faced by clients undergoing head and neck surgery. The client who will use a dental prosthesis must learn to remove, clean, and replace the prosthesis. Client implications are summarized in Table 21–2.

Nursing Implications

Preoperative Care
The client and family members (or significant others) must be informed of the expected change in physical appearance. The extent of the change will vary depending on the location and extent of the neoplasm. Some clients benefit from meeting a well-adjusted client who has experienced the same type of surgery, while others will not.

The nurse should make sure that family members, as well as the client, understand that the ability to swallow and speak will be impaired. The client's primary communication immediately after surgery may be via writing or gesturing.

Postoperative Care
The nurse's approach to the client, family members, and significant others can make a tremendous difference in their emotional adjustment. The nurse should encourage self-care as soon as possible, instructing the client in oral care, oral suctioning, and self-administration of tube feedings. Care must be taken not to damage suture lines when the pharynx has been reconstructed. Interact with these clients in ways that communicate an acceptance of the client's altered appearance. Refer to Table 21–4 for specific nursing interventions. Encourage the client to ambulate in the hallway, unless contraindicated for medical reasons. Do not assume that clients understand (or want to understand) any specific aspect of their condition, or that clients have enough knowledge to judge how much they can do without harm.

Inspect the suture line for any signs of infection, such as inflammation and drainage. Cleansing with a solution of hydrogen peroxide and the application of antibiotic ointment are often prescribed. Nursing care of the recipient and donor sites of skin grafts and flaps is discussed later in this chapter. Nursing implications following removal of the orbit of the eye are discussed in Chapter 72.

If extensive portions of oral structures are removed in conjunction with a maxillectomy, a tracheotomy will be performed to ensure a patent airway. Nursing care of the client who has undergone a tracheotomy is discussed later in this chapter.

Discharge Teaching
Clients using a dental prosthesis need to know how to remove and replace it and how to keep it clean. The removable prosthesis should be removed and cleansed after each meal; if it is not, there is a high probability of irritation of the surrounding tissue. Instruction should include the importance of frequent brushing of teeth and use of mouthwash. Clients should be encouraged to return for follow-up evaluations to assess healing and to check for recurrence of cancer. The dental prosthesis will have to be adjusted as healing continues and the size of the cavity is altered.

Some clients will find speaking difficult even with the dental prosthesis. They should be referred to a speech therapist on an outpatient basis. Mental health counseling can help clients come to terms with altered appearance and function.

ETHMOIDECTOMY

An ethmoidectomy is the removal of one or more of the ethmoidal air cells that lie between the frontal and maxillary sinuses. There may be 15 or 20 of these air cells on

Table 21−3 Physiological Complications of Head and Neck Surgery

Complication	Nursing Intervention
Carotid artery rupture Rupture (blowout) of the external carotid artery occurs after destruction of the outer, middle, and inner layer of the vessel. It is a complication of radical neck dissection, caused by damage from infection, exposure during surgery, and treatment with radiation and chemotherapy. The most common factor contributing to carotid artery blowout is previous irradiation. Carotid artery rupture will rapidly result in death unless the bleeding is stopped, the circulatory volume replaced, and a patent airway maintained. The blood may flow outward, away from the neck, or into the tracheostoma or pharynx. Attempts are not always made to save the terminally ill client who develops a carotid artery rupture. The client, family members, and the physician may have agreed that no heroic measures to save the client are to be performed.	Observe for signs that could indicate the client is at increased risk for carotid artery rupture: • Presence of blood in drainage from overlying area • Exposure of the carotid artery after wound breakdown Control of bleeding when rupture occurs: • Call for assistance and have the physician notified immediately. • Carotid "blowout" tray containing necessary equipment should be kept at the bedside. • Suction source and catheter should be at bedside. • Exert pressure on the point from which bleeding occurs. Bleeding may be controlled by finger pressure at the site. Abdominal pads may be used to absorb blood. • To prevent aspiration from external bleeding, turn client to the side. If the client has a tracheostomy, inflate the cuff. • If bleeding occurs into the pharynx or a tracheostoma, suction via mouth or stoma. Assist with physiologic support of the client: • Administer intravenous fluids and blood as prescribed. • Administer oxygen. • Assist surgeon if ligation of artery is attempted. This may be performed in the client's room or the operating room depending on the situation. Provide psychological support for the client and significant others: • Remain with the client. • Interact with the client and significant others calmly. • Briefly explain your actions. • Administer sedatives or pain medication as prescribed. • Have clergyman contacted if client wishes.
Chyle leak During a radical neck dissection, the thoracic duct may be damaged; chyle may leak into the underlying tissues, causing wound breakdown. Small lesions may close spontaneously, although drainage may occur for weeks. A firm pressure dressing should be applied to the area for 5−7 days. Suturing of the vessel may be necessary to control the leak (Nora, 1980).	Report signs and symptoms of a chyle leak: • White, milky secretions (chyle) from drains • Swelling of the area of the clavicle Perform measures to aid in resolution of the leak and support the client's physical condition: • Apply pressure dressing as needed. • Report abnormal electrolyte and protein levels. • Administer prescribed dietary supplements. • Maintain pressure dressing as needed.
Facial edema Any surgery of the head and neck involving significant manipulation may result in facial swelling. The edema develops because the lymphatic vessels are disturbed and the jugular vein is ligated, impairing the drainage of venous blood and lymph from the head. Facial edema is present in varying degrees after a radical neck dissection.	Minimize the development of facial edema: • Elevate the head of the bed at least 30°. • Apply cold compresses after facial surgery if prescribed.
Fistula formation Fistula formation is more likely when the client has undergone extensive surgery and has received radiotherapy to the area. It tends to occur about 5−10 days after surgery (Nora, 1980). An *orocutaneous* fistula is a connection between the oral cavity and the skin. A *pharyngocutaneous* fistula is a connection between some part of the	Report signs of fistula formation: • Drainage from wound • Elevated temperature Prevent secretions from fistula from irritating skin, contaminating suture lines, or entering tracheostoma: • Apply dry gauze dressing.

(continued)

Table 21–3   Physiological Complications of Head and Neck Surgery *(continued)*

Complication	Nursing Intervention
pharynx and the skin. Both types result in drainage of saliva onto the skin. Enzymes in the saliva irritate the skin and can prevent wound healing. If a large fistula is present, a catheter may be placed in the opening and attached to continuous suction.	• Maintain suction to catheter placed in opening of fistula (if utilized). • Change gauze frequently to keep area dry and clean.
Hemorrhage Because of the richness of the vascular supply, bleeding is a potential problem in all head and neck surgeries.	Monitor vital signs and report significant changes: • Elevated pulse • Decreased blood pressure Observe the area for: • Swelling • Drainage of blood from incision lines, drains, tracheostoma (if present), and oral cavity
Infection Infection after head and neck surgery is relatively rare because of the vascularity of the area. However, meningitis may occur after surgery of the paranasal sinuses (an existing infection may gain direct access to the meninges because of anatomic proximity).	Observe for and report symptoms and signs of an infection: • Inflammation • Redness • Tenderness • Purulent drainage or secretions • Persistent temperature elevation • Tachycardia • Stiff neck (meningitis) Perform wound care: • Cleanse around tracheostoma. • Cleanse tracheostomy or laryngectomy tube. • Cleanse suture line with one-half strength hydrogen peroxide followed by sterile water or normal saline and apply antibiotic ointment (may vary among surgeons). Suction oral cavity to remove secretions; avoid traumatizing suture lines. Suction bronchial tree as necessary.
Innominate artery-tracheal fistula An infrequent but profound complication of placement of a tracheostomy tube is a fistula from the innominate artery to the trachea. A tube that is sharply angled may cause pressure to the tracheal wall and eventual erosion of the innominate artery. Erosion may sometimes be prevented by placement of a shorter tube. Hemorrhage from the artery will cause death if not stopped. Placement of a cuffed endotracheal tube with packing may be used to control bleeding until surgery can be performed.	Notify the physician immediately if a pulsating movement of the tracheostomy tube is noted. Assist with physiologic support of the client if fistulization occurs: • Suction blood from the airway. • Administer oxygen. • Administer replacement intravenous fluids as prescribed. Provide emotional support of client and significant others (refer to carotid artery rupture).
Residual nerve damage Various cranial nerves may be purposefully resected or inadvertently damaged during surgery of the head and neck. The accessory nerve (CN XI) is usually resected during a radical neck dissection. Ramifications are discussed in the section on radical neck dissection.	Assess cranial nerve function. (Refer to Chapter 35 for a review of functions of the cranial nerves.)
Skin flap necrosis Necrosis, or breakdown of the tissue of the flap, often results from impairment of the vascular supply to the flap. Factors that predispose to flap necrosis include irradiation to the area, tension on the suture line, hematoma, and infection. Treatment involves debridement of the area. Sterile wound irrigation and packing may also be required.	Prevent excessive tension on the tissue from feeding tubes, tracheostomy ties, oxygen, and humidification tubing. Assess the area and report signs indicating damage such as: • Poor capillary refill • Decrease in warmth of tissue • Change in color (ideally, should be pink) • Separation of flap from underlying tissue • Drainage from underneath the flap

Complication	Nursing Intervention
Tracheal stenosis Tracheal stenosis or narrowing of the tracheostoma is a long-term complication that usually arises as a result of scar tissue at the site of the tracheostomy tube. Treatment consists of tracheal dilation, although surgical removal of the stenosed section and reanastomosis of the trachea may be required (DeWeese & Saunders, 1982).	Prior to discharge, the client should be told to report air hunger as well as obvious narrowing of the tracheostoma.
Tracheoesophageal fistula Tracheoesophageal fistula is an abnormal connection between the trachea and the esophagus. It may occur as a result of pressure from an inflated cuff on a tracheostomy tube. This complication has become less common since the introduction of low-pressure cuffs.	Prevent excessive pressure on the walls of the trachea and esophagus (refer to care of the client with a cuffed tracheostomy tube in Chapter 18). Report symptoms and signs that might indicate the presence of a fistula: • Food or liquids in tracheal secretions • Decreased exhalation volume when the client is assisted by a mechanical ventilator

either side of the head between the eye and the nose. They can be removed through the nose (intranasally) or through an incision around the inner canthus of the eye (external ethmoidectomy). The external approach is preferred.

An ethmoidectomy may be performed for the following reasons:

- Removal of polyps
- To eradicate chronic infection of the ethmoid cells resulting from impaired nasal drainage
- To approach tumors of the frontal, ethmoid, and sphenoid sinuses
- To repair cerebrospinal fluid leaks
- As an extracranial approach when performing a hypophysectomy

Surgical Procedure

An intranasal ethmoidectomy is usually performed under local anesthesia. The middle turbinate is fractured and may be partially removed to allow better access to the sinuses. The infected tissue and ethmoid cells are then removed, and the nose is packed.

An external ethmoidectomy may be performed under local or general anesthesia. The approach is made through an incision around the inner canthus (Figure 21–2). After the underlying tissue and periosteum are incised, the ethmoid air cells, infected tissue, and a portion of the lateral wall of the nose are removed. If the sphenoid and frontal sinuses are involved, they can be approached through this area. The operative area is packed, and one end of the packing is placed into the nose to assist in removal of the gauze postoperatively. The soft tissues and skin are approximated with sutures (Paparella & Shumrick, 1980).

Implications for the Client

Physiological and Psychosocial/Lifestyle Implications

The client will experience some degree of discomfort and will require medication. Varying degrees of swelling and ecchymosis usually occur. Infection is a potential complication. Diplopia may be present initially, but will subside if the superior oblique muscle was not damaged. Blindness can result from damage to the optic nerve (CN II), vessels, or the globe itself. Bleeding is often considerable (Paparella

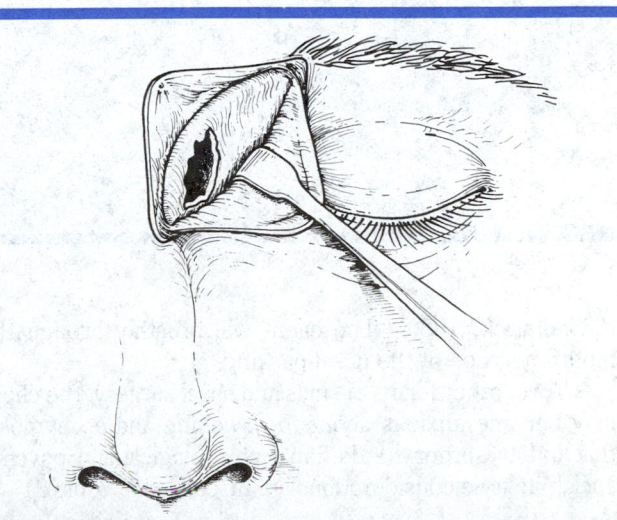

Figure 21–2

External ethmoidectomy. An external ethmoidectomy can be done under better visualization as cell by cell can be carefully removed. This approach can be used to gain access to the ethmoid, frontal, and sphenoid sinuses.

Table 21–4 Psychosocial Concerns Following Head and Neck Surgery	
Concern	**Nursing Intervention**
Feeling of loss of control over the future A great many of those who need surgery of the head and neck face a diagnosis of cancer and a low 5-year survival rate. Also, surgical therapies can cause extensive alteration in the client's lifestyle. As a result, clients may feel as though they have no control over what will happen.	Assist the client to regain a sense of control: • Encourage self-care as soon as possible after surgery. Instruction that begins in the preoperative period implies that the client will have control. • Encourage clients to make decisions about aspects of their own care. • Encourage significant others to become involved in the care of the client.
Altered body image Any surgical intervention of the head and neck can alter the way clients view themselves. Changes may be temporary, as in ecchymosis from nasal surgery, or permanent, as with a total laryngectomy. Inability to adjust to a temporary change may not pose any problem; inability to adjust to a permanent change will. The reaction of family members and significant others to the client's altered appearance and/or function is important and may influence the client's rehabilitation. Family members may require as much support as the client, or even more. The client will gradually begin to deal with the change. The initial steps may include talking about the disfigurement and taking a first look at it. Clients who continue to refuse to see themselves in a mirror may need specialized professional help in accepting the results of the surgery and the disease process.	Provide emotional support and encouragement for the client, family, and friends: • Approach the client in a manner that indicates acceptance of the disfigurement or altered function. • Maintain direct eye contact when interacting with the client. • Spend time with the client and significant others after completing nursing care. This provides nonverbal reassurance that the nurse considers the client, family, and friends important. It also offers a chance to find out about misconceptions and fears. • Provide honest answers to questions. • Focus on the client's strengths rather than weaknesses.
Fear of sexual activity An alteration in body image will affect clients' conceptions of their sexuality. Some clients will shy away from asking the nurse questions of this nature.	Assist clients to reintegrate their conception of sexuality into an altered self-view: • Be alert for statements or questions indicating that the client or significant others are ready to discuss concerns about sexual function. • If the client has a tracheostomy, suggest suctioning the stoma beforehand to remove mucus and wearing a stoma cover or other clothing to avoid expelling mucus during sexual activity. • When prior customary forms of sexual activity are made difficult, it may be appropriate to provide information regarding other means of sexual gratification including different positions, oral sex, masturbation. • Be sensitive that great age (or sex) differences between nurse and client may make an ordinary discussion inappropriate in the client's view.

& Shumrick, 1980). The client will breathe through the mouth because of the nasal packing.

As in other forms of sinus and nasal surgery, the client may become anxious about the swelling and ecchymosis that follow surgery. Additional physiological and psychosocial/lifestyle considerations are discussed in Table 21–2.

Nursing Implications

Postoperative Care

After the external approach, make sure that the client's head remains elevated to minimize edema and ecchymosis.

A pressure dressing (eye pads and fluffs held in place by an elastic bandage) is applied from the client's forehead to the cheek for 1 or 2 days. Assess the client's neurological status with particular attention to visual changes that might occur.

After an intranasal ethmoidectomy, the packing is removed in 1 or 2 days. Packing after the external approach is removed in 2 to 5 days. Fibrin clots and mucus are removed frequently until the sinus cavity has healed. The client should be instructed to return for evaluation and removal of fibrin clots to prevent infection and the formation of adhesions.

FRONTAL TREPHINATION

This procedure creates an opening in the bone of the frontal sinus. It is used in cases of acute frontal sinusitis when conservative measures fail to establish normal drainage through the frontonasal duct.

Surgical Procedure

Frontal trephination may be performed under local or general anesthesia. An incision is made under the medial end of the eyebrow. The thin bone of the sinus floor is perforated with a burr or a gouge and hammer, and the opening is enlarged to inspect the sinus. A drainage tube is inserted and sutured in place.

Implications for the Client

Physiological and Psychosocial/Lifestyle Implications

The client usually experiences some discomfort and may require pain medication. Localized edema occurs. Potential complications include the spread of infection, which could result in osteomyelitis of the skull, meningitis, or a brain abscess (Paparella & Shumrick, 1980).

The client may experience some anxiety both because of the discomfort and because of the presence of the drain. See Table 21–2.

Nursing Implications

Postoperative Care and Discharge Teaching

Observe the client for any signs of spread of the original infection. Irrigate the wound with warm sterile saline 2 to 4 times a day until the fluid return from the nose is clear. Initially, pain medication may be administered.

Upon discharge from the hospital, the client should be told how to recognize signs that might indicate recurrence of the infection or blockage of drainage from the area, and the importance of prompt reporting.

OSTEOPLASTIC FLAP

Surgical Procedure

This operation, which eliminates diseased mucosa from a frontal sinus, is performed only after other attempts to eradicate infection within the frontal sinus have failed. General anesthesia is employed. An incision is made either through the eyebrow and across the bridge of the nose or above the hairline. The surgeon then raises the scalp and uses a bone saw to cut into the sinus above and on each side, exposing the interior of the sinus for the removal of the mucosa. The next step is to remove a plug of fat from the abdominal wall and place it in the cavity. The bony wall

of the frontal sinus (the osteoplastic flap) is then replaced and the incision sutured (DeWeese & Saunders, 1982).

Implications for the Client

Physiological and Psychosocial/Lifestyle Implications

The client will experience some pain, but more discomfort may be caused from the abdominal incision than the skull incision. A drain is often in place and a dressing applied to absorb drainage. Potential complications include blood accumulation under the scalp flap and meningitis (DeWeese & Saunders, 1982).

If the scalp incision is used, the client's head is shaved before surgery, which results in a temporary alteration of body image. See Table 21–2 for a summary of psychosocial/lifestyle implications.

Nursing Implications

Preoperative Care

To prepare for a scalp incision, the client's head is shaved. The client could be advised to purchase a hair piece if this will pose a significant problem.

Postoperative Care and Discharge Teaching

After the operation, the nurse will administer pain medication at regular intervals if necessary for the particular client. Observe the client for the formation of a hematoma and meningitis (stiff neck, fever, and headache). The physician usually removes the drain after 2 days. Nursing care includes care of the dressing applied to absorb drainage and to hold the scalp firmly against the skull. The abdominal wound should be inspected for signs of infection, and may need cleansing.

Before being discharged, the client should be encouraged to report signs of infection in either wound site and informed of what to look for.

SPHENOIDOTOMY

Incision of the deep-lying sphenoid sinus—sphenoidotomy—may be approached as for an external ethmoidectomy or through the nasal septum. Indications for this procedure are:

- Removal of primary disease within the cavity or removal of purulent material resulting from chronic sinusitis
- Surgery on the pituitary gland

Surgical Procedure

Access to the sphenoid sinus is gained by external ethmoidectomy (already described) or an intranasal approach that usually requires removal of a portion of the nasal septum for adequate exposure. The sphenoid sinus is opened and diseased tissue removed. The sphenoidethmoidal cavity is packed; the packing is left in place for approximately 6 days. The nasal cavity is also packed (Paparella & Shumrick, 1980). (Chapter 45 describes surgery of the pituitary gland.)

Client and Nursing Implications

The physiological, psychosocial, and nursing implications are the same as those for ethmoidectomy. They are summarized in Table 21–2.

Section III: Surgical Approaches to Maxillofacial Trauma

As mentioned in the Chapter 19 discussion of trauma to the maxillofacial area, surgical intervention may be needed. A variety of procedures, depending on the nature and extent of the injury, may be used.

Surgical Procedure

Surgical repair consists of removal of debris, suturing lacerations, and performing closed and open reduction of fractured bones. Attention is first directed toward repair of soft tissue wounds. Reduction of fractures can be delayed up to 2 weeks if the client is unstable or has other complications, but the fractures are not easily corrected after 2 weeks. Interdental wiring (see Chapter 19) is often necessary to correct fractures of the maxilla and mandible. Some clients will require intubation or tracheotomy to maintain an adequate airway. If the injuries are accompanied by cervical fractures, Crutchfield tongs (or a similar device) may be applied to stabilize the head (see Chapter 39). Severely injured clients will often require repeated surgery to obtain results that are both functionally and cosmetically acceptable.

Implications for the Client

Physiological Implications
The client's experience of discomfort or pain will depend on the extent of the trauma. Some clients will experience little more than facial swelling and lacerations that require minimal treatment. At the other extreme are clients who experience alteration in their level of consciousness and multiple fractures and lacerations that require extensive surgical revision. Damage to cranial nerves will result in altered motor or sensory function. The client's ability to swallow and speak may be affected. An injury may result in altered respiratory function so that the client requires mechanical ventilation.

Psychosocial/Lifestyle Implications
The client will experience alteration in body image because of the change in appearance. This may be short-lived or long-term because of a permanent disfigurement. The client may have feelings of helplessness because of being dependent on equipment and the nursing staff for respiratory or nutritional support. Table 21–5 summarizes the client implications for maxillofacial repair.

Nursing Implications

Preoperative and Postoperative Care
The nurse plays an important part in the assessment and stabilization of these clients. Specific preoperative nursing measures are discussed in Chapter 19.

Appropriate postoperative nursing measures depend on the specific situation. Factors that should be considered in formulating the nursing care plan include: maintenance of pulmonary function and cardiac output, maintenance of fluid and electrolyte balance, prevention of infection, facilitation of wound healing, prevention of skin breakdown, and emotional support.

Discharge Teaching
Clients who sustain nasal fractures or require interdental wiring should receive specific instructions (refer to Chapter 19). Clients need to know when to report for follow-up evaluation and therapy.

Table 21–5 Repair of Maxillofacial Trauma: Implications for the Client	
Physiological Implications	**Psychosocial/Lifestyle Implications**
Facial swelling and ecchymosis	Alteration in body image from change in physical appearance
Discomfort	
Interdental wiring	Anxiety because of inability to speak or swallow
Alteration in sensory and motor function (ie, inability to speak and swallow)	

Note: The implications will vary depending upon the extent of injury.

Section IV: Surgical Approaches to Disorders Affecting the Oropharynx and Trachea

TONSILLECTOMY

Tonsillectomy, or removal of the palatine tonsils, is among the most common operations. Physicians disagree about indications for removal of the tonsils. Indications that remain acceptable are:

- Repeated attacks of acute tonsillitis
- Peritonsillar abscess (quinsy)
- Hypertrophy of the tonsils resulting in dysphagia and loss of weight
- Biopsy of the tonsil for suspected malignancy
- Development of cor pulmonale as a result of chronic airway obstruction from tonsillar hypertrophy
- The client who is a diphtheria carrier
- Relationship between attacks of tonsillitis and exacerbations of rheumatic fever, asthma, arthritis, or iritis (DeWeese & Saunders, 1982)

Surgical Procedure

In adults, local anesthesia is preferred, supplemented by premedication. The local anesthetic (either Novocain 1% or Xylocaine 1%) is injected into the peritonsillar tissues and the anterior and posterior pillars. Epinephrine 1:100,000 is commonly administered with either drug (DeWeese & Saunders, 1982).

If a local anesthetic is used, the client is most likely to be in a semisitting position. During the procedure, the client may become faint. If this occurs, the nurse should lower the client's head.

Dissection and snare are the most common approaches to tonsillectomy. Initially, the tonsil is grasped with the forceps, the capsule is incised at its base, and the snare is placed over the tonsil. Closing the snare removes the tonsil. Pressure is applied to the area with gauze for several minutes. Electrocoagulation may be used to control some of the bleeding.

Implications for the Client

Physiological and Psychosocial/Lifestyle Implications

The client will experience a sore throat for 5 or 6 days. Possible complications include immediate or delayed hemorrhage. Adults often complain of more discomfort than children. Initially, a liquid and soft, bland diet is best tolerated.

Psychosocial implications for the client include missing work for several days because of a sore throat.

Nursing Implications

Preoperative Care

The client is usually admitted the day before the surgery is to be performed. That evening, explanations of the procedure and what to expect postoperatively are often given to the client and significant others. The client should have nothing to eat or drink after midnight.

Check the results of laboratory tests and report abnormal findings to the surgeon. Of particular concern would be abnormal clotting times, low platelet count, low hemoglobin and hematocrit values, and an elevation in the number of leukocytes. These findings could result in postponement of the operation to prevent complications. Tonsillectomy is contraindicated in individuals who have blood dyscrasias, uncontrolled systemic disease, or an acute infection.

Postoperative Care

When general anesthesia is used, the client is placed in a side-lying modified Trendelenburg position. This allows for easy removal of secretions without aspiration. It is important not to injure the operative area with the oral suction catheter; trauma to the area could precipitate bleeding. As soon as clients are alert, fluids or ice chips are encouraged. Once liquid is tolerated, ice cream is permitted. Analgesics are administered as needed. An ice collar may provide temporary comfort. Aspirin and codeine usually provide sufficient relief. Some physicians prefer acetaminophen because aspirin can interfere with platelet aggregation.

Bleeding may occur a few hours after the surgery. Suspect bleeding if there is frequent swallowing. Habitual coughing and throat clearing after surgery may increase the chance of hemorrhage. The surgeon should be notified immediately of any excessive bleeding or large amounts of emesis positive for occult blood. If pressure and the application of vasoconstrictors do not stop the bleeding, the client will need to have the blood vessels resutured.

Delayed bleeding may occur if the white scab that forms over the operative area separates prematurely. Separation may be caused by an infection or trauma, as when rough food is swallowed. Delayed bleeding is most common from day 5 to day 10 after surgery; usually, the bleeding is from capillaries, but sometimes a large blood vessel is involved. Even so, delayed bleeding is rarely dangerous unless ignored, but it can fatal if not treated. Treatment often involves removal of a small clot that may have formed in the tonsil fossa. Epinephrine, mild caustics, or local pressure may be used to control the bleeding (DeWeese & Saunders, 1982).

Diluted saline or peroxide mouthwashes will make the client more comfortable and decrease unpleasant breath odor. Monitor and inspect the back of the throat regularly for bleeding. Any persistent elevation in temperature should be reported.

Discharge Teaching

Unless complications occur, the client can be discharged the day of surgery or 24 hours after surgery. It is helpful

Box 21–1 **Instructions for Clients Who Have
Had a Tonsillectomy**

Food: Eat only liquids and very soft foods (custard, ice cream, milk) the first day home. Lukewarm liquids tend to be less irritating than cold ones. Avoid straws. On the second day, soft foods such as mashed potatoes can be tolerated. The fourth day after discharge, solid foods (but not burnt meat, raw carrots, crunchy peanut butter) can be added. For several days, rough foods and acidic fluids (eg, orange juice) should be avoided. Rough foods may cause bleeding, and acidic juices will sting the throat.

Activity: Avoid overexertion. Resting in bed or in front of the TV may be appropriate the first day home. Activity should be gradually increased as tolerated by the individual.

Care of the Healing Area: Avoid coughing and vigorous nose-blowing. Gargle with lukewarm diluted salt water at frequent intervals, perhaps as often as every 2 hours the first day. Dilute salt water is made by adding 1 teaspoon of salt to 1 pint of water. White membranes will develop where the tonsils were removed. These are normal; they function like a scab. Be careful not to scrape or injure this scab as it may cause bleeding. If soreness is a problem at mealtime, chew Aspergum 15 minutes before eating.

Complications

• Heavy bleeding is possible but not likely, and is dangerous only if ignored. Slight bleeding often occurs. Lie down and gently spit out the blood. Gargle gently using ice water. If bleeding is not readily stopped, call a physician immediately.

• Ear pain may be present for several days after the surgery.

• A persistent elevation of temperature above 100.4°F or 38°C orally may indicate an infection; tell your physician.

• Return for your follow-up examination after 1 week (DeWeese & Saunders, 1982).

to give the client written as well as verbal instructions prior to discharge, such as those provided in Box 21–1.

TRACHEOTOMY

Tracheotomy, an incision into the trachea, is performed to obtain a temporary opening into the trachea. If the trachea is brought to the skin and sutured there to make a permanent opening, it is a tracheostomy.

The surgical technique is performed to provide access for aspiration of the bronchial tree or to relieve upper airway obstruction. It is often employed when the client is unable to cough effectively and expel secretions. Indications for a tracheotomy include:

• Mechanical ventilation that will be required for more than 7 to 10 days

• When an artificial airway is required, but the client is not a candidate for orotracheal or nasotracheal intubation (eg, because of severe facial injuries)

• To reduce the work of breathing for a weak or critically ill client by decreasing the amount of dead space

• A neurological disorder paralyzing the chest muscles and diaphragm

• In conjunction with certain procedures such as a radical neck dissection or laryngectomy

• To bypass an obstructed upper airway caused by a tumor of the trachea or pharynx

Surgical Procedure

A tracheotomy is commonly performed under local anesthesia. When permissible, the neck is hyperextended to place the trachea in a more superficial position. The surgeon may use either a transverse or vertical incision. The deep tissues are divided in the midline to expose the trachea. It is sometimes necessary to retract or divide the thyroid isthmus to complete the exposure. A vertical incision is made into the trachea through the second and third or third and fourth tracheal rings (Figure 21–3), and the tracheostomy tube is inserted. Care must be taken to avoid rupturing the inflated cuff of the tube on a calcified tracheal cartilage. Some surgeons place stay sutures on both sides of the opening to facilitate changing the tube in the early postoperative period. A tracheotomy is not recommended in an emergency; instead, a cricothyroidotomy should be performed.

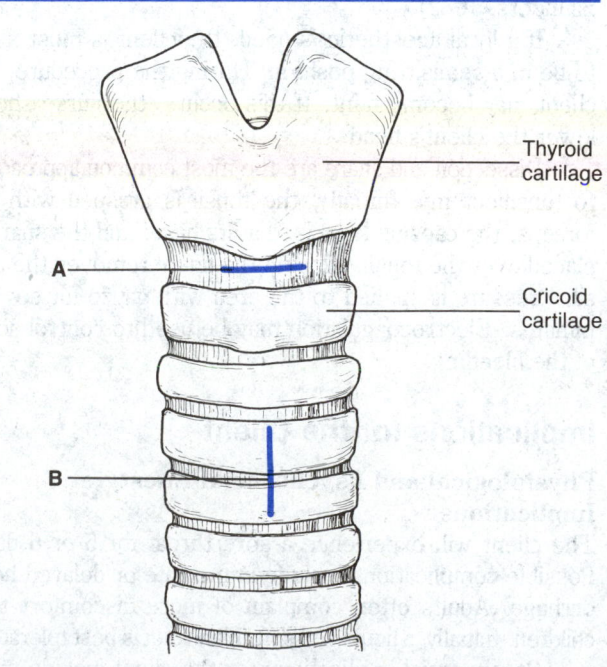

Figure 21–3

A. Area of incision for cricothyroidotomy. **B.** Area of incision for tracheotomy. (This illustrates incision at the second and third tracheal rings. It can also be performed at the level of the third and fourth tracheal rings.)

Other complications are fistula from the innominate artery to the trachea, tracheal stenosis, and tracheoesophageal fistula. These complications and their related nursing interventions are discussed in Table 21–3.

Implications for the Client

Physiological Implications

Some clients are unable to swallow effectively and may require the placement of a nasogastric feeding tube. This is true even when the cuff of the tracheostomy tube is deflated. After the surgery, they will experience mild discomfort and may require analgesics. Narcotics should be administered judiciously to prevent respiratory depression. Because inspired air does not have the advantage of humidification, warming, and filtering by the nose, clients require humidified air or oxygen to prevent irritation of the mucosal lining. Even so, an increase in mucus production is likely.

Complications associated with this procedure in the early postoperative period include: hemorrhage, tear of the trachea, extratracheal intubation (ie, placement of the tube anterior to the trachea in a false passage), and subcutaneous emphysema.

Psychosocial/Lifestyle Implications

Clients may fear suffocation by inadvertent closure of the opening, as by a plug of mucus in the trachea. Clients may also fear that the opening (stoma) will become occluded by blankets or clothing during sleep. Clients will be unable to speak unless the opening is occluded. Client implications are summarized in Table 21–6.

Nursing Implications

Preoperative and Postoperative Care

The client should be prepared for the effects of the operation—breathing through the stoma in the neck and loss of ability to speak while the stoma is open.

Frequently assess respiratory rate and breathing patterns after the tracheotomy is performed. Humidification may be provided by humidified air or oxygen via a tracheal mask. It can also be achieved by placing a piece of 4 × 4 gauze moistened with sterile normal saline or water over the stoma. Tracheal suctioning should be performed as needed, depending on the status of the client. The nurse determines the need for suctioning by auscultation of lung sounds or by the degree of the client's respiratory distress. Other indications are arterial blood gas results and chest x-rays. Cleansing of the area around the stoma and the tracheostomy tube will be necessary. (Chapter 18 describes suctioning technique and care of the client with a tracheostomy tube.)

Discharge Teaching

Clients who have a tracheotomy will need to learn how to care for themselves at home (Chapter 18). The client and at least one family member should demonstrate competence at suctioning and cleansing the tube prior to discharge. Clients should be assured that occlusion of the opening by clothing (as when sleeping) would awaken them. Water poses a risk, however; clients should be reminded to cover the stoma when taking a shower. Some physicians advise against all water sports; others indicate that clients can engage in certain water sports if cautious. Stress that drowning can occur rapidly and that clients must be extremely cautious if they choose to engage in boating or fishing.

CRICOTHYROIDOTOMY

This procedure consists of making an opening between the thyroid and cricoid cartilages into the trachea to establish an airway. Cricothyroidotomy is the procedure of choice in an emergency when orotracheal or nasotracheal intubation is not possible.

Cricothyroidotomy is appropriate when emergency establishment of an airway is necessary, as in complete obstruction of the upper airway. Occasionally, it may be done electively for a client who requires the altered route of airflow for a short period of time. This procedure is not without risk and should not be attempted by an unqualified individual.

Table 21–6 Tracheotomy: Implications for the Client

Physiological Implications	Psychosocial/Lifestyle Implications
Lack of humidification, warming and filtering of inspired air	Body image problems due to presence of stoma
Difficulty swallowing (experienced by some)	Inability to produce voice unless stoma is covered
Increase in amount of mucus production (experienced by some)	Fear of suffocation
Decreased amount of dead space in respiratory system	Inability to participate in water sports

Surgical Procedure

The emergency room of a hospital is a common setting for this technique, which must often be done without anesthesia because there is no time for administration of medication. If the procedure is elective, local anesthesia is given. A short transverse incision is made in the neck immediately below the thyroid cartilage to expose the cricothyroid membrane. A stab wound is made through this membrane (Figure 21–3), and a small tracheostomy tube is inserted to establish the airway. If the client will require intubation for more than a few days, the cricothyroidotomy should be converted to a standard tracheotomy (DeWeese & Saunders, 1982). The implications for the client are the same as for a tracheotomy; refer to Table 21–6.

Section V: Surgical Approaches to Disorders Affecting the Larynx

Laryngeal surgery may be performed to remove benign or malignant neoplasms, or to repair damage resulting from trauma to the neck. Growths such as vocal nodules and laryngeal polyps can be removed using indirect or direct laryngoscopy, as discussed in Chapters 18 and 19. Laser surgery to eradicate benign laryngeal lesions and early localized laryngeal neoplasms is increasingly common.

This section will focus on the four types of surgical intervention for carcinoma of the larynx: excision via suspension laryngoscopy, partial laryngectomy using a laryngofissure approach, supraglottic laryngectomy, and total laryngectomy.

EXCISION VIA SUSPENSION LARYNGOSCOPY

This is a version of direct laryngoscopy performed for removal of a growth. An attachment holds the laryngoscope, which frees the surgeon's hands. An operating microscope magnifies the area. This technique is indicated for the removal of carcinoma in situ or other lesions that are minimally invasive.

Surgical Procedure

This operation may be performed under general or local anesthesia. The client is placed in a supine position. The surgeon grasps the vocal cord with forceps and removes the diseased portion using a knife or scissors. When the procedure is performed carefully, the client's voice will be essentially normal postoperatively (DeWeese & Saunders, 1982).

Implications for the Client

Physiological and Psychosocial/Lifestyle Implications

Passage of the laryngoscope may produce soreness or irritation of the throat. Initially, the client should avoid coughing, clearing the throat excessively, and talking, which may further traumatize the area.

Because the client is encouraged to rest the voice, the ability to communicate will be impaired. Client implications are summarized in Table 21–7.

Nursing Implications

Postoperative Care

Observe the client for signs of respiratory distress, bleeding, and return of gag reflex. The airway could be compromised by spasm or edema of the vocal cords. Hemoptysis, vomiting of blood, or an increase in heart rate may indicate bleeding from the area. A liquid diet may be tolerated best.

Discharge Teaching

Information should be reinforced concerning prevention of irritation to the area. Family members should understand why they must support the client's need for voice rest for the next few days.

PARTIAL LARYNGECTOMY

The removal of a portion of the larynx encompasses a number of different operations. One of the most common is the laryngofissure approach, discussed here.

Partial laryngectomy using the laryngofissure approach is recommended for clients in whom the cancerous growth is limited. The ideal client is one who has an early growth confined to one vocal cord or to the anterior section of the larynx. As the malignant process advances, the likelihood of obtaining favorable results with this procedure declines.

Surgical Procedure

This procedure is accompanied by a high cure rate. It has the advantages of preserving the normal airway and the client's ability to speak.

Either local or general anesthesia can be used. For the laryngofissure approach, the surgeon makes an incision in the midline of the neck and splits the larynx open (much like a clamshell). The cancerous tissue and a margin of normal tissue are removed in an attempt to obtain all of the malignant cells. This may include excising only the true cord; however, a larger lesion may necessitate removal of the true cord, ventricle, and false cord on one side. A tracheotomy is performed to ensure a patent airway in the early postoperative period in the event of edema or hemorrhage. Occasionally, a hemilaryngectomy may be performed, removing half of the thyroid cartilage and soft

Table 21–7 Laryngeal Surgery: Implications for the Client		
Surgery	**Physiological Implications**	**Psychosocial/Lifestyle Implications**
Excision via suspension laryngoscopy	Sore throat	Rest voice for a few days
Partial laryngectomy (laryngo-fissure approach)	Temporary tracheostomy; difficulty swallowing while tracheostomy is present	Inability to produce voice while tracheostomy is present; fear of recurrence of malignancy
Supraglottic laryngectomy	Temporary tracheostomy; difficulty swallowing; nutritional intake via nasogastric tube or intravenous infusion temporarily	Inability to produce voice while tracheostomy is present; dependent on nurse initially to administer nasogastric feeding; frustration while learning to swallow
Total laryngectomy	Permanent tracheostomy; presence of drains under skin in early postoperative period; anosmia; initially may experience some difficulty swallowing; feeding via nasogastric tube in early postoperative period; loss of ability to perform glottic Valsalva's maneuver, blow nose, or drink through a straw	Loss of ability to produce voice via normal mechanism; need for clients to learn to care for themselves (ie, stoma, laryngectomy tube, suctioning); possible need for job change, creating financial difficulties; depression not unusual

tissue on the inside of the larynx (DeWeese and Saunders, 1982).

Implications for the Client

Physiological Implications

For 2 or 3 days after surgery, the client has a tracheostomy tube in place and must deal with the associated problems. The amount of mucus increases, slight bleeding may occur from the tracheostomy, and clients will be unable to talk unless the tube is occluded. Clients may experience incisional discomfort; they usually experience difficulty swallowing during the first few days. The potential for aspiration of fluids and food into the airway is present. Occasionally, subcutaneous emphysema may occur in the neck and face to the point where the client's eyes are swollen shut. Postoperative bleeding is also a potential complication. Healing results in scar tissue, which fills the area where the diseased cord was removed. Usually, the remaining vocal cord is close enough to the scar tissue to allow voice production. The scar tissue does not compromise the airway (Saunders et al., 1979).

Psychosocial/Lifestyle Implications

The client will have to deal with the diagnosis of cancer and will probably experience a great deal of anxiety over the diagnosis and fear of recurrence. Clients also have impaired ability to communicate for the first few days. Client implications are summarized in Table 21–7.

Nursing Implications

Postoperative Care

Initially, the nurse should direct the most attention to promoting respiratory function. A tracheal mask should be used to humidify the air the client breathes. Tracheal suctioning is performed when appropriate (suctioning technique is described in Chapter 18). The client should be provided with lint-free gauze wipes to cover the stoma when coughing and to wipe away secretions. (Lint could be aspirated through the stoma.) Inspect periodically around the tracheostomy. Puffiness of the skin or a crackling sensation when touching the skin of the neck or face indicates subcutaneous emphysema.

Since clients may find swallowing difficult, be alert for symptoms and signs of aspiration, such as coughing during or immediately after drinking or eating. Check tracheal secretions for the presence of food and liquids, which may spill over into the trachea and out the opening. If aspiration occurs, perform tracheal suctioning and notify the physician. Some clients will tolerate soft foods better than liquids, since the soft foods do not tend to spill over into the trachea. A client who has aspirated may also become febrile. The client may require intravenous or nasogastric feedings until the swallowing difficulty subsides. The nurse must cleanse the tracheostomy tube and the skin around the area (tube cleansing is discussed in Chapter 18).

Reminding the client that the tracheostomy tube will be removed 2 to 3 days after surgery and that the client will regain the ability to talk helps to reduce anxiety.

Discharge Teaching

The hospital course for partial laryngectomy clients lasts from 5 to 7 days. Clients should be told to report signs of infection, such as drainage from the incisional area or a persistent temperature elevation, and should be encouraged to return for follow-up examination to assess healing of the area. Smoking should be discouraged. Remind clients addicted to smoking that the nicotine is now gone from their systems and that not returning to smoking is the one thing they can do that may prevent a recurrence.

SUPRAGLOTTIC LARYNGECTOMY

This procedure, removal of the portion of the larynx above the true vocal cords, has also been referred to as a *horizontal* or *conservation* laryngectomy. Supraglottic laryngectomy is performed on clients who have carcinoma of the epiglottis and adjacent structures above the true vocal cords.

Surgical Procedure

The supraglottic area consists of the epiglottis, false cords, arytenoid cartilages, and arytenoepiglottic folds in addition to the preepiglottic and paraepiglottic spaces. The surgical procedure involves a horizontal cut that passes just above the vocal cords to excise the malignant and damaged tissue. A tracheostomy provides an adequate airway. The surgeon often does a unilateral neck dissection in conjunction with this type of laryngectomy.

Implications for the Client

Physiological Implications

Clients who undergo a supraglottic laryngectomy experience great difficulty swallowing for the first 2 or 3 weeks. Discomfort will be present. Removing the epiglottis and false vocal cords means that the normal protective mechanism against aspiration is absent, so food and especially fluids tend to flow directly into the trachea. The client may be fed intravenously or by nasogastric tube for 2 to 3 weeks. The client must learn how to swallow effectively. Clients must also deal with the presence of the tracheostomy tube for the first week or so, and with voice loss while the tracheostomy tube is in place. The true vocal cords remain intact; thus, the client's voice is "conserved." Possible complications include: hemorrhage, fistula formation, and carotid artery rupture. The last two are more likely if a neck dissection was also performed (see the discussion of radical neck dissection later in this chapter) (Saunders et al., 1979).

Psychosocial/Lifestyle Implications

Initially, the client must deal with the diagnosis of cancer and the fear of recurrence. The client also must depend on the nurse in the early postoperative phase to administer nasogastric feedings and care for the tracheotomy. If a radical neck dissection was performed, there will be a greater (and perhaps unexpected) alteration in body image. After the nasogastric tube is removed, the client must learn to swallow again; this may be frustrating, since swallowing previously required little or no concentration. After healing occurs, the client's voice is usually normal. Client implications are summarized in Table 21–7.

Nursing Implications

Postoperative Care

The nurse is responsible for pulmonary toilet and care of the tracheostomy tube. The tracheostomy will be kept open until adequate healing occurs and the client can learn to swallow effectively.

After approximately 2 weeks of nasogastric tube feeding, healing should be sufficiently advanced to permit the nurse to start instructing the client in how to swallow (Box 21–2). A client can usually swallow best after the tracheostomy tube and nasogastric tube have been removed. Waiting until the tracheostoma is almost closed before starting means that pressure can build up to assist in swallowing. Start oral feedings with semisolid foods such as custard, gelatin, and mashed potatoes. Avoid fluids initially because they tend to be aspirated. Record the type of food and fluid best tolerated, the amount consumed, the weight pattern of the client, signs of aspiration, and any signs of possible fistula formation. Some clients learn rapidly, whereas others have a great deal of difficulty. Encouragement and patience on the part of the nurse will facilitate the learning process. Supplemental intravenous feeding is often necessary.

The degree of motivation greatly affects client success. Learning and maintaining deglutition (swallowing) after surgical resection require strenuous effort. Debilitated or elderly clients may need considerable time to gain strength before they can swallow effectively. When aspiration continues, the nasogastric tube should be reinserted and the client sent home for several weeks to be maintained on tube feedings. *If a client pulls out the nasogastric tube or it is accidentally removed after a laryngectomy or other type of pharyngeal reconstruction, do not attempt to reinsert it.* Attempts to replace the tube could result in damage to tissue and the creation of a fistula.

Discharge Teaching

Clients who have a great deal of difficulty swallowing may benefit from a therapist who specializes in this type of

---

Box 21–2   Learning to Swallow After a Supraglottic Laryngectomy

Instruct the client in the following method of swallowing, which facilitates closure of the epiglottis:

- Take a deep breath and hold it, keeping the neck flexed forward.
- Put the food on the back of the tongue.
- Swallow three times while continuing to hold the breath, and then cough.
- Any food that has been aspirated will be coughed out through the tracheostomy tube or through the opening where the tube had been.

rehabilitation. The dietitian and nursing staff should reinforce nutritional information. The client should be told to contact the physician if signs of infection occur. Clients should be encouraged in efforts not to smoke and referred to a stop smoking program or to the literature for helpful suggestions. (See the resources list at the end of Chapter 18.)

TOTAL LARYNGECTOMY

This surgical procedure involves the removal of the entire larynx. A person who undergoes this type of surgery is referred to as a *laryngectomee*. Total laryngectomy is appropriate for the removal of neoplasms too extensive to be removed by a partial or supraglottic laryngectomy.

Surgical Procedure

The surgeon generally removes the hyoid bone, the preepiglottic space, the strap muscles, and one or more of the tracheal rings in addition to the larynx. Removing the larynx severs the connection between the trachea and the pharynx, so the trachea is sutured to the skin of the neck, forming a permanent tracheostomy (Figure 21–4). A radical neck dissection often accompanies this surgery. A case study for the client with cancer of the larynx is presented at the end of Chapter 19.

Implications for the Client

Physiological Implications

Unlike the partial and supraglottic laryngectomy, a total laryngectomy results in permanent changes in the client's airway and speech. During ventilation air enters through the tracheostoma instead of the nose. This results in absence of the sense of smell (*anosmia*) and lack of humidification. Since the sense of taste depends on the sense of smell, clients may experience a permanent alteration of taste. Some clients do regain partial olfactory function. Potential complications include: hemorrhage, nerve damage, fistula formation, and carotid artery rupture.

Mucus secretion is often copious after surgery. The client cannot cough effectively because there is no glottis to close to increase intrathoracic pressure. Clients can still expel secretions (often forcefully) through the stoma, however. Clients can no longer blow their noses or use a straw when drinking. Clients may experience difficulty swallowing initially, but this usually subsides after healing. The change that affects individuals the most is the loss of the ability to talk. Clients will experience varying degrees of discomfort.

Psychosocial/Lifestyle Implications

These clients not only have the diagnosis of cancer and fear of death to deal with, but also permanent changes that alter body image and interactions with others. Some clients

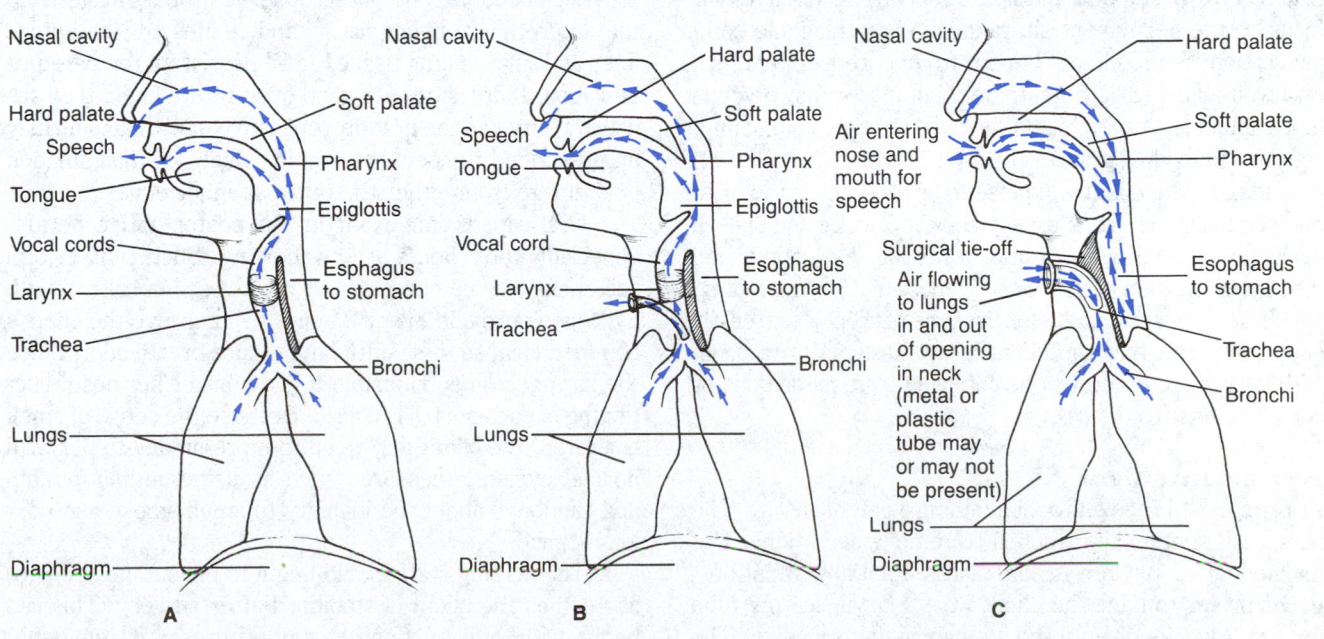

Figure 21–4

A. Normal anatomy. **B.** Anatomy after tracheotomy. **C.** Anatomy after total laryngectomy.

find the production of mucus and the accompanying odor through the stoma offensive. Some think that the quality of sound produced by some of the communication aids is too "mechanical" or "abnormal." People are social beings; the fear of not being able to communicate can cause a great deal of anxiety. Voice is an integral part of body image and is often given sexual characteristics ("sexy voice," "sounds like a real man"). Voice quality is essential in many occupations. Clients may have to consider a job change that can cause additional psychological and financial problems.

Clients may not come to terms with the reality of the situation until after the immediate postoperative period. This is when the nurse may first notice signs of depression, such as the refusal to look in the mirror or the lack of participation in self-care. A client who remains severely depressed over an extended time is reacting abnormally and should be seen by a mental health professional such as a psychiatric nurse. Client implications are summarized in Table 21–7.

Nursing Implications

Preoperative Care
Preparation of the client and family members or significant others for the results of the surgery is of paramount importance. How much the client wants to know varies among individuals; therefore, the members of the health care team must use their judgment. An array of professionals may work with the client to provide comprehensive care, including surgeons, nurses, the speech therapist, social worker, and psychiatrist. Radiologists and chemotherapy specialists may be part of the team, since these clients may receive multimodal therapy. Preoperative teaching will focus on the permanent alterations in breathing and communication. Some clients benefit from a preoperative visit by a well-adjusted laryngectomee, but others may become more anxious. When planning preoperative counseling, consider individual differences.

Ideally, the client will be seen by a speech pathologist preoperatively. Sessions usually consist of voice and speech evaluation and tape recording, a hearing evaluation, and time for discussion of the consequences of a laryngectomy.

The room assignment for this type of client is extremely important. See that the client is not assigned to a room with a laryngectomee who is suffering from metastasis or complications from surgery.

Postoperative Care
Priority must be given to maintaining a patent airway. The nurse will suction the trachea to remove secretions. Humidified air or oxygen is administered initially. Most surgeons prefer to have the client wear a laryngectomy tube for 1 to 2 weeks or until the stoma maintains its size. The surgeon changes the tube the first time. The nurse then changes and cleans the tube, and teaches the client to do so. (Chapter 18 describes care of laryngectomy tubes.)

After the tube has been permanently removed, the client should wear a lightweight stoma covering or bib. This allows movement of air into and out of the stoma, yet prevents dust particles or insects from entering the stoma. If the bib is moistened with sterile normal saline, it provides some humidification.

If thick secretions are a problem, the nurse teaches the client to instill a few drops of normal saline into the stoma, followed by suctioning; this will remove tenacious secretions. A mucous plug that obstructs the trachea can usually be removed by suctioning, which stimulates the client to cough. If these measures are unsuccessful, notify the physician.

A nasogastric tube will often be in place after surgery. In the immediate postoperative period, it may be connected to low suction to prevent nausea and vomiting. However, the nurse will start the client on feedings soon, beginning with a small amount of water or dietary supplement to see how well the client tolerates it. If no problems arise, feedings are given every 2 to 3 hours. Moving or disturbing the feeding tube risks trauma to the pharyngeal suture lines, which could result in fistula formation. Discontinue intravenous fluid administration when the client's intake is adequate. Physicians differ about when the feeding tube should be discontinued and the client started on an oral diet. No one who has undergone a total laryngectomy can aspirate easily because there is no longer a connection between the trachea and esophagus. The only way a laryngectomee will aspirate is if a fistula forms to connect the esophagus and trachea or if material is inhaled through the tracheostoma.

Nursing measures should promote wound healing and prevent infection. The nurse observes for drainage from the suture lines, inflammation and redness of the suture lines and surrounding tissue, and a persistent temperature elevation. If dressings are used over suture lines, they are usually removed the first postoperative day. Cleansing may be prescribed. Inspect the stoma closely for inflammation or drainage from either the outer or inner edges.

Oral care is important in the postoperative period, especially until clients are swallowing. Suctioning of oral secretions may be necessary. A mouthwash of half-strength hydrogen peroxide every 2 hours will improve the client's comfort, cleanse the mouth, and reduce breath odor. Since the laryngectomee is unable to blow his or her nose, suctioning of each nostril is useful. Because the sense of smell is altered, the client may need to be reminded to perform normal hygienic measures such as using antiperspirants and cautioned about the inability to smell smoke and noxious stimuli.

The nursing staff should begin to encourage self-care as soon as the client is stabilized after surgery. This can begin with oral suctioning and progress to removing, cleaning, and replacing the laryngectomy tube. The withdrawn client should be encouraged to walk in the hallway rather than avoid social contact. Include the significant others in the client's care. Family members may be more disturbed than the client and need a great deal of information and support. See also Table 21–4.

Discharge Teaching

Make certain the laryngectomee understands changes in personal habits that are necessary. For example, the stoma should be covered when taking a shower to avoid aspiration. A shower head below the level of the neck is recommended. When washing the hair, the client should bend over a sink or bathtub and use a spray hose to direct the spray. Some otolaryngologists warn laryngectomees to avoid all water sports, whereas others condone fishing if the client is cautious. Remind the client that drowning can occur rapidly with a laryngectomy. A scarf or high collar can be worn for warmth and for prevention of foreign body aspiration. The client should be encouraged to carry a wallet card or bracelet indicating that he or she is a laryngectomee.

Self-care understanding and technique should be reinforced and checked at intervals. Arrange for the client to demonstrate suctioning, cleansing the stoma, and the like to ensure that the client maintains proper technique. Feedback should be provided for clients concerning their alaryngeal speech. Most clients will return as outpatients for continued instruction and evaluation of the method they choose for voice production. Smoking should be discouraged.

Communication After Total Laryngectomy

Clients may or may not be exposed to alaryngeal methods of communication prior to surgery. In the early postoperative period, the individual may rely on writing or gesturing. A special problem is posed by the client who is blind, deaf, or cannot read or write. The options available to laryngectomees other than nonverbal communication include: esophageal speech, artificial speech aids, and surgical-prosthetic voice restoration. These methods are discussed below.

A patient and understanding nurse can do much to support the client during speech rehabilitation. It is crucial that clients who are trying to communicate by writing or alaryngeal speech not be rushed. Impatience adds to their anxiety and frustration. Explain to others why they should not attempt to finish the sentence for clients or pretend to understand them when they have not. Family members often need guidance in this area so they can be a source of support for the client. Films, slide strips, and written material are available through community resources such as the American Cancer Society. The Lost Chord or Nu Voice Club is sponsored by the American Cancer Society. Clients, family members, and significant others often find affiliation with these resource groups helpful. Specific information is included in the resources list at the end of Chapter 18.

Box 21–3 Artificial Larynx Devices

The oral device transmits an electronically-produced tone into the mouth by a tube, which is attached to a tone generator. The client introduces the plastic tube 1 or 2 in into the side of the oral cavity, presses the tone generator, and modifies the tone into meaningful sounds (Figure 21–5A). The oral device does not interfere with suture lines or dressings and can be used as soon as the client is alert after surgery.

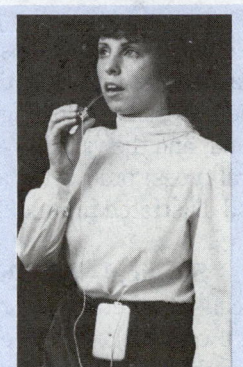

The neck-type aid consists of a diaphragm, circuitry, and a battery. When the client switches the device on, it produces a buzzing sound. The device diaphragm is placed against the neck. The sound is transmitted through the neck tissue and modified by the client into meaningful sounds (Figure 21–5B).

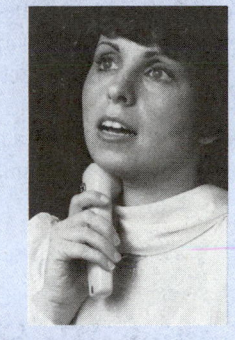

The pneumatic aid consists of a reed (or diaphragm) in a metal housing. Air from the stoma is directed through a funnel placed over the stoma during voice production. The air then passes into the mouth via the plastic tubing, and sound is modified by the speech musculature (Figure 21–5C). This type of device produces a more natural sound and is relatively inexpensive.

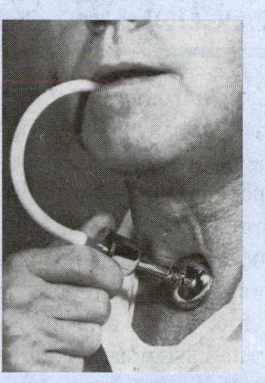

Figure 21–5

Artificial larynx devices. **A.** Cooper–Rand electrolarynx. **B.** Western Electric electrolarynx. **C.** TOKYO speech aid.

Esophageal Speech. In the past, speech rehabilitation was directed almost exclusively toward learning esophageal speech. The esophageal voice is produced by trapping air inside the mouth and forcing it down the esophagus. Air in the esophagus is quickly forced out, causing the walls of the upper esophagus and lower pharynx to vibrate similar to a belch. The sound is then modified by the tongue, lips, and teeth. Learning this type of speech requires weeks to months, and not all succeed. (It has been suggested that fewer than half of all laryngectomees learn esophageal speech.)

Artificial Speech Aids. Artificial speech aids are also available. The "artificial larynx" devices can be used to communicate very soon after surgery and may be useful while the client learns to produce an esophageal voice. The device will remain the primary mode of speech for some people. Disadvantages of these devices include the machinelike quality of the voice, the cost of maintenance, the necessity of holding and operating the device with one hand, and the visibility of the device. There are three general types: oral, neck, and pneumatic. They are described and illustrated in Box 21–3, Figure 21–5.

Surgical–Prosthetic Voice Restoration. Surgical–prosthetic voice restoration consists of the creation of a connection between the esophagus and trachea. Air can then be directed from the lungs and trachea to the esophagus and into the pharynx, resulting in tissue vibration much like that of traditional esophageal speech. This is performed on selected clients who, for one reason or another, were unable to develop adequate esophageal speech. Aspiration is a problem because food and fluids can flow from the esophagus into the trachea, resulting in aspi-

ration. One-way valve prostheses have been developed that allow air to pass from the trachea to the esophagus, but prevent aspiration.

The Blom–Singer or "duckbill" prosthesis consists of a silicone tube that projects through the stoma into the esophagus. When the stoma is occluded with a finger, air from the lungs passes into the esophagus through a small opening. The opening is closed when the client swallows to prevent aspiration. A disadvantage is that the prosthesis must be worn at all times and must be removed and cleaned every day (Ryan, 1982).

The Panje prosthesis, or "voice button," is a small silicone one-way valve prosthesis that can be worn up to several weeks without changing. It is not easily dislodged by coughing or retching (Knapp & Panje, 1982).

Various forms of laryngeal reconstruction are being attempted. In one type, the surgeon uses an arm or leg tendon and rib cartilage to create vocal cords and a thyroid cartilage. The resulting voice is reported to be of good quality (Ryan, 1982).

Section VI: Surgical Approaches to Radical Neck Dissection

Lymph from most of the areas in the head and neck where carcinomas may develop drains into the lymph nodes of the neck. These nodes constitute a fairly efficient barrier to malignant cells from the head and neck. Even after cancer spreads to the nodes, distant metastasis may not occur for months. A radical neck dissection, removal of a large portion of the contents of the neck, can be useful because removing the area of "localized metastasis" can often prevent dissemination of the cancer to other parts of the body. Neck dissections are classified as unilateral or bilateral and elective or therapeutic.

A radical neck dissection is appropriate when a client has palpable cervical lymph nodes secondary to a primary tumor of the head and neck when the tumor has been controlled by previous therapy or can be potentially controlled. In this instance, the procedure is classified as a *therapeutic neck dissection*. A second situation is that of a client who does not have palpable nodes but has a type of malignancy that has a high incidence of microscopic nodal metastasis. This is referred to as an *elective neck dissection*.

Surgical Procedure

The surgery is always done under general anesthesia. The anatomical boundaries of a neck dissection are the clavicle, mandible, trapezius muscle, and the anterior midline of the neck. The structures removed include the sternocleidomastoid muscle, the omohyoid muscle, the external jugular

vein, and generally the internal jugular vein. The accessory nerve (CN XI) is frequently resected. All of the nodes in the anterior and posterior triangle superficial to the deep fascia are removed. The carotid artery, vagus (CN X) and phrenic nerves, and the sympathetic ganglion are spared. The surgeon frequently places drains connected to continuous suction (Figure 21–6) to prevent a hematoma that could compromise the airway and disrupt wound healing (Paparella & Shumrick, 1980).

Depending on the extent of the cancer, the surgeon may perform other procedures in conjunction with the neck dissection, such as a total or supraglottic laryngectomy, hemiglossectomy (removal of a portion of the tongue), or hemimandibulectomy (removal of part of the lower jaw).

Because malignant cells spread, cancer of the head and neck may require extensive surgical revision that can create significant disfigurement in this visible part of the body. The otolaryngologist or plastic surgeon will try to remove the diseased tissue, yet leave the client with results that are functionally and cosmetically acceptable.

The use of flaps and grafts enables the surgeon to repair the surgically created defects (eg, for reconstruction around the oral cavity and maxillary sinus). A *graft* is an area of tissue that is disconnected from one part of the body and placed on another. For example, a dermal graft may be removed from the thigh and placed over the neck to prevent exposure (and subsequent rupture) of the carotid artery.

A *flap* is a section of tissue that is rotated or advanced from one part of the body to another without being completely detached. For example, a deltopectoral flap is swung from the deltoid and pectoral muscles to the neck. It can also be used to create a new pharynx and cervical esophagus. These additional procedures place the client at increased risk for complications and prolong the time required for rehabilitation.

Implications for the Client

Physiological Implications

The discomfort experienced by the client is less than would be expected considering only the extent of tissue removed. This is because the nerves that supply sensation to the cervical neck are resected as part of the dissection. The client may experience a pounding and persistent headache because of ligation of the jugular vein, which results in a rise in spinal fluid pressure. Potential complications include: hemorrhage, nerve damage, fistula formation, flap necrosis, and carotid artery rupture. Refer to Table 21–3 for explanation of these complications and related nursing interventions.

Any surgery of the head and neck that entails significant manipulation can result in facial edema, or swelling of the face. The edema develops because the lymphatic vessels are disturbed and the jugular vein is ligated, both of which impair the drainage of venous blood and lymph from the head.

The client is able to resume oral intake of fluids after having fully recovered from the general anesthesia. The advance to a regular diet can take place the first or second postoperative day. If pharyngeal construction or laryngectomy is performed, the client's intake will be altered as previously discussed.

A tracheotomy is *not* routinely performed during a radical neck dissection unless other procedures accompany the operation. Thus, the client does not have to deal with an altered breathing mechanism.

Drains are present and may cause the client some aggravation. They must be disconnected from wall or machine suction prior to ambulation and reconnected afterward. The Hemovac will provide adequate suction while the client is out of the room. In fact, some surgeons will use the Hemovac routinely rather than wall or machine suction. In the early postoperative period, the Hemovac may be connected to wall suction to obtain additional suction.

The trapezius muscle is innervated by the accessory nerve. Because this nerve is sacrificed during surgery, the trapezius muscle will atrophy. In addition, because the sternocleidomastoid muscle is removed, the client will experience shoulder drop, limited abduction, and discomfort in the shoulder area for several months. Accidental damage to the mandibular portion of the facial nerve (CN VII) will result in weakness of the upper lip.

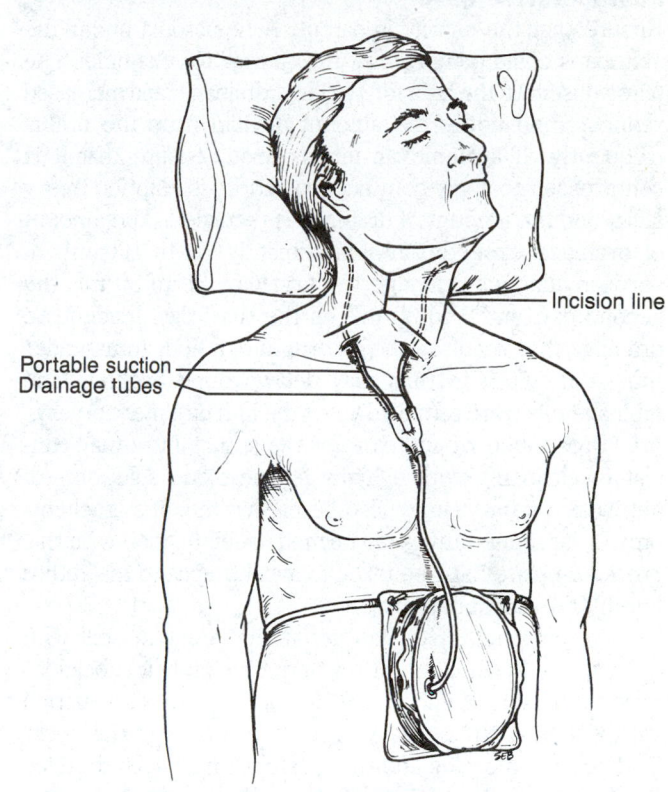

Portable suction
Drainage tubes

Incision line

Figure 21–6

The incision line and drainage system for radical neck dissection.

Psychosocial/Lifestyle Implications

The standard radical neck dissection is well tolerated by many. If complications do not occur, the client is out of bed in 1 day and ready for discharge in 1 week (Nora, 1980).

The procedure does not result in extensive physical disfigurement, although the client will have to deal with facial edema, the suture lines, and the presence of drains. A dressing may be used during the first day, but is usually removed after that time.

The client may be anxious that malignant cells have, or may have, spread to the neck. Fear of recurrence of cancer and death is real. Client implications are summarized in Table 21–8.

Nursing Implications

Preoperative Care

Many clients believe that the disfigurement resulting from a neck dissection is much greater than it actually is. This is particularly true when they have seen others who have undergone extensive surgery in conjunction with neck dissection. The nurse should not only explain, but listen to the client and make sure any misconceptions are clarified.

Postoperative Care

Ensure that the airway is patent. A hematoma under the skin flaps could compromise the airway, for example. The nurse observes the area for swelling, drainage, and increased redness, and notes the amount of fluid from the drains frequently. If a Hemovac unit is used, ensure that it is compressed to apply continuous suction, is emptied every shift, and the amount of drainage is recorded. The amount of drainage expected is approximately 70 to 100 mL of serosanguineous drainage the first day, 30 to 50 mL the second day, and 0 to 30 mL on the third day. Inadequate drainage may result in the formation of a hematoma under the skin, which in turn may delay wound healing. The drainage tubes are removed about the fifth day after surgery.

Prescribed wound care for the suture lines may consist of cleansing with a hydrogen peroxide solution. An antibiotic ointment may also be prescribed. If a tracheotomy or laryngectomy is performed in conjunction with this procedure, care must be taken to avoid trauma to the suture line by the tracheostomy ties.

Nursing measures can assist the client to deal with the loss of the function of the trapezius and sternocleidomastoid muscles. The sternocleidomastoid in conjunction with CN XI is the primary flexor and rotator of the neck. The scalene muscles and the small intrinsic neck muscles are secondary flexors and rotators. These muscles can be strengthened by gentle, gradual neck and shoulder ROM exercises, with and without resistance. Neck ROM with resistance is shown in Figure 21–7. Exercises should not be attempted until the wound is healed. Shoulder exercises are discussed under thoracic surgery.

If the client has a skin flap or graft, it is important to prevent damage to the newly placed flap or graft and pro-

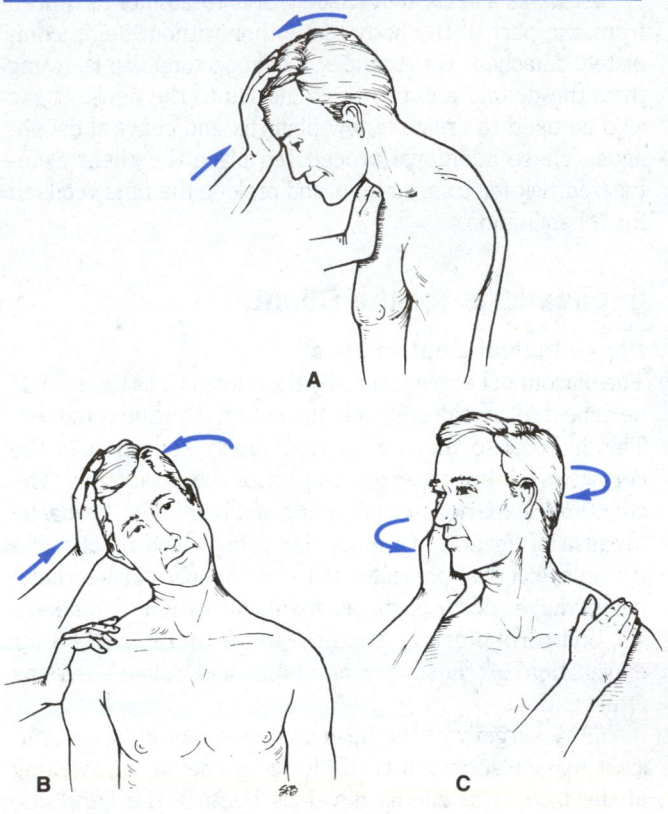

Figure 21–7

Neck range-of-motion with resistance. **A.** Neck flexion. **B.** Lateral bending. **C.** Lateral rotation.

mote healing of the donor site. Tension and pressure should be avoided over the flap or graft. Bed linen and clothing should also be kept off the donor sites. A bed cradle may be useful for this purpose.

Skin flap necrosis may result when surgical skin flaps are used. Necrosis, or breakdown of the tissue of the flap, is often caused by impairment of the vascular supply to the flap. Factors that predispose a client to flap necrosis include irradiation to the area, tension on the suture line, hematoma, and infection. Treatment entails debridement, which may be followed by sterile wound irrigation and packing.

The donor site for a graft or flap should be observed for signs of infection. Some surgeons apply a layer of petrolatum gauze at the donor site of a split-thickness skin graft and leave it in place until it falls off. Others may apply a fine mesh type of gauze. As the tissue heals, the gauze lifts off the periphery of the wound. The elevated portion can be trimmed with scissors until the gauze is removed. Some donor sites for flaps can be closed, and others require a skin graft. The treatment and care prescribed vary widely among surgeons. A more comprehensive discussion of skin grafting appears in Chapter 80.

Table 21–8	Radical Neck Dissection: Implications for the Client	
Physiological Implications	**Psychosocial/Lifestyle Implications**
Presence of drains under skin flaps	May experience temporary alteration in body image from facial edema and neck incisions
Resection of accessory nerve (CN XI) and sternocleidomastoid muscle: • Shoulder drop • Limited abduction • Discomfort of shoulder	Should perform exercises to compensate for muscle function loss
Interruption of lymphatic and venous drainage: • Facial edema • Headache	

Section VII: Surgical Approaches to Disorders of the Thorax

Thoracic surgery refers to any surgical procedure of the chest wall or any organ between the diaphragm and clavicles. This section will deal specifically with surgery of pulmonary structures; Chapter 25 describes cardiovascular procedures. Client and nursing implications are similar for each operation; they are discussed with pulmonary resections at the end of this chapter.

A variety of incisions may be employed in thoracic surgery: the posterolateral and anterolateral approaches are used often in general thoracic surgery, whereas median sternotomy is employed for certain cardiothoracic procedures (Figure 21–8).

CLOSED TUBE THORACOTOMY

Closed tube thoracotomy or thoracostomy refers to percutaneous insertion of a chest tube into the intrapleural space. Placement of a chest tube is used to evacuate blood or other fluid from trauma, surgery, malignancy, or infection or to reexpand the lung in clients who have a pneumothorax with more than 10% collapse.

Surgical Procedure

The surgeon may insert a chest tube at the bedside in an emergency, such as when a client suffers a spontaneous pneumothorax and is in significant respiratory distress. Some hospital policies require that the procedure be performed in the operating room if at all possible to decrease the risk of infection.

If it is not contraindicated, the client should be recumbent. If the tube is to remove air, it is placed anteriorly in the midclavicular line in the second to fifth intercostal space. If the tube is to remove fluid, it is inserted posteriorly in the lower chest, usually in the sixth to eighth intercostal space. Thoracentesis and/or x-ray may be used to determine the specific site of insertion. Figure 18–20 illustrates the placement of chest tubes for both purposes.

An oral or parenteral analgesic may precede the insertion of a chest tube, which is painful. The skin is cleansed with an antiseptic such as povidone-iodine, and a topical anesthetic is infiltrated to anesthetize the skin, intercostal area, and pleura. A skin incision of approximately 2 cm (1 in) is made. A hemostat may be used to spread the entrance into the pleural space. Firm pressure is applied to advance the chest tube, which is tunneled subcutaneously to an intercostal space several centimeters from the opening. Sutures should be securely placed at the entrance site. Traditionally, petrolatum gauze is wrapped around the tube at the insertion site to prevent air from leaking into the intrapleural space. (If the tubes are placed subcutaneously and are secured, air leakage should not be a problem.) An occlusive dressing is applied to prevent inadvertent removal

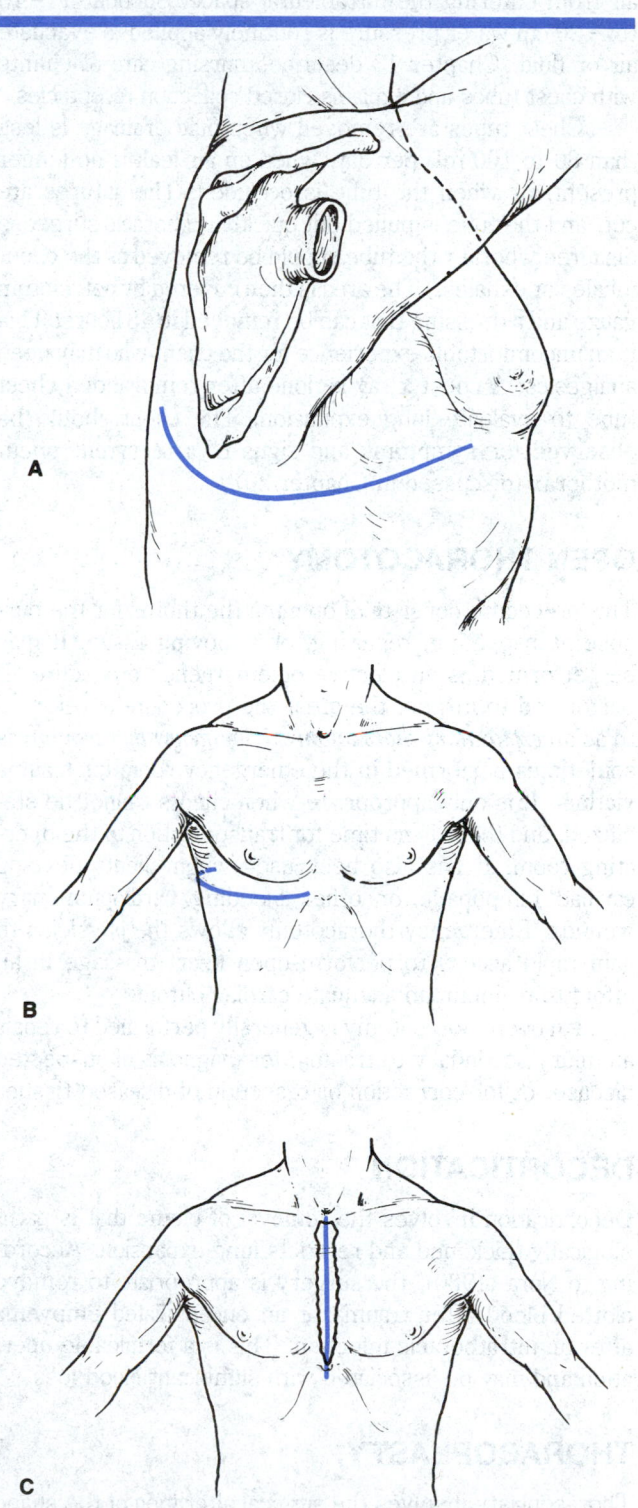

Figure 21–8

A. Incision for posterolateral thoracotomy. **B.** Incision for anterolateral thoracotomy. **C.** Incision for median sternotomy.

of the tube. The surgeon then connects the chest tube to a closed water-seal collection receptacle, which prevents air from entering the intrapleural space. Suction of − 15 to − 20 cm water pressure is routinely applied to evacuate air or fluid. Chapter 18 describes nursing care of clients with chest tubes and explains closed collection receptacles.

Chest tubes are removed when fluid drainage is less than 80 to 100 mL per day, when an air leak is no longer present, or when the tube is occluded. The sutures are cut, and the tube is pulled out quickly. (Thoracic surgeons disagree whether the tube should be removed as the client inhales or exhales.) The area is then covered by petrolatum gauze and a dressing that can be removed in 48 hours. This is an uncomfortable experience for the client who may need analgesics. A chest x-ray is done after removal of a chest tube to evaluate lung expansion. The client should be observed for symptoms and signs of a recurrent pneumothorax (discussed in Chapter 20).

OPEN THORACOTOMY

This procedure consists of opening the thorax for the purpose of inspecting, repairing, or removing tissue. It may be performed as an elective or emergency procedure. If performed to inspect the area, the procedure is referred to as an *exploratory thoracotomy*. *Emergency thoracotomy* is sometimes performed in the emergency room for trauma victims. It is only appropriate when clients cannot be stabilized, and there is no time for transportation to the operating room. It has also been used when clients develop cardiac tamponade or other bleeding cardiopulmonary wounds. Emergency thoracotomy allows the physician to gain rapid access to perform open heart massage in an effort to maintain an adequate cardiac output.

An open thoracotomy is generally performed to repair an injury secondary to trauma, for diagnosis of suspected disease, or for correction or resection of diseased tissue.

DECORTICATION

Decortication involves the removal of pleura that is pathologically thickened and restricts lung expansion. According to Nora (1980), the surgery is appropriate to remove clotted blood after trauma or an encapsulated empyema after an intrathoracic infection. This is a formidable operation and may be associated with significant blood loss.

THORACOPLASTY

Thoracoplasty involves the surgical alteration of the shape of the thoracic cage by removing sections of ribs. The purpose of the procedure is to collapse a diseased portion of a lung. Thoracoplasty was the principal surgical procedure for treatment of pulmonary tuberculosis until about 1935. The use of this surgery has declined considerably since the development of drugs effective against tuber-

culosis. It is rarely performed but may be indicated in the following situations (Glenn, 1983): (1) a client with tubercle bacilli consistently present in sputum cultures who is resistant to drugs but is not a candidate for pulmonary resection; (2) to obliterate an empyema cavity; or (3) to obliterate a noninfected residual pleural space.

LUNG TRANSPLANTATION

Lung transplantation is the removal of diseased lung tissue and replacement with lung tissue from a donor. Between 1963 and 1980, 38 people received lung transplants as treatment for end-stage pulmonary disease. Only two of them survived longer than 6 months after surgery (but not longer than 10 months). Since 1980, an immunosuppressive drug, cyclosporine, has contributed to progress; one person has survived transplantation for more than 1 year. Techniques have been developed to transplant one lung, both lungs, and the heart with both of the lungs. The optimal amount of lung tissue to transplant remains questionable (Veith, Kamholz, Mollenkopf, & Montefusco, 1983).

PULMONARY RESECTIONS

The nature and extent of the disease and the condition of the client determine the type of pulmonary resection to be done. As little tissue as possible is removed to retain maximal pulmonary function. This section discusses several procedures, beginning with removal of the entire lung.

Types of Pulmonary Resection

Pneumonectomy
Pneumonectomy refers to the removal of a lung. A radical pneumonectomy also includes the removal of anterior and posterior mediastinal lymph nodes and excision of the tracheobronchial nodes on the involved side. Removal of an entire lung may be indicated to treat carcinoma of the lung or destruction of lung tissue as a result of extensive pleural disease (ie, tuberculosis). The phrenic nerve on the affected side is crushed or severed to paralyze the diaphragm in an elevated position. This reduces the size of the thoracic cavity on the operative side.

Lobectomy
Lobectomy is the term used to describe the removal of one lobe of either the right or left lung (the right lung has three lobes and the left has two). A lobectomy may be indicated for removal of diseased tissue as a result of bronchiectasis, an emphysematous bleb, carcinoma of the lung, or cysts.

Segmental Resection
The removal of a portion of a lobe of the lung is also referred to as a segmentectomy. A segmental resection may be employed to remove tissue if bronchiectasis, tuberculosis,

well-localized primary or metastatic malignant neoplasm, or an emphysematous bleb has affected only a small portion of the lung.

Wedge Resection

This surgical technique consists of removing a small section or "wedge" of the lung. A wedge resection is appropriate to remove small lesions on or near the surface of the lung. Notable examples include: to remove benign or inflammatory lesions, to obtain a biopsy from a client with diffuse lung disease, to remove metastatic growths, or to obtain tissue when lung cancer is suspected.

Surgical Procedure

The surgeon makes an incision (see Figure 21–8), spreads the ribs apart with a retractor, transects the bronchus or bronchiole, and ligates vessels to the area. The area is inspected, and lung tissue is removed or repaired as appropriate.

Opening the thorax obliterates the normal negative pressure in the intrapleural space, allowing the lung to collapse. During surgery, the loss of negative intrapleural pressure is compensated for; the client is intubated and mechanically ventilated. Chest tubes must be placed prior to closure of the thorax, however, to restore the negative intrapleural pressure and assist in reexpansion of the lungs. After most pulmonary resections, a tube (sometimes more than one) is placed to allow for drainage of blood and fluid from the intrapleural space, and another for the removal of air. After placement of the chest tubes, the chest is closed.

Implications for the Client

Physiological Implications

The client who undergoes thoracic surgery will experience significant discomfort. The degree of pain varies with the type of incision. Because of the pain, clients will tend to guard the area and hypoventilate, which predisposes them to the development of atelectasis (collapse of a section of the lung).

When pulmonary resection is performed, the client's body will have to adjust to the decrease in pulmonary function. The degree of adjustment required by the body depends on the amount of functional lung tissue removed. The pulmonary status of the client may improve postoperatively, especially if the tissue removed had significant perfusion without ventilation.

Complications following thoracic surgery are hemorrhage, hypotension, infection, atelectasis, cardiac dysrhythmias, respiratory failure, pulmonary edema, subcutaneous emphysema, residual pleural space, persistent air leak, bronchopleural fistula, and empyema. These complications and the related nursing care are discussed in Table 21–9.

Psychosocial/Lifestyle Implications

Some clients who have thoracic surgery must cope with the fear of cancer recurrence and death. Those who undergo lung transplants have an additional reason to be anxious: if the surgery is unsuccessful, they will die. They are also aware that lung transplantation is a relatively new procedure and that clients who have survived the surgery have not lived for a long period of time.

Nursing Implications

Preoperative Care

Many of those who undergo thoracic surgery have impaired pulmonary or cardiac function. Most are cigarette smokers and are at least in middle age. Those being treated for cancer may be debilitated by the disease process. Clients are usually admitted for extensive evaluation to determine if they can withstand the stress of thoracic surgery. In addition to routine preoperative tests, clients undergo an evaluation of nutritional status and of cardiac, pulmonary, and renal function. The results of pulmonary function tests and arterial blood gas analyses allow evaluation of respiratory status. (Chapter 18 describes pulmonary function studies and arterial blood gas values.)

If evaluation indicates it will help, aggressive measures may be employed in an attempt to improve the client's nutritional or pulmonary status. This may involve the administration of hyperalimentation or enteral (tube) feedings (see Chapters 8 and 47). IPPB treatments containing bronchodilators may be prescribed to improve respiratory status. Ideally, the client should not smoke. The administration of antibiotics may be necessary in the preoperative period.

Preoperative teaching is of extreme importance since client compliance will greatly affect progress following thoracic surgery. Family members should be included in preoperative preparation. Thoracic surgery is painful because of the incision and presence of chest tubes. Clients will be asked to breathe deeply, to ambulate, and to perform shoulder exercises after surgery. Thoracic surgery affects several muscles that act on the shoulder—the trapezius, the rhomboideus major, the serratus anterior, and the latissimus dorsi. These muscles abduct, adduct, rotate, extend, elevate, and lower the shoulder.

Arm and shoulder exercises prevent stiffening of the shoulder and loss of muscle strength. For abduction and external rotation of the affected arm, ask clients to reach behind their heads and try to touch the opposite scapula. For internal rotation and adduction, ask clients to reach over their chests and touch the opposite acromion and also to reach behind their backs and touch the lower edge of the opposite scapula (Figure 21–9).

The client should be taught (and should demonstrate) the shoulder exercises and the proper technique for coughing and deep breathing. Tell the client that pain medication will be available and not to hesitate to ask for it.

Table 21–9 Physiological Complications of Thoracic Surgery

Complication	Nursing Intervention	Complication	Nursing Intervention
Atelectasis The most common cause of atelectasis is retained bronchial secretions from ineffective coughing. This results in collapse of a portion of the lung distal to the obstruction; infection may develop in the collapsed area.	Refer to nursing measures in the section on promoting optimum pulmonary ventilation.	biotics. For some clients, open drainage and debridement may be necessary. The open wound is packed several times each day. If that is not effective, a decortication may be necessary.	
Bronchopleural fistula A bronchopleural fistula, or opening between the bronchus and the pleural space, may occur during the first week after surgery. It can be signaled by hemoptysis, fever, subcutaneous emphysema, or an extensive air leak. If the fistula develops after pulmonary resection, thoracotomy is usually performed to reclose the bronchial stump; a pneumonectomy is occasionally required.	Assess for and report symptoms and signs that may indicate the presence of a bronchopleural fistula: hemoptysis, fever, subcutaneous emphysema, extensive air leak.	**Hemorrhage** Abnormal bleeding may be caused by a variety of factors. These include inadequate hemostasis at the time of surgery or inadequate coagulation mechanisms.	Monitor vital signs and report significant changes: • Increased pulse • Decreased blood pressure Observe for presence of blood on dressing. Monitor drainage from chest tubes and record hourly.
Cardiac dysrhythmia This is a common complication of thoracic surgery, especially sinus tachycardia, premature atrial contractions, premature ventricular contractions, atrial fibrillation, and atrial flutter.	Monitor the client's status continuously via ECG for a prescribed period. Note the presence of cardiac dysrhythmias. Take appropriate measures to alleviate side effects from the particular dysrhythmia.	**Hypotension** Clients may become hypotensive after thoracic surgery because of a decreased cardiac output. This may result from fluid or blood loss, a myocardial infarction, or cardiac tamponade.	Refer to nursing intervention in the section on maintaining adequate cardiac output.
		Infection Wound infections at the site of a lateral thoracotomy occur but are fairly uncommon.	Assess and report symptoms and signs of infection: inflammation, redness, tenderness, purulent drainage, tachycardia, persistent temperature elevation.
Empyema Empyema, or the presence of pus in a body cavity, is a fairly common complication of pulmonary resection, where the body cavity involved is the intrapleural space. Empyema is more likely to develop if the pleural space is not obliterated, and serosanguineous fluid collects in it. Most clients who develop empyema can be successfully treated with pleural drainage (chest tubes) and systemic anti-	Assess and report symptoms and signs that could indicate the presence of an empyema: • Fever • Pleuritic pain • Dullness on percussion of the area Perform dressing change as needed. If the client is discharged with the wound still open, either the client or a family member or friend should be taught to change the dressing.	**Persistent air leak** Most of the openings in the lung parenchyma through which air can leak close spontaneously by the second or third day after surgery. An air leak that persists may be treated by injecting a sclerosing agent such as tetracycline into the pleural space and, if that is ineffective, by surgery (Glenn, 1983).	Assess the client's respiratory status. Monitor chest tube drainage; bubbling in the under-water seal chamber from the chest tube signals an air leak.
		Pulmonary edema Pulmonary edema is a grave complication that results when fluid from the pulmonary capillaries effuses into the interstitial spaces and into the	Assess for symptoms and signs of acute respiratory failure: • Tachypnea • Restlessness • Cyanosis

Complication	Nursing Intervention	Complications	Nursing Intervention
alveoli. A common cause of pulmonary edema after thoracic surgery is hypervolemia from overinfusion of fluids. Contributing factors may include myocardial infarction, decreased serum protein, and injury to pulmonary capillaries from sepsis or oxygen toxicity. The goal of treatment is to remove fluid from the pulmonary interstitial spaces and improve blood gas exchange. This may entail administration of diuretics and inotropic agents to improve cardiac output. Morphine sulfate may be prescribed to reduce the client's anxiety and peripheral vascular resistance. Oxygen is administered. Other therapeutic measures include rotating tourniquets and phlebotomy. Mechanical ventilation assistance may be needed (Glenn, 1983).	Assess for signs and symptoms of pulmonary edema: • Rales on auscultation of the lungs • Productive cough • Diastolic gallop Observe for cardiac dysrhythmias that may accompany impaired blood gas exchange. Administer oxygen and medication as prescribed. Provide for safety of client requiring rotating tourniquets (see Chapter 24).	mediastinum, and elevation of the diaphragm. If these do not occur, treatment may involve thoracoplasty using muscle tissue to fill the pleural space. **Respiratory failure** Respiratory failure is a potential complication whose etiology is not always clear. An inability to get rid of bronchial secretions and pulmonary edema seem to be contributing factors. **Subcutaneous emphysema** Subcutaneous emphysema is the presence of air under the skin; it occurs because of disruption of the respiratory tract. An occluded chest tube, for example, prevents the escape of air through the tube; the air travels under the skin instead. An air leak may also cause subcutaneous emphysema.	Refer to Chapter 19 for nursing interventions. Assess for signs of subcutaneous emphysema: • Swelling or puffiness of the skin • Presence of crepitation (a crackling sensation as if touching wrinkled cellophane) on light palpation of the area Assess progression or resolution of subcutaneous emphysema: • Note and record daily the anatomical areas involved • Note the degree of swelling of the areas Provide comfort for the client by avoiding physical irritation of affected areas by sheets or equipment.
Residual pleural space Residual pleural space is a complication that can affect respiratory status. When a portion of a lung is removed, the pleural space should be obliterated by further inflation of the remaining lung tissue, shifting of the	Monitor the client's respiratory status.		

Psychological preparation of the client and family may include a preoperative visit to the intensive care unit. Such a visit may decrease anxiety. The client must be prepared for the presence and function of the tubes (including chest tubes) that will be inserted during surgery. For chest tubes, it should be sufficient to say that they allow drainage of fluid or air so the lungs can function as they should.

Postoperative Care

Clients who have thoracic surgery are initially transported to a recovery room or intensive care unit for continuous observation. They should remain in the unit until they are stabilized. The client may arrive from surgery with an endotracheal tube, pulmonary artery catheter (Swan–Ganz catheter), central venous pressure line (CVP), arterial line, peripheral intravenous lines, chest tubes connected to a closed water-seal drainage system, and a urinary catheter.

Nursing goals for the thoracic surgical client in the postoperative period include: maintenance of adequate cardiac output, promotion of optimal pulmonary ventilation, maintenance of normal fluid and electrolyte balance, relief from pain, promotion of optimal wound healing, promotion of recovery without residual dysfunction, and emotional support and encouragement.

Maintaining Adequate Cardiac Output. Immediately upon arrival from surgery, the client's blood pressure should be obtained and electrodes fixed to the chest

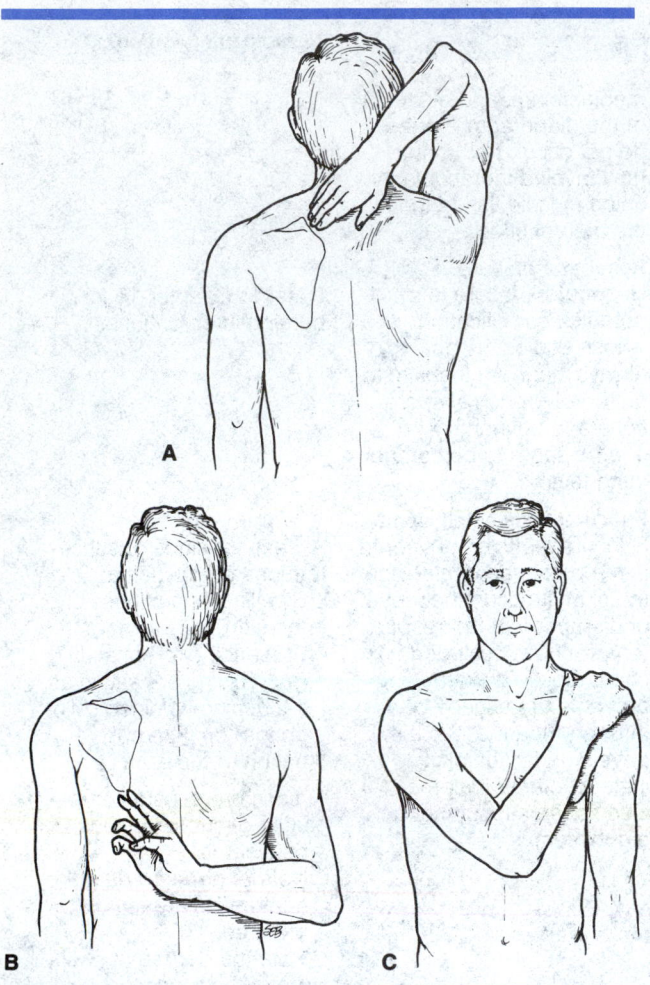

Figure 21–9

Arm and shoulder exercises for the post-operative thoracotomy client. **A.** External rotation and abduction. **B, C.** Internal rotation and adduction.

to facilitate continuous monitoring of the cardiac rhythm. Connect the Swan–Ganz catheter and arterial line to the transducers that transform the pressure into continuous readings of pulmonary artery pressures and systemic blood pressure on the oscilloscopes. Monitor respiratory rate and heart rate every 15 minutes until stable and then hourly, along with the client's temperature.

Take CVP readings hourly. Pulmonary capillary wedge pressures may be ordered every 1 or 2 hours. This reading indirectly reflects the function of the left ventricle, whereas the CVP is an indication of right ventricular function. The nursing care of clients with a Swan–Ganz catheter, arterial line, and CVP line is discussed in Chapter 23.

A change in body temperature alters the metabolic requirement and, thus, affects the cardiac output. If the client's temperature is greater than 102°F (39°C), an antipyretic is prescribed. If the temperature rises above 104°F (40°C), the client is placed on a cooling pad. A hypothermic client, conversely, is placed on a heating mattress and covered with blankets (Glenn, 1983).

Drainage from the chest tubes must be monitored hourly. In the immediate postoperative period, it is wise to note the amount every 15 minutes. Persistent drainage of more than 200 mL per hour may require reexploration to achieve hemostasis. Clients should be encouraged to move their legs frequently while in bed to promote venous return to the heart and prevent the formation of clots.

Promoting Optimal Pulmonary Ventilation. Most thoracic surgery clients can have the endotracheal tube removed immediately after surgery. Some, however, require assisted mechanical ventilation because of complications. Humidified oxygen is administered either by endotracheal tube or by mask to prevent hypoxia and liquify secretions. Assess the client's color, respiration, and other vital signs. Auscultate the chest. Frequent analysis of arterial blood gas samples may be necessary.

The nurse must ensure that chest tubes remain in the intrapleural space, are patent, and connected to a closed water-seal collection receptacle. (Refer to Chapter 18.) Carefully observe the amount and character of the chest tube drainage. The client who undergoes a pneumonectomy, however, may not have chest tubes; a majority of surgeons now elect *not* to place them after this surgery. The residual space gradually fills with fluid the first few days after surgery, but this fluid eventually solidifies. Some surgeons place a chest tube for the first 2 or 3 postoperative days, but keep it clamped, ordering it opened periodically to evacuate residual air (Nora, 1980). The nurse caring for a client who has a pneumonectomy must observe for symptoms and signs of a mediastinal shift (discussed in Chapter 20).

As soon as the client regains consciousness, encourage coughing and deep breathing every hour for the first 24 hours. Coughing is more effective if the client is assisted to a sitting position with the feet resting on a chair. The incision should be supported anteriorly and posteriorly to minimize pain (Figure 21–10). Diaphragmatic breathing and postural drainage may be prescribed, depending on the amount of pulmonary secretions. (They are described in Chapter 18.)

The client should change position every 1 to 2 hours. Special precautions are usually ordered for clients after a pneumonectomy. Opinions differ among surgeons. In general, however, it is recommended that the client not be turned to the unoperative side. This is to allow maximum ventilation of the remaining lung. Many physicians specify that clients who undergo lobectomy or a segmental resection be positioned so their operated side is up, to facilitate expansion of the remaining tissue in the lung. After 1 or 2 days, these clients can usually be turned to either side (Johanson, Dungca, Hoffmeister, & Wells, 1981). Clients who undergo other types of thoracic surgery can usually be turned from their back to each side.

If other measures are unsuccessful in the removal of pulmonary secretions, nasotracheal suctioning may be required (discussed in Chapter 18).

The client may dangle the legs at the bedside the evening of surgery and should ambulate with assistance the first day after surgery, unless contraindicated for medical reasons.

Maintaining Normal Fluid and Electrolyte Balance. Several measures can assist in determining the client's fluid status. Daily weights are obtained. The urine output is closely monitored and should amount to at least 30 mL per hour. Some clients will require a urinary catheter, but others will not. Elevated CVP readings can indicate that the client is hypervolemic and a reading below normal suggests hypovolemia. The normal reading is 5 to 12 cm of water. Intravenous fluid replacement is prescribed at specific rates by the physician. Administering fluids too rapidly, however, can lead to complications such as pulmonary edema.

If the abdominal cavity was not entered during surgery, clients can take fluids by mouth as soon as they are alert. Clients should be encouraged to drink a minimum of 1500 to 2000 mL of fluid each day unless contraindicated for medical reasons. The client can usually be advanced to the prescribed diet by the third postoperative day.

Relief From Pain. A narcotic analgesic such as meperidine or morphine is prescribed to be given every 2 to 3 hours as needed. Caution should be used when administering narcotic analgesics since they can lead to respiratory depression. Later, oral medication such as codeine, aspirin, or acetaminophen should be sufficient.

Pain medication should be administered 30 to 40 minutes before the client is asked to perform exercises that cause discomfort. This may increase client cooperation. Intercostal nerve blocks have been effective in reducing the pain in some clients.

Promoting Optimal Wound Healing. In the operating room, a light dressing is usually applied to the wound and secured with elastic adhesive tape. It may be taken off the first postoperative day to expose the wound to air. Bloody drainage on the chest dressing is unusual and should be reported to the surgeon. Cleansing of the wound may be necessary at regular intervals. The specific technique varies among surgeons and institutions. Sutures may be removed approximately 1 week after surgery.

Promoting Recovery Without Residual Dysfunction. As a result of anterolateral and posterolateral approaches in which nerve and muscle tissues are transected, the client may experience atrophy of the distal end of the transected muscle. In addition, altered sensation around the wound can last for months. The client will tend not to move the arm on the affected side because of the discomfort it causes. To combat these factors, the client is taught arm and shoulder exercises. Passive ROM exercises should be performed a few hours after surgery. The client should progress to active ROM exercises despite the discomfort they cause. Clients often need a great deal of encouragement to carry out these exercises.

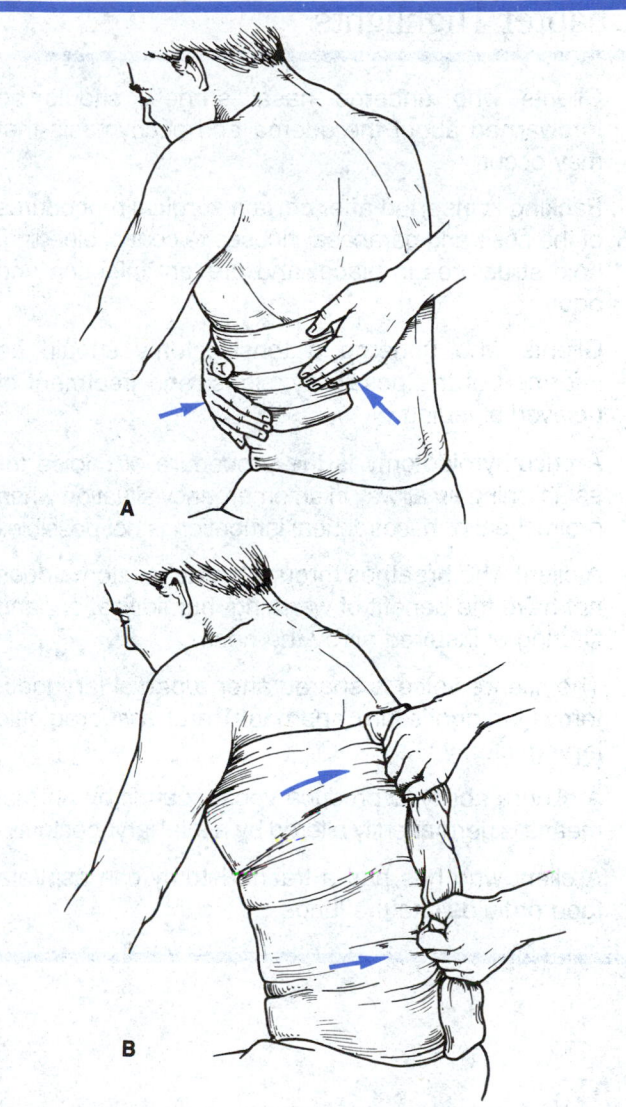

Figure 21–10

Support of a thoracotomy incision during coughing.

Emotional Support and Encouragement. The environment, the presence of numerous tubes, and the pain can drain the client emotionally. The client and family members (and significant others) will require explanations and reassurance.

Discharge Teaching

Prior to discharge from the hospital, clients should be able to care for themselves. They should know to report any symptoms and signs of a respiratory tract infection such as persistent fever, increased sputum production, and shortness of breath. They should understand why it is important to continue exercising the affected arm. Encourage clients to return for follow-up evaluation; this consists of assessment of the degree of wound healing and respiratory status. If the client was diagnosed as having cancer, an assessment will be made for recurrence or progression of the disease.

Chapter Highlights

Clients who undergo nasal surgery should be forewarned about the edema and ecchymosis that may occur.

Packing is inserted after certain surgical procedures of the nose and paranasal sinuses to control bleeding, hold structures in place, and prevent infection and odor.

Clients who undergo a tonsillectomy should be informed of the possibility, signs, and treatment of delayed bleeding.

A cricothyroidotomy is the procedure of choice for establishing an airway in an emergency situation when orotracheal or nasotracheal intubation is not possible.

A client who breathes through a tracheostoma does not have the benefit of warming, humidification, and filtering of inspired air by the nose.

The client's voice is spared after a partial laryngectomy (laryngofissure approach) and a supraglottic laryngectomy.

A client's ability to produce vocal sounds by normal means is permanently altered by a total laryngectomy.

A client who has had a tracheostomy can aspirate food or fluids into the lungs.

It is anatomically impossible for a client who has had a total laryngectomy to aspirate unless a fistula forms between the trachea and esophagus or fluid enters through the stoma.

Entrance into the intrapleural space results in obliteration of the negative intrapleural pressure and collapse of the lung.

During thoracic surgery, the loss of negative intrapleural pressure is compensated for by intubating and mechanically ventilating the client.

Chest tubes are placed after most thoracic surgical procedures to restore the negative intrapleural pressure by allowing exit of air and fluid.

Vigorous pulmonary care is necessary in the postoperative period after thoracic surgery to prevent complications.

In general, clients who undergo pneumonectomy should *not* be placed on their unoperative side.

Thorough preoperative teaching of the client undergoing thoracic surgery is essential to ensure client and family cooperation in the postoperative period.

Observation for early symptoms and signs of potential complications of thoracic surgery is a major part of nursing care.

Bibliography

Conlee D: Put a new face on your care of cosmetic surgery patients. *Nursing '81,* 1981; 11:90–95.

DeWeese D, Saunders W: *Textbook of Otolaryngology,* 6th ed. St. Louis: Mosby, 1982.

Gates G (editor): *Current Therapy in Otolaryngology—Head and Neck Surgery.* Trenton, NJ: Decker, 1982.

Glenn W (editor): *Thoracic and Cardiovascular Surgery.* 4th ed. Norwalk, CT: Appleton-Century-Crofts, 1983.

Johanson B et al: *Standards for Critical Care.* St. Louis: Mosby, 1981.

Kane KK: Carotid artery rupture in advanced head and neck cancer patients. *Oncol Nurs Forum* (Winter) 1983; 10(1): 14–18.

Katz LE: Postoperative complications of thoracic surgery: Their recognition and treatment. *AANA J* (June) 1980; 48(3): 222–228.

Knapp B, Panje E: A voice button for laryngectomees. *AORN J* 1982; 36:183–191.

Nora P (editor): *Operative Surgery, Principles and Techniques.* Philadelphia: Lea & Febiger, 1980.

Paparella M, Shumrick D (editors): *Otolaryngology* Vol. 3. Philadelphia: Saunders, 1980.

Ryan J: *The Nurse and the Communicatively Impaired Adult.* New York: Springer, 1982.

Saunders, W: Surgery of the inferior nasal turbinates. *Ann Otol Rhinol Laryngol* 1982; 91:445–447.

Saunders W et al: *Nursing Care in Eye, Ear, Nose, and Throat Disorders.* St. Louis: Mosby, 1979.

Veith FJ et al: Lung transplantation–1983. *Transplantation* (April) 1983; 35(4):271–278.

Suggested Readings

Baker BM, Cunningham CA: Vocal rehabilitation of the patient with a laryngectomy. *Oncol Nurs Forum* (Fall) 1980; 7(4):23–27. This comprehensive article contains information about client rehabilitation after a laryngectomy. It is divided into preoperative and postoperative counseling, assessment of the client, and specific techniques of vocal rehabilitation.

Larsen G: Rehabilitation for the patient with head and neck cancer. *Am J Nurs* (Jan) 1982; 82(1):119–120. The author describes the various problems clients encounter after head and neck surgery. Information is presented that the nurse can use to help the client.

McCormick GP et al: Artificial speech devices. *Am J Nurs* (Jan) 1982; 82(1):121–122. The authors give specific information about artificial speech aids. Information on electronic talking machines (speech synthesizers) is also presented.

Pilcher L: Carbon dioxide lasers in laryngeal surgery. *AORN J* (June) 1981; 33(7):1402–1406. The author provides a good explanation of laser surgery. Nursing implications of the use of the laser in the operating room are discussed. Client complications are presented.

The Client With Cardiovascular System Dysfunction

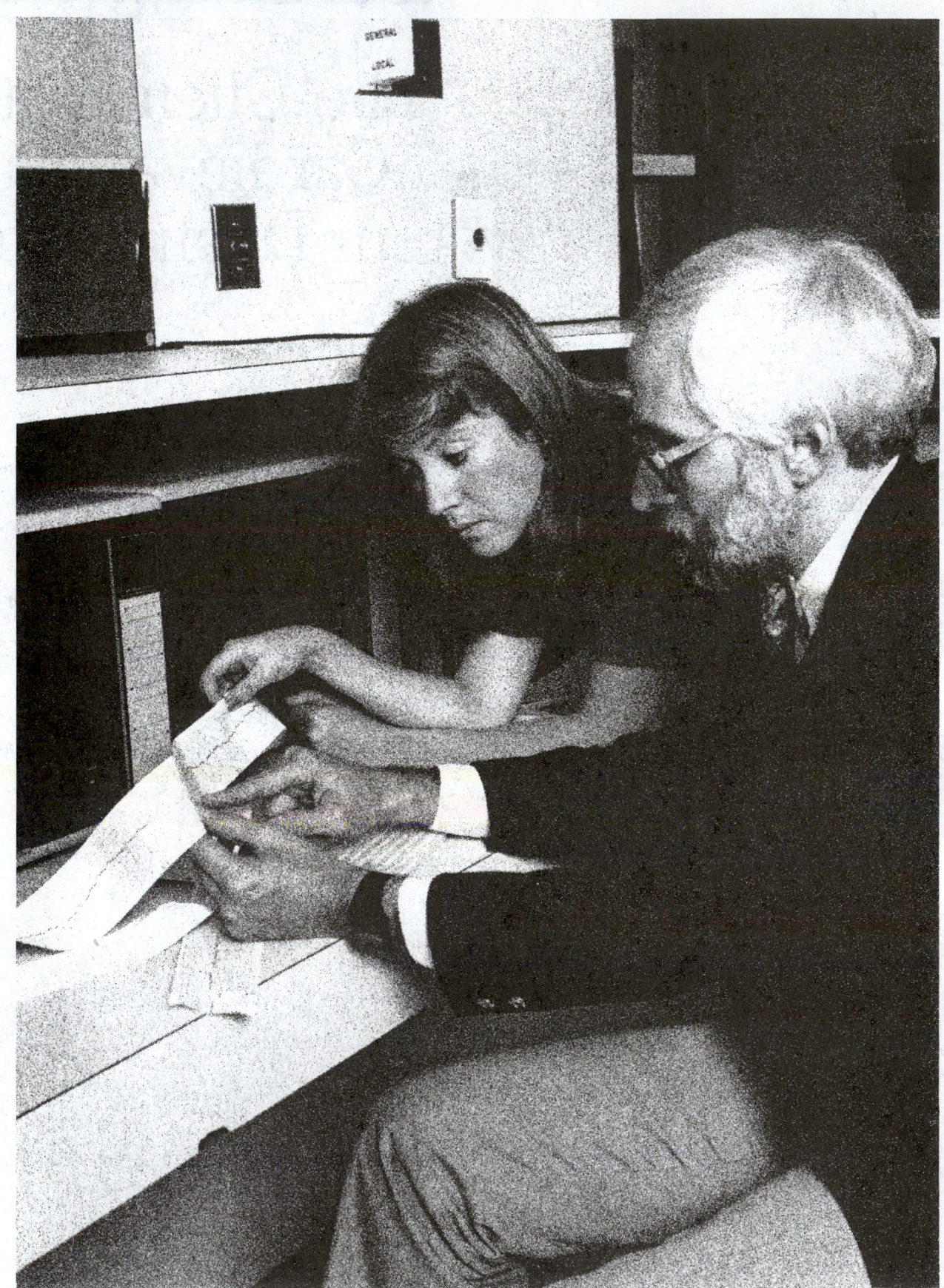

Chapter 22

The Cardiovascular System in Health and Illness

Constance A. Settlemyer
Linda Rae Belsky

Objectives

When you have finished studying this chapter, you should be able to:

List the purposes of the circulating blood.

Trace the blood flow through the heart, the pulmonary circulation, and the systemic circulation.

Trace the normal conduction of an electrical impulse through the heart and relate it to muscular activity and blood flow through the heart and major vessels.

Identify the types of blood vessels and their functions.

Describe the functions of the lymphatic system.

Identify the formed elements of the blood and their purposes.

Discuss the regulatory influences on the cardiovascular system.

Explain the sequence of events when tissue is deprived of adequate blood flow.

Identify the pathological conditions that promote decreased blood flow and the mechanisms by which they inhibit cellular nutrition.

Discuss internal and external factors that influence bone marrow function.

Differentiate disorders of the erythrocytes, thrombocytes, and leukocytes and their general effects on the client.

Recognize the consequences for other body systems of problems with the cardiovascular or blood-forming system.

Anticipate the psychosocial/lifestyle adjustments that an individual with a cardiovascular problem or bone marrow dysfunction may need to make and discuss the impact on the client and family or significant others.

This chapter will review the anatomy and physiology of the heart, blood vessels, lymphatic system, and blood components in relation to aspects of nursing care most significant for adult clients. Pathological changes will be discussed in relation to their interference with cardiovascular function. The psychosocial aspects will be discussed in relation to the effects of pathological cardiovascular changes on the client's lifestyle.

Section I: Structural and Functional Interrelationships

The heart, which actually functions as two pumps, contracts and generates pressures to push the blood through the entire vascular system and back. Figure 22–1 traces the blood flow through pulmonary and systemic circuits. The right side of the heart generates the pressures required to pump blood through the capillaries of the lungs (where exchange of gases, primarily oxygen and carbon dioxide, occurs) and to the left side of the heart. The left side of the heart generates pressure to push the blood throughout the systemic circulation (where nutrients, waste products,

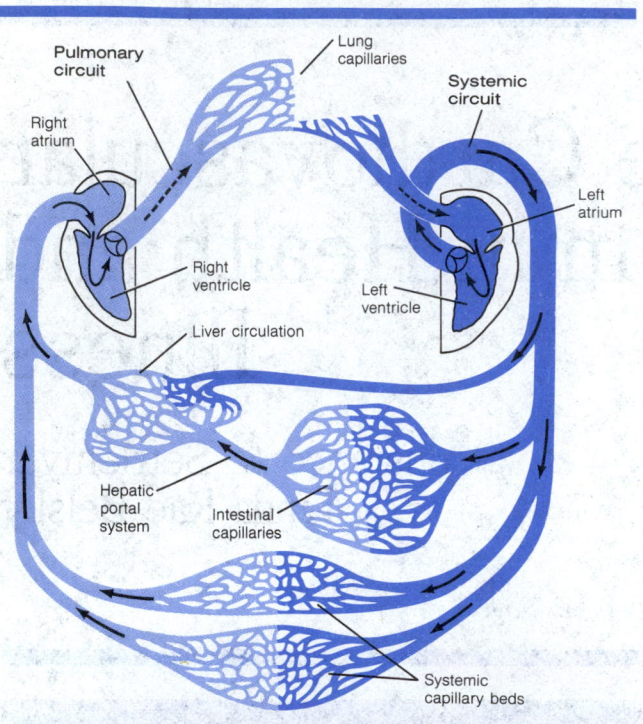

Figure 22–1

Blood circulation through the pulmonary and systemic circuits.

SOURCE: Spence AP, Mason EB: *Human Anatomy and Physiology.* Menlo Park, CA: Benjamin/Cummings, 1983, p. 482.

and a variety of other chemical substances are exchanged between the capillaries and interstitial spaces or the cellular internal environment) and back to the right side of the heart, where the process is repeated.

The vascular system consists of arteries, arterioles, capillaries, venules, and veins, which provide the conduit for blood flow. The arteries promote blood flow throughout the system and divert it to the capillaries. There the blood provides nutrients or body defense substances when and where needed and picks up waste by-products from the cellular environment. The arteries also route the blood to areas where nutrients, body defense substances, and chemicals are picked up to be distributed elsewhere in the body. They transport the blood to areas where waste products either can be reprocessed or removed, such as the liver and kidneys. The arteries contribute to body temperature regulation by diverting blood to the skin where heat can be released or diverting blood away from the skin so body heat can be conserved. An artery less than 0.5 mm in diameter is called an *arteriole*. Small arteries and arterioles are called resistance vessels because by dilation or constriction they regulate the volume and pressure in the arterial system and blood flow into the capillary bed.

Venules, which receive their blood from the capillaries, converge to form veins of progressively larger diameters. The veins carry the blood back to the right side of the heart (or to the left side from the lungs). They also serve

as a reservoir for blood when the body needs are reduced. The *capillaries* serve not only as conduits for blood flow but also as sites for the exchanges between the interstitial spaces and the blood.

The lymphatic system acts as an accessory circulation for the fluids and particles that leave the capillaries and do not return by the same route. The lymphatics pick up excess fluid and larger particles such as proteins and return them to the circulatory system. The lymphatics also protect the body against infection.

The blood consists of erythrocytes (red cells), leukocytes (white cells), thrombocytes (platelets), clotting factors, water, oxygen, carbon dioxide, electrolytes, vitamins, minerals, sugar, proteins, fats, hormones, and other chemical substances, as well as waste products. The quality and quantity of the blood determine whether the circulatory system can fulfill its purpose.

In studying cardiovascular dynamics, the nurse should understand and be able to apply some laws of physics. Probably the most important is **Poiseuille's law,** which holds that the flow rate of a fluid through a tube is proportional to pressure differences and the diameter of the tube in relation to the length of the tube and the viscosity of the fluid. In the cardiovascular system, the heart generates the pressure, the diameter and length of the tubes are determined by the blood vessels, and the blood has a certain viscosity. To visualize the application of this law, imagine giving an injection. The more pressure applied to the plunger, the faster the fluid flows; the smaller the diameter and the longer the needle, the greater the pressure needed to make the fluid flow; and the more viscous the fluid, the greater the pressure needed to make the fluid flow. Factors that hinder flow involve *resistance,* which in this case is determined by the diameter and length of the tube as well as the viscosity of the fluid. In addition, the pressure depends on the amount of fluid in the container.

THE HEART

The **cardiac output,** or the amount of blood the heart pumps per minute, is determined by the amount of blood the heart pumps with each stroke (**stroke volume**) and the number of strokes per minute (**heart rate**). The heart pumps about 70 mL of blood with each stroke at an average rate of 72 beats per minute; this accounts for an average of over 5000 mL of blood per minute. The heart can increase this quantity of blood by about four times by increasing its rate, the amount of blood it pumps with each stroke, or both. The heart's ability to do this depends on its ability to time contractions, its ability to contract, and the amount of blood available to pump. These capabilities of the heart first will be described in an overall presentation of blood flow through the heart, contractility of the heart, electrical conduction in the heart, and coronary circulation in relation to anatomy and physiology. Factors outside the heart that influence these variables will be discussed later in the chapter in relation to their influence on the whole system.

Blood Flow Through the Heart

The heart, a four-chambered structure about the size of a fist, is located in the mediastinum of the chest just beneath the sternum. The upper chambers are called the *atria* and the lower, the *ventricles*. The chambers are separated by valves. The valve separating the right chambers, with three cusps, is called the *tricuspid valve*. The valve separating the left chambers is called the *bicuspid* or *mitral valve* and has two cusps. Both are referred to as the *atrioventricular (A-V) valves*. Two other valves in the heart open when blood leaves the ventricles: the *pulmonic valve* on the right and the *aortic valve* on the left. They are named for the arteries into which they open. These valves are often referred to as the *semilunar valves*.

A key point to keep in mind while tracing blood flow is that fluids move from an area of higher pressure to one of lower pressure (Figure 22–2). Blood flows from the venous system (which averages about 10 mm Hg pressure)

into the right atrium (which averages about 0 mm Hg pressure) via the venae cavae and coronary sinus. While the right ventricle is in relaxation, or diastole, blood continues to flow through the tricuspid valve and into the right ventricle. When the right ventricle is about 70% to 75% full, the right atrium contracts (causing a rise in pressure) and fills the right ventricle about 25% to 30% more. Shortly after the right atrium completes its contraction (right atrial systole), the right ventricle begins to contract (right ventricular systole) and generates enough pressure (about 22 mm Hg) to cause the tricuspid valve to close, the pulmonic valve to open, and blood to flow into the pulmonary artery. While the right ventricle is in systole, the right atrium is in diastole and collects blood from the venous system.

Simultaneously, similar activity is happening in the left side of the heart. Blood flows freely into the left atrium and through the mitral valve into the left ventricle during left ventricular diastole, as the blood pressure in both chambers is near 0 mm Hg. When the left ventricle is about

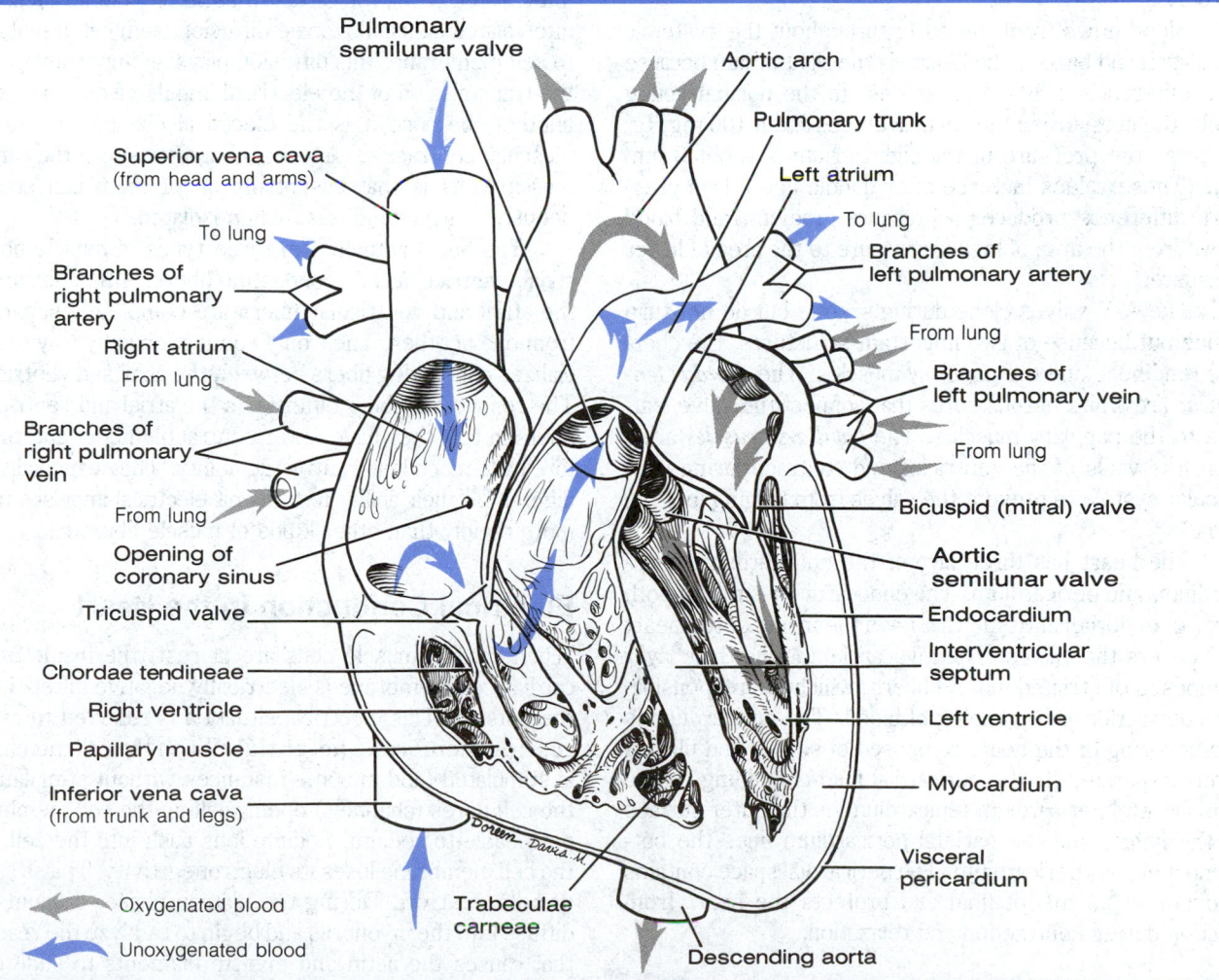

Figure 22–2

Frontal section of the heart. The arrows indicate the path of the blood flow through the chambers, the valves, and the major vessels. Note that the branches of the right pulmonary vein pass behind the heart and enter the left atrium.
SOURCE: Spence AP, Mason EB: *Human Anatomy and Physiology.* Menlo Park, CA: Benjamin/Cummings, 1983, p. 478.

70% to 75% full, the left atrium contracts to fill the left ventricle another 25% to 30%. Shortly after left atrial systole, the left ventricle begins to contract (left ventricular systole) and generates enough pressure (about 120 mm Hg) to cause the mitral valve to close, the aortic valve to open, and blood to flow into the aorta to be carried into the systemic circulation. As the ventricles relax (ventricular diastole), the pressure drops, and blood attempts to flow backward through the semilunar valves. Because these valves are shaped like cups, blood fills them up and closes the valves. This is important because the arteries that feed the heart muscle are located near the cusps of the aortic valve and fill during diastole.

The left ventricle generates a higher pressure than the right; this is logical, because the left side of the heart needs to pump the blood a greater distance. The left ventricle has a greater work load, needs more muscle mass, and therefore has a thicker muscular wall. If the arterial diastolic pressure rises, promoting more resistance to flow as it does in hypertension, the left ventricle must work harder.

Blood flows from the aorta throughout the systemic circulation and back to the heart via the right atrium because of a difference in blood pressures. In the normal young adult, the pressure in the aorta averages about 100 mg Hg, whereas the pressure in the right atrium is about 0 mm Hg. (These values increase after middle age.) This pressure difference produces a pressure gradient, and blood flows from the area of higher pressure to the area of lower pressure.

The A-V valves close during systole but do not turn inside out because of two important structures, the chordae tendineae and the papillary muscles. The *chordae tendineae* are white fibrous cords that connect the valve leaflets to the papillary muscles. The *papillary muscles* arise from the walls of the ventricles and contract during ventricular systole to prevent the valves from bulging into the atria.

The heart has three layers: the endocardium, myocardium, and pericardium. The endocardium is the smooth layer of endothelial tissue that lines the inside of the heart and covers the valves. The myocardium is the thick layer composed of striated muscle fibers, which are responsible for contraction and pumping of blood. The pericardium is the covering of the heart composed of serous and fibrous layers separated by the pericardial fluid-containing space. The visceral pericardium (epicardium) is the outer surface of the heart, and the parietal pericardium lines the outermost fibrous pericardium. The pericardial space contains about 5 to 20 mL of fluid and protects the heart from friction during contraction and relaxation.

Contractility of the Heart

Within its physiological limits, the heart is able to pump all the blood returning to it without allowing it to back up into the veins. Because the body tissues regulate their own blood flow according to their needs, the amount of blood returning to the heart varies from moment to moment, and the heart is able to accommodate these changes. The muscle fibers of the heart act similarly to skeletal muscle fibers when stretched. The more they are stretched within physiological limits, the greater the force of contraction. The myocardial fibers stretch with increased amounts of returning blood during diastole and contract with greater force during systole (called the Frank Starling law of the heart). **Preload** is the term that refers to the degree of stretch of myocardial fibers before contraction. **Afterload** is the term that refers to the tension the ventricles must develop in systole to pump against pressure in the aortic valve, aorta, and to resistance in the systemic and pulmonary arterioles.

The cardiac muscle fibers are similar to skeletal muscle fibers in that they have actin and myosin protein filaments that slide along one another, producing contraction. They are different from skeletal muscle fibers in that the cardiac muscle cells are separated from one another by intercalated disks, the cardiac muscle cell membranes. The intercalated disks allow free diffusion from cell membrane to cell membrane; this diffusion plays an important part in the transmission of the electrical impulse from one cell to another, because it is the electrical change that signals muscular contraction. Another characteristic of the cardiac muscle cells is that essentially all of them can spontaneously contract and relax when isolated.

The heart actually has three types of muscle fibers: atrial, ventricular, and conducting fibers. Although similar, the atrial and ventricular fibers are completely separated from one another. Their only connection is by way of specialized conducting fibers between the atria and ventricles. The conducting fibers differ from the atrial and ventricular fibers in that they have fewer contractile fibers and therefore have much less contractile ability. They especially are different in their ability to transmit electrical impulses much more rapidly than other kinds of muscle fibers can.

Electrical Conduction in the Heart

When cardiac muscle cells are at rest, the inside of the cardiac cell membrane is electrically negative in relation to the outside. This electrical situation is referred to as the **resting membrane potential.** When the cell membrane is stimulated (and in some instances without stimulation), the cell pores (channels) open, making the cell membrane permeable to sodium. Sodium ions rush into the cell, and the cell membrane loses its electronegativity. This is called **depolarization.** During the plateau phase, calcium ions diffuse into the myofibrils and begin to catalyze the reaction that causes the actin and myosin filaments to slide over one another to effect contraction. Suddenly, the cell membrane becomes impermeable to sodium ions and permeable to potassium ions. Potassium ions rush out of the cell and promote the return to the resting membrane potential, or **repolarization.** After repolarization, the calcium ions diffuse out of the myofibrils, causing muscular relaxation. This entire process of depolarization and repolarization is called the **action potential.**

This electrical activity in the heart can be visualized by putting electrical sensors on the surface of the skin and recording the activity by use of the electrocardiograph (ECG). Imagine the cells in a resting state as dominoes that are standing up side by side waiting to be knocked down. When a domino falls, it depolarizes; when it automatically gets up and is capable of falling down again, it is repolarized. These are special dominoes, because when one domino falls, it can knock down all the dominoes close to it—ahead, behind, or to the side of it—and all of them at the same time. The influx of sodium causes the dominoes to fall and subsequently causes the next dominoes to fall. Realize that a domino can knock down any adjacent domino, but it knocks down those near the intercalated disk faster. Some domino pathways are faster, and some take longer. The fast pathways are through the specialized conductive tissue; going through muscle mass takes longer. The only way the atrial dominoes can knock down the ventricular dominoes is to go through the specialized con-

ductive tissue between atria and ventricles. Think of an electrical sensor (the ECG) detecting the direction in which the dominoes (cells) are falling (depolarizing) and getting up (repolarizing).

The fast conductive fibers that are important in understanding impulse transmission through the heart include the sinoatrial (S-A) node, the A-V node, the bundle of His, the right and left bundle branches, and the Purkinje fibers (see Figure 22–3). Essentially all the cells of the heart are believed capable of automaticity (spontaneous depolarization without external stimulation). The S-A node, located in the right atrium medial to the junction of the right atrium and the superior vena cava, has the fastest intrinsic rate for spontaneous depolarization. The S-A node normally spontaneously depolarizes between 70 and 80 times per minute. The fast conductive fibers in the area of the A-V node, located just beneath the septal wall of the atria, have an intrinsic rate of about 40 to 60 spontaneous depolarizations per minute. The bundle of His is continuous with the A-V node, the left bundle branch (which runs along the left interventricular septum), the right bundle branch (which runs along the right interventricular septum), and the ter-

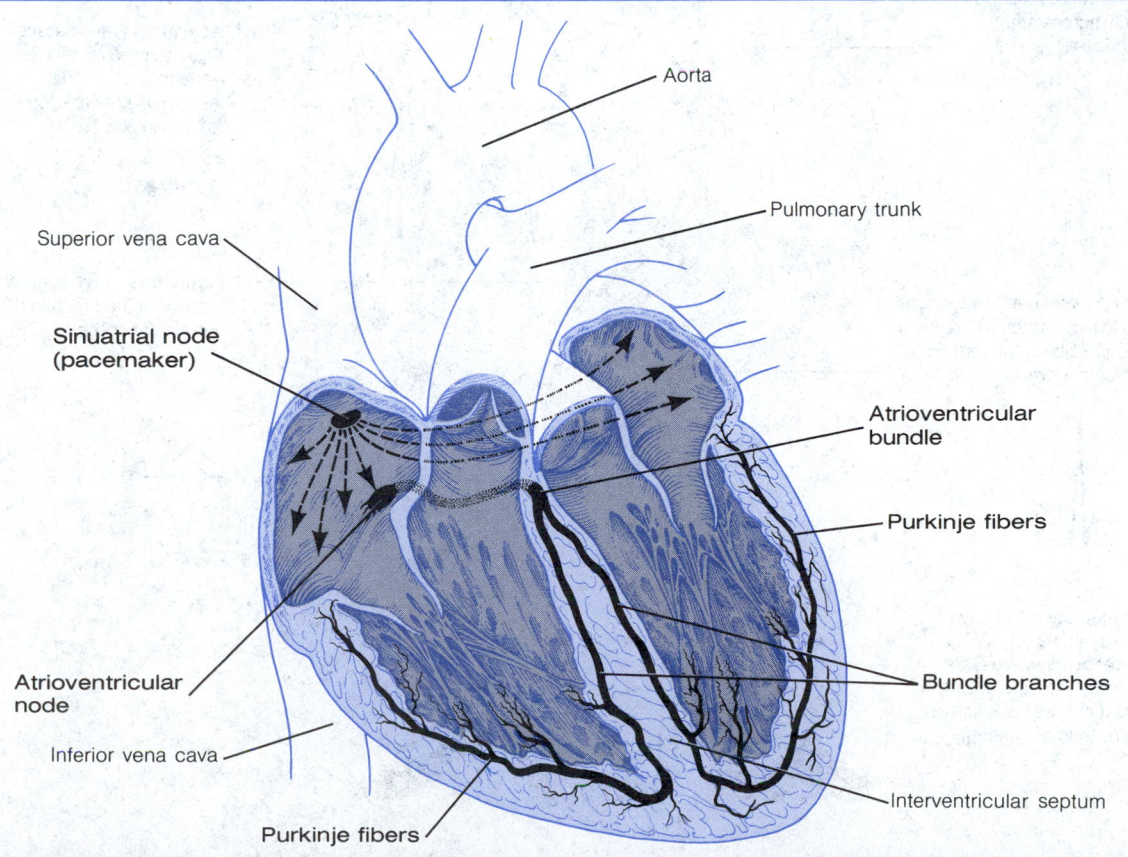

Figure 22–3

The excitation and conduction system of the heart. The dashed arrows indicate the stimulatory impulse from the S-A node as it travels through the myocardia of both atria.

SOURCE: Spence AP, Mason EB: *Human Anatomy and Physiology.* Menlo Park, CA: Benjamin/Cummings, 1983, p. 485.

minal Purkinje network (which penetrates the heart muscle). The Purkinje fibers have an intrinsic rate of between 15 and 40 spontaneous depolarizations per minute.

The S-A node is called the "pacemaker of the heart" because its depolarization wave spreads throughout the heart and causes depolarization of the heart cells before any other cells spontaneously depolarize. Normally, the depolarization wave spreads rapidly through these extremely fast fibers and spreads less quickly through the muscle walls, signaling the muscle's cells to contract.

Figure 22–4 shows the electrical events and the ECG inscription described as P, Q, R, S, and T waves. The S-A node initiates the impulse, which is spread throughout the atria and into the A-V node, where the impulse is delayed while the atria contract to fill the ventricles completely. This produces a P wave on the ECG, signifying transmission of the depolarization wave through the atria. (The wave is written upright, because the sensor is near the apex of the heart.) There is a period of no electrical activity (signified by a straight line on the ECG) while the ventricles are filling (called the PR interval). Suddenly, the wave spreads through the bundle of His and into the ventricular septum (from left to right), which causes the inscription of the Q wave (the first negative deflection). The depolarization wave spreads rapidly through the right and left ventricles. Because the left ventricle has many more cells, the electrical sensor draws an upward R wave. The last part of the ventricle to depolarize is the left upper

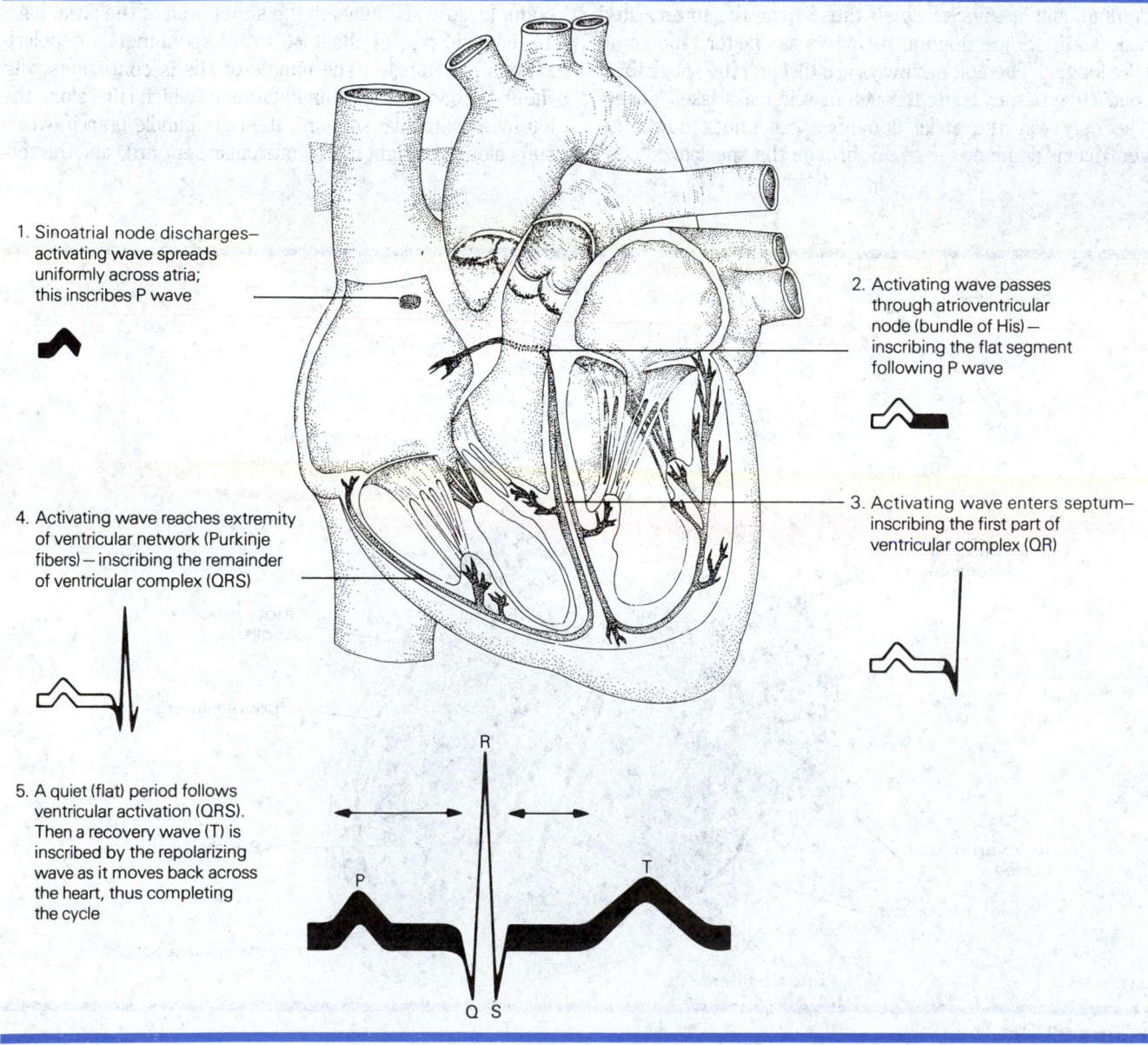

1. Sinoatrial node discharges—activating wave spreads uniformly across atria; this inscribes P wave

2. Activating wave passes through atrioventricular node (bundle of His)—inscribing the flat segment following P wave

3. Activating wave enters septum—inscribing the first part of ventricular complex (QR)

4. Activating wave reaches extremity of ventricular network (Purkinje fibers)—inscribing the remainder of ventricular complex (QRS)

5. A quiet (flat) period follows ventricular activation (QRS). Then a recovery wave (T) is inscribed by the repolarizing wave as it moves back across the heart, thus completing the cycle

Figure 22–4

Correlation between the ECG and electrical activity of the heart.

SOURCE: Saxton DF et al.: *The Addison–Wesley Manual of Nursing Practice.* Menlo Park, CA: Addison–Wesley, 1983, p. 166.

wall of the left ventricle, which causes the sensor to draw a small downward deflection, called the S wave. Atrial repolarization cannot be seen on the normal ECG because it occurs during ventricular depolarization and is hidden in the QRS complex. Another straight line signifies no electrical activity. Shortly thereafter, a T wave forms, which the sensor records when the ventricular muscle cells repolarize. Because ventricular repolarization occurs in a different sequence than depolarization, the T wave is upright.

There are normal time limits for these events to occur. During the ECG recording, the paper marked with light and dark horizontal lines moves under the writing instrument at a standard rate. The distance of five dark lines (counting the origin would make six) equals 1 second. The distance between two dark lines equals 0.2 seconds. Figure 23–2 shows the details of the normal ECG. The time necessary for the depolarization wave to be conducted through the various parts of the heart is significant in evaluating abnormalities of the heartbeat.

Coronary Circulation

Like the other cells of the body, the heart needs blood flow to maintain cellular life and perform its work. It receives its blood supply from the left and right coronary arteries, which originate in the root of the aorta just above the left posterior and anterior cusps of the aortic valve (Figure 22–5). Blood flows into these arteries during ventricular diastole, when the aortic valve is closed by blood pushed backward by the recoil of the aorta at the beginning of ventricular diastole. The duration of ventricular diastole is important to ensure that the heart cells get sufficient blood supply. Note that when the heart cells contract, the contraction exerts pressure against the coronary vessels and inhibits blood flow.

The left coronary artery primarily supplies the left atrium and the majority of the left ventricle. This artery branches into the left anterior descending artery and the circumflex artery. In most persons, the left anterior descending artery and its branches supply the interventricular septum and surrounding myocardium. The circumflex artery and its branches supply the lateral wall and some of the posterior wall of the left ventricle (Figure 22–6A). The right coronary artery supplies the right atrium; the right ventricle; and, in most persons, the A-V node and the inferior and posterior portions of the left ventricle (Figure 22–6B).

Most cardiac veins empty into the coronary sinus, which drains directly into the right atrium. Some of the veins empty directly into all chambers of the heart.

BLOOD VESSELS

The blood vessels carry the blood from the heart, provide an area for exchange of substances between the blood and interstitial spaces, and carry the blood back to the heart to be recirculated. Generally, the arteries and arterioles carry the blood to the capillaries (or sinusoids, which are larger and more irregular small tubes such as those found in the endocrine glands, liver, bone marrow, and spleen). There exchange takes place, and the venules and veins carry the blood back to the heart for recirculation. (Some exchange takes place in the capillary ends of the venules.)

All the blood vessels except the capillaries are innervated by sensory and vasomotor nerves and have three layers of tissue. The inner layer, lined with a smooth layer of endothelial cells supported by a layer of connective tissue, is called the *tunica intima;* the middle layer of fibromuscular tissue is called the *tunica media;* the outer layer of collagen and elastin fibers is called the *tunica adventitia.* The vessels have small nutrient vessels (vasa vasorum) that run into the tunica adventitia and the tunica media, and most have lymphatic vessels. The size of the blood vessels and the amount of muscular tissue vary according

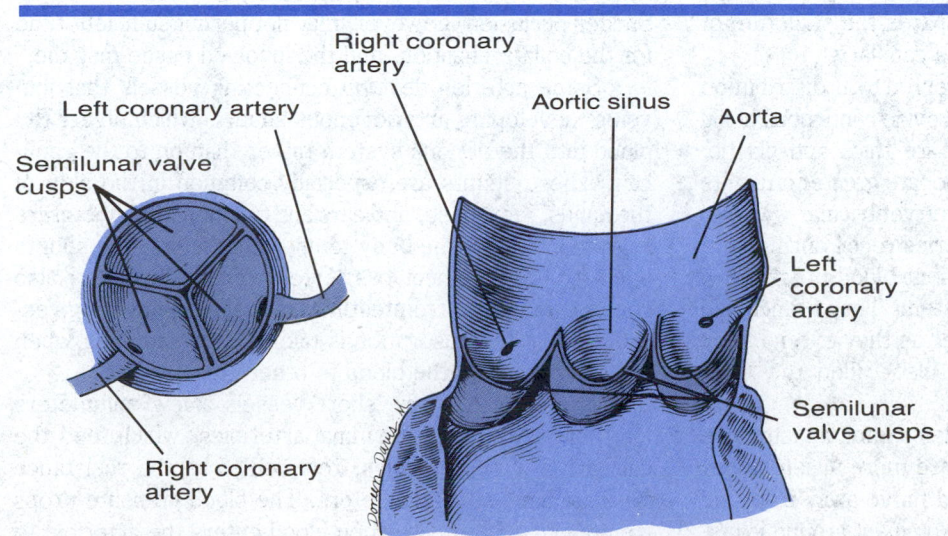

Left coronary artery

Semilunar valve cusps

Right coronary artery

Aortic sinus

Aorta

Left coronary artery

Semilunar valve cusps

Right coronary artery

Figure 22–5

Origin of the coronary arteries: **A.** A closed aortic valve viewed from above. **B.** An aortic orifice cut and opened to show the semilunar valves.
SOURCE: Spence AP, Mason EB: *Human Anatomy and Physiology.* Menlo Park, CA: Benjamin/Cummings, 1983, p. 480.

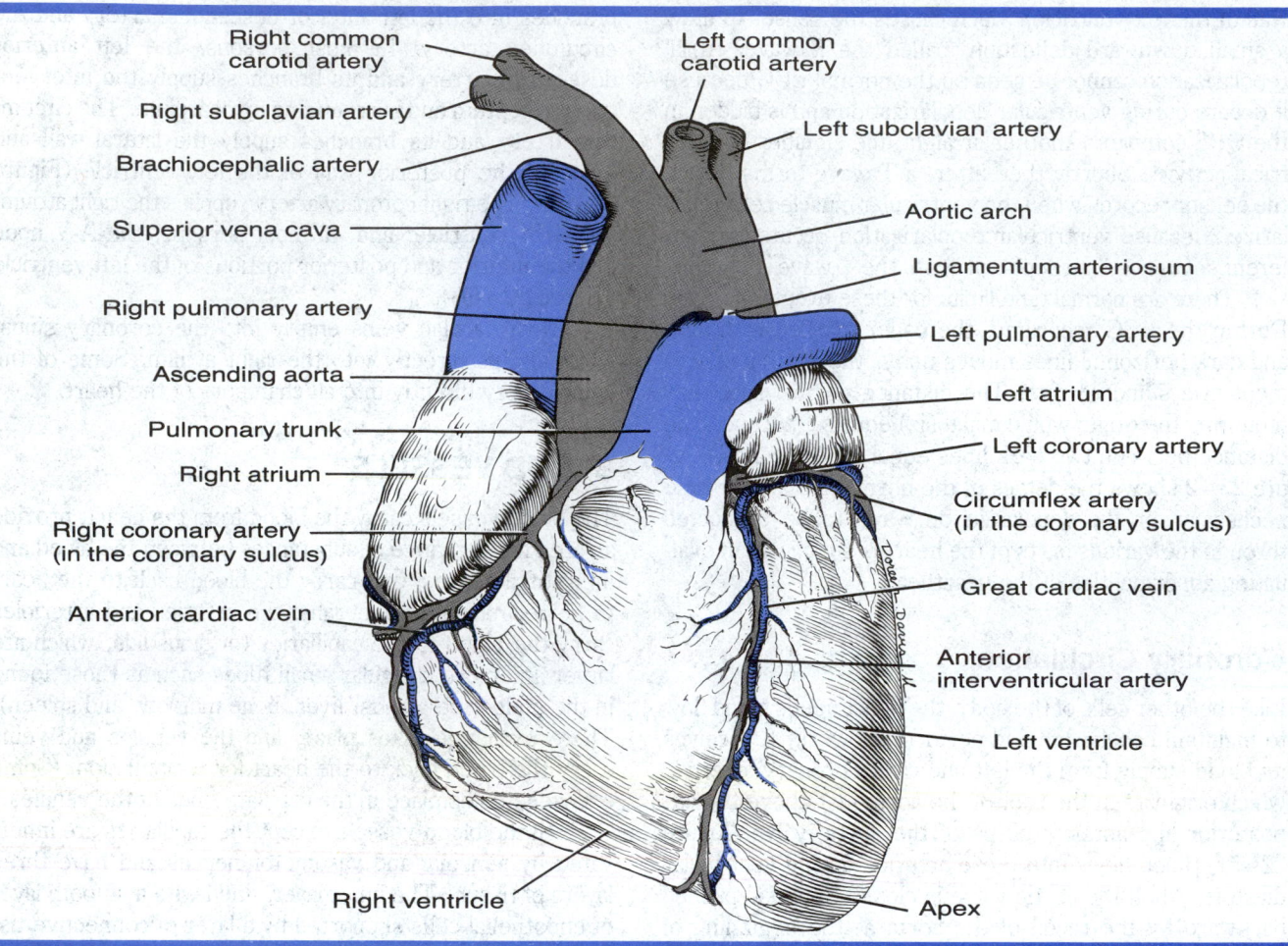

Figure 22–6

A. Blood vessels of the anterior surface of the heart.

SOURCE: Spence AP, Mason EB: *Human Anatomy and Physiology*. Menlo Park, CA: Benjamin/Cummings, 1983, p. 476.

to the blood pressures within the vessels. The capillaries consist of a single layer of endothelial cells covered by a glucoprotein layer that merges into an adventitious layer of fine reticular tissue. The structure of the vessels is related to their function. Figure 22–7 compares the structure of a vein, an artery, an arteriole, and a capillary.

The arteries are sometimes referred to as distribution or conduction vessels because they provide continuous blood flow to the periphery. Their walls are thick and elastic, enabling them to stretch to accommodate greater amounts of blood under high pressure during ventricular systole. Because of their elasticity, the arteries recoil during ventricular diastole and maintain sufficient blood pressure to promote blood flow through the system. They branch like a tree, and the branches get smaller as they extend away from the heart. The arteries are also called the *high-pressure blood vessels*.

Not all arteries end in arterioles. Some anastomose (unite) with other arteries. There are more anastomoses as the arteries decrease in size and move away from the heart. Anastomoses are especially prominent around joints, where external pressure during movement momentarily

interrupts circulation. The anastomosed artery provides the intermittent blood supply. When blood supply is compromised for a time from disease or injury, the anastomosed artery enlarges to provide collateral circulation. Sudden occlusion, however, may not permit sufficient time for the collateralization, and the involved tissue may die.

Some arteries develop connecting vessels that join veins, developing arteriovenous shunts, which divert the blood into the venous system rather than on to the capillary. These shunts are especially common in the skin of the hands, feet, nose, and ears and function in temperature regulation. When the body temperature is low, the shunts open and promote heat loss. Arteriovenous shunts are also common in the gastrointestinal tract. The connecting vessels close when absorption is taking place and open when it is not, shunting the blood to other areas.

The arterioles are short vessels a few millimeters long that branch into terminal arterioles, which feed the capillaries. The arterioles, referred to as the resistance vessels, have small diameters. The blood pressure drops from about 85 mm Hg when blood enters the arteriole to about 30 mm Hg at the beginning of the capillary.

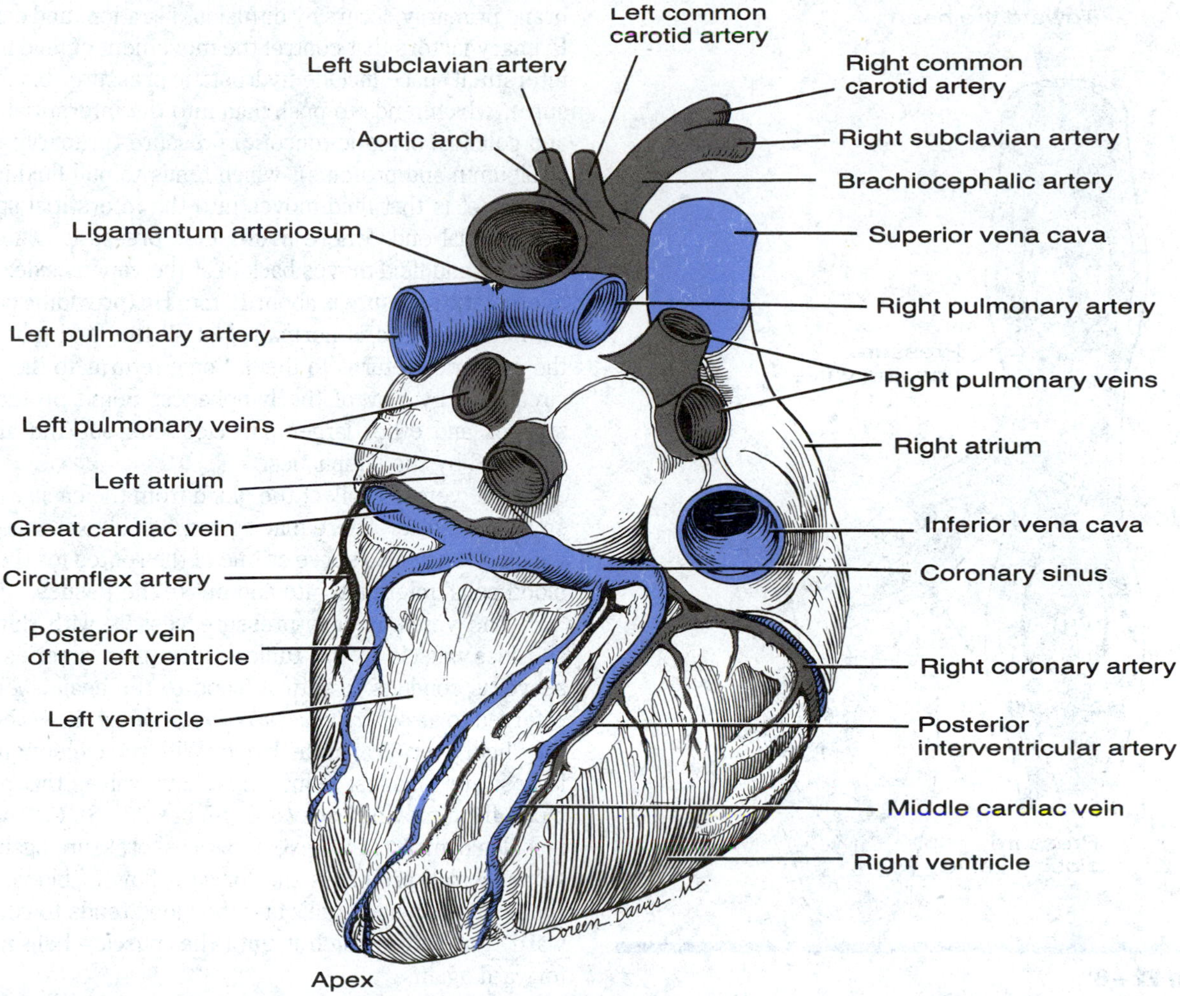

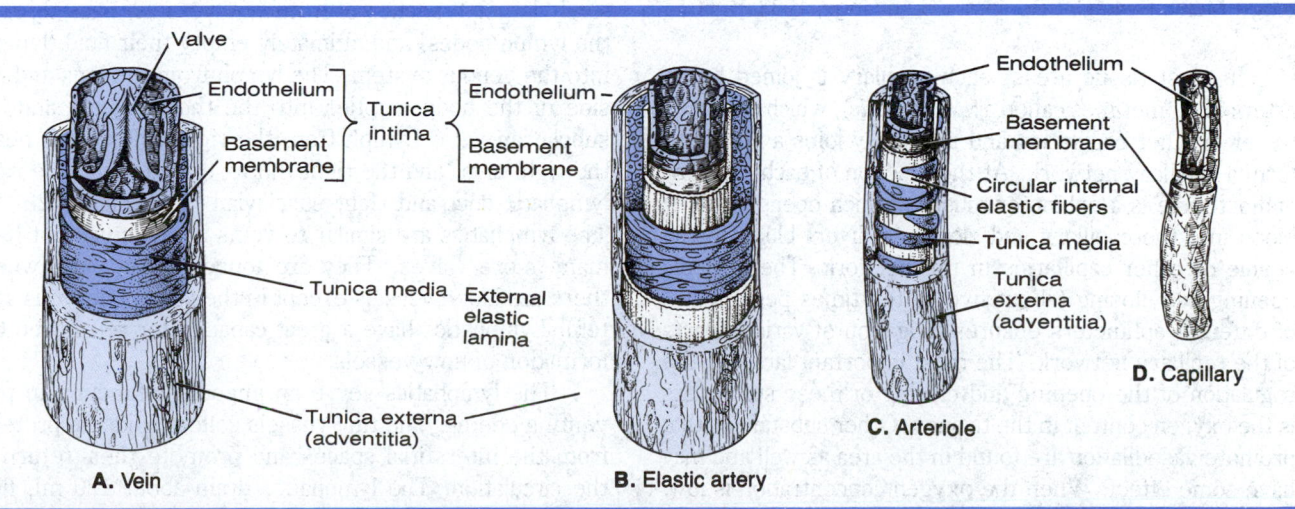

Left common carotid artery

Left subclavian artery

Aortic arch

Right common carotid artery

Right subclavian artery

Brachiocephalic artery

Ligamentum arteriosum

Superior vena cava

Left pulmonary artery

Right pulmonary artery

Left pulmonary veins

Right pulmonary veins

Left atrium

Right atrium

Great cardiac vein

Inferior vena cava

Circumflex artery

Coronary sinus

Posterior vein of the left ventricle

Right coronary artery

Left ventricle

Posterior interventricular artery

Middle cardiac vein

Right ventricle

Apex

Doreen Davis, M.

Figure 22–6 *(continued)*

B. Blood vessels of the posterior surface of the heart.
SOURCE: Spence AP, Mason EB: *Human Anatomy and Physiology.* Menlo Park, CA: Benjamin/Cummings, 1983, p. 477.

Valve

Endothelium

Tunica intima

Basement membrane

Endothelium

Basement membrane

Endothelium

Basement membrane

Circular internal elastic fibers

Tunica media

External elastic lamina

Tunica media

Tunica externa (adventitia)

Tunica externa (adventitia)

Tunica externa (adventitia)

A. Vein

B. Elastic artery

C. Arteriole

D. Capillary

Figure 22–7

Comparison of the structure of (**A**) a vein, (**B**) an artery, (**C**) an arteriole, and (**D**) a capillary.
SOURCE: Spence AP, Mason EB: *Human Anatomy and Physiology.* Menlo Park, CA: Benjamin/Cummings, 1983, p. 504.

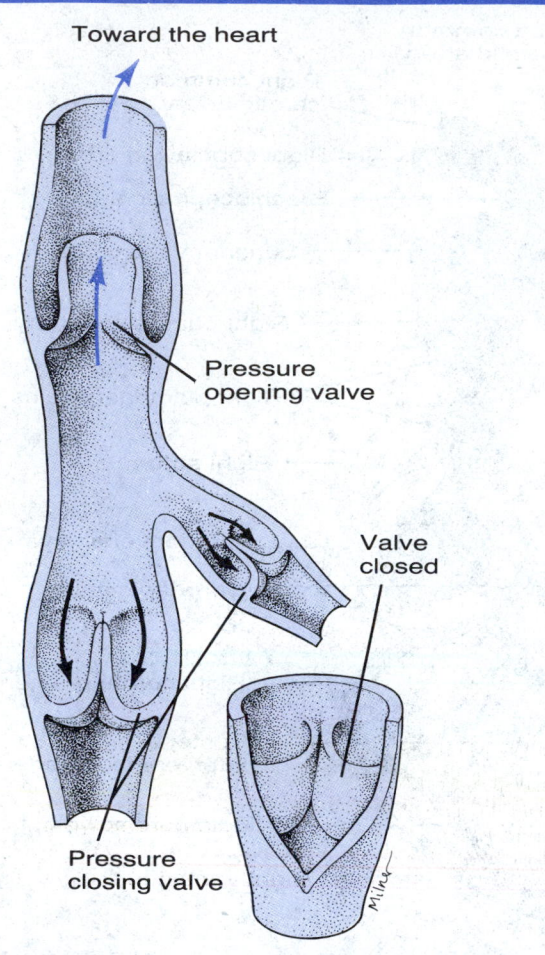

Figure 22–8

Valves of a vein. The arrows indicate that the valves are forced open by pressure from below and shut by pressure from above. This arrangement of valves allows blood to move in only one direction—toward the heart.
SOURCE: Spence AP, Mason EB: *Human Anatomy and Physiology*. Menlo Park, CA: Benjamin/Cummings, 1983, p. 507.

In most tissue areas, each capillary is joined by an arteriole (sometimes called a *metarteriole*), which branches to serve other capillaries and ultimately joins a venule to form a capillary network. At the junction of each capillary and arteriole is a sphincter muscle, which opens to allow blood into the capillary and closes to divert blood to the venule or other capillaries in the network. The periodic opening and closing (about five to ten times per minute) of different sphincters ensures irrigation of various parts of the capillary network. The most important factor in the regulation of the opening and closing of these sphincters is the oxygen content in the tissues. Other substances that promote vasodilation are found in the area as well and may have some effect. When the oxygen concentration is low, the sphincters open more often and permit more blood flow, resulting in more oxygen and nutrients to the area (autoregulation of blood supply).

Exchange takes place in the capillaries. The move-

ment of substances both ways across the capillary membrane primarily occurs by diffusion, filtration, and osmosis. Primary factors that control the movement of fluid into the interstitial space include hydrostatic pressure (blood pressure), which tends to push fluid into the interstitial space, and colloidal osmotic (oncotic) pressure (primarily related to albumin and proteins), which tends to pull fluid in. The net effect is that fluid moves into the interstitial space at the arterial end, where hydrostatic pressure is about 30 mm Hg, and fluid moves back in at the venous side, where hydrostatic pressure is about 10 mm Hg (providing colloidal osmotic pressure is normal). Not all the fluid that leaves the capillaries returns to them. Some returns to the venous circulation by way of the lymphatics. Some protein substances and other larger particles leak out and are also returned by the lymphatics.

The venules collect the blood from the capillaries and small arterioles. There may be some fluid exchange in the venules. They also serve as one of the routes for the white blood cells' migration into and out of the tissues.

The veins are low-pressure vessels with thin walls and less muscle in the tunica media than arteries. They serve as conduits to return blood to the heart. Veins are referred to as *capacitance* or *reservoir blood vessels* because they hold over 60% of the blood. With the exception of the largest and smallest veins, most have valves that prevent blood from moving backward (Figure 22–8). As the body muscles contract, they exert external pressure against the veins, which promotes the forward flow of blood. When the venous pressure falls and the blood tends to run backward, the valves catch it until the muscles help move it forward again.

THE LYMPHATIC SYSTEM

The lymphatics begin blindly in the tissue spaces as tiny vessels a little larger than capillaries, empty into progressively larger branches of lymphatic vessels, pass through the lymph nodes, and ultimately empty their fluid (lymph) into the venous system. The lymph from the legs and left side of the body empties into the thoracic duct and left subclavian vein. Lymph from the right side of the head, the right arm, and the right thorax empties into the right lymphatic duct and right subclavian vein (Figure 22–9). The lymphatics are similar to veins in structure but have many more valves. They are found almost everywhere there are blood vessels except in the central nervous system. Lymphatics have a great capacity for repair and the formation of new vessels.

The lymphatics serve an important function in preventing edema. The tiny vessels collect fluid and proteins from the interstitial spaces and promote their return to the circulation. The lymphatics drain about 120 mL fluid per hour and can drain about 20 times that much if necessary. They also collect the larger digested fat particles (chylomicrons) from the digestive system and empty them into the circulation.

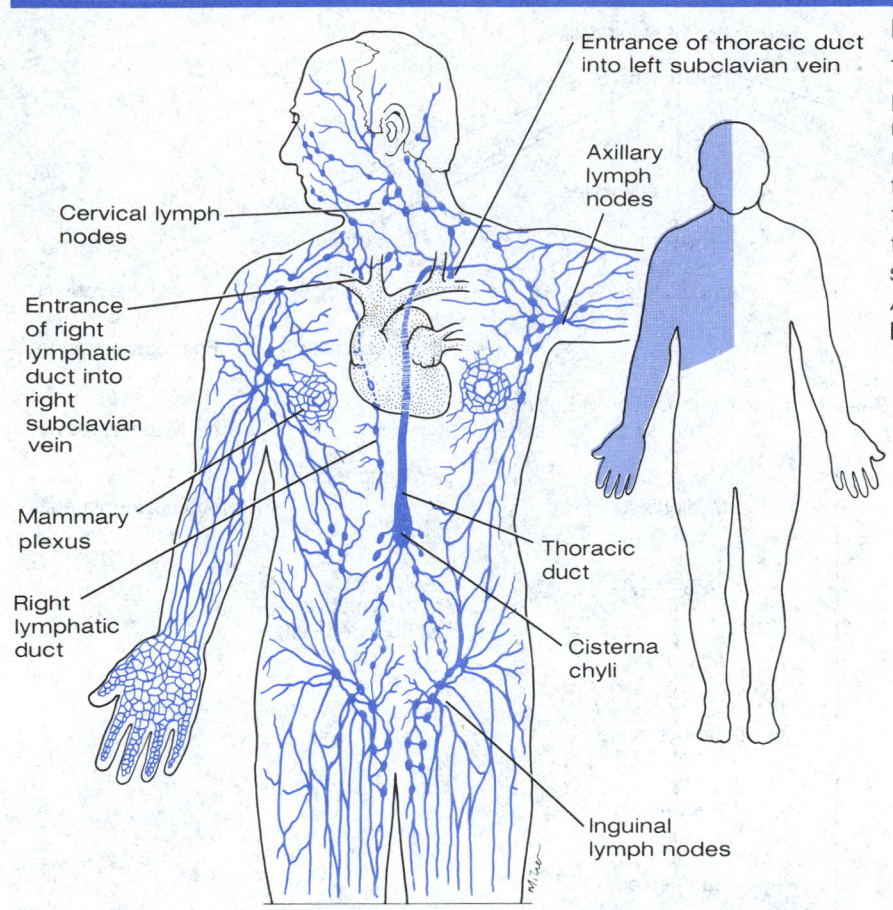

Figure 22–9

The lymphatic system. **A.** Major lymphatic vessels and groups of lymph nodes. **B.** Lymph from the colored area returns to the blood vascular system through the right lymphatic duct. Lymph from the remainder of the body travels through the thoracic duct.
SOURCE: Spence AP, Mason EB: *Human Anatomy and Physiology.* Menlo Park, CA: Benjamin/Cummings, 1983, p. 544.

Labels: Entrance of thoracic duct into left subclavian vein; Axillary lymph nodes; Cervical lymph nodes; Entrance of right lymphatic duct into right subclavian vein; Mammary plexus; Right lymphatic duct; Thoracic duct; Cisterna chyli; Inguinal lymph nodes

In addition, the lymphatics play a key role in the body's defense against microorganisms. They collect microorganisms in the interstitial spaces and carry them along with the fluid into the lymph nodes (small masses of lymphoid tissue), where the lymphocytes and macrophages remove bacteria and other foreign substances from the lymph before sending it into the venous system.

THE SPLEEN

The spleen is the largest lymphatic organ and is highly vascular. It is located in the left upper abdomen directly below the diaphragm, posterior and lateral to the fundus of the stomach. The spleen functions as a blood filtration system, trapping foreign particles and destroying bacteria and viruses. It also serves as a blood reservoir.

The spleen contains two types of pulp, red and white. The red pulp, which contains lymphocytes, macrophages, and erythrocytes, is the most abundant. Old erythrocytes are destroyed in the red pulp. Masses of white pulp, which surround the arterioles, are scattered throughout the red pulp. White pulp produces lymphocytes and sequesters lymphocytes, macrophages, and antigens.

THE BONE MARROW

Bone marrow, contained inside all bones, collectively is one of the largest organs of the body. Hematopoiesis, or the formation of blood cells, is its primary function. There are two kinds of bone marrow: red and yellow bone marrow. Hematopoiesis is carried out by red (functioning) marrow. By adulthood, red marrow is confined to the pelvis, sternum, ribs, cranium, ends of the long bones, and the vertebral spine. Yellow (fatty) bone marrow is red marrow that has changed to fat. It is found in the remaining bones and does not contribute to hematopoiesis.

All the blood components start as stem cells. These differentiate and become committed to one cell line—erythrocytes, leukocytes, or thrombocytes. They mature through orderly stages and are normally released into the bloodstream when they reach maturity (Figure 22–10). On occasion, when the demand for a particular blood cell is high, the bone marrow may respond by releasing the needed blood component too early. The nurse needs to know the functions of the blood components to interpret the clinical significance of abnormal findings of the blood count appropriately.

THE BLOOD

The purpose of the cardiovascular system is to circulate the blood to bring it into proximity with the body cells. Blood is the substance of life because it carries materials necessary to provide the correct environment in which the body cells can do their work.

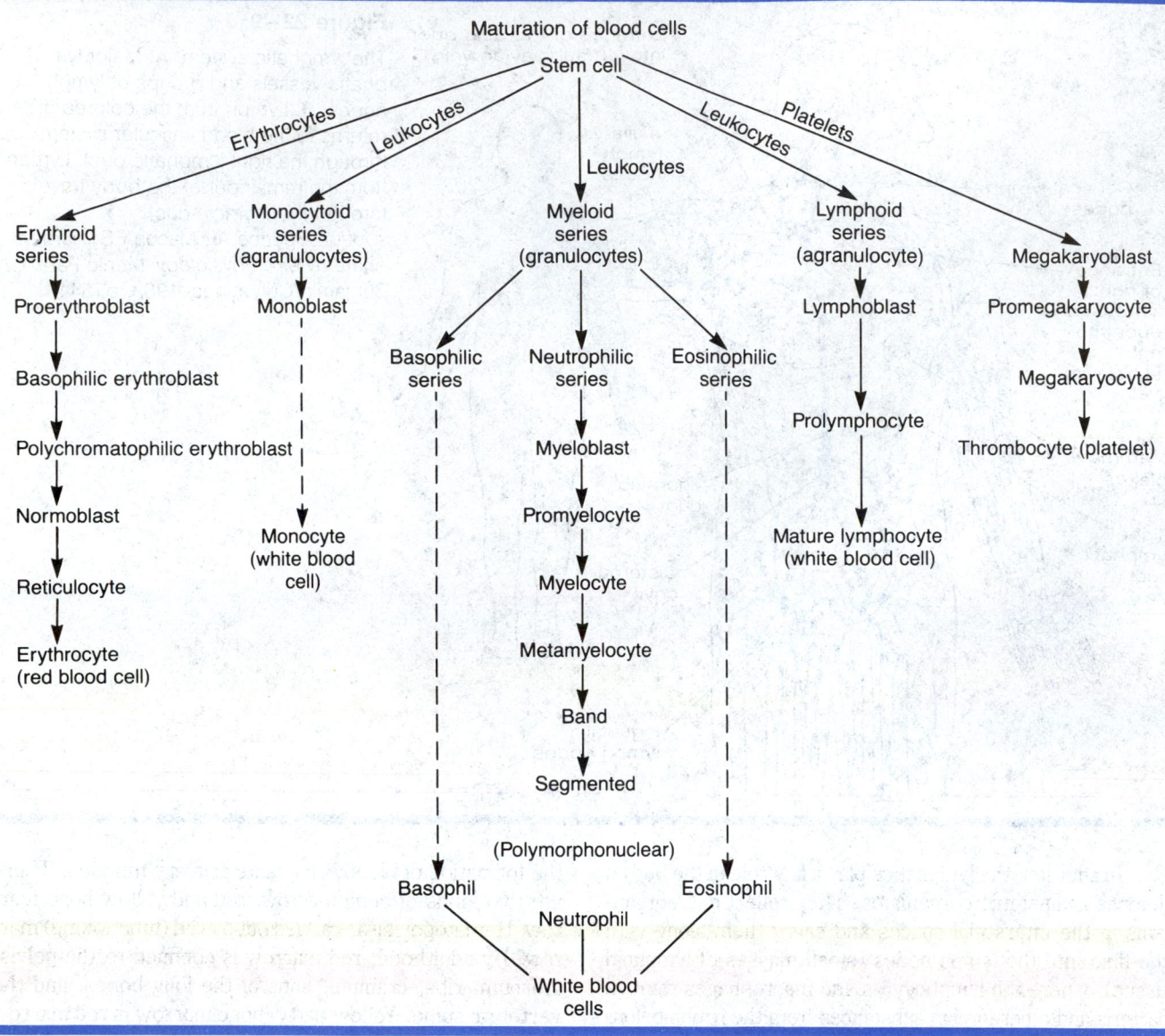

Figure 22–10

Maturation of blood cells. Dotted lines indicate that the maturation sequence is similar to that of the neutrophilic series.

When blood is centrifuged in a test tube, the erythrocytes form the bottom layer, the leukocytes and thrombocytes form the middle layer, and a clear fluid called *plasma* is on the top. The erythrocytes constitute about 45% of the volume and the plasma, about 55%; the volume of the leukocytes and the thrombocytes is negligible. The blood cells just mentioned are often referred to as the *formed elements of the blood,* or the *blood components.*

Erythrocytes

The erythrocytes (red blood cells) number about 5 million/mL, carry about 14 g of hemoglobin per deciliter, and occupy about 45% of the blood volume. They are formed in the bone marrow and released in an immature form called *reticulocytes* because they still contain some of their endoplasmic reticulum, which they used in forming hemoglobin while maturing in the bone marrow. The endoplasmic reticulum is lost in 1 to 2 days, and the cell becomes an erythrocyte. Because the life span of the erythrocyte is about 120 days, and the usual production of erythrocytes approximately equals the loss, the normal number of reticulocytes in the blood can be used to measure overall bone marrow activity. The reticulocyte count is expressed as a percentage with a range of approximately 0.5% to 1.5%. Values less than 0.5% may signal bone marrow suppression or failure, depending on the disease process involved. Conversely, values greater than the normal range can signal bone marrow recovery or increased activity. The stimulus prompting reticulocytosis varies from one client to another, depending on the underlying disease process.

The erythrocytes are vital to survival. They contain

hemoglobin, which transports oxygen picked up in the lungs to the capillaries near the cells, where it is diffused for use by the cells. The erythrocytes also contain a large amount of carbonic anhydrase, which catalyzes the chemical reaction between carbon dioxide and water. This makes it possible for the blood to carry large amounts of carbon dioxide in solution; thus, the carbon dioxide can be picked up in the capillaries near the cells and carried to the lungs to be converted back to the gas form and exhaled. The erythrocytes also are important in maintaining an acid–base balance in the blood and are responsible for about 70% of the blood-buffering power.

The normal erythrocyte has a biconcave shape, like a doughnut without the hole. The biconcavity of the erythrocyte allows flexibility, pliability, and distortion without destruction. Flexibility and pliability are necessary to traverse the microcirculation. For the erythrocyte to survive, it must be able to squeeze through the smallest capillary, release its oxygen to adjacent cells, and reenter the venous circulation. Alterations in the normal biconcave shape (poikilocytosis) can cause increased erythrocyte fragility, increased splenic sequestration of erythrocytes, and anemia. Spherocytosis is a genetically transmitted erythrocyte shape disorder (see Chapter 29).

The mean corpuscular volume (MCV) of the erythrocyte ranges from 82 to 92 μm^3. Clients with anisocytosis (variations in erythrocyte size) may have erythrocytes larger than normal (macrocytic), smaller than normal (microcytic), or both. The anemias in particular are characterized by abnormal sizes of the erythrocyte (see the discussion about the blood in Section III).

As already mentioned, the erythrocyte contains the hemoglobin molecule. The adult hemoglobin molecule is composed of a heme (iron) portion and a globin (protein) portion. The protein portion is composed of two alpha and two beta polypeptide chains. Variations of the structure of these protein chains alter the hemoglobin molecule and

create problems in oxygen transport. Sickle cell anemia and thalassemia are two such disorders in hemoglobin synthesis (see Chapter 29).

The erythrocytes contribute significantly to the viscosity of the blood and therefore influence the heart's ability to perform its function. When the quantity of erythrocytes is high, as in polycythemia, the heart must work harder to overcome the increased viscosity that impedes blood flow. The viscosity of the blood is measured by the packed cell volume (PCV), or hematocrit. The hematocrit is expressed as a percentage of the total blood volume and should be three times the hemoglobin concentration.

The erythrocytes carry antigens, of which over 50 have been identified. These antigen types are inherited (see Table 22–1). The most important to nursing are the ABO and Rh blood types because individuals produce antibodies against antigens other than the antigens they carry on their own erythrocytes. For instance, persons with type O erythrocytes have neither the type A nor B antigen and develop antibodies against them. If they receive a blood transfusion from persons with type A, B, or AB, their antibodies will attach to the donor's erythrocytes and cause agglutination (clumping). Because type O blood lacks antigens, it can be transfused into clients without causing reactions and is known as the **universal donor.** Persons with type A erythrocytes develop antibodies against type B blood and therefore cannot receive type B or AB blood; persons with type B erythrocytes develop antibodies against type A blood, which results in agglutination with type A and AB erythrocytes. Persons with type AB erythrocytes have both A and B antigens and therefore can receive erythrocytes from any of the other three types. Type AB blood is known as the **universal recipient.**

Erythrocytes are also Rh positive or Rh negative, meaning that they either have the Rh antigen or they do not, respectively. The Rh system is different from the ABO system. Individuals who are Rh negative do not have

Table 22–1 ABO Genetics and Blood Types

Blood Type (Phenotype)	Genotype	Antigens on RBCs	Antibodies in Serum	% of Humans Who Have Blood Type	Compatible Donor Blood Types
A	AA	A	B ⎫		A, O
A	AO	A	B ⎬	41	A, O
B	BB	B	A ⎫		B, O
B	BO	B	A ⎬	9	B, O
AB	AB	AB	None	3	A, B, AB, O (universal recipient)
O	OO	None	A, B	47	O (universal donor)

SOURCE: Reprinted with permission from Vick RL: *Contemporary Medical Physiology.* Menlo Park, CA: Addison–Wesley, 1984, p. 367.

antibodies against Rh-positive erythrocytes but develop them if Rh positive blood comes in contact with their blood.

Thrombocytes

The thrombocytes (platelets) are fragments of the megakaryocytes formed in the bone marrow and released into the bloodstream, where they are completely replaced over a 10-day period. They are important to the blood-clotting mechanism and clot retraction. Thrombocytes are especially important to the vascular system because they plug the many small ruptures that occur in small vessels daily. Without thrombocytes to plug the ruptures, blood leaks out and causes small hemorrhagic areas (petechiae) in the skin.

The thrombocytes swell, become sticky, and begin to adhere to one another when they come in contact with rough surfaces or are in areas of blood stasis. This characteristic is known as *platelet adhesion. Platelet aggregation* refers to the ability of thrombocytes to be mobilized to a site of injury and plug the leak. Adequate platelet numbers are necessary to promote the release of serotonin, which causes local vasoconstriction at the injury site and reduces the amount of bleeding following injury.

The thrombocytes are also important in clot retraction. A few minutes after a clot is formed, it retracts into the vessel and expresses fluid called *serum* over the next hour. This causes the ends of the damaged vessel to come together and promotes hemostasis.

Clotting Cascade

In addition to thrombocytes, a number of coagulation factors have been identified in the blood that contribute to hemostasis. The majority of these factors are produced in the liver. Table 22–2 lists the clotting factors and their site of production. Collectively, these clotting factors are referred to as the *clotting cascade.*

The term clotting cascade denotes an interdependent and orderly relation among these clotting factors, resembling a cascade or waterfall. A deficiency or defect of any one factor may contribute to a tendency to bleed in a par-

Table 22–2 The Coagulation System

Factor Number	Name(s)	Function	Site of Production
I	Fibrinogen	Protein acted on by thrombin to produce fibrin polymer, which forms structure of clot	Liver
II	Prothrombin	Precursor of thrombin	Liver (vitamin-K dependent)
III	Thromboplastin	Lipoprotein derived from tissue. In extrinsic coagulation cascade, interacts with other factors to produce prothrombinase	Thromboplastic activity present in most tissues
IV	Calcium	Necessary for function of extrinsic cascade, intrinsic cascade, and common pathway	
V	Proaccelerin (labile factor)	Accelerates plasma thromboplastin generation in stage I; speeds conversion of prothrombin in stage II	Liver
VII	Proconvertin	Interacts with thromboplastin and Ca^{2+} to activate factor X in *extrinsic* cascade	Liver (vitamin-K dependent)
VIII	Antihemophilic factor	Interacts with other factors to activate factor X in *intrinsic* cascade	Uncertain
IX	Plasma thromboplastin component, Christmas factor	Interacts with other factors to activate factor X in *intrinsic* cascade	Liver (vitamin-K dependent)
X	Stuart–Prower factor	Accelerates and amplifies prothrombin activation; point of *convergence* of *extrinsic* and *intrinsic* systems	Liver (vitamin-K dependent)
XI	Plasma thromboplastin antecedent	Activated by factor XII; accelerates thrombin formation in *intrinsic* cascade	Uncertain
XII	Hageman factor	Plasma factor activated by contact with negatively charged surfaces (collagen, glass, kaolin, fatty acids); activates factor XI to initiate *intrinsic cascade*	Uncertain
XIII	Fibrin stabilizing factor	Cross-links fibrin to make it stronger and less soluble	Liver

SOURCE: Adapted from Byrne CJ et al: *Laboratory Tests: Implications for Nursing Care,* 2nd ed. Menlo Park, CA: Addison–Wesley, 1986, p. 537–542; Vick RL: *Contemporary Medical Physiology.* Menlo Park, CA: Addison–Wesley, 1984, p. 392.

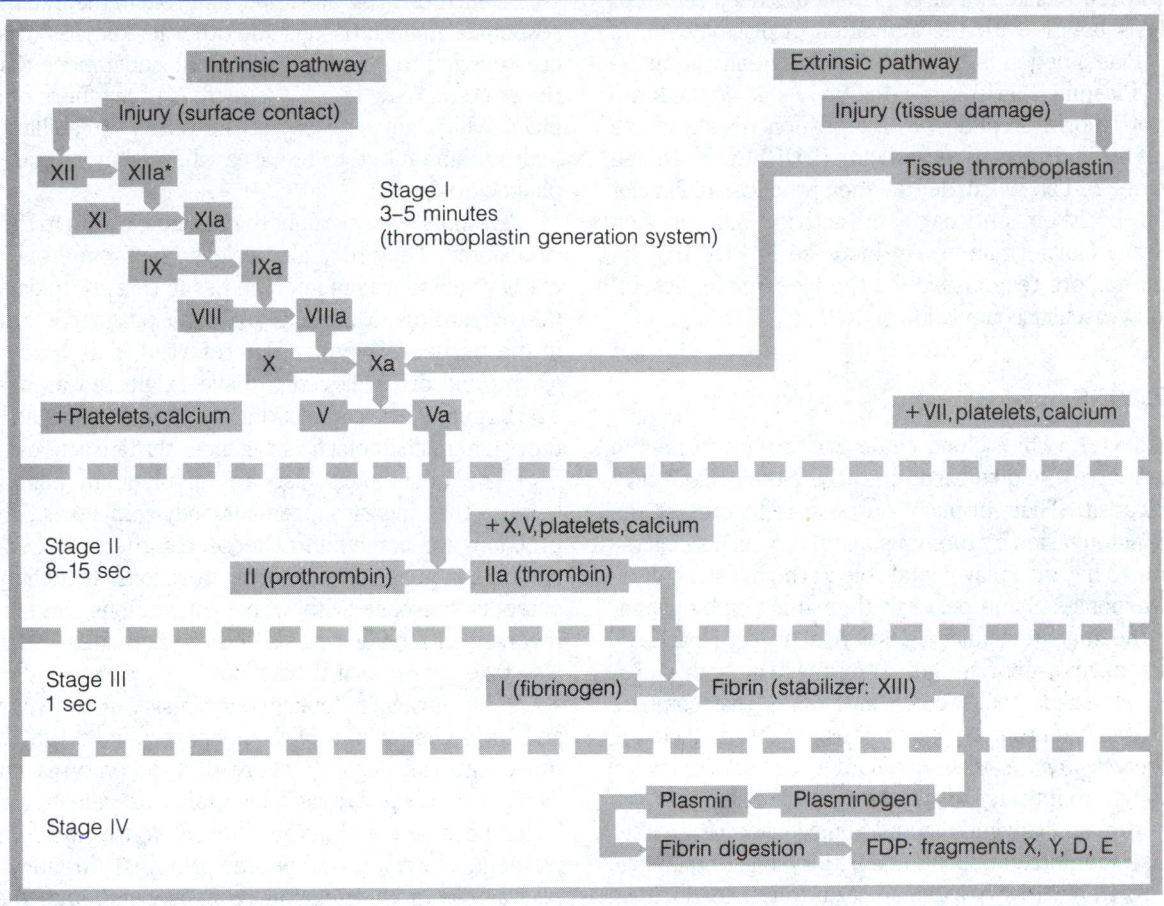

Figure 22–11

The four stages of the coagulation sequence. Letter *a* signifies the activated form of the factor.
SOURCE: Byrne CJ et al.: *Laboratory Tests: Implications for Nurses and Allied Health Professionals*. Menlo Park, CA: Addison–Wesley, 1981, p. 85.

ticular client. Clot formation is not a random and haphazard event. The sequence of events leading to the formation of a fibrin clot is progressive and orderly. Clotting occurs in four stages, which are illustrated in Figure 22–11.

Coagulation is initiated with injury to the wall of a blood vessel. Two pathways are activated. The *intrinsic pathway* describes events inside the injured blood vessel. The clotting events that occur on the outside of the blood vessel are called the *extrinsic pathway*. In Figure 22–11, Roman numerals represent the clotting factors. Roman numerals are used more often today than the factor names (see Table 22–2) to prevent confusion. The letter *a* in Figure 22–11 signifies the activated form of the clotting factor. The clotting factors II, V, VII, IX, X, XI, and XII are continuously present in an inactive form in the circulation. When a vessel is injured, the clotting factors are transformed to their activated states, promoting clot formation. Stage I includes both the intrinsic and extrinsic pathways. The mechanism for activation of these pathways is injury. The *intrinsic pathway* is a sequence of events in which the next reaction is stimulated by the preceding one.

In other words, injury initiates factor XII to stimulate factor XI, which converts factor IX to its activated form and so on. For successful progression of events, calcium and platelets must also be present.

The *extrinsic pathway* occurs simultaneously with the intrinsic pathway. With tissue injury, tissue thromboplastin is released. In the presence of factor VII, platelets, and calcium, tissue thromboplastin activates factors X and V, and the coagulation process continues.

Stage II of the clotting cascade consists of the conversion of prothrombin to thrombin by the plasma and tissue thromboplastin generated in stage I. Factors X, V, calcium, and platelets are vital to the successful completion of stage II.

Stage III begins with the action of thrombin on fibrinogen. Thrombin acts like an enzyme and splits fibrinogen into fibrin strands. The fibrin strands have the ability to mesh together side by side and end to end to form a clot. Factor XII (fibrin stabilizing factor) acts upon the fibrin clot, making it stronger, "more stable," and insoluble.

Stage IV is fibrinolysis, or the breakdown of the fibrin

clot. This occurs once the blood vessel has been repaired. Fibrinolysis begins with the activation of plasminogen to plasmin. Plasminogen is normally found within the insoluble clot. Plasmin is an enzyme that breaks down the fibrin in the clot. Fibrin breakdown or digestion results in the release of fibrin degradation products (FDP) (X, Y, D, and E in Figure 22–11). Fibrin degradation products inhibit clot formation by their anticoagulant activity and prevent unnecessary clot formation. An increase in FDP may be one of the factors responsible for the bleeding in disseminated intravascular coagulation (DIC).

Leukocytes

The leukocytes (white blood cells, WBCs) are formed in the bone marrow and released into the blood, which they use for transit. Their primary purpose is to protect the body against invasion by foreign substances such as microorganisms. They also play a vital role in the normal inflammatory response. Some perform their function by phagocytosis, the ingestion and digestion of foreign particles (microorganisms), debris, and sometimes the body's own cells. Some leukocytes secrete antibodies that combine with antigens and promote phagocytosis. Some leukocytes secrete *complement,* a substance sometimes necessary for the leukocyte to interact with a foreign substance, such as in the antigen–antibody interaction. Some leukocytes secrete chemicals (chemotactic substances) that signal other leukocytes to move to a particular tissue area to do their work. Some interact with others, such as by helping them or by secreting substances that affect the others' growth. Some are able to move out of the capillaries by squeezing through the pores in a process known as **diapedesis.** Leukocytes can perform many different functions that contribute to the body's defense.

Leukocytes are classified as either granulocytes or agranular leukocytes (see Figure 22–10). Granulocytes consist of the neutrophils, basophils, and eosinophils. These have similar stem-cell origins and contain granules that cause different staining reactions, which give them their names. Neutrophils stain a purplish hue; basophils, a bluish hue; and eosinophils, an orange color.

The neutrophils make up the largest number of the leukocytes and are most important to the body in defense against bacteria. Neutrophils include both a mature variety (segmented neutrophils, or segs) and an immature variety (bands). If not used by the body, bands mature to become segs. Neutrophils have the ability to phagocytize (engulf and digest) up to 25 bacteria before they die and are then phagocytized by larger macrophages. The number of neutrophils in the blood rises rapidly with the onset of bacterial infection, as does the WBC count. The differential count (a count of the number of each type of leukocyte in the blood) then demonstrates an increased percentage of segs and bands. An elevation of the percentage of bands above the normal level, referred to as a *shift to the left,* indicates the likelihood of a bacterial infection.

Neutrophils play an important role in the inflammatory response. Injured tissues and other leukocytes (basophils) are believed to secrete chemotactic substances that signal the bone marrow to release increased numbers of neutrophils, which squeeze out of the pores of capillaries (diapedesis) and move to the area where they are needed for phagocytosis.

Basophils are thought to prevent clotting in the microcirculation. They may also release histamine and inflammatory substances in infected tissue that are toxic to many microorganisms. Mast cells are larger phagocytic cells found in the tissues. They are also referred to as *tissue macrophages* and are believed to have originated as basophils. The basophils also play a part in the allergic response because they secrete chemotactic substances that attract eosinophils.

The eosinophils also are involved in phagocytosis because they ingest antigen–antibody complexes. They also probably are involved in allergic disorders, because their numbers increase during allergic reactions. In addition, their numbers increase with worm infestations, and they are involved with phagocytosis of these parasites. Eosinophils also take part in clot retraction.

The agranular leukocytes consist of the monocytes and the lymphocytes. The monocytes have the ability to move into the tissues, where they become macrophages capable of phagocytosis. They also secrete a variety of substances involved in the body's defense (including complement, enzymes, and plasma proteins). Monocytes also play a role in the immune response, although the exact mode of action is not known.

The lymphocytes are agranular leukocytes that have attracted great interest since the advent of organ transplantation. They are formed in the hematopoietic organs, including the bone marrow, before birth, and migrate to a variety of body tissues before the birthing process begins. Lymphocytes continuously proliferate and travel throughout the body. Their cell division proceeds at much higher rates during invasion by viruses and foreign cells.

There are two kinds of lymphocytes: T-lymphocytes and B-lymphocytes. The T-lymphocytes travel from the bone marrow to the thymus before birth for storage, where they develop the ability to distinguish normal body tissue from foreign substances. T-lymphocytes are responsible for cellular immunity. They adhere to cells identified as foreign and secrete cytotoxic substances, killing the cells. The B-lymphocytes also migrate from the bone marrow before birth. The exact storage and processing place for B-lymphocytes in human beings is unknown. In a species of birds, they are found in the bursa of Fabricius (a part of the gastrointestinal tract). The B-lymphocytes are involved in humoral immunity; in the presence of an antigenic response, they produce antibodies. B-lymphocytes are also responsible for immunoglobulin production.

Both T-lymphocytes and B-lymphocytes can divide upon stimulation by antigens, producing different types of cells such as memory cells, regulatory cells, and effector cells. Memory cells contain all the information from the lymphocyte that divided. Regulatory cells consist of the suppressor and helper cells, which either suppress or help the immune process and assist in the protection of the body. Effector cells are the T-lymphocyte killer cells and the B-lymphocyte plasma cells.

REGULATORY FUNCTIONS OF THE CARDIOVASCULAR SYSTEM

The ability of the body cells to function depends on the ability of the heart to pump blood, the ability of the blood vessels to carry the blood for transportation of substances across capillary walls, the ability of the lymphatics to carry some of the interstitial substances back into the system, and the quantity and quality of the blood. The cardiovascular system needs a communications system to let it know how well it is performing its function in relation to the whole body to determine priorities or make moment-to-moment adjustments. The vasomotor center located in the pons and medulla oblongata receives messages from the periphery and sends signals through the autonomic nervous system to the cardiovascular structures indicating what they are to do. These immediate adjustments are referred to as *autonomic reflexes*. To understand how these reflexes work, knowledge of the chemical mediators and the cardiovascular structural responses to them is necessary.

The postganglionic parasympathetic nerve fibers primarily secrete acetylcholine and are referred to as *cholinergic*. The postganglionic sympathetic nerve fibers, which secrete norepinephrine, are referred to as *adrenergic*. The sympathetic chemical transmitters to the sweat glands and a few blood vessels are cholinergic. (This helps explain why sweating is increased with strong sympathetic discharge.)

The heart is innervated by both parasympathetic and sympathetic nerve fibers. The parasympathetic fibers are primarily found in the atria, especially the S-A and A-V nodes. They are sparse in the ventricles. Parasympathetic stimulation to the heart results in a decreased heart rate (a negative chronotropic response) and decreased force of contraction (a negative inotropic response). The sympathetic fibers innervate the same areas as the parasympathetic fibers, but there is a greater number of sympathetic fibers in the ventricles. The heart responds to sympathetic stimulation by increasing its rate (a positive chronotropic response) and increasing its force of contraction (a positive inotropic response). Sympathetic stimulation increases metabolism in the heart and therefore creates the need for a greater blood supply.

The blood and blood vessels essentially respond to autonomic nervous system stimulation of the sympathetic nervous system. The blood responds to sympathetic stimulation by increasing coagulation. The blood vessels, including the arteries, arterioles, venules, and veins, respond by either constricting or dilating. The capillaries neither constrict nor dilate in response to sympathetic stimulation.

The heart and blood vessels have two types of adrenergic receptors, alpha and beta. Blood vessels with alpha receptors constrict when stimulated by adrenergic chemicals, and those with beta receptors dilate when stimulated by adrenergic chemicals. This helps explain why some vessels (such as those in the abdomen and skin) constrict during strong sympathetic stimulation, whereas those in other areas (such as muscles) dilate.

The sympathetic nervous system affects the amount of blood circulating by influencing the heart rate and the force of cardiac contraction, as well as by changing the diameter of the blood vessels. These factors influence blood pressure and peripheral vascular resistance, which in turn affects blood flow. Several peripheral receptors send messages to the vasomotor center, which in turn promotes autonomic nervous system responses to regulate blood flow by influencing blood pressure. Some of these receptors are the baroreceptors, chemoreceptors, and atrial stretch receptors.

Baroreceptors are nerve receptors that respond to changes in blood pressure. This response is important to adjustments needed when changing positions, such as from lying to standing. The baroreceptors are stimulated by increases in blood pressure and send signals to the vasomotor center, which inhibits vasoconstriction and stimulates a parasympathetic response. This results in less vasoconstriction, a slower heart rate, less force of cardiac contraction, and lower blood pressure. When the blood pressure decreases, these receptors send fewer signals to the vasomotor center, which results in more vasoconstriction, increased heart rate, and a greater force of contraction, which raises blood pressure.

The baroreceptors are found in most of the large arteries in the chest and neck. Of greatest clinical importance are the baroreceptors in the bifurcation of the carotid artery. When the heart rate is very fast, this area may be massaged, stimulating the baroreceptors to send more signals to the vasomotor center, indicating that they sense the blood pressure to be very high. The vasomotor center responds by decreasing the heart rate.

Chemoreceptors sensitive to arterial oxygen, carbon dioxide, and hydrogen ion concentration are located in the carotid bifurcation *(carotid bodies),* and at the aortic arch *(aortic bodies).* When the hydrogen ion content is high, carbon dioxide content is high, and oxygen content is low, they send messages that excite the vasomotor center, resulting in sympathetic discharge in an effort to increase blood flow.

Stretch receptors in the atria send signals to the vasomotor center when the atrial pressure is high, indicating that blood is damming up in the heart. The vasomotor center responds by causing dilation of the peripheral arterioles, which results in less peripheral resistance and increases the ability of the heart to pump blood. When the arterioles to the kidney dilate, not only is renal filtration increased, but signals are sent to the hypothalamus, which results in a decreased secretion of antidiuretic hormone and a subsequent increase in urine production. This effectively decreases the circulating blood volume and subsequently decreases the blood pressure.

The vasomotor center responds with a powerful sympathetic response when it does not have enough blood supply (when the systolic blood pressure falls below 50 mm Hg); the response becomes stronger as the blood pressure is lowered below this point. This response is called the central nervous system ischemic response.

The activated sympathetic nervous system stimulates the adrenal medulla to secrete norepinephrine and epinephrine. These catecholamines have an effect on the blood vessels and heart that activates the sympathetic nervous system responses. Other organs, such as the kidneys and hypothalamus, also contribute their secretions to influence vasomotor activity.

This discussion has described responses to short-term changes in blood pressure. The receptors adapt as the blood pressure remains relatively stable over time (hours to days). The kidneys regulate longer term blood pressure and blood flow by regulating the body fluids.

Proper bone marrow functioning and hence integrity of the hematopoietic system are vital to the client's survival. Many factors have been identified that contribute to the regulation of hematopoiesis.

Erythropoiesis is influenced by the client's nutritional status, activity, age, chemical or radiation exposure, and drug therapy. Nutritional deficiencies in iron, vitamin B_{12}, and folic acid tend to decrease erythrocyte production and interfere with red cell maturation. Overall, the sedentary client has relatively less erythrocyte production. As previously stated, the sites of bone marrow activity change as the client ages. In the adult client, the sites of bone marrow activity are confined to the pelvis, sternum, ribs, cranium, and ends of the long bones and vertebral spine. This decrease in functional bone marrow mass may account in part for some of the anemias in the elderly population. Chemical and radiation overexposure may cause bone marrow damage and interfere with production of red cells, white cells, and platelets. Drug therapy of any kind can also influence the production of all blood cell components.

Tissue anoxia has been identified as causing an increase in erythropoiesis. Tissue anoxia stimulates the production of erythropoietin, a hormone made in the kidneys and liver. Erythropoietin stimulates the bone marrow to increase red cell production. Increases in altitude tend to increase erythrocyte production. At high altitudes, the amount of oxygen in the inspired air is diminished. This decrease in the amount of oxygen increases red cell production.

As already mentioned, chemical and radiation overexposure and drug therapy may interfere with all blood component production. Leukopenia may result in these situations. Leukocyte production is also influenced by chemotactic substances during an inflammatory response. These substances signal the bone marrow to increase the release of white cells necessary for a normal inflammatory response. Lymphocytes continuously travel throughout the body. Their proliferation is stimulated during the invasion of viruses and foreign substances (antigens).

Thrombocytopenia may result from overexposure to chemicals and radiation. Drugs may cause a decrease in platelet production. Hormones, especially estrogen and corticosteroids, tend to diminish the production of platelets.

Section II: Pathophysiological Influences and Effects

A major purpose of the circulatory system is to supply blood to the tissues via the capillaries and to return the blood to the heart for recirculation. An adequate supply of blood is necessary for the body cells to do their work. Therefore, any problem that interferes with adequate blood supply may have serious consequences. Inadequate blood supply, or ischemia, usually produces pain. Temporary ischemia may do no damage; however, the cells may not be able to perform their functions as well as usual. Continued ischemia injures the cells. The injury may be reversible if blood flow increases sufficiently to meet the tissue demands. If ischemia continues and irreversible damage occurs, the cells of the involved tissues or organs die. Tissue death is often referred to as *infarction, necrosis,* or *gangrene.*

THE HEART

Within physiological limits, the heart pumps all the blood that returns to it. The difference between the cardiac output at rest and the cardiac output when the physiological limit is reached (which may be more than four times the resting state) is called the **cardiac reserve** and varies according to the condition of the heart and factors that may interfere with the heart's ability to pump effectively. When the physiological limits are exceeded, heart failure results. When the cardiac reserve is used up, the body tissues become ischemic. The heart itself also becomes ischemic, which may result in injury or death to some of its tissues and a further reduction in its ability to pump blood.

Cardiac reserve is essential for adjustment to the normal changes in body activity and stresses that increase tissue demands, as well as for adjustment to changes in the environment. During increased activity, the tissue demands increase as the cells need more oxygen and nutrients to do their work. When the environmental temperature is low, the cells increase their metabolic rate to maintain body temperature and therefore need a greater blood supply. When the environmental temperature is high (especially when the humidity is high, reducing the effectiveness of sweating), blood is shunted to the skin to promote loss of body heat; this requires a greater cardiac output. Pregnancy, a normal physiological process, requires a much greater cardiac output than the nonpregnant state.

Cardiac reserve is reduced by factors that increase the work load of the heart or decrease the heart's ability to pump blood. The work load of the heart increases when cardiac output increases and when the heart has to pump against increased resistance. Factors that decrease the heart's ability to pump blood include those that decrease blood return to the heart and the heart's ability to work.

Some disease conditions increase the tissue demands for oxygen and nutrients, resulting in increased cardiac output. For example, hyperthyroidism results in increased cellular metabolism, which requires a greater cardiac output. Infections also require a greater cardiac output because the phagocytes have a high oxygen demand, and vasodilation occurs in the area of the infected tissues. In addition, these conditions raise body temperature, which promotes increased metabolism and the need to release the increased body heat; this further increases the cardiac output.

Abnormal shunting of blood from arteries to veins requires an increase in cardiac output because the shunted blood does not meet tissue demands for nutrients. Abnormal arteriovenous shunts may be a result of surgery or trauma. These shunts, as well as abnormal congenital arteriovenous shunts, may not cause difficulties until combined with other problems that put additional strain on the heart.

Another cause of increased cardiac output related to increased blood returning to the heart is *volume overload*. The increased blood volume may relate to increased fluid retention by the kidneys or overload of IV fluids.

The overall condition of the blood also affects cardiac output. Anemic states resulting from such conditions as loss of blood, inadequate nutrition for erythrocyte maturation, poisoning, or hereditary disease create a situation in which the blood is unable to carry enough oxygen and nutrients to meet cellular demands. Consequently, the cardiovascular system circulates the blood more often, increasing cardiac output. Increased output also may result from lack of availability of enough oxygen or nutrients for the blood to carry, as occurs in pulmonary disease, nutritional deficiencies, and liver disease.

Under some conditions, the heart pumps enough blood with each stroke, but some of it goes in the wrong direction. This happens with a ventricular septal defect after myocardial infarction, when blood is pumped from the left ventricle into both the aorta and right ventricle. The same situation exists with incompetent valves that do not close tightly, causing tricuspid, mitral, pulmonic, or aortic regurgitation. Some of the blood, instead of moving forward, flows back through the incompetent valve. The heart has to pump the regurgitated blood again, increasing its work load.

When resistance to blood flow increases, the heart must create more pressure, increasing its work load and, subsequently, its need for more nutrients and a greater blood supply. When the resistance increases, the total amount the heart is capable of pumping diminishes, affecting the amount of cardiac reserve. A common condition that places additional strain on the left ventricle is diastolic hypertension. (When the left side of the heart generates enough pressure to ensure flow into the aorta, it must overcome the pressure in the aorta for blood to flow.) Other factors that increase the resistance against which the left ventricle has to pump include stenosis (narrowing) of the aortic valve or the narrowing of the blood vessels from conditions such as coarctation of the aorta and atherosclerosis. Increased pulmonary resistance, which is observed with some lung diseases and pulmonic stenosis, increases resistance for the right ventricle. Other conditions that cause resistance to blood flow through the pulmonary vessels include pulmonary emboli that block some of the vessels and increased viscosity of the blood; this occurs with polycythemia vera, a disorder characterized by an increased number of erythrocytes.

Decreased blood return to the heart means the heart is unable to pump enough blood to meet the body's needs and possibly its own. Inadequate blood volume occurs with dehydration and massive hemorrhage. Insufficient blood return to the heart occurs with massive vasodilation promoted by ineffective sympathetic control in conditions such as loss of nervous innervation by accident or surgery and sympatholytic drugs or chemicals. The constriction of the heart by the pericardium in constrictive pericarditis and pericardial tamponade prevents sufficient blood from entering the heart. Mitral and tricuspid valvular stenosis inhibit ventricular filling during diastole and subsequently affect cardiac output. Disturbances in the heart's rhythm (**dysrhythmias** or arrhythmias) also may prevent the heart from having enough time to fill the ventricles completely.

Inadequate blood supply to the myocardium caused by diseases such as coronary artery disease decreases the heart's ability to pump blood and therefore reduces the cardiac reserve. Nutritional diseases of the heart as well as the cardiomyopathies, infections, and trauma also reduce the heart's ability to pump blood.

THE BLOOD VESSELS

Blood flow through the vessels depends on the vascular integrity and the ability of the blood vessels to perform their functions. To meet changing tissue demands for blood flow, the blood vessels must be able to change their diameters in response to normal local regulatory substances, temperature, vasoactive substances in the blood (eg, vasopressin, angiotensin, epinephrine), and the sympathetic nervous system. The arteries need to stretch during systole to accommodate the blood pumped from the heart and to recoil during diastole to move it on. The veins depend on muscular movement and the action of their valves to move the blood on. Disturbances in these functions result in the inability of the blood vessels to supply blood to the tissues properly, which results in ischemia.

Arterial Disorders

The blood vessels may lose integrity from trauma or disease processes that destroy their walls. The ultimate result is bleeding. If the vessel cannot contain the blood, it cannot fulfill its function to move the blood forward.

A common problem that inhibits the arteries' ability to stretch and recoil properly is atherosclerosis. In this disease process, atheromatous plaques, usually of lipid origin, develop in the tunica intima. The resultant inability to stretch and recoil places additional strain on the heart.

Atheromatous plaques may become larger, progressively narrowing the arteries, causing atherosclerotic occlusive disease. As an artery narrows, it is unable to carry sufficient blood to the tissues it feeds, resulting in ischemia that may lead to tissue death. Sometimes an artery is able to handle enough blood during relative inactivity when tissue demands are low. When activity increases or tissue demands are higher, however, the narrowed artery is unable to accommodate enough blood flow, and the tissues become ischemic. In addition, a hemorrhage may occur in the area of the plaque, causing formation of a blood clot and the complete blocking of the artery. This results in no blood flow to the tissues and certain death of the tissues unless sufficient collateral circulation has developed.

Other diseases may obstruct blood flow in the arteries. Some obstruction results from inflammatory processes such as thromboangiitis obliterans, commonly called *Buerger's disease*. Some diseases, such as Raynaud's disease, cause arterial spasms that decrease blood flow and may result in ischemia.

External pressures in excess of the arterial diastolic pressure inhibit arterial blood flow, and pressures that surpass the arterial systolic blood pressure stop blood flow through the artery. Common causes of obstruction to blood flow include tumors and swelling from injuries, such as body burns. Clothing, bandages, or casts may tighten with swelling from bleeding or edema and obstruct blood flow. The constant weight of the body tissues on a vessel without intermittent relief of pressure may also obstruct blood flow.

Venous Disorders

The inability of the veins to move the blood on is called *venous insufficiency*. The most common cause is valves that do not function properly and promote damming up of blood in the veins. The hydrostatic pressure in the veins increases and causes edema in the tissues from which the blood empties into the involved vein. Complications of chronic venous insufficiency include thrombophlebitis, hemorrhage, stasis dermatitis, stasis cellulitis, and stasis ulcers.

Other factors that may inhibit venous flow, contribute to venous insufficiency, and result in edema include any event that causes enough pressure against the veins to inhibit blood flow. External pressure is commonly caused by garters or elastic used to hold stockings or socks up. Tumors or hematomas within the tissues may exert pressure against veins. Lack of the use of muscles that assist venous flow promotes venous stasis. Pressure on the veins from maintaining a constant position (eg, crossing the legs at the knees) also inhibits venous flow.

Embolus Formation

An *embolism* is the obstruction of a blood vessel by a blood clot or foreign substance such as air or fat. Emboli can occur in both the arteries and the veins. The most common type of embolus is a blood clot (thrombus) that forms in the heart or a blood vessel. The thrombus or a piece of it becomes dislodged and travels (then called a *thromboembolus*) until it gets to a vessel so small that it cannot move any farther; it then blocks any flow ahead of it. If the embolus is in a vein (or the right side of the heart), it travels through larger and larger vessels until it arrives in the heart, where it moves through the right atrium and ventricle and into vessels in the lungs, which get smaller and smaller. When the embolus reaches a pulmonary vessel too small for it to pass through, it stops. It is then called a *pulmonary embolus*. When a blood clot breaks off in the left side of the heart or an artery, the thromboembolus travels through smaller and smaller arteries. When it comes to one smaller than itself, it stops and obstructs the blood flow ahead of it. The artery in which it stops may be anywhere in the systemic circulation (the brain, the legs, the arms, or the internal organs). The ultimate result may be death to the tissues ahead of it. Other types of emboli include fat, air, cholesterol, and pieces of tumors.

THE LYMPHATIC SYSTEM

The lymphatics remove fluid and particulate matter such as proteins and organisms from the interstitial spaces; carry these substances, which form the lymph, through the lymphatic vessels and into the lymph nodes for digestion by phagocytic cells; and return the processed lymph to the circulatory system. When the net amount of fluid remaining in the interstitial spaces exceeds the capability of the lymphatic vessels to remove it, edema results. Edema also may result from increased venous pressure when lymphatic drainage is normal. It also occurs with normal venous pressure if the lymphatics are diseased. Edema that results from improper function of the lymphatics is called **lymphedema.**

The lymphatics may function improperly because of primary or secondary problems. Primary lymphedema results from lack of formation of lymphatic vessels or distortion of the vessels. Secondary lymphedema is caused by the obstruction or surgical removal of the lymphatic vessels. Obstruction most commonly results from the pressure of tumors or from infections. Inflamed lymphatic vessels occur in **lymphangitis.** When the lymph nodes are involved and become swollen, the condition is called **lymphadenopathy.** In **lymphadenitis** the involved lymph nodes are inflamed.

THE BONE MARROW

The bone marrow is a delicate organ and must be healthy to function properly. Bone marrow function is influenced by many internal and external factors.

Internal factors might include the client's age and nutritional status. As the client ages, extramedullary hematopoiesis no longer occurs; the primary site becomes the bone marrow. Nutritional deficiencies can lead to improper or inadequate bone marrow function. Pernicious anemia illustrates the delicate interrelation between the bone marrow and proper nutrition (see Chapter 29).

External factors influencing normal hematopoiesis are chemical exposure, radiation exposure, and drug therapy. Overexposure to chemical agents, radiation, or drug therapy can cause bone marrow suppression or failure, depending on the kind of agent the client is exposed to, the dose of the agent delivered during exposure, and the length of exposure. Chemical agents that interfere with bone marrow function include herbicides, pesticides, industrial solvents, and industrial cleaners. Radiation overexposure is a risk to workers in nuclear power plants or nuclear arms factories. Drug therapy also can interfere with proper bone marrow function. Although antineoplastic agents are the drugs most often thought to interfere with bone marrow function, any medication can adversely affect bone marrow integrity. Both prescription and over-the-counter agents may have either general or specific suppression effects on the bone marrow. In other words, the side effects of one drug may be listed as bone marrow suppression; a second drug may have neutropenia (decrease in neutrophils) listed as a side effect; and a third drug may cause thrombocytopenia (decrease in platelets).

Any of these factors can disrupt the normal production of leukocytes, erythrocytes, and thrombocytes, making the client prone to developing infections, alteration in the oxygen-carrying capacity of the blood, and bleeding. Proper bone marrow function is necessary for life.

THE BLOOD

The major purpose of the erythrocytes is to carry hemoglobin and subsequently oxygen to the capillaries for diffusion into the cells. Any condition that decreases the amount of hemoglobin, the number of erythrocytes, or the ability of the erythrocytes to flow through the capillaries decreases the oxygen supply to the tissues and may result in ischemia. In polycythemia ("many red cells"), the blood becomes viscous and cannot flow easily. This condition is caused by the bone marrow's high output of erythrocytes in response to tissue hypoxia. Anemia, a decrease in the number of erythrocytes or their ability to carry oxygen, may result from the inability of the bone marrow to produce enough erythrocytes, conditions that promote the rapid destruction of erythrocytes, or loss of blood through hemorrhage. Abnormalities of the erythrocytes that reduce their ability to carry oxygen include insufficient nutrients (such as vitamins and iron) or abnormal genetic material resulting in the production of defective erythrocytes or synthesis of abnormal hemoglobin.

The thrombocytes are necessary for blood to clot properly. Increased thrombocyte production is called *thrombocytosis*, and decreased or defective thrombocyte production is called *thrombocytopenia*. When thrombocytes are insufficient or defective, the client has an increased potential for bleeding.

The leukocytes protect the body from invasion by pathogenic organisms through phagocytosis and the immune response. The number of leukocytes normally increases (leukocytosis) in response to infection or tissue destruction. When a particular type of leukocyte increases in number, the condition is named according to cell type (eg, granulocytosis, neutrophilia). A decrease in the number of leukocytes (leukopenia) results in the inability of the body to defend itself against invasion of pathogenic organisms. This condition also is named by cell type (eg, agranulocytosis, lymphopenia).

Disorders in leukocyte production and maturation make the client prone to overwhelming infection by invading microorganisms (bacteria, viruses, fungi, and protozoa). The abnormal proliferation of immature leukocytes is called *leukemia*. Immature leukocytes cannot defend the body against invasion by foreign substances, as mature leukocytes do. In addition, immature leukocytes require nutrients for survival. Disease that involves the abnormal proliferation of leukocytes essentially robs the normal cells of their required nutrients, which prevents them from adequately performing their functions.

Section III: Related System Influences and Effects

All systems of the body rely on the cardiovascular system and blood-forming organs to supply them with the blood needed to perform their functions. Thus, a problem with the cardiovascular or blood-forming system may result in devastating consequences for the other systems. The other body systems also influence the ability of the cardiovascular and blood-forming systems to perform their functions.

Without a healthy nervous system, the blood vessels would not be able to respond to changes in a person's activity and position. The baroreceptors, as well as the other reflexes discussed earlier in the chapter, would not transmit messages to meet the moment-to-moment need for changes in blood flow. The temperature regulatory function of the cardiovascular system depends on communication between the vasomotor center and the hypothalamus, as well as the integrity of the skin.

The cardiovascular system depends on the respiratory system to make the necessary oxygen available to be picked up and to remove carbon dioxide from the blood. Without the necessary oxygen, the cardiovascular system would not be able to meet tissue needs. Lung-related problems may also increase the work of the heart, because they may promote increased resistance to blood flow as the heart responds to tissue hypoxia.

The cardiovascular system would not be able to pick up and deliver nutrients necessary for cellular function without proper intake of food and water and proper function of the gastrointestinal tract or the liver in metabolism (in processing and storing nutrients, as well as secreting substances necessary for digestion). Without the liver's role in the formation of blood-clotting factors, the integrity of the cardiovascular system would not be sustained.

The blood must be relatively free of waste products to provide the proper environment for the cells. Cellular health depends on the ability of the liver and kidneys to excrete waste products. In addition, the failure of the kidneys to excrete excess water—whether due to a problem with the kidneys, hypothalamus, or pituitary gland—would result in circulatory overload. This might stress the heart and promote an electrolyte imbalance, which would destroy the blood cells.

The proper function of the musculoskeletal system is essential to the ability of the bone marrow to produce the blood cells to be carried by the cardiovascular system. The most important role of the musculoskeletal system is the muscular activity that returns blood to the heart for recirculation.

The endocrine system, through its secretions, affects the entire body metabolism. Problems with hyperthyroidism and its effect on increasing cardiac output have already been discussed. The role of the pituitary gland in secretion of antidiuretic hormone and the role of the adrenal glands in secreting aldosterone affect the cardiovascular system by regulating water and sodium balance. The adrenal glands are most important in the secretion of epinephrine and norepinephrine in times of need to assist the sympathetic nervous system in promoting vasoconstriction. The pancreas plays its role in glucose metabolism.

Section IV: Psychosocial/Lifestyle Influences and Effects

A major physiological problem caused by a disorder of the cardiovascular system, the blood, or the blood-forming organs is the inability to provide adequate nutrients to the cells. This disorder generally results in the client's need to reduce the metabolic demands of the body by decreasing activity levels. The adjustment to decreased activity may be temporary until the disease process is resolved, or it may involve a permanent change in lifestyle. A decrease in activity may not be compatible with the client's responsibilities for home or career. For some persons, a planned exercise program as part of rehabilitation also may be difficult.

Clients encounter other major physiological problems with leukopenia and thrombocytopenia. The client with leukopenia must take special precautions to prevent infection. Once established, infection can be fatal; therefore, client education should be geared toward prevention. Clients may need to change their usual routine, especially during periodic leukopenic episodes. The client may need to avoid crowds or people with upper respiratory tract infections. Even a simple trip to the grocery store may be contraindicated during leukopenic episodes. The client and family or significant others may find this difficult to cope with.

Thrombocytopenia has its own set of restrictions to which the client must adjust. The client must be knowledgeable about measures to prevent serious bleeding episodes during thrombocytopenic periods. Lack of knowledge about the prevention of infection or bleeding episodes may make the client more prone to developing these complications. Decreasing the likelihood of these complications necessitates that clients take responsibility for learning about their disease processes and treatments. Taking responsibility for their own health care may be too stressful for some clients, however.

Adjustments may be needed in nutritional needs. Taking medications also may create an adjustment problem for some. Together, the changes in activity level, the changes in nutritional habits, the need to take medications, and the added responsibility of learning about a disease process and its treatment require adjustments in developmental and cultural aspects of living.

The nurse as counselor should assist clients by discussing their lifestyles in relation to the effects on the

Nursing Research Note

Bohachick P: Progressive relaxation training in cardiac rehabilitation: Effect on psychologic variables. *Nurs Res* 1984; 33:283–287.

The effects of relaxation training for stress management in cardiac clients were studied. One group of subjects was given relaxation training and exercise therapy, and the control group was given exercise therapy. Both groups were tested before and after their course of therapy. The results indicated that the experimental group receiving relaxation training had a significantly lower self-report of symptoms, interpersonal sensitivity, anxiety, and depression.

Incorporating relaxation training into cardiac rehabilitation programs may help to reduce psychological distress. Nurses can set up relaxation training programs to begin this process and closely assess their effectiveness.

cardiovascular and blood-forming organs. Studies have shown that the level of compliance in both preventive and curative situations is low. A review of the literature by Dracup and Meleis (1982) found that about one-third to one-half of all clients studied did not follow suggested positive health practices. Even though not all clients will respond to recommendations, they all have the right to information so they can make informed decisions about lifestyle changes.

DEVELOPMENTAL INFLUENCES

Developmental tasks that adults must perform include those related to their vocational, family, home, social, and leisure time responsibilities. Depending on the capabilities of the cardiovascular system and blood-forming organs, clients may need to make some changes in these responsibilities. Discuss the possibility of the client's returning to work. The need for alterations in activities of daily living to accomplish the responsibilities in the home also should be explored.

Consider whether the client will need to make changes in sexual activity. The client's participation in the usual family activities also may need to change. Activities such as family outings, sporting activities, and shopping trips may be physiologically too stressful or may put the client at an increased risk for developing serious infections if there is bone marrow dysfunction. In addition, some changes may be needed in living arrangements. For example, whether the client will be required to climb steps is important.

Discuss community activities in relation to the need for energy expenditure and the possible risk of infection. Some activities, such as being a volunteer fire fighter or participating in preparing dinners and bake sales, may be stressful to the cardiovascular and blood-forming systems and may need to be eliminated. Others, such as making telephone calls or stuffing envelopes for an organization, may be acceptable.

Leisure time activities also should be considered. Some persons use their leisure time in sedentary activities and may need to make no adjustments during the recovery period. Others who participate in activities requiring a high energy expenditure (eg, skiing and camping) may have difficulty adjusting. Some persons who have no hobbies or leisure time activities find having time on their hands stressful.

In some cases, eliminating an activity may be more stressful to the client than establishing a new leisure regimen. Probably the most important issue in counseling the client about a change in activity level is the importance the activity has for the client. Counseling may help clients decide what is most important for them. Some activities may need to be eliminated, some may be continued if they are spaced, and some may need no adjustment at all.

CULTURAL INFLUENCES

What a person believes is important plays a significant role in the development of cardiovascular diseases as well as in his or her compliance with rehabilitation and treatment for both cardiovascular and blood disorders. These beliefs are related to personality attributes. The role of the personality in heart disease has received considerable attention. The type A person, who is competitive, impatient, ambitious, tense, and aggressive, may be more prone to myocardial infarction than the type B person, who is relatively easygoing. Although emotional stress is neither good nor bad, observations indicate that it does have a physiological effect on heart rate, blood pressure, and respiration. The extent to which a person is stressed is an individual matter, and the effect of the stressor is related to its significance to the individual.

The culture in which a person lives greatly determines the significance of emotional and physiological stressors. For example, smoking has been a culturally acceptable behavior identified as a major risk factor in the development of cardiovascular disease. The importance a person places on such areas as family, work, eating, social activities, and health care is also related to cultural values.

DIETARY FACTORS

Diet is important in all diseases. Without the proper nutrients, the cells cannot function properly. Certain dietary habits are associated with cardiovascular disease. A high blood cholesterol level has been determined to be a major risk factor in the development of atherosclerosis. Clients can control high cholesterol levels by changing to a diet low in saturated fat and cholesterol. Being overweight is a problem for many. Changing the dietary habits of one member of the family usually effects changes in the diets of others as well, which may place stress on the entire family. Dietary changes also have the potential for improving the entire family's health.

Nursing Research Note

Sloan R: Achieving compliance to a reduced sodium diet. *Nurse Pract* (Feb) 1985; 10:25–26.

This research describes use of urinary chloride titrator sticks to evaluate client compliance to low-sodium diets, often prescribed in the treatment of hypertension. Test subjects were taught to use the chloride sticks on first morning urine specimens. Readings greater than +2 indicated noncompliance to sodium restrictions. Readings less than +2 demonstrated adherence to a dietary sodium intake of less than 85 mEq/day or a 2-g sodium restriction. Results suggest that with dietary instruction and use of chloride sticks, clients were able to adjust daily salt intake and monitor their own dietary restrictions with greater accuracy.

Chloride sticks may be an effective tool for nursing intervention. Results of daily chloride stick use can provide feedback to both the nurse and the client.

ECONOMIC AND OCCUPATIONAL FACTORS

Changes in diet, occupation, activity level, and living arrangements, as well as the need for medication and the cost of health care may cause a severe economic burden for the client and family. In addition, persons with cardiovascular or blood disorders may have difficulty obtaining insurance because they pose a greater economic risk for health and life insurance companies than the general population. Consequently, insurance costs may be prohibitive, but the lack of insurance reduces economic security and brings more stress.

The client with a cardiovascular or blood disease may or may not be able to return to work. Job requirements may need to be adjusted, which can produce stress between the client and peers over work load. Workmen's compensation insurance may be available if the cardiovascular problem is related to the job. In cases of complete disability, the client may be eligible for Social Security compensation.

ENVIRONMENTAL FACTORS

Environmental threats to the person with cardiovascular and blood problems include terrain and climate. Walking up an incline requires much more energy expenditure than walking on level ground. Environmental temperature extremes place an additional burden on the cardiovascular and blood systems. Cold temperature promotes vasoconstriction and shivering to generate body heat, and a person with an already diminished blood flow may experience ischemia. Shivering increases the metabolic needs and cardiac output. Hot temperature promotes dilation of the vessels near the skin, which also requires an increased cardiac output.

SEXUAL EXPRESSION

Clients with angina and those recovering from myocardial infarction or coronary artery bypass surgery often have fears about the resumption of sexual activity. The spouse may also be anxious, which can interfere with a satisfying intimate relationship. Males with hypertension may be taking antihypertensive medications that cause impotence, failure to ejaculate, or decreased libido.

The nurse can be instrumental in identifying clients who have been unable to resume a satisfying sexual relationship because of fear of worsening their cardiac status or those with sexual dysfunction resulting from drug therapy. Careful history taking and a sensitive approach can pave the way for identifying sexual problems for which something can be done.

Chapter Highlights

The purpose of the cardiovascular system is to supply the body tissues with the nutrients and other substances they need, remove the waste products from the cellular environment, and circulate body defense substances.

Blood flows from an area of higher pressure to one of lower pressure, and the heart generates the pressure to promote blood flow.

Because of their elasticity and recoil, the arteries are able to continue blood flow during ventricular diastole.

The exchange of substances between the blood vessels and the interstitial spaces occurs in the capillaries.

The veins are capacitance vessels that serve as a reservoir for blood.

The lymphatics prevent edema.

The erythrocytes carry oxygen to the cells.

The thrombocytes (platelets) are essential to the blood-clotting mechanism and clot retraction.

The granulocytes (neutrophils, basophils, and eosinophils) are primarily involved in phagocytosis.

The agranular leukocytes (monocytes and lymphocytes) are primarily involved in the immune response.

The autonomic nervous system influences heart rate and contraction. Parasympathetic activity slows the heart, and sympathetic activity speeds it up.

The sympathetic nervous system controls the diameter of the blood vessels. Some vessels dilate and some constrict in response to sympathetic activity.

The baroreceptors, chemoreceptors, and atrial stretch receptors monitor moment-to-moment changes in blood pressure and communicate with the vasomotor center.

Inadequate blood supply or decreased quality of the blood may produce ischemia of the cells, which in turn may lead to cellular death.

The abnormal proliferation of immature leukocytes (leukemia) may rob the normal cells of their nutrients and cause cellular death.

All the body systems depend on the cardiovascular system and blood-forming organs to supply their needs.

A problem with another body system will ultimately affect the cardiovascular and blood-forming systems.

An individual's lifestyle may contribute to the development of cardiovascular disease, and persons with cardiovascular problems may need to make changes in their lifestyles.

After a major cardiac event, both the client and sexual partner may be fearful about resuming sexual activity.

Bibliography

Byrne CJ et al: *Laboratory Tests: Implications for Nursing Care,* 2nd ed. Menlo Park, CA: Addison–Wesley, 1986.

Chesnewy MA, Rosenman RH: Type A behavior: Observation on the past decade. *Heart Lung* 1982; 11:12–19.

Dracup KA, Meleis AI: Compliance: An interactionist approach. *Nurs Res* 1982; 31:31–36.

Glenn WL et al: *Thoracic and Cardiovascular Surgery,* 2nd ed. Norwalk, CT: Appleton–Century–Crofts, 1983.

Guyton AC: *Textbook of Medical Physiology,* 6th ed. Philadelphia: Saunders, 1981.

Heart Facts 1983. Dallas: American Heart Association, 1982.

Hurst JW et al: *The Heart,* 5th ed. New York: McGraw–Hill, 1982.

Lee BY et al: *Handbook of Noninvasive Diagnostic Techniques in Vascular Surgery.* New York: Appleton–Century–Crofts, 1981.

Saxton DF et al: *The Addison–Wesley Manual of Nursing Practice.* Menlo Park, CA: Addison–Wesley, 1983.

Spittell JA (editor): *Clinical Vascular Disease.* Philadelphia: Davis, 1983.

Stites DP et al: *Clinical Immunology,* 4th ed. Los Altos, CA: Lange, 1982.

Williams PL, Warwick R: *Gray's Anatomy,* 36th ed. Philadelphia: Saunders, 1980.

Williams WJ et al: *Hematology,* 3rd ed. New York: McGraw–Hill, 1983.

Wilson HS, Kneisl CR: *Psychiatric Nursing,* 2nd ed. Menlo Park, CA: Addison–Wesley, 1983.

Suggested Readings

Bailey JC: The electrophysiologic basis for cardiac electrical activity: Normal and abnormal. *Heart Lung* 1981; 10:455–464. The heart's action potential is clearly explained in this article.

Conroy KM: Anergy: The hidden danger. *Heart Lung* 1982; 11:85–92. This article discusses cellular immunity.

Erickson R: Tube talk: Principles of fluid flow in tubes. *Nurs 82* (July) 1982; 12:54–61. Fluid flow is discussed in this article.

King NH: Controlling bleeding when the platelet count drops. *RN* (Aug) 1984; 47(8):25–27. Factors contributing to abnormal function of thrombocytes or abnormal numbers of them are discussed, along with related nursing care.

Mansen TJ: Does that CBC spell trouble? *RN* (July) 1984; 47(7):48–51. Quick and easy-to-understand guidelines are presented for interpretation of the complete blood count with the differential count.

Chapter 23

The Nursing Process for Clients With Heart and Major Blood Vessel Dysfunction

Frances L. Stier

Objectives

When you have finished studying this chapter, you should be able to:

List the components of the cardiovascular health history.

Identify the principal symptoms of heart disease.

Explain the characteristics of chest pain of cardiac origin.

Discuss the common emotional responses of both client and significant others to a cardiac event.

Identify the cardiovascular risk factors.

Determine specific physical assessment approaches in evaluating clients with cardiovascular dysfunction.

Describe the diagnostic tests used in assessing cardiovascular dysfunction and the nursing implications for each test.

Anticipate common nursing diagnoses for clients with cardiovascular dysfunction.

Develop a nursing care plan for clients with cardiovascular dysfunction.

Evaluate the effectiveness of the nursing care plan and modify it as necessary to meet the client's needs.

This chapter discusses the information to be obtained in a cardiovascular history, physical assessment of the cardiovascular system, and the common diagnostic tests used. Sections II and III describe the nursing diagnoses specific to clients with cardiovascular dysfunction and related nursing care. The final step in the nursing process, the evaluation of care, is discussed in Section IV. A sample nursing care plan is provided at the end of the chapter.

Section I: Nursing Assessment: Establishing the Data Base

SUBJECTIVE DATA

Obtaining a cardiovascular health history from the client is the first and most important step in cardiovascular assessment. Selection of diagnostic tests, interpretation of test results, and prescription of therapy all depend on the client's history. Most clients fear heart disease and often understate their symptoms. By carefully observing their nonverbal gestures, their reactions to questions, the words they use to describe symptoms, and their overall attitudes, the nurse can evaluate clients' emotional responses. Assessment of clients' emotional support systems is also beneficial, especially if invasive procedures must be performed or long-term disability is a possible outcome. Taking the time to get to know both clients and their families or significant others helps the nurse to correlate behavioral and emotional factors with the onset of cardiac symptoms.

The principal symptoms of heart disease are dyspnea, chest pain, palpitation, and syncope. Other common symptoms are fatigue and cough. The nurse should attempt to gain information about these symptoms, evaluating them according to the level of activity that precipitates the symptom. Clients may not experience any problems with minimal activity, but the symptoms may appear with exertion. This is the classic situation with cardiovascular dysfunction.

Dyspnea

Dyspnea, the most common symptom of both cardiac and pulmonary disease, is the condition of difficult or labored breathing. Clients report that it is difficult to breathe, that there is not enough air, or that they become short of breath with any activity. In heart disease, the dyspnea usually occurs with exertion: clients cannot seem to get enough air into their lungs. In pulmonary disease, the dyspnea occurs both at rest and with exertion, and clients feel more difficulty during exhalation. The differentiation between cardiac and pulmonary dyspnea is difficult; the two diseases often coexist.

Dyspnea should be evaluated in relation to the extent of activity it takes to bring on the symptom. Ask clients if they can perform their normal daily activities without difficulty in breathing. If they have no problems with these activities, ascertain the highest level of activity they can attain without dyspnea—eg, the ability to climb two but not three flights of stairs without difficulty. Dyspnea associated with exertion is known as dyspnea on exertion (DOE). DOE is an early symptom of congestive heart failure (CHF).

Paroxysmal Nocturnal Dyspnea
Paroxysmal nocturnal dyspnea (PND) occurs during sleep. The client usually awakens suddenly, breathing with difficulty and having a sensation of suffocation. This usually occurs 2 to 5 hours after the onset of sleep and happens only once during the night.

PND occurs in clients with CHF and is due to pump failure of the left ventricle, which leads to fluid accumulation in the lungs. PND is relieved by sitting upright with legs over the side of the bed or by walking around the room. It usually subsides within 20 minutes without aftereffects, and the client can sleep the remainder of the night.

Orthopnea
Orthopnea is the form of dyspnea that develops when the client lies down. It is relieved within minutes by sitting up or standing. The client uses several pillows at night to elevate the head and prevent nocturnal breathlessness. In fact, the severity of the condition is often measured by the number of pillows the client needs. As heart disease advances and CHF progresses, the number of pillows required to provide relief increases. In severe heart failure, the client is unable to lie down and usually sleeps in a chair. To obtain information about this symptom, ask the client, "How well do you sleep?" Find out how many pillows the

client normally uses and whether the number of pillows has increased to provide breathing comfort during the night.

Chest Pain

By far the most frightening cardiovascular symptom is chest pain. Because chest pain may have a variety of causes, the main objective in evaluating chest pain is to determine the origin. The most common origins are cardiac, pleuropulmonary, musculoskeletal, gastric, or psychosomatic. Pain originating from the heart is due to **ischemia** (deficiency of blood due to a constricted or obstructed blood vessel). Ischemic pain is referred to as either angina or myocardial infarction (MI) pain. The diagnosis depends on the client's history and subsequent physical examination.

The most serious cause of chest pain is pain from an MI. This cause should be considered first and, when the diagnosis of MI is ruled out, then questioning can be directed to other causes. When obtaining information about chest pain, assess the following aspects: the onset, location, radiation, duration, quality, alleviating and aggravating factors, and associated symptoms (see Chapter 7).

Chest pain due to MI is often described as a crushing substernal pain. The client may say, "It felt as if a ton of bricks was on my chest." A common gesture clients use is a tight fist over the center of the chest. The pain is usually associated with dyspnea, diaphoresis, and (less frequently) nausea and vomiting. The onset is acute and not

Nursing Research Note

Winslow EH, Lane LD, Gaffney FA: Oxygen uptake and cardiovascular response in control adults and acute myocardial infarction patients during bathing. *Nurs Res* 1985; 34(3):164–169.

This study examined oxygen consumption, peak heart rate, after-bath rate pressure product (systolic BP × HR ÷ 100), dysrhythmias, ST changes, perceived exertion while bathing, and bath preference in groups of stable myocardial infarction (MI) clients and normal adults. These variables were studied during basin baths, tub baths, and showers.

The findings indicate that stable post-MI clients had significantly lower oxygen consumption than normal adults. Post-MI clients had higher peak heart rates, often exceeding discharge target heart rate. Bath type did not influence peak heart rate or number of dysrhythmias in either group. Post-MI clients had no cardiovascular symptoms during the three bath types. The post-MI group had higher after-bath rate pressures than the control group. The post-MI group disliked basin baths and felt all forms of bathing were light exertion.

The findings suggest that physiologic cost is similar in all three bathing forms. The implications of this research for nursing practice lie in careful nursing assessment of activity tolerance of stable post-MI clients. Nurses must assess for orthostasis, weakness, obesity, client stability, air and water temperature, medications, and other existing medical conditions. Bathing must be carefully monitored in early recovery to ascertain the degree of exertion and physiologic response.

associated with a precipitating event. The pain lasts longer than 5 minutes; nothing relieves it. Often, the pain radiates to the left or right arm, into the neck, or to the jaw. Occasionally, the client may have only radiating pain.

Like MI pain, angina is a constricting, pressure type of pain. Angina differs from the pain of an MI in that it is episodic and temporary, usually lasting less than 5 minutes. Also, the onset is associated with exertion, emotion, eating, or exposure to cold. Acute episodes are relieved by nitroglycerin and/or rest. For long-term management, angina is controlled by other cardiac medications, usually a beta-adrenergic inhibitor. If angina is uncontrollable and the client is unable to maintain an adequate lifestyle, coronary bypass surgery may be required.

Other serious causes of chest pain are pulmonary embolus and dissecting aortic aneurysm. Pain from a pulmonary embolus is described as knifelike shooting pain. The pain increases with inspiration and is often associated with a sudden onset of dyspnea, tachycardia, hypotension, diaphoresis, rales, and hemoptysis.

Pain from a dissecting aortic aneurysm is characterized as a sudden, tearing, intense chest pain with radiation to the back, flanks, and legs. Usually, the client has a history of hypertension.

Chest pain well localized to a specific area of the chest wall is usually due to a musculoskeletal problem. Tenderness in response to palpation is often present. An example is chest pain due to inflammation of the costochondral junctions of the ribs and sternum.

Stress and anxiety may also cause chest pain. This type of pain is usually localized in the left chest wall and does not radiate. The history assists in determining whether the chest pain is related to stress and anxiety.

Palpitation

Palpitation is an unpleasant awareness of the heartbeat. The client often describes a fluttering feeling in the chest or says that the heart seems to jump, race, pound, stop, or skip beats. Palpitations are most often due to rhythm disturbances such as premature contractions, atrial fibrillation, or sinus tachycardia. A variety of causes produces rhythm disturbances, however. Anxiety, stress, fatigue, or cardiac stimulants such as caffeine and nicotine are factors that precipitate palpitations. Detailed questions about the onset, relation to exercise, presence of associated symptoms such as shortness of breath or syncope, relieving factors such as stooping or breathholding assist in determining the significance of the palpitation. Drug toxicity may also cause palpitations. Therefore, a medication history, which includes asking *how* the client takes the medication, is necessary.

Syncope

Syncope, a transient loss of consciousness, is associated with muscle weakness and an inability to stand. It is due

to inadequate blood flow to the brain, which may be a result of a cardiac rhythm disturbance or decreased cardiac output from valvular disease. Dizziness with an inability to maintain an upright posture is referred to as *near syncope.* The client should describe the circumstances that lead to dizziness or fainting. Syncope that occurs with exercise may be related to aortic or subaortic valve stenosis. This condition is serious and requires further documentation, usually through noninvasive testing.

A sudden loss of consciousness due to a heart block is known as a Stokes–Adams attack. This type of syncope commonly occurs in elderly clients and is followed by breathlessness and absence of pulse, usually lasting only seconds. Cardiac arrest may occur if respiration and circulation are not restored.

The elderly client may also develop another type of syncope caused by hypersensitivity of the carotid sinus bodies. The carotid sinus bodies are located in the carotid artery below the jawline. Pressure applied to the carotid artery may stimulate a vagal response that decreases the blood pressure and heart rate; exaggerated vagal response may produce syncope. The client may report episodes of fainting while shaving or buttoning a tight collar. Digitalis appears to increase carotid sinus sensitivity, making the client susceptible to syncope. Bilateral palpation of the carotids should never be performed.

Fatigue

Fatigue is a frequent complaint of clients suffering from cardiovascular dysfunction. Clients describe muscle weakness and an inability to complete normal daily activities. They often need one to two naps a day to function. The fatigue is probably related to a combination of physical and emotional factors. Physically, the fatigue is thought to be related to insufficient blood flow to the tissues, the result of inadequate cardiac output. Depression may also cause fatigue. Fatigue is assessed by the level of activity tolerance.

Cough

Cough associated with cardiovascular disease is due to fluid accumulation in the lungs. The cough is described as dry, irritating, spasmodic, and nocturnal. Clients may cough after episodes of dyspnea. A productive cough with colored sputum may indicate a pulmonary problem.

Psychosocial Response

The heart's functioning is associated with life itself. A serious disruption of cardiovascular function can be a significant emotional and physical threat. The onset of heart disease is often considered a major life crisis. The life of a client who has a cardiac event (eg, an MI or cardiac surgery) may be either immediately threatened or altered.

Survival cannot be guaranteed; former support systems may be diminished; roles as spouse, parent and worker may be interrupted; and future plans often need revision. Central to this crisis is the fear of death, pain, disability, and physical dependence. Most clients respond to these fears by developing anxiety.

Anxiety can be manifested through a variety of physical, emotional, and behavioral responses. In cardiovascular assessment, it is important to appreciate that the physical responses to anxiety are similar to those of cardiovascular dysfunction: tachycardia, increased blood pressure and respiratory rate, fatigue, diaphoresis, or palpitations. Emotional and behavioral responses may include fear, apprehension, nervousness, crying, irritability, or withdrawal.

Anxiety may also be a result of the client's assessment of personal body image. An acute event poses a great threat to body integrity and function. The personal meaning of the heart to the client and the impact of the event on body image will greatly influence the client's convalescence. Client role responsibilities, knowledge of the severity of the disease, and the reaction of significant others are important components to assess.

To cope with anxiety and fear, the client may use denial. In the acute care setting, denial is used for defensive coping and serves to protect the client from perceived threats. As an effective coping mechanism decreasing the physical and emotional outcomes of anxiety, denial is beneficial in the acute phase of illness. Sustained denial, however, is maladaptive. The nurse must assist the client in identifying effective coping mechanisms.

Past Health History

After obtaining information about the client's symptoms, review the client's past health history, paying particular attention to information about previous hospitalization for cardiac problems. Ask the client whether any episodes of chest pain resulted in hospitalization. If cardiac surgery was performed, document the date, the type of surgery, number of bypasses, and any complications. If valvular surgery was performed, include the type of valve used (eg, porcine, ball and cage, or tilting disk). If a cardiac pacemaker was implanted, the client should know the type and have the model number available. Previous diagnostic procedures performed, such as ECGs, exercise stress testing, or cardiac catheterizations, add to the client's history.

Certain childhood diseases predispose the client to cardiovascular dysfunction. Childhood rheumatic fever can cause valvular disease that becomes evident in adulthood. Untreated streptococcal throat infections may also cause valvular disease. Maternal exposure to rubella in the first 2 months of pregnancy is associated with congenital heart defects. Many children who have had corrective surgery for congenital heart defects are now living through adulthood; therefore, information regarding the childhood cardiac problem should be obtained.

Medication and Dietary History

A medication history including prescribed and over-the-counter (OTC) medications should be obtained. OTC drugs may precipitate cardiac symptoms. Many antihistamines, decongestants, and antitussives contain sympathomimetic amines, which may cause palpitations or transient hypertension. Some antacid preparations contain large amounts of sodium, which may cause fluid retention and subsequent increase in blood pressure. If the client is taking a prescribed medicine, ask how the client is taking it, specifying the time of day and the amount.

A dietary history assists the nurse in evaluating the client's understanding of the relation between food and heart disease. Assess the eating of red meat, salt, dairy products, and sugar and estimate caloric intake. Evaluate the client's weight compared with the recommended ideal weight.

Risk Factors

An important component in cardiovascular assessment is evaluating the client's cardiovascular risk factor profile. Risk factors are personal characteristics and habits that increase the client's chances of developing coronary artery disease (CAD). The risk factors are divided into unalterable and alterable factors. The unalterable risk factors are sex (male) and a family history of heart disease or hypertension. Alterable risk factors include hypercholesterolemia, smoking, diabetes mellitus, obesity, physical inactivity, and oral contraceptive use. Personality may also

Table 23–1	Classification for Diastolic and Systolic Hypertension
Diastolic Blood Pressure (mm Hg)	**Category**
<85	Normal blood pressure
85 to 89	High normal blood pressure
90 to 104	Mild hypertension
105 to 114	Moderate hypertension
≥115	Severe hypertension
Systolic blood pressure (mm Hg); when DBP <90 mm Hg	
<140	Normal blood pressure
140 to 159	Borderline isolated systolic hypertension
≥160	Isolated systolic hypertension

SOURCE: Reprinted from *1984 Report of the Joint National Committee on Detection, Evaluation, and Treatment of High Blood Pressure*. US Department of Health and Human Services. NIH Publication No 84-1088, June 1984.

contribute to CAD. A behavior pattern called type A behavior, characterized as competitive, compulsive, hard driving, and time oriented has been associated with twice the normal risk of developing CAD. The most prominent risk factors are hypertension, a high blood cholesterol level, and cigarette smoking.

Hypertension

Unequivocally, hypertension, either systolic or diastolic, increases the risk of developing CAD; the higher the blood pressure, the greater the risk. Hypertension causes coronary, cerebral, and renal vascular disease. It is the leading cause of death and disability among adults. The standard most often used to establish a diagnosis of diastolic or systolic hypertension is given in Table 23–1.

Symptoms often attributed to hypertension include headache, epistaxis, tinnitus, dizziness, and fainting. Unfortunately, uncomplicated hypertension is usually asymptomatic until significant organ damage occurs. Therefore, frequent screening is required.

Cholesterol

In evaluating cholesterol, ask about the client's previous history of elevated cholesterol levels and the therapeutic and preventive regimens the client is following. Ascertain how much the client knows about the role of cholesterol in developing CAD and whether the client understands the role of diet, exercise, and weight in controlling cholesterol levels. A diet low in saturated fats, high in polyunsaturated fats, and low in cholesterol is beneficial. A reduction in calories is usually recommended, especially if the client is overweight. Aerobic exercise appears to increase the high-density lipoprotein (HDL) levels, which appear to retard the development of CAD (see Diagnostic Studies). The optimal goal of client management is to achieve a serum cholesterol level below 200 mg/dL with a level of HDL higher than low-density lipoprotein (LDL). Values for adults at moderate or high risk of heart disease according to age and cholesterol level are shown in Table 23–2. The client should limit the daily intake of cholesterol to less than 300 mg/day.

Smoking

The principal cause of death in cigarette smokers is CAD, not lung cancer. The risk is directly related to the number of cigarettes smoked per day. Smoking a pack or more a day increases the risk of heart disease at least threefold. How long smokers have been smoking and whether they inhale smoke do not appear to be significant. The risk can be reduced by discontinuing smoking. Within a year, the former smoker has the same risk as the nonsmoker. The client should understand this encouraging fact.

When cigarette smoking is combined with oral contraceptives, the risk of CAD and MI is extremely high. Smokers who have hypertension and/or diabetes mellitus are also at greater risk.

Table 23–2	Cholesterol Values for Adults at Moderate or High Risk of Heart Disease	
Age	Moderate Risk	High Risk
20–29	≥ 200 mg/dL	≥ 220 mg/dL
30–39	≥ 220 mg/dL	≥ 240 mg/dL
40 and over	≥ 240 mg/dL	≥ 260 mg/dL

SOURCE: Reprinted from National Institutes of Health: *Lipid Research Clinics Population Study Data.* Vol. I, NIH Publication No. 80–1527, July 1980.

After explaining the effect of cigarette smoking, offer the client assistance in smoking cessation. Group classes are effective, but if the client prefers individual help, the American Lung Association provides a written program. The health care provider should carefully review this program with the client. Informing the client of other community resources increases the client's chances of smoking cessation.

Physical Inactivity

Exercise appears to be effective in preventing CAD by reducing other risk factors such as stress, obesity, and elevated cholesterol levels. Physically fit individuals are more likely to survive a cardiac event than sedentary individuals.

Clients should be encouraged to incorporate exercise into their lifestyle as a routine. Walking is usually recommended as an easy type of exercise that can be done anywhere. The amount and duration of exercise are prescribed *after* clients undergo a complete history and physical examination.

Alcohol and Caffeine Use

Excessive alcohol consumption causes an increase in serum lipid levels and caloric intake. Both effects contribute to CAD. A moderate consumption of alcohol (one glass of wine per day) has been associated with increased HDL levels, which may be positive. Documentation of the alcohol intake should include the client's pattern of drinking as well as the amount and type of alcohol consumed.

Caffeine is a cardiovascular stimulant causing tachycardia and dysrhythmias. It may contribute to other risk factors such as hypertension. Determine the client's intake of caffeine including coffee, tea, chocolate, and carbonated soft drinks. More than 16 oz per day is often considered excessive. Some clients who are especially sensitive to caffeine may experience symptoms with lesser amounts.

OBJECTIVE DATA
Physical Assessment

The physical assessment of the cardiovascular system begins with a general examination of the client. Whereas cardiac dysfunction may directly affect other body systems, systemic illnesses often have cardiac manifestations. For these reasons, a thorough examination of the client is necessary.

First, observe the general appearance of the client—physical build, skin color, pallor or cyanosis—and the client's emotional status. Assess whether the client appears to be in pain. The client experiencing pain may have overt signs. Typically, the client with angina sits quietly, whereas the client with acute MI pain is uncomfortable and moves continuously. With pericarditis, the client assumes a sitting position, leaning forward.

Tall clients with long extremities and arm spans exceeding their height may have Marfan's syndrome, which is associated with a variety of cardiac disorders. Note chest contour: some thoracic deformities, such as kyphoscoliosis, pectus carinatum, and pectus excavatum, can affect the position of the heart and possibly cardiac function.

The general description is followed by detailed inspection. Note abnormal facial appearance, particularly facial edema, color, and skin texture. Rheumatic heart disease with severe mitral stenosis may cause cyanotic lips and jaundice. Constrictive pericarditis causes fluid retention, which can result in swelling of the face.

A funduscopic exam is performed on all clients. Changes caused by hypertension, such as A-V narrowing, exudate, and hemorrhage formations, are seen on the fundi. A thin grayish white circle, an arcus, in the iris is seen in clients with hypercholesterolemia.

Skin color and temperature are important indicators of circulation. Pallor and cyanosis are key signs in assessing skin color. *Pallor* is the absence of the normal pink skin color. One cause of pallor is vasoconstriction, which decreases blood flow to the skin. In clients with deeply pigmented or dark skin, the conjunctivae and oral mucosa are examined for skin color changes.

Cyanosis is a blue tinge to the skin that appears when hemoglobin oxygen saturation is reduced. Cyanosis can take the form of central cyanosis or peripheral cyanosis. Central cyanosis is assessed in the lips, mucous membranes, and nail beds; peripheral cyanosis is found in the extremities. With prolonged central cyanosis, clubbing of fingers and toes can occur.

The nails are a good source of information regarding cardiovascular status. Circulation can be evaluated in the nail beds by applying pressure to the distal part of the fingernail and noting the pallor as the capillary blood flow is temporarily halted. When the fingernail is released, the color returns by capillary refill. The original color should be restored within 1 to 2 seconds or by the time the words *capillary refill* are said. The nail beds are also inspected for hemorrhagic areas resembling splinters, which can be seen in clients with bacterial endocarditis.

Temperature of the skin and extremities also reflects circulation. Cool, pale, wet, blue-tinged skin often indicates a decrease in circulation. This condition is seen in clients with an acute MI when the cardiac output is suddenly reduced. Warm and flushed skin appears in clients with a high cardiac output, as in hyperthyroidism.

Some skin lesions have also been associated with cardiac dysfunction. **Petechiae,** small red macules on the skin or mucous membranes, are observed in clients with infective endocarditis. **Xanthomas,** cholesterol-filled papules, are found on the eyelids or within the orbit of the eyes. These skin lesions are associated with hyperlipoproteinemia.

Edema

Edema is a local or general accumulation of excess fluid in the body tissues. Edema in any dependent area such as the extremities, the sacrum, or the abdomen is important to recognize. Edema is distinguished as pitting or nonpitting. Pitting edema is considered more serious than nonpitting edema, but the presence of either type is significant. The depth of pitting and the extent and location of edema indicate the severity of the condition. Bilateral edema is associated with heart disease. Some cardiovascular causes of edema include CHF and constrictive pericarditis. Ask the client if shoes, rings, or clothes are getting uncomfortably tight. Tightness may reflect fluid retention in those areas. Changes in body weight also reflect fluid status. A weight gain in a short period may be due to fluid retention. Sudden increases in weight may indicate cardiac failure.

Pulses

Arterial pulses provide significant information regarding cardiac output. Cardiac output, which depends on stroke volume and heart rate, can be assessed by the pulse rate and the quality of the pulse. Pulses should be examined bilaterally and include the carotid, brachial, radial, ulnar, femoral, popliteal, dorsalis pedis, and posterior tibial pulses. The rate, rhythm, and force are assessed. A pulse rate greater than 100 beats per minute (**tachycardia**) is considered abnormal for healthy adults. Although a variety of factors may cause tachycardia, the long-term effect is usually decreased cardiac output. A pulse rate below 60 beats per minute (**bradycardia**) is considered abnormal except in clients with well conditioned hearts (eg, marathon runners). In the diseased heart, bradycardia causes a decrease in cardiac output, possibly indicating heart block. An irregular pulse is associated with cardiac dysrhythmias. The quality of the pulse or force is assessed on a scale of 4 with 0 equal to unpalpable or absent and 4+ equal to full and bounding. A normal pulse is designated as 4+.

The absence of a pulse may be a normal variation, particularly the popliteal, ulnar, or posterior tibial pulses. A diminished or absent carotid pulse, however, usually indicates arterial disease. When a pulse is not palpable, a more distal pulse is assessed; eg, the dorsalis pedis pulse is assessed when the popliteal pulse is not palpable, and the radial pulse is assessed when the brachial pulse is not palpable. If distal pulses are felt, adequate circulation is present. If absent, other assessment parameters are noted such as skin temperature, skin color, and sensation.

Pulses are assessed bilaterally (eg, right radial and left radial). Asymmetric or unequal bilateral pulses are abnormal and may indicate a serious circulatory problem. An exception: the carotid arteries should never be palpated bilaterally. Palpation can overstimulate the pressure sensors (carotid sinus bodies), which will decrease heart rate and may result in syncope. As mentioned previously, the elderly client is especially susceptible.

The arteries are also assessed by auscultation. A **bruit** is an abnormal sound heard in arteries that have some occlusion causing turbulence of blood flow. A carotid artery bruit may be due to occlusion or may actually be a referred systolic murmur from aortic valve disease.

The quality of the pulse can also be assessed according to the shape of the waveform, which can be palpated or displayed and measured by an arterial pressure monitor. Pulse waves that alternate in strength, every other beat being weaker than the preceding beat, are known as *pulsus alternans*. This condition is common in clients with severe arterial hypertension and/or left ventricular failure. A small, weak pulse that seems to have a delay in the beginning (upstroke) and a delay in the ending (downstroke) is called *pulsus parvus* and is found in aortic stenosis, mitral stenosis, constrictive pericarditis, and cardiac tamponade. A strong, bounding pulse with a rapid upstroke and downstroke, *pulsus magnus*, is seen in clients with hypertension, thyrotoxicosis, or aortic insufficiency. A double-beating pulse, called *pulsus bisferiens*, is found in aortic insufficiency and aortic stenosis.

The effect of respiration on the pulse pressure can be assessed by use of the sphygmomanometer. Normally, the pulse pressure decreases approximately 10 mm Hg with inspiration; if the pulse pressure drops more than 10 mm Hg, it is abnormal. This condition, referred to as a *pulsus paradoxus,* is often found in clients with pericardial effusion, constrictive pericarditis, and severe pulmonary emphysema.

Blood Pressure

Blood pressure is routinely assessed in all clients. The indirect method is used, employing a sphygmomanometer, aneroid or mercury gauge, cuff, and stethoscope. The blood pressure is a good indicator of cardiovascular health. It reflects not only the physical state of the client but also the psychological effect on the physical state.

Blood pressure is initially obtained in both arms with the client in supine, seated, and standing positions. The blood pressure in both arms should be comparable: a difference of more than 10 mm Hg is abnormal. The readings are recorded as shown in Table 23–3.

The cuff size is an important factor in obtaining accurate blood pressure. The cuff should be 20% wider than the diameter of the arm and cover two-thirds of the upper

Table 23–3	Recording Blood Pressures		
Client Position		Right Arm*	Left Arm*
Supine		120/80	122/84
Seated		126/80	130/84
Standing		130/80	136/86

*Use legs and arms when taking initial blood pressures of clients with a history of hypertension or vascular disease; use prone position for leg pressures.

arm. If the cuff is too small, the reading will be elevated. Conversely, a cuff too large will artificially lower the reading. Positioning of the cuff and the level of the brachial artery are also important. The bladder of the cuff should be centered over the brachial artery with the lower edge 1 to 2 in. above the antecubital space. The arm should be positioned so that the brachial artery is at the level of the heart; if below that level, the blood pressure will be artificially increased; if above that level, the blood pressure will be artificially decreased. These factors apply to any artery used.

Clients with a history of vascular disease or hypertension should also have initial blood pressure readings performed on both legs. Blood pressure in the legs is normally higher than in the arms. Lower blood pressure in the legs may indicate an abdominal aortic obstruction or coarctation of the aorta.

A large cuff is usually needed for leg blood pressures. The cuff is placed around the thigh, and the popliteal artery is auscultated. Leg pressures are best obtained with the client in the prone position.

Body position may have a significant effect on blood pressure in clients who take diuretics or who may have a fluid volume deficit. Standing up quickly from a supine position causes a drop in blood pressure. A slight drop in systolic pressure (less than 10 mm Hg) is normal. A drop in the diastolic pressure is abnormal.

Korotkoff sounds (ie, arterial vibrations) are indicators of blood pressure (Figure 23–1). As the blood pressure cuff is deflated, note (1) the onset of the first sound, (2) the muffling point of the sound, and (3) the disappearance of the sound. The onset of the first sound is the systolic pressure; the muffling point and the disappearance of sound have both been used as the diastolic pressure reading. In normal adults, the cessation of sound may best approximate the diastolic pressure. In hypertensive clients, there may be a silent interval between the systolic and diastolic pressure, known as the **auscultatory gap.** Noting the muffled sound may be more appropriate in these clients.

Most clinicians consider the systolic blood pressure elevated when the reading is greater than 140 mm Hg; diastolic blood pressure is elevated when the reading is

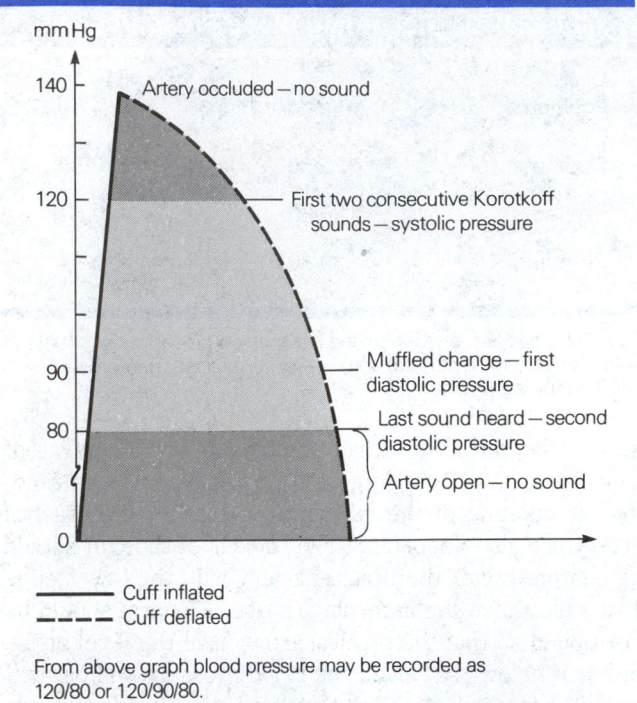

mm Hg

Artery occluded — no sound

First two consecutive Korotkoff sounds — systolic pressure

Muffled change — first diastolic pressure

Last sound heard — second diastolic pressure

Artery open — no sound

——— Cuff inflated
- - - - Cuff deflated

From above graph blood pressure may be recorded as 120/80 or 120/90/80.

Figure 23–1

Korotkoff sounds heard on auscultation of the blood pressure.

SOURCE: Saxton DF, et al.: *The Addison–Wesley Manual of Nursing Practice*. Menlo Park, CA: Addison–Wesley, 1983, p. 158.

greater than 90 mm Hg. Systolic hypertension is seen often in elderly clients, usually due to atherosclerosis. Increased cardiac output from conditions such as thyrotoxicosis, anemia, anxiety, and aortic regurgitation can also cause systolic hypertension. Diastolic hypertension is associated with essential hypertension, arteriosclerosis, and renal disease. Low blood pressure or hypotension may be seen in clients with MI, shock, or hypovolemia.

Pulse pressure, the difference between the systolic and diastolic pressures, is also an indicator of cardiovascular status. The normal pulse pressure is between 30 and 40 mm Hg. A value greater than this is referred to as a widened pulse pressure. A widened pulse pressure can occur in conditions such as hypertension, aortic regurgitation, and thyrotoxicosis. A pulse pressure less than 30 mm Hg is called a narrowed pulse pressure and may occur in shock, pericardial effusion, severe aortic stenosis, and constrictive pericarditis.

Venous pressure is estimated by inspecting the jugular vein and measuring the height of pulsation from the sternal angle. This technique is discussed in the section on examination of the heart.

Examination of the Heart

In addition to the basic cardiac assessment and evaluation of the neck veins discussed in Chapter 7, certain other factors need to be assessed. During inspection, observe the precordial pulsations in the following areas: sternoclavicular, aortic, pulmonic, right ventricular, apical, epigastric, and the ectopic area overlaying the wall of the left ventricle (Figure 7–26). Ventricular dysrhythmias, such as premature ventricular contractions (PVCs), may be seen as pulsations in the ectopic area.

After inspection, palpate the same precordial areas to confirm the previous observations. If there is a pulsation, evaluate its location, size (whether diffuse or discrete), timing, and duration in relation to the cardiac cycle. Note the presence of low-frequency, purring vibrations (referred to as **thrills**). Thrills are associated with valvular disease and can be felt especially with aortic stenosis. Note the timing of the thrill as systolic, diastolic, or both.

During auscultation, a normal physiological splitting of the first heart sound (S_1) and the second heart sound (S_2) may be heard. The normal splitting of S_1 is more difficult to hear, although it may be heard occasionally in the tricuspid area. An easily heard S_1 splitting is abnormal. Often the sound is actually a diastolic S_4 heart sound.

The S_2 is a physiological split sound because of the differences in the intracardiac pressures between the left heart and right heart. The split can be augmented by having the client breathe deeply. The normal physiologic split occurs only during inspiration; to hear it during expiration is abnormal. S_2 splitting that disappears with inspiration is referred to as paradoxical splitting, and the finding may signify heart disease. *Fixed splitting* (ie, wide splitting during both respiratory cycles) is often seen with atrial septal defects and right ventricular failure.

A high-pitched sound occurring after S_2, very early in diastole, is known as an opening snap. It is heard best at the apex with the client in the left lateral decubitus position. An opening snap is often associated with a stenotic mitral or tricuspid valve. Occasionally, an opening snap may be heard in clients with a high cardiac output, which causes a rapid, high-frequency sound.

Extra heart sounds heard during systole (ie, between S_1 and S_2) are referred to as clicks. Clicks are high pitched and may be heard at any auscultatory site. The sound may occur in early, middle, or late systole. Generally, there are two types of clicks: ejection and nonejection. The ejection click occurs in early systole as the blood rushes through the semilunar valves and into the aortic and pulmonic arteries. The sound is thought to be caused either by the bulging of a stenotic valve or the vibrations in a dilated vessel wall.

The nonejection click occurs in middle to late systole. It is high pitched and heard best in the mitral area. The sound is associated with prolapse of the mitral valve. All clicks are abnormal, but the severity varies with each client.

Clients with pericarditis may develop a friction rub. The sound usually occurs throughout the cardiac cycle but appears to have three components corresponding to atrial contraction, ventricular contraction, and ventricular filling. With inflammation, the friction rub is produced by the two layers of the pericardial sac rubbing against each other.

The sound is scratchy like sheets of sandpaper rubbing together or like new leather creaking. The rub is high pitched and heard best with the client leaning forward. The location is variable but often heard best at Erb's point or the third left intercostal space (LICS). Pericarditis is a frequent complication of myocardial infarction. A friction rub from the pericarditis may be detected. Pericardial infections also produce a rub.

Murmurs heard in midsystole or throughout systole are usually associated with valvular disease. Midsystolic ejection murmurs are caused by either aortic or pulmonary stenosis. Aortic stenosis is a common result of rheumatic fever or congenital disease. The sound is best heard in the aortic area, second RICS, with the client sitting upright. The murmur is high pitched and blowing and radiates to the neck and apex. Many older adults have calcification of the aortic valve, which often causes a murmur.

Pulmonary stenosis is less common than stenosis but, when present, may be associated with other congenital defects such as tetralogy of Fallot. In adults, the pulmonic systolic ejection murmur is usually due to pulmonary hypertension. This murmur is high pitched and harsh, is best heard at the second and third LICS, and radiates toward the left shoulder.

Murmurs heard throughout systole are referred to as holosystolic or pansystolic. These murmurs are associated with either mitral or tricuspid regurgitation or with a ventricular septal defect. Mitral regurgitation is the most common of these and can be caused by rheumatic heart disease, mitral valve prolapse, calcification, or left ventricular failure. Left ventricular failure is the most common cause. This murmur is loud, high pitched, and blowing; is heard best at the apex; and radiates to the left axilla.

Tricuspid regurgitation is most often due to right ventricular failure. Right ventricular failure may be secondary to pulmonary hypertension, left heart failure, mitral stenosis, or cor pulmonale. Rheumatic fever may have a direct effect on the tricuspid valve. The tricuspid regurgitant murmur is high pitched, is heard best at the lower left sternal border, and is associated with a parasternal lift.

Diastolic murmurs, although less common than systolic murmurs, are almost always associated with heart disease. Murmurs during diastole are caused either by mitral or tricuspid stenosis or by aortic or pulmonic regurgitation. Mitral stenosis and aortic regurgitation are the most common diastolic murmurs.

Mitral stenosis usually results from rheumatic fever, but calcification can also cause narrowing. The murmur occurs in middle to late diastole and has a characteristic "rumble" sound that is long and low pitched. It is best heard at the apex with the client in the left lateral decubitus position. There is little radiation of this murmur, unlike the murmur of mitral regurgitation. The murmur is also associated with an opening snap and a diastolic thrill in the mitral area. Chronic mitral stenosis usually causes left atrial enlargement and hypertrophy and subsequent right ventricular hypertrophy or failure.

Tricuspid stenosis is similar to mitral stenosis in both timing and quality and is usually a result of rheumatic fever. It is rare to have only tricuspid stenosis. This murmur is heard best at the lower left sternal border with the client in a recumbent position.

Aortic regurgitation is an early diastolic murmur. This murmur is high pitched and blowing and is heard best at the second RICS and at Erb's point with the client seated and leaning forward. Like other valvular disease, aortic regurgitation is most often a result of rheumatic fever. Other conditions such as endocarditis, hypertension, or arteriosclerosis may also cause this murmur, however.

Marked pulmonary hypertension may cause pulmonic valve regurgitation, another diastolic murmur. Best heard at the second and third LICS, it is medium to high pitched, rough, and brief.

Diagnostic Studies

The assessment of the client with suspected cardiovascular dysfunction requires the examination of the blood and urine for abnormalities. Tests are performed to establish a diagnosis (eg, MI), to obtain general screening information, to assess risk factors, or to detect concurrent disease. The most common tests are serum lipids, serum cardiac enzymes, serum glucose, coagulation studies, complete blood count, electrolytes, urinalysis, and arterial blood gases. Normal values and expected abnormal findings in cardiovascular disease are listed in Table 23–4.

Serum Lipids

The association between serum lipid levels (cholesterol, triglycerides, and lipoproteins) and CAD has been studied extensively. An elevated serum cholesterol level is directly related to the development of CAD: the higher the cholesterol level, the greater the risk. The inverse (ie, the lower the level, the lower the risk) is not true, however. Whether an elevated serum triglyceride level is a coronary risk factor is unclear. Some studies have documented an association between CAD and elevated triglyceride levels, but this association appears to be less predicative than the association of an elevated cholesterol level and CAD.

Cholesterol and triglyceride are bound to plasma proteins and transported in the blood as lipoproteins. The major lipoproteins are classified as chylomicrons, very low-density lipoproteins (VLDL), low-density lipoproteins (LDL), and high-density lipoproteins (HDL). The densities of lipoproteins vary according to the proportion of protein to fat and correspond to the protein portion of the lipoprotein (eg, HDL contains more protein than fat).

Each of the lipoproteins contains varying proportions of cholesterol, triglyceride, protein, and phospholipid. Chylomicrons and VLDL are composed primarily of triglyceride; LDL is predominantly cholesterol; an intermediate between VLDL and LDL called intermediate-density lipoprotein (IDL) contains a combination of triglycerides

Table 23-4 Laboratory Tests Common to the Cardiovascular System

Laboratory Test	Normal Expected Value	Disease State	Expected Abnormal Findings
Serum lipids			
Total lipids	400–800 mg/dL	Atherosclerosis	Increased
Cholesterol	144–275 mg/dL (range increases with age)	Atherosclerosis	Increased
Triglycerides	10–140 mg/dL (range increases with age)	Atherosclerosis	Increased
Serum cardiac enzymes			
Creatine kinase (CK) or creatine phosphokinase (CPK)	Women: 10–70 μ/mL Men: 25–90 μ/mL (varies by method)	Heart disorders: acute MI, cardiac surgery, acute myocarditis, heart transplant rejection	Increased
CK$_3$(MM)	90%–100% of total CK	Heart disorders above	Normal or increased
CK$_2$(MB)	0%–5% of total CK	Heart disorders above	Increased
CK$_1$(BB)	0%–3% of total CK	Heart disorders above	Normal
Lactic dehydrogenase (LDH)	80–120 Wacker μ (varies by method)	MI	Increased
LDH$_1$	16%–33% of total LDH	MI	Increased
LDH$_2$	28%–40% of total LDH	MI	Increased
LDH$_3$	16%–30% of total LDH	MI	Normal
LDH$_4$	5%–16% of total LDH	MI	Normal
LDH$_5$	2%–20% of total LDH	MI	Normal
		MI with liver congestion	Increased
Serum glucose	80–120 mg/dL	MI, coronary thrombosis	Mildly elevated
Partial thromboplastin time	40–100 s	Heparin therapy	1.5–2.6 times normal is the therapeutic range
Prothrombin time	11–15 s	Anticoagulant therapy (heparin or dicumarol)	2–2.5 times normal is the therapeutic range
		MI	Decreased
Complete blood count			
Hemoglobin	Men: 14–18 g/dL	Cardiac decompensation	Decreased
	Women: 12–16 g/dL	Excessive intravenous fluids	Decreased
Red blood cells	Men: 4.5–6.2 million/μL	Anoxia	Increased
	Women:	Cardiovascular disease	Increased
	4.0–5.5 million/μL	Excessive intravenous fluids	Decreased
White blood cells	4500–11,000 mL		
Neutrophils	54%–75%	Endocarditis	Increased
		MI	Increased
Lymphocytes	25%–40%	Heart failure	Decreased
Monocytes	2%–8%	Subacute bacterial endocarditis	Increased
Electrolytes			
Sodium	135–145 mEq/L	CHF (dilution hyponatremia)	Decreased
		Excessive intravenous water	Decreased
		Excessive intravenous sodium	Increased

Laboratory Test	Normal Expected Value	Disease State	Expected Abnormal Findings
Potassium	3.6–5.0 mEq/L	CHF Diuretic therapy	Decreased Decreased
Carbon dioxide	22–34 mEq/L (venous) 21–30 mEq/L (arterial)	Alkalosis (hypoventilation) Acidosis	Increased Decreased
Chloride	95–108 mEq/L	Cardiac conditions Diuretic therapy	Increased Decreased
Calcium	8.5–10.5 mg/dL or 4.3–5.3 mEq/L	Diuretic therapy	Increased
Phosphorus	3.0–4.5 mg/dL or 1.8–2.6 mEq/L	Heparin therapy Phenytoin therapy Adrenalin administration	Increased Increased Decreased
Magnesium	1.8–3.0 mg/dL or 1.5–2.5 mEq/L	Diuretic therapy	Elevated
Urinalysis			
Specific gravity	1.001–1.040	Heart failure	Increased
pH	4.6–8	Heart failure (hyperventilation)	Alkaline
Protein	10–20 mg/dL	Heart failure	Increased
Red blood cells	2–3 HPF	Subacute bacterial endocarditis Anticoagulant therapy	Increased Increased
Red blood cell casts	Few	Subacute bacterial endocarditis	Increased
Granular casts	None	CHF	Present
Arterial blood gases			
pH	7.35–7.45	Uncompensated CHF	Decreased or increased
PCO_2	35–45 mm Hg	Congenital CV defect Uncompensated CHF Cardiogenic shock Acute MI	Increased Increased Decreased Decreased
Bicarbonate (CO_2)	22–34 mEq/L (venous) 21–30 mEq/L (arterial)	Uncompensated CHF	Increased
PO_2	80–100 mm Hg	Congenital CV defect CHF, cardiogenic shock, MI	Decreased
O_2 saturation	95%–98%	Uncompensated CHF	Decreased

and cholesterol. HDL contains mostly protein but also has 20% cholesterol.

Elevated LDL levels are positively correlated with atherosclerosis. Therefore, clients with increased LDL are at risk for developing vascular disease. Elevated HDL is negatively correlated with atherosclerosis, however. In fact, studies demonstrate that elevated HDL levels appear to prevent plaque formation by converting cholesterol to a less active form. Elevated HDL levels may be a protective factor.

A total serum cholesterol level does not distinguish between LDL and HDL. Clients' health care management depends on this differential. A lipoprotein electrophoresis provides the information.

Cardiac Enzymes
Cardiac enzyme studies are performed primarily to document acute myocardial damage. The enzyme levels most commonly obtained are creatine kinase (CK), CK isoenzymes, lactic dehydrogenase (LDH), LDH isoenzymes, and (less commonly) serum glutamic-oxaloacetic transaminase (SGOT).

Enzymes are catalytic proteins that accelerate biochemical reactions within cells. Each organ or tissue of the body contains specific enzymes, often similar enzymes, but in varying concentrations. Under normal conditions, the intracellular concentration of enzymes is high, and the extracellular or serum concentration is low. Serum enzyme concentrations increase when cell damage occurs and the enzyme leaks into the blood. Thus, cardiac muscle damage can be detected by measuring serum levels of enzymes specific to the heart. The severity of the damage can be assessed by the amount and duration of the elevation.

Found in high concentrations in both skeletal and heart muscle, CK is the most useful enzyme in the early diagnosis of MI. When the myocardium is injured, the serum CK level rises 3 to 6 hours after the event, peaks at 24 hours, and usually returns to normal within 72 to 96 hours. The specificity of CK activity is increased with the identification of the three CK isoenzymes: CK-MM, CK-MB, and CK-BB. CK-MM predominates in skeletal muscle, with small amounts in cardiac muscle. CK-BB is found primarily in brain and nervous tissue. The CK-MB has the highest concentration in the cardiac muscle, making this isoenzyme specific to the heart. Elevation in CK-MB level is diagnostic of MI and appears within 4 to 6 hours after the onset of chest pain, peaks within 24 hours, and returns to normal within 48 to 72 hours. If the client is not hospitalized within 24 hours from the onset of chest pain, the rise and peak of CK-MB may not be detected. CK-MM also increases and persists for approximately 5 days. Serial documentation of CK and CK isoenzymes provides a continuous assessment of myocardial necrosis.

LDH is found in most tissues of the body. The highest concentrations are in the heart, liver, brain, skeletal muscle, kidneys, and red blood cells. The specificity of LDH is improved when the LDH isoenzymes (LDH_1 through LDH_5) are measured. LDH_1 and LDH_2 are found primarily in the heart, red blood cells, and brain. Normally, LDH_2 is proportionally higher than LDH_1 in the serum ($LDH_2 > LDH_1$), but after a myocardial infarction, the ratio is reversed, and LDH_1 is higher ($LDH_1 > LDH_2$). This "flipped ratio" increases specificity in diagnosing MIs.

The LDH level is usually elevated within 8 to 12 hours after myocardial infarction, peaks within 24 to 48 hours, and remains elevated for 10 to 14 days. Because the LDH level remains elevated much longer than CK, it provides a significant diagnostic benefit in documenting MIs more than 35 hours old.

SGOT, now called aspartate aminotransferase (AST), was one of the original enzymes used in documenting cardiac muscle, liver, pancreas, kidneys, brain, testes, and spleen. SGOT isoenzymes have not been identified, so SGOT activity remains relatively nonspecific for myocardial damage. It is rarely used.

Serum Glucose

Elevated serum glucose and persistently abnormal glucose tolerance tests are associated with increased risk of developing CAD. Although uncontrolled diabetes mellitus is recognized as a precursor of vascular disease, the physiologic mechanism remains unclear. Relations among hyperglycemia and hyperlipidemia, obesity, platelet aggregation, and coagulation abnormalities are being investigated. Also being studied is the effect of certain oral hypoglycemic agents and insulin regimens on the vascular changes in diabetes.

Transient hyperglycemia is found during periods of emotional and physiological stress. It is a common finding in clients with an MI.

Blood Coagulation Studies

The major purposes of blood coagulation studies are to monitor the effectiveness of anticoagulant therapy and to detect deficiencies in serum clotting factors. Anticoagulant therapy with heparin is evaluated by obtaining the partial thromboplastin time (PTT). The therapeutic range is 1.5 to 2.5 times the normal value of PTT. The prothrombin time (PT) is used to monitor the effectiveness of therapy with an oral anticoagulant such as warfarin sodium. The therapeutic PT range is 2 to 2.5 times the normal value. Oral anticoagulants take 3 to 5 days to reach therapeutic levels; therefore, heparin and warfarin sodium are given in combination until the PT is prolonged.

Anticoagulant therapy may be used in clients with acute MI complicated by CHF to prevent clot formation. Clients who receive prosthetic valves often require chronic warfarin therapy to prevent clot formation on the valve. Certain medications may interact with the anticoagulants and potentiate or lessen the effect. For example, quinidine, salicylates, and adrenocorticosteroids increase PT; antihistamines, barbiturates, and chloral hydrate decrease PT. Pharmacologic resources should be consulted, and a complete medication history should be obtained and reviewed when anticoagulant therapy is used.

Complete Blood Count

The complete blood count (CBC) includes the red blood cell count (RBC), corpuscular indices, white blood cell count (WBC), differential white cell count (Diff), hemoglobin (Hb), and hematocrit (Hct). The detection of anemia is important in clients with heart disease. Anemia, which decreases the oxygen-carrying ability of the blood, can aggravate CHF and precipitate chest pain. The anemia may also be secondary to hemolysis caused by a prosthetic heart valve. The WBC level is often elevated in clients with infections or injuries of the heart. The differential count, which includes neutrophil and lymphocyte counts, is also useful in assessing clients' cardiovascular condition: neutrophils increase with bacterial endocarditis and MI; lymphocytes decrease with heart failure.

Electrolytes

Cardiac function depends in part on the body's electrolyte balance. Myocardial muscle requires adequate stores of calcium to maintain the force of contraction; potassium is needed to facilitate the myocardial cell's response to stimuli. Cardiovascular clients' most common electrolyte abnormality is potassium imbalance. Depletion of potassium can result from vomiting, diarrhea, diuretics, cardiac bypass surgery, and renal disease. Hypokalemia predisposes the client to dysrhythmias, particularly premature ventricular contractions and ventricular fibrillation, and contributes to digitalis toxicity. A high serum potassium level is usually a result of renal failure but may be caused by excessive potassium intake. Hyperkalemia slows the heart rate and may result in asystole or ventricular fibrillation.

Clients with CHF or an acute MI are most susceptible to electrolyte imbalance. Depletion of sodium, potassium, magnesium, calcium, and phosphorus may occur. Clients often complain of weakness, fatigue, and occasionally, muscle cramps. Serum electrolyte levels and ECG changes should be routinely monitored.

Urinalysis

The retention of fluid by the kidneys is a compensatory response in acute heart failure and results in decreased output of urine, but that urine has a high specific gravity. Nocturia is a frequent symptom of clients with CHF, and the nighttime urinary volume is often twice the daytime volume. Red blood cells may be present in the urine when the client is receiving anticoagulant therapy. Urinary myoglobin is often present in clients with acute MI; however, it is not specific to the diagnosis.

Arterial Blood Gases

Arterial blood gas (ABG) values are usually monitored when the client is acutely ill. The acid–base balance (pH) and oxygenation (PO_2) are the parameters observed. Although ABGs are not performed routinely in cardiovascular assessment, they are useful for detecting the acid–base imbalances and hypoxemia often found in unstable cardiac clients. Uncompensated CHF may result in hypoxemia and either respiratory alkalosis or respiratory acidosis. Cardiogenic shock may cause hypoxemia and metabolic acidosis. Clients with acute MI tend to hyperventilate; hyperventilation can lead to respiratory alkalosis and hypoxemia. Large doses of morphine for MI pain may depress respirations and cause respiratory acidosis.

Chest X-ray

Significant information in the diagnosis of cardiac disease can be obtained through examination of the routine chest x-ray. The silhouette of the heart, cardiac chambers, and great vessels is observed, and the size and contour of the heart can be measured. Assessments are made by comparing the radiographic densities of the heart to those of surrounding structures such as the lungs. In addition to cardiac enlargement, calcifications in the coronary arteries and great vessels can be seen. Pulmonary involvement from CHF and other cardiac dysfunctions may be detected from x-ray examination. Pulmonary venous congestion and dilation of the pulmonary veins and artery may be observed.

A specific procedure called a cardiac series enhances the routine chest x-ray. The contrast in the x-ray film is increased by administering barium to the client. The esophagus is filled with barium, which makes it more opaque. Chamber enlargement or aortic dilation can be detected by noting the displacement of the esophagus.

Electrocardiogram

The ECG graphically represents the electrical activity of the heart. Cellular activity of the cardiac muscle generates electrical impulses that flow through the heart, causing cardiac contraction and relaxation. The flow of electrical impulses that leads to contraction is called *depolarization*. Electrical recovery of the heart muscle is referred to as *repolarization*. This electrical activity of the heart muscle can be measured by a system of electrodes placed at specific points on the body surface. Only electrical activity generated by the atria and ventricles can be recorded by the body-surface ECG. The specialized conducting tissues within the heart do not provide enough voltage to be detected by the body-surface electrodes.

The ECG displays the electrical activity as waveforms, which are arbitrarily named (Figure 23–2). As the electrical impulses travel through the atria, depolarization of the atria occurs. The ECG displays this activity as a *P wave*. The impulses continue through the heart to the ventricles. Ventricular depolarization is represented by a three-wave complex called a *QRS complex*. Since there are more muscle cells in the ventricles, the electrical recovery of the ventricles can be measured. A *T wave* is inscribed, representing ventricular repolarization.

For the standard ECG, electrodes are placed on each limb and on six sites across the precordium. The basic 12-lead ECG system is divided into bipolar leads, which have a positive ($+$) and negative ($-$) pole, and unipolar leads, which have only a positive pole. Waves are inscribed on the graph with a positive (upward) deflection when the direction of depolarization is moving toward the positive pole and a negative (downward) deflection when depolarization is receding. The wave of depolarization in a normal heart flows from the base to the apex, slightly right, then left. Positive electrodes placed inferiorly to the apex and across the left precordium generally record positive deflections.

Three categories of leads compose the 12-lead ECG: the bipolar limb leads, lead I, II, and III; the unipolar augmented limb leads, aV_R, aV_L, and aV_F; and the unipolar precordial leads V_1 to V_6. Each lead or combination of electrodes records the electrical activity of the entire cardiac cycle from slightly different perspectives. The bipolar limb leads and the unipolar augmented limb leads measure the electrical potentials in the frontal plane (ie, the direction of the electrical impulse, right and left, superior and inferior). The precordial leads measure the electrical potentials in the horizontal plane: right and left, anterior and posterior.

The bipolar limb leads, leads I, II, III, measure the difference in electrical activity between two selected limbs:

Lead I = difference between the left arm (LA) and the right arm (RA)

Lead II = difference between the left leg (LL) and the right arm (RA)

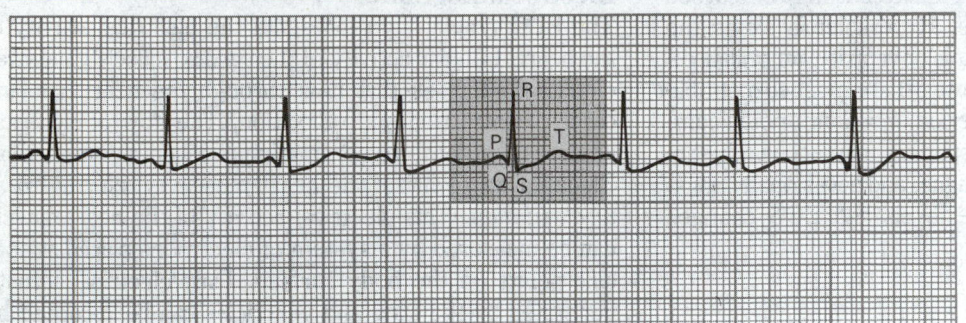

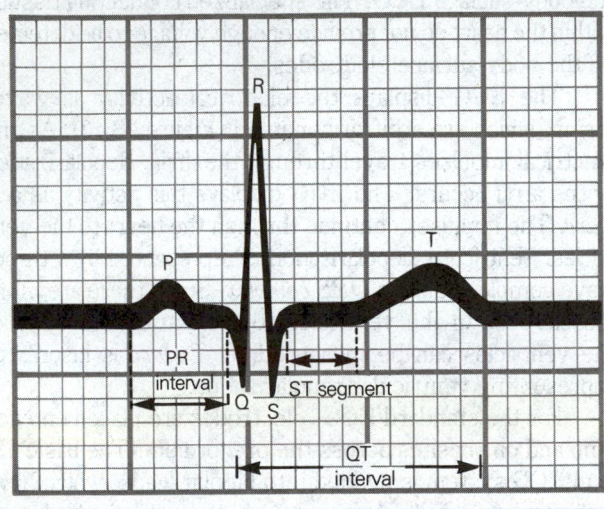

Figure 23–2

The normal electrocardiogram. **A.** Regular sinus rhythm. **B.** Detail of ECG. SOURCE: Saxton DF, et al.: *The Addison–Wesley Manual of Nursing Practice.* Menlo Park, CA: Addison–Wesley, 1983, p. 164.

P wave	= 0.04–0.08 sec
PR interval	= 0.12–0.20 sec
QRS complex	= 0.04–0.08 sec

Time: small squares	= 0.04 sec
1 large square	= 0.20 sec
5 large squares	= 1.00 sec

Lead III = difference between the left arm (LA) and the left leg (LL)

The unipolar augmented limb leads, aV_R, aV_L, aV_F are measurements of the electrical potential of each limb rather than the difference between two limbs. The height of the waveforms produced by these leads is small and therefore requires augmentation for easier reading. The ECG machine automatically augments the waves by increasing the size by 50%. The sites of the three augmented limb leads are:

aV_R = right arm

aV_L = left arm

aV_F = left leg (foot)

The precordial leads, V_1 to V_6, are unipolar leads that record the electrical potential of each site in the horizontal plane. Six sequential positions across the anterior chest are used (Figure 23–3):

V_1 = fourth intercostal space at the right sternal border

V_2 = fourth intercostal space at the left sternal border

V_3 = midway between V_2 and V_4

V_4 = fifth intercostal space at the midclavicular line

V_5 = fifth intercostal space at the anterior axillary line

V_6 = fifth intercostal space at the midaxillary line

The ECG recording is a valuable aid in cardiovascular assessment. Not only does it illustrate the rate and rhythm of the heart and conduction through the heart; it also indicates enlargement of the atrial and ventricular chambers,

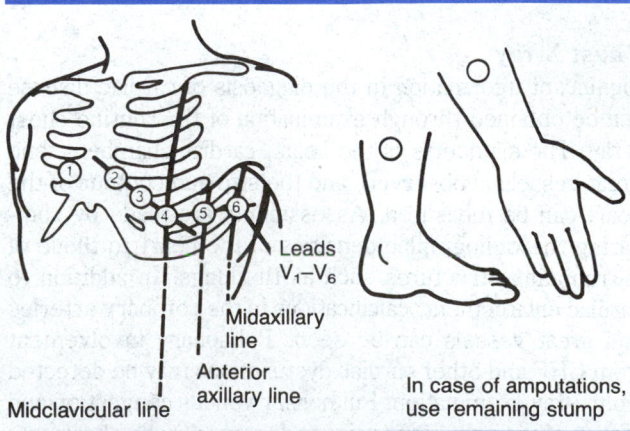

Figure 23–3

Standard 12-lead ECG electrode positions. **Left.** Unipolar chest leads. **Right.** Bipolar limb leads. SOURCE: *Operation and Self-Training Guide for the ECG Technician,* HP 4700A Cardiograph, 1981, p. 71. Hewlett-Packard Medical Products Group.

inflammation of the pericardium, or damage to the myocardium. Any influence on the heart's ability to contract and relax can be documented by the ECG. In a normal physical exam, the 12-lead ECG reading is obtained for baseline information. To monitor effectiveness of cardiac drugs, serial ECGs may be performed.

The standard 12-lead ECG provides only a 1-minute recording of the heart's rhythm; irregularities of the cardiac cycle that require longer recordings may not be detected. A rhythm strip, a recording of one to three selected leads, may be obtained for a longer recording.

A major limitation is that a normal ECG may be recorded even with significant CAD. The ECG can be combined with other tests such as Holter monitoring (see next section) to increase the diagnostic ability. In any clinical setting, ECG interpretations should be made in conjunction with the client's history and physical exam.

Nursing Implications. The ECG is a noninvasive test that can be performed by a trained individual in any clinical setting. The nurse should prepare clients for the test by informing them about the purpose, procedure to be used, and the risks involved. Explain to clients that the ECG provides a graphic description of the heart rhythm, which yields information about their cardiac status and such matters as the effectiveness of their heart medicine.

The ECG is performed with the client in a supine position; the client's chest is exposed for placement of electrodes. If hair is present, the electrode sites may need to be shaved. A conducting medium (creme, gel, or saline pads) is applied to the electrode sites if suction cups or metal plates are used. Adhesive electrodes are prepackaged with conducting gel. Ten electrodes are applied to the standard sites and attached to lead wires that connect to the ECG machine (Figure 23–4). A 12-lead ECG reading is obtained by selecting the indicators on the machine. The ECG is completed in less than a minute.

The client does not need to follow prior dietary restrictions, but occasionally certain medications are discontinued before testing. The client's watch may need to be removed if electrical interference is noted.

The risks are minimal: possible ecchymoses from the suction cups and a rare electrical hazard if proper electrical safety precautions are not followed. A written consent is not necessary, but the client should give verbal consent.

Ambulatory Electrocardiography (Holter Monitoring)

A client's heart rhythm during daily activities can be evaluated by applying a portable ECG recorder that the client wears for a specific length of time, usually 24 hours. The ECG is recorded onto a tape, and the client documents in a diary daily activities as well as any symptoms occurring with the activity. After completion of the test period, the

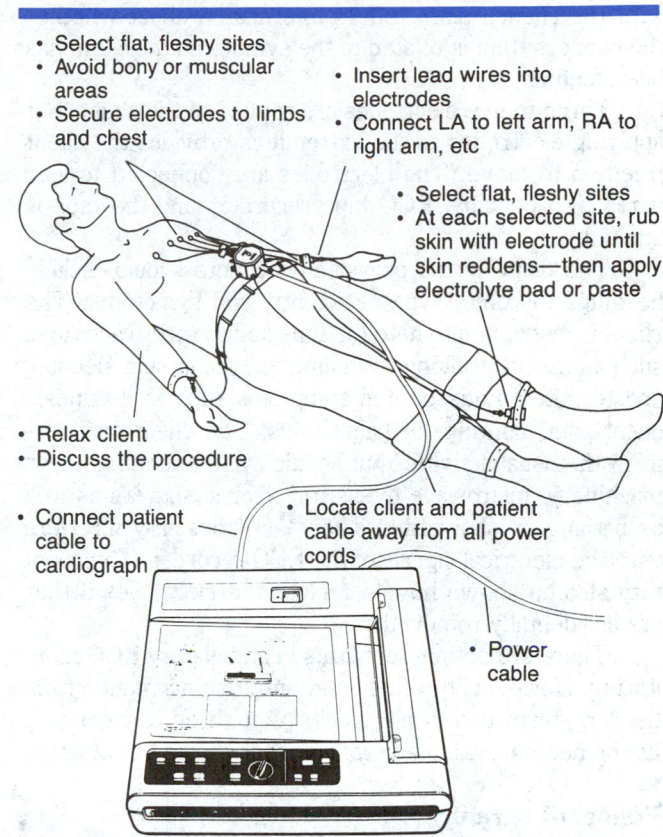

- Select flat, fleshy sites
- Avoid bony or muscular areas
- Secure electrodes to limbs and chest

- Insert lead wires into electrodes
- Connect LA to left arm, RA to right arm, etc

- Select flat, fleshy sites
- At each selected site, rub skin with electrode until skin reddens—then apply electrolyte pad or paste

- Relax client
- Discuss the procedure

- Connect patient cable to cardiograph

- Locate client and patient cable away from all power cords

- Power cable

Figure 23–4

Attaching the client to a 12-lead ECG.
SOURCE: *Operation and Self-Training Guide for the ECG Technician,* HP 4700A Cardiograph, 1981, p. 67. Hewlett-Packard Medical Products Group.

tape is translated into a standard graphic ECG reading by an electrocardioscanner. The ECG is reviewed, and the client's documentation is correlated with the interpretation. This technique of ambulatory ECG recording is often referred to as Holter monitoring.

Ambulatory ECG monitoring is used most often with clients whose symptoms may include episodes of dizziness, chest pain, fainting, or palpitations. This long-term monitoring permits a better correlation between the client's subjective information and objective findings. Clients who have had open heart surgery or an MI can be monitored for 24 hours prior to discharge to detect latent dysrhythmias or abnormal hemodynamic responses. The effects of therapy (drug, exercise, or diet) can also be evaluated with this test.

Nursing Implications. Ambulatory monitoring is a noninvasive test similar to the standard ECG. The nurse should provide instructions to the client regarding the client's involvement in the procedure: the Holter monitor provides a recording of the heart rhythm for 24 hours, which, along with the client's diary, offers information about whether the heart rhythm is related to the symptoms the client has been feeling.

Three to five electrodes are applied to the chest. Not applying electrodes to the extremities provides the client freedom to move. The electrodes are connected to lead wires of a portable ECG tape recorder, and the tape is started.

The diary forms provided to clients should include headings for time, type of activity, and symptoms. The client is instructed to note the time and to record activities such as eating, walking, watching television, and sleeping and to note any associated symptoms such as dizziness, chest pain, fainting, or palpitations. The client may perform the usual activities but should avoid operating heavy machinery, microwave ovens, or electric shavers as well as bathing or showering. These activities may interfere with the electrical signals of the ECG recorder. The client may also be shown how to replace the electrodes if they are accidentally removed.

There are no inherent risks in ambulatory ECG monitoring. However, the client may suffer skin irritation from the long-term use of electrodes. A written consent may not be necessary, but a verbal consent should be obtained.

Echocardiography

The motion and dimensions of the cardiac structures can be measured by using high-frequency sound waves (ultrasound) and graphically recording the reflected sound (echo). This technique is called echocardiography. A sound-emitting transducer is applied to the client's chest and focused at the heart. As the sound transects the various structures, echoes are produced and recorded. There are two methods for obtaining information: the M-mode and the two-dimensional (2-D) mode.

The M-mode, the original technique, uses a narrow beam of sound and is described as giving an ice-pick view of the heart. The 2-D mode, also referred to as the cross-sectional mode, transmits a wider sound beam. Thus, the images produced by the 2-D have both motion and shape, whereas the M-mode images have only motion. The images, along with those of the ECG, are usually videotaped. The tape can be reviewed, and cardiac measurements that require comparison of several images can be obtained. Chamber size, ejection fraction, and flow gradient across the valves are some routine measurements. **Ejection fraction,** a measure of left ventricular wall function and contractility, is the percentage of left ventricular end-diastolic volume that is pumped.

Echocardiography, frequently used in clinical cardiology, is a valuable tool in documenting valvular and congenital heart disease. In addition, the recording of cardiac movement permits objective assessment of cardiomyopathy, pericardial effusion, and ventricular aneurysm.

Nursing Implications. Echocardiography is a noninvasive test that can be performed in any clinical setting that has an ultrasound machine. The nurse should explain to the client that the echocardiogram will provide a recording of the movement of the heart valves and ventricular walls, which can be used to measure the functional ability of the heart valves and the heart as a pump.

The client is placed in the recumbent position. A transducer, lubricated with a gel to facilitate movement and conduction, is applied to the client's anterior chest. As the transducer moves over the chest, images of the cardiac structures in motion are viewed. The images and the ECG are recorded. The client can expect the procedure to take about an hour.

Ultrasonography is a relatively new technology and, at this time, there are no proven risks. A verbal consent should be obtained; a written consent is not necessary. Echocardiography has some limitations: the procedure for obtaining good images is difficult, and clients who have a large, thick chest and those with a small heart are especially problematic. The procedure is also time consuming.

Exercise Testing (Stress Test)

In the exercise test, the ECG is recorded during prescribed exercise. A motorized treadmill or a bicycle ergometer provides the method of exercise, and the work load is gradually increased to a prescribed level of stress. The objective of the test is to document the level of stress necessary to produce symptoms or signs. During the exercise, the ECG is monitored for changes: ST-segment depression, ventricular dysrhythmias, conduction defects, or severe heart-rate changes. Alterations in blood pressure are also monitored. The client is observed for symptoms of fatigue, chest pain, or shortness of breath.

The exercise test is noninvasive and is used primarily in the prognosis and diagnosis of CAD. The results of the test are best used in documentation of risk factors rather than as a statement of whether disease is present. General indications for exercise testing include evaluation of dysrhythmias provoked by exercise; differentiation in the diagnosis of chest pain; identification of probable causes of nontypical angina; assessment of functional physical capacity and exercise levels in cardiac rehabilitation; and evaluation of therapeutic interventions such as drug, exercise, or surgery.

Unlike the resting 12-lead ECG and the Holter monitor, the exercise test has several contraindications: any unstable cardiac condition such as unstable angina, uncontrolled dysrhythmias, acute MI, uncompensated CHF, or severe hypertension. In general, the test is contraindicated for any client who has a condition that could be aggravated by vigorous exercise. The client must be interviewed and examined thoroughly before testing.

Limitations are to be considered when using an exercise test. The correlations between positive (abnormal) exercise tests and the presence of CAD have been poor. There is a high degree of false-positive and false-negative results in the diagnosis of ischemic heart disease. Clients with significant CAD may have a negative test, but clients with no CAD may have a positive test. When the exercise test is performed in conjunction with myocardial perfusion studies, the correlation with CAD increases.

Nursing Implications. Exercise testing is noninvasive, but because risks are associated with exercising until cardiovascular symptoms appear, the client should be thoroughly informed and a written consent obtained. The exercise test is performed with a cardiologist or physician present. Safety of the procedure depends primarily on adherence to the contraindications, termination of the exercise when the client exhibits untoward symptoms and signs, and availability of personnel and equipment to manage complications.

The client's understanding of the procedure and the importance of cooperation during the test are essential to successful exercise testing. To be adequately prepared, the client should know the purpose, the procedure, and the risks involved. The purpose of the test is to evaluate the effect of activity on the heart as exercise on a moving treadmill is performed. Heart rhythm, blood pressure, and the client's symptoms and signs are continuously monitored.

The client should either fast overnight or have only a light meal no later than 2 hours before testing. Certain cardiac medications may be discontinued before testing (eg, digitalis or propranolol). The exercise test is performed on a motorized treadmill or bicycle ergometer. The client should wear loose-fitting clothes and supportive shoes. A cardiovascular history and physical exam are obtained along with a resting 12-lead ECG which is examined by the physician for any abnormalities (eg, evidence of ischemia or serious dysrhythmia) that would preclude exercise testing. Several protocols for exercise testing have been developed and, depending on client characteristics and physician preference, one protocol is chosen. The Bruce protocol for the treadmill, the most common, consists of several stages of increasing speed and slope, with each stage lasting 3 minutes. With the Bruce test, the maximum speed is 6 mph with an elevation of 22%.

After the client is instructed to report any untoward symptoms and shown how to walk on the treadmill, the exercise test is started. The client exercises until one of the following occurs: a predetermined heart rate is reached and maintained; symptoms such as fatigue, chest pain, or dysrhythmias appear; or significant ST-segment depression occurs.

In the postexercise period, the ECG and blood pressure continue to be monitored until the client is completely recovered. The test is usually completed in approximately 20 minutes.

The risk of an exercise test is small if contraindications and safety precautions are understood. A client with preexisting cardiovascular disease has the highest risk.

Phonocardiography
Phonocardiography, the graphic recording of heart sounds heard during auscultation, is an extension of the physical exam. The heart sounds are translated into electrical impulses, amplified, and recorded by a microphone. Each component of the heart sound and murmurs can be documented. External pulse recordings of either the carotid artery, jugular vein, or apical pulse are taken at the same time as the ECG, which provides a timing reference for the heart sound.

The client is placed in the normal auscultatory positions. A pressure-sensitive transducer is applied to the selected pulse, and the ECG reading is usually obtained through the standard limb leads. A special microphone, used in the same manner as a stethoscope, is applied to the various auscultatory points. A phonocardiography machine connects the three extensions and graphically records simultaneously the pulse wave, ECG, and heart sounds.

The phonocardiogram is most useful in documenting heart sounds and murmurs that are almost inaudible with the ordinary stethoscope. The phonocardiogram's multiple-sound recordings, correlated with the ECG-timed pulse measurements, facilitate interpretation of the sounds.

Often, phonocardiography is also helpful in teaching auscultation of heart sounds to students. Even though the test is an extension of auscultation, the client should be informed of the procedure's purpose and risk, which are the same as an ECG. Of course, if students are observing, the client's permission should be obtained.

Cardiac Fluoroscopy
The movements of cardiac structures, the lungs, and coronary vessels may be viewed by fluoroscopy, permitting assessment of the degree of dysfunction of calcified heart valves and coronary vessels. In the past, the radiation exposure from this procedure was high, but now, with the use of image intensifiers and computers, the hazard is greatly reduced. The quality of the images has also improved.

Cardiac fluoroscopy is of less diagnostic value than the more sophisticated procedures now available, but it carries fewer risks and therefore may be used as a screening tool. Fluoroscopy is still used for guiding the placement and positioning of temporary pacemakers and intracardiac catheters.

Nursing Implications. Although the roentgenographic procedures are essentially noninvasive, the client should be informed about the radiation exposure. No prior preparation is necessary unless barium is used. Roentgenographic procedures should be avoided during pregnancy.

Nuclear Cardiology
Using radioactive tracer substances, cardiovascular abnormalities can be viewed, recorded, and evaluated. The use of radionuclide techniques in cardiovascular assessment is called nuclear cardiology. Radionuclides are unstable isotopes which, as they decay to a stable form, emit energy as gamma rays. The gamma rays are detected by a scintillation camera and converted to electrical impulses, which are then displayed and recorded.

The radionuclide techniques facilitate the evaluation of CAD, MI, ventricular wall function, valvular disease, and intracardiac shunts. The most commonly used radionuclides in nuclear cardiology are thallium (^{201}Tl), technetium pyrophosphate (^{99m}Tc-PYP), and ^{99m}Tc-labelled red blood cells. Each of the radionuclides has different individual properties that contribute to the cardiovascular assessment. In general, two kinds of studies are performed in nuclear cardiology: the myocardial perfusion/imaging study and the cardiac function/performance study.

A myocardial perfusion study assesses the blood supply in the various regions of the myocardium. Thus, this study shows the effect of CAD on myocardial perfusion. The most commonly used radionuclide in perfusion studies is ^{201}Tl, a potassium analogue. Like potassium, thallium readily diffuses across the cell membrane and accumulates in myocardial cells. Thallium uptake depends on coronary blood flow and ability of the myocardial cell membrane to extract the thallium from the blood. In CAD or coronary spasm where the coronary blood flow is decreased, the quantity of thallium reaching the myocardium is reduced, and the uptake of thallium within the cells is low. If myocardial cell membranes are destroyed or nonfunctional, as in an MI, the thallium is not extracted from the blood into the cell; hence, there is no thallium uptake.

The assessment of CAD has been greatly enhanced by combining exercise stress testing and thallium scintigraphy. Thallium is given intravenously during peak exercise, and the scan is performed immediately after the exercise test. This method permits detection of regions that may be perfused normally at rest but have reduced blood flow during exercise. A follow-up scan, about 2 hours after the first scan, is performed to assess the redistribution of blood into the regions that were previously underperfused. Redistribution indicates that the myocardium is viable.

Thallium scintigraphy is also used to evaluate the effect of pharmacological agents on coronary blood flow. Perfusion studies performed before or after coronary artery bypass assess the ability of the grafts to increase coronary blood flow. Thallium may be used to detect acute MI, but the scan, to be sensitive, should be performed within 6 to 8 hours after the onset of symptoms. Collateral blood flow interferes with the interpretation.

Technetium pyrophosphate (^{99m}Tc-PYP), which concentrates in zones of necrosis, is used in imaging MIs. The mechanism of the uptake, although not yet clear, appears to be related to the calcium deposits in the infarct zones. Apparently, calcification may facilitate the extraction and concentration of pyrophosphate.

Although pyrophosphate detects necrosis, the uptake still depends on coronary blood flow. The infarct zone must have 30% to 40% of normal blood flow for the radionuclide to reach the region. Abnormal scintigrams appear 10 to 12 hours after infarction. Any heart condition that results in myocardial cell damage (eg, cardiac tumors, viral myocarditis, or cardiomyopathy) may be assessed with ^{99m}Tc-PYP.

Ventricular function measurements including ejection fraction and cardiac output can be obtained through radionuclide angiography. The radionuclide used is sodium pertechnetate ^{99m}Tc, which attaches to red blood cells. Red blood cells labeled with ^{99m}Tc are large bodies that remain within the vascular system and thus provide for visualization of the vessels and cardiac chambers. Information from these studies is essentially the same as from contrast studies. However, radionuclide angiography is less invasive, requires less time, permits repeated studies, and has fewer inherent risks. Also, both right and left ventricular performance can be assessed at the same time.

Two techniques are used in radionuclide angiography: *first pass* and *gated blood pool studies*. In first-pass angiography, the initial passage of the injected radionuclide is followed through the circulation with the scintillation camera, and images of the vessels, chambers, and volume waves are viewed. The study is completed within 30 seconds. The images are processed further by a computer, and a series of pictures is produced. The presence of intracardiac shunts is determined, the ventricular ejection fraction and chamber volumes are calculated. In clinical situations in which contrast studies are contraindicated, radionuclide angiography could be performed.

In gated blood pool studies, the radionuclide is injected and allowed to mix until an equilibrium of distribution is achieved. The ECG or echocardiogram is used to time the cardiac cycle. By using the ECG as a physiologic signal, images are recorded during selective portions of the cardiac cycle. Dividing the cardiac cycle into time periods and recording measurements during these sequences is referred to as gating. Images are obtained at contraction (end-systole) and relaxation (end-diastole). With gated blood pool studies, measurements of ventricular ejection fraction, ventricular volumes, and ventricular wall motion may be obtained. The study can be performed at rest and during exercise.

Nursing Implications. Radioisotope cardiovascular assessment is relatively noninvasive; the radiation exposure and risks are minimal. Because a radioisotope is used, there is no chemical toxicity. The studies do not require hospitalization or prior preparation. Nevertheless, the client should be given information regarding the purpose of the study, and the procedure should be fully explained. The radioisotope is injected intravenously and the client is asked to lie still during the test. A written consent is obtained.

Cardiac Catheterization. The most invasive but the most definitive test in the diagnosis of cardiac disease is cardiac catheterization. A catheter is passed into the right or left side of the heart to obtain information on cardiac pressures, cardiac output, oxygenation, and competency of intracardiac structures. When contrast dye is used to view the cardiac structures, the procedure is referred to as angiography. Most cardiac catheterizations are combined with angiography.

Right-heart catheterization is performed by inserting

a catheter through either the basilic vein, superior vena cava, femoral vein, or inferior vena cava. With continuous cardiac pressure monitoring and fluoroscopy, the catheter is advanced into the right side of the heart. Intracardiac pressures (right atrial, right ventricular, pulmonary artery, and pulmonary wedge pressures) are obtained. Blood samples are also withdrawn. Contrast dye is usually injected to detect any regurgitation from the pulmonic or tricuspid valves or to detect cardiac shunts.

The left-heart catheterization procedure is more invasive. The heart is approached either by passing the catheter from the right heart through the atrial septum, using a special needle to puncture the septum, or by retrograde insertion, which is performed by advancing the catheter from the brachial or femoral artery up the aorta, across the aortic valve, and into the left ventricle. This approach is used when coronary artery angiography will be performed during the study. As with right-heart catheterization, pressure readings and blood samples are obtained. Pressures in the left atrium, left ventricle, and aorta and mitral and aortic valve status are evaluated. In addition, a ventriculogram (contrast dye injected into the ventricle) is performed, and calculations are made of end-systolic volume, end-diastolic volume, stroke volume, and ejection fraction.

For coronary arteriography, the catheter is advanced into the aortic arch and positioned selectively into the right and left coronary arteries. Contrast dye is injected, and cineangiographic films are taken. Observing the flow of the dye through the coronaries provides information about the site and severity of coronary lesions. Drugs such as ergonovine and nitroglycerin may be administered during the study to evaluate the cardiovascular response.

With the more sophisticated noninvasive tests available, the need for cardiac catheterization has decreased slightly. Nevertheless, when either valvular or vascular cardiac surgery is indicated, a cardiac catheterization is performed to confirm the diagnosis and to evaluate the surgical approach.

There are no absolute contraindications to cardiac catheterization. However, the client must be physically able to tolerate the procedure and subsequent cardiac surgery if necessary. Evidence of acute MI, uncompensated CHF, or severe dysrhythmias may be contraindications. The risks and the benefits are evaluated before the procedure is performed.

Nursing Implications. Because cardiac catheterization is an invasive test, it is often frightening to the client. The client's psychosocial readiness should be assessed. Often the client knows someone who has had the procedure or heard stories of the procedure. The accuracy of the client's knowledge is important. Nursing assessment and teaching are essential for the client to have a positive experience.

The purpose of the procedure should be explained to the client. Explain that the information obtained by this procedure will facilitate the client's treatment, and only a cardiac catheterization can provide this information. The client is admitted to the hospital for the procedure, and the length of hospitalization varies depending on the outcome. Standard preoperative tests are usually performed: chest x-ray, ECG, CBC, and urinalysis. The client receives nothing by mouth after midnight or has only a liquid breakfast if the cardiac catheterization is scheduled for the afternoon. A mild sedative is usually given before the test. Nursing assessment includes the client's vital signs, evaluation of peripheral pulses, and auscultation of heart and lung sounds. The site of catheter insertion is prepared, the area is shaved if necessary, and usually a hexachlorophene scrub is done.

The client should be told how long the procedure usually takes, who will be present while it is going on, and what kind of physical environment it is done in. The client will be kept in a supine position, which may become uncomfortable. The injection of the dye often causes a warm feeling throughout the body—often compared to "hot flashes"—that the client may find disagreeable.

Postcatheterization care involves monitoring vital signs q. 15 min. ×4; then q. 30 min. ×2 or until stable; then q. 4 h. Peripheral pulses and possible bleeding at catheter insertion sites should be assessed with the vital signs. An intravenous line for medication and fluid replacement is usually required. The client is kept on bed rest 8 to 12 hours following the procedure.

The risks of cardiac catheterization, which are usually explained by the cardiologist, vary according to the client's physical status and the procedures to be performed. Coronary arteriography, the most hazardous, may involve risk of death. Other risks include MI, cerebrovascular accident, arterial bleeding, arterial thromboembolism, and development of lethal dysrhythmias. Intracardiac trauma from the catheter may also occur. Right-heart catheterization has the least risk. A written informed consent from the client is necessary.

Digital Subtraction Angiography

Digital subtraction angiography (DSA) is a new approach to the traditional angiograms. Instead of injecting contrast dye directly into an artery, dye is injected into the venous system via the superior vena cava so it circulates through the heart and into the arterial system. A fluoroscopic image-intensifier displays the vessels and focuses (intensifies) the image. A computer then converts images into numbers. The first image obtained before the injection of the contrast dye is subtracted from the postinjection images. The image obtained from the computer subtraction is an enhanced image of the arterial system. Several vessels rather than one vessel can be evaluated with one injection of contrast dye.

This technique has many advantages. It is less invasive than the conventional angiograms and requires less contrast dye, less time, and less radiation exposure, yet it provides better images. It requires no hospitalization and can be performed on high-risk clients.

Hemodynamic Monitoring

Intracardiac pressures can be measured and monitored continuously at the bedside in many critical care units. A balloon-tipped, flow-directed catheter is inserted percutaneously or by a venous cutdown into a large vein such as the internal jugular, subclavian, femoral, or brachial veins. The catheter (the Swan–Ganz catheter is the most common) is slowly advanced toward the right atrium; when it enters the right atrium, the balloon is inflated. Then the flow of blood carries the catheter through the tricuspid valve, the right ventricle, and the pulmonary valve into the pulmonary artery. The balloon finally wedges into a branch of the pulmonary artery. A pressure reading, the *pulmonary artery wedge pressure* (PAWP), is obtained, and the balloon is quickly deflated. The catheter floats back into the pulmonary artery and remains in this position for continuous monitoring. The pressures routinely monitored are the pulmonary artery systolic pressure (PASP) and diastolic pressure (PADP), PAWP, and the cardiac output. The PASP represents the pressure generated by the contraction of the right ventricle, whereas the PADP represents the filling pressure of the right ventricle. These pressures are monitored to assess right-sided heart function and pulmonary resistance. In the absence of lung dysfunction and mitral valve stenosis, the PAWP reflects left atrial pressure and left ventricular end-diastolic filling pressure. Thus, the function of the left heart can be assessed.

Catheters with a special temperature-sensing device, a thermistor, can be used to measure cardiac output by the thermodilution technique. A bolus of a solution with a known temperature is injected into the proximal port of the catheter, and the thermistor at the distal end measures the temperature change of the diluted solution. A bedside cardiac output computer connected to the catheter records the data, calculates the temperature curve, and displays the cardiac output.

These intracardiac pressure readings are valuable aids in the assessment of the critically ill client. Serial readings assist in evaluating the effectiveness of the therapeutic plan.

Nursing Implications. As an invasive procedure, hemodynamic monitoring carries several risks. The catheter site, and subsequently the blood, may become infected. Endocarditis may occur but can be prevented by using sterile technique and observing the client for early signs of infection. Other serious complications include thromboembolism from blood clotting to the catheter; air embolism from balloon rupture, faulty line connections, or improper procedure; ventricular dysrhythmias due to ventricular irritation from the tip of the catheter floating back into the right ventricle; and pulmonary artery rupture from

Nursing Research Note

Patacky M, Garvin BJ, Schwirian P: Intra-aortic balloon pumping and stress in coronary care units. *Heart Lung* 1985; 14(2):142–148.

The intra-aortic balloon pump (IABP) is a cardiac assisting device that increases myocardial oxygenation, diminishing left ventricular workload and increasing cardiac output. The relation between clients' perceptions of psychological stress and the use of the IABP in the coronary care unit (CCU) was the focus of this study. Stress levels were compared for clients on the pump, clients not on the pump but in the CCU when it was used, and clients not in the same environment when the pump was used and not requiring the pump themselves.

The sample consisted of 27 subjects in the CCU of a teaching hospital. The subjects were subdivided into three groups: the IABP group consisted of 7 subjects who were on the pump; 10 subjects who were in the CCU when the pump was used made up the second group. The third group consisted of 10 subjects admitted to the CCU when the IABP was not used. Stress was measured with the coronary care stress measurement tool, and data were collected in structured interviews.

Stress levels for clients on the IABP were significantly higher than those for clients not on the pump but in the CCU. There was no significant difference between stress levels of clients on the pump and clients without the IABP who were present or between the groups who were not on the pump. Overall, being admitted to the CCU was the most stressful situation. The next most stressful situations were not knowing about or understanding the illness and its seriousness and the inability to move freely in bed because of equipment.

According to this study, admission to the CCU is the greatest stressor for all clients. Nurses must realize that stress and anxiety reduce the ability to comprehend and retain information; therefore, information must be repeated frequently to client and family. Because immobility provokes anxiety, nurses must reassure clients that it is temporary and necessary. Communication is essential. Encouraging the client to vent feelings may help reduce stress. Providing information to clients regarding health status and why certain therapies are necessary may alleviate the fear of the unknown and uncertainty about health status. Intensive care nursing is challenging, and client problems are unique. Nurses must be sensitive to the stressors of intensive care units and offer creative alternatives for stress reduction.

overdistention of the balloon or from the tip of the catheter piercing through the artery.

The client needs to be prepared for the procedure and the continuous presence of the catheter, intravenous line, and monitors. Explain that the situation is temporary and the information obtained will assist in the overall treatment plan. The family should also be informed. A written consent is necessary, but often, because the situation is critical and the client barely conscious, obtaining a written consent from the client may not be feasible. In this situation, the family may give a written consent.

Section II: Nursing Diagnosis

The client with a cardiovascular dysfunction may have several needs requiring nursing intervention. Information gathered from the client's health history, physical examination, and diagnostic studies is used to determine nursing diagnoses and plan of care. Not every client will have the same needs. The most common nursing diagnoses related to clients with cardiovascular dysfunction are presented in the next section. A list of these diagnoses appears in Box 23–1.

FEAR AND ANXIETY

Clients who undergo a major cardiac event are under the stress of a life-threatening illness and are often consumed by the fear of death, pain, disability, physical dependency, and inactivity. Lack of knowledge and of effective emotional support may be fundamental to this fear. The client may use the call light frequently, ask many questions, and appear restless. If fear is unrelieved, the client will be at risk for developing anxiety that can lead to physical complications.

Anxiety is the most common emotional response of clients who are hospitalized for a coronary event. The physical responses to anxiety, which result from stimulation of the central nervous system, are likely to manifest themselves clinically as increases in pulse rate, blood pressure, and respiration, perhaps accompanied by heart rhythm irregularities or recurrent chest pain. This anxiety-induced

physical stimulation may be detrimental to the client's already compromised cardiac status.

On the other hand, the client may not exhibit overt signs of anxiety and may camouflage true feelings by false cheerfulness. Denial of the seriousness of the cardiac event is a coping mechanism often used to diminish fear and anxiety.

DISTURBANCE IN SELF-CONCEPT

Clients who have had a cardiac event (MI, cardiac surgery, or heart transplant) may feel betrayed by their bodies because they can no longer do what they used to do. Most clients also subscribe to the culturally accepted view that the heart is not simply a mechanical pump but is also a person's vital center. Because of this psychosocial view, the impact of cardiac dysfunction on clients' lives depends to a large extent on clients' own ideas about what is happening to them.

Clinical manifestations of disturbances in self-concept are varied and often subtle. Each client reacts differently to the situation. In addition, there is often a time lag between the actual body change and the client's acceptance of this change. Often, this is displayed as denial, which is protective in the early phase of illness but a problem in convalescence.

To assess clients' self-concepts, find out how they feel about health problems in general, how they perceive the significance of this illness, and how well they are able to cope with their normal responsibilities. Some objective clues that may indicate a disturbance in self-concept include a lessening of the client's ability or willingness to make appropriate decisions, passive response to limitations, retrogression from well-role to sick-role behavior, and unwillingness to discuss problems or participate in cardiac rehabilitation classes. The client's assessment of the reaction of significant others to the cardiac event and their ability to be supportive is also important.

ALTERATION IN COMFORT: PAIN

The client with cardiac dysfunction may develop acute chest pain from inadequate myocardial perfusion. Decrease in perfusion is most commonly a result of CAD. Myocardial ischemia or infarction may develop if inadequate perfusion persists. With acute myocardial pain, cardiac functioning is usually diminished, and a reduction in cardiac output may be noted. The client may experience shortness of breath; dizziness; weakness; nausea; vomiting; and changes in heart rate, rhythm, and blood pressure.

Some clients, who may not be surgical candidates or who may have decided against surgery, may have long-term chest discomfort called stable angina. Angina pain is usually infrequent and associated with precipitating factors

---

Box 23–1 Nursing Diagnoses Commonly Related to Heart and Major Blood Vessel Dysfunction

Diagnoses Directly Related to Heart and Major Blood Vessel Dysfunction

Fear and *Anxiety*

Self-concept, disturbance in

Comfort, alteration in: pain

Sexual dysfunction

Cardiac output, alteration in: decreased

Additional Potential Nursing Diagnoses

Tissue perfusion, alteration in: cardiopulmonary

Activity intolerance

Powerlessness

Coping, ineffective individual

Coping, ineffective family: compromised

Fluid volume, alteration in: excess

such as exertion or stress. Stable angina usually lasts no longer than 30 minutes and is most often relieved with rest.

SEXUAL DYSFUNCTION

Most clients who have cardiovascular disease experience a change in their sexual function. The most common cause of sexual dysfunction in these clients is lack of knowledge that results in fear. Clients may believe that sexual intercourse will cause another heart attack or that the stitches of new coronary blood vessels might rip apart. Their sexual partners may also fear inducing a cardiac event. Both clients and partners should be given guidelines regarding sexual activity. Previous marital or sexual problems may be exacerbated by the stress of the cardiac event.

Fatigue, pain, and shortness of breath due to cardiovascular disease also may cause sexual dysfunction. Because sexual intercourse induces elevated heart rate and blood pressure, clients must be physically ready to tolerate this stress. The energy expended during sexual activity, including orgasm, is equivalent to the energy required in moderate activity such as climbing stairs or walking 4 to 5 miles per hour (Braunwald, 1980). A stair-climbing test may be given to the client to determine physical readiness. Many antihypertensive agents can alter sexual functioning. Reserpine, clonidine, propranolol, and methyldopa are commonly reported to cause impotence, decrease libido, and decrease vaginal lubrication. Chronic use of potent diuretics such as furosemide and ethacrynic acid may also cause impotence.

ALTERATION IN CARDIAC OUTPUT: DECREASED

Numerous systemic and cardiac factors affect the ability of the heart to pump blood adequately throughout the body. Only the direct cardiac factors will be discussed here.

Box 23–2   Symptoms of Inadequate Cardiac Output

Dyspnea	Fatigue
Paroxysmal nocturnal dyspnea	Dizziness
Orthopnea	Low urine output
Cough	Cool, clammy skin
Edema	Weak pulse

The most common cause of inadequate cardiac output is a reduction in myocardial contractility, usually a result of myocardial ischemia secondary to CAD. Myocardial contractility may also be influenced by certain medications (eg, beta-adrenergics). Electrolyte imbalance such as calcium depletion can also decrease the cardiac output.

Any condition causing a decrease in ventricular filling (eg, mitral and tricuspid valvular stenoses) can cause a decrease in cardiac output. In these conditions, impeded blood flow through the valves causes ventricular pulmonary congestion, shortness of breath, edema, distended neck veins, tachycardia, dizziness, and fatigue.

Chronic ventricular overload also causes a decrease in cardiac output by decreasing the strength of myocardial contraction. Respiratory symptoms of heart failure are pronounced. The client often complains of severe shortness of breath, PND, orthopnea, and cough.

Abnormal cardiac rhythm and conduction disturbances can affect the cardiac output. In atrial fibrillation, atrial contraction is absent. This subsequently reduces ventricular filling, decreasing cardiac output. A very slow or fast heart rate may also be a precipitating factor. Box 23–2 summarizes the cardiovascular symptoms associated with an inadequate cardiac output.

Section III: Planning and Implementation

A sample nursing care plan for clients with dysfunction of the heart and major blood vessels is presented in Table 23–5. The following section discusses the objectives of care.

RELIEVING FEAR AND ANXIETY

To reduce fear, offer the client information and reassurance. Knowledge and reassurance diminish anxiety and fear by enhancing the client's coping skills. The client is able to rehearse information mentally and formulate expectations. The following items should be thoroughly explained: room arrangements, use of equipment, monitoring procedures, routine hospital activities, visiting practices, purpose of diagnostic tests, and progression of self-care activ-

ities. Liberal visiting for family and significant others should be allowed.

In the acute setting, a mild sedative may be prescribed to relax the client. Diazepam (Valium) is often given. As the client's condition stabilizes, the nurse assists the client in recognizing the anxiety and the conditions that precipitate it. Reassurance and comfort are offered by conveying understanding, supporting the client's present coping mechanisms (which may include denial), and providing a calm environment. As anxiety diminishes, the client is assisted in identifying the threats and more effective coping mechanisms. The client's support systems are identified and included in providing emotional comfort to the client. Both the client and family are encouraged to attend cardiac rehabilitation classes.

Table 23–5   Sample Nursing Care Plan for Clients With Heart and Major Blood Vessel Dysfunction

Nursing Diagnosis	Client Care Goal	Plan/Nursing Implementation	Expected Outcome
Fear and anxiety	Recognize situations that produce fear and anxiety; use effective coping mechanisms; achieve psychological comfort and ability to rest quietly	Provide reassurance and comfort; use diazepam as ordered; support present coping mechanisms until acute anxiety and fear subside; clarify misconceptions; orient client and family to the environment, care routines, procedures, and expected steps in convalescence (ie, transfer from CCU); eliminate ineffective coping and teach client and family effective coping skills; allow liberal visiting by family within client's tolerance; teach stress reduction	Client and family exhibit effective coping and are comfortable
Self-concept, disturbance in	Improve body image; assume role responsibilities	Assign a primary nurse who can establish a trusting relationship with client and family; encourage client and family to express feelings and concerns; clarify misconceptions; encourage participation in group cardiac rehab classes; discuss physical progression and return to work; provide or obtain guidance in career alternatives if client unable to return to work	Client will show increased self-confidence and exhibit well behavior
Comfort, alteration in: pain	Rest comfortably; progressively increase activity without pain; reduced incidence of angina	Use morphine sulfate or other pain medications as prescribed; reduce precipitating factors: excessive anxiety, fear, or activity; apply oxygen 2 L by nasal cannula as ordered; provide quiet and calm environment; teach client and family methods to reduce the incidence of pain, ie, plan activity, modify risk factors, and use prophylactic measures	Client rests comfortably without severe pain; able to sleep; client performs ADL without pain; client modifies alterable risk factors
Sexual dysfunction	Resume normal sexual function; achieve satisfaction in sexual relationship	Provide information about normal recovery process from a cardiac event and the resumption of sexual activity; discuss use of exercise stress test in determining a safe activity level; clarify misconceptions; ascertain whether impotence is caused by medications; obtain a sexual history from the client and partner; discuss methods to minimize adverse cardiovascular responses to sexual intercourse; include use of prophylactic medications, eg, nitroglycerin	Client is able to discuss fears and problems; client achieves satisfying sexual relationship
Cardiac output, alteration in: decreased	Achieve cardiac tolerance of increased activity	Organize client care and provide undisturbed rest periods; establish gradual increases in activity; monitor client's response to increased activity; teach client to monitor pulse rate; assess the client's ability to provide self-care, especially in taking medications; identify the client's risk factors and suggest modifications: smoking cessation, weight reduction, stress reduction, etc; provide activity guidelines	Client is able to perform ADL; client will modify risk factors; client is able to identify factors that increase cardiac work load; adverse CV responses are reduced

IMPROVING SELF-CONCEPT

To encourage the client's development of a positive self-concept, the nurse needs to establish a trusting relationship with the client. In the acute care setting, primary nursing works effectively. Providing information to the client and significant others during each phase of the condition clarifies misconceptions and promotes understanding of the plan of care.

As soon as possible, the client and significant others

Nursing Research Note

Mills G, Barnes R, Rodell D, Terry L: An evaluation of an inpatient cardiac patient/family education program. *Heart Lung* 1985; 14(4):400–406.

Client knowledge, general intelligence and problem-solving abilities, dysfunctional behavior parameters (motivation), and demographic information were examined as potential predictors of compliance behavior in clients with ischemic heart disease who had been involved in a cardiac education program. An extensive statistical analysis revealed that a documented increase in knowledge can be attributed to client education programs. The clients themselves and how they are taught were found to be as important as the content. Although not definitive, some findings suggested that client education programs may motivate clients to be more compliant.

Because motivation correlates with compliance, nurses must identify techniques that enhance client motivation and incorporate these into client education programs. Programs for cardiac clients are highly desirable and useful for the knowledge gained by clients. Therefore, all nurses should encourage clients to attend these programs and should help reinforce the knowledge presented.

should be included in classes and encouraged to socialize with other cardiac clients and families. Whether the client will be able to return to work needs to be evaluated. If clients are unable to return to their former occupations, counseling should be provided. Career alternatives may be possible. Guidance regarding the disability is offered.

Community resources are extremely helpful in the convalescent phase. Support group information for the client and significant others is available through the American Heart Association.

RELIEVING PAIN

The client's history is the most important factor in the assessment of cardiac pain. With MI pain, the client is hospitalized. Intravenous morphine sulfate and nasal oxygen are usually given. If the pain is not relieved, other medications such as intravenous nitroglycerin, propranolol, or a calcium antagonist may be used. Activities are restricted until pain is controlled. As perfusion of the myocardium improves, the pain subsides.

Stable angina is usually controlled by medication such as propranolol. Proper use of medication, identification of precipitating factors, and an evaluation of risk factors are important components in the client's management of pain. The following recommendations are usually offered: smoking cessation, weight reduction to ideal body weight, stress reduction, exercise for cardiac fitness, and proper diet. Blood pressure and serum lipids are monitored periodically. Teaching the client to recognize potential precipitating factors and to use prophylactic measures will assist in reducing recurrent pain.

PROMOTING SEXUAL FUNCTION

Sexual counseling of the client and partner begins before the client is released from the hospital and becomes part of the routine assessment in the long-term care of the client with cardiovascular dysfunction. An exercise stress test using a treadmill or stairs assesses the level of activity the client can safety achieve. Usually, the client who has had an uncomplicated MI may resume sexual activity in 5 to 8 weeks. Clients recovering from coronary artery bypass surgery may resume sexual activity in 3 to 6 weeks.

The first step in sexual counseling is the clarification of misconceptions regarding cardiovascular physiology and sex. A sexual history from the client and partner provides information on previous patterns and desires. The history taking may be the first opportunity the client and partner have had to express their sexual needs. Provide instruction and discussion about the physiological and psychological stress of sexual intercourse and interventions to minimize the physical impact of this stress.

Sexual intercourse should be planned to reduce its adverse effects. The client should wait at least 2 hours postprandial and should avoid excessive alcohol intake before intercourse. Prophylactic nitroglycerin or additional doses of propranolol may be used to prevent angina. The client is given written guidelines and instructed to report the following symptoms: chest pain during or after intercourse, persistent rapid heart rate, or persistent fatigue (Sadler, 1984).

Changes in sexual function in clients who take antihypertensive agents should be routinely assessed. If the client has developed side effects, the physician may alter the dosage or prescribe another medication. Clients rarely volunteer information about their sexual function; therefore, direct questions are required.

IMPROVING CARDIAC OUTPUT

Factors that increase cardiac work load (ie, activities that increase heart rate and blood pressure) need to be identified. Stress, smoking, obesity, excessive activity, and fluid retention may be contributing factors.

Nursing strategies are focused on reducing or eliminating precipitating factors. The management of underlying cardiac dysfunction is achieved with medical management.

The level of activity is increased as cardiac performance improves. An exercise stress test before the client's discharge will determine a safe level of activity. Planned activity with gradual increases and frequent rest periods is prescribed. Clients are instructed in monitoring their pulse rate to evaluate the cardiac response to activity: decreases in pulse rate during activity, resting pulse rate greater than 110, an irregular pulse, or pulse rate failing to return to normal within 3 minutes following the cessation of activity should be reported. Clients should report any symptoms such as shortness of breath, dizziness, or excessive fatigue. Clients are instructed to stop activity immediately and notify their health care provider if unrelieved chest pain and/or severe dyspnea occurs.

Psychological stress may also contribute to a decrease in cardiac output. The client's understanding of the effects of stress on the heart's performance should be evaluated. Stress reduction techniques should be taught to clients and families.

Section IV: Evaluation

Evaluation is the final step in the nursing process. The client's response to the interventions is assessed, and adjustments are made if the client care goals have not been achieved. The next section discusses potential client responses to the nursing diagnoses specific to cardiovascular dysfunction. These responses also appear in the sample nursing care plan (Table 23–5).

FEAR AND ANXIETY

As the client's fear subsides, physical and behavioral symptoms return to normal. The client rests more comfortably and uses the call light less frequently. The client copes effectively and can identify personal needs. As the family's fear diminishes, they may show a readiness to learn and participate in cardiac rehabilitation classes.

The client becomes able to recognize anxiety and use effective coping mechanisms to control its adverse effects. The client stops using denial as a coping mechanism and accepts the cardiac event. As the client becomes more knowledgeable, the conditions that previously precipitated anxiety diminish. The family or significant others are able to provide effective emotional support because they have become emotionally secure themselves.

DISTURBANCE IN SELF-CONCEPT

As self-concept improves, the client openly discusses the personal adjustments to be made and offers realistic goals for resuming career and family responsibilities. The client readily participates in classes and maintains the prescribed level of activity. Significant others can easily discuss future plans with the clients.

ALTERATION IN COMFORT: PAIN

Pain is relieved when the client can rest comfortably and physiological responses to pain have resolved. The client is able to sleep without discomfort.

For clients who have chronic angina, the incidence of acute pain is reduced. The client follows precautions to avoid chest pain. Planned activity is the key component. Through planned activity and prophylaxis, the client shows the ability to perform the activities of daily living.

SEXUAL DYSFUNCTION

The majority of clients with a cardiovascular dysfunction are able to resume sexual function. Clients who have achieved satisfaction often exhibit improvement in self-confidence and have a positive outlook in maintaining a healthy lifestyle.

ALTERATION IN CARDIAC OUTPUT: DECREASED

With an adequate cardiac output, the client can increase activity without cardiovascular side effects, and the physical examination will not reveal signs of inadequate myocardial perfusion. After recovery from the cardiac event, the client can maintain the lifestyle of a healthy person. The client understands risk factors, is able to identify personal risk factors, and can make necessary modifications to alter the risk.

Chapter Highlights

The client's health history is the most important source of information in cardiovascular assessment.

The principal symptoms of heart disease are dyspnea, chest pain, palpitation, and syncope. Other symptoms often associated with heart disease include fatigue and cough.

An important component in cardiovascular assessment is evaluating the client's risk-factor profile. Risk factors are personal characteristics and habits that increase the client's chance of developing CAD.

Clients who experience a major cardiac event are under the stress of a life-threatening illness and are often consumed by fear and anxiety.

Elevated serum cholesterol levels are directly related to the development of CAD: the higher the cholesterol

(continued)

Chapter Highlights *(continued)*

level, the greater the risk. The inverse is not true. The relation of an elevated serum triglyceride level and CAD is unclear. An elevated HDL level appears to protect against the development of atherosclerosis. Conversely, an elevated LDL level is associated with increased risk of developing CAD.

Cardiac enzymes—CK and its isoenzymes and LDH and its isoenzymes—are elevated when the client has had a myocardial infarction.

Diagnostic studies commonly used in cardiovascular assessment include the ECG, the ambulatory ECG (Holter) monitor, echocardiography, exercise stress test, phonocardiography, cardiac fluoroscopy, radionuclide studies, cardiac catheterization, and digital subtraction angiography.

Nursing diagnoses common to clients with cardiovascular dysfunction include fear and anxiety, disturbance in self-concept, pain, sexual dysfunction, and decreased cardiac output. The nurse's primary role in the care of clients with cardiovascular dysfunction is to facilitate physical and emotional adjustment. Modification of alterable risk factors is the major goal in the client's management.

Bibliography

Braunwald E (editor): *Heart Disease: The Textbook of Cardiovascular Medicine*. Vol 2. Philadelphia: Saunders, 1980.

Cantwell J: Exercise and coronary heart disease: Role in primary prevention. *Heart Lung* 1984; 13:6–13.

Carpenito L: *Nursing Diagnosis*. Philadelphia: Lippincott, 1983.

Chobanian A, Loviglio L: *Heart Risk Book*. Toronto: Bantam, 1982.

Criss E: Digital subtraction angiography. *Am J Nurs* 1982; 82:1706–1707.

Goldberg L, Elliot DL: The effect of physical activity on lipid and lipoprotein levels. *Med Clin North Am* 1985; 69(1):41–55.

Goldschlager N: Use of the treadmill test in the diagnosis of coronary artery disease in patients with chest pain. *Ann Intern Med* 1982; 97:383–388.

Hackett T, RosenBaum J: Emotion, psychiatric disorders and the heart. In: *Heart Disease: The Textbook of Cardiovascular Medicine*. Vol 2. Braunwald E (editor). Philadelphia: Saunders, 1980.

Kannel WB, McGee D, Gorden TA: A general cardiovascular risk profile: The Framingham study. *Amer J Cardiol* 1976; 38:46.

Levy R, Feinleib M: Risk factors for coronary artery disease and their management. In: *Heart Disease: The Textbook of Cardiovascular Medicine*. Vol 2. Braunwald E (editor). Philadelphia: Saunders, 1980.

Pantaleo N et al: Thallium myocardial scintigraphy and its use in the assessment of coronary artery disease. *Heart Lung* 1981; 10:61–71.

Papadopoulos C: Sexuality of women after myocardial infarction. *Med Aspects Human Sexual* 1985; 19:215–223.

Roberts R: Diagnostic assessment of myocardial infarction based on lactate dehydrogenase and creatinine kinase isoenzymes. *Heart Lung* 1981; 10:486–506.

Sadler D: *Nursing for Cardiovascular Health*. Norwalk, CT: Appleton–Century–Crofts, 1984.

Saul L: Heart sounds and common murmurs. *Am J Nurs* 1983; 83:1680–1689.

Scheidt S: Basic electrocardiography: Abnormalities of electrocardiographic patterns. *Ciba Clin Symp* 1984; 36(6):2–32.

Thomas S et al: Denial in coronary care patients: An objective reassessment. *Heart Lung* 1983; 12:71–80.

Tilkian A, Conover M: *Understanding Heart Sounds and Murmurs*. Philadelphia: Saunders, 1979.

Tilkian S, Conover M, Tilkian A: *Clinical Implications of Laboratory Tests*. St. Louis: Mosby, 1983.

Tobis J, Nalcioglu O, Henry W: Cardiovascular applications of digital subtraction angiography. *Mod Concepts Cardiov Dis* 1984; 53:31–36.

US Department of Health and Human Services. National Institutes of Health: *1984 Report of the Joint National Committee on Detection, Evaluation and Treatment of High Blood Pressure*. NIH Publication No 84-1088, June 1984.

US Department of Health and Human Services. National Institutes of Health: *Lipid Research Clinics Population Study Data*. Vol. I. NIH Publication No. 80–1527, July 1980.

Willerson J et al: Recent advances in nuclear cardiology. (Part I & part II) *Postgrad Med* 1981; 70(3):55–64, 69–72.

Suggested Readings

Daily E, Schroeder J: *Techniques in Bedside Hemodynamic Monitoring*. St. Louis: Mosby, 1981. Excellent reference book on invasive monitoring. The procedures are described in detail: the equipment to be used, client preparation, and the physiological parameters for each procedure.

Duncklee J: Protocol: Congestive heart failure. *Nurse Pract* 1984; 9(9):15–24. This article offers a protocol for nursing management of congestive heart failure. It provides guidelines for assessment and a flow sheet to document the ongoing assessment.

Fowler N: Diagnosis: Guide to interpretation of chest pain. *Hosp Med* (Jan) 1981; 12–14, 19–23, 30–34. This article describes succinctly various types of chest pain using many illustrations.

Kuller L: Risk factor reduction in coronary heart disease. *Mod Concepts of Cardiov Dis* 1984; 53:7–11. This article briefly discusses the recent trends in cardiovascular risk factors and mortality.

Resources

SELF-HELP GROUPS AND OTHER ORGANIZATIONS

American Heart Association
7320 Greenville Ave.
Dallas, TX 75231
Phone: (214) 750-5300

Local chapters are run by over 2 million volunteers. This association offers information, support groups, financial counseling, and classes related to heart ailments, hypertension, and stroke, and sponsors hypertension screening clinics in many communities in the US. Members are interested private citizens and professionals. Produces books, pamphlets, and audiovisual aids on heart disease for the public and for health professionals; a catalog is available.

Heartlife/AHP (Association of Heart
    Patients), Inc.
PO Box 54305
Atlanta, GA 30308
Phone: (404) 523-0826

This organization provides health education information on heart disease and offers its members a discount drug program, a life insurance program, and a quarterly magazine.

International Association of Pacemaker
    Patients
610 Equitable Building
100 Peachtree
Atlanta, GA 30303
Phone: (404) 659-0919

This nonprofit organization supports the emotional needs of clients with pacemakers and their families through group discussions, provides information about pacemaker technology and usage, and publishes a newsletter ("Pulse"). It provides many other useful services including a nationwide directory of pacemaker clinics, ID bracelets for clients, and a low cost telephone service that allows the client to check whether the pacemaker is functioning properly without leaving home.

Mended Hearts, Inc.
721 Huntington Ave.
Boston, MA 02115
Phone: (617) 732-5609

This nonprofit organization maintains chapters throughout the US and in some foreign countries. Members are persons who have undergone heart surgery. Volunteers share their personal experiences with others who will have or have had heart surgery. A volunteer will visit in the hospital or the home (with the physician's permission) and bring educational materials.

National Heart, Lung, and Blood
    Institute
(See resources listing in Chapter 29.)

US Government High Blood Pressure
    Information Center
120/80 National Institutes of Health

Bethesda, MD 20205
Phone: (703) 558-4880

This federal program serves as a clearinghouse for information on hypertension.

In Canada

Canadian Heart Foundation
1 Nicholas St., Suite 1200
Ottawa, Ontario, Canada K1N 7B7

Hundreds of chapters are available throughout Canada which further prevention and relief of cardiovascular diseases through research and professional and public education.

Mended Hearts, Inc.
℅ Dr. Paul S. Gomori
601–99 Wellington Crescent
Winnepeg, Manitoba, Canada I3M 0A2

Provides information of local chapters of the Mended Hearts (see earlier description) throughout Canada.

HOT LINES

Heartlife/AHP
Phone: (800) 241-6993
    in Georgia (404) 523-0826, collect

Sponsored by Heartlife/AHP (Association of Heart Patients), Inc., this hot line provides up-to-date information on heart disease.

Help for Patients with Pacemakers
Phone: (414) 659-0910

This hot line, sponsored by the International Association of Pacemaker Patients, offers information about nearby medical services for pacemaker clients who are traveling.

MEDICAL EQUIPMENT

Cardiac Card
Lutheran Medical Center
Harney & 26th St.
PO Box 3434
Omaha, NE 68103

A laminated waterproof card that contains the names of the client, the client's physician, cardiac history, current medications, and a 12-lead ECG strip with date and interpretation are available for a cost of $8.50.

Life Alert
6710 Varial Ave.
Canoga Park, CA 91303

This company provides a laminated wallet-size card that gives the client's complete history, name, address, blood type, medical problems, insurance information, and an ECG strip on an ECG card if desired. Lifetime individual and family memberships are available for $15 and $25 respectively.

HEALTH EDUCATION MATERIAL

From: American Heart Association

"After a Heart Attack," a booklet that answers commonly asked questions about returning to normal activity after a heart attack.

"Available Products for the Fat-Controlled Diet," a list of commercial products that can be used on a fat-controlled diet.

"Inside the Cardiac Care Unit: A Guide for the Patient and His Family," a booklet describing the monitoring equipment and health personnel found in a cardiac care unit.

"Recipes for Fat-Controlled, Low Cholesterol Meals," a recipe book.

"Reduce Your Risk of Heart Attack," a brochure to help analyze health habits, determine risk of heart attack, and modify lifestyle.

"Varicose Veins," a booklet describing the signs, symptoms, potential complications, and treatment of varicose veins.

From: Consumer Information Center
Pueblo, CO 81009

"What Every Woman Should Know About High Blood Pressure," a booklet on the relation between hypertension and being a woman who is black, pregnant, past menopause, or on birth control pills.

From: National Heart, Lung, and
  Blood Institute
Public Inquiries and Reports Section
9000 Rockville Pike
Bethesda, MD 20014

"A Handbook of Heart Terms," a booklet defining many of the medical terms used in discussing the heart and heart disease.

"Fact Sheet: Congestive Heart Failure," a pamphlet explaining the causes and methods of preventing heart failure.

"Fact Sheet: Heart-Lung Machines," a pamphlet explaining the function of this machine and describing the surgeries in which it is used.

"High Blood Pressure: Facts and Fiction," a booklet exploring common myths about hypertension.

"If You're Black, Here Are Some Facts You Should Know About High Blood Pressure," a brochure describing the special problem of high blood pressure in the black population.

Chapter 24

Specific Disorders
of the Heart

Constance A. Settlemyer
Frances L. Stier
SueAnn Wooster Ames

Objectives

When you have finished studying this chapter, you should be able to:

Identify risk factors that promote the development of heart disease.

Describe the subjective and objective findings in clients with hypertension, dysrhythmias, coronary artery disease, myocardial infarction, valvular disease, and heart failure.

Explain the expected physiological actions of common pharmacological agents used in the treatment of clients with heart problems.

Apply specific nursing measures to decrease the oxygen demands of the heart.

Discuss common medical interventions for clients with heart disease.

Anticipate the psychosocial/lifestyle implications of disorders of the heart on clients and significant others.

Specify appropriate nursing interventions for clients with cardiac dysfunction.

Over 42 million Americans have one or more forms of heart or blood vessel disease, according to 1980 statistics from the American Heart Association. One out of every four adults is estimated to have high blood pressure. Cardiovascular disease is responsible for over 50% of all deaths, with myocardial infarction being the leading cause of death.

As these statistics indicate, a large proportion of a nurse's clients have heart or blood vessel disease or the potential for it. In all clients the nurse cares for, the probability of death from cardiovascular disease is at least one out of two. Nurses who have a good understanding of the cardiovascular system and associated problems are in a position to help prevent premature death from cardiovascular disease by providing nursing care and education. This chapter provides basic information about common heart problems and their nursing implications.

Section I: Congenital Disorders (Clients Over Age 16)

Significant congenital disorders of the heart are usually identified and corrected early in life. Some persons reach adulthood without having had their congenital abnormality diagnosed or treated, perhaps because of inadequate medical care as a child or a lack of symptoms.

The two most common congenital heart problems in the adult are atrial septal defect, which may not produce symptoms until the fourth or fifth decade, and bicuspid aortic valve, which may never produce symptoms. Other congenital heart abnormalities found in adults, which may or may not have been diagnosed in childhood, include ventricular septal defect, pulmonic stenosis, coronary artery anomalies, and congenital heart block. For further information on congenital heart problems treated early in life, refer to a pediatric textbook. Congenital disorders diagnosed later in life are treated much the same as acquired defects discussed in this chapter.

A significant problem for adults who have had congenital problems diagnosed and treated early in life is obtaining health insurance. Because of the high cost of care that these persons may need, insurance rates are prohibitive. In addition, employers may be reluctant to hire individuals with a history of congenital heart disease because of the possible impact on an employer's group health insurance plan. Lack of adequate health insurance may discourage some clients from seeking needed care.

Section II: Disorders of Multifactorial Origin

Disorders of multifactorial origin that involve the heart may result from physiological changes in the body, environmental influences, genetic characteristics, or psychosocial/lifestyle factors. Symptoms range from minor discomfort that is easily tolerated to life-threatening emergencies. Because these disorders are influenced by environmental and psychosocial/lifestyle factors, they are often preventable to some extent by changes in lifestyle.

GENERAL NURSING IMPLICATIONS

Nurses can play a crucial role in the prevention of some of these cardiac disorders by educating the public. A person who understands the disease process and its effect on quality and length of life can make informed decisions regarding changes in lifestyle that will promote health. Education about the effects of diet, exercise, and smoking may promote healthier living. Educating the public about warning signs of heart attack may save lives. Detection and treatment of high blood pressure may prevent serious consequences of heart disease.

In the clinic and on the medical–surgical unit, nurses who are knowledgeable about abnormal assessment findings can refer clients for prompt medical evaluation. Astute detection of heart problems can mean the difference between life and death for clients who have been hospitalized for other reasons. For clients who are recovering from a heart problem, nurses can provide psychological support to help them adjust to their new health status, to follow a rehabilitation program, and to make the changes in lifestyle that may minimize the effects of the disease.

Nursing assessment for stable clients with suspected heart disease involves a thorough history to identify risk factors including:

- Age and sex (Incidence of coronary artery disease increases with age and is higher in men than in women.)
- Family history of cardiovascular disease
- Cigarette smoking
- Elevated blood pressure
- Elevated blood lipid levels
- Obesity
- Diabetes mellitus
- Abnormal glucose tolerance
- Gout
- Use of oral contraceptives

- Sedentary lifestyle
- Emotional factors

The role of emotional factors such as stress is still not completely understood. In 1974, Friedman and Rosenman described what they called the type A personality, which has been linked with coronary artery disease. Among the characteristics of the type A person are a compelling sense of time, compulsiveness, aggressiveness, and an extreme dedication to achievement. Type B personalities, on the other hand, are more easygoing.

Their observations have been both confirmed and denied. In 1981, a panel sponsored by the National Institutes of Health concluded that type A behavior was an independent risk factor for coronary disease. More recently, studies have questioned the role of these emotional factors. Comparing type As and type Bs, Case et al. (1985) found no relation between type A behavior and the long-term outcome of acute myocardial infarction. More research is needed on the influence of personality on heart disease.

Complete assessment and care planning for the cardiac client are described in Chapter 23. This chapter focuses on care of the ambulatory client or the client on a medical unit. For care given in the coronary care unit, refer to a cardiovascular nursing text.

HYPERTENSION

High blood pressure, or hypertension, is a widespread chronic disease and a major health problem in North America. The incidence in blacks is twice that of whites. It is a significant cardiovascular risk factor and is the leading cause of cerebral vascular accident (CVA, or stroke). The mortality associated with hypertension is directly proportional to the diastolic and systolic blood pressures. As these pressures rise, mortality increases. Hypertension is usually detected between the ages of 20 and 40 years. Complications of hypertension are most prevalent after the age of 40.

According to most authorities, hypertension exists when the diastolic blood pressure is greater than 90 mm Hg. The systolic pressure may be normal or elevated. Isolated systolic hypertension is common in adults over 65 years of age and is most often due to atherosclerosis.

Hypertension is classified as either essential or secondary hypertension. Essential hypertension is the most common and affects approximately 90% to 95% of clients. The cause of the elevated blood pressure is unknown, although there are often many contributing factors (eg, high-salt diet, obesity). Secondary hypertension, affecting approximately 5% of clients, is caused by a disease entity such as pheochromocytoma, renovascular disease, primary aldosteronism, or coarctation of the aorta. Oral contraceptives may also cause hypertension. Although the probability of secondary hypertension is low, the client's initial examination should always consider the possibility.

Clinical Manifestations

Hypertension has been called the silent disease or silent killer because clients are often asymptomatic until a CVA, myocardial infarction (MI), renal failure, or sudden death occurs. Persistent uncontrolled hypertension whether mild, moderate, or severe causes some degree of target organ damage to the heart, brain, or kidneys.

Cardiac manifestations of hypertension include angina, acute MI, left ventricular hypertrophy, acute pulmonary edema, congestive heart failure (CHF), and sudden coronary death. Renal involvement may initially present as nocturia or proteinuria. More advanced renal damage leads to azotemia and renal failure. Cerebral strokes and transient ischemic attacks are often directly related to systolic hypertension. In fact, hypertension is a more potent risk factor for developing a CVA than coronary or renal disease.

Symptoms reported by clients that may be due to hypertension include dizziness, palpitations, chest pain, weakness, epistaxis, hematuria, and brief episodes of memory loss (transient ischemic attacks). Less frequently, severe hypertension may cause occipital headaches that are present when the client awakens in the morning and subside spontaneously within hours. Most often, clients are asymptomatic.

Essential hypertension is often described as mild diastolic elevation (90 to 104 mm Hg), moderate diastolic elevation (105 to 114 mm Hg), or severe diastolic elevation (>115 mm Hg). Because of increased morbidity in clients with diastolic pressures of 85 to 89 mm Hg, a high-normal category has recently been added to the classification.

When the average of two or more blood pressure readings shows a diastolic pressure greater than 90 mm Hg or systolic pressure greater than 160 mm Hg in three visits, the diagnosis of essential hypertension is confirmed. To ensure accurate measurements, the equipment (cuff and sphygmomanometer), environment, and the client's physical and psychological state must be optimal.

Therapeutic Measures

To reduce the morbidity and mortality associated with hypertension, nonpharmacological and pharmacological therapies are used. The client's condition is evaluated, and therapy is prescribed according to the severity of the blood pressure elevation, the client's symptoms, and the risk-

Nursing Research Note

Harper D: Application of Orem's theoretical construct to self-care medication behaviors in the elderly. *ANS* (April) 1984; 6:29–45

Orem's conceptual framework was applied to self-medication behaviors among elderly black hypertensive clients. Two groups were used. One participated in a medication self-care program. The other participated in a hypertension teaching program. The self-care group received intervention about purpose, side effects, dosing, scheduling, adminstration, and safety factors for medications. The teaching program group received intervention about hypertension, including pathology and risk factors.

The findings suggest that the self-care group evidenced a greater degree of knowledge about medication and self-care behaviors; they also felt in more control over their own health. Postexperimental testing, however, indicated a decrease in this knowledge over time.

This sutdy points out the need for frequent assessment and monitoring of elderly individuals who have acquired new knowledge and skills. Periodic evaluation may help to reduce a decrease in knowledge. More research is required to determine follow-up and reinforcement techniques. This study links nursing practice with nursing theory, strengthening both clinical expertise and nursing science.

factor profile. High-normal and mild hypertension are initially treated with a nonpharmacological approach that includes weight reduction, dietary sodium restriction, moderation of alcohol intake, regular exercise, smoking cessation, stress reduction, and serum cholesterol reduction if needed.

Weight Reduction

Clients who are overweight (ie, 20% over their ideal body weight) are often hypertensive. Although the actual relation between obesity and hypertension is unclear, many studies have demonstrated that weight reduction can result in blood pressure reduction. In general, a 1 kg (2.2 lb) weight loss is associated with a 1.5 mm Hg decrease in diastolic pressure and a 2.5 mm Hg reduction in systolic pressure (McMahon, 1984).

Sodium Restriction

In some clients, excessive salt/sodium intake correlates with the development of hypertension. Moderate restriction of sodium intake (2 g Na or 5 g NaCl) has lowered blood pressure in some, but not all, hypertensive clients. A combination of weight reduction and sodium restriction may provide the most benefit. Foods with low, medium, and high sodium content are listed in Table 24–1. Many OTC medications also contain sodium. Clients should be encouraged to read drug and food labels carefully.

Alcohol Moderation

Moderate alcohol intake may offer a protective effect in the development of cardiovascular disease. However, heavy

Table 24–1   Foods With Low, Medium, and High Sodium Content

Foods Low in Sodium (less than 100 mg per serving) Emphasize These:	Foods Medium in Sodium (100–400 mg per serving) Use in Moderation:	Foods High in Sodium (over 400 mg per serving) Beware of These:
Unsalted seasonings:	*Lightly salted seasonings:*	Salt
Basil	Barbecue sauces	*Highly salted seasonings:*
Bayleaf	Catsup	Bouillon
Cinnamon	Chili sauce	Lemon-pepper marinade
Cloves	Gravies	Salted meat tenderizers
Curry	Mayonnaise	Salt/salt substitute mixtures
Dill	Mustard	Salted spices (garlic salt, onion salt, seasoned salt)
Dry mustard	Monosodium glutamate (MSG)	Soy sauce
Oregano	Prepared salad dressings	Teriyaki sauce
Paprika	Steak sauce	
Pepper	Tomato puree or sauce	
Thyme	Worcestershire sauce	
Bitters		
Garlic (fresh or powdered)		
Mint		
Onion (fresh or powdered)		
Parsley		
Tabasco sauce		
Tomato (fresh or paste)		
Vanilla		
Vinegar		
Most salt substitutes (check with your physician)		
Unsalted grain products:	*Grain products made with small amounts of salt, baking powder, or baking soda:*	*Highly salted grain products:*
Low-sodium breads and crackers	Breads and rolls	Commercially prepared spaghetti and pasta dishes
Flour	Dry cereals	Instant hot cereal
Hot cereals (except instant)	Biscuits and muffins	Pretzels
Matzoh	Cakes	Salted crackers and chips
Noodles	Cookies	Salted popcorn
Puffed rice or wheat	Pastries	
Rice	Pies	
Shredded wheat	Doughnuts	
Corn tortillas	Pancakes and waffles	
Unsalted popcorn	*Baking soda and baking powder contain sodium; avoid using large amounts; baked products using yeast are good alternatives*	
Whole grains		
Baked products made without salt, baking powder, or baking soda		
Fruits	Beet greens	*Highly salted vegetables:*
Fruit juices	Celery	All pickled vegetables
Unsalted vegetables (except as noted)	Chard	Olives and pickles

Foods Low in Sodium (less than 100 mg per serving) Emphasize These:	Foods Medium in Sodium (100–400 mg per serving) Use in Moderation:	Foods High in Sodium (over 400 mg per serving) Beware of These:
	Lightly salted vegetables:	Sauerkraut
	Canned vegetables	Vegetable juices
	Frozen lima beans	Vegetables with seasoned sauces
	Frozen peas	
Fresh meat prepared without salt:	Fresh shellfish	*Smoked, cured, or pickled products:*
Beef and veal	Salted nuts	Bacon
Fish	Salted peanut butter	Corned beef
Lamb		Dried meat or fish
Poultry		Ham
Pork		Luncheon meats
Dried beans cooked without salt or salt pork		Sausages and frankfurters
Eggs		Fish or meat canned with salt
Unsalted nuts		Frozen dinners
To control fats, choose lean meats, poultry, fish, and beans		Most commercially prepared entrees
		Packaged or canned soups
Cream cheese	Milk	American cheese
Gruyere cheese	Buttermilk	Blue cheese
Ricotta cheese	Cheese (except as noted)	Cottage cheese
Swiss cheese	Custard	Parmesan cheese
Unsalted cheese	Ice cream	Roquefort cheese
Cream	Pudding	Processed cheese products
Unsalted butter or margarine	Salted butter and margarine	
Sherbet	Yogurt	
To control fat, choose low-fat dairy products; limit butter, margarine, and cream		
Beer, liquor, and wine (moderation advised)	Milk	
Carbonated beverages	Buttermilk	
Coffee and tea		
Most mineral waters (check with supplier)		

SOURCE: Reprinted with permission from American Heart Association, Alameda County Chapter, Oakland, CA.

alcohol consumption (ie, more than three to four hard-liquor drinks per day) is associated with increased blood pressure.

Smoking Cessation

Cigarette smoking is a major risk factor in the development of cardiovascular disease. Nicotine causes constriction of both small and large blood vessels. When smoking is combined with hypertension, the risks are significantly increased. Although a cause-and-effect relation between cigarette

smoking and the development of hypertension has not been documented, short-term nicotine use is known to increase both systolic and diastolic blood pressure.

Exercise

Regular isotonic exercise such as walking, jogging, or swimming promotes cardiovascular fitness. Exercise facilitates weight reduction and promotes relaxation, which may result in lowering of the blood pressure. Clients who exercise regularly appear to have a lower incidence of cardiovascular disease than clients who remain sedentary or exercise irregularly.

If nonpharmacological therapy is ineffective in lowering the blood pressure, or if faster results are desired, pharmacological intervention is also prescribed. Clients with moderate or severe hypertension are usually treated immediately with both interventions.

Pharmacologic Therapy

Most health care providers use the *stepped-care* program in prescribing pharmacologic therapy. This approach has four steps (see Table 24–2).

Clients with mild hypertension who fail to respond to nonpharmacologic methods are routinely started at *step 1*, diuretic therapy. The diuretic works on the renal tubules, causing a sodium diuresis and subsequent volume depletion. A thiazide diuretic is usually selected, using the lowest effective dose.

Common side effects of diuretic therapy include hypokalemia, hyperuricemia, and carbohydrate intolerance. Cardiac dysrhythmias may develop if hypokalemia is present. Clients with a serum potassium level below 3.5 mEq/L may require a potassium supplement. Clients with gout often require treatment with probenecid or allopurinol.

If the diastolic blood pressure remains above normal (ie, >90 mm Hg), treatment is advanced to *step 2*. An antiadrenergic agent is added to the diuretic. The drugs in this group act on a variety of sites—centrally on the vasomotor center, peripherally by modifying catecholamine release, or on target tissue by blocking adrenergic receptor sites. Beta-adrenergic blocking agents (eg, propranolol) are the most commonly used agents in step 2. Recently, drugs that block the movement of calcium within smooth and cardiac muscle and drugs that inhibit the enzyme that converts angiotensin I to angiotensin II have been added to step 2.

Side effects of the drugs are often dose related. The therapeutic goal is to achieve hypertension control with the lowest dose and the fewest side effects. Therefore, a second drug is often substituted rather than using the maximum dose of a drug that may precipitate side effects. Sexual dysfunction is frequently reported by clients who are taking antihypertensive medication, especially adrenergic blocking agents. The mechanism of dysfunction is unclear, however. Psychological factors, age, or other illnesses may contribute to the problem.

Step 3 is used when a variety of step 2 drugs combined with a diuretic have not achieved blood pressure control. The medications in step 3 are vasodilators that cause relaxation of smooth muscle, lowering peripheral resistance and blood pressure. The most common medication prescribed is hydralazine. Vasodilator therapy may cause a sympathetic reflex response (increased heart rate and cardiac output); therefore, an adrenergic blocking agent and a diuretic are often used in conjunction with the step 3 medication.

In severe hypertension or uncontrolled moderate

Table 24–2 Stepped Care Program: Antihypertensive Agents*	
Antihypertensive Drug	**Daily Dose Range**
Step 1: Diuretic therapy	
Thiazides	
Chlorothiazide (Diuril)	250–500 mg
Hydrochlorothiazide (Oretic, HydroDIURIL, Esidrix)	25–50 mg
Sulfonamide diuretics	
Chlorthalidone (Hygroton)	25–50 mg
Loop diuretics	
Furosemide (Lasix)	40–120 mg
Ethacrynic acid (Edecrin)	50–200 mg
Potassium-sparing agents	
Spironolactone (Aldactone)	25–100 mg
Triamterene (Dyrenium)	50–100 mg
Step 2: Adrenergic inhibitors	
Beta-adrenergic blockers	
Atenolol (Tenormin)	25–100 mg
Metoprolol (Lopressor)	50–300 mg
Nadolol (Corgard)	20–120 mg
Propranolol (Inderal)	40–480 mg
Timolol (Timoptic)	20–60 mg
Central adrenergic inhibitors	
Clonidine (Catapres)	0.2–1.2 mg
Methyldopa (Aldomet)	500–2000 mg
Peripheral adrenergic inhibitor	
Reserpine (Serpasil)	0.05–0.25 mg
Alpha-1 adrenergic blocker	
Prazosin (Minipress)	1.0–20.0 mg
Angiotensin-converting enzyme inhibitors	
Captopril (Capoten)	37.5–150.0 mg
Slow-channel calcium-entry blocking agents	
Nifedipine (Procardia)	30–180 mg
Verapamil (Isoptin, Calan)	240–480 mg
Step 3: Vasodilators	
Hydralazine (Apresoline)	50–300 mg
Minoxidil (Loniten)	5–100 mg
Step 4: Peripheral adrenergic antagonist	
Guanethidine (Ismelin)	10–300 mg

*Most commonly used drugs

hypertension, *step 4* is used. The approach in step 4 is substituting a step 2 agent for a peripheral adrenergic blocking agent. Guanethidine is frequently used. Side effects are common, however, and often contribute to poor client compliance. Some of the side effects include impotence, retrograde ejaculation, diarrhea, fatigue, weight gain, and edema.

The stepped-care program appears to be effective for most clients, but the client's history and clinical condition should be evaluated. A flexible, individualized plan is the most effective approach.

Specific Nursing Measures

Early detection, education, and promoting adherence to therapy are key factors in controlling blood pressure. The nurse's role is instrumental in each.

Early Detection
The nurse is often the health care provider who takes the initial blood pressure on the client. Accurate measurement depends on the technique used (see Chapter 23). The client should be calm, quiet, and relaxed before obtaining the blood pressure. Restrictive clothing should be removed. If the initial reading is elevated, two more measurements 1 to 5 minutes apart should be obtained with the client in the supine position. The mean of the three readings is reported as the blood pressure.

Screening for hypertension may be performed at a variety of public events such as community programs, club meetings, company activities, fairs, or church functions. When nurses obtain elevated readings at these screening programs, they should urge affected clients to see their health care providers for a follow-up blood pressure check.

Education
Perhaps the most significant factor in controlling blood pressure is the client's understanding of the disease and the treatment plan. Client education usually begins with the definition and cause of hypertension and the complications and risks associated with uncontrolled hypertension. The nonpharmacological approach to hypertension management is initially emphasized.

After reviewing the client's health history and cardiovascular risk appraisal, an individualized nonpharmacological approach is planned. Weight reduction and proper nutrition are the primary interventions. The client should be given written guidelines such as a list of foods to avoid (ie, those high in sodium and cholesterol) and a calorie reduction diet. Assisting the client in menu planning is effective. Both the client and family may need additional nutritional counseling. A referral to a nutritionist may be helpful.

Clients who use antihypertensive medications need additional education. The purpose, dosage, and possible side effects of the medication should be explained. If more than one medication is used, the client must understand that each drug acts differently; therefore, substitution is inappropriate and dangerous. Skipping doses and discontinuing medication may cause rebound hypertension and possibly provoke a CVA or MI. Unpleasant side effects often result in poor drug compliance. Therefore, nurses need to investigate carefully any side effects the client experiences. Hypokalemia is a common side effect of diuretic therapy. The symptoms and signs include muscle weakness, apathy, hypotension, cardiac dysrhythmias, and pro-

longed Q-T interval on the ECG. Clients should be given a list of foods containing potassium to counterbalance the potassium loss (see Box 24–1). Occasionally, clients need a potassium supplement. Clients should be informed that if side effects occur, the drug dose may be altered to minimize the problem, or an alternative drug can be prescribed.

Adherence to Therapy
The predominant problem in controlling high blood pressure is the client's adherence to therapy. The nonpharmacological approach requires personal lifestyle changes, and the pharmacological approach may cause unacceptable side effects. Also contributing to poor compliance is the chronicity of hypertension, the asymptomatic nature of the disease, and the long-term management.

Involving the client in establishing the short-term and long-term goals of therapy is important in obtaining client cooperation. Clients are more likely to adhere to the hypertension regimen if they are active participants. Both nonpharmacological and pharmacological interventions should be instituted gradually, and a nonauthoritarian approach should be used. Management decisions may include negotiation between the client and health care provider. The client may decide on a weight reduction goal and select the foods to be sacrificed. For example, the client may negotiate for a daily beer but offer to give up salty pretzels. The nurse may also influence the client to consume "light" beer which is lower in calories and sodium.

Box 24–1	Foods High in Potassium	
Almonds	Grapefruit juice	Potato chips
Apricots	Honeydew melon	Potatoes (baked or boiled)
Artichokes	Meat (especially veal)	Poultry
Avocados	Milk	Prune juice
Bananas	Molasses (dark or light)	Prunes
Beans (lima, navy, pinto)	Nectarines	Pumpkin
Bran cereal	Nuts (Brazil, cashew, chestnuts, peanuts, pecans, pistachio, walnuts)	Raisins
Bread (whole and grain)		Rhubarb
Broccoli		Rhutabaga
Brussel sprouts	Orange juice	Scallops
Cantaloupe	Oranges	Shrimp
Chocolate	Papaya	Soybeans
Cocoa	Parsnips	Squash (winter)
Coffee (instant or percolated)	Peaches	Tangerines
	Pears	Tomato juice
Dates	Pineapple	Tomatoes
Figs	Pineapple juice	Vegetable juice
Fish	Pomegranate	Wheat germ
Grapefruit		Yams

Lack of adherence to antihypertensive medications may be from side effects, a dosage schedule of more than once a day, or expense. The client's satisfaction with the medication as well as blood pressure response should be assessed at every visit.

DYSRHYTHMIAS

Disturbances in heart rate or rhythm are commonly referred to as cardiac dysrhythmias (arrhythmias). Dysrhythmias range from the common insignificant dysrhythmias found in persons with normal hearts to life-threatening dysrhythmias. The disturbance may be either in the automaticity of the cardiac cells or in the conduction of the impulses. Thinking of the pacemaker cells as dominoes falling, imagine dominoes that should fall automatically falling (depolarizing) either too frequently or not frequently enough, disturbing automaticity. Examples of disturbances in automaticity include an abnormal pacemaker site and **ectopic beats** (cardiac impulses originating outside the SA node). With a disturbance in conduction, a conducting heart cell (domino) may not depolarize (fall) when it is stimulated and completely "block" the conduction of the impulse ahead of it. The conducting cells to the sides of it conduct normally, but the conducting cell waits until the impulse is transmitted through abnormal pathways and propagated backwards. The cell then depolarizes (falls), permitting the impulse to reenter the same abnormal pathway and set up an abnormal tachydysrhythmia. This is referred to as "reentry phenomenon."

Cardiac dysrhythmias are usually assessed by coronary care or critical care nurses using electronic monitoring equipment and ECG rhythm strips. However, all nurses routinely assess clients for the presence or absence of dysrhythmias by taking the pulse. A basic understanding of common disturbances in cardiac rate and rhythm as diagnosed from rhythm strips is helpful to nurses in the care of clients who may be susceptible to dysrhythmias or those who are being medically treated for prevention of cardiac dysrhythmias.

Etiology

Dysrhythmias have many causes. Ischemia or injury to cardiac cells is a frequent cause. Enlargement of the chambers of the heart sometimes affects normal conduction, resulting in dysrhythmias. Many drugs, including caffeine, nicotine, and alcohol, can be responsible for dysrhythmias. Disturbances in electrolyte balance or the normal physiological environment of the cardiac cells may sometimes cause disturbances in rhythm. Some dysrhythmias are not abnormal but a normal physiological response. Some common examples of normal physiological response include sinus tachycardia associated with increased activity level and sinus bradycardia, which is quite often seen in athletes at rest.

Clinical Manifestations and Therapeutic Measures

Because the clinical manifestations and treatment of dysrhythmias depend on the type of rhythm disturbance, common cardiac dysrhythmias will be discussed individually. Normal sinus rhythm will also be presented for comparison. A review of the section on conduction in Chapter 22 may be helpful. Because dysrhythmias are named for their site of origin (sinus, atrial, atrioventricular [A-V], junctional, ventricular, etc) they will be presented in that order. Keep in mind that the rhythm strip alone does not provide sufficient information to make an unequivocal diagnosis of dysrhythmia. Often, several experts make different diagnoses from the same rhythm strip.

Drugs used to treat dysrhythmias reduce automaticity of ectopic foci, alter conduction velocity or cardiac membrane responsiveness (class 1 drugs), inhibit the effects of circulating catecholamines—beta-adrenergic blockers—(class 2 drugs), prolong action potential (class 3 drugs), or inhibit the influx of calcium ions—calcium channel blockers—(class 4 drugs). These drugs are discussed in detail in Table 24–3.

Normal Sinus Rhythm

Under normal circumstances, the heart beats at a rate of between 60 and 100 beats per minute. The atria are electrically stimulated; these recorded electrical signals produce a P wave on the ECG (Figure 24–1; refer also to Figures 22–3 and 22–4). The impulse is slowed in the A-V node before being conducted through the ventricles and forming the QRS complex. The slowing permits the atria to contract and fill the ventricles with more blood before they contract. The amount of time from the beginning of the P wave to the beginning of the QRS complex is between 0.12 and 0.20 seconds, or 3 to 5 small squares (0.04 seconds each) on the paper. Every P wave is followed by a QRS in normal sinus rhythm. Normal sinus rhythm has the following characteristics:

- P waves occur regularly. The distance between P waves is the same; ie, the distance between the first and second P waves is the same as the distance between the second and third P waves.

- P waves occur at a rate of between 60 (25 small squares between P waves) and 100 (15 small squares between P waves).

- Every P wave is followed by a QRS complex.

- The PR interval is the same for all cycles and is between 0.12 and 0.20 seconds. (It takes at least 0.12 seconds for an impulse to travel from the atria to the ventricles; therefore, what may appear to be a normal sinus rhythm may be an atrial rhythm.)

- The duration of the QRS complex is between 0.06 and 0.12 seconds (unless conduction is abnormally slow

(continued on p. 770)

Table 24–3   Antidysrhythmic Drugs

Classification (Generic Name, Trade Name)	Route of Administration and Dosage	Action and Uses	Side Effects and Other Considerations	Nursing Implications
Class 1	IV, IM, SC	The class 1 antidys-rhythmics primarily interfere with the action potential by affecting the transfer of sodium or potassium through the fast channels; class 1 drugs also have anticholinergic effects	Side effects: CNS disturbances are side effects of all drugs in this class; GI disturbances are side effects of some drugs in this class, predominantly those with anticholinergic effects Other considerations: Na and K levels as well as drugs affecting Na and K influence the activity of these drugs	
Quinidine sulfate (Cin-Quin, Quinidex, Quinora) Quinidine polygalacturonate (Cardioquin) Quinidine gluconate (Duraquin, Quinaglute)	Oral; 200–800 mg q. 2–3 h until desired effect; then 100–300 mg 3–6 times per day Oral: 275–825 mg q. 3–4 h; then gradually increase to desired effect IV, IM, PO IV: 300 to 750 mg at rate of 1 mL/min of dilute solution IM: 600 mg initially; then 400 mg up to 12 times/day PO: 200 to 300 mg q. 8 h	Quinidine affects the action potential by influencing Na transfer; it suppresses automaticity by decreasing the rate of phase 4 diastolic depolarization and also prolongs the effective refractory period in atrial and ventricular tissue Use: Supraventricular premature complexes; atrial flutter; atrial fibrillation; ventricular premature complexes; long-term control of ventricular tachycardia and fibrillation	CNS: Disturbances in orientation: confusion, visual disturbances, tinnitis, headache, fever, tremor GI: Nausea, vomiting, diarrhea, abdominal pain CV: Hypotension, pallor, ECG changes Other: Rash, thrombocytopenia, hemolytic anemia, anaphylaxis Other considerations: Quinidine's vagolytic (anticholinergic) effect promotes conduction through the junctional area and may promote a fast ventricular response with atrial flutter or atrial fibrillation; digitalis, propranolol, or verapamil are usually given before quinidine to control this effect May cause bleeding when given with oral anticoagulants; phenobarbital and phenytoin may shorten the duration of action; may increase digitalis blood levels	Assess effects and side effects; give with food; observe use of other drugs: • Digitalis: Assess for digitalis toxicity • Phenytoin and phenobarbital: Increased dosage of quinidine may be ordered Client and family teaching, which includes: name of drug; dosage prescribed; reason drug is prescribed; side effects; take with food When to notify physician: If side effects develop; for advice when taking other drugs

(continued)

Table 24–3	Antidysrhythmic Drugs (continued)			
Classification (Generic Name, Trade Name)	**Route of Administration and Dosage**	**Action and Uses**	**Side Effects and Other Considerations**	**Nursing Implications**
Procainamide hydrochloride (Pronestyl, Procan SR)	Oral: One 250-, 375-, or 500-mg tablet or capsule q. 4–6 h to suppress dysrhythmias; sustained-release capsules (250, 500, and 750 mg): 500–1000 mg q. 6 h as maintenance after dysrhythmia is interrupted with use of standard procainamide hydrochloride IM: 500–1000 mg IM q. 4–8 h until oral therapy is possible IV: 100 mg q. 5 min at rate of 50 mg/min until life-threatening dysrhythmia is suppressed or 500 or 600 mg is given; 500–600 mg of diluted solution to be given over 25 min followed by a maintenance infusion of 2–6 mg/min	Resembles quinidine in its actions; procainamide HCl depresses excitability in the atria and ventricles; slows conduction and the effective refractory period; anticholinergic effects are less than those of quinidine and disopyramide Use: Supraventricular and ventricular dysrhythmias, including paroxysmal atrial tachycardia, atrial fibrillation, premature ventricular contractions, and ventricular tachycardia	CNS: Giddiness, hallucinations, depression, psychosis CV: Dysrhythmias, hypotension GI: Nausea, vomiting, diarrhea, abdominal pain Skin: Rash Other: Agranulocytosis, purpura, syndrome resembling lupus erythematosus, myalgias, anemia Contraindications: Hypersensitivity to the drug; myasthenia gravis; second- or third-degree A-V block in the absence of a ventricular pacemaker Other considerations: Anticholinergic effect may promote conduction through the junctional area and may promote a fast ventricular response with atrial flutter or atrial fibrillation; prior digitalis administration reduces this danger; caution in clients with renal and liver disease because drug may accumulate	Constant monitoring of ECG pattern during IV administration; assess effects and side effects Client and family teaching, which includes: name of drug; dosage prescribed; reason drug is prescribed; side effects; need to have periodic blood studies When to notify physician: If side effects develop; if upper respiratory infection develops; if sore mouth, gums, or throat develop; if fever develops; for advice when taking other drugs
Disopyramide phosphate (Norpace)	Oral: Immediate release: one 100- or 150-mg capsule q. 6 h; 300 mg in continuous-release-capsule form (100 and 150 mg) q. 6 h	Similar actions to quinidine and procainamide; disopyramide lengthens conduction time in normal and depolarized Purkinje fibers Use: Premature ventricular contractions and ventricular tachycardia	CNS: Nervousness, dizziness, headache, depression, insomnia CV: Hypotension, ECG changes, dysrhythmias, heart failure, dyspnea, edema, weight gain GI: Nausea, vomiting, diarrhea, anorexia GU: Urinary frequency, urgency, retention, impotence Skin: Rash Other: Blurred vision; dry mouth, nose, and throat; fatigue; weakness; hypoglycemia Contraindications: Cardiogenic shock, second- or third-degree A-V block in	Assess effects and side effects Client and family teaching, which includes: name of drug; dosage prescribed; reason drug is prescribed; side effects When to notify physician: If side effects develop

Classification (Generic Name, Trade Name)	Route of Administration and Dosage	Action and Uses	Side Effects and Other Considerations	Nursing Implications
			absence of a ventricular pacemaker, hypersensitivity to the drug, glaucoma, myasthenia gravis, urinary retention Other considerations: Anticholinergic effect may promote a fast ventricular response with atrial flutter or atrial fibrillation; prior digitalis administration reduces this danger; caution with clients with renal and liver disease because drug may accumulate Drug interactions: When taken in conjunction with phenytoin, level of disopyramide will be reduced	
Lidocaine (Xylocaine)	IM: 300 mg in deltoid muscle, aspirating frequently to avoid intravascular injection (100 mg/mL solution); switch to IV infusion as soon as possible IV: Single bolus, 50–100 mg under ECG monitoring at a rate of 25–50 mg/min; may be necessary to repeat in 5 min; no more than 200–300 mg should be given in 1 h Continuous infusion: 1 to 4 mg/min of a diluted solution (1 to 4 mg/mL)	Attenuates phase 4 diastolic depolarization of Purkinje fibers and decreases automaticity Use: Acute management of ventricular dysrhythmias	CNS: Nervousness, dizziness, paresthesia, euphoria, confusion, drowsiness, visual disturbance, convulsions, coma CV: Bradycardia, hypotension Contraindications: Hypersensitivity to local anesthetic agents of the amide group; heart block in the absence of a ventricular pacemaker; caution in clients with liver or renal disease because drug may accumulate	Constant monitoring of ECG pattern; assess effects and side effects; have resuscitative equipment and drugs available
Phenytoin (Dilantin)	Oral: 400–600 mg/day in one or two doses IV: 50–100 mg every 5–10 min up to 1000 mg	Believed to depress automaticity in Purkinje fibers by increasing potassium conductance Use: Treatment of atrial and ventricular dysrhythmias caused by digitalis toxicity; treatment of ventricular dysrhythmias unresponsive to lidocaine or procainamide	CNS: Nystagmus, ataxia, drowsiness, slurred speech, confusion, coma, nervousness, headache GI: Nausea, constipation, anorexia Skin: Rash Other: Gingival hypertrophy, megaloblastic anemia, peripheral neuropathy, lymph node hyperplasia, hyperglycemia, hypoglycemia, drug-induced systemic	Constant monitoring of ECG pattern during IV administration; assess effects and side effects Client and family teaching, which includes: name of drug; dosage prescribed; reason drug is prescribed; side effects; importance of good dental care; need to have periodic blood studies to determine levels

(continued)

Table 24–3   Antidysrhythmic Drugs (continued)

Classification (Generic Name, Trade Name)	Route of Administration and Dosage	Action and Uses	Side Effects and Other Considerations	Nursing Implications
			lupus erythematosus Contraindications: Hypersensitivity to drug, sinus bradycardia, heart block Other considerations: Interactions are common with numerous drugs; therefore, serum levels should be obtained to determine therapeutic level	When to notify physician: If side effects develop, for advice when taking any other drugs
Class 2: Beta-adrenergic blocking agents				
Propranolol (Inderal)	Oral: 10–30 mg three or four times daily before meals and at bedtime; IV for life-threatening dysrhythmias: 1–3 mg IV at a rate of 1 mg/min under constant ECG monitoring	Beta-adrenergic blocking agents inhibit the effects of circulating catecholamines on the beta-adrenergic receptors. Their effect is greatest during surges of sympathetic activity; only propranolol, which is a nonselective beta-adrenergic blocking agent having both beta 1 and beta 2 blocking effects, is currently approved in the US for treatment of dysrhythmias Blocking effects vary, depending on type of beta receptor affected: Beta 1 blocking effects: heart has decreased contractility, conduction velocity, automaticity; Beta 2 blocking effects: vasoconstriction, bronchoconstriction, decreased coronary blood flow Use (not all agents in class approved for all uses): Treatment of hypertension: actual mechanisms causing decreased blood pressure not known but may be related to decreased cardiac output, central effect resulting in decreased	CNS: Mental depression sleep disturbances, dizziness, weakness CV: CHF, bradycardia, heart block, arterial insufficiency, coldness of the extremities, hypotension, paresthesia, prolongs myocardial ischemia in clients with Prinzmetal's angina Respiratory: Bronchospasm, respiratory distress GI: Nausea, vomiting, diarrhea, cramping, constipation Skin: Rash, alopecia Hematologic: Agranulocytosis, purpura Contraindications: Beta 1 blockade: cardiac failure, cardiogenic shock, bradycardia, greater than first-degree heart block; Beta 2 blockade: bronchial asthma Other considerations: Beta blockade impairs defense of insulin-induced hypoglycemia; beta blockade impairs signs and symptoms of thyrotoxicosis; abrupt withdrawal may have a rebound effect, which may result in acute angina; drug interac-	Thorough drug history; assess effects and side effects Client and family teaching, which includes: name of drug; dosage prescribed; reason drug is prescribed; side effects; if diabetic, may need to have medical plan of care adjusted; drug must be discontinued over several weeks (should not stop taking it) When to notify physician: If side effects develop; for advice when taking any other drug; if planning to have an anesthetic for surgical procedures

Classification (Generic Name, Trade Name)	Route of Administration and Dosage	Action and Uses	Side Effects and Other Considerations	Nursing Implications
		sympathetic outflow to the periphery, suppression of renin activity Treatment of angina pectoris due to coronary atherosclerosis: decreases oxygen requirements of the heart Treatment of supraventricular and ventricular cardiac dysrhythmias, particularly those induced by catecholamines Prophylaxis of migraine (mechanism not established) Management of hypertrophic subaortic stenosis; control of stress-induced angina, palpitations, and syncope; adjunctive therapy for the control of tachycardia with pheochromocytoma; prevention of cardiac mortality post-MI	tions: may have additive effect when given with catecholamine-depleting drugs	
Class 3	(See individual drug)	Class 3 drugs prolong action potential; only bretylium is currently approved for use in the US; other drugs in this class under investigation include amiodarone bethanidine and sotalol		
Bretylium (Bretylol)	IV for life-threatening dysrhythmias: 5 mg/kg given rapidly; may increase to 10 mg/kg and repeat as necessary IV maintenance: Constant IV infusion of 1–2 mg/kg/min of solution diluted to no more than 10 mg/mL *or* infuse diluted solution containing total content of 5 mg/kg over at least 8 min and repeat every 6 h IM: 5 to 10 mg/kg; may repeat in 1 or 2 h; maintenance 5 to 10 mg/kg q. 6 h	Bretylium acts as a chemical sympathectomy; first causes norepinephrine release; then prevents its release by depressing adrenergic nerve terminals Use: Prophylaxis and treatment of ventricular fibrillation; treatment of life-threatening dysrhythmias when other drugs have failed to control them	CNS: dizziness, confusion, anxiety, lethargy CV: Transient hypertension, postural hypotension, bradycardia, dysrhythmias, flushing, shortness of breath, angina GI: Hiccups, abdominal pain, nausea Skin: Rash Other: Diaphoresis, nasal stuffiness, generalized tenderness, conjunctivitis Contraindications: None; may aggravate digitalis toxicity; caution in clients with	Constant monitoring of ECG pattern; monitor blood pressure; keep in supine position if possible and watch closely for hypotension; assess effects and side effects; observe for postural hypotension for several days after therapy; rotate IM injection sites and take special care not to inject near major nerve

(continued)

Table 24-3	Antidysrhythmic Drugs (continued)			
Classification (Generic Name, Trade Name)	Route of Administration and Dosage	Action and Uses	Side Effects and Other Considerations	Nursing Implications
			renal disease: dosage may need to be reduced	
Class 4: Calcium channel blockers				
Verapamil (Calan, Isoptin)	IV: 5–10 mg slowly over at least 2 to 3 min; may repeat with 10 mg after 30 min	Calcium channel blockers inhibit influx of calcium ions during depolarization of the membranes of cardiac and vascular smooth muscles; antidysrhythmic effect is believed to be related to the effect on the slow channels in the cardiac conductile system; calcium channel blocking agents slow A-V conduction and can interfere with the sinus node impulse; of the calcium channel blockers, only verapamil is currently approved for the treatment of dysrhythmias Use: Treatment of supraventricular tachycardia	CNS: Headache, dizziness CV: Hypotension, bradycardia, tachycardia, dysrhythmias, worsening of heart failure GI: Abdominal discomfort Contraindications: Severe hypotension or cardiogenic shock; second- or third-degree A-V block and sick sinus syndrome in absence of ventricular pacemaker; severe CHF unless etiology is supraventricular tachycardia; should not be given within a few hours of administration of IV beta blockers because both depress A-V conduction and have a negative inotropic effect; not recommended to be used with disopyramide because risk of heart failure increases Other considerations: Because effect may be prolonged in clients with renal or hepatic problems, caution must be taken with repeat injections	Constant monitoring of ECG pattern and blood pressure during IV administration; assess effects and side effects; have resuscitative equipment and drugs available

through the ventricles, as occurs with a bundle-branch block, which may produce a longer QRS complex).

Sinus Dysrhythmia

Sinus dysrhythmia is different from normal sinus rhythm only in the variation in the distance between the P waves (Figure 24–2). Most frequently, sinus dysrhythmia is seen in normal persons with slower heart rates that vary with respiration. The rate increases during inspiration and decreases with expiration. The P waves (and associated QRS complexes) are closer together during inspiration and further apart during expiration. Sinus dysrhythmia causes the pulse rate to vary slightly with breathing. There is no treatment for sinus dysrhythmia.

Sinus Tachycardia

The electrocardiographic difference between sinus tachycardia (Figure 24–3) and normal sinus rhythm is in the rate. The distance between P waves (and associated QRS complexes) is less than 15 small squares, which produces a heart rate of over 100.

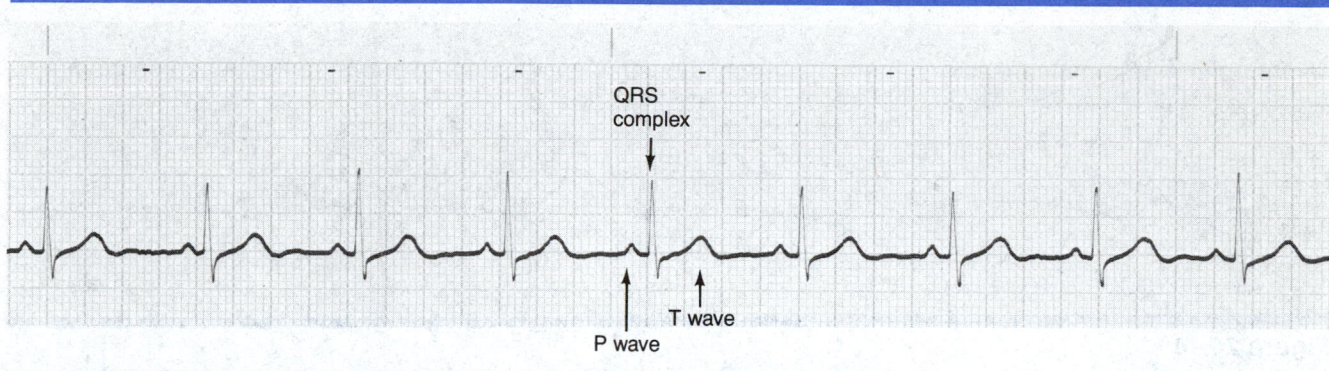

Figure 24–1

Normal sinus rhythm.

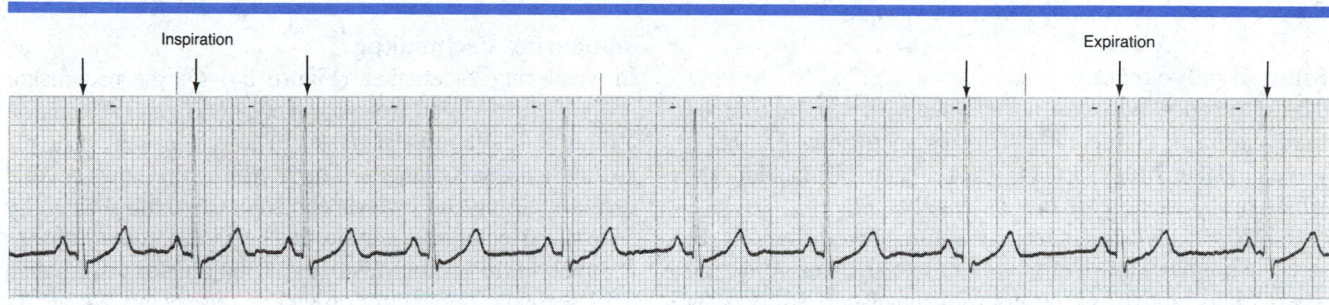

Figure 24–2

Sinus dysrhythmia. The heart rate varies with respiration, increasing during inspiration and slowing during expiration. Check the distance between the first three arrows and the last three arrows.

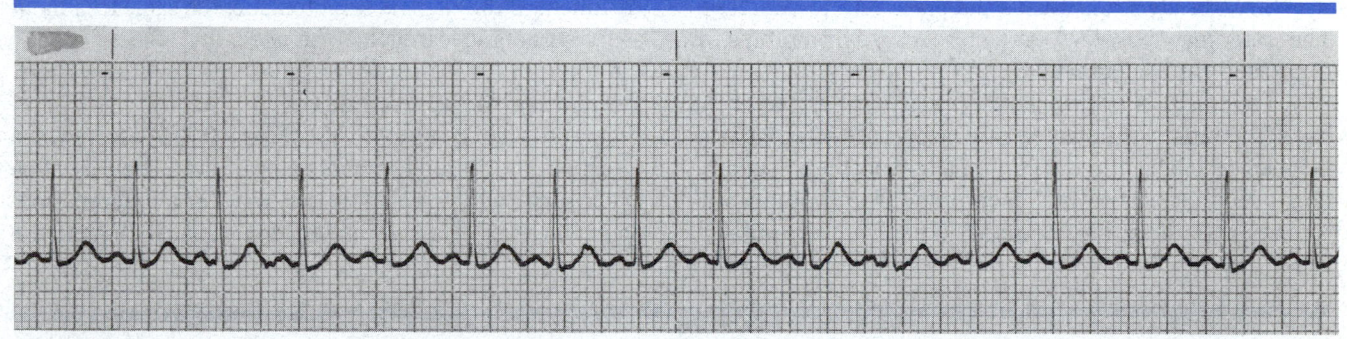

Figure 24–3

Sinus tachycardia. The heart rate is 130 beats per minute. Each complex has a P wave and QRS indicating a sinus tachycardia.

Normally, the most common cause of sinus tachycardia is physical exercise. Depending on age and physical condition, an individual may increase the heart rate as high as 160 to nearly 200 beats per minute without problems. In the diseased heart, as the heart rate is increased past the physiological limit, the ventricles do not have sufficient time to fill with blood, and cardiac output decreases. Decreased output may result in myocardial ischemia and lead to more serious dysrhythmias. Other causes of sinus tachycardia include removal of parasympathetic stimulation (such as with atropine and other vagolytic drugs); increase

in sympathetic nervous system stimulation such as with fear or with administration of adrenergic drugs; use of stimulants such as nicotine, caffeine, and alcohol; and pathological conditions such as fever, anemia, hypovolemia, and heart failure.

Sinus tachycardia causes the pulse rate to increase. In the diseased heart as the rate increases to the point that cardiac output is diminished, a weak pulse will reflect the decreased stroke volume.

Treatment is usually to remove the cause. In some cases, such as when the client is symptomatic, drugs may

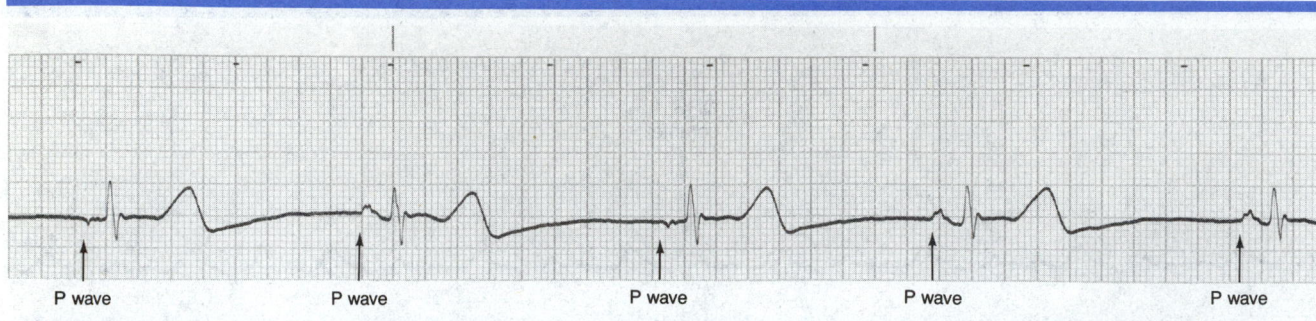

Figure 24—4

Wandering pacemaker. P wave changes are seen in height and direction. The PR interval also varies.

be used (eg, propranolol, which blocks the effects of beta-adrenergic activity, or verapamil, a calcium channel blocker that decreases automaticity in the S-A node).

Sinus Bradycardia

The difference between normal sinus rhythm and sinus bradycardia is in the rate. The distance between the P waves in sinus bradycardia is greater than 25 small blocks, which produces a heart rate of less than 60.

Sinus bradycardia normally occurs in well-trained athletes, who may have heart rates as low as 35 or 40 during sleep. Sinus bradycardia occurs with stimulation of the vagus nerve, such as during vomiting or straining at defecation, as well as with the administration of parasympathetic drugs, beta-adrenergic blocking drugs, and calcium channel blocking drugs. It also occurs with increased intracranial or intraocular pressure as well as in some disease states.

Sinus bradycardia causes the pulse rate to decrease. The rate may be slow enough to cause symptoms of decreased cardiac output.

Treatment is not usually necessary unless the client has symptoms of insufficient cardiac output. Atropine may be used to inhibit the effects of parasympathetic stimulation, which slows the heart. Isoproterenol or another sympathomimetic drug may be used. When the sinus brady-

cardia is chronic and the client has symptoms, a pacemaker may be indicated.

Wandering Pacemaker

In wandering pacemaker (Figure 24—4), the pacemaker shifts back and forth from the sinus node to an area in the atrium or the junctional tissue. The rate usually changes as the pacing site changes. The rhythm strip shows several cycles meeting the criteria for sinus rhythm followed by several cycles of a slower rhythm, with different or absent P waves with PR intervals that may be greater or less than 0.12 seconds, depending on where the pacing site is. As the heart rate increases, the pacing site reverts to the sinus node.

A wandering pacemaker may be normal in the very young or very old and in athletes when the heart rate is slowed from increased vagal tone. Generally, there is no treatment. If the client is symptomatic, the same treatment as for sinus bradycardia may be used.

Premature Atrial Complexes

Premature atrial complex (PAC) (Figure 24—5) occurs when an area in the atrium promotes a premature depolarization of the atria, which results in a P wave of a different configuration than P waves of the dominant rhythm. If the

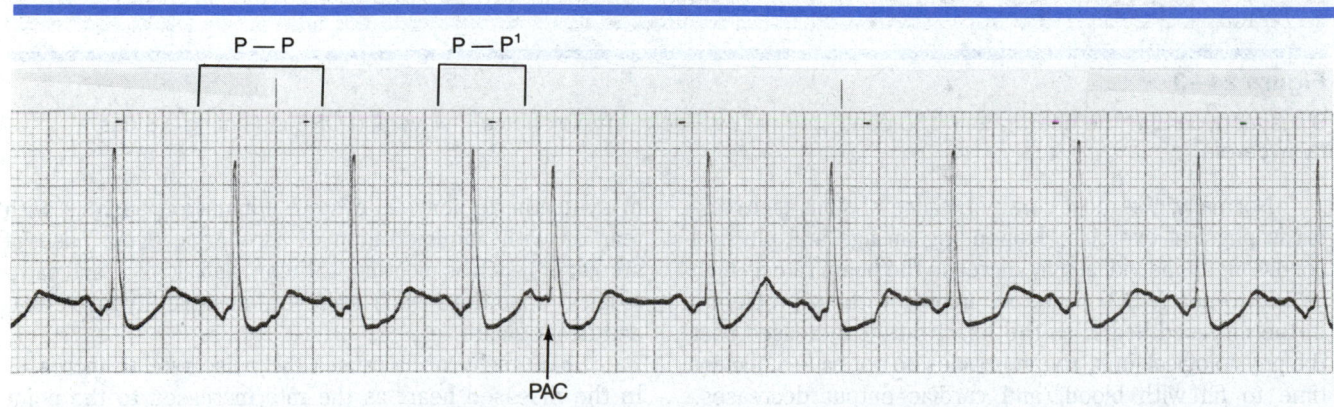

Figure 24—5

Premature atrial complexes. The 5th beat is a premature atrial contraction. Note that the P–P' interval is shorter than the P–P interval. The P' wave is partially buried in the preceding T wave. The QRS is normal.

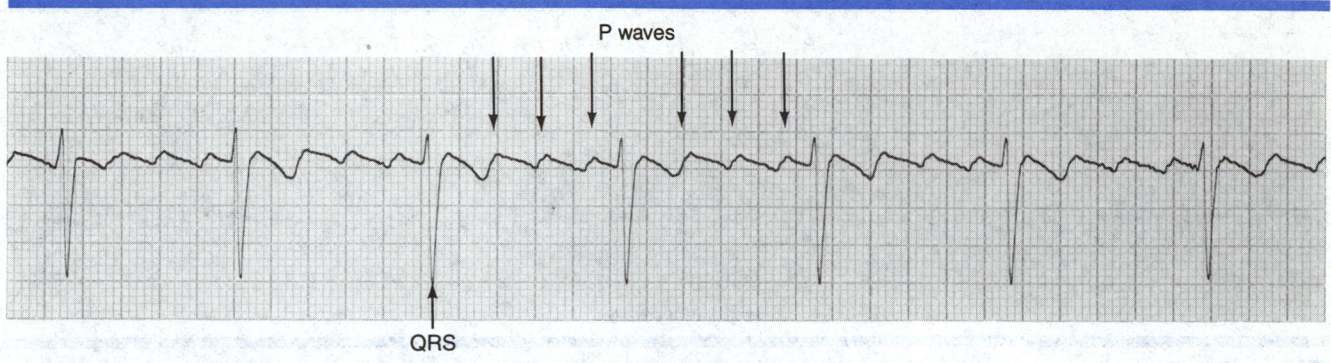

Figure 24-6

Atrial flutter. In atrial flutter the ECG forms a sawtooth pattern of P waves on the baseline.

impulse is conducted through the A-V junctional area, resulting in a QRS complex to follow, the PR interval is greater than 0.12 seconds. Because PACs usually result in depolarization of the sinus node, the sinus node has to reset its rhythm, and the subsequent normal sinus impulse comes later than expected. There is a pause after the premature P wave. Because the pause is usually not long enough for the normal P wave to occur where it originally would have, the pause is called *noncompensatory*. Sometimes, PACs are not conducted through the A-V junctional tissue and are called blocked PACs.

The etiology of PACs is the same as those of many dysrhythmias, including ischemia, drug effects, stimulants, and stretching of the atrial tissue. Persons with normal hearts may have PACs and note palpitations from them. With PACs, the major concern is that they sometimes promote the development of more severe dysrhythmias, including supraventricular tachycardia and atrial fibrillation. Treatment is not usually necessary. If prone to supraventricular tachycardia, the client may be given digitalis, which slows conduction through the A-V node; propranolol, which inhibits the effects of sympathetic stimulation; or verapamil, which slows conduction through the A-V node. Other drugs used to decrease conduction and automaticity in atrial tissue include quinidine, procainamide, or disopyramide (see Table 24-3).

Atrial Flutter

Atrial flutter (Figure 24-6) is characterized by sawtooth or flutter P waves. The atrial rate (P wave rate) is usually between 250 and 350 beats per minute. Because the A-V node has a physiological limit that will not usually conduct more than 200 impulses per minute, atrial flutter causes a physiological block, resulting in every other flutter wave being conducted through the A-V node. If the problem is untreated, the rate of the QRS complex is one-half that of the atrial rate. If treated, the flutter rate may be less than 250. The rate of impulses conducted will usually be an even number such as 2:1 or 4:1.

Persons with normal hearts experience occasional atrial flutter, but persistent atrial flutter is usually indicative of heart disease. Causes of atrial flutter include conditions that cause the atria to stretch, such as mitral or tricuspid stenosis or regurgitation, pulmonary emboli, MI, or ventricular failure. Other conditions such as thyrotoxicosis, alcoholism, and pericarditis may cause atrial flutter.

The goals of therapy include terminating the rhythm or controlling the ventricular response as well as determining and treating the cause of the dysrhythmia. Direct current (DC) synchronous cardioversion is often effective in terminating the rhythm or converting it to atrial fibrillation, which is less dangerous because of a slower ventricular response. Drugs that block conduction through the A-V node (eg, digitalis, verapamil, and propranolol) may be used to control the ventricular response. Long-term management of atrial flutter includes the use of class 1 antidysrhythmic drugs, including quinidine, procainamide, or disopyramide in combination with digitalis (see Table 24-3).

Atrial Fibrillation

Atrial fibrillation (Figure 24-7) is characterized by an irregularly irregular QRS rhythm with QRS complexes occurring at a rate of between 100 and 150 in the untreated client. P waves are indistinguishable and may be represented by an undulating baseline or fine fibrillatory waves. The atrial rate is between 350 and 600, is chaotic, and does not support complete atrial contraction.

Atrial fibrillation may be experienced by persons with normal hearts, but chronic atrial fibrillation is usually indicative of heart disease. The causes of atrial fibrillation are the same as those of atrial flutter. Atrial fibrillation is considered less dangerous because it will not support as rapid a ventricular rate as atrial flutter. The stimulation of the A-V node is chaotic, and most stimulations are not capable of propagating an impulse because of the physiological limits of the A-V node. Atrial fibrillation does not support atrial contraction. Therefore, because of the nature of the blood flow through the atria, clot formation and subsequent release of emboli when the rhythm is corrected are potential problems. The treatment of atrial fibrillation is much the same as for atrial flutter.

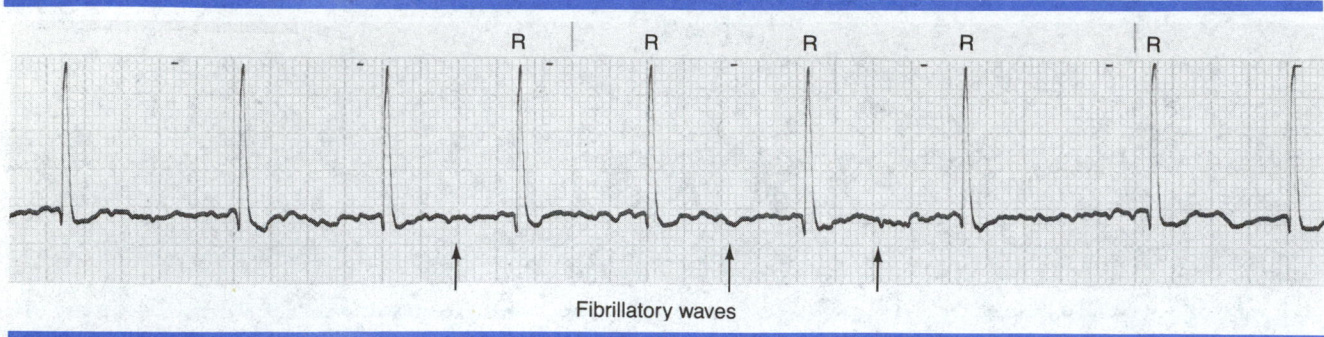

Fibrillatory waves

Figure 24–7

Atrial fibrillation. Atrial activity is manifested as fibrillatory waves—rapid, small, irregular waves. Note the varying R–R intervals. The ventricular rhythm is irregular.

Supraventricular Tachycardia

Supraventricular tachycardia includes any tachycardia in which the tissue responsible for pacing the heart is above the ventricles (above the bifurcation of the bundle of His). Supraventricular tachycardia promotes a ventricular rate between 150 and 250. The classification of supraventricular tachycardia includes sinus, atrial, and junctional tachycardia as well as tachycardia resulting from atrial flutter or atrial fibrillation. A tachycardia originating in the S-A node or atria should have a P wave before every QRS complex and a PR interval greater than 0.12 seconds. Junctional tachycardia may produce a P wave before the QRS complex with a PR interval less than 0.12 seconds. Or the P wave might be buried in the QRS complex or come after the QRS complex. This classification is useful because extremely fast rates may cause the P wave to be buried in the T wave or QRS complex in atrial tachycardia, and a P wave that comes after the QRS in a tachycardia originating in the junctional tissue may look like an atrial P wave. Other maneuvers or specific ECG studies may be done to determine the origin of the tachycardia. The differentiation of supraventricular tachycardia from ventricular tachycardia becomes a problem when the conduction through the ventricles is slowed and the QRS complex becomes longer than 0.12 seconds.

Although persons with normal hearts may experience supraventricular tachycardia, most supraventricular tachycardia is associated with heart disease. The causes of supraventricular tachycardia are the same as those described under atrial flutter and sinus tachycardia.

The goals of therapy are to terminate the rhythm if possible or to slow down the ventricular response. The physician might massage the carotid sinus or apply pressure to the eyeballs to increase parasympathetic activity to terminate the rhythm, or decrease the ventricular response. The client might be encouraged to promote vagal nerve stimulation by gagging or simulating a diving reflex by dipping the head into cold water. Other treatment includes all the modalities discussed under atrial flutter: DC synchronous cardioversion to terminate the rhythm and administration of digitalis, verapamil, propranolol, quinidine, procainamide, or disopyramide. Sometimes a pacemaker is inserted, and in some cases, surgery is performed to remove accessory pathways (see Chapter 25).

Premature A-V Junctional Complexes

Premature A-V junctional complexes (PJCs) (Figure 24–8) may originate in tissues other than in the atria, as described for PACs. If they originate in the junctional tissues, which include the low atrium, A-V node, or bundle of His, they

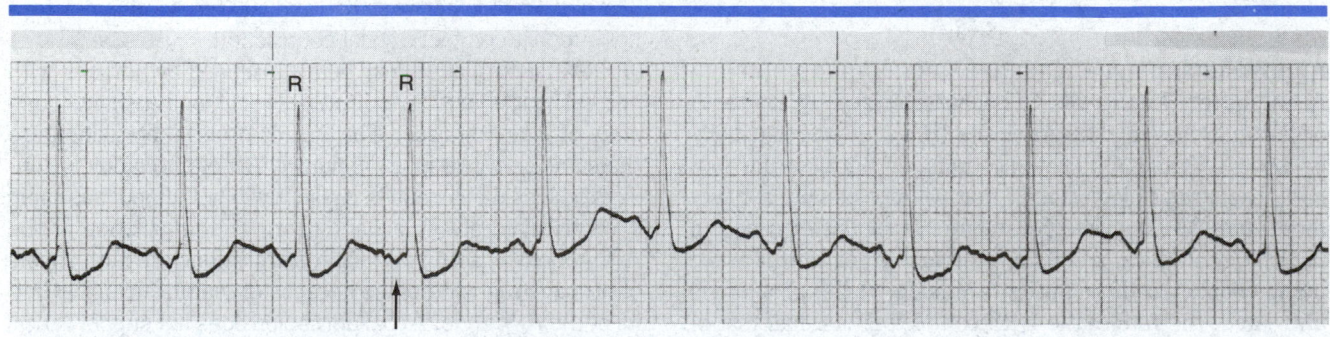

Figure 24–8

Premature A–V junctional complexes. The 4th beat is a premature A–V junctional beat. Note the atrial wave is inverted with a short PR interval. The R–R interval is short, indicating the premature beat.

are called premature A-V junctional complexes. PJCs, like PACs, cause an irregularity in the pulse. The PJC may produce a pulse wave that is less full and earlier than expected. The PJC may occur early enough in the cardiac cycle so the heart does not have sufficient time to fill and the cardiac contraction does not eject sufficient blood to produce a pulse wave. The pulse wave following the PJC may be much fuller because of sufficient time to fill the heart between the premature contraction and the contraction that follows.

The major ECG feature distinguishing PJCs from PACs is the P wave and the PR interval. If the PJC stimulates retrograde (backward) conduction through the atria, it will produce a retrograde P wave on the rhythm strip and interrupt the sinus mechanism, producing a noncompensatory pause as the sinus mechanism is reset. If the PJC does not promote retrograde conduction, the normal sinus mechanism will not be interrupted, and a compensatory pause will occur after the PJC; ie, the next sinus-stimulated complex will occur at the time it normally should. If the PJC does produce retrograde conduction, the P wave may precede, be buried in, or come after the QRS complex. If the P wave comes before the QRS complex, the PR interval will be less than 0.12 seconds.

PJCs are much less common than PACs and premature ventricular complexes both in persons with and without heart disease. They usually require no treatment unless they initiate ventricular dysrhythmias such as ventricular tachycardia. If they do initiate ventricular tachydysrhythmias, the ventricular dysrhythmia is treated.

A-V Junctional Rhythm

The A-V junctional tissue may take over the pacemaking activity of the heart when the sinus node fails as a pacemaker, sinus node rate is less than the automatic rate of depolarization of the junctional tissue, or the sinus impulses are blocked from passing through the A-V junctional tissue. The junctional rate is normally between 35 and 60 beats per minute. A-V junctional rhythm (Figure 24–9)

may normally occur in response to the effects of vagal tone or in disease states that produce sinus bradycardia or A-V block. The pulse rate with A-V junctional rhythm is between 35 and 60 beats per minute.

The ECG features of A-V junctional rhythm include a fairly regular QRS rate between 35 and 60 with a normal QRS configuration. Normal P waves may be present and may occur at a rate faster or slower than the QRS rate. If the A-V junctional complexes produce retrograde conduction, the P waves produced may precede, be buried in, or come after the QRS complexes. If the P wave comes before the QRS complex, the PR interval will be less than 0.12 seconds. The P waves resulting from the junctional pacemaker may interrupt the rhythm of the P waves produced by the sinus mechanism.

Treatment is not necessary unless the client has symptoms of insufficient cardiac output. Atropine may be used to increase the heart rate by decreasing parasympathetic (vagal) activity. If atropine is not successful, isoproterenol (a sympathomimetic drug) may be used. If atropine and isoproterenol are unsuccessful or contraindicated, an artificial pacemaker may be inserted.

Premature Ventricular Complexes

When an area in the ventricle promotes a premature depolarization of the ventricles, it is called a premature ventricular complex (PVC) (Figure 24–10). PVCs, like PJCs and PACs, cause an irregularity in the pulse. The PVC may also produce a pulse wave that is less full and earlier than expected. The PVC may also occur early enough in the cardiac cycle so the heart does not have sufficient time to fill and the heart contraction does not eject sufficient blood to produce a pulse wave. The pulse wave that follows the PVC may be much fuller because of sufficient time to fill the heart between the premature contraction and the contraction that follows.

The major ECG feature distinguishing PVCs from PJCs and PACs is a wide, bizarre-looking QRS complex (greater than 0.12 seconds), not preceded by a P wave, with a T

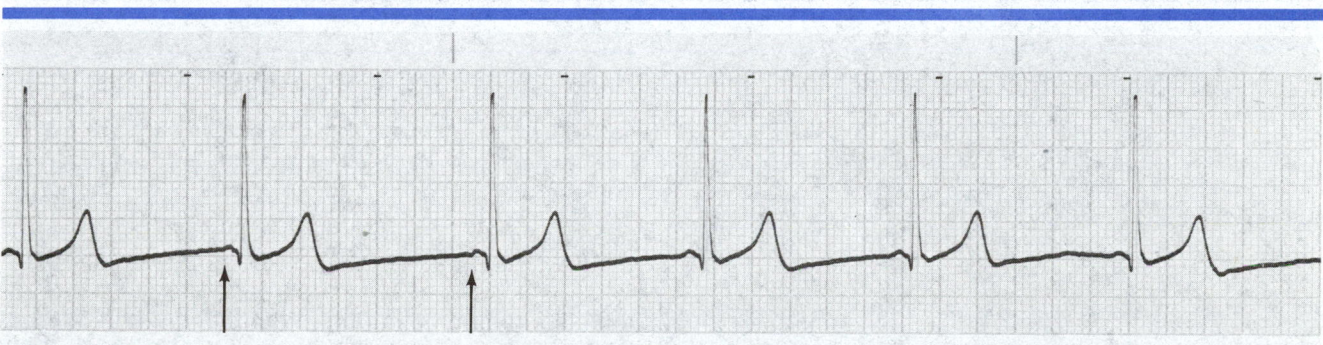

Figure 24–9

A–V junctional rhythm. The PR interval is 0.05 sec indicating a retrograde atrial conduction. Note that the QRS complexes are normal since ventricular conduction follows the normal pathways. The heart rate is 48 beats per minute, which is within the inherent pacemaker rate for the junctional tissue.

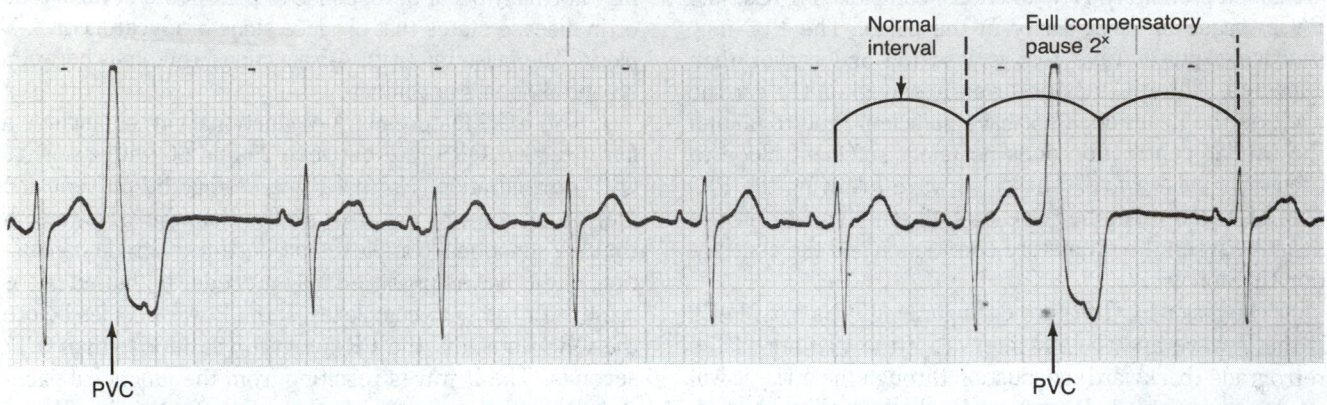

Figure 24–10

Premature ventricular complexes. The second and ninth beats are PVCs. Note that the QRS is greater than 0.12 sec, the R–R interval is shorter than the following beats, atrial depolarization follows the wide QRS, and a complete compensatory pause is present. A complete compensatory pause exists when the R–R interval containing the PVC is two times the R–R interval of the basic rhythm.

wave that usually is inscribed in the opposite direction of the major deflection of the QRS. PVCs recorded on a rhythm strip cannot be distinguished with certainty from either PJCs or PACs that are conducted aberrantly through the ventricles and also produce wide, bizarre QRS complexes. Generally, the PVC does not travel retrograde through the atria. As a result, the pause following the PVC is usually compensatory because the normal sinus node is not interrupted and maintains its rhythmicity. Sometimes the PVC does stimulate retrograde (backward) conduction through the atria and produces a retrograde P wave on the rhythm strip, interrupts the sinus mechanism, and produces a noncompensatory pause as the sinus mechanism is reset. If the PVC produces retrograde conduction, the P wave may precede, be buried in, or come after the QRS complex. If the P wave comes before the QRS complex, the PR interval will be less than 0.12 seconds.

PVCs are the most common type of rhythm disturbance and occur both in health and disease. They may cause discomfort in the neck or chest or palpitations. The frequency of PVCs increases with age. The causes of PVCs include ischemia, injury, drugs, caffeine, nicotine, alcohol, electrolyte imbalance, and extremes in heart rate. PVCs are of most concern in clients in the coronary care unit because they often presage more dangerous ventricular dysrhythmias.

Treatment may be to increase or decrease the heart rate if the PVCs are associated with extremes in heart rate. The initial therapy for PVCs in hospitalized clients is intravenous lidocaine. Other antidysrhythmic agents include procainamide, quinidine, disopyramide, propranolol, and phenytoin (see Table 24–3).

Ventricular Tachycardia

When three or more PVCs occur in a row at a fairly regular rate of 110 to 250, the dysrhythmia is called ventricular tachycardia (Figure 24–11). Ventricular tachycardia may occur in people with healthy hearts and produce no symp-

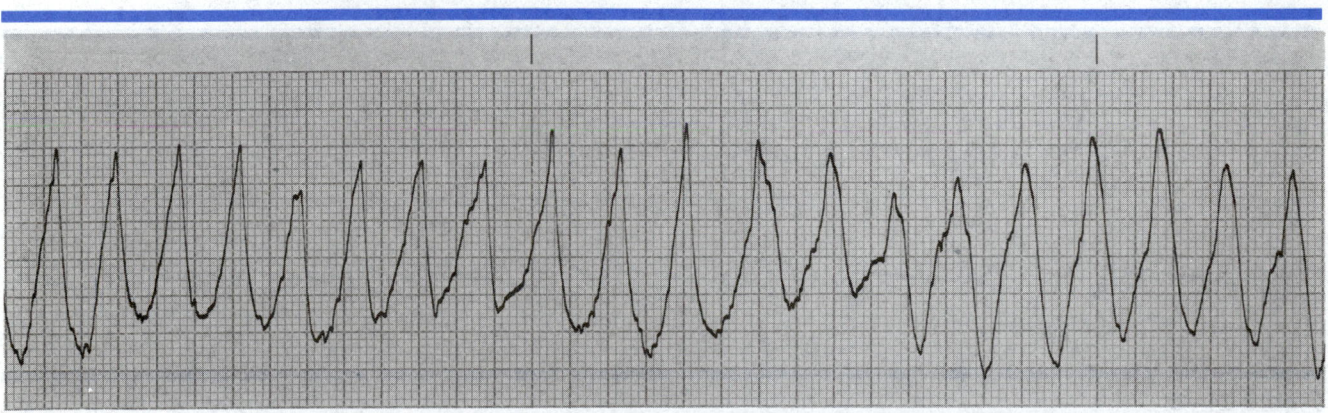

Figure 24–11

Ventricular tachycardia. With ventricular tachycardia a rapid succession of ventricular ectopic beats is seen on the ECG. The QRS complexes are wide and bizarre.

toms. Ventricular tachycardia may be a life-threatening dysrhythmia in people with heart disease, especially if the dysrhythmia is sustained.

Persons who have ventricular tachycardia that is not sustained and produces no symptoms are not treated pharmacologically but are followed closely by their physician. The usual first line of therapy for persons with ventricular tachycardia who have heart disease or are symptomatic is intravenous lidocaine. Procainamide or bretylium may be used if lidocaine is unsuccessful (Table 24–3). An artificial pacemaker is inserted if pharmacological therapy is unsuccessful (see Chapter 25). DC countershock may be used if the client is hemodynamically unstable.

Ventricular Fibrillation

Ventricular fibrillation (Figure 24–12) is a chaotic rhythm in which the ventricles produce completely disorganized depolarization and repolarization waves. Ventricular fibrillation is usually a terminal event associated with coronary artery disease. It may also be caused by ischemia, pharmacological agents, electrical shock, and other dysrhythmias. The ECG features of ventricular fibrillation include irregular waveforms that vary in size. There are no distinguishable P waves, QRS complexes, ST segments, or T waves.

Because of the electrical disorganization, the ventricles do not contract as a unit, and there is no cardiac output. Ventricular fibrillation is a life-threatening dysrhythmia and usually will result in death if it is not treated within 3 to 5 minutes. DC countershock should be instituted as soon as possible. Cardiopulmonary resuscitation should be performed until the equipment is ready and continued as long as there is no effective rhythm.

First-Degree A-V Block

First-degree A-V block (Figure 24–13) is a delay in the transmission of impulses from the atria to the ventricles. All of the impulses reach the ventricles, which distinguishes first-degree block from the other forms of A-V heart block. The delay may be in the A-V node or the tissues beneath the A-V node.

First-degree A-V block may be observed in normal persons. Causes of first-degree heart block include pharmacological agents, heart disease, hypoxia, congenital heart disease, lesions or calcifications of the conducting system, and other diseases affecting the heart.

The ECG feature that indicates first-degree heart block is a PR interval greater than 0.20 seconds with a QRS following every P wave. There is usually no treatment for first-degree A-V block, but attention is given to determining the cause and observing for progression to second- or third-degree heart block.

Second-Degree A-V Block

Second-degree A-V block (Figures 24–14 and 24–15) is characterized by some impulses being conducted from the atria to the ventricles and some impulses not being conducted. The client may notice skipped heart beats. The

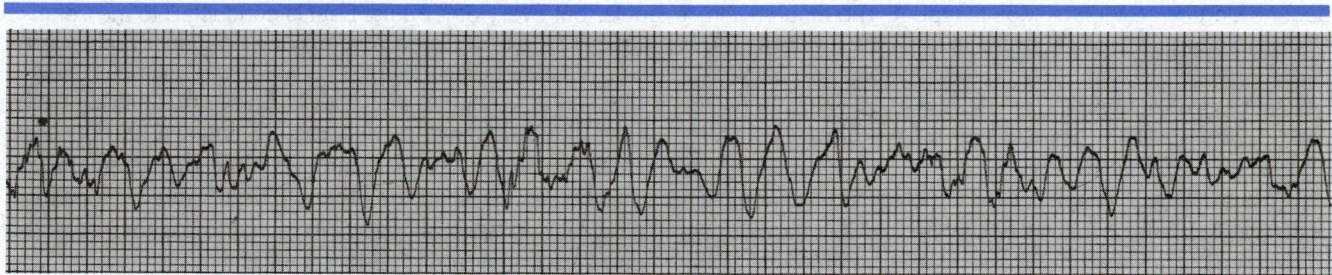

Figure 24–12

Ventricular fibrillation. Irregular wave forms occur that vary in size. There are no distinguishable P waves, QRS complexes, ST segments, or T waves. The rhythm is chaotic.

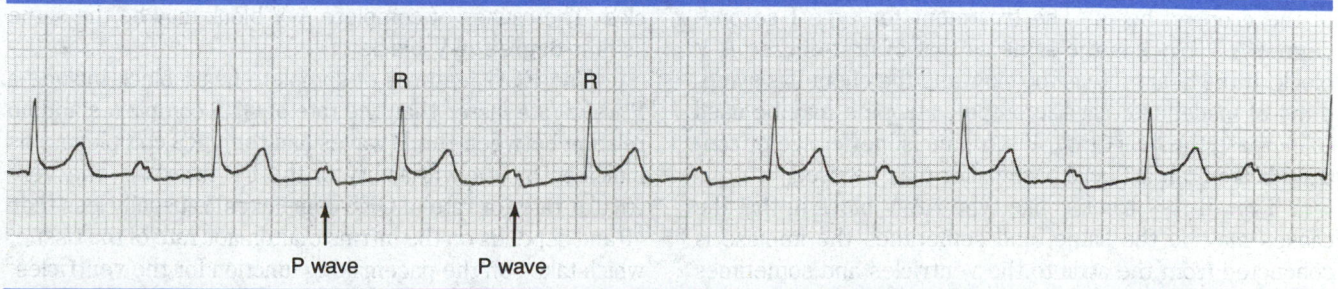

Figure 24–13

First degree atrioventricular (A–V) block. The PR interval is prolonged (0.40 sec). Each complex has a P wave and QRS. The rhythm is regular.

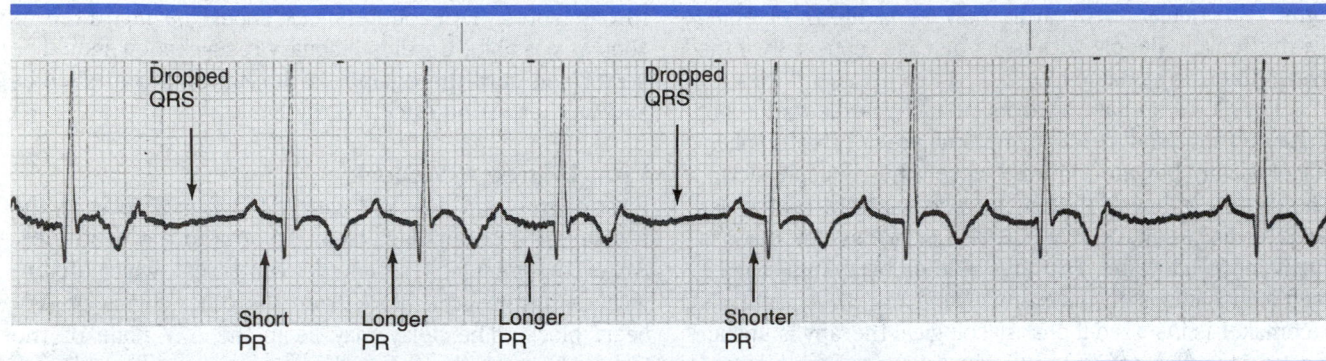

Figure 24–14

Second degree A–V block Mobitz type I. The atrial rhythm is regular, the P–P intervals are equal, but every fourth atrial beat is blocked and a ventricular beat (QRS) is dropped. The PR interval becomes progressively longer until the ventricles fail to beat. Then the cycle begins again.

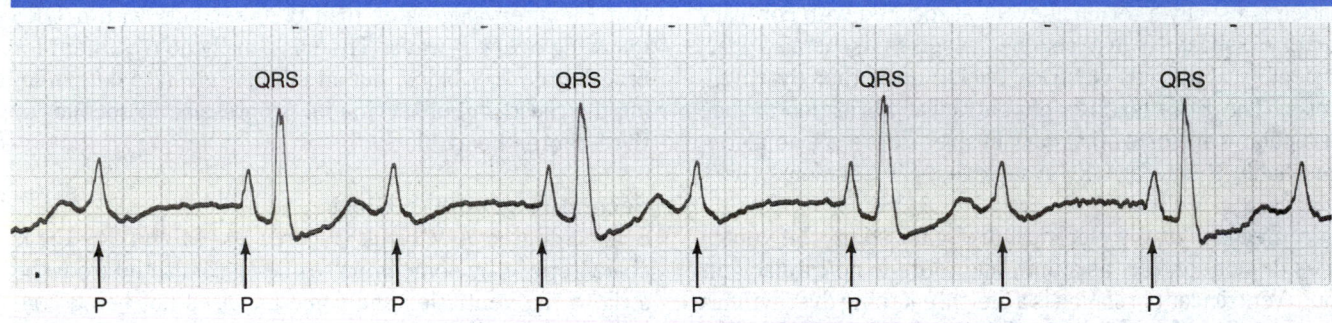

Figure 24–15

Second degree A–V block Mobitz type II. The atrial rhythm is regular but every other atrial beat is conducted to the ventricles. Therefore, every QRS complex has two P waves. The PR interval of the conducted beat may be normal or prolonged.

causes of second-degree A-V block are the same as those of first-degree block. Second-degree A-V block is divided into type I and type II.

Mobitz type I A-V block, also referred to as Wenckebach, is the most common of the two. ECG characteristics of type I include a progressive lengthening of the PR intervals (the PR interval gets longer and longer with each cycle) and a progressive shortening of the RR intervals (the distance between QRS complexes gets closer from one complex to the next) followed by a P wave with no subsequent QRS complex (a dropped beat). The P rate is regular, and the QRS rate is less than the P rate because of the dropped beats. The treatment for type I second-degree A-V block is the same as that of first-degree A-V block. If the heart rate is too slow and the client has symptoms of inadequate cardiac output, atropine may be used to increase the heart rate. If atropine is ineffective or contraindicated, an artificial pacemaker may be used.

Type II A-V block is like type I A-V block in that the causes may be the same, and sometimes the impulse is conducted from the atria to the ventricles and sometimes it is not. Type II block is different from type I in that type II is considered more serious because the block is usually lower in the conductive system and more frequently pro-

gresses to complete A-V block. Electrocardiographically, type II is different in that the PR interval is constant, except that the first PR interval after the dropped beat may be shorter than the others. The RR interval does not change as it does in type I. An artificial pacemaker is the usual treatment for type II A-V block.

Complete A-V Block

Complete A-V block (Figure 24–16), sometimes referred to as third-degree A-V block, occurs when none of the impulses conducted through the atria reaches the ventricles. The causes of complete A-V block may be the same as first-degree A-V block.

The ECG features of complete heart block include a P wave rate faster than the rate of QRS complexes and no relation between the P waves and the QRS complexes, as indicated by the variability of the PR interval. The ventricular rate (or rate of QRS complexes) is usually less than 40 and depends on the intrinsic automatic rate of the tissue, which takes on the pacemaking function for the ventricles. Emergency treatment of complete heart block may be the administration of atropine or isoproterenol to increase the heart rate until an artificial pacemaker can be inserted.

Specific Nursing Measures

When assessing the client for a dysrhythmia, the nurse's major concern is whether the client has a sufficient heart rate to maintain cardiac output. The nurse determines this by the pulse rate; the critical care nurse gathers additional information by assessing on the ECG monitor the QRS complex that immediately precedes the pulse wave. Too fast a rate, or a tachycardia, may be dangerous because the heart may not have enough time to fill. Too slow a rate may be dangerous because cardiac output is determined by stroke volume and heart rate. Any time cardiac output is insufficient, the heart may not be able to supply its own muscle with sufficient nutrients, which may result in more severe dysrhythmias and heart failure.

If the rate is sufficient and the client is relatively stable, further assessment can take place. The nurse determines the regularity of the rhythm and the volume of the pulse. Is the volume of the pulse sufficient? An apical and radial pulse taken simultaneously might show a pulse deficit. An assessment of the radial pulse alone might reveal that some pulse waves are fuller than others. A perceptive nurse might associate these pulse findings with the probability of a rhythm disturbance.

Ask the client how he or she feels. Evaluate level of consciousness and mentation to determine adequacy of cerebral perfusion. Assess capillary refill, skin color and temperature, and pedal pulses to determine adequacy of peripheral circulation.

Several questions may be helpful in assessing the cardiac rhythm from a rhythm strip. Is the rate sufficient for adequate cardiac output? This is determined by the number of QRS complexes per minute, assuming that a pulse wave probably follows each QRS. If not, check the client before proceeding with further assessment because action may be required. If the rate is sufficient and the client is relatively stable, continue with the assessment. To determine origin of the heart rhythm and the atrial contribution to ventricular filling, ask:

- Are there P waves?
- What is their rate?
- What is their rhythm?
- Are the P waves related to the QRS complexes?
- What is the PR interval?
- Is the rhythm one that may decrease cardiac output or lead to serious dysrhythmias?

CORONARY ARTERY DISEASE

The coronary arteries that supply blood to the heart muscle may become diseased and fail to supply sufficient blood to enable the heart to perform its work. Disease of the coronary arteries usually results in obstruction to blood flow. The proximal sections of the major coronary arteries with as much as 80% blockage may continue to supply adequate blood to the heart when a person is at rest (Hurst et al., 1982). Further narrowing or increased activity usually results in ischemia to the heart muscle, however.

Etiology

Coronary artery disease (CAD) resulting from atherosclerosis is the most commonly recognized cause of myocardial ischemia (Hurst et al., 1982). Lipoproteins (substances consisting of both fat and protein) have an important role in the development of atherosclerosis. There are five types of lipoproteins: the chylomicron, very low-density lipoprotein (VLDL), intermediate-density lipoprotein (IDL), low-density lipoprotein (LDL), and high-density lipoprotein (HDL). Chylomicrons and VLDL are composed mainly of triglycerides. LDL is predominantly cholesterol, and IDL is a combination of triglycerides and cholesterol. HDL are composed mainly of protein and are thought to serve a protective function against the development of CAD.

Although the complete cause of atherosclerosis is not known, empirical study has identified risk factors associated with the development of atherosclerosis. Factors that cannot be changed include heredity, sex (males are more prone), and increasing age. Other risk factors include cigarette smoking, elevated blood pressure, hyperlipidemia,

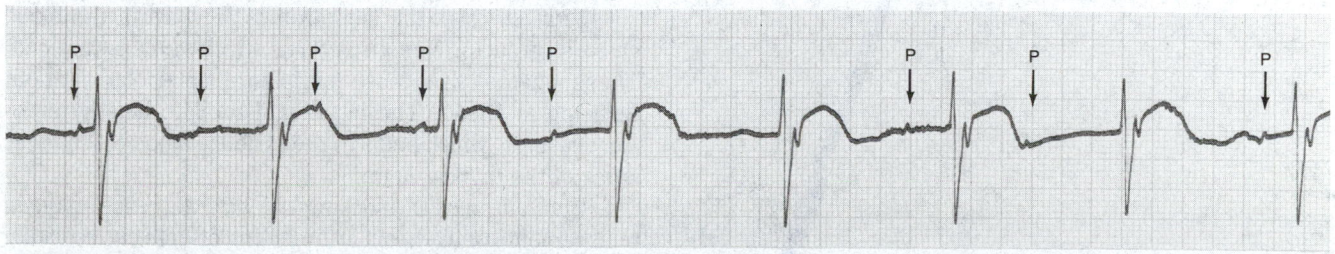

Figure 24–16

Complete A–V block. The atrial rhythm is regular but the P waves appear unrelated to the QRS and often are buried in the T wave or QRS. The QRS is wide (0.12 sec) and the ventricular rate is 52 sec. The underlying rhythm may be a junctional escape rhythm.

obesity, diabetes mellitus, abnormal glucose tolerance, gout, use of oral contraceptives, and a sedentary lifestyle. The relation between personality and CAD is controversial. Other causes of CAD include coronary artery spasms, congenital anomalies, thrombosis, embolism, trauma, inflammation, and external compression, such as that from tumors.

Clinical Manifestations

The person with CAD may never have symptoms of the disease until having a fatal MI. Some persons experience symptoms of heart failure and decrease their activity level. The most common symptom of CAD is **angina,** or chest pain that results from myocardial ischemia.

The pain of angina may last from 30 seconds to 30 minutes. The description of angina differs among individuals. It may be described as a heaviness; a squeezing, viselike pain; or crushing pain over or near the sternum. The pain may radiate into the arms, neck, or jaws. Most commonly, it radiates down the left arm on the side of the little finger (Figure 24–17). Difficulty in breathing may accompany the pain. Angina usually occurs with increased activity or exposure to a cold environment when myocardial oxygen need increases.

Angina is classified into three types: stable (chronic), unstable, and variant (Prinzmetal's) angina. The terms *chronic* or *stable angina* describe angina following increased

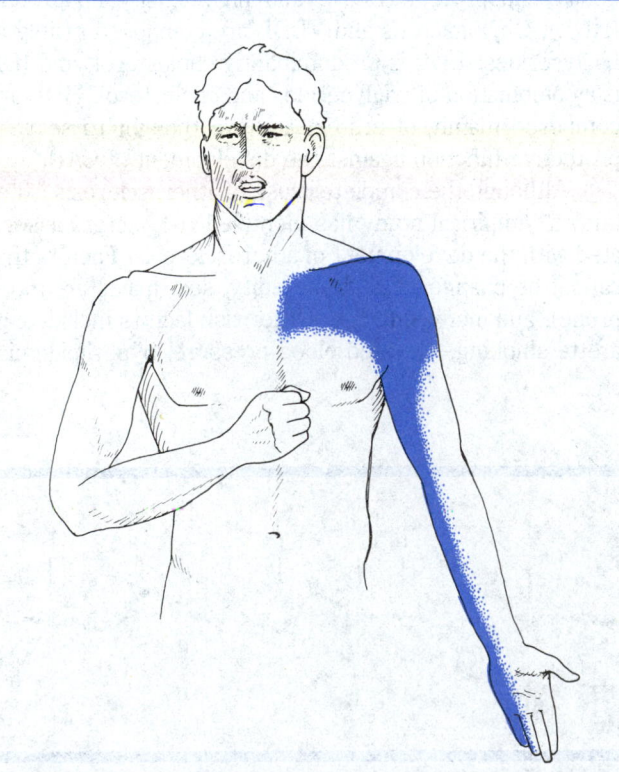

Figure 24–17

Typical pattern of anginal pain, radiating down the left arm on the side of the little finger.

activity, and the symptoms are relatively the same with each occurrence. *Unstable angina* refers to new or worsening angina. Variant or **Prinzmetal's angina** differs from stable angina in that it occurs at rest. Prinzmetal's angina differs from the other forms in that spasms of the coronary arteries occur at the time of the angina. Persons with Prinzmetal's angina may or may not have atherosclerosis of the coronary arteries. Persons with stable and unstable angina usually have atherosclerosis of the coronary arteries.

Persons with severe atherosclerosis or other forms of CAD may have normal resting ECGs. Those with angina usually have changes in the ST segment and the T wave of the ECG either during anginal attacks, as in the case of Prinzmetal's angina, or during stress electrocardiograms in the other forms. Stress ECGs are not usually performed when the client has pain.

After electrocardiographic diagnostic studies, other diagnostic tests may be performed to determine the cause of the angina and the extent of the CAD (see Chapter 23). The ECG may be followed by chest x-ray, cardiac enzyme laboratory studies, thallium perfusion scan, echocardiography, and cardiac catheterization with coronary arteriography and ventriculogram.

Therapeutic Measures

There are six types of hyperlipidemia, also called hyperlipoproteinemia. Dietary management is directed to the specific elevated blood lipid. Table 24–4 summarizes the six hyperlipidemias and the suggested dietary management for each type.

Persons with new angina or worsening angina are admitted to the hospital for treatment of their symptoms and diagnosis of their problems. Because CAD may progress to MI and/or heart failure, the plan of care is directed at relieving symptoms and preventing progression of the disease as well as complications. Management may be medical, surgical, or a combination. Whether the client is treated with medication or surgery, lifestyle modification to diminish risk is of major importance.

Pharmacological management includes the use of nitrates, beta-adrenergic blocking agents, and calcium channel blockers (Table 24–5). The drugs may be used separately or in combination.

Nitrates relax the smooth muscle walls of the blood vessels, reducing venous return, which reduces preload. These agents also cause peripheral arteriolar dilation, reducing afterload. The nitrates also dilate healthy coronary vessels, which helps to redistribute blood to ischemic areas of the myocardium.

Beta-adrenergic blocking agents decrease oxygen requirements of the heart by inhibiting effects of circulating catecholamines on the beta-adrenergic receptors. Propranolol is the best known beta-blocking agent. Blocking effects vary depending on the type of beta receptor

(continued on p. 787)

Table 24–4 Dietary Management of Hyperlipidemia

Type of Hyperlipidemia	Lipoprotein Involved	Lipid Component	Dietary Restriction
I	Chylomicrons	Triglyceride	Reduce total fat intake to less then 20% of total calories; avoid alcohol
IIa	LDL	Cholesterol	Reduce saturated fats, keep cholesterol intake below 300 mg/day
IIb	LDL, VLDL	Cholesterol, triglyceride	Reduce carbohydrate intake to 40% of total calories, avoid sweets; reduce fat intake to 40% of total calories; reduce saturated fats; keep cholesterol intake below 300 mg/day
III	IDL	Triglyceride, cholesterol	Same as for IIb
IV	VLDL	Triglyceride, cholesterol	Reduce carbohydrate intake to 45% of total calories; avoid sweets; reduce saturated fats; keep cholesterol intake between 300 and 500 mg/day
V	Chylomicrons, VLDL	Triglyceride, cholesterol	Reduce carbohydrate intake to 50% of total calories; avoid sweets; reduce saturated fats; reduce total fat intake to less than 30% of total calories; keep cholesterol intake between 300 and 500 mg/day; avoid alcohol

Table 24–5 Antianginal Drugs

Classification (Generic Name, Trade Name)	Route of Administration and Dosage	Actions and Uses	Side Effects and Other Considerations	Nursing Implications
Glyceryl trinitrate, nitroglycerin		Relaxes smooth muscle; reduces venous return which reduces preload; causes peripheral arteriolar dilation which reduces afterload; results in decreased myocardial oxygen consumption		
Sublingual (Nitrostat)	Smallest effective dose (see below by route of administration) One tablet (0.15, 0.30, 0.40, or 0.60 mg) at onset of pain and q. 5 min times 3 if needed; one tablet 5–10 min before engaging in activity likely to result in angina	Use: Prevention, treatment, and management of angina pectoris due to CAD Intravenous forms are used for angina not responsive to other forms; also used for treatment of CHF associated with MI, controlled hypotension during surgical procedures, and control of perioperative hypertension	CNS: Transient headache, faintness, dizziness CV: Hypotension, flushing, increased heart rate GI: Nausea Contraindications: Hypersensitivity to the drug, severe anemia, increased intraocular pressure, increased intracranial pressure; discontinue if blurred vision or drying of mouth occur Drug interactions: May cause hypotension when taken with alcohol	Assess for side effects Client and family teaching, which includes: name of drug; reason drug is prescribed; side effects; need to replace drug supply every 3 mo; need to remove cotton from container (drug is absorbed by cotton); need to keep drug in a cool, dark place; take sublingual form while in a sitting position; take sublingual form at onset of pain and every 5 min until pain is relieved or
Oral (Nitro-Bid capsules, Nitroglyn tablets, Nitrolin capsules, Nitrong tablets, Nitrospan capsules)	One tablet or capsule (2.5, 2.6, 6.5, or 9 mg) two or three times daily			

(continued)

Table 24–5 Antianginal Drugs (continued)

Classification (Generic Name, Trade Name)	Route of Administration and Dosage	Actions and Uses	Side Effects and Other Considerations	Nursing Implications
Transdermal ointments (Nitrol, Nitrong, Nitrostat)	½ in to 4 or 5 in spread on skin q. 8 h; start with ½ in and increase by ½ in with each dose until effective response; average dose is 2 in			three doses are taken; if no relief, notify physician; take sublingual form 5 to 10 min before engaging in activities likely to precipitate angina (eg, sexual intercourse); take oral forms on empty stomach; that alcohol may cause hypotension
Infusion systems (Nitro-Dur, Nitrodisc)	Apply adhesive patch or disc (containing 16, 26, 32, 51, 77, or 104 mg) to a nonhairy or shaved area of the skin; remove and repeat q. 24 h			When to notify physician: If side effects develop; if vision is blurred; if mouth becomes dry
Intravenous (Nitro-Bid, Nitrostat, Tridil)	Dilute (5, 8, 25, or 50 mg/mL) concentrated form to desired strength in 5% dextrose or normal saline solution; start administration of 5 μg/min by infusion pump; titrate by increasing by 5 μg q. 3–5 min up to 20 μg/min; then increase every 3–5 min by 10 μg/min until desired response or change in blood pressure			Intravenous administration: Use glass bottle and special infusion set; if plastic is used, dosage needed will increase significantly because nitroglycerin migrates into plastic; constant hemodynamic monitoring will provide information concerning effects; blood pressure and pulse rate must be assessed to titrate drug
Isosorbide dinitrate				
Sublingual (Isordil, Sorbitrate, Sorate)	One tablet (2.5, 5, or 10 mg) at onset of angina; one tablet 5–10 min before engaging in activity likely to result in angina; one tablet q. 2–3 h to control angina	Relaxes vascular smooth muscle; mechanism of action to reduce anginal pain not known Use: Prevention, treatment, and management of angina pectoris	CNS: Headache, dizziness, faintness CV: Hypotension, flushing Skin: Rash Contraindications: Hypersensitivity to the drug Drug interactions: Can act as a physiological antagonist to norepinephrine, acetylcholine, histamine, and other agents; alcohol may promote hypotension; tolerance to drug and cross-tolerance to nitroglycerin may occur	Assess for side effects Client and family teaching, which includes: name of drug; reason drug is prescribed; side effects; take sublingual or chewable form at onset of pain while in a sitting position; take other oral forms on an empty stomach; that alcohol may cause hypotension When to notify physician: If side effects develop
Chewable (Isordil, Sorbitrate, Sorate)	One tablet (5 or 10 mg) as above for sublingual forms			
Tablets (swallow) (Isordil, Sorbitrate)	One tablet (5, 10, 20, 30, or 40 mg) q.i.d. before meals and at bedtime			
Sustained-release cap-	One tablet or capsule (40 mg) q. 6–12 h			

Classification (Generic Name, Trade Name)	Route of Administration and Dosage	Actions and Uses	Side Effects and Other Considerations	Nursing Implications
sules (Angicon, Iso-Bid, Isordil, Sorate, Sorbide, Sorbitrate)				
Pentaerythritol tetranitrate				
(Peritrate, Duotrate, Pentritol, PETN)	One tablet (10, 20, or 40 mg) before meals two or three times daily One sustained-release capsule (30, 45, 60, or 80 mg) q. 12 h or b.i.d. on empty stomach	Slow-acting nitrate relaxes vascular smooth muscle; mechanism of action not known Use: Prophylactic treatment of angina pectoris	CNS: Headache, faintness, dizziness CV: Hypotension GI: Nausea Skin: Rash Contraindications: Hypersensitivity to the drug; glaucoma Drug interactions: Can act as a physiological antagonist to norepinephrine, acetylcholine, histamine, and other agents; alcohol may promote hypotension; tolerance to drug and cross-tolerance to nitroglycerin may occur	Assess for side effects Client and family teaching, includes: name of drug; reason drug is prescribed; side effects; take on an empty stomach; that alcohol may cause hypotension When to notify physician: If side effects develop, if visual disturbance develops
Erythrityl tetranitrate				
(Cardilate)	One oral/sublingual (5 or 10 mg) tablet sublingually or one chewable (10 mg) tablet 5–10 min before events that precipitate angina One oral/sublingual (5 or 10 mg) tablet swallowed on an empty stomach q. 2–3 h as needed	Relaxes vascular smooth muscle; mechanism of action to reduce angina pain not known Use: Prophylactic and long-term treatment of clients with frequent or recurrent anginal pain	CNS: Headache, dizziness, faintness CV: Hypotension, flushing GI: Nausea Skin: Rash Contraindications: Hypersensitivity to the drug; caution should be taken in clients with severe liver or renal disease Drug interactions: Alcohol may promote hypotension; tolerance to drug and cross-tolerance to nitroglycerin may occur	Assess for side effects Client and family teaching, which includes: name of drug; reason drug is prescribed; side effects; take sublingual or chewable form at onset of angina while in a sitting position; swallow oral/sublingual form on an empty stomach; that alcohol may cause hypotension When to notify physician: If side effects develop
Beta-adrenergic blocking agents		Beta-adrenergic blocking agents inhibit the effects of circulating catecholamines on the beta-adrenergic receptors. Their effect is greatest during surges of sympathetic activity. Some drugs in this class are		

(continued)

Table 24–5	Antianginal Drugs (continued)			
Classification (Generic Name, Trade Name)	**Route of Administration and Dosage**	**Actions and Uses**	**Side Effects and Other Considerations**	**Nursing Implications**
		called cardio-selective because their effects are primarily on the beta 1 receptors in the heart and have less of an effect on the beta 2 receptors Blocking effects vary depending on the type of beta receptor affected. Beta 1 blocking effects: decreased contractility, conduction velocity, and automaticity. Beta 2 blocking effects: vasoconstriction, bronchoconstriction, decreased coronary blood flow		
	(See individual drugs)	Use (not all agents in class approved for all uses): Treatment of hypertension: actual mechanisms causing decreased blood pressure not known but may be related to decreased cardiac output, central effect resulting in decreased sympathetic outflow to the periphery, suppression of renin activity Treatment of angina pectoris due to coronary atherosclerosis: Decreases oxygen requirements of the heart Treatment of cardiac dysrhythmias: Particularly those induced by catecholamines Prophylaxis of migraine (mechanism not established) Management of hypertrophic subaortic stenosis: Control of stress-induced angina, palpitations and syncope; adjunctive therapy for control of tachycardia with pheochromocytoma; prevention of cardiac mortality post-MI	CNS: Mental depression, sleep disturbances, dizziness, weakness CV: CHF, bradycardia, heart block, arterial insufficiency, coldness of the extremities, hypotension, paresthesia, prolongs myocardial ischemia in clients with Prinzmetal's angina Respiratory: Bronchospasm, respiratory distress GI: Nausea, vomiting, diarrhea, cramping, constipation Skin: Rash, alopecia Hematologic: Agranulocytosis, purpura Contraindications: Beta 1 blockade: cardiac failure, cardiogenic shock, bradycardia, greater than first-degree heart block; Beta 2 blockade: bronchial asthma Other considerations: Beta blockade impairs defense of insulin-induced hypoglycemia; beta blockade impairs signs and symptoms of thyrotoxicosis; abrupt withdrawal may have	Thorough drug history; assess effects and side effects Client and family teaching, which includes: name of drug; dosage prescribed; reason drug is prescribed; side effects; if diabetic, may need to have medical plan of care adjusted; drug must be discontinued over several weeks (should not stop taking it abruptly) When to notify physician: If side effects develop; for advice when taking any other drug; if planning to have an anesthetic for surgical procedures

Classification (Generic Name, Trade Name)	Route of Administration and Dosage	Actions and Uses	Side Effects and Other Considerations	Nursing Implications
			rebound effect, which may result in acute angina Drug interactions: May have additive effect when given with catecholamine-depleting drugs	
Propranolol (Inderal)	Oral: One 10- or 20-mg tablet three or four times daily before meals and at bedtime; increase dosage every 3 to 7 days until optimal response; usual total daily dosage is 160 mg/day (comes in 10-, 20-, 40-, 60-, 80-, and 90-mg tablets) Long-acting capsules: One 80-mg capsule daily; increase dosage every 3 to 7 days until optimal response; average is 160 mg daily (comes in 80-, 120-, and 160-mg capsules)	Nonselective beta-adrenergic blocking agent has both beta 1 and beta 2 blocking effects Use: All described above	As above	As above
Nadolol (Corgard)	Oral: One 40-mg tablet daily; increase by one tablet every 3 to 7 days until the heart rate slows (comes in 40-, 80-, 120-, and 160-mg tablets)	Nonselective beta-adrenergic blocking agent has both beta 1 and beta 2 blocking effects Use: Management of hypertension, long-term management of angina pectoris	As above	As above
Calcium channel blockers		Calcium channel blockers inhibit the influx of calcium ions during depolarization of the membranes of cardiac and vascular smooth muscles Exact mechanism of action is not known but actions that relieve angina are related to: dilation of main coronary arteries and arterioles; dilation of peripheral arterioles reducing total peripheral resistance and decreasing myocardial work and oxygen requirements		

(continued)

Table 24–5   Antianginal Drugs (continued)

Classification (Generic Name, Trade Name)	Route of Administration and Dosage	Actions and Uses	Side Effects and Other Considerations	Nursing Implications
		Calcium channel blocking agents also slow atrioventricular conduction and can interfere with the sinus node impulse		
	(See individual drugs)	Use: Management of chronic stable angina and resting angina	CNS: Headache, dizziness, nervousness, mood changes CV: Hypotension, flushing, weakness GI: Nausea Other: Muscle cramps, peripheral edema not related to heart failure Drug interactions: May increase digitalis levels; may have an additive effect on lowering blood pressure when given with antihypertensive agents Contraindications: See individual drugs	Monitor blood pressure; monitor heart rate; assess for side effects Client and family teaching, which includes: name of drug; reason drug is prescribed; side effects When to notify physician: If side effects develop
Verapamil (Calan, Isoptin)	Oral: One 80-mg tablet q. 6–8 h; 240–480 mg daily; increase at daily or weekly intervals until optimal response (comes in 80- and 120-mg tablets)	As above	As above Contraindications: Left ventricular dysfunction, hypotension, second- or third-degree A-V block, sick sinus syndrome in absence of ventricular pacemaker	As above
Diltiazem (Cardizem)	Oral: One 30-mg tablet three or four times daily before meals and at bedtime; increase dosage gradually at 1- or 2-day intervals until optimum response or total daily dose of 240 mg (comes in 30- and 60-mg tablets)	As above; actions similar to verapamil)	As above Contraindications: Hypotension, second- or third-degree A-V block, sick sinus syndrome in absence of ventricular pacemaker	As above
Nifedipine (Procardia)	Oral: One 10-mg capsule three or four times daily; may be increased to 20 or 30 mg three or four times daily until desired effect; usual dose up to 120 mg daily; over 180 mg not recommended	As above; most potent vasodilator of three calcium channel blocking drugs listed; concentration required to produce effects on conduction tissue is not reached because the powerful vasodilating effects are reached first	As above Contraindications: Hypersensitivity to drug	As above

Classification (Generic Name, Trade Name)	Route of Administration and Dosage	Actions and Uses	Side Effects and Other Considerations	Nursing Implications
Other				
Dipyridamole (Persantine)	Oral: One 25-, 50-, or 75-mg tablet three times a day at least 1 h before meals	Increases coronary artery blood flow by selective dilation of the coronary arteries	CNS: Headache, dizziness, syncope CV: Flushing GI: Mild upsets Skin: Rash Other: Weakness Contraindications: None	Assess effects and side effects Client and family teaching, which includes: name of drug; dosage prescribed; reason drug is prescribed; side effects When to notify physician: If side effects develop

affected—beta 1 receptors (cardiac) or beta 2 receptors (bronchial and vascular smooth muscles). The effects of propranolol on the heart include decreased contractility, conduction velocity, and automaticity.

Calcium channel blockers inhibit the influx of calcium ions during depolarization of the membranes of cardiac and vascular smooth muscles. Although the exact mechanism is not known, the drugs have certain actions related to the relief of angina. Among these are dilation of main coronary arteries and arterioles and dilation of peripheral arterioles, which reduces peripheral resistance and decreases myocardial work and oxygen requirements. Calcium channel blocking agents also slow A-V conduction and can interfere with the sinus node impulse.

Surgical treatment depends on several factors including the age, psychological status, and general health of the client. Also considered are diagnostic findings indicating the extent of the disease, the number of coronary arteries involved, the amount of tissue they supply, the placement of the lesions within the coronary artery, and the prognosis for the client with or without surgery.

When only one or two of the coronary arteries are involved and the lesions are easily accessible, percutaneous transluminal coronary angioplasty (PTCA) may be performed. The procedure involves the insertion of a balloon dilation catheter under fluoroscopic guidance into the coronary artery to the site of the lesion. The balloon is then inflated and compresses the plaque. PTCA is discussed in detail in Chapter 25. Sometimes the procedure is not successful, and emergency coronary bypass surgery must be done. The client is prepared for this possibility before the procedure. Coronary bypass surgery is discussed in Chapter 25.

Specific Nursing Measures

Assessing the client's cardiovascular status to determine the effectiveness of medical management and any changes indicating deterioration is essential. Major nursing respon-

sibilities include providing physical and psychological comfort and security; keeping the client and family informed of all treatment approaches, diagnostic studies, and client progress; and providing health teaching and counseling to assist the client and family to adjust to changes in lifestyle that may be necessary for reducing risk factors. Teaching should include information about cigarette smoking, elevated blood pressure, hyperlipidemia, obesity, diabetes mellitus, abnormal glucose tolerance, gout, use of oral contraceptives, sedentary lifestyle, and emotional factors.

The client should be well informed regarding the purpose of medications, side effects, and when to seek medical help. (Nursing implications of antianginal drugs are summarized in Table 24–5.) Clients should be taught to take their nitroglycerin before strenuous activity and before sexual intercourse. Over-the-counter drugs such as diet

Nursing Research Note

Kirby J, Woods S: A study of variation in measurement of doses of nitroglycerin ointment. *Heart Lung* 1981; 10(5): 814–820.

Differences in measuring nitroglycerin ointment were examined. Forty-eight registered nurses participated in the study; each measured out 16 doses of nitroglycerin.

There were statistically significant variations in measurement of doses of nitroglycerin. The influence of fullness was statistically significant only at the ½ in dose level. The difference in brand of ointment in measurement also was statistically significant at all dose levels. One brand was applied more heavily than the other. The results indicate there is an unacceptable variation in measurement of nitroglycerin doses.

Nitroglycerin ointments are manufactured in time-released paper and patches and are good for 24 hours. Nevertheless, some clients still use the ointment at intervals during the day, requiring frequent measurement. Guidelines should be developed for application that incorporate pharmaceutical recommendations and hospital procedure. For maximum effectiveness of the drug, nurses must be consistent in applying nitroglycerin ointment.

pills and decongestants must be avoided because they often will increase the heart rate. No drugs other than those specifically prescribed should be taken without consulting with the physician or pharmacist.

Encouraging the client to follow dietary guidelines requires careful instruction and follow-up. Clients will be instructed to avoid overeating and to eliminate or reduce salt and fat consumption; they may also be advised to lose weight. For clients who feel they cannot eat food without salt, advise them to avoid highly salted foods such as potato chips and ham. Suggest that they remove the salt shaker from the table. Caffeine should also be avoided because it may increase the heart rate.

Encourage obese clients to lose weight slowly according to a reasonable food plan, such as that outlined in Chapter 9. Advise them to avoid crash diets and to strive for nutritional balance. Help them to set a weight goal and to monitor their progress.

Teach clients to avoid any activity that precipitates angina. Moderate mild exercise is encouraged as long as pain is not induced and the exercise periods are balanced with periods of rest. Clients should avoid exercise after meals.

Because nicotine causes vasoconstriction, cigarette smoking is contraindicated and should be discontinued. Extreme cold should also be avoided because of vasoconstriction.

Provide emotional support for these changes in lifestyle. Empathize with the client and indicate that feelings of depression and discouragement are common reactions to changes in health status. Enlist the support of family and significant others in helping the client understand and cope with the condition.

MYOCARDIAL INFARCTION

When blood supply to a portion of the myocardium is inadequate, the cells become ischemic and are injured. If blood supply remains low, the cells die. The death of myocardial cells is the condition called myocardial infarction (MI), or heart attack. The American Heart Association estimates that over one-third of Americans who have heart attacks will die, and most of them will die before they reach the hospital. The average victim does not seek help for about 3 hours after symptoms develop. Many deaths are from disturbances in heart rhythm, or dysrhythmias, that commonly occur within the first few hours after MI.

The vast majority of clients with MI that nurses see will have their MI in the left ventricle. Most MIs occur in the left ventricle and may involve the septum. About one-third of those occurring on the diaphragmatic surface of the left ventricle also involve the right ventricle. About 3.5% of autopsies reveal isolated infarction of the right ventricle. Atrial infarctions sometimes occur with left ventricular infarction and are observed in 7% to 17% of autopsies done for MI. The right atrium is involved more frequently than the left (Braunwald, 1984).

MIs usually result from atherosclerotic CAD. Only about 4% of persons who have an acute MI have no evidence of atherosclerosis of the coronary arteries (Braunwald, 1984). In most clients with MI resulting from atherosclerosis, blood clots form on or adjacent to the atherosclerotic lesion. These clots cause MI by contributing to the occlusion of the coronary arteries (Braunwald, 1984).

Clinical Manifestations

The signs and symptoms of MI include those described for CAD (newly developed chest pain, which may occur with rest or activity; chest pain lasting longer than 5 minutes or not relieved by three tablets of nitroglycerine taken 5 minutes apart; or chest pain accompanied by sweating, shortness of breath, nausea or vomiting, or a feeling of weakness). Some persons have an MI without ever having symptoms (a silent MI).

The diagnosis of an acute MI is made from at least two of the three usual findings: chest pain, ECG changes indicative of MI (newly developed abnormal Q waves), and enzymatic changes in creatine kinase (CK) and lactic dehydrogenase (LDH), discussed in Chapter 23. The location of the Q waves are diagnostic for the location of the infarction. Leads II, III, and aV_F indicate an inferior wall MI of the left ventricle. An extensive anterior wall MI of the left ventricle may produce Q waves in the anterior leads I, aV_L, and V_1 through V_6. When only a portion of the anterior wall is involved, only some of the anterior leads will record Q waves. Abnormal Q waves indicate an MI that is transmural or through the entire wall of the chamber. The location of an MI that does not extend through the entire wall (nontransmural or subendocardial) is diagnosed by ST segment and T wave changes in the same ECG leads when there is also evidence of MI, as indicated by the presence of chest pain, and diagnostic changes in the cardiac enzyme studies.

Therapeutic Measures

Because elevated serum cholesterol and triglyceride levels are important risk factors for atherosclerosis, and atherosclerosis is the main cause of CAD and MI, careful attention to diet is essential. If dietary restriction does not reduce serum cholesterol and/or triglyceride levels, a 2-month trial of a hypolipidemic drug may be prescribed. Table 24–6 reviews the common hypolipidemic drugs.

When the client has an MI, therapeutic management is aimed at relieving client discomfort, preventing and treating complications, promoting healing of the damaged myocardium, and promoting rehabilitation. More recently, in selected persons of those who seek help early enough, early therapeutic management is directed to opening the blocked coronary artery or bypassing the blocked artery to enable enough blood to get to the ischemic area before extensive amounts of myocardial tissue die.

Table 24–6	Hypolipidemic Drugs			
Classification (Generic Name, Trade Name)	Route of Administration and Dosage	Actions and Uses	Side Effects and Other Considerations	Nursing Implications
Nicotinic acid, niacin (Nicolar, Nicobid)	Oral; 1–2 g t.i.d.; start with smaller dose (100 mg t.i.d.) and increase every few days if side effects do not develop	Decreases synthesis of cholesterol and triglycerides; exact mechanism not known Use: When hyperlipidemia is not responsive to diet and weight loss	CNS: Headache GI: Nausea, diarrhea, activation of peptic ulcer, jaundice, liver abnormalities CV: Hypotension Skin: Pruritus, rash, dryness Other: Gout, decreased glucose tolerance	Thorough drug history; assess for side effects Client and family teaching, which includes: name of drug; dosage prescribed; reason drug is prescribed; side effects; need to have liver function and blood glucose laboratory studies done frequently during early therapy When to notify physician: If side effects develop; for advice when taking any other drug
Clofibrate (Atromid-S)	Oral; 2 g daily in divided doses; 1 g b.i.d	Lowers serum lipids; reduces VLDL rich in triglycerides and LDL rich in cholesterol by inhibiting synthesis; exact mechanism not known Use: Treatment of hyperlipidemia when diet and exercise are not effective	CNS: Headache, fatigue, dizziness, weakness GI: Diarrhea, flatulence, cholelithiasis, hepatomegaly, hepatotoxicity Skin: Rash, urticaria, pruritus, dry and brittle hair CV: Chest pain, dysrhythmias GU: Renal toxicity Contraindications: Pregnancy, lactation, hepatic dysfunction, renal dysfunction Interactions: Potentiates action of anticoagulants	Thorough drug history; assess for side effects Client and family teaching, which includes: name of drug; dosage prescribed; reason drug is prescribed; side effects; that drug will be discontinued if not effective within 3 mo; diet and exercise; need to have laboratory studies done periodically to monitor effects of drug; drug contraindicated in pregnancy and lactation When to notify physician: If side effects develop; for advice when taking any other drug
Gemfibrozil (Lopid)	Oral; 600 mg b.i.d. before morning and evening meals	Lowers serum triglyceride levels; lowers VLDL cholesterol concentrations and elevates HDL levels; mechanism of action not firmly established Use: Treatment of persons with very high triglyceride levels when diet and exercise are not effective	CNS: Headache, dizziness, blurred vision, vertigo, insomnia, paresthesia, tinnitis GI: Abdominal pain, epigastric pain, diarrhea, nausea, vomiting, dry mouth, constipation, liver function abnormalities Skin: Rash, dermatitis, pruritus, urticaria	Thorough drug history; assess for side effects Client and family teaching, which includes: name of drug; dosage prescribed; reason drug is prescribed; side effects; that drug will be discontinued if not effective within 3 mo;

(continued)

Table 24–6	Hypolipidemic Drugs (continued)			
Classification (Generic Name, Trade Name)	**Route of Administration and Dosage**	**Actions and Uses**	**Side Effects and Other Considerations**	**Nursing Implications**
			Other: Muscle and joint pain Contraindications: Hepatic dysfunction, renal dysfunction, gallbladder disease Interactions: Potentiates action of anticoagulants	diet and exercise; need to have laboratory studies done periodically to monitor effects of drug; drug interactions When to notify physician: If side effects develop; for advice when taking any other drug
Cholestyramine (Questran)	Oral: 9 g t.i.d. or q.i.d. in a preferred beverage	Lowers serum cholesterol by absorbing and combining with bile acids in the intestines and forming an insoluble complex excreted in the feces; this inhibits cholesterol in the bile acid from being reabsorbed Use: As an adjunct to diet therapy to reduce serum cholesterol in persons with hypercholesterolemia not controlled by diet alone	CNS: Headache, anxiety, dizziness, weakness, syncope, tinnitis GI: Constipation, aggravated hemorrhoids, impaction Skin: Urticaria Respiratory: Shortness of breath Hematologic: Bleeding tendencies Other: Muscle and joint pain, may prevent absorption of fat-soluble vitamins A, D, and K; hyperchloremic acidosis Contraindications: Biliary obstruction Interactions: May interfere with absorption of digitalis glycosides, anticoagulants, thyroxine	Thorough drug history; assess for side effects Client and family teaching, which includes: name of drug; dosage prescribed; reason drug is prescribed; to take other oral drugs 1 h before or 4 h after cholestyramine; to take vitamin supplements; diet and exercise; need to have laboratory studies done periodically to monitor effects of drug When to notify physician: If side effects develop; for advice when taking any other drug
Colestipol (Colestid granules)	Oral: 15–30 g/day in two or four divided doses taken mixed in a preferred beverage	Lowers serum cholesterol by absorbing and combining with bile acids in the intestines and forming an insoluble complex excreted in the feces; this inhibits cholesterol in the bile acid from being reabsorbed Use: As an adjunct to diet therapy to reduce serum cholesterol in persons with hypercholesterolemia not controlled by diet alone	CNS: Headache, dizziness, drowsiness GI: Constipation, aggravated hemorrhoids, impaction, flatulence, abdominal pain, nausea, vomiting, diarrhea Skin: Urticaria Respiratory: Shortness of breath Hematologic: Bleeding tendencies Other: Muscle and joint pain; may prevent absorption of fat-soluble vitamins A, D, and K; hyperchloremic acidosis Interactions: May delay absorption of other drugs being taken	Thorough drug history; assess for side effects Client and family teaching, which includes: name of drug; dosage prescribed; reason drug is prescribed; to take other oral drugs 1 h before or 4 h after cholestipol; to take vitamin supplements; diet and exercise; need to have laboratory studies done periodically to monitor effects of drug When to notify physician: If side effects develop; for advice when taking any other drug

Classification (Generic Name, Trade Name)	Route of Administration and Dosage	Actions and Uses	Side Effects and Other Considerations	Nursing Implications
Dextrothyroxine (Choloxin)	Oral: 4–8 mg daily; start with 1–2 mg daily and increase by 1 or 2 mg daily after each 1 mo of therapy	Stimulates the liver to increase catabolism and excretion of cholesterol, which results in lowered blood cholesterol Use: Adjunct to diet and other measures to reduce serum cholesterol in persons who are euthyroid and are without evidence of organic heart disease	CNS: Headache, insomnia, tremors, nervousness, dizziness, visual disturbances, paresthesia GI: Nausea, vomiting, indigestion, diarrhea, constipation Skin: Acneform eruption CV: Palpitations, dysrhythmias, ischemia, angina, sweating, flushing Other: Muscle pain, menstrual irregularities, iodine poisoning, coryza, salivation, foul breath, weakness Contraindications: Organic heart disease; hypertension; liver disease; kidney disease; pregnancy and lactation Interactions: Potentiates action of anticoagulants	Thorough drug history; assess for side effects Client and family teaching, which includes: name of drug; dosage prescribed; reason drug is prescribed; side effects; need to have laboratory studies done periodically to monitor effects of drug; diet and exercise; drug interactions; effects with pregnancy and lactation When to notify physician: If side effects develop; for advice when taking any other drug
Probucol (Lorelco)	Oral: 250 mg b.i.d.; 500 mg b.i.d.	Increases LDL catabolism and lowers LDL lipoprotein cholesterol; exact mechanism not firmly established Use: Treatment of hypercholesterolemia when diet and exercise are not effective	CNS: Headache, dizziness, paresthesia, syncope GI: Diarrhea, flatulence, abdominal pain, nausea, vomiting Skin: Infrequent CV: Prolongation of Q-T interval, chest pain Hematologic: Eosinophilia Contraindications: Evidence of recent or progressive myocardial damage; not recommended with pregnancy or lactation	Thorough drug history; assess for side effects Client and family teaching, which includes: name of drug; dosage prescribed; reason drug is prescribed; side effects; that drug will be discontinued if not effective within 3 mo; diet and exercise; need to have laboratory studies done periodically to monitor effects of drug; need to have periodic ECG When to notify physician: If side effects develop; for advice when taking any other drug

Of about every 150 persons admitted to coronary care units for suspected MI, only 100 have an MI (Marriott, 1982). The initial goal of promoting comfort is started when the client is first seen, which may be in the ambulance, clinic, or emergency room. Oxygen is provided by nasal cannula at about 2 to 4 L/min, the client is positioned for comfort, and nitroglycerin and morphine or another analgesic are ordered for pain control. Management is then directed to making the diagnosis while preventing complications, monitoring the client for indications of complications, and treating complications early when they occur.

Before the establishment of coronary care units, almost half (47%) of the 30% to 40% of hospital deaths from MI were from dysrhythmias; 43% were from circulatory failure; and the others were from embolism and ruptured ventricle. With coronary care units and ability to control dysrhythmias, the number of inhospital deaths has been reduced by about one-half. The majority of deaths are due to heart failure, cardiogenic shock, cardiac rupture, and papillary muscle dysfunction (Trevino & Massey, 1983). Therapeutic management continues to be directed at the early detection and treatment of dysrhythmias as well as early detection and treatment of the other complications.

Because in many instances, thrombosis is responsible for the complete occlusion of the coronary artery that produces the symptoms, newer therapies attempt to remove the clot as soon as possible after symptoms develop and before ischemia is prolonged enough to cause extensive infarction. Clients who have recently developed symptoms (less than 6 hours), may be candidates for parenteral or intracoronary streptokinase infusion if they have not had recent surgery, are not pregnant, have not had a recent cerebrovascular accident, have no bleeding disorders, and do not have severe hypertension. Streptokinase promotes fibrinolysis and essentially dissolves blood clots.

The client may be taken to the cardiac catheterization laboratory for this procedure. A cardiac catheterization is performed including a left ventriculogram and angiography of the coronary artery not involved. Then nitroglycerin is infused into the involved artery to ensure that the complete occlusion is not the result of coronary artery spasm rather than a blood clot. Streptokinase is then infused into the involved coronary artery first by a bolus and then by continuous infusion. The effects are observed through coronary arteriography about every 10 to 15 minutes. The therapy is completed in about 1 hour and is effective if the coronary artery is opened and left ventricular performance is improved. The atherosclerotic lesion remains at the site. When indicated by coronary anatomy and evaluation of the extent of the CAD, angioplasty may be carried out before transferring the client to the coronary care unit (angioplasty is discussed in Chapter 25). In the coronary care unit, bleeding is a major concern in addition to the usual complications of MI.

In some institutions, the streptokinase is given intravenously, and the client is closely monitored. Later, cardiac catheterization is performed for further diagnosis and treatment.

In some cases, coronary artery bypass surgery may be indicated. The client may be taken to the operating room after the effects of the streptokinase have worn off (several hours) so there is minimal danger of bleeding.

Immediate use of streptokinase with or without angioplasty or coronary artery bypass surgery is not always indicated. These procedures must be done early to prevent extensions of the infarction. The possible benefits must be weighed against the risks for the individual client. When these procedures are not done, the extent of the CAD is either diagnosed just before discharge or about 6 weeks after the MI, depending on the attending physician's determination. In some cases, the CAD involves only one area,

and there is no further myocardial tissue to preserve, so further treatment is not indicated. In other cases, the disease involves other areas of the coronary arteries, and coronary artery bypass surgery may be indicated to prevent further damage. In all cases, measures to prevent progression of CAD are essential.

The usual course of treatment for clients with uncomplicated MI who do not have surgery involves admission to the coronary care unit, bed rest, liquid diet, and continuous monitoring for dysrhythmias and complications. The client and significant others are kept fully informed of the plan of care. During the first day, blood pressure is recorded every hour, and a cardiac assessment for evidence of complications such as heart failure is performed every 2 hours. By the second day, the client is given a soft diet and permitted to use the bedside commode and sit in a chair. Clients are closely observed during increases in activity for any signs of complications.

On the third or fourth day, when the threat of complications is significantly decreased, clients are transferred to a stepdown unit where they may continue to be monitored for dysrhythmias or to a regular medical surgical unit. By this time, a rehabilitation program has usually been started, and clients continue to increase activity while their tolerance to the activity is carefully assessed. Usually, clients are discharged within 10 to 14 days and are allowed to continue a gradual increase in their activity. Clients are usually permitted to return to work part time about 8 to 12 weeks after the MI.

Specific Nursing Measures

The goals of nursing care for a client with MI include relieving discomfort; preventing, detecting, and treating complications; promoting healing; and assisting in the rehabilitation program. The nursing care described under CAD is also applicable to the client with an MI.

The most common complications of MI include dysrhythmias, congestive heart failure, extension of the MI, rupture of a papillary muscle, ventricular septal defect, ventricular aneurysm, pericarditis, and thromboembolism. Thromboembolism can be prevented by having clients move their legs and feet while in bed and push their feet against a footboard. The nurse should be aware of the clinical manifestations of all potential complications and report significant findings to the physician so the medical treatment plan can be adjusted.

By the time clients have reached the general medical unit, their condition is usually stable, and a rehabilitation program has been started. Be especially observant of the client's response to increased activity. Spacing of activities and preventing physical stress are important.

Clients find the move to the unmonitored unit encouraging but also frightening because they are used to constant monitoring. Take extra care to provide an environment in which the client feels safe.

Straining at bowel movements should be avoided by

providing bulk in the diet and use of stool softeners. Foods high in potassium are important because most clients are on diuretics. A diet low in carbohydrates and low in saturated fats may also be necessary, depending on the client's type of hyperlipidemia. Sodium should be restricted for clients with symptoms of heart failure. These dietary modifications are instituted during the client's hospitalization. Most of them will be continued throughout the client's life.

Clients should be given specific exercise instructions for home use based on pre-discharge exercise testing, clinical status, and activity level prior to the MI and during hospitalization. A progressive, individualized program is both physiologically and psychologically beneficial.

Walking is the major component of the early convalescent program. Teach clients to take their own pulses so they can monitor their own heart rate response to exercise. If the client has not had exercise testing prior to discharge, the pulse rate should not exceed 110 to 120 beats per minute with exercise.

In preparing clients for walking activities, tell them to walk on level ground and to avoid hills and steps, walking against the wind, and walking during periods of extreme heat, cold, or high humidity. They should wait at least 2 hours after eating before exercise.

Readiness to resume sexual activity following an MI is often gauged by the client's ability to climb two flights of stairs or walk vigorously around the block without symptoms such as chest pain or tachycardia. Sexual relations must be planned so that sexual activity after alcohol ingestion or after meals is avoided. Nitroglycerin can be used sublingually 5 to 10 minutes before sexual intercourse to prevent angina.

Teaching the client the importance of smoking cessation is another major nursing responsibility. Clients are usually anxious to do all they can to prevent another MI and are willing to embark on any program to improve their health. Nurses should use this opportunity and work to help both client and significant others understand the important lifestyle modifications to prevent future cardiac events. A case study for the client with MI is presented at the end of this chapter.

VALVULAR DISEASE

Diseases of the heart valve result in either stenosis of the involved valve, incompetency of the valve, or a combination. A stenotic valve impedes blood flow forward. An incompetent valve does not close after blood has entered the chamber ahead of it, permitting blood to flow back into the chamber when it should be moving forward. Both stenotic and incompetent valves may lead to heart failure.

Clinical Manifestations and Therapeutic Measures

Most valvular problems require surgical treatment eventually, depending on the client's problems. The American Heart Association recommends secondary prophylaxis for prevention of streptococcal infections for persons who have had rheumatic fever, a common cause of valvular abnormalities. When rheumatic fever is a cause of the valvular problem, the client should take antibiotics continuously. Persons with valvular disease are also given antibiotic therapy for prophylaxis against infective endocarditis before and after dental procedures associated with bleeding, surgery, or procedures involving instrumentation of the genitourinary or gastrointestinal tracts. Specific treatment depends on the valvular abnormality.

Tricuspid Stenosis

Although tricuspid stenosis is usually caused by rheumatic fever, other causes include systemic lupus erythematosus, right atrial tumors, metastatic carcinoid lesions of the tricuspid valve, and congenital malformations. The most common symptoms of tricuspid stenosis include dyspnea and fatigue. Because blood is hindered from flowing from the right atrium into the right ventricle during diastole, a diastolic murmur is heard best at the left sternal border or tricuspid area. Atrial fibrillation may also be present. Medical management includes sodium restriction and diuretics. Eventually, surgical repair or replacement of the valve is indicated.

Tricuspid Insufficiency

The most common cause of tricuspid insufficiency is a dilated right ventricle from right ventricular failure. Congenital malformations may also cause tricuspid insufficiency. The clinical manifestations are those of right ventricular failure and include distention of the jugular veins, hepatomegaly, jaundice, and peripheral edema. Because blood flows through the incompetent tricuspid valve into the right atrium during systole, a systolic murmur is heard at the left sternal border. Atrial fibrillation is usually present. Medical management centers on treating the cause of the tricuspid insufficiency.

Pulmonic Stenosis

The most common cause of pulmonic stenosis is congenital malformation. Other causes include rheumatic fever and metastatic carcinoid lesions of the pulmonic valve. Pulmonic stenosis is usually tolerated well and does not cause symptoms. When the problem is severe, the clinical manifestations are those of right heart failure. Because blood is hindered from flowing from the right ventricle into the pulmonary artery, a systolic murmur is heard at the pulmonic area or upper left sternal border. Persons with pulmonic stenosis usually require no therapy. Surgical repair may be necessary if the lesion is severe.

Pulmonic Insufficiency

Pulmonic insufficiency is usually caused by pulmonary hypertension, infective endocarditis, or congenital malformations. Pulmonic insufficiency rarely causes symptoms unless severe enough to cause right heart failure. Because blood that is pumped into the pulmonary artery during systole regurgitates into the right ventricle during diastole, a diastolic murmur is heard in the pulmonic area (upper left sternal border). If the client develops problems related to pulmonic insufficiency, the treatment is aimed at the cause. Sometimes valve replacement is necessary.

Mitral Stenosis

Mitral stenosis in the adult is usually the result of previous rheumatic fever. Other causes of mitral stenosis in the adult are rare. Mitral stenosis impedes blood flow from the

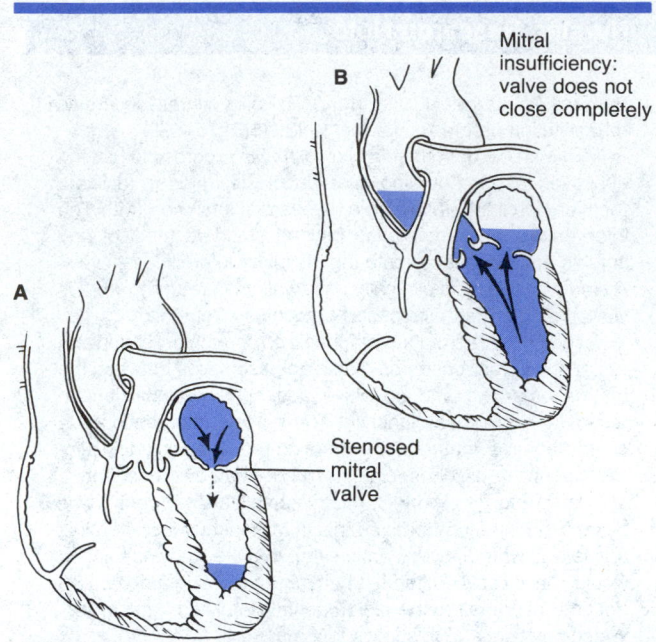

Figure 24–18

Mitral stenosis and mitral insufficiency. **A.** Mitral stenosis: during diastole, blood flow from the left atrium to the left ventricle is impaired because the valve leaflets are diseased and do not open completely. **B.** Mitral insufficiency: normally during systole, all blood from the left ventricle is ejected through the aortic valve into the aorta. With mitral insufficiency, some of the blood flows backward through the incompetent mitral valve.

left atrium into the left ventricle during diastole and produces a diastolic murmur, which is best heard at the apex (Figure 24–18A). The client usually does not develop a murmur or symptoms until several years after having had rheumatic fever. The most common symptoms are dyspnea and fatigue. As the stenosis increases, the symptoms become more severe and are related to pulmonary hypertension and right ventricular heart failure. Atrial fibrillation frequently accompanies mitral stenosis.

Medical management includes treatment of atrial fibrillation with digitalis or antidysrhythmic drugs and anticoagulant therapy for prevention of blood clots and systemic emboli. Surgical therapy includes reconstruction or valve replacement.

Mitral Insufficiency

The most common causes of mitral insufficiency in the adult are rheumatic heart disease and mitral leaflet prolapse. Other causes include dilatation of the left ventricle, CAD, papillary muscle dysfunction, and congenital problems. Because mitral insufficiency results in blood flowing through the incompetent mitral valve into the left atrium during systole, a systolic murmur may be heard at the apex (Figure 24–18B). The clinical manifestations of mitral insufficiency vary depending upon the cause. Mitral insufficiency from rheumatic heart disease may cause no difficulties for many years and then produce manifestations associated with heart failure.

The medical management depends upon the clinical manifestations and the cause. Management of the client with heart failure is discussed later in this chapter. The management of dysrhythmias has been previously discussed. Surgical treatment involves valve replacement.

Mitral Valve Prolapse. Mitral valve prolapse, also called mitral leaflet prolapse, and Barlow's syndrome, deserves special mention because it is a common and usually benign clinical syndrome. It occurs more frequently in women and has a familial tendency. On auscultation at the apex, a mid- or late systolic click may be heard, sometimes accompanied by a late systolic murmur with a whooping sound.

Most clients with mitral valve prolapse never have clinical symptoms. Dysrhythmias, palpitations, syncope, and vague chest pain can occur, however. Treatment generally involves reassurance and propranolol for troublesome chest pain.

Aortic Stenosis

The most frequent causes of aortic stenosis in the adult are congenital malformations; degenerative calcifications in the valve; and less frequently, the sequelae of rheumatic fever. The clinical manifestations of aortic stenosis depend upon the severity of the stenosis. Because blood flow is hindered from flowing into the aorta from the left ventricle during systole, a systolic murmur can be heard in the aortic area or right upper sternal border (Figure 24–19A). Left ventricular hypertrophy (Figure 24–20) develops and can

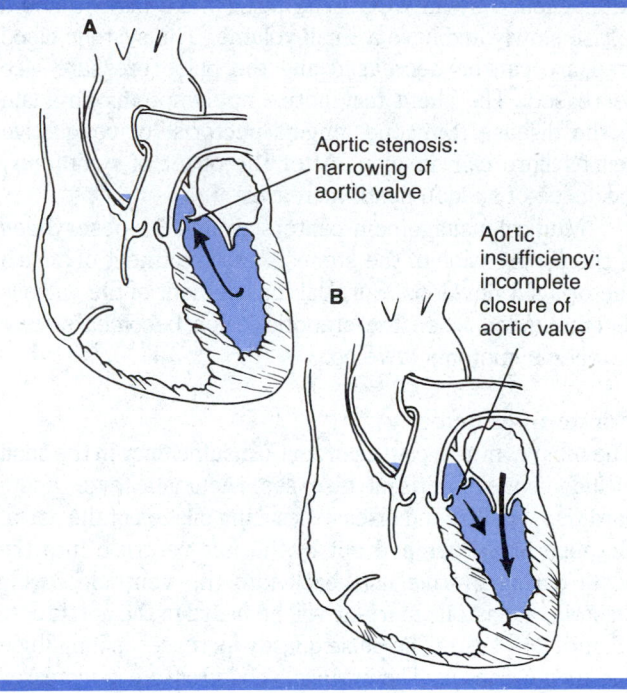

Figure 24–19

Aortic stenosis and aortic insufficiency. **A.** Aortic stenosis: during systole, blood flow from the left ventricle through the aortic valve is impaired because of the stenotic aortic valve. **B.** Aortic insufficiency: during diastole, some of the blood ejected through the aortic valve during systole flows backward through the incompetent aortic valve.

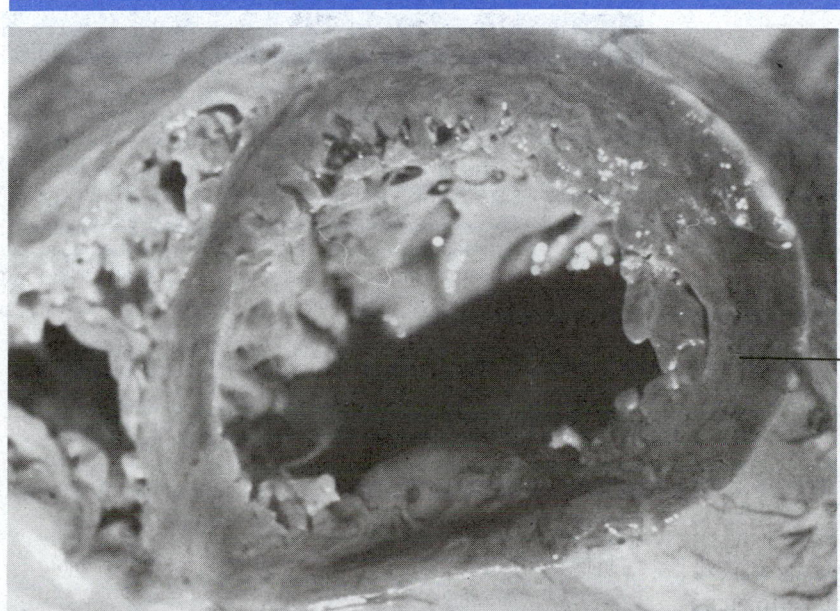

Figure 24–20

Left ventricular hypertrophy. With aortic stenosis, the impairment to outflow results in increased work for the left ventircle. The myocardial fibers hypertrophy to generate more pressure and maintain peripheral perfusion. (Courtesy of Millard Fillmore Hospital, Buffalo, NY)

Hypertrophy of the left ventricle

be diagnosed by an ECG. The pulse wave may be noted to rise slowly and have a small volume. The systolic blood pressure can be decreased and the pulse pressure also decreased. The client may notice no symptoms until late in the disease. Syncope, angina pectoris, or congestive heart failure can develop. After the onset of symptoms, incidence of sudden death increases.

Medical management centers around the observation of the progression of the stenosis and treatment of angina pectoris if it develops. Surgical replacement of the valve is recommended when the stenotic lesion becomes severe or when symptoms develop.

Aortic Insufficiency

The most common causes of aortic insufficiency in the adult include connective tissue diseases, rheumatic fever, endocarditis, syphilis, and diseases causing dilation of the aorta. Because blood pumped out of the left ventricle into the aorta during systole falls back into the ventricle during diastole, a diastolic murmur will be heard in the aortic area (Figure 24–19B). The pulse quickly increases in amplitude and then collapses. The systolic blood pressure is increased and the diastolic blood pressure decreased.

The client often has no symptoms for many years after the murmur is first heard. Later, as the regurgitation progresses, clients may notice a gradual increase in heart palpitations, palpitations in the neck, flushing, sweating, and chest pain. After development of symptoms, the person's condition usually rapidly deteriorates.

Medical management aims at following the client and observing for progression of valvular disease. Surgical replacement of the valve is recommended when the early symptoms develop, before the valvular problem becomes severe.

Specific Nursing Measures

Nursing management centers on teaching the client about the need for prophylactic antibiotics while the condition is being managed medically. Clients who have had rheumatic fever are encouraged to take their antibiotics daily. Clients who have any type of valvular disease should be reminded to inform dentists and physicians planning invasive procedures about the valvular problem. Nursing responsibilities for clients having cardiac diagnostic studies were discussed in Chapter 23. Nursing implications of cardiac surgery are discussed in Chapter 25.

HEART FAILURE

Heart failure indicates that the heart has failed to perform adequately its function of pumping blood throughout the circulatory system. Perhaps the best definition of heart failure is that of Hurst et al. (1982), who define heart failure as a condition in which the heart is no longer able to pump an adequate supply of blood to meet the metabolic needs

of the body when there is an adequate venous return. The terms *forward* and *backward* heart failure have been used to indicate the symptoms the person exhibits as a result of heart failure. Forward failure produces symptoms related to low cardiac output, and backward failure produces symptoms related to increased venous pressure.

Left heart failure and *right heart failure* are terms describing the side of the heart that has the primary impairment. It is sometimes helpful to think of heart failure as left or right sided because the symptoms and signs may provide clues to the location of the primary problem. Keep in mind, however, that failure of one side of the heart usually leads to failure of the other side.

Heart failure may be acute or chronic. A person may not have any indication of heart disease and develop heart failure suddenly. A good example is the asymptomatic person with CAD who has an MI and develops acute heart failure with pulmonary edema. Chronic heart failure may also develop as a result of CAD as well as other forms of heart disease. The affected person may progressively reduce activity as the failure increases but attribute the decrease in activity to other causes such as normal aging.

Heart failure may be described as latent, compensated, and intractable. Latent heart failure implies that the heart is able to handle the circulatory needs at rest but fails with increased stress. Compensated heart failure is heart failure that was previously present, but cardiac output has been maintained at a normal level by therapy or by compensatory mechanisms. Intractable heart failure implies that heart failure persists when all therapies have been used.

Congestive heart failure is a state in which abnormal circulatory congestion occurs as the result of heart failure, and compensatory mechanisms are brought into play (Hurst et al., 1982). CHF may be classified as mild, moderate, or

---

Nursing Research Note

Sanders JB, Cunningham SG, Knowlton C: A comparison of plasma renin activity levels in patients with and without congestive heart failure after myocardial infarction. *Heart Lung* 1985; 14(1):1–6.

This study assessed plasma renin activity in clients immediately after myocardial infarction. These levels were then used to compare clients who developed congestive heart failure (CHF) and/or cardiogenic shock with those who did not develop complications.

Data suggested that clients with higher plasma renin activity did develop complications. Thus, treatment with an angiotensin-converting enzyme inhibitor may be appropriate.

Caregivers need to monitor decreased sodium levels because these may also mean a severe level of myocardial damage. Nurses should also increase their knowledge about angiotensin-converting enzyme inhibitors because their use is increasing. Fear, anxiety, heat, stress, and pain must be minimized when caring for clients with CHF because these factors can also increase levels of renin and antidiruretic hormone.

severe, based on the development of dyspnea in relation to activity. With mild CHF, dyspnea occurs with moderate activity; with moderate CHF, dyspnea occurs with mild activity; and with severe CHF, dyspnea occurs at rest (Hurst et al., 1982).

Etiology

The causes of heart failure include conditions that overload the heart, affect cardiac rhythm or conduction, or decrease the ability of the heart to contract. The heart may become overloaded by decreased or increased preload and increased afterload. Examples of conditions that *increase preload* include increased venous return, incompetent valves that cause blood to be regurgitated back into the heart chamber to be pumped again, and shunts or openings between chambers that promote the flow of blood from one side of the heart to the other. Conditions that *decrease preload* include insufficient blood return to the heart from bleeding or dehydration. When venous return is adequate, preload may be decreased by reduced ability of the ventricles to fill because of stenosis of the mitral or tricuspid valves or constriction of the pericardium, as in pericardial tamponade. Conditions that *increase afterload* include increased pulmonary or systemic blood pressure and stenosis of the valves through which the heart has to pump the blood, as in aortic or pulmonic stenosis.

Examples of disturbances in heart rhythm and electrical conduction include extremely fast or slow heart rate, fibrillation, and cardiac arrest. Conditions that decrease the ability of the heart to pump blood include diseases of the heart, toxic substances in the heart, and conditions that deprive the heart of oxygen. Examples of diseases of the heart muscle include MI and infections of the heart. Toxic substances include drugs and alcohol. Conditions that deprive the heart of oxygen include inadequate blood supply to the heart, as in CAD, or inadequate quality of the blood from anemia and other systemic diseases.

Left-sided heart failure occurs with pressure or volume overload of the left ventricle. Pressure overload can result from systemic hypertension, aortic stenosis, or coarctation of the aorta. Volume overload occurs with aortic or mitral regurgitation.

Left-sided heart failure can progress to pulmonary edema. In left heart failure, the left ventricle cannot pump out all of its blood, increasing the residual volume in the ventricle. Accumulating blood backs up into the left atrium, pulmonary veins, and the pulmonary capillary bed. *Pulmonary edema,* engorgement of the pulmonary vasculature with subsequent excessive accumulation of fluid in the interstitial spaces and alveoli of the lung, results.

Right-sided heart failure occurs with pressure or volume overload of the right ventricle. Pressure overload can result from pulmonary hypertension or stenosis of the pulmonic valve. Volume overload can result from an atrial septal defect.

Clinical Manifestations

The clinical manifestations of heart failure depend on the severity of the failure and the side of the heart that is predominantly affected. Depending on the severity, the client may notice difficulty in breathing; coughing of blood-tinged frothy sputum; fatigue; edema; nocturia; oliguria; weight gain; cerebral symptoms such as dizziness and syncope; or gastrointestinal symptoms such as anorexia, bloating, and abdominal pain. Table 24–7 lists common subjective and objective findings in left-sided and right-sided heart failure.

A chest x-ray may reveal an enlarged heart and pleural effusion. Although there are no ECG findings diagnostic of heart failure, the ECG probably will be abnormal because persons with heart failure generally have some form of heart disease.

Therapeutic Measures

The medical plan of therapy for heart failure is generally based on goals that include:

- Determining and eliminating or controlling the cause.
- Determining and treating the condition(s) that precipitated the heart failure.
- Improving the ability of the heart to pump blood by:
  - Decreasing the work load of the heart by:
    1. Decreasing the body demands.
    2. Decreasing preload.

Table 24–7	Subjective and Objective Findings in Left and Right Heart Failure	
	Subjective	**Objective**
Left heart	Dyspnea	Rales
	Orthopnea	S₃ gallop
	Paroxysmal nocturnal dyspnea	Pleural effusion
	Cough	Peripheral cyanosis
	Fatigue	↑ Respirations; Cheyne–Stokes respirations
Right heart	Abdominal pain	Distended neck veins
	Anorexia, nausea	
	Bloating	Hepatojugular reflux
	Fatigue	Hepatomegaly
		Ascites
		↑ CVP
		S₄ gallop
		↓ urine output
		Peripheral edema

3. Decreasing afterload.
- Improving the ability of the heart to contract.

Eliminating the cause of heart failure depends on the disease process and the available treatment modalities. Keep in mind that all forms of heart disease have the potential to lead to heart failure.

The condition that precipitated the heart failure may be readily apparent and immediately treatable, such as inadvertent rapid administration of fluids, stresses of emergency surgery for another condition, or in the case of mild failure, the increase of sodium in the diet. Other stressors, such as other systemic diseases, may be less amenable to control. Decreasing the body demands to decrease the work load of the heart and subsequently improve its ability to pump blood may be accomplished by helping the client to decrease activity and, in some cases, by promoting improvement of the quality of the blood being pumped.

The person with chronic heart failure may need only to regulate the amount of physical activity to be free of symptoms. Sometimes discontinuing an activity is distressing to the individual, and spacing activities that cause symptoms may be appropriate. If the client is overweight, measures should be encouraged to reduce weight to decrease body demands for blood flow.

Clients with acute and severe heart failure may be confined to bed. They may be positioned in a sitting position to help them decrease the work of breathing. Oxygen may be administered by nasal prongs at 4 to 6 L/min if arterial oxygen saturation is low. Morphine sulfate may be given intravenously over a period of time to help decrease the work of breathing, decrease psychological distress, and decrease the effects of sympathetic stimulation of the arteries and veins causing pooling of blood in the extremities so less blood is returned to the heart.

Control of the heart rate and rhythm to improve the ability of the heart to pump blood is managed by the use of antidysrhythmic agents, which were discussed in the section on dysrhythmias. In some cases, the use of an artificial pacemaker may be indicated (see Chapter 25).

In most cases, heart failure is related to increased preload, and measures to decrease preload will improve the heart's ability to contract. The severity of the heart failure will determine the measures necessary to decrease preload. When clients have a mild form of failure, preload can be decreased by reducing sodium intake. The physician will probably prescribe a mild diuretic such as one of the thiazides. Antianginal drugs such as nitroglycerin and isosorbide dinitrate (see Table 24–5) may also be prescribed to reduce preload through their vasodilating effects. Actions of the major types of antianginal drugs were described in the section on CAD.

With severe heart failure, the use of the more potent diuretics such as ethacrynic acid or furosemide is necessary. In addition to antianginal drugs, antihypertensive agents such as nitroprusside, prazosin, or captopril may

be used to promote pooling of blood in the veins. Nitroprusside and agents with properties that promote arterial dilation also decrease afterload. Additional measures such as rotating tourniquets or phlebotomy may also be necessary.

If the cause of heart failure is decreased preload, the treatment may be the administration of blood or fluids, depending on the cause. Use of this therapy may seem confusing because rapid fluid administration is contraindicated in most types of heart failure. To understand the rationale, consider that, if there is not enough blood to pump, the heart will pump it faster to meet body demands and subsequently become overloaded and fail. In these relatively infrequent instances, fluid administration is proper.

Measures to decrease afterload in a person with mild heart failure include therapies for control of high blood pressure. Antianginal drugs also decrease afterload by causing peripheral arteriolar dilation. As heart failure progresses, more potent drugs are used to promote arterial dilation. Hydralazine, minoxidil, phenoxybenzamine, and phentolamine are specific drugs for arterial dilation. Drugs such as nitroprusside, prazosin, and captopril that promote arterial dilation and venous dilation may also be used and will also decrease preload.

Digitalis glycosides are inotropic agents used for many years to improve the contractility of the heart (Table 24–8). Digitalis preparations are usually prescribed for persons who have mild heart failure to promote better contraction of the heart and increase cardiac output. As heart failure progresses, the dosage of digitalis may be adjusted. In acute, severe heart failure, other inotropic drugs are used temporarily. These include catecholamines such as epinephrine, norepinephrine, isoproterenol, dopamine, dobutamine, and amrinone.

When these therapies are ineffective in relieving the symptoms of heart failure, mechanical assistive devices such as the intra-aortic balloon pump may be instituted. Cardiac transplantation or mechanical hearts may be employed (see Chapter 25).

Specific Nursing Measures

Nursing care involves continuous assessment of the client's cardiac status and the effects produced by drug therapies. Changes in the client's status indicating further deterioration should always be reported to the physician immediately so the medical plan of care can be adjusted.

When CHF progresses to pulmonary edema, the client should be assisted to a high Fowler's position with the legs dependent to decrease venous return. Support the lower arms on pillows to reduce strain and fatigue. Oxygen and IV morphine sulfate and IV diuretics may be ordered. Sometimes rotating tourniquets, by sphygmomanometer cuffs or automatic rotating-tourniquet machine, are applied to further reduce the volume of venous blood returning to

(continued on p. 803)

Table 24-8 Inotropic Drugs

Classification (Generic Name, Trade Name)	Route of Administration and Dosage	Actions and Uses	Side Effects and Other Considerations	Nursing Implications
Digitalis glycosides	IM use avoided because of associated pain; other considerations depend on form of digitalis as listed			
Deslanoside (Cedilanid-D)	IV slowly; used for loading (dosage required for therapeutic effect, previously referred to as digitalization); 1.2–1.6 mg divided over 24-h period	Same for all forms Inhibits Na, K-ATPase; results in Na accumulation in the cells causing greater amount of intracellular Na, which promotes more free Ca to interact and increase force of contraction	Same for all forms Side effects may indicate digitalis toxicity: anorexia, nausea, vomiting, diarrhea, headache, and other CNS disturbances, visual disturbances, dysrhythmias	Same for all forms Assess for previous use of digitalis glycosides before initiation of therapy; do not substitute one preparation of digitalis for another (dosages, absorption rates, and
Ouabain, G-strophanthin	IV slowly; used for loading; 0.25–0.5 mg initially; then 0.1 mg q. 30 min or h until therapeutic effect reached (no more than total of 1 mg in 24 h)	Effects: Increased force and strength of heart contraction; decreased conduction through A-V node Use: CHF, atrial tachycardia, atrial flutter, atrial fibrillation	Potential for digitalis toxicity increases with: hypokalemia; hypomagnesemia; hypercalcemia; renal disease; concomitant use of quinidine, calcium channel blockers, diuretics, sympathomimetics	duration of effects differ among drugs and among the same drugs with different brand names) Before administering prescribed drug, note recent laboratory findings: digitalis level, electrolytes; assess apical–radial pulse for
Lantoside C (Cedilanid)	Oral: Loading dose of 8 mg divided over several days; then 0.5–1.5 mg daily			rate, rhythm, and pulse deficit; if substantial change: do not give drug, take blood pressure, report findings
Digoxin (Lanoxin, Masoxin, Lanoxicaps, Digoxin)	Oral and IV (dosages differ) Oral: Loading dose of 1.0 mg divided over 24 h; then maintenance with 0.125–0.5 mg daily IV: ½ to ⅔ oral dosage			Client and family teaching, which includes: name of drug; dosage prescribed; reason drug is prescribed; side effects; how to assess pulse for rate and rhythm
Digitoxin (Crystodigin)	Oral and IV (same dosage): Loading dose of 1.2–1.6 mg divided over 24 h; then 0.1 mg daily			When to notify physician: If pulse rate not within prescribed rate or rhythm changes,
Gitalin (Gitaligin)	Oral: Loading dose started with 2.5 mg; then 0.75 mg q. 6 h until therapeutic effect; then 0.25–1.25 mg daily			side effects develop, advice for use of OTC drugs
Digitalis leaf (Digifortis)	Oral: Loading dose of 1.2–1.8 g divided over 24 h; then 100 mg daily			

(continued)

Table 24–8   Inotropic Drugs (continued)

Classification (Generic Name, Trade Name)	Route of Administration and Dosage	Actions and Uses	Side Effects and Other Considerations	Nursing Implications
Sympatho-mimetics		Beta receptor stimulation; effects vary depending on amount of stimulation and type of beta receptor: beta 1 effects: increased contractility, increased heart conduction velocity, increased automaticity; beta 2 effects: vasodilation, bronchodilation, increased coronary blood flow Alpha receptor stimulation; promotes peripheral vasoconstriction; decreases coronary blood flow	Side effects: See individual drugs Other considerations: Beta effects may be counteracted by use of beta-adrenergic blocking agents such as propranolol Alpha effects may be counteracted by use of alpha-adrenergic blocking agents such as phentolamine (Regitine)	Beta stimulation: Assess heart rate for increase; assess pulse and/or ECG pattern for dysrhythmias Alpha stimulation: Assess blood pressure for increase General: Monitor infusion rate, urinary output Other: Assess recent use of other drugs
Epinephrine (Adrenalin chloride)	Cardiac arrest: IV or intracardiac use—0.5 mL of 1:1000 solution diluted to 10 mL with normal saline; 3–5 mL (1:10,000 solution) are injected IM or SC: 0.2–1 mL (1:1000)	Very strong alpha- and beta 1-receptor activator; mild beta 2-receptor activator Cardiac uses: Cardiac arrest: may generate spontaneous contraction; in fine ventricular fibrillation, promotes more vigorous fibrillation, which is more responsive to defibrillation Other uses: Relieve respiratory distress due to bronchospasm; relief of hypersensitivity reactions; as a hemostatic agent	CNS: Headache, anxiety, dizziness, agitation CV: Tachycardia, dysrhythmias, palpitations, increased blood pressure, angina GI: Nausea, vomiting Respiratory: Dyspnea, dry mouth Other considerations: Tricyclic antidepressants and some antihistamines may potentiate effects; use with cyclopropane or halothane anesthesia is contraindicated because of increased risk of cardiac dysrhythmias; potency affected by light; incompatible with alkaline solutions	As above Keep solution in light-resistant containers Do not use if solution is brown or contains a precipitate Discard solution within 24 h after mixing Do not mix with alkaline solution
Norepinephrine (Levophed bitartrate)	IV (4 mg in 1000 mL): Start at 2–3 mL/min (8–12 μg); titrate to maintain a low-normal blood pressure; usual maintenance is about 0.5–1 mL/min or 2–4 μg/min	Very strong alpha- and beta 1-receptor activator; at low doses, beta 1 effects predominate; at high doses, alpha effects predominate Use: Restoration of blood pressure in the following hypotensive states: MI, pheo-	CNS: Headache CV: Bradycardia, hypertension Local: Necrosis if drug extravasates Other considerations: MAO inhibitors and some tricyclic antidepressants potentiate effects; use with cyclopropane or halo-	As above Observe client constantly during administration; assess blood pressure every 2 min until desired blood pressure attained and then every 5 min; adjust rate of flow accordingly Observe IV site for

Classification (Generic Name, Trade Name)	Route of Administration and Dosage	Actions and Uses	Side Effects and Other Considerations	Nursing Implications
		chromocytomectomy, sympathectomy, spinal anesthesia, septicemia, blood transfusion, drug reactions, cardiac arrest	thane anesthesia is contraindicated because of increased risk of cardiac dysrhythmias	infiltration; use large arm vein Avoid extravasation; have phentolamine (Regitine) on hand for use if extravasation occurs Reduce rate of administration gradually
Isoproterenol (Isuprel)	IV: 1 mg in 500 mL (2 μg/mL) 0.5–5 μg/min (0.25–2.5 mL/min) IM: 2 μg SC: 2 μg Intracardiac: 2 μg	Very strong beta 1- and beta 2-receptor activator; essentially no alpha-receptor activation Use: Shock, cardiac arrest, carotid sinus hypersensitivity, A-V block	CNS: Headache, tremor, nervousness, insomnia, weakness, dizziness CV: Tachycardia, palpitations, dysrhythmias, angina, flushed face GI: Nausea, vomiting, dry mouth Skin: Sweating Other considerations: Isoproterenol produces increased myocardial work and oxygen consumption; when isoproterenol is given in sufficient amount to raise the heart rate to more than 130, ventricular fibrillation may occur	As above Observe client constantly during administration Adjust infusion rate on basis of heart rate, ECG, hemodynamic measurements, and urine flow Consider reducing rate if heart rate exceeds 110
Dopamine (Intropin)	IV only: 200 mg in 250 mL; 800 μg/mL 2–5 μg/kg/min; titrate by increasing by 5–10 μg/kg/min every 10 to 30 min; may need more than 50 μg/kg/min	Very strong alpha- and beta 1-receptor activator; mild beta 2-receptor activator; also stimulates dopaminergic receptors, which promotes renal and mesenteric blood flow; as dosage increases, alpha effects predominate; less increase in myocardial oxygen consumption than with isoproterenol Use: To correct hemodynamic imbalance in shock syndrome in MI, trauma, endotoxic septicemia, open heart surgery, chronic cardiac decompensation	CNS: Headache, nervousness CV: Tachycardia, bradycardia, palpitations, dysrhythmias, hypertension, hypotension, anginal pain, numbness and tingling of fingers and toes GI: Nausea, vomiting Respiratory: Dyspnea Local: Necrosis if drug extravasates Other considerations: MAO inhibitors potentiate effects Use with cyclopropane or halothane anesthesia warrants extreme caution because of increased risk of cardiac dysrhythmias; incompatible with alkaline solutions	As above Observe client constantly during administration Adjust infusion rate on basis of heart rate, ECG, hemodynamic measurements, and urine flow Observe IV site for infiltration; use large arm vein Avoid extravasation; have phentolamine on hand for use if extravasation occurs Observe color of extremities

(continued)

Table 24–8   Inotropic Drugs (continued)

Classification (Generic Name, Trade Name)	Route of Administration and Dosage	Actions and Uses	Side Effects and Other Considerations	Nursing Implications
Dobutamine (Dobutrex)	IV: 250 mg in 250 mL (1000 μg/mL); 250 mg in 500 mL (500 μg/mL); 250 mg in 1000 mL (250 μg/mL); 2.5–10 μg/kg/min; up to 40 μg/kg/min	Very strong beta 1-receptor activator; moderately strong beta 2 activator; and weak alpha-receptor activator; promotes less increase in heart rate and decrease in peripheral vascular resistance than isoproterenol Use: Short-term treatment for cardiac decompensation	CNS: Headache CV: Increased heart rate, dysrhythmias, palpitations, increased blood pressure, anginal pain, shortness of breath GI: Nausea No significant adverse effects with other cardiac stimulants; incompatible with alkaline solutions	As above Observe client constantly during administration Adjust infusion rate on basis of heart rate, ECG, hemodynamic measurements, and urine flow
Bipyridines		New class of positive inotropic agents that do not affect Na or K-ATPase or the adrenergic receptors; does inhibit myocardial cAMP phosphodiesterase activity and increases cellular levels of cAMP		
Amrinone (Inocor)	IV: (100 mg in 20 mL); dilute with normal saline or half normal saline to yield 1–3 mg/mL; start with bolus of 0.75 mg/kg over 2–3 min; usual maintenance is about 5–10 μg/kg/min; diluted solutions should be used within 24 h	Positive inotropic agent with vasodilator activity; action not fully understood Use: Short-term management of CHF in clients who have not responded to other therapies	GI: Nausea, vomiting, abdominal pain, anorexia, hepatotoxicity CV: Chest pain, hypotension Other: Burning at IV site, thrombocytopenia Contraindications: Hypersensitivity to amrinone or bisulfites Other considerations: Limited clinical experience with the drug indicates that concomitant use of disopyramide is contraindicated because it may result in hypotension; not recommended for use in pregnancy or lactation	Do not dilute in solution containing dextrose because it inactivates the drug over time; may be given through a Y-connector through which a dextrose solution is being administered Discard solution within 24 h after mixing Keep solution in light-resistant container Do not use if solution is discolored or contains particulate matter Monitor heart rate and blood pressure Fluid and electrolytes and renal function will be monitored; report results Assess for improvement; increase in cardiac output, reduction in pulmonary capillary wedge pressure, lessening dyspnea Slow rate of infusion if blood pressure lowers significantly Observe for side effects

the heart. Important nursing responsibilities in applying rotating tourniquets are:

- Measure and record a baseline blood pressure and take pulses in each extremity, marking their location.
- Apply stockinette to all extremities to protect the skin.
- Apply sphygmomanometer cuffs as high as possible on three extremities pumping them to 40 mm Hg of pressure. (Make every effort to find cuffs of the appropriate size to the client's extremities.)
- Use a flow sheet; rotate the tourniquets every 15 minutes in a fixed sequence (eg, clockwise), leaving one extremity unobstructed (Figure 24–21).
- Check arterial pulses frequently to be sure arterial flow is not impeded; check blood pressure in the unobstructed limb.
- If an IV is in place, a tourniquet should not be used on that extremity.
- When the treatment is discontinued, the sphygmomanometer cuffs should be removed gradually, one every 15 minutes, so as not to suddenly overload the venous system.

Explain the treatment in detail to the client and significant others. Prepare them for the discoloration of the peripheral skin while the tourniquets are in use, and assure them that arterial blood flow to the hands and feet will continue. Monitor urinary output. An increase in urine output is one measure of a decrease in blood volume.

Independent nursing action should be compatible with the goals of the medical plan of care. A major nursing measure is to provide an environment where clients feel safe and are assured of receiving proper care, whether in an acute care or outpatient facility. Clients may be frightened, and attention to their needs may increase or decrease the anxiety. Letting clients know that nurses will be assessing them frequently to determine the effects of the medical plan of care may be reassuring if they are told that this is routine and does not mean their condition is worsening.

Adjusting activity level may be a problem for many persons. In the acute care situation, the nurse should observe for untoward symptoms and signs as daily activities increase. Spacing activities to allow time for the heart to rest will promote a pattern of behavior that can be carried through to discharge. Involving clients by instructing them to be aware of symptoms with increased activity and planning for rest periods and activity periods should help them to be more aware of activity tolerance after discharge. Clients should be attentive to activities that bring on symptoms and avoid them if possible. If it is impossible to avoid some activities such as climbing steps, the activity should be spaced to allow for rest periods. If activity is severely compromised, nursing measures associated with care of clients with immobility are appropriate.

Correctly taking the prescribed medications is sometimes a problem. The client should be taught the reasons for each medication, the possible side effects, and the possible consequences if the medications are not taken.

Compliance with dietary advice is also difficult for clients. A low-salt diet is unpalatable to some, and a low-calorie diet is distressing to those who enjoy eating rich food. Knowledge of the long-term effects of noncompliance sometimes helps clients to comply. The nurse may be most effective in counseling the client to avoid very salty foods such as potato chips, ham, pretzels, and condiments. Clients

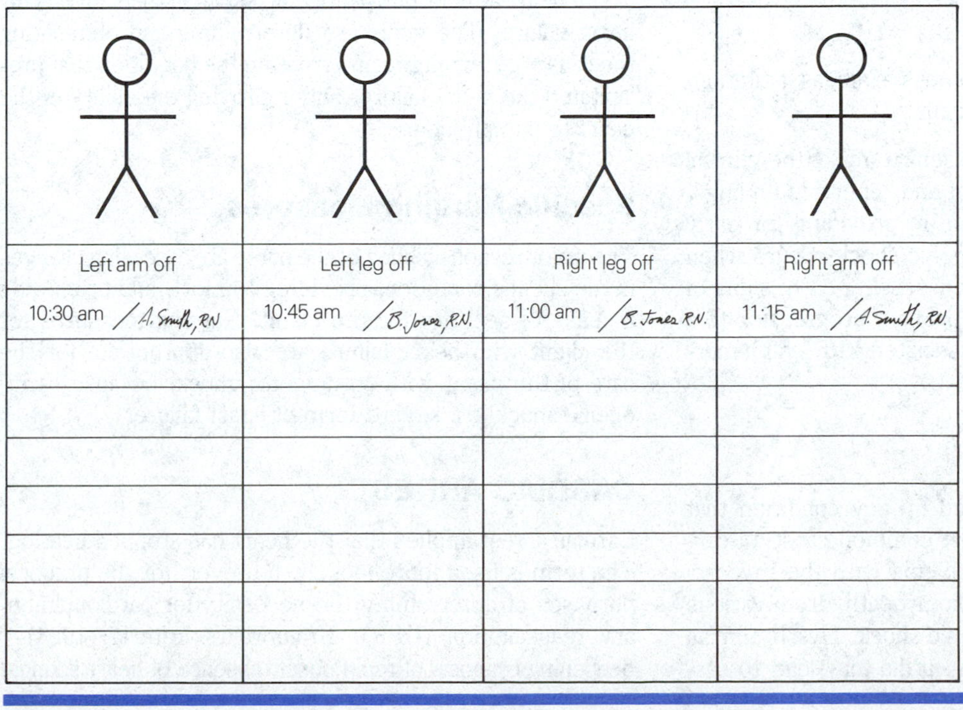

Figure 24–21

Rotating-tourniquet flowsheet. SOURCE: Saxton DF, Pelican PK, Nugent PM, Hyland PA: *The Addision–Wesley Manual of Nursing Practice*. Menlo Park, CA, 1983, p. 1146.

Left arm off	Left leg off	Right leg off	Right arm off
10:30 am / A. Smith, RN.	10:45 am / B. Jones, R.N.	11:00 am / B. Jones R.N.	11:15 am / A. Smith, RN.

will be more likely to follow this approach than a strict no-salt diet. Removing the salt shaker from the table also helps because salting food is sometimes more of a habit than a real need.

Losing weight is a problem for most persons who need to lose it. Clients should be encouraged to lose weight slowly (refer to Chapter 9). They should be reminded that rapid weight loss or gain is usually related to fluid balance. Weighing themselves daily or weekly will help them to assess the effectiveness of the plan of therapy.

Depression may be a problem, as it is with most persons who lose their health or are forced to change their lifestyles. Acknowledging that these feelings are common may help. The family or significant others may also be helpful in providing the encouragement necessary for clients to be able to live with a disability.

CARDIOGENIC SHOCK

Shock occurs when tissue anoxia develops from insufficient blood flow to vital organs because cardiac output is decreased and/or blood flow is impaired. Shock is described according to its degree as preshock, reversible shock, or irreversible shock. Preshock implies that the client is in a stage that will progress to shock if not treated. Reversible shock is treatable; in irreversible shock, all available therapies fail, and the client has no hope for recovery. In cardiogenic shock, heart failure is the cause of the shock.

Most authorities refer to shock as a syndrome or group of symptoms and signs. Hurst et al. (1982) outline the signs of shock as:

- Decreased urinary output of less than 30 mL/h with less than 30 mEq of sodium per liter of urine
- Cool and moist skin
- Auscultated systolic blood pressure of less than 90 mm Hg
- Metabolic acidosis
- Impaired state of consciousness such as agitation, somnolence, confusion, or coma

Any two of the signs must be present to make the clinical diagnosis. By assessing the client and reporting findings, the nurse plays an important role in providing for early diagnosis and treatment. Cardiogenic shock occurs when there is severe heart failure. By assessing early signs of heart failure, the nurse can help prevent progression to a severe state of shock, which is associated with a high mortality rate.

Etiology

Cardiogenic shock may be caused by any condition that causes the heart to fail. The most common cause of cardiogenic shock is MI. Other problems with the myocardium, such as myocarditis or cardiomyopathy from various causes, may also lead to cardiogenic shock. Dysrhythmias that produce bradycardia or tachycardia may lead to car-

diogenic shock, as previously described. Mechanical factors that impair blood flow through the heart, such as valvular problems, rupture of the interventricular septum, ventricular aneurysm, and papillary muscle rupture, may lead to cardiogenic shock. Trauma involving the heart may also produce cardiogenic shock.

Clinical Manifestations

The clinical manifestations of heart failure, which have been previously described, are important for the nurse to assess so medical intervention and nursing intervention can be instituted in the preshock state. Clinical manifestations typically observed in cardiogenic shock are produced by sympathetic activity or occur over a period of time. The client may have mental symptoms such as restlessness, confusion, or stupor. The body temperature will be decreased. The skin will become moist and cool. The pulse will be rapid and weak. The blood pressure, pulse pressure, and urinary output will decrease.

Therapeutic Measures

The medical plan of therapy is based on the cause of the cardiogenic shock. If the cause is mechanical, such as ventricular septal defect, papillary muscle dysfunction, or ventricular aneurysm, immediate surgery may be indicated. Sometimes an attempt will be made to stabilize the client by using an intra-aortic balloon pump to provide assistance to the heart. The balloon is placed in the descending aorta and inflated during diastole to assist pushing the blood forward to the peripheral circulation and backward to fill the coronary arteries. The balloon is deflated during systole, which reduces the resistance against which the heart has to pump.

The treatment of cardiogenic shock is the same as for heart failure. The goals are determining and eliminating the cause, determining and treating the condition that precipitated the heart failure, and improving the ability of the heart to pump blood.

Specific Nursing Measures

The major responsibilities of the nurse are assessing changes in the client's condition, providing comfort, and promoting a sense of security for the client. Nursing measures for the client with heart failure are also appropriate for the care of the client with cardiogenic shock, because cardiogenic shock is a severe form of heart failure.

CARDIAC ARREST

Cardiac arrest implies that the heart has stopped beating. The term is used more loosely, however, for the practical purposes of determining the necessity for cardiopulmonary resuscitation (CPR). Braunwald's criteria (1984)—deepening cyanosis of rapid onset, absence of heart sounds, and a lack of detectable pulses in the major vessels—are sufficient findings to diagnose cardiac arrest. Most cardiac arrests occur before the victim reaches the hospital. Because so many deaths occur before hospitalization, the American Heart Association and the American Red Cross have developed a community effort for education and training in CPR for the public as well as professionals.

Cardiovascular disease is the most common cause of sudden death or death within 24 hours of onset of symptoms. The most common causes of sudden cardiac death are ventricular fibrillation, ventricular tachycardia, severe bradycardia, and asystole (McIntyre & Lewis, 1981).

Therapeutic Measures

The initial approach to cardiac arrest depends on whether the client is monitored. Hospitals and other health agencies have trained teams of personnel and developed guidelines to follow in the event of a cardiac arrest. The American Heart Association and the American Red Cross are the most common information sources in developing a cardiac arrest protocol. All personnel are trained in basic cardiac life support, and special teams are trained in advanced cardiac life support. When cardiac arrest occurs, basic cardiac life support is initiated, and the emergency plan developed by the agency is activated.

If the client is monitored and the cause of the arrest is ventricular fibrillation, a precordial thump is attempted to terminate the dysrhythmia. The client is thumped sharply on the midportion of the sternum to provide an electrical stimulus to restore a heart beat. If successful, lidocaine therapy is initiated. If unsuccessful, electrical countershock is performed. (Countershock involves application of an electrical current to the heart through the chest wall with a defibrillator.) If countershock is unsuccessful, CPR is initiated (see Chapter 13), and the procedure for unmonitored ventricular fibrillation is followed. If these procedures are successful, lidocaine or other antidysrhythmic therapy is initiated.

If ventricular fibrillation is diagnosed and confirmed by ECG after CPR has been initiated, countershock is used as soon as the equipment is available. If countershock is unsuccessful, an endotracheal tube is usually inserted and oxygen therapy initiated. An intravenous line is established, epinephrine is administered intravenously or through the endotracheal tube, and defibrillation by countershock is attempted again. Sodium bicarbonate may be administered, depending on the length of time after cardiac arrest

---

Box 24–2 Cardiopulmonary Resuscitation for the Unmonitored Client

Establish unresponsiveness (shake and shout).

Call for help.

Position the victim.

Open the airway.

Establish breathlessness (look, listen, feel).

Begin rescue breathing.

Check for foreign body airway obstruction.

Establish presence or absence of pulse.

Activate emergency medical system.

Begin chest compressions if pulse is absent.

---

and the probability of acidosis. Defibrillation by countershock is attempted again.

If the cause of the arrest is ventricular tachycardia, synchronized cardioversion (application of an electrical current at the time of the QRS complex in the cardiac cycle) is performed. Less current is used than for defibrillation by countershock.

If cardiac arrest resulted from ventricular asystole, or ventricular asystole resulted from other causes of cardiac arrest, CPR is initiated or continued, an endotracheal tube is inserted, oxygen therapy is initiated, and an intravenous infusion is started. Drug therapy is started to initiate a rhythm. Drugs may include epinephrine, sodium bicarbonate, atropine, calcium chloride, and isoproterenol. A temporary pacemaker may be inserted to attempt to restore a cardiac rhythm. The prognosis for successful resuscitation of cardiac arrest from asystole is poor.

Specific Nursing Measures

All nurses should have special training in basic cardiac life support with an annual review. The steps of CPR are described in Chapter 13 and should be reviewed periodically. Review the emergency plan in the agency, and be prepared for emergency action. In case of cardiac arrest in any setting, perform CPR according to the standards of the American Red Cross or the American Heart Association. The steps outlined by the American Heart Association for treating an unmonitored client are in Box 24–2.

Section III: Infectious Disorders

Infections of the heart frequently follow systemic infections. These may be serious infections that if undiagnosed can result in death. When infections of the heart are treated,

clients may have prolonged recovery periods and are prone to future heart problems. Infections may involve the endocardium (endocarditis), the myocardium (myocarditis), the pericardium (pericarditis), or a combination of these three layers. Involvement of all three layers, as frequently occurs with rheumatic fever, is called pancarditis.

ENDOCARDITIS

Endocarditis may result from invasion of the lining of the heart by organisms or from injury to the lining of the heart, a noninfective cause. Infective endocarditis involves the endocardium of the heart valves more frequently than the endocardium of the heart chambers. Infectious endocarditis may be acute, developing over a period of less than 2 weeks, or subacute, developing over several months. Although infectious endocarditis occurs in persons with no previous heart disease, it is most frequent in those with previous heart disease. In persons with no previous heart disease, infectious endocarditis is often observed in drug abusers and in children under 2 years of age. In those with heart disease, it is associated with rheumatic heart disease, congenital heart disease, previous cardiac surgery, and previous endocarditis (Hurst et al., 1982).

Microorganisms enter the bloodstream and lodge on the endocardial surface. They multiply and produce thrombosis, which stimulates the deposit of fibrin around the bacteria. This results in the formation of vegetations. On healing, the vegetations are covered by endothelium and calcium deposits. The endocardium becomes scarred, and the surface is susceptible to reinfection.

Although infectious endocarditis usually involves the left side of the heart, it also may involve the right side, especially in drug abusers. The most common complications include heart failure and embolization. If the right side of the heart is involved, emboli travel to the pulmonary circulation. If the left side is involved, emboli travel to the arterial circulation.

Etiology

The organisms usually responsible for infective endocarditis are streptococci and staphylococci, although other organisms are sometimes responsible. The most common procedures providing portals of entry for the organisms include dental procedures that cause gingival bleeding, such as occurs with brushing of teeth; oral surgery; upper respiratory tract surgery; genitourinary and gastrointestinal surgery; and cardiac surgery. Intra-arterial and intravenous catheters are excellent avenues of entry for organisms, which may cause nosocomial infective endocarditis. Drug abusers are at risk because of contamination during drug use.

Clinical Manifestations

In the subacute form, the clinical manifestations persist over several weeks before the diagnosis is made. In the acute form, the clinical manifestations usually lead to hospitalization within a few days. The symptoms are usually described as flulike and include fever, chills, sweats, anorexia, fatigue, weakness, headache, and musculoskeletal aches and pains. Most persons develop cardiac murmurs during the course of the disease, and the pulse rate may be rapid. If heart failure develops, the clinical manifestations of heart failure will be apparent. If vegetations dislodge from the endocardium, there may be clinical manifestations of embolization. The client may have symptoms of microembolization originating in the left side of the heart, such as petechiae in the skin or mucous membranes or splinter hemorrhages under the nails. Other manifestations of larger arterial emboli might include decreased or absent arterial pulses in an extremity, cerebrovascular symptoms related to a stroke, abdominal pain related to infarctions of the spleen or bowel, back pain related to infarction of the kidney, or chest pain related to infarction of the myocardium. There may be clinical manifestations of pulmonary embolism, including increased respiratory and pulse rates, fever, pleuritic pain, or cough, if embolization originates in the right side of the heart.

Because the clinical manifestations are common to many types of illnesses, laboratory studies are important to medical diagnosis. Some important findings include anemia, an elevated erythrocyte sedimentation rate, hematuria, isolation of the organism from blood culture, ECG changes, detection of valvular lesions by echocardiography, and evidence of CHF by chest x-ray.

Therapeutic Measures

Medical management is critical because infective endocarditis is usually fatal if untreated. The primary goal is to kill the infecting organisms as quickly as possible. If the organism is known, the antibiotic is chosen based on the sensitivity of the organism. When the organism is not known, nafcillin, ampicillin, and gentamicin are often used in combination therapy. Prolonged antibiotic therapy may be indicated for at least 4 weeks but may be extended for 8 weeks or longer to achieve a cure. Treatment for complications may also be necessary. Surgery to correct structural lesions may be indicated if heart failure becomes severe enough or if the client develops significant arterial emboli. Anticoagulant warfarin therapy for embolization is sometimes cautiously undertaken. The use of heparin is avoided.

Specific Nursing Measures

Nursing measures during the acute phase center around care related to infections and close assessment and reporting of subjective and objective findings that may indicate complications described previously. Because the client and family may be anxious, nursing approaches to decrease anxiety through careful explanation are important. Implement measures to preserve energy while promoting sufficient activity to prevent complications, as the client's condition indicates. Spacing of activities as well as other measures described for heart failure are appropriate.

The nurse can assist the client to prevent further episodes of endocarditis through health teaching about prophylactic antibiotic therapy. Explain that the client is prone to future episodes of endocarditis because the scars usually remaining on the heart lining can trap bacteria and promote bacterial growth. With this information, the client may be more likely to comply with prescribed prophylactic antibacterial therapy when undergoing invasive procedures such as dental surgery.

MYOCARDITIS

Myocarditis is an inflammatory process involving the myocardium caused by infectious agents, radiation, chemicals, pharmacological agents, or metabolic disorders. Infectious myocarditis, which may be acute or chronic, frequently goes unrecognized. Most persons recover completely, although acute myocarditis is a common cause of acute dilated cardiomyopathy (previously called acute congestive cardiomyopathy). Several months or years after the initial myocarditis, an individual may develop clinical manifestations of CHF with ventricular enlargement and dysfunction. Progressive deterioration is usually followed by death within 4 years (Braunwald, 1984).

Etiology

Any infectious agent may cause myocarditis. In North America, viruses are the most common cause, especially coxsackievirus B. Some common viral infections that have been identified as causing myocarditis are mumps, influenza, viral hepatitis, and infectious mononucleosis. Rickettsial, bacterial, spirochetal, fungal, protozoal, and metazoal infections can also cause myocarditis.

Clinical Manifestations

The clinical manifestations of myocarditis vary from no symptoms to symptoms of severe CHF. The manifestations are indistinguishable from those of systemic infection. The pulse rate may be higher than expected with the degree of temperature elevation. Transient ECG abnormalities may occur, including ST segment changes, T wave changes, and dysrhythmias, although these are also observed in clients with infections without myocardial involvement. Diagnosis is based on identification of the systemic infection and is suspected when ECG changes are present. When the client has CHF without an identifiable cause, a biopsy of the right ventricle may be diagnostic.

Therapeutic Measures

Medical management centers around treating the client for the clinical manifestations. Antibiotic therapy may also be instituted against some organisms. The client should be observed closely for ECG changes and appropriately treated for dysrhythmias. Drugs, such as beta-blockers, which cause a negative inotropic effect are usually avoided in the treatment of dysrhythmias. If the client develops CHF, the treatment is similar to that previously described. Because persons with myocarditis are especially sensitive to the effects of digitalis, they should be observed closely for the development of digitalis toxicity. Adequate rest and oxygenation are also indicated.

Specific Nursing Measures

Nursing measures during the acute phase involve care of the client with an infection and assessment and reporting of cardiac dysrhythmias and signs of CHF. Because systemic infections may result in myocarditis, stress the importance of rest and provide supportive care of the client who has a systemic infection. The nursing care of clients with dysrhythmias and CHF have been previously described.

PERICARDITIS

Pericarditis is an inflammation of the pericardium, the sac surrounding the heart. The infection, which may be acute or chronic, is frequently not properly diagnosed and sometimes results in death. Pericarditis may be caused by trauma, tumors, anticoagulants, bleeding disorders, systemic diseases, MI, and drugs, as well as infectious agents. Pericarditis is frequently observed in clients who have had open heart surgery. Acute pericarditis is often misdiagnosed as pleurisy, MI, bronchopneumonia, or pulmonary embolism. Pericarditis may cause the life-threatening emergency of **cardiac tamponade,** an accumulation of a large amount of fluid in the pericardial sac, which prevents the heart from filling and consequently reduces cardiac output dramatically. Cardiac tamponade usually requires pericardiocentesis, an immediate surgical procedure to empty the pericardial sac. Pericarditis may also result in constrictive pericarditis, which may develop over months or years with the development of fibrosis of the pericardial sac. Constrictive pericarditis requires surgical removal of the pericardium, and recovery may require months.

Etiology

Infectious pericarditis is most commonly caused by viral, bacterial, tuberculous, fungal, or parasitic organisms. Coxsackievirus B is a common viral cause, although mumps, influenza, poliomyelitis, varicella, hepatitis B, and viruses causing infectious mononucleosis are sometimes implicated. Bacterial pericarditis most commonly occurs by spread of intrathoracic infections. Common organisms include staphylococci, streptococci, gram-negative bacilli, *Neisseria, Salmonella,* and others. Fungal pericarditis usually develops from extension of infections of the lungs from inhalation of *Histoplasma* or *Coccidioides* organisms. Histoplasmosis is most common in the western Appalachian region and the Ohio and Mississippi Valleys, and coccidioidomycosis is most common in the Southwest. *Aspergil-*

lus, Blastomyces, and *Candida* may also be responsible organisms. Unusual infectious causes of pericarditis include the parasites *Entamoeba histolytica* and *Echinococcus granulosus.*

Clinical Manifestations

Chest pain, a pericardial friction rub, and serial ECG abnormalities are characteristic findings in the client with acute pericarditis. The chest pain is variable among clients and is sometimes indistinguishable from an MI. The chest pain can also be unlike MI pain, however. The pain is aggravated by lying supine, respiratory movements, and swallowing. It may be relieved somewhat by sitting up and leaning forward. The pericardial friction rub may have one or more of the three components of the friction rub sounds occurring during atrial systole, ventricular systole, and early diastole. The friction rub may be heard intermittently or may last as long as a week or more with some types of pericarditis. The sound is usually heard best at the left lower sternal border with the client sitting up and leaning forward upon inspiration and full expiration. The grating sound is similar to that of rubbing hairs together near the ear or squeaking leather. The ECG changes are ST and T wave changes. The client may also have dyspnea and manifestations of systemic infection including fever, chills, and sweating.

Constrictive pericarditis caused by fibrosis and calcification of the pericardium restricts filling of the heart and produces manifestations of systemic venous congestion including increased jugular venous pressure, edema, and abdominal swelling and discomfort related to liver congestion. Manifestations of pulmonary venous congestion including dyspnea, cough, and orthopnea may be present.

When pericarditis results in a **pericardial effusion** or accumulation of fluid in the pericardial sac, the clinical manifestations of cardiac tamponade occur. Pulsus paradoxus, diminished pulse pressure, distant heart sounds, and jugular venous distention may be present. *Pulsus paradoxus* is an exaggeration of the normal decrease in amplitude of the pulse and decrease in arterial blood pressure during inspiration. With severe tamponade, the palpated pulse may completely disappear during inspiration. The manifestations of tamponade may occur in the acute stage or after constrictive pericarditis has developed. The diagnosis of constrictive pericarditis is made after pericardiocentesis. Pericardiocentesis will not restore normal hemodynamics in constrictive pericarditis, and surgical removal of the pericardium is eventually necessary. The cause of the pericarditis is sometimes identified through laboratory examination of the pericardial fluid.

The client with acute pericarditis caused by a viral infection will usually report a recent cold or the flu and sudden development of precordial pain. A pericardial friction rub is usually present and may last up to a week. The client with pericarditis caused by a bacterial infection will usually have a history of fever, chills, night sweats, and dyspnea of a few days duration before seeking medical assistance. The client may have a pericardial friction rub but usually does not have the typical chest pain. Because bacterial pericarditis usually results in a pericardial effusion, the manifestation of cardiac tamponade from the development of purulent fluid in the pericardium will be apparent. Clients with fungal infections may develop a pericardial effusion rapidly or over a period of several months. Usually, they seek medical help for manifestations related to systemic infection. Those with pericarditis resulting from tuberculosis are usually not diagnosed as having pericarditis until the constrictive state, when the major symptoms are dyspnea and heaviness in the chest. A pericardial friction rub may or may not be heard in clients with all types of pericarditis.

Therapeutic Measures

Medical management of the client with acute pericarditis includes hospitalization, rest, and close observation for the development of cardiac tamponade as well as treatment for the underlying problem. Nonsteroidal anti-inflammatory agents such as aspirin or indomethacin are used to control the pain. Sometimes they are not effective, however, and steroids may be necessary to control the pain. Specific antibiotic therapy is employed, when indicated, against the causative organism. When the client has constrictive pericarditis, surgical resection of the pericardium is usually performed.

Specific Nursing Measures

Nursing management includes providing an environment conducive to rest and the control of pain. The client is assessed for the development of cardiac tamponade as described previously.

Section IV: Neoplastic and Obstructive Disorders

Many disorders can obstruct blood flow within the heart. Lack of blood flow to any tissue, including the heart, results in ischemia, injury, and infarction. With the advent of open heart surgery and better diagnostic studies, the obstructive problems of hypertrophic cardiomyopathy and tumors within the heart are diagnosed and treated with increasing frequency. Nurses are beginning to see persons with these problems more often in the clinical setting.

HYPERTROPHIC CARDIOMYOPATHY

Hypertrophic cardiomyopathy has more than 50 names. In the United States, it has most frequently been called idiopathic hypertrophic subaortic stenosis (IHSS). In Canada, it has been known as muscular subaortic stenosis. As these terms imply, the disease was once thought to involve hypertrophy of the ventricular septum, causing a stenotic obstruction to blood flow in the left ventricle during systole at an area beneath the aortic valve opposite the anterior leaflet of the mitral valve. More recently, the term has been changed because it has been found that not all persons have systolic obstruction to blood flow in the subaortic region.

The term *hypertrophic cardiomyopathy* is more appropriate because it indicates that the entire heart is enlarged even though the septum is more enlarged. Although the heart is enlarged, the ventricular chambers are small. Because of the hypertrophy, the ventricles are resistant to filling during diastole. The atria compensate for this by expanding. Hypertrophic cardiomyopathy is important to nurses because many of the therapies for heart problems are contraindicated in its treatment; in addition, the condition is frequently observed in young adulthood, and sudden death is common, especially during strenuous exercise and most commonly from dysrhythmias. Some persons have a long life with few or no symptoms, but many die within 10 years after the symptoms begin. The cause of hypertrophic cardiomyopathy is not known, but it is thought to be genetically transmitted, because many persons have relatives with the problem or a familial history of sudden death.

Clinical Manifestations

Although many persons experience no symptoms of the disease and die suddenly, dyspnea is the most common symptom that prompts the client to seek medical assistance. Because there is resistance to diastolic filling, the left ventricular end diastolic pressure rises, and the client becomes dyspneic. Because of inadequate cardiac output, especially during strenuous exercise, angina, fatigue, and syncope may also occur. Exertion tends to bring on the symptoms. The ECG is usually abnormal with ST and T wave abnormalities and ventricular hypertrophy evidenced by large QRS complexes. Dysrhythmias are common. The chest x-ray may be abnormal or show left atrial enlargement or general cardiac enlargement. Echocardiography, radionuclide imaging, and phonocardiography are performed to assist in the diagnosis. Angiocardiography is often definitive.

Therapeutic Measures

The goals of medical management center on attempts to minimize the consequences of hypertrophic cardiomyopathy. Because sudden death is the major problem, the client should avoid strenuous exercise, tachycardia, and hypotension, which increase likelihood of sudden death. Inotropic drugs such as digitalis and the sympathomimetics as well as hypotensive agents such as nitroglycerin should be avoided. Major therapeutic agents for the control of dysrhythmias include beta blockers or calcium channel blockers. Pacemaker therapy is sometimes indicated.

Atrial fibrillation is considered an emergency, and therapy is directed at prevention of the formation and embolization of blood clots through heparinization and cardioversion. If the client develops CHF, the usual therapy is digitalis and diuretics for those clients who do not have the obstructive component associated with hypertrophic cardiomyopathy. Use of the drugs may promote problems if the client has obstruction to blood flow, however. Antibiotic prophylaxis is prescribed for invasive procedures, because clients with hypertrophic cardiomyopathy can develop infective endocarditis of the aortic valve, mitral valve, or septum. Surgery is sometimes performed, replacing the mitral valve or removing a wedge of the hypertrophied myocardium from the left ventricular septum.

Specific Nursing Measures

The most important aspects of nursing care are client teaching and counseling. Clients are often hospitalized for the diagnostic procedures, and the nurse can provide support by preparing the client for changes in lifestyle that might be needed. Many persons with hypertrophic cardiomyopathy are young adults who have been active but must now avoid strenuous activity. Concerns regarding having children must be discussed. Although women with the condition seem to do remarkably well throughout pregnancy and delivery, the familial tendencies regarding the disease should be considered, especially if there is a strong history on both sides. Because there is a possibility of sudden death, families and significant others should be encouraged to learn basic life support.

Clients should be counseled regarding the drug regimen and the necessity to avoid inotropic and hypotensive agents. Any physician, dentist, or anesthesiologist treating the client for other problems should be alerted to avoid these drugs. Antibiotic prophylaxis is indicated during invasive procedures, because of the tendency to develop infective endocarditis.

TUMORS

Tumors of the heart may be primary or secondary, malignant or benign, and they may affect the endocardium, myocardium, or pericardium. Tumors occur in any chamber of the heart and obstruct blood flow. About 75% of primary tumors of the heart are benign, the majority being myxomas or lipomas. The majority of primary malignant tumors of the heart are angiosarcomas, rhabdomyosarcomas, and fibrosarcomas. Secondary metastatic tumors that invade the heart are more frequent than primary tumors.

Clinical Manifestations

Tumors of the heart frequently cause systemic manifestations that may be attributed to collagen vascular disease, infections, or malignancy of other organs. They can cause fever, weight loss, arthralgia, rashes, anemia, bleeding disorders, or pulmonary and systemic embolization. The cause of the systemic manifestations is not known but has been attributed to secretions by the tumor or to necrosis.

Cardiovascular manifestations are related to the anatomical position of the tumor. Tumors in the pericardium produce manifestations of pericarditis. Those in the myocardium produce dysrhythmias, heart block, angina, infarction, or CHF, depending on their size and location. Tumors within the heart cavity produce manifestations related to their size and location and may be affected by body position, which affects the obstruction.

Tumors of the right atrium and right ventricle produce symptoms of right heart failure including increased venous pressure, peripheral edema, enlargement of the liver, and ascites. Tumors of the left atrium and ventricle frequently produce manifestations of left heart failure including dyspnea, orthopnea, pulmonary edema, cough, hemoptysis, fatigue, and peripheral edema. Tumors within the chambers of the heart frequently produce manifestations of valvular disease.

The diagnosis of cardiac tumors is made from x-ray, radionuclide imaging, computed tomography, and echocardiography. Cardiac catheterization with angiography is sometimes performed to provide additional information before surgery.

Therapeutic Measures

The treatment for cardiac tumors is surgical removal, which results in cure for most benign tumors. Surgery is usually not an effective cure for primary malignant tumors of the heart. Chemotherapy and radiation therapy alone or in combination are used for treatment of both primary and metastatic cardiac tumors. Surgery is sometimes a palliative treatment for primary and metastatic cardiac tumors.

Specific Nursing Measures

Nursing measures center around assisting the client through diagnostic procedures while assessing cardiovascular status. Preparation for surgery and postoperative management are discussed in Chapter 25. Nursing management related to radiation and chemotherapy is discussed in Chapter 12.

Section V: Traumatic Disorders

With the development of emergency medical services and rapid transportation, more persons with trauma to the heart are reaching hospitals alive. Injuries to the heart are not readily observed because there may be no apparent trauma to the chest. Nurses aware of the manifestations of cardiac trauma can play a significant role in the care of these clients.

Nonpenetrating trauma, sometimes referred to as blunt trauma, may not produce evidence of external chest trauma. The pericardium, myocardium, valves, or coronary arteries may be involved. The injuries can be lacerations or contusions, which may heal without complications or may cause inflammation, aneurysms, rupture, bleeding, cardiac tamponade, or emboli.

Nonpenetrating trauma results from direct force, such as when a person is kicked by a horse or hit by a flying object; crushing or bidirectional force, such as when a person is caught between a steering wheel and car seat; indirect force, such as when the abdomen is compressed; and decelerative force, such as when a person is thrown from a moving vehicle and suddenly stopped by a stationary object such as a tree.

Penetrating injuries of the heart may damage any of the structures of the heart, but the right ventricle is most likely to be involved because of its anterior position. The injury may involve only the pericardium or may penetrate the cardiac chambers. Penetrating wounds of the heart frequently accompany injuries to the lungs and other organs.

The usual penetrating objects are bullets, knives, ice picks, and sharp internal structures such as a fractured rib or sternum.

Clinical Manifestations

The clinical manifestations depend on the structures of the heart that are injured. Injury to the pericardium produces manifestations of pericarditis and may result in cardiac tamponade. Contusion of the myocardium is a common injury that may produce no symptoms and go unrecognized or may cause pain identical to that of MI. Other manifestations are similar to those of MI, including ECG and serum enzyme changes. Dysrhythmias are also a common complication.

Damage to the valves or papillary muscles produces murmurs. Lacerations of the aortic or mitral valve may produce the manifestations of CHF. Diagnosis is confirmed by echocardiographic, phonocardiographic, and angiographic studies.

Rupture of the ventricular septum may also produce a murmur and the manifestations of CHF. Diagnosis is confirmed by cardiac catheterization and ventricular angiography. Rupture of a chamber of the heart usually results in instant death, although immediate surgical treatment has been successful in some cases. Clinical manifestations of penetrating injuries include cardiac tamponade, hemorrhage into the pleural space, or a combination.

Therapeutic Measures

Medical management of pericardial injuries is similar to that of pericarditis. If the pericardium is lacerated and tamponade occurs, pericardiocentesis is usually followed by surgical repair.

Contusions of the myocardium are managed the same as MI. The major difference between the management of MI and myocardial contusion is that the client with a myocardial contusion does not have underlying heart disease and has a much better long-term prognosis. Injuries to the valves, papillary muscles, or ventricular septum usually require surgical repair.

If the client has a penetrating injury with a hemothorax, a chest tube is inserted, blood is replenished, and surgery is performed as soon as possible. If the clinical manifestations are those of cardiac tamponade, a pericardiocentesis is done, and blood is replenished. Emergency surgery is usually indicated.

Specific Nursing Measures

Nurses should carefully assess clients who have been involved in accidents that could have resulted in cardiac injuries and report any clinical manifestations to the physician immediately so the medical plan of care may be adjusted accordingly. Nursing management for the care of clients having cardiac surgical procedures is discussed in Chapter 25. The management otherwise is similar to that previously described under pericarditis, myocardial infarction, and CHF.

Chapter Highlights

Any disease affecting the heart may promote the development of heart failure.

Heart problems can result from congenital problems, multifactorial causes, degenerative changes, infections, tumors, trauma, and systemic diseases.

Heart disease may develop as a result of physiological changes within the body, environmental factors, genetic characteristics, or psychosocial/lifestyle factors affecting the individual.

Avoidance of risk factors may retard the development of some forms of heart disease.

Avoidance of risk factors usually means that clients will need to change their lifestyles.

Heart problems can result in long-term problems requiring lengthy medical treatment and adaptation to changes.

The emotional status of a client with heart problems may be affected because of loss of independence and self-esteem, changes in body image, and alterations in sexual function.

Bibliography

Braunwald E: *Heart Disease,* 2nd ed. Philadelphia: Saunders, 1984.

Case RB et al: Type A behavior and survival after acute myocardial infarction. *N Engl J Med* 1985; 312:737–741.

Cooley DA: *Techniques in Cardiac Surgery,* 2nd ed. Philadelphia: Saunders, 1984.

Craig H: Accuracy of indirect measures of medication compliance in hypertension. *Res Nurs Health* 1985; 8:61–66.

Dawson C: Hypertension, perceived clinician empathy, and patient self-disclosure. *Res Nurs Health* 1985; 8:191–198.

Friedman M, Rosenman RH: *Type A Behavior and Your Heart.* New York: Knopf, 1974.

Glenn WWL et al: *Thoracic and Cardiovascular Surgery,* 4th ed. Norwalk, CT: Appleton–Century–Crofts, 1983.

Haun AB, Barkin RL, Oestreich SJK: *Pharmacology in Nursing.* St. Louis: Mosby, 1982.

Heart Facts 1983. Dallas: American Heart Association, 1982.

Hurst JW et al: *The Heart,* 5th ed. New York: McGraw–Hill, 1982.

Leon AS: Physical activity and coronary heart disease: Analysis of epidemiologic and supporting studies. *Med Clin North Am* 1985; 69(1):3–20.

Margolis JR, Wagner GS: *Coronary Care: Arrhythmias in Acute Myocardial Infarction.* Dallas: American Heart Association, 1976.

Marriott HJ, Gozensky C: Arrhythmias in coronary care: A renewed plea. *Heart Lung* 1982; 11:33–39.

McIntyre KM, Lewis AJ: *Textbook of Advanced Cardiac Life Support.* Dallas: American Heart Association, 1981.

McMahon F: *Management of Essential Hypertension. The New Low-Dose Era,* 2nd ed. Mount Kisco, NY: Futura, 1984.

McMahon M, Palmer R: Exercise and hypertension. *Med Clin North Am* 1985; 69(1):57–70.

New guidelines for hypertension management. *Am J Nurs* 1984; 84:976–978.

Nissen MB: Streptokinase therapy in acute myocardial infarction. *Heart Lung* 1984; 13:233–230.

Pender N: Effects of progressive muscle relaxation training on anxiety and health locus of control among hypertensive adults. *Res Nurs Health* 1985; 8:67–72.

Purcell JA: Shock drugs: Standardized guidelines. *Am J Nurs* 1982; 82:965–973.

Purcell JA, Holder CK: Intravenous nitroglycerine. *Am J Nurs* 1982; 82:254–259.

Runions J: A program for psychological and social enhancement during rehabilitation after myocardial infarction. *Heart Lung* 1985; 14:117–125.

Sloan R: Achieving compliance to a reduced sodium diet. *Nurse Pract* (Feb) 1985; 10:24–26.

Standards and guidelines for cardiopulmonary resuscitation (CPR) and emergency cardiac care (ECC). *JAMA* (Aug) 1980; 453–509.

Stanford JL, Felner JM, Arensberg D: Antiarrhythmic drug therapy. *Am J Nurs* 1980; 80:1288–1295.

The 1984 report of the Joint National Committee on detection, evaluation, and treatment of high blood pressure. *Nurse Pract* (July) 1985; 10:9–14, 19–26, 31–34.

Trevino S, Massey J: Risk factors for arrhythmias after myocardial infarction. *Heart Lung* 1983; 12:240–247.

Wessman JP: Preventing ventricular dysrhythmia following myocardial infarction. *Dimensions Crit Care Nurs* (Jan–Feb) 1985; 4:24–32.

Winslow EH, Lane LD, Gaffney FA: Oxygen uptake and cardiovascular responses in control adults and acute myocardial infarction patients during bathing. *Nurs Res* 1985; 34:164–169.

Suggested Readings

Bohachick P, Rongaus AM: Hypertrophic cardiomyopathy. *Am J Nurs* 1984; 84:320–326. This article reviews the clinical manifestations, physical assessment, diagnostic studies, and therapeutic management of hypertrophic cardiomyopathy. The focus of nursing is client education and counseling regarding necessary lifestyle adjustments to maintain optimal health.

DeVon HA, Powers MJ: Health beliefs, adjustment to illness, and control of hypertension. *Res Nurs Health* 1984; 7:10–16. In this study, a significant relation was found between adjustment to hypertension and complexity of the hypertensive medication regimen. Uncontrolled hypertensives had greater psychosocial adjustment problems related to their illness. Adjustment to the disease and compliance with the plan of care were found to be inversely related.

The Client With a Myocardial Infarction

I. Descriptive Data

Mr Gary Holzerland, a 42-year-old white male, arrived by ambulance at the medical center emergency department with acute substernal chest pain radiating to the left arm. He was admitted to the CCU with the diagnosis of possible myocardial infarction (MI). His wife was notified immediately.

II. Personal Data

Date and Time:	December 22, 1986; 3 PM
Full Name:	Gary Holzerland
Address:	143 Victoria Pl, Buffalo, NY
Sex:	Male
Age:	42
Birthdate:	4-30-44
Race/Culture:	Caucasian
Occupation:	Computer systems analyst
Usual Health Care Providers:	Dana Hanavan, NP; Matthew Sigman, MD
Social Security Number:	000-00-0000
Telephone:	Home: 000-0000
	Work: 000-0000
Marital Status:	Married
Religion:	Protestant

III. Health History

Source of Information:	Client and wife
Reliability of Informant:	Mr Holzerland and his wife appear reliable
Chief Concern:	Unrelieved substernal chest pain

History of Present Illness:

During a business meeting, Mr Holzerland developed substernal chest pain, radiating to the left arm, associated with shortness of breath and diaphoresis, lasting longer than 5 minutes. He describes the pain as crushing, "like someone was sitting on my chest." Severity decreased with rest, but heaviness was constant. He denies palpitations, syncope, dizziness, or nausea and vomiting. Coworkers called an ambulance.

Mr Holzerland states that during the last 6 months he has experienced intermittent chest pain 1–2 times/wk, usually following a stressful encounter. The pain subsided with rest. He describes the pain as heavy, dull, nonradiating, and lasting less than 1 minute. Occasionally, he experiences "chest tightness" while playing racquetball, which is relieved if he stops playing. He feels the accompanying shortness of breath and tachycardia are related to the exercise. He denies DOE, othopnea, PND, cough, wheezing, and hemoptysis; has 2–3 URIs every winter, of brief duration.

Mr Holzerland experiences burning epigastric pain following stressful situations, relieved with antacid; appetite and bowel pattern normal; no diarrhea, constipation, melena, or hematemesis; no history of peptic ulcer disease; has gained 15 lb in last 2 years; has a sedentary job.

Mr Holzerland has a history of mild hypertension × 8 yr. He received no pharmacological therapy for his blood pressure but was told to stop smoking, lose weight, reduce salt intake, and exercise regularly. He exercises 1–2 times/wk, watches his

(continued)

Case Study written by Frances L. Stier.

The Client With a Myocardial Infarction

salt intake, has not lost weight, and smokes 1 pack of cigarettes per day × 20 yr. Last health evaluation was 2 years ago; his ECG, chest x-ray, and blood work were normal, and his blood pressure was "slightly" elevated at that time. He did not consult his physician about his chest pain because he believed it to be related to stress at work and his sedentary lifestyle.

Past Health History:

Childhood: Had usual childhood diseases—chickenpox, mumps, rubella; no history of strep throat, scarlet fever, or rheumatic fever

Immunizations: Had routine childhood immunizations; tetanus booster (1980); received flu vaccine last winter

Medical Problems: Mild hypertension × 8 yr, no medications

Surgeries: Vasectomy, 1980

Transfusions: None

Special Diagnostic Procedures: None

Trauma: None

Allergies: No known allergies to medications, food, or environmental elements

Medications: No prescribed medication. Takes aspirin 600 mg q.d. for headache as needed; antacid 30 mL 3 times p.r.n./wk for "acid stomach"

Family History:

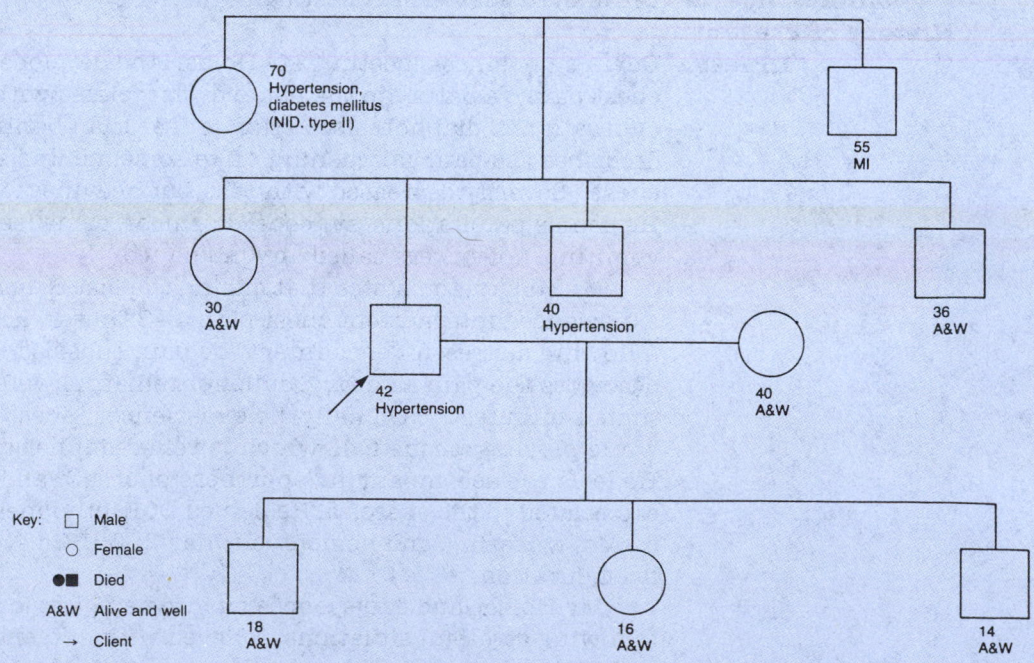

Key:
☐ Male
○ Female
●■ Died
A&W Alive and well
→ Client

Personal/Social History: The client is married (20 years) and lives with his wife and three children in their home, which they own; is a college graduate with an MBA and works as a computer systems analyst with a well-known firm; usually works 10 hours a day, 5 days a week; states he has no time for hobbies. His wife works at home and participates in community volunteer programs. Mr Holzerland states his children are "good kids" with the normal adolescent problems; his eldest child will be attending a private university next year; he expresses concern over their financial status if he is unable to work.

Habits: Mr Holzerland sleeps 6 hr/night without difficulty; he tries to follow a low-salt diet; eats two meals a day—lunch and dinner; admits to a heavy caffeine intake—6–10 cups of coffee/day; has an occasional martini at lunch and usually two martinis before dinner.

Review of Systems:
General: Feels "out of shape"; increased fatigue the last 6 months
HEENT: Experiences daily occipital headaches and stiff neck, relieved with aspirin, 600 mg; denies syncope, vertigo, blurred, or double vision
Respiratory: See HPI
Cardiovascular: See HPI
Genitourinary: Denies dysuria, incontinence, penile discharge, lesions, or impotence; no history of UTIs or kidney stones; no sexual problems
Musculoskeletal: Denies muscle weakness, joint swelling, or limitations in movement
Neurological: Denies fainting, dizziness, loss of balance, weakness, or paresthesia
Endocrine: Denies heat or cold intolerance, history of goiter, excessive sweating, polydipsia, polyphasia, or polyuria; no difficulty in concentration
Psychological: Often feels anxious and tense; states work is stressful but wife and family are supportive; expresses concern about missing work because "this is a busy time of year."

IV. Physical Assessment

Height: 5 ft 11 in
Weight: 200 lb
Vital Signs: Temperature 100°F (37.7°C); P. 100 apical, irregular; R. 24; BP RA 150/100, LA 145/98 (both supine); RA 154/100, LA 150/100 (both seated)

Client is a 42-year-old white male in acute distress with unrelieved chest pain; appears anxious and restless

Relevant Organ Systems:
Thorax and Lungs: Thorax symmetrical, lungs resonant; breath sounds normal, no adventitious sounds
Cardiovascular: PMI @ 5th LICS, 8 cm from sternal border, 2 cm in diameter; no thrills, lifts, or heaves; apical HR 100 irregular, S_1 nl, S_2 split, S_4 present @ apex, no S_3 or Ⓜ; carotid pulses = bilat, no bruit; JVP flat @ 30° angle; extremities: pale, cool, no edema; peripheral pulses 2+ = bilat
Abdomen: Bowel sounds active, no bruit; palpable abdominal aortic pulse; no organomegaly
Neurological: DTRs 2+ = bilat
Mental Status: Alert but restless and apprehensive; responds appropriately

V. Diagnostic Data

12-Lead ECG: Sinus tachycardia, elevated ST segment in leads V_1–V_4 and incomplete right bundle branch block (RBBB)
Serum Enzymes: Elevated CK and CK-MB isoenzyme; LDH and LDH_1 slightly elevated
Arterial Blood Gases: Shows a respiratory alkalosis and slight hypoxemia
Technetium 99m Pyrophosphate Scan: Increased uptake in the anterior surface of the heart
Echocardiogram: Indicates decreased contractility in the anterior surface

(continued)

The Client With a Myocardial Infarction

	including the septum; heart valves normal; delayed closure of the aortic and pulmonic valves; no ventricular aneurysm seen
Chest X-ray:	wnl
CBC:	WBC slightly elevated
Electrolytes:	wnl
Urinalysis:	Specific gravity elevated

VI. Summary
The history, physical assessment, and diagnostic studies indicated that Mr Holzerland suffered an anterior-septal MI. The plan is to keep Mr Holzerland in the CCU until his condition is stable and then transfer him to an intermediate acute care unit.

VII. Nursing Care Plan

Nursing Diagnosis	Client Care Goals	Plan/Nursing Implementation	Expected Outcome
Comfort, alteration in: pain	Reduce or eliminate chest pain	Bed rest until pain is relieved; continuous bedside monitoring; use morphine sulfate or other pain medication as prescribed; administer 2–4 L of O_2 by nasal cannula; monitor vital signs at onset, before and after medication, and after pain is relieved; notify MD if pain is unrelieved by prescribed medication; provide a quiet, calm environment; offer reassurance to client and family; refrain from nonessential procedures; obtain ECG as ordered	Client will be pain free; postinfarction angina is controlled; client will be able to perform activities without pain
Anxiety and fear	Achieve psychological comfort and rest quietly	Facilitate client's coping mechanisms: provide relevant information and orientation to CCU routines, equipment, and procedures; offer reassurance to client and family; encourage expression of feelings regarding hospitalization, diagnosis, and sequelae; clarify misconceptions; identify a primary nurse for client and family; offer spiritual support; use diazepam as ordered; allow liberal visiting by family within client's tolerance	Diminished anxiety and fear within 48 hr; client and family will demonstrate effective coping mechanisms
Coping, ineffective individual: related to denial	Accept diagnosis of MI; use effective coping mechanisms	Assess denial: specific etiology, ie, fear of death, disability, loss of control, altered body image; do not reinforce denial or force client acceptance; for active denial (ie, disregards activity restrictions), assess consequences—are they detrimental? Convey concern and allow the client more control; assist client in identifying coping mechanisms that worked effectively in previous stressful events; utilize supportive resources: family, social services, or spiritual advisor	Client's use of denial decreases; client exhibits interest in learning about the heart attack and the rehabilitation process Client will perform activities within prescribed limits
Self-concept, disturbance in: related to altered body image	Accept alteration in body image over time; assume role responsibilities	Assign a primary nurse who can establish a trusting relationship with client and family; encourage client to express feelings; provide atmosphere of acceptance; clarify misconceptions; emphasize client's progress; encourage socialization with other cardiac clients and families; encourage participation in cardiac rehabilitation classes	Client expresses feelings about altered self-concept

Nursing Diagnosis	Client Care Goals	Plan/Nursing Implementation	Expected Outcome
Gas exchange, impaired: related to decreased cardiac output	Breathe comfortably at normal rate	Administer O_2 at 2–4 L as ordered; monitor ABGs; gradually increase client's activity	Vital signs will remain wnl with absence of dyspnea
Cardiac output, alteration in: decreased	Perform ADL without risk; identify factors that increase cardiac work load	Organize client's care and provide undisturbed rest; monitor client's response to activity: vital sign changes, pain, shortness of breath, pallor, cyanosis, disequilibrium, confusion, development of dysrhythmias; establish gradual increases in activity; prophylactic medication prior to activity (eg, nitroglycerin); use of O_2 during periods of increased activity	Cardiac tolerance to increased activity will gradually improve
Bowel elimination, alteration in: potential for constipation	Maintain normal bowel elimination pattern	Administer stool softener as prescribed; assist client to commode daily after breakfast; explain why straining should be avoided; encourage activity within prescribed limits; within dietary restrictions, encourage client to consume bran, fruit, and fluids; arrange environment, food, and client comfort to maintain the client's appetite	Bowel movement every 1–2 days without straining; client states why straining should be avoided
Knowledge deficit: related to MI	Acute phase: demonstrate understanding of CCU equipment and routines	Explain CCU routines and procedures client will encounter; assist client in feeling safe; prepare client and family for procedures, advancement of activities, and transfer from CCU	Client will be able to relax and experience less anxiety
	Convalescent: identify personal cardiovascular risk factors	Discuss risk factors for CAD with client and emphasize the risk factors client can control; encourage client and family to participate in rehabilitation classes; offer nutritional counseling services; teach relaxation techniques to client and family; document teaching and evaluate client's learning	Client participates in learning and can identify own risk factors; client verbalizes plan to modify risk factors
	Distinguish between angina and MI pain	Teach client and family how to differentiate angina from MI pain; offer written information and instruction	Client will state differences between angina and MI pain and give recommended treatment for each
	State the names of prescribed medications, dosage, and administration	Discuss medications the client will be taking at home	Client and family will be able to identify each drug and state dosage and administration
	Maintain supply of medications	Discuss importance of refilling drugs and to avoid "running out"; discuss resources available to client to cover expenses	Client and family will know how to obtain medication refills; client will be helped with sources to defray the cost of medications, if necessary
	Explain prescribed activity levels	Discuss activity levels and why levels are progressed in steps; teach client to monitor the CV response by obtaining pulse rate and observing signs of fatigue, palpitations, or DOE; discuss the importance of adequate rest periods between activities	Client will state what activities are allowed within a given level; client progresses in activities within the cardiac rehabilitation guidelines; client will be able to monitor his own CV response

Chapter 25

Surgical Approaches to Heart and Major Blood Vessel Dysfunction

Leslie S. Kern

Objectives

When you have finished studying this chapter, you should be able to:

Discuss the indications for surgical treatment of coronary artery disease, valvular heart disease, ventricular aneurysm, cardiomyopathy, thoracic aortic aneurysm, aortic dissection, and cardiac dysrhythmia.

Identify the nonsurgical technique, client implications, and nursing care involved in percutaneous transluminal coronary angioplasty.

Provide a brief description of the surgical procedures used in treating heart and major blood vessel dysfunction.

Recognize the physiological implications of these surgical procedures on the client.

Describe the impact of these surgical procedures on the client's psychosocial adaptation and lifestyle.

Specify the content to be covered in the preoperative and postoperative teaching of the cardiac surgery client.

Describe the preoperative and postoperative nursing care required of the heart surgery client.

Explain the nurse's role in the prevention of complications of cardiac surgery.

The care of the client requiring heart surgery is a fascinating and challenging area of nursing. Often the client's condition has reached life-threatening limits, and immediate surgery is required. In other cases, the disease process has slowly developed into a phase in which symptoms limit the client's activities and affect lifestyle.

In either situation, heart surgery is one of the most serious operations clients can undergo. During heart surgery, extensive physiological changes occur, increasing the risk for complications in the early postoperative period.

Because of this, the nursing needs of these clients are complex and demanding. During the acute phase, the nurse constantly monitors for multiple complications that can suddenly appear. In the subacute phase, clients continue to be closely monitored and guided as they begin to recover. Finally, at discharge, the nurse educates clients for home recovery and a lifestyle that helps prevent a recurrence of the disease process. This chapter focuses on the nursing care of clients who have undergone surgery of the heart and major blood vessels.

Section I: Surgical/Nonsurgical Approaches to Disorders Affecting the Coronary Arteries

When pharmacologic treatment of coronary artery disease (CAD) with nitrates, beta-adrenergic blocking agents, or calcium channel blockers is unsuccessful, surgical treat-

ment of CAD is considered. Surgical treatment was initially aimed at the relief of debilitating angina. In the early 1900s, this was accomplished by sympathectomy (surgical interruption of the sympathetic nervous pathways), and procedures were developed later to increase coronary blood flow. In one such procedure, asbestos or talcum powder was placed on the surface of the heart to stimulate the development of adhesions that irritated the epicardial tissue and stimulated increased coronary blood flow. Implantation of the internal mammary artery directly into the myocardium was first performed in 1945. This procedure was common until 1962, when the first coronary artery bypass surgery was performed. Since then, coronary artery bypass surgery has been the primary surgical technique for the treatment of CAD.

Through research, investigators are attempting to develop treatments less traumatic than coronary artery bypass surgery, which requires a 4- to 8-week convalescence and costs up to $40,000. Percutaneous transluminal coronary angioplasty (PTCA) is one such technique. Both coronary artery bypass surgery and PTCA are discussed here. An experimental technique, excimer laser angioplasty, which uses a "cool" laser to vaporize the blockage without burning a hole in the blood vessel, has been used on human cadavers and also appears promising.

CORONARY ARTERY BYPASS SURGERY

In coronary artery bypass surgery, a graft consisting of the saphenous vein, internal mammary artery, or both brings a new blood supply to the distal position of the stenotic coronary artery. The surgeon connects the saphenous vein graft to the aorta proximally and to the coronary artery distally. Blood flowing into the aorta then passes through the new graft to the coronary artery, restoring the blood supply to the ischemic myocardium. The internal mammary artery graft is based on the same principle; the difference is that the artery remains connected at its point of origin and is simply brought down to the stenotic coronary artery. The advantage is a greater longevity than the vein graft. With either type of bypass graft, stenosis of the new graft is always a potential problem, particularly during the first year after surgery (Chesebro et al., 1982).

The indications for coronary artery bypass surgery are controversial. Studies continue to delineate the criteria for surgical intervention. All clients with suspected significant CAD are evaluated with coronary angiography before surgery. The decision for surgery is based on the client's symptoms and angiography results. The indications for coronary artery bypass surgery are:

- Stable angina pectoris with greater than 50% blockage of the left main coronary artery.
- Stable angina pectoris in the presence of three-vessel coronary artery disease.
- Unstable angina pectoris with three-vessel disease or severe two-vessel disease.
- Recent myocardial infarction (MI) (less than 30 days), after which the client continues to experience angina pectoris (Rogers et al., 1981).
- Ischemic heart failure with cardiogenic shock.

- Signs of ischemia or impending MI in a postangioplasty client.

Surgical Procedure

During heart surgery, the client requires constant hemodynamic and laboratory monitoring and cardiopulmonary bypass using the *heart–lung machine*. Most clients have a Swan–Ganz catheter or other thermodilution catheter inserted. A radial artery catheter measures arterial pressure. Urine output is monitored closely, as are blood electrolyte and blood oxygen levels.

The coronary artery bypass graft procedure begins with removal of the saphenous vein from the leg. The incision is made on the medial aspect of the leg along the saphenous vein. The vein is removed by blunt dissection; usually 20 cm is removed for each graft (Figure 25–1). The vein branches are tied off and the vein flushed with heparinized saline. The wound is flushed with an antibiotic solution and then closed with nylon sutures and adhesive strips.

While one surgeon prepares the vein graft, a second makes a medial sternotomy incision in preparation for placing the client on the heart–lung machine. The sternum is divided using an electric saw. Cautery controls bleeding, and bone wax is applied to the bone edges. The pericardium is incised and opened for clear heart exposure.

The cannulas for the heart–lung machine are then placed in the venae cavae or the right atrium and ascending aorta (Figure 25–2). The blood is diverted from the body through the venae cavae cannulas; it circulates through a bubble oxygenator and is then pumped back into the body through the ascending aorta cannula. **Cardiopulmonary bypass** using the heart–lung machine allows the heart to be stopped during the surgery and helps maintain a bloodless field. The procedure maintains minimal circulation and tissue perfusion, and the body is in a shocklike state. In addition, the body is cooled to reduce the metabolic tissue needs. As a result of this abnormal state, intravascular volume and electrolytes fluctuate during and after the surgery. Moreover, the mechanical components of the

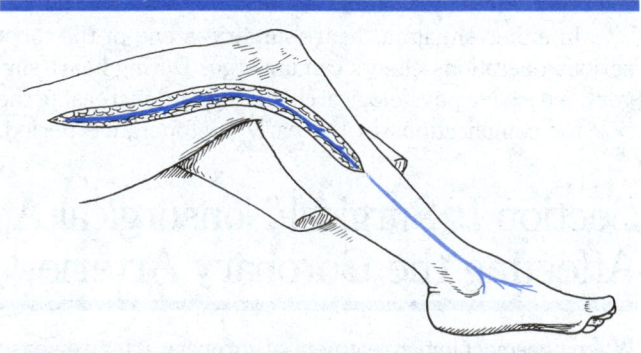

Figure 25–1

Removing the saphenous vein.

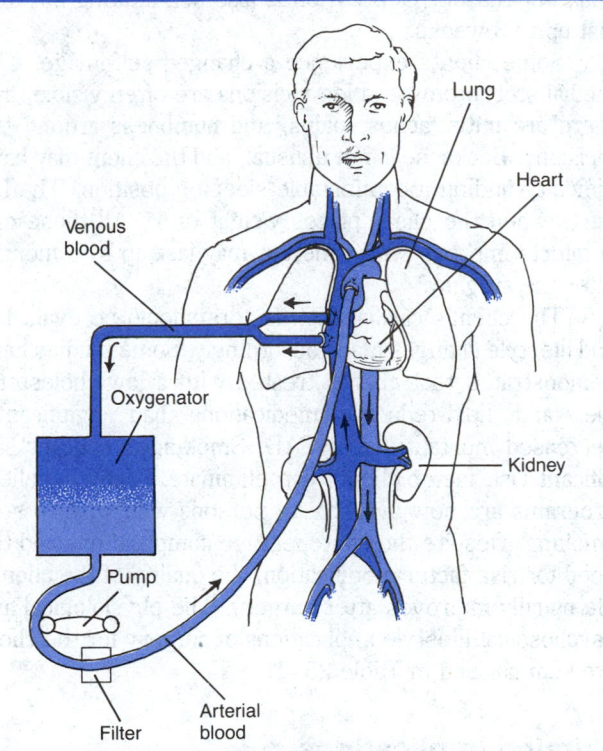

Figure 25–2

The heart–lung machine. Blood is diverted to the heart–lung machine through the cannulas in the superior and inferior venae cavae. Oxygen is bubbled through the blood in the oxygenator, and blood is then returned to the body through the arterial cannula in the ascending aorta.

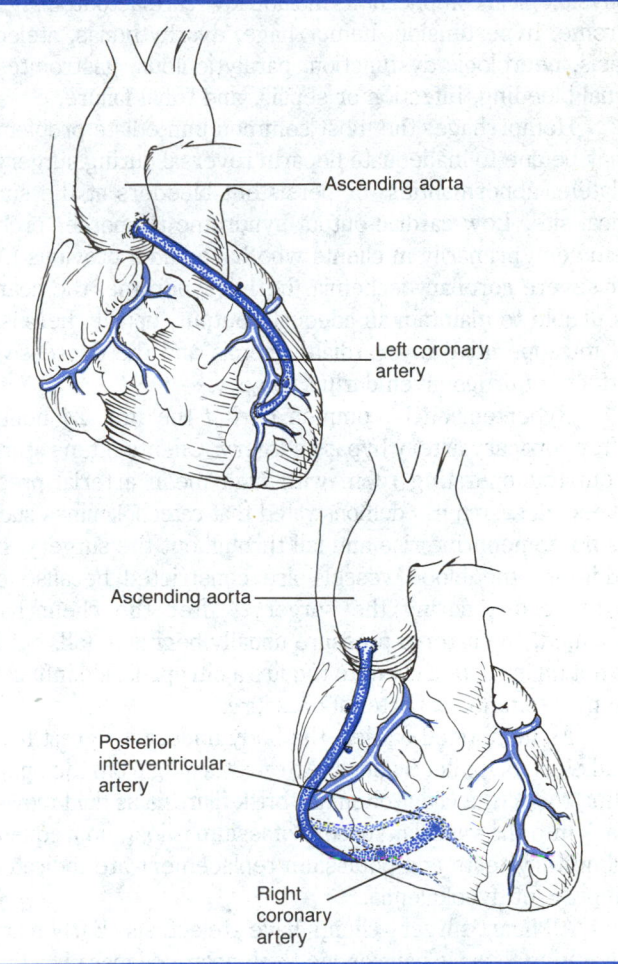

Figure 25–3

Coronary artery bypass grafts using the saphenous vein. **Top.** A single graft from the ascending aorta to the left coronary artery on the anterior surface of the heart. **Bottom.** A sequential graft from the ascending aorta to the right coronary artery and the posterior interventricular artery on the posterior surface of the heart.

heart–lung machine injure red blood cells and platelets, causing hemolysis and abnormal platelet function.

After the client is on the heart–lung machine, the graft or grafts can be anastomosed to the coronary artery distal to the stenosis. Following distal anastomosis, the graft is sutured onto the ascending aorta. Single or sequential grafts may be performed. In a single graft, one vein is used to bypass one blockage. A sequential graft is one vein graft that supplies two or more vessels; the graft requires less vein, and the suturing takes less time (Figure 25–3).

When the grafts are in place and tested for patency, the client is gradually removed from the heart–lung machine. This is a critical time in the surgery, because the heart must begin beating on its own. During weaning from the machine, dysrhythmias may appear, and the heart's contraction may be depressed from surgical medications or ischemic injury during surgery. If weaning is difficult, inotropic drugs or calcium may be given to stimulate contractility. Dysrhythmias are treated with the usual antidysrhythmic drugs (see Chapter 24).

After the bypass cannulas are removed, pacing wires are placed in the atria and ventricles and brought out through the skin. These wires are connected to an external pacing generator and placed in a demand mode. If the heart rate slows below the preset rate, the pacer automatically begins pacing the heart.

Anterior and posterior chest tubes are placed in the mediastinum and connected to a closed drainage system so drainage can be measured hourly. Free drainage through these tubes prevents the accumulation of blood around the heart and the development of life-threatening cardiac tamponade.

Closed with stainless steel wire, the sternum heals after approximately 6 weeks. The wires remain permanently and are always visible on x-ray examination. The skin is closed with subcutaneous sutures, and the wound is dressed. The client is then taken to the recovery room or intensive care unit (ICU).

Implications for the Client

Physiological Implications

The client usually spends 2 days in the ICU. Complications are most likely during the first 24 hours. Early physiological complications include low-cardiac-output syndrome, hypertension, hemorrhage, dysrhythmias, atelectasis, neurologic dysfunction, paralytic ileus, gastrointestinal bleeding, infection or sepsis, and renal failure.

Hemorrhage, the most common immediate problem, may be due to inadequate heparin reversal during surgery, platelet abnormalities, or persistent bleeders at the surgical site. Low-cardiac-output syndrome is another problem seen primarily in clients who have had a previous MI or severe coronary ischemia. In this syndrome, the heart is unable to maintain an adequate output, usually because of intraoperative myocardial ischemia and the depressive effects of drugs given during surgery.

Hypertension is common during the first 24 hours after coronary artery bypass surgery. Clients often return from the operating room with high mean arterial pressures. Research has demonstrated that catecholamines such as norepinephrine rise and fall throughout the surgery. In addition, the blood vessels are constricted because of hypothermia during the surgery. After the client has warmed, the arterial pressure usually begins to fall, but it is not unusual for a client to require a nitroprusside infusion to maintain normal arterial pressure.

As mentioned earlier, the body undergoes great fluid and electrolyte fluctuations. After returning from the operating room, the client often has brisk diuresis as fluid moves back into the vascular space. Potassium is lost, so frequent laboratory tests and potassium replacement are indicated to prevent hypokalemia.

All heart surgery clients have atelectasis. Early postoperative fever is usually due to alveolar collapse. For this reason, clients must perform deep-breathing and coughing exercises.

Late complications of coronary artery bypass surgery include wound infection, postpericardiotomy syndrome, and late cardiac tamponade. Despite these possible complications, most clients benefit from the surgery in improved heart pumping action, relief of anginal pain, relief of the signs and symptoms of heart failure, and improved quality of life (Jenkins, Stanton, Savageau, Denlinger, & Klein, 1983). The client may be concerned about the effects on leg circulation of removal of the saphenous vein. This is a superficial vein; deep veins perform the majority of the work of returning blood to the heart. About 6 weeks is required for the deeper veins to take over; until then, the client may have temporary leg edema.

To prevent graft closure, the client will probably have antiplatelet therapy (325 mg of aspirin a day, 75 mg of dipyridamole [Persantine], or both) for a time that varies according to the physician.

Psychosocial/Lifestyle Implications

The client in the ICU may become confused and experience delirium and hallucinations (sometimes called *ICU psychosis*). These conditions usually resolve when the client leaves intensive care. Depression may begin on the third or fourth postoperative day, and clients may cry for no apparent reason. Depression is also self-limiting but may last up to 3 weeks.

Some clients experience a changed self-image. The medial sternotomy and leg incisions are often visible, and there are initial aches, pains, and numbness around the incisions. Backache is not unusual, and the client may have difficulty finding a comfortable sleeping position. The leg hurts when the client places weight on it. All these discomforts improve with time but may last up to 6 months after the surgery.

The client's cardiac risk factors should be evaluated and lifestyle changes made accordingly. Some studies have demonstrated that clients treated with a low-cholesterol diet and lipid-reducing medications had significantly decreased mortality from CAD. Smoking is another significant risk factor clients can eliminate. Many excellent programs are now available to persons who wish to stop smoking. Despite the postoperative complications and the need for risk factor modification, the quality of the client's life usually improves after surgery. The physiological and psychosocial/lifestyle implications of surgery for the client are summarized in Table 25–1.

Nursing Implications

Preoperative Care

The nurse's most important role in the preoperative period is to prepare the client physically and psychologically for coronary artery bypass surgery. Physical preparations include ensuring that the client's nutritional state is

Table 25–1 Coronary Artery Bypass Surgery: Implications for the Client	
Physiological Implications	**Psychosocial/ Lifestyle Implications**
Possible early complications of low-cardiac-output syndrome, hypertension, hemorrhage, dysrhythmias, atelectasis, neurologic dysfunction, paralytic ileus, GI bleeding, infection or sepsis, renal failure, and diuresis	Intensive care unit psychosis
	Postoperative depression
	Changed self-image
Postpericardiotomy syndrome or possible late cardiac tamponade	Risk-factor modification (change in diet, possible medications, elimination of smoking)
Improved heart pumping action	Improved quality of life
Relief of anginal pain	
Relief of the signs and symptoms of heart failure	
Need for antiplatelet therapy	

optimal, preparing the skin by shaving and showering, cleansing the bowel with an enema, assessing preoperative laboratory values to ensure normal ranges (especially blood-clotting values), and assessing the client for any risk factors that would interfere with a smooth operation. A history of smoking increases the risk of pulmonary complications. Although smoking is not a contraindication for surgery, nurses should be alerted to this risk factor so that they can give special pulmonary care.

The value of preoperative teaching in psychological preparation has been well documented and is included in the standard care of the heart surgery client. The client should thoroughly understand the normal heart anatomy and the heart problem. A heart model is helpful in giving these explanations. Clients often have misconceptions about the exact nature of their heart problems. They are often relieved to learn that their heart surgery is not as complicated as they envisioned.

When describing the tubes that will be present after surgery, also explain the sensations the client will experience. For example, the endotracheal tube is uncomfortable, and clients may feel they are not getting enough air. Some clients also experience a gagging sensation with this tube. Explain that this is a temporary discomfort and that the client will be getting sufficient air from the mechanical ventilator. A nurse will be with the client at all times while the tube is in place. The client also should know that the pain after heart surgery is an achiness and soreness that is especially felt with deep breathing. The pain is not sharp and unbearable, as some may think, and analgesics will be available.

Deep-breathing and coughing exercises are extremely important for the first 5 days following heart surgery. (See the discussion and illustrations in Chapter 14.) Before surgery, the client should practice these exercises and the use of the incentive spirometer.

Postoperative Care

In the early postoperative period, the nurse must constantly assess the client because of the many physiological changes with cardiopulmonary bypass surgery. Arterial pressure, pulmonary artery pressures, heart rate, and heart rhythm are evaluated every 15 minutes until the valves have stabilized. Chest drainage and urinary flow are measured hourly. Blood counts, clotting studies, and arterial blood gas measurements are performed regularly. The nurse carefully assesses the client's neurovascular, abdominal, and pulmonary functions and the circulatory function of the operated leg.

The goal of nursing care in the immediate postoperative period is the prevention or early identification of the complications of cardiac surgery. In addition to a comprehensive nursing assessment, the nurse checks daily weights and chest x-rays to help monitor the client's fluid and pulmonary statuses. A weight gain of 1 kg in 24 hours is considered significant and may indicate the need for diuretic therapy. The nurse can identify atelectasis in the early

Nursing Research Note

Whiteside S: Patient education. *J Psychosoc Nurs Mental Health Serv* 1983; 21(10):17–20.

This study investigated the effect of a client educational program that included both a one-to-one information exchange and written material on medications the client was taking. The sample included 28 cardiac clients who also had mental health problems. In a quasi-experimental design, the control group received no education, whereas the experimental group received education about their medications. Both groups were pre- and post-tested. In the educational experimental group, clients were able to answer questions correctly about their medications. The control group showed no significant improvement in medication knowledge.

This study demonstrates that client educational programs are effective. In this case, education was also beneficial to clients with mental health problems. The findings underscore the importance of client teaching.

postoperative period by decreased breath sounds and fever. When clients have been extubated, they should perform deep-breathing and coughing exercises every 2 hours. In many institutions, clients use an incentive spirometer hourly.

Clients on bed rest should perform range-of-motion (ROM) exercises and mild calisthenics. They gradually increase their activity until they are able to bathe and dress themselves and ambulate 400 ft unassisted and with minimal symptoms. A progressive exercise program is recommended; as clients are advanced to the next level, evaluate them for activity tolerance using heart rate, blood pressure, and heart rhythm as indicators (LaForge et al., 1984). Ambulation is often begun within the first 48 hours.

Adequate nutrition is important for any surgical client, particularly the heart surgery client. These clients are often nauseated and anorexic the first few days following surgery. Taste-bud function diminishes because the endotracheal tube rubs on the tongue surface. Fluid retention may necessitate a sodium-limited diet. Offer tasty high-protein foods in frequent small feedings. Custards, puddings, and milk shakes provide calories as well as protein. The dietitian should assist in planning individualized, attractive meals.

Discharge teaching begins the fifth or sixth postoperative day. Make sure the client and family or significant other clearly understand what normal recovery includes and what signs and symptoms to report. Clients must learn the dosages and side effects of medications. They must understand that they should not discontinue any medications without the physician's approval. If there is any wound drainage or separation, give clients dressing supplies, and instruct them in how to change dressings. All clients should know the signs of wound infection.

Activity depends on the client's response to exercise. Walking is encouraged, but the client should avoid lifting heavy objects for 6 weeks and driving a car for 3 weeks. Diet instructions depend on special needs, but all cardiac surgery clients should follow a diet of no added salt for the first month because the body is undergoing changes in its fluid balance. Adequate intake of nutrients is also essential for proper wound healing, so the client should eat a diet high in protein, vitamins, and minerals. Eventually, a diet low in cholesterol and saturated fat can be followed.

The surgical leg tends to be edematous, so instruct the client to wear antiembolism support stockings during the day and to remove them at night. The operated leg should be elevated on a footstool when the client sits until the swelling has subsided.

PERCUTANEOUS TRANSLUMINAL CORONARY ANGIOPLASTY

Percutaneous transluminal coronary angioplasty (PTCA) is an invasive but nonsurgical technique used in the treatment of CAD. A balloon catheter is introduced into a vessel, and the balloon is positioned at the site of the atherosclerotic plaque. The balloon is inflated, compressing the plaque and reestablishing blood flow to the ischemic myocardium. This procedure is only a few years old but is being performed worldwide. The ideal candidate for this procedure has had angina pectoris for less than 1 year, has not benefitted from medical therapy, is a candidate for bypass surgery, and does not have left main coronary artery stenosis.

Procedure

PTCA is done in a cardiac catheterization laboratory using fluoroscopy. The insertion site can be the femoral or brachial arteries. Heparin is given during the procedure to prevent thrombosis, and nitroglycerin is given to prevent coronary artery spasm. A guide catheter is first inserted and advanced to the coronary arteries (Figure 25–4). The balloon dilatation catheter is advanced through the guide catheter and positioned within the stenosis. Angiography documents the degree of stenosis. The balloon is then inflated under pressure, using a solution of saline and contrast material, and inflation is maintained for 3 to 5 seconds to compress the plaque. The angiography is repeated to observe for lumen patency. Coronary artery and arterial pressures are measured throughout the procedure. The client is then transferred to the coronary care unit to be continuously monitored for complications.

Implications for the Client

PTCA has been well received by clients and insurance companies. Hospitalization is for 2 or 3 days, and there are significantly fewer complications than with bypass surgery. The current success rate is 60% to 70%.

Physiological Implications

Complications of this procedure include cardiac tamponade, MI, dysrhythmias, hemorrhage, heart failure, hematoma formation, and thrombus formation at the insertion

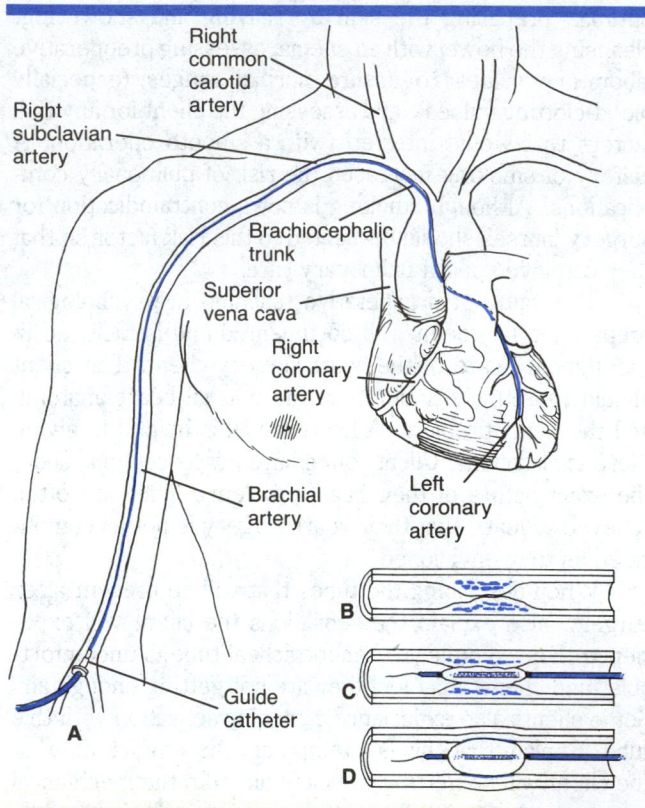

Figure 25–4

Percutaneous transluminal coronary angioplasty procedure. **A.** The guide catheter is threaded through the brachial artery to the blocked left coronary artery. **B.** An inside view of the blocked artery. **C.** The balloon dilation catheter is positioned in the artery so the balloon is within the obstruction. **D.** The inflated balloon flattens the obstruction against the vessel wall.

site. Of the successful angioplasties, 5% of clients have developed acute MI. Of the unsuccessful dilatations, a reported 20% have developed this complication (Levy et al., 1981). About 20% of PTCA clients experience recurrences within 6 months; however, the recurrence rate after a second PTCA drops to as low as 5%.

To assist in maintaining the patency of the newly opened lumen, antiplatelet drugs are prescribed. The two most common drugs are aspirin and dipyridamole. These drugs are taken indefinitely and will continue to be prescribed until newer therapies are developed.

Psychosocial/Lifestyle Implications

The value of PTCA for the client is avoiding the trauma of a major operation. Successful angioplasty relieves anginal pain and eliminates the threat of an imminent heart attack. The risk of MI is always present, of course, but is significantly reduced. The client should be evaluated for cardiac risk factors and should work toward controlling factors such as smoking, diet, and exercise. Table 25–2 summarizes the physiological and psychosocial/lifestyle implications for the angioplasty client.

Table 25–2   Percutaneous Transluminal Coronary Angioplasty: Implications for the Client

Physiological Implications	Psychosocial/Lifestyle Implications
Possible complications of cardiac tamponade, myocardial infarction, dysrhythmias, hemorrhage, heart failure, hematoma formation, and thrombus formation at the insertion site	Relief of anginal pain
	Elimination of the threat of immediate myocardial infarction
Indefinite use of antiplatelet drugs	Risk-factor modification (change in diet, elimination of smoking, need for exercise)

Nursing Implications

Preoperative Care

The client is usually admitted the day before angioplasty. Preangioplasty diagnostic tests include: coronary angiogram, treadmill stress test, chest x-ray, ECG, blood chemistries, complete blood count, and glucose levels. Each client is blood typed and screened in preparation for possible heart surgery. Medications are started, including aspirin, dipyrimadole, nifedipine (Procardia), and nitroglycerin. A complete heart surgery preparation is done, and the client is placed on NPO status after midnight.

The nursing assessment is an important activity in the preoperative period. The client's cardiovascular assessment is documented in the nursing notes for reference in the early postoperative period. Client education for this procedure is just as important as it is for heart surgery. Explain the coronary anatomy, the atherosclerotic process, the angioplasty procedure, and complications that can occur, particularly the potential need for heart surgery.

Postoperative Care

The most important aspect of postangioplasty nursing care is observing the client for signs of coronary artery occlusion, including chest pain, ECG changes, dysrhythmias, and hypotension. These episodes may be treated with morphine sulfate for pain, IV or sublingual nitroglycerin, or a calcium antagonist such as nifedipine. If symptoms continue, coronary artery bypass surgery may be indicated.

Postangioplasty nursing assessment also includes monitoring vital signs every 15 minutes for an hour and then every 30 minutes until stable; taking a 12-lead ECG every 8 hours (three times in all); and continuous ECG monitoring. Assess the client's peripheral circulation (color, warmth, pulses, sensation, and mobility) every hour (four times), then every 2 hours (four times), and finally every 4 hours. Assess the catheter insertion site for bleeding, hematoma, or infection every hour (four times), then every 2 hours (four times), and finally every 4 hours. Monitor the client's urinary output every hour and breath sounds every 2 hours.

Maintain 5 to 10 lb of pressure on the catheter insertion site until all bleeding has ceased, and keep the head of the bed below 30°. Push fluids to assist in the elimination of contrast material.

Upon discharge, clients must understand the need for antiplatelet drugs and the necessity that they not be discontinued without the physician's consent. Clients also need instruction on signs and symptoms to report; these include new chest pressure or heaviness, recurrence of angina pectoris, dizziness, or light-headedness.

Section II: Surgical Approaches to Disorders Affecting the Heart Valves

Valvular heart disease can be medically managed as long as the client remains asymptomatic. When the client develops fatigue, dyspnea, orthopnea, palpitations, or angina pectoris, however, surgical treatment is usually indicated. Types of surgery include annuloplasty, mitral valve commissurotomy, and valve replacement.

ANNULOPLASTY

Annuloplasty involves the surgical repair of a native valve. This procedure is usually performed on the insufficient or regurgitant valve instead of valve replacement. The surgeon decides to perform an annuloplasty at the time of surgery. Some believe it is better to maintain the client's original valve than to replace it, because artificial and tissue valves carry inherent risks and require significant lifestyle changes.

Surgical Procedure

A medial sternotomy incision is made, and the client is placed on the heart–lung machine. The left atrium is entered for mitral valve annuloplasty, and the ascending aorta for aortic valve annuloplasty. Using interrupted silk sutures, the surgeon gathers the valve annulus, much like a skirt, and makes it smaller so that the valve leaflets are in apposition. The atriotomy or aortotomy is closed, and the client is weaned from the heart–lung machine. The wound is closed in the same manner as for bypass surgery.

Table 25–3 Annuloplasty: Implications for the Client	
Physiological Implications	**Psychosocial/ Lifestyle Implications**
Complications and improvements similar to those of bypass surgery (see Table 25–1)	Postoperative confusion or depression
Abnormally high preload until ventricle adjusts to smaller volume	Temporary need for antidysrhythmic drugs
Susceptibility to pulmonary congestion	

Implications for the Client

Physiological Implications

The client's postoperative course is similar to that of the bypass client. The left ventricle has become accustomed to an increased volume because of the regurgitant valve. Therefore, as the excess volume is relieved, the client requires a higher-than-normal preload (pulmonary artery wedge pressure) to maintain adequate heart output until the ventricle has adjusted to a smaller volume.

The complications of this surgery are similar to those of bypass surgery. The client with valvular disease is more susceptible to pulmonary congestion, however, and should be observed closely for signs of pulmonary edema, pleural effusion, or both.

Psychosocial/Lifestyle Implications

The psychological responses following bypass surgery can also be observed after annuloplasty. Postoperative periods of confusion or depression are not unusual. In the early postoperative period, atrial dysrhythmias are common, so the client may temporarily require antidysrhythmic drugs. Table 25–3 summarizes the implications for the annuloplasty client.

Nursing Implications

Preoperative Care

The preoperative instructions for annuloplasty clients are similar to those given before bypass surgery, except no leg incision need be discussed. It is often helpful to show clients a heart model and discuss the location of the heart valves. Clients are often relieved to see that there is more than one valve and that they are not unique in requiring the repair of two or sometimes three valves. The physical preparations of the client are identical to those for bypass surgery.

Postoperative Care

The postoperative nursing care of the annuloplasty client is the same as for any client who has undergone heart

surgery (see the discussion of bypass surgery for a summary of this care). Valve surgery always carries a higher risk for the development of pulmonary complications, as has been described. Carefully evaluate daily weights and 24-hour intake and output. Diuretic therapy is initiated for any signs of fluid retention. The client's fluid intake is limited to as little as 1200 mL per day, and sodium is restricted. Atrial dysrhythmias may be present because of left atrial enlargement or because of myocardial edema at the surgical site. Usually, digitalis is given first, followed by procainamide hydrochloride (Pronestyl) or quinidine (Cardioquin, Quinidex). The client's activity should progress according to how he or she is feeling. Discharge instructions on wound care, activity limitations, medications, and diet are similar to those for bypass surgery.

MITRAL VALVE COMMISSUROTOMY

When a client has mitral stenosis, the valve leaflets are stiffened and fused together by vegetative or calcific deposits. In commissurotomy, an alternative to valve replacement, the valve leaflets are cut free from one another.

When the mitral valve is open in the normal adult heart, the blood flows through an area of 6 cm^2. As the valve becomes stenotic, the opening for blood flow becomes smaller; blood flow is impeded when the valve opening is narrowed by 50% (3 cm^2). With severe narrowing to less than 2 cm^2, signs of congestive heart failure appear. If mitral valve stenosis goes untreated, the left atrium enlarges to compensate for the increased force necessary to push blood through the stenotic valve. Atrial fibrillation often appears, and stasis of blood in the left atrium can result in clot formation and emboli thrown off to the brain or body. Some clients have systemic embolization with mitral stenosis and atrial fibrillation. Surgery is therefore indicated for (1) any symptomatic client with mitral stenosis, (2) any client with New York Heart Association (NYHA) class II or III disease (see Chapter 24), and (3) any client with recurrent thromboembolism.

Surgical Procedure

A medial sternotomy incision is made, and the client is placed on the heart–lung machine. The left atrium is excised and the valve exposed. The left atrium is examined for clots and the commissure (the junction of the valve leaflets) identified. The commissurotomy is then performed using a right-angle clamp. The surgeon assesses leaflet mobility and looks for any residual regurgitation. The client is weaned from the heart–lung machine. The wound is closed with chest tubes, and pacing wires are placed.

Implications for the Client

Physiological Implications

In the immediate postoperative period, the client is prone to pulmonary complications and fluid overload as described

Table 25–4	Mitral Valve Commissurotomy: Implications for the Client
Physiological Implications	**Psychosocial/Lifestyle Implications**
Pulmonary complications and fluid overload in immediate postoperative period	Intensive care unit psychosis
	Postoperative depression
	Changed self-image
Continuation of preoperative atrial dysrhythmias	Risk-factor modification (change in diet, antidysrhythmic drugs, elimination of smoking)
Possible recurrence of symptoms and need for valve replacement	
Need for antiplatelet therapy	Improved quality of life

in the section on annuloplasty. Preoperative atrial dysrhythmias continue in the postoperative period. Some clients take sodium warfarin (Coumadin) or aspirin, particularly if they have a history of thromboembolism.

A drawback of commissurotomy is that symptoms may recur, necessitating valve replacement. For this reason, commissurotomies are not performed as often as in the past.

Psychosocial/Lifestyle Implications

Changes in the client's psychosocial function and lifestyle parallel those described for bypass surgery. The client must learn the dosages and side effects of the antidysrhythmic drugs prescribed. The client follows a diet of no added salt for the first month at home. Table 25–4 summarizes the physiological and psychosocial/lifestyle implications for the client with mitral valve commissurotomy. The preoperative and postoperative nursing care of the mitral valve commissurotomy client is covered in the next section on valve replacement.

VALVE REPLACEMENT

Valve replacement involves the removal of the native valve and the insertion of a prosthesis. Three general categories of valves can be used: allografts, or human valves; xenografts, or animal valves; and artificial valves. Allografts are no longer in general use because they are difficult to obtain and offer no advantages over other valves.

Xenografts originate from a pig (porcine valve) or cow (bovine valve) and are specially prepared for human use. The tissue valve has little risk of clot formation on the leaflets—a major advantage, because artificial valves are prone to clot formation and require that clients take sodium warfarin the rest of their lives. Tissue valves lack longevity, however. They begin to deteriorate after 5 to 10 years and too often require replacement.

Artificial valves are generally used in the young client, where valve longevity is important (Figure 25–5). Other factors are also considered when choosing a valve, such as bleeding history and plans for pregnancy. For example, if a client has a history of peptic ulcers or other bleeding problems, a tissue valve is preferred so sodium warfarin will not be needed. For a young female client who wishes to become pregnant, a tissue valve is also preferable because of the bleeding risk with sodium warfarin. Indications for valve replacement include:

- Symptomatic mitral stenosis
- Debilitating mitral regurgitation
- Severe aortic stenosis and ventricular hypertrophy
- Repeated syncope or heart failure from aortic stenosis
- Symptomatic aortic regurgitation
- Combined valve and coronary artery disease

Surgical Procedure

A medial sternotomy incision is performed, and the client is placed on the heart–lung machine. With mitral valve replacement, the papillary muscles and chordae tendineae are removed with the valve leaflets. Precautions are taken to avoid injuring the nearby aortic valve and atrioventricular (A-V) node. Interrupted sutures are placed around the annulus and in the new valve, which is steadied with a special valve holder. The valve is lowered into place and the sutures tied off. The left atrium is closed with all air expelled.

With aortic valve replacement, the surgeon makes an incision in the ascending aorta. Often the aortic valve is calcified, so it must be removed carefully to avoid releasing emboli into the brain or nearby coronary arteries. Sutures

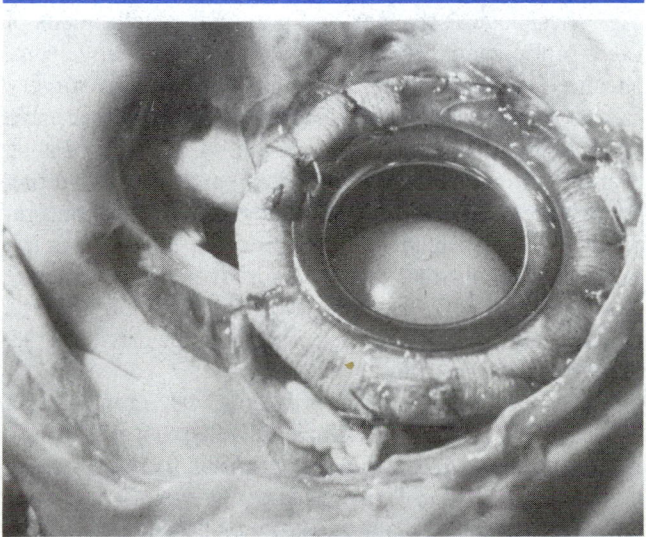

Figure 25–5

The plastic and metal Starr–Edwards artificial mitral valve in place. (Courtesy of Millard Fillmore Hospital, Buffalo, NY)

Nursing Research Note

Quinless FW, Cassese M, Atherton N: The effect of selected preoperative, intraoperative and postoperative variables on the development of postcardiotomy psychosis in patients undergoing open heart surgery. *Heart Lung* 1985; 14(4): 334–340.

These researchers examined the relations between physiologic, environmental, and psychological factors and the development of postcardiotomy psychosis. The most significant results occurred with the factors observed during the intraoperative period. They found that systolic blood pressure, perfusion time, and anesthesia time were all significantly correlated with the development of postcardiotomy psychosis. Of these, a low systolic blood pressure was most significant. It was interesting however, that all study participants developed some degree of postcardiotomy psychosis.

Nurses should be aware that postcardiotomy psychosis is common. They should educate their cardiac clients about the transient effect common to this type of surgery. The authors suggest that some type of checklist be developed so nurses can readily identify clients at risk for postcardiotomy psychosis—those having prolonged anesthesia and perfusion times along with hypotensive reactions.

are placed below the coronary ostia and through the prosthesis, which is lowered into place. The aortic incision is closed and air removed.

Tricuspid valve replacement is uncommon. The procedure is similar to mitral valve replacement except that entry is through the right atrium. One, two, or three valves can be replaced at once, and the valve surgery can be combined with other heart repairs.

Implications for the Client

Physiological Implications

The physiological changes and potential complications of valve replacement are numerous. The postoperative complications discussed for coronary artery bypass surgery can also occur after valve replacement. The artificial valve creates additional risks. First, even with anticoagulation therapy, thromboembolism is a risk, particularly if clotting studies are not closely monitored and the client is noncompliant in taking sodium warfarin. Second, hemorrhage is a risk while taking this drug. Third, over time, turbulent blood flow through the valve may result in hemolysis of red blood cells. Finally, any valve replacement carries a risk of bacterial endocarditis.

Despite these potential problems, valve replacement has advantages. Ventricular and atrial hypertrophy diminishes, and the vascular changes of pulmonary hypertension slowly reverse. These changes improve exercise tolerance and diminish shortness of breath.

Psychosocial/Lifestyle Implications

Lifestyle changes are related to the need for sodium warfarin therapy (with the artificial valve), as well as endo-

carditis prophylaxis. Sodium warfarin increases the blood-clotting time, so clients who injure themselves should apply pressure to the bleeding site. They should wear gloves when gardening and be careful when using sharp knives or power equipment. Weekly clotting studies are performed initially, and the drug dosage is altered accordingly to maintain a prothrombin time that is 1½ times the control value. The client should report any dietary changes to the physician, because an increase or decrease in vitamin K consumption can alter clotting times.

Endocarditis prophylaxis is indicated for anyone with valve disease or valve surgery. The American Heart Association provides a card that lists antibiotics to be taken before and after dental work (including teeth cleaning), endoscopic examinations, or surgery. Clients should not undergo any dental work for the first 6 months after valve replacement surgery.

The client who has a valve replacement should reduce sodium intake as a lifelong change; a 2-g sodium diet makes food palatable (see Chapter 24). The dietitian can help educate these clients.

The psychological response to valve surgery is similar to that after bypass surgery. In addition, the client must adjust to the soft but audible clicking sound of the artificial valve. The sound can be extremely annoying at times, can be heard by others nearby, and can inhibit the client's social life. The nurse may need to spend time with clients while they verbalize their feelings about the new valve. Overall, the client enjoys an improved quality of life. The physiological and psychosocial/lifestyle implications for the valve replacement client are given in Table 25–5.

Table 25–5 Valve Replacement: Implications for the Client

Physiological Implications	Psychosocial/Lifestyle Implications
Same possible postoperative complications as bypass surgery (see Table 25–1)	Need for precautions related to increased clotting time caused by sodium warfarin
Thromboembolism	Need for endocarditis prophylaxis
Hemorrhage with sodium warfarin (Coumadin)	
Possible hemolysis of red blood cells	Need for reduction of sodium intake
Risk of bacterial endocarditis	Annoying clicking of artificial valve
Diminished ventricular and atrial hypertrophy	Improved quality of life
Reversal of vascular changes of pulmonary hypertension	
Improved exercise tolerance	
Diminished shortness of breath	

Nursing Implications

Preoperative Care

The preoperative preparations for valve replacement are similar to those discussed in the section on coronary artery bypass surgery. In preparing the valve surgery client, the nurse's teaching should include valve pathology, types of replacement valves, the need for sodium warfarin, and special emphasis on deep-breathing and coughing exercises. Other instructions and information are given in the discussion of bypass surgery.

Postoperative Care

After valve surgery, the client requires the detailed assessment and monitoring described for the bypass client. Adequate fluid and IV intake to maintain adequate heart preload is important to ensure normal cardiac output. At the same time, an overinfusion of fluids can result in heart failure.

Atrial dysrhythmias are common. Occlusion or damage to the coronary arteries during valve replacement may result in ventricular dysrhythmias or acute MI. Continuous ECG monitoring provides early detection of these dysrhythmias.

Section III: Surgical Approaches to Disorders Affecting the Myocardium

VENTRICULAR ANEURYSMECTOMY

The surgical removal of a ventricular aneurysm is termed ventricular aneurysmectomy. The procedure is considered when the client exhibits angina pectoris, heart failure, ventricular tachycardia, or systemic emboli (Cosgrove & Loop, 1983).

Surgical Procedure

A medial sternotomy incision is made, and the client is placed on the heart–lung machine. The surgeon excises the aneurysm and inspects the ventricular chamber for clots. The myocardial edges are brought together and sutured, using a Teflon felt reinforcement. The ventricle is vented of any air and the client weaned from the heart–lung machine. Temporary pacing wires and mediastinal drainage tubes are placed.

Implications for the Client

Physiological Implications

Clients often experience some decrease in cardiac output and dysrhythmias in the immediate postoperative period. Ventricular aneurysmectomy clients are at risk for the complications of heart surgery listed in the discussion of bypass surgery. The postoperative progression in activity also parallels that of bypass surgery.

The long-term results of ventricular aneurysmectomy are likely to be favorable. Ninety percent of clients with symptoms of angina pectoris and heart failure have significant improvement with surgery (Cosgrove & Loop, 1983). It is always hoped that cardiac function will improve following removal of a ventricular aneurysm, but this may not always be the case. If a large area of scar tissue is removed, the client may be left with too little functioning myocardium, and symptoms may worsen after surgery.

Psychosocial/Lifestyle Implications

The client undergoes no significant lifestyle changes other than adjustment to the surgery if a small aneurysm is

removed. If left with insufficient functional myocardium after surgery, the client will require both pharmacologic and rehabilitative support in reaching maximum physical potential. This is often a gradual process that requires a few months of outpatient rehabilitation. In this instance, significant changes in lifestyle are experienced, particularly the ability to engage in physical activity. Table 25–6 summarizes the client implications for ventricular aneurysmectomy.

Nursing Implications

Preoperative Care

The preoperative preparations for ventricular aneurysmectomy clients are the same as described for coronary artery bypass surgery. One difference may be the preoperative presence of an intra-aortic balloon pump. The pump is a mechanical-assist device composed of a sausage-shaped balloon inserted into the thoracic aorta that inflates and

Table 25–6 Ventricular Aneurysmectomy: Implications for the Client	
Physiological Implications	**Psychosocial/ Lifestyle Implications**
Decrease in cardiac output and dysrhythmias in immediate postoperative period	No significant lifestyle modifications usually necessary
Possible complications similar to those of bypass surgery (see Table 25–1)	Pharmacologic and rehabilitative support and reduction in physical activity if insufficient functional myocardium remains
Improvement in angina pectoris and heart failure	
Improvement in exercise tolerance	
Risk of being left with insufficient functional myocardium	

deflates with the heartbeat. The counter-pulsation of the balloon effectively decreases the cardiac work load and increases coronary artery perfusion. If present, the balloon remains in place during surgery as well as 1 to 2 days postoperatively. The care of the client with a pump requires specialized nursing skills, usually provided by a critical care nurse.

Postoperative Care

Postoperatively, the client requires comprehensive, frequent assessment and monitoring of arterial pressure, pulmonary pressures, heart rates and rhythm, urinary output, chest tube drainage, laboratory tests, chest x-ray films, neurovascular status, and gastrointestinal and pulmonary function. As in coronary artery bypass surgery, the major goal of nursing care in the early postoperative period is the prevention of complications (see Table 25–1). Following ventriculotomy, the heart muscle recovers slowly, and low cardiac output syndrome is common. Ventricular dysrhythmias may also continue until myocardial edema has subsided.

Activity should progress with the nurse's help until the client can ambulate 200 to 400 ft unassisted and provide self-care. Discharge instructions are the same as for any adult cardiac surgery client (see the section on coronary artery bypass surgery).

HEART TRANSPLANTATION

Heart transplantation is reserved for the client with intractable cardiac disease when all forms of medical treatment have been exhausted—NYHA class IV disease, which involves extensive loss of ventricular function, severe CAD not amenable to bypass surgery, cardiomyopathy, severe valvular disease with cardiomyopathy, and congenital heart disease. Clients with symptomatic cardiomyopathy and decreased myocardial contractility have a 50% 2-year survival rate. Medical therapy is beneficial in a few cases but does not effectively improve the client's lifestyle. For this reason, heart transplantation is an option. Recently, heart transplantation clients have had a 60% to 80% 1-year survival rate and a 30% to 50% 5-year survival rate (Copeland, 1984).

The client selection criteria are strict:

• Under 55 years of age
• Emotional stability
• Good psychological support system
• Absence of insulin-dependent diabetes mellitus
• Absence of hyperlipidemia
• Normal pulmonary vascular resistance (less than 8 Woods units)
• Absence of other significant systemic disease

Surgical Procedure

The donor heart is usually from a brain-dead person of body size similar to the recipient's. The donor must be less than 35 years old and without any history of cardiac disease, cardiac trauma, serious infection, or malignancy. There must be ABO compatibility between donor and recipient and a negative lymphocyte crossmatch to minimize the possibility of rejection. The donor heart must be harvested, transported, and preserved for no more than 4 hours. Special consent from the donor's family is always required.

The first successful human transplant was performed by Christiaan Barnard in 1967. In this *heterotopic transplant*, the original heart was left in place, and the donor heart was transplanted on top of it. *Orthotopic transplant*, the removal of the recipient's heart and insertion of the donor heart, is the primary type of transplant performed in North America today. This simple procedure uses only three suture lines.

A median sternotomy incision is made, and the outflow cannulas of the heart–lung machine are placed in the posterior right atrium. The recipient's body is cooled using hypothermic techniques. The recipient's heart is resected at the atrial walls, the atrial septum, and the great vessels. The posterior atrial walls and atrial septum are left intact (Figure 25–6). The donor atria are sutured into place and the great vessels anastomosed. Air is evacuated from the heart, and blood is allowed to flow through the coronary arteries. Resumption of cardiac contraction is usually spontaneous, but defibrillation may be necessary. As the use of the heart–lung machine is discontinued, inotropic drug therapy may be needed as the donor heart faces new (and often elevated) pulmonary and systemic vascular resistance. Isoproterenol (Isuprel) is the most commonly used inotropic drug following heart transplantation. Temporary pacing wires and mediastinal drainage tubes are placed. A direct pulmonary artery or direct left atrial pressure line may also be placed and passed through the chest wall.

Implications for the Client

Physiological Implications

The transplanted heart is denervated (see the implications in the section on postoperative care). The recipient's transplanted heart has two P waves on the ECG, a higher resting heart rate than normal, and a slower heart response to exercise.

Infection is the primary cause of death after heart transplantation; the risk is highest the first 3 months after surgery. Rejection, the second cause of death, may be acute or chronic. Acute rejection involves changes in the myocardial cells and disarray of the cell components. There are few clinical signs, so diagnosis is made by myocardial biopsy.

Chronic rejection is a slow, degenerative process primarily involving the graft's vessels. There is an accelerated atherosclerotic process in the coronary arteries of the cardiac allograft. Over time, abnormal growth and changes in the structure of the endothelial cells narrow the vessel

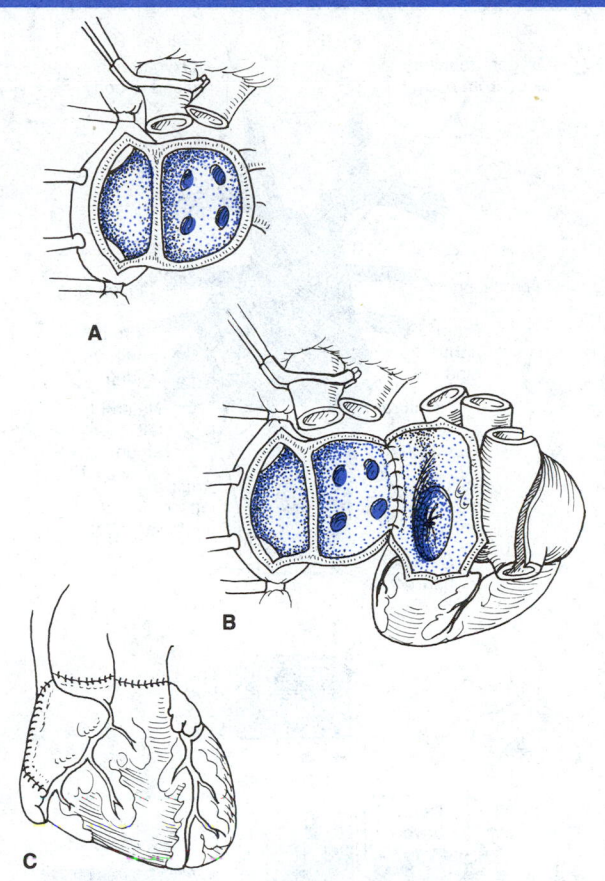

Figure 25–6

Orthotopic heart transplant. **A.** The posterior wall of the right and left atria and a ridge of atrial septum remain after the recipient's heart has been removed. **B.** The transplantation is begun by anastomosing the left atrium of the donor heart to the residual left atrial wall of the recipient. **C.** Transplantation is complete when the atrial walls, atrial septum, and great vessels have been joined.

lumen and cause eventual myocardial ischemia. The exact mechanism for chronic rejection is unknown, but humoral immune mechanisms may be responsible.

CAD can develop in the transplanted heart and is more common in clients with chronic rejection. Surgeons now prescribe aspirin and dipyridamole postoperatively, along with a low-cholesterol diet to prevent CAD in the new heart. Lymphoma has been linked to the immunosuppressive drug cyclosporine, which clients must take the rest of their lives (see discussion of postoperative care).

Psychosocial/Lifestyle Implications

The lifestyle changes of heart transplantation clients are demanding. They must learn the signs and symptoms of infection as well as precautions to prevent it. They will take immunosuppressive drugs for a lifetime and may experience any number of side effects. These clients must have regular biopsies and laboratory tests. A diet low in saturated fat and cholesterol must be followed. The client may

need to live close to the hospital both before, and a few months after surgery which disrupts family functioning.

In addition, heart transplantation recipients must cope with a changed body image. They may experience depersonalization or guilt at having someone else's heart. They may also feel better and begin to resume a somewhat normal lifestyle; 90% have an improved quality of life and normal rehabilitation (Copeland, 1984). As a result, family members or significant others may have to adjust to new roles. The client's health is no longer in the precarious state it was before surgery, and it may be difficult for family members to withdraw protective responses. The client implications of heart transplantation are summarized in Table 25–7.

Nursing Implications

Preoperative Care

Cyclosporine is administered to the client before surgery. The usual heart surgery preparations apply (see the discussion of coronary artery bypass surgery).

Postoperative Care

The heart transplantation recipient requires the intensive nursing care necessary after any heart operation. One major difference with this operation is that the heart is denervated and therefore does not respond to vagal or sympathetic stimulation. Thus, atropine cannot be administered if the client has a bradydysrhythmia because the drug affects the heart rate via the vagus nerve (cranial nerve X). The client with myocardial ischemia also does not experience

Table 25–7	Heart Transplantation: Implications for the Client
Physiological Implications	**Psychosocial/Lifestyle Implications**
Denervation (no anginal pain or response to atropine)	Need to take precautions against infection
Two P waves in ECG	Lifelong need for immunosuppressive drugs
Higher resting heart rate	Drug side effects
Slowing of heart's response to exercise	Need for frequent physician visits
High risk for infection	Low-fat, low-cholesterol diet
Possible rejection	
Risk of coronary artery disease	Change in body image
Risk of malignancy from cyclosporine	Guilt or depersonalization
	Improved quality of life
	New roles for client and family members or significant others

angina pectoris. Therefore, ischemic changes must be detected by ECG or myocardial enzyme studies.

Immunosuppressive drug therapy begins immediately after surgery. Conventional therapy uses azathioprine (Imuran), prednisone, and antithrombocytic globulin to prevent rejection. In 1979, the drug cyclosporine was discovered to have potent immunosuppressive properties. Cyclosporine can curb tissue rejection without inhibiting the body's infection-fighting mechanisms. This drug has been found to be highly effective and has facilitated early client rehabilitation.

The nurse must monitor the client for the side effects of immunosuppressive drugs and report them to the physician. Side effects of cyclosporine include abdominal discomfort, nausea, vomiting, hirsutism, headache, tremor, lymphoma, hypertension, and renal dysfunction. Corticosteroids can cause osteoporosis, muscle weakness, sodium retention, glucose intolerance, increased appetite, increased infection risk, fragile skin, peptic ulcers, and mood swings. With corticosteroid use, the nurse must observe the client's blood glucose levels for elevation. Oral hygiene also becomes extremely important to prevent dental and gum disease that could be an infection source. The diet should be as high in protein as the drug regimen allows to encourage normal healing.

Protective isolation is maintained the first few weeks after surgery. Special precautions to prevent infection include inserting a suprapubic urinary catheter, using strict sterile technique with suctioning and dressing changes, washing all equipment with a bactericidal solution, observing wounds for early signs of infection, and auscultating the lungs for early signs of pulmonary congestion.

The nurse also monitors signs of rejection. With conventional therapy, the signs include heart failure and diminishing QRS voltage. With cyclosporine therapy, clinical changes are not observed, and only myocardial biopsy is diagnostic. If rejection occurs after discharge, the client must be rehospitalized. Treatment usually consists of higher doses of corticosteroids or antithrombocytic globulin.

Discharge instructions are essential to successful rehabilitation. The client must have knowledge of:

- The purpose, dosages, and side effects to report of all medications and the need not to discontinue taking them without the physician's orders.
- Situations to avoid that increase the risk of infection.
- Good health care habits for teeth, skin, and so on.
- Early signs of infection.
- Treatment of injuries.
- A diet low in saturated fat and cholesterol.
- Activities allowed.
- Clinic follow-up appointments.
- Need for carrying a medical information tag or card.

ARTIFICIAL HEART IMPLANTATION

The artificial heart (Figure 25–7) is an experimental device that is indicated for the client with intractable heart failure

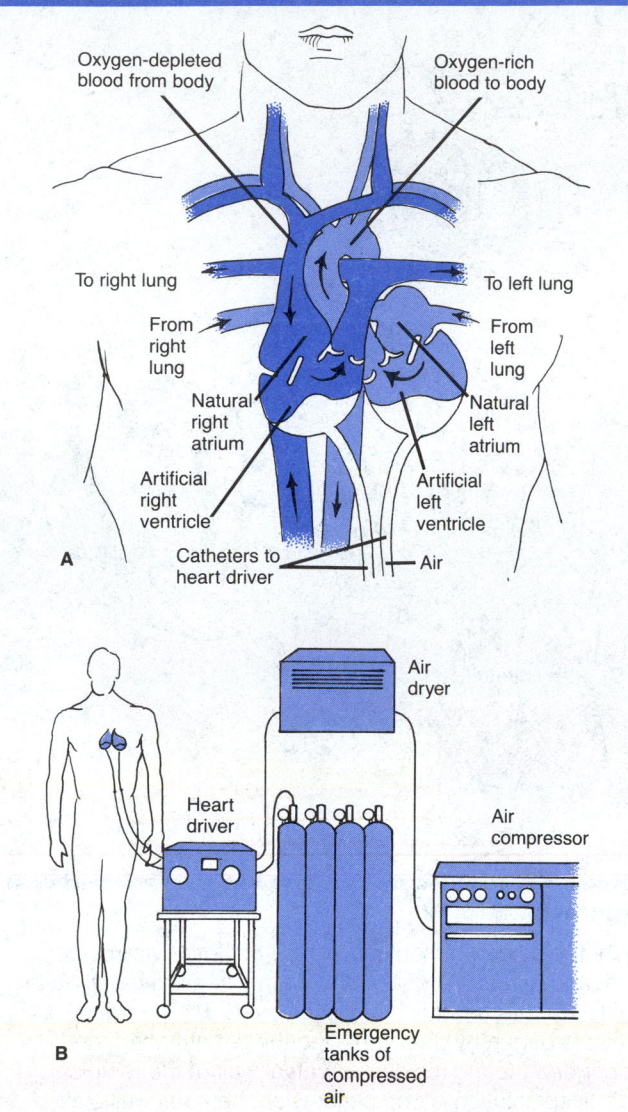

Figure 25–7

The artificial heart **A.** The implant. **B.** The support system.

resistant to all known therapeutic measures. This type of heart failure occurs in individuals with severe CAD or cardiomyopathy. It is estimated that up to 60,000 people annually could benefit from what is called the total artificial heart (even though it actually consists of only two artificial ventricles). This procedure is done in only a few centers.

Surgical Procedure

The surgical implantation of the artificial heart is technically simple compared with other heart surgeries. The client is placed on cardiopulmonary bypass, and the client's ventricles are excised, leaving the atria intact. The cuffs from the artificial heart are sutured onto the client's atria and great vessels. The artificial ventricles are then separately snapped into place and joined together by a strip of Velcro. Special connecting lines, called tethers, are brought out through the abdominal wall and connected to the drive unit, which sends compressed air in and out of the heart. Researchers are exploring alternatives to the air-driven artificial heart.

Implications for the Client

Physiological Implications
The physiological changes associated with the artificial heart are not fully understood. Clients who have undergone this surgery have had a variety of major complications—stroke, bleeding, emboli, hemolysis of red blood cells, and infection.

Psychosocial/Lifestyle Implications
The major adjustment for the client receiving an artificial heart is that he or she will always be connected to a drive unit that must be carried at all times. A shoulder-bag-style drive unit is available. Development of alternative drive units is continuing. In the future, the size of the drive unit might be reduced significantly so it could be worn as a belt.

The client must also adjust to the change in body image and to lifelong dependence on a mechanical device. So far, clients have experienced a variety of emotional reactions to the implantation, primarily depression. Careful and regular ongoing health care is a necessity and often requires living near the medical center.

The family must be willing to move near the hospital and make the necessary role changes. They must be able to support the client through the uncertainty of the postoperative period and be prepared for any complications. The implications of artificial heart implantation for the client are summarized in Table 25–8.

Nursing Implications

Preoperative Care
The preoperative preparations are similar to those for coronary artery bypass surgery (see the earlier section in this chapter). A team of physicians, nurses, and social workers evaluates the client for a stable psychological profile and ability to comply with the medical regimen and postoperative follow-up care. The client is also evaluated to be sure there is a stable home environment because living alone is not possible.

Postoperative Care
The care of postoperative artificial heart recipients is a new challenge for critical care nurses. Not only does the client have the many tubes and lines present after any major heart operation, but he or she must also be monitored for any problems of mechanical failure. An ECG cannot be recorded from the artificial heart. The heart rate can be controlled with the drive unit console. A compressed-air exhaust curve represents the shuttling of air to and from the heart. The nurse must be familiar with this curve and recognize changes in its pattern that represent mechanical failure or heart malfunction. For example, the spike on the

Table 25–8	Artificial Heart Implantation: Implications for the Client	
Physiological Implications	**Psychosocial/Lifestyle Implications**
Implications not yet fully understood	Lifelong dependence on a mechanical device
Major complications are stroke, bleeding, emboli, hemolysis of red blood cells, and infection	Drive unit must be transported with client at all times
	Body image change
	Emotional responses such as anxiety and depression during the uncertainty of the postoperative period
	Regular ongoing health care requires client and family to move near the medical center
	Role changes for client and family

curve becomes more rounded if the client is hypovolemic. A loss in pressure and a dampening of the curve may indicate bladder rupture of the heart or inadequate air pressure. A technician trained to troubleshoot these problems is usually at the bedside.

The hemodynamics and fluid management of the client are also different from that of other cardiac surgery patients. If cardiac output falls, the drive pressure or heart rate is increased. Inotropic drugs cannot be used.

After the client is discharged from the ICU, the problem of mobility arises. The nurse must be creative in developing ways for the client to move while maintaining the integrity of the tethers. Rehabilitation must be individualized according to the client's response to surgery.

VENTRICULAR ASSIST IMPLANTATION

Ventricular assist devices (VADs) are mechanical pumps that can be used temporarily or over the long term to provide assistance to an overburdened or poorly functioning ventricle. Temporary assist is indicated for ventricular dysfunction where recovery of the myocardium is anticipated. Temporary devices have also been used for support of the collapsed circulation prior to cardiac transplantation. Long-term assist is indicated for permanent damage to the myocardium.

There are many types of VADs available. Some devices are extracorporeal with the pump located outside the body and some are intracorporeal and implanted into the thoracic or abdominal cavity. VADs have the capability of supporting the left ventricle, right ventricle, or both ventricles simultaneously. They can be as simple as a roller pump or as sophisticated as an electrically-actuated pump.

No matter what type of device is used, the principles remain the same. Blood is diverted away from the ventricle being assisted, passes through the pump and is returned to the corresponding major vessel, i.e., pulmonary artery or aorta. Although the client's natural ventricle still contracts while the VAD device is in place, its load is much lighter since the blood is routed through the VAD. Permanent VADs are being developed. Powered by an electric motor about the size of a coffee mug, they do not require outside tubing nor tethers to an air-driven machine. Permanent VADs are expected to be approved for clinical testing in clients in 1986 and are expected to have wider practical application than the artificial heart.

PACEMAKER IMPLANTATION

Many heart dysrhythmias can be treated successfully with pharmacologic therapy. Medications are not helpful for treatment of chronic bradydysrhythmias, however. For the client with a bradydysrhythmia, the treatment with lasting results is the implantation of a permanent **pacemaker,** a device that supplies electrical impulses to the heart muscle to stimulate the heartbeat. The pacemaker is powered by batteries that last from 8 to 10 years. Because of recent advances in pacemaker technology, an estimated 100,000 persons per year worldwide will benefit from cardiac pacing (Kruse et al., 1982).

The pacemaker system has two components: (1) a pulse generator, which contains the electrical circuitry and batteries and is implanted in the chest or abdomen, and (2) the pacemaker electrodes, which are connected to the heart. Many different types of pacemakers are produced and can be programmed to stimulate the heart in a variety of pacing modes. For example, a pacemaker can pace only the atria, only the ventricles, or both. The pacemaker can pace continuously (fixed-rate pacing), or it can be programmed to pace the heart when needed (demand pacing). Newer self-adjusting units alter pulse rates slowly and smoothly like the natural heart does. Pacemakers also can be used temporarily with an external pulse generator or can be permanently implanted.

The indications for permanent cardiac pacing include complete heart block, Adams–Stokes syndrome, symptomatic sick sinus syndrome, symptomatic A-V block, and symptomatic tachydysrhythmias. More emphasis has been placed on the presence of symptoms, regardless of the type of dysrhythmia. The person with an Adams–Stokes attack (a syncope due to cardiac standstill), dizziness, or neurologic symptoms that occur with documented bradydysrhythmia is a candidate for a permanent pacemaker. Temporary pacemakers are usually indicated for life-threatening situations in which the heartbeat cannot be stimulated by drugs or cardiopulmonary resuscitation.

Automatic implantable defibrillators for clients known to be at risk for fibrillation are also available in some medical centers. The defibrillator device, about the size of a deck of cards and weighing 1½ lb, was given Food and Drug Administration approval in late 1985.

Surgical Procedure

Transvenous Endocardial Pacing

Local anesthesia is used during electrode insertion for either permanent or temporary transvenous endocardial pacing. Vein routes for the electrode include cephalic, internal jugular, and external jugular routes. The cephalic vein is the most common site, because only one incision is required over the deltopectoral area for transvenous electrode and pacing generator box insertion under the skin (Figure 25–8). For temporary pacing, no incision is needed. An introducing sheath is placed into the vein, and the pacing electrode is passed through this sheath into the heart. The electrode is then connected to an external pulse generator.

Epicardial Pacing

In epicardial pacing, the heart is stimulated to beat by an electrode sutured or screwed onto the epicardium. This method of insertion is used for permanent pacing. The most commonly used epicardial electrode is the flat lead, which is sutured to the surface of the heart, usually over the apex. A thoracotomy approach is required so the heart is in view for the suturing (Figure 25–9A).

The second type of myocardial electrode is a screw-in lead inserted into the myocardium by three clockwise

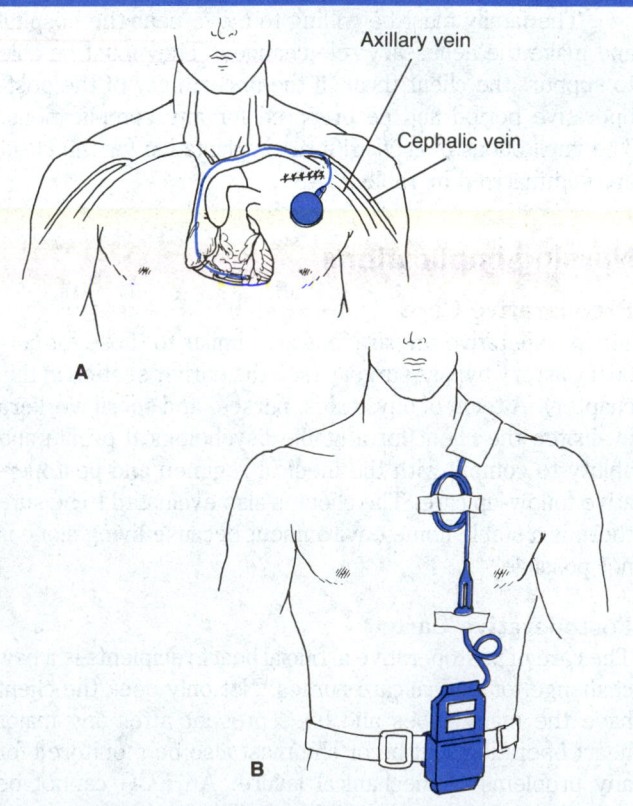

Figure 25–8

Transvenous endocardial pacing. **A.** Transvenous endocardial pacing using the cephalic vein with a pulse generator pocket on the anterior chest wall. **B.** External pulse generator for temporary pacing.

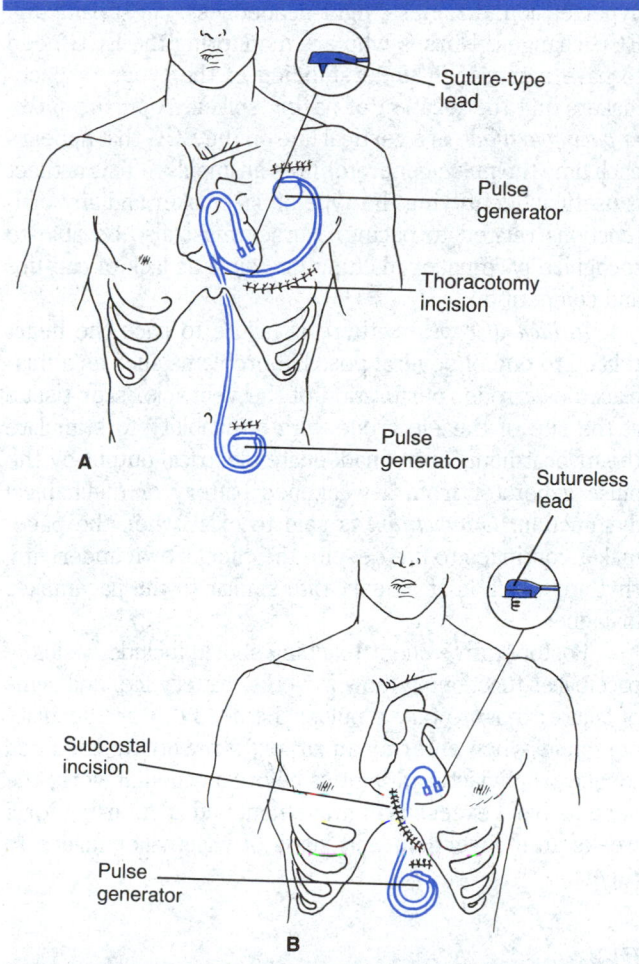

Figure 25–9

Epicardial pacing. **A.** The electrode is sutured to the surface of the heart. The pulse generator pocket can be on the anterior chest wall or on the abdomen. **B.** The electrode is screwed into the myocardium. The pulse generator pocket is on the upper abdomen.

turns. The advantage is that a thoracotomy approach is not required for insertion. An incision can be made in the subcostal area; the electrodes are slipped under the ribs and screwed into the myocardium (Figure 25–9B). Another advantage is that this lead is easily repositioned during implantation.

Implications for the Client

Physiological Implications

The pacemaker supplies the client with a regular heartbeat at a rate that meets the body's needs for tissue perfusion. Therefore, the symptoms of bradydysrhythmia should disappear.

In the period immediately following pacemaker insertion, there is potential for pacemaker malfunction and the recurrence of the dysrhythmia. Any pacemaker malfunction is usually easily rectified, however. Pain at the insertion site is common. Bleeding and infection may also occur

there. If the electrode perforates the myocardium or the client has a thin-walled ventricle, twitching of the diaphragm could develop; the client would be aware of this problem.

Psychosocial/Lifestyle Implications

Before pacemaker insertion, clients often fear their hearts will stop. Pacemaker insertion diminishes this fear but creates concerns about the surgical procedure and the changes the pacemaker will make in clients' lives. They hear rumors about what pacemaker clients can or cannot do.

Thus, clients must have a good understanding of where their pacemakers are located, how they work, and the location of the electrodes. They must be able to recognize the signs and symptoms of pacemaker failure—decreased heart rate, chest pain, dizziness, fainting, hiccups, undue fatigue, and shortness of breath. They need to learn to determine their own heart rates and report a heart rate below the set pacemaker rate. Clients should always have an identification card that tells the type of pacemaker implanted. Clients must also be aware that pacemakers set off airport alarms. Therefore, they should warn security personnel before entering the airport x-ray machine.

Clients should avoid excessive arm movements and reaching for 5 weeks postoperatively to avoid dislodging the pacing electrode. Finally, clients should take antibiotics before and after dental work, including cleaning. Clients with pacemakers, particularly transvenous ones, are at risk for bacterial endocarditis. The client implications for cardiac pacing are summarized in Table 25–9.

Table 25–9	Pacemaker Implantation: Implications for the Client
Physiological Implications	**Psychosocial/Lifestyle Implications**
Bradydysrhythmia no longer present Possible pacemaker malfunction Pain, bleeding, or infection at insertion site Diaphragm twitching	Need to recognize signs of pacemaker failure (decreased heart rate, chest pain, dizziness, fainting, hiccups, undue fatigue, and shortness of breath) Need to carry an identification card and to alert airport security personnel to presence of pacemaker Avoidance of excessive arm movements and reaching 5 weeks postoperatively Need to take antibiotics before and after dental work to avoid bacterial endocarditis

Nursing Implications

Preoperative Care

Because clients often fear pacemaker insertion, nursing interventions should focus on reassuring the clients and explaining the need for the pacemaker. Explain to clients in simple terms how the heart is stimulated to beat and talk about the heart's conduction system. Clients must also understand where the incision is to be made; how the pacemaker will appear under the skin; and the fact that there will be a large, bulky dressing.

The procedure will take 30 minutes to 2 hours, depending on the approach. Warn clients that fluoroscopy will be used during the procedure. Also, blood pressure, heart rate, and heart rhythm will be continuously monitored. Restraints may also be necessary during the procedure. The client is kept NPO before pacemaker insertion. A shave of the upper chest is also performed.

Postoperative Care

After insertion, pacemaker function is closely monitored on the ECG, and vital signs are assessed frequently. The client remains in bed for 12 to 24 hours to allow for pacemaker electrode stabilization. The nurse should check the wound every 30 minutes for signs of bleeding. Record fluid intake and output to ensure that the client is well hydrated. Give medication for pain relief as needed.

Be especially alert for signs of pacemaker failure:

hypertension, dizziness, light-headedness, chest pain, and ECG changes. Nurses who are monitoring the ECG need to have a thorough understanding of the types of pacemakers and the location of pacing spikes. A *pacing spike,* or *pacing artifact,* is a vertical line on the ECG that appears each time the pulse generator fires an impulse. This artifact is useful in identifying the type of pacemaker and any malfunctions related to pacing. Nurses must also be able to recognize pacemaker malfunction, such as lack of capture and competition.

In *lack of capture,* there is failure to pace the heart related to one of several possible problems such as a misplaced electrode, perforation of the ventricle, scar tissue at the site of the electrode with an inability to stimulate the myocardium, or an inadequate electrical output by the pulse generator from a weakened battery or mechanical dysfunction. *Competition* is said to exist when the pacemaker continues to fire despite the client's own underlying rhythm, which is at a heart rate similar to the pacemaker or higher.

Postoperative client teaching should include basics of pacemaker functioning (how it works, battery life, and signs of failure); how to take a pulse; the need to warn security personnel when entering an airport x-ray booth; the need to take prophylactic antibiotics before any dental work; the need to avoid excess arm movement and arm raising for 5 weeks after insertion; and signs of pacemaker failure to report.

Section IV: Surgical Approaches to Thoracic Aortic Aneurysms and Dissections

In the past, aortic aneurysms and dissections had a high mortality rate with little hope for client survival. Studies have found that 50% of clients with acute dissections die within 48 hours if untreated (Kouchoukas & Karp, 1983). With current surgical techniques, however, more persons are surviving. Surgery is done in the following situations: progressive aortic regurgitation associated with an ascending aortic aneurysm, evidence of aneurysm enlargement on x-ray, all aneurysms of the transverse and thoracic aorta, expansion or perforation of an aortic dissection, or compromise of a major vessel by an aneurysm or dissection.

Surgical Procedure

Ascending Aortic Aneurysm

The goals of surgical treatment for an ascending aortic aneurysm are removal of the aneurysm and correction of aortic regurgitation, if present. A medial sternotomy incision is made, and the client is placed on the heart–lung machine. In one method of repair, the aortic valve is replaced, and a separate Dacron tube graft is used to replace the ascending aorta. In the second method, a composite graft and aortic valve are inserted as a single unit.

Transverse Aortic Aneurysm

A transverse aortic aneurysm presents a great challenge to the surgeon. Repair requires inserting a Dacron graft into the aorta and suturing the brachiocephalic vessels directly onto the graft. The graft is then anastomosed proximally and distally to the aorta, and the aorta is closed around the graft.

Descending Thoracic Aortic Aneurysm

The surgical treatment of a descending thoracic aortic aneurysm uses a lateral thoracotomy approach; use of the heart–lung machine is rarely necessary. The aorta is simply closed around the graft.

Aortic Dissections

The heart–lung machine is used for all aortic dissections. With type 1 dissections (where the initial tear is in the ascending aorta) the aortic valve is replaced if necessary; a tube graft is placed within the dissected portion of aorta. All sutures are reinforced with Teflon strips, and the aorta and false lumen are then closed around the graft. The same procedure is used for type 2 (where the dissection originates and remains in the ascending aorta) and type 3 dissections (where the dissection originates within the descending aorta and may progress in either direction).

Implications for the Client

Clients with an expanding aneurysm or dissection have little choice about surgery. Nevertheless, it is difficult for them to be informed of the complications and implications of this surgery.

Physiological Implications

Bacterial infection, or prosthetic endocarditis, is a potential problem with any implanted artificial material, especially when implanted as a part of the bloodstream. Bacteria can enter the blood from the mouth via the gums or through a break in any mucous membrane. Once in the bloodstream, the bacteria can start an infection inside the heart or great vessels that can destroy any prosthetic material used with the surgery.

Complete heart block and other dysrhythmias may occur because of cardiac edema after surgery. The heart–lung machine cannulas placed in the right atrium during surgery can lead to conduction disturbances. The client with aneurysmal disease usually also has CAD. The low blood flow maintained during the surgery may predispose the client to myocardial ischemia with the risk of infarction, lethal dysrhythmias, or both. MI makes the client prone to postoperative congestive heart failure.

Vocal cord palsy, due to edema of the recurrent laryngeal nerve, is usually a temporary problem. Stroke may occur as a result of emboli that reach the brain during surgery. These emboli may be from clots within the aneurysm or air emboli from the heart–lung machine pump.

Paraplegia from spinal cord ischemia is one of the most dreaded complications. Flow in the lumbar artery feeding the spinal arteries may be interrupted during thoracic aorta resection. Prolonged occlusion of the aorta or hypotension during surgery place the client at risk for this complication.

Renal failure or respiratory insufficiency can develop after any heart operation. Clients with aneurysmal disease of the great vessels often have other medical problems preoperatively and a history of heavy smoking. Therefore, they are usually at high risk for developing these complications.

Psychosocial/Lifestyle Implications

The client who has had an aortic repair procedure has the same psychological responses as any heart surgery client (see the section on coronary artery bypass surgery). Postoperative delirium and confusion may be observed during recovery in the ICU. Stroke and paraplegia are potential complications that require great psychological adjustments.

When the client is past the acute phase of recovery, other adjustments center around lifestyle changes. The control of high blood pressure is a mandatory change. The client must adhere to a sodium-restricted diet and maintain an adequate calcium intake. Antihypertensive drugs must

Table 25–10	Repair of Thoracic Aortic Aneurysms and Dissections: Implications for the Client
Possible Physiological Implications	**Psychosocial/ Lifestyle Implications**
Possible complications of	
Prosthetic endocarditis	Postoperative delirium or confusion
Complete heart block	
Conduction disturbances	Adjustment to stroke or paraplegia if present
Myocardial ischemia with risk of myocardial infarction, lethal dysrhythmias, or both	Sodium-restricted diet and adequate calcium intake
Congestive heart failure	
Temporary vocal cord palsy	Need for antihypertensive and anticoagulation medications
Thromboembolism	
Stroke	
Paraplegia	Need to stop smoking
Renal failure	
Respiratory insufficiency	Prophylaxis against bacterial endocarditis or graft infection

be taken religiously and not stopped without a physician's order. Clients who smoke should be directed to a program to assist them in stopping (see resources in Chapter 18). Anticoagulation medications may be prescribed, and the client must then watch for bleeding problems.

If artificial material has been used in the surgical repair, the client must take precautions against bacterial endocarditis and graft infection. These precautions include taking prophylactic antibiotics before any dental work or any endoscopic examination. The implications for the client undergoing repair of thoracic aortic aneurysm or dissections are listed in Table 25–10.

Nursing Implications

Preoperative Care

The nurse prepares the client preoperatively as described in the discussion of coronary artery bypass surgery. Surgical preparations are usually rushed. The client is often anxious, because the symptoms appeared suddenly, and the decision to have surgery was made quickly. The goal of nursing care at this time is to stabilize the client's blood pressure with nitroprusside and offer emotional support to the client and family or significant other.

Postoperative Care

The client is usually unstable in the immediate postoperative period and requires constant monitoring of arterial pressure. The goal of nursing care is to maintain a pressure high enough for tissue perfusion but not so high that stress is placed on suture lines.

Nursing assessment includes evaluating circulation to the extremities, assessing for stroke, monitoring hourly urine output for decreased kidney perfusion, monitoring clotting studies to prevent coagulopathy, monitoring the ECG for signs of complete heart block after aneurysm resection and MI, assessing breath and heart sounds, and monitoring pulmonary and right atrial pressures for signs of hypovolemia or heart failure. Vasodilating agents are given intravenously to control arterial pressure. Give analgesics liberally, especially if a thoracotomy incision was used. Finally, emphasize breathing exercises with any thoracic or cardiac surgery client.

Chapter Highlights

The coronary artery bypass graft is the most common surgical technique to treat coronary artery disease.

Many surgical procedures of the heart and major blood vessels use the heart–lung machine, and close client monitoring is needed by the nurse in the early postoperative period.

Early complications of heart surgery include low cardiac output syndrome, hypertension, hemorrhage, dysrhythmias, atelectasis, neurologic dysfunction, paralytic ileus, gastrointestinal bleeding, infection, and renal failure. The client benefits from improved heart pumping action, relief of anginal pain, relief of signs and symptoms of heart failure, and improved quality of life.

Heart surgery clients often experience intensive care unit psychosis, confusion, and depression; a changed self-image; and the need to modify risk factors by dietary changes, medication, and the elimination of smoking.

A relatively new nonsurgical approach to coronary artery disease in worldwide use is percutaneous transluminal coronary angioplasty.

Surgical approaches to disorders affecting the heart valves include annuloplasty; mitral valve com-missurotomy; and valve replacement using xenografts, allografts, and artificial valves.

Ventricular aneurysmectomy, heart transplantation, artificial heart implantation, and ventricular assist devices are used to treat disorders of the myocardium. Transplantation and artificial heart implantation entail significant psychosocial adjustment, including the need for dietary changes, feelings of guilt and depersonalization, and new roles for the client and family or significant other.

The client with an artificial heart is a new challenge in nursing because of the need for special monitoring of the drive unit and air compressor waveforms. Nurses must also be able to provide support to artificial heart recipients and their families while they undergo major life adjustments.

Bradydysrhythmias are successfully treated by cardiac pacemakers, devices that supply electrical impulses to the heart muscle to stimulate the heartbeat. Surgical implantation procedures depend on the type of pacemaker.

Surgical techniques are improving the mortality rate for clients with thoracic aortic aneurysms and aortic dissection.

Bibliography

Brzenski TS: Pacemakers: Pulse of life. *AORN J* 1980; 32:967–976.

Chesebro JH et al: A platelet-inhibitor drug trial in coronary-artery bypass operations. *N Engl J Med* 1982; 307:73–78.

Cisar NS, Morphew SF: Preoperative teaching: Aortocoronary bypass patients. *Focus* 1983; 10(1):21–25.

Copeland JG: Cardiac transplantation today. *J Cardiovasc Med* 1984; 30:528–536.

Cosgrove DM, Loop FD: Aneurysms of the heart. In: *Thoracic and Cardiovascular Surgery*. Glenn WL (editor): Norwalk, CT: Appleton–Century–Crofts, 1983.

Guzzetta CE, Dossey BM: Cardiovascular nursing: Bodymind tapestry. St. Louis: Mosby, 1984.

Jenkins CD et al: Coronary artery bypass surgery: Physical, psychosocial, social and economic outcomes six months later. *JAMA* 1983; 250:782–788.

Kern LS: Mechanical support of the failing heart. In: *Congestive Heart Failure*. Michaelson CR (editor). St. Louis: Mosby, 1983.

Kern LS: Surgical treatment of underlying heart disease: Coronary artery bypass, heart valve replacement, heart transplant. In: *Congestive Heart Failure*. Michaelson CR (editor). St. Louis: Mosby, 1983.

Kern LS, Gawlinski A: Stage-managing coronary artery disease. *Nurs 83* 1983; 13:34–40.

Kouchoukas NT, Karp RB: Aneurysms of the ascending aorta. In: *Thoracic and Cardiovascular Surgery*. Glenn WL (editor). Norwalk, CT: Appleton–Century–Crofts, 1983.

Kruse I et al: A comparison of the acute and long-term hemodynamic effects of ventricular inhibited and atrial synchronous ventricular inhibited pacing. *Circulation* 1982; 65:846–855.

LaForge R et al: Cardiac rehabilitation programs: The Sharp Memorial Hospital Cardiac Rehabilitation Program. *J Cardiac Rehabil* 1984; 4(1):6–9.

Levy RI et al: Percutaneous transluminal angioplasty: A status report. *N Engl J Med* 1981; 305:399–400.

Owen P: Defibrillating pacemaker patients. *Am J Nurs* 1984; 84(9):1129–1130.

Quaal SJ: *Comprehensive Intra-Aortic Balloon Pumping.* St. Louis: Mosby, 1984.

Rogers WJ et al: Coronary revascularization surgery: Feasibility after myocardial infarction. *Postgrad Med* 1981; 69(1):36–49.

Shank J: Postpericardiotomy syndrome. *Cardiovasc Nurs* 1983; 19(3):11–14.

Suggested Readings

Guzzetta CE, Dossey BM: *Cardiovascular Nursing: Bodymind Tapestry.* St. Louis: Mosby, 1984. This text has a strong nursing focus covering all aspects of the care of the cardiac client. See particularly Chapters 13, 20, and 22 on pacing, valvular heart disease, and heart surgery.

Kern LS: Surgical treatment of underlying heart disease: Coronary artery bypass, heart valve replacement, heart transplant. In: *Congestive Heart Failure.* Michaelson CR (editor). St. Louis: Mosby, 1983. This chapter provides a critical care focus on the nursing management of the adult heart surgery client that supplements this text. Specific examples of client care protocols, client education guides, and nursing care plans are provided.

Levy RI et al: Percutaneous transluminal angioplasty: A status report: *N Engl J Med* 1981; 305:399–400. This editorial summarizes controversies surrounding this new technique. The article provides food for thought and answers to questions that may be asked by clients undergoing this procedure.

Purcell JA, Burrows SG: A pacemaker primer: For CE credit. *Am J Nurs* 1985; 85:553–568. This continuing education feature discusses the basics of how pacemaker systems work and their insertion and care. Potential client care problems are discussed along with nursing intervention in a comprehensive two-page table. Another table discusses troubleshooting pacemaker problems.

Chapter 26

The Nursing Process for Clients With Vascular System Dysfunction

Janice Lech Dusek
SueAnn Wooster Ames

Objectives

When you have finished studying this chapter, you should be able to:

Specify the subjective data to be obtained in the history of a client with a disorder of the peripheral vascular system.

Discuss the physical examination of a client with a peripheral vascular system disorder.

Compare and contrast arterial insufficiency and venous insufficiency.

Identify diagnostic studies used to assess the peripheral vascular system.

Explain common nursing diagnoses for clients with peripheral vascular diseases.

Anticipate the psychosocial/lifestyle implications of peripheral vascular dysfunction for clients and their significant others.

Develop a nursing care plan for a client with peripheral vascular disease.

Evaluate the effectiveness of the nursing care plan and modify it as necessary to meet client needs.

Nurses can play an instrumental role in the care of clients with peripheral vascular disease. A thorough nursing assessment aids in determining the extent of the circulation problem. Nursing interventions are effective in ameliorating the disease and may contribute to saving a client's limb. This chapter deals primarily with nursing care for arterial and venous insufficiency. For nursing implications of surgical treatment of vascular system dysfunction, refer to Chapters 25 and 30.

Section I: Nursing Assessment: Establishing the Data Base

Peripheral vascular disease can be readily detected through a precise, logical nursing assessment. The client's reports of particular kinds of pain, for example, may indicate vascular symptoms that can be confirmed through physical assessment and diagnostic studies.

SUBJECTIVE DATA

Begin the nursing assessment by taking a complete history that elicits the client's chief concern, current symptoms, past health history, habits, occupation, and lifestyle. Explore factors that can lead to peripheral vascular disease (eg, cigarette smoking, oral contraceptive use, hyperlipidemia, hypertension, diabetes mellitus, and genetic predisposition).

History of Present Illness

Intermittent Claudication

Intermittent claudication, the most common symptom of arterial insufficiency, is a cramping pain in a muscle brought on by exercise and relieved by rest. The pain usually develops in the legs after the client has walked a specific distance (eg, two blocks) and is relieved after leg rest of a few minutes. The client then can walk two more blocks and must rest again. Although the client experiences cramping pain in the muscle, the muscle is flaccid when palpated.

The cause of intermittent claudication is unknown but is thought to be due to the accumulation of toxic metabolites (lactic acid) in the tissues or to the release of histamine or other chemicals into the tissues near the nerve endings. It is probably not due to ischemia of the contracting muscle. The client who has calf pain usually has a blockage of the superficial femoral artery. Thigh pain may indicate a blockage in the iliac artery.

Rest Pain

Rest pain occurs in clients who have advanced chronic arterial occlusive disease. This pain, which often occurs when the client is resting in bed at night, is usually experienced as a constant burning in the distal portion of the leg. Awakened from sleep, the client obtains relief by sitting up in a chair or allowing the legs to be dependent. The dependent position allows the arterial pressure in the legs to increase.

Blockage of a vessel by a thrombus or embolus, or severe arterial disease, may cause rest pain. These pathological problems decrease the supply of blood to the surrounding tissues, resulting in ischemic pain. Ischemia, in turn, allows metabolites (lactic acid) to build up in the tissue and causes more pain (Figure 26–1).

Rest pain should not be confused with night leg cramps, which do not necessarily indicate a pathological condition. Leg cramps can be brought on by just stretching the leg or foot quickly while asleep. Clients who are hypocalcemic may also experience cramping leg pain.

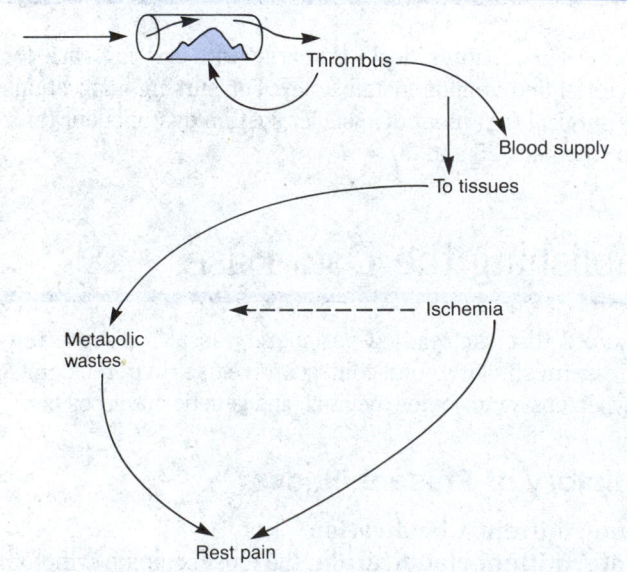

Figure 26–1

Sequence of events in rest pain.

Additional Symptoms

The functional ability or appearance of an extremity may change in conjunction with a gradual decrease in arterial circulation to the legs, which leads to atrophy of the muscles of the extremities. The male client with an occlusion of the aortic or femoral trunks may also complain of sexual impotence (Leriche's syndrome).

The client may have delayed healing after cuts or abrasions or complain of a cold and pale extremity. When the blood flow is insufficient so the supply of nutrients is deficient, the extremities look pale, feel cool, and heal poorly. When a client says a limb is cold in a warm environment, suspect arterial insufficiency. The client may also report aching, tiredness, and a feeling of fullness in the legs following long periods of standing or sitting. These symptoms are associated with venous insufficiency and are relieved when legs are elevated for a short time.

Medication History

Obtain a history of current and past use of medications, both prescription and over the counter. Ask the client specifically about the use of ergotamine and oral contraceptives.

Ergotamine preparations, used to treat migraine headache, are vasoconstrictors. Although ergotamine is an excellent drug for migraine, it must be used carefully in limited amounts to avoid causing vasoconstrictive complications. Ergotamine preparations are contraindicated in peripheral vascular disease.

Oral contraceptives have been associated with thromboembolic complications, including thrombophlebitis in an extremity, pulmonary embolism, and myocardial infarction (MI). The cause of these complications is not known, although some abnormalities in clotting are suspected. Cigarette smoking with oral contraceptive use markedly increases the risk of cardiovascular side effects.

Habit History

Cigarette Smoking

Obtain a detailed history of the client's smoking habits. Cigarette smoking is absolutely contraindicated in clients with vascular disease. Smoking causes constriction of both small and large blood vessels and damages intimal cells. Nicotine also increases the aggregation of platelets (Miller & Roon, 1982).

Diet Patterns

Nutritional assessment should include complete information on the daily diet of the client. Because elevated cholesterol and triglyceride levels are major risk factors for atherosclerosis, a diet high in calories, saturated fat, and cholesterol increases the client's risk for vascular disease. In a client with hypertension or a strong family history of hypertension, it is important to assess salt intake as well as ingestion of saturated fats and cholesterol.

Obese clients with peripheral vascular disease often

have less claudication pain after they lose weight. A careful history that explores symptoms related to weight gain, which leads to a sedentary lifestyle and still greater weight gain, often helps the client make the association between increased weight and increased pain.

A complete dietary history should also be obtained from clients with diabetes mellitus or a strong family history of diabetes mellitus. A diabetic client with poor dietary control is at greater risk for vascular disease. Diabetics are more prone to leg and foot injuries because of peripheral neuropathy, are at greater risk for infection with resulting tissue destruction, and have amputation rates four times greater than nondiabetic clients with peripheral vascular disease (Miller & Roon, 1982).

OBJECTIVE DATA
Physical Assessment

Inspection

Observe the color of the extremities in a comfortably warm environment because skin responds to changes in external temperature. Begin the examination of skin color by having the client walk barefoot. Foot pallor indicates vasodilation of the arteries in the muscles. With ambulation, the muscles of the legs and hips receive increased blood flow, and blood flow to the feet and skin is compromised.

Trophic changes in peripheral vascular disease occur because of ischemia and malnutrition of tissues. In looking for trophic changes, begin by looking at the symmetry and size of each limb and normal or decreased muscle mass. Inspect the groin, buttocks, and feet. Look for decreased muscle mass in the gluteal muscles, which is commonly seen in Leriche's syndrome. Inspect for loss of hair, especially on the toes and feet. Check for smooth, thin, shiny skin and thickened, blackish brown nails.

To check for arterial deficiency in the lower extremities, ask the client to elevate both legs to 45°. With arterial insufficiency, the legs are markedly pale, especially in the soles of the feet, toes, and heels. Called *pallor on elevation*, this occurs because the circulatory system cannot pump enough blood into the capillary system against gravity. In a client with a healthy vascular system, blood continues to perfuse the elevated extremities, although mild pallor does occur.

Another indication of arterial insufficiency is *dependent rubor*. Have the client elevate the legs for 60 seconds, then sit with the legs in a dependent position. Normally, color returns to the extremity within 10 seconds or less. When there is a delay in color return, arterial insufficiency is suspected. The appearance of a reddish blue color after a few minutes may indicate peripheral vessel damage. Rubor develops because of ischemia to the tissue. The dependent rubor sign usually indicates a 90% loss of blood flow (Doyle, 1981).

While examining arterial status, also note venous filling. Venous filling is assessed with the feet in the dependent position. After 15 or 20 seconds of dependency, the veins of the dorsum of the leg should fill. With ischemia, there may be a delay of 40 to 60 seconds before the vein fills. With varicose veins, there is rapid venous filling as blood flows backward unchecked by the incompetent valves.

Test *capillary refill* for assessment of the circulation to the foot. Normally, compressing the nail beds or the sole of a foot causes blanching, which is followed by rapid return of normal color. In the ischemic foot, the return to normal color after blanching takes much longer, signifying a delay in capillary filling.

Leg ulcers or cellulitis may be present. Arterial ischemic leg ulcers are caused by chronic occlusion of small arterioles and arteries, resulting in skin breakdown and ulceration. In venous stasis ulcers, the venous blood pools in the tissues of the extremities. This pooling of venous blood provides an excellent medium for bacterial growth, causing skin lesions and infections.

Arterial ulcers have a pale base, are very painful, and usually occur on the lateral lower leg above the lateral malleolus. Venous ulcers are usually moderately painful and usually involve the medial aspect of the ankle.

Pregangrene and frank gangrene are present in the client with chronic arterial insufficiency. Gangrene develops first in the most distal part of the legs. Gangrene results from severe and prolonged ischemia to an area, usually caused by a complete or almost complete blockage of blood flow. In pregangrene, which is reversible, the skin has a purple-black color that does not change when pressure is applied. Frank gangrene, characterized by skin that is black, shriveled, hard, and dry, is irreversible. Table 26–1 and Figures 26–2 and 26–3 compare the common findings in arterial and venous insufficiency.

Palpation

Assessment of all peripheral pulses is essential in clients with possible peripheral vascular disease. Pulses are evaluated according to their:

- Absence or presence
- Rate and rhythm
- Quality and strength
- Symmetry

Pulses are described according to a numerical classification from 0 (absent pulse) to 4+ (a normal full, bounding pulse) (see Chapter 7).

Palpate the *carotid pulse* in the neck just below the mandible and anterior to the sternocleidomastoid muscle. Take care not to palpate the carotid sinus, which is located in the upper portion of the carotid artery just above the bifurcation between the internal and external carotid arteries at the angle of the mandible. Palpating the carotid sinus area sends impulses from the carotid sinus stretch receptors that increase parasympathetic nervous activity and decrease sympathetic nervous activity. Within 3 to 4 seconds, a parasympathetic effect of decreased heart rate and

Table 26–1	Comparison of Findings in Arterial and Venous Insufficiency	
Assessment	**Arterial Insufficiency**	**Venous Insufficiency**
Skin changes	Smooth, shiny, thin; loss of hair over the toes and foot; thickened blackish brown nails	Rough, thickened, brown pigmentation around ankles; stasis dermatitis
Skin color	Pallor on elevation and dependent rubor	Feet normal or slightly cyanotic in a dependent position
Skin temperature	Cool	Warm
Pulses	Absent or decreased; a bruit may be heard over an arterial plaque or aneurysm	Normal; no bruits
Pain	Sharp pain that increases with walking; resting helps relieve pain	Heavy aching, tiredness, and feeling of fullness; elevation of legs helps
Edema	Absent	Present; worse at end of day
Ulcers of ankles and feet	Very painful pale base; occur on lateral lower leg above the lateral malleolus and on the toes; also occur in areas of trauma	Moderately painful, pink base; occur on medial aspect of ankle
Gangrene	May develop Pregangrene: skin purple-black (reversible) Frank gangrene: skin black, shriveled, hard, and dry (irreversible)	Does not develop

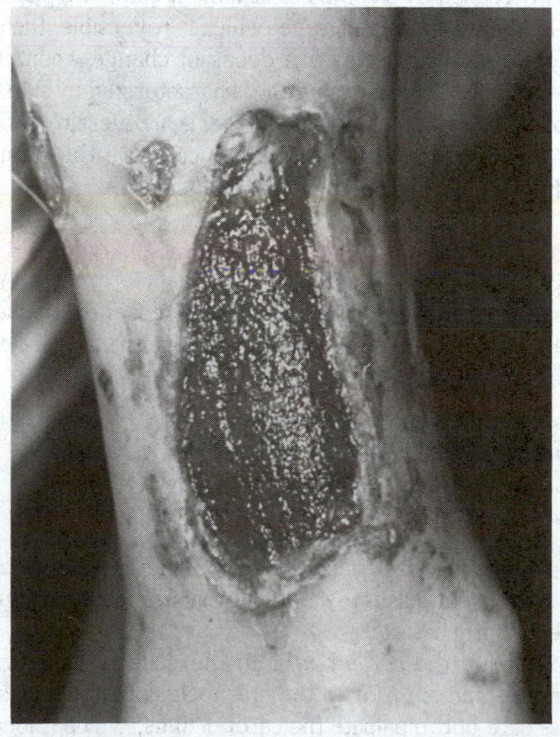

Figure 26–2

Leg ulcer in a client with arterial insufficiency. Ulcer is located on lateral lower leg above malleolus. Note smooth, shiny skin and hair loss. (Courtesy of Millard Fillmore Hospital, Buffalo, NY)

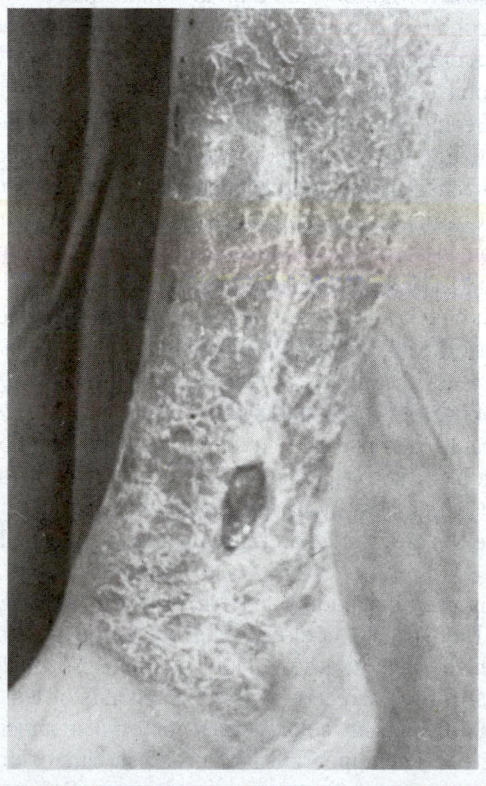

Figure 26–3

Leg ulcer in a client with venous insufficiency. Ulcer is located just above medial malleolus. Note rough, thickened, pigmented skin. (Courtesy of Millard Fillmore Hospital, Buffalo, NY)

vasodilation will occur and can lead to significant cerebral hypotension, with resulting syncope (Fetzer–Fowler, 1983).

Palpation of the *ulnar* and *radial* pulses provides information about circulation to the hands and fingers. Allen's test (Figure 26–4) can also be used to evaluate the patency of the radial and ulnar arteries. The *brachial* pulse is assessed in conjunction with the radial and ulnar pulses to evaluate arterial blood flow to the arms and hands.

Palpation of the *aorta* in the upper abdomen may detect a prominent pulsation with lateral expansion, which may indicate an abdominal aortic aneurysm. Diminished, unequal, or absent *femoral* pulses suggest aortoiliac occlusive disease. An increase in the pulse's amplitude may be due to an increase in energy of the pulse wave, which is rebounding laterally at the point of occlusion (Taggart, 1977).

Palpate the *popliteal* pulse deep in the popliteal fossa, posterior to the knee. The client should be supine with the knee slightly bent. Use the fingertips of both hands to locate the popliteal artery. This pulse is usually more difficult to find than other pulses. If it is absent, the superficial femoral artery may be occluded.

Palpate the *posterior tibial* pulse in the groove between the medial malleolus and the Achilles tendon and the *dor-*

salis pedis pulse on the dorsum of the foot. Although the congenital absence of one of these pedal pulses is considered normal, both pulses should not be absent on the same foot. If both are impalpable, the branches of the popliteal artery or the anterior tibial artery may be occluded.

During palpation of the peripheral pulses, assess the skin temperature. The areas to be checked should be exposed and at rest for several minutes. Compare the temperature of each limb with the other in similar surroundings. To detect differences in temperature, use the dry, cool dorsum of the fingers rather than the warm, moist palmar surface of the fingers.

Diminished motor sensory ability may result from poor blood supply to distal nerve fibers. Assess motor function by having the client flex and extend the toes, and evaluate sensory function by asking the client to identify the part of the foot the nurse is touching (Doyle, 1981).

Palpate each calf for signs of deep phlebitis. Tenderness and increased firmness and tension suggest thrombophlebitis. If phlebitis is suspected, palpate for tenderness or palpable cords and feel for warmth accompanied by redness or discoloration, which indicate superficial thrombophlebitis. Palpate for varicose veins by checking for thickened walls and tortuous veins.

The client with thrombophlebitis may have a positive *Homans' sign*, which is elicited by forcefully dorsiflexing the client's foot with the knee bent. Pain in the calf may indicate deep-vein thrombophlebitis (DVT). Homans' sign is a common clinical assessment for DVT but is not a sensitive or specific test. More specific approaches to evaluation include assessing the client for pain, aching, or a full sensation in the leg; inspecting and palpating the leg for swelling, tenderness, discoloration, increased heat, and dilated superficial veins; and unexplained tachycardia and fever (Miller & Roon, 1982).

Auscultation

Auscultate over the aorta and the carotid, iliac, and femoral arteries for bruits. In addition, auscultate arteries in any area of suspected arterial disease or decreased perfusion. Bruits over the carotid artery suggest arterial narrowing. Bruits of the aorta in older clients suggest abdominal aortic aneurysm.

Diagnostic Studies

Common diagnostic studies used in evaluation of the peripheral vascular system are discussed in this section. The studies are also described in Table 26–2.

Skin Temperature Studies

Skin temperature of the extremities can be evaluated in a variety of ways. Immersing one extremity in warm water while observing the other extremity gives a gross evaluation of arterial disease. In the healthy client, the temperature in an unimmersed arm will rise with the temperature in the immersed arm because of reflex vasodilation. In

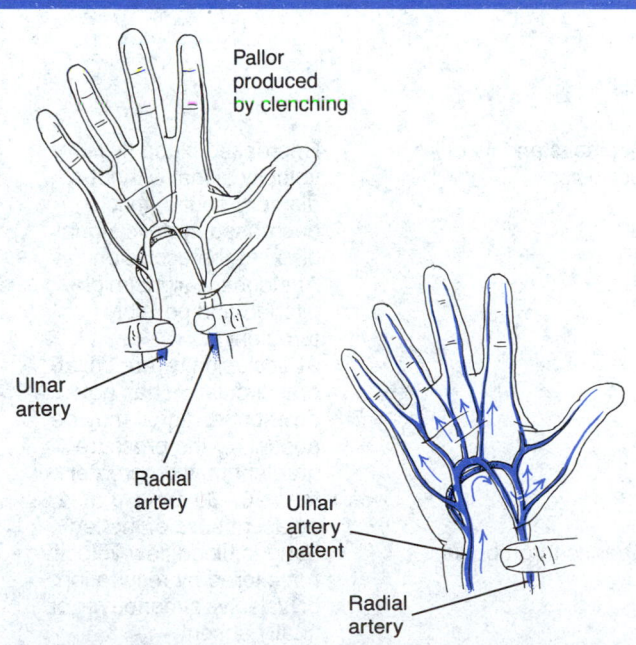

Pallor produced by clenching

Ulnar artery

Radial artery

Ulnar artery patent

Radial artery

Figure 26–4

Allen's test. Position the client's arm on a flat surface. Compress both the radial and ulnar arteries while the client clenches the fist tightly. After 1 minute, the client extends the fingers quickly while the examiner releases pressure on the ulnar artery but continues compression of the radial artery. If there is adequate ulnar circulation, color will return promptly. Persistent pallor indicates occlusion of the ulnar artery (Bates, 1983). This maneuver is repeated, maintaining compression of the ulnar artery while releasing pressure on the radial artery. In this instance, persistent pallor indicates radial artery disease.

Table 26-2   Diagnostic Studies Common to the Peripheral Vascular System

Diagnostic Study	Normal Expected Value	Disease State	Expected Abnormal Findings
Skin temperature studies			
Immersion test: one extremity is immersed in warm water, and the other is observed	The temperature of the unimmersed limb will rise slowly due to reflex vasodilation	Arterial disease	Skin temperature will scarcely change in the opposite extremity
Cold pressure test: The client's BP and pulse pressure are taken before and after immersion of the hand in ice water	Increase of 25 mm Hg pressure in BP; no change in pulse pressure	Arterial occlusive disease	BP rises 40 mm Hg; pulse pressure increases by 20 mm Hg
Direct skin temperature readings	Normal skin surface temperature ranges 14–16°F (−10 to −9°C) below normal body temperature; it also varies on different parts of the body	Arterial disease	Lower skin temperature in the extremities than in other body areas
Cold stimulation test: a thermistor in direct contact with each of the client's fingers is used to record normal temperature; hands are immersed in ice water for 20 s, then temperature is recorded every 5 min until the pretest temperature is reached	Digital temperature returns to pretest level within 15 min	Raynaud's phenomenon or disease	Digital temperature return to pretest level takes more than 20 min
Doppler ultrasound: a noninvasive test used to measure blood flow in the major veins and arteries; sound frequency is proportional to blood flow and velocity	Artery: multiphasic signals with prominent systolic component and one or more diastolic sounds Vein: intermittent signal of lower pitch than that of arterial flow; varies with respiration and Valsalva's maneuver	Arterial stenosis or occlusion	Decreased blood flow velocity signal without a diastolic sound; much decreased systolic signal distal to the occlusion At stenosis: signal high-pitched and possibly turbulent At occlusion where collateral circulation has not developed: signal may be absent, or the pressure gradient may be greater than 20–30 mm Hg at adjacent sites of the leg Venous blood flow velocity not altered by respiration or Valsalva's maneuver or totally absent
	Ankle–arm pressure index (API): ≥1	Venous thrombosis	
	Proximal thigh pressure 20–30 mm Hg higher than arm pressure; pressures in adjacent sites almost identical	Varicose veins and chronic venous insufficiency Mild vascular insufficiency, claudication, rest pain, and pregangrene symptoms	Flow-velocity signal may be the reverse Abnormal API readings
Exercise (treadmill) test for intermittent claudication: client remains supine for 10 min while Doppler studies are done of the ankle pressures; client then begins walking on the	Arm and ankle pressures rise during exercise	Peripheral vascular disease	Ankle pressure falls with exercise

Diagnostic Study	Normal Expected Value	Disease State	Expected Abnormal Findings
treadmill until claudication pain develops; client returns to supine position, and Doppler pressures are again recorded			
Impedence plethysmography: electrodes are applied to client's leg to measure changes in electrical resistance that result from blood-volume variations; a blood pressure cuff is inflated around the thigh to 60 mm Hg to occlude venous return	When cuff is inflated, venous blood volume increases; when cuff is deflated, there should be rapid venous outflow	DVT	When cuff is inflated, venous blood volume increase is less than normal; deflation of cuff produces less than normal venous outflow
Lumbar sympathetic block: procaine hydrochloride injected into the sympathetic ganglia blocks sympathetic vasomotor nerve tracts of a limb on side of the injection, resulting in vasodilation	Drying and warming of the skin of the leg show increased circulation to the limb	Peripheral vascular disease	Increase in drying and warming of the skin of the ischemic leg as circulation improves to the limb, indicating that circulation in the limb may be improved by a sympathectomy (Chapter 30); adverse reaction may be shock due to sudden fluid shift from vital organs into peripheral circulation
Lower limb venography (phlebography): radiographic examination of deep leg veins	Normal venogram shows opacity of all veins (deep and superficial) without deficits in filling	DVT Deep vein valvular incompetence Congenital venous abnormalities Venous insufficiency	Filling defects; abrupt termination of contrast medium Unfilled major deep veins Diversion of flow through collateral circulation
Radionuclide venography: ^{125}I fibrinogen is injected in a muscle on the distal side of a suspected thrombus; a scintiscanner records the clearance of the isotope	Less than 20% radioactivity in sites in legs	DVT	Increase of more than 20% radioactivity in any area in leg suggests DVT; an abnormality present for more than 24 h definitively confirms DVT
Angiography: a contrast medium injected into the femoral artery shows the extent of occlusive arterial lesions and available collateral circulation	Normal blood flow through the arteries	Atherosclerosis obliterans Aneurysms or arteriovenous malformation	Decreased blood flow; increased or decreased collateral circulation Aneurysm formation; vascular anomaly; increased or decreased collateral circulation; small leakage or hemorrhage from site

clients with arterial disease, no reflex vasodilation is detected.

In a cold pressure test, the client's normal blood pressure and pulse pressure are compared to pressures taken after immersion of the hand in ice water. The healthy client has a slight increase in blood pressure and no increase in pulse pressure, whereas the client with occlusive arterial disease has a significant increase in both blood and pulse pressures.

Excessive variations in skin-surface temperatures may indicate arterial disease. Skin temperatures are normally in the range of 14 to 16°F (−10 to −9°C) below normal body temperatures. Lower temperatures in the extremities than in the trunk may indicate impeded arterial flow. Direct skin thermometers (thermistors) are used to measure skin surface temperature.

In the cold stimulation test, normal finger temperature is recorded by skin thermometers. The hands are then immersed in ice water for 20 seconds. Digital temperature should return to normal within 15 minutes. If the return to normal temperature takes 20 to 40 minutes, the client is exhibiting Raynaud's phenomenon, attacks of severe pallor in the fingers or toes (sometimes also the ears and nose) brought on by cold or sometimes by emotion. Raynaud's phenomenon is usually linked to arterial insufficiency but sometimes appears by itself without causal disease. In that case, it is called Raynaud's disease. Thus, the cold stimulation test does not conclusively indicate arterial insufficiency.

Doppler Ultrasonography

The Doppler ultrasonography test is so named because it makes use of the Doppler effect—the alteration of sound by contact with a moving body. The transducer of the test instrument placed on the skin sends out bursts of ultra-high-frequency (UHF) sound; between bursts, it picks up echoes of the UHF sound that have been changed by bouncing off red blood cells flowing in a vein or artery. The difference between the transmitted and received UHF signals is an audible signal, the nature of which indicates the condition of the vein or artery. The sound also indicates blood pressure in areas of low blood flow. The ankle-arm pressure index (API), the ratio of ankle to brachial systolic pressure, provides information about vascular sufficiency, as do pressure gradients at adjacent sites. See Table 26–2 for a list of test results and their interpretations. Because the test is noninvasive, involving only the moving about of the transducer on the skin, the nurse usually needs only to explain the procedure to allay clients' fears.

Treadmill Test for Intermittent Claudication

The treadmill test aids in discriminating between clients with true intermittent claudication and those with conditions that mimic claudication. ECG monitoring is often done concomitantly.

The Doppler probe is used to measure the systolic pressure at the dorsalis pedis and posterior tibial arteries. The client then walks on the treadmill until claudication develops. Foot and ankle pressures are again obtained. In peripheral vascular disease, these pressures fall with exercise.

Impedance Plethysmography

Impedance plethysmography is a noninvasive test to measure the venous flow in the extremities. It is helpful in detecting DVT in the popliteal and iliofemoral systems.

The impedance plethysmograph works on the principle that electrical resistance in a vein is proportional to blood volume. The plethysmograph is used in conjunction with a blood pressure cuff to discover whether a blockage in a vein prevents the normal buildup and release of venous blood in response to temporary vascular occlusion by the cuff.

Lumbar Sympathetic Block

With the client in a prone position, procaine hydrochloride is injected into the sympathetic ganglia that innervate the lumbar spine at the level of the second or third lumbar vertebra. Successful blocking of the sympathetic tracts results in increased circulation with drying and warming of the skin of the extremity on the side of the block.

Nursing Implications. Clients experience initial discomfort with needle insertion and tingling and warmth in the extremity for several hours after the procedure. Postprocedure nursing care includes careful assessment for shock, which can result from sudden fluid shift into the peripheral circulation.

Lower Limb Venography

Lower limb venography (also called phlebography) assists in determining patency of the tibial–popliteal, superficial femoral–common femoral, and the saphenous veins. A contrast medium is injected into the superficial and/or deep veins of the extremity. X-rays are taken while the legs are placed in a variety of positions. Venography is the definitive test for DVT and also is used to locate a vein for possible arterial bypass grafting. The test is expensive and may cause localized clotting.

Radionuclide Venography

Radionuclide venography using ^{125}I fibrinogen is used to detect thrombi in the leg veins; it is not a good test for thrombi in the pelvis and groin. It is less expensive and less hazardous than venography with a contrast medium and may be used for clients who are too ill to undergo contrast venography or are sensitive to the dye. The ^{125}I fibrinogen is incorporated into thrombi when present. The initial scan is done 12 hours after injection and repeated in 24 hours to verify the findings.

Angiography

Angiography (arteriography) is the radiographic examination of one or more arteries after injection of a contrast medium (such as Hypaque) into an artery. For visualization of the arteries in the lower extremities, the contrast medium is injected into the femoral artery. Several x-rays are taken during the last few seconds of the injection, and another series is taken immediately after the injection. Concentrations of radioactivity, or "hot spots," indicate arterial blockage.

Nursing Implications. Angiography is an invasive diagnostic procedure. A consent form is required. Ask the client about iodine allergy because the contrast medium contains iodine. Tell clients undergoing angiography that they will experience a burning sensation at the injection site and a flushing warm feeling in the extremity (and sometimes in the whole body) that lasts a few seconds.

Following the procedure, the client is on bed rest, and vital signs are monitored every 15 minutes until stable. Check the injection site for local inflammation and internal and external bleeding. Ecchymosis is an indication of internal bleeding. Assess the peripheral pulses each time vital signs are taken and evaluate the affected extremity for skin color, warmth, numbness, and pain. Encourage the client to drink plenty of fluids to assist the kidneys in excretion of the contrast medium.

Section II: Nursing Diagnosis

The subjective and objective data collected during the assessment phase of the nursing process are analyzed to make pertinent nursing diagnoses. Nursing diagnoses common to clients with peripheral vascular disorders are listed in Box 26–1.

ALTERATION IN PERIPHERAL TISSUE PERFUSION

Decreased peripheral tissue perfusion can be related to vasoconstriction from cold temperatures, medications such as ergotamine, cigarette smoking, or Raynaud's phenomenon. Decreased perfusion can also result from plaque formations that have narrowed peripheral blood vessels, as in atherosclerosis. Altered tissue perfusion leads to inflammation and hypoxia, which can lead to skin breakdown and client discomfort.

IMPAIRMENT OF SKIN INTEGRITY

Clients with peripheral vascular disorders have changes in skin integrity. With poor arterial circulation, tissues lack adequate oxygen and nutrients and may become ulcerated or necrotic as a result. A decrease in circulating blood to the periphery and trauma to an extremity already lacking adequate perfusion can lead to inflammation (cellulitis), skin breakdown (ulcers), and necrosis (gangrene).

Box 26–1 Nursing Diagnoses Commonly Related to Vascular System Dysfunction

Diagnoses Directly Related to Vascular Dysfunction

Tissue perfusion, alteration in: peripheral
Skin integrity, impairment of: actual
Comfort, alteration in: pain

Additional Potential Nursing Diagnoses

Fear
Knowledge deficit
Self-concept, disturbance in: body image
Sexual dysfunction

ALTERATION IN COMFORT: PAIN

Clients with disorders of the peripheral vascular system experience various degrees of pain. Arterial occlusion, increased levels of tissue hypoxia and tissue necrosis, and stress are all sources of pain. Inflammation directly contributes to pain because the inflammatory process irritates and compresses nerve endings. Pain can interfere with recovery by discouraging the client from remaining ambulatory. Immobility interferes with activities of daily living and contributes to further circulatory stasis.

FEAR

Many clients with peripheral vascular complications are anxious and stressed. They fear potential emboli, obstruction, occlusion, and limb loss. The pain clients experience intensifies their anxiety level, causing sympathetic stimulation, which further constricts peripheral vessels.

KNOWLEDGE DEFICIT

The client with a peripheral vascular disorder may deny the existence of the disease, lack knowledge about the disease process, or fear inability to cope with the facts of the disease. Assess the client's knowledge level and then promote activities to increase knowledge and understanding to maximize quality of life.

DISTURBANCE IN SELF-CONCEPT: BODY IMAGE

Depending on its severity, peripheral vascular disease causes a number of body changes. Any of these changes can affect a client's self-concept and relationships with significant others. Skin-color changes, muscle atrophy, swelling, leg ulcers, and amputation all have the potential to affect the client's body image negatively.

SEXUAL DYSFUNCTION

An unsightly extremity, pain, or fear of injury to the affected limb may cause the client or the sexual partner to avoid sexual intercourse. This change in an intimate relationship will add to the client's poor self-image and may increase anxiety and fear.

Inability to have an erection can result from occlusive vascular disease. Impaired penile blood supply in Leriche's syndrome occurs with obstruction of the distal aorta at the bifurcation of the common iliac arteries.

Section III: Planning and Implementation

Nursing interventions for clients with disorders of the peripheral vascular system should be geared toward resolving the problems identified in the assessment and analysis phases of the nursing process. A sample nursing care plan for clients with peripheral vascular disease is presented in Table 26–3.

PROMOTING PERIPHERAL TISSUE PERFUSION

Inadequate tissue perfusion may be related to arterial or venous thrombus formation and obstruction, vasoconstriction, or inflammatory effects. The major goal of care is to maximize tissue perfusion by reducing risk factors, maintaining a proper environment, wearing nonconstrictive clothing, balancing rest and exercise, and doing specialized exercises.

Smoking Cessation

Smoking is one of the major contributing factors in the development of peripheral vascular disease. The importance of decreasing, or preferably eliminating, smoking cannot be overemphasized. Nicotine causes vasospasm and constriction of the arteries and also increases the heart rate, which increases the work load of the heart and cir-

Table 26–3 Sample Nursing Care Plan for the Client With Vascular System Dysfunction

Nursing Diagnosis	Client Care Goals	Plan/Nursing Implementation	Expected Outcome
Tissue perfusion, alteration in: peripheral	Reduce or stop smoking; maintain proper diet; maintain comfort and warmth of extremities	Encourage client to stop smoking and provide information on "stop smoking" programs; if client is obese, prescribe weight-reduction diet; instruct client and family about maintaining a comfortable environmental temperature; encourage use of extra clothing to provide warmth; encourage participation in ADL (balanced exercise and rest periods); teach client proper foot care and use of foot cradles or foot board; encourage adequate fluid intake to prevent dehydration and increased viscosity of blood, which leads to decreased O_2 to tissues	Adequate tissue perfusion; participation in ADL; can describe reasons for proper foot care and exercise; client who smokes will stop smoking
Skin integrity, impairment of: actual	Describe hazards of skin breakdown and injury to extremities; remain protected from injury and infection; monitor skin changes correctly	Assess skin for signs of breakdown; instruct client and family about skin changes such as thickening, drying, cracking, and areas of ulceration; monitor skin color, temperature, and peripheral pulses; keep skin clean and dry; instruct client and family about the importance of protecting extremities from exposure to extremes in temperature and from trauma; instruct client and family about the importance of physical exercise	Skin integrity is normal; shows no signs of breakdown or infection
Comfort, alteration in: pain	Experience a decreased level of pain	Ascertain the source of pain and eliminate, if possible (eg, by administration of analgesics as ordered); provide distraction (eg, reading, television, visitors); position extremities to relieve pressure; instruct client not to sit or stand for long periods, not to sit with legs crossed, to elevate feet (venous insufficiency), or provide a flat position for feet (arterial insufficiency); provide for balanced exercise and rest periods; provide warmth to extremities by controlling environmental temperature; instruct client on the importance of nonconstrictive clothing; administer analgesics as ordered	Client comfortable and free of pain

culatory system. The carbon monoxide that is inhaled by the smoker decreases the oxygen-carrying capacity of the hemoglobin so less oxygen is delivered to the tissues.

Smoking is extremely difficult for many clients to give up. Provide the client with information about smoking cessation programs, self-help groups in the community, and nicotine chewing gum as a temporary aid for clients with a high nicotine dependence who are also attempting behavior modification. Clients with peripheral vascular disease who do not quit smoking face serious sequelae including gangrene and amputation.

Dietary Management

Dietary instruction is essential for clients with peripheral vascular disease. Obesity increases stress on the heart and increases venous congestion, impeding proper nutrition to body cells. A properly balanced weight-reduction diet should be prescribed and carefully monitored by the nurse or physician.

When serum lipid levels are elevated, dietary management is directed to the specific elevated serum lipid. Clients with an elevated cholesterol level are given a low-cholesterol diet. Clients with an increase in the triglyceride level are given a diet low in saturated fats and low in carbohydrates. More specific diets for the six types of hyperlipidemia are described in Chapter 24. Clients with hypertension are placed on a diet low in sodium.

Environmental Temperature and Wearing Apparel

A warm environment is important for a client with peripheral vascular disease because it causes vasodilation, which in turn increases blood supply to the extremities. Warm clothing such as bed socks or long underwear achieve the required warmth. Direct heat applied to the extremities is not advisable: most clients with peripheral vascular disease suffer from peripheral neuropathy, which diminishes the ability to sense heat accurately, predisposing the client to burns. Clients should understand the importance of checking bathwater temperature with the arm rather than the foot because of peripheral neuropathy.

Clients should avoid constrictive clothing such as elastics, garters, girdles, knee-high nylon socks, and tight waistbands. Such items compromise circulation to the already deficient areas. Shoelaces should not be tied too tightly.

Clients should wear thermal underwear, heavy socks, and gloves in cold weather. Chilling of the feet and/or body causes vasoconstriction, which leads to inadequate circulation to the extremities.

Exercise and Position Change

The client with peripheral vascular disease must understand the importance of daily exercise. Exercise provides necessary muscle contraction for movement of arterial blood to the peripheral areas of the body, for return of venous blood to the heart, and for the development of collateral

Nursing Research Note

Ventura M et al: Effectiveness of health promotion interventions. *Nurs Res* 1984; 33(3):162–167.

The purpose of this research was to determine whether participation in a health promotion program for clients with peripheral vascular disease would improve their level of exercise, reduce smoking, and enhance foot care. The sample size was 84 with a study group of 44 subjects, and a control group of 40 subjects. The study group received three booklets about exercise, living with peripheral vascular disease, and foot care and a pamphlet about smoking reduction. The control group received no special intervention.

There was no significant difference between the control group and experimental group in smoking and foot care, although there was a trend toward reducing smoking and improving foot care. Members of the experimental group who chose to increase their activity showed greater increases over the control group in frequency, distance, and length of exercise. Overall, there was no difference between groups in blood pressure indices after intervention, nor was there a change in symptoms.

This study demonstrates that health promotion activities have some benefit. Client education, support, and encouragement may facilitate behavior modification with improved health outcomes.

circulation. The exercise regimen must begin gradually, and a moderate daily exercise program must be continued. Excessive exercise increases the metabolic demands of the body, increasing the work load of the circulatory system.

Clients should rest after exercise periods. Elevating the feet above heart level is helpful to the client with venous insufficiency. Clients with arterial insufficiency should rest lying flat; raising the legs increases the work of the arterial system and impedes perfusion to the legs.

Clients should not maintain one position for too long. Sitting for long periods with knees bent or crossed causes undue pressure on the popliteal vessels, which decreases circulation to and from the area and results in leg swelling and pain. Standing for long periods also causes venous congestion because the veins have to work against gravity to return blood to the heart.

The best form of moderate exercise to increase blood flow to the legs is walking. Rest periods are important during the walking regimen. If pain develops with walking short distances, rest at regular intervals should become part of the exercise program. Clients should be aware of their level of pain tolerance; those with a high tolerance need to be careful not to walk too much at one time; clients with low tolerance may have to push themselves to get enough exercise.

MAINTAINING SKIN INTEGRITY

Clients with peripheral vascular disease suffer from decreased blood supply to the extremities, particularly the feet. Therefore, clients must learn to protect skin integrity through generalized foot care and to promote skin integrity by stimulating increased blood flow to the skin.

Clients should take meticulous care of their feet. They should wash their feet daily with mild soap and warm water and rinse them thoroughly. They must dry the feet completely, using a patting motion. Rough drying of the feet can cause tissue trauma. The feet should be kept soft by use of lanolin lotions to prevent drying and cracking between the toes, which leads to infection. If drying and itching occur on the feet or legs (especially in the elderly), clients should take fewer baths and use lanolin or superfat soaps. Hard, scaly areas; discoloration; or swelling of the legs must be reported to the physician.

Corn and callous removers or other chemicals should not be used. Toenails should be cut straight across after a bath has softened them. If there is a problem with hard, overgrown nails, a podiatrist should cut the nails routinely.

Fungal infections of the feet can be prevented by keeping the feet dry. The client who perspires may use foot powder judiciously. Clients should change their socks daily (or more often, if indicated). Leather-soled shoes are preferable to rubber soles because rubber impedes evaporation of moisture and provides a dark, moist area in which fungi can breed.

The feet should always be protected by socks and slippers or shoes. The client should not walk barefoot. Shoes should not be constricting, and new shoes should be broken in slowly. All these measures diminish the potential for trauma to the feet. Trauma, no matter how minor, requires physician consultation.

Clients should not scratch itchy spots on the feet or legs because scratching can break down the skin, and broken skin can progress to leg ulcers. Calamine lotion may be used on itchy areas.

Even with meticulous care of the legs and feet, some clients will develop leg ulcers. Preventing infection in the ulcerated area is essential. Whether the client remains at home or is hospitalized, strict aseptic technique is required with ulcer care because the impaired circulation to the extremity decreases the availability of nutrients to promote fast healing. Wet dressings are applied with sterile gloves and allowed to dry before removal to facilitate removal of the necrotic tissue. Protective agents such as zinc oxide or petrolatum are used in dressings.

Dressing or soaking the ulcer can be painful. Pain medication should be administered 30 minutes before ulcer care.

Clients with chronic ulcers learn to be meticulous in their care when they understand that infection is potentially limb threatening. Severe leg ulcers may need skin grafting. A visiting community health nurse can assist the client and family with proper ulcer care.

PROMOTING COMFORT

In peripheral vascular disorders, pain may result from the inflammatory response that produces tissue edema and pressure on nerve endings and/or from tissue hypoxia. Analgesics may be ordered for symptomatic relief. Tranquilizers may help reduce anxiety, which can increase pain perception. Vasodilators may be used to increase blood supply to the ischemic area.

Nursing measures to alleviate pain include isolating the source of the pain and taking measures to diminish it, providing distraction for the client, and promoting relaxation and comfort. Teach clients about the action, expected therapeutic effect, dosage, frequency of administration, and potential side effects of any medication prescribed.

IMPROVING KNOWLEDGE AND SELF-CONCEPT

Peripheral vascular disease is usually a chronic, lifelong problem. Treatment is often slow with frequent setbacks, which add to the discouragement and frustration of clients and significant others. Fears of chronic disease and becoming a burden to the family are not unrealistic. Clients feel a loss of control over their disease and their lives. The nurse should assist both clients and families to express these fears.

Teach the client about the disease process and the symptoms and signs that should be reported to the physician. Realistically and honestly encourage the client when progress is made. Involve the client and significant others in the plan of care, so that a realistic plan for living with peripheral vascular disease can be made. Involve the client in all decision making, which is essential for maintaining feelings of self-worth. Encourage the client and sexual partner to discuss any fears they have about resumption of sexual intercourse. Suggest positions they can try that will be sexually satisfying and yet avoid trauma to the extremity.

Section IV: Evaluation

In evaluation, the last phase of the nursing process, the nurse ascertains whether the goals of care have been met and whether the expected outcomes have been achieved. If they have not been achieved, the nurse and client must reassess the client care goals, decide whether the plan of care was appropriate, and, if necessary, revise the care plan.

PERIPHERAL TISSUE PERFUSION

The following expected outcomes demonstrate the client's understanding of measures to promote tissue perfusion:

- Demonstrates an active interest in smoking cessation programs

- Shows a decrease in the number of cigarettes smoked in a cigarette count
- Discusses the importance of maintaining the prescribed diet and proper weight
- States reasons for avoiding direct application of heat
- Explains importance of preventing exposure to extremes in temperature and use of warm clothing in winter
- Describes proper wearing apparel for avoiding vasoconstriction
- Lists ambulation requirements
- Explains balance of rest and activity throughout the day
- States rationale for avoiding prolonged standing, sitting in one position, crossing legs, and elevating legs

SKIN INTEGRITY

The following expected outcomes demonstrate the client's understanding of measures to maintain skin integrity:

- Explains reasons for washing feet and changing socks daily and for keeping feet dry
- Demonstrates foot care including patting rather than rubbing feet dry
- Discusses approaches to avoiding trauma to legs and feet
- Demonstrates the proper care of leg ulcers
- Lists symptoms and signs of infection
- Specifies symptoms and signs that require medical attention

COMFORT

The following expected outcomes demonstrate the client's understanding of measures to promote comfort:

- Explains the balance of rest and activity
- Specifies pain-relief approaches following exercise
- States dosage, action, side effects, and frequency of administration of prescribed pain medication

Chapter Highlights

Nursing assessment to determine the adequacy of peripheral circulation includes evaluation for color, temperature of extremities, the presence of pulses, and trophic changes.

Tissue perfusion may be altered by degenerative changes, trauma, infection, and inflammation.

A diet with large amounts of cholesterol or saturated fats, a family predisposition to atherosclerosis or diabetes mellitus, and high stress levels can cause alterations in circulation.

Clients with peripheral vascular disorders often have edema, symptoms of intermittent claudication, and/or pain in the extremity.

Peripheral vascular disease can result in long-term degenerative changes requiring extended medical treatment and adaptation to changes.

Quality of ambulation, perfusion to the extremities, and venous and arterial competency are important criteria in the assessment of peripheral vascular disorders.

Smoking is absolutely contraindicated in clients with peripheral vascular disease. Clients cannot hope to achieve improvement in symptoms unless they abandon their cigarette habit.

Oral contraceptives and drugs containing ergotamine (often used for clients with migraine headaches) are also contraindicated in vascular disease.

The most important goals of a nursing care plan for a client with peripheral vascular disease are to increase perfusion of tissues, to maintain skin integrity, and to keep the client comfortable.

Bibliography

Bates B: *A Guide to Physical Examination,* 3rd ed. Philadelphia: Lippincott, 1983.
Doyle J: If your patient's legs hurt, the reason may be arterial insufficiency. *Nurs 81* (April) 1981; 11:74–78.
Durbin N: The application of Doppler techniques in critical care. *Focus Critical Care* (June) 1983; 10:44–46.
Eddy M: Teaching patients with peripheral vascular disease. *Nurs Clin North Am* (March) 1977; 12:151–159.
Fetzer–Fowler S: Carotid sinus massage. *Critical Care Nurse* (July–Aug) 1983; 3:26–30.

Hale E: Deep vein thrombosis: Tying the knot. *Nurs Mirror* (Feb) 1981; 152:42–43.
Hinnant JR, Stallworth MJ: Simplified surgery for varicose veins. *AORN J* 1981; 34:135–150.
Hudson B: Sharpen your vascular assessment skills with the Doppler ultrasound stethoscope. *Nurs 83* (May) 1983; 13:55–57.
Kim MJ, Moritz DA: Classification of nursing diagnosis. In: *Proceedings of the Third and Fourth National Conferences.* New York: McGraw–Hill, 1982.
Martin I: Varicose ulcers 1: Breaking down in vein. *Nurs Mirror* (July) 1981; 153:34–35.
Martin I: Varicose ulcers 2: Rewarding remedies. *Nurs Mirror* (Aug) 1981; 153:34–35.

Miller DC, Roon AJ: *Diagnosis and Management of Peripheral Vascular Disease.* Menlo Park, CA: Addison–Wesley, 1982.

Petersdorf RG et al: *Harrison's Principles of Internal Medicine,* 10th ed. New York: McGraw–Hill, 1983.

Raab D: Peripheral vascular disease: How to recognize it, how to treat it. *Can Nurse* (Sept) 1982; 78:30–33.

Seville RH: Leg ulcers. *Nurs Times* (July) 1981; 77:1249–1253.

Taggart E: The physical assessment of the patient with arterial disease. *Nurs Clin North Am* (March) 1977; 12:109–117.

Suggested Readings

Bastarache MM et al: Assessing peripheral vascular disease: Noninvasive testing. *Am J Nurs* 1983; 83:1552–1556. The authors review noninvasive techniques to evaluate arterial, venous, and extracranial cerebrovascular insufficiencies. Doppler studies, pulse-volume waveform analysis, segmental limb pressures, treadmill testing, and plethysmography are discussed.

Baum PL: Heed the early warning signs of PVD. *Nurs 85* (March) 1985; 15:50–57. A case study approach is used to compare acute and chronic arterial disease and acute and chronic venous disease. Assessment of the client with peripheral vascular disease and client and family education are also covered.

Peterson FY: Assessing peripheral vascular disease at the bedside. *Am J Nurs* 1983; 83:1549–1551. Peripheral vascular problems may be acute or chronic, arterial or venous, and are difficult to diagnose. This article discusses the assessment of clients with peripheral circulatory problems, including client teaching and preventive approaches.

Chapter 27

Specific Disorders of the Peripheral Circulation

Janice Lech Dusek
SueAnn Wooster Ames

Objectives

When you have finished studying this chapter, you should be able to:

Describe the pathophysiology, clinical manifestations, and nursing care of clients with coarctation of the aorta and congenital arteriovenous fistula.

Identify the clinical manifestations and nursing care of clients with Raynaud's disease, Raynaud's phenomenon, and Buerger's disease.

Discuss the pathophysiology, clinical manifestations, and nursing care of clients with abdominal, thoracic, peripheral, and dissecting aortic aneurysms.

Specify nursing approaches in the care of clients with varicose veins and venous leg ulcers.

Describe the pathophysiology, clinical manifestations, and management of polyarteritis nodosa and aortic arch syndrome.

Discuss the pathophysiology, clinical manifestations, and management of arterial and venous occlusive disease and of lymphedema.

Explain the major types of traumatic injuries to the peripheral circulation and discuss the nursing implications related to the care of these clients.

Specific disorders of the peripheral circulation may involve any condition of the vascular system that alters circulation through the aorta, arteries, veins, and lymphatic vessels.

The alteration in circulation may be due to a congenital, multifactorial, degenerative, immunologic, infectious, obstructive, or traumatic disorder.

Section I: Congenital Disorders

This section discusses coarctation of the aorta and arteriovenous fistulas that are present at birth. This chapter discusses the care of adult clients with these disorders.

COARCTATION OF THE AORTA

Coarctation of the aorta is a localized narrowing of the aorta; the narrowing is most common slightly beyond the origin of the left subclavian artery or slightly distal to the insertion of the ligamentum arteriosum (Figure 27–1).

Coarctation can be an isolated defect but can also occur with a bicuspid aortic valve.

The cause of coarctation is not known. The most common theory is that the coarctation is an abnormal extension of the same fibrotic process that converts a patent ductus into a ligamentum arteriosum. Coarctation is one of the most common congenital abnormalities. It occurs in 10% to 15% of clients with congenital heart disease. It is twice as common in males as in females (Schwartz et al., 1979).

The narrowing of the aorta obstructs blood flow,

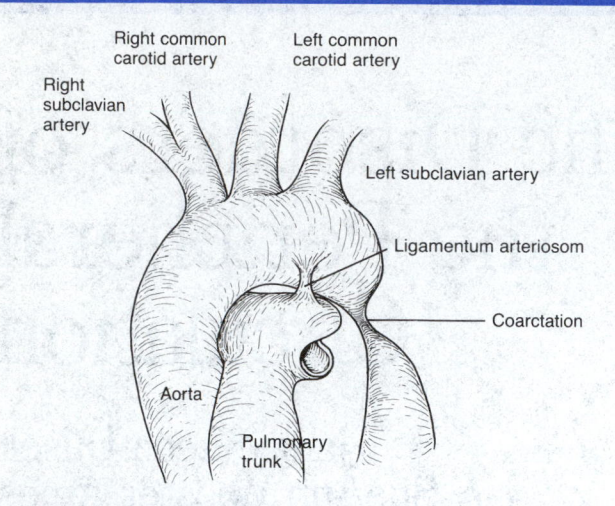

Figure 27–1

Coarctation of the aorta immediately beyond the ligamentum arteriosum and the origin of the left subclavian artery, which tends to become dilated because of an increase in blood pressure in the region.

increasing the left ventricular pressure and cardiac work load. Collateral circulation develops around the stenosis (Figure 27–2). These collateral vessels arise from the subclavian arteries and anastomose with the intercostal and epigastric vessels that enter the distal aorta, which supplies blood to the lower extremities.

Clinical Manifestations

Many children are asymptomatic for long periods. If coarctation is asymptomatic in infancy, it usually remains so throughout adolescence. Growth and development are unremarkable. On the other hand, severe hypertension and progressive degenerative changes may occur in the aorta. When symptoms occur, they include headache, dizziness, and epistaxis (the most common symptoms), dyspnea on exertion (DOE), chest pain, and (infrequently) claudication pain in the lower extremities.

When a child is hypertensive in the arms and has absent or greatly reduced pulses in the legs, aortic coarctation should be suspected. The adult may have diminished blood pressures in the lower extremities and be hypertensive in the arms. Normally, the blood pressure in the legs is slightly higher than in the arms. There are marked pulsations in the neck and in the muscles of the shoulder girdle. A bruit may be auscultated over these pulsating areas. A chest x-ray may show a prominent aorta and may depict bilateral notching of the ribs. The ECG may show signs of left ventricular hypertrophy. Cardiac catheterization is done to evaluate collateral circulation and to determine pressures in the heart and aorta. Aortography locates the site and the degree of coarctation.

Therapeutic Measures

The treatment of choice is surgery. In adults, surgery is complicated by the degenerative process in the arteries. The surgery involves resection of the coarcted segment and end-to-end anastomosis or graft. Refer to Chapter 30 for details of the surgical procedure and postoperative care.

Specific Nursing Measures

Carefully assess any client with dyspnea, claudication, and epistaxis for possible coarctation. When checking vital signs, auscultate the apical pulse and listen for murmurs and additional heart sounds. Look for any visible pulsations. Palpate the peripheral pulses. The blood pressure may show resting systolic hypertension and a wide pulse pressure. The client who is diagnosed as having coarctation needs an explanation of the disorder, reasons for compliance with medical therapy, and the probability of surgery.

ARTERIOVENOUS FISTULA

Arteriovenous fistulas, which are usually congenital but infrequently develop after trauma, are uncommon lesions. As the name indicates, there is an abnormal communication between arteries and veins, but a single communication is rare. The lesion may be localized in a foot or a finger or it may be diffuse and involve an entire arm or leg. Multiple lesions may indicate a basic defect in the peripheral vas-

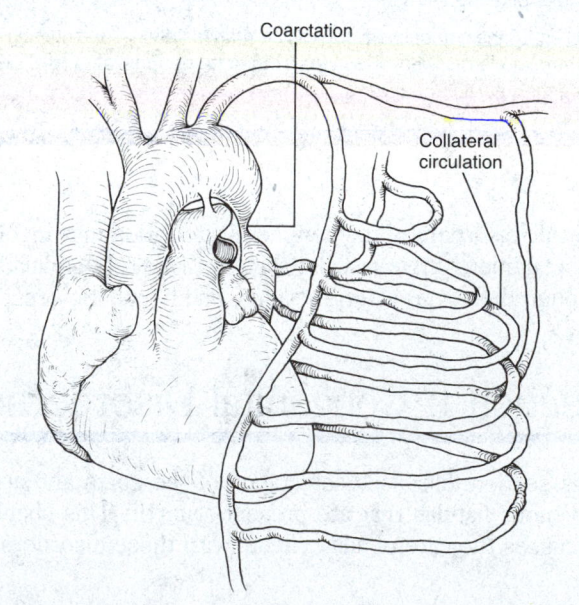

Figure 27–2

Development of collateral circulation in coarctation of the aorta. Collateral vessels develop to bypass the occluded aortic lumen and can be seen on x-ray as notching of the ribs.

cular system that allows arteriovenous fistulas to develop throughout life.

Clinical Manifestations

Multiple dilated veins (venous angiomas) seen during physical examination often suggest varicosities. If the dilated veins are located in unusual areas (eg, the head and neck), arteriovenous fistulas must be considered. A continuous bruit over the mass establishes the diagnosis. If the fistulas involve the entire extremity, a bruit may not be heard. Digital compression that eliminates a bruit suggests a single arteriovenous fistula, often of traumatic origin. Multiple bruits that cannot be eliminated by digital compression suggest a congenital origin.

Arteriovenous fistulas are also associated with symptoms and signs of venous insufficiency (ie, edema of the extremity and darkened, mottled skin). Dilated veins tend to enlarge gradually, causing difficulty from occasional external bleeding and rupture. If the digits are involved, ischemic pain may occur, and gangrene of fingertips is a possibility.

Arteriography, which is indicated to confirm the diagnosis, shows many tortuous arteries with rapid opacification and numerous dilated veins. Ultrasonography is also used in diagnosis (Schwartz et al., 1979).

Therapeutic Measures

Arteriovenous fistula is best treated conservatively (eg, with support stockings). An operation should only be undertaken when the lesion is large enough to cause ulceration or bleeding, because surgical excision is considered palliative in most clients. Lesions involving the head, neck, pelvis, and flank are difficult to treat. A favorable response has been achieved with intra-arterial embolization in which arterial injection of an agent such as polyvinyl alcohol sponge occludes the major feeding vessels of the fistula (Miller & Roon, 1982).

Specific Nursing Measures

Emotional support of the client and significant others is essential. Many clients must have several en bloc excisions of soft tissue or entire digits; excision of an isolated fistula is rarely possible. Schwartz et al. (1979) describe a case of fistula that had been operated on several times and still was not eradicated; amputation of an ear was finally necessary to prevent hemorrhage. When the cartilage of the ear was divided adjacent to the skull, numerous arteries adherent to the cartilage were resected. Yet, only a year after surgery, bruits were audible over and around the operative area. As this example illustrates, surgery is often palliative.

Education of the client and family about the disease process and the potential complications is also a nursing responsibility. The importance of routine medical follow-up should be stressed.

Section II: Disorders of Multifactorial Origin

Disorders of multifactorial origin involving the peripheral vascular circulation can cause symptoms ranging from mild discomfort to severe pain and loss of sensation. Alteration in circulation to the extremities can lead to poor nutrition and oxygenation of tissues; ulceration and subsequent loss of digits or an entire extremity may result. Conditions discussed in this section include Raynaud's disease, Raynaud's phenomenon, and Buerger's disease.

RAYNAUD'S DISEASE AND RAYNAUD'S PHENOMENON

Raynaud's disease is an idiopathic benign disorder characterized by vasospasm of the peripheral small arteries and arterioles of the upper extremities, especially the hands; the feet are rarely affected. The disease is more common in women than in men and often begins in the late teens.

The cause of Raynaud's disease is unknown, but the following theories have been suggested: (1) excessive adrenergic stimulation, selective to the arms, resulting in the constriction of small arteries and arterioles, which causes the characteristic changes in color, temperature, and sensation of the fingers; (2) intrinsic vascular-wall hyperactiv-

ity to cold and emotional stresses; or (3) an antigen–antibody immune response. The latter is the most likely theory because abnormal immunologic test results usually accompany the disease.

Raynaud's phenomenon is also characterized by vasospasm of the arteries, but the vasospasm is secondary to another underlying condition. Raynaud's phenomenon is seen with connective-tissue disease (especially scleroderma); thoracic outlet syndrome; exposure to polyvinyl chloride, lead, arsenic, or ergot; continuous trauma such as that with typing, piano playing, or jackhammer use; and drug therapy (mainly ergotamine, methysergide, and propranolol).

Clinical Manifestations

When the client is exposed to cold or a stressor, the fingers first blanch and turn completely white (the *pallor* phase); the fingers next become blue (the *cyanotic* phase); finally, the fingers turn red (the *rubor* phase). In the pallor phase, the fingers become cold. They begin to warm in the rubor phase. Numbness and tingling may occur during these phases. The thumbs are often not involved. If the disease is severe or long-standing, trophic changes, skin ulcerations, and gangrene may develop.

Therapeutic Measures

Drugs that interfere with the action of sympathetic nerves by blocking vasoconstriction are often used in Raynaud's disease. These drugs include reserpine, guanethidine (Ismelin), methyldopa (Aldomet), phenoxybenzamine (Dibenzyline), or prazosin (Minipress). Nifedipine (Procardia), a calcium channel blocking agent with a peripheral vasodilating effect, has been used experimentally in Raynaud's disease.

Temporary cervicothoracic sympathetic block may be done to assess the amount of vasodilation that could be gained by a cervicothoracic sympathectomy. Cervicothoracic sympathectomy is performed in severe cases of Raynaud's disease to reduce vasospasm and pain. In some instances, gangrenous fingers are amputated to remove necrotic tissue. Medical treatment of Raynaud's phenomenon is directed toward the underlying disease process.

Specific Nursing Measures

Teaching clients to abstain from smoking and to avoid exposure to cold are the major nursing responsibilities for clients with both Raynaud's disease and Raynaud's phenomenon. Urge the client to stop smoking, explaining that nicotine, a vasoconstrictor, aggravates the disease process. Encourage and support the client in these efforts and involve significant others. Teach approaches that have been helpful to others in giving up cigarettes—smoking clinics, self-help groups, behavior modification, biofeedback, hypnosis, and nicotine gum. Some persons can quit "cold turkey," but many cannot. Clients may have to experiment with several approaches before they find the one that works for them. Many of these methods are costly; however, continuing to smoke costs more in the long run, not only in health and health-related expenses but also in the actual cost of cigarettes. Significant others who live with the client should also give up cigarettes to help the client become and remain a nonsmoker. Health-care providers who do not smoke are also good role models.

Warn clients against exposing hands to cold. Measures to prevent chilling, such as wearing adequate clothing for total body warmth and use of warm gloves and socks in cold weather, are essential. Also urge clients to use gloves when handling frozen foods or when cleaning the freezer or refrigerator. Clients with Raynaud's disease or Raynaud's phenomenon should avoid jobs that expose them to constant cold. Teach clients to avoid applying heat directly to cold extremities; burns can result.

Teach clients to avoid secondary causes of vasospasm, such as occupational use of pneumatic tools or exposure to toxins and vasoconstricting drugs. Explain the need to avoid constrictive clothing such as tight cuffs and elastic wristbands.

Clients on vasodilating drugs should be taught the action, expected therapeutic effect, dosage, frequency of administration, and any side effects of the drug. Women with Raynaud's disease or Raynaud's phenomenon should not use oral contraceptives because of the danger of thromboembolism.

BUERGER'S DISEASE

Buerger's disease (thromboangiitis obliterans) is an inflammatory, obstructive, nonatheromatous disease that affects small and medium arteries and veins (unlike atherosclerosis, which involves only arteries). Diminished blood flow to the legs and feet from thrombus development and vessel spasm results in leg ulceration and gangrene. Arteries of the upper limbs may also be involved.

Buerger's disease is an idiopathic disease, occurring mainly in men from 20 to 40 years of age. There is a high incidence of the disease among smokers.

Clinical Manifestations

The chief symptom in Buerger's disease is pain. Intermittent claudication of the arch of the foot is common. There may also be rest pain, which signifies that ischemia is increasing in severity. When the feet are exposed to cold, there is a cold feeling of the extremity, followed by cyanosis and numbness, and later by reddening and hot, tingly sensations. There may be ulceration and gangrene of fingers and toes. There may also be migratory superficial thrombophlebitis manifested as painful, red, swollen lumps under the skin. In the later stages of the disease, the limbs may become red and/or cyanotic in a dependent position. Muscle atrophy, ulceration, and gangrene around the nails and toes can occur.

Findings on physical examination are (Petersdorf et al., 1983):

- Intense rubor of the feet
- Absent foot pulses in the presence of normal femoral and popliteal pulses
- Absent or reduced radial and/or ulnar pulses

Therapeutic Measures

Vasodilating drugs such as tolazoline (Priscoline) or papaverine (Pavabid) may be used with some clients. The only effective treatment approach is complete abstinence from tobacco, however.

Temporary lumbar sympathetic block may be done to assess the amount of vasodilation that might be gained by a lumbar sympathectomy. Lumbar sympathectomy (see Chapter 30) is performed to reduce vasospasm and pain and to increase collateral circulation. Gangrenous digits may have to be amputated to remove necrotic tissue.

Specific Nursing Measures

Encourage the client to stop smoking. This is the single most important aspect of care. Refer to the discussion of smoking under Raynaud's disease.

Educate the client about the importance of keeping the extremities warm, wearing adequate clothing for total body warmth, and avoiding constricting clothing. Keeping room temperature at 71°F (21°C) aids in maintaining a stable body temperature. Clients should avoid all situations that exacerbate vasoconstriction, such as exposure to cold water, refrigerators, freezers, cold weather, vibrating tools, oral contraceptives, beta-adrenergic blocking agents, and ergotamine preparations.

Educate the client about the importance of not remaining in one position, either standing or sitting, for too long. Explain the necessity for leg movement, ankle rotation, and knee bending on long trips to stimulate circulation. Reinforce the importance of not crossing the legs and not sitting too close to the chair edge, which can compromise popliteal circulation. Elevating the head of the client's bed a few inches (eg, by putting blocks under it) may enhance circulation to the extremities.

Encourage the client to drink fluids to increase vascular volume and decrease blood viscosity. Reinforce the exercise regimen prescribed by the physician. Walking is recommended unless pain is severe. Trauma to the extremities must be avoided because of the danger of lesions that will not heal, infection, and gangrene.

Educate the client and significant others about foot care, including the use of warm water, mild soaps, rinsing well, and patting rather than rubbing dry. Also reinforce the importance of applying lotions to keep skin moist, preventing drying and cracking. Encourage the client to wear supportive slippers and properly fitted shoes to minimize trauma to feet. Demonstrate how to check the extremities for symptoms and signs of decreased blood flow, such as a change in color or temperature of the limb, cuts that do not heal, cracking skin, and thickening of the nails.

Section III: Degenerative Disorders

The degenerative disorders of the peripheral circulation affect both the arterial and the venous systems. This section discusses aneurysms of the aorta, peripheral arterial aneurysms, and venous insufficiency with resultant varicose veins and venous leg ulcers.

sclerosis, which weakens the arterial wall and gradually distends the arterial lumen at the weakened area. Infections, congenital defects, syphilitic aortitis, and cystic medial necrosis associated with Marfan's syndrome or hypertension are other causative factors (Petersdorf et al., 1983).

AORTIC ANEURYSM

An aneurysm is a sac or dilatation of the arterial vessel wall that develops because of a weakness in the arterial wall. It can be localized or diffuse. Aneurysms occur most often in the aorta and the cerebral arteries, but they may develop in any artery.

There are many types and shapes of aneurysms (Figure 27–3). A true aneurysm is the outpouching or dilatation of all three layers of an artery. Involvement of the entire circumference of the artery is called a *fusiform aneurysm,* the most common type. A *saccular aneurysm,* an outpouching involving one side of the artery, looks like a sac or pouch and is attached by a small neck. A *false aneurysm* is actually a pulsating hematoma. A disruption in the arterial wall allows an accumulation of blood to be held in place by the surrounding tissue.

A *dissecting aneurysm* occurs when blood between the medial and intimal layers of the arterial wall begins to split the arterial layers. This can lead to rupture of the artery and death from internal hemorrhage and shock.

Aneurysms are also classified according to the specific blood vessel and the area of that vessel they involve (eg, a femoral aneurysm, an aneurysm of the aortic arch, and an abdominal aortic aneurysm). Very small aneurysms resulting from infection are called mycotic aneurysms.

The most common cause of an aneurysm is athero-

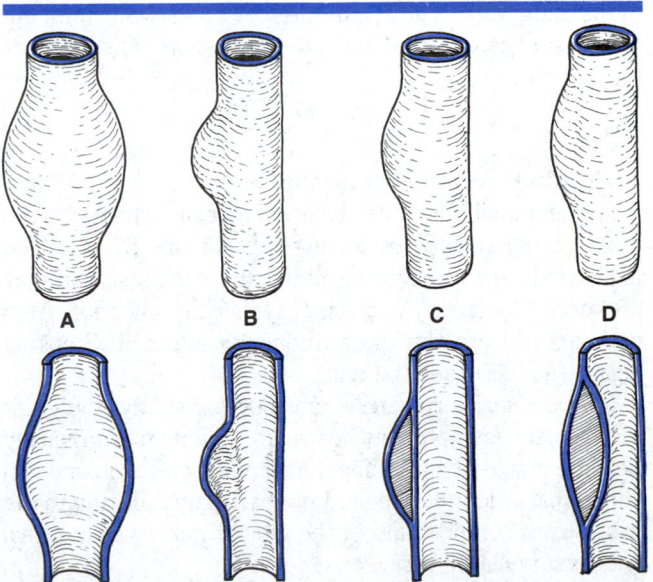

Figure 27–3

Types of aortic aneurysms. **A.** Fusiform: a spindle-shaped expansion of the entire circumference of the artery. **B.** Saccular: an outpouching involving one side of the artery. **C.** False: a pulsating hematoma, often mistaken for an abdominal aneurysm. **D.** Dissecting: a hemorrhagic separation between the medial and internal arterial layers.

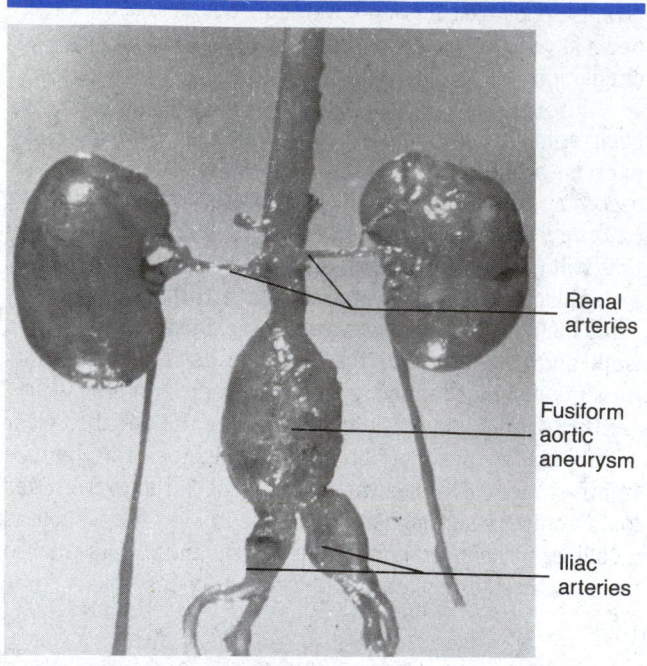

Figure 27-4

Abdominal aortic aneurysm. A fusiform aneurysm of the abdominal aorta beginning just below the renal arteries and involving the iliac arteries. (Courtesy of Millard Fillmore Hospital, Buffalo, NY)

Clinical Manifestations

The specific manifestations are associated with the location of the aneurysm. The symptoms may not develop until the aneurysm has enlarged and exerts pressure on surrounding organs.

Abdominal Aortic Aneurysm

The abdominal aorta just below the renal arteries is the most common site for aneurysms (Figure 27-4). The aneurysms are usually caused by atherosclerosis but may also occur secondary to trauma, syphilis, or infection. Men over age 60 are the most frequently affected. Smoking cigarettes increases the risk.

Abdominal aortic aneurysms develop slowly; the client may remain asymptomatic for years. Clients may gradually become aware of a prominent abdominal pulsation and dull abdominal or low-back pain. Low-back pain radiating to the groin from compression of the lumbar nerves may signal aneurysm enlargement.

Physical findings include an expansile pulsating mass in the midabdomen, usually slightly to the left of midline. Bimanual palpation can aid in identifying the lateral borders of the aneurysm. A systolic bruit is heard with auscultation. Peripheral pulses may be decreased.

Often, abdominal aortic aneurysms are detected on an abdominal x-ray, which demonstrates a curvilinear calcification in the wall of the aneurysm. Ultrasonography can confirm the diagnosis. The size and shape of the aneurysm

and presence of thrombi can be detected on ultrasonography. Aortography also demonstrates the size and shape of the aneurysm as well as the condition of blood vessels proximal and distal to the aneurysm.

When an abdominal aortic aneurysm ruptures, the client experiences persistent severe abdominal and back pain; the pain is sometimes not unlike renal colic. Because the retroperitoneal space contains the rupture, a tamponade effect sometimes occurs, temporarily preventing further hemorrhage. These clients may remain stable for several hours before developing signs of shock such as weakness, tachycardia, and hypotension. Without immediate surgical intervention, these clients will die of exsanguination.

Thoracic Aortic Aneurysm

The thoracic aorta (the section of the descending aorta within the thoracic cavity distal to the origin of the left subclavian artery) is the second most likely location for aortic aneurysms (Zimmerman & Ruplinger, 1983). Thoracic aneurysm (Figure 27-5) is usually caused by atherosclerosis or trauma.

Thoracic aneurysms may cause dysphagia as a result of esophageal compression or hoarseness from pressure on the recurrent laryngeal nerve. The client may also experience dyspnea. A deep aching pain that increases in the supine position is a common symptom.

Physical assessment of the client may reveal dilated superficial veins on the chest, neck, and arms; edema of

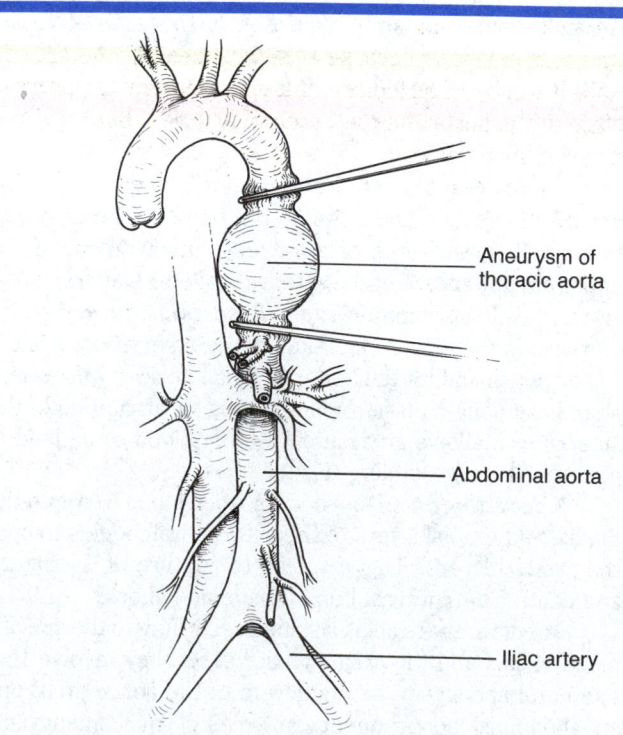

Figure 27-5

Thoracic aortic aneurysm.

the chest wall; cyanosis; aortic murmur; discrepancy in radial pulses; and an abnormal pulsation on the chest wall over the region of the aneurysm. Blood pressure may vary between arms.

A comparison of a current chest x-ray with a previous one can demonstrate widening of the aorta. Aortography can show the location and the size of the aneurysm. An ECG can help distinguish the chest discomfort of thoracic aneurysm from that of myocardial infarction (MI).

Dissecting Aortic Aneurysm

Dissecting aortic aneurysm, which is caused by degenerative disease of the aortic tunica media and intima, is not a true aneurysm. The more appropriate term is *dissecting hematoma* because of the hemorrhagic separation of the arterial layers (Figure 27–6).

Causes include hypertension and Marfan's syndrome. Dissecting aneurysms can also be iatrogenic (eg, from arterial lines or intra-aortic balloon insertion) (Zimmerman & Ruplinger, 1983).

Clients with dissecting aortic aneurysm experience an abrupt onset of excruciating pain that almost immediately reaches a peak of intensity—very different from the gradually increasing intensity of an MI. Pain can be felt in both the anterior and posterior chest. The pain has a tendency to migrate as the dissection progresses.

The client is pale, diaphoretic, and in acute distress. Syncope may occur. There may be associated neurologic defects (ie, weakness, paraplegia). Diagnostic tests include an ECG to distinguish between MI and dissecting aneurysm of the aorta. A chest x-ray may show a widening mediastinum or left pleural effusion from extravasation of blood. An aortogram is the most definitive diagnostic test; it can show the aneurysm's size and location.

Peripheral Arterial Aneurysm

Aneurysms of the femoral and popliteal arteries are usually of the fusiform (Figure 27–7) or saccular types. Fusiform aneurysms are more frequent. They may be singular or multiple segmental lesions. Fusiform lesions can affect one leg or both legs (25% of clients), and may accompany aneurysms of the abdominal aorta. They affect mostly males aged 50 to 70. Hypertension is present in 40% to 50% of clients.

Peripheral aneurysms usually occur secondary to atherosclerosis but also may be caused by trauma, infection, or previous vascular surgery. These aneurysms tend to progress rapidly to embolization and gangrene because of the intermittent compression of the aneurysm by flexion of the knee (Schwartz et al., 1979).

Some clients are asymptomatic. Others notice a vigorous pulse in the popliteal region or upper thigh. The aneurysm rarely enlarges sufficiently to cause local pain and tenderness. Rupture seldom occurs (Schwartz et al., 1979). Venous distention may be seen secondary to compression of adjacent veins.

There may be symptoms of ischemia in the leg or foot due to acute thrombosis in the aneurysmal sac or embol-

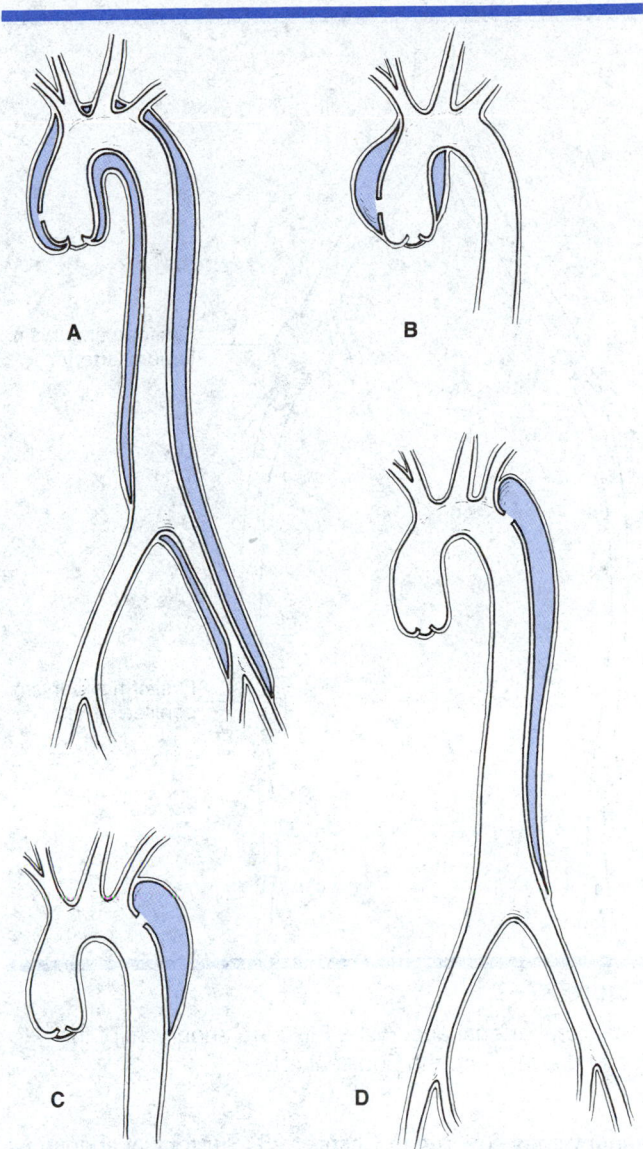

Figure 27–6

Dissecting aortic aneurysm. **A.** Dissecting aneurysm that begins in the ascending aorta near the aortic valve and extends to the external iliac arteries. **B.** Dissecting aneurysm limited to the ascending aorta. **C,D.** Dissecting aneurysms beginning distal to the left subclavian artery. **C** is a localized aneurysm, whereas **D** extends into the abdominal aorta.

ization of a thrombus fragment. After arterial occlusion, there is severe pain, loss of pulse and color, coldness, and eventually, gangrene.

Bilateral palpation reveals a pulsating mass in the region of the inguinal ligament. A firm, nonpulsating mass can be palpated when pooling of blood in the aneurysmal sac causes thrombosis. Ultrasonography and arteriography are helpful in diagnosis.

Therapeutic Measures

The usual treatment of choice for aneurysms is surgery to prevent rupture and thrombosis. Surgery of thoracic aortic

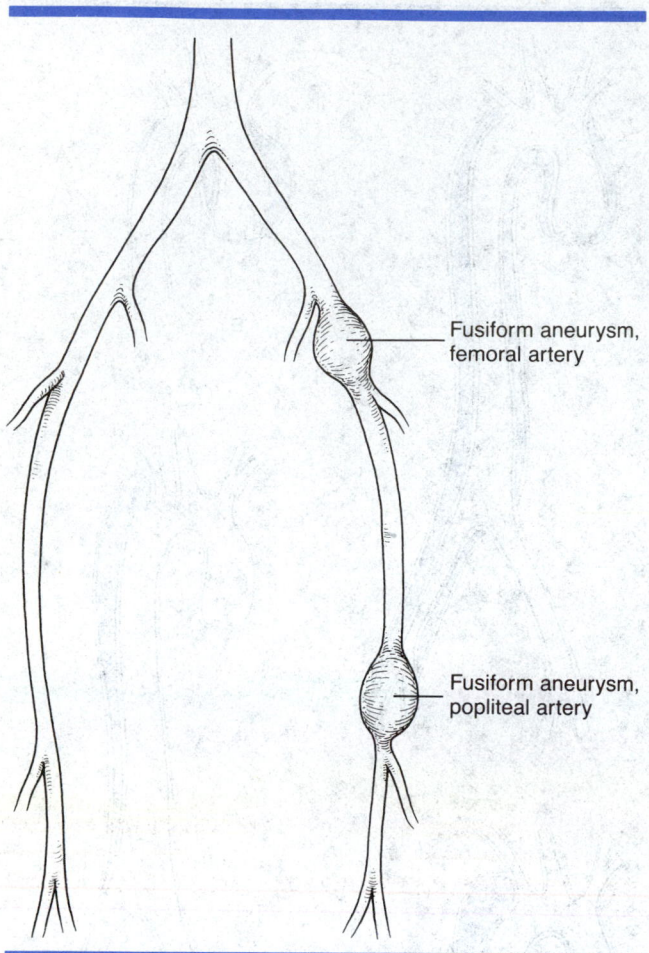

Figure 27–7
Peripheral arterial aneurysm. Fusiform aneurysm of the femoral artery and the popliteal artery.

aneurysm is covered in Chapter 25. Surgery of abdominal aortic aneurysm and femoral popliteal aneurysm is covered in Chapter 30.

Specific Nursing Measures

Nursing management is aimed at providing emotional support and health teaching if surgery is not immediately indicated. Teach the client and family to watch for early symptoms and signs of changes in vascular function, such as alteration or discrepancy in pulses and color changes in the extremities. Also warn the client to avoid Valsalva's maneuver—bearing down during a bowel movement or holding the breath while moving up in bed. The nurse also assists clients to prepare emotionally for surgery.

Make sure that the client and significant others understand the potential complications of an untreated aneurysm. Periodic physical examination and abdominal x-ray or ultrasonography can demonstrate expansion of the aneurysm. Electing to have an expanding aneurysm surgically repaired while the client is in relatively good health is better than having emergency surgery when the aneu-

rysm is leaking or has ruptured. Although the surgery is major and not without risk, morbidity and mortality are considerably lower when aneurysms are surgically repaired under elective rather than emergency conditions.

VARICOSE VEINS

Varicose veins are dilated, tortuous, elongated branches of the greater and lesser saphenous veins. Resulting from incompetent valves (Figure 27–8), they are a major cause of venous insufficiency. Varicose veins are common in persons whose occupations require long periods of standing (eg, waitresses, nurses). Heredity is also a factor.

It is not known whether the valvular incompetence of varicose veins is caused by dilation of the veins or whether the dilation of the valvular ring occurs first and then causes secondary valvular incompetence. During pregnancy, varicosities may appear because of hormonal changes, increased pelvic venous blood flow, or increased intra-abdominal pressure of the enlarged uterus, which prevents good venous return.

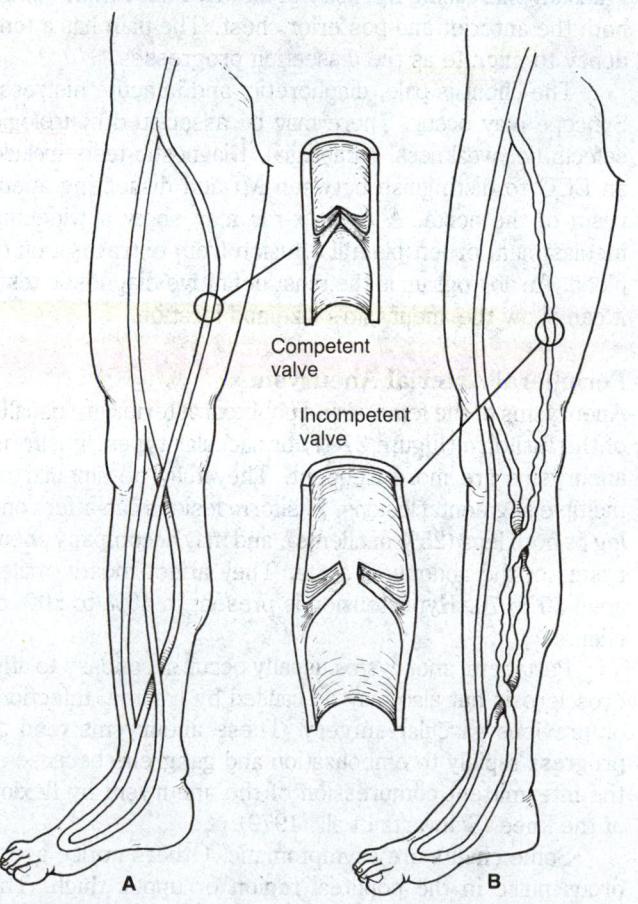

Figure 27–8
A. Competent valves with normal blood flow patterns (arrows). No backflow of blood occurs. **B.** Incompetent valves with backflow of venous blood.

Infections and trauma to the veins with accompanying thrombophlebitis may also lead to varicose veins. Poor posture with sagging abdominal organs, obesity, systemic disease (ie, portal hypertension), and chronic constipation with straining at stool all contribute to venous engorgement in the legs and eventually to varicose vein formation.

Clinical Manifestations

Clients with superficial varicosities are often asymptomatic. Their varicosities are dark, tortuous, raised veins that become more prominent when they stand or cross their legs. Over time, dilation of the veins produces venous stasis with edema and fibrotic changes in fatty tissue and changes in the skin pigmentation.

Symptoms vary from minimal to incapacitating, depending on the location and severity of the varicosities. Nodular protrusions occurring along the veins as a result of sclerosed valves may result in disfigurement of the leg. Clients may report dull aching, heaviness, pain, and muscle cramping as well as a generalized tiredness and discomfort in the legs that tends to increase in hot weather and with prolonged standing.

Therapeutic Measures

Treatment approaches range from conservative medical treatment to surgical intervention for severe varicosities. Medical management is aimed at decreasing the amount of blood pooling in the veins of the lower extremities and decreasing the venous pressure in the superficial veins. Compression of the superficial veins by nylon support hose or elastic bandages decreases the volume of venous pooling.

A client with mild symptomatic varicosities may gain relief of symptoms and edema with nylon support hose and leg elevation. A client with severe venous insufficiency requires regular periods of foot elevation and use of elastic bandages.

Surgical ligation and stripping of the greater or lesser saphenous veins is indicated for clients with recurrent leg ulcers. This surgical procedure and related nursing care are discussed in Chapter 30.

Specific Nursing Measures

Nursing intervention is directed toward client education to decrease intra-abdominal pressure, promote venous return, and maintain skin integrity. Teach the client to avoid sitting or standing for long periods, to keep the legs uncrossed, and to use low chairs that are not too deep so the feet can touch the floor to avoid putting pressure on the popliteal fossae. Tight, restrictive clothing, such as girdles, binders, garters, and elastics, must be avoided. Constipation can be managed with bran, fresh fruits and vegetables, psyllium seed, and exercise. When obesity is a contributing factor, the client should be on a weight-reduction diet.

Support stockings or elastic bandages should be donned before getting out of bed. If this is inconvenient (eg, if the client always showers in the morning), the client should resume the supine position and elevate the legs before applying the stockings. Support stockings and elastic bandages are applied from the toes upward, providing greater support to the lower leg, with a gradual decrease in pressure in the knee, thigh, and groin areas. Venous pooling is increased with constriction at the knee or groin. The ankle should be flexed several times to promote venous return before stockings or elastic bandages are applied. Clients should walk at least once each hour and elevate the legs above heart level four to six times a day or more, depending on symptoms.

Teach the client the importance of preserving skin integrity. The feet should be carefully cleaned with mild soaps, rinsed well, and patted (not rubbed) dry. Moisturizing creams or lotions should be applied to the dry skin of the lower legs and feet. The client should maintain a well-balanced diet that includes vitamins, proteins, and minerals.

VENOUS LEG ULCERS

Venous leg ulcers result from incompetent valves in the perforating veins. Venous ulcers are found in the lower third of the lower leg and are common posterior and superior to the medial and lateral malleoli. These ulcerations are shallow and have a rim of bluish discoloration and erythema. They can penetrate to the level of the deep fascia or tendons but not through them. They may also erode through veins or arteries. Occasionally, the ulcers encircle the leg. Before ulceration, a firm edema is present that decreases slowly and minimally when the client's legs are elevated. A brown pigmentation of the lower leg is observed in a client with long-standing venous insufficiency. It can frequently be found around healed ulcers. This brown pigmentation is secondary to hemosiderin in the subcutaneous tissue, derived from the breakdown of extravasated blood (Schwartz et al., 1979).

Venous leg ulcers may appear spontaneously or following trauma. The underlying problem is venous insufficiency. Postphlebotic syndrome (discussed later in this chapter) and stasis account for most leg ulcers. Ulcerations are more common in clients with deep vein abnormalities and incompetent perforating veins than in clients with varicose veins alone. In venous insufficiency, the tissue of the lower legs has a decreased resistance to infection. Thus, trauma and abrasions may result in ulcer formation.

Clinical Manifestations

Because of high venous pressure, localized varicosities and edema occur, with an increase in deposition of fibrous tissue. With long-standing venous insufficiency, the edema, initially soft and pitting, becomes firmer and may decrease only slowly and minimally upon elevation. The edema then acquires a "woody" feeling, termed **brawny induration** because of increased connective tissue in the subcutaneous tissue (Schwartz et al., 1979). Ulcer formation is preceded by a localized area of redness, tenderness, and brawny induration.

The diabetic client is prone to ulcer formation because of vascular changes that occur in diabetes mellitus. The diabetic's leg ulcers heal slowly, and skin grafting is often required.

Therapeutic Measures

To stimulate ulcer repair and maintain skin integrity around the ulcer, a semirigid boot of paste (eg, Unna's paste) may be applied to the client's ulcerated leg. These boots are used for the ambulatory client to provide stability, support, and protection to the ulcerated area as well as to promote healing. The Unna's paste boot is somewhat inconvenient to apply; an elastic bandage over a layer of foam rubber and a medicated dry gauze may be applied instead. These protective ulcer dressings are left in place for several days but may be changed as necessary, depending on the drainage from the ulcer.

There are different approaches to the pharmacologic management of leg ulcers. Some physicians avoid application of local medications and debriding agents. Others use enzymatic debriding agents such as fibrinolysin or collagenase to clear away necrotic tissue. Debridement provides a clean layer of granulation tissue to serve as a base for optimal healing. Dextranomer (Debrisan), a nonenzymatic agent, is effective for draining wounds. Dextranomer is available as small spherical beads that absorb secretions by exerting a suctionlike force on exudates and tissue particles. The bead layer changes color according to the infecting organism. A grayish yellow color indicates the beads have become saturated and should be completely removed. Irrigation or whirlpool treatments may be nec-

essary to remove residual patches of saturated dextranomer. Beads can be reapplied every 12 hours or more often if necessary.

Topical antibiotics are rarely used. Systemic antibiotics are prescribed according to wound culture and sensitivity results.

Specific Nursing Measures

Nursing intervention is directed toward promoting healing of ulcers, preventing infection, and educating clients to maintain optimal health of the extremities. While engaged in client care, continually reinforce proper ulcer-care technique and make clear the rationale for the care regimen.

Cleanse the extremities with mild soap and warm water and apply moisturizing lotion to the unaffected skin. Using aseptic technique, debride the ulcer as prescribed (ie, irrigate the ulcer with sterile normal saline and/or dilute hydrogen peroxide and use enzymatic debriding agents or dextranomer). Another approach is to use wet-to-dry dressings for debridement of the ulcer. First, apply wet sterile saline dressings. When they are dry, gently remove the dressings, which bring with them devitalized tissue.

Instruct the client and significant others to elevate the client's extremities above heart level for 30 minutes at least every 2 hours. Teach proper application of supportive stockings or bandages. Encourage as much regular exercise as the client can tolerate to stimulate venous return. Encourage a high-protein diet with adequate vitamin C and E to aid in healing and connective-tissue repair. If the client is obese, a weight-loss diet is indicated. The dietitian can help plan a diet to meet the client's particular needs. As in all disorders of the peripheral circulation, clients should eliminate constrictive clothing from their wardrobes, be attentive to proper foot care, avoid trauma, and abstain from smoking.

Section IV: Immunologic Disorders

Immunologic disorders of the peripheral circulation develop as a result of a deficit in the immune system. Polyarteritis and aortic arch syndrome, rare disorders of adulthood suspected to be of immunologic origin, are discussed in this section.

POLYARTERITIS NODOSA

Polyarteritis nodosa is a rare disorder that produces widespread necrotizing segmental inflammation in the medium and small arteries, adjacent veins, and occasionally, the arterioles and venules. Only part of the vessel circumference is affected, often in areas of arterial bifurcation. Capillaries are not involved. Initially, lesions develop in the

tunica media of the artery and then progress into the adventitia and intima. Palpable nodules can occur along the artery. These arterial wall changes result in occlusion, thrombosis, aneurysm formation, ecchymosis, ulceration, and gangrene of the extremities.

Polyarteritis nodosa, though usually a disease of adulthood, can occur at any age. It affects men more than women. The onset of the disease is variable but has been associated with hepatitis B, acute serous otitis media, other upper respiratory tract infections, and drug reactions.

The cause of polyarteritis nodosa is unknown, although evidence suggests an immunologic cause. Research has shown a deposition of immune complexes of foreign antigens and antibodies in the necrotic areas of the arteries.

Clinical Manifestations

The early symptoms of polyarteritis nodosa are weakness, weight loss, anorexia, myalgia, and arthralgia. Progression of the disease brings widespread organ involvement. Renal vascular lesions lead to hypertension, proteinuria, hematuria, and eventually, renal failure. Disease of the mesenteric arteries leads to abdominal pain, nausea, vomiting, diarrhea, and gastrointestinal bleeding. Liver and gallbladder involvement can cause jaundice, ascites, hepatomegaly, hepatic infarction, and cholecystitis. Chest pain, pericarditis, and MI can result from cardiac involvement. Muscle weakness, sensory and motor deficits, headache, and retinal hemorrhages and exudates are additional manifestations of widespread vascular disease.

Diagnosis is based on subjective and objective findings. There is no specific laboratory test for polyarteritis nodosa. Tissue biopsy is necessary for diagnosis.

Therapeutic Measures

The prognosis is poor when multiple organ systems are involved. Treatment is directed mainly at symptoms. Pharmacologic management includes use of corticosteroids, which are most effective during the early course of the disease. Immunosuppressive drugs have been used experimentally and may be considered when other treatment approaches have been exhausted. Antihypertensives, digitalis, and antibiotics are used in selected clients. Death usually results from uremia or hypertension.

Specific Nursing Measures

Nursing care involves support of the client and care of the client's symptoms. Give analgesics and corticosteroids as prescribed to control pain and the inflammatory process. Monitor vital signs, especially blood pressure and temperature. Observe the client for signs of infection such as fever and chills, keeping in mind that steroids can mask infection. Assess the client for subcutaneous nodules, and auscultate the heart and lungs for pulmonary and cardiac changes.

Advise the client to rest when the disease process is active. Position the client with arthralgia or myalgia comfortably to decrease pain. If bedridden, the client should be put through daily range-of-motion (ROM) exercises.

Emotional support for client and family is essential. They must be helped to cope with the disease process and the effects of steroid therapy. One way to decrease anxiety levels is to explain all treatments and drugs consistently. Advise the client to avoid sulfonamides, iodides, and penicillins, all of which may exacerbate polyarteritis. Discuss the side effects of steroid therapy (ie, moon face, hirsutism, buffalo hump, weight gain, acne, masking of infections) with client and family so they may better cope with the treatment. Encourage the client and family to talk about their feelings, and work with them as they deal with their fears and expectations.

AORTIC ARCH SYNDROME

Aortic arch syndrome, also called Takayasu's disease or pulseless disease, is a progressive inflammatory disorder of the aortic arch and its branches. Fibrosis of tissue in the tunica intima leads to thrombus development and aortic arch blockage with loss of pulse in both arms and carotid arteries. The syndrome leads to a diminished blood supply to the upper half of the body with ischemia of the nervous system, hypertension, and heart failure.

Aortic arch syndrome occurs most often in Oriental women in their second or third decades but has occurred in children and in the elderly. It occurs in women nine times as often as in men.

Aortic arch syndrome is thought to be an autoimmune disease because laboratory tests show elevated gamma and alpha globulins and a positive complement fixation. The clinical and serologic information suggest a relation to systemic lupus erythematosus or to rheumatoid disease.

Clinical Manifestations

Before the pulseless stage of the disease, clients may have fever, night sweats, malaise, weight loss, anorexia, arthralgia, anemia, nausea, and vomiting. Physical assessment shows absent or diminished pulse(s) in the neck and/or arm(s) and low blood pressure in one or both arms, depending on the extent of involvement of the subclavian and carotid arteries. Bruits may be auscultated over the affected vessels. Blood pressure is frequently elevated in the lower extremities. Aortic arch syndrome has been called reversed coarctation because it produces the effect of coarctation (ie, symptoms of constriction) in the opposite half of the body.

As the disease progresses, ocular symptoms (ie, blurred vision, retinal defects, cataracts, and blindness) are common. Headache, syncope, and mental confusion also accompany progressive obstruction of the carotid arteries. Subclavian obstruction leads to loss of upper extremity pulses, paresthesia, and arm pain.

Therapeutic Measures

The life expectancy of clients with aortic arch syndrome is 5 to 10 years. Anticoagulants and corticosteroids can improve the prognosis slightly if major organs have not become involved.

Surgical approaches to relieve the symptoms of aortic arch syndrome include bypass grafting and thromboendarterectomy. Although none of these approaches improves life expectancy, treatment may improve the quality of the client's life.

Specific Nursing Measures

Nursing care of the client with aortic arch syndrome mainly involves supportive care. Clients must be helped to understand the disease process in relation to their symptoms. They should know that the disease follows a relentless course, and death usually occurs in 5 to 10 years. Psychological support is important. Encourage the client and significant others to express their fears and concerns. Referral to a psychiatric nurse clinician or other mental health professional may be of great assistance.

Explain all procedures and tests to decrease the client's level of anxiety. For clients on corticosteroids or antico- agulants, provide information about the action, expected therapeutic effect, and potential side effects of the drugs. Warn clients on anticoagulant therapy to avoid using aspirin to decrease the incidence of bleeding. Also explain signs of anticoagulant overdose such as bleeding gums, ecchymoses, hematuria, continuous oozing from small cuts, and excessive menstrual bleeding. Prothrombin times must be carefully monitored in both hospitalized clients and those who return home on anticoagulants. Clients should not abruptly discontinue anticoagulants or corticosteroids. Doses are usually tapered off gradually over a period of weeks or months.

Section V: Infectious Disorders

Infectious disorders of the peripheral circulation include syphilitic aortitis and lymphadenitis. These disorders result from the entrance into the body of microorganisms that are capable of altering or destroying tissue. Some microorganisms cause temporary inflammation, swelling, and tenderness, which resolve after treatment with antibiotics. Other microorganisms alter the tissue permanently and destroy its functional capability as well. Even with antibiotic therapy, the changes are irreversible.

SYPHILITIC AORTITIS

Syphilitic aortitis usually begins before the fifth decade of life. Cardiovascular syphilis develops about a decade after an initial infection of untreated syphilis. Approximately 10% of untreated clients develop cardiovascular complications (Price & Wilson, 1982). Fibrosis of the elastic tissue of the aorta leads to aortitis in the ascending and transverse sections of the aortic arch. Cardiovascular syphilis may be asymptomatic or may cause weakening of the aorta with aneurysm formation. Syphilitic aortitis is caused by the untreated syphilitic infection, in which the spirochetes attack the aorta. Syphilitic aortitis should soon be a disease of the past because of the marked decrease in syphilis in North America.

Clinical Manifestations

Upon exertion, the client may experience substernal pain associated with constriction of the aorta at the orifices of the coronary arteries. Thromboembolism occurs as the aorta becomes dilated and calcium plaques are deposited. The calcium plaques provide a roughened surface for thrombus formation, which can lead to emboli that, in turn, bring on cerebral or myocardial infarction.

An aneurysm may go undetected until the linear calcification along the ascending aorta appears on x-ray. As the aneurysm expands, it may encroach on surrounding organs and cause dyspnea and pain by putting pressure on the trachea and intercostal nerves.

Therapeutic Measures

The overall goal is to treat all persons with syphilis before they develop cardiovascular disease. If primary syphilis is detected, it can be halted, but once the aorta has been affected, care is aimed at treating the client symptomatically.

Penicillin is the drug of choice in the treatment of the client with syphilitic aortitis. Penicillin destroys any active spirochetes *(Treponema pallidum)* and promotes healing. The client should be reminded that already damaged tissue will not heal. If the client is allergic to penicillin, tetracycline or erythromycin may be used.

If an aneurysm is present, the client should avoid strenuous activities (eg, Valsalva's maneuver, heavy lifting, and bending over) that may suddenly increase aortic pressure. The aneurysm may be surgically resected if its location and the client's overall state of health permit.

Specific Nursing Measures

Nursing care of the client with syphilitic aortitis includes education and emotional support. At this stage of syphilitic infection, the client should know that treatment will not restore damaged aortic tissues and that severe scarring is already present. However, it is important to follow through with pharmacological therapy—either penicillin G benzathine or penicillin G procaine—to destroy any active spirochetes.

The client who receives penicillin on an outpatient basis should be aware of the Jarisch–Herxheimer reaction, which can occur within hours of the penicillin injection and subsides within 24 hours. Symptoms include chills, headache, fever, and malaise. This reaction is due to a rapid release of antigenic material after spirochetes are killed by penicillin (Price & Wilson, 1982). All clients must be observed for 30 minutes following a penicillin injection because of the danger of an anaphylactic reaction.

Clients may react to the diagnosis of syphilitic aortitis with a variety of emotions, such as denial, shame, guilt, or anger. Encourage the client and sexual partner to talk

Table 27–1	Causes of Lymph Node Enlargement
Region of Lymphadenopathy*	**Suspected Cause**
Occipital nodes	Ringworm of scalp, seborrheic dermatitis, pediculosis capitis
Posterior auricular nodes	Rubella, infections of the auricle
Anterior auricular nodes	Lesions of the conjunctivae and eyelids, keratoconjunctivitis, ophthalmic herpes zoster
Cervical lymph nodes	Upper respiratory infections, oral or dental infections, mononucleosis, tuberculosis, coccidioidomycosis, lymphoma, leukemia
Supraclavicular lymph nodes**	
Right side	Malignancy of the lungs or esophagus
Left side	Malignancy of the stomach, kidney, ovary, or testis
Axillary lymph nodes	Local infections, metastatic breast cancer
Epitrochlear nodes	Local infections in the area of drainage
Inguinal nodes	Vaginitis, urethritis, urinary tract infections, herpes, syphilis, chancroid, malignancy

*Generalized lymphadenopathy involving three or more lymph node groups often occurs in rubella, rubeola, mononucleosis, scabies, leukemia, Hodgkin's disease, lymphosarcoma, systemic lupus erythematosus, sarcoidosis, dermatomyositis, and amyloidosis.

**Enlargement of the supraclavicular nodes is always considered abnormal.

about their feelings. Support and counseling should be available for the couple as the reality of sexual activity outside of their relationship, even though it happened many years ago, is addressed.

Client education is also aimed at activities of daily living. The client and significant others should understand the importance of protecting the damaged aorta. The risk of aortic rupture or dissection are ever present. Provide guidance in planning the client's daily activities to avoid energetic movements that could stress the damaged aorta. Prophylactic antibiotic therapy is recommended before dental care and any invasive procedures.

LYMPHANGITIS AND LYMPHADENOPATHY

Lymphangitis is an acute or chronic inflammation of the lymphatic vessels generally caused by a streptococcal infection of an extremity. Lymphadenopathy or lymph node enlargement can be generalized or regional. Table 27–1 lists the suspected causes of lymph node enlargement by region and conditions associated with generalized lymphadenopathy.

Clinical Manifestations

Lymphangitis is characterized by red, warm, tender streaks spreading up an arm or leg toward the regional lymph nodes from a focal point of infection. Chills, fever, and generalized malaise usually occur. The regional lymph nodes become enlarged and tender.

Lymph node characteristics in lymphadenopathy, whether regional or general, provide important clues to diagnosis. Nodes may be tender or painless, firm or rock

hard, movable or fixed, discrete or matted together. The location, size, and characteristics of the enlarged nodes should be carefully documented.

Although lymph node enlargement is often clinically significant, some people have a chronically enlarged node that remains palpable after an infection resolves. Such nodes are not usually problematic. Change in the node should be checked by the client's health-care provider, however.

Therapeutic Measures

Therapeutic approaches are aimed at treating the cause. Antibiotics, fluids, rest, warm soaks, and drainage of infected areas are all possible approaches, depending on the cause of the inflamed lymph vessels and lymph nodes.

Specific Nursing Measures

Nursing care for clients with lymphangitis is aimed at promoting drainage of the lymph nodes by elevating the extremity and applying warm moist packs to the inflamed area. Nurses often have opportunities to advise clients with lymph node enlargement in normal daily contact with family, friends, and neighbors. Those with cervical lymph node involvement accompanying a viral upper respiratory infection (URI) do not need to be referred to a care provider unless the URI persists for several weeks. Those currently under treatment for an infection (eg, vaginal) in the region of lymph node enlargement (eg, inguinal) need an explanation of the function of lymph nodes and why they enlarge. All others should be referred to a care provider, because the node enlargement may signal an infection that requires treatment, or the lymphadenopathy could herald a more serious health problem.

Section VI: Obstructive Disorders

Obstructive disorders of the peripheral circulation develop as a result of changes that occlude the normal pathway of circulation. Circulatory occlusion may cause gradual or sudden changes in tissues, resulting in ischemic ulcerations, gangrene, and/or edema. Acute and chronic arterial occlusive disease, thrombophlebitis, chronic venous insufficiency, and lymphedema are discussed in this section.

ACUTE ARTERIAL OCCLUSION

Acute arterial occlusion is a sudden interruption of the blood supply to all or a part of an extremity. The clinical manifestations depend on the location and extent of the occlusion as well as on the availability of collateral circulation. The major causes of acute arterial occlusion are embolism, thrombosis, and injury.

Embolization of a thrombus from the heart is the most frequent cause of an acute arterial occlusion in the upper extremities. These emboli develop as a result of a prosthetic heart valve, atrial fibrillation, or MI. Emboli are carried from the left side of the heart through the circulatory system until they reach an artery too small to allow passage. Arterial thrombus formation also occurs in an atherosclerotic vessel where there is a rough surface. Emboli break off from the thrombus formation and lodge in the arterial system. In the lower extremities, over half of the emboli lodge in the superficial femoral or popliteal artery.

Clinical Manifestations

Severe pain and loss of both motor and sensory function are the symptoms of acute arterial embolism. If acute arterial occlusion involves a critical segment of the arterial tree where there is poor collateral circulation, the initial complaint is pain in the most distal part of the limb, which is then quickly followed by pallor, coldness, and a sensation of numbness. In the first hour, cutaneous sensation is lost. After 6 hours, ischemic muscular contractures, focal gangrene, and subcutaneous hemorrhage develop. Table 27–2 lists clinical manifestations for obstructions in different arterial systems.

When the artery is not completely blocked and allows sufficient blood flow to prevent tissue death, there may be only loss of pulses distal to the occlusion, decreased skin temperature, decreased systolic pressure in the distal portion of the limb, and ischemic pain at rest. Active or passive ROM of the limb increases the pain. If there is adequate collateral circulation, the client may experience only numbness or weakness of the limb.

Table 27–2 Sites of Occlusion in the Arterial System	
Site of Occlusion	**Clinical Manifestations**
Carotid arterial system (including the external and internal carotids)	Neurologic dysfunctions (ie, transient ischemic attacks, or TIAs) that occur because of reduced cerebral circulation, which also produces sensory or motor dysfunction; transient monocular blindness; transient hemiparesis, aphasia, dysarthria; decreased mental ability; confusion and headache; possible bruit over the carotids; manifestations may last for a few seconds or 5 to 10 min and may be present for up to 12 h; 20% of clients with TIAs suffer a stroke (Petersdorf et al., 1983)
Innominate (brachiocephalic) artery	TIAs of brain stem and cerebellum (visual disturbances, vertigo, falling down without loss of consciousness, and dysarthria); claudication of the right arm and a bruit over the right neck
Subclavian artery	TIAs with visual disturbances, vertigo, falling down without loss of consciousness, and dysarthria; arm claudication after exercise, with potential gangrene of the fingers
Mesenteric artery (including the superior mesenteric artery, which is most often affected, the celiac axis, and inferior mesenteric)	Sudden acute abdominal pain, nausea, and vomiting; bowel ischemia, necrosis, and gangrene because of a possible infarct; leukocytosis and shock
Aortic bifurcation (saddle occlusion), considered a medical emergency	Muscle weakness, numbness, paresthesia and paralysis; ischemic signs of sudden pain, cool pale legs, and absent or diminished pulses
Iliac artery (Leriche's syndrome)	Claudication of buttocks and legs (relieved by rest), diminished or absent leg pulses, bruit over the femoral arteries, and impotence; atrophy of the lower extremities is a late manifestation
Femoral and popliteal artery	Intermittent claudication of the legs, ischemic pain, leg coolness and pallor; potential gangrene

Therapeutic Measures

Remember that acute arterial occlusion is a life-threatening medical emergency. If the embolus or thrombus blocks off a major artery, immediate embolectomy is performed under local anesthesia (see Chapter 30). Intravenous heparin therapy is instituted immediately to reduce emboli formation and expansion. Analgesics are administered for relief of pain. Morphine sulfate may be used not only for its analgesic effect but also for decreasing the client's anxiety level.

Thrombolytic agents such as streptokinase or urokinase may be given IV for lysis of intravascular deposits of fibrin. The danger of hemorrhage is increased when thrombolytic agents are given concurrently with an anticoagulant. Aspirin and indomethacin therapy should also be avoided during thrombolytic treatment because of the potential for bleeding.

Specific Nursing Measures

Nursing care of clients with an acute arterial occlusion involves monitoring vital signs and frequently assessing the extremities. The client should be on bed rest in a warm room. The involved extremity should be protected from injury (eg, from hard surfaces and tight or heavy bed covers) by a bed cradle. The extremity should be kept level or just slightly dependent. Analgesics should be administered as necessary (as ordered) to improve client comfort. Sedatives may be given concurrently, if needed.

On admission the client may be prepared for emergency surgery. The client should understand that immediate surgery is necessary to preserve viability of the extremity. Both client and significant others will be anxious and fearful. Pain can alter the client's ability to think clearly and respond calmly to the situation. Be sensitive to the fears and frustrations of both client and significant others, explaining all treatments and medications clearly, while completing surgical preparations in a timely and sensitive manner. Continuous assessment for bleeding is important when anticoagulants or thrombolytic agents are used.

ARTERIOSCLEROSIS OBLITERANS

Arteriosclerosis obliterans is a chronic arterial occlusive disease of the extremities. It can involve the aorta, the common iliac artery, the superficial femoral artery (Figure 27–9), the posterior tibial artery at the ankle, and the anterior tibial artery at its origin. The lesions are segmental and localized, often obstructing one section of the artery and leaving other sections uninvolved.

Arteriosclerosis obliterans is most often seen in older men. Clients with diabetes mellitus develop the disease at an earlier age and have greater involvement of the lower leg.

Clinical Manifestations

Clinical manifestations occur because progressive arterial obstruction prevents oxygen and nutrients from being supplied to the tissues. Pain is the most common symptom—both intermittent claudication and rest pain. There may be numbness and tingling of the digits and coldness in the digits or feet on exposure to cold. Tissue necrosis and/or gangrene in the terminal digit can occur.

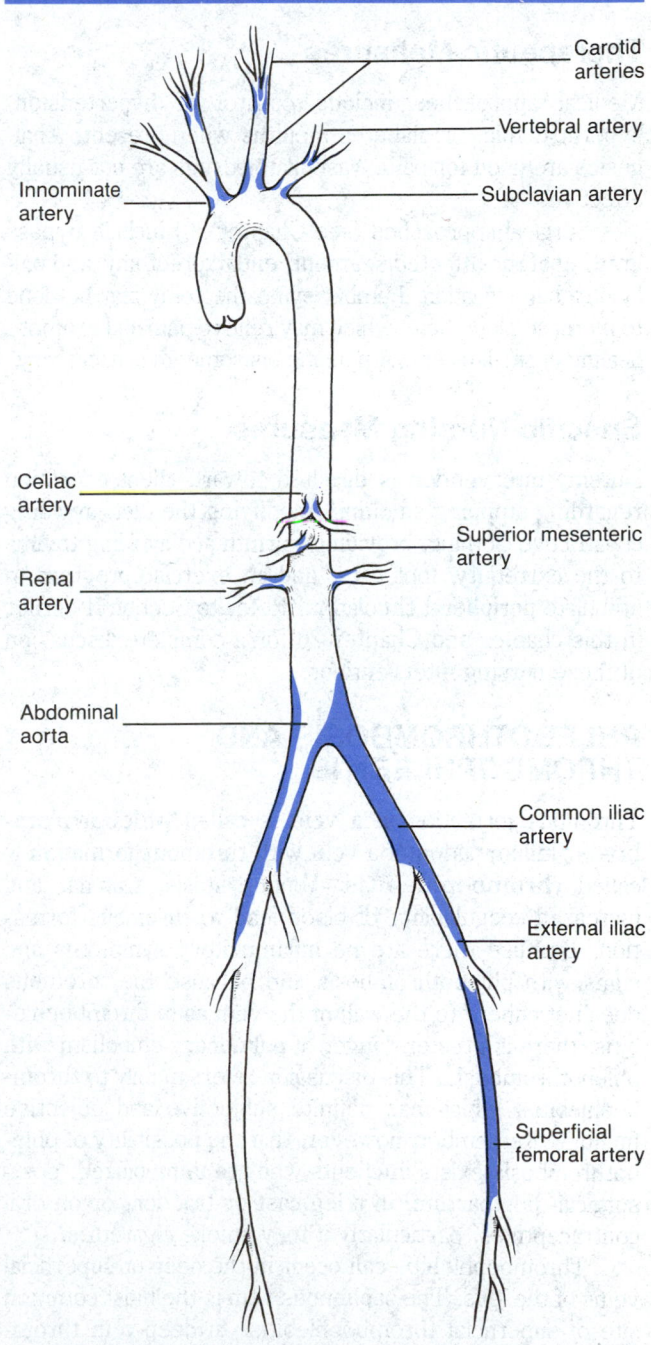

Figure 27–9

Arteriosclerosis obliterans. Typical locations and extent of occlusion in this chronic arterial occlusive disease.

Other manifestations include thin, pale, shiny, taunt skin with loss of hair on the lower part of the legs. In severe cases, cyanosis, dependent rubor, and edema of the feet and legs can occur.

Leriche's syndrome (caused by slowly progressive atherosclerotic occlusion of the terminal aorta and the iliac vessels) has a characteristic cluster of manifestations, which depend on the location and extent of the plaque formation. Intermittent claudication in the lower back, buttocks, thigh, calf, or foot occurs with exercise and is relieved by rest. Impotence, muscle atrophy, and leg weakness also occur.

Therapeutic Measures

Medical approaches include control of hypertension, hyperlipidemia, or diabetes mellitus when present. Analgesics are used for pain. Vasodilator drugs are not usually effective.

Surgical approaches (see Chapter 30) include bypass grafting of the affected segment, endarterectomy, and balloon catheter dilation. Lumbar sympathectomy may be done to increase blood flow, which may relieve pain and promote healing of small ulcers. Amputation is sometimes necessary.

Specific Nursing Measures

Nursing intervention is directed toward client education regarding stopping smoking, modifying the diet, avoiding constrictive clothing, providing warmth and avoiding trauma to the extremity, foot care, and an exercise program to stimulate peripheral circulation. Refer to Section II earlier in this chapter and Chapter 26 for a complete discussion of these nursing interventions.

PHLEBOTHROMBOSIS AND THROMBOPHLEBITIS

Thrombus formation in a vein is called **phlebothrombosis.** Inflammation of a vein with thrombus formation is called **thrombophlebitis.** Venous stasis, trauma, and increased coagulability of blood lead to thrombus formation. Because there are no inflammatory symptoms and signs with phlebothrombosis and because the thrombus does not adhere to the wall of the vein as in thrombophlebitis, there is greater danger of pulmonary embolism with phlebothrombosis. This discussion refers mainly to thrombophlebitis, which has definite subjective and objective findings. Remember, however, that the possibility of phlebothrombosis exists in clients who are immobilized, postsurgical, postpartum, in a leg cast or traction, or on oral contraceptives, particularly if they smoke cigarettes.

Thrombophlebitis can occur in the deep or superficial veins of the legs. The saphenous vein is the most common site of superficial thrombophlebitis. In deep-vein thrombophlebitis (DVT), the iliofemoral vein, popliteal segments, or small veins of the calf are most often involved. DVT can also cause distention of the superficial veins because of the backflow of blood through communicating veins.

Clinical Manifestations

In both deep-vein and superficial-vein thrombophlebitis, clinical manifestations vary with the site and length of the disease process. With inflammation of the endothelial lining of the vein, redness, swelling, and increased warmth occur along the path of the vein. Temperature may also be elevated.

As the thrombus enlarges causing greater reduction in blood flow, there is pain, dependent cyanosis, a positive Homans' sign, and an increase in the circumference of the extremity. The client may experience muscle cramping.

Inflamed superficial veins feel like firm cords when palpated. Palpation may elicit tenderness over the involved segment. Frequent, deep palpation must be avoided because of the possibility of dislodging a thrombus. Pulmonary embolism is not a danger with superficial thrombophlebitis but is a definite concern with DVT.

Diagnosis of thrombophlebitis is aided by noninvasive tests such as Doppler ultrasonography and impedance plethysmography. The ^{125}I-labeled fibrinogen test may help in detecting the thrombus. Contrast venography may also be done. See Chapter 26 for a description of these tests.

Therapeutic Measures

Anti-inflammatory agents such as ibuprofen or indomethacin are usually prescribed for superficial thrombophlebitis. Anticoagulants are seldom used. Anticoagulants are indicated if the thrombosis progresses proximally or if the

---

Nursing Research Note

Vanbree N, Hollerbach A, Brook G: Clinical evaluation of three techniques for administering low-dose heparin. *Nurs Res* 1984; 3(1):15–19.

The effect of methods of administering low-dose heparin on the incidence of postinjection abdominal bruising was investigated. Three techniques were compared. All three methods were the same in site, preinjection skin preparation, skin holding, drug dose and packaging, angle of needle insertion, needle withdrawal, and postinjection skin preparation. Differences in techniques were: (1) during technique 1, the roll of tissue was released after needle insertion, and the plunger was aspirated; (2) in technique 2, the roll of tissue was not released, and the plunger was not aspirated; (3) in technique 3, the tissue roll also was not released, and the plunger was not aspirated, but 0.2 mL of air was injected after injection.

There was no significant reduction in incidence of abdominal bruising regardless of the technique used. Women 60 years and older had the most numerous and largest bruises compared with other subjects.

Nurses must continue to investigate different approaches to low-dose heparin therapy that may reduce bruising. Care must be taken with current technique to minimize tissue trauma. Because older women are at highest risk for bruises, nurses must take extra care in technique.

involved segment of the superficial thrombosis is near the deep venous system at the groin.

For DVT, intravenous heparin is the treatment of choice. The partial thromboplastin time (PTT) should be maintained at about two times the control time. Oral anticoagulation with warfarin sodium is prescribed for 4 to 6 weeks after the acute stage of DVT in uncomplicated clients. Oral anticoagulation may be extended when the popliteal, femoral, or iliac vessels are involved. The prothrombin time (PT) of clients on warfarin sodium must be carefully monitored and kept at about twice the control time.

Intravenous thrombolytic (fibrinolytic) therapy with streptokinase may be helpful in dissolving the clot, preventing damage to the valves of the vein, and preventing development of chronic venous insufficiency and postphlebitic syndrome. Bleeding is a danger with streptokinase treatment, especially if the client is also on anticoagulants.

Specific Nursing Measures

Clients with superficial thrombophlebitis are usually cared for at home. They or their significant others must be taught to elevate the affected limb for 15 minutes every 3 to 4 hours, to apply moist heat, and to use anti-inflammatory agents. Clients should wear support stockings during ambulation.

The client with DVT should be on complete bed rest for at least 7 days, with the affected limb elevated above heart level. Elastic bandages or stockings are applied from the toes up with even support along the entire leg (Figure 27–10). They should be removed daily for inspection and gentle cleansing of the skin. When pillows are used for leg elevation, they should support the entire length of the leg to prevent compression of the popliteal space. Continuous applications of moist heat will reduce the inflammation and decrease pain. The client should do exercises in bed by pressing the foot against a footboard. The unaffected leg should be exercised more actively.

Measure and record the circumference of the extremity daily and compare with the initial measurement. Make an identifying mark on the extremity to ensure that each nurse measures in the same place. Monitor the PTT in clients on heparin therapy and the PT in clients on warfarin sodium.

Observe the client for any signs of bleeding—hematuria; bleeding gums; dark, tarry stools; coffee ground emesis. Be alert to symptoms and signs of pulmonary embolism—restlessness, sudden pleuritic pain and dyspnea, hypotension, tachycardia, and hemoptysis.

Home care of clients with DVT involves instructing them about periodic leg elevation, use of support hose at all times when ambulatory, and frequent walking, which aids in emptying the leg veins. Clients should not sit or stand for long periods. Instruct clients who return home on warfarin sodium to have a weekly PT to monitor the level of anticoagulation. Clients on anticoagulants should not take any other medication without first checking with

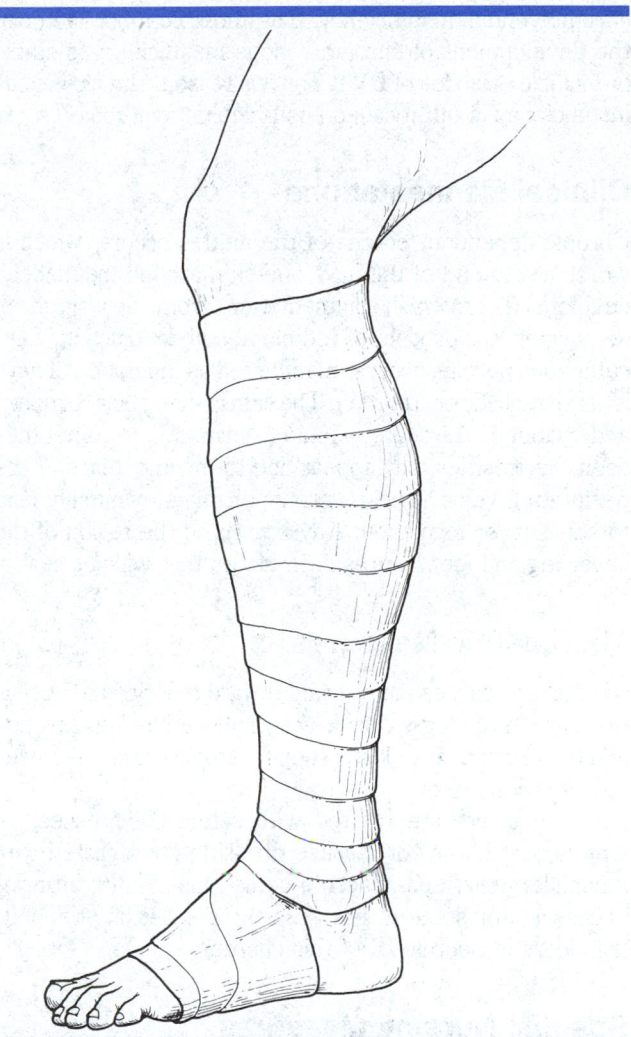

Figure 27–10
Elastic bandages applied from the toes up with even support along the entire leg.

their physician or pharmacist. Aspirin and nonsteroidal anti-inflammatory drugs such as indomethacin must be avoided because they increase anticoagulant activity that could lead to bleeding.

Assisting clients to prevent future episodes of thrombophlebitis is a major nursing responsibility. Periodic leg elevation above heart level, elastic stockings, walking, not crossing the legs, and avoiding periods of prolonged sitting or standing are beneficial approaches. Obesity and constipation, which increase intra-abdominal pressure and promote venous stasis, should be avoided. Instruct clients about weight loss and high-fiber diets as appropriate. Adequate hydration will prevent concentration of blood. Clients should never take ergotamine preparations or oral contraceptives. They also should not smoke.

CHRONIC VENOUS INSUFFICIENCY

Destruction of the venous valves, which leaves the deep veins of the legs functionally inadequate, is the cause of chronic venous insufficiency. The most common factor in the development of chronic venous insufficiency is single or multiple episodes of DVT. For this reason, chronic venous insufficiency is often called postphlebitic syndrome.

Clinical Manifestations

Chronic dependent edema of the ankles occurs, which is worse at the end of the day. The skin around the malleoli develops a brownish pigmentation from deposition of hemosiderin, a product of red blood cell destruction. Subcutaneous fibrosis occurs, manifested as induration. There is also lymphatic obstruction. The skin is thin, shiny, atrophic, and cyanotic. An acute weeping dermatitis is sometimes seen. Varicosities may appear due to incompetence of the perforating veins. These chronic changes eventually lead to stasis ulcer formation. Any trauma to the region of the lower leg and foot can result in ulcers that will not heal.

Therapeutic Measures

Medical approaches are directed toward reducing the venous pressure in the legs. This is accomplished by leg elevation and the use of heavy elastic support stockings or pneumatic compression boots.

Leg ulcers are treated with saline compresses, an Unna's paste boot, or a gauze dressing impregnated with a nonallergenic, self-adhering compound. Skin grafting is necessary for some ulcers. See the discussion of venous leg ulcers in Section III of this chapter.

Specific Nursing Measures

Instruct the client to keep the legs elevated above heart level at night. The legs should also be elevated intermittently during the day. Close-fitting, heavy-duty elastic support stockings are essential. Clients must understand that failure to wear the stockings will contribute to increasing edema and ulceration, which markedly interfere with ambulation and quality of life. Also refer to nursing responsibilities discussed under preventing future episodes of thrombophlebitis.

LYMPHEDEMA

Lymphedema is swelling of a part of the body as a result of insufficient lymph drainage. There is stasis of lymph with resultant chronic swelling, which can vary from mild to severe. The severity of the edema is directly related to the degree of obstruction and protein concentration in the interstitial spaces.

Lymphedema is caused by interference with the flow of lymph from an extremity. It can result from trauma, infection, allergy, malignancy, or the congenital absence of a developed lymphatic system.

When the normal outflow of lymphatic fluid is obstructed, the pressure in the lymphatic vessels builds up as the lymph begins to flow backward. Valves become incompetent, and protein accumulates in the interstitial spaces. This protein begins to draw or retain fluid that would normally be reabsorbed by the bloodstream.

Clinical Manifestations

The swelling in lymphedema is initially manifested as a soft edema, which then progresses and becomes harder, due to fibrosis. In later stages, skin becomes thick and brown.

Therapeutic Measures

There is no cure for lymphedema. Measures used to control the manifestations of the disease include application of a pneumatic cufflike apparatus and regular light massage to the affected limb to enhance lymph drainage. Elastic support stockings are prescribed to help drain the legs and for cosmetic reasons.

Thiazide diuretics are sometimes prescribed to prevent fluid retention. Antibiotics may be used if there is any evidence of infection.

Specific Nursing Measures

Weigh the client twice a week and measure the circumference of the extremity. Seeing whether fluid retention is increasing, decreasing, or stabilizing allows for evaluation of therapy. The involved extremity should be examined (ie, pulses, skin color, and temperature) daily. Teach the client to observe for changes in the extremity and to notify the physician if there is an increase in limb size; an absence in pulse; or a change in skin color, temperature, or texture.

Another nursing objective is to increase client comfort and promote lymph return. Elevation of the affected limb or limbs during sleep and several times during the day should be emphasized. The foot of the bed can be raised on a chair or blocks. Teach the client the hazards of a prolonged dependent limb position.

Demonstrate the correct method of massaging the extremity to client and significant others. The extremity should be massaged gently, using lotions, from the most distal point to the lymph nodes that drain the area (ie, from toes upward to the inguinal nodes).

The client should be correctly measured for elastic support hose and taught the proper way to don these stockings. Also, the correct procedure for application and use of the pneumatic cuffs should be taught. A number of pneumatic pumping devices is available for intermittent compression of the extremity. The pressure used is 30 mm Hg for the deeper lymphatic vessels and 20 mm Hg for the more peripheral lymphatic vessels. Pneumatic pumping therapy is evaluated by measuring the extremity before and after therapy.

Nutritional management includes instruction about sodium restriction to decrease fluid retention. The client may also be on diuretic therapy and should maintain an adequate potassium intake to counterbalance the potassium loss caused by diuretics. A well-balanced weight-reduction diet is appropriate for clients who are obese because elevated intra-abdominal pressure interferes with lymph return.

Emphasize meticulous hygiene to the skin and nails of the involved extremities and avoidance of trauma (eg, cuts and burns) that can lead to infection. The client should also understand the importance of regular medical examinations.

The physician should order a regular exercise program that can be implemented by the nurse. If an exercise program is not suggested, the nurse should ask the physician about the possibility of instituting one.

The nurse must be able to provide emotional support to the client who feels disfigured or who feels rejected because of an unshapely extremity. The client needs to be able to express feelings of exasperation and anger because of the body change and its effect on relationships and lifestyle. Withdrawal and depression can occur. The client's active involvement in making decisions about care can foster greater independence and control over the disease process and its management. The nurse must listen, encourage, and aid both the client and significant others in learning to cope effectively with this chronic disease.

Section VII: Traumatic Disorders

The aorta and peripheral arteries can suffer penetrating and nonpenetrating traumatic injuries. A penetrating injury is the sort produced by a knife or bullet. Nonpenetrating injuries result from physical force delivered to the external body, as in a hammer blow to a thumb or a sudden slam against the dashboard or windshield in an automobile accident.

Traumatic injuries to blood vessels are frequently complicated by fractures that can obstruct or compress the vessel. Blunt injuries to extremities can cause contusions of vessels with resultant thrombosis.

PENETRATING AND NONPENETRATING WOUNDS OF THE AORTA

Penetrating wounds of the aorta and/or vena cava are a common cause of death from hemorrhage with chest injuries. These penetrating injuries usually result from stabbing or missile penetration.

Nonpenetrating injury of the aorta, which occurs following blunt trauma, is important to recognize because surgery can most often save these clients. The great majority usually die quickly from exsanguination, but 15% to 20% survive the initial insult. Rupture can be delayed, with some clients forming aneurysms several months or years after the traumatic injury.

Rupture from blunt trauma is usually an indirect result of acceleration–deceleration forces generated in automobile accidents, vehicle–pedestrian accidents, aircraft accidents, and falls from great heights, but it occasionally results directly from a hard blow to the chest. In 70% to 75% of clients, laceration occurs just distal to the left subclavian artery (Schwartz et al., 1979); the descending thoracic aorta and the aortic arch decelerate at different rates because of differences in anatomic structure and produce a transverse tear in the aorta. The tear (Figure 27–11), can involve one or all of the layers of the aorta and part or all of the circumference of the aortic wall. Immediate fatal hemorrhage is prevented in some clients because the tunica adventitia is not torn.

Clients who survive longer than 2 months after injury usually develop a false aneurysm of the aorta and then proceed through an uneventful course. They may remain asymptomatic for many years until massive enlargement occurs. Calcification develops at different times during development of the aneurysm, and the first clue of aneurysm formation is often seen on x-rays of the chest.

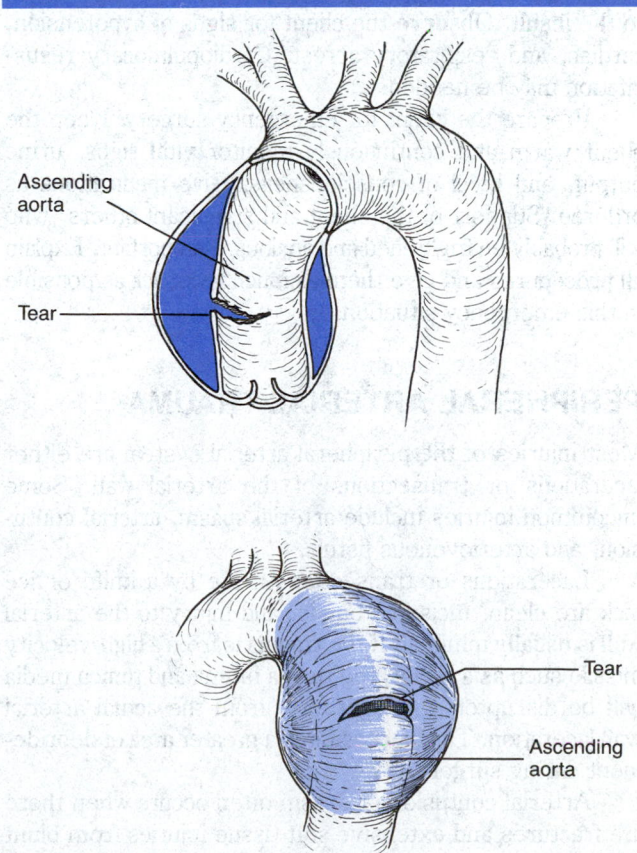

Figure 27–11

Aortic tear in blunt trauma.

Clinical Manifestations

Clients who survive a penetrating injury are first seen with symptoms and signs of massive intrathoracic bleeding and severe shock. Later, however, an aneurysm may be discovered when a chest x-ray is done. If the aneurysm begins to expand, the symptoms and signs are those of the organs it compresses.

Therapeutic Measures

With penetrating injuries, the treatment is immediate thoracotomy and reanastomosis of the aorta. An arterial prosthesis may be necessary. Care of the client with aortic surgery is described in Chapter 25.

Therapeutic approaches to nonpenetrating wounds of the aorta include resection and graft replacement of the traumatized area. Many physicians advocate resection of all trauma-induced aneurysms. If the aneurysm is leaking, a chest x-ray shows widening of the mediastinal area.

Specific Nursing Measures

Nursing care of the client with a penetrating wound or suspected blunt wound of the aorta includes assessment of the client's circulatory status and the body's response to the insult. Observe the client for signs of hypotension, cardiac, and respiratory arrest. Cardiopulmonary resuscitation may be needed.

Prepare the client for emergency surgery. Keep the client warm and continuously monitor vital signs, urine output, and level of consciousness. Give medications as ordered. Support of the client and significant others, who will probably be frightened and anxious, is important. Explain all procedures and give them as much feedback as possible in this emergency situation.

PERIPHERAL ARTERIAL TRAUMA

Most injuries of the peripheral arterial system are either lacerations or transections of the arterial wall. Some uncommon injuries include arterial spasm, arterial contusion, and arteriovenous fistula.

Lacerations or transections made by a knife or ice pick are clean, incised wounds, and injury to the arterial wall is usually minimal. If the trauma is from a high-velocity missile such as a bullet, the tunica intima and tunica media will be disrupted some distance from the actual arterial wall laceration. This necessitates a greater area of debridement during surgery.

Arterial contusion or spasm often occurs when there are fractures and extensive soft tissue injuries from blunt trauma (Figure 27–12). Multiple injuries often obscure the arterial injury. Arterial spasm occurs most frequently in response to a brachial artery injury accompanying a fractured humerus.

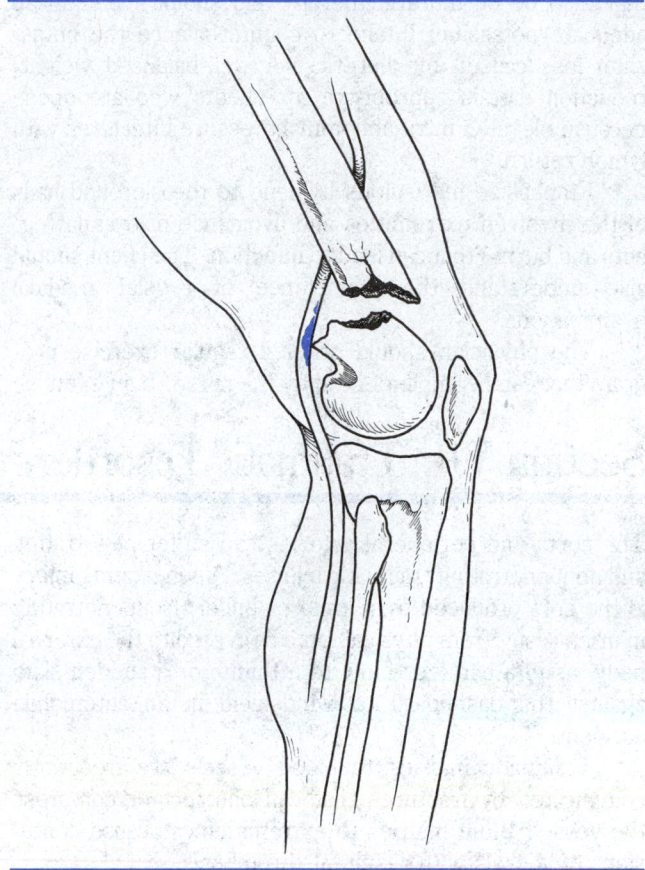

Figure 27–12

Arterial contusion accompanying a fracture.

Arterial contusion from a blunt injury is characterized by multiple areas of breakage in the arterial wall with intramural hemorrhage. The tunica intima becomes separated and prolapses into the lumen, obstructing arterial flow. The typical bumper injury (Figure 27–13) produces contusion of the popliteal artery.

Most arterial injuries result from penetrating wounds that partially or completely disrupt the arterial wall. Nonpenetrating injuries are not as common but carry a serious prognosis, partially because of possible crushing injury to the arterial wall and because of the potential delay in diagnosis (Schwartz et al., 1979).

Clinical Manifestations

Loss of blood predisposes 50% of clients to shock. Hemorrhaging results from the arterial injury itself or from associated body injuries. With profound shock, severe peripheral vasoconstriction may conceal the arterial injury.

In blunt trauma, there is usually multiple organ injury. If an extremity suffers either blunt injury or penetrating wounds, fractures and nerve trauma often occur. When femoral artery injury is associated with a fractured femur,

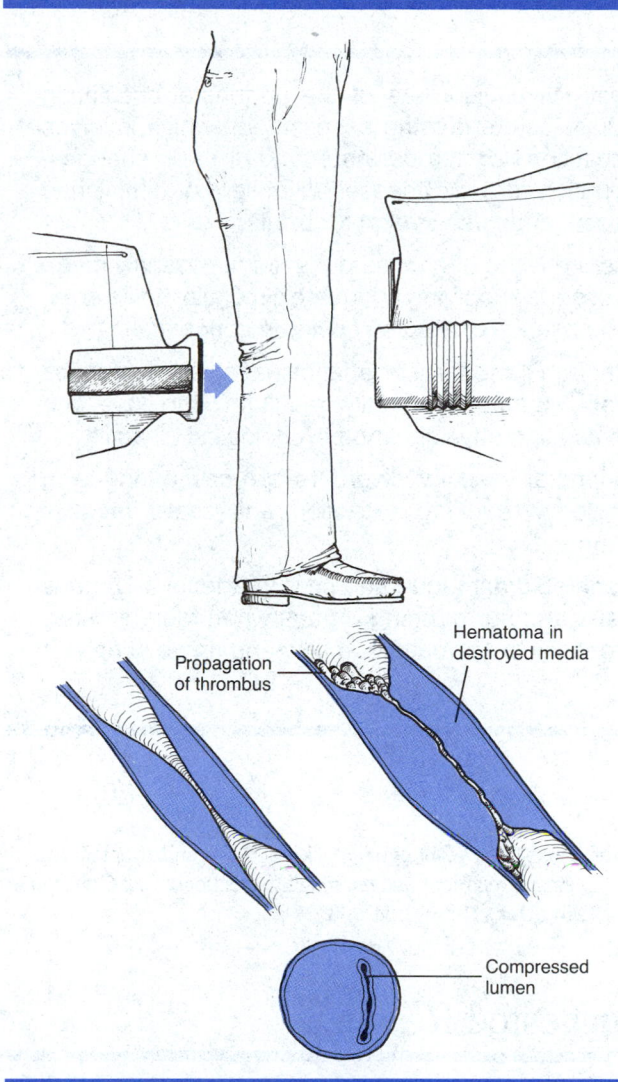

Figure 27–13

Popliteal artery damage from blunt injury (bumper of a car compressing artery).

the incidence of gangrene is high (Schwartz et al., 1979).

In the extremity, arterial injury often produces four abnormal findings. They are best remembered as the "4 Ps"—paralysis, paresthesia, loss of pulses, and pallor. Of these, paralysis and paresthesia are the most important clinical manifestations because loss of neurological function indicates tissue ischemia, which slowly progresses to gangrene unless the arterial blood flow is improved. Absence of pulse in one extremity and a normal pulse in the opposite extremity indicate arterial injury. (Keep in mind that there could also be a congenital absence of a pedal pulse. This possibility reinforces the importance of documenting pulses on a routine physical exam.) The presence of a peripheral pulse does not exclude the possibility of arterial injury. A lacerated arterial wall could be sealed with a blood clot, and arterial blood could still flow.

Bright red pulsatile bleeding, even in small quantities, is highly suggestive of arterial injury. On the other hand, bleeding may be totally absent, but a tense hematoma (from extravasation of blood into the fascia) may be palpated around the wound. A systolic bruit may also be audible over the traumatized artery.

Remember that arterial injury may be present if there is a penetrating wound near a major artery. Unrecognized secondary hemorrhage, a false aneurysm, or an arteriovenous fistula may develop.

Therapeutic Measures

The most urgent problem is control of bleeding, which is accomplished by tightly packing the wound with gauze and then applying a pressure dressing. Tourniquets increase the risk of permanent injury to a peripheral nerve and should be avoided. Because of shock, rapid infusion of fluid is instituted until the systolic blood pressure rises to 80 mm Hg. After this, additional fluids may be given gradually. A total of 1000 to 2000 mL of fluid is necessary. Whole blood or volume expansion with Ringer's lactate solution, dextran, or plasma is also used (Schwartz et al., 1979). Tetanous toxoid is given prophylactically, and antibiotics are often started.

Specific Nursing Measures

Nursing care of the client with peripheral arterial trauma is aimed at evaluation of the extremity according to the "4 Ps." Assess the extremity for paralysis and paresthesia: loss of neurological function suggests tissue ischemia. Without surgical intervention, gangrene will develop. Carefully assess the pulses. Pulse assessment must be continuous because a pulse may be present even though there is arterial injury. Palpate the extremity for a hematoma formation, which may be a manifestation of extravasation of blood into the fascia. Be alert for bright red bleeding and aid in controlling the bleeding by applying a pressure dressing.

Assessment of all vital signs is important in detecting any changes in systemic status. The client may be ashen or pale and shiver due to peripheral vasoconstriction. If there is marked blood loss, the client's level of consciousness may be altered. The client may be anxious, irritable, confused, or comatose. As shock progresses, heart rate and rhythm vary. Initially, tachycardia occurs, followed by bradycardia as shock progresses.

Hypotension will be seen if 25% of the blood volume has been lost from the vascular tree. A reflex hypertensive state may be noted in shock. This is due to sympathetic and adrenal stimulation.

Preparation of the client for surgery involves insertion of an intravenous infusion and, in hypotensive states, volume expansion. A pulmonary artery catheter or central venous pressure line may be inserted before surgery.

Chapter Highlights

Alteration in the anatomy and physiology of the peripheral vascular tree can disrupt vascular flow to a specific area, resulting in limited motion, pain, and/or deformity.

Blood flow may be disrupted by congenital malformations, tumors, infection, obstruction, trauma, or rupture of the vessel.

Emotional stress, inactivity, degenerative changes, infection, and trauma may lead to ischemic changes in the periphery.

The emotional status of a client with peripheral vascular disease may be affected because of loss of independence and self-esteem, changes in body image, and alterations in sexual functioning.

Blood flow to and from the extremities can be aided by client education regarding diet, exercise, wearing apparel, care of the feet, avoidance of cold, and smoking cessation.

Obstructive disorders of the peripheral circulation require astute nursing assessment, which involves inspection for temperature and trophic changes, palpation for hard masses or absent or diminished pulses, and auscultation for bruits.

The presence of a pulse does not necessarily mean a vessel is supplying adequate circulation to an area, and absence of a pulse could be congenital.

Although peripheral arterial disease seldom causes death, it may eventually result in limb loss and devastating physical and psychological disability.

Peripheral vascular disorders can cause long-term problems requiring extended and costly medical treatment.

Irreparable damage can occur to arterial or venous tissue and surrounding organs when there is interference with normal blood flow and nerve supply.

Bibliography

A single syndrome for Raynaud's disease: *Emerg Med* (May) 1982; 14:175–176.

Foley WT et al: *Advances in the Management of Cardiovascular Diseases.* Chicago: Yearbook Medical Publishers, 1982.

Goldberger E: *Textbook of Clinical Cardiology.* St. Louis: Mosby, 1982.

Jackson DS Jr: Varicose veins: Often neglected, eminently treatable. *Female Patient* (July) 1981; 6:46–51.

Malseed R: *Pharmacology: Drug Therapy and Nursing Considerations.* Philadelphia: Lippincott, 1982.

Martin I: Varicose ulcers. 1: Breaking down in vein. *Nurs Mirror* (July) 1981; 153:34–35.

Martin I: Varicose ulcers. 2: Rewarding remedies. *Nurs Mirror* (Aug) 1981; 153:34–35.

Miller DC, Roon AJ: *Diagnosis and Management of Peripheral Vascular Disease.* Menlo Park, CA: Addison–Wesley, 1982.

Petersdorf RG et al: *Harrison's Principles of Internal Medicine,* 10th ed. New York: McGraw–Hill, 1983.

Price SA, Wilson LM: *Pathophysiology: Clinical Concepts of Disease Processes,* 2nd ed. New York: McGraw–Hill, 1982.

Schwartz S et al: *Principles of Surgery.* New York: McGraw–Hill, 1979.

Taylor DL: Thrombophlebitis: Physiology, signs, and symptoms. *Nurs 83* (July) 1983; 13:52–53.

Thompson DA: Teaching the client about anticoagulants. *Am J Nurs* 1982; 82:278–281.

Wyngaarden JB, Smith L: *Cecil Textbook of Medicine,* 16th ed. Philadelphia: Saunders, 1982.

Zimmerman TA, Ruplinger J: Thoraco-abdominal aortic aneurysms: Treatment and nursing interventions. *Crit Care Nurse* (Nov–Dec) 1983; 3:54–63.

Suggested Readings

Baum L: Abdominal aortic aneurysm? *Nurs 82* 1982; 12:34–41. The author uses the SOAP method to assess a client with an abdominal aortic aneurysm. The article discusses mortality and complications, classifies abdominal aortic aneurysms, and describes history taking and laboratory studies.

Craven RE, Curry TD: When the diagnosis is Raynaud's. *Am J Nurs* 1981; 81:1007–1009. The authors discuss the pathophysiology, course, prognosis, and treatment of clients with Raynaud's disease. A section is included on controlling vasospasm.

Fahey VA, Finkelmeier BA: Iatrogenic arterial injuries. *Am J Nurs* 1984; 84:448–451. Types of arterial injuries secondary to procedures involving arterial cannulation are discussed. Prompt evaluation of complications and approaches to management are reviewed.

Raab D: Peripheral vascular disease: How to recognize it, how to treat it. *Can Nurse* 1982; 78:30–33. This article contains information about the etiology, clinical manifestations, and nursing care of clients with arterial vascular disease. It includes a chart that describes the common types of arterial blockage and surgeries for each.

The Client With Varicose Veins

I. Brief Descriptive Data

Mr Eric Osterhaut, a 59-year-old male, comes to the general medical clinic with concerns about aching and tiredness in his legs. He has a history of varicose veins.

II. Personal Data

Date:	July 2, 1986
ID Number:	000-00-0000
Full Name:	Eric Osterhaut
Address:	18 Huxley Rd, Toronto, Ontario, Canada
Telephone:	Home: 000-0000
	Work: 000-0000
Sex:	Male
Marital Status:	Married
Age:	59
Birthdate:	4-14-27
Religion:	Catholic
Race/Culture:	Caucasian
Occupation:	Owner and manager of a motel
Primary Health Care Provider:	Marguerite Drummond, MD

III. Health History

Source of Information:	Client
Reliability of Informant:	Good
Chief Concern:	Pain and tiredness of the lower extremities, which are interfering with his daily activities

History of Present Illness:

Mr Osterhaut has had frequent episodes of dull aches with feelings of heaviness in the legs, which do not seem to diminish with leg elevation. He has noticed increased pain and muscle cramping as well as fatigue of his leg muscles in hot weather. The pain has been aggravated by the long hours he is on his feet in the summer running his motel business.

Mr Osterhaut has had varicose veins "for as long as I can remember." In 1970, he underwent bilateral saphenous vein ligation. He also had several sclerosing procedures in which a sclerosing agent was injected into distended superficial veins to obliterate the distended segments. However, he developed an allergic reaction to the sclerosing agent. He has never had a leg ulcer or thrombophlebitis.

In the past, Mr Osterhaut wore elastic bandages on his legs. For the past few years, he has not worn any type of support stocking or bandage. "They are much too hot," he says. He does try to elevate his legs periodically during the day, although he admits this is difficult during heavy tourist seasons. He is never constipated but has had a gradual weight increase of 20 to 30 lb over a 5-year period. He has never smoked cigarettes. His mother had severe varicose veins and always wore heavy support stockings.

Past Health History:

Childhood:	Chickenpox
Immunizations:	Tetanus toxoid, 1983, dog bite
Medical Problems:	None
Surgeries:	Tonsillectomy, 1950; bilateral vein ligation, 1970

(continued)

Case Study written by Janice Lech Dusek and SueAnn Wooster Ames.

The Client With Varicose Veins

Trauma:	None
Allergies:	None
Medications:	None
Family History:	Father, died age 56, hypertension, CVA
	Mother, age 82, hypertension, varicose veins
	Brothers ×3, ages 62, 58, 55, all A&W; eldest with Type II DM
	Wife, age 55, A&W
	Son, died age 18, automobile accident
	Daughters ×2, ages 38 and 40, A&W; eldest with varicose veins following pregnancy
	No positive FHx of MI or malignancy
Personal/Social History:	Mr Osterhaut took over the family motel business in 1965 when his father died. His youngest brother works with him. The business is fairly successful. Mr Osterhaut and his wife live on the property. During the heavy tourist season, she also works at the motel.
	He has no formal exercise program—"just work." He eats a well-balanced diet, enjoys fresh fruits and vegetables, and avoids salt because of his father's hypertension and CVA. He attributes his weight gain to his increased beer intake over the past 4 years—three to four glasses per day and a six-pack on Saturday and Sunday. In the past, he never drank beer during the week and would have only one to two glasses on the weekend. He drinks no other alcoholic beverages.
Review of Systems:	
Skin:	Has noted no changes in the skin of the extremities; no areas that do not heal easily; no bruising
Respiratory:	Sinus trouble in the spring and fall with nasal stuffiness and frontal headache; pneumonia once in 1977
Heart:	No chest pain, palpitations, DOE; ECG in 1977 was normal
Genitourinary:	No dysuria, frequency, nocturia, decrease in stream, or urgency; able to achieve and maintain an erection s̄ difficulty
Extremities:	States varicose veins both legs have markedly increased with visible knots; they are tender to touch as well as causing him much pain when legs are dependent
IV. Physical Assessment	
Weight:	185 lb
Height:	5 ft, 10 in
Vital Signs:	T. 98.6°F (37°C); P. 72; R. 16; BP 114/68
	WD/WN 59-year-old w/m, appears younger than his stated age, in NAD
Relevant Organ Systems:	
Skin:	Temperature nl; mild cyanosis both ankles and feet; left ankle appears somewhat edematous when compared to right; edema does not pit
Thorax and Lungs:	Expansion = bilat; clear to percussion and auscultation
Heart:	Apical rate 72; regular; no ⓜ
Abdomen:	ō bruits; soft; nontender; no palpable masses or groin nodes; bilateral well-healed scars groin area from previous vein ligation

Vascular:

Pulses	Radial	Carotid	Femoral	Popliteal	Dorsalis Pedis	Posterior Tibial
Right	4+	4+	4+	4+	4+	4+
Left	4+	4+	4+	4+	4+	4+

Large, bulging varicose veins lateral aspect both legs, extending from knees to ankles; veins in left leg larger and more tortuous than right

V. Summary

Mr Osterhaut was scheduled for a stripping and ligation of his varicose veins

VI. Nursing Care Plan

Nursing Diagnosis	Client Care Goals	Plan/Nursing Implementation	Expected Outcome
Mobility, impaired physical	Maintain mobility; reduce or eliminate possibility of postoperative complications such as edema, thrombophlebitis; reduce intra-abdominal pressure through weight loss	Prepare client for surgery; postoperatively, keep legs elevated 18 out of 24 h to decrease edema formation; check pulses and circulation every 2 to 4 h; within 24 to 48 h after surgery, encourage client to get up and walk several minutes of every hour to promote circulation; teach the correct method of applying elastic bandages—from toes upward; prepare client for discharge by teaching importance of continuous support of the legs with elastic stockings; this will be a lifelong necessity to prevent venous insufficiency; also explain need for periodic leg elevation and walking at least 5 min of every hour during the day; encourage weight reduction by decreasing alcohol intake and maintaining a well-balanced high-fiber diet; instruct client to avoid standing or sitting for long periods and not crossing the legs	Expresses an understanding of the disease process; can explain the preventive measures to decrease the incidence of venous complications
Comfort, alteration in: pain	Prevent discomfort in extremities	Apply elastic bandages from toes to groin, assuring an even tension and even spacing of evolutions, taking care to avoid creases; administer analgesics as necessary; elevate legs at regular intervals throughout the day	Will apply elastic bandages and elevate legs as instructed; will have no pain and no apparent swelling in legs

The Nursing Process for Clients With Disorders of the Blood and Blood-Forming Organs

Linda Rae Belsky
Janice Lech Dusek
Carol Ren Kneisl

Objectives

When you have finished studying this chapter, you should be able to:

Specify the subjective data to be obtained in the nursing assessment of a client with a disorder of the blood or blood-forming organs.

Describe methods used in the physical examination of clients with disorders affecting the blood and blood-forming organs.

Identify diagnostic studies common to clients having disorders of the blood or blood-forming organs.

Anticipate the nursing diagnoses common in the care of a client with disorders of the blood or blood-forming organs.

Determine the goals to be attained by a client with a disorder of the blood or blood-forming organs.

Develop a nursing plan of care for a client with a disorder affecting the blood or blood-forming organs.

Discuss the expected outcomes of care for a client with a blood disorder.

Anticipate the physiological and psychosocial needs of clients donating blood or undergoing phlebotomy.

Implement nursing interventions specific to clients having a transfusion of blood or a blood component.

Clients with disorders of the blood and blood-forming organs have special needs, partly because a disturbance in blood production or bone marrow functioning can affect every organ system. These disorders can produce symptoms that become life threatening. Many clients' lives become uncertain in a number of ways—bleeding is often a constant threat; discomfort can evolve into severe pain; recurrent infections that are resistant to treatment can be life threat-ening; and weakness can become incapacitating fatigue. There may be little energy to devote to family, friends, job, school, or recreation. Therefore, both physiological and psychosocial support are essential nursing measures. The nurse caring for these clients must first assess them thoroughly. Planning and implementing care for such clients must be broad in scope, considering all potential problems and plans of action.

Section I: Nursing Assessment: Establishing the Data Base

Dysfunction of the blood or blood-forming organs can affect every organ system. For this reason, presenting symptoms can be varied and widespread.

SUBJECTIVE DATA

Initially, clients may report nonspecific symptoms such as weakness, fatigue, or malaise. Encourage clients to describe these and other symptoms in their own words and to explain how the symptoms affect their daily activities.

Bruising and Bleeding

Ask clients if they have bruised easily lately or had larger bruises than normal; this fact may signal problems either with platelet production or consumption or with a clotting factor. Ask about the nature of the bruises: What causes them? Do they appear without injury? Also obtain information about when the client first noticed the bruising.

Petechiae, red to brownish pinpoint hemorrhages in the skin, may go undetected; clients may or may not spontaneously report them. Without biasing or influencing the client's response, ascertain whether there are petechiae, which may indicate platelet dysfunction. For example, ask, "Have you noticed any pinhead-sized reddish discolorations on your skin, especially where clothes fit snugly, such as at your belt line?"

Thrombocytopenia is the most frequent cause of bleeding and can accompany the leukemias, the lymphomas, or idiopathic thrombocytopenic purpura. Thrombocytopenia can also be a side effect of the chemotherapeutic treatment of any malignancy. Bleeding commonly occurs in a number of body systems. For example, clients may experience epistaxis and/or bleeding from the gums. Epistaxis may cause significant blood loss. Bleeding from the gums can also interfere with the client's sense of taste; clients may report that nothing tastes good.

Gastrointestinal bleeding, appearing as hematemesis and melena, may occur with thrombocytopenia or gastrointestinal tumors. Frequently, the blood loss in the gastrointestinal tract is occult and can only be detected through chemical testing.

Female clients with thrombocytopenia may have menorrhagia, resulting in severe blood loss. When interviewing the female client about blood loss during menses, be specific and thorough in the questioning. Ask about color and amount of menstrual flow. Amount of menstrual flow can be documented by the number and size of the sanitary pads or tampons the client uses per day.

Ask about bleeding in other organ systems the client may have observed. Has the client noticed any hematuria? If so, what is the extent of the bleeding? Is the urine pink tinged, or is it grossly bloody? Determine also whether the client has noticed any bleeding into the sclera or any pulmonary bleeding.

Lymphadenopathy

Clients sometimes report a painless mass in the area of the cervical lymphatic chain. Enlargement of the lymph nodes of the neck is most common in Hodgkin's disease but may also accompany non-Hodgkin's lymphoma or the leukemias. Clients may also report swelling in the groin or edema of the lower extremities. This may occur in clients with lymphoma (Hodgkin's and non-Hodgkin's) who have inguinal lymph node involvement that impedes the normal flow of lymphatic fluid.

Pain

Clients with hematopoietic dysfunction are also subject to pain. Although severe eye pain and impairment of visual acuity may occur in sickle cell anemia, clients are more likely to experience pain in the joints, bones, or abdomen.

Hemarthroses (bleeding into the joints) may accompany bleeding disorders such as hemophilia and result in joint pain. Other hematologic dysfunctions—the leukemias, the lymphomas, multiple myeloma, and sickle cell anemia—may be accompanied by bone pain. High uric acid levels sometimes found in the hematologic malignancies may initiate a painful gouty arthritis.

Abdominal tenderness may be due to splenomegaly, though splenomegaly is not always accompanied by abdominal tenderness. Abdominal pain may have many causes. It may be due to intestinal obstruction caused by invasion of lymphoma into the gastrointestinal tract. Abdominal pain may be experienced during crisis by the client having sickle cell anemia. Clients taking the Vinca alkaloids vincristine and vinblastine are prone to paralytic ileus, which can be painful.

Determine whether the client has a sore tongue. Severe iron deficiency anemia, pernicious anemia, and vitamin deficiencies commonly cause this symptom.

Integumentary Changes

Frequently, clients having disorders of the blood and blood-forming organs have abnormalities in skin texture, appearance, or color. As the largest organ of the body, the skin provides valuable information about clients' bone marrow functioning.

Clients should be asked about changes in skin color. Have they or their significant others noticed pallor or flushing? Pallor, especially if it occurs over weeks or months, may not be noticed by either clients or their significant others. Jaundice is a color change clients usually easily recognize as abnormal. Jaundice may represent a hemolytic process involving erythrocytes, with or without accompanying hepatic dysfunction. Determine when change in color was first noticed. Approximations may have to suffice—eg, "Did you notice you were first becoming jaundiced around Christmas or Thanksgiving?" Correlate changes in skin color with the onset of fatigue or decreased activity tolerance. Ask clients whether they noticed a change in skin color at about the same time their tolerance to activity changed.

Pruritus may or may not be present, depending on the disorder; it frequently accompanies Hodgkin's disease and non-Hodgkin's lymphoma, although the exact cause of the pruritus is unknown. Clients tend to regard pruritus as a nuisance and not to associate it with the blood disorder. Questions about pruritus should focus on the approximate time the client first noticed pruritus, what aggravates it, and what home remedies seem to relieve the itching.

Ask also about the condition of the skin of the lower extremities. The lower extremities seem to be especially vulnerable to blood abnormalities. Adult clients with sickle cell disease frequently have leg ulcers.

Neurologic Changes

Headache is a common complaint of clients with hematologic disease. Its causes are varied. Headache may accompany anemia or polycythemia vera. It may be present with central nervous system (CNS) involvement in leukemia or lymphoma, as a result of CNS infection, or with CNS hemorrhage secondary to thrombocytopenia.

Alterations in vision may accompany the blood disorders and be related to neurological changes. The client can experience diplopia or blurred vision with CNS involvement of the leukemias or from retinal hemorrhage.

Numbness and tingling of the extremities may be present in pernicious anemia. With modern therapeutic measures, however, neurologic complications of pernicious anemia are rare.

Loss of deep tendon reflexes frequently accompanies the use of vincristine and vinblastine. Loss of the reflex in itself causes no problem for the client. However, gait abnormalities, gross or fine motor uncoordination, footdrop, or slurred speech while clients are taking plant alkaloids may indicate neurologic toxicity of the drug. If neurologic toxicity is suspected, use of the drug is discontinued.

Dizziness or light-headedness may be experienced with any of the anemias. If the blood loss has been gradual, extending over weeks or months, the client's body may have adapted to the decreased oxygen-carrying capacity of the blood. Gradual blood loss does not cause the fluid volume deficits that occur in sudden major hemorrhaging such as from motor vehicle injuries.

Other more severe changes in neurologic status (ie, disorientation and loss of consciousness) may occur with various hematologic disorders. Clients with sickle cell anemia may be prone to CNS infarction with a possible consequent change in level of consciousness. Clients who have idiopathic thrombocytopenic purpura or leukemia with profound thrombocytopenia may have an altered consciousness level because of a cerebral hemorrhage.

Cardiovascular and Respiratory Changes

Clients with anemia may complain of tachycardia, palpitations, or chest pain. They may even seek medical treatment because of congestive heart failure. The degree of effect of the anemia on the cardiovascular system is related to the amount and the rapidity of blood loss. With the chronic anemias, the client may have no cardiovascular symptoms because of the body's ability to adapt to small blood losses over a long time.

Clients with anemia sometimes complain of shortness of breath or dyspnea, usually with exertion. Sometimes, however, clients have difficulty breathing even at rest. The effect of anemia on the respiratory system is similar to its effects on the cardiovascular system: the client's symptoms depend on the amount and the rapidity of blood loss.

Gastrointestinal Changes

Clients with disorders of the blood and blood-forming organs frequently have gastrointestinal symptoms. Some symptoms such as anorexia, nausea, and vomiting are relatively nonspecific to the disease process, whereas other symptoms pinpoint the hematologic deficit. For example, clients with chronic iron deficiency may report difficulty swallowing due to atrophy of the oral mucous membrane. The sore tongue of clients with certain anemias or vitamin deficiencies was discussed earlier, as was the anorexia of clients with gingival oozing or epistaxis.

Ulcerations of the oral mucosa or the mucosa elsewhere in the gastrointestinal tract can result from the side effects of chemotherapeutic agents used in the treatment of the leukemias and the lymphomas, placing clients at risk for bleeding, infection, and changes in elimination. Clients who are immunosuppressed are more likely to have infections of the oral mucosa such as candidiasis (discussed in Chapter 48). Clients taking Vinca alkaloids may also be constipated.

Drug Use and Chemical and Radiation Exposure

Because many drugs interfere with normal hematologic functioning, the history should make note of any prescribed or over-the-counter (OTC) medications the client takes. Antineoplastic drugs as well as some antibiotics such as chloramphenicol cause bone marrow suppression. Sedatives, hypnotics, analgesics, laxatives, and aspirin may cause or worsen hematologic abnormalities. (These drugs are discussed in Chapter 29.)

The use of aspirin is so common that both the client and the nurse can overlook or disregard its significance. Aspirin reduces platelet aggregation (the ability of platelets to be called to an injury site), increasing the potential for bleeding, especially in clients with compromised hematologic functioning. Thus, determining the client's use of aspirin and noting when the client last used aspirin are especially important.

Alcohol consumption must also be assessed. Alcohol abuse damages the liver; liver damage alters the production of clotting factors.

Exposure to chemicals increases the incidence of hematologic disorders. Clients may come into contact with chemicals through their jobs or avocations, by living in a contaminated area, or by using certain cosmetics. At increased risk for developing hematologic disorders are clients who are continuously exposed to asbestos, asphalt, industrial dyes, lead, and dry-cleaning fluid. Dyes used in fabrics and even on the client's own hair may cause hematologic injury. Clients living close to industrial plants are also at increased risk.

Exposure to radiation also increases the incidence of hematologic disorders. Clients who live close to nuclear power plants or work with radioactive materials may be at increased risk, as are clients who have been accidentally exposed to high amounts of radiation or purposely exposed for therapeutic purposes.

Health History

Elicit the client's health history. Allergies, preexisting medical conditions such as liver disease, and knowledge about past immune response should be documented. Note previous diagnoses of blood disorders such as anemia or mononucleosis or gastrointestinal malabsorption problems. Determine how many and what kinds of infections the client has had. What part of the body has been affected? Do the infections recur? Do they respond to treatment? What symptoms are evident (ie, Is the temperature elevated? Is there a pattern? Does the client have night sweats?)?

Ask about the client's bleeding tendencies after injury, surgery, or dental extraction: Has the client had any problems with abnormal bleeding or bruising? The client's history of receiving blood transfusions—the number of transfusions, why they were administered, and whether there were any complications during or following the transfusion—should be documented.

Ask about the client's surgical history. In particular, the fact that a client has undergone a splenectomy or surgical resection of the duodenum may give valuable information about blood dyscrasias. For example, knowing that a client has a past history of splenectomy might also reveal the reason for the splenectomy (usually trauma or spherocytosis). Removal of the stomach and duodenum interferes with the client's ability to properly absorb vitamin B and sets the stage for a surgically induced pernicious anemia. Information about the client's postoperative healing may give clues to the client's bone marrow integrity and competence of immune response.

Dietary History

The dietary history may provide important clues about the causes of some hematologic disorders. Information about intake of iron, vitamin B_{12}, and folic acid may be revealed in clients' listings of the kinds of foods they eat regularly. High alcohol intake may suggest why a client has a diminished appetite or vitamin deficiencies. A dietary history that reveals low intake of foods high in iron may indicate the cause of the client's anemia; knowing that a client takes vitamin B injections suggests the possibility of pernicious anemia. Although dietary history alone cannot diagnose hematologic abnormalities, it can aid in both the diagnosis and management of disorders of the blood and the blood-forming organs.

Family Health History

Certain hematologic disorders and other hematologic dysfunctions tend to run in families. The family history should include any history of anemias, jaundice, liver dysfunctions, red blood cell disorders, sickle cell disease, clotting disorders, and malignancies.

OBJECTIVE DATA

Physical Assessment

The collection of objective data begins with a complete physical examination, which requires the skills of inspection, palpation and, to a lesser extent, auscultation and percussion. The physical assessment is organized according to areas of the body from the head to the toe.

Skin
Inspection and palpation of the skin can give valuable information about the status of the client's hematologic system. Clients with hepatic or biliary disease with elevated bilirubin levels may have a hemolytic anemia (destruction of erythrocytes), which manifests itself as jaundice. Clients having reduced hemoglobin levels may be cyanotic. Clients with polycythemia vera frequently have ruddy complexions.

Color of the client's skin depends not only on the level of the client's hemoglobin but also on the amount of pigmentation in the skin. If clients have darkly pigmented skin, disorder-induced color changes may be obscured by the client's natural skin tones or hues. Hence, skin color cannot be used as the sole indicator of overall oxygenation of body tissues. To assess skin color properly in these situations, closely inspect the client's oral mucosa, conjunctivae, and the fingernail beds. Another good way to assess oxygenation to tissues without interference from skin pigmentation or hemoglobin level is to inspect the color of palmar creases. Have the client open the hand with fingers fully extended. If oxygenation to the body tissues is adequate, the palmar creases should be pink.

Clients having problems with platelets—production, life span, or function—and those with clotting-mechanism dysfunction have alterations in skin integrity that can be observed on physical examination. Frequently, the nurse observes purpura (redness), ecchymoses, or petechiae. **Ecchymoses** (hemorrhagic spots larger than petechiae) may be dark purplish, brown, yellow, or greenish, depending on the age of the lesion, and they may or may not be precipitated by a bump or injury. Lesions can be flat or elevated and may be painful or tender to palpation (Figure 28–1). Petechiae are most common when clients have disorders of platelet function, life span, or decreased platelet numbers. Petechiae can occur over any part of the skin but are most common where pressure has been applied to a body part (eg, after application of a tourniquet or blood pressure cuff). Petechiae are usually flat, nontender lesions that do not blanche with pressure.

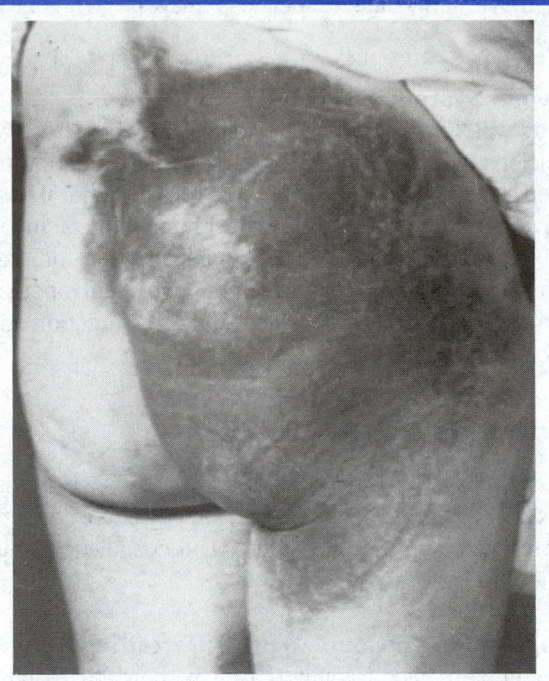

Figure 28–1

A large and painful ecchymosis in a client with a coagulation disorder. (Courtesy of Millard Fillmore Hospital, Buffalo, NY)

Pruritus in clients with Hodgkin's disease or non-Hodgkin's lymphoma may be so severe that the skin is excoriated from scratching. Leg ulcers in clients with sickle cell anemia are most frequent over the medial and lateral malleoli. Ulcerations may be present at the time of the physical examination, or the nurse may observe healed scars over the lower extremities.

Eyes

Jaundice of the sclera may accompany jaundice of the skin. Retinal or scleral hemorrhages may be observed with thrombocytopenia. Conjunctival pallor can be seen in many of the anemias.

Mouth

Tissue oxygenation also may be assessed using the gingivae of the mouth as the guide. With optimal tissue oxygenation, the gingivae appear pink, but pallor indicates inadequate oxygenation.

The tongues of clients with pernicious anemia and iron deficiency anemia may be smooth. Nutritional deficits, in general, may cause the tongue to become red and smooth (see Table 8–4 in Chapter 8).

Bleeding or oozing from the gums or teeth may occur in any client having a bleeding disorder, whether due to platelet abnormalities or clotting-factor deficiencies. Infections and lesions of the oral mucosa frequently develop in clients with leukopenia. Inspect the client's mouth daily, noting any of these alterations in skin integrity.

Lymph Nodes

The lymph nodes make up part of the lymphoreticular system, which is responsible for the body's defense against invading pathogens. Lymph node enlargement is frequent among clients with hematologic and lymphoreticular disorders, particularly malignant ones. In physical assessment, it is important to note whether the lymph nodes (Figure 28–2) are mobile or fixed, tender or painless, or enlarged upon palpation.

Thorax

Sternal tenderness or pain upon palpation may accompany the leukemias and the lymphomas in the presence of a mediastinal mass. Auscultation of heart sounds may reveal tachycardia and cardiac murmurs if the client is severely anemic. The tachycardia and murmur usually resolve following the administration of packed red blood cells.

Auscultation of the lungs may reveal diminished or absent breath sounds that may be related to a malignant pleural effusion or tumor obstruction. The presence of adventitious sounds (described in Chapters 7 and 18) may indicate pulmonary bleeding, pulmonary edema, or pneumonia. Decreased diaphragmatic excursion (movement) may be due to splenomegaly or hepatomegaly.

Abdomen

Clients with disorders of the blood and blood-forming organs frequently have hepatomegaly, splenomegaly, or both. The size of these organs can be ascertained using the skills of percussion and palpation of the liver and spleen, discussed in Chapter 7.

With percussion, the liver heights are 4 to 8 cm in the midsternal line and 6 to 12 cm in the right midclavicular line. When the liver is enlarged, the span of liver dullness is increased.

The spleen can also be identified and splenic size estimated from percussion. The spleen is palpated as a small oval area of dullness over the tenth rib and posterior to the midaxillary line. An enlarged area of dullness may indicate increased splenic size.

Liver and spleen size can also be assessed using palpation. An increase in liver size, with or without tenderness, is a significant finding in the blood disorders. The spleen normally is not palpable in the adult client. The finding of splenomegaly or simply palpating the tip of the spleen in the adult client is significant because splenomegaly is present in many hematologic disorders such as chronic granulocytopenic leukemia.

Musculoskeletal System

Musculoskeletal system abnormalities are not uncommon in clients with disorders of the blood and blood-forming organs. Visible joint deformities are present in clients with the hemophilias and sickle cell disease. Limitation of the normal range of motion may accompany the joint deformity. The client may experience either active or passive pain

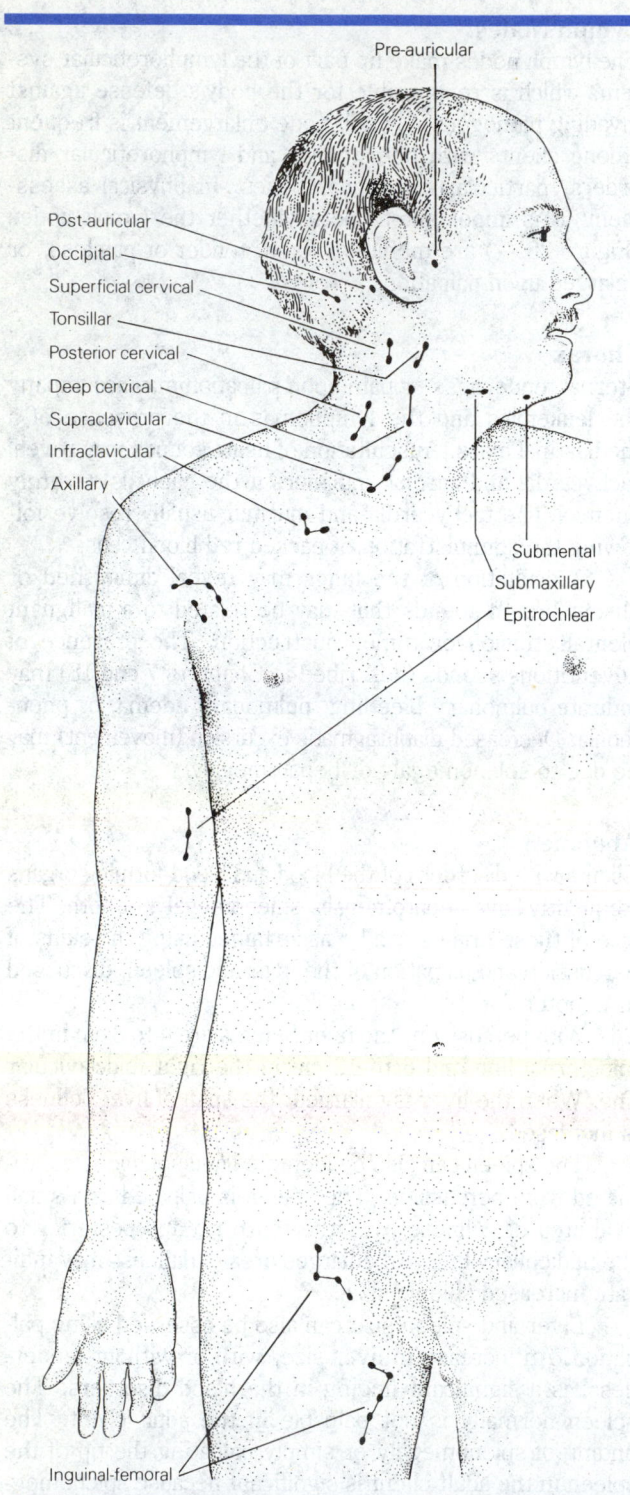

Figure 28–2

Palpable lymph node chains.
SOURCE: Saxton DF, Pelikan PK, Nugent PM, Hyland PA: *Addison–Wesley Manual of Nursing Practice*. Menlo Park, CA: Addison–Wesley, 1983.

with movement, and tenderness may be triggered by palpation.

Nervous System

Clients with vitamin B_{12} deficiency, such as those with pernicious anemia, can have neurologic dysfunction manifested as cerebral, spinal cord, or peripheral nerve involvement. Leukemic clients with meningeal involvement may have headache, visual impairment, or cranial nerve involvement. Clients who have neutropenia or thrombocytopenia may have neurologic dysfunction due to CNS infection or bleeding.

Diagnostic Studies

Three kinds of laboratory tests are routinely done to assess the client's hematologic status: erythrocyte measurements, leukocyte measurements, and coagulation studies (Table 28–1).

Complete Blood Count With Differential

The complete blood count (CBC) with white blood cell (WBC) differential (Diff) is one of the most important tests for evaluating the status of the client's hematologic system; the CBC with Diff provides a measure of the blood's ability to carry and transport oxygen (erythrocyte measurements) and to resist invading infectious organisms (leukocyte measurements). The CBC with Diff usually requires approximately 7 mL of venous blood.

The CBC erythrocyte measurements consist of a red blood cell count, hemoglobin, hematocrit, various erythrocyte indices (such as mean corpuscular volume, mean corpuscular hemoglobin, and mean corpuscular hemoglobin concentration), and a stained red cell examination (film or peripheral blood smear). The CBC leukocyte measurement includes a WBC count. In addition to the total WBC count, the CBC with Diff determines the various types of leukocyte cells (neutrophils, basophils, eosinophils, lymphocytes, and monocytes). These erythrocyte and leukocyte measurements are discussed individually. In some laboratories and institutions, a platelet count is considered part of the CBC. The platelet count is discussed later in this chapter in the section on coagulation measurements.

Red Blood Cell Count. The red blood cell count (RBC), or erythrocyte count, is the measurement of the number of erythrocytes circulating in 1 μL of whole blood. Factors or disease states that result in an elevation of the erythrocyte count are high altitude; hemoconcentration resulting from shock, trauma, or hemorrhage; anoxia; and polycythemia vera. The erythrocyte count may be decreased in anemia, Hodgkin's disease, or the leukemias.

Hemoglobin. Hemoglobin (Hb) is the main component of the erythrocyte or RBC. Disease states or pathologic conditions that contribute to an elevation in the hemoglobin level include polycythemia or erythrocytosis,

Table 28–1 Laboratory Tests Common to Disorders of the Blood and Blood-Forming Organs	
Laboratory Tests	**Normal Expected Value**

Laboratory Tests	Normal Expected Value	
Complete blood count with differential:		
Red blood cell count	Males 4.5–6.0 million/µL	
	Females 4.0–5.5 million/µL	
Hemoglobin	Males 14–18 g/dL	
	Females 12–16 g/dL	
Hematocrit	Males 40%–54%	
	Females 37%–47%	
Erythrocyte indices:		
Mean corpuscular volume	76–100 fL	
Mean corpuscular hemoglobin	25–35 pg	
Mean corpuscular hemoglobin concentration	30%–38%	
White blood cell count:	4500–11,000/µL	
Differential white-cell count	*% of total WBC*	*Cells/µL*
Neutrophils (segmented)	54–75	3000–7500
(banded)	3–8	150–700
Lymphocytes	25–40	1500–4500
Monocytes	2–8	100–500
Eosinophils	1–4	50–400
Basophils	0–1	25–100
Erythrocyte sedimentation rate	0–20 mm/h (varies with sex, age, and test method)	
Erythrocyte osmotic fragility	Initial hemolysis at 0.40%–0.46% saline; complete hemolysis at 0.30%–0.35% saline	
Reticulocyte count	25,000–75,000/µL	
Coagulation measurements		
Platelet count	150,000–400,000/µL	
Bleeding time	1–3 min (Duke), 1–7 min (Ivy)	
Prothrombin time	11–15 s	
Partial thromboplastin time	40–100 s	

SOURCE: Normal expected values from Byrne CJ et al: *Laboratory Tests: Implications for Nursing Care,* 2nd ed. Menlo Park, CA: Addison–Wesley, 1986.

hemoconcentration in shock or immediately after hemorrhage, and high altitude. Hemoglobin levels are decreased in anemia resulting from increased blood destruction or decreased RBC production.

Hematocrit. The hematocrit (Hct) or packed cell volume (PCV) measures the percentage of a given volume of whole blood occupied by erythrocytes. Disorders that result in an elevated hematocrit are polycythemia vera and hemoconcentration from shock, surgery, or hemorrhage. A decrease in hematocrit can be caused by anemia resulting from diminished blood production or increased red blood cell destruction, the leukemias, and the lymphomas. If hematocrit is done separately from the CBC, a sample of blood may be obtained by a finger prick.

Erythrocyte Indices. The erythrocyte indices are three different values that examine the size, weight, and

hemoglobin content of the average erythrocyte. These three values—mean corpuscular volume (MCV), mean corpuscular hemoglobin (MCH), and mean corpuscular hemoglobin concentration (MCHC)—reflect red cell morphology. Abnormalities in the erythrocyte indices in conjunction with the stained red cell examination provide a way of classifying anemias and suggesting their possible causes. Values are increased in folate or vitamin B_{12} deficiency, liver disease, alcoholism, sprue, and antimetabolite therapy. Values are decreased in anemia from chronic blood loss, iron deficiency anemia, pernicious anemia, and thalassemia.

Stained Red Cell Examination. The stained blood smear is examined to determine abnormalities in the size, shape, or structure of erythrocytes as well as the staining properties. This microscopic examination helps in the diagnosis of anemia, leukemia, and thalassemia and in determining harmful effects of chemotherapy and radiation.

White Blood Cell Count and Differential. The total WBC count, or leukocyte count, determines the number of circulating white blood cells in 1 μL of whole blood. An elevated WBC (or leukocytosis) can accompany anoxia, anemia, infections, mononucleosis, the leukemias, polycythemia vera, and transfusion reactions and may also occur immediately following trauma or hemorrhage. Leukopenia, or a decreased WBC, may accompany agranulocytosis, anemia, hypersplenism, and the leukemias.

The differential WBC count (Diff) determines the distribution of the kinds of WBCs. The Diff count is usually reported in percentages, which should add up to 100. The Diff classifies leukocytes as monocytes, lymphocytes, or granulocytes. Granulocytes are further classified as neutrophils, eosinophils, or basophils. Neutrophils are divided into and reported as either banded (a juvenile form) or segmented (the mature neutrophil). The Diff not only reports leukocyte morphology but also identifies and reports immature or atypical leukocytes. An increase in the number of immature leukocytes, often called "a shift to the left," is discussed in Chapter 22.

A rise in the percentage of neutrophils (neutrophilia) may occur in any malignancy, crushing injury, the leukemias, malignant lymphoma, polycythemia vera, the hemolytic anemias, and hemolysis due to transfusion reaction. The percentage of circulating neutrophils (neutropenia) can be decreased in infectious mononucleosis, agranulocytosis, the leukemias, aplastic anemia, pernicious anemia, multiple myeloma, and vitamin B_{12} deficiency. Most leukocytes are neutrophils.

Lymphocytosis, an elevation in the percentage of lymphocytes, accompanies the lymphocytic leukemias, infectious mononucleosis, agranulocytosis, aplastic anemia, multiple myeloma, and lymphosarcoma. Lymphopenia, or a decreased number of lymphocytes, may be present in Hodgkin's disease and in the acute leukemias. An elevation of monocytes, or monocytosis, may be the bone marrow's response to agranulocytosis, Hodgkin's disease, monocytic leukemia, non-Hodgkin's lymphoma, and hemolytic anemia. Eosinophilia (elevated eosinophils) accompanies eosinophilic leukemia, Hodgkin's disease, pernicious anemia, polycythemia vera, and sickle cell anemia in some clients. Basophils may be elevated (basophilia) in chronic myelogenous leukemia, the hemolytic anemias, Hodgkin's disease, and polycythemia vera.

Erythrocyte Sedimentation Rate

The erythrocyte sedimentation rate (ESR) is the rate at which erythrocytes in anticoagulated whole blood settle to the bottom of a tube. The ESR's great value is to indicate the presence of an active inflammatory disease process. The ESR is elevated in leukemia, malignant lymphoma, Hodgkin's disease, severe anemia, and agranulocytosis but may be within the normal range in polycythemia and sickle cell anemia.

Erythrocyte Osmotic Fragility

The erythrocyte osmotic fragility test measures the erythrocytes' ability to resist hemolysis in a hypotonic solution. Cells that hemolyze in a relatively high concentration of saline (barely hypotonic) have an increased osmotic fragility. Disease states accompanied by an increased osmotic fragility are acquired hemolytic anemia, hemolytic disease due to blood-type incompatibility, pernicious anemia, symptomatic hemolytic anemia due to Hodgkin's disease, and leukemia. Iron deficiency anemia, polycythemia vera, sickle cell anemia, and thalassemia major are accompanied by a decreased osmotic fragility.

Reticulocyte Count

The reticulocyte count is considered the most useful test in the evaluation of anemia and is a good index of effective erythropoiesis and bone marrow response to anemia. Reticulocytes are nonnucleated, immature RBCs capable of oxygen transport. They remain in the blood for 24 to 48 hours, after which they are mature. An elevated reticulocyte count, or reticulocytosis, occurs in disease states or conditions that cause a relative anoxic or hypoxic state in the client. Elevated reticulocyte counts are seen in acquired autoimmune hemolytic anemia, acute posthemorrhagic anemia, sickle cell anemia, thalassemia major, treatment of iron deficiency anemia, and treatment of vitamin B_{12} and folic acid deficiency.

A decreased reticulocyte count, or reticulocytopenia, occurs in disease states or conditions in which the bone marrow's ability to respond to hypoxic or anoxic states by an outpouring of reticulocytes has been impaired. Disease states and conditions accompanied by reticulocytopenia are aplastic anemia, aplastic crisis of hemolytic anemia, malignant disorders involving the bone marrow, untreated iron deficiency anemia, and untreated megaloblastic anemia. Reticulocytopenia also occurs in clients receiving antineoplastic chemotherapeutic agents that cause bone marrow suppression.

Coagulation Measurements

There are a wide variety of measurements of coagulation function. Some of the most common are discussed here.

Platelet Count. The platelet count measures the number of circulating platelets, or thrombocytes, per μL of whole blood. Platelet values may be altered by many of the disorders of the blood and blood-forming organs. Thrombocytosis, or an elevation in the number of platelets, can be present in acute blood loss, chronic granulocytic leukemia, idiopathic thrombocytopenic purpura, iron deficiency anemia, and polycythemia vera. Thrombocytopenia, or decreased platelet numbers, may accompany acute granulocytic leukemia, acute lymphocytic leukemia, chronic lymphocytic leukemia, monocytic leukemia, multiple myeloma, pernicious anemia, idiopathic thrombocytopenic purpura, and aplastic anemia.

Platelets are usually reported as adequate, low adequate, or high adequate. In some of the hematologic disorders, such as the leukemias or idiopathic thrombocytopenic purpura, a quantitative platelet determination is performed. This test is a more accurate determination of the platelet level. Quantitative platelets are reported as specific numbers such as 50,000, 150,000, or 300,000. The normal quantitative platelet range is 150,000 to 400,000/μL.

Bleeding Time. The bleeding time, a test that records the duration of active bleeding, provides information on vascular response to injury and helps to evaluate platelet function. The two principal methods of performing the bleeding time are Duke's and Ivy's methods. In Duke's method, bleeding time is measured by observing active bleeding after a puncture on one of the client's ear lobes. Ivy's method, preferred because it is less liable to variation among testers, measures the bleeding time after two small punctures on the client's forearm. Pressure is applied by inflating a blood pressure cuff up to 40 mm Hg. The client's bleeding time may be prolonged in any of the leukemias, aplastic anemia, disseminated intravascular coagulation (DIC), idiopathic thrombocytopenic purpura, infectious mononucleosis, multiple myeloma, and pernicious anemia. Bleeding time is also used in the diagnosis of von Willebrand's disease.

Tourniquet Test. The tourniquet test, or Rumpel–Leede capillary fragility test, measures capillary strength and may be used to identify platelet defects or deficiencies. It is, however, one of the least scientific of the coagulation studies. This test utilizes a blood pressure cuff inflated to midway between the systolic and diastolic pressures (to a maximum of 100 mm Hg) and sustained for 5 minutes. The number of petechiae on the forearm within a 5 cm circle at least 1 in from the cuff are then counted. The scale of normal values is as follows (Byrne et al., 1986):

- Grade 1+, 0–10 petechiae
- Grade 2+, 10–20 petechiae
- Grade 3+, 20–50 petechiae
- Grade 4+, more than 50 petechiae

Clot Retraction Test. Clot retraction estimates the quantity and quality of platelets and fibrinogen. A clot normally retracts or pulls away partially from the sides of a test tube in 1 to 2 hours, and completely retracts in 12 to 24 hours, expressing serum as it shrinks. When platelet numbers are low, platelet quality is poor, or fibrinogen level low or poorly functioning, clot retraction is slowed. This test can be useful in the diagnosis of disorders of platelet dysfunction or deficiency and in diseases involving low fibrinogen levels or increased destruction of fibrinogen. Examples of these disorders are the acute leukemias, the thrombocytopenias, hypofibrinogenemia, and aplastic anemia.

Prothrombin Time. Prothrombin time (PT) evaluates stages II and III in the coagulation cascade. An increased PT may be present in the acute leukemias, DIC, factor VII or X deficiency, polycythemia vera, and multiple myeloma. This test is also used to regulate warfarin therapy.

Partial Thromboplastin Time. The partial thromboplastin time (PTT) is a general evaluation of the entire coagulation system except for factors VII, XIII, and platelets and can also be used to regulate heparin therapy. A prolonged PTT can occur in DIC and in deficiencies of factors V, VIII, IX, X, XI, or XII.

Coagulation Factors Assay. Coagulation factors assay or profile is a combination of selected coagulation studies that assists in evaluating all the stages in the clotting cascade and helps to pinpoint the area in which the clotting deficiency or problem occurs. Institutions vary in what is included in a coagulation profile, but a typical profile might contain bleeding time, platelet count, clot retraction, partial thromboplastin time, and prothrombin time, all previously described.

Factor VIII Activity. Factor VIII$_{AHF}$ (antihemophilic factor) activity is the test for classic hemophilia or hemophilia A. Clients with little or no factor VIII are classified as severe hemophiliacs; those with 1% to 5% of normal values are called moderate hemophiliacs; and those with values between 6% and 30% of the normal are termed mild hemophiliacs. Clients with von Willebrand's disease have deficiencies in both factor VIII$_{AHF}$ and factor VIII$_{VWF}$ (von Willebrand factor). Deficiency of factor VIII$_{VWF}$ may range anywhere from 0% to 50% of normal.

Other disease processes or changes in health status may interfere with the amount of available factor VIII for normal coagulation. Childbirth, penicillin allergy, and certain antibodies in the blood may interfere with factor VIII activity. Disease processes that inhibit factor VIII activity include lupus erythematosus, multiple myeloma, rheumatoid arthritis, and cancer.

Immunoglobulin Studies
Immunoglobulin studies evaluate the amount and types of immunoglobulin—IgG, IgA, IgM, IgD, IgE—present in the client. A sample of blood is collected and examined under immunoelectrophoresis. Each immunoglobulin has its own unique pattern. Abnormal levels occur in many hematologic disorders. Any immunizations or vaccinations that the client may have received within the previous 6 months may affect the results. These should be documented and reported to the laboratory; testing may need to be delayed.

Serum Ferritin Level
Serum ferritin determinations evaluate the amount of iron stored in body tissues. Depleted iron supplies depress the

synthesis of ferritin. Clients experiencing iron deficiency states, such as iron deficiency anemia, have decreased serum ferritin levels. The test helps to distinguish between iron deficiency anemia and anemias associated with chronic disease.

Total Iron-Binding Capacity

Total iron-binding capacity (TIBC) measures the amount of available transferrin (a protein that binds with iron and transports it throughout the body) in the blood. TIBC increases as iron levels and iron stores decrease. Elevated TIBC is found in iron deficiency states, infancy, pregnancy, and blood loss. Decreased TIBC is found in iron overload states such as hemochromatosis, chronic hemolytic anemias such as pernicious anemia, and blood transfusion overload.

Gastric Analysis

Gastric analysis measures the acidity of secretions in the stomach. It is used in the diagnosis of pernicious anemia. Its use in the diagnosis of disorders of the stomach is discussed in Chapter 47.

Gastric analysis can be performed in two ways. Nasogastric intubation allows the collection of gastric secretion specimens. The client should be NPO after midnight the evening before and should not smoke the morning of the test until all specimens have been obtained. Gastric secretions are collected every 15 minutes for 1 hour, and labeled consecutively as #1, #2, and so on. These are called basal acid secretion specimens. Once basal acid secretion specimens have been collected, the client is given a gastric acid stimulant, usually histamine, parenterally. Gastric contents are then collected every 15 minutes for 1 hour and labeled appropriately. These specimens are called maximal acid secretion specimens. Monitor the client following histamine administration for adverse side effects such as increased pulse, decreased blood pressure, headache, flushing, dyspnea, vomiting, diarrhea, and shock.

The tubeless method determines the presence or absence of gastric acid without a quantitative measure of acid production. The client must refrain from all foods and medications after the evening meal the night before the test but may have water at any time. The client voids upon awakening or immediately before the test is begun, and the specimen is discarded. The client ingests a gastric acid stimulant such as caffeine and is instructed to void again. This specimen is labeled #1. Once the first urine specimen is obtained, the client is given an oral resin–dye complex. This resin–dye complex is excreted in the urine and, in the presence of hydrochloric acid, turns the urine blue. Two hours after ingesting the resin–dye complex, the client voids again; this specimen is labeled #2. Encouraging the client to drink water will facilitate collecting the urine samples. Inform the client that the urine may continue to be blue for several days.

Both methods of gastric analysis require the client's cooperation to be completed successfully. Prepare the client for the procedure and provide encouragement and support.

Schilling Test

The Schilling test is used in the differential diagnosis of pernicious anemia. This test, and its nursing implications, are discussed in Chapter 47.

Sickle Cell Test

The sickle cell test, or Sickledex, screens the presence of hemoglobin S (Hb S) in the client suspected of having sickle cell anemia or the client suspected of being a carrier of the sickle cell trait. The client with sickle cell anemia has 90% or greater Hb S. Individuals having 50% or less Hb S are known as carriers of the disease; the remainder of their hemoglobin is the normal adult hemoglobin (Hb A). Normally, the erythrocyte contains no hemoglobin S.

Bone Marrow Examination

Examination of the client's bone marrow, one of the most common hematologic diagnostic tests, provides information about the character, integrity, and production of the client's erythrocytes, leukocytes, and thrombocytes. Bone marrow examination can be done either by aspiration or biopsy.

Bone marrow aspiration is usually performed when only a small amount (less than 5 mL) of marrow is needed for diagnosis. Bone marrow aspiration is used to diagnose and evaluate clients having any of the anemias, the acute leukemias, neutropenia, or thrombocytopenia and as part of the staging process for some of the solid tumor malignancies such as Hodgkin's disease, multiple myeloma, and non-Hodgkin's lymphoma. Bone marrow biopsy, a surgical procedure usually performed under local anesthesia, is done when a larger amount of bone marrow is required to aid diagnosis or evaluation. The most common sites for bone marrow examination in the adult are the sternum and the iliac crest (especially the posterior iliac crest) (Figure 28–3).

Nursing Implications. Bone marrow aspiration is routinely performed in clients' rooms or in a treatment room on the nursing unit. Prepare clients for the aspiration procedure by educating them and their families about the reasons for the aspiration and by generally describing what to expect during the aspiration. In particular, prepare the client for a sharp but brief pain (suction pain) when bone marrow is aspirated into the syringe.

For a bone marrow aspiration using the iliac crest, the client should be lying on either side with hips and knees flexed at 90° angles if the anterior iliac crest is used, or prone if the posterior iliac crest is used. When the sternum is used for sampling, the client can be supine. The skin site for puncture is prepared in a circular fashion using an iodine cleansing agent, and the overlying skin, subcutaneous tissue, and periosteum are anesthetized. When anesthesia is obtained, an aspiration needle with stylet is advanced through the skin and tissue until it meets bone.

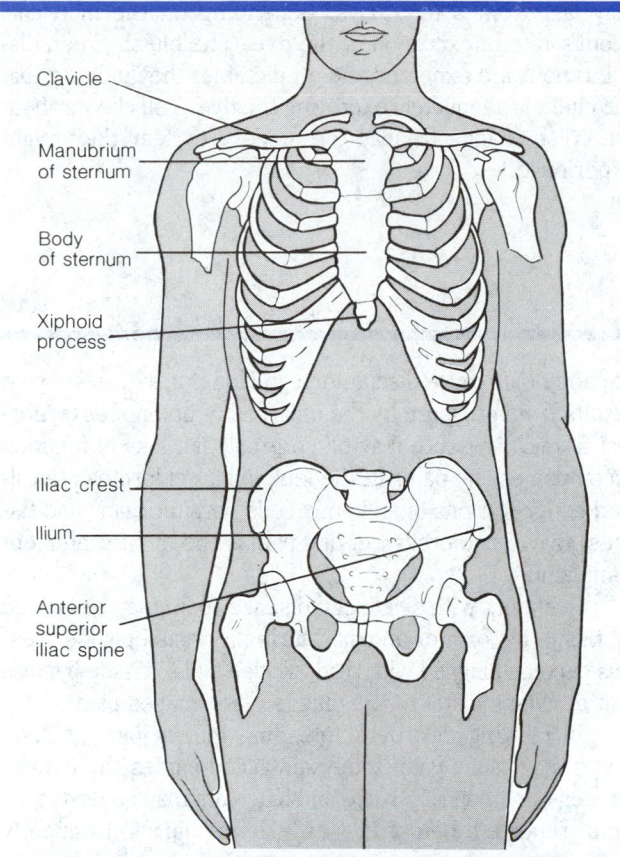

Figure 28–3

Common sites for bone marrow aspiration or biopsy. The sternum and iliac crest are used most often.
SOURCE: Kozier B, Erb G: *Fundamentals of Nursing: Concepts and Procedures,* 2nd ed. Menlo Park, CA: Addison–Wesley, 1983.

Penetration of the periosteum requires a twisting motion. As the aspirate is withdrawn into a syringe, clients may experience the suction pain and hear a crunching or grinding sound. Clients need to be taught that, to avoid mechanical injury, they must hold completely still during the aspiration. This may be difficult for some clients. Be prepared to support them emotionally and gently restrain them when necessary. Once the bone marrow sample is obtained, the needle is removed, and immediate pressure is applied using a sterile gauze sponge. When hemostasis is assured, an adhesive bandage or small sterile dressing should be applied. A pressure dressing may be applied if the client is prone to bleeding or is thrombocytopenic. Encourage clients to resume the same kinds of activities they were performing before aspiration. Analgesic medication is usually not indicated following the procedure. Assess the aspiration site for signs of hemorrhage and for signs and symptoms of infection.

For *bone marrow biopsy,* clients are treated as surgical clients. A small incision (3 mm to 4 mm) is made through the skin overlying the bone to be used, and a wedge specimen or a large needle specimen of bone marrow is obtained.

Clients undergoing an open biopsy may require analgesic medication. Care of the incision includes keeping it clean and dry and assessing the wound for signs of hemorrhage and for signs and symptoms of infection. Clients are usually able to resume their normal activities following the biopsy but are asked to leave the dressing in place and avoid getting it wet for 48 hours.

Lymphangiography

Lymphangiography is the radiographic examination of the lymphatic system. Radiopaque dye is injected into the lymphatic chains in the client's feet. First, a blue dye to stain the lymphatic vessels is injected intradermally between each of the first three toes of each foot. The dorsum of each foot is then anesthetized. An incision is made into the dorsum of the foot between the second and third toes, and the lymph nodes are identified and isolated. The lymphatic chain is then cannulated, and the radiopaque dye is injected. X-ray films (lymphangiograms) are taken immediately and as the contrast dye moves up the lymphatic chain to the level of the third and fourth lumbar vertebrae, when the injection is discontinued. A second set of films is taken 24 hours later when the contrast medium has filled the lymph nodes. The dye remains in the lymphatic chains up to 6 months following its initial injection, so subsequent x-rays and follow-up can determine disease status without the need to repeat dye injection. Lymphangiography is performed for clients with edema due to an obstruction in lymphatic drainage and for clients suspected of having Hodgkin's disease or non-Hodgkin's lymphoma.

Normally, the lymphatic system shows complete filling with the dye on the initial set of films. Twenty-four hours later, the lymph nodes are shown as opaque, well-defined nodes. With a metastatic process, filling defects and lack of opacification are demonstrated. Primary lymphedema shows fewer shortened lymphatic vessels on x-ray films. Secondary lymphedema appears as abruptly terminating vessels.

Nursing Implications. Client and family education is the primary responsibility of the nurse whose client is undergoing lymphangiography. The procedure is lengthy, ranging from as little as 2 hours to as long as 8 hours, depending on the skill of the radiologist and the ease with which the lymphatic chain is identified and isolated. Clients must lie supine and hold completely still.

When clients are returned to the nursing unit after the procedure, the incisions on the dorsum of the feet should be watched for signs and symptoms of bleeding, infection, and inflammation. Clients may resume normal activities but must keep their feet dry. Clients should not get their feet wet when bathing until after the sutures are removed—usually about 5 days after the procedure. Pain or discomfort at the incision sites ordinarily does not require analgesic medication nor interfere with ambulation. To minimize discomfort that could result from shoes rubbing against the incisions, clients should wear soft shoes, such as moccasins or slippers.

Although expected, one of the most alarming side effects of the lymphangiogram is a bluish green discoloration on the dorsal skin of the feet, in the urine, and in the veins of the lower extremities. Some clients have even reported that their feces turn bluish green. This color change may last from 2 to 5 days, depending on the individual client's rate of excretion of the dye. The bluish green discolorations are expected and predictable; they indicate that the client is adequately excreting the dye. Tell clients about the color change to allay the anxiety or fear they might experience.

Section II: Nursing Diagnosis

Nursing diagnoses common to clients with disorders of the blood and blood-forming organs are listed in Box 28–1. The following sections discuss their implications for the client and the nurse.

ALTERATION IN COMFORT

In the malignant disorders of the blood and blood-forming organs, pressure of the tumor on surrounding tissues of the body may cause discomfort. In Hodgkin's disease, pain results from pressure by the enlarged lymph nodes on normal tissue. Pressure may be so great that loss of function accompanies the pain. In the leukemias, chloromas (localized congregations of leukemic cells within organs and tissues) may cause pressure, and pain is the most prominent complaint.

In clients with sickle cell disease, pain may be caused by tissue hypoxia or anoxia. During a crisis episode, vessels become plugged with rigid, sickled cells. Tissue hypoxia that develops distal to the plugged site causes pain.

In clotting disorders, bleeding into a joint or body cavity may cause pain. Joint pain accompanies the hemarthroses of hemophilia. Knee and hip joints may be destroyed from repeated hemarthroses. Hemophiliacs frequently experience pain on movement or with weight bearing.

Hyperuricemia, which frequently accompanies malignant disorders, may precipitate a goutlike joint pain. Hyperuricemia occurs when there is rapid cell metabolism and when there is an accumulation of cellular wastes after cytotoxic drug therapy.

> **Box 28–1   Nursing Diagnoses Commonly Related to Dysfunction of the Blood and Blood-Forming Organs**
>
> **Diagnoses Directly Related to Disorders of the Blood and Blood-Forming Organs**
>
> *Comfort, alteration in:* pain
>
> *Gas exchange, impaired,* related to sickling, low hemoglobin concentration, disruption in coagulation, or red blood cell dysfunction
>
> *Mobility, impaired physical,* related to weakness, dyspnea on exertion, pain, or decreased endurance
>
> *Skin integrity, impairment of: potential,* related to chemotherapy
>
> *Nutrition, alteration in: less than body requirements,* related to nutrient deficiency
>
> *Knowledge deficit*
>
> *Coping, ineffective individual*
>
> *Coping, ineffective family: compromised*
>
> **Additional Potential Nursing Diagnoses**
>
> *Fluid volume deficit, potential*
>
> *Tissue perfusion, alteration in: cerebral*
>
> *Oral mucous membrane, alteration in:* related to immunosuppression
>
> *Activity intolerance,* related to imbalance between oxygen supply and demand
>
> *Self-care deficit*
>
> *Injury: potential for,* related to altered clotting factors, etc.

IMPAIRED GAS EXCHANGE

Any interference with normal erythrocyte production, function, or activity may impair oxygen transport and exchange to body tissues. For example, when sickling occurs in sickle cell anemia, tissue hypoxia develops distal to the site of sickling. In any anemic client, the oxygen-carrying capacity of the blood is reduced by a low hemoglobin concentration or a decreased number of circulating erythrocytes or both.

Gas exchange may be impaired in disease processes disrupting coagulation. Whether the bleeding is caused by a coagulation abnormality, such as the hemophilias, or by thrombocytopenia, such as occurs in the leukemias, blood loss may be severe enough that the oxygen-carrying capacity of the blood is diminished or impaired.

IMPAIRED PHYSICAL MOBILITY

Fatigue, weakness, or dyspnea on exertion (DOE) may accompany the anemias; the client may limit physical movement to avoid these symptoms. In bleeding disorders, such as idiopathic thrombocytopenic purpura and the hemophilias, actual bleeding into the joints may destroy joints, with loss of joint motion and function.

Clients having malignancies such as multiple myeloma and leukemia frequently have bone pain. Pain may limit the client's mobility.

IMPAIRED SKIN INTEGRITY AND POTENTIAL FOR INFECTION

Clients with disorders of the blood and blood-forming organs frequently have problems with impaired skin integrity. Whenever leukocyte production, function, or activity is interfered with or interrupted, the client has an increased risk for developing infection.

Leukemic clients tend to be subject to frequent infections. Clients with multiple myeloma frequently have a history of infections, particularly pneumonia, during the prodromal phase. Clients with pernicious anemia are at risk for infection because of defective leukocyte production.

Clients with malignancies such as leukemia, lymphoma, Hodgkin's disease, and multiple myeloma are likely to undergo chemotherapy or radiation therapy at some point during their illnesses. These treatments leave the client leukopenic. Research has documented that as the neutrophil count decreases, the infection rate increases. The oral and gastric mucosa are sites of irritation and ulceration from chemotherapy. These sites may be portals of entry for potentially harmful microorganisms.

In clients with sickle cell anemia, decreased circulation to the peripheral tissues results in leg ulcers. The relative tissue hypoxia in sickle cell anemia makes healing of these ulcers difficult. Frequently, the ulcers become infected.

ALTERATION IN NUTRITION

Anorexia and weight loss are frequently symptomatic of hematologic disorders. Anorexia, nausea, vomiting, and weight loss may accompany antineoplastic drug treatment of the blood disorder, further compromising and altering the client's nutritional status.

Stomatitis, mucositis, or other oral lesions may limit the client's ability to chew and swallow food in adequate amounts. Alterations in the client's sense of taste may make mealtime and eating unpleasant. In addition, the client's tumor burden may be so large that the normal food intake has become inadequate.

Whereas clients with malignant disorders have general nutritional deficits, clients with anemia have nutrient deficiencies specific to the anemia. For example, clients having iron deficiency anemia have different nutritional needs than those with pernicious anemia. The nutritional support program for each of these clients must take into account the individual's deficiency. (These specific nutrient deficiencies are described in Chapter 29.)

KNOWLEDGE DEFICIT

Clients with disorders of the blood and blood-forming organs often do not know much about the disease process and treatment programs. This group of disorders is complex and may seem overwhelming to clients or their significant others. Frequently, clients are asked to manage their disease processes and to seek medical and nursing intervention when appropriate. To take on this responsibility, clients must understand the disease process, the function of the blood-cell components, medications, and signs and symptoms indicating a need for medical and nursing interventions.

INEFFECTIVE COPING

Clients with blood disorders may have to alter their lifestyles temporarily or permanently. These alterations may require that the client learn new methods of coping with living.

For the adult client with leukemia, the poor long-term prognosis is the issue facing the client and family. Grieving may accompany the diagnosis, and the client and family may begin to cope ineffectively. The client may try to be strong for the family's sake, and the family may be overly solicitous toward the client.

Clients with disorders like Hodgkin's disease, which primarily affects young individuals, may be anxious and fearful about whether they can attain career and personal goals and about the effect of antineoplastic agents on future fertility.

Clients may be anxious about diagnostic procedures that may discover an incurable illness. They may also be anxious because they lack knowledge or have misconceptions about the disease process and the effects of therapy and how these may affect family and business matters.

Section III: Planning and Implementation

Nursing interventions for clients with disorders of the blood and blood-forming organs should be geared toward resolving the problems identified in the previous phases of the nursing process. A sample nursing care plan is presented in Table 28–2.

PROMOTING COMFORT

As noted in the previous section, pain accompanying disorders of the blood and blood-forming organs may have many causes—the disease process itself, which results in

Table 28–2   Sample Nursing Care Plan for Clients With Disorders of the Blood and Blood-Forming Organs

Nursing Diagnosis	Client Care Goals	Plan/Nursing Implementation	Expected Outcome
Comfort, alteration in: pain	Remain comfortable throughout the therapy and the disease process	Administer analgesics for pain p.r.n. as ordered (nonaspirin products); aid pain relief by comfortable positioning of client; aid client in position changes; use pillows for support and change position q. 2 h; provide good mouth care: mouthwashes, gentle teeth care, and soft diet to relieve discomfort of oral ulcerations; use topical anesthetics p.r.n. and a.c.; relieve rectal and anal discomfort from ulceration by providing meticulous perineal care, sitz bath, and preventing constipation and relieving diarrhea; use distraction and diversional activities; offer antianxiety agents; gently rub back; spend unhurried time with client every day; encourage activity but provide client with frequent rest periods as needed	Clients will remain pain free, will independently perform own ADLs when appropriate, will state they are comfortable; skin warm and dry; relaxed body posture; vital signs within normal limits
Gas exchange, impaired	Optimal gas exchange	Restrict activity as needed; balance rest and exercise periods throughout the day; administer blood, blood components, or blood substitutes as ordered and observe for any untoward reactions; assess daily laboratory reports for decrease in blood's oxygen-carrying capacity (Hb and Hct); assess client's ability to tolerate activity and adjust activity order as indicated; monitor vital signs q. 4 h; listen to the client's subjective concerns (ie, SOB, dyspnea); assess skin color, temperature and moisture; elevate the head of the bed 35° to 40°; administer O_2 as ordered; teach the rationale for blood transfusions (eg, "This blood will make you feel better by relieving the work load on your heart and lungs"); encourage foods high in iron; provide iron supplements as needed	No complaints of fatigue or weakness; vital signs within normal limits; oriented ×3; skin pink, warm, and dry
Mobility, impaired physical	Function independently and maintain mobility	Encourage frequent rest periods and adequate sleep time; assist client in moving if necessary but maintain independence as much as possible; aid client in self-care management; administer nonaspirin analgesics p.r.n. if pain is interfering with client's mobility; encourage active ROM if ambulation is not possible and consult with physical therapy to set up a program and schedule for exercises; if active ROM is not possible, help client perform passive ROM to maintain joint mobility	Maintain independent functioning; no decrease in activity tolerance; able to perform ADL without help
Skin integrity, impairment of: potential for infection	Maintain skin integrity and infection-free state	Encourage client to avoid exposure to infectious persons, excessive fatigue, or an inadequate diet; assess temperature and BP at regular intervals; maintain optimum oral hygiene and carefully examine mouth q.d.; mouth washes q. 2–4 h; adequate oral fluid intake; maintain strict aseptic technique when medical procedures invade integument barrier; isolate client from others with infectious disease; use good hand-washing technique; administer antibiotics as ordered and watch for toxic effects of antibiotics with high doses; reverse isolation as needed; explain rationale for reverse isolation (ie, to protect the client from sources of infection); monitor the client's WBC and assess	Skin intact and client infection free (ie, normothermic); no purulent drainage; skin pink, warm, and dry

Nursing Diagnosis	Client Care Goals	Plan/Nursing Implementation	Expected Outcome
		count for neutropenia; assess all portals of entry (eg, access devices) for signs and symptoms of infection; listen to the client's verbalizations of discomfort (eg, tenderness or pain that may signal infectious process); administer granulocytes as ordered; initiate infection-preventing measures (ie, assist client to ambulate as tolerated); encourage turning, coughing, and deep-breathing exercises; assess skin integrity, including integrity of mucous membranes; assess integrity of bony prominences and turn and reposition q. 2 h	
Nutrition, alteration in: less than body requirements	Maintain optimum nutritional status	Initiate dietary consult; inquire about client's food preferences, remembering that neutropenic clients are not allowed fresh fruits and vegetables because of potential infection; offer small, frequent feedings (ie, breakfast, mid-morning snack, lunch, midafternoon snack, supper, bedtime snack); avoid temperature extremes in foods served if oral ulcers present; serve meals attractively and remove unpleasant stimuli from surroundings at mealtime; assist client in selecting easily chewed foods that meet requirements from the basic four food groups; maintain daily calorie count; weigh client q.d. at 7:30 AM; administer antiemetics when client is receiving chemotherapy—do not wait until client becomes nauseated or vomits before giving the antiemetic; perform oral hygiene daily using soft toothbrush/gauze/sponges for oral care; assess client's mouth for stomatitis or other oral lesions (eg, candidiasis) twice daily; note condition and integrity of ginginvae, buccal mucosa, tongue; observe characteristics of saliva (ie, thin, abundant or stringy, scant; encourage frequent rinsing of mouth with cool water to keep mucous membranes moist; apply lubricant to lips as needed	Eat ¾ of meals, snacks served; maintain stable weight; feel energetic
Knowledge deficit	Understand disease process and treatment used	Encourage both client's and significant others' involvement in discharge plans; help client and significant others to ask questions of health care professionals; actively listen to verbalization of fears/anxieties; assess readiness to learn (eg, do client and significant others ask questions about disease process, treatment, diagnostic tests? Do they ask questions/make statements about disease's effect on previous lifestyle?); teach at client's level of readiness to learn: disease process, functions of blood cells, treatment regimen, signs and symptoms indicating need for medical/nursing intervention; remember client and family will need review of teaching periodically throughout the hospitalization; contact the outpatient nurse and establish a relationship between the client and the outpatient nurse before discharge; give client inpatient and outpatient nurses' telephone numbers and encourage the client to call with questions	Correctly recall information taught; verbalize feelings of anxiety openly; begin to make decisions about health care; feel comfortable about or look forward to going home

(continued)

Table 28–2	Sample Nursing Care Plan for Clients With Disorders of the Blood and Blood-Forming Organs (continued)		
Nursing Diagnosis	**Client Care Goals**	**Plan/Nursing Implementation**	**Expected Outcome**
Coping, ineffective individual and family	Regain sense of control	Establish therapeutic relationship between client and nurse and between significant others and nurse; spend "quality" time with client every day—15 min to ½ h daily with client doing what client wants to do; answer questions honestly but do not destroy client's defense mechanisms—allow client to express denial (it may be the client's only defense mechanism in coping with disease process/diagnosis); assess client's and family's coping ability, note any clues to ineffective coping (eg, giddiness/inappropriate joking about diagnosis, reluctance to begin learning about home care needs) and effective coping (eg, asking questions regarding illness, alterations in lifestyle from illness, denial, crying, asking questions about death/dying)	Make decisions about health care and ask questions about disease process; open lines of communication between nurse and client, nurse and family, and client and family

tissue changes; pressure on body organs; or tissue hypoxia. Nursing measures as adjuncts to the administration of analgesics for the relief of pain may be offered in the form of comfort measures (eg, position changes, back massages) and distraction.

Discomfort may be caused by gastrointestinal ulcerations or inflammation secondary to the administration of chemotherapy or radiation. These lesions may be oral (stomatitis) or can extend along the gastrointestinal tract and manifest as rectal or oral ulcerations. The nurse should provide good mouth care by using nonalcoholic-based mouth rinses and gentle teeth cleansing by using soft-bristled brushes or sponge or gauze tooth cleaners. A soft diet may relieve the discomfort of oral ulcerations. Topical anesthetics may be used as needed and before meals to decrease the discomfort associated with mastication when ulcers are present. Rectal and oral discomfort of ulceration resulting from chemotherapy, radiation therapy, and disease can be relieved by providing meticulous perineal care and sitz baths and relieving diarrhea or preventing constipation.

Touch denotes acceptance and caring to most clients. Back rubs should be given, keeping this principle in mind. Not only may back rubs improve circulation and promote relaxation but they may also promote a sense that the nurse accepts and cares about the client; this sense may relieve pain. The amount and quality of the time the nurse spends with the client daily assist in fostering a trusting nurse–client relationship. Trust creates a bond that promotes comfort.

Clients with blood disorders may be anxious enough that their perception of pain is altered. Antianxiety drugs may aid in the overall plan to promote client comfort.

Nonpharmacologic measures that may promote comfort should be used as much as possible. Clients should be encouraged to keep up interests they pursue when not hospitalized. Some clients have sedentary vocations or avocations (eg, paperwork, sketching, knitting) that can be done while hospitalized. These interests and activities may serve as distractions from pain.

PROMOTING OPTIMUM GAS EXCHANGE

The interventions for both anemia and bleeding problems are geared toward increasing the total oxygen-carrying capacity of the client's blood. Nursing intervention begins with interpretation of the results of the most recent blood work (RBC, Hb, and Hct). This information provides a basis for planning care and developing observational criteria.

The nurse's assessments of clients' responses to decreases in oxygen-carrying capacity are important. Assess clients' skin color, temperature, and moisture. For example, one client will have pallor and shortness of breath with an Hb value of 9.0 g/dL, but another client with a similar Hb may be asymptomatic. It is essential to listen to clients' complaints of shortness of breath or difficulty in breathing, headache, and dizziness. Monitor the client's vital signs, especially noting changes reflecting decreased oxygen-carrying capacity such as tachycardia and tachypnea and also assessing for orthostatic hypotension. Note the client's tolerance to activity and adjust the client's activity level appropriately. With impaired gas exchange, the client needs to have balanced periods of rest and activity and may need assistance to complete activities of daily living.

When giving a transfusion, be alert for possible allergic reactions and administer antihistamines before transfusion if necessary. Clients receiving transfusion therapy need to be educated about the use of blood products. For more information about transfusion therapy and care of the client receiving a blood transfusion, see Section V in this chapter.

Besides transfusion therapy, clients may also require iron supplements and an iron-rich diet to enhance the formation of hemoglobin. Client education must accompany the use of iron supplements and food sources rich in iron (see discussion in Chapter 29 under iron deficiency anemia). In general, self-medication with OTC iron supplements should be discouraged.

Oxygen therapy may be administered to further promote gas exchange. Elevating the head of the client's bed facilitates downward movement of the diaphragm, allows greater lung expansion, and increases the volume of air taken into the lungs, promoting a better gas exchange.

PROMOTING INDEPENDENT FUNCTION AND MAINTAINING MOBILITY

Clients who often become tired should be encouraged to take frequent rest periods. Strenuous activity should be minimal. Adequate rest and time for sleep are important.

Because of clients' feelings of weakness, fatigue, and lack of energy, self-care activities become difficult. The nurse may need to help clients complete activities of daily living while allowing clients to do as much as they can without compromising overall energy levels. As clients regain energy, an increase in exercise may begin with the resumption of their self-care activities. Activity should be planned to prevent overexertion.

Problems of immobility must be counteracted by range-of-motion (ROM) exercises and frequent position changes. If clients cannot perform active ROM, the nurse should initiate and perform passive ROM. A physical therapist may help clients maintain mobility. Ambulation of the client as soon as possible, within limits, is important to prevent the hazards of immobility. To prevent pulmonary involvement caused by immobility, encourage the client to perform turning, coughing, and deep-breathing exercises.

Because pain severely alters clients' tolerance to movement, plan a course of action to determine the extent of the client's activity. For instance, activity in a client with multiple myeloma reverses the negative calcium balance caused by skeletal degeneration and can prevent spinal cord compression. Maintain an effective analgesia regimen and assess the client's tolerance to activity provided by the analgesia.

MAINTAINING SKIN INTEGRITY AND PREVENTING INFECTION

Clients with blood disorders are predisposed to decubitus ulcer formation and poor wound healing. When clients are on prolonged bed rest, frequent turning and positioning are essential. Continued assessment of the skin for redness on bony prominences and pressure areas is required along with good skin care techniques and ambulation whenever possible.

Clients are often predisposed to oral sores and bleeding. The mucous membranes should be evaluated each day

---

Box 28–2 Calculating the Absolute Neutrophil Count

1. Convert the percentage of neutrophils from the white blood count differential to a decimal. **(A neutrophil count of 25% becomes 0.25)**

2. Multiply the total white blood cell count by the converted neutrophil percentage. **(If the client's WBC is 2300/mm³ then: 2300 × 0.25 = 575)**

3. The product (575) is the absolute neutrophil count (ANC).

---

and every 8 hours in clients who are neutropenic or thrombocytopenic. The use of soft-bristled toothbrushes or cotton swabs, as well as the use of soothing nonalcohol mouthwashes every 2 to 4 hours, should be recommended for mouth care. Tell these clients not to use toothpicks or dental floss.

Predisposition to infection can be managed by monitoring the vital signs, especially the temperature, every 4 hours. At the first sign of infection, obtain blood, urine, throat, and stool cultures for the identification of the organism. Because these clients may lack the ability to form pus or may have an altered ability to produce an inflammatory response, the typical signs and symptoms of infection may be absent. Therefore, it is important always to listen to the client's concerns. Antibiotic therapy will be administered whenever infection is suspected; the dosage ordered and administered may be high. Toxic reactions to antibiotic therapy need to be assessed. Look for electrolyte abnormalities such as hypokalemia, hypomagnesemia, and hypocalcemia (described in Chapter 5), oliguria, hearing loss, and the more common symptoms of nausea, vomiting, and diarrhea. Granulocytes may be ordered as supportive therapy when the client's total WBC is exceedingly low.

The incidence of infection and the absolute neutrophil count (ANC) are inversely related: as ANC falls, the incidence of infection rises. Box 28–2 is a guide to calculating ANC. The client having an ANC less than 500 is at increased risk for developing an infection. Institute infection-preventing measures, such as good hand-washing technique and isolation and aseptic technique with any invasive procedure. It is important that both nurse and client practice good hand-washing techniques. Isolation of the client is controversial. The client should be educated to avoid contact with individuals with known infections, with recently immunized individuals, and with large crowds.

PROMOTING OPTIMUM NUTRITIONAL STATUS

Nursing interventions should promote an optimum nutrition intake. Seek the advice and suggestions of a dietitian or nutritionist. A calorie count may be recommended. Subtle weight losses may go undetected, so it is advisable to weigh the client daily. Inquire about the client's food preferences, recalling that fresh fruits and vegetables may not be allowed for severely neutropenic clients because these food items are a potential source of infection. (This practice varies from institution to institution.) Clients should be offered small, frequent feedings to avoid expending unnecessary energy while eating and digesting meals. Meals should be served attractively; unpleasant stimuli, such as bedpans and emesis basins, should be removed in an attempt to entice the client into eating.

For clients with oral ulcerations, avoid temperature extremes in foods served. Warm or cool foods are better than hot or cold ones. Choose foods that are easily chewed and meet the requirements of the basic four food groups. Performing oral hygiene before meals stimulates the secretion of the salivary glands, the first step in digestion.

Clients receiving chemotherapy frequently experience nausea and vomiting from the effect of chemotherapeutic agents on the gastrointestinal mucosa and on the chemoreceptor/emetic-trigger zone in the brain. Nausea and vomiting can be effectively controlled in the majority of cases. The antiemetic should be administered before chemotherapy and subsequently on a regular schedule until the client is nausea free. An as-necessary regimen usually does not curb nausea effectively. In any case, try to anticipate the client's needs and do not wait until the client becomes nauseated or vomits before giving the ordered antiemetic (see also Chapter 12).

PROMOTING UNDERSTANDING OF DISEASE PROCESS AND TREATMENT

Encourage both the client and significant others to become involved in all health teaching sessions. Listen actively to the client and the significant others discuss fears and anxieties, and support the client and significant others when they ask questions.

Assess the client's and significant others' ability and readiness to learn. Consider whether they ask questions about the disease process, diagnostic tests, treatments, or the effect of the disorder on lifestyle. These assessments might indicate the client's readiness to learn.

Remember to teach the client at the client's level and when the client is ready. General content includes the disease process, functions of the blood cells, and the treatment regimen. It is always helpful to list signs and symptoms that indicate a need for medical or nursing intervention.

Remember that all clients need review and reinforcement of content taught. Clients with blood disorders tend to need frequent reteaching. Once diagnosed, these clients are taught about the disease process, pharmacologic and dietary management, home care management, alterations in lifestyle, and the signs and symptoms that warrant immediate intervention. The amount of information given to the client in a relatively short period is enormous and often overwhelming. It is unrealistic to expect the client to comprehend and manage this large amount of information and the associated instructions during one hospitalization period or clinic visit. Continual reassessment of the client's knowledge level and reteaching when indicated are essential nursing functions. Consider providing phone numbers for the client to call when questions arise after discharge and including outpatient caregivers in the client's care before discharge. A well-thought-out teaching program also promotes effective coping.

PROMOTING EFFECTIVE COPING

Initially, the nurse needs to establish a therapeutic relationship with the client and significant others. Spend "quality" time with the client each day. This may involve planning a 15-minute period of each day with the client, doing whatever the client wishes.

Assess the client's and family's coping ability. Note any clues to ineffective coping, such as giddiness or inappropriate joking about the diagnosis. Effective coping may be demonstrated when the client asks questions about the illness or alterations in lifestyle imposed by the disorder.

Honesty promotes trust and aids the establishment and maintenance of a therapeutic nurse–client relationship. Temper this principle with knowledge about the protective qualities of defense mechanisms. Answer the client's questions honestly but without destroying the client's defense mechanisms. This balance is difficult to achieve, because defense mechanisms may be the client's or family's only method of coping with the disease process. Demonstrate acceptance of the defense mechanisms and support the client's attempts to cope positively with the illness. An example is the client with a diagnosis of leukemia who uses denial to cope with the diagnosis. Denial may serve to protect the client from a reality too difficult to face. In this situation, support the client's attempts to deal with the reality of the diagnosis, but do not destroy or take away the client's use of denial before the client has given evidence of being ready to give it up. (See also Chapter 6.)

Section IV: Evaluation

Specific and realistic expected outcomes for clients with dysfunction of the blood and blood-forming organs are discussed below. Outcomes are also listed in Table 28–2.

COMFORT

Clients should remain as pain free as possible and able to perform their own activities of daily living independently when appropriate. Attempt to elicit clients' subjective statements about the amount of pain and examine clients' vital signs, noting especially any tachycardia, tachypnea, or rise in systolic blood pressure above baseline measurements. Clients having pain frequently demonstrate nonverbal clues in response to painful stimuli (eg, facial grimacing, diaphoresis, and muscle tension). The response the nurse sees depends largely on the client's attitudes toward pain.

GAS EXCHANGE

To evaluate whether clients are exchanging gas optimally, assess complaints of fatigue and weakness; vital signs; level of consciousness; and the color, temperature, and moisture of the skin. Clients who are exchanging gas optimally do not complain of fatigue or weakness, have vital signs within the normal limits established for them; remain oriented to time, place, and person; and have skin that is pink, warm, and dry. Determine whether other factors influence this goal. For example, sleep deprivation or nutritional deficiencies may cause fatigue; infection may elevate the body temperature; hypovolemia may decrease the blood pressure; and orientation to time, place, and person may be affected by drugs.

INDEPENDENT FUNCTION AND MOBILITY

Expected outcomes include activity tolerance. The client also should be able to carry out activities of daily living without nursing assistance.

SKIN INTEGRITY AND INFECTION

Skin should be intact. Breaks in the skin, ulcers in the oral mucosa or elsewhere, and reddened areas over the bony prominences indicate that this client-care goal is not being met. Because clients with blood disorders may have altered inflammatory and immune responses, fever is one of the best indicators of infection. Therefore, the client who is normothermic is probably infection free.

NUTRITION

Expected outcomes indicating clients are getting adequate nutrition include subjective statements about the way they feel, the amount of food they eat daily, and their weight. Clients who are improving or maintaining an optimum nutritional status should feel energetic, eat at least three-fourths of the food offered, and maintain a stable weight or, in the case of improving nutritional status, gain weight.

KNOWLEDGE DEFICIT

After implementing the teaching plan, evaluate how much clients and their families have learned. Ask clients to repeat or recall the content in their own words. In addition, observing clients making decisions about their health care based upon principles or content taught suggests that they have learned. Clients' stating that they feel comfortable about the prospect of going home, or at least look forward to going home, indicates that self-care and home management of the disorder are not troublesome to them because they have learned how to manage their disease state.

COPING

Expected outcomes indicating that the client and the client's family have achieved a sense of control are the kinds of communication techniques used by the client and family, the questions they ask, and their ability to make decisions about health care. Open communication between the nurse and client, between the nurse and family, and especially between the client and family demonstrate positive coping behaviors. The fact that the client and family ask questions pertinent to the disease process and treatments prescribed indicate an attempt to deal with the altered health patterns. Clients who can make decisions about health care offered to them are demonstrating effective coping mechanisms.

Section V: Blood and Blood Component Administration

Blood and blood components are administered primarily to provide adequate tissue oxygenation. The other purposes are to restore circulatory blood volume or to restore coagulation factors. With current methods, clients need only receive the missing components, avoiding unneeded blood products that may cause a transfusion reaction or circulatory overload. Nurses may be involved in providing care to donors as well as to recipients. These nursing roles are discussed below.

ASSESSING BLOOD DONORS

Prospective donors are carefully screened before donating blood to protect the health and safety of both donor and recipient. Nurses often have responsibility for screening donors according to criteria established by the American Association of Blood Banks and the Centers for Disease Control.

Subjective Data

Blood donors should be in good health, and suspicion of disease should disqualify a potential donor. Other aspects of a client's health history may also disqualify a potential donor. These factors and their rationales are listed in Table 28–3.

Table 28-3 Factors Disqualifying Potential Blood Donors

Factor	Rationale
History of heart, respiratory, kidney, or liver disease; abnormal bleeding tendencies; seizures	Potential donor at risk
Exposure to infectious disease within the past 3 weeks or current infection	Risk of transmission to the recipient
Allergies (including asthma)	Hypersensitivity may be passively transferred to the recipient
Cancer	Transmission factors are unknown
Pharmacologic treatment with drugs such as anticoagulants, antimicrobials, anticonvulsants, antiparkinsonian agents, digitalis, hormones, steroids	May indicate current disease in donor, placing donor at risk; recipient may also be at risk from donor's current disease or presence of pharmacologic agent in the blood product
History of viral hepatitis at any time or history of close contact with a person having hepatitis or receiving hemodialysis within the past 6 months	Risk of transmission of hepatitis to the recipient (potential donor may be a carrier)
Drug abuse with injectable drugs (includes not only IV injection but also subcutaneous injection)	Risk of transmission of hepatitis to the recipient (hepatitis carrier rates are high among substance abusers who self-inject drugs)
Recent tattoo	Risk of hepatitis transmission to the recipient
Tooth extraction or oral surgery within the past 72 hours	Infection and bacteremia are often associated with recent dental and oral procedures
History of syphilis	Risk of transmission to the recipient
Untreated malaria or treatment with antimalarials during the past 3 years	Risk of transmission to the recipient
Recent immunizations (receiving live, attenuated organisms within 2 weeks; rubella within 2 months; rabies within 1 year)	Risk of transmitting live organisms to the recipient
Donation of whole blood within the past 8 weeks	Donors need time to reconstitute blood components and may be at risk if donating too quickly
History of receiving whole blood or a blood component other than gamma globulin or serum albumin within the past 6 months	Risk of transfusion reaction increases as the number of previous transfusions increases
Pregnancy within the past 6 months	Pregnant or recently pregnant potential donors have high nutritional demands and need iron stores
History of acquired immune deficiency syndrome (AIDS) or being at risk for exposure to AIDS virus	Risk of transmission to the recipient

Objective Data

A potential donor's temperature, pulse, respirations, and blood pressure should be within normal limits. Donors should be between 17 and 65 years of age and weigh at least 110 lb (50 kg) for a standard 450 mL donation. Less than the standard 450 mL is taken from donors who do not meet the weight minimum. A hemoglobin screening test should identify that the donor's hemoglobin level is within normal limits for sex.

PHLEBOTOMY

A phlebotomy, or venesection, the rapid withdrawal of blood from a peripheral vein, is the method used to obtain blood from donors. A phlebotomy may also be a therapeutic measure for clients with polycythemia vera because it reduces the circulating blood volume and the red blood cell mass. (Polycythemia vera is discussed in Chapter 29.) Phlebotomy is also sometimes used in the treatment of clients with acute pulmonary edema to reduce the venous return to the heart, decreasing congestion of the pulmonary vessels and lung capillaries. (Pulmonary edema is discussed in Chapter 20.)

Procedure and Nursing Implications

The donor assumes a comfortable semirecumbent position to prevent vertigo or syncope. The skin over the antecubital fossa is cleansed and prepared, usually with an iodine preparation. A tourniquet (or a blood pressure cuff inflated to approximately 100 mm Hg) is applied to the arm and a venipuncture performed. If the purpose of the phlebotomy is to treat polycythemia or pulmonary edema, the groin is an alternate venipuncture site. The standard amount of donor blood withdrawn is 450 mL into a 500 mL sterile closed system containing 63 mL of anticoagulant and preservative. If the purpose of the phlebotomy is to treat polycythemia or pulmonary edema, the blood is not preserved as donor blood and a full 500 mL can be removed. The withdrawal of the blood takes approximately 15 minutes.

After the required amount of blood has been withdrawn, the tourniquet (or blood pressure cuff) is removed before the needle is removed. The client's arm should be elevated and firm pressure applied to the venipuncture site for at least 2 or 3 minutes, or longer if bleeding has not stopped. The venipuncture site is dressed with a firm bandage. The client should remain in the semirecumbent position for 5 minutes before being allowed to walk. If the client is able to tolerate an upright position, the donor can move to a sitting area and be observed for 15 minutes before leaving the facility. Foods and fluids are given because the donor is asked to fast before donating blood in order to reduce the risk of allergy to the recipient.

Faintness, dizziness, diaphoresis, tachycardia, or hypotension may be caused by a vasovagal reaction, fasting, or emotional factors such as anxiety. Decrease in blood volume itself may be enough to precipitate orthostatic hypotension when the client moves from a lower to a higher or more erect position. Should this occur, assist the client to assume a recumbent position or to sit down and lower the head between the knees. Remain with the client for another 30 minutes.

Instruct clients to keep the dressing on, to avoid heavy lifting with the involved arm, and to avoid smoking and drinking alcoholic beverages for 3 to 4 hours after the phlebotomy. Fluid intake should be increased for at least 2 days after the phlebotomy, and clients should remember to pay special attention to their nutrition for the next few weeks.

All donated blood is typed and tested for the hepatitis B antigen, for specific antibodies to confirm the ABO grouping, for syphilis, and recently, for acquired immune deficiency syndrome (AIDS). Testing for exposure to AIDS in blood donors began in response to situations in which persons have contracted AIDS after blood transfusions. Detection of this antibody does not indicate that the donor has or will develop AIDS. It does mean that the donor has, at some point in time, been exposed to the AIDS virus. Blood containing this antibody is not used for donation. It is speculated that tests for exposure to the AIDS virus are not yet sophisticated enough to be able to detect its presence early. Potential donors are also screened to determine if they are at increased risk for AIDS (see Chapter 29 for a description of risk categories). Individuals found to be at risk are not considered for donation and are dis-

couraged from donating blood in the future. Research into the development of more specific determinations of AIDS exposure is ongoing. Although the number of blood donors has decreased because donors fear contracting the disease during blood donation, this has not been proven to occur. Fear of contracting AIDS from blood transfusion has led to an increased use of autologous blood transfusion (discussed later in this chapter).

ADMINISTRATION OF BLOOD OR BLOOD COMPONENTS

A guide to the types of blood products that can be transfused is given in Table 28–4. Before a transfusion, the nurse verifies the type of blood or blood component the client is to receive, the number of units to be given, the date of infusion, and the rate of infusion. Be sure also to check with the client and the client's chart for previous transfusion reactions. Clients with a history of transfusion reactions may need diphenhydramine (Benadryl) and prednisone before receiving blood.

The nurse then follows hospital policy to obtain the blood from the blood bank. The blood bank may send only one unit at a time, especially if the product requires refrigeration to prevent any breakdown of blood components. Refrigeration also decreases the risk for growth of bacteria. (See Table 28–4 for specifics.)

Ascertain that the intravenous infusion was started using an 18- or 19-gauge needle. In pediatric clients or elderly clients, a 21-gauge needle can be used. Assure that the priming solution is 0.9% NaCl and that this setup remains until the transfusion is completed. The IV 0.9% NaCl provides a continuous route for flushing purposes, does not result in clotting of citrated blood, and also is necessary as a maintenance route in case of a transfusion reaction.

After obtaining the blood component, check the label on the blood bag with another nurse against the requisition form for:

- The client's name and hospital number
- The physician's name
- The client's blood group and Rh factor
- The donor's blood group and Rh factor
- VDRL (Venereal Disease Research Laboratories) results
- The expiration date

Ask the client to identify herself or himself by name and check the blood bag label against the client's identification band. Also check the bag for air bubbles or discoloration. If these conditions are present, do not use the blood and send the unit back to the blood bank.

A baseline set of vital signs should be obtained before the unit of blood is piggybacked into the 0.9% NaCl solution

Table 28–4 Guide to Blood Products

Product	Uses	Approximate Volume	Specifics for Administration
Whole blood	Acute hemorrhage, hypovolemic shock	450–500 mL	Use standard blood set with 170 μ filter
Fresh whole blood: stored less than 24 h	Exchange transfusions, multiple transfusions, postoperative transfusion of clients transfused extracorporally with banked blood, clients bleeding actively with hemorrhagic disorders	450–500 mL	Use standard blood set with 170 μ filter
Packed red blood cells	Infant transfusion, anemic clients with normal blood volume, clients at risk from congestive heart failure	225–250 mL	Use standard blood set with 170 μ filter; administer through large-bore needle at slower flow rate than for whole blood
Washed red cells	Clients who are immunosuppressed or highly allergic or who have a history of transfusion reaction; 93% free of white cells, plasma proteins, and plasma potassium	Variable	Use standard blood administration set, but exercise caution inserting spike into doughnut-shaped blood bag because it is made of fragile plastic
Fresh frozen plasma (FFP): removed from a unit of blood and frozen at −30°C	Clotting deficiencies, especially those involving factors V and VIII; blood volume expansion in treatment of burns or shock	200 mL	FFP must be thawed in water bath at 37°C; use immediately because it remains viable for only 2 h after defrosting; use standard blood set with 170 μ filter
Granulocytes: obtained from ABO-compatible donor by leukapheresis	Agranulocytosis, especially in oncology clients who are bone marrow suppressed and highly subject to infection, granulocyte count below 500	Variable (50–100 mL)	Administer soon after donation to provide maximum granulocyte viability; use standard blood set with 170 μ filter; administer over 2–4 h; take vital signs before beginning transfusion; take temperature upon completion and 1 h later; if shaking, chills, and temperature elevation occur, administer acetaminophen ½ h before subsequent transfusions and reduce flow rate
Platelets: usually harvested from 4–6 units of donor blood or by platelet pheresis from single donor; usually frozen and then thawed for use; not usually refrigerated	Clients who are bleeding and thrombocytopenic due to bone marrow depression or as a result of massive transfusions of banked blood, platelet count of 20,000/mm³ or less	30–50 mL	Administer as soon as possible to provide for maximum viability; infuse within ½ h using cryoprecipitate/platelet infusion set; monitor temperature and pulse throughout infusion
Cryoprecipitate: gelatinous precipitate obtained when fresh plasma is rapidly frozen and slowly thawed; contains factors I and VIII	Hemophilia, von Willebrand's disease, fibrinogen deficiency	25–50 mL	Administer immediately to avoid losing factor VIII; use cryoprecipitate/platelet infusion set for administration; rate of administration is usually 1 unit in 5 min
AHF concentrate: factor VIII superconcentrated, lyophilized, prepared from large pools of fresh human plasma	Classical hemophilia. AHF has many advantages over FFP and cryoprecipitate in treating severe hemophilia: 1. Higher potency, less volume 2. More accurate dosage—each vial labeled for AHF content	Usually about 40 mL	Read manufacturer's instructions for reconstitution; administer immediately after reconstitution by IV push or IV infusion; take vital signs before administration and at intervals throughout; client may experience headache, urticarial reactions,

Product	Uses	Approximate Volume	Specifics for Administration
	3. Easier storage—powder may be stored under refrigeration for prolonged period 4. Easy administration; reconstitutes quickly and may be given by IV push or infusion 5. Low incidence of adverse reactions because of low protein content		and vasomotor reactions; if client complains of dyspnea, chest pain, abdominal or leg pain during infusion, infusion should be stopped and physician notified
Factor IX complex: lyophilized, prepared from pooled human plasma; contains concentrated factors II (prothrombin), VII (proconvertin), IX (antihemophilic factor B), and X (Stuart–Prower factor)	Christmas disease (hemophilia B); deficiencies of clotting factor II, VII, or X; coumarin-derivative overdose; has same advantages over plasma as AHF concentrate	Usually about 20 mL	Read manufacturer's instructions for reconstitution; administer immediately after reconstitution by IV push or IV infusion; take vital signs before administration and at intervals throughout; client may experience vasomotor reactions and should be watched for signs of intravascular clotting such as vital sign changes, dyspnea, cough, and chest pain; factor IX complex is contraindicated in the presence of liver disease where fibrinolysis is suspected
Plasma protein factor (PPF): selected plasma proteins in a buffered saline solution; osmotically equivalent to equal amount of plasma	Hypovolemic shock, protein replacement, prevent hemoconcentration and electrolyte imbalance in burned patients, supplement to packed cells when whole blood needed but unavailable	250 mL	Administer with standard blood administration set; if supplied in glass bottle, vented tubing must be used
Fibrinogen: fractionated from pooled plasma; high risk of hepatitis transmission because it cannot be heat treated	Hypofibrinogenemia	200 mL	Use standard blood administration set; if supplied in glass bottle, venting needle must be used
Albumin (25%): albumin fraction of plasma in concentrated form, stored at room temperature	Blood volume expansion, hypoalbuminemia, prevention and treatment of cerebral edema	50 mL	Use standard blood administration set; if supplied in glass bottle, vented tubing must be used; rate of administration of undiluted albumin to clients with normal blood volume is 1 mL/min; more rapid administration is used for blood volume expansion; use extreme caution when administering to client with cardiac or pulmonary embarrassment because rapid administration draws 3.5 times its volume into the intravascular compartment within 15 min; vital signs should be taken before, during, and after infusion; allergic reactions may occur because of individual client sensitivities to plasma protein

SOURCE: Adapted with permission from Saxton et al: *Addison–Wesley Manual of Nursing Practice*. Menlo Park, CA: Addison–Wesley, 1983.

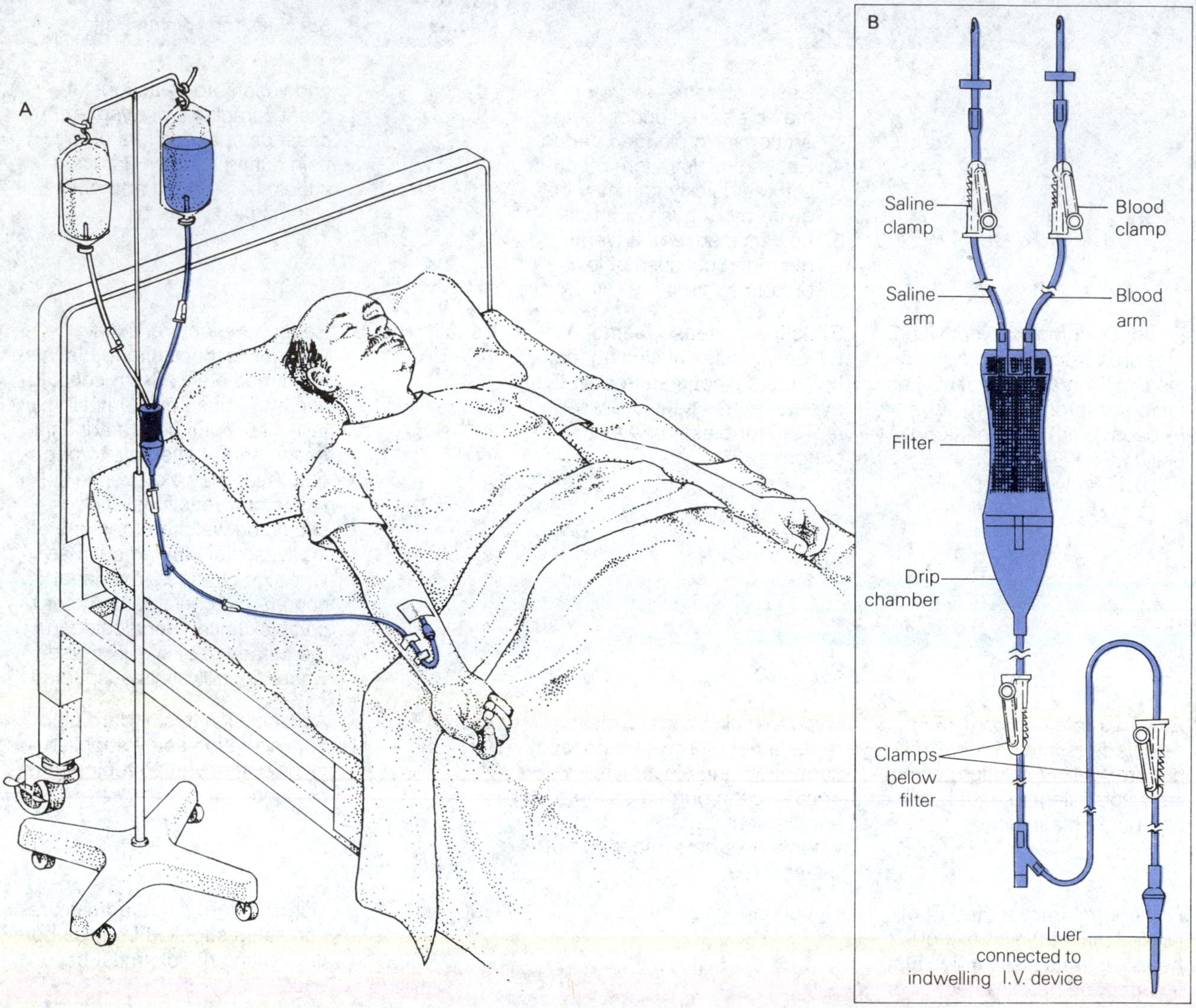

Figure 28–4

Blood or blood component administration. **A.** Client with standard Y-type blood administration set. **B.** Detail of standard Y-type blood administration set.
SOURCE: Saxton DF, Pelikan PK, Nugent PM, Hyland PA: *Addison–Wesley Manual of Nursing Practice.* Menlo Park, CA: Addison–Wesley, 1983.

already hung. Figure 28–4 illustrates the equipment used. The blood should infuse slowly at first (20 to 30 drops/minute). Remain with the client for the first 15 minutes of the infusion to evaluate the client's response to the blood infusion; the symptoms of an adverse reaction usually occur during this first 15-minute period. After the first 15 minutes, the flow rate is adjusted to allow for infusion in 1 to 2 hours; if the client cannot tolerate this rate of infusion, the flow may be slowed still further. The rate of infusion of whole blood and red cell components should not exceed 4 hours because of the potential for bacterial growth. Elderly clients and clients with heart disease may need slower infusions.

To discontinue the infusion, flush the tubing with 50 mL of 0.9% NaCl and remove the IV device. Return a completed blood form with the empty blood bag wrapped in a plastic bag to the blood bank. Documentation in the client's chart should include the blood component delivered and the blood unit number, the starting and completion time, and the client's response to the transfusion.

When transfusing a client with a blood product, keep several important points in mind. No medications of any kind should be infused with the blood because of possible incompatibility and the potential for contamination. In addition, a filter is required for blood or blood-component administration to prevent infiltration of fibrin clots and other blood debris. A cryoprecipitate-platelet infusion set (Figure 28–5) is used to provide for complete component infusion. If longer tubing is used for small-volume products, some of the components may be lost to the client because they are trapped in the longer tubing.

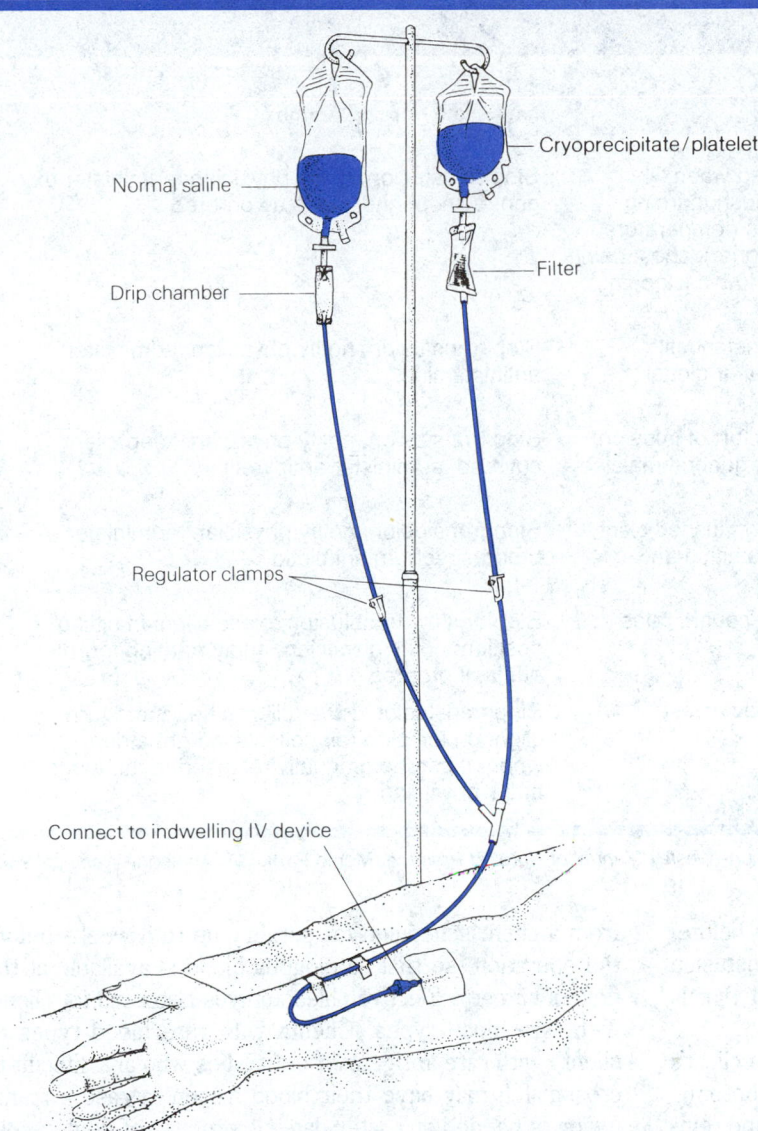

- Normal saline
- Cryoprecipitate/platelet
- Drip chamber
- Filter
- Regulator clamps
- Connect to indwelling IV device

Figure 28–5

Cryoprecipitate/platelet infusion set.
SOURCE: Saxton DF, Pelikan PK, Nugent PM, Hyland PA: *Addison–Wesley Manual of Nursing Practice*. Menlo Park, CA: Addison–Wesley, 1983.

TRANSFUSION REACTIONS

Whenever administering any blood or blood component, be aware that, because blood is a protein substance, it has the potential for initiating an antigen–antibody reaction (a transfusion reaction). A reaction to the delivered blood can occur even with the best type-and-crossmatch results. Be on guard whenever administering a blood product.

The types of transfusion reactions are outlined in Table 28–5. These reactions may be mild enough to go unnoticed, or they may be severe enough to result in anaphylaxis. In general, the greater the number of transfusions the client receives, the greater the risk for developing antibodies against blood or blood products. Because of the large number of transfusions received by sickle cell anemia or oncology clients, be especially attuned to their increased risk for developing a reaction. With any reaction during a transfusion:

- Stop the infusion of blood.
- Switch the infusion to the 0.9% NaCl solution.
- Take vital signs every 5 minutes.
- Notify the physician.
- Notify the blood bank of a possible transfusion reaction.
- Obtain urine specimens for examination.
- Send the remaining blood in the blood bag back to the blood bank with the transfusion reaction form attached.

Institutions may vary in the steps to follow in a suspected transfusion reaction. This information is only a basic guideline. Become familiar with the institution's specific protocol.

AUTOLOGOUS BLOOD TRANSFUSION (AUTOTRANSFUSION)

Autotransfusion is the process for removing whole blood from a client, storing it, and then reinfusing it into the same client at a later date. Autologous transfusion has several advantages for the client who has had or will have a 1000-mL or greater blood loss. Such great blood loss can

Table 28–5 Transfusion Reactions

Type of Reaction	Clinical Observation	Immediate Nursing Actions
Hemolytic	Immediate onset (may be delayed when Rh incompatibility involved); facial flush, burning sensation along vein, fever, chills (temperature elevation to 40.6°C [105°F] or higher); chest pain, labored respirations; headache; low-back pain; shock	Stop transfusion; notify physician; administer oxygen, epinephrine; fluids as ordered
Allergic	Urticaria, rash, pruritus; in rare instances, asthma, pulmonary edema, facial or glottal edema; anaphylactic shock	Stop transfusion; notify physician; administer antihistamine
Febrile	Fever and chills about 1 h after start of infusion; headache, flushing, tachycardia, general malaise; symptoms persist for 8–10 h	Stop transfusion; notify physician; keep client covered; administer antipyretic
Bacterial	Chills and fever; hypotension; dry, flushed skin; abdominal and extremity pain; vomiting and bloody diarrhea	Stop transfusion; notify physician; administer broad-spectrum antibiotic
Circulatory overload	Chest constriction, dyspnea, dry cough, rales at base of lung, pulmonary edema	Stop or slow transfusion; place client in sitting position; notify physician; apply rotating tourniquets, if ordered
Air embolism	Cyanosis, dyspnea, shock, cardiac arrest	Stop transfusion; lower client's head and turn client on left side (air collects in right atrium where it can be gradually released to the lungs); notify physician

SOURCE: Adapted with permission from Saxton et al: *Addison–Wesley Manual of Nursing Practice*. Menlo Park, CA: Addison–Wesley, 1983.

occur in trauma cases (with massive hemorrhage) or before, during, or after cardiothoracic surgery. Autotransfusion can also be used in clients who have rare blood that is difficult to crossmatch.

The five methods for collecting and reinfusing a client's own blood are (Emminizer, 1981): elective phlebotomy, perioperative phlebotomy, intraoperative salvage and reinfusion, postoperative mediastinal collection, and collection and reinfusion from a client with a traumatic hemothorax. The advantages, disadvantages, and contraindications for autotransfusions are outlined in Table 28–6.

Elective phlebotomy is the withdrawal of the client's own blood for use at a later date. Blood may be collected from a client scheduled for surgery up to 8 weeks before the operation, so that autologous blood is available at the time of surgery. Elective phlebotomy is also used for clients with rare blood types. Clients with rare blood types or clients with rare antigens or antibodies who are difficult to crossmatch may have their blood frozen in case a transfusion is needed at a later date. A process of deglycerolization decreases the possibility of allergic and febrile reactions and preserves the red blood cells.

A second type of autotransfusion is perioperative phlebotomy with concomitant hemodilution. This technique is usually carried out just after the client has been anesthetized but before the surgery is performed. One or

Table 28–6 Advantages, Disadvantages, and Contraindications to Autotransfusion

Advantages	Disadvantages	Contraindications
Reduced usage of blood from blood bank	Potential contamination with gastrointestinal secretions if abdominal wound blood used	If contamination with gastrointestinal secretions occurs
Decreased cost to client	Potential for air embolus if air not aspirated from donating system	If abdominal wound is more than 4 h old
Eliminate transfusion reaction		If there is cancerous lesion in cavity from which blood is taken
Eliminate transmission of hepatitis, syphilis, and AIDS through blood transfusion		
Avoid religious conflicts		

two units of blood are withdrawn while 500 to 1000 mL of crystalloid or colloid is infused.

Intraoperative salvage or reinfusion of shed blood is the third type. The blood is collected and filtered during surgery in a commercially available autotransfusion system. Anticoagulants are then added, and the blood is reinfused into the client.

Postoperative collection of blood from mediastinal tubes from cardiac surgical clients is another type of autotransfusion. An autotransfusion collection system is attached to the client's mediastinal tubes at the completion of surgery, and the blood is collected by gravitational flow. The blood from the mediastinum does not require anticoagulation because of defibrination. Defibrination occurs as a result of the mechanical action of the heart and lungs as well as contact with the pericardial surface.

Collection and reinfusion of blood in the emergency department from a client with a traumatic hemothorax can also be used as an autotransfusion. Because there is no need to anticoagulate blood collected from the chest, an autotransfusion unit that works with chest tubes is attached, and the blood is rapidly reinfused.

APHERESIS

Apheresis is the process of separating whole blood into its major components—plasma, thrombocytes, erythrocytes, and leukocytes—and removing one of these components for use. Apheresis is used to replace cell components that are defective or insufficient.

Four types of apheresis may be performed. *Plasmapheresis* (plasma exchange) removes multiple liters of plasma that contain abnormal substances (ie, antigen–antibody complexes) and replaces this amount with a similar plasma solution. It is used in the treatment of hemolytic anemia, Goodpasture's syndrome, myasthenia gravis, renal transplant rejection syndrome, systemic lupus erythematosus, rheumatoid arthritis, multiple myeloma, biliary cirrhosis, hyperlipedemia, familial hypercholesterolemia, and cancer states in which substances in the plasma interfere with the client's immune system (Lopez & Hausz, 1982).

Lymphapheresis (leukapheresis), removal of abnormal or excessive WBCs, is used in the treatment of chronic lymphatic leukemia, rheumatoid arthritis, and multiple sclerosis. *Platelet pheresis* removes abnormal or excessive platelets and is instituted in treatment of thrombocytosis. *Red cell pheresis,* removal of abnormal or excessive erythrocytes, is used in the treatment of polycythemia vera and sickle cell anemia (Lopez & Hausz, 1982).

Although not a cure for the majority of these diseases, apheresis is a way of interfering with the disease process or preventing further pathophysiologic changes. Apheresis is used in conjunction with routine therapy and is a last resort to control the disease process.

Apheresis can be accomplished manually or mechanically. Manual apheresis requires centrifuging one unit of blood at one time, removing the wanted components, and reinfusing the remaining blood. Because this laborious and time-consuming process must be repeated several times, it is impractical. Mechanical apheresis, a more practical procedure, involves a continuous or noncontinuous process using a cell separator that allows large volumes (4 L) of the client's blood to be processed. Blood is withdrawn from the client (from a needle in one arm) and routed into a continuous-flow centrifuge machine, which separates the blood into four components and returns the wanted blood components back to the client through a needle in the opposite arm.

During the procedure, the client is confined for from 1 to 6 hours. If arm veins are used, the client must be aided in moving the arms during the procedure. If the femoral route is used, free movement of the legs is prevented. The client is requested to eat and void before the procedure because of the restriction on movement during the apheresis. (A bedpan may be used during the procedure.)

Immediately after the procedure, assess the client for bleeding and hematoma formation, electrolyte imbalance, edema secondary to hypoproteinemia, orthostatic hypotension due to hypovolemia, signs of fluid overload, and problems related to depleted erythrocyte stores. Also be alert for signs of a pyrogenic reaction.

Psychological support before, during, and after apheresis is necessary. Be aware of the client's and family's concerns and fears and be available for constant reassurance, clarification, and education.

BLOOD SUBSTITUTES

The search for a blood substitute has focused on the replacement of the oxygen-carrying capacity of erythrocytes. The experimental replacement for erythrocytes has fallen into three categories: perfluorochemicals, stroma-free hemoglobin, and oxygen-binding chelates.

Perfluorochemicals

Perfluorochemicals are synthetic compounds related to Teflon and Freon. Perfluorochemicals dissolve 40% to 60% oxygen per unit volume, approximately three times the capacity of blood, and also have a carbon-dioxide-carrying capacity three times greater than their ability to carry oxygen.

In their pure form, perfluorochemicals cannot act in the body unless they are emulsified, allowing for diffusion into cells and capillaries. In emulsion, larger particles are excreted more quickly (6 days) than smaller particles (up to 900 days). The process of emulsification and the size of particles is important because particles not excreted tend to aggregate in the liver and spleen. The effect on the liver and spleen is still unknown.

Fluosol-DA is a rapidly excreted perfluorochemical that was developed in Japan and has been used there. Over 200 Japanese clients have received the infusions without observable ill effects, but because no systematic studies have been done in Japan, Fluosol-DA is available only as an investigational drug in the United States and in Canada.

Perfluorochemicals have four major limitations. Perfluorochemical therapy requires the concomitant administration of 70% to 100% oxygen because perfluorochemicals do not extract oxygen from the air as hemoglobin does. This high oxygen administration exposes the client to oxygen toxicity (Leser, 1982). Another limitation of perfluorochemicals is the potential for thrombus formation, especially in the lungs, caused by alteration of platelet membranes. The lungs are a prime target because perfluorochemicals are excreted mainly by respiration. A third limitation is the lack of clotting factors, which are not replaced by perfluorochemicals. Despite this lack, bleeding has not been a problem in any subject, which may be explained by the hypothesis that a cut end of a capillary will constrict when there is a lack of blood. Infection could be a serious limitation because leukocytes are not replaced by perfluorochemical therapy. Thus, prophylactic antibiotics may need to be added to the perfluorochemicals.

Perfluorochemical therapy has several advantages. A unit of Fluosol-DA may be transfused immediately; there is no need to crossmatch or type because there are no antigens. Although frozen, refrozen, and autoclaved, perfluorochemicals will last indefinitely. There is a decreased risk of hepatitis. Perfluorochemicals are valuable in the treatment of carbon monoxide poisoning because they do not carry carbon monoxide. In the treatment of sickle cell crisis, they allow more carbon dioxide to be used and act as an antisickling agent. Because of their low viscosity, these agents are able to penetrate vessels occluded by sickled cells, perfusing the hypoxic areas (Leser, 1982).

Nurses must evaluate clients on this experimental product for four potential problems. Be aware of potential spleen and liver damage by assessing for organ enlargement and enzyme change. Oxygen toxicity and lung damage, which can occur from platelet aggregation, must be assessed when the client demonstrates coughing, nasal congestion, a sore throat, and substernal discomfort. Careful monitoring of vital signs, lab values, and wound sites aid in the detection of bleeding and infection (Leser, 1982).

Stroma-Free Hemoglobin

Stroma-free hemoglobin uses human hemoglobin stripped of the elements that clog capillaries. The substance has several advantages over other synthetic blood products: it functions well at low levels of oxygen, it has a colloidal osmotic effect and thus works as a plasma expander, it has a universal compatibility, and it can be stored indefinitely. Stroma-free hemoglobin also has several disadvantages: it can only be obtained from human donors; when it is metabolized, iron accumulates and iron toxicity develops; it will not solve problems related to agents that are toxic to hemoglobin (ie, carbon monoxide) because it will most likely be affected as well; and because it is a volume expander, the client with anemia who has an adequate circulating blood volume but a poor hemoglobin value must be monitored carefully for fluid overload (Leser, 1982).

Oxygen-Binding Chelates

Oxygen-binding chelates are erythrocyte substitutes that contain elements that act like hemoglobin—ie, they bind oxygen to themselves. Because these products use iron, they are subject to the same difficulties as stroma-free hemoglobin, particularly the development of iron toxicity. Also, this chelate requires storage temperatures of $-45°C$ to $-40°C$ and is therefore impractical to use (Leser, 1982).

Chapter Highlights

Disorders of the blood and blood-forming organs have the potential for causing widespread bodily changes, placing every other body system at risk for dysfunction.

Tissue changes make clients with disorders of the blood and blood-forming organs especially prone to alterations in comfort level.

Information regarding the client's tendency for bleeding episodes is an important part of establishing a thorough data base.

A detailed account of the client's exposure to drugs and chemicals is an important part of the nursing assessment because many drugs and chemicals may interfere with normal hematologic functioning.

Nursing assessment to determine abnormalities in blood-forming organs includes, but is not limited to,

assessment of organ enlargement and tenderness. The nurse's assessment of the client includes evaluation of color changes in the skin and mucous membranes and changes in circulatory integrity, such as capillary hemorrhages.

In physical assessment, changes in skin pigmentation and integrity, eyes and oral mucosa, range of motion and condition of the joints, and neurological functioning may provide clues about the progress of the disorder.

The CBC and WBC differential are the most important laboratory tests in diagnosing disorders of the blood and blood-forming organs. In bleeding disorders, coagulation studies are also important.

Client care problems to watch for in making the nursing diagnosis and care plan are alterations in comfort, impaired gas exchange, changes in mobility and ability to function independently, skin integrity, nutrition less than the client's bodily needs, lack of knowledge about the disease and its treatment, and impaired ability of clients and their significant others to cope with the impact of the disorder.

Blood or blood-component transfusions are indicated for provision of adequate tissue oxygenation, restoration of circulatory blood volume, and restoration of coagulation factors.

The nurse administering blood or blood components must ensure that the correct protocol is followed. This includes assessment of the client before the transfusion and close monitoring of the client during and after transfusion therapy.

Autotransfusion eliminates the possibility of a transfusion reaction and the transmission of hepatitis, syphilis, and AIDS.

Apheresis is not a cure for diseases such as hemolytic anemia, systemic lupus erythematosus, and leukemias but a way of interfering with pathophysiologic changes of the disease process.

Nursing evaluation of clients on synthetic blood products should include assessment for any organ enlargement or enzyme changes.

Bibliography

Bahu GAB: Administering blood safely. *AORN J* 1983; 37:1073–1077+.

Bates B: *A Guide to Physical Examination,* 3rd ed. Philadelphia: Lippincott, 1983.

Byrne JC et al: *Laboratory Tests: Implications for Nursing Care,* 2nd ed. Menlo Park, CA: Addison–Wesley, 1986.

Centers for Disease Control: Possible transfusion-associated acquired immune deficiency syndrome (AIDS). *MMWR* 1982; 31:652–654.

Centers for Disease Control: Prevention of acquired immune deficiency syndrome (AIDS): Report of interagency recommendations. *MMWR* 1983; 32:101–103.

Dyer KE: Lymphangiography. In: *Diagnostics.* Springhouse, PA: Intermed, 1982.

Emminizer S et al: Autotransfusion: Current status. *Heart Lung* 1981; 10:83–87.

Freedman ML: New thoughts on old blood. *Emerg Med* (July 15) 1982; 14:148–150+.

Fox LS: Granulocytopenia in the adult cancer patient. *Cancer Nurs* (April) 1980; 3:101–104.

Habel M: What you need to know about infusing plasma expanders. *RN* (Aug) 1980; 43:30–33.

King C: Exploring the neck and lymphatics. *RN* (June) 1982; 45:48–55.

Kirsch CM: Reticulocyte count. In: *Diagnostics.* Springhouse, PA: Intermed, 1982.

Leser DR: Synthetic blood: A future alternative. *Am J Nurs* 1982; 82:452–455.

Lopez JA, Hausz M: Therapeutic apheresis. *Am J Nurs* 1982; 82:1572–1578.

Rutman R, Miller W (editors): *Transfusion Therapy: Practices and Procedures,* 2nd ed. Rockville, MD: Aspen, 1985.

Smith LG: Reactions to blood transfusions. *Am J Nurs* 1984; 84:1096–1101.

Woods ME, Mazza I: Blood and component therapy. *Nurs Clin North Am* 1980; 15:629–646.

Suggested Readings

Bahu GAB: Administering blood safely. *AORN J* 1983; 37:1073–1077. This article gives thorough guidelines for administering blood safely to clients. The author describes the function and composition of blood, the ABO system, Rh typing, and type and crossmatching. She also gives a detailed and thorough description of transfusion reactions and associated nursing responsibility and intervention.

Benson ML, Benson DM: Autotransfusion is here—Are you ready? *Nurs 85* (March) 1985; 15:46–49. This brief article includes a valuable three-page illustrated guide of 14 photographs that demonstrate setting up an autotransfusion system.

King NH: Controlling bleeding when the platelet count drops. *RN* (Aug) 1984; 47:25–27. This brief article focuses on identifying thrombocytopenia early and taking steps to prevent or control bleeding. Two useful tables are included—drugs that can cause thrombocytopenia and when to monitor platelets.

Masoorli ST, Piercy S: A step-by-step guide to trouble-free transfusions. *RN* (May) 1984; 47:34–42. This article describes precautions to increase the safety of clients receiving transfusions. It also discusses the use of pumps and includes a sequence of photographs showing how to set up a piggyback transfusion line.

Resources

SELF-HELP GROUPS AND OTHER ORGANIZATIONS

American Association of Blood Banks
1828 L St., NW
Washington, DC 20036
Phone: (202) 872-8333

    This organization maintains a registry (National Clearinghouse for Blood Donation and Rare Donor File) to match blood demand with blood supply in collaboration with almost 2000 hospitals and blood banks throughout the country. It also provides information on blood and blood banking.

Cooley's Anemia Foundation, Inc.
420 Lexington Ave., Suite 1644
New York, NY 10017
Phone: (212) 697-7750

This organization provides educational programs, assistance with drugs and equipment, and referral programs to families affected by Cooley's anemia. Sponsors referral services to specialized centers for the diagnosis and treatment of Cooley's anemia and to screening programs for the detection of the trait. Publishes a monthly newsletter called *Lifeline*.

Leukemia Society of America, Inc.
211 E. 43rd St.
New York, NY 10017
Phone: (212) 573-8484

Supports research, client assistance, and public and professional education about leukemia and allied disorders including the lymphomas and Hodgkin's disease. This organization also provides financial assistance and maintains a list of state and local agencies that also offer financial assistance to leukemia clients as well as to those with Hodgkin's disease or non-Hodgkin's lymphoma.

National Association for Sickle Cell Disease, Inc.
945 S. Western Ave., Suite 206
Los Angeles, CA 90006
Phone: (213) 731-1166

This is an association of community groups involved in sickle cell programs throughout the United States and in the Bahamas. The organization is involved in the education of the public, health professionals, and government officials and helps to develop sickle cell testing and counseling programs.

National Foundation–March of Dimes
1275 Mamaroneck Ave.
White Plains, NY 10602
Phone: (914) 428-7100

This organization is concerned with preventing birth defects and genetic diseases such as sickle cell anemia and thalassemia. It disseminates information, sponsors research, and provides referrals for genetic counseling and treatment centers.

National Hemophilia Foundation
2 W. 39th St.
New York, NY 10018
Phone: (212) 869-9740

This voluntary health organization has over 50 chapters throughout the United States that provide information and services and sponsor research into the causes of and treatments for hemophilia or other related blood-clotting disorders. Local chapters can provide referrals to health specialists, treatment centers, and blood banks. Some local chapters have volunteers to help with inhome transfusions or transportation to local clinics or hospitals. Publishes the *Hemofax* newsletter.

National Leukemia Association
Roosevelt Field, Lower Concourse
Garden City, NY 11530
Phone: (516) 741-1190

This organization raises funds to help clients and their families with the costs of laboratory tests, radiation therapy and chemotherapy, blood transfusions, and related expenses not covered by the client's health insurance plan.

National Rare Blood Club
164 Fifth Ave.
New York, NY 10010
Phone: (212) 243-8037

This organization maintains a list of individuals who donate their rare blood without charge whenever needed. Membership information is in their brochure entitled *National Rare Blood Club of the Associated Health Foundation*.

In Canada:

Canadian Hemophilia Society
PO Box 2085
Hamilton, Ontario, Canada L8N 3R5
Phone: (416) 523-6414

This organization operates in all provinces and supports research, education, treatment, and client care services related to hemophilia and other coagulation disorders. Local phone books list branches.

Canadian Sickle Cell Society
1076 Bathurst St., Suite 305
Toronto, Ontario, Canada M5R 3G9
Phone: (416) 537-3475

This organization also has chapters in Alberta, Nova Scotia, and Quebec and publishes a quarterly, *Sickle Cell Digest*.

Families Leukemia Association
Canadian Cancer Society
130 Bloor St., W., Suite 1001
Toronto, Ontario, Canada M5S 2V7
Phone: (416) 961-7223

Support groups and support services for families of leukemia clients. No dues or fees. Semimonthly meetings and newsletter. See also Chapter 12 for organizations related to leukemia, lymphoma, Hodgkin's disease, and multiple myeloma.

HOT LINES

AIDS Hot Line
Phone: (800) 342-AIDS (Mon-Fri, 8:30 AM to 5:30 PM EST)

Sponsored by the US Public Health Service, this hot line gives a recorded informational message on AIDS. If the caller stays on the line, someone will be available to answer questions or respond to concerns.

National Gay Task Force Crisis Line
Phone: (800) 221-7044. In New York, call (212) 807-6016; 12 PM to 6 PM EST

Provides up-to-date information on AIDS.

HEALTH EDUCATION MATERIAL

From: AIDS Project
937 N. Cole Ave., Suite 3
Los Angeles, CA 90038
    This organization sponsors the International AIDS Archives. A complimentary AIDS reference list is available.

From: American Association of Blood Banks
    Questions and Answers About Blood and Blood Banking. This booklet contains answers to common questions about blood, blood components, blood transfusions, blood donation, and blood banking.

From: Kaposi's Sarcoma Research and
Educational Foundation
PO Box 14227
San Francisco, CA 94114
    A bibliography and information on Kaposi's sarcoma and AIDS are available.

From: National Hemophilia Foundation
    Educational Material List. An annotated catalog of books, articles, and special reports on all aspects of hemophilia is available to the general public and health education professionals.
    State and Federal Resources Guide for Hemophiliacs. A state-by-state listing of hemophilia programs and their eligibility requirements.

From: National Heart, Lung, and Blood
    Institute
Public Inquiries and Reports Branch
9000 Rockville Pike
Bethesda, MD 20014
    HEW Fact Sheet: Cooley's Anemia. Describes the causes, effects, diagnosis, and treatment of Cooley's anemia and summarizes related research.
    Special Report: Hemophilia. A brochure describing the most common types of hemophilia including classic hemophilia, von Willebrand's disease, and Christmas disease.

From: National Library of Medicine
Literature Search Program
Reference Section
8600 Rockville Pike
Bethesda, MD 20209
    A bibliography on AIDS is available. Include name and address typed on a gummed label (no return postage is necessary).

See also Chapter 12 for health education material on leukemia, lymphoma, multiple myeloma, and Hodgkin's disease.

Chapter 29

Specific Disorders of the Blood and Blood-Forming Organs

Linda Rae Belsky

Objectives

When you have finished studying this chapter, you should be able to:

Identify congenital disorders of the blood and blood-forming organs and the general nursing implications involved in dealing with these clients.

List the drugs that interfere with coagulation and discuss instructions nurses should give clients with hematologic disorders about taking medication.

Discuss the treatment measures for multifactorial hematologic disorders, including aplastic anemia, pernicious anemia, iron deficiency anemia, disseminated intravascular coagulation (DIC), idiopathic thrombocytopenic purpura (ITP), and granulocytopenia.

Identify the clinical manifestations and tests involved in the detection of immunologic disorders of the blood and blood-forming organs.

Describe the role of prevention in nursing interventions related to clients with acquired immune deficiency syndrome (AIDS).

Discuss the nursing interventions common to the care of clients with neoplastic disorders of the blood and blood-forming organs.

Differentiate among the types of leukemia and describe therapeutic measures used with them.

Explain the clinical staging method commonly used to classify Hodgkin's disease and non-Hodgkin's lymphoma (NHL) and the application of this method in treatment of these disorders.

Disorders of the blood and blood-forming organs pose complex problems for clients, their families, and nurses. Many of these disorders disrupt the immune system, reduce the ability to fight infection, and interfere with the ability to maintain vascular integrity and transport oxygen to the tissues. Thus, these conditions not only compromise health, they also threaten life. In addition to these physiologic problems, clients must cope with interrupted career plans, altered family roles, genetic counseling, changes in lifestyle, and possibly the uncertainty of their future.

Section I: Congenital Disorders

Congenital disorders of the blood and blood-forming organs include disease processes that affect the body's erythrocyte, leukocyte, and coagulation mechanisms. These disorders are present at birth and may be transmitted as autosomal dominant, autosomal recessive, or sex-linked traits.

General Nursing Implications

The role of the nurse is to educate the client to avoid or eliminate situations that may further compromise an already deficient bone marrow. The nurse must individualize client instruction according to the types of cells involved in the disease process. The nurse's role also includes providing psychosocial support to the client and family or significant others during genetic and career counseling. Parents of children with congenital disorders may experience guilt about causing their children's discomfort or poor prognosis. The nurse should assist the client and family members in expressing their feelings about the genetic nature of these disorders.

SICKLE CELL ANEMIA

In sickle cell anemia, the hemoglobin of sickle cells easily releases oxygen, and with deoxygenation, the erythrocyte takes on a sickle shape (Figure 29–1). Local hypoxia develops; sickling continues, leading to the plugging of vessels. In a sickle cell crisis, rigid sickled cells cause vaso-occlusion,

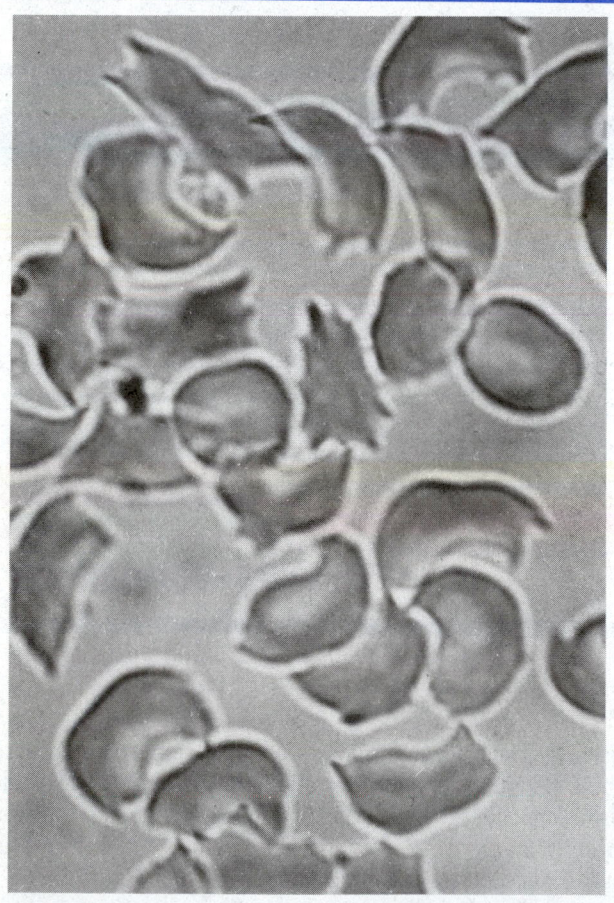

Figure 29–1

Unstained red cells containing hemoglobins incubated under reduced oxygen tension. Hemoglobin 5 crystallizes when the oxygen tension is reduced, causing red cells to assume bizarre sickle and holly-leaf shapes.

SOURCE: *Introduction to Human Disease*, by Leonard V. Crowley. Copyright © 1983 by Wadsworth, Inc. Reprinted by permission of Wadsworth Health Sciences Division, Monterey, CA and the author. Photo provided by Dr. Crowley.

which in turn leads to tissue anoxia and tissue death. Sickling usually occurs in areas prone to vascular hemostasis because of a relative hypoxia in these tissues. Once vaso-occlusion occurs, the cycle is repeated. Sickling syndromes include sickle cell–hemoglobin C disease, sickle cell–hemoglobin D disease, sickle cell–beta-thalassemia disease, and sickle cell anemia. This discussion centers around sickle cell anemia because it is the most prevalent and the most severe.

Sickle cell anemia, a genetic hemoglobinopathy, is inherited as an autosomal dominant trait. Individuals with sickle cell anemia are homozygous for the sickle cell gene. Those who are heterozygous for the gene have sickle cell trait; they do not have sickle cell anemia but are carriers (see Figure 29–2 for a diagram of the genetic transmission of sickle cell anemia). In the United States, sickle cell anemia is almost exclusively confined to the black population. An estimated one in nine US blacks has the sickle cell trait, and one in every four black infants born in the United States has sickle cell anemia (Williams et al., 1983). The incidence for sickle cell trait is highest in Africa where the frequency is usually about 20%.

Clinical Manifestations

Clinical manifestations of sickle cell anemia appear primarily as crises, which can involve any organ. The symptoms vary, depending on the area or areas involved. Pain is the most common clinical manifestation of a vaso-occlusive sickle cell crisis. Because each client manifests a sickling event in a unique way, it is important to become familiar with the variability of clinical manifestations.

Prime target organs are the spleen, bones, chest, and abdomen. The spleen is the most common target organ for sickling early in life. By adolescence, the client usually has had repeated crises leading to fibrosis and markedly decreased function of the spleen (autosplenectomy). Other target areas are the brain; eyes (particularly the retinas); ankles; liver; urinary system; and in the older sickle cell client, the lower extremities. Priapism (sustained penile erection) caused by sickling, venous congestion, and vascular stasis can be prolonged and painful. Scleral jaundice, occurring with liver involvement, may become exaggerated. Both sickle cell anemia and sickle cell trait are diagnosed by the sickle cell test (see Chapter 28).

Factors Precipitating a Crisis

Tissue hypoxia contributes to or precipitates a sickle cell crisis, as described. Some areas are normally relatively hypoxic. Tissue hypoxia also can be caused by general anesthesia, high altitudes, and air travel. Most commercial aircrafts are pressurized, but sickle cell anemia clients must avoid unpressurized aircraft cabins.

Environmental temperature also can precipitate a sickle cell crisis, so the client should avoid overexposure in both cold and hot weather. Cooling of a body part or cold weather can cause venous stasis with subsequent sickling. Hot weather also can precipitate a crisis by caus-

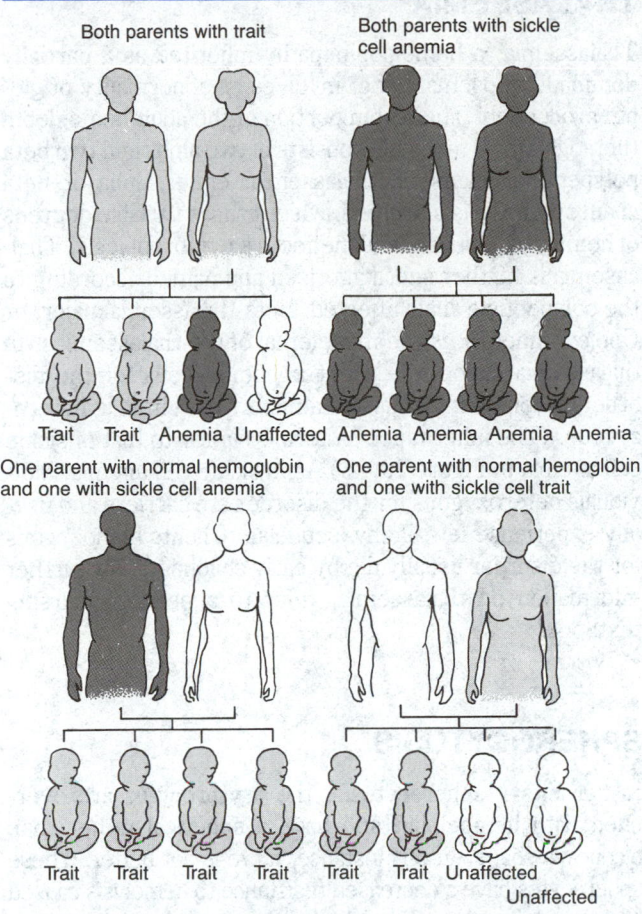

Figure 29–2

Inheritance of sickle cell anemia and sickle cell trait.

ing dehydration and, consequently, hyperviscosity of the blood. Hyperviscosity causes stasis of blood flow and resultant hypoxia. Hyperviscosity of the blood also can be caused by the relative high hematocrit levels in clients with sickle cell anemia.

Metabolic acidosis tends to contribute to sickle cell crises. Acidosis hastens the deoxygenation of the erythrocyte, causing sickling, and the sickled erythrocyte predisposes the client to vaso-occlusion and a crisis (Williams et al., 1983).

Infections, especially of the lungs, also can cause sickle cell crises. The crisis in pulmonary infection may be related to concurrent fever, hypoxia, and acidosis (Williams et al., 1983). For both the adult and pediatric sickle cell anemia population, pneumococcal pneumonia and pulmonary infarction are common. Distinguishing between the two complications is difficult because the signs and symptoms (fever, leukocytosis, chest pain, and pulmonary infiltrates) may be identical. Fever, leukocytosis, and pulmonary infiltrates usually indicate pneumonia, the most common cause of hospitalization for the sickle cell anemia client. In adults, the most common organisms causing pneumonia are *Staphylococcus aureus* and *Hemophilus influenzae*, whereas in children the most common cause is *Diplococcus pneumoniae*. Both adults and children with sickle cell anemia can develop mycoplasmal pneumonia.

Infectious Complications

The sickle cell anemia client is prone to other infectious complications as well. The homozygous client has an increased risk for bacterial infections from *Streptococcus pneumonia, Salmonella, Hemophilus influenzae, Escherichia coli,* and *Klebsiella.* Deficient splenic activity and an ineffective immune system may play a role in this increased risk (Landsman, Rao, & Ahonkhai, 1982).

Central Nervous System Complications

Central nervous system (CNS) complications can be life threatening. Cerebral infarction, the most common and dangerous, has an overall incidence in sickle cell clients of 6% to 7% (Sarnaik & Lusher, 1982). Usually, cerebral infarction occurs without warning signs, but the most common sign is sudden hemiparesis. Transient visual disturbances, seizures, or both may accompany the cerebral infarction. Aphasia is common if the dominant cerebral hemisphere is infarcted. A CNS infarction is diagnosed by the clinical signs and symptoms, by examination of the cerebrospinal fluid by spinal tap, and by computerized tomography (CT) scan.

Another CNS complication is intracranial hemorrhage. Sickling is thought to damage the blood vessel walls, causing thinning, dilation, and eventual rupture of the vessel. Intracranial hemorrhage may occur alone or with other altered health states such as pneumonia, painful sickle cell crisis, or pregnancy. The overall incidence of intracranial hemorrhage in sickle cell anemia is 1.5% to 2.7% (Sarnaik & Lusher, 1982). Clinical manifestations include a change in the level of consciousness, headache, vomiting, and signs and symptoms of meningeal irritation. Diagnosis is made by lumbar puncture and CT scan.

Therapeutic Measures

The treatment of vaso-occlusive crisis includes transfusion therapy, usually with packed red blood cells (RBCs). The goal of transfusion is to dilute the percentage of sickled cells, improve circulation, enhance oxygenation, and dislodge the sickled cells. Concomitant hydration with IV fluids is also performed. Analgesics provide pain relief, with narcotic analgesics prescribed for severe pain. Oxygen is administered in an attempt to decrease the hypoxia. Bed rest decreases the metabolic demands of all body tissues. Affected joints may be splinted to decrease pain.

Simple transfusion therapy, partial exchange transfusion, or both improve the course of many other complications of sickle cell anemia, including pulmonary crisis with or without pneumonia, **splenic sequestration** (the trapping of sickled erythrocytes by the spleen), and priapism. Transfusion therapy can also control or alter chronic illnesses associated with sickle cell anemia, such as leg ulcers, blindness, recurrent painful sickle cell crises, and heart disease. Transfusion therapy is also used for sickle cell clients undergoing surgery and general anesthesia to decrease the risk of general anesthesia precipitating hypoxia and hyperviscosity. Preoperative preparation with simple exchange transfusions decreases the percentage of sickled cells (Schmalzer, Chien, & Brown, 1982).

A CNS infarction is treated with either a simple transfusion or a partial exchange transfusion and adequate hydration. These two measures decrease the percentage of circulating hemoglobin S erythrocytes; improve oxygenation to the CNS; and, it is hoped, improve circulation in the infarcted area. Assess the client for seizure activity and attempt to control the increased intracranial pressure associated with the infarction. CNS infarction can recur, and the death rate is high with repeated episodes.

CNS infarction is easier to prevent than treat, so prophylactic transfusion therapy is recommended for clients with one episode. Transfusions are administered to maintain a hemoglobin level between 11 and 12 g/dL, keeping the hemoglobin S population at less than 25% of the total circulating blood volume (Sarnaik & Lusher, 1982). Preventive transfusion programs carry the risks of viral hepatitis, transfusion reactions, irregular erythrocyte antibody production, iron overload, infection, and hyperviscosity.

Specific Nursing Measures

The overall nursing goal with sickle cell anemia clients is to prevent crises through extensive teaching and to reinforce and assess compliance with both the medical and nursing regimens. The client and family or significant others should be taught about the maintenance of hydration, prevention of infection, avoidance of temperature extremes of cold and heat, and career and genetic counseling. A sedentary career is necessary, because these clients have decreased oxygen-carrying capacity and exercise tolerance. They should not be inactive, however, and should be encouraged to develop regular exercise habits that include activities such as walking, bicycling, bowling, or swimming. They should avoid contact sports or vigorous exercise.

Continually assess and monitor all areas of the client's body for physical signs and symptoms indicating a sickling episode. During a painful crisis episode, monitor the client's serum pH, assess for acidosis (see Chapter 5), provide adequate hydration in the form of IV and oral fluids, and administer analgesics for pain relief. Packed RBCs may be administered in circumstances such as CNS infarction, priapism, lung or liver involvement, and hepatitis. Monitor hemoglobin and hematocrit values during transfusion therapy and observe for hyperviscosity (ie, increased signs and symptoms of sickling). Normothermia is maintained to decrease the client's oxygen demands. The nurse may administer oxygen therapy during the acute period of sickle cell crisis.

THALASSEMIA

Thalassemia, a hemoglobinopathy inherited as a partially dominant autosomal gene, involves an abnormality of globin production. The globin portion of the adult hemoglobin (hemoglobin A) molecule consists of two alpha and two beta polypeptide chains. In thalassemia, either alpha or beta chain synthesis is disrupted, which causes variable degrees of hemolysis, anemia, and ineffective erythropoiesis. Thalassemia is further subcatagorized and named according to the polypepticle chain affected. Beta-thalassemia major, or Cooley's anemia, is the most lethal of the thalassemias. In thalassemia major, the client is homozygous for the disorder, whereas in thalassemia minor, the client is heterozygous. (The inheritance pattern is similar to that of sickle cell anemia in Figure 29–2.) As in sickle cell anemia, individuals heterozygous for the disorder are carriers and usually experience few, if any, sequelae. Clients homozygous for the disorder usually die by early childhood. For further information on thalassemia, refer to a pediatric nursing textbook.

SPHEROCYTOSIS

In hereditary spherocytosis, the erythrocytes are overfilled with hemoglobin and have a spherical rather than biconcave shape. In this instance, more is not better. These spherocytes have a decreased resistance to hemolysis caused by hypotonic solutions, a shortened erythrocyte life span, and increased splenic sequestration—characteristics that can lead to anemia.

When anemia occurs, the bone marrow compensates by undergoing hyperplasia. The peripheral blood count demonstrates reticulocytosis and an elevation of the mean corpuscular hemoglobin concentration. Crises can also arise from a temporary inhibition of erythropoiesis. Life-threatening crises, signaled by a dramatic drop in the hemoglobin concentration, are rare. The majority of clients experience no complications of the disorder and lead relatively healthy lives.

Hereditary spherocytosis is transmitted as a mendelian-dominant trait; therefore, one of the parents is also affected. To date, all individuals affected with hereditary spherocytosis have been heterozygous for the defect. Most clients can trace their ancestry to northern or western European countries.

Clinical Manifestations

Spherocytosis may go undetected. The most prominent clinical feature is chronic anemia demonstrated by pallor. Mild to moderate splenomegaly may also be present. In addition to the changes in the bone marrow and peripheral blood already mentioned, hyperbilirubinemia is also present.

Therapeutic Measures

Splenectomy is recommended for all clients diagnosed as having hereditary spherocytosis. The procedure does not correct the erythrocyte defect but rather removes the major organ responsible for the destruction and removal of the spherocyte from the circulation, avoiding dramatic decreases in RBCs. The rationale for splenectomy is the inability to predict which clients will undergo spontaneous, life-threatening crises. For clients with little or no anemia, the risk of surgery may seem too great. Splenectomy is a relatively safe surgical procedure for clients over 4 years of age, however.

Specific Nursing Measures

The initial goal of nursing management of the client with spherocytosis is adequate education. At diagnosis, thoroughly explain the disease process, including the signs and symptoms indicating anemia and crises. Teach the client to seek medical attention immediately whenever the symptoms of anemia appear or worsen. See Chapter 30 for nursing care for the splenectomy client.

GLUCOSE-6-PHOSPHATE DEHYDROGENASE DEFICIENCY

Glucose-6-phosphate dehydrogenase (G-6-PD) deficiency is a hereditary intrinsic disorder of the erythrocytes resulting in hemolysis under certain conditions such as infection, the administration of certain drugs, and exposure to fava beans. The enzyme deficiency results in a usually mild and self-limiting anemia; in the presence of these special conditions, however, the anemia may have a sudden, dramatic onset.

The incidence of G-6-PD deficiency varies by ethnic and racial background. Among whites, the incidence ranges from 1 in 1000 among northern European descendants to 50% among Kurdish Jews. The disorder is also found in Southeast Asians and the Chinese (Williams et al., 1983). Sickle cell anemia clients may also have G-6-PD deficiency.

The sex-linked hereditary disorder is passed from mother to son, never from father to son. Because females heterozygous for this disorder have one normal and one abnormal gene, they vary in their genetic expression of this disease.

Clinical Manifestations

The most frequent manifestation of a hemolytic episode of G-6-PD deficiency is anemia. The client may become pale and, in severe hemolysis, have shortness of breath and abdominal or back pain. The urine may turn dark and even black.

The laboratory diagnosis of G-6-PD deficiency is made by a simple blood test to determine the level of G-6-PD.

The normal value varies according to the actual laboratory procedure used, but usually G-6-PD is present in substantial amounts. Individuals with levels below what is considered normal for that laboratory are considered G-6-PD deficient.

Therapeutic Measures

Because most episodes of hemolysis are self-limiting, no intervention is usually necessary. No specific drug therapy is indicated for G-6-PD deficiency, but clients should *avoid* certain drugs, including analgesics (eg, acetanilid, aspirin, and phenacetin), sulfonamides, sulfones, antimalarials, nitrofurantoin (Furadantin), chloramphenicol (Chloromycetin), furazolidone (Furoxone), aminosalicylate sodium (para-aminosalicylic acid [PAS]), ascorbic acid (vitamin C), naphthalene, methylene blue, and phenylhydrazine (Williams et al., 1983). A complete list of these drugs can be obtained from any pharmacy. Clients should avoid ingestion of fava beans. If hemolysis is severe, transfusion therapy with packed RBCs may be administered.

Specific Nursing Measures

The nursing management of the client with G-6-PD deficiency consists of providing information on the disease process, including stimuli initiating a hemolytic episode and signs and symptoms indicating hemolysis. Send a list of agents causing hemolysis home with clients and encourage them to read labels of all over-the-counter (OTC) drugs to avoid the accidental ingestion of these compounds.

HEMOPHILIA

Hemophilia is a hereditary disorder of coagulation in which increased bleeding tendencies are caused by a deficiency of coagulation factors VIII and IX. Recall from Chapter 22 that the blood's ability to form a fibrin clot depends on platelets and clotting factors. In hemophilia, the decrease of available factors VIII and IX makes severe bleeding episodes more likely.

The two classes of hemophilia are hemophilia A and hemophilia B. Hemophilia A is the more common, and the ratio of the occurrence of hemophilia A to hemophilia B is approximately 7:1. Hemophilia A, often referred to as *classic hemophilia* or simply *hemophilia*, involves a deficiency of factor VIII. Hemophilia B, also known as *Christmas disease*, results from a deficiency of factor IX. Clinically, hemophilia A and B are identical.

In hemophilia A, the severity of the bleeding tendency closely correlates with the amount of factor VIII available. Hemophilia A can be subdivided into three groups representing the different levels of available factor VIII. Clients with mild hemophilia A have 6% to 30% of factor VIII; moderate hemophilia A clients have 1% to 6% of factor VIII; those with severe hemophilia A have less than factor VIII. The level of factor VIII rarely fluctuates from person to person within the same affected family or within the affected client (Williams et al., 1983).

Hemophilia A and B are genetically transmitted as a sex-linked recessive trait; transmission is from mother to son. In rare instances, hemophilia can be transmitted to a daughter when the mother is a carrier and the father has the disease. It is possible to detect female carriers of the disease through laboratory serum studies.

Because hemophilia occurred in the genes of the ruling families in Russia, Spain, and Germany, it was known as the royal disease. The disorder was originally transferred from Queen Victoria of England (in the 1800s) who was believed to be the first carrier in her family, through her daughters who married members of royalty in other European countries. England's reigning family, beginning with Queen Victoria's son Edward VII, escaped the disorder. Today, hemophilia is far more widespread than the descendants of these royal families. In the United States alone, it is estimated that 1 in 7000 males is born with hemophilia, and the number of hemophiliacs is estimated at 20,000 (Couric, 1984).

Clinical Manifestations

Clinical manifestations of severe factor VIII or IX deficiency may be detected during the neonatal period following circumcision. Milder forms of hemophilia may not be detected until childhood or adolescence, when prolonged bleeding follows a tooth extraction. The most common clinical manifestation is hemarthrosis (bleeding into the joint) in the knee; however, the hip, ankle, shoulder, elbow, and wrist also can be affected. The client frequently has a history of only mild trauma to the involved joint, which becomes painful, swollen, tender, and stiff. Later complications of hemarthrosis include loss of joint motion, contracture formation, muscle atrophy, and joint degeneration and deformity.

Hematomas may form with only slight trauma. Bleeding, most commonly subcutaneous or intramuscular, primarily involves the lower extremities. Enough blood may be lost into a thigh to cause symptoms of shock. Petechiae do not accompany ecchymotic areas. Other manifestations of hemorrhage include epistaxis, hematuria, swelling of the tongue (from accidentally biting it while eating), paresthesias (from pressure on a nerve by bleeding into tissues), and ischemia (from pressure on blood vessels). The most life-threatening complication of hemophilia is intracranial hemorrhage. Superficial cuts usually do not cause undue problems.

Hemophilia is diagnosed by laboratory serum determinations. Tests include serum calcium, prothrombin time (PT), partial thromboplastin time (PTT), quantitative platelets, coagulation factors assay, and antibody directed against factor VIII (for hemophilia A). Serum calcium level, PT, and platelet count are normal in hemophilia, and PTT prolonged.

Therapeutic Measures

Drug therapy is not used in the management of hemophilia, except possibly to treat joint pain, which may become severe enough to require narcotics. The major emphasis is on the client avoiding all drugs that increase bleeding time. These include anticoagulant drugs such as heparin sodium and warfarin; fibrinolytic agents such as streptokinase and urokinase; nonsteroidal anti-inflammatory drugs (NSAIDs) such as indomethacin (Indocin), and phenylbutazone (Butazolidin); antineoplastic agents; and miscellaneous drugs affecting platelet function such as aspirin, sulfinpyrazone (Anturane), dipyridamole, IV dextran, and guaifenesin. Because many OTC preparations contain aspirin or aspirin products, encourage clients to read medication labels before ingestion. Ideally, the client should avoid all OTC preparations to avoid accidental aspirin ingestion.

The maintenance or promotion of optimal nutritional status ensures good dental hygiene. Because hemophiliacs bleed excessively after dental extractions, preventing dental cavities and, ultimately, tooth extraction is the goal of nutritional management.

Administration of the appropriate factor concentrate is an important treatment measure prophylactically as well as during episodes of acute bleeding. The administration of factor concentrate is discussed in the section on specific nursing measures.

Specific Nursing Measures

The nursing management of hemophilia can be divided into three phases: the diagnostic phase, acute bleeding episodes, and the home setting.

In the diagnostic phase, assess all clients for prolonged bleeding following minor surgical procedures. Clients with this characteristic need further medical investigation.

Nursing management during an acute bleeding episode involves the IV administration of the deficient factor—either factor VIII AHF human (Factorate, Factor VIII, Hemofil, Hemafac) or factor IX human (Koȳne, Proplex) (see Chapter 28). With joint pain and hemarthrosis, splinting or casting the involved joint may be indicated. Whenever a client with hemophilia is admitted to the hospital, nursing assessments are directed toward the prompt recognition of hemorrhage.

Factor concentrates make surgery possible for clients with hemophilia. These clients still carry a considerably increased risk, however, so surgery should be performed only when absolutely necessary to save life.

Many hemophiliacs administer factor concentrate prophylactically at home, usually several times weekly. The advantages of home management include fewer episodes of hospitalization for major bleeding episodes, a decreased incidence of major bleeding episodes and subsequent orthopedic complications, better school and work attendance, and a sense of control. The home administration of factor concentrate is not without risks, however; poor administration technique can lead to sepsis and vessel damage. Not all clients or families are appropriate candidates. The responsibility and accountability may prove too stressful for some. Moreover, a home care program for hemophiliacs does not end the responsibility of medical or nursing professionals. Close monitoring and assessment of the client's understanding and performance of IV venipuncture and factor concentrate administration must continue.

Regardless of whether clients undertake home administration of factor concentrate, adequate client education is necessary. The client and family or friends must recognize early signs and symptoms necessitating medical interventions. Superficial cuts, which usually do not cause undue bleeding, can be treated in the home using cold compresses or ice bags. Clients with hemophilia should be told to wear a medical identification bracelet indicating the kind of hemophilia they have.

Clients with hemophilia may have an increased risk for developing acquired immune deficiency syndrome (AIDS) because of contamination of factor concentrate with the virus suspected of causing AIDS. Heat treatment of factor concentrate destroys the virus. Through recombinant DNA technology, a factor concentrate is being developed that may eliminate the risk for developing AIDS. Furthermore, new quality controls will ensure a more potent, reliable product while lowering costs.

Encourage clients with hemophilia to seek career counseling. Because hemarthrosis is the most frequent cause of hospitalization for the hemophiliac, clients clearly should avoid jobs requiring physical exertion. The National Hemophilia Foundation may prove beneficial and informative for some clients (see the resources list at the end of Chapter 28).

VON WILLEBRAND'S DISEASE

Von Willebrand's disease is a hereditary disorder of coagulation involving a dysfunction of thrombocytes and a deficiency of factor VIII. Von Willebrand's disease is diagnosed by a battery of diagnostic tools that determine the client's bleeding time. Included are tests on platelets, PT, PTT, factor VIII (antihemolytic factor) activity, factor VIII$_{AGN}$ (antigen) activity, and factor VIII$_{VWF}$ (von Willebrand's factor) activity.

Factor VIII$_{AHF}$, which is deficient in clients with von Willebrand's disease, seems to be necessary for proper platelet functioning. Factor VIII$_{AGN}$ activity indicates the presence of an antigen that is precipitated by a rabbit antibody to factor VIII. Clients having severe forms of von Willebrand's disease totally lack this antigen. Specifically, factor VIII$_{VWF}$ is necessary for platelets to adhere to sites of vascular injury and plug the leak. A deficiency of factor VIII$_{VWF}$ seems to be responsible for the prolonged bleeding time associated with von Willebrand's disease.

Von Willebrand's disease is inherited as an autosomal dominant trait. Unlike hemophilia, how von Willebrand's disease is expressed varies among affected individuals within the same family. The level of factor VIII and platelet dysfunction also varies at different times for the same individual.

Clinical Manifestations

As in hemophilia, abnormal bleeding in von Willebrand's disease begins in early childhood. Epistaxis and ecchymoses are common, whereas petechiae are not. Fatal bleeding episodes occur but are extremely rare. The hemarthrosis in von Willebrand's disease differs from that in hemophilia. Hemarthrosis is not common in von Willebrand's disease, and joint damage is not permanent. In contrast, hemarthrosis is common in hemophilia. Hemophiliac clients have repeated episodes of hemarthrosis involving the same joint, whereas von Willebrand's clients do not. Although excessive bleeding following surgery can be a problem, it can be managed with the infusion of factor VIII concentrate. Von Willebrand's disease decreases in severity as the client ages; hemophilia does not.

Therapeutic Measures

Encourage the client to read labels on all medications and to avoid all OTC preparations, if possible. All medications that interfere with bleeding time, such as aspirin, should be avoided. See the discussion of hemophilia for a list of drugs that interfere with coagulation.

Specific Nursing Measures

Specific nursing measures for von Willebrand's disease are similar to those for hemophilia clients. The primary aim is to avoid major bleeding episodes. The client and family or significant others need thorough explanations of the disease process and the manifestations that warrant medical interventions. These include prolonged or excessive bleeding from the nose, gastrointestinal tract, or subcutaneous tissue. One of the most common indications of gastrointestinal bleeding is black, tarry stools. Painful or swollen joints may signal hemarthrosis. All minor and major surgery necessitates prophylactic therapy with factor VIII concentrate. Advise clients to wear a medical identification bracelet stating they have von Willebrand's disease.

Section II: Disorders of Multifactorial Origin

Multifactorial disorders of the blood and blood-forming organs may be precipitated by (1) a nutritional deficiency, (2) environmental or chemical toxins, (3) other disease processes, or (4) no known cause. Any of the bone marrow elements may be involved, resulting in an inability of the body to resist infectious organisms, a deficiency in the blood's ability to coagulate, or an alteration in the body's ability to transport oxygen to tissues. Some acquired hematologic diseases interfere in only one of these functions; in others, the entire bone marrow may fail.

General Nursing Implications

The role of the nurse in the management of acquired hematologic disorders includes client education on the disease process and assessment of client compliance with prescribed medications. Include instruction on avoiding situations that an ineffective bone marrow cannot master, such as resisting infection, maintaining vascular integrity, or sustaining adequate tissue oxygenation. Provide emotional support to clients having disorders with poor prognoses. A strong trusting relationship between the client and family or significant others and the nurse provides emotional support, and consistent caregivers can initiate and maintain a therapeutic trusting relationship. Primary nursing is an ideal way to achieve these goals.

APLASTIC ANEMIA

Aplastic anemia can be an acquired or congenital hematologic disorder. The disorder is characterized by a decrease in the hematopoietic tissue, its replacement by fatty bone marrow, and marked pancytopenia. The three hallmarks of aplastic anemia are *leukopenia, anemia,* and *thrombocytopenia.*

The etiology of aplastic anemia can be classified as idiopathic or secondary. Idiopathic aplastic anemia has no known cause and can be further classified as either congenital (Fanconi's anemia) or acquired. Secondary aplastic anemia involves the client's prior exposure to stimuli such as chemicals (eg, benzene or dichlorodiphenyltrichloroethane [DDT]), radiation, environmental toxins, drugs (eg, chloramphenicol or cytotoxic drugs), or immunologic injury. Aplastic anemia may also be related to a defect in the regulation of blood cell production by the bone marrow, a defect of the bone marrow tissue themselves, or both. Regardless of the etiology, the overall result is a decrease in the amount of functional bone marrow.

Clinical Manifestations

Clinical manifestations of aplastic anemia are related to the pancytopenia. Clients have symptoms of severe bone marrow depression: pallor, tiredness, repeated infections, malaise, and bleeding tendencies. Bleeding tendencies may be occult or conspicuous; major or minor, such as gastrointestinal bleeding versus gingival oozing; or in the form of purpura or petechiae. Hepatosplenomegaly is usually not present at diagnosis.

Diagnosis is made by bone marrow aspiration, bone marrow biopsy (discussed in Chapter 28), or both. The bone marrow is found to contain primarily hypocellular fatty deposits.

Therapeutic Measures

Supportive therapy is prescribed to help the client maintain as normal a life as possible. Therapy includes blood and platelet transfusions. Infections are treated aggressively, especially when the client is symptomatic. Reverse isolation may be used, possibly including a laminar air flow unit to purify the air.

Bone marrow transplantation (see Chapter 30) is effective for clients with aplastic anemia. Bone marrow can be transplanted from identical twins or human leukocyte antigen (HLA)-compatible siblings. Bone marrow-stimulating agents also may be used. Steroids stimulate hematopoiesis. Androgens increase erythropoiesis, possibly by increasing the release of erythropoietin and the bone marrow's response to it. Both steroids and androgens hold promise for the treatment of children but not adults.

Clients with aplastic anemia need a high-fiber diet to allow easy defecation, because straining at stool can precipitate a bleeding episode. Clients undergoing bone marrow transplantation also need nutritional support.

Specific Nursing Measures

The client receiving androgens needs psychological support. Assess the feelings of the client and significant others toward body image changes caused by androgen and prednisone therapy. (These body image changes are discussed in Chapter 41.) Be aware of the nonverbal messages others send to the client and strive to demonstrate a personal acceptance of the client's altered body appearance. The client and significant others should be encouraged to express their feelings.

Assessment of the aplastic anemic client should include gathering data relating to the client's progress in school or work, noting particularly any difficulty in developing and maintaining peer relationships. The client with aplastic anemia may be prohibited from engaging in sexual intercourse because severe leukopenia and thrombocytopenia increase the possibility of infection or bleeding. Suggest sexual counseling or refer the client to a sex counselor when indicated. Maintaining existing relationships between the client and family members and significant others should be a primary goal guiding nursing care. Include family members and significant others in the client's care and education whenever possible. Securing close contact and involvement with family members and significant others can provide the client needed affection and a feeling of belonging.

Collect data on hobbies; activities of daily living; exposure to chemical agents in the home, school, or work environment; and possible exposure to radiation. Also thoroughly investigate the client's use of prescription and OTC drugs. Pay particular attention to the client's safety; avoid infection and prevent bleeding episodes. This means not using intramuscular injections or straight-edged razors. Special soft toothbrushes and stool softeners may be needed.

Blood component therapy in the form of packed RBCs, platelets, and granulocytes may be administered.

PERNICIOUS ANEMIA

Pernicious anemia is characterized by a metabolic defect involving the absence of intrinsic factor (IF), a protein (possibly a globulin) secreted by the gastric mucosa. (Intrinsic factor is discussed in Chapter 46.) Its chief purpose is to combine with extrinsic factor (vitamin B_{12}) for transport to the ileum. Once deposited in the ileum, vitamin B_{12} can be absorbed. In the absence of IF, vitamin B_{12} deficiency develops.

Vitamin B_{12} is necessary for proper growth and maturation of all body cells; but cells of the bone marrow, the gastrointestinal tract, and the central nervous system are especially vulnerable to deficiencies in this vitamin. Vitamin B_{12} deficiency affects normal erythropoiesis and granulocytopoiesis, but the major impact of vitamin B_{12} deficiency is on the erythrocyte. The erythrocyte demonstrates both anisocytosis (abnormal size)—in this case, it is abnormally large—and poikilocytosis (abnormal shape). The membrane of the vitamin B_{12}-deficient erythrocyte is also extremely fragile and ruptures easily. The effect on the erythrocyte is so profound that anemia develops.

Vitamin B_{12} also plays a major role in the proper formation of myelinated nerves. Vitamin B_{12} deficiency causes widespread demyelination of nerves and degeneration of white matter. Untreated pernicious anemia has a progressive and usually terminal course. Spontaneous remissions have been known to occur but are rare.

Pernicious anemia is thought to be caused by a single autosomal dominant defect. It occurs predominantly in light-skinned, blue-eyed people of northwest European, Scandinavian, or British descent. The disorder seems to involve a predisposition for atrophy of the secreting glands of the gastric mucosa (found on postmortem examination). Along with this atrophy, IF, pepsin, and hydrochloric acid are absent in the gastric juices. Other causes of pernicious anemia include gastrectomy, gastric cancer, infestation by fish tapeworms, and malabsorption problems involving the ileum.

Clinical Manifestations

Because of vitamin B_{12} therapy, the classic clinical manifestations of pernicious anemia are rare today. However, because vitamin B_{12} has such profound effects on hematopoiesis and the normal structure and function of the nervous system, a review of these manifestations is warranted.

The onset of pernicious anemia occurs in late middle adult life. The first clinical manifestations are usually those of anemia. Clients demonstrate pallor with slight icterus, as well as lassitude and weakness disproportionate to the degree of existing anemia. Most red cell indices of the peripheral blood count are abnormal. Quantitative erythrocyte counts may be as low as 2 million μL; the hemo-globin level is approximately 8 g/dL; and mean corpuscular volume (MCV) is elevated. Only the mean corpuscular hemoglobin count (MCHC) is normal. As already stated, the peripheral blood smear demonstrates anisocytosis and poikilocytosis. These changes demonstrate the impact of vitamin B_{12} on normal erythrocyte maturation.

Neurologic manifestations of pernicious anemia also show the important role of vitamin B_{12} on nerve structure and subsequent nerve function. Demyelination of nerves and degeneration of white matter occur in vitamin B_{12}-deficient states. The loss of vibratory sense may be the first clue in the diagnosis of pernicious anemia. Numbness and tingling of the extremities can follow. As demyelination and degeneration continue, paralysis and psychosis may develop. Once neurologic damage has occurred, neurologic function may not be regained.

The stomach atrophies and loses its acid- and enzyme-secreting abilities, developing achlorhydria and achylia. The remainder of the intestinal tract enlarges, and digestion becomes difficult as the disease progresses.

Pernicious anemia is diagnosed by the Schilling test. Gastric analysis may also be used. In addition, multiple laboratory studies are performed on the peripheral blood both before and after the initiation of vitamin B_{12} therapy. Examination of the bone marrow rules out any other existing hematologic disorders. A thorough neurologic examination, including a test of vibratory sense, should be part of the client's history and physical examination.

Therapeutic Measures

Treatment of pernicious anemia once consisted of daily feedings of raw or rare liver. Later, crude liver extract was developed, but it lost major potency when administered orally. Liver extract was painful when administered IM, stained tissues, and sometimes caused tissue necrosis. Finally in 1948, the red cystalline factor now known as vitamin B_{12}, or cyanocobalamin, was discovered. This vitamin has all the antianemic principles of crude liver extract and is the elusive extrinsic factor. Current treatment of pernicious anemia includes regular injections of vitamin B_{12}.

Specific Nursing Measures

Nursing management of pernicious anemia includes client support and education during the diagnostic phase, client education about the disease process and the importance of compliance with lifelong vitamin B_{12} therapy, and assessment and rehabilitation of clients with neurologic changes. The client with pernicious anemia will need assistance to complete activities of daily living until the lassitude and weakness are resolved. Encourage these clients to rest frequently and make every effort not to tire them by long and vigorous days of testing.

After the diagnosis of pernicious anemia and the initiation of vitamin B_{12} therapy, the client's hemogram quickly returns to normal. Results of the peripheral blood smear may begin to improve as early as 4 days after the initiation of vitamin therapy. In addition, a dramatically increased sense of well-being accompanies the hematologic improvement. The client with pernicious anemia is committed to a lifetime of vitamin B_{12} therapy. Noncompliance causes the return of symptoms and possibly more dramatic consequences, such as neurologic involvement. Thus, these clients must understand the rationale for vitamin B_{12} therapy and comply completely with the chemotherapeutic regimen. Vitamin B_{12} therapy administered before the onset of neurologic signs and symptoms is ideal. When these signs and symptoms have already appeared, prompt and accurate diagnosis and treatment are imperative. Physical therapy may help restore some use and function, but residual neurologic damage may persist for life.

IRON DEFICIENCY ANEMIA

Iron deficiency anemia is a microcytic, hypochromic disorder of the erythrocyte; in other words, the erythrocyte is small and pale because of a reduction in hemoglobin concentration. The causative factor is usually inadequate dietary intake of foods containing iron. Clients at high risk for iron deficiency anemia are menstruating, pregnant, and lactating females. Blacks have a higher incidence of iron deficiency anemia than whites.

Clinical Manifestations

Clinical signs and symptoms of iron deficiency anemia depend on the condition's severity. The client feels chronically tired and may be pale. The erythrocyte is microcytic and hypochromic. Laboratory studies indicate a hemoglobin level of less than 12 g/dL, decreased serum ferritin levels, increased total iron-binding capacity, and decreased iron stores in the bone marrow. Clients with severe anemia may have malaise, tachycardia, and shortness of breath on exertion.

Therapeutic Measures

Iron supplementation may be given by a parenteral or oral route. The injectable iron preparation is often painful and may lead to necrosis if misplaced into fatty tissue, so the oral route is preferred. Clinical improvement is seen in 2 to 4 weeks. The client should eat a diet high in iron.

Specific Nursing Measures

The focus of nursing measures is client education regarding the importance of adequate iron for optimum body function. Education is important in gaining client compliance with iron therapy. Initiate a dietary referral and give the client a list of foods high in dietary iron for home use. Explain the side effects of iron therapy. The most common are gastrointestinal and include constipation or diarrhea, abdominal cramping, and gastric distress. Stool color will change from normal brownish to either a dark green or black. Warn the client to keep all iron preparations out of the reach of children.

Administer oral iron preparations with citrus juice to enhance absorption. If parenteral iron therapy is prescribed, use the Z-track method with a 20-gauge, 2- to 3-in needle injected in the dorsogluteal site only (see a nursing fundamentals text).

DISSEMINATED INTRAVASCULAR COAGULATION

Disseminated intravascular coagulation (DIC) is an acute abnormal stimulation of the normal hemostatic mechanism. The normal coagulation process, or clotting cascade, is a series of enzymatic reactions that follows a specific sequence—a finely tuned balance between clot formation and clot dissolution. In DIC, this balance is disrupted. The abnormal stimulation of coagulation is explosive, resulting in widespread thrombi formation that eventually exhausts clotting factors and platelets. The existing degree of clotting activates the fibrinolytic process. These two events can result in major bleeding episodes.

DIC does not exist alone; it coexists with a variety of other acute disease processes that damage cells in some way and thus potentiate stimulation of the normal hemostatic mechanism. Disorders or situations associated with DIC include malignancies, sepsis, shock, abruptio placentae, postextracorporeal bypass, respiratory distress syndrome, malaria, and venomous bites. Mismatched blood and fat emboli can initiate DIC by releasing excessive factor XII.

Clinical Manifestations

In DIC, consumption of platelets and clotting factors is preceded by deposition of fibrin in the microcirculation. The client with DIC may have bleeding tendencies, tissue damage from ischemia, erythrocyte damage, and hemolysis with a potential for shock. These problems have either occult or overt signs and symptoms. Signs and symptoms of bleeding include epistaxis; petechiae; ecchymosis; bleeding from surgical sites, placental detachment areas, or old sites of injury; positive findings of blood in the stool or emesis; fall in blood pressure; postural hypotension; tachycardia; decreased packed red cell volume; and restlessness.

Manifestations of thrombosis depend on the specific organ or body system affected. The kidneys are a prime target organ, and hematuria is the most common clinical evidence that the renal system is affected. Thrombosis also can affect the central nervous system; changes in the level of consciousness may signal interruption in cerebral blood flow. Characteristic skin changes such as acrocyanosis, in which the client experiences generalized sweating with cold, mottled toes and fingers, also occur.

A battery of laboratory analyses is used in the diagnosis of DIC in conjunction with the client's signs and symptoms. These tests measure the client's coagulation. Platelet counts are decreased; PT and PTT are prolonged. Fibrinogen levels are decreased, and levels of fibrin degradation products (fibrin split products) are elevated. A protamine sulfate test is strongly positive, and coagulation factor assay demonstrates a reduction in factors II, V, and VII.

Therapeutic Measures

The pharmacologic management of DIC is controversial. Currently, heparin, or blood components such as packed RBCs, platelets, plasma, and factor replacements, or both are used. Some think that DIC is best managed by no treatment at all, because treating the client's signs and symptoms may worsen the clotting–bleeding phenomenon. The overall goal of therapy is removing the stimulus that initiated the DIC process.

Specific Nursing Measures

The nursing management of DIC clients is complex. The overall nursing goal is to protect them from bleeding by applying pressure to bleeding sites, avoiding intramuscular injections, keeping the client's nails trimmed, and having both male and female clients shave with an electric razor instead of a straight-edged razor.

The client undergoing heparin sodium or blood component therapy needs additional support and explanations. Heparin may be given either continuously or intermittently by IV drip, and the nurse must closely monitor the prescribed flow rate. The client receiving heparin must be assessed continuously for bleeding. Blood component therapy, although prescribed to replace depleted coagulation factors consumed by the systemic clotting phenomenon, may stimulate additional clotting. Changes in the client's level of consciousness, pallor or cyanosis of body parts, or oliguria or anuria may indicate additional clotting. Notify the physician immediately if these changes occur so the medical management of the client can be adjusted.

Clients with DIC have multiple disease processes simultaneously. They may have a malignancy, cardiovascular disease, sepsis, or be pregnant. Therefore, the stress levels of the DIC client and significant others are high. The client and family or friends require thorough teaching and psychosocial support to cope effectively with this complex, confusing disease.

IDIOPATHIC THROMBOCYTOPENIC PURPURA

Idiopathic thrombocytopenic purpura (ITP) is characterized by a decrease in the number of circulating platelets with resultant purpura. The disorder occurs in all age groups. Congenital thrombocytopenic purpura occurs in the neonate. Acute ITP is primarily a disorder of childhood, whereas chronic ITP occurs primarily in adults.

The exact etiology of ITP is unknown and may differ depending on the kind of ITP and the client's age. Regardless of the cause, an immunologic response results in a decrease in circulating platelets, an alteration in thrombocyte life span, and bleeding tendencies. Splenic sequestration further contributes to the thrombocytopenia. The stimulus precipitating the immunologic response may be a virus, bacteria, environmental toxin, or chemical (eg, in drug-induced ITP).

Clinical Manifestations

Clinical manifestations of ITP result from thrombocytopenia. The client is prone to hemorrhagic episodes. Bleeding tendencies may be minor—involving small petechial hemorrhages of the skin and mucous membranes—but the platelet count may fall low enough to allow central nervous system hemorrhage. The client may also experience hematuria, hematemesis, melena, gingival oozing, and epistaxis. The female client who is still menstruating may experience menorrhagia.

Physical assessment of the client usually reveals scattered petechiae over all body parts; these may be so abundant that they coalesce to form ecchymoses. The ecchymotic, purpuric, and petechial areas occur spontaneously. Close examination of these lesions does not reveal inflammatory changes indicating trauma. The liver and spleen tip may be palpable, but hepatosplenomegaly is uncommon. Traumatic hemorrhages manifested by painful hemarthrosis or hematomas may be evident if the client has been injured. Significant bleeding may cause pallor and fatigue. The client may have diminished tolerance to activity and shortness of breath on physical exertion.

Diagnostic tests indicate low platelet numbers and alterations in bleeding times. The physician may order a CBC, including quantitative platelet determinations, as well as bone marrow examination to determine the nature of platelet production (megakaryocytopoiesis). Other diagnostic procedures may include determination of bleeding time, Rumpel–Leede capillary fragility test (the tourniquet test), and studies of coagulation time and clot retraction.

Therapeutic Measures

Most clients with acute ITP recover spontaneously and never have a recurrence. Clients with chronic ITP rarely undergo spontaneous remission. After a diagnosis of chronic ITP, steroid therapy is initiated in an attempt to decrease or diminish the immunologic (antigen–antibody) response of the reticuloendothelial system and decrease sequestration of thrombocytes by the spleen. The client continues steroid therapy for several weeks to several months. If the circulating platelet count does not improve, splenectomy may be performed; this procedure usually restores platelet counts to normal or near-normal levels by removing the primary organ involved in platelet destruction and the removal of platelets from the circulation.

If the client is anemic from severe blood loss, a diet high in protein and iron should be implemented. Small, frequent meals may be more manageable for the anemic client.

Specific Nursing Measures

Hospitalization is required for diagnosis of ITP. Nursing care is aimed at both preventing bleeding episodes and promoting client education about the disease process and the diagnostic procedures. The most common and life-threatening problem is hemorrhage. During hospitalization, monitor the client continuously for signs or symptoms of hemorrhagic shock. The central nervous system is particularly vulnerable during thrombocytopenia. Therefore, make every effort to provide a safe environment for the thrombocytopenic client. Suggested nursing interventions during hospitalization include testing urine, stools, and emesis for occult blood; providing footwear for the ambulating client; avoiding rectal temperature determination, intramuscular injections, and rectal medications; administering platelet concentrates, if needed; and offering mouth rinses composed of hydrogen peroxide and water or normal saline in lieu of routine oral hygiene using toothbrushes.

Nursing assessments during hospitalization are related to the thrombocytopenia. The progression or resolution of petechial and purpuric hemorrhages needs close monitoring; daily documentation of these lesions by a consistent caregiver is ideal. Pallor or paresthesia of an extremity distal to ecchymotic areas or to hematomas may signal loss of vascular integrity and compromised tissue oxygenation to that extremity. Assess the client's level of consciousness regularly, and immediately report subtle changes in orientation or personality to the physician.

The majority of clients with acute ITP have spontaneous remission and may be discharged when platelet counts are greater than 50,000. Circulating platelets are then regularly assessed (in an outpatient clinic or health provider's office) until the platelet count is normal. Stress that protective headgear (football or hockey helmets) may be needed while the client plays or rides in a car. Teach the signs and symptoms of relapse (eg, increased tendency to bruise, recurrence of petechiae, and epistaxis). Consult a pediatric nursing textbook for further information.

Chronic ITP requires even more challenging nursing management. In addition to the nursing assessments and interventions already mentioned, client education about steroid therapy is needed. Explain the rationale for its use and the side effects common to steroid consumption. Tell the client that compliance with the prescribed dose and frequency is of utmost importance in avoiding dangerous or life-threatening complications. Have the client seek medical attention immediately if for any reason he or she cannot continue taking the medication orally.

When conventional conservative steroid therapy is contraindicated, splenectomy is recommended. See Chapter 30 for information on the preparation of splenectomy clients. Additionally, steroid therapy (if the client is not already weaned) is continued throughout the postoperative period to promote adaptation to the stress of surgery. Platelet concentrates are administered throughout the intraoperative and postoperative periods to decrease the likelihood of major hemorrhagic episodes. After discharge, the client's platelet level is monitored closely to detect the return to normal levels. Thrombocytopenia usually does not recur following splenectomy, but discharge teaching following surgery should include signs and symptoms indicating a relapse.

GRANULOCYTOPENIA

In granulocytopenia, the quantity of circulating granulocytes is dramatically reduced. The absolute granulocyte count in these clients is less than $500/\mu L$ (Williams et al., 1983). Although neutrophils, eosinophils, and basophils are all granulocytes, the clinically significant affected cell type is the neutrophil. Neutrophils seem to be the granulocyte most important in fighting bacterial infections. An inverse relation has been demonstrated between the percentage of neutrophils and the rate of bacterial infection; that is, as the percentage of neutrophils decreases, the infection rate increases. (See Box 28–2 in Chapter 28 for information on calculating the absolute neutrophil count.) Agranulocytosis involves the same defect, although the condition is more severe. Granulocytopenia and agranulocytosis predispose the client to repeated, sometimes overwhelming infections. Granulocytopenia may be acute or have a more chronic pattern. Chronic granulocytopenia usually does not carry as large a risk of bacterial infection as the acute variety, but infection is a lifelong threat.

Granulocytopenia may be caused by either decreased production of granulocytes, increased utilization of granulocytes, or both. In addition, a shortened granulocyte life span may further depress the number of granulocytes.

One of the most frequent causes of granulocytopenia is medication. Antineoplastic chemotherapeutics predictably cause bone marrow suppression and resultant granulocytopenia. Examples of these medications are the antimetabolites (6-mercaptopurine and methotrexate), alkylating agents (nitrogen mustard and cyclophosphamide), and plant alkaloids (vincristine sulfate). Other common medications—gentamicin, chloramphenicol, benzene and benzene-derivative drugs, phenothiazines, diphenylhydantoins, and colchicine—also cause granulocytopenia, although in a less predictable manner. Other causes of granulocytopenia include radiation overexposure, hypersplenism, sepsis, and alcohol abuse, among others.

Clinical Manifestations

A major problem for the client with granulocytopenia is the accurate recognition and diagnosis of infection because its signs and symptoms in the presence of granulocytopenia are unpredictable. Clients with acute granulocytopenia have the most life-threatening infections. Total WBC counts may dip to less than $500/\mu L$, the percentage of neutrophils drop, and overwhelming bacterial and fungal sepsis can develop.

Fever is present during infection, but the usual signs and symptoms are not typical. An inflammatory response with the production of purulent matter may not be present, and the usual natural elevation of leukocytes is not found. Thus, granulocytopenia clients present a difficult diagnostic picture.

Therapeutic Measures

Suspected infection is treated aggressively with broad-spectrum antibiotic therapy. Antimicrobial treatment is initiated as soon as cultures have been taken. Once the microorganism has been identified, the antibiotic regimen can be altered as needed to conform to the sensitivity tests. Multiple antibiotics are usually prescribed, and IV delivery is the route of choice.

In acute granulocytopenia, bone marrow recovery is usually rapid after the removal of the offending stimulus. The peripheral blood count may show some atypical (immature) forms during the recovery phase, but recovery is usually complete and sustained. In chronic granulocytopenia, androgens and corticosteroids can restore the normal hematologic picture. These agents have not been found useful in the management of acute granulocytopenia, however. Granulocytes may be administered during the initial stages of acute granulocytopenia.

Specific Nursing Measures

The nurse must identify clients at risk for developing granulocytopenia and have knowledge of medications with potential side effects or adverse reactions of blood dyscrasias. Granulocytopenia is not preventable nor predictable, but anticipation of potential problems may save the client's life.

Once infection is suggested, the stimulus precipitating the granulocytopenia is removed, if possible. The most likely cause is a medication, which should be stopped immediately. The client should be isolated from potential carriers of infection. Visitors may need to be screened. Staff members with bacterial or fungal infections should not come into contact with these clients, and even staff members with minor viral infections should not care for them. Clients with severe granulocytopenia are sometimes placed in protective or reverse isolation. This practice is controversial, however.

As already mentioned, the usual signs and symptoms of infection are not reliable with granulocytopenia. Nevertheless, the nurse should monitor the client's temperature frequently. Continuously assess potential sites of infection, such as the skin and mucous membranes, lungs, ears, mouth, and gastrointestinal and genitourinary tract. Above all, listen to the client who may provide the best clues to the source of infection.

Nursing management of the client experiencing acute granulocytopenia is similar to that of the client with leukemia experiencing leukopenia.

Clients with chronic granulocytopenia on steroid and androgen therapy need emotional support to deal with the body-image side effects of this therapy. Educating them on the potential masculinization effects of both drugs may help them cope when these side effects appear.

Additional client education centers around recognizing signs and symptoms of infection until hematologic recovery occurs and avoiding potential sources of infection. Instruct clients on the method of measuring body temperature using the oral or axillary route, as well as the specific signs and symptoms of infection. In addition, instruct them to seek medical attention immediately with any manifestations of infection. Typically, infections in these clients are from their own normal flora; however, they should still be encouraged to avoid large crowds and contagious people whenever possible.

Section III: Immunologic Disorders

Immunologic disorders of the blood and blood-forming organs affect the body's ability to resist infectious agents. These disorders may be congenital or acquired. Without an adequate immune system or a competent bone marrow, the client is prone to life-threatening infections. There have been recent advances in the medical management of immunologic disorders. For example, children with severe combined immunodeficiency (a genetically inherited immune disorder) usually die by 2 years of age; however, recently one boy survived until 12 years of age in a special protective environment. Continued research into the immune

system may discover new advancements in treatment for severe immunologic disorders.

General Nursing Implications

The nurse's role in the management of immunologic disorders of the blood and blood-forming organs involves (1) client and family education on the disease process and potential measures to avoid contact with infectious agents, (2) psychosocial support during genetic counseling, (3)

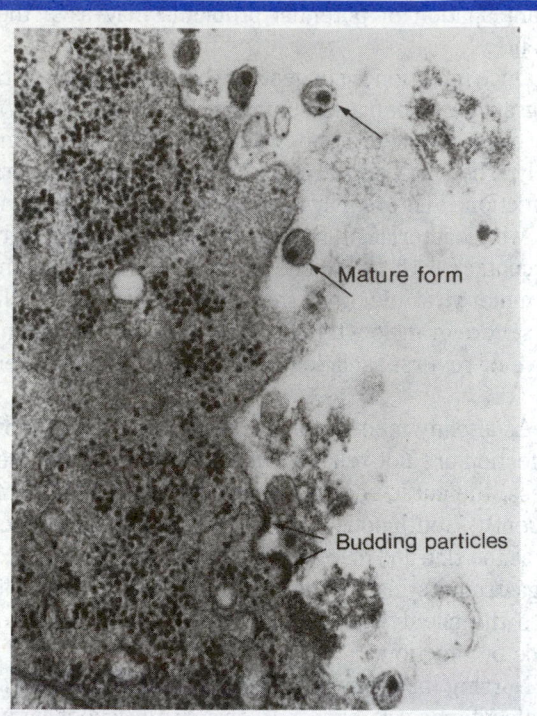

Mature form

Budding particles

Figure 29–3

HTLV-III/LAV-type virus found in a hemophiliac patient who developed AIDS. (Magnification of virus particles ranges in size from 90–120 nm.) (Courtesy Centers for Disease Control, Atlanta, GA)

emotional support when the prognosis is poor, and (4) assessment of the client for signs and symptoms of infection.

Nursing assessment of the client with an immunodeficiency involves close monitoring for signs and symptoms of infection. Because their immune systems are not competent, these clients are highly susceptible to viral, fungal, bacterial, and protozoal infections of all body systems. Their systems usually cannot halt even the most innocuous virus, so infections fulminate easily.

Whether the client is in the hospital or at home, the nurse is responsible for preventing the spread and occurrence of infections. Hospitalized clients may need reverse or protective isolation. At home, teach the client and family or significant others to avoid crowds or large gatherings to lower the likelihood of contracting an infection. Also instruct these clients to seek medical attention immediately at the first sign of infection.

ACQUIRED IMMUNE DEFICIENCY SYNDROME

Acquired immune deficiency syndrome (AIDS) is a specific defect in immunity against disease. Clients with this immune system defect are unable to defend against disease and are prone to debilitating, often fatal opportunistic infections.

The causative agent of AIDS is a retrovirus known in the United States as the human T-lymphotropic virus type III (HTLV-III) and in France as the lymphadenopathy-associated virus (LAV). This is thought to be the same virus

isolated in two independent laboratories. Figure 29–3 is a photomicrograph of the HTLV-III virus. These viruses tend to seek out and reproduce in T-lymphocytes and, in so doing, injure and kill the lymphocytes. This activity accounts for the severe decrease in the number of T-lymphocytes in AIDS clients.

Mode of Transmission

The presence of the AIDS virus has thus far been demonstrated in blood, semen, saliva, and tears. Whether it can be transmitted through saliva and tears is not yet known.

Sexual transmission, especially homosexual transmission among men through receptive anal intercourse, is the most common. Semen can carry infected lymphocytes that are transferred through minute breaks in the rectal mucosa that occur during anal intercourse. The question of transmission by oral–genital contact remains unanswered.

The AIDS virus can also be transmitted parenterally by using contaminated needles or through contaminated blood and blood products such as whole blood, cellular components, plasma, and clotting factor concentrates that have not been heat treated. Thus far, other blood products such as immune globulin, albumin, plasma protein fraction, and hepatitis B vaccine have not been implicated (Bennett, 1985). AIDS can also be transmitted by an infected mother to a fetus or newborn infant.

Incidence and Risk Factors

The first cases of AIDS appeared simultaneously in New York City and Port-au-Prince, Haiti, in 1978 (Bennett, 1985). The Centers for Disease Control (CDC) first began publishing incidence reports in June 1981 related to these first cases of AIDS as well as others diagnosed in San Francisco and Los Angeles. Since then the number of AIDS cases has escalated in geometric proportions—reported cases have doubled about every 10 months. At least half of these persons have died, most within 2 years of diagnosis. The rapid progress of the disease is thought to be related to the tremendous speed with which the HTLV-III virus reproduces. The number of AIDS cases reported by the CDC by January 1986 are illustrated by state in Figure 29–4. The CDC has predicted a continuing alarming rise in the incidence of AIDS, estimating that there will be approximately 200,000 cases on record by 1988. In the Americas, the countries other than the United States with the highest number of reported cases were Haiti, Canada, and Brazil (Curran et al., 1985).

Several groups have been identified in the United States as being at high risk of developing AIDS: homosexual/bisexual men represent approximately three-quarters of all AIDS cases; parenteral drug users are the category with the second highest incidence; and hemophiliacs and blood transfusion recipients have the third highest rate. Female sexual partners of bisexual men and children of AIDS clients are also at high risk. At one time, Haitian-born immigrants to the US were also listed as a high-risk group. This clas-

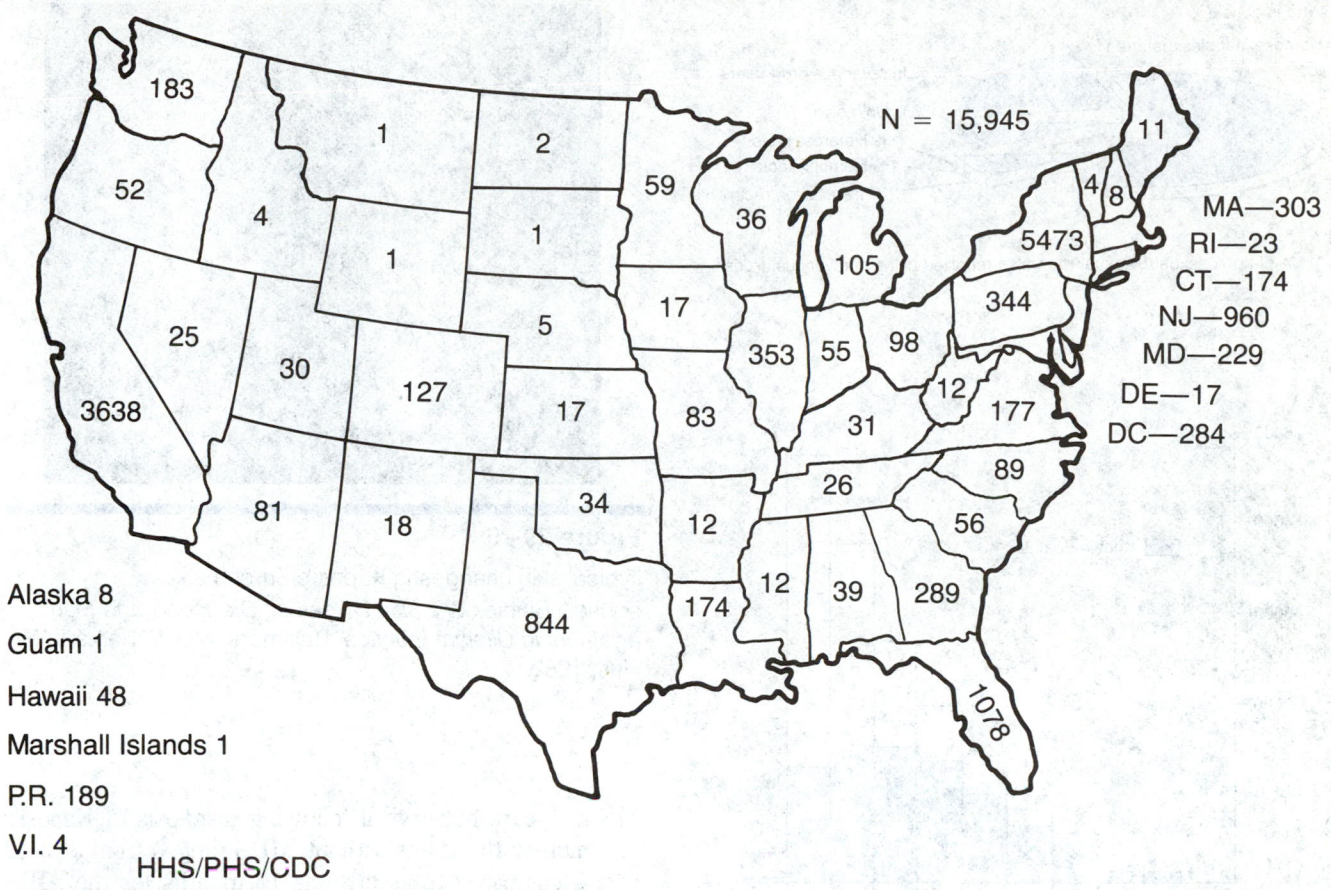

Figure 29–4

AIDS cases reported to the CDC, by state, through January, 1986.
SOURCE: Centers for Disease Control, Atlanta, GA

sification was abandoned in mid-1985 when it became apparent that the designation inaccurately pointed to a single risk factor in this ethnic group. It has now been determined that the risk for Haitians is related to the risk factors discussed previously and not to ethnicity. Only 9% of cases have occurred outside the two highest risk groups. Of this number, 6% are categorized as unknown.

The incidence among heterosexuals in the US is approximately 1%. In Africa, however, AIDS occurs about equally among men and women. This has led to speculation that AIDS, which has been largely confined to homosexual and bisexual men, will spread to and among the general population. Figure 29–5A illustrates the risk factors for specific populations in the United States, and Figure 29–5B shows the geometric rise in new cases.

Clinical Manifestations

The incubation period for AIDS is unknown. The time between exposure to the virus to onset of symptoms ranges from about 6 months to 5 years. In transfusion-associated cases, the mean is 2 years (Benenson, 1985). The onset of AIDS is usually insidious. Early in the disease, clients have nonspecific symptoms such as fatigue and weakness,

lymphadenopathy, anorexia and weight loss, recurrent diarrhea, pallor, fever, and night sweats. This group of symptoms has been termed AIDS-related complex (ARC) when it occurs in persons who have had the symptoms for at least three months and test positive for the HTLV-III virus. Not everyone who has ARC develops full-blown AIDS. The symptoms gradually increase in severity, usually until the client becomes ill with an opportunistic disease. The unusual occurrence of *Pneumocystis carinii* pneumonia or Kaposi's sarcoma in clients who have not had a past diagnosis of an immune disorder and have not received immunosuppressive therapy is the single most important piece of data suggesting AIDS. Although the line that separates AIDS from ARC is unclear, a person is usually considered to have AIDS once the client develops a life-threatening infection.

Pneumocystis carinii pneumonia is a rare parasitic protozoan lung infection otherwise almost always seen in cancer clients or transplant recipients who have received immunosuppressive agents. This serious, often fatal lung infection is characterized by shortness of breath and fever. The shortness of breath may be so profound that the client may experience air hunger. The infection begins insidiously; possibly the only symptoms are fever, sore throat,

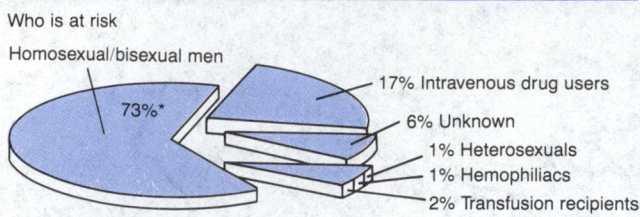

Who is at risk

Homosexual/bisexual men

73%*

17% Intravenous drug users
6% Unknown
1% Heterosexuals
1% Hemophiliacs
2% Transfusion recipients

*11% of homosexual/bisexual men also reported using intravenous drugs.

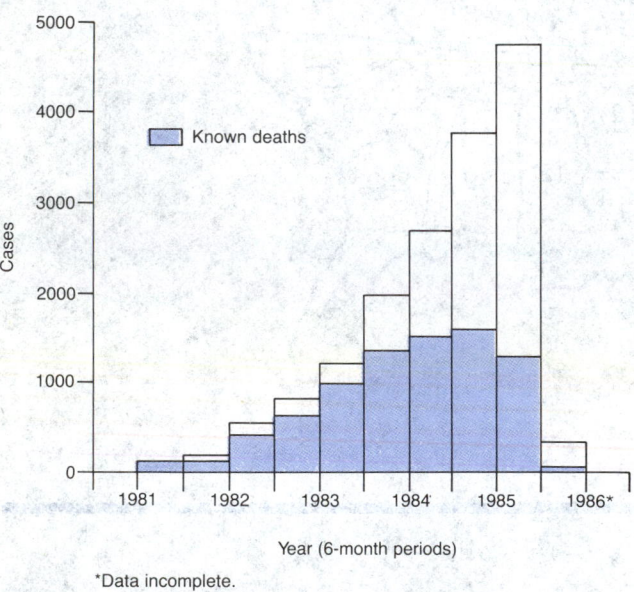

Year (6-month periods)

*Data incomplete.

Figure 29–5

AIDS in the United States. **A.** Populations at risk. **B.** Geometric increase in new cases.
SOURCE: Centers for Disease Control, Atlanta, GA

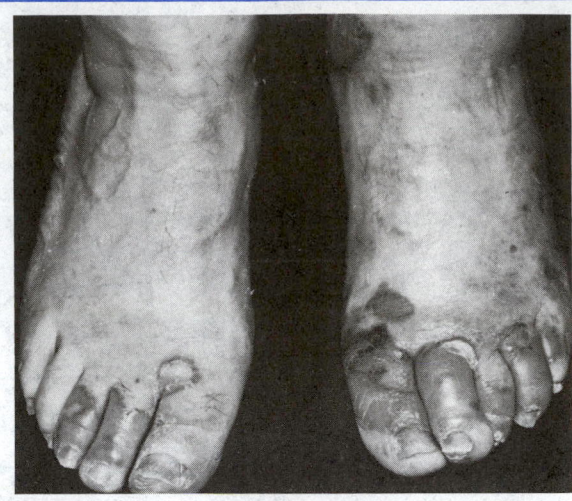

Figure 29–6

Typical skin changes in Kaposi's Sarcoma.
SOURCE: Binnick SA: *Skin Diseases: Diagnosis and Management in Clinical Practice.* Baltimore, MD: Williams & Wilkins, 1982.

chills, and a nonproductive cough. Within months, the infectious process becomes so extensive that dyspnea, cyanosis, painful respiration, and air hunger become pronounced. High fever with night sweats may also be present (Allen & Mellin, 1982). By this time, the protozoa have invaded lung tissue and created cystic pockets that impede the oxygen-carbon dioxide exchange across the alveolar membrane. Clients may require oxygen administration via an artificial ventilation device. (For a discussion of pneumonia, see Chapter 20.)

Kaposi's sarcoma is a rare, usually mild skin cancer that occurs in males over 60 years of age with a Mediterranean ancestry. Typical skin changes include dark purplish, sometimes ulcerating lesions that usually appear over the lower extremities (Figure 29–6). Kaposi's sarcoma is rarely fatal in clients without AIDS. In the AIDS client, the disease is virulent and invasive, often involving internal organs; mucous membranes; and the face, arms, and chest.

Median years of survival following diagnosis of Kaposi's sarcoma for the client without AIDS ranges from 8 to 13 years, compared to as little as 15 months for the AIDS client (Allen & Mellin, 1982).

Although there is no one laboratory or diagnostic test to determine whether a client has AIDS, a blood test to screen for the HTLV-III virus was approved for use in March 1985 by the US Food and Drug Administration. This screening test was originally intended to determine potential blood donors who had been exposed to the HTLV-III virus. Having antibodies to the virus does not indicate that the person has AIDS or even that the person will, with any certainty, develop AIDS in the future. Demonstrating antibody formation to the virus simply means that the person has been exposed to the virus and has developed antibodies in response to it. This finding allows blood donation centers to screen out potential donors who might possibly be incubating the disease. There is some concern that persons infected with the AIDS virus may not test positive in the early stages. Other laboratory findings are lymphopenia, hypergammaglobulinemia, and diminished reactivity to antigens. In early 1986, the FDA noted that a positive test could be linked to AIDS antibodies found in most of the USA's gamma globulin supply. The virus itself has not been found in those supplies.

Once the diagnosis is made, the course of AIDS is predictable. Repeated, life-threatening opportunistic infections (eg, *Pneumocystis carinii* pneumonia and overwhelming candidiasis, cytomegalovirus infection, or disseminated herpes simplex infection, among others) requiring hospitalization are the rule. The nonspecific early

Box 29–1 Prevention Strategies for AIDS

Avoiding sexual contact with persons *known* to have AIDS

Avoiding sexual contact with persons *suspected* to have AIDS

Practicing "healthy sex" (no exchanges of body fluids including semen, urine, saliva, feces, or blood; no contact of body fluids with mucous membranes)

Avoiding unnecessary transfusions of blood or blood products

Encouraging autologous transfusions for elective surgery whenever possible

Administering only heat-treated coagulation factor to hemophiliacs

Screening all potential blood donors carefully

Encouraging AIDS clients and persons at high risk not to donate blood, plasma, organs for transplantation, or semen for artificial insemination

Advising parenteral drug users to use only clean, disposable needles and syringes and not to share drug equipment

Recommending that seropositive women delay pregnancy

Providing educational programs on AIDS for the public and school children

Using appropriate blood/body fluid precautions with known or suspected AIDS clients

symptoms described earlier increase in severity along with the progression of the disease. Central nervous system changes have been observed in later stages of the disease.

Therapeutic Measures

AIDS has no known cure, and the death rate is 100%. Immunotherapy with interferon has been used for clients with Kaposi's sarcoma. Although interferon treatment has had some success, it does not correct the immune defect in AIDS. Interleukon-2 may help fight the severe immunodeficiency by increasing the ability of the impaired lymphocytes of AIDS clients to fight infection. The substance has been shown to improve infection-fighting activity in the test tube; it is not yet shown to work in vivo. Clinical trials now test interleukon-2 activity in AIDS clients.

Experimentation is also under way to develop drug therapy for AIDS. A drug developed in France that interferes with the virus's multiplication, HPA-23, was approved for experimental use in the United States in late 1985. Another experimental agent that appears to prevent viral multiplication and is less toxic than HPA-23 is azidothymidine, also known as Compound S. A third drug, available in Europe, Mexico, and Canada but not in the United States, is isoprinosine. This drug reportedly stimulates the immune system and has also been used for herpes genitalis, hepatitis B, and genital warts. Another drug that seems to stimulate the immune system and also increases the body's production of interferon and interleukon-2 (natural antiviral agents) is ABPP, an experimental drug for cancer clients, soon to be tested in AIDS clients. Researchers are also

investigating the potential uses of other drugs such as suramin sodium (Antrypol, Germanin), used to treat African sleeping sickness caused by a protozoal parasite spread by the tsetse fly; and ribavirin (Virazole), an antiviral agent said to be effective in certain forms of influenza and in herpesvirus infections. Complicating drug treatment is the fact that the HTLV-III virus also attacks the brain, which is difficult for drugs to reach.

Antibiotic therapy is used for clients with infection. For example, *pneumocystic carinii* infections are treated with either a combination of trimethoprim and sulfamethoxazole or with pentamidine isethionate (Lomidine). Refer to the other specific disorders chapters for treatment of other infections.

Research into the development of a vaccine is ongoing. Vaccine development could, however, be a slow process. For example, although the hepatitis B virus was identified as early as 1968, an effective vaccine did not become available until 1983. The development of a vaccine is likely to be a difficult task. The virus behaves much like the influenza virus, changing its structure frequently. It would be difficult to develop a vaccine that would be effective against all forms of the virus.

Specific Nursing Measures

Prevention is the focus of AIDS nursing measures today. Prevention strategies for AIDS are given in Box 29–1. Nurses can play an important role in educating clients, their significant others, and the public in risk-reduction strategies and in identifying individuals at risk.

In caring for clients with AIDS, the CDC (1983) recommends that blood–body fluid precautions be instituted. (These isolation guidelines are discussed in detail in Chapter 11 in Box 11–4.) Equipment contaminated with blood, excretions, or secretions should be disinfected concurrently. Body fluids and body tissues should be handled with caution. In addition, if the client has an opportunistic infection, other isolation precautions specific to the infectious disease should be observed. The likelihood of transmission to health care personnel if precautions are observed is small.

Clients with AIDS have many emotional needs. They often are rejected by significant others, leading to increasing isolation. Families or friends of homosexual AIDS clients may have abandoned the clients before they became ill because of the stigma still associated with homosexuality. When they confront a diagnosis of AIDS, these clients may truly be isolated and alone.

Fear surrounds AIDS clients because of the increasing incidence of AIDS and the yet-unknown factors that influence its transmission. Health care personnel may be fearful of caring for AIDS clients and reject clients because of the diagnosis or because the clients may be homosexual. Giving holistic care to AIDS clients requires a nonjudgmental and accepting approach that promotes open communication. These clients can be very ill and require skilled physiologic and psychosocial nursing care.

Because AIDS is universally fatal, AIDS clients may demonstrate signs of depression, grief, and mourning, along with other adaptations to death and dying discussed in Chapter 16. Assess these clients for these psychosocial alterations and intervene appropriately. Inform clients as more support groups for AIDS clients form (see the resources list at the end of this chapter).

Because anorexia and weight loss accompany AIDS, it is important to promote optimal nutritional intake while monitoring the client's nutritional status. A palatable diet that is high in calories and proteins, served attractively, and easily digestible is ideal for AIDS clients. Flexibility in menu planning and meal time is advised. Small frequent meals may be easier for the client to eat.

Other nursing care measures depend on the specific opportunistic diseases affecting the client. These are discussed in the appropriate chapters in this text.

AGAMMAGLOBULINEMIA

Agammaglobulinemia, an acquired or inherited depression in gamma globulin synthesis, renders the client susceptible to recurrent episodes of infection. Males and females are equally affected. The cause of most cases of acquired agammaglobulinemia is unknown. Likewise, there is no definite pattern of inheritance in the genetic variety. However, the incidence of immunologic disorders seems to be increased in family members of clients with primary agammaglobulinemia (Williams et al., 1983).

Clinical Manifestations

The client with acquired agammaglobulinemia has recurrent pyogenic infections, especially sinusitis and pneumonia (Williams et al., 1983). A sruelike syndrome is also frequent. The majority of adults with agammaglobulinemia have diarrhea, steatorrhea (fatty stools), protein-losing enteropathy, and malabsorption problems. Another clinical feature is noncaseating granulomas of the liver, spleen, skin, and lungs. Hepatosplenomegaly may be present. Furthermore, these clients have a markedly increased incidence of autoimmune disease, and their immunoglobulin G (IgG) levels are low.

Therapeutic Measures

Steroid therapy is useful in treating agammaglobulinemia. Immunoglobulin therapy is given to clients with a severe antibody deficit. Metronidazole (Flagyl), an effective amebicide, is prescribed for clients with the sruelike syndrome. Clients with this syndrome take a diet free of milk, milk products, and gluten. See Chapter 48 for a list of foods to be avoided in a gluten-free diet.

Specific Nursing Measures

The nursing management of acquired agammaglobulinemia centers around client teaching. Topics should include signs and symptoms of infection that necessitate health care; diet and medication instruction for clients having the sruelike syndrome; and detailed instructions on steroid therapy.

Section IV: Neoplastic Disorders

Neoplastic disorders of the blood and blood-forming organs include the leukemias, lymphomas, and multiple myeloma. These disease processes can involve infiltration and disruption of normal bone marrow function and alteration of the usual protective mechanism of the immune system.

Neoplastic disorders render the client susceptible to invasion and attack by infectious agents, prone to life-threatening bleeding episodes, and unable to tolerate normal daily activities. Furthermore, the diagnosis of cancer interrupts the client's normal psychosocial equilibrium. Fears and uncertainty about all matters of everyday life place great strain on the client, client's family unit, and significant others.

General Nursing Implications

The nurse's role in the management of clients with neoplastic disorders of the blood and blood-forming organs includes education of the client and family or friends regarding the disease process and medical treatment. Continued reinforcement of teaching is essential. The client with a malignancy also needs emotional support from the nurse. National support groups have local affiliates that attempt to reassure the cancer client that the experience need not be endured alone. (See Chapter 12, and the resources at the end of Chapter 28 for lists of support groups.)

The nurse needs to collect a detailed nursing data base and thoroughly assess all body systems. Pay particular attention to skin color; petechiae; bruising; occult or gross bleeding; liver, splenic, lymph node, or joint enlargement; vital signs; and any complaints of shortness of breath or alterations in comfort.

Signs and symptoms of neoplasia of the blood and blood-forming organs depend on the kind of malignancy. The leukemias can be thought of as liquid tumors primarily involving the bone marrow. Therefore, pallor, fatigue, fever, recurrent infections, petechiae, purpura, and gross bleeding may be present at the time of diagnosis. Clients with solid tumors of the blood and blood-forming organs, such as the lymphomas, may initially have an enlarged lymph node or mediastinal mass causing dyspnea.

Nursing interventions attempt to alter the client's adaptations to anemia, leukopenia, and thrombocytopenia. The diagnostic period may be long, so explain the need for multiple diagnostic examinations and provide emotional support to help clients cope.

Once diagnosis has been established and therapy has begun, teach the client about the disease process and therapy. The goal during the treatment phase is to help the client maintain as normal a life as is possible. Client teaching promotes independence in performing activities of daily living and gives the client a feeling of control over life. See Chapter 12 for the care of clients receiving radiation therapy and chemotherapy.

LEUKEMIA

Leukemia is characterized by an accumulation and proliferation of abnormal cells in the bone marrow. The leukemic cells are initially confined to the bone marrow but subsequently invade other organs and tissues as well as the peripheral blood. The accumulation of the leukemic cells in the bone marrow prevents normal hematopoiesis. The result is functionally incompetent bone marrow. The client's peripheral WBC count is generally greater than 50000/μL. It is possible, however, to have a WBC count near or below normal limits and still have leukemia. See Figure 22–11 in Chapter 22 for a review of the normal maturation of blood cells.

The exact cause of any of the leukemias is not known, although the pathogenesis is clearly multifactorial. Review of the literature reveals possible chemical, viral, radiation, and genetic stimuli preceding the development of leukemia. It is nearly impossible, however, to identify the causative factor or factors for individual clients diagnosed as having leukemia.

Types of Leukemia

Leukemia occurs in acute forms (involving proliferation of immature cells) and chronic forms (involving proliferation of mature cells) and can affect the erythrocyte or any of the white cell precursors. This discussion focuses on the four most common types of leukemia: acute lymphocytic leukemia (ALL), chronic lymphocytic leukemia (CLL), acute myelogenous leukemia (AML), and chronic granulocytic leukemia (CGL). Hematology textbooks describe more unusual varieties. The principles guiding nursing management are similar for all the leukemias. A case study of a client with leukemia is presented at the end of this chapter.

Acute Lymphocytic Leukemia

Acute lymphocytic leukemia is a malignant disorder involving the lymphoid series. The abnormal leukemic cell resembles an immature lymphocyte or lymphoblast. The leukemic lymphoblast cell is morphologically similar to the normal lymphoblast cell but does not mature. Instead, leukemic lymphoblasts accumulate in the bone marrow, crowding out precursors for normal myelopoiesis, erythropoiesis, and megakaryocytopoiesis.

Acute lymphocytic leukemia is predominantly a disorder of children. It is the most common malignancy in childhood and ranks as the second leading cause of death

in that age group. The peak incidence is between the ages of 2 and 10 years. A second rise in incidence occurs during middle and older adulthood.

Chronic Lymphocytic Leukemia

Chronic lymphocytic leukemia is a proliferative disorder of lymphoid tissues. Abnormal and incompetent lymphocytes initially are found in the lymph nodes; the disease progresses to involve the reticuloendothelial system (liver and spleen) and invade the bone marrow. The abnormal and incompetent lymphocytes accumulate in the blood. Eventually, the lining of the respiratory and gastrointestinal tracts, as well as the skin, are infiltrated by leukemic cells. As the disease process continues, abnormal lymphocytes eventually replace normal bone marrow elements. This process interferes with normal myelopoiesis, erythropoiesis, and megakaryocytopoiesis.

Unlike ALL, the lymphocytes in CLL are immunologically incompetent. Hypogammaglobulinemia is a characteristic of the late stages of the disease. The defect seems to involve immunoglobulin-producing B-lymphocytes.

Chronic lymphocytic leukemia has an insidious onset and is usually found by accident upon routine blood count examination. It is the most common leukemia of the Western Hemisphere and primarily affects the elderly population.

Acute Myelogenous Leukemia

Acute myelogenous leukemia is a malignant disorder involving the myeloid cell line of the bone marrow. Other marrow elements can be affected as well. The terminology for the varieties of AML is confusing, but remember that the descriptors identify cell line precursor affected. Examples of varieties or types of AML include acute granulocytic leukemia (AGL), acute promyelocytic leukemia (AProL), acute myelomonocytic leukemia, and erythroleukemia. Myelomonocytic leukemia, AGL, and erythroleukemia differ morphologically but are clinically similar. Clients with the rare AProL often develop DIC with hemorrhagic tendencies during relapse. When AProL is controlled by chemotherapeutic agents, it resembles the more common varieties.

Acute granulocytic leukemia is the most common variety of the AMLs. Often the terms AML and AGL are used interchangeably. Acute granulocytic leukemia involves abnormal proliferation and accumulation of immature granulocytes in the bone marrow. The immature granulocytes may proliferate slower or faster than normal granulocytes. Regardless of the speed of cell division, however, the abnormal leukemic cells eventually crowd out normal myelopoiesis or granulopoiesis, erythropoiesis, and megakaryocytopoiesis. Normal hematopoiesis is impaired.

The incidence of AGL peaks at several ages. The majority of acute leukemias diagnosed during the neonatal period and early infancy are AGL, and a second peak incidence occurs in the eighth and ninth decades of life. Approximately one-third of all clients are over 60 years old.

Chronic Granulocytic Leukemia

Chronic granulocytic leukemia is a malignant disorder characterized by an abnormal and excessive accumulation and overgrowth of mature granulocytes in the bone marrow, blood, and spleen. These abnormalities are associated with a unique chromosomal abnormality, the Ph^1 (Philadelphia) chromosome. The granulocytes also seem to have lengthened life spans and may or may not retain their ability to fight infection through phagocytosis.

The onset and progression of CGL are insidious. Remission may last for as long as 4 years, but almost 70% of clients undergo an acute transformation, or "blast crisis." In this stage, the leukemia resembles AGL but is not amenable to chemotherapy; death usually occurs within months.

Approximately 20% of all leukemias in the Western hemisphere are CGL. The disease occurs in adolescence but it is more likely to occur between the ages of 25 and 60 years with the peak incidence in the fourth decade of life. In the neonate, CGL tends to have a rapid progression of infiltration and invasion.

Clinical Manifestations

The clinical manifestations of leukemia are related to the lack of normal hematopoiesis in the bone marrow. As already mentioned, bone marrow dysfunction results in varying degrees of anemia, thrombocytopenia, and leukopenia. Anemia can appear as pallor, fatigue, malaise, shortness of breath, dyspnea, or decreased activity tolerance. Thrombocytopenia frequently has symptoms of petechiae, easy bruising, bleeding gums, occult hematuria, or retinal hemorrhages. There is an inverse relation between the number of thrombocytes and the incidence of severe bleeding episodes. When present, leukopenia leaves the client at risk for infection from bacterial, viral, fungal, or protozoal organisms. As in thrombocytopenia, there is an inverse relation between the number of leukocytes—particularly granulocytes—and the incidence of infection. Infection is suspected in the presence of fever (greater than 38.5°C or 101.5°F) and is treated aggressively using broad-spectrum bactericidal agents.

Other manifestations of leukemia include lymphadenopathy, joint swelling and pain, weight loss, anorexia, and varying degrees of hepatosplenomegaly. Sternal tenderness is frequent in CGL, and gingival hyperplasia frequently accompanies AGL.

Meningeal involvement is more common in children than adults, especially in children with ALL. Central nervous system involvement is possible in any of the leukemias, however. Meningeal involvement causes increased intracranial pressure. Its signs and symptoms include irritability, nausea and vomiting, headache, personality changes, blurred vision, cranial nerve dysfunction involving CN III and CN IV, and changes in the level of consciousness. Papilledema can be visualized on ophthalmoscopic examination.

Therapeutic Measures

Antineoplastic drug therapy varies with the type of leukemia. Drug therapy also depends on the stage of treatment (remission-induction, remission-consolidation, and remission-maintenance phases).

The aim of the remission-induction phase, which begins upon diagnosis, is to destroy as many leukemic cells as possible and to return the bone marrow to a functionally "normal" state. At diagnosis, an estimated 1 million to 100 trillion cells are leukemic. At this time, leukemia cells are present in the bone marrow, the peripheral blood, the organs, and the tissues. Upon remission, the estimated number of leukemic cells is less than 100 million, found predominantly in the bone marrow.

The remission-induction phase of drug therapy cannot destroy all leukemic cells present upon diagnosis. This inability to destroy leukemic cells completely is best explained by the theory that there are two pools, or populations, of leukemic cells. The first pool is actively dividing and has approximately 1×10^3 or 1×10^4 leukemic cells. These leukemic cells are found in the bone marrow, in tissues and organs, and in the peripheral blood. The second, quiescent pool of leukemic cells of 1×10^8 or 1×10^9 cells is primarily in the bone marrow. Because these cells are not actively replicating, they are difficult to kill. It is hoped that over a 2- to 3-year period these cells will become active and therefore amenable to treatment.

Drugs to treat ALL and AML during the remission-induction phase are used in combination. Single-agent drug therapy has been less effective than combinations of antineoplastic agents. Combinations of vincristine sulfate and prednisone are most commonly used in ALL. Often a third drug—frequently asparaginase (Elspar) or daunorubicin (Cerubidine)—is added. Chances of complete remission for adults and children with ALL is good. The complete remission rate for adults is approximately 75%; in children, complete remission is being achieved in 80% to 90% of all cases. AML has not been as amenable to remission-induction therapy as ALL. Most commonly, vincristine sulfate, prednisone, cytosine arabinoside, cyclophosphamide, and 6-thioguanine are used in various combinations. With more aggressive chemotherapeutic protocols, the remission-induction success rate for AML approaches 75% in some studies.

A second phase of antineoplastic drug therapy, the remission-consolidation phase, is sometimes employed to reduce the leukemic cell population further. This phase is usually short, averaging about 3 or 4 days. Drugs commonly used in the remission-consolidation phase for the acute leukemias are methotrexate, cyclophosphamide, hydrocortisone, cytosine arabinoside, asparaginase, and 6-thioguanine.

The remission-maintenance phase is instituted when remission is established and is continued for 2 to 3 years after diagnosis. Research strongly suggests that continuing chemotherapy beyond a 2- to 3-year period does not alter the relapse rate. The goal of this phase is to destroy the leukemic cell population further. Drugs used most commonly to treat the acute leukemias include 6-mercaptopurine, 6-thioguanine, cyclophosphamide, vincristine sulfate, cytosine arabinoside, and hydroxyurea. In ALL, methotrexate and 6-mercaptopurine appear to be the most important drugs in maintaining remission.

The chronic leukemias require a somewhat different pharmacologic approach. Remission is never completely established; instead, the chronic leukemias are more or less controlled for as long as possible. The drugs of choice for CLL are chlorambucil and cyclophosphamide. CLL is also treated with apheresis and interferon. In chronic granulocytic leukemia, busulfan, melphalan, and uracil mustard are used. Treatment is aggressive in an attempt to eradicate the Philadelphia chromosome to try to delay the onset of "blast crisis." The usefulness of autologous bone marrow transplantation is being investigated. Blood counts, especially quantitative leukocyte determinations, are carefully monitored, and dosages of medications are adjusted accordingly. Drug therapy for the chronic leukemias may be administered intermittently or continuously.

In both children and adults, the central nervous system (CNS) acts as a sanctuary for leukemic cells. The exact mode of CNS invasion by abnormal cells is not exactly known, but once it occurs, conventional routes of chemotherapy are not successful because systemic treatment does not adequately penetrate the blood-brain barrier. Therefore, the intrathecal route is used in CNS treatment. This approach necessitates an initial lumbar puncture, dilution of the antineoplastic agent with cerebrospinal fluid or preservative-free saline or water, and instillation of the medication. Intrathecal instillation is not without risk and should never be performed by an inexperienced practitioner. Transient and permanent neurologic abnormalities (paresthesias or paralysis) have been known to occur with improper placement of the lumbar puncture needle or if the needle is dislodged by sudden movement of the client. The following drugs are used for CNS treatment of leukemia: methotrexate, cytosine arabinoside, aminopterin, and hydrocortisone. Because vincristine sulfate is extremely neurotoxic, it is never administered intrathecally. Some treatment protocols combine intrathecal medication with cranial irradiation; others use intrathecal medication only. Regardless of the protocol, the purpose remains the same: to eradicate leukemic cells from the sanctuary of the CNS.

Specific Nursing Measures

Nursing care of all leukemic clients centers around potential or actual neutropenia, anemia, and thrombocytopenia caused by replacement of the normal bone marrow cellular elements by leukemic cells or destruction by antineoplastic chemotherapy. Chemotherapeutic treatment also can lead to bone marrow suppression. The nurse must help the leukemic client deal with pain, develop coping skills, and accept body image changes. Clients receiving chemotherapy need special nursing attention.

Infection

Infections can be fatal for the leukemic client. During the remission-induction phase, the most common infections are caused by bacterial and fungal organisms, and mortality from both is high. The most common kind of infection during the remission-maintenance phase is viral. Infection is related to the degree of granulocytopenia. As previously stated, the number of neutrophils and the risk for developing infection are inversely related—as the neutrophil count decreases, the infection rate increases.

It is the nurse's responsibility to prevent infection. Clients should be isolated when leukopenic. Several different techniques may be used. Some institutions have laminar airflow units; some use protective isolation or reverse isolation techniques. Regardless of the isolation technique, the purpose is to protect the client against infection. In addition, screen all visitors, and staff members who are even mildly ill should avoid caring for these clients. Once remission has been established and the client is discharged, teach the client to avoid large crowds and contact with contagious persons.

Avoid taking rectal temperatures and administering enemas and suppositories whenever possible to avoid damage to the rectal mucosa and consequent contamination by the gastrointestinal flora. Also avoid intramuscular injections, which compromise the skin integrity and create a portal for bacterial invasion and abscess formation.

Clients may have an altered inflammatory response and may not exhibit the usual signs of inflammation and infection, such as purulent discharge. For this reason, frequently assess the leukemic client for indicators of infection. An elevated temperature signals a potential infection, so monitor the client's temperature frequently. Client complaints should be taken seriously and investigated quickly. Whenever infection is suggested in a leukopenic client, take cultures of the blood, urine, throat, and other sites (see Chapter 11) in an attempt to identify the location of infection and the causative organism. Granulocytes and broad-spectrum antibiotics are given.

Clients on a chemotherapeutic regimen are immunosuppressed. Therefore, they should not receive immunizations of any kind during this time. It is the nurse's responsibility to be aware of immunosuppressed clients and to refrain from administering immunizations to them.

Anemia

The leukemic client may demonstrate pallor, shortness of breath, tachycardia, and limited activity tolerance in response to anemia. These clients frequently need replacement transfusion therapy in the form of packed RBCs. Facilitate breathing by elevating the head of the client's bed. To decrease the client's energy requirements, help the client perform activities of daily living as needed. Offer frequent rest periods throughout the waking hours to prevent exhaustion.

Hemorrhage

Thrombocytopenia resulting in hemorrhage can be life threatening to the leukemic client. Nursing care centers around preventing major hemorrhagic episodes. Leukemic clients with thrombocytopenia need safe, gentle nursing care with continuous assessment of signs or symptoms of hemorrhage. Changes in level of consciousness (intracranial bleeding), hematemesis, and epistaxis may occur with or without injury.

Not all bleeding is apparent or life threatening. Frequently, the leukemic client has occult bleeding in the form of petechiae and ecchymoses. Gingival oozing may occur after brushing the teeth or eating. Occult hematuria is common. Nursing assessment includes observing for these signs of occult bleeding and testing stools, emesis, and urine for occult blood. Carefully assess clients who have had an invasive procedure such as arterial blood gas determinations, oral suctioning, NG tube insertion, or bone marrow aspiration or biopsy.

Nursing management is also directed toward preventing injury. Rectal temperatures, enemas, rectal suppositories, and intramuscular injections are avoided because they can cause severe hemorrhagic episodes. Encourage clients to wear protective foot coverings whenever ambulating. They should use soft toothbrushes and electric razors instead of blades. Platelet concentrates may be given.

Anticoagulants, aspirin or aspirin-containing products, and medications containing guaifenesin should not be administered to the client with leukemia because they interfere with adequate platelet function. Aspirin is found in many OTC cold and influenza medications, and guaifenesin is in OTC cough suppressants. Febrile episodes are controlled with acetaminophen (rather than aspirin) and antibiotics, if needed. Remind clients that anticoagulants, aspirin, and guaifenesin should be avoided and discourage self-medication with OTC drugs.

Pain

The leukemia client may have pain, most commonly in the bones and joints, because of pressure caused by the infiltration and accumulation of leukemic cells in the bone marrow. Hemarthrosis may also occur and can be painful. The nurse may administer narcotics to control the pain, or chemotherapy may be administered when the pain is thought to be caused by leukemic infiltration.

Ineffective Coping Skills

The client with leukemia may have ineffective coping skills and require the support of family members, friends, and national or local support groups. Continuously assess the client's coping ability and offer support when needed by initially establishing a one-to-one relationship with the client and significant others. Spending time with the client regularly demonstrates concern about the client's welfare.

Assess the client's knowledge of the disease process and treatment, and begin teaching about the disorder and therapy to offer the client some sense of control. Answer the client's questions honestly, but do not destroy defense mechanisms that protect the client from an intolerable reality. For example, the nurse who notices that the client occasionally demonstrates denial but complies with the medical and nursing prescriptions should allow the client to express the denial, because it may be the client's only way to cope with the disease process.

Body Image Changes

Body image changes caused by chemotherapy or radiation therapy interfere with the client's ability to cope positively with the disease process. Emphasize that alopecia is only a temporary consequence of treatment. Until the client's hair does grow back, wigs, toupees, decorative scarfs, or caps can promote a positive self-concept (refer to Chapter 12).

Client Teaching

The leukemic client and family or significant others need extensive teaching with information on the leukemic disease process, procedures during the diagnostic and maintenance phases of treatment, radiation therapy, antineoplastic drug therapy, signs and symptoms warranting medical intervention, precautions needed for home care, restrictions on activities of daily living and employment, community resources, and OTC medications to be avoided. Teaching must be planned carefully to avoid overwhelming the client. Coordination of the teaching between the acute care and ambulatory care settings is most important.

Chemotherapy

Clients receiving chemotherapy may experience anorexia, weight loss, nausea, vomiting, and stomatitis. Children and adolescents may experience slowed growth. These adaptations may be related to the disease process or to side effects of treatment. Height and weight should be measured routinely, using height and weight growth curves to monitor children and adolescents. Weight losses, weight gains (from fluid retention while taking corticosteroids), or slowing of growth in height should be noted and acted upon quickly. With delayed growth or weight loss, a diet high in proteins and calories is needed. Supplemental high-protein, high-calorie feedings may need to be added to the client's 24-hour regimen. Fluid retention caused by corticosteroids can be decreased by a reduced-sodium diet. Because these clients frequently may continue corticosteroid therapy after discharge from the hospital, they may need instruction not only about a sodium-restricted diet but also about the preparation of foods without salt.

HODGKIN'S DISEASE

Hodgkin's disease is a malignant disorder of the lymph nodes characterized by the presence of Reed–Sternberg cells on histopathologic examination. Reed–Sternberg cells are giant binucleated malignant reticulum cells having prominent nucleoli. Hodgkin's disease metastasizes predominantly via the lymphatics along predictable, contiguous pathways. This disease represents 40% of all malignant lymphomas. Hodgkin's disease occurs in persons of all ages, but one-half of all clients are between the ages of 20 and 40. Less than 10% of all cases occur before 10 years of age. The overall incidence of Hodgkin's disease is higher in the male population, and males have a poorer prognosis (Bakemeier et al., 1983).

The exact etiology of Hodgkin's disease is unknown. Both genetic and environmental factors seem to be predispositions. Family members are at increased risk, but the disease does not seem to be contagious.

Clinical Manifestations

The usual clinical presentation of Hodgkin's disease is painless lymph node enlargement that may be accompanied by fever, night sweats, pruritus, weight loss, and malaise. Usually, enlarged nodes are above the diaphragm; the cervical nodes are most commonly involved (Figure 29–7).

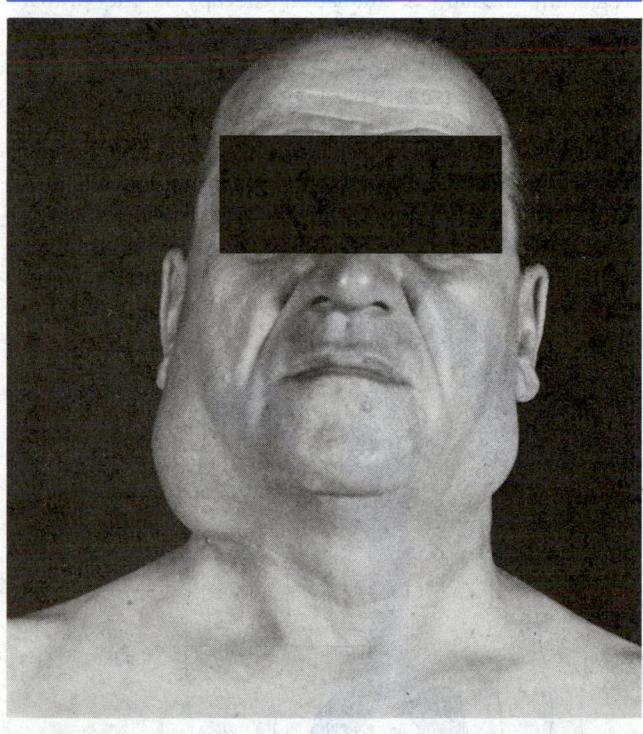

Figure 29–7

Enlargement of cervical lymph nodes due to malignant lymphoma.

SOURCE: *Introduction to Human Disease,* by Leonard V. Crowley. Copyright © 1983 by Wadsworth, Inc. Reprinted by permission of Wadsworth Health Sciences Division, Monterey, CA and the author. Photo provided by Dr. Crowley.

Other supradiaphragmatic nodes that can be involved are the axillary and mediastinal nodes. Signs and symptoms associated with axillary and mediastinal lymphadenopathy include cough, dyspnea, and superior vena cava obstruction. Less commonly, subdiaphragmatic lymphadenopathy is present, most likely in the inguinal nodes. Mesenteric nodes are rarely involved.

Other clinical manifestations may include retroperitoneal lymph node enlargement, hepatosplenomegaly, and bone involvement. These usually occur later, as the disease becomes more generalized. However, a small number of clients may have generalized disease at the time of diagnosis.

Classifications

The four classifications of Hodgkin's disease are based on the histopathologic findings of lymph node biopsy: (1) lymphocyte predominance, (2) nodular sclerosis, (3) mixed cellularity, and (4) lymphocyte depletion. Lymphocyte predominance, which represents approximately 16% of all Hodgkin's disease cases, has the best prognosis with a 90% 5-year disease-free survival rate. Nodular sclerosis has a 70% 5-year disease-free survival rate and represents approximately 35% of all cases of Hodgkin's disease. Mixed cellularity represents approximately one-third of all Hodgkin's disease and has a 4% 5-year disease-free survival rate. Lymphocyte depletion represents approximately 16% of all Hodgkin's disease cases (Bakemeier et al., 1983). This form is usually associated with extensive disease at the time of diagnosis and has a poor overall prognosis.

Staging

Hodgkin's disease is also staged by performing a staging work-up to detect the extent of the malignancy at the time of diagnosis. Clinical staging dictates the treatment modality that will provide the client with the greatest chance for long-term survival and cure. Which clinical staging method to use is controversial. The current method, first introduced in 1971, relies on clinical signs and symptoms along with tissue sampling usually performed during laparotomy. The recommended stages are (Bakemeier et al., 1983):

- Stage I: Involvement of a single node region (stage I) or of a single extralymphatic organ or site (stage IE).

- Stage II: Involvement of two or more nodes on the same side of the diaphragm (stage II) or localized involvement of an extralymphatic organ or site and of one or more lymph node regions on the same side of the diaphragm (stage IIE). (An alternate method uses a subscript of the number of lymph node regions involved; eg, stage II_3.)

- Stage III: Involvement of lymph nodes on both sides of the diaphragm (stage III) and possible involvement of an extralymphatic organ or site (stage IIIE), splenic involvement (stage IIIS), or involvement of both (stage IIISE).

Box 29–2 Essential Diagnostic Tests for Hodgkin's Disease

Complete physical examination, including a pelvic examination in females

Laboratory procedures:

Complete blood count, including a reticulocyte count

Erythrocyte sedimentation rate

Direct Coomb's test

Serum alkaline phosphatase level

Serum albumin level

Serum globulin level

Serum immunoglobulin level

Serum uric acid level

Serum creatinine level

Bone marrow biopsy

Radiologic procedures:

Chest x-ray; possibly tomography or CT scan of chest in the presence of hilar lymphadenopathy

IV pyelography to detect any renal obstruction or ureteral deviation brought about by lymph node enlargement

Bipedal lymphangiography

Abdominal CT scan

Surgical procedures:

Lymph node biopsy

Laparotomy and splenectomy are controversial

• Stage IV: Diffuse, disseminated disease with or without lymph node enlargement. Dissemination usually involves one or more extralymphatic sites identified as follows: H+ = liver (hepatic), L+ = lung, M+ = marrow, P+ = pleura, O+ = bone (osseous), and D+ = skin (dermis).

Each stage is further subdivided either as A or B. *A stage* designates that the client is without certain symptoms or is symptom free. *B stage* denotes that the client has certain symptoms: weight loss of greater than 10% of body weight 6 months before diagnosis, unexplained fever greater than 38°C (100.4°F), and night sweats (Bakemeier et al., 1983).

Diagnostic Tests

Extensive testing is required to diagnose and stage Hodgkin's disease properly. Because the client's clinical stage dictates the treatment modality, these tests are necessary to provide the best chance for cure. Essential diagnostic tests for Hodgkin's disease are listed in Box 29–2.

The performance of laparotomy and splenectomy is controversial. Splenectomy carries a risk in itself, and the splenectomized client, especially the child, has an increased risk for infection. Although laparotomy can identify unsus-

pected nodal and splenic metastasis not found on radiologic examination, it is currently recommended only when the results may influence the choice of therapeutic approach.

Another important diagnostic procedure is lymph node biopsy, which establishes the diagnosis of Hodgkin's disease by the presence of Reed–Sternberg cells. In addition, lymph node biopsy enables the pathologist to classify Hodgkin's disease.

Characteristic patterns in laboratory specimens have been established. Neutrophilic leukocytosis may be present, as well as a mild normocytic, normochromic anemia and eosinophilia. Both Coomb's positive and Coomb's negative hemolytic anemia may be present. Elevations in leukocyte count, alkaline phosphatase level, serum copper level, and erythrocyte sedimentation rate are often associated with exacerbations of the disease. An elevation of the serum alkaline phosphatase level may signal liver and bone metastasis. Hypergammaglobulinemia is common, and hypogammaglobulinemia may occur with advanced disease.

Therapeutic Measures

To develop the best therapeutic program for the client with Hodgkin's disease, the hematologist-oncologist, radiologist-oncologist, and surgeon-oncologist must collaborate about treatment modalities. Radiation therapy is the primary treatment for Hodgkin's disease stages I, II, and IIIA (Bakemeier et al., 1983). Figure 29–8 illustrates the radiation fields used in the treatment of lymph nodes both above and

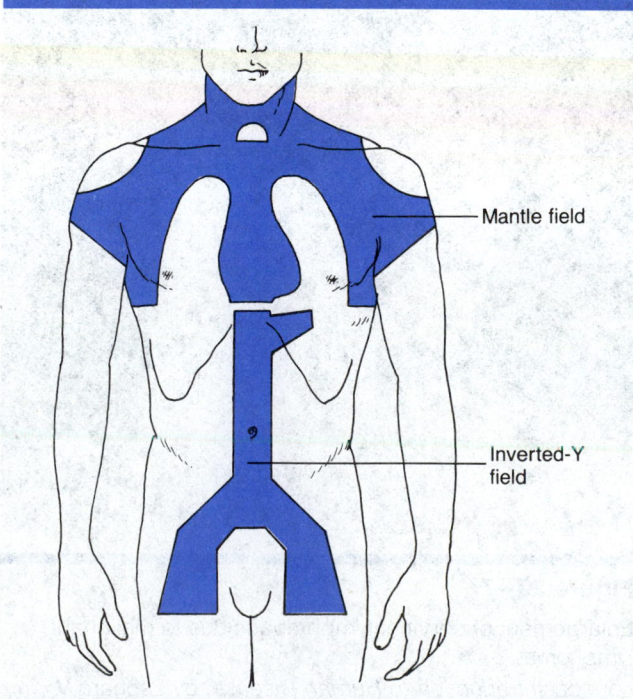

Mantle field

Inverted-Y field

Figure 29–8

The standard mantle and inverted-Y radiation therapy fields for Hodgkin's disease.

below the diaphragm. Subtotal nodal irradiation, which includes fields I and II, is the most common radiation treatment for stages IA and IIA laparotomy-negative clients.

Chemotherapy has its place in the management of more disseminated disease, ie, Hodgkin's disease stages IIIB and IV. Even clients with widespread disease at the time of diagnosis and those with evidence of cross-resistance to one chemotherapeutic protocol still have a chance for long-term survival. Today the major chemotherapeutic protocols involve combinations of antineoplastic drugs. These combinations are listed in Box 12–4 of Chapter 12.

Radiation therapy and chemotherapy also can be combined to give the client the greatest chance for long-term sustained remission. Maintenance-phase chemotherapy has not been useful, however.

Clients who have had a weight loss of greater than 10% of body weight before diagnosis need special nutritional considerations and testing. Serum protein studies may be indicated; if total serum protein and albumin levels are low, a diet high in protein and carbohydrates is needed. Nutritional supplements also may be administered. These clients should consider food part of the medical prescription.

Specific Nursing Measures

Nursing management of the client with Hodgkin's disease is complex. Emotional support and client education are important in all phases of care. Even clients with disseminated disease have a chance for long-term disease-free periods, and those with localized disease have an excellent chance for cure.

During the diagnostic phase, the client may seem overwhelmed by the number and invasiveness of the diagnostic procedures. Explain all procedures thoroughly to the client and family or significant others. Be alert to the need to have questions clarified and to ventilate feelings.

The remission-induction phase brings new challenges to the client, the client's family or friends, and the nurse. These clients are prone to the same problems as anyone receiving radiation therapy or chemotherapy. Because the majority of Hodgkin's disease clients are between 20 and 40 years of age and are receiving radiation therapy, chemotherapy, or both, reproduction may be impaired. Sperm banking offers the male client the possibility of fathering normal offspring at a later time. Especially troublesome are problems caused by nausea and vomiting, bone marrow suppression, and alopecia. The client with nausea and vomiting is prone to developing disturbances in electrolyte balance. Thus, antiemetics should be given routinely, and IV fluids must be regulated to maintain homeostasis.

Bone marrow suppression can lead to leukopenia, anemia, and thrombocytopenia. These conditions make the client prone to the problems of infection, deficits of oxygen transport, and major and minor bleeding episodes. Monitor the client's complete blood count and note when the values are low.

During leukopenic episodes, the major nursing goal is prevention of infection. Clients should avoid crowds and frequently assess themselves for signs and symptoms of infection. This self-assessment necessitates detailed instruction by the nurse.

Oxygen transport problems may be caused by anemia or a large mediastinal mass. Clients with these problems should be encouraged to alternate activity with rest periods. Use of a Fowler's or semi-Fowler's position for resting or sleeping may relieve dyspnea. Monitoring the client's heart and respiratory rates before and after activity may provide clues to the client's ability to tolerate activity. When anemia is severe, administer blood component therapy in the form of packed RBCs.

Overt or occult bleeding episodes are another client problem caused by bone marrow suppression. Special oral hygiene using soft toothbrushes may be needed to prevent gingival oozing. Straight-edged razors and drugs interfering with platelet function are contraindicated.

Body image changes may be difficult for the client to endure and may damage self-esteem. Clients 20 to 40 years old—the age group most commonly affected by Hodgkin's disease—undergo many changes. They are establishing intimate relationships, planning families, and attaining career goals. This is one of the most productive periods of life. The diagnosis of Hodgkin's disease, even with its good chance for cure, still brings the fears associated with cancer. Fertility may be impaired for the client receiving radiation therapy or antineoplastic chemotherapy. These therapies are teratogenic (see Chapter 12); they cause an increased rate of spontaneous abortion or genetically defective offspring. Feelings of loss of control, rejection, and isolation may overwhelm the client.

The nurse is in a prime position to offer these clients emotional support, restored feelings of control, and relief from some of the feelings of rejection and isolation. Establish a trusting relationship as early as possible in the diagnostic phase. Use a calm, unhurried, reassuring approach whenever interacting with these clients. Provide accurate information about Hodgkin's disease, radiation therapy, and chemotherapy, and correct misconceptions about the disease process. Allow clients to make decisions about their schedules whenever possible. Attempt to meet any physical and emotional needs they may have.

NON-HODGKIN'S LYMPHOMA

Included in the classification non-Hodgkin's lymphoma (NHL) are all malignant lymphomas that cannot be classified as Hodgkin's disease. This wide variety of malignant lymphomas differs histologically from one another and is subdivided into two main classes: lymphocyte malignancies and histiocyte malignancies. This discussion considers the NHLs collectively.

In NHL extranodal involvement, unpredictable metastasis and wide dissemination of malignancy are present early in the disease process and usually are encountered at the time of diagnosis. The exact etiology is unknown.

Theories of causality center around viruses and immunosuppression.

There are approximately 15,000 new cases of NHL annually. Most likely to develop the condition are clients 50 to 70 years old, but NHL is not limited to the adult population. Males carry a slightly higher risk for NHL than females.

Clinical Manifestations

The clinical manifestations of NHL are similar to those of Hodgkin's disease: painless lymph node enlargement with or without fever, sweating, weight loss, malaise, and pruritus. There are also differences between NHL and Hodgkin's disease. Extranodal involvement occurs early in the course of NHL and is frequently present upon diagnosis. Manifestations may include involvement of the skin, gastrointestinal tract, bone, and bone marrow. Transformation to leukemia occurs in approximately 13% of NHL cases with high peripheral lymphocyte counts (Bakemeier et al., 1983).

The staging of NHL is identical to that of Hodgkin's disease, and the diagnostic procedures and staging work-up are also similar. As with all malignancies, diagnosis of cell type is based on histopathological tissue sampling.

Therapeutic Measures

As with Hodgkin's disease, collaboration among the hematologist-oncologist, radiologist-oncologist, and surgeon-oncologist is needed to develop the best treatment plan for the individual NHL client. Therapeutic management depends on the clinical stage, histologic type, age of the client, and bone marrow integrity at the time of diagnosis.

The primary purpose of surgery in the treatment of NHL is the diagnosis and clinical staging of the disorder. Radiation therapy is the primary treatment modality in localized disease (stages I and II). In advanced disseminated disease, radiation therapy is combined with adjuvant chemotherapy. For advanced lymphoma (stages III and IV), chemotherapy is prescribed. Multiagent regimens carry the best chances for long-term disease-free survival. Combinations of cyclophosphamide (Cytoxan), vincristine sulfate, prednisone, procarbazine hydrochloride, doxorubicin hydrochloride, and bleomycin are used for disease control. Single-agent treatment programs used in the past led to only short-lived remissions. Nutritional management of clients with NHL is similar to that in Hodgkin's disease.

Specific Nursing Measures

Nursing management of NHL clients is similar to the nursing management for Hodgkin's disease and multiple myeloma. Oncological emergencies occur more frequently in NHL than in Hodgkin's disease, however (see Chapter 12). Superior vena cava obstruction and spinal cord compression are two of the most common. Other complications of NHL include CNS involvement, infections, the development of other primary malignancies, bone involvement, and joint effusions.

The prognosis for the client with NHL is variable. Favorable outcomes are increasingly frequent for localized disease (stages I and II), and long periods free of disease are becoming more common for clients with disseminated disease (stages III and IV). The development of less toxic, more effective chemotherapeutic treatment protocols holds great promise for NHL clients.

MULTIPLE MYELOMA

Multiple myeloma, also called plasma cell myeloma (PCM), is a malignant disorder characterized by the proliferation of abnormal plasma cells in the bone marrow. Single or multiple tumors containing abnormal plasma cells are found throughout the marrow, and immunoglobulin synthesis is disturbed. Multiple myeloma is disseminated throughout the body, ultimately involving the lymph nodes, liver, spleen, and kidneys.

Multiple myeloma occurs exclusively in people over 40 years old. The peak incidence is in the sixth decade of life, and the male-to-female ratio is 2:1. The exact etiology is unknown, but research data suggest a genetic stimulus.

Clinical Manifestations

The onset of multiple myeloma is insidious. A presymptomatic phase may last from 5 to 20 years. During this time, the client's only complaint may be frequent infections, particularly pneumonia. The earliest initial and most frequent complaint is bone pain. Spontaneous pathologic fractures may also occur. Skeletal changes are caused by loss of calcium from bone tissue resulting in hypercalcemia, as well as by invasion of the bone marrow by abnormal plasma cells.

Anemia, fatigue, repeated infection, and bleeding tendencies (such as purpura and epistaxis) represent dysfunction or impairment of bone marrow function. Anorexia, nausea, vomiting, weight loss, and confusion also may be presenting signs and symptoms.

About half of clients have renal insufficiency. Renal function is impaired by hypercalcemia, hyperviscosity of the blood caused by proteinemia, and hyperuricemia. Most commonly, the disease affects the renal tubules, resulting in proteinuria. Characteristic of multiple myeloma is the loss in the urine of a light-chain protein, the Bence–Jones protein.

Diagnosis involves multiple tests. A complete history and physical examination are performed. Complete blood counts with quantitative platelet determinations may demonstrate granulocytopenia, anemia, and thrombocytopenia. Serum studies show hypercalcemia, hyperuricemia, and proteinuria. Prothrombin time and partial thromboplastin times may be altered. The erythrocyte sedimentation rate is elevated. Quantitative immunoglobulin assays indicate a monoclonal immunoglobulin abnormality. Radiologic studies of the ribs, spine, skull, and pelvis show a characteristic "punched-out" or "honeycombed" appearance. A 24-hour urinalysis may demonstrate Bence–Jones protein. The diagnosis of multiple myeloma is confirmed by bone marrow biopsy. Normally, the plasma cell concentration in the bone marrow is approximately 5%; in multiple myeloma, abnormal plasma cell proliferation may range between 30% and 95%.

Therapeutic Measures

Antineoplastic agents are used to induce and maintain a remission in multiple myeloma. The alkylating agents melphalan (Alkeran) and cyclophosphamide are most commonly used. Prednisone may be added to the client's chemotherapeutic program. Remission-induced rates currently approach 60%, and survival is approximately 2 to 5 years.

Supportive pharmacologic management may enhance renal function and promote an optimal level of comfort. Diuretics, particularly furosemide (Lasix), may prevent complications such as congestive heart failure secondary to impaired renal function. This drug also enhances the excretion of calcium ions and therefore is useful in controlling or reducing hypercalcemia. Oral phosphate drugs also promote calcium ion excretion by binding with free calcium ions and aiding excretion via the kidneys. Oral phosphate agents must be used with caution in clients already having renal impairment, however. Allopurinol (Zyloprim) reduces uric acid formation by inhibiting xanthine oxidase formation, preventing uric acid nephropathy caused by hyperuricemia prevalent in multiple myeloma. Narcotic analgesics used in conjunction with muscle relaxants control the pain associated with malignant invasion of the bone marrow by plasma cells.

Clients with multiple myeloma can experience severe anorexia, weight loss, nausea, vomiting, diarrhea, or constipation related to the disease process itself, the effects of chemotherapy and radiation therapy, or immobility. The nurse should attempt to make meals enjoyable. Antiemetics should be used as a forethought, not an afterthought. Offer a diet high in proteins, vitamins, minerals, and carbohydrates. The client may more easily tolerate small, frequent meals (perhaps six a day).

Dehydration can become a life-threatening complication because of renal shutdown. Acute renal failure can be precipitated by the accompanying hyperuricemia, proteinemia, hypercalcemia, and increased viscosity of the blood. Clients with multiple myeloma have a fluid need requirement above the maintenance need, and 1½ to 2 times the normal fluid requirements (approximately 4 to 5 L/day) should be forced. Urine output should show the appropriate increase. At no time should these clients have a sustained period without fluid intake. If an NPO status is necessary for diagnostic procedures, an IV route with an appropriate flow rate is warranted. Renal disease is easier to prevent than treat. If renal shutdown occurs, hemodialysis may be necessary.

Specific Nursing Measures

The two foremost goals of nursing management for clients with multiple myeloma are maintaining optimal hydration and promoting optimal physical activity. Ambulation must be maintained because the activity increases circulation, decreases demineralization of bones by slowing the loss of calcium, and can reduce the occurrence of spontaneous fractures. Use assistive devices such as splints, canes, or walkers to reduce the discomfort and fear associated with full weight bearing. Before expecting cooperation with ambulation, make sure the client is relatively comfortable by administering non-narcotic analgesics and muscle relaxants. Accompany clients taking these drugs whenever they are ambulating.

Bone marrow suppression results from infiltration and destruction of bone marrow tissue, and is also a side effect of the radiation and antineoplastic drug therapy. For a description of the nursing care of the client receiving radiation therapy and chemotherapy, see Chapter 12. Monitor the client's blood counts for values indicating leukopenia, anemia, or thrombocytopenia. Severe bone marrow suppression is indicated by pallor, a tendency toward fatigue, shortness of breath, petechiae, purpura, epistaxis, melena, or fever. Administer blood component therapy (packed RBCs, or platelets) when warranted. Use safe, gentle nursing techniques when thrombocytopenia and anemia are present. Refer to the discussion of care of the leukemic client with thrombocytopenia and anemia.

The client with multiple myeloma has complex psychosocial needs. Because the peak incidence is middle adulthood, the client is likely to be facing financial responsibilities of a mortgage and college tuition for children, other family monetary responsibilities, unemployment, divorce, or death of a spouse. Middle adulthood also can be a time of career success. Complications of disease progression and the side effects of treatment may alter the client's self-esteem and feeling of control. Provide an environment that promotes self-esteem and gives the client a sense of control over the body. Establish a trusting relationship, maintain open and honest communication, encourage the client and family or significant others to participate in care as much as possible, and provide a sense of control through client education. A teaching plan for the client with multiple myeloma includes education about the disease process, the significance of antineoplastic drug and radiation therapy, the importance of ambulation and adequate hydration, and pain management.

POLYCYTHEMIA VERA

Polycythemia vera is a myeloproliferative disorder characterized by panmyelosis. Panmyelosis is characterized by marked erythrocytosis, leukocytosis, and thrombocytosis.

Splenomegaly is also present. The erythrocytosis is so massive that hypervolemia and hyperviscosity of the blood result. The red blood cell mass may be two to three times normal without a concurrent rise in plasma volume. The hyperviscosity and thrombocytosis set the stage for the development of thrombi, which can affect every organ system of the body.

Overt or occult bleeding episodes also accompany this disorder. Hypervolemia is thought to damage the walls of veins. Once damaged, veins may rupture from overdistension.

Polycythemia vera has an insidious onset and a lengthy, progressive course. Eventually, the bone marrow undergoes myelofibrotic and osteosclerotic changes, anemia occurs, and immature granulocytes appear in the bloodstream. Extension and infiltration of erythrocytes primarily, and to a lesser extent, leukocytes and platelets, into the spleen, liver, and lymph nodes can develop. Transformation of polycythemia vera into leukemia and other myeloproliferative disorders has been reported.

This disorder is primarily a disease of the middle-aged and older adult. Incidence is slightly higher in males, but there is no known geographic or regional distribution. The exact etiology is unknown. A viral agent has been implicated in mice, but polycythemia vera is not transmitted by contact with clients or their blood.

Clinical Manifestations

The basic pathologic changes associated with polycythemia vera are caused by hypervolemia and hyperviscosity of the blood from erythrocytosis. Because this disorder is systemic, clinical manifestations are varied and may not suggest the underlying disease process. Any organ system may be involved.

Clients have alterations in their peripheral blood counts. The hemogram shows elevated levels of hemoglobin, circulating erythrocytes, hematocrit, and reticulocytes. Leukocytosis and thrombocytosis are also present.

As in many myeloproliferative disorders, the basal metabolic rate is elevated without any evidence of alteration in thyroid function. Hyperuricemia and hyperuricosuria are also evident in the presence of leukocytosis. Symptoms of gouty arthritis may become apparent if uric acid levels are left untreated.

The skin takes on a characteristic ruddy appearance, especially over the face and hands. Pruritus and eczema-like dermatologic changes may also be present. In addition, these clients may be sensitive to extremes of hot and cold, as in bath water temperature.

Clients may have an elevated systolic and diastolic blood pressure, left ventricular hypertrophy, palpitations, and angina in response to the increased work load on the heart. Other cardiovascular signs and symptoms include dizziness, exertional dyspnea, and peripheral edema.

Sluggish circulation with resultant thrombi formation may precipitate infarctions of the spleen, heart, and brain.

CNS symptoms are the most frequent. Disturbances in cerebral blood flow may cause headaches, vertigo, tinnitus, and visual problems such as diplopia and blurred vision. Hypervolemia and consequent venous distention can cause esophageal varices and hemorrhoids. As already mentioned, hemorrhage can ensue when vessels are weakened and damaged. Some hemorrhages, such as bleeding esophageal varices, may be life threatening. Other bleeding may be minute, such as petechiae and ecchymoses. Epistaxis is common.

Peptic ulcer disease is 10 times more common in polycythemia vera clients than in the general population. The exact reason for this increased incidence is unknown. The predilection may involve thrombi formation to the stomach and ileum, or a disequilibrium between the gastric mucin and hydrochloric acid secretion may leave the gastric and intestinal mucosa unprotected by mucin.

Therapeutic Measures

Phlebotomy is often used to return the hemogram rapidly to relative normalcy. Once the peripheral blood count is normalized, radiation therapy or chemotherapy is begun. Radioactive phosphorus (^{32}P) is a safe, easy, and effective mode of inducing myelosuppression in the client with polycythemia vera. Recently, alkylating agents have been shown to effect myelosuppression as well; these include busulfan (Myleran), cyclophosphamide, chlorambucil (Leukeran), and melphalan (Williams et al., 1983). The introduction of ^{32}P and antineoplastic agents to the treatment program of polycythemia vera has lengthened the average survival time to approximately 13 years.

The control of hyperuricemia and the treatment of gouty arthritis are discussed in Chapter 59. Peptic ulcer disease is discussed in Chapter 49.

The client with polycythemia vera who has an increased basal metabolic rate may have lost weight before diagnosis. Small, frequent, high-calorie, high-protein meals should be served. Dietary supplements high in calories and proteins may need to be added to the client's nutritional regimen. The nurse should make mealtime pleasant and productive and monitor the client's weight carefully.

Regardless of whether there is an elevated basal metabolic rate or peptic ulcer disease, maintaining adequate hydration is essential for these clients. Dehydration compounds the hyperviscosity of polycythemia vera and may precipitate thrombotic episodes.

Specific Nursing Measures

Nursing management of polycythemia vera clients centers around reducing hypervolemia and hyperviscosity. As already stated, the use of ^{32}P or alkylating agents to attain myelosuppression may follow phlebotomy. Phlebotomy is not without risk. Volume loss may precipitate signs and symptoms of shock, so the assessment of vital signs and the signs and symptoms of hypovolemia during phlebotomy is crucial. Repeated phlebotomies may be necessary to reduce the viscosity of the blood adequately, and iron deficiency anemia can result. Supplemental iron can correct this deficiency. Phlebotomy does not correct the panmyelosis of this disease; it only reduces hypervolemia and hyperviscosity. Phlebotomy is further discussed in Chapter 28.

When chemotherapeutic agents are administered, assess their adverse or toxic effects. Close monitoring of the peripheral blood count is necessary. Hyperuricemia can result from a dramatic and rapid reduction in leukocytes. A decreasing urinary output seen while accurately measuring the client's intake and output may be the first indication of uric acid nephropathy. Hydration and dietary requirements are discussed in the section on therapeutic measures.

Stress the need for adequate activity to promote vascular integrity, prevent stasis, and promote a sense of control over life. Because these clients have a life expectancy of approximately 13 years after diagnosis, it is essential for them to return to their usual patterns of everyday life.

Client education is another important aspect of nursing management to improve compliance with the medical and nutritional regimens. In addition, client education may foster autonomy and a sense of control over the disease process. Instruction should include explanations of the disease process, the rationale for phlebotomy and radiation therapy or chemotherapy, the importance of compliance with the dietary prescription and fluid needs, and the effectiveness of maintaining optimum activity levels. Encourage clients who smoke to reduce their smoking or stop altogether. Over a long time, smoking increases the hematocrit level, increasing the viscosity of the blood.

Chapter Highlights

Congenital disorders of the blood and blood-forming organs affect the body's erythrocyte, leukocyte, and coagulation mechanisms. Clients with these disorders require the nurse's support and instruction during genetic and career counseling.

Included in the congenital disorders are sickle cell anemia, thalassemia, spherocytosis, glucose-6-phosphate dehydrogenase (G-6-PD) deficiency, hemophilia, and von Willebrand's disease.

Multifactorial hematologic disorders may involve interference in one or a combination of the following functions of the bone marrow elements: resistance to infectious organisms, coagulation, or the transportation of oxygen to tissues.

These multifactorial disorders include aplastic, pernicious, and iron deficiency anemia; disseminated intravascular coagulation (DIC); idiopathic thrombocytopenic purpura (ITP); and granulocytopenia.

The nurse's role in the management of clients with immunologic disorders of the blood and blood-forming organs includes education on the disease process and avoiding contact with infectious agents, providing support during genetic counseling or when the prognosis is poor, and assessing the client for signs and symptoms of infection.

Immunologic disorders include acquired immune deficiency syndrome (AIDS) and agammaglobulinemia.

Neoplastic hematologic disorders—the leukemias, lymphomas, and multiple myelomas—involve infiltration and disruption of normal bone marrow function and an alteration in the usual protective mechanism of the immune system.

Nursing care of the client with leukemia centers around leukopenia, anemia, and thrombocytopenia. In addition, the client may need help in dealing with pain, ineffective coping skills, body-image changes, and the side effects of chemotherapy.

Both Hodgkin's disease and NHL affect clients at a period of life when their major concerns involve raising a family and establishing and maintaining a career.

The nursing care of clients with multiple myeloma includes promoting comfort and preventing spontaneous fractures and renal shutdown.

Nursing management of polycythemia vera clients centers around reducing hypervolemia and hyperviscosity, providing client education, promoting vascular integrity, and preventing stasis.

Bibliography

Acquired immunodeficiency syndrome (AIDS) update: United States. *MMWR* 1983; 32:309–311.

Allen J, Mellin G: The new epidemic: Immune deficiency, opportunistic infections, and Kaposi's sarcoma. *Am J Nurs* 1982; 82:1718–1722.

American Cancer Society: *Facts and Figures.* New York: American Cancer Society, 1985.

Bakemeier RF et al: The malignant lymphomas: Hodgkin's disease and non-Hodgkin's lymphoma, multiple myeloma, and macroglobulinemia. In: *Clinical Oncology for Medical Students and Physicians.* Bakemeier RF (editor). Rochester, NY: American Cancer Society, 1983.

Bank AJ, Mears G, Ramirez F: Disorders of human hemoglobin. *Science* 1980; 27:486–493.

Benenson AS: *Control of Communicable Disease in Man,* 14th ed. Washington, DC: American Public Health Association, 1985.

Bennett JA: AIDS epidemiology update. *Am J Nurs* 1985; 85:968–972.

Bleyer WA: Acute lymphoid leukemia. *Pediatr Ann* 1983; 12(4):277–292.

CDC: Update: Prospective evaluation of health-care workers exposed via parenteral or mucous-membrane route to blood or body fluids from patients with acquired immunodeficiency syndrome. *MMWR* 1985; 34:101–103.

Cloak MM, Levitt DZ: Cancer chemotherapy: The nurse can make the difference. *Critical Care Update* (April) 1982; 7–18.

Couric JM: Hemophilia has outlasted the czars. *FDA Consumer* (June) 1984; 18:18–23.

Curran JW et al: The epidemiology of AIDS: Current status and future prospects. *Science* 1985; 229:1352–1357.

Dampier C, Chilcote RR: Acute non-lymphoid leukemia. *Pediatr Ann* 1983; 12(4):293–305.

Kayser SR: Thrombosis. In: *Applied Therapeutics: The Clinical Use of Drugs,* 3rd ed. Katcher BS, Young LY, Koda–Kimble, MA (editors). San Francisco: Applied Therapeutics, 1983; 333–360.

Landsman SH, Rao SP, Ahonkhai VI: Infections in children with sickle cell anemia. *Am J Pediatr Hematol/Oncol* 1982; 4:407–415.

Masoorli ST, Piercy S: A step-by-step guide to trouble-free transfusions. *RN* (May) 1984; 47:34–42.

Price DM, Scimeca AM: The epidemic of the 80s: AIDS. *Canc Nurs* 1984; 7(4):283–290.

Reich P: *Hematology: Physiopathologic Basic for Clinical Practice,* 2nd ed. Boston: Little, Brown, 1984.

Rodman MJ, Smith DW: *Clinical Pharmacology in Nursing,* 2nd ed. Philadelphia: Lippincott, 1984.

Sarnaik SA, Lusher JM: Neurological complications of sickle cell anemia. *Am J Pediatr Hematol/Oncol* 1982; 4:396–394.

Schmalzer E, Chien S, Brown A: Transfusion therapy in sickle cell disease. *Am J Pediatr Hematol/Oncol* 1982; 4:395–403.

Spivak J (editor): *Fundamentals of Clinical Hematology,* 2nd ed. Philadelphia: Harper & Row, 1984.

Update: Acquired immunodeficiency syndrome (AIDS): United States. *MMWR* 1983; 32:389–391.

Williams WJ et al: *Hematology,* 3rd ed. New York: McGraw–Hill, 1983.

Yasko JM: *Guidelines for cancer care: Symptom management.* Reston, VA: Reston, 1983.

Suggested Readings

Caza B, Ross CA: Living with leukemia. *Can Nurse* (Sept) 1981; 77:32–36. Description of the early work-up and diagnostic period of a young registered nurse with leukemia. Article focuses on the nurse–client's feelings.

Ersek MT: The adult leukemia patient in the intensive care unit. *Heart Lung* 1984; 13:183–193. The author reviews the disease, its treatment, and major complications, and focuses on the nursing role in infection and hemorrhage. The article includes a detailed discussion of the stress to client, family, and nurse.

Levitt DE: Multiple myeloma. *Am J Nurs* 1981; 81:1345–1347. This article describes the pathophysiology, diagnosis, and treatment of multiple myeloma. Additional suggestions are given for preventing complications.

Maxwell MB: When the cancer patient becomes anemic. *Cancer Nurs* 1984; 7:499–503.. This article includes assessments and nursing care for the cancer client who becomes anemic.

Pack B (editor): Symposium on sickle cell disease. *Nurs Clin North Am* 1983; 18:129–229. The entire issue is devoted to sickle cell disease, including pathophysiology, the pain experience, antisickling agents, psychosocial considerations, and complications of sickle cell disease.

Price DM, Scimeca AM: The epidemic of the 80s: AIDS. *Cancer Nurs* 1984; 7:283–290. This article investigates the impact and complications of AIDS. A major premise supports the viewpoint that AIDS is moving from a disorder of homosexual males to a heterosexual disorder.

Slaff JI, Brubaker JK: *The AIDS Epidemic: How You Can Protect Yourself and Your Family—Why You Must.* New York: Warner, 1985. This soft-cover book is addressed to both the heterosexual and homosexual communities and is available at local bookstores. Written by a medical investigator at the National Institutes of Health and a medical writer, it discusses practical personal precautions and answers questions on transmission.

The Client With Leukemia

I. Brief Descriptive Data

Mr Jones, a 45-year-old Caucasian male, made an appointment to see his physician because of fatigue, weakness, fever, aching "all over," and bone and joint pain for 2 months. Mr Jones was admitted to the hospital for further work-up.

II. Personal Data

Date: April 4, 1986

Full Name: Martin J. Jones

Address: 4831 Pine St., Belleville, IL 60935

Telephone: Home: 000-0000

Work: 000-0000

Sex: Male

Age: 45

Birthdate: 2-17-41

Marital Status: Married

Religion: Baptist

Occupation: Architect

Usual Health Care Provider: Lonny Tiedman, MD

III. Health History

Source of Information: Client

Reliability of Informant: Reliable, good historian

Chief Concern: Fatigue, weakness, fever, and bone and joint pain for last 2 months

History of Present Illness: Mr Jones states that over the past 2 months, he has become increasingly tired and weak. "It's so bad sometimes that I can hardly make it through the day." Mr Jones has noticed periodic episodes of pain, "especially in my joints." He has also been anorexic and lost 10 lb in the past month. Mr Jones' wife has noticed that he seems rather pale.

Over the past 2 months, has noticed a change in his sleep patterns; now sleeping at least 10 hours a night. "I just can't get enough sleep; sometimes I come home from work and nap before supper; I fall asleep a lot while watching television." Denies use of alcohol, except an occasional beer once or twice a month. Does not smoke.

No indigestion, dysphagia, food intolerance, diarrhea, constipation, nausea, or vomiting. Stools are brown—have never been black. States he has had a "chest cold" for the past month that he "can't seem to shake." No SOB, DOE, PND. Has an occasional nonproductive cough. No chest pain, no palpitations, no ankle edema.

Has noticed no lymph node enlargement in the neck, axilla, or groin regions. Recently has noted easy bruising and bleeding gums after teeth brushing; no epistaxis, nocturia, or rectal bleeding.

Has occasional episodes of severe joint pain, especially in the knees and hips; no swelling of joints. No hx of joint trauma or arthritic problems. No hx of recent infections except for his cold. Takes no medications except an occasional aspirin for headache. Has had no exposure to radiation or toxic chemicals.

(continued)

The Client With Leukemia

Past Health History:	
Childhood:	Usual childhood illnesses; measles, mumps, chickenpox
Immunizations:	Unsure of date of last Td; otherwise thinks immunizations are current
Medical Problems:	None
Surgeries:	Appendectomy as a child; left inguinal hernia repair, 1972
Transfusions:	None
Trauma:	None
Allergies:	None known to medications, foods, or environmental allergens
Medications:	None
Family History:	Father, died age 60, massive MI
	Mother, age 73, alive; has IDDM
	Siblings, none
	Wife, age 42, A&W, no health problems
	Sons × 2, ages 18 and 20, A&W, no health problems
	No positive FHx of hypertension, CVA, malignancy, or hematologic problems
Personal/Social History:	Lives with wife and two sons in suburban community; owns own home; financially secure; has a master's degree; employed full time as senior architectural engineer for large architectural firm. Average day spent either in office working on designs or on location at construction site overseeing progress of construction work. Wife is a lawyer.
	States he and wife have not had sexual intercourse for at least 1 month. "I'm just too tired." Denies any problems with sexual functioning. Previously played tennis weekly with college roommate; hasn't played tennis for at least 2 months. States wife and he communicate easily. "Evelyn usually reads me like a book"; wife can usually get client to verbalize feelings.
	Usually skips breakfast; lunch is eaten in restaurants or fast-food chains; supper is eaten at home with wife and sons. "We all pitch in to help with supper—it's about the only time we all get to see other other."
Review of Systems:	
Overall Health:	Until the past 2 months, has been in good health. Has an annual physical exam and states he's always gotten "a clean bill of health."
Skin:	Denies any past problems related to the skin; denies jaundice or pruritus
Eyes:	No changes in visual acuity; doesn't wear corrective lenses
Ears:	Denies any hearing problems
Nose and Sinuses:	No olfactory changes; no recent problems with sinus infections
Mouth and Teeth:	Denies any gustatory changes; has full set of teeth; last dental examination 8 months ago
Throat and Neck:	See history of present illness
Chest/Heart:	See history of present illness
Genitourinary:	No frequency, urgency, trouble starting or stopping urinary stream

Neurologic:	Denies any headaches, dizziness, fainting spells, difficulty concentrating
Psychologic:	Denies any psychological problems. States: "Things have been going really well for us. I just want to find out why I'm so tired all the time."

IV. Physical Assessment

Weight:	185 lb
Height:	5 ft 11 in
Vital Signs:	Temperature 101.7°F (38.7°C); pulse 110; respirations 36; blood pressure 116/86, rt arm, supine
Relevant Organ Systems:	
Skin:	Pale, warm, and dry; bruises and petechiae noted, particularly over the lower extremities; one large (6 × 7 cm) ecchymotic area, right elbow
Neck:	Solitary 3 × 3 cm lymph node palpable in rt cervical chain; slightly tender; no other lymphadenopathy
Axillae:	s̄ nodes
Mouth:	Mucous membranes pale, gums hypertrophied
Respiratory:	Bibasilar rhonchi both anteriorly and posteriorly; other lung fields clear
Cardiovascular:	PMI at 5th LICS at MCL; heart rate regular; no murmurs heard
Abdomen:	Bowel sounds hypoactive; abdomen soft, flat; liver palpated 3 cm below RCM; tip of spleen palpable; no palpable groin nodes
Musculoskeletal:	No obvious joint deformities or swelling noted; resisted full ROM left hip; maintains left hip in 20° flexion; lies on right side
Psychological:	Oriented to time, place, and person; good recent and remote memory; logical thought pattern; asks and answers questions appropriately

V. Diagnostic Data

The following diagnostic studies were done:

- CBC with differential: WBC 50.0; RBC 2.0; Hb 8.0; platelets 45,000; polymorphonuclear neutrophils 0; bands 3%; lymphs 2%; basophils and eosinophils 0; monocytes 0; blasts 95%
- Urinalysis: Specific gravity: 1.028; protein: negative; glucose: negative; blood: moderate
- Myeloperoxidase positive
- Sudan black stain positive
- Plasma fibrinogen normal
- Prothrombin time (PT), 11.5 seconds (normal)
- Partial thromboplastin time (PTT), 32 seconds (normal)
- Fibrin degradation products, 7 µg/mL (normal)
- Blood cultures: *Pseudomonas aeruginosa*
- Bone marrow aspiration: Demonstrated replacement of the bone marrow cellular elements with myeloblasts; Auer bodies visualized
- Chest x-ray: Bibasilar consolidation with atelectasis

VI. Summary

Following bone marrow aspiration, the diagnosis of *acute granulocytic leukemia* was established. Remission-induction phase was initiated using the following drugs: Cytosine arabinoside (Cytosar-U), prednisone, vincristine (Oncovin), doxorubicin (Adriamycin). In addition, the client was given carbenicillin, gentamicin, and oxacillin intravenously for the Pseudomonas septicemia. The following nursing care plan was developed for the remission-induction phase of Mr Jones's illness

(continued)

The Client With Leukemia

VII. Nursing Care Plan

Nursing Diagnosis	Client Care Goals	Plan/Nursing Implementation	Expected Outcome
Comfort, alteration in: pain related to proliferation of bone marrow elements	Remain free of pain	Place client in a position of comfort, use pillows for support, change position every 2 h; use distraction or diversional activities p.r.n.; administer analgesic medication as prescribed; back rub gently p.r.n.; spend unhurried time with client every day; encourage activity but provide client with frequent rest periods as needed	Decrease in joint and bone discomfort; client will independently perform ADL when appropriate
Injury: potential for infection related to incompetent bone marrow and immunosuppressive effects of chemotherapeutic regimen	Recover from current infection; remain afebrile; prevent additional infections	Reverse isolation: use good handwashing; no fresh fruits or vegetables, fresh cut flowers, or plants in room; explain rationale to client (ie, to protect the client from sources of infection); monitor temperature q. 4 h, monitor for any signs/symptoms of infection, including symptoms of septic shock; assess respiratory status (ie, dyspnea, cough, SOB); administer granulocytes as ordered; assess urinary status (ie, burning, frequency, urgency with urination); administer antibiotics as ordered; watch for toxic effects of antibiotics; monitor WBC level and differential count; begin client teaching about the function of WBCs; assess all portals of entry (eg, intravenous sites) at least every shift	Client will have increased energy and improved interest in what is happening to him; current infection will be resolved, and no new infections will occur
Injury: potential for bleeding related to incompetent bone marrow and immunosuppressive effects of chemotherapeutic regimen	Be alert to symptoms and signs of bleeding; remain free from major bleeding episodes	Monitor pulse and BP q. 4 h; note any signs/symptoms of hypovolemic shock; test urine, stool, emesis for blood; use soft toothbrush or gauze sponge for oral hygiene; do oral hygiene q.i.d.; note gingival oozing after oral hygiene; apply topical thrombin if gingival oozing persists; offer foods soft and easy to chew; note occurrence and spread of petechiae and bruising; caution client to be careful when up; no straight-edged razors, IM injections, aspirin or aspirin products, or rectal temperatures; monitor platelet levels; teach client to read all OTC medication labels and to avoid taking products containing aspirin; encourage client to seek medical advice before self-medicating with OTC drugs	Client will tell care provider of any symptoms or signs of bleeding; client will avoid aspirin products and all OTC medications; client will not have any major bleeding episodes
Nutrition, alteration in: less than body requirements; related to side effects of chemotherapeutic regimen	Maintain optimum nutritional status; maintain normal weight level	Initiate dietary consult; inquire about client's food preferences, remembering that fresh fruits and vegetables are not allowed because they are potential sources of infection; offer small, frequent feedings (ie, breakfast, midmorning snack, lunch, midafternoon snack, supper, H.S. snack); avoid extremes of temperature in foods served (hot and cold); serve meals attractively; remove unpleasant stimuli	Client will eat well-balanced meals without causing bleeding of oral mucosa; client will become knowledgeable about nutrition and select appropriate foods when at home; client will maintain normal weight; client will feel more energetic

Nursing Diagnosis	Client Care Goals	Plan/Nursing Implementation	Expected Outcome
		from surroundings at mealtime; assist client in selecting easily chewed foods that meet requirements from the basic food groups; maintain daily calorie count; weigh client every other day at the same time each day; administer antiemetics as ordered; do not wait until client becomes nauseated or vomits before giving antiemetic	
Oral mucous membrane, alterations in	Maintain healthy oral mucosa; remain free from oral infections	Perform oral hygiene p.r.n.; use soft toothbrush/gauze/sponges for oral care; assess client's mouth for stomatitis or other oral lesions (candidiasis) twice daily; note condition and integrity of gingiva, buccal mucosa, tongue; observe characteristics of saliva (ie, thin, abundant or stringy, scant); encourage frequent rinsing of mouth with cool water to keep mucous membranes moist; apply lubricant to lips as needed	Client will feel confident in assessing mouth for lesions, infection—and will notify the health care provider if they occur; client will manage oral hygiene effectively
Knowledge deficit, related to disease process and treatment	Understand disease process and treatment used; return home with confidence	Assist client and wife to ask questions of health professionals; listen to their expression of fears/anxieties; teach at client's level of readiness to learn about: disease process, function of blood cells, chemotherapy, predictable side effects of chemotherapy; remember client and significant others will need review periodically throughout the hospitalization; encourage involvement of client and significant others in discharge plans; contact the outpatient nurse and establish a relationship between the client and the outpatient nurse before discharge; give the client a copy of the inpatient and outpatient telephone numbers and encourage the client to call when questions arise	Client will express feelings of anxiety openly; client begins to make decisions about health care; client states he feels comfortable about going home or looks forward to going home; client is able to state in own words what was taught
Coping, ineffective individual and family: related to severity of diagnosis and potential fatal outcome (long term)	Regain a sense of control	Establish therapeutic relationship with client and significant others; answer questions honestly, but do not destroy client's defense mechanisms; acknowledge client's feelings; be nonjudgmental and accepting if the client demonstrates anger, fear, or denial; support the client's defense mechanisms; recognize use of anger, fear, denial are defense mechanisms needed by the client to cope with this disease	Client will make decisions about health care and ask about disease process

(continued)

The Client With Leukemia

VII. Nursing Care Plan *(continued)*

Nursing Diagnosis	Client Care Goals	Plan/Nursing Implementation	Expected Outcome
Self-concept, disturbances in: related to body-image changes with chemotherapy and isolation secondary to immunosuppressive effects of chemotherapy	Maintain positive self-concept	Do not avoid client or avoid making eye contact with client; spend "quality" time with client each shift; if allowed, encourage other staff members to make client visits; encourage family members to visit frequently; if allowed, encourage friends to visit; instruct family members and friends about the rationale for and proper technique of isolation (if implemented); encourage client to continue work-related activities when able (eg, phone calling, memo writing); if permissible, encourage the client to pursue hobbies while hospitalized; involve client in decisions about daily care routines; be flexible in scheduling care; encourage client to ventilate feelings about diagnosis and treatment; explore with the client how he feels about present situation	Client will express that body-image changes are temporary; client will make decisions about health care needs; client will become involved in daily care routines

Chapter 30

Surgical Approaches to Vascular and Blood Dysfunction

Janice Lech Dusek
Carol Ren Kneisl

Objectives

When you have finished studying this chapter, you should be able to:

Define and describe the surgical procedures for peripheral vascular disease and disorders of the blood and blood-forming organs.

Apply an understanding of the physiological and psychosocial/lifestyle implications of each procedure to the nursing care of the client.

Identify the preoperative and postoperative nursing implications of each procedure.

Explain the similarities in the care of clients having surgery for peripheral vascular disease.

Describe the nursing care of the bone marrow donor and the bone marrow recipient.

The preoperative and postoperative care of clients undergoing surgical intervention for vascular or blood-forming organ dysfunction offers a challenge to nursing. Many clients are hospitalized for long periods and are at risk for major complications associated with these types of surgeries—bleeding, occlusion of blood vessels, and infection. Astute nursing care is essential to prevent, detect, and minimize these complications as well as to enhance the client's recovery and adaptation to any long-term lifestyle changes.

Section I: Surgical Approaches to Disorders Affecting the Arteries and Veins

This section discusses a wide variety of surgical procedures. Some procedures involve the direct removal, replacement, or manipulation of a blood vessel; others require diversion of blood flow; and still others, such as lumbar sympathectomy, indirectly affect blood flow.

Many clients having these surgeries have a long history of peripheral vascular disease. In addition to the specific preoperative and postoperative nursing measures described below, remember to implement the nursing measures, health teaching, and lifestyle changes recommended in Chapter 27 where peripheral vascular disorders are discussed in detail. In some instances, clients with advanced peripheral vascular disease may require amputation of an extremity. Amputation is discussed in Chapter 60.

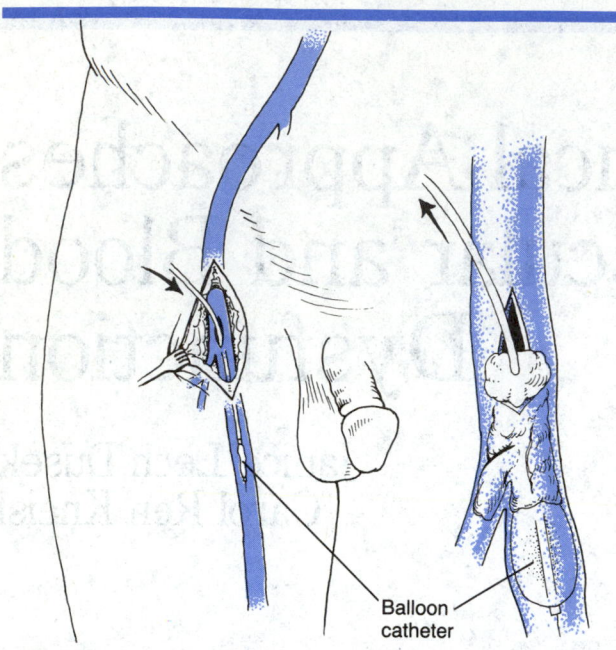

Figure 30–1
Embolectomy. **A.** The balloon catheter is inserted into the common femoral artery. **B.** The catheter is withdrawn along with the embolus.

EMBOLECTOMY

An embolectomy is the removal of an occluding embolus from an artery by means of a surgical incision into a blood vessel with the aim of restoring normal blood flow. Embolectomy is the procedure of choice when a major vessel to an extremity is occluded. This procedure is most effective in acute arterial occlusion if it is performed within 6 hours of the occlusion, because tissue damage is progressive and often reaches an irreversible stage by the sixth hour. After this time, saving the extremity may be impossible, and amputation may become necessary.

Surgical Procedure

An initial incision exposes the occluded artery. The obstructed artery and its branches are then controlled above and below the point of embolic occlusion. A balloon catheter such as a Fogarty catheter is passed beyond the point of clot attachment. The balloon is then inflated, and the catheter is withdrawn along with the embolus (Figure 30–1). This may have to be repeated, to ensure embolus removal. After the operative area is closed, pressure dressings to prevent bleeding are usually applied.

Implications for the Client

Physiological Implications

Embolectomy alleviates the severe pain associated with vasospasm and ischemia secondary to arterial obstruction and, if performed soon enough, maintains the viability of the affected extremity. Potential major complications are bleeding and emboli. Following an embolectomy, clients require long-term anticoagulant therapy because the surgical area and the site of the occlusion provide a rough surface for potential platelet aggregation and thrombus formation.

Psychosocial/Lifestyle Implications

A successful embolectomy alleviates the client's fear of losing an extremity to amputation. However, clients may be anxious about the possibility of thrombus formation at the operative site or development of another embolus, especially if the client is prone to atheromatous plaques. To help prevent stasis, the client must become accustomed to a daily exercise routine designed to stimulate circulation to the extremity. Avoiding long periods of sitting or pressure on peripheral vessels is essential. The physiological and psychosocial/lifestyle implications are listed in Table 30–1.

Nursing Implications

Preoperative Care

Before surgery, measures are essential to prevent fragmentation of the embolus that would result in occlusion of distal vessels. These measures include keeping the client on bed rest and protecting the extremity from trauma. A bed cradle keeps linens off the extremities, avoiding pressure and providing protection. A soft pillow between the legs helps to prevent the client from accidentally bumping the affected extremity. Family and nursing personnel should also be reminded to avoid bumping or jarring the extremity or the client's bed. Do not elevate the affected extremity; it should be kept level or in a slightly dependent position.

Obtain baseline vital sign measurements for comparison in the postoperative period. Preoperative vascular assessment will help to determine postoperative changes. Obtain peripheral pulses distal to the occlusion, noting their

Table 30–1	Embolectomy, Thrombectomy, and Endarterectomy: Implications for the Client	
Physiological Implications	**Psychosocial/Lifestyle Implications**
Alleviates pain from vasospasm and ischemia; maintains viability of affected extremity	Alleviates fear of losing extremity to amputation
Potential complications of bleeding, thrombus, or embolus	Anxiety over possibility of thrombus or embolus
Long-term anticoagulant therapy	Regular daily exercise; avoidance of long periods of sitting or pressure on peripheral vessels

presence or absence and pulse strength. Measurements should be obtained for both extremities. It may be necessary to use a Doppler flow-meter (see Chapter 26). Note and record the color, temperature, and sensation in both extremities. Administer anticoagulants, thrombolytics, analgesics, and antispasmodics as necessary.

Postoperative Care

The client is maintained on bed rest for 8 to 10 hours postoperatively. Monitor vital signs and compare them to their preoperative baselines. The blood pressure should not vary significantly from preoperative levels; variations predispose the client to thrombus formation.

Assess vascular status, paying particular attention to the pulses palpable distal to the site of the occlusion and to the color, temperature, and sensation in the affected extremity. Be alert to any changes. Observe the pressure dressings for evidence of bleeding and be aware of potential signs of hemorrhage such as increased pulse, decreased blood pressure, restlessness, and pallor. Renal function is an excellent indicator of vascular perfusion: if hemorrhage occurs, oliguria follows shortly.

As with any postoperative client, encourage coughing and deep breathing every hour and observe for indications of cardiac, renal, and pulmonary complications as well as infection. Range-of-motion (ROM) exercises are especially important in preventing stasis. Encourage the client to turn and move in bed to stimulate circulation to the affected extremity. Other activities and ambulation are determined mutually with the surgeon.

In addition to administering analgesics, attempt to create a comfortable environment for the client when performing ROM exercises and while deep breathing and coughing. Administer anticoagulants or thrombolytics as ordered.

Before discharge from the hospital, clients will need information on the daily exercise routine and the anticoagulant therapy regimen they are to follow. Health teaching for clients undergoing anticoagulant therapy is discussed in Chapter 24.

THROMBECTOMY

A thrombectomy is the removal of a thrombus from a vessel. The objectives of a thrombectomy are to reduce venous insufficiency and to minimize postphlebotic disability. Clients with iliofemoral involvement or recent onset of thrombosis are candidates for this procedure.

Surgical Procedure

The procedure for a thrombectomy is similar to that for an embolectomy: a catheter is passed on the uninvolved side and inflated to prevent pulmonary embolization; another catheter is passed on the involved side, inflated, and pulled back to the point of insertion, bringing the thrombus with it. Figure 30-2 shows the technique used in an iliofemoral thrombectomy.

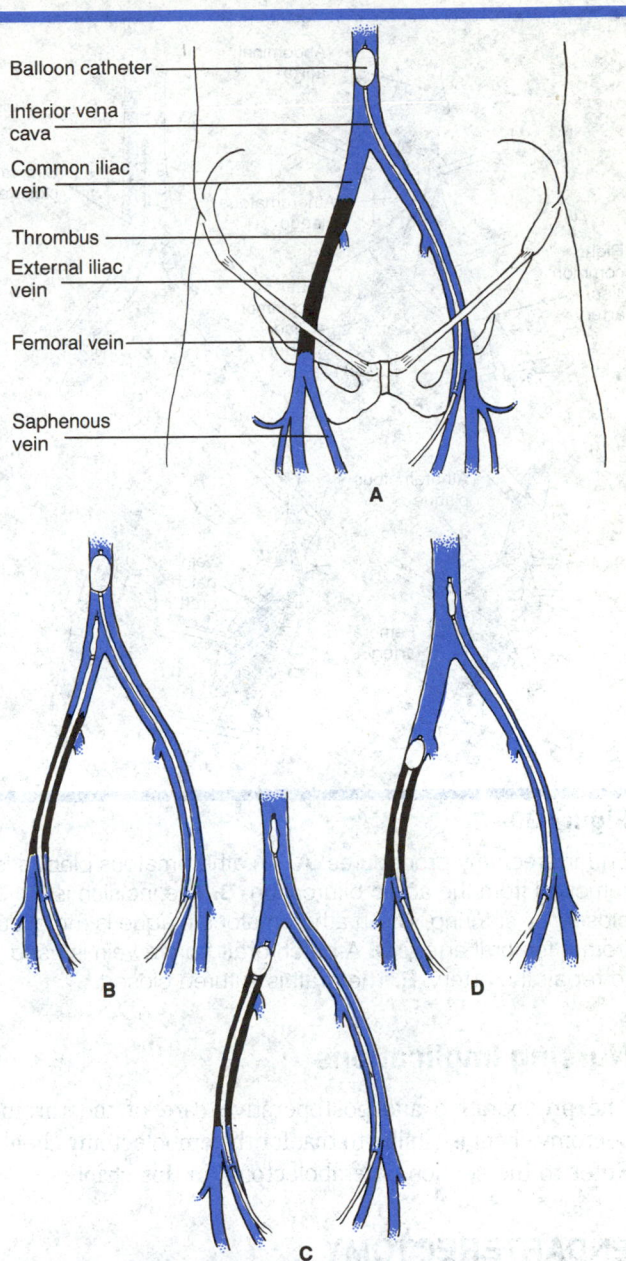

Figure 30-2

Iliofemoral thrombectomy. **A.** A balloon catheter is passed into the inferior vena cava through the saphenous vein on the uninvolved side and is inflated to prevent pulmonary emboli. **B.** A second balloon catheter is passed through the involved side. **C.** Inflating this second balloon and pulling it back into the common iliac vein allows deflation of the balloon in the inferior vena cava. **D.** The inflated balloon is pulled back through the common iliac vein, bringing the thrombus with it.

Implications for the Client

The physiological and psychosocial/lifestyle implications for the client having a thrombectomy are similar to those for the client having an embolectomy. They were discussed earlier and summarized in Table 30-1.

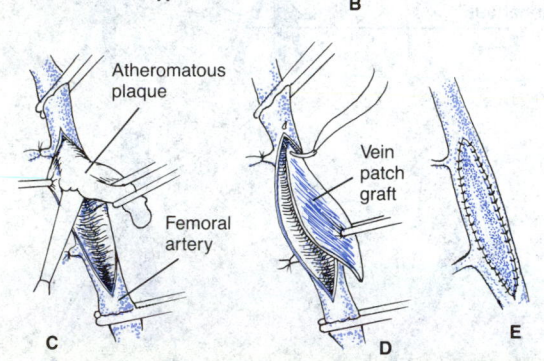

Figure 30–3

Endarterectomy procedures. **A.** An atheromatous plaque is removed from the aortic bifurcation. **B.** The incision is closed by suturing. **C.** An atheromatous plaque is removed from a femoral artery. **D.** A patch graft from a vein is used to repair the artery. **E.** The graft is sutured closed.

Nursing Implications

The preoperative and postoperative care of the thrombectomy client is similar to that for the embolectomy client. Refer to the section on embolectomy in this chapter.

ENDARTERECTOMY

An endarterectomy involves surgically incising an artery to remove an obstruction such as a progressive atheroma. This procedure is most often indicated for lesions of the femoral artery, the aortic bifurcation, or the carotid artery. (The carotid endarterectomy is discussed in Chapter 39.)

Surgical Procedure

The operation is performed through longitudinal incisions in the involved arteries, and the occlusive atherosclerotic tissue is removed using sharp and blunt dissection. Simple closure is performed in large vessels. In smaller vessels, the incision is closed by inserting patch grafts, usually from a client's own vein. Figure 30–3A illustrates an endarterectomy of aortic bifurcation with simple closure. Figure 30–3B illustrates a femoral endarterectomy with a patch graft.

Implications for the Client

The client implications for endarterectomy are similar to those for embolectomy. Refer to the discussion of embolectomy and to Table 30–1.

Nursing Implications

The nursing implications for a client undergoing endarterectomy are similar to those for a client undergoing embolectomy. (See the earlier discussion of embolectomy.) If the endarterectomy involves the aortic bifurcation, the nurse needs to also monitor the client for abdominal distention or rigidity and to assess the client's bowel sounds.

PERCUTANEOUS TRANSLUMINAL ANGIOPLASTY

Percutaneous transluminal angioplasty (PTA), using a balloon-tipped catheter to dilate a partially occluded artery and thus reestablish blood flow, was first performed in 1964 to improve the patency of femoral arteries narrowed by atherosclerosis. Currently, this procedure is preferred to bypass surgery for reperfusion of an area.

Procedure

The most common peripheral vascular angioplasties are the aortoiliac and femeropopliteal. Iliac artery dilations are generally the easiest and most likely to be successful in the long term (Waltman, 1980). A complete discussion and illustration of this surgical approach is in Chapter 25 in the section on percutaneous transluminal coronary angioplasty.

Implications for the Client

The physiological and psychosocial/lifestyle implications are similar to those for coronary percutaneous transluminal angioplasty. These implications are discussed in Chapter 25.

Nursing Implications

Preoperative Care
Obtain and record vascular assessments of the extremity—color, warmth, presence and strength of pulses, sensation, and mobility. Use of a Doppler flow-meter to assess circulation may be vital. These preoperative baseline measurements are important indicators of postoperative progress. Prepare the client to expect frequent assessments of vital signs and vascular status and restriction of activity and mobility in the early postprocedure period.

Postoperative Care
Care of the client after a PTA includes assessing the vital signs and vascular status. Color, temperature, and pulses distal to the operative site are monitored for presence and

strength every 15 minutes the first hour, then hourly for the next 4 hours. The client should be kept flat in bed for 8 hours and instructed to keep the catheterized extremity in an extended position to minimize bleeding potential. Inspect the operative area for evidence of hematoma formation or bleeding.

After the first 8 hours on bed rest, the client can have the head of the bed elevated to a semi-Fowler's position. An increase in the client's activity level is usually permitted within 24 hours, beginning with sitting at the side of the bed or sitting up in a chair on the evening following the procedure.

An anticoagulation regimen is instituted postoperatively and continued indefinitely. Explain to the client the importance of taking this medication as directed upon discharge as well as the need for follow-up visits.

ARTERIAL BYPASS

An arterial bypass is a diversion of blood flow to bypass or circumvent a thrombosed arterial segment. An anastomosed autogenous graft or a graft made of synthetic material such as Teflon or Dacron is used to reestablish the blood flow. Coronary artery bypass surgery is described and illustrated in Chapter 25. This chapter will discuss arterial bypass surgery for lower extremity ischemia.

Four common types of surgeries have the ability to bypass occlusive lesions causing lower extremity ischemia: femoropopliteal bypass, aortofemoral bypass, femorofemoral bypass, and axillofemoral bypass. Today every effort is made to salvage an ischemic limb by arterial bypass surgery, provided the client has a lesion that can be bypassed and is not considered a poor surgical risk. The decision for surgery is made after angiographic studies to determine the extent of the occlusion.

Surgical Procedure

Femoropopliteal Bypass
A bypass in which a graft extends from the femoral to the popliteal arteries (Figure 30–4A) is indicated when occlusion of the superficial femoral artery results in claudication with moderate exercise, along with trophic changes in the extremity. The autogenous saphenous vein graft is used as the bypass material. The saphenous vein is dissected from the client and prepared for anastomosis. When the distal point of anastomosis has been selected, a tunnel is made to house the graft. The more difficult distal anastomosis is always done before the proximal anastomosis. The types of distal bypass routes are illustrated in Figure 30–4B.

Aortofemoral Bypass
A graft extending from the aorta down to the femoral arteries (Figure 30–5) is indicated with Leriche's syndrome when an aortogram shows occlusion of the distal aorta and proximal iliac arteries. An incision in the groin is made for the purpose of assessing the status of the femoral arteries. If

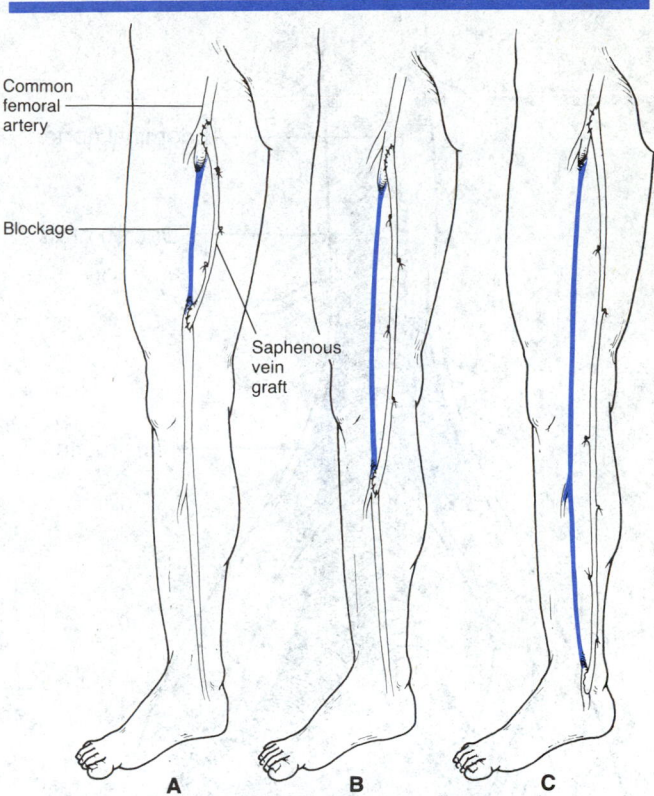

Figure 30–4

Femoropopliteal bypass. **A.** Bypass to proximal popliteal artery. **B.** Bypass to tibioperoneal trunk. **C.** Bypass to ankle.

severe arteriosclerosis is evident, surgery is not practical, and the client has been spared an abdominal incision. If the femoral arteries are in satisfactory condition, the aorta is exposed, a Dacron graft is selected, and an aortic anastomosis followed by a distal anastomosis is made. The graft is thoroughly heparinized during this procedure.

Femorofemoral Bypass
An **extra-anatomic bypass** (EAB), in which a Dacron graft extends from one femoral artery to the other (Figure 30–6), is indicated in cases of femoral blockage with decreased circulation to the leg. In this surgery, an incision is made in each groin to expose the femoral arteries. A subcutaneous suprapubic tunnel is created. The graft is anastomosed to the femoral artery that has good vascular flow, passed through the suprapubic tunnel, and then anastomosed to the inadequately perfused femoral artery.

Axillofemoral Bypass
A second type of EAB, in which a graft placed subcutaneously on the side of the chest extends from the axillary artery to the femoral artery (Figure 30–7), is indicated in peripheral vascular disease when the client has no suitable site on the thoracic aorta or is at high risk. In the axillofemoral bypass, the axillary artery is exposed by an inci-

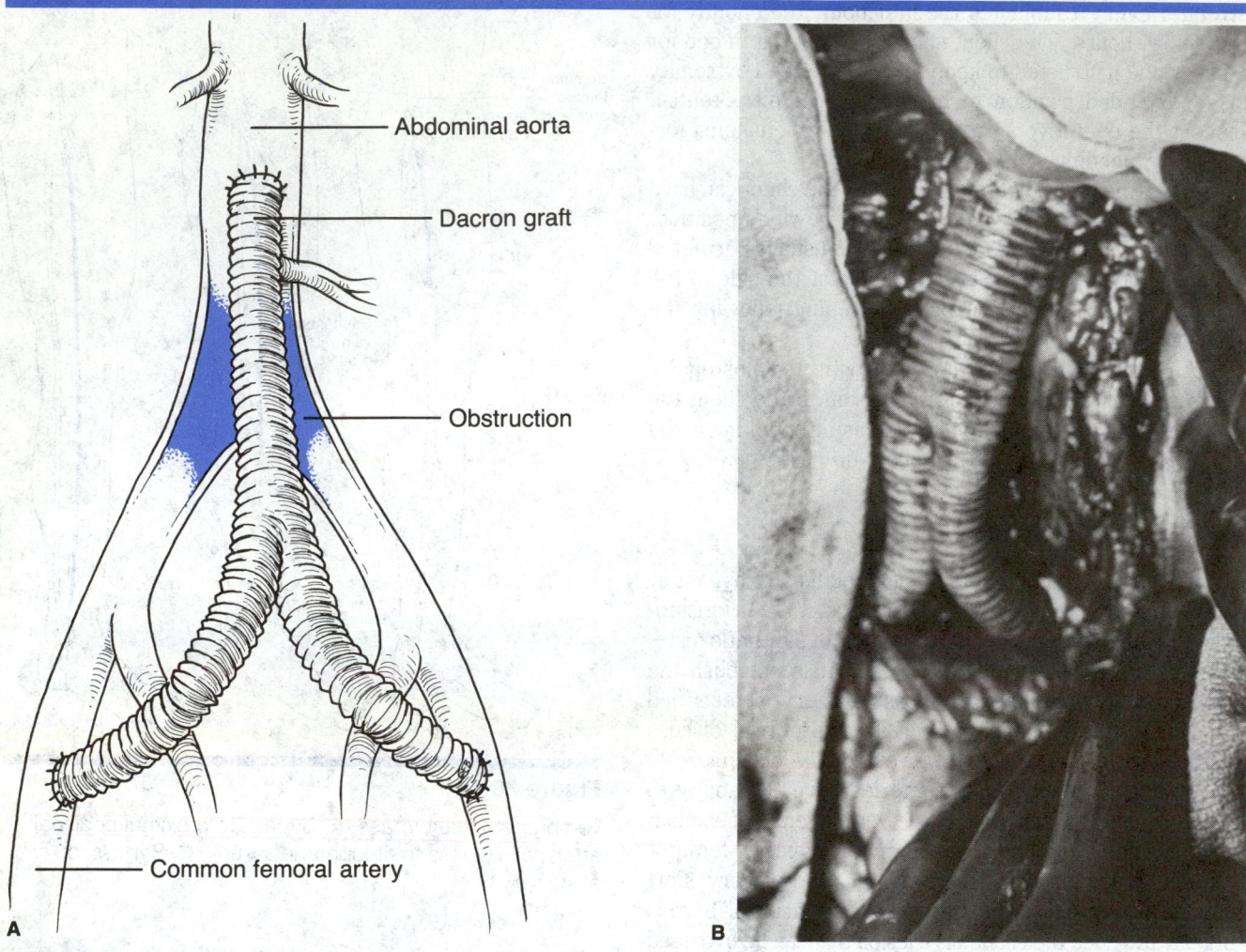

Figure 30-5

A. Aortoiliac bypass. **B.** Dacron graft in place during surgery. (Photo courtesy of Millard Fillmore Hospital Buffalo, NY)

sion below the clavicle, and the graft is sutured to this artery. A tunnel is created between the axillary and femoral sites. The graft is passed through this tunnel and anastomosed to the poorly perfused femoral artery.

Implications for the Client

Physiological Implications

As with the surgeries previously discussed, the trauma of surgery itself and the creation of anastomoses provide a rough surface for platelet aggregation and thrombus formation. Thrombosis is a potential early postoperative complication. The formation of emboli, often from portions of thrombi, can be a major complication. Because of their arterial disease, these clients are also at high risk for postoperative myocardial infarction. Bleeding from an anastomosis site is another potential complication.

Rejection of the graft or failure of the graft itself are other possible major postoperative complications. An addi-

tional complication is impotence, which may result from the prolonged clamping of arteries that supply the pelvis during surgery. Intestinal ischemia from clamping of the mesenteric artery during surgery is another potential complication. Also, clients who have had an axillofemoral or femorofemoral bypass have a subcutaneous tunnel for the bypass graft that is susceptible to injury. Anticoagulant therapy may be necessary for an indefinite time.

Psychosocial/Lifestyle Implications

Bypass surgery requires a number of lifestyle changes. Clients must avoid body positions (especially those involving flexion) that may kink the graft and decrease the blood flow. For example, the client who has had a femorofemoral bypass should not cross the legs or sit for long periods. These activities cause kinking of the graft and pooling of blood, potentiating thrombus formation and possibly leading to closure of the bypass itself. The client with an axillofemoral bypass should not lie on the side with the graft;

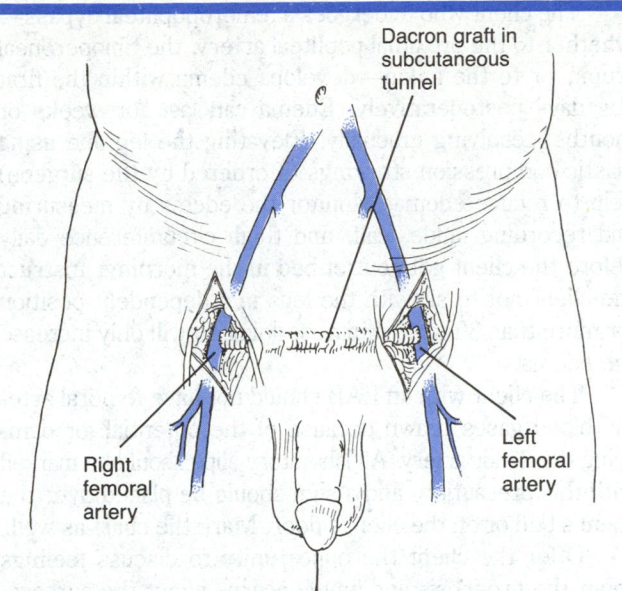

Figure 30-6

Femorofemoral bypass.

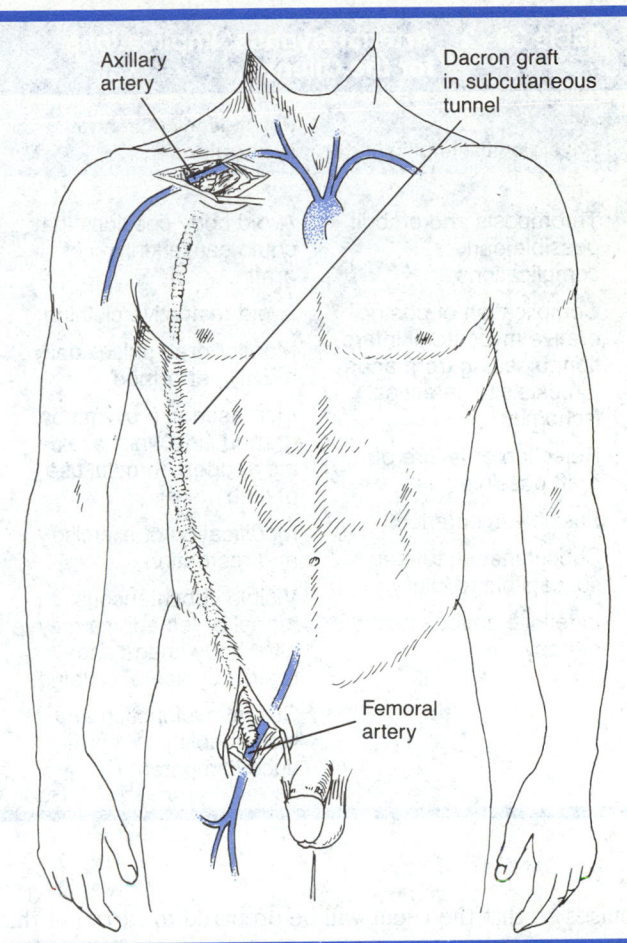

Figure 30-7

Axillofemoral bypass.

the client with a bilateral axillofemoral bypass must lie supine. Clients with either type of femoral bypass should not flex the hip to 90°. Clothing worn over the graft should not be restrictive or cause pressure. Clients who have had an EAB must monitor their graft pulses daily to be sure the graft is functional. (The specifics are discussed later in nursing implications.)

Use of the limb on the grafted side should be increased to prevent stasis, but sudden, forceful use of the limb on the grafted side should be avoided. In addition, a daily exercise program is necessary to prevent stasis. Exercise and recreational activities may need modification to protect the easily accessible subcutaneous tunnel from injury.

The client's body image and self-esteem may be altered with arterial bypass surgery. The visible subcutaneous tunnel may alter the client's body image. Choice of clothing may be restricted because the client wishes to conceal the subcutaneous tunnel. If impotence occurs, the client's self-esteem is likely to be diminished, and finding an alternate means of sexual expression and reproduction will be necessary. Client implications are summarized in Table 30-2.

Nursing Implications

Preoperative Care

Nursing implications for the client having arterial bypass are similar to those for the vascular surgeries discussed earlier. Baseline measurements are necessary for postoperative comparison. Inform the client that postoperative discomfort in the operative area is due to manipulation of tissue in order to perform the bypass, and that analgesics will be available for pain relief.

Postoperative Care

Careful vascular assessments hourly for the first 12 hours (refer to the earlier discussion in the section on embolectomy) and at least once per shift thereafter, are crucial for the client having had arterial bypass surgery. Thrombi broken off by an increase in blood pressure or blood velocity can become emboli, a major complication of this surgery. Signs of embolization of a major arterial supply to an extremity could include rapid, severe pain; pallor; cyanosis; coolness; and the absence of pulses distal to the site of the obstruction. If the embolus has lodged in a small vessel, warmth and function may return to the extremity.

Vital signs must also be carefully monitored because hypotension increases the potential of thrombus formation and clotting of the graft. Also, leakage of blood around the anastomosis of the graft may be minimal or can occur as a steady leak, both of which can lead to hemorrhage.

When checking pulses of the client with an EAB, check the arterial pulses in the donor arm, in the axillofemoral graft itself, or the femorofemoral graft as it passes above the prominence of the symphysis pubis, and in the revascularized legs. Teach the client how to check the graft

Table 30–2	Arterial Bypass: Implications for the Client	
Physiological Implications	**Psychosocial/Lifestyle Implications**
Thrombosis and emboli possible early complications	Avoid body positions that could cause kinking of graft
Complication of postoperative myocardial infarction, bleeding from anastomosis site, intestinal ischemia	Avoid restrictive clothing
	Monitor graft pulses daily if EAB performed
Rejection or failure of graft possible	Increased use of limb on grafted side while avoiding sudden, forceful use of limb
Possible impotence	
Subcutaneous tunnel susceptible to injury	Modification of exercise and recreation
Indefinite anticoagulant therapy	Visible subcutaneous tunnel or leg edema may alter body image and restrict choice of clothing
	Sexual dysfunction and lack of ability to reproduce if impotent

pulses so that the client will be prepared to carry out this procedure independently after discharge from the hospital.

Monitor the color and clarity of the urine as well as the urine output postoperatively because perfusion to the kidneys may have been decreased during surgery. Assess the incision lines for healing and the presence of infection; signs of infection should be reported to the surgeon immediately.

Clients who have had bypass surgery are restricted to bed for usually the first 48 hours. Assisting the client to change positions at regular intervals and using supportive devices will increase the client's comfort. After the first 48 hours of bed rest, the client is assisted to ambulate slowly. Although ambulation is encouraged, actual knee or hip flexion for longer than 30 to 45 minutes is discouraged. Joint flexion may cause kinking of the graft and thrombus formation. If there have been no complications, the client may sit up in the chair on the third postoperative day. Because the client should not flex the hip to 90°, a reclining chair is preferable. On the fourth postoperative day, the client may be assisted to the bathroom and may increase mobility as tolerated on the fifth day. Liberal administration of analgesics during these first few days after surgery will help the client to ambulate and decrease discomfort.

Carry out abdominal assessments on the client who has had an aortofemoral bypass. These include measurement of the abdominal girth each shift, assessment of bowel sounds, and monitoring nasogastric tube losses so fluid replacement needs can be determined.

The client who undergoes a femoropopliteal bypass— whether to the proximal popliteal artery, the tibioperoneal trunk, or to the ankle—develops edema within the first few days postoperatively. Edema can last for weeks or months, resolving gradually. Elevating the leg and using elastic compression stockings (if ordered by the surgeon) help to reduce edema. Monitor the edema by measuring and recording ankle, calf, and thigh circumference daily before the client gets out of bed in the morning. Instruct the client not to sit with the legs in a dependent position for more than 30 to 45 minutes; doing so will only increase the edema.

The client with an EAB should not have femoral arterial blood gases drawn because of the potential for damaging the donor artery. All laboratory slips should be marked with this precaution, and a sign should be placed over the client's bed or on the client's door. Mark the chart as well.

Offer the client the opportunity to discuss feelings about the prognosis and any concerns about the surgery, its effects, or the change in self-image. Clients may understandably be worried about graft rejection. Graft rejection, although rare, can occur with synthetic grafts. Carefully assess perfusion to the grafted area. Sometimes, however, a body rash and elevated temperature may be the only cues to graft rejection. Encourage the involvement of significant others in the client's care, providing them the opportunity to express their concerns and anxieties as well.

REPAIR OF ABDOMINAL AORTIC AND PERIPHERAL ANEURYSMS

An abdominal aneurysm repair, like the ventricular and aortic aneurysm repairs discussed in Chapter 25, is a resection of the aneurysm and restoration of normal blood flow through replacement of the damaged section with a Dacron or Teflon graft. If abdominal aortic aneurysms are larger than 4 to 5 cm, surgery is indicated. Hypothermia is induced during surgery to decrease the need for oxygen at the tissue level and to decrease the production of metabolic waste products. Aneurysms may also occur in the peripheral arteries and may be repaired by synthetic grafts or natural grafts using a portion of a vein.

Surgical Procedure

Abdominal aneurysm resection involves ligation of the inferior mesenteric artery, clamping of the iliac arteries, and cross-clamping of the aorta at the neck of the aneurysm. The aneurysm is then cut longitudinally, and the thrombus is removed from its interior (Figure 30–8A). The synthetic bifurcation graft, which has been heparinized and trimmed to the correct size, is anastomosed end to end to the aorta; then one distal limb of the graft is anastomosed. Blood flow is permitted through this portion of the graft for a brief time to check the functioning of the graft. The second distal anastomosis is then done (Figure 30–8B), and the flow of blood through the graft is rechecked.

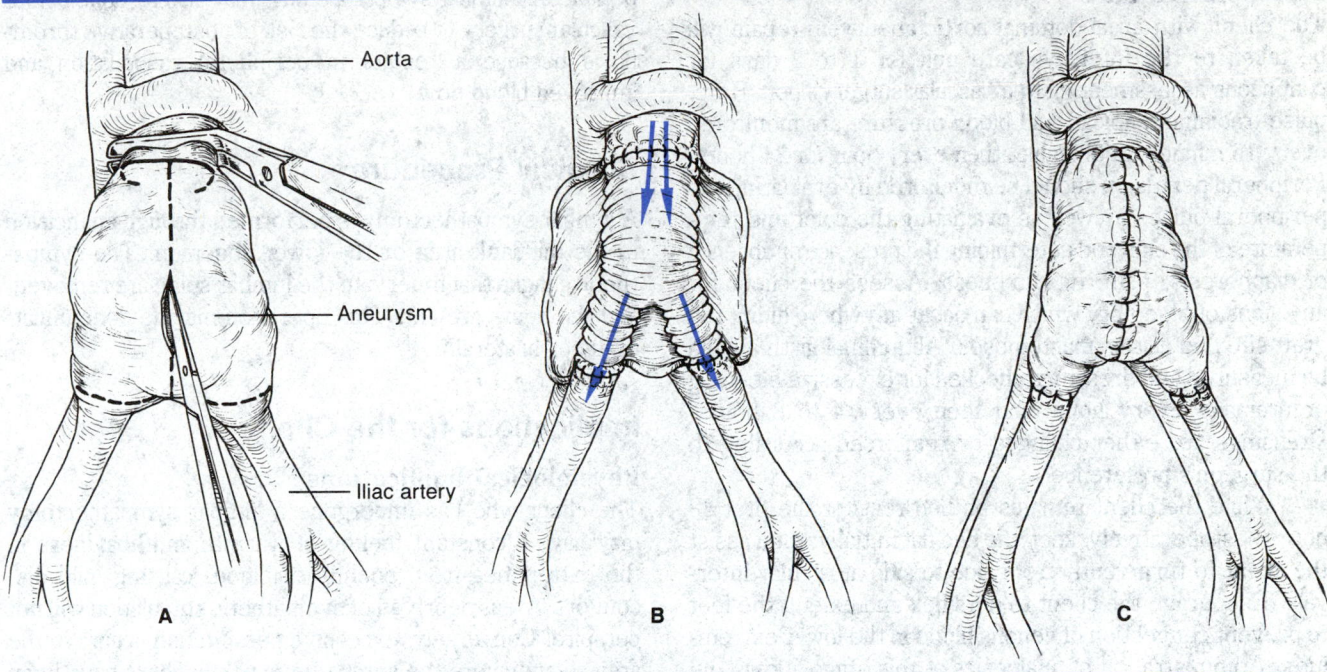

Figure 30–8

Abdominal aortic aneurysm repair. **A.** The aneurysm is resected. **B.** The synthetic graft is anastomosed to the aorta and the iliac arteries. **C.** The aneurysm is then sutured over the graft itself.

After this, the aneurysm itself is sutured over the graft (Figure 30–8C) to provide added support to the graft. Surgery for peripheral aneurysms involves resection of the aneurysm and its replacement with a vein or prosthetic graft.

Implications for the Client

Physiological Implications

Platelet aggregation and thrombus formation are possible complications of aneurysm repair because of trauma from the surgery and because the anastomoses provide rough surfaces. In abdominal aneurysm repairs, other possible complications arise from clamping off the aorta and its tributary arteries during surgery. The clamping of the renal, mesenteric, and celiac arteries may cause undue tissue damage and ultimately cause malfunction of the tissues and organs that they normally supply with blood. Aneurysm repair does not preclude the future development of other aneurysms. Other aneurysms may still occur because of trauma, infections, or factors associated with arteriosclerosis.

Psychosocial Implications

The psychosocial implications are similar to those of bypass surgery. Clients need to undertake a program of regular exercise and to avoid situations that could produce trauma or cause infections. Lifestyle modifications (such as those discussed in Chapter 24) to decrease the risk factors associated with atherosclerosis are important. Regular health

care supervision following surgery will be necessary. The implications of aneurysm repair are summarized in Table 30–3.

Nursing Implications

Preoperative Care

Nursing implications for the preoperative care of the client is similar to that of the bypass surgeries discussed earlier. Baseline measurements of vital signs and vascular status are important and serve as a basis for evaluating postoperative progress.

Table 30–3	Repair of Abdominal Aortic and Peripheral Aneurysms: Implications for the Client
Physiological Implications	**Psychosocial/Lifestyle Implications**
Possible thrombi or emboli	Regular exercise and avoidance of situations that could produce trauma or infection
Clamping of aorta and tributary arteries may cause tissue malfunction	Lifestyle modifications to reduce risk of atherosclerosis (see Chapter 24)
Possibility of future aneurysms	Regular health care supervision

Postoperative Care

The client with an abdominal aortic aneurysm repair will be taken to the intensive care unit for 1 to 2 days for continuous assessment or to a vascular surgery floor. Here, pulse (radial and apical) and blood pressure are monitored every 15 minutes until stable, then every hour for 24 hours. Peripheral perfusion should be monitored by evaluating the peripheral pulses as well as evaluating the color and temperature of the skin and determining the presence or absence of diaphoresis, pain, or numbness. Assess the client for any signs of bleeding, which can occur anywhere along the graft site and at the anastomoses. Abdominal girth should be measured and dressings checked for excessive bleeding or drainage every hour, and then every 4 to 8 hours. Dressings are either changed or reinforced according to the surgeon's preference.

While the client remains on bed rest for the first 48 hours postoperatively, keep the bed flat initially; then assist the client to turn gently from side to side at regular intervals. Encourage the client to dorsiflex and extend the feet to prevent congestion of venous blood in the lower extremities. Administration of analgesics at this stage allows the client to move with less distress and helps to make coughing and deep breathing easier. Determine the location and the severity of any pain. Back pain may indicate retroperitoneal hemorrhage or thrombus at the graft site.

Assist the client with initial ambulation and guard the client against any injury. The client must remain erect when ambulating to prevent kinking and tension of grafts. Monitor the client for any signs of infection, such as elevated temperature or redness at the incision line, so appropriate treatment measures can be taken early.

The client with an abdominal aortic aneurysm repair will have a nasogastric tube. Note the quality and amount of the nasogastric tube losses and monitor electrolyte levels daily.

The client is likely to have a number of fears and anxieties about the surgery itself, restrictions on activity, the change in self-image, possible loss of the limb, and death. Create an environment that facilitates discussion of these fears and concerns. Encourage the family to become involved in the client's postoperative care and provide them with opportunities to ask questions and discuss their concerns. The general nursing care of the client having abdominal aortic or peripheral aneurysm repair is similar to that discussed for bypass surgery.

LUMBAR SYMPATHECTOMY

A lumbar sympathectomy is the severing of the sympathetic nerve fibers supplying the peripheral vessels. This severing causes relaxation of the small vessels and collateral channels of the legs, resulting in peripheral vasodilation and improved blood flow. A lumbar sympathectomy is often used in clients who are at high risk for corrective vascular surgery. This procedure is indicated only in clients whose vessels are elastic and only mildly or moderately occluded. A lumbar sympathectomy may also be done before vascular surgery to reduce the risk of postoperative thrombosis because it results in peripheral vasodilation and improved blood flow.

Surgical Procedure

A lumbar sympathectomy is performed through an incision in the midflank area or the lower abdomen. The sympathetic ganglia that innervate the lumbar spine are removed, and the fibers are cut. This operation may be done unilaterally or bilaterally.

Implications for the Client

Physiological Implications

The client who has undergone a lumbar sympathectomy may have a constant feeling of warmth and heaviness in the extremities from pooling of blood, causing mild discomfort. Areas deprived of sympathetic stimulation will not perspire. Conversely, excessive perspiration occurs in the area above where the sympathetic nerve fibers have been severed. An important physiological implication for the male client is the possibility of being unable to ejaculate after a bilateral lumbar sympathectomy that includes the first or second lumbar ganglion (Rutherford, 1984).

Psychosocial/Lifestyle Implications

Discomfort in the extremities from pooling of blood may require the client to wear elastic support hose during waking hours. Sterility and sexual dysfunction are possible after bilateral lumbar sympathectomy. Lifestyle modifications such as those described earlier for clients with peripheral vascular disease will also be required. Implications for lumbar sympathectomy are summarized in Table 30–4.

Nursing Implications

Preoperative Care

Prepare the client for what to expect in the postoperative period and provide the usual preoperative care. Because the client will be prone to postoperative orthostatic hypotension, instruct the client to request assistance for ambulation, especially in the early postoperative period.

Postoperative Care

After this procedure, the client is positioned on one side, and vital signs are taken every 15 minutes until they have stabilized. A complication to be especially alert for is shock: the dilated vessels of the extremities and lower abdomen will provide for pooling of blood.

As with any surgical procedure, the client must be carefully assessed for urinary retention and abdominal distention; because of the nature of this surgery, these problems are more likely. An in-dwelling urinary catheter and a rectal tube may be necessary to relieve these symptoms.

Table 30−4	Lumbar Sympathectomy: Implications for the Client	
Physiological Implications	**Psychosocial/Lifestyle Implications**
Mild discomfort from constant warmth and heaviness in extremities	Need to wear elastic support hose during waking hours
Chance of inability to ejaculate after bilateral sympathectomy	Sexual dysfunction and sterility possible after bilateral sympathectomy
	Lifestyle modifications related to peripheral vascular disease

Reposition the client every hour and encourage coughing and deep-breathing exercises. Assist the client to ambulate with assistance the day after surgery. Be alert for orthostatic hypotension and take measures to ensure the client's safety. Apply elastic support hose before the client gets out of bed to sit. This will decrease pooling of blood in the legs.

Clients are usually discharged in 5 days. Instruct the client to balance exercise with rest at home and to elevate the extremities frequently during the day. Support hose worn during the first few weeks or months at home may increase comfort. Also instruct the client not to take hot baths; they may cause further vessel dilatation leading to hypotension.

VEIN LIGATION AND STRIPPING

Ligation and diversion of a vein above the varicosity and removal of varicosed veins are carried out on enlarged tortuous veins that cause great discomfort. This procedure prevents secondary edema, ulceration, pain, and fatigue in the affected extremity.

Surgical Procedure

The great saphenous vein is ligated close to the femoral vein (Figure 30–9A) through a groin incision. A second incision is made in the medial aspect of the ankle. The vein is stripped (pulled) by a plastic or metal vein stripper which is threaded through the lumen of the vein from the ankle to the groin and then pulled downward, bringing the vein with it. The bleeding that occurs as these tributaries are broken off can usually be controlled in surgery by pressure, elevation of the extremity, and electrocautery.

The procedure is more complex when the saphenous vein is extremely tortuous or when incompetent perforating veins are also involved. In these cases, other smaller incisions have traditionally been used to resect the veins involved. A more recent approach uses a cauterization probe introduced into a small incision (1 to 2 mm) every 1 to 3

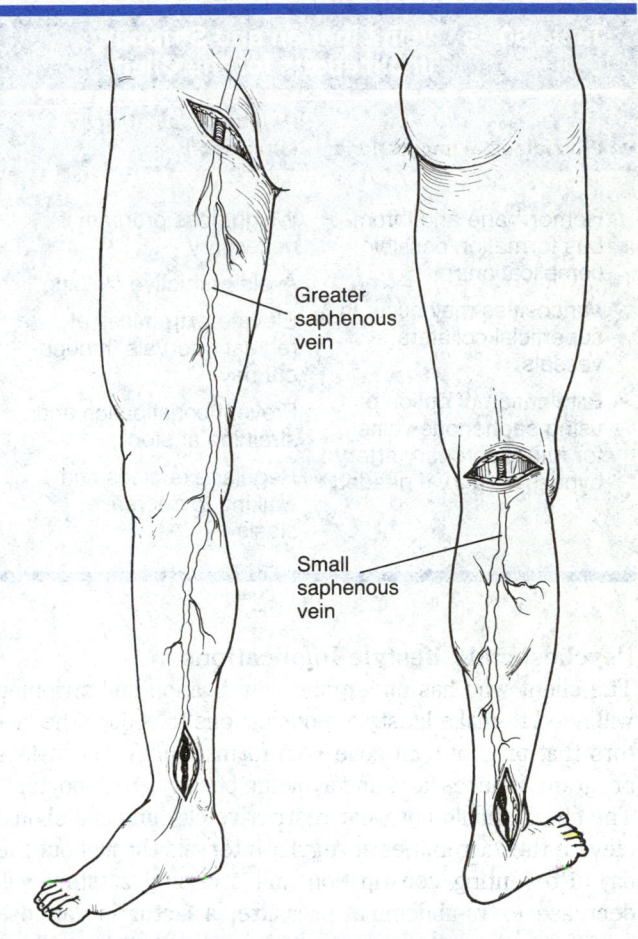

Figure 30–9

Incisions for vein ligation and stripping for varicosities of the great and small saphenous veins.

cm to cauterize small sections of a varicose vein. Because these tiny incisions are not sutured closed, there are no visible scars (Hinnant & Stallworth, 1981). The cautery approach requires less operating time—less than 1 hour compared with 2 to 4 hours for the traditional procedure. Because there are fewer and smaller incisions, the infection rate is minimal. After the groin is sutured, sterile dressings are applied along the incisions, and compression bandages are applied from the foot to the groin. See Figure 30–9B for an illustration of incision sites for the small saphenous vein.

Implications for the Client

Physiological Implications

Hemorrhage and thrombus formation are possible postoperative complications. Varicose veins may reoccur if the superficial collateral vessels become engorged and tortuous. Removal of the saphenous veins eliminates the option of using saphenous veins in coronary artery bypass surgery if it should be needed.

Table 30–5	Vein Ligation and Stripping: Implications for the Client	
Physiological Implications	**Psychosocial/Lifestyle Implications**
Hemorrhage and thrombus formation possible complications	Weight-loss program if necessary
Varicosities may occur in superficial collateral vessels	Avoid restrictive clothing
	Elevate extremities at regular intervals throughout day
Elimination of option of using saphenous veins for future coronary artery bypass surgery if needed	Prevent constipation and straining at stool
	Regular exercises and walking to decrease stasis

Psychosocial/Lifestyle Implications

The client who has undergone vein ligation and stripping will need to make lifestyle modifications to reduce the factors that promote varicose vein formation. A weight-loss program, if necessary, and avoiding obesity are important. The client should not wear restrictive clothing and should elevate the extremities at regular intervals throughout the day. Preventing constipation and straining at stool will decrease extra-abdominal pressure, a factor in varicose vein formation. A regular exercise program and walking help to decrease venous stasis. The client implications are summarized in Table 30–5.

Nursing Implications

Preoperative Care

In addition to routine preoperative preparation, instruct the client in the importance of early ambulation, frequent walking, avoiding sitting for long periods, and elevation of the limbs to prevent venous stasis. Sometime during the evening before surgery, the surgeon will mark the client's veins with a felt-tip pen while the client is in a standing position. Inform the client that the purpose is to aid the surgeon to identify the veins to be operated on. Since the client will be lying on the operating table, the varicosities may appear less prominent and more difficult to locate without markings.

Postoperative Care

In addition to the usual postoperative care, the client who has had a vein ligation and stripping should be assessed for bleeding every 2 hours. If hemorrhage occurs, apply pressure over the area, elevate the foot, and notify the vascular surgeon immediately. For the first 4 hours after surgery, the client should be kept recumbent with the foot of the bed elevated to promote venous return to the heart.

Ambulation is encouraged the day of surgery and short, frequent walks the following days. Early ambulation is important in preventing thrombus formation in the remaining veins of the extremities. Ambulating after vein ligation and stripping is painful, so administering analgesics approximately 30 minutes before ambulation will increase the client's comfort and willingness to ambulate. Assist the client with ambulating and guard against trauma to the legs. Check the compression bandages after each ambulation to make sure they remain snug and in place.

Clients are usually discharged from the hospital after 2 or 3 days. Instruct clients to elevate the extremities routinely for 10 to 18 hours each day during the first week at home and not to stand or sit for long periods. By the third and fourth week, the client may slowly resume normal activities modified by the necessary lifestyle changes.

INSERTION OF INTRACAVAL FILTER/ PLICATION OF INFERIOR VENA CAVA

The intracaval (umbrella) filter is a tiny device that partially occludes the inferior vena cava. An intracaval filter is used when a client has deep vein thrombophlebitis (DVT) or pulmonary emboli and is unable to withstand anticoagulants because of blood dyscrasias, hemorrhage, hepatic dysfunction with alteration in the clotting mechanism, major visceral injury, or a history of cerebrovascular accident or other neurologic conditions. The procedure is also indicated if the client cannot withstand major surgery.

Plication (partial occlusion) of the inferior vena cava is also performed to prevent movement of pulmonary emboli through the inferior vena cava. It is a major surgical procedure and is used less often than insertion of the intracaval filter.

Surgical Procedure

The umbrella filter is inserted under local anesthesia in a cardiac catheterization laboratory. The filter is passed through a small incision into the right internal jugular vein. The umbrella filter is attached to a stylet and folded inside a capsule (Figure 30–10A). Under fluoroscopic guidance, the capsule is passed into the right atrium and out through the inferior vena cava to the level of the third or fourth lumbar vertebra, distal to the renal veins. When correctly situated, the stylet is pushed forward to eject the umbrella from the capsule. The capsule then springs open, and the spokes fix to the wall of the vein (Figure 30–10B). After fluoroscopic confirmation that the filter is placed correctly, the stylet and catheter are removed, and the incision is closed.

The left internal jugular vein or the femoral vein may be used if the filter cannot be inserted into the right internal jugular vein because of obstruction or tortuosity. Femoral insertion is usually done in the operating room because it is necessary to repair the vein surgically after the procedure.

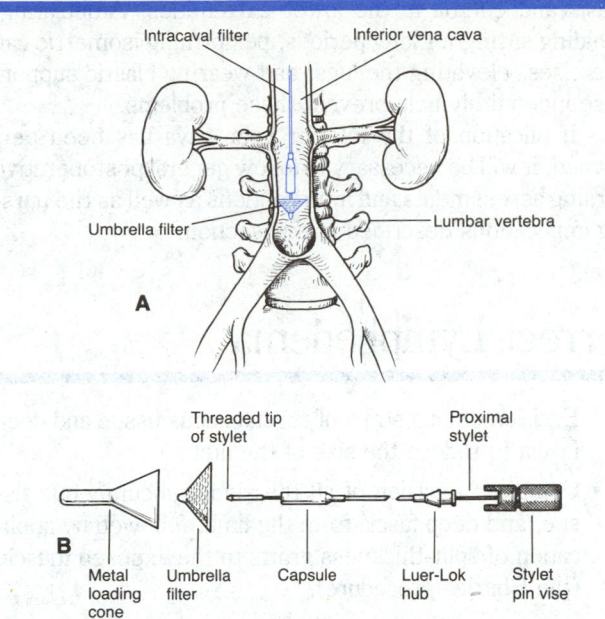

Figure 30–10
Insertion of intracaval filter. **A.** The intracaval filter in place. **B.** The components of the umbrella filter.

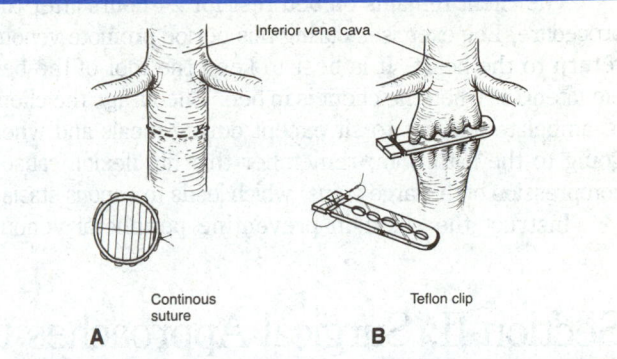

Figure 30–11
Plication of the inferior vena cava. **A.** Strainer formed by a continuous suture. **B.** Strainer formed by a Teflon clip.

Plication of the inferior vena cava is carried out in an operating room under a general anesthetic. Two heavy sutures are passed around the vena cava, which is tied above or below the lumbar vein. The vena cava is not cut; suture ligaments or Teflon clips are used to strain the blood or partition the inferior vena cava (Figure 30–11).

Because the intracaval filter is used more often than plication, the following discussion focuses on intracaval filter insertion. The principles can be applied to the care of the client who has had a plication.

Implications for the Client

Physiological Implications
Clots trapped in the filter may cause stasis of the peripheral veins and edema in the lower extremities. Peripheral vein stasis may lead to thrombi formation. Interruption of the inferior vena cava by the filter itself may decrease the venous return. It is also possible for air embolism to develop and for the filter to migrate into the vascular system.

Psychosocial/Lifestyle Implications
To prevent stasis and subsequent clotting, clients must walk regularly and frequently. Clients who can tolerate it will receive long-term anticoagulant therapy; all clients can expect to wear support hose indefinitely. If clotting obstructs the filter, or if the filter migrates, surgical replacement or correction may be necessary. The implications of these procedures for the client are listed in Table 30–6.

Nursing Implications

Preoperative Care
Because this procedure is carried out while the client is awake, the client's anxiety level is likely to escalate. Thorough preparation of the client before the procedure will aid in decreasing anxiety levels and increasing cooperation during the procedure. The client should be told why this procedure is being done, what the filter looks like and what it does, and what sensations to expect during the procedure.

Postoperative Care
Vital signs should be monitored every half hour until they return to a stable level, usually after 3 hours. Assessment of the insertion site is important: hematoma development may indicate jugular bleeding, which requires immediate notification of the physician. Daily dressing changes with a bactericidal ointment are often recommended until the sutures are removed.

Table 30–6	Insertion of Intracaval Filter/Plication of Inferior Vena Cava: Implications for the Client	
Physiological Implications	**Psychosocial/Lifestyle Implications**
Trapped clots may cause stasis of blood and edema in lower extremities	Regular and frequent walking to prevent stasis
Possible formation of thrombi or emboli	Long-term anticoagulant therapy
Air embolism or filter migration into vascular system possible	Indefinite wearing of support hose
	Surgical correction if filter clots or migrates

The client remains on bed rest for 24 hours after the procedure. Leg exercises during this period promote venous return to the heart. It is best to keep the foot of the bed elevated 15° when the client is in bed. Encourage the client to ambulate and not to sit except during meals and when going to the bathroom; remember that hip flexion causes compression of the large veins, which leads to venous stasis.

Instruct the client in preventing peripheral venous stasis and edema in the lower extremities. Ambulating, avoiding sitting for long periods, performing isometric calf exercises, elevating the legs, and wearing elastic support hose indefinitely help prevent these problems.

If plication of the inferior vena cava has been performed, it will be necessary to follow general postoperative nursing assessments and interventions as well as the nursing implications described in this section.

Section II: Surgical Approaches to Correct Lymphedema

Surgical treatment for **lymphedema** (edema of the extremities caused by stasis of lymph) is indicated for only a small percentage of clients with lymphedema. The major indications for surgery are excessive edema, interference with activities of daily living because of the excessive weight and bulk of the limb, recurring cellulitis, recurring inflammatory episodes, or the desire for cosmetic improvement of the limb to enable the client to wear attractive clothing and footwear. Surgery for cosmetic reasons alone should be carefully considered; there will always be some disproportion in size of the two limbs, and the scars from the surgery will also call attention to the appearance of the limb. The success of these procedures is controversial.

Surgical Procedure

Surgical approaches to lymphedema are numerous. Among approaches are:

- Insertion of silk threads or polyethylene tubing into the subcutaneous tissue to drain edema fluid into normal tissue.
- Removal of long strips of fascia to promote the formation of new anastomoses between the superficial and deep lymphatics.
- Construction of pedicle grafts from the edematous limbs to the trunk to bypass obstructed lymphatics.

- Excision of long strips of subcutaneous tissue and deep fascia to reduce the size of the limb.
- Complete excision of all the skin, subcutaneous tissue, and deep fascia from the limb, followed by application of split-thickness grafts to the exposed muscle (the Charles procedure).

The most radical and complicated approach, the Charles procedure, is thought by some to be the most effective in reducing the size and weight of the limb and decreasing the incidence of cellulitis and lymphangitis because edematous subcutaneous tissue has been removed. Others have found it less effective (Brunner, 1982).

Implications for the Client

Physiological Implications
Because the lymph system has potential regenerative abilities, potential return of lymphedema is a risk. Lymphedema may also result from the trauma of the surgery itself. Other physiological implications are determined by the type of procedure. See Chapter 80 for a discussion of the physiological implications of skin grafting.

Psychosocial/Lifestyle Implications
Surgery does not totally restore normal limb appearance, and the client will need to adapt to the body image and to possible changes caused by pedicle grafts or split-thickness skin grafts. Lifestyle modifications such as preventing trauma to the limb and elevating the limb at regular intervals are necessary. The psychosocial and lifestyle implications of grafting are discussed in Chapter 80. Prevention of trauma to a lymphedematous limb is discussed in Chapter 65 in the section on mastectomy. The physiological and psychosocial/lifestyle implications for surgery to reduce lymphedema are briefly summarized in Table 30–7.

Nursing Implications

Preoperative Care
In addition to the usual preoperative care, prepare the client according to the type of surgery the client will have. If grafting or tissue transplantation is involved, refer to Chapter 80.

Table 30–7 Surgical Treatment for Lymphedema: Implications for the Client

Physiological Implications	Psychosocial/Lifestyle Implications
Lymphedema may return or result from surgery itself (see Chapter 80 for implications of skin grafting)	Adjustment to body image change, especially with grafting
	Preventing trauma and elevating limb are necessary (see Chapter 65)

Postoperative Care

Assess the limb postoperatively for edema, hematomas, cellulitis, cysts, abscess formation, or the presence of necrotic areas. The limb must be constantly elevated while the client is in bed or sitting up in a chair. Aseptic technique must be used during dressing changes. Antibiotics are usually administered in the postoperative period for infection control. Drains have usually been placed in the limb; monitor the type and amount of drainage and assess the efficiency of the drain apparatus.

The length of hospitalization and recovery are determined by the type of surgery and the client's health status. Discharge teaching should include dressing changes and measures for preventing or reducing lymphedema and avoiding trauma to the limb (see Chapter 65).

Section III: Surgical Approaches to Disorders of the Blood and Blood-Forming Organs

SPLENECTOMY

Splenectomy, the surgical removal of the spleen, is usually performed for a spleen ruptured by trauma (eg, automobile accidents, knife or bullet penetration, or blows to the spleen) or because of severe hypersplenism. Because of recent evidence that the immune system may be compromised by spleen removal, splenectomy is usually reserved for life-threatening circumstances.

Surgical Procedure

The spleen is removed through an upper midline incision after the ligaments have been divided and the blood vessels ligated. Drains may be inserted if adhesions or clotting abnormalities are present.

Implications for the Client

Physiological Implications

The immune systems of clients having splenectomies may be compromised; the client may be at greater risk of infections, particularly pneumococcal infection, and antibody development may be adversely affected. Thrombosis because of an elevated platelet count in the early postoperative period (approximately the first 7 days) is possible, and thrombophlebitis is a frequent complication. Abdominal distention because of organ manipulation or thromboses in the portal system is possible. Subphrenic abscess and atelectasis of the left lower lobe with pneumonia are other possible complications.

Psychosocial/Lifestyle Implications

A temporary regimen of anticoagulant therapy will be necessary. The client should maintain adequate rest, adequate nutrition, and contact a health care provider if any signs of infection are present or if the client has been exposed to an infectious disease. The client may need to have prophylactic antimicrobial treatment and periodic pneumococcal vaccine (Pneumovax; see Table 11–7 in Chapter 11). Implications of splenectomy are listed in Table 30–8.

Nursing Implications

Preoperative Care

The client about to undergo a splenectomy because of trauma may be in shock from blood loss. A major responsibility is to monitor the client's vital signs and undertake preparations for surgery as soon as possible. Anxiety may accompany the urgent nature of the client's condition as well as result from tissue hypoxia related to blood loss. Support and reassurance of the client and family are important in the preoperative period.

Postoperative Care

Routine postoperative care for abdominal surgery is performed along with monitoring for hemorrhage and potential shock. The client with idiopathic thrombocytopenic purpura has an increased tendency for hemorrhage because the platelet level is decreased from its preoperative level. Platelet transfusion may aid in reducing this threat. The traumatized client is also a potential candidate for hemorrhage from trauma to other body sites.

Table 30–8	Splenectomy: Implications for the Client	
Physiological Implications	**Psychosocial/Lifestyle Implications**
Compromised immune system with greater risk of infections and adverse effect on antibody development	Temporary anticoagulant therapy
	Adequate rest and nutrition
Thrombosis is early complication	Stop smoking
Abdominal distention possible	Contact with health care provider necessary for infection or exposure to infectious disease; may require prophylactic antimicrobial therapy and periodic pneumococcal vaccine (Pneumovax)
Subphrenic abscess and atelectasis of the left lower lobe with pneumonia are possible complications	

Because the platelet count automatically rises after surgery up to five times the normal level before subsiding within about 7 days after surgery, the client is at risk for thrombosis and thromboembolic phenomena. Take measures to reduce the risk of postoperative thrombosis and assess the client regularly to detect possible thrombophlebitis. Insertion of an intracaval filter or plication of the inferior vena cava may be necessary in some clients.

Assess for abdominal distention and apply abdominal binders snugly to decrease distention and increase the client's comfort. Monitoring for abdominal distention is important in determining the possibility of thrombi being lodged in the portal system.

Monitor the client's temperature carefully. Temperature elevation (38.3°C or 101°F) for 7 to 10 days postoperatively may be related to thrombosis of the splenic vein. Temperature elevation may also occur in conjunction with the development of a left subphrenic abscess. Assessment of respiratory status and respiratory distress are also indicated and give clues to the possibility of subphrenic abscess.

Before discharge, instruct the client on avoiding situations with high infection risk and explain the lifestyle modifications necessitated by removal of the spleen. Remind the client of the need for regular health care follow-up.

BONE MARROW TRANSPLANTATION

A bone marrow transplantation (BMT) is the replacement of diseased or deficient bone marrow with healthy marrow from a donor. It is done primarily to reconstitute hematologic and immunologic function in clients with leukemia, severe combined immunodeficiency, or aplastic anemia. BMT is also being used on a trial basis for clients with thalassemia (Nuscher et al., 1984).

Matching Donor and Recipient

Before BMT can be performed, a suitable matched donor must be found. Two tests of histocompatibility must be performed to determine whether a donor candidate is a suitable match. The first test consists of tissue typing. Specific tissue type is determined by the human leukocyte antigen (HLA), the antigen complex on the surface of human cells, which can be detected most easily on lymphocytes. Four types of cell surface antigens—HLA-A, HLA-B, HLA-C, and HLA-D—appear to constitute the strongest barriers to tissue transplantation. When two persons are found who have the same four antigens, they are HLA matched. These persons might be identical twins, siblings, or nonsiblings. Identical twins are ideal donors because they are genetically similar. There is a 25% chance that a nontwin sibling will be identical in HLA composition. When a client has more than one sibling, the chances of a match increase to 35% to 40% (Nuscher et al., 1984). Siblings are the most common donors. Parents can be only half-matched because an individual inherits one antigen from each parent.

The second test for histocompatibility is the mixed lymphocyte culture (MLC). In this test, T-lymphocytes (which mediate tissue rejection) from the BMT candidate and the potential donor are mixed. If, after 7 days, the cells show no immune reactivity, the suitability of the HLA-matched donor is confirmed.

Four basic types of BMTs can be performed. *Syngeneic transplants* are those in which there is a perfect match between donor and recipient (such as might occur in identical twins), and a successful transplant is assured. *HLA-matched allogeneic transplants* are those between compatible donors and recipients. Transplants between mismatched donors and recipients, *HLA-mismatched transplants*, are a new approach that allows half-matched parents to be donors. *Autologous transplants* are those that result from transplantation of the client's own cryofrozen bone marrow obtained before chemotherapy or radiation therapy (Nuscher et al., 1984).

Surgical Procedure

The surgical procedure is brief. The donor is given either spinal or general anesthesia, and multiple bone marrow aspirations are taken from the anterior and posterior iliac crests (similar to the bone marrow aspiration procedure discussed in Chapter 28) over 30 to 40 minutes. Altogether, about 100 needle aspirations consisting of about 700 mL of bone marrow are obtained. The donor bone marrow is mixed with an anticoagulant and strained to remove fat and bone particles, mixed with heparinized saline, cultured, and transferred to blood bags. The bone marrow is infused in the recipient through a central vein over a 4-hour period.

Although the procedure is brief, the preparations for bone marrow transplantation are complicated and lengthy. The recipient receives both chemotherapy and radiation therapy. These procedures are discussed in the section on nursing implications.

Implications for the Client

In BMT, there are a number of clients to consider—the donor, the recipient, and the donor's significant others. The implications for all these persons are discussed next.

Physiological Implications for Donor
There are no known long-term effects from bone marrow donation. Bone marrow is replaced naturally within the body within a few weeks after surgery. Some donors may choose to have their own blood removed by venipuncture and stored for replacement during the surgery to prevent postoperative anemia. (See Chapter 28 for a discussion of autologous blood transfusion.) Oral iron replacement therapy may be ordered for a few weeks following the donation.

The donor experiences soreness at the aspiration sites for approximately 1 week. Pressure dressings are applied to the aspiration sites in the operating room and are changed to bandages the day after the surgery. Infection is a possible complication because of the numerous aspiration sites. The donor is also subject to the same risks of any client undergoing surgery and anesthesia.

Physiological Implications for Recipient

The recipient's tissue-rejection potential must be suppressed before the transplantation. This is accomplished by chemotherapy and total body irradiation, which are discussed under nursing implications. Total body irradiation causes sterility in men. Clients who wish to father children may arrange for sperm banking before total body irradiation (see Chapter 12).

Pulmonary overload and allergic reactions are possible during the bone marrow infusion. Infection is the most common complication because the client is granulocytopenic; even normal body flora can cause opportunistic infections. The major cause of death following BMT is interstitial pneumonia caused by *Pneumocystis carinii* or cytomegalovirus. The potential for infection persists for 12 to 18 months after BMT until the client regains normal immune activity. Bleeding is another common complication that results from the drastically reduced platelet count that is the aftermath of immunosuppressive therapy. Infusions of platelets and packed red blood cells may be required.

Graft-versus-host disease (GVHD), a tissue incompatibility syndrome in which competent T-lymphocytes from the donor circulate and attack host tissue primarily in the skin, liver, and gastrointestinal tract, is also a common complication. GVHD threatens graft success. The disorder usually develops within 1 to 2 weeks after BMT, the most critical period, but may develop as late as 2 to 12 months after the transplant. The incidence of GVHD is reported to be 30% to 70% of clients transplanted with bone marrow from other than identical twins, despite measures to prevent GVHD (Hutchinson & Itoh, 1982; Nuscher et al., 1984). Transplant failure leads to eventual relapse.

Veno-occlusive disease, another complication of BMT, usually occurs in the first 3 weeks after transplantation and is fatal in about one-third of these clients. This condition, which occurs in up to 25% of clients, affects the liver (Nuscher et al., 1984). Symptoms of veno-occlusive disease include:

- Ascites
- Hepatomegaly
- Heart failure
- Encephalopathy
- Elevated serum bilirubin

This complication is most common in clients who have undergone intensive radiochemotherapy before BMT. In some instances, the syndrome resolves without major aftereffects. On the positive side, BMT has a lifesaving purpose in restoring hematologic and immune functioning.

Psychosocial/Lifestyle Implications for Donor

The donor can achieve great satisfaction in knowing that a personal gift of healthy bone marrow has provided a life-saving opportunity. The uncertainty following BMT is often a period of high stress for the donor who often feels personally responsible for the transplant's success. If the BMT is unsuccessful, the donor may experience sadness, anger, or a sense of failure and may need to mourn the loss. There are no lifestyle changes other than the possible need to take oral iron preparations temporarily.

Psychosocial/Lifestyle Implications for Recipient

BMT and its aftermath can be harrowing for clients and their significant others. The client will require lengthy hospitalization for pretransplantation preparation as well as posttransplantation care in a specially regulated environment. The length of the client's hospitalization depends on the client's condition and response to the treatment as well as on the protocol of the institution. Sometimes clients are kept in the transplant unit for 14 to 16 weeks after the BMT; other clients are discharged to home or to an apartment near the transplant center 3 to 6 weeks after the BMT.

Extreme susceptibility to infection makes it necessary that the client be isolated during the posttransplan-

Table 30–9	Bone Marrow Transplantation: Implications for the Client	
Physiological Implications	**Psychosocial/Lifestyle Implications**
Donor:	
No known long-term effects	Satisfaction in providing gift of bone marrow
Possible need for blood transfusion or iron replacement	Period of high stress while success of transplant is uncertain
Soreness at aspiration sites for first week	Sadness, anger, sense of failure, and need to grieve if graft is not successful
Infection possible	
Recipient:	
Sterility from total body irradiation	Lengthy hospitalization and posttransplantation care
Infection is common complication for 12 to 18 months; bleeding and veno-occlusive disease possible	Isolation and restriction of visitors and mobility
	Lifestyle modifications to avoid infection
Graft may fail	Loss of control with dependence on family and health care providers
Hematologic and immune functioning restored	
Extreme discomfort from side effects of chemotherapy and total body irradiation	Alteration of family roles
	Anxiety and stress until graft is known to be successful

tation period, restricting visitors and mobility. Even after this period is over, clients and their families need to be constantly aware of the potential for late infection (possibly for as long as 100 days after the transplant) and to modify their lifestyles accordingly. (These modifications are discussed under nursing implications.) It is not unusual for clients and their families to fear leaving the hospital to live in what is perceived to be an unprotected home environment.

Some clients will receive total parenteral nutrition (TPN) while in the hospital and may be discharged on home parenteral administration. This means that the client and family must learn to take care of the TPN catheter and the tubing, bottles, and pumps used to deliver the TPN.

Extensive body image changes from chemotherapy and total body irradiation lead to alterations in self-image. (See Chapter 12 for a discussion of these implications for the client.) Contending with complications such as GVHD, or with the threat of it, is anxiety provoking, and clients and their families fear a relapse or death.

Clients often feel as if they have lost control over their lives because of dependence on health care personnel and significant others. Regulated and controlled follow-up by a variety of health care personnel including dentists and dietitians is necessary. Family members often feel a loss of control over their own lives as well. They take an active role in the client's care, and family roles may be altered temporarily or permanently. The client, the family, or both may perceive this as a burden. The implications of bone marrow transplant for donor and recipient are given in Table 30–9, previous page.

Nursing Implications

Preoperative Care of the Donor
The donor will probably be admitted to the hospital the day before the transplant so any preoperative preparation, including an anesthesia assessment, can be completed. It is likely that a complete history and physical, chest x-ray, electrocardiogram, and blood studies will have been done on an outpatient basis before this time.

The donor should also be offered the opportunity to discuss concerns about the BMT. The nurse's role is supportive during this time but also includes reinforcing or clarifying the information the donor has previously received.

Postoperative Care of the Donor
Check the donor's pressure dressings for bleeding on the first day. Use aseptic technique when removing the pressure dressings and replacing them with bandages on the following day. Instruct the donor to observe for and report any signs of infection—tenderness, swelling, redness, purulent drainage, or acute pain—and to take showers rather than baths until the bone marrow aspiration sites have healed. The donor will probably be discharged from the hospital on the second or third postoperative day to wait out the results of the BMT. Remind the persons who

constitute the donor's support system that the donor may be anxious during the postoperative period and worried about whether the donated bone marrow is "good enough" to act as a lifesaver for the recipient. The donor will need their understanding support during this period.

Preoperative Care of the Recipient
Before admission to a transplant unit, the client has a central venous catheter inserted into either the cephalic vein or the subclavian vein to facilitate the administration of parenteral drugs, blood products, TPN, and the bone marrow infusion. The central venous catheter is also used to draw venous samples (except coagulation screens because heparin sodium is often instilled in the central venous catheter).

The BMT recipient may be cared for in a number of environments—reverse isolation in a single room, a clean environment in a laminar airflow unit, or a germ-free environment in a laminar airflow unit—depending on the protocol in the institution. The client is in this environment for 5 to 7 days before the BMT takes place while efforts focus on suppressing the recipient's tissue-rejection potential by destroying bone marrow function and destroying all malignant cells.

Once the client has been immunosuppressed, the client is at risk of infection from normal body flora, so steps are taken to protect the client from this source of infection before immunosuppression. Baths and showers with an antimicrobial skin cleanser such as chlorhexidine gluconate (Hibiclens) are instituted, and the client receives antibiotics to sterilize the gastrointestinal tract. Female clients receive antimicrobial creams for instillation in the vagina. A pretransplant medication schedule often includes the administration of trimethoprin-sulfamethoxazole (Bactrim, Septra) to inhibit the growth of *P. carinii*, the organism that most often causes posttransplantation interstitial pneumonia. Some protocols also include the oral administration of antifungal agents and the topical application of antifungal powders to the axilla, groin, and other **intertriginous areas** (apposed surfaces of the skin), such as the creases of the neck and beneath pendulous breasts, to prevent fungal infection.

The two components of the immunosuppressive regimen are chemotherapy and total body irradiation. In some centers, the chemotherapy is done first; in others, it follows total body irradiation. The most common agent used for chemotherapy is cyclophosphamide (Cytoxan), 40 to 60 mg/kg IV per day for 2 to 4 days. Total body irradiation is also administered in varying dosages; the usual range is 1000 rads in 1 day or up to 1575 rads in fractionated doses over a 4- to 7-day period (Hutchinson & Itoh, 1982; Nuscher et al., 1984). The variations in dosage for both chemotherapy and total body irradiation depend on the reason for the bone marrow transplantation (clients with leukemia and Hodgkin's disease receive the higher doses) and the protocol of the institution. Once the immunosuppressive regimen has been completed, the bone marrow transplant is performed, usually after a day of rest for the client.

Restrictions are begun in the pretransplant period and continued throughout the client's hospitalization. Personnel and family members dress in sterile garb, and visitors other than the family are discouraged. Food and liquids are sterilized before being served if the client is able to tolerate an oral diet. Again, the extent of these restrictions depends on the protocol in the transplant unit.

Both the pretransplant and the posttransplant periods are times of great discomfort and stress for the client. There are numerous uncomfortable and discouraging effects of both chemotherapy and total body irradiation, including nausea, vomiting, diarrhea, stomatitis, weakness, anorexia, and alopecia. Refer to Chapter 12 for the nursing care for clients undergoing chemotherapy and radiation therapy.

Postoperative Care of the Recipient

Engraftment (the appearance of normal erythrocytes, leukocytes, and thrombocytes in the bone marrow) takes from 2 to 4 weeks after BMT. While without a functioning bone marrow, the client is subject to infection and bleeding. Chemotherapy and total body irradiation cause the client to feel worse rather than better, and the nurse is constantly challenged to find ways to reduce the client's discomfort. During hospitalization, bone marrow aspirations are usually done weekly to assess bone marrow function. The uncertainty of whether the transplant will be successful remains a concern of clients, family, and the transplant team.

Infection. The suppression of the client's bone marrow makes the client granulocytopenic. Protecting the client from infection is essential to the client's survival. Change IV tubing, central venous catheter dressings, and the client's bed linen and clothing daily. Daily baths with antimicrobial soaps should remain a part of the routine. Monitoring pulmonary hygiene; protecting skin integrity; and avoiding urinary drainage catheters, IM injections, and rectal medication help to prevent infection. Weekly cultures monitor the client's germ-free status and detect colonization before it becomes infection.

Assess the client's skin, mouth, throat, axilla, perineum, and rectum for signs of infection; check all body fluids and excreta for color and consistency; and obtain cultures if infection is suspected (see Box 11–2 in Chapter 11). Monitor vital signs and assess the lungs every 4 hours. The possibility of interstitial pneumonia, a frequent complication in immunosuppressed clients, warrants these continuous 4-hour assessments. A temperature of 38°C (100.4°F) or greater should be investigated by cultures with sensitivity determinations, chest x-ray, and urinalysis. IV wide-spectrum antibiotic therapy is instituted until the results of the cultures and sensitivities are obtained, after which specific antimicrobial therapy can be given.

Daily infusions of granulocytes are often given to the client with a granulocyte count below 500 μL and with a fever that fails to respond to antimicrobial therapy. In some institutions, granulocytes are administered routinely as a prophylactic measure. Granulocytes and all blood products are irradiated before infusion to eliminate any T-lymphocytes that could contribute to GVHD. Side effects and nursing measures with blood and blood product infusion are discussed in Chapter 28.

Stomatitis. The management of stomatitis (discussed in Chapter 12) is always aimed toward increasing the client's comfort and oral intake. Additional goals with the BMT client are to decrease bacterial and fungal superinfections and to decrease mucosal ulcerations that may cause bleeding in this client whose platelet count is low. The frequency of mouth care will need to increase as mucosal deterioration increases.

Bleeding. Assessing for petechiae, gastrointestinal bleeding, and conjunctival and cerebral hemorrhage is essential because the BMT client's low platelet counts may lead to these conditions. If platelet counts are below 20,000 μL, the hemoglobin level below 10 g/dL, or the hematocrit below 30%, infusions of platelets or packed red blood cells are given (see Chapter 28). Encourage family members to donate their blood for this purpose. Avoid IM and SC injections and rectal temperatures. Clients should not shave to avoid bleeding from cuts and nicks as well as impairment of skin integrity.

Nutrition. Clients are usually started on TPN 24 hours after the last dose of chemotherapy. TPN provides vitamins, minerals, trace elements, amino acids, carbohydrates, and fats in the necessary amounts to prevent or reverse the catabolic state of malnutrition (Layton et al., 1981). The amounts to be infused are determined weekly by a nutritional support team, of which the nurse is often a member. The amounts are based on monitoring electrolytes, minerals, liver function, kidney function, and hematologic tests. Optimal nutritional status is essential during BMT. Anorexia, gastrointestinal and metabolic changes, and increased need for nutrients during periods of infection and fever combined with malnutrition increase the incidence of morbidity and mortality in BMT clients. Encourage as much oral intake as possible.

Graft-Versus-Host Disease. Because GVHD can occur despite the measures to prevent it discussed earlier, low-dose methotrexate or cyclosporine may be administered for 4 to 6 months after BMT. The onset of GVHD is serious because it signals the possibility that grafting has not been successful. At present, there is no known cure for GVHD, although the administration of high doses of corticosteroids has sometimes proven helpful. Clients who do not respond to steroid therapy may receive antithymocyte globulin (Nuscher et al., 1984).

Be alert for the development of both early onset and late onset GVHD. An early sign is impairment of skin integrity characterized by a rubellalike rash that begins on the face, palms of the hands, and the soles of the feet, eventually progressing to the trunk and the rest of the limbs. The skin may become dry and scaly, progressing to blistering and eventual desquamation (peeling). In some clients, the condition progresses to a chronic form in which inelasticity of the skin leads to contractures, scarring, impaired physical mobility, possible skin ulceration, and muscle wasting (Brown & Kiss, 1981). Some clients do not have the early signs but rather begin with the chronic form up to 1 year after the transplant.

GVHD may also involve the gastrointestinal tract, causing nausea and vomiting, abdominal cramping, malabsorption, and bleeding. Clients can lose from 500 mL to 6 L of fluid per day in severe diarrhea that is a dark green-brown (Nuscher et al., 1984). Hepatic involvement causes pruritus, jaundice, ascites, and fatigue. The liver is enlarged and the serum bilirubin, alkaline phosphatase, and serum glutamic-oxaloacetic transaminase (SGOT) levels are elevated.

Assess the extent, nature, and location of the client's discomfort and administer analgesics accordingly. Topical creams and soothing oatmeal baths may help relieve the discomfort of pruritus. Petrolatum gauze may be used to cover blistered or desquamated areas. Keep the client's perianal area clean after each bowel movement. Soothing ointments may help irritated skin and also help to promote skin integrity.

Not only does GVHD cause physical discomfort, it also causes emotional distress. Clients who develop GVHD and their families may experience depression, anger, and fear of death. As clients lose hope, they may become reluctant to participate in self-care or refuse medical treatment. Sometimes clients withdraw from interaction by sleeping or refusing visitors. Explaining this behavior to family members will help them to understand it, tolerate it, and be supportive of the client. It is important to serve as an anchor for clients as well as their families by encouraging self-care, joining with them in the hope that symptoms will subside, pointing out any subtle signs of improvement, and sustaining them through despair and discouragement.

Planning for Discharge. Discharge planning begins approximately 2 weeks after BMT. At least 2 weeks before discharge, the client and family should begin to perform the required care under nursing supervision. Instruct the family in skills such as caring for the central venous catheter, administering TPN, and administering medications. Advise them to prevent infection by proper hand-washing, avoiding contact with the client if they are ill, and remaining healthy. The client should avoid contacts with crowds and animals for at least the first 100 days after the transplant. Teach the client and family about the early signs of infection and GVHD.

Emphasize the importance of continued health care and assessments by dentists and dietitians because late-developing GVHD is a possibility. Until the immune system has regained normal function, the client is susceptible to infection, especially viral infection. Referral to a visiting nurse service is a resource for both client and family. Encourage clients and their families to identify the support systems available to them—other family members, friends, neighbors, community services, self-help groups, mental health counselors—and to plan to use them after discharge.

Chapter Highlights

Embolectomy uses a balloon catheter to clear an obstructed artery, preferably within 6 hours of occlusion.

Thrombectomy is the removal of a thrombus from a vessel with the aim of reducing venous insufficiency and minimizing postphlebotic disability.

Endarterectomy removes occlusive atherosclerotic material from arteries.

Following embolectomy, thrombectomy, or endarterectomy, the nurse must assess the client for the principal complications of vascular surgery: bleeding and thrombus formation. Clients need long-term anticoagulant therapy and regular exercise to prevent thrombus formation.

Percutaneous transluminal angioplasty is an option for removing blood vessel obstructions in clients who are poor surgical risks.

Surgical bypass of an obstructed artery may be necessary; the four types of bypasses are the femoropopliteal, the aortofemoral, the femorofemoral, and the axillofemoral. Following surgery, clients must exercise regularly and take anticoagulants. With the last two types of bypass, clients must be careful to avoid trauma to the subcutaneous tunnel made for the graft and to avoid positions which might kink the graft.

Abdominal aortic aneurysms are repaired with a Dacron or Teflon graft. Peripheral aneurysms are bypassed with a synthetic or vein graft.

Lumbar sympathectomy improves peripheral circulation by severing the sympathetic nerve fibers that cause the peripheral vessels to constrict. The procedure is usually used for clients who are at risk for corrective surgery.

Vein ligation and stripping remove painful, enlarged varicose veins. After surgery, clients should lose weight if necessary, avoid venous stasis, and keep the extremities elevated 10 to 18 hours a day.

An intracaval filter (umbrella filter) may be inserted into the inferior vena cava of clients whose vessels contain thrombi or emboli but who cannot withstand anticoagulation therapy or surgical intervention. This procedure can be done in a cardiac catheterization laboratory under local anesthesia and has largely replaced plication of the inferior vena cava, which requires general anesthesia and major surgery.

Surgical treatment for lymphedema is rare; it is used only when the weight and bulk of an edematous limb interfere with daily life and cause recurrent inflammation and cellulitis.

Splenectomy is almost always an emergency procedure performed to control bleeding from a ruptured spleen, although it is sometimes done in hypersplenism.

Bone marrow transplant is a lifesaving measure used when other treatments for aplastic anemia, severe immunodeficiency, leukemia, and Hodgkin's disease have failed. The BMT client experiences severe physical and emotional discomfort. Providing effective nursing care for these clients and their families is challenging.

Bibliography

Brown MH, Kiss ME: Standards of care for the patient with "graft-versus-host disease" post bone marrow transplant. *Canc Nurs* 1981; 4:191–198.

Brunner UV: Clinical lymphedema. In: *Advances in the Management of Cardiovascular Disease.* Vol 3. Foley WT (editor). Chicago: Yearbook Medical Publishers, 1982.

Charters AC, Stewart N: The management of trauma. In: *AACN's Clinical Reference for Critical Care Nurses.* Kinney MR (editor). New York: McGraw–Hill, 1981.

Ekers MA, Satiani B: EAB: A new route for vascular rehabilitation. *Nurs 82* (Nov) 1982; 12:34–41.

Ford R et al: Veno-occlusive disease following marrow transplantation. *Nurs Clin North Am* 1983; 18(9):563–568.

Gruendemann BJ, Meeker MH: *Alexander's Care of the Patient in Surgery,* 7th ed. St. Louis: Mosby, 1983.

Hinnant JR, Stallworth JM: Simplified surgery for varicose veins. *AORN J* 1981; 34:135–150.

Hutchinson MM, Itoh K: Nursing care for the patient undergoing bone marrow transplantation for acute leukemia. *Nurs Clin North Am* 1982; 17(12):697–711.

Jasinkowski NL: The unique needs of a distal bypass patient. *RN* (March) 1982; 45:44–47, 122.

Layton PB et al: Nutritional assessment of allogeneic bone marrow recipients. *Canc Nurs* 1981; 4:127–135.

Logan J, Ziebell E: Axillofemoral artery bypass for lower limb ischemia. *Can Nurse* (Sept) 1982; 78:25–29.

Nuscher R et al: Bone marrow transplantation. *Am J Nurs* 1984; 84:764–772.

Raab D: Peripheral vascular disease: How to recognize it, how to treat it. *Can Nurse* (Sept) 1982; 78:30–33.

Rutherford RB: Lumbar sympathectomy: Indications and technique in vascular surgery. In: *Vascular Surgery,* 2nd ed. Rutherford RB (editor). Philadelphia: Saunders, 1984.

Strandness, DE: Vascular diseases of the extremities. In: *Harrison's Principles of Internal Medicine,* 10th ed. Petersdorf RG et al (editors). New York: McGraw–Hill, 1983.

Thomas ED: Bone marrow failure and bone marrow transplantation. In: *Harrison's Principles of Internal Medicine,* 10th ed. Petersdorf RG et al (editors). New York: McGraw–Hill, 1983.

Waltman AC: Percutaneous transluminal angioplasty: Iliac and deep femoral arteries. *AJR* 1980; 135:921–925.

Suggested Readings

de la Montaigne M, DeMao J: Standards of care for the patient with "graft-versus-host disease" post bone marrow transplantation. *Canc Nurs* (June) 1981; 14:199–205. A brief review of basic immunology introduces the reader to graft-versus-host disease (GVHD), followed by a description of its pathophysiology, stages, and treatment. A well-organized nursing care plan for the GVHD client is included.

Doyle JE: The intracaval filter: New nursing challenge. *RN* (May) 1980; 43:38–42. This article gives an overview of the indications for and purposes of the umbrella filter, the insertion process, and preoperative and postoperative care of the client who undergoes its insertion.

Hinnant JR, Stallworth JM: Simplified surgery for varicose veins. *AORN J* 1981; 34:135–150. This article discusses a method of treating varicose veins by high-frequency cautery to destroy venous tributaries. This procedure reportedly results in reduced scarring of the legs.

Jasinkowski NL: Aortic bypass: Trimming the postop risks. *RN* (June) 1983; 46:41–45. The nursing care for a client with a leaking abdominal aortic aneurysm is followed from admission to the emergency department through the perioperative period, including a stay in the ICU. Photographs and illustrations of abdominal aortic aneurysm, abdominal aortogram, and the Doppler probe are included.

Logan J, Ziebell E: Axillofemoral artery bypass for lower limb ischemia. *Can Nurse* (Sept) 1982; 78:25–29. This article discusses the perioperative care of the client having an axillofemoral bypass. The nursing role in research and data collection is interwoven.

Nuscher R et al: Bone marrow transplantation. *Am J Nurs* 1984; 84:764–772. This comprehensive article was written by the nursing staff of a bone marrow transplant unit in a large oncology center. It discusses donor and recipient matching, the transplant unit environment, the procedure, complications, and the related nursing care of the bone marrow recipient. The section on complications is especially thorough.

Raab D: Peripheral vascular disease: How to recognize it and how to treat it. *Can Nurse* (Sept) 1982; 78:30–33. This article follows a client through various surgical interventions for peripheral vascular disease. It includes a chart of the types of surgeries, their indications, and the importance of the nursing role in the physiological and emotional support of client and family.

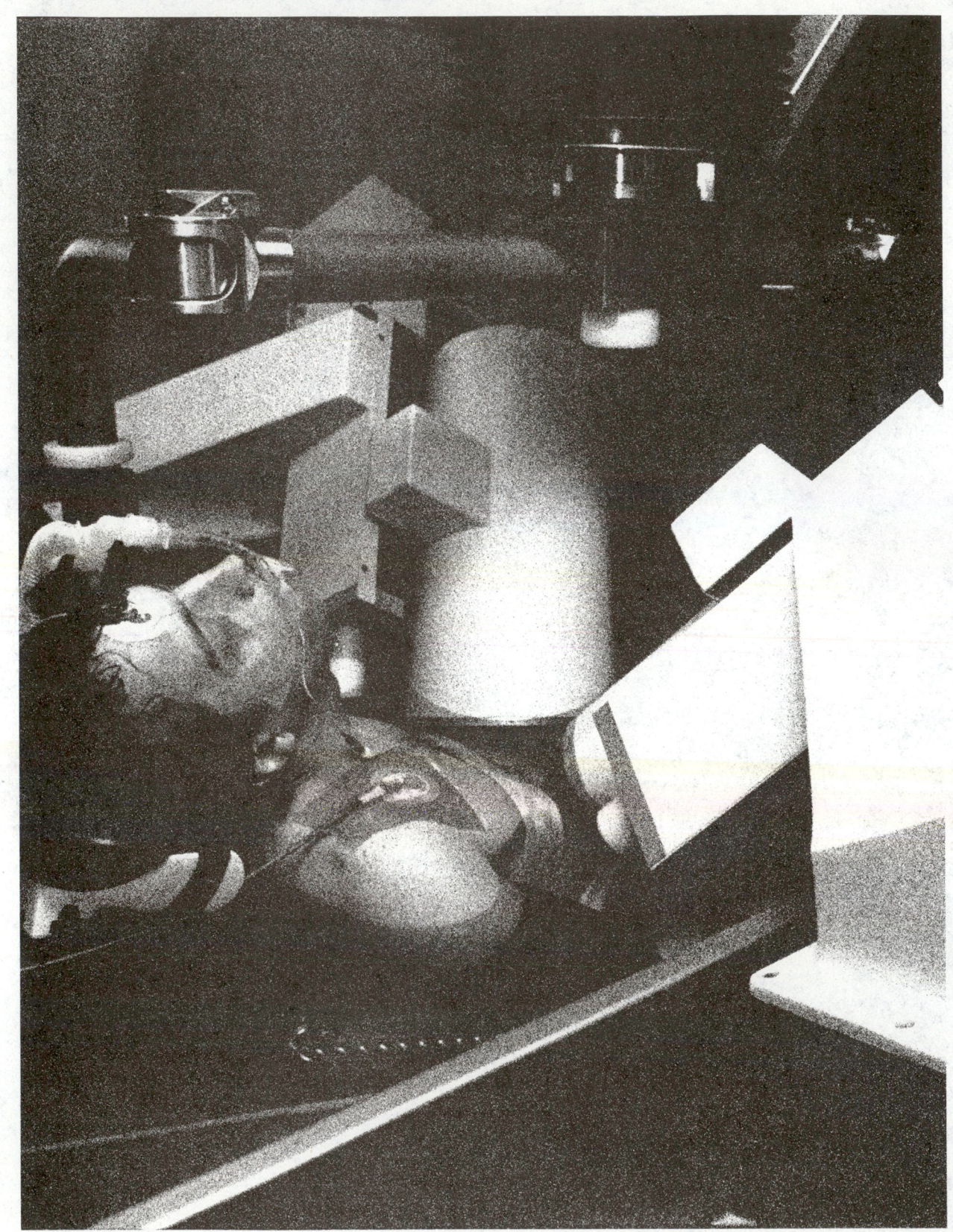

UNIT 5

The Client With Urinary System Dysfunction

Chapter 31

The Kidneys and Urinary System in Health and Illness

Jane Hokanson Hawks
Jeanette K. Chambers

Objectives

When you have finished studying this chapter, you should be able to:

Describe the structural components of the urinary tract and their major anatomic relationships.

Identify the functions of the nephron.

Explain the major circulatory variables that contribute to renal function.

Describe renal–hormonal mechanisms for maintaining fluid balance and regulating blood pressure.

Trace the pathway for the formation and excretion of urine.

Identify the primary electrolyte and acid–base abnormalities associated with failure of renal regulation.

Describe the general effects of uremia.

Discuss general psychosocial and cultural considerations relevant to the kidneys and urinary system.

The urinary system includes the kidneys, ureters, urinary bladder, and urethra. Although this system has as a major function the removal of waste products from the body, it actually accomplishes much more than that. The urinary system is also essential to the maintenance of homeostasis. The kidneys rid the body of a variety of metabolic waste products as well as conserve or excrete fluid and electrolytes as needed to maintain the internal balance of these substances. To do so, the kidneys filter a volume equivalent to all of the blood plasma in the body every 5 minutes. A person can live with only one kidney. If both kidneys fail, however, many of these waste products cannot be removed from the body. To prevent death in these cases, a kidney transplant or dialysis is necessary. The importance of the ureters, bladder, and urethra must not be overlooked. They transport urine, and the bladder also stores it. All structures function together to accomplish these important tasks.

Section I: Structural and Functional Interrelationships

The urinary system consists of two kidneys, which produce urine; two ureters, which carry urine to the urinary bladder, where it is temporarily stored; and the urethra, which transports urine to the outside of the body (Figure 31–1). Because of the prostate gland's proximity to the urinary bladder and urethra in the male, it will be considered briefly in this unit as well. For a more detailed discussion of the prostate gland, refer to Chapter 62.

STRUCTURE OF THE KIDNEYS

An adult normally has two kidneys, which are reddish brown and bean shaped. Their size varies with the size of the individual. The length of the average kidney is about 11 cm, the thickness about 2.5 cm, and the width about 5 cm. The weight of a single kidney averages 150 g. The kidney's lateral border is convex, whereas the medial border is con-

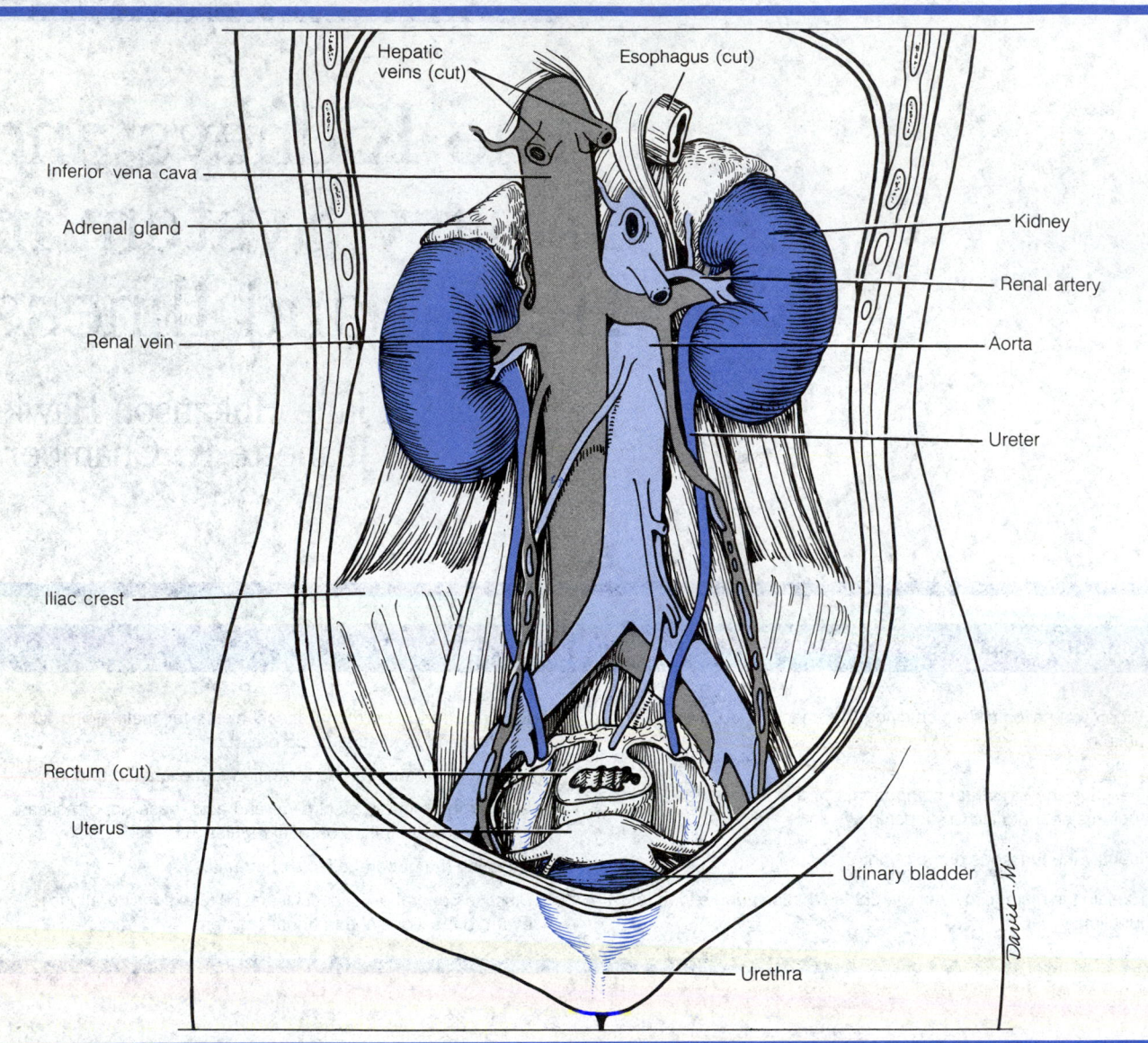

Figure 31–1

Organs of the urinary system (anterior abdominal wall and most abdominal organs are absent).
SOURCE: Spence AP, Mason EB: *Human Anatomy and Physiology,* 2nd ed. Menlo Park, CA: Benjamin/Cummings, 1983.

cave and indented in a depression called the renal hilus. All related structures enter or leave the kidney at the hilus.

The kidneys lie in the retroperitoneal space of the posterior abdominal cavity. Thus, a surgeon can expose them without opening the peritoneal cavity. One kidney lies on either side of the vertebral column. Layers of muscle surround the posterior surfaces of the kidneys, and abdominal organs surround their anterior surfaces. The peritoneal membrane covers most of the anterior surface of each kidney.

The kidneys are protected and supported by renal fascia and layers of perirenal fat. Posteriorly, the psoas, quadratus lumborum, and transversus abdominis muscles provide support (Figure 31–2). The position of the kidneys is not fixed but varies somewhat with a person's position.

When the client is in the supine position, the kidneys lie between the 12th thoracic and 3rd lumbar vertebrae. When the client is standing, the kidneys may descend to the top of the iliac crest. For a client in Trendelenburg's position, the kidneys ascend to the 10th intercostal space.

The left kidney, which lies near the tail of the pancreas and the splenic flexure of the colon, is normally slightly longer and narrower than the right kidney. The right kidney is lower in the abdomen than the left because of the presence of the liver in the right upper quadrant. The superior pole of the right kidney lies beneath the liver in an area referred to as the *renal bed.* The right kidney's anterior surface is adjacent to the hepatic flexure of the colon, the duodenum, and the liver. The lower portion of each kidney descends beneath the lower portion of the rib cage. The

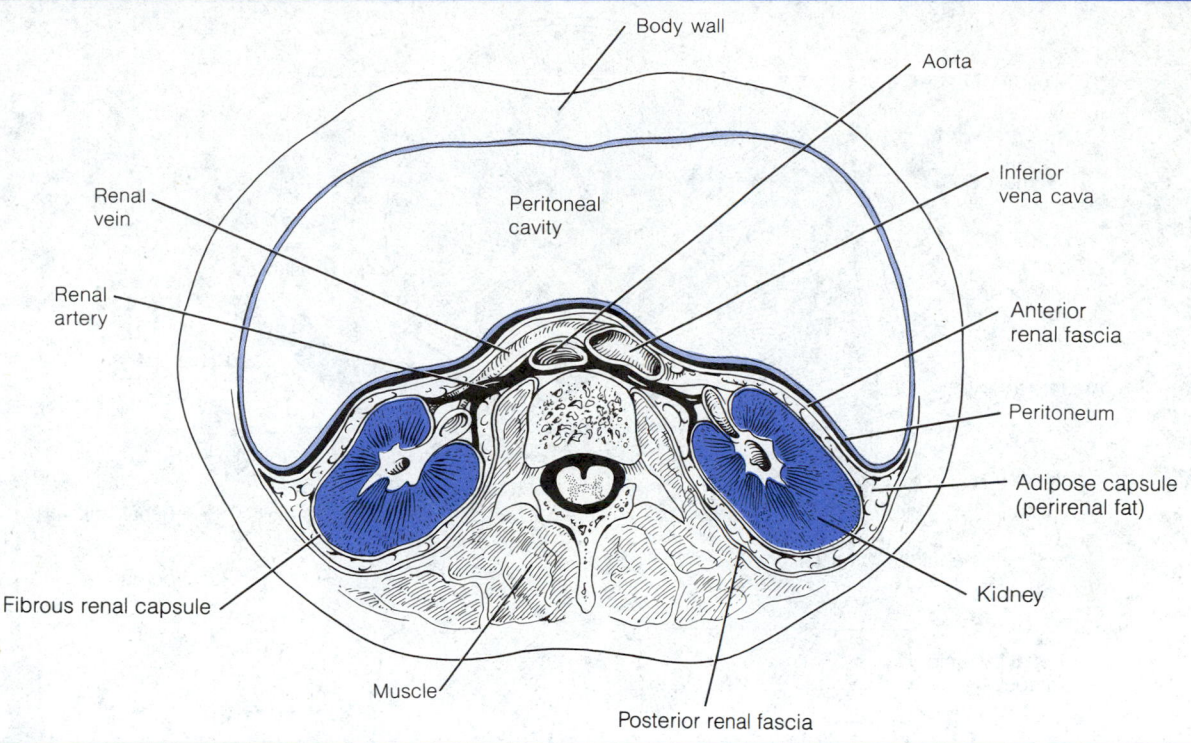

Figure 31–2

Transverse section of body showing retroperitoneal location of kidneys and renal fascia surrounding them.
SOURCE: Spence AP, Mason EB: *Human Anatomy and Physiology,* 2nd ed. Menlo Park, CA: Benjamin/Cummings, 1983.

angle formed between the lower rim of the rib cage and the vertebral column is referred to as the costovertebral angle (CVA).

Each kidney is surrounded by three layers of tissue (Figure 31–2). The fibrous renal capsule, the innermost layer, covers the surface of the kidney. The adipose capsule, a mass of perirenal fat, surrounds the renal capsule. The third layer, the renal fascia, surrounds and encloses the kidney and adipose capsule and anchors the kidney to the posterior abdominal wall.

The cross-sectional view in Figure 31–3 shows three general regions of each kidney: the cortex, the medulla, and the pelvis. These structures are located inside the renal capsule; two of them, the cortex and the medulla, are often referred to as the *renal parenchyma.* The cortex is directly beneath the renal capsule. This highly vascularized area of tissue is very sensitive to changes in blood flow. The medulla, located deep in the cortex, consists of 8 to 18 triangular renal pyramids. The renal pyramids are composed of collecting ducts that drain urine into the calyces. The cortex covers the bases of the pyramids, and the tips (or papillae) project toward the renal pelvis. Cortical tissue known as *renal columns* dips into the medulla to separate the pyramids, and blood vessels that supply the cortex and medulla pass through these columns. Urine flows from the papillae into a minor calyx, and several of the funnel-shaped minor calyces emerge to form a major calyx. The major calyces join to form the renal pelvis, which is the expanded upper end of the ureter.

The Nephron

The nephron, the functional unit of the kidney, is primarily responsible for most of the mechanisms that provide internal homeostasis. Each kidney contains approximately 1.25 million nephrons, and each nephron in turn is composed of a vascular and tubular system that allows for the formation of urine. The nephrons are located in the renal parenchyma. Most nephrons are in the cortex (cortical nephrons), but juxtamedullary nephrons begin in the cortex and extend deep into the medulla (Figure 31–4).

The vascular system of the nephron consists of the glomerulus and Bowman's capsule, both located in the cortex of the kidney. The glomerulus is composed of a knot of capillaries. Bowman's capsule, or the glomerular capsule, surrounds the glomerulus. The glomerulus derives its blood flow from the renal artery of the abdominal aorta. Each renal artery branches into segmental arteries and increasingly smaller interlobar, arcuate, and interlobular arteries, which supply progressively smaller areas of renal parenchyma. The smallest branch, the afferent arteriole, feeds blood to the glomerulus. After passing through the capillaries in the glomerulus, the blood exits the glomerulus, not through a venule but via the efferent arte-

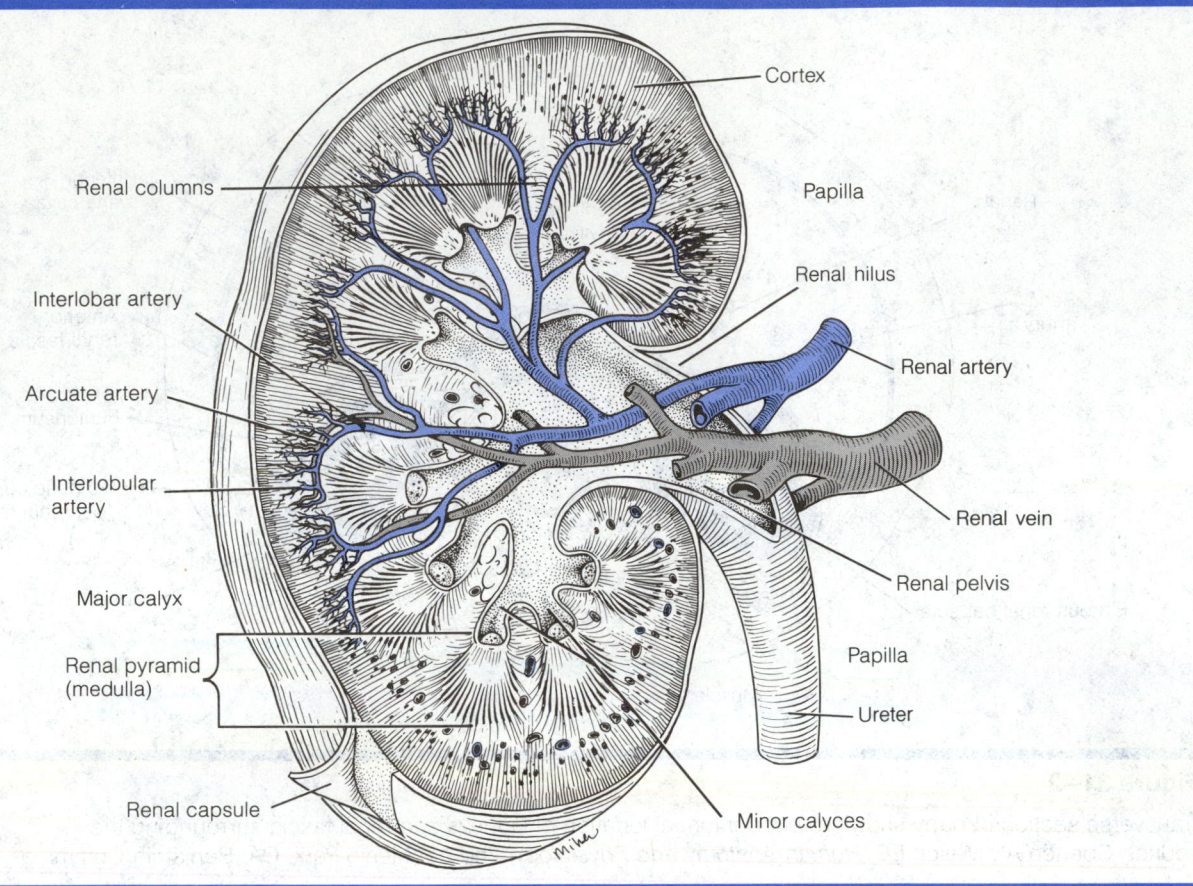

Figure 31–3

Longitudinal section of kidney showing internal structure.
SOURCE: Spence AP, Mason EB: *Human Anatomy and Physiology,* 2nd ed. Menlo Park, CA: Benjamin/Cummings, 1983.

riole. From the efferent arteriole, the blood enters the peritubular capillaries of the cortical nephron or the vasa recta of the juxtamedullary nephron. This plexus of capillaries surrounds the proximal tubule, Henle's loop, and the distal tubule. Finally, from either the peritubular capillaries or the vasa recta, blood enters the venous system and returns to the general circulation through a series of renal venules and veins that drain all portions of the kidney. The renal vein of each kidney returns blood into the inferior vena cava (Figure 31–5).

The tubular system of the nephron begins with Bowman's capsule, which is invaginated around each glomerular tuft to form a sac. Bowman's capsule narrows into the proximal convoluted tubule, which changes direction many times until it straightens into the descending limb of Henle's loop and angles downward toward the pelvis of the kidney. The hairpin loops of tubular tissue are much longer in juxtamedullary nephrons than in cortical nephrons and are contained within the pyramids of the medulla. The ascending limb of Henle's loop then becomes the distal convoluted tubule. The distal convoluted tubules of several nephrons enter a collecting duct within a pyramid of the medulla; these ducts are responsible for the drainage of formed urine from the nephrons. Pyramids then are drained into

the calyceal system of the renal pelvis through the tips of the papillae.

Renal Circulation

The important relation between the kidneys and the blood vascular system becomes apparent in considering the large size of the renal arteries that supply the kidneys. At rest, these vessels carry about 20% of the total cardiac output to the kidneys, or approximately 600 mL of blood per minute through each kidney. Little of this blood supplies the nutritive needs of the kidneys; the large blood flow actually is related to the fact that the kidneys can maintain homeostasis of the blood only if a large amount of the blood passes through them.

The vascular supply to the kidneys consists of several microcirculations:

- Glomerular capillaries, where plasma filtration occurs
- Peritubular capillaries, which encircle the proximal and distal convoluted tubules, where water, electrolytes, glucose, amino acids, and protein are reabsorbed, and some substances are secreted
- Medullary circulation (vasa recta), which aids in the concentration of urine

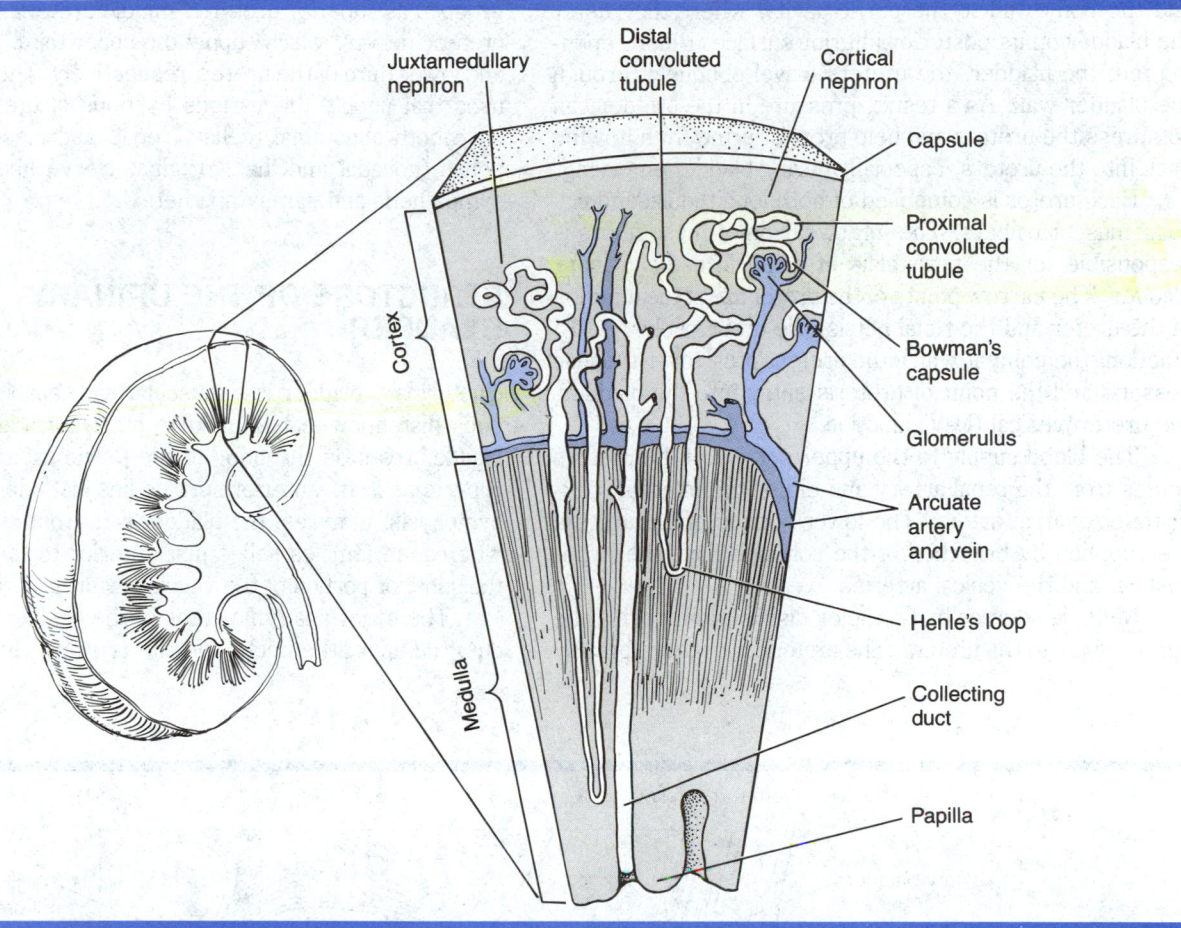

Figure 31–4

Longitudinal section of kidney showing location of cortical and juxtamedullary nephrons.
SOURCE: Spence AP, Mason EB: *Human Anatomy and Physiology,* 2nd ed. Menlo Park, CA: Benjamin/Cummings, 1983.

STRUCTURE OF THE URETERS

Urine drips from the collecting tubules into the minor calyces and then the major calyces which, in turn, join the renal pelvis. From the renal pelvis, ureters transport urine to the urinary bladder. Each kidney normally has a single ureter, which is responsible for emptying the urine formed by that kidney. Although the ureter's size varies with the size of the individual, an average ureter is around 30 cm (almost a foot long). The ureter's diameter ranges from 2 to 8 mm at various points in its structure.

The ureters descend between the parietal peritoneum

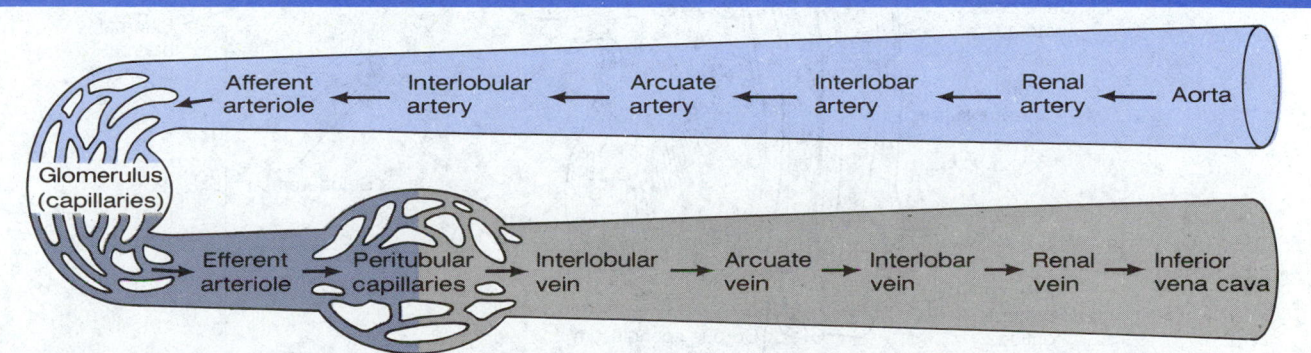

Figure 31–5

Summary of pathway of blood through kidney.
SOURCE: Spence AP, Mason EB: *Human Anatomy and Physiology,* 2nd ed. Menlo Park, CA: Benjamin/Cummings, 1983.

and the body wall to the pelvic cavity, where they enter the bladder on its posterior inferior surface. Before opening into the bladder, the ureters travel obliquely through the bladder wall. As a result, pressure in the bladder can compress the ureters and help prevent urine from flowing back into the ureters, especially during bladder emptying.

Each ureter is composed of both longitudinal and circular muscular fibers. The interweaving of these fibers is responsible for the peristalsis of urine into the urinary bladder. The narrow points of the ureter are at the junction of the ureter and the renal pelvis, the ureteropelvic (U-P) junction; the point at which the ureters cross over the iliac vessels; and the point of ureteral entry into the bladder, the ureterovesical (U-V) junction.

The blood supply to the upper portion of the ureters comes from the renal artery and either the internal spermatic or ovarian artery. The lower portion of the ureters are supplied by branches of the common iliac, the hypogastric, and the vesical arteries.

Multiple sources in a complex distribution provide the nerve supply to the ureters. The ureteric nerves are broadly grouped as superior ureteric, middle ureteric, and inferior ureteric nerves, which supply the upper third, middle third, and lower third of the ureter, respectively. The nerve plexuses that supply the various portions of ureteric nerves have both abdominal (celiac, renal, and mesenteric) and pelvic (gonadal and iliac) origins. Nerve fibers are both sympathetic and parasympathetic.

STRUCTURE OF THE URINARY BLADDER

The urinary bladder is a muscular sac capable of tremendous distention that is used to store formed urine. The bladder rests on the floor of the pelvic cavity and is retroperitoneal. Its anterior surface lies just behind the pubic symphysis. In males, the bladder is in front of the rectum, whereas in females it lies just anterior to the uterus and the superior portion of the vagina (Figures 31–6 and 31–7).

The major anatomic areas of the bladder are the fundus, the apex, the neck, and the **trigone** (Figure 31–8).

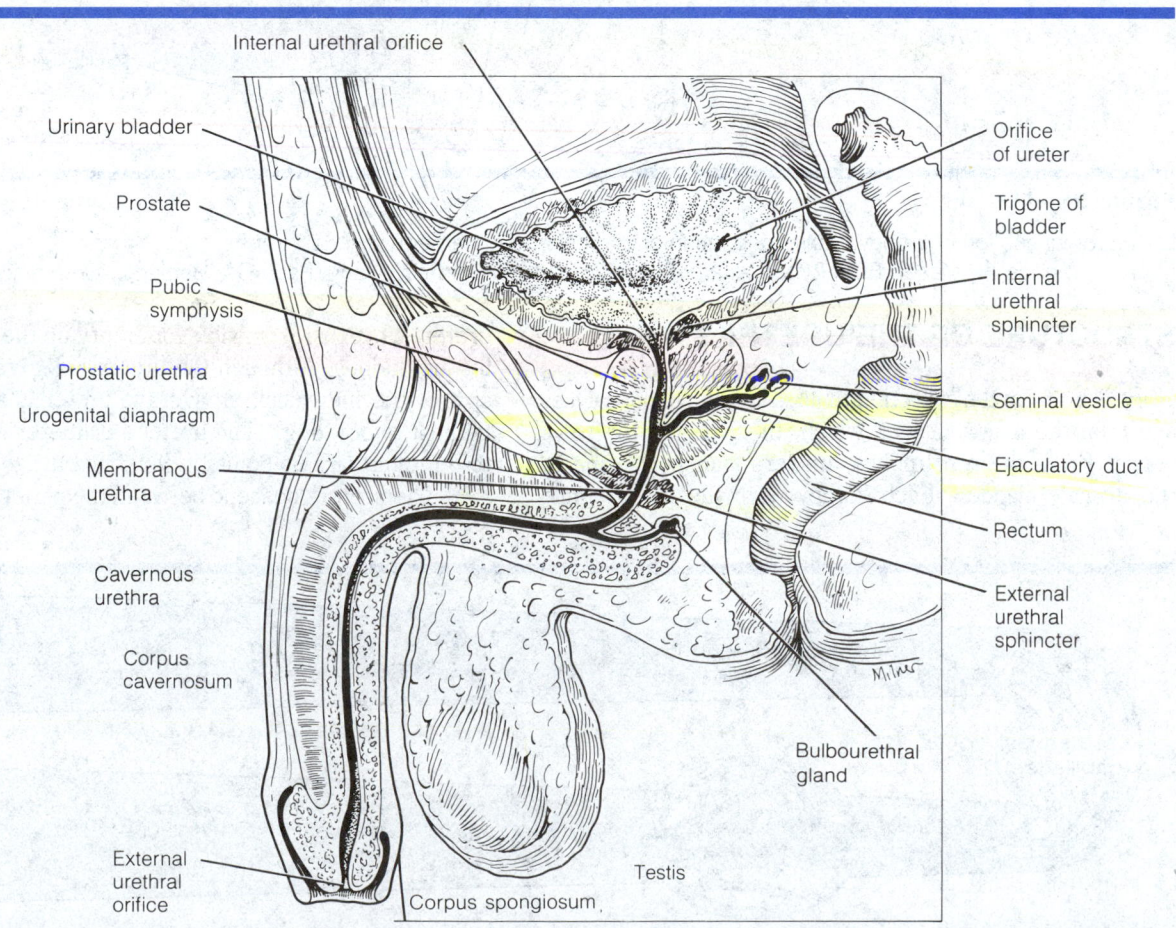

Figure 31–6

Urinary bladder and urethra in the male.
SOURCE: Spence AP, Mason EB: *Human Anatomy and Physiology*, 2nd ed. Menlo Park, CA: Benjamin/Cummings, 1983.

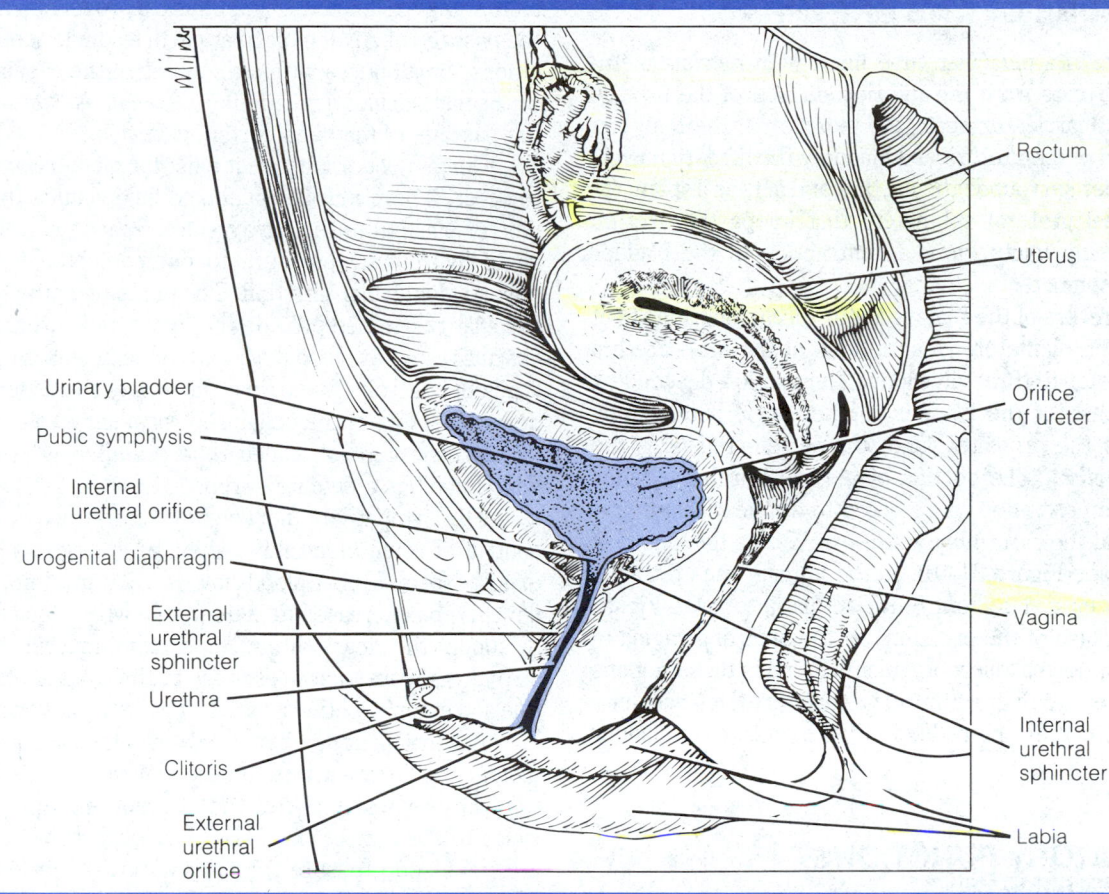

Figure 31–7

Urinary bladder and urethra in the female.
SOURCE: Spence AP, Mason EB: *Human Anatomy and Physiology,* 2nd ed. Menlo Park, CA: Benjamin/Cummings, 1983.

The fundus is the upper portion of the bladder, and the apex is the bottom portion of the bladder closest to the pelvic floor. The bladder neck is the most inferior portion of the bladder and contains the internal sphincter. It is actually a group of thickened fibers of the detrusor muscle, which evolves into the smooth muscle of the urethra. The trigone is an area of the posterior wall of the bladder defined by the urethra and the two ureteral slits, where the ureters enter the bladder. Special characteristics of this area of muscle are responsible for separating the upper urinary tract from the lower urinary tract during normal micturition.

As the bladder fills with urine, its internal pressure increases somewhat initially and then remains fairly constant up to a volume of about 300 to 400 mL. Beyond this point, the pressure rises rapidly. The bladder can hold 600 to 800 mL of urine, but it is generally emptied before it reaches this capacity (Spence & Mason, 1983).

The nerve supply to the bladder is both sensory and motor. Sympathetic, parasympathetic, and somatic nerves carry sensations to the central nervous system. Sympathetic fibers arise from T-9 through L-2, and parasympathetic and somatic nerves arise from S-2 through S-4. The motor nerve supply to the bladder involves parasympathetic supply to the detrusor muscle and sympathetic supply to the trigone. The pudendal nerves, which are under voluntary control, supply the external sphincter and the muscles of the pelvic floor.

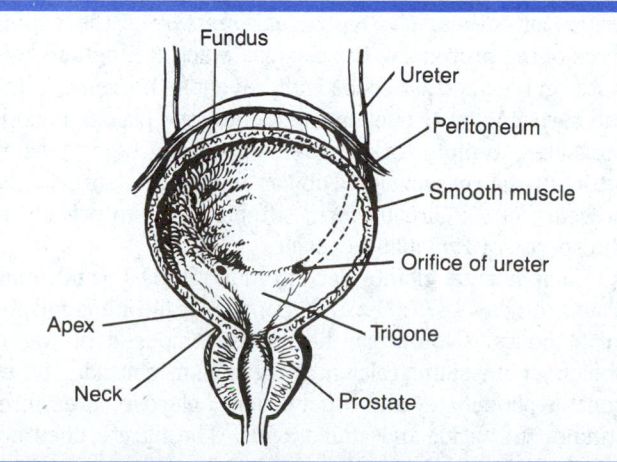

Figure 31–8

Opened male urinary bladder showing trigone.
SOURCE: Vick RL: *Contemporary Medical Physiology.* Menlo Park, CA: Addison-Wesley, 1984.

STRUCTURE OF THE URETHRA

The urethra is a muscular tube lined with mucous membranes that exits from the inferior surface of the urinary bladder and carries urine to the exterior of the body. At the junction of the urethra and bladder, the smooth muscle of the bladder surrounds the urethra and acts as a sphincter (the internal urethral sphincter) that keeps the urethra closed. During micturition, a contraction of the bladder opens the sphincter.

The urethra of the male is about 21 cm long and about 8 to 9 mm in diameter. Descriptions of the male urethra generally refer to three divisions. The urethra descending from the base of the bladder to the pelvic floor is surrounded by the prostate gland; this is referred to as the *prostatic urethra*. The portion of the urethra that extends through the pelvic floor is referred to as the *membranous urethra*, and the *cavernous urethra* traverses the length of the penis (see Figure 31–6). In the female, the urethra is about 4 cm long and about 8 mm in diameter (see Figure 31–7). Because of the proximity of the anus and vagina to the urethra, normal microorganisms found in those regions may more easily migrate into the bladder. This accounts for why women are more likely than men to have bladder infections.

REGULATORY FUNCTIONS OF THE KIDNEYS

The kidneys and urinary system maintain internal homeostasis of body fluids and their composition. A variety of mechanisms maintain this fluid and electrolyte balance, and the end result is the production of urine. This final product represents the work of the kidneys and results in the removal of nitrogenous waste products, as well as the regulation of fluid, electrolyte, and acid–base balances. In addition, the kidneys produce hormones and additional substances that influence other metabolic and chemical processes.

Formation of Urine

The basic function of the nephron is to cleanse the blood of unwanted substances as it passes through the kidney. This results in the formation of urine and is accomplished through three specific processes that occur in the nephron: glomerular filtration, tubular reabsorption, and tubular secretion. Each process occurs dynamically in the kidneys' continuous efforts to maintain internal equilibrium.

Glomerular Filtration

Glomerular filtration is the ultrafiltration of blood across a semipermeable membrane in which fluid, electrolytes, and certain nonelectrolytes are filtered but plasma proteins remain. Glomerular filtration occurs within the glomerulus, across the glomerular capillary membrane. This capillary membrane has anatomic and physical properties that allow the passage of small molecular particles under certain conditions. Small pores within the lining of the capillary loops of the glomerulus (called the *basement membrane*) allow the passage of fluid and certain particles.

Certain conditions must exist for glomerular filtration to occur. There must be adequate fluid volume (blood volume or plasma) in the intravascular space, as well as adequate hydrostatic pressure to overcome the forces that oppose glomerular filtration. The pumping of the heart and vascular resistance provide the hydrostatic pressure. The vascular tone, or blood flow, within the kidney is under two types of control: (1) extrinsic factors such as sympathetic nerve fibers from the celiac and renal nerve plexuses and (2) intrinsic control, called *autoregulation of renal blood flow*. Each has a definite purpose (Guyton, 1981).

The sympathetic nervous system provides extrinsic control of renal blood flow when an emergency situation exists. Normal renal blood flow is 1200 mL/min, but this flow may be decreased to 200 mL/min when blood is needed to supply the heart, brain, or skeletal muscle. This is a strong vasoconstrictor response to the release of epinephrine and norepinephrine by the sympathetic nervous system.

Autoregulation of blood flow maintains a constancy of glomerular filtration through the kidney's unique ability to regulate the resistance of the afferent and efferent arterioles to the flow of blood. Because of this autoregulation, arterial blood pressure can vary widely—between 80 and 180 mm Hg—while renal blood flow and glomerular filtration remain basically unchanged.

The product of glomerular filtration is glomerular filtrate. As long as the various mechanisms that regulate renal blood flow maintain adequate hydrostatic pressure, glomerular filtrate will form. However, forces that oppose the formation of glomerular filtrate—plasma oncotic pressure and tubular filtrate pressure (Guyton, 1981)—must be overcome. Understanding plasma oncotic pressure is essential to appreciate the shift of body fluids and the formation of edema. *Plasma oncotic pressure* is the pulling force of the proteins in the plasma, which attempts to hold water in the vascular space and prevent its movement into the surrounding tissue. In the kidney, the plasma oncotic pressure attempts to keep the water from being pushed into Bowman's capsule. Tubular filtrate pressure is the pressure of the already formed tubular filtrate present in the spaces of Bowman's capsule.

The normal glomerular filtration rate is 130 mL/min. Thus, roughly 187,000 mL of glomerular filtrate is formed in 24 hours. Glomerular filtrate is composed of water, sodium, potassium, calcium, magnesium, chloride, bicarbonate, phosphate, and other anions; glucose; urea; creatinine; uric acid; and amino acids. The filtrate does not contain protein, because the glomerular membrane is almost completely impermeable to all plasma proteins. For all practical purposes, glomerular filtrate is the same as plasma except it has no significant amount of plasma proteins. If all these substances were excreted as urine, death would occur immediately. Therefore, much of the filtrate is returned to the blood via tubular reabsorption.

Tubular Reabsorption

In tubular reabsorption, the initial refinement process, water, and specific electrolytes and nonelectrolytes from the tubular filtrate are reabsorbed into the plasma of the peritubular capillaries or vasa recta. Tubular reabsorption occurs throughout the tubular system of the nephron, but much of it occurs within the proximal convoluted tubule.

The tubules have a limited capacity for reabsorption of some substances. For example, the threshold for reabsorption of glucose may be limited when the blood level of glucose is exceedingly high or when renal tubular surfaces are altered through injury. Reabsorption is primarily accomplished through passive and active transport mechanisms of diffusion. In *passive transport,* the development of a pressure gradient causes the movement of molecules or particles. In this case, simple *diffusion* occurs (molecules move from an area of greater to lesser concentration or greater to lesser pressure). With some substances, however, expenditure of energy may be necessary to move the molecules. *Active transport* occurs through this expenditure of energy—basically, the release of adenosine triphosphate (ATP). Active transport is required when there is not a pressure gradient yet a substance must be moved to another area (Guyton, 1981).

Normally, reabsorption from the tubular filtrate into the blood is sufficient to maintain normal serum levels of the various electrolytes. However, reabsorption of some nonelectrolytes (eg, urea, creatinine, and uric acid) is not readily accomplished. The organism benefits from this because these substances are removed or cleared from the body.

Reabsorption of water is by **osmosis,** the movement of water across a semipermeable membrane from an area of lesser concentration to greater concentration of solute. Water is reabsorbed primarily in the proximal convoluted tubule. If greater water reabsorption is needed to maintain balance, however, the permeability of the distal tubule and collecting duct may be increased.

This reabsorption of water reflects the kidneys' ability to concentrate or dilute the urine as necessary. Sensitive osmoreceptors in the hypothalamus direct antidiuretic hormone (ADH) as follows. The supraoptic and paraventricular nuclei of the hypothalamic area sense the plasma **osmolality,** the concentration of particles (electrolytes and nonelectrolytes) in the plasma. When plasma osmolality is out of the normal range of 280 to 295 mOsm/L, the osmoreceptors detect this abnormality and trigger responses to return the osmolality to normal.

Only slight alterations in the osmolality of the blood are required to trigger appropriate regulatory mechanisms. A combined response by the neuroendocrine system and the kidneys will ensure that the serum osmolality is returned to the normal range by the release of ADH from its storage area in the posterior pituitary. The ADH alters the permeability of the distal convoluted tubules and collecting ducts so more or less water can be reabsorbed as needed. When ADH secretion increases, so does the reabsorption of the water in the tubules; when ADH secretion decreases, more water is excreted by the kidneys. Maintenance of intravascular volume is always the primary goal of the homeostatic mechanism. Thus, normally functioning kidneys concentrate or dilute urine to maintain normal serum osmolality.

Tubular Secretion

The third major process in urine formation is tubular secretion, the process by which ions in the tubular cells are secreted into the lumen of the tubule to be excreted in the end product, urine. Tubular secretion of potassium and hydrogen regulates the serum potassium level and serves as the kidneys' acid–base balancing mechanism.

The kidneys regulate acids and bases in conjunction with other body regulatory mechanisms (ie, the blood buffers and the lungs). The kidneys are responsible for the secretion of the fixed acids of normal metabolism, whereas the lungs excrete the volatile acids. The blood buffers provide moment-to-moment regulation. The fixed acids derive primarily from the metabolism of protein. The kidneys regulate their excretion by conserving bicarbonate, excreting sodium in exchange for the secretion of hydrogen, and secreting ammonia.

Thus, the processes of filtration, reabsorption, and secretion create the end product, urine. Urine is composed primarily of water, sodium, potassium, chloride, urea, creatinine, and uric acid. The volume of urine is normally about 1500 mL per 24 hours, but it depends on the amount of solute that must be excreted.

Blood Pressure Control

The kidneys regulate blood pressure through the maintenance of fluid volume and the release of the hormone renin, which stimulates powerful vasoconstrictive responses. Fluid volume in the extracellular compartment, and specifically the plasma, is controlled by the kidneys' ability to concentrate or dilute urine in response to the serum osmolality. Thus, hypertonic plasma stimulates the release of ADH, the reabsorption of water, the expansion of intravascular volume, the decrease of urine output, and the elevation of blood pressure. This primary mechanism of volume expansion is partially responsible for the regulation of blood pressure.

The renin–angiotensin system is the other kidney-controlled hormonal mechanism that can result in blood pressure elevation in certain situations. This mechanism is activated when there is low serum sodium level, decreased cardiac output, or ischemia to the kidneys. Any of these situations can stimulate the release of renin from the juxtaglomerular cells of the afferent arteriole of the glomerulus. It is believed that the macula densa of the distal convoluted tubule is sensitive to both the sodium content and the volume of the tubular filtrate and that this sensing mechanism stimulates the release of renin (Schrier, 1980). Renin release influences blood pressure. When renin is liberated from the juxtaglomerular cells it acts on angiotensinogen, a glycoprotein made in the liver and normally found in plasma, converting it to angiotensin I. Another converting enzyme in the pulmonary capillary bed acts on angiotensin I to change it to angiotensin II, a powerful vasoconstrictor that elevates blood pressure through peripheral vasoconstriction. Angiotensin II also triggers the release by the adrenal cortex of aldosterone, a mineralocorticoid that helps control sodium utilization. With the release of aldosterone, the distal convoluted tubule of the nephron reabsorbs sodium, and water reabsorption follows the sodium reabsorption increasing plasma volume. Thus, angiotensin II has two main effects that help to elevate blood pressure; peripheral vasoconstriction and plasma volume expansion. When ADH production increases, aldosterone production usually does as well.

When cardiac output is severely decreased because of loss of circulating blood volume, vasoconstriction within the kidneys will severely limit intrarenal blood flow and maintain flow to more vital organs, the heart and brain. This is an excellent example of the kidneys' role in the preservation of the whole organism because if renal vasoconstriction is not abated, death of the renal parenchyma results.

Recently, substances have been identified that may be useful in helping overcome severe renal vasoconstriction. These **prostaglandins** are believed to have vasodilation capabilities. Part of their antihypertensive effect is through the inhibition of norepinephrine and angiotensin II (Nasjletti & Malik, 1981).

Miscellaneous Hormonal and Metabolic Controls

Several other metabolic and hormonal functions of the kidneys have been identified, including the production of **erythropoietin,** the production of 1,25-dihydroxycholecalciferol, and the breakdown of insulin. Erythropoietin is a glycoprotein produced in the kidneys that influences red blood cell production. Neither the site of erythropoietin production nor the site for its storage in the kidney has been identified (Rose, 1981), but the effects of bilateral nephrectomy and the subsequent decrease in erythropoiesis have been observed. Erythropoietin seems to increase both the rate of production and the rate of release of new red blood cells from the bone marrow and the spleen.

The kidneys also produce 1,25-dihydroxycholecalciferol, the active component of vitamin D. Without this substance, calcium cannot be absorbed properly from the intestines, so calcium levels decrease. The complexities of calcium metabolism are discussed in more detail in Chapter 55.

The kidneys also break down and excrete insulin. Failure to excrete insulin results in an increased availability of insulin (Rose, 1981), which has important consequences for the management and control of diabetic clients. Most clients with Type I diabetes mellitus have a decreased need for insulin as renal failure progresses. The reliability of urine testing to calculate insulin needs is also severely limited, as the renal threshold changes constantly with decreasing renal function.

Process of Micturition

Micturition, also called *urination* or *voiding,* is a complex physical process under a variety of neural controls. For the toilet-trained person, urination is under voluntary control and can be interrupted or initiated upon cerebral command, as long as motor and sensory nerve pathways are intact. Micturition normally is a painless function that occurs five to six times a day and possibly once at night. The average person voids a total of about 1500 mL of urine per 24 hours. This amount is affected by fluid intake, the ingestion of diuretics, sweating, temperature, vomiting, and diarrhea (Smith, 1981).

The adult usually perceives an initial desire to empty the urinary bladder when about 150 mL of urine has accumulated there. However, the bladder can distend to a much larger capacity, and it often does before there is a feeling of bladder fullness. Since urine accumulates gradually in the bladder, the slow distention of the muscular sac accommodates larger and larger quantities of urine. The capacity of the urinary bladder has been calculated at 450 mL, but much larger amounts may accumulate if there is obstruction to outflow (Smith, 1981).

Micturition involves a number of responses that occur almost simultaneously. Initially, there is the felt need to void and an assessment of the environment. The individual must determine that the environment is appropriate to the release of urine, or urination will be prevented.

After the person has determined that conditions are satisfactory, a series of nerve impulses are activated to allow the release of urine. First, the muscles of the pelvic floor are relaxed, which relaxes the urethral opening and allows the descent of the urinary bladder. Next, the trigone contracts, which ensures closure of the ureterovesical junction and prevents the reflux of urine into the ureters. Trigonal contraction also causes contraction of the bladder neck, which makes the bladder more funnel shaped. Finally, the detrusor muscle of the bladder, which is continuous with the urethral lining, contracts. Detrusor contraction increases the pressure within the bladder and results in bladder emptying (Smith, 1981).

The cerebral control mechanism can interrupt the voiding process at any point identified as appropriate. When the bladder is empty, the detrusor muscle relaxes, the bladder neck closes, the trigone assumes its normal tone, and the perineal muscles resume their normal tone.

Section II: Pathophysiological Influences and Effects

Alterations in urine formation and excretion have profound effects on homeostasis. Failure to maintain the chemical balance of the fluids of the various fluid compartments will result in death unless the balance is restored. Manifestations of alterations in urine formation and excretion may include changes in the clearance rates of substances, changes in the amount and composition of the urine and the pattern of its excretion, elevated blood pressure, decreased maturation of red blood cells, and changes in the excretion of metabolic waste products. Pathophysiological changes commonly seen in urinary dysfunction are discussed below. Chapter 33 will present special influences and effects of specific illnesses.

ENLARGEMENT OF THE KIDNEYS AND RELATED STRUCTURES

Enlargement of one or both kidneys is most commonly related to the invasion and multiplication of neoplastic cells. If a mass becomes very large, it can put pressure on abdominal nerves or displace other abdominal organs and cause discomfort or pain.

The kidneys may also become enlarged because of a blockage of the ureters, and occasionally the urethra, by either a stone, tumor, or enlargement of the prostate. In these instances, urine backs up into the renal pelvis, causing the enlargement. The ureters and urethra also may enlarge in diameter as they fill with urine that cannot be voided because of an obstruction. If the urethra is blocked or nerve intervention is interrupted, the bladder also can become overdistended with urine.

ATROPHY OF THE KIDNEY

In most chronic diseases of the kidneys, the kidneys eventually atrophy because of the destruction of the renal parenchyma. In some instances, the cortex is most affected, whereas in others, the medulla is most affected. The kidneys often shrink to less than one-fifth of their normal size.

ALTERATIONS IN FLUID VOLUME

A major goal of renal function is the maintenance of fluid volume to ensure that metabolic and perfusion processes occur. With renal dysfunction, the inability to control fluid volume may have a variety of sequelae. For example, a loss of the ability of the kidneys to concentrate urine may be the earliest observation of renal pathology. Continuous loss of dilute urine in turn may result in volume depletion and thus low blood pressure. *Hypovolemia,* or inadequate circulating blood volume, will eventually alter renal function, because adequate blood volume is required to establish a pressure gradient so that glomerular filtration can occur.

Although the kidneys have the capacity for some autoregulation of blood flow, they also will deprive the renal parenchyma of necessary blood volume if the organism demands are greater elsewhere. This capacity to limit severely renal blood flow to supply the heart or skeletal muscles is observed in severe shock or stress states. Fluid deficits can also occur with abnormal decreases in the ingestion of water or excessive water losses from diarrhea, vomiting, or rapid dehydration.

Failure of the kidneys to excrete water and thus maintain normal fluid volume also has serious consequences for the overall functioning of the body. *Hypervolemia,* an increase in circulating and total body water, puts severe strain upon the cardiovascular system. Hypervolemia manifests itself in the elevation of blood pressure, increased cardiac workload, and the development of fluid in the interstitial spaces and alveoli of the lungs or other body tissues. Hypertension will cause long-term problems related to ventricular hypertrophy and increased peripheral vascular resistance. More immediate changes that are due to fluid shifts, particularly into the lungs, will impair adequate diffusion of gases and can cause severe hypoxia.

The response to ischemia of any renal tissue is the liberation of renin and the stimulation of the renin–angiotensin–aldosterone system. The release of renin is triggered to increase renal blood flow in response to hormonal mechanisms, but it is also associated with increased volume retention and volume expansion. Particularly, this can happen in kidney tissue damage that affects the normal formation of urine, but aldosterone and ADH are being produced normally. Therefore, overhydration is more common as the client reaches end-stage renal disease.

ELECTROLYTE IMBALANCES

Failure of the kidneys to regulate the internal milieu has major metabolic effects. The kidneys, in conjunction with various endocrine mechanisms, control the appropriate balance of electrolytes in body fluids. Excesses and deficits of various electrolytes result in serious problems in the maintenance of normal nerve transmission and muscle conduction. The kidneys also maintain the normal osmolality of body fluids. Sodium, potassium, calcium, and magnesium are the major cations under the regulation of the kidneys. The anions such as chloride and bicarbonate, as well as other anions such as sulfates, phosphates, and proteinate, are also under renal direction. Electrolyte imbalance is discussed in Chapter 5.

Of the various electrolytes, potassium—the primary intracellular cation—has the most potential for causing death. Failure of the kidneys to excrete potassium will disturb the conduction system of the heart and, if untreated, will terminate myocardial contraction. *Hyperkalemia is* the most frequently encountered imbalance in chronic renal failure. The kidney tubules also may fail to conserve potassium correctly and thus excrete large amounts. *Hypokalemia* may also result in altered cardiac muscular contraction. Hypokalemia will also alter the medullary interstitium of the kidney and impair renal function.

Sodium excesses *(hypernatremia)* can occur in clients with end-stage renal disease when urine volume drops to very low levels. In these cases, even a restricted salt intake results in sodium and water retention with edema and pump failure. Since sodium conservation occurs primarily in the renal medulla, deterioration of this area produces excessive sodium loss, or *hyponatremia,* which leads to decreased extracellular fluid. As the circulating blood volume decreases, the glomerular filtration rate decreases, and renal function is further compromised.

Imbalances of calcium and phosphorus are related to the reciprocal relationship between the electrolytes and the effect of parathormone, which regulates serum calcium levels. When the glomerular filtration rate decreases to around 30 mL/min, the renal excretion of phosphate also decreases (Rose, 1981). With increases in the serum phosphate level *(hyperphosphatemia),* the body attempts to lower the phosphate level through binding phosphate with calcium. The resultant calcium phosphate ($CaPO^4$) may then precipitate in various tissues. However, the body's response to hyperphosphatemia causes the calcium level (nonprotein bound or ionized) to decrease. *Hypocalcemia* (decreased serum calcium level) occurs because calcium is bound to phosphate. In response to the low calcium level, the parathyroid glands release parathormone. Parathormone stimulates the release of calcium from stores in bone in an attempt to increase the circulating calcium level in the serum. In renal insufficiency, a second problem exists: The kidney is unable to produce 1,25-dihydroxycholecalciferol, the active component of vitamin D, which is necessary for the intestinal absorption and utilization of calcium in the diet. Without it, calcium cannot be utilized. This further contributes to the development of hypocalcemia.

The ongoing process of hyperphosphatemia and hypocalcemia with subsequent production of parathormone results in secondary hyperparathyroidism. Untreated, this leads to serious bone pathology known as *renal osteodystrophy* (discussed later in this chapter).

When urine output is low and a normal magnesium intake continues, *hypermagnesemia* can occur. It may also be aggravated by the administration of magnesium-containing laxatives and antacids.

METABOLIC ACIDOSIS

The kidneys are responsible for excreting the acids produced by the metabolism of amino acids. The excretion of hydrogen ions by the kidneys, or the metabolic pathway, is accomplished by the conservation of bicarbonate, the secretion of ammonia, and the excretion of hydrogen in exchange for sodium. The kidneys work with the blood buffers and the pulmonary system to maintain a normal pH

of the blood of 7.35 to 7.45. Blood buffers maintain this narrow range of acceptability; they almost instantaneously convert acids for either pulmonary excretion as carbon dioxide or for renal excretion through the conservation of bicarbonate or the exchange of sodium or potassium for hydrogen.

Without the renal regulation of hydrogen ion excretion, a diminished amount of bicarbonate is available to buffer the fixed acids. In addition, the ability to excrete hydrogen as ammonia or with phosphoric acid is limited. Thus, unless the pulmonary reserve compensates, the pH will fall, and metabolic acidosis will result. (See also Unit 3.)

IMPAIRMENT OF GAS EXCHANGE

Several factors related to renal failure cause impaired gas exchange. The problems of fluid overload previously discussed cause pulmonary edema, ventricular hypertrophy, and hypertension, which can lead to impaired gas exchange in the lungs and at the cellular level. Potassium imbalances can cause cardiac arrhythmias, which also can lead to impaired gas exchange. The lungs of a client in metabolic acidosis have to work hard to correct the acidosis; if they are not able to do so, gas exchange is again impaired. Anemia results from a decrease in erythropoietin produced by the kidney, and this deficiency of erythrocytes makes gas exchange more difficult. Furthermore, clients encounter bleeding problems as a result of decreased aggregation ability from a defect in platelet factor III.

IMPAIRMENT OF ANTI-INFECTIOUS FUNCTIONS

Clients with impaired renal function have an increased number of infections as a result of impaired immune responses. They also may have delayed hypersensitivity to antigens.

ACCUMULATION OF UREMIC TOXINS

The kidneys remove nitrogenous waste products derived from protein metabolism. The kidneys must continually filter and excrete creatinine and urea nitrogen, whether it is from endogenous protein sources (such as the metabolism of the amine creatinine in skeletal muscle) or from primarily exogenous sources (such as dietary protein).

Azotemia is the accumulation of uremic toxins (urea, uric acid, and creatinine) in the blood. **Uremia** refers to azotemia with clinical symptoms. The accumulation of uremic toxins in renal failure can result in neurological complications, gastrointestinal bleeding, and skin changes resulting from urochrome pigments deposited in the skin. This pigmentation, combined with anemia, results in the pale yellow-gray color characteristic of clients with renal failure. Pruritus, also common, is thought to be the result of a buildup of the urochrome pigments in the skin as well as the crust of urate crystals that accumulates on the skin (called **uremic frost** because it is similar in appearance to frost on a window on a cold morning). Recent theories cite increased parathormone production as a possible cause of pruritus.

The accumulation of uremic toxins also causes neurological changes that range from fatigue, decreased ability to concentrate, irritability, and insomnia to depression, peripheral neuropathy, and retinopathy. Coma, convulsions, and death can occur if the toxins are not removed.

ALTERATIONS IN NUTRITION-RELATED FUNCTIONS

Uremic toxins and gastrointestinal bleeding cause nutrition-related problems. The gastrointestinal tract becomes inflamed and irritated because of the uremic toxins. This results in loss of appetite, nausea, vomiting, and diarrhea—problems that further complicate fluid and electrolyte imbalances. The irritability of the gastrointestinal tract, compounded by altered platelet function, causes the

gastrointestinal bleeding so common in clients with impaired kidney function. The buildup of ammonia in the body results in a characteristic **uremic fetor**—a urinelike odor of the client's breath accompanied by a bad taste in the mouth (described by some as metallic)—which greatly alters the appeal of food. Associated pancreatitis may also impair digestion.

ALTERATIONS IN URINE OUTPUT

Urine output may greatly increase in certain situations, such as in the diuretic phase of acute renal failure. However, a decreased urine output is the more common alteration. This may be temporary, as with the oliguric phase of acute renal failure, benign prostatic hyperplasia, or kidney stone obstruction of the urethra, or it may be a longterm sequela common with acute tubular necrosis and chronic renal failure. Alterations in the pattern of urination result from the underlying pathological conditions. Alterations, their definitions, and related medical problems are discussed in Chapter 32.

Section III: Related System Influences and Effects

Since the kidneys and urinary system perform multiple functions related to the performance of many body systems, impairment of renal function can affect other body systems to varying extents.

INTEGUMENTARY SYSTEM

Dry, pale, yellow-gray skin is characteristic of renal failure. Nails and hair are also brittle and dry. Increased parathormone secretion, uremic frost, and urochrome pigments cause pruritus, which may become so severe that clients scratch until they bleed. This break in skin integrity increases the client's susceptibility to infection. (Pruritus and the itch-scratch cycle are discussed in Unit Thirteen.) Edema from sodium and water retention, as well as poor nutritional status, can also make the skin highly susceptible to breakdown. Decubitus ulcers may form within hours if clients are not frequently repositioned.

CARDIOVASCULAR SYSTEM

The cardiovascular complications that may occur after a loss of renal function and the resulting uremia include pericarditis, accelerated atherosclerosis, fluid overload, anemia, and the potential for arrhythmias because of potassium abnormalities.

Uremic pericarditis is fairly common for clients with end-stage renal disease. Although this condition usually develops within 12 months of the initiation of dialysis, a later onset has certainly been observed. The cause of this inflammatory response is believed to be related to nitro-

genous waste products not removed by dialysis (Rose, 1981). Fluid accumulates within the pericardial sac, called a *pericardial effusion*. With increased membrane irritability and the platelet aggregation problems that occur in the uremic environment, the effusion may be serosanguineous. Massive pericardial effusions (greater than 2000 mL) may accumulate over a period of days to weeks, seriously altering cardiovascular hemodynamics. *Cardiac tamponade* (compression of the heart from excessive fluid in the pericardial sac) will result in death unless medical intervention, surgical intervention, or both relieve the fluid accumulation.

Accelerated atherosclerotic processes have been observed in clients with chronic renal failure. An increased incidence of death from coronary artery disease seems to be associated with the effects of chronic essential hypertension, ventricular hypertrophy, and possible alterations in lipid metabolism associated with uremia (Rose, 1981). In addition, diffuse atherosclerotic processes that include cerebral, aortic, and peripheral vessels are not uncommon. Clients with these conditions frequently develop renal failure as a result of chronic glomerulonephritis, nephrosclerosis, renal artery stenotic lesions, or atheromatous embolization.

Uncontrolled hypertension, either from volume or hormonal response, greatly increases peripheral vascular resistance in small blood vessels throughout the body. The loss of elasticity of the arterioles in the kidney as well as other organs, such as the retina of the eye and the small vessel circulation of the brain, will seriously affect the long-term functioning of those organs. The problems of fluid overload, anemia, and the potential for potassium abnormalities have been previously discussed.

RESPIRATORY SYSTEM

The interrelation of the renal and respiratory systems is important in maintaining an acid–base balance in the long-term management of the client with renal failure. Although this balance is partially restored by medication and control of diet, these conservative measures can accomplish only so much. Dialysis may assist, but the lungs must help to control this narrow range of imbalance minute to minute. Clients with obstructive lung disease have carbon dioxide retention with respiratory acidosis. Thus, when renal and respiratory diseases exist simultaneously, the ability to combat metabolic acidosis is severely impaired because of the already present respiratory acidosis. Gas exchange is further hampered by pulmonary edema and anemia states.

NEUROLOGICAL SYSTEM

The neurological manifestations of uremia include a generally described *uremic encephalopathy* and peripheral neuropathy associated with azotemia and metabolic acidosis. Uremic encephalopathy (the development of altered mentation and intellectual processes, speech manifestations, and the presence of tremors and myoclonus) is characteristically associated with the onset of uremic manifestations. **Asterixis**, a flapping tremor of the hands (described in Chapter 32), is an early manifestation of increased irritability of the central nervous system from elevated serum ammonia levels. This symptom is important, since grand mal seizures may develop if the encephalopathic process is not corrected.

Peripheral neuropathies are common in the client with end-stage renal disease who requires chronic dialysis. These neuropathies are neither clearly understood nor easily treated. Their improvement with dialysis is uncertain, and leg weakness and difficulty with ambulation and maintenance of comfort are problems. Transplantation offers more hope for the relief of these symptoms.

MUSCULOSKELETAL SYSTEM

Musculoskeletal manifestations of renal failure are collectively referred to as **renal osteodystrophy**. A variety of problems, including osteomalacia, osteoporosis, and osteitis fibrosa cystica, may result from the chronic stimulation for release of parathormone because of elevated phosphorous levels and decreased calcium levels in the serum. Bone pain, increased tendencies for fractures, and metastatic calcifications throughout the body result from this chronic imbalance.

HEMATOPOIETIC SYSTEM

Hematologic effects of uremia include a chronic anemia and disorder of platelet aggregation. Each of these alterations can have a variety of effects on the client who has lost kidney function. Clients with renal failure have a chronic normochromic, normocytic anemia. Hematocrit values fall to 20% to 30%, and hemoglobin values drop to 7 to 8 g/dL. The result of the anemia is chronic fatigue. Clients respond differently, however, and some adjust reasonably well. For clients with coronary artery disease, decreased circulating red blood cell mass may exacerbate anginal attacks or increase tendencies to develop arrhythmias, particularly if hypoxia occurs.

Platelet dysfunction is usually described as a problem with platelet aggregation. The platelet count is normal, and there is no alteration in the ability to produce platelets. In the uremic environment, however, the platelets do not promote the clotting mechanism as well. The results of other clotting tests are normal (eg, the prothrombin time and the partial thromboplastin time). However, bleeding time may be prolonged (Rose, 1981). Impaired platelet function in the uremic environment is believed to be responsible for the frequent and easily induced bleeding into the skin and mucous membranes of the client with either acute or chronic renal failure. Irritations to mucous membranes, particularly of the gastrointestinal tract, along with the frequent presence of occult blood detectable through a variety of methods, supports the evidence that a uremic environment persists in spite of dialytic therapy.

GASTROINTESTINAL SYSTEM

Uremia profoundly affects the gastrointestinal system. Anorexia, nausea, and vomiting are generally the most annoying and uncomfortable symptoms. The inability to eat or to retain food results in loss of weight and a breakdown of muscle and fat. Uncorrected, profound debilitation

Nursing Research Note

Numan I, Barklind K, Lubin B: Correlates of depression in chronic dialysis patients: Morbidity and mortality. *Res Nurs Health* 1981; 4:295–297.

The authors studied the mortality and morbidity rates related to depression in a population of end-stage renal disease (ESRD) outpatients. Using a sample of 74 ESRD outpatients, depression scores were obtained using the Depression Adjective Check List (DACL).

Clients with high scores on the DACL, indicating depression, had the highest number of hospital admissions in 1 year. These results were statistically significant.

Clients who died during that period also had higher scores on the depression list. Again, this was statistically significant. These findings indicate that depression is associated with higher morbidity and mortality rates.

Nurses must carefully assess clients for evidence of depression; early detection is essential. When depression is diagnosed, counseling may help reduce morbidity and mortality.

results, because the client is less able to combat infections and make appropriate immune responses.

The effects of uremia may be observed throughout the gastrointestinal system. As has been described, the client will notice a bad taste in the mouth (described by some as metallic) and a urinelike odor to the breath. Alteration in taste sensation, known as *hypogeusia*, involves both loss of acuity and loss of ability to discriminate tastes. Thus, with significant changes in the ability to taste foods, eating is less pleasurable.

Parotitis, gastritis, pancreatitis, and colitis may occur at varying stages in the development of uremia. The parotid glands may become infected and cause much discomfort. Irritation of the gastric and intestinal mucosa often is accompanied by vague discomfort, nausea, vomiting, eructation, and diarrhea. Bleeding from the mucous membrane lining the gastrointestinal tract is common because platelet abnormalities alter the clotting mechanism. The bleeding generally is occult, but gross bleeding with severe gastritis is also common.

REPRODUCTIVE SYSTEM

The loss of renal function and the development of uremia also affect the reproductive systems of both men and women. Both experience a loss of libido, and men frequently become impotent. Fertility is affected as well: Men have lower testosterone levels and a decrease in sperm formation, whereas women ovulate and menstruate less often, if at all. Successfully carrying a pregnancy to term is rare (Rose, 1981).

Section IV: Psychosocial/Lifestyle Influences and Effects

The urinary system both influences and is influenced by psychosocial factors. This section discusses factors having a generalized effect. Factors related to specific disorders or therapies are discussed in subsequent chapters.

SEX

Sex influences the structure of the urinary system in an important way. As has been discussed, because the urethra is shorter in women, they are more prone to cystitis (bladder infection) than men. Stress urinary incontinence is not uncommon in women who have experienced relaxation of the pelvic muscles as a result of pregnancy.

DEVELOPMENTAL INFLUENCES

Urination is important in our daily routines. In fact, people who have stopped urinating almost completely because of renal failure frequently describe the absence of this physical act from the habits of a usual day as odd, unusual, and difficult to get used to.

Our society has specific values and attitudes toward the organs associated with the urinary tract, as well as toward urination itself. Most young children learn that control is probably the most important aspect related to urination. Urine should also be delivered into appropriate receptacles, not bedding or clothing.

Associated with this developmental process known as *toilet training* is the use of selected language for reference to urination. "Pee-pee," "number 1," and "making water" are a few terms adults use as they teach their children the proper control of urine and use of the toilet. Adults rarely use the word *urine* themselves. Some may be both unfamiliar and uncomfortable with the correct terminology. The biological terms are more commonly encountered in discussions of the topic with health professionals.

CULTURE

The proximity of the urethral orifices to the genitalia further contributes to the difficulties some people encounter in talking about these areas of the body. Cultural and soci-

Nursing Research Note

Hilbert G: An investigation of the relationship between social support and compliance of hemodialysis patients. *AANNTJ* (April) 1985; 12:133–136.

This study tested the hypothesis that higher levels of social support would be associated with higher levels of compliance in hemodialysis clients. The results indicated that age, income, educational level, and time hospitalized did not significantly affect compliance. Compliance was greatest when support was by directive guidance. Such guidance was given by a significant other and consisted of information and feedback and telling the client what to do.

Compliance was found to be greatest for the medication regimen, followed by fluid restriction, and diet. In addition, length of time on dialysis and compliance were inversely related; as the length of time on dialysis increased, compliance decreased. Clients on hemodialysis for 5 years or longer were less compliant than clients on dialysis for less than 5 years.

Because social support increased compliance to medications, diet, and fluid restriction, nurses may need to assess client support systems when planning care and evaluating compliance. Including supportive individuals in teaching and client care may enhance overall compliance. Nurses can also guide these individuals in how to provide support for the end-stage renal disease client. Actions such as offering information, giving positive feedback, and reminding the client to follow prescribed regimens can be beneficial in overall compliance. Because this research found that compliance declines as time on hemodialysis increases, nurses may need to reassess this group more frequently and more closely for compliance. Re-education may be helpful; including supportive individuals may also help.

etal attitudes toward these "private parts" create a challenge in nursing interventions with clients who have problems associated with the genitourinary system. Identifying the language in which to talk about the problems and creating an accepting emotional environment are the general goals.

Other aspects of sociocultural background and lifestyle also greatly influence people's health care practices. A concern for and awareness of preventive measures during the early years can help people avoid lifelong problems related to kidney and urinary tract function; eg, females should be taught to wipe from front to back. Although routine guidance from health professionals regarding health maintenance is commonly recommended, many people actively avoid doctors and hospitals unless a crisis occurs.

DIETARY HABITS AND MEDICATIONS

Dietary habits also can affect the kidneys and urinary system. For example, a high-salt diet can contribute to the development of hypertension, which can lead to renal disease. For people with diagnosed renal problems, salt and protein restrictions may limit the pleasure of eating. They can avoid certain foods and beverages in their own homes with some discipline, but visiting friends or dining in restaurants presents difficulties that may not be controlled so easily. Many social functions involve sharing food and drink. People who must strictly limit fluid intake may feel pressure to explain why they must avoid fluids. Thus, the altered health state is always a part of life. Participation and sharing are social expectations, and some people prefer to avoid these situations rather than not do what is expected.

Among medications that may have a toxic effect on the kidneys are a number of antibiotics including penicillin, neomycin, kanamycin, and amphotericin. Probably the most nephrotoxic category of antibiotics, however, is the aminoglycosides (gentamicin, tobramycin). Other nephrotoxic drugs include the sulfonamides, salicylates, thiazides, and furosemide.

ECONOMIC FACTORS

The costs of renal dialysis and transplantation are high. Although the government pays for most of the costs, minor expenses add up to thousands of dollars. Moreover, a loss of income may result if the client is a wage earner.

OCCUPATION AND AVOCATION

Exposure to nephrotoxic chemicals may be related to occupation or hobbies. Carbon tetrachloride, used in dry cleaning and various industrial processes, is nephrotoxic, as are methyl alcohol, phenols, and ethylene glycol. Several metals used in the fabrication of jewelry and some electronic components are nephrotoxic, including gold, lead, copper, uranium, arsenic, mercury, and cadmium.

The development of kidney disease may severely influence the client's occupational performance. Jobs that require travel, flexible hours, or physical energy may prove difficult to maintain. The need to change careers or develop new skills, in addition to coping with physical illness, may be an enormous challenge or too much to cope with for the client with kidney disease.

ROLES AND RELATIONSHIPS

For the client with serious kidney dysfunction, as in end-stage renal disease, the psychosocial effects are numerous. Lifestyle, family life, and work commitments usually are interrupted, often in substantial ways. The client usually must make major adjustments in various roles. Stress accompanies the effort to maintain the existing lifestyle in the face of vast uncertainty about the future, and both clients and all those near them are affected (especially spouses and children). Powerlessness, helplessness, and hopelessness are all components of the newly experienced dependency created by renal failure.

SEXUAL EXPRESSION AND REPRODUCTION

Disorders of the urinary system may profoundly affect the expression of sexuality. Surgical procedures such as urinary diversion may require the client to wear an appliance on the abdomen to collect urine, and clients with such appliances may be reluctant to participate in sexual activity. They and their partners may find it necessary to alter their sexual behaviors to accommodate the appliance, a catheter, or a dialysis fistula. Clients and their sexual partners may have to discuss and experiment with alternate positions for sexual intercourse, and intercourse may be somewhat unpleasant or even uncomfortable or painful.

The client's reproductive ability may also be altered. For example, certain surgical procedures (such as radical cystectomy in men) may cause impotence. Because hormone levels are not regulated in the presence of chronic renal failure, many female clients have amenorrhea and are unlikely to become pregnant. In men, low testosterone levels and decreased sperm formation significantly reduce the ability to fertilize an ovum. Active prevention of pregnancy in women receiving dialysis is indicated for a number of reasons. For one, pregnancy increases the circulating blood volume. In addition, the low hemoglobin values of most chronic renal failure clients are inadequate to support a healthy fetus. Attempting to have a baby while on dialysis can be harmful to both mother and fetus.

If the renal problem is genetically transmitted, as in polycystic kidney disease, reproduction may be discouraged.

BODY IMAGE AND SELF-CONCEPT

Because where and how we urinate is essentially culturally prescribed, it is intimately linked to our view of ourselves and to our self-concept. A person faced with the problem of disposing of a plastic bag full of urine, or who finds that passing flatus means that urine is likely to leak over the body or clothing, may feel dirty and out of control of basic body functions. The person may also worry about being offensive to others because of odor.

To conceal urinary diversion appliances or drainage tubes, a client may find the choice of clothing limited to nonrestrictive and comfortable styles. Not being able to wear a preferred style of clothing—in other words, sacrificing fashion for comfort—may provoke anxiety in peo-

ple who highly value being fashionable. Being unclothed and seen in the nude may also cause great discomfort to the client concerned about body changes.

The client with a transplanted kidney may have to deal with concerns about having another person's organ within his or her own body. The knowledge that a related donor has sacrificed a healthy kidney for the client's benefit may become a burden of guilt. The guilt may be increased if the donor kidney is rejected by the client's body.

Chapter Highlights

The nephron is the functional unit of the renal parenchyma, and each kidney has over 1 million nephrons.

Glomerular filtration, tubular reabsorption, and tubular secretion are the processes that remove nitrogenous waste and maintain electrolyte and acid–base balances.

The glomerular filtration rate requires adequate intravascular volume and hydrostatic pressure to effect the clearance of creatinine and urea nitrogen.

Tubular reabsorption moves water and electrolytes from tubular filtrate into the plasma.

Tubular secretion regulates potassium and hydrogen ion levels.

Blood pressure may be described as either volume or renin dependent.

Erythropoietin production by the kidneys is necessary for the production of red blood cells in the bone marrow and spleen.

Insulin breakdown and excretion are partially a renal mechanism.

Control of micturition is voluntary as long as motor and sensory nerve pathways are intact.

The inability of the kidneys to excrete phosphate and

produce 1,25-dihydroxycholecalciferol, the active form of vitamin D, results in hypocalcemia and secondary hyperparathyroidism.

The failure to excrete nitrogenous waste products and middle molecules creates the uremic environment.

Uremia, or azotemia with clinical symptoms, affects all body systems.

The major uremic symptoms affect the gastrointestinal system (anorexia, nausea, and vomiting), the neurological system (muscle cramps, lethargy, and inability to concentrate), and the integumentary system (severe pruritus).

Hypervolemia in renal failure may result in hypertension and peripheral or pulmonary edema.

Developmental and psychosocial forces are influential in the formation of attitudes and values about urination.

The proximity of urinary system organs to the organs of reproduction and sexuality influences the adult client's attitude toward urinary system dysfunction.

Dysfunction in the urinary system may affect the client's modes of sexual expression and may limit reproductive ability.

Changes in the urinary system may alter the client's body image and self-concept.

Bibliography

Guyton AC: *Textbook of Medical Physiology,* 6th ed. Philadelphia: Saunders, 1981.

Nasjletti A, Malik KU: Interrelationships among prostaglandins and vasoactive substances. *Med Clin North Am* 1981; 65(4):881.

O'Brien ME: *The Courage to Survive.* New York: Grune and Stratton, 1983.

Pickering L, Robbins D: Fluid, electrolyte, and acid–base balance in the renal patient. *Nurs Clin North Am* 1980; 15(3):577–592.

Rose BR: *Pathophysiology of Renal Disease.* New York: McGraw-Hill, 1981.

Schrier RW: *Renal and Electrolyte Disorders.* Boston: Little, Brown, 1980.

Smith DR: *General Urology.* Los Altos, CA: Lange, 1981.

Spence AP, Mason EB: *Human Anatomy and Physiology,* 2nd ed. Menlo Park, CA: Addison-Wesley, 1983.

Suggested Readings

Artinian BM: Role identities of the dialysis patient. *Nephrology Nurse,* 1983, pp 10–14. This research study reports on five role identities assumed by dialysis clients: the worker role, the waiter role, the emancipated role, the undecided role, and the true dialysis client role. Nursing interventions for each role identity are suggested.

Orr ML: Cost containment and patient choice in the end-stage renal disease program. *AANNT J* 1982; 9(Dec):11–15. A discussion of the costs of various alternatives for ESRD clients, how costs can be curtailed, and the importance of client choice in program participation.

Symposium on chronic renal disease. *Nurs Clin North Am* 1981; 16(3). [Entire issue.] Several articles by various authors on the topic of chronic renal failure.

Taylor DL: Renal hypertension: Physiology, signs and symptoms. *Nurs 83* 1983; 13(10):44–45. Brief article with illustrations that discusses the physiology and signs and symptoms associated with renal hypertension.

Chapter 32

The Nursing Process for Clients With Kidney and Urinary Dysfunction

Jane Hokanson Hawks
Jeanette K. Chambers

Objectives

When you have finished studying this chapter, you should be able to:

Discuss the significant subjective data to be obtained from a client with alterations in the pattern of urination.

Describe the objective data collected when assessing the client with urinary system dysfunction.

List the diagnostic tests used to assess renal function and discuss the nursing implications for each test.

Discuss nursing diagnoses and their applications to the client with problems of renal function or urinary flow.

Discuss the plans of care and expected outcomes for each nursing diagnosis listed for the client with kidney and urinary tract disorders.

Identify the causes of prerenal, renal, and postrenal acute renal failure.

Describe the four phases of acute renal failure.

Describe the three stages of chronic renal failure.

Define the principles of dialysis.

Identify and define the various types of dialysis.

Discuss nursing interventions for hemodialysis and peritoneal dialysis.

The nursing process with problems of the kidneys and urinary tract encompasses a wide range of assessments and interventions. This chapter discusses nursing responsibilities generally applicable to kidney and urinary system dysfunction. Chapters 33 and 34 discuss nursing measures applicable to specific disorders and surgical approaches.

Section I: Nursing Assessment: Establishing the Data Base

SUBJECTIVE DATA

Consideration of the client's normal pattern of urination and the discussion of changes in this pattern involve questioning the client about the urinary volume, timing characteristics, micturition control, and appearance of urine. Clients often experience anxiety in discussing this aspect of their daily activities. Urination is a culturally established act performed in privacy. Language referring to the process frequently involves colloquial expressions or terminology unique to a particular family or group, and medical or biological terms may not be familiar to the client. Thus, communication about the exact nature of the problem may be difficult. In addition, the proximity of the urinary tract to the organs of sexual functioning may cause further embarrassment or anxiety during the assessment process. The nurse's calm, confident approach to the interview and examination may make the client more comfortable.

The nurse should question the client about any changes in micturition. What color is the urine? Is there pain with urination? Does the client have frequency, urgency, or hesitancy with voiding? Are there problems with incontinence? Does the client void excessive amounts? Only a little? At night? These questions will elicit information about the various alterations in micturition discussed in Table 32–1), and this information will provide clues to the client's underlying problem.

Are there changes in the color of urine? Changes in the urine's appearance may have caused the client to seek medical advice. Hematuria may be a serious sign because it may indicate cancer of the urinary system. It also may be related to anticoagulant therapy, excessive exercise, infection, or trauma. If the urine is alkaline, clients may describe their urine as being bright red or coffee colored. If the urine is acidic, blood gives the urine a cloudy or smoky appearance. Cloudy urine, however, is usually related to pus in the urine (pyuria). In severe pyuria, the urine may be malodorous. Almost colorless urine usually results from excessive fluid intake, chronic renal disease, diabetes insipidus, or diabetes mellitus. Dark yellow-orange urine suggests dehydration or ingestion of medications or foods that discolor the urine. Table 32–2 lists possible color changes of urine and their causes. It is important to know when a change in urine color began and if it is related to other events, is constant, or is intermittent.

Pain is not always present with disorders of the kidneys and urinary tract; it is more common in acute conditions. The client's history must include descriptions of the character, location, distribution, onset, duration, and frequency of the discomfort. Is it related to voiding? What brings it on? What relieves it?

Pain from within the kidney is described as a dull ache.

In most cases, the pain is always present and not interrupted with position change. The client will point to the **flank** region (the part of the body between the ribs and the ileum) and say the pain also extends into the lower abdomen or the umbilical area (Smith, 1981). Renal colic and ureteral colic cause severe, excruciating pain of sudden onset. The pain, located in the flank area and radiating to the groin, is accompanied by nausea, vomiting, and paralytic ileus (Figure 32–1).

Bladder pain in the suprapubic area is usually the result of bladder spasms, which can be contractions of the detrusor muscle responsible for normal micturition (Smith, 1981). Urgency and burning on urination are also common in clients with cystitis or urethritis (irritation of the urethra). Cystitis may produce burning both during and after urination, whereas urethritis usually causes burning during urination only. Strangury (see Table 32–1) often accompanies severe bladder infection.

Some women with symptoms of burning on urination may actually have a vaginal infection. Ask the client about any signs of vaginal discharge. Has she noted any vaginal or perineal itching or dyspareunia (pain with sexual intercourse)? Pain at the urethral orifice or meatus results from bladder neck irritation or trauma, or infection of the urethra. Scrotal pain is attributed to inflammation and swelling of the testicle or epididymis. Rectal and perineal fullness and pain suggest prostatitis. Metastasis of prostatic cancer to the pelvis can cause leg and back pain.

Questions regarding micturition frequency, dribbling, hesitancy, and incontinence are important. How many times a day does the client void? Is there trouble initiating the stream or difficulty holding the urine? Does the client get up at night to void? How many times? When did this begin? Stress incontinence is a common problem for women. A weakness can develop in the bladder–urethral sphincter mechanism through the stretching of pelvic muscles during childbirth or the pressure of the uterus on the bladder during pregnancy. In the elderly (especially those who have had babies), relaxation of pelvic musculature also contributes to the incontinence. Frequent catheterizations and the use of forceps during delivery increase the chances for development of stress incontinence. When questioned, many women state that they have to wear sanitary pads, adult diapers, or even plastic pants at all times to prevent embarrassment.

Does the client maintain an adequate fluid intake (1500 to 2000 mL a day) to help prevent urinary tract infections (UTIs) and renal calculi? Does the client have an excessive intake of milk and vitamin D, which could lead to hypercalciuria? What are the client's exercise habits? Proteinuria, hematuria, or both can be a normal finding in people who exercise excessively. Immobility because of a frac-

Table 32–1   Altered Patterns of Micturition

Pattern	Definition	Related Disorder
Hematuria	Red blood cells in urine; smoky or cloudy appearance if urine is acid or red appearance if urine is alkaline	Cancer, trauma, excessive exercise, anticoagulant therapy
Pyuria	Pus in urine; cloudy appearance of urine	Infection
Polyuria	Large amounts of urine voided at one time, with the total 24-h volume exceeding 3000 mL	Diabetes mellitus, diabetes insipidus, chronic renal disorders, excessive fluid intake, use of diuretics
Oliguria	Small volume of urine output (100–400 mL/24 h)	Shock, trauma, blood transfusion reaction, poisoning, acute and chronic renal failure, decreased renal perfusion or ischemia
Anuria	Urine output less than 100 mL/24 h	Same as for oliguria; more common in acute cortical necrosis and complete obstruction of urinary tract
Dysuria	Painful or difficult voiding	Many causes (broad term)
Urgency	Strong desire or need to void	Prostatitis in men, cystitis, urethritis
Strangury	Slow and painful voiding of small amounts of urine; possible presence of blood	Cystitis
Burning on urination	Burning pain that can occur during or after urination	Urethritis, cystitis, vaginal infection in women, venereal disease
Frequency	Increase in number of voidings per day or frequent voiding of small amounts of urine	Anxiety, stress
Hesitancy	Delay and difficulty in initiating urination	Prostatic enlargement, neurogenic bladder, compression of the urethra, outlet obstruction
Dribbling	Incomplete urination	Prostatic enlargement, prostatic surgery
Incontinence	Involuntary loss of urine from the bladder	Neurogenic disease (see specific definitions below)
Overflow incontinence	Incontinence that occurs when the bladder is distended but outflow of urine is obstructed	Renal calculi, prostatic hypertrophy, neoplasms, blood clot at internal urethral orifice
Urgency incontinence	Strong urge to pass urine that overrides cerebral control of urine passage	Voiding delayed for a long time
Enuresis	Loss of urine during sleep	Psychological origin, obstructive disease process
Stress incontinence	Intermittent, involuntary leakage of urine, usually initiated by coughing, lifting, laughing, or sneezing	Weakness of bladder–urethral sphincters related to aging, pregnancy, multiple deliveries, frequent catheterizations
Nocturia	Awakening to void two or more times per night	Decreased bladder capacity as in pregnancy or in presence of a tumor, bladder irritability, kidney disease, heart disease
Pneumaturia	Passage of gas with urine while voiding	Surgery for cancer in pelvic area; bowel problems such as ulcerative colitis or regional enteritis, in which fistulas develop between GU and GI tracts

ture, thrombophlebitis, or surgery can predispose the client to the development of renal calculi.

A medication history is essential, because many drugs can damage the kidney. Has the client taken any prescrip-tion drugs recently? What OTC (over-the-counter) medications does the client routinely take? The client also may be exposed to nephrotoxins on the job or with certain hobbies. See Box 32–1 for a list of nephrotoxic substances.

Table 32–2   Color and Appearance of Urine

Appearance	Cause	Appearance	Cause
Almost colorless (very pale greenish yellow)	Alcohol ingestion Chronic kidney disease Diabetes insipidus Diabetes mellitus Large fluid intake Nervousness Severe iron deficiency		Phenolphthalein-containing products such as Ex-Lax (in alkaline urine) Phenindione Phenolsulfonphthalein (PSP) dye (in alkaline urine) Phenytoin sodium (Dilantin) Porphyrin
Yellow	Anisindone (Miradon [in alkaline urine]) Cascara sagrada Food color Nitrofurantoin (Furadantin) Phenacetin (Fiorinal) Phenindione (Hedulin [in alkaline urine]) Quinacrine hydrochloride (Atabrine, Mepacrine) Riboflavin Sulfasalazine (Azulfidine [in alkaline urine])		Pyrvinium pamoate (Povan) Rhubarb, santonin, senna (in alkaline urine) Sulfobromophthalein sodium (Bromsulphalein dye or BSP [in alkaline urine])
		Green or blue-green (often blue mixed with yellow urine)	Amitriptyline hydrochloride (Elavil) Azuresin (Diagnex Blue) Bilirubin-biliverdin Blutene Evans blue Guiacol Indican Indigo-carmine Methocarbamol (Robaxin) Methylene blue *Pseudomonas toxemia* Vitamin B complex Yeast concentrate
Orange	Azo Gantrisin (a combination of sulfisoxazole and phenazopyridine hydrochloride) Bilirubin Carotene Concentrated urine Excess sweating Fever Food color Furazolidone (Furoxone) Nitrofurantoin (Furadantin) Phenazopyridine hydrochloride (Pyridium) Restricted fluid intake Rhubarb, senna, santonin, cascara (in acid urine) Sulfonamides Urobilin in excess	Brown or black	Alkapton bodies (homogentisic acid) Bilirubin-biliverdin Cascara Chloroquine hydrochloride (Aralen) Iron compounds (injectable) Lysol poisoning Melanin Methemoglobin Phenol Porphyrin
Pink, red, or reddish orange	Azo Gantrisin Beets Cascara (in alkaline urine) Chlorpromazine hydrochloride (Thorazine) Chromogenic bacteria *(Serratia marcescens)* Danthron (Modane) Emodine (in alkaline urine) Food color Hemoglobin Methemoglobin Myoglobin	Cloudy	Bacteria Calculi "gravel" Clumps, pus, tissue Fecal contamination Leukocytes Mucin, mucus threads Phosphates, carbonates Prostatic fluid Red cells (smoky) Spermatozoa Urates, uric acid
		Milky	Fat (lipuria, opalescent; chyluria, milky) Pyuria

Adapted from Byrne CJ et al: *Laboratory Tests: Implications for Nursing Care,* 2nd ed. Menlo Park, CA: Addison-Wesley, 1986, p 8.

The client's health history may be significant. Has the client ever had problems that could lead to nephropathy, such as frequent streptococcal infections, recurrent UTIs, renal calculi, hyperuricemia (as occurs in gout), or hypercalcemia (as occurs in hyperparathyroidism, sarcoidosis, or metastatic bone disease)? Has the client ever had an indwelling catheter, cystoscopy, or x-rays of the renal system? Is there a history of trauma?

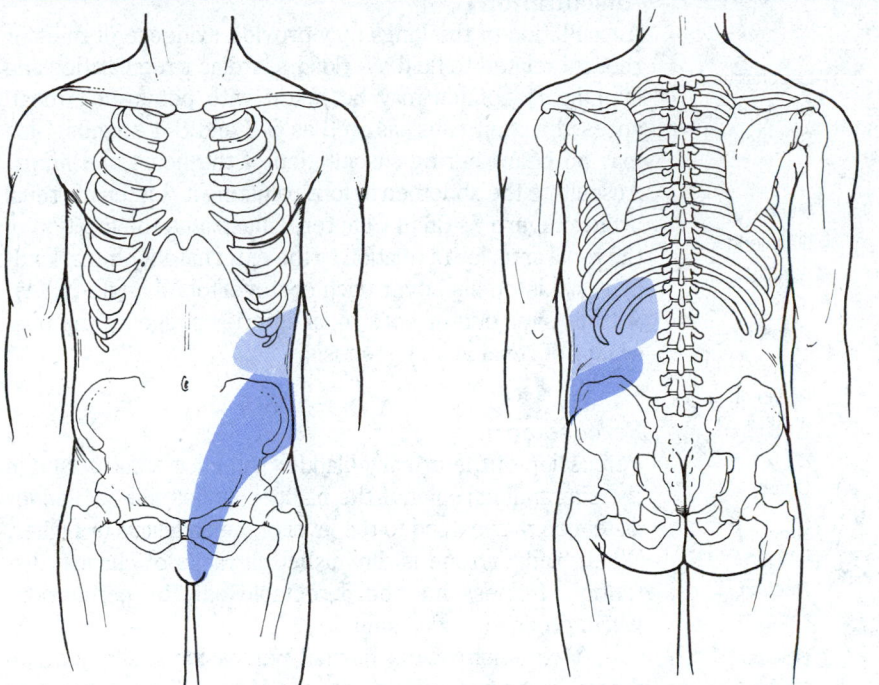

Figure 32–1

Referred pain from kidney (lightly shaded areas) and ureter (darker shaded areas).

Is there a family history of any congenital disorders such as polycystic kidney or congenital malformations of the urinary tract? A strong family history of diseases such as diabetes mellitus or hypertension is also significant because these diseases tend to run in families and can cause renal problems.

Because of common autonomic and sensory nervous system innervation between the gastrointestinal and urinary tracts, as well as the anatomic proximity of the organs of the two systems, gastrointestinal symptoms often accompany urinary system and kidney conditions (Figure 32–2). Some of these symptoms are nausea, vomiting, diarrhea, abdominal pain, hemorrhage of the gastrointes-

tinal system, and paralytic ileus. Conversely, urinary symptoms may accompany gastrointestinal conditions.

OBJECTIVE DATA

Physical Assessment

Objective data are obtained in the physical assessment of the client through inspection, auscultation, percussion, and palpation. Objective data are also obtained through a variety of diagnostic studies. The physical assessment skills and diagnostic studies specific to the kidneys and the urinary system are discussed below; general information has been discussed in Chapter 7.

Inspection

The first stage of data collection is inspection of the client. Examination of the skin is important; uremic clients have a characteristic ashen, yellow skin coloring, and uremic frost may be visible. The eyes of uremic clients are often sunken and give the client a wasted appearance that is exaggerated with muscle wasting and edema. The edema associated with renal failure is generalized rather than dependent. Bruises are common.

The integument also provides clues to renal involvement in clients not yet diagnosed as having urinary system problems. In a hypernatremic state, the skin is dry and flushed, and the body temperature is elevated. Examination of the mucous membranes of the nose and mouth is

---

Box 32–1 Nephrotoxic Substances

Phenacetin* (usually combined with aspirin)

Some antibiotics (especially the aminoglycosides)

Nonsteroidal anti-inflammatory agents (ibuprofen and fenoprofen)

Anesthetics (methoxyflurane)

Radiographic contrast media

Carbon tetrachloride

Lead

Cadmium

*Although this product is no longer available, clients may experience problems related to past use.

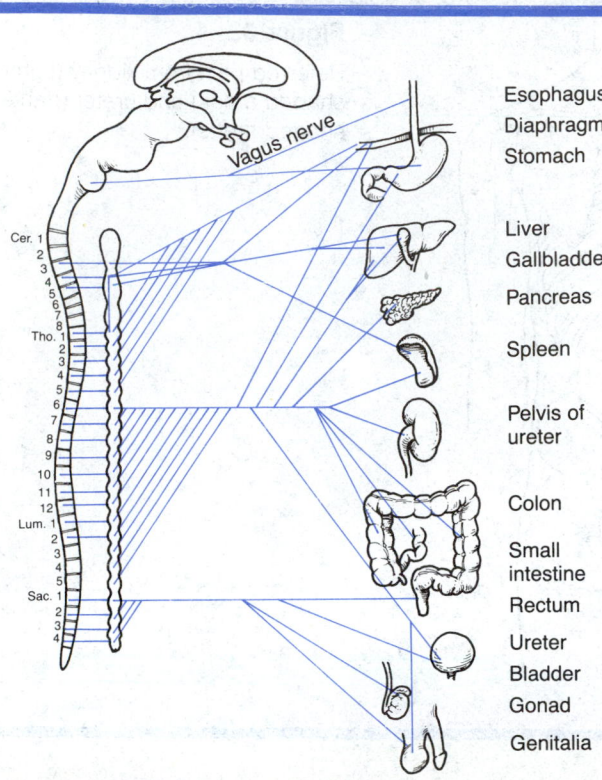

Figure 32–2

Sensory nerves of the gastrointestinal and genitourinary tracts. Note the common innervation.

important. With hypernatremia, the mucous membranes are dry and sticky, and the tongue is rough and dry. Tetany including carpopedal spasms occurs with hypocalcemia. Observe for other signs of various electrolyte imbalances. For example, skin turgor provides an important assessment of the client's hydration status.

Respirations should be observed. Rapid respirations suggest metabolic acidosis, infection, or fluid overload. Kussmaul's respirations (described in Chapter 18) are common with metabolic acidosis. Shallow respirations and shortness of breath may be signs of hypokalemia. Shortness of breath may also suggest pulmonary edema, congestive heart failure, or both.

Inspection of the abdomen will reveal some important findings with many clients. Scars may represent surgical procedures or trauma. There may be urinary or fecal diversions or cutaneous fistulas. The abdominal contour may be altered if the bladder is distended or the kidneys are enlarged, as with polycystic kidney disease. With significant bladder distention, the umbilicus may be displaced toward the client's head. In the male, the penis should be inspected for lesions, scars, or discharge.

The urine should be inspected for blood, color, cloudiness, and precipitates. If any discharge is present at the urinary meatus, a specimen should be obtained before the client gives a urine sample.

Auscultation

Auscultation of the lungs may provide evidence of rales or rhonchi related to fluid overload. Cardiac irregularities and faint heart sounds may be heard with potassium imbalances. Friction rubs, as well as S-3 and S-4 sounds, also may be heard during auscultation of the heart and lungs. Auscultate the abdomen before palpating it. Listen for renal bruits; Figure 7–36 in Chapter 7 illustrates the location of the renal arteries in relation to the external abdominal landmarks. Listen also over each costovertebral angle (CVA). A bruit over one or both renal arteries suggests the possibility of renal artery stenosis.

Percussion

Percussion of the urinary bladder will elicit a dull sound in the suprapubic region if the bladder is distended. Bladder distention may extend to the level of the umbilicus or higher. When bladder tone is diminished because of chronic distention, fullness may be detectable only by percussion, which produces a dull sound.

A variation of the normal percussion technique can detect discomfort or pain over the kidney. Tenderness over the CVA suggests infection in the kidney or perinephric area. The client should assume a sitting position, and the nurse should quickly and sharply strike each CVA with the heel of the hand. This should be done gently, because it can cause the client a great deal of pain.

Palpation

Palpation can define the borders, and thus the size and contour, of internal organs. Palpation of normal-sized kidneys is difficult except in individuals who are thin or have poorly developed muscles. The right kidney is more readily palpable because it is normally lower in the abdomen and slightly more anterior than the left kidney.

Figure 32–3 illustrates the technique for kidney palpation. Deep palpation is necessary to identify the kidney. In this method, the lower pole of the right kidney may be palpated when the client takes a deep breath. In another method of kidney palpation, called *capturing*, hand placement is the same, but the right hand exerts greater pressure. The client is asked to exhale and then to stop breathing. If the kidney has been captured, it will be felt as the pressure of the fingers is released. The client may feel this procedure, but it is not painful.

If abdominal masses are present and are thought to be enlarged kidneys, perform only gentle and light palpation, because tumor cells may be liberated with manipulation if the masses are hypernephromas. Furthermore, if the masses are polycystic kidneys, palpation may aggravate bleeding. Examiners in doubt about the nature of the mass should eliminate this aspect of the examination.

The prostate of men should be palpated during the rectal examination. In women, pathological conditions in the reproductive organs may encroach upon the urinary

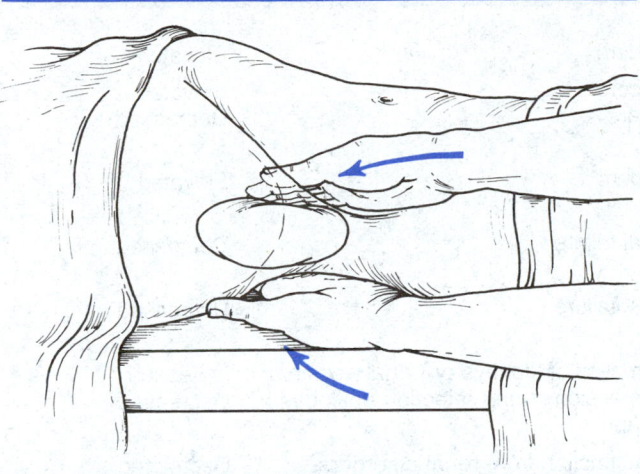

Figure 32–3

Technique for kidney palpation.

tract and alter its function. The pelvic and rectal examinations must not be overlooked when assessing clients with kidney and urinary system dysfunction (see Chapter 7).

Diagnostic Studies

A wide variety of diagnostic studies used to assess kidney and urinary system dysfunction are discussed in the following pages. Laboratory tests on both urine and blood are also summarized in Table 32–3.

Hematologic Studies

The tests most often used to assess kidney function include the serum creatinine test, the blood urea nitrogen (BUN) test, and the creatinine clearance test (to be discussed later). These tests are referred to as *renal function studies*.

Serum Creatinine. Serum creatinine measurements primarily reflect the ability of the kidneys to excrete creatinine, the waste product of skeletal muscle metabolism derived from the breakdown of phosphocreatine. The normal serum creatinine level is 0.6 to 1.5 mg/dL (Byrne et al., 1986), but it varies with sex and individual muscle mass characteristics (women generally having less muscle mass). Serial changes in serum creatinine levels are significant in evaluating and interpreting renal function, because this substance is excreted entirely by the kidney and is therefore directly proportional to excretory function. Unlike the BUN level, the serum creatinine level normally remains constant and is not influenced by other variables such as dehydration, malnutrition, or hepatic function. Only renal disorders will cause an abnormal elevation in creatinine. Therefore, serum creatinine levels are more accurate than BUN levels in assessing renal function. Refer to the section on creatinine clearance for further discussion.

Blood Urea Nitrogen (BUN). The BUN level is a general indicator of renal ability to excrete urea nitrogen. The normal BUN level is 6 to 20 mg/dL (Byrne et al., 1986). Urea nitrogen is synthesized by the liver using protein sources for the conversion, so a functioning liver is required for this test. Because dietary proteins form the primary source of urea nitrogen, a diet high in proteins will increase BUN levels, especially in the presence of renal disease. The metabolism of hemoglobin also results in the production of urea nitrogen.

Nearly all primary renal diseases cause BUN levels to rise, as do certain medications such as steroids, tetracyclines, tobramycin, gentamicin, and chemotherapeutic drugs. Hydration changes such as hemoconcentration or hemodilution also alter the BUN level. In dehydration, a decreased renal blood flow leads to decreased excretion of urea nitrogen and increased serum BUN levels. The BUN levels also may rise when excessive amounts of protein are available for hepatic catabolism or when there is gastrointestinal bleeding. Since urea synthesis depends on the liver, the BUN level may be normal in hepatorenal syndrome or any time there is combined liver and kidney disease. The BUN level is normal not because the renal excretory function is good, but because hepatic function is poor, and BUN formation is therefore decreased.

Uric Acid. Uric acid is a nitrogenous product derived from urine metabolism. Purines are produced by the metabolism of cellular nucleic acids and complex dietary proteins. Elevated uric acid levels in the serum may indicate renal dysfunction or a defect in purine metabolism. The normal uric acid level in the serum is 2.1 to 7.5 mg/dL in men; the range for women is 2.0 to 6.6 mg/dL (Byrne et al., 1986).

Other Tests. Hemoglobin and hematocrit values of clients with chronic renal failure are low (hemoglobin of 7 to 8 g/dL and hematocrit of 20% to 30%) because of decreased erythropoietin production. White blood cell counts are elevated when infectious processes of the urinary system are present.

Serum potassium and phosphorus levels are elevated with acute renal failure and uremia. Hyperkalemia and metabolic acidosis are especially common in clients with acute renal failure. Elevated phosphorus levels also occur with chronic renal failure. Serum calcium is also decreased in renal failure.

Methods of Urine Collection

Direct examination of the quantity and quality of the urine produced by the kidneys can offer much information about the overall status of the kidneys and urinary tract. Proper collection of the specimen, with consideration of the factors that can impair the value of the data, is an important

Table 32−3   Laboratory Tests Common in Diagnosis of Urinary System Dysfunction

Laboratory Test	Normal Expected Value	Disease State	Expected Abnormal Findings
Serum creatinine	0.6−1.5 mg/dL	Renal disorders	Elevated
Blood urea nitrogen (BUN)	6−20 mg/dL	Renal disorders Liver disorders	Elevated Decreased
Uric acid	Male 2.1−7.5 mg/dL Female 2.0−6.6 mg/dL	Renal disorders	Elevated
Hemoglobin	Male 14−18 g/dL Female 12−16 g/dL	Chronic renal failure	Decreased
Hematocrit	Male 40%−54% Female 37%−47%	Chronic renal failure	Decreased
White blood cells	4500−11,000 μL	Infectious process of kidneys or urinary system Immunosuppression during rejection episodes after transplant	Increased Decreased
Creatinine clearance	Male 107−141 mL/min Female 87−132 mL/min	Loss of renal function from renal disorders, chemotherapy, medications	Decreased
24-h urine	Depends on tests being done: to check creatinine clearance, concentration of urine, or composition of urine; to diagnose hypertension secondary to pheochromocytoma		
Urinalysis: pH	4.6−8	Phenylketonuria, high meat protein diet, metabolic acidosis, respiratory acidosis, tuberculosis of kidneys	Low pH
		High intake of vegetables and citrus fruits, metabolic and respiratory alkalosis, urinary tract infection, constant diuretic therapy, Cushing's syndrome	High pH
Color	Yellow-amber	Refer to Box 32−1	Refer to Box 32−1
Specific gravity	1.016−1.022, but can range from 1.001−1.040	Glycosuria, proteinuria, pituitary tumor, decreased fluid intake, fever, heart failure, Dextran or albumin administration, x-ray contrast media, urine preservatives, renal artery stenosis	Over 1.020
		Acute renal failure, alkalosis, diabetes insipidus, hypercalcemia, increased fluid intake, pyelonephritis, polycystic kidney disease, hydronephrosis	Less than 1.009
Protein	2−8 mg/dL	Glomerulonephritis, lupus erythematosus, nephrotic syndrome, acute infectious diseases, drug therapy (Orinase, penicillin, Gantrisin), hepatic disease, nephrosclerosis, pyelonephritis, septicemia, toxemia of pregnancy, toxic irritation of the kidney, polycystic kidney disease, exposure to cold, stress, dehydration	Increased
Ketones	None	Incomplete metabolism of fats, diabetes, high-protein and low-carbohydrate diet, dehydration, excessive aspirin consumption	Present
Glucose	0−15 mg/dL	Aging, pregnancy, diabetes mellitus, excitement and stress, hyperthyroidism, acromegaly, Cushing's syndrome, renal tubular damage	Increased
Blood	None	Blood transfusion reactions, hemolytic anemias, burns, crushing injuries, ingestion of poison (mushrooms, etc)	Present
Bilirubin	0.02 mg/dL	Liver disorders	Increased

nursing intervention. Specimen collection is generally done by the nurse directly, by assistants under the nurse's supervision, or by the client. Many times, it is acceptable to collect a specimen without considering specifics such as time of day. The instances in which other factors must be considered are outlined below.

The Clean-Catch (Midstream) Specimen. The clean-catch (midstream) urine specimen is the collection method usually used for routine urinalysis, examination of urinary sediment, and culture and sensitivity. Most institutions have a protocol for the collection of the clean-catch urine specimen. General principles include:

- Cleansing the urethral meatus with an antiseptic solution such as povidone-iodine (Betadine).
- Initiating voiding with the urethral meatus exposed.
- After the stream of urine has started, directing the urine into the container that will be taken to the laboratory.
- Completing urination in the toilet or elsewhere but not in the specimen container.

To cleanse the urethral meatus properly, a man must retract the foreskin, if present. The woman must understand the need to separate the labia completely to expose the urethral meatus. Then, using a new cotton ball for each cleansing stroke, the client makes three or four downward wipes over the urethral meatus.

Collecting the urine specimen midstream will eliminate any residual bacteria, pus, or cleansing solution. After the specimen has been collected, the cover should be securely closed and the container properly labeled. The specimen should be delivered to the laboratory within 2 hours to prevent disintegration of formed elements, bacterial overgrowth, or both. The specimen should be refrigerated if delay is anticipated; refrigeration may help retard disintegration and cell growth.

The First Voided Morning Specimen. A first voided morning urine specimen is generally regarded as the one that will provide the most consistent information, since it is the most acidic and most concentrated urine formed. Adjustments will have to be made for persons who work during the night. The best collection time for them would be after arising from their sleep period. Random specimens may be requested for the analysis of electrolytes or if urinary tract infection is a newly suspected problem. When infection is suspected, the specimen must be collected for culture and sensitivity before an antibiotic is administered. Unless there are other requests, the next available specimen rather than the next day's first morning specimen should be sent for culture and sensitivity.

The 24-Hour Specimen. A 24-hour collection of urine is a challenging procedure for both the hospitalized client and the staff. A complete and properly collected specimen is essential for accurate interpretation of the data obtained. Any delays in collection are extremely costly, not only because of the delay in the diagnostic process, but also in cost, considering the expense of a single day of hospitalization.

When a 24-hour specimen of urine is requested, determine what preservative is required and whether the specimen needs to be iced or refrigerated. Refer to the institution's laboratory manual for specific directions about the container to be used.

Next, instruct the client to empty the bladder completely. Note the time; this marks the beginning of the 24-hour period. From this time until 24 hours later, all urine produced by the client should be included in the collection bottle. At the same time, 24 hours later, ask the client to empty the bladder and include this in the collection; this will complete the 24-hour collection. Promptly deliver the properly labeled container to the laboratory, or refrigerate it in the case of delay. Documentation of the collection completes the procedure; protocol of the institution dictates how to do this.

A number of potential problems make collection of the 24-hour specimen a challenge. Remembering to collect all the urine is a major problem for the staff, the client, or the client's family. Thorough client and family instruction, as well as frequent reminders and discussion with staff, are essential. A teaching sheet similar to that in Box 32–2 may make collections more successful. The nurse should place signs indicating that a 24-hour collection is in process in bathrooms near toilets to remind anyone involved in emptying urine.

Urinary or fecal incontinence, diarrhea, or diagnostic tests that require bowel preparation all may impede the collection of a 24-hour specimen. If any of these conditions exist, the collection may be easier if it is postponed or if a Foley catheter is used.

Small samples of urine often are needed for sugar, acetone, or electrolyte examination during the 24-hour collection process. Remove only the minimal amount needed; then carefully measure the amount removed, and note the amount as an addition to the total volume. This will allow calculations based on the total volume of urine produced. In some situations, collection of the specimen by the client as an outpatient may be easier and more economical. The nurse should provide the client with a thorough discussion and instruction in such instances.

Creatinine Clearance Test

The best test to measure overall renal function is the creatinine clearance test, a mathematical calculation that compares the amount of creatinine filtered in a 24-hour urine collection (the preferred length of time for urine collection) with the amount of creatinine that remains in the serum. Because almost all creatinine is excreted, and other variables do not influence muscle metabolism and renal excretion, creatinine clearance is regarded as the best indicator of renal function. Although a 24-hour collection is preferred, a 12-hour or shorter collection may be acceptable in some situations.

The normal creatinine clearance value for men is 107 to 141 mL/min; for women it is 87 to 132 mL/min. For practical purposes, a rate of 100 mL/min may be considered normal to allow a comparison of the clearance to a percentage value. For example, a creatinine clearance value of 100 mL/min is 100%, or normal. A creatinine clearance value of 50 mL/min suggests that 50% renal function is lost and 50% remains. After the initial calculation, subsequent increases of the serum creatinine level imply that renal function is deteriorating; in other words, the kidneys are clearing less creatinine, and the serum level is increasing. If a creatinine clearance were calculated, it would be decreasing, because less creatinine would be measured in the urine as more accumulated in the serum. The trend is what is significant. The serum level will not increase until at least 50% of renal function has been lost.

Dialysis or transplantation generally is not required until the creatinine clearance values drop below 5 mL/min. Occasionally, however, symptoms may dictate that dialysis be started before the levels get that low.

Routine Urinalysis

A routine urinalysis is a urologic screening test to assess the nature of urine produced. It includes:

- Measurement of color, pH, and specific gravity
- Determination of the presence of glucose, protein, blood, and ketones
- A microscopic examination of the urine sediment for cells, casts, bacteria, and crystals

Abnormal findings require further delineation and confirmation.

The pH and the presence of protein, glucose, ketones, or blood in the urine can be detected easily using reagent strips. A plastic stick to which several separate reagent strips are affixed for testing various substances is most common. Completely immerse the reagent strip in well-mixed urine and remove it immediately to avoid dissolving the reagents. Hold the strip in a horizontal position to prevent possible mixing of the chemical reagents, and compare it with the test chart at the specified time.

Urinary pH. Urine is normally slightly acidic, because the kidneys excrete hydrogen ions. The first voided morning specimen is generally most acidic because of alterations in ventilation during sleep. Food usually results in the production of a more alkaline urine. The range of urinary pH is 4.6 to 8, averaging around 6.

Color. The color of urine ranges from pale yellow to amber because of the pigment urochrome. The color indicates the urine's concentration and varies with the specific gravity. Dilute urine is straw colored, and concentrated urine is a deep amber. Abnormally colored urine can result

---

Box 32–2 Instructions for 24-Hour Urine Collection

Patient Instructions: 24-Hour Urine Collection

Your physician has requested that you participate in the collection of a 24-hour urine specimen. The information obtained from various 24-hour collections will assist in diagnosis and/or evaluation of therapy.

Your test is scheduled to begin at _____
on _____ .

The collection of *all* urine passed during this period is extremely important. Therefore, if some urine is spilled, or lost, please notify a nurse so that the test can be restarted. This is essential for accurate test interpretation by your doctor.

The procedure for accurate urine collection is as follows:

1. At the time the collection is to begin, empty your bladder and note the time. Do not save this specimen, unless you are otherwise instructed.

2. The exact time of bladder emptying is considered as the test starting time.

3. Please save all urine for the next 24 hours.

4. Occasionally a preservative is added to the bottle. *This can be caustic.* Therefore:
   a. Do not urinate directly into the bottle.
   b. Do not pour anything out of the bottle.
   c. Do not sniff the bottle.
   d. Do not smoke while filling the bottle.
   e. Use containers provided to empty urine into the bottle, or ask one of the nursing personnel to do this.

5. The urine collection will be kept in your bathroom in a container of ice. If you notice that the ice has melted, please notify one of the nursing personnel.

6. Each time you urinate, the amount will be measured and recorded by a member of the nursing staff. You will be notified if this is not necessary.

7. 24 hours after the test was started, empty your bladder and *include this specimen* in the collection.

from the ingestion of certain foods or medicines or from a pathological condition.

Specific Gravity. Specific gravity, a measure of the concentration of particles in the urine, reflects the ability of the kidney tubules to concentrate or dilute urine. The normal specific gravity is 1.016 to 1.022, but it can range from 1.001 to 1.040. The specific gravity increases in clients with:

- Dehydration, because the kidneys absorb all available free water, which makes the excreted urine very concentrated
- Pituitary tumor that causes the release of excessive amounts of ADH, resulting in excessive water absorption

- Decrease in renal blood flow, as in hypotension, heart failure, or renal artery stenosis
- Glucosuria and proteinuria, because of the increased number of particles in the urine

In contrast, the specific gravity decreases in clients with:

- Overhydration
- Diabetes insipidus, in which there is inadequate secretion of antidiuretic hormone (ADH), which decreases water reabsorption
- Chronic renal failure, because the kidney has lost its ability to concentrate urine through water reabsorption

In clients with chronic renal failure, the specific gravity is usually stable at about 1.010 despite changes in intake because the kidney can no longer respond to changes.

Specific gravity can easily be measured with a hydrometer. First, place the urine in a clean, dry cylinder. Second, suspend or float a weighted hydrometer in the cylinder of urine (the concentration of the urine determines the depth at which the hydrometer will float). Third, read the depth measured on the calibrated scale on the hydrometer to determine the specific gravity reading (Figure 32–4).

Protein (Albumin). The normal protein content of urine is less than 8 mg/dL. The first voided morning specimen is preferred to detect the presence of protein in the urine. Since the client has not been up and exercising, orthostatic and transient proteinuria generally can be ruled out. Stress and cold weather exposure over time also can contribute to transient proteinuria, however. Higher-than-average protein levels found on routine analysis should be evaluated further for total protein by a 24-hour collection. Most protein excreted in the urine is albumin and may be referred to as *albuminuria*. Other abnormal proteins may be identified, however, and require investigation by other methods, such as urine electrophoresis.

Ketones. Normally, there are no ketones in the urine. *Ketonuria*, or ketones in the urine, occurs when there is incomplete metabolism of fats. This condition may be observed in diabetic ketoacidosis. However, nondiabetic clients who follow a diet high in protein and low in carbohydrates in an effort to lose weight quickly will form ketones. Ketonuria also may be seen in the presence of dehydration, starvation, or excessive aspirin consumption.

Glucose. Normal urine contains only small amounts of glucose—usually less than 15 mg/dL. *Glucosuria*, or glucose in the urine, occurs when the renal threshold for reabsorption of glucose is exceeded. The ability of the renal tubule cells to reabsorb glucose is exceeded when the blood glucose level is about 180 mg/dL, but this varies with individuals. When the renal tubules are impaired, glucosuria will occur at lower blood glucose levels. Aging, pregnancy, and diabetes mellitus of several years duration will increase the renal threshold for glucose (Rose, 1981).

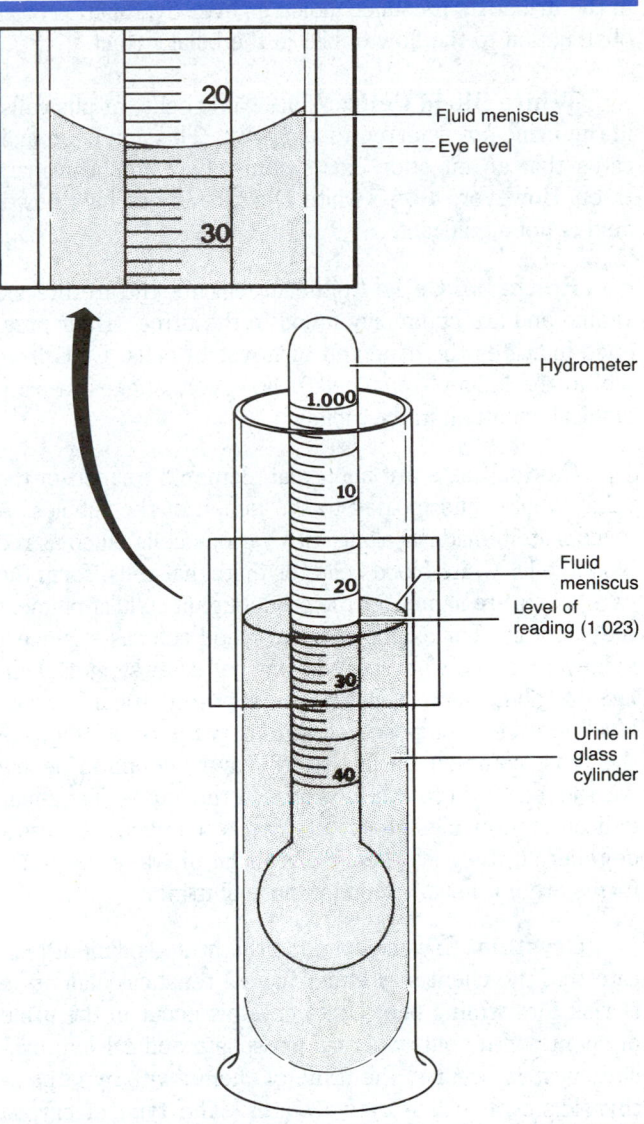

Figure 32–4

Reading specific gravity.
SOURCE: Holloway N: *Nursing the Critically Ill Adult: Applying Nursing Diagnosis,* 2nd ed. Menlo Park, CA: Addison–Wesley, 1984, p. 286.

Blood. Any disruption in the blood–urine barrier, whether at the glomerular or tubular level, will cause blood cells to enter the urine. *Hematuria* occurs when more than two to three red blood cells are found in the sediment of urine on microscopic examination. Hematuria and its causes were discussed earlier in this chapter. Hemoglobinuria, or free hemoglobin in the urine, is an abnormal finding. Hemolysis of red blood cells that results in hemoglobinuria may occur in various hemolytic anemias and following some blood transfusion reactions.

Bilirubin. *Bilirubinuria*, or bilirubin in the urine, should be suspected when the color of the urine is dark gold or brown. Normally, there is no detectable bilirubin in the urine. Its presence indicates liver dysfunction or an obstruction to the flow of bile in the biliary tract.

White Blood Cells. White blood cells, or pus cells, in the urine are referred to as *pyuria*. This condition indicates that an infection exists somewhere in the urinary tract. However, 4 to 5 white blood cells per high power field is not significant.

Epithelial Cells. Epithelial cells line the urethra and vagina and are commonly found in the urine. Their presence indicates the expected turnover of cells. Cells from within the kidney (renal cells), however, suggest a pathological condition in the kidney.

Casts. Casts are abnormal elements formed in the renal tubules and molded to the lumen of the tubules. A mucoprotein material along with various cells, such as red blood cells, white blood cells, or epithelial cells, form the cast. Casts are named for the predominant cellular element they contain. For example, white blood cell casts suggest kidney infection, whereas red blood cell casts suggest damage to glomerular capillaries or ruptured tubular walls. Hyaline casts, composed of various types of protein, are the most common. In fact, they may be found in people with fever or those who exercise strenuously. They may indicate the mildest form of tubular damage. As casts degenerate, they may become granular or waxy, but these forms are not usually found in normal urine.

Crystals. Crystals found in the urine sediment indicate that the client may either have a renal calculus or be at risk for forming one. Urate crystals occur in the urine of clients with gout, whereas phosphate and calcium oxalate crystals occur in the urine of clients with hyperparathyroidism of malabsorptive states. The type of crystal found varies with urine pH. Urate crystals are in acidic urine, and calcium oxalate crystals are in alkaline urine.

Bacteria. Few if any bacteria are normally present in urine, and large numbers of bacteria suggest infection in the urinary tract. Normal urine contains less than 1000 bacteria per mL of urine. A count greater than 100,000 colonies per mL of urine indicates a urinary tract infection. Some debate exists about the minimal colony count at which there is evidence of infection and not contamination. Many experts have accepted a count of 100,000 colonies per milliliter of urine as indicating infection, but Smith (1981) states that this level is too high and that infections will be missed using this criterion.

Urinary Electrolytes and Osmolality
Urinary electrolytes and osmolality can be measured using a random sample of urine or 24-hour collection. The random sample yields a quick analysis of the urine content, especially when the client is oliguric or anuric. The 24-hour collection for analysis of total urinary excretion of certain electrolytes will provide more information regard-

ing the specific nature of the renal problem. Sodium, potassium, chloride, and calcium are electrolytes commonly measured in 24-hour collections. The amount present in the urine reflects how well the kidney is excreting or conserving these electrolytes.

Urinary osmolality reflects the ability of the kidneys to concentrate or dilute urine to maintain the osmotic balance between cells, tissues, and plasma. Urine osmolality is interpreted in comparison with the plasma osmolality. For example, if the plasma osmolality is elevated, the kidneys should reabsorb water and excrete a more concentrated and smaller volume of urine. In contrast, if the plasma osmolality is low, the kidneys should excrete a less concentrated and larger volume of urine. This maintains the proper osmotic balance among cells, tissue, and plasma. The ratio of urine osmolality to plasma osmolality should be greater than 1:1. Urine osmolality may range from 300 to 1090 mOsm/kg, depending upon sex and activity (Byrne et al., 1986). Variations in urinary osmolality also depend on the amount of solute to be excreted.

Ultrasonography
Ultrasonography of the kidney can locate renal cysts, differentiate renal cysts from solid renal tumors, demonstrate renal or pelvic calculi, and guide a percutaneously inserted needle for cyst aspiration or removal of a biopsy specimen (Pagana & Pagana, 1982).

Nursing Implications. The test is best performed prior to any barium contrast studies, or all barium must be removed first with cathartics. No preparation for the client is required other than to advise the client to not empty the bladder prior to ultrasonography. A full bladder enhances organ and tissue delineation. Instruct the client to lie quietly in the prone position for about 15 minutes. If a biopsy is done at the same time, 30 minutes may be necessary (refer to the section on renal biopsy). Warn the client about the copious amounts of lubricant that will be applied to the skin to enhance transmission of the sound waves. Nonhealing open wounds may be a deterrent to the placement of the lubricant but do not necessarily make the test impossible to perform. After the procedure, remove the lubricant from the client's back.

Kidneys, Ureters, Bladder X-ray
An abdominal flat-plate x-ray of the abdomen is called a KUB or plain film. This simple x-ray does not involve any client preparation or injection of contrast media; the client is in the supine position. The KUB will generally determine the presence of two kidneys, as well as provide a general outline of the kidneys, from which their size may be grossly determined. The left kidney is normally about 0.5 cm longer than the right. Thus, if the left kidney is not slightly larger, it may represent a pathological condition on that side. The KUB may also identify tumors, malformations, and calculi. The study is contraindicated in the pregnant client.

Nursing Implications. Explain the KUB x-ray to clients and reassure them that it will not hurt. It should be scheduled before any barium studies to ensure adequate visualization.

Intravenous Pyelography

An intravenous pyelogram (IVP) is a frequently employed fluoroscopic examination that involves the IV injection of a contrast medium, which is carried through the blood into the kidneys and then filtered and excreted into the ureters and bladder. The IVP will give some information on function of the kidneys, as reflected by the uptake and excretion of dye. Well-functioning kidneys take up and excrete the dye rapidly, whereas delayed uptake and excretion indicate a decrease in functioning. The IVP also provides information about the presence or absence of kidneys; the pole-to-pole size of the kidneys; the depth of the renal cortex; the integrity or contour of the calyces; the size of the renal pelvis; the presence of stones in the pelvis, the ureters, and the bladder; and the size of the ureters and their patency (Figure 32–5). Complications of IVP include allergic reaction, infiltration of the contrast agent, and renal shutdown and failure.

The IVP films yield the best information when the bowel has been cleansed of stool, air, and fluid. Therefore, clients are usually given a laxative the evening before the procedure, and preparatory enemas or suppositories are generally administered. In addition, the client is usually assigned NPO status until after the films have been taken. After the dye has been administered intravenously, x-ray films are exposed at 1-, 5-, 10-, 15-, 20-, and 30-minute intervals (and sometimes longer). The client is then asked to void, and another film is exposed to assess bladder emptying.

Nursing Implications. Explain the purpose and procedure of the test and that it takes about 45 minutes. Emphasize that it will not hurt except for the placement of the IV needle. Give cathartics as ordered the evening preceding the examination, and keep the client NPO after midnight. Assess the client for allergy to iodine. Explain that the dye can cause flushing of the face, a feeling of warmth, and a salty taste in the mouth. Assess the IV site for infiltration. Observe for anaphylaxis after the dye has been administered. Encourage fluids after the test has been completed.

In clients with known renal insufficiency (ie, elevation of the serum creatinine level above 1.5 mg/dL), diabetes mellitus, or multiple myeloma tests using contrast media are contraindicated. Other renal diagnostic tests are recommended, if possible. The elderly client is also a candidate for these additional tests because of the deterioration of renal function associated with age.

Cystoscopy

A cystoscopy is a procedure in which a cystoscope is inserted into the bladder via the urethra to visualize directly the internal bladder wall and the contents of the bladder. A cystoscopy is indicated to identify the origin of hematuria as well as to diagnose and remove tumors, stones, or any other foreign material. The application of electrical current to the lesion (fulguration) to remove bladder tumors may be carried out during the cystoscopic examination. A cystoscope also can be used to implant radium seeds into a

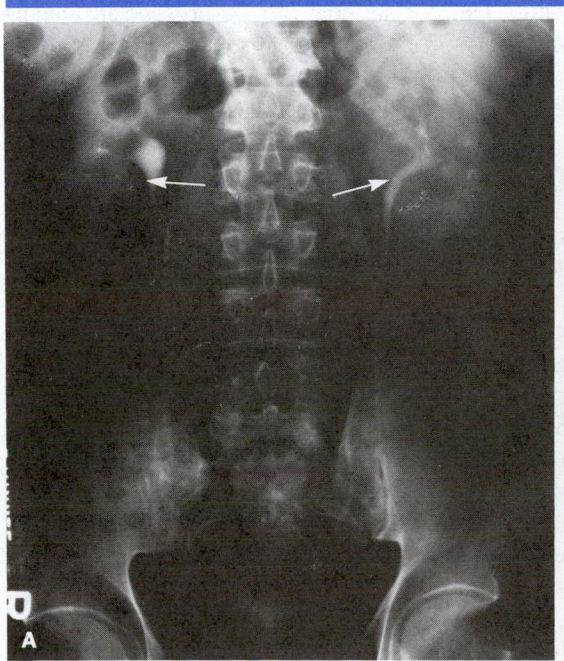

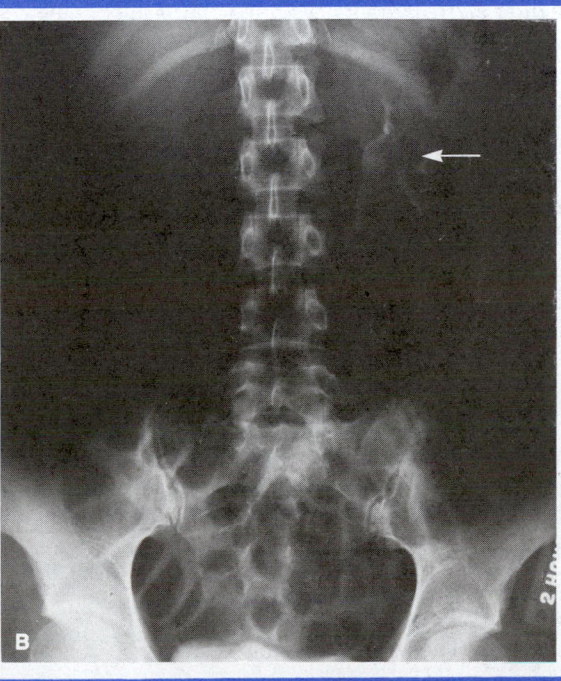

Figure 32–5

Intravenous pyelogram. **A.** The renal pelves and calyces fill normally on both sides, and both ureters are visualized. **B.** After 2 hours, the ureter and kidney on the right are not visualized; they are functioning normally and the dye has cleared. A calculus in the left ureter causes dilation of the calyx shown here.

tumor, place catheters in the ureters to drain the renal pelvis, and coagulate bleeding areas.

A cystoscopy is performed under general or local anesthesia. During the procedure, the client is supine, with the legs and feet supported in a lithotomy position. Strict aseptic technique is essential during the examination. The cystoscope is available in a variety of sizes from 12 to 26 F. Its wide-angle lens allows viewing of the interior bladder surfaces. A panendoscope will be used to examine the urethra visually, because its lens is more directly in line with the instrument. Retrograde pyelography, which involves the direct injection of dye into each ureter through the cystoscope, also may be performed during cystoscopy. It is indicated if obstruction is suspected in the ureters or the renal pelvis. Because the dye is not directly injected into the bloodstream, this procedure avoids the risk of an allergic reaction to the contrast media.

Nursing Implications. In explaining the procedure to clients, tell them the cystoscope is inserted into the bladder in the same manner as a catheter (Figure 32–6). Because it is rigid and not flexible as a catheter would be, the procedure may cause mild to moderate discomfort. Give enemas as ordered to clear the bowel. Keep the client NPO if general anesthesia is to be used. A liquid breakfast may be given if local anesthesia is to be used. Administer pre-procedure sedatives as ordered to help reduce anxiety as well as bladder spasms.

Postoperatively, record careful measurement of urinary output. Measure vital signs at least every 4 hours and report any elevation in temperature immediately. Urinary instrumentation is a major cause of nosocomial urinary tract infections, but prompt detection and treatment may prevent complications such as sepsis and acute renal failure. Hematuria is a common postprocedure finding, but it will gradually decrease over 24 to 48 hours. Carefully note and monitor the presence of large blood clots as they may result in obstruction of the urinary drainage system. To avoid this problem, a catheter that permits irrigation and drainage may have been inserted during the cystoscopy.

The client may experience back pain, bladder spasms, urinary frequency, and burning on urination. Warm sitz baths and mild analgesics may be ordered and given. Sometimes belladonna and opium (B & O) suppositories are given to relieve bladder spasms. Encourage fluids. Occasionally, antibiotics are ordered 1 day before and 3 days after the procedure to reduce the incidence of bacteremia.

Cystogram and Voiding Cystourethrogram

The cystogram outlines the contour of the bladder and identifies any reflux of urine from the bladder into the ureters toward the kidney (ureterovesical or U-V reflux). For this test, a catheter is inserted into the urinary bladder, and dye is injected through the catheter into the bladder. No reflux should occur, but if it does, it will be detected when the dye is injected. The voiding cystourethrogram (VCU or VCUG) is performed in a similar manner. It pro-

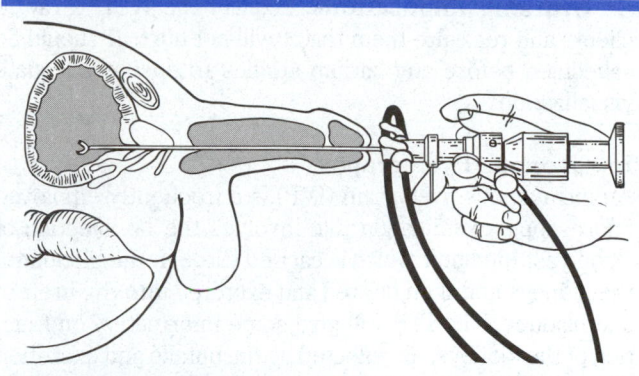

Figure 32–6
Cystoscope insertion.

vides additional information about strictures or urethral disorders as the client is observed voiding. This test is particularly embarrassing to the client so it requires some psychological preparation. It is important that the client have the opportunity to discuss and understand thoroughly why the test is necessary and how it will help in the diagnostic process. Assurance that there will be as much privacy as possible may help diminish concerns. However, most clients thoroughly dread this test.

Urodynamic Studies

Urodynamics is a relatively new field of study that involves the physiology of micturition. A variety of tests is available to study known or suspected problems related to nerve innervation of the bladder, incontinence, or variations in the urinary pattern.

The uroflometer measures the rate of urine flow during voiding. The normal flow rate, expressed in volume (milliliters) per second, for a man is 20 to 25 mL/s; for a woman it is 25 to 30 mL/s. A decreased flow rate may be observed with obstruction or decreased innervation.

Cystometrography. In cystometrography, a cystometrogram measures changes in pressure within the bladder. A catheter is inserted into the urinary bladder, water is instilled into the bladder via the catheter, and measurements of the internal pressure are recorded. Since part of the test is to determine how the client feels as bladder pressure increases, the client is asked to note when bladder fullness is detected and when the urge to void is felt. The normal bladder capacity is 400 to 500 mL, and the urge to void is felt at around 50 to 100 mL below the capacity. Bladder pressure increases when the client is told to urinate and decreases when urination is completed. This increase in pressure is related to the contraction of bladder musculature during the voiding process.

Urethral Pressure Profile. Pressures within the urethra can be measured and calculated in a variety of combinations. The primary measurements determine the peak pressure in the urethra and the pressure upon closure of the urethra. Variations in pressure and pressure distribution help identify the type of incontinence being experienced.

Electromyography. A component of urodynamic studies, electromyography (EMG) determines alterations in the voluntary control of urination as maintained by the external sphincter. Normally, when the bladder is filling and the external sphincter is relaxed, there is electrical activity in the muscles; EMG records this. With voiding, the pelvic muscles relax, the external sphincter (the detrusor muscle) contracts, and there is an absence of electrical activity. Various methods may be used to measure this muscle activity. Cutaneous electrodes, needle electrodes, an anal catheter, or an anal plug (sometimes called a *rectal plug*) may be used.

Determine which method has been selected before initiating client instruction. A great deal of explanation is needed for the client, because needle electrodes are quite uncomfortable. The needle electrode is placed near the urethra in the female client and through the perineum in the male client. Needle placement is difficult, and information may be hard to obtain. The anal plug is generally preferred for overall perineal muscle evaluation and produces only a slight sensation of pressure.

Nephrotomography

Nephrotomography provides radiographic visualization of the kidney using the tomographic technique, usually following the IV injection of radiopaque dye. Tomographic techniques involve x-ray films of various planes of the kidney. Taking pictures at varying depths of kidney tissue permits detailed study of alterations in structure. Refer to the discussion on IVP earlier in the chapter for nursing implications associated with nephrotomography.

Computerized Tomography

A computerized tomography (CT) scan of the abdomen is often done to identify kidney size and structural alterations within the urinary system. It may be done with or without contrast media. The scan picks up images at varying levels—from 3 to 13 mm apart—so small lesions, tumors, or defects can be pinpointed precisely. In addition to the kidneys, the retroperitoneal space, adrenals, bladder, and prostate can be visualized well. The IV injection of contrast media may be contraindicated for the same reasons as the IVP. A CT scan without contrast media may provide detail adequate for the diagnostic process, however.

Nursing Implications. Clients must lie motionless throughout the CT scan. Explain the procedure, show the client a picture of the machine if possible, and encourage the client to verbalize fears (eg, some clients may suffer claustrophobia when their bodies are enclosed in the machine). Keep the client NPO for 4 hours before the test to prevent food in the stomach or duodenum from confusing the final picture.

Renal Scan

The renal scan, a nuclear medicine procedure, demonstrates blood flow to each kidney following the IV administration of a small amount of radioisotope. A variety of isotopes may be used for the imaging. Pictures are taken immediately following injection of the isotope and at various intervals thereafter.

The renal scan is used to:

1. Show the size, shape, and location of the kidneys
2. Detect localized infections
3. Detect renal infarctions
4. Detect renal arterial atherosclerosis or trauma (uptake of the isotope is delayed on the affected side)
5. Monitor rejection of a transplanted kidney (in chronic rejection, uptake is delayed)
6. Detect primary renal disease (uptake is delayed)
7. Detect pathological renal conditions in clients who cannot have an IVP because of dye allergies

Some examiners request that Lugol's solution be administered before the isotope injection and for several days following the scan to block the uptake of the isotope by the thyroid gland. The client is unsedated and nonfasting when the radionucleotide (^{131}I or ^{125}I) is given. It takes only minutes for the isotope to be concentrated in the kidneys. A gamma-ray detecting device then is passed over the kidney area, and the uptake is recorded on either x-ray or Polaroid film. The test is contraindicated in pregnant women.

Nursing Implications. Explain the procedure to the client, and encourage the verbalization of concerns. Assure clients that they will not be exposed to large amounts of radioactivity, and tell them there will be no pain during the procedure except the discomfort of starting an IV. Also explain that the procedure usually takes about 1 hour.

Nurses should take precautions with the urine of a client who has had a renal scan. The ambulating client may use the toilet without concern for disposal of the isotope. Wear gloves when caring for an incontinent client, and bag linens for special handling. Pregnant health care providers should avoid contact with the client for at least 24 hours.

Renal Angiography

Renal angiography is a test that allows further study of kidney structure. It specifically delineates the vascular supply. Intravenous injection of radiopaque contrast media is followed by a series of films as the dye is taken up by the kidneys. Delays in uptake, alterations in contour of the kidney, and vessel abnormalities provide useful information about renal function. Stenosis (narrowing) of the renal artery is best demonstrated with this study.

During the procedure, a local anesthetic is injected into the femoral area, and a catheter is threaded through the femoral artery into the aorta. From there, it is directed into each renal artery, and dye is subsequently injected. The client may experience an intense burning feeling throughout the body that dissipates in seconds. This test can identify stenosis of the renal artery, localize aneurysms, and can also show vascular tumor masses or infarcted areas of renal parenchyma in detail. Renal arteriography may be contraindicated in clients with dye allergies, atherosclerosis, and physiological instability. Concerns during the procedure include sensitivity to dye, dislodgment of thrombi, and excessive bleeding at the catheterization site.

Nursing Implications. Explain the procedure being sure to show where the catheter will be inserted, and prepare the client for the burning feeling that occurs when the dye is injected. Encourage the client to verbalize concerns regarding the angiography. Question the client about iodine allergies. Ensure that a written and informed consent form is on the chart as this is an invasive procedure and carries some risk. Bowel cleansing with enemas and/or cathartics prior to the procedure helps to ensure adequate visualization of the kidneys. Keep the client NPO after midnight on the day of the study, and administer preprocedure medication as ordered. Have the client void immediately before the procedure.

Postprocedure care includes the frequent assessment of vital signs and inspection of the catheter insertion site for bleeding or hematoma formation. In addition, the color, temperature, and nature of pulses in the extremity involved should be assessed along with a basic check of neurological function. Apply cold compresses to the puncture site as needed, to reduce swelling and discomfort. Force fluids after the procedure to prevent dehydration from the osmotic diuretic effects of the dye.

Symptoms of abdominal or flank pain may indicate that significant bleeding is occurring. Because bleeding is the major complication, changes in vital signs, abdominal pain, or flank pain should be reported immediately to the physician. The client is kept in bed for 12 to 24 hours, and the IV infusion normally in place following the procedure is maintained for the duration of bed rest. Since dehydration increases the risk of renal damage, the IV line may be kept open for a longer period. Urine output and serum creatinine levels should be monitored for at least 5 to 7 days after the procedure, particularly in the high-risk client.

Renal Biopsy

A biopsy of kidney tissue may be necessary to determine the exact nature of renal pathology. Direct tissue examination allows assessment of the glomeruli—particularly the cellular elements of the glomeruli, the glomerular basement membrane, and the supporting tissue for the glomerular tuft. In addition, biopsy permits examination of the tubules and interstitium for evidence of inflammatory responses, fibrosis, or scarring. Renal biopsy is almost always indicated when unexplained proteinuria or hematuria are evident. Biopsy can identify the cause of the proteinuria or hematuria and thus allow the prescription of appropriate treatment.

A renal biopsy may use either open or closed technique. An open renal biopsy is a surgical procedure in which a flank incision is made and a piece of kidney tissue obtained by direct visualization of the kidney. Direct visualization permits greater control of potential bleeding and thus minimizes related risks. However, the need for general anesthesia and the time involved in postoperative recovery make the open biopsy a major procedure. The open biopsy is indicated for clients with only one kidney or when other abdominal surgery is necessary.

A closed, or *percutaneous,* renal biopsy is relatively easy to perform. However, significant postprocedure bleeding is possible, although rare. Furthermore, tissue may not always be obtained. A closed biopsy may be performed with the kidney visualized under fluoroscopy or by ultrasonography. Some nephrologists may use the "blind" technique, in which they have previously determined the kidney location. This technique is often done in the client's room, and the nurse may assist the nephrologist with the procedure.

In any kind of closed renal biopsy, the client assumes the prone position. A rolled blanket is placed under the lower abdomen to angle the kidney closer to the surface and to straighten the spine. Clients with lung disease or difficulty breathing may not be able to tolerate this position for the time required, which varies from 30 to 45 minutes. The client must be reasonably alert and cooperative as well as able to respond to requests to alter the breathing pattern; this is essential because changes in the level of the diaphragm will alter the position of the kidney. The client must be able to take a deep breath and hold it while the needle is introduced into the renal cortex. The left kidney is chosen for renal biopsy, since the right kidney is so near the liver.

The procedure involves thorough cleansing of the skin with povidone-iodine and draping the area around the site where the needle will be introduced. A local anesthetic is injected cutaneously and then into progressively deeper layers of tissue. A spinal needle determines the depth of the kidney beneath the surface of the skin. The biopsy needle then is inserted as close as possible into the spinal needle's path. After the biopsy needle has been placed into the kidney, just beneath the capsule, the client's breathing pattern is observed. When the needle is properly positioned to obtain kidney tissue, the needle's angle with the skin will go back and forth with respiration. When tissue is obtained, the client is asked to take a deep breath and hold it to minimize kidney movement. Usually three pieces of tissue are needed for the stains and tests that will be used to identify the exact pathological conditions.

Nursing Implications. The nurse must prepare clients for a kidney biopsy both intellectually and emotionally. Most clients immediately fear cancer when they hear the word *biopsy*. They should be assured that cancer is rarely a consideration when a renal biopsy is performed; usually its purpose is to evaluate conditions leading to renal failure.

The client's participation and cooperation are necessary during the closed biopsy, so allow adequate time for discussion of the procedure and what is expected of the client during the biopsy. Although this discussion may not totally eliminate anxiety, it will facilitate the client's ability to cope with the situation and to participate actively with greater control.

Prebiopsy physical preparation involves ensuring that clotting studies (prothrombin time, partial thromboplastin time, and platelet count) are normal. It is also important that hypertension be controlled, because uncontrolled high blood pressure increases the bleeding potential. Depending on when the biopsy is scheduled, clear liquids may be allowed. The client is usually kept NPO for 5 to 6 hours prebiopsy. Assess vital signs prior to the procedure for baseline comparison.

After the biopsy, apply pressure over the site for about 5 minutes, and apply a bandage or a Band-Aid. Measure the client's vital signs immediately and then every 15 minutes for an hour, every half hour times 2, and hourly for 6 hours. The client should lie flat in bed with a sandbag or blanket roll under the flank to provide direct pressure. The head of the bed may be raised slightly. Bed rest is maintained for 24 hours. The client may take food and fluids

immediately. Hemoglobin and hematocrit are usually checked about 6 and 24 hours after the procedure.

Serious bleeding after a renal biopsy is extremely rare when the biopsy is performed by experienced and well-trained nephrologists. However, changes in vital signs or flank pain that radiates into the front of the abdomen may signify that bleeding is occurring, so notify the physician immediately if this develops. In this case, expect to start an IV infusion to restore intravascular volume; normal saline and possibly blood transfusions will be administered. Bleeding that cannot be controlled with volume or blood replacement may necessitate surgical intervention for control. The most serious consequence of uncontrolled bleeding would be the loss of the kidney. Pink-tinged urine or small amounts of frank blood are not uncommon for 24 hours after the biopsy. Tell the client to expect this to prevent undue alarm. Large amounts of blood in the urine are not expected, however. Advise the client to avoid heavy exercise, activity, or athletic endeavors for 1 to 2 weeks after the biopsy.

The time required to process the tissue specimens varies, depending on laboratory facilities. Almost all processing requires at least 48 to 72 hours; however, the results of some stains may not be available for a week or longer. Since the results of the tissue examination may determine treatment or provide evidence of disease progression or remission, waiting for the results of the biopsy is an anxious time for the client. Nursing support during this waiting period can assist the concerned client and family.

Section II: Nursing Diagnosis

A variety of nursing diagnoses may apply to the client with disturbances in the structure and function of the kidneys and the urinary tract. Nursing diagnoses directly and indirectly related to renal and urinary system disturbances are listed in Box 32–3. The following section discusses the nursing diagnoses most directly related to disturbances of the kidneys and urinary system.

ALTERATIONS IN COMFORT

Pain

Clients with renal or ureteral calculi commonly experience excruciating pain. Renal abscesses and infections of the urinary tract, including cystitis and urethritis, produce moderate pain. Tumors, enlarged polycystic kidneys, and a distended urinary bladder also result in discomfort for the client.

Pruritus

Mild or severe generalized itching accompanies end-stage renal failure and the development of uremia. The production and elimination of urate crystals by the skin and the

increased production of parathormone are believed to be the causes of the intense pruritus. Dry skin or perspiration and other moisture will worsen the pruritus.

POTENTIAL FOR IMPAIRMENT OF SKIN INTEGRITY

A number of factors contribute to the potential development of alterations in skin integrity. Poor nutrition, chronic anemia, and pruritus with associated scratching are all present in uremic clients with end-stage renal failure. In addition, edema, immobility, alteration in skin sensation, and decreased mental alertness and responsiveness may contribute to problems of skin breakdown. Slowed wound healing has been observed in uremic clients and thus further contributes to the potential for impairment of skin integrity. Decubitus ulcers can develop within 12 to 24 hours.

POTENTIAL FOR INFECTION

Clients with stones in the kidneys, ureters, or bladder may develop infections; the stones are a continuing nidus of bacterial growth. Indwelling urinary catheters, stents, ureteral tubes, and nephrostomy tubes (to be discussed in Chapter 34) also may contribute to the client's potential for the development of infection. Urinary stasis associated with a neurogenic bladder is an excellent medium for ascending urinary tract infections, which may become systemic bacteremic episodes. Any urinary instrumentation required for diagnosis or treatment, such as a cystoscopy, may cause infection. In clients who are uremic from either acute renal failure or end-stage renal disease, altered immune processes further contribute to the potential for infection.

ALTERATION IN FLUID VOLUME

Fluid Volume Deficit

Loss of fluid or blood volume through the use of diuretics, infectious processes, hemorrhage, or fluid shift to the interstitial space (which occurs in the nephrotic syndrome) may result in a fluid volume deficit. For clients with normal renal function, this may contribute to decreased renal perfusion and the development of prerenal azotemia. Clients who undergo hemodialysis or peritoneal dialysis also may have too much fluid removed during the treatment and experience a fluid volume deficit (hypovolemia).

Fluid Volume Excess

Excess circulating fluid volume, or hypervolemia, occurs when the client is oliguric because of renal failure. This problem may occur acutely with sudden loss of renal function or develop as end-stage renal failure progresses. Excesses in fluid volume contribute to cardiopulmonary decompensation and must be corrected. Furthermore, after renal transplant surgery, large volumes of IV fluid are infused at the same rate that urine is produced. This amount often exceeds 4000 mL/h the first day.

ALTERATION IN THOUGHT PROCESSES

Changes in the sensorium, inability to concentrate, and impaired memory for recent events are common manifestations of uremia. Nitrogenous waste products accumulate because of impaired renal excretion, metabolic acidosis occurs because of inadequate acid excretion and a bicarbonate deficit, and electrolyte disturbances arise with renal failure. These biochemical alterations cause a progressive deterioration in mental functioning. Clients become increasingly lethargic and drowsy until dialysis can correct the metabolic alterations. Dietary alterations may temporarily slow the development of these altered mental functions. The use of potent diuretics also can contribute to electrolyte imbalances and altered thought processes.

POTENTIAL FOR NUTRITIONAL DEFICIT

The client with acute or chronic renal failure always has altered nutritional status. Nausea, vomiting, and anorexia are common manifestations of each of these processes in

Box 32–3	Nursing Diagnoses Commonly Related to Dysfunction of the Kidneys and Urinary System

Diagnoses Directly Related to Renal and Urinary System Dysfunction

Comfort, alteration in, related to pain

Comfort, alteration in, related to pruritus

Skin integrity, impairment of, potential

Infection, potential for

Fluid volume alteration, deficit or excess, actual or potential

Thought processes, alteration in

Nutritional deficit, actual or potential

Gas exchange, impaired

Self-concept, alteration in, related to body image changes or role performance disturbance

Urinary elimination, alteration in pattern of

Sexual dysfunction

Tissue perfusion, alteration in, renal, cerebral, and cardiac

Additional Potential Nursing Diagnoses

Bowel elimination, alteration in continence related to urinary diversion

Knowledge deficit, actual or potential

Noncompliance, actual or potential

Grieving, anticipatory

Injury, potential for, related to uremic toxins

Sensory perceptual alterations related to uremic toxins

Self-care deficit related to severe renal failure

which there is azotemia. In addition, clients commonly experience a metallic taste in the mouth, and some foods may no longer taste good to them. Hypogeusia is a common problem for clients with end-stage renal failure. Dietary modifications (low-salt, low-potassium diets) that are prescribed for clients with renal failure complicate efforts to maintain a good nutritional status. The loss of proteins via peritoneal dialysis and loss of water-soluble vitamins via either peritoneal dialysis or hemodialysis further complicate the maintenance of a good nutritional status. Clients with altered renal function who are acutely or critically ill from sepsis or other problems will also experience nutritional deficits.

IMPAIRMENT OF GAS EXCHANGE

The impairment of oxygen–carbon dioxide exchange leading to inadequate oxygenation may be caused by several problems related to renal disorders or surgical interventions. If the kidneys fail to excrete hydrogen ions and regenerate adequate bicarbonate, the lungs must compensate for the increased load of metabolic acids by increasing the rate and depth of breathing, also known as Kussmaul's respirations. Respiratory fatigue from continued compensation may lead to decreased oxygenation, especially if infection or cardiac problems are present. Chronic lung disease severely limits pulmonary compensation for metabolic acidosis and becomes a life-threatening problem. In oliguric or anuric clients with either acute or chronic renal failure, hypervolemia that accompanies congestive heart failure and results in pulmonary edema also may impair gas exchange. Flank incisions or thoracoabdominal approaches for renal or urologic surgery also may limit respiratory movements. Hypoventilation following these surgical interventions may precipitate atelectasis or hypostatic pneumonia. Chronic anemia also impairs gas exchange and results in increased cardiac workload (noted by an increased heart rate).

ALTERATION IN SELF-CONCEPT

Altered kidney and urinary tract function causes a variety of body image changes. Urinary diversions may result in cutaneous stomata and necessitate the client's wearing an external pouch. Indwelling urinary catheters or a suprapubic tube may also be used to provide permanent or temporary urinary drainage. If chronic renal failure develops, dialysis will require some major adjustments. Vascular access or permanent peritoneal catheter placement will alter the client's body image. In addition, chronic dialysis clients often cease to produce much urine. Not urinating, after a lifetime of this habit, commonly causes a significant change in body image. Furthermore, dependence upon a machine for the preservation of life is a major alteration in self-concept and often precipitates crises in role relationships and sexuality. Finally, the amount of time required for dialysis per week (12 to 15 h/wk for hemodialysis and 32 to 48 h/wk for peritoneal dialysis) may necessitate job changes or collection of disability insurance. Changes in customary family roles may also occur.

Several body image changes also accompany renal transplantation. Having a part of someone else's body creates emotional turmoil. Also, the use of steroids following transplantation results in many body changes such as softening of skin, thinning of hair, osteoporosis, moon face, buffalo hump, and weight gain. (Refer to Unit Seven for an in-depth discussion of the use of steroids.)

ALTERATION IN URINARY ELIMINATION PATTERN

Alteration Related to Urinary Diversion

An ileal or colon conduit will result in diversion of the urinary stream. Clients with an ileal conduit or other cutaneous urinary diversion must wear a pouch to collect urine.

Urinary diversions into the sigmoid colon will result in a loss of urine during defecation. A continent vesicostomy will require catheterization for the evacuation of urine.

Alteration Related to Incontinence

Urinary incontinence is fairly common in aging women, especially the multiparous and obese. Incontinence may be total, related to stress, or associated with urinary retention with overflow.

Alteration Related to Retention

Retention of urine occurs when there is an obstruction to its outflow. It may result from bladder neck obstruction, as may occur in prostatic hypertrophy. The resulting bladder distention may lead to hydroureter or hydronephrosis. These conditions also may be caused by obstruction above the bladder. Neurogenic bladders also result in urinary retention and, thus, in alteration of the urination pattern.

Alteration Related to Polyuria, Oliguria, or Anuria

Clients with acute or chronic renal failure may experience a variety of changes in the pattern and amount of urine produced. Decreased renal concentrating ability, such as occurs with progressive renal insufficiency, results in the client's experiencing polyuria. Oliguria or anuria may occur acutely, with sudden loss of renal function. Clients who progress to end-stage renal failure often notice that virtually all urine production ceases after the initiation of dialytic therapy.

SEXUAL DYSFUNCTION

Alterations in sexuality for clients with altered kidney and urinary system function may occur because of a variety of factors. Loss of libido commonly accompanies chronic illnesses. Changes in hormonal production lead to loss of libido in both female and male clients with chronic renal failure. Some men with neurogenic bladders or end-stage renal disease may experience impotence. Many couples have difficulty coping with the possibility of sterility in chronic renal failure or with recommendations to avoid pregnancy because of the strain it imposes in renal function.

ALTERATION IN TISSUE PERFUSION

Severe blood loss, dehydration, or a shift of fluid from the intravascular fluid compartment may cause a decrease in renal tissue perfusion. This alteration in hemodynamics may result in the development of prerenal azotemia. If uncorrected, acute renal failure may result. Clients with chronic renal failure have decreased production of erythropoietin, which results in decreased red blood cell mass. Because the decrease is gradual, the situation is not life threatening unless this value suddenly drops further because

of hemorrhage. Uremic states also result in a decreased life span of red blood cells and an increased number of immature red blood cells.

Section III: Planning and Implementation

A nursing care plan for the client with dysfunction of the kidneys and urinary system is presented in Table 32–4. Objectives of care are discussed in this and the following section.

PROMOTING COMFORT
Pain Relief

The pain of renal colic experienced by clients with renal or ureteral calculi will require narcotic analgesics for relief. Morphine sulfate is generally given intravenously to provide immediate pain relief, and subsequent doses may be given subcutaneously until the stone is passed or removed. Non-narcotic analgesics, urinary antiseptics, antibiotics, and increased fluid intake may be prescribed to control the discomfort associated with infectious processes. Analgesia may also be needed to relieve the bone pain associated with the hypocalcemia of renal failure. Clients with polycystic kidney disease should avoid aspirin and aspirin-containing compounds because of the potential for bleeding within the cysts.

Pain associated with surgical incisions will require narcotic analgesia during the initial 24 to 48 hours, and extensive surgical incisions may be quite uncomfortable for a longer period. Belladonna and opium suppositories may relieve the pain of bladder spasms following prostate surgery, bladder surgery, and kidney transplant surgery (because the new ureter is surgically placed through the bladder wall).

Pruritus Relief

Pruritus in uremic clients with end-stage renal disease is often not relieved by starting dialytic treatments. Interventions that may provide comfort include keeping the client's fingernails short and avoiding agents known to dry the skin (eg, soaps and lotions that contain alcohol). Bathing without soap will remove the uremic frost that compounds itching, but note that the bath water will be yellow because of the urochrome pigments. Oil-based lotions and soaps containing lanolin or high fat content should be encouraged. In addition, clients should be encouraged to control phosphorus levels through taking phosphate-binding agents as prescribed. Control of the phosphorous–calcium balance will moderate the production of parathormone, which is believed responsible for pruritus in uremic clients.

The aluminum hydroxide antacids (Nutrajel, ALternaGel, Alu-Cap, Amphojel, Basaljel) promote phosphate excretion. They should not be administered with iron

because they combine with iron, preventing its absorption. Vitamin D and calcium supplements should also be given to correct the calcium deficit once the hyperphosphatemia has been normalized. Observations that may indicate the presence of hypocalcemia are sore feet, muscle weakness, joint pain, generalized bone aching, and spontaneous fractures. Medications such as trimeprazine tartrate (Temaril) may provide relief from the itching. Diphenhydramine hydrochloride (Benadryl) may also afford comfort but often causes excessive drowsiness. Furthermore, because it is excreted by the kidney, the dosage must be cut down to avoid the development of toxicity in the body. Ultraviolet light treatments in the sunburn range given three times a week may control severe pruritus. Phototherapy results in a more rapid turnover of epithelial skin cells and therefore may control itching. Parathyroidectomy may be required if excessive parathormone production and pruritus cannot be controlled with more conservative measures.

MAINTAINING AND IMPROVING SKIN INTEGRITY

The alleviation of pruritus will promote the maintenance of skin integrity through decreasing the scratching that is difficult to control. Uremic clients who become immobilized for any reason are prone to the development of decubitus ulcers, so they should be turned every 1 to 2 hours and positioned to relieve pressure on edematous areas. A low-sodium diet, fluid restriction, and diuretic therapy or perhaps dialysis may be prescribed to lessen edema. The regulation of parathormone secretion will also decrease pruritus. Other fundamental nursing measures should be implemented to prevent skin breakdown.

Nutritional measures may promote healing and improve skin integrity. Improving the nutritional status of the client with kidney and urinary system dysfunction is discussed in a following section on the improvement of nutritional intake.

PREVENTING INFECTION

Infections increase the workload of the kidneys, and the prevention of infection at surgical sites or where urinary diversions exist is a challenge. Maintain sterile technique during dressing changes and at sites where catheters have been inserted into the blood or urinary system. Intermittent catheterization is preferable to the placement of a continuous indwelling urinary catheter. If continuous urinary catheter drainage is necessary, however, the continuity of

Table 32–4   Sample Nursing Care Plan

Nursing Diagnosis	Client Care Goals	Plan/Nursing Implementation	Expected Outcomes
Alteration in comfort related to pain	Ambulation without undue discomfort; ability to rest comfortably	Avoid nephrotoxic analgesics and administer analgesics as prescribed; perform nursing comfort measures	Client performs ADL without undue pain; rests comfortably; has relief from pain
Alteration in comfort related to pruritus	Ability to rest comfortably, understand the cause of pruritus, and be free of itching	Maintain good diet, rest, ventilation; change wet sheets; avoid drying products on the skin; use oil-based emollients; keep client's nails short; administer Benadryl and phosphate-binding agents; teach about pruritus	Client performs ADL without scratching; rests comfortably; has relief from itching; describes cause of pruritus
Potential impairment of skin integrity	Maintenance of skin integrity	Provide well-balanced diet that adheres to fluid, sodium, potassium, and protein restrictions; relieve pruritus; turn client every 1–2 h; relieve pressure on edematous areas with positioning; perform dialysis	Normal skin integrity; evidence that client is following diet restrictions and maintaining a well-balanced diet
Potential for infection	Prevention of infection	Use sterile technique when inserting catheters, changing dressings, and providing care of vascular access sites; utilize strict aseptic technique during dialysis	Absence of infection
Alteration in fluid volume	Normal fluid volume balance; understanding of fluid restrictions	Administer diuretics and albumin carefully; record I & O; assess skin turgor, daily weights; instruct client on fluid restriction; make accurate estimate of client's dry weight; perform dialysis to remove fluid excess; follow fluid restrictions closely when administering medications	Good skin turgor; I & O measurements that indicate correction of fluid volume alterations; absence of problems with fluid deficit or overload during dialysis; client follows fluid restrictions
Alteration in thought processes	Maintenance and improvement of thought processes	Perform dialysis for removal of excess electrolytes and nitrogenous waste products and correction of metabolic acidosis; follow protein restrictions; assess for asterixis; take safety measures and seizure precautions	Client oriented to person, place, and time; absence of asterixis; absence of injury for falls or seizures
Potential for nutritional deficit	Improvement of nutritional intake; ingestion of balanced diet; understanding of diet restrictions	Provide low-salt, low-potassium diet with fluid restrictions; increased protein diet for peritoneal dialysis and nephrosis clients; low-protein diet for hemodialysis clients; well-balanced diet; good oral hygiene; small frequent feedings; antiemetics; diet teaching; dialysis	Client adheres to diet restrictions and consumes a balanced diet; client lists foods that are to be avoided because of high potassium and sodium levels
Impaired gas exchange	Adequate O_2/CO_2 exchange	Provide oxygen as needed; perform dialysis to correct acidosis and remove excess fluid; administer diuretics as ordered and blood transfusions as needed	Client performs ADL without use of O_2; increased activity levels; absence of dyspnea with rest and activity
Alteration in self-concept	Improvement in self-concept; acceptance of urinary diversion or chronic renal failure	Listen to client and encourage verbalization of feelings; suggest clothing colors that tone down yellow skin; assist client in accepting problem	Ventilation of feelings; acceptance of problem

(continued)

Table 32–4 Sample Nursing Care Plan (continued)

Nursing Diagnosis	Client Care Goals	Plan/Nursing Implementation	Expected Outcomes
Sexual dysfunction	Acceptance of altered sexual functioning or restoration of sexual satisfaction; identification of alternatives for sexual pleasure	Explore factors contributing to impotence or loss of libido; suggest alternatives for sexual expression; recommend sex counselor	Satisfying sexual expression
Alterations in tissue perfusion	Adequate tissue perfusion	Monitor vital signs and urinary output; perform dialysis for fluid overload; administer packed red blood cells and O_2 as needed; correct electrolyte imbalances that may result in arrhythmias	Blood pressure of no more than 140/80; hemoglobin values around 7–8 g/dL, absence of arrhythmias or fluid excess
Alteration in urinary elimination pattern related to:			
1. Urinary diversion	Ability to care for and acceptance of urinary appliance or alternate means of voiding	Instruct client in self-care of various urinary diversions (see Chapter 34); discuss implications of urinary diversion	Client demonstrates self-care of urinary appliance or urinary diversion
2. Incontinence	Ability to maintain urinary continence	Instruct client in care following procedures to correct incontinence problems (refer to Chapter 34)	Improvement in urinary incontinence
3. Retention	Absence of urinary retention	Instruct client in care following procedures to correct urinary retention (Chapter 34)	Client voids in a normal manner; bladder is not distended
4. Polyuria, oliguria, or anuria	Acceptance of altered urinary elimination patterns	Explain reasons for altered elimination patterns (such as anuria with end-stage renal disease, or polyuria when concentrating ability of kidneys cease)	Client manages alteration in urinary elimination without difficulty

the system must not be disrupted; the tubing and bag must remain below the level of the bladder to ensure that urine does not ascend into the upper urinary tract. Vascular access routes for hemodialysis and catheters for peritoneal dialysis should all be cared for meticulously. For shunt care, some medical centers use clean technique, whereas others employ aseptic technique (refer to the sections on hemodialysis and peritoneal dialysis). All institutions use sterile technique for insertion or cannulation of access sites to prevent the development of bacteremic infection, a common problem.

Preventing infection from an indwelling catheter is the most successful and easy way to prevent infection in clients with urinary disorders. A closed drainage system (one that is closed to outside air) including the catheter connecting tube and collection bag must be maintained. The catheter must be secured to prevent movement and injury to the urethra. For female clients, the drainage tubing should be taped horizontally to the thigh. For male clients, the catheter should be secured by taping it horizontally to the thigh or the abdomen. The client should be assessed for signs and symptoms of urinary tract infection such as fever, chills, and bloody or cloudy urine. The ure-

thral meatus should also be observed for drainage or irritation.

The following principles apply to the care of a client with a closed urinary drainage system.

- Never disconnect the tubing or contaminate any part of the collecting bag or drainage tube.
- Do not allow the collecting bag to rest on the floor.
- Keep the collection bag and drainage tubing below the level of the bladder at all times to prevent reflux of urine into the bladder.
- Prevent kinking or twisting of the drainage tubing.
- Drain the collection bag at least every 8 hours.
- Be sure to use different receptacles for each client, and always wash hands between clients when obtaining outputs.
- Gently wash the urethral meatus with a nonantiseptic soap at the time of the daily bath.
- Do not apply antimicrobial solutions at the meatal–catheter junction.

A liberal fluid intake will help dilute the urine and discourage encrustation and infection. A good rule of thumb is: No client should be catheterized unless it is absolutely necessary.

RESTORING NORMAL FLUID VOLUME
Fluid Volume Deficit

Oral or IV fluid replacement will be necessary if the client becomes fluid-depleted from diuretic therapy, surgical drainage loss, or dialysis. Blood or plasma expanders also may be given to restore intravascular volume. Careful measurement of intake and output, the client's weight, and vital signs is essential to assess fluid volume status. In addition, the client's dry weight may need to be reevaluated. Dry weight is weight after dialysis without evidence of edema and with the client's blood pressure in the normal range; refer to the discussion of dialysis.

Fluid Volume Excess

Fluid volume excess may be avoided in dialysis clients if they understand the need to control fluid volume intake. Instruct clients to restrict fluid intake to the amount of urinary output in 24 hours plus 600 mL. If there is no urine output, fluid should be limited to no more than 1000 mL and perhaps to no more than 500 mL per day. Intravenous infusions should be administered with microdrip tubing to avoid excessive fluid administration. Medications administered piggyback are generally dissolved in the smallest possible volume of fluid, thus decreasing the amount of fluid administered.

A plastic glass with lines marking the amount of fluid will help the client control fluid intake. Also helpful is a list of the amount of fluid held in common containers found on the hospital tray. Fluid restriction may be prescribed as a guideline; however, the client eventually will need to assume responsibility for control of thirst and fluid intake and thus may impose his or her own fluid restriction. Staff members may assist the client to control fluid intake by not placing the usual full water pitcher at the bedside. Intake and output, weight, and blood pressure should be monitored to assess the client's fluid status. Clinical manifestations of fluid excess include edema, hypertension, or shortness of breath at rest or with exertion.

MAINTAINING AND IMPROVING THOUGHT PROCESSES

For the uremic client, removal of nitrogenous waste products and control of metabolic acidosis usually improves thought processes. Hemodialysis or peritoneal dialysis is usually necessary when thought processes are impaired. In addition, modifying the diet to restrict protein intake may decrease cognitive impairment. If the client has impaired mental functioning, explanations should be short and concise. Because of impaired memory for recent events, the client will need frequent reinforcement of previous explanations. The nurse should assure clients and family members that the loss of clear thought processes is temporary and will be normalized with adequate dialysis.

In addition to assessing the client's level of orientation to person, place, and time, the nurse should assess the extent of uremic encephalopathy by observing for slurred speech, tremors, and myoclonus. The presence of asterixis also should be assessed. Asterixis may be evaluated by asking the client to extend the arms, hyperextend the hands, and spread the fingers. Inability to maintain the position or visible flapping indicates the presence of high levels of nitrogenous waste products. The client with uremic encephalopathy is vulnerable to seizures, so safety precautions should be initiated. Siderails should be padded, and the client should be assisted when ambulating or out of bed. The nurse should monitor the client for drug toxicity that can occur because of limited renal excretion of drugs.

IMPROVING NUTRITIONAL INTAKE

The diets of clients with altered renal function generally require modification or restriction (eg, special diets may be prescribed for clients with calculi or infections). Clients with hypertension should be given a diet of no added salt, which is restricted to 4 g of sodium. If severe hypertension or heart failure is also present, the dietary sodium content may be restricted to 2 g/day.

Protein allowances also may be adjusted. Clients who are losing excessive protein, such as clients with nephrotic syndrome who have proteinuria or peritoneal dialysis clients who may lose up to 70 g/wk of protein in the dialysate, need a high-protein diet of 100 g/day or more. In contrast, clients with end-stage renal failure who are becoming uremic or are undergoing chronic hemodialysis generally are prescribed a diet restricted in protein (around 40 to 60 g/day for clients who have not yet started dialytic therapy; 50 to 70 g/day for dialysis clients). Protein in foods should be of high biological value (ie, contain a high proportion of essential amino acids) to ensure that essential amino acids are provided (Box 32–4). Adequate protein and calories must be provided so the client's own muscle mass is not catabolized as a source of energy.

When clients stop excreting urine, potassium intake also must be restricted, because fatal cardiac arrhythmias will occur with excessively high serum potassium levels. The nurse should routinely observe for signs of hyperkalemia. Muscle weakness, which can result in a flaccid paralysis of the extremities and cardiac arrhythmias, is one symptom. The earliest effect of hyperkalemia on cardiac function is an elevated T wave on the ECG, commonly detectable when the serum potassium level is greater than 6.0 to 7.0 mEq/L. Progressive ECG changes include widening of the QRS complex, a prolongation of the PR interval, and flattening or absent P waves. Premature ventricular contractions may be present, and asystole may result.

The potassium allowance is generally equivalent in milliequivalents to the grams of protein. For example, a 60-g protein diet and a 60-mEq potassium diet would be compatible. Each gram of protein provides a milliequivalent of potassium; therefore, potassium may not be more restricted than protein. Refer to Chapter 23 for a list of foods with a high potassium content.

Often, the dietary restriction of potassium is not enough to prevent hyperkalemia. To lower dangerously high potassium levels, sodium polystyrene sulfonate (Kayexalate) may be administered in addition to dialysis. Kayexalate is a cation-exchange resin in which sodium is exchanged for potassium, and the potassium is excreted in the stool. One gram of Kayexalate will decrease the serum potassium level by 1.0 mEq/L. It may be administered orally, by nasogastric tube, or rectally, and its effectiveness is enhanced by retention in the bowel for at least 6 hours. Because it causes constipation, Kayexalate often is administered with sorbitol and water. A 30-mL Foley catheter with the balloon inflated distal to the anal sphincter has proven helpful in enhancing rectal retention. This procedure can, however, be extremely uncomfortable for the client.

If hyperkalemia is severe, more rapid measures, such as 50% dextrose with regular insulin, IV push, may be used. The insulin increases the permeability of the cell membrane and returns the potassium to the intracellular space. The glucose prevents the development of hypoglycemia. This method generally is reserved for times when there are ECG changes, usually when the potassium exceeds 7.0 mEq/L. It lowers serum potassium levels immediately, but its effect is temporary, and other means for permanent reduction must also be used.

Calcium gluconate may also be given when there is ECG evidence of hyperkalemia. Calcium stabilizes the cardiac membranes and restores the normal threshold for excitation. Calcium should be administered when the client is on continuous ECG monitoring, since arrhythmias may result from calcium administration.

The general caloric recommendation for clients maintained on chronic dialysis is about 35 kcal/kg of ideal body weight. Chronic dialysis clients who become ill with other problems or require surgery usually have dietary limitations temporarily removed so that nutritional needs may be met through more liberal choice of food intake. This is to ensure healing and prevent further debilitation from infection or stress. Nutritional supplements may be offered, such as milk shakes made with a high-carbohydrate and high-fat additive. Potassium restrictions, however, are not removed.

Severely debilitated or critically ill clients in severe need of adequate nutrition will be fed via parenteral or enteral alimentation. In general, protein intake is not restricted when these methods of feeding are required. If necessary, more frequent dialysis can control fluid and BUN levels. With parenteral or enteral alimentation and concurrent dialysis, frequent examination of the client's serum is necessary to monitor electrolyte levels. Rapid imbalances

---

Box 32–4	**Protein Foods of High and Low Biological Value**

Proteins of High Biological Value Are Found in:

Meat

Fish

Poultry

Eggs

Cheese

Proteins of Low Biological Value Are Found in:

Potatoes

Rice

Spaghetti

Bread

Other vegetable products

---

of electrolytes may produce critical situations if careful monitoring is not part of the routine.

Promoting a well-balanced diet for a client who often has no appetite or a metallic taste in the mouth is a challenge for the nurse, especially if the previously mentioned restrictions must be followed. Appetite may be improved by providing oral hygiene and fresh air, minimizing movement, and administering prescribed antiemetics. A mouthwash of sodium acid phosphate will relieve the uremic fetor (ammonialike breath). Sucking on hard candy can also relieve the bad taste. Work with the dietitian to provide appetizing meals, perhaps in small, frequent feedings supplemented by nourishing snacks. The mealtime environment should be pleasant and free of unpleasant odors. The client's food preferences as elicited in the nursing history should be considered, and explaining the rationale underlying the diet may encourage the client to eat more.

IMPROVING GAS EXCHANGE

For clients with metabolic acidosis from acute or chronic renal failure, oxygen–carbon dioxide exchange may be improved with the administration of sodium bicarbonate or with the institution of dialysis. Sodium bicarbonate may also be administered to treat hyperkalemia, because correcting metabolic acidosis helps to correct hyperkalemia. Correction of metabolic acidosis and the lowering of serum potassium levels are an important part of stabilizing the client with acute renal failure. Sodium bicarbonate may be administered orally in tablet form or intravenously. The major risk associated with IV administration of sodium bicarbonate is that it may further expand extracellular fluid volume and worsen problems of hypervolemia, if they are present. Since the correction of acidosis can lead to calcium deficits, it is important to observe for signs of tetany. The dialysate used for either peritoneal dialysis or hemodialysis contains acetate, which converts to bicarbonate when absorbed. Thus, dialysis will provide for the replacement of depleted bicarbonate stores.

Decreased oxygenation due to fluid accumulation in the lungs may impair gas exchange; thus ventilation should improve when dialysis removes fluid from the lungs. Respiratory rate, pulse rate, and arterial blood gases should be monitored to prevent cardiopulmonary arrest.

In addition to sodium bicarbonate and dialysis, oxygen will usually be prescribed for administration via a cannula. Ensure that the airway is patent and help the client into a semi-Fowler's position to ease respiratory effort. Moderately or completely unresponsive clients should be positioned on their sides to prevent aspiration of secretions or stomach contents. Clients who hypoventilate because their surgical incision makes breathing painful should receive analgesics before coughing and deep-breathing exercises. After the procedure, assist the client into a comfortable position and instruct him or her in how to splint the incision. Splint the incision until the client is able to do so alone.

IMPROVING SELF-CONCEPT

Nursing interventions to improve the client's self-concept as a result of alterations in body image require time for listening to the client's concerns and anxieties. Verbalizing feelings about urinary diversion procedures or the need for vascular or catheter access for dialysis is essential in nursing care for these clients. After the initial period of shock passes, opportunities to talk with other clients who have successfully managed these adjustments may be helpful. Nurses who patiently support clients learning new self-care practices will promote feelings of confidence and ease the burdens associated with changed body image.

Suggest that changes in skin color—the ashen-yellow appearance—may be partially masked by colors such as bright red or blue that tone down the yellow. Orange, green, yellow, and white should be avoided. Severe edema may be hidden by loose-fitting clothing. Gain the client's confidence, however, before discussing these sensitive subjects. Explaining the physiological changes that contribute to body changes will help the client cope.

The client having a kidney transplant also has special needs. Professional counseling and ventilation of feelings with the nurse will help the client learn to live with the fact that his or her kidney once was in someone else. The client also will need guidance in adjusting to the long-term effects of immunosuppressive therapy (moon face, buffalo hump, osteoporosis, thinning of hair, etc).

The development of renal failure may necessitate several changes in a client's roles. The client may have to quit working entirely, change jobs, or work part-time. Feelings of not being worthwhile are common. Someone may need to be hired to carry out household tasks, or other family members will have to take on additional responsibilities. All these changes require crisis intervention by the health care team, because they may seem insurmountable at first. Government aid for the care of renal failure clients may ease the financial burden.

MAINTAINING URINARY CONTINENCE

A variety of interventions may be chosen for the client with an alteration in urinary pattern either because of incontinence, a neurogenic bladder, or urinary diversion. Incontinent men may elect to wear an external catheter (also called a *condom catheter*), which is preferable to continuous internal catheter drainage. The major drawback of this catheter is that the penis may become excoriated and painful if the area is not kept clean. Even with good hygiene, skin breakdown can occur. A satisfactory external catheter does not exist for women. A detailed discussion of nursing interventions for clients with incontinence or neurogenic bladder is presented in Chapter 33. Nursing interventions for clients with urinary diversions are presented in Chapter 34.

Nursing Research Note

Hume M: Factors influencing dietary adherence as perceived by patients on long-term intermittent peritoneal dialysis. *Nurs Papers* 1984; 16(1):38–53.

This research examined factors that clients on intermittent peritoneal dialysis perceive as influencing dietary adherence. The sample consisted of 25 subjects ages 29 to 79 years.

Clients' self-reports and clinical measures were approximately the same in estimating dietary adherence. The subjects reported more positive than negative influence on dietary adherence. Health beliefs and values were positively related to compliance when the individual perceived the importance of diet to health, held health as a value, and when the dialysis team communicated the importance of diet modification. Factors that negatively affected adherence were dietary habit changes, thirst, diet difficulty, and poor appetite.

Almost all subjects described the illness as having disrupted their social role; almost all subjects perceived the severity of their illness. Nineteen subjects stated that this perceived severity encouraged them to comply with the diet. Almost all subjects stated they were compliant because diet was essential to physical health.

Situational factors such as family support, duration of the diet regimen, and interactions with the health team supported adherence. Nineteen subjects stated that changing the diet interfered with adherence; 14 of the subjects thought that adherence increased with time.

In nursing intervention with end-stage renal disease clients, education of family and clients will help to facilitate an understanding of the seriousness of their illness. Consistent dietary communication about the need for compliance may enhance compliance. In addition, maintaining one diet, decreasing negative factors (eg, thirst and diet difficulty), and increasing nursing involvement in diet adherence and assessment may encourage compliance with dietary restrictions.

PROMOTING SEXUALITY

Clients with urinary diversions may have problems with sexuality. The presence of stomata and appliances to collect urine may embarrass clients who may feel they are no longer sexually attractive to their partners. The partners, in turn, may feel unable to cope with the clients' alterations and may need counseling before being able to offer support. If a client feels wanted by the partner, adjustment will be easier. Suggestions by the nurse or a sexual counselor on alternate sexual intercourse positions may be helpful and can encourage the couples to experiment in determining what is best for them.

Alterations in sexual functioning also occur in clients with end-stage renal disease. The problems include infertility, loss of libido, inability to have an erection, cessation of menstruation, and decrease in vaginal lubrication. Clients on immunosuppressants following renal transplant may develop some characteristics of the opposite sex, such as softening of skin and hair loss in men or, occasionally, development of facial hair in women.

The client may be reluctant to share information and concerns about loss of libido or loss of potency. For clients in the child-producing years, the nurse may initiate discussions about sexual functioning through discussion about birth control practices or routine health practices, such as the annual pelvic examination, PAP test, or breast self-examination. Comments from men about altered masculinity may provide opportunity for discussions about sexuality. Be supportive and nonjudgmental when the client shares these highly personal feelings. The client must be confident that the communication is kept confidential.

At the same time that significant physiological changes such as hormonal secretion alterations contribute to problems of impotence, sterility, and decreased libido in uremic clients, alterations in their self-concept, self-esteem, body image, and role performance also contribute to emotional concerns regarding sexual expression. If free communication and trust have been established between the client and the nurse, discussions may explore these concerns. For example, they may discuss alternative methods for sexual expression and satisfaction, including use of sexual appliances (eg, vibrators), penile implants, oral and manual stimulation of the genitals, and cuddling and massaging by the couple. Sexual counseling may interest the client and spouse, and the nurse should identify resources, if appropriate.

MAINTAINING TISSUE PERFUSION

Nursing interventions during a period of impaired tissue perfusion include careful monitoring of the client's vital signs and urinary output. Fluid volume or blood replacement should occur at the prescribed rate, and the nurse should promptly report to the physician any inability to administer the fluid as prescribed. If severe hemorrhage is causing the lack of renal tissue perfusion, the client will need to be prepared for potential emergency surgery.

For clients with renal failure, severe hemorrhage or fluid volume loss may significantly affect cardiac and cerebral tissue perfusion. The blood count of the client with end-stage renal failure is chronically low. Because the hemoglobin and hematocrit usually are in the range of 7 to 8 g/dL and 20% to 30% respectively (decreased erythropoietin), the available hemoglobin for tissue perfusion is greatly reduced. Although clients experience chronic fatigue, vital processes normally are not impaired. If further hemoglobin loss occurs, however, cardiac dysrhythmias, angina, and hypotension may develop. Expect to administer packed red blood cells and oxygen, monitor cardiac and neurologic status, and immediately report any dysrhythmias or change in the level of consciousness.

Nonacute correction of impaired tissue perfusion may be achieved through the administration of iron supplements, folic acid, anabolic steroids, and judicious administration of blood transfusions.

Section IV: Evaluation

Expected outcomes for the client with kidney and urinary tract dysfunction are presented in Table 32–3. The following information supplements the data in the table. If data collected do not substantiate these expected outcomes, nursing plans must be revised.

COMFORT

Nursing interventions related to comfort are successful if the client is resting, moving, or sleeping comfortably. Facial expressions and body movements should be relaxed and without tension. Relief from pruritus is successful if the client does not constantly scratch or ask to be scratched on the back or if skin is free of excoriation from frequent scratching.

SKIN INTEGRITY

Data supporting the maintenance of skin integrity include healed surgical incisions without redness or drainage, absence of excoriation from scratching, the absence of decubitus ulcers from pressure, and evidence that the client is eating the prescribed diet.

ABSENCE OF INFECTION

Evaluation of the absence of infection includes the measurement of normal body temperature, a normal white blood cell count, and the absence of chills. In addition, the client should not have foul-smelling urine or wound drainage, and catheter and vascular sites should be free of erythema, drainage, or tenderness.

FLUID VOLUME

Blood pressure recorded at the client's normal level verifies successful interventions for stabilization of fluid volume. In addition, the client should have a stable body weight reflective of his or her dry weight. The client should demonstrate knowledge of the fluid allowance, how to calculate fluid intake and loss, and how to compare weight changes with feelings of physical well-being. For example, the client who suddenly becomes short of breath should be able to suspect that the dry weight has been exceeded and the blood pressure will be elevated. Other manifestations of normal fluid volume include absence of cerebral manifestations such as syncope or light-headedness with changes in posture. The client should not feel nauseated or thirsty; peripheral edema should be minimal, and there should be no rales or congestion in the lung fields.

THOUGHT PROCESSES

Successful correction of altered mental functioning may be determined through orientation to person, place, and time, clarity of the client's speech, improved alertness and ability to remember explanations, and the absence of asterixis. No tremors or myoclonus should occur.

NUTRITION

Improvement of nutritional status may be assumed if the client is eating the prescribed diet without nausea and vomiting. Over a period of several weeks to months, laboratory values for albumin, total protein, and electrolytes should become normal. Other evidence of adequate nutrition includes healing of wounds and maintenance of skin integrity.

GAS EXCHANGE

Indications that oxygenation is adequate include arterial blood gases that give evidence of a pH between 7.35 and 7.45, a carbon dioxide content of 38 to 42 mg/dL, and an oxygen level greater than 60%. In addition, the client should have no subjective feelings of respiratory distress and should perform normal exercise without undue respiratory embarrassment. Slight tachypnea is common in clients who use respiratory compensation for metabolic acidosis, but the client usually is not aware of the increased respiratory rate.

SELF-CONCEPT AND SEXUAL FUNCTION

Successful nursing interventions result in the client's ability to verbalize freely feelings related to self-concept, self-esteem, changes in body image, altered performance of roles, and altered sexuality. If the client fails to discuss feelings in all areas, however, nursing interventions have not necessarily failed. Respect for appropriate timing and sensitivity to the client's need for delay or denial of feelings to cope with other stressors is another successful nursing intervention. The transplant recipient should demonstrate increasing ability to cope with having a donor kidney and with the effects of immunosuppressants.

URINARY PATTERN

The client with altered urinary elimination patterns should not have bladder distention or incontinence and should be able to manage the alteration in urine flow without difficulty.

TISSUE PERFUSION

Adequate tissue perfusion may be verified through the measurement of blood pressure and pulse in the client's normal range. In addition, the client should not experience chest pain or arrhythmias with activity. The client should demonstrate orientation to person, place, and time.

Section V: Renal Failure

The previously mentioned nursing diagnoses, plans of care, and evaluations are appropriate for clients with various disorders associated with the kidneys and urinary system, including chronic and acute failure. The specific disorders that lead to acute and chronic renal failure will be discussed in the next chapter. Acute and chronic renal failure must be discussed in some detail here, however, as an introduction to the discussion of dialysis.

Acute renal failure that is reversible occurs rapidly over a period of hours or days. Causes of acute renal failure are divided into three categories: prerenal, renal, and postrenal. *Prerenal causes* diminish renal perfusion but do not cause tubular damage unless prolonged. Examples are shock, severe hemorrhage, severely diminished cardiac output, and renal artery stenosis or thrombosis. Damage to the renal parenchyma (glomeruli and tubules) characterizes *renal causes,* which result from acute glomerulonephritis or acute tubular necrosis (ATN). *Postrenal* causes include any cause of urinary tract obstruction, such as bilateral ureteral stones, benign prostatic hypertrophy, or carcinoma. Therefore, in prerenal and postrenal causes the kidney is normal, but with renal causes the kidney is damaged. About 75% of all acute renal failure is caused by ATN (Holloway, 1984). Despite the cause, clients with acute renal failure cannot excrete waste products or regulate fluid, electrolyte, and acid–base balances.

The four phases of acute renal failure are: onset, oliguric, diuretic, and recovery (Table 32–5). The onset phase can be as short as 24 hours or as long as one week. Detection of acute renal failure and prevention of further renal damage are the priorities during this period. In the oliguric phase, urine output falls below 400 mL/day. This phase usually begins within 48 hours of the renal insult and may last up to 2 weeks. During this phase serum creatinine and BUN levels rise steadily. The diuretic phase begins when urine output rises above 400 mL/day, but BUN and creatinine levels continue to increase. Regeneration of kidney tubules occurs during this phase, which generally lasts about 2 weeks. During the recovery phase, which lasts about 4 to 12 months, laboratory values begin to stabilize and return to normal. The actual and potential nursing diagnoses previously discussed are especially appropriate during the oliguric and diuretic phases. Hyperkalemia is the most common and serious problem. Dialysis will most likely be required if uremia develops, and it should continue until the client stabilizes in the recovery phase.

Chronic renal failure, which is irreversible, is a slow, gradual loss of renal function that develops over a period of months or years. Causes of chronic renal failure will be discussed in Chapter 33. Chronic renal failure is characterized by three stages: diminished renal reserve, renal insufficiency, and uremia. Renal damage occurs in the *diminished renal reserve stage*. Nitrogenous wastes do not accumulate, however, because 50% of renal function still exists. With *renal insufficiency*, nitrogenous wastes in the blood increase slightly, but the kidneys function well enough to sustain life. Metabolic or physiological stresses may be difficult for the kidneys to handle, however. During the *uremic stage*, the creatinine clearance value falls below 10 mL/min. Nitrogenous wastes and fluid, electrolyte, and acid–base imbalances may necessitate dialysis or renal transplantation to sustain life. The nursing diagnoses previously discussed apply to chronic renal failure. A case study for the client with chronic renal failure is presented at the end of Chapter 33.

Section VI: Dialysis Interventions

When conservative treatment of renal failure is no longer effective, and renal function has deteriorated to the point where death will ensue, dialysis therapy must be started. Kidney transplantation, another alternative for clients with chronic or end-stage renal disease, will be discussed in Chapter 34.

Principles and Types of Dialysis

The combination of three principles—diffusion, osmosis, and filtration—permits the removal of metabolic wastes and excess electrolytes and fluids from the client with renal failure by artificial means. Dialysis involves the differential *diffusion* of substances (solute) across a semipermeable membrane that separates two fluid compartments containing substances of different concentrations. The pressure gradient produced results in the flow, or diffusion, of substances to the less concentrated area. This process continues until the concentrations are equal on each side. *Osmosis*, the movement of fluid or solvent from a lower concentration to a higher one, also occurs during dialysis. *Filtration*, the movement of both solvent and solute across a semipermeable membrane under force, also occurs. An increase in hydrostatic pressure on one side of the membrane used for dialysis drives fluid and dissolved substances into the opposite side.

Indications for Dialysis

In acute renal failure, dialysis is usually begun when acidosis, hyperkalemia, and other uremic symptoms no longer can be controlled. In chronic renal failure clients, dialysis should be started before the appearance of symptoms of uncontrolled hypertension and acidosis, bone disease, peripheral neuropathy, uremic encephalopathy, and severe anemia. This is generally when creatinine clearance values fall below 5 mL/min and serum creatinine levels are greater than 10 mEq/L (Saxton et al., 1983). Clients who begin dialysis before these problems arise are more likely to remain complication-free and sustain normal life activities than clients who begin dialysis after these symptoms arise.

Dialysis affects only fluid, electrolyte, and acid–base imbalances (and only during the time it is performed), so it cannot completely substitute for renal functions such as the production of erythropoietin and renin; detoxification of drugs; and intermediary metabolism of glucose, insulin, and vitamin D.

There are two types of dialysis: **peritoneal dialysis** and **hemodialysis.** In peritoneal dialysis, the client's own peritoneal lining serves as the semipermeable membrane, whereas in hemodialysis, an artificial kidney contains the semipermeable membrane. These two procedures will be discussed in greater detail in the next sections. Refer to Table 32–6 for a comparison of the advantages of the two types of dialysis.

Table 32–5 Stages of Acute Renal Failure

Stage	Duration	Laboratory Data	Urine Output	Fluid Allowance	Dietary Modification
Onset	24 h–1 wk	↑ Creatinine ↑ BUN	Normal or decreasing	No restriction	None
Oliguric/anuric	8–15 days (average)	↑ Creatinine ↑ BUN ↑ Potassium ↑ Phosphorous ↓ Calcium ↓ Bicarbonate	Oliguria: <400 mL/24 h Anuria: <100 mL/24 h	600 mL + urine output for previous 24 h	Restricted potassium; low protein to control BUN; high-calorie, high-carbohydrate diet and fat to meet nutritional needs; parenteral or enteral nutrition may be needed; no added salt if hypertensive
Diuretic Early	Variable	↑ Creatinine ↑ BUN ↑ Potassium ↑ Phosphorus ↓ Calcium ↓ Bicarbonate	Greater than 400 or 100 mL/24 h; may reach 2 or 3 L per day	At least equal to urinary output plus 600 mL/24 h	Continue as above; monitor lab data
Late	Variable	↑ ↓ Creatinine ↑ ↓ BUN ↑ ↓ Potassium ↑ ↓ Phosphorous ↓ ↑ Calcium ↓ ↑ Bicarbonate	Usually stabilizes between 2 and 3 L/24 h	As above	Protein and potassium no longer restricted; high caloric needs remain
Recovery	Up to 12 m	Creatinine and BUN levels stabilize near preinsult normal	Around 1500 mL/24 h	Normal	Normal diet; sodium not restricted unless high blood pressure remains

Client Implications in Dialysis

The client usually decides the mode of dialysis to be used, and the health care team gives support and recommendations. Factors that influence this decision include answers to the following questions: What aspects of the client's lifestyle, work goals, or travel considerations may influence the method of dialysis selected? Is the client capable of self-care? Continuous ambulatory peritoneal dialysis (CAPD) may be the best alternative for a motivated, active person. What social support system does the client have? Family members often can be taught to carry out dialysis at home, although the training program is extensive and usually requires 8 to 12 weeks. Do physical complications or limitations make one mode of dialysis less than ideal or contraindicated? (Contraindications of each type of dialysis will be discussed in their respective sections.) The client should participate actively in the selection of the method for chronic dialysis or the client may choose to have no dialysis at all. Some clients may prefer to die rather than to face chronic dialysis or renal transplantation.

Because of the enormous cost of dialysis or transplantation, Public Health Law 92-603 was enacted in 1972 to fund dialysis or transplantation treatment for clients with end-stage renal disease who were eligible for Medicare. It also provided assistance to eligible clients' dependents. In 1974, this coverage was extended to cover the care of all US citizens. Hence, the government now pays for approximately 90% of all treatment for end-stage renal disease. However, the high cost of the program makes it the subject for constant review and reconsideration. About 60,000 clients are now being maintained on dialysis; each year about 6,800 new clients begin dialysis, and another 5,600 clients receive transplants. At least another 6,000 persons could receive a transplant if a kidney was available. The annual cost of the program has stabilized at about a billion dollars for

Table 32–6 Advantages of Hemodialysis and Peritoneal Dialysis

Hemodialysis	Peritoneal Dialysis
1. Requires 12–15 h/wk compared to up to 48 h with peritoneal dialysis 2. Can be used when peritoneal dialysis is contraindicated because of abdominal lesions 3. Causes rapid reversal of fluid and electrolyte imbalances 4. Does not result in protein loss	1. Can be started in 1 h (this includes time for catheter placement) 2. Is a simple procedure 3. Because it is slow, there are fewer distressing symptoms 4. Coagulants are not necessary 5. Does not cause blood loss 6. Includes CAPD, which is less expensive and allows client flexibility

approximately 60,000 clients. With this large population, obviously the prevention of renal failure and cost-effective treatment are necessary. The cost of peritoneal dialysis and hemodialysis for one client ranges from about $25,000 to $30,000 per year with somewhat lower figures for home dialysis. A kidney transplant costs about $20,000. Medical costs after kidney transplant range from $1,000 to $2,000 per year.

HEMODIALYSIS

Hemodialysis removes nitrogenous waste products, excess electrolytes, and excess fluid from the blood via a specially processed, cellophanelike dialyzing membrane. The membrane, housed in a dialyzer in the artificial kidney machine, maintains sterility and integrity. A vascular access (to be discussed later) provides a route for blood to exit the body and then return to the vascular system.

While outside the body, the blood is pumped through the artificial kidney machine, composed of a pump, a semipermeable membrane, and a source of dialysate solution for the removal of waste products from the blood. In addition to these basic components, a variety of devices monitor and ensure the safety of the system. Regulation of the pump adjusts the rate of blood flow; the goal for blood flow is usually 200 to 300 mL/min. The most common semipermeable membrane is a hollow-fiber kidney that serves as a negative pressure dialyzer. Its hollow fibers are made of synthetic materials that are permeable to water, electrolytes, and nitrogenous waste products but impermeable to plasma proteins and red blood cells. The hollow fibers are encased in a plastic cylinder, which also contains portals for entry and exit of the dialysate. Other types of dialyzers include the coil (positive pressure), the Hoeltzenbein (negative pressure), and the parallel or flat plate (negative pressure) types.

The client is heparinized before dialysis is initiated, the machine is loaded with a heparinized solution before

blood is sent through the dialyzer, or both. Blood flows from the client's body through plastic tubing into the hollow fibers and returns to the client's vascular system through plastic tubing.

Dialysate is a solution composed of water, glucose, sodium, chloride, potassium, calcium, and acetate or bicarbonate. It contains varying amounts of substances to help remove as much or as little water, electrolytes, and waste products from the blood as are indicated by the client's laboratory values. While blood is pumped through the semipermeable hollow fibers, dialysate is delivered into the plastic cylinder containing the fibers. The flow of dialysate thus continuously surrounds the fibers, but the dialysate does not come in direct contact with the blood inside them. While the dialysate is in contact with the hollow fibers, waste products and excess electrolytes diffuse into it from the blood. The dialysate exit is at the end of the plastic cylinder opposite the blood entry point, which minimizes the possibility of the waste products being reabsorbed.

Removal of water is by osmosis and filtration. Because the glucose concentration in the dialysate is greater than the glucose concentration in the blood, water moves from the blood into the dialysate by osmosis. The higher the glucose concentration of the dialysate, the more water is removed by osmosis. If water were removed only by this method, however, the time required for the process would be very long. Therefore, more water may be removed by increasing the hydrostatic pressure applied to the blood as it flows through the dialyzer, resulting in the ultrafiltration of the blood. Another method of pressure application to increase removal of water is the use of negative pressure, or suction. Negative pressure is applied to the membrane, and water is pulled from the blood as it passes through the dialyzer.

Dialyzers are available in a variety of sizes. Larger dialyzers provide a greater surface area for removal of waste products, but they also require a larger volume of blood to fill the hollow fibers; this can lead to hypotension, one of the complications of hemodialysis. Complications will be discussed in a later section. The blood is also warmed after dialysis before it returns to the client.

Indications/Contraindications

Hemodialysis can treat acute or chronic renal failure. Because it corrects hyperkalemia, metabolic acidosis, or hypervolemia in 1 to 2 hours, it is the dialysis of choice in emergency situations. Hemodialysis is preferred over peritoneal dialysis whenever there is a hypercatabolic state, a diaphragmatic leak, severe respiratory insufficiency, a large abdominal wound, intra-abdominal cancer, abdominal adhesions or scar tissue, peritonitis, or critical volume excesses such as pulmonary edema or pericardial friction rub. Hemodialysis is contraindicated when there are clotting disorders, circulatory instability, or cardiovascular disease. Some treatment centers think that diabetes is also a contraindication to hemodialysis because of the possibility that large amounts of heparin may result in blindness for the diabetic client. The blindness may also be the result of the natural progression of diabetic retinopathy.

Requirements/Routines

Hemodialysis requires a vascular access. A variety of vascular accesses are available: the **arteriovenous** (AV) **fistula;** vessel substitutes such as the bovine graft, or synthetic graft materials such as the Gore-Tex graft; the cannula, an external **arteriovenous shunt;** and catheters for subclavian or femoral placement. Other experimental devices are being used with varying degrees of success. For clients with chronic renal failure, the AV fistula is the preferred access. An AV fistula is the internal anastomosis of an artery to a vein, and for hemodialysis the nondominant forearm usually is chosen (Figure 32–7). After 8 to 12 weeks, the vein wall becomes thickened and more muscular, resembling an artery. The fistula also distends and becomes prominent. At this point, the fistula is considered mature and is expected to be able to withstand frequent venipunctures and to provide adequate blood flow for the hemodialysis procedure (nursing care will be discussed later). The average lifetime of a fistula is about 3 to 4 years.

A bovine graft is a section of a blood vessel from a cow that has been treated to avoid contamination. It is implanted with one end in an artery and the other in a vein. Like the fistula, it is internal (Figure 32–8). If possible, at least 1 week should elapse between the bovine graft surgery and use of the graft. This type of access is used in the same way as the AV fistula.

A Gore-Tex graft is a synthetic tube used in place of a bovine graft or fistula. It is placed in the same manner as the bovine graft: One end of the tube is attached to an artery and the other, to a vein. Two weeks should elapse

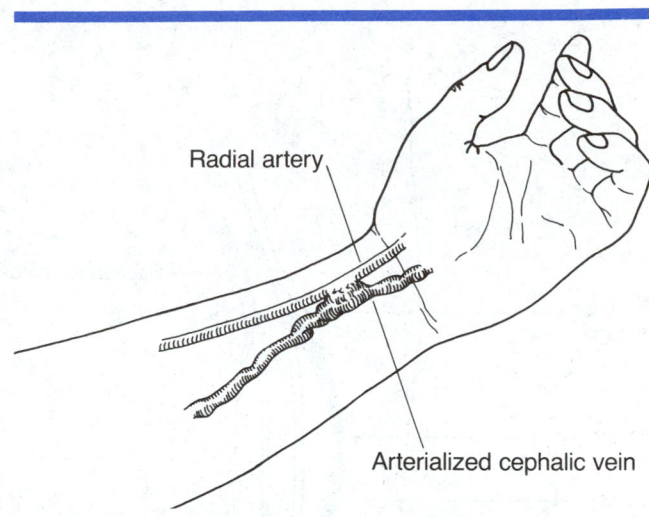

Figure 32–7

Arteriovenous (AV) fistula for hemodialysis.
SOURCE: Holloway N: *Nursing the Critically Ill Adult: Applying Nursing Diagnosis,* 2nd ed. Menlo Park, CA: Addison–Wesley, 1984, p. 299.

from the time of surgery to the time of dialysis. This access also is used in the same way as the fistula.

A cannula, or arteriovenous shunt, is another form of vascular access used for hemodialysis. It is an external connection of an artery to a vein in which two pieces of synthetic tubing form a loop (Figure 32–9). One limb of tubing is sutured into an artery, and the other is sutured into a vein. The two limbs of shunt tubing are joined by either a t-connector or a straight connector. The t-connector has the advantage of allowing blood to be withdrawn, or fluids or medication to be administered intravenously via the cannula, thus avoiding venipuncture. In some centers, a straight connector is used, especially when a cannula has a tendency toward clotting. It is thought that a disadvantage of the t-connector is increased resistance to blood flow through the slightly narrowed diameter of its lumen. A straight connector is generally preferred for outpatients with a cannula. Their external junction may be disconnected and attached to tubing to accomplish extracorporeal blood flow through the artificial kidney machine. Cannulas are considered temporary forms of vascular access because they can be used immediately. For this reason, they may be appropriate for acute renal failure clients or for chronic renal failure clients while a fistula develops. The lifetime of a cannula is usually less than 1 year. The cannula is typically placed in the dominant forearm, although the other arm, a thigh, or an ankle may be selected. The dominant forearm is preferred as a temporary site so that when a permanent access is developed, the client will have the more usable hand and arm for activities during the dialysis treatment.

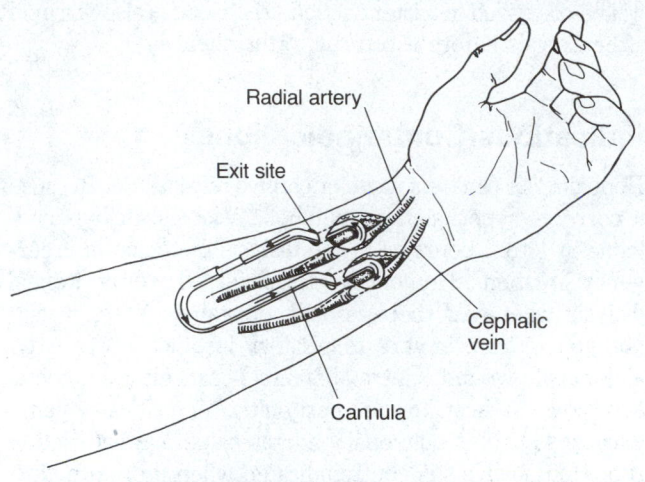

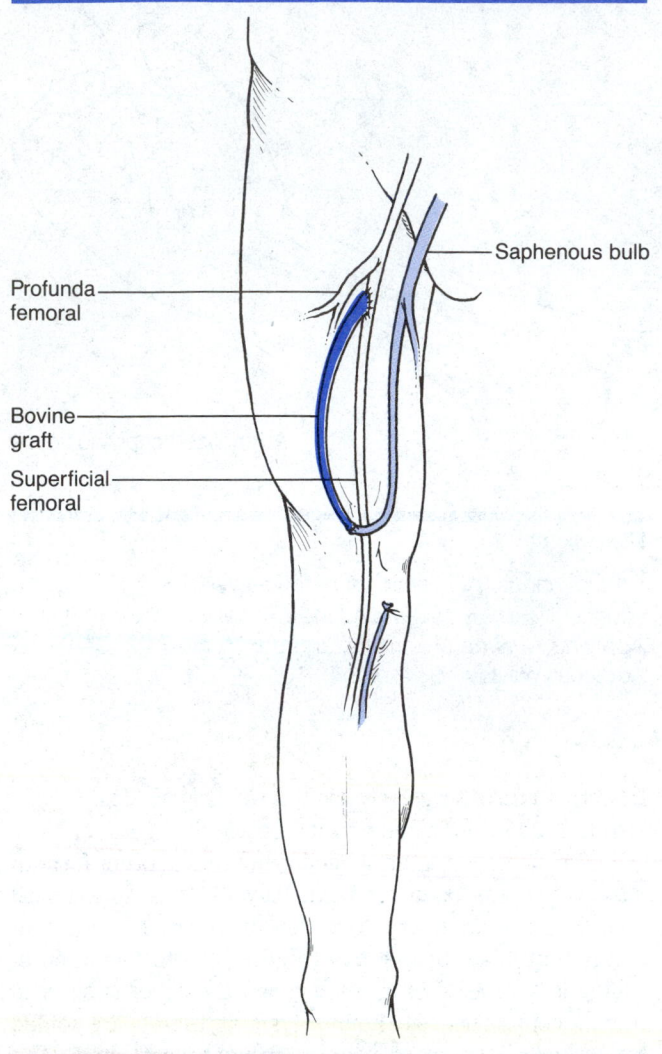

Figure 32–8

Bovine graft between the superficial femoral artery and saphenous vein, forming an AV fistula.

Figure 32–9

Standard AV shunt (cannula) for hemodialysis.
SOURCE: Holloway N: *Nursing the Critically Ill Adult: Applying Nursing Diagnosis,* 2nd ed. Menlo Park, CA: Addison–Wesley, 1984, p. 296.

Complications

The potential problems with hemodialysis include air emboli, angina, arm pain, bleeding fistula, blood transfusion reaction, blood vessel spasm, bone disease, cardiac dysrhythmias, clotting in dialyzers, cramps, dyspnea, eye changes, fever and chills, headache, hepatitis, hemolysis, hypertension, infection, nausea and vomiting, neuropathy, and pruritus, as well as the most common problems of hypotension, seizures, and blood loss (Cairoli & Voyce, 1982). Refer to Table 32–7 for a summary of the causes, assessments, nursing interventions, and expected outcomes for each of these potential problems.

Nursing Implications

Hemodialysis treatments are not without risk to the client. Because the artificial kidney machine or its monitoring system can malfunction and cause death, it is necessary to obtain informed consent from the client or guardian prior to initiating the treatment. The physician explains the benefits and risks of the procedure, and the nurse frequently obtains the signature and, if there is lack of client understanding, initiates further teaching.

The client receiving hemodialysis treatment requires close nursing supervision. Check the blood pressure at the beginning of the treatment and at least every 30 minutes throughout. Hemodialysis treatments for the client with end-stage renal failure commonly last 4 hours three times a week. However, the client with acute renal failure who is extremely catabolic, requires parenteral nutrition, or both, may require hemodialysis more frequently to maintain fluid

Special catheters also have been developed for placement in blood vessels with a large blood flow. Subclavian and femoral catheters have been used successfully when immediate hemodialysis is needed, and no other form of vascular access exists.

There are a limited number of vessels in which cannulas can be placed or fistulas established. Stenosis or thrombosis of a vascular access often result in its permanent loss as an access site. However, advances in vascular surgery techniques and the increased availability of synthetic grafts have resulted in the ability to create alternate blood flow patterns in the same limb. For example, synthetic grafts may be tunneled subcutaneously to bypass the area of stenosis or clotting. In addition to the forearms and thighs, the upper arms, and even the anterior chest wall, have been used as access sites.

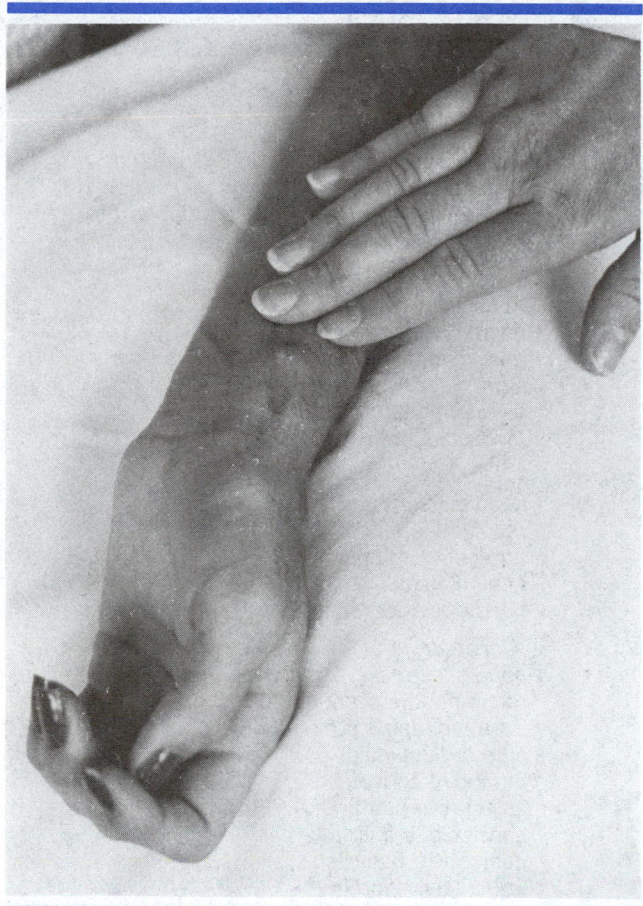

Figure 32–10

Palpating an AV fistula.

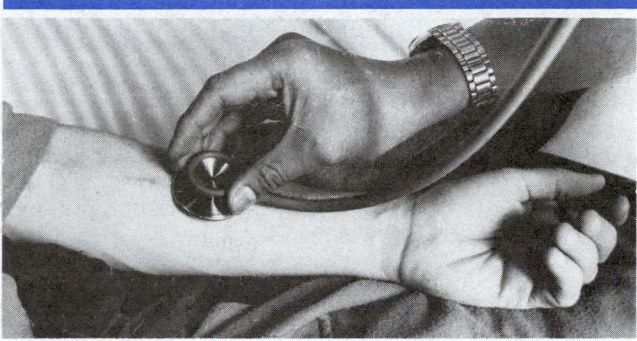

Figure 32–11

Listening for bruits.

and electrolyte balance and remove nitrogenous waste products.

Monitor the vascular access for patency, absence of infection, and absence of bleeding. The cannula and fistula should be checked for patency every hour for the first 24 hours after insertion and then at least every 4 hours by palpation of the thrill and auscultation of the bruit. A thrill is a rippling sensation palpable on the venous side of the cannula or fistula. It is usually more readily palpable in a fistula than a cannula (Figure 32–10). The bruit, heard through the stethoscope, is a rushing or roaring noise or "swoosh" timed with each heartbeat (Figure 32–11). Failure to detect a thrill or bruit when either was previously present suggests loss of patency, usually because of clotting of the access. A properly trained nurse should declot a cannula immediately, as time is critical. Clotted fistulas may require surgical intervention. In either case, once patency has been established, measures to prevent reclotting—continuous heparin infusions, administration of Low Molecular-Weight Dextran (LMD), and antiplatelet agents such as dipyridamole (Persantine)—should be considered.

The client and significant others should be instructed in checking patency of the access so they can do so at least

every 4 hours. Some medical centers suggest checking every 1 to 2 hours, especially following dialysis. The client with a fistula should be taught to:

- Keep the arm elevated and extended at first
- Avoid lying on the access (such as having the arm curled under the head while sleeping)
- Avoid wearing constricting clothing or jewelry on the affected extremity
- Allow no venipunctures or blood pressure cuffs or tourniquets to be placed around the extremity
- Watch for signs of infection

The nurse should also follow these rules when caring for a client who has had surgery for a fistula, as well as check for capillary refill in the extremity. In some centers, clients receive specific instructions on exercises or activities to increase the strength of the vessel walls until the fistula is mature and ready to be used (ie, for approximately 8 to 12 weeks). Emphasize to the client that the vascular access is a lifeline and should be protected as such. A fistula does not require a dressing, since it is internal.

The client with a cannula requires slightly different care. Because the cannula can be used immediately, no exercises are needed. The client with a cannula should also be taught to check for patency, as previously discussed. In addition, advise the client that the blood should be bright red. If the blood is dark or if clots can be seen in the tubing, the cannula must be declotted immediately. Although the cannula is wrapped in gauze to prevent separation or infection, a small loop of tubing should be made easily accessible by lifting up a piece of the gauze. This permits visualization of the blood in the tubing and can be assessed for the warmth characteristic of the tubing of a patent cannula. The same restrictions apply to the cannula as to the fistula, for example, no blood pressure cuffs or tourniquets, no restrictive clothing or jewelry, and no lying on the access.

The subclavian and femoral catheters do not have an arterial-to-venous flow so there is no thrill or bruit. Pat-

Table 32—7   Nursing Care for Complications of Hemodialysis

Complication	Cause	Assessments	Nursing Interventions	Expected Outcomes
Air embolus	Nonfunctioning air detector; air leak in tubing; careless fluid administration	Presence of dyspnea or chest tightness; presence of cyanosis; foam in blood tubing	Clamp blood line; lower client's head and turn client to left side; notify physician	No dyspnea; no cyanosis or cough; no cardiac arrest
Angina	Anxiety; hypotension	Presence of chest pain	Administer oxygen; decrease blood flow rate; monitor EKG; start IV; provide sedative or antianginal medications	No chest pain
Arm pain	Prolonged immobility; needle position; trauma at needle site	Presence of pain, numbness, or throbbing in arm	Avoid traumatic needle insertion; readjust needle and arm position; apply heat; consider needle replacement	No pain
Bleeding fistula	Overheparinization; prolonged clotting time; too little pressure at puncture site; trauma; aneurysm at site	Bleeding or formation of hematoma at puncture site	Avoid trauma at needle insertion; rotate needle sites; if bleeding, apply pressure and topical thrombin; consider giving IV protamine; check clotting time during next dialysis and adjust heparin dose	No bleeding after 10 min
Blood loss	Dialyzer leak; blood line separation; fistula needle replacement	Leaking at needle sites; blood detector alarm activated; air in blood lines	Depends on type of dialyzer; give blood transfusion as needed	Resolution of blood loss
Blood transfusion reaction		See Chapter 28		
Blood vessel spasm	Irritation of blood by cold normal saline or albumin	Presence of cold along vessel path	Avoid giving cold IV solutions; apply heat to affected area	No evidence of vessel spasm
Bone disease	Calcium–phosphate imbalance; hyperphosphatemia; impaired vitamin D metabolism; decreased calcium absorption; excess parathyroid hormone	Evidence of bone degeneration from x-ray, pathological fractures, or elevated serum phosphate levels; pain; altered gait	Increase phosphate binders and calcium in dialysate; evaluate client's diet and medication regimen; assure client compliance with phosphate binders and increase dosage if necessary; add calcium to dialysate after serum phosphorus is normalized	No evidence of bone degeneration on x-ray; client verbalizes correct diet and medication regimen
Cardiac dysrhythmias		See Chapter 23		
Cramps	Fluid depletion; ischemia; sodium shift	Presence of tingling sensation or cramps	Apply local heat and massage area; decrease blood flow; give quinine sulfate prior to dialysis; give	Minimal cramps or none

Complication	Cause	Assessments	Nursing Interventions	Expected Outcomes
			mannitol, glucose 50%, or concentrated saline IV push if indicated	
Dyspnea	Fluid excess; air embolus; dialyzer content returned too rapidly at end of dialysis	Difficulty breathing; tightness in chest; cyanosis; rapid and labored respirations	Administer oxygen; remove excess fluid; observe for air in system	Diminished respiratory distress or comfortable breathing
Eye changes (red eye syndrome, band keratopathy, hypertensive retinopathy)	Diabetes; hemodialysis	Decreased visual acuity; retinal hemorrhages	Reduce heparin during dialysis; assist client as needed; client may need surgery or laser treatment; promote safety	Improvement or stabilization of eyesight
Fever/chills	Transfusion reaction; diffusion of bacterial toxin into blood across membrane	Headache; itching; chest pain; fever; chills; hypotension; hives; dyspnea	Send blood cultures to lab; check temperature and blood pressure often; give antipyretic drugs if ordered, after all necessary cultures have been obtained; stop dialysis	Absence of symptoms
Headache	Hypertension; disequilibrium; emotional problems	Headache; nausea	Slowly increase blood flow and ultrafiltration; medicate as ordered; treat hypertension; provide shorter treatments more often	Absence of headache
Hepatitis	Exposure to hepatitis virus(es); frequent blood transfusions; failure to minimize client contact with blood of other clients; failure to follow procedures to prevent transmission of hepatitis	Monitor for signs and symptoms; check blood of client and health care workers often	Thoroughly cleanse and properly dispose of equipment; wear gloves, meticulously wash hands; clean up blood spills	Absence of hepatitis
Hypertension	Volume overload from too much salt and water; anxiety	Blood pressure elevated above client's normal; weight gain above client's normal; headache, nausea	Initiate vigorous ultrafiltration; begin antihypertensive therapy; monitor blood pressure	Normotension; weight at estimated dry weight
Hypotension	Congestive heart failure; eating; fluid depletion; presence of two access sites; gastrointestinal bleeding	Nausea; blurred vision; loss of consciousness; seizures; abnormally low blood pressure	Monitor blood pressure; weigh client every 2 h on dialysis; provide small or no meals during dialysis; give normal saline	Weight not below dry weight; normotension
Infection	Decreased immunocompetence; failure to use aseptic technique in caring for	Drainage, redness, or swelling at exit site; elevated temperature and WBCs	Obtain cultures and CBC; administer antibiotics; review technique for dialysis	No symptoms of infection

(continued)

Table 32–7   Nursing Care for Complications of Hemodialysis (continued)

Complication	Cause	Assessments	Nursing Interventions	Expected Outcomes
	vascular access; failure to use aseptic technique when inserting catheters or needles or attaching or disconnecting blood lines			
Nausea and vomiting	Hypotension (frequently the earliest symptom); physical or emotional disequilibrium; GI upset	Nausea; vomiting	Monitor client's potassium level; decrease blood flow rate and remove ultrafiltration; medicate as ordered; prevent if possible by preventing hypotension and keeping client NPO during dialysis	No nausea; no evidence of vomiting
Neuropathy	CNS disorders; inadequate dialysis	Burning, pain, or weakness in extremities; leg weakness	Reassess type and size of dialyzer; consider increasing frequency or duration of dialysis treatment	Freedom from pain; burning or weakness in extremities
Pruritus	Transfusion or drug reaction; inadequate dialysis; uremia; reaction to hollow-fiber dialyzer	Itching, scratching by client	Increase dialysis time; give antipruritic drugs; stop drugs or blood transfusion; instruct client to use fatty soaps (such as BASIS) and avoid lotions with alcohol content	No scratching or itching
Seizures	Hypotension; epilepsy; mechanical dysfunction; disequilibrium	Presence of aura or muscle twitching; petit mal or grand mal seizures	Prevent hypotension; take seizure precautions; administer antiseizure medications; prevent injury to client; note characteristics of seizure	Control or absence of seizures

Adapted from: Cairoli OM, Voyce PK: *Memory Bank for Hemodialysis.* Pacific Palisades, CA: Nuresco, 1982, p 198.

ency of these catheters is maintained through intermittent irrigations with a dilute heparin-saline solution or by the intermittent instillation of a heparinized saline solution.

Infection at the insertion site and, subsequently, the bloodstream is a common problem and source of concern for the client with vascular access. Frequent manipulations and the presence of foreign materials in the blood make the cannula, the subclavian catheter, and the femoral catheter all likely sites for infection. Employ aseptic technique whenever the tubings are disconnected and blood exposed, such as when attaching or disconnecting bloodlines or placing a t-connector or straight connector. The skin over the fistula puncture sites should be prepared carefully with a bactericidal solution.

Since the cannula is external, preventing infection is particularly important. Thoroughly cleanse the cannula site after washing the hands. Wear sterile gloves when opening the cannula. Do not pull or tug on the tubing. Some health care centers suggest scrubbing the client's skin with bactericidal soap and rinsing the area with sterile saline, whereas others recommend swabbing exit sites with hydrogen peroxide. Next, apply a bactericidal ointment at the exit sites, and put dry, sterile gauze under the tubing. It is important to keep the tubing from touching the skin, so wrap the area with gauze, and cover the tubing lightly with gauze. Leave some tubing accessible to check patency, however.

Bleeding is another complication of the vascular access. With the cannula, the two options for joining the limbs of the tubing are the t-connector and the straight connector discussed earlier. Regardless of which option is selected, care should be taken to prevent disconnection. Taping a bridge prevents the pulling apart of the cannula tubing and minimizes the chances of hemorrhage. If a cannula pulls apart, the client can bleed to death in minutes; for this reason, bulldog or alligator clamps should be attached to the plastic wrap or elastic bandage that covers the gauze around the cannula. This way, the cannula tubings can be clamped off immediately should they become disconnected. The fistula, bovine graft, or Gore-Tex graft require direct pressure over the two venipuncture sites to control hemorrhage. Blood clots at each site will form in about 10 minutes. If new bleeding develops, direct pressure over the site for about 10 minutes will usually result in hemostasis. If bleeding occurs around the subclavian or femoral catheter insertion site, direct pressure, topical hemostatic agents (such as thrombin), or a pressure dressing may be required to stop it.

The client receiving hemodialysis treatments, either acutely or chronically, needs extensive physical care. The client's emotional needs are just as great. Because peritoneal dialysis and hemodialysis create essentially the same psychological stresses, the psychological implications of both types will be described after the following discussion of peritoneal dialysis. Figure 32–12 illustrates the components of hemodialysis nursing care.

PERITONEAL DIALYSIS

During peritoneal dialysis the peritoneal membrane, which lines the abdominal cavity and is richly supplied with small capillaries, serves as the semipermeable membrane for dialysis. The peritoneal membrane allows the diffusion of small molecules such as electrolytes, urea, creatinine, uric acid, and glucose, all of which have molecular weights below 200. It is impermeable to large molecules such as blood cells and proteins, which have molecular weights greater than 50,000.

During peritoneal dialysis, a catheter (a common one is the Tenckhoff catheter) is placed into the abdominal cavity (Figure 32–13). A temporary or permanent catheter may be inserted at the client's bedside, but the permanent catheter generally is inserted in surgery. Dialysate is then instilled through the catheter into the abdominal cavity. Through diffusion and osmosis, excess electrolytes, nitrogenous waste products, and fluid are transported from the blood into the dialysate. The dialysate is then drained, and new, pure dialysate is instilled.

A complete cycle involves new fluid running in (inflow phase), sitting for diffusion and osmosis (dwell time), and being drained out (outflow phase). The length of each cycle affects the efficiency of dialysis. During the inflow phase, which usually lasts about 5 to 10 minutes, about 2 L of dialysate are allowed to flow into the abdominal cavity after it has been warmed to enhance diffusion and minimize discomfort. During the dwell phase of about 30 minutes, dialysis

takes place. Initially, the exchange rate is rapid, but it slows down in later cycles, when dialysate and blood composition are similar. The outflow phase, which lasts about 20 minutes, begins when the dialysate flows out of the abdomen. These cycles may be accomplished manually, with the aid of an automatic peritoneal dialysis machine, or through continuous ambulatory peritoneal dialysis (CAPD).

With manual peritoneal dialysis, the fluid is exchanged every 60 minutes for 30 to 40 hours. This method is slow and inefficient, but it effectively clears waste products and removes fluid when rapid decreases are not required.

With an automatic peritoneal dialysis machine, the cycling and the amount of dialysate to be infused are preset. Pressure alarms inform the nurse of any problems with inflow or outflow. About 10 to 16 hours of treatment are necessary two or three times a week. Intermittent peritoneal dialysis (IPD) by machine is relatively easy to learn, and many clients do this form of therapy at home. Clients who select IPD for use at home usually require the assistance of a second person. Midway through the procedure, eight new 2-L bottles of dialysate must be added to the system. The bottles are cumbersome, and the tubing that connects the machine to the peritoneal catheter is not long. Therefore, the client generally has limited freedom to move about. Furthermore, reaching up to place the bottles on the hangers above the machine requires more strength and mobility than many home IPD clients have.

The client using CAPD enjoys greater freedom and independence. The same permanent peritoneal catheter is used, but dialysate is always present in the abdominal cavity. The dialysate is drained into a bag attached by tubing to the peritoneal catheter four times a day, every day of the week (Figure 32–14). Exchanges are timed to occur about every 4 to 5 hours and at bedtime. This lack of machine dependency is appealing to many people who want to maintain as normal a lifestyle as possible. With CAPD, the client assumes responsibility for all aspects of the dialysis procedure. For those unable to assume responsibility for the procedure, the significant other can receive training to help provide this treatment. Many clients who have experienced other modes of therapy report that they feel better more consistently with this form of continuous dialysis.

Indications/Contraindications

Peritoneal dialysis, a relatively simple procedure, may be used when hemodialysis is not available. It is often chosen over hemodialysis for acute renal failure clients when immediate results are not crucial. Some advantages of peritoneal dialysis are that it can be used for clients with clotting disorders, cardiovascular disease, exhausted vascular access sites, inadequate veins (the very young and very old), and diabetes, as well as for clients who refuse blood transfusions.

Peritoneal dialysis is contraindicated in clients with active pathological conditions in the abdomen, including

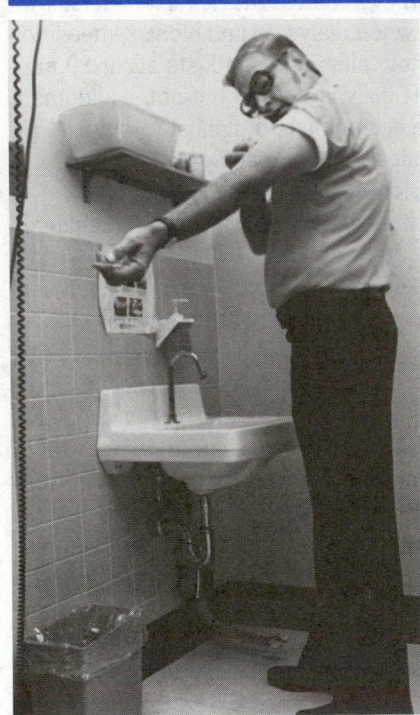

A. Client participates in care by taking baseline temperature before beginning treatment while cleansing the access site.

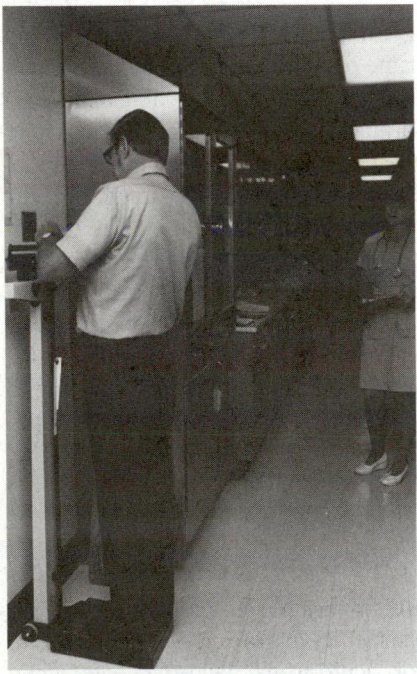

B. Client weighs in before dialysis. Weight determines how much fluid has been gained since last treatment and how much needs to be removed.

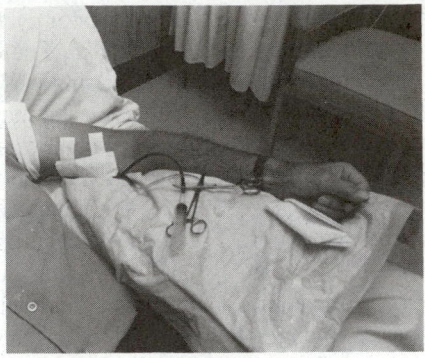

C. Needles have been placed in the fistula prior to connection to extracorporeal blood tubing. The arterial line has blood in it; the other is the venous line.

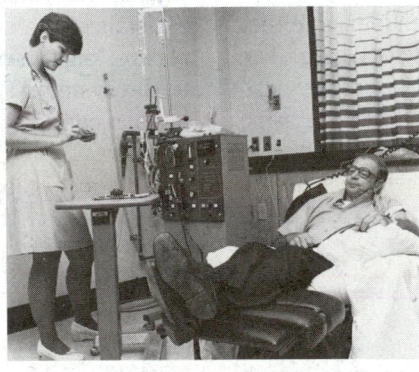

D. Nurse uses a calculator to determine the machine settings for removing the desired amount of fluid. Client's legs are elevated to promote hemodynamic stability.

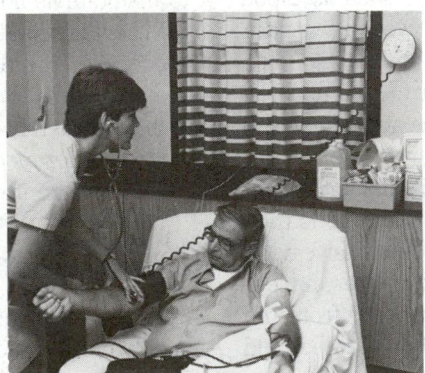

E. Monitoring the client's blood pressure during dialysis treatment.

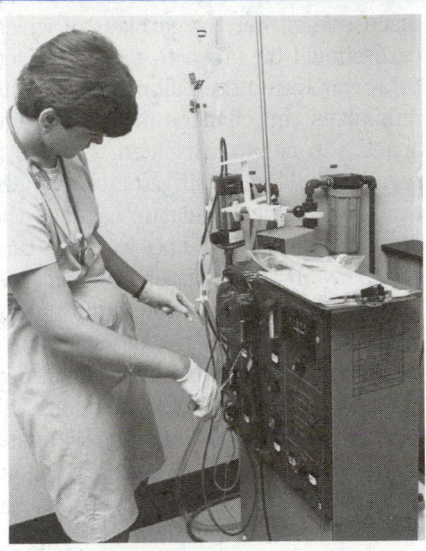

F. Nurse prepares for treatment of hypotension by volume replacement with IV normal saline.

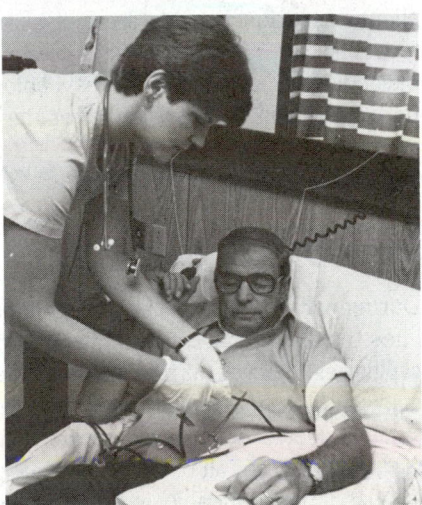

G. Disconnecting the client at the end of treatment.

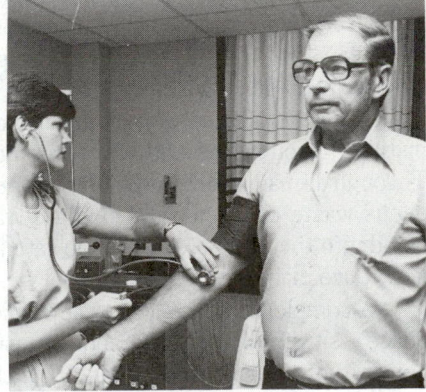

H. Obtaining a standing blood pressure reading after dialysis treatment to verify that too much blood has not been removed.

Figure 32–12

Hemodialysis unit and components of nursing care.

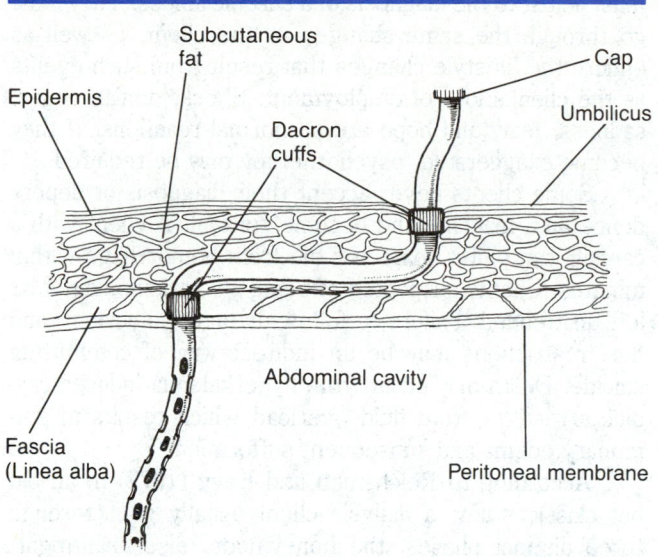

Figure 32–13

Catheter placement for peritoneal dialysis. The permanently implanted catheter exits from a point different than the insertion site through a subcutaneous tunnel.

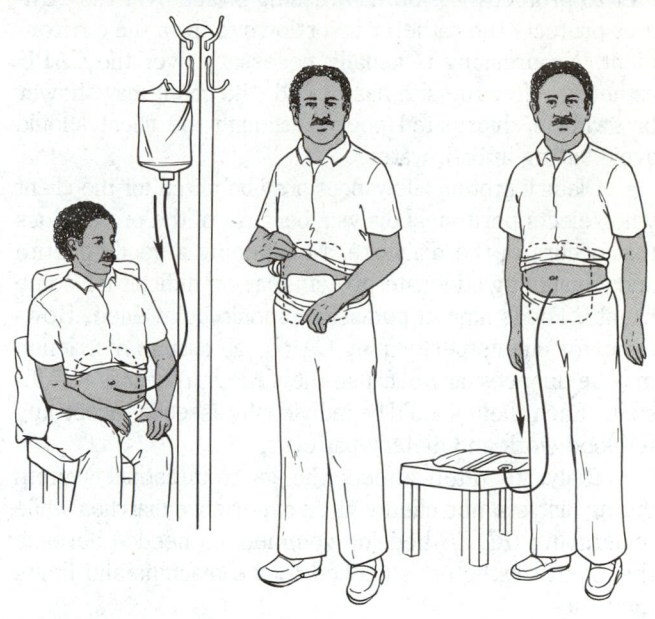

Figure 32–14

Client performing CAPD at home.

diaphragmatic leaks, abdominal wounds, abdominal cancer, abdominal adhesions, or infected abdominal wall, as well as for respiratory insufficiency or a hypercatabolic state.

Complications

The primary complication of peritoneal dialysis is peritonitis or infection of the catheter and the tunnel of tissue through which the catheter enters the abdominal cavity. Instruct the client to report any abdominal discomfort or change in the appearance of the peritoneal fluid. Normally, the peritoneal fluid returned is clear and uncolored. Cloudy, discolored, or bloody fluid suggests that infection is present, and appropriate treatment is required without delay. Other symptoms of infection include fever and abdominal tenderness. Instillation of antibiotics into the peritoneal cavity accompanied by several peritoneal flushings may effectively treat infection. If the peritonitis persists, catheter removal may be necessary to eradicate the infection. Multiple episodes of peritonitis are believed to result in the development of scar tissue in the peritoneal membrane, which decreases the surface area available for clearance of waste products.

Hyperglycemic and hyperosmolar syndromes may occur during the procedure, especially when the dialysate contains high glucose levels. The blood absorbs solute at the same time that water flows out of the blood by osmosis, which causes an increased solute concentration in the blood. These changes can lead to hyperosmolar coma with hypovolemia that can lead to shock. Treatment involves monitoring serum glucose levels and administering insulin to reverse the high serum glucose levels. Occasionally, salt-

poor albumin may be required to increase the amount of interstitial fluid movement into the plasma.

Protein loss is unavoidable during peritoneal dialysis; this necessitates an increased dietary intake of high-quality protein such as eggs, meat, fish, and poultry, which contain all the essential amino acids. Other complications include perforation of the bowel, bladder, or major blood vessel during catheter insertion; respiratory distress, especially at the onset of dialysis; and outflow obstruction by either a change in the client's position, peritonitis, or formation of a fibrin clot.

Nursing Implications

Nursing care of the client during peritoneal dialysis procedures includes monitoring blood pressure, pulse rate, temperature, and body weight. The specific method of peritoneal dialysis and the stability of the client determine the frequency of monitoring. Obtain all measurements prior to beginning the dialysis treatment and at its conclusion.

After the peritoneal catheter has been placed, the catheter site and the dressing should be kept clean and dry. The dressing should be occlusive. Temporary catheters are usually removed after the completion of the treatment and replaced if necessary. If more than one or two peritoneal dialysis treatments are anticipated, a permanent peritoneal catheter is generally placed. The Dacron Teflon cuffs on the permanent catheter stabilize the catheter in the subcutaneous tissue and form a partial barrier to the entrance of bacteria (see Figure 32–13).

The IPD catheter is capped at the end of the dialysis treatment. After capping, gauze is placed under the catheter to protect the skin. A dressing placed over the catheter protects the catheter insertion site from the environment. No dressing is usually necessary over the CAPD catheter. After the site has healed, the client may shower or swim in chlorinated pools, although the client should avoid sitting in bath water.

Dietary protein allowances are liberalized for the client who selects peritoneal dialysis because of the protein loss that occurs in the dialysate. Maintaining a good appetite and consuming adequate protein may be difficult for some clients. Foods high in potassium should be avoided. However, for clients performing CAPD, potassium restriction may be unnecessary because the CAPD process is so efficient. Each client should be individually assessed according to blood work and dietary patterns.

Dialysate often affects the gastrointestinal system during dialysis, and clients often experience diarrhea while undergoing IPD. A bedside commode is needed because the client's catheter is hooked to the machine and limits movement.

Although peritoneal dialysis generally offers some increased independence (particularly CAPD), many clients experience significant changes in body image. The permanent peritoneal catheter and/or the presence of 1 to 3 L of dialysate in the peritoneal cavity both alter body contour. Although the tube and drainage bag can be concealed reasonably well, a slim waist and flat abdomen are not possible. Thus, the client may need to alter clothing selection. If possible, the client should discuss clothing style preferences with the surgeon prior to placement of the catheter, since the identification of the normal waistline or belt line can enhance comfort after surgery.

PSYCHOSOCIAL IMPLICATIONS OF DIALYSIS

Although the physiological aspects of both hemodialysis and peritoneal dialysis are numerous, the psychosocial ones are also. The psychosocial implications of both types of dialysis are similar and are discussed together here.

Clients with chronic renal failure must adjust to the fact that they have a chronic and terminal illness. Life can be prolonged with dialysis or transplantation, but death may occur any time complications arise. For instance, if the peritoneal lining becomes infected, peritoneal dialysis is no longer possible. If all four limbs have exhausted vascular accesses, hemodialysis is not possible. Therefore, clotting or infection is a serious threat to these clients.

Adjusting to a chronic illness involves phases similar to the changes that occur with the death of loved ones. First, people are shocked to hear the news. Then they become angry and depressed or deny the existence of death. Acceptance finally occurs, it is hoped. Thus, certain psychological reactions are normal and expected, and the nurse should help the client work through these feelings and offer support (see Chapter 16). The client's family also

must adjust to the diagnosis of a chronic illness. They must go through the same changes as the client, as well as endure the lifestyle changes that result from such events as the client's loss of employment. Shock, denial, anger, sadness, fear, and hope are all normal reactions. If they become exaggerated, psychotherapy may be required.

Some clients never accept their diagnosis or dependence on a machine and become suicidal. A client with a cannula can pull it apart and die from hemorrhage within minutes. Clients suspected of being suicidal should not be left unattended. Failure to follow dietary (potassium) and fluid restrictions may be an indirect way of committing suicide. Death may occur from hyperkalemia-induced cardiac arrest, or from fluid overload which results in pulmonary edema and subsequent suffocation.

According to Reichsman and Levy (1972) in an old but classic study, a dialysis client usually goes through three distinct phases: the honeymoon, disenchantment, and long-term adaptation phases. Euphoria characterizes the honeymoon stage, which begins during the first weeks of dialysis and can last up to 6 months. Emotional and physical states markedly improve. The disenchantment phase begins 3 to 12 months after dialysis is begun; the client becomes depressed over the change-related stresses. The client finally begins to accept and cope with dialysis in the long-term adaptation phase, which begins 6 to 15 months after the initiation of dialysis. Remember, however, that responses vary. Not everyone experiences these phases in the same way.

During adjustment, most clients display responses such as regression, anxiety, hostility, or depression. Regression occurs because of increasing dependency on others. Anxiety is common because of the fears of death, dialysis, uremia, physical and socioeconomic changes, and altered family relationships. This reaction intensifies if impotence becomes a problem. Hostility, which is directed toward family and staff members, is related to all the restrictions on the client. Finally, the client becomes depressed, realizing that the previous lifestyle must change to allow for diet modifications and hours spent in dialysis.

The client's family may experience similar reactions. Roles and relationships must withstand severe strains. New marriages or marriages in trouble are usually more affected than stable, long-term ones. A family that was close before dialysis probably will become more supportive and helpful. A family that was not close, however, may dissolve. The family can greatly affect the client's attitude toward dialysis.

Since acceptance of the dialysis treatment and compliance with the dietary and medical regimen are important to the client's well-being, the nurse must help the client and significant others adjust to all the stresses. If this cannot be accomplished, the inability to cope can lead to a deterioration in physical status that may result in death. Chapter 16 discusses strategies that the nurse can employ in working with dying clients. Support systems for both clients and nurses are discussed in Chapter 4.

Chapter Highlights

Subjective symptoms that prompt the client with kidney or urinary system problems to seek health care are usually related to a change in the amount or general appearance of urine or alterations in comfort.

Because of anxiety related to renal and urinary functioning and proximity to external genitalia, clients may have difficulty communicating their concerns.

Previous difficulties of the renal and urinary system may recur and cause long-term problems.

Creatinine clearance and serum creatinine values are the best indicators of renal function.

A urinalysis will provide many clues to the cause of the client's symptoms.

Diagnostic studies used for clients with urinary dysfunction include x-rays, ultrasonography, dye clearance studies, nephrotomography, radionucleotide scanning, computerized tomography, renal angiography, intravenous pyelography, cystoscopy, cystography, renal biopsy, and urodynamic studies.

For the client with alteration in comfort related to pain, promoting comfort includes administering analgesics appropriate to the source and severity of pain, avoiding nephrotoxic analgesics, and providing other nursing comfort measures.

Nursing measures to relieve pruritus for the client with urinary dysfunction include keeping the client's fingernails short, avoiding agents that dry the skin, removing urochrome pigments on the surface of the skin, using oil-based lotions, controlling the phosphorous–calcium balance, administering antipruritic medications, and using ultraviolet light.

Nursing measures related to the maintenance of skin integrity include providing a nutritious diet that follows the limitations placed on the client, relieving pruritus, repositioning and turning the client with edema every 1 to 2 hours, and providing good skin care.

Restoration of fluid volume involves fluid restrictions, diuretics, and dialysis for fluid volume excesses or the administration of fluids with appropriate electrolytes for fluid deficits.

Helping the client maintain satisfactory mentation involves performing dialysis to remove nitrogenous wastes and control metabolic acidosis; giving simple, repeated instructions; and promoting safety.

Nursing measures to overcome nutritional imbalances include encouraging the intake of a well-balanced diet that is low in sodium and potassium for renal failure clients, high in protein for clients who have proteinuria or are undergoing peritoneal dialysis, low in protein for clients undergoing hemodialysis, or specially ordered for clients with recurrent infections or calculi.

Promoting adequate oxygen–carbon dioxide exchange in the client with urinary dysfunction involves correcting metabolic acidosis with dialysis and the administration of sodium bicarbonate, removing excess fluid with dialysis, encouraging surgical clients to cough every hour, and administering oxygen as needed.

Nursing measures to improve the client's self-concept and sexuality involve listening to the client and encouraging ventilation of feelings related to ostomies, dialysis, transplantation, and role changes.

Acute renal failure has four phases: onset, oliguric, diuretic, and recovery. Detection of acute renal failure and prevention of further renal damage are priorities.

Dialysis to cleanse the blood of uremic toxins, excess water, and electrolytes is begun in acute renal failure clients when the symptoms can no longer be controlled and in chronic renal failure clients when the creatinine clearance value falls below 5 mL/min or when uremic symptoms are problematic.

Dialysis works on the principles of diffusion, osmosis, and filtration.

With hemodialysis, a vascular access is necessary, the time involved is about 12 to 15 hours a week, and an artificial kidney contains the semipermeable membrane across which waste products flow.

With peritoneal dialysis, the peritoneal membrane serves as the semipermeable membrane, there are fewer risks, and up to 48 hours a week are involved in treatment.

Bibliography

Binkley LS: Keeping up with peritoneal dialysis. *Am J Nurs* 1984; 84:729–733.

Byrne CJ et al: *Laboratory Tests: Implications for Nursing Care.* 2nd ed. Menlo Park, CA: Addison-Wesley, 1986.

Cairoli OM, Voyce PK: *Memory Bank for Hemodialysis.* Pacific Palisades, CA: Nuresco, Inc, 1982.

Holloway NM: *Nursing the Critically Ill Adult: Applying Nursing Diagnosis.* Menlo Park, CA: Addison-Wesley, 1984.

McConnell EA, Zimmerman MF: *Care of Patients With Urologic Problems*. Philadelphia: Lippincott, 1983.

Pagana KD, Pagana TJ: *Diagnostic Testing and Nursing Implications: A Case Study Approach*. St. Louis: Mosby, 1982.

Perras ST, Mattern ML, Zappacosta AR: Presentation of treatment modalities for the ESRD patient: Peritoneal dialysis. *AANNT J* 1984; 11: 43–46.

Reichsman F, Levy NB: Problems in adaptation to maintenance hemodialysis: A four-study study of 25 patients. *Arch Intern Med* 1972; 130: 859–865.

Rose BD: *Pathophysiology of Renal Disease*. New York: McGraw-Hill, 1981.

Saxton DF et al: *Addison-Wesley Manual of Nursing Practice*. Menlo Park, CA: Addison-Wesley, 1983.

Sims TN, Ulrich B: Successful utilization of subclavian catheters for hemodialysis and apheresis access. *AANNT J* 1983; 10:41–44.

Smith DR: *General Urology,* 19th ed. Los Altos, CA: Lange Medical, 1981.

Suggested Readings

Chambers JK: Bowel management in dialysis patients. *Am J Nurs* (July) 1983; 83:1051–1052. The author discusses the treatment measures renal dialysis patients must follow that contribute to constipation and then offers suggestions for modifying the usual guidelines nurses give for managing the problem of constipation.

Criss E: Digital subtraction angiography. *Am J Nurs* (Nov) 1982; 82:1706+. Discussion of digital subtraction angiography (DSA), an innovative alternative to traditional arteriography in the evaluation of arterial occlusive disease. The DSA involves the placement of a catheter into the brachial vein and injecting contrast media into it. The advantage of DSA is the decreased risk to the client and the capability of the test's being done without admission to the hospital.

Denniston DJ, Burns KT: Home peritoneal dialysis. *Am J Nurs* (Nov) 1980; 80:2022+. Discussion of advances in catheters for permanent placement and machinery for dialysate delivery that have permitted the development of systems for home peritoneal dialysis. Criteria for client selection and components of the training program are described in this article.

Fleming LM, Kane J: Step-by-step guide to safe peritoneal dialysis. *RN* (Feb) 1984: 44–47. The pages of this article are filled with colorful photographs that illustrate the steps needed to connect and disconnect the catheter from the cycler and dress the catheter site.

Jaskula SJ et al: *An Exercise Program for the Person With Chronic Renal Disease*. St. Louis: The National Kidney Foundation of Eastern Missouri and Metro East, Inc, 1982. Description and illustration of five levels of exercise. Simple explanations, large print, and clear drawings make this booklet an excellent reference for staff and clients.

Kjellstrand CM: Current problems in long-term hemodialysis. *Dialysis and Transplantation* 1980; 9(4):295+. Includes acute problems of hypotension, hypertension, nausea, vomiting, muscle cramps, and headache. Chronic problems include arteriosclerosis, infection, and peripheral neuropathies. This article also describes new methods of treatment and some of the potential benefits.

Whitson SE: Nursing care of the chronic renal failure patient with sexual dysfunction. *AANNT J* (Oct) 1982; 9:48–49, 58. The pathophysiological and psychological bases for sexual dysfunction in CRF clients and helpful nursing interventions are discussed.

Resources

SELF-HELP GROUPS AND OTHER ORGANIZATIONS

American Council on Transplantation (ACT)
4701 Willard Ave.
Suite 222
Chevy Chase, MD 20815
Phone: (301) 652-0994

The American Council on Transplantation (ACT) was formed in 1984 to address the multiple issues of concern related to organ and tissue donation and transplantation. ACT is a federation of member organizations such as the ANA, NATCO, AHA, and AMA, as well as individual lay and professional members. The purposes of ACT are to promote public and professional education about the need for increased availability of donated organs and tissues and the advances in the successful transplantation of organs and tissues. A major focus of the federation is to work for coordinated voluntary efforts to assure equitable access and distribution of donated organs and tissues. A quarterly newsletter is published, an annual business and educational meeting is held, and a hot line is available.

Help For Incontinent People
PO Box 544
Union, South Carolina 29379

This newly organized nonprofit organization is designed to promote national interest in the problem of incontinence. The organization publishes a quarterly newsletter, "The HIP Report," and other resources of interest to the public and health professionals.

National Association of Patients on Hemodialysis
   and Transplantation (NAPHT)
505 Northern Blvd.
Great Neck, NY 11021
Phone: (516) 482-2720

This organization, made up largely of clients, promotes the well-being of clients with kidney dysfunction and provides education for lay persons and professionals on kidney disease and treatment. There are several local chapters. They publish a newsletter and several pamphlets and brochures. Kidney client ID card available.

National Kidney Foundation
116 E. 27th St.
New York, NY 10016
Phone: (212) 889-2210

This voluntary agency is concerned with the prevention and treatment of kidney diseases. It sponsors a national program of organ donors, research, education, and client services through local chapters. Publications on the organ donor program, kidney functioning, and kidney disease are available. Persons interested in donating their kidneys should contact a local affiliate for information.

United Network for Organ Sharing (UNOS)
PO Box 5303
2024 Monument Ave.
Richmond, VA
Phone: (800) 446-2726

> A computer network that lists the names of persons waiting for a kidney transplant as well as their blood and tissue types. About 110 local affiliates are associated with transplant programs while another 41 function independently and contract with transplantation centers for organ procurement and placement.

United Ostomy Association, Inc.
1111 Wilshire Blvd.
Los Angeles, CA 90017
Phone: (213) 481-2811

> Persons who have had urostomies, colostomies, or ileostomies belong to this national organization through its almost 500 local chapters in the United States and Canada. It provides local support groups and also serves as an educational resource and publishes pamphlets and brochures.

In Canada: Calgary Ostomy Society
210 86th Ave., SE, Apt. 91
Calgary, Alberta, Canada T2H 1N6

> A Canadian chapter of the United Ostomy Association. For information on other Canadian affiliates write to the national headquarters listed above.

HOT LINE

American Council on Transplantation
Phone: (800) ACT-GIVE

> This national phone number is maintained to answer questions about organ and tissue donation and transplantation.

Information Clearinghouse for Dialysis and Transplant Patients
(National Association of Patients on Hemodialysis and Transplantation)
Phone: (516) 482-2120 (24-hr hotline)

> Provides information on kidney dialysis, transplant, or chronic disease. Makes a resource file available and offers referrals to state and local agencies for further services.

HEALTH EDUCATION INFORMATION

American Cancer Society
(local chapters or national headquarters)
> "Urinary Ostomies: A Guidebook for Patients," second edition
> "Living With Your Urostomy"

These are available at no charge to clients or health professionals.

Jeanette K. Chambers, RN, MS
Renal Clinical Nurse Specialist
Dialysis Unit
Riverside Methodist Hospital
3535 Olentangy River Road
Columbus, OH 43214

> "Living with Kidney Failure," 44 pages, illustrated. $8.00 each. (Discounts for multiple copies.) Books mailed postpaid. Send check or money order payable to Riverside Methodist Hospital.

National Association of Patients on Hemodialysis and Transplantation (NAPHT)
> "Dialysis Worldwide for the Traveling Patient"
> "Living With Renal Failure"
> "Na-K-Counter"
> "Renal Failure and Diabetes"
> "Transplant Kidneys—Don't Bury Them"

SPECIALTY ORGANIZATIONS

American Nephrology Nurses Association (ANNA)
Box 56
Pitman, NJ 08071
Phone: (609) 589-2187

> The goal of this organization is to provide education and support for nurses involved in the care of clients with kidney disease. Sponsors regional meetings and a national conference and publishes the ANNA journal, a bimonthly publication.

American Urological Association, Allied
6845 Lake Shore Drive
Raytown, MO 64133
Phone: (816) 358-3317

> Membership in this organization is composed of RNs, LPNs, and any allied care workers who have completed an approved course of instruction and are actively engaged in urology. Dues, $50 new members; $45 renewals.

Council of Nephrology Nurses
and Technicians
National Kidney Foundation

> Membership in the council is open to nurses interested in nephrology nursing. An annual educational program and business meeting coincides with the meeting of the National Kidney Foundation.

International Association for Enterostomal
Therapy, Inc.
505 N. Tustin Ave. Suite 282
Santa Ana, CA 92705
Phone: (714) 972-1720

> This organization provides care and rehabilitation to persons with abdominal stomas, and to those with incontinence. Members are enterostomal therapists and interested others who are licensed to practice medicine or nursing. Dues, $65.

North American Transplant Coordinators
Organization (NATCO)
% Mark Reiner
J-286 Department of Surgery
J.H. Miller Health Center
Gainesville, FL 32610
Phone: (904) 392-3741

> The major purposes of NATCO are to provide a forum for discussion of issues common to transplant coordinators and to educate new transplant coordinators. The organization also maintains a donor registry. Membership is open to all transplant coordinators, many of whom are RNs. An annual meeting and periodic training courses are conducted.

Chapter 33

Specific Disorders of the Kidneys and Urinary System

Jeanette K. Chambers
Jane Hokanson Hawks

Objectives

When you have finished studying this chapter, you should be able to:

Discuss the clinical manifestations and nursing interventions for reflux nephropathy and polycystic kidney disease.

Identify treatment measures and nursing implications for acute tubular necrosis, urinary incontinence, and neurogenic bladder.

Describe clinical manifestations, medical treatment, and nursing measures for clients with analgesic abuse nephropathy, nephrosclerosis, renal artery stenosis, and diabetic glomerulopathy.

Discuss the clinical manifestations and treatments for membranous nephropathy, nephrotic syndrome, and acute and chronic glomerulonephritis.

Describe the clinical manifestations and nursing implications for the client with infectious processes in the urinary tract (urethritis, cystitis, acute and chronic pyelonephritis, and renal abscess).

Explain the circumstances associated with renal cell and bladder cancer and interventions for clients with these disorders.

Discuss risk factors, signs and symptoms, and nursing care of clients with renal or ureteral calculi.

Identify types of trauma of the urinary system and the nursing care involved for the client with trauma to the kidneys, bladder, and ureters.

Specific disorders of the kidneys and urinary system include life-threatening illnesses with long-term implications. Disorders of the urinary system may be generally classified as congenital, multifactorial in origin, degenerative, immunologic, infectious, neoplastic and obstructive, and traumatic.

Section I: Congenital Disorders

Congenital disorders of the kidneys and urinary system are present at birth, although they may not be apparent or symptomatic until adulthood. These disorders may result from inherited genetic disturbances or a birth deformity. Some congenital disorders are treatable by surgical intervention in infancy or early childhood. The goal of these surgical interventions is to prevent deterioration of renal function that would result in the client's death. Other inherited disorders are not treatable, however, so renal function will deteriorate over a period of years. For these clients, dialysis or transplantation will be required to prevent death from uremia. Nurses must provide clients with education and emotional support to promote the maintenance of health and appropriate self-care measures. In addition, young adults with a family history of inherited renal disease should be encouraged to receive genetic counseling.

REFLUX NEPHROPATHY

Reflux nephropathy, also called ureterovesical (U-V) reflux or vesicoureteral (V-U) reflux, develops when urine from the bladder is *directed back* toward the renal pelvis through the ureters during voiding. The bladder normally contracts to expel urine, and the U-V junction of each ureter closes tightly. With reflux, however, this ureteral closure is incomplete. There may be reflux of urine into the ureter or into the pelvis of the kidney (intrarenal reflux). Since the renal pelvis of the adult holds only 5 to 10 mL of urine, intrarenal reflux will damage the renal parenchyma. Damage may occur with or without infection present (Rose, 1981).

Reflux may result from poor development of the bladder muscle or abnormal placement of the ureters. Normally, the ureters enter the urinary bladder on the posterior surface in the trigone (an area of bladder musculature bounded by the two ureteral orifices and the bladder neck). When the bladder contracts to empty urine, the trigone also contracts. Thus, during normal voiding, the portions of the ureters contained in the bladder wall are closed. A weak bladder muscle may result in incomplete ureteral closure, which can reflux urine into the ureters. If one or both ureters develop outside the trigone, there may also be incomplete closure because of the length of the ureter or the absence of enough smooth muscle to close the ureter.

The U-V reflux may be demonstrated by a voiding cystourethrogram; the excretory urogram may be normal and show that the lower portion of the ureter is dilated (Smith, 1981). Renal parenchymal damage may also be manifested by tissue scarring. The calyceal system is blunted, so the edges are not clearly demarcated. In addition, the renal cortical tissue atrophies.

Clinical Manifestations

Symptoms of reflux generally appear only when infection is present. With acute infection, there may be burning with urination, fever, chills, and flank pain. With chronic infection, however, symptoms may be absent so the client is unaware of this process. In the absence of infection or symptoms noticeable to the client, progressive damage to kidney tissue and eventual chronic renal failure may result. With progressive renal deterioration, fatigue, weakness, and hypertension may be the initial manifestations. A history of urinary tract infections as a child is often associated with reflux.

Therapeutic Measures

The primary objective of U-V reflux treatment is to ensure the sterility of the urinary tract. When reflux has not disappeared in the adult client, antibiotics will be prescribed if there is acute infection and may also be used for long-term suppression of bacterial growth. In the adult with renal insufficiency, ampicillin, cephalexin, or trimethoprim-sulfamethoxazole (Bactrim) may be required (Rose, 1981). A urinary antiseptic such as sulfamethoxazole may not be filtered into the kidney if there is significant renal insufficiency. In this case, potentially nephrotoxic antibiotics may be needed to kill the bacteria. Drug levels must be monitored to determine if the blood level is therapeutic. Serum creatinine levels also need to be monitored to detect worsening renal function.

Periodic evaluation of the urine for bacterial growth is recommended, especially after each course of antibiotics. Vesicoureteroplasty, to correct abnormal placement of the ureters, will be discussed in Chapter 34. Surgical intervention for repair of the reflux in adults with elevated serum creatinine levels has not been demonstrated to be effective in slowing the deterioration of renal function (Rose, 1981).

Specific Nursing Measures

Nursing interventions are primarily directed toward the education of the client or significant others about the treatment plan. The client should thoroughly understand the importance of taking the antibiotics for the prescribed period of time. The client should consume between 2500 and 3000 mL of fluids but should avoid more liberal fluid intake to prevent excessive dilution and too rapid excretion of the antibiotics. A nutritious diet should be followed; dietary restrictions will not be prescribed unless there is evidence of hypertension or severe renal failure. Dietary modifications for these problems are discussed in Chapter 32. The client should understand the need for frequent voiding to empty the bladder and minimize the stasis of residual urine.

POLYCYSTIC KIDNEY DISEASE

Polycystic kidney disease (PCKD or PKD) is an inherited disorder in which cysts form within the nephrons (Figure 33–1). These grapelike clusters of cysts are filled with fluid from tubular filtrate and thus are composed of water and electrolytes (Rose, 1981). The disease has two forms— one affecting adults and the other affecting children. The adult form is a regular autosomal dominant hereditary disorder, whereas the childhood form is an autosomal recessive disorder. Both kidneys are involved in both disorders. Because the disorder may affect the renal medulla, salt wasting or sodium loss may be a problem that requires sodium replacement. Weakness of cerebral blood vessel walls with resultant intracranial bleeding is also associated with PCKD.

Clinical Manifestations

Symptoms in the adult form generally are not present until the client is at least 30 years of age, and more commonly 40 to 50. Initial symptoms often include flank pain and hematuria. Hypertension also is common, because polycystic kidneys lose their ability to regulate sodium balance. As the size of the kidneys increases over the years, the client may notice the abdomen enlarging. Polycystic kidneys become palpable with depression of abdominal tissue. Palpation should be done gently, however, to prevent discomfort and possible bleeding. Accompanying urinary tract infections and hematuria are common. Uremia develops gradually.

Therapeutic Measures

Treatment of the client with PCKD is supportive and determined by the problems that develop. Heat and analgesics may be useful in controlling the discomfort from the enlarged kidneys. If bleeding occurs, heat should not be used, however, and bed rest should be instituted in an attempt to control the hemorrhage. Because the cysts often rupture and bleed, blood transfusions may be needed to stabilize the hemodynamic status of the client if significant bleeding develops. Aminocaproic acid (Amicar) may control bleeding that does not stop spontaneously. In addition, the client with bleeding into the cysts should be observed carefully for the development of acute renal failure from obstruction by clots or sloughed tissue.

If necessary, antibiotics will be prescribed to eradicate infection which develops in the cysts. Antihypertensives

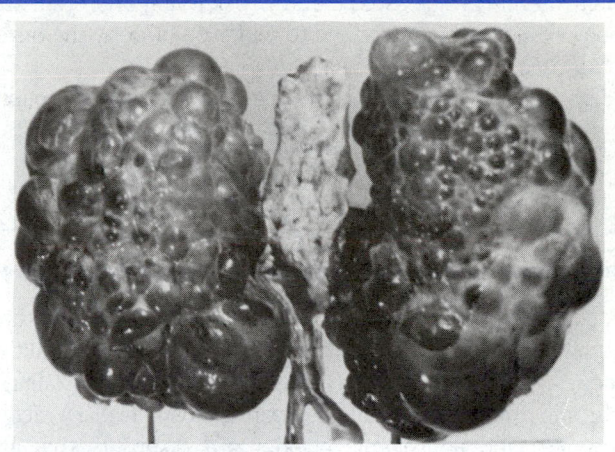

Figure 33–1

Polycystic kidneys. (Courtesy of Millard Fillmore Hospital, Buffalo, NY)

and diuretics will be prescribed as renal function deteriorates. A sodium supplement may be required if there is severe salt wasting from damage to the medulla. Because end-stage renal disease may develop, the client should avoid known nephrotoxic agents, which may compromise renal function prematurely.

A unilateral or bilateral nephrectomy may be required if conservative medical therapy cannot control bleeding or infection (see Chapter 34). Surgical intervention is delayed as long as possible, however, since erythropoietin production and water excretion still occur despite the formation of the cysts.

Specific Nursing Measures

Nursing interventions for the client with PCKD, like the therapeutic measures, depend on the specific problems encountered. Client education to maximize understanding of the disease and self-care management is an important consideration. If bleeding develops, the vital signs and blood count must be monitored closely. Observe and carefully measure urinary output, because acute renal failure may develop. Analgesics should be administered to control discomfort from the cysts. The monitoring of temperature and white blood cell counts also is important, because infection is a potential problem.

The client should understand the methods prescribed to help control hypertension. For example, sodium restriction may be recommended as part of the dietary modification if the client is retaining sodium. Clients with PCKD will need 24-hour urine collections to determine the amount of sodium excreted (Rose, 1981). Careful assessment is important, because restricting sodium in a client who is losing sodium may result in the development of renal insufficiency from volume depletion and lack of renal perfusion. Furthermore, if the renal medulla is affected, clients will need to take in more sodium to correct for the salt wasting.

As azotemia progresses, dietary restriction of protein and potassium may be prescribed to minimize or delay the onset of uremic symptoms.

With the progression of renal insufficiency, the client and significant others will need information about dialytic alternatives and transplantation. The age at which end-stage renal failure develops for the client with PCKD will vary, but it is usually after 50 years.

Section II: Disorders of Multifactorial Origin

A combination of alterations, because of exposure to toxins or altered vascular or neurological function, may result in kidney or urinary tract dysfunction. Acute renal failure, chronic renal failure, acute tubular necrosis, urinary incontinence, and neurogenic bladder are disorders that are commonly of multifactorial origin. Because *acute renal failure* and *chronic renal failure* refer to the result of the pathological condition rather than to disorders per se, they were discussed in Chapter 32. This chapter discusses disorders that potentially can result in acute and chronic renal failure (end-stage renal disease).

ACUTE TUBULAR NECROSIS

Acute tubular necrosis (ATN) represents about 75% of the cases of acute renal failure (Richard, 1981). In this condition, intrarenal problems result in an abrupt, sudden deterioration in renal function in which nitrogenous waste products accumulate in the blood. Acute renal failure and *acute tubular necrosis* are sometimes used interchangeably, but distinction may be made as follows: All ATN produces acute renal failure, but not all acute renal failure is from ATN.

The causes of ATN are generally grouped as postischemic, nephrotoxic, or pigment-related. Postischemic causes include all mechanisms that result in ATN. For example, hypotension due to hemorrhage or lack of cardiac pumping ability may alter renal blood flow and cause subsequent renal damage.

Nephrotoxic causes of ATN include exposure to antibiotics, contrast media, organic solvents, or other drugs that result in inflammatory responses. The aminoglycosides—gentamicin, tobramycin, streptomycin, and amikacin sulfate—are among the drugs that have the greatest nephrotoxic potential. Drugs that may result in inflammatory or hypersensitivity responses within the kidney causing ATN include the nonsteroidal anti-inflammatory agents such as indomethacin (Indocin), as well as the penicillins, sulfonamides, and diuretics (Henrich, 1983). Nonsteroidal analgesics prescribed to clients with arthritis may result in acute deterioration of renal function.

Contrast media—the dyes injected during diagnostic procedures such as intravenous pyelography (IVP), arteriography, cholecystography, and computerized tomography (CT) scans—represent another potential nephrotoxic cause of ATN. Clients at particularly high risk for contrast-induced ATN include those with known renal insufficiency, the elderly, diabetics, and those with multiple myelomas

(Porter & Bennett, 1980; Schrier, 1980). The risk of ATN from contrast media increases if there are elevation of the serum creatinine level, dehydration (volume depletion), or both. In these cases, alternative diagnostic procedures may need to be selected.

The heme pigments hemoglobin and myoglobin may also cause ATN. Hemoglobin injury to renal tubules is possible when there is hemolysis of red blood cells, as in a transfusion reaction. In rhabdomyolysis, the breakdown of skeletal muscle causes the release of myoglobin, a large molecule that cannot be removed adequately by the tubules. Rhabdomyolysis can develop in many situations, including in severe crushing injuries, with prolonged and extensive exercise, following seizure activity, with viral syndromes affecting the muscles, and when large muscles are deprived of adequate blood and oxygen for a time (Frank & Admire, 1982).

Clinical Manifestations

Clinical manifestations of ATN depend on several factors. One consideration is the cause of ATN. With contrast-induced and aminoglycoside ATN, the client is usually non-oliguric; he or she continues to excrete normal volumes of urine, but BUN and serum creatinine levels are elevated. Oliguric clients may have hypertension, peripheral edema, and pulmonary edema as a result of fluid retention. Hyperkalemia (with possible ECG manifestations), hyperphosphatemia, hypocalcemia, and metabolic acidosis are also common. With metabolic acidosis, hyperkalemia is intensified, and thus life-threatening arrhythmias are possible.

Characteristics of rhabdomyolysis include oliguria, rapid onset of azotemia, and hyperkalemia. Urine may be dark brown or black, although the color change is transient and may not be detected. Serum creatinine phosphokinase (CPK) levels are greatly elevated in clients who have rhabdomyolysis and may reach levels of 30,000 to 40,000 units. Serum aldolase also is elevated, and myoglobin is found in the urine.

Uremic manifestations also may be present in clients with ATN, particularly as azotemia and metabolic acidosis worsen. The BUN and serum creatinine levels increase daily. Uremic symptoms include nausea, vomiting, anorexia, muscle cramps, pruritus, and lethargy. Examination of the urine produced by a client with ATN reveals the presence of brown cellular casts and many cells of the tubular epithelium (Schrier, 1980). Clients with ATN pass through the same four phases as those with acute renal failure discussed in Chapter 32: onset, oliguric, diuretic, and recovery phases.

Therapeutic Measures and Specific Nursing Measures

Both therapeutic and specific nursing measures are similar to those for the client with acute renal failure discussed in Chapter 32.

URINARY INCONTINENCE

The client with urinary incontinence is unable to control the flow of urine, and urine leaks spontaneously. Loss of urinary control may result from increased intra-abdominal pressure, relaxation of pelvic muscles, trauma to the external sphincter, cystitis, decompensation of the bladder, or impairment in cerebral blood flow.

Clinical Manifestations

These contribute to four types of incontinence. In *true,* or *total, incontinence,* the client experiences a constant loss of urine via the urethra. In *stress incontinence,* the client loses urine in upright positions when coughing, laughing, sneezing, or otherwise increasing the intra-abdominal pressure. *Urgency incontinence* is characterized by a strongly felt need to void followed by loss of urine; this can occur in any position. *Paradoxical incontinence,* also called overflow incontinence, is primarily manifested by constant dribbling.

Therapeutic Measures

If cystitis is causing the symptoms of incontinence, appropriate antibiotics should be prescribed. Pharmacological agents may be prescribed for the treatment of stress incontinence that is not corrected by perineal exercises before surgical intervention is attempted. Agents that increase contraction of urethral smooth muscle, such as phenylpropanolamine hydrochloride (Ornade), an alpha-adrenergic stimulant, also may be prescribed. If upper motor neuron disease has resulted in increased detrusor muscle irritability, parasympatholytic agents such as dicyclomine hydrochloride (Bentyl), propantheline bromide (Pro-Banthine), or methantheline bromide (Banthine) may decrease the irritability and promote continence (McConnell & Zimmerman, 1983).

Surgical interventions may repair a vesicovaginal fistula, suspend the bladder (Marshall–Marchetti–Krantz procedure), remove bladder tumors, or insert an artificial sphincter device. In addition, urinary diversion may be necessary to preserve the function of the upper urinary tract. See Chapters 34 and 65.

Nursing Research Abstract

Pierson C: Assessment and quantification of urine loss in incontinent women. *Nurse Pract* 1984; 9(12):18–30.

A method is described for measurement of urine loss in incontinent women. Termed the pad test, the method is a successful and objective means for quantifying urine loss. The test has two versions, the 1-hour pad test done in the office or clinic and the 12-hour home test. The test consists of wearing a preweighed sanitary pad for a period of time and engaging in certain activities. The pads are later reweighed, and urine loss is measured and correlated with activities. This test has been found useful for diagnosing stress incontinence and correlating triggering factors with incontinence.

Specific Nursing Measures

Nursing care of the client who has urinary incontinence requires patience, understanding, and concern for the preservation of the client's dignity. Because urinary incontinence is associated with infant and toddler behavior, it is disturbing to the adult's self-esteem, self-concept, and self-image. Embarrassment about the problem may delay the client's seeking medical treatment. There may be concern about altered sexual functioning if surgical intervention is necessary. Nursing support with appropriate preparation for diagnostic procedures may be helpful to the adult client.

If perineal exercises (Kegel exercises) are prescribed, the nurse should explain the proper method (see Chapter 64). Obese clients with stress incontinence should be advised that weight loss may improve muscle compliance and promote continence. The client with incontinence should know that adequate fluid volume—2000 to 3000 mL/day—should be consumed, because inadequate fluid intake may further decrease the functional capacity of the bladder. Wearing incontinence pads or specially designed undergarments helps preserve the client's dignity.

Nursing Research Abstract

Burns P, Marecki M, Dittmar S, Bullough, B: Kegel's exercises with biofeedback therapy for treatment of stress incontinence. *Nurse Pract* 1985; 10(2):28–34.

Two case studies described the effectiveness of Kegel exercises when combined with biofeedback therapy in reducing symptoms of urinary stress incontinence. Kegel exercises were found to be effective in decreasing incontinence episodes. Biofeedback therapy was found to be beneficial in assisting clients to identify the pubococcygeal muscle as well as providing immediate feedback and reinforcement of muscle activity.

Kegel exercises have important implications for nurses working in the area of women's health. These exercises, which can be easily taught in the primary care setting and in the hospital, offer the client hope for relief of incontinence symptoms.

NEUROGENIC BLADDER

A neurogenic bladder occurs in clients whose normal neural innervation of bladder contraction is interrupted. The result may be sensory disruption, motor disruption, or both. A neurogenic bladder may have a variety of causes. Diabetes mellitus may result in autonomic neuropathy resulting in a sensory deficit. Neurological disease such as multiple sclerosis or amyotrophic lateral sclerosis also may result in a neurogenic bladder. Another cause is spinal cord injuries or tumors that interrupt normal nerve transmission. One method of describing the neurogenic bladder is to consider the origin of the problem as either lower motor neuron (sacral) or upper motor neuron (suprasacral).

Clinical Manifestations

The client with a lower motor neuron neurogenic bladder will have lost the perception of bladder fullness and not experience a desire to urinate. As a result, overflow incontinence occurs because of greatly extended bladder capacity. The distended bladder may be palpated and percussed. The client with an upper motor neuron neurogenic bladder will also experience spontaneous voiding when the bladder is stimulated. However, the bladder is hyperirritable, and voiding is not complete.

The client with a neurogenic bladder is more susceptible to the development of a UTI because of ineffective bladder emptying and also because catheterization carries increased risk. Repeated infections put the client at risk of developing chronic renal failure. In addition, the risk of urinary tract obstruction from struvite kidney stones increases in the client with a neurogenic bladder.

Therapeutic Measures

Parasympathomimetic agents may be prescribed for the client with a lower motor neuron neurogenic bladder to improve the contraction of the detrusor muscle. Examples include bethanechol chloride (Urecholine) and neostigmine (Prostigmin). For clients with an upper motor neuron neurogenic bladder, other pharmacological agents may be prescribed. Bladder spasms or contractions may be inhibited with medications such as the parasympatholytics, which include propantheline bromide (Pro-Banthine) and methantheline bromide (Banthine). Sympathomimetic agents such as ephedrine sulfate, phenylpropanolamine hydrochloride (Ornade), or imipramine hydrochloride (Tofranil) also may be useful in contracting the bladder neck and improving continence (McConnell & Zimmerman, 1983). Muscle relaxants such as diazepam (Valium) may reduce skeletal muscle spasms. Lethargy and profound muscle weakness are common and undesirable side effects, however.

In addition to pharmacological agents, voiding or catheterization programs may be prescribed. For the client with lower motor neuron neurogenic bladder, bladder massage (Credé's maneuver) or intermittent catheterization may be used. Clients with upper motor neuron neurogenic bladders may be able to stimulate bladder contraction by reflex contraction of the spastic bladder, which may be precipitated by stroking the abdomen, genitalia, or thighs. Digital rectal stimulation also may result in reflex voiding. These methods are used in conjunction with intermittent catheterization.

Transurethral bladder neck resection with or without external sphincterotomy may be performed for the client with lower motor neuron neurogenic bladder. Depending on the type of procedure required, it may not be possible to preserve continence. Surgery may convert the spastic bladder into a flaccid bladder. This procedure, bilateral anterior/posterior sacral rhizotomy, commonly results in impotence.

Specific Nursing Measures

Emotional support and educational interventions are extremely important nursing measures for the client with a neurogenic bladder. Complex interrelations and combinations of manifestations are common. The nurse must understand details of management and the underlying pathological process before offering education and counseling. Concern for preservation of the client's dignity and privacy should accompany all diagnostic and therapeutic interventions.

Teach the client to perform Credé's maneuver on the bladder to promote emptying (Figure 33–2). These instructions include how to place the palm of the hand on the lower part of the abdomen over the bladder. The palm of the hand is flattened, and gradually increasing pressure is applied as the palm is rotated. The client should sit on the toilet while performing Credé's maneuver.

The nurse also will teach intermittent self-catheterization to many of these clients. A clean technique of intermittent self-catheterization is adequate and will not result in an increased incidence of urinary tract infection. The male client will be able to see his own urethra readily. For the female client, the nurse must hold a mirror to assist the client, and a method may need to be created to allow the client to do this by herself at home. Reusable catheters generally are soaked in a solution of povidone-iodine (Betadine) and water when not being used. The client washes his or her hands before beginning the technique and then cleans the urinary meatus and surrounding area with a solution such as Betadine prior to the catheter insertion. At the beginning, the schedule for intermittent catheterization is every 2 hours. The time between catheterizations may increase gradually, usually by ½ to 1 hour increments (McConnell & Zimmerman, 1983). The final schedule usually requires catheterization every 4 hours. Maximizing fluid intake before 6 PM will minimize problems with nocturnal incontinence or the need for awakening at night for self-catheterization.

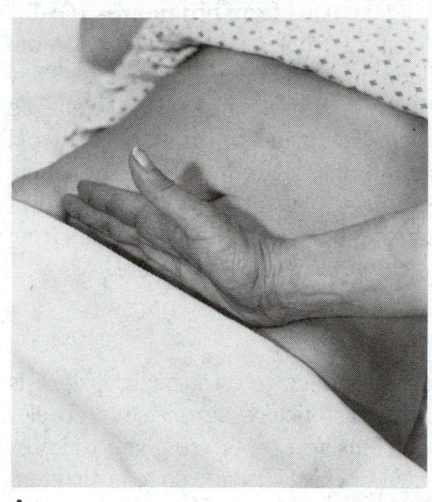 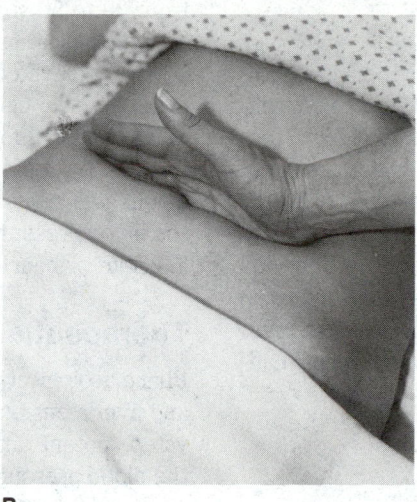

A   B

Figure 33–2

Credé's Maneuver. **A.** Manual pressure applied to the bladder can be employed to facilitate the removal of urine for clients whose bladders are irreversibly flaccid (eg, clients with neurogenic bladders). Usually the procedure is performed every 4 to 6 hours to prevent the bladder from becoming overly distended. **B.** When the client is in a comfortable position, place the ulnar surface of your hand at the umbilicus. Instruct the client to bear down with the abdominal muscles, if possible. Press downward and sweep your hand onto the suprapubic area, using a kneading motion to initiate urination. Continue the maneuver every 30 seconds until urination ceases. SOURCE: Swearingen PL: *Addison–Wesley Photo-Atlas of Nursing Procedures*. Menlo Park, CA: Addison–Wesley, 1984, p. 474.

Section III: Degenerative Disorders

Degenerative disorders of the renal parenchyma are frequently described in reference to their structural alterations. Degenerative changes may occur in the glomeruli, the tubules, or in the blood vessels that supply the kidney. Glomerular disorders will be discussed in the next section, because much of the recent research links glomerular pathology to immunologic processes.

In the early stages of renal deterioration, there are few indications of the loss of renal function. Degenerative processes occur over a long time—often 20 or 30 years or longer—and the client is usually unaware that these changes are taking place. Over a period of years, degeneration of renal function generally results in end-stage renal failure.

General Nursing Implications

Nursing interventions for the client with degenerative disorders of the renal parenchyma primarily are related to educating the client in the measures necessary to control the effects of the pathological condition. Control of high blood pressure and electrolyte and acid–base disturbances are two major therapeutic objectives. Client understanding of the rationale for the prescribed medications and the need for adequate follow-up is particularly important to long-term health maintenance.

ANALGESIC ABUSE NEPHROPATHY

Analgesic abuse nephropathy, a tubular interstitial disorder, is caused by the chronic ingestion of phenacetin-containing compounds or agents that combine aspirin or acetaminophen with phenacetin. Whether injury to tubular tissue results from prostaglandin inhibition or from direct toxic effects of metabolites is not known at this time (Rose, 1981). Phenacetin-containing compounds have been removed from the US market in both prescription and non-prescription medications. However, because the effects may not be seen for a number of years, nurses still see clients with this condition. There are many cases of analgesic abuse nephropathy in the southern states where many people took "headache powders" (containing phenacetin) regularly. Although the long-term effects of aspirin continue to be controversial, many physicians and scientists do not believe aspirin alone results in nephropathy. Aspirin–acetaminophen combinations, however, have been demonstrated to cause renal tubular damage similar to that caused by phenacetin-containing compounds.

Clinical Manifestations

A client with a history of a chronic pain disorder is the most likely to develop analgesic abuse nephropathy. Headaches, back pain, and chronic problems with arthritis are common in these clients' histories. Some clients who have a history of difficulty coping with stress have sought relief from these analgesic agents.

Necrosis of the papillae may result in the sloughing of papillary tissue into the ureters. There may be flank pain and hematuria. Other manifestations may include symptoms of uremia—anorexia, nausea, vomiting, muscle cramps, and pruritus—if there is a significant decrease in the creatinine clearance.

Therapeutic Measures

Therapeutic interventions that prevent further deterioration are a priority in the management of the client with analgesic abuse nephropathy. Agents to control hypertension and infections are often administered, but the client must stop taking analgesic agents that cause deterioration of renal function to prevent further deterioration. Alternative therapies for the control of pain must be identified (see Chapter 5), or the client must be assisted to learn new methods for coping with the discomfort or the stress. Dialysis or transplantation will be necessary when end-stage renal failure with uremia develops.

Specific Nursing Measures

Nursing management for the client with analgesic abuse nephropathy should focus largely on educational efforts to help the client alter practices harmful to his or her long-term health status. The client must thoroughly understand the implications of continued abuse of analgesics that are harming residual renal function. Alternative methods for coping with and controlling pain, such as relaxation or biofeedback, must be explored. If end-stage renal disease has developed, the client and family or significant others will need emotional and educational support about the dialytic alternatives and possibilities for renal transplantation.

NEPHROSCLEROSIS

Nephrosclerosis results from untreated or uncontrolled systemic hypertension acting on the vascular supply of the kidney. It may be classified as benign or malignant according to the severity of the rise in diastolic blood pressure. With benign nephrosclerosis, the diastolic reading is less than 115 mm Hg, whereas malignant nephrosclerosis is found with diastolic readings greater than 130 mm Hg (Rose, 1981). The renal tissue deterioration is caused by a combination of the thickening of the walls of the blood vessels and the resulting ischemia to the interstitium. The tubules are particularly sensitive to the decreased blood supply. Fibrosis also occurs.

Clinical Manifestations

Benign nephrosclerosis is associated with aging and usually affects clients over 60. It is less often fatal than the malignant form because it progresses more slowly. In this condition, the urine has a low specific gravity that is fixed, as well as a small amount of protein. Renal insufficiency and end-stage renal disease arise late in the disease process as more glomeruli are damaged. The client will be hypertensive unless the hypertension is well controlled with antihypertensive agents. The client with well-controlled

hypertension is much less likely to develop end-stage renal disease from nephrosclerosis.

The client with malignant nephrosclerosis is usually from 30 to 50 years of age. This form progresses rapidly. The client will first identify problems related more to the severely elevated blood pressure than the kidneys. They include visual disturbances, severe headaches, or altered neurological functioning. The urine will contain blood and protein. As renal function falls, BUN and serum creatinine values will rise. Death may occur in a few months and, if the blood pressure cannot be lowered, usually results from a stroke or heart attack rather than renal failure.

Therapeutic Measures

Pharmacological agents are used to treat nephrosclerosis and hypertension. If the diastolic pressure is severely elevated, potent antihypertensive agents are given to lower the blood pressure rapidly. This is usually done in an intensive care unit to allow close monitoring. First, fast-acting powerful vasodilators such as sodium nitroprusside (Nipride) and diazoxide (Hyperstat) are administered. Then agents for long-term management are administered to control the hypertension and prevent cardiovascular, cerebral, and renal complications. Unfortunately, the control of blood pressure may result in a decreased blood supply to the kidney and, subsequently, decreased renal function. However, uncontrolled hypertension places a tremendous burden on cardiac function and stresses cerebral blood vessels. Dialysis or transplantation will be necessary for the client with end-stage renal failure.

For clients with severe malignant hypertension and malignant nephrosclerosis, bilateral nephrectomy may be necessary to control the hypertension (see Chapter 34). This surgical intervention is used rarely, only when all known methods for blood pressure control have been tried without success. Chronic dialysis (Chapter 32) or transplantation (Chapter 34) would then be necessary to prevent death from uremia.

Specific Nursing Measures

Administering the agents necessary to control hypertension in the acute phase and monitoring the client to prevent or detect complications are major nursing objectives. Thromboembolic phenomena may cause deterioration of cardiac or cerebral functioning as a result of severe hypertension, so frequent measurement of blood pressure through conventional cuff measurements or by arterial line monitoring in the intensive care unit (if indicated) will be necessary. With uremia, the client will require monitoring and preparation for eventual dialysis. Health teaching for self-care should address the appropriate methods of taking the antihypertensive agents prescribed, as well as other drugs such as diuretics, and include blood pressure assessment. If dialysis is necessary, provide educational and emotional support of the client and family or significant others. Refer to Chapter 32 for specific recommendations.

RENAL ARTERY STENOSIS

In renal artery stenosis, the narrowing of the lumen of the renal artery or arteries results in diminished blood flow to the kidney, the release of renin, and the stimulation of the renin–angiotensin system. It may occur unilaterally or bilaterally. Severe high blood pressure, as well as ischemia to the renal interstitium and tubules, results. The cause of renal artery stenosis is diffuse atherosclerosis that includes the renal vasculature.

Clinical Manifestations

The onset of mild, moderate, or severe hypertension before the age of 30 or after the age of 50 is characteristic of renal artery stenosis (Rose, 1981). An abdominal bruit over one or both renal arteries may also be heard, but this does not occur consistently.

Therapeutic Measures

In general, interventions are designed to control blood pressure and improve blood supply to the kidney. In determining the appropriate plan for a specific client, factors to consider are age, other existing health problems, and relative risks and benefits of the available options.

If hypertension is severe as a result of renal artery stenosis, a hypertensive crisis may result. Pharmacological measures and bed rest are essential to prevent a cerebral vascular accident. Since these clients characteristically have an increased production of renin, an agent such as captopril (Capoten) that blocks the normal renin–angiotensin–aldosterone system is ideal. Without angiotensin formation and release, there usually is a profound decrease in blood pressure. An acceptable pharmacological regimen for lifetime control of the high blood pressure is essential for the long-term health of the client.

Percutaneous transluminal renal angioplasty is an option that may be increasingly available to clients with renal artery stenosis. A ballon-tipped catheter is used to dilate the renal artery at the point of narrowing to increase renal blood flow, improve renal function, and decrease blood pressure (Sos et al., 1983). Potential complications associated with renal angioplasty include perforation of the renal artery with the catheter tip and acute renal failure associated with the contrast media required during the arteriography that precedes the angioplasty. A risk associated with this procedure is that renal failure may not reverse if significant underlying renal dysfunction is already present. In this case, renal angioplasty may be the only alternative to prevent the eventuality of dialysis.

Renal vascular surgery may be performed to restore blood flow to the renal parenchyma, as discussed in Chapter 34. For the young client who faces a lifetime of taking oral antihypertensive agents, the choice of surgery may be relatively easy. For the older client with significant vascular disease affecting other organs or other systemic diseases, the choice of renal artery bypass surgery may be less clearcut. For both groups, renal artery bypass surgery may not totally eliminate the need for medications; however, it may lessen considerably the complexity of the medical regimen. Finally, for the client with a significant decrease in renal blood supply, renal artery bypass surgery may be necessary to prevent a total loss of renal function. A severely atrophic kidney (less than 9 to 10 cm) is not generally considered for revascularization. However, this atrophic kidney may be a major source of renin production, so nephrectomy may be indicated.

Specific Nursing Measures

Regardless of the treatment method selected, nursing interventions will be directed toward physical and emotional support of the client. Since a variety of risks and benefits are associated with any method, the client will be anxious during decision making. The nurse must understand the rationale for the various alternatives that will be explained to the client, because supportive discussion that clarifies and validates the client's understanding is important. Postoperative nursing care is discussed in Chapter 34.

DIABETIC GLOMERULOPATHY

Nephropathies that develop because of diabetes mellitus usually result from one of several pathological processes. Diabetic nephropathy (a noninflammatory disease of the kidney) may take the form of glomerulosclerosis caused by alterations in the mesangium, the support structure of the glomerular loops. This diffuse form of glomerulosclerosis may be present alone, or nodules also may be present on the capillary loops. Nodular glomerulosclerosis is called Kimmelstiel–Wilson syndrome.

The cause of diabetic nephropathy has not been conclusively established. Excellent blood glucose control can help preserve renal function. The glomerular changes that develop with diabetes mellitus are believed to result from abnormal deposition of protein in the glomerular basement membrane, which may be due to the altered metabolic processes associated with insulin deficiency.

Clinical Manifestations

The clinical manifestations of diabetic glomerulosclerosis include proteinuria, hypertension, and edema. Retinal vascular changes and peripheral neuropathies of diabetes mellitus also are often present. Current estimates are that 50% of clients with Type I diabetes mellitus and 6% of clients with Type II diabetes mellitus will develop end-stage renal failure (Rose, 1981). In most instances, it will develop within 3 to 5 years after the onset of azotemia (Schrier, 1980).

Nursing Research Abstract

Baldree KS, Murphy SP, Powers M: Stress identification and coping patterns in patients on hemodialysis. *Nurs Res* 1982; 31(2):107–112.

Technologically effective hemodialysis treatments for end-stage renal disease (ESRD) have imposed new stressors on clients dependent on such treatments. This study designed and tested an instrument to evaluate and grade stressors and to determine coping strategies.

Fluid restriction, muscle cramps, fatigue, and uncertainty about the future were defined as the greatest stressors. There was no significant difference between the degree of physiological and psychosocial stress. Stressors were not related to age, sex, marital status, or education. A trend was found in that clients on dialysis for less than 12 months and for 37 to 48 months had fewer stressors than clients on treatment for 13 to 36 months and for longer than 48 months. Problem-oriented coping skills were used significantly more than affective problem solving. Most frequently used coping skills included hope, control maintenance, prayer, trust in God, objectively looking at one's problem, worry, and acceptance.

In planning care for chronic renal clients, nurses can strengthen coping mechanisms by allowing individuals to take an active role in organizing treatments and medications. They can teach them about their treatment so they are knowledgeable about their medical regimen. Nurses can offer emotional support and allow them independence and autonomy. By encouraging clients and allowing them some control over treatment, nurses can help reduce psychological stressors. ESRD client management requires a team approach so individuals are assessed physiologically and psychosocially.

Therapeutic Measures

The major objectives of pharmacological interventions are to support the client as renal function deteriorates and to prevent further damage from potentially nephrotoxic agents. Antihypertensives and diuretics may be prescribed to control hypertension and fluid retention. As the glomerular filtration and creatinine clearance rates decrease, the dosage schedules of drugs that are primarily excreted via the kidneys (eg, antibiotics) will need to be modified by increasing the interval between doses. In addition, the insulin needs of the Type I client will usually decrease as the renal function deteriorates.

The medical management of the client with renal manifestations of diabetes mellitus is directed toward control of the hypertension and its effects upon the kidney and other organs. In addition, a primary objective is to protect the client from further renal damage from a variety of other causes. Risks to renal reserve include the use of contrast media for diagnostic testing and the threat of infection, which may be worsened in the diabetic client who has the potential for development of a neurogenic bladder from autonomic neuropathy.

Once uremia develops, dialysis or transplantation will be necessary to maintain life. Although these mechanisms assume the primary responsibilities of the kidneys, they do not eliminate the problems of decreasing vision; increasing peripheral and visceral neuropathies; and altered vascular supply to the heart, brain, and periphery.

Surgical management involves renal transplant surgery (refer to Chapter 34) for the client with end-stage renal disease from diabetes mellitus. Both longevity and quality of life are better with transplantation than with dialysis, and the heparin required for hemodialysis further complicates the already present retinopathy.

Specific Nursing Measures

Educational efforts to increase the client's understanding and management of the changes developing as renal function deteriorates are a major nursing objective. Particularly important is the client's need to understand the changes occurring in the need for insulin. The client may interpret the decreased need for insulin as evidence that the diabetes mellitus is improving; however, the renal breakdown and excretion of circulating insulin actually is impaired with decreasing renal function. As a result, the client will experience episodes of hypoglycemia and changes in insulin requirements.

Monitoring blood glucose levels becomes the primary method for assessing degree of control, because as renal function becomes significantly compromised, the use of urine to assess for glycosuria and ketonuria is much less reliable. This is particularly important for clients who have autonomic neuropathy affecting bladder emptying.

Nursing care of the client with diabetes mellitus and impaired renal functioning has an overall primary objective of preventing the development of any kind of infection. Uremia enhances the increased susceptibility to infection associated with diabetes, as both conditions result in a generalized immune suppression. Nursing interventions to actively prevent the client from developing acute renal failure in the presence of already compromised renal reserve may be a major factor in the preservation of renal function (Chambers, 1983).

The client and family or significant others will require emotional support as end-stage renal disease ensues. They must decide between transplantation and dialysis. Often the client, although as young as 30, may be blind or have severe nephropathies by this time. In some instances, both transplantation and dialysis may be necessary.

Section IV: Immunologic Disorders

Advances in electron microscopy and techniques of analyzing tissue obtained from renal biopsy have enabled increasingly accurate diagnosis of the pathological processes resulting in glomerulonephritis (the term referring to all glomerular disorders). For this reason, the term *glomerulonephritis* has only limited application to specific diseases; most glomerular disorders are identified by the immunologic processes that cause them. Diabetes mellitus, which also affects glomerular integrity, is an exception and is not considered an immunologically based disorder.

Pathophysiologically, the loss of glomerular integrity is the result of immune (antigen–antibody) complexes that circulate and are deposited in the glomeruli (Rose, 1981). The size of each immune complex and the number of complexes formed influence the development of disease. Another pathological process may be the combination of antibodies with antigens that have been previously deposited in the glomeruli. A third immunologic mechanism is the development of antibodies to the glomerular basement membrane (anti-GBM antibodies). These three processes activate the complement system, movement of leukocytes to the glomerulus, platelet aggregation, and fibrin deposition. Necrosis and fibrosis of tissue lead to end-stage renal failure if the process is not reversed.

Current classification describes glomerulonephritis, or all glomerular disorders, as glomerulopathies or glomerulonephridities (interchangeable terms). The effects on the client are variable, depending on the etiology and whether there is response to treatment. There may be spontaneous reversal, progression to total deterioration, or stabilization of the current situation. Glomerulopathies may be associated with infectious processes, malignancies, specific organ diseases, multisystem diseases, and hereditary metabolic disorders.

General Nursing Implications

The client's history is important in detecting a possible cause for the glomerular disorder. Systemic disease, a recent history of upper respiratory tract infection or gastroenteritis, the use of pharmacological agents, or pregnancy are all potential contributing factors.

Ask the client about changes in urinary output or in the appearance of the urine. A urine sample should be obtained and sent to the laboratory for urinalysis. A major component of the assessment process will be a 24-hour urine collection for quantitation of protein and calculation of the creatinine clearance rate. If edema, hypertension, or uremic symptoms are present, assess how the client is feeling in general and whether essential physiological balance is being maintained.

General nursing interventions for the client with immunologic disorders are similar to those suggested for clients with degenerative disorders. Urine specimens should be collected according to accepted techniques so that accurate data can be obtained. Careful measurement of intake and output, daily weights, and blood pressure are all important sources of data for these clients. In addition, the nurse should initiate client education about the various diagnostic tests. Emotionally, this may be a time of great uncertainty for the client and the client's family or significant others

because many of the immunologic disorders may progress to end-stage renal disease, in which chronic dialysis or transplantation will be necessary to maintain life.

NEPHROTIC SYNDROME

Nephrotic syndrome, or nephrosis, occurs in any condition that seriously damages the glomerular capillary membrane, thus allowing increased permeability of the membrane to plasma proteins. A variety of glomerular diseases, such as chronic glomerulonephritis, lupus nephritis, poststreptococcal nephritis, Kimmelstiel–Wilson syndrome, toxic nephropathy, and membranous nephropathy, can result in the nephrotic syndrome. The primary cause of nephrotic syndrome, however, is membranous nephropathy.

Membranous nephropathy may develop from malignancies or endogenous antigens such as DNA; DNA antigens and antibodies to DNA occur in systemic lupus erythematosus and may result in lupus nephritis. Exogenous antigens that may result in membranous nephropathy include hepatitis B virus, gold, and penicillamine.

Clinical Manifestations

Nephrotic syndrome is characterized by renal losses of protein that exceed 3.5 g/24 hours, hypoalbuminemia, edema, hyperlipidemia, and a hypercoagulable state (Rose, 1981). The client will notice the development of edema, primarily in dependent areas. The client may notice periorbital or facial edema upon awakening, and edema in the legs and feet will be apparent as the day progresses. Urinalysis will reveal the presence of protein. In addition, plasma albumin levels decrease, and plasma lipid levels of cholesterol and triglycerides increase. Although the mechanisms are unclear, increased incidences of arterial and venous thrombosis have been noted in clients with nephrotic syndrome (Rose, 1981).

Therapeutic Measures

If renal biopsy has identified an immunologic basis, corticosteroids, cytotoxic agents, or both are prescribed for clients with glomerular disorders leading to nephrotic syndrome. These substances decrease the large amounts of protein lost by decreasing the immunologic response. Corticosteroids may be given as bolus therapy (eg, 1 g intravenously every day for 3 to 5 days). Then, during the active stages of immunologic activity, the client may receive 1.0 to 1.5 mg/kg/day of prednisone (Rose, 1981). With stabilization, the dosage of prednisone is converted to alternate-day therapy in an attempt to decrease the incidence and severity of side effects. Cytotoxic agents such as azathioprine (Imuran) and cyclophosphamide (Cytoxan) may also be prescribed for some forms of immunologic processes that have led to the nephrotic syndrome.

Numerous side effects are associated with both the corticosteroids and the cytotoxic agents. Suppression of bone marrow production of leukocytes, thrombocytes, and erythrocytes leads to increased susceptibility to infection, increased bleeding potential, and problems with anemia. Gastrointestinal bleeding is a relatively frequent side effect, and antacids are commonly prescribed prophylactically. Known gastrointestinal irritants should be eliminated when possible. Cytoxan is associated with hemorrhagic cystitis; clients taking this agent should be instructed to drink large volumes of water and empty their bladders frequently because urine that remains static in the bladder contains drug metabolites that can irritate the bladder's mucosal lining.

Antiplatelet drugs and anticoagulant therapy have been tried in some instances to counteract the effects of increased platelet aggregation and fibrin deposition. However, bleeding problems generally make these therapeutic modalities useless.

If renal deterioration is not responsive to pharmacological management, plasmapheresis may be attempted. For some immunologically based disorders, this effectively removes the circulating immune complexes or the antigens and antibodies. If renal deterioration continues, however, dialysis or transplantation is necessary.

Specific Nursing Measures

Many clients with nephrotic syndrome require considerable nursing care. Profound edema is common in these clients (Figure 33–3) so meticulous skin care is essential. Difficulties with skin breakdown and immobility are also common; thus, devices to prevent skin breakdown, such as mattresses that provide pressure relief, should be used. Routinely inspect dependent parts for evidence of erythema and the need for pressure relief. Immobility from edema, as well as the hypercoagulable state associated with nephrotic syndrome, make the client susceptible to the development of thromboembolic phenomena. Instruct the

client to do hourly leg and toe exercises to increase circulation, as well as institute range-of-motion (ROM) activities unless contraindicated by the known presence of thrombotic processes. Hourly position changes for the client confined to bed, chair activity, and ambulation (if allowed) should be encouraged, and the client should be supported in attaining alterations in activity. The eyes of clients with periorbital edema may swell shut and need to be irrigated with sterile normal saline.

Nutritional management may include a diet high in protein foods because renal losses of protein are extensive (see Box 32–5). When massive edema is present, fluid restriction may be prescribed. Since edema occurs in the lining of the gastrointestinal tract as well as the periphery, clients frequently experience anorexia and feelings of abdominal fullness. Smaller and more frequent servings may be more appealing. Monitoring daily weights and measuring fluid intake and urinary output will help determine the effectiveness of diuretics prescribed.

Many opportunities will arise in which the nurse can help the client understand the rationale for medications and other interventions. This is important, because many clients will continue with these pharmacological and dietary interventions for some time. Clarify the purpose and methods of self-care procedures to facilitate the client's assuming responsibility for this facet of care.

ACUTE GLOMERULONEPHRITIS

Acute glomerulonephritis (postinfectious glomerulonephritis or acute nephritic syndrome) generally has a sudden onset and causes changes in the urine such as proteinuria and hematuria. It is commonly associated with a recent infectious process, and the etiology is exposure to an exogenous antigen to which antibodies are formed and subsequently deposited in the glomerulus. For example, the group A beta-hemolytic streptococcus organism has certain strains that are associated with the ability to evoke a glomerulonephritis. Not all group A beta-hemolytic streptococcal infections will cause acute glomerulonephritis, however.

Clinical Manifestations

The client usually reports having had a recent upper respiratory tract infection, often with a sore throat. The urine may be the color of cola. There may be evidence of decreased urinary output, peripheral and periorbital edema, and hypertension. The urine contains protein and red blood cell casts.

Therapeutic Measures

Hypertension related to decreased glomerular filtration and the hypervolemic state may need to be controlled. The administration of diuretics and antihypertensive agents is often required during the acute phase of illness as well as for a while into the recovery phase or if permanent renal

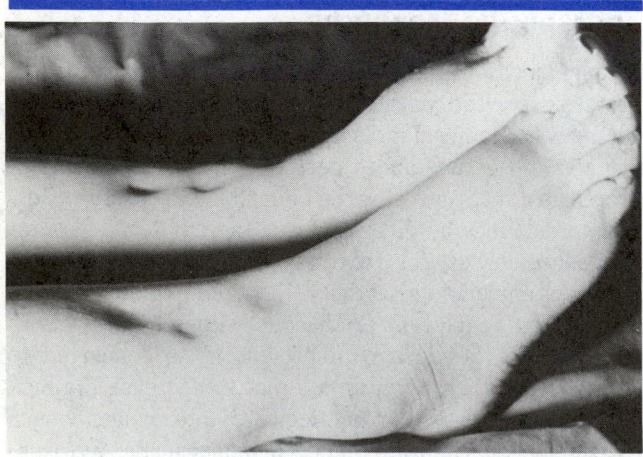

Figure 33–3

Severe pitting edema in a client with nephrotic syndrome. (Courtesy of Millard Fillmore Hospital, Buffalo, NY)

insufficiency results. Corticosteroids have not been demonstrated effective in the treatment of this condition.

Short-term hemodialysis or peritoneal dialysis may also be necessary if acute renal failure develops. There is evidence that this syndrome is progressive in a number of adult clients. Continued follow-up for the treatment of hypertension and careful management to prevent further renal insufficiency from developing are indicated.

Specific Nursing Measures

During the period of acute illness, the client should be kept in bed if there are severe symptoms of volume overload, heart failure, or severe hypertension. Otherwise, encourage modest activity that includes ambulation. Supportive measures to increase comfort and allow the time needed for healing are important. The nursing care plan should include careful monitoring of fluid status during the period of oliguria, daily weighing, and measurement of intake and output.

Fluid restrictions will be prescribed to correlate with the amount of urine produced, plus about 600 mL to account for insensible losses. If blood chemistry measurements indicate an elevated BUN level, dietary protein may be restricted. Sodium intake may be limited if hypertension is present. In any case, a nutritious diet is important during the acute phase of this syndrome. The client and family or significant others must understand the need for consistent follow-up after the acute illness is past; it is estimated that progressive renal deterioration occurs in 50% or fewer of clients, often depending on other factors involved in their overall health status.

CHRONIC GLOMERULONEPHRITIS

In chronic glomerulonephritis, glomerular disorders have resulted in chronic renal failure or end-stage renal disease. Renal deterioration has usually been a long, slow process, and the client generally is unaware of this loss of function. The cause of chronic glomerulonephritis is usually not known although it is thought to be the result of repeated antigen–antibody reaction or autoimmune response. Because the kidneys are atrophic, little is gained from biopsy; the amount of kidney tissue that could be obtained would only demonstrate scarring. The client is past the time

when the disease might have been reversed; loss of renal function is permanent.

Clinical Manifestations

Protein, red blood cells, leukocytes, and waxy casts are often present in the urine of clients with chronic glomerulonephritis. Urine specific gravity fixates at about 1.010 because the nephrons lose their urine-concentrating ability. Hypertension and the nephrotic syndrome also may be present. Significant renal deterioration commonly occurs before the client is aware of it. Eye changes, sudden nose bleeds, elevated blood pressure, or uremic manifestations of chronic renal failure (anorexia, nausea, vomiting, muscle cramps, pruritus, fatigue, and lethargy) may be initial symptoms.

Once the condition is diagnosed, the client may have good health for 10 to 30 years or may develop end-stage renal disease in 1 to 2 years. The client's state of health is determined by the extent of glomerular necrosis, the extent of renal vasculature sclerosis, and the extent of the autoimmune activity. As the disease progresses, the client will develop severe headaches, shortness of breath, angina, edema, dry skin, nocturia, and polyuria. Eye changes from retinal artery thickening include seeing black spots or flashes of light, as well as dimness of vision.

Therapeutic Measures

Specific medications prescribed for the client with chronic glomerulonephritis include diuretics and antihypertensives. These agents control the fluid retention and elevated blood pressure that result from renal deterioration. When renal function deteriorates to a level at which diuretics are no longer effective, dialysis or transplantation are necessary to prevent death from uremia.

Specific Nursing Measures

Attend to the cardiac system and infections, using the same interventions described in Chapter 32 for any client with chronic renal failure. Dietary modifications, fluid restriction, prevention of skin breakdown, control of electrolyte and acid–base balances, and removal of waste products are also required.

Section V: Infectious Disorders

Infections within the urinary tract are a common clinical problem and may occur anywhere in the urinary tract. They may be localized to a specific anatomical structure or become a systemic process through infection of the blood.

The routes of infection in the urinary tract include the blood (hematogenous route), the lymphatic system (lym-

phatogenous route), or ascending or descending routes (eg, traveling up the urinary tract from urethra to bladder, or traveling down the urinary tract from kidney to bladder). The routes of infection are shown in Figure 33–4. Indwelling or suprapubic catheters placed for the control or facilitation of urinary drainage are often associated with the

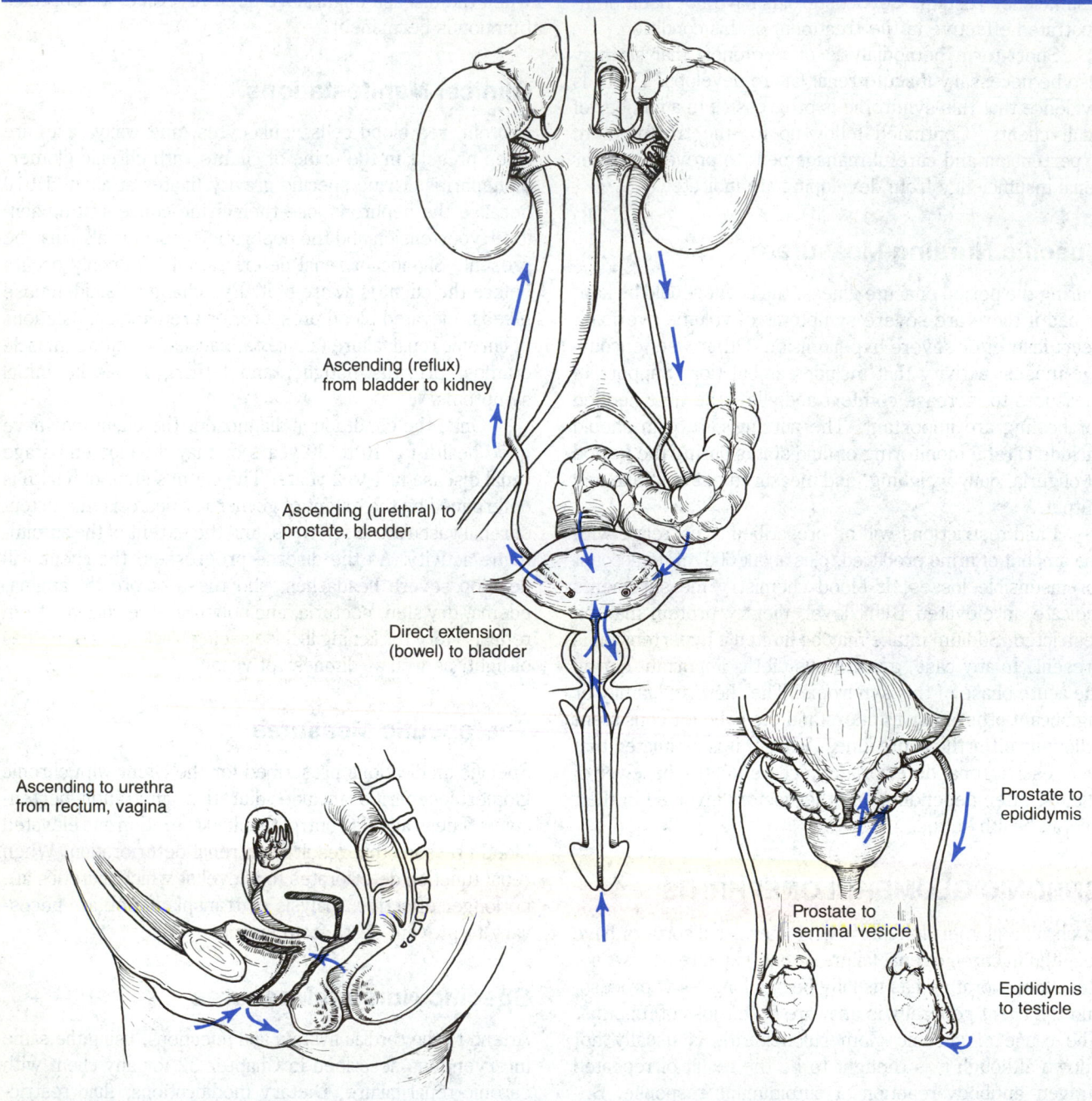

Ascending (reflux)
from bladder to kidney

Ascending (urethral) to
prostate, bladder

Direct extension
(bowel) to bladder

Ascending to urethra
from rectum, vagina

Prostate to
epididymis

Prostate to
seminal vesicle

Epididymis
to testicle

Figure 33–4

Routes of urinary infection.

development of infections; Table 33–1 shows the estimated annual incidence. Urinary tract infections are the most significant of hospital-acquired infections: 41% of the nosocomial infections are within the urinary tract (the highest of any category), and invasion of the urinary tract by either a catheter or other instrument precedes 75% to 100% of the hospital-acquired infections (Garibaldi, 1981). Urinary tract infections produce significant discomfort. When urine outflow is obstructed or there is a continuous site of infection, end-stage renal failure may develop from the infection and associated scarring.

General Nursing Implications

An alteration in the pattern of urination is one of the earliest manifestations of infectious processes within the urinary tract. Frequency, burning, incontinence, or urination of small amounts may signal such disturbances. Infection in the urinary tract may cause a general elevation of body temperature.

Interventions for the client with a urinary tract infection involve eliminating the cause of infection and killing the residual organisms. During the infectious period, it is

Table 33–1 Estimate of the Annual US Incidence of Catheter-Associated Urinary Tract Infections and Their Consequences

Population	%	Number
Clients admitted to acute care hospitals	—	40,000,000
Clients catheterized	10	4,000,000
Catheterized clients who acquire bacteriuria	15	600,000
Bacteriuric clients who become bacteremic	1	6000
Bacteremic clients who die of sepsis	30	1800

Adapted from: Garibaldi RA: Hospital acquired urinary tract infection. In: *CRC Handbook of Hospital Acquired Infections.* Wenzel RC (editor). Boca Raton, FL: CRC Press, 1981, p. 514.

important to maintain a large fluid intake to facilitate the flow of urine; 3 L/day is usually recommended. Ensure that the client has a nutritious diet and gets adequate rest.

Most infections are of bacterial origin. Antibiotic administration should ensure that blood levels remain within the therapeutic range 24 hours a day and that antibiotics are taken for the entire prescribed time. The client should avoid fluid intake greater than 3 L/day because this will dilute antibiotic levels in the blood and increase the rate of renal excretion; therapeutic blood levels will not be maintained.

Major nursing implications involve the management and education of clients for prevention of urinary tract infections. Proper postdefecation hygiene practices should be taught at an early age so they become a lifelong habit. Women, who are particularly vulnerable to contamination of the urethral orifice with bacteria from the vaginal and anal orifices, should be taught to wipe from front to back after voiding or defecation. Women also should be encouraged to void before and after sexual intercourse. The routine use of indwelling catheters for care of incontinent clients should be avoided whenever possible. Frequent voiding programs to retrain the client to achieve bladder control should be instituted as early as possible.

URETHRITIS

Urethritis, or inflammation of the urethra, may result from bacterial infection, traumatic irritation, or hypersensitivity to detergents or bubble bath. Bacterial causes of urethritis include *Chlamydia trachomatis* and *Neisseria gonorrhoeae.* The herpes simplex virus type 2 also may cause urethritis (McConnell & Zimmerman, 1983).

Clinical Manifestations

The client usually complains of discomfort with urination. Female clients also may experience generalized discomfort in the labial tissues. The urethra may be red, but there is generally no drainage. Examination of urine will show pus in the first morning specimen and the absence of pus or white blood cells in the specimen collected immediately following.

Therapeutic Measures

Bacterial urethritis is treated with antibiotics appropriate to the eradication of the pathogens. Postmenopausal women may experience symptoms similar to bacterial urethritis; these respond to the topical application of estrogen preparations. Urethritis may result in the inability to expel urine from the bladder. In such cases, the flow of urine must be reestablished to prevent deterioration of renal parenchyma. If strictures develop, gradual dilatation with progressively larger instruments or direct internal repair of the stricture will be required.

Specific Nursing Measures

Instruct clients about taking the prescribed antibiotics, the proper application of topical ointments or creams, the need for women to wipe from front to back after urination or defecation, and the need for the uncircumcised man to clean beneath the foreskin routinely. Urethritis may occur from sexual activities resulting in transmission of bacteria between partners. Reinfection frequently results when one partner is not adequately treated, so treatment of both is necessary.

CYSTITIS

Cystitis, or inflammation of the urinary bladder, usually is the result of bacterial contamination. It also can be caused by a fungal infection or fibrosis of the bladder wall. Bladder calculi, urinary diverticuli, or an indwelling urethral or suprapubic catheter will increase the likelihood of cystitis developing. Because of the relatively short female urethra and its proximity to the rectum and vagina, women are much more susceptible than men to cystitis. Recent literature suggests that sexual intercourse, as a single variable, does not cause urinary tract infection (Rose, 1981). In healthy subjects, bacteriuria increases following sexual intercourse; however, this increase is transient and does not produce the symptoms commonly referred to as "honeymoon cystitis."

Clinical Manifestations

The client with cystitis generally experiences a burning discomfort upon urination. There may also be frequency, urgency, nocturia, bladder spasms, or incontinence. The urine may be cloudy or cola colored from the presence of red blood cells, white blood cells, or both. Other symptoms may include fever, general feelings of fatigue, and pelvic and abdominal discomfort. When cystitis is associated with urinary tract obstruction at the bladder neck, the client may have symptoms of urinary obstruction and/or acute renal failure resulting in uremia.

Therapeutic Measures

If cystitis has resulted in obstruction or acute renal failure, the obstruction must be removed immediately and the infection treated and eradicated. Failure to remove the obstruction and treat the infection may result in permanent renal damage. Antibiotics effective in eradicating the bacteria causing the cystitis will be prescribed. Any infected foreign bodies such as calculi must be removed to eradicate the source of the infection.

Clients with cystitis should have a liberal fluid intake of at least 3 L/day. The nurse should encourage the client to void frequently, even if it is uncomfortable, to help wash out contaminating microorganisms. Surgery to remove obstructions resulting in cystitis or acute renal failure may be indicated and will be discussed in Chapter 34.

Specific Nursing Measures

Nursing interventions for the care of clients with cystitis are supportive and educational. Methods to promote comfort may include sitz baths for local comfort and the administration of mild analgesics as prescribed; phenazopyridine hydrochloride (Pyridium) is often given for the first 2 to 3 days to lessen the pain and bladder spasms. Warn the client that this drug colors the urine red or orange and may stain fabrics. Warm compresses or sitz baths as well as opium and belladonna suppositories may assist the client in achieving adequate relaxation for natural micturition. Oil of peppermint held near the urethra also has been useful. Avoid urethral catheterization whenever possible, since additional contamination may result from the procedure. The administration of antibiotics is essential to the supportive management. Fluids should be available and offered frequently. The continued monitoring of renal function involves measurement and recording of fluid intake and output.

Include several specific points in the client's education. An important point is that moisture around the urethral meatus provides a medium that enhances bacterial growth and puts the client at risk for an ascending urinary tract infection that travels up the urethra to the bladder. Cotton briefs are more absorbent than nylon and do not trap moisture. The client should avoid nylon panty hose or other tight clothing, if possible. If the client's urine is routinely alkaline, the goal should be to acidify the urine to inhibit bacterial growth; drinking cranberry or prune juice will help. Urine may become alkaline through the ingestion of juices such as tomato, orange, grapefruit, or apple.

PYELONEPHRITIS

Pyelonephritis, or inflammation of the renal pelvis, may occur bilaterally or unilaterally. It may be a short-term phenomenon or become a long-term health problem with serious sequelae in terms of maintaining renal function. Acute pyelonephritis is the result of bacterial invasion of the renal pelvis and medulla—usually an infection that has ascended from the lower urinary tract. In chronic pyelonephritis, infectious processes tend to persist or recur, resulting in renal parenchymal deterioration from scarring (Figure 33–5). However, biopsies of kidney tissue without infection have demonstrated scarring patterns and tissue changes similar to those in chronic pyelonephritis. Most authorities believe that bacteriuria alone does not cause renal failure, but that structural alterations along with the infection produce serious renal deterioration. A major cause of chronic pyelonephritis is believed to be ureterovesical reflux, in which infected urine ascends into the ureters and, consequently, the renal pelvises due to inadequate closure of the U-V valves during voiding (Smith, 1981).

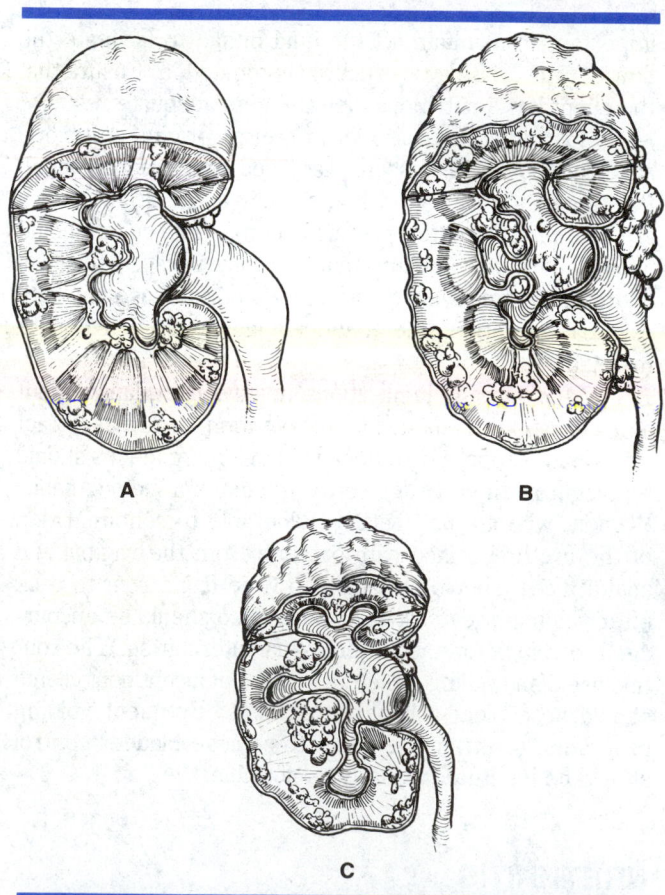

Figure 33–5

Progressive kidney changes in pyelonephritis. **A.** Early parenchymal scarring in periphery and irregular pitting of surface. **B.** Progressive scarring with calyceal dilation and narrowing of the nicks of the calices. **C.** End stage with kidney atrophy.

Clinical Manifestations

Acute Pyelonephritis
The client with acute pyelonephritis is usually quite ill with fever, chills, nausea, and vomiting. Severe pain or constant dull aching over the kidney in the flank area may be present unilaterally or bilaterally.

Chronic Pyelonephritis
Unless there is an acute episode of a new infectious process, the client generally is unaware of chronic pyelonephritis. If the client notices anything, it may be only bladder irritability, chronic fatigue, or a slight aching over one or both kidneys. Eventually, the client develops hypertension, and the kidneys atrophy. Salt wasting occurs when the medulla is damaged.

Therapeutic Measures

Acute Pyelonephritis
Antibiotics to which the bacteria are sensitive must be administered to eradicate the infectious process. Follow-up cultures must be obtained to ensure that the urine is sterile. Recurrence of the infection necessitates reculturing to ensure that another organism has not invaded the urinary tract or that a resistant strain has not developed. Antispasmodics may be prescribed to alleviate bladder spasms. Rest, nutrition, and adequate fluid intake are necessary for the client's condition to improve. Any obstruction must be surgically removed (refer to Chapter 34).

Chronic Pyelonephritis
In addition to appropriate antibiotics for the treatment of bacterial infections, agents that suppress the formation of new bacteria are generally prescribed. Urinary antiseptics such as the sulfonamides or nitrofurantoin may be administered. Antihypertensive agents also may be necessary. The major goal of medical management of chronic pyelonephritis is to prevent further damage to the renal parenchyma. Surgical correction of structural abnormalities should be considered when possible. If end-stage renal failure develops, dialysis or transplantation will be necessary to maintain life.

Specific Nursing Measures

Acute Pyelonephritis
Nursing measures for the client with acute pyelonephritis are directed toward support during the period of illness and education about the self-care measures necessary to attain or maintain health. Assist the client with such basic care needs as hygiene, nutrition, elimination, rest, and sleep—important components in the healing process. Fluid balance should be monitored and recorded accurately. Antibiotics should be administered to ensure that appropriate 24-hour blood levels are achieved.

Education about self-care in the convalescent phase of acute pyelonephritis should include discussion about how to take the prescribed medications. The client, family, or significant others should thoroughly understand the need to take all the medications prescribed and the need to finish the prescribed amount even if the client is feeling much better. Appropriate follow-up to evaluate the effectiveness of therapy is essential. Likewise, it is extremely important that the client seek assistance if a new infection is suspected.

Chronic Pyelonephritis
Nursing interventions for the client with chronic pyelonephritis should include educational efforts to maximize understanding about self-care needs. The appropriate administration of prescribed medications, adequate fluid intake to ensure removal of metabolic wastes, and adequate nutrition for continued health are all components of the nursing care plan. If significant renal deterioration has occurred, the client and family or significant others will need support in understanding the dialytic or transplantation options available.

RENAL ABSCESS

A renal abscess is an infection that develops within the kidney. Single or multiple sites of bacterial abscess may be present. Renal abscesses are most common in clients with a history of pyelonephritis, chronic obstruction, or calculous disease. Staphylococcal skin infections may also spread to kidney parenchyma and result in an abscess.

Clinical Manifestations

The client usually has pain in the costovertebral angle, fever, and chills. Physical examination may reveal edema and a palpable mass.

Therapeutic Measures

Penicillin-type antibiotics must be given immediately. If the infection is associated with chronic pyelonephritis, other broad-spectrum antibiotics may be necessary. Medical treatment aims at supporting the client while the antibiotics eradicate the infection. For example, IV fluid administration may be required. If severe bacteremia develops, septic shock may follow and cardiopulmonary support may be required. Surgical drainage of the abscess may be necessary. Partial or complete nephrectomy may be required if significant renal deterioration has occurred. Refer to Chapter 34 for a discussion of nephrectomy care.

Specific Nursing Measures

The client with a renal abscess is acutely and possibly critically ill. Administration of the prescribed antibiotics is a priority nursing action. Anticipate IV administration of the antibiotics to ensure adequate absorption of the drug. In addition, parenteral fluid replacement may be necessary if the client is not able to tolerate fluids and food. Nursing interventions also include careful monitoring of vital signs, including temperature. Changes in level of consciousness, along with hypotension, may signify that the infection is becoming systemic. Measurement of intake, output, and daily weights should be part of the nursing care plan. The

client will often be weak from the infection and require temporary assistance with hygienic measures. In addition, the client may be susceptible to problems of immobility, such as atelectasis, skin breakdown, and thrombophlebitis. Initiate appropriate interventions to prevent the sequelae of these problems.

Section VI: Neoplastic and Obstructive Disorders

Neoplastic and obstructive disorders of the kidneys and urinary tract are fairly common in the adult client. Although cancer in general is discussed in Chapter 13, this chapter will include a specific discussion of the neoplastic disorders most common in the kidneys and urinary system.

The most common nonmalignant obstructive disorders of the kidneys and the urinary system result from the formation of calculi or the effects of their obstruction, or from hyperplasia of prostatic tissue (benign prostatic hyperplasia). Calculi are discussed later in this section; prostatic disorders are discussed in Chapter 67.

A variety of terms are used to describe the types of tumors that arise in the kidney and urinary tract. Most tumors are malignant. Malignant tumors are generally renal cell carcinomas (adenocarcinomas), squamous cell carcinomas, or transitional cell carcinomas. Sarcomas of the renal urinary tract are rare.

Approximately 60,000 new cases of cancer in the urinary system were estimated for 1985, while deaths were estimated at 19,000. Of these new cases, over 40,000 would be bladder cancers with 10,000 deaths and over 19,700 cancers of the kidneys or other urinary organs with 8900 deaths (American Cancer Society, 1985). Because these tumors tend to develop in later life (the fifth, sixth, and seventh decades and beyond), clients with neoplastic disorders of the kidneys and urinary tract may already have other health alterations that require management. Consequently, the individual client must be carefully assessed so that the therapeutic interventions selected will maximize the quality of life.

General Nursing Implications

A considerable number of nursing implications exist in the care of clients with neoplastic disorders of the kidneys and urinary tract. In addition to the implications discussed in Chapter 12, the client often recognizes the nurse as a potential confidant for the disclosure of early symptoms, so referral to a physician for appropriate diagnosis and treatment is essential. Because seeing blood in the urine produces tremendous anxiety, the client may delay seeking treatment. Encourage the client to seek immediate medical assistance for evaluation of the problem, since a delay will only intensify the anxiety surrounding the unknown situation. Emotional support and educational interventions are important nursing interventions throughout the referral, diagnostic, therapeutic, and rehabilitative phases.

The health history should identify alterations in urinary output, with particular emphasis on altered patterns of urination and the appearance of the urine. Clients commonly report intermittent hematuria. If the neoplastic process is in the lower urinary tract or if the client has only one kidney, there may be alterations in urinary output related to obstruction. Percuss for suprapubic dullness as evidence of bladder distention. There may be some loss of urinary continence upon palpation or percussion of the bladder. The client may report a feeling of bladder or lower abdominal fullness or dull flank pain. Loss of weight, feelings of fatigue, and anorexia may accompany the neoplastic process.

In general, nursing interventions for the client with neoplasia of the kidneys or urinary tract include providing comfort; providing emotional support during the diagnostic, therapeutic, and convalescent period; and educating the client in self-care and optimal decision making. In addition, the nurse must continually assess the client to prevent complications associated with the therapeutic interventions or the disease process. The prevention of problems such as infection, urinary tract obstruction, and acute renal failure depends on constant assessment for their potential development. The client and family or significant others should be involved throughout. Emotional support and educational counseling of the family or significant others should facilitate the posthospitalization convalescence and rehabilitation.

RENAL CELL CARCINOMA

Renal cell carcinomas, also referred to as *hypernephromas* or *adenocarcinomas*, account for about 80% of renal tumors and occur in men about 66% more often than in women (Smith, 1981). The age of appearance is generally in the 50s or 60s. The renal cell carcinoma usually occurs in the pole of a single kidney and has a capsule. There may be hemorrhage or necrosis within the capsule, and enlargement of the kidney from the tumor. Because the tumor frequently grows for months before detection, the tumor may be quite large before the client seeks medical assistance. The tumor typically spreads to other structures by blood or lymph. The liver, lungs, long bones, and other kidney are the most common sites of metastasis.

The term *hypernephroma* was used in the past when this tumor was thought to arise from the proximity of the adrenal gland and the kidney. The current viewpoint is that tumors in the renal tubules or benign adenomas in the renal parenchyma result in this pathological condition. Cytological evidence from renal biopsy indicates that the malignant cells are similar to renal tubular cells. Various hormonal secretions have been identified from these neoplastic cells, including ACTH, gonadotropins, erythropoietin, and hormones that resemble parathormone and insulin (Smith, 1981).

Clinical Manifestations

Gross hematuria is the most common manifestation of a renal cell carcinoma. The client may identify dull flank pain, but this is generally a late symptom that develops as the tumor enlarges and presses upon adjacent structures. Occasionally, the client identifies a mass in the flank region, but this is rare. Other manifestations of a renal carcinoma may include nausea or vomiting, which result from the direct involvement or displacement of abdominal contents. Metastatic symptoms include weakness, loss of weight, and bone pain.

Therapeutic Measures

In general, the renal cell carcinoma is not responsive to available chemotherapeutic agents or radiation therapy. The treatment of pulmonary metastases with vinblastine sulfate (Velban), however, may lead to successful remission (Smith, 1981). Hormonal therapies may be useful for hormone-producing tumors. Recent research indicates that interferon may be useful in the treatment of renal malignancies (see Chapter 12).

The intentional embolization of the involved kidney by purposefully occluding the renal artery may be performed prior to surgical intervention. This procedure, sometimes referred to as a *medical nephrectomy*, decreases the blood supply to the kidney with the tumor and facilitates the technical aspects of surgery. In addition, renal artery embolization may be performed to control hemorrhage (Smith, 1981).

Surgery is the primary intervention for treatment of a renal cell carcinoma, and the surgical procedure of choice is a nephrectomy. Ideally, the procedure is a radical one that also removes the perirenal fat, fascia, accompanying adrenal gland, adjacent lymph nodes, and posterior parietal peritoneum. Because spontaneous remission of renal carcinomas has occurred, surgical debulking of the tumor mass is indicated even if obvious metastases are present. Nephrectomy is discussed in Chapter 34.

Specific Nursing Measures

Care for the client with a renal cell carcinoma is the same as with any diagnosis of cancer as discussed in Chapter 13 and the preceding discussion under general nursing care for neoplastic disorders. Most care revolves around the surgical intervention as discussed in Chapter 34.

BLADDER CANCER

Bladder malignancies are the most common tumors of the genitourinary tract, with the exception of prostatic tumors (Smith, 1981). The majority are found in men over 50. The bladder tumor commonly involves the ureteral orifices or bladder neck. The tumor cells are usually transitional cells and are judged according to degree of differentiation (described by staging) and depth of penetration. The staging of cell type is important when therapeutic interventions are considered. Grade 1 tumors of the bladder are primarily papillary and well differentiated. Grade 2 tumors are also papillary but are less differentiated and may have invaded deeper tissue layers. Both grade 1 and 2 bladder tumors are curable by transurethral fulguration, but they are not responsive to radiation therapy. Grade 3 and 4 bladder tumors are generally nodular, invasive, and not differentiated. The cells are responsive to radiation and require surgical removal. Bladder neoplasms commonly metastasize to the organs supplied by the lymph nodes of the bladder and to the hypogastric, common iliac, and lumbar vessels.

Considerable evidence shows that exposure to certain compounds is associated with increased incidence of bladder cancer. For example, there is a well-established link between prolonged exposure to industrial compounds such as the aniline dyes and development of bladder cancer. A variety of substances have been described as potentially carcinogenic to the bladder, and suspected carcinogens have been identified in the urine of clients with bladder cancer. Cancer is thought to occur through liver metabolism of various substances followed by renal excretion of the metabolites. Tryptophan and the tars of smoking have been strongly linked with bladder cancer, but the evidence is not unequivocal.

Clinical Manifestations

Painless hematuria is the primary clinical manifestation of bladder cancer. The hematuria is intermittent, so the client may ignore the earliest manifestation of the pathological process. Obstruction of the urinary tract by the tumor may alter the outflow of urine, causing intermittent anuria and polyuria; there also may be bladder distention. Infection may cause symptoms of dysuria, such as burning, frequency, or urgency. Other urinary flow alterations may include a decrease of the force or volume of the urinary stream.

Therapeutic Measures

Considerable research continues in the administration of various chemotherapeutic agents for the treatment of bladder cancers. Methods of administration include direct bladder instillations, intra-arterial infusions, IV infusion, and oral ingestion. Many chemotherapeutic agents (including 5-fluorouracil, methotrexate, bleomycin, mitomycin-C, and hydroxyurea) have been used in an attempt to demonstrate a significant clinical response. More recently, doxorubicin and cyclophosphamide or cisplatin have been tried; reports of effectiveness are variable, and results are not conclusive. Because of the high association of tryptophan metabolites with bladder cancer, Smith (1981) recommends the administration of pyridoxine to those with a confirmed diagnosis, because pyridoxine neutralizes tryptophan metabolites.

Bladder malignancies may be treated by transurethral removal, partial cystectomy, or radical cystectomy. Urinary diversion procedures also may be necessary; these procedures are discussed in Chapter 34.

Specific Nursing Measures

Nursing care for the client with bladder cancer is the same as for anyone diagnosed as having cancer. The care required following the various surgical procedures is discussed in Chapter 34.

NEPHROLITHIASIS AND UROLITHIASIS

Nephrolithiasis and *urolithiasis* refer to the presence of **calculi** (stones) in the urinary tract. Calculi in the urinary tract are a relatively common problem, especially for men. They usually occur within the same family but are rare in black persons. There is a high incidence of recurrence; the incidence of a second calculus within 2 years is reported to be as high as 40%. Renal calculi are extremely painful, and the individual is incapacitated during an acute episode. Napoleon III was defeated at Sedan in the Franco–Prussian War when he was felled by a kidney stone. When associated with infection or obstruction, renal calculi may be life threatening.

The majority of calculi originate in the renal parenchyma (nephrolithiasis) and are passed out into the ureters or bladder (urolithiasis). Most calculi are composed of calcium salts (calcium oxalate or calcium phosphate; Figure 33–6), uric acid, or struvite (magnesium ammonium phosphate, a triple salt; Figure 33–7). Cystine calculi are uncommon. A number of factors contribute to the formation of calculi. The primary factors influencing calculi formation are the degree to which the urine is supersaturated with an element normally excreted, the pH of the urine, the presence of substances that inhibit the formation of crystals, the stasis of urine, and a special preexisting environment.

Clients with pathological conditions in which large amounts of calcium phosphate or uric acid are excreted may develop calculi. A dietary excess of foods containing calcium or purine, immobilization, primary hyperparathyroidism, hypervitaminosis D, and renal tubular acidosis may result in hypercalciuria (Smith, 1981). Medications taken in excess, such as the antacids or vitamin C, may also result in hypercalciuria or excess calcium oxalate. However, most cases of calculus formation are idiopathic.

The pH of the urine may also influence calculus formation. Normally, urine is slightly acidic with a pH of 5 to 6. With infection, the urine is slightly alkaline (pH above 7). Uric acid and cystine calculi will form in acidic urine; calcium phosphate calculi will dissolve in acidic urine; and calcium oxalate calculi are not influenced by the pH of the urine. Struvite calculi are associated with infection from urea-splitting bacteria. Bacteria such as the *Proteus* strains convert areas to ammonia, and the alkaline urine contributes to the formation of struvite calculi.

Figure 33–6

A. Calcium oxalate stone. **B.** Calcium phosphate stone. (Courtesy of Millard Fillmore Hospital, Buffalo, NY)

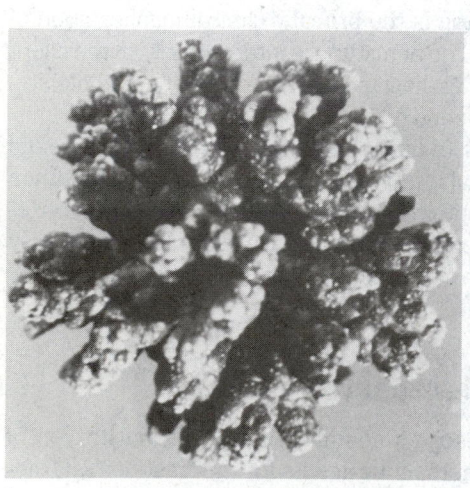

A

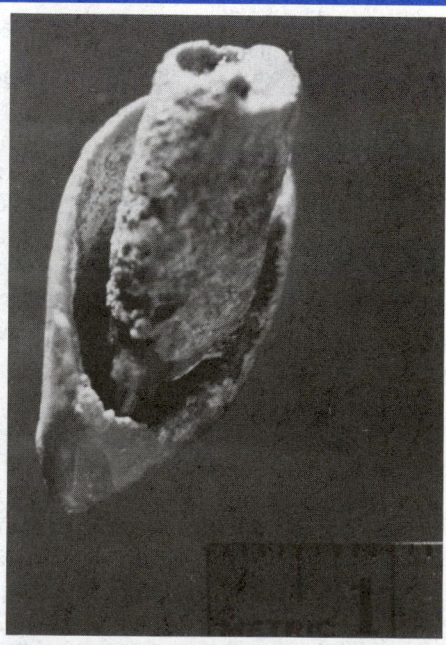

B

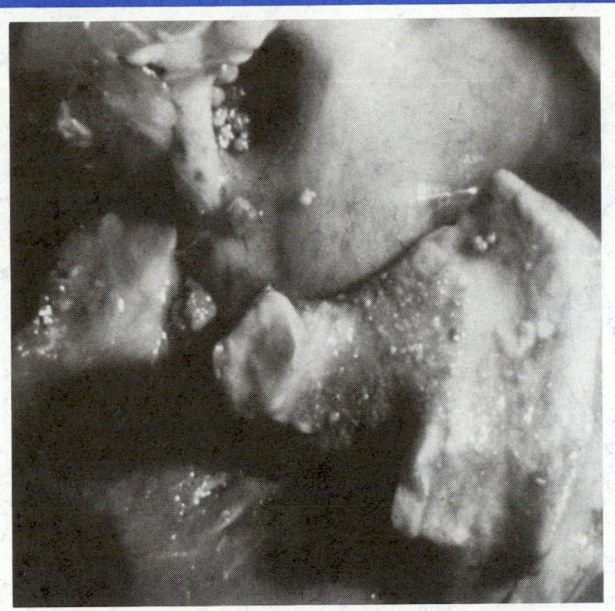

Figure 33–7

Staghorn calculus composed of struvite. (Courtesy of Millard Fillmore Hospital, Buffalo, NY)

Exactly how calculi form is not clearly understood. However, certain substances that the kidney excretes (pyrophosphate, magnesium, and citrate) are believed to inhibit the formation of calculi, and decreases in the levels of these substances have been associated with calculus formation. In contrast, calculus formation is enhanced when there are old scars (either from infection or surgical procedures in the urinary tract) or when urinary stasis or urinary crystallization is already present.

Clinical Manifestations

The primary clinical manifestation of nephrolithiasis or urolithiasis is pain, and its location may suggest the location of the calculus (eg, the client may describe a calculus in the kidney pelvis as dull, intermittent flank pain). In some situations there may be no discomfort at all. However, if the calculus moves down into the ureter, the client may describe the pain as excruciatingly severe. Some clients describe the pain as an 11 on a scale of 10. The ureteropelvic junction, the uretero-iliac bend, and the U-V junction—the narrowest points in the ureter—are the sites at which the calculus is most likely to become lodged (Figure 33–8). Severe intermittent pain results as the musculature of the ureter goes into spasm (**colic**) in an attempt to move the calculus out of the ureter by peristalsis. The pain of ureteral colic may traverse along the route of the ureter and extend into the lower abdomen, the vulva, or the testes. The client commonly experiences nausea and perhaps vomiting. He or she may also report the presence of blood in the urine and, if infection is present, chills and fever.

Therapeutic Measures

Narcotics are generally necessary for relief of the pain associated with renal or urinary calculi. Antispasmodics may also be prescribed to relax the ureteral musculature. If infection is present or if instrumentation is necessary to remove the calculus, antibiotics will be prescribed. Other agents may be prescribed to alter the urinary pH to create the desired environment; for example, sodium acid phosphate, potassium acid phosphate, or ascorbic acid will promote the formation of an acidic urine. Thiazide diuretics have been demonstrated to increase calcium reabsorption and thus may be prescribed for clients who form calcium calculi. However, these diuretics may cause hyperuricemia, so agents to manage the excess uric acid may also be necessary. For example, allopurinol (Zyloprim) decreases the formation of uric acid. For clients who need to have an alkaline urine, 50% sodium citrate may be prescribed (Smith, 1981).

The long-term management of the client identified as a calculus-former should emphasize obtaining a high-volume, dilute urine. The client may achieve this goal by consuming 4 L fluid per day; water is the ideal liquid. It is important to void before bedtime and to consume fluids so the client will awaken in the middle of the night to empty the bladder. When awakened, the client should drink more water to ensure a constant dilution of urine.

Dietary modifications depend on the chemical content of the calculus. A low-calcium diet is recommended only for clients who have active hypercalciuria. Decreasing calcium absorption from dietary intake increases calcium oxalate absorption to maintain a balance, so the total amount of calcium oxalate is unchanged. Thus, if calcium intake is decreased, calcium oxalate intake also must be decreased. Dietary modifications may also be suggested for clients who are hyperuricosuric and form uric acid calculi. These clients may benefit from a diet of foods low in purines. The intake of meat, fish, and poultry, which are high in purines, should be reduced. Struvite calculi, which form from bacteria, contain phosphate; therefore, a diet that limits phosphate intake may reduce struvite calculi. Medications that alter urine composition are given to prevent calculus development and are more effective than dietary modifications.

Clients with calculi too large to pass spontaneously may be able to avoid urological surgery for calculus removal through a technique called *lithotripsy*. In this treatment, the client is supported and suspended in a large tank of water (Figure 33–9). An extracorporeal shock wave lithotripter sends shock waves through the water to the calculus, which shatters and is excreted within several days (Wickham & Miller, 1983). Clients liken the feeling of the shock waves to having a rubber band snapping their backs.

Lithotripsy is expected to be used in the near future in 60% to 80% of all cases where large calculi cannot be voided without assistance. Kidney stones can also be broken down with ultrasound vibrations and flushed out of the kidney with water. Ultrasound treatment requires a small

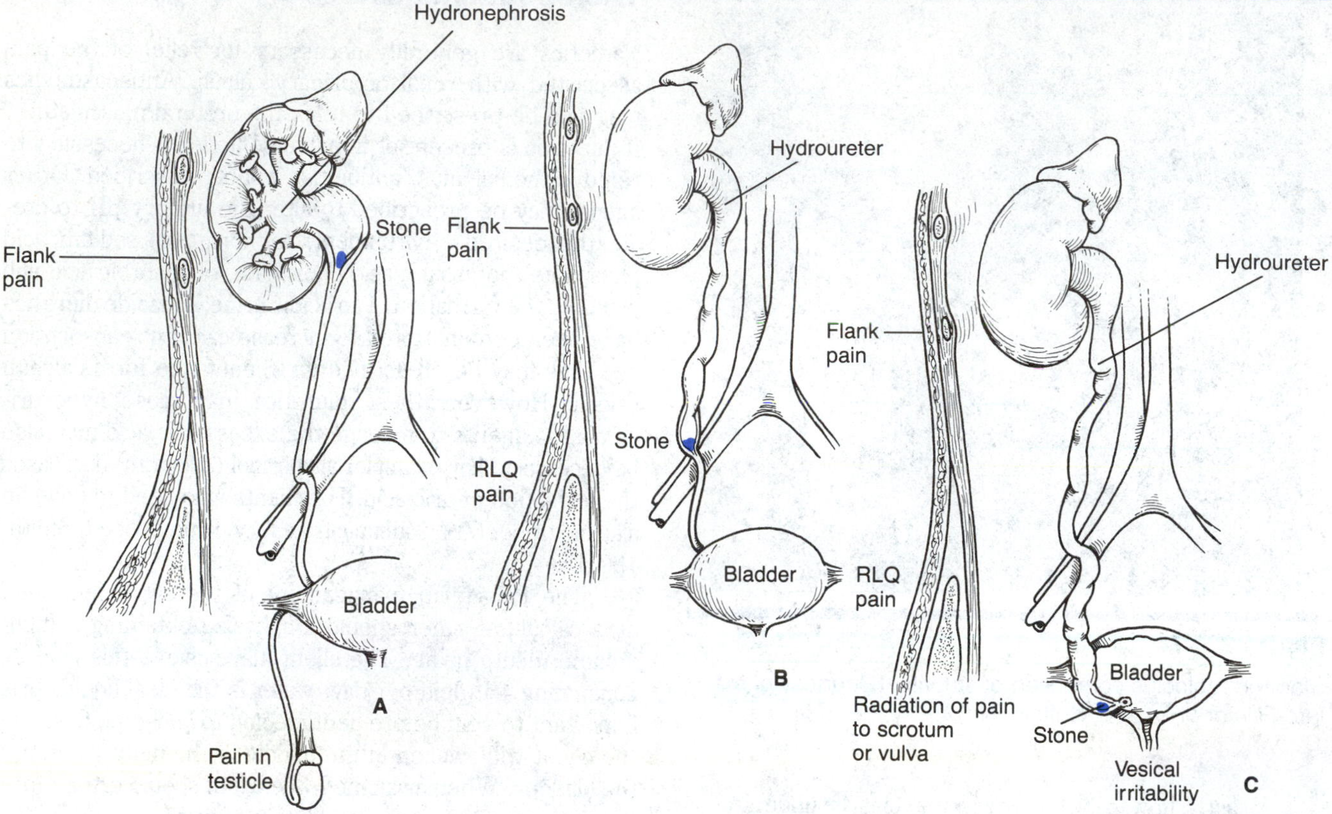

Figure 33–8

Radiation of pain and location of lodged calculi. **A.** Calculus lodged at the ureteropelvic junction. Distention of the renal pelvis and renal capsule causes severe costovertebral angle pain. Hyperperistalsis of smooth muscle of the ureter causes pain to radiate along the course of the ureter and into the testicle, which is hypersensitive. **B.** Calculus lodged at the iliac bend (the point at which the ureter crosses over the iliac vessels). Pain symptoms are like those in A with the addition of pain in the lower quadrant of the abdomen. **C.** Calculus lodged at the ureterovesical junction. Pain symptoms are like those in A and B with the addition of pain radiating into the bladder, scrotum, or vulva. Urgency, frequency, and burning on urination may result from inflammation of the bladder wall around the ureteral orifice.

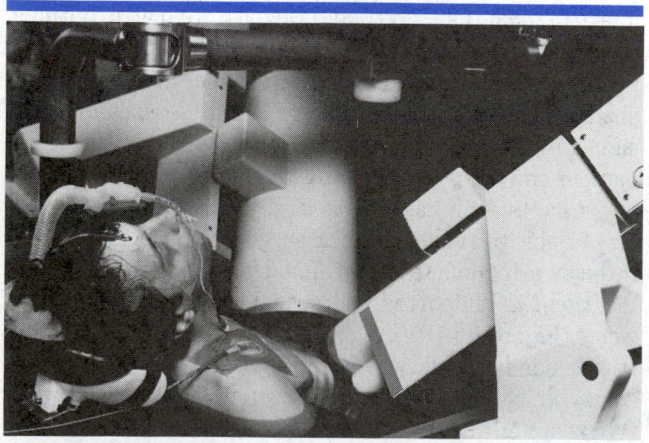

Figure 33–9

Client receiving lithotripsy treatment. The client is anesthetized and immersed in water where he will receive up to 1000 shock waves over a period of 30 to 45 minutes.

incision, about ⅓ in long. It shares the major advantage of lithotripsy—making major surgery a thing of the past for clients with kidney stones. However, if the calculus does not pass spontaneously or if there is intractable pain, persistent infection, or obstruction, surgical removal of the calculus will be necessary. A variety of surgical procedures may be used to remove the calculus; the method selected depends somewhat on its location. Surgical interventions are discussed in Chapter 34.

Specific Nursing Measures

Care of the client with renal or urinary calculi presents challenges to the maintenance of comfort and the prevention of infection. The goal for client education is the prevention of recurrence, if possible. In addition to measuring intake and output carefully, an essential nursing intervention is the straining of all urine through a fine mesh gauze contained in a funnel-shaped container. The goal of the straining procedure is to obtain a calculus or calculus fragments that may be analyzed by the laboratory for chemical characteristics.

The prescribed medications should be administered to afford the client relief from pain. Initially, the client may require IV administration of morphine sulfate to obtain relief. Antibiotics should be administered as prescribed to ensure that bacterial growth ceases. The client should drink fluids liberally, attaining the goal of 3 to 4 L per day (Figure 33–10). Intravenous fluids may be required if the client cannot take them orally. A high fluid intake of 3 to 4 L/day is usually recommended for the remainder of the client's lifetime. If surgery is necessary, nursing care will depend on the method chosen. Table 33–2 summarizes the types of calculi and the goals of treatment and nursing care.

HYDROURETER AND HYDRONEPHROSIS

A *hydroureter* is an enlargement of the lumen of the ureter as the result of obstruction distal to the point of the enlargement (see Figures 33–8B and C). Unilateral hydroureter might occur as a result of an obstruction within the ureter from a calculus at the U-V junction, whereas bilateral hydroureter might occur from an obstruction at the bladder neck or within the urethra. When obstruction to the urinary outflow causes the accumulation of fluid under pressure in the renal pelvis, it results in distention of the renal pelvis and calyces. This condition, known as *hydronephrosis,* is accompanied by severe atrophy of the renal parenchyma (see Figure 33–8A). Hydroureter and hydronephrosis are known to always occur during pregnancy and to persist for some time afterward because of two factors—the enlarged uterus obstructs the ureters, and high progesterone levels cause muscular relaxation (Price & Wilson, 1982).

Clinical Manifestations

Pain is a common manifestation as the ureteral musculature enters a spasm. In bilateral hydroureter, symptoms will include a decrease in or absence of urinary output. Bladder distention may also be present if the obstruction is distal to the bladder neck, as would be the situation in prostatic hyperplasia. With hydronephrosis there may be dull flank pain, local tenderness, and vomiting or gastrointestinal upset as the distended kidney presses on the stomach. Infection or renal failure develops if the problem is not corrected quickly.

Therapeutic Measures

Medical treatment includes diagnostic testing to identify the cause of the obstruction and pharmacological treatment to manage the symptoms:

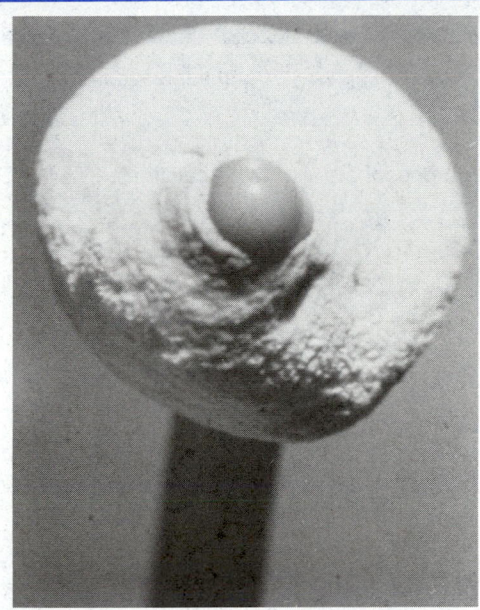

Figure 33–10
Balloon of Foley catheter encrusted with calcium phospate. Keeping the urine pH acidic could have prevented this problem. (Courtesy of Millard Fillmore Hospital, Buffalo, NY)

- Narcotics for relief of pain
- Antispasmodics to relieve ureteral spasm
- Antibiotics and urinary antiseptics to prevent or treat infection
- Antiemetics to control nausea and vomiting

Urinary catheterization will be necessary if there is urinary retention with bladder distention. An indwelling catheter may be required to continue urinary drainage and prevent recurrence of the obstruction. A nephrostomy tube may be used to drain urine from the renal pelvis. Antibiotics may be prescribed if infection is present. Surgical interventions may be required, such as ureterolithotomy or cystoscopy with prostatic resection or fulguration of bladder tumors, or nephrectomy if irreparable kidney damage has occurred. These are discussed in Chapter 34.

Specific Nursing Measures

Take careful measurements of the client's intake, output, and weight. Providing adequate pain relief is essential. Educational preparation for diagnostic tests and emotional support for proposed procedures will be necessary. The client is likely to have concerns about permanent alteration in kidney function and thus may be quite anxious. Other measures depend on the type of pharmacological management or surgical intervention selected.

Table 33–2 Urinary Calculi: Nursing Considerations

Type	Conditions Promoting Formation	Dietary Modifications	Medications	Goal of Urinary pH
Calcium phosphate	Hypercalciuria	Decrease dietary calcium if normally a high calcium intake; increase fluid intake	Cellulose phosphate; thiazide diuretics (eg, Diuril, Hydrodiuril); avoid antacids that contain calcium; use aluminum hydroxide antacids that bind with phosphorus	Less than 6
Calcium oxalate	Hyperoxaluria	Increase fluid intake; decrease calcium oxalate intake (avoid tea, cocoa, colas, instant coffee, and beer); avoid citrus fruits, grapes, cranberries, beans, spinach, apples, mushrooms, beets, turnips, and most nuts	Cholestyramine, pyridoxine, and methylene blue; avoid antacids that contain calcium	Less than 6
Uric acid	Hyperuricemia and uricosuria	Low purine diet may help; increase fluid intake; limit intake of ham, beef, halibut, trout, and salmon	Allopurinol; avoid uricosuric agents such as the thiazide diuretics and aspirin; give sodium bicarbonate to increase urine pH	Greater than 6.5
Struvite (triple phosphate or magnesium ammonium phosphate)	Presence of *Proteus* bacteria strains in the urinary tract: bacterial splitting of urea results in high-ammonia, highly alkaline urine	Encourage eggs, meat, poultry, fish, and cereals; increase fluid intake	Antibiotics (long term); methionine; ascorbic acid	Between 5.5 and 6.2

Section VII: Traumatic Disorders

Direct or indirect injury to the organs of the urinary system usually interrupts the structural integrity of the kidney or kidneys, the ureter or ureters, or the bladder. A major interruption of vascular supply may occur concomitantly. Traumatic injuries are commonly classified as either penetrating or nonpenetrating (blunt).

Injuries to the kidneys, ureters, or bladder may significantly affect the client's overall health. Preservation of renal function is the primary goal. Loss of a single kidney from trauma may not be life threatening assuming the other kidney is functioning adequately, but it can have serious consequences (see client implications for nephrectomy in Chapter 34). In addition, clients who experience renal trauma are often victims of other abdominal trauma that may be life threatening.

The dissemination of information to the general public could prevent many injuries to the urinary tract. The proper use of seat belts and safety straps in automobiles and other vehicles should be included in basic safety education programs. Health educators should stress the importance of avoiding delayed bladder emptying; for example, amusement park rides commonly involve wearing safety straps over the lower abdomen and may result in injury if the bladder is distended.

General Nursing Implications

The history of the client with a traumatic disorder is often the most significant part of the diagnosis. Gunshot or stab wounds are quite obvious, but only the history may disclose less obvious traumatic events. Physical sports involving heavy direct contact, such as football or ice hockey, may result in injuries that did not seem significant at the time. Other sports generally not labeled as contact sports, such as baseball, basketball, snow skiing, tobagganing, and horseback riding, all may involve heavy blows to the back or ribs. A history of rib fractures, chest injuries, or abdominal injuries should always suggest the potential for renal trauma. Physical assessment includes the collection of a urine specimen to determine the presence of blood. Flank pain or suprapubic tenderness may or may not be present. Alterations in urinary output and patterns of voiding are very important.

The client and family or significant others need education about the diagnostic procedures to be performed. For example, abdominal ultrasonography and a computerized tomography (CT) scan are commonly performed. If significant bleeding is suspected, a renal arteriogram with subsequent surgical intervention should be anticipated. However, conservative management is recommended when possible including bed rest, comfort measures, assessment to detect complications of bed rest, and interventions to prevent these complications. Vital signs, intake, and urinary output need regular monitoring. A Foley catheter will be placed if the client is unable to urinate. Blood and IV fluids may be prescribed to maintain intravascular volume if bleeding is active.

Evaluation of the effectiveness of the nursing interventions involves an assessment of the physical and emotional responses of the client and family or significant others. Major physical responses include continued renal function and the establishment of urinary tract integrity. In addition, the client should be free of infection and other postoperative complications. On the emotional level, the client and family or significant others should be able to verbalize feelings related to the accident that produced the trauma and the effects of the trauma and the treatment required. Feelings may include anger, sadness, loss, and guilt. If the return of renal function is questionable and the client needs permanent dialysis or transplantation or experiences a major interruption in normal body image, feelings may change and require months or years for adaptation or resolution.

RENAL TRAUMA

The kidneys are well protected from injury because of their structural placement partially within the rib cage and under the strong muscles of the back and spine. However, about 50% of all injuries involving the urinary system are reported to involve the kidneys. Renal injuries are generally described as minor, major, or critical (injuries to the renal pedicle) (Figure 33–11). Minor injuries include contusions, hematomas, and simple lacerations of the cortex. Major injuries involve significant laceration of the renal parenchyma, loss of renal parenchyma, or injury to a major branch of the renal artery. Critical injuries involve lacerations of the renal artery, renal vein, or renal pelvis (McConnell & Zimmer-

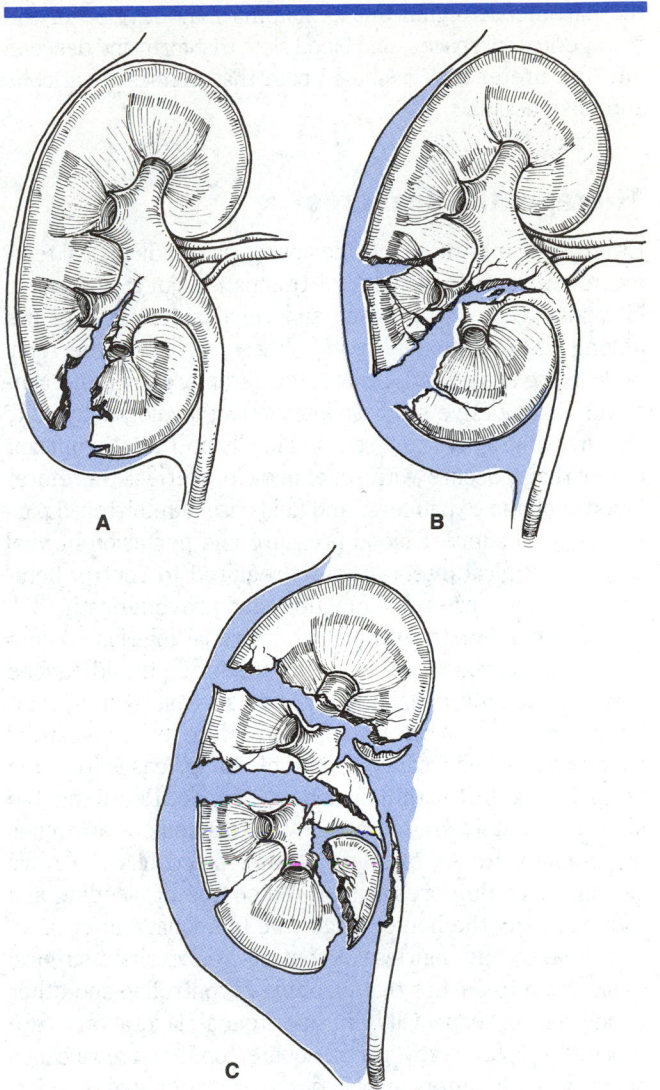

Figure 33–11

Classification of renal trauma. **A.** Minor. **B.** Major. **C.** Critical.

man, 1983). A transplanted kidney is not as well protected from injury, so abdominal injuries to the transplant recipient may result in significant renal trauma. Other abdominal trauma is common in clients who experience renal trauma.

Injuries of the kidney usually occur from either penetrating or nonpenetrating (blunt) trauma. Abdominal gunshot or stab wounds may affect either or both kidneys. Automobile accidents, automobile–pedestrian accidents, motorcycle accidents, or injuries from sporting events may result in blunt trauma. All levels of involvement—minor, major, or critical—may occur.

Clinical Manifestations

Gross or microscopic hematuria, flank pain, abdominal pain, or a combination are the most common manifestations of renal trauma. Flank pain may be related to the direct force of the injury or to bleeding in the parenchyma or under the capsule. A significant hematoma may develop in the retroperitoneal spaces, and blood clots that form and descend into the ureter may result in pain that mimics renal colic and obstruction.

Therapeutic Measures

Emergency measures include appropriate radiological testing to evaluate the extent of traumatic injury; abdominal ultrasonography, CT scan, and renal arteriography are among the most useful tests. When injuries to the renal pedicle are suspected, renal arteriography is most informative. Risks of dye studies, intravenous pyelography, CT, and arteriography are discussed in Chapter 32. Significant hemorrhage occurs with renal pedicle injuries; therefore, blood, volume expanders, and fluids are administered parenterally to support blood pressure and perfusion of vital organs. Surgical intervention is required to control hemorrhage, preserve renal function, and prevent death.

For nonpenetrating and minor renal injuries, a conservative approach is generally accepted, including bed rest; monitoring of laboratory data such as hemoglobin, hematocrit, serum creatinine, and BUN levels; and careful evaluation of fluid balance. Minor bleeding ceases from the tamponade effect within the kidney capsule. Recall that the kidney is contained in a capsule that expands or stretches only minimally. As bleeding occurs, blood fills the renal capsule, exerting pressure on the source of bleeding and thus stopping the hemorrhage (the tamponade effect).

Penetrating injuries, in contrast, necessitate surgical exploration to ensure that bleeding is controlled and other tissue tears, especially intraperitoneal lacerations, are repaired. Nephrectomy, partial nephrectomy, and renal bench surgery with autotransplantation are potential surgical interventions for renal trauma. These are discussed in Chapter 34. Antibiotics are generally prescribed for clients with penetrating renal trauma. Gunshot and stab wounds often perforate the peritoneum and abdominal organs such as the intestine, so analgesics are required to control the pain. Antibiotic dosages must be adjusted appropriately when compromise of renal function is present or the development of toxicity is evident.

Specific Nursing Measures

Monitor urine output and vital signs hourly, laboratory values (eg, hemoglobin, hematocrit, BUN, and electrolytes), and fluid balance. Observe the client for hypovolemic shock that may occur because of hemorrhage or peritonitis from urine leaking into the peritoneum. The administration of blood, fluids, volume expanders, antibiotics, and medications for pain relief is a primary nursing responsibility. Preoperative and postoperative nursing care (see Chapter 34) should be followed when surgery is required for the control of hemorrhage or kidney repair.

URETERAL TRAUMA

Ureteral injuries are relatively rare, because the ureters are deep and well protected. When it occurs, however, injury to the ureter or ureters is significant because of the resulting loss of continuity for urinary drainage. The majority of ureteral injuries result from penetrating trauma such as gunshot or stab wounds or from accidental ligation or unintentional incision during another surgical procedure.

Clinical Manifestations

Alteration in urinary output is the most common manifestation of ureteral trauma. Anuria is common, and abdominal pain, fever, and chills may be present if peritonitis develops from the leakage of urine into the peritoneum. In addition, if there is an abdominal incision, urine may leak to the surface or exit via a drain.

Therapeutic Measures

Recognition of ureteral injury should be followed by surgical measures to reconstruct the continuity of the urinary tract (refer to Chapter 34). Peritonitis, if present, should be treated without delay by antibiotics. In addition, analgesics will promote comfort. Renal function and fluid replacement must be monitored carefully until the integrity of the ureter has been reestablished.

Specific Nursing Measures

Assess urine output and observe the client for symptoms of peritonitis (elevated temperature, abdominal discomfort, and tenderness). Preoperative and postoperative nursing care is described in Chapter 34.

BLADDER TRAUMA

Injuries to the urinary bladder, like those to the kidneys and ureters, may also be described as penetrating or nonpenetrating. Nonpenetrating injuries are usually contusions, whereas penetrating injuries result in rupture with leakage of urine. Although the bladder is somewhat protected by its position in the lower pelvis, bladder injury is common with pelvic fractures. A full bladder is at increased risk to injury from perforation during a traumatic or compression injury. Gunshot and stab wounds may penetrate the urinary bladder. Automobile injuries, especially from seat belt placement over a distended bladder, and automobile–pedestrian accidents are common causes of bladder trauma. The risk of bladder injury from seat belt use is minimized by keeping the bladder nondistended. The overall value of the use of seat belts is well established and should be encouraged.

Clinical Manifestations

Manifestations of bladder injury include hematuria, difficulty with voiding, or absence of urine output. Suprapubic pain or tenderness is common, as is scrotal or perineal swelling from the extravasation of urine into these tissues.

Therapeutic Measures

The immediate recognition and treatment of bladder rupture are important in saving the client's life. Conservative treatment—rest and constant drainage via a Foley catheter—is used for bladder contusions. A suspected bladder tear or laceration, however, requires surgical exploration. Surgical intervention also is needed to repair penetrating bladder trauma. These procedures are discussed in Chapter 34. Antibiotics are usually required to treat the infection that occurs with leakage of urine into the peritoneum or other tissues.

Specific Nursing Measures

Major nursing implications include recognizing symptoms that may identify a previously undetected bladder rupture; for example, persistent, unidentified fever may result from leakage of urine. The client will be given IV fluids postoperatively. Monitor intake and output to ensure that fluid balance is achieved. Alterations in urinary output should be detected as soon as possible so corrective measures may be initiated. Drains and catheters should be cared for aseptically to prevent infection. Initiate measures to prevent complications associated with stasis of pulmonary secretions or venous congestion in the extremities. In addition, appropriate health teaching and emotional support should be provided, because the client and family or significant others will be concerned about normalization of urinary function. In addition, they may have concerns about sexuality or sexual function.

Chapter Highlights

Clients with congenital disorders of the kidneys and urinary system may require adequate education in self-care and health maintenance, surgical intervention, and other general measures to preserve renal function, along with emotional support and genetic counseling.

Acute tubular necrosis (ATN) is the most common cause of acute renal failure, the sudden deterioration in renal function. It may present a life-threatening situation that requires prompt intervention and management.

Clients with urinary incontinence have physical discomfort, as well as social and emotional embarrassment.

A neurogenic bladder may increase the client's potential for the development of infection, obstruction of the urinary tract, or chronic renal failure.

Degenerative disorders of the urinary system and kidneys, which include analgesic abuse nephropathy, nephrosclerosis, renal artery stenosis, and diabetic glomerulopathy, result in changes in the renal parenchyma or blood vessels that supply the kidney.

Loss of glomerular integrity as the result of immune (antigen–antibody) complexes in the bloodstream that are deposited in the glomeruli occurs with nephrotic syndrome and acute and chronic glomerulonephritis.

Urinary tract infections account for more than 40% of all nosocomial infections. Treatment of these infections involves the correct administration of antibiotics, ingestion of about 3 L/day of fluid, and client education about hygiene measures to help prevent the development of future infections.

Management of clients with malignant tumors of the urinary tract includes care appropriate to any client with a malignancy, emotional support regarding altered sexuality, and preservation of the remaining function of the urinary system.

Clients with a tendency toward formation of renal and urinary calculi must have them analyzed before dietary changes or medications may be prescribed for treatment. All calculi-forming clients should avoid dehydration and maintain a liberal fluid intake.

Most common traumatic occurrences interrupt the structural integrity of the kidney or kidneys, ureter or ureters, or bladder, as well as the vascular supply to these structures.

Bibliography

Chambers JK: Save your diabetic patient from early kidney damage. *Nurs 83* 1983; 13(5):58–64.

Frank LI, Admire RC: Rhabdomyolysis. *Urol Clin North Am* 1982; 9(2):267–273.

Garibaldi RA: Hospital acquired urinary tract infection. In: *CRC Handbook of Hospital Acquired Infections.* Wenzel RC (editor). Boca Raton, FL: CRC Press, 1981.

Hart M, Adamek C: Do increased fluids decrease urinary stone formation? *Geriat Nurs* 1984; 5:245–248.

Henrich WL: Nephrotoxicity of non-steroidal anti-inflammatory agents. *Am J Kidney Dis* 1983; 2(4):278–284.

McConnell EA, Zimmerman MF: *Care of Patients With Urologic Problems.* Philadelphia: Lippincott, 1983.

McConnell J: Preventing urinary tract infections. *Geriat Nurs* 1984; 5:361–362.

Porter GA, Bennett WM: Nephrotoxin-induced acute renal failure. In: *Contemporary Issues in Nephrology, Vol 6, Acute Renal Failure.* Brenner BM, Stein JH (editors). New York: Churchill Livingstone, 1980.

Price S, Wilson L: *Pathophysiology: Clinical Concepts of Disease Processes,* 2nd ed. New York: McGraw-Hill, 1982.

Richard C: Management of patients with renal and genitourinary disorders. In: *ACCN's Clinical Reference for Critical Care Nursing.* Kinney M, et al (editors). New York: McGraw-Hill, 1981.

Rose BD: *Pathophysiology of Renal Disease.* New York: McGraw-Hill, 1981.

Rubin P (editor): *Clinical Oncology for Medical Students and Physicians: A Multidisciplinary Approach.* New York: American Cancer Society, 1983.

Schrier RW: *Renal and Electrolyte Disorders,* 2nd ed. Boston: Little, Brown, 1980.

Smith DR: *General Urology,* 10th ed. Los Altos, CA: Lange, 1981.

Sos FA et al: Percutaneous transluminal renal angioplasty in renovascular hypertension due to atheroma or fibromuscular dysplasia. *New Engl J Med* 1983; 309:274–279.

Suggested Readings

Brown RO: Nutritional support in acute renal failure. *AANNT J* 1983; 10:25–29. Article discussing diet alterations and nutritional support for the client with acute renal failure.

Chambers JK: Save your diabetic patient from early kidney damage. *Nurs 83* 1983; 13(May):58–64. Diabetic clients are particularly vulnerable to a variety of factors commonly encountered during a routine hospitalization. Nursing knowledge of factors that contribute to decreased renal function may help prevent the diabetic client from developing renal failure and the need for dialysis.

Dugan JS: Winning the battle against incontinence. *Nurs 84* 1984; 14(6):59. One-page description of how confused elderly patients can learn to become continent again.

Freed SZ: Urinary incontinence in the elderly. *Hospital Practice* 1982; 10(March):81 +. Article describing the importance of determining the reason for urinary incontinence in elderly clients. The author emphasizes that urinary incontinence is not inevitable with advancing age. Various diagnostic tests and methods of treatment are described.

Harcum P: Renal nutrition for the renal nurse. *ANNA J* 1984; 11:38–44. Thorough, concise article detailing the caloric and nutrient needs of the adult hemodialysis and CAPD client. Overviews electrolyte, vitamin, and mineral supplementation for long-term nutritional management.

Orr ML: Drugs and renal disease. *Am J Nurs* 1981; 81(May):969 +. Article describing the pharmacological considerations necessary for clients with impaired renal function. This article includes how alterations in drug absorption, distribution, metabolism, and excretion influence the dosage schedules and methods of administration. In addition, specific pharmacological concerns of clients receiving dialysis treatments are reviewed.

The Client With Chronic Renal Failure

I. Descriptive Data	Mrs Ethel Redding, a 73-year-old black woman, is currently undergoing outpatient peritoneal dialysis 3 days a week for end-stage renal disease secondary to hypertensive nephrosclerosis. She is hypertensive, weak, and anorexic.

II. Personal Data

Date and Time:	Sept 5, 1986, 11 AM
Full Name:	Ethel Joy Redding
Social Security Number:	000-00-0000
Address:	700 Third Ave., Waverly, Kan
Telephone:	Home: 000-0000
Sex:	Female
Age:	73
Birthdate:	4-5-13
Marital Status:	Widowed
Race:	Black
Religion:	Lutheran
Occupation:	Retired post office employee
Usual Health Care Provider:	Dr John Hoak

III. Health History

Source of Information:	Client
Reliability of Informant:	Reliable
Chief Complaint:	Extreme tiredness and inability to eat
History of Present Illness:	Mrs Redding has had severe hypertension for 12 years. A low-sodium diet and antihypertensive drugs failed to control her blood pressure adequately. In November 1982, she went into renal failure secondary to hypertensive nephrosclerosis. She was placed on hemodialysis. She had several fistula failures and revisions in both arms and the left leg. Following the clotting of the last fistula in her right arm, a Tenckhoff peritoneal catheter was inserted (October 1984). She has been on peritoneal dialysis since that time. During peritoneal dialysis, she has episodes of cramping, nausea, and diarrhea. She associates her decrease in appetite with the peritoneal dialysis procedure.

In October 1983, Mrs Redding had a pacemaker inserted because of an arrhythmia and was placed on disopyramide (Norpace) 100 mg q.d. and digoxin 0.125 mg Mon, Wed, and Fri. She also takes a stool softener, iron, folate, thiamine, and a multivitamin. Mrs Redding is on a 2 g Na, 50–60 g protein, 50 mEq K^+ diet. However, she lives alone, cooks for herself, and finds it difficult to follow the dietary restrictions.

Past Health History:

Childhood:	Measles, mumps, chickenpox
Immunizations:	Td, 1982
Surgeries:	Pacemaker, Oct 1983; various access (fistula) procedures from 1982–1984
Transfusions:	Approximately 5 during hemodialysis
Pregnancies:	None
Trauma:	None
Allergies:	None

Current Medications:

Multivitamin, $\frac{-}{i}$ q.d.

Thiamine tablet, $\frac{-}{i}$ q.d

Folate, mg $\frac{-}{i}$ q.d.

Disopyramide, 100 mg q.d.

Digoxin, 0.125 mg M,W,F

Ferrous gluconate, 325 mg t.i.d.

Surfak, q.d.

(continued)

Case Study written by Jane Hokanson Hawks.

Case Study (continued)

The Client With Chronic Renal Failure

Family History:

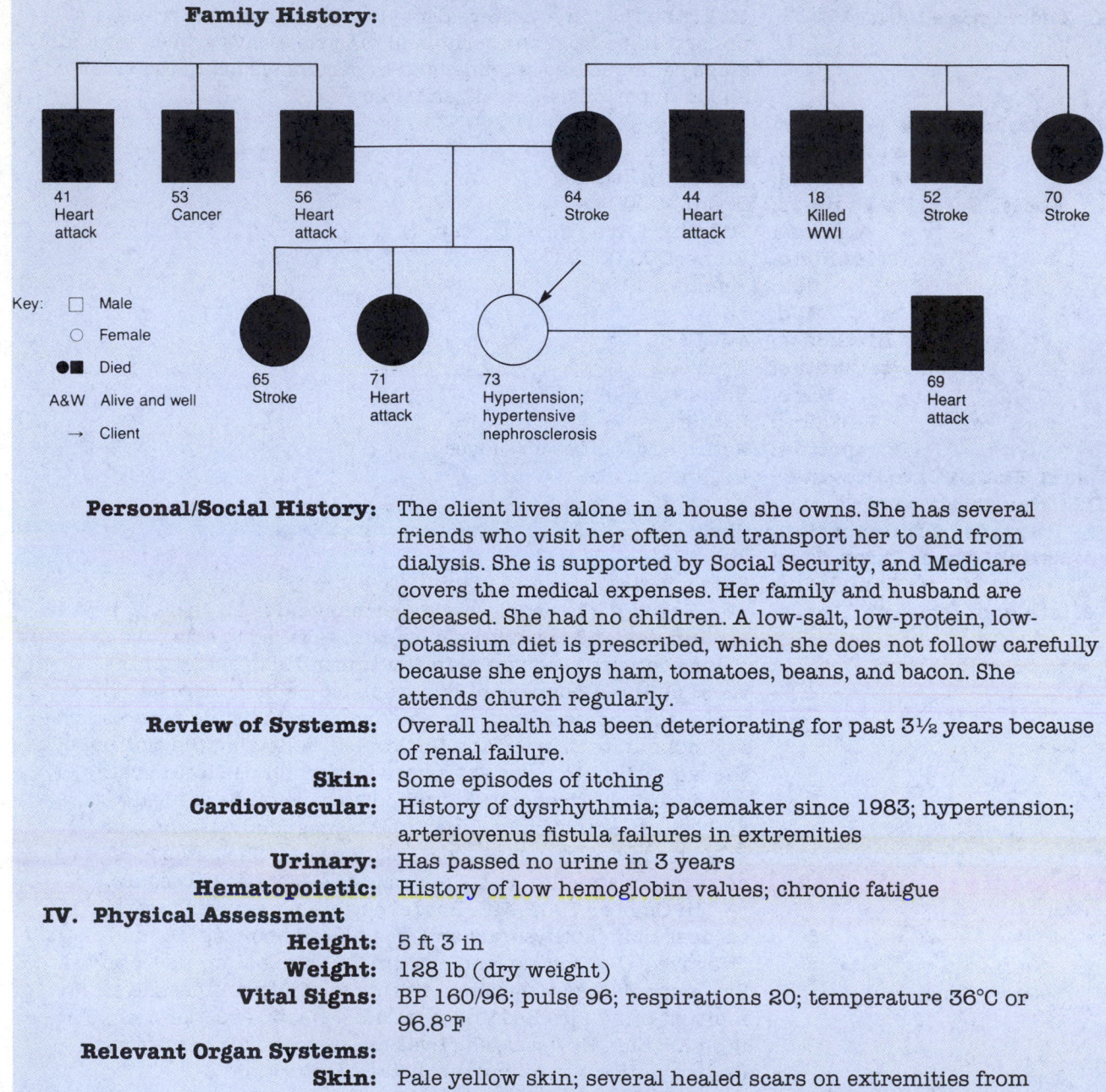

Key:
- □ Male
- ○ Female
- ●■ Died
- A&W Alive and well
- → Client

Personal/Social History: The client lives alone in a house she owns. She has several friends who visit her often and transport her to and from dialysis. She is supported by Social Security, and Medicare covers the medical expenses. Her family and husband are deceased. She had no children. A low-salt, low-protein, low-potassium diet is prescribed, which she does not follow carefully because she enjoys ham, tomatoes, beans, and bacon. She attends church regularly.

Review of Systems: Overall health has been deteriorating for past 3½ years because of renal failure.

Skin: Some episodes of itching

Cardiovascular: History of dysrhythmia; pacemaker since 1983; hypertension; arteriovenus fistula failures in extremities

Urinary: Has passed no urine in 3 years

Hematopoietic: History of low hemoglobin values; chronic fatigue

IV. Physical Assessment

Height: 5 ft 3 in

Weight: 128 lb (dry weight)

Vital Signs: BP 160/96; pulse 96; respirations 20; temperature 36°C or 96.8°F

Relevant Organ Systems:

Skin: Pale yellow skin; several healed scars on extremities from previous fistulas, pacemaker site; Tenckhoff catheter present; generalized edema

Chest: Shortness of breath on exertion and during fill stage of dialysis; rales in lower lobes bilaterally

Cardiovascular: Pacemaker set for 72 beats to fire as necessary; generalized edema predialysis; predialysis weight of 134 lb (dry weight is 128)

Gastrointestinal: Eats ⅛ of food on tray; severe abdominal cramping and diarrhea during dialysis; Tenckhoff catheter with abdominal placement

Urinary: Anuric

Musculoskeletal: Some neuromuscular irritability; fatigue

Psychological: Sometimes she feels life isn't worth living; feels she is a burden to her friends who take her and pick her up from dialysis 3 days a week; dietary restrictions eliminate all her favorite foods,

1066

		although often she goes off her diet because food is one of her main enjoyments in life	
V. Diagnostic Data		Present predialysis abnormal laboratory results showed decreased hemoglobin and hematocrit and elevated blood urea nitrogen, creatinine, potassium, and triglyceride values	
VI. Medical Regimen		Diet, 2 g Na, 50–60 g protein, 50–60 mEq K^+	
		Dialysis: 15 h/week, Mon, Wed, Fri	
		Use a 30% solution if 0–3 lb above dry weight	
		Use a 50% solution if 4–5 lb above dry weight	
		Add 250 mL of D50 in water if more than 6 lb above dry weight	
		4000 U heparin per 2000 mL dialysate	
		40 mEq KCl to every bottle of dialysate	

VII. Nursing Care Plan

Nursing Diagnosis	Client Care Goals	Plan/Nursing Implementation	Expected Outcomes
Fluid volume, alteration in: excess, related to kidney failure and non-compliance with fluid and dietary restrictions	Will discuss feelings about her illness and the dietary and fluid restrictions; compliance with dietary and fluid restrictions will improve	Nonjudgmental, supportive approach to client; attempt to understand how disease and necessary restrictions affect her life; work with client regarding foods; methods of food preparation; seasonings that limit sodium, protein, and potassium. Consider more frequent meals. Involve nutritionist; help client understand process of fluid retention and its relation to diet, energy levels, and breathing; since depression is an additional cause of fatigue, consider referral to a mental health nurse clinician; assess predialysis weight and lung sounds; change fill time and dialysate amounts as needed to minimize diarrhea and cramping; encourage and praise client appropriately	Has improved understanding of reasons for fatigue, shortness of breath; feels comfortable verbalizing her feelings of frustration; improved compliance with diet restrictions, absence of cramping and diarrhea during dialysis; weight gain of no more than 8 lb between dialysis treatments; improved breathing pattern
Impaired gas exchange and activity intolerance related to low hemoglobin	Decreased fatigue; normal bowel function	Administer ferrous gluconate after dialysis and not with antacid; explain that iron turns stools black and also causes constipation; encourage continuing use of stool softener; monitoring of bowel function	Will take iron and stool softener as prescribed; will not become constipated; improved energy level
Skin integrity, impairment of: potential for, related to itching and edema	Client will be more comfortable; decrease in or absence of itching	Dialysis to remove excess fluid; explain causes of itching to client	Increase in client comfort; maintenance of skin integrity
Skin integrity, impairment of: potential for infection related to peritoneal catheter	Will recognize signs and symptoms of infection; understands and is comfortable with home care of peritoneal catheter	Use sterile technique when hooking up catheter to dialysis machine; teach client signs and symptoms of infection; teach correct home care of abdominal skin and peritoneal catheter	Client will recognize symptoms and signs of infection; will care for abdominal skin and catheter without problems

Chapter 34

Surgical Approaches to Kidney and Urinary System Dysfunction

Jeanette K. Chambers
Jane Hokanson Hawks

Objectives

When you have finished studying this chapter, you should be able to:

Identify the indications that necessitate the surgeries of nephrectomy, nephrolithotomy, pyelolithotomy, renal revascularization, renal transplantation, ureterolithotomy, ureteroplasty, partial and radical cystectomies, ileal and colon conduits, ureterosigmoidostomy, ureterostomy, and continent vesicostomy.

Describe the surgical procedures involved in these surgeries.

Discuss the physiological and psychosocial/lifestyle considerations of these surgeries.

Discuss the preoperative and postoperative nursing implications for these surgeries.

Discuss the nursing implications for ureteral stent and nephrostomy tube care.

Identify the signs and symptoms of the three types of kidney transplant rejection.

Discuss alterations in body image encountered by clients requiring urinary diversion and their relationship to self-image, sexuality, and role relationships.

Surgical interventions for dysfunction of the kidneys and the urinary system may be used for palliative effects or to achieve a cure. In many disorders, surgery is reserved for cases in which more conservative medical treatment has not proven effective.

Section I: Surgical Approaches to Disorders Affecting the Kidney

NEPHRECTOMY

A nephrectomy is a surgical procedure in which a kidney is removed. It may be indicated in instances of chronic infection, trauma, hemorrhage, tumor, hypertension refractory to treatment, an infected calculus, or a desire to donate a kidney to a relative. A radical nephrectomy includes the removal of a kidney, adjacent perinephric fasciae and fat, the superior adrenal gland, and nearby lymph nodes. This procedure is indicated when there is renal cell carcinoma. A partial nephrectomy may be performed in clients with significant renal deterioration as evidenced by an elevated serum creatinine level or decreased 24-hour creatinine clearance rate, or in clients who have only one kidney. If a tumor is present, however, removal of the entire kidney is necessary, and a partial nephrectomy may not be possible.

Surgical Procedure

General anesthesia is required for a nephrectomy. The position of the client during the surgery depends on the site selected for the incision. In general, one of three surgical approaches will be selected. For a healthy client requiring a simple nephrectomy, a lumbar–flank incision

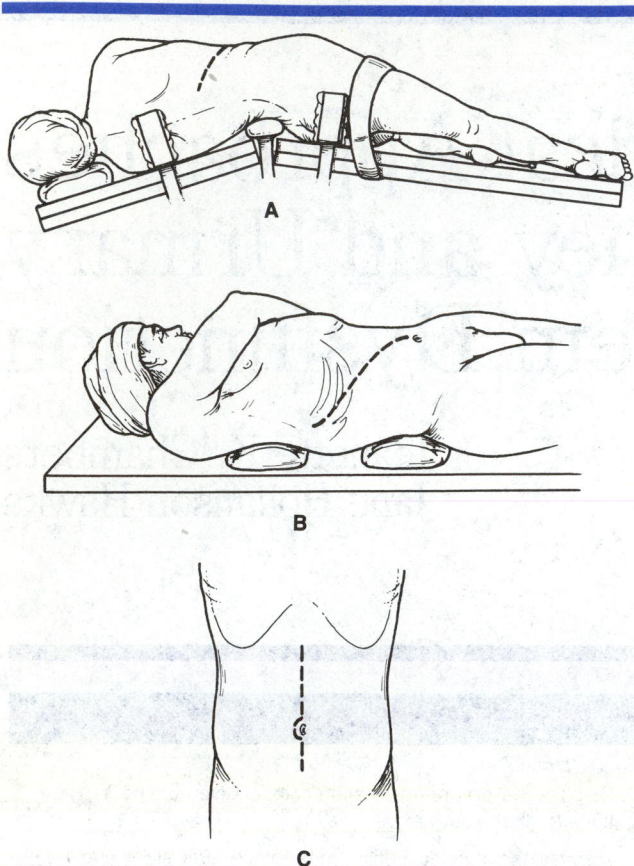

Figure 34–1

Positioning and incision sites for nephrectomy.

may be selected; the client assumes a hyperextended side-lying position (Figure 34–1A). The thoracoabdominal approach is preferred for the client requiring a radical nephrectomy, because the operative area with this approach permits wide visibility so the malignant mass may be totally removed. The thoracoabdominal approach places the client in a recumbent position with the side of the incision elevated about 40° (Figure 34–1B). This approach should be avoided if the client has decreased pulmonary reserve. The third approach, the transabdominal approach, is preferred for the client with pulmonary insufficiency who also requires wide visualization for removal of tissue. This approach places the client in a supine position (Figure 34–1C).

Implications for the Client

Physiological Implications

Preoperative considerations for the nephrectomy client include the evaluation of overall renal function to determine whether postoperative kidney function is adequate to sustain life without dialysis or transplantation.

In addition to the usual preoperative considerations identified in Chapter 14, others are important for the client facing a nephrectomy. Remaining renal function should be preserved and protected. The client should be adequately

hydrated to maximize the removal of metabolic wastes and minimize the effects of decreased perfusion. Toxic agents—especially the known nephrotoxic antibiotics and the contrast media required for various diagnostic tests—should be used minimally with caution or avoided entirely if possible. Since kidney infection may be present, bacteremia is a possibility. If the client has a history of bruising, hemorrhage may be a problem. Electrolyte imbalances should be corrected to prevent cardiac arrest. Pneumonia is a major postoperative concern, because pain following surgery may hinder coughing and deep breathing. Adrenal insufficiency may occur if a radical nephrectomy is performed.

Psychosocial/Lifestyle Implications

If the remaining kidney is normal, the client need not have major concerns regarding overall kidney function and physiological stability for a normal life span. However, clients requiring nephrectomies for cancer experience tremendous emotional upheaval and concern related to tumor metastasis and long-term prognosis. Clients with decreased renal reserve or with only one kidney will find the potential or actual need for chronic dialysis or transplantation alarming and disturbing. Thus, clients and their families or significant others will need emotional support during the perioperative and convalescent periods.

Lifestyle alterations may be immediate if dialysis is needed (refer to Chapter 32). The nurse should fully inform the client with a single remaining kidney about the risks of sports requiring vigorous body contact. Although the client is responsible for making decisions about his or her own life, these decisions should be based on full knowledge of the implications of accidental trauma to the remaining kidney. The client also should be aware that untreated infections of the remaining kidney may result in its removal and the need for dialysis. The client may return to work and other activities in about 8 weeks but may need to avoid heavy lifting for a longer period of time. Client implications of a nephrectomy are summarized in Table 34–1.

Nursing Implications

Preoperative Care

Evaluate overall renal function and ensure that it is optimum. Nephrotoxic agents should be avoided if diagnostic tests are performed. Adequately hydrate the client to promote the excretion of waste products before surgery. A complete blood count (CBC) and coagulation profile (prothrombin time, partial thromboplastin time, and platelet count) should be obtained, and any problems should be corrected prior to surgery. Electrolyte values should also be monitored and corrected as necessary. Teach clients how to splint an incision to ensure that coughing and deep breathing will be done postoperatively. The measurement of BUN and serum creatinine levels preoperatively will allow comparison with postoperative values.

Table 34–1 Nephrectomy: Implications for the Client

Physiological Implications	Psychosocial/Lifestyle Implications
Dialysis or transplantation if inadequate kidney function remains	Need for emotional support
Decreased perfusion	Need for assurance of possibility to live with one healthy kidney
Avoidance of nephrotoxins	Dialysis implications
Infection and bacteremia	Avoidance of contact sports
Hemorrhage	Return to activities in 8 weeks
Electrolyte imbalance	Avoidance of heavy lifting for at least 8 weeks
Pneumonia	
Adrenal insufficiency	
Pain	

Postoperative Care

Postoperative nursing care for the client having a nephrectomy or partial nephrectomy follows the general principles described in Chapter 32. In addition, several specific nursing interventions are required. A major objective of postoperative nursing care is to ensure adequate oxygenation and the prevention of postoperative pulmonary complications. A temperature elevation to more than 100° F (37.7° C) after the first 24 hours suggests the development of these complications. Atelectasis and pneumonia are significant possibilities; because lumbar–flank incisions involve the accessory muscles of respiration, postoperative discomfort is a major deterrent to deep breathing and coughing exercises. Medications administered liberally will facilitate relief of pain and maximum relaxation. In turn, the client who is relaxed and reasonably comfortable (but not oversedated) can more easily perform breathing exercises. Incentive spirometry or other respiratory therapy techniques may also promote maximum respiratory excursion. Splinting of the incision will decrease pain upon coughing. Finally, ambulation on the first postoperative day improves pulmonary function.

If the pleural cavity has been entered, a chest tube will be in place. Refer to Chapter 18 for discussion of client care when a chest tube is present.

Alterations in gastrointestinal function, including paralytic ileus, intestinal obstruction, or hemorrhage, is common following renal surgery. Fluids and foods should not be taken orally until active peristalsis, identified by the return of bowel sounds and the passage of flatus, is present. Paralytic ileus is the most common complication. To treat it, a nasogastric tube generally is placed, and the client is kept NPO. Encourage ambulation if the client is able. Intestinal obstruction may develop if there was significant manipulation of the bowel during surgery. Hemorrhage in the gastrointestinal tract may result from generalized stress. A more detailed discussion of these complications is presented in Unit Eight.

Wound care is another important postoperative nursing objective. The type of incision and the nature of the surgery determine whether drains will be placed. For example, a lumbar–flank incision does not usually require drain placement. In any case, the use of aseptic or clean technique (protocol differs among institutions) is essential when caring for the incision or drains. Keep the dressing and incisional site clean and dry. A temperature greater than 100° F (37.7° C) may signal wound infections. Dehiscence and evisceration are rare with the lumbar–flank incision but are potential complications with abdominal approaches.

Postoperative renal function is assessed through the careful measurement of intake and output; monitoring of serum creatinine, BUN, and electrolyte levels; and the measurement of urine specific gravity. The nurse also may take central venous line measurements, especially if large amounts of fluids are infused. Hourly outputs often are recorded, and IV infusions of an amount equal to the output may promote perfusion of the remaining kidney. In this case, hourly CVP readings are often recorded as well to avoid overhydration. Recording daily weights also is useful in assessing the client's hydration status.

Intraoperative hemorrhage, dehydration, and altered hemodynamics (associated with the hyperextended position) may alter renal perfusion. Consequently, the detection of the prerenal azotemia that may develop is important.

Discharge planning includes the provision of emotional support and education about activities related to self-care. The client should avoid lifting and other major activities for at least 8 weeks, depending on the specific surgical procedure and the client. Thus, the involvement of the family and significant others in posthospital plans is valuable. The client should receive information regarding the injuries that may be sustained in contact sports. If radiation, chemotherapy, or chronic dialysis are needed, the nurse should provide referrals to appropriate clinical nurse specialists, social workers, and nutritionists.

NEPHROLITHOTOMY

A nephrolithotomy is any surgical procedure in which the parenchyma of the kidney is incised for the removal of a calculus or small tumor or the correction of altered anatomic structure and vascular abnormalities. Although *lith* literally means "stone," this procedure may be performed to correct any intrarenal abnormality. Special skills and techniques are required for this surgical intervention that can preserve functioning renal parenchyma. The use of high-energy shock waves to shatter calculi or ultrasound to disintegrate them are recently developed alternatives to traditional surgery. They are discussed in Chapter 33.

Surgical Procedure

With the client under general anesthesia, the surgeon makes a lumbar–flank incision. This type of incision is preferred because it requires less overall body hypothermia from the cooling solution, facilitates intraoperative radiological evaluation, and prevents the need for entry into the peritoneum (Rose, 1981). For a discussion of physiological, psychosocial, and nursing implications of nephrolithotomy, refer to the sections on nephrectomy and pyelolithotomy.

PYELOLITHOTOMY

In a pyelolithotomy, an incision is made into the renal pelvis, generally to remove a calculus from it. This procedure is indicated when a calculus is infected and the infection cannot be eradicated, or when an obstruction to the outflow of urine results in hydronephrosis.

Surgical Procedure

A pyelolithotomy is performed with the client under general anesthesia, usually through a transabdominal approach. Depending on the location of the stone, the incision may be made into the renal pelvis or into the upper third of the ureter. Postoperatively, one or two wound drains are placed as well as a ureteral catheter.

Implications for the Client

Physiological Implications

Physiological implications for the pyelolithotomy client are similar to the implications for the client requiring a nephrectomy: possibility of infection, pneumonia, pain, and electrolyte imbalances. However, this client should not have a loss of renal parenchymal tissue from surgical removal; the objective is to repair the problem and prevent further deterioration of renal tissue. Postoperatively, the major concern is to control or prevent infection.

Psychosocial/Lifestyle Implications

Education is the major psychological and lifestyle consideration for the client who requires a pyelolithotomy for removal of a calculus in the kidney or proximal ureter. If possible, the nurse should advise the client of methods to minimize the likelihood of future calculus formation. These instructions regarding diet, fluid intake, testing of urinary pH, and medication administration are discussed in Chapter 32. Implications for the client with a pyelolithotomy are summarized in Table 34–2.

Nursing Implications

Preoperative Care

Preoperative care is the same as is described for the nephrectomy client.

Postoperative Care

Postoperative nursing implications are similar to those indicated for the client requiring a nephrectomy. Although the pyelolithotomy client will not have lost a portion of renal parenchyma, maximizing renal reserve is still important. Use meticulous aseptic techniques for the proper care of the ureteral catheter that will be in place along with a Foley catheter. The ureteral catheter ensures that local edema in the ureter will not result in hydronephrosis after the calculus is removed, and it must not be dislodged.

The dressing will need to be changed frequently during the first 24 hours after surgery. Drainage via the Penrose drain is frequently copious and sanguineous in the

---

Table 34–2 Pyelolithotomy: Implications for the Client

Physiological Implications	Psychosocial/Lifestyle Implications
Infection	Education on diet, fluid intake, testing of urinary pH, and medication administration in attempt to prevent further calculi development (see Chapter 32)
Pneumonia	
Pain	Avoidance of heavy lifting for 6–8 weeks
Electrolyte imbalance	
Hemorrhage	
Avoidance of nephrotoxins	

early postoperative period. The amount will diminish and the color will return to clear amber, usually within 48 hours. Infection is a potential postoperative problem. Elevated temperature or an abnormal odor of the drainage may indicate an infection in the urinary tract. The nursing care plan should include careful measurement and recording of intake and output and daily weights to detect changes in urinary output and fluid imbalances, as well as prompt collection of specimens. Monitor laboratory work for changes in the serum creatinine level and any evidence of leukocytosis. In addition, the client should be monitored for the development of hemorrhage, wound infection, atelectasis, and sepsis.

Postoperative respiratory complications such as atelectasis or pneumonia are a major consideration for the client who has had a lumbar–flank incision. The client who guards against the use of respiratory muscles may limit deep breathing and adequate postoperative coughing to clear secretions. Sufficient pain relief will facilitate the necessary coughing and deep breathing exercises. Direct external support also may assist the client with these exercises. In addition, liberal fluid intake will loosen and thin secretions and facilitate expectoration. Acute renal failure from obstruction or sepsis is another possible complication.

A nephrostomy tube may be placed if fragments of the calculus remain. This U-shaped or circular tube inserted directly into the kidney is attached to closed gravity drainage or to a urostomy appliance. Its purpose is to divert urine temporarily or permanently or to instill irrigating fluid.

Care of the nephrostomy tube includes evaluating for bleeding at the site, ensuring that the catheter drains freely, and never clamping the tube (any blockage of the tube will result in acute hydronephrosis). Encourage a large fluid intake to dilute both urine and elements that form calculi. An acidic urine also will prevent calculus formation. The tube can be irrigated (usually by the physician) to flush out fragments using small amounts (10 mL or less) of a solution with an acid pH, such as renacidin or hemiacidrin. Irrigations are controversial because they are potential causes of renal damage or infection (Rose, 1981).

If there is a nephrostomy tube from each kidney, maintain separate output records for each. Leg bags permit the ambulatory client to move about. A nephrostomy tube may also be placed percutaneously.

RENAL REVASCULARIZATION

In situ revascularization of the renal parenchyma is indicated when there is renal artery stenosis or renovascular hypertension. With renal artery stenosis, the narrowed renal artery decreases the renal blood flow. Consequently, kidney tissue is ischemic and vulnerable to eventual necrosis unless blood supply is restored. Stimulation of the renin–angiotensin–aldosterone system results in severely high blood pressure, which over a long period endangers the function of target organs such as the heart, eyes,

and kidneys. Revascularization procedures are commonly used to restore renal function, or at least to prevent further deterioration, or to regain control of high blood pressure.

Surgical Procedure

In situ revascularization procedures include endarterectomy, resection and end-to-end anastomosis, and renal artery bypass graft. The endarterectomy and resection with anastomosis are less common and have less chance of long-term patency than the renal artery bypass graft. If the aorta is severely damaged from atheromatous disease, a splenorenal graft using the hypogastric artery will be used to repair some left renal arteries (Glenn, 1983). The renal artery bypass procedure is performed under general anesthesia with a transabdominal approach. The graft is sutured into the aorta and then into the renal artery distal to the site of stenosis. The graft material may be a portion of saphenous vein or made of a synthetic material. Newer developments in the quality and long-term patency of synthetic materials have made the synthetic graft increasingly common.

Renal bench surgery (ex vivo surgery) and autotransplantation are indicated when there are complicated disorders of the renal artery and one or more of its branches that would require a lengthy period of surgery and anesthesia. Renal bench surgery involves removing the kidney, placing it on the table, repairing the renal vasculature, and reimplanting the kidney into the right iliac fossa after adequate blood flow is ensured (Glenn, 1983). Hypothermia of the kidney prevents damage to the kidney parenchyma by depressing renal metabolic activity and preventing ischemia to the tissue. Bench surgery can repair aneurysms that involve the renal artery and one or more of its branches. This technique also may be used in cases of complicated nephrolithiasis or trauma.

Implications for the Client

Physiological Implications

Preserving and restoring renal function and controlling the blood pressure within normal limits are the most important goals. Because the client who undergoes renal vascular repair often has compromised renal function with an elevated serum creatinine level and a decreased creatinine clearance rate, renal function may be further compromised in the preoperative period. Contrast media or nephrotoxic antibiotics may have been used. Intravascular volume may be decreased, so adequate hydration through fluids will be necessary. Severe postoperative hypotension may result in closure of the graft, whereas severe postoperative hypertension may result in leakage at the sites of anastomoses. Either extreme may necessitate surgical exploration for correction. The client's hydration balance and adequate renal perfusion should result in an acceptable flow of urine; the client should urinate at least 30 to 50 mL/h.

Temporary dialysis may be required in the immediate postoperative period, depending on the individual client's overall condition.

Psychosocial/Lifestyle Implications

For surgical repairs that do not necessitate temporary dialysis, the postoperative period for recovery will be 4 to 8 weeks. Other clients or clients with other chronic disease states usually require longer recovery periods. The client will generally need assistance with shopping, transportation, and general household requirements during recovery. The support of family and friends during this period is similar to that needed by any client following major surgery.

If the client needs temporary dialysis, appropriate plans for its continuance on an outpatient basis must be made. Lifestyle alterations may be similar to those described in Chapter 32 for clients requiring chronic dialysis. Although these clients are usually expected to regain sufficient renal function so they will not require chronic dialysis permanently, this period of uncertainty is understandably distressing. Table 34–3 summarizes client implications for renal revascularization surgery.

Nursing Implications

Preoperative Care

The avoidance of contrast media or nephrotoxic antibiotics is essential whenever possible before surgery to avoid further compromising renal function. Intravenous fluids may be required to correct fluid volume deficit, and electrolyte imbalances also should be corrected. The management of hypertensive crises is described in Chapter 24.

Postoperative Care

Monitor the client's postoperative urine output and vital signs at least hourly. Daily weights provide information regarding overall hydration. Hemodynamic monitoring with a flow-directed, balloon-tipped catheter such as a Swan–Ganz catheter may be needed temporarily to determine the

intravascular volume. An arterial line may also be placed intraoperatively and continued postoperatively to facilitate the control of blood pressure. The physician should clearly delineate the desired blood pressure parameters for the nurse, who should report deviations immediately to the physician. The physician also should clearly specify fluid replacement and urine flow parameters, and exceptions to these should also be reported promptly.

In addition to hemorrhage and acute renal failure, the client is at risk to develop thromboembolic phenomena and infection. Thus, institute turning, coughing, and deep breathing immediately after surgery. Ambulation, or at least sitting at the bedside and standing, should occur within the first 24 to 48 hours. In the interim, institute leg exercises, elastic support stockings, and positioning that avoids circulatory stasis.

Meticulous aseptic treatment of all invasive lines and catheters is essential to prevent the development of local infections that could become systemic and place the kidneys under greater stress. Good nutrition also is important to the healing process, so encourage the client to eat well. Daily monitoring of serum creatinine levels and electrolytes should continue during the postoperative period. Other blood tests that should be performed regularly are hemoglobin, hematocrit, and white blood cell (WBC) counts. Leukocytosis and temperature elevation should be promptly assessed.

During this time, the client needs to be encouraged about progress being made, because the healing process is seemingly slow. The client should receive instructions to limit activities for 4 to 8 weeks.

RENAL TRANSPLANTATION

Renal transplantation is a surgical procedure in which the kidney of one person (the donor) is placed into the body of another person (the recipient). The donor may be a relative from the immediate family (a living-related donor or LRD), or a cadaver (CAD). For clients with end-stage renal disease (chronic renal failure), a renal transplantation is nec-

Table 34–3 Renal Revascularization: Implications for the Client	
Physiological Implications	**Psychosocial/Lifestyle Implications**
Possible improvement in the quality of life by restoring blood supply and renal function, preventing further deterioration in renal function, or helping control hypertension	Limit activity 4 to 8 weeks
	Possible need for assistance at home
Hydration through IV fluids if intravascular volume is decreased	Possible lifestyle alterations for dialysis (see also Chapter 32)
Severe postoperative hypotension causing graft closure	
Severe postoperative hypertension causing bleeding at the sites of anastomoses	
Temporary dialysis possible	

essary to maintain life without the need for chronic dialysis. Chapter 33 discusses a number of diseases that can result in end-stage renal disease.

Recipient Selection

Renal transplantation should be considered for the client whose renal function has deteriorated to a creatinine clearance rate of 5 mL/min. When the creatinine clearance rate has reached this level, the client typically has multiple systemic effects of uremia. Some clients will have these systemic effects even before reaching this creatinine clearance rate. Therefore, clinical assessment of the client is more important than the specific results of laboratory tests.

Clients with severe cardiovascular problems, connective tissue disorders (eg, systemic lupus erythematosus, diabetes, malignancies), or immune problems (eg, AIDS) are not the best transplant candidates. These disorders can cause the same kidney destruction in a transplanted kidney. Most transplant centers no longer use the age limit of 55 as a criterion; instead, staff evaluate each client individually for the potential benefit from transplant surgery. After a complete physical examination, a psychiatric evaluation also is conducted to be sure the client is mentally able to withstand the procedure and the idea of having someone else's kidney in his or her body.

Donor Selection

Potential LRDs include full-blooded mothers, fathers, sisters, brothers, sons, or daughters over the age of 18. An identical twin provides the best possible match. First, the donor relative's ABO blood compatibility with the recipient must be established. Following the determination of ABO blood compatibility, HLA testing is done. A four-antigen HLA match is the best possible. If less than a four-antigen match is achieved, the donor may still be considered an acceptable match, but further evaluation and treatment may be required. HLA testing is discussed further in Chapter 30.

Before surgery, the donor client is given an in-depth physical examination, and a health history is taken to ensure excellent health. Renal function is evaluated by two 24-hour urine collections to determine creatinine clearance rate, an intravenous pyelogram, and a renal arteriogram. In addition, blood chemistries and electrolytes are evaluated, and a glucose tolerance test is performed. The donor's ability to live without one kidney must be established. The thoroughness of assessment of relatives prior to graft donation has contributed to high survival statistics for LRDs.

The names of clients without potential LRDs are placed on a national computer network, the United Network for Organ Sharing (UNOS), that lists all clients and describes their blood types and HLA requirements. This network enables transplant centers to communicate a client's transplant needs and the availability of CAD kidneys and is described in the resources listing at the end of Chapter 32.

The CAD must have met established criteria for brain death. Some states have legislation that determines these criteria, and most institutions have established definitions and criteria for brain death. In general, brain death may be determined by two or more flat EEGs at least 24 hours apart (Irwin, 1983). The proposed CAD is examined to determine the absence of systemic diseases, including generalized infection, diabetes mellitus, hypertension, renal disease, malignancies, or systemic lupus erythematosus. Normal kidney perfusion and renal function also must be established. The CAD's age generally is restricted to 18 through 55, but this varies by institution.

Once brain death and other criteria for donation have been established, renal perfusion must be maintained. Hydration and control of electrolyte and acid–base balances are necessary during the time prior to the donor nephrectomy. After the next of kin has signed a consent form, the donor nephrectomy is performed by the transplant recovery team, which also arranges for the transport and preservation of the donated kidney. Two techniques are available for organ preservation: hypothermia with saline flushing and pulsatile perfusion. The primary advantage of pulsatile perfusion (using a pump to perfuse the kidney in much the same way a heart would) is the length of time the kidney may remain viable; this technique may ensure adequate perfusion for 24 hours or longer. In fact, some successful transplants have been done within 3 days with graft survival.

Many centers now administer at least 10 units of packed red blood cells to recipients before including them on the cadaver list. This practice increases the survival of the graft at 12 months from 40% to 70%.

Surgical Procedure

The procedure for donor nephrectomy is similar to the surgical procedure for nephrectomy discussed earlier in this chapter. The left kidney of the donor is preferred, because the left renal vein is longer. In addition, the ureter of the donor is also removed and included in the transplantation procedure.

The kidney transplant recipient's own kidneys are not removed unless chronic infection is present. However, the kidneys may have been removed previously because of problems with hypertension or infection. A splenectomy may be performed in some cases to improve the client's tolerance to azathioprine (Imuran) and to reduce the incidence of leukopenia and thrombocytopenia. If not previously performed, an appendectomy also should be done during the nephrectomy to avoid appendicitis, which may be confused with a very tender rejecting renal allograft (transplant), in the right lower quadrant.

Unless a CAD kidney is used, adjacent operating rooms are essential, with the donor in one room and the recipient in the other. The renal transplant is placed in the right lower quadrant, generally in the anterior iliac fossa (Figure 34–2). The peritoneal cavity is not incised, so the kidney

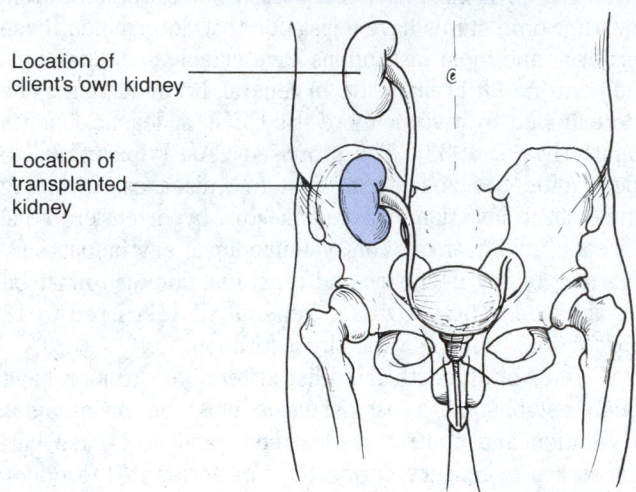

Location of client's own kidney

Location of transplanted kidney

Figure 34–2

Location of transplanted kidney in the anterior iliac fossa.

is placed retroperitoneally. Three anastomoses are necessary to ensure that the transplanted kidney will be able to function normally: The renal artery is usually anastomosed to the hypogastric artery or internal iliac artery; the renal vein is anastomosed to the iliac vein; and the ureter must be anastomosed to a ureter or the bladder.

Ureteroneocystostomy, in which the ureter is placed directly into the bladder wall via suturing and tunneling, is the preferred method of ureteral anastomosis (Figure 34–3). Urinary leakage with this method is minimal.

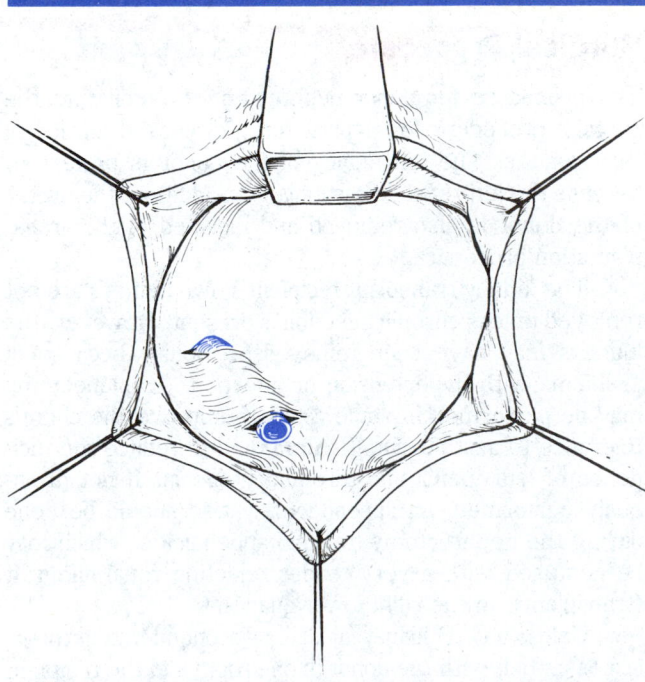

Figure 34–3

Ureteroneocystostomy.

Implications for the Client

Physiological Implications

Implications for an LRD are discussed in the earlier section on nephrectomy. The following discussion refers mainly to the recipient. In preparation for renal transplantation, the client must be in the best possible physical condition. Dialysis may be required to correct fluid, electrolyte, and acid–base imbalances, as well as to remove metabolic waste products. The client must be free of infection and gastrointestinal bleeding preoperatively, because these are the most common postoperative complications. Last-minute HLA tissue typing is needed to minimize the risk of rejection. Blood transfusions and exposure to or having a cold or the flu can cause additional antigens and antibodies that might trigger a rejection episode.

Potential postoperative complications include pneumonia, gastrointestinal bleeding (from large steroid doses to prevent rejection), and rejection of the transplanted kidney. Symptoms of rejection include elevated blood pressure and temperature, weight gain, tenderness over the allograft, enlargement of the allograft, decreased urinary output, elevated serum creatinine level, anorexia, and drowsiness. Following successful transplantation, urine output may range from massive diuresis to total anuria. As much as 200 mL/h of urine has been reported. Anuria is seen most frequently with CAD kidneys in which the ischemic period was long. The anuria in this case results from acute tubular necrosis. Dialysis may be necessary, because adequate renal function may not return for 5 weeks. Partial function of the transplanted kidney but inadequate output usually is the result of rejection.

Other physiological changes for the client result from the immunosuppressive therapy, which will be administered for the life of the kidney. Continuous doses of steroids cause systemic effects including moon face, thinning of hair, osteoporosis, redistribution of body fat, buffalo hump, muscle wasting, fragility of blood vessels, softening of skin, and so on. In addition, immunosuppressive therapy increases the client's risk of infection. Refer to Chapter 44 for an in-depth discussion of steroid use.

If the client has previously been on dialysis and the transplant has been successful, many of the adaptations associated with dialysis will be corrected. For example, serum creatinine and BUN levels will decrease and then stabilize at or near normal. Hematocrit and hemoglobin levels also will return to normal. The yellow-ashen skin color will disappear, and food will taste good again.

Psychosocial/Lifestyle Implications

The LRD makes a conscious, voluntary decision to donate a kidney to a family member. To help a loved one, he or she takes on the restrictions associated with living with one kidney, such as avoiding all contact sports. This individual and family decision is different from the circumstances that surround the gift of an organ from a CAD, who voluntarily indicated the desire to have his or her organs used in the event of death or whose next of kin made the decision to donate. At the same time, the donor's family must agree to honor the expressed wishes of the brain-dead donor. Difficult decisions in a time of crisis— accepting the unexpected death of a loved one and agreeing to the organ donation—may be facilitated through nursing counseling and education. The dignity and level of care provided for the donor client should be of the highest level throughout the entire period. The donor client's family, while coping with the grief of the loss of a loved one, may feel a sense of satisfaction and some happiness that the organ donation will help another person to live without the restriction of chronic dialysis.

The psychiatric evaluation of the transplant recipient should reveal no major psychological problems. The client must also come to terms with having a kidney from someone else. Family roles often change, either temporarily or permanently, because of transplantation surgery. Housekeeping, income production, or the discipline of children may have to be redistributed among others in the family. The use of steroids may lead to altered mental states, mainly euphoria but sometimes depression, however. Although clients are no longer dependent on dialysis after transplantation, they still have limitations. They must always take immunosuppressants as ordered (usually every day or every other day). Because of the increased risk of infection associated with immunotherapy, they should avoid crowds, particularly in the cold and flu season. If the client cannot avoid shopping malls, theaters, and the like, a surgical mask should be worn to limit inhalation of foreign particles. The client may have difficulty adjusting to the body changes that accompany immunosuppressive therapy. Furthermore, these clients constantly worry about the possibility of rejection developing at any time.

Economic considerations are great; the cost of the surgery is $20,000 and up. The government pays most of the expenses, but other expenses remain, such as housing near the transplant center after dismissal from the hospital and before the client returns home. Table 34–4 lists client implications related to renal transplant.

Nursing Implications

Preoperative Care

Transplant recipients need a great deal of emotional care before and after surgery. Answer their questions honestly but avoid terrifying them with possible difficulties. Good preoperative teaching can help the client understand the preparation necessary for surgery, as well as what to expect during and after surgery. The client is usually dialyzed the day before surgery to correct the fluid, acid–base, and electrolyte imbalances, as well as to remove urea and other dialyzable body wastes. For the CAD transplant recipient, dialysis is done a few hours before surgery if the client has not been dialyzed that day.

Blood is drawn to determine leukocyte counts and prothrombin time, as well as hemoglobin, hematocrit, serum bilirubin, creatinine, and electrolyte values. Typing and crossmatching of leukocyte-poor blood is also done. A sample is sent for final tissue type crossmatch. A physical examination, chest x-ray, and ECG are completed, along

Table 34–4 Renal Transplant: Implications for the Recipient Client	
Physiological Implications	**Psychosocial/Lifestyle Implications**
Preoperative dialysis to correct imbalances and remove wastes	Altered mental states from steroids
Should be free of GI bleeding and infection preoperatively	Immunosuppressive drugs taken for life of kidney
Postoperative complications: pneumonia, GI bleeding, rejection of kidney, elevated blood pressure and temperature, weight gain, tenderness and enlargement of allograft, decreased urine output, elevated serum creatinine level, anorexia, drowsiness, massive diuresis or anuria (CAD kidney)	Need to avoid crowds to prevent infection
	Body image changes associated with immunosuppressants
	Adjustment to someone else's kidney
Symptoms of immunosuppression: moon face, buffalo hump, thinning hair, osteoporosis, redistribution of body fat, muscle wasting, fragility of blood vessels, softening of skin, and so forth	Constant fear of rejection
	Financial concerns
Eventual correction of dialysis adaptations (normalization of serum BUN, creatinine, and the erythropoietin response)	Changes in family roles
Increased risk of infection from immunosuppressant therapy	

with other usual preoperative measures. The nurse should weigh the client before surgery.

The client will receive IM or PO antibiotics and IV push methylprednisolone sodium succinate (Solu-Medrol) in the afternoon preceding surgery. Azathioprine (Imuran) is given 2 days before surgery when possible, and 5000 units of heparin is given 1 hour before surgery. Usually IV antibiotics, Solu-Medrol, and azathioprine are sent to the operating room with the client in the appropriate dosage. A 0.5% solution of neomycin also may be sent with the client for bladder irrigation before surgery.

Postoperative Care

Upon the client's arrival from the operating room, weigh the client on the bed scale before assisting the client into bed. Any bedclothes must be weighed separately once the client is in bed and their weight subtracted. The nurse then weighs the client every morning. The daily weight is compared to the baseline weight to determine whether the client is retaining fluid or diuresing following the transplant surgery. The usual postanesthetic checks are carried out, and blood pressure, pulse, respiration, and CVP are monitored at least hourly. Temperature is recorded every 4 hours. Urine output is recorded (a Foley catheter is placed during surgery), and urine specific gravity and sugar are checked hourly. The urine should be clear or light pink, indicating that clots are not developing. Take extreme caution to avoid blockage of the catheter patency: no clots, no kinking or twisting, no pressure, and direct gravitational flow. Obstruction and bladder distention can result in excessive tension upon the sutures of the ureteral anastomosis and can seriously jeopardize the success of the surgical procedure. A backup of urine may also cause an infection to develop.

Monitor urine and blood specimens at intervals of 4 to 6 hours to furnish a guide to electrolyte replacement and possible insulin requirements. In addition, monitor serum creatinine and BUN levels daily. Other routine laboratory work includes daily evaluation of sodium, potassium, white blood cells, hemoglobin, and prothrombin time. Serum calcium and phosphorus levels are checked weekly and creatinine clearance is often performed twice weekly. Chest x-rays also are done weekly. Urinalysis and cultures for bacteria and fungus are performed when the urinary catheter is removed, when the temperature is 101° F (38° C) or above, and weekly.

If oliguria or anuria develops, the cause must be identified and corrected as soon as possible. Postoperative anuria suggests an acute rejection process or a blockage of the catheter. Oliguria may result from hypovolemia or ischemic injury that causes acute tubular necrosis (ATN).

At least two IV lines are used for IV and fluid therapy: a central venous line and a peripheral line. Some institutions prefer a flow-directed, balloon-tipped catheter. Full replacement of urine output with D5/0.5NS is carried out for urine outputs of 250 mL/h or less, and supplemental potassium is administered in accordance with urine and serum values. It is often unnecessary to give as much potassium as the measured urinary loss; two-thirds replacement is usually adequate for outputs of 250 to 500 mL/h, and half replacement should suffice for outputs greater than 500 mL/h. This order may vary according to the physician. When a deficit of 1500 mL is reached, volume-for-volume replacement is usually resumed until midnight, when records begin. When the client starts to take fluids orally, the amounts are included in the replacement. Keep in mind that IV medications are also part of the replacement. The protocols for fluid replacement may vary from center to center.

Analgesics are prescribed on a p.r.n. basis for the client after surgery. Transplant recipients may not have pain as great as other abdominal surgical clients because the transplanted kidney is in the retroperitoneal space. Nevertheless, they do have pain. The nurse must assess the client's need for analgesics and offer them. The bladder spasms that are quite severe and common following surgery can be relieved by belladonna and opium suppositories. Keeping the client comfortable will make coughing, ambulating, and sleeping easier. Do not gatch the bed at the knee or elevate the foot of the bed. Both of these actions may increase the potential for thrombosis.

Pneumonia is a major concern in the renal transplant client. Thus, the nurse must maintain pulmonary function through rigorous attention to postoperative turning, coughing, and deep breathing exercises. Adequate hydration will assist in the mobilization of secretions. Incentive spirometry is commonly prescribed to decrease alveolar hypoventilation. Other measures, such as intermittent positive-pressure breathing treatments or the administration of medications through nebulization may be needed to ensure adequate clearance of pulmonary secretions.

Initiate ambulation as soon as possible, preferably the first postoperative day. Ambulation assists in the return of gastrointestinal function, the prevention of thromboembolic phenomena, and improved ventilation.

Immunosuppressive agents increase the possibility of infection, particularly from cytomegalovirus (CMV) or from the parasite *Pneumocystis carinii*. However, practices regarding isolation of the renal transplant client have undergone considerable change in the last decade. Strict isolation was formerly employed, but modified reverse isolation or no isolation are the current general practices. Although isolation practices have changed significantly, the nurse should recognize the client's vulnerability. Aseptic technique for appropriate procedures, hand washing before and after each client contact, and use of common sense to avoid unnecessary exposure to persons with upper respiratory tract infections are essential. Persons with upper respiratory tract infections who must be in contact with the transplant recipient should wear a mask and follow strict hand washing techniques.

The client may have a nasogastric tube attached to low suction until peristalsis of the gastrointestinal tract returns. Often the client is merely kept NPO and started on liquids as peristalsis returns. Routinely check nasogastric drainage and stool for blood, because gastrointestinal bleeding is a major risk in the transplant client given high doses of immunosuppressants after surgery to avoid or treat rejection. Other factors that contribute to gastrointestinal bleeding include the stress of surgery and the alteration in platelet aggregation associated with uremia. Consequently, antacids are commonly prescribed as often as hourly; low-magnesium, low-sodium, phosphate-binding antacids are the most common. Laxatives may be needed if antacids are taken every 2 hours or more.

Transplantation Rejection

Rejection is the result of the whole body's reaction to foreign tissue. It cannot be prevented completely, but with proper management rejection can usually be reversed and renal function returned. If rejection is irreversible, the graft is removed. Rejection is a continuing threat. Early diagnosis of kidney rejection is mandatory. The nurse must maintain a close, constant observation of the client to detect symptoms such as a swollen and tender kidney, weight gain, elevated temperature and blood pressure, decreased urine output, anorexia, drowsiness, and elevated serum creatinine values.

Rejection of the transplanted organ may be one of three kinds. Hyperacute rejection occurs immediately after the kidney is implanted. The transplanted kidney appears pale, because tissue perfusion is not achieved. There is no treatment for hyperacute rejection, and a transplant nephrectomy is performed immediately. Ischemia and death of the transplanted kidney occur immediately as cytotoxic antibodies invade the graft. Next, acute rejection may develop within 1 week or as long as 2 years after the transplant surgery. The symptoms are similar to those of acute renal failure with oliguria. Steroid medications are increased, and the client is supported until the rejection passes. An episode or two of acute rejection occurs for almost all clients. Most episodes reverse, but some do not. Finally, chronic rejection occurs gradually, generally over months to years. Its onset is detected by gradually worsening renal function as determined by elevation of the serum creatinine and BUN levels. Other electrolyte abnormalities may also be present, such as elevated phosphorous and decreased bicarbonate. Edema and hypertension may be increasing. No treatment for chronic rejection exists, and the graft eventually is lost.

For increasing graft survival, a number of centers now use donor-specific transfusions (DSTs). This procedure involves the administration of 200 mL of fresh blood from a specific donor to the proposed LRD recipient every 2 weeks for three transfusion administrations.

Treatment of rejection includes the administration of large doses of steroids; doses of 1000 to 2000 mg are common. Methylprednisolone sodium succinate (Solu-Medrol) should never be given quickly; it is given over 20 to 30 minutes for 6 to 7 days, depending on the duration of the rejection and the age of the client. Such high doses require antacids to prevent gastrointestinal bleeding; 30 mL of an antacid is given every 2 hours if the client is receiving 1 g of Solu-Medrol, and 30 mL every hour if the client is bleeding or receiving 2 g of Solu-Medrol. Furosemide (Lasix) IV should not be given within 2 hours of Solu-Medrol infusions to prevent cardiac arrhythmias. Ambulation helps to prevent the muscle atrophy that accompanies high-dose steroid therapy.

Immunosuppressive agents facilitate the development of infection, so prevention and early detection of infection are major nursing goals. In the past, reverse isolation was used to reduce this threat, but the cause of most infections resulted from the client's own flora. Thus, today reverse isolation is used only if the WBC count falls below 800. Meticulous hand washing, pulmonary exercises, and aseptic wound and catheter care are important.

After removing the client's urinary catheter, the nurse should instruct the client to void hourly while awake and to awaken the client every 4 hours at night to void. This prevents pressure in the bladder, which could disrupt the anastomosis of the ureter to the bladder.

Blood is not administered unless the client's hemoglobin falls below 4 g. The client may receive only leukocyte-poor blood. Premedication with Solu-Medrol 30 minutes before the transfusion helps to prevent rejection.

Discharge Care and Teaching

Client education about the pharmacological regimen that will be prescribed to prevent the rejection of the graft is extensive. The client should be advised to wear identification jewelry that clearly notes that the client is a transplant recipient and requires immunosuppressive agents. Inform the client that therapy normally taken may not be adequate if excessive physiological or emotional stress occurs. The stress of trauma, surgery, or infection may precipitate an adrenal crisis if it precipitates adrenal insufficiency. Refer to Chapter 44 for a discussion of the management of adrenal insufficiency and its clinical manifestations.

Pharmacological agents are prescribed for the renal transplant recipient to suppress the normal immunologic response that occurs in the presence of foreign tissue. Those commonly prescribed include prednisone, azathioprine (Imuran) and cyclophosphamide (Cytoxan), usually in combination. Prednisone is administered with either azathioprine or cyclophosphamide. Cyclosporine which became available in 1983, appears to be a drug that will alter many pharmacological regimes. It is also administered in combination with corticosteroids.

Complications with long-term steroid use in transplant clients include the ever-present potential for infection, bone demineralization with necrosis of the femoral head or pathological fractures, cataract formation, gastritis with bleeding, hyperglycemia with insulin deficiency, and psychological alterations that may result in psychotic behavior. In addition, each drug has its own side effects.

Prednisone, a corticosteroid, is an anti-inflammatory agent that stabilizes the cell membrane and thus prevents the entry and infiltration of leukocytes into the tissue during rejection. Prednisone also suppresses the formation of antibodies and immune complexes. Numerous side effects accompany the use of prednisone, however. Because lifetime therapy is required, the dose is decreased as soon as possible to a maintenance level. Alternate-day therapy is recommended in an attempt to minimize complications.

Azathioprine blocks the formation of antibodies by altering DNA and RNA synthesis. This therapy is also required for the life of the graft. Side effects of azathioprine include bone marrow depression with leukopenia and thrombocytopenia, as well as altered liver function. If these complications develop with the use of azathioprine, cyclophosphamide may be substituted. Cyclophosphamide suppresses antibody and lymphocyte formation. Its side effects include bone marrow suppression, alopecia, and hemorrhagic cystitis.

Cyclosporine is administered to clients at high risk for the development of rejection or in whom rejection has been detected. Prior to the availability of cyclosporine, transplantation might not have even been tried in these high-risk clients, or the amount of immunosuppressive drugs required to save the graft would have resulted in death to the client from infection. Cyclosporine's action is apparently related to its ability to block the formation of T-lymphocytes, which have a role in cell-mediated immunity. There is no bone marrow suppression, but side effects may include nephrotoxicity, hepatotoxicity, and the development of lymphoma or other malignancy. Blood levels must be monitored and dosage adjusted if these side effects are detected.

Immune suppression also may be achieved by the use of antilymphocyte and antithymocyte preparations to provoke the formation of antibodies to the antigens administered in the agent. These agents are largely experimental and may be in the form of a serum or a globulin. Problems include hypersensitivity reactions, the possibility of anaphylaxis, and the development of opportunistic infections (Irwin, 1983).

The need for the client to understand the importance of taking the prescribed medications cannot be overemphasized. Clients must understand that doses cannot be missed. If they have the flu and cannot take the medication by mouth, the client should seek medical care and receive it intravenously. Emergency IM administration of prednisone should be taught to the client, family, or significant others. Clients should also be instructed about any other medications they may take, such as anticoagulants or antihypertensives (see Chapter 23).

In addition to teaching the client about the importance of the medication therapy, the nurse should also help the client learn the signs and symptoms of rejection. Many transplant centers have the client keep a log of daily weights, blood pressure, and temperature measurements to help the physician monitor the client's progress. Regular creatinine values, WBC counts, and prothrombin times are often recorded in the log as well. Compliance increases when the client understands the rationale for treatments. In some transplant centers, selected clients, under nursing supervision, give themselves their own medications and record weight, vital signs, and laboratory values.

The client should understand the need to avoid crowds and any risk of infection. Follow-up visits for the evaluation of renal function and overall health status are equally important.

The client must also receive psychological and emotional support from the nurse to adjust to the psychosocial and lifestyle changes previously discussed. Renal transplant clients always live in fear of rejection. If hyperacute or acute rejection occurs, the joy of receiving the new kidney quickly becomes sorrow. If irreversible rejection occurs later, the loss of the kidney means returning to dialysis, awaiting retransplantation, or both.

Section II: Surgical Approaches to Disorders Affecting the Ureters

URETEROLITHOTOMY

A ureterolithotomy is a surgical procedure in which the ureter is incised to remove a calculus that is not passing spontaneously. This procedure is indicated when obstruction to the flow of urine results in hydroureter or hydronephrosis. If the obstruction is not removed, an increase in the diameter of the ureter and resulting urine collection in the small renal pelvis may cause deterioration of renal parenchyma and loss of functioning tissue. Another indication for surgical intervention is an infection in which the calculus provides a nidus for continued infection.

Surgical Procedure

Ureterolithotomies are performed under general anesthesia. The site of the incision depends on the location of the calculus in the ureter. For calculi lodged in the upper third of the ureter, the surgeon selects a lumbar–flank incision. For calculi lodged in the midureter or the lower third of the ureter, the incision will be lower in the abdomen. (Figure 34–4 illustrates potential sites for these incisions.) A Penrose drain is placed to drain any urine or blood that may leak and collect around the site of the ureteral incision. A ureteral catheter or stent is also commonly placed to

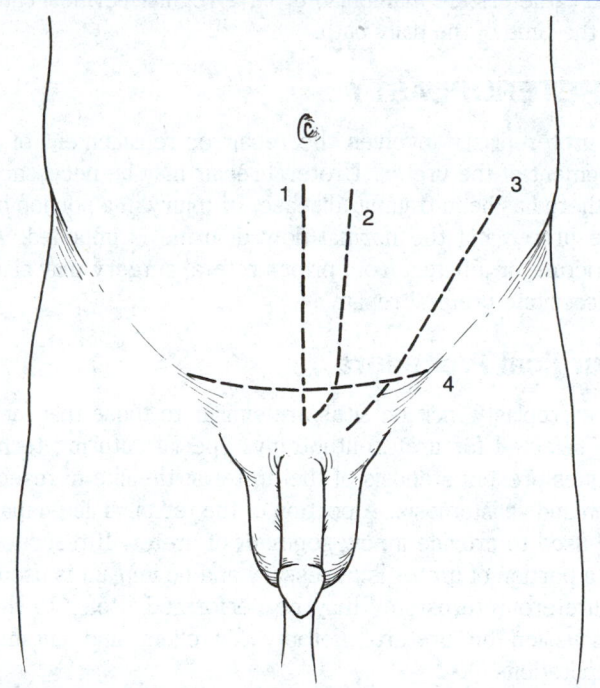

Figure 34–4

Sites for ureterolithotomy when stone is lodged in lower third of ureter or lower portion of middle third. Stones lodged in the upper third or upper portion of the middle third are approached through a lumbar–flank incision.

ensure patency of the ureter during the period of ureteral tissue healing. Without the catheter, edema of local tissue in the ureter could result in ureteral obstruction.

A ureteral **stent** is a hollow tubelike device made of soft, flexible silicone that is placed within a ureter to maintain ureteral flow in clients with ureteral obstruction, to restore kidney function, to divert urine, to promote healing, and to maintain ureteral patency after surgery (Figure 34–5). The stent may be used temporarily or permanently to open a closed or narrowed ureter to permit the flow of urine. In addition, stents allow tissues to heal without stricture or fistula formation. The stent may be inserted via a cystoscope, through a nephrostomy tube, percutaneously, or by open surgery. The double-J ureteral stent prevents movement of the stent without restricting the client's activities. Nursing care involves monitoring for bleeding and purulent drainage from the stent, measuring output, and observing for stent dislodgement (colicky pain and decreased urine output).

Implications for the Client

Physiological Implications

Preservation of renal function is a goal of ureterolithotomy. The procedure will remove the obstruction and relieve the client of the severe, colicky pain associated with a calculus or infection. Renal function can be restored once the problem has been eliminated, so further damage that might

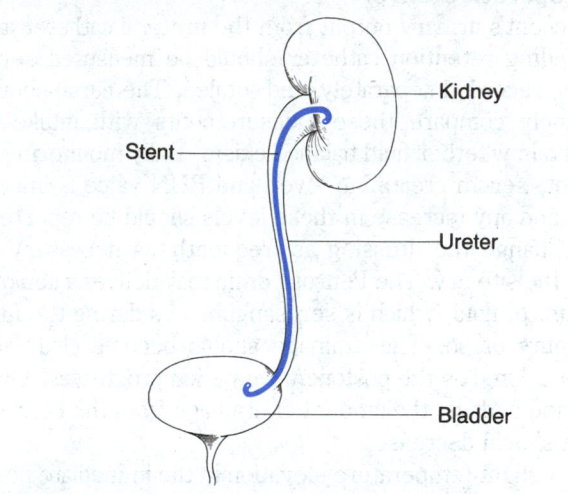

Figure 34–5

Double-J ureteral stent.

result in renal failure can be avoided. If the obstruction is caused by malignancy, the changes associated with advanced cancer will be present.

Psychosocial/Lifestyle Implications

Excessive physical activity will probably be restricted for 6 to 8 weeks, and the client should make appropriate plans for self-care during the posthospital period. The long-term education of the client should include measures to prevent the formation of additional calculi (see Chapter 33). If a malignancy is the cause of the problem, a stent may be permanently placed. If the procedure was done to remove a calculus, the limitations will be temporary, so no long-term changes are required other than lifestyle alterations to prevent new calculus formation. Table 34–5 lists client implications associated with ureterolithotomy.

Nursing Implications

Preoperative Care

Preventing further renal damage is a key goal. General preoperative teaching and interventions for all clients undergoing surgery are recommended (see Chapter 14).

Table 34–5	Ureterolithotomy: Implications for the Client	
Physiological Implications	**Psychosocial/Lifestyle Implications**
Goal to preserve or restore renal function, remove sources of severe pain	Restricted activity for 6 to 8 weeks Changes in lifestyle to prevent calculus formation (see Chapter 32)

Postoperative Care

The client's urinary output from the ureteral catheter and indwelling retention catheter should be measured separately, recorded separately, and totaled. The nurse should routinely compare these measurements with intake to ascertain whether fluid balance exists. Daily monitoring of weight, serum creatinine level, and BUN value is important, and any increase in these levels should be reported.

Change the dressing as frequently as necessary to keep the site dry. The Penrose drain may deliver a copious amount of fluid, which is serosanguineous during the first 24 hours or so. The drainage should become clear and straw colored as the postoperative period progresses. Over a period of days, the amount of drainage from the Penrose drain should decrease.

A slight temperature elevation in the immediate postoperative period is commonly associated with the effects of surgery and anesthesia, but a continued fever or sudden temperature elevation may indicate infection. A wound infection may be present in the area of the surgery and drain site, or there could be infection within the kidney. Aseptic technique is necessary when dressings are changed and catheters are manipulated. Give regular perineal care at the time of the daily bath.

URETEROPLASTY

A ureteroplasty involves the repair or replacement of a segment of the ureter. Ureteral repair may be necessary if there has been trauma, disease, or injury in a portion of the ureter and the normal flow of urine is impeded. A stricture or a fistula from prior ureteral surgery may also necessitate ureteral repair.

Surgical Procedure

Ureteroplasty incision sites are similar to those that may be selected for ureterolithotomy. Special suturing techniques prevent stenosis of the ureter at the site of resection and anastomosis. A portion of the terminal ileum may be used to provide a new segment of ureter. If resection of a portion of ureter is necessary and no implant is used, a ureteroureterostomy may be performed. Refer to the discussion on ureterolithotomy for client and nursing implications.

Section III: Surgical Approaches to Disorders Affecting the Bladder

PARTIAL CYSTECTOMY

A partial cystectomy involves the surgical incision of a portion of the urinary bladder. This procedure generally is indicated only when there is a single, primary tumor too large for transurethral resection. Small superficial tumors may be removed by transurethral resection via cystoscopy. Operative risks related to age, cardiovascular disease, or pulmonary disease may make a partial cystectomy preferable to a total or a radical cystectomy. The surgical intervention is chosen after individual client evaluation.

Surgical Procedure

The surgeon makes an incision into the lower abdomen of the client under general anesthesia. The tumor and adjacent bladder muscle are resected and the size of the urinary bladder decreased.

Implications for the Client

Physiological Implications

A common reason for partial cystectomy is a malignancy. If preoperative treatment with external radiation or chemotherapy has been prescribed, the client may be in a compromised physiological state at the time of surgery.

Because the surgery decreases the size of the bladder, constant urinary drainage is necessary after surgery to prevent excessive tension on the sutures of the bladder. The bladder will gradually return to its normal size in about 6 months. A major concern of the immediate postoperative period is the potential for the development of infection from surgery and the indwelling catheter.

Psychosocial/Lifestyle Implications

Emotional preparation for surgical intervention is important for this client. Bladder capacity will be diminished initially, creating minor lifestyle changes. Although the bladder is expected gradually to return to its normal capacity, the small volume of urine that may be held comfortably at first will necessitate that the client void frequently to avoid embarrassing accidents. The client will also need to plan for frequent cystoscopy—every 3 months for 2 years—to evaluate the effectiveness of treatment (Glenn, 1983). Psychosocial considerations for any malignancy apply in this case as well. Table 34–6 summarizes client implications for a partial cystectomy.

Nursing Implications

Preoperative Care

Prior to surgery, the goal is to have the client in the best possible state of health. The client who has had radiation therapy or chemotherapy has had some time to adjust to the diagnosis of cancer. However, all clients and family need a good deal of support and time to ask questions or ventilate feelings.

Postoperative Care

Postoperatively, the client will generally have an indwelling and a suprapubic catheter. Accurate measurements and

Table 34–6 Partial Cystectomy: Implications for the Client	
Physiological Implications	**Psychosocial/Lifestyle Implications**
Compromised state from preoperative chemotherapy or radiation-related malignancy	Diminished capacity of bladder that requires frequent voidings to avoid embarrassing accidents
Decreased bladder size postoperatively	Cystoscopy every 3 months for 2 years
Stress on sutures if too much urine	Changes associated with diagnosis of cancer
Bladder's gradual return to normal size in about 6 months	
Risk of postoperative infection from surgery and indwelling catheter	

recording of intake and urinary output are important. Catheter drainage will be continued until all identifiable urinary leakage has ceased (Glenn, 1983). The nurse should note drainage from each catheter. The suprapubic catheter will be removed as drainage ceases.

Fluid intake after surgery should be at least 2000 mL per day, but advise the client to limit fluid intake prior to sleeping or when toilet facilities are not readily available. The return to a normal bladder capacity of about 400 mL will require about 6 months. Until bladder capacity is normal, instruct the client to void frequently. He or she should identify the location of toilet facilities in advance of the need to urinate to prevent embarrassment from urinary incontinence. The nurse should offer support to the client, family, and significant others during any further cancer treatment.

RADICAL CYSTECTOMY

A radical cystectomy involves the removal of the urinary bladder and adjacent structures; it necessitates permanent urinary diversion. Indications for a radical cystectomy include malignancies not treatable with less conservative measures.

Surgical Procedure

General anesthesia is required for a radical cystectomy. The client is placed in a supine position, and the surgeon makes an incision into the midline of the abdomen from about 4 cm above the umbilicus and extending to the symphysis pubis. In the man, a radical cystectomy involves the removal of the urinary bladder, pelvic peritoneum, prostate, seminal vesicles, and pelvic lymph nodes; removal of the urethra remains controversial (Glenn, 1983). In the woman, a radical cystectomy includes removal of the urinary bladder, pelvic peritoneum, urethra, uterus and broad ligaments, and part of the anterior vaginal wall. Pelvic lymph nodes are also removed (Glenn, 1983). Urinary diversion is necessary with a radical cystectomy.

Implications for the Client

Physiological Implications

The type of urinary diversion procedure determines the physiological implications. These procedures—ureteroileal urinary conduit, colon conduit, ureterosigmoidostomy, ureteroileosigmoidostomy, cutaneous ureterostomy—are discussed later in this chapter. Preoperative radiation therapy may result in infection or prolonged decreased healing at the surgical site because healthy tissue is also affected by radiation. The surgeries in which the flow of urine is diverted into the colon or small intestine carry with them the risk of ascending urinary tract infection. Pelvic congestion may result from the surgery itself and the healing process. Surgical removal of the pelvic lymph nodes also causes pelvic congestion as well as peripheral edema and increases the client's discomfort. Peripheral edema, surgical manipulation in a highly vascular area, lymph node removal, and decreased mobility all increase the risk of thrombus or embolus.

Psychosocial/Lifestyle Implications

The psychosocial implications for each form of urinary diversion are discussed later in this chapter. The diagnosis of cancer and the poor prognosis associated with a radical cystectomy create fear and anxiety. The financial burdens associated with chemotherapy and radiation therapy cause added stress. The body image is altered and sexual dysfunction occurs (see the discussion in Chapter 32 and later in this chapter). In the woman, most of the reproductive organs are removed. The man is impotent because of the removal of reproductive organs. Table 34–7 summarizes client implications associated with radical cystectomy.

Nursing Implications

Preoperative Care

Measures to place the client in an optimal state of health prior to surgery are important, especially if radiation was begun preoperatively. The client will need assistance in

Table 34–7 Radical Cystectomy: Implications for the Client	
Physiological Implications	**Psychosocial/Lifestyle Implications**
Urinary diversion procedures necessary (see Tables 34–8 and 34–11)	Dependence on urinary diversion selected
Decreased healing related to preoperative radiation	Fear and anxiety associated with cancer
Pelvic congestion and peripheral edema from removal of lymph nodes	Altered body image and sexuality from urinary diversion (see specific urinary diversion procedures)
Thromboembolic phenomena	
Infection	

deciding which type of urinary diversion is most suitable, so thorough discussion of diversion procedures is necessary. Diversion procedures are discussed next. The client also should be informed of his or her right to refuse treatment. Considerations for malignancy in general should also be included.

Postoperative Care

Postoperatively, encourage the client to perform routine coughing, deep breathing, and turning. Leg exercises and early ambulation will promote good circulation, particularly venous return. This is particularly important because of the lymph node removal and the tendency to develop congestion and edema. Thrombosis with embolization is another potential complication following this surgical procedure. Bowel sounds and gastrointestinal motility should return in 3 to 5 days after surgery. The client will be NPO and receiving IV fluids until peristalsis returns. Carefully measure intake, and output, and vital signs during the postoperative period. Other postoperative care depends on the type of urinary diversion selected.

URETEROILEAL URINARY CONDUIT

Ureteroileal urinary conduit, ileal conduit, ileal bladder, ileal loop, Bricker's procedure, or ureteroileostomy are terms describing the same basic procedure. A portion of the ileum is resected and used as a new receptacle for the collection of urine. The open end of the resected segment is brought to the surface of the skin in the form of a stoma. This is one type of urinary diversion that can be used when the bladder has been removed or when the urine outflow is obstructed.

Surgical Procedure

With the client under general anesthesia, a portion of the ileum is resected from the small intestine. Blood supply to this segment is maintained, and one end is closed. The remaining segments of the bowel are anastomosed. The ureters are implanted into the side of the isolated segment, and the open end of the ileal segment is brought out onto the surface of the skin as a stoma (Figure 34–6).

Implications for the Client

Physiological Implications

The ileum's surface has excellent absorptive properties for water and electrolytes. This may become a problem postoperatively, because water and electrolytes may be reabsorbed from the urine as it passes through the ureteroileal urinary conduit. Therefore, the segment of ileum must be as short as possible but long enough to prevent excessive tension on the stoma. Renal function and electrolyte balance must be monitored carefully and problems corrected when necessary. The lengthy time required for this procedure, particularly when performed with a radical cystectomy, increases the client's risk for postoperative deep vein thrombosis and embolization. Peristalsis usually will not return before 3 to 5 days, before which parenteral fluid and electrolyte replacement are required.

The skin around the stoma is highly sensitive to urine, so skin care and the correct application of an appliance for urine collection are important in preventing skin breakdown. Another problem is the congealing of mucus in the stoma; a high fluid intake will help prevent this. Other complications include wound infections and dehiscence, ureteral and small bowel obstructions, and stomal gangrene. Renal calculi and pyelonephritis also may occur.

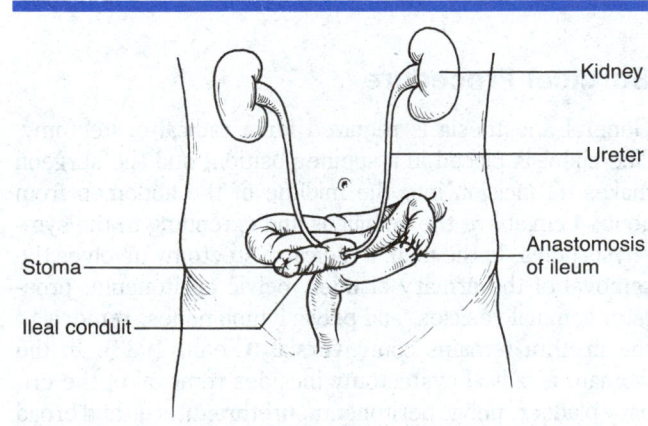

Figure 34–6

Ureteroileal urinary conduit.

Urine odor and leaking around the stoma may embarrass the client.

Psychosocial/Lifestyle Implications

The ureteroileal urinary conduit or other forms of urinary diversion force the client to make major emotional adjustments. The external stoma creates a change in body image, along with potential alterations in self-concept, self-esteem, and sexual identity. Learning to adjust to pouch drainage, odor control, and skin irritation prevention and management requires considerable effort and perseverance. Close personal contact, including sexual intimacy, may be difficult for the client to resume. The lack of privacy in health clubs or other locker facilities may cause the client to avoid previous recreational activities; clients often prefer to isolate themselves socially rather than risk embarrassment. Assisting the client in learning self-care and adjusting to changes in body image requires time, patience, and continuous support from the family or significant others and the health care team. Table 34–8 summarizes physiological and psychosocial/lifestyle implications for the client with a ureteroileal urinary conduit.

Nursing Implications

Preoperative Care

Preoperatively, the client should receive thorough explanations about the need for evaluation of the intestinal tract. The client should assist in selecting a comfortable site for stoma placement (generally in the upper right lower quadrant of the abdomen). The surface of the skin at the site should be free of scars and deep tissue folds. In addition, the site should be readily accessible to the client. Having the client wear a pouch filled with water for several days during the preoperative period may help ensure that the site selected is optimally functional and comfortable, as

---

Nursing Research Note

Williamson M: Reducing post-catheterization bladder dysfunction. *Nurs Res* 1982; 31:28–30.

This study determined the effect of bladder reconditioning before removal of an indwelling catheter on bladder dysfunction postcatheterization. One group of women had their indwelling catheters clamped for 3 hours with a 5-minute drain period for a total of 9 hours. The control group had no conditioning, and the indwelling catheter was just removed.

Those clients who underwent reconditioning resumed normal bladder elimination significantly sooner than the control group. Residual urine volumes for both groups did not differ significantly. However, for the control group, residual urine volumes after the first normal micturition following catheter removal were 10 times the mean baseline residual volume. The group with reconditioning had residual volumes 1.3 times the mean baseline.

This study suggests an intervention to assist clients to return to normal urinary elimination sooner after catheterization. Reconditioning was found to shorten the amount of time needed to resume normal micturition. It also reduced residual urine volumes after the first normal voiding and therefore may help to reduce bladder infection.

---

well as help with the postoperative adjustment by helping the client know what to expect. Several different pouches may be tried to ensure comfort and compatibility with normal clothing. An enterostomal therapist is invaluable for all preoperative teaching.

Preoperative bowel preparation is achieved through a low-residue diet, a laxative or enemas, or oral neomycin to reduce the risk of infection. Three days is generally needed for bowel preparation procedures. Cardiovascular evaluation is also important in determining whether the client can withstand the lengthy surgery.

Table 34–8 Ureteroileal Urinary and Colon Conduits: Implications for the Client

Physiological Implications	Psychosocial/Lifestyle Implications
Reabsorption of water and electrolytes from conduit leading to imbalances	Altered body image and sexual identity related to stoma and appliance
Deep vein thrombosis and embolization	Embarrassment from drainage and odor from stoma leading to social isolation
No peristalsis for 3 to 5 days	
Skin irritation around stoma	
Mucus congealing at stoma	
Wound infection and dehiscence	
Obstruction of ureter and small bowel	
Stomal gangrene	
Renal calculi	
Pyelonephritis	
Odor and leaking from stoma appliance	

Postoperative Care

The goals of postoperative nursing management are to preserve renal function and assist the client in adapting to an altered body image. The client will have a nasogastric tube inserted until bowel motility returns (usually in 3 to 5 days). Urine will flow into a pouch placed over the stoma at the time of surgery. Lack of urine flow during the first 12 to 18 hours may be the result of edema at the site of ureteral implantation (McConnell & Zimmerman, 1983). A catheter may be gently inserted to check for stasis or residual urine from a tight stoma. The nurse must carefully measure and record intake and output, as well as monitor renal function through daily measurement of serum creatinine and BUN values. Electrolyte balance should also be assessed by daily laboratory data.

Early ambulation will prevent venous stasis and the development of atelectasis, as well as promote the return of peristalsis. The administration of narcotic analgesics in the early postoperative period will achieve pain control.

Preserving renal function depends upon proper stoma care and the absence of infection. If the area is kept clean, infection probably will not develop. Stoma care involves several factors. Assess the stoma for adequate vascular supply; it should be red or pink. If the stoma becomes purple, surgical intervention may be required to correct the blood supply to the stoma. The choice of the correct appliance promotes proper stoma care and functioning. Clients may choose disposable or reusable appliances. The appliance should be $\frac{1}{16}$ in larger than the diameter of the stoma. After about 1 month, the stoma size should stabilize.

The collecting appliance should be changed every 4 to 5 days or whenever it is leaking. Instruct the client to remove the face plate and then bend over quickly and remain that way for a minute to allow the conduit to empty completely. The client then washes and rinses the skin, taking care to dry the skin before reapplying the appliance. A gauze wick or tampon inserted at the stoma will absorb urine and keep the skin dry during appliance application. The client should apply a skin barrier or protectant if needed. Next, gentle pressure applied around the appliance removes air bubbles and secures the adhesive or cement and the appliance to the skin. Taping around the appliance will give extra security.

Clients often wear leg bags to be sure the collecting bag at the stoma does not get too full and empty itself. An adapter attaches the drainage apparatus to the leg bag and tubing. At night the client may prefer to snap a tubing with dependent drainage to a collection bottle to have uninterrupted sleep.

Odor control may be a challenge for the client with a ureteroileal urinary conduit. Foods that give urine a strong odor, such as tomatoes and asparagus, should be avoided. Wearing an appliance too long without cleaning it will also create an odor. Ascorbic acid intake will help suppress odors, as will white vinegar introduced into the drain spout at the bottom of the pouch. After rinsing the bag in warm water, soak it in a vinegar-and-water solution for 30 to 60 minutes. After the bag is rinsed, dried (avoiding sunlight), and powdered with cornstarch, it can be stored until the next use. Other tips on caring for the appliance and managing odor control may be obtained from the local ostomy association.

Helping the client adapt to an altered body image is not easy. Refer to the discussions on altered body image and sexual dysfunction in Chapter 32.

COLON CONDUIT

The colon conduit, or sigmoid conduit, is a type of urinary diversion in which a portion of the sigmoid colon is resected and used to hold urine. The ureters are implanted into the resected segment, and a stoma is formed with the open end of the segment. The procedure is indicated in clients with neurogenic bladders and normal upper urinary tracts, those requiring temporary diversions, or those undergoing pelvic exenteration. Active bowel disease, such as diverticulitis, is a contraindication to this form of diversion. The colon conduit is not generally recommended for use following radical cystectomy because of the potential for impaired healing. Delayed healing also may occur as a result of irradiation or disrupted circulation.

The colon conduit has two advantages over the ureteroileal urinary conduit. First, because the diameter of the sigmoid is larger than the diameter of the ileum, there are fewer problems with stoma stricture. Second, the colon conduit permits the development of an antireflux mechanism, decreasing the likelihood of eventual renal deterioration from infection (Glenn, 1983).

Surgical Procedure

The colon conduit is created via a midline incision with the client in a supine position and under general anesthesia. This procedure follows cystectomy, if cystectomy is required. To create the conduit, the surgeon resects a portion of sigmoid colon and anastomoses the remaining segments of the bowel. The vascular supply to the isolated segment remains intact. One end of the sigmoid segment is closed, the ureters are tunneled into the mucosa of the side of the sigmoid segment, and the open end of the segment is brought through the left lower quadrant to form a stoma. Refer to Figure 34–7.

Implications for the Client

Physiological Implications

The postoperative absorption of water and electrolytes is possible through the surface of the colon conduit, as it is through the ureteroileal urinary conduit. Like the ureteroileal urinary conduit, the colon conduit should not be a storage area but instead provide for rapid passage of the urine into the pouch. Other physiological implications for the client are similar to those discussed in the previous section on the ureteroileal urinary conduit and summarized in Table 34–8.

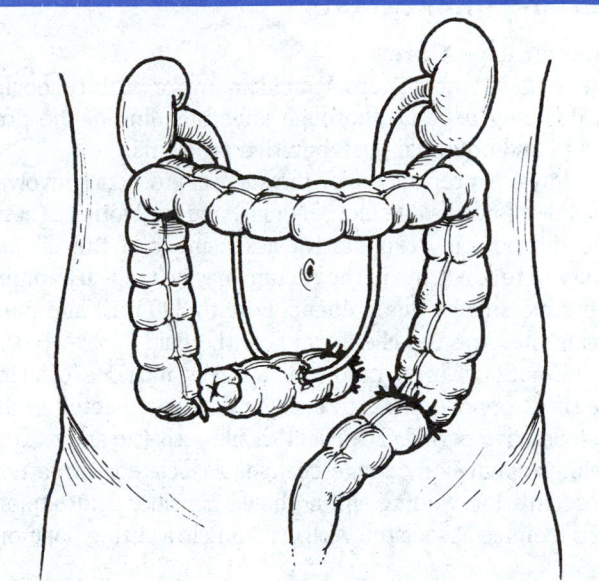

Figure 34–7

Colon conduit.

Psychosocial/Lifestyle Implications

Refer to the discussion of psychosocial and lifestyle considerations for the client having a ureteroileal urinary conduit and to Table 34–8.

Nursing Implications

Nursing implications are similar to those detailed in the discussion for clients who have a ureteroileal urinary conduit. The major exception is that the site for the stoma of the colon conduit will be the left lower quadrant.

URETEROSIGMOIDOSTOMY AND URETEROILEOSIGMOIDOSTOMY

Ureterosigmoidostomy and ureteroileosigmoidostomy are urinary diversions in which the flow of urine is directed into the rectum. A ureterosigmoidostomy, which is usually done for the client with small bowel disease, involves the implantation of the ureters into the sigmoid colon. Clients with rectal incontinence, impaired renal function, active colon disease, liver dysfunction, or a history of pelvic irradiation should consider other urinary diversion procedures. A ureteroileosigmoidostomy is done for the client who is not a candidate for other urinary diversions, but who, because the small bowel is healthy, is able to have a portion of it used to form a pouch that attaches to the colon. This procedure minimizes the spread of bacteria and reflux of urine back to the kidneys because the ureters are attached to a section of the ileum rather than directly to the sigmoid colon.

These procedures do not require an external pouch because urine is passed via the rectum. In addition, the ureteroileosigmoidostomy is believed to minimize urinary

reflux and thus avoid destruction of renal parenchyma from pyelonephritis.

Surgical Procedure

The ureterosigmoidostomy is performed under general anesthesia, via a midline incision, with the client in a supine position. Each ureter is freed from the bladder and inserted into the sigmoid colon (Figure 34–8). In the ureteroileosigmoidostomy, a segment of ileum is resected, and the remaining segments of the small bowel are anastomosed (the isolated segment of the ileum is anastomosed to the sigmoid colon on one side and closed on the other end). The ureters are then inserted into the isolated segment of the small bowel. Other aspects of the procedure are similar to those described for the ureterosigmoidostomy.

Implications for the Client

Physiological Implications

Because the client's urine exits via the rectum, any fecal incontinence that develops and the expulsion of flatus will result in urinary incontinence. The perianal area may become excoriated from contact with feces and urine if diarrhea or incontinence develops.

The presence of the urine in the rectum results in electrolyte (sodium, chloride, and hydrogen) absorption. At the same time, bicarbonate diffuses into the bowel lumen, resulting in hyperchloremic metabolic acidosis. The physiological response to the hyperchloremic metabolic acidosis is the loss of potassium from intracellular spaces; thus, hypokalemia also develops. A magnesium deficit may also occur. Diarrhea will worsen these electrolyte abnormalities. Serum electrolytes should be monitored on a regular basis.

Bone mobilization of calcium also occurs, and the resultant hypercalcemia predisposes the client to the for-

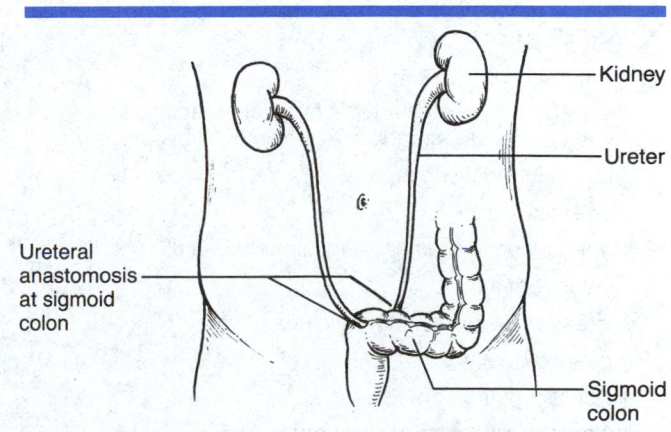

Kidney

Ureter

Ureteral anastomosis at sigmoid colon

Sigmoid colon

Figure 34–8

Ureterosigmoidostomy.

mation of renal or urinary calculi. Acute or chronic pyelonephritis may develop from urinary reflux. If sterilization of the urinary tract is not possible, an alternate method of urinary diversion may be necessary for long-term preservation of renal function. Absorption of urinary ammonia may result in increased blood levels of ammonia, particularly in clients with hepatic cirrhosis. Encephalopathy may result. Pyelonephritis, ureteral obstruction, and tumors in the colon have been demonstrated to occur frequently (Glenn, 1983). These complications have made these procedures of questionable value for young clients with a normal life expectancy. Furthermore, adenocarcinoma of the colon is more likely to develop following these procedures.

Psychosocial/Lifestyle Implications

The major advantage of these types of urinary diversions is that no external pouch is required, and urinary continence may be maintained most of the time. Clients will have an altered body image, however. Men should understand that they will have to sit to urinate after this procedure, and both men and women should understand that the passage of flatus will result in expulsion or leakage of urine. Thus, embarrassment is common. Clients will need to empty the rectum every 2 to 3 hours to minimize problems of electrolyte reabsorption. Adherence to prescribed medications and dietary modifications (high-potassium, low-chloride, and low-calcium consumption) will also be essential in preventing long-term complications from electrolyte imbalances. Even so, these complications may be unavoidable.

Table 34–9 summarizes physiological and psychosocial/lifestyle implications for the client with ureterosigmoidostomy or ureteroileosigmoidostomy.

Nursing Implications

Preoperative Care

The client having ureterosigmoidostomy or ureteroileosigmoidostomy needs a thorough understanding of the procedure and potential postoperative problems.

Physical preparation for the surgical procedure involves a liquid or low-residue diet, enemas, and antibiotics to sterilize the bowel. Preoperative assessment of the client's ability to retain urine in the rectum may be made by administering a small-volume enema (200 to 300 mL) and measuring the time the client can hold the fluid.

Emotional preparation for surgery includes offering the client opportunities to discuss what is expected in the postoperative period. The client should verbalize and explore feelings about body image changes associated with a new procedure for voiding. Men should consider and explore their feelings associated with urinating in a sitting position.

Postoperative Care

A rectal tube is placed postoperatively for the collection and measurement of urinary output. Gentle irrigations with small amounts of normal saline may be required to prevent obstruction from stool or mucus. In addition to the rectal tube, two ureteral catheters, which serve as stents to keep the ureters patent at the site of anastomosis, will also exit the rectum and drain into one collection bag. The rectal tube will empty into another bag. Careful measurement of fluid intake and output is important. Intravenous fluids and electrolytes will be necessary until intestinal motility returns. The client will be NPO and may have a nasogastric tube in place initially. The nurse must provide regular skin care to the anal area and keep the area as dry as possible.

Table 34–9 Ureterosigmoidostomy and Ureteroileosigmoidostomy: Implications for the Client	
Physiological Implications	**Psychosocial/Lifestyle Implications**
Urinary incontinence with expulsion of flatus or fecal incontinence	No external pouch
Anal irritation	Altered body image
Reabsorption of electrolytes and fluid leading to hyperchloremia, metabolic acidosis, and hypokalemia	Male's need to adjust to sitting to urinate
Magnesium deficit	Embarrassment if incontinent
Hypercalcemia	Frequent emptying of colon
Hypercalcemia predisposing client to calculi	Need to make diet adjustments to prevent complications (high potassium, low chloride, low calcium)
Pyelonephritis	
Increased serum ammonia levels	
Encephalopathy	
Ureteral obstruction	
Increased risk of colon adenocarcinoma	
Usually not considered for long-term diversion	

Infection in the urinary tract is always a potential problem. The development of fever and flank pain indicates infection in the urinary tract. Sudden decreases in urinary output may occur with infection or obstruction of the catheters or rectal tube.

Following the acute postoperative period, nursing care will revolve around educating the client for maximum self-care in the future. The client should understand that dietary modifications will be necessary to provide a high-potassium, low-chloride, and low-calcium intake. Chloride intake may be reduced if salt intake is limited. High-potassium foods include the citrus fruits (oranges, grapefruit, and so on) and their juices; strawberries; potatoes; tomatoes and tomato juice; bananas; and green vegetables, such as green beans and lima beans. Calcium, which occurs in milk and dairy products, should be consumed in limited quantities. In addition, medications may be prescribed to supplement potassium and bicarbonate consumption.

Foods that readily produce gas should be avoided (eg, beans, cabbage, cauliflower, brussels sprouts, prunes, and raisins). Gum chewing, using straws, and smoking, which increase flatus production causing air to be swallowed, also should be avoided.

The client also needs to understand the rationale for prescribed medications. The client should avoid enemas, laxatives, diagnostic enemas, and activities that would increase intrarectal pressure; an increase in intrarectal pressure will result in reflux and possible infection of the urinary tract. Because the urine flows into the stool, constipation is generally not a problem. A liberal fluid intake of 2 to 3 L per day should be consumed. The client should get up once or twice at night to empty the rectum of urine.

CUTANEOUS URETEROSTOMY

In the cutaneous ureterostomy, another form of urinary diversion, the ureters are brought to the surface of the skin for drainage. This procedure may be indicated for clients who have obstruction of the urinary tract, usually because of pelvic or abdominal malignancies. The extensive fibrosis of pelvic tissue that results in ureteral obstruction might necessitate ureteral diversion as well. Specifically, the cutaneous ureterostomy is indicated for clients who have a dilated ureter or those with a poor prognosis (Glenn, 1983).

Surgical Procedure

Several types of cutaneous ureterostomies may be performed, and they may be considered temporary or permanent urinary diversions. The procedure is not recommended for long-term diversion, however, because of infection and progressive narrowing of the stomas. The bilateral (or double-barreled) cutaneous ureterostomy involves each ureter's surfacing onto the skin with a stoma for urine drainage. The unilateral cutaneous ureterostomy

involves a single ureteral stoma. A ureteroureterostomy involves the anastomosis of one ureter into the side of the other; one ureter is brought to the surface (Figure 34–9A).

Typically, the bilateral ureteral stomas are placed at the midline, or sometimes on the lateral aspects of each side of the abdomen (Figure 34–9B). A single stoma is created for the ureteroureterostomy or unilateral cutaneous ureterostomy.

Implications for the Client

Physiological Implications
Cutaneous urinary diversions require a minimal amount of surgical and anesthesia time in comparison with the more extensive forms of ureteral diversion. This aspect of the procedure may make it more appropriate for elderly and debilitated clients. After the diversion has been created, major physiological considerations include the prevention of infection and protection of the skin to prevent irritation.

Psychosocial/Lifestyle Implications
Clients who require cutaneous urinary diversion undergo body image changes and their accompanying alterations in self-concept and self-esteem. Clients must learn to care

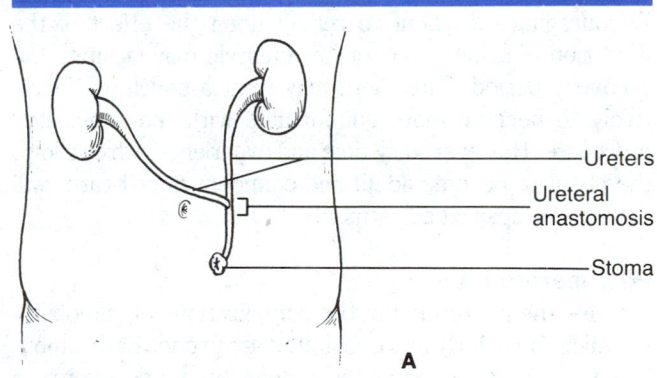

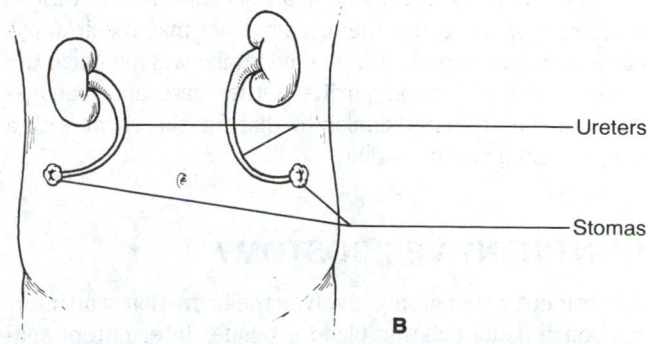

Figure 34–9

Sites for cutaneous ureterostomy. **A.** Ureteroureterostomy. **B.** Bilateral cutaneous ureterostomy.

Table 34–10	Cutaneous Ureterostomy: Implications for the Client	
Physiological Implications	**Psychosocial/Lifestyle Implications**
Little surgical time; good for debilitated clients	Altered body image, self-concept, and self-esteem
Infection	Possible social isolation because of pouch leakage and odor
Skin irritation	Need for self-care assistance

for the pouch. Embarrassment from pouch leakage or suspected odor contribute to self-imposed social isolation. Because clients are often elderly or in poor general health, assistance with self-care and altered teaching and learning strategies may be indicated. Table 34–10 summarizes the implications for the client with a cutaneous ureterostomy.

Nursing Implications

Preoperative Care

Offer the client opportunities to express concerns and clarify expectations about the proposed urinary diversion. Encouraging the client to reflect upon the effect of the diversion of urine on his or her lifestyle may facilitate the recovery period. The client may wear a pouch preoperatively to become more comfortable with the anticipated procedure. However, only time and experience, which allows the client to become adept and confident in self-care, will ensure the desired adjustment.

Postoperative Care

Plan for the prevention of the complications of immobility to which the elderly and debilitated are prone. Early ambulation, turning, coughing, and deep breathing exercises should be instituted. Routine postoperative measurement of intake and output, daily weights, and vital signs is essential. Early detection of infection also is imperative, because the direct opening into the urinary tract may result in pyelonephritis or sepsis. A high fluid intake will minimize the development of pyelonephritis. Other care and management of the stoma is similar to that for the client with a ureteroileal urinary conduit.

CONTINENT VESICOSTOMY

A continent vesicostomy involves the formation of an internal pouch using existing bladder tissue. Intermittent self-catheterization through a nipple valve that exits the skin provides for urinary drainage. The continent vesicostomy is indicated for the client with a neurogenic bladder.

Surgical Procedure

For the continent vesicostomy, existing bladder musculature is molded into an internal pouch. The vesicostomy stoma, formed from bladder tissue, will initially have a catheter in place for drainage. After surgery, a suprapubic catheter is in place for drainage until local edema and tissue healing take place.

Implications for the Client

Physiological Implications

Any infection of the urinary tract should be eradicated preoperatively. Since the client already has a neurogenic bladder, several physiological situations, such as infection, incontinence, and self-catheterization, will have already been faced. The client will have to learn how to catheterize the nipple of the vesicostomy. The nurse must carefully monitor renal function to prevent any damage to the kidneys from infection or urine backing up into the kidney. High-fluid intake will decrease the chances of infection.

Psychosocial/Lifestyle Implications

Body image changes and associated concerns related to sexual identity and expression, self-esteem, and self-concept will be among the primary general concerns of the client who undergoes a continent vesicostomy. The client with a neurogenic bladder often has already encountered a number of problems and concerns related to long-term health alterations and limitations. However, new techniques of self-management will be required with this procedure, including self-catheterization. A summary of implications for the client with a continent vesicostomy appears in Table 34–11.

Nursing Implications

Preoperative Care

Any infections of the urinary tract should be eradicated preoperatively. Encourage and facilitate the client's clari-

Table 34–11	Continent Vesicostomy: Implications for the Client	
Physiological Implications	**Psychosocial/Lifestyle Implications**
Need to self-catheterize nipple	Altered body image
Careful monitoring of renal function	Altered sexual identity, self-esteem, and self-concept
High fluid intake to decrease chances of infection	Need to learn self-catheterization

fication of postoperative expectations, including feelings and concerns related to changes in self-concept, body image, and sexuality. Antibiotics may be given preoperatively to sterilize the urinary tract.

Postoperative Care

Postoperative considerations include careful monitoring of renal function and the prevention of infection. Closed urinary drainage systems for the suprapubic and stomal catheters should be ensured to prevent the introduction of infectious microorganisms. Intravenous fluid and electrolyte replacement will be required until normal intestinal motility returns. Careful measurement of fluid intake and output is important. Meticulous skin care should be done daily or as needed to keep the skin dry and free from irritation.

Catheter irrigation will be required by the client at home for about a month after surgery, until each catheter is removed. Intermittent self-catheterization may be done with clean technique at home. The client should be instructed to drink a normal amount of fluids and carry or wear identification indicating the presence of the vesicostomy. Clients may avoid embarrassing leakage of urine during sexual intercourse if they empty the bladder in advance.

Chapter Highlights

The postoperative care of most clients who have undergone urological surgery focuses on maintenance of renal function, maintenance of fluid and electrolyte balances, prevention of pulmonary complications and infection, and adaptation to altered body image and sexual functioning.

A lumbar–flank approach is preferred for surgeries involving the kidney and upper one-third to one-half of the ureter; a mid- to lower-abdominal approach is preferred for surgeries involving the lower two-thirds to one-half of the ureters, bladder, and urethra.

A nephrectomy is the surgical removal of a kidney that is indicated when there is chronic infection, trauma, hemorrhage, tumor, uncontrolled hypertension, an infected calculus, or a desire to donate a kidney to a relative.

A nephrolithotomy involves the incision into the renal parenchyma in order to remove a calculus or small tumor or correct altered anatomic structures and vascular abnormalities.

A pyelolithotomy is a surgical procedure which involves an incision into the renal pelvis in order to remove a calculus.

Renal artery stenosis and renovascular hypertension are indications for renal revascularization surgeries which include endarterectomy, renal artery bypass graft, and resection and end-to-end anastomosis.

A ureteral calculus is removed through an incision into the ureter during the procedure known as a ureterolithotomy.

A ureteroplasty involves the replacement or repair of a segment of the ureter that may be needed if there has been trauma, disease, or injury to a portion of the ureter which interrupts the normal flow of urine.

A cystectomy involves the surgical excision of all (radical) or part (partial) of the urinary and is indicated when a large tumor is present.

A urinary diversion procedure is required after a radical cystectomy and may include a ureteroileal conduit, colon conduit, ureterosigmoidostomy, ureteroileosigmoidostomy, or cutaneous ureterostomy.

For the ileal or colon conduit a portion of either the ileum (ileal conduit) or colon (colon conduit) is used as a new receptacle for urine collection.

Ureterosigmoidostomy and ureteroileosigmoidostomy are urinary diversions in which the flow of urine is directed into the sigmoid colon directly or via a portion of ileum anastomosed to the sigmoid colon.

With the cutaneous ureterostomy urinary diversion is accomplished by bringing the ureters to the surface of the skin for drainage of urine into a collection bag or appliance.

A continent vesicostomy, which involves the formation of an internal pouch from existing bladder tissue that can be catheterized via a nipple, is indicated for clients with a neurogenic bladder.

A kidney transplant is an alternative to dialysis for clients with chronic renal failure.

Signs and symptoms of kidney transplant rejection include elevated blood pressure, temperature, and serum creatinine value; decreased urine output; a swollen and tender kidney; drowsiness; anorexia; and weight gain.

Bibliography

Barrett N: Continent vesicostomy: The dry urinary diversion. *Am J Nurs* 1979; 79(3):462–464.

Cockett ATK, Koshiba K: *Manual of Urologic Surgery.* New York: Springer-Verlag, 1980.

Glenn JF (editor): *Urologic Surgery,* 3rd ed. Philadelphia: Lippincott, 1983.

Irwin BC: Renal transplantation: Advances in immunology. A nursing perspective. *AANNT J* 1983; 10(4):11–15,22.

McConnell EA, Zimmerman, MF: *Care of Patients With Urologic Problems.* Philadelphia: Lippincott, 1983.

Rose BD: *Pathophysiology of Renal Disease.* New York: McGraw-Hill, 1981.

Woods JE: *Clinical Organ Transplantation in Surgical Immunology,* Munster A (editor). New York: Grune & Stratton, 1976.

Suggested Readings

Cain L, Bigongiari L: The percutaneous nephrostomy tube. *Am J Nurs* 1982; 82:296–298. Description of the percutaneous nephrostomy tube procedure. Postprocedure nursing care and discharge teaching are presented in a case study.

Do More With Your Life Than Just Cope With It: Managing Your Urostomy. Libertyville, IL: Hollister, 1983. Descriptive booklet about urinary diversions and their management, written for clients.

Fairman JA: Sexual concerns of the renal transplant patient in the ambulatory care setting: A format for nursing intervention. *AANNT J* 1982; 9(Dec):45–48. Describes alterations in fertility and sexuality in the ESRD client, and the potential for reversal after kidney transplant. Interview guidelines for obtaining a sexual history are a valuable aspect of the article.

Hinkle MT, Bowditch RW: The great stent mystery: Can you solve it? *Nurs 81* 1981; 11(April):94 + . Article describing the nursing implications for ureteral surgery clients who have stents placed.

Robbins KC et al: Donor-specific transfusions as pretreatment for living related donor transplants and implications for nursing. *Nephrol Nurse* 1983; 5(May/June):4 + . Article describing the background, client selection, protocol, and implications for nursing of donor-specific transfusions to living related transplant recipients.

Vogel CH: Keeping patients alive in spite of postobstructive diuresis. *Nurs 79* 1979; 9(March):50 + . Detailed description of the appropriate management and nursing interventions essential during the period following removal of an obstruction.

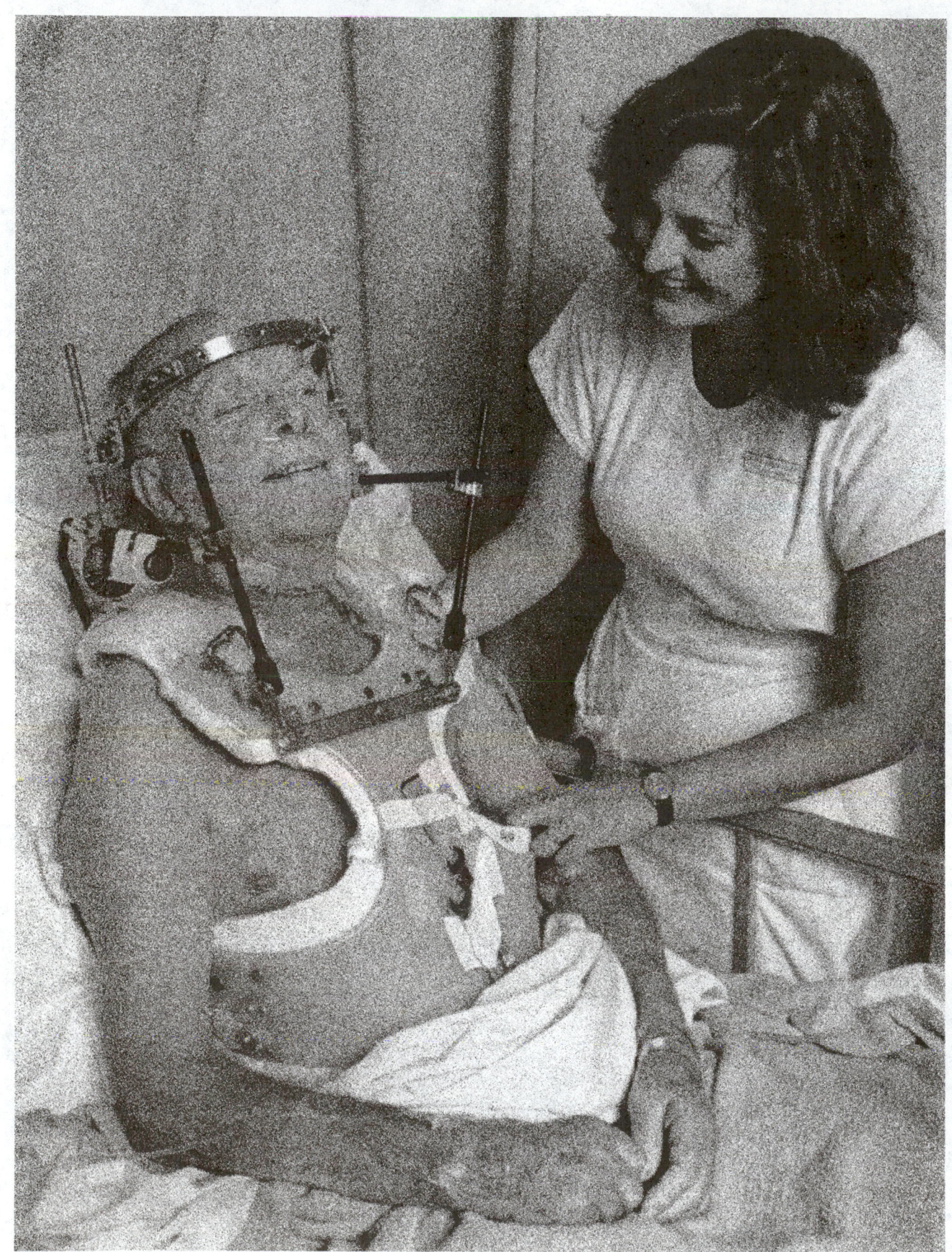

The Client With Nervous System Dysfunction

Chapter 35

The Nervous System in Health and Illness

Martha Firth Markarian

Objectives

When you have finished studying this chapter, you should be able to:

Describe the major structural and functional components of the nervous system.

Identify elements in the nervous system's structure that predispose the system to pathology.

Discuss neurons' construction and their roles in message transmission throughout the body.

Explain the functions of cells responsible for the maintenance and support of the nervous system.

Describe the nervous system's intricate vascular network including its strengths and weaknesses.

Trace the nerve tracts involved in motor and sensory activities.

Delineate the locations, divisions, and functions of the autonomic nervous system.

Discuss alterations in nervous system structure and function that can affect the body's homeostatic state.

Give examples of biochemical alterations that can interfere with effective nervous system function.

Describe structural alterations of the nervous system and their effect on neurologic function.

Identify developmental factors to be considered when providing care for clients with neurologic deficits.

Recognize biopsychosocial approaches to be considered when assisting the client with altered neurologic function.

Identify other body systems that contribute to the maintenance of the integrity and effective function of the nervous system.

Every physical, mental, and emotional aspect of a person's existence is influenced by continually changing internal and external environments. To deal with these changes effectively, the nervous system must perceive and interpret the changes and then quickly and continuously initiate, coordinate, and modulate body responses. The nervous system is always "on alert." Its job is endless because the environment is never static. Consider just a few common internal and external changes: Among internal changes are the process of aging, anabolic and catabolic activities, and psychological states; external changes include ambient temperatures, light, noise levels, and colonies of microorganisms. Many more can easily be identified.

The nervous system not only plays a key role in the management of body functions; it also depends on other body systems. Indeed, the nervous system quickly malfunctions if its sources of nourishment, its waste management systems, or its protective mechanisms are lost or even impeded.

Section I: Structural and Functional Interrelationships

An understanding of neurologic structure and function and the interdependence of body systems is an essential part of the nurse's knowledge base. With this knowledge, the nurse can effectively assess and plan care for the client with central nervous system (CNS) dysfunction.

STRUCTURE OF THE NEURON

Neurons (nerve cells) are primary components of the nervous system. Working alone or as units, they detect environmental changes and initiate body responses needed to maintain homeostasis. Each neuron is composed of a cell body, an axon, and a varying number of dendrites. Both axons and dendrites vary in size and shape. The *axons*, ranging in length from miniscule to over a meter, transmit messages throughout the central and peripheral nervous systems. Each cell has only one axon, but axonal branching is common and allows for broader dissemination of neuronal transmissions. *Dendrites*, the processes of neurons that conduct electrical impulses to the cell body, also have varying branching patterns. These characteristics allow for efficient transmission and reception of impulses throughout the body.

Many central and peripheral axons are wrapped in insulating sheaths of a white fatty substance called *myelin*. The myelin is encased in special cells lying end to end along the axons. Junctures, known as nodes of Ranvier, occur where these cells abut, allowing for more rapid transmission of electrical impulses. Axons often branch at these nodes.

Two distinct types of cells cover axons of the CNS and peripheral nervous system (PNS). Those located in the CNS are known as oligodendrocytes. These cells and the neurons they protect cannot be replaced or repaired if damaged. On the other hand, Schwann's cells, which surround PNS myelinated and unmyelinated axons, form the neurilemma, the outer membrane that supports and protects PNS axons and sometimes facilitates the healing of damaged axons.

Groups of neurons called nuclei provide routes for the transmission of complex afferent and efferent impulses. Clusters of neurons in the PNS are referred to as ganglia. *Fasciculi* are bundles of neurons encased in a covering called perineurium, whereas groups of fasciculi, encased in a covering called epineurium, are referred to as *nerves*. Most nerves are mixed nerves that contain afferent (toward the CNS) and efferent (from the CNS) fibers.

Structurally distinct neurons are responsible for receiving and sending specific messages to the brain about the body's internal and external environment. There are five major types of sensory receptors: *mechanoreceptors*, which receive impulses related to pressure, touch, and mechanical deformation of the receptor; *thermoreceptors*, which respond to heat and cold; *nociceptors*, which receive messages about pain caused specifically by physical or chemical damage; *electromagnetic receptors*, which respond to light on the retina; and *chemoreceptors*, which sense flavors, odors, oxygen levels, osmolality of body fluids, and the concentration of carbon dioxide.

Each type of receptor is sensitive to the particular stimulus it is designed to receive and almost nonresponsive to other types of stimuli. For example, a nociceptor can be stimulated by electricity, heat, crushing, or other tissue damage that will be experienced as pain. The nociceptor will not, however, respond to light. Each sensory nerve terminates at specific points in the CNS where the message is interpreted.

CNS and PNS neurons cannot function independently.

Their nutritional and physical support and protection are provided by other cells commonly referred to as glial cells. Glial cells, unlike neurons, are able to undergo mitosis. *Astrocytes,* star-shaped cells with many projections, are the largest and most numerous glial cells. They provide structural support and nutrition to neurons and maintain a biochemical environment supportive of nerve impulse transmission and synaptic activity. If nervous tissue is destroyed, astrocytes multiply in a process called gliosis to fill in the area or line a cavity. *Microglia,* considered the phagocytes of the CNS, are classified as part of the body's reticuloendothelial system. They remove dead tissue and foreign matter. *Ependymal* cells are involved in cerebrospinal fluid (CSF) system function. They line the choroid plexuses of the ventricular system, the ventricles, and central canal of the spinal cord. *Oligodendrocytes* and *Schwann's* cells, previously considered for their roles in the encasement and protection of axons, are also classified as neuroglia.

Table 35–1 Embryonic Divisions of the Brain With Corresponding Adult Brain Structures

Embryonic Division	Subdivision	Adult Brain Structure
Prosencephalon (forebrain)	Telencephalon	Cerebral hemispheres (cerebrum) Cerebral cortex Limbic system Basal ganglia Caudate Lenticular (putamen and globus pallidus) Claustrum Amygdala Olfactory bulbs and tracts
	Diencephalon	Epithalamus Thalamus Subthalamus Hypothalamus
Mesencephalon (midbrain)	Mesencephalon	Corpora quadrigemina Tegmentum Red nucleus Substantia nigra
Rhombencephalon (hindbrain)	Metencephalon	Cerebellum Pons
	Myelencephalon	Medulla oblongata
Spinal cord	Spinal cord	Spinal cord

CENTRAL NERVOUS SYSTEM STRUCTURES

The brain is structurally divided into components according to its embryological development. These components, known as the forebrain (prosencephalon), midbrain (mesencephalon), hindbrain (rhombencephalon), and spinal cord, are further divided according to their location within the adult brain. Knowing these subdivisions is useful because they are often referred to when several structures are involved in a CNS function or pathology (Table 35–1).

The Cerebral Cortex

The outer area of the cerebral cortex is composed of gray matter in complex folds called *gyri* or convolutions separated by deep depressions called *fissures* and shallow depressions called *sulci*. These folds make the surface area much greater. The patterning of gyri and sulci is similar in all individuals. The following well-marked fissures are distinguishable in all brains (Figure 35–1): the longitudinal fissure, which separates the right and left hemispheres of the brain; the central sulcus (fissure of Rolando), which extends outward and downward over each hemisphere; and the lateral fissure (fissure of Sylvius), which begins on the underside of the brain and moves out and around the brain along its side.

Each hemisphere of the cerebral cortex is divided into lobes. The names of the bones of the skull correspond to the lobes of the brain that they protect. The *frontal lobe* is located anterior to the central sulcus and above the lateral fissure. The *parietal lobe* is positioned behind the central sulcus. The *temporal lobe* is located below the frontal and parietal lobes (ie, below the lateral fissure) and merges

posteriorly with the occipital lobe. The *occipital lobe* extends from the parieto-occipital sulcus inferiorly around the base of the cerebrum. The insula (island of Reil or *central lobe)* lies within the lateral cerebral fissure. The cerebellum, which lies below the occipital lobe, is separated by the deep transverse fissure into which a dural fold, called the tentorium cerebelli, extends.

Nerve fiber tracts establish connections between areas within the brain. The *corpus callosum* consists of fibers extending between the right and left hemispheres. The commissural tracts of the corpus callosum, located deep in the longitudinal fissure, extend from one convolution to a corresponding one in the opposite hemisphere. The internal capsule (Figure 35–2) also allows networking between areas within the brain. The internal capsule comprises two distinct sections referred to as anterior and posterior limbs. Here afferent and efferent fibers extend from an extensive fanlike radiation of fibers in the cerebrum to link it with the brain stem and spinal cord. Association tracts consist of short and long tracts. Short association fibers extend from one convolution to another in the same hemisphere. Long association tracts interconnect cortical regions in different lobes of each hemisphere.

The *basal ganglia* (see Figure 35–2), bodies of gray matter, are located within the white matter of the cerebral hemispheres. This area contains the caudate nucleus, putamen, globus pallidus, thalamus, subthalamus, substantia nigra, and the red nucleus. These structures have many and varied functions including sensory and motor activities and transmission of afferent and efferent signals to appropriate parts of the nervous system. The *hypothalamus*, a small but extremely important area of the brain, is situated just below the thalamus. It receives input from all parts of

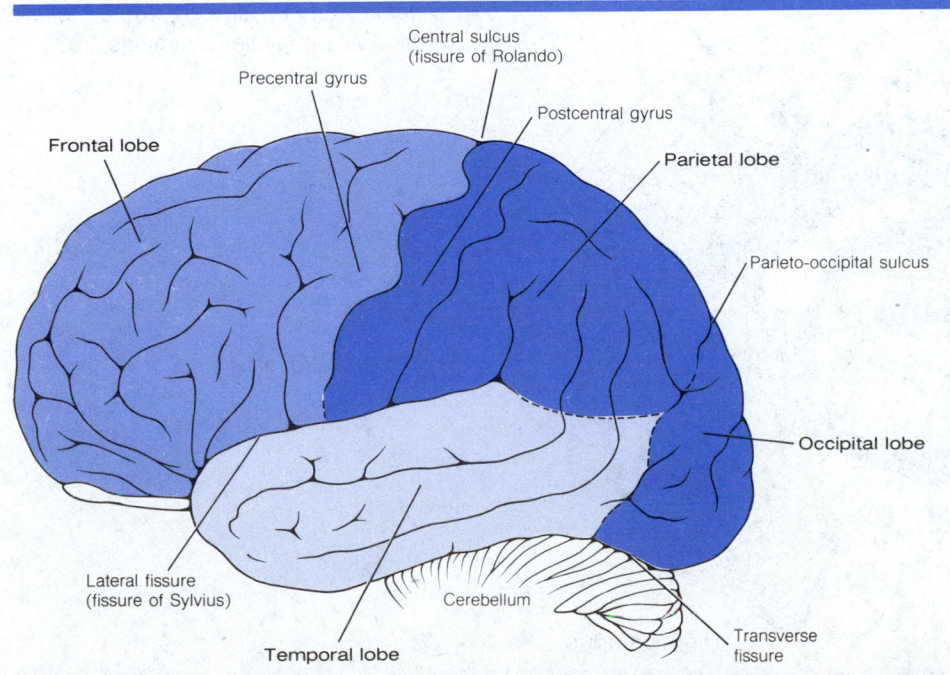

Figure 35–1

Division of the cerebral hemispheres into lobes by specific fissures and sulci.

SOURCE: Spence AP, Mason EB: *Human Anatomy and Physiology*, 2nd ed. Menlo Park, CA: Benjamin/Cummings, 1983

Central sulcus (fissure of Rolando)
Precentral gyrus
Postcentral gyrus
Frontal lobe
Parietal lobe
Parieto-occipital sulcus
Occipital lobe
Lateral fissure (fissure of Sylvius)
Cerebellum
Transverse fissure
Temporal lobe

the body both by neuronal transmission and its blood supply. The hypothalamus, in turn, influences body functions via these sames routes.

The *limbic system* comprises a group of structures including the olfactory bulbs, septum pellucidum, fornix, cingulate gyrus, parts of the basal ganglia including the amygdaloid nucleus, hippocampus, uncus, mammillary bodies, and various thalamic and hypothalamic nuclei (Figure 35–3). This system's multiple interconnections with brain structures influence behavior and responses to stim-

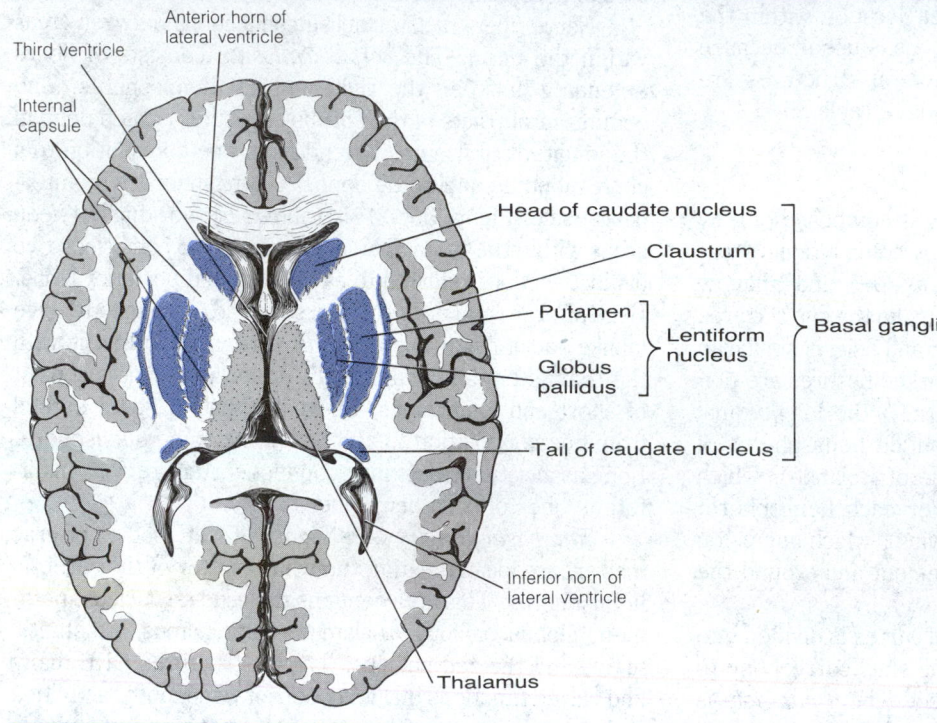

Figure 35–2

A transverse section through the brain showing basal ganglia and thalamus.

SOURCE: Spence AP, Mason EB: *Human Anatomy and Physiology*, 2nd ed. Menlo Park, CA: Benjamin/Cummings, 1983.

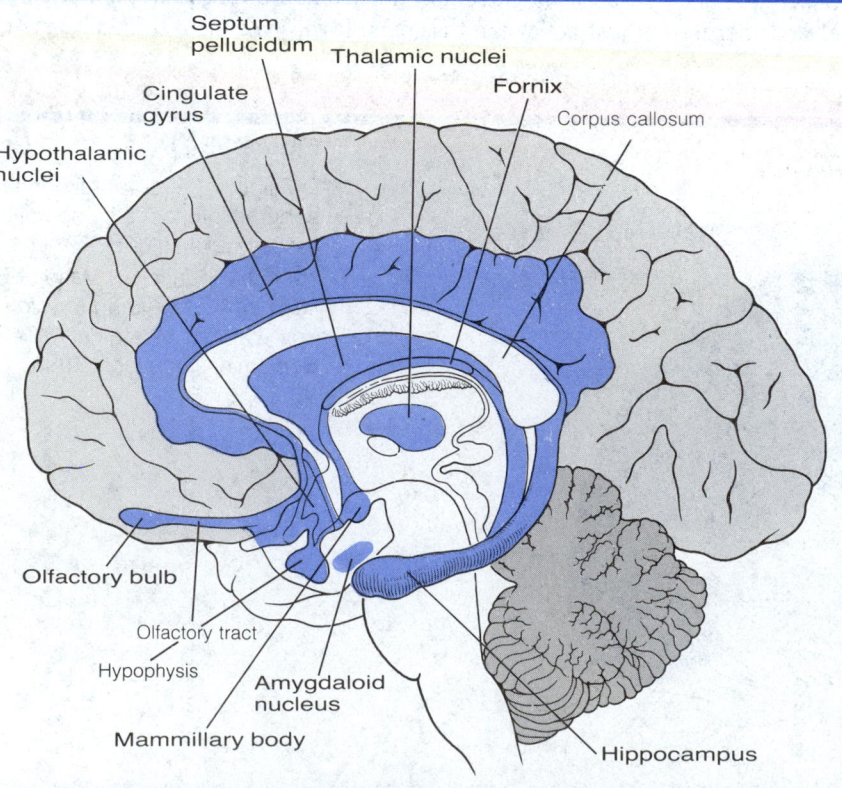

Figure 35–3

The structures of the limbic system.

SOURCE: Spence AP, Mason EB: *Human Anatomy and Physiology*, 2nd ed. Menlo Park, CA: Benjamin/Cummings, 1983.

uli. For example, the sensory system, cerebral cortex, and limbic system are involved in the stimulation of visceral and somatic effectors, which result in psychological expressions of behavior and emotions (Carpenter & Sutin, 1983).

The *brain stem*, which lies between the diencephalon and the spinal cord, has three sections—the midbrain (superior portion), pons (center portion), and the medulla oblongata. The medulla oblongata joins the spinal cord at the foramen magnum located at the base of the skull. The brain stem contains many fiber tracts that transmit messages to and from the brain. It also serves as a relay station between the cerebellum and brain. Ten of the twelve cranial nerves (CN) located here function much like peripheral nerves (spinal nerves). With the exception of CN IV, the trochlear nerve, they are unlike peripheral nerves in that they innervate tissues ipsilaterally—that is, on the same side of the body (Figure 35–4).

The *reticular activating system* is composed of a diffuse system of neurons extending through the medulla, pons, midbrain, diencephalon, and cortex. Afferent and efferent connections also exist between the cerebellum and spinal cord.

The Cerebellum

The cerebellum lies below the tentorium cerebelli in the posterior inferior portion of the cranial vault. It is made up of two hemispheres connected in the center by a structure called the vermis. The superficial area of the cerebellum is composed of gray matter, which lies in even, horizontal folds forming fissures and sulci. White fiber tracts lying below the gray matter provide extensive afferent and efferent connections with the brain stem, cortex, thalamus, and basal ganglia. The cerebellum receives afferent signals via the spinal cord and brain stem. Cerebellar efferent signals travel to the brain stem, thalamus, and motor cortex.

The Spinal Cord

The spinal cord is continuous with the brain stem. It begins at the foramen magnum and descends through the vertebral canal to the level of the first or second lumbar vertebrae. Nerve roots known collectively as the *cauda equina* extend off the base of the spinal cord and travel for some distance before exiting at the appropriate intervertebral foramina (Figure 35–5).

The spinal cord contains neuronal cell bodies, ascending sensory tracts, and descending motor tracts. A cross section of the cord shows a gray center shaped like a capital H surrounded by white fibers. The gray area is made up of neuronal cell bodies, internuncial neurons, neuroglial cells and synapses. Within the center of the gray matter lies the central canal, which is continuous with the fourth ventricle. It may contain CSF but is often filled with cellular debris.

The white fiber area of the cord contains myelinated and unmyelinated fiber tracts, which transmit the many

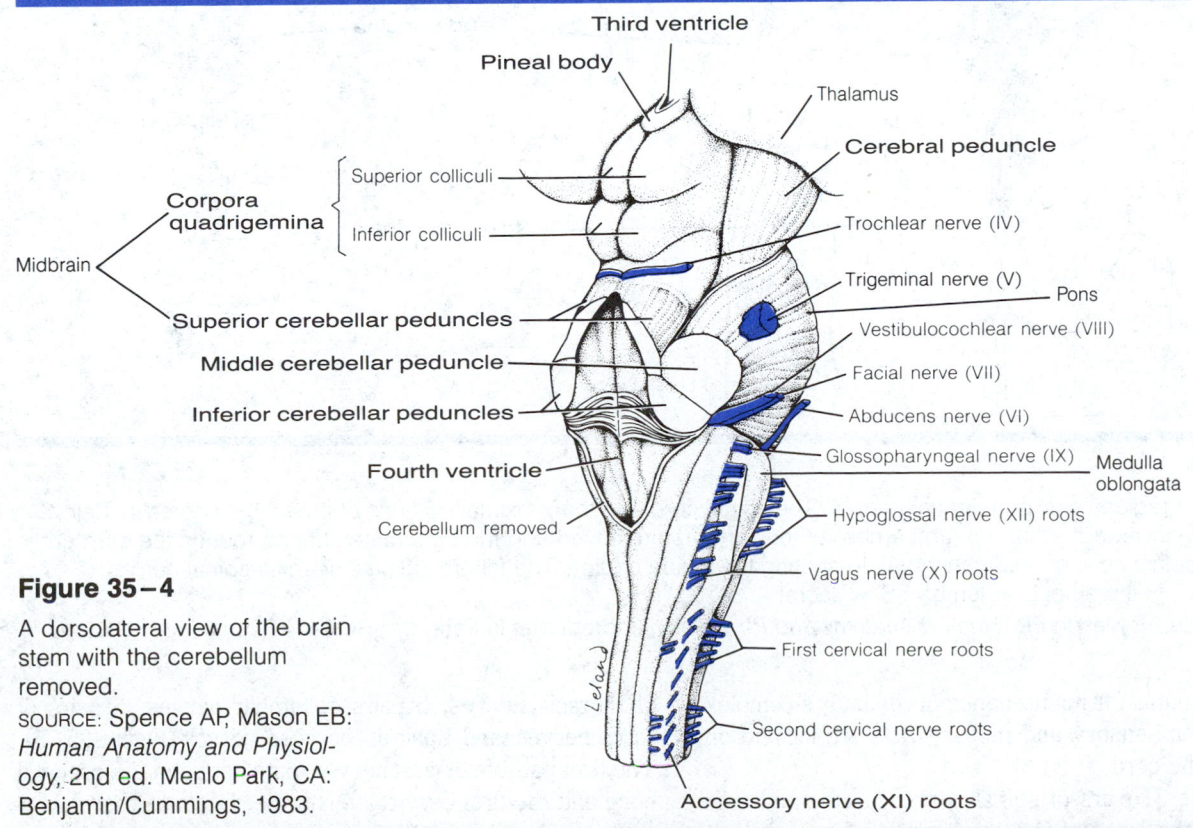

Figure 35–4

A dorsolateral view of the brain stem with the cerebellum removed.

SOURCE: Spence AP, Mason EB: *Human Anatomy and Physiology*, 2nd ed. Menlo Park, CA: Benjamin/Cummings, 1983.

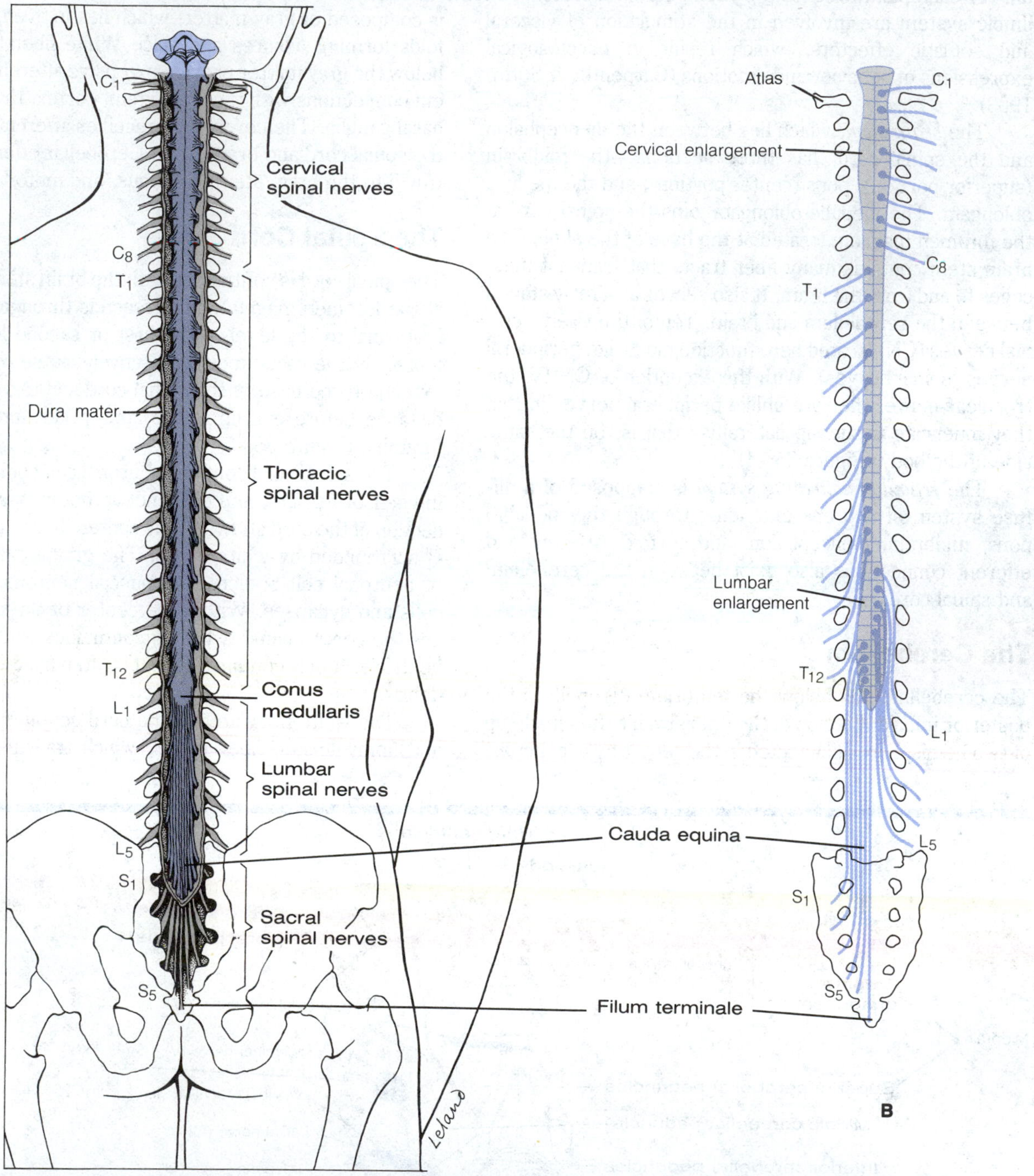

Figure 35–5

The spinal cord regions and principal nerves. **A.** The spinal cord and the proximal portions of the spinal nerves in their normal positions, viewed with the neural arches of the vertebrae removed and the dura mater that surrounds the cord cut open. **B.** The spinal cord and spinal nerves illustrating the cauda equina. The letters indicate specific spinal nerves: C = cervical; T = thoracic; L = lumbar; S = sacral.

SOURCE: Spence AP, Mason EB: *Human Anatomy and Physiology,* 2nd ed. Menlo Park, CA: Benjamin/Cummings, 1983.

messages essential for maintenance of the body's complex functions. Both sensory and motor tracts are located on each side of the cord.

There are 31 pairs of spinal nerves, each numbered according to the level of the cord section from which it originates. There are 8 pairs of cervical nerves, 12 pairs

of thoracic nerves, 5 pairs of lumbar nerves, 5 pairs of sacral nerves, and 1 pair of coccygeal nerves (Figure 35–5). The first pair of cervical nerves exits between the occipital bone and the first cervical vertebrae. Because there are 8 cervical nerves and only 7 cervical vertebrae, spinal lesions are identified according to the cord level rather than the vertebral level. Generally, each cord segment is named for the vertebral body below its exit point. (Note the numbering system for the spinal nerves outlined in Figure 35–5.)

Peripheral nerve trunks extend from anterior and posterior roots, which unite in the intervertebral foramina. Upon emerging from the vertebral foramina, they form mixed nerves, which divide into anterior and posterior branches and extend into the periphery to skeletal muscles and skin. Also present are white rami containing autonomic nervous system fibers. The posterior rami divide into smaller nerves connected to the muscles and skin of the posterior surface of the head, neck, and trunk. Anterior rami (except for the thoracic nerves) divide to supply fibers to the skel-

etal muscles, skin of the extremities, and the anterior and lateral surfaces. Subdivisions of the anterior rami form three complex networks or plexuses, which contain fibers from many nerves. These plexuses are the *cervical plexus, brachial plexus,* and *lumbosacral plexus.* Smaller nerves emerge from these plexuses and continue to subdivide to innervate distal regions of the extremities.

The Autonomic Nervous System

The autonomic nervous system (ANS) comprises two efferent subsystems—the sympathetic and parasympathetic subsystems. Organs influenced by the ANS are controlled by one of the two subsystems (Figure 35–6).

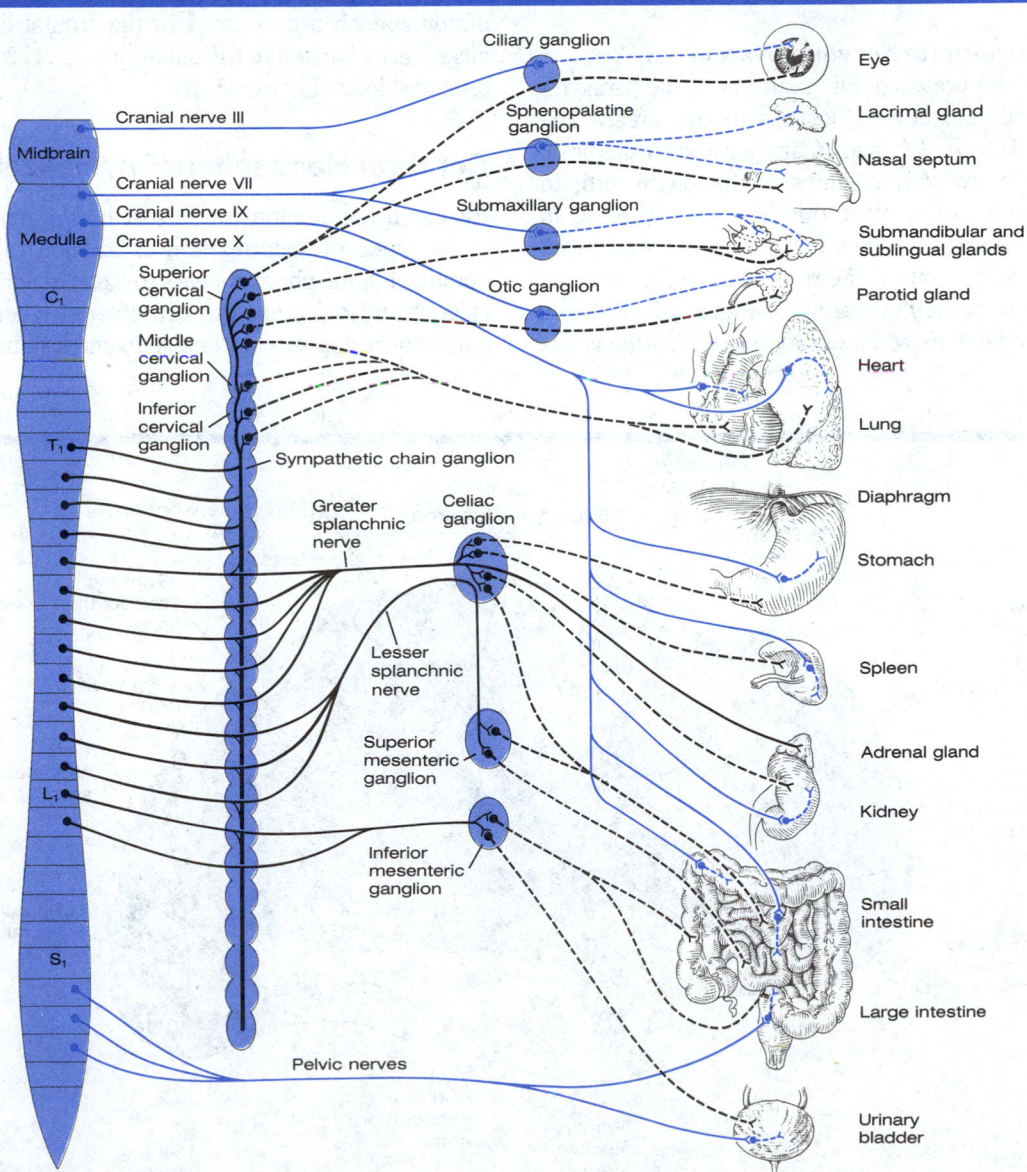

Figure 35–6

Components of the autonomic nervous system. The parasympathetic division is shown in blue; the sympathetic division is shown in black. The solid lines indicate preganglionic nerve fibers; the dotted lines indicate postganglionic nerve fibers.
SOURCE: Spence AP, Mason EB: *Human Anatomy and Physiology*, 2nd ed. Menlo Park, CA: Benjamin/Cummings, 1983.

The Sympathetic Nervous System

Sympathetic nervous system impulses are transmitted to the periphery by tracts of sympathetic fibers containing cell bodies and dendrites that extend within the intermediolateral gray horns of the spinal cord from thoracic spinal nerve 1 to lumbar spinal nerve 2. Because of its location, the sympathetic nervous system is often referred to as the *thoracolumbar division*. Axons leave the cord with the anterior roots of the thoracic and first four lumbar spinal nerves. After exiting, they quickly join the sympathetic trunk via white rami. The sympathetic trunks located on both sides of the cord extend from the second cervical vertebrae to the coccyx. The axons, upon entering the trunks, extend branches up and down the chain. The sympathetic nervous system preganglionic axons terminate on many postsynaptic ganglia present in organs.

The Parasympathetic Nervous System

Cell bodies of the preganglionic neurons of the parasympathetic nervous system are located in two areas. The nuclei of CN III, VII, IX, and X are located in the brain stem and the lateral gray columns of the sacral cord. In the sacral region, parasympathetic axons are present in spinal nerves. Because of these anatomical locations, the parasympathetic nervous system is often referred to as the *craniosacral division* of the ANS. Figure 35–6 shows the complex and extensive innervation of CN X (the vagus nerve), which supplies parasympathetic fibers to the heart, lungs, esophagus, stomach, small intestine, proximal half of the colon, liver, gallbladder, pancreas, spleen, and kidneys.

Speech Centers

About 95% of the population have their speech centers in the left hemisphere of the cerebral cortex. Speech centers in the remaining 5% are in the right hemisphere or (rarely) in both. There is a relation between the preferred hand and the hemisphere controlling speech: most *right-handed* persons' speech centers are in the *left hemisphere; left-handed* persons' speech centers tend to be in the *right hemisphere*. The term *cerebral dominance* refers to the hemisphere containing the speech centers. Two areas within the brain concerned with speech and language are Broca's motor speech area located in the frontal lobe and Wernicke's area located in the superior posterior aspect of the temporal lobe (Figure 35–7).

Cerebral Hemisphere Specialization

Research has demonstrated that both hemispheres have many types of specialization in addition to speech. The dominant hemisphere appears to excel in mathematical calculation and logical analysis of problems, whereas the other hemisphere appears better able to understand complex vis-

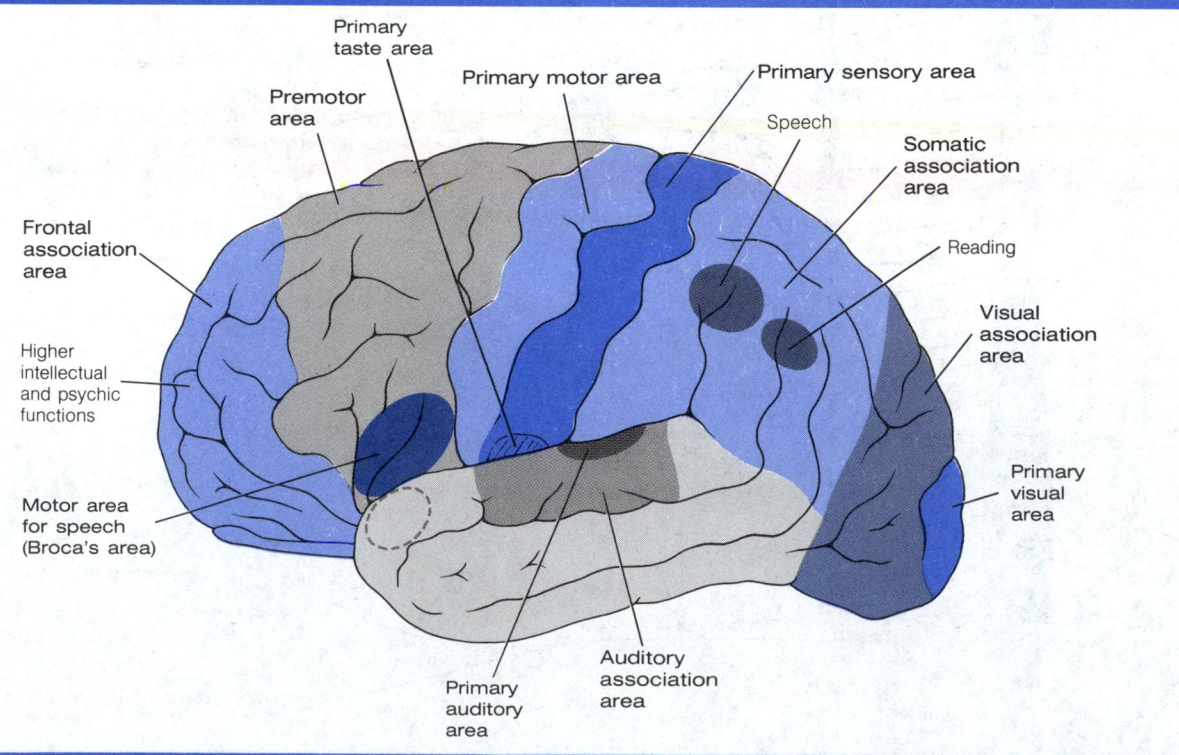

Figure 35–7

Major functional areas of the cortex.

SOURCE: Spence AP, Mason EB: *Human Anatomy and Physiology*, 2nd ed. Menlo Park, CA: Benjamin/Cummings, 1983.

ual patterns and spatial relations and to appreciate music. Development and effective use of these special skills require that the fibers connecting the hemispheres be intact.

The Blood–Brain Barrier

The blood–brain barrier theory stems from observations that only water, oxygen, carbon dioxide, and alcohol can readily enter or leave the capillaries of the CNS. Large molecules penetrate slowly through special systems or not at all. This protective barrier is believed to prevent sudden, extreme fluctuations in the composition of CNS tissue fluid while allowing nutrients to pass. The blood–brain barrier is thought to be formed within the capillaries by a continuous layer of endothelial cells connected by tight junctions. The basement membrane surrounds the endothelium. Astrocytes that lie in close apposition are no longer considered part of this barrier (Carpenter & Sutin, 1983).

The blood–brain barrier protects most of the brain and cord tissue. Exceptions are the pineal body and the posterior lobe of the hypophysis, among others, which are believed to be nourished by vessels with fenestrated endothelia that provide specific sites for the transfer of proteins and solutes irrespective of molecular size and lipid solubility. Tight junctions at the intracellular clefts of the choroid epithelium serve as the blood–brain barrier in the vascular choroid plexuses of the CSF system (Carpenter & Sutin, 1983).

FUNCTION OF THE NERVOUS SYSTEM

Neuronal Function

Functionally, neurons are recognized as being *motor* (efferent) neurons, *sensory* (afferent) neurons, or *internuncial* neurons (transmitters of messages from neuron to neuron). Neuronal messages are transmitted through electrical impulses. The necessary voltages are created by positive and negative forces produced when ions line up inside and outside the cell's plasma membrane. When a nerve is in a resting state (known as a resting membrane potential), the electrical charge outside the wall is positive; inside, the charge is negative.

The principal extracellular cation is sodium; the main intracellular anion is potassium. With adequate stimulation of the cell, the charge is reversed as sodium moves into the cell and potassium moves out. This reversal results in a flow of electric current (Figure 35–8). With sufficient stimulation, the reversal of polarity travels along the entire axon. This process, known as an *action potential,* requires only a few milliseconds. Quickly, electrical forces and ion concentration forces reestablish the resting membrane potential. If a stimulus is not sufficient to produce an action potential, and another stimulus occurs before the membrane has completely stabilized, depolarization will be facilitated.

Information is transmitted from one neuron to another at *synapses* following the initiation of an action potential. In

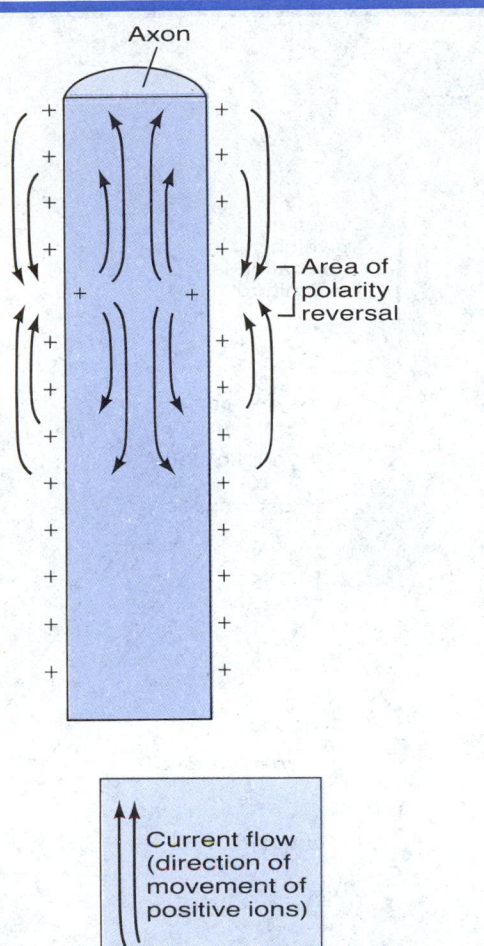

Figure 35–8

Current flow between an area of polarity reversal and adjacent areas of the axonal membrane during an action potential.

SOURCE: Spence AP, Mason EB: *Human Anatomy and Physiology*, 2nd ed. Menlo Park, CA: Benjamin/Cummings, 1983.

humans, chemical synapses initiate almost all action potentials. These synapses, located where axons and dendrites meet (Figure 35–9), employ various neurotransmitters, which are stored in and released from the axon terminal following an action potential. Action potentials are believed to increase the permeability of the axon terminal to calcium, allowing it to move into the axon terminal to stimulate the release of neurotransmitters into the synaptic cleft. The neurotransmitter diffuses across the cleft and attaches to postsynaptic receptors.

The influence of neurotransmitters on the postsynaptic receptor depends on the combination of impulses received. This combination is derived from the total number and frequency of impulses received over a period of time from one or multiple synapses. Strong stimuli activate a greater number of neurons. Myelinated fibers speed the

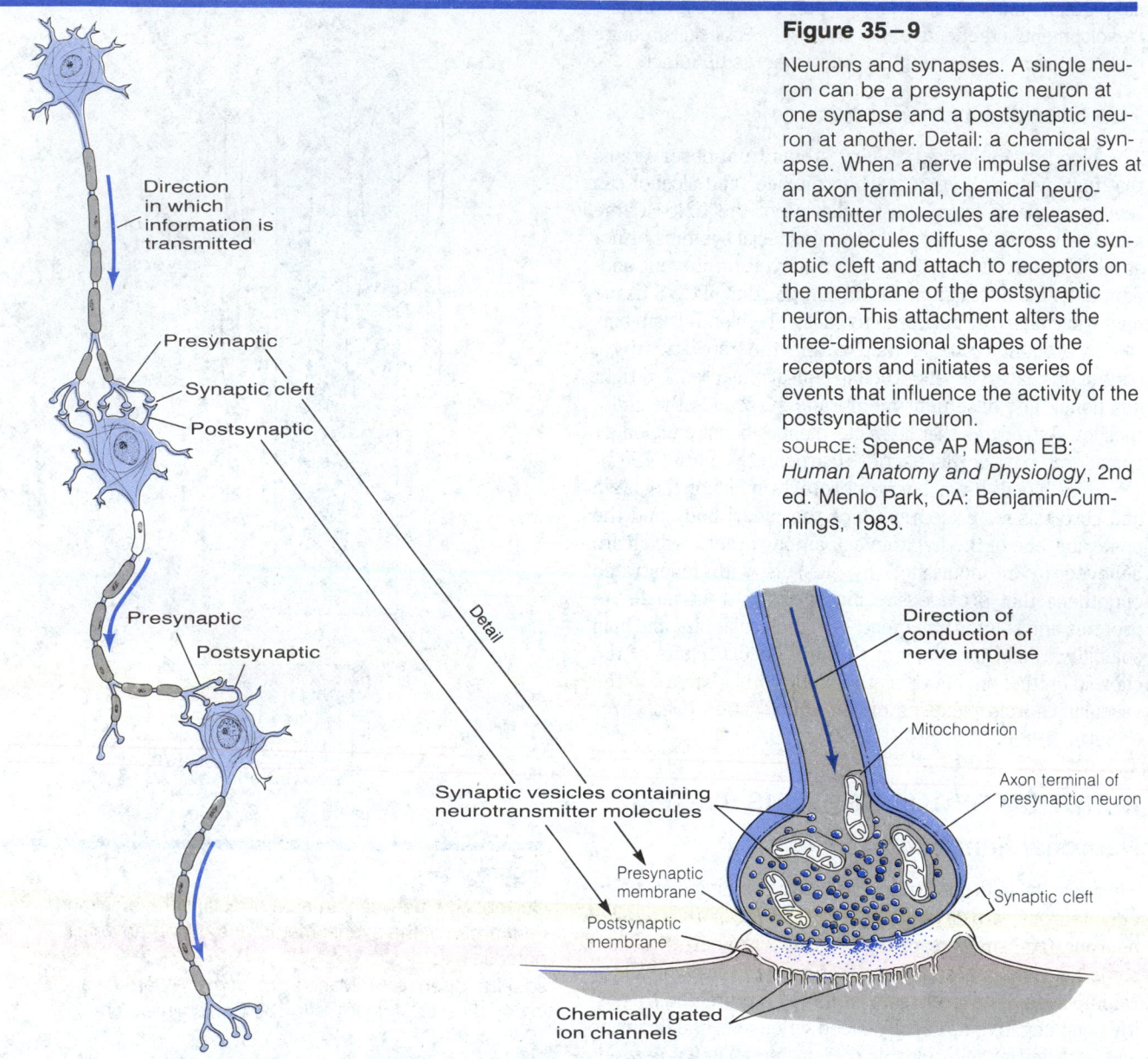

Figure 35–9

Neurons and synapses. A single neuron can be a presynaptic neuron at one synapse and a postsynaptic neuron at another. Detail: a chemical synapse. When a nerve impulse arrives at an axon terminal, chemical neurotransmitter molecules are released. The molecules diffuse across the synaptic cleft and attach to receptors on the membrane of the postsynaptic neuron. This attachment alters the three-dimensional shapes of the receptors and initiates a series of events that influence the activity of the postsynaptic neuron.

SOURCE: Spence AP, Mason EB: *Human Anatomy and Physiology*, 2nd ed. Menlo Park, CA: Benjamin/Cummings, 1983.

transmission of impulses. Inhibitory impulses also influence the postsynaptic receptors' response. Through these combinations, the nervous system "fine tunes" synaptic activity needed to manage the body's complex functions. Nerve impulses are binary (ie, either "on" or "off"), so the CNS must discriminate among stimuli by interpreting variations in strength, frequency, and number of stimuli received.

Synapses between neuron effector junctions such as neuromuscular junctions are similar to chemical synapses between two neurons. A review of the events that produce skeletal muscle contraction serves as a good example of how these synapses work. Following depolarization of the axon terminal and movement of calcium into the terminal, acetylcholine is released. It diffuses across the synaptic cleft at the neuromuscular junction to the plasma membrane of the muscle cell and attaches to the receptor sites, causing an increased permeability of the muscle fiber membrane to sodium and potassium ions (Figure 35–10). If the impulse, known as an endplate potential, is sufficient to depolarize the muscle-fiber membrane, a propogated action potential leads to contraction of the muscle fiber. At the cleft site, a small portion of acetylcholine diffuses away, but most is quickly inactivated by the enzyme cholinesterase, located on the muscle-cell membrane, which prevents continued excitation of the muscle fibers.

There are many other neurotransmitters. About 30 are known or suspected to play a role in nerve-impulse transmission. Some have multiple actions. For example, norepinephrine is involved in the maintenance of arousal and dreaming sleep and regulation of moods; dopamine has roles in the regulation of emotional responses and control

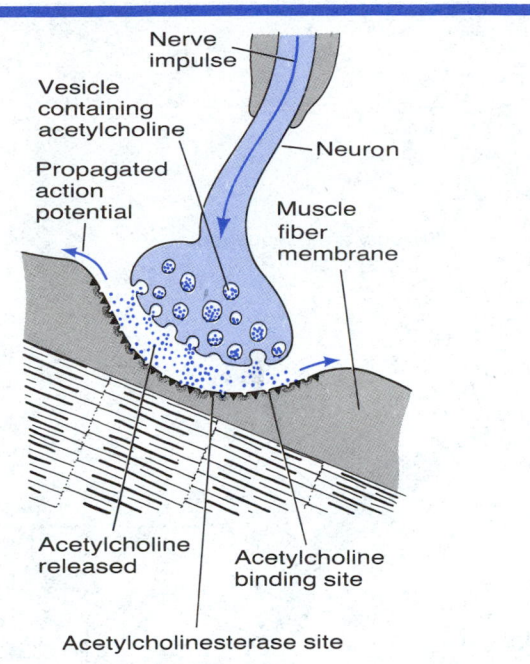

Figure 35–10

A neuromuscular junction. When a nerve impulse arrives at the axon terminal, acetylcholine is released. The acetylcholine binds with receptors on the muscle cell membrane at the junction. This binding leads to a change in the membrane's permeability to sodium and potassium ions and produces a propagated action potential that travels along the membrane.
SOURCE: Spence AP, Mason EB: *Human Anatomy and Physiology*, 2nd ed. Menlo Park, CA: Benjamin/Cummings, 1983.

of complex movements; and endorphins and enkephalins are believed to be involved in the perception and integration of pain and emotional experiences.

Cerebral Function

The Frontal Lobes
The frontal lobes are involved in mental, emotional, and physical functions. Anterior portions have major roles in the control of conscious and unconscious behaviors such as personality, social behavior, judgment, and complex intellectual activity. The central and posterior portions of the frontal lobes control motor function. The primary motor areas, located in precentral gyri, control voluntary movement via the pyramidal tracts. The premotor areas control and coordinate complex, learned movements such as typing, writing, scanning eye movements, conjugate deviation of the eyes, and movement of the head. These activities are effected via the extrapyramidal tracts and described in the following section on function of the central nervous system. Pyramidal and extrapyramidal centers control movements on the opposite side of the body. The dominant

frontal lobe also contains Broca's motor speech area (Figure 35–7).

The Parietal Lobes
The parietal lobes interpret sensory input. The postcentral convolutions, organized similarly to the major motor strip (Figure 35–11), receive conscious sensory input. Sensations perceived on one side of the body are interpreted by the contralateral parietal lobe. Somatic sensations perceived are pain, temperature, touch, pressure, and proprioception (awareness of position in space and muscle activity). The parietal lobes contain the somatesthetic association areas, which lie in the superior portion of the lobes and extend to the medial surface of the hemisphere. Many other connections within the parietal lobe allow for interpretation of sensory input such as stereognosis (perceiving and understanding an object by touch and relating the sensations to experience and knowledge). Awareness of body parts and the establishment of body image also take place here. The angular gyrus located in the parietal lobe of the dominant hemisphere is responsible for interpretation of written language (Price & Wilson, 1982).

The Insula
The insula, thought by some to be a fifth lobe of the brain, lies deep within the lateral fissure where it is covered by portions of the frontal, temporal, and parietal lobes (Spence & Mason, 1983). It is believed to be involved in visceral activities related to intra-abdominal sensations and visceral motility (Angevine & Cotman, 1981). Little information is available regarding function.

The Temporal Lobes
The temporal lobes receive input from three senses—hearing, taste, and smell—and have a role in memory processes. Association fibers, especially in the dominant lobe, allow the comparison of sensory input with past experiences. Association fibers, particularly those of the dominant lobe, interrelate somatesthetic visual and auditory stimuli to give them meaning (Conway–Rutkowski, 1982). Wernicke's area, also located on the dominant side, is involved in the hearing component in speech and in the formulation of language.

The Occipital Lobes
The occipital lobes contain the primary visual areas and visual association areas (refer to Figure 35–7). The primary visual areas receive information and perceive color. The visual association areas give visual input meaning and have a role in visual reflexes for fixing the eyes on a stationary or moving object. To appreciate the function of the association areas, consider the problems that arise when the areas are damaged. Injury to the medial surface on the dominant side can result in loss of the ability to recognize objects and know their function, although recognition of faces still is possible. A consequence of damage to the nondominant side may be the inability to recognize faces

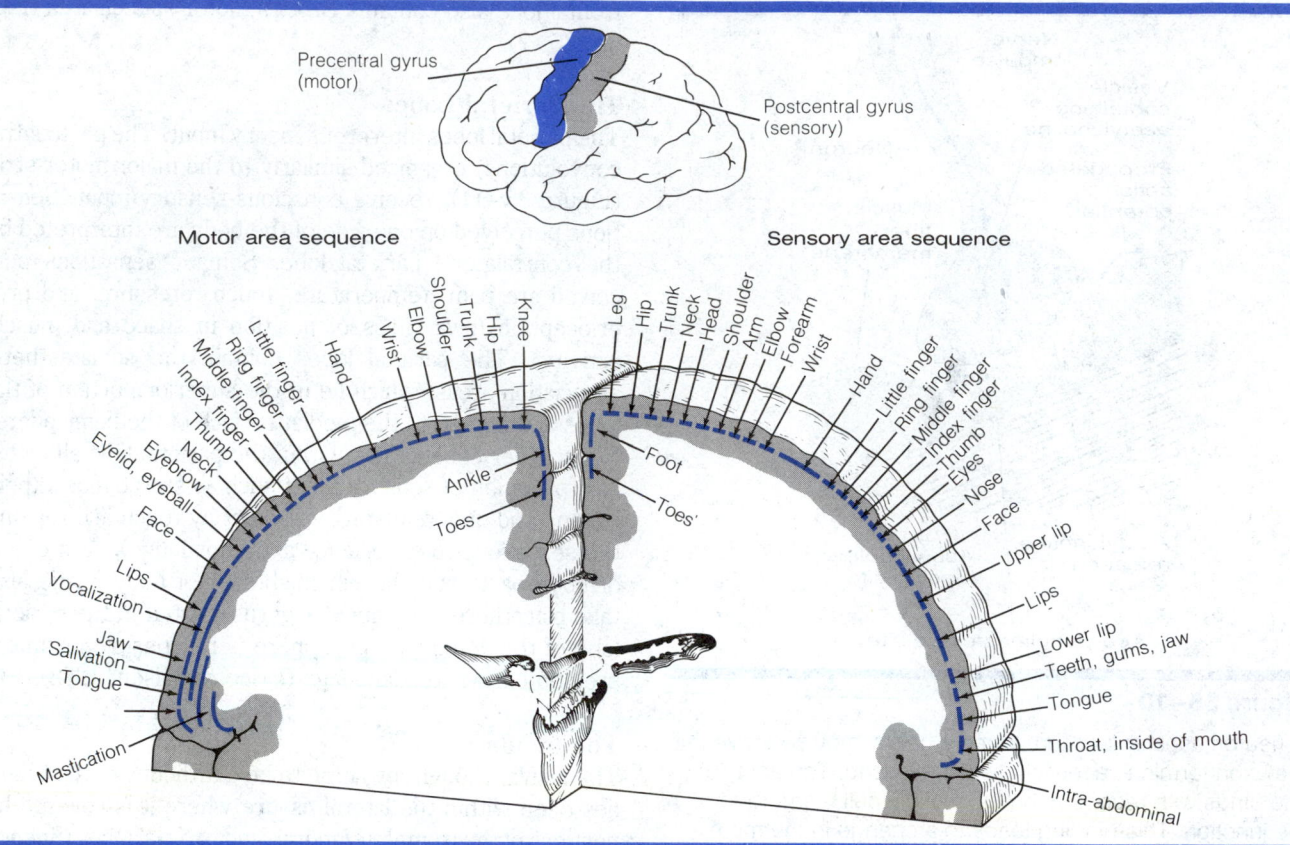

Figure 35-11

Frontal section of the cerebrum. **Left.** Through the precentral gyrus, showing the locations of neurons within the cerebral cortex that control voluntary motor movement of specific structures. **Right.** Through the postcentral gyrus, showing the locations of regions of the cerebral cortex that receive sensory nerve impulses from specific body structures.
SOURCE: Spence AP, Mason EB: *Human Anatomy and Physiology*, 2nd ed. Menlo Park, CA: Benjamin/Cummings, 1983.

and differentiate various forms of life such as horses and elephants (Price & Wilson, 1982).

The Thalamus

The thalamus, a large ovoid gray mass, surrounds the third ventricle. Specific areas within the thalamus receive axons from the cord, brain stem, cerebellum, basal ganglia, and various parts of the cerebellum. These connections allow it to influence motor function and have a role in arousal, alerting mechanisms, and reflex movements.

The thalamus influences the motor cortex through its connections with the pyramidal tract neurons. It is involved with the initiation of movement, control of muscle tone, and regulation of cortical reflexes through connections with the cerebellum, globus pallidus, and substantia nigra (Carpenter & Sutin, 1983). The thalamus interprets and relays sensory impulses from all parts of the body except the olfactory nerve. Recognition of crude sensations such as pain, temperature, and touch also takes place here. Sensory impulses that the thalamus is unable to interpret are relayed by it to appropriate primary sensory and association nuclei in the cerebral cortex (refer to Figure 35-7).

The thalamus is even involved in emotional responses, interpreting sensations as pleasant or unpleasant.

The Hypothalamus

The hypothalamus, a small but extremely important area of brain tissue situated just below the thalamus, plays a major role in the maintenance of many homeostatic functions. Numerous regulatory activities initiated here are effected through the pituitary gland and the ANS.

The pituitary gland, also known as the hypophysis, lies below the hypothalamus in the sella turcica. Hypothalamic nuclei influence pituitary gland function through neural and endocrine activity (see Chapter 40).

The hypothalamus receives input from all parts of the body. ANS activity is initiated in response to input received from areas within the thalamus, medulla oblongata, spinal cord, and limbic system. The influence of the hypothalamus on ANS activity includes the regulation of heart rate, blood pressure, and body temperature. In temperature regulation, the ANS lowers body temperature through the activation of vasodilation and sweating. It raises temperature by initiating (through shivering, vasoconstriction, and piloerection) increases in heart rate, basal metabolic rate, and mobilization of carbohydrate reserves.

The limbic system, important in emotions and behavior, surrounds the hypothalamus and has connections with it. Hypothalamic connections with the thalamus, which interprets feelings of pleasantness and unpleasantness, and with the reticular activating system, which influences wakefulness, provide additional input to which the hypothalamus responds.

Many hypothalamic activities are initiated by changes in the perceived composition of its blood supply. For example, specific areas within the hypothalamus are sensitive to changes in water balance, glucose, and insulin levels. The hypothalamic response to an increase in osmotic pressure illustrates this sensitivity: with a loss of body fluid, the hypothalamus detects an increase in osmotic pressure. In response, it initiates the release of antidiuretic hormone by the posterior pituitary gland to concentrate the urine and stimulate the thirst center to increase the oral intake of fluid.

Other centers within the hypothalamus regulate appetite. Specific nuclei credited with the initiation of feeding behavior and satiety have been identified. These centers are reciprocal in their inhibition of one another. (See Chapter 9.) The hypothalamus also influences gastrointestinal function and sexual activity.

The Limbic System

The limbic system (refer to Figure 35-3) influences memory, drives, motivation, visceral functions, and interactions with the environment. Emotional expressions believed to evolve from this complex group of structures include rage, placidity, fear, and attack reactions.

Research with animals has demonstrated that the limbic system contains centers of reward and punishment with both serving as important motivators of behavior and affecting memory (Guyton, 1982). The *hippocampus* is thought to be involved in the transfer of short-term memory into long-term memory, especially with events related to elements perceived in the environment.

The *amygdala* is thought to have major responsibilities for the control of behavior in social and environmental circumstances. It is also believed to influence visceral responses to emotions and various movements related to posturing and eating (Guyton, 1982).

The Brain Stem

The brain stem comprises the midbrain, pons, and medulla oblongata. Each of these structures has unique responsibilities, but the three function as a unit to serve as a conduit for impulses passing to and from the cerebral cortex and the spinal column (Figure 35-4). The midbrain (mesencephalon), the uppermost portion of the brain stem, contains afferent and efferent nerve tracts that travel to and from the cerebral hemispheres. It also houses the red

nucleus, which serves as a relay station for coordination of impulses traveling between the cerebellum and cerebral hemispheres, and the corpora quadrigemina (see Figure 35-4), which are involved in reflex responses to visual stimuli and the relay of auditory impulses.

The *pons* sits between the midbrain and the medulla oblongata and anterior to the cerebellum. It contains nerve fiber tracts that provide communication between upper and lower levels of the CNS and the cerebellum. The lower third of the pons contains respiratory reflex centers influenced by the carbon dioxide levels of the blood and spinal fluid. The pons also influences vasomotor activity.

The *medulla oblongata* (myelencephalon) forms the inferior portion of the brain stem. The pyramids for the motor tracts are located on its ventral surface. Sensory tracts ascend through the medulla to the thalamus. Major reflex centers in the medulla influence respiratory and cardiovascular function.

The Reticular Activating System

The reticular activating system regulates spinal motor activity as well as voluntary and reflex muscle activity. Projections to the diencephalon and cortex effect and maintain arousal and alerting states (Figure 35-12). In addition to maintaining wakefulness, this system also participates in the regulation of sensory input from the periphery, regulation of respirations, and vasomotor activity.

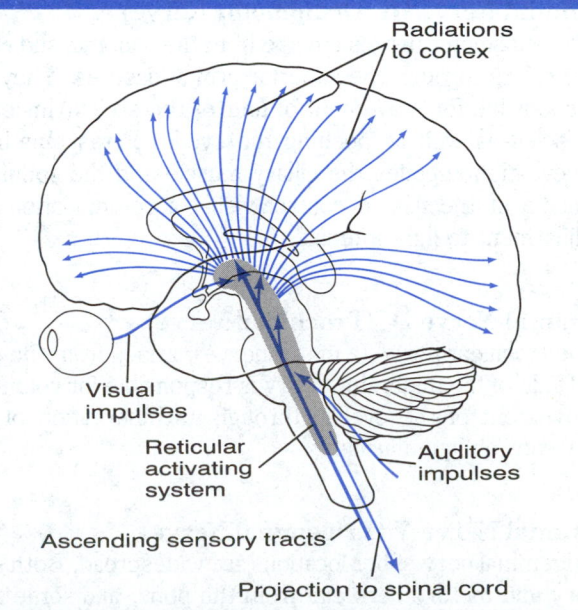

Figure 35-12

The reticular formation. The arrows indicate input to and output from the reticular activating system.

SOURCE: Spence AP, Mason EB: *Human Anatomy and Physiology*, 2nd ed. Menlo Park, CA: Benjamin/Cummings, 1983

The Cranial Nerves

The functions of cranial nerves vary; some are motor, some sensory, and others mixed. Motor nerves are innervated with proprioceptive (sensory) branches. The parasympathetic branch of the ANS provides a visceral component for some cranial nerves. The 12 pairs of cranial nerves, identified by Roman numerals, are ordered by their position within the skull.

Cranial Nerve I (Olfactory Nerve)

These nerves, made up of sensory receptor cells within the epithelial lining of the nasal mucosa, are responsible for the perception of odors. Nerve impulses originating here are transmitted to the temporal lobes for interpretation.

Cranial Nerve II (Optic Nerve)

The optic nerves (sensory nerves), which are actually nerve tracts, originate in the retina of the eye and enter the cranium via the optic foramina. Nerve impulses are transmitted to the occipital lobe, where vision is perceived. Optic nerves projecting back from the orbits meet at the optic chiasm. Here each tract divides, the inner halves joining with fibers from the opposite orbit. Hence, from this point, each tract carries fibers from both eyes. Some fibers, important for visual reflexes, synapse in the midbrain. Most travel to the thalamus to synapse with neurons that form pathways called optic radiations. These fibers terminate in the visual cortex of the occipital lobe.

Cranial Nerve III (Oculomotor Nerve)

The oculomotor nerves emerge from the midbrain and enter the orbits through the superior orbital fissures. They are responsible for movement of four of the six extrinsic eye muscles as well as opening the eyelid. Parasympathetic innervation supplies the ciliary muscle and the sphincter muscle of the iris to control visual accommodation and adjustment to light intensity.

Cranial Nerve IV (Trochlear Nerve)

The trochlear nerve (a motor nerve), arises from the dorsal side of the midbrain. CN IV is responsible for voluntary movement of the eyeball through its innervation of the superior oblique muscle.

Cranial Nerve V (Trigeminal Nerve)

Trigeminal nerve fiber locations are widespread. Both sensory and motor fibers exit from the pons, and some sensory nuclei are located in the medulla. Deep and superficial sensory fibers innervate the face and anterior portion of the head through the ophthalmic, maxillary, and mandibular branches. Sensory fibers for pain, light touch, and proprioception can be readily identified. The motor components of this nerve are responsible for mastication.

Cranial Nerve VI (Abducens Nerve)

These cranial nerves exit from the medulla just below the pons and enter the orbits with CN III and IV. Their function is to roll the eyes outward.

Cranial Nerve VII (Facial Nerve)

These cranial nerves project from the lower edge of the pons. They supply motor neurons for the facial and scalp muscles. Sensory fibers supply the taste buds for sweet, sour, and salt on the anterior two-thirds of the tongue. Parasympathetic fibers supply the lacrimal glands and the submandibular and sublingual salivary glands. (The location of CN VII and its relations to these structures is illustrated in Figure 76–5 in Chapter 76.)

Cranial Nerve VIII (Vestibulocochlear Nerve)

There are two sensory divisions to these cranial nerves, an auditory division and a vestibular division. Both originate at inner-ear receptors located in the petrous portion of the temporal bones. The two divisions, enclosed in a single sheath, pass to the brain stem just below the pons. Some of the vestibular fibers travel directly to the cerebellum. Auditory impulses are transmitted to the temporal lobes for interpretation.

Cranial Nerve IX (Glossopharyngeal Nerve)

The nuclei for these cranial nerves, located in the medulla oblongata, innervate the tongue and pharynx. The motor component is important in swallowing. Sensory responsibilities include perception of bitter taste on the posterior one-third of the tongue; sensory awareness for the mucous membranes of the pharynx, tonsils, and middle ear cavity; carotid body receptor sensitivity to serum oxygen and carbon dioxide levels; and baroreceptor information regarding blood pressure. Parasympathetic neurons innervate the parotid gland.

Cranial Nerve X (Vagus Nerve)

The vagus nerve nuclei, also located in the medulla, carry motor impulses to the pharynx and larynx and sensory impulses from them. Extensive parasympathetic nerve fibers innervate the pharynx, larynx, and trachea and extend into the thorax and abdomen. Thoracic and abdominal vagal branches influence the function of the esophagus, lungs, aorta, stomach, gallbladder, spleen, small intestine, kidneys, and upper two-thirds of the large intestine.

Sensory fibers from the vagus nerve related to visceral functions generally operate at an unconscious level. An exception is nausea which is perceived via the vagus nerve.

Cranial Nerve XI (Accessory Nerve)

These motor nerves actually are formed by two nerves. One projects from the medulla; the other, projecting from the fifth or sixth cervical segment of the spinal cord, is actually a spinal nerve. Fibers from the cranial portion join with the vagus nerve to supply muscles of the larynx and pharynx. Fibers from the spinal component innervate the trapezius and sternocleidomastoid muscles.

Cranial Nerve XII (Hypoglossal Nerve)

The hypoglossal nerves (motor nerves) exit from the medulla oblongata and pass through the hypoglossal canals located beneath the tongue. These nerves are responsible for tongue movement.

The Cerebellum

The cerebellum modulates and coordinates skeletal muscle activity and maintains body posture and muscle tone. It controls movement with both excitatory and inhibitory signals, which fine tune movements in ways the cerebral cortex is incapable of carrying out. Each hemisphere influences the movement on the ipsilateral side of the body. It modifies activity initiated elsewhere in the body. There is no conscious input.

Activities of the cerebellum derive from the multiple inputs from the CNS and PNS. Afferent fibers travel to the cerebellum from the cerebral cortex by way of the corticocerebellar tracts and the pons. Peripheral afferent impulses from muscle spindles, Golgi tendon organs, skin, and joint receptors travel to the cerebellum via the ventral and dorsal spinocerebellar tracts. (See Table 35–2 and Figure 35–13 for more information on these tracts.) The reticular substance of the brain stem and vestibular tracts also provide the cerebellum with information.

Cerebellar efferent impulses are sent to the motor cortex via the thalamus. Additional efferent signals are transmitted to the basal ganglia, red nucleus, reticular for-

Table 35–2   Major Ascending and Descending Tracts of the Spinal Cord

Spinal Cord Tract	Responsibilities	Crossover Point
Sensory Tract— Ascending		
Fasciculus gracilis	Carry information to parietal lobe regarding lower limb movement and position; sensations of fine touch from receptors located in the muscle, joint, and skin.	Cross in medulla
Fasciculus cuneatus	Carry information about upper extremities, trunk, and neck. Proprioception—conscious stereognosis (being able to perceive and understand objects by touch) from receptors located on muscle, joint, and skin. Synapse in thalamus—ascend to sensory cortex in parietal lobe.	Cross in medulla
Spinothalamic:		
• Lateral	Convey impulses of pain and temperature from surface and viscera.	Cross in spinal cord
• Ventral	Convey impulses of crude touch and pressure, itch, and tickle. Synapse in thalamus—ascend to sensory cortex in parietal lobe.	Cross in spinal cord
Spinocerebellar:		
• Dorsal	Unconscious proprioception from neuromuscular receptors.	Uncrossed—directly to cerebellum
• Ventral	Sensory information originates in muscle spindles and Golgi tendon apparatus; coordination of posture and limb movement.	Uncrossed—directly to cerebellum
Motor Tract— Descending		
Corticospinal:		
• Lateral	Volitional movements, especially in distal parts of extremities.	Cross in medulla
• Ventral	Innervate muscles of upper extremities and neck.	Cross where they synapse with lower motor neurons
Tectospinal (includes reticulospinal tracts)	Optic relay centers—mediate reflex postural movements in response to visual and perhaps auditory stimuli.	Cross in the brain stem
Rubrospinal (includes reticulospinal tracts)	Control muscle tone in flexor muscle groups. Require an intact cerebellum.	Some cross in brain stem; some uncrossed
Vestibulospinal	Influence derived from vestibular nuclei and cerebellum. Exert facilitory influence on reflex activity in the spinal cord and spinal mechanisms that control muscle tone.	Uncrossed
Olivospinal	Role unclear; may serve as relay centers from basal ganglia to spinal motor nerves.	Cross in the brain stem

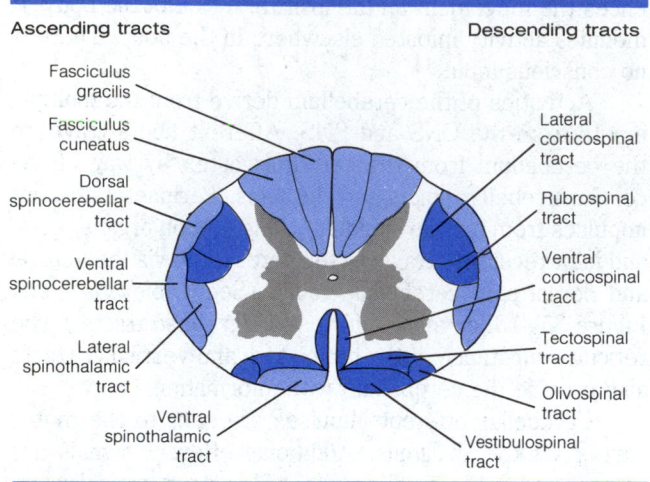

Ascending tracts   Descending tracts

Fasciculus gracilis
Fasciculus cuneatus
Dorsal spinocerebellar tract
Ventral spinocerebellar tract
Lateral spinothalamic tract
Ventral spinothalamic tract

Lateral corticospinal tract
Rubrospinal tract
Ventral corticospinal tract
Tectospinal tract
Olivospinal tract
Vestibulospinal tract

Figure 35–13

Main fasciculi of the spinal cord. The ascending (sensory) tracts are labeled only on the left side. The descending (motor) tracts labeled only on the right side.
SOURCE: Spence AP, Mason EB: *Human Anatomy and Physiology*, 2nd ed. Menlo Park, CA: Benjamin/Cummings, 1983.

mation of the brain stem, and vestibular nuclei. The connections with the vestibular nuclei integrate changes in the direction of body movement and posture. The semicircular canals of the inner ear perceive these changes and transmit this information to the cerebellum via the vestibular nerve and the brain stem. Balance is maintained through the modification of muscle tone. The cerebellum has no direct influence on lower motor neurons.

The cerebellum is also involved with predictively coordinating visual clues with bodily motion. For example, the cerebellum provides persons with input on how rapidly they are approaching an object. The findings of an experiment on monkeys illustrate the value of this function. In this experiment, when the portion of the cerebellum involved in vision was removed, the monkey could not judge distance from a corridor wall, and repeatedly charged into the wall (Guyton, 1982).

The Spinal Cord

The spinal cord is a conduit for messages to and from the higher levels within the CNS and participates in reflex motor activities. Descending pathways within the cord carry motor instructions to the anterior horn (ventral roots) from the cerebral cortex, brain stem, and cerebellum. Impulses synapse in the anterior horn (motor gray area) just before leaving the cord. This synaptic activity involves upper motor neurons, located within the cord, and lower motor neurons, which extend beyond the cord. Ascending (dorsal) roots transmit sensory impulses from the skin and viscera to the cord and CNS. Synaptic activity necessary for transmission of signals occurs at various levels within the cord. Dermatome charts provide a "map" of the area of skin

supplied by the dorsal root of each spinal nerve (see Figure 36–1 of Chapter 36).

Specific sensory and motor tracts have been identified within the spinal cord. These tracts, located within the white matter, are identified as anterior, lateral, and posterior funiculi. These funiculi, further divided into tracts called fasciculi, carry similar types of nerve impulses to specific destinations (Figure 35–13). (For ease in identifying the ascending and descending tracts, each is identified on only one side of the diagram.)

Motor Function

Effective skeletal muscle function involves many components of the CNS and PNS. Muscle function requires the perception and interpretation of sensory stimuli for movements and an intact motor system to initiate and carry out muscle contraction. Areas of the nervous system involved in motor function include the premotor cortex, the primary motor area, pyramidal and extrapyramidal tracts, basal ganglia, thalamus, brain stem, spinal cord, and cerebellum.

The premotor cortex (associative cortex), positioned just anterior to the major motor strip, is involved in muscle activities that produce hand skills, voluntary eye movements, eyelid blinking, and vocalization. To appreciate the complexity of the functions carried out by the premotor cortex, consider the many coordinated activities needed to speak. Speaking requires groups of muscles in the tongue, larynx, pharynx, and chest (for breathing) to contract and relax in carefully programmed sequences. Function of the premotor area requires intact connections with the sensory association areas of the parietal lobe, the temporal lobe, frontal lobe, occipital lobe, components of the basal ganglia, primary motor cortex, thalamus, brain stem, and spinal cord.

The primary motor area is believed responsible for the initiation of movement by individual groups of muscles such as those involved in the movement of fingers, toes, and mouth. The cross section of the precentral gyrus (Figure 35–11) illustrates specific areas of the primary motor area identified as initiating willed movement by various muscles. Note the large amount of gray matter (nerve cells) allocated to muscle groups involved in complex movements of the hands and mouth.

Nerve cells of the major motor strip and their conducting fibers make up the *pyramidal* (corticospinal) motor system. Nerve fibers descend from the motor strip through the internal capsule, midbrain, and pons to the medulla oblongata where the pyramidal fibers cross. After crossing, the fibers descend in the spinal cord to appropriate levels. Most pyramidal fibers descend via the lateral corticospinal tracts to ventral horns of gray matter in the cord. Some motor fibers travel via ventral corticospinal tracts.

Extrapyramidal motor tracts (those that exclude the pyramidal tract) are more complex in their arrangement and synaptic activity in the cerebrum and brain stem. A functional, rather than an anatomic unit, the extrapyramidal tracts are involved in maintaining balance and posture by facilitating some muscle movements and inhibiting others. Movements initiated in one hemisphere influence movements on the opposite side of the body. The basal ganglia, bodies of gray matter deep within the white matter of the cerebral hemispheres, are part of the extrapyramidal tract. Specifically, they are the caudate nucleus, putamen, and the globus pallidus. In addition, the thalamus, subthalamus, substantia nigra, and red nucleus have roles in motor function. Multiple connections exist among all of these areas. A second pathway allows for feedback control of extrapyramidal motor activity.

The basal ganglia have three motor functions. A major responsibility of the basal ganglia as a whole is believed to be the inhibition of postural muscle tone. The caudate nucleus and putamen, collectively referred to as the *striate body*, are thought to initiate and regulate gross intention movements such as body posture and major arm movements. This regulation involves pyramidal and extrapyramidal pathways. The globus pallidus is believed to provide background muscle tone for intended movements initiated by the striate body or the cerebral cortex (eg, the muscle contractions needed to support the arm and trunk while using a typewriter or a tennis racket).

Final pathways for extrapyramidal signals into the cord are the reticulospinal tracts that lie in both the ventral and lateral tracts of the cord. Also involved in transmission to a lesser degree are the rubrospinal, tectospinal, vestibulospinal, and possibly the olivospinal tracts.

Reflex Movements

Reflexes differ from voluntary muscle activity in that they are automatic, stereotypic movements that do not require cortical processing. Reflex actions may involve skeletal, smooth, and cardiac muscles and glands. *Monosynaptic and polysynaptic* reflexes are carried out through neural pathways known as spinal reflex arcs. They are initiated by various noxious stimuli such as pain, rapid stretch, and fear.

Monosynaptic reflexes involve a sensory receptor, an afferent neuron to carry impulses to the cord, and a synapse within the spinal cord between the afferent neuron and the efferent neuron, which transmits the impulse to the effector. A common example of a monosynaptic impulse is the knee jerk, elicited by tapping a tendon with a reflex hammer (see left side of Figure 35–14). In this example, the stretching of the patellar tendon causes a reflex contraction of the quadriceps muscle.

A polysynaptic reflex response involves an additional activity, a synapse with an internuncial neuron within the cord (see right side of Figure 35–14). With this reflex, muscle (or other sensitive tissue) subjected to a noxious stimulus produces a polysynaptic reflex. This activity can be complex, with signals sent to neurons above, below, and on to the opposite side of the spinal cord. These additional synapses are part of the automatic actions designed to initiate actions to protect the body.

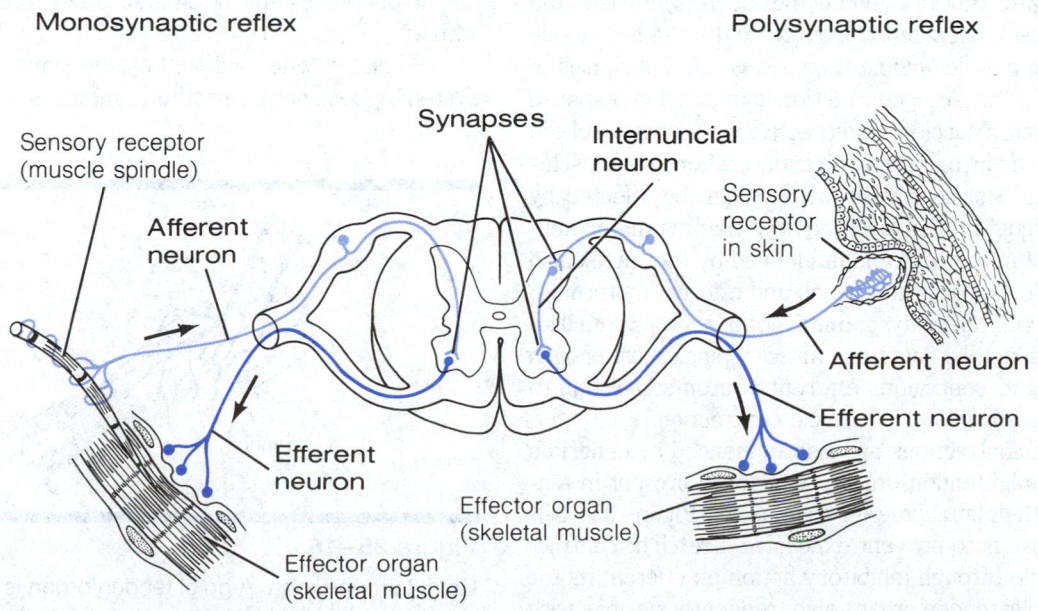

Monosynaptic reflex   Polysynaptic reflex

Synapses

Sensory receptor (muscle spindle)

Afferent neuron

Internuncial neuron

Sensory receptor in skin

Afferent neuron

Efferent neuron

Efferent neuron

Effector organ (skeletal muscle)

Effector organ (skeletal muscle)

Figure 35–14

The components of a spinal reflex arc. The left side of the diagram illustrates a monosynaptic reflex; the right side shows a polysynaptic reflex.

SOURCE: Spence AP, Mason EB: *Human Anatomy and Physiology*, 2nd ed. Menlo Park, CA: Benjamin/Cummings, 1983.

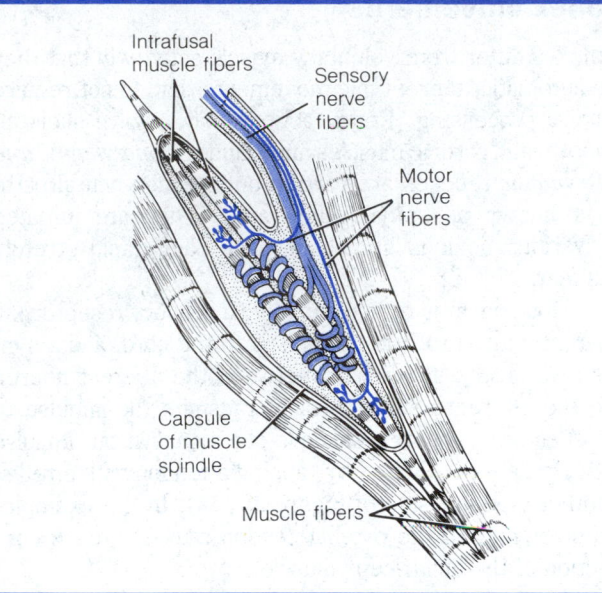

Figure 35–15

A muscle spindle.

SOURCE: Spence AP, Mason EB: *Human Anatomy and Physiology*, 2nd ed. Menlo Park, CA: Benjamin/Cummings, 1983.

The quality of reflex responses and the effectiveness of muscle contractions are influenced by muscle sensory receptors, muscle fiber stretch, and spinal cord activity. Sensory receptors known as muscle spindles are wrapped around special intrafusal muscle fibers located within the muscle (Figure 35–15). When muscle is stretched, the intrafusal muscle fibers tense and stretch the attached muscle spindle. The muscle spindle then sends afferent signals to the spinal cord where a contraction is initiated in response to the stretch. Muscle spindle activity also has a role in maintaining even muscle contraction whenever muscles are working. Muscle spindle activity can be affected by physical fatigue and cortical activity. Gamma motor neurons present in the cord and influenced by the cortex also affect muscle response to stretch and efferent motor neuron stimulation. Normally, gamma motor neurons stimulate the intrafusal muscle fibers and muscle spindles just enough to cause slight, continuous efferent neuron stimulation to produce a small amount of muscle contraction.

Muscle contractions are also influenced by dendrites known as Golgi tendon organs, which are present in tendons near their attachments to muscle (Figure 35–16). Their purpose is to prevent excessive stretch or contraction of muscle through inhibitory action on efferent motor neurons. Golgi tendon organs also frequently synapse with neurons that initiate the contraction of antagonist muscles, helping to reduce further the tension on the involved muscles.

With both monosynaptic and polysynaptic reflexes and

Golgi tendon organ reflexes, messages are sent via internuncial fibers to apprise the brain stem, cerebellum, and cortex of activities. Reflexes occur in isolation only when the cord is damaged and unable to transmit the impulses.

The Autonomic Nervous System

Autonomic nervous system activity is initiated by centers in the spinal cord, brain stem, hypothalamus, and limbic system. This system helps to regulate visceral functions, maintain homeostasis, and combat stress. Afferent messages reach these centers via sensory nerve transmission. The ANS usually operates at an unconscious level.

Sympathetic and parasympathetic activities are effected by preganglionic and postganglionic fibers that stimulate target organs. Two neurotransmitters, acetylcholine and norepinephrine, are required for impulse transmission. Acetylcholine is the transmitter for parasympathetic preganglionic and postganglionic synapses and preganglionic sympathetic synapses. Norepinephrine is the transmitter required for almost all sympathetic postganglionic synapses.

The sympathetic nervous system helps the body to respond quickly to emergencies. Its network of branching axons provides for extensive and rapid stimulation of the sympathetic chain when quick responses are needed. Fear or rage can stimulate the sympathetic nervous system to produce an increase in heart rate, dilation of blood vessels, a rise in blood sugar, and secretion of epinephrine and norepinephrine to reinforce and prolong the body's response to the stress. (See the section on anxiety in Chapter 6.) Parasympathetic nervous system activity primarily maintains body functions under normal conditions. For example, it decreases the heart rate and promotes digestive activity.

Some activities initiated by the sympathetic nervous system oppose parasympathetic impulses—eg, countering

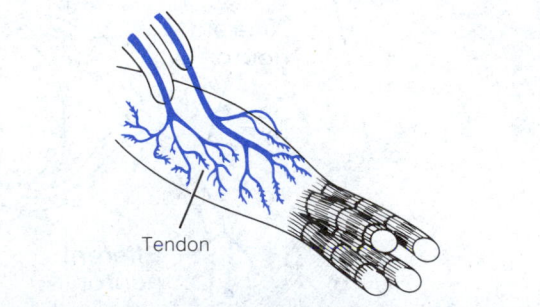

Figure 35–16

Golgi tendon organ. A golgi tendon organ is composed of dendrites that divide into many small branches in the tendon, near its junction with a muscle.

SOURCE: Spence AP, Mason EB: *Human Anatomy and Physiology*, 2nd ed. Menlo Park, CA: Benjamin/Cummings, 1983.

the parasympathetic nervous system's slowing effect on the heart by increasing the rate and force of contraction. It also slows peristalsis and increases the tone in sphincters, thereby slowing digestion and absorption of nutrients.

The sympathetic nervous system, the major regulator of blood pressure, always maintains some tone within the vessel walls. Blood pressure is decreased when sympathetic nervous system activity is reduced. Parasympathetic fibers do not innervate the smooth muscles of blood vessels. The only way the system can decrease the blood pressure is by slowing the heart rate and decreasing the force of cardiac contraction.

PROTECTION AND MAINTENANCE OF THE NERVOUS SYSTEM

Understanding the complex and wonderful capabilities of the nervous system helps in appreciating the system's means of protection and maintenance. Recognizing the safeguards of the bony cranial vault and vertebral column is easy. Less obvious but also valuable is the protection provided by the hair, skin, scalp, fascia, muscle, meninges, fluid cushioning, and complex vascular supply. The superficial structures help to limit injuries from external trauma, and the ventricular and vascular systems provide an environment for optimal neuronal function.

The *meninges* within the cranial vault and vertebral column protect the CNS from physical harm and support the cerebrospinal fluid system and the circulation. The *dura mater,* the outermost layer of meninges, forms a double layer over the brain tissue. Its outer layer forms an inner periosteal lining for the skull and vertebral canal. In the cranium, the inner layer of dura, for the most part fused with the outer layer, helps to secure the brain to the cranial vault. To provide extra support and protection, the inner layer of dura separates in areas, dipping down between the longitudinal fissure, between the cerebellar hemispheres, and between the cerebrum and cerebellum and passing over the pituitary gland nestled in the sella turcica. In other areas, dura layers separate to form venous sinuses that collect and carry venous blood away from the brain. Arachnoid processes (villi) project into the dural sinuses.

In the spinal cord, the inner layer of dura is continuous with the spinal dura mater. The spinal dura extends to the second sacral vertebrae where it joins with the external filum terminale and attaches to the back of the first segment of the coccyx (Figure 35–5). The middle layer of the meninges, the *arachnoid,* is a thin, fibrous membrane that adheres closely to the inner surface of the dura allowing only a narrow space between the two. The inner layer of the meninges, the *pia mater,* adheres so closely to the brain that it follows the contour of the fissures and sulci. The space between the pia mater and arachnoid is bridged with weblike strands of arachnoid called trabeculae. A rich network of pial blood vessels extends into the brain. The area between the arachnoid and pia mater is called the *subarachnoid space.* Located here are arteries, veins, arachnoid trabeculae, and CSF. Within the spinal cord, fibrous bridges join the pia mater with the arachnoid and dura mater. These bridges, known as denticulate ligaments, help to stabilize the cord within the spinal canal.

The Cerebrospinal Fluid System

The CSF protects the brain and spinal cord by supporting the tissues, acting as a shock absorber, and serving as a medium in the transfer of elements from the bloodstream to nervous system tissues. CSF flows through an elaborate ventricular system located within the brain and through the subarachnoid space surrounding the brain and spinal cord (Figure 35–17). Two large ventricles are positioned within each cerebral hemisphere. Their central portions extend into the parietal lobes. The anterior horns project into the frontal lobes, the inferior horns extend into the temporal lobes, and the posterior horns project into the occipital lobes. A small third ventricle lies below and communicates with each lateral ventricle via a small channel known as the foramen of Monro. The thalamus forms the lateral walls of the third ventricle. The third ventricle is connected via the cerebral aqueduct to the fourth ventricle, which lies below. The pons and medulla are positioned below the fourth ventricle. The cerebellum lies above.

CSF flows from the ventricular system to the arachnoid space of the brain and spinal cord by way of the lateral apertures (foramina of Luschka) and the median aperture (foramen of Magendie). CSF is constantly being produced by capillary tufts, called choroid plexuses, located in the ventricles. Arachnoid villi, projecting into the dural sinuses, provide routes for the reabsorption of CSF into the venous circulation.

Central Nervous System Circulation

The viability and functioning of the CNS depend on a rich and continuous blood supply. Major arteries supply oxygenated blood to the arterioles, which branch into capillaries where actual uptake of oxygen and nutrients occurs. The brain utilizes approximately 20% of the body's oxygen supply and requires about 400 kcal of glucose per day. The average cerebral blood flow is about 750 mL per minute.

Two major arteries branch directly off the arch of the aorta to establish the blood supply to the head—the brachiocephalic artery and the left common carotid artery. The brachiocephalic artery divides into the right common carotid artery and the right subclavian artery. The two common carotid arteries move up the neck along the trachea where they separate into the internal and external carotid arteries. *Carotid sinus baroreceptors*, sensitive to changes in blood pressure, are located at this point of separation. *Carotid bodies*, also located here, monitor changes in the blood's oxygen, carbon dioxide, and pH levels.

The external carotid arteries supply the scalp and parts

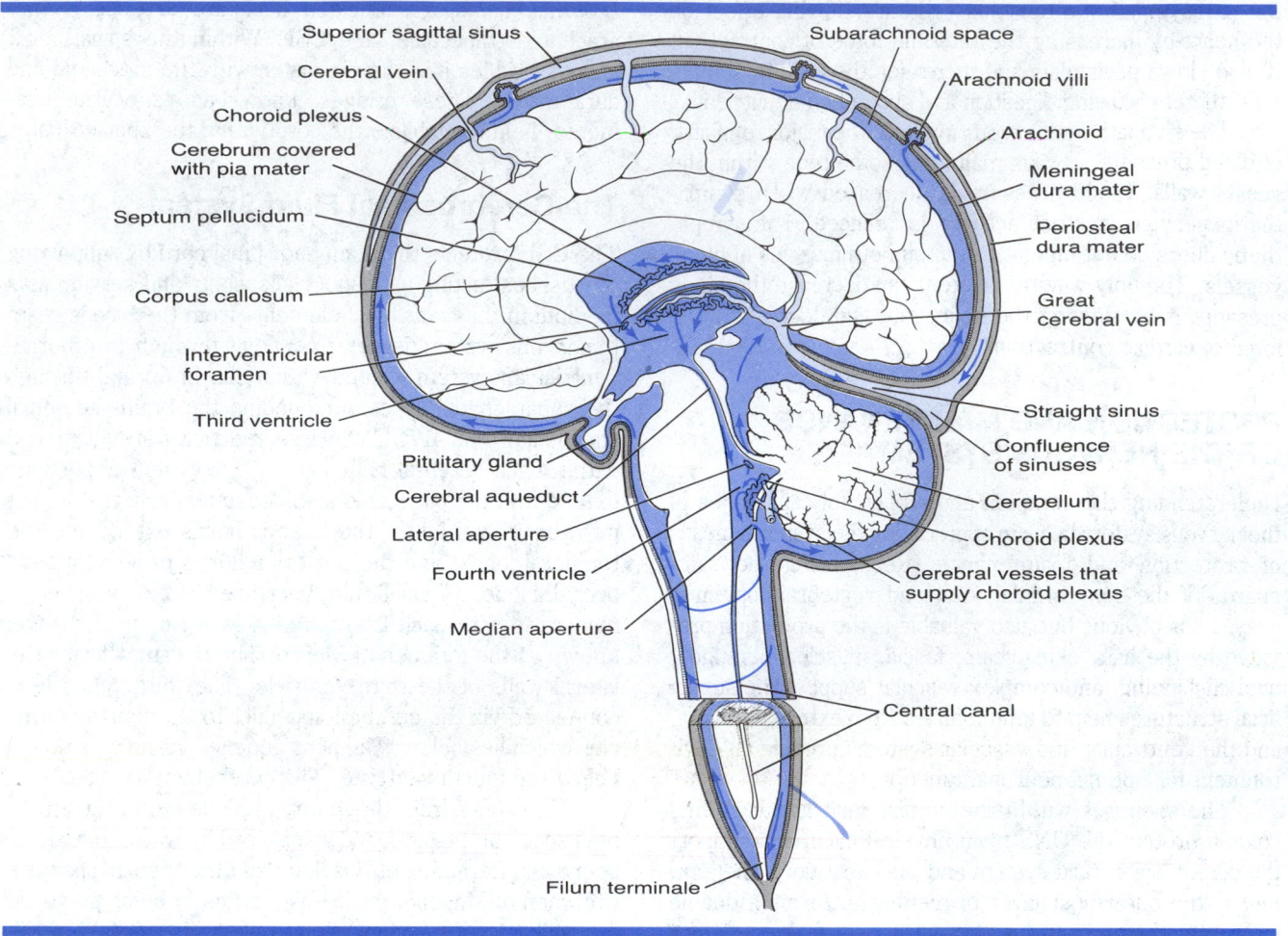

Figure 35–17

The location of the cerebrospinal fluid (blue) surrounding the brain and spinal cord. The arrows indicate the direction of the fluid's flow. Blood is shown in light blue.

SOURCE: Spence AP, Mason EB: *Human Anatomy and Physiology*, 2nd ed. Menlo Park, CA: Benjamin/Cummings, 1983.

of the head and neck. Secondary branches of the external carotids, the middle meningeal arteries, supply blood to the meninges of the brain. The right and left internal carotid arteries, after passing through the carotid canals, branch into the anterior cerebral arteries and middle cerebral arteries at the level of the optic chiasm. The right and left anterior cerebral arteries are connected by the small anterior communicating artery to form the anterior portion of the circle of Willis (Figure 35–18). Anterior cerebral arteries perfuse the caudate and putamen nuclei of the basal ganglia, portions of the internal capsule, corpus callosum, and portions of the frontal and parietal lobes. The middle cerebral arteries are the major suppliers of blood to the precentral and postcentral gyri and feed portions of the temporal, parietal, and frontal lobes.

The vertebral arteries, whose source is the subclavian artery, travel to the brain via the foramina of the cervical vertebrae and the foramen magnum. At the level where the medulla and pons meet, the vertebral arteries join to form the basilar artery. The basilar artery separates

at the rostral border of the pons, forming the posterior cerebral arteries. Posterior communicating arteries extending back from the internal carotid arteries complete the anastomosis with the posterior cerebral arteries to form the circle of Willis. This anastomosis, intended to maintain circulation to the brain tissue if one of the vessels closes, is not always functional (Eliasson, Prensky, & Hardin, 1979). Other vessels providing collateral circulation are vessels at the base of the brain; small pial anastomotic branches on the surface; external carotids to the eyes; and anterior, middle, and posterior cerebral anastomoses on the surface of the brain.

Passage of venous blood from surface and deep brain tissue takes place via thick veins lacking valves. The blood flows into the dural sinuses and then drains into the internal jugular veins. Three dural sinuses are of particular importance. The *superior sagittal sinus* serves as a major route for the removal of the constantly forming CSF. The *cavernous sinus* drains blood from the eye, orbit, and face. The *transverse sinus* lies close to the ear.

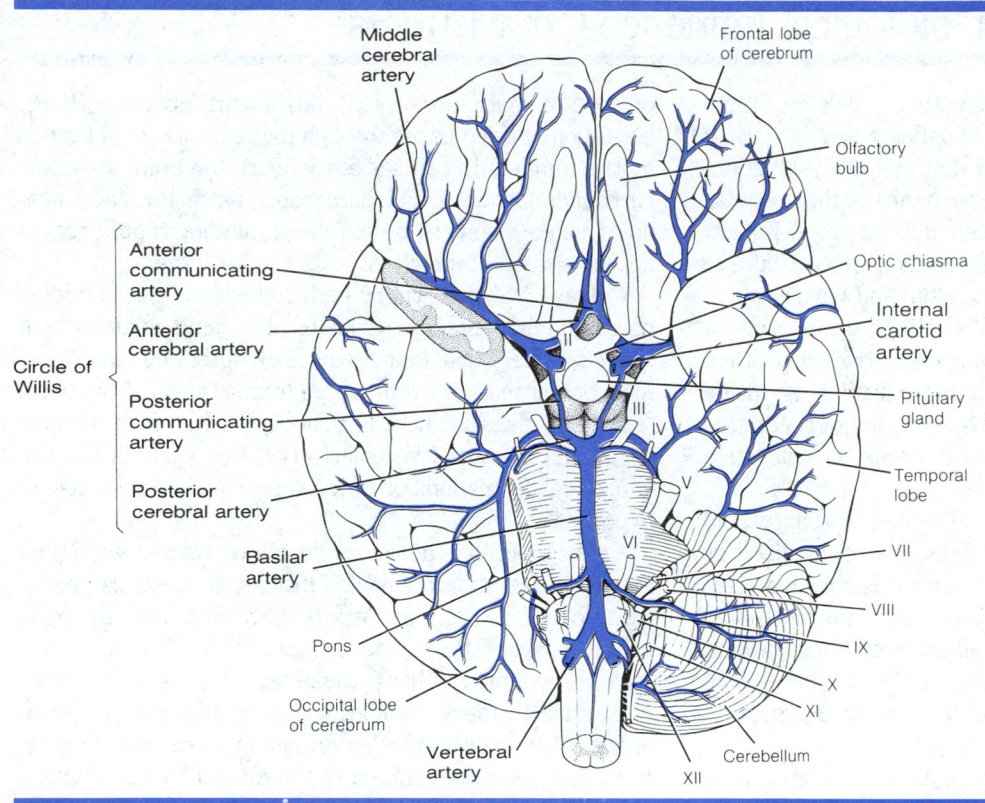

Middle cerebral artery

Frontal lobe of cerebrum

Olfactory bulb

Anterior communicating artery

Optic chiasma

Anterior cerebral artery

Internal carotid artery

Circle of Willis

Posterior communicating artery

Pituitary gland

Posterior cerebral artery

Temporal lobe

Basilar artery

VII

Pons

VIII

IX

Occipital lobe of cerebrum

X

XI

Vertebral artery

Cerebellum

XII

Figure 35–18

Arteries of the base of the brain, forming the circle of Willis around the pituitary gland. To provide an unobstructed view, part of the right temporal lobe and the right cerebellar hemisphere have been removed. Roman numerals indicate cranial nerves.
SOURCE: Spence AP, Mason EB: *Human Anatomy and Physiology*, 2nd ed. Menlo Park, CA: Benjamin/Cummings, 1983.

Regulation of Cerebral Blood Flow

Control of blood flow in the CNS is essential for viability and optimal function. The body can use several built-in mechanisms to maintain effective circulation.

Three major factors that have a direct and potent effect on cerebral blood flow by producing vasodilation are elevations in carbon dioxide concentration, hydrogen ion concentration, and oxygen concentration. (Elevated carbon dioxide levels lead to an increase in hydrogen ion concentration.) The increase in hydrogen ion concentration causes vasodilation of the cerebral vessels. Vasomotor reflex responses that affect the body's general vascular perfusion also affect the perfusion of blood in the CNS. Vasomotor centers in the pons and medulla maintain vascular tone through impulses transmitted via the spinal cord to all blood vessels in the body. The reticular areas of the brain stem and hypothalamus have both excitatory and inhibitory effects on vasomotor activity. The hypothalamus also influences vasoconstriction activity through excitatory or inhibitory action on the vasomotor centers. It also helps to regulate total body water and therefore blood pressure by increasing or decreasing the release of antidiuretic hormone.

A severe drop in blood pressure to 50 mm Hg or less will result in ischemia in the vasomotor center. The resulting local increase in concentration of carbon dioxide causes a profound stimulation of the sympathetic nervous system, which initiates the constriction of blood vessels—some to the point of occlusion. This response, meant to shunt the blood to the CNS, is known as the ischemic response.

Cushing's phenomenon occurs when an increase in pressure in the CSF system equals the pressure in the cerebral vascular bed, hampering the flow of blood to the brain. At this point, the CNS ischemic response is initiated to raise the CNS blood pressure above the CSF pressure to facilitate blood flow to the brain (Guyton, 1982).

Spinal Cord Circulation

Multiple arteries feed the spinal cord. The vessels join, forming a complex network that supplies the vertebrae, periosteum, and dura. Branches supply the ventral and dorsal roots and penetrate deeply into the cord. Anterior and posterior spinal arteries extending the length of the cord originate from the carotid and vertebral arteries.

The venous system of the spinal cord is a rich network. The internal vertebral venous plexus, located between the dura mater and vertebral periosteum, is made up of anterior and posterior venous channels that extend from the skull to the sacral region. Thoracic, abdominal, and intercostal veins as well as the external vertebral venous plexus have connections with the internal vertebral plexus at each intervertebral space. There are no valves in this venous network. As a result, blood flow varies depending on pressure. With elevation of intra-abdominal pressure, venous blood from the pelvic plexus passes into the vertebral venous channels. If the jugular vein is occluded, blood from the skull can drain via the vertebral channels. On the other hand, this venous plexus is believed to provide potential routes for metastasis of neoplasms (Carpenter & Sutin, 1983).

Section II: Pathophysiological Influences and Effects

The nervous system's complex structure and diverse functions predispose it to a multitude of pathologies, each capable of causing varying types and degrees of dysfunction. The protective structures and mechanisms discussed in the preceding section are obviously not fail proof. In fact, these protective structures often produce or contribute to nervous system trauma. The rigid skull and vertebral column allow little room for neuronal swelling, tumor growth, or circulatory congestion. Trauma may also occur when external forces drive the nervous tissue against the inside of the bony structures. Fractures and bony degenerative processes can perforate or crush neurons or supportive tissues.

The elaborate CSF system, designed to support and cushion the CNS, is subject to risks from a localized or generalized buildup of CSF if reabsorption is impeded. This extensive fluid system also provides routes for the spread of infection. Foramina of the skull and vertebral column, serving as avenues for the passage of blood vessels and nerves traveling to and from the periphery, also provide routes for microorganisms into the CNS.

Meningeal tissues, too, present hazards as well as protection. With increases in intracranial pressure (ICP), herniation of brain tissue through the tentorial notch formed by the tough dura can seriously injure the brain stem and surrounding tissues. The dura mater, pia mater, and arachnoid tissues also provide extensive, uninterrupted routes for the spread of infection.

The CNS's circulatory bed, so important in providing nourishment, presents risks to the same structures it serves. The circulation provides routes for migrating microorganisms and even tumors from all parts of the body. Additional risks include an increase in ICP from hemorrhage and abnormal vascular structures such as arteriovenous malformations or reflex vasodilation in response to hypoxia.

The neurons, nerves, and nerve tracts, with their long communication chains and multiple connections needed for effective afferent and efferent activity, form the most complex part of the nervous system. Because of their presence throughout the body, these neurologic structures are vulnerable to many pathological elements including alterations in the biochemical environment, structural damage from disease, degeneration of the myelin sheath, trauma, and neurotransmitter abnormality.

The functions of specific structures within the nervous system vary greatly. Some, such as the hypothalamus, are known to contain nuclei responsible for the regulation of certain body functions. Other structures, such as the cerebellum, pyramidal, and extrapyramidal systems, must effect regulatory activity in concert with other nervous system structures joined via complex fiber linkages. Supportive structures such as glial cells and interneurons are required to allow nervous system management of body functions.

Various pathological changes can damage any or many of the components of the nervous system. Diagnosis of cause or area affected is often difficult because of the interdependence of structures and their dependence on nerve fibers and neurotransmitters to carry signals to organs outside the CNS. Each component of a system and its innervated organs are possible causes of a particular symptom or deficit.

Nervous system damage often produces complex physical and mental disabilities. A stroke, for example, may produce spasticity rather than flaccid limbs. Sometimes the spasticity is useful, but it often results in severe positioning problems and contractures. Personality changes can occur from physical deficits produced by the stroke or from psychological stressors stemming from the disability.

INFLAMMATION AND INFECTIOUS PROCESSES

Inflammatory processes affecting nervous tissue alter the metabolism and thus the tissue's nutritional and immune

Nursing Research Note

Mathis M: Personal needs of family members of critically ill patients with and without acute brain injury. *J Neurosurg Nurs* 1984; 16(1): 36–44.

Using the theoretical framework of systems theory and self-concept theory, Mathis explored the personal needs perceived by family members of critically ill persons without acute brain injury and of those with acute brain injury. This descriptive study was in part a replication of Molter's study and incorporated her interview guide of 45 declarative statements that listed specific needs that may be perceived by family members of critically ill persons. Eight need statements of family members listed as "very important" were to:
- Have questions answered honestly.
- Believe hospital personnel cared about the relative.
- Know exactly what was being done for the relative.
- Believe there was hope.
- Have specific facts concerning the relative's progress.
- Be reassured the best care possible was being given.
- Know they would be called at home if there were changes.
- Receive information about the relative's condition at least once a day.

Although there was a difference between needs of family members of critically ill persons with brain injury and of those without brain injury, it was suggested that some needs may be applied to all family members of critically ill persons. The basic difference was the degree of importance of each need.

The needs listed should be considered when planning nursing care of critically ill persons. The individuality of all ill persons and their family members must always be paramount. Special consideration should be provided when there is brain injury, because neurological dysfunction causes further separation between the family and the ill person.

processes. Infectious processes destroy tissue through the toxins released by the organisms. The CNS becomes inflamed with trauma, lumbar punctures, and infectious processes such as meningitis. Meningitis illustrates well the response of the CNS to inflammation. This infection of the pia mater and arachnoid membranes can be caused by a variety of microorganisms. Its symptoms—headache, fever, stiffness in the back and neck, as well as pain when the neck is forcefully moved—reflect the inflammatory response of the meninges. The infectious process may cause alterations in the level of consciousness, behavior, and motor and sensory function as well as convulsions. Severe cases, unresponsive to antibiotics, may cause death.

Inflammatory processes are known to attack the spinal cord's gray matter. Inflammation can occur in response to acute infections such as measles or pneumonia or can be part of a primary infectious process such as poliomyelitis. The inflammatory processes can cause necrosis, emboli, or thrombotic complications. Sensory and motor deficits may result. In herpes zoster (shingles), an acute unilateral and segmental inflammation of the dorsal root ganglia results from reactivation of the chickenpox virus. It produces localized vesicular lesions, confined to one dermatome. Severe pain is experienced in the peripheral areas innervated by the inflamed ganglia. (See Chapter 37.)

TRAUMA, TUMORS, AND COMPRESSION

Trauma to the nervous system may result from external forces or elements within the nervous system. The skull and vertebral bodies make it difficult to discover, locate, and assess trauma or physical changes. Symptoms indicating progressing damage are sometimes subtle or lacking until the condition is too advanced to treat effectively.

At times, the system's response to the trauma causes more damage than the insult itself. This secondary damage occurs when edema, bleeding, and increased ICP destroy nervous tissue by compression or restriction of circulation. Edema results from trauma associated with contusions and laceration, trauma to capillary walls, or from hematomas or tumors that obstruct venous blood outflow. The obstruction causes the blood to back up and fluid to move out of the capillaries. Expanding tumors not only cause an increase in ICP and edema; they may also cause bleeding by damaging vessels. All these elements, which cause an increase in ICP, carry the hazard of herniation through the tentorial notch or foramen magnum.

Spinal injuries may cause many of the same problems as cranial injuries, but the complexity of the vertebral column's structure and the concentration of neural tracts at all levels of the cord present special concerns. Injuries to the spinal cord (refer to Figure 35–5) are more common in areas of greater mobility such as the lower cervical spine (C-4, C-5, C-6, C-7, T-1) and the lumbar juncture (T-12, L-1, L-2). Vertebral injuries can cause compression of nerve roots by bone, ligaments, extruded disk material, hematomas, and disruption or overstretching of the neural tis-

sue. Edema caused by trauma can compromise cord function.

Peripheral nerves are responsible for all input for somatic sensations and somatic reflex activity and for all output for the control of striated muscle and other peripheral effector structures. Damage to peripheral nerves will result in loss of sensory or motor functions below the site of the lesion. Some severed peripheral nerves may heal and function may be restored if the integrity of the tissue can be maintained and the nerve ends surgically aligned. Peripheral nerve damage may result from compression of nerves by ruptured disks or by compression from anatomical structures, as in carpal tunnel syndrome. In this syndrome, inflammation or fibrosis of the tendon sheath compresses the median nerve as it passes through the tunnel at the wrist. The compression causes loss of motor and sensory function in the area of the hand innervated by this nerve. (See Chapter 59.)

Another peripheral nerve disease that affects sensory and motor nerves is Guillain-Barré syndrome (discussed in Chapter 38); the cause is unknown but is suspected to be a cell-mediated immunologic attack. The process usually begins in the lower extremities and quickly progresses up the spine, causing muscle weakness or flaccid quadriplegia. Cranial nerves may be affected. Respiratory failure, increased ICP, and autonomic involvement causing bladder and bowel incontinence occurs in some individuals. Assessment of spinal nerve segments is important in this disease because sensory loss at T-8 or higher indicates that respiratory function will probably be impaired.

DEGENERATIVE PROCESSES

Many nervous system diseases can be categorized as degenerative. Their causes vary, as do their severity and influence on lifestyle. Upper and lower motor neuron diseases are examples of degenerative processes manifested in the nervous system. Progressive muscular atrophy follows degeneration of lower motor neurons in the spinal

Nursing Research Note

Power DJ, Craven RF: ALS and aging: A case study in autonomy and control. *Image* (Winter) 1983; 15:22–25.

The clinical case study is one approach in qualitative research. This case study of a client with amyotrophic lateral sclerosis (ALS) in a long-term care setting assessed the client's balance between ADL and coping resources and support systems. The authors discuss the physiology of aging and the pathophysiology of ALS. Proposed nursing interventions, their rationale, and their expected and actual outcomes are presented.

The authors learned that the demands of daily living stimulated collaboration between the client and the nurse to develop an individualized plan of care. The case study suggests that the maintenance of autonomy and control is basic to attaining a high quality of life.

cord because the muscles are no longer stimulated to contract. The disease amyotrophic lateral sclerosis (ALS) is manifested by degeneration of the upper motor neurons in the medulla oblongata and lower motor neurons in the spinal cord. Its cause is unknown. The symptoms and signs of this disease are fasciculations, atrophy, and weakness, particularly in the muscles of the forearms and hands. The upper motor neuron degeneration leads to impaired speech, chewing, swallowing, and breathing.

HEREDITARY AND CONGENITAL DISEASES

Hereditary diseases result from inborn errors that affect development, maturation, or aging. These illnesses present varying degrees of risk to offspring both in the threat of developing the disease and carrying it on to another generation. For example, Huntington's chorea, a hereditary disease that causes mental and physical deterioration,

is transmitted as an autosomal dominant trait. Each child born of a parent with this trait has a 50% chance of developing the disease. The disease usually becomes apparent between the ages of 25 and 55. By the time the disease appears, affected persons often have already had children.

Congenital defects causing CNS abnormalities or malfunctions may occur alone or in combination. Causes include a hereditary tendency, intrinsic factors such as inadequate circulation for the embryo, and in-utero exposure to infectious diseases such as rubella. Neurofibromatosis is a congenital disorder characterized by multiple tumors of the spinal or cranial nerves and the skin, and by cutaneous pigmentation. The disease results from abnormal cortical cellular migrations occurring primarily during the earliest weeks after conception. This condition is not usually life threatening, but surgery may be required for cranial nerve or spinal root lesions. In addition, bone changes and overgrowth of tissue may cause hypertrophy of the tongue, face, and extremities.

Section III: Related System Influences and Effects

The nervous system orchestrates activities to maintain body functions and homeostasis. The central nervous system's control over other major bodily systems has already been discussed. A brief discussion of other system activities that support CNS function will help complete the picture.

Each major system has a role in maintaining homeostatic activity through the regulation of the body's biochemical environment. Alteration in system functions by disease or trauma can result in abnormal neuronal activity or tissue destruction within the CNS. For example, effective pumping by the heart is essential to nourish the CNS and remove waste. Along with the respiratory system, the heart provides the oxygen necessary for function. Failure of these systems quickly results in neuronal death.

The kidneys serve several functions to support the nervous system. They participate in the maintenance of water balance and thus blood pressure. The kidneys also are important in maintaining electrolyte and acid–base balance. They even have a role in ensuring an adequate oxygen supply through the manufacture of erythropoietin, the

hormone that stimulates the production of oxygen-carrying red blood cells.

Gastrointestinal absorption maintains an adequate nutritional level of food elements, vitamins, and minerals. The liver also helps by maintaining an effective level of blood glucose and other nutrients. Detoxification of drugs and other foreign substances are other ways in which the liver helps to maintain homeostasis.

An example of the influence of abnormal liver function on CNS function is hepatic coma. With this condition, the liver is unable to convert ammonia, the end product of amino-acid metabolism, into urea. As a result, the ammonia concentration becomes elevated and may reach toxic levels. Alterations in mental function and coma can occur.

The endocrine system, which has multiple roles in the regulation of body function, influences metabolism, utilization of foods, heart rate, water balance, and mental function. Pathology within this system can cause a variety of neurologic abnormalities or deficits.

Section IV: Psychosocial/Lifestyle Influences and Effects

DEVELOPMENTAL FACTORS

Changes with aging are the result of alterations in effector tissues, receptor systems, and impairment of the body's homeostatic regulatory system. Athletic ability usually peaks in the late teens or early 20s and gradually declines with age. There is also a gradual decline in such skills as finger

tapping and other activities requiring rapid sensory and motor coordination. Isometric muscle strength usually peaks at about age 18 and is maintained through the fifth decade, after which there is a gradual decline related to a decrease in the number of muscle fibers and muscle atrophy. The rate of decline accelerates in the mid-50s. Loss of muscle mass, especially in the thigh, calf, and intrinsic hand muscles occurs even in the active elderly (Katzman & Terry, 1983). Gait changes, such as slowing of step, widening of base, and shuffling are believed to be related to a decrease in muscle mass, loss of large motor nerve fibers regulating motor function, stiffening of joints, and proprioceptive impairment. The capacity of a 70-year-old to do physical work is half that of a 20-year-old (Kenney, 1982).

These facts seem discouraging, but research reports have also presented some encouraging data. Epidemiologic studies indicate that physical exercise contributes to longevity by decreasing the incidence of heart disease. Studies suggest that exercise may reverse or retard age-related changes in synaptic function and nerve-conduction velocity. Physical training in the elderly has been found to improve heart rate, cardiac output, blood pressure, and joint mobility and to decrease stiffness, although it has not improved pulmonary function. Research has also shown that those who are active physically can outperform younger sedentary individuals.

Intellectual function is also a concern for the aged, those who interact with them, and those who are aging. Intellectual performance as measured by vocabulary and information comprehension peaks between 20 and 30 years of age and is maintained through life or until the mid-70s, in the absence of disease. Mental dexterity, especially learning and memory, shows some deficit, especially after age 70. As with physical activity, individuals who continue to be active mentally can perform better than some 20-year-olds. However, the speed of central processing for mental functioning is impaired with age (Katzman & Terry, 1983).

Sensory deficits have been identified in the aged. The loss of vibratory perception in the lower extremities usually begins at about age 50. Touch becomes significantly diminished due to skin changes and a decrease in the number of sensory receptors. (This fact may be particularly significant to nurses during neurological assessments.) Corneal sensitivity, an accurate measurement of sensory perception, shows a decrease in sensitivity in the aged. One study has even documented a significant decrease in corneal sensitivity between 30 and 40 years of age (Katzman & Terry, 1983). Visual, auditory, gustatory, and olfactory senses are also diminished.

Cortical size and blood flow decrease over time. The weight of the brain peaks in the early 20s and then undergoes a slow decline. Along with the weight loss, the cortical area is reduced with a broadening of sulci and a flattening of gyri. Cerebral blood flow in the adult is about 50 to 60 mL per minute per 100 g of tissue. (The base requirement for normal cortical function is a little less than 40 mL per minute per 100 g.) Between 30 and 70 years of age, the rate of flow decreases about 20% (Kenney, 1982). Alterations in blood flow from atherosclerosis, structural changes such as the positioning of vessels in the vertebral column, and heart disease can easily decrease the oxygen supply, compromising neuronal function.

Changes in autonomic nervous system function in the elderly can be seen in the deterioration of pupillary, cardiovascular, thermal, and secretory functions. It is not clear whether these changes are the result of peripheral or CNS changes.

The elderly face the threat of altered homeostasis due to health problems unrelated to neurologic pathology such as cardiac, respiratory, kidney, and gastrointestinal disturbances. If an imbalance occurs, the nervous system can be affected. Even psychological reactions to stress can alter neurologic function.

SOCIOCULTURAL AND LIFESTYLE INFLUENCES

Neurologic disease processes frequently force clients and their significant others to deal with devastating and wide-ranging alterations in lifestyles. These alterations may include the shattering of hopes and dreams for themselves and perhaps for their offspring. Neurologic disease may cause tremendous financial strain and perhaps even the need to seek public assistance. Clients may suddenly be forced to become receivers rather than contributors to life, family, and community.

Depending on the time of onset of the disease, educational or professional aspirations may be interrupted. Many neurologic diseases strike early, leaving deficits or a slowly progressing loss of function. Alterations in function from diseases such as stroke, amyotrophic lateral sclerosis, poliomyelitis, multiple sclerosis, and cerebral palsy are often accompanied by changes in physical appearance. These changes may include awkward gait, drooling, distorted facial expression, tremors, and being wheelchair-bound.

Mental function may also be altered, affecting interaction with others. Common problems include confusion and changes in intellect. Mental function may be further compromised by alteration in sensory perceptions such as vision, hearing, touch, and smell. These changes in function as well as the experience of the disease contribute to a negative change in the individual's body image. Many characteristics valued by society may be lost.

Even though society has become more accepting toward persons who are different from others or from the images created by advertisers, interactions with the disabled may still be strained. Perhaps part of this discomfort is the result of conscious or unconscious concern about one's own susceptibility to illness. The physical, mental, and emotional deficits often experienced by persons with neurologic diseases, along with society's difficulty in relating to them, can cause clients and their loved ones to become isolated from others. The alteration in physical function and body image, as well as self-consciousness and possibly depression, can result in self-imposed isolation. Clients may have limited opportunities for environmental or social interaction. This physical and mental isolation affects how clients feel, live, work, and play.

Society has taken steps to help individuals with neurologic or other types of physical and psychological disabilities by establishing private, voluntary, and governmental agencies with special responsibilities. These groups are working to assist the handicapped and chronically ill, to educate members of the public, and to teach them how to help. Public and private groups are also developing programs to educate the public about lifestyles that can lead

to or contribute to neurologic impairment. Of special interest are smoking and drug abuse. The chronically ill and disabled are also helping themselves by seeking rehabilitative programs and becoming more assertive in seeking their rights in the community and workplace. They are also contributing to the community by sharing their problems so that others will learn from their experiences.

Chapter Highlights

Neurons, the cells that regulate intricate and gross body functions, require a homeostatic biochemical environment and an extensive system of support and protection to function effectively.

Central nervous system neurons cannot be repaired or replaced. Some peripheral neurons may be repaired.

Complex intercommunication among individual neurons and neurons within functional units and hemispheres of the brain is required for nervous system function and body function.

Specialized areas of function have been identified within the nervous system. Effective function is based upon neurotransmitter presence and amount and complex intercommunication among parts of the nervous system.

The limbic system, upon receiving multiple input from the internal and external environments, influences physical and emotional responses.

The autonomic nervous system, composed of the sympathetic and parasympathetic nervous systems, regulates visceral functions, maintains homeostasis, and combats stress.

Nervous tissue requires constant nourishment and removal of waste products.

Cerebrospinal fluid is constantly being produced and must be reabsorbed to prevent excessive pressure within the central nervous system.

Many of the nervous system's structural components protect vital brain tissue but are subject to pathology, which may harm brain tissue.

Blood vessels and peripheral nerves provide routes for foreign elements to enter the central nervous system.

The effects of pathology on nervous system function depend on the size of the lesion, its location, and the reaction of the system to the insult.

The nervous system is subject to harm when other body systems fail.

For many, keeping active mentally and physically can slow the aging process.

Deficits caused by neurologic disease can alter all aspects of life.

Planning care for clients with neurologic problems requires assessment for psychosocial and lifestyle problems as well as for physical deficits.

Bibliography

Angevine JB, Cotman CW: *Principles of Neuroanatomy.* New York: Oxford, 1981.

Anthony CP, Thibodeau GA: *Textbook of Anatomy and Physiology.* St Louis: Mosby, 1983.

Carpenter MB, Sutin J: *Human Neuroanatomy.* Baltimore: Williams & Wilkins, 1983.

Chusid JG: *Correlative Neuroanatomy and Functional Neuroanatomy,* 19th ed. Los Altos, CA: Lange, 1985.

Conway–Rutkowski BL: *Carini and Owens' Neurological and Neurosurgical Nursing,* 8th ed. St Louis: Mosby, 1982.

Diseases. Springhouse, PA: Intermed, 1983.

Eliasson SG, Prensky AL, Hardin WB: *Neurological Pathophysiology.* New York: Oxford, 1979.

Goldberg S: *Clinical Neuroanatomy Made Ridiculously Simple.* Miami: MedMaster, 1979.

Groër ME, Shekleton ME: *Basic Pathophysiology: A Conceptual Approach,* 2nd ed. St Louis: Mosby, 1983.

Guyton AC: *Human Physiology and Mechanisms of Disease.* Philadelphia: Saunders, 1982.

Katzman R, Terry R: *The Neurology of Aging.* Philadelphia: Davis, 1983.

Kenney RA: *Physiology of Aging: A Synopsis.* Chicago: Year Book Medical Publishers, 1982.

Price SA, Wilson LM: *Pathophysiology: Clinical Concepts of Disease Processes,* 2nd ed. New York: McGraw–Hill, 1982.

Spence AP, Mason ER: *Human Anatomy and Physiology,* 2nd ed. Menlo Park, CA: Benjamin/Cummings, 1983.

Chapter 36

The Nursing Process for Clients With Nervous System Dysfunction

Martha Firth Markarian

Objectives

When you have finished studying this chapter, you should be able to:

Discuss how the complexity of the nervous system and its influence on other body systems complicate the identification of disease processes.

Identify components of the nursing assessment that provide information about the central nervous system's influence on mental and physical function.

Recognize how abnormalities observed during physical assessment are related to CNS dysfunction.

Explain factors that can influence a client's subjective reports.

Describe the importance of initial and ongoing assessment of clients with neurologic deficits.

Specify how diseases of other body systems can affect nervous system function.

Identify the nursing implications of diagnostic studies commonly used in evaluating neurological disease.

Formulate nursing diagnoses common to clients with neurologic problems.

Discuss general nursing interventions for clients with neurologic conditions.

Anticipate the psychosocial/lifestyle implications of nervous system dysfunction for the client and significant others.

The pervasive influence of the central nervous system (CNS) on mental and physical functions often complicates the analysis of neurologic symptoms. Identification of nervous system pathology can be difficult because symptoms are often far removed from the source. For example, a cerebrovascular accident (CVA) can result in weakness in a lower extremity. Furthermore, because of similar symptoms and signs some diseases of the CNS can confound the diagnosis; eg, subarachnoid hemorrhage, stroke, and hydrocephalus all create symptoms of increased intracranial pressure (ICP).

Section I: Nursing Assessment: Establishing the Data Base

The rewards from neurologic assessment are many. Symptoms and signs may be identified in time to prevent serious or extensive neurologic damage. A neurologic assessment also provides an opportunity to teach the client about body function and health and adds to the nursing knowledge needed to develop a comprehensive care plan.

SUBJECTIVE DATA

Collection of subjective data from clients with CNS diseases can be especially difficult because the disease often compromises the client's ability to provide reliable information. In some instances, the client will be unresponsive, unconscious, or unreliable as a historian. At these times, family members, friends, or persons who were present when the problem arose should be consulted.

The fear or apprehension that often accompanies possible diagnosis of neurologic disease can limit client disclosure. The nurse's expressed interest in the client's problems along with appropriate teaching and support while collecting the data can comfort the client and family, build confidence in the nurse, and increase willingness to share symptoms and concerns.

Essential to a neurologic assessment is a review of the client's long-term and recent health history because neurologic problems (peripheral neuropathy) can result from diseases affecting other systems (diabetes mellitus). Neurologic problems are also sometimes misdiagnosed as psychiatric problems. Other health problems must also be considered in planning treatments or care. For example, plans for diet, medications, and intravenous therapy will be more complex if the client with neurologic dysfunction also has diabetes, cirrhosis, or renal disease.

Communication with the client during the assessment must be well planned. Keep in mind that terminology describing neurologic problems can be foreign to individuals without a health care background. Therefore, when seeking information from the client, use lay terminology or descriptive terms to avoid miscommunication or intimidation. For example, when describing sensations, use the words *numbness* and *tingling* rather than *paresthesia*. Encourage more thorough disclosure by giving examples of symptoms. Consider this approach: "Mrs Smith, do you have any difficulty in seeing, such as blurred vision or spots or lines in your vision?" This approach helps clients understand what kind of information is sought.

Skin, Nails, and Hair

Integumentary changes are important symptoms in many neurologic disorders. Ask about changes in the skin, hair, and nails. Hair loss can signal nutritional deficiencies related to the inability to eat because of dysphagia, depression, or altered level of consciousness. The client with syringomyelia (a disease of the spinal cord) has many integumentary changes including glossiness of skin, deep skin fissures, and nail changes.

Question the client about skin changes or overgrowths of skin, port-wine stains, or nevi. **Café au lait spots**, spots of light brown patchy skin pigmentation, and disfiguring overgrowths of skin resembling polyps are seen in neurofibromatosis. Because these growths can also occur in the CNS, it is important to inquire about other symptoms of an enlarging CNS mass such as headache, sensory

changes, alteration in level of consciousness, mood changes, and alteration in motor function.

Head and Neck

Client symptoms related to the head and neck should be carefully reviewed during the history of the present illness (HPI). Headaches are common in a variety of health problems, including stress, tumors, meningitis, or one of the many diseases causing increased ICP.

The history or presence of earache accompanied by diminished hearing and possibly ear drainage often suggests otitis. Ear infections can spread into the brain via adjacent blood vessels and the mastoid bone of the skull. Infections of the scalp, paranasal sinuses, and the nasopharynx also present the risk of meningitis or encephalitis because of their proximity to venous sinuses, blood vessels, and foramina. These channels facilitate the spread of infection into the CNS.

Reported hearing loss may be the result of a conduction problem or of damage to CN VIII or to cortical tissue. Question the client about **tinnitus** (ringing or buzzing in the ears). If emotional or behavioral changes are reported, ask whether the client has been having auditory hallucinations, which can result from temporal lobe lesions. Keep in mind that damage to the auditory receptive area in the temporal lobe of the dominant hemisphere can also cause difficulty in understanding the communication of others. Dizziness and vertigo are significant symptoms of tumors or degenerative changes in the vestibular branch of CN VIII, the brain stem, or the cerebellum.

Uncontrolled head movements are significant for Parkinson's disease, other extrapyramidal disease processes, and multiple sclerosis. A partial loss of motor function of the face can be the result of Bell's palsy, CVAs, or pathology affecting the nuclei of the brain stem. Loss of smell from insult to the olfactory bulbs or tracts can be related to shearing trauma, orbital fractures, or tumors.

A loss of taste, perceived by CN V and CN IX, can suggest local or CNS pathology. On the other hand, many older clients comment on loss of taste or decreased taste without the presence of pathology.

Visual changes can result from many elements affecting CN II, its optic radiations, the occipital lobe, CN III, CN IV, CN VI, and their related nuclei in the brain stem. Diseases causing visual changes include multiple sclerosis, myasthenia gravis, stroke, tumors, and trauma.

CN IX, X, and XII direct muscle activity related to talking, chewing, and swallowing. A deficit may be evident during the history. Many disease processes affect these cranial nerves including stroke, tumor, myasthenia gravis, amyotrophic lateral sclerosis (ALS), and multiple sclerosis. Help the client to identify problems by inquiring about difficulty in chewing, swallowing, a need for conscious effort to chew or swallow, choking, excessive accumulation of saliva or food in the mouth, and fatigue from chewing, which may even limit intake and result in weight loss. Speech problems stemming from pathology in these areas may include difficulty in formulating words and in articulation.

Bowel and Bladder

Bowel and bladder function is controlled by various components of the autonomic nervous system. Thoroughly review symptoms such as constipation, urinary retention, and fecal and urinary incontinence.

The client may be unable to expel stool if thoracic spinal cord segments T-1 through T-12 are injured. This problem occurs because voluntary control of abdominal contraction, important in the contraction of the rectal wall, can be lost. In addition, spinal cord injury or disease above or involving sacral nerves S-3, S-4, and S-5 can result in incontinence because of the loss of sphincter tone and reflex activity. Diseases of the cerebral cortex that interfere with mental function can also cause fecal incontinence.

Urinary bladder dysfunction can occur with diseases affecting the cerebral cortex; parasympathetic fibers of S-2, S-3, and S-4; sympathetic fibers from T-11 and T-12 and L-1 and L-2; and peripheral nerve fibers. Examples of CNS diseases are tumors, ruptured disks, and tabes dorsalis. Incontinence or urinary retention can also stem from peripheral nerve damage from diabetes and herpes zoster (Samuels, 1982). Transient urinary retention can follow lumbar puncture or lumbar myelography.

Sexual Function

Occasionally, clients mention concern about sexual dysfunction. Careful and sensitive questioning is needed to establish that problems exist. Sexual dysfunction can occur in men and women who have had insults to the parasympathetic fibers from spinal cord segments S-2, S-3, and S-4; sympathetic fibers from the lumbar spine; or peripheral nerves from these segments. For clients who report sexual dysfunction, take a careful and thorough medication history because many medications have been implicated in impotence. These include anticholinergic agents; drugs with significant anticholinergic side effects such as tricyclic antidepressants, phenothiazines, and antivertigo drugs; narcotic stimulants or psychedelic drugs; drugs that induce depression such as reserpine, methyldopa, propranolol, and other antihypertensive drugs; and ethyl alcohol.

Motor Function

Changes in motor function are often unique to a disease process. Inquiry into changes in motor function should include thorough questioning about localized or generalized weakness. Asking specifically about difficulty arising from or turning in bed; flopping of ankles during walking; and difficulty in moving legs to go up and down steps or in lifting objects, brushing teeth, or keeping eyes open will help clients explain their symptoms better.

Attend to reports of widely separated areas of motor deficit as well as isolated or continuous areas, because disseminated patches of deficit often occur in multiple sclerosis. Symptoms of **ataxia** (lack of muscle coordination) should raise concern about degeneration of the posterior tracts of the spinal cord or cerebellar dysfunction. Uncontrolled movements stemming from faulty basal ganglion function may herald the development of Parkinson's disease, Huntington's chorea, or other diseases affecting the basal ganglia. Reports of uncontrolled movement can also be related to seizure activity.

Spasticity of muscles (increased resistance to passive stretch with rapid extension or flexion of a joint) occurs with CVAs or multiple sclerosis, which release muscles from upper motor neuron control. In contrast, **flaccidity** (decreased or absent muscle tone) can result from isolation of muscles from neuronal impulses. This pathology occurs when anterior horn motor neurons are destroyed, as in poliomyelitis or ALS. Flaccidity may also be seen with peripheral nerve damage from trauma or peripheral nerve inflammation as in Guillain–Barré syndrome. Reports of weakness can be attributed to a variety of disease processes such as entrapment of nerves, as seen in carpal tunnel syndrome (see Chapter 59), or as a weakness that increases with exertion, as with myasthenia gravis.

Twitching (localized, spasmodic contraction of a single muscle group) of the trapezius muscle may occur with lesions in the nucleus of CN XI. Twitching may also occur in other muscles affected by poliomyelitis, spinal cord disease, motor root and peripheral nerve disease, ALS, and muscular dystrophy (Chusid, 1985). Diseases affecting sternocleidomastoid functions are muscular dystrophy, polyneuritis, and poliomyelitis. **Fasciculations** are fine, rapid, twitching movements originating in small groups of muscle fibers. Fasciculations in muscles that are becoming atrophied indicate lower motor neuron disease.

Reports of other abnormal movements include spasm of a muscle or muscle groups (**myoclonus**) as in Creutzfeldt–Jakob disease (Samuels, 1982). Tremors, paucity of movement, and rigidity of movement occur in Parkinson's disease. **Dyskinesias** (defects in voluntary movement) including facial and limb **chorea** (involuntary twitching of the limbs or facial muscles), **athetosis** (slow, twisting, snakelike movements in the upper extremities), and **dystonia** (intense, irregular torsion muscle spasms) can result from antipsychotic medications such as chlorpromazine hydrochloride (Thorazine) and haloperidol (Haldol), among others, or from Huntington's chorea.

Sensory Function

Diseases of the spinal cord's sensory tract can alter or even prevent transmission of stimuli to the brain for interpretation. Symptoms of pathology causing alteration in transmission include numbness, tingling, pain, increased or decreased sensitivity to touch, and alteration in perception of cold and heat. The loss of these sensations may be partial

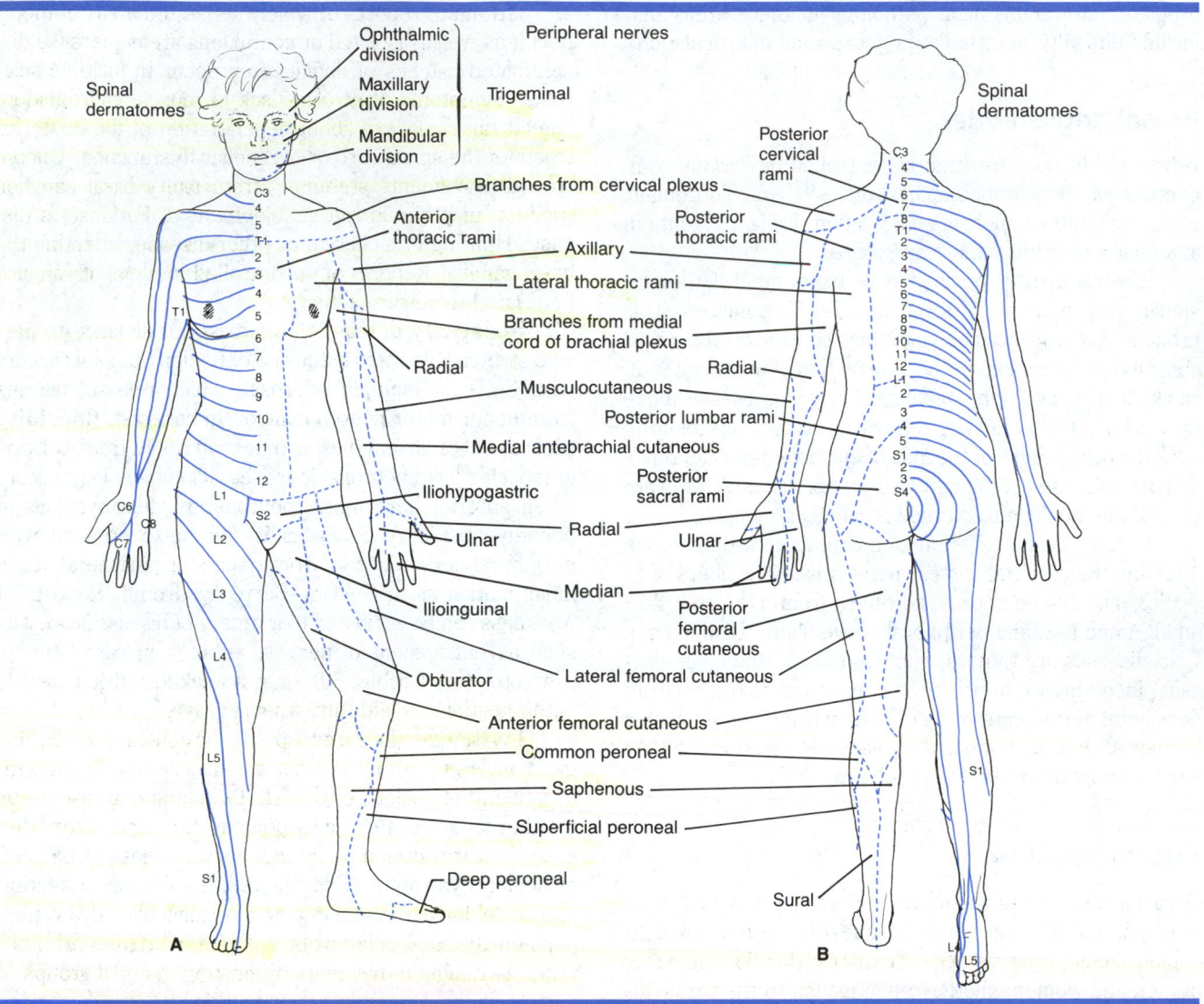

Figure 36–1

Patterns of peripheral and spinal nerve distribution to the skin. Spinal nerve distribution occurs in uniform regions called dermatomes. **A.** Anterior body surface. **B.** Posterior body surface.

or complete. In addition, clients often show evidence of trauma and burns, incurred because of the absence of a sensory warning of impending injury. Many sensory deficits result from peripheral neuropathy and follow peripheral nerve distribution patterns. Knowledge of the cutaneous distribution of spinal nerves makes it possible to locate the spinal cord injury level by mapping areas of decreased sensation (Figure 36–1).

Common sensory disturbances include neuritis, neuralgia, root pain, and herpes zoster. **Neuritis**, characterized by pain and tenderness along the course of the nerve, results from inflammation, trauma, or infection. It can progress to complete loss of sensory and motor function. Reflexes may be diminished or lost (Chusid, 1985). **Neuralgia**, an uncomfortable, painful, burning sensation, may occur spontaneously or from unintentional stimulation of

"trigger zones." Trigeminal neuralgia is typical of this process. **Root pain** occurs with lesions of the dorsal roots of the spinal nerves. The pain is sharp and lightninglike. Coughing and sneezing increase the pain. The pain may result from ruptured disks, cord tumors, fractures, inflammatory diseases of the vertebrae, or meninges. Herpes zoster, a viral inflammatory process, is characterized by painful blisters that follow the cutaneous nerve roots. Transient motor paralysis may accompany the condition.

Clients may also report sensory changes following peripheral nerve damage from trauma, metabolic diseases such as pernicious anemia and diabetes, and entrapment of nerves as in carpal tunnel syndrome. Reports of enlarging joints or loose joints may be given by clients with diabetic neuropathy, syringomyelia, spinal cord disorders, and peripheral nerve injuries. Joint deterioration results when the joints, lacking sensation, are repeatedly injured (Chussid, 1985).

OBJECTIVE DATA

A thorough neurologic assessment of clients with probable nervous system disease is important initially and often throughout the nurse–client interaction. Comprehensive baseline data assist in effective evaluation of the client's changing status. In addition to the formal assessment, frequent contact with the hospitalized client during treatments and activities of daily living will allow close observation of client actions.

Physical Assessment

Mental Status

Keep in mind when assessing mental function that many clients and family members view the brain with awe. Their concern over the diagnosis of a disease affecting the brain can cause fear. In addition, some tests may seem to be a test of intelligence and may cause misunderstanding and apprehension. Therefore, the purpose of the exam should be explained and the testing carried out in a nonthreatening and supportive manner in a quiet and private environment.

The client's mental status is an important component of the neurologic assessment, providing valuable insights into the cause of disease and its effect on the body. Determination of level of consciousness is often used to evaluate improvement or decline of health status in clients with brain trauma or tumors. See Chapter 7 for a sequential approach to the mental status exam.

Assessment of level of consciousness begins with noting the degree of alertness. Is the client awake and alert? If sleeping, is the client aroused by verbal stimuli or tactile stimulation such as touch or gentle shaking, or does the client respond only to a noxious stimulus? After arousal, is alertness maintained once the stimulus is removed? Does the client appear drowsy, restless, irritable, or combative? Question the client regarding time, place, person, and self. If the client is becoming disoriented, awareness of time will usually be lost first, then place, then person, and last self. Inappropriate responses to such questioning may not necessarily indicate mental dysfunction. The client may fail to respond appropriately because of a language barrier, impaired hearing or vision, or some degree of expressive or receptive dysphasia. The trauma client may be confused about time or place because of a period of unconsciousness or the rapidity of events. The client transferred from another hospital or even from another unit may have trouble keeping up with the changes. This is especially true of the elderly.

Long periods of hospitalization can easily cause a client, even without a neurologic problem, to lose track of the date. An extended stay in an intensive care unit, where there is round-the-clock activity, can readily lead to confusion about time of day. Ask the client to follow simple commands, such as "squeeze my hand," "hold up your arm," "wiggle your toes." The response permits assessment of motor function as well as mental function. If the client does not respond to verbal or tactile stimulation, a noxious or painful stimulus may be needed. As a general rule, the stimulus should be the least that will elicit a response and yet not inflict damage. Even in the unconscious client, noxious stimuli may cause a precipitous rise in blood pressure.

Charting should include the stimulus used as well as a description of the client's response to it. Responses are usually classified as appropriate, inappropriate, or absent. In an appropriate response the client localizes the unpleasant stimulus and attempts to withdraw from it or push it away. An inappropriate response involves random or purposeless movements and decerebrate or decorticate posturing. In extreme situations no response can be elicited and the client remains flaccid. Because subtle changes in level of consciousness can be significant, precise documentation and clear communication are essential. Avoid words like confused, stuporous, and comatose. Instead describe the clients behavior, what is said, and what can or cannot be done. At change of shift, it may be especially beneficial for the nurse coming on duty and the nurse reporting off duty to do an assessment together. In this way, the nurse about to assume responsibility for the client has a clearer picture of the client's condition. Subtle or minor changes that may be significant are less likely to be missed or misinterpreted.

Nursing Research Note

Wells P, Geden E: Paraplegic body support pressure on convoluted foam, waterbed and standard mattresses. *Res Nurs Health* 1984; 7:127–133.

Research assessed the amount of pressure placed on the four bony prominences common for pressure sore development by three types of hospital mattresses—waterbed, convoluted foam, and the standard hospital mattress. The four pressure sites studied were occiput, scapula, sacrum, and heels. The researchers found that pressures greater than 20 to 30 mm Hg resulted in reduced capillary perfusion, leading to tissue ischemia and tissue necrosis.

The findings suggest that the water mattress produced the least amount of pressure on all four areas. Waterbeds exerted pressure between 27 and 28 mm Hg on the occiput and heels at prescribed interval readings. The convoluted foam mattress produced less pressure on all four sites than the standard mattress. The foam mattress resulted in readings of 40 to 42 mm Hg over the sacral and occiput prominences at timed intervals. The standard mattress had the highest pressure readings at all four areas. The highest readings were found at the occiput and sacrum where readings were greater than 50 mm Hg.

The researchers concluded that prevention of pressure sores consists of appropriate mattress selection and regular position changes. Nurses play a major role in prevention and must be actively involved in assessment, diagnosing, planning, and evaluating effects of these preventive measures.

Table 36–1	Levels of Consciousness: Glasgow Coma Scale	
Faculty Measured	**Response**	**Score**
Eye opening	Spontaneous	4
	To verbal command	3
	To pain	2
	No response	1
Motor response	To verbal command	6
	To painful stimuli:	
	• Localizes pain	5
	• Flexes and withdraws	4
	• Assumes decorticate posture	3
	• Assumes decerebrate posture	2
	• No response	1
Verbal response (arouse client with painful stimuli, if necessary)	Oriented, converses	5
	Disoriented, converses	4
	Uses inappropriate words	3
	Makes incomprehensible sounds	2
	No response	1

SOURCE: Adapted from Teasdale G, Bennet B: Assessment of coma and impaired consciousness: A practical scale. *Lancet* 1974; 2(7872):81.

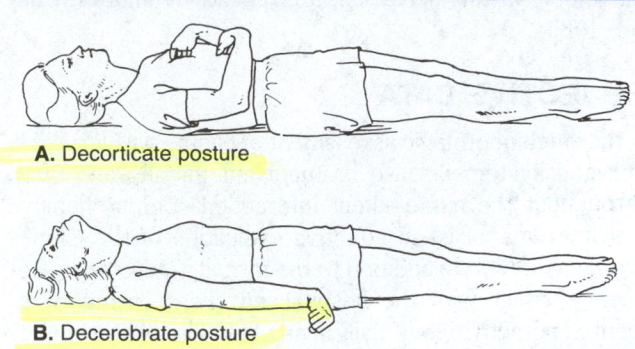

A. Decorticate posture

B. Decerebrate posture

Figure 36–2

Decorticate and decerebrate posturing. **A.** Decorticate posture: the client's arms are adducted with elbows and wrists in rigid flexion, the hands rotated internally and fingers flexed; the lower extremities are hyperextended. **B.** Decerebrate posture: the client has hyperextended upper and lower extremities; **opisthotonos** (head extended, body arched) is an exaggerated decerebrate posture seen in tetanus, when the body may be supported on the back of the head and the feet during a convulsion.

The Glasgow Coma Scale is an objective measure of level of consciousness that can also be somewhat predictive of recovery (Table 36–1). Coma is defined as a score of 7 or less. With a score of 3 or 4, there is an 85% chance of dying or remaining vegetative. A score above 11 is associated with an 85% chance of moderate disability or good recovery.

Station and Gait

Observation of the client's **station** (manner of standing) and gait will give many clues. Postures can be influenced by mental and physical problems. The degree of decrease in the level of consciousness affects posture, which can vary from slouching to flaccid with no response to stimuli. Two types of posture in unresponsive clients can be significant in identifying the level of CNS involvement, giving evidence of decortication or decerebration. The postures can occur spontaneously or in response to a stimulus such as testing for reflexes.

With **decorticate posturing** (Figure 36–2A), the client demonstrates hyperflexion of the upper extremities and hyperextension of the lower extremities. Lesions on the cerebral hemisphere or internal capsule are believed to cause decorticate postures by interrupting the corticospinal pathways. With **decerebrate posturing** (Figure 36–2B), both the upper and lower extremities are hyperextended. Decerebrate posture is believed to result from rostral to caudal deterioration, which can occur when a diencephalic lesion of the hemisphere extends, causing midbrain and upper pontine damage (Hickey, 1981).

Unusual gait, stance, or sitting posture can result from motor or sensory deficits as in stroke or tabes dorsalis. Clients with Parkinson's disease have a typical shuffling and propulsive (**festination**) gait. The normal arm swing is also lost.

Skin and Hair

Trophic changes on the face and extremities are often noticeable at the beginning of the exam. Café au lait spots, frequently accompanied by subcutaneous nodules, are seen on any part of the body in neurofibromatosis (Recklinghausen's disease). Angiomatous lesions such as port-wine stains on the face are associated with Sturge–Weber syndrome (Conway–Rutkowski, 1982). Autonomic nervous system (ANS) abnormalities are suspected with abnormal colorations ranging from erythema to cyanosis; temperature changes, either coolness or increased warmth; and variations in skin moisture, either dryness or sweating. Melanomas—malignant skin tumors—metastasize to the CNS. Burns and bruises of the extremities suggest decreased sensation.

Decreased sensory awareness can result in decubitus ulcers. In the spinal and posterior fossa areas, look for tufts of hair and abnormal pigmentation, suggesting underlying neural tube deformity.

Baldness can result from nutritional disorders, anxiety, or chemotherapy. Pluckable or shedding hair and brittle hair are signs of nutritional deficiency (see Chapter 8).

Chemotherapy may temporarily affect the hair follicle, causing hair loss. A client with nervous dysfunction may show signs of patchy baldness from pulling out hair without being aware of doing so; thus, the baldness may suggest sensory dysfunction. Baldness may also suggest nutritional deficiency, which can result from neurologically based dysphagia, depression, or dulled consciousness.

Head and Neck

A major portion of the neurologic exam focuses on the head and neck because of the concentration of nervous tissue in this area. Keep in mind that, although the skull protects the brain, foramina are portals for organisms and can be obstructed by tumors and calcifications. Palpation can reveal trauma, tender areas, and bony elevations, which can range from the serious—eg, meningiomas—to the insignificant (Conway–Rutkowski, 1982). If the history includes a report of severe and often unpredictable facial pain, like that of tic douloureux (trigeminal neuralgia), avoid palpating or stimulating an identified trigger zone. Asymmetry in facial muscles can indicate a deficit in motor function. Observe for deep furrows on the forehead and prominent superficial arteries in the temporal region, which can indicate temporal arteritis or migraine headache (Conway–Rutkowski, 1982).

Auscultation over the closed eyes may reveal bruits (murmurs) stemming from a variety of vascular changes such as arteriovenous malformation, stenosis of the carotid arteries or aorta, dilation of vessels to meet the increased nutritional needs of a vascular meningioma, or distortion of blood vessels by a space-occupying lesion (Conway–Rutkowski, 1982). With arteriovenous malformations or aneurysms of the temporal lobe, bruits may be heard directly over the site.

Cranial Nerves

Assessment of the individual cranial nerves is essential when pathology is suspected in the head, neck, and shoulders. The widespread influence of CN X must be considered with the general assessment.

Assessment of an individual's ability to smell is a test of CN I. Loss of smell (**anosmia**) can result from a shearing force with a blow to the head or pressure from a tumor on the olfactory bulb or tract.

Visual changes provide a vast array of information about the function of CN II, III, IV, and VI. The extension of CN II from its exit site on the retina (optic disk) to the occipital lobe makes it vulnerable to a variety of lesions (see Figure 69–5 in Chapter 69). Identifying problems of visual acuity and loss of peripheral vision can help to establish the location of the pathology (see Figure 37–1 in Chapter 37). For example, partial loss of visual field suggests injury to the optic tracts. Loss of vision can occur with occipital lobe trauma; the inability to interpret visual input can occur with parietal lobe trauma. Ophthalmoscopic examination of the optic disk can give valuable information

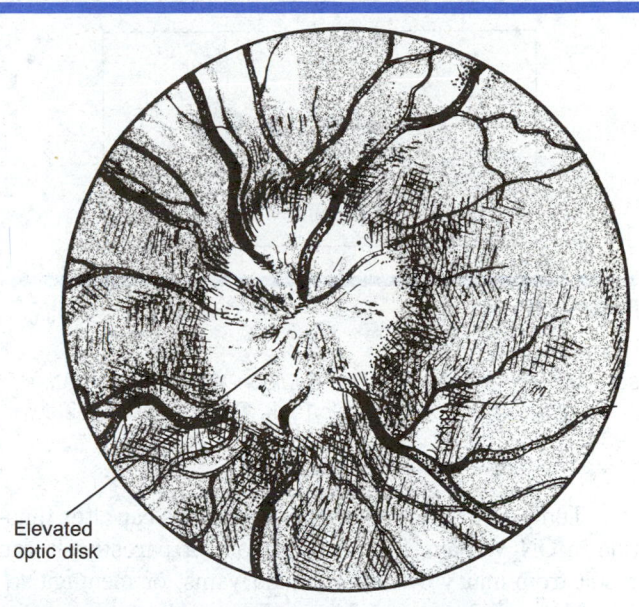

Elevated optic disk

Figure 36–3

Papilledema. The disk margins are obliterated because of the swelling of the optic nerve head.

about its integrity. A white disk indicates atrophy of the optic nerve, which can occur with tabes dorsalis. **Papilledema** (edema and inflammation of the optic nerve at its point of entrance into the eye ball—also called choked disk) results from increased ICP (Figure 36–3).

Cranial nerves III, IV, and VI are responsible for eye movements needed for focusing. CN III controls eye movement medially, upward, and downward. Diseases affecting CN IV will result in loss of the ability to look down and laterally in the involved eye. Deficits in CN VI function will be evidenced by the loss of ability of the affected eye to look laterally. With any of these deficits, the client might have double vision (**diplopia**) or dizziness. Observe also for nystagmus, which can be physiological or due to central or labyrinthine lesions. It can also occur with certain drugs, for example, phenytoin (Dilantin), bromides, barbiturates, and alcohol (Chusid, 1982). Squinting or tilting the head to facilitate focusing are additional signs of pathology. A lack of conjugate movement can occur in multiple sclerosis (Conway–Rutkowski, 1982).

Cranial nerve III also controls elevation of the eyelid. Ineffective closure of the lid is a common problem in myasthenia gravis and in pathology in the brain stem as in stroke or head injury. Parasympathetic fibers traveling with CN III are responsible for constriction of the pupil. Pupillary size and reaction (or lack of reaction) to a light stimulus are significant in various neurologic diseases. Pupillary change is of special concern when increased ICP or brain stem pathology is suspected. Using an assessment guide similar to that in Figure 36–4 will aid in measuring pupil size.

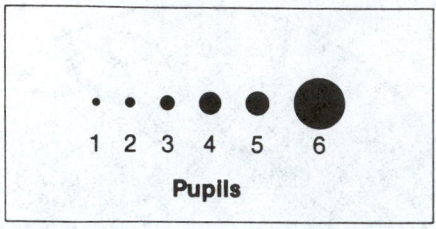

Figure 36–4

Pupil gauge.

SOURCE: Swearingen PL: *The Addison-Wesley Photo-Atlas of Nursing Procedures*. Menlo Park, CA: Addison-Wesley, 1984.

Tumors, injury, and disease processes can alter function in CN V. Pain, loss of sensation, or paresthesia can result from injury by tumors, aneurysms, or meningitis.

Motor and sensory abnormalities of the face can also be seen with CN VII pathology. The motor component of this nerve innervates all facial muscles. Its sensory component perceives taste on the anterior two-thirds of the tongue. Bell's palsy, a fairly common disease process, illustrates well the motor control of CN VII. With Bell's palsy, the client experiences unilateral drooping of the mouth, collection of food between cheek and gum, tearing of the eye, loss of deep sensation (position and vibratory sense),

Nursing Research Note

Feroli–Lord K, McGinty–Maquire M: Toward a more objective approach to pupil assessment. *J Neurosurg Nurs* 1985; 7(5):309–312.

This descriptive study examined the differences between a hand-held tongue depressor pupil gauge and a printed millimeter scale sheet to assess pupillary size. The tongue depressor was held next to the client's eye and moved up and down until it best correlated with pupil size. The printed millimeter tool was on a sheet of paper, and size was compared to scaled drawings and diagrams of millimeter circles. Forty-two pairs of nurses were randomly assigned to either the tongue depressor pupil tool or the printed millimeter sheet tool. An investigator watched as each pair of nurses individually assessed pupil size with the tools. Twenty-eight pairs were in the tongue depressor group, and 14 pairs were in the standard pupil measurement group. There was no significant difference between measurements in either group. However, the tongue depressor group had higher interrater reliability, indicating that different nurses using the tool measured pupil size the same.

This research indicates that millimeter pupil gauges that can be held near the client's eye provide a more consistent and reliable measure of pupil size for nursing practice; using such a tool decreases subjective pupil measurement. The tool must be placed near the eye for best measurement. Developing such a tool on a tongue blade is inexpensive, convenient, and disposable.

and inability to close the eye). With stroke or trauma affecting unilateral upper motor neurons, a partial loss of motor function can result. Examination reveals a flatness of the nasolabial fold and weak closure of the eyes when the eyebrows are raised. Forehead movement will not be affected. The eyebrows will raise, and the forehead will wrinkle bilaterally. Loss of taste on the anterior two-thirds of the tongue can be experienced with pathology in the nucleus or sensory fibers of CN VII (Conway–Rutkowski, 1982).

Pathology involving CN VIII causes hearing loss (cochlear branch) or disturbances in balance (vestibular branch). (Hearing assessment is discussed in Chapter 7.) Assessment of vestibular function involves special caloric testing by a physician (see Chapter 74).

Cranial nerves IX and XII can be affected by tumors, trauma, hemorrhage, ALS, and bulbar diseases. Aspiration of food or saliva is a serious threat to clients when these cranial nerves are affected. Other signs of involvement include the collection of food or saliva in the mouth, choking, loss of weight, and a poor nutritional state. The client's gag reflex and ability to chew, to form a bolus of food, and to swallow must be carefully assessed.

Cranial nerves IX and X also have a major role in perception of pain, touch, and temperature. All are important for safe chewing and swallowing. Loss of sensitivity in the pharynx, tonsils and fauces, together with the loss of taste on the posterior one-third of the tongue, occur with CN IX pathology.

Cranial nerve XII controls motor function of the tongue. Lesions affecting its movement can result from unilateral or bilateral upper or lower motor neuron lesions. Signs of CN XII pathology include deviation of the tongue upon protrusion, flaccid or spastic paralysis, atrophy, and fasciculations. Supranuclear lesions result in spastic paralysis with deviation to the side opposite the lesion. Nuclear or medullary lesions result in fasciculation and sensory disturbances. If the lesion is bilateral, dysphagia (difficulty in swallowing), **dysarthria** (poorly articulated speech), and difficulty in chewing will be present. CN XII is also harmed in poisoning by lead, alcohol, arsenic, and carbon monoxide (Chusid, 1985).

Cranial nerve XI is subject to a number of diseases that can limit contraction of the sternocleidomastoid and trapezius muscles. These diseases include multiple sclerosis, syphilis, meningitis, poliomyelitis, and muscular dystrophy. Alteration of muscle function can result from pathology in the medulla, in the cervical cord and its peripheral nerves, and from cortical lesions. Signs of CN XI pathology include atrophy of muscle, inability to rotate the head to the healthy side, unequal strength in pushing against resistance, inability to shrug the involved shoulder, or dropping of this shoulder. Look for the involved scapula to be displaced downward. Bilateral nuclear or peripheral lesions cause difficulty in rotating the head or raising the chin. The head droops forward. Atrophied trapezius muscles give the shoulder a square appearance. Central paralysis causes similar limitations in movement but no atrophy.

Muscles are spastic. Unilateral central involvement can result in **torticollis** (tilting of the head to one side in response to muscle contraction) (Chusid, 1985). Fasciculation in involved muscles may be observed, felt, or heard on auscultation. Pain with rotation of the head suggests cervical arthritis.

Motor Function

Alteration in motor function can result from cortical, cerebellar, spinal cord, or peripheral nerve pathology as well as psychiatric disturbances. Observed changes in motor function provide valuable information about the disease process and nursing care needed.

Assessment of motor function includes examination of the physical structure of muscles and their ability to function normally. The structure of muscles gives information about their innervation, strength, and nutritional status as well as about the type of physical activity usually undertaken. Muscle mass and bulk are influenced by age, sex, and heredity. Syringomyelia, poliomyelitis, and peripheral nerve disorders are examples of diseases that waste muscle. Muscular dystrophy also results in muscle wasting, but the enlargement of muscle with connective and fatty tissue can be deceiving. Clients with myasthenia gravis, a disease of the neuromuscular junction, demonstrate a greater degree of weakness during exercise.

Muscle tone, the response of a limb to movement, can be increased or decreased by disease. Increased tone can be seen in extrapyramidal tract disorders such as Parkinson's disease or in upper motor neuron damage as in stroke. A pronounced increase in tone is referred to as **rigidity**. Rigidity can be increased when the individual concentrates on movement and when another limb is moved (Snyder, 1983). In **cogwheel rigidity**, seen in Parkinson's disease, the examiner feels predictable fluctuations in the intensity of muscle tone. Spasticity is seen in pyramidal tract disease. Joint contractures are often seen in clients with a history of spasticity. Flaccidity of muscle (**hypotonia**) is observed with lesions of the sensory and motor components of the reflex arc (Conway–Rutkowski, 1982). Fasciculation can be seen with denervation of muscle, with drug therapy, dietary deficiencies, fever, and uremia.

Other abnormal movements such as chorea, athetosis, dystonia, and tremor can be seen in extrapyramidal tract dysfunction. Choreic movements are rapid, jerky, and semipurposeful. In athetosis, less purposeful movements are slower, sinuous, and continuous. They are exaggerated with voluntary movements or emotional stimuli. These movements do not occur during sleep but can interfere with speech, eating, smooth respiration, and other activities (Conway–Rutkowski, 1982). Dystonia is characterized by intense, irregular torsion muscle spasms that twist the client's trunk, shoulders, and pelvis out of shape. Although myoclonus and ataxia are seen in Creutzfeldt–Jakob disease, myoclonic jerks occur in normal individuals with drowsiness and light sleep.

Cerebellar control of coordination, balance, and the judgment of distance can be limited or destroyed by a number of pathologies such as trauma, congenital deficits, disease, and medications. Signs, which may be subtle or obvious, include tremor, ataxia, exaggerated arm swing, hypotonia, and impaired posture without loss of motor power (Conway–Rutkowski, 1982).

Useful in diagnosing lumbar disease is *Lasègue's sign*, which assesses pain and limitation in motor function. For this test the client lies supine and is asked to do straight leg raises. With lumbar disk disease, leg raising on the affected side will be limited. Root pain can occur on the affected side when the opposite leg is raised. If a lesion is present in the upper lumbar area, pain is increased when the hip is hyperextended (Conway–Rutkowski, 1982).

Sensory Function

Sensory changes, significant in all disease processes, are especially important in neurologic problems; they are often the first or only symptom of a disease or disease progression. Neurologic sensory changes call for careful planning to ensure client safety and maintenance of optimal function because lack of attention to symptoms of pain or paresthesia (eg, with clients who have spinal cord or root injuries) could lead to a permanent loss of motor and sensory function. Sensory changes can result from disease or trauma of the parietal lobe, thalamus, brain stem, spinal cord, and peripheral nerves. They include alteration or loss of touch, pain, or temperature sensitivity and the loss of vibratory and position sense.

Assessment of sensory function is covered in Chapter 7. Assessment includes testing of superficial sensation (light touch, pain, and temperature) and deep sensation (position and vibratory senses). Sensory evaluation for higher integrative functions includes testing for two-point discrimination, stereognosis, and graphesthesia. The absence of sensory changes when motor deficits are present can help to confirm a diagnosis. In both Guillain–Barré syndrome and ALS, profound motor deficits occur while sensation remains unchanged.

Superficial and Deep Tendon Reflexes

Reflex changes provide valuable information about diminished sensations or paralysis in the conscious and unconscious client. These changes can provide early warning of pathology involving the corticospinal pathways, anterior horn cells, their axonal projections, and the afferent sensory component of muscles. Reflex responses also help to localize the level of a spinal cord injury.

When assessing deep tendon reflexes (DTRs), view asymmetry and diminished, increased, or absent reflexes in light of other neurologic findings. Superficial reflexes such as the abdominal and cremasteric responses are of limited value because of the superimposed cortical pathway. Therefore, lesions of either the cortical tract or the lower motor neuron can result in abnormal reflexes (Conway–Rutkowski, 1982). Furthermore, when checking

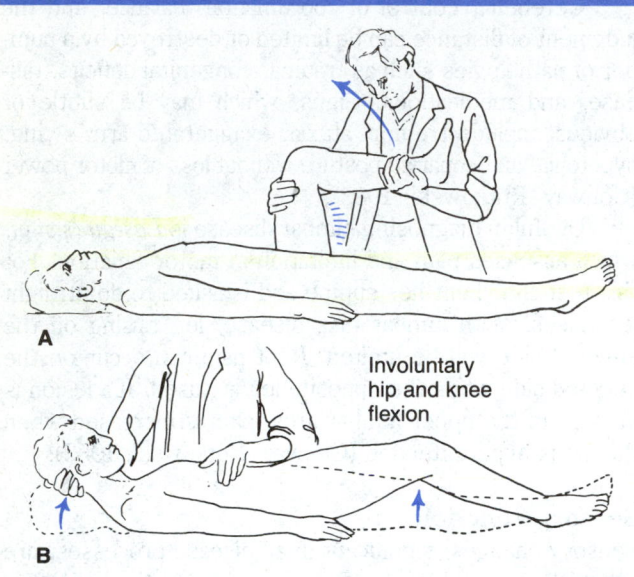

Involuntary
hip and knee
flexion

Figure 36–5

Kernig's sign and Brudzinski's sign—two signs of meningeal irritation. **A.** Kernig's sign: with client supine, flex hip and knee to about 90°; then attempt to extend the knee. **B.** Brudzinski's sign: with client supine and legs extended, passively flex the client's neck.

these reflexes, keep in mind that lesions above the decussations (crossings) of the corticospinal tract result in loss or diminished reflexes on the opposite side of the body. Lesions below this level result in a loss of reflexes on the same side as the lesion (Hickey, 1981).

A superficial reflex frequently used for discovering an upper motor neuron lesion is **clonus**, a continued rapid flexion and extension of the foot. This reflex is elicited by quickly dorsiflexing the foot. The wrist and patella can also be tested. Note that if the clonus stops quickly, it may be a normal response (Chusid, 1985).

Meningeal Irritation

Assessment for nuchal (neck) rigidity, Kernig's sign, and Brudzinski's sign aid in diagnosing meningeal irritation as in meningitis or subarachnoid hemorrhage. In nuchal rigidity, the client is unable to place the chin on the chest because neck flexion is limited by involuntary muscle spasm.

To test for Kernig's and Brudzinski's signs, the client is in the supine position. For Kernig's sign, one hip is flexed to 90° with the knee also flexed to 90° (Figure 36–5A). If meningeal irritation is present, the client in this position will be unable to extend the knee past 90° without pain (Hickey, 1981). To test for Brudzinski's sign, the client is supine with the legs extended. When the examiner flexes the client's neck, if meningeal irritability is present, the hips and knees will spontaneously flex to avoid the accompanying pain (Figure 36–5B).

Diagnostic Studies

Diagnosis is often complicated because the central nervous system is contained within the skull and vertebral canal. For this reason, most diagnostic studies for neurologic disease are invasive. Careful client preparation is needed for all diagnostic studies. The invasiveness of neurologic tests and the consequences of misdiagnosis increase the importance of client teaching and nursing care both before and after diagnostic studies.

Most laboratory studies specific for assessment of neurologic function are based on the contents of the cerebrospinal fluid (CSF) or its pressure within the CNS. Other laboratory studies, such as analysis of blood samples, are used to determine whether malfunction of other body systems compromises nervous system function. Some examples are blood tests for anemia that could reduce the brain's oxygen supply and tests for fluid and electrolyte imbalances that could alter neuronal function.

Skull Films

These x-rays are used as a basic noninvasive screening for trauma and neoplasms. They can reveal pathological changes such as pituitary gland tumors. They can detect calcified abnormalities, such as aneurysms, or abnormal position of the calcified pineal gland (calcification is normal in the adult).

Nursing Implications. Explain the purpose for the procedure and steps involved. Comb tangled or braided hair, and remove pins and wigs. Glass eyes can produce confusing shadows in a radiograph, so their presence should be noted (Snyder, 1983).

Spinal Films

Radiography may reveal changes in spinal bones resulting from fractures, tumors, or infections. It may also show the bony ridges and spur formations characteristic of osteoarthritis and help to identify congenital defects.

Electroencephalography

Electroencephalography (EEG) is essentially a noninvasive test that records a portion of the brain's electrical activity. The EEG is valued for its ability to reveal abnormal brain-wave patterns that help in diagnosing seizure disorders, brain tumors, abscesses, and psychological disorders. The analysis of brain waves is possible because specific types of normal and abnormal brain waves have been identified. Diagnosis is made by evaluating patterns and characteristics of brain waves recorded, along with the client's clinical state. An absence of brain waves establishes brain death. Note, however, that acute drug intoxication or severe hypothermia resulting in a loss of consciousness can also cause a flat EEG.

The client is placed in a bed or on a lounge chair in a quiet secluded area. Surface electrodes, or occasionally needle electrodes, are positioned on or in the scalp. The

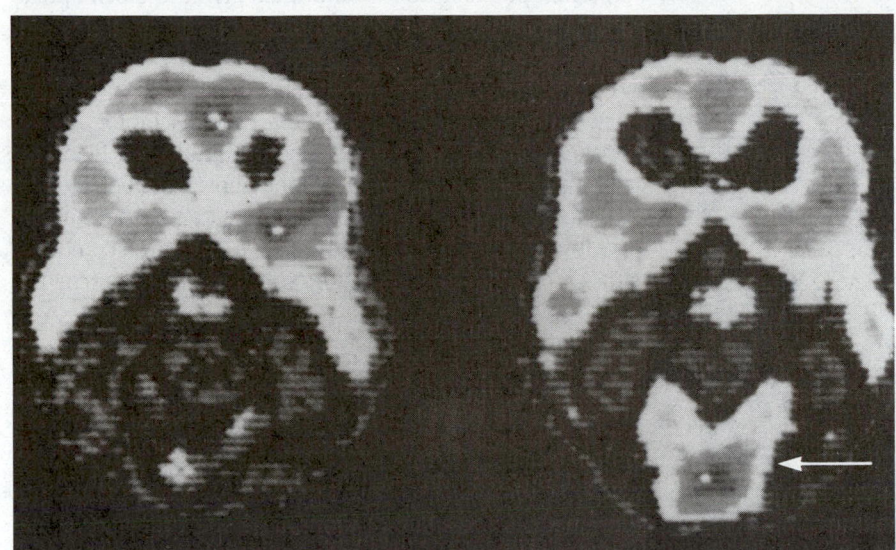

Figure 36–6

PET Scan. **Left,** client has eyes closed. **Right,** client has eyes open. A marked increase in glucose utilization in the visual cortex (arrow) is seen in the scan on the right. (Courtesy of Leonard I. Malis, MD, The Mount Sinai Hospital, Neurosurgery Department, New York, NY)

client is instructed to close the eyes, relax, and rest quietly. Various stimuli are introduced to determine whether seizure activity can be produced. The client may be asked to hyperventilate for 3 minutes, to watch a flashing light, to endure a sensory stimulus such as a minor electrical shock, to observe a black-and-white checkerboard, and to listen to sounds through earphones. The client must be observed carefully and protected if seizure activity occurs. If a sleep EEG is requested, the client will be instructed to stay awake the night before the test. A sleeping medication may be given to promote sleep.

Nursing Implications. Instruct the client to eat meals as usual with the exception of coffee, tea, cocoa, and cola, which the physician may want withheld because of their stimulant effect. Medications that may influence the test are often withheld. These include anticonvulsants, tranquilizers, barbiturates, or sedatives. Be sure the hair is clean and free from oils, sprays, or pins.

An explanation of the procedure and its purpose, the function of the electrodes, and the length of the test will help the client relax. The test usually takes 40 to 60 minutes with pretest and posttest care taking another hour.

Following test completion, assist clients in removing the electrode paste from the hair. At the same time, observe them for seizures and recovery from any sedation given during the test. The physician's order for resumption of medications is reviewed with the client. Check vital signs and neurologic signs as appropriate.

Computerized Tomography
Computerized tomography (CT) scanning is used to diagnose intracranial and spinal cord lesions. Scans are also used to monitor the effects of surgery, radiotherapy, or chemotherapy on tumors and to reveal vascular displacement, hematomas, cerebral atrophy, infarction, edema, and hydrocephalus. An iodinated contrast dye is sometimes administered to make large blood vessels visible or to define lesions. Administered intravenously, the dye increases the blood density and delineates intracranial masses.

Nursing Implications. Explain the purpose of the exam. If no contrast medium is to be used, restriction of food and drink is not necessary. With use of dye, the client fasts for 4 to 6 hours to prevent emesis if nausea occurs. Before administering a contrast dye, identify any allergies to shellfish, iodine, or contrast media because use of the dye may be contraindicated. Skin testing to determine allergy is sometimes done.

Explain details about the procedure including special positioning, noise emitted by the machine, and length of the test. Some machines require the client to be strapped to the table, which moves into a gantry during the test. Loud clacking noises are normally emitted during this time. The test takes 15 to 30 minutes if no dye is used; with dye, the time is doubled. Clients receiving the dye should know that it is normal to feel flushed and warm and that sometimes a headache or salty taste or nausea occurs.

Positron Emission Tomography
Positron emission tomography (PET) is a noninvasive nuclear-imaging technique available in large medical centers. It is used to study oxygen uptake, blood flow, and glucose utilization in clients with cerebrovascular disease, seizure disorders, cardiovascular disease, and some degenerative disorders. With PET, viable tissue can be discriminated from nonviable tissue and the amount of nutritional blood flow to an area can be identified (Figure 36–6). PET is combined with computerized tomography. See nursing implications for CT scanning.

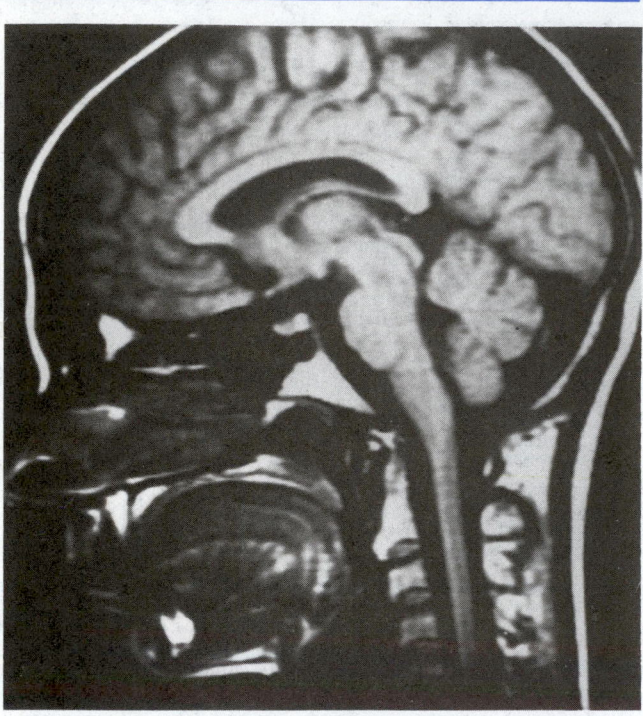

Figure 36–7

MRI imaging. The MRI scan shows a normal midsagittal view and demonstrates the amount of detail possible to obtain with this diagnostic test. (Courtesy Leonard I. Malis, MD, The Mount Sinai Hospital, Neurosurgery Department, New York, NY)

Magnetic Resonance Imaging

Nuclear magnetic resonance (MRI) imaging is based on the fact that the hydrogen nuclei in abnormal tissues behave differently in a magnetic field. A computer can manipulate these differences into a detailed picture of the organ under study (Figure 36–7). This noninvasive study does not require contrast media or exposure to radiation.

The client lies supine in a huge doughnut-shaped magnet. Bone tissue is not visualized with MRI but soft tissue close to bone is easily viewed. This enhances the use of MRI for problems of the skull and spine.

Radionuclide Scan of the Brain

The radionuclide scan detects intracranial masses; vascular lesions; and areas of ischemia, infarction, and hemorrhage. A radionuclide, usually administered intravenously, accumulates in affected areas if the blood–brain barrier has been compromised. Oral or intra-arterial administration can also be used. Some scans also include oscilloscope scanning of the carotid and cerebral blood flow. After the radioactive isotope has circulated for at least 1 hour, a scanner records the accumulation of isotopes. Another scan can be done 3 to 4 hours after injection.

Nursing Implications. Ask about allergies to the isotope. No dietary or fluid restrictions are required.

Potassium perchlorate is sometimes given to block uptake of the isotope by the thyroid, choroid plexus, and salivary glands (Conway–Rutkowski, 1982). Discuss the steps of the procedure and its time requirements, and inform the client that the injection will be the only discomfort. Have the client remove all jewelry and metal objects from the head and neck. To prevent client apprehension, explain that the radioisotope is harmless to self and others and is quickly excreted from the body. This test is often combined with CT scanning and angiography to help confirm the diagnosis.

Cerebral Angiogram

The cerebral angiogram is used to diagnose intracranial lesions. A radiopaque contrast medium is injected into blood vessels of the head and neck to allow visualization of intracranial and extracranial vessels (Figure 36–8). The cerebral angiogram can reveal aneurysms; arteriovenous malformations; and displacement of vessels by masses, edema, or herniation. The test is also used during surgery to check the position and integrity of aneurysm clippings.

The contrast material can be injected into a variety of sites. The most common are the carotid, brachial, and femoral arteries. Catheters are used in the more distal sites. Injection is done under local or general anesthesia in a special procedures area where resuscitation equipment is available or in the operating room. This test is contraindicated in clients with renal, hepatic, thyroid, or clotting disorders as well as in those who are hypersensitive to iodine or contrast materials.

Nursing Implications. Client education includes review of the procedure's purpose. The physician explains the risks, which include CVA, thrombus, allergic reactions, seizures, pulmonary emboli, and visual disturbances (Hickey, 1981). A consent must be signed. To reduce apprehension, inform the client that a supine position, with the head secured to prevent movement, will be required throughout the test, which lasts approximately 2 hours. In addition, tell the client that periodic assessment of heart function and blood pressure are routine.

Careful explanation of sensations expected when the dye is injected is essential to reduce fear, because having the contrast medium injected into the blood vessels of the head can be painful. The sensations vary from warmth to severe burning behind the eyes and in the jaw, teeth, tongue, and lips. Even fillings in the teeth can feel warm (Hickey, 1981). The sensation of heat lasts 4 to 6 seconds after the dye is injected. More than one injection may be needed.

Nursing care also includes collection of baseline data and preparation of the client. Record vital signs and neurologic status. Mark pulses distal to the puncture site to facilitate assessment after the procedure. If the carotid site is used, document the neck measurement to allow comparison after the test (Snyder, 1983). Hairpins, nets, and dentures must be removed. The client should also void.

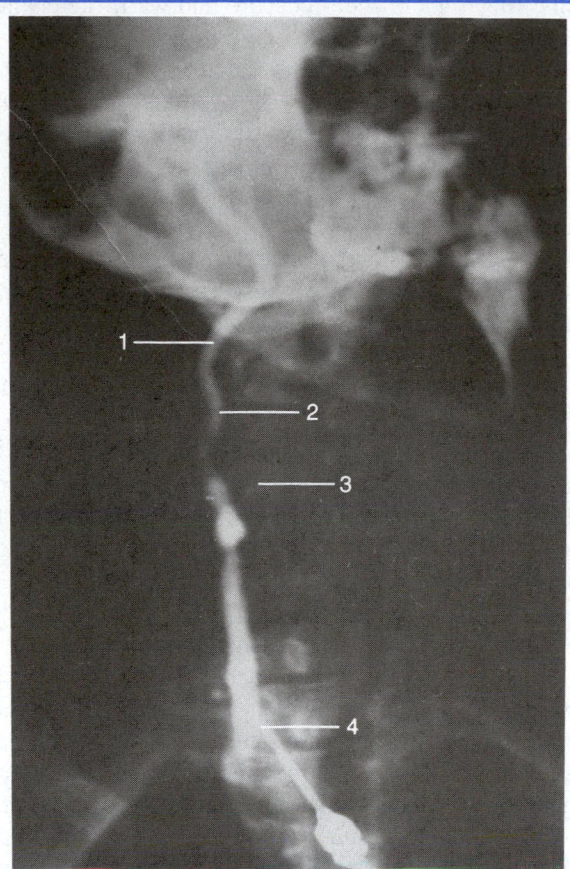

Figure 36–8

Cerebral angiogram performed through the carotid artery. 1, External carotid artery; 2, region of carotid bifurcation; internal carotid artery cannot be seen because of atheromatous plaques occluding the lumen; 3, superior thyroid artery; 4, needle in the common carotid. (Courtesy of Millard Fillmore Hospital, Buffalo, NY)

Preprocedure medications can include phenobarbital, to help the client relax, and atropine sulfate, to protect against a reflex response (hypotension, syncope, and bradycardia) by the carotid artery (Hickey, 1981). The client should be well hydrated to promote clearance of the dye by the kidneys but should fast for 6 to 8 hours before the test. Shave the injection site and prepare it with an antiseptic solution. Local anesthetic is usually given before insertion of the catheter or needle.

Immediately following the removal of the needle or catheter from the artery, apply pressure to the puncture site for 15 minutes to prevent hemorrhage and development of a hematoma. Record vital signs and neurologic checks every hour for 4 hours, then every 4 hours for 24 hours. Also record intake and output.

Carefully monitor the puncture site, surrounding areas, and the distal extremity. Examine the puncture site for redness, swelling, and superficial or deep hematoma. A pressure dressing and ice bag may decrease the risk of bleeding and discomfort. When the carotid artery is used, monitor the client for respiratory distress and swallowing difficulty, which may indicate excessive edema or an expanding hematoma. For femoral or brachial sites, monitor pulses in the distal limb for 12 hours. Maintain the limb in an extended position and observe it for normal temperature, color, and sensation. Do not monitor blood pressures in the involved arm. Notify the physician immediately of any untoward effects. The client should rest quietly in bed for 12 to 24 hours, with diet and medications given as tolerated.

Pneumoencephalography

Pneumoencephalography (PEG) is a radiographic study to detect small tumors of the cerebral ventricles, cisterns, and intraspinal and intracranial subarachnoid spaces and to visualize the pituitary gland, which is positioned below the ventricles. PEG is seldom used now because less painful and less dangerous tests are available. PEG is contraindicated if there is risk of herniation or if a lumbar puncture (LP) has been done within the last 9 days (Conway–Rutkowski, 1982).

PEG is carried out in a special procedures room. The client is strapped into a motorized chair that can be moved in various directions. A contrast gas (oxygen, room air, or other gas) is injected into the subarachnoid space via an LP or via a cisternal or ventricular tap if LP is contraindicated. Clients are normally sedated during the procedure; those who cannot remain still because of anxiety or motor dysfunction are anesthetized.

Initially, a small amount of gas is injected and a radiogram taken to make the brain stem visible. Then small amounts of CSF are removed and gas injected until 25 to 30 mL of CSF have been replaced. With each injection of gas, the client's chair is somersaulted to help move gas into the ventricles. (Some institutions do not use a chair but have the client assume various positions on an examination table.) The needle is removed, and a series of radiograms is taken. The study takes 1 to 2 hours.

Nursing Implications. A written consent must be secured by the physician. Discuss with the client and the family the purpose and steps of PEG; the length of time required; and the common side effects of nausea, vomiting, and headache. Further teaching includes the purpose of sedation or anesthesia, postprocedure treatment, and discomfort. Headache, nausea and vomiting, photophobia, and syncope can be severe and are not unusual after PEG.

Client preparation includes fasting for 8 hours before the test; dressing in a hospital gown, pajama bottoms, and slippers; and removing dentures, partial plates, hair pins, hair nets, and jewelry. Nails must be free of polish and long hair secured with gauze. Record baseline vital signs and neurologic checks. Ask the client to void before administering preprocedure sedatives.

One or two nurses may attend the client during PEG to monitor vital signs, provide reassurance, and assist the physician. Responses of the client during PEG often include pallor, diaphoresis, a weak and rapid pulse, and a slight drop in blood pressure.

The client should be positioned flat or at no more than 30° elevation for 12 to 24 hours after PEG. The room should be quiet and dark. If the client is sedated or prone to seizures, siderails should be up and suction equipment at hand. Seizure precautions also require an airway at the bedside. Record vital signs and neurologic status, including nuchal rigidity, every 15 minutes for 2 hours, then every hour for 4 hours, and finally every 4 hours for 24 hours. Report abnormalities immediately. Positioning from side to side at least every 2 hours facilitates gas absorption and reduces the hazards of immobility. Encourage oral fluids (unless contraindicated) as soon as nausea and vomiting are controlled and monitor urinary output. Administer pain medications and antiemetics according to the client's needs, as ordered. Gradually elevate the head of the bed, beginning 12 to 24 hours after PEG. The client may begin to resume usual activities on the second day.

Electromyography and Nerve Conduction Studies

Electromyography (EMG) records electrical activity in muscle at rest and during contraction. Findings allow differentiation of muscle disease from lower motor neuron dysfunction. Recorded electrical patterns can be specific to various diseases such as myositis, dystrophy, and myasthenia gravis. EMG can be used to assess function in the spinal cord, nerve root, nerve plexus, peripheral nerves, or myoneural junction. The test can detect and measure regeneration of nerve and muscle before clinical signs appear. This information can be used to predict recovery (Snyder, 1983).

A nerve conduction test is often administered along with an EMG. This test measures the strength and speed of conduction in the sensory and motor fibers of peripheral nerves. Motor conduction studies are valued for assessing nerve damage when minor symptoms of motor weakness or atrophy exist. Sensory fiber conduction rates are especially useful for diagnosing neuropathies in clients with diabetes, alcoholism, metabolic and nutritional disorders, and trauma. Sensory nerve fiber conduction is assessed with a single electrical stimulus. The action potential is recorded by an electrode placed on the skin where the nerve is close to the surface. The recorded conduction time is compared with established norms for healthy nerves (Hickey, 1981).

Nursing Implications. Fluid or food intake is not restricted for this test. The physician may, however, request that cigarettes, coffee, tea, cola, or medications be restricted before the test. A written consent is obtained.

Educate clients about the time EMG takes (1 hour or more), steps of the procedure, the need to insert a needle into the muscle, and the changing of needle position that will probably cause discomfort. In addition, stress the need for client cooperation in flexing and relaxing muscles during the test. To prepare a client for a nerve conduction test,

outline the steps of the procedure and warn the client to expect mild electrical shocks.

Treat residual pain after the test with warm compresses and prescribed analgesics. Consult with the physician to determine whether medications withheld for the test should be resumed.

Lumbar Puncture

Lumbar puncture is an invasive procedure to obtain samples of CSF, to measure fluid pressure, and to reduce pressure in conditions such as subarachnoid hemorrhage. Lumbar puncture is also done to instill antibiotics; steroids; and dye, air, or oxygen for diagnostic studies and to evaluate CSF flow.

Lumbar puncture can be done at the bedside or in the diagnostic lab. The procedure is done with the client positioned to one side with head and knees flexed toward the abdomen. The client is assisted in maintaining this position, which separates the vertebrae, allowing the needle to enter the subarachnoid space at the level of L-3 and L-4 (Figure 36–9). Aseptic technique is required.

Contraindications for LP include skin lesions in the lumbar area, epidural infection or abscess, or lumbar deformity near the puncture site. LP is also contraindicated with increased ICP because of the risk of brain compression or herniation through the tentorial hiatus when the spinal fluid pressure is lowered. In some circumstances, such as when meningitis is suspected, it is crucial to establish a diagnosis despite the danger of the procedure, and LP may be justified.

Complications of LP include headache, transitory low back pain and root irritation, and meningitis or abscess. Headache is believed to result from the loss of CSF at the puncture site, which lowers the spinal fluid pressure and places tension on the intracranial structures.

Nursing Implications. Carefully explain the purpose of the test and steps of the procedure because clients often fear this test. Emphasize the importance of lying still in the flexed position during the LP. Inform the client of the brief episodes of pain when the anesthetic and spinal needle are inserted. A discussion of postprocedure activity is also helpful. Have the client void before the LP.

After an LP, most physicians require the client to remain flat in bed for 4 to 24 hours, but turning should be encouraged. Forcing fluids will help to promote replacement of withdrawn spinal fluid. Headaches, experienced by many, can be treated with prescribed analgesics. Carefully monitor vital signs and neurologic status including signs of increased ICP and root pain radiating down the back of the leg. Observe for signs of meningitis and drainage or discharge at the puncture site. Report abnormal findings to the physician.

Cisternal Puncture

Cisternal puncture is an alternative procedure for obtaining CSF used when lumbar puncture is contraindicated. For

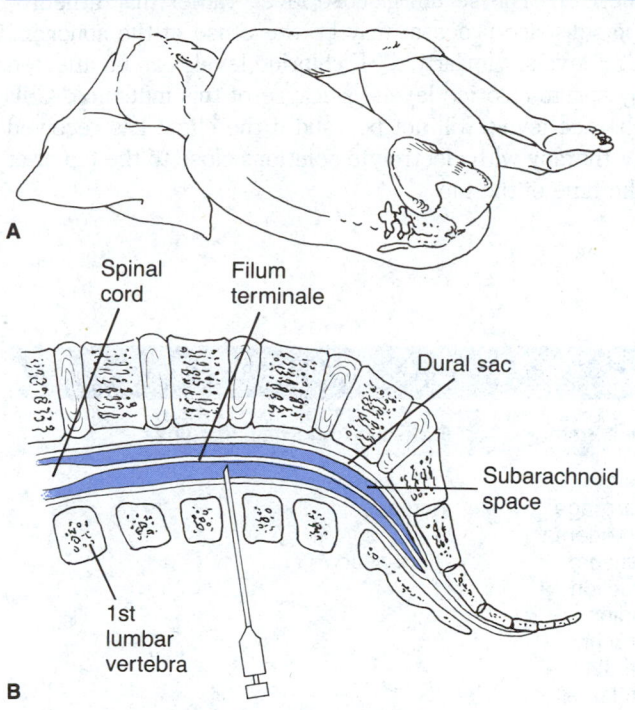

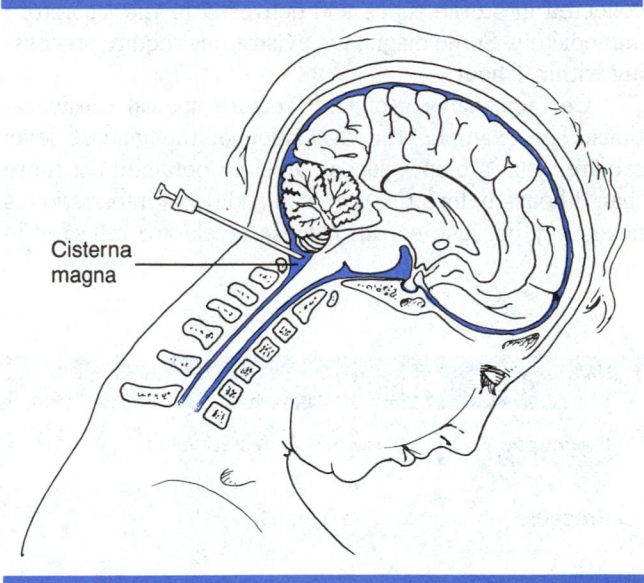

Figure 36–10

Cisternal puncture showing position of the needle.

Figure 36–9

Lumbar puncture. **A.** Client position for lumbar puncture with neck and hips flexed to increase space between the vertebrae. **B.** Position of the spinal needle in the subarachnoid space, below the termination of the spinal cord.

this test, the client's head should be flexed forward so it touches the chest. A short beveled needle is inserted into the subarachnoid space of the cisterna magna (Figure 36–10). Cisternal punctures are hazardous because of the closeness of the brain stem.

Nursing Implications. Preprocedure care is the same as for lumbar puncture. Bed rest is usually maintained for several hours after the procedure. Observe respiratory and cardiac function frequently because of the puncture's proximity to medullary centers controlling these functions. Headaches are uncommon.

Myelogram

In a myelogram, fluoroscopy and radiography are combined to study the subarachnoid space, spinal cord, and vertebral bodies. The test reveals spinal cord tumors, herniated or ruptured intervertebral disks, and nerve root injury. In this study, a spinal tap is used to replace a small amount of CSF with a radiopaque dye or gas. The client is positioned on a movable table that tilts to various positions to allow the flow of dye through the subarachnoid space. Abnormalities in flow provide the diagnostic information.

Nursing Implications. Explain the procedure and postprocedure routine. Determine any client allergies to iodine, shellfish, or radiographic dye, and obtain a written consent from the client. Maintain the client in a fasting

state for 4 to 8 hours, and record baseline vital signs and neurologic status. Administer a cleansing enema to reduce x-ray shadows, a sedative to relax the client, and atropine to reduce secretions, as ordered.

Client education should cover information about the procedure including the length of time (1 hour or more); the purpose of the LP (or cisternal puncture if lumbar deformity or skin infection is present); the usual response to the dye, which includes flushing, a warm sensation, a salty taste, headache, nausea and vomiting; the positioning and strapping to the table with the head hyperextended to prevent the dye from entering the cranium; and the need to tilt the table during the study and to remove the dye.

After the procedure, position the client's head to keep the dye from entering the cranium. The physician should order a specific head position for a prescribed period of time depending on whether an iodized oil or a water-soluble iodine contrast was used. In addition, monitor vital signs and neurologic status including nuchal rigidity, nausea and vomiting, and reports of back pain and spasms for at least 24 hours or as indicated by the institution's policy. Headache can be treated by positioning and analgesics. Encourage plenty of fluids and monitor intake and output as well as the ability to void.

Cerebrospinal Fluid Analysis

Because CSF is in contact with the components of the CNS, CSF is valuable in the diagnosis and evaluation of disease progression or healing processes. CSF is colorless and consists of water and traces of protein, glucose, sodium, chloride, and potassium (Table 36–2). The average volume in adults ranges from 100 to 150 mL. CSF pressure in the supine client ranges from 7 to 20 cm/H_2O.

The collection and handling of CSF must be carefully controlled to ensure proper analysis. The fluid must be collected in sterile tubes and delivered to the laboratory immediately. Some diagnostic evaluations require processing within 1 hour.

Certain analyses of CSF require special considerations. For example, the evaluation of the glucose level requires that a blood glucose level be obtained not more than 3 hours before the tap. The additional information is necessary because serum glucose levels are reflected in the CSF. The serum glucose level, rather than a neurologic disease process, may be the cause of the abnormal CSF levels. Similarly, CSF chloride levels can be affected by serum chloride levels. Because of this influence, CSF chloride levels will not be valid if the client has received IV therapy with electrolyte solutions close to the tap or at the time of the tap.

Table 36–2 Diagnostic Tests of Cerebrospinal Fluid

Diagnostic Test	Normal Expected Value	Disease State	Expected Abnormal Findings
Pressure	7–20 cm/H_2O	Hemorrhage, tumor, edema	Increased
		Spinal cord obstruction occluding subarachnoid space above spinal tap site	Decreased
Appearance	Clear/colorless	Presence of infection, ie, meningitis	Turbid
		Bleeding within the CNS or traumatic spinal tap	Brown, orange, or yellow 3–28 days after blood intrudes into CSF
Protein	15–40 mg/dL (albumin/globulin ratio may be useful in differential diagnosis)	Blood in CNS, meningeal irritation, viral disease, CNS syphilis, spinal block by tumor	Elevated
Glucose	45–80 mg/dL	Brain tumor, postinfectious encephalitis, systemic hyperglycemia	Increased
		Meningitis, brain abscess, subarachnoid hemorrhage	Decreased
Cell count	0–10 WBC/μL	Encephalitis and other infections, latent syphilis, demyelinating disease	Increased
VDRL	Nonreactive	Neurosyphilis	Positive (may remain positive even after effective treatment)
Chloride	113–133 mEq/L	Bacterial meningitis, decreased serum chloride concentration, tubercular meningitis	Decreased

Section II: Nursing Diagnosis

The nervous system's varied and subtle influences on other body systems may make neurologic nursing diagnoses difficult. Careful gathering and analysis of client information, physical findings, and diagnostic data will be needed. Following is a discussion of nursing diagnoses common to clients with neurologic diseases. A list of nursing diagnoses related to neurologic disorders appears in Box 36–1.

INEFFECTIVE AIRWAY CLEARANCE

Patency of the respiratory tract depends on a person's ability to maintain proper positioning, effective functioning of the muscles of respiration, and healthy respiratory tract mucosa. Neurologic diseases often cause dulled consciousness, confusion, and decreased motor function. Clients may not be able to assume positions independently that keep the tongue from obstructing the airway. Disease processes such as myasthenia gravis or ALS that affect cranial nerve function, as well as conditions affecting level of consciousness, can make it difficult to swallow or cough to clear the airway of sputum, foreign objects, or vomitus.

Ingestion of adequate fluids can be a problem for clients with various neurologic problems. Those with mental limitations may forget to drink. Those with communication problems may not be able to tell of their thirst or dry mouth. Those who are limited physically may not be able to obtain or safely ingest liquids. These situations can result in dehydration, drying, and crusting of the mucosal tissue in the oropharyngeal area and respiratory tree with damage to mucous cells and cilia. This damage compromises the individual's normal phagocytic action and ability to expel organisms, increasing the risk of respiratory tract infections.

ALTERATION IN BOWEL ELIMINATION: CONSTIPATION

Many neurologic diseases can cause constipation. Neurologic alterations can result in decreased fluid intake, decreased physical activity, inability to monitor bowel patterns, inability to initiate changes in diet to correct constipation, limitations in using toilet facilities, and increased dependence resulting in a lack of privacy.

Diseases such as stroke, myasthenia gravis, and ALS often produce paralysis of the lips, tongue, mouth, pharynx, and larynx (**bulbar paralysis**). The resultant difficulty in swallowing frequently reduces fluid intake. Stools become hard and difficult to pass.

Immobility from motor neuron damage or decreased level of consciousness limits abdominal muscle contraction, and bowel activity slows. More water is absorbed from the stool, making its passage difficult. Positioning constraints, as with spasticity or contractures, are often outcomes of neurologic diseases. These limitations can prevent a client

Box 36–1 Nursing Diagnoses Commonly Related to Nervous System Dysfunction
Diagnoses directly related to neurologic dysfunction
Airway clearance, ineffective
Bowel elimination, alteration in: constipation
Bowel elimination, alteration in: incontinence
Breathing pattern, ineffective
Cardiac output, alteration in: decreased
Communication, impaired
Mobility, impaired physical
Nutrition, alteration in: less than body requirements
Self-care deficit: feeding, bathing, hygiene, dressing, grooming, toileting
Sensory perceptual alteration: visual, auditory, kinesthetic, gustatory, tactile, olfactory
Sexual dysfunction
Urinary elimination, alteration in pattern of

from assuming positions that facilitate defecation. For example, being confined to bed for treatment of a lumbar disk problem often causes constipation brought about by both immobility and positioning constraints.

Aphasia often accompanies neurologic disease that damages the cerebral cortex. Because communication is impaired, clients may be unable to make their needs known, so they become constipated.

The client's loss of toilet privacy frequently accompanies the physical disabilities of weakness, paralysis, and immobility. Embarrassment over exposure during toilet activities and related helplessness can hamper normal defecation.

ALTERATION IN BOWEL ELIMINATION: INCONTINENCE

Bowel incontinence may accompany a wide variety of disease processes. Sphincter control can be lost because of cortical, spinal cord, or peripheral nerve damage. Recovery of control may or may not be possible. Clients whose personalities change following brain trauma may have temporary or chronic loss of bowel continence. Aphasia predisposes some clients to incontinence because they cannot express their need to defecate. Tube feedings and medications may cause diarrhea, which the physically or mentally compromised client may not be able to control.

INEFFECTIVE BREATHING PATTERNS

Changes in body functions from neurologic diseases can cause ineffective breathing that interferes with the brain stem's regulation of respiratory function. Neurologically based changes in body function—eg, decreased level of consciousness, immobility, obstruction of airway, and aspiration—can result in decreased ventilation, decreased gas exchange, and hypoxia. Hypoxia presents two threats: anoxia in vital neurons and dilation of cerebral vessels leading to an increase in ICP.

Pathological conditions producing an increase in intracranial pressure can lead to herniation, damaging respiratory centers in the brain stem. This trauma and other pathologies involving the brain stem, such as stroke or tumor, alter the rate, depth, and rhythm of respirations. Diseases, injuries, or infections affecting phrenic innervation of the diaphragm can result in loss of stimulus for breathing.

Hyperventilation can result from physical problems such as encephalitis, drug overdose, and hypoxia. It can also be initiated by psychological stress or pain, both common in neurologic diseases.

ALTERATION IN CARDIAC OUTPUT: DECREASED

Impairment of cardiac output can follow injury to the brain stem's vasomotor center, which influences cardiac function via the ANS. The brain stem's vasomotor center also controls blood pressure. With sharp elevations in blood pressure initiated to perfuse a severely edematous brain, the vasomotor center initiates reflex slowing of the heart, reduces contractility, and produces vasodilation (Price & Wilson, 1982). Cardiac output can also be compromised by anoxia stemming from alterations in respiratory function, as discussed earlier.

Decreases in vasomotor tone with various neurologic problems can affect cardiac function because of the decrease in blood returning to the heart. In addition, spinal cord injuries producing spinal shock severely decrease vasomotor tone. Orthostatic hypotension after long periods of bed rest is also the result of a loss of vasomotor tone.

IMPAIRED COMMUNICATION

Strokes, gunshot wounds, and carbon monoxide poisoning are just a few causes of damage to speech centers located in the dominant hemisphere. If Broca's area or the nerve fibers connecting Wernicke's area and Broca's area are damaged, speech may be severely limited, but understanding of one's own and others' speech will be intact. If Wernicke's area is damaged, speech may be fluent but nonsensical.

Speech can also be impaired if cranial nerves responsible for movement of the lips, tongue, oral pharynx, and larynx are injured. Damage to spinal nerves that control respirations also affects verbal communication.

Destruction or swelling of neuronal tissue in the parietal, occipital, and temporal lobes impairs perception and interpretation of stimuli including touch, sight, and hearing. All aspects of awareness needed for communication can be altered.

Limitations in motor function will also impair nonverbal forms of communication. These include writing as well as gesturing, facial expressions, and various postures that add expression to oral communication. Impaired nonverbal communication also influences the receiver's interpretation of communications because gestures, facial expressions, and posturing enhance oral communication.

IMPAIRED PHYSICAL MOBILITY

Hemiplegia from strokes, tumors, spinal cord injuries and motor deficits from peripheral nerve injury may be obvious or subtle. Subtle limitations such as decreases in range of motion (ROM), lesser involvement in activities of daily living, or unsteady gait are often first identified by the nurse, especially in clients with progressive diseases. In extrapyramidal tract diseases, which frequently complicate movement, the impairment in mobility may be difficult to detect. Nevertheless, careful analysis can reveal the clumsiness and limitations in movement resulting from tremors and rigidity.

Mobility may also be compromised by cerebellar dysfunction, alterations in sensory perception, changes in mentation, and changes in mood and energy level. Cerebellar dysfunction can produce ataxia, uncoordinated movements, and limitations in depth perception.

Damage to the parietal, temporal, and occipital lobes as well as to the sensory tract impairs an individual's ability to perceive and interact with the environment to varying degrees. Limitations from sensory deficits can often be difficult to determine and measure. Careful observation and diagnostic testing are necessary.

Activity levels frequently increase or decrease with alterations in mental function. Both states are potentially dangerous. Immobility affects all body systems. Unfortunately, the restless and confused client may also suffer from immobility if restraints are used to ensure safety. Body image changes that accompany neurologic diseases frequently lead to depression, fatigue, decreased participation in daily activities, and fewer interactions with the environment.

ALTERATION IN NUTRITION: LESS THAN BODY REQUIREMENTS

The physical, psychological, and social influences accompanying neurologic diseases can have a profound effect on an individual's nutritional status. Common physical problems that may limit intake include lack of exercise, which stimulates the appetite; inability or awkwardness in self-feeding; social isolation; difficulty in chewing and swallowing; fear of choking; and limited energy for eating.

For the individual at home, physical and mental deficits can make buying food and preparing meals challenging. A limited income (eg, because of illness-related unemployment) can also influence the amount and type of food available. As a result, the quality and quantity of food consumed may be reduced.

Sight, smell, taste, and touch—all important to an interest in eating—are altered by many neurologic diseases. In addition, mental changes from injury to the cerebral cortex or the psychological response to disease can diminish interest in eating.

SELF-CARE DEFICIT

Neurologic diseases predispose clients to many types and degrees of self-care deficits. Planning effective care depends on determining how the following factors influence the treatments and activities planned for or by the client: cause of the illness, its current and expected degree of influence on self-care, the prognosis and expected outcomes for the treatments anticipated by health care providers, the client's personality and response to deficits, and the family's interest and ability to support the client mentally and physically.

ALTERATION IN SENSORY PERCEPTION

Central and peripheral nervous system dysfunction can change one's perception of the environment and of the body's spatial relations. Parietal, occipital, and temporal lobes all have major roles in the interpretation of messages received from peripheral nerves. The interdependence of these areas within the cerebral cortex as well as with the cerebellum, subcortical areas, brain stem, and peripheral nerves influence the client's physical and mental interaction with the environment. Perceptual changes and deficits predispose the client to injury, depression, confusion, fear, and isolation.

SEXUAL DYSFUNCTION

Sexual dysfunction can result from spinal cord trauma, peripheral nerve trauma, or diseases that damage the peripheral nerves necessary for sexual activities. Medication regimens can also produce sexual dysfunction. Mental changes stemming from brain damage may result in inappropriate sexual behaviors.

ALTERATION IN URINARY ELIMINATION

Urinary retention or urinary incontinence can result from diseases affecting the cerebral cortex, spinal cord, and peripheral nervous system. With CNS dysfunction, the client often has both a dimished awareness of bladder fullness and a decreased ability to empty the bladder (Hickey, 1981). Alterations in consciousness from trauma, electrolyte imbalance, anoxia, and disease processes can produce temporary or permanent urinary incontinence.

Section III: Planning and Implementation

Clients who have neurologic health problems often require long periods of treatment and time to adapt to the changes in their lives brought on by the disease. These adaptations may involve many physical and mental changes, including the reorganization of their self-image and the adjustment of their expectations of life. Specific nursing interventions depend on when care is sought for the disease process and how the individual responds physically and mentally to the illness. A sample nursing care plan for clients with nervous system dysfunction is in Table 36–3.

PROMOTING AIRWAY CLEARANCE

For the physically impaired or **obtunded** (lethargic, drowsy) client, careful positioning with pillows and special devices promotes drainage of secretions, maintains a patent airway, and reduces the risk of aspiration. This includes careful positioning during meals, supplemental oral intake, nasogastric feedings, and oral care. A suction machine should be at hand if choking is a risk or secretions are unmanageable. Active or passive ROM exercises and frequent position changes help to promote mobilization of secretions. In

an emergency, the nurse may need to initiate the Heimlich maneuver (see Chapter 13) or oxygen therapy if obstruction is suspected.

Steps to ensure adequate hydration promote healthy respiratory function both by promoting the elimination of secretions and the destruction of organisms. Careful, ongoing assessment of the oropharyngeal mucosa, breath sounds, and ability to manage secretions are necessary because the client's condition may change quickly, and the change may not be obvious.

PREVENTING CONSTIPATION

Special nursing techniques for the client with limited motor function who needs to increase fluid intake to keep stools moist include special positioning and the use of special cups, straws, and other adaptive devices. Recognizing the client's physical and mental deficits allows for effective planning and assistance. If the client's communication is limited, family or friends may be able to suggest favored fluids and foods that will increase fluid intake and bulk to relieve or prevent constipation.

Table 36–3 Sample Nursing Care Plan for Clients With Nervous System Dysfunction

Nursing Diagnosis	Client Care Goals	Plan/Nursing Implementation	Expected Outcome
Communication, alteration in	Interact safely with environment; express needs/feelings; improve communication through speech or alternate forms of communication; adapt to alteration in lifestyle and self-image	Assess client's ability to perceive and integrate sensations; confer with other health professionals to prevent progression of communication impairment and to promote recovery; prepare and support client during diagnostic studies and treatment approaches; work with speech pathologist to develop a program to be used by health care team and family to improve communication with client; record in care plan techniques for client to use and avoid; assess client's ability to understand communications of others; record results and incorporate them in care plan; provide a safe and supportive environment that prevents sensory overload, promotes independence, limits frustration, and promotes communication efforts and adaptation of body image and lifestyle; teach client and significant others about cause of communication problems and about techniques and tools to overcome these limitations; establish a therapeutic relationship that allows time for client/family to talk about frustrations and concerns; determine client and family expectations; initiate actions to prevent sensory deprivation and isolation; support client efforts with communication by: acknowledging attempts and positive results; attending to communication; refraining from interrupting client; making short, concise statements; and using facilitative techniques, gestures and alternate communication systems when appropriate; plan for follow-up services after discharge	Communicates effectively regarding physical, intellectual, and emotional needs; attends to communications of self and others; functions effectively in the environment
Sensory perceptual alterations	Participate in activities to maintain safety and integrity of involved sensory systems and systems compensating for deficit; use compensatory methods to ensure safety and optimize interactions with the environment; make use of support from health care system and family; function at optimal safe level of independence	Assess client's ability to perceive and integrate by senses; determine effects of deficit on lifestyle (physical and psychosocial); seek therapies for control of pain (Chapter 5); consult with health team to determine cause, extent of limitations, prognosis, and therapies; provide a safe and supportive environment that allows periods of activity and rest; determine and implement techniques to preserve and enhance use of remaining senses; promote independence by teaching the use of other senses and tools	Alteration in sensory function is corrected or compensated for; no additional dysfunction occurs; pain is managed; psychological issues are resolved; client perceives the environment in an enriching and realistic manner; client develops and maintains an optimal level of function after discharge

Nursing Diagnosis	Client Care Goals	Plan/Nursing Implementation	Expected Outcome
		that can compensate for deficits; confer with OT and PT to coordinate client care goals and gain an understanding of their approaches that can be reinforced during nurse–client interactions; provide emotional support by teaching client and family about deficits; offering reassurance through explanations of therapies, adaptive devices, and available support systems; involving them in problem-solving activities to deal with deficits and crises; anticipating distress and supporting client during adaptation to changing lifestyle and body image	
Mobility, impaired physical	Actively plan and participate in activities to maintain or improve ROM; express frustrations and adapt to necessary alterations in lifestyle; seek out community groups to interact with others and gain new information regarding illness and assistance available	Assess and record ROM; evaluate potential for development of limitations in light of diagnosis, such as upper or lower motor neuron disease; plan therapies to improve or maintain current ROM through activities planned by PT, OT, and nursing and through use of splints and positioning techniques; periodically reevaluate ROM to determine effectiveness of program; confer with PT and OT regarding how spasticity may facilitate mobility or hamper positioning; assess limitations in movements resulting from tremors, rigidity, or other uncontrolled movements. Confer with OT regarding adaptive devices such as tools to facilitate dressing, weighted cups and utensils, special clothing, and self-care items to optimize levels of independence despite spasticity, rigidity, or uncontrolled movements; confer with physician regarding effectiveness of medications used to control spasticity, rigidity, or uncontrolled movements; provide emotional support, taking into account the long-term effects of illness; optimize opportunities to interact with environment in spite of limitations through activities that promote independence and feelings of usefulness and improved self-esteem; assist client and significant others in problem solving and identifying strengths and support systems; plan for discharge; teach importance of follow-up care; provide information on self-help groups, common interest groups, and community organizations	No contractures or limitations in motor function will occur, *or* Exercises and adaptive equipment will be used to limit loss of motor function or compensate for limitations in mobility; client will maintain interactions with the environment to greatest possible extent; client will share feelings about loss of mobility and will adapt lifestyle; family and community will support client physically and emotionally; client will describe purpose and side effects of medications

Privacy can often be provided to reduce embarrassment and feelings of helplessness. A Posey vest might allow safe positioning so the client can be left alone to use the toilet. A padded toilet seat or bedpan may increase comfort and promote defecation, especially for the client who has mobility problems or who is very thin. For the immobile client who is hesitant to ask for the bedpan or assistance, offering help regularly demonstrates acceptance of the client's needs and a willingness to help. If the client is unable to report symptoms or signs of constipation because of confusion, forgetfulness, or communication problems, daily monitoring of bowel function allows early treatment and prevention of constipation and impactions.

REDUCING BOWEL INCONTINENCE

Bowel incontinence presents profound psychosocial as well as physical problems. The client's frame of reference and responses must be considered. The client's unique problems determine what actions are needed.

Keep in mind that time is needed after CNS trauma for the edema to resolve and the intact neurons to resume normal activity. With time, communication can be established with aphasic clients. Precious moments are gained by having a clean bedpan in the bed and an over-the-bed trapeze available to help the client get onto the pan alone. A bedside commode is another possible solution for the client who has some warning of an impending bowel movement. The staff's strategies for prompt answering of the call light help to meet the client's physical and psychological needs. Evaluation of dietary or medication regimens and consultation with the physician and dietitian can assist in locating and eliminating bowel irritants that hamper control. Education of the client, staff, and family on the potential for control and the purpose of bowel training programs promote commitment and effort by all. A consulting psychologist may assist in developing a behavior modification program for the client with mental dysfunction.

Throughout the process of regaining bowel control, or when efforts to regain control are exhausted, the nurse must use techniques (physical and psychological) to maintain the client's dignity and self-esteem. Special underpants can keep moisture and other irritants away from the skin and control odor. These pants may allow a fairly normal lifestyle.

IMPROVING BREATHING PATTERN

Many neurologic diseases and injuries of the CNS predispose clients to ineffective respiratory function. Care for clients who are not breathing effectively may include oxygen therapy or ventilator assistance. In some instances, the equipment should be on standby in case it is needed suddenly. Notify the physician immediately if the breathing pattern becomes tachypneic, bradypneic, or markedly irregular suggesting a worsening of the client's condition.

Clients may be placed on a ventilator soon after the onset of the illness or trauma, or the ventilator may be used in the future if their disease progresses. In both instances, psychological support and special planning for client communication are needed. (Care of the client on a ventilator is discussed in Chapter 18.)

Nursing care for clients having trouble breathing because of apprehension or pain is focused on determining the cause and planning interventions. Analgesics should be given as ordered if positioning and other comfort measures are not effective and if vital signs are stable.

IMPROVING CARDIAC OUTPUT

Nurses must be knowledgeable about disease processes that threaten cardiac output, such as brain stem trauma or ANS dysfunction, to provide comprehensive monitoring of clients at risk. Nursing actions must focus on the assessment of heart rate, rhythm, and effectiveness of beat to anticipate decreases in output that could threaten the integrity of both cardiovascular and CNS function. Because of the influence of high and low blood pressures on cardiac function, blood pressure must also be carefully monitored and treatments provided to maintain a safe range. To ensure oxygenation of the heart muscle, attend to neurologic deficits hindering respiratory function. Anticipate the need for resuscitation when spinal shock (discussed in the section on spinal cord injury in Chapter 37) or other events produce hypotension.

IMPROVING COMMUNICATION

Fear, apprehension, and frustration are common feelings among clients whose ability to communicate has been impaired, no matter how long they have lived with the deficit. Focus on these client concerns and seek to optimize safe and effective communication.

Clients with sudden aphasia are frequently frightened and confused. Nursing approaches should be directed toward reducing fear and promoting communication. Working out a communication system can be a challenge for both nurse and client. Let clients know the nursing staff will keep them comfortable and informed and will be sensitive to their needs.

The nurse and all those in contact with communication-impaired clients should speak slowly and avoid lengthy questions and responses. Do not talk down to clients or treat them as if they were children. Communication can be enhanced by gestures, pantomime, writing, and other visual cues. Do not avoid talking in the client's presence because hearing conversation is thought to be therapeutic for aphasic clients.

Nursing care for the client with motor deficits hindering nonverbal communication requires a sensitivity for each client's unique limitations in sharing feelings and needs through body expression. Some examples are the masklike face common in Parkinson's disease, the loss of hand gestures with quadriplegia, and the loss of posturing in the client with ALS. After deficits are recognized, alternate routes of expression are identified and encouraged.

Nursing care for the client with verbal impairment and/or diminished or altered sensory function should focus on the promotion of understanding through senses that are still functional. Consultation with the physician and speech pathologist is helpful to determine the most effective therapy.

IMPROVING PHYSICAL MOBILITY

Nursing actions must focus on both the physical and psychological needs of clients with impaired mobility. Approaches must consider the extent of limitations, the cause of the disability, the prognosis, the client's physical and emotional strengths, and the availability of family and community support.

Assess the client's gait deficit (eg, the spastic gait of a client with hemiplegia) or lack of muscle coordination (ataxia), both of which can cause postural instability. Consult with the physical therapist in developing a plan for maximum client mobility. Arrange for an evaluation of the client's home environment. Are there stairs to be climbed? Is the bathroom on the same floor as the bedroom? Are there safety hazards (eg, throw rugs or cords extending across floors)? Is there a shower, or will the client have to use a bathtub? These factors influence the client's rehabilitation program.

IMPROVING NUTRITION

Physical problems of neurologic origin—eg, weakness, limited ability to feed oneself, or a decreased level of consciousness—frequently mean clients have difficulty eating. Adaptive devices to facilitate cutting and eating food, supplemental feedings, arranging for someone to assist the client with food shopping and meal preparation, and contact with organizations like Meals-on-Wheels may help correct the nutritional problems.

Depression, isolation, and fear are common psychosocial problems that often contribute to a disinterest in food. Plans to correct such situations consider each client's needs. Plans might include encouraging involvement of the family at mealtime, arranging for the client to eat with others on the unit, or providing music and special positioning at mealtime.

IMPROVING SELF-CARE ABILITY

At times, the seriously ill or physically impaired client needs the nurse or family members to provide what are normally self-care activities. Meeting these needs in a supportive manner promotes feelings of safety and security that can foster recovery or adaptation to a change in lifestyle.

If and when a client is able to begin to participate in self-care, the nurse's role gradually changes to that of facilitator to encourage the client's effort and to reduce frustration in learning to overcome physical impairments. Nursing actions must be specific for each client's needs. When possible, work closely with the occupational therapist to encourage the client to apply skills learned during therapy and during nurse–client interactions.

IMPROVING SENSORY PERCEPTION

Nursing interventions must be based on each client's specific changes or deficits in sensory perception. Often, there are multiple sensory deficits that, depending on the diagnosis, will decrease or extend rapidly.

Nursing assessment of the client's ability to interact effectively with the environment as well as diagnostic studies and evaluation by the occupational therapist are guides for planning care. Interventions should focus on client safety, optimal awareness of the environment, and therapies to help the client learn to use remaining senses to live with the deficit and to function at the highest possible level of independence, both in the hospital and at home.

Psychological support will be needed for the client and significant others because even one area of sensory loss produces major changes in lifestyle. The nurse, too, may need to seek support, because caring for a client with severe deficits may be difficult to cope with if recovery is slow or limited.

IMPROVING SEXUAL FUNCTION

Nursing care for the client with sexual dysfunction seeks to create an atmosphere in which clients feel comfortable in expressing their concerns. The nurse can facilitate discussion by maintaining a professional and matter-of-fact approach toward body functions. If inappropriate behaviors result because of mental changes, maintain a professional approach. Behavior modification or psychotherapy may be needed. Consultation with a mental health–psychiatric nursing clinical specialist can be helpful to clients, family members, and nursing staff.

IMPROVING URINARY ELIMINATION

Work closely with the physician to determine the cause of the incontinence and the client's potential for regaining control. Diagnostic procedures, such as cystometrography (see Chapter 32) may be needed.

Bladder training programs consisting of regularly scheduled attempts to void help many clients with cortical injury to relearn bladder control. Partial control of function may keep the client continent if steps are taken to provide frequent toileting or access to toilet equipment. Intermittent self-catheterization may be an option for some clients with urinary retention.

Special pants for incontinent clients that protect the skin and control odor may be helpful for the client who is unable to regain control. These pants reduce the need for dependence on an in-dwelling catheter.

There is a potential for urinary retention after sur-gery, myelogram, or LP, which increases the risk of urinary tract infections and reflux into the ureters. Carefully monitor client voiding patterns after any of these procedures and accurately record urine output.

Section IV: Evaluation

Recovery from neurologic diseases or adaption to changes from these conditions is often a long process with small successes and setbacks. In some instances, care will be planned to support the dying client. In any case, care should be designed to allow optimal client involvement in decision making about his or her life.

Clients' responses to the plan of care vary. Some responses are easily recognized; others are subtle or hidden. In seeking to promote the client's achievement of care goals, carefully monitor the client's responses to identify effective and ineffective nursing interventions. Prompt identification of ineffective approaches is essential so new interventions can be developed to support vital neuronal tissue, to maintain the client's physical and mental capabilities, and to control energy-draining frustration.

Nursing care plans will be revised frequently because of the nervous system's complex influence on body functions and clients' unique responses. Patience, perseverance, determination, creativity, and hope must be woven into each client care goal and nursing intervention.

Chapter Highlights

A major focus of nursing care for the client with neurologic disease is to prevent the disease from progressing, because damaged neurons are irreparable.

The nervous system is predisposed to a wide variety of diseases and traumas because of its complex and widespread structures.

The nervous system is vulnerable to diseases affecting other body systems.

The nervous system's influence over other body systems may produce symptoms suggesting malfunction of other systems.

Physiological and psychosocial lifestyle influences affect the client's response to neurologic disease during all stages of the illness.

Although some deficits from neurologic disease processes do not cause obvious structural changes, they may produce severely limiting disabilities that last a lifetime.

Clients require support when diagnostic studies are ordered because most neurologic tests are invasive, lengthy, and frightening; they often produce considerable discomfort and involve some risk to the client.

Nursing assessment must be an ongoing process for clients with neurologic disease because improvement or decline in their condition will require prompt changes in the plan of care.

Nursing interventions for clients with neurologic diseases often involve supportive measures for other body systems the nervous system can no longer effectively control.

Family members and significant others of clients with neurologic disease are often presented with monumental physical and psychosocial challenges.

Bibliography

Assessment. Springhouse, PA: Intermed, 1982.

Bates B: *A Guide to Physical Examination*, 3rd ed. Philadelphia: Lippincott, 1983.

Chusid JG: *Correlative Neuroanatomy & Functional Neurology*, 19th ed. Los Altos, CA: Lange, 1985.

Conway–Rutkowski BL: *Carini and Owens' Neurological and Neurosurgical Nursing*, 8th ed. St Louis: Mosby, 1982.

Diagnostics. Springhouse, PA: Intermed, 1982.

Goldberg B, Chiverton P: Assessing behavior: The nurse's mental status exam. *Geriatr Nurs* (March-April) 1984; 94–98.

Hackett C: Limbering up your neurovascular assessment technique. *Nurs 83* (March) 1983; 13:40–43.

Hickey J: *Clinical Practice of Neurological and Neurosurgical Nursing.* Philadelphia: Lippincott, 1981.

Kallail KJ, Hemphill MK: Notes from a young aphasic patient in a nursing home. *Nurs Health Care* 1985; 6:379–381.

Price SA, Wilson LM: *Pathophysiology: Clinical Concepts of Disease Processes*, 2nd ed. New York: McGraw–Hill, 1982.

Samuels MA: *Manual of Neurologic Therapeutics*, 2nd ed. Boston: Little, Brown, 1982.

Snyder M (editor): *A Guide to Neurological and Neurosurgical Nursing*. New York: Wiley, 1983.

Whitney FW: Guidelines for neurological consultation. *Nurse Pract* (July-Aug) 1982; 7:13–18.

Suggested Readings

Konikow NS: Alterations in movement: Nursing assessment and implications. *J Neurosurg Nurs* (Feb) 1985; 17(1):61–65. This article discusses assessment, pathophysiology, implications for daily living, and nursing implications for selected functional aspects of movement: seeing, eating, speaking, facial expressions, moving, and walking.

Ozuna J: Alterations in mentation: Nursing assessment and intervention. *J Neurosurg Nurs* (Feb) 1985; 17(1):66–70. This article discusses assessment, pathophysiology, implications for daily living, and nursing interventions for selected functional aspects of mentation: language, memory, and performing learned movements.

Resources

ORGANIZATIONS

Alzheimer's Disease and Related Disorders Association (ADRDA)
360 N Michigan Ave
Chicago, IL 60601
Phone: (800) 621–0379; in Illinois (800) 572–6037
   This organization provides information to the public and to health professionals, advocates and aids research, provides emotional support to family and friends, and makes referrals to other appropriate services.

American Parkinson's Disease Association
116 John St
New York, NY 10038
   Thirteen satellite centers throughout the United States maintain extensive information for the public and health professionals, and offer diagnostic and treatment services.

Committee to Combat Huntington's Disease
250 W 57th St
New York, NY 10019
Phone: (212) 757–0443
   This organization of family, friends, health professionals, and researchers sponsors educational programs and raises funds for research.

Epilepsy Foundation of America
4351 Garden City Dr
Suite 406
Landover, MD 20785
   This voluntary organization provides information on seizure disorders, referrals, advocates the civil rights of persons with seizure disorders, monitors related legislative activity, and sponsors self-help groups for clients and their families. Members are eligible for discount prescription drugs and life insurance at group rates.

Muscular Dystrophy Association
810 Seventh Ave
New York, NY 10019
Phone: (212) 586–0808
   Comprehensive free client care programs are offered by this voluntary health agency. It also sponsors a worldwide research program.

Myasthenia Gravis Foundation, Inc
15 E 26th St
New York, NY 10010
Phone: (212) 889–8157
   Chapters throughout the United States provide education, raise funds for research, and sponsor low-cost diagnostic and treatment clinics and discount drug plans.

National ALS (Amyotrophic Lateral Sclerosis) Foundation Inc
185 Madison Ave
New York, NY 10016
Phone: (212) 679–4016
   The ALS maintains an information bureau, recommends neurologists who specialize in the treatment of ALS, directs clients and families to manufacturers of aids and appliances, and raises funds for research. Volunteers with personal experience are available to answer letters and telephone calls. A free outpatient clinic operates out of Mount Sinai Medical Center in New York City.

National Ataxia Foundation
6681 Country Club Dr
Minneapolis, MN 55427
Phone: (612) 546–6220
   This organization sponsors a network of clinics for persons with ataxia and offers referrals for medical, social, emotional, and financial support.

National Huntington's Disease Association
128A E 74th St
New York, NY 10021
Phone: (212) 744–0302
   This agency maintains a comprehensive listing of specialists and is actively engaged in supporting research.

National Migraine Foundation
5214 N Western Ave
Chicago, IL 60625
Phone: (312) 878–7715
   This nonprofit organization makes information available and offers referrals to health professionals who are members of the American Association for the Study of Headache.

National Multiple Sclerosis Society
205 E 42nd St
New York, NY 10017
Phone: (212) 986–3240
   Chapters throughout the United States sponsor diagnostic and treatment clinics, group recreation programs, personal counseling by trained volunteers, and free loan of equipment and appliances.

National Paraplegia Foundation
333 N Michigan Ave
Chicago, IL 60601
Phone: (312) 346–4779
   This voluntary health agency encourages research and helps paraplegics through self-help, counseling, and information services. Volunteer counselors help clients adjust to wheel-

chair living. Offers referral to sources that provide special equipment.

Parkinson's Disease Foundation
William Black Medical Research Building
Columbia University Medical Center
640–650 W 168th St
New York, NY 10032
Phone: (212) 923–4700

Offering information and referral for persons with Parkinson's Disease and other diseases of the basal ganglia, this organization serves as a clearinghouse for clients, families, and health professionals.

US Government
National Institute of Neurological and Communicative Disorders and Stroke
Bethesda, MD 20205
Phone: (301) 496–5751

In Canada:

Canadian Paraplegic Association
520 Sutherland Dr
Toronto, Ontario M4G3V9
Phone: (416) 423–5690

Multiple Sclerosis Society of Canada
130 Bloor St W, Suite 700
Toronto, Ontario M5S1N5
Phone: (416) 924–4406

Migraine Foundation
390 Brunswick Ave
Toronto, Ontario M5R2Z4
Phone: (416) 920–4916

HOT LINES

Counseling for families and friends of those with Alzheimer's disease and related diseases (Alzheimer's Disease and Related Disorders Association)
Phone: (612) 830–1043

Counseling for psychological support for clients with amyotrophic lateral sclerosis (National ALS Foundation)
Phone: (212) 679–4016

NURSING ORGANIZATIONS

American Association of Neuroscience Nurses
22 S Washington St, Suite 203
Park Ridge, IL 60068
Phone: (312) 823–9850

Members include RNs actively engaged or primarily interested in neurological or neurosurgical nursing. Dues, $53 a year.

Association of Rehabilitation Nurses
2506 Gross Point Rd
Evanston, IL 60201
Phone: (312) 475–7530

Members include RNs interested in rehabilitative nursing practice. Dues, $40 a year.

Chapter 37

Specific Disorders Affecting the Central Nervous System

Susan Nevins

Objectives

When you have finished studying this chapter, you should be able to:

Explain the transmission mechanism and types of muscular dystrophy and list the priorities of nursing care.

Describe the manifestations of Huntington's chorea and the nursing care needed as the disease progresses.

Describe the clinical manifestations of neurofibromatosis (NF) and the role of the nurse in working with clients and their significant others.

Identify the mechanisms by which vascular abnormalities affect CNS functions.

Enumerate the nursing precautions with clients having possible subarachnoid hemorrhage from a ruptured cerebral aneurysm.

Anticipate the nursing interventions for clients with seizures.

Compare and contrast the common types of headache and their management.

Identify the risk factors for cerebrovascular accident and discuss the role of the nurse in stroke prevention.

Distinguish among Alzheimer's disease, Parkinson's disease, and amyotrophic lateral sclerosis and describe nursing care priorities for each.

Compare and contrast myasthenia gravis and multiple sclerosis and describe nursing care priorities for each.

Specify the routes by which pathogens gain access to the CNS and possible clinical manifestations of an infection of the meninges or brain tissue.

Describe the problems that occur from compression of cranial or spinal structures by tumors.

Discuss the principal types of head trauma and spinal injuries, their treatment, and specific nursing responsibilities.

Diseases of the central nervous system include those of congenital, multifactorial, degenerative, immunologic, infectious, neoplastic, and traumatic origin. Because of the complexity of the nervous system, symptoms and signs associated with malfunction are multiple and varied. Many of the disorders in this chapter (eg, Alzheimer's disease, cerebrovascular accident, and spinal cord injuries) cause severe physiological and psychosocial/lifestyle problems for clients* and their significant others and present a tremendous challenge to the health care team.

Section I: Congenital Disorders

A congenital disorder of the central nervous system (CNS) can be defined as a developmental defect. A variety of these defects may be present at birth. Although the causes of maldevelopments are often unknown, a majority are considered to result from the hereditary transmission of a

---

*The term client has been used here and in Chapter 38 in referring to the person receiving care, even though it is inconsistent with my professional philosophy. In the setting in which I practice, recipients of care are considered patients. S. Nevins

chromosomal abnormality or are secondary to embryonic damage from teratogenic agents.

The developing CNS in the fetus is particularly vulnerable to radiation effects, anoxia, metabolic diseases, and infections in the mother. The range of prenatal, perinatal, and postnatal factors will be illustrated in this section in the discussion of cerebral palsy and seizure disorders. Prenatal developmental defects will be discussed with diseases of the vascular system such as intracranial aneurysms and cerebral arteriovenous malformations.

Neurologic development in the fetus occurs early, often before women have recognized or confirmed their pregnancies. If prenatal care and appropriate health information are not provided early enough, risk for exposure to teratogenic agents is greater. The nurse can assume a major role in helping to prevent developmental defects through health teaching. Important aspects of teaching include dietary instructions, discussion of the effects of harmful agents, alterations in activities during pregnancy, and early and continuous prenatal care (Conway-Rutowski, 1982).

CEREBRAL PALSY

Cerebral palsy (CP) is not a disease entity per se but a variety of neuromotor disorders resulting from cerebral hypoxia or damage to the nervous system in utero, at birth, or in early life. CP occurs most often in infants born prematurely or after a difficult labor, at the rate of about 2 cases per 1000 live births (Merrit, 1979). The incidence has decreased because of better prenatal and obstetrical care but may increase because improved neonatal care has improved the survival rate of affected individuals.

CP affects primarily control of the voluntary motor system, involving various areas of the brain including the basal ganglia, motor cortex, cerebellum, and sometimes the sensory cortex. Paralytic symptoms in infancy or childhood are categorized into five types: spastic, athetoid, ataxic, rigid, and tremorous. They account for the largest single cause of crippling in children.

Causal factors can be divided into four groups:

- Genetic defects associated with chromosomal abnormalities.
- Prenatal factors including maternal infections (eg, rubella, cytomegalovirus, and toxoplasmosis), irradiation, harmful drug intake, malnutrition, toxemia, and diabetes during pregnancy. Rh and ABO blood incompatibilities may affect prenatal and postnatal states.
- Perinatal factors causing anoxia of the brain, such as difficult breech and midforceps deliveries, improper anesthesia during labor and delivery, premature birth, and low birth weight.
- Postnatal factors including injury to the neonate's brain by cerebral vascular lesions, infections, trauma, and malnutrition; prolonged convulsive seizures may produce severe brain damage if anoxia is extensive.

CP can afflict anyone during fetal development, birth, or the neonatal stage. Although maternal age, race, and economic status have not been correlated with cerebral palsy, developmental disorders are more frequent in infants of mothers in their teens or over age 35. The most recent data from computerized tomography (CT) scanning confirm that perinatal and/or postnatal cerebral vascular bleeding is the major cause.

The symptoms and signs of cerebral palsy are variable, ranging from mild muscle incoordination to a severe spasticity. Cerebral atrophy accounts for clinical findings. In addition to the range of motor deficits, there may be signs of injury to the somatic sensory cortex, optic pathways, or speech centers. Resultant sensory deficits are agnosia, apraxia, and hemianopia. Dysphasias may be manifestations of sensory or motor impairments. Intellectual performance is often hampered by seizures, speech, visual, hearing, and motor impairments. Because of these deficits, individuals with CP often develop serious emotional and social problems. In addition, at least half have mental retardation as a primary aspect of the disorder.

CP is usually diagnosed within the first year of a client's life. For more information about its diagnosis and treatment consult a pediatric text. Because many clients with CP live into adulthood and develop other health problems, the nurse working in adult health settings should have some knowledge of physiological and psychosocial/lifestyle effects of CP.

MUSCULAR DYSTROPHY

Muscular dystrophy is a hereditary, degenerative neuromuscular disorder characterized by chronic, progressive wasting and weakness of voluntary muscles. The Muscular Dystrophy Association estimates there are 4 to 9 cases per 100,000 population in the United States, or 200,000 identified clients (Panel of Neuromuscular Disorders: HEW, 1979). Far more common in men than women, the disease affects both children and young adults.

Recent research on muscular dystrophy has shown that the surface membrane of muscle cells are abnormally permeable. Defective cells leak proteins and other molecules that should be retained. Electron microscopy shows interruptions in surface membranes, and a new technique called "freeze-fracture" enables the internal surface of these membranes to be examined.

Recognizing the biochemical abnormalities in muscular dystrophies is advantageous. Carriers of the gene could be better identified, improving genetic counseling. Affected infants could be identified in utero through amniocentesis. Most beneficial would be the development of biochemical repair treatments for affected individuals, similar to insulin therapy for diabetics.

The five different types of muscular dystrophy vary in the age of onset, rate of symptom progression, and clinical manifestations. All types exhibit degenerative changes in the muscle fibers. The myofibrils are destroyed, and striated muscle is replaced by connective tissue and fatty deposits. Muscles appear hypertrophic or pseudo-hypertrophic, varying greatly in size (normal muscles are uniform). *Pseudohypertrophic muscular dystrophy,* also known as the Duchenne type, is an X-linked recessive disorder with a high mutation rate transmitted by unaffected females (carriers). The disease affects only males, usually in the first 4 years of life. There is a 50% chance that any son of a female carrier will be affected and a high risk that any daughter will become a carrier. *Facioscapulohumeral* muscular dystrophy is inherited as an autosomal dominant trait that can be transmitted by either parent and affects both sexes equally. About 50% of the offspring may inherit the disease. Although onset varies, it usually manifests itself in adolescence. *Limb-girdle* muscular dystrophy is usually transmitted as an autosomal recessive trait to the children of parents who both carry defective genes. The offspring will be 50% carriers, 25% affected, and 25% free of hereditary defect (Conway-Rutowski, 1982). This type affects males and females, with onset usually in adolescence. *Myotonic* muscular dystrophy is inherited as an autosomal dominant trait affecting both sexes but is more common in males. Its frequency is one-fourth that of Duchenne dystrophy. *Ocular* muscular dystrophy is a rare form of the disease that can be inherited as either a dominant or recessive autosomal trait. The usual onset is in later middle years; more rarely, it occurs in adolescence.

Clinical Manifestations

Pseudohypertrophic (Duchenne) muscular dystrophy is the most common (50%) and the most severe form, marked by a rapid course. Bilateral muscle weakness occurs involving proximal muscles. There is a progressive involvement of all voluntary muscles with confinement to a wheelchair expected in the second decade. Failure of cardiac or respiratory musculature usually leads to death in the second or third decades of life. Paradoxically, the affected muscles suggest strength because they are enlarged by excess fat. Muscles primarily affected are the deltoid, quadriceps, and gastrocnemius. The disability is often first noted by parents who observe the child's difficulty walking, running, and climbing stairs. A waddling gait, lordosis, and marked difficulty rising from the supine to standing position *(Gowers' sign)* occur. The increasing disability is hard to understand when the muscles appear so well "developed." As the disease progresses, facial, oropharyngeal, and respiratory muscles become involved. Incidence of mental retardation is high in this type.

The major diagnostic tests include serum creatine kinase (CK), electromyography (EMG), muscle biopsy, and electrocardiogram (ECG). The CK is markedly elevated to 1000 or 2000 units. The EMG shows typical myopathic changes. The muscle biopsy finds wide variations in muscle size as well as enlargement and wasting. Finally, an ECG demonstrates changes in the cardiac musculature as the disease progresses (Wilson, 1979).

Facioscapulohumeral muscular dystrophy affects the muscles of the face, shoulder girdle, and upper arms, as its name suggests. The disease is most pronounced in the shoulder girdle. Later it can involve all voluntary muscles. Because its onset is later than the Duchenne type and its progression is slow, clients usually have a much longer life span. Muscle biopsy and EMG show typical degenerative changes. The CK, however, might be normal because of the slow progression.

Limb-girdle muscular dystrophy has a slow course, involving the shoulder or pelvic girdle first. The disease either ascends or descends as it progresses. The disability is noted with activities of daily living such as combing hair, dressing, and climbing stairs. The symptoms may be minimal, persisting for years, a particular characteristic of clients who start with shoulder-girdle involvement. The diagnostic tests are the same as for the Duchenne type.

In myotonic muscular dystrophy the onset of symptoms is often difficult to detect because the myotonia usually appears in childhood, but the muscular wasting develops later in the teens or early 20s. Another form of myotonia starts in infancy, producing marked sucking and swallowing difficulties. Mental retardation may be severe, although there is a lack of limb weakness and peripheral myotonia. Clinical signs of later onset include facial diplegia, ptosis, myotonia, and dysarthria. There is a marked wasting of face, neck, and shoulder. Facial muscles may also be weak, especially the orbicularis oculi muscle of the eye. Eventually the eyes may become fixed in midline. Clients may also develop dysphagia. In later stages, the trunk and extremities are affected. The most characteristic sign is the failure of muscles, especially hand muscles, to relax fully after a strong contraction. There is a high frequency of cataracts and mental retardation. Males have early baldness and impotence. Females have early menopause. The disease runs a slow course, often with great longevity; it is not uncommon to find clients who are bedridden, incapacitated, and institutionalized. Diagnosis is based on family history of the disease with signs of glandular dysfunction, alopecia, and cataracts. The EMG shows marked myopathy. CK is only of value when muscle wasting is significant. ECG abnormalities are common, evidenced by atrioventricular conduction problems.

Ocular muscular dystrophy is characterized by degenerative changes in the eye muscles and lids. Clinical findings include progressive ptosis, diplopia or strabismus, and restrictions in eye movements.

Therapeutic Measures

There is no cure for the muscular dystrophies. Accurate diagnosis is essential, however, to rule out similar muscle diseases for which effective treatments are available.

Muscular dystrophy clients can be helped with supportive interventions. Physical therapy may enable clients to gain optimal use of affected muscles. Muscle stretching helps prevent contractures. Tendon-lengthening surgeries have varying degrees of success. Assistive devices are invaluable.

Specific Nursing Measures

The major nursing priority for the muscular dystrophy client is the management of the progressive impairments in mobility. The client must be assisted to remain physically active as long as possible. Physical therapy regimens are essential; stretching and resistive exercises preserve joint range of motion (ROM), prevent or minimize contractures, decrease atrophy, and promote mobility. Exercises should be done at least twice a day for the outpatient and four times a day for the hospitalized client. Each joint should be put through its normal arc of motion as tolerated. Avoid moving a joint beyond the point of resistance. Never apply force, and stop the exercises whenever the client has pain. The body should be in proper alignment before beginning exercises. All motions should be gentle, slow, and rhythmic. Each sequence is done three times, unless otherwise prescribed.

Clients with muscle spasticity experience an increased tonus in a weak muscle. The nursing objective is to promote muscle relaxation and prevent complications such as contractures, muscle atrophy, pressure sores, and urinary tract infections. When a spastic limb is initially guided through ROM, it is more resistive to stretching than at the end of an exercise when there is a sudden loss of resistance. Changes in position also can be helpful. Teach clients and their families to avoid stimuli that can increase spasticity such as fatigue, tightening of muscles, maintaining one position for too long, and cold temperatures.

Braces may be needed to stabilize the lower limbs and trunk. They must be light enough for weakened muscles to support. Assistive devices to recommend are bed trapezes, handrails, and raised toilet seats for home use. A wheelchair may be necessary.

Many clients who develop muscular dystrophy in late adolescence and early adulthood have had good health until onset of the disease. These clients may develop anticipatory grieving related to the progressive loss of mobility. The nurse can be a major support in helping clients accept the fact that there is no cure for their disability at present and that they will always have to cope with its problems.

Handicapped individuals are often overprotected by their immediate families and friends. An overprotective attitude may result from feelings of guilt, anger, and pity. Help the family to recognize these feelings are normal and expected. Otherwise, ineffective family coping patterns may develop that further disable the client.

Individuals with muscular dystrophy may have to develop more realistic role performance goals such as developing skills in verbal, visual, and auditory communication and identifying other alternatives when physical disabilities increase.

Management of alteration in nutritional intake is another nursing priority. The physical inactivity of these clients may contribute to overweight. It is crucial to provide for optimal energy needs while preventing unnecessary weight gain. Although clients have limited mobility, they can gain independence through decision making. The goal is to promote independence as long as possible.

Control of nutritional patterns is one goal they can realistically achieve. Clients can participate in planning menus, preparing grocery lists, or finding new recipes. Foods to emphasize include citrus fruits, green leafy and deep-yellow vegetables, milk, poultry, and fish. Clients can plan meal schedules that permit smaller, more frequent meals. Evaluation of weight patterns and energy requirements help clients to maintain or adjust plans.

HUNTINGTON'S CHOREA

Huntington's chorea is a rare hereditary disease of the CNS. The disorder is progressive, degenerative, and fatal. The disease is characterized by severe choreiform movements and mental deterioration. Although the disease was recognized as a clinical entity over 100 years ago, public awareness lagged. Afflicted persons were often concealed by their families. The disorder was poorly understood and misdiagnosed. Insanity and suicide were not uncommon outcomes for its sufferers. In the late 1960s, public attention was finally focused on the disease when Woody Guthrie, a prominent folk singer and composer, died from its effects. His wife founded the Committee to Combat Huntington's Disease (CCHD).

Huntington's chorea is inherited through an autosomal dominant gene with full penetrance. Therefore, 50% of the children of affected individuals eventually inherit the disease. Either the male or female parent can transmit the disease, which does not skip generations. Those who have not inherited the disease cannot transmit it. Rarely, new mutations occur.

Documenting the incidence of Huntington's chorea is difficult because of the reluctance of family members to report cases. The disorder affects all ethnic groups and occurs worldwide. The CCHD claims an incidence of 50,000 in the United States.

Clinical Manifestations

The disorder usually develops insidiously and runs its course over 15 to 20 years. Onset is usually in middle life (ages 35 to 40). The earlier the age of onset, the more rapid the deterioration. The primary signs include chorea and dementia combined with a positive family history.

The choreiform movements are the most striking characteristics. They begin slowly, usually first in the face and upper extremities. Facial grimacing and jerking limb movements occur. Over time, movements become frequent, erratic, and violent. The trunk and legs become involved. A twisted, prancing gait is a hallmark finding. Communication becomes poor with increasing dysarthric, unintelligible speech. Volitional activity becomes limited because of the severity of involuntary movements and incoordination.

The mental aberration resembles the organic dementias. Early behavioral changes include periods of irritability, labile mood swings, and impulsiveness. Periods of apathy, elation, depression, and aggression can be expected. Progressive memory impairment, inattention to personal hygiene, and decreased intellectual capacity accompany the personality changes. Poor judgment results. Increased supervision is required for activities of daily living. Some clients become overtly psychotic.

Additional neurologic findings include muscular rigidity and seizures in the end stages of classic Huntington's chorea. Abnormal plantar responses and hyperactive deep tendon reflexes (DTRs) may be observed. Death is usually from cardiac or respiratory failure, extreme systemic exhaustion, or suicide.

Diagnosis is best made by the classic symptoms mentioned earlier. Diagnostic findings include diffuse abnormalities on electroencephalogram (EEG) and a CT scan of the brain, showing enlargement of the ventricles and degenerative changes in the caudate nucleus. Urine, blood, and cerebrospinal fluid (CSF) studies are normal; plasma growth hormone levels are abnormal (Merritt, 1979).

Therapeutic Measures

Treatment is difficult. There are no known methods of arresting the disease. Current research indicates a defect in metabolism of gamma-aminobutyric acid (GABA) and an increased amount of dopamine compared to acetylcholine. Precursors have been used to elevate GABA levels by inhibiting its catabolism.

Drug regimens have been generally unsuccessful. Low doses of bromocriptine have been used to achieve dopamine blocking, with outcomes similar to those with phenothiazines. Choreiform movements have been symptomatically controlled with phenothiazines or butyrophenones. These antipsychotic medications must be carefully balanced to decrease chorea symptoms but not worsen depression or promote tardive dyskinesia (continued movements of the lips, tongue, and face that occur late in the course of drug treatment).

More promising is choline, a precursor of the neurotransmitter acetylcholine. Choline lessens aberrant movements without causing the side effects of the neuroleptic drugs. Drug therapy is only an adjunct to the supervised management of the client's activities of daily living as mental deterioration progresses.

Specific Nursing Measures

The chronic, disabling nature of this disorder requires nursing interventions that are preventive, protective, and supportive. These clients are at high risk for injury. As the choreiform movements become more abnormal, a safe physical environment must be maintained, with precautions similar to those for seizures. Restraints are not recommended because they may increase the risk of injury and heighten abnormal movements. The client's immediate environment should be monitored for any objects that pose a safety threat. If the client becomes bedridden, padded siderails can prevent falls from the bed when spasms are severe.

Subtle stages of mental deterioration may occur before alterations in cognitive function. Slight alterations in personality may be the first clues: clients find fault with family members and complain about them. They may soon become irritable, suspicious, eccentric, and unpredictable. Behavioral outbursts may show poor self-control, such as temper tantrums and sexual or alcohol abuse. Astute observations of personality changes are crucial. The risk of suicide increases when apathy and depression worsen, but clues to risks may not be obvious because of mental status changes.

Cognitive deficits invariably follow. One of the first signs is memory loss, especially recall of names of common objects. Inattention becomes evident. Gradually, signs of generalized dementia occur, accompanied by apraxia and agnosia.

As mental and cognitive capacity deteriorate, the nurse and family need to assume more responsibility for the client's self-care—daily hygiene, nutrition, and elimination. Particular patience and sensitivity are required. Schedules of care must be flexible and changed frequently to adjust to the client's labile moods and problems with memory and concentration. The nurse must become particularly sensitive to the emotional needs of both the client and the family. Helping clients learn new ways to communicate requires creativity. The most difficult task, however, may be learning to cope with their fear and anxiety, especially with the recognition that institutionalization may become their only alternative. Family members may find this process even more painful because they recognize the client's continual deterioration. Families should be directed to CCHD groups for crisis mediation and ongoing support. Genetic counseling is crucial to screen families whose children may later develop the disease, to counsel these families against having more children, and to support other family members carrying the gene.

NEUROFIBROMATOSIS

Neurofibromatosis (NF) is a hereditary disorder with an autosomal dominant mode of inheritance. Neurofibromatosis is characterized by a variety of congenital abnormalities. The skin, PNS, CNS, bones, endocrine glands, and sometimes other organs are affected. Usually, some form of benign tumor is the typical finding. The disorder is most commonly classified according to what parts of the nervous system are affected: peripheral, central, or both. The first definitive account of its clinical and pathologic features is credited to von Recklinghausen in 1882, and NF is therefore also known as von Recklinghausen's disease. The poignant portrayal of John Merrick in the movie *The Elephant Man* brought this disorder into public awareness, although fibrous dysplasia accounted for more of Merrick's disfigurement than NF.

Neurofibromatosis is one of the most common hereditary disorders. According to the National Neurofibromatosis Association, the incidence is approximately one case per 3000 live births. In the United States, there are an estimated 100,000 cases. NF occurs in all races and nationalities. Although it can affect both sexes equally, the disease is slightly more common in males. Each child of an affected parent has a 50% chance of inheriting the gene and developing NF. NF can also result from a new or spontaneous mutation of a dominant gene.

Clinical Manifestations

The earliest signs of NF are usually light to dark brown patches of cutaneous pigmentation called café au lait spots. The spots vary in diameter from several millimeters to centimeters. The patches are an early diagnostic clue because they are rarely associated with other pathologic states. Any individual with six or more café au lait spots is considered at risk for NF. Diagnosis is based on the presence of six or more café au lait spots of 0.5 cm or more in conjunction with neurofibromas. Another clinical manifestation is diffuse axillary pigmentation (axillary freckling).

Café au lait spots commonly increase during childhood, and skin tumors typically increase in number and/or size during puberty and pregnancy. For some, the disorder stabilizes during adulthood, but in others, the symptoms progress usually between the late teens and early 20s and again in the 60s. The course of the disease is not easy to predict.

About a third of all NF clients are asymptomatic and diagnosed incidentally. That is, the clinical manifestations are observed during a routine physical examination when the individual is being evaluated for symptoms of another disorder. These clients have mild cutaneous abnormalities.

In the peripheral form of NF, multiple cutaneous and subcutaneous nodules occur. Cutaneous tumors are located in the dermis as discrete, soft, or firm papules. Their size varies from millimeters to centimeters. They also vary from flat to conical or lobular. If pressed, these soft nodules feel like a seedless grape, which aids in distinguishing lesions of NF from other tumors.

Subcutaneous tumors are usually multiple, assuming two forms. The first group is discrete, firm nodules that attach to the peripheral portion of a nerve. These nodules may cause neurologic or paresthetic pain on pressure and rarely cause weakness, atrophy, or sensory loss in the distribution of the affected nerve. The number of nodules varies from a few to thousands and varies from pea-sized to orange-sized. The second type is plexiform neuromas, which are an overgrowth of subcutaneous tissue. Because they reach enormous sizes, the condition is frequently called "elephantous neuromatosis." The face, scalp, chest, and neck are affected with growths that feel like a "bag of worms" when palpated. The hypertrophy is highly disfiguring and often accompanied by underlying bone abnormalities.

These peripheral tumors undergo malignant changes in 2% to 5% of cases (Merritt, 1979). Peripheral degeneration sometimes results in sarcomas. Clients with NF also have a high incidence of CNS tumors, including tumors of the meninges (meningiomas), tumors of the glial cells (astrocytomas, ependymomas, glioblastomas), and a high incidence of neurofibromas of cranial and spinal nerves. In many cases, clients have a variety of these tumors.

A form of central NF involving bilateral acoustic neuromas (CN VIII, the vestibulocochlear nerve) may be the only central finding. Clinical symptoms usually are progressive hearing loss accompanied by tinnitus. There is also a primary hereditary disorder in which bilateral acoustic neuromas appear in the absence of NF. Neuromas of the trigeminal nerve, causing facial pain and numbness, are also common. These tumors, if large enough, can cause increased intracranial pressure (ICP) and brain stem compression. With the presence of small neurofibromas on spinal roots or even larger ones in the cauda equina there may be no clinical symptoms. Large neurofibromas that compress the cervical or thoracic spinal cord may cause symptoms and signs of transverse lesions (Brown–Séquard syndrome). Regardless of the form of central NF, there are usually few skin lesions.

Developmental abnormalities of bone associated with NF include bone hypertrophy, pathologic fractures, and bone cysts. There may be enlargement of the foramen magnum, inadequate articular facets of the vertebra, and scoliosis.

In hypertensive clients, pheochromocytoma is a possibility because it can be associated with NF. Hypertension in NF is more commonly associated with an abnormality in the vasculature of the renal arteries. Instead of one main renal artery supplying each kidney, several splayed branches are present. Calcifications often occur within them, severely thickening and narrowing the vessels, leading to severe hypertension.

Therapeutic Measures

NF has no cure. The most promising approach is surgery for removal of symptomatic lesions. In cases of multiple CNS lesions, the decision to have surgery depends on the severity of symptoms, risk for survival, and the quality of life. Some have advocated aggressive plastic surgical treatment for cosmetic reasons or for removing lesions that might degenerate into sarcomas. Radiotherapy is not justified because of unsatisfactory results and the risk of x-ray exposure.

Treatment decisions involve ethical issues that frequently require a multidisciplinary approach including the client and significant others, neurosurgeons, nursing staff, a psychiatrist, a social worker, and a chaplain. After this group has thoroughly explored the issues, the client and family will be in a better position to decide on treatment.

Specific Nursing Measures

The client with NF is often unaware of the implications of the diagnosis. Initial reactions of shock and disbelief can be intensified by stereotypes like "the elephant man." Help the client recognize that there are many variants of the disease and that no two individuals have the same course and prognosis. Erroneous ideas should be dispelled. Explain the current extent of the illness and possible treatment strategies. Emphasize support for the client's right to make decisions regarding treatment choices.

A difficult task is helping the client recognize the uncertainty of the disease course and prognosis. Inform clients that lesions can change from asymptomatic to symptomatic at any time, that new ones can develop spontaneously without warning, and that others may remain dormant for long periods; in fact, clients may experience symptom-free periods. The nurse may play a key role in teaching the client and family to live one day at a time and to resume as normal a lifestyle as possible. Emphasize the importance of reporting new symptoms immediately and seeking medical attention early.

CEREBRAL ANEURYSMS

A cerebral aneurysm is an abnormality of the wall of a cerebral artery caused by a structural weakness in the vessel. Most common is a focal deficit in a vessel wall that results in a saccular dilation. As pressure in the artery increases, adjacent nervous tissue is compressed and/or arterial rupture and hemorrhage occurs. The majority of cerebral aneurysms are called *berry* aneurysms because of their saccular appearance. Others appear as a ballooning or puckering of a vessel without a distinct neck. Cerebral aneurysms vary from 2 mm to 3 cm with an average size of 8 to 10 mm.

Most cerebral aneurysms occur in the anterior circle of Willis. The circle of Willis is crucial to total brain circulation because it forms an anastomosis between the internal carotids and the vertebral–basilar system providing a means of collateral circulation. About 85% of cerebral aneurysms occur in the anterior cerebral and anterior communicating arteries, the internal carotid and posterior communicating arteries, and the middle cerebral artery at its trifurcation. The most frequent sites are the posterior communicating and internal carotid arteries. The incidence of aneurysms in the vertebral–basilar system is only about 15% (Hickey, 1981). Most cerebral aneurysms occur at vessel bifurcations, where there is potential for weakness. A classification for intracranial aneurysms is shown in Box 37–1.

When an aneurysm ruptures, it can bleed into the subarachnoid space or into the cerebral tissue. In first incidents, blood usually escapes from the aneurysm dome into the subarachnoid space (the space between the arachnoid and pia layers of the meninges where CSF circulates). Bleeding into this area is a *subarachnoid hemorrhage* (SAH), whereas bleeding into cerebral tissue causes an intracerebral hematoma. More than 70% of spontaneous subarachnoid hemorrhages are caused by ruptured cerebral aneurysms. Ruptured cerebral aneurysms cause three major medical complications: rebleeding, cerebrovasospasm, and communicating hydrocephalus. The major cause of death in the unoperated client is rebleeding within the first 2 weeks following the initial bleed.

Although the exact etiology of cerebral aneurysms is unknown, several theories have been proposed. One well-known explanation suggests that aneurysms arise from congenital defects in the media of arterial walls. Another theory suggests that aneurysms develop from remnants of pre-existing fetal vessels. A third possibility is that aneurysms follow arteriosclerotic changes in blood vessels and hypertensive effects. Research continues because these theories are not yet conclusive.

Clinical Manifestations

The majority of clients with cerebral aneurysms are asymptomatic until an aneurysm ruptures. Rupture is the most prevalent diagnosis among clients between ages 35 and 65 years. Although premonitory signs of subarachnoid hemorrhage are common, clients sometimes ignore them. The most common symptom of a ruptured cerebral aneurysm is the *sudden* onset of a severe headache, often described as "explosive." The headache may be associated with nausea and vomiting, visual disturbances, motor deficits, and a loss of consciousness. All of these signs can be related to an intense rise in ICP. In addition, meningeal irritation often occurs, causing nuchal rigidity, positive Kernig's and Brudzinski's signs, photophobia, blurred vision, irritability, restlessness, and a low-grade fever. Meningeal signs diminish as the blood clears from the CSF.

Fewer than a third of clients with cerebral aneurysms seek health care before rupture. These clients usually show

---

Box 37–1 Classification of Cerebral Aneurysms

Berry aneurysms are thought to be congenital defects in arterial wall development. The aneurysms may rupture because of hypertension, exercise, and sexual intercourse.

Giant aneurysms are designated as 2 cm or larger. Their massive compression of cerebral tissue results in neurologic deficits.

Mycotic aneurysms are rare, occur in the younger population, and are related to septic emboli.

Charcot–Bouchard aneurysms are microscopic and occur primarily in the brain stem and basal ganglia. They have been associated with hypertension.

Traumatic aneurysms are usually associated with head trauma.

signs of oculomotor nerve pressure or compression from an aneurysm in a posterior communicating artery. Clinical signs include an eyelid ptosis; a dilated and sluggish or nonreactive pupil; and a restriction of extraocular movement in upward, inward, and downward gaze.

Regardless of the symptoms and signs, the client's condition is grave and the prognosis guarded. To interpret clinical findings, a grading system is employed. The most widely adopted system is the Botterel scale (Table 37–1). The criteria provide baseline data for future comparison and a method for determining prognosis and suitability for neurosurgical intervention. On admission, clients are assigned to one of the categories and their status revised with changes in condition.

Many institutions are now using an adaptation of the Botterel scale known as the Hunt and Kosnick scale. The major changes include the addition of a Grade 0 for unruptured aneurysm and the division of Grade I into Grade I and I-a. Grade I means "no neurologic deficits and slight nuchal rigidity," and Grade I-a is "no meningeal irritation but a fixed neurologic deficit."

Lumbar puncture (LP) was a major diagnostic tool in confirming a subarachnoid hemorrhage before the CT scan. The classic lumbar puncture findings are a grossly bloody spinal tap from a recent bleed and a xanthochromic one from a bleed occurring 6 to 12 hours before the spinal tap. Xanthochromic or straw-colored CSF results from the release of bilirubin during the breakdown of red blood cells. An elevated CSF cell count and protein level are expected in these clients.

The CT scan has had a major impact on the diagnosis and management of clients with a SAH. A CT scan without contrast enhancement can verify the presence of blood in the cisterns (enclosed spaces or CSF reservoir cavities), which indicates a SAH. The CT scan also rules out a subdural or intracerebral hematoma. Lumbar puncture is contraindicated in these conditions. In cases of hematomas, the elevated ICP and the negative pressure created by lumbar puncture could cause a brain shift, which could lead to brain compression and herniation through the tentorial hiatus. A CT scan can also demonstrate the presence of communicating hydrocephalus and, with contrast, may indicate the location of the aneurysm itself.

An LP is done when a CT scanner is unavailable or when a CT scan is not confirmatory. The spinal tap may demonstrate elevated ICP above 250 mm H_2O pressure or higher. Even with the increased pressure, the risk of herniation is markedly decreased because of the nature of the increased pressure. The initial increase in CSF pressure is not due to an absorption problem, but there is the potential for developing communicating hydrocephalus later.

The cerebral angiogram is most valuable in outlining the vasculature and identifying abnormality and displacement of vessel lumina. Because of the high incidence of multiple aneurysms (in 10% to 15% of clients), four-vessel angiography is the procedure of choice. This study examines complete anterior-posterior cerebral circulation by assessing both the carotid and vertebral arteries.

Angiography is also the primary diagnostic tool for identifying vasospasm, a major complication of aneurysm rupture. The procedure can identify clients with vasospasm who have no clinical signs. Vasospasm is a process in which the lumen of the parent and adjacent vessels to the aneurysm becomes narrowed. The narrowing decreases cerebral blood flow to brain tissue supplied by the affected arteries and their branches. Cerebrovasospasm is thought to be related to the vasoactive effects of the blood-bathing arteries in the subarachnoid space.

Symptoms of acute vasospasm occur 1 to 3 hours after initial aneurysm rupture. Chronic vasospasm occurs 3 to 4 days later. Its onset is often slow and insidious. Symptoms vary depending on the severity of the vasospasm and its effects on cerebral blood flow. Other considerations include cerebral perfusion pressure and the degree of autoregulation maintained. Regional alterations may cause focal neurologic deficits such as aphasia or hemiparesis. Diffuse alterations result in level of consciousness changes. Neurologic deterioration in the absence of headache, raised systolic blood pressure, or increased meningeal signs usually suggests development of or increase in cerebrovasospasm.

On the other hand, a deterioration or change in neurologic status may be related to an aneurysm bleed. The major cause of death in the unoperated client is *rebleeding*

Table 37–1	The Botterel Scale for Grading Ruptured Cerebral Aneurysms	
Category	**Criteria**	**Survival Rate**
Grade I (minimal hemorrhage)	Client alert, neurologically intact, with a minimal headache and slight nuchal rigidity	65%
Grade II (mild hemorrhage)	Client alert with minimal neurologic deficits, such as CN III palsy (eg, ptosis, diplopia), with a mild to severe headache and nuchal rigidity	55%
Grade III (moderate hemorrhage)	Client has definite change in level of consciousness, is drowsy or confused; nuchal rigidity is present with mild focal deficits	45%
Grade IV (moderate to severe hemorrhage)	Client stuporous or semicomatose with mild to severe hemiparesis, nuchal rigidity, and possible early decerebration	30%
Grade V (severe hemorrhage)	Client decerebrate, comatose, with a moribund appearance	5%

for the 2 weeks following initial aneurysm rupture. The risk of rebleeding is greatest within 24 hours and again 7 to 10 days after the initial bleed. When the aneurysm first ruptures, a fibrin clot forms over the rupture, sealing the dome. Seven to 10 days later, the fibrin clot undergoes lysis, leaving the aneurysm vulnerable to rebleeding.

Some clients with a SAH have ECG changes. A sinus bradycardia is often seen, related to elevated ICP. A change in S-T segment and T-wave pattern is also observed. Although the exact etiology is unknown, one proposed explanation is that ischemia to the hypothalamus has caused alterations in the ECG. In any event, it is important to differentiate normal SAH changes on an ECG from classic ones seen in myocardial infarction.

Therapeutic Measures

Therapy is based on the clinical and neurodiagnostic findings. The primary focus of medical care after initial aneurysm rupture is to prevent rebleeding. Aminocaproic acid (Amicar) prevents destruction of the clot that has sealed the dome of the aneurysm following initial rupture; it also enables endothelial repair and fibrous tissue development to take place. Extended use (3 weeks or more) of aminocaproic acid has been associated with thrombophlebitis and pulmonary embolism.

Cerebrovasospasm is treated by a number of protocols:

- Calcium channel blockers such as verapamil (Calan) and nifedipine (Procardia) have been employed in an attempt to prevent, reverse, or inhibit vasospasm. These drugs are thought to prevent calcium from entering vascular smooth muscle, reducing vasospasm.
- Kanamycin sulfate (Kantrex) and reserpine (Serpasil) have been used together to prevent cerebrovasospasm. Kanamycin sulfate inhibits serotonin levels in the gastrointestinal tract. Reserpine depletes brain norepinephrine and serotonin. There is no evidence that this protocol is effective once angiography diagnoses vasospasm.
- Isoproterenol (Isuprel) and aminophylline combined relax vascular smooth muscle. Dysrhythmias can develop with this regimen; therefore, cardiac monitoring is advised.
- Isoproterenol (Isuprel) and lidocaine (Xylocaine) are used in combination. Isoproterenol dilates vascular smooth muscle, and lidocaine prevents potential dysrhythmias.

A more controversial protocol is hypertensive therapy to maintain cerebral perfusion. It is preferable for clients who undergo hypertensive therapy to be placed in a special care unit with appropriate monitoring devices. The client is placed in a hypertensive state with various fluid regimens, atropine, and dopamine. The blood pressure is raised 40 to 60 mm Hg above the normotensive range and as high as 180 to 200 mm systolic if ischemia develops. The dif-

ficulty with such a protocol is achieving an adequate level of cerebral perfusion without causing aneurysm rupture.

A more common protocol is to expand blood volume and to assist cerebral perfusion by using colloids (albumin) and packed red blood cells to maintain a hematocrit of 35% to 45%. A central venous pressure catheter or ICP monitor can be used to modify fluid therapy. The ICP must be kept below 15 to 20 mm Hg; serum sodium and osmolality levels are carefully monitored to prevent water intoxication. Management of postoperative cerebrovasospasm with hypertensive therapy is less dangerous because the aneurysm is surgically repaired and in no danger of rebleeding.

Communicating hydrocephalus, the third most common complication of SAH, can occur with the bleed or weeks later. It is caused by a malabsorption or blockage of CSF from the arachnoid villi into the venous sinuses. The drainage of the arachnoid villi is blocked by the breakdown products of blood resulting from the initial subarachnoid hemorrhage. Hydrocephalus should be suspected if any of these signs appears:

- Mental status changes
- A decrease in level of consciousness
- Dementias
- Flat affect
- Urinary incontinence
- Disturbances in gait

Hydrocephalus is confirmed by a CT scan that shows an enlargement of the ventricles and a decrease in CSF space due to a decreased absorption of CSF. Surgery may be required if clients do not recover spontaneously. Ventricles can be drained by ventriculosubgaleal shunt to manage the problem for 2 to 3 weeks. Long-term management requires a ventriculoperitoneal shunt (see Chapter 39).

Surgical repair that includes clipping of the aneurysm neck is the best treatment of a ruptured intracranial aneurysm. This procedure is recommended for clients who are neurologically stable. The appropriate timing for surgery is controversial. Early operation is sometimes advocated, 24 to 48 hours after rupture, in clients who are asymptomatic. The rationale is to treat the client before the peak risk of rebleeding and before cerebrovasospasm increases and communicating hydrocephalus develops. This group of clients, however, constitutes only a small number. Those who demonstrate more extensive signs of meningeal initiation or neurologic deficit may be at greater risk if operated on during the first week following aneurysm rupture. Despite the continuing interest in early surgery, there is not enough statistical evidence to indicate that it has merit except in asymptomatic clients.

Specific Nursing Measures

Unfortunately, about 40% to 50% of clients with subarachnoid hemorrhage due to ruptured intracranial aneurysms die from catastrophic bleeds before receiving medical attention. For those who do have medical care, mortality and morbidity rates can be greatly reduced with careful nursing and medical management. The acute care of such clients presents the nurse with a formidable challenge. Nursing care is aimed at preventing rebleeding, the most life-threatening complication for these clients. Subarachnoid aneurysm precautions are instituted to manage actual or potential alterations in neurologic status from rebleeding (Box 37–2).

The majority of clients are in good health and independent until the aneurysm rupture. The unexpected hospitalization and impending surgery may be difficult for clients to cope with, and their first reaction may be denial. Assist clients to acknowledge their concerns without forcing them into acceptance. During a period when the client's denial is beneficial, the nurse can respond by listening empathi-

---

Box 37–2 Nursing Precautions for Clients With Ruptured Cerebral Aneurysms

Provide a quiet, dark environment with complete bed rest.

Assess neurologic and vital signs every hour for 24 hours, then every 2 to 4 hours if client is stable. Report any changes in vital signs, especially elevations in systolic blood pressure above 120 mm Hg or a 20 mm Hg rise above baseline.

Report immediately to the physician any new or worsening neurologic deficits. Important signs to watch for are restlessness, confusion, and a decrease in level of consciousness. Cardinal symptoms and signs of rebleeding include increased or severe headache, significant increase in systolic blood pressure, and increased signs of meningeal irritation. Other neurologic signs to watch for are motor weakness, change in pupillary size and function, and dysphasia. Document all changes and nursing actions taken.

Administer complete hygiene and feed the client.

Restrict visiting privileges to significant others as designated by the client. Provide brief periods for visitation and instruct client and significant others about the importance of precautions to prevent rebleeding.

Avoid external stimuli that can increase stress—eg, telephone, television, smoking.

Caution client to avoid straining on defecation. Administer stool softeners and mild laxative as ordered.

Give no enemas.

Keep the head of the client's bed elevated at 30° to decrease intracranial pressure.

Administer sedatives and/or anticonvulsant medications as ordered and monitor serum drug levels.

Medicate clients with mild analgesics for headaches only as ordered.

Administer antifibrinolytic agent (aminocaproic acid) via continuous intravenous infusion pump or orally, as ordered. Observe clients for side effects such as thrombophlebitis, diarrhea, and rash.

Be aware that these protocols may have to be modified in some cases by the physician to decrease clients' anxiety and agitation.

---

cally and reflecting accurately the client's comments. Demonstrate an accepting attitude toward the client's concerns, establish a regular time for sharing feelings, and maintain consistency in nursing management.

Clients may feel a loss of self-control and independence because of the subarachnoid hemorrhage precautions. Offer clients whatever choices are available and assist them to identify alternatives. Give ongoing updates of their neurologic condition and prepare them in advance for any diagnostic tests.

Neurologic status can also be altered by cerebrovasospasm. Potential neurologic deficits to watch for are described in the earlier clinical manifestations section. Report and document all changes as well as nursing actions taken. Maintain adequate client hydration. The intravenous fluid rate is usually titrated according to serum osmolality, blood pressure, and/or CVP measurement. Keep a strict intake and output record during acute changes in neurologic status. Calcium channel blockers may be administered.

Clients' cardiovascular status may change because of hypothalamic dysfunction. A common cardiac change in a client with a subarachnoid hemorrhage is sinus bradycardia with ST-segment or T-wave changes. These alterations should be differentiated from those of a myocardial infarction. Monitor ECG pattern and vital signs with the neurologic assessment.

ARTERIOVENOUS MALFORMATIONS OF THE BRAIN

An arteriovenous malformation (AVM) is characterized by the direct shunting of arterial blood into veins. An AVM is thought to arise from fetal maldevelopment of the vascular plexus and primitive capillary system. Instead of normal capillaries developing between arteries and veins, the arteries drain directly into venous structures. The developing malformation is fed by an arterial blood supply consisting of normal arteries in the area plus collateral ones. Venous drainage of the anomaly also occurs via normal venous channels plus collateral ones. Over time, however, normal vessels become thick or thin, dilated, and tortuous. The vessels supplying the malformation continue to enlarge, shunting blood from surrounding areas. Eventually, a conglomeration of abnormal vessels is formed that resembles a "bag of worms." The cerebral tissue that would normally be perfused and oxygenated is deprived of circulation shunted to the malformation. Chronic ischemia results with cerebral atrophy or localized infarction. In addition, parenchymal tissue degenerates within the lesion and proximal to it. Minor hemorrhages also occur, leaving hemosiderin deposits in and around the malformation.

Arteriovenous malformations vary greatly in size. Some are small enough to be obliterated after a bleed; others may affect a large portion of a hemisphere. Most malformations appear as many tortuous blood vessels of varying diameters. They often extend from the duralike cones or wedges into subcortical areas of the brain. The cone-shaped base is near the surface of the cerebral cortex, and the apex is pointed inward. The apex frequently extends to the ventricular wall. Of all these malformations, approximately 75% are found on the lateral surface of the brain. Of the remaining 25%, about half are on the medial surface, and the remainder are in deep structures such as the ventricles or in the posterior fossa (Malis, 1982).

Both sexes are about equally at risk for cerebral AVMs. Two-thirds of all clients with intracranial AVMs experience symptoms before age 30. Noteworthy is the relation between AVMs and intracranial aneurysms. About 1 in 20 clients with AVM have aneurysms, whereas only 1 intracranial aneurysm client in 75 has an associated AVM (Malis, 1982).

Potential for bleeding does not necessarily correlate with the size or site of the malformation. A larger, deeper lesion in the hemisphere may cause more progressive neurologic deficits. Malformations rarely enlarge rapidly. More commonly, they become relatively stable over time.

Clinical Manifestations

Clinical findings depend on the size and location of malformation as well as the additional consequences of cerebral ischemia, compression, hemorrhage, and hydrocephalus. Clinical manifestations include seizures, hemorrhage, headaches, motor and sensory deficits, organic mental impairments, visual dysfunction, syncopal episodes, and bruits. The most common are seizure activity and hemorrhage.

About half of all clients have seizure activity—focal (partial) seizures that often progress to generalized seizures over time. These seizures are most common with frontal and parietal lesions. They develop from ischemia due to shunting of blood away from normal brain tissue to the site of the AVM. Psychomotor seizures are observed with temporal lesions.

The majority of the remaining clients initially have bleeds. Of these, SAH is the most common type (15%), although they are generally less severe than SAH from aneurysm rupture (see the section on cerebral aneurysms). Severe intracerebral bleeds can also occur from these malformations. Presenting symptoms and signs include vomiting, intractable headache, and loss of consciousness. Less severe AVMs of this type can cause aphasias and hemiparesis. Ten to fifteen percent of clients experience sudden, severe paralysis after seizure. An equal percentage develops a progressive rather than sudden hemiparesis. Sizable bleeds in the brain stem can lead to coma and death.

About half the AVM clients have frequent headaches on the side of the malformation, termed "atypical migraine." Visual disturbance and vomiting often accompany the headache. In about 20% of clients, headaches become intractable and disabling. Ischemia of cerebral tissue adjacent to the malformation can account for mental deterioration or paresis.

Other symptoms might include transient episodes of syncope, fainting, and dizziness. Bruits are a rare sign today because earlier diagnosis detects lesions before obvious bruits develop. When a bruit occurs, it is related to a bleed from the internal carotid artery into the cavernous sinus. Associated signs include a pulsating exophthalmos, retinal bleeding, and papilledema.

Therapeutic Measures

Complete excision of the AVM is the treatment of choice to eliminate the possibility of rebleeding. Few clients are in the high-risk or inoperable category. This is a major change brought about by microneurosurgery, better methods of controlled ventilation, and accurate blood pressure monitoring and control during surgery. Microneurosurgical technique permits the removal of most lesions, regardless of size and depth. The purpose of surgery is the removal of the shunt. Feeding arteries and draining veins are not removed.

Generally, microneurosurgery is an elective procedure. A subdural (or intracerebral) hematoma that requires early treatment is an exception. Otherwise, those with subarachnoid hemorrhage need a recovery period before surgery to permit careful evaluation of neurodiagnostic studies. Angiography is essential to visualize the circulation of the malformation and inspect collateral and redistributed cerebral circulation.

Embolization, a treatment choice for surgically inaccessible lesions, has had mixed results. Particulate matter (eg, Gelfoam pellets) is injected into the vessel feeding the malformation. The technique has failed because collateral circulation develops around embolized feeders. More recently, the injection of glue directly into the nidus of the malformation has been successful. This technique continues its development.

Specific Nursing Measures

Assessment of initial symptoms and signs usually related to either seizures or hemorrhage is one of the most important aspects of nursing care for the client with a cerebral AVM. Nursing care of clients with seizures is covered in the next section. Although a SAH with an AVM is generally less severe than a ruptured cerebral aneurysm, many of the symptoms will be the same. Intracerebral hemorrhage can occur. Be alert for vomiting, intractable headache, or loss of consciousness. Report any deterioration in level of consciousness to the physician immediately. Aphasia and hemiparesis can also accompany hemorrhage. To prevent masking any symptoms or signs of neurologic deterioration, only mild analgesics should be given. It is important to identify the rate of progression of any mental status changes that might occur.

Transient episodes of syncope, fainting, and dizziness increase the client's risk for injuries from falls. Instruct clients to assume a safe position, and call for assistance at the initial onset of any of these symptoms. Carefully document any episodes that occur. Provide a safe environment for hospitalized clients and instruct clients and their families about safety measures in the home.

SEIZURE DISORDERS

Seizures are generally defined as sudden, involuntary abnormal discharges of electrical energy in the neurons of the brain. These discharges are usually rapid and excessive with the foci of disturbance in the cerebral cortex. Seizures may be a primary disorder or secondary to CNS disease. Seizures occur in all races, generally have no geographic predilection, and have an equal distribution between sexes. The term *epilepsy* is used to indicate that an individual experiences seizures. "Fit" and convulsion are other common synonyms. It has been estimated that approximately 1% of the population in the United States suffer from epilepsy (Conway-Rutowski, 1982). Seizures can be classified according to etiology, clinical signs, and EEG patterns. The "International Classification of Epileptic Seizures" is a common classification (Box 37–3).

Some seizure disorders originate from antenatal, per-

Box 37–3   International Classification of Epileptic Seizures

I. Focal or partial seizures

Simple (general without an impairment of level of consciousness)
- Motor (eg, Jacksonian seizures)
- Sensory or somatosensory
- Autonomic

Complex (the spread of simple or partial to a generalized convulsive form such as temporal lobe or psychomotor)

II. Generalized seizures (without a local onset, bilaterally symmetric)

Absences (petit mal)

Tonic-clonic (grand mal)

Infantile spasms

Bilateral massive myoclonus

Clonic seizures

Tonic seizures

Atonic seizures

Akinetic seizures

III. Unilateral seizures

IV. Unclassified seizures (when complete data is not available)

V. Classification of paroxysmal forms

Benign febrile seizures

Convulsive equivalent syndrome

Breath-holding spells

Nursing Research Note

Tucker C: Safety assessment for the postictal confusional phase following complex partial seizure. *J Neurosurg Nurs* 1985; 17(1):201–207.

The efficacy of an orientation tool in determining client safety after a complex partial seizure was examined. The Level of Safety Tool includes six orientation questions that test ability to recall name, year, place, month, day, and city. After answering all the questions correctly, clients were instructed to stay in their rooms for 30 minutes. The sample of 20 subjects was tested after each seizure for a total of two separate seizure events for each subject.

For the first seizure, 100% of the sample answered all orientation questions correctly in times ranging from 3 to 300 seconds. For the second seizure, approximately 70% or 14 subjects answered the questions correctly within 3 to 300 seconds. The remaining six subjects were not tested because of lack of an investigator. After the first seizure, all of the 20 subjects stayed in their rooms for 30 minutes after orientation testing. All 14 subjects tested after the second seizure also remained in their rooms for the designated time. Therefore, clients who were able to respond correctly to the questions during postictal confusion were safe for 30 minutes following testing.

This research suggests that clients are no longer confused when they can answer orientation questions. It can be assumed they would be safe when left alone. Such orientation tools need further testing as a means of predicting client safety following seizure activity. Nurses must closely assess each client to assure postseizure safety. Injuries during this time can be potentially life threatening when the client is confused and disoriented. Reorientation and close monitoring are essential.

inatal, or postnatal problems. Seizures can occur with conditions that cause vascular hemorrhage or hypoxia such as vascular malformations, neuroinfective diseases, trauma, or hereditary diseases. Seizures can be a prominent feature of cerebral palsy and cerebral arteriovenous malformations. Febrile periods during infancy and childhood that involve vascular accidents can lead to seizures. Seizures may also develop during the course of a degenerative disease. Sometimes the etiology of seizures is unknown.

The onset of a majority of seizure disorders occurs before the second decade. Those occurring later that are unrelated to trauma, are usually caused by a cerebrovascular or neoplastic disease. Less commonly they are caused by neuroinfective disorders such as meningitis or encephalitis. Seizures can develop during withdrawal from alcohol, sedatives, tranquilizers, and antidepressants. Toxic intoxication from heavy metals or carbon monoxide may induce seizures. Certain cardiac, liver, and kidney diseases may cause seizures.

Factors that can precipitate seizures in clients predisposed to them include nutritional deficiencies, emotional stress, alcohol abuse, and excessive fatigue. Noncompliance with anticonvulsant drug therapy places a client at risk for seizures.

Clinical Manifestations

Partial or focal seizures usually affect a specific body part. The symptoms of an attack depend on where the cerebral focus is. For example, the Jacksonian or focal motor seizure occurs in the motor strip of the cerebral cortex. It is also known as the Jacksonian march because the seizure usually begins in an extremity or the facial muscles with tonic-clonic activity that spreads over the same side of the body. Seizure activity will occur on the opposite side of the body from the irritable cerebral foci. When the seizure activity spreads to involve the other side of the body, it is then considered generalized and may involve a loss of consciousness. Usually a tumor or irritant such as scar tissue causes the attack. Another type of focal seizure is Todd's paralysis, in which convulsive twitching of an affected side of the body is followed by a temporary paralysis of the involved side.

Partial seizures may involve only sensory symptoms like numbness or tingling of a body part. Clients may experience dizziness or visual, auditory, gustatory, or olfactory symptoms. More complex partial seizures involve cognitive signs including a feeling of "deja-vu" (a feeling that things are all very familiar), fear, unreality, anxiety, or a dreamy state. Psychomotor seizures usually cause a sudden change in behavior. Motor automatisms can occur in which purposeful patterned activity is carried out by the client with no memory of the behavior. Clients may do something that is out of character or inappropriate to the situation. The behavior may be preceded by various hallucinations such as olfactory, visual, or gustatory. These episodes are not usually related to an environmental stimulus. A common phenomenon is the "uncinate" fit. These are olfactory seizures with unusual odors or tastes that are unpleasant experiences for the client. Seizures involving visual hallucinations are described as flashes of light or a formed image. Those involving auditory hallucinations may involve a nondescript noise or a well-developed sound. It is important to recognize that hallucinatory seizures may be the aura phase preceding a generalized seizure. Any partial seizure can become generalized if the seizure activity spreads from the original focus to other parts of the brain. However, most focal seizures do not become generalized nor do they involve a loss of consciousness.

Generalized seizures are most commonly described as convulsions, or grand mal seizures. This type usually consists of three phases: an aura, an ictal, and a postictal state. The aura is a warning sign of the convulsive, or ictal, phase of a seizure, and the postictal phase represents the period after a convulsion during which the client may be dazed, confused, or asleep. It is not uncommon for generalized seizures to have a marked focal component. This may be demonstrated during any phase of the seizure. Auras that involve very descriptive neurophysiological phenomenon can suggest a cortical focus. Some examples include paresthesias, auditory hallucinations, or a vivid remembrance of a former experience.

Petit mal attacks are a special type of minor epileptic seizures. They are idiopathic with an onset in childhood or adolescence. They rarely continue into adulthood. Petit mal is known as an absence attack. Attacks usually last from a few seconds to less than a minute. The frequency of the seizure can be as high as several hundred per day. The seizure usually consists of a short staring episode in which there is a pause in the child's conversation. Words may be skipped or repeated. Head nodding and eyelid fluttering may occur during an attack. These absence attacks can be accompanied by myoclonic jerks. Some clients have akinetic petit mal attacks that involve a brief duration of sudden falling to the floor or dropping of objects. They can last only a fraction of a second.

The diagnosis of a seizure disorder is based on a detailed client and family history, electroencephalograms (EEG), and the accurate assessment of seizure activity as reported by the client and observed by the family and/or health team members. An EEG is often the most valuable diagnostic test.

Therapeutic Measures

Seizure disorders caused by CNS disease are treated by removing the causative agent (eg, a craniotomy may be done to remove a brain tumor or a burr hole drilled to evacuate a subdural hematoma). Follow-up includes the use of anticonvulsants for about one year or longer depending on whether or not the client remains seizure free.

The primary medical treatment for idiopathic seizure disorders includes various anticonvulsant drug regimens. The objective is to reduce the excitation threshold of the neurons to a level that requires a much higher stimuli than normal to initiate a seizure. Choice of drug therapy depends on an accurate diagnosis of the type and frequency of seizures. The goal is to achieve optimal seizure management using the lowest dose of anticonvulsants with the least side effects.

For grand mal, or generalized major motor, seizures, the hydantoins are especially useful. The most common is phenytoin (Dilantin) 100 mg b.i.d. or t.i.d. This is often combined with phenobarbital, 30–60 mg b.i.d. or t.i.d. If the major seizures have a focal onset, primidone (Mysoline), 250 mg t.i.d., and carbamazepine (Tegretol), 100–200 mg t.i.d., are used. This combination is also recommended in the treatment of partial complex (psychomotor) seizures. For generalized petit mal seizures, the drug choice is the succinimides. This is followed by the benzodiazepines of which diazepam (Valium) is one. Diazepam has a very short half-life and has limited use in the oral form. IV diazepam is the drug of choice for status epilepticus (rapid succession of seizures without regaining consciousness). It is usually given at a rate of 1 mg per minute up to 10 mg in most cases followed with IV phenytoin or phenobarbital drips (see therapeutic measures for CVA).

One of the newest anticonvulsant medications is valproic acid (Depakene). It is most effective in managing petit mal seizures. It is less effective for focal motor seizures. Sometimes phenobarbital is added to valproic acid to treat petit mal because many children will progress from petit to grand mal.

The treatment of epilepsy requires a precise regulation of drug dosage. Long term management requires determination of therapeutic drug levels as well as actual or impending drug toxicity. Subtherapeutic drug levels can be caused by noncompliance or by problems with drug absorption. For example, drug absorption can be affected by gastrointestinal or liver dysfunction depending on where the drug is metabolized. Correcting specific organic problems can help. Sometimes drug doses may be increased or administered in a more soluble form. Serum drug levels must be used as reasonable guides for drug regulation, because clients may remain seizure-free with slightly higher or lower than therapeutic drug levels. With long-term use and high drug doses, various symptoms can occur. An acnelike rash can develop, especially with barbiturates (eg, phenobarbital). Drowsiness may occur with barbiturates or primidone.

The administration of high levels of the hydantoins can cause cerebellar signs such as an ataxic gait, slurred speech, and intention tremors. Nystagmus and blurred vision can also occur. A common side effect of phenytoin is a diffuse red patchy rash, especially over the trunk area. Phenytoin can also cause severe gingival hyperplasia (see Figure 48–7 in Chapter 48). Valproic acid may cause gastrointestinal irritation. The drug can be given with meals. The most serious complications of anticonvulsant therapy are blood dyscrasias and liver dysfunction. The hydantoins are the most responsible for these complications. Clients must be well informed about action, dosage, side effects, and toxicity of the drugs.

Surgical interventions may be recommended for clients who are intractable to various anticonvulsant regimens. Candidates for surgery must be carefully evaluated. The goal is to remove part or all of the seizure focus. Surgery can be done to excise scar tissue in post-traumatic epilepsy or to remove part of the temporal lobe in temporal lobe epilepsy. Surgery may also create scar tissue that can become a potential future focus for seizure activity.

Specific Nursing Measures

Help the client and family to understand epilepsy by using an analogy. The brain may be referred to as the biological equivalent of a computer. That is, brain cells connect and communicate through tiny electrical components that are similar to the interconnections found in a computer. When there is an abnormal burst of electrical energy, a computer may shut down whereas the brain may experience a physical reaction known as a seizure. A seizure may be described as a temporary period during which the brain is "overcome" by intense, rapid spurts of electrical energy.

The primary goal of nursing care during a seizure is to prevent client injury and to protect the client's airway.

Place the client in a lying position on a flat surface (eg, bed or floor). The side-lying position will promote drainage of secretions and prevent the tongue from falling back and obstructing the airway. Breathing can be facilitated by loosening the client's clothing, especially anything tight around the neck. At the onset of a generalized major motor or grand mal seizure, place a firm soft object between the teeth to prevent biting the tongue. Wash cloths, handkerchiefs, or a padded tongue blade are recommended. Force should *never* be used in placing the object. Do not attempt to open a clenched jaw. Remove all potentially harmful objects around the client. Protect the client's head from injury by cradling the head or placing a soft object under it. *Never* restrain the client during a seizure. Call for help, report the seizure to the physician immediately, record all symptoms and signs of an attack, and administer anticonvulsant drugs as ordered. Place all clients with a history of seizures on seizure precautions, including the following:

- Keep an oral airway, padded tongue blade, and oropharyngeal suction equipment at the client's bedside.

Box 37–4   Seizures—General Assessment Guidelines

A. Ictal (convulsive phase)

Note date, onset, time, duration, and cessation of seizure activity.

Describe the course of the seizure: site of focal onset (thumb, mouth, toe), progression, and sequence of spread.

Evaluate pupillary size and reaction to light.

Assess status of entire body:
- Did the client cry out, lose consciousness, fall to the ground?
- Did the eyes or head deviate to one side?
- Did tonic-clonic movements of the extremities occur?
- Did nystagmus occur?
- Did eyelids flicker or eyeballs roll, close, or open?
- Was there clenching of teeth or jaw?
- Did the client bite the tongue or cheek?
- Was there any drooling or frothing from the mouth?
- Were there any tremors or marked jerking of limbs?
- Was client incontinent of urine and/or feces?
- Were there changes in speech, color, or breathing pattern?
- Were there changes in body posture (stiffening, relaxation, twisting)?
- Was skin diaphoretic?

What was the level of consciousness? Was client confused, irritable, excited?

B. Postictal (after seizure ceases)

Assess the client for memory impairment; depression; headache; muscle aching; sleepiness; change in level of consciousness, respirations, or heart rate.

Evaluate the client for possible injury during the seizure (eg, bruises, lacerations).

Check for paresis or paralysis of extremities.

Question the client about activity at the onset of the seizure and whether an aura occurred.

- Maintain the client's bed in the lowest position and pad the siderails.
- Provide a protected environment free of potentially harmful objects in the event of a seizure.
- Indicate on the Kardex and nursing care plan that the client is on seizure precautions.

One of the most important nursing actions when caring for a client with an active seizure disorder is accurate observation of seizure symptoms and signs. General assessment guidelines are found in Box 37–4.

Teach clients and their significant others approaches to managing any future seizures. Provide written information. Assist them to react to the diagnosis and ventilate their feelings. The long-term management of epilepsy requires courage and acceptance by the client and family. Compliance with medication regimens is essential. Teach the client about drug side effects and the need for continuous monitoring of blood levels. Encourage clients to avoid factors that might precipitate seizures such as infections, stress, and trauma.

Section II: Disorders of Multifactorial Origin

Central nervous system disorders of multifactorial origin can be associated with lifestyle factors, trauma, environmental toxins, and inherited defects, to name a few. Health problems in this section include dystonia, headaches, trigeminal neuralgia, and cerebrovascular disease.

DYSTONIA

Dystonia is an abnormality of involuntary movement (dyskinesia). The abnormality can involve a single, focal muscle group or can be a diffuse neurologic syndrome in which multiple muscle groups are involved. A number of factors cause dystonia. Two different genetic types have been implicated. The inherited dominant trait affects primarily a non-Jewish population, whereas the recessive form appears to prevail among the Ashkenazic (Eastern European) Jews.

Current research suggests that an enzyme deficiency may occur in recessively inherited dystonia, and there may be a structural abnormality in a protein in dominant gene mutations. Other research suggests a malfunction of a neurotransmitter or a disturbance in function or metabolism of catecholamines.

Secondary dystonic syndromes have been associated with a number of hereditary neurologic diseases such as Wilson's disease and Huntington's chorea. In addition, a number of specific environmental insults or factors have been associated with dystonia. These include perinatal cerebral injury, infections (eg, encephalitis due to measles, Reye's syndrome), head trauma, brain tumors, toxins, and focal cerebral vascular injury. Dystonic states are thought to occur either coincidentally with an environmental insult or upon recovery from an acute neuroinfective or vascular problem. These states are usually not progressive and have a milder presentation than hereditary dystonias.

Clinical Manifestations

Dystonic states may become manifest after a period of normal early development. Onset usually occurs before age 15 and is commonly associated with more severe clinical signs. Later onset is rare and more benign. Dystonia is observed as a slow, sustained, involuntary twisting of affected muscles of the trunk, limbs, neck, and face. When the movements are rapid, they are called "dystonic spasm" and are jerky, repetitive, and ticlike. Movements may be focal or generalized.

Dystonia is not usually present during sleep. During waking periods, dystonic movements can be continuous or initiated by a voluntary condition called "action dystonia." Dystonic movements can intensify with stress or fatigue and can be alleviated by relaxation or sleep. Occasionally, dystonia causes fixed posturing of the affected site with potential for contractures.

Therapeutic Measures

A primary treatment choice for clients with intractable dystonia has been surgery. The main objective is to improve overall motor function rather than eliminate all abnormal movement. The more dramatic abnormal movements are eliminated without increasing functional impairments in other areas. Results of such procedures have been inconsistent.

A more common treatment is a wide range of medication regimens. Anticholinergic drugs have been beneficial in reversing acute symptoms of dystonia induced by antipsychotic drugs. Trihexyphenidyl (Artane) is usually the first-line anticholinergic drug. In adults who develop blurred vision and confusion, an alternative is ethopropazine (Parsidol). Adjunctive drug therapies include anticonvulsants, dopamine agonists, antispasmodics, antidepressants, serotonin agonists, antihistamines, norepinephrine, calcium channel blockers, sedatives, and hypnotics. Antipsychotic drugs are rarely used because of the risk of tardive dyskinesia.

Specific Nursing Measures

The effect of dystonia on the muscles may be reduced by stretching exercises. These are described in the specific nursing measures section on muscular dystrophy.

HEADACHE

Headache symptoms account for a large proportion of phone calls and visits to physicians. A number of pain-sensitive structures and mechanisms can be involved in headache, including the skin and periosteum over the outer skull; the dura with its venous sinuses and tributaries; branches of CN V, CN IX, and CN X; and branches of large arteries at the brain's base. Headache can result from compression, traction, displacement, or inflammation of these structures. Pain can be referred from other cranial structures such as the scalp, neck, and extraocular muscles as well as the paranasal sinuses and air cells of the mastoid (Forster, 1978).

Tension headaches, characterized by a sustained constriction of scalp and neck muscles are the most common form. Tension headaches occur by themselves or as the residual effect of a migraine. These headaches are usually caused by tension or poor posture; they may or may not have a vascular component.

The classic *migraine headache* is a clinical condition recognized for centuries. Although the exact cause is unknown, attacks are thought to be precipitated by chemical changes in and around affected blood vessel walls. One common theory is that migraine results from spasm of intracranial blood vessels and a dilation of extracranial blood vessels. The spasm sometimes produces an aura, or warning of an attack, and the dilation leads to headache. Several biochemical agents have been considered in causality—norepinephrine, serotonin, and bradykinin. Migraines have a familial tendency, occurring in a 3:1 ratio on the maternal side. They have also been associated with a history of allergic disorders within the same family—asthma and eczema being common ones (Bickerstaff, 1980). Migraine attacks have been associated with stress, fatigue, overwork, the menstrual cycle, dietary intake (eg, chocolate, cheese, wine), and the letdown of weekends or vacations. They are more common in women, beginning in the teens and often occur in clients with perfectionistic personalities.

Cluster headaches, also known as atypical migraines, are more common in men. The term *cluster* refers to the tendency for a rapid succession of attacks over days or weeks followed by a remission. They were previously considered to be caused by histamine sensitization but are now thought to have a vascular cause.

Temporal arteritis causes severe, unremitting headaches in the region of the temporal artery. An inflammation of this artery causes a tenderness and palpable thickness, and the site sometimes becomes nodular. Temporal arteritis affects men and women about equally but occurs most often among the elderly. It is not a common cause of headache but requires prompt diagnosis and treatment. If untreated, the condition can affect the ophthalmic artery and lead to blindness. Involvement of the intracranial arteries can lead to stroke syndromes.

The headache associated with mild hypertension is usually not characteristic and is similar to a tension head-

ache. Frequent, intense headaches may be associated with severe hypertensive episodes and can be similar to those caused by intracranial lesions.

Ocular headaches can be caused by acquired or congenital conditions. Glaucoma is a common cause of intense headache from increased intraocular pressure. Sharp pain radiates over the ophthalmic branch of the trigeminal nerve. Contraction of scalp and neck muscles causes occipital headaches. Ocular headaches can also be caused by hyperopia, astigmatism, and an imbalance of ocular muscles. Myopia rarely causes severe ocular headaches.

A number of *ear, nose,* and *throat* diseases have been implicated in headache. Mucous membranes of the nasal and paranasal sinuses are more pain sensitive than the sinuses themselves. Inflammations of the superior sinuses can cause pain in the anterior head and between the eyes; an inflammation of the inferior sinuses generally leads to discomfort in the teeth, jaws, and temples.

Lumbar puncture headache is caused by a traction on the structures at the base of the brain after the removal of CSF via the lumbar subarachnoid space. The mechanism is similar to that in increased ICP.

Meningitis also can result in severe headache and nuchal rigidity. Meningeal irritation is caused by blood or pus mixing with CSF (see infectious disorders).

Headaches of intracranial origin are related to a distortion of pain-sensitive structures in early stages of organic disease. During later stages, increased ICP may displace pain-sensitive structures at a location distal from the specific site of the problem. Etiology may include space-occupying lesions, cerebral trauma, cerebral edema, hydrocephalus, or vascular anomaly. (Refer to sections on cerebral aneurysms and neoplasms.)

Supratentorial headaches result from stimulation of pain receptors above the tentorium. Pain impulses travel via CN V, causing headaches in the front half of the head. On the other hand, infratentorial or posterior fossa headache problems cause "occipital" headaches, or pain in the back of the head. Pain receptors are stimulated by CN II in these clients.

Clinical Manifestations

Tension headaches are often mistaken for migraine. Involvement of the scalp muscles leads to more prolonged pain sensation. The pain is often described as a "pressure" or tightness around the head and neck. Tension headaches usually have no aura, cause no alterations in sleep patterns, and are not accompanied by vomiting.

The classic characteristics of migraine headache include throbbing and the tendency of attacks to alternate sides of the head and to be unilateral. Unilateral headaches always occurring on the same side may indicate a serious neurologic problem, especially a vascular anomaly. The initial symptoms of a migraine are caused by the specific blood vessels that go into spasm. Some attacks are preceded by an aura type of visual disturbance. One common aura includes teichopsia (flashing lights zigzagging across the visual fields) and fortification (colored patterns with a dark center and jagged edges). Clients may have visual field defects such as homonymous hemianopia (loss of half of the visual field) and bitemporal hemianopia (loss of the peripheral visual fields) (Figure 37–1). Scotomas (blind gaps in the visual fields) are patchy losses or complete loss of vision. Less common is unilateral numbness of the face or extremities. Some clients experience vertigo, tinnitus, extremity tingling, and dysarthria. The type of aura depends on which cerebral blood vessels are in spasm. Symptoms last from several minutes to an hour, followed by the headache. At this point, some clients briefly lose consciousness. Migraine headaches are associated with nausea and vomiting, accounting for the popular term "sick headache." A migraine headache can persist for as long as 2 days.

Common signs of cluster headache are nasal stuffiness, facial flushing, sweating, and sometimes edema of the affected side. Cluster headaches are sustained, occur in rapid succession, and may have an onset during sleep. Intense, unilateral pain in the orbital and temporal region is not uncommon. Attacks last from 30 to 90 minutes. Unlike other forms of migraine, they usually have no aura or warning preceding onset.

With temporal arteritis, the client has severe localized headache, anorexia, and fever. Visual disturbances can develop, such as visual field defects or sudden blindness. The disorder is diagnosed by clinical symptoms, artery palpation, an elevated erythrocyte sedimentation rate, and leukocytosis. In some clients, a temporal artery biopsy may be performed.

Hypertensive headaches can be pulsatile and are characterized by pallor, nausea, vomiting, and tachycardia. They tend to occur on arising. When associated with vomiting, they are similar to headaches related to intracranial lesions. Hypertensive headaches can signify a pheochromocytoma (adrenal cortex tumor).

The symptoms and signs of ocular headaches vary according to their cause. A common symptom is orbital pain that radiates to the occiput. Ocular headaches do not usually awaken a client, are more frequent with eye use, and may be alleviated by rest. Constant eye strain precipitates attacks.

Headaches related to increased ICP are usually worse when the client first awakens. These headaches are related to an irritation, traction, or compression on dural sinuses or cerebral blood vessels. If the client has slept on a flat bed, the headache may be intensified by a decrease in central venous drainage by gravity. These headaches vary from mild to excruciating and from generalized to localized, depending on tumor location, type, and growth rate. Usually, the headache is reported as not severe and intermittent. It may be associated with vomiting, papilledema, or visual disturbances.

Therapeutic Measures

Muscle tension headaches may be treated by increasing circulation to the affected area, relaxing neck and shoulder muscles. Circulation can be stimulated by applying moist or dry heat, improving posture, performing stretching and ROM exercises, and using acupressure. Acupressure relieves pain through a technique of applying pressure to stimulate certain body points. Biofeedback has been used to help clients learn to control muscle contraction and relaxation. Muscle relaxation drugs may be helpful for clients who do not respond to other measures. In some cases, local anesthetic may be injected into muscle trigger points to relieve pain and spasm.

There is no panacea for migraine headaches, but a number of medications are more or less effective. Acute attacks are commonly treated with ergot preparations, (cranial vasoconstrictors), which if given during the aura stage, may prevent the headache. A physician sometimes uses dihydroergotamine mesylate (DHE 45) during a probable migraine attack to confirm the diagnosis.

At headache onset, ergotamine tartrate 2 mg orally may be given, followed by 1 mg every half hour to a maximum of six tablets per attack. If the client is vomiting, a rectal suppository or inhalation form of the drug can be given. Another alternative may be dihydroergotamine

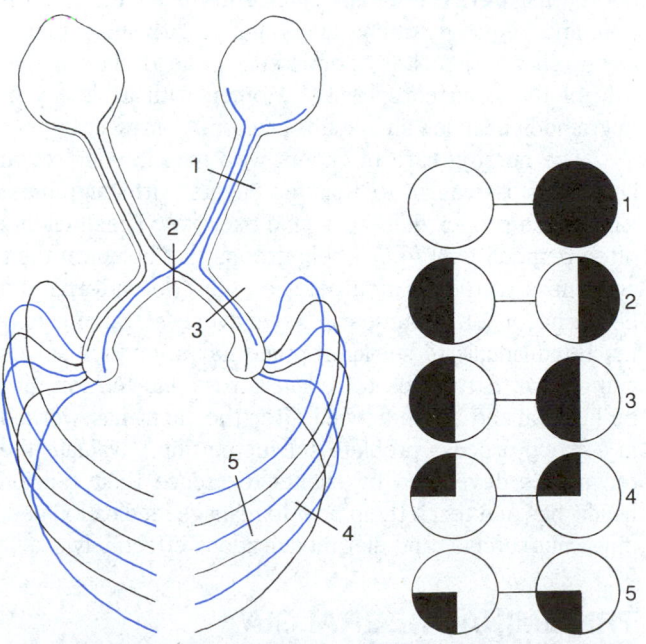

Figure 37–1

Visual field defects caused by lesions in the visual pathways. 1. Right optic nerve lesion results in blindness of the right eye. 2. Lesion at the optic chiasm causes bitemporal hemianopia. 3. Lesion in the right optic tract causes left homonymous hemianopia. 4. Partial lesion of optic radiation; homonymous left upper quadrant defect. 5. Partial lesion of optic radiation; homonymous left lower quadrant defect.

mesylate 0.5 mg to 1 mg IM with a repeat dosage 1 hour later as needed to a maximum of 3 mg. Some clients need an antiemetic such as dimenhydrinate (Dramamine) to prevent gastrointestinal side effects. Long-term overuse of ergot preparations can result in mild malaise and chronic headache, symptoms sometimes mistaken for an actual migraine. Ergot preparations are best reserved for severe attacks, cannot be used frequently, and are not recommended as preventive treatment. Ergot preparations should not be used by clients with peripheral vascular disease, coronary artery disease, hypertension, or impaired hepatic or renal function. Pregnant women should not take ergot.

Caffeine products are also cranial vasoconstrictors and are a household remedy for migraines. A compound of caffeine 100 mg and ergotamine tartrate 1 mg (Cafergot) is effective for some clients. Usually, two tablets are given at headache onset, followed by one tablet every half hour, not to exceed six tablets per attack or ten per week.

Methysergide maleate (Sansert), a serotonin antagonist, has been used to prevent attacks and treat intractable cases of migraine headache. Long-term use is not recommended because it may cause retroperitoneal fibrosis or peripheral vascular insufficiency. The drug should be given for no longer than several continuous months and be stopped slowly to prevent untoward effects. Short-term therapy with methysergide maleate may alter the pattern of migraine frequency enough to permit smooth drug reduction and discontinuation.

Propranolol (Inderal) has been effective for migraine prophylaxis but has no effect on a headache that has already started. The dosage is individualized. Amitriptyline (Elavil) has also been used in migraine prevention. Its ability to offset headache does not seem to be related to its antidepressant effect.

Some clients obtain a prophylactic effect by using minor tranquilizers or barbiturates to decrease levels of stress and anxiety that tend to precipitate their migraines. Clients who understand their predisposition to headaches and take appropriate precautions (eg, avoiding a glass of wine at the time of the menses) can participate in their normal activities without much difficulty. The frequency of attacks tends to decrease with age and may subside for menopausal women. On the other hand, hypertension or use of oral contraceptives may induce, intensify, or prolong an attack.

Although cluster headaches differ from migraines, they also respond to the vasoconstrictive effects of ergot preparations. The previous restrictions and precautions also apply. Some clients with cluster headaches respond well to indomethacin (Indocin). This drug should be employed for short-term therapy only and clients monitored closely for gastrointestinal side effects and blood dyscrasias. Indomethacin should be administered with meals or milk and the client's blood count periodically evaluated.

Temporal arteritis requires prompt diagnosis and early treatment. Steroid therapy with ACTH or cortisone acetate relieves pain and prevents involvement of other arteries, especially the ophthalmic artery. The condition often responds to drug therapy over time. Sometimes surgical division of the temporal artery is recommended.

Hypertensive headaches are treated with antihypertensive drug therapy. Persistent ocular headaches may require evaluation by an ophthalmologist to detect or treat astigmatism, hyperopia, or muscle imbalance. Avoiding continuous activities that cause eye strain may help to prevent attacks. For headaches of intracranial origin, refer to the sections on cerebral aneurysms, meningitis, and neoplasms.

Specific Nursing Measures

Obtaining a complete history and a description of headache characteristics is important to identify factors that precipitate the migraine headache. Nursing care is directed toward assisting the client to develop strategies to decrease the frequency and duration of migraine attacks. One strategy is to maintain a headache log to document duration of headaches, intervals between them, and probable precipitants. A log enables clients to recognize the patterns of their headaches. Some clients need to be assisted to identify and avoid dietary factors that induce headache. Decreasing intake of cheese, wine, and chocolate may be helpful. Eliminating salt for several days before menstruation is beneficial in some cases. Client education about drug regimens is crucial to avoid untoward side effects. Tell clients to notify their physician of any change in the severity, duration, and frequency of migraines. Particularly important is having clients report any persistence of headaches on one side of the head consistently. Women with a history of migraine headaches should not take oral contraceptives.

The nursing care of clients with muscle contraction headaches is similar to that for clients with migraines. Emphasize proper diet, rest, and exercise. These clients often respond well to self-help groups that heighten their awareness of the relation between lifestyle patterns and headache onset. Courses in assertiveness training may teach individuals to set appropriate limits for themselves and others. Strategies to reduce stress and tension may be internalized and practiced after the client has worked in a group process problem-solving setting. Evaluate the techniques developed by clients to reduce their tension headaches and teach them how to manage medication use, physical exercise, and diet modifications effectively.

TRIGEMINAL NEURALGIA

Trigeminal neuralgia (tic douloureux) is the most common neurologic disorder to affect CN V and is also the most frequent of the neuralgias. The etiology can be associated with other neurologic disorders such as MS, tumors, or aneurysms. Often the cause is unknown. Paroxysms of recurrent excruciating, sharp, stabbing pain of short duration along one or more branches of the trigeminal nerve characterize this disorder. The intensity of the pain often causes clients to wince; thus the word "tic" is used to describe the condition. Recurrent episodes of pain are not only disabling, but are anticipated with fear and anxiety. Although trigeminal neuralgia can occur at any age, the onset is most often between the fourth and sixth decades of life.

Clinical Manifestations

An attack of trigeminal neuralgia is often described as paroxysms of excruciating pain with a lightninglike stab that burns. The onset is usually abrupt and related to a precipitating event that irritates a "trigger" point. Dental caries, sinusitis, trauma, and hot or cold temperatures or fluids can stimulate a trigger point. The usual sites for these sensitive spots are the mouth, lips, cheek, tongue, face, or nose. Movements such as speaking, brushing the teeth, washing the face, shaving, laughing, and facial movements in the maxillary and mandibular divisions of CN V can precipitate an attack. An important diagnostic point is that during or following an attack there is no objective loss of cutaneous sensation. Diagnosis is usually made on the history of facial pain as well as the client's ability to identify any precipitants.

Therapeutic Measures

A plethora of medication regimens have been used to treat trigeminal neuralgia over the years but most have been unsuccessful. Standard analgesics are ineffective. Morphine provides some relief but is contraindicated because of its addictive properties. Sometimes phenytoin (Dilantin) is given intravenously to prevent an acute attack although long term use of oral phenytoin is not effective in treating paroxysms of trigeminal neuralgia. Carbamazepine (Tegretol), an anticonvulsant, has controlled the disorder in some clients. Clients on carbamazepine must carefully be monitored for blood dyscrasias.

Injections of absolute alcohol into the gasserian ganglion have been used with clients intractable to other medication therapies. When effective, it causes a loss of sensation in the affected divisions of the trigeminal nerve. The length of symptom remission is variable. Surgical interventions have also been attempted involving resection of the retrogasserian rootlets, causing a permanent facial anesthesia in the sectioned branch. Sometimes the rootlets are decompressed and manipulated to retain sensory function. Several microneurosurgical techniques to relieve pressure on CN V are currently being used in major neurosurgical centers with more promising results.

Specific Nursing Measures

Preventing attacks of trigeminal neuralgia is the priority of nursing care. Document a detailed history of precipitating factors and describe the client's trigger points on the nursing care plan. Place clients in an environment that avoids exposure to drafts or excessive heat or cold.

Encourage ambulation between attacks to prevent hazards of immobility. Assist clients to anticipate their own needs and help them with hygiene and meals as needed to prevent precipitating an attack. Give prescribed medications on time to promote adequate blood levels. Document the client's response to all medications given.

Clients often lose weight because they fear that chewing movements will precipitate an attack. Encourage food choices that avoid excessive chewing. Teach clients to chew on the unaffected side and to avoid liquids and solids of extreme temperatures. Frequent, small feedings are often helpful. For some clients, temporary intravenous therapy, or hyperalimentation may be necessary.

Fearing an attack of pain, clients may avoid washing their faces, performing mouth care, and shaving. Recommend tepid tub baths. Mild mouth wash can be used for oral hygiene. For clients with loss of corneal sensation, teach special eye care to avoid complications. Refer to nursing measures in Bell's palsy (Chapter 38) for specifics of eye care.

Clients may develop ineffective coping patterns due to the disabling and extremely painful nature of trigeminal neuralgia. Use a kind, understanding approach. Reassurance, support, and comfort measures to minimize attacks are essential. Review preventive measures with the client and significant others.

CEREBROVASCULAR ACCIDENT

Cerebrovascular accident (CVA), or stroke, is a syndrome in which cerebral circulation is interrupted. CVA causes sudden onset of neurologic deficits that vary according to the location and extent of vascular interruption. As a result, cerebral ischemia and infarction may occur. A CVA may or may not be preceded by warning signs.

CVAs account for more than 10% of all deaths in the United States each year, making them the third leading cause of death. An additional two million individuals are disabled, making CVAs the second most common cause of chronic disability.

Stroke tends to run in families. It is more frequent in men than in women and in blacks than in whites. (The higher incidence in blacks is considered related to their greater incidence of hypertension, a predisposing factor in stroke.) The highest incidence of stroke is among those between 75 and 85 years old. On the other hand, about one out of seven individuals under age 65 sustains a stroke.

CVA is divided into two major types: ischemic and hemorrhagic. In an *ischemic* episode, cerebral blood flow is suddenly impaired and no longer sufficient to enable affected brain cells to function adequately. In hemorrhagic stroke, the rupture of a cerebral blood vessel causes bleeding into the subarachnoid space or directly into brain tissue (intracerebral hemorrhage). (See the previous section on ruptured intracranial aneurysms and cerebral AVMs).

Cerebral thrombosis accounts for at least half of all CVAs. A cerebral thrombosis is caused by a shortage of cerebral blood supply, commonly because of an *atheroma,* a hard, fatty degenerative plaque that forms on the inner wall of an artery. Atherosclerosis is the most common cause of an ischemic CVA. Thrombotic stroke usually is a progression from partial to complete occlusion of the vessel, with an initial transient ischemic attack (TIA) or warning sign, the reversible ischemic episode, stroke in evolution, and the completed stroke. Clients may experience one, several, or all syndrome stages.

In an embolic stroke, the clot usually forms outside the brain in the heart, neck, or thorax. Usually, a segment of the original clot breaks off and travels via the bloodstream to the brain. The embolus eventually lodges in a vessel too small to permit passage. The process is known as cerebral embolism with causation. The neurologic deficits are similar to those with thrombotic stroke. Embolic stroke develops within a few seconds to minutes without warning signs. The risk factors for cerebrovascular occlusive disease are listed in Box 37–5.

A cerebral thrombosis may be specifically attributed to a number of conditions, the most frequent being atherosclerosis and inflammatory disease processes that damage arterial walls. An intracranial mass can also mechanically constrict cerebral arteries. Hematologic disorders and diseases that increase coagulation can lead to thrombus formation. Conditions causing inadequate cerebral perfusion such as hypotension and dehydration may increase the risk of thrombosis, as may problems of prolonged vasoconstriction such as malignant hypertension. Trauma, on the other hand, only occasionally causes cerebral thrombosis.

Cerebral embolism also has specific risk factors. The most common causes are myocardial infarction, myocarditis and endocarditis, rheumatic heart disease, postcardiac surgical procedures, atrial–septal defects, and atrial dysrhythmias. (The risk of embolic stroke for clients with atrial dysrhythmias is five times greater than for those without.) Another major risk is a disorder of the aortic, carotid, or vertebral–basilar circulation. Less frequent contributors to embolic stroke are air, fat, tumors, and foreign objects. A major risk of posterior fossa surgery in the sitting position is an air embolism; fat emboli are usually associated with fractures of long bones. Finally, any condition that increases coagulation, such as taking oral contraceptives or diseases such as sickle cell anemia or polycythemia vera, potentiates the risk for embolic stroke.

Clinical Manifestations

The clinical symptoms and signs of occlusive stroke vary according to which cerebral blood vessel and its branches are involved. Symptoms and signs also depend on the site, size, and degree of occlusion or infarction. The syndromes that result from thrombotic and embolic strokes frequently overlap (see Box 37–6).

Involvement of the middle cerebral artery is the most common form of all cerebral occlusions. A massive infarction of the affected hemisphere occurs with an occlusion of the main stem of this vessel. CVA of the posterior cerebral artery constitutes less than 4% of all cerebral occlusions. Even less common is a CVA in the anterior cerebral artery.

An occlusion of the internal carotid artery may not be evident if collateral circulation is sufficient. When symptoms do occur, they are similar to those caused by middle cerebral artery occlusion. An internal carotid artery occlusion is considered when the client has repeated TIAs. Atheromas of the internal carotid artery in the neck may lead to embolic occlusions of the middle cerebral artery.

The clinical diagnosis of the cause of a CVA can be difficult. The client's history should investigate risk factors and trace symptoms and signs. The physical exam focuses on neurovascular and neurologic status. Neurovascular assessment includes vital signs, cardiac rhythm, blood pressure, and pulses. The heart and great vessels are assessed for bruits. Funduscopic examination evaluates the vasculature of the retina. Some clinicians attempt to determine the effects of precipitant events such as body position changes on blood pressure; head turning; carotid sinus massage; and Valsalva's maneuver.

CSF analysis is important to distinguish cerebral thrombosis from hemorrhage. The CSF is normal in the majority of clients with cerebral thrombosis and bloody in a large proportion of clients with hemorrhagic stroke.

Angiography is valuable in the definitive diagnosis of arterial stenosis, occlusion, or hemorrhage. A femoral angiogram, which permits selective catheterization of the aortic arch, is the procedure of choice. This study visualizes extracranial and intracranial circulation. It also avoids directly puncturing an atheromatous vessel, eliminating risk of precipitating an occlusion. Digital venous angiography is another accepted method for differentiating between a stenosis and occlusion.

Box 37–5 Risk Factors for Cerebrovascular Occlusive Disease

Atherosclerosis

Hypertension

Diabetes mellitus

Obesity

Elevated serum cholesterol, lipoprotein, triglyceride, and uric acid levels

Cigarette smoking

Sedentary lifestyle

Hypothyroidism

Use of oral contraceptives

Sickle cell anemia

Coagulation disorders

Polycythemia vera

Dehydration, especially combined with any of above conditions

Box 37–6   General Symptoms and Signs of Occlusive CVA

I. CVA involving the anterior cerebral artery:

Mental status impairments
• Confusion
• Amnesia
• Perseveration
• Personality changes: flat affect, apathy
• Cognitive changes: short attention span, slowness
• Deterioration of intellectual function

Urinary incontinence (long duration)

Contralateral hemiparesis or hemiplegia; sensory impairments; foot and leg deficits greater than arm deficits

Footdrop

Apraxia on affected side

Expressive aphasia (for dominant hemisphere involvement)

Deviation of eyes and head toward affected side

Albulia (inability to make decisions or perform voluntary acts)

Gait dysfunction

II. CVA involving the middle cerebral artery:

Dysphasia (dominant hemisphere involvement), dyslexia, dysgraphia

Contralateral hemiparesis or hemiplegia

Contralateral hemisensory disturbances

Rapid deterioration in consciousness from confusion to coma

Vomiting

Homonymous hemianopia

Denial or lack of recognition of a paralyzed extremity

Inability to turn eyes toward affected side

III. CVA involving the posterior cerebral artery:

Peripheral Signs
• Visual disturbances:
  - Homonymous hemianopia
  - Cortical blindness
  - Lack of depth perception
  - Failure to see objects not centered in the field of vision
  - Visual hallucinations
• Memory deficits
• Perseveration
• Dyslexia

Central Signs
• Thalamic or subthalamic nuclei involvement: diffuse sensory loss, mild hemiparesis, intentional tremor
• Cerebral peduncle involvement: contralateral hemiplegia, oculomotor nerve deficits
• Brain stem involvement: pupillary dysfunction, nystagmus, loss of conjugate gaze (Hickey, 1981)

IV. CVA involving the internal carotid artery:

Contralateral hemiparesis with facial asymmetry

Contralateral sensory deficits, especially paresthesia

Hemianopia

Ipsilateral episodes of visual blurring or amaurosis fugax (temporary blindness)

Dysphasia (dominant hemisphere involvement)

Carotid bifurcation bruit

Mild Horner's syndrome

V. CVA involving the vertebral–basilar system:

Dysarthria, dysphagia

Vertigo, nausea, and syncope

Memory loss, disorientation

Ataxic gait

Dysmetria

Visual symptoms: double vision, homonymous hemianopia

Tinnitus, hearing loss

Ocular signs: nystagmus, conjugate gaze paralysis, ophthalmoplegia

Akinetic mutism (locked-in syndrome when basilar artery occlusion occurs)

Numbness of tongue

Facial weakness, alternating motor paresis

Drop attacks

VI. CVA involving the anterior–inferior cerebellar artery (inferior lateral pontine syndrome):

Contralateral signs
• Horizontal nystagmus
• Sensory impairments, mainly of trunk and limbs

Ipsilateral signs
• Horner's syndrome
• Tinnitus and deafness
• Ataxia and nystagmus
• Facial paralysis and loss of tactile sensation

VII. CVA involving the posterior–inferior cerebellar artery:

Dysarthria, dysphagia, dysphonia

Vertigo, nystagmus, unsteady gait

Ipsilateral Horner's syndrome

Sensory changes—ipsilateral face and contralateral body

Hiccoughs, vomiting

Paralysis of larynx and soft palate

Wallenberg syndrome: sudden onset of:
• Vertigo, horizontal nystagmus, ataxia
• Nausea and vomiting
• Dysphagia
• Horner's syndrome (ipsilateral)
• Pain and temperature loss on trunk and limbs (contralateral)
• Balance loss on affected side
• Pain and temperature loss on face (ipsilateral)

The CT scan is valuable for detecting signs of cerebral infarction as early as the first day of a CVA. The scan readily distinguishes thrombosis from hemorrhagic embolic infarction. In cases of TIA, the CT scan is generally normal. Doppler studies of the neck are done to evaluate extracranial circulation as well as to detect a possible carotid lesion in the neck.

Cerebral blood flow is sometimes evaluated for

decreased regional perfusion by radionuclide studies. Serial isotope scanning examinations may be done. In cases of vascular lesions, uptake around the infarct will be increased. Repeated investigation demonstrates an improving condition, suggesting a vascular lesion rather than a tumor.

An ophthalmodynamometry study may be performed to detect an occlusion. This exam measures the amount of global pressure required to temporarily obliterate retinal circulation. Ocular pressure compared with brachial blood pressure should measure two-thirds of the systolic and one-third of the diastolic. This noninvasive study can demonstrate an occlusion of the carotid artery beneath the origin of the ophthalmic artery. A positive finding shows a decrease in ocular values on the side opposite the clinical signs.

Ocular testing may include an ophthalmologic examination with the pupils dilated. The retinal vessels are checked for emboli, which could be fragments of an ulcerated plaque or of thrombotic origin. Laboratory tests usually include the complete blood count with platelets, electrolytes, glucose level, blood urea nitrogen and creatinine, uric acid, and cholesterol level.

Therapeutic Measures

Treatment of cerebrovascular occlusive disease varies according to etiology. Routine treatment for TIAs with aspirin to prevent platelet aggregation has been more effective in men than women. Anticoagulants help to alleviate microembolism; however, an underlying atheromatous process may continue to progress. Complete occlusion of the affected vessel may result.

It is crucial for the physician to establish whether the source of cerebral ischemia is carotid disease of the neck or intracranial vessel disease. Clients undergoing surgery for carotid stenosis who have not had a CVA should have their diagnosis confirmed by angiography. Candidates for surgery include those who have had one or more temporary strokes, including TIAs. Surgery is usually more urgent for a client who has bilateral carotid artery disease and impairment in the vertebral or basilar system. However, the best surgical results are in clients with minimal or no permanent neurologic deficits and in those where cerebrovascular disease only affects one of the major vessels with an obstruction of approximately 80% of the lumen (Forster, 1978). The procedure of choice for clients with carotid disease of the neck is a carotid endarterectomy (see Chapter 30). The operation involves the surgical excision of the thickened, atheromatous tunica intima of the affected vessel.

Cerebrovascular occlusive disease caused by emboli is best treated by identifying and controlling the foci for the emboli. Varicosities in the lower extremities may require a high saphenous vein ligation. Cardiac problems such as atrial fibrillation or mitral stenosis may be treated with anticoagulants. Digitalis preparations are given to treat atrial dysrhythmias. Vasculitis related to collagen diseases can be managed with steroid therapy.

Clients who sustain completed strokes receive supportive therapy. Comatose clients require various life-sustaining interventions such as airway maintenance, fluids, electrolytes, and measures to prevent complications. In some cases, artificial airways are required. Although intermittant catherization is preferred, in-dwelling urinary catheters or condom catheters may be used. Continuous collection of urine helps prevent decubiti.

The acute onset of a completed stroke may be accompanied by marked cerebral edema that can lead to brain stem compression. The client is at risk for potential herniation. Signs of impending herniation include pupil dilation, deterioration in level of consciousness, irregular respiratory pattern, hiccoughs, and motor deficits. Aggressive therapy is required to reduce increased ICP. Bolus infusions of mannitol and dexamethasone (Decadron) are often used. Urea solutions may be given IV if no signs of hemorrhage accompany increased ICP.

Cerebral vasodilating agents may also be used in the acute phase. The most potent cerebral vasodilator in current use is an inhalation mixture of 5% CO_2 and 95% O_2. The mixture can be given via mask every hour for 15 minutes during the first 48 hours after a completed stroke. In some clients, however, vasodilators may increase cerebral blood flow by shunting blood away from an ischemic site.

Anticoagulant therapy is best used in clients with an evolving stroke caused by thrombi or emboli. Its use is contraindicated in clients with hypertensive states or blood dyscrasias. When indicated, heparin is the drug of choice during the acute phase and warfarin sodium (Coumadin) for long-term management. Heparin therapy is best monitored by checking the partial thromboplastin time or clotting time; warfarin anticoagulation is assessed by checking the prothrombin time.

During acute phases of a stroke, convulsive episodes can be managed with phenytoin (Dilantin), diazepam (Valium), and phenobarbital. Loading doses of intravenous phenytoin must be given slowly in divided doses to prevent cardiac dysrhythmias. Phenytoin is only compatible in solution with normal saline. Clients require careful cardiac monitoring during the loading time. Diazepam cannot be diluted in an intravenous Soluset solution. It should be given as prepared by the manufacturer. For clients who are hypertensive, antihypertensive medications should be used to decrease the systolic blood pressure to 150 to 160 mm Hg.

Therapeutic measures for clients with cerebrovascular occlusive disease include prevention. Women taking birth control pills high in estrogen content have an increased incidence of cerebral thrombosis. Risk for cerebral thrombosis is also greater in women with a history of hypertension, severe migraines, and venous thrombosis. For men, cardiovascular disease, obesity, sedentary lifestyle, and poor dietary habits constitute the greatest risk factors.

Specific Nursing Measures

The first nursing priority in acute stroke is to prevent ineffective airway clearance and to manage increased ICP.

Clients are at risk for obstructed airways and hypoxia. A patent airway and adequate ventilation are essential to prevent atelectasis, pneumonia, respiratory arrest, and increased ICP. Assess the depth and rate of respirations frequently and auscultate the chest for adventitious sounds. For clients with marked deterioration in level of consciousness, an oral airway should be inserted and a side-lying position maintained. For specific respiratory protocols, refer to the nursing management sections for ALS, myasthenia gravis, and head trauma in this chapter. Respiratory treatments should not be instituted vigorously, or the ICP may elevate proportionately.

Standard measures for managing increased ICP are:

- Elevating the head of the bed at least 30° to promote central venous drainage.
- Maintaining a patent airway to help prevent an accumulation of CO_2. (An elevated partial pressure of carbon dioxide [PCO_2] causes vasodilation of cerebral blood vessels that can lead to increased ICP.)
- Providing gentle respiratory care and avoiding straining at defecation.
- Frequent monitoring of neurologic signs and reporting promptly changes from the baseline.
- Avoiding frequent head rotation. (Neck muscles can compress the jugular veins, impeding central venous drainage. Turn clients with head and shoulders as a unit to avoid this problem.)

Recognize the rationale for medication regimens used to treat stroke in evolution and their side effects. These regimens are discussed under therapeutic measures.

Maintenance of skin integrity and the management of immobility are major nursing care objectives that influence future rehabilitation. Circulation can be impaired if the paretic or paralyzed side is not carefully positioned. Affected limbs should be supported with splints and elevated to prevent or treat dependent edema. Motor deficits are usually accompanied by sensory loss. The client will not be able to report circulatory impairments on the affected side. Check peripheral pulses in the hands and feet periodically.

Good skin care and maintaining clean, dry, and wrinkle-free linen decrease interruptions in skin integrity. Carefully schedule active and passive ROM exercises as well as repositioning in the side-lying and prone positions to decrease problems of immobility. Hip flexion contractures can be avoided with a prone position, and footdrop can be prevented with footboards for side-lying and supine positions.

After respiratory dysfunction, the second major complication of immobility is thrombophlebitis and pulmonary embolism. Thigh-high elastic stockings and ROM exercises are ordered as preventive measures. Be alert for client complaints of calf stiffness, aching, or pain and check for Homan's sign. Also check for local signs of calf or thigh redness, swelling, and increased temperature. Measure calf and thigh circumferences every shift and document the comparisons. Watch for respiratory distress such as shortness of breath or chest pain that could indicate a pulmonary embolism. Other signs are tachycardia; a decreased PO_2 on arterial blood gas analysis; and in some cases, inverted T-waves on an ECG.

Alteration in communication patterns is one of the most distressing problems for a client with stroke. Receptive and/or expressive dysphasia may be present. Establish effective communication by written or visual cues and provide an appropriate type of call bell for the unaffected extremity. A trusting relationship can develop if the nurse treats the client with respect and demonstrates a knowledge of the deficit. Speak to the client directly in a slow, patient manner. Remember that hearing is intact. Listen carefully, allow the client time to answer, and offer appropriate cues. These measures conserve the client's energy and avoid frustration. Discuss the communication problem and plans for rehabilitation with the client and significant others. This is particularly helpful for those with expressive aphasia (the inability to formulate and use expressive language). Place objects within easy reach of the unaffected side. Clients with receptive aphasia (the inability to comprehend and integrate receptive language) need frequent reorientation and a safe environment.

Alterations in elimination patterns are a potential problem for the stroke client. Plan a regular voiding pattern for continent clients. Offering the bedpan every 2 or 3 hours and using Credé's maneuver can assist the client to void. (Credé's maneuver is discussed in Chapter 33 and illustrated in Figure 33–2.) Stroke clients may develop constipation or fecal impaction. Administer stool softeners, cathartics, and suppositories as ordered. Encourage adequate fluid intake including water and fruit juice. Auscultation of bowel sounds is important to detect any signs of a paralytic ileus. See specific nursing measures for clients with multiple sclerosis for additional guidelines for bladder and bowel management.

Alterations in visual function can accompany a CVA. Assess the client's visual acuity, visual fields, and extraocular eye movements. Approach clients on the side of best visual perception and teach them to use the best field of vision. Be alert for diplopia or nystagmus. Alternate eye patching can correct diplopia.

Section III: Degenerative Disorders

Degenerative CNS disorders are those with an unknown etiology that have an insidious onset and involve atrophy of neurons and nerve fibers. It is not uncommon for degenerative diseases to occur after a long period of normal nervous system functioning. The disease course is gradual and progressive over many years.

ALZHEIMER'S DISEASE

Alzheimer's disease is a progressive, degenerative disorder that causes cerebral atrophy. The disorder was first identified in 1906 by a German neurologist, Alois Alzheimer. The disorder develops insidiously, marked by progressive organic mental changes and language dysfunction. *Dementia,* the deterioration of intellectual capacity, is characteristic of Alzheimer's disease. Alzheimer's disease is thought to account for at least half of all cases of dementia in the elderly (McKinstry, 1982). Afflicting 1.5 to 2 million persons a year (Kolata, 1982), Alzheimer's is the fourth or fifth leading cause of total disability in the United States.

The cause of Alzheimer's disease is unknown, although several theories have been proposed. One theory suggests that the disease is the result of the brain's generalized reaction to a number of harmful processes. Another suggests that a specific agent such as a toxin, slow virus, genetic deficit, metal deposit, or an immunologic dysfunction causes the disorder (McKinstry, 1982). Current research is aimed at identifying a genetic marker responsible for Alzheimer's disease. Evidence of a familial pattern supports this area of investigation. Researchers expect to find a biological marker unique to the disease such as a peripheral abnormality, a specific sensory organ change, or a diagnostic blood test. Another research focus has been on the role of neurotransmitters. The most substantial finding has been the deficiency of acetylcholine in the brain of affected clients. This finding has encouraged further research into acetylcholine precursors as a potential treatment, similar to the use of L-dopa in Parkinson's disease. These studies involve the role of lecithin and choline in treating Alzheimer's disease. Findings have been inconclusive.

Alzheimer's disease research poses legal and ethical dilemmas. The major issue is obtaining an informed consent from demented clients. The most controversial area, whether an invasive procedure such as a brain biopsy should be done to confirm the diagnosis, raises the issue of therapeutic benefit to the client. Recent practice has been to arrive at a "presumptive" diagnosis.

Clinical Manifestations

The clinical diagnosis of Alzheimer's disease is presumptive. A confirming diagnosis is best made by microscopic examination in a postmortem to identify the characteristic neuronal degeneration. Therefore, diagnosis is made by exclusion. First, the signs of dementia are established. Then identification of the pathology is attempted: is it curable and reversible, or is it irreversible? Treatable causes of dementia may include general paresis, myxedema, normal pressure hydrocephalus, intracranial masses, avitaminosis, and depression. Other irreversible causes of dementia include alcoholism, Huntington's chorea, and multiple cerebrovascular infarction.

The diagnostic work-up for Alzheimer's disease should be exhaustive because the psychosocial/lifestyle implications of the diagnosis can be devastating for both client and family. A widely accepted diagnostic screening tool is shown in Box 37–7.

Symptoms have been divided into three stages. The first stage is marked by memory loss caused by the patchy loss of neurons throughout the cerebral cortex. Judgment and logic compensate for memory deficits as long as enough frontal lobe neurons remain intact. As the disease progresses, judgment and logic decline, and disorientation and global aphasia occur. The aphasia includes motor and expressive speech deficits (Broca's aphasia) and sensory comprehension deficits (Wernicke's aphasia). Speech deficits are more difficult to assess because the pattern is different than in other neurologic problems such as cerebrovascular disease. The neuronal damage in Alzheimer's disease is symmetrical, preventing the opposite hemisphere compensation common in hemorrhagic stroke. Other aspects of first-stage Alzheimer's disease are irritability, mood swings, flattening of affect, and agitation.

The second stage usually occurs between 2 and 4 years after the first, depending on the extent and location of lesions. Loss of frontal and temporal lobe function increases. Clients forget learned, socially acceptable behaviors. They neglect hygiene and develop inappropriate eating habits and poor elimination patterns. Clients lose portions of their ability to see, to hear, and to feel pain. A common sensory deficit is **agnosia,** the inability to recognize familiar objects in the environment through the senses of touch and vision. Clients may have seizures. Behavioral problems include **perseveration** (repetition of a motor or verbal action) and **hyperorality** (an insatiable need for oral stimulation by chewing or tasting objects). This second stage varies from 2 to 12 years; regression is more rapid in younger persons and men.

The third or terminal stage is the impaired confusional stage, marked by the progression of both generalized and focal deficits. The client eventually becomes mute and unresponsive and has anorexia and **apraxia** (the inability to carry out a learned, voluntary act when motor function is intact).

Therapeutic and Specific Nursing Measures

In planning care, consider that the adjustments and compensations the client develops at an early stage of the disease will not remain for future use. Clients need increased supervision and manipulation of the environment.

During the first stage, families of Alzheimer's clients often experience shock, disbelief, and a degree of social isolation from friends. Anticipatory grieving is essential at this time. The client focuses on compensating for memory deficits and adjusting to fear and uncertainty. Mutual recognition of these concerns should be encouraged.

Tension and restlessness are common problems that can lead to sleep-pattern disturbances in the client. Pre-

Box 37–7 University of Washington Research Diagnostic Criteria for Primary Neuronal Degeneration of the Alzheimer's Type

Clinical Features for Inclusion

A deterioration of general cognitive functions from a previously higher performance level compromising the ability to adapt to the environment including:

A. Onset   Yes   No

Gradual progression   ___ ___

Duration of at least 6 months   ___ ___

B. Impairment of at least two of the following abilities (on the basis of performance on the Mini-Mental Status, the Wechsler Adult Intelligence Scale, or WAIS)

	Absent	Mild	Moderate	Severe
Learning	___	___	___	___
Attention	___	___	___	___
Memory	___	___	___	___
Orientation	___	___	___	___

C. Impairment on at least one of the following cognitive skills (on the basis of performance on the WAIS and Mini-Mental Status)

	Absent	Mild	Moderate	Severe
Calculation	___	___	___	___
Abstraction and judgment	___	___	___	___
Comprehension	___	___	___	___

D. Problems in at least one of the following areas (on the basis of the psychosocial examination)

	Absent	Mild	Moderate	Severe
Ability to work	___	___	___	___
Ability to relate to family	___	___	___	___
Ability to relate to peers	___	___	___	___
Ability to function socially	___	___	___	___

E. Indication of cerebral dysfunction on at least one of the following:

	Yes	No
Cerebral atrophy on CT scan	___	___
Abnormal EEG (see also exclusion criteria)	___	___

F. Ischemic score 4 (modified from Hachinski, 1978)

Feature:	Possible Score	Real Score
Abrupt onset	2	___
Stepwise deterioration	1	___
Fluctuating course	2	___
Nocturnal confusion	1	___
Emotional lability	1	___
History of hypertension	1	___
History of strokes	2	___
Evidence of associated atherosclerosis	1	___
Focal neurologic symptoms	2	___
Focal neurologic signs	2	___

SOURCE: Reprinted from Eisendorf, Cohen: Diagnostic criteria for primary neuronal degeneration of the Alzheimer's type. *Journal of Family Practice* 1980; 11(4):553–557.

cautions to prevent injury for clients with sleep disturbances include using night lights; keeping stairway doors closed; and using communication devices, such as a bell to alert family members when a client wanders into hazardous areas. Exercise programs—walking, dancing, playing a simple sport—can help reduce tension and restlessness. Exercise may also reduce the need for tranquilizers and sleeping medications. Daily schedules need to be flexible to accommodate the client's memory loss and mood swings.

During the second stage, the family may become intolerant. Their feelings of helplessness, anger, and guilt must be recognized as normal reactions. The client will have marked communication and perceptual deficits as well as behavioral problems. The nurse can best assist families by helping them identify effective coping strategies, assess support systems, and seek legal and financial counseling.

The client is not well attuned to the present, but reminiscing can be supportive because long-term memory is more intact. Encourage the family to help the client reminisce about familiar persons and events. Reminiscing is comforting and increases the client's self-confidence. Communication strategies are important. Conversation should be clear and simple, using short words and sentences that are readily understood. Repetition is required. Keeping a log of effective techniques can be helpful. Clients frequently refuse treatment during this stage. Never pressure them. Reapproach a task when the client is more receptive.

During the final stage, comprehensive, supervised care is required. Maintaining a safe environment is a major priority. Suggestions for protective measures include:

- Providing an identification necklace or bracelet with the client's name, address, and telephone number for those with a tendency to wander

- Securing hazardous areas by installing safety locks that are difficult for clients to reach or use

- Keeping toxic fluids and firearms locked up and preventing access to lighters and burners

- Providing an uncluttered environment to prevent falls

- Keeping objects in the same place to decrease client confusion

Help families to recognize the need for skilled care and think about alternative placement for the client. Appropriate referrals to social service agencies assist families in investigating the chronic care facilities. Families need support in dealing with the anxiety and guilt of separation from the client as well as the change in their own roles and responsibilities.

PARKINSON'S DISEASE

Parkinson's disease is a degenerative process of nerve cells in the extrapyramidal system: basal ganglia, thalamus, substantia nigra, red nucleus, and reticular formation. The disorder was first described in 1917 by James Parkinson as the "shaking palsy." Later it became known as "paralysis agitans." The disease has a slow, gradual course. Parkinsonism is one of the most common neurologic disorders, affecting both men and women over age 30.

The causes of Parkinson's disease are not known. The condition may result from an accelerated aging process or from a virus causing gradual destruction of dopaminergic neurons, or it may be an inherited genetic defect. Several forms of the disease have been described according to etiology:

- Idiopathic (in which the cause is unknown)
- Arteriosclerotic (related to a defective blood supply to the basal ganglia)
- Postencephalitic (occurring after encephalitis)
- Post-traumatic (following an ischemic episode to the brain)
- Toxic (following inhalation of carbon monoxide, manganese, or mercury)
- Neurosyphilitic (as a complication of syphilis, now rare)
- Drug induced (pseudoparkinson's disease, related to high doses of antipsychotic drugs)

Of these, the postencephalitic form is of special interest. In 1919, a pandemic of encephalitis occurred. Over the next 40 years, the incidence of Parkinson's disease was markedly higher.

The most promising research has been in biochemistry. Studies have demonstrated a deficiency of dopamine and homovanillic acid (HVA), a metabolite of dopamine, in the basal ganglia of affected clients. Dopamine influences purposeful movement. In the absence of dopamine's inhibitory effect on movements controlled by the motor cortex, rhythmic spontaneous movements cannot occur (Wilson, 1979).

Clinical Manifestations

Diseases of the basal ganglia are clinically manifested as disturbances of movement: tremor, rigidity of muscles, and dyskinesias. Dyskinesias involve a problem in initiating or performing a movement quickly. Clients report feeling stiff and sore in the joints and are slow in performing activities of daily living.

Tremor is the most common initial symptom. Classic signs of tremor in clients with Parkinson's disease include pill rolling of the thumb and forefingers at rest, to-and-fro head tremors, and tremulous voice quality. The involuntary resting tremors differ from the intention tremors of clients with cerebellar disease. In parkinsonism, tremors vary from mild to severe to incapacitating. They are aggravated by fatigue and stress and dissipate when the client sleeps or performs a purposeful activity. After the hands, the larger joints and the lower extremities become involved. Eventually, tremors are so marked that it is impossible for a client to control or conceal them.

Rigidity occurs either at the same time as tremors, or long before, as the only sign of the syndrome. Muscular rigidity has been described in three ways: the rhythmical jerking interruption of passive ROM as "cogwheel" rigidity, mild resistance as "plastic" rigidity, and total resistance as "leadpipe" rigidity.

Hypokinetic features include paucity of movement and hypertonicity of antagonistic muscles despite client attempts to relax. These signs are caused from the irregular, asynchronous pattern of neuronal discharges. Bradykinesia is observed as difficulty initiating voluntary movement marked by episodes of "freezing" of movement. Facial expression becomes masklike (masklike facies) with a fixed stare and paucity of facial movement. Clients assume a bent-forward, stooped position, and adjustments are uncoordinated. The gait consists of small, short shuffling steps that are slowly initiated. Movements become propulsive with an acceleration in gait. Clients lose their armswing when walking and have difficulty ceasing motion. The feet fail to move before a change in position from sitting to standing and vice versa. Clients also lose finesse of movement. Their bodies tend to turn all at once (like a statue) rather than in the normal sequence.

Handwriting is cramped and small (**micrographia**) with signs of tremor; the voice tends to be a monotone with no range. Speech becomes rapid, unpunctuated, and incomprehensible. **Pallalia** (involuntary sentence repetition) and **echolalia** (parrotlike repetition of words spoken by others) may be heard.

Other symptoms include insomnia, dysphagia, weight loss, and drooling (sialorrhea); shiny, oily skin with scalp seborrhea; and involuntary rapid eyelid blinking (blepharospasm). Oculogyric crisis can occur—sudden, forceful spasms of the eye muscles in which the eyeballs deviate and jump up and down. There is also evidence that parkinsonism affects the sensory system. Tingling, numbness, and crawling sensations of the extremities have been reported. The client's intelligence is not affected. Other distressing symptoms include alterations in mood, paranoid ideations, and depression.

Therapeutic Measures

The diagnosis is based on the history, neurologic examination, electromyography, clinical signs, handwriting

Box 37–8 Stages in Parkinson's Disease

Stage I: Unilateral involvement

Stage II: Bilateral involvement

Stage III: Bilateral involvement with impaired posture and mild imbalance; disability is mild; client independent

Stage IV: Bilateral involvement with postural instability; client requires considerable assistance

Stage V: Fully developed, severe disease; client confined to wheelchair or bed

SOURCE: Hoehn M, Yahr, M: Parkinsonism: onset, progression and mortality, *Neurology* 1967; 17:433.

analysis, and an HVA analysis. HVA is diminished in urine and in the cerebrospinal fluid. The disease is best classified by the scale in Box 37–8. Therapeutic measures include drug therapy and physical therapy.

During the past decade, the treatment of choice has been to increase available dopamine. A derivative of dopamine, such as levodopa (L-dopa), taken orally, is converted into dopamine in the brain. The drug compensates for the client's deficit and is most effective for those with an akinetic form of the disease. The masklike facies should disappear. The client can initiate, turn, stop, and accelerate movements better. Tremor is usually less responsive to the drug but may decrease on prolonged therapy. The rapid appearance and disappearance of symptom relief (the "on-off" phenomenon) can be avoided by prescribing smaller amounts of L-dopa in divided doses. In some cases, a drug "holiday" may be required.

Because most L-dopa taken by mouth is destroyed before reaching the brain, carbidopa (Sinemet) is also given. A smaller dose of L-dopa is needed, more levodopa is available to the basal ganglia, and peripheral side effects are reduced. Dyskinesia remains a major side effect, but some clients prefer this reaction to their original akinesia. Bromocriptine mesylate (Parlodel) is a dopamine agonist that decreases dopamine turnover. It allows a reduction of levodopa dosage for clients experiencing dyskinesias.

The antiviral drug amantadine (Symmetrel) was accidentally found to prevent neuronal reuptake of natural dopamine. Amantadine improves rigidity but has little effect on tremor and is best used for clients with minimal symptoms.

Anticholinergic drugs may be used early in the disease when tremor is a predominant problem. These drugs reduce cholinergic activity by decreasing the excitation effects of acetylcholine. Then an attempt is made to restore the balance between the dopaminergic and cholinergic systems in the basal ganglia. Common drug choices include benztropine mesylate (Cogentin), ethopropazine (Parsidol), and trihexyphenidyl (Artane). These drugs indirectly control rigidity, tremor, and drooling.

Although antihistamines have only a minimal effect on Parkinson's symptoms, they can be combined with anti-

cholinergic drugs for clients unable to tolerate other combinations. Diphenhydramine (Benadryl) is the most commonly used antihistamine. For sedation, diazepam is preferred over barbiturates or hypnotics that could cause an excitation of symptoms.

The major objective of physical therapy for parkinsonian clients is to prevent contractures and atrophy while reducing muscular rigidity. Physical therapy can maximize the level of functioning. A basic program for clients includes general ROM of all joints as well as walking, sitting, and stretching maneuvers. Exercises should be done to improve speech and facial expression.

Severe tremor may be resistant to medical treatment. Surgery for clients whose condition is intractable interrupts the extrapyramidal pathways. The most common procedure is thalamotomy. Criteria for this stereotaxic surgery are severe unilateral tremor that is a manifestation of nondominant hemispheric disease; no signs of lip, chin, and tongue involvement in clients under 65; good general health; and freedom from atherosclerotic disease. A bilateral thalamotomy can result in speech disturbances, memory deficits, and poor urinary control. L-dopa has greatly reduced the use of stereotaxic surgical procedures.

Specific Nursing Measures

The goal of nursing care is to assist the client to manage self-care deficits and to handle alterations in body image. Mobility must be maintained. Purposeful activity can reduce or eliminate tremors, whereas bed rest can lead to contractures and muscular atrophy. Gait training includes teaching the client to walk by placing each foot down as heel, ball, and toe instead of shuffling. Pivotal heel maneuvers can aid turning. Ambulation may require supervision.

Help clients to recognize that feelings of depression and frustration may result from alterations in body image and loss of independence. Nursing approaches should assist clients to share their feelings, recognize their reaction as a realistic coping mechanism, and encourage and support as much independence as possible.

Teach clients to perform activities of daily living with minimal assistance to foster self-confidence. Assistive devices may be required to maintain a safe environment. Guardrails in bathtubs and hallways may prevent falls because of client tremors and loss of protective reflexes. Showers can be taken with a special chair. Other self-help devices include clothing that is easier to wear (eg, with Velcro fasteners instead of zippers and slip-on instead of laced shoes).

Interruption in skin integrity is a potential problem because of drug therapy and autonomic dysfunction. Daily or as-necessary bathing can reduce excessive perspiration and seborrhea.

There is a potential for altered nutrition and elimination patterns. Weight loss may result from difficulty in eating related to tremors and the diuretic effect of drug therapy. Constipation is a common problem caused by immobility and anticholinergic drug effects. Recommendations include use of psyllium, stool softeners two or three times a day, a daily glycerin or bisacodyl (Dulcolax) suppository, and increased bulk in the diet. Monitor the client's weight pattern, maintain a high-calorie and controlled protein diet, and provide small frequent feedings and assistive eating devices.

Recognize the effects of diet on drug absorption. Ineffective drug absorption is a potential problem because of obesity, alcohol intake, and diet. Obesity increases vascular problems, decreases mobility, and affects levodopa regulation. (Fat cells absorb and release levodopa erratically.) Reducing diets are best planned with nutritional counseling. Teach clients to avoid or limit alcohol intake to no more than two glasses of wine or beer with dinner. Alcohol antagonizes the effects of L-dopa and can also increase the risk of depression. A high-protein intake may also block the effects of L-dopa, an amino acid, by competing for intestinal and blood-brain barrier absorption with other protein by-products. Protein intake should be decreased by 50%. Include limiting protein products such as milk, poultry, fish, meat, cheese, nuts, eggs, soybean products, sunflower seeds, and whole grain in client and family teaching. Also emphasize limitation of caffeine intake because caffeine promotes the development of abnormal body movements.

Document the client's baseline symptoms—especially tremor, rigidity, and dyskinesia—before medications are initiated. Therapeutic effects are measured against the baseline.

The common side effects of prescribed medications should be recognized. These include dryness of the mouth, nausea, postural hypotension, and dysrhythmias such as sinus tachycardia. Frequent mouth care alleviates dryness related to anticholinergic drug effects. For nausea, give antiemetics such as trimethobenzamide (Tigan) or metoclopramide (Reglan). Phenothiazines—eg, prochlorperazine (Compazine)—should be avoided because they interfere with dopamine metabolism. For postural hypotension, assist the client to make gradual position changes, apply antiembolism stockings, and record standing and supine blood pressures at least twice a day. Monitor and report heart rate changes.

Drug therapy can also precipitate abnormal involuntary movement. Clients and significant others are taught what choreiform and athetoid movements look like. Abnormal movements to report are head nodding, tongue protrusion, facial grimacing, exaggerated gestures, and unusual breathing patterns. Drug dosages must be reduced to prevent the "on-off" phenomenon.

Medication may also have to be adjusted if clients exhibit behavioral problems. Observe and report the following symptoms: irritability, outbursts of anger, hostility, delirium, hallucinations, and paranoid ideation. A safe environment must be maintained.

Give the client and significant others a list of symptoms and signs to report to the physician when the client returns home. A discharge plan should include instructing the client and family in the factors decreasing medication absorption, potential side effects of medication, how to maintain a safe environment, and a plan for daily living.

AMYOTROPIC LATERAL SCLEROSIS

Amyotrophic lateral sclerosis (ALS) is a progressive degenerative CNS disease with a relentless, fatal course. The term *amyotrophic* refers to the muscle atrophy from the degeneration of ventral horn cells. *Lateral sclerosis* pertains to the demyelination of the corticospinal tract. The disease affects both upper and lower motor neurons of the pyramidal tracts of the CNS. The three major aspects of the motor neuron disease are progressive muscle atrophy, progressive bulbar palsy, and upper motor neuron deficits.

The course of ALS varies from 1 to 4 years. The survival rate is 5 years for 20% of clients and 10 years for another 10%. Men are more frequently affected than women in a ratio of about 2:1. Disease onset occurs between ages 40 and 70, most frequently in the fifth and sixth decades. The cause of ALS is unknown. Researchers are currently investigating viral, metabolic, infectious, toxic, immunologic, and specific life events as possible causes.

Clinical Manifestations

To make a differential diagnosis in ALS, disorders whose symptoms resemble ALS must be ruled out—cervical stenosis or osteoarthritis, spinal cord tumors, syringomyelia, polyneuritis, muscular dystrophy, multiple sclerosis, and neurosyphilis. A myelogram is often performed to rule out any other degenerative disease or treatable condition. Diagnosis in early stages of ALS can be difficult if no signs of lateral sclerosis are evident and when only one aspect of the spinal cord or brain stem is involved. A characteristic finding is absence of sensory signs.

Diagnostic studies include a history and complete physical and neurologic examination. Electromyography demonstrates muscle wasting, atrophy, fasciculations, and fibrillations. Nerve biopsy is normal, whereas a muscle biopsy may demonstrate degenerative fibers interspersed with normal ones. Laboratory tests find normal CSF and a continuous elevation of serum enzyme levels: aldolase, SGPT, and especially CK.

Clinical manifestations vary and are related to the anatomical areas of involvement. ALS usually includes a combination of the syndromes of progressive muscle atrophy, bulbar palsy, and primary lateral sclerosis. Initial symptoms include skeletal muscle weakness and atrophy that progresses from distal to proximal and unilateral to bilateral involvement in the upper extremities. These symptoms are accompanied by fasciculations and a decrease or absence of DTRs.

Signs of progressive bulbar palsy are caused by damage to cranial nerves. Damage to CN IX and CN X lead to dysphagia and aphonia. Swallowing problems affect eating, drinking, and swallowing of saliva. Vagus nerve involvement can also cause dyspnea and bradycardia. Damage to CN XII causes difficulty with tongue movements during swallowing and speech. Speech becomes slurred (dysarthric) and sounds nasal. Tongue fatigue, atrophy, and tremor are noted. Damage to CN VII leads to the loss of facial expression, especially the ability to blow the nose and yawn. In the late stage of ALS the trapezius and sternocleidomastoid muscles atrophy because of damage to CN XI. The ability to shrug the shoulders and turn the head laterally is lost.

Primary lateral sclerosis results in upper motor neuron signs: spastic paresis of extremities, positive Babinski's reflex, and hyperactive DTRs. Progressive muscle spasm may cause pain because of intact afferent nerve fibers. Most clients remain mentally clear, showing signs of emotional lability only when the corticobulbar tract becomes involved.

With total paralysis and lower cranial nerve involvement, the "locked-in syndrome" occurs. Clients are fully conscious of the environment and themselves, but "locked in" by a paralyzed body. All movement and ability to verbalize are absent. The client may only be able to communicate by eyelid movement and blinking. The immediate cause of death is often respiratory muscle weakness and bulbar palsy causing respiratory failure.

Therapeutic Measures

There is no specific or effective treatment for this relentless, progressive disease. Supportive symptomatic therapy is recommended to improve and, in some cases, extend life. The quality of life should be a primary consideration when planning treatment.

Drug researchers have advocated the administration of guanidine HCl and small amounts of detoxified snake venom to arrest disease progression, although no conclusive evidence supports this regimen. Symptomatic drug therapy includes diazepam, baclofen (Lioresal), and dantrolene sodium (Dantrium) to control spasticity. Neostigmine methylsulfate (Prostigmin) is used temporarily to manage bulbar weakness. Analgesics are used to control pain. Short-term use of anticholinergic drugs is helpful in relieving sialorrhea. Invasive measures for sialorrhea have included neurectomy and salivary gland irradiation. Alternate feeding methods are solutions to swallowing problems. Efforts are made to prevent infections, especially of the respiratory tract. In many cases, tracheostomy and mechanical ventilation are mandatory to maintain respiratory function. Regardless of treatment, the prognosis is poor, and survival is brief for most clients.

Specific Nursing Measures

Nursing priorities for the client with ALS vary depending on the stage of disease. A common problem is ineffective communication patterns related to muscular weakness, dysarthria, and respiratory complications. Provide adequate time to anticipate client needs, offer explanations of care, identify client problems, and encourage client participation in decisions about nursing care. Alternate communication methods may be necessary: the use of an alphabet and number board, writing, common object cards, and eye blinking. The client must be assisted to use whatever method is most feasible and least likely to cause fatigue.

Monitor any alteration in nutritional status due to swallowing and chewing impairments. Some management suggestions include small, frequent feedings to prevent fatigue and choking. Provide a soft diet high in calories, protein, and carbohydrates with an adequate daily fluid intake. When feeding clients with ALS, elevate the head of the bed, keep oropharyngeal suction equipment nearby, and allow adequate time for meals. To evaluate nutritional status of hospitalized clients, obtain weights three times a week, check calorie counts, and review serum albumin and protein levels. Tube feedings may be necessary for some clients.

Alterations in mobility accompany increased motor paresis. To keep clients independent as long as possible, active and passive ROM exercises and physical and occupational therapy are helpful. Assistive devices may be necessary for daily activities. Clients should remain out of bed and up in a chair as long as their condition permits. Treatments and rest periods should be coordinated to avoid excessive fatigue. Changing the client's position with supportive devices provides comfort and minimizes the hazards of immobility. These interventions and antispasmodic drugs should reduce spasticity. For management of bladder and bowel incontinence, refer to specific nursing measures for clients with multiple sclerosis.

Management of ineffective breathing patterns related to muscle weakness or aspiration often becomes a nursing priority. Aspiration may occur from dysphagia and excessive salivation. Preventive measures include monitoring the client during eating, suctioning if necessary, assessing respiratory patterns around meal times, and administering anticholinergic drugs as ordered. Good oral hygiene must be provided.

When respiratory involvement progresses, the maintenance of a patent airway and adequate ventilation become the nursing priorities. Assess respiratory function every 1 to 2 hours including observation of rate, depth, and rhythm of respirations and auscultation of breath sounds. Encourage frequent coughing and deep breathing. Monitoring of tidal volume, vital capacity, and arterial blood gases becomes crucial. Chest physical therapy including postural drainage may be required as well as nasotracheal and oropharyngeal suctioning every hour and as necessary. Keep intubation and ventilatory equipment on standby.

A major nursing concern should be the management of anticipatory grieving related to the terminal nature of this disease. The most difficult nursing task often becomes helping the client and significant others to accept the seriousness of the condition. The nursing objective should be to facilitate client–family communication of anxieties and fears to assist them in their grieving process, and to help identify support systems such as social services, mental health liaisons, and community agencies. Communicate to the client and family that nursing care is available to promote optimal client comfort and safety.

SPINAL STENOSIS*

Spinal stenosis can occur in older persons with a history of osteoarthritis of the spine or chronic disk degeneration, or it can be a congenital problem. The cervical and lumbar spine are most affected.

Cervical Stenosis

The client with a stenotic cervical canal has spinal cord compression by the bony pincers of the back of the vertebral body above and the arch of the lamina below whenever the head is extended. The client gradually has spastic quadraparesis or paraparesis that is frequently accompanied by fasciculations (coarse, involuntary twitching of individual muscle fiber groups) and atrophy in the upper extremities.

Cervical stenosis is diagnosed by measuring the bony distance between the vertebral body and the laminar arch on CT scan or plain lateral x-ray films. On CT scan, a mesurement of 7 mm or 8 mm or less indicates severe stenosis. Because plain x-ray films have about a 30% magnification factor, a measurement of 10 mm or 11 mm indicates stenosis because, on x-ray, the normal diameter of the cervical canal is about 16 mm. Myelography often demonstrates a complete block to the flow of contrast material when the client's head is in extension.

When the total bony canal is stenotic, posterior decompression laminectomy is indicated. On the other hand, stenosis due to large arthritic spur formations may occur at only one or two levels. Then it may be treated by the anterior approach with removal of the disk and resection of the bony spurs. Because the cord dysfunction may have been long-standing, the degree of cord recovery is often limited. If dysfunction is not too severe, a considerable amount of improvement will take place. If it is severe, at least the progression of symptoms may be halted.

Lumbar Stenosis

Unlike cervical stenosis, lumbar stenosis is manifested mainly by pain. There is no cord damage or spasticity although there may be considerable numbness and weakness of the lower extremities. More often, the syndrome is manifested by spinal claudication. The client has rapidly developing severe pain on walking any distance. Unlike vascular claudication, the client with spinal claudication obtains relief by bending forward because this maneuver widens the anterior–posterior diameter of the spinal canal. Lumbar stenosis rarely affects L-1; it is usually limited to L-2, L-3, L-4, and L-5. It is often accompanied by marked hypertrophy of the articular facets. Diagnosis of lumbar stenosis is confirmed by spine films, CT scanning, and myelography.

Clients with lumbar stenosis usually do remarkably well following laminectomy. Despite considerable incisional pain, they are usually ambulating on the first postoperative day. Generally, clients are out of the hospital by the end of 1 week and back to their normal activities by the end of a month.

Therapeutic and Specific Nursing Measures

Surgery is the main treatment approach to spinal stenosis. Care of the client with laminectomy is discussed in Chapters 39 and 60.

Section IV: Immunologic Disorders

Myasthenia gravis, a disorder affecting the neuromuscular junction, and multiple sclerosis, a demyelinating disease, are both thought to have an autoimmune component. These are both covered here although the exact etiology of each disease remains unknown.

MYASTHENIA GRAVIS

Myasthenia gravis is a chronic neuromuscular disorder that affects voluntary (striated) muscles. The disease is characterized by fluctuating muscle weakness that becomes worse with use and shows some improvement with rest.

The course of the disease is variable. Onset is usually gradual, marked by either a stable period or rapid progression of symptoms. Respiratory infections and emotional stress may greatly exacerbate symptoms. The highest mortality rate is seen in the first year of the disease.

The disease is common, with incidence estimated at 1 in 10,000. Peak incidence is between the second and third decades; onset is rare in the first decade of life or after age 70. Under age 40, females are affected approximately two to three times as often as males. In later life, the incidence is about equal (Hickey, 1981).

This disorder usually persists for life, although there may be periods of spontaneous improvement for weeks or months followed by worsening. This disease is not hereditary, but 15% of the infants born to myasthenic mothers

*This section contributed by Dorothy A. Kaminski.

have a transient case of the disease. With treatment, infants recover fully in 2 to 3 months.

Despite numerous theories and a great deal of research, the cause of myasthenia gravis remains unknown. There is general agreement that the defect occurs at the neuromuscular junction, and myasthenia gravis is now considered an autoimmune disease. In the normal individual, there are approximately 38 million acetylcholine receptors at each neuromuscular junction. In the client with myasthenia gravis, acetylcholine receptors are reduced by about 20%. An autoimmune reaction is now known to cause the acetylcholine receptor deficiency.

The autoimmune attack is directed against acetylcholine receptors. Immunoglobulin G (IgG) antibodies, detected in the serum of 90% of myasthenic clients, react against the acetylcholine receptors. These autoantibodies cause two different types of adverse effects: they can prevent receptors from responding to acetylcholine, and they can cause receptor portions of a muscle cell to degenerate rapidly. Both conditions cause fewer receptors to be available at the neuromuscular junction.

The thymus gland is also considered to be involved in myasthenia gravis. The thymus gland, located beneath the sternum, plays an important role in normal immunity. Active from birth until puberty, the gland is thought to initiate the body's immune response and to cease functioning after puberty. In about 85% of myasthenic clients, however, the thymus gland is abnormal and remains active. An autoimmune reaction is probably triggered by the lymphocyte or musclelike cell abnormalities of the thymus gland.

Myasthenia gravis has been associated with thymic hyperplasia in 80% of affected clients (Hickey, 1981), whereas thymoma has a 15% to 20% incidence in older male clients. There is also a 5% association between myasthenia gravis and other autoimmune disorders such as lupus erythematosus, rheumatoid arthritis, polymyositis, and thyroid toxicosis. The high incidence of myasthenia gravis in females with its characteristic pattern of remissions and exacerbations, lends empirical support to an autoimmune basis for the disease.

Clinical Manifestations

The most characteristic finding in myasthenia gravis is an increasing weakness of certain voluntary muscles with activity, and some improvement with rest. The muscles of the eyes are often most affected. The eyelids droop (ptosis), the eyes squint, and there may be double vision (diplopia). The ptosis may be unilateral or bilateral and intensifies when the client attempts to gaze upward. The extraocular movements of the eyes are controlled by CN III, CN IV, and CN VI. Pupillary response to light and accommodation remain normal.

Other muscles affected are those of facial expression, chewing, swallowing, and speech. The facial nerve (CN VII) is responsible for all components of facial expression. The mobility and expression of the face is altered in myasthenic clients. Their attempts to smile look like a snarl. The affect is flat, and the jaw muscles hang loosely. Chewing (mastication) is controlled by the trigeminal nerve (CN V). When chewing, clients with myasthenia gravis often become fatigued and must rest.

The gag reflex and the swallowing reflex are controlled by the glossopharyngeal nerve (CN IX) and the vagus nerve (CN X). Clients with CN IX and CN X deficits experience problems with managing saliva, choking, and nasal regurgitation. Speech deficits include a weak voice that fades with conversation and diminishes to a whisper. Speech becomes nasal, monotonous, and dysarthric.

The shoulder and neck muscles are often affected. The head tends to fall forward, and clients have difficulty holding their arms above the head, so reaching for an object and fixing the hair are difficult. The muscles for fine hand movements can also be affected, resulting in difficulty in writing, serving, and moving the hands to the mouth. The most life-threatening situation occurs when the intercostal and/or diaphragm muscles are affected. An early sign of respiratory involvement is breathlessness. Respiratory weakness can develop rapidly.

A generally accepted classification system for myasthenia gravis is outlined in Box 37–9. Classification is based

---

Box 37–9 Classification System to Determine Severity of Myasthenia Gravis

Ocular: Only ocular muscles involved (ptosis and diplopia)
- No mortality; remission often spontaneous
- Medication usually ineffective

Mild generalized: Slow onset, usually ocular; then advances to bulbar and skeletal muscles
- Remission possible
- Mortality rate low
- Response to medication favorable

Moderate generalized: Gradual onset, usually ocular, progressing to more bulbar symptoms and a more generalized skeletal muscle involvement
- Remission possible
- Activities of daily living restricted
- Mortality rate low
- Response to medication less favorable

Acute fulminating: Rapid onset of bulbar and skeletal muscle involvement with early respiratory symptoms
- Deterioration rapid
- Mortality rate high
- Crises frequent (myasthenic and cholinergic)

Late severe: Symptoms developing at least 2 years after onset of ocular or generalized myasthenia
- Marked bulbar involvement
- Course either gradual or marked by sudden deterioration
- Mortality rate high
- Response to medication poor

Muscle atrophy: Begins as generalized myasthenia but develops atrophy as early as 6 months into the course
- Prognosis and mortality rate depend on clinical signs

on symptom severity. The diagnosis of myasthenia gravis is based on the history of voluntary muscle weakness, a physical exam that identifies muscle fatigability on repetitive action, and the clinical signs previously described.

The Tensilon test is the most discriminating diagnostic study. Tensilon is a short- and rapid-acting cholinergic drug that dramatically improves the muscle strength of a myasthenic client. This test can distinguish between myasthenic and cholinergic crises.

Other diagnostic tests include thyroid function tests (T_3 and T_4) to rule out thyroid etiology. (Hyperthyroidism occurs in 3% to 8% of all myasthenic clients.) Positive serum antibody titers against acetylcholine receptors are found in 90% of affected clients. Laboratory evaluations of antinuclear antibodies, serum protein electrophoretic pattern, and lupus erythematosus cell test are done.

Radiologic studies include CT scans to reveal thymomas and thymus scans to reveal hyperplasia or a thymoma. Chest x-ray and mediastinal tomograms may also reveal a thymoma.

In myasthenia gravis, the EMG shows that the amplitude of the evoked muscle's action potentials decreases rapidly. This reaction can be diminished or prevented with a single 2-mg IV dose of Tensilon.

Therapeutic Measures

Drug therapy is the first line of treatment. The drugs—pyridostigmine bromide (Mestinon), neostigmine bromide (Prostigmin), and occasionally ambenonium chloride (Mytelase)—act by inhibiting anticholinesterase, preventing the rapid destruction of the neurotransmitter acetylcholine. Although this effect does not change the basic abnormality, it increases the amount of acetylcholine available, partially compensating for symptoms of a defective neuromuscular transmission.

There are no set rules for determining the amount of anticholinesterase medication a client may need. Drug dosage must be individualized to provide the greatest symptom relief and the fewest side effects. Pyridostigmine usually provides a smoother action with fewer gastrointestinal side effects. The usual dosage is 60 to 80 mg orally every 3 to 4 hours. Neostigmine is given 15 to 30 mg orally every 3 to 4 hours. Pyridostigmine timespan capsule 180 mg is usually given at bedtime because it slowly releases medication and maintains the client's drug level throughout the night. Small doses of atropine sulfate may be given to reduce parasympathetic side effects. Atropine sulfate is the antidote for anticholinesterase drugs.

Corticosteroids are sometimes prescribed for clients who do not respond well to anticholinesterase drugs. Current practice recommends giving prednisone 100 mg every other day for 10 days. Clients are hospitalized for close observation during the initial treatment period on full-dose therapy. Symptoms intensify at 7 to 10 days of treatment but improve after treatment ends. This treatment is given with anticholinesterase therapy. As improvement is shown, the steroid is reduced slowly to the lowest effective dose. The effectiveness of immunosuppressive drug therapy for these clients has not been conclusively established.

The surgical removal of the thymus gland (thymectomy) is indicated for clients with thymomas and hyperplasia of the gland. The procedure is most effective for young women within the first 2 years of diagnosis and least effective for older men with thymomas. The removal of the thymus gland without an associated tumor produces a high rate of improvement or remission of symptoms in clients with early onset.

Plasmapheresis is usually performed on clients whose disease is refractory to standard treatments. Potential complications such as loss of clotting factors, hemolysis, and fluid and electrolyte imbalances must be considered. Clients undergoing this procedure remain on their medication in adjusted lower doses.

Specific Nursing Measures

The care of clients with myasthenia gravis presents a formidable challenge. What was once a catastrophic disease with a high mortality and morbidity rate has become, in many cases, a treatable condition. Careful nursing assessment, management, and evaluation can make a major difference in treating clients in crisis. Nursing priorities for myasthenic clients depend on whether the client is stable or in crisis. For clients in crisis, ineffective breathing patterns can be a life-threatening problem.

In myasthenic crisis, the client experiences an abrupt exacerbation of motor weakness, usually from undermedication. The neuromuscular junction is no longer responsive to drug therapy. This crisis may also occur in a myasthenic client receiving no medication.

Cholinergic crisis is caused by overmedication with cholinergic (anticholinesterase) drugs. Excessive medication results in a depolarization block. An acute exacerbation of myasthenic muscle weakness also occurs in this crisis. Symptoms and signs of myasthenic and cholinergic crises are listed in Table 37–2.

Baseline assessments of the client are important. Evaluate ineffective breathing patterns by taking serial vital capacity measurements. (Vital capacity, which equals the respiratory capacity plus expiratory reserve volume, represents the largest gas volume a client can exhale after maximum inspiration.) Testing can be done at the client's bedside with a respirometer attached to a mouthpiece, face mask, tracheostomy or endotracheal tube. The client should be in an upright position to promote maximum chest expansion. Emergency respiratory equipment must be available for clients in crisis, including intubation equipment, suction apparatus, an Ambu bag with an oxygen source, and a ventilator.

Another important function to evaluate is the client's ability to swallow. Check this by gently placing a hand over the anterior neck and instructing the client to attempt "dry" swallowing. This maneuver is preferable to giving the client

Table 37-2 Symptoms and Signs of Myasthenic and Cholinergic Crises

Myasthenic Crisis	Cholinergic Crisis
Sudden marked crisis in blood pressure and pulse	*Generalized weakness
*Extreme restlessness and apprehension	*Dysphagia
*Increased diaphoresis, secretions, and lacrimation	Dysarthria
	*Dyspnea
	Nausea and vomiting
*Severe cyanosis and dyspnea that may lead to respiratory arrest	Abdominal cramps and diarrhea
	Miosis, pallor
*Dysphagia (difficulty swallowing)	*Increased copious secretions: salivation, lacrimation, phlegm, perspiration
Absent cough reflex	
Urinary and fecal incontinence; urinary output	Blurred vision
	Muscle twitching
*Dysarthria (difficulty speaking)	*Apprehension
*Generalized muscle weakness	

*Indicates that dyspnea, dysphagia, dysarthria, generalized weakness, increased secretions, and apprehension are common to both myasthenic and cholinergic crises.

liquids that might induce choking or aspiration. If the swallowing reflex is intact, test the gag reflex. Suction apparatus should be available during testing.

The strength of several other muscle groups should also be assessed. Check ocular muscles by testing the six extraocular movements of cardinal gaze (see Chapters 7 and 69). Ocular movements can also be timed for duration of a particular gaze and number of times blinking occurs.

Test upper extremity strength by asking the client to do a repetitive act such as squeezing and releasing an object placed in the hand and flexing and extending the elbow. Assess lower extremity strength by having the client alternate dorsiflexion and plantar flexion of the feet repeatedly or flex and extend the knees. Baseline assessment of the various muscle groups of the client in crisis is essential for future comparisons, diagnosis of the problem, and intervention.

For clients who develop respiratory failure, endotracheal intubation creates an emergency airway. Long-term management includes a planned tracheostomy. A volume-cycled ventilator should be used during periods of acute respiratory insufficiency. During the acute phase, current practice recommends discontinuing all anticholinesterase medication to allow a "rest period" for the neuromuscular junction. Once the client's condition stabilizes, small doses

of anticholinesterase medication can be restarted. During this period, the client is generally fed by nasogastric tube. To prevent aspiration, check for proper tube placement before each feeding, check the amount and type of stomach aspirant, and feed the client in the upright position with an inflated tracheal or endotracheal cuff. Aspiration of feedings can lead to major complications for myasthenic clients with bulbar paralysis.

Intensive chest physiotherapy should be carried out during crises to prevent respiratory complications. In addition, a bedside physical therapy program should be instituted to prevent muscle atrophy or contractures. Adequate hydration and antiembolism support stockings should be used to prevent thrombophlebitis.

The most difficult nursing challenge for a client in crisis is how to handle ineffective coping patterns that result from the client's complete dependency. The crisis may persist for a long time, placing a great emotional strain on the client. The nurse must be able to anticipate the client's needs while helping the client to identify concerns and preferences for care. Clients with chronic illnesses often become well informed about their diseases and treatment approaches. They want to participate in decision making for their care as well as identify successful techniques they have developed.

To develop an accurate, detailed plan of care, an effective communication system must be provided. Ordinary communication devices are not usually effective for clients in crisis. Alternatives may include a bell tied to the client's ankle and wrist, a light touch bell under the client's shoulder, or a special communication device that requires head turning or forehead movement.

Myasthenic clients often experience fear and anxiety because of the disease sequelae. The client needs constant help to express fears and establish realistic goals. Ensure sufficient time for ventilation of the client's feelings and avoid frustration-producing conditions.

Clients with myasthenia gravis often experience long-term muscle weakness that worsens with activity and fatigue. Anticholinesterase drugs should always be administered *exactly on time.* Assess the client's strength and motor ability with drug administration, and observe and report side effects. Give medications with milk or food to prevent gastrointestinal irritation. Give the medication at least 45 minutes before meals to ensure optimal muscle strength during meals. In addition, plan nursing care to provide rest periods and prevent excessive fatigue. Teach alternative methods of communication such as lip reading; writing; and use of erasable boards, pictures, and gestures. Be sure to provide adequate listening time.

Alterations in protective mechanisms can occur, such as incomplete eyelid closure. Corneal abrasion or ulceration is a potential problem. Provide routine eye care with normal saline every 4 to 6 hours and as necessary. Lubricate the cornea with artificial tears every 2 hours and as appropriate; provide a protective eye shield if necessary. Eye patching may be alternated every 2 to 4 hours and clients taught compensatory techniques. Clients may have diplopia and require assistance with daily activities.

Clients on long-term anticholinesterase drug therapy may have periods of altered gastrointestinal function. Common concerns include nausea, diarrhea, abdominal cramping, and constipation. The type and frequency of discomfort should be monitored. Gastrointestinal symptoms may indicate anticholinesterase toxicity. Anticholinergics (atropine sulfate) should be administered as ordered and small frequent feedings given. Antiemetics and antidiarrheal agents may also be necessary. For clients with constipation, enemas should be avoided to prevent a crisis. Mild cathartics and suppositories can be used. Alterations in diet and fluid regimen may be helpful. Educate clients about actions of drugs and specific factors that might precipitate an increase in muscle weakness.

MULTIPLE SCLEROSIS

Multiple sclerosis (MS) is a degenerative disease with a chronic course, marked by variable periods of remission and exacerbation. The disorder is the most common neurologic condition causing demyelination of the CNS. Myelin sheaths and nerve conduction pathways are affected. Myelin can be destroyed anywhere in the CNS white matter, followed by the development of patches of plaques (scars), a recovery period, and subsequent degeneration. Plaques may develop in the cerebral hemispheres, brain stem, cerebellum, and in the spinal cord. The PNS is not involved per se. Eventually remyelination becomes less likely, and neurologic deficits result from permanent sclerosis (Bickerstaff, 1980). In early stages of the disease, it is more common to have periods of both remission and exacerbation. Later, exacerbations are more common, longer, and more severe.

Approximately 500,000 cases of multiple sclerosis occur in the United States per year. Although females are affected slightly more often than males, the difference is not significant. Because at least two-thirds of all cases occur between the ages of 20 and 40 (Foster, 1978), MS is known as the "crippler" among young adults. MS tends to occur more frequently in cold, damp climates.

The cause of multiple sclerosis is unknown. Most theories involve a viral or immunologic cause. Many theories postulating a vascular, traumatic, nutritional, allergic, or infectious cause have been tested, but none has adequately explained the etiology. It had been thought that a slow virus identical to or similar to the measles virus might be responsible for MS. Now attention is focused on the age of onset of measles because MS incidence is higher in clients who had measles later than in infancy or early childhood. Those with MS have a high level of measles specific antibody in their serum. This finding lends support to an immunologic explanation for MS. An autoimmune reaction might occur in which a person develops antigens that act against normal antibodies.

Serologic studies have identified a much higher-than-normal incidence of certain antigens. These include the histocompatibility antigens known as HLA-Dw2, HLA-A3, and HLA-B7, the most significant of which is the HLA-Dw2. Also important is the B-lymphocyte alloantigen. The significance of these findings is not clear, but it suggests that these antigens might be markers for a "susceptibility" gene that is possibly an immune-response gene. The presence of an immunogenetic determinant might identify individuals at greater risk for developing MS because of exposure to certain environmental factors. The presence of these antigens might also be correlated with disease frequency, expression, and course.

Clinical Manifestations

Symptoms differ among clients, depending on the areas of the CNS affected, duration of disease, and disease expression. Some clients have only mild exacerbations, long remission periods, and minimal disabilities, whereas others have frequent relapses with increasing residual deficits followed by deterioration. The symptoms are discussed according to the clients' subjective concerns and objective clinical findings. The most common initial symptoms are fatigue, visual disturbances, and motor weakness.

All symptoms tend to subside after white matter degenerates initially. Relapses increase as sclerosis becomes more extensive during subsequent exacerbation periods. The diagnosis of MS is presumptive based on report of the symptoms, with an emphasis on remission and exacerbation, the neurologic exam, and CSF analysis.

The examination of CSF is diagnostically significant. The CSF shows an elevation of gamma globulin in two-thirds of clients with MS. Lange's test has a distinctive gold-colloid color, especially in clients with chronic disease. Sensitive radioimmunoassay has demonstrated varied levels of myelin basic protein in the CSF of clients with MS. The level is high during an acute exacerbation; lower in slower, progressive courses; and normal during disease remission (Cohen et al., 1976). CSF protein levels vary, with some normal, others low, and about 25% showing an increase. A major diagnostic finding is abnormal brain stem auditory-evoked, somatosensory-evoked, and visual-evoked response studies. Abnormalities occur in a high percentage of clients with MS.

Several factors can precipitate disease onset as well as cause an exacerbation. Infections, pregnancy, and trauma can precipitate the onset of MS or a relapse. Menstruation, extreme cold or heat, fatigue, and stress can cause an exacerbation of symptoms.

Visual Symptoms and Signs

The client describes visual disturbances as double and blurred vision, decreased acuity, loss of peripheral vision, and blind spots. Clinical examination often reveals optic neuritis. This common early sign accounts for the blurring and loss of vision as well as orbital pain. Nystagmus occurs in almost three-fourths of all clients. Pupillary response is slowed in the affected eye. A sign strongly suggestive of MS is internuclear ophthalmoplegia (paralysis of ocular muscles) on lateral gaze.

Motor Symptoms and Signs
The client usually reports stiffness, weakness, and clumsiness of the extremities, which are initially more frequent in the legs than arms. Limbs become heavy and spastic, causing a "jumping" of affected limbs, especially at night. Clients may also report a decrease in motor strength after a hot bath or shower; strenuous exercise can also decrease motor strength. The clinical exam finds muscular weakness, spasm, and spasticity.

Reflex Changes
On clinical exam, DTRs are found to be hyperactive. Clonus occurs as well as Babinski's sign. The abdominal reflex, a superficial reflex, is frequently absent in MS.

Sensory Alterations
Common client concerns include numbness and tingling (paresthesia) of the face and affected extremities. Disturbing symptoms are feelings of burning or crawling (formications) and shocklike sensations. Clients may report loss of position sense, which is often accompanied by feelings of extremity swelling and tightness. Clinical examination shows paresthesia, decrease or loss of position sense, and vibration. *Lhermitte's sign,* transient sensations of electriclike shock extending bilaterally down the arms, back, and trunk, is evoked on neck flexion.

Cerebral Deficits
Frontal lobe involvement can lead to emotional lability and deterioration of intellectual function. Clients feel irritable and apathetic, have a short attention span, and have difficulty doing calculations and thinking abstractly. They report lapses in memory and inappropriate episodes of laughing or crying. They sometimes report seizures. Neurologic examination shows deficits of memory, affect, judgment, and reasoning. Later signs include confusion, disorientation, and depression. The CT scan demonstrates nonspecific ventricular enlargement and/or cortical atrophy in approximately 40% of clients with MS. An abnormal EEG and neuropsychological deficits can be observed.

Brain Stem Signs
Clients are often concerned about speech impairments, which are a result of spastic weakness in the muscles responsible for speech. Initially, speech is slurred; later, speech becomes garbled, staccatolike, and unintelligible. **Scanning speech**—speech that is slow and deliberate, punctuated with pauses between syllables—is a common characteristic of MS. Other brain-stem signs include reports of dizziness, vertigo, nausea, diplopia, tinnitus, dysphagia,

facial weakness, and loss of sensation and (much less commonly) hearing loss. Physical examination findings include nystagmus; ophthalmoplegia; dysarthric, scanning speech; and trigeminal neuralgia.

Cerebellar Deficits
Cerebellar involvement is more frequent in later stages of the disease. Clients note clumsiness, loss of balance and coordination, and tremors. Clinical exam reveals truncal ataxia, **dysmetria** (inability to measure distance properly in muscular acts), and intention tremors. The ability to perform alternating movements is impaired. Head tremors are observed in the final stage of the disease.

Bladder and Bowel Problems
Clients often have urinary hesitancy, urgency, frequency, dysuria, nocturia, retention, or reflex emptying. Constipation and incontinence are common problems.

Sexual Problems
Men may be impotent or have difficulty sustaining erections. Women report absence of sexual desire and decreased vaginal secretions.

Therapeutic Measures

Because numerous treatment protocols have been tried over the last several decades, clients are often confused about long-term treatment and prognosis. There is no curative treatment for MS. Intervention is supportive according to symptoms. The drugs of choice are corticosteroids, which reduce edema and inflammation at sites of demyelination. High doses of ACTH can shorten an acute exacerbation if given early enough and can produce clinical improvement in some cases. Steroids do not alter the course of the disease however; the drugs are considered ineffective in the long term and do not prevent relapses.

Recently, public attention has focused on diet in the treatment of MS. Previously, low-fat diets were encouraged because incidence of MS has been low during wars when famine prevailed. Gluten-free diets and diets high in linoleic acid (sunflower seed oil) are still being investigated. The consensus among most neurologists is that no statistically valid controlled studies have demonstrated the value of any special diet.

Physical therapy is aimed at maintaining function and preventing complications of immobility. Muscle spasms can be treated with muscle relaxants such as diazepam and dantrolene sodium. These drugs must be carefully regulated to prevent increased muscle weakness.

Clients with severe symptoms that do not respond to drug therapy are sometimes considered for palliative surgical procedures. Thalamotomies can be done to eliminate intention tremors of cerebellar origin. It should be recognized, however, that this is a destructive procedure with variable results. Clients with severe swallowing problems might require a gastrostomy.

Plasmapheresis is a new treatment aimed at removing autoantibodies, similar to its use in myasthenia gravis. It is important to consider potential complications such as the loss of clotting factors, hemolysis, and fluid and electrolyte imbalances.

Specific Nursing Measures

Clients with multiple sclerosis must recognize that they may experience various stages of loss and acceptance as the disease progresses. Although the symptoms may be minimal at disease onset, there is a tendency for neurologic deficits to progress. Teach clients strategies to cope with periods of symptom exacerbation and progression. Symptoms and signs of relapse should be identified early. Instruct the client to avoid extreme fatigue, emotional stress, and infection. Clients should adjust daily schedules to include regular exercise, rest periods, and proper dietary habits. Also assist clients to reach realistic goals and potentials during periods of remission.

During periods of exacerbation, steroids may be used (ACTH, prednisone, or dexamethasone). Medication selection depends on the severity of the client's symptoms. The objectives of the medication regimen are to reduce the acute inflammatory response, expedite a remission, and promote the level of recovery. Clients may require bed rest at this time in a relaxed, quiet environment. It is crucial to prevent any secondary infections from steroids or restricted activity. Side effects of steroids to be alert for include fluid retention, hypertension, electrolyte imbalance, and gastric irritation. To prevent gastric irritation, antacids may be given with steroids or between meals if medication is given with meals. Hypokalemia is not uncommon. Therefore, potassium supplements are given or high-potassium foods increased. Although vitamins have not been proven effective, some clients feel better taking them. Linoleic acid may have an effect on myelin formation.

A common problem is alteration in elimination patterns. Urinary incontinence or urinary retention and constipation may occur. For bladder problems, in-dwelling catheters with a closed drainage system may be required. Catheter care should be done at least twice a day. Clients can be taught to clean their own catheters with warm water and soap using hydrogen peroxide for encrustations. If unusual or foul-smelling drainage is noted around the meatus or in the urine, notify the physician. Encourage fluid intake to about 3 L per day. Cranberry juice (200 mL) given four times a day can keep the urine pH acidic and possibly decrease the incidence of urinary tract infections. In-dwelling catheters are changed every 10 to 14 days or once a month, depending on the client's urinary status. Intermittent catheterization is recommended because of the lower incidence of bladder infections and the potential for increasing bladder tone between catheterizations. To prevent or manage constipation, administer a suppository daily or as necessary at the same time of day, give stool softeners as prescribed, and provide bulk in the diet. Establish a regular schedule for bowel movements.

Impairment in mobility is another common problem. Loss of motor strength and coordination are the most frequent concerns. The degree of deficit varies. Approaches to prevent disuse atrophy and increase muscle strength include resistive exercises and muscle stretching and active and passive ROM every 4 to 6 hours. Assistive devices (eg, braces, walkers) may be required to prevent injury. Encourage as much ambulation as the client can tolerate. Handrails may be needed in bathrooms and halls and on stairways. Hand controls may be necessary in the client's automobile. Encourage clients to maintain as normal an activity level as possible.

Clients may also experience a loss of protective mechanisms because of sensory deficits. Caution clients to avoid extreme temperatures and hazards because they may not feel the pain associated with such injuries. Compensatory mechanisms can include the use of eye-hand coordination when manipulating objects.

Alterations in sensory perception are common, especially visual disturbances such as decreased visual acuity and diplopia. To combat visual loss, organize objects for easy reach and orient the client to new settings. A magnifying glass and large-print reading material can be invaluable. For diplopia, alternate patching of the eye with a dark cloth eyepatch can correct this disturbing problem.

Self-care deficits can occur because of intention tremors and spasticity. To manage intention tremors, avoid fatigue and place objects within easy reach. Clients can be helped to learn how to anticipate their needs and reorganize their environments. Otherwise, they may experience unnecessary frustration. A number of interventions can diminish spasticity. In addition to exercises mentioned under impaired immobility, muscle relaxants, warm tub baths, and sleeping prone can help. Hot baths must be avoided because they can increase the metabolic rate, causing more weakness. Flexor spasms can diminish with position changes, such as sleeping in the prone position.

Alterations in body image and self-esteem can lead to depression and a sense of hopelessness. It is crucial for both clients and their families to have an accurate understanding of the disease and to use appropriate resources, especially the National Multiple Sclerosis Society. Clients need to function to the level of their ability and tolerance, to continue socialization, and to find diversional activities that decrease anxiety and fatigue.

Clients may have periods of emotional lability that do not appear appropriate to a given situation. Teach family members to be understanding when the client has changes in mood. Open communication in families is essential for optimal coping patterns to develop, especially in chronic illness. Foster a positive attitude to maintain as near a normal lifestyle for the client as possible.

Section V: Infectious and Inflammatory Disorders

The nervous system's parenchyma, blood vessels, and protective coverings may be infected by many of the pathogenic microorganisms that affect other organs of the body. CNS infections cause various neurologic responses. Diffuse inflammatory reactions such as meningitis, encephalitis, and myelitis, as well as localized neuroinfective processes such as brain abscesses are included in this section. The effects of herpes viruses on the CNS and an example of a slow neurovirus, Creutzfeldt–Jakob disease, are also covered.

There are four major routes by which pathogens gain access to the CNS. The most common route is the bloodstream (hematogenous) from a septicemia or a septic embolus from endocarditis, lung infections, or pelvic abscesses. Direct invasions can be traumatic or nontraumatic. The traumatic sources include skull fractures, penetrating wounds, and operative procedures. Nontraumatic infections can occur from otitis media, mastoiditis, sinusitis, and osteomyelitis. Pathogens may enter in a retrograde manner via nerve trunks (eg, rabies) or through the cerebrospinal route from lumbar puncture or ventricular tap.

In addition to mechanisms of entry, host factors contribute to neuroinfective disorders. Major host factors include:

- Dental abscess
- Congenital heart disease
- A decrease in polymorphonuclear function
- Immunoglobulin deficiency
- Malignancy (eg, reticuloendothelial system)
- Long-term radiation treatment
- Chemotherapeutic agents (eg, immunosuppressives or antimetabolites)
- Debilitation due to age, chronic illness, or malnutrition
- Diabetes mellitus
- Renal failure
- Alcoholism

MENINGITIS

Meningitis is an inflammation of the meninges caused by a viral, bacterial, or fungal organism. It is classified according to the location of CNS involvement. *Pachymeningitis* refers to an inflammation of the dura; *leptomeningitis* involves an inflammation of the arachnoid and pia layers of the meninges. The term meningitis more commonly refers to leptomeningitis, because pachymeningitis is rarer. Another type, *basal meningitis,* describes an infectious process occurring mostly at the brain's base. Meningoencephalitis is an inflammation that is more extensive, involving not only the meninges but also cerebral tissue.

There are three major types of meningitis—aseptic, septic, and tuberculous. *Aseptic* meningitis is thought to occur from viral inflammation or meningeal irritation. Meningeal irritation results from a brain abscess, encephalitis, leukemias, lymphoma, or the presence of blood in the subarachnoid space. *Septic* purulent meningitis is caused by infection of the pia and arachnoid from a pus-forming bacteria (eg, meningococcus, pneumococcus, staphylococcus, or the influenza bacillus). The third major type is *tuberculous* caused by the tubercle bacillus.

The pathophysiology of meningitis can best be described by tracing the route of the causative organism throughout the CNS. Once the pathogen enters the subarachnoid space, the infection spreads because of the open communication over the brain's convexity. Arachnoid cells become edematous from the inflammatory process. The infection extends along the blood vessels of the pia and then penetrates the sulci. It is not uncommon for affected blood vessels to become engorged, leading to thrombosis or rupture. The accumulation of exudate over the convexities, in the cisterns or the ventricles, can cause obstruction of CSF flow. The exudate may extend to involve the spinal cord. If the brain surface adjacent to the meninges becomes involved, secondary encephalitis and neuronal degeneration can occur (Core Curriculum of Neuroscience Nursing, 1983).

Clinical Manifestations

The clinical course can be acute, subacute, chronic, or recurrent. Headache, fever, meningeal irritation, and mental status changes are the most common. Clients will complain of severe headaches, the worst they have ever experienced. Meningeal signs will include nuchal rigidity; opisthotonic positioning (extensor rigidity with legs hyperextended, forming an arc with the trunk); photophobia; and pain down the back and limbs. Generalized hyperirritability with hypersensitivity/hyperalgesia, alterations in mental status, decreased level of consciousness, restlessness, confusion, hallucinations, and delirium can occur. There may be generalized seizures and increased ICP due to cerebral edema and communicating hydrocephalus. There also may be medullary signs such as vomiting, respiratory difficulties, and a weak, rapid pulse. Cranial nerve involvement causes visual disturbances, ptosis, pupil abnormalities, strabismus, deafness, nystagmus, and vertigo.

In meningococcal meningitis there can be a skin rash, evidenced by petechiae in which skin stroking yields tache cerebrale (meningitis streak). The onset of tuberculous meningitis is less acute. The client may have vague symptoms with a progressive listlessness and headache. Eventually, similar symptoms and signs as in other types of meningitis occur. The onset of viral meningitis is less severe with symptoms comparable to the previous general description.

Diagnosis is based on history of prior infection or exposure, symptoms and signs of an existing infection, clinical neurologic signs, and diagnostic tests. Skull x-rays are ordered to look for fractures, and infected sinuses or mastoids. Chest x-rays are checked for pneumonia and lung abscesses. CSF studies reveal increased CSF pressure from 200 to 700 mm/water. The appearance of the CSF varies according to the organism. In bacterial infection, the CSF is turbid to purulent. In tubercular infection, the CSF is clear, xanthochromic, or like ground glass. In viral infection, the CSF is usually clear. An important differential diagnosis is the glucose level, which is low in bacterial and tubercular infections but normal in viral infections.

Therapeutic Measures

The diagnosis of bacterial meningitis is confirmed by lumbar puncture. CSF pressure will be increased; the fluid will be milky or cloudy, with many polymorphonuclear leukocytes and a low glucose level. Culture confirms the type of bacteria, and results of sensitivity tests indicate appropriate drug therapy. The drugs of choice for the major bacterial types are:

- *Meningococcus*—Penicillin G, chloramphenicol
- *Pneumococcus*—Penicillin G
- *Staphylococcus*—Oxacillin, methicillin
- *Streptococcus*—Penicillin G, chloramphenicol
- *Klebsiella*—Gentamicin, kanamycin
- *Pseudomonas*—Gentamicin, carbenicillin
- *Proteus*—Gentamicin, kanamycin
- *H. Influenzae*—Chloramphenicol, ampicillin

Prognosis is good with antibiotic therapy.

In the acute phase of meningococcal meningitis, it is possible to infect others. It is spread by nasopharyngeal and droplet secretions from the respiratory tract. This organism is usually controlled within 24 hours of antibiotic therapy. Isolation procedures to protect others should be maintained until cultures are negative.

In tuberculous meningitis the CSF shows fewer cells and low glucose and chloride levels. Tuberculous meningitis was fatal in the past. Prognosis has improved with a prolonged course of drug therapy including streptomycin injections together with oral isoniazid (INH) and rifampin. Streptomycin is given intrathecally (via lumbar puncture) in some clients. Drug treatment should be continued for a minimum of 3 months.

Specific Nursing Measures

The major priority in the care of a client with meningitis is management of the acute phase of infection. Frequently assess level of consciousness and neurologic signs. Maintain appropriate infection control precautions according to institution and infection control guidelines. Clients with meningococcal meningitis or meningitis of unknown etiol-ogy are kept in isolation. Administer antibiotics on a strict schedule to maintain blood levels.

Clients will have a febrile period. Monitor the client's temperature every 1 to 2 hours if higher than 101°F (38°C). Give tepid sponge baths, axillary and groin compresses, and antipyretic drugs as ordered. Hypothermia blankets are used for temperatures above 102 to 103°F (39°C). A cooling blanket reduces fever by conduction and radiation. Provide frequent skin care with a lanolin lotion. If shivering develops during hypothermia treatments, the temperature could increase. Chlorpromazine (Thorazine) is sometimes used to counteract shivering.

Fluid volume deficits can occur due to fever and inadequate intake. The body metabolism increases 7% for every 1°F elevation in body temperature, raising the caloric requirement by 50% with high fevers (Wilson, 1979). During pyrexic states, potassium; sodium; vitamin A, B complex, and C are lost. Requirements for protein, carbohydrates, and fat increase. Fluid administration at a minimum of 3000 mL/24 hours is required to replace fluid lost by evaporation or urinary output. A balance must be achieved that will provide enough fluid to maintain hydration without increasing ICP. Monitor serum electrolytes daily during febrile periods and maintain strict intake and output. Give oral fluids, intravenous fluids, and/or tube feedings as needed. Intermittent or in-dwelling bladder catheterization may be necessary for clients with impaired levels of consciousness.

Sensory perceptual alterations can occur because of photophobia, hyperalgesia, and hyperirritability. Maintain a quiet, dark, nonstimulating environment to reduce photophobia. Hyperirritability may be caused by hypoxia or bladder distention, which should be ruled out before considering it a neurologic problem. Plan nursing care to minimize overstimulating the client. Restricted visiting hours may be necessary to promote rest.

For headache management, keep the head of the bed elevated unless contraindicated. Maintain good body alignment and position the client every 2 hours. Provide cold compresses and avoid overstimulation. Salicylates and codeine, the drugs of choice, are usually ordered.

ENCEPHALITIS

Encephalitis is an infection of brain tissue caused by viruses, pyogenic bacteria, fungi, or parasites. Viruses are the most common. Epidemic encephalitis begins in a reservoir and is transmitted to humans (eg, equine encephalitis begins in squirrels, horses, wild birds, chickens, or garter snakes; a mosquito or tick bites the reservoir animal and transmits the virus to a human host). Incubation periods vary according to the host's susceptibility, reaction to, and strength of the pathogen.

Encephalitis begins with the pathogen gaining access to the CNS. This occurs via the bloodstream or along peripheral and cranial nerves. The cortex, white matter, and meninges develop a nonsuppurative inflammation. There is a degeneration and destruction of cortical neurons with demyelination. Patches of hemorrhage, necrosis, and cavitation can occur, depending on the type of pathogen involved. Diffuse cerebral edema results.

Viruses are the most common pathogens. Type I herpes simplex virus has the potential to cause acute encephalitis in the adult and Type II can cause neonatal encephalitis from vaginal delivery of a mother with genital herpes. Other latent viruses that can cause encephalitis include herpes zoster, cytomegalovirus, Epstein–Barr virus, mumps, rabies, and measles. Arboviruses (Eastern and Western equine, St. Louis, Japanese B viruses), and enteroviruses (polio, ECHO, and coxsackie viruses) have also been implicated. Other miscellaneous pathogens causing encephalitis are bacteria and spirochetes, fungi, malaria, toxoplasmosis, and amebas. The severity of encephalitis depends on the pathogen.

Clinical Manifestations

A prodromal illness often precedes neurologic signs. Usual symptoms are headache, fever, malaise, sore throat, and vague aches and pains. This is often followed by marked alteration in level of consciousness from lethargy to coma. Confusion and disorientation with abrupt behavioral disturbances may occur. Objective signs include motor and sensory deficits, tremor, and ataxia. Hyperirritability, meningeal signs, seizures, and cranial nerve palsies are possible.

Diagnosis depends on a number of factors. The health history may reveal a preceding infection or related precipitating factor. The client may have symptoms and signs of an existing infection. Serum and urine laboratory studies may be of little value because they demonstrate findings consistent with a number of infectious diseases. Elevated CSF pressure with a xanthochromic appearance of CSF occurs with hemorrhage. CSF may also show elevated protein, decreased glucose, and an elevated WBC. A CT scan identifies edematous tissue areas and a brain shift.

It is essential to make a quick and accurate diagnosis. Isolation of the organism is not always possible. The only conclusive diagnostic method is by special fluorescent antibody studies and viral culture of cerebral tissue from a brain biopsy.

Therapeutic Measures

Medical approaches are mainly symptomatic and supportive. There is no effective drug to treat encephalitis. The use of steroids such as dexamethasone (Decadron) combats cerebral edema. Potent antiviral drugs (eg, adenine arabinoside or Ara-A) have been used for the treatment of viral strains. Antiviral drugs in combination with steroids may prevent a fatal outcome. All clients do not recover completely, however. Those surviving an acute episode can have residual neurologic deficits including seizures, dysphasia, memory deficits, or personality changes.

Specific Nursing Measures

Nursing priorities for the client with encephalitis are similar to those outlined for meningitis with several major differences. Clients with acute encephalitis have more marked alterations in level of consciousness and behavioral manifestations. Restlessness, agitation, and dementia are more severe. There are also sleep pattern disturbances in which the sleep–wake cycle is less predictable. Minimal stress will increase agitation and hostility. Carefully control environmental stimuli; set limits; and provide a safe, supervised environment. Use a calm, soothing approach because the client's behavior may be unpredictable. Education of significant others is crucial to increase their awareness and guide them in their interactions with the client.

Neurologic deficits may increase rapidly due to cerebral edema and necrosis. Assess neurologic signs frequently during the acute stage, and report changes promptly. There is potential for fluid volume overload related to intravenous antiviral drug administration. Administer these drugs on a strict time schedule as ordered. Maintain accurate intake and output. Observe for possible drug side effects, including nausea, vomiting, diarrhea, weight loss, and transient alterations in blood cell and liver function tests. Other nursing measures include elevating the head of the bed and monitoring electrolytes and respiratory and cardiac status. Explain all procedures and tests to the client and family; allow time for verbalization of anxieties; and encourage participation in care planning.

CREUTZFELDT–JAKOB DISEASE

Creutzfeldt–Jakob disease (CJD) is a fatal neuroinfective disorder presumed to be caused by an unidentified "slow" virus. Slow viruses have been considered sequelae of viral diseases (eg, measles, rubella), prophylactic inoculations, or obscure illnesses of viral origin. The incidence of previous eye or brain surgery in clients who develop CJD is unusually high (Petersdorf et al., 1983). CJD is a progressive degeneration of the cerebral cortex, basal ganglia, and spinal cord. Symptom onset usually occurs in middle or late life, culminating in death within a few months or years.

Clinical Manifestations

Pyramidal and extrapyramidal signs gradually develop. Pyramidal signs include weakness, stiffness of the extremities, and reflex changes. Extrapyramidal signs include rigidity, tremors, dysarthria, and slow movements. Mental deterioration is extreme with psychotic manifestations. Myoclonus and convulsive seizures occur in a large number of clients. Muscular atrophy and cerebellar dysfunction may also be present.

Therapeutic Measures

There is no specific treatment for CJD; therapy is aimed at providing supportive measures. The drug Isoprinosine is currently under investigation to treat slow viral infections. Preventive measures for human transmission include maximum caution in the handling of CSF, blood, and tissue specimens from clients with CJD.

Specific Nursing Measures

Assess the client for alterations in thought processes and anticipate behavioral disturbances. Assist the client to continue normal activities in a protective environment and help the client and family understand the reasons for the client's lack of self-control. A gentle, firm nursing approach is indicated. Attempt to anticipate anxiety-provoking situations a client might encounter such as the absence of significant others, personnel and environmental changes, and fear of new tasks or procedures.

Myoclonus and increasing spasticity create a potential for mobility impairments. Maintain a safe environment. With myoclonus, it may be necessary to pad side rails, remove sharp objects, and apply a waist restraint when sitting. Provide activities and recreation that require minimal motor coordination. With spasticity, maintain ROM; give antispasmodics as ordered; and avoid rapid movements. Clients are at risk for alterations in nutritional patterns because of dysphagia. Monitor gag and swallowing reflexes. Keep suction equipment at the bedside for use as needed. The diet should be high caloric, and soft or pureed. Ensure proper positioning and provide supervision during meals. A nasogastric or gastrostomy feeding tube may be necessary.

The client and family are usually frustrated and confused by the diagnosis and progression of symptoms. Help them by explaining the clinical manifestations and setting realistic goals. Reinforce physician explanations; assist in developing coping strategies to deal with the long process; and provide psychosocial support and referrals to appropriate resources. Because CJD is a potentially transmissible viral dementia, be certain that all health care personnel use strict precautions with injections, venipunctures, and specimens of blood, CSF, and tissue.

MYELITIS

The term *myelitis* refers to an inflammation of the spinal cord. At one time, the term also referred to a number of diseases affecting the spinal cord, including those causing trauma and compression. Myelitis currently applies to a group of infective and noninfective inflammatory processes affecting the spinal cord. This discussion is limited to the three major types of myelitis: that related to viruses, that of unknown etiology, and that secondary to meningeal inflammation.

The most common viral diseases causing myelitis are poliomyelitis and herpes zoster. Unknown etiologies include possible postinfection or postvaccination myelitis or myelitis related to an exacerbation of multiple sclerosis. Myelitis associated with meningeal inflammation may be trig-

gered by various organisms such as the tubercle bacillus, funguses, or parasites. Myelitis can also be related to epidural spinal abscesses and spinal arachnoiditis.

Clinical Manifestations

The viruses that cause myelitis usually have an affinity for motor and sensory neurons rather than spinal tracts. Neurons of the anterior horn are affected by poliomyelitis; those of the dorsal root ganglion are affected by herpes zoster. In most cases, inflammations involving motor and sensory tracts are not viral in origin. Myelitis developing after an infection is commonly associated with measles, varicella, and gonorrhea and less frequently with mumps, rubella, and influenza. The vaccinations most commonly related to onset of myelitis are cowpox and antirabies. In this group, neurologic symptoms and signs develop over a few days and may involve both the brain and spinal cord or primarily the spinal cord. Following an isolated attack, the degree of recovery is variable over several weeks. Acute multiple sclerosis can be confused with myelitis because of manifestations similar to those that occur after a viral infection. Symptoms and signs develop more insidiously in acute MS, however. In addition, there is less evidence of a definite relation between a previous infection or vaccine.

Clinical findings in clients experiencing spinal cord involvement include paresis, numbness of the feet and legs more than arms, dysuria, and sometimes headache and stiff neck. As the skin rash related to the initial infection fades, neurologic symptoms and signs develop, progress, stabilize, and then recede. CSF analysis demonstrates an elevated lymphocyte count with normal glucose and a normal or slightly elevated protein level. Neurologic involvement can extend to the brain stem, cerebellum, cerebrum, and optic nerves in some clients. In myelitis related to vaccines, the PNS may be more involved than the CNS.

Inflammatory conditions of the meninges can lead to a myelitis. This type of myelitis is often a sign of generalized disease. The disease can involve the epidural space, the dura (pachymeningitis), or the pia and arachnoid (leptomeningitis). These are discussed in more detail in a previous section.

The diagnosis of myelitis includes evidence of an acute infection with a history of sudden motor paresis accompanied by other neurologic deficits. The CSF analysis may be within normal limits, and assessments such as Queckenstedt's test may demonstrate no blockage.

Therapeutic Measures

Treatment is supportive but usually without therapeutic value. If an autoimmune disorder is responsible for the myelitis, steroids are recommended (ACTH or prednisone). Generally, the prognosis is guarded because of the variability among cases. Some clients make remarkable recoveries; some sustain severe and irreversible deficits.

A certain proportion of clients who have relapses have multiple sclerosis as the underlying disease.

Specific Nursing Measures

Nursing care is aimed at preventing hazards of immobility and alterations in comfort. Bed rest is usually indicated during the acute phase of the illness. It is important that rehabilitation measures be instituted early. (Refer to nursing measures under muscular dystrophy for rehabilitation objectives and CVA for immobility measures.)

BRAIN ABSCESSES

An abscess may form around or within the brain as a result of a local or systemic foci of infection. Brain abscesses are purulent collections that are usually encapsulated. Although abscesses can form anywhere in the brain, the most common sites are the temporal lobes, frontal lobes, and the cerebellum. Brain abscesses tend to become deeply situated within the hemispheres, because the infection has a tendency to spread into the white matter.

Most brain abscesses comprise a core and layers of encapsulation. The core is filled with debris and organisms, and the capsule contains fibrous tissue. The disorder is accompanied by cerebral edema and congestion. Over several weeks, single or multiple areas of cavitation may occur. The normal healing process occurs toward the center. In some cases, however, a diffuse cerebritis can develop without capsule formation; this happens when a potent organism causes the abscess.

Most brain abscesses develop secondarily to a primary source of infection. Of these, at least 40% are caused by a mastoiditis, otitis media, or sinusitis. Approximately a third are hematogenous, resulting from a septic focus in the pulmonary system or, less often, from a cardiac or pelvic source. In about 20% of cases, no source is identified. A smaller percentage results from direct invasion by traumatic injury, such as gunshot wounds, basilar skull fractures, and compound skull fractures with dural tears.

Clinical Manifestations

During the initial stage of organism invasion of the brain, the client experiences chills, fever, malaise, and appetite loss. The most common presenting symptom of an intracranial abscess is headache, which may be associated with vomiting and papilledema. Other common presenting symptoms are alterations in level of consciousness, especially drowsiness and confusion, and partial or generalized seizures. Focal neurologic deficits vary according to the anatomic location of the abscess. These include various motor, sensory, and speech disturbances.

In contrast, a subdural abscess tends to produce even more profound symptoms than brain abscesses. A subdural abscess affects the cortical blood vessels, causing thrombosis, arteritis, and eventually ischemia. The abscess usually arises from an acute sinusitis. A headache occurs with a rapid deterioration in neurologic status including seizures, hemiplegia, and dysphasia.

Brain abscesses in the early stages can have an insidious onset and progress through suppurative encephalitis accompanied by edema. Without treatment, brain compression or abscess rupture into the ventricle or subarachnoid space can be fatal.

Diagnosis is usually made by history of a previous infection, neurologic exam, and CT scan. A lumbar puncture is not recommended because a brain abscess acts as a mass lesion. The negative pressure created by the procedure can lead to a brain shift and herniation. When meningitis is the presumptive diagnosis, however, a lumbar puncture may be justified. The most important diagnostic test is the CT scan, which can demonstrate displacement of the lateral ventricles from a cerebral abscess or dilation from an abscess in the posterior fossa. The CT scan usually isolates an abscess, which is observed as an area of decreased density (Jennett & Galbraith, 1983). Cerebral angiography may be recommended in the absence of CT scanning in clients whose clinical picture is unclear.

Therapeutic Measures

Intervention is aimed at diagnosing and managing the primary infection source, providing for abscess drainage, and administering an effective antibiotic regimen. The most crucial aspect of treatment is drainage and elimination of the abscess by neurosurgical intervention. Most cerebral abscesses can be drained via a burr hole aspiration. Some may require more than one aspiration. Traumatic and cerebellar abscesses cannot be eliminated by this method, however. Antibiotic therapy is given for at least 6 weeks to reduce virulence of the organism, eliminate the pathogen, and penetrate the cavity. Prognosis is usually good after an effective regimen of antibiotics and/or surgery.

Specific Nursing Measures

Management of the acute infection is a priority of nursing care. Administer antibiotics on a strict schedule to maintain therapeutic blood levels. Carefully inspect intravenous sites and rotate them every 48 to 72 hours to prevent thrombosis or phlebitis. During antibiotic therapy, watch for the development of opportunistic infections. The growth of other organisms results from imbalances in natural flora, especially in the mouth and gastrointestinal tract.

Monitor the client for alterations in level of consciousness. Sudden increases in ICP can result from cerebral edema that may surround an acute abscess. Frequent assessment of neurologic and vital signs, head of bed elevation to 30°, restricted fluid intake, and avoiding any stimulant that can raise intracranial pressure are necessary components of care.

Monitor clients for potential seizures. Administer anticonvulsants as ordered with periodic checking of serum blood levels. During actual seizures, protect the client from self-injury and maintain a patent airway. A careful description of seizure onset, course, and duration may assist the physician in localizing the abscess site. Interventions for headache include providing a quiet environment, changing position to promote comfort, and administering mild analgesics as ordered. Reduce knowledge deficits by preparing clients psychologically and physically for surgery for aspiration of the abscess and intrathecal medication. Discharge teaching should include methods of preventing future abscesses if caused by an infected tooth, ear infection, or sinus problem.

HERPES ZOSTER

Herpes zoster (shingles) is a viral disorder that affects the posterior root ganglia. The disease is characterized by cutaneous eruptions of vesicles along the distribution of involved spinal or cranial nerve roots. The highest percentage of cases involves spinal ganglia. Herpes zoster occurs mainly in adults; the incidence is higher in women than men and during the spring and fall.

Herpes zoster develops from reactivation of the virus responsible for chickenpox, the varicella virus. In fact, children can develop chickenpox if exposed to an adult with shingles. Adults with shingles have all had chickenpox in the past. There also seems to be a relation between herpes zoster and certain systemic infections, spinal diseases, neoplasms, and immunosuppressive therapy. Probably, these conditions reactivate the virus.

Clinical Manifestations

Mild to severe neuralgic pain in the affected nerve root distribution is the most common presenting symptom. The pain may be burning, tingling, sharp, or dull. Pain may be concurrent with or followed by skin reddening and an eruption of vesicles. Over the next 1 or 2 weeks, these lesions become pustules and then develop a crust. After healing, a pigmented scar may appear. If an infection or ulceration accompanies the vesicles, the scarring may be permanent.

Less often, sensory and motor dysfunctions develop in the affected nerve root. With meningeal involvement, nuchal rigidity, headache and changes in level of consciousness can occur. The virus rarely causes an encephalopathy.

Diagnosis is usually based on the sudden onset of root pain followed by the characteristic distribution of shingles. The lesions are unilateral and do not cross the midline of the body. They follow a characteristic bandlike distribution that follows nerve root lines; therefore, they are transverse on the hemithorax and vertical on an extremity. If lesions are widespread, diagnosis may be difficult.

There are potential complications from an attack of herpes zoster. The main ones are scarring of the skin, facial palsies, and postherpetic neuralgia. In elderly or debilitated clients, the neuralgia can persist for months or years. The skin may also be hypersensitive to touch. Unfortunately, this variant does not respond well to treatment. Less commonly, some individuals develop Guillain–Barré syndrome following herpes zoster.

Therapeutic Measures

No specific antiviral treatment is effective. Zoster immune globulin is not helpful during an attack but may be preventive. Most treatment is aimed at giving local care to the vesicles. Topical corticosteroids can alleviate local pain and itching and may shorten the stage of vesicle eruption. Antibiotics may be administered to prevent or treat secondary infections related to shingles. During the acute phase, bed rest and analgesics can be supportive.

Postherpetic neuralgia is a difficult condition to treat. Intractable cases may require neurosurgical sectioning of affected nerve roots or occasionally irradiation to the site. Treatment results are variable.

Specific Nursing Measures

The primary objective of nursing management is care of interruptions in skin integrity. Instruct clients to avoid scratching vesicles to prevent spreading the lesions and promoting infection. Skin eruptions can be treated with topical applications of corticosteroids. Open vesicles require wet-dry saline and povidone-iodine compresses. Systemic steroid therapy may be used. Be alert for side effects of steroids. Clients experience alterations in comfort due to localized pain and itching. Comfort measures include positioning techniques (especially during bed rest), skin treatments, and analgesics as ordered.

Section VI: Neoplastic and Obstructive Disorders

Tumors within the cranium can be either primary or metastatic. Primary tumors are classified as primary intracranial intracerebral tumors or primary intracranial extracerebral tumors. Primary intracerebral tumors arise from the supporting cellular elements of the brain, such as glial cells (Figure 37–2). Primary extracerebral tumors arise outside the substance of the brain. Metastatic tumors are found predominantly within the substance of the brain, which they reach through the systemic circulation. The histologic appearance of a metastatic tumor is identical to the organ of tumor origin.

Tumors produce symptoms by invasion or compression of surrounding neural structures. The neurologic symptoms and signs of any tumor affecting the brain depend on the location of the tumor and its rate of growth. Disruption of neural structures by the tumor can cause an insidious deterioration of neurologic function or an acute neurologic disturbance. In the latter instance, the client may have a seizure without any previous history of neurologic symptoms. In some cases, hemorrhage within the tumor results in an acute deterioration of neurologic status.

Besides directly disrupting neural structures, tumors may produce symptoms as a consequence of the resulting edema in the brain surrounding the tumor. The edema contributes to the mass effect of the tumor and can result in ICP elevations and concomitant cerebral herniation. In addition, tumor obstruction of the CSF pathway may result in symptoms usually attributed to hydrocephalus.

Preoperative evaluation of a client suspected of having a brain tumor relies principally on neuroradiologic studies. CT scanning and, more recently, magnetic resonance imaging (MRI) are the usual initial diagnostic studies. The size and anatomic location of the tumor can frequently be determined from these studies. In a CT scan, intravenous contrast agents aid in determining the extent of tumor vascularity. In some institutions, positron emission tomography (PET) enables the clinician to evaluate the metabolic activity of the tumor. Cerebral angiography defines the blood supply of the tumor and aids in preoperative diagnosis. In addition, angiography contributes valuable information in planning the neurosurgical removal or elimination of these lesions.

Spinal cord tumors can cause spinal cord compression. As with brain compression, the clinical picture is similar regardless of whether compression is due to tumor,

abscess, or other pathological process (Jennett & Galbraith, 1983). The pathophysiology depends on the interruption of the transmission of impulses via the ascending (sensory) or descending (motor) fiber tracts within the spinal cord.

PRIMARY INTRACRANIAL INTRACEREBRAL TUMORS

Astrocytoma

About 25% of cerebral gliomas are astrocytomas. These tumors arise from astrocytes, and their potential for growth can usually be determined histologically by the amount of mitosis and the lack of differentiation of cell structure. Astrocytomas may be found in the cerebrum, cerebellum, brain stem, hypothalamus, and optic nerve. They may be associated with cystic cavities. These tumors may be slow growing and surgical resection can result in cure. Astrocytomas have the potential to transform into more aggressive tumors with time. The more benign tumors of this group may show a low density on CT scan that may not be enhanced with contrast media. Angiography frequently demonstrates displacement of cerebral vessels; the more aggressive type of astrocytoma demonstrates a vascular blush.

Glioblastoma Multiforme

Glioblastoma multiforme accounts for approximately 55% of all glial tumors. The most malignant of the glioma group, this tumor has a propensity for rapid growth. Pathologically, the tumor demonstrates frequent mitosis, necrosis, and hypervascularity. These tumors often reach large proportions and may cross the midline along fiber tracts such as the corpus callosum. Glioblastomas are highly vascular lesions that appear on CT scan as dense lesions following the administration of contrast medium. They may be associated with a cystic cavity or necrotic cavity and may appear as a ring lesion on CT scan. Angiography may be diagnostic for glioblastoma multiforme when it reveals a vascular blush, early draining veins, and abnormal arterial blood vessels. Clients with a confirmed diagnosis of glioblastoma multiforme and surgical removal without any additional treatment have a median survival of 14 weeks. The addition of radiation and chemotherapy prolongs median survival to approximately 1 year.

Oligodendroglioma

An oligodendroglioma arises from oligodendroglia cells, which function similar to Schwann's cells in the PNS. Oligodendrogliomas constitute 5% of all intracranial gliomas. The most common location for these tumors is in the frontal lobes. They are slow-growing tumors and frequently contain calcium. If the tumor has areas with the histologic appearance of an astrocytoma, it is referred to as a mixed glial tumor. CT scan may demonstrate calcium and an area of low density. A contrast medium may increase the den-

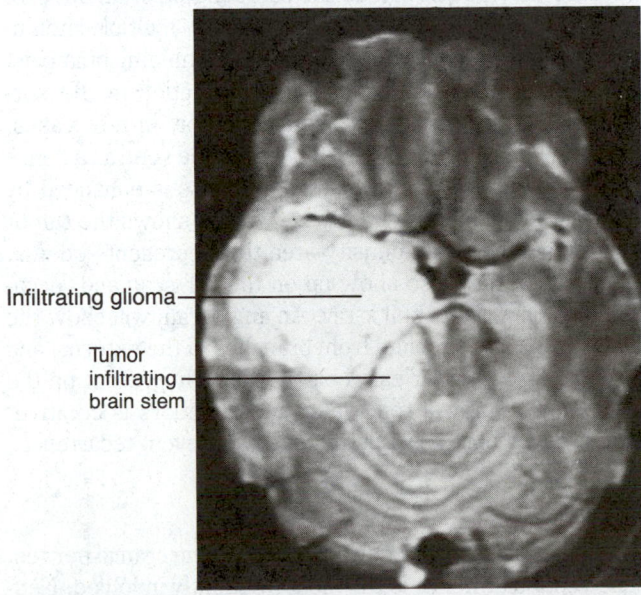

Infiltrating glioma

Tumor infiltrating brain stem

Figure 37–2

MRI showing a large, infiltrating glioma of the temporal lobe invading the brain stem. (Courtesy of Leonard I. Malis, MD, The Mount Sinai Medical Center, New York, NY)

sity of the lesion. Angiographic findings can be similar to those in astrocytomas.

Ependymoma

Ependymomas are tumors that arise from the ependymal lining of the ventricular surface and consequently are more common in the ventricular system. These tumors are most frequent in children, usually arising from the floor of the fourth ventricle. Their position in the fourth ventricle often leads to hydrocephalus because of obstruction of the CSF pathways. The tumor is grayish and friable. In some cases, the tumor may grow out of the lateral recesses into the cerebellopontine angle. A more aggressive form of the tumor is referred to as ependymoblastoma. Aggressive tumors may spread along CSF pathways and seed to other areas of the CNS.

On CT scan, these tumors may be seen as midline lesions occupying the vermian area of the cerebellum. (The vermis is the midline structure in the cerebellum that connects the two lateral cerebellar hemispheres.) A contrast medium may enhance the lesion. When these tumors arise in lateral ventricles, they must be differentiated from meningiomas, gliomas, and choroid plexus papillomas. Angiography frequently demonstrates separation of the posterior inferior cerebellar arteries and the vermian veins, an indication of the midline preference of these tumors.

Surgical removal of the entire tumor, including the attachment, results in cure. With the more invasive type of tumor, postoperative radiation is required after surgical excision to prevent seeding.

Medulloblastoma

Medulloblastomas arise from primitive neural cells of the cerebellum. Nearly as frequent as astrocytomas of childhood, they constitute approximately 20% of all childhood brain tumors. Because of their preference for the midline cerebellum and the age when they occur, these tumors are frequently difficult to differentiate diagnostically from ependymomas. Medulloblastomas arise from the inferior surface of the vermis and project into the fourth ventricle. There is a significant incidence of seeding through the CSF to other areas of the CNS. They may produce hydrocephaluslike ependymomas because of obstruction of CSF pathways at the fourth ventricle. CT scan and angiographic findings are similar to ependymoma, except that in medulloblastomas, the scan may show the tumor arising from the vermis rather than the floor of the fourth ventricle. Surgical removal followed by total radiation is the therapy. The results depend on the extent of tumor removal and its sensitivity to radiotherapy.

Papilloma of the Choroid Plexus

Papillomas arise on the choroid plexus of the ventricular system. They are found most frequently in the lateral ventricles (in children) and fourth ventricle (in adults). The tumor can produce hydrocephalus either by blocking the flow of CSF within the ventricular system or possibly by an oversecretion of CSF.

Colloid Cyst of the Third Ventricle

Colloid cysts of the third ventricle are thought to represent embryonic structures. These tumors usually occur in adults. The tumor is cystic and lined by ciliated cuboidal cells. Found at the area of the foramen of Monro, they produce symptoms by occluding outflow of CSF from the lateral ventricle into the third ventricle. On CT scan, the lateral ventricles are usually enlarged, but the remainder of the ventricular system is of normal size. In rare cases, the tumor may have an enhancing ring with contrast medium. Surgical removal of these lesions leads to cure.

Ganglioglioma

A ganglioglioma is a rare tumor made up of both neural and glial elements. The neural elements probably represent neuroblasts, whereas the glial component of the tumor is an astrocytoma. These tumors are slow growing and usually found in children or young adults. Surgical removal results in a good prognosis.

PRIMARY INTRACRANIAL EXTRACEREBRAL TUMORS

Meningioma

Meningiomas account for approximately 25% of the primary intracranial tumors. They arise from the arachnoid layer and are well circumscribed and encapsulated. Meningiomas are usually slow growing and occur frequently around the parasagittal area. They are considered benign because they do not invade the surrounding brain but produce symptoms by compression. Rarely, multiple meningiomas form, a condition referred to as meningiomatosis. Sometimes, the tumor may form a reaction in the surrounding bone manifested as sclerosis or, in rare cases, erosion. On CT scan, these tumors may be seen as a dense mass without contrast medium; the mass is enhanced by contrast medium. Frequently, a CT scan shows the tumor surrounded by a low-density area that represents edema. Calcification may also show up on the CT scan and, occasionally, on a plain skull x-ray. An angiogram will show the lesion is usually supplied from branches of the external and internal carotid arteries. A blush is usually present on the angiogram. Surgical removal of these tumors is curative. Any involved bone must be removed to prevent recurrence.

Neuroma

Neuromas arise from Schwann's cells of the cranial nerves. The vestibular nerve is the most frequently involved. Neuromas are usually solitary lesions, but they can occur on multiple cranial nerves in neurofibromatosis. Their clinical presentation depends on the particular cranial nerve involved.

An acoustic neuroma is a benign lesion arising from

the superior vestibular portion of CN VII. As it grows it expands within the auditory canal and meatus and extends to the cerebellopontine angle (the anatomic meeting between the mid and lower brain stem and cerebellum). The most common clinical symptoms are a unilateral hearing loss accompanied by tinnitus. The client often notices this deficit while using a telephone on the affected side. Although facial nerve compression occurs early within the auditory canal, rarely does the client experience CN VII dysfunction. Alterations in blink and taste may be identified on electromyography however. In cases of a larger tumor, clients may have deficits in CN V such as loss of the corneal reflex and sensory loss on the affected side of the face. Cerebellar compression can develop causing ataxia and dysmetria. Late signs can include evidence of increased ICP such as nausea, vomiting, double vision, and papilledema. Neurodiagnostic testing includes a complete clinical neurologic examination, CT scan, cerebral angiography, skull x-rays, electromyography, caloric testing, audiometry, and tomograms of the petrous bones.

Pituitary Tumors

Tumors in the region of the pituitary fossa can cause endocrine disturbances, visual dysfunction, cranial nerve deficits, or obstructive hydrocephalus (Figure 37-3). Historically, pituitary tumors were classified according to cell type. More recent classifications divide them into two groups: nonsecreting tumors and secreting tumors. The nonsecreting type, commonly known as chromophobe adenomas, account for 90% of pituitary tumors. Nonsecreting tumors produce no hormones, but invade and destroy the rest of the pituitary gland. Secreting pituitary tumors produce various endocrine hormones. See Chapter 44 for a discussion of pituitary disorders caused by pituitary tumors.

Craniopharyngiomas

Craniopharyngiomas are not tumors of the pituitary gland but occur in the suprasellar region. They are thought to be congenital tumors; the majority are cystic, at least in part. They contain a dark brown engine-like oil that is full of cholesterol crystal that illuminates. They can cause an obstructive hydrocephalus from upward tumor extension to the hypothalamus and third ventricle. In addition to signs of increased ICP, clients often have headache, visual problems, hypopituitarism, and diabetes insipidus.

Pinealomas

The majority of pineal tumors are atypical teratomas that resemble seminomas of the testicle. Pineal gland tumors have a higher incidence in men between ages 15 and 25. Even though many grow slowly, due to their location clients have a life expectancy of 2 to 5 years. Survival rate can vary according to histology and the client's response to treatment. Pinealomas can occlude the aqueduct of Sylvius causing obstructive hydrocephalus. Pineal tumors are usually radiosensitive and respond to radiation therapy and shunting for hydrocephalus. Serial CT scans can monitor response to radiotherapy. Surgical intervention may be indicated for tumors that respond poorly to radiotherapy. The anatomic location of these tumors generally makes them inaccessible to surgical treatment and even more difficult to resect following radiotherapy.

Hemangioblastoma

Hemangioblastomas are derived from blood vessel tissue. They are comprised of endothelial cells and some fibroblastic cells and most commonly develop in the cerebellum. A cystic tumor forms that appears cherrylike, encased in a cyst filled with clear, yellowish fluid. Hemangioblastomas can be multiple and have a familial tendency. If so, angiomas may be seen in the retina and tumors and cysts may develop in the kidneys and pancreas. Polycythemia vera can also occur and is cured by surgical removal of the tumor (Jennett & Galbraith, 1983).

Epidermoid Tumors

Epidermoid tumors are congenital, pearly-type tumors. A cholesteatoma is an epidermoid tumor. It consists of epithelial residue that collects within a thin capsule. This capsule has a "mother-of-pearl" type appearance due to cells forming shiny flakes within. Cholesteatomas most frequently develop in the basal subarachnoid cisterns. They can occur near the sella or within the cerebellopontine

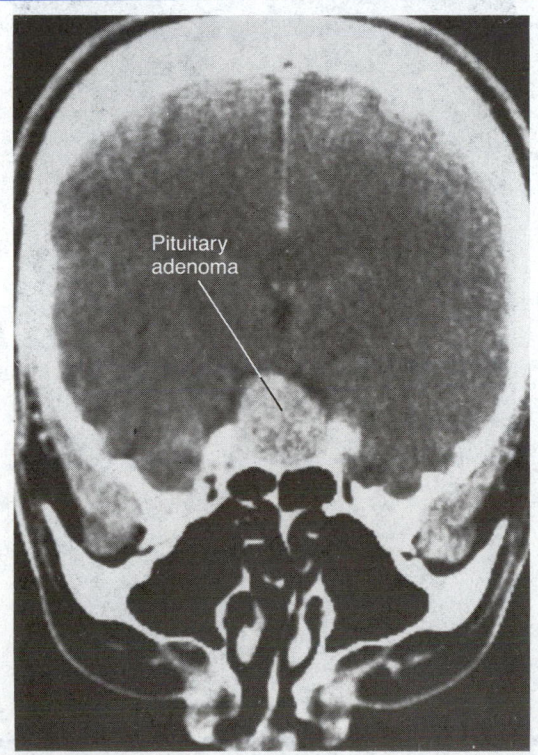

Figure 37-3

CT scan, coronal view, showing a pituitary adenoma. (Courtesy of Leonard I. Malis, MD, The Mount Sinai Medical Center, New York, NY)

angle. Although the tumor is a noninvasive type, its consistency causes it to adhere to surrounding surfaces making total surgical removal difficult.

Dermoid Tumors

Dermoid tumors also develop as a congenital defect. In this case, the capsule contains dermal elements and sebaceous material such as oily fluid and hair. The location of these can vary from pericranial, orbital, to posterior fossa regions. Pericranial tumors develop and erode bone near the anterior fontanelle in children. Orbital tumors slowly arise from the lateral roof resulting in erosion of bone and a proptosis that is painless. The most variable and serious form occurs within the posterior fossa.

Therapeutic and Specific Nursing Measures

The therapeutic and specific nursing approaches to the care of clients with brain tumors, including the care of clients undergoing neurosurgical procedures, are covered in Chapters 39, 44, and 45. General care of the client with a malignancy is found in Chapter 12.

SPINAL CORD TUMORS*

Spinal cord tumors are classified not only by their histological type but by their relation to the dura and spinal cord. They are of two principal kinds:

- Extradural tumors, which lie outside the dura, are usually metastatic.
- Intradural tumors are subdivided into extramedullary (within the dura but not within the spinal cord itself) and intramedullary (within the substance of the spinal cord.

Metastatic tumors of the spine cause epidural compression of the spinal cord. Metastases rarely occur to the cord itself or to the epidural tissue but generally occur in the vertebrae. They cause compression either by progressive growth with gradual cord compression or by destruction of the vertebrae with sudden collapse and sudden compression of the cord. With the sudden compression, paraplegia or quadraplegia occurs within hours, or even instantaneously depending on the level of the lesion. Pain at the site of the collapse is often agonizing. Sometimes the symptoms develop over hours or days but may have been preceded by a week or so of backache.

Total motor and sensory loss with sudden vertebral collapse is rarely recoverable, regardless of the treatment, and surgical intervention is not usually indicated. On the other hand, slowly progressive paralysis from continued tumor growth is usually diagnosed while some function

remains, and appropriate treatment may lead to significant recovery. The most frequently affected site is the thoracic spine, and the most common lesions are from lung, breast, and prostate cancers. Some clients have no known primary malignant lesion. Even after histologic confirmation and extensive diagnostic investigation, evidence of the primary site may not become evident before their death (Hayward, 1980).

Meningiomas and neurofibromas are the most common *intradural extramedullary* tumors. Meningiomas are most frequent in the thoracic region and much more prevalent in women (Figure 37–4). Less common is the foramen magnum meningioma. Lumbar meningiomas are virtually unheard of. Neurofibromas can occur at any level. Because they arise from the nerve root, they can be intradural, extradural, or a combination. In some instances, the tumor grows out through the intervertebral foramen and expands outside the spine. Because of their appearance, these are referred to as dumbbell neurofibromas. The extraspinal portion may present as a lump in the neck or as a shadow in the posterior mediastinum, which is often discovered on routine chest x-ray. Occasionally, these tumors require a combined approach in a two-stage procedure to remove both the intraspinal and extraspinal portions of the tumor.

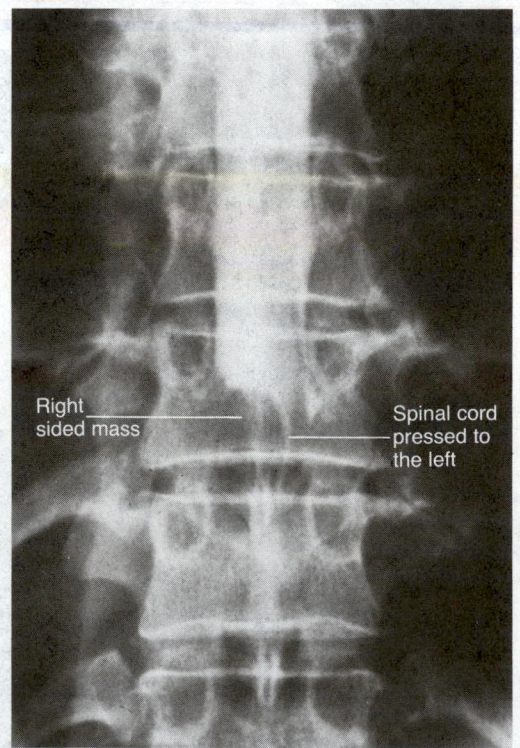

Figure 37–4

Myelogram showing block due to intradural extramedullary thoracic spinal meningioma. The cord is pressed to the left by the right-sided mass. (Courtesy of Leonard I. Malis, MD, The Mount Sinai Medical Center, New York, NY)

---

*This section contributed by Dorothy A. Kaminiski.

Both meningiomas and neurofibromas are benign, slow growing and most prevalent in the fourth through sixth decades of life. They grow between the spinal cord and dura and slowly displace the cord, after forming a deep cup or groove into it as they grow into what is usually a smooth, encapsulated, oval-shaped mass. The symptoms are root pain and progressive paresis, usually with a partial Brown-Séquard syndrome (ie, loss of vibration and position sense below the level of the lesion ipsilaterally and loss of the perception of pain and temperature contralaterally), when they occur in the cervical and thoracic regions.

Lumbar neuromas often present a clinical picture similar to that of a herniated disk. Because of slow growth, symptoms may develop over years before treatment is sought. The diagnosis is confirmed by CT scan, myelography, or both. In the client with neurofibromatosis, the possibility of multiple tumors, both meningiomas and neurofibromas as well as intramedullary lesions, should be considered. A full laminectomy is done and usually extends a level above and below the lesion.

Neuromas usually arise from the posterior root and sometimes from only a few fascicles (bundles of nerve fibers) of the root. With microscope visualization, it is usually possible to spare the uninvolved fascicles. Even if the entire root is involved and has to be sacrificed, there is usually enough sensory overlap from the nerve roots above and below so there is no significant deficit. Motor roots have less in the way of overlap, but fortunately, they are rarely involved by neuromas.

Intramedullary cord tumors are relatively rare (Figure 37–5). The majority of these tumors arise from the connective tissue cells of the CNS, particularly the ependymal cells that line the central canal of the spinal cord and the astrocytes (Hayward, 1980). Ependymomas may be totally intramedullary, usually forming an encapsulated, well-demarcated lesion that expands the cord, or they may involve the cauda equina. Astrocytomas vary in their degree of malignancy and resectability. Some are reasonably well demarcated whereas others infiltrate between all the viable fibers of the cord. Infiltrating tumors are unresectable because, unlike the brain where certain areas of nervous tissue can be sacrificed without causing significant damage, no such leeway exists within the spinal cord (Jennett & Galbraith, 1983).

As these tumors grow, they enlarge the cord and interfere with its function by destroying cord parenchyma from within or by pressure on surrounding normal cord. They usually first damage the sensory fibers of the spino-

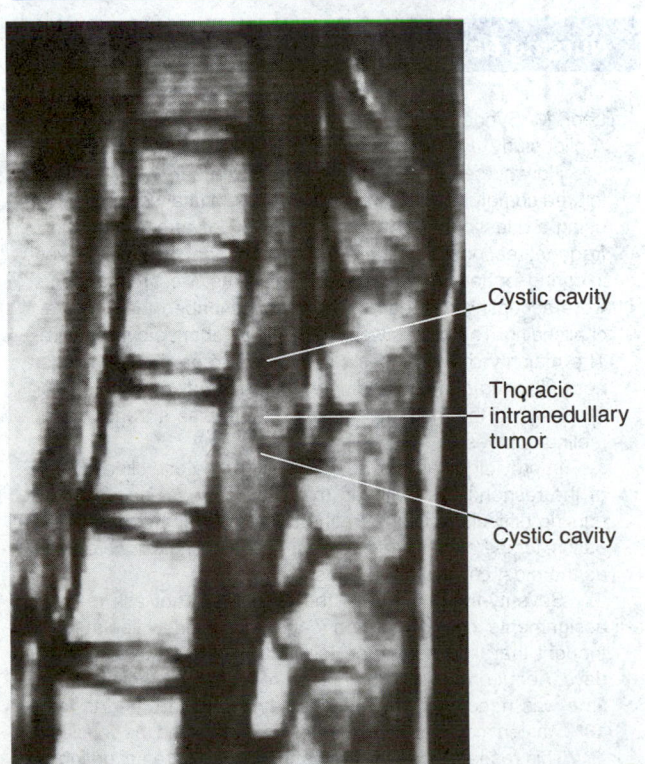

Cystic cavity

Thoracic intramedullary tumor

Cystic cavity

Figure 37–5

MRI showing a thoracic intramedullary spinal cord tumor with a cystic cavity above and below. (Courtesy of Leonard I. Malis, MD, The Mount Sinai Medical Center, New York, NY)

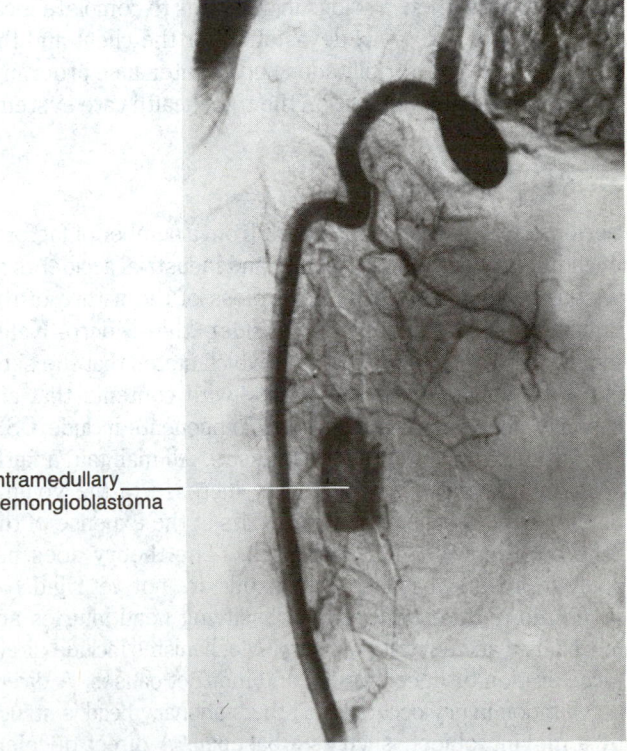

Intramedullary hemongioblastoma

Figure 37–6

Intramedullary hemangioblastoma. The tremendous vascularity is demonstrated on the spinal angiogram. (Courtesy of Leonard I. Malis, MD, The Mount Sinai Medical Center, New York, NY)

thalamic tract, which crosses in the center of the cord, producing a band of sensory loss in the cutaneous distribution corresponding to the level of the lesion. The client loses the appreciation of pain and temperature, whereas the sensation of light touch, which travels in the uncrossed tracts of the dorsal columns, remains intact. As the lesion enlarges, it interferes with the vertically running fiber tracts within the cord and causes motor weakness, which is of an upper motor neuron type. Bladder function is often preserved until a late stage (Hayward, 1980).

The diagnosis is usually made by myelography, which demonstrates the widened cord. As these tumors are frequently associated with the collection of cystic fluid above and/or below the tumor which also contributes to the widened cord, CT scanning and MRI are often useful in determining the exact location and extent of the tumor. Unfortunately, no diagnostic method can determine whether the tumor is an ependymoma or an astrocytoma or predict the degree of resectability. If the lesion is especially vascular, spinal angiography may also be performed to rule out or confirm the diagnosis of hemangioblastoma (Figure 37–6). This tumor is totally resectable but because of its vascular supply requires special operative techniques.

Therapeutic and Specific Nursing Measures

Care of the client undergoing spinal surgery is covered in Chapter 39. General care of the client with a malignancy is found in Chapter 12.

Section VII: Traumatic Disorders

Craniocerebral trauma is the major cause of death in persons between the ages of 1 and 44 years and contributes to more deaths than strokes in persons aged 45 to 64. Close to 6.5 million head injuries occur yearly in the United States (Friedman, 1983). There are approximately six to nine thousand new clients with spinal cord injury in the United States. The highest incidence occurs in young, previously healthy men. Serious injury leads to complete incapacitation and emotional devastation for the client and the cost of long-term rehabilitation and maintenance programs have a tremendous impact on the total health care system.

HEAD TRAUMA

Serious cerebral injury can result from a number of factors, including motor vehicle, sports, and industrial accidents as well as assaults and falls. Regardless of the nature of the injury, it is important to consider the Monro–Kellie hypothesis (closed-box theory), which states that the skull is a rigid sphere filled to capacity with contents that are basically noncompressible. These components include CSF, the vascular system, and brain tissue. All maintain a fairly constant volume. Therefore, any increase in the volume of one intracranial component occurs at the expense of the others; otherwise, ICP increases. (The theory does not apply to infants, because their skulls are not yet rigid.)

Among the methods for classifying head injuries are mechanism and severity of injury. Mechanisms include direct (acceleration or deceleration) and indirect causes. A direct acceleration injury occurs when the stationary head is struck by a moving object, such as a baseball. A direct deceleration injury occurs when the head in motion strikes an immovable object, such as when a person falls from a bicycle onto the pavement. In an indirect injury, the traumatic force is not directly applied to the head but is usually transmitted through an impact to the neck or buttocks.

Another major classification is closed and open head injury, referring to whether the skull and the dura mater are intact. A closed head injury is a nonpenetrating, blunt injury with no break in the integrity of the skull and dura mater. Severity ranges from slight to moderate to severe. Injuries include scalp bruises or lacerations, depressed

Nursing Research Note

Leon M, Synder M: Care of the long-term comatose patient: A pilot study. *J Neurosur Nurs* 1980; 12(3):134–137.

How nurses feel about and deal with caring for a head-injured comatose client was investigated. Data were collected using a questionnaire with a sample of 91 nurses. The most frequent responses concerned the great deal of work involved in caring for head-injured comatose clients. Most respondents were accepting of these clients and described their care as challenging. The nurses were not anxious about providing care. The majority of responses were neutral regarding hopelessness, discouragement, and whether the client would be "better off dead." In the majority, however, there was a trend toward feeling hopeless.

In providing care for head-injured comatose clients, 67% of the respondents believed that physical care needs made nursing difficult. Copious tracheal secretions, a hopeless situation, temperature spikes, restlessness, and rigidity were listed as the most common problems.

Seventy-five percent of the nurses did not ask to have assignments changed when caring for these clients; 36% thought that the assignment should be rotated every 2 to 3 days. About one-third (31%) of the respondents thought more time was needed to read and study the client's charts, and 18% wanted more resource material to understand the condition.

This research demonstrates that nurses are accepting of the comatose client and see the nursing care as challenging. The demands of physical care can be balanced by assignment rotation. Continuing education focusing on the anatomy and physiology of the nervous system can enhance care and acceptance. The specific demands of physical care require more research in approaches to effective management.

fractures with no dural tears, and linear fractures that are undisplaced. Brain concussions (jarring), contusions (bruising), and lacerations (tearing) may occur (Wilson, 1979). Closed head injuries can also result in hemorrhage, cranial nerve injury, and cerebral edema.

An important phenomenon in closed head injury is coup–contrecoup. The *coup injury* is bruising of the brain directly below the point of injury resulting from impact to the skull; there are visible signs of injury. *Contrecoup* refers to the rebound effect of injury, the mass movement of the brain opposite to the site of impact. For example, a blow to the frontal region (coup) causes damage to the occipital region (countrecoup) of the brain. Injuries include lacerations and hemorrhage causing sensory and motor dysfunctions.

In open head trauma, a penetrating injury breaks the integrity of the skull or dura. Cerebral contusions or lacerations occur. The most frequent fractures are linear, at the base of the skull. Depressed and comminuted fractures are less frequent but more serious because of dural tears and lacerations of brain tissue. Infection is a high risk in open head injuries.

Clinical Manifestations

Skull Fractures

Clinical findings are related to specific types of skull fractures and brain injuries. The location of a skull fracture is most crucial for determining damage to the underlying structures: the meninges, blood vessels, and the brain itself. Distinction is made between fractures of the cranial vault and the base of the skull. Fractures are classified as linear, comminuted, depressed, compound, and basilar.

Linear skull fractures are usually simple breaks in bone continuity anywhere in the skull. A simple crack or several straight lines appear. Both the outer and inner table of the skull can be affected. These fractures usually cause no problem, but those in the temporal bone can damage the middle meningeal artery and cause epidural bleeding. *Comminuted skull fractures* are multiple fragmentations of the bone. When these involve the inner table of the skull, bone fragments can be driven into the dura or brain. These structures may be compressed or torn. This finding is referred to as a depressed fracture. *Depressed skull fractures* are caused by trauma from sharper, penetrating injuries. Brain lacerations and infections are common. Less serious forms of these fractures are caused by blunter objects that do not fragment the inner table of the skull. A *compound skull fracture* is a scalp laceration along with a depressed skull fracture. Debris (hair, dirt, and foreign material) penetrates into the wound. The dura may or may not be torn. A *basilar skull fracture* involves injury to the base of the skull. The middle and anterior fossa are more often affected than the posterior fossa. The most common type involves the extension of a linear fracture into the base of the skull. These fractures usually involve the petrous

portion of the temporal bone. Basilar skull fractures can indicate severe trauma and should be suspected in any significant head injury.

Concussions, Contusions, and Lacerations

Brain injury is classified as a concussion, contusion, or laceration that may or may not be associated with vascular rupture and cranial nerve damage. A cerebral *concussion* is considered the most benign form of brain injury. A concussion is characterized by a loss of consciousness for 5 minutes or less and memory loss of events preceding and following trauma. Other symptoms may include dizziness, spots before the eyes, and a dazed state. In the past, a concussion was believed to cause no structural brain damage. Current data indicate conclusively that there is microscopic damage in virtually all cases. Residual deficits are clinically observable if carefully sought and may be long lasting.

A cerebral *contusion* is a bruising of the brain. There may be petechial hemorrhage of cortical tissue and white matter with tearing of the pia mater. Contusions are commonly found beneath depressed skull fractures and around penetrating injuries of the frontal and temporal lobes. Contusions cause unconsciousness that persists for longer than 5 minutes. An initial period of shock is followed by signs of cerebral irritability.

A cerebral *laceration* is a tearing of the brain tissue followed by intracerebral bleeding. Prolonged unconsciousness, immediate neurologic deficits, and a deterioration in condition can be expected.

Epidural, Subdural, and Intracerebral Hematomas

The major vascular hemorrhages from trauma include epidural, subdural, and intracerebral hematomas. An *epidural* hematoma is a life-threatening hemorrhage in the epidural space, which is between the inner table of the skull and the dura. Trauma to the temporal bone from a linear fracture constitutes the most common form. The fracture causes tearing of the middle meningeal artery and its branches. Most epidural hematomas are from arterial bleeds. Classically, the trauma causes an initial loss of consciousness, followed by a lucid interval. Unconsciousness follows that is both rapid and often unexpected. Epidural hematomas require prompt surgical intervention.

Subdural hematomas are collections of blood from clots in the subdural space between the arachnoid and dura that usually involve venous bleeding. The three types include acute, subacute, and chronic hematomas, referring to the time interval between initial injury and symptom development. Acute hematoma occurs within 48 hours; subacute, within 2 weeks; and chronic, more than 2 weeks after injury. Subdural hematomas can develop over an entire hemisphere. Chronic subdural hematomas can increase in size over time, probably due to rebleeding.

Acute subdural hematomas are often associated with massive cerebral or brain-stem injury. Although bleeding is mostly venous, it develops quickly with rapid onset of symptoms. Common clinical symptoms and signs are headache, drowsiness and confusion, slow responses, and restlessness. These worsen over time. A critical sign of deterioration is an ipsilateral dilation of the pupil that becomes unreactive.

Subacute subdural hematomas usually develop 7 to 10 days after injury and are associated with less severe brain contusions. The course is slower with a much better survival rate. Persistent cerebral pressure causes prolonged alteration in level of consciousness.

Chronic subdural hematomas commonly occur from more trivial injuries. At first, a small hemorrhage fills the subdural space. Several weeks later, a vascular membrane forms around the collection, which slowly enlarges. Symptoms may not occur for several weeks or months. Because of this time lapse, the initial injury may not be recalled. Progressive headache, confusion and drowsiness, slow responses, and seizures occur. Pupillary changes and motor deficits result, similar to those in subacute subdural hematomas. Papilledema may develop as well.

An intracerebral hematoma, a collection of blood in brain tissue, is a complication in a small percentage of all head traumas. The hematoma may accompany the contrecoup phenomenon. Most are related to contusions and occur in frontal and temporal areas. Lesions can be single or multiple. They may occur deep within the hemispheres but are rare in the cerebellum. Symptoms may be delayed because of slow bleeding or delay in onset.

Therapeutic Measures

The treatment of head trauma includes medical or surgical therapy or both. The initial management of head trauma clients not only includes diagnosis of head injury but also an awareness of potential respiratory problems or injury to other systems. These other problems are important, because anoxia or shock may complicate the initial head injury. The survival rate has improved with central head trauma units. Standards ensure that clients have immediate stabilization of vital signs, that further injury is prevented, and that intracranial edema is reduced. The primary focus is on maintenance of a patent airway. In these centers, the conditions requiring surgery, such as epidural hematomas, are diagnosed, and surgical intervention is prompt. In a large group of clients with closed head injury, no surgery is necessary. Client management depends on neurologic care that includes maintenance of airway and blood pressure, monitoring of ICP, and appropriate antibiotic therapy as necessary. Treatment of cerebral edema includes use of dehydrating agents such as mannitol, which withdraw water from intracranial tissue. High-dose steroid therapy is usually administered although studies show no benefit. Hyperventilation therapy is employed in clients with severe head trauma to decrease PCO_2, reducing cerebral vasodilation and thereby decreasing ICP. Although controversial, current data indicate that these procedures are beneficial for the brain-injured client. Assessment approaches such

Nursing Research Note

Parson LC, Peard–Smith AL, Page MC: The effects of hygiene interventions on the cerebrovascular status of severe closed-head injured persons. *Res Nurs Health* 1985; 8:173–181.

This study measured physiologic responses by the severe closed-head injured client to three nursing interventions: oral care, body hygiene, and in-dwelling catheter care. The physiologic responses measured were heart rate, mean arterial blood pressure, mean intracranial pressure, and cerebral perfusion pressure.

All three interventions produced increases in heart rate, mean arterial pressure, mean intracranial pressure, and cerebral perfusion pressure. Oral care and body hygiene produced a greater rise in all four measures than did catheter care. These elevations all returned to baseline within 1 minute following completion of the care. Although the nursing interventions raised physiologic measures, the cerebral perfusion pressure was never less than 50, the minimal pressure needed to perfuse the brain adequately.

The results indicate that these nursing measures can be performed safely on clients with severe closed-head injuries. The interventions help to reduce associated complications of immobility, oral decay, and urinary tract infection.

as the Glasgow Coma Scale are beginning to permit institutions to compare data about modes of therapy and outcomes.

Specific Nursing Measures

The initial nursing priority for the care of the client with acute head injury must be maintenance of effective airway clearance and breathing pattern. Respiratory control may be interrupted by direct trauma to the cerebrum or brain stem. Compromised respiration leads to increased ICP, which causes ischemia to respiratory centers. An inadequate airway or ventilation may be caused by a number of factors. Mechanical complications include upper airway obstruction and poor pulmonary toilet. Gag reflex absence, phrenic nerve damage, or aspiration can compromise pulmonary status. Clients with alterations in level of consciousness are at greatest risk for hypoventilation because of shallow respiration and potential for respiratory failure or arrest. Specific monitoring includes checking for airway patency and adequate pulmonary toilet and assessing, reporting, and documenting breathing patterns and breath sounds.

Be sure that the client's head and neck are immobilized and *not* manipulated until cervical injury is ruled out by cervical spine x-ray or CT scan. Avoid neck hyperextension, flexion, and rotation. Manipulation can cause an airway obstruction or can seriously complicate a cervical injury. If respiratory resuscitation is required, the jaw thrust maneuver can be used. Do *not* suction nasal passages until basal skull fractures and dural tears have been ruled out. Clear the mouth and oropharynx of foreign bodies. Gentle oropharyngeal suctioning can be done to maintain an effective airway. If the airway is not patent, endotracheal intubation or a tracheostomy will be indicated. If an artificial airway is created, use standard precautions when suctioning. These precautions and the nursing care of clients with an artificial airway are discussed in Chapter 18.

Clients with potential for respiratory complications may be repositioned after the cervical spine is stabilized. The semiprone lateral position facilitates drainage of secretions, or the client can be turned from side to side. Position should be changed at least every 2 hours. Assess respiratory rate, rhythm, and pattern every 1 to 2 hours or as necessary. Evaluate chest excursions and breath sounds at the same interval. Arterial blood gases are monitored initially, after 4 hours, and subsequently as necessary. Neurologic dysfunction can cause specific changes in respiratory patterns: Cheyne–Stokes respirations; central neurogenic hyperventilation; and apneustic, cluster, or ataxic breathing. Teach conscious clients to do deep breathing exercises.

Assess the neurologic status of the client with acute head trauma immediately after respiratory airway patency is established. The level of consciousness is the single most important aspect of the clinical nursing observation, because it is maintained by the normal functioning of the cerebral cortex and the ascending reticular activating system of the brain stem. Consciousness is assessed on a continuum from full reaction to no reaction to various kinds of stimuli. At present, no levels of consciousness terms are universally accepted. Therefore, it is best to describe the stimulus given and the response obtained (see Glasgow Coma Scale in Chapter 36).

Care of clients with basal skull fractures includes assessment for "raccoon" eyes or bilateral periorbital ecchymosis and hemorrhage; Battle's sign, an ecchymosis of the mastoid region; and hemotympanum, blood behind the eardrum. Cerebrospinal fluid leaks may occur as rhinorrhea or otorrhea. Never probe or irrigate the nose or ear when a CSF leak is suspected. If drainage occurs, collect the fluid in a test tube and test it with a Dextrostix for the presence of glucose. A glucose positive result can confirm a CSF leak, since glucose is present in CSF but not in mucus. If drainage cannot be collected for testing, carefully inspect the client's gown and linen. The halo sign, a combination of bloody or darker drainage encircled by a lighter yellowish stain, signifies a bloody leakage of CSF. Basal skull fractures are considered serious head injuries due to the proximity of the fracture site to vital brain stem areas. Brain stem edema can result in severe respiratory and cardiac dysfunction. Assess the client frequently for any alterations in neurologic, respiratory, or cardiac status.

SPINAL CORD INJURY

The vast majority of spinal pathology results from traumatic injury. The highest incidence is in young men in the second and third decades of life. Spinal injury usually results from a sudden catastrophic event in a previously healthy individual. The leading causes in the United States are car and motorcycle accidents, sports accidents (football, diving), and penetrating injuries (gunshot or stab wounds).

Fracture-dislocations can occur anywhere along the spine. The mechanisms of injury vary according to the area of the spine involved. Cervical injuries, the most common, are usually related to flexion–extension maneuvers during a traumatic injury. Fracture-dislocations in the thoracic and lumbar areas usually arise from compression injuries, as in falls from high places. Spinal column fracture-dislocations may also result from pathological bone processes: metastatic, infectious, or degenerative disease. This discussion focuses on traumatic injuries to the cervical spine because of its potential to cause the most extensive neurologic deficits.

Dislocation fractures of the high cervical vertebrae (C-1 to C-2) can occur as a result of fractures or congenital defects of the odontoid process or from arthritic changes that weaken the ligaments in this area. A forward movement of the skull and C-1 and C-2 vertebrae can compress the cervical cord. These fractures can occur in the body or posterior elements of the spine causing a forward or backward dislocation of cervical vertebrae and compromising the neural canal. Additional compression can result from bony fragments or disk material that impinges on the spinal cord.

Instability is often observed on cervical spine radiographs where a misalignment is seen. This situation is exemplified by "locked facets," in which an upper cervical vertebra is dislocated forward on the adjacent lower vertebra. The vertebra is held in position because of slippage of the upper facet on the lower facet. In some cases, however, the spine appears to be aligned although the spinal cord is actually or physiologically severed (transection). At the time of injury, damage to the support structures of the spine results in a vertebral subluxation that compresses neural elements and then returns to a normal position. The position of the vertebra is unstable, however, and any movement can result in dislocation or transection.

Clinical Manifestations

The extent of a client's functional loss depends on the degree of spinal cord injury. *Complete* spinal cord transection causes a total loss of motor and sensory function below the level of injury with irreversible spinal cord damage.

In the cervical area, millimeters can be crucial for spinal nerve-root function. With cervical cord transection, **quadriplegia** (paralysis of all four extremities) results, with varying degrees of respiratory and arm paralysis, depending on the injury level. Cord transection of the thoracic spine through L-1 and L-2 causes **paraplegia** (paralysis of both legs) (Figure 37–7). A common classification system relating neurologic deficits to anatomic level of injuries is outlined in Table 37–3.

The classification in Table 37–3 is more helpful in evaluating spinal-cord injury than one based on structural

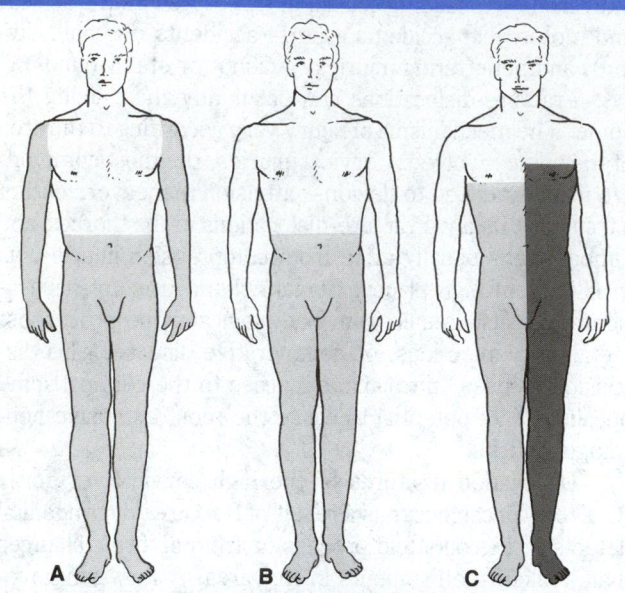

Figure 37–7

Spinal cord injury with paralysis. **A.** Quadriplegia—paralysis of all four extremities. **B.** Paraplegia—paralysis of both legs. **C.** Brown–Séquard syndrome—the client with an injury to the left cord has motor paresis and loss of vibration and proprioception on the left with loss of pain and temperature sensation on the right, one to two segments below the level of injury.

Table 37–3	Classification of Neurologic Deficits According to Level of Spinal-Cord Injury
Level of Injury	**Neurologic Deficit**
Cervical C-1 to C-2	Quadriplegia: no respiratory function with an immediate respiratory arrest if untreated
C-3 to C-4	Quadriplegia: loss of phrenic nerve innervation to the diaphragm causing absence of respirations
C-4 to C-5	Quadriplegia: no motor power in the arms
C-5 to C-6	Quadriplegia: gross motor function in the arms only
C-6 to C-7	Quadriplegia: no triceps function; biceps spared
C-7 to C-8	Quadriplegia: no intrinsic muscle function in the hands; triceps spared
Thoracic T-1 to T-12 and Lumbar L-1 to L-2	Paraplegia; arm function preserved; some loss of intercostals; loss of bladder, bowel, and sexual function
L-2 and below	Cauda equina damage: a combination of loss of sensory, motor, bowel, bladder, and sexual function; degree of injury depends on which nerve roots are involved
Sacral	Loss of bowel, bladder, and sexual function

changes in the cord. For example, a complete cord transection can cause visible damage to cord tissue or only minimal gross structural change. In either, the individual sustains an immediate flaccid paralysis, loss of sensation, and usually loss of reflexes below the level of injury. Some reflexes may be intact initially, then disappear within a few days, indicating "spinal shock," or the loss of all reflex activity below the level of injury. The loss can last for days, for weeks, or several months. As paralysis subsides, reflexes usually return, and flaccidity changes to involuntary spastic movement. Recovery of any motor or sensory function is rare when there is complete paralysis of these functions for several days after injury.

With incomplete spinal-cord injuries, degrees of sensory and motor deficit below the level of damage vary, resulting in one of several spinal cord syndromes. The most common is *anterior-cord syndrome,* caused by acute flexion injuries to the cervical spine. The anterior spinal artery and/or ventral part of the spinal cord is injured. Complete loss of motor function occurs with preservation of dorsal column sensation, known as "sacral sparing." Below the level of injury, there are hyperesthesia and hypalgesia with some preservation of position sense as well as vibration, pressure, and touch sensation.

The *central-cord syndrome* usually involves hyperextension injuries, primarily in the elderly with osteoarthritic spines. The central gray matter is the main site of injury. Central-cord syndrome is characterized by a greater loss of motor power in the arms than in the legs accompanied by varying degrees of sensory and bladder dysfunction. A flaccid paralysis at the site of injury and a spastic involvement below the level of injury occur.

The *Brown–Séquard syndrome,* also known as a hemisection of the spinal cord, usually follows penetrating injuries of a rotation-flexion nature. On the ipsilateral side of cord injury, motor paresis and loss of vibration and proprioception occur. On the contralateral side of the injury, one to two segments below, there is loss of pain and temperature sensation (Figure 37–7). Clients who sustain injuries to the lower spinal cord, conus medullaris, and cauda equina may experience signs of both upper and lower motor neuron dysfunction.

A number of factors are examined to assess the degree of spinal cord damage. The first consideration may be the mechanism of injury. A compression of the cord can occur from ligaments, bone, herniated disk material, or hematomas. A contusion causes a bruising of the cord. In transection injuries, the spinal cord is actually or physiologically severed. A hemorrhage known as hematomyelia can occur within the cord substance.

Another important factor influencing the degree of spinal injury is the diameter of the spinal canal, the amount of space the spinal cord has to move within to avoid compression. This factor is especially crucial in the cervical area. This space tends to be wider in children and narrower in persons with various congenital anomalies, arthritic changes, and conditions such as spondylosis.

Neurons do not regenerate within the cord substance. Spinal cord necrosis can result from a number of factors such as disturbances in circulation causing poor cord perfusion, edema, and progressive hemorrhage of central gray matter.

Therapeutic Measures

The first priority in initial treatment of an acute spinal cord injury is handling of the client's spine with extreme caution. Proper handling can prevent further dislocation of fractured or already dislocated bone. At the scene of injury, the client should be moved with the head and neck immobilized. There should be no movement of the cervical spine, especially flexion. The client should be placed supine on a rigid frame or stretcher with sandbags (or other firm objects) applied to both sides of the head and neck. Place a firm roll under the nape of the neck. Any life-threatening injury to another body system or signs of systemic shock should be treated immediately. For emergency life support, the neck should *not* be hyperextended. The jaw-thrust maneuver can be used for mouth-to-mouth resuscitation.

Formerly, clients with acute spinal trauma had prompt surgery to "decompress" their injured cord. Today the immediate goal of trauma care is to stabilize bony malalignments and ligamentous instability. Stabilization is usually achieved in cervical injuries with the application of skeletal traction by Crutchfield or Gardner–Wells tongs. (Crutchfield tongs are illustrated in Figure 58–12 in Chapter 58.) Realignment may be achieved with skeletal traction or an open reduction later. In most trauma units, early fixation and spinal traction have replaced decompression laminectomies.

Another goal of therapy is to reverse the effects of vertebral body fractures. Neurosurgery replaces the injured vertebra with bone, acrylic, or a combination. The advantage of acrylic is early mobilization for the client, whereas bone fusion requires some internal fixation. For clients who remain unstable, a halo frame and body jacket vest are applied for several months until stabilization is achieved. In the lower thoracic and lumbar areas, internal fixation can be achieved using rods.

Spinal-cord-injured clients are at greatest risk in the first week to 10 days after trauma. During this time, shock, pulmonary dysfunction, infection, and paralytic ileus can be major problems. Clients who sustain quadriplegic injuries require intensive total medical and nursing management. The post-traumatic care of paraplegic clients mainly involves management of bladder and bowel dysfunctions, skin care, nutrition maintenance, and physical therapy.

Specific Nursing Measures

The most intensive nursing care is required for clients with acute, unstable cervical fractures resulting in quadriplegia. The first objective for the nurse admitting these clients to an ER, ICU, or trauma unit is absolute immobilization of the head and neck with sandbags and a firm roll under the nape of the neck. Once the client is placed in tongs and cervical traction, follow physician's orders for client positioning. Pin sites must be cared for once per shift. The tong sites are cleansed with hydrogen peroxide and saline to remove exudate. Culture unusual or foul-smelling drainage and report it to the physician. After cleansing the sites, apply povidone-iodine ointment as ordered around pin sites. Maintain the integrity of the tongs and skeletal traction. If the tongs come out, keep the client's head in a neutral position, remain with the client, and call for immediate help. Caution the client to avoid any head and neck movement.

The client with an acute cervical injury should not be turned until the fracture is reduced and stabilized. Turning the client requires an explicit order from the physician. When a turning order has been verified, a minimum of three staff members is required to logroll the client. One person is assigned to support the client's head. Carefully explain the turning or transferring procedure to the client and provide reassurance. In some institutions, Stryker frames or circle beds are used to care for clients. More recently, the Rota Rest bed has been recommended to provide safe stabilization and reduce the hazards of immobility.

Continuous monitoring of the client's neurologic status including respiratory, motor, and sensory function is essential. Assess the client's level of consciousness and evaluate pupillary response. Report the progression of any neurologic deficit immediately.

With high cervical lesions, there will be ineffective airway clearance and alterations in breathing patterns. Assess the adequacy of respiration and ventilation. Specific assessment includes the rate, depth, and rhythm of respirations. Periodically check tidal volumes and arterial blood gas values. Many clients require endotracheal or tracheostomy tubes with ventilatory support. Oxygen administration will be ordered by tracheostomy tube, tracheostomy collar, or ventilator. For respiratory care and respiratory toilet, refer to specific nursing measures for amyotrophic lateral sclerosis, head trauma, and Chapter 18.

High cervical injuries frequently cause respiratory arrest. During this emergency, the neck *must not* be hyperextended. Instead, the jaw thrust maneuver is used for mouth-to-mouth resuscitation. The client then requires careful nasotracheal intubation or an emergency tracheostomy. For clients admitted with respiratory function intact, observe respiration carefully. During spinal shock, it is not uncommon for the level of injury to ascend one or two levels above actual damage due to massive spinal cord edema. When this occurs, clients with high cervical injuries may develop respiratory dysfunction and/or arrest even if they did not have the problem initially. This group of clients is at high risk for pulmonary complications such as pneumonia and atelectasis.

To alleviate early spinal-cord edema, large doses of intravenous or intramuscular dexamethasone (Decadron) may be given. Steroids may cause gastric distress as well as other side effects such as behavioral changes, elevated glucose levels, and an acnelike rash.

Clients are also at risk for abdominal distention and paralytic ileus. Keep the client NPO until bowel sounds return. Use a rectal tube if not contraindicated to relieve abdominal distention. Carefully monitor the client for gastrointestinal bleeding from stress ulcers related to steroid therapy. For clients with ulcer histories, cimetidine (Tagamet) may be ordered with the steroids. Remind the physician if the client has an ulcer history. If gastrointestinal bleeding is suspected, test gastric secretions and stool specimens for occult blood. A nasogastric tube may be passed if signs of a gastric ulcer are identified. Protocols for irrigation vary (eg, continuous iced saline, room temperature saline, or vasopressin drips for gastrointestinal bleeding). Obtain immediate complete blood counts and specimens for blood typing and crossmatching.

In developing a plan of care to prevent hazards of

immobility, emboli, skin breakdown, and bowel and bladder dysfunction, refer to specific nursing measures for clients with stroke. In addition, it is helpful to begin a bowel management program by administering a cleansing enema. To establish a bowel reflex, provide a combination of bulk in the diet, stool softeners, prune juice, and daily suppositories. Abdominal massage and digital stimulation can help. Establish a schedule for defecating and administer the daily suppository at the same time each day.

Assess the client for symptoms and signs of thrombophlebitis and pulmonary embolism because the client cannot give subjective reports of calf pain. When managing skin care, consider the type of bed the client is in. A Rota Rest bed is preferred. If unavailable, a circle bed or Stryker frame can provide sufficient turning capability to assess and care for all skin areas. Changing clients to a prone position may evoke fear and anxiety about falling or suffocation. Assess vital signs, tidal volume, or vital capacity before turning. These clients have a potential for hypoxia, hypotensive episodes, and vagal reflexes.

The most sensitive area of nursing care is the client's psychological reaction to paralysis. Body image and the client's entire future have been suddenly and irrevocably altered. Assess available support systems, prevent sleep deprivation and sensory overload, and provide time to talk with clients or just be with them.

Understand and prepare significant others for the client's angry outbursts or other behaviors that reflect attempts to cope (refer to Chapter 6). These behaviors are healthy and cathartic. Recognize the range of emotion the client experiences, with the goal of supporting the client in progressing toward eventual acceptance and resolution. Encourage clients to make as many decisions about their care as possible to help them regain a sense of control over self and environment.

The acceptance of permanent disability may take a long time. Acknowledge client concerns without forcing acceptance. Denial can be beneficial for a time. Be an empathic listener who can accurately reflect the client's comments and feelings. A consistent, supportive approach is essential.

Sometimes clients develop an extreme dependence on the acute care setting, the care providers, and ventilatory support. The client experiences varying degrees of anxiety about separating from a stable group of caregivers and support systems. A careful, well-planned approach is required for the task of separation. Provide simple explanations for ventilatory weaning. It is helpful to discuss the criteria for weaning from ventilation and the client's achievement of the appropriate goals. Remain with the client being weaned and check vital signs and respiratory status at intervals. Institute short periods of weaning initially and have all backup equipment available and functioning. (Weaning clients from ventilatory support is discussed in Chapter 18.) Prepare clients for any setbacks and reinforce their progress. Clients' confidence levels can improve by encouraging them to assume responsibility for

Nursing Research Note

Aadelen SP, Kahn–Stroebel F: Coping with quadriplegia. *AJN* 1981; 81: 1471–1478.

This case study examined how one person coped with quadriplegia using Hoon's concept of adaptive mechanisms. Hoon grouped adaptive mechanisms into three processes. The coping process is purposeful, reality oriented, and involves choice. The defense process distorts reality, is rigid, and is often based on a degree of magical thinking. The fragmentation process is unresponsive to reality, repetitive, and ritualistic. Hoon believes that persons will cope if they can, defend if they must, and fragment if they are forced.

The article traces the person's use of these adaptive processes during her long recovery and rehabilitation from injury. Also examined is the husband's adaptive response, which ultimately led to the couple's divorce. Because the subject was permanently disabled, the study describes the need for her to repeat the developmental tasks of young adulthood. Learning to maximize her physical potential, developing autonomy, and reestablishing identity were tasks to be reworked and remastered.

The authors state that the ability to cope with the stress of spinal cord injury is based on intrinsic biopsychological processes, ego strength, family structure and extrinsic environmental support. Intrinsic biopsychological coping is aided by interdisciplinary care. Family and individual coping is also aided by such care and is supported by educational programs at all levels of rehabilitation. Nursing care that is based on preventive health care and health promotion provides the external support system and resources to facilitate coping.

timing of certain treatments and reminding the staff of the schedule.

Once vertebral fractures fuse, clients can be transferred to stretcher chairs. Hypotension and dizziness may occur, so mobilization must be done progressively. Abdominal binders and antiembolism stockings can be used to decrease hypotensive episodes and periods of dizziness.

Sexual dysfunction is a major concern that clients may or may not verbalize during the acute stage of injury. Factors that determine future potential for sexual function are the anatomic level of injury, the client's personality and former sexual experiences, and the effectiveness of sexual counseling. The most important fact to convey is that a caring, loving relationship is possible with another individual. The majority of female clients can physically participate in intercourse. Assistive information about technique, positions, and catheter taping is helpful. Male clients have greater sexual potential when they have a high cervical or thoracic lesion because of reflexogenic ability. Lumbar and sacral injury can destroy the reflex arc, decreasing the potential for an erection. For these clients, prosthetic devices such as penile implants (see Chapter 68) can be used.

Clients may give cues that signal appropriate timing for discussion of sexual issues. If they do not, the nurse should initiate the discussion.

Anticipate autonomic dysreflexia with quadriplegics and paraplegics who sustain high thoracic lesions. Autonomic dysreflexia results from exaggerated autonomic responses to stimuli. Bladder or bowel distention or skin stimulation can trigger the response. Autonomic dysreflexia is an emergency that may lead to increased ICP and severe hypertension. Assess the client for severe headache, flushing, bradycardia, elevated blood pressure, and diaphoresis. When symptoms occur, elevate the client's head to lower blood pressure, assess patency of the in-dwelling catheter, and check for a fecal impaction. Anesthetic ointment can be topically applied in the rectum before feces are removed to decrease the stimulation of manual removal. Antihypertensive drugs may be necessary—eg, hydralazine hydrochloride (Apresoline). The nurse can help prevent episodes of dysreflexia by preventing conditions that result in stimulus overload, eg, fecal impaction or bladder distention.

Chapter Highlights

Ataxia is the most common symptom of cerebral palsy.

All forms of muscular dystrophy are inherited.

Clients are at high risk for potential injury in later stages of Huntington's chorea.

Knowledge deficits are common for clients with neurofibromatosis and their significant others because of the uncertainty of the diagnosis.

An explosive headache is the most common symptom of a client with rupture of an intracranial aneurysm. Clients with ruptured intracranial aneurysms should not be given enemas or any form of stimulus that can increase ICP.

The most common presenting signs of a cerebral AVM are seizure activity and hemorrhage.

Never restrain a client having a major generalized motor (grand mal) seizure. Never use force to insert an oral airway into a client having a grand mal seizure.

Migraine headaches usually change location during different attacks from one side of the head to another.

Trigeminal neuralgia is characterized by excruciating paroxyms of facial pain.

Occlusive cerebrovascular disease is caused by a thrombus or embolus. Hemorrhagic cerebrovascular disease is caused by an aneurysm rupture or AVM bleed.

The most common initial symptom of Parkinson's disease is tremor.

Amyotrophic lateral sclerosis usually has a fatal outcome.

Medication for treating myasthenia gravis must be given at the exact time ordered.

Multiple sclerosis is characterized by remission and exacerbation of symptoms.

Clients with meningococcal (bacterial) meningitis must be isolated until therapeutic antibiotic levels are achieved. Diagnosis of viral encephalitis has greatly improved with electron microscopy.

Cruetzfeldt-Jakob disease is presumed to be caused by a slow virus.

Teach clients to seek medical treatment for dental caries, ear infections, and sinusitis to prevent development of a brain abscess.

There is a relationship between the chicken pox and herpes zoster virus.

A client's head and neck must be immobilized and not manipulated if cervical trauma is suspected. Use the jaw thrust maneuver to resuscitate a client with cervical injury.

(continued)

Chapter Highlights *(continued)*

Never suction the nasal passage ways of a client with head trauma until basal skull fractures and/or dural tears have been ruled out.

Basal skull fracture is characterized by Battle's sign, ecchymosis of the mastoid region, and hemotympanum.

Spinal shock following an acute spinal cord injury can increase the functional level of injury for weeks after injury.

Bibliography

Adams RD, Victor M: *Principles of Neurology,* 2nd ed. New York: McGraw-Hill, 1981.

American Association of Neuroscience Nurses: *Core Curriculum for Neuroscience Nursing.* Chicago: The American Association of Neuroscience Nurses, 1983.

Bickerstaff E: *Neurology,* 3rd ed. London: Hodder and Stroughton, 1980.

Cohen S et al: Radioimmunoassay of myelin basic protein in spinal fluid. *New Engl J Med* 1976; 295:1455.

Conway-Rutowski: *Carini and Owens' Neurological and Neurosurgical Nursing.* St. Louis: C.V. Mosby, 1982.

Eisendorf, Cohen: *J Fam Pract* 1980.

Eldridge R, Fahn S (editors): *Advances in Neurology,* Vol. 14. Dystonia, NY: Raven, 1976.

Forster FM: *Clinical Neurology,* 4th ed. St. Louis: C.V. Mosby, 1978.

Friedman W: Head injuries. *Clinical Symposia* 1983; 35(4):2–32.

Hakim AM, Mathieson G: Basis of dementia in Parkinson's disease. *Lancet* 1978; 2:729.

Hayter J: Patients who have Alzheimer's disease. *Am J Nurs* 1974; 8:1460–1463.

Hickey J: *The Clinical Practice of Neurological and Neurosurgical Nursing.* Philadelphia: Lippincott, 1981.

Hoehn M, Yahr M: Parkinsonism: Onset, progression and mortality. *Neurology* 1967; 17:427–433.

Jennett B, Galbraith S: *An Introduction to Neurosurgery,* 4th ed. Chicago: Year Book, 1983.

Kaminski, D: Air embolism during surgery in the sitting position: Prevention, detection and treatment. *Neurosurg Nurs* 1975; 7(2):65–71.

Kolata G: Alzheimer's research poses. *Science* (Jan) 1982; 215.

Malis LI: Arteriovenous malformations of the brain. In: *Neurological Surgery,* Vol. 3. Yomans JR (editor). Philadelphia: W. B. Saunders, 1982.

McKinstry D: Diagnosis, cause and treatment of Alzheimer's disease. *Research Resources Reports* (June) 1982; VI(6).

Merritt HH: *A Textbook of Neurology,* 6th ed. Philadelphia: Lea & Febiger, 1979.

Mulford E: Degenerative diseases or "slipped" disc? The clues are clear-cut. *RN* (Feb) 1981.

Panel of Neuromuscular Disorders. Washington, D.C.: Department of Health, Education, and Welfare, 1979.

Plum F, Posner JB: *The Diagnosis of Stupor and Coma.* Philadelphia: F.A. Davis, 1980.

Wehrmaker S, Wintermute J: *Case Studies in Neurological Nursing.* Boston: Little Brown, 1978.

Wilson S: *Neuro-Nursing.* New York: Springer Publications, 1979.

Zervas T: Early management of subarachnoid hemorrhage due to ruptured cerebral aneurysms. *Neurol and Neurosurg* 1979; 2:10.

The Client With Head Trauma

I. Brief Descriptive Data:	Joseph Holmlund, a 32-year-old certified public accountant and father of two young daughters, was brought unconscious to the emergency department following a head injury. The injury resulted from being hit with a baseball during a ball game.

II. Personal Data

Date and Time:	June 25, 1986; 6:15 P.M.
Full Name:	Joseph Stephen Holmlund
Social Security Number:	000-00-0000
Address:	16 Juliet St., Warren, Ohio
Telephone:	Home: 000-0000
	Work: 000-0000
Sex:	Male
Age:	32
Birthdate:	2/6/54
Marital Status:	Widower
Race:	Caucasian
Religion:	Born-again Christian
Occupation:	Certified Public Accountant
Usual Health Care Provider:	Geraldine Kostusiak, M.D.

III. Health History

Source of Information:	Two members of the baseball team, who were present when the injury occurred, and Mr. Holmlund's fiancee, Donna Shipman.
Reliability of Information:	Reliable
Chief Concern:	Unresponsive 32-year-old man who sustained a head injury 7 hours ago.
History of Present Illness:	During a baseball game 7 hours ago, Joe was accidently hit on the right side of his head by a hardball traveling at high speed. He fell to the ground and lost consciousness for several minutes. He awakened somewhat dazed, with a headache, but felt well enough to remain at the game. Later, while lying on his couch at home watching TV, he fell asleep; his fiancee was unable to arouse him. She called the paramedics and Joe was rushed to the emergency room.
	His fiancee states that his general health has been excellent. He has never had surgery or been treated for a medical problem. To her knowledge he has not had a previous head injury. He takes no medications; does not smoke or drink; no known allergies.
Past Health History:	Unknown except for fiancee's report.
Family History:	Daughters × 2—ages 4 and 7; both A&W.
	Wife died, age 28—automobile accident.
	Brother—age 39, A&W; lives in Nevada.
	His parents are both dead, cause unknown.
	Nothing known about other blood relatives.
Personal/Social History:	Joe lives in a condominium with his 2 daughters; his youngest attends a day care center and the oldest is in second grade. They have had some difficulty adjusting to the tragic death of Mrs. Holmlund 2 years ago. Joe recently joined the baseball team to get some exercise and recreation. Donna has known Joe for 8 months—they became engaged 6 weeks ago.
Review of Systems:	Unknown

(continued)

Case Study written by Susan Nevins.

The Client With Head Trauma

IV. Physical Assessment

Height	6 ft 2 in
Vital Signs:	BP 100/60; pulse 106; resp. 22; temperature 98°F (36.7°C)
Relevant Organ Systems:	
Head:	boggy swelling, right occiput.
Neurologic:	Cerebral function—no response to painful stimuli with absence of gag, cough, and corneal reflexes.

Cranial nerves:

I: Not tested

II: Fundi benign

III, IV, VI: Ptosis of right eyelid with fully dilated, fixed pupil unresponsive to light; left pupil reacting somewhat sluggishly to light

V: Corneal reflex absent; no response to painful stimuli

VII: Facial muscles appear symmetrical; lacrimation adequate

VIII: Caloric testing done confirming deep coma

IX, X: Gag reflex absent

XI: Not tested

XII: No atrophy or deviation of tongue noted

Motor system: No atrophy or tremors; spastic paralysis of the left extremities noted

Sensory system: No response to deep, painful stimuli

Reflexes: DTRs hyperactive

V. Diagnostic Data

A stat CT scan was done, revealing a right epidural hematoma; an emergency craniotomy was scheduled. The surgeon contacted Mr. Holmlund's brother, Leon, in Nevada (his closest living relative), explaining the gravity of the situation. Leon agreed to wire permission for the procedure.

VI. Preoperative Regimen

Mr. Holmlund was intubated and given hyperventilation therapy to maintain PCO_2 between 25–30 mm Hg (by decreasing PCO_2, cerebrovasodilation is reduced causing a decrease in ICP)

Dexamethasone (10 mg) given IV bolus followed by 4 mg IV q. 6 hrs.

Mannitol 1 Unit given IV stat

An in-dwelling catheter was inserted

VII. Surgery:

An emergency craniotomy was performed down to the base of the skull; the right middle meningeal artery was isolated at the foramen spinosum; a large right epidural hematoma was evacuated, arterial bleeders were coagulated, and a Hemovac was inserted

Mr. Holmlund was transferred from the OR to the Intensive Care Unit

VIII. Nursing Care Plan:

Nursing Diagnosis	Client Care Goal	Plan/Nursing Implementation	Expected Outcome
Airway clearance, ineffective: potential for	Prevent respiratory arrest and aspiration	Maintain patent airway by removing debris from mouth and throat; check to be sure tongue is not obstructing airway; monitor	No signs of respiratory arrest, aspiration, or respiratory distress

Nursing Diagnosis	Client Care Goal	Plan/Nursing Implementation	Expected Outcome
		baseline and ongoing ABGs; assist with intubation; suction endotracheal tube prn; maintain functional ambu with O_2 source, suction machine, and ventilator at bedside; provide source of humidification for ET tube	
Gas exchange, impaired	Reduce cerebral edema	Administer hyperventilation therapy via ventilator as ordered; maintain PCO_2 between 25–30 mm Hg as ordered	Maintain state of respiratory alkalosis; cerebral edema will decrease
Communication, impaired verbal	Reduce anxiety levels for comatose client by recognizing hearing is intact	Explain all procedures to the client and provide reassurance despite comatose state	Client will not experience anxiety or fear related to knowledge deficits
Injury: potential for	Prevent further deterioration in client's neurologic status	Perform accurate baseline neurologic assessment for further comparison; continue to monitor all neurologic parameters q. 15 min until stable, then q. ½–1 hr	Comparison of neurologic assessment to a baseline aids in documenting client progress
	Assess neurologic status according to which parameters may change first	Critical aspects of assessment are level of consciousness, pupil signs, and motor function; document neurologic findings on standard assessment sheet as designated by institution;	Neurologic status will be assessed accurately and any changes recognized early
	Prevent unrecognized deterioration in neurologic status	Report any new or worsening signs of neurologic deterioration to the physician immediately; anticipate emergency neurodiagnostic procedures, especially CT scan; prepare to accompany client to procedures; maintain ongoing rapport with significant others; provide psychological support; give explanations and rationale for therapeutic measures; anticipate emergency surgical interventions	All changes in the client's neurologic condition will be reported promptly Significant others will have decreased anxiety
	Prevent meningitis related to CSF leak	Never suction head trauma clients through nasal passageways until ordered by the physician	Meningitis will not develop
Fluid volume, alteration in: excess	Decrease ICP Promote central venous drainage	Administer steroids and osmotic diurectics as ordered; Maintain HOB at 30° elevation; avoid any unnecessary stimuli; keep ventricular tap set on standby; avoid positioning with any neck compression	Increased ICP will not develop

(continued)

The Client With Head Trauma

VIII. Nursing Care Plan: *(continued)*

Nursing Diagnosis	Client Care Goal	Plan/Nursing Implementation	Expected Outcome
	Ensure adequate urinary output	Maintain and monitor strict I&O and patency of foley catheter; also check lab values for problems with function	Renal function will be maintained; urinary output wn1

Chapter 38

Specific Disorders of the Peripheral Nervous System

Susan Nevins

Objectives

When you have finished studying this chapter, you should be able to:

Identify the area within the nervous system mainly affected in adults with lead poisoning.

Discuss priorities of nursing care for the client with acute lead poisoning.

Name the most common form of polyneuritis.

Name the two different functions of the facial nerve usually affected in Bell's palsy.

Explain several nursing interventions to prevent corneal abrasions in clients with Bell's palsy.

Specify the most common neurologic sign in pellagra.

Describe the onset and progression of symptoms in Guillain-Barré syndrome.

Specify the most common disease of the peripheral nervous system in the world.

Discuss at least three risk factors that predispose a client to peroneal nerve injury.

Anticipate factors that predispose a client to radial nerve injury.

The causes of disease in the peripheral nervous system (PNS) include hereditary defects, neurotoxic agents such as lead and arsenic, nutritional deficiency, autoimmune disease, neoplasms, and trauma. A client with PNS dysfunction can face a major disruption in lifestyle. Recovery may require long periods of rehabilitation, straining support systems and personal finances. Accurate diagnosis is often difficult, contributing to client frustration and coping problems.

Section I: Congenital Disorders

A congenital disorder of the PNS can also be defined as a developmental defect. The causes for these maldevelopments are often unknown. A majority of congenital defects of the PNS develop from a hereditary chromosomal abnormality. These defects are assumed to occur according to laws of mendelian inheritance. A variety of these defects can be seen from birth to late adolescence: peroneal muscular atrophy, progressive hypertrophic neuropathy, and hereditary sensory neuropathy. These defects are rare, and because of their early onset, discussion of them properly belongs in a pediatrics text.

Section II: Disorders of Multifactorial Origin

Some disorders of multifactorial origin involving the PNS are caused by toxic substances such as metallic elements and drugs. There are two types of toxic substances: exogenous toxins, which are from a source outside the body, and endogenous toxins, which develop within the body. The mechanisms of their effects on nervous tissue are varied. Toxins that have an affinity for peripheral nervous tissue include lead, arsenic, and alcohol. Intoxication with large amounts of these harmful agents can result in various forms of neurologic dysfunction. In the peripheral nerves, symptoms and signs can include atrophy and weakness of legs and arms, loss of reflexes, loss of sensation, numbness and tingling in hands and feet, and various cranial-nerve deficits. Such losses can make it difficult for the affected individual to perform activities of daily living, maintain a job, and participate in recreational activities. Bell's palsy, an inflammation of CN VII, is also a disorder of multiple causation.

General Nursing Implications

The primary objective for nurses is prevention. Public health nurses have an opportunity to discover clients who have been inadvertently or intentionally exposed to neurotoxins. In addition to immediate care measures, nurses should take follow-up action by sending recommendations to public officials and employers on occupational hazards. Nurses can also develop plans to teach industrial workers about potential hazards of toxic agents. In cases of intentional overdoses, causes of ingestion should be investigated and attempts made to prevent recurrences. This process will require a multidisciplinary cooperative effort.

LEAD POISONING

The most common form of heavy metal intoxication is lead poisoning. Lead poisoning is much less frequent in adults than children. Two kinds of lead toxicity affect the CNS: peripheral neuropathy and encephalopathy. Peripheral neuropathy affects mainly adults. Exposure to industrial processes that produce fumes from remelting of lead or dust from inorganic lead salts presents the greatest occupational hazard to adults.

Clinical Manifestations

Colic, anemia, and peripheral neuropathies constitute the usual presenting symptoms and signs of lead poisoning in adults. Colic is in the form of severe abdominal pain and muscular rigidity. These symptoms are not associated with leukocytosis or temperature elevation. Mild anemia usually develops. Peripheral neuropathy involves mainly motor nerves innervating the arm muscles. Wristdrop often

develops. Alterations in sensation are rare. Diagnosis includes an analysis of urine, feces, and serum for levels of lead toxicity.

Therapeutic Measures

Therapy is aimed at mobilizing ingested lead so it can be excreted from the body. Chelating agents, which are used for this purpose, combine with lead to form a nontoxic substance. These agents are also water soluble and can readily be eliminated by the kidneys. The agent of choice is calcium disodium edetate given IM. After lead absorption ceases, these agents remove lead only from soft tissue, not from bone. Most of the lead is stored in bone; therefore, any subsequent disorder causing bone demineralization can cause a relapse, and symptoms recur. That is why it is crucial to identify and attempt to remove agents in the environment that cause lead poisoning.

Adjunctive therapy includes measures to ensure adequate kidney function. Careful regulation of fluid intake and administration of diuretics can ensure an adequate urinary output. In some cases in which diagnosis is difficult, a mobilization test can be performed. A chelating agent is given, and urinalysis is done to detect lead in the urine.

Specific Nursing Measures

In an acute care setting, the nurse's major objective is to prevent alterations in protective mechanisms. The nurse can help to decrease lead absorption by offering the client large quantities of milk. Milk helps promote the formation of an insoluble lead salt that has poor intestinal absorption and will heighten the deposit of lead in the bone. The next priority is to promote the removal of lead from the bone. This removal is accomplished by administering calcium disodium edetate as ordered. Because this drug has an affinity for lead, it combines with lead to form a nontoxic compound that can be excreted by the urine. The preferred route of administration is by intramuscular injection. A rapid parenteral infusion of calcium disodium edetate can be lethal; the drug can markedly increase ICP in clients with cerebral edema. The dosage is adjusted according to body weight and given in divided doses for at least 5 days. Observe for signs of an untoward reaction—rash, lethargy, vomiting, shock, and tetany. These signs are more frequent with intravenous administration.

Monitor the client for alterations in fluid volume. Calcium disodium edetate should not be administered to dehydrated clients, and overhydration should be prevented. Check the urine daily for blood and protein. Check serum BUN and creatinine to assess kidney function.

Alterations in comfort can occur from edetate injections. To minimize local pain at the injection site, mix 1 mL of 1% procaine with each 1 mL of edetate concentrate as ordered. Rotate injection sites and document them on the chart. If muscle soreness develops at injection sites, apply warm compresses.

Dimercaprol (BAL) helps to remove lead from tissues by forming a stable, nontoxic compound that can be excreted. Be aware that untoward effects may occur 10 to 15 minutes after an injection and subside 1 or 2 hours later. These symptoms include nausea and vomiting, headache, and an increase in secretions—tears, salivation, and sweat. A burning sensation can develop in the lips, mouth, and throat. Muscular aches and fever may occur. The most distressing symptom is the sensation of constriction in the chest associated with tachycardia.

Recognize factors that can interfere with the absorption of lead in the bones. Two of the major factors are infections and alterations in electrolyte balance. Infections can reactivate the mobilization of lead, causing a recurrence of lead poisoning symptoms. Acidosis can also interfere with the deposit of lead in the bone.

Inform clients about the seriousness of reexposures. Initiate a visiting nurse referral to follow up on continued lead exposure. Assist the client to identify sources of lead exposure and propose methods to eliminate contact. One preventive measure is to place literature explaining harmful effects of lead in places where risk of occupational exposure is high. Stress the importance of long-term follow-up. Teach the client to avoid exposure to sources of infection. Infection not only can cause symptom recurrence but can also increase serum iron levels greatly and cause additional nervous system damage. Be aware of the complications of encephalopathy, evidenced by high blood pressure, bradycardia, papilledema, and convulsions.

ARSENIC INTOXICATION

Arsenic poisoning is a major metallic intoxication affecting the nervous system. Ingestion of an organic compound of arsenic usually causes peripheral neuropathies; a parenteral infusion of an inorganic compound can result in encephalopathy. With toxic ingestion of arsenic, fulminating gastrointestinal symptoms develop. These symptoms can be followed quickly by convulsions, circulatory collapse, and even death if the level of intoxication is high enough. Polyneuritis can develop several weeks after acute intoxications in surviving clients, or it can result from chronic ingestion of arsenic.

In the past, the treatment of syphilis with Fowler's solution (potassium arsenite) or organic lead arsenical compounds was a frequent cause of arsenic intoxication. Today, accidental or intentional ingestion of insecticides, rat poisons, or certain occupational products are common causes of arsenic poisoning. Arsenic produces its toxic effect by interacting with certain enzymes necessary for cellular metabolism.

Clinical Manifestations

Arsenic poisoning usually causes gastrointestinal and nervous system symptoms, depending on the form and amount of the compound ingested. A painful polyneuritis is the most common form of nervous system dysfunction. Cranial nerves can be affected, especially CN VIII (the vestibulocochlear nerve). Less commonly, optic nerve irritation occurs. Arsenical poisoning is demonstrated by levels of arsenic in hair and urine specimens. After several weeks of exposure, the drug will be found in the hair. Arsenic is slowly excreted via urine and feces. It can remain within hair and bones for long periods.

Therapeutic Measures

Acute arsenic poisoning requires immediate treatment with gastric lavage. Adjunctive therapy includes fluid replacement, the use of vasopressor drugs, and the administration of dimercaprol (BAL). Dimercaprol is given according to body weight at 3 mg/kg. Drug injections should be given at 4-hour intervals for the first 48 hours, four times a day for another day, then twice a day for 1 to 2 days. The drug is given twice daily for the next 7 to 10 days or longer as the client's condition warrants (Merritt, 1979). Dimercaprol can decrease gastrointestinal and CNS symptoms; however, peripheral neuropathies do not respond well to the drug and usually subside gradually over time. During acute intoxication, a combination of milk and eggs may be given orally. If the client recovers from the initial crisis, causes of ingestion should be investigated and remedies planned.

Specific Nursing Measures

The first priority of emergency nursing care is to assist with gastric lavage. The stomach contents are aspirated via a nasogastric tube. Then water is instilled, followed by a continual siphoning of gastric contents. Lavage is repeated 10 to 15 times or until returns are clear. A lavage usually requires 1000 to 2000 mL of water. The samples from the first several washings can be saved for possible analysis. At the completion of a lavage, the stomach can be left empty, an antidote instilled and left in the stomach, and/or a cathartic may be given. The choice depends on the type and severity of poisoning.

During removal of the nasogastric tube, the tube is clamped or pinched or suction is applied to prevent aspiration. Keep the client's head positioned down and to the side. Close observation is required for 24 hours. The type of poisoning should be documented, as well as the client's condition before, during, and after the procedure. Once the client is stable enough to have oral feedings, large quantities of milk and eggs can be given to decrease arsenic levels. For nursing measures for the administration of dimercaprol, see nursing measures for lead poisoning.

Alterations in comfort can result from painful peripheral involvement. Provide comfort measures such as mild analgesics, physical therapy regimens, assistive devices, and emotional support.

ALCOHOL- AND VITAMIN-INDUCED POLYNEURITIS

Alcohol- and vitamin-induced polyneuritis is the most common form of polyneuritis, occurring much more often in men than women. Incidence is highest between the ages of 40 and 70. The outcome depends on the degree of accompanying CNS dysfunction or other systemic problems. Recovery can be prolonged; the client may be confined to bed for months.

This form of polyneuritis is observed most frequently in chronic alcoholics. Poor vitamin and dietary intake is common in this population. When polyneuritis develops in alcoholics, it is difficult to determine whether the nerve damage is caused by the toxic effects of alcohol, nutritional deficiencies, or both.

Clinical Manifestations

Symptoms usually develop slowly, beginning with leg pains accompanied by numbness and tingling in hands and feet. Then atrophy and weakness of the legs occur, followed by arm involvement with loss of deep tendon reflexes (DTRs). There can be more extensive sensory deficits along with some cranial nerve dysfunction. Clients' skin alterations are similar to those with pellagra or vitamin A deficiency—drying, flaking, and pigmentation on the wrists and dorsal surface of the hands.

Some laboratory findings include moderate leukocytosis, anemia, and presence of alcohol in serum and cerebrospinal fluid (CSF). CSF pressure may be elevated, and protein is present in the CSF of a small number of clients.

In alcoholic polyneuritis related to nutritional deficiencies, muscular weakness and atrophy become severe if treatment is delayed or not given. Legs will be affected more than arms. Footdrop, ataxic gait, and eventually inability to walk will occur.

Without treatment, muscular pain and paresthesia can intensify to the point that there is severe pain to touch, especially in the feet. Vibratory sense is impaired. Reflexes are absent in the legs and sometimes the arms. In severe cases, an optic neuritis and facial paresis develop. Urinary and rectal sphincter tone may be lost. Tachycardia can persist without other changes in vital signs.

There is a prolonged disease course in which symptoms initially become more severe, even with treatment. Overall prognosis is affected by the degree of dementia accompanying the polyneuritis, whether alcohol consumption continues, and future dietary and vitamin intake. Occasionally, a hemorrhagic form of polioencephalitis occurs

that can prove fatal. Most clients who recover do so only after months of confinement.

Specific Nursing Measures

The primary nursing goal is to help correct alterations in nutritional intake and to develop strategies to control alcohol consumption. A specific balanced diet should be prescribed as well as daily vitamin supplements. Dietary instructions should be in a written plan with printed menus and charts of food groups. Review these plans with a family member who can support and reinforce them.

Bed rest will be required during acute phases of illness. Prevent hazards of immobility such as footdrop and wristdrop by frequent repositioning, support devices, and ROM exercises. Analgesics and hygiene measures can relieve pain.

Management of psychosocial problems is the most crucial aspect of nursing care. Help provide a secure, structured environment for the client to ventilate feelings. Involvement of significant others can be beneficial. See Chapter 10 for specific approaches to treatment of alcoholism.

BELL'S PALSY

Bell's palsy is the most common neurologic condition to affect the facial nerve, CN VII. An inflammatory, edematous reaction is thought to occur in or around CN VII resulting in nerve compression, which is characterized by an abrupt onset of a flaccid facial paralysis. There is a loss of facial expression on the affected side, an inability to close the eyelid on the ipsilateral side, and a deviation of the mouth toward the contralateral side. Bell's palsy occurs most often between the third to fifth decades of life with an equal distribution between sexes. Most clients with Bell's palsy recover without residual neurologic deficits. The period of recovery varies and can range from several weeks to as long as a year, however.

Previous infection, prolonged exposure to cold temperatures, and psychological trauma have been suggested as possible causes of Bell's palsy. Concurrent herpetic vesicles in the external auditory meatus of some clients with Bell's palsy suggest a viral cause (Conway-Rutowski, 1982). Bell's palsy usually has no identifiable precipitant, however. The facial nerve can be affected by many other conditions such as brain tumor, traumatic injury, meningitis, middle ear infection, intracranial hemorrhage, or demyelinating disease.

Clinical Manifestations

Bell's palsy often begins with pain behind the ear followed within several hours or 1 to 2 days by a flaccid facial paralysis. The client is unable to wrinkle the forehead, close the eyelid, whistle, blow out the cheek, or smile (Figure 38–1). The affected eye may tear excessively and saliva may drool from the affected side of the mouth. Impairment of taste in the anterior two-thirds of the tongue can occur. Bell's phenomenon refers to the upward and slightly inward positioning of the eyeball that occurs when the client attempts to close the eyelid. The corneal reflex is usually absent. **Hyperacusis** (abnormal sensitivity to sound) can result from nerve involvement to the stapedius muscle. There is usually a loss of deep facial sensation and hypesthesia occurs in some clients.

Therapeutic Measures

Treatment is symptomatic, supportive, and aimed at preventing complications. Protection of the cornea is a priority when the client cannot voluntarily close the eyelid. Electrical stimulation with a weak galvanic current can be done to massage and stimulate facial muscle tone and prevent atrophy. Steroids may be given to reduce facial nerve inflammation. Less commonly vasodilating drugs are given to stimulate circulation and restore blood supply to the affected area. The application of moist heat several times a day for 15 to 30 minutes is a more conservative method of stimulating circulation and may also decrease facial pain. A facial sling is sometimes recommended to prevent muscle stretching and sagging, improve muscle tone, facilitate eating, and improve lip alignment. When spontaneous recovery does not occur over time, surgical procedures may be done. This involves either an end-to-end suturing of the affected nerve or an anastomosis of CN XI or CN XII to the facial nerve.

Specific Nursing Measures

The priority of nursing care is to prevent alterations in protective mechanisms related to loss of the corneal reflex. Cover the affected eyelid with a clear plastic eye bubble or a cloth patch. Avoid gauze patches that can cause corneal scratching. Taping of the eyelid is an effective alternative. Instill artificial tears every 2 to 4 hours and more often as necessary to clear mucus and debris from the eye. This prevents eyeball dryness when the client is unable to produce tears spontaneously. Teach client to manually close the affected eyelid during the period of recovery. As eyelid movement begins, teach client to practice progressive movement toward lid closure. Clients should wear protective glasses during the day and an eye patch or eye tape at night.

A second objective is to prevent alterations in protective mechanisms related to sensorimotor changes until paralysis subsides. Instruct the client to chew on the unaffected side to prevent food from collecting and lodging in the paralyzed side. This also prevents the client from biting

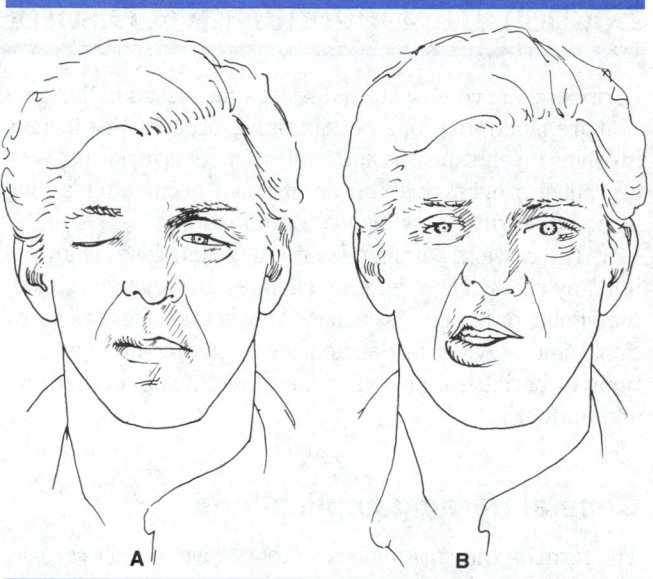

Figure 38–1
A client with left-sided Bell's palsy—paralysis of CN VII. **A.** Note the sagging of the left side of the face and inability to close the left eyelid. **B.** Note that when the client smiles only one side of the face moves.

the mucous membranes inadvertently where sensation is absent. Give frequent mouth care to prevent the development of parotitis. Instruct the client to avoid extreme temperatures of foods to prevent injuries to areas lacking sensation. Privacy for clients during meals avoids embarrassment because of drooling and awkward chewing.

Maintain facial muscle tone by applying a facial sling to prevent stretching of weakened muscles and improve lip alignment, which facilitates eating and drinking. Stimulate circulation to affected muscles with warm, moist compresses. Teach clients to massage facial muscles three to four times a day from the chin upward on the affected side. When return of facial movement occurs, have the client practice various facial expressions in a mirror.

Clients may have alterations in body image related to changes in facial appearance and function. Assist the client and family to be realistic about the length of facial dysfunction. In 80% of clients with Bell's palsy, recovery is complete in several weeks to months. During the regenerative period, teach the client the rationale for protective measures and techniques in activities of daily living to support the natural course of recovery. Help the client to understand that there is not much that can be done to hasten nerve regeneration. Provide clients with opportunities to verbalize feelings about changes in appearance and give positive reinforcement as they progress.

A case study of a client with Bell's palsy is presented at the end of this chapter.

Section III: Degenerative Disorders

Peripheral nervous system diseases discussed in this section are illustrative of a degenerative process that usually involves myelin sheaths and axons. Onset is insidious, with a gradual progressive course and can occur after a long period of normal nervous system function.

The cause of peripheral nerve degeneration is unknown in many cases. Degenerative changes are related to toxic, metabolic, or infectious causes. This section reviews nutritional and/or vitamin deficiencies resulting in degenerations of peripheral nerves. Classic examples are pellagra and beriberi.

General Nursing Implications

The term *degenerative* implies a progressive, usually chronic, loss of nerve function. Anticipate that peripheral nerve changes will include varying degrees of motor, sensory, and reflex changes. A major priority of nursing care involves assisting the client to remain as independent as possible during rehabilitation. Recovery is often variable. Clients may experience alterations in body image, self-esteem, and sensory perception. Modifications in patterns of daily living may be indicated. Emphasize nutritional objectives to promote nerve regeneration and prevent recurrences. The nurse has an important opportunity to do health teaching with clients who have nutritional disorders. Pellagra and beriberi can be complicated by alcoholism. An intensive multidisciplinary approach is required to treat underlying chronic alcoholism.

PELLAGRA

Pellagra, a disease caused by a dietary deficiency of niacin, occurs in most parts of the world. At the turn of the century, pellagra was epidemic in the United States. Its prevalence has greatly decreased over the last 45 years. There are two forms of pellagra: one simply related to a deficiency state and another associated with chronic alcoholism. Pellagra is most common in the fourth and fifth decades of life, and incidence is equally distributed between the sexes. The form associated with alcoholism is more prevalent in men, however.

Clinical Manifestations

Pellagra mainly affects the gastrointestinal tract, skin, and nervous system. Diarrhea can occur secondary to inflammation of mucosal surfaces in the gastrointestinal tract. Stomatitis and glossitis may also be present. Skin manifestations include a characteristic dermatitis in areas exposed to sun.

Paresthesias and polyneuritis are the most common

neurologic findings. Clients may express concern about their extreme fatigue, nervousness, irritability, insomnia, and depression. Acute confusion and memory loss can also occur. Spinal cord involvement is sometimes less distinguishable because of difficulty in making an accurate assessment in a client with mental status changes.

About 50% of clients have some degree of anemia and achlorhydria. The course of the disease varies according to the degree of symptom progression and rapidity of treatment.

Therapeutic Measures

Therapy is primarily directed toward correcting dietary deficiencies. The recommended regimen is large supplements of nicotinic acid and thiamine orally or parenterally with a well-balanced nutritional intake. The skin and gastrointestinal symptoms respond well to treatment, as do the minor neurologic symptoms. With long-term dementia, permanent mental status changes can be expected. Severe signs of peripheral neuritis (eg, motor, sensory, and reflex changes) respond slowly to treatment. Note that peripheral neurologic symptoms respond better to thiamine therapy; cutaneous and gastrointestinal symptoms respond well to nicotinic acid.

Specific Nursing Measures

The major objective of nursing care is to prevent alterations in nutritional patterns. Individuals need to consume adequate amounts of milk, eggs, and wheat products. These foods have a tryptophan-containing protein that decreases the risk of a niacin deficiency.

Other sources of niacin deficiency should be identified. Problems that can increase the incidence of pellagra are alcoholism, cirrhosis of the liver, long-term use of intravenous dextrose without vitamin supplements, and chronic diarrhea.

Be aware that clients with CNS involvement may have disturbances in memory and orientation, may be confused, and may fill memory gaps with imagined experiences that have no basis in fact (**confabulate**). These symptoms can be preceded by an elevated temperature, state of delirium, or prolonged administration of dextrose without vitamins. A simultaneous deficiency of thiamine should be suspected in clients with peripheral neuritis and/or spinal cord involvement. Certain precipitating factors can be avoided through careful nursing intervention.

There is no definitive diagnostic test for pellagra. The nurse can aid in diagnosis by careful history taking and reporting of characteristic symptoms and signs found during assessments.

BERIBERI

Beriberi is a nutritional disorder that affects the cardiac and peripheral nervous systems, either separately or concurrently. This disease has been divided into two forms: wet and dry (with edema and serous effusion and without). Cardiac symptoms vary greatly, ranging from tachycardia and exertional dyspnea to acute, rapid heart failure. Beriberi is principally a degenerative disease of the PNS, however. Neurologic signs usually have an insidious onset; progress slowly from distal to proximal; and involve sensory, motor, and reflex changes. Fatalities have occurred in tropical forms of untreated beriberi. Generally, recovery from beriberi is slow. Residual deficits may include muscular weakness and atrophy.

Beriberi involves a nutritional deficiency of vitamin B_1, or thiamine. The disorder causes degeneration of axons along with destruction of myelin sheaths and axons. Segmental demyelination occurs. The most extensive degeneration is in myelinated fibers in the cranial and brachial nerves. Advanced cases can also involve anterior and posterior nerve roots and the vagus and phrenic nerves.

Clinical Manifestations

Usual clinical findings include muscle weakness, pain, and paresthesias. Legs are affected earlier and more extensively than arms. Symptoms vary from dull, constant aching pains to sharp and severe pain. Muscle tightness and cramping occur in the feet and calves. Some clients report their feet feel cold. More characteristic is heat or a burning sensation in the soles of the feet, associated with varying degrees of pain and paresthesias. Hyperesthesia is a frequent finding in affected areas. Clients may lose DTRs in the legs and develop footdrop and wristdrop. Mobility can be impaired from contractures of the ankles and knees. With involvement of peripheral sympathetic fibers, excessive sweating occurs involving the fingers and the soles of the feet. Neurologic deficits are usually limited to the limbs. Occasionally, cranial nerves are affected with resulting hoarseness and dysphagia. Nerve conduction studies show a decrease in sensory and motor velocities.

Therapeutic Measures

A balanced diet supplemented with vitamin B complexes, especially vitamin B_1, is essential. Parenteral feedings are required for clients with gastrointestinal problems that interfere with eating. Vitamins are administered by intravenous or intramuscular routes. Analgesics such as aspirin are given for pain and paresthesias. Occasionally, oral codeine sulfate may be required. Generally, addictive drugs should be avoided because the disease is chronic. For clients with causalgia (severe burning pain) of the feet, lumbar sympathetic blocks may be done. Recovery can be a slow, tedious process.

Specific Nursing Measures

Be aware of factors that interfere with thiamine absorption or increase requirements for it—pregnancy, lactation, fever, and thyroid dysfunction. Conditions such as diarrhea, alcoholism, and liver disease also impair thiamine absorption.

Clients experience alterations in sensation. In severe cases of dysesthesia, clients have such severe causalgia in their feet that they cannot even tolerate bed linens touching them. Use bed cradles to alleviate this pressure and give analgesics as ordered.

Clients are at risk for alterations in mobility. The combined effect of muscle cramps, stiffness, weakness, and aching can cause limitations in mobility. Contractures and "frozen" joints must be avoided. Progressive physical therapy should be instituted as soon as the pain is under control. Assistive devices can help, such as footboards to prevent shortening of the heel cords and splints for arms and legs. Pressure points can develop at knees and elbows if splints are not properly padded.

Alterations in coping patterns are not uncommon for clients recovering from chronic disabling diseases. Motor function may be restored within a few weeks or many months. In cases of more extensive peripheral nerve damage, clients need to be prepared to wait several months to ambulate unassisted. For alcoholic clients, continued drinking greatly hampers recovery. They require intensive counseling.

Section IV: Immunologic Disorders

GUILLAIN–BARRÉ SYNDROME

Guillain–Barré syndrome, also known as acute infectious polyneuritis, causes a demyelination and degeneration of peripheral nerves and anterior and posterior spinal nerve roots. The disease is characterized by acute, rapid ascending symmetrical motor and sensory deficits. Cranial nerve involvement can occur. There is a potential for respiratory failure. Symptom progression occurs within about 2 weeks of the initial signs, and progression can cease at any time.

Guillain–Barré syndrome can affect any age group, race, or sex; however, it is more common in young adults and more severe in pregnant women and the very young or old. The pathophysiological signs include an inflammation of peripheral nerves and infiltration of them by perivascular lymphocytes. The inflammatory process is marked by edema and exudate that leads to compression of nerve roots. Segmental demyelination causes an ascending bilateral pattern of paresthesias and paralysis along with cranial nerve dysfunction.

Guillain–Barré syndrome is a disease of unknown etiology. The major theories propose an infective, viral, or immunologic cause. About half of diagnosed clients have had a mild respiratory or gastrointestinal infection 1 to 3 weeks before the onset of polyneuritis. Additional preceding events are other viral illnesses, certain surgical procedures, lymphomatous diseases (particularly Hodgkin's disease), and the influenza vaccine. In 1976, national attention was focused on Guillain–Barré syndrome when swine flu immunizations were suspended. More than 100 individuals in different states developed symptoms of the disease after receiving swine flu immunization. Epidemiologic investigations failed to either confirm or conclusively rule out a link between the syndrome and immunization.

Current research efforts have focused on Guillain–Barré syndrome as an autoimmune disease. The syndrome may represent an autoimmune response to antibodies formed in reaction to damage of body tissue. Whether this is a response to a prodromal illness, an immunization, or unknown agent remains to be established. An alteration in cell-mediated immunity may be responsible for the hypersensitivity reaction of tissue in this disease.

Clinical Manifestations

Clinical signs and disease course help to distinguish Guillain–Barré syndrome from other forms of polyneuritis. An acute onset of symptoms with a rapid progression of motor weakness and paralysis are characteristic findings. The bilateral progression of symptoms from distal to proximal in an ascending pattern is common.

The disease is usually characterized by a history of a preceding respiratory or gastrointestinal infection, a latent period of about 2 weeks, and then symptom onset. Paresthesias and weakness of proximal, distal, and trunk muscles occur. The absence of atrophy is significant. There is an abrupt onset of flaccid motor paralysis from involvement of the anterior roots of lower motor neurons. Symptoms ascend symmetrically from lower extremities and can stop at any level of the CNS. Respiratory distress can result from diaphragm and intercostal muscular weakness. Cranial nerves may become involved. Bladder and bowel sphincter function usually remains intact.

The cardinal signs include paresthesias, paralysis, and CSF findings. Symptoms progress over several days to 2 months, with an average duration of intensive symptoms for about 10 days. Recovery usually takes several weeks to a year. Relapse is infrequent.

The major diagnostic tests are the examination of CSF and nerve conduction tests. The CSF findings include the unusual finding of a high protein level without cellular abnormality, the so-called albuminocytologic dissociation. The protein count is initially normal (15 to 50 mg/mL), then shoots up (often to over 250 mg/100 mL), and grad-

ually returns to normal. Protein is released into the CSF by meningeal capillaries and damaged spinal nerves. Physicians may perform serial lumbar punctures to determine the relation between elevations in CSF protein and the degree of the client's clinical signs.

Nerve conduction studies usually demonstrate a slowing of conduction time. A serum leukocytosis may develop early in the course of the syndrome. Sedimentation rates are usually normal.

Therapeutic Measures

The acute care of clients with Guillain–Barré syndrome consists of maintaining a patent airway. Clients are best cared for in a hospital where potential respiratory and cardiac complications can be detected and monitored. Respiratory insufficiency is high because of dysfunction of the phrenic nerve (affecting diaphragm excursion) or the vagus nerve (affecting laryngeal function), or thoracic nerve root damage. Hypoxia is a common complication that requires endotracheal intubation or a tracheostomy with ventilatory support. Aggressive respiratory protocols should be instituted to prevent complications.

Controversy persists regarding steroid therapy. Prednisone or ACTH given during acute stages of the illness is thought to speed recovery. Steroids are considered to have little therapeutic value when given in later stages. When steroids are given, clients must be monitored for fluid retention, gastrointestinal irritation, and electrolyte imbalance. Potassium replacement is often indicated. Dosages are usually tapered to prevent an acute episode of adrenal insufficiency.

Throughout the illness, proper nutrition should be maintained by nasogastric or gastrostomy tube when the oral route cannot be used. Physical therapy programs can be instituted once the client's condition has stabilized. Motor strength should be frequently evaluated because return of function is not always symmetrical. It is important to prevent back problems from premature ambulation of clients with asymmetric muscle function. When respiratory muscle function begins to return as paralysis recedes, the client should be slowly weaned from the ventilator. The tracheostomy may be closed through the decannulation process.

Specific Nursing Measures

The priority of nursing care is to maintain effective airway clearance and breathing patterns. See specific nursing measures under head trauma and amyotrophic lateral sclerosis as well as in Chapter 18.

Clients with Guillain–Barré syndrome have a potential for alterations in cardiovascular status related to autonomic dysfunction. During the acute phase, vital signs must be frequently evaluated. In some cases, clients are placed on cardiac monitoring.

Potential neurologic deficits usually include alterations in mobility and function of cranial nerves. Measure clients for antiembolism stockings, change their position at least every 2 hours, and perform passive ROM exercises for 15 minutes four times a day. When repositioning the client, assess respiratory function and handle extremities gently because of change in pain sensation. Cranial nerve dysfunction can occur in CN VII, CN IX, CN X, and CN XII. Important assessments for the facial nerve (CN VII) include checking all facial movements, lacrimation, and the anterior two-thirds of the tongue for taste. In addition, some clients lose corneal sensation from trigeminal nerve (CN V) dysfunction. Care of eyes is essential to prevent drying and corneal abrasion. Normal saline eye care twice a day, administration of artificial tears every 2 to 4 hours, and the use of a plastic eye bubble (see Figure 39–4) will protect the eyes. The glossopharyngeal nerve (CN IX) and the vagus nerve (CN X) must be assessed by checking the gag, cough, and swallowing reflexes. Oropharyngeal suction setups and alternate methods of feeding must be available. Other changes clients may manifest are inability to shrug their shoulders or turn their heads to the extreme lateral position from deficit of the accessory nerve (CN XI). Dysfunction of the hypoglossal nerve (CN XII) will manifest as paresis and deviation of the tongue.

A major concern of clients with Guillain–Barré syndrome is alteration in comfort. Clients require complete maintenance of hygiene needs not only during the acute phase of illness but also for varying periods during convalescence. Maintenance of basic hygiene and cleanliness fosters better self-esteem and a more positive body image. Provide good mouth care and prevent interruption in skin integrity.

Clients' knowledge deficits may cause them fear and anxiety. The fact that Guillain–Barré syndrome strikes swiftly and clears slowly largely accounts for the alterations in coping patterns. Be supportive, provide a safe environment, and acknowledge to the client any signs of neurologic improvement. Clients must be given sufficient opportunity to help plan their nursing care so they can begin to regain control and reduce their feelings of powerlessness. Psychosocial support systems can aid in optimal client rehabilitation, goals, and plans.

Section V: Infectious Disorders

Polyneuritis is a general term describing the clinical syndrome of multiple peripheral neuritis. Syndromes of polyneuritis are generally caused by toxic agents or metabolic factors. Degenerative changes occur in peripheral nerves as a result of polyneuritis. The exact cause is often unknown. In lupus erythematosus and diabetes mellitus, blood flow to the nerves may be impaired. Metabolic disturbances that impair nerve nutrition and cause a polyneuritis are vitamin and dietary deficiencies, debilitating diseases such as chronic lung problems or cancers, acute infections, or some endocrine problems. Polyneuritis can occur in systemic conditions such as mononucleosis, viral hepatitis, and diphtheria. Polyneuritis associated with deficiency states such as beriberi and pellagra has already been discussed. Polyneuritis related to leprosy will be discussed in this section.

Most cases of polyneuritis involve a noninflammatory degeneration of peripheral nerves. An initial edema and fragmentation of myelin occur. The process of nerve destruction can occur in a retrograde manner. Sometimes, when there is no evidence of damage to the myelin sheath or axons, recovery is rapid. If damage involves the myelin sheaths and axons, recovery is slow.

Although polyneuritis can occur at any age, incidence tends to be higher in middle-aged men. Symptoms and signs can develop slowly over several weeks, or the onset can be sudden with infection or allergy.

LEPROSY

Leprosy, or Hansen's disease, a classic example of an infectious polyneuritis, is considered the world's most common peripheral nervous system disease. The acid-fast bacillus *Mycobacterium leprae* causes leprosy. This organism has an affinity for the skin and PNS, causing sensory loss with trophic changes. The face, hands, and feet are mutilated from the sloughing of skin and bone. The degree of disease progression depends on the resistance of the host.

Children are more susceptible to the disease than adults. Leprosy has an equal sex distribution in children but among adults is somewhat more frequent in men. From 10 to 20 million persons worldwide are stricken with leprosy. The disease is most frequent in tropical and subtropical climates (ie, South and Central America, India, Africa, and China). Most clients diagnosed in North America have come from India and the Middle East. In the United States, the disease is mainly confined to Texas, Florida, Hawaii, Louisiana, and California (Merritt, 1979).

There are two major clinical types of leprosy, lepromatous and tuberculoid. Tuberculoid leprosy is characterized by initial cutaneous lesions followed rapidly by pronounced disease of the peripheral nerves. In lepromatous leprosy, cutaneous lesions are extensive with minimal neurologic involvement. Leprosy has a low contagion rate, contrary to general assumptions. Leprosy is transmitted by direct, intimate contact with an affected individual for a long period. The incubation period in children is at least 3 years; it is even longer in adults. *M. leprae* is thought to enter the body through interruptions in skin integrity or the mucous membranes.

Clinical Manifestations

The earliest manifestation of tuberculoid leprosy is an innocuous-looking macule or papule that lacks pigmentation and sensation. The lesion enlarges by peripheral extension with an affinity for the ulnar, auricular, tibial, or popliteal nerves. Common cranial nerves affected are the trigeminal and facial nerves. Related neurologic deficits occur in a patchy distribution. Loss of facial sensation, which commonly occurs in the first division of the trigeminal nerve, can lead to corneal abrasions and keratitis. The facial nerve is usually affected in the upper half of the face, causing facial asymmetry and inability to close the eyelid.

The muscles innervated by affected peripheral nerves can become weak and atrophied. Muscle wasting begins in the hands and feet, which eventually assume a clawed appearance. The late stage of the disease is characterized by wristdrop and footdrop. Sensory loss more frequently involves superficial cutaneous sensation and assumes a glove-and-stocking type distribution. Deep tendon reflexes have a better rate of preservation in leprosy than in other polyneuropathies.

There is **anhidrosis,** absence of sweat in the areas of sensory loss. Hands and feet become cyanotic, develop ulcers, and undergo a resorption of bone. Fingers are especially affected, beginning in the terminal phalanges and proceeding upward. Eventually, the digits shrink, and the nails actually recede and attach to the stumps of limbs.

Therapeutic Measures

Treatment involves long-term use of sulfones (chemical relatives of the sulfonamides). Dapsone, the sulfone of choice for all forms of leprosy, has a bacteriostatic effect. For clients with sulfone-resistant bacilli, drug choices include rifampin or clofazimine (Lamprene). Sulfones have the potential to arrest leprosy and offer hope of a cure.

Specific Nursing Measures

The main objective in the care of clients with leprosy is to help them adjust to deformities that may have developed.

Clawing of hands or feet is the most common. Late manifestations include wristdrop and footdrop. Clients, who have to adapt to both disfigurement and loss of function, go through a grieving process like all clients with progressive, degenerative disorders. Clients with leprosy have an additional emotional burden—the stigma associated with leprosy. Although the contagion level is low, most persons are unaware of this fact. Nurses can educate the general public to help dispel misconceptions. They can explain that leprosy has a long incubation period and is only transmitted in cases of intimate, prolonged contact.

Clients with leprosy require intensive rehabilitation programs that include physical and occupational therapy, as well as assistive devices such as splints for wristdrop and footdrop and various adaptive devices for ADL. The degree of disability varies according to the type of leprosy and the level of host immunity. The prognosis for clients with the neural form is usually better than for those with the cutaneous form. Death can occur in 1 to 2 decades for clients with the cutaneous type. Those with the neural form can have a spontaneous arrest of the disease, or the disease can be controlled by long-term therapy with dapsone.

The client's protective mechanisms may be altered related to sensory impairments. Impairments can involve a nerve or root distribution but are more in a glove-and-stocking type of distribution. Superficial cutaneous sensations are more affected than deep sensation, pressure pain, and appreciation of position sense and vibration. Teach the client to use visual and auditory cues to compensate for tactile ones in identifying potential or actual sources of injury. Instruct clients to cook with protective mitts and to use assistive utensils when handling objects that are extremely hot or cold. Teach clients the importance of smoke detectors and periodic testing of their function. Emphasize the use of thermometers to gauge water temperature for bathing and drinking. Explain the need for protective measures for outdoor temperature changes, such as appropriate clothing, sunscreens, and sunglasses. Extreme temperatures should be avoided. If an injury occurs, teach the client and family to cleanse the wound carefully and seek medical attention. Explain the importance of seeing a health care provider for periodic assessment of the extent of sensory loss, because motor loss often follows sensory loss.

To prevent knowledge deficits, teach the client the importance of adhering to the sulfone therapy regimen. Clients should not stop their therapy regimen when symptoms seem to have been arrested.

Section VI: Neoplastic Disorders

Peripheral nervous system tumors develop in cranial and spinal nerve roots. These tumors are composed of some of the cellular components that encase axons of the periph-eral nerves as they leave the CNS. These components include Schwann's cells, fibroblasts, and specialized cells.

Usually, tumors are divided into those affecting the

nerve sheath and those of the nerve cell. The former group includes schwannomas, neurofibromas, and malignant nerve sheath tumors. The latter group includes chemodectomas (paragangliomas), pheochromocytomas, and neuroblastomas.

Peripheral nerve tumors may have a wide-ranging effect. They can be relatively benign or highly malignant, cause minor dysfunction or major disability, and result in little or extensive cosmetic changes.

SCHWANNOMAS

Schwannomas, tumors arising from Schwann's cells, usually envelop peripheral nerve root axons as they exit from the CNS. Peripheral schwannomas are usually isolated, encapsulated lesions that attach to one nerve trunk fascicle. The lesions can occur at any age, and incidence by sex is equal.

Clinical Manifestations

Usually schwannomas appear as well-circumscribed palpable masses. They tend to appear on the flexor aspect of extremities: the wrists, elbows, and knees. They are usually present for a long time with little change in size or shape. Pain is not a major symptom.

Therapeutic Measures

The treatment is usually microsurgical removal. High-powered magnification is helpful during the dissection of the tumor from the remaining nerve. In most cases, the tumor can be removed without impairing function.

Specific Nursing Measures

The primary nursing objective is to prevent impairment of skin integrity from wound breakdown. Check integrity of dressings and assess for unusual drainage or signs of localized heat, pain, or redness. When the operative wound is healed, institute progressive ROM. Sutures are removed approximately 7 days postoperatively. Encourage a diet high in calories, proteins, and vitamin C to promote optimal wound healing and rehabilitation.

MALIGNANT TUMORS OF PERIPHERAL NERVES

Malignant tumors of peripheral nerves are characterized by the sudden, rapid increase in their size. Peripheral neurofibromas can degenerate into malignant tumors (eg, sarcomas). Malignant PNS tumors are a primary source of metastasis to the lung. Many arise from intercostal nerves and become situated on the proximal aspect of nerves they affect. Age of onset varies, with tumors occurring more

often during the third decade in women and the fourth decade in men.

The tumors arise from the nerve sheath of peripheral nerves. The degree of malignancy can be altered by endocrine changes such as those occurring during puberty, pregnancy, and adolescence.

Clinical Manifestations

Specific sensorimotor and reflex changes vary according to which nerve roots are affected. In addition to clinical neurologic signs, the client is checked for pulmonary signs, an elevated erythrocyte sedimentation rate, and other nervous system involvement if neurofibromatosis is present.

Therapeutic Measures

A biopsy of affected nerves is performed for frozen sections. Usually, proximal and distal ends are excised, helping to determine the degree of neurosurgical resection needed. When the tumor is highly malignant, more radical resection is required. Radiation and chemotherapy are important adjunctive therapies. About 30% of clients undergoing radical resection have a 5-year survival rate.

Specific Nursing Measures

Clients may experience ineffective coping patterns and anticipatory grieving because of the prognosis and the degree of disability. Expect the client to go through the stages of grieving while attempting to accept the loss of body function and possible death. Clients often go through the grieving process faster than their significant others. Nursing care must also include support and intervention with the client's significant others.

CHEMODECTOMAS

Chemodectomas (paragangliomas) are rare, insidious tumors that arise from elements of the chemoreceptor system. One form is the carotid body tumor which arises at the bifurcation of the common carotid artery and usually spreads to the pharynx, cervical plexus, and CN XI. Another form of chemodectoma is the glomus jugulare tumor which is a secondary tumor of the CNS.

Clinical Manifestations

Carotid body tumors can be asymptomatic. A mass develops in the upper central portion of the neck resulting in syncopal attacks and peripheral nervous system dysfunction. Tracheal pressure can cause hoarseness, dyspnea, and cough. Paralysis of the muscles innervated by the accessory nerve (CN XI) can occur. Middle ear symptoms occur with the glomus jugulare tumor. These include pain in the ear, deafness, and otorrhea (CSF leak from the ear).

The external auditory meatus often develops a red, fleshy, hemorrhagic mass.

Therapeutic Measures

Angiography is a valuable neurodiagnostic tool for differential diagnosis. The recommended treatment is surgical excision. Radiation is sometimes used with the glomus jugulare tumor.

Specific Nursing Measures

A priority of nursing care for clients with carotid body tumors is assessment of alterations in cranial nerve function, especially CN IX, CN X, and CN XI. Assess the client's airway for any respiratory embarrassment due to tracheal pressure. Check the client's voice quality, gag reflex, and ability to swallow. Also assess the client's ability to shrug the shoulders and turn the head from side to side. The client is at risk for alterations in protective mechanisms related to potential injury during a syncopal attack. Teach clients to maintain an environment free of obstacles and harmful objects and to be alert for warning signs of an attack so they can protect themselves.

Section VII: Traumatic Disorders

The peripheral nerves can be injured by a number of different conditions, including pressure, compression, constriction, stretching, or traction on affected nerves. More specifically, nerves can be damaged by skeletal fractures, perforating wounds, lacerations, cuts, or stabbing or gunshot wounds. Single or multiple nerve injury can occur from an injection of a metabolic or toxic substance into the nerve. Injury can be the result of an intramuscular or intravenous injection into the nerve.

The extent of peripheral nerve injury ranges from a mild contusion to a complete severing of the nerve. Within the PNS, the afferent and efferent nerve fibers are surrounded by myelin sheaths and encased in neurilemma. These myelin sheaths permit regeneration of neuronal fibers after destruction, in a process called wallerian degeneration, in which the nerves undergo internal reorganization.

The degree of nerve regeneration within the PNS is affected by a number of factors. The closer a severed peripheral nerve to the CNS, the poorer the chances for regeneration. The more developed and specialized the function of a peripheral nerve, the less likely that functional integrity will be effectively restored. Even under optimal conditions, regeneration proceeds at an approximate rate of 1.0 to 1.5 mm/day. A limiting condition can be the distance between the distal and proximal ends of a severed nerve. If the distance is more than a few millimeters, regenerating fibrils may fail to connect with the neurilemma of the distal stump. This situation can result in development of a painful neuroma (scar tissue) at the site of nerve damage. Surgical reanastomosis will be indicated to reestablish nerve function. Included in this section is a discussion of syndromes such as common peroneal, radial nerve, axillary, brachial plexus, and ulnar nerve injuries. Carpal tunnel syndrome is the most recognized entrapment neuropathy (see Chapter 59).

General Nursing Implications

The nurse should be aware of a number of factors that can impede regeneration of peripheral nerves—a poor state of health, wound infection, or any constriction that interrupts the nutrition to healing tissue. Initiate appropriate dietary measures to promote optimal nerve healing. Although the degree of neurologic deficits, length of disability, and functional outcome vary greatly, strive to help reestablish, support, and maintain client independence.

Recognize that traumatic injuries to peripheral nerves may initially appear to entail more extensive neurologic involvement than is actually the case. Maximum recovery can take 1 to 2 years—a major point to reinforce during preoperative and discharge teaching.

COMMON PERONEAL NERVE INJURY

The peroneal nerve is an extension of the sciatic nerve that innervates the extensor muscles of the ankles and toes and the abductors of the feet; the nerve also provides cutaneous sensation to the outer and lower anterior surface of the legs and the dorsal aspect of the feet. The common peroneal nerve (external popliteal nerve) is most frequently injured. Because the common peroneal nerve is located near the head and neck of the fibula, it is vulnerable to pressure injuries. Any compression or prolonged traction on the lateral aspect of the knee can cause peroneal nerve injury. Injury is especially likely in a sleeping, anesthetized, or intoxicated individual. High-risk factors for injury include lower-leg casts, prolonged positioning during an operative procedure, gunshot injuries, or ganglion cysts at the head of the fibula.

Clinical Manifestations

Peroneal nerve injury can result in footdrop, foot eversion, and numbness of the anterior aspect of the foot. Injury causes a steppage gait characterized by an overflexion of the knee and slapping of the foot. The sensory loss described involves only a partial distribution of the nerve, which is common. The affected area can become swollen, discolored, and anhidrotic.

Therapeutic Measures

Clients usually partially or fully recover when the nerve sustains only transient, short-term pressure. The main intervention will be intensive physical therapy. For peroneal palsy (footdrop), the client will be fitted for an orthopedic brace.

Specific Nursing Measures

Clients are at risk for alterations in protective mechanisms because of the steppage gait described earlier. The affected foot may also have sensory alterations such as numbness. The combined sensorimotor deficits can lead to falls or other injuries. Retrain the client to walk with the support of a foot brace. Encourage the client to progress from a walker to a cane.

Impairments of skin integrity can occur from circulatory changes, especially edema, which often accompanies damage to the peroneal nerve. The foot may also become discolored. Check the quality of distal pulses (dorsalis pedis and posterior tibial) frequently. Assess capillary refilling time in the nail beds by briskly depressing the toenail and then releasing it to time how quickly normal circulation is restored.

Before discharge, prepare the client for potential impairments in home maintenance. Also retrain the client for stair climbing and driving if the right foot is affected.

RADIAL NERVE INJURY

The radial nerve is mainly a motor nerve arising from cervical roots (C-5 to C-8) at the end of the brachial plexus. The nerve innervates a number of muscles in the upper arms, including the brachioradial, triceps, and supinator muscles as well as the finger, wrist, and forearm extensor muscles. The nerve's sensory distribution is found between the thumb and index finger of the hand and in the posterior forearm.

The radial nerve is subject to several forms of pressure injuries, particularly vulnerable at its groove around the humerus. Injury at this site has been called "Saturday night palsy" or "bridegroom palsy" because pressure is

exerted from a fractured humerus or during sleep. Crutch walking compresses the axilla and can also result in radial nerve injury. The nerve can also be damaged by lead intoxication, cuts, or gunshot wounds.

Clinical Manifestations

Complete injury to the radial nerve results in varying degrees of the following motor deficits: inability to extend the wrist, fingers, elbow and thumb; inability to supinate the forearm or abduct the thumb; and limitation in elbow flexion. Sensory impairments occur in the radial aspect of the dorsum of the hand and posterior forearm.

Therapeutic Measures

Radial nerve palsy causes wristdrop. Surgical intervention includes tendon transplants to increase the functional use of the hands. Results are variable. Once the client recovers from the immediate postoperative period, intensive physical therapy is required to prevent disuse atrophy and contractures. A supportive splint is used.

Specific Nursing Measures

Knowledge deficits may result if the client has an unrealistic expectation of surgical outcome. Assist the client to recognize that the surgery is done to increase hand function and cannot restore function to a preinjury state. Reinforce the purpose of the surgery and expected outcome during preoperative teaching. After postoperative wound healing, an intensive program of physical therapy will be instituted. An assistive hand splint is provided for wrist support. Occupational therapy can assist in preparing the client for alterations in home maintenance. The unaffected extremity should be developed by teaching the client to use it during rehabilitation of the affected hand. Reinforce prescribed exercise regimens with the client before discharge and make appropriate follow-up referrals for necessary home care.

AXILLARY NERVE INJURY

The axillary nerve is a branch of the posterior cord of the brachial plexus arising from C-5 and to a lesser degree from C-6 nerve roots. The nerve innervates the deltoid muscles and has a sensory distribution involving a small region of the lateral shoulder.

The axillary nerve can be injured by fractures of the head of the humerus and dislocations at the shoulder joint. This type of injury is usually related to trauma to the brachial nerve plexus. Axillary neuritis can develop following vaccination, especially from tetanus toxoid.

Clinical Manifestations

Axillary nerve damage is characterized by a weakness or paralysis of the deltoid muscle limiting the range of arm movement in outward, backward, and forward positions. There is a slight loss of sensation over the outer aspect of the affected shoulder.

Therapeutic Measures

In cases of fracture or dislocation, the primary orthopedic problem is treated first with immobilization, reduction, and casting. When fracture union has occurred, rehabilitation regimens begin. Neuritis induced by a serum or vaccination may require pain management. Physical therapy is geared toward increasing the abduction and rotation of the arm.

Specific Nursing Measures

The client is at risk for future injury to the axillary nerve until diagnosis is made. Suspected injuries to this area are kept immobile until the cause is determined. If nerve injury is not related to a fracture or dislocation, the local neuritis is treated. Progressive passive ROM is done to increase arm abduction and rotation, and active exercises are slowly introduced. Tolerance for the type of exercise, degree of shoulder joint and elbow rotation, and amount of exercise time is gradually increased. Some clients need an arm sling to support the shoulder during the healing process.

BRACHIAL PLEXUS INJURIES

The brachial plexus develops from the anterior and posterior cervical roots (C-5 to C-8) and the first thoracic nerve root (T-1). These nerve roots form three main branches from which a further distribution of nerve fibers arises. Injuries to the brachial plexus can result in a number of syndromes.

Brachial plexus damage occurs in traction injuries that separate the shoulder or in injuries in which there is an extreme abduction of the arm. Brachial plexus injury can be associated with a difficult delivery during childbirth. Compression injuries to the brachial plexus may occur with neoplasms, aneurysms, skeletal abnormalities, or fascial bands. Other causes of brachial plexus injury include direct trauma from lacerations or gunshot wounds or injections of foreign agents (serum or vaccine).

Clinical Manifestations

A broad range of neurologic deficits results from brachial plexus injuries. A total avulsion of the nerve roots from the cord causes a paralysis of the entire arm. The arm dangles uselessly at the client's side (flail arm). A brachial plexus stretch injury that causes proximal arm paralysis in a neonate is known as Erb's palsy. Complete lesions of the brachial plexus cause extensive sensory loss diagonally from the shoulder to the arm's middle third. Biceps and triceps reflexes are absent.

In intermediate lesions, sensory and motor loss varies depending on which nerves are affected—median, ulnar, and/or radial nerves. Minor injuries may result in only transient loss of function.

Therapeutic Measures

Interventions for the syndrome of brachial neuropathy depend on the etiology and the extent of neurologic deficits. Generally, all treatment regimens involve rest for the affected site. Analgesics, procaine injections to tender areas, slings, local heat, and diathermy are used for clients with acute neuritis. Immobilization is provided by cervical collar or a cast in some cases. The collar is usually preferred because it can be easily adjusted and removed at intervals. Immobilization usually continues for several weeks after neuralgia has subsided. Conservative measures are effective in many cases. Intractable cases have been treated by a number of surgical interventions to relieve pressure on nerve roots—simple decompression procedures; removal of causative problems such as disk herniations; and in some cases, fusion of the involved area. Most surgeons operate only when they can correct an obvious underlying problem.

Specific Nursing Measures

Many degrees of brachial plexus nerve injuries require intervention. Flail arm or paralyzed arm is the most distressing to the client and requires the most intervention. Passive ROM exercises are done to prevent joint contractures and circulatory impairments. As soon as possible, teach the client to use the unaffected arm to perform active exercises on the paralyzed arm. Clients need to learn that they must become the "eyes" for the injured extremity (ie, they must prevent it from dangling by using a splint or sling or by manually repositioning it, especially crossing the arm over the chest when sitting). Retraining in activities of daily living and vocational rehabilitation may be necessary. The greatest impact of this disability is on body image and self-esteem.

ULNAR NERVE INJURY

The ulnar nerve, which arises from C-8 to T-1 segments, is the main branch of the brachial plexus's secondary trunk. Motor innervation is extensive, including finger abductors and adductors, thumb adductors, wrist ulnar flexors, and the ulnar half of deep finger flexors, muscles of the hypothenar eminence, and the third and fourth lumbricals. Sensory innervation involves the skin on the palm and dorsal surface of the little finger and inner half of the ring finger plus the hand's ulnar side.

A complete lesion of the hand results in a claw hand deformity. In some cases, ulnar involvement is delayed. Some time after trauma, a tardy ulnar palsy may develop.

Joint fracture or dislocation at the elbow most commonly causes ulnar nerve injury. The ulnar nerve can also be compressed at the elbow during sleep or from prolonged resting on the elbow. Ulnar injury can result from fractures, gunshot wounds, or stabs to the lower end of the humerus or head of the radius. A cervical rib can compress the nerve in the axilla.

Clinical Manifestations

Characteristics of clawing of the hand include wrist weakness of adduction and flexion, ring and little finger flexion weakness, paralysis of finger abduction and adduction, and thumb adduction. Hypothenar muscle atrophy occurs with sensory loss in ring and index fingers. Diagnosis can readily be made from claw hand posturing. These signs are most pronounced when the median and ulnar nerves are compressed. Froment's paper sign is characteristic: when the client tries to hold an object such as paper between the thumb and index finger, there is a flexion of the thumb's terminal phalanx. Injuries to the ulnar nerve are not usually accompanied by causalgia (intense burning pain). Pain is usually the result of an irritative lesion.

Therapeutic Measures

For complete lesions of the ulnar and median nerve causing a claw hand, the client loses a considerable amount of hand function. Interventions are mainly supportive. The goal is to assist the client to attain the maximum level of function through physical therapy programs and use of self-help devices to assist in activities of daily living.

Specific Nursing Measures

Alterations in body image should be anticipated. The client must adjust to a deforming injury that has both cosmetic and functional effects. The degree of alterations in daily activities depend on whether the dominant hand is affected or not. To improve self-esteem, assist clients to assess their overall appearance and help them to develop other aspects of their appearance and personality. Help clients to recognize that how they present themselves in total has the most impact on others. Teach clients strategies to cope with the reactions of strangers. For example, if someone stares because of concern, an honest, short explanation of the problem can be helpful. Clients need nursing and family support to learn to deemphasize the injury and focus on their strengths and potential.

Chapter Highlights

Lead poisoning is the most common form of heavy metal intoxication. Usual symptoms and signs of lead poisoning are colic, anemia, and peripheral neuropathy.

Chelating agents are used to mobilize lead from the body. The nurse should carefully monitor kidney function in clients with lead poisoning.

Arsenic poisoning is a metallic intoxication affecting the nervous system. Immediate treatment for arsenic poisoning is gastric lavage.

The most common form of polyneuritis is induced by excessive alcohol intake.

Bell's palsy is characterized by a flaccid facila paralysis. The priority of nursing care for clients with Bell's palsy is protecting the cornea.

Guillain–Barré syndrome often develops after a respiratory or gastrointestinal illness. The onset is characterized by ascending symmetrical sensory and motor deficits.

Leprosy is a classic example of an infectious polyneuritis. It has a low contagion rate and transmission requires prolonged, intimate contact.

The common peroneal nerve is the most frequent nerve to sustain injury within the body. Injury causes a steppage gait characterized by overflexion of the knee and slapping of the foot.

A total avulsion of the brachial plexus results in a flaccid arm.

Bibliography

Adams RD, Victor M: *Principles of Neurology*, 2nd ed. New York: McGraw-Hill, 1981.

American Association of Neuroscience Nurses: *Core Curriculum for Neuroscience Nursing*. Chicago: The American Association of Neuroscience Nurses, 1983.

Bickerstaff E: *Neurology*, 3rd ed. London: Hodder and Stroughton, 1980.

Conway-Rutowski: *Carini and Owens' Neurological and Neurosurgical Nursing*. St. Louis: C.V. Mosby, 1982.

Forster FM: *Clinical Neurology*, 4th ed. St. Louis: C.V. Mosby, 1978.

Hickey J: *The Clinical Practice of Neurological and Neurosurgical Nursing*. Philadelphia: J.B. Lippincott, 1981.

Jennett B, Galbraith S: *An Introduction to Neurosurgery*, 4th ed. Chicago: Year Book, 1983.

Merritt HH: *A Textbook of Neurology*, 6th ed. Philadelphia: Lea & Febiger, 1979.

Wehrmaker S, Wintermute J: *Case Studies in Neurological Nursing*. Boston: Little Brown, 1978.

Wilson S: *Neuro-Nursing*. New York: Springer Publications, 1979.

The Client With Bell's Palsy

I. Brief Descriptive Data	Ms Lois Champlin, age 45, arrived at the emergency room, accompanied by her 16-year-old son. The reason for her visit was the sudden development of a right-sided facial paralysis.

II. Personal Data

Date and Time:	February 24, 1986; 9:00 PM
Full Name:	Lois Champlin
Social Security Number:	000-00-0000
Address:	19 Record Ave, Punxsutawney, PA
Telephone:	000-0000
Sex:	Female
Age:	45
Birthdate:	2-18-41
Marital Status:	Divorced
Race:	Caucasian
Religion:	Unitarian
Occupation:	School crossing guard
Usual Health Care Provider:	Clarice Walsh, RN, NP Katherine McKaig, MD

III. Health History

Source of Information:	Client
Reliability of Informant:	Very reliable
Chief Concern:	Inability to close the right eyelid and sagging of the right side of the face.
History of Present Illness:	Lois Champlin is a divorced, 45-year-old mother of two teenage sons, employed as a crossing guard for a local elementary school. Today while on duty she noticed a persistent, annoying pain behind her right ear and assumed it was related to the cold temperature. After work she took two aspirin tablets and a nap. Later she looked in the mirror and noticed that the right side of her face and the corner of her mouth were sagging. When she could not close her right eyelid, she became frightened. She soon realized that she could not perform any usual facial functions on the right side. Her older son drove her to the emergency room of a local hospital. States her general health has been excellent. She has had no recent infections, no trauma, no headache, no back pain; no visual problems or any symptoms or signs of problems in the head or neck region until now. Her blood pressure has always been normal; takes no medications except OTC calcium carbonate. She does not have considerable exposure to cold in the winter months.
Past Health History:	
Childhood:	Rheumatic fever age 6, chicken pox age 10
Immunizations:	None since childhood
Medical Problems:	Duodenal ulcer 1978 (during divorce); no recurrence
Surgeries:	T&A age 4; D&C age 38
Pregnancies:	P_2 G_3 Miscarriage T
Trauma:	Psychological—divorce 1978
Allergies:	To sulfa (skin eruptions)
Medications:	OTC—calcium carbonate 1,000 mg qd to prevent osteoporosis

Case Study written by Susan Nevins.

Family History:	Father—age 68; A&W
	Mother—died age 48; Ca breast
	Brothers × 2—ages 50, 43; A&W; youngest c̄ ↑ BP
	Sons × 2—ages 16, 14; A&W
	No ⊕ FHx, DM, MI, CVA, TBC
Personal/Social History:	Lives in an apartment with her two sons. Has some difficulty "making ends meet" and is concerned about being able to send her sons to college and "hopes they'll both get scholarships." She feels she has adjusted well to being a single parent and although "worse off financially" is "better off emotionally." Does not smoke or drink alcohol. Is active in the PTA and involved in youth activities in the church because of the positive influence these programs have on her sons. Enjoys her job and has several close women friends; does not date.
Review of Systems:	Unremarkable

IV. Physical Assessment

Height:	5 ft 9 in
Weight:	148 lb
Vital Signs:	BP 130/70; pulse 80; respirations 16; temperature 98.8°F (37°C). Attractive, articulate 45-year-old w/fe with obvious sagging of right face and inability to close the right eyelid.
Relevant Organ Systems:	HEENT: wnl
Neurologic:	Cerebral function: alert and responsive, memory and orientation intact; appropriate behavior and speech noted.
	Cranial Nerves:
	I: Smell intact
	II: Vision 20/20 both eyes; color intact; visual fields by gross confrontation, normal; fundi benign
	III, IV, VI: EOMS intact, no ptosis; no nystagmus; pupils small, equal, reacting briskly to light
	V: Deep facial sensation absent, jaw closure normal; corneal sensation absent in right eye
	VII: Facial muscles asymmetrical; right side of face c̄ complete facial weakness and loss of all facial functions (unable to close eyelid, wrinkle forehead, whistle, smile, blow out cheek on right side); no lacrimation on right
	VIII: Hearing wnl; hyperacusis noted (abnormal sensitivity to sound); Weber and Rinne tests normal
	IX, X: Swallowing and gag reflex intact
	XI: Head movement and shrug of sholders normal
	XII: Tongue protrudes in midline, no tremor
	Cerebellar function: Finger to nose, heel to shin coordination intact; Romberg negative; gait normal
	Motor system: No atrophy, tremors, or weakness
	Sensory system: Intact to touch, vibration, pin-prick, hot–cold temperature
	Reflexes: wnl

V. Diagnostic Data

Ms Champlin was diagnosed as having Bell's palsy based on the history and physical assessment findings. She was placed on oral steroids to reduce facial nerve inflammation and fitted for a facial sling. An outpatient appointment was scheduled for electrical massage to the right facial muscles. Ms Champlin was upset about the potential duration of the paralysis but was reassured knowing she did not have a more serious health problem. The nurse in the emergency department instructed her in home care.

(continued)

The Client With Bell's Palsy

VI. Nursing Care Plan

Nursing Diagnosis	Client Care Goals	Plan/Nursing Implementation	Expected Outcome
Sensory-perceptual alteration: visual, potential for	Prevention corneal abrasion or ulceration Lubricate eye and keep it clear of mucus and debris; prevent infection; practice progressive exercise	Cover affected eye with a clear plastic eye bubble or a cloth patch; instill artificial tears q 2–4 hrs; clean debris from eye by gently wiping from inner to outer canthus; as eyelid movement begins, teach client how to progressively work toward eyelid closure; when lid can close ¾ of the way—teach client to wear sunglasses during daytime (outdoors) and the eyepatch at night	No corneal abrasion or ulceration, no eyeball dryness, and no infection of eye will develop Eyelid movement will progressively improve
Injury: potential for	Prevent tongue, cheek injury from biting an insensitive area; prevent parotitis from poor oral hygiene	Instruct client to chew foods on the unaffected side and to avoid extreme food temperatures; teach client to begin with a soft diet and progress as tolerated; explain that diet supplements and vitamins in liquid form can be used; encourage frequent oral hygiene	The oral mucous membranes remain intact; parotitis does not develop
Mobility, impaired physical: related to facial muscles	Prevent loss of facial muscle tone	Instruct in use of moist compresses t.i.d. 15–30 min to stimulate circulation (Avoid any extreme temperatures) Teach manual facial massage 3–4 × a day; work from chin upward on the affected side; encourage client to practice facial expressions as motor function returns; have client practice in front of a mirror	Facial circulation will remain at optimal levels Assumes responsibility for own recovery
Self-concept, disturbance in: body image	Maintain self-esteem and a positive body image; remain independent; reduce anxiety	Assist client to be realistic about duration of facial dysfunction; review rationale for protective measures and techniques for ADL; encourage ventilation of feelings about condition; encourage family to point out and reinforce all signs of improvement in facial function	Will be realistic in estimating length of recovery period; will follow self-care regimen; anxiety will resolve as symptoms improve

Chapter 39

Surgical Approaches to Nervous System Dysfunction

Dorothy A. Kaminski

Objectives

When you have finished studying this chapter, you should be able to:

Identify the indications that necessitate cranial and intracranial surgeries such as placement of a Burr hole, craniotomy, craniectomy, cranioplasty, and creation of a ventricular shunt.

Identify the indications that necessitate spinal surgeries such as microlumbar diskectomy, anterior cervical diskectomy, and multilevel posterior laminectomy.

Provide a brief description of the surgical procedures used in treating nervous system dysfunction.

Discuss the physiological implications of these surgeries for clients and their families.

Anticipate the psychosocial/lifestyle implications of these surgeries for clients and their families.

Describe the preoperative and postoperative nursing implications in caring for these clients.

Surgical intervention for neurologic disorders is broad in scope and complex. Not only is neurologic surgery performed to treat diseases and disorders of the central, peripheral, and autonomic nervous systems; it also occasionally is done to treat general medical conditions. A detailed discussion of all neurosurgical procedures is beyond the scope of this textbook. Basic approaches to the structures of the nervous system will be described and the implications for nursing care outlined.

The significance of a neurosurgical procedure is not necessarily indicated by the operation listed on the OR schedule. The schedule may state only the operative method for reaching the area of the pathology and not the definitive treatment. For example, craniotomy is only the means for exposing the intracranial contents. A laminectomy, though, may constitute a surgical remedy if the client's* problem stems from bony compression of the spinal cord or its nerve roots. On the other hand, if the client has a spinal-cord tumor, laminectomy is only the means for exposing that lesion. This distinction is important because, although general nursing considerations apply to each of the basic approaches, the specific nature, location, and extent of the pathology have considerable bearing on the plan of care and its implementation. In this chapter, the general nursing considerations for each of the basic surgical approaches are described before discussing the specific implications of a particular anatomical area or disease entity.

Section I: Cranial and Intracranial Surgery

BURR HOLE

A burr hole is simply a hole drilled into the skull. This simple procedure has numerous diagnostic and therapeutic indications. It is often used to gain access to one of the lateral ventricles. Air or contrast material can be intro-

*The term client has been used herein in referring to the person receiving care, even though it is inconsistent with my professional philosophy. In the setting in which I practice, recipients of care are considered patients. D. Kaminski

1227

duced into the ventricular system for diagnostic studies (ventriculography), although these studies are virtually obsolete because of computerized tomography (CT) scanning. Ventricular puncture may be an emergency measure when the intracranial pressure (ICP) needs to be reduced. In such cases, the removal of cerebrospinal fluid (CSF) via lumbar puncture (LP) is usually contraindicated because of the danger of herniation. Fluid can usually be safely removed from the ventricles, however, because they are above the area of occlusion. Placement of a burr hole and insertion of a ventricular catheter are also initial steps in a ventricular shunting operation. In addition, a catheter may be left in the ventricle (ventriculostomy) for intermittent or continuous drainage of CSF, for instillation of antibiotics or chemotherapeutic agents, or for monitoring of intracranial pressure. Ventricular shunting procedures are discussed later in this chapter.

A burr hole may be adequate for the drainage of some intracranial cysts, abscesses, hematomas, and hygromas, avoiding a major craniotomy. A burr hole may be used to obtain samples of dura, cortex, or neoplastic tissue for histologic examination, although the site of the pathology must be fairly accurately localized. In head trauma, rapid drilling of a burr hole in the temporal area may be life saving if the brain is severely compressed by a rapidly accumulating epidural hematoma secondary to tearing of the middle meningeal artery. A burr hole is sometimes all that is required to elevate a section of bone in a depressed skull fracture, relieving pressure on the underlying brain.

Surgical Procedure

Because a burr hole is usually a short and relatively simple procedure, preparation is usually minimal. It is advisable to start an intravenous infusion in case medications are necessary during the procedure. Cardiac monitoring is also recommended because changes in ICP or intraventricular pressure or fluid dynamics may precipitate significant changes in heart rate and rhythm. A burr hole is often drilled under local anesthesia, although if the client is restless or unable to cooperate, general anesthesia may be preferred. General endotracheal anesthesia ensures control of the airway so the client can be hyperventilated to reduce cerebral congestion. When a burr hole's purpose is to drain a hematoma or an enlarged ventricle in a comatose client, the client may awaken after the pressure has been relieved. A short-acting anesthetic agent may be given to prevent restlessness while the wound is being closed.

The location of the burr hole often depends on the area of pathology. There are instances in which the location of the hole does not matter (ie, ventricular drainage). In such cases, the hole is usually placed on the nondominant side to avoid possible damage to the speech area. For this reason, most ventricular punctures are done on the right side.

Usually, the client is supine with the head turned so the operative side is uppermost. Special devices for head stabilization are not usually necessary. Because the skin incision is small, little hair removal is necessary. (Some surgeons or clients may prefer to have the entire scalp shaved.)

After the usual antiseptic preparation and draping, a small semicircular or straight-line scalp incision is made and retracted. The periosteum covering the area of bone to be drilled is incised and scraped back out of the way. The skull is then penetrated with a manual or power-driven burr. The bone is irrigated during drilling to wash away the bone fragments and to minimize the heat produced by the friction of the drill. The sizes of holes may vary slightly, depending on the size of the burr used. In most instances, the hole is less than 12 mm in diameter (about the size of a dime). The edges of the inner table of the bone may be enlarged with a curet, and the dura is separated from the bone with a blunt dissector. From this point, the procedure varies, depending on the reason for the procedure. Hemostasis is always achieved before the dura is opened and before the wound is closed.

When an abscess or hematoma is drained, a catheter may be inserted into the cavity to allow pus, clots, or necrotic material to be washed out. In case of a depressed skull fracture, the burr hole is usually placed adjacent to the depressed area, a blunt elevator is placed in the hole, and leverage is used to elevate the depressed piece of bone. This maneuver may not always be successful, or there may be dural or cortical damage, necessitating a craniotomy or craniectomy to repair the damage.

Implications for the Client

Physiological Implications
In most instances, placement of a burr hole involves little or no manipulation of the intracranial contents or trauma to the tissue, and postoperative incisional pain is usually minimal. Intraoperative blood loss is usually minimal. Except for head trauma where there may be profound blood loss from an arterial tear or extensive scalp lacerations, the need for a transfusion is unusual. Nevertheless, the procedure is not without risks, depending on the manipulations carried out through the burr hole and the condition for which it was performed. The neurologic condition can decline for a variety of reasons. Hemorrhage can occur as a result of damage to cerebral vessels from instrumentation through the burr hole. After a burr hole is placed for a biopsy, the neurologic state may deteriorate due to swelling in the operative area. This swelling must be differentiated from bleeding and hematoma formation. As with any operative procedure, postoperative infection is always a danger.

Although the risks are usually minimal, the potential complications are the same as those for a craniotomy or craniectomy because the burr hole enters the cranial vault. Therefore, the client must be carefully observed postoperatively for any subtle or sudden decline in neurologic status. The potential complications include hemorrhage, increased ICP, seizure activity, and infection.

Psychosocial/Lifestyle Implications

Because the indications vary, the implications for the client depend on the reason for surgery. If the burr hole was done for diagnostic purposes (eg, ventriculogram, biopsy), the client and family face uncertainty regarding the diagnosis, treatment, and ultimate outcome of the disease. Even when frozen sections are done, the results are often inconclusive. Because the prognosis depends on the underlying pathological condition, the days before the diagnosis is certain are a time of great stress and anxiety. The client and family may realize further treatment will be necessary. In other circumstances, the studies may show a disease for which no treatment is available (eg, Alzheimer's disease) or a metastasis from a distant, undetected, and often asymptomatic primary tumor. When a burr hole has been drilled to permit ventricular puncture to reduce ICP, the neurologic picture may immediately and dramatically improve. The nature of the lesion responsible for the increased pressure greatly influences the ultimate outcome. The physiological and psychosocial/lifestyle implications for the client having a burr hole are summarized in Table 39–1.

Nursing Implications

Although a burr hole is usually considered a minor surgical procedure, the preoperative preparation is generally the

Table 39–1 Drilling of Burr Holes: Implications for the Client	
Physiological Implications	**Psychosocial Implications**
Usually involves minimal manipulation of the intracranial contents	Depend on the underlying pathological condition
Postoperative pain is usually minimal	With head trauma, numerous factors influence recovery. The most significant factor is the extent of brain damage inflicted at the time of the initial injury
Intraoperative blood loss is usually minimal	
Because the cranial vault has been entered, possible complications are similar to those for craniotomy or craniectomy and include: hemorrhage, increased intracranial pressure, seizure activity, infection	When a burr hole is done for diagnostic purposes, several days of anxiety and uncertainty follow before the diagnosis is confirmed
Neurologic deterioration can be subtle and/or sudden	Need to adjust to the diagnosis and/or the need for further treatment may significantly alter lifestyle

same as for any intracranial procedure. Nursing observations and interventions are discussed in detail in the following section on craniotomy and craniectomy. Only measures specific to the client with a burr hole are included in this section.

Remember that the client's fears and level of anxiety may be out of proportion to the scope of the surgical procedure. Although health care personnel consider the surgery minor, the client may have fears of death, disability, or disfigurement. Provide opportunities for the client and family to express their fears and to ask questions. If the procedure is to be done under local anesthesia, the client must be prepared for what to expect. If the client is comatose, disoriented, or confused, preparation may be impossible but should be attempted.

In some instances, a burr hole may not achieve the goal of surgery (eg, drainage of subdural hematoma or elevation of depressed skull fracture), and a craniotomy or craniectomy may be necessary. The client and significant others should be prepared for that possibility.

Many surgeons prefer and hospital policy may dictate the precaution of crossmatching a unit of blood. If a more involved operative procedure might be necessary, additional blood will be reserved, the preoperative scalp preparation will be more extensive, and additional intraoperative monitoring may be employed.

Mild analgesics are usually sufficient to relieve headache. Narcotics are avoided because of their depressant effect on the central nervous system and respiratory system and because their effect may mask changes in neurologic status. In the trauma client who exhibits signs of postoperative hypovolemia or shock, be alert to the possibility of blood loss from other sources (eg, intra-abdominal bleeding). Take care to maintain the integrity of any tubes or drains. The type and quantity of drainage should be noted. Meticulous care must be taken to maintain the sterility of any external drainage or monitoring system because an intraventricular infection can be especially devastating. Specific nursing measures will be discussed in the section on ventricular shunting procedures.

CRANIOTOMY AND CRANIECTOMY

A craniotomy or craniectomy is the means of exposing or gaining access to the brain and cranial nerves so intracranial disease can be surgically treated. These diseases include tumors, abscesses, hematomas, and vascular lesions. The cranium may also be opened to excise an area of cortex or disrupt various nerves and fiber tracts for the relief of pain, seizures, tremors, spasms, or severe mental disturbances that do not respond to pharmacologic therapy. Craniotomy or craniectomy is often indicated in the treatment of skull fractures and other traumatic head wounds, not only to repair the bony defect but to repair dural tears; decompress the underlying brain; inspect for bleeding or cortical damage; and, in some instances, to debride the brain of foreign material. CSF leaks, occurring spontaneously or as a result of trauma or surgery, may also require intracranial repair.

If a neoplasm is present, the goal of surgery is usually the total removal of the pathology while preserving the normal neural and vascular structures. When this is not possible, the surgeon must decide whether to risk possible neurologic impairment or to leave a tumor that will regrow. Many factors influence this decision. A few considerations are the age and preoperative condition of the client; histology of the lesion, its rate of growth, and its proximity to vital structures; the amount of disability that may be induced; and the client's ability to cope. This section deals primarily with the client with a supratentorial lesion. Special considerations for the client with an infratentorial lesion are discussed in the following section on suboccipital craniectomy.

Surgical Procedure

Because of the size and extreme delicacy of the structures that must be dissected and manipulated during many neurosurgical procedures, it is imperative that the operative site remains relatively immobile and that any chance of inadvertant movement is eliminated. Immobilization and proper alignment are usually accomplished by means of a pinned head rest device (see Figure 39–1).

A *craniotomy* is an incision or opening into the cranial cavity. A flap of bone is cut in the skull and secured back in place after the intracranial portion of the procedure. Depending on the site of the bone opening, the surgeon may elect to turn either a free flap or an osteoplastic flap. With a free flap, a portion of bone is completely removed.

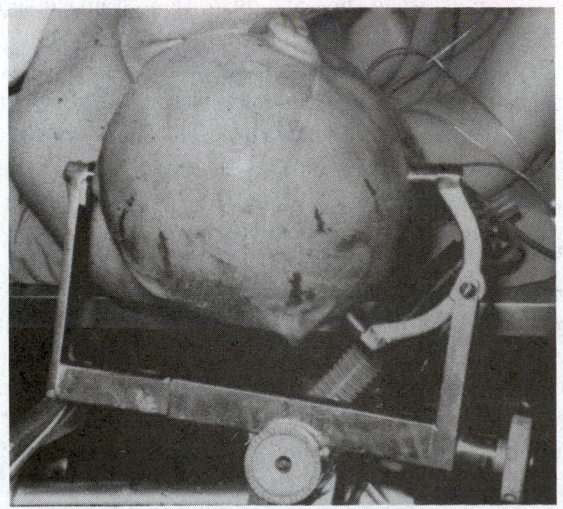

Figure 39–1

Head supported in pinned headrest device prior to draping. The clamp is applied to the head and tightened until the pins penetrate the outer table of the skull. (Courtesy of Leonard I. Malis, MD, The Mount Sinai Medical Center, New York, NY)

In an osteoplastic flap, the bone is not completely removed but is hinged to a pedicle of adjacent muscle. This method, which offers the advantage of providing blood supply to the bone flap, is most frequently used in the frontal, temporal, and occipital areas where there are adequate muscle layers overlying part of the bone flap.

On the other hand, *craniectomy* involves permanent removal of bone. In an area where a layer of muscle is sufficient to provide postoperative protection to the underlying brain, the surgeon may prefer a piecemeal removal of the bone to turning a flap. This type of opening is used primarily for posterior fossa operations (suboccipital craniectomy; discussed later in this chapter) because the posterior neck muscles provide good protection. It may also be employed for the subtemporal approach to the middle fossa because the bone in this area is extremely thin, and temporalis musculature is heavy enough to provide safe coverage. Craniectomy may also be indicated in the presence of infection, when the bone is invaded by tumor, or when the ICP is elevated to an extent that replacement of the bone flap would compress the brain.

The location of the skin incision and bone flap depends on the location of the pathological condition. The location and dimensions of the opening are carefully planned in advance so it can be kept small and placed accurately. The size of the opening may not correspond with the size of the lesion. The overall aim is to provide optimal exposure with as little brain retraction as possible. For a good cosmetic result, with few exceptions the skin flaps are placed in the area covered by the hair. Unfortunately, little can be done cosmetically for the bald client or when trauma dictates the area of the incision.

Whenever possible, the cortical incision is placed to avoid damage to the cortex, eg, through a sulcus. When nondestructive approaches are not possible, a corticotomy (incising an area of overlying cortex) may be necessary to reach the lesion.

Benign tumors are regularly removed piecemeal. The inner portion of the tumor is removed to achieve an internal decompression. As the tumor is shrunk, it tends to fall away from the surrounding brain and neural and vascular structures. This technique facilitates safer tumor removal (Figure 39–2). Carcinomas and abscesses are usually removed in one piece if possible to prevent the dissemination of tumor cells or infectious agents to the surrounding brain or into the subarachnoid space where disease can spread via the CSF circulation.

When the bone is to be replaced, small holes are drilled into the bone flap and in the surrounding cranium, and the bone flap is sewn or wired back into place. A drain is often left in the wound and may be placed in the tumor bed or the subdural, extradural, or subgaleal space (under the galea aponeurotica, the broad flat tendon that lies against the top of the skull). Any open drain can become a migratory pathway for microorganisms, so a closed drainage system such as a Hemovac is preferred to an open drain such as a Penrose.

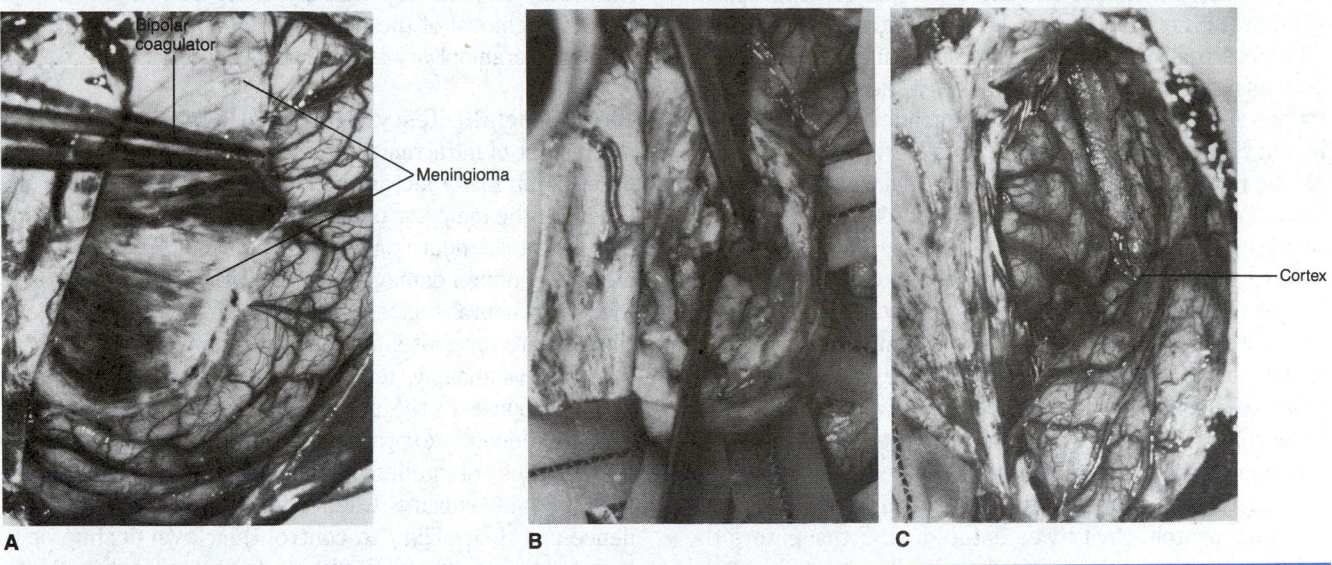

Figure 39–2

Craniotomy for removal of a meningioma. **A.** The meningioma on the right has been exposed and the vessels along its surface are being sealed with a bipolar coagulator. **B.** The interior of the tumor is resected to reduce the tumor size and permit it to fall away from the brain. **C.** The tumor has been removed atraumatically. (Note the vascularity of the underlying cortex.) (Courtesy of Leonard I. Malis, MD, The Mount Sinai Medical Center, New York, NY)

Implications for the Client

Physiological Implications

An intracranial operation can be considered a planned head injury, and the complications are similar. Postoperatively, the degree of neurologic impairment depends on the extent of damage to neural tissue inflicted by the lesion and/or the surgical manipulations. Damage may be transient or permanent.

Cerebral edema is the normal reaction to manipulation and retraction of brain tissue. Swelling is often proportional to the amount of manipulation and retraction. Periorbital edema and ecchymosis are usually noted following frontal and/or temporal craniotomy, usually appearing the day after surgery. The eyelids swell in varying degrees, probably reflecting individual susceptibility and anatomy rather than the extent or trauma of the procedure. However, swelling is often marked when a postoperative clot is developing (Jennett & Galbraith, 1983).

Cerebral and periorbital swelling usually reach their peak between 48 and 72 hours and then begin to subside. The degree of periorbital edema is often a clue to intracranial swelling. Focal motor deficits may result from cerebral edema. In this instance, the deficits are transitory. Permanent focal motor deficits may be a direct and predictable consequence of the surgical procedure itself or the result of a complication such as stroke or other brain or peripheral nerve damage.

Development of a postoperative hematoma is the most devastating and dreaded complication. The clot may be extradural, intradural, or both and usually is caused by a single bleeding vessel rather than a generalized oozing from numerous minute bleeding points. Bleeding can occur from the remaining portion of a partially resected infiltrating tumor or in the walls of the empty space left after tumor removal. Following decompression of the brain by tumor removal or decrease in ventricular size, the dura overlying the brain can strip away from the bone, causing epidural bleeding.

Postoperative discomfort such as headache is usually expected following cranial surgery; however, it is usually minimal and can ordinarily be controlled with mild analgesics. Hyperthermia may occur following operations in the region of the upper brain stem and hypothalamus, a condition requiring vigorous treatment (Jennett & Galbraith, 1983). Infection is a risk with cranial surgery. The risk is greater following head trauma in which the skin, bones, or dura are breached or if a CSF leak is present preoperatively (if fluid can exit the skull, organisms can enter). Surgery that enters the paranasal sinuses or the mastoid cavity may also involve a higher-than-normal risk. An externalized ICP monitoring device also predisposes clients to infection, with the intraventricular-catheter type carrying the highest risk.

Any manipulation of the supratentorial cortex predisposes the client to postoperative seizures. The risk is related to the underlying pathological condition and the degree of cortical damage caused by the surgery. The incidence of seizures seems to be higher following surgery in the frontotemporal region and in clients who had seizures preoperatively. Seizures may also precipitate the complication of intracranial bleeding. Jennett and Galbraith (1983) state that if a seizure occurs in the first week after operation, there is greater risk of epilepsy as a late complication.

Diabetes insipidus and the syndrome of inappropriate antidiuretic hormone (SIADH) are contrasting endocrine disorders that can follow intracranial surgery. Either can be transient or permanent. Although the clinical manifestations are almost opposite, either condition unchecked can be life threatening because of the severity of the fluid and electrolyte imbalance it precipitates. Diabetes insipidus is probably more common and is frequent following head injury or surgery in the area of the pituitary or hypothalamus (These two conditions are discussed in Chapter 44).

A CSF leak may occur immediately following surgery but more often appears later in the postoperative course. It may become apparent with seepage of fluid from the wound edges. Leaks are more likely when the dura has been resected or left open and pressure is high. CSF rhinorrhea or otorrhea is frequent with basal skull fractures but may also occur following surgery in which the frontal sinus or mastoid cavity was entered. CSF that enters the mastoid cavity can drain into the nasopharynx and into the nose via the eustachian tube. Fluid entering the frontal sinus drains into the nose via the frontonasal duct. Rhinorrhea may also be seen following resection of some tumors of the anterior portion of the skull base. Any opening that allows for the leakage of CSF also provides an entry route for microorganisms, predisposing the client to meningitis. Further surgery may be necessary to repair the leak.

The olfactory nerves are extremely sensitive to pressure. Anosmia (loss of sense of smell) is frequent following head injury or frontal craniotomy. Unilateral loss often is unnoticed by the client. Bilateral loss of smell invariably occurs following bifrontal craniotomy for subfrontal lesions, because the olfactory nerves that run along the base of the frontal lobes are sectioned in the exposure. Bilateral loss of smell markedly decreases the ability to appreciate flavor. If blindfolded, the client with complete anosmia cannot distinguish the taste of an apple from a raw potato.

Damage to an optic nerve causes visual loss in that eye. Chiasmal involvement produces bitemporal loss. Damage posterior to the chiasm produces a homonymous hemianopia (ie, a loss of vision to the side opposite the lesion, in both eyes). Injury to CN III sequentially leads to ptosis, with loss of medial, upward, and downward gaze, and then pupillary dilation and loss of reaction. With damage to the optic nerve, the eye is blind and the response to direct light is lost, but the consensual reflex remains intact. With damage to the oculomotor nerve, both the direct and consensual light reflexes are absent.

Hydrocephalus may develop as a result of postoperative adhesions secondary to blood sealing the subarachnoid space or to postoperative meningitis. Hydrocephalus is not unusual after successful aneurysm surgery and is usually the result of arachnoid scarring caused by the initial subarachnoid hemorrhage.

Late complications also include abscess formation in the operative site and osteomyelitis of the bone flap. Treatment of the abscess may require re-exploration of the craniotomy or aspiration via burr hole. Osteomyelitis is usually refractory to antibiotic therapy alone and almost always requires removal of the bone flap to achieve a permanent cure (see cranioplasty later in this chapter).

Psychosocial/Lifestyle Implications

The impact of intracranial surgery varies greatly. The effect depends on many factors including but not limited to the extent of the injury or underlying disease, the degree and duration of the neurologic impairment before surgery, the amount of neural damage during surgery (eg, resection of functional neural tissue, damage to cranial nerves), and the ultimate prognosis for the underlying disease.

Understandably, fear is often the predominant emotional response to the prospect of major cranial surgery. Clients frequently express fears of death, disability, disfigurement, loss of intellectual function, and loss of self (personality) or sexuality. Clients fear losing their independence and their ability to control their own destiny or to care for themselves and provide for their families. Many clients fear surviving in a vegetative state and being a financial and emotional burden to their loved ones. Unfortunately for some, their fears have a firm basis in reality.

Even if uncomplicated, hospitalization for a craniotomy or craniectomy is a significant interruption in a person's life. The average craniotomy client remains in the hospital for at least a week to 10 days following surgery. In many cases, the preoperative diagnostic work-up is extensive, time consuming, and costly. In addition, many clients may require a period of rehabilitation following surgery. On the average, it is about 4 to 6 weeks before clients are able to return to their previous occupation, assuming the preoperative deficits were minimal and the surgical outcome is favorable. The financial impact is often devastating, even to the client with full insurance coverage.

Temporary or permanent postoperative sequelae may require clients to modify their lifestyles significantly. If their ability to perform activities of daily living is lost or impaired, radical changes may have to be made in family roles, responsibilities, and routines as well as in future plans. Changes in body image and loss of self-esteem may result from the loss of hair or functional ability (eg, hemiplegia) or from a visible neurologic deficit (eg, facial paralysis). Postoperative seizures may inflict serious social consequences. Laws in some areas prohibit a person with a seizure disorder, or even a history of seizures, from driving a motor vehicle. This may severely limit the person's travel to activities outside the home, inflict a degree of dependence on others, or even necessitate a change of occupation. In addition, clients need prophylactic anticonvulsant therapy for 1 year after surgery.

Clients may require a period of mourning before they can accept the loss of bodily function or for some, even the loss of their hair. A period of profound depression, frequently on the second or third postoperative day, usually lasts for 2 or 3 days. The degree of depression is often totally unrelated to the surgical outcome and prognosis; it is seen even in clients with perfect surgical results. The depression is believed to be physiological rather than psychological in origin and is probably due to a hormonal imbalance precipitated by the stress of the surgery. It usually resolves without treatment. In severe cases, mood-elevating drugs may be used.

Varying degrees of personality changes related to steroid therapy may occur. Some clients may experience symptoms such as hyperactivity, inability to sleep, inappropriate behavior, and in severe cases, paranoid delusions and signs of overt psychosis. Tapering of the steroid dose results in prompt and complete reversal of symptoms.

In addition to the normal range of emotional reactions, the craniotomy client may also exhibit a wide range of personality changes and emotional disturbances directly attributable to organic brain disease or damage. Syndromes of disorientation and denial are seen with diffuse or bilateral cerebral lesions, such as bifrontal or bitemporal

contusions, or with meningitis or subarachnoid hemorrhage. In some instances, subtle preoperative mental changes noted by the family have been interpreted as signs of mental illness. Such assumptions, coupled with the unwarranted stigma of mental illness, usually delay seeking diagnosis and treatment. In such cases, family members often have feelings of extreme guilt after the organic nature of the disturbance has been discovered. The physiological and psychosocial/lifestyle implications for the client undergoing a craniotomy or craniectomy are summarized in Table 39–2.

Nursing Implications

Preoperative Care
The amount and type of nursing care depend on the underlying disease process, the neurologic manifestations of that

Table 39–2 Craniotomy/Craniectomy: Implications for the Client

Physiological Implications	Psychosocial/Lifestyle Implications
Pre-existing health problems may adversely affect the pre-, intra-, or postoperative course. Respiratory status is especially important because of its relation to intracranial pressure	Impact of surgery varies and is influenced by numerous factors, including, but not limited to, the following: extent of the injury or underlying disease; degree and duration of the preoperative neurologic impairment; degree of neural damage resulting from the surgery; ultimate prognosis for the underlying disease; financial factors; available support systems
Postoperative cerebral edema, and periorbital edema and ecchymosis reach their peak between 48 to 72 hours and influence the neurologic status	
Postoperative pain (headache) is usually minimal	Common concerns are fear of death, paralysis, disfigurement, personality changes, loss of independence, survival in a vegetative state, becoming a burden to family, and financial worries
Mild hyperpyrexia and neck pain in the first 48 hours may be expected as a result of the introduction of blood into the subarachnoid space	
Potential complications include: intracranial hemorrhage/hematoma; increased intracranial pressure/herniation; seizures; infection; CSF leak; fluid/electrolyte and/or metabolic/hormonal imbalance such as diabetes insipidus or SIADH; hydrocephalus; complications related to the hazards of immobility and/or a depressed level of consciousness	Hospitalization requires possibly extensive, time-consuming, and costly preoperative diagnostic workup; 7–10 days postoperative hospitalization; and 4–6 weeks of rehabilitation
	Depression in the first postoperative week is common even with a favorable surgical outcome and good prognosis; it is thought to be physiological rather than psychological in origin
Risk of postoperative seizures, especially after surgery in the frontotemporal region or in clients with seizures preoperatively	Postoperative sequelae may be transient or permanent; client may require assistance with ADL, a period of rehabilitation therapy, and significant alteration in lifestyle
Postoperative impairment will depend on the location and extent of neural damage and may be transient or permanent. Deficits may include: impaired level of consciousness; mental status changes; focal motor and/or sensory impairment; language disturbances; cranial nerve dysfunction, eg, anosmia, visual deficits, oculomotor palsies	Seizures may require limitation of activities, travel, driving a motor vehicle, or a change in occupation; prophylactic anticonvulsant therapy usual for one year following surgery
	Visible deficits can result in significant changes in body image and loss of self-esteem
Abscess formation in the operative site and osteomyelitis of the bone flap are potential late complications	Personality changes, emotional disturbances, or conceptual disorders related to organic brain damage or disease can be very difficult for family to handle
	Language disturbances can be extremely frustrating for the client and family and frequently cause depression

disease, and any coexisting medical problems. One of the most important nursing measures is the assessment and documentation of the baseline neurologic status to provide a standard by which postoperative progress or deterioration can be measured. Assessment should include:

- Mental status
- Level of consciousness
- Responsiveness
- Behavior
- Speech
- Motor, sensory, and cranial nerve function
- Pupillary size, position, response to light, and any abnormality of extraocular movements

In documenting the client's status, avoid the use of labels (eg, stuporous, hemiplegic, dysphasic) and describe the client's behavior (eg, responds by withdrawal to painful stimulus, is able to walk but drags right leg, speech is garbled but intelligible). The frequency of preoperative neurologic assessment depends on the condition of the client and the physician's orders. If any decline in neurologic status is observed—no matter how slight or subtle—increase the frequency of neurologic and vital sign assessments and promptly report and record changes.

Preoperative recordings of vital signs are important in assessing postoperative cardiovascular and respiratory status. The documentation of the client's preoperative weight may be extremely important if the client develops postoperative diabetes insipidus or SIADH. It may also be valuable in assessing the nutritional status of a client with a depressed level of consciousness who is unable to take oral feedings.

Any significant existing health problems such as hypertensive, renal, cardiac, or respiratory disease should be documented. Such health problems may adversely affect the intraoperative and postoperative course by interfering with optimal cerebral perfusion, oxygenation, and metabolic processes, and should be corrected or controlled whenever possible. These system abnormalities and the current medication regimen (eg, insulin, antihypertensive medication) should be communicated to nurses in the OR, recovery room, and intensive care unit (ICU). Laboratory values should be checked and any abnormality promptly reported.

Hyperglycemia may occur while intravenous glucose is being administered or with large doses or prolonged administration of glucocorticosteroids. If hyperglycemia continues or is accompanied by ketonuria, diabetic fractional testing of urine may be ordered. Unless ketosis occurs, treatment is not usually indicated, and the glucose level usually falls as the steroid dosage is decreased.

The client's blood should be typed and crossmatched. The number of units placed on reserve depends on the nature of the lesion. Preoperative hemoglobin and hematocrit values are useful in assessing blood loss and in determining the need for replacement. Because hemostasis within the brain is critical, the prothrombin time is often ordered.

Some surgeons prefer that a complete coagulation workup be done to rule out a coagulation disorder. Clients, especially those with a history of headaches, should be questioned regarding the use of aspirin. In general, they should take acetaminophen (Tylenol) instead to avoid possible increased bleeding.

Assuming that the client is alert and cooperative, preoperative teaching includes demonstration and practice of deep-breathing techniques. Vigorous coughing is usually not encouraged because it increases ICP. Vigorously encourage stopping smoking even for a few days before surgery to reduce respiratory complications. Teach leg exercises and explain the use of antiembolism stockings.

Be sensitive to the fears of the client and family regarding the impending surgery. Assigning one nurse consistently to the client so rapport can be established is extremely helpful. Provide the client and family with opportunities to express their fears and concerns and to ask questions. Whenever possible, accompany the physician during discussion of the surgery with the client and family to be able to clarify and reinforce the information given and to provide support. Learning about possible complications can be emotionally devastating for the client and family. Also determine the level of understanding and the perceptions regarding the surgery and its expected outcome. Reinforce accurate perceptions and correct misconceptions. Realistic positive expectations should be emphasized.

Remember that as the day of surgery approaches, the stress level of the client and family is likely to increase, and their displaced anger, frustration, or inability to cope may be directed toward nursing staff. Involvement of the liaison mental health nurse or social worker early in the preoperative period may be beneficial. A visit by a priest, minister, rabbi, or other clergy can provide a great deal of comfort and support for many persons.

Because fear of the unknown is a significant stress factor, prepare the client for what to expect in the perioperative period. Explain the preoperative routines, such as the placement of a peripheral IV line, a central venous pressure (CVP) line, and an in-dwelling catheter. Familiarize the client with postoperative routines (eg, pupil checks, motor testing) and expected sensations (eg, headache, the sensation of having to void produced by the in-dwelling catheter).

Also prepare the client for the hair removal procedure. The amount of hair removed depends on the area to be exposed, the extent of the incision, and the surgeon's preference. Some surgeons prefer that the entire head be shaved to facilitate the preparation and maintenance of the sterile field. Other advantages are that the head dressing is easier to apply and keep in place, regrowth is more even, and wigs may fit better. Encourage the client to discuss the extent of hair removal with the surgeon preoperatively. Often a compromise can be struck. Allowing the client to participate is important because it provides some degree of control over the situation.

When the operating room suite does not have a separate induction or preparation room, it may be necessary to clip clients' hair before they enter the operating room. In some hospitals, this can be accomplished in an adjacent holding area, but it may be necessary to do it while the client is still on the preoperative unit. Because hair loss is often traumatic for client and significant others, it is preferable to shave the scalp after the client is anesthetized. This also spares the client discomfort. It is also preferable to do the shave as close to the time of incision as possible to reduce the time bacteria have to colonize in skin nicks or cuts. After the shave, the entire area is thoroughly washed with an antibacterial agent and painted with an antiseptic solution. Some surgeons may also prescribe a shampoo with povidone-iodine, hexachlorophene, or other antimicrobial soap the night before surgery to reduce the bacteria on the skin.

Clients' reactions to the loss of hair vary. Many clients, both male and female, are devastated by it, but others consider it relatively trivial. Often, if the hair is long enough, sections can be combed and secured away from the operative site. The remaining hair may be adequate to cover the shaved area. In the case of posterior fossa surgery, the hair loss often is not even apparent from the front.

The client and family should be made aware that the client will be transferred to the recovery room or intensive care unit from the operating room. Depending on the client's condition, the emotional state of client and family, and the policies of the institution, a visit to the postoperative unit may be arranged. It may also be possible to introduce the client and/or family to the nurse who will be responsible for the client's postoperative care.

Be sure the family understands that the surgery is long and explain how to get information about the client's condition and the progress of the surgery. They should also know when they can expect to talk with the surgeon and see the client following surgery. Because this is such a stressful time, a written form with the necessary information is helpful. The family should be alerted to the array of infusion lines and monitoring devices that will be in place as well as the presence of the head dressing and wound drain. Stress that these are normal measures and do not indicate a problem or complication. If there is any possibility that the client will remain intubated and on a respirator, explain this in advance. The family should also be made aware of the significance and importance of assessing vital signs and neurologic status because these are often perceived as cruel or inconsiderate disturbances.

Postoperative Care

Ideally, postoperative nursing care begins before the client arrives in the recovery room or intensive care unit. The nurse on the postoperative unit should obtain a thorough report from the operating room nursing staff before receiving the client. In some instances, it may be supplemented by information from the surgeon or the anesthesiologist.

This report prepares the postoperative nursing staff for what to expect, increases their ability to set priorities and formulate a plan of care, and alerts them to possible complications.

Information regarding the surgical procedure should include the site of the cranial opening, the underlying pathology, and specific information regarding the operation (eg, Is there a bone flap? Was the tumor completely or partially removed? Was the aneurysm clipped or wrapped? Was brain tissue resected? Were cranial nerves damaged or sacrificed?) Knowledge of the status of the dural closure, the quality of hemostasis, and the degree of brain swelling help in anticipating problems, and postoperative positioning is influenced by the presence or absence of a bone flap.

The postoperative nurse should also be alerted to any untoward events that may have occurred intraoperatively (eg, excessive bleeding, air embolism) and the client's tolerance of the procedure. Information about the client's preoperative neurologic and medical status is also crucial to formulating a plan of care. The report should include the preoperative mental status, level of consciousness, any focal deficits and/or existing medical problems, and information regarding the short-term prognosis (eg, When is the client expected to awaken from the anesthetic? Are specific deficits expected?) Intraoperative medications as well as specific anesthetic agents and techniques (eg, induced hypotension, hypothermia) may influence postoperative care and should be communicated.

Monitoring lines and devices usually include a central venous catheter and an arterial line but may also include a Swan–Ganz catheter and/or an intracranial pressure monitoring device. Because respiratory status is important, the nurse should know if and why the client will remain intubated, whether ventilatory support will be necessary, and current blood gas values.

A report of the cardiovascular status should include heart rate and the presence or absence of any rhythm abnormalities. In addition to knowing the range of blood pressure, it is also important to know whether vasopressor or vasodilator drugs are being used to control blood pressure. In many instances, the surgeon prescribes a range within which the mean arterial pressure is to be maintained postoperatively. The drugs necessary for manipulation of blood pressure should be prepared and available at the bedside before the client arrives. The report should also include an approximation of intake and output, an estimate of blood loss, and whether blood has been replaced.

The client's body temperature should also be reported so the nurse can anticipate measures to raise or lower it. Because shivering increases ICP as well as the metabolic need and rate of oxygen consumption, attempt to have the client at a normothermic level before emergence from anesthesia. Cardiac irritability is also increased at low temperatures, predisposing the client to cardiac dysrhythmias. Unless the recovery room or intensive care unit is immediately adjacent to the operating room, transfer is unwise until the client can be rewarmed to at least 95°F (35°C). If the temperature is lower than 97°F (36°C), place a warming blanket on the postoperative bed before the client arrives.

As soon as possible after the client is admitted to the postoperative unit, assess the client's neurologic status, including level of consciousness, pupillary reaction and eye signs, motor function, and vital signs. This initial baseline postoperative assessment will serve as a basis for determining subsequent progress or deterioration. Compare the findings with preoperative findings. Auscultate breath sounds bilaterally.

Observe the site and type of wound drain as well as the quantity and characteristics of the drainage. Check the head dressing to be sure it is dry and intact. A blood-stained area remote from the operative site is not unusual; it is usually the result of oozing from the site of a skull pin used for intraoperative fixation of the head. Note the size of the stain and reinforce the dressing. In most instances, this bleeding will stop on its own or respond to mild pressure applied to the site for a few minutes. Occasionally, a skin stitch may be required.

During the critical 24 to 48 hours following intracranial surgery (in some cases this period may be extended), the nurse's main task is to recognize promptly any potential complications and to implement preventive measures. Changes in neurologic condition are often related to changes in ICP. Acute changes in ICP postoperatively are most likely to result from intracranial bleeding or severe edema. Regardless of the cause, markedly increased pressure can cause irreversible damage or death if not controlled. It is important to recognize the change early so appropriate therapy can be instituted.

Level of Consciousness. Level of consciousness is the most sensitive indicator of ICP and, in most instances, provides the first clue to a deteriorating condition. Assessment of level of consciousness is described in Chapter 36 (see also the Glasgow coma scale in Table 36–1).

Eye Signs. Assessment of pupillary activity includes observation of their size, shape, equality, and reactivity to light. Normal pupils are round, usually at midposition, and have a diameter ranging from 1.5 to 6 mm. Most pupils are equal in size. Remember, however, that in a small percentage of the normal population, the diameter of the pupils varies by a millimeter or two. When recording pupillary size, be specific: terms like *pinpoint* or *partially dilated* are less useful than a millimeter measurement. (see Figure 36–4 in Chapter 36).

Assess each pupil for direct and consensual reaction to light. Note whether the pupil reacts briskly, sluggishly, or not at all. A pupil that previously reacted briskly and now reacts sluggishly could be an early sign of increasing ICP and should be reported promptly. A sudden dilated and nonreactive pupil is an ominous sign of impending uncal herniation and requires immediate attention. Eye movements should also be assessed. In the client without neurologic damage, the eyes usually move conjugately and

without abnormal movements such as nystagmus. If alert, the client can be asked to follow the nurse's finger to test the vertical and horizontal movements to determine CN III, CN IV, and CN VI function.

Abnormality of eye movements or pupillary response may have causes other than neurologic ones. Check the client's history for previous eye surgery or trauma. Various drugs administered intraoperatively may also affect pupil size and reactivity, but this reaction is bilateral. Atropine and scopolamine, which are frequently given preoperatively, dilate the pupil. Pupils may become bilaterally dilated and fixed following a seizure, but they usually recover within minutes. In the trauma client, recent ingestion of drugs or alcohol may be a factor. The surgical procedure or the underlying pathological condition may have damaged the optic nerve or any of the cranial nerves responsible for eye movements (eg, an aneurysm of the posterior communicating artery often compresses CN III, resulting in a dilated pupil and oculomotor palsy). In these circumstances, deficits are to be expected. (See Physiological Implications for the Client section in this chapter.)

Motor Function. In testing motor function, check for the presence or absence of movement, assess the strength and symmetry of movement, and observe for abnormal or inappropriate movements. In the conscious client, motor strength of the upper extremities is best tested by assessing grip strength and presence of pronator drift. Grip strength tests the function of distal muscles and is assessed by asking the client to squeeze the examiner's fingers as tight as possible. Both hands should be tested simultaneously and the grip strength compared. Proximal muscle strength can be tested by asking the client to close the eyes and hold both arms out forward with the palms up. If one arm gradually drifts down or turns inward (pronator drift), it may be an early indication of hemiparesis. In the lower extremities, subtle changes are best detected if the client is asked to dorsiflex, plantar flex, and leg raise against the resistance of the examiner's hand (Smith & Geist, 1978).

Focal motor deficits not present before the surgery may be the result of edema in the operative area. These deficits are often transient, and severity may vary in relation to the degree of swelling. In many instances, the deficit is a direct and predictable consequence of the surgical procedure. If the deficit, which can be sensory as well as motor, does not correlate anatomically with the operative site (eg, left-leg weakness should not occur following left-sided brain surgery), the possibility of vascular or peripheral nerve injury or brain damage remote from the operative area (eg, intraoperative stroke) should be considered and investigated.

In the comatose client or in one whose level of consciousness prevents active participation in the examination, begin the assessment by observing general posture and the presence of any spontaneous movements. Stimulate the client to elicit a response. Apply the stimulus, which should be the least that will elicit a response, to both sides of the body. Movements in response to a noxious stimulus are usually graded as either purposeful (or appropriate), inappropriate, or absent. Note that many unresponsive clients exhibit a grasp reflex that can be misinterpreted as a response to command. To distinguish a grasp reflex from a voluntary motor activity, ask the client to grip and release repeatedly. Inappropriate movements, which can occur spontaneously or in response to a stimulus, include decorticate and decerebrate posturing (see Figure 36–2 in Chapter 36). These responses are usually bilateral but can occur unilaterally or in combination. The total absence of response to a noxious stimulus is viewed as a grave sign (see the Glasgow coma scale in Table 36–1 in Chapter 36 for an objective measure). When assessing motor function, consider preoperative deficits as well as factors that may limit movement such as pain, armboards, or intravenous lines or monitoring equipment.

Intracranial Pressure. Prevention of increased ICP is one of the most important aspects of nursing care of the postcraniotomy client. Untreated increased ICP can result in shifting of the intracranial contents and displacement of a portion of the brain through or around linings or openings within the intracranial cavity. This herniation can be lifethreatening unless promptly recognized and treated (AANN Core Curriculum, 1984). As uncontrolled pressure increases, the medial temporal lobe, known as the uncus, is pushed downward through the tentorial hiatus. CN III is compressed, causing the pupil on that side to dilate. Pressure on the midbrain affects the transmission of impulses passing through the reticular activating system, and the level of consciousness is progressively impaired. If pressure is unchecked, the herniation of the uncus fills the tentorial hiatus along the midbrain. This obstructs the downward flow of CSF through the aqueduct and the upward flow of subarachnoid CSF toward the absorptive pathways, rapidly and progressively increasing the compression and ICP. The process reaches its catastrophic irreversible conclusion when midbrain hemorrhage is produced by venous obstruction.

Increased ICP secondary to cerebral edema can often be prevented or at least limited by various medical and nursing interventions. Unless otherwise ordered, the head of the bed should be kept elevated to at least 30°. This position enhances venous drainage from the head. Make certain the client does not slide down in bed, lowering the degree of head elevation. Avoid any position that allows for neck flexion because this can impede venous outflow through the jugular veins.

Steroids are almost routinely ordered. Because these drugs cause gastric irritation, they are usually administered with an antacid and/or cimetidine (Tagamet). Dehydration is another method frequently employed to minimize swelling. Oral fluid intake may be severely restricted, and intravenous infusions may be limited to the minimal rate required to keep the vein open or to administer medica-

tions. The surgeon frequently orders a range of serum osmolality (usually 300 to 315) at which the client is to be maintained. In the alert client, thirst can be the major discomfort. Frequent mouth care and moist, cold gauze applied to the lips and tongue provide some degree of comfort. Often the surgeon allows the client to suck on ice chips periodically. Lollipops provide relief without adding to fluid intake if the client is alert enough to suck on them safely. If the neurologic condition is stable and the client is alert and thirsty, the surgeon frequently allows more liberal fluid intake on the second postoperative day.

Intracranial pressure and central venous pressure may be monitored. Measure urine output carefully to assure that renal perfusion is adequate. This monitoring is especially important when dehydration and hypotensive techniques are employed. Output should be at least 30 mL per hour.

Monitor respiratory status carefully because anoxia and hypercarbia result in cerebral vasodilation, increasing ICP. Hypoventilation may occur as a result of the prolonged effects of the anesthetic agents or may be secondary to a depressed level of consciousness. Assess breath sounds and respiratory rate. Encourage deep breathing as soon as the client is alert enough to cooperate. In the extubated client, oxygen via face mask or nasal cannula is usually administered for the first 12 to 24 hours. Humidification is often added to decrease the viscosity of secretions. Suction the intubated client every 2 hours or as necessary. Avoid vigorous suctioning because it increases ICP. As a general rule, limit suctioning to 15 seconds or less. In many institutions, the procedure for suctioning a neurosurgical client includes hyperventilation and hyperoxygenation with 100% oxygen via Ambu bag both before and after suctioning to reduce the risk of hypercarbia. In other facilities, the Ambu bag is avoided to prevent the venous pressure increase that its positive cycle induces. For the same reason, vigorous coughing, IPPB, and postural drainage are avoided. Arterial blood gases are periodically monitored. Ideally, the PO_2 should be kept in the 80 mm- to 90 mm-Hg range, and the $PaCO_2$ should not exceed 45 mm Hg.

Stool softeners are often administered to prevent straining. Assist clients in turning or changing position to avoid straining or Valsalva's maneuver. Attempt to keep the client normothermic because shivering increases ICP as well as the metabolic needs and oxygen consumption of the brain. Surgery in or around the hypothalamus can disturb temperature regulation mechanisms, and wide fluctuations in temperature may occur. In such cases, it might be advantageous to prepare the postoperative bed with a hyper/hypothermia mattress before the client arrives. Regardless of the cause, hyperthermia should be treated with antipyretic medications, cooling blanket or mattress, and/or alcohol or ice water sponge baths. Chlorpromazine (Thorazine) may be administered to prevent shivering.

Headache following cranial surgery is expected and usually can be relieved by mild analgesics such as aspirin

Nursing Research Note

Watson C, Ross J, Ramsey M: Identification of neurosurgical patients susceptible to pulmonary infection. *J Neurosurg Nurs* 1984; 16(3):123–127.

This research tested the effectiveness of a tool to identify clients at high risk for development of pulmonary infection and to investigate the efficacy of a pulmonary protocol in preventing infections in this group.

Using a quasi-experimental design, the researchers identified two groups of high-risk clients using a tool they had developed—the Pulmonary Infection Risk Assessment Tool. The first group identified during a pilot study served as the control, whereas a second group received the pulmonary protocol. This protocol consisted of a pulmonary assessment every 4 hours; turning every hour or out of bed four times daily; incentive deep breathing every 2 hours; pulmonary physical therapy every 2 hours; suctioning of tracheostomy clients or those with altered levels of awareness; humidified oxygen or compressed air; forced fluids to 2500 mL daily; and, in alert clients, effective breathing technique training.

The results indicated that the tool overidentified clients at high risk for pulmonary infection; 35% of the control group and 33% of the experimental group developed infections. The pulmonary protocol did not significantly reduce infection. The incidence of infection was higher in the experimental group. In both groups, clients who had diminished levels of consciousness, pre-existing chronic obstructive pulmonary disease, were receiving steroids, had undergone lengthy surgery, or had paralyzed palates, exhibited the greatest incidence of infection. The authors note that nursing actions were not consistently implemented unless the client showed clinical evidence of pulmonary compromise.

When providing nursing care to neurologically impaired clients, the risk for pulmonary complications must be assessed. When these clients are identified, consistent and aggressive nursing intervention should be planned and implemented to prevent such complications. Consistent and regular intervention is necessary.

or acetaminophen. Occasionally, codeine is required for adequate comfort. More potent narcotics are contraindicated because their CNS depressant effect may mask changes in level of consciousness. In addition, they may depress respirations, contributing to increased ICP. Elevating the head of the bed and maintaining a quiet, dark environment is often helpful. Any change in the severity or pattern of headaches may indicate rising ICP and should be reported. Other early and frequently subtle signs of increasing ICP may include visual disturbances, nausea with or without vomiting, restlessness, irritability, or the tendency to fall asleep under circumstances that previously had kept the client awake. If the client exhibits any signs of increased ICP, the surgeon should be promptly notified.

Anticipate the administration of furosemide (Lasix) or mannitol and hyperventilation with oxygen via Ambu bag or mechanical respirator to reduce the intracranial volume. A CT scan may be done to differentiate between edema, hydrocephalus, and hematoma formation as the causative factor. Hypothermia or barbiturate therapy (the adminis-

tration of phenobarbital or pentobarbital in doses sufficient to produce complete unresponsiveness) may also be instituted in an attempt to reduce the metabolic demands. The therapy requires complete mechanical respiration with an endotracheal tube or cuffed tracheostomy. If medical interventions fail to reduce the ICP adequately, surgery is likely. The procedure may include placement of an intraventricular catheter or shunting system for the removal of CSF, removal of the bone flap, or possible lobectomy to relieve pressure.

A postoperative hematoma results in a marked and often extremely rapid rise in the ICP that can be devastating to neurologic function and life threatening. Take care to maintain the blood pressure within the prescribed parameters. In some instances, this can be an extremely difficult task involving the manipulation of several drugs such as propranolol (Inderal), nitroprusside (Nipride), and nitroglycerin, alone or in combination. With pharmacological manipulation of the blood pressure, continuous monitoring of the mean arterial pressure via arterial catheter is strongly recommended. Whenever direct arterial pressure monitoring is employed, the monitoring system should be regularly checked for accuracy. Take great care to maintain the integrity of the monitoring lines as well as the wound drain. Check the amount and type of drainage hourly, and promptly report any sharp increase in amount. Restless or uncooperative clients may require mitts to prevent inadvertent disruption of monitoring or infusion lines. Restraints may occasionally be necessary but should be used only as a last resort. Because restlessness or combative behavior may be an early manifestation of increased ICP, be alert to any decline in level of consciousness, motor strength, or pupillary response.

If a hematoma is suspected, measures are taken to reduce ICP. A CT scan is often done to confirm the diagnosis and assess the location (which may be epidural, subdural, intracerebral, or intraventricular) and extent of the hemorrhage. If the client's condition is rapidly deteriorating, be prepared for the surgeon to forgo the scan and return the client directly to the operating room for reexploration and evacuation of the hematoma. Examination of the wound may reveal elevation of the bone flap. In cases where there is no bone flap, the wound may appear tense and bulging. In rare instances, where minutes may make the difference between life and death, the surgeon may elect to open the wound in the recovery room or intensive care unit to decompress the brain stem. Occasionally, the situation progresses so rapidly that the surgeon does not have enough time to provide adequate explanation to the family or to even obtain consent for the surgery. Needless to say, this is a period of confusion and extreme anxiety for the family. It may be especially difficult for them to understand if the client was doing well initially before a sudden deterioration in condition. Offer support and provide as much explanation and information as possible.

Changes in vital signs from increased ICP are usually a late sign and most often signal impending herniation. With any decline in level of consciousness, motor function, or pupillary reactivity, pay careful attention to respiratory rate and pattern. The particular respiratory pattern may provide a clue to the area of the brain or brain stem being compressed. Some fluctuations in vital signs usually occur long before the appearance of the classic Cushing's reflex. *Cushing's reflex*, which includes a rising blood pressure, bradycardia, and respiratory irregularity, is a compensatory mechanism and an ominous sign of impending intracranial crisis. This stage is followed, often rapidly, by the late decompensatory stage in which blood pressure falls; the pulse becomes rapid, irregular, and thready; and the respiratory pattern becomes increasingly irregular and includes periods of apnea. If the rising ICP is not checked and the client is allowed to deteriorate to this point, intervention is likely to be ineffective.

Endocrine Function. Diabetes insipidus and SIADH can complicate the postoperative course of any craniotomy/craniectomy client especially following head trauma or surgery in the area of the pituitary gland and hypothalamus. Although the symptoms for each of these syndromes appear to be opposite, both carry the danger of severe fluid and electrolyte imbalance. Therefore, the nursing measures are similar for both.

Even in the alert client, the in-dwelling catheter should remain in place to facilitate precise monitoring of urinary output. Fluid loss or retention is reflected in the body weight; therefore, daily weights are an essential part of evaluation of the effectiveness of the therapy. Assess mental status frequently because electrolyte imbalance, especially hyponatremia or hypernatremia, can impair cerebral function. Fluid and electrolyte imbalances may also alter cardiac function. Continuous monitoring of cardiac function is indicated until the client is stabilized. The most effective and important monitor of the client's condition is the serum osmolality. As long as the osmolality is close to the normal range, there is no great risk. If it is elevated, the dehydration may be disastrous; if it is low, water intoxication may be catastrophic. Care of clients with diabetes insipidus and SIADH is discussed in Chapter 44.

If either condition is permanent or long lasting, the client and family require extensive teaching before discharge. Include the following: the nature of the dysfunction; the administration of appropriate medications, including side and toxic effects; measurement of urinary output and specific gravity; and the need for appropriate fluid intake (diabetes insipidus) or restriction (SIADH). Advise clients to wear or carry some form of medical alert identification.

Infection. The use of prophylactic antibiotics is controversial and unresolved. The head dressing should be kept clean, dry, and intact and should be reinforced as necessary if drainage is noted. Strict adherence to aseptic technique is essential when the dressing is changed, when the drain or sutures are removed, and when the wound-drainage reservoir is emptied. Care should be taken to maintain the integrity of any wound drain because blood collecting within the surgical wound provides an excellent culture medium for the growth of microorganisms. Restless or confused clients may attempt to remove their head dressings and, even if they fail, can introduce organisms into the incision line. Mitts or restraints may be necessary to protect the wound from contamination.

If infection at the operative site is suspected, a specimen of any drainage or exudate should be sent for culture and sensitivity testing. Blood samples should also be drawn to determine the white cell count, including differential, and the erythrocyte sedimentation rate. A slight elevation in temperature (to 100°F or 38°C), with or without some mild neck stiffness, is not uncommon about the second or third postoperative day and is the result of the introduction of blood into the subarachnoid space at the time of surgery. Persistent or spiking temperatures, especially accompanied by severe headaches or the tendency to keep the neck immobile and in an extended position, are the classic signs of meningitis and are cause for concern and prompt therapeutic measures. Clients with meningitis usually have severe pain when they attempt to flex the head to the chest. Other symptoms may include photophobia, restlessness, hyperirritability, a decline in the level of consciousness, and the appearance of focal neurologic deficits or worsening of existing deficits. If not treated or if inadequately treated, confusion, delirium, or disorientation may progress to coma and seizures. Anticipate a lumbar puncture will be done to confirm the diagnosis and to obtain a specimen for culture and sensitivity testing to identify the offending organism and determine the appropriate antibiotic therapy. The tap may also have a therapeutic effect by lowering the ICP.

Infection from extracranial sources also seriously threatens neurologic function and life. Comatose clients or those with limited mobility are especially prone to pneumonia and urinary tract infections. In addition, invasive monitoring and infusion lines predispose clients to bacteremia and septicemia. The incidence of infection seems to rise sharply if the catheter is left in place for more than 72 hours.

If infection occurs, prompt, adequate, and appropriate antibiotic therapy is essential. The administration schedule must ensure an adequate and consistent blood level. Treat the temperature elevation and headache as previously described in the section on intracranial pressure. Carefully monitor input and output and serum electrolyte levels. Attempt to maintain an adequate fluid and caloric intake. To protect staff and other clients, observe appropriate infection control precautions. If there is any drainage of infectious material, the client should be isolated.

Seizures. Seizure precautions should be instituted on all clients following supratentorial craniotomy or craniectomy. In many clients, the risk is minimal but should always be anticipated if the client is known to have any history of seizure activity, if the surgery involves the frontotemporal area, or if there has been a large amount of cortical manipulation or resection. Trauma, especially if cortical damage was inflicted, and subarachnoid or intracerebral hemorrhage may also increase the likelihood of a postoperative seizure. A seizure in the early postoperative period may signal an intracranial complication such as meningitis or a hematoma.

Anticonvulsant medications are almost routinely ordered postoperatively, and administration is often instituted preoperatively to ensure an adequate blood level during the period immediately following surgery. When a loading dose is administered, be aware that it may precipitate a slight decline in the level of consciousness. If a seizure should occur, the client should be protected from injury and attempts should be made to ensure an adequate airway. If possible, administer oxygen.

Observations regarding the nature of the seizure activity should be documented and immediately reported to the physician. Following the seizure, check for possible injuries and provide support and reassurance. The neurologic status should be carefully monitored. If the client does not make a gradual improvement from the immediate postictal condition, this should be promptly reported to the physician. The seizure, which results in increased venous and arterial blood pressure and ICP, may precipitate an intracranial hemorrhage. For more specific details on care of the client with seizures, see Chapter 37.

Cerebrospinal Fluid Leakage. Leakage of CSF from the wound or from the nose or ear is a serious threat because microorganisms can enter the skull through whatever opening allows the escape of CSF. If fluid leaks from the ear or nose, attempt to obtain a sample of the fluid. CSF is glucose positive and can easily be tested with a chemical reagent strip used to check the glucose content of urine. For the test to be valid, the fluid sample should be free of blood, because blood also tests glucose positive.

If fluid is leaking from the wound edges, reinforce or change the dressing as necessary to keep it dry and prevent contamination. Conservative management includes measures to decrease ICP in the hope that the leak will seal spontaneously. The head of the bed is usually kept elevated to at least 30° and activity may be restricted and the client kept on bed rest. Fluid intake may also be limited, and frequent or daily spinal taps may be done to drain CSF and keep the ICP low. Acetazolamide (Diamox), 250 to 500 mg every 6 hours, may be given to decrease CSF production. Caution the client against blowing the nose and avoid any straining such as Valsalva's maneuver. Do not place packs in the ear or nose. If endotracheal suctioning is required, do it via the mouth rather than the nose. Because of significant risk of infection, be alert to any rise in temperature, neck stiffness, or increased headache. Additional skin and/or galeal sutures may be required to stop leakage. Many leaks seal without the need for surgery. When leakage persists following an adequate trial of conservative

therapy, re-exploration of the wound may be necessary to repair the dural defect.

Later Postoperative Care. The postoperative client without any serious neurologic sequelae usually progresses through the postoperative phase much as any client who has undergone a major general surgical procedure. Diet is usually increased as tolerated, and most clients are taking a regular diet by the second postoperative day. Ambulation is begun early, with many clients out of bed in a chair on the day after surgery. Monitoring devices and lines as well as intravenous infusions are usually discontinued after 48 hours. The urinary catheter is removed as soon as the client is able to use a bedpan, commode, or toilet. Because postoperative edema usually reaches its peak between 48 and 72 hours, reduction of the steroid dosage is begun on about the third or fourth day. Clients undergoing postoperative radiation therapy usually remain on steroids during treatment because the radiation often results in cerebral edema. The average postoperative hospital stay is between 7 and 10 days, and the client can often return to work in 4 to 6 weeks. While still hospitalized, the client's level of physical activity will gradually increase.

Discharge Teaching. Discharge teaching should include a warning regarding too rapid an increase in activity. During the first week or so at home, the client will tire easily and need a nap or rest by late afternoon. Reassure the client that this is normal, that strength and endurance will increase daily, and that it may take a few weeks before a feeling of well-being returns. Advise clients to do as much as they feel up to. Their own fatigue will be the limiting factor that protects them from any harmful overexertion. Involve the family and include both oral and written instructions in discharge teaching. Ideally, the client and family should be able to verbalize an adequate understanding of discharge therapies, safe activities, and the schedule for follow-up.

Skin sutures are usually removed on the seventh day, and the hair can usually be shampooed 3 to 4 days later. To protect the incision line, the client should wear a hat in full sunlight. Direct heat (eg, a hairdryer or hot curlers) should be avoided until the hair has regrown to a reasonable length. Mild headaches may persist for a while and can usually be controlled by standard over-the-counter pain relievers. Usually no restrictions are placed on sexual activity, but very strenuous exercises such as tennis or jogging should be avoided for a few weeks.

If the steroid taper has not been completed before discharge, the client should be given specific written instructions regarding dosage. Too rapid a taper or missed doses can precipitate adrenocortical insufficiency. Also warn the client and family that severe stress (physical or emotional) may increase the need for steroids and that they should consult the physician to determine whether the dosage needs to be increased or therapy reinstituted to cover the period of increased stress. Teach the client to take the steroid with an antacid or food.

Prophylactic anticonvulsant therapy is frequently maintained for a full year following supratentorial intracranial surgery, even if the client has never had a seizure. Stress the importance of compliance and follow-up. Periodic blood tests should be done to assure that an adequate serum level is being maintained and to detect any toxic effects that may result from long-term anticonvulsant therapy. The client and family should know the side effects and signs of toxicity of the medications as well as the signs of late infection and hydrocephalus. Alcoholic beverages may have an exaggerated effect and should be taken cautiously.

For clients with transient or permanent neurologic impairment and those with complicating events the recovery period is usually prolonged. Discharge planning depends on clients' capacity to care for themselves or the family's ability to provide the needed care.

In assessing a client's potential for future adjustment, remember adjustment largely depends on the extent of the impairment. Adaptation to disability does not really begin until after the person returns home and makes the necessary adjustments. Often the involvement of the social worker and other allied health professionals is necessary to make appropriate referrals and arrangements to ensure a smooth transition from hospital to home or other health-care facility.

SUBOCCIPITAL CRANIECTOMY

A suboccipital craniectomy involves the removal of a portion of the posterior occipital bone. Because the muscles of the neck are thick enough to protect the underlying brain, the bone is usually removed and discarded. Depending on the size and location of the lesion, the exposure may be unilateral or bilateral, midline or paramedian. It may include removal of the posterior rim of the foramen magnum and the arch of atlas.

This approach is indicated for lesions involving the infratentorial portion of the brain, those structures that lie beneath the tentorium. It allows access to the contents of the posterior fossa including the cerebellum, brain stem, fourth ventricle, and the lower cranial nerves. The approach is also used to expose and treat aneurysms and vascular malformations involving the vertebral arteries and the posterior branches of the circle of Willis. CN V through CN XII can be visualized, and tumors arising from or surrounding them can be excised. These nerves can be decompressed or interrupted for the relief of pain or spasm (eg, trigeminal or glossopharyngeal neuralgia or hemifacial spasm).

A midline suboccipital craniectomy may be combined with an upper cervical laminectomy to approach lesions at the cervicomedullary junction (the area where the medulla joins the cervical spinal cord) or to treat congenital malformations that compress posterior fossa structures and obstruct the normal flow of CSF (eg, Arnold–Chiari mal-

formation). A lateral craniectomy may include resection of the mastoid to facilitate exposure of the cerebellopontine angle (the junction area between the cerebellum and pons). In some instances, such an opening may be combined with an occipital or temporal craniotomy for a combined supratentorial and infratentorial approach to lesions that extend along the clivus (eg, meningioma or chordoma) or into the middle fossa (eg, neuroma of CN V).

Surgical Procedure

The suboccipital craniectomy is frequently performed with the client in the sitting position (Figure 39–3) but may also be done in a prone or a modified lateral position (see Figure 39–9 later in this chapter). If ICP is markedly elevated, supratentorial drainage may be instituted by drilling an occipital burr hole and placing an in-dwelling catheter or cannula in the lateral ventricle at the beginning of the procedure. Using this technique, fluid can be drained as necessary.

Most often a vertical skin incision is used rather than turning a skin flap. The muscles are divided and freed from their bony attachments. The skin and muscles are retracted, and a burr hole is drilled. After the dura is freed from the inner table of bone, the suboccipital bone is removed piecemeal with a power cutter or a bone-biting instrument known as a rongeur.

During lateral exposures, mastoid air cells are frequently encountered. These cells must be plugged with bone wax because they not only provide a route for the entry of air and bacteria into the cranium but also allow for CSF leakage into the middle ear, eustachian tube, and posterior pharynx if the dura cannot be closed at the conclusion of the intracranial procedure. The dura is opened to expose one or both of the cerebellar hemispheres. At this point, the arachnoid layer that forms the posterior wall of the cisterna magna is frequently opened and CSF is

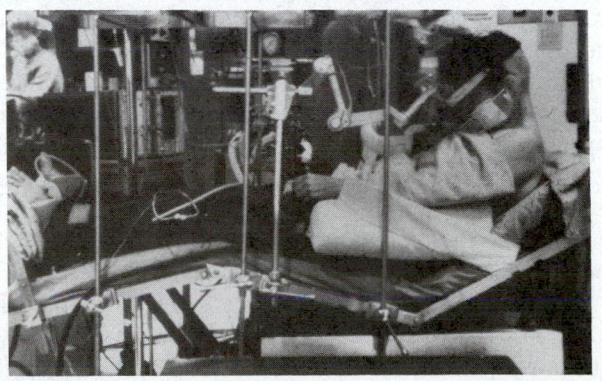

Figure 39–3

Client in the semi-sitting position with pressure suit, pinned headrest, monitoring equipment, and overhead tables for instrumentation. (Courtesy of Leonard I. Malis, MD, The Mount Sinai Medical Center, New York, NY)

allowed to escape, providing additional decompression and better exposure.

Lesions within the cerebellum are usually approached by incising the cerebellar cortex directly over the area of suspected pathology. The fourth ventricle is reached by splitting the vermis (the midline cerebellar structure) and retracting both cerebellar hemispheres. Lesions of the cerebellopontine angle (eg, acoustic neuroma) are usually approached by elevating the cerebellar hemisphere of the affected side.

Approaches to the tentorial margin or neurovascular decompression of the trigeminal nerves may be carried out through a unilateral operation with division of the veins on the superior surface of the cerebellum. This approach allows the cerebellum to fall away from the tentorium and provides reasonable access for a microsurgical procedure. Carried out as a bilateral exposure, the midline visualization permits removal of pineal area tumors by a subtentorial supracerebellar approach.

Implications for the Client

The absence of seizures and the preservation of normal intellectual function are the two most important features that differentiate the client with a posterior fossa syndrome from one with forebrain dysfunction. General client implications for supratentorial craniotomy or craniectomy were discussed in Table 39–2. The specific implications and potential complications related to the anatomical structures within the posterior fossa will be discussed in this section and are summarized in Table 39–3.

Physiological Implications

Although the posterior fossa contains only about a quarter of the intracranial contents, the concentration of vital structures in this small area makes surgery especially hazardous. During the operative procedure, it is frequently necessary to manipulate the cerebellum, cranial nerves, and the structures adjacent to the brain stem.

Specific cranial nerve deficits may be present preoperatively or may occur postoperatively as a result of damage or manipulation during the surgical procedure. The dysfunction may be permanent or transient, depending on the condition of the nerve. Some degree of functional impairment is anticipated following any surgical manipulation of the cranial nerves. Often the surgeon can make a reasonable prediction regarding expected function by ascertaining the integrity of the nerves at the end of the operative procedure before the wound is closed.

Dissection of CN VI (the abducens nerve) often results in diplopia that may take several months to clear. Dysfunction may also result from damage to nuclei within the brain stem. Damage to CN III (the oculomotor nerve) and CN IV the trochlear nerve is unusual but may occur.

Decreased or lost corneal sensation secondary to trigeminal nerve (CN V) dysfunction can soon lead to irreparable keratitis if proper corneal care is neglected. This situation is especially dangerous when accompanied by facial nerve damage that prevents elevation of the lower lid and results in the loss of lacrimation. This combination of a partially open, dry, anesthetized eye and the loss of the protective corneal blink reflex make the affected eye especially vulnerable to corneal abrasion and ulceration that can lead to a permanently blind eye.

Manipulation of branches of the trigeminal nerve or the ganglion may be followed postoperatively by herpes simplex eruptions in the cutaneous distribution of the disturbed branch (Stern, 1982). The blisters are unilateral, most usual in the second division, and resemble herpes zoster (shingles), which they are not. The painless, noninfectious lesions require no treatment. Irritation or damage to the trigeminal nerve may also be manifested by either pain or numbness on the affected side of the face. Often the numbness is unnoticed by the client and is only detected on sensory testing. Section of this nerve (eg, rhizotomy for relief of trigeminal neuralgia) may occasionally result in an extremely distressing and untreatable condition known as anesthesia dolorosa, in which the client's pain is replaced by severe dysesthetic sensations such as burning, itching, or the feeling of insects crawling under the skin. Damage to the motor branch of CN V can result in weakness of the muscles of mastication on the affected side.

Because CN VII (the facial nerve) and CN VIII (the vestibulocochlear nerve) are close together, manipulation of either nerve may result in some degree of dysfunction of the other. Tinnitus, vertigo, or alteration of space perception may result from irritation of the vestibular portion of CN VIII and usually disappear as nerve damage progresses, although they may persist indefinitely, even following surgical sectioning of the nerve.

CN VIII seems to be especially sensitive. When complete neural hearing loss occurs, it is nearly always permanent. In clients with an acoustic neuroma, the tumor almost invariably arises from one vestibular branch of the nerve; therefore, if the client can hear preoperatively, there is a chance that hearing can be preserved if adequate perfusion of the nerve has been maintained, and if the nerve itself has been preserved. Hemotympanum (blood or fluid behind the eardrum) may interfere with normal sound conduction. This condition, frequently seen following surgery involving the opening of mastoid air cells (eg, acoustic neuroma surgery), is self-limiting and usually resolves without treatment within a week or two.

Although not the most debilitating of the cranial nerve deficits, facial paralysis is often the most distressing for the client. The risk of damage to the facial nerve depends on the location of the lesion and, as in the acoustic neuromas, is often directly proportional to the size of the tumor. If the nerve is known to be anatomically intact, the surgeon can usually reassure the client that function will return. Unfortunately, it is difficult and sometimes impossible to predict the rate of recovery. Electromyography may offer some degree of predictability but if no reaction is recorded, may lead to undue pessimism.

Table 39-3 Sub-Occipital Craniectomy: Implications for the Client

Physiological Implications	Psychosocial/Lifestyle Implications
The implications are similar to those for a supratentorial intracranial procedure (see Table 39-2) except that in a suboccipital craniectomy, seizures are absent and normal intellectual function is preserved.	
The high concentration of vital structures within a small area make posterior fossa surgery especially hazardous	Ataxia may impair mobility and necessitate rehabilitation, ambulatory aids, and assistance with ADL. Bilateral damage may prove incapacitating
Permanent or transient ipsilateral dysfunction can be caused by the lesion itself or operative manipulation of the cerebellum, brain stem, or specific cranial nerves	Clients with damage to CN V need to protect and care for the affected eye
Some degree of cranial nerve dysfunction is to be anticipated following surgical manipulation. It can be permanent or transient, depending on the condition of the nerve	The deformity from CN VII paralysis, whether transient or permanent, often has a profound effect on body image. Some degree of depression can be expected. Following anastomosis or nerve grafting, retraining exercises may be required
CN V dysfunction results in lost or decreased corneal sensation that predisposes the client to keratitis	Bilateral loss of hearing from damage to CN VIII causes significant lifestyle changes; bilateral damage to the vestibular branches of CN VIII may be incapacitating
Manipulation of CN V or its ganglion can result in painless, noninfectious herpes simplex eruptions on the affected side of the face	In the elderly, loss of CN IX and CN X function may lead to permanent dependence on tracheostomy and/or gastrostomy. This requires significant lifestyle alterations for client and family. It may also interfere with placement of the client in a rehabilitation center or nursing home
Damage to the motor branch of CN V results in weakness of the muscles of mastication	
Dissection of CN VI results in diplopia that may last several months	
If CN VII is anatomically intact, function almost always returns: if not, plastic surgery may be required. Recovery rate is variable and may take up to 2 years	
CN VIII is especially sensitive and neural hearing loss is usually permanent; tinnitus, vertigo, or alteration of space perception are usually transient	
Loss of CN IX, CN X, and CN XII function that occurs in younger clients or is gradual is usually compensated for well. Dysphagia and loss of the gag reflex predispose the client to aspiration	
Lateral exposures, which involve opening the mastoid cavity, carry a higher risk of CSF leak	
The risk of GI hemorrhage is somewhat higher following posterior fossa surgery	
Damage during surgery to the anterior inferior cerebellar artery carries a significant risk of fatal brain stem infarction	
Compression of the respiratory center in the brain stem (ie, by edema or hematoma) can result in respiratory arrest that occurs with little or no warning and without a decline in the level of consciousness	
Potential complications include: hemorrhage/hematoma; increased ICP; herniation resulting in respiratory arrest; infection; CSF leak; hydrocephalus; GI hemorrhage; ataxia	

If intracranial anastomosis of the cut ends of the facial nerve is necessary, recovery may take as long as 2 years, and the client often becomes discouraged. If prolonged recovery is expected, the client may benefit from a face lift or facial sling procedure performed by a plastic surgeon.

Such procedures offer good immediate cosmetic results, but over time, atrophy of facial musculature results in progressive sagging.

When the facial nerve is lost or sacrificed at surgery, a reasonable degree of facial symmetry and function can be restored by anastomosis of the distal extracranial branch of the facial nerve to proximal extracranial branches of the accessory (CN XI) or hypoglossal nerve (CN XII). Often the procedure is performed a day or two before the planned discharge date, or it may be done as an elective ambulatory surgical procedure following discharge. Clients learn to control their facial movements by moving their shoulder in the case of a facial-accessory nerve anastomosis, and by moving their tongue in the case of a facial-hypoglossal anastomosis. Following either procedure, a reasonable degree of muscle tone and facial symmetry at rest can be expected. Movement will never be perfectly symmetrical. Clients will need to practice in front of a mirror until they learn to control their facial movements. Some electromyographic feedback training techniques have been helpful.

The inability to raise the lower lid and completely close the eye predisposes the eye to corneal damage and can be especially dangerous if the facial paralysis is accompanied by decreased or absent corneal sensation. Damage to the facial nerve also results in decreased lacrimation and a poor blink reflex. If function is not expected to return within a short time, a lateral tarsorrhaphy is performed to unite the outer eyelid edges to reduce the width of the palpebral tissue. If the nerve is known to be lost completely, the surgeon may elect to perform the procedure before the client leaves the operating room. Often, it is performed at the bedside using local anesthesia. The outer third of the lid margins are made raw by slicing off a thin margin of the edge, and a single mattress suture is tied over thin rubber tubing (Jennett & Galbraith, 1983). The stitches are left in place until the closure is secure, usually 12 to 18 days. If facial function returns, the lid adhesions can easily be lysed with little or no cosmetic deformity.

The glossopharyngeal (CN IX), vagus (CN X), accessory, and hypoglossal nerves are anatomically close to one another. Lesions or surgical manipulation of these cranial nerves often result in varying degrees of cardiac irregularity or impairment of swallowing and speech. Dysphagia and depressed gag reflex may also be secondary to damage at the brain stem. The client's ability to compensate for the loss of these nerves is related to rate of loss of function as well as the client's age. Gradual loss of function, usually seen with many of the slow-growing lesions that occur in this area, is compensated for surprisingly well. On the other hand, sudden loss as a result of a surgical procedure usually is devastating, especially for the elderly client. Tracheostomy and nasogastric tube feedings are often necessary to prevent aspiration and maintain nutrition. Occasionally, reconstructive pharyngeal and esophageal surgery may be performed to improve swallowing. These procedures are usually complex and may require multiple-staged operations. Some clients benefit from a relatively simple procedure in which the fibers of the cricopharyngeal muscle in the neck are incised (cricopharyngeus myotomy). This procedure relaxes the pharyngeal musculature to facilitate swallowing.

Lateral exposures for tumors of the cerebellopontine angle frequently involve opening the mastoid cavity, either intentionally or inadvertently. Unless the mastoid air cells are adequately sealed, the client is at considerable risk of developing a CSF rhinorrhea or otorrhea. If conservative treatment fails, re-exploration to repair the leak is usually necessary to prevent meningitis.

Gastrointestinal hemorrhage following the stress of a major intracranial procedure is always a danger, especially in any client with a history of gastric hyperirritability. The risk may be increased by steroids. Cushing's stress ulcer is more common following posterior fossa surgery than supratentorial surgery especially if it involves manipulation of the floor of the fourth ventricle.

Damage to the anterior inferior cerebellar artery and its branches by thrombosis or accidental clipping, cutting, or coagulation is one of the most significant dangers associated with operations in the posterior fossa, and especially in the cerebellopontine angle. This artery, which has an irregular anatomical course, is a critical source of blood to the lateral portion of the brain stem. Damage to this artery carries a significant risk of brain stem infarction and can be fatal.

Edema or a postoperative hematoma within the posterior fossa is even more dangerous than when it occurs within the cerebral hemispheres because of the vital local structures. Pressure from a mass within the posterior fossa can cause upward displacement of the upper part of the vermis through the tentorial hiatus, compressing the dorsal midbrain; this is known as upward herniation. Another possibility is that the compressive lesion will push the structures nearest to the foramen magnum downward into the cervical canal. When pressure reaches the critical level, the cerebellar tonsils, which normally lie just above the foramen magnum, are pushed downward and may descend to the level of the first or second cervical vertebra (tonsilar herniation). As the tonsils become firmly impacted within the bony rim of the foramen magnum (known as foraminal impaction), they compress the brain stem where the centers for respiration are located. Because the area of compression is below the level of the reticular formation, these clients may become apneic with little or no warning and without decline in the level of consciousness (Hayward, 1980).

Psychosocial/Lifestyle Implications

The impact of the surgery depends on the prognosis for the underlying disease process and on the nature and degree of disability or functional impairment. Ataxia may impair mobility and interfere with the ability to perform some of the necessary activities of daily living. The significance of cranial nerve dysfunction varies according to the nature, severity, and duration of the impairment.

Unilateral hearing loss does not usually significantly alter lifestyle. In certain occupations, however, the ability to hear with both ears is critical (eg, orchestra conductor, cardiologist), and even unilateral loss can have serious consequences. A person who is already deaf in one ear and requires surgery in the area of the opposite CN VIII faces the prospect of total deafness. Persons with the central form of neurofibromatosis (von Reckling-hausen's disease) also may become deaf because they commonly develop bilateral acoustic neuromas.

The loss of one vestibular branch of CN VIII is usually compensated for well and in most instances goes unnoticed by the client. Ballet dancers, tightrope walkers, some construction workers, and others whose jobs require precise balance may have to change occupations. Bilateral loss can be reasonably compensated for as long as clients can orient themselves through visual clues, but it can severely incapacitate a blind or severely visually impaired person.

Damage to CN V, which results in corneal anesthesia, necessitates minor changes in lifestyle. Once established, a routine for protection and care of the affected eye should have little impact. Contact lenses are contraindicated because of the inability to recognize potentially harmful irritation. For the person who has previously worn contacts, the need instead to wear protective eyeglasses may affect body image.

Facial nerve paralysis can disrupt lifestyle in varying degrees, ranging from minimal to profound. How the individual deals with this alteration in body image depends greatly on self-image. The person's personal and social profile, general attitude toward life, previous coping mechanisms, and the presence or absence of support systems are all important factors. Another important consideration is whether the condition is temporary or permanent. The client is also affected by others' reactions to the deformity. For the client whose lifestyle or livelihood depends largely or totally on physical appearance (eg, actress, model, salesman), drastic lifestyle changes may be necessary. Following nerve graft or anastomosis, the degree of recovery depends largely on the client's motivation and willingness to work at retraining exercises. Even when the deformity is temporary, most clients become depressed to some degree. If depression is severe or prolonged, psychological or psychiatric consultation may be helpful.

Unilateral dysfunction of CN IX and CN X with resulting impaired ability to swallow usually prolongs the hospital stay considerably. Recoverability of lower cranial nerve function depends on the damage inflicted by the lesion or the surgical manipulation, the rate at which the damage occurred, and the client's age. The young client may recover function within a few weeks. In the very young, permanent unilateral loss may be compensated for within a few months. As a general rule, the older the client, the slower the recovery. Elderly persons are often permanently dependent on a tracheostomy for management of secretions and a gastrostomy for adequate nutritional intake.

Nursing Implications

Preoperative Care
Specific nursing measures for clients undergoing suboccipital craniectomy depend on the neurologic manifestations of the disease. The general nursing interventions outlined in the previous section on supratentorial craniotomy also apply.

The preoperative assessment focuses on determining cerebellar and brain stem function as well as detecting specific cranial nerve deficits. Cerebellar function can often be assessed without formal testing. Observe the client's gait and routine activities of daily living (eg, eating, bathing). Is the gait broad based? Is the client steady? Is there a tendency to walk close to a wall or a nearby steady object in case support is needed? Can the person rise from a lying position without difficulty? Evaluate the smoothness or accuracy with which tasks are performed. Look for abnormal movements such as tremors, tics, or exaggerated arm swings. Care must be taken when testing tandem walking or Romberg's sign. Never attempt such testing unless someone is available who can support the client's weight in case the client becomes unsteady and begins to fall. Teach clients with any degree of ataxia or vertigo to get up slowly, to avoid any sudden head movements, and to seek help when necessary. Assistive devices (eg, tripod cane, walker) may be necessary to allow for safe ambulation. Determine whether it is safe for the person to walk without supervision or assistance. When sitting, the client's balance may be improved by placing both feet firmly on the ground (or on a chair or stool if the client is short or is dangling the legs off the side of the bed). Pressure on the soles of the feet stimulates the posterior columns and helps maintain orientation in space.

Depending on the size, location, and nature of the posterior fossa lesion, clients require varying degrees of vigilance for respiratory status. Lesions that compress or distort the brain stem or produce hydrocephalus place the client at greater risk of sudden medullary compression. Vascular lesions also present a special danger because a sudden episode of bleeding can precipitate respiratory failure. Clients with cerebellar hemangioblastomas may also be at risk because the size of these cystic lesions tends to fluctuate. The preoperative unit should be equipped with equipment for emergency intubation and ventilatory support. The client at risk should be placed on an apnea monitor as a precaution.

Size; consistency; vascularity; proximity to surrounding structures; and the degree of adherence of the lesion to the brain stem, arteries, and cranial nerves are important factors in determining the operative risks (Horowitz & Rizzoli, 1982). Many of these factors are impossible to determine preoperatively. As a general rule, the outcome and risks can be directly correlated with the size and location of the lesion and the client's preoperative condition.

Both client and family need to be prepared for what may be a complicated postoperative course. Although an informed consent has been granted, remember that information may not be heard or may be misinterpreted. Accompany the surgeon during discussions of the surgical procedure and the expected outcome. Try to determine the level of understanding. Accurate perceptions should be reinforced, misconceptions clarified, and realistic expectations stressed. Because of the lesion's proximity to the brain stem, the surgeon or anesthesiologist may elect to keep the client intubated and mechanically ventilated during the immediate postoperative period. The client and family should be prepared for this possibility.

If surgical manipulation in the area of the internal auditory canal is anticipated (as with many of the lesions of the cerebellopontine angle or approaches to the trigeminal nerve), clients should be prepared for possible loss of hearing and facial paralysis on the operative side. Stress that when the nerve is left anatomically intact, function nearly always returns. Also assure clients that if the nerve is lost, grafting procedures, which are relatively minor operations, allow for the return of a reasonable degree of function and symmetry.

The male client with a beard should be encouraged not to shave it off, because the beard will, to some extent, disguise or conceal a postoperative facial weakness or paralysis. Confusion and difficulty may occasionally arise because many anesthesiologists request that the client be clean shaven to facilitate securing the endotracheal tube to the face. The surgeon and anesthesiologist may not have discussed this option before the anesthesiologist makes the preoperative visit. The nurse may need to explain the rationale for keeping the beard to the anesthesiologist and to reassure the client that other methods for securing the endotracheal tube are available.

Some clients with benign lesions may be admitted for a diagnostic work-up and readmitted later for surgery. When elective posterior fossa surgery is planned, it can be suggested that the male client grow a beard and that the female client allow her hair to grow as long as possible before the surgery. Often, hair not directly in the operative field can be secured out of the way. Postoperatively, the hair will cover the operative scar and the shaved area. This improvement in appearance may be especially helpful to the client suffering a severely altered body image as a result of facial paralysis.

The lesion or surgical dissection of CN IX and CN X may interfere with phonation and swallowing. If the dysfunction is severe or prolonged, a tracheostomy and some alternative means of feeding (nasogastric tube, gastrostomy, or hyperalimentation) may be necessary to protect the tracheobronchial tree and to provide adequate nutrition. Documentation of the preoperative body weight is important in assessing caloric intake.

The client with lost or impaired hearing on one side who is now at risk of losing hearing on the other side needs to be prepared for the possibility of total deafness. Alternative means of communication should be established and practiced during the preoperative period. Faced with deafness, some clients endeavor to learn lip reading or sign language. Some are successful, but in most cases, the client does not really become proficient until after hearing is actually lost. Magic slates, signs, or letter boards can be used to communicate. If the nurse and the client can invent gestures or signals for common words, phrases, or questions and practice them during the preoperative period, both are likely to have more success in using them postoperatively.

Postoperative Care

Except for seizure precautions, all of the nursing measures outlined in the previous section on supratentorial craniotomy/craniectomy are generally applicable. An intraoperative ventricular tap constitutes a supratentorial operation, however. It may, therefore, carry a minimal risk of postoperative seizures and bleeding within the cerebral hemisphere.

In the immediate postoperative period, the focus of nursing intervention is the same as for a client who has undergone a supratentorial craniotomy—the prompt recognition of complications and measures aimed at their prevention. The report from the operating room should include all of the information outlined in the previous section dealing with the postoperative care of the craniotomy client. Specific attention should be given to the status of the cranial nerves and the degree of function or dysfunction that can be expected in the immediate postoperative period. The amount of dissection or manipulation of the brain stem and its arterial supply are also important in anticipating the need for respiratory support.

Hemorrhage or edema within the posterior fossa is even more dangerous than in the cerebral hemisphere because of the vital local structures. Because rapid herniation can occur with little or no warning and without decline in the level of consciousness, vigilant monitoring of respiratory status is imperative. Carefully observe the respiratory rate and pattern and monitor blood gases regularly. Any irregularity, especially slowing of the rate with periods of apnea, may be evidence of impending respiratory arrest and should be reported immediately. An apnea monitor is advisable following operative manipulation of the brain stem or the anterior–inferior cerebellar artery or when posterior fossa surgery is combined with any dissection of the upper cervical spinal cord. This painless, noninvasive technique provides an early warning system if the respiratory rate decreases or becomes irregular.

Be alert to other warning signs, which may include neck pain or stiffness and tingling in the arms on neck extension as a result of pressure on the cervical cord. Some clients may faint if they move the head too far. This movement probably raises pressure by completing the block to CSF circulation in addition to causing pressure directly on the medulla (Jennett & Galbraith, 1983). Headache, especially with vomiting, may also be a warning sign. Hiccups may be an early sign of medullary irritation, especially if associated with respiratory irregularity, such as sighing. Equipment for emergency intubation and ventilatory support should be readily available. Because respiratory arrest is frequently rapidly followed by cardiac arrest, a defibrillator and the necessary drugs and solutions should also be accessible, and the staff should be familiar with their location and use.

Also be prepared for the possibility of a ventricular tap to reduce ICP. Because edema, hemorrhage, hydrocephalus, and infarction are often clinically indistinguishable, a CT scan is usually done as soon as the condition stabilizes enough to transport the client safely.

In the early postoperative period, if the wound appears tense and bulging, hematoma is usually suspected. The surgeon is likely to re-explore the wound to decompress the brain stem and achieve hemostasis. Edema is treated with the measures outlined in the previous section. Ventricular drainage may be instituted or a ventricular shunting system inserted to relieve hydrocephalus.

Unless otherwise ordered, the head of the bed should be elevated to at least 30°. Turn the client every 2 hours. Although the bone has been removed, the neck muscles provide sufficient protection for the underlying brain, and there are usually no special positioning precautions or restrictions.

These clients may have more postoperative pain than clients who have undergone a supratentorial operation because of the incision through the neck muscles. Head movement can be painful during the first few days. Take care to maintain the head in alignment when turning the body and to provide support for the neck area when the client is moving or turning. Mild analgesics usually provide sufficient relief, and the client is usually reasonably comfortable as long as movements of the head and neck are limited.

Cardiac irregularity in the early postoperative period may be the result of manipulation of CN IX or CN X or may be secondary to a central venous catheter within the right atrium. The location of the tip of the catheter can usually be determined by chest x-ray. The irregularity can often be reversed almost immediately if the catheter is withdrawn a few inches.

To protect the tracheobronchial tree, no oral intake should be permitted until the gag reflex can be checked. Once the gag reflex, swallowing, and cough have been assessed, the initial intake should be supervised by the physician or an experienced nurse. Suction apparatus should be immediately available. Swallowing should first be tested by a small sip of water so that if aspiration occurs, it will cause little harm.

Because of the delicacy of neural tissues, some degree of paresis is always anticipated when the surgical procedure involves manipulation of cranial nerves. Paresis occurs despite the neurosurgeon's improved visualization of anatomical structures with the operating microscope and despite microsurgical techniques and instrumentation permitting precise dissection. The degree and duration of the dysfunction greatly influence the nursing care plan.

Because of its anatomical location, damage to CN III is unusual but may be seen following dissection of lesions that extend high along the tentorial margin. Isolated dysfunction of CN IV is relatively rare but is difficult to rec-

ognize clinically. When dysfunction occurs, the diplopia is usually mild. The client can learn to compensate for it by tilting the head slightly so the visual images fuse. Damage to CN VI (the abducens nerve) interferes with outward movement of the eye. Diplopia is most severe with lateral gaze to the affected side. If the nerve is anatomically intact, recovery is usually complete but may take several months. Treatment consists of alternating eye patches to eliminate one visual image. If there is a CN III palsy, no cover will be necessary as long as ptosis is present. If diplopia is accompanied by damage of CN V or CN VII, the affected eye will be patched rather than using alternating patches.

Cotton ophthalmic eyepatches are contraindicated for the client with damage to the ophthalmic division of CN V: the client without corneal sensation may be unable to detect a partially opened lid, and the cotton gauze irritates or abrades the cornea. Instead, the eye should be taped closed or covered with a cone of stiff paper or other material that covers the eye without actually touching it. A piece of exposed x-ray film is a suitable material.

The Guibor Expo Bubble Bandage® manufactured by Concept, Inc (Figure 39–4), designed by an ophthalmologist, is commercially available and offers several advantages. The bandage provides a sterile, safe, convenient (adhesive-backed), transparent coverage for the eye that allows for binocular vision as well as assessment of pupillary function and extraocular movements. It also traps moisture, providing an additional degree of protection and comfort for the eye. These features can be especially beneficial when the client also has a facial nerve paresis or paralysis that markedly decreases lacrimation and the inability to raise the lower lid to close the eye adequately. For the client with diplopia, an opaque eye covering that eliminates one visual image may be preferable. In such cases, tape can be placed on the outside of the Guibor shield to render it opaque. If facial nerve function is intact and the

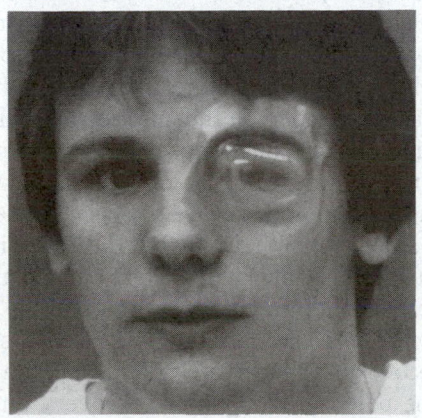

Figure 39–4

The Guibor bubble protects an exposed cornea. (Courtesy of Leonard I. Malis, MD, The Mount Sinai Medical Center, New York, NY)

client has adequate lid closure, the eye need only be shielded or taped closed during sleep or if the level of consciousness is depressed.

Lubricate the eye with artificial tears or some other ophthalmic lubricant every 4 hours, and inspect it for redness or signs of irritation or infection. If the condition is expected to be long term or permanent, teach the client to inspect the eye with a mirror every morning and evening and to seek medical attention if any redness is noted. The client will need to tape the eye closed or wear a shield for sleep. Eyeglasses that incorporate a side piece (moist chamber) should be worn outdoors to protect the eye from foreign bodies.

Most clients soon learn to compensate for the chewing difficulty that results from damage to the motor portion of CN V by chewing on the opposite side. In the initial recovery period, foods that require extensive chewing should be avoided. Loss of sensation from the sensory portion of CN V can predispose the client to injury to the tongue, lips, and buccal mucosa. After the client eats, check the mouth for pockets of food retained on the anesthetized side. Frequent mouth care is essential, and the mouth should be inspected daily for any signs of ulceration or infection. Teach the client to continue these practices at home. Regular dental care is also imperative because tooth decay and periodontal disease can go undetected because of the lack of pain.

Following operations that involve manipulation of the gasserian ganglion (eg, CN V decompression or neuroma), cutaneous lesions of herpes simplex can be expected about the fourth postoperative day. Reassure the client that they are painless, noninfectious, and will resolve in a week or so without scarring or any other sequelae and will not recur. Also reassure family members, other clients, and staff members that these lesions are not contagious and that there is no need to isolate or otherwise restrict the client.

Damage to CN VII with resulting facial paralysis causes the mouth to droop on the affected side and causes difficulty with eating and drinking. Liquids often present the greatest problem. Most clients learn to compensate by tilting the head slightly and using the unaffected side. The impaired taste sensation on the anterior two-thirds of the affected side of the tongue and decreased salivation are often not troublesome enough to disturb the client or interfere with adequate nutritional intake. Speech may be slightly slurred because of mouth droop, but the deficit is mild and compensated for quickly. Faint flickers of movement of the lower lid can sometimes be observed when the client forcibly attempts to close the eye. This usually signals the start of recovery of function. If the flickers are observed early in the postoperative period, recovery often occurs rapidly (within days or weeks) and provides encouragement for the client.

In the early postoperative period, it may be difficult to assess damage to CN VIII because of hemotympanum. The client with hemotympanum usually feels fullness or

stuffiness in the ear and speech sounds are muffled. The process is self-limiting and requires no treatment. Caution the client against forceful nose blowing. Nasal decongestants may increase comfort by reducing the stuffiness. If hearing is present, it will usually improve as the fluid is absorbed. If blood or fluid drains from the external canal, allow it to drain freely. Packs or irrigation should never be used. Examination with an otoscope may predispose to infection. As a general rule, the ear should be left alone for at least 6 weeks, after which crusting or exudate can be gently cleaned and the eardrum adequately inspected.

Stressing realistic expectations for hearing is important. Neural hearing loss is almost always irreversible. Cochlear implants do not function if CN VIII is absent and offer no hope in this situation. When any amount of hearing is present preoperatively, testing is usually done to provide a baseline for postoperative comparison. Hearing loss secondary to neural damage is most often characterized by loss by speech discrimination rather than loss of volume. Often, the person may be unaware of gradual loss. These clients often find they have switched the ear with which they use the telephone without even realizing it. Strategies to use when talking with hearing-impaired clients are discussed in Chapter 74.

Clients with tinnitus can be referred to hearing specialists who can recommend devices designed to mask tinnitus. Occasionally, the problem is so distressing that the surgeon will re-explore the wound and intentionally section the nerve. Unfortunately, in some instances the tinnitus persists even after the nerve has been cut.

Encourage clients who have lost the vestibular portion of CN VIII to use touch and sight to compensate for the loss. Teach them to avoid quick head turns or sudden movements. The elderly client or one with any degree of visual impairment or cerebellar ataxia may need help with ambulation. Handrails may be helpful, and the home should be cleared of clutter to protect the client from injuries. Bilateral vestibular loss can usually be managed as long as the person is able to maintain visual orientation to the environment. To prevent injury, a night light should be left on or within easy reach at the bedside.

The degree of dysfunction resulting from impaired function of CN IX, CN X, and CN XI may vary. The client may require only a period of relearning following edema of the cranial nerves, or function may be completely lost following tumor resection (Hargrove, 1980). The combination of functional impairment of the pharynx and vocal cords results in the loss of adequate airway protection and makes the client especially susceptible to spillage of pharyngeal contents into the trachea. A primary goal of nursing management is to prevent aspiration. Suction apparatus should be available at the bedside at all times. Once the client is able to participate in self-care, the suction should be kept within easy reach and the client encouraged to suction the mouth as often as necessary.

A client with swallowing difficulty should always be fed in the upright position and supervised closely the entire time. Fluids are generally more difficult to handle. Most clients are better able to manage soft or semisolid foods because these stimulate the swallowing reflex (Hargrove, 1980). Foods that require a great deal of chewing should be avoided. Instruct the client to place the food on the unaffected side and to tilt the head in that direction. Provide a calm, comfortable, nondistracting environment and allow the client as much time as necessary. Care should be taken that the client does not become overtired because fatigue makes swallowing more difficult. Unfortunately, foods that are easiest to swallow are not always the most nutritious (Hargrove, 1980).

Monitor input and output and daily weight and evaluate the caloric and nutritional adequacy of oral intake. If caloric or nutritional intake is not adequate, nasogastric feedings or hyperalimentation may be necessary. If the deficit is expected to be long term or permanent, gastrostomy may be considered. Follow oral feedings with mouth care and inspect the mouth carefully because food tends to be trapped on the affected side.

Clients with severe or long-lasting deficits may require tracheostomy to facilitate adequate pulmonary toilet. The combination of tracheostomy and upper gastrointestinal feeding can be especially hazardous. To prevent soiling of the tracheobronchial tree, the cuff on the tracheostomy tube should be inflated. The client should be maintained in an erect position during feeding and for at least 30 minutes afterward to lessen the danger of gastric regurgitation and aspiration.

Because phonation depends on the action of the musculature of the tongue, lips, pharynx, larynx, and soft palate, many clients also experience varying degrees of dysarthria. Speech is often slurred and indistinct. Damage to the vagus nerve may result in vocal cord paralysis that results in a hoarse, raspy, and sometimes barely audible voice. The person with a long-standing deficit needs to be treated with genuine concern by the nursing staff as well as family and significant others. Recognize the client's frustration and be accepting of anger or depression. Maintain a calm, relaxed, and unhurried environment. Remember that comprehension is usually intact. Although communication should be kept brief and simple, treat the person as an adult and avoid using ''baby talk.'' Encourage clients' efforts to speak and praise them for any success, regardless how small. Use alternative methods of communication discussed earlier as necessary. Speech therapy is often helpful but as a general rule should not be instituted until the person expresses readiness. The client and family can also be taught environmental management, support behavior, and behaviors to enhance communication (Boss, 1984).

Ataxia is frequently aggravated by surgery and may interfere with early ambulation. On the other hand, recovery, especially in younger clients, is often remarkable, and the condition is usually temporary. For other clients, some degree of disability may be permanent. For them, physical therapy is usually necessary. Rehabilitation is directed at the restoration of mobility and self-care.

Antacids and cimetidine should be administered with steroids because of the risk of Curling's stress ulcer and gastrointestinal hemorrhage. Carefully monitor blood pressure, hematocrit, and hemoglobin levels. Frequent or daily examination of stool for occult blood may detect gastrointestinal bleeding early.

The incidence of CSF leaks is higher in clients in whom dural closure was not accomplished and following lateral exposures when mastoid air cells are entered. CSF accumulation in the tissues of the operative area is easily recognizable: the wound appears to bulge and is soft and fluctuant to touch. If pressure builds until the operative site is tense, there is a danger of wound breakdown and secondary infection. Repetitive spinal taps or closed lumbar drainage may reduce the pressure. Direct puncture to aspirate the fluid from the wound is less desirable because of the danger of introducing organisms into the wound. The therapeutic and nursing measures are described in the previous section on craniotomy and craniectomy. If conservative measures fail, the wound may have to be re-explored and the mastoid air cells sealed with bone wax or a fat, muscle, or fascia graft. In some instances, a small amount of fluid may continue to leak for a few days following the repair until adequate sealing takes place. Spinal taps may be done to keep the ICP low and to hasten sealing of the graft.

In the absence of complications, the usual postoperative course is similar to that of the client undergoing a supratentorial intracranial operation. Late complications may include infection, hydrocephalus, CSF leak, and tumor recurrence. Discharge teaching should include alerting the client and family to the possible clinical manifestations of these complications.

CRANIOPLASTY

Cranioplasty is the surgical correction of a defect in the cranial vault. This procedure usually involves insertion of a substitute material that has been prepared and shaped to fit into or over the defective area. Cranioplasty is most often done to protect the intracranial contents or to improve the client's appearance. The necessity for a cranioplasty is often determined by the size and location of the defect. The procedure is most often indicated when there is a supratentorial bony defect.

A cranial defect, especially if it is difficult to conceal, can have a major effect on a client's lifestyle. Besides the obvious alteration in body image, many of these clients fear damage to the underlying brain. This may severely limit their activities. Often, these restrictions are self-imposed and out of proportion to the danger. A change of occupation is rarely necessary. Occasionally, a suboccipital craniectomy client with a defect in a well-protected area will be so apprehensive that the surgeon does a cranioplasty so the client will resume normal activities. When the defect is especially large or in a highly vulnerable area or if the client's condition is such that an injury may not always be avoidable (eg, a client is prone to seizures or is confused or agitated), a football helmet or other protective headgear may be worn. Caring for such clients can be considerably stressful for family caregivers.

The procedure may also be performed to relieve headaches, vertigo, and the local tenderness and throbbing that sometimes occurs when the bone flap has been left out after craniectomy. Small defects that are not cosmetically unattractive usually do not require repair; the neck muscles protect the posterior fossa contents and hide the bony defect.

Repair of a bony defect may be indicated following extensive or comminuted skull fractures. Osteomyelitis or radiation necrosis may necessitate removal of the bone flap. In fact, these complications may occur several years after the original surgical procedure or radiotherapy. Erosion or invasion of the bone by tumor, frequently seen with convexity meningiomas and some metastatic lesions, may necessitate removal of all or part of the bone flap. When markedly increased ICP precludes replacement of the bone flap, a secondary cranioplasty is often required. Cranioplasty may also be indicated to repair certain congenital malformations of the skull or for improved cosmetic results following craniectomy for craniostenosis (premature closure of one or more of the cranial sutures).

Surgical Procedure

Cranioplasty may be done as part of the closure of a craniostomy or as a separate secondary procedure. If the wound is clean, ICP is under control, and the extra operative time required for the repair will not put the client at risk, the cranioplasty is usually done at the time of the original craniectomy. When infection exists (eg, removal of an osteomyelitic bone flap) or is suspected or expected (eg, following compound skull fracture), no attempt at cranioplasty should be made for at least 6 months. Some surgeons prefer to wait a full year to ensure that the wound is free of organisms so a foreign body can be tolerated without causing reinfection.

Opinions vary about the ideal material for cranioplasty. Some surgeons favor use of the client's own bone flap and place it in a sterile container at the time of the original surgery. The flap is then kept frozen until the client is ready for cranioplasty. An autogenous graft of bone or cartilage may be used. Rib grafts are especially common in children. In most instances, however, a foreign substance is used. A wide variety of materials is available. The important consideration is that the substance be inert and not rejected by the body. In the past, metal plates of stainless steel, tantalum, or Vitallium were common. These plates were commercially available in a wide variety of sizes and shapes but usually required cutting and molding to fit the particular defect and to achieve the desired contour. In some instances, the original bone flap was retained and used preoperatively as a template for molding the replacement plate.

Metal plates are fixated with screws to the surrounding skull. The metal alloys in the plate must be identical to those of the screws. Incompatibility of these metals can lead to an electrolytic reaction that eventually erodes the bone and can erode through the scalp. Metal plates are also radiopaque, which presents difficulties if the client requires radiological studies or if the lesion necessitates follow-up with x-ray or CT scanning. Because of their magnetic properties, these plates preclude use of magnetic resonance imaging (MRI) as a diagnostic tool. If metal plates are used, they should be nonmagnetic, or the client should be warned never to have an MRI scan.

Methyl methacrylate, a synthetic acrylic substance that is inert and causes no tissue reaction, has simplified cranioplasty procedures. A small ledge is usually carved around the edge of the bony defect to provide support for the plate. The methyl methacrylate is then prepared by mixing the liquid monomers with the powdered polymer. The doughy mass can then be molded to the desired shape, contour, and thickness. This plate is placed over the defect and allowed to harden. After hardening, holes are drilled in the plate and the surrounding skull, and the plate is secured in the same fashion that a bone flap would be attached. These plates are radiolucent so they do not interfere with radiological studies.

A modification of this procedure uses a sheet of wire mesh (usually stainless steel) that is cut, molded, and secured to the prepared bone edge and then impregnated with methyl methacrylate (Figure 39–5). Another technique, frequently used for small defects, consists of criss-crossing strands of wire across the defect before applying the doughy acrylic mixture. The principle involved in both of these methods is similar to that used when concrete is reinforced with steel mesh or rod. The metal provides added strength to the acrylic. Radiological studies are possible because the mesh allows a reasonable degree of lucency.

Implications for the Client

When a cranioplasty is part of a more extensive intracranial procedure (eg, meningioma removal, metastatic tumor removal), the implications for the client include those covered in the previous section on craniotomy and craniectomy as well as those for the specific underlying disease process. A cranioplasty itself usually involves little or no manipulation of the intracranial contents and is therefore considered relatively minor. The implications are outlined in Table 39–4.

Physiological Implications

Most cranioplastic procedures involve little or no manipulation of the cerebral cortex, so a decline in the neurologic status is not usually anticipated. Blood loss is usually minimal and transfusion rarely required. If dura was previously resected or if infection occurred, the brain may adhere to the overlying muscle or galea, and a great deal of dissection may be required to free it. The dissection may cause cortical damage or swelling. The resulting neurologic symp-

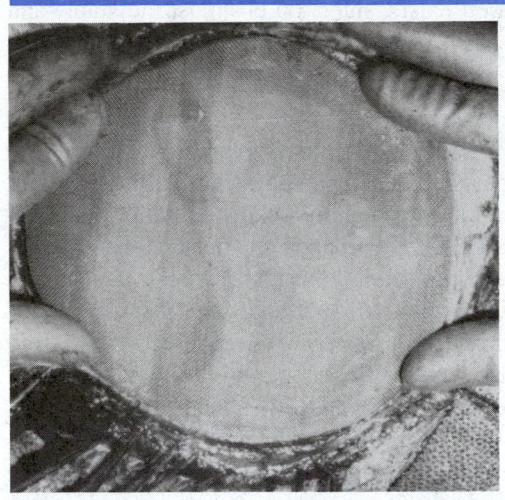

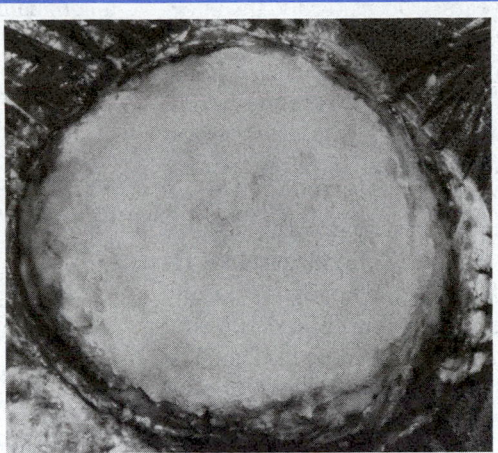

tomatology depends on the area involved and the degree of damage.

The incidence of mortality and morbidity following cranioplasty is low. The most frequent complication is infection, which is ordinarily local but which may lead to meningitis. Factors that predispose to wound breakdown and infection include thin or poorly vascularized skin over the plate, poorly fitting or inadequately secured plates, and nonperforated plates that prevent proper fluid absorption (Horowitz & Rizzoli, 1982). Plates placed in proximity to an air sinus (eg, the frontal sinus) may have minute communications with the sinus undetected at surgery that can result in infection of the plate, cellulitis, or osteomyelitis of the surrounding bone. In many instances, breakdown or infection may not occur or become evident for several years following implantation of the plate. (Infection has

Table 39-4 Cranioplasty: Implications for the Client

Physiological Implications	Psychosocial/Lifestyle Implications
When a cranioplasty is done as part of a more extensive procedure the implications outlined in Table 39-2 will also apply.	
Because the cranial cavity is entered but there is usually little or no manipulation of the intracranial contents, edema and an accompanying decline in neurologic status should not be expected unless extensive dissection was required	Relief of apprehension and enhanced self-esteem
	Occasionally a client not at risk following craniectomy may require cranioplasty to relieve the apprehension associated with the cranial defect to be able to resume normal activities
Mortality and morbidity is low	
The most frequent complication is infection, which is usually local but can lead to meningitis	Postoperative cranioplasty infection can prove very disruptive because of the need for prolonged antibiotic therapy, repeat hospitalization, and reoperation
Resection of dura and/or a foreign body reaction may lead to the development of a subgaleal fluid collection over the cranioplasty site	Need to wait 6-12 months following infection to replace the cranioplasty plate can severely disrupt lifestyle, exhaust financial reserves, and often results in some degree of depression
Autogenous bone may undergo some degree of absorption	
Clients with metal plates may experience headaches associated with extremes of heat or cold	Cosmetic results may not always live up to the client's expectations resulting in disappointment and depression
A blow of sufficient force to shatter bone will also shatter acrylic plates; reinforcement with wire adds strength to the acrylic plate and reduces the risk of breakage	Disappointment if preoperative symptoms such as headache, throbbing, or local tenderness do not subside following cranioplasty
Repeated operations in the same area may result in devascularization of the skin flap necessitating skin grafting or extensive plastic surgical repair	Concern over long-term effects of repeated operations

been reported as late as 15 years.) Occasionally, the infection can be cured by appropriate systemic antibiotics, alone or in combination with local instillation of the drug. In most instances, however, the infection is only temporarily controlled and tends to flare up periodically. Complete and permanent cure usually requires removal of the cranioplastic plate.

Clients with cranioplastic plates sometimes develop subgaleal fluid collections in the area. This accumulation is probably a form of localized foreign body reaction. In many clients, it is probably also related to resection of the dura (eg, in meningiomas of the convexity). In all likelihood, it is a combination of both factors. Often the fluid collection is worse in the morning and lessens or disappears completely as the day goes on. This phenomenon probably is related to position, because pressure rises and fluid accumulates during sleep. The accumulation is unsightly and annoying but is usually painless and often subsides gradually without treatment. Treatment is required only if swelling threatens the integrity of the suture line.

The use of autogenous bone eliminates the problems of implantation of a foreign substance but has disadvantages. In most instances, the operative procedure is longer because two operative sites are frequently involved. Pain at the donor site is often considerable. Pneumothorax is a danger when a rib graft is taken.

Properly stored autogenous bone is not altered in morphology, but the process kills osteophytes and prevents actively forming new bone after grafting (Horowitz & Rizzoli, 1982). Bone that has been steam sterilized (eg, to kill tumor cells or to sterilize a bone flap accidentally dropped during surgery) becomes a well-tolerated foreign body. The bone usually does not cause infection, but there is a risk of aseptic necrosis and partial absorption. Instances of complete absorption have been documented by x-ray follow-up over a period of years. Some degree of absorption may also affect fresh autogenous bone but usually to a lesser degree. The risk of infection may be greater when bone has been stored.

Clients with metal plates frequently complain of annoying pain or headache associated with extremes of heat or cold. This is especially true if the client is bald or does not wear a hat. An improperly fitting plate that moves may have an edge erode through the skin. Metal incompatibility can lead to erosion of the surrounding skull with progressive mobility of the plate. A direct blow can dent the plate.

Acrylic plates carry no risk of absorption, are easy to shape, and are suitable for filling large defects. Allergic reaction or rejection is rare. A blow of sufficient force to shatter bone also shatters acrylic. One disadvantage is that acrylic fragments cannot be seen on x-ray and may be difficult to locate (Horowitz & Rizzoli, 1982). The addition of wire or wire-mesh reinforcement adds to the strength of the plate and greatly reduces the risk of breakage. Extreme care must be taken when using acrylic in any area that may communicate with air cells (eg, mastoid, frontal sinus). If

a communication exists, infection is almost inevitable and could necessitate removal of the cranioplasty.

Psychosocial/Lifestyle Implications

An infection after a cranioplasty can be extremely disruptive, especially if the client appears to have recovered from the original surgery and resumed a normal lifestyle. An infection almost always requires rehospitalization for intravenous antibiotic therapy. Long-term antibiotic therapy may result in side effects and toxicity that may necessitate changing drugs. Often, this extends the hospital stay or requires readmission. This can be an extremely frustrating and depressing time for the client and family, especially if conservative therapy fails and the plate has to be removed.

Waiting 6 to 12 months to replace the plate is also distressing and disruptive. Occasionally, even following an extended period, the surgeon may find evidence of infection when the wound is opened; if so, the cranioplasty cannot safely be performed. The delay may exhaust the emotional and financial reserves of clients and families. In addition, repeated operations may lead to devascularization of the skin flap, necessitating skin grafting or extensive plastic surgical repair.

For most clients, cranioplasty offers relief by protecting their brain as well as enhanced self-esteem resulting from their improved physical appearance. For some, though, the cosmetic result may not live up to their expectations, and the postoperative period is one of disappointment and depression. The client who has suffered from headaches or other post-traumatic symptoms may also be disappointed because these distressing symptoms may not always resolve following cranioplasty.

Nursing Implications

Preoperative Care

Preoperative preparation is basically the same as for a client undergoing a craniotomy or craniectomy although usually not as extensive. As with any intracranial procedure, a baseline neurologic assessment should be performed and well documented to assess the postoperative condition adequately. The client's blood should be typed and possibly crossmatched. Clients, especially those with a history of headaches, should be questioned regarding aspirin use. Report any recent use to the physician. Encourage the client to express fears and expectations. Reinforce realistic expectations about relief of symptoms and cosmetic results. Defects in the frontal area may be especially difficult to repair, especially if rebuilding of the orbital ridge is necessary.

Intraoperative monitoring is usually minimal. Unless there are existing medical problems (eg, heart, pulmonary, or renal disease), arterial and central venous lines are not often used. Because little or no brain retraction is usually required and because it is desirable to maintain the normal contour of the brain, osmotic diuretics are often withheld. If the surgery is expected to be lengthy, an in-dwelling urinary catheter may be inserted for the operative and immediate postoperative period.

Postoperative Care

Postoperatively, cranioplasty clients usually do not require intensive care management unless there are serious underlying medical problems. Because the cranial vault has been entered, however, the usual vital signs and neurologic status should be monitored for at least 24 hours. The urinary catheter can usually be removed as soon as the client is awake and alert. Steroids and anticonvulsants may be ordered. Seizure precautions should be observed if the client has a history of seizures or if the surgery involved the frontal or temporal area.

Because infection is the main danger, attention to aseptic technique is imperative in any aspect of wound care such as suture removal and caring for the wound drain. The postoperative course progresses rapidly, and the client can usually be discharged within a week. Because the operation involves reopening a previous incision line, the skin sutures are left in place longer than usual—about 2 weeks. Sutures can be removed in the physician's office or the outpatient department. Discharge teaching should include symptoms and signs of infection. Any inflammation, tenderness, or wound drainage should be reported to the physician.

VENTRICULAR SHUNTING PROCEDURES

Ventricular shunting creates an alternative pathway for removing CSF from the ventricular system. In most instances, the goal is to divert the CSF into another part of the body where it can be absorbed. Since the turn of the century, many diversionary procedures have been used with varying degrees of success. The two methods that currently are widely used are the *ventricular–atrial shunt,* in which excess CSF is shunted into the vascular system (Figure 39–6), and the *ventricular–peritoneal shunt,* in which the fluid is diverted into the peritoneal cavity (Figure 39–7).

Ventricular shunting is indicated when increased intracranial volume or pressure, usually due to hydrocephalus, interferes with or threatens normal neurologic function. Occasionally, shunting is indicated as a temporary measure to stabilize a client whose neurologic condition is rapidly deteriorating because of increased ICP. This is often the case when an intracranial lesion obstructs the flow of ventricular fluid. The treatment of choice is removal of the lesion creating the blockage. Temporary shunting may relieve intraventricular pressure and stabilize the client until the corrective operative procedure can be performed and normal CSF circulation is restored. Temporary shunting may also "buy time" for the client with a resectable lesion who requires additional diagnostic studies or time for the medical or nutritional status to improve. Following head injury or during radiation therapy to the brain, temporary decompression of the ventricular system may dramatically improve the clinical picture by providing a degree of additional intracranial space during the period of acute brain swelling. For the client with a CSF leak, the goal of

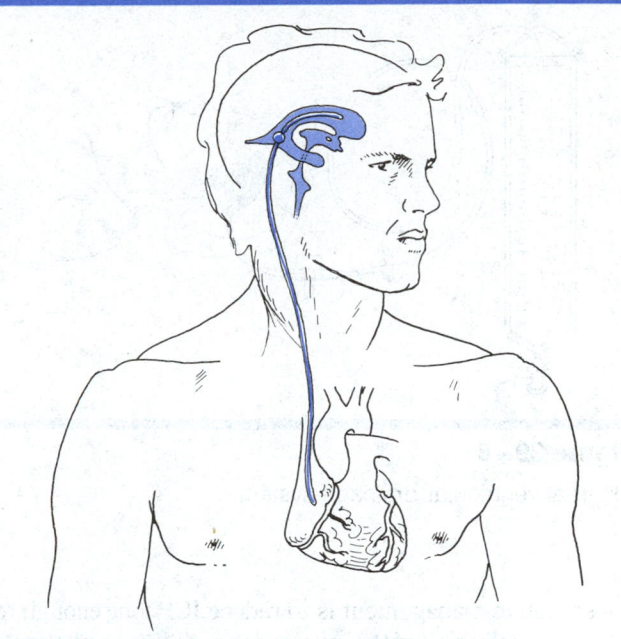

Figure 39–6
Ventricular–atrial shunt.

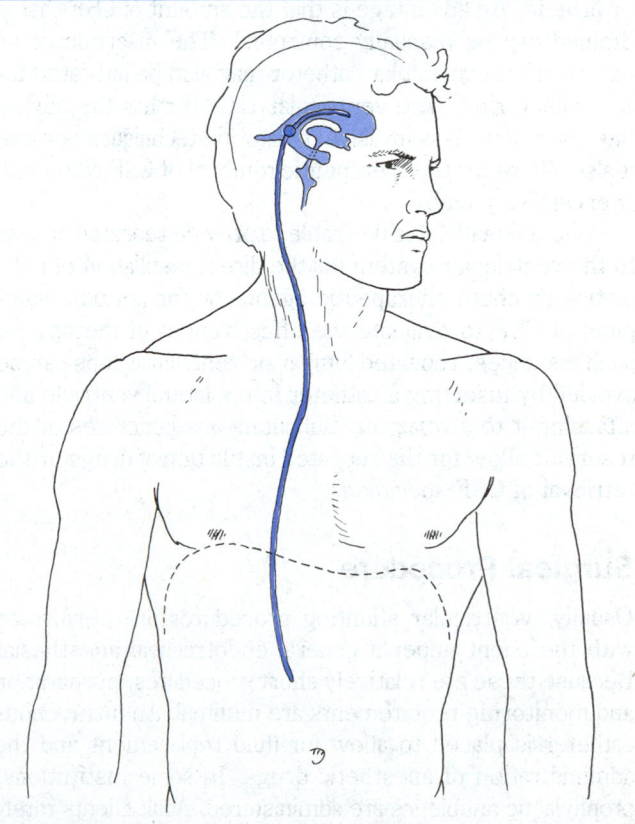

Figure 39–7
Ventricular–peritoneal shunt.

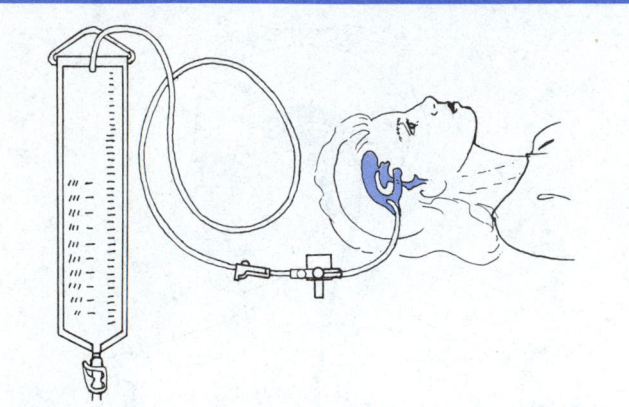

Figure 39–8

External ventricular drainage system.

conservative management is to reduce ICP long enough to allow for sealing off of the involved area. Temporary shunting may accomplish that goal.

One temporary measure is the shunting of CSF to an *external drainage* system (Figure 39–8). This technique is used if the shunting of CSF into the peritoneal cavity or vascular system is contraindicated. This is the case when infection within the ventricular system is present or suspected or when the CSF contains large amounts of blood or protein. An advantage is that the amount of CSF that is drained can be manually controlled. The insertion of an externalized ventricular catheter may also be indicated for ICP monitoring. The ventricular catheter has the advantage over other less invasive monitoring techniques because it also allows for the therapeutic removal of CSF when ICP is excessively high.

Occasionally, it is desirable to provide repeated access to the ventricular system for the direct instillation of antibiotics or chemotherapeutic agents or for periodic sampling of CSF to evaluate the effectiveness of therapy. In such instances, repeated lumbar or ventricular taps can be avoided by inserting a catheter into a lateral ventricle and attaching it to a *reservoir*. Subcutaneous punctures of the reservoir allow for the repeated instillation of drugs or the retrieval of CSF specimens.

Surgical Procedure

Usually, ventricular shunting procedures are performed with the client under a general endotracheal anesthesia. Because these are relatively short procedures, preparation and monitoring requirements are minimal. An intravenous catheter is placed to allow for fluid replacement and the administration of anesthetic drugs. In some institutions, prophylactic antibiotics are administered. Adult clients rarely need blood replacement, but many surgeons prefer having a unit of blood crossmatched and available. Continuous cardiac monitoring is carried out because changes in ventric-

ular pressure may precipitate changes in heart rate and rhythm.

The client is usually supine with the head slightly elevated and turned so that the operative side is uppermost. Special supports and fixation devices are not usually necessary. In most instances, the ventricular puncture is made on the right side to avoid traversing the cortex of the dominant hemisphere. The amount of hair shaved depends on the surgeon's preference and the client's wishes. For a ventricular–atrial shunt, the antiseptic preparation of the skin includes the neck as well as the head and is extended down to include the chest and abdomen when a peritoneal shunt is planned.

Shunt components are made of a medical-grade elastomer that is nonreactive in body tissue and fluids. These components are commercially available in a wide variety of designs, sizes, and pressure ranges. Although one-piece systems have become available, many surgeons prefer the original technique of inserting and connecting components to meet the needs of each client. Most shunt catheters include some type of radiopaque marker to aid in determining their exact position by x-ray. Many are also reinforced with a wire coil that prevents collapse or kinking of the catheter.

A shunt system consists of a ventricular catheter and a distal catheter, which usually is placed either in the right atrium of the heart or the peritoneal cavity. All shunt systems include a valve system, which is designed to open and drain ventricular fluid when the pressure in the tube exceeds that set by the manufacturer. When the pressure in the ventricle falls below the specified level, the valve remains closed, and no drainage or backflow occurs. Valves are manufactured in a wide variety of pressure ranges. They may be incorporated into the distal catheter or may consist of a separate unit placed between the ventricular and distal catheters.

Usually, a reservoir is also inserted between the ventricular and distal catheters. The reservoir can be punctured through the scalp to irrigate the shunt system, to allow insertion of medication or contrast material into the ventricular system or to obtain a CSF sample. External digital compression can also be applied to the reservoir to flush the shunt system or to check its patency. If the reservoir compresses easily and then quickly returns to its original shape, the shunt system is assumed to be functioning.

Ventricular–Atrial Shunt

Ventricular–atrial shunting diverts CSF from the lateral ventricle into the right atrium of the heart (Figure 39–6). This procedure is contraindicated when meningitis, ventriculitis, bacteremia, septicemia, or skin infection are present or suspected anywhere along the shunt. An atrial shunt should also be avoided if there is any evidence of cerebrovascular or cardiopulmonary disease.

The ventricular catheter can be placed in either the frontal or the occipital horn of the lateral ventricle. A small

Nursing Research Note

Williams M: Arteriovenous malformations: Complications of surgical intervention and implications for nursing. *J Neurosurg Nurs* 1985; 17(1):14−21.

Arteriovenous (A-V) malformations are congenital anomalies between arterial and venous vessels most often seen in young adults. Case studies examined complications resulting from surgery. Over 20 months, 24 clients with A-V malformations were seen. Treatment included either embolization via angiography or surgical resection of the malformation using microsurgical resection. There were no deaths in the group receiving embolization; one death occurred in the group having microsurgical resection. Preoperative hemorrhage occurred in 54% of the embolized group and 61% of the surgical group. After 1 year, there was no hemorrhaging in either group. Preoperative seizures occurred in 73% of the embolized group and 61% of the surgical group. Neither group had seizure activity at the 1-year follow-up. Thirty-six percent of the embolized group had preoperative hemiparesis, 36% had speech deficits, and 18% had visual disturbances. For the surgical group, 46% had hemiparesis, 23% had speech deficits, and 39% had visual problems. At 1-year follow-up, 36% of the embolized clients still had hemiparesis, 27% had visual abnormalities, and 9% had speech deficits. Twenty-three percent of the surgical clients had hemiparesis, 39% had visual problems, and 16% had speech deficits. Combining both groups, 29% had no post-treatment sequelae, and 37% were deficit-free after 1 year.

In providing nursing care for clients with A-V malformations, it is essential to assess for and try to prevent impaired pulmonary status, cerebral tissue ischemia, confusion, alterations in fluid and electrolyte balance, memory and thought process impairment, and fear of role disturbances in the family unit.

skin incision is made above and behind the ear when the catheter is to be placed in the occipital horn or behind the hairline, adjacent to the coronal suture to catheterize the frontal horn. A burr hole is made in the skull large enough for insertion of the catheter and placement of a reservoir.

For the other end of the shunt, a small incision is made in the neck along the medial border of the clavicle. The sternocleidomastoid muscle is separated and retracted to expose the facial or jugular vein. A small incision is made into the vein, and the distal end of the cardiac catheter is threaded into the vein to a premeasured distance. Proper positioning of the tip of the catheter in the right atrium is verified by image intensifier fluoroscopy or chest x-ray. The position can also be confirmed by attaching a sterile ECG electrode to a blunt needle filled with hypertonic saline. Characteristic ECG changes are noted as the catheter passes into the right atrium. Once localization is verified, the catheter is secured with a purse-string suture.

A subcutaneous tunnel is created extending from the burr hole to the neck incision using a tunneling device. The proximal end of the atrial catheter is threaded through the tunneling device to the burr hole where it is cut to size

and secured to the valve or reservoir. The neck and scalp wounds are checked for hemostasis and then closed.

Ventricular−Peritoneal Shunt

Because of complications associated with an intracardiac catheter, especially in children and adolescents (see Physiological Implications), the relatively safe and simple technique of ventricular−peritoneal shunting has gained favor. In many institutions, it is the operation of choice for hydrocephalus.

The ventricular portion of this operation is the same as for an atrial shunt. After placement of the ventricular catheter, a small incision is made just below the costal margin, and the muscles are retracted to expose a small area of peritoneum. The peritoneum is lifted away from the abdominal viscera, and a purse-string suture is placed. A small incision is made within the boundaries of the purse-string suture, and the distal end of the catheter is threaded into the abdominal cavity to the desired length. The purse-string is pulled closed to hold the catheter securely. Some surgeons prefer not to open the peritoneum surgically but instead to insert the catheter by passing it through a percutaneously placed trocar.

The tunneling device is then passed from the burr hole under the superficial tissue of the neck and chest to the abdominal incision, and the peritoneal catheter is threaded up to the ventricular puncture site. In some instances, the tunneling instrument is not long enough to reach the burr hole site, and a small supraclavicular incision is necessary to advance the catheter up to the burr hole. The peritoneal catheter is then attached to the ventricular catheter with or without an intervening reservoir or valve system (Figure 39−7).

External Ventricular Drainage

The procedure is usually done using local anesthesia. In emergencies, it may even be performed at the bedside. Access to the lateral ventricle is obtained via a burr hole or twist drill. The distal end of the catheter is externalized, often via a separate stab wound to reduce the risk of introducing organisms from the skin, and attached to a sterile collecting system. Several commercial drainage systems are available. A makeshift system can be devised using IV tubing and a collection bag or bottle. The main advantage of commercial systems is that most have a one-way valve that prevents reflux of fluid or air into the ventricles (Figure 39−8).

Implications for the Client

Physiological Implications

Although relatively minor, a ventricular shunting procedure involves entering the cranial cavity. Therefore, many of the implications of craniotomy and craniectomy also apply. The most common complications are increased ICP secondary to shunt malfunction and infection. Although relatively rare, postoperative subdural and intracerebral hemorrhage can also occur. Most other complications are the direct result of the implantation of a foreign object in human tissue (Horowitz & Rizzoli, 1982).

Shunt malfunction is probably the most common reason for removal or revision (Horowitz & Rizzoli, 1982). The malfunction can occur at the ventricular catheter, at the distal catheter, or at the valve or reservoir. It can also be the result of kinking or disconnection of any of the system components. Disconnection is often evidenced by swelling or fluid accumulation anywhere along the path of the subcutaneous catheter. Causes of blockage of the ventricular catheter are numerous, and including obstruction of the tip of the catheter by the choroid plexus, a blood clot, or high-protein CSF. Blockage also occurs if the tip of the catheter is resting in brain tissue rather than within the ventricle. This condition, easily identified on CT scan, may be the result of faulty initial placement of the catheter. Often, following correct placement, the tip may migrate out into brain tissue because successful shunting markedly reduces ventricular size. Valve malfunction is most often the result of blood within the valve itself or disconnection from the ventricular or distal catheter.

Problems related to the distal catheter are less frequent with peritoneal shunts than with atrial catheters. The atrial catheter, because of its location within the vascular system, is more susceptible to blockage. Most other complications are the result of a foreign substance within the cardiovascular system. Venous thrombosis associated with embolization into the pulmonary arterial system can occur. Although rare, cardiac perforation and pericardial tamponade secondary to the accumulation of CSF have been reported and can be life threatening if not promptly recognized and repaired. A disconnected atrial catheter can migrate into the ventricle and pulmonary artery. If left in place, it can result in cardiac dysrhythmia, perforation, septicemia, and embolization (Horowitz & Rizzoli, 1982).

Peritoneal catheter tip blockage most often results from obstruction by a piece of omentum. Insufficient absorption or complete failure of absorption may occur secondary to the formation of pseudocysts (probably a foreign body reaction) within the peritoneal cavity. Disconnection may result in the catheter being lost within the abdominal cavity. Though not common, perforation of the bowel, diaphragm, and pelvic organs have been reported.

Shunt revision is frequently required in children and may be required in adolescents because of somatic growth but is rarely necessary in adults, especially when the distal catheter is placed in the peritoneal cavity. The ventricular-atrial shunt may need revision because the cardiac catheter tends to become obstructed by thrombotic material.

Shunt failure in the shunt-dependent client is a special problem. These ventricles may not dilate despite shunt obstruction because of the loss of compliance of the surrounding brain tissue. The clinical condition may deteriorate rapidly from an acute increase in ICP.

Though rare, intracerebral hemorrhage can result from injury to blood vessels within the brain as the ventricular

catheter passes through the brain tissue. During revision, avulsion of choroid plexus that has become adherent to the catheter can cause intraventricular hemorrhage (Horowitz & Rizzoli, 1982). Subdural bleeding and subsequent hematoma formation are thought to be caused by an acute drop in ICP. As the ventricles are decompressed, the brain tends to shrink away from the dura, placing traction on the bridging veins that run between the dura and the cortex. Tearing of these veins results in the formation of a subdural hematoma, which may develop insidiously. Clients thought to be at particular risk are those with long-standing hydrocephalus, very high ICP, or extensive cortical atrophy (Arsenault, 1983). Another critical factor may be the rapid change in pressure. The minimal loss of CSF at the time of ventricular puncture plus maintenance of the recumbent position in the immediate postoperative period to reduce siphonage are believed to allow for a slow decompression that tends to minimize the risk (Horowitz & Rizzoli, 1982).

Overdrainage of CSF can cause persistent low-pressure headaches. If fluid loss is pronounced, headaches may be accompanied by nausea, tachycardia, and diaphoresis. Overdrainage is most frequently associated with external ventricular drainage because the amount of fluid drained is determined by the height of the drainage bag in relation to the ventricle. Overdrainage with a peritoneal or atrial shunt may necessitate revision to change the valve pressure either at the reservoir or the distal catheter so it closes at a higher pressure, maintaining a higher intraventricular volume.

Psychosocial/Lifestyle Implications

External ventricular drainage is used only for temporary control of ICP. The client remains hospitalized until permanent control can be achieved either by placement of a permanent shunt or removal of the cause. The effects of a ventricular–atrial or ventricular–peritoneal shunt on lifestyle depend on the underlying disease. Is the shunt the definitive treatment (as in normal-pressure hydrocephalus, aqueductal stenosis, or hydrocephalus secondary to a subarachnoid hemorrhage)? Or is it intended to control pressure until permanent relief can be obtained by tumor removal, radiation, or other form of therapy? Is the underlying disease process curable? These factors have more bearing on the situation than the shunting procedure itself.

Children must be relatively sedentary to avoid shunt disruption. For the adult, shunting should not place severe limitations on lifestyle. Often, the only limitation is avoiding vigorous contact sports because they may strain the subcutaneous portion of the catheter, leading to breakage or disconnection.

Clients who are shunt dependent need to be alert for signs of increasing ICP. Shunt failure can precipitate a rapid deterioration in the neurologic condition and can result in death if not properly corrected. An awareness of this danger can be a source of stress and anxiety for both the client and family. For such clients, travel may be limited because it is advisable always to be near adequate medical attention

Table 39–5 Ventricular Shunting Procedures: Implications for the Client

Physiological Implications	Psychosocial/Lifestyle Implications
Implications will depend on the underlying disease process necessitating shunting and the type of shunt procedure performed	External ventricular drainage offers only temporary control of ICP; need to remain hospitalized until permanent shunt is placed or cause is removed
Since the cranial cavity is entered, the implications outlined in Table 39–2 also apply	With the exception of avoidance of vigorous contact sports, shunting should not significantly interfere with lifestyle
Complications include increased intracranial pressure secondary to shunt malfunction and infection, possible subdural or intracerebral hemorrhage, tissue reactions to implantation of foreign material	Anxiety over possible need for shunt revision
Overdrainage of CSF is frequently associated with external ventricular drainage and can cause headaches, nausea, tachycardia, and diaphoresis	Travel may be somewhat restricted or limited to areas where medical facilities are readily available should shunt failure necessitate urgent intervention
Shunt revision to compensate for body growth may be required in adolescents	
Ventricular-atrial shunts may require revision if cardiac catheter becomes obstructed	

and surgical facilities. Client implications of shunting operations are summarized in Table 39–5.

Nursing Implications

Preoperative Care

Preoperative preparation and teaching are much the same as for any neurosurgic procedure. Provide specific information about the shunting procedure and postoperative routines. Assess client's and family's knowledge of the dynamics of hydrocephalus, the underlying disease entity, and the reason for shunting.

Postoperative Care

As with any intracranial procedure, frequent postoperative evaluation of the neurologic status is imperative. Promptly report and accurately document any indication of increasing ICP.

Specific nursing measures vary according to the type of shunt. The client with an externalized catheter usually has the head of the bed elevated. For the client with an internal shunting system, the head is kept flat or elevated only slightly to prevent siphonage via the distal catheter, which is well below the level of the ventricles. How long the head is kept flat and how soon the client is allowed to return to the full upright position depend on the physician's orders and the response of the client to progressive elevation.

Dehydration techniques are not usually employed, and diet can often be resumed after bowel sounds have returned. Observe the client for signs of infection—neck stiffness, fever, irritability or redness, or swelling or tenderness anywhere along the shunt pathway. Disconnection is often evidenced by subcutaneous fluid along the course of the

tubing. Because a subdural hematoma may occur as a late complication and shunt malfunction can occur at any time, be alert to subtle behavioral changes that may indicate deterioration—drowsiness, lethargy, apathy, change in orientation, irritability, or restlessness. Regardless of the cause of the shunt malfunction, prompt recognition of the symptoms and signs of increased ICP is imperative.

Discharge teaching should include the potential complications and their symptoms and signs. Both client and family should be able to explain the signs of increasing ICP as well as understand the need for prompt medical attention if they occur. Stress the importance of follow-up care.

For the client with an external ventricular drain, the major dangers are overdrainage, which can lead to ventricular collapse and/or subdural hematoma; underdrainage, with increased ICP; and infection.

Specific nursing measures are aimed at the prevention of these complications. Maintain the drainage bag or bottle at the level prescribed by the physician (usually at the level of the ventricles). Check the amount and characteristics of the drainage every hour. In addition, check the tubing for kinks, cracks, or leakage. Maintenance of the sterility of the system is essential. Exercise care when turning the client to avoid any tension on the tubing. If the tube accidentally becomes disconnected, do not reconnect it. Clamp it close to the client's head and notify the physician. Usually, the entire drainage system will be changed. It is wise to keep a spare drainage system available at all times.

To avoid overdrainage or underdrainage, never change the level of the head of the bed without making a corresponding change in the level of the drainage bag. It may be advisable to disconnect the plug on an electric bed or to tape over the manual controls to prevent accidental change in the head level. Some physicians may order that the tube be clamped during change of position, ambulation, or the client's absence from the unit for diagnostic studies. Extreme care must be taken to prevent the backflow of fluid from the drainage bag into the client's ventricular system. (Most commercial shunt systems have a one-way valve that prevents reflux, but it is wise to take no chances.) Notify the physician if drainage stops or accumulates rapidly. Drain-

age usually ranges between 150 and 250 mL in 24 hours. If the catheter is irrigated to maintain patency, use strict sterile technique and only sterile saline without preservatives. CSF samples may be obtained periodically. In addition, the serum sodium should be monitored because sodium is lost in the CSF and may result in hyponatremia.

Section II: Spinal Surgery

The major spinal operation is a *laminectomy*. This procedure involves the removal of one or more of the vertebral laminae to expose the spinal cord and its adjacent structures. In recent years, laminectomy has become a more general term, encompassing procedures that are not truly laminectomies, such as laminotomies and interlaminar procedures.

Most neurosurgery of the spine is aimed at relieving *compression*. Although the most frequent spinal operation is the resection of a herniated lumbar disk, there are numerous other congenital and acquired conditions for which a laminectomy is performed. These include the treatment of injuries such as fractures, dislocations, subluxations, and instability of the posterior elements; excision of tumors and vascular malformations; drainage of abscesses and hematomas; correction of deformity or disease of the vertebral bodies; repair of congenital malformations or acquired disorders of the spinal cord such as syringomyelia and Arnold–Chiari malformation; and bony compression of the cord or nerve roots due to narrow canal syndrome or arthritic bone-spur formation. Although less common, laminectomy may also be performed for the insertion of a subarachnoid shunt, for lysis of arachnoidal adhesions, and for the treatment of intractable pain by the sectioning of posterior nerve roots (rhizotomy) or the interruption of spinothalamic fiber tracts within the cord (cordotomy).

The traditional laminectomy for the treatment of herniated lumbar disk is discussed in Chapter 60. In recent years, the large laminectomies and fusions have given way to progressively smaller procedures such as hemilaminectomy and hemilaminotomy. In many institutions, these procedures have been replaced by a microsurgical approach.

MICROLUMBAR DISKECTOMY

Surgery for the removal of a herniated lumbar disk is the most common spinal operation and the eighth most common operation in the United States. Approximately 200,000 operative disk procedures are done annually (Maroon & Abla, 1985).

Microlumbar diskectomy is the microsurgical technique used in the treatment of a lumbar disk. Although techniques vary slightly, the main emphasis is the removal of the disk with minimal alteration of the lumbar spine. This procedure does not involve a laminectomy, and dis-

section of the paravertebral muscles is minimal. Access to the disk is gained via a small hemilaminotomy. Advantages over standard techniques include a much smaller incision, less soft tissue and muscle dissection, and the maintenance of the stability of the lumbar spine. The operating microscope allows for direct visualization of the nerve root as well as the herniated disk and extruded fragments. If necessary to further decompress the nerve root, foraminotomy can also be performed via the same exposure. In addition, the same amount of disk material can be removed as with the standard larger procedures.

Surgical removal of a herniated lumbar disk is indicated when conservative therapy has failed or when there is evidence of progressive CNS involvement, either motor or sensory. A trial of conservative therapy, often lasting at least 3 to 4 weeks, usually includes bed rest and the administration of analgesics and muscle relaxants. Applications of heat, physical therapy, pelvic traction, and back bracing may also be tried. Most herniated disks are amenable to conservative measures. More than 80% of clients with a confirmed herniation get well without surgery. Many clients have long remissions or suffer only one attack (Jennett & Galbraith, 1983).

The only two indications for urgent surgery on a herniated disk are sudden loss of bowel or bladder function or an acute total or almost total footdrop. Loss of bowel and bladder function is usually caused by cauda equina compression secondary to a massive disk extrusion. If not relieved within a few hours, the impairment will be permanent. With footdrop, if pressure on the nerve root is not relieved within a day or two, the footdrop is likely to be permanent.

Surgical Procedure

Most clients are given a general endotracheal anesthetic. Because this is a relatively short procedure, spinal anesthesia may also be used. The client may be positioned prone, lateral, at a 45° oblique angle (Figure 39–9), or in a modified knee-chest position. Regardless of the position, the chest and abdomen must be free of compression. Having the abdomen hang free not only reduces venous congestion and epidural bleeding, but also provides an added degree of safety. If the abdominal viscera, aorta, vena cava, iliac arteries, or ureters are compressed against the ante-

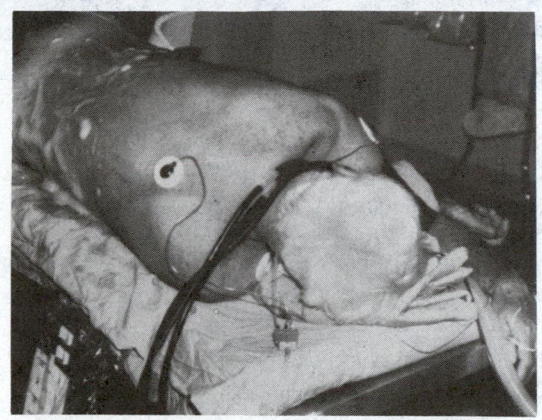

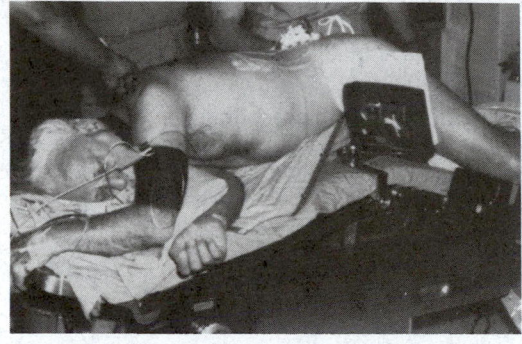

Figure 39–9

A. Client in 45° prone-oblique position. **B.** Proper supporting of the client in the prone-oblique position. (Courtesy of Leonard I. Malis, MD, The Mount Sinai Medical Center, New York, NY)

rior surface of the vertebrae, inadvertant injury by a surgical instrument could be catastrophic.

Because the skin incision is small, it must be placed precisely over the involved interspace. Often, a needle is inserted into the interspace or the spinous process above or below it, and a preoperative x-ray is taken to ensure that it is at the desired level. A 1-inch incision is made along the junction of the spinous process and carried down unilaterally to the interlaminar space. Complete emptying of the disk space is controversial. Some surgeons think it is necessary to remove only the extruded portion of the disk. Others think recurrence is more likely because fragments of the remaining disk material can herniate through the opened portion of the anulus fibrosis. When desired, the interspace can be as widely emptied with this microsurgical procedure as through a major laminectomy. The nerve sheath and dura are not opened. When disk removal is complete, a few sutures are placed in the deep fascia, and a few subcuticular sutures are placed in the superficial fascia. Most often, skin sutures are not used. Instead, the wound edges are approximated and held together with sterile wound tapes. Blood loss is ordinarily less than 50 mL.

Implications for the Client

Physiological Implications

Following surgery, recovery of function and relief of pain vary depending on the degree and duration of preoperative compression. As a general rule, the longer the preoperative symptomatology, the less favorable the outcome. In some clients, whose sciatica has persisted for years before surgery, the nerve root may be so damaged that some degree of pain, sensory loss, and decreased deep tendon reflexes may persist indefinitely. Following major preoperative cauda equina compression, motor recovery is usually slow, continuing over 18 months or more. Control of bladder function is regained slowly and is often incomplete (Jennett & Galbraith, 1983).

The overall success rate of microlumbar diskectomy is high: 80% to 90% of clients recover completely. Often clients awaken from the anesthetic and remark that their back and leg are free of pain. Continued pain is not necessarily cause for alarm, however. It is probably due to inflammatory changes in the compressed root, which may take considerable time to resolve. Persistence or recurrence of sciatic pain following initial postoperative relief may indicate migration of an additional piece of remaining disk material. Repeat radiological investigation and reoperation may be necessary to decompress the root.

Incisional pain is usually minimal because only a small amount of muscle dissection and retraction are performed. Stability of the spine remains intact because there is only a minor alteration in lumbar spine structure. In fact, the area of bone removal is often difficult to detect on x-ray. Because of immediate ambulation, the general postoperative complications related to immobility are rare.

Postoperative complications include hematoma, disk-space infection, CSF leak due to dural perforation, and recurrence. Hematoma, infection, and CSF leaks are rare. Pain or a complete disk syndrome recur in a small percentage of clients, sometimes several years after successful surgery and complete freedom from symptoms. Recurrence is usually due to recurrent herniation at the operative site or at a previously unaffected level (Jennett & Galbraith, 1983).

Psychosocial/Lifestyle Implications

For most clients, microlumbar diskectomy requires no alteration of lifestyle. Often lifestyle is enhanced by the relief of chronic or recurrent back and sciatic pain. Most clients require little or no analgesic and are allowed to ambulate freely following recovery from the anesthetic. They are usually discharged on the second or third postoperative day and allowed to return to their normal activities within a few weeks.

No restrictions are placed on sexual activity. Progressive athletic activities, such as swimming, are encouraged as soon as the wound has healed. Some surgeons prescribe muscle strengthening exercises. Heavy manual labor or strenuous sports may be restricted for a month or

Table 39–6 Microlumbar Diskectomy: Implications for the Client

Physiological Implications	Psychosocial/Lifestyle Implications
Following diskectomy, relief of pain and recovery of function vary depending on the degree and duration of preoperative compression; when sciatica has persisted for years, the nerve root may be so damaged that some degree of pain, sensory loss, or decreased DTRs may persist indefinitely	Lifestyle is usually enhanced by the relief of chronic or recurrent back and sciatic pain
Following cauda equina compression, motor recovery is gradual but often continues over a period of 18 months or more; control of bladder function is regained slowly and recovery may be incomplete	Most clients require no analgesics, can ambulate immediately, and are discharged on the second or third postoperative day
80%–90% of clients make a complete recovery	Sexual activities are not restricted; progressive athletic activities are encouraged
Inflammatory changes in the compressed nerve root may continue to cause postoperative pain before it resolves; persistence or recurrence of sciatic pain after initial postoperative relief may indicate recurrent herniation	Muscle-strengthening exercises may be required
Incisional pain is minimal and stability of the spine remains intact	Heavy manual labor and strenuous sports may be restricted for a month or so
Immediate ambulation lowers the risk of complications associated with immobility	Long-term follow-up is not necessary
Potential complications include hematoma, infection, CSF leak due to dural perforation, and recurrent disk herniation	Obese clients should be encouraged to begin a weight control program
	Clients with long-term preoperative restriction of activities may need physical therapy or a program of exercises to increase strength and develop supportive musculature

so; after that, no restrictions are usually necessary. Long-term follow-up is not usually indicated. Client implications are summarized in Table 39–6.

Nursing Implications

Preoperative Care

Preoperative preparation includes the standard measures and teaching appropriate for any surgical client. A thorough assessment of motor and sensory function as well as the characteristics and distribution of the pain should be documented for postoperative comparison. Analgesics and muscle relaxants are frequently prescribed, and steroids may also be administered to reduce the nerve root irritation. Because straining aggravates pain by increasing intrathecal pressure, stool softeners are often ordered. Because most clients have pain, they should be asked about prolonged or recent use of aspirin.

Postoperative Care

Some surgeons prefer to have the client remain flat in bed for 2 hours postoperatively to promote hemostasis. Most allow the client to assume whatever position is most comfortable and to be out of bed as soon as completely recovered from the anesthesia. Immediate assessment includes motor and sensory testing and comparison of the findings with the preoperative status. Question the client about the relief

or persistence of back and leg pain. Monitor vital signs as for any postsurgical client.

Although damage to the great vessels is rare and is usually discovered at surgery, it can cause retroperitoneal hematoma that may not be detected for several hours until the client develops a mass or exhibits signs of shock. Although impairment of blood supply to the lower extremities is also rare, assess vascular status of the legs. Check the dressing for any sign of bleeding or CSF leakage.

Assess the bladder for distention. Notify the physician if the client does not void within 6 hours following surgery. Allowing the male client to stand to void or encouraging the female client to get out of bed and use the toilet is often sufficient to stimulate voiding. If not present preoperatively, bladder dysfunction is rare following disk surgery but can occur as a result of manipulation of the cauda equina nerve roots and is usually transient. Ongoing assessment depends on the physician's orders and the condition of the client. As with any neurosurgical client, any decline in function from the immediate postoperative status or any acute increase in pain should be promptly reported.

Most clients have less pain after the operation than before. Narcotic pain medications are rarely necessary unless the client has a psychological or physiological dependence on them. Because the stability of the spine has not been affected, logrolling (turning the client as a unit) is not necessary. Clients are often apprehensive about movement, fearing that they can do damage or that movement will precipitate pain. They need to be reassured and encouraged to ambulate as soon as possible.

A full regular diet can be resumed as soon as bowel sounds have returned. Ambulation and activities are progressively increased, but some surgeons prefer that the client lie flat while in bed. This measure is taken because the semisitting position with the head of the bed elevated often precipitates muscle spasms in the lower back. Therefore, it is preferable to have clients dangle their legs at the side of the bed or sit in a straight-backed chair.

Most clients are discharged on the third postoperative day. Skin sutures can be removed in the physician's office or the outpatient department. When adhesive strips have been used for skin closure, the client is often instructed to shower after about a week, when the tapes can be removed.

Discharge teaching includes proper body mechanics. Encourage obese clients to begin a program for weight control. Some clients, especially those with long-term preoperative restriction of activity, may require physical therapy or an exercise program to increase strength and develop supportive musculature.

ANTERIOR CERVICAL DISKECTOMY

Herniated disks also occur in the cervical region, most commonly at C-5 to C-6 and C-6 to C-7. As with herniated lumbar disks, conservative therapy is recommended after x-rays demonstrate the absence of vertebral disease. Progressive weakness or failure of conservative therapy to relieve the pain are indications for future intervention.

Surgical Procedure

A number of surgical approaches are used. The classic cervical laminectomy is now rarely performed. If a posterior approach is used, an incision is made much like that described for the microlumbar diskectomy. Most often, cervical disks are approached anteriorly.

This surgery is performed with the client supine under general endotracheal anesthesia. Care must be taken during intubation to avoid hyperextension of the neck. Because the anterior–posterior diameter of the cervical spinal canal is narrowed when the head is extended, such a maneuver could compress the cord, because the room within the canal has been compromised by the extruded disk fragment.

As with microlumbar diskectomy, identification of the operative level is essential and may be accomplished by taking an x-ray with a marker at the operative level. Image intensifier fluoroscopy may be used preoperatively and during the procedure to identify bony landmarks. A unilateral incision is made parallel to the clavicle and carried through the platysma muscle. An incision is then made along the anterior border of the sternocleidomastoid muscle and carried down medial to the carotid sheath and lateral to the trachea and esophagus. A cervical vertebra spreader is inserted into the interspace and all of the disk material is removed.

Implications for the Client

Physiological Implications

Following surgery, the rate and degree of recovery depend on the degree and duration of spinal cord or nerve root compression. Clients have virtually no postoperative pain. Postoperative hoarseness may be the result of retraction of the trachea or unilateral vocal cord paralysis secondary to stretching of the recurrent laryngeal nerve. In most instances, unless the nerve has been severed, the condition resolves without treatment within a few days. Transient dysphagia can also occur from prolonged retraction of the esophagus. Esophageal perforation is a rare complication. Bleeding and hematoma formation is the main danger: tracheal compression and distortion can severely compromise respirations. Because bone removal is minimal, the stability of the cervical spine is not affected unless multiple levels are involved. Spontaneous fusion usually occurs within 6 months.

Psychosocial/Lifestyle Implications

Psychosocial/lifestyle implications are also similar to those for the client who has undergone removal of a herniated lumbar disk. Clients may be discharged from the hospital by the third day. Neck movements are not restricted. Initially, however, activities that excessively strain or stretch the cervical spine (eg, driving a car) may be restricted for a few weeks. For the client with a long history of pain, surgery usually means freedom from analgesics and muscle relaxants as well as the unsightly and often uncomfortable cervical collar. Activities are gradually increased and are usually unrestricted by the end of a month or 6 weeks. Unless occupational or leisure time activities impose a severe strain on the cervical spine, no change in lifestyle is usually necessary. Client implications are summarized in Table 39–7, on following page.

Nursing Implications

Preoperative Care

Preoperative medical management and nursing care are similar to those for the client with a lumbar herniated disk. The client should avoid excessive flexion, extension, and rotation of the head. Often a cervical collar is worn preoperatively to maintain the neck in alignment and to reduce pain by limiting movement. As with any neurosurgical client, document a baseline motor and sensory assessment. Record the history and description of the pain syndrome. In addition, evaluate the client for muscle wasting or atrophy and difficulty in performing activities of daily living.

Postoperative Care

Postoperatively, following a baseline assessment of motor and sensory function, assess neurologic status and vital

Table 39–7   Anterior Cervical Diskectomy: Implications for the Client

Physiological Implications	Psychosocial/Lifestyle Implications
The implications are similar to those outlined in Table 39–6 for microlumbar diskectomy.	
Herniated cervical disk may cause spinal cord compression as well as nerve root pressure; recovery depends on the degree and duration of compression	Discharge from the hospital by the third day is likely
Pain is usually minimal	Activities that involve straining or stretching of the cervical spine (such as driving a car) may be restricted for a few weeks
Hoarseness may result from retraction of the trachea or stretching of the recurrent laryngeal nerve; usually resolves within a few days	Activities are usually unrestricted by the end of a month to 6 weeks
Transient dysphagia can occur because of prolonged retraction of the esophagus	Freedom from analgesics, muscle relaxants, and cervical collar
Bleeding and hematoma formation can cause tracheal compression and compromise respirations; esophageal perforation is a rare complication	Unless occupational or leisure activities impose severe strain on the cervical spine, no change in lifestyle is necessary
Since bone removal is minimal, the stability of the spine is not affected unless multiple levels are involved	
Spontaneous fusion usually occurs within 6 months	
Early ambulation lessens the risk of complications related to immobility	

signs as ordered or as indicated by the client's condition. In most instances, these assessments decrease in frequency as the client's condition improves and are often discontinued or reduced to once per shift after the first 24 hours. Assess swallowing and speech. Inspect the dressing frequently for signs of bleeding, and monitor the neck area closely for swelling or shift in the position of the trachea. Because tracheal compression can be life threatening, have emergency respiratory support equipment available. Report any decline in function or sharp increase in pain to the physician.

Pain is usually minimal, but steroids, mild analgesics, and muscle relaxants may be necessary. Often, a cervical collar is prescribed for a few days to provide support and minimize muscle movements of the neck. Most often, the client is permitted to ambulate the evening of surgery or the following day. Activities are gradually increased, and the client often is discharged within 3 days.

Activities that involve excessive stretching or straining of the cervical spine (eg, driving, tennis) are restricted for a few weeks, but normal lifestyle can almost always be resumed without restrictions. As with lumbar diskectomy, the client who has had a long period of restricted activity preoperatively may require general muscle-strengthening exercises to achieve optimal function and well-being.

MULTILEVEL POSTERIOR LAMINECTOMY

Multilevel posterior laminectomy is the removal of one or more of the vertebral laminae. Because most indications

for this procedure involve compression of the spinal cord on its nerve roots because of conditions such as stenosis of the cervical or lumbar canal, spinal cord tumors, or a metastatic lesion from elsewhere in the body, many physiological, psychosocial/lifestyle, and nursing care implications are similar regardless of the underlying pathology. Spinal stenosis and spinal cord tumors are used as examples.

Surgical Procedure

The location, nature, and extent of the lesion determine the operative position as well as the type and amount of intraoperative monitoring. When the lesion is confined to the cervical region, the client is often placed in a sitting position. For the remainder of the spine, the prone or a side-lying position is usually used.

Because these procedures can be lengthy, an in-dwelling catheter is often inserted. When the lesion is expected to be extensive or highly vascular, an arterial line may be inserted for precise blood pressure monitoring. A CVP line or Swan–Ganz catheter may also be used when excessive blood loss is anticipated, when the client has significant cardiac or pulmonary disease, or when the sitting position is used.

Preoperatively, the area of the bone removal may be localized by x-ray (Figure 39–10) and the skin marked at the appropriate levels. A linear midline skin incision is made over the spinous processes for the desired length of the exposure and carried down through the deep fascia bilaterally to expose the tips of the spinous processes.

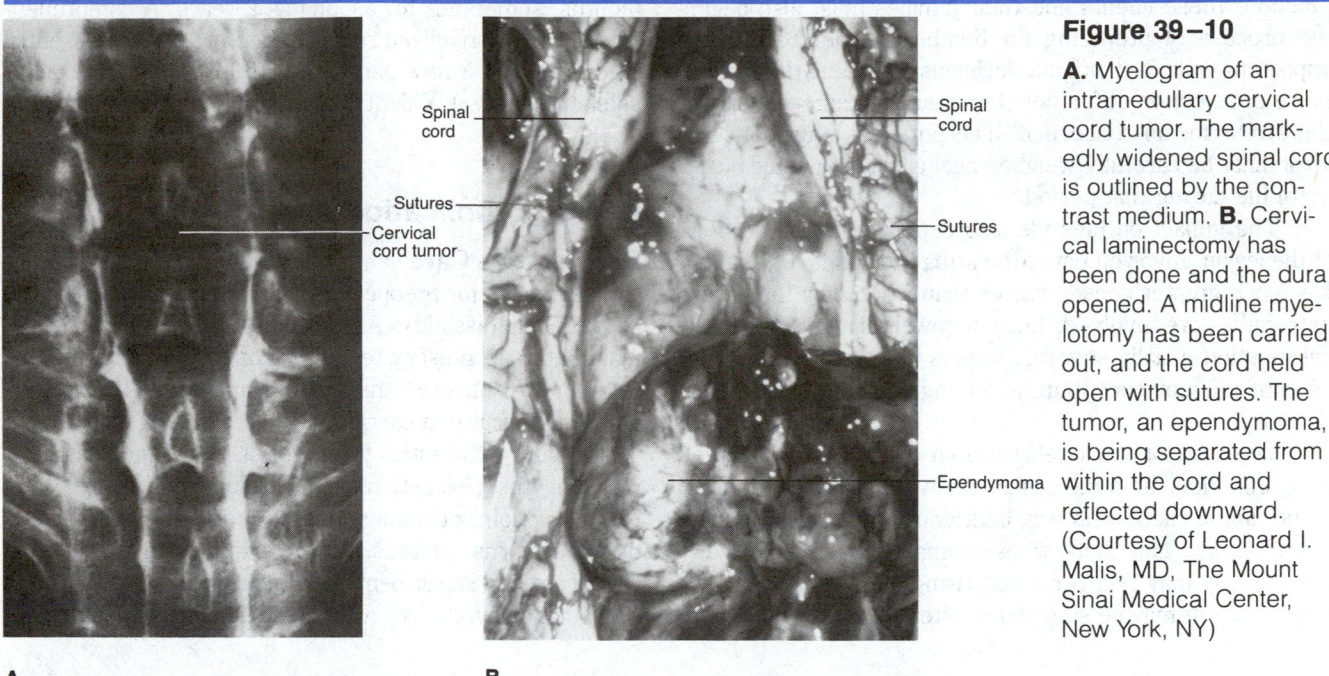

Figure 39–10

A. Myelogram of an intramedullary cervical cord tumor. The markedly widened spinal cord is outlined by the contrast medium. **B.** Cervical laminectomy has been done and the dura opened. A midline myelotomy has been carried out, and the cord held open with sutures. The tumor, an ependymoma, is being separated from within the cord and reflected downward. (Courtesy of Leonard I. Malis, MD, The Mount Sinai Medical Center, New York, NY)

When the laminectomy is performed for the treatment of spinal stenosis, bone removal is all that is required to treat the condition. Bone removal permits the dural sac to expand backward and eliminate compression of the cord. When underlying pathology is to be treated, the procedure varies from this point on, depending on the lesion and its resectability.

The exposed dura may be covered with a sheet of absorbable gelatin sponge (Gelfoam). Frequently, a wound drain is left in place. Subcutaneous and skin closure is done with separate suture layers. This closure is remarkably strong. After healing is complete, the scar provides adequate protection for the spinal cord, so the absence of the bony structure does not lead to damage or injury. Also remarkable is the fact that this extensive bone removal does not produce significant instability, providing either the anterior or lateral structures are intact. Accordingly, no fusion or stabilization is required. If adequate hemostasis has been maintained throughout the procedure, blood loss is often below the amount that requires replacement.

Implications for the Client

Physiological Implications

The spinal cord turns, twists, stretches, and moves to a great degree. The one stress the spinal cord cannot tolerate is compression. Spinal cord compression causes a transverse lesion that affects to some extent all cord function (motor, sensory, and autonomic) below that level (Jennett & Galbraith, 1983).

Recovery depends on the level of the lesion, the degree and anatomic distribution of the compression, the rate at which the compression develops, and the timeliness of the surgical intervention. Following decompression, function may return to a surprising degree, even after years of partial cord compression. Specifics in terms of recovery of function are discussed in the Psychosocial/Lifestyle Implications section that follows. The ultimate prognosis depends on the underlying disease process.

Clients are likely to experience severe incisional pain that gradually decreases by the third postoperative day. Possible complications include hemorrhage, CSF leak, and infection.

Psychosocial/Lifestyle Implications

With the spinal stenosis and the benign intradural tumors, surgery halts neurologic deterioration and offers the hope of recovery of function, which may be partial or complete.

The outlook for the client with a metastatic lesion is often bleak. If performed early enough, surgical decompression often allows for return of function and the maintenance of bowel and bladder control. Frequently, the spinal lesion is only part of a malignant disease process that has already severely disrupted the lifestyle of both client and family. When the spinal tumor is the first indication of an additional, as yet undetected, malignant lesion elsewhere in the body, the implications are far more devastating. The client and family must cope not only with the impact of the current situation but also with the consequences of the primary lesion. The diagnostic work-up to locate the primary tumor is often time consuming, expensive, painful, and frightening as well as physically and emotionally exhausting. The stress associated with fear of the unknown is often exacerbated by frustration and anger if early studies fail to track down the malignant source. In addition to grieving over the possible loss of neurologic function, these clients and their families must also begin the process of preparing for death. The need to make important and often difficult decisions regarding the acceptance or rejection of further therapeutic measures adds to the stress for all concerned. The potential length of survival must be carefully weighed against the expected quality of life during that period.

The impact on lifestyle also depends on the location of the lesion. Involvement of the arms and hands, of course, has much greater consequences than when only the lower extremities are involved. Loss of bowel, bladder, and sexual function usually severely affects body image and self-esteem and may contribute to feelings of helplessness and despair.

The need for active rehabilitation varies with the degree of dysfunction. In some cases, recovery is rapid and dramatic, and a client who was bedridden walks again within a few weeks. The client whose complete paralysis developed slowly may recover a surprising degree of function. Improvement may be slow, but it often continues for many

months, sometimes for as long as 2 years. A comprehensive and well-organized rehabilitation program is essential when there is severe paralysis with loss of sensation and sphincter control. Client implications are summarized in Table 39–8.

Nursing Implications

Preoperative Care

Clients' needs for preoperative care vary with the degree of functional disability. Assessment can begin before formal motor and sensory testing is done. If the client is able to ambulate, observe the posture and gait. Note impairment or difficulty in carrying out activities of daily living. Test all four extremities for motor strength and sensation, including the perception of pinprick, temperature, light touch, and joint position sense. Examine the skin for evidence of burns, bruises, or scars that might indicate an area of sensory impairment. Document any area of decreased sensation or hyperalgesia (excessive sensitivity) and com-

Table 39–8 Multilevel Posterior Laminectomy: Implications for the Client

Physiological Implications	Psychosocial/Lifestyle Implications
Recovery depends on: location, nature, and extent of underlying disease; degree and duration of neurologic impairment; ultimate prognosis for the underlying disease	Loss of bowel, bladder, and sexual function greatly affects body image and self-esteem; depression and despair are common
For spinal stenosis and benign intradural tumors, surgery will halt the progress of neurologic deterioration; recovery of function may be partial or complete	The need for and type of active rehabilitation varies with the location and degree of dysfunction
For the client with a metastatic lesion, decompression, if performed early enough, may allow for return of function and maintenance of bowel and bladder control	Profound lifestyle changes may be required, especially when the onset of dysfunction is sudden and unexpected (ie, trauma, metastatic disease), or when the cervical cord is involved
Recovery for the client with an intramedullary tumor varies with the malignancy of the tumor and the degree of resectability	Grieving over loss of function, regardless of cause, or possibility of death from an as yet undetected malignancy elsewhere in the body
The client with a slowly developing paralysis (even when complete) may recover a surprising degree of function; improvement may be slow but continues for many months	
Postoperative pain is severe for about the first 3 days because of extensive muscle dissection	
Bladder and/or bowel function may be temporarily or permanently impaired; respiratory function may be impaired, depending on the level of the lesion	
Clients with foramen magnum or high cervical lesions may develop sleep apnea due to bilateral damage in the area of C-1, which interferes with the normal respiratory response	
Possible complications include: hemorrhage; infection; CSF leak; complications in clients with spinal cord lesions are related to the hazards of immobility or specific motor or sensory deficits	

municate the findings to other staff members. Appropriate precautions can then be taken to avoid injury to an insensitive area and to protect the client from unnecessary pain or discomfort when a hyperalgesic area needs to be touched.

Care needs to be taken with the temperature of bath or shower water because decreased sensation can predispose the client to thermal injuries. For the client with a cervical or high thoracic lesion, pay special attention to the status of respiratory function. Question the client about any existing pulmonary problems that might complicate intraoperative or postoperative management. If respiratory insufficiency exists or might be anticipated in the postoperative period (eg, following removal of a high cervical intramedullary tumor), a baseline measurement of vital capacity and tidal volume may be helpful in assessing postoperative function. Also assess bowel and bladder function. Question the client about urinary frequency, urgency, dribbling, or retention; constipation or diarrhea; and fecal or urinary incontinence. Male clients may report impotence or difficulty in attaining or maintaining an erection.

The frequency of motor and sensory testing depends on the physician's orders and the client's condition. As with any neurologic condition, any deterioration should promptly be reported. Although it is relatively rare, be aware that a spinal tap, performed for removal of CSF for diagnostic purposes or for the instillation of contrast material for myelography, can precipitate an acute deterioration in the client's neurologic condition. Deterioration occurs because of alterations in the CSF dynamics; the reduction of pressure below blocks the circulation of CSF within the thecal sac. Immediate surgical decompression is often necessary to prevent catastrophic loss of function.

Preoperative teaching should prepare the client and family for expected postoperative sensations, devices, and routines (eg, monitors, cervical collar, motor and sensory testing). Warn them that incisional pain will be severe, but adequate medication will be provided to maintain comfort. Help them to understand that pain is to be expected and is not an indication of any problem or complication. Also reassure them that the stability of the spine will not be affected and that turning and ambulation, although painful, will not be harmful.

Postoperative Care

A baseline assessment of motor and sensory function is done as soon as the client is awake enough to cooperate and to answer questions. Even before this, observe the client's ability to move the extremities, either spontaneously or in response to a stimulus. Response to stimulus also gives some indication of sensory function.

Severe incisional pain is apparent almost immediately after the client's emergence from the anesthetic, and adequate analgesia is needed. If respiratory status is not compromised, intravenous or intramuscular meperidine (Demerol) or morphine may be administered every 3 to 4 hours. With adequate monitoring of blood pressure and respiratory status, a continuous intravenous infusion of morphine may be administered. Using this method, a surprising degree of relief can be achieved with significantly smaller doses than when the drugs are administered intermittently. The dosage is gradually reduced over 2 to 3 days, when oral analgesics are usually sufficient. Steroids are often prescribed to prevent or minimize the cord and nerve-root swelling that results from surgical manipulation.

After a client has undergone surgery in the cervical area, emphasize the assessment of respiratory status. Often, these clients are left intubated until adequate spontaneous respirations can be assured. Following extubation, remain vigilant because edema or bleeding at the operative site can lead to respiratory failure. After the excision of a tumor at the foramen magnum or C-1 to C-2 level, an apnea monitor is advisable because these clients may develop sleep apnea (also known as Ondine's curse). They breathe adequately while awake, but when they fall asleep their respirations become irregular and they may fail to breathe. The exact mechanism for this phenomenon is unclear, but it is known that the syndrome results from bilateral damage in the C-1 area of the cord, which interferes with the normal respiratory response to a rising blood CO_2 level.

Often, an in-dwelling catheter is left in the bladder during the initial postoperative period. Following its removal, assess bladder function and notify the physician if the client fails to void within 6 hours or if distention occurs. Bladder dysfunction may be transient or permanent and may necessitate the continued use of an in-dwelling catheter, a schedule for intermittent catheterization, or use of Crede's method to expel urine. Bethanechol chloride (Urecholine) may be administered to stimulate the bladder.

When bowel sounds have returned following anesthesia, the client is usually allowed to begin oral intake. Diet is progressed as rapidly as tolerated, and a high-protein, high-vitamin, high-bulk diet is encouraged. Stool softeners or a daily bowel regimen may be necessary to facilitate elimination.

If mobility is impaired, position clients to prevent complications and turn them every 2 hours. Perform active or passive range-of-motion exercises regularly to stimulate circulation, maintain muscle tone, prevent contractures, and maintain joint mobility. Because the stability of the spine has not been impaired, many surgeons do not think that logrolling is necessary. Because movement is painful, however, spinal alignment should be maintained. Clients with extensive incisions may benefit from logrolling in the initial postoperative period. A turning sheet facilitates turning. Unless the client is receiving continuous intravenous pain medication, turning and other potentially painful activities should be scheduled, as much as possible, to coincide with the time when pain medication is at maximum effectiveness. During changes in position, examine the skin for any signs of breakdown and massage areas prone to decubiti to stimulate circulation.

Often the client is ambulated with assistance, if only for a short time, on the first postoperative day. Ambulation, participation in self-care, and other activities progress according to the location and extent of the neurologic dysfunction. When neurologic damage is limited, the client can often be discharged within a week and may resume normal activities within a month to 6 weeks.

A decline in the neurologic condition may indicate a postoperative hemorrhage. A drop in the hemoglobin and hematocrit or changes in vital signs may help to differentiate bleeding from deterioration secondary to swelling or ischemia. Prompt detection is essential so the hematoma can be evacuated and the cord decompressed before permanent damage occurs. In the cervical area, the prompt detection of any decline in respiratory status can be life saving because a hematoma can result in sudden respiratory collapse.

Although the leakage of CSF through the wound is infrequent, the potential for this complication is increased when the dura has not been closed. A CSF leak may be evidenced by frank seepage of fluid through the suture line or by swelling at the operative site. Often, the fluid collection is only apparent when the client is up and about and subsides or disappears completely when the client lies in bed.

Infection can occur early or late and can be superficial and localized, or the client may exhibit symptoms and signs of meningitis. Most other complications in clients with spinal cord tumors are related to the hazards of immobility or the client's specific motor or sensory deficit. They can be prevented or minimized by aggressive measures.

Chapter Highlights

The significance or extent of a neurosurgical procedure is not necessarily indicated by the name of the surgical procedure; the specific nature, location, and extent of the pathology have considerable bearing on the plan of care for the client.

Postoperative neurosurgical clients must be carefully observed for any subtle or sudden decline in neurologic status.

The prognosis and recovery of many neurosurgical clients is based on the extent of damage to neural tissue inflicted by the lesion and/or the surgical manipulations.

Most neurosurgical clients and their families fear that death, disability, disfigurement, loss of intellectual function, and personality changes will result from the surgical procedure.

Neurosurgical approaches attempt to remove or correct underlying pathology while preserving neural and vascular structures to the extent possible.

Rapid drilling of a burr hole may be a life-saving measure in instances of rapid intracranial bleeding.

Cerebral edema and periorbital edema are expected reactions to manipulation and retraction of brain tissue.

A postoperative hematoma is the most devastating and dreaded complication of intracranial surgery.

One of the most important nursing measures is the assessment and documentation of the baseline neurologic status to provide a standard by which postoperative progress or deterioration can be measured.

The nurse on the postoperative unit should obtain a thorough report from the operating room nursing staff before receiving the client in order to set priorities, formulate a plan of care, and become alert to possible complications.

Level of consciousness often provides the first clue to a client's deteriorating neurologic condition.

Seizure precautions should be instituted on all clients following supratentorial craniotomy or craniectomy.

Suboccipital craniectomy is especially hazardous because of the concentration of vital structures in this small area.

Defects in the cranial vault can be corrected by cranioplasty.

Ventricular shunting creates an alternative pathway for removing CSF from the ventricular system.

Most neurosurgery of the spine is aimed at relieving compression. Recovery of function and relief of pain depend on the degree and duration of spinal cord or nerve root compression and the nature of the underlying pathology.

Bibliography

Arsenault L: Delayed onset symptomatic hydrocephalus related to aqueductal stenosis. *J Neurosurg Nurs* 1983; 15(5):291–298.

Bell M, Rekate HL: Cerebrospinal fluid dynamics. *J Neurosurg Nurs* 1978; 10(2):46–48.

Boss BJ: Dysphasia, dyspraxia and dsysarthria: Distinguishing features, Part I. *J Neurosurg Nurs* 1984; 16(3):151–160.

Boss BJ: Dysphasia, dyspraxia and dysarthria: Distinguishing features, Part II. *J Neurosurg Nurs* 1984; 16(4):211–216.

Hargrove R: Feeding the severely dysphagic patient. *J Neurosurg Nurs* 1980; 12(2):102–107.

Hayward R: *Essentials of Neurosurgery*. London: Blackwell, 1980.

Horowitz NH, Rizzoli HV: *Postoperative Complications of Intracranial Neurological Surgery.* Baltimore: Williams & Wilkins, 1982.

Jennett B, Galbraith S: *An Introduction to Neurosurgery,* 4th ed. London: William Heinemann, 1983.

Malis LI: *Intramedullary Spinal Cord Tumors in Clinical Neurosurgery.* Kenner EB (editor). Baltimore: Williams & Wilkins, 1978; 512–539.

Maroon JC, Abla A: Microdiscectomy versus chemonucleolysis. *Neurosurg* 1985; 16(5):644–649.

Michenfelder JD, Gronert GA, Rehder K: *Anesthesia in Neurological Surgery.* Youmans, JR (editor). Philadelphia: Saunders, 1982.

Rhodes PR (editor): *Core Curriculum for Neurosurgical Nursing in the Operating Room.* Chicago: American Assn Neurosurgical Nurses, 1980.

Ricci M: Neurologic assessment: Keeping it ongoing. In: *Coping With Neurological Problems Proficiently.* Robinson J (editor). Hosham, PA: Intermed Communications, 1979.

Ricci M (editor): *Core Curriculum for Neuroscience Nursing.* Park Ridge, IL: American Assn Neuroscience Nurses, 1984.

Smith J: Nursing management of diabetes insipidus. *J Neurosurg Nurs* 1981; 13(6):313–317.

Smith J, Geist B: Evaluation and care of the acute craniotomy patient. *J Neurosurg Nurs* 1978; 10(3):102–111.

Stern WE: Preoperative evaluation; complications, their prevention and treatment. In: *Neurological Surgery.* Youmans, JR (editor). Philadelphia: Saunders, 1982.

Stewarts MLK: When the patient has the "other" diabetes. *RN* (May) 1985; 54–58.

Swift-Bandini, N: *Manual of Neurological Nursing,* 2nd ed. Boston: Little Brown, 1982.

Wilkins RH, Odom GL: General operative technique. In: *Neurological Surgery.* Youmans JR (editor). Philadelphia: Saunders, 1982.

Suggested Readings

Jennett B, Galbraith S: *An Introduction to Neurosurgery,* 4th ed. London: William Heinemann, 1983. While not specifically intended for nurses, this text provides an excellent overview of current management of the neurosurgical client. It follows a logical and easy to understand sequence and includes a wide variety of conditions. Each section includes discussion of pathophysiology, symptoms and signs, diagnostic measures, management approaches, and possible complications.

Rhodes PR (editor): *Core Curriculum for Neurosurgical Nursing in the Operating Room.* Chicago: The American Association of Neurosurgical Nurses, 1980. The step-by-step descriptions of specific operative procedures and the rationale for each step are helpful in developing an understanding of the intraoperative phase. Most of the commonly performed procedures are covered and include a discussion of the underlying pathology, appropriate diagnostic measures, the objectives of surgery, preoperative physical and psychological preparation, considerations for the immediate postoperative period, and possible late and early complications. Excellent illustrations.

Ricci M (editor): *Core Curriculum for Neuroscience Nursing.* Park Ridge, IL: The American Association of Neuroscience Nurses, 1984. The Core is "designed to complement the learner's existing fundamental knowledge." The nursing process is used as a framework for presenting the most common neurologic and neurosurgical concepts. Behavioral objectives, comprehensive care plans, expected outcome criteria, and specific nursing interventions are included for each set of concepts discussed.

Potts DJ: How can I reassure my patient if I've never been in surgery. *Neurosurg Nurs* 1981; 13(4):211–216. This article describes the various routine medical and nursing interventions undertaken for the client undergoing a craniotomy and explains the rationale for each measure. Includes the pre-, intra-, and postoperative phases. Also provides the reader with an understanding of the role of the operating room nursing team.

Smith J, Geist B: Evaluation and care of the acute craniotomy patient. *J Neurosurg Nurs* 1978; 10(3):102–111. Provides a comprehensive guide for the care of the adult craniotomy client in the acute postoperative phase. It includes assessment of neurologic status, initial postoperative management, complications encountered, and the psychosocial aspects of care.

Youmans JR (editor): *Neurological Surgery,* (3 volumes). Philadelphia: Saunders, 1982. While this extensive three-volume text was not written for nurses, it is an excellent reference source regarding current concepts in the management of the most commonly encountered conditions treatable by neurologic surgery. Each chapter is written by a recognized expert in that particular field.

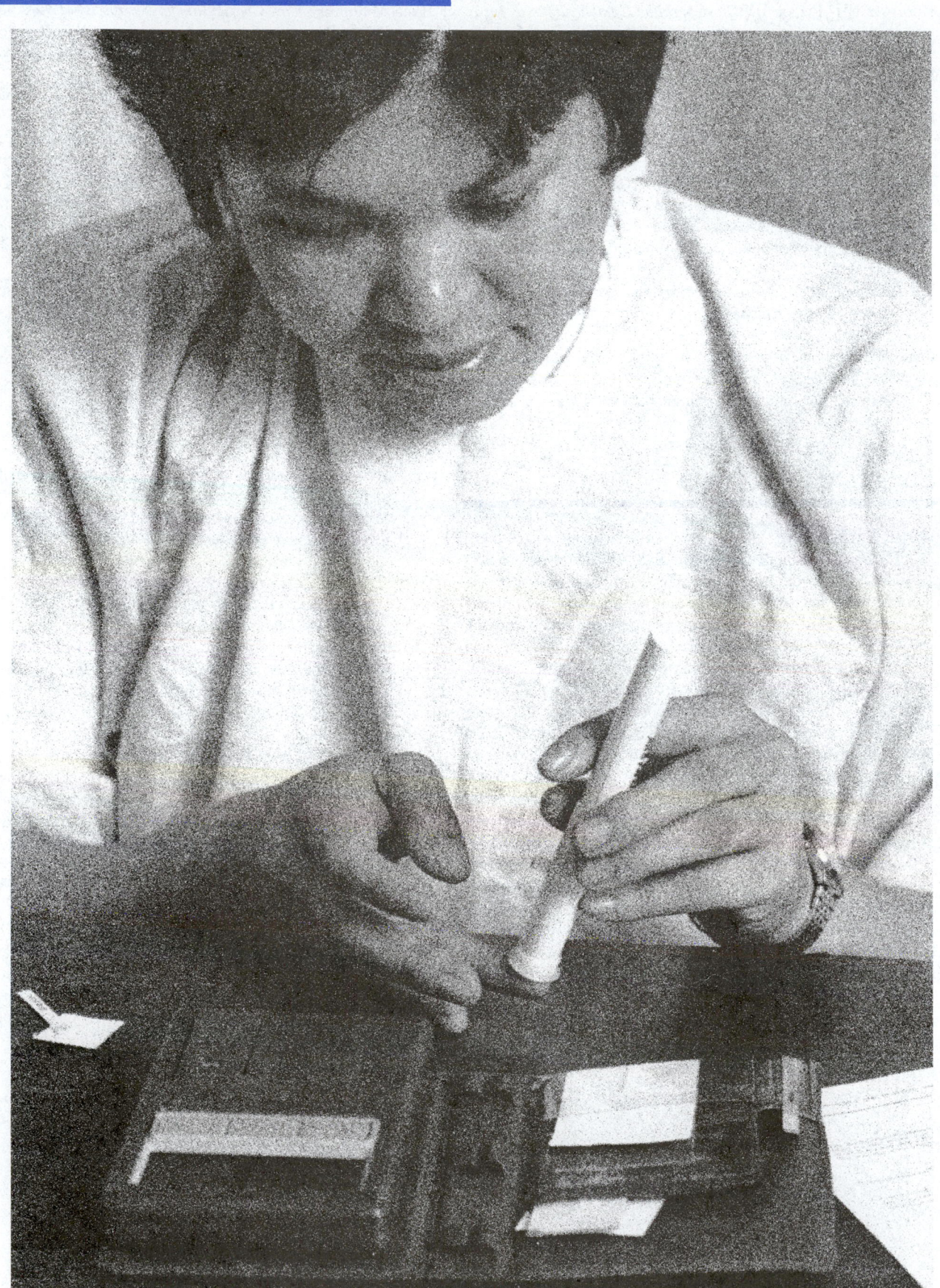

The Client With Endocrine System Dysfunction

Chapter 40

The Endocrine System in Health and Illness

Anne Herrstrom Skelly

The endocrine system can be thought of as a communications system that links all other body systems and affects nearly all physiological aspects of life. The system functions as an interrelated unit with the nervous system to maintain homeostasis. This interrelation is the subject of a new field of interest and study—neuroendocrinology.

Endocrinology often seems a complex and vast subject, but it is an exciting and challenging field because of the impact of the endocrine system on day-to-day functioning. Endocrinology is a rapidly expanding area of practice for nurses, as evidenced by the appearance of diabetic nurse clinicians and nursing specialists in endocrinology.

Section I: Structural and Functional Interrelationships

The endocrine system is a complex of glands that are not anatomically continuous but are interrelated so they function as an organ system. Traditionally, the endocrine system has been defined as a system of glands that secrete hormones directly into the bloodstream. In contrast, the exocrine glands secrete their hormones through ducts or directly into the intestinal lumen or onto the skin.

The principal functional units in the system are the endocrine glands: the pituitary, thyroid, parathyroid, adrenal, and pineal glands; the cells of the islets of Langerhans in the pancreas; the gonads (ovaries and testes); and the thymus (Figure 40–1). The kidneys also perform an endocrine function. Some of these glands are solely endocrine in function, whereas others form parts of larger organs

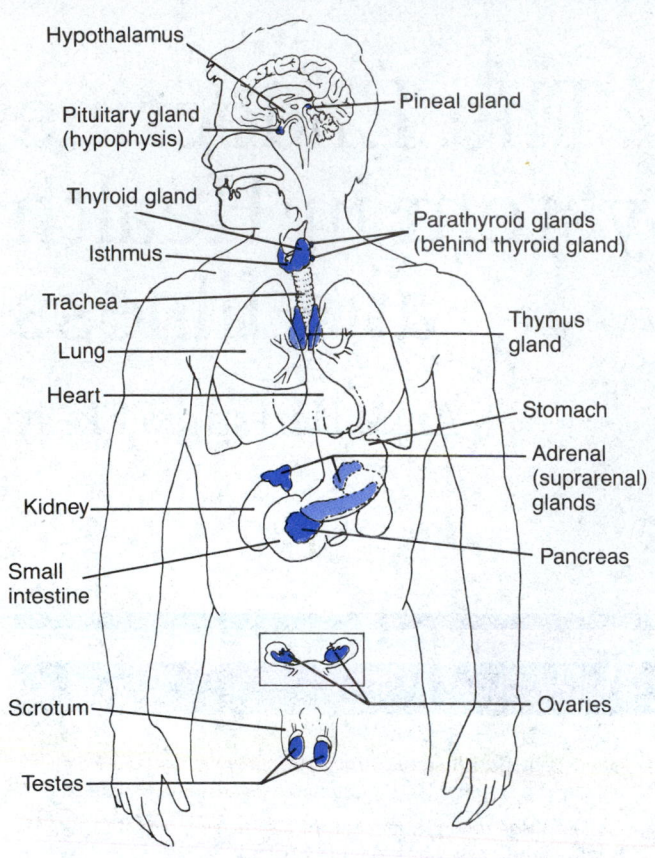

Figure 40–1

The endocrine glands and related structures.

that may have both endocrine and nonendocrine functions. For example, the pituitary, thyroid, parathyroid, pineal, and adrenal glands have distinct endocrine functions, whereas the pancreas has both an endocrine and an exocrine function. The gonads are involved in the production of germ cells as well as hormones. The thymus, besides producing hormones, is involved in the body's immune processes. The kidneys produce two hormones and an enzyme.

STRUCTURE OF THE ENDOCRINE GLANDS

Pituitary Gland

The pituitary gland (hypophysis) is located in the sella turcica at the base of the skull. It lies just below the hypothalamus and is connected to it by a stalk containing blood vessels and nervous tissue. The pituitary gland is composed of an anterior and posterior lobe (**adenohypophysis** and **neurohypophysis,** respectively), each of which performs specific functions, and a rudimentary intermediate lobe.

Thyroid Gland

The thyroid gland lies in the anterior central portion of the neck below the larynx. It is composed of two lobes joined by a strip of tissue called the *isthmus*. The thyroid gland lies anterior to the trachea and receives an abundant blood supply. Knowing the proximity of the thyroid gland to the recurrent laryngeal nerve, which innervates the larynx, is critical for postoperative care. Damage to the recurrent laryngeal nerve during surgery can affect the client's breathing and voice production.

Parathyroid Glands

The parathyroid glands are paired and usually total four, although the actual number may vary; some persons have two glands and others, as many as six. They are usually located on the posterior surface of the thyroid gland, beneath the capsular covering. The parathyroid glands may actually be embedded in the tissue of the thyroid; because of their minute size and variability in number and location, they are often hard to locate. This can result in their accidental excision during thyroid surgery, causing temporary hypoparathyroidism if more than three glands are affected. If this should occur, one gland can produce the necessary amount of hormone if it is able to increase in size sufficiently to meet the increased demand.

Adrenal Glands

The adrenal glands are paired and located in the retroperitoneal space at the upper pole of the kidney. Because of this position, they may be referred to as the *suprarenal glands*. Each adrenal gland consists of an outer portion (the cortex) and an inner portion (the medulla), which differ in both anatomic structure and function.

The adrenal cortex is composed of three zones, or groups of different cells: the zona glomerulosa (the outer layer of cortical cells that secretes the mineralocorticoids), the zona fasciculata (the middle layer of cortical cells that secrete the glucocorticoids), and the zona reticularis (the layer of cortical cells proximal to the medulla that secretes the adrenal sex hormones, androgens and estrogen).

The adrenal glands receive an abundant blood supply. The medulla of the adrenal gland functions as part of the sympathetic nervous system, whereas the cortex has only minimal nervous system innervation.

Pancreas

The pancreas lies transversely deep in the abdomen along the posterior aspect and can be found in the epigastric area and left upper quadrant. Both sympathetic and parasympathetic nerve fibers innervate it. The pancreas performs both endocrine and exocrine functions. The islets of Langerhans are involved in endocrine function and contain at least three types of hormone-secreting cells: alpha, beta, and delta. The alpha cells are thought to secrete glucagon; the beta cells, insulin; and the delta cells, somatostatin. Refer to Chapter 46 for a discussion of the exocrine functions of the pancreas.

Gonads

The gonads—the testes and the ovaries—are the organs of reproduction. The gonads are discussed in Chapters 61 and 62.

Thymus

The thymus is a flat structure consisting of two symmetrical lobes located in the mediastinal cavity anterior and superior to the heart. The size of the thymus varies with age. Compared with body size, it is the largest at birth and for the first 2 years of life; it then grows slowly until puberty, when it begins to atrophy.

Pineal Gland

The pineal gland (epiphysis cerebri) has a characteristic pinecone shape and is attached to the posterior portion of the third ventricle of the brain. It is composed of an anterior and posterior lobe and secretes a substance that acts as a base for calcium deposits within the gland. Calcification of the pineal gland starts at age 19, and by age 60, most pineal glands are partially calcified. The relation of this process to the actual function of the pineal gland in adults has led to much discussion and research.

FUNCTION OF THE ENDOCRINE SYSTEM

Generalized functions of the endocrine system include (Williams, 1981):

- Maintenance of the body's internal environment
- Response to internal and external challenges (stress, infection, and trauma)
- Growth and development
- Sexual reproduction

To describe how the endocrine glands perform these functions, it is necessary to review hormones and their roles briefly.

Hormones

A **hormone** may be defined as a "chemical substance synthesized by an endocrine gland and secreted into the bloodstream, which carries it to other sites in the body where its actions are exerted" (Vander, Sherman, & Luciano, 1980). Hormones may function independently, in conjunction with other hormones, or as a step in a series of related actions. They may influence the action, metabolism, synthesis, and/or transport of another hormone—one of the integrative aspects of the endocrine system.

Hormones can be differentiated into two major categories: Local hormones have specific local effects (eg, secretin, cholecystokinin–pancreozymin [CCK–PZ], and other gastrointestinal hormones). General hormones, in contrast, are transported by the circulation to distant sites, where they have a physiological effect (eg, cortisol). The endocrine hormones are summarized in Table 40–1.

Mechanism of Hormonal Action

Hormones travel throughout the body via the bloodstream, yet the body's response to them is highly specific. Only certain cells, known as **target cells,** have the capability to respond to a specific hormone in a characteristic way. Their response depends on the presence of specific receptors for a particular hormone. This response is called **hormone–target cell specificity,** and the process is known as **hormone–receptor binding.** The initial interaction between a hormone and its target cell receptor initiates a chain of biochemical events that eventually provokes a cellular response. This often involves a hormone-induced change in the activity of a specific enzyme found in the target cell that might change the rate of reactions within the cell, change the growth of the cell, or control the cell's secretion. Because cells are exposed to many hormones, complex hormone–hormone interactions can occur in target cells. These interactions may be inhibitory, synergistic, or permissive (ie, one hormone, by its presence, potentiates the effect of the second hormone). Vander et al. (1980) have postulated that many of these complex interactions are the result of the influence of one hormone on the other's number or affinity of receptors.

Hormone Structure and Receptors

Hormones include steroid, polypeptide, amino acid, catecholamine, or iodothyronine structures. The steroidal hormones are aldosterone, cortisol, and the estrogens and androgens. The receptors involved in hormone–receptor binding differ for steroidal and nonsteroidal hormones. The receptors for most nonsteroidal hormones are located on the outer surface of the plasma membrane of the target cells, whereas the receptors for the steroidal hormones are soluble proteins within the cytoplasm of the target cell. Possibly, several of the nonsteroidal hormones also have receptors within the cytoplasm of the cells. The physiology of hormone receptors is a rapidly expanding area of research in endocrinology.

Circulation of Hormones

Most hormones are not secreted at a constant rate. After secretion into the bloodstream, they circulate in a free form or are bound to proteins. Polypeptide hormones and the catecholamines are essentially unbound in the circulation. These free hormones are directly available to the target

Table 40–1 The Major Hormones: Their Sources and Effects

Endocrine Gland, Organ, or Organ System	Hormone	Target	Effect
Hypothalamus	Thyrotropin releasing factor (TRF)	Anterior pituitary	Secretion of TSH
	Corticotropin releasing factor (CRF)	Anterior pituitary	Secretion of ACTH
	Growth hormone releasing factor (GRF)	Anterior pituitary	Secretion of GH
	Somatostatin	Anterior pituitary	Inhibition of the secretion of GH, prolactin, and TSH
	Luteinizing hormone releasing factor (LRF)	Anterior pituitary	Secretion of LH and FSH
	Luteinizing hormone inhibiting factor (LIF)	Anterior pituitary	Inhibition of the secretion of LH and FSH
	Prolactin releasing factor (PRF)	Anterior pituitary	Secretion of prolactin
	Prolactin inhibiting factor (PIF)	Anterior pituitary	Inhibition of the secretion of prolactin
Anterior pituitary gland (adenohypophysis)	Thyroid-stimulating hormone (TSH)	Thyroid	Secretion of T_4, T_3, and calcitonin
	Adrenocorticotropic hormone (ACTH)	Adrenal cortex	Secretion of glucocorticoids (cortisol), mineralocorticoids (aldosterone), and sex hormones
	Growth hormone, or somatotropic hormone (GH, or STH)	Bones, muscles, organs	Promotion of growth and metabolism
	Luteinizing hormone (LH)	Ovarian follicle	Formation of corpus luteum; production of estrogen
	Interstitial cell-stimulating hormone (ICSH)	Testes	Production of testosterone
	Follicle-stimulating hormone (FSH)	Ovaries or seminiferous tubules	Development of ovarian follicle; secretion of estrogen; production of sperm
	Prolactin, or luteotropic hormone (LTH)	Corpus luteum, breasts	Maintenance of corpus luteum; secretion of progesterone; stimulation of milk secretion
Intermediate pituitary gland	Melanocyte-stimulating hormone (MSH)	Skin	Pigment deposition
Posterior pituitary gland (neurohypophysis)	Antidiuretic hormone (ADH), or vasopressin	Distal tubules of kidney	Reabsorption of water
	Oxytocin	Uterus, breasts	Stimulation of uterine contraction; secretion of milk; uterine motility; facilitation of movement of sperm in fallopian tubes
Thyroid gland	Thyroxine (T_4), triiodothyronine (T_3)	Widespread targets	Increase in metabolic rate; energy metabolism; regulation of growth; stimulation of gluconeogenesis; mobilization of fats; effect on protein metabolism
	Calcitonin	Skeleton	Decrease in plasma calcium levels

Endocrine Gland, Organ, or Organ System	Hormone	Target	Effect
Parathyroid glands	Parathyroid hormone (PTH) or parathormone	Bones, kidneys, GI tract	Increase in plasma calcium levels; regulation of phosphorus excretion
Adrenal cortex	Glucocorticoids (eg, cortisol)	Widespread targets	Effect on carbohydrate, fat, and protein metabolism; promotion of gluconeogenesis; mobilization of amino acids; suppression of inflammation; response to stress; effect on plasma glucose levels; lipolysis
	Mineralocorticoids (eg, aldosterone)	Distal renal tubules	Maintenance of fluid balance; reabsorption of sodium; excretion of potassium
	Sex hormones (eg, androgens, estrogen, progesterone)	Gonads	Influence on development of secondary sex characteristics and growth
Adrenal medulla	Epinephrine, norepinephrine	Widespread targets	Vasoconstriction; increase in blood pressure; gluconeogenesis (plasma glucose); sympathetic response to stress; stimulation of metabolism; secretion of ACTH
Pancreas	Insulin	Widespread targets	Decrease in plasma glucose aids glucose transport into cells; decrease in protein catabolism
	Glucagon	Liver, muscle, adipose cells	Increase in plasma glucose via glycogenolysis, gluconeogenesis, and lipolysis
	Somatostatin, or growth hormone inhibiting factor (GIF)	Pancreas, stomach	Inhibition of the secretion of insulin and glucagon
Gonads:			
Female ovaries	Estrogen	Reproductive tissues	Development of secondary sex characteristics; maturation of sexual organs; sexual functioning
	Progesterone	Uterus, breasts	Development of mammary tissue; maintenance of pregnancy; preparation of endometrium
Male testes	Testosterone	Widespread targets	Anabolism; development of secondary sex characteristics; maturation of sexual organs; sexual functioning
Kidneys	Renin	Renin substrate	Angiotensin I (regulation of blood pressure)
	Erythropoietic stimulating factor (ESF)	Bone marrow	Red blood cell production
	1,25-dihydroxycholecalciferol	Kidneys	Serum calcium levels
Gastrointestinal tract	Gastrin	Stomach	Increase in gastric secretion and motility; production of pepsin and intrinsic factor

(continued)

Table 40–1   The Major Hormones: Their Sources and Effects (continued)

Endocrine Gland, Organ, or Organ System	Hormone	Target	Effect
	Secretin	Stomach, pancreas	Decrease in gastric secretion
	Cholecystokinin–pancreozymin (CCK–PZ)	Pancreas	Decrease in gastric motility
	Gastric inhibitory peptide (GIP)	Gallbladder, stomach	Secretion of enzymes
	Somatostatin		
Thymus	Thymosin	Immune system	Lymphocyte development
	Thymopoietin	Immune system	Probable blocking of neuromuscular transmissions
Pineal gland	Melatonin	Hypothalamus, midbrain, gonads	Inhibition of GH secretion; decrease in plasma LH; increase in sleepiness; possible increase in well-being; sexual maturity

tissues, and only they can affect the target cells. The protein-bound forms are thought to represent a hormonal reserve, because the protein binding may prevent excretion of the hormone by the kidney. The amount of circulating free hormone is usually quite small and exists in equilibrium with the bound fraction.

Regulation of Hormones

There are five major influences on the secretion of hormones by the endocrine glands: the hypothalamus, hypothalamic releasing factors, anterior pituitary hormones, the autonomic nervous system, and nutrient and ion concentrations in the plasma (Vander et al., 1980). The hypothalamus affects hormone secretion by secreting a series of peptides called *releasing factors (RFs)*, which stimulate or inhibit the release of hormones by the anterior pituitary gland. The hypothalamus also directly manufactures oxytocin and antidiuretic hormone (ADH), or vasopressin. This relationship is shown in Figure 40–2.

The hypothalamic releasing factors cause the anterior pituitary gland to secrete growth hormone (GH), prolactin, thyroid-stimulating hormone (TSH), the gonadotropic hormones follicle-stimulating hormone (FSH) and luteinizing

Box 40–1   Summary of the Control of Hormone Secretion*

In response to neural, hormonal, or metabolic inputs, hypothalamic neurons themselves release:
   Oxytocin
   Antidiuretic hormone } (From the posterior pituitary)
   Hypothalamic releasing hormones

Hypothalamic releasing hormones directly control the release from the anterior pituitary of:
   Growth hormone
   Thyroid-stimulating hormone
   Adrenocorticotropic hormone
   Gonadotropic hormones (FSH and LH)
   Prolactin

Anterior pituitary hormones directly control the release of:
   Thyroid hormone
   Cortisol (from adrenal cortex)

Gonadal hormones
   (Female: estrogen and progesterone)
   (Male: testosterone)

Autonomic neurons directly control the release of:
   Epinephrine and norepinephrine (from adrenal medulla)
   Renin (from kidney)
   Insulin and glucagon (from pancreas)
   Gastrointestinal hormones
   ?Others

Plasma concentrations of ions or nutrients directly control the release of:
   Parathyroid hormone
   Insulin and glucagon (from pancreas)
   Aldosterone (from adrenal cortex)
   Calcitonin (from thyroid glands)

*This table does not necessarily list all the controls of each hormone.

SOURCE: Reproduced with permission from Vander AJ, Sherman JH, Luciano DA: *Human Physiology: The Mechanisms of Body Function*, 3rd ed. New York: McGraw–Hill, 1980, p. 201.

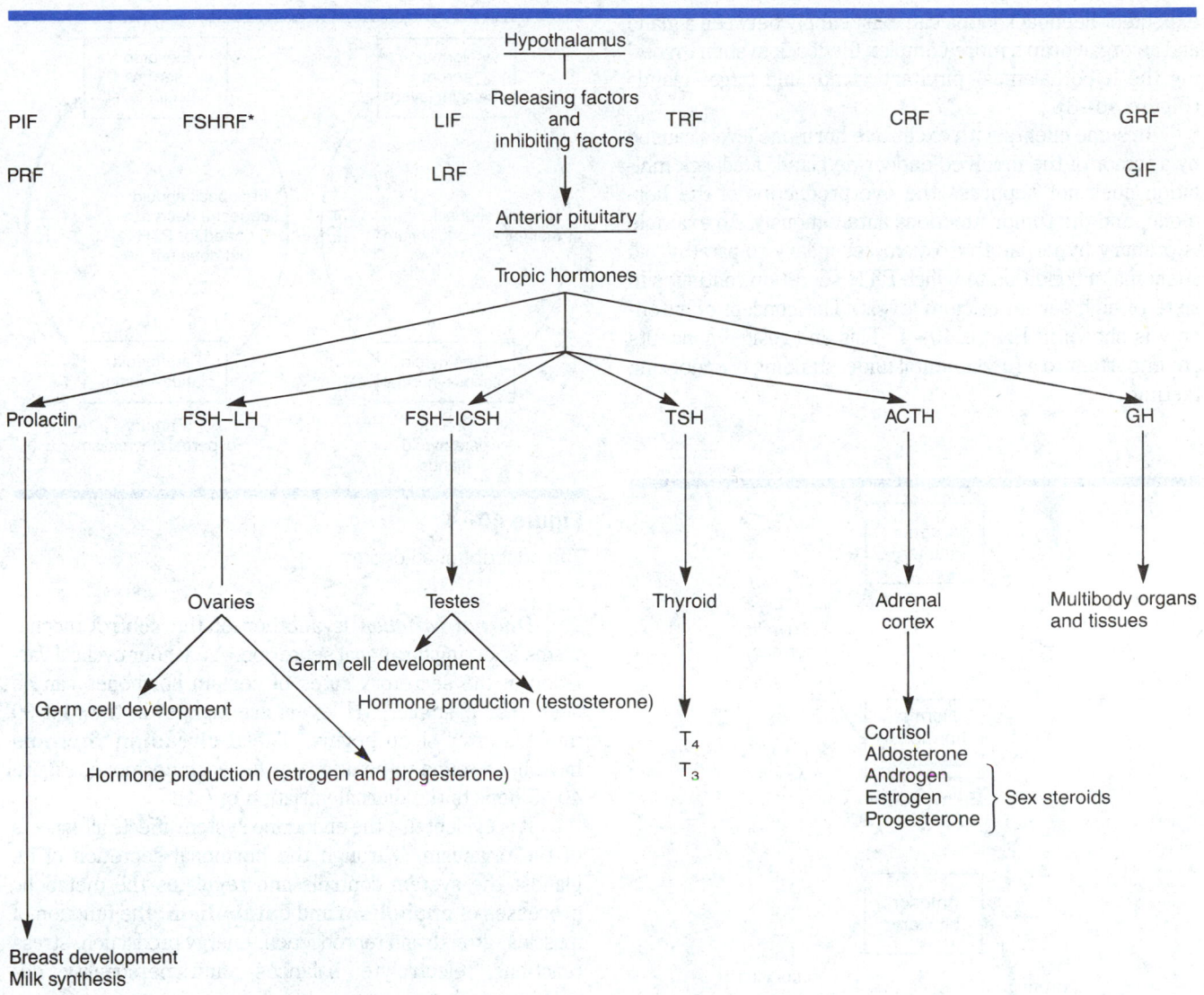

Figure 40–2

The relationship of the hypothalamus, anterior pituitary gland, and target organs.

hormone (LH), and adrenocorticotropic hormone (ACTH). The anterior pituitary hormones directly control the release of thyroid hormone (T_3 and T_4), cortisol, testosterone in the male, and estrogen and progesterone in the female.

The release of epinephrine and norepinephrine from the adrenal medulla, the gastrointestinal hormones, insulin and glucagon from the pancreas, and renin from the kidney are under the direct control of the autonomic nervous system. The adrenal medulla and posterior pituitary are under neural influence and function as part of the autonomic nervous system.

The secretion of parathyroid hormone (PTH), insulin, glucagon, aldosterone, and thyrocalcitonin is directly controlled by the amount of these hormones in the serum. Other controls of hormonal secretion are summarized in Box 40–1.

Feedback, Autonomy, and Diurnal Variation in Hormonal Regulation

Feedback mechanisms are also involved in the regulation of hormone secretion. For example, the anterior pituitary gland secretes TSH, which stimulates the thyroid to secrete thyroxine (T_4) and triidothyronine (T_3). As the serum levels of T_4 and T_3 rise, the secretion of TSH by the anterior pituitary gland is suppressed. If the serum levels of T_4 and T_3 fall, the anterior pituitary gland increases its secretion of TSH.

To apply this concept to a clinical situation, consider primary hypothyroidism and hyperthyroidism. In a client with primary hypothyroidism (low circulating levels of T_4), high serum levels of TSH are expected. Conversely, in a client with hyperthyroidism, low serum levels of TSH are expected. Feedback loops can exist simply between a gland and an organ or in a more complex feedback system involving the hypothalamus, pituitary gland, and target glands (Figure 40–3).

In some clients with excessive hormone levels caused by a tumor of the involved endocrine gland, feedback inhibition does not suppress the overproduction of the hormone, and the tumor functions autonomously. An example is primary hyperparathyroidism secondary to parathyroid adenoma, a condition in which PTH secretion continues in spite of high serum calcium levels. The concept of autonomy is shown in Figure 40–4. This and related concepts are important to a fundamental understanding of endocrine testing.

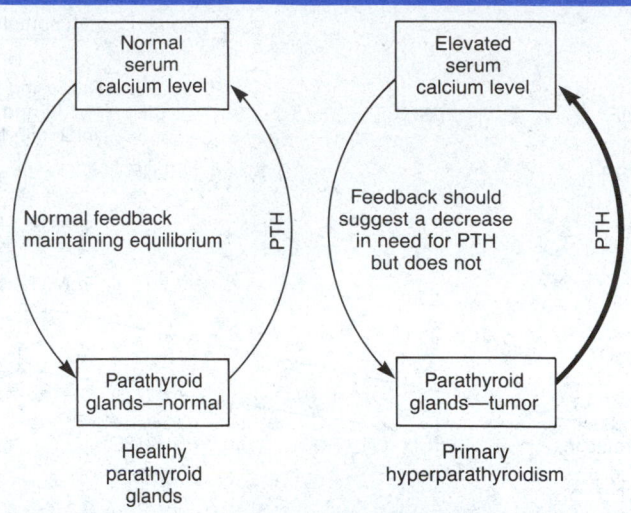

Figure 40–4

The concept of autonomy.

Diurnal variation is another of the control mechanisms affecting hormonal secretion. A 24-hour cyclical variation in the secretory rates of certain hormones can be seen. For example, GH levels are highest in the first 90 minutes after sleep begins. These **circadian rhythms** have been found to be different for each hormone. Figure 40–5 depicts the diurnal variation of GH.

It is evident that the endocrine system affects all aspects of the organism. Through the hormonal secretion of its glands, the system controls and regulates the metabolic processes of **anabolism** and **catabolism,** the function of muscles, growth and reproduction, energy production, stress reactions, electrolyte balances, and personality development.

REGULATORY FUNCTIONS OF THE ENDOCRINE SYSTEM

Hypothalamus

The hypothalamus functions as an integral part of both the endocrine and nervous systems. In its neural role, it receives and processes innervations from the thalamus, cerebral cortex, spinal cord, and brain stem. This results in the control of such bodily functions as temperature, respiration, arterial blood pressure and circulation, and metabolism. The hypothalamus also controls certain behavioral functions, including the emotional states of fear, anxiety, anger, rage, pleasure, and pain, as well as the states of sleep, wakefulness, and alertness. The hypothalamus, as it is influenced by the autonomic nervous system, affects all the unconscious activities of the body.

In its endocrine role, the hypothalamus has two regulatory functions:

- Regulating the anterior pituitary gland by producing and secreting releasing factors

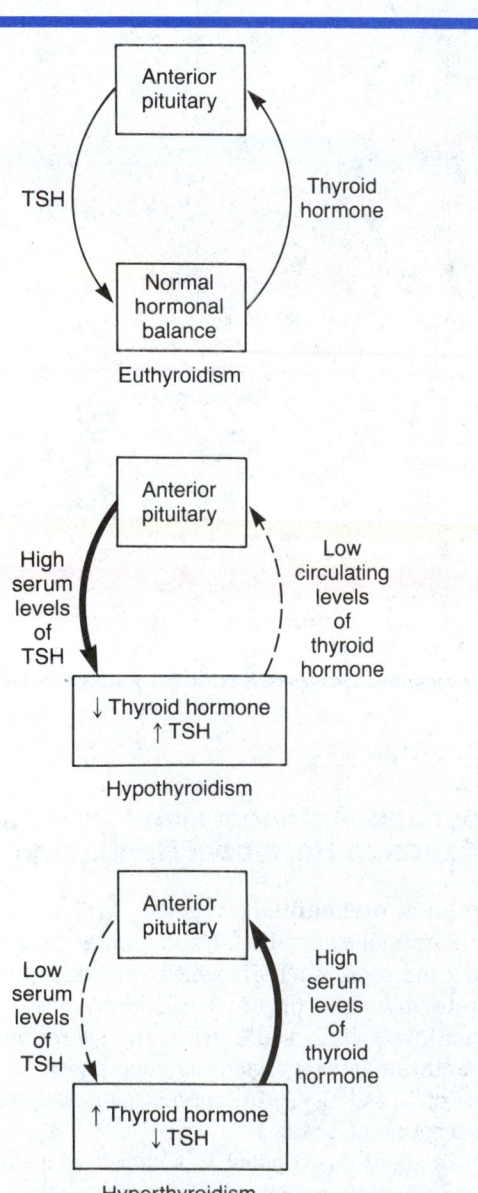

Figure 40–3

The concept of feedback.

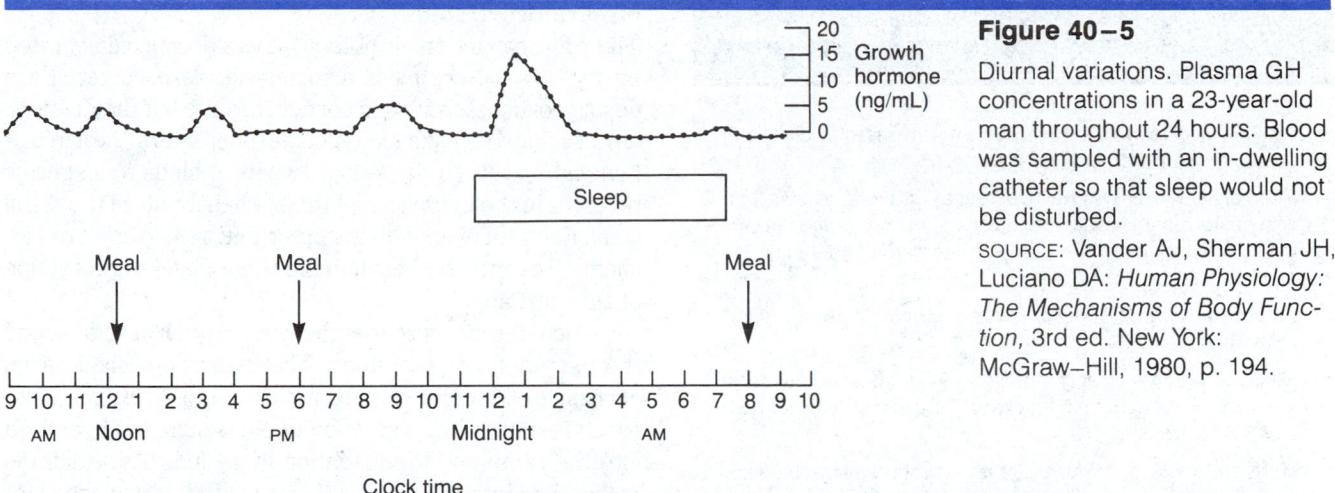

Figure 40−5

Diurnal variations. Plasma GH concentrations in a 23-year-old man throughout 24 hours. Blood was sampled with an in-dwelling catheter so that sleep would not be disturbed.

SOURCE: Vander AJ, Sherman JH, Luciano DA: *Human Physiology: The Mechanisms of Body Function,* 3rd ed. New York: McGraw−Hill, 1980, p. 194.

- Producing and secreting two hormones, oxytocin and ADH, which are stored in the posterior pituitary gland

The hypothalamic releasing factors are proteins that act on the anterior pituitary gland to stimulate or inhibit the release of tropic hormones (THs). Both inhibiting factors (IFs) and releasing factors (RFs) have been identified; it is thought, although still unproven, that the hypothalamus may produce both an inhibiting and a releasing factor for each of the anterior pituitary hormones.

The release or inhibition of these hypothalamic hormones is controlled by various neurotransmitters such as serotonin, acetylcholine, norepinephrine, and dopamine (Ryan, 1980). The THs released from the anterior pituitary gland then act upon a target gland or tissue to produce a specific response (Figure 40−2). In regulating the secretion of these releasing factors, the hypothalamus processes input from both the circulatory and nervous systems. The releasing factors are secreted into the pituitary portal venous system and transported to the anterior pituitary gland. This hypothalamic−pituitary link is shown in Figure 40−6.

The hypothalamus also secretes the hormones oxytocin and ADH. The storage and release of ADH are influenced by such factors as plasma osmolality, blood volume, physiological and psychological stress, and input from the central nervous system (Box 40−2). ADH is produced in the hypothalamus and then transported to the posterior pituitary gland where it is stored. In the posterior pituitary gland, oxytocin and ADH are bound to the protein neurophysin and released into the circulation in response to specific physiological stimuli.

Anterior Pituitary Gland

In response to the releasing factors from the hypothalamus, the anterior pituitary gland secretes several hormones, some of which control hormonal secretion by other glands. Some of the effects of the hypothalamic factors on the anterior pituitary gland are inhibitory, such as those of

prolactin inhibiting factor (PIF), luteinizing hormone inhibiting factor (LIF), and growth hormone inhibiting factor (GIF), and some stimulate secretion.

The anterior pituitary hormones secreted include TSH, ACTH, GH, and LH—also called interstitial cell-stimulating hormone (ICSH) in men—FSH, and prolactin. In general, GH, ACTH, and TSH are concerned with metabolic activities, whereas LH, FSH, and prolactin are concerned with reproduction. ACTH, TSH, FSH, and LH exert their effects on target glands, either increasing their size or their secretions. Prolactin and GH directly affect the metabolism of specific target tissues. (See Table 40−1 for a summary of the major hormones.)

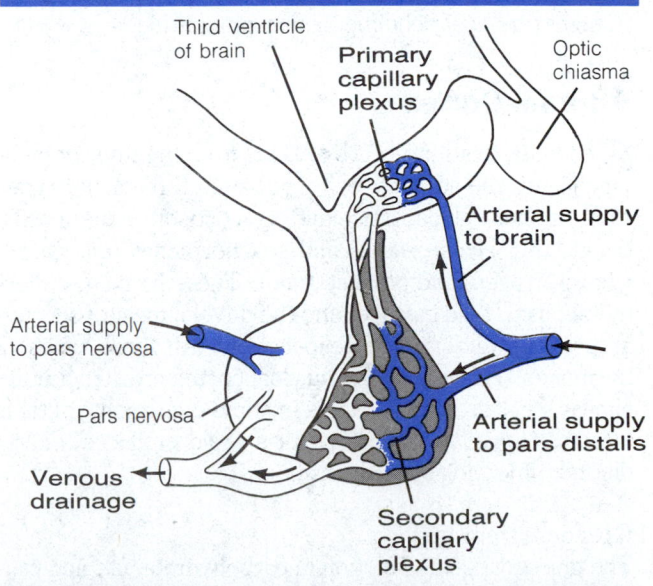

Figure 40−6

The circulatory link between the hypothalamus and the adenohypophysis of the pituitary gland.

SOURCE: Spence AP, Mason EB: *Human Anatomy and Physiology,* 2nd ed. Menlo Park, CA: Benjamin/Cummings, 1983, p. 431.

Box 40–2 **Factors Influencing the Secretion of ADH**

Plasma osmolality. Increased concentrations of sodium and potassium stimulate the release of ADH.

Circulating blood volume. Decreases in blood volume (eg, with hemorrhage) initiate the release of ADH, possibly through the actions of the baroreceptors in the carotid artery and left atrium.

Blood pressure. Reduced cardiac output increases ADH secretion.

Nausea. Nausea is accompanied by an intense release of ADH; this is thought to be the result of a reflex from the medullary vomiting center.

Emotional stress. Emotional stress and pain can stimulate ADH secretion, possibly through their effect on the nervous system.

Thirst. The sensation of thirst arises from the hypothalamus and can be induced by hyperosmolality (as in dehydration) or by severe hemorrhage. The thirst mechanism and the control of ADH secretion are integrated and are thought to be activated by the same hypothalamic osmoreceptors.

Posterior Pituitary Gland

The posterior pituitary gland does not produce any hormones; it stores and releases the two hypothalamic hormones, ADH and oxytocin. The hypothalamus mediates the release of these hormones from the posterior pituitary gland into the circulation when stimulated by the neurotransmitters acetylcholine or norepinephrine.

Adrenal Cortex

In response to stimulation by ACTH from the anterior pituitary gland, the adrenal cortex secretes three major types of hormones: glucocorticoids (eg, cortisol), mineralocorticoids (eg, aldosterone), and sex hormones (eg, androgens, estrogen, and progesterone). These hormones affect metabolism, fluid balance, and the development of secondary sex characteristics, respectively. All three types of hormones secreted by the adrenal cortex are structurally similar steroids, which results in some overlapping of their effects. However, each type of steroid produces a fairly distinct physiological response.

Glucocorticoids

The glucocorticoids function in carbohydrate, fat, and protein metabolism and play an important role in the body's response to stress and emotional well-being. The principal glucocorticoid secreted by the adrenal cortex is cortisol, which constitutes 95% of cortical production. Corticosterone and cortisone are also produced. Cortisol has many physiological actions and affects many tissues of the body (Box 40–3).

Mineralocorticoids

The principal and most potent mineralocorticoid secreted by the adrenal cortex is aldosterone. Also secreted are desoxycorticosterone and corticosterone, but their actions are of minor importance. Aldosterone enters the circulation and travels to the kidney, where it binds to a specific receptor in the cytoplasm of the epithelial cells of the distal convoluted tubules. This receptor initiates a series of biochemical events that result in the major physiological action of aldosterone.

Aldosterone increases the reabsorption of sodium and the excretion of potassium. This is accomplished as an exchange of sodium ions for potassium or hydrogen ions, which results in the excretion of potassium and hydrogen into the urine and the retention of sodium. As sodium is reabsorbed into the blood, it brings with it water and chlorides, which mechanically increases the blood volume. This action of aldosterone is vital to the maintenance of the extracellular fluid volume. Aldosterone also promotes sodium reabsorption to a lesser degree from the sweat glands, salivary glands, and gastrointestinal tract.

Aldosterone is an important factor in the maintenance of circulatory blood volume homeostasis through its effect on the electrolyte balance and its control of blood volume. It is the most potent hormonal regulator of electrolyte excretion.

The secretion of aldosterone is regulated by three (or possibly four) major mechanisms: the renin–angiotensin system, ACTH, plasma potassium levels, and perhaps prostaglandins. The renin–angiotensin system is thought to represent the chief control of aldosterone secretion. Renin, an enzyme produced by the kidney, acts upon renin substrate and converts it into angiotensin I. Angiotensin I is then rapidly converted into angiotensin II by specific "converting" enzymes in the lung. Angiotensin II circulating in the blood directly stimulates the adrenal cortex to secrete aldosterone. Aldosterone then acts on the kidney to increase the reabsorption of sodium and water, causing the expansion of the extracellular fluid volume. This action of aldosterone indirectly suppresses the secretion of renin, completing a long feedback loop (Figure 40–7). Stimuli for the release of renin include:

- Decreased intra-arterial volume, decreased blood flow to the kidneys (as seen in renal artery stenosis), or both
- Neural input from the sympathetic nervous system via the increased secretion of epinephrine or norepinephrine
- Decreased serum sodium levels

Although chiefly affecting the secretion of cortisol, ACTH is also thought to affect aldosterone production for short periods. This appears related to crises, when ACTH causing the increased secretion of glucocorticoids also stimulates the production of aldosterone. This effect of ACTH is thought to be minor and secondary to that of the renin–angiotensin system and serum potassium levels.

Box 40–3 Physiological Actions of Cortisol

Protein metabolism. Cortisol's effect on protein is catabolic; ie, it breaks down protein and inhibits its synthesis in the bone, skin, muscle, and connective tissue. This action promotes a negative nitrogen balance and results in an increased amino acid concentration in the blood. It also provides a mechanism by which amino acids may be obtained in times of stress.

Glucose metabolism. Cortisol blocks the use of glucose by tissues and stimulates gluconeogenesis by the liver. It is antagonistic to insulin. These actions, in excess, contribute to a rise in plasma glucose levels and are the basis for the diabetogenic effect of the glucocorticoids. In normal amounts, these actions contribute to glucose homeostasis in the body.

Fat metabolism. Cortisol promotes lipolysis, thereby increasing the concentration of fatty acids in the bloodstream. This also contributes to the diabetogenic action of glucocorticoids, because these fatty acids can be used for energy rather than glucose. If adequate insulin is not present in this instance, ketosis may result.

Permissiveness. Cortisol is permissive to many physiological processes; ie, it must be present for the processes to occur. For example, it plays a role in the secretion of digestive enzymes by gastric cells, as well as in the excitability of the nervous system and the myocardium.

Maintenance of normal blood pressure. Cortisol, along with aldosterone and the catecholamines from the adrenal medulla, contributes to the maintenance of a normotensive state. Although the exact role of the glucocorticoids is not known, it is thought to involve permissiveness of catecholamine effectiveness and enhancement of sodium and water retention.

Regulation of fluid and electrolyte balance. Cortisol acts on the kidney by stimulating the glomerular filtration rate and decreasing water reabsorption, increasing the flow of urine. The decrease in the reabsorption of water is thought to be secondary to an inhibition of ADH secretion. When cortisol is secreted in excess, it stimulates the reabsorption of sodium in the distal tubules in exchange for potassium. This can result in hypokalemia and hypertension secondary to the retention of sodium.

Normal function of muscles. Although the exact effect of cortisol on muscle function is unknown, muscle weakness is seen in both cortisol deficiency and excess.

Hematopoietic effect. Cortisol is thought to stimulate red blood cell formation and possibly platelet formation, although the exact mechanism of action is not well understood. With an increased administration of cortisol, leukocytosis has been seen with neutrophilia, lymphopenia, and eosinopenia.

Lymphatic effect. Cortisol appears to be necessary for the development of the thymus and lymph nodes.

Immune effect. Excesses of glucocorticoids suppress both the inflammatory and immune responses of the body. They inhibit the formation of scar tissue and interfere with cell-mediated immunity (decreased T-lymphocyte involvement). When given in large doses, glucocorticoids also may suppress antibody formation by the plasma cells.

ACTH feedback mechanism. Cortisol regulates the secretion of ACTH by the anterior pituitary gland via a feedback mechanism.

Effect on emotional status. Cortisol either directly or indirectly influences the personality and emotional stability of the individual.

Combating stress. Cortisol is one of the physiological mechanisms of defense used by the body to combat stress. Emotional or physiological stress results in a response by the sympathetic nervous system (and thereby the adrenal medulla) and the release of glucocorticoids. Glucocorticoids are essential in the management of stress. Although their exact role is not known, it is thought to involve permissiveness to the catecholamine role. In addition, in stressful situations glucocorticoids rapidly mobilize amino acids (protein catabolism) and fats (lipolysis) for conversion to other substances or use in energy production.

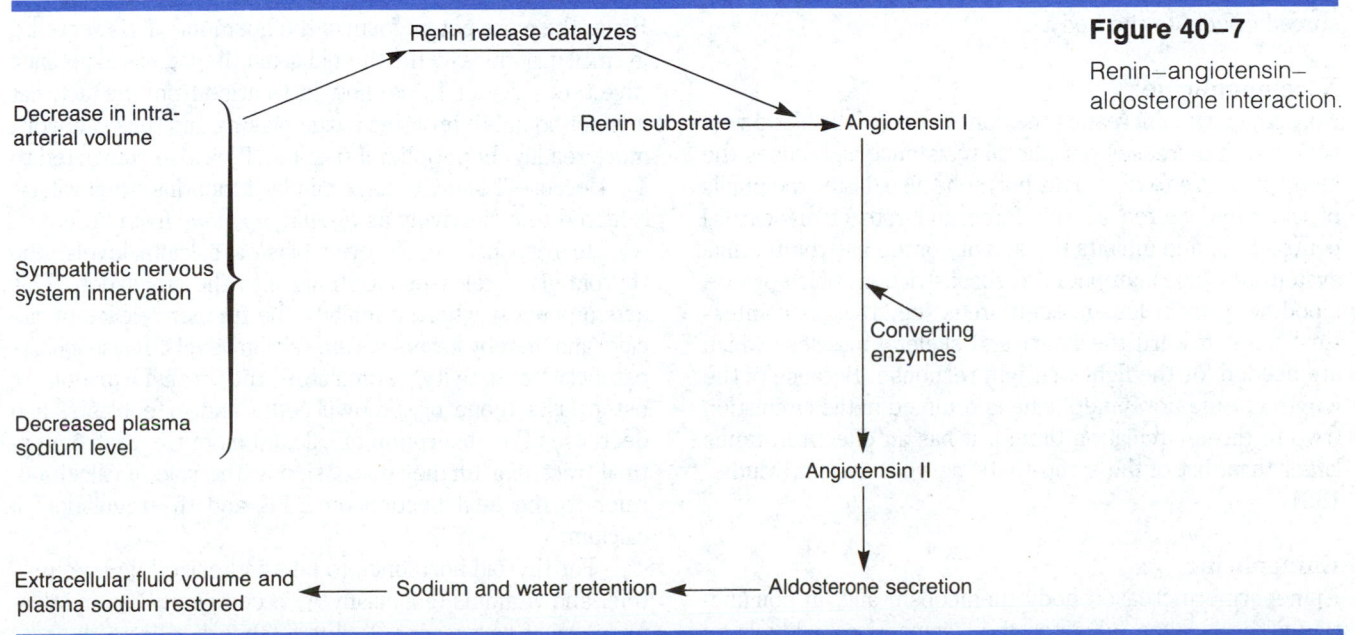

Figure 40–7

Renin–angiotensin–aldosterone interaction.

The ratio of serum sodium levels to serum potassium levels is another important regulator of aldosterone secretion. If the serum potassium level rises or the serum sodium level decreases, changing the sodium–potassium ratio, the adrenal cortex will be stimulated to produce aldosterone. Prostaglandins are also thought to be involved in aldosterone secretion (Williams, 1981) through the regulation of sodium and water excretion and the release of renin.

Sex Hormones

The sex hormones produced by the adrenal cortex are the androgens and smaller amounts of estrogen and progesterone. This group of hormones has less physiological impact than the other adrenal hormones but does affect reproductive function.

Adrenal Medulla

The adrenal medulla is considered a part of the sympathetic division of the autonomic nervous system, which controls the secretion of its hormones. Because the functions of the sympathetic nervous system and the functions of the hormones of the adrenal medulla are the same, they can compensate for each other. Thus, the medullary hormones are not essential to life but play an important role in the body's response to stress. About 15% of the hormonal secretion by the adrenal medulla is norepinephrine, and 75% is epinephrine. The nerve endings in the sympathetic nervous system also secrete norepinephrine.

Epinephrine is considered chiefly a hormone, whereas norepinephrine functions as both a hormone and a neurotransmitter. Although constant amounts of norepinephrine and epinephrine are secreted into the bloodstream, stress triggering the sympathetic nervous system can dramatically increase their output. The overall effect of the adrenal medullary hormones is to prepare the individual physiologically to function during an emergency. They have widespread effects in the body.

Norepinephrine

Norepinephrine increases the contraction of the blood vessels, which increases peripheral resistance and causes the blood pressure to rise. This hormone also dilates the pupils of the eyes, increases the force and rate of myocardial contraction, and inhibits the activity of the gastrointestinal system. It causes peripheral vasoconstriction, which diverts blood away from less-needed areas (eg, the gastrointestinal tract) toward the heart and skeletal muscles, which are needed for the fight-or-flight response. Because of the length of time norepinephrine is retained in the circulation (two to three circulation times), it has an effect ten times larger than that of the sympathetic nervous system (Muthe, 1981).

Epinephrine

Epinephrine increases body metabolism and, in conjunction with glucagon, elevates the plasma glucose levels by **glycogenolysis** (the conversion of glycogen to glucose). Epinephrine also inhibits the secretion of insulin and elevates blood lipid levels by promoting **lipolysis** (the breakdown of fat). All these actions provide the body with a plasma glucose source for increased energy expenditure. Epinephrine is also able to constrict the arterioles of the skin selectively (causing pallor) while dilating the blood vessels of the heart and skeletal muscles. This effect increases the blood flow to these structures, which also is vital to the stress response.

Epinephrine exerts a stronger effect on glycogenolysis than norepinephrine. Both have equivalent effects on increasing the metabolic rate and producing hyperlipidemia, however (Muthe, 1981). It is important to remember the permissive role of the glucocorticoids with respect to catecholamines. In the absence of cortisol, the vasoconstrictive and metabolic responses mediated by norepinephrine and epinephrine will not occur.

Regulation of Secretion

Through innervation from the sympathetic nervous system, the secretion of the adrenal medullary hormones is influenced by emotional stresses (fear, anxiety, and isolation) and physiological stresses (childbirth, burns, cold, hypoxia, immobilization, and physical exercise). The relation between the psychological–emotional state and the endocrine system is one of the body's major homeostatic mechanisms for protecting the individual from harm and physiological stresses in a way that preserves integrity.

Thyroid Gland

In response to stimulation by TSH, the thyroid gland secretes two types of hormones: iodinated (T_3 and T_4) and noniodinated (calcitonin). The ratio of T_4 to T_3 in the circulating blood is approximately 20:1. These hormones have similar functions but differ in the rapidity and degree of action. By far the more potent form of the hormone, T_3 is secreted in small quantities by the thyroid gland. Its increased potency (five times that of T_4) is thought to arise from the fact that it is not bound to proteins in the plasma and thus can work more readily. In peripheral tissues, T_4 is also converted to T_3. Because T_4 and T_3 have similar functions, they will be referred to collectively as *thyroid hormone* from here on.

In response to elevated plasma calcium levels, the thyroid gland releases calcitonin into the circulation. This acts on bones, where it inhibits the further release of calcium and thereby lowers serum calcium levels. It also inhibits osteoclastic activity, stimulates the transformation of osteoclasts (bone breakdown cells) and osteoblasts, and decreases the absorption of calcium from the gastrointestinal tract. For further discussion of the role of calcitonin, refer to the next section on PTH and the regulation of calcium.

For thyroid hormones to be synthesized, iodine, protein, and vitamins (especially A, B complex, B_{12}, and thiamine) must be present. Iodine is absorbed from the gastrointestinal tract and transported via the bloodstream in the form of inorganic iodine. Through a special mechanism known as the *iodine pump,* the thyroid gland is able to absorb and concentrate the iodine and convert it to form thyroid hormone. The thyroid gland is thought to need about 2 mg of ingested iodine each week. Normally, the thyroid stores enough thyroid hormone to maintain circulating plasma levels for several weeks. It is the only endocrine gland that is able to do this.

About 99.94% of thyroid hormone circulates in the plasma-bound proteins, the major protein being thyroxine-binding globulin (TBG). Protein-bound hormones are not biologically active. To exert their effect, they must be separated from the proteins to which they are attached. In contrast, the small amount of free-circulating hormone (free T_4 and T_3) is readily available for use by the tissues.

Thyroid hormone has widespread physiological actions that involve all body systems and affect many tissues and organs. Its major effects are on metabolic activities and the activities of other body tissues (Box 40–4). Thyroid hormone has both extracellular and intracellular effects. The response to thyroid hormone is based on both the dosage and state of the recipient target cells.

Thyroid hormone also affects red cell production; milk

production during lactation; regulation of fertility and the menstrual cycle; mental processes and development of the central nervous system; maintenance of cardiac rate, force, and output; maintenance of normal muscle and skin tone; maintenance of GH secretion, skeletal maturation, and tissue development; and maintenance of secretions from the gastrointestinal tract.

Parathyroid Glands

The parathyroid glands produce and secrete one hormone, parathyroid hormone (PTH). The basic function of PTH is the regulation of serum calcium and phosphorus, which is also regulated by vitamin D and calcitonin. Calcium is the chief cation of the body and is necessary for the integrity of the bony structures and many neuromuscular and metabolic activities.

The three target sites for PTH are the kidneys, the bones, and the gastrointestinal tract. Vitamin D obtained through the diet must be present for PTH to be effective at these three sites. In the kidneys, PTH acts directly on the renal tubules to increase the reabsorption of calcium and increase the excretion of phosphate in the urine. This maintains a normal serum calcium level. Parathyroid hormone also is necessary for the conversion of vitamin D_3 (cholecalciferol) into its active form in the kidney.

The bones of the skeletal system are the main source of calcium in the body. When serum calcium levels are low, PTH causes the release of calcium from the bone into the circulation. High serum calcium levels reduce PTH secretion, causing either movement of the excess calcium back into the bones or excretion. It is thought that PTH accomplishes this activity by increasing osteoclast activity and acting on the osteoblasts to convert them to osteoclasts. This increases bone breakdown and absorption. In the normal state, this relation between breakdown and buildup remains equal.

In the gastrointestinal tract, PTH directs the absorption of calcium and phosphorus from the duodenum and jejunum through active and passive transport. Vitamin D is essential for this process. Vitamin D is thought to be permissive to the transport of calcium through the intestinal mucosa, and decreases in serum calcium may be found in clients with a vitamin D deficiency.

Parathyroid hormone also affects the level of phosphorus in the serum. Phosphorus is normally absorbed from the gastrointestinal tract and excreted by the kidneys. Increased levels of circulating PTH stimulate an increase in phosphorus excretion by the kidneys.

Calcitonin counterbalances the effects of PTH by protecting against hypercalcemia through its ability to lower serum calcium levels. This hormone affects the same target tissues as PTH (ie, the bones, kidneys, and gastrointestinal tract) and tends to promote hypocalcemia by the initiation of bone resorption and decreased calcium absorption from the small intestine. Both mechanisms reduce the rate of movement of calcium into the extracellular fluid and

---

Box 40–4 Major Functions of Thyroid Hormone

Metabolic effects. Thyroid hormone increases the rate of both protein synthesis and catabolism. The anabolic action of T_4 promotes growth; this hormone also enhances the synthesis of enzymes. Intracellularly, thyroid hormone increases substrate availability, metabolic energy, and the synthesis of the structural and functional components of the cell.

Carbohydrate metabolism. All processes of carbohydrate metabolism are affected by T_4. It stimulates gluconeogenesis and the utilization of glucose by the cells. It also potentiates the effect of insulin on glycogen synthesis and increases the absorption of glucose and galactose by the gut. Thyroid hormone also regulates the magnitude of the effect of epinephrine and norepinephrine on carbohydrate metabolism. In excess, T_4 interacts with insulin as an insulin antagonist to reduce its effectiveness by breaking it down quickly. In reduced doses, such as in hypothyroidism, it may cause a slower breakdown of insulin, so the individual may need less insulin.

Fat metabolism. T_4 affects the synthesis, mobilization, and breakdown of fats, with its greatest effect being on fat degradation. It stimulates cholesterol synthesis and the mechanisms that remove cholesterol from the circulation. It regulates the conversion of carotene to vitamin A in the liver, stimulates lipid turnover, and stimulates the release of free fatty acids.

Metabolic rate. Thyroid hormone regulates the metabolic rate of all cells and increases the body's overall consumption of oxygen and depth of respiration. It increases heat production and regulates the heat-dissipating mechanism. This function of T_4 (ie, its effect on metabolism) is used as a criterion for estimating thyroid activity in a procedure known as measuring the basal metabolic rate.

thus promote hypocalcemia. In the kidneys, calcitonin initially increases the excretion of calcium and phosphorus.

Calcitonin is valuable where there is an acute excess of calcium because of its ability to produce an effect in less than an hour. Although it is able to lower the serum levels of calcium rapidly, it does not have PTH's prolonged effect. The homeostatic mechanisms used to maintain normal serum calcium levels are shown in Figure 40–8.

PTH secretion is regulated through a negative feedback mechanism between the serum levels of calcium and the parathyroid glands. High circulating serum levels of calcium inhibit the secretion of PTH by the parathyroid glands, and low serum levels of calcium stimulate PTH secretion. Recent research has shown that magnesium also can affect the secretion of PTH. High levels of magnesium have been found to inhibit the secretion of PTH in a way similar to the action of calcium (Williams, 1981).

Gonads

The ovaries produce estrogen and progesterone, which affect reproduction and the development of secondary sex characteristics in the female. The testes produce testosterone, which affects reproduction and the development of secondary sex characteristics in the male. For a detailed discussion of the function and regulation of secretion of the gonadal hormones, refer to Chapters 61 and 62.

Pancreas

The pancreas has both endocrine and exocrine functions. For a discussion of the exocrine functions, refer to Chapter 46. The endocrine function of the pancreas involves the secretion of three hormones. The major pancreatic hormones, insulin and glucagon, are secreted by the beta and alpha cells of the islets of the pancreas, respectively. The delta cells of the pancreas secrete a third hormone, somatostatin, also called growth hormone inhibiting factor (GIF). The function and regulation of the secretion of insulin and glucagon will be discussed here in detail, with an overview of the function and regulation of somatostatin.

Insulin

Insulin is a protein secreted by the beta cells of the pancreas that directly affects the metabolism of carbohydrates, proteins, and lipids. This anabolic hormone promotes the synthesis, storage, or both, of carbohydrates, fats, proteins, and nucleic acids. Insulin affects many tissues, but its most important sites of action are fat, muscle, and liver cells. The brain, renal tubule cells, intestinal mucosa, and erythrocytes do not require insulin for the uptake of glucose.

Insulin is thought to act by altering the permeability of the cell membrane, increasing the plasma membrane transport of glucose, other monosaccharides, certain amino acids, certain fatty acids, potassium, and magnesium. After binding to a receptor in the plasma membrane, insulin transmits a signal to the interior of the cell via a "second messenger." This second messenger influences the enzymatic processes in the involved cells. Unlike other cellular processes involving second messengers, cyclic AMP is not involved here. The precise nature of this substance is still under study (Williams, 1981).

Insulin also promotes the movement of potassium and magnesium into the cell. Potassium is an important factor in the regulation of enzymes and affects the membrane potential of the cell. Magnesium is involved in the activation of certain cellular enzymes. Insulin is degraded by the liver, kidney, and pancreas; 80% of this process is accomplished by the liver and kidneys. The major functions of insulin are summarized in Box 40–5.

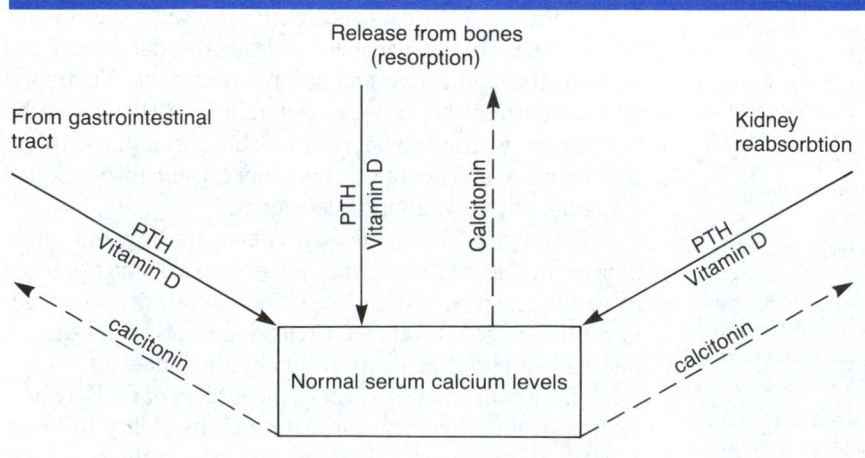

Figure 40–8

Mechanism of calcium homeostasis.
SOURCE: Jubiz W. *Endocrinology: A Logical Approach for Clinicians.* New York, McGraw–Hill, 1979, p. 195.

Many factors inhibit and stimulate the secretion of insulin, including:

- Circulating levels of glucose, amino acids, and fatty acids
- Gastrointestinal hormones
- The influence of the sympathetic nervous system
- The influence of other hormones and neurotransmitters
- The influence of drugs

Glucagon

Glucagon is secreted by the alpha cells of the islets of Langerhans in the pancreas as well as by the cells of the upper intestinal tract. The major site for the action of glucagon is the liver, where it promotes gluconeogenesis (the formation of glucose from noncarbohydrate substances such as fat and proteins), lipolysis, and glycogenolysis. All these actions increase serum glucose levels, which is the major function of glucagon. This hormone also stimulates the release of catecholamines, which increase the serum level of glucose.

Glucagon stimulates the secretion of insulin by a direct effect on the beta cells of the pancreas (Muthe, 1981). This appears to be a contradiction in function but when

---

Box 40–5   Major Functions of Insulin

Carbohydrate metabolism. The major effect of insulin on carbohydrate metabolism is to increase the uptake and utilization of glucose by the muscle and adipose cells. Insulin also regulates the synthesis of glycogen in the liver (glycogenesis) and inhibits the breakdown of glycogen to glucose (glycogenolysis) and of amino acids to glucose (gluconeogenesis). All these actions reduce serum glucose levels.

Fat metabolism. Insulin is required for the transport of glucose across the cell membrane from the circulation into the adipose cell. This hormone enhances the uptake and storage of free fatty acids by the adipose cells and the synthesis of lipids (primarily triglycerides). These actions in turn promote lipogenesis and inhibit lipolysis. Insulin decreases the oxidation of free fatty acids and inhibits ketone formation.

Protein metabolism. Insulin assists the movement of amino acids into the cells and the conversion of amino acids into protein, thereby depositing more protein into muscles. Growth and nitrogen retention are promoted by insulin, whereas proteolysis (the catabolism of protein) is inhibited.

Effect on the liver. The liver plays an important role in the regulation of serum glucose levels. When these levels are elevated, glucose is stored as glycogen in the liver, muscles, or other tissues. When serum glucose levels are low, the liver is able to break down glycogen, lipids, and proteins to glucose and thereby restore the blood glucose levels to normal. It does this through glycogenolysis, lipolysis, and proteolysis.

Effect on fluid and electrolyte balances. Besides decreasing serum glucose levels, insulin decreases the serum levels of potassium by increasing its intracellular transport. Insulin also increases the transport of magnesium and phosphorus into the cell.

Effect of nucleic transformation. Insulin stimulates the formation of DNA, RNA, and adenosine triphosphate (ATP).

---

looked at in its entirety, the process is a mechanism for the control of normal serum glucose levels. For example, in hypoglycemia, the decrease in serum glucose levels caused by insulin stimulates the secretion of glucagon, which then raises glucose levels by stimulating glycogenolysis and gluconeogenesis. Because glucagon has the net effect of raising serum glucose levels, it stimulates the secretion of insulin, which then lowers the level of glucose in the serum. These specific actions of glucagon are under study for the management of type I diabetes mellitus, which is often hard to control. Clients often fluctuate between episodes of hypoglycemia and hyperglycemia, and a glucagon deficiency is thought to play a role.

The secretion of glucagon is stimulated by decreased serum glucose levels, increased levels of amino acids, and decreased serum levels of fatty acids. It is inhibited by increased serum levels of fatty acids. In general, there is an inverse relationship between serum glucose levels and the output of glucagon.

Somatostatin

Somatostatin, or GIF, is secreted by the hypothalamus, the delta cells of the pancreas, and cells in the upper portion of the small intestine and gastric mucosa. Because of these multiple sites of secretion, somatostatin has proven difficult to study; at present little is known about its exact nature and role in metabolism.

Somatostatin's major function is to inhibit the release of GH, and it also inhibits the release of thyrotropin releasing factor (TRF). Locally, it appears to inhibit the release of insulin and glucagon by the pancreas and to suppress the secretion of gastrin and other secretions from the gastrointestinal tract, although this role is not clear. Somatostatin is also thought to play a role in body weight, especially in obesity.

Thymus

Although little is known about the thymus, it is thought to be an endocrine gland and to produce at least two hormones—thymosin and thymopoietin—which exert their principal effect on the body's immune system. Thymosin stimulates the maturation of T-lymphocytes, which are necessary in the cellular response to infection and influence the production of lymphocytes by peripheral areas of the body. Thymosin also contributes to the development of B-lymphocytes, which are involved in the antigen–antibody response (Muthe, 1981; Williams, 1981). Thymopoietin is thought to block neuromuscular transmissions and has been implicated as a factor in myasthenia gravis. Decreased or absent circulating levels (specific to age) may be seen in combined immunodeficiency states.

Pineal Gland

The pineal gland is thought to secrete many hormones, the most studied and first identified of which is melatonin. This hormone seems to exert its effects on the pituitary, hypothalamus, midbrain, and gonads. In the laboratory, melatonin has been found to have the following effects (Williams, 1981):

- Inhibition of GH secretion
- Decrease in serum LH levels
- Increase in sleepiness and an increase in REM (rapid eye movement) sleep
- Selectively, an increase in the sense of well-being, mild elation (increase in alpha waves), or both
- In animals, skin lightening (not shown to affect human skin pigmentation)

Other substances associated with the pineal gland are histamine, norepinephrine, dopamine, and serotonin.

Kidneys

The major functions of the kidneys are excretion of urine and the regulation of water, electrolyte, and acid–base balances. The kidneys also perform an endocrine function through production of renin, erythropoietin, and 1,25-dihydroxycholecalciferol. The kidneys control the production of erythropoietin, the hormone that regulates red blood cell production. They also produce renin, an enzyme that functions as an integral part of the renin–angiotensin system. This system is vital to the maintenance of the body's extracellular fluid volume. In the presence of PTH, the kidneys produce 1,25-dihydroxycholecalciferol from 25-hydroxycholecalciferol. The compound 1,25-dihydroxycholecalciferol is the major active form of vitamin D, which is necessary for the maintenance of calcium in the body.

Gastrointestinal Tract

Several hormones work in conjunction with the nervous system to control digestion and the absorption of foodstuffs. These hormones are produced in the walls of the stomach, in the upper intestine, and at various sites throughout the bowel. The hormones that have been isolated and studied are gastrin, secretin, and CCK–PZ. Others currently being researched include gut glucagon, somatostatin, and gastric-inhibitory peptide (GIP).

Section II: Pathophysiological Influences and Effects

Pathophysiological changes commonly seen in endocrine dysfunction are discussed in this section. More specific influences and effects of dysfunction in individual endocrine organs are presented in Chapters 42, 43, and 44.

ANTERIOR PITUITARY GLAND

Most of the disorders affecting the pituitary gland originate in the anterior lobe. The effects of pathology on the anterior pituitary gland can be broadly summarized as hyperpituitarism and hypopituitarism.

Hyperfunction of the Anterior Pituitary Gland

The most common cause of *hyperfunction* of the anterior pituitary gland is a neoplastic secreting tumor, usually a benign adenoma. Tumors of the pituitary gland exert their effects through two major mechanisms:

1. Pressure on structures in the brain (eg, the optic tract), which causes visual symptoms and headaches
2. Excessive secretion of one or more of the anterior pituitary hormones, which results in increased stimulation of one or more target glands

One of the pathophysiological manifestations of these tumors is hypersomatotropism (excess GH), which can result in acromegaly in adults and gigantism in children. Other pathophysiological effects of excessive GH secretion include **goiter** (from GH stimulation of the thyroid tissues) and diabetes mellitus secondary to the diabetogenic effect of GH. Cardiomegaly and hypertension can also occur. Visual impairment and eventual blindness are possible because of compression of tissue by the expanding tumor. Amenorrhea in women and loss of libido and potency in men may occur because compression from the expanding tumor leads to gonadal deficiencies from loss of healthy gonadotropin-producing cells.

Hypofunction of the Anterior Pituitary Gland

Hypofunction of the anterior pituitary gland can arise from many causes. It can be secondary to pathology of the anterior pituitary gland or to injury to the hypothalamus resulting in a decrease or absence of the hypothalamic releasing factors. Hypopituitarism may be manifested by isolated hormonal deficiencies or by a deficiency of both the anterior and posterior pituitary hormones (panhypopituitarism). The exact hormonal deficit and its etiology are important to an understanding of a client's symptoms and signs. The causes of hypofunction of the anterior pituitary gland are listed in Box 40–6.

The symptoms of hypopituitarism, like those of hyperpituitarism, depend on the number and type of hormones involved. Approximately 70% to 80% of the pituitary gland must be destroyed before symptoms and signs of deficiency are apparent. This loss of function is seen in the gonadal target tissue first; this is followed by signs of thyroid deficiency and, lastly, adrenal cortex insufficiency.

POSTERIOR PITUITARY GLAND

The two hormones of the posterior pituitary gland are synthesized in the hypothalamus; the posterior pituitary gland simply serves as a site of storage and release. Therefore, damage to the posterior lobe does not affect the synthesis of these hormones. However, if the hypothalamus or hypothalamic–hypophyseal pathways were damaged, changes in the secretions of ADH and oxytocin would result. Only the pathophysiological influences of ADH will be discussed in this section. The effects of oxytocin imbalances are described in Chapter 61.

The pathophysiological effects involving the hypothalamus and posterior pituitary gland can be summarized broadly as a deficiency and inappropriate secretion of ADH hormone. A deficiency of ADH results in diabetes insipidus.

Deficiency of Antidiuretic Hormone

Deficiencies of ADH may be primary or secondary. In primary diabetes insipidus, a defect is thought to be inherent in the posterior pituitary gland itself. The etiology may be congenital or **idiopathic** (accounting for 30% to 40% of cases). In secondary diabetes insipidus, the symptoms are the result of pathology in the hypothalamic–pituitary pathways. Causes of secondary diabetes insipidus are shown in Box 40–7. Nephrogenic diabetes insipidus arises from an inherited defect in which the kidney tubules are unresponsive to ADH. Its causes include electrolyte disorders (chronic potassium depletion and chronic elevated serum calcium levels), chronic renal disease, and drugs (methoxyflurane, lithium, and demeclocycline). Pathophysiological changes with diabetes insipidus include copious excretion (5 to 15 L/day) of a dilute urine (specific gravity ranges from 1.002 to 1.004) causing intense thirst and dehydration.

Inappropriate Secretion of Antidiuretic Hormone

Hypothalamic–posterior pituitary pathology also can result in a syndrome of inappropriate ADH (SIADH). The secretion of ADH normally is controlled by a feedback mechanism that monitors the osmolality of the plasma. For example, as the osmolality of the plasma rises, ADH secretion is stimulated. As it falls (hypo-osmolality), the secretion of

ADH is suppressed. In SIADH, a persistent secretion of ADH occurs unrelated to the osmolality of the plasma. Causes of SIADH include tumors, trauma, infections, porphyria, drugs, and stress.

THYROID GLAND

Pathophysiological influences on the thyroid gland result in hyperfunction, hypofunction, or enlargement of the gland. The results are hyperthyroidism, hypothyroidism, or goiter. **Euthyroidism** refers to a normal state of thyroid functioning.

Hyperfunction of the Thyroid Gland

Hyperfunction of the thyroid gland is characterized by an excessive secretion of thyroid hormones T_3 and T_4, resulting in a condition known as hyperthyroidism. The causes of hyperthyroidism include ingestion of exogenous thyroid hormones (factitious thyrotoxicosis); Graves' disease; Hashimoto's thyroiditis; subacute and chronic thyroiditis; nodular hyperthyroidism; ovarian carcinoma (struma ovarii); and overproduction of TSH, chorionic gonadotropin, or both. Increased thyroid hormone production affects many body systems as well as the body's basal metabolic rate and energy production. The circulatory, nervous, and endocrine systems are affected, as is the gastrointestinal tract. The pathophysiological symptoms are generally related to the increase in body metabolism.

Hypofunction of the Thyroid Gland

Hypofunction of the thyroid gland, or hypothyroidism, results in a deficiency of T_3 and T_4 or both. Hypothyroidism can be congenital or acquired. In this condition, the rate of metabolic processes decreases, which affects both mental and physical functions.

Congenital etiologies of hypothyroidism include the absence of the thyroid gland and defects in the enzymes responsible for the synthesis of thyroid hormone. **Cretinism** is a condition of severe congenital hypothyroidism characterized by retardation of both growth and mental development. It is related to a deficiency of thyroid hormone in fetal life and usually occurs in areas where there is a dietary deficiency of iodine and where goiters (enlargements of the thyroid gland) are prevalent.

Acquired causes of hypothyroidism include surgical removal of the thyroid gland, chronic thyroiditis, irradiation of the thyroid gland or therapy using radioactive iodine, decreased secretion of TSH from the anterior pituitary gland secondary to hypothalamic or pituitary damage, idiopathic atrophy of the thyroid, and drugs that inhibit the synthesis or release of thyroid hormone.

In the adult, a severe deficiency of thyroid hormone results in **myxedema,** which may be primary (from a pathological condition within the gland itself) or secondary (from a pathological condition in the anterior pituitary gland). A severe form of untreated hypothyroidism with depression of the sensorium is called *myxedema coma.*

Enlargement of the Thyroid Gland

An enlarged thyroid gland, or *goiter,* may be fibrous or cystic and may contain nodules or be composed of an increased number of follicular cells. Goiters may be associated with hyperthyroidism, hypothyroidism, or euthyroidism. Goiters associated with normal thyroid function are called *nontoxic goiters.* Clients with hyperthyroidism may have diffusely enlarged glands (Graves' disease) or multinodular glands (toxic nodular goiters). Goiters are often thought to represent an increase in the size of the thyroid gland to compensate for decreased thyroid hormone synthesis. The stimulus for the enlargement of the gland is the increased secretion of TSH that occurs as a result of the low circulating T_4 levels.

PARATHYROID GLANDS

Pathology of the parathyroid glands results in their hyperfunction and hypofunction. Resulting conditions are *hyperparathyroidism* and *hypoparathyroidism.*

Hyperfunction of the Parathyroid Glands

Hyperfunction of the parathyroid glands leads to an excessive secretion of PTH. This condition, known as hyperparathyroidism, can be classified as primary, secondary, or tertiary.

Primary hyperparathyroidism arises from intrinsic pathology in the parathyroid glands. Causes of primary hyperparathyroidism include a benign adenoma of the gland (90% of all cases), hereditary factors, multiple adenoma of the gland, a parathyroid carcinoma, and hyperplasia and hypertrophy of the gland. Radiation also has been associated with primary hyperparathyroidism.

Secondary hyperparathyroidism is the result of a compensatory mechanism to overcome low serum calcium levels (hypocalcemia). The causes of secondary hyperparathyroidism include nephrosis, renal tubular acidosis, osteomalacia, rickets, intestinal malabsorption syndrome, and chronic renal disease (Williams, 1981). Secondary hyperparathyroidism may evolve into primary hyperparathyroidism over a long period.

Tertiary hyperparathyroidism is caused by an excessive secretion of PTH from an ectopic source. Carcinomas of the lungs and kidneys are implicated in the ectopic production of PTH.

Hypofunction of the Parathyroid Glands

Hypofunction of the parathyroid, or hypoparathyroidism, results in a deficiency in PTH secretion or a decrease in the peripheral action of PTH. This condition is characterized by low levels of PTH, resulting in low circulating serum levels of calcium (and high serum levels of phosphorus). The elevated serum phosphorus levels maintain the calcium phosphate salts in the bone and bind calcium in the gut. This reduces the absorption of calcium and the effectiveness of vitamin D, which serves to perpetuate the low serum levels of calcium.

Causes of hypoparathyroidism include familial or hereditary hypoparathyroidism, pseudohypoparathyroidism, autoimmune disorders, and iatrogenic causes. The clinical manifestations of hypoparathyroidism may be acute or chronic. Severe untreated hypoparathyroidism is manifested by marked hypocalcemia with tetany.

ADRENAL GLANDS

Pathophysiological influences on the adrenal glands result in either hyperfunction or hypofunction. The clinical manifestations seen in these clients represent the effects of an excess or deficiency of the adrenal hormones on their target tissues or glands.

Adrenal Cortex

Adrenal Cortex Hyperfunction

Hyperfunction of the adrenal cortex results in the increased secretion of glucocorticoids, mineralocorticoids, and sex hormones. The overall symptoms and signs are most representative of the excess secretion of cortisol (hypercortisolism). The primary causes of hypercortisolism, originating from within the adrenal cortex itself, include neoplasia and bilateral hyperplasia. In **iatrogenic** hypercortisolism, an exogenous source, such as prolonged use of glucocorticoids or ACTH, is responsible for the hypercortisolism. The normal adrenal glandular tissue may be atrophic, and ACTH levels are suppressed.

It has been hypothesized that a pathological condition (such as a tumor) originating in the hypothalamus may stimulate the release of excessive amounts of corticotropin releasing factor (CRF). The CRF acts upon the anterior pituitary gland to stimulate the release of ACTH, which then acts upon the adrenal cortex to cause a hypersecretion of cortisol. The increased ACTH levels may cause hyperplasia of the adrenal tissue. Increased ACTH production by the pituitary gland that is due to hypoplasia or tumor also may cause adrenal hyperfunction. Pituitary tumors or hyperplasia is responsible for approximately 60% to 80% of all cases of adrenal hyperfunction. Ectopic ACTH-producing tumors include carcinomas of the lung or the gastrointestinal tract.

Hyperfunction of the adrenal cortex results in three major disorders:

1. Cushing's syndrome, characterized by an excessive secretion of the adrenal glucocorticoids.

2. Primary aldosteronism (Conn's syndrome), a disorder characterized by an excessive secretion of mineralocorticoids, particularly aldosterone.

3. Excessive production of the sex hormones characterized by virilizing changes in women, feminizing changes in men, and precocious sexual development in children. These physiological changes often cause serious psychological problems (eg, of self-esteem and body image) for the client and family or significant others.

Adrenal Insufficiency

Hypofunction of the adrenal cortex, or adrenal insufficiency, results in a decreased secretion of glucocorticoids, mineralocorticoids, and sex hormones. The causes of adrenal insufficiency can be grouped into two categories: primary (based on pathology occurring within the gland itself) and secondary (arising from an undersecretion of ACTH from the anterior pituitary gland, which may be due to pathology in the pituitary gland or the hypothalamus). Primary causes may be acute or chronic.

Primary adrenal insufficiency, or Addison's disease, is characterized by a failure of the adrenal cortex to produce sufficient corticosteroids (glucocorticoids, mineralocorticoids, and sex hormones). Acute severe symptoms of Addison's disease are referred to as *addisonian crisis*. A major difference between primary and secondary causes of adrenal insufficiency is that secondary failure is not usually associated with a marked deficiency of aldosterone.

Adrenal Medulla

Pathophysiology of the adrenal medulla is rare and is usually associated with hyperfunction. The clinical manifestations seen in hyperfunction of the adrenal medulla are related to the excessive secretion of epinephrine and norepinephrine.

A pheochromocytoma is the most common cause of adrenal medulla hyperfunction. This tumor secretes excessive amounts of epinephrine and norepinephrine, resulting in increased metabolism, hypertension, and hyperglycemia. Other disorders associated with hyperfunction of the adrenal medulla include neurofibromatosis, carcinomas (eg, of the thyroid), and hyperparathyroidism.

PANCREAS

In its role as an endocrine gland, the pancreas is responsible for the production of at least three hormones: insulin; glucagon; and somatostatin or growth inhibiting factor (GIF). When there is a deficiency of insulin (diabetes mellitus), the blood glucose level rises. In the diabetic state, the normal insulin mechanism has been disrupted. Factors that may be involved in this include insufficient production of insulin, increased insulin requirements by the body, a decrease in the availability of insulin receptors, a decrease in the effectiveness of the available insulin, and increased destruction of insulin by the liver and other tissues.

Chronic hyperlipidemia often occurs in diabetics because of increased lipolysis. This abnormality, combined with the other derangements of glucose and protein metabolism seen in diabetes mellitus, often results in pathological changes affecting both large and small blood vessels. Peripheral vascular insufficiency and ulcerations may occur secondary to the development of atherosclerosis. The atherosclerotic lesions are the same as in the nondiabetic population but occur at an earlier age, with a greater frequency, and with a more rapid progression because of greater infiltration by these glycoproteins into the arterial walls. Changes in the small vessels of the body (microangiopathy) affect primarily the eyes and kidneys. This leads to retinal damage (diabetic retinopathy), and damage to the vessels of the kidney (nephropathy).

Section III: Related System Influences and Effects

The endocrine system affects and is affected by many other organ systems through the action of its hormones. Of special importance is the interrelatedness of the endocrine and central nervous systems mediated through the actions of the hypothalamus and adrenal medulla. The endocrine system also interrelates with the sensory (eye and ear), cardiovascular, renal, gastrointestinal, integumentary, musculoskeletal, and reproductive systems. These interactions maintain homeostasis as well as the ability to withstand episodes of stress. The evaluation of a symptom or sign requires not only a careful assessment of the endocrine system, but also an assessment of the related systems influenced by endocrine dysfunction.

CENTRAL NERVOUS SYSTEM

The interrelation between the central nervous system and the endocrine system lies between the adrenal medulla and the hypothalamic–pituitary axis. The hypothalamus, which is under the control of higher neurologic centers and circulating endocrine hormones, maintains a close relationship with the pituitary gland through the hypothalamic–pituitary portal system (Figure 40–6).

Central nervous system symptoms and signs that may indicate endocrine dysfunction include ataxia (myxedema), seizures (hypoglycemia, hyperglycemia, hypocalcemia, and acromegaly), headache (pituitary tumors and pheochromocytomas), fatigue (hypoglycemia, adrenocortical insufficiency, hypothyroidism, and hyperthyroidism), coma (diabetic ketoacidosis, hyperglycemia, hypoglycemia, hypercalcemia, myxedema, and hyponatremia), and paresthesia (diabetes mellitus, hypocalcemia, acromegaly, and myxedema).

SENSORY SYSTEM

Clients with myxedema may experience deafness and tinnitus. Those with diabetes mellitus and hyperthyroidism may have diplopia, and those with pituitary tumors may exhibit hemianopia (blindness in half the field of vision).

CARDIOVASCULAR SYSTEM

Cardiovascular symptoms and signs that may reflect endocrine dysfunction include hypertension (aldosteronism, pheochromocytoma, Cushing's syndrome, hypercalcemia, and acromegaly), tachycardia or atrial fibrillation (pheochromocytoma and hyperthyroidism), congestive heart failure (Cushing's syndrome and thyrotoxicosis), deep venous thrombosis (hypercalcemia), hypotension (adrenal insufficiency), bradycardia (hypothyroidism), and pericardial effusions (myxedema).

RENAL SYSTEM

Renal calculi are sometimes seen in hyperparathyroidism, acromegaly, and Cushing's syndrome. Polyuria and polydipsia may be attributable to pituitary tumors, diabetes mellitus, hypercalcemia, and hyperparathyroidism.

GASTROINTESTINAL SYSTEM

Gastrointestinal symptoms and signs that may indicate endocrine pathology include anorexia (adrenal insufficiency, myxedema, and hypercalcemia), indigestion (adrenal insufficiency, myxedema, and hypercalcemia), weight loss (adrenal insufficiency, hyperthyroidism, and pheo-

chromocytoma), diarrhea (diabetes mellitus, hyperthyroidism, adrenal insufficiency, and hypocalcemia), constipation (myxedema, hypercalcemia, and pheochromocytoma), peptic ulcer formation (hyperparathyroidism), ascites (myxedema), and abdominal pain (adrenal insufficiency and hyperparathyroidism).

INTEGUMENTARY SYSTEM

Clients with diabetes mellitus, hyperthyroidism, or both often have pruritus. Excessive hair growth may be seen on clients with adrenal hyperplasia or tumor. Clients with acromegaly, hypoglycemia, pheochromocytoma, or hyperthyroidism may exhibit hyperhidrosis. Facial flushing may be seen in clients with pheochromocytoma, and coldness of the skin may be seen with hypothyroidism. Vitiligo is possible in clients with diabetes mellitus, hyperthyroidism, hypothyroidism, Hashimoto's thyroiditis, and adrenal insufficiency. Clients with Addison's disease and hyperthyroidism may have hyperpigmentation of the skin, and those with Cushing's syndrome may have ecchymosis and purplish striae on their abdomens.

MUSCULOSKELETAL SYSTEM

The endocrine system can affect the musculoskeletal system by causing fractures (Cushing's syndrome and hyperparathyroidism), bone pain (hyperparathyroidism), arthralgias (myxedema and acromegaly), and muscle weakness and fatigability (hyperparathyroidism, hyperthyroidism, acromegaly, and Cushing's syndrome).

REPRODUCTIVE SYSTEM

The endocrine system can cause major changes in an individual's reproductive function. A loss of libido and potency is seen in clients with hypogonadism, diabetes mellitus, acromegaly, and hypothyroidism. Menorrhagia is often associated with hyperthyroidism and metrorrhagia, with hypothyroidism. Amenorrhea can be caused by a pituitary tumor, hyperthyroidism, hypogonadism, acromegaly, or Cushing's syndrome.

Section IV: Psychosocial/Lifestyle Influences and Effects

The endocrine system has far-reaching effects on both physiological and psychological function, so endocrine dysfunction can contribute to major developmental and psychosocial crises. To provide comprehensive client care, the nurse should be aware of these potential crises and their manifestations.

The client with endocrine dysfunction may have to face the reality of coping with chronic illness or an acute life-threatening situation. Anger, fear, guilt, and denial are common initial reactions to a new diagnosis. Individual responses to this challenge vary according to the client's past experiences, attitudes toward health and illness, past

coping patterns, and support system strength. It is not unusual to find clients with several years' history of a disease (eg, diabetes mellitus) still working through their anger and denial over the initial diagnosis. In working with diabetic children, recognize that they must deal with the parents' feelings of guilt as part of a total plan of care.

Lifestyle changes may be necessary because of changes in the ability of the client with an endocrine disorder to perform normal activities of daily living, to tolerate stress, to meet economic obligations, or to continue with usual dietary patterns. The simple fact that these changes are necessary often confirms to the client and family or significant others that the illness is serious and that all of their lives will be affected.

SELF-CONCEPT AND SELF-ESTEEM

The client with endocrine dysfunction may have to deal with a change in self-concept and a loss of self-esteem arising from changes in body image, decreased functional abilities, limitations to intimacy, restrictions in autonomy, and limitations in decision-making processes. Changes in self-concept and the loss of self-esteem may interfere with the client's ability to carry through with the treatment plan and accept the diagnosis and its implications. For example, body image significantly affects how people view and feel about themselves. A client who is a pituitary dwarf must adjust to a world structured for taller people. Clients with Cushing's syndrome have to adjust to the cosmetic implications of the moon face, buffalo hump, and truncal obesity seen with that disorder. Those with Addison's disease must protect themselves from stressful situations, and clients with hypothyroidism suffer from easy fatigability and sometimes a slowing in mental functions. These pathophysiological changes affect the client's ability to function in normal situations, causing further stress and anxiety.

Certain endocrine disorders, including pituitary tumor, dysfunctions of the adrenal cortex and medulla, and thyroid dysfunction, cause emotional lability and personality change. This presents serious concerns for the client, who often states, "I can't control myself" or "What is the matter with me?" The nurse can help both client and family understand the relation between the physiological problem and the psychological changes.

SEXUAL EXPRESSION AND REPRODUCTION

Often in thyroid disorders, as well as in disorders affecting the secretion of the adrenocortical sex hormones, changes in libido and sexual potency concern clients and their sexual partners. Sensitive intervention by the nurse may relieve anxiety in the couple.

OCCUPATIONAL AND ECONOMIC FACTORS

Occupational implications of endocrine disorders include the possibility of changing occupations or limitations in working because of a physical disability. Clients with visual loss or changes in mentation often must make significant occupational adjustments. The client may need to move to a different area to be closer to a source of health care, need a special living environment, and need adaptive equipment. This could necessitate changing jobs or even occupations. Economic factors that might cause a change in lifestyle include the need for lifelong medications and medical supervision along with the burdens of the increasing costs of diagnostic tests and hospitalizations.

DIETARY FACTORS

The adjustment to new dietary requirements is a major challenge for clients with endocrine disease. Clients who previously gave little thought to nutrition or balanced meals may now require fluid restrictions, special diets, and dietary supplements. These clients are often asked to weigh and measure each portion of their meals and keep an accurate intake record. These dietary changes not only add extra strain to an already stressful situation but also create an economic burden. In addition, the client who previously gained psychological satisfaction from eating must now consciously think about not only the content of the foods to be ingested but also the spacing of meals throughout the day. This is especially true for diabetes, where the variables of nutrition, insulin, and exercise must be balanced carefully.

The nurse must recognize the importance of these psychosocial influences and understand how they affect the client and significant others. Take ample time to explore with clients the effects of these influences on them and their implications for an improved state of health. In planning care for clients with endocrine disorders and for all clients, psychosocial influences on health are as important as the pathophysiological factors.

Chapter Highlights

The major glands of the endocrine system are the anterior and posterior pituitary glands, thyroid gland, parathyroid glands, gonads, adrenal glands, and the pancreas.

The thymus and pineal glands also function as part of the endocrine system, although their exact mechanism of action is still under study. The kidneys and gastrointestinal tract perform an endocrine function, along with other functions.

Hormones are the chemical substances secreted by the endocrine glands directly into the circulation. Their effects may be local or generalized.

Each hormone secreted by an endocrine gland exerts a characteristic effect on its target tissue.

Hormones may be regulated by the hypothalamus, hypothalamic releasing factors, anterior pituitary hormones, the autonomic nervous system, serum nutrient and ion concentrations, feedback mechanisms, autonomous functioning, or diurnal variation.

The effects of pathology on the anterior pituitary gland are hypersecretion (hyperpituitarism) or hyposecretion (hypopituitarism). The symptoms of hyperpituitarism

(continued)

Chapter Highlights *(continued)*

and hypopituitarism depend on the number and type of hormones involved.

Pathological conditions of the posterior pituitary gland do not affect the synthesis of oxytocin and ADH, because these hormones are produced by the hypothalamus and merely stored and released by the posterior pituitary gland.

The two major endocrine effects related to pathological conditions of the hypothalamic–posterior pituitary region are deficiency of ADH (which results in diabetes insipidus) and inappropriate secretion of ADH (which results in a syndrome of inappropriate secretion of ADH).

Pathophysiological influences on the thyroid gland can produce hyperfunction, hypofunction, or enlargement of the gland.

A deficiency of thyroid hormone in fetal life results in cretinism in the infant. In the adult, myxedema is a severe form of hypothyroidism.

A goiter is an enlarged thyroid gland and may be associated with hyperthyroidism, hypothyroidism, or euthyroidism. Goiters are thought to represent an increase in the size of the thyroid gland to compensate for decreased thyroid hormone synthesis.

Pathological conditions of the parathyroid glands result in hyperfunction of the gland (hyperparathyroidism) or hypofunction of the gland (hypoparathyroidism).

The three major disorders resulting from hyperfunction of the adrenal cortex are Cushing's syndrome (adrenal glucocorticoid excess), primary aldosteronism (mineralocorticoid excess), and reproductive disorders related to excessive amounts of adrenal sex hormones.

Hypofunction of the adrenal cortex (adrenal insufficiency) can be primary or secondary. Primary adrenal insufficiency results in Addison's disease.

Pathological conditions of the adrenal medulla are rare and usually associated with hyperfunction. Pheochromocytoma is the most common cause of adrenal medulla hyperfunction.

The major disorder associated with endocrine dysfunction of the pancreas is diabetes mellitus (characterized by high serum glucose levels).

The endocrine system interrelates with many other organ systems of the body to maintain homeostasis and help the organism withstand stress.

Because the endocrine system has far-reaching effects on both the biological and psychological organism, dysfunction in this system can cause major developmental and sociocultural crises. Lifestyle changes are often necessary because of changes in abilities to perform the activities of daily living; changes in tolerance to stress; economic, environmental, and occupational factors; and special nutritional needs.

Bibliography

DeGroot L et al: *Endocrinology.* New York: Grune & Stratton, 1979.

Diabetes Mellitus, 8th ed. Indianapolis: Eli Lilly, 1980.

Dimmond M, James SL: *Chronic Illness Across the Life-Span.* Norwalk, CT: Appleton–Century–Crofts, 1983.

Jubiz W: *Endocrinology: A Logical Approach for Clinicians.* New York: McGraw–Hill, 1979.

Kaye D, Rose LF (editors): *Fundamentals of Internal Medicine.* St. Louis: Mosby, 1983.

Miller JF: *Coping With Chronic Illness.* Philadelphia: Davis, 1983.

Muthe NC: *Endocrinology: A Nursing Approach.* Boston: Little, Brown, 1981.

Ryan WG: *Endocrine Disorders: A Pathophysiological Approach.* Chicago: Year Book Medical Publishers, 1980.

Vander AJ, Sherman JH, Luciano DA: *Human Physiology: The Mechanisms of Body Function.* New York: McGraw–Hill, 1980.

Williams RH (editor): *Textbook of Endocrinology,* 6th ed. Philadelphia: Saunders, 1981.

Wilson HS, Kneisl CR: *Psychiatric Nursing,* 2nd ed. Menlo Park, CA: Addison–Wesley, 1983.

Suggested Readings

Sanford SJ: Dysfunction of the adrenal gland: Physiologic considerations and nursing problems. *Nurs Clin North Am* 1980; 15:481–498. This article is an in-depth presentation of the adrenal hormones and their physiological effects.

Solomon BL: The hypothalamus and the pituitary gland: An overview. *Nurs Clin North Am* 1980; 15:435–451. A basic discussion of the role of the hypothalamus and the physiological effects of the major pituitary hormones is presented.

Taitano–Hoffman JT, Newly–Bond T: Hypercalcemia in primary hyperparathyroidism. *Nurs Clin North Am* 1980; 15:469–480. A detailed discussion of calcium metabolism in the body is provided, along with the role of PTH and thyrocalcitonin.

Wake–Musante M, Brensinger JF III: The nurse's role in hypothyroidism. *Nurs Clin North Am* 1980; 15:453–467. This article is an excellent presentation of the role of thyroid hormone in the body and the effect of insufficient production on homeostasis.

Chapter 41

The Nursing Process for Clients With Endocrine System Dysfunction

Anne Herrstrom Skelly

When you have finished studying this chapter, you should be able to:

Explain the parts of the health history especially relevant to a client with a problem in the endocrine system.

Specify the areas routinely assessed in the client with endocrine dysfunction.

Discuss the common diagnostic approaches used in evaluating clients with endocrine disease.

List the common nursing diagnoses used in caring for clients with endocrine problems.

Identify nursing considerations relevant to the planning of care for clients with endocrine dysfunction.

Outline nursing care plans that include client care goals, nursing interventions, and expected outcomes for clients with endocrine dysfunction.

The application of the nursing process to the care of clients with endocrine dysfunction is a challenge because of the complexity of the endocrine system and its interrelation with other body systems. This chapter discusses assessment of the client with suspected endocrine problems, relevant diagnostic studies, and the development of nursing care approaches based on the nursing diagnosis.

Section I: Nursing Assessment: Establishing the Data Base

One of the most important nursing responsibilities in working with clients having endocrine dysfunction is the establishment of a comprehensive data base with both subjective information (client symptoms and historical data) and objective information (physical signs and laboratory data). Because of the widespread effects of endocrine dysfunction, thoroughness and accuracy are essential in the collection of this data. Many different organ systems and tissues are involved, so a knowledge of normal endocrine physiology is required as well as a basic understanding of how endocrine pathophysiology can manifest itself in other body systems.

Based on a careful evaluation of the data base, the nurse can arrive at nursing diagnoses that reflect the client's major health problems and needs. These diagnoses then provide the framework for an individualized, client-centered plan of care.

SUBJECTIVE DATA

Document any history of endocrine disease (eg, thyroid disease or diabetes mellitus). Has the client ever been evaluated for any endocrine disorder? If so, when and where? What was the outcome? Has the client undergone any head trauma, neck surgery, or head and neck radiation? Has the client ever taken any medication for an endocrine disorder? If so, what type, why, and for how long? Obtaining the places and dates of former treatments is invaluable in obtaining medical records later. In addition to specific questions on history of endocrine dysfunction, ask about past diagnosed related system disorders such as hypertension, seizure disorders, autoimmune dysfunction, reproductive problems, cardiac disease, and central nervous system disorders.

Inherited patterns can occur in some endocrine disorders, so pay careful attention to a family history of pituitary, adrenal, pancreatic, thyroid, parathyroid, or gonadal dysfunction. Question clients about a family history of glucose intolerance. If the family history is positive, determine the nature of the family relationship, as well as the degree of severity of the relative's condition (eg, maternal aunt, age 35, Type I diabetes mellitus, blind × 10 years; paternal grandfather, age 82, Type II diabetes mellitus × 5 years). Knowledge of the family's general state of health gives the nurse an opportunity to identify health problems that may have an immediate or future effect on the client's well-being.

Endocrine dysfunction may produce psychological as well as physiological changes. In addition to coping with a possibly life-threatening situation, the client may need to adjust to the probability of living with a chronic disorder that requires major lifestyle changes. A psychosocial history should cover the client's previous responses to ill health, including coping patterns, support system, and cultural and religious influences.

Psychological problems may arise from the disease process itself and the client's perception of the actual diagnosis and response to it. Although the relation of endocrine dysfunction to psychological well-being is not well understood, certain psychological changes have been observed in specific endocrine disorders. For example, clients with hypothyroidism may be lethargic and confused, have slowing of their cognitive processes, and occasionally even experience psychotic episodes. Clients with hyperthyroidism may exhibit increasing irritability, anxiety, and emotional lability. Families or friends may say that the client "never acted this way before." The history can indicate the client's general cognitive abilities. If a question exists, cognition can be tested formally as part of the mental status examination.

Because endocrine disorders can have such widespread effects, the nurse must evaluate clients for the impact of the present problems on their lives. An occupational history should be obtained, including current occupation, type of duties, length of time employed, and ability to perform required tasks. Have any limitations been imposed by the employer because of the client's physical or mental status? How satisfied is the client with his or her present position? Has the client's illness affected the present economic status? Is the client's income adequate to meet current and future needs?

Other questions include: What is the client's educational background? Is the client able to read and write? What is the client's present living arrangement? Are there supportive people in the client's life, or is the client living in an environment filled with conflict and hostility? If someone other than the client cooks the meals, would that person be willing to come in and talk with the care provider about dietary restrictions necessary for the client?

A review of systems (ROS) attempts to elicit any health problems not mentioned during the preceding history. The ROS pertinent to endocrine disorders includes:

- **General**   Sudden or unexplained changes in height or weight; unexplained increase in hand or foot size; change in head size; episodes of weakness or fatigue; fevers or sweats; frequent colds, infections, or illnesses; intolerance to heat or cold
- **Skin and hair**   Excessive hair growth or loss, excessive sweating, facial flushing, changes in skin pigmentation and temperature, ecchymoses, pruritus, changes in skin texture, abnormalities in hair distribution, **vitiligo** (skin patches that lack pigment)
- **HEENT**   Tinnitus, changes in hearing acuity, visual loss or changes in visual acuity, diplopia, hemianopia, exophthalmos (unilateral or bilateral), nasal congestion, excess cerumen, changes in size of neck, pressure sensations in throat, difficulty swallowing, goiter
- **Cardiovascular**   Hypertension, hypotension, dysrhythmias, tachycardia, atrial fibrillation, bradycardia, congestive heart failure, pericardial effusions, venous thromboses
- **Gastrointestinal**   Polyphagia, anorexia, diarrhea, constipation, weight loss or gain, abdominal pain, ascites, indigestion, ulcer
- **Urinary**   Polydipsia, polyuria, renal calculi
- **Reproductive**   Amenorrhea, oligomenorrhea, dysmenorrhea, menorrhagia, metrorrhagia, changes in sexual function and libido
- **Musculoskeletal**   Weakness, fractures, joint and bone pain
- **Neurologic**   Headaches, fatigue, changes in cognitive ability, changes in mood or behavior, ataxia, somnolence or coma, seizures, **paresthesia**

OBJECTIVE DATA

The nurse gathers objective data through a thorough physical assessment of the client and a careful review of all pertinent laboratory data. Assess those systems directly related to the chief concern. The information from the subjective and objective assessments enables the nurse to formulate and rank a list of client problems.

Because the effects of endocrine pathology are so widespread, often several organ systems must be examined. In general, the areas to be assessed in most clients suspected of having endocrine problems include vital signs;

general appearance; hair and nails; skin; eyes; neck; heart; lungs; abdomen; genitals; and the musculoskeletal and neurologic systems. In addition, if a client has a specific complaint (eg, menstrual irregularities or costovertebral angle pain), thoroughly examine the system related to that complaint (in this case, the reproductive or urinary systems, respectively).

Physical Assessment

Vital Signs
Assess the client's height and weight and compare them with growth charts. A careful developmental and familial growth history may help in the interpretation of abnormalities. Assess the blood pressure in both arms initially and in at least two positions (supine and seated). Determine the apical and radial pulse rates, rhythm, and quality, along with the client's respiratory rate, rhythm, and depth. Take the client's temperature.

General Appearance
Note whether clients appear to be close to their chronological age. Are the body parts symmetrical and in proportion? Are any limbs missing or malformed? What is the client's stature and **habitus** (physical appearance)? How is the weight distributed? Are there any abnormal movements of the extremities or face, eg, spasms or twitching of facial muscles (Chvostek's sign)? Does the face appear normal in configuration and color? A **plethoric** (round, erythematous), moon face suggests Cushing's syndrome, whereas puffiness of the face suggests hypothyroidism.

Assessment of the Skin, Hair, and Nails
Endocrine dysfunction often affects the temperature and texture of the skin. Temperature changes are associated with myxedema (cool, dry skin) and pheochromocytoma (increased skin temperature with sweating). It is important to note the presence of any skin lesions. Ecchymoses often accompany Cushing's syndrome, and vitiligo has been seen in clients with adrenal insufficiency, hyperthyroidism, and hypothyroidism. Other skin lesions include skin infections (furuncles and carbuncles); ulcerations; and, in clients with diabetes, candidiasis, diabetic dermopathy ("spotted leg" or pigmented patches in the pretibial area), and diabetic xanthoma.

What is the texture and distribution of the body hair? Is there **hirsutism** (excessive hair growth) or hair loss? Are the eyebrows present and in a normal distribution? (In hypothyroidism there is often a loss of the lateral third of the eyebrow.) Has the hair prematurely grayed? Are any abnormalities of the nails present (eg, pitting or moniliasis of the nails)?

Assessment of the Eyes
Pay careful attention to any periorbital swelling (hypothyroidism), **proptosis** (hyperthyroidism), **ptosis** of the eyelids, or demonstrable lid lag. Assess the visual acuity and

visual fields for any defects. The optic disk, macula, retinal vessels, and retinal background should be examined with an ophthalmoscope. Diabetes mellitus often is accompanied by characteristic changes in the retina, including retinal edema, **microaneurysms,** retinal hemorrhages, and exudates. New vessel formation or fibrous proliferation of blood vessels (**neovascularization**) is found in a malignant form of **retinopathy,** proliferative retinopathy. Clients with these conditions need immediate referral to an ophthalmologist to preserve their sight. Figure 41–1 shows hard exudates and retinal edema in the fundus of a diabetic client.

Assessment of the Neck
Inspect the neck for any asymmetry, which can be seen in clients with goiters and other masses. Does the enlargement appear symmetrical or asymmetrical? Carefully palpate the thyroid gland. Note its size, degree of symmetry, and consistency. Assess for the presence of any bruits, tenderness, or nodules.

Cardiorespiratory Assessment
Evaluate the client's heart rate and rhythm and detect the presence of any murmurs or extra heart sounds. In thyrotoxicosis and pheochromocytoma, elevated blood pressure readings, tachycardia, and atrial fibrillation may be noted. Thyrotoxicosis and Cushing's syndrome often lead to congestive heart failure as manifested by increasing shortness of breath, dyspnea on exertion, paroxysmal nocturnal dyspnea, and cough. Bradycardia and pericardial

Nursing Research Note

Baun M et al: Physiological effect of human/companion animal bonding. *Nurs Res* 1984; 33(3):126–129.
This study investigated the difference in the physiological reactions of persons petting a dog with whom they had established a companion bond, petting a dog without a bond established, and quietly reading a book. Twenty-four subjects were included in the study. Physiological responses measured included heart rate, respiratory rate, and blood pressure.
There was a significant drop in overall systolic and diastolic blood pressure readings when subjects petted their own dogs. However, when they started to pet their dog, a greeting response occurred in which they had a significant elevation in blood pressure readings. This elevation subsequently decreased. Heart rate dropped significantly when subjects sat quietly and read a book. When the subject petted an unknown dog, heart rate was elevated. Heart rate drop when petting one's own dog was similar to that of reading a book. Respiratory rates fell significantly in all three situations, but the largest drop occurred when petting one's own dog.
This study supports the belief that pets have a positive effect on health. Physiological responses for petting one's own dog and quietly reading were about the same, both producing a relaxation effect. Studies on the effect of pets on individuals' health should be continued. Pet therapy offers an approach to treating certain health problems.

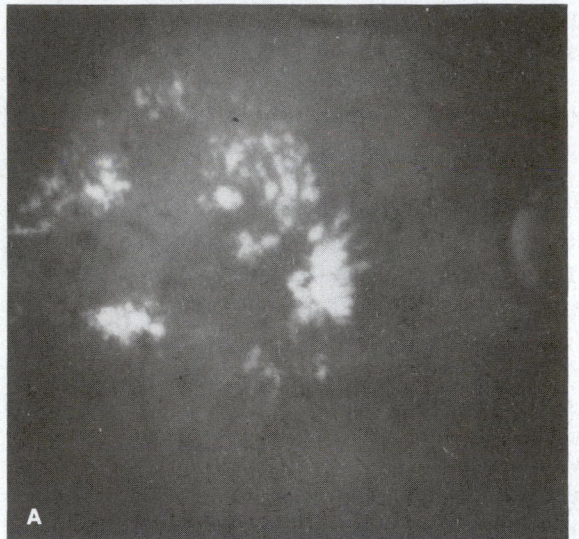

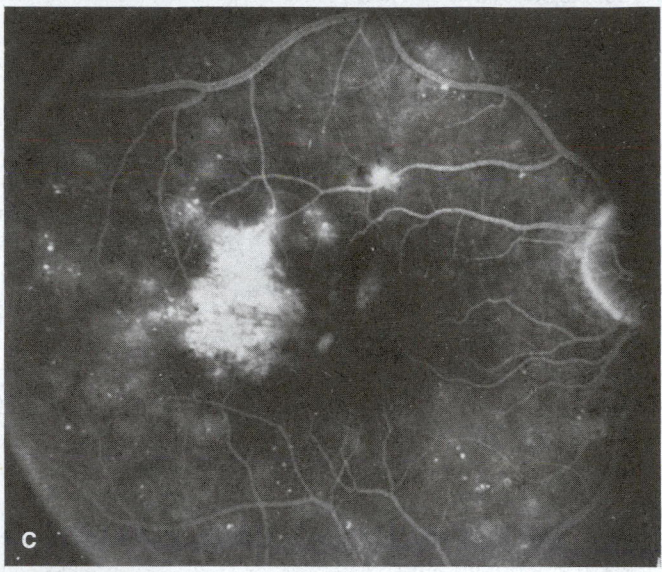

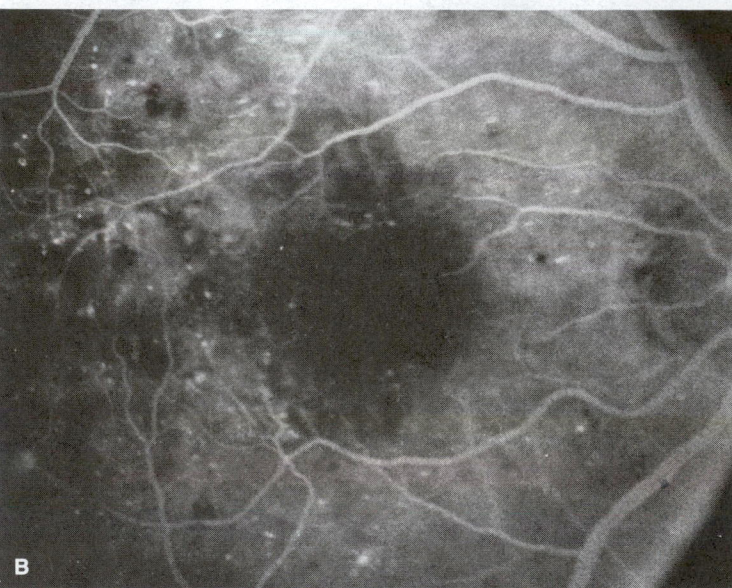

Figure 41–1

Diabetic retinopathy. **A.** Intense hyperfluorescence of edematous retina. **B.** Fluorescein angiogram demonstrates multiple leaking microaneurysms within area of edema. **C.** Intense hyperfluorescence of edematous retina noted in later phase angiogram.

SOURCE: **A & B.** Retina Unit, Pacific Presbyterian Medical Center, courtesy of Dr. Everett Ai. **C.** National Institutes of Health, Dept. of Health and Human Services, courtesy of Dr. Frederick L. Ferris.

effusions may result from the insufficient production of T_4 in myxedema. Hypertension can accompany Cushing's syndrome, and hypotension can accompany adrenal insufficiency.

Because of the interrelation between the cardiac and respiratory systems, cardiac pathology often produces changes in the lungs (eg, pleural effusions or congestive heart failure). Therefore, assess the lungs for any abnormal breath sounds, rales, rhonchi, wheezes, or pleural friction rubs.

Assessment of the Abdomen and Genitals

Inspect the abdomen for any asymmetry that might indicate ascites, enlargement of an organ, or a mass. Auscultate the abdomen to detect bruits (especially over the renal arteries) and palpate to determine if the client has any abdominal pain. Epigastric pain, often accompanying peptic ulcer, can be associated with hyperparathyroidism. Abdominal pain can also be present in clients with adrenal insufficiency.

Assessment of the genitalia is important in the evaluation of clients with endocrine dysfunction, because changes in sexual development and reproductive function often occur. Note the appearance of the client's genitals and any abnormalities. Do the genitals appear appropriate for the client's age and sex? Are there secondary sex characteristics? Does there appear to be agreement between the genital, hormonal, and psychological sex of the client?

Neuromuscular Assessment

Examine the musculoskeletal system for fractures (seen in Cushing's syndrome and hyperparathyroidism), bone pain, joint pain (seen in myxedema and acromegaly), and generalized muscle weakness (seen in hyperthyroidism, acromegaly, hyperparathyroidism, and Cushing's syndrome). The neurologic and endocrine systems work closely together to maintain the homeostasis of the internal environment and to help the person withstand stress. Therefore, pathology in the nervous system often affects endocrine function (eg, a benign tumor of the pituitary gland can cause hypersecretion of anterior pituitary hormones), and pathology in the endocrine system can be reflected in the nervous system (eg, hypothyroidism can dull mentation).

Conduct a careful neurologic evaluation, including assessment of mental status, cranial nerves (dysfunction of cranial nerves I and II—the olfactory and optic nerves—is associated with enlargement of the pituitary gland), motor and sensory function (neuropathy is seen in advanced diabetes mellitus), the cerebellum, and deep tendon and superficial reflexes. Ataxia can be seen in myxedema. Paresthesia is commonly associated with diabetes mellitus

but also can occur in hypocalcemia, acromegaly, and myxedema. Thoroughness in examination and accuracy in recording findings are essential. Report all abnormal findings to the physician for further evaluation.

Diagnostic Studies

Single measures of endocrine function are rarely sufficient to support a diagnosis but nevertheless should be an integral part of the whole data base. In endocrine testing, be aware of the importance of client preparation and adhere strictly to the testing protocols. Client and environmental influences that might modify the test results are other important nursing considerations. Diagnostic studies common to the endocrine system are summarized in Table 41–1.

(continued on p. 1302)

Table 41–1 Diagnostic Studies Common to the Endocrine System

Laboratory Test	Normal Expected Value	Disease State	Expected Abnormal Findings
Anterior pituitary			
Serum growth hormone (GH) RIA	0—8 ng/mL	Increased GH secretion in acromegaly, gigantism, hypoglycemia, exercise, stress	Above 8 ng/mL
		Decreased GH secretion in pituitary dwarfism, hyperglycemia, use of glucocorticoids	Below 8 ng/mL
Insulin tolerance test (ITT or GH stimulation test)	Serum cortisol above 7 μg/dL with peak at 20 μg/dL GH above 20 ng/mL Prolactin above 10 ng/mL (doubling baseline)	Adrenal–hypothalamic–anterior pituitary deficiency	Failure to respond to hypoglycemic challenge indicates a defect in the hypothalamus or anterior pituitary gland
GH suppression test	Basal level 10 ng/mL; suppressed below 5 ng/mL sometime during test	Excess GH (acromegaly, gigantism)	In active acromegaly or gigantism: basal level 5 ng/mL; no suppression below 5 ng/mL during test
		Renal failure, cirrhosis, starvation	Nonsuppression of GH
Radiologic testing			
X-ray and CT scan of skull with attention to sella turcica	Negative	Anterior pituitary dysfunction	Possible widening of sella turcica with anterior pituitary tumor
Posterior pituitary *Routine screening tests*			
Urine	Specific gravity 1.016–1.022	Diabetes insipidus	Low morning urine specific gravity (below 1.007)
	Urinary sodium (24 h) 100—260 mEq/24 h	SIADH	Increased urinary sodium

(continued)

Table 41–1   Diagnostic Studies Common to the Endocrine System (continued)

Laboratory Test	Normal Expected Value	Disease State	Expected Abnormal Findings
		Diabetes insipidus	Increased sodium concentrations in both urine and serum
Serum	Serum sodium 135–148 mEq/L	SIADH	Decreased sodium and chloride concentrations in serum
	BUN 6–20 mg/dL	Diabetes insipidus	Normal range
	Creatinine 0.6–1.5 mg/dL		
	Potassium 3.6–5.0 mEq/L		
	Hematocrit M 40%–54%; F 37%–47%	SIADH	Decreased hematocrit (increased MCV and decreased MCHC) secondary to hemodilution
	Mean corpuscular volume (MCV) 76–100 fL		
	Mean corpuscular hemoglobin concentration (MCHC) 30%–38%		
Osmolality tests			
Urine	M 390–1090 mOsm/kg or mOsm/L	Diabetes insipidus	Decreased urine osmolality
	F 300–1090 mOsm/kg or mOsm/L	SIADH	Increased urine osmolality
Serum	275–300 mOsm/kg	Diabetes insipidus	Increased serum osmolality
		SIADH	Decreased serum osmolality
Water deprivation test	Urine osmolality over 800 mOsm/kg	Diabetes insipidus (pituitary–hypothalamic etiology)	Serum osmolality greater than 300 mOsm/kg
	Urine osmolality greater than serum osmolality		Urine osmolality less than serum osmolality
	No change in serum osmolality over course of test		Response to vasopressin: greater increase in urine osmolality than serum osmolality
	No change in serum sodium levels over course of test	Nephrogenic diabetes insipidus	Serum osmolality greater than 300 mOsm/kg
			Urine osmolality less than serum osmolality
			No response to vasopressin
Water-loading test	Decrease in urinary volume due to stimulation of ADH	Diabetes insipidus (pituitary)	No antidiuresis; no change in urine osmolality (less than 400 mOsm/L)
	Urine osmolality equal or greater than 600 mOsm/L	Nephrogenic diabetes insipidus	No antidiuresis; no change in urine osmolality (less than 400 mOsm/L)
Thyroid gland			
Serum T_4	4–12 µg/dL	Hyperthyroidism	Increase
		Hypothyroidism	Decrease

Laboratory Test	Normal Expected Value	Disease State	Expected Abnormal Findings
Serum T_3	80–100 ng/dL	Hyperthyroidism	Increase (greater proportionately than T_4)
		Hypothyroidism	Decrease
Thyroxine-binding globulin (TBG)	10–26 μg/dL	Pregnancy, estrogen administration	Increased TBG and T_4, decreased RT_3U (resin T_3 uptake)
		Hypoproteinemia, androgen therapy, use of salicylates	Decreased TBG and T_4, increased RT_3U
Thyrotropin-stimulating hormone (TSH)	<5 μU/mL	Primary hypothyroidism	Increased TSH and TRF
		Secondary hypothyroidism	Decreased TSH and TRF
Thyroid circulating antibody (thyroid autoantibody, or TAA)	Usually absent	Graves' disease, Hashimoto's thyroiditis	Increased antibody levels
		Most other thyroid disorders; also pernicious anemia, myasthenia gravis, and Type I diabetes mellitus	Decreased antibody levels
Radiologic testing			
Thyroid scanning using radioactive ^{131}I uptake (RAIU)	Serum: 2 h, 4%–12% uptake; 6 h, 6%–15% uptake; 24 h, 8%–30% uptake	Hyperthyroidism	Serum: Increased ^{131}I with early high peak
		Hypothyroidism	Decreased ^{131}I with consistent low peak
	Urine: 40%–80% [131]I excreted in first 24 h		Urine: Less than 40% excretion (hyperthyroidism)
			More than 80% excretion (hypothyroidism)
Ultrasonography of the thyroid gland	Normal size, shape, and location of thyroid gland	Nonfunctioning thyroid nodules	Can differentiate between cystic and solid nodules; used in following the effect of treatment on thyroid masses
Thyroid stimulation test	Increase in T_4 and RAIU uptake	Primary hypothyroidism	Less than 10% increase in RAIU or less than 1.5 μg/dL increase in T_4
		Secondary hypothyroidism	At least 10% increase in RAIU and 1.5 μg/dL increase in T_4
Thyroid suppression test	25% decrease in second RAIU finding (suppression)	Primary hyperthyroidism (Graves' disease)	No suppression
Serum calcitonin	Undetectable	Medullary carcinoma of thyroid gland	More than 100 pg/mL
Parathyroid glands			
Serum calcium	Adult 8.5–10.5 mg/dL	Primary hyperparathyroidism	Increased serum calcium
		Hypoparathyroidism	Decreased serum calcium
Serum phosphorus	Adult 3.0–4.5 mg/dL	Hyperparathyroidism, rickets, osteomalacia	Decreased serum phosphorus
		Primary and secondary hypoparathyroidism, uremia, alkalosis	Increased serum phosphorus

(continued)

Table 41–1   Diagnostic Studies Common to the Endocrine System (continued)

Laboratory Test	Normal Expected Value	Disease State	Expected Abnormal Findings
Serum PTH	Less than 2000 pg/mL	Hyperparathyroidism	Increased PTH
		Hypoparathyroidism	Decreased PTH
Qualitative urinary calcium (Sulkowitch's test)	1+ −2+ or negative (scale from negative to positive)	Hyperparathyroidism	Increased urinary calcium
		Hypoparathyroidism	Decreased urinary calcium
Quantitative urinary calcium	50−300 mg/24 h	Hyperparathyroidism	Increased urinary calcium
		Hypoparathyroidism	Decreased urinary calcium
Adrenal cortex			
Serum cortisol	8−10 AM: 5−25 μg/dL 4 PM−midnight: 2−18 μg/dL	Cushing's disease, Cushing's syndrome	Increased serum cortisol
		Addison's disease, hypopituitarism	Decreased serum cortisol
Serum aldosterone	Normal sodium intake: 8 AM (recumbent) 3−9 ng/dL 9 AM (upright) 4−30 ng/dL	Primary aldosteronism (Conn's syndrome), secondary aldosteronism	Increased serum aldosterone
		Addison's disease, Sheehan's syndrome	Decreased serum aldosterone
Serum ACTH	8 AM (fasting) 20−100 pg/mL 4 PM (nonfasting) 10−50 pg/mL	Primary Addison's disease, ectopic ACTH-producing tumors, stress	Increased serum ACTH
		Cushing's disease secondary to pituitary-dependent adrenal hyperplasia	High-normal to low-normal serum ACTH
		Hypopituitarism, Cushing's syndrome secondary to adrenal adenomas or carcinomas	Decreased serum ACTH
Urinary 17-hydroxycorticosteroids (17-OHCS)	M 5−15 mg/24 h F 2−13 mg/24 h	Hyperfunction of the adrenal gland (Cushing's syndrome)	Increased 17-OHCS
		Hypofunction of the adrenal gland (Addison's disease)	Decreased 17-OHCS
Urinary 17-ketosteroids (17-KS)	M 8−25 mg/24 h F 5−15 mg/24 h	Hyperfunction of the adrenal gland; testosterone or estrogen-secreting tumors of the adrenal gland, ovaries, or testes; adrenogenital syndromes	Increased 17-KS
		Hypofunction of the adrenal gland	Decreased 17-KS
Urinary free cortisol	0−10 μg/24 h	Cushing's syndrome	Increased urinary free cortisol
Urinary aldosterone	2−26 μg/24 h	Primary and secondary aldosteronism	Increased urinary aldosterone
		Addison's disease, Sheehan's syndrome	Decreased urinary aldosterone
Dexamethasone suppression test	Low dose: More than 50% reduction in urinary 17-OHCS levels	Bilateral adrenal hyperplasia (Cushing's syndrome)	Low dose: no change; high dose: more than 50% reduction

Laboratory Test	Normal Expected Value	Disease State	Expected Abnormal Findings
	High dose: More than 50% reduction in urinary 17-OHCS levels	Adrenal adenoma or carcinoma	Low dose: no change; high dose: no change
		Ectopic ACTH-producing tumors	Low dose; no change; high dose: no change
ACTH stimulation test (modified Thorn test, ACTH provocative test, ACTH infusion test)	Serum cortisol 40 μg/dL after 24-h infusion	Cushing's syndrome secondary to bilateral adrenal hyperplasia	Increased serum cortisol
		Cushing's syndrome secondary to autonomic hyperfunctioning adrenal tumors	No change in serum cortisol
		Addison's disease secondary to pituitary hypofunction (secondary adrenal insufficiency)	Serum cortisol 10−40 μg/dL
		Addison's disease secondary to primary adrenal insufficiency	No change in serum cortisol
Metyrapone test	24-h level of 17-OHCS double the baseline	Cushing's syndrome secondary to bilateral adrenal hyperplasia	Double the baseline or higher urinary 17-OHCS
		Cushing's syndrome secondary to autonomous hyperfunctioning adrenal tumors	No change in urinary 17-OHCS
Adrenal medulla			
Serum catecholamines (fractionated)	Epinephrine: supine, 0−150 ng/L; standing, 0−150 ng/L Norepinephrine: supine, 103−193 ng/L; standing, 293−489 ng/L	Pheochromocytoma, neuroblastoma, ganglioneuroblastoma, ganglioneuroma	Increased serum catecholamine
Urinary vanillylmandelic acid (VMA)	0.5−8 mg/24 h	Tumors of adrenal medulla (eg, pheochromocytoma)	Increased urinary VMA
Urinary homovanillic acid (HVA)	More than 15 mg/24 h	Neural crest tumor (neuroblastoma or ganglioneuroma)	Increased urinary HVA
Total urinary catecholamine	Less than 100 μg/24 h (varies with activity)	Pheochromocytoma	No increase in urinary HVA
		Tumors of adrenal medulla	Increased total urinary catecholamines
Pancreas (endocrine function)			
Urinary glucose and ketones	Negative	Diabetes mellitus, Cushing's syndrome, acromegaly, stress, HHNK coma	Increased urinary glucose
		Diabetes mellitus, high-fat and low-carbohydrate diet, starvation, febrile and toxic illnesses	Increased urinary acetone
Fasting serum glucose	80−120 mg/dL	Diabetes mellitus, HHNK coma, Cushing's syndrome, acromegaly, stress, acute pancreatitis, and numerous drugs	Increased serum glucose

(continued)

Table 41–1   Diagnostic Studies Common to the Endocrine System (continued)

Laboratory Test	Normal Expected Value	Disease State	Expected Abnormal Findings
		Advanced liver disease, Addison's disease, islet cell adenoma, impaired glucose tolerance, spontaneous hypoglycemia	Decreased serum glucose
2-hour postprandial glucose	145 mg/dL; over age 60, less than 160 mg/dL	Diabetes mellitus, HHNK coma, Cushing's syndrome, acromegaly, stress	Increased 2-hour postprandial glucose
Glycosylated hemoglobin (HbA$_{1c}$)	4.82%–5.09% of total hemoglobin	Hyperglycemia	Increased HbA$_{1c}$
		Hemolytic states (secondary to loss of hemoglobin)	Decreased HbA$_{1c}$
24-h urine test for quantitative glucose levels	No glucose in urine in a 24-h period	Diabetes mellitus	Increased urinary glucose
Glucose tolerance test (GTT)	Serum glucose levels peak within 30 min to 1 h in a range of 160–180 mg/dL, return to normal range within 2–3 h; urine negative for glucose throughout test	Diabetes mellitus, Cushing's syndrome, pheochromocytoma, CNS lesions, hemochromatosis	Decreased glucose tolerance curve (sharp peak with curve that returns slowly to baseline)
		Insulinoma, Addison's disease, hypothyroidism, hypopituitarism, malabsorption states	Increased glucose tolerance curve (peak at less-than-normal levels)
Serum insulin	4–24 μU/mL	Insulinoma	Increased serum insulin and glucose
		Diabetes mellitus (with insulin resistance), idiopathic functional hypoglycemia, conditions causing reactive hypoglycemia	Increased serum insulin
		Diabetes mellitus (no insulin resistance)	Decreased serum insulin
Tolbutamide tolerance test (TTT, insulin tolerance test, insulin stimulation test)	After infusion, serum glucose levels drop to approximately half the fasting level in 30 min and return to pretest levels within 1½ to 3 h	Hyperinsulinism	Results same as in normal individuals
		Insulinoma	Marked drop in glucose with a return to normal in 3 h or more
		Diabetes mellitus	Prolonged time of return to pretest levels; slow initial drop in serum glucose

Anterior Pituitary Function

Three common tests for evaluating selective function of the anterior pituitary gland in adults are the serum growth hormone (GH) radioimmunoassay (RIA), the insulin tolerance test (ITT), and the GH suppression test. X-rays and CT scans are also used.

Serum Growth Hormone Radioimmunoassay. The serum GH RIA is used to evaluate clients who are suspected of having either excesses or deficiencies of growth hormone. Although the function of GH in adults is not well understood, information about the serum level of this hormone can be used as a guide in evaluating pituitary function. Normal levels of GH vary widely; they may be less than 3 ng/mL or undetectable. Because of this, the samples should be drawn in the early morning when the levels are higher.

Nursing Implications. The client should be NPO for 8 hours before the serum growth hormone RIA. The client should remain at rest for 30 minutes before the venipuncture to avoid an increase in GH secretion because of exercise.

Insulin Tolerance Test (Growth Hormone Stimulation Test). The insulin tolerance test (ITT)— also called the GH stimulation test—is used to evaluate clients with suggested deficiencies in GH, prolactin, or the adrenal–hypothalamic–anterior pituitary network. These deficiencies may be evaluated singly or simultaneously. The ITT is based on the principle that insulin-induced hypoglycemia will stimulate the release of cortisol, prolactin, and GH and that the elevations in these serum concentrations can be measured directly. Substances other than insulin may be used to stimulate a response; for example, glucagon, tolbutamide, vasopressin, and L-dopa are also used in stimulation tests and may be combined with other agents to provoke a maximal response.

Because the normal basal secretion level of GH is so low, a stimulation test is often required to rule out the possibility of hypopituitarism. Because they stress the system, stimulation tests also provide information about the reserve capacity of GH and the ability of the pituitary gland to respond to increased need. The ITT is contraindicated in clients with a history of myocardial infarction, ischemic heart disease, cerebrovascular disease, and epilepsy. The physician should be present during testing, especially if the client is suspected of having adrenal insufficiency, because profound hypoglycemia may occur in these clients.

Nursing Implications. The client is on bed rest and NPO after midnight the night before the ITT. A heparinized in-dwelling needle is inserted in the client's arm vein. Ask the client to rest for 30 minutes. Samples are drawn to measure serum glucose and/or cortisol, GH, and prolactin levels. Administer regular insulin intravenously in the dosage determined by the physician. If the serum glucose level fails to go below 40 mg/dL or clinical signs of hypoglycemia do not appear after 45 minutes, the insulin dose may need to be repeated.

Blood samples of serum glucose and/or cortisol, GH, and prolactin are drawn 30, 45, and 60 minutes after the administration of insulin. In addition, at 90 minutes after injection, samples of GH and cortisol are drawn. After drawing the last sample, give the client breakfast promptly. Observe the client for symptoms and signs of severe hypoglycemia. An IV bottle of 50 mL of 50% dextrose should be at the bedside for use in an emergency.

Growth Hormone Suppression Test. The GH suppression test is used to evaluate clients suspected of having acromegaly or gigantism. It is based on the principle that levels in the serum decrease in response to the administration of glucose.

Nursing Implications. The client should be on bed rest and NPO after midnight. To perform the test, serum GH level is determined to establish a baseline. The client is then given 100 g of glucose orally. A serum GH level is again determined 60 minutes after the glucose load.

Radiological Testing. The diagnostic investigation of anterior pituitary dysfunction often involves an x-ray or computerized tomography (CT) scan of the skull. A cerebral flow brain scan or echoencephalogram also may be used. In the presence of a pituitary tumor, a widening of the sella turcica (the bony seat of the pituitary gland) can sometimes be seen. To further detect the presence of a brain tumor, a complete neurologic evaluation may be done, including assessment of the client's visual fields.

Posterior Pituitary Function
Laboratory tests used to evaluate the function of the posterior pituitary gland include routine screening tests, serum and urine osmolality tests, the water deprivation test, and the water-loading test. Routine screening tests are described in Table 41–1.

Osmolality Tests. Osmolality, the measurement of the number of dissolved solute particles in a unit of solution, is the best measure of body fluids because it represents a constant weight-to-weight ratio. Specific gravity, in contrast, depends on both the quality and precise nature of the particles and is influenced by the presence of glucose, protein, and temperature. Osmolality varies with the temperature of the solution and fluid volume.

Assessment of urine osmolality provides information on (1) the ability of the kidney tubules to concentrate or dilute urine and (2) the presumptive presence or absence of antidiuretic hormone (ADH). It also indicates what the serum osmolality might be. Osmolality tests use the first-voided morning urine specimen, which is thought to represent the maximum concentration ability of the kidneys.

Water Deprivation Test. A water deprivation test is done when the client's symptoms suggest diabetes insipidus. This test is based on the principle that withholding fluid stimulates ADH secretion.

Nursing Implications. Other conditions such as diabetes mellitus, hyperkalemia, or hypercalcemia should be ruled out before the water deprivation test is attempted. The client is NPO from midnight until the conclusion of the test and should be instructed to abstain from fluids, because fluid intake could invalidate the test. The client is weighed at midnight; serum osmolality, serum sodium levels, urine volume, and urine osmolality are checked. At 8 AM the client is weighed again and the laboratory studies repeated. Urine osmolalities may be checked every hour. If an inadequate concentration of the urine is seen or the diagnosis of diabetes insipidus is suggested, 5 units of aqueous vasopressin may be ordered to be given subcutaneously. Urine osmolalities are then measured on each voided specimen for the next 4 to 6 hours. Observe the client carefully for signs of serious dehydration (loss of 10% of body weight), which could result in vascular collapse.

Water-Loading Test. The principle of the water-loading test is that ADH release will be stimulated by a rise in serum osmolality, and the effect of this increased secretion can be determined in the urine. The indication for a water-loading test is symptoms that suggest diabetes insipidus. It is also thought to be useful in the diagnosis of the syndrome of inappropriate ADH secretion (SIADH) but may be extremely dangerous if clients have serum sodium concentrations less than 125 mEq/L (Treseler, 1982).

Nursing Implications. Clients may take food and fluids as desired until the test begins. They should remain in bed throughout the procedure. A urinary catheter is sometimes inserted to obtain samples.

Obtain samples for serum osmolality, urine volume, and urine osmolality as a baseline. Then ask the client to drink 20 mL/kg of water in 15 minutes. Alternatively, an IV line of 5% dextrose in water (D5W) is started at a controlled rate of 8 to 10 mL/min to establish diuresis. After 30 minutes, change the IV to 2.5% saline infused at a rate of 0.25 mL/kg/min. This is run for approximately 45 minutes; then changed back to D5W for 2-minute periods to replace the urine volume lost in each preceding 15-minute period. A vasopressin challenge may be given to differentiate between pituitary and nephrogenic diabetes insipidus.

Clients with cardiac disease are at risk of developing congestive heart failure during the test. Serum sodium levels should be evaluated before this procedure, because sodium replacement may be necessary before testing is attempted. The minimal safe level is 125 mEq/L.

Thyroid Function

Tests of thyroid function are used to diagnose hyperthyroidism and hypothyroidism and to evaluate thyroid nodules, thyroiditis, and goiters. Serum tests, serum RIA, scintillation scanning, and specialized tests are used. Measurement of serum T_4 is sufficient in most cases except borderline situations. The measurement of TSH is the most useful in diagnosing primary hypothyroidism, particularly in clients with borderline T_4 levels.

In the past, thyroid function was inferred from measurements of protein-bound iodine and basal metabolic rates. Today more direct and accurate methods are available.

Serum Thyroxine and Triiodothyronine Levels. Serum concentrations of T_4 and T_3 are measured to confirm a diagnosis of hyperthyroidism or hypothyroidism. The test uses a nonfasting sample of venous blood.

In general, both T_4 and T_3 levels are increased in hyperthyroidism and decreased in hypothyroidism. T_4 levels may be decreased in chronic thyroiditis and Hashimoto's thyroiditis, as well as in conditions that decrease the concentration or binding capacity of thyroxine-binding globulin (TBG) (eg, increased plasma steroid levels, acute illness, and chronic illness). Drugs that may decrease T_4 levels include androgens, salicylates, sulfonamides, reserpine, and heparin. T_4 levels increase in acute and subacute thyroiditis and in conditions that increase the concentration of binding capacity of TBG (eg, pregnancy, use of oral contraceptives, certain liver diseases, and acute intermittent porphyria).

Nursing Implications. Question clients carefully for a history of medication use and the possibility of pregnancy. Also ask clients whether they had an intravenous pyelogram, gallbladder studies, or CT scan within the past year. Depending on the type of contrast medium used, these tests can distort the outcome of a serum T_4 level.

Thyroxine-Binding Globulin Concentrations. Abnormalities in TBG concentrations can affect the levels of T_4 and T_3 in the serum, often causing inaccuracies in diagnosis. The many factors that can affect TBG levels are mentioned in the previous discussion of serum T_4 and T_3 levels.

Thyrotropin-Stimulating Hormone Level. Measurement of serum TSH helps differentiate primary from secondary hypothyroidism. In primary hypothyroidism, where the deficit is in the thyroid gland itself, there is a compensatory rise in both TSH and thyrotropin releasing factor (TRF). In secondary hypothyroidism, where the deficit is either in the hypothalamus or the pituitary gland, the serum levels of TSH and TRF are very low.

Thyroid Circulating Antibody Test (Thyroid Autoantibody Test). The thyroid circulating antibody test, or thyroid autoantibody (TAA) test, is based on the fact that the immune system plays a role in certain thyroid dysfunctions, particularly Graves' disease and Hashimoto's thyroiditis. The immunoglobulins produced in these conditions are thought to act as antibodies to the TSH receptor. In human thyroiditis, four separate antibody–antigen systems have been identified to date. Thyroid circulating antibody tests are used to diagnose these autoimmune thyroid conditions.

Thyroid Scanning. Thyroid scanning with a scinti-scanner measures radioactive ^{131}I uptake (RAIU) and can be used to assess the size, position, shape, and function of the thyroid gland. The use of radioactive iodine in thyroid scanning is based on the thyroid's ability to trap and retain ^{131}I and its eventual excretion in the urine. Use of the gamma-ray detector after the administration of the ^{131}I enables the examiner to determine the percentage of ^{131}I taken up by the gland over specified periods of time. Increased uptake of ^{131}I is seen in hyperthyroidism; and decreased uptake, in hypothyroidism.

Thyroid scanning is used for clients with undiagnosed masses in the neck, thyroid nodules, metastatic disease, thyroid cancer, and hyperthyroidism. It is especially invaluable in diagnosing thyroid nodules. Depending on how they assimilate the radioactive substance, nodules are classified as hot (functioning) or cold (nonfunctioning) (Figure 41–2). Hot nodules include localized toxic goiter and benign adenoma. Cold nodules might represent carcinoma, a cyst, a nonfunctional adenoma or goiter, a lymphoma, or thyroiditis (Pagana & Pagana, 1982).

The test can be influenced by several factors, such as

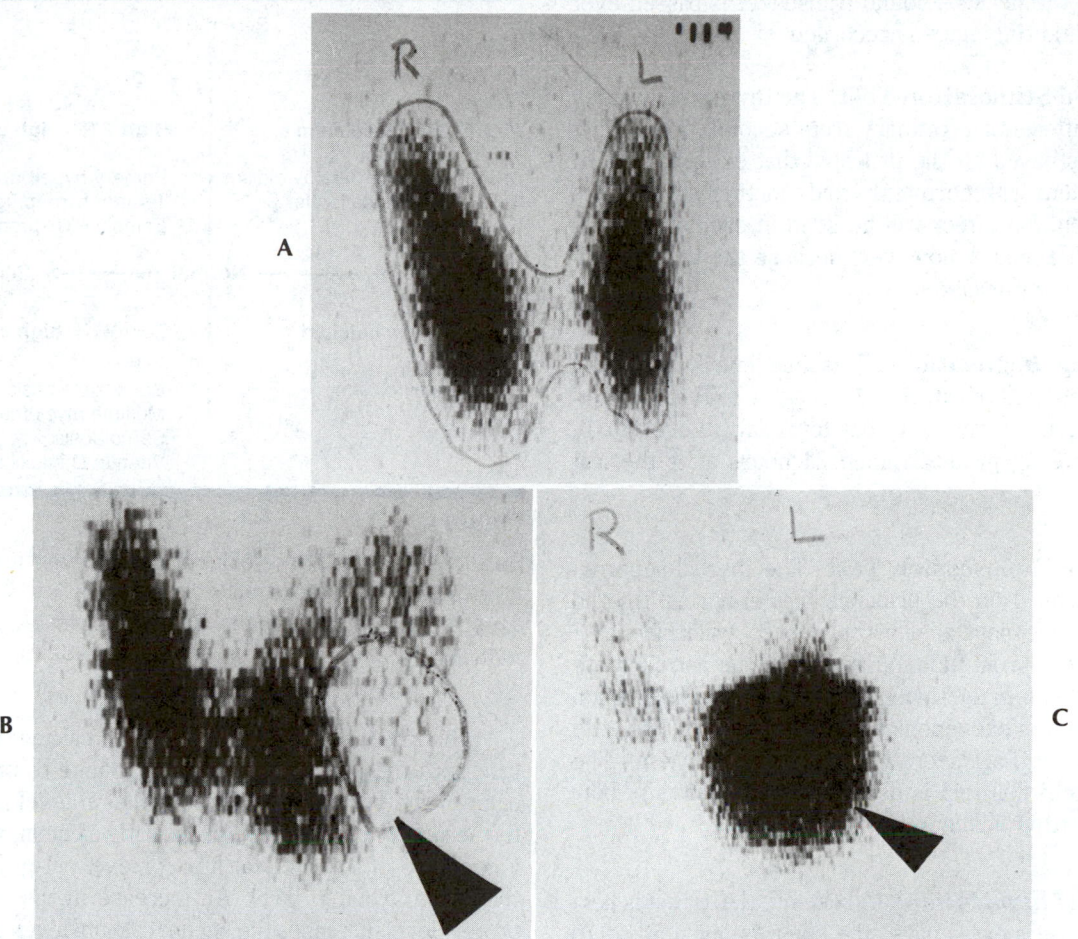

Figure 41–2

Thyroid scintiscan. **A.** Normal thyroid. **B.** Cold area (arrowhead). **C.** Hot area (arrowhead).
SOURCE: Pagana KD, Pagana, TJ: *Diagnostic Testing and Nursing Implications,* 2nd ed. St. Louis: Mosby, 1986.

iodine deficiency in the client; the previous administration of thyroid medication, antithyroid medication, or iodine; and diarrhea. It is contraindicated in clients who are pregnant, who had recent radioactive or x-ray dye studies, who are receiving iodine preparations, or who have a history of taking antithyroid or thyroid medication.

Nursing Implications. Take a thorough history before the administration of ^{131}I. Ask about use of thyroid or antithyroid drugs, estrogen, barbiturates, or TSH; the intake of any iodine preparations (eg, saturated solution of potassium iodide [SSKI], Lugol's solution, or tolbutamide); a history of any diagnostic studies using an iodine contrast material within the past 5 to 10 years (eg, gallbladder studies or intravenous pyelography); and the intake of any iodine-containing foods (shellfish or fish). The client should not take any iodine or thyroid preparations for 1 week before the test.

A 24-hour urine specimen collection is begun. The client is then given an oral dose of ^{131}I and asked to return to the laboratory in 2 to 24 hours, depending on the care provider. The RAIU is routinely measured at 24 hours, although measurement at different times (eg, 30 minutes and 6 hours) can evaluate several aspects of thyroid function. Measurement at 24 hours reflects the maximal uptake of ^{131}I by the thyroid gland.

On returning to the laboratory, the client is placed in the supine position, and a scintillation counter is passed over the thyroid gland to measure the amount of ^{131}I that has accumulated. The RAIU is stated as a percentage of the thyroid uptake compared with the total administered dose.

Ultrasonography of the Thyroid Gland. Ultrasonography of the thyroid gland uses reflected sound waves to assess the gland's size, location, and shape. It can distinguish cystic from solid thyroid nodules and follow the progress of a thyroid mass under treatment.

Nursing Implications. For ultrasonography of the thyroid, the client is placed in the supine position, and gel is applied to the neck. A sound transducer is passed over the thyroid and the image is recorded.

Thyroid Stimulation Test. The thyroid stimulation test helps differentiate primary from secondary hypothyroidism. It is based on the principle that exogenous TSH given to a client with normal thyroid function will increase T_4 production. No effect will be seen in clients with primary hypothyroidism, however, because the thyroid cannot respond to stimulation.

Nursing Implications. Baseline levels of T_4 and RAIU are obtained. Next, 5 to 10 units of TSH are administered intramuscularly every day for 3 days. Levels of T_4 and RAIU are again determined 24 hours after the last injection.

Thyroid Suppression Test. The thyroid suppression test is based on the principle that in normal thyroid function, an exogenous administration of T_4 will inhibit TSH secretion and thyroid function as part of the normal feedback mechanism. In the hyperthyroid state, TSH secretion is minimal, so the exogenous administration of T_4 has little or no effect on TSH secretion or thyroid function. The thyroid suppression test is useful in the diagnosis of borderline hyperthyroidism.

Nursing Implications. A baseline RAIU test is performed. For the next 7 days, the client is given 50 to 70 µg of T_4 orally. At the end of this period, the RAIU test is repeated. Take a careful history to determine previous high iodine intake, which can invalidate the test results.

Serum Calcitonin Level. Calcitonin plays an important role in calcium and phosphorus homeostasis. Serum levels of the hormone are consistently elevated in clients with medullary carcinoma of the thyroid glands. Elevated calcitonin levels have also been seen in clients with acute pancreatitis.

Parathyroid Function

The parathyroid glands secrete parathyroid hormone (PTH) in response to low serum calcium levels. PTH raises serum calcium levels by increasing bone resorption of calcium, increasing the reabsorption of calcium by the kidney tubules, increasing the absorption of calcium from the intestines, and increasing the excretion of phosphorus.

Serum phosphorus levels are in an inverse relationship to serum calcium levels; ie, an increase in phosphorus levels can result in a decrease in calcium levels. Both hyperparathyroidism and hypoparathyroidism are manifested by changes in serum calcium and phosphorus levels. Figure 41–3 summarizes the relationship of serum calcium and PTH levels to hyperparathyroidism and hypoparathyroidism.

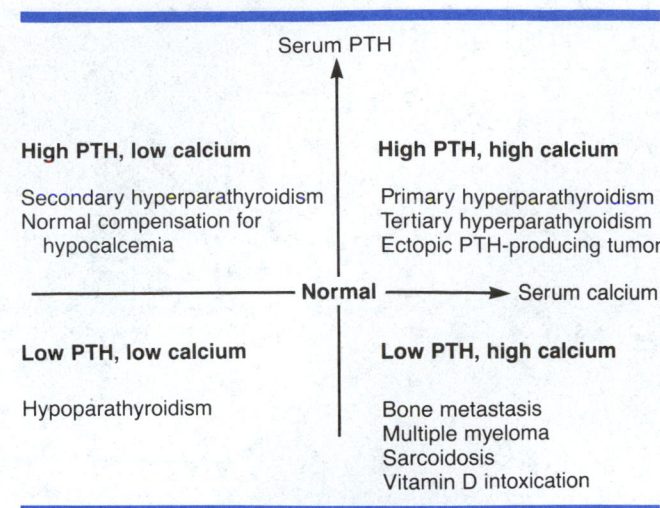

Figure 41–3

Relationship of serum calcium and PTH levels to hyperparathyroidism and hypoparathyroidism.
SOURCE: Pagana KD, Pagana TJ: *Diagnostic Testing and Nursing Implications.* St. Louis: Mosby, 1982, p. 203.

Serum Calcium Level. Serum calcium levels indicate both the ionized and inactive (bound to protein) calcium in the serum. The serum calcium level depends on the serum levels of protein, particularly albumin, and reflects a decrease of 1 mg of calcium for every 1-g decrease in the serum albumin level. An increase in the total serum protein level increases the serum calcium level. Therefore, in evaluating serum calcium results, it is important to consider the total protein levels in the serum as well as the serum phosphorus levels.

Serum calcium levels are elevated in primary hyperparathyroidism, increased concentrations of total protein, conditions characterized by an increase in bony resorption, excessive intake of vitamin D, carcinoma with metastasis to the bone, ectopic PTH-producing tumor, and milk–alkali syndrome. Serum calcium levels may be depressed in primary and secondary hypoparathyroidism, renal disease, conditions characterized by increased bone-building activity, and long-term phenytoin therapy.

Serum Phosphorus Level. An adverse relationship exists between serum calcium and serum phosphorus levels; it is maintained by the reabsorption or excretion of phosphorus by the kidney tubules under the direction of PTH.

Serum phosphorus levels are increased in primary and secondary hypoparathyroidism; chronic renal failure; conditions characterized by an excess of GH; and prolonged or massive use of antacids, vitamin D, heparin, and tetracycline.

Serum phosphorus levels are decreased in all the conditions characterized by an increase in serum calcium; in women during their menses; immediately after meals; and in clients receiving insulin, epinephrine, or aluminum hydroxide. They are also decreased in clients who have recently received a general anesthetic (Treseler, 1982).

Serum Parathyroidhormone Level. PTH levels in the serum can now be measured directly using RIA. When evaluated with the serum calcium levels, PTH levels provide the basis for a diagnosis of hyperparathyroidism. Therefore, the serum calcium level needs to be measured along with a serum PTH. The specimen should be placed on ice during transport to the laboratory.

PTH levels increase in primary, secondary, and tertiary hyperparathyroidism, as well as in conditions where there is a nonparathyroid, ectopic PTH-producing tumor (tumors of bronchi, kidney, ovary, and colon). Increased PTH levels also exist in conditions resulting from a normal compensatory response to hypocalcemia (eg, renal failure or vitamin D deficiency).

Levels of PTH may be depressed in hypoparathyroidism and as a response to hypercalcemia in clients with metastatic bone tumors. Decreased PTH levels also may be seen transiently following a thyroidectomy or parathyroidectomy. They may be lower in the morning because of a diurnal rhythm in their secretion.

Qualitative Urinary Calcium Level. The qualitative urinary calcium level measurement (Sulkowitch's test) is based on the principle that urinary calcium concentrations reflect serum calcium levels in the normal physiological state. When the serum calcium level falls below 7.5 mg/dL, no calcium is excreted in the urine. Urinary calcium levels may increase in hyperparathyroidism, hyperthyroidism, renal tubular acidosis, vitamin D intoxication, osteolytic bone disease, and osteoporosis. They also are associated with concentrated urine. Decreased urinary calcium levels may occur in hypoparathyroidism, vitamin D deficiency, malabsorption syndromes, and dilute urine (Treseler, 1982).

Quantitative Urinary Calcium Level. The quantitative urinary calcium test is used when quantification of the exact amount of calcium excreted is required. It involves the collection of a 24-hour urine specimen.

Nursing Implications. Clients are placed on a controlled diet of 100 mg of calcium for 3 days before the test is taken. They should be instructed to keep the 24-hour urine container at room temperature to keep the calcium sediment from precipitating. The nurse and client should be careful when pouring urine into the specimen bottle, because hydrochloric acid is added as a preservative.

Adrenocortical Function

The adrenal glands are composed of two distinct anatomic and physiological parts: the adrenal cortex and medulla. Each secretes several hormones essential to life and well-being. Serum and urine levels of these hormones are important in evaluating adrenal and pituitary disorders.

Serum Cortisol Level. Cortisol, the major hormone of the adrenal cortex, has a diurnal rhythm in its secretion. One of the earliest signs of adrenal dysfunction may be the loss of this diurnal variation. Cortisol levels measured in the serum can be used to evaluate adrenal activity.

Serum cortisol levels are increased in Cushing's syndrome and Cushing's disease. Increased levels may also be a physiologic response to obesity or stress. False increases in serum cortisol levels can occur in kidney and liver disease (secondary to decreased metabolism and excretion) and with increased serum estrogen levels. Decreased serum cortisol levels are seen in Addison's disease, in hypopituitarism, and in individuals receiving long-term androgen or phenytoin therapy.

Nursing Implications. Obtain a sample of venous blood at 8 AM after the client has had a full night's sleep. Send it to the laboratory for RIA analysis; label the laboratory request slip with the time of the venipuncture. A second specimen may be drawn around 4 PM to try to identify the variation in the cortisol levels. (Although the lowest level of cortisol is usually seen around midnight, this time may not be convenient for many laboratories.)

Because serum cortisol levels have a definite diurnal variation, screen the client for long-term deviations from the normal sleeping pattern (eg, working nights and sleeping days). Serum cortisol levels also can be affected by both chronic and acute stress, so it is important to screen the client carefully for any symptoms and signs of physical or emotional stress.

Serum Aldosterone Level. To facilitate interpretation of findings, the determination of a serum aldosterone level is usually accompanied by a urinary sodium test to rule out a sodium deficit in the body, which might falsely elevate the aldosterone level. A sample to determine the serum renin level is frequently drawn at the same time as the aldosterone sample to help differentiate between primary and secondary hyperaldosteronism.

Serum aldosterone levels increase in both primary aldosteronism (Conn's syndrome) and secondary aldosteronism. They also increase physiologically in clients with sodium restrictions or increased potassium intake. Clients receiving diuretic therapy (especially furosemide), estrogen, or drugs that are known to increase the serum renin levels also have an elevated serum aldosterone level.

Serum aldosterone levels decrease in clients with Addison's disease, Sheehan's syndrome, or destruction to the adrenal cortex. Levels are also decreased physiologically in clients following high-sodium diets or those who have decreased their potassium intake. Position changes affect serum aldosterone levels. Prolonged standing increases the level, whereas resting in a recumbent position decreases it.

Nursing Implications. The client should be restricted from food for at least 8 to 12 hours before testing. All steroids and diuretics should be discontinued 2 weeks before testing. Clients should receive an established sodium intake (135 mEq daily) for 2 weeks prior to testing. Hypertensive clients should be carefully evaluated for any evidence of sodium depletion (despite normal serum sodium levels) before the test is attempted. Advise clients to avoid licorice or licorice products, which produce an aldosteronelike effect.

Clients should remain recumbent until 30 minutes before the test and then ambulate until the sample is taken. Some laboratories may require one sample taken while the client is recumbent and another taken after ambulation to check the effect of changes in position.

Serum Adrenocorticotropic Hormone Level. A serum ACTH level can be measured via RIA to help determine the etiology of either Cushing's syndrome or Addison's disease. The interpretation of a serum ACTH level requires familiarity with the negative feedback system between the adrenal and the anterior pituitary gland (see Chapter 40). It is also important to remember that ACTH, like cortisol, is characterized by a diurnal variation in secretion. Serum ACTH levels are used to establish a baseline before adrenal suppression tests are done.

Serum ACTH levels increase in primary Addison's disease, nonpituitary ectopic ACTH-producing tumors (usually in the lung, pancreas, thymus, or ovary), and stress conditions (secondary to the increased release of glucocorticoids). High normal to low normal serum ACTH levels occur in clients with Cushing's disease secondary to pituitary-dependent adrenal hyperplasia. In this instance, ACTH does not show a diurnal variation and may remain elevated during the day.

Decreased ACTH levels occur in clients with hypopituitarism or Cushing's syndrome secondary to adrenal adenomas or carcinomas (which increase the serum level of cortisol and thereby suppress ACTH production). Clients receiving glucocorticoid therapy also have decreased levels.

Nursing Implications. A fasting blood sample is usually drawn between 8 and 10 AM. Obtain a sample of approximately 20 mL of venous blood using a chilled plastic heparinized syringe. Put the sample on ice, and send it immediately to the laboratory for RIA.

The client may be required to abstain from food for 8 hours before the test. This requirement may be modified, however, if a 4 PM sample is needed.

Urine Tests for 17-Hydroxycorticosteroid and 17-Ketosteroid. Urine tests for 17-hydroxycorticosteroid (17-OHCS) and 17-ketosteroid (17-KS) indirectly measure adrenal function. They reflect the levels of hormone precursors found in a 24-hour collection of urine. The 17-KS, the newer of the two tests, is thought to be more sensitive to pregnanediol, a glucocorticoid derivative, which

is not picked up by the 17-OHCS test and is seen in adrenogenital syndromes.

Urine 17-OHCS levels increase when there is hyperfunction of the adrenal gland, whether from hyperplasia of the adrenal cortex (Cushing's syndrome), adrenal or pituitary tumor, or ectopic ACTH production. Elevations of urinary 17-OHCS levels are also seen in clients with polycystic ovaries, those receiving estrogen therapy, in clients in the late stages of pregnancy, and in those under extreme stress.

Urinary 17-OHCS levels decrease with hypofunction of the adrenal gland, such as Addison's disease and hypopituitarism. Decreased levels may rarely be seen in pancreatitis and eclampsia (Treseler, 1982). Decreased levels of 17-OHCS also occur in clients with adrenal suppression secondary to prolonged steroid therapy.

Elevated urinary 17-KS levels appear in any condition that increases the serum levels of cortisol. They frequently occur in clients with adrenal hyperplasia; tumors of the adrenal gland, ovaries, or testes that secrete testosterone or estrogen; and adrenogenital syndromes. Decreased urine 17-KS levels are seen in any conditions with hypofunction of the adrenal glands, in clients who have had their ovaries or testes removed, and in Klinefelter's syndrome when there is a decrease in testosterone production.

Nursing Implications. Withhold all medications if possible, for several days before the test. The client may have a normal diet and fluids during the collection period unless contraindicated.

Urine is collected over a 24-hour period because of the diurnal variation in cortisol levels. The specimen should be refrigerated during collection. A preservative is added for the 17-KS test.

Obtain a history to detect consumption of the following products that might influence the test results: aspirin, acetaminophen, paraldehyde, chloral hydrate, nitrofurantoin, coffee, morphine, barbiturates, reserpine, furosemide, thiazides, monoamine oxidase (MAO) inhibitors, colchicine, sulfonamides, quinine, propoxyphene, spironolactone, cloxacillin sodium, and licorice. Because both emotional and physical stress can increase the activity of the adrenal gland, observe the client closely and report any evidence of stress to the physician.

Urinary Free Cortisol Level. A urinary free cortisol level measures the amount of free cortisol excreted by the kidneys in 24 hours. Because the urinary free cortisol levels correspond to serum cortisol levels, this test is a highly sensitive indicator of increased adrenal activity and is considered one of the most important tests for hypercortisolism. It has not been found to be a reliable indicator of decreased adrenal activity, however.

Increases in the level of urinary free cortisol are seen in Cushing's syndrome, with severe emotional stress (increases from 50% to 250%), in pregnancy, and with estrogen therapy. Decreases in urinary free cortisol levels are not considered clinically significant and do not necessarily indicate hypofunction of the adrenal cortex.

Nursing Implications. Collect a 24-hour urine specimen and send it to the laboratory for analysis. Refrigerate the specimen or place it on ice during collection. Carefully screen clients for any history of the use of steroids, reserpine, phenothiazine, morphine, or amphetamines—substances that can falsely elevate cortisol levels.

Urinary Aldosterone Level. Urinary aldosterone levels are useful in the diagnosis of primary and secondary aldosteronism. This test uses RIA and is evaluated in conjunction with serum electrolyte and renin levels.

Urinary aldosterone levels are elevated in primary and secondary aldosteronism. Decreased levels of urinary aldosterone are seen in Addison's disease and Sheehan's syndrome, in congenital adrenocortical hyperplasia when there is a loss of salt, and occasionally in toxemia of pregnancy.

Nursing Implications. Carefully screen all medications that might influence the test results (antihypertensive drugs, diuretics, and steroids). Instruct the client to maintain a normal sodium diet (135 mEq/day) before the test and to avoid foods with a high sodium content. Failure to follow these instructions can influence test results. The client also should avoid stressful situations and vigorous physical exercise.

Collect a 24-hour urine specimen, and send it to the laboratory for analysis. The specimen should be refrigerated or kept on ice during collection.

Dexamethasone Suppression Test. The dexamethasone suppression test investigates the negative feedback system between the pituitary and adrenal glands. It provides the physician with essential information about the cause of adrenal hyperfunction and often makes possible a distinction between hyperplastic and neoplastic causes.

This test is an important tool in the diagnosis of Cushing's syndrome. In normal situations, an increase in the serum levels of cortisol suppresses ACTH secretion by the anterior pituitary gland. Conversely, as serum cortisol levels decrease, ACTH secretion is stimulated. This feedback mechanism does not function as expected in Cushing's syndrome. In clients with Cushing's syndrome secondary to hyperplasia of the adrenal glands, the pituitary gland only responds to very high levels of cortisol. Therefore, serum ACTH levels are often in the normal to low normal range. Clients with Cushing's syndrome secondary to adrenal adenoma or carcinoma may have a very low level of serum ACTH. This is due to the increased secretion of cortisol by the autonomous tumors, which suppress ACTH production. In clients with Cushing's syndrome secondary to a nonpituitary ectopic ACTH-producing tumor, ACTH levels are often high despite high serum cortisol levels.

Correct interpretation of the results of the dexamethasone suppression test is based on this knowledge of the defects in the pituitary–adrenal feedback mechanism. The test is based on the principle that the administration of a small amount of dexamethasone (Decadron) in a normal individual will suppress the pituitary secretion of ACTH. This results in decreased stimulation to the adrenal glands, which is reflected in a 50% or more drop in the serum cortisol and urinary 17-OHCS levels.

In clients with Cushing's syndrome secondary to adrenal hyperplasia, the pituitary gland does not suppress the secretion of ACTH, because it is accustomed to high levels of glucocorticoids. Therefore, no changes in the urinary levels of 17-OHCS are seen on low-dose testing, but a 50% reduction can be seen when high-dose suppression is administered. In clients with adrenal adenoma or carcinoma, there will be no changes in the levels of the urinary 17-OHCS with either low- or high-dose testing, because pituitary ACTH is already suppressed. In cushingoid clients with ectopic ACTH-producing tumors, there will be no changes in the levels of 17-OHCS with either low- or high-dose testing.

Nursing Implications. There are many forms of the dexamethasone suppression test, including an overnight single-dose test, a low-dose test, and a high-dose test. The classic form takes 6 days and usually requires hospitalization.

On the first and second days, baseline urinary 17-OHCS levels are determined. On the third and fourth days, a low dose of dexamethasone is administered every 6 hours, and a 24-hour collection of urine for 17-OHCS is obtained. On the fifth and sixth days, a high dose of dexamethasone is administered every 6 hours, and another 24-hour urine collection is obtained for analysis of the urinary 17-OHCS levels. Creatinine levels are often measured in the 24-hour urine samples to check the accuracy and adequacy of the collection; the overall amount of creatinine in the sample should not vary from day to day. The urine sample of 17-OHCS should not contain a preservative and should be refrigerated during the collection period.

Carefully assess clients for signs of stress, which can affect the test results (stress increases the secretion of ACTH). The administration of dexamethasone with milk or an antacid prevents irritation of the gastric mucosa. Evaluate the client for any untoward symptoms and signs of steroid therapy. Check the urine for glucose, evaluate serum potassium levels, and watch for changes in the psyche. Finally, assess the client for factors that might interfere with the normal suppression responses; eg, estrogen therapy, hyperthyroidism, phenytoin therapy, obesity, or mental depression (possibly related to a biochemical phenomenon).

Adrenocorticotropic Hormone Stimulation Test. The ACTH stimulation test (also called the modified Thorn test, the ACTH provocative test, or the ACTH infusion test) is used to evaluate clients with adrenal dysfunction. It is based on the principle that in the normal individual, the exogenous administration of a 24-hour infusion of ACTH should cause a rise in the serum cortisol levels (greater than 40 μg/dL).

Clients with Cushing's syndrome secondary to bilateral hyperplasia of the adrenal glands will have increased serum cortisol levels that may persist beyond a 24-hour period. Those with autonomous hyperfunctioning adrenal tumors will exhibit little or no change in serum cortisol levels, because they are relatively insensitive to changes in ACTH secretion.

For clients with Addison's disease, the ACTH stimulation test can be a valuable diagnostic tool in differentiating between primary and secondary adrenal insufficiency. In secondary adrenal insufficiency due to pituitary hypofunction, the serum cortisol levels should be between 10 and 40 ng/dL after ACTH infusion. This shows that the adrenal glands are capable of functioning if stimulated. In primary adrenal insufficiency, no changes are seen in the serum cortisol levels after a 24-hour infusion of ACTH. Clients experiencing adrenal suppression secondary to the long-term administration of steroids may have a delayed response to the ACTH stimulation test.

Nursing Implications. Carefully obtain a history of factors that might influence the test results (refer to the discussion of serum cortisol levels). To perform the test, a baseline serum cortisol level is obtained. An IV infusion of ACTH is then administered to the client over a 24-hour period. After 24 hours, the laboratory analyzes serum cortisol levels. The ACTH stimulation test can also be performed by comparing the 17-OHCS levels excreted in the urine (normal levels are 25 mg/24 hr). A rapid form of this test, the rapid ACTH stimulation test, uses an intramuscular injection instead of the IV infusion.

Metyrapone Test. The metyrapone test differentiates between adrenal hyperplasia and ectopic ACTH production as a cause of Cushing's syndrome. Both clinical entities have increased serum ACTH levels. This test is based on the principle that the administration of metyrapone (Metopirone) normally results in decreased cortisol production because of its ability to block necessary enzymes to produce cortisol. This decrease in cortisol production should stimulate ACTH secretion by the pituitary gland. The inability to synthesize cortisol in response to ACTH stimulation will result in the excretion of cortisol precursors, which can be measured in the urine using the urinary 17-OHCS test. The metyrapone test also can assess the reserve of the pituitary gland and is similar in principle to the ACTH stimulation test.

In clients with Cushing's syndrome secondary to bilateral adrenal hyperplasia, the levels of urinary 17-OHCS are increased more than in normal clients. In clients with Cushing's syndrome secondary to autonomous hyperfunc-

tioning adrenal tumors, there is no increase in urinary 17-OHCS levels.

Nursing Implications. The metyrapone test may be conducted overnight or over a 2-day period. No special fluid or food limitations are required. First, a baseline 24-hour urine collection is obtained to determine 17-OHCS levels. An oral dose of metyrapone (approximately 500 to 750 mg) is then administered every 4 hours for 24 hours. During and 24 hours after the administration of metyrapone, 24-hour urine samples for 17-OHCS levels are collected.

Carefully evaluate the client for symptoms and signs of addisonian crisis, which can be precipitated in clients with Addison's disease because of the inhibition of cortisol synthesis. Addisonian crisis is a medical emergency that requires prompt assessment and intervention (see Chapter 44).

X-ray Studies, Arteriography, Venography, CT Scanning. Tumors of the pituitary can cause Cushing's syndrome. In this case, Cushing's syndrome occurs because of hyperfunction of the anterior pituitary, which in turn causes bilateral adrenal hyperplasia with excess cortisol production. Deviations in the normal sella turcica, such as enlargement or destructive changes, can be seen on x-ray examination.

Adrenal arteriography and venography are used to study the vasculature of the adrenal arteries and veins. Adrenal arteriography is similar to renal angiography. Adrenal venography is similar to other venous study procedures and is especially useful in differentiating unilateral from bilateral pheochromocytoma as well as unilateral adrenal tumors from the bilateral adrenal hyperplasia of Cushing's syndrome.

Computerized tomography (CT) of the adrenal glands is a noninvasive method for detecting very small tumors, such as adrenal adenomas, pheochromocytomas, or carcinomas. Some radiologists believe that by using the density coefficients of the CT scan, it is possible to differentiate among these tumors, detect bilateral adrenal hyperplasia, and identify areas of adrenal hemorrhage.

Adrenal Medullary Function
The hormones of the adrenal medulla, epinephrine and norepinephrine, are called *catecholamines* and have a sympathomimetic action. Clinical symptoms and signs of adrenal medullary dysfunction include hypertension, signs of increased metabolism (such as diaphoresis, heat intolerance, weight loss, and cardiac dysrhythmias), and postural hypotension. The clinical findings in adrenal medullary dysfunction are more prominent than the laboratory findings, so they should be carefully assessed and correlated with the diagnostic test results.

Because epinephrine inhibits the release of insulin, it is not unusual to find increased serum glucose levels and glycosuria in clients with disorders of the adrenal medulla.

Free fatty acids are also increased in the serum secondary to (1) the increased levels of epinephrine and (2) an increase in the metabolism of fats because of the lack of insulin.

Measurement of Serum Catecholamine Levels (Fractionated). The serum levels of individual catecholamines (norepinephrine and epinephrine) are not measured routinely. Unlike the measurement of urinary vanillylmandelic acid (VMA) and total urinary catecholamines, this test yields levels for individual catecholamines that are useful in determining whether pheochromocytoma is adrenal or extraadrenal. An adrenal tumor secretes both epinephrine and norepinephrine, whereas an extraadrenal tumor usually secretes only norepinephrine.

High serum catecholamine levels occur in clients with pheochromocytoma, ganglioneuroma, neuroblastoma, and ganglioneuroblastoma. However, elevations in serum catecholamine levels also occur in cardiac disorders, hypoglycemia, and thyroid dysfunction as well as in clients after electroshock therapy and those in shock from hemorrhage, infections, or anaphylaxis.

Nursing Implications. Obtain a careful history of all variables that may affect test results (radioactive scan within 1 week or the ingestion of epinephrine, amphetamines, phenothiazines, levodopa, sympathomimetics, decongestants, tricyclic antidepressants, and reserpine). The client should rest in bed in a quiet environment for at least 30 minutes before the test. He or she should be kept warm and relaxed. The diet before testing should contain a normal sodium intake. The client should abstain from amine-rich foods (cheese, coffee, tea, cocoa, beer, bananas, and avocados) for at least 48 hours before testing to avoid distorting the test results. The client should refrain from smoking for at least 15 minutes before the test.

The test requires two venous blood samples, usually taken in supine and standing positions. Use chilled tubes containing ethylenediamine tetra-acetic acid (EDTA) solution to collect the samples. After obtaining the specimens, roll the tubes slowly between the palms to mix the blood with the EDTA. Then pack the tubes in crushed ice, and send them immediately to the laboratory. Observe clients for any symptoms and signs of stress, because catecholamine secretion is influenced by position, activity, and stress.

Urinary Vanillylmandelic Acid Test. VMA is the principle urinary metabolite of the catecholamines (dopamine, epinephrine, and norepinephrine). The urinary VMA test measures the amount of VMA in a 24-hour collection of urine.

Urinary VMA increases with tumors of the adrenal medulla that cause increased secretion of epinephrine and norepinephrine. It also can increase in some muscular disorders, such as muscular dystrophy and myasthenia gravis; in thyrotoxicosis; in Cushing's disease; in Cushing's syndrome; and in clients with myocardial infarction, hemolytic anemia, and burns. Urinary VMA levels can be elevated in clients with malignant hypertension.

Urinary VMA levels may be falsely decreased in clients taking clofibrate or those with familial dysautonomia. False increases in urinary VMA also can occur in clients with uremia who have been tested using a fluorescent-based method and in clients taking medications that produce fluorescent primary products (eg, aspirin, methyldopa, tetracyclines, MAO inhibitors, levodopa, large doses of vitamin B complex, and epinephrine).

Nursing Implications. Ask the client to restrict any food containing vanilla, coffee, tea, citrus fruits, bananas, nuts, and chocolate for 3 days before the collection of the urine specimen to avoid distorting the test results. Screen clients for a history of conditions leading to false increases or decreases in urinary VMA levels.

To perform the test, obtain a 24-hour urine specimen starting and ending at 8 AM. Refrigerate it during collection; then send it to the laboratory for an analysis of its VMA content.

Urinary Homovanillic Acid Test. Homovanillic acid (HVA) is an indicator of the breakdown of dopamine, a precursor of norepinephrine. The urinary HVA test measures the amount of HVA excreted in the urine in a 24-hour period and can distinguish neural crest tumors from pheochromocytoma. Increases in urinary HVA levels occur in clients with a neuroblastoma or ganglioneuroma. Urinary HVA levels do not rise in pheochromocytoma, because this tumor mainly secretes epinephrine, which is metabolized to VMA (not HVA).

Nursing Implications. There is no restriction of diet, but counsel clients to use moderation in their intake of coffee, alcohol, salty foods, food containing vanilla, or food rich in vitamin B before the test. The client also should avoid all drugs affecting the test for 3 to 7 days before testing (aspirin, quinine, diazepam, disulfiram, reserpine, levodopa, tranquilizers, nerve blockers, and diuretics). Carefully assess clients for emotional stress and caution them against excessive physical activity, both of which will falsely elevate HVA levels in the urine.

A 24-hour urine sample is obtained and sent to the laboratory for analysis of urinary HVA. The specimen should be refrigerated during collection.

Total Urinary Catecholamine Levels. Approximately 1% to 5% of norepinephrine and epinephrine is excreted into the urine unchanged. The rest is broken down and forms the derivatives metanephrines and VMA. The total urinary catecholamine measures the 1% to 5% of norepinephrine and epinephrine that is excreted unchanged in the urine and correlates well with the assay of serum catecholamines. Total urinary catecholamine levels are elevated in clients with tumors of the adrenal medulla that result in the increased secretion of epinephrine and norepinephrine.

Nursing Implications. Counsel the client to avoid vigorous exercise before and during the collection of the sample. Obtain a 24-hour urine specimen. Refrigerate the sample during collection; then send it immediately to the laboratory after the test is concluded for analysis of total urinary catecholamines.

Pancreatic Function

The laboratory evaluation of pancreatic endocrine function is primarily concerned with the levels of glucose in the serum and urine, although cholesterol and triglycerides are also important. The two major types of pancreatic dysfunction are hyperglycemia and hypoglycemia.

Urinary Glucose and Ketone Tests. Urine is examined for the presence of glucose and ketones as part of a routine urinalysis. This relatively inexpensive screening tool can be used quickly in almost any setting. It is based on the principle that as the serum glucose level rises, it may exceed the reabsorptive threshold of the kidney, resulting in the excretion of the excess glucose into the urine. This usually occurs at 170 mg/dL, the renal threshold for glucose.

The principle underlying urine testing for ketones is that as the body starts to accumulate excess ketone bodies as a result of increased lipolysis, they will be excreted into the urine because of the body's inability to metabolize them completely. The kidneys have a low threshold for ketones. In clinical states where there is an increasing mobilization of fats for use as fuel, the serum ketone levels may rise from 0.5–1.5 mg/dL to 20 to 30 mg/dL.

Positive test results for urinary glucose can be seen in any condition in which the serum glucose levels exceed the renal threshold. Examples of this are diabetes mellitus, Cushing's syndrome, acromegaly, hyperthyroidism, stress responses to acute injury or extreme emotion, hyperglycemic hyperosmolar nonketotic (HHNK) coma, pheochromocytoma, and chronic pancreatitis. Positive test results can also be seen in clients with defects of the renal tubules and, occasionally, during pregnancy. False positive test results occur in clients taking certain antibiotics (eg, cephalosporins) or salicylates. False positive results are also seen in some postgastrectomy clients and those who have just ingested a large amount of carbohydrates. False negative results may be seen in older clients who are diabetic (the renal threshold increases with age) and in clients taking large doses of ascorbic acid (vitamin C). Positive test results for urinary ketones can be seen in clients on high-fat, low-carbohydrate diets; in diabetes mellitus; in starvation; in febrile and toxic clinical states; and in glycogen storage disease.

Nursing Implications. Obtain a careful history of all factors that might influence test results. As a screening test, this procedure can be done on almost any sample of freshly voided urine. If it is to be done on a known diabetic to regulate insulin dosage, a double-voided specimen is required. Although studies have proven the efficacy of single-voided specimens, at present the double-voided specimen is still considered the best method, especially for early morning samples. For routine screening, obtain a midstream specimen of urine. Using meticulous technique, test the sample for glucose and ketones.

Most errors in urine testing are caused by poor technique, not the test itself. To ensure reliability, check the testing materials for the date of expiration and make sure they are properly stored in a cool, dry area. Use the testing material immediately after removal from its container and take care not to contaminate it. Completely cover the reagent area with the urine, but avoid prolonged dipping, which can skew the test results. The test should be carefully timed and the results read at the exact moment specified. In comparing the test results to a color chart, always use the appropriate company's guide and read in direct daylight, if possible. Always indicate on the laboratory slip and the chart whether a fasting or random specimen is used.

Clients with a positive urinary glucose and/or ketone result should be referred for further evaluation. This might include 2-hour postprandial or fasting serum glucose tests; glucose tolerance testing; and 24-hour urine tests for glucose, and serum sodium, and serum potassium levels.

Fasting Serum Glucose and 2-Hour Postprandial Glucose Tests. The fasting serum glucose test (also called *fasting blood sugar,* or *FBS,* test) estimates the body's use of glucose. The 2-hour postprandial glucose test provides information about how the body utilizes and disposes of a glucose load. In the normal individual, the blood glucose level rises and peaks about ½ to 1 hour after a meal. These changes are not reflected in the urine until 2 hours or more later. The normal value of the 1-hour sample may range from 100 to 140 mg (venous whole blood), but rarely will the blood glucose level go above 150 mg in a nondiabetic. In 2 hours in normal persons, the blood glucose levels should be between 80 and 120 mg. Serum glucose levels are usually about 15% higher than whole blood levels.

Serum glucose levels are elevated in diabetes mellitus, stress responses to acute injury, hemorrhage, extreme emotion, severe pain, Cushing's syndrome, acromegaly, hyperthyroidism, HHNK coma, pheochromocytoma, and acute pancreatitis. Drugs known to elevate serum glucose levels include acetaminophen, dextran, thiazide diuretics, furosemide, chlorthalidone, triamterene, oral contraceptives, benzodiazepines, phenothiazines, phenytoin, lithium, epinephrine, diazoxide, and large doses of corticosteroids. Low serum glucose levels may be seen in advanced liver disease, Addison's disease, islet cell adenoma, malnutrition, postgastrectomy states, impaired glucose tolerance, and spontaneous hypoglycemia of unknown etiology. In addition to oral hypoglycemic agents and insulin, drugs known to lower serum glucose levels include the MAO inhibitors, propranolol, ethanol, and clofibrate.

Nursing Implications. Keep the client NPO for 8 hours before the fasting serum glucose test. Withhold insulin from any diabetic before testing. Obtain a venous sample of blood. Refrigerate or send the sample to the laboratory immediately, because glycolysis from failure to keep the sample chilled can result in a false negative test result.

Keep the client NPO for 8 hours preceding the 2-hour postprandial glucose test. Draw a fasting serum glucose level. Then give the client approximately 100 g of glucose orally. Draw a second serum glucose level 2 hours later. Test values of greater than 160 mg/dL are indicative of diabetes mellitus.

If insulin has been withheld prior to testing, the client should receive insulin and a meal immediately after taking the test. Observe the client carefully for symptoms and signs of hypoglycemia, hyperglycemia, or both.

Glycosylated Hemoglobin Assay. Glycosylated hemoglobin (HbA_{1c}) is found in everyone. In diabetics, however, it may be elevated two to three times the normal level. Levels increase at a slow but constant rate throughout the 120-day life span of the erythrocyte. Because increased blood glucose levels increase the rate of glycosylation, the HbA_{1c} assay is an index of the average blood glucose levels during the preceding months. Therefore, it provides valuable information about long-term control of diabetes mellitus. Levels of HbA_{1c} are only increased in hyperglycemia. They are decreased in hemolysis secondary to actual loss of hemoglobin. As diabetes becomes well controlled, the HbA_{1c} levels begin to fall into the normal range.

Levels of HbA_{1c} have also provided information on the pathology of diabetes mellitus. Relationships have been shown between increased levels of HbA_{1c} and the incidence of infection, thrombosis, lipoproteinemia, thickening of the basement membrane, and abnormalities in platelet and leukocyte production.

Glycosylated hemoglobin assay has the following advantages over serum glucose monitoring: Serum glucose monitoring requires repeated venipunctures. The results represent only the time when the sample was taken. Monitoring of HbA_{1c} can be done on a 6- to 8-week basis and reflects the blood glucose levels over a period of 2 to 3 months. Levels of HbA_{1c} are more stable, because they reflect the glucose level within the erythrocyte rather than the serum glucose level, which is more susceptible to other metabolic influences.

Nursing Implications. There are no food or fluid restrictions for this test. Advise the client to maintain a normal diet and medication regimen. To perform the test, collect a venous sample of blood. Roll the tube slowly between the palms to mix the sample and anticoagulant; failure to do so will affect the test results. Send the sample to the laboratory for analysis.

Self Blood Glucose Monitoring. Self blood glucose monitoring (BGM) has become an important diagnostic

tool in the control of diabetes mellitus. Using this technique, clients can monitor their own blood glucose fluctuations and thereby achieve better control of their diabetes. It also allows clients to become direct participants in their own care and to see the relationship between diet, medication, exercise, and blood glucose levels (see Chapter 42).

Twenty-Four Hour Urine Test for Quantitative Glucose Levels. The 24-hour urine test quantifies the amount of glucose excreted in the urine in 24 hours. Some care providers use it to measure control of diabetes mellitus; good regulation is equivalent to no loss in the urine of greater than 5% of the total carbohydrate intake for the day. Any finding of glucose in the urine is considered abnormal and requires further evaluation.

Nursing Implications. There are no fluid, food, or medication restrictions. A 24-hour specimen of urine is collected. The first voided specimen is usually discarded, and the first voided specimen of the next morning is included. The specimen is then sent to the laboratory for quantification of urinary glucose levels.

Glucose Tolerance Test. The glucose tolerance test (GTT) assists in the evaluation of impaired glucose tolerance. It is not routinely used in clients with documented fasting blood glucose levels over 140 to 150 mg/dL or postprandial glucose levels above 180 mg/dL. The GTT also can aid in the diagnosis of hypoglycemia and malabsorption syndrome.

The oral GTT evaluates absorption of carbohydrate after an oral administration of glucose. It is based on the principle that in the normal individual, after a glucose load, serum glucose levels peak within 30 minutes to an hour and then return to a normal range after 2 to 3 hours in response to the increased secretion of insulin. In the diabetic, however, even though fasting serum glucose levels may be within the normal range, an insufficient secretion of insulin may cause the serum glucose levels to rise sharply and return to normal values much more slowly.

An intravenous method of performing the GTT is also available and is used for clients with suspected impairment of absorption (sprue, celiac disease, Addison's disease, or hypothyroidism). IVGTT is often employed when the results of the oral GTT are unclear.

Depressed glucose tolerance curves, which peak sharply and fall slowly, are seen in diabetes mellitus. However, these curves also occur in clients with Cushing's syndrome, pheochromocytoma, central nervous system lesions, and hemochromatosis.

Increased glucose tolerance curves, which peak at less than normal levels, are seen in insulinoma, Addison's disease, hypothyroidism, hypopituitarism, and malabsorption states. Figure 41–4 shows glucose tolerance curves seen clinically.

The relationship of age to changes in glucose tolerance curves is well recognized, and a correction factor can prevent the misdiagnosis of diabetes in the elderly. The suggested adjustments for age are an increase of 10 to 15 mg/dL for clients in their 60s and an increase of 20 to 30 mg/dL for those in their 70s.

Nursing Implications. Obtain a careful history of all medications that might elevate or depress serum glucose levels (large amounts of salicylates, oral contraceptives, large doses of ascorbic acid, thiazide diuretics, phenytoin, and steroids). A history of other factors that might influence the test results also should be obtained (eg, pregnancy, prolonged inactivity, surgery, trauma, acute illness, and infectious disease). In addition, clients who have been on a low-carbohydrate diet before the test may show an abnormal glucose tolerance curve because of an inability of the pancreas to respond to a high-carbohydrate load.

Instruct the client to maintain a high-carbohydrate diet (150 g of carbohydrate) for 2 to 3 days and then fast for 8 to 12 hours before the test begins. Strenuous exercise, smoking, or coffee or alcohol intake in the 8 hours before the test will affect the test results. Withhold all medications that might affect the test results. Teach clients the symptoms and signs of hyperglycemia and hypoglycemia and instruct them to report these immediately.

Obtain a fasting serum glucose and fasting urine specimen between 7 and 9 AM. Administer the test load of oral glucose and record the exact time. Encourage the client to take all the glucose load within 5 minutes and to drink water during the test to promote adequate urination. Collect serum glucose and urine specimens at 30 minutes, 1 hour, 2 hours, and 3 hours. If hypoglycemia or malabsorption syndrome is being evaluated, levels may be monitored for an additional 2 to 3 hours. All samples should be properly labeled and either refrigerated or sent to the laboratory immediately.

Observe the client closely for symptoms and signs of hyperglycemia or hypoglycemia, and report them immediately to the physician. If symptoms of severe hypoglycemia develop, discontinue the test, obtain a blood sample and label it with the exact time, and administer treatment immediately.

Serum Insulin Level. Serum insulin levels measured using RIA are of diagnostic value in the evaluation of fasting hypoglycemia. They are not used to diagnose diabetes mellitus and have not been found valuable in the evaluation of postprandial or reactive hypoglycemia because of the variability in normal response. Serum insulin levels are often used in conjunction with the GTT and may show characteristic curves in given conditions (eg, Type I diabetes mellitus).

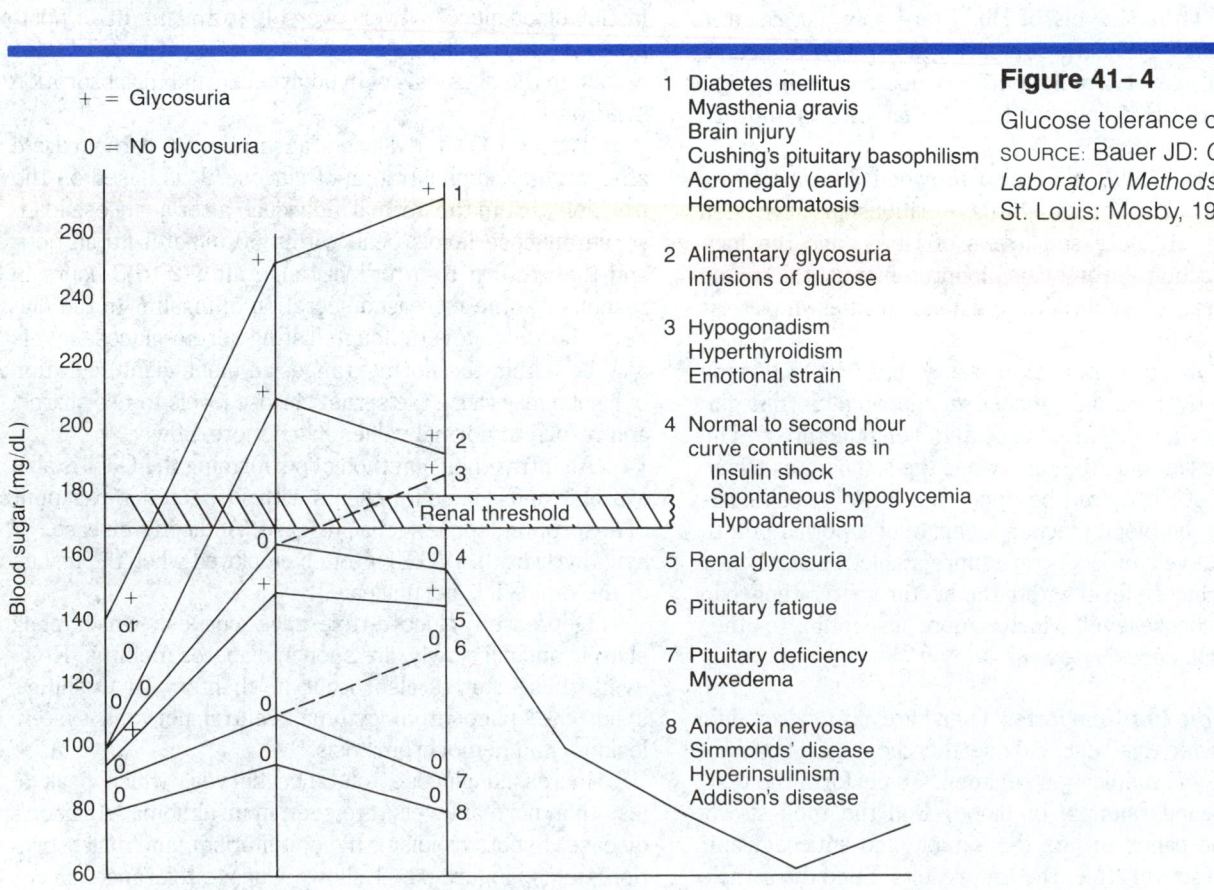

1 Diabetes mellitus
Myasthenia gravis
Brain injury
Cushing's pituitary basophilism
Acromegaly (early)
Hemochromatosis

2 Alimentary glycosuria
Infusions of glucose

3 Hypogonadism
Hyperthyroidism
Emotional strain

4 Normal to second hour
curve continues as in
Insulin shock
Spontaneous hypoglycemia
Hypoadrenalism

5 Renal glycosuria

6 Pituitary fatigue

7 Pituitary deficiency
Myxedema

8 Anorexia nervosa
Simmonds' disease
Hyperinsulinism
Addison's disease

Figure 41–4

Glucose tolerance curves.
SOURCE: Bauer JD: *Clinical Laboratory Methods*, 9th ed. St. Louis: Mosby, 1982, p. 477.

Nursing Implications. Take a careful history of all medications that might interfere with the test results (steroids, ACTH, oral contraceptives, epinephrine, or thyroid hormone). The client should fast for 10 to 12 hours before the test and remain relaxed and recumbent for 30 minutes because excitement can affect insulin levels.

To perform the test, a venous sample for glucose and another for insulin are collected. Pack the sample of insulin on ice and send it to the laboratory immediately along with the sample of serum glucose. Observe clients closely during the test, because it may precipitate severe hypoglycemia in clients with an insulinoma. Keep a solution of 50% IV glucose at the client's bedside for emergency use.

Tolbutamide Tolerance Test. The tolbutamide tolerance test (TTT, insulin tolerance test, or insulin stimulation test) is used to diagnose mild diabetes mellitus and insulinoma and to rule out conditions of functional hyperinsulinism. It is based on the principle that an IV infusion of tolbutamide will stimulate the beta pancreatic cells and certain tumors to secrete insulin. In the normal individual, serum levels of glucose will fall rapidly (usually to about half the fasting level) and return to baseline levels in 1½ to 3 hours. Abnormalities in insulin secretion can be detected during this test by evaluating the serum glucose levels.

Evaluating the results of the TTT involves assessing the degree and duration of the hypoglycemia. In insulinoma, there is a marked initial drop in the serum glucose level with a return to pretest levels in 3 hours or more. Clients with hyperinsulinism have findings similar to those of normal individuals. In diabetes mellitus, the initial drop in serum glucose levels is slow, and there is a prolonged return to pretest levels. This test is contraindicated in clients with fasting serum glucose levels below 50 mg/dL and in those with a sensitivity to sulfonylureas.

Nursing Implications. Instruct the client to maintain a high-carbohydrate diet (150 to 180 g of carbohydrate) for 3 days before the test. Keep the client NPO for fluid and food 8 to 12 hours before the test and make sure he or she refrains from smoking both before and during testing.

To avoid multiple venipunctures, a keep-open IV infusion with normal saline solution or a heparin lock is inserted. A fasting serum glucose level is drawn and the time noted. A preparation of 1 g of tolbutamide and 20 mL of sterile water is infused over 2 to 3 minutes. If insulinoma or hyperinsulinism is suspected, blood samples are drawn at 15, 30, 45, 60, 90, 120, 150, and 180 minutes. If the client is being evaluated for diabetes mellitus, samples are drawn at 20 and 30 minutes.

Keep in mind the following precautions. The tolbutamide solution must be used within an hour of preparation. If the client develops any signs or symptoms of severe hypoglycemia, discontinue the test and notify the physician. A sample of blood for glucose should be obtained immediately and sent to the laboratory, noting the time it was drawn. If the client develops any anaphylactic symptoms, notify the physician immediately and administer epinephrine subcutaneously or intramuscularly.

Obtain a careful history of all substances that might enhance the action of tolbutamide (salicylates, MAO inhibitors, sulfonamides, phenylbutazone, chloramphenicol, and methandrostenolone). False positive test results have occurred in clients with adrenal insufficiency, liver disease, obesity, functional hypoglycemia, alcoholism, and starvation. False negative test results occur in approximately 50% of clients with insulinoma (Treseler, 1982). Use the test with caution in clients in the last trimester of pregnancy; in the elderly; and in clients with a history of heart disease, chronic illness, or severe acute illness.

Section II: Nursing Diagnosis

The nursing diagnosis forms the basis of the plan of care for the client and provides guidelines for its implementation and evaluation. Because endocrine dysfunction has such widespread effects, many nursing diagnoses can be used in caring for these clients. Box 41–1 lists those most frequently used and reflects the most common types of problems seen in clients with endocrine dysfunction. The client's actual problem is unique, however, and requires a skillful assessment by the nurse. The recognition of the specific client problem and its etiology is integral to a comprehensive, well-executed nursing care plan.

INEFFECTIVE INDIVIDUAL COPING

Because of the profound physiological and psychosocial stresses on clients with endocrine disorders, it is not unusual for them to be fearful and unable to cope. Their nervousness and anxiety can be directly related to the disor-

der (as in hyperthyroidism or pheochromocytoma) or exogenous, resulting from vague feelings of unexplained apprehension about the situation.

Endocrine disorders often require the client and significant others to make major changes in their lifestyles. Clients with endocrine dysfunction must often depend on medication for life and usually require lifelong medical and nursing supervision. They also may face the possibility of major surgery. The client may have some degree of transitory or permanent sensory loss.

ALTERATION IN THOUGHT PROCESSES

Central nervous system involvement may produce a variety of problems in the endocrine client, ranging from headaches and lethargy (hypoglycemia or pheochromocytoma) to outright psychoses (thyrotoxicosis, Cushing's syndrome, or hyperparathyroidism). Alterations in thought

cushingoid clients because of changes in the fragility of the capillaries. Facial flushing may be seen in clients with pheochromocytoma. Hirsutism is a problem for clients with adrenal tumor or hyperplasia and is an especially troublesome body image problem for women.

Clients with endocrine disorders are often unable to manage self-care or maintain their home environment. They are at increased risk for injury because of weakness, fatigue, and visual disturbances. For example, weakness of the musculoskeletal system is seen in clients with acromegaly, Cushing's syndrome, hyperparathyroidism, and hyperthyroidism. Clients with hyperparathyroidism and Cushing's syndrome have an increased incidence of fractures. Fatigue often accompanies endocrine disorders, including adrenal insufficiency, hypoglycemia, hyperthyroidism and hypothyroidism, and acromegaly. Clients with pituitary tumors, diabetes mellitus, and hyperthyroidism often have some visual impairment.

Sexual dysfunction may occur as loss of libido (acromegaly, diabetes mellitus, and hypothyroidism) or impotence (diabetes mellitus). Menstrual problems such as menorrhagia (hyperthyroidism), and amenorrhea (hyperthyroidism, hypothyroidism, Cushing's syndrome, acromegaly, and pituitary tumors) are not uncommon.

ALTERATION IN NUTRITION

Alterations in nutrition occur in clients with hypothyroidism (hypometabolism or weight gain). Anorexia and weight loss are common in clients with adrenal insufficiency, pheochromocytoma, and hypercalcemia. Clients with hyperthyroidism often lose weight even though they have an insatiable appetite.

ALTERATION IN BOWEL ELIMINATION

Alterations in bowel elimination, specifically diarrhea, may be seen in clients with hyperthyroidism (because of the increased metabolic rate and hypocalcemia), diabetes mellitus (because of autonomic nervous system involvement), and Addison's disease. Constipation can occur in clients with hypothyroidism, hypercalcemia, and pheochromocytoma.

ALTERATION IN FLUID VOLUME

Actual or potential fluid volume deficits occur in clients with diabetes mellitus and posterior pituitary disorders. In addition, clients with hypothyroidism and Cushing's syndrome may develop congestive heart failure. Ascites and pericardial effusions may occur secondary to hypothyroidism. Clients with hypercalcemia and hyperaldosteronism may have polydipsia and polyuria.

processes and perception pose difficulties not only for clients but for their families and friends as well.

ALTERATION IN COMFORT

Many clients with endocrine dysfunction have problems with thermal regulation. For example, clients with hyperthyroidism often complain of intolerance to heat, and those with hypothyroidism are exquisitely sensitive to cold. Clients with pheochromocytoma, hyperthyroidism, and hypoglycemia often experience excessive sweating. Pruritus is often a problem for clients with diabetes mellitus and hyperthyroidism. Those with hypothyroidism and acromegaly often have joint pain.

DISTURBANCE IN SELF-CONCEPT

Changes in the skin and hair occur in clients with endocrine dysfunction and frequently contribute to disturbances in body image. Increases in skin pigmentation may occur in clients with Addison's disease. Ecchymoses increase in

Section III: Planning and Implementation

Many of the problems that result from endocrine dysfunction are also caused by dysfunction in other organ systems

(eg, constipation). Refer to the appropriate chapter for specific interventions related to these problems. Table 41–2, a sample nursing care plan for clients with endocrine dysfunction, reviews the nursing care for the following nursing diagnoses: alteration in nutrition: more than body requirements (secondary to hypothyroidism); alteration in bowel elimination: diarrhea (secondary to Addison's disease); potential fluid volume deficit (due to possible diabetes insipidus); and actual fluid volume deficit (due to diabetic ketoacidosis or DKA). The next section discusses nursing interventions for endocrine clients to improve coping abilities, maintain and improve thought processes, promote comfort, and improve self-concept.

Table 41–2 Sample Nursing Care Plan for Clients With Endocrine Dysfunction

Nursing Diagnosis	Client Care Goals	Plan/Nursing Implementation	Expected Outcomes
Nutrition, alteration in: more than body requirements (related to hypothyroidism)	Reduce weight to normal range within 1 yr with consistent initial loss of 1–2 lb/wk; maintain prescribed diet, adequate fluid intake, and exercise regimen	Assess state of control of client's hypothyroidism (signs and symptoms of hypothyroidism; medication regimen; results of last T_4 and T_3 uptake tests; any signs of cardiac or respiratory complications); weigh and measure client; compare results to actuarial tables to arrive at a proper goal; use skinfold assessment as needed; obtain a 3-day diet diary from client; assess client's food preferences and dislikes; assess client's activity level and general plan of daily activities; assess client's level of understanding regarding hypothyroidism, obesity, and their relation; if client appears to be well controlled on thyroid medication, secure a diet prescription from the physician and nutrition consultant (if available); if hypothyroidism is not well controlled, refer client for medical evaluation; work with client to plan an appropriate weight-loss regimen based on caloric restriction, adequate fluid intake, and exercise; consider client's food likes and dislikes, as well as any cultural or economic influences; encourage clients to weigh themselves only once weekly at same time of day (usually in morning) while wearing the same amount of clothes; explain that weight may plateau and the reasons for it; encourage client to keep a daily log of what is eaten and any influencing factors (depression, eating out, etc); provide ongoing follow-up (to encourage adherence to diet) via telephone consultation or weigh-ins every 2 wk; refer client to weight-loss or behavior modification groups, if indicated; remember that obesity is often a lifelong disorder and may require considerable lifestyle adjustments; provide support and honestly compliment client for pounds lost	Client consistently loses 1 to 2 lb weekly; client within normal range for weight and height within 1 yr; client able to explain the prescribed diet accurately and discuss importance of fluid intake and exercise in successfully meeting the weight goal; client maintains weekly telephone contact with the care provider and weighs in regularly at the prescribed intervals

(continued)

Table 41–2 Sample Nursing Care Plan for Clients With Endocrine Dysfunction (continued)

Nursing Diagnosis	Client Care Goals	Plan/Nursing Implementation	Expected Outcomes
Bowel elimination, alteration in: diarrhea (related to Addison's disease)	Maintain a normal electrolyte balance; exhibit no signs of dehydration; prevent skin breakdown in perineal/anal area; reduce or eliminate symptoms of diarrhea	Monitor vital signs q.i.d. or p.r.n., blood pressure, pulse, respirations, temperature; weigh client daily and report results; measure intake and output and quantify sodium intake; provide a quiet, restful, stress-free environment; force fluids to 3000 mL/24 h; maintain high-sodium, low-potassium diet or as ordered (diet may need between-meal supplements); inspect anal area for signs of breakdown and irritation; provide basin with soap and water for client to wash hands after defecation; lubricate anal area with water-soluble lubricant as needed; keep anal area clean and dry; initially assist client with daily care as needed	Client maintains a normal electrolyte balance, as shown by laboratory results; no signs of dehydration, as shown by good skin turgor, moist mucous membranes, normal vital signs, normal intake and output, hematocrit, and urine specific gravity within normal limits; perianal area free of erythema, excoriation, tenderness, or discomfort; resolution of diarrhea
Fluid volume deficit, potential (due to possible diabetes insipidus)	Reduce or eliminate symptoms of weakness, ice water thirst, and polyuria in 24 h; no fluid volume deficit or electrolyte imbalance	Provide fluids for client (cold water is usually preferred); measure intake and output (output plus 100 mL may be replaced q.h. when ordered); parenteral therapy may be ordered; provide easy access for frequent urinary elimination; weigh client daily at same time; provide diet as ordered; assist with diagnostic tests as ordered, and explain all procedures to client; observe client closely for signs and symptoms of dehydration; administer medications as ordered; teach client to avoid substances that increase diuresis (alcohol, coffee, and tea)	Blood pressure and all vital signs maintained in normal range for client's age and body build; urine specific gravity in range of 1.016–1.022; serum electrolytes within normal limits; hemoglobin and hematocrit maintained within normal range; client maintains good fluid intake and avoids diuretic substances
Fluid volume deficit, actual (due to diabetic ketoacidosis)	Restore normal fluid and electrolyte balance; restore blood glucose and urine levels to acceptable levels; discuss signs and symptoms of DKA and the factors that produce it	During acute episode: Obtain electrolyte, serum glucose, carbon dioxide, BUN, hematocrit, and urine specimens stat as ordered; indwelling catheter may be inserted; set nasogastric tube to low suction, as ordered; gastric lavage may be done; administer parenteral fluids as ordered (normal saline or sodium lactate solution is usually given initially); possibly replace 1000 mL in first hour and then 300–500 mL/h, depending on the fluid deficit; replace electrolytes [K] as ordered; administer parenteral sodium bicarbonate as ordered if blood ph 7.0 or below; administer insulin as ordered ($\frac{1}{3}$ of initial dose of regular insulin IV, $\frac{2}{3}$ of initial dose SC, all remaining doses SC); monitor client carefully for signs and symptoms of hypoglycemia, especially 12–24 h after treatment has begun; monitor client carefully for hypokalemia, especially if vomit-	Restoration of normal fluid balance (urine specific gravity 1.016–1.022; urine output 800–2000 mL/24 h; blood pressure, respirations, pulse, and temperature all within normal range; no signs of dehydration); serum electrolytes within normal range; urine negative for glucose and ketones; client alert and oriented; client asymptomatic for signs and symptoms of hyperglycemia, hypoglycemia, hyperkalemia, and hypokalemia

Nursing Diagnosis	Client Care Goals	Plan/Nursing Implementation	Expected Outcomes
		ing or diarrhea occurred; obtain ECG as ordered: hypokalemia will show depressed T waves and hyperkalemia, peaked T waves; measure intake and output every hour; test urine hourly for glucose and ketones; check blood pressure, respirations, and apical heart rate every ½–1 h; assess LOC every ½–1 h; observe for signs and symptoms of circulatory collapse (maintain open airway and elevate the lower extremities as needed); be prepared for seizure measures if needed; client is usually more comfortable in Fowler's position; turn and position client every hour; administer skin care as needed	
		During recovery from acute episode: Assess client's understanding of acute episode of DKA; review signs and symptoms of hypoglycemia and DKA; discuss when and how to treat emergency situations and need to call physician immediately; based on client's level of understanding, review diet, medications, exercise, infection management, and self-care skills; involve a member of client's family or a significant other in the client teaching sessions; assess, if possible, the home situation for factors influencing ability to maintain a safe and healthy diabetic regimen	Client able to discuss signs and symptoms of ketoacidosis and the factors that contribute to it; client and family or friends seem confident about managing future problems

IMPROVING COPING ABILITIES

Clients with endocrine problems often have anxiety related to the disease process. The nurse, although unable to alter the actual disease, can support and reassure clients, as well as educate them about what is occurring. By careful environmental manipulation, the nurse can reduce the internal and external stressors that contribute to a negative outcome. Clients need to be aware that their anxiety is related to what is happening in their bodies and that the treatment is expected to help. Provide opportunities for clients to express what they are feeling and, if appropriate, encourage activities that provide physical release of energy. Organize the environment to provide minimal stimulation and to promote relaxation. Counsel visitors and families to avoid topics that may cause an increase in symptoms. Families or friends need to be reassured that the symptoms and signs they observe in the client reflect the underlying endocrine pathology and are expected to resolve with treatment.

MAINTAINING AND IMPROVING THOUGHT PROCESSES

Of equal concern to clients and their significant others are the changes in cognitive ability and the mood swings that accompany certain endocrine disorders. Explain the etiology of these changes to the client and significant others and provide interventions based on the client's current level of functioning. For example, for clients with hypothyroidism characterized by mental slowing, interactions should be simple and direct, with explanations geared to the client's present level of understanding. Help clients understand that the changes they are experiencing should be relieved by treatment. Extend teaching and counseling to the client's family or friends, who are often troubled by the dramatic changes they see in their loved one.

The erratic mood swings of cushingoid clients and clients with hyperthyroidism pose another challenge to the nurse. Although the etiology of these fluctuations is pathology in the endocrine system, nursing interventions should be directed toward the symptoms. These clients and their significant others require support and reassurance about the basis of these changes. Clients often respond well to a simple restructuring of their environment to reduce stimulation. For example, turning the lights down, playing soft music on the radio, limiting visitors or avoiding anxiety-producing topics during a visit, and providing soothing baths or back rubs often encourage clients to relax.

PROMOTING COMFORT

The client with hyperthyroidism who is highly sensitive to heat often benefits from a cooler room temperature, fewer blankets with frequent linen changes, and cool back rubs. The client with hypothyroidism generally needs a warmer room temperature, more bed linens, and layers of clothing in cold weather. Clients experiencing excessive perspiration need repeated clothing and bed linen changes, more frequent bathing, and liberal use of deodorants and body powder.

Manage joint pain with rest and heat or cold, depending on which is most effective for the individual client. Aspirin or nonsteroidal anti-inflammatory agents may be ordered if they are compatible with the rest of the client's medical regimen.

IMPROVING SELF-CONCEPT

One of the most disabling problems for clients with endocrine disorders is the change in body image and its effect on how they perceive themselves. Some of the body image changes include changes in skin texture and pigmentation, loss of hair or change in hair texture, coarsening of facial features, changes in body fat distribution, protrusion of the eyes, enlargement of the neck, and gross change or lack of change in stature. Many of these changes are amenable to treatment (although the effects often require time to resolve), but some are not. Be sensitive to the needs of these clients and provide opportunities for them to discuss their feelings and concerns. Although interventions such as makeup or skin creams may have minimal effect, they should not be overlooked, especially if the client and family find them valuable.

Sexual dysfunction and menstrual irregularities often are resolved when the client's specific endocrine problem is brought under control. Remember to ask about changes in these areas, however, because clients are often hesitant to bring them up. If there is no improvement, the drug therapy may be contributing to the problem. Bring these concerns to the physician's attention.

Section IV: Evaluation

If the goals of care have not been met, reevaluation is required. The nurse and client should jointly review the nursing diagnosis, client care goals, and plan of care. Based on their findings, new objectives may need to be formulated; other nursing interventions may be added or modified; or the evaluation may show that more time is required to meet the objectives.

Chapter Highlights

The carefully collected data base is the foundation for developing nursing diagnoses as well as for the planning, implementation, and evaluation of nursing care for endocrine clients. The data base enables the nurse to use a scientific approach in making judgments about changes in client status.

The review of systems pertinent to an endocrine client involves questions about the head and neck, visual, auditory, integumentary, cardiovascular, gastrointestinal, urinary, reproductive, musculoskeletal, and neurologic systems.

The areas routinely assessed in a client with endocrine disease are the vital signs; general appearance; skin, hair, and nails; eyes; neck; heart; lungs; abdomen; genitals; and musculoskeletal and neurologic systems.

Studies used to diagnose clients with endocrine dysfunction include screening tests, serum and urine tests, radiologic studies, and special testing procedures.

The nursing diagnoses are a logical outgrowth of a careful analysis of the data base. Because endocrine dysfunction manifests itself in a variety of physiological and psychosocial changes, a wide variety of nursing diagnoses are employed.

The nursing diagnoses most relevant to the care of clients with endocrine disease are ineffective individual coping, alteration in thought processes, alteration in comfort, disturbance in self-concept, alteration in nutrition, alteration in bowel elimination, potential fluid volume deficit, and actual fluid volume deficit.

In planning the nursing care for clients with endocrine dysfunction, consider that clients may have a sensory loss; they may be facing the prospect of serious surgery; endocrine disorders often result in significant lifestyle changes for clients and their families; clients often depend on medication and require lifelong medical supervision; and clients may have symptoms that inhibit their coping and adaptation to normal life situations.

The nursing care plan for clients with endocrine

problems should be individualized and client centered as well as reflect methods to meet the client care goals arising from the nursing diagnoses.

The evaluation of nursing care is an important nursing responsibility keyed to the construction of client-centered goals or objectives. If the objectives have been met, the evaluation is complete. If the objectives have not been met, the nurse and client should review the care plan and make the necessary revisions.

Bibliography

Bates B: *A Guide to the Physical Examination,* 3rd ed. Philadelphia: Lippincott, 1983.

Bolli G et al: Simultaneous central venous and arterial blood sampling for catecholamine assay in pheochromocytoma. *Lancet* 1981; 2(8245):526–527.

Byrne CJ, et al: *Laboratory Tests: Implications for Nursing Care,* 2nd ed. Menlo Park, CA: Addison–Wesley, 1986.

Cohen S, Harris E: Programmed instruction: Mental status assessment. *Am J Nurs* 1981; 8:1493–1518.

Diagnostics. Nurse's Reference Library. Springhouse, PA: Intermed, 1983.

Feng CA: Laboratory tests in diabetes mellitus. *New York State J Med* 1981; 81(9): 1328–1331.

Fields WL, McGinn–Campbell KM: *Introduction to Health Assessment.* Reston, VA: Reston, 1983.

Grimes J, Iannopollo E: *Health Assessment in Nursing Practice.* Monterey, CA: Wadsworth, 1982.

Hall R, Evered D, Greene R: *Color Atlas of Endocrinology.* Chicago: Yearbook Medical Publishers, 1979.

Honigman RE: Deciphering diagnostic studies: Thyroid function tests. *Nurs 82* (April) 1982; 12:68–71.

Kaye D, Rise LF (editors): *Fundamentals of Internal Medicine.* St. Louis: Mosby, 1983.

Malasanos L et al: *Health Assessment.* St. Louis: Mosby, 1981.

Maree SM: The endocrine system. Preoperative evaluation and physical assessment of the patient. *J AANA* 1981; 49:389–404.

Pagana KD, Pagana TJ: *Diagnostic Testing and Nursing Implications: A Case Study Approach.* St. Louis: Mosby, 1982.

Sana JM, Judge RD (editors): *Physical Assessment Skills for Nursing Practice,* 2nd ed. Boston: Little, Brown, 1982.

Saxton DF, et al: *The Addison–Wesley Manual of Nursing Practice.* Menlo Park, CA: Addison–Wesley, 1983.

Tamai H et al. Triiodothyronine suppression and TSH-releasing hormone tests before and after ^{131}I therapy for Graves' disease. *J Nuclear Med* 1980; 21:240–245.

Thompson JM, Bowers AC: *Clinical Manual of Health Assessment.* St. Louis: Mosby, 1980.

Treseler KM: *Clinical Laboratory Tests: Significance and Implications for Nursing.* Englewood Cliffs, NJ: Prentice–Hall, 1982.

Watts NB, Keffer JH: *Practical Endocrine Diagnosis,* 3rd ed. Philadelphia: Lea & Febiger, 1982.

Suggested Readings

Gotch PM: Teaching patients about adrenal corticosteroids. *Am J Nurs* 1981, 81(1):78–81. The author reviews the major adrenocortical hormones and discusses the approaches to corticosteroid therapy. Dosage schedules, management of stress states, and long-term effects are presented.

Harris E: The dexamethasone suppression test. *Am J Nurs* 1982; 82(5):784–785. This article discusses the use of the dexamethasone suppression test with depressed clients to identify those who would most likely respond to antidepressants. The test also has the potential for monitoring recovery from depression. The physiology, test procedure, and conditions that alter the test are included.

Metzger MJ: A new test for blood sugar: Hemoglobin A. *Am J Nurs* 1983; 83(5):763–764. Testing for glycosylated hemoglobin reflects average blood sugar levels over a period of time. The article discusses the advantages of the test in working with insulin-dependent diabetics.

Resources

SELF-HELP GROUPS AND OTHER ORGANIZATIONS

American Diabetes Association
National Service Center
1660 Duke Street
PO Box 25757
Alexandria, VA 22313
Phone: (800) 232-3472

> A national organization with state and local units that seeks to improve the well-being of persons with diabetes and their families and promotes the search for preventive approaches or a cure for diabetes. Consult the ADA for the address and telephone number of the state affiliates. Consult the state affiliate for addresses and telephone numbers of local chapters.

Division of Diabetes Control
Center for Prevention Services
Centers for Disease Control
Atlanta, GA 30333
Phone: (404) 329-1851

> The CDC, a division of the Public Health Service, administers diabetes control programs through the health departments of 20 states.

International Diabetes Center
5000 W. 39th St.
Minneapolis, MN 55416
Phone: (612) 927-3393

> The center conducts educational, clinical care, outreach, and clinical research programs. Its diabetes education programs, print materials, and audiovisual aids are available for health professionals and persons with diabetes.

Juvenile Diabetes Foundation International
23 E. 26th St.
New York, NY 10010
Phone: (800) 223-1138

This international organization focuses on promoting the health of children and their families. The organization actively supports basic medical research.

Michigan Diabetes Research and Training Center
University of Michigan Medical School
Ann Arbor, MI 48109
Phone: (313) 763-0200

The center annually publishes the "Recommended Audiovisual Resources for Diabetes Education" and "Recommended Print Materials for Diabetes Patient Education." These useful catalogs describe diabetes educational materials, including a brief evaluation of current resources and how they can be obtained.

National Diabetes Information Clearinghouse
NIH–NIADKK
Box NDIC
Bethesda, MD 20892
Phone: (301) 468-2162

The clearinghouse publishes annotated bibliographies on diabetes topics and the Diabetes Dateline that reports diabetes education and research activities.

Also:

Canadian Diabetes Association
123 Edward St., Suite 601
Toronto, Ontario, Canada M5G 1F2

Joslin Diabetes Foundation
15 Joslin Rd.
Boston, MA 02215

National Pituitary Agency
210 W. Fayette St., Suite 150
Baltimore, MD 21201
(301) 837-2552

HOT LINE

American Diabetes Association
Phone: (800) 232-3472

Members of the client education staff will answer questions.

SPECIALTY ORGANIZATIONS

American Association of Diabetes Educators
500 N. Michigan Ave., Suite 1400
Chicago, IL 60611
Phone: (312) 661-1700

A multidisciplinary organization of health professionals interested in diabetes education. AADE provides educational opportunities for health professionals and promotes quality diabetes education for consumers. Consult AADE for addresses and telephone numbers of local chapters.

Dietitians in Diabetes Care and Education
Practice Group

American Dietetic Association
430 N. Michigan Ave.
Chicago, IL 60611
Phone: (312) 280-5000

This practice group within the ADA includes registered dietitians involved in diabetes education and management.

HEALTH INFORMATION MATERIAL

Publications of the American Diabetes Association

Diabetes Care. A bimonthly clinical research and care journal for health professionals.

Clinical Diabetes. A bimonthly newsletter for primary care health professionals in clinical practice.

Diabetes Forecast. A bimonthly publication for the person with diabetes that provides up-to-date information on nutrition, clinical advances, and research.

Diabetes. A quarterly newsletter for the person with diabetes that provides basic information.

Publications of the International Diabetes Center

A complete series of single-concept brochures and booklets is available for use by health professionals for client education. Included in the series are: *What is Diabetes?, Diabetes and Brief Illness, Fast Food Facts, Convenience Food Facts, Diabetes and Exercise, Diabetes and Alcohol, Recognizing and Treating Insulin Reactions, Gestational Diabetes, Meal Planning for Type II Diabetes, Adding Fiber to Your Diet,* and *A Guide to Healthy Eating.*

Publications of the American Association of Diabetes Educators

The Diabetes Educator. A quarterly publication of the association that focuses on educational and clinical issues in diabetes management.

Tupling H et al: *You've Got to Get Through the Outside Layer: A Handbook for Health Educators, Using Diabetes as a Model.* Diabetes Education and Assessment Programme of the Royal North Shore Hospital of Sydney and the Northern Metropolitan Health Region of the Health Commission of New South Wales. Reprinted by the American Association of Diabetes Educators. Available from: Outside Layer, PO Box 802, South Bend, IN 46624. A succinct, well-written, and practical discussion of educational and emotional issues in diabetes and other chronic diseases. Includes examples, case studies, and sample teaching exercises.

Publications of the American Dietetic Association

Wheeler M (editor): *Diabetes Mellitus and Glycemic Responses to Different Foods: A Summary and Annotated Bibliography.* Published by the Diabetes Care and Education Practice Group of the American Dietetic Association, 1983.

Chapter 42

Specific Disorders of Glucose Regulation

LeAnn McNeil
Marion J. Franz

The most common disorder of glucose regulation is diabetes mellitus, a chronic disease characterized by abnormal metabolism of carbohydrate, protein, and fat. Reactive hypoglycemia, in which blood glucose concentrations fall to symptomatic levels several hours after a meal, is another glucose regulation disorder. Nursing care is a critical aspect in the control of both conditions.

Section I: Diabetes Mellitus

Diabetes mellitus results from (1) an absolute lack of insulin, (2) impaired secretion of insulin by the pancreas, or (3) cellular resistance to the action of secreted insulin. Diabetes mellitus is both a metabolic and a vascular disease. Hyperglycemia results from the absolute or relative lack of insulin. Then, as the disease progresses, small blood vessels in the retina and kidney and larger vessels in the heart and peripheral circulatory system deteriorate.

Diabetes mellitus is a major health problem, affecting an estimated 66 million people worldwide (Dolan–Heitlinger & Antle, 1983). An estimated 12 million Americans have diabetes; in nearly half of them, the disease remains undiagnosed. Diabetes, with its complications, is the third leading cause of death by disease in the United States. Persons with diabetes are 25 times more likely than the general population to develop blindness, 17 times more likely to develop kidney disease, 5 times more likely to develop gangrene, and 2 times more likely to develop heart disease and stroke. Excluding its complications, diabetes costs more than $10 billion annually in health care costs and lost productivity (National Diabetes Data Group, 1981).

CLASSIFICATION OF DIABETES MELLITUS

For more than a century, two forms of diabetes mellitus have been recognized—one with its onset primarily in childhood and the other beginning primarily in adulthood. More recent evidence has made it apparent that diabetes is a more heterogeneous disease. This knowledge has stimulated revisions of the categories of diabetes and of the criteria used for diagnosing the disease.

In 1979, the National Diabetes Data Group, an international panel of experts in diabetes sponsored by the National Institutes of Health, proposed the current classification (Tables 42–1 and 42–2). The three categories—diabetes mellitus, impaired glucose tolerance, and gestational diabetes—are of primary interest to health professionals in clinical practice. The statistical risk categories—previous abnormality of glucose tolerance (PrevAGT) and

potential abnormality of glucose tolerance (PotAGT)—were created for research purposes. This revised classification system eliminated such vaguely defined terms as *juvenile-onset, adult-onset,* and *borderline diabetes*.

DIAGNOSTIC CRITERIA

The diagnosis of diabetes mellitus is confirmed by the presence of an elevated serum glucose level. The definition of normalcy for the serum glucose level may depend on factors such as age and pregnancy, however. Therefore, the revised system in Box 42–1 specifies diagnostic criteria for children, pregnant women, and nonpregnant adults. The criteria are stringently defined to prevent overdiagnosis of diabetes mellitus.

This chapter will focus on the two most common clinical types of the disease—Type I, or insulin-dependent diabetes mellitus (IDDM), and Type II, or noninsulin-dependent diabetes mellitus (NIDDM). The chapter will emphasize diabetes in the adult. Although Type I diabetes first appears in childhood, it becomes a disease of adulthood as the person ages. Type II, formerly called *adult-*

Table 42–1 Types of Diabetes Mellitus and Other Categories of Glucose Intolerance

Clinical Classes	Distinguishing Characteristics
Diabetes mellitus Type I, or insulin-dependent diabetes mellitus (IDDM)	Clients may be of any age, are usually thin, and usually have abrupt onset of symptoms and signs with insulinopenia before age 40. These clients often have strongly positive urine glucose and ketone tests and are dependent on insulin to prevent ketoacidosis and to sustain life.
Type II, or noninsulin-dependent diabetes mellitus (NIDDM) (obese or nonobese)	Clients are usually older than 40 years at diagnosis, obese, and have relatively few classic symptoms. They are not prone to ketoacidosis except during periods of stress. Although not dependent on exogenous insulin for survival, they may require it for stress-induced hyperglycemia and hyperglycemia that persists in spite of other therapy.
Other types of diabetes mellitus	Clients with other types of diabetes mellitus have certain associated conditions or syndromes (see Table 42–2).
Impaired glucose tolerance (IGT) (obese or nonobese)	Clients with impaired glucose tolerance have serum glucose levels that are higher than normal but not diagnostic for diabetes mellitus.
Other types of impaired glucose tolerance	Clients with other types of impaired glucose tolerance have certain associated conditions or syndromes (see Table 42–2).
Gestational diabetes mellitus (GDM)	Clients with gestational diabetes mellitus have onset or discovery of glucose intolerance during pregnancy.
Statistical Risk Classes*	
Previous abnormality of glucose tolerance (PrevAGT)	Persons in this category have normal glucose tolerance and a history of transient diabetes mellitus or impaired glucose tolerance.
Potential abnormality of glucose tolerance (PotAGT)	Persons in this category have never experienced abnormal glucose tolerance but have a greater-than-normal risk of developing diabetes mellitus or impaired glucose tolerance.

*Used for epidemiologic and research purposes

SOURCE: Adapted with permission from Rifkin H (editor): *The Physician's Guide to Type II Diabetes (NIDDM): Diagnosis and Treatment.* New York: American Diabetes Association, 1984, p. 4. Adapted from classification developed by an international workgroup sponsored by the National Diabetes Data Group, National Institutes of Health. National Diabetes Data Group: Classification and diagnosis of diabetes mellitus and other categories of glucose intolerance. *Diabetes* 1979; 28:1039–1057.

Table 42-2 Other Types of Diabetes Mellitus and Impaired Glucose Tolerance	
Secondary to:	**Examples**
Pancreatic disease	Pancreatectomy, hemochromatosis, cystic fibrosis, chronic pancreatitis
Endocrinopathies	Acromegaly, pheochromocytoma, Cushing's syndrome, primary aldosteronism, glucagonoma
Drugs and chemical agents	Certain antihypertensive drugs, thiazide diuretics, glucocorticoids, estrogen-containing preparations, psychoactive agents, catecholamines
Associated With:	**Examples**
Insulin-receptor abnormalities	Acanthosis nigricans
Genetic syndromes	Hyperlipidemia, muscular dystrophies, Huntington's chorea
Miscellaneous conditions	Malnutrition

SOURCE: Adapted with permission from Rifkin H (editor): *The Physician's Guide to Type II Diabetes (NIDDM): Diagnosis and Treatment.* New York: American Diabetes Association, 1984, p. 6. For a more complete list, see National Diabetes Data Group: Classification and diagnosis of diabetes mellitus and other categories of glucose intolerance. *Diabetes* 1979; 28:1039–1057.

onset diabetes, is the more prevalent form of the disease and will become even more predominant as the percentage of older adults in the population increases.

General Nursing Implications

The role of the nurse in diabetes mellitus management is to help the client and significant others adapt to the lifelong challenge of living well with diabetes. Few diseases have as many physiological, emotional, and social implications. Diabetes presents major challenges not only as a multisystem disease but also as a condition that affects issues such as self-image, diet, participation in exercise and sports, sexuality, childbearing, parenting, employment, and insurability.

Diabetes is best approached from a wellness perspective. To best serve diabetic clients, health care providers should help them make decisions that will encourage a full, productive, and healthy life. Client education requires an understanding of the principles of management of the numerous effects of diabetes.

Diabetes education is a lifelong process that can be divided into three phases. Immediate education begins upon diagnosis and is designed to provide the basic knowledge necessary for immediate management of diabetes. Illness and the emotional impact of the diagnosis often impede learning. To avoid overwhelming the client, educational objectives at this stage should be limited. The content includes a diabetes overview, glucose and ketone monitoring, basic meal planning, insulin or oral hypoglycemic agent administration, and management of hypoglycemia and ketosis. This education occurs in ambulatory care and inpatient settings. If the client is ill, hospitalization is necessary. For the well client, however, immediate diabetes education in an ambulatory setting is preferable.

The second phase, in-depth education, maximizes the client's ability to incorporate diabetes into a healthy lifestyle. Within several months of diagnosis, the demands of living with a chronic disease become evident both to the client and significant others. Thus, this is a period of readiness and motivation to learn. The in-depth curriculum focuses on establishing diabetes self-management, developing and maintaining motivation, and using the health care system. A 4- to 5-day in-depth program in an ambulatory setting is optimal.

The third phase, continuing education, renews previous learning and updates the client's knowledge. The periodic health care visit is a good time for continued learning. Objectives are mutually determined by the client and the health professional and may range from reviewing a basic skill to discussing research advances. Membership in diabetes education and support groups, attendance at continuing education programs, and periodic enrollment in in-depth programs are other means for renewing the client's learning and motivation.

DIABETES MELLITUS TYPE I (IDDM)

Type I diabetes mellitus (IDDM) is distinct from Type II diabetes mellitus (NIDDM) in its etiology, onset, and clinical course. Although IDDM has received more attention from health professionals and the public, it accounts for less than 10% of all cases of diabetes. The key difference between IDDM and NIDDM is that in IDDM, the pancreas does not produce enough insulin to sustain life. Therefore, individuals with IDDM depend totally on exogenous insulin. Because of the absence of insulin production, persons with IDDM are prone to **ketosis** secondary to hyperglycemia. In ketosis, the lack of insulin leads to the body's inability to metabolize glucose for energy. As a result, fatty acids are used as a fuel source. Fatty acids are incompletely oxidized, leading to an accumulation of ketones.

The onset of IDDM can occur any time from infancy to middle adulthood as a result of pathogenic causes; it can also occur at any age as a result of traumatic damage to the pancreas. It usually occurs in persons of normal body weight, unlike NIDDM, which is more frequent in the overweight or obese.

The etiology of IDDM is unclear and may be multifactorial. A genetic role is conceivable, because there is an

---

Box 42–1 Diagnostic Criteria for Diabetes Mellitus, Impaired Glucose Tolerance, and Gestational Diabetes Mellitus

Nonpregnant Adults

Criteria for diagnosis of diabetes mellitus

Diagnosis of diabetes mellitus in nonpregnant adults should be restricted to those who have *one* of the following:

- A random serum glucose level of 200 mg/dL or greater *plus* classic symptoms and signs of diabetes mellitus including polydipsia, polyuria, polyphagia, and weight loss.
- A fasting serum glucose level of 140 mg/dL or greater on at least two occasions.
- A fasting serum glucose level of less than 140 mg/dL *plus* sustained elevated serum glucose levels during at least two oral glucose tolerance tests. The 2-hour sample and at least one other between 0 and 2 hours after the 75-g glucose dose should be 200 mg/dL or greater. Oral glucose tolerance testing is not necessary if the client has a fasting serum glucose level of 140 mg/dL or greater.

Criteria for diagnosis of impaired glucose tolerance

Diagnosis of impaired glucose tolerance in nonpregnant adults should be restricted to those who have *all* of the following:

- A fasting serum glucose of less than 140 mg/dL
- A 2-hour oral glucose tolerance test serum glucose level between 140 and 200 mg/dL
- An intervening oral glucose tolerance test serum glucose value of 200 mg/dL or greater

Pregnant Women

Screening for gestational diabetes

- By glucose measurement in serum.
- 50-g oral glucose load, administered between the 24th and 28th week and without regard to time of day or time of last meal to all pregnant women who have not been identified as having glucose intolerance before the 24th week.
- Venous serum glucose is measured 1 hour later.
- A value of ≥140 mg/dL (7.8 mmol/L) in venous serum indicates the need for a full diagnostic glucose tolerance test.

Pregnant Women (continued)

Diagnosis of gestational diabetes mellitus

- 100-g oral glucose load, administered in the morning after overnight fast for at least 8 hours but not more than 14 hours, and after at least 3 days of unrestricted diet (≥150 g carbohydrate) and physical activity.
- Venous serum glucose is measured fasting and at 1, 2, and 3 hours. Subject should remain seated and not smoke throughout the test.
- Two or more of the following venous serum concentrations must be met or exceeded for positive diagnosis:
  Fasting, 105 mg/dL (5.8 mmol/L)
  1 h, 190 mg/dL (10.6 mmol/L)
  2 h, 165 mg/dL (9.2 mmol/L)
  3 h, 145 mg/dL (8.1 mmol/L)

Children

Criteria for diagnosis of diabetes mellitus

Diagnosis of diabetes mellitus in children should be restricted to those who have *one* of the following:

- A random serum glucose level of 200 mg/dL or greater *plus* classic symptoms and signs of diabetes mellitus, including polyuria, polydipsia, ketonuria, and rapid weight loss.
- A fasting serum glucose level of 140 mg/dL or greater on at least two occasions *and* sustained elevated serum glucose levels during at least two oral glucose tolerance tests. Both the 2-hour serum glucose and at least one other between 0 and 2 hours after the glucose dose (1.75 g/kg ideal body weight up to 75 g) should be 200 mg/dL or greater.

Criteria for impaired glucose tolerance: The diagnosis of impaired glucose tolerance in children should be restricted to those who have *both* of the following:

- A fasting serum glucose concentration of less than 140 mg/dL.
- A 2-hour oral glucose tolerance test serum glucose level of greater than 140 mg/dL

SOURCE: Reprinted with permission from Rifkin H (editor): *The Physician's Guide to Type II Diabetes (NIDDM): Diagnosis and Treatment.* New York: American Diabetes Association, 1984, p. 10.
Section on gestational diabetes from the Summary and Recommendations of the Second International Workshop-Conference on Gestational Diabetes Mellitus. *Diabetes* 34, suppl. 2, June 1985, 123–126.

---

increased frequency of certain antigens of the human leukocyte antigen (HLA) system, part of the body's immune mechanism. Some researchers speculate about the likelihood of a distinct diabetogenic gene. Further, there may exist an autoimmune mechanism that triggers the production of antibodies to destroy pancreatic islet cells. Such antibodies are found in a large percentage of persons at the time of diagnosis of IDDM. The role of immunosuppressive drugs in preserving islet cell function is under investigation. Viral agents, specifically coxsackievirus B, also may damage pancreatic islet cells (Freinkel, 1981).

None of these theories is sufficient to explain the etiology of IDDM. It may be that in the person with a genetic susceptibility, an environmental agent such as a virus may stimulate an autoimmune response, which in turn provokes IDDM.

Clinical Manifestations

The symptoms and signs of IDDM often occur abruptly and include the characteristic three "polys"—polyuria, polydipsia, and polyphagia. The absence of insulin prevents cellular metabolism of glucose. Thus, blood glucose levels rise while fat and protein stores are metabolized for energy, causing weight loss and ketosis. Weight loss continues despite hunger and excessive eating.

Rapid shifts in fluid and acid–base balance also occur. Hyperglycemia produces cellular dehydration and a profound diuresis. Dramatic fluid losses through urination can occur within hours. Hyperglycemia and dehydration accelerate the development of metabolic acidosis. If the disease is untreated, coma and death result.

Therapeutic Measures

Following the diagnosis of IDDM, the immediate and ongoing goal of therapy is the correction of hyperglycemia and the restoration of normal carbohydrate, fat, and protein metabolism to prevent long-term vascular complications. The degree of control over blood glucose levels necessary to prevent the microvascular kidney and retinal complications of IDDM has long been a source of controversy (Cahill, Etzwiler, & Freinkel, 1976). Proponents of rigorous, or tight, control cite evidence that these complications are directly related to blood glucose levels. Opponents argue that microvascular complications can occur independently of blood glucose control and may be hereditary.

In 1976, after careful review of the evidence, the American Diabetes Association published a position paper that urged optimal control of blood glucose levels, particularly in young and middle-aged persons, who are at greatest risk for developing long-term complications (Cahill, Etzwiler, & Freinkel, 1976). The National Institutes of Health are currently conducting a major 10-year study, the Diabetes Control and Complications Trial, to determine the relation between blood glucose levels and microvascular complications.

Insulin

Insulin is the foremost regulator of energy production, conversion, and storage. It is necessary for the metabolism of carbohydrate, protein, and fat. Metabolism of food carbohydrate begins when it is absorbed across the intestinal mucosa in the form of glucose. Insulin stimulates the entry of glucose into the cells, allowing it to be used for energy. Insulin is also necessary for **glycogenesis**—the synthesis of **glycogen** (stored carbohydrate) from glucose—and for the storage of glycogen in the muscles and liver. When insulin levels are low, *glycogenolysis*, the reconversion of glycogen to glucose, occurs to supply energy.

Food protein is absorbed across the intestinal mucosa as amino acids. Insulin lowers blood amino acid levels along with blood glucose levels. It also facilitates the incorporation of amino acids into tissue protein, allowing for growth and maintenance of body tissues.

Food fat is absorbed across the intestinal mucosa and carried in the lymphatic system in the form of **chylomicrons,** or particles of lipids, which are mostly triglycerides. Excess carbohydrates and amino acids are converted to fat in the liver. Without insulin, the enzyme lipoprotein

lipase is not released, and fat cannot be stored. Insulin also inhibits the breakdown of triglyceride from adipose cells.

Hormones that are counter-regulatory to insulin include glucagon, epinephrine, cortisol, and growth hormone (GH). All have the general effect of increasing blood glucose levels. Glucagon stimulates hepatic glucose production through glycogenolysis and gluconeogenesis and inhibits hepatic glucose uptake. It also increases lipolysis, the splitting up of fat.

In the normal state, blood glucose levels are maintained in a limited range by a delicate balance between insulin and the counter-regulatory hormones. In IDDM, this balance is jeopardized. The goal of insulin therapy in IDDM is to replace endogenous insulin so normal blood glucose levels can be maintained.

Classification of Insulin. Insulin has been greatly improved since it was first administered in 1922. Insulin may be classified by source, purity, concentration, formulation, and time activity:

- *Source and purity.* Bovine and porcine pancreata are the most common sources of insulin. Standard animal insulins have steadily improved in purity, ie, freedom from antigenic proteins. Purified animal insulin contains less than 10 ppm of **proinsulin,** a precursor to insulin that is its chief impurity. Purified animal insulins are indicated for children and adults who are beginning insulin therapy, for short-term insulin therapy, and for situations in which complications arise from the use of standard animal insulin.

  Human insulin, developed in the early 1980s, is produced by recombinant DNA technology or by chemical modification of porcine insulin. It is less antigenic than animal insulin. The DNA generated insulin also provides a continuing supply independent of meat consumption trends. It is indicated for the same reasons as purified animal insulin and may someday replace it.

- *Concentration.* The standard concentration, or number of units per milliliter of fluid, used for insulin therapy in the United States is U100. Several other strengths have been used but discontinued to avoid dosage errors.

- *Formulation and time activity.* Many insulin formulations are available; the common preparations are listed in Table 42–3. Insulin is classified as short, intermediate, or long acting on the basis of onset, peak, and duration of action. These characteristics are also listed in Table 42–3.

Complications of Insulin Therapy. Insulin therapy may involve several complications. Lipoatrophy, the loss of fat at injection sites, occurs more often in women and is thought to be caused by an immune response to insulin impurities. The treatment is injection of purified porcine insulin into affected areas until they fill out, usually

Table 42–3	Time Activity of Insulin Formulations		
Formulation	Onset	Peak	Duration
Short-acting			
Regular	15–30 min	2–4 h	5–7 h
Semilente	30–60 min	2–8 h	12–16 h
Intermediate-acting			
NPH	1–2 h	6–12 h	24–28 h
Lente	1–2 h	6–12 h	24–28 h
Long-acting			
Ultralente	4–6 h	18–24 h	32–36 h

SOURCE: Adapted from Karam J: Insulins 1983: Overview and outlook. *Clinical Diabetes.* New York: American Diabetes Association, 1983, p. 7.

in 4 to 6 weeks. Lipohypertrophy, the overgrowth of fat at injection sites, occurs more often in men and results from repeated injection into the same site. It can be prevented by rotating injection sites.

Occasionally, local or systemic allergic responses to insulin occur. Local allergies are often transient and may not require treatment. Systemic allergy, ranging from hives to anaphylactic shock (a rare reaction) responds to desensitization. Interrupted therapy with standard animal insulin increases the likelihood of allergy. Therefore, whenever temporary insulin therapy is necessary, as in gestational diabetes mellitus or other stress states, human insulin should be prescribed.

Insulin resistance occurs when blood glucose levels are unaffected by daily doses exceeding 200 units. Obesity is a common cause of insulin resistance, but insulin antibodies may also bind injected insulin and diminish its effect. Treatment in nonobese clients consists of transferring them from standard to human insulin. Hypoglycemia, an acute complication of insulin therapy, is discussed later in this section.

Administration of Insulin. Insulin regimens meet the body's requirement for insulin at meals and during the remainder of the day. Conventional therapy consists of one daily injection of intermediate-acting insulin alone, or in combination with short-acting insulin, or two daily injections of a combination of short- and intermediate-acting insulin.

When conventional regimens do not result in adequate control, *intensive therapy* is an option. Intensive regimens include multiple daily injections of three or more doses of short-acting insulin in combination with intermediate- or long-acting insulin. Another method of intensive therapy involves continuous subcutaneous insulin infusion (CSII) by a battery-powered external pump (Figure 42–1). The pump delivers a basal level of insulin throughout the day and extra doses, or boluses, before meals. In theory,

intensive regimens more nearly mimic insulin secretion of the pancreas.

Nutritional Management

Nutritional management is the foundation of therapy for IDDM (as well as NIDDM). It is essential to convey to the person with diabetes mellitus both the goals and the means of nutritional management through the development of an individualized diet prescription, initial nutrition education, and ongoing nutrition counseling.

The overall goal of nutritional management in both types of diabetes is to normalize blood glucose and blood lipid levels while maintaining good nutrition and health. The nutritional guidelines for achieving this goal are excellent for the whole family, because they are what anyone should eat to remain healthy. With the current focus on control of blood glucose levels, normalization of blood lipid levels must not be forgotten. Approximately 80% of the deaths of diabetic Americans are associated with atherosclerotic lesions, but these need not be an inevitable result of diabetes. Persons with diabetes in Japan and Hong Kong have only about one-fourth the incidence of coronary artery disease as their counterparts in Western societies when matched for age, average blood glucose level, duration of diabetes, and blood pressure (Keen & Jarrett, 1979). Some researchers suggest that diets low in saturated fat protect against coronary artery disease even when diabetes mellitus is present (West, 1978).

Specific Nursing Measures

Nutritional Approaches

The overall nutritional goal is the same for IDDM and NIDDM, but it is important to understand goals especially important to each type. IDDM therapy involves three goals:

1. Prevent the acute complications of hypoglycemia and hyperglycemia by balancing food intake with insulin

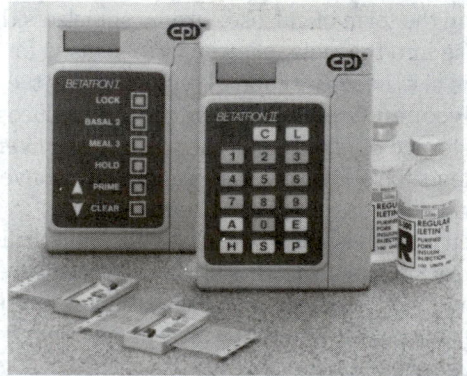

Figure 42–1

Two insulin pumps for continuous subcutaneous insulin infusion (Betatron I, Model 9205; Betatron II, Model 9200). (Courtesy of Cardiac Pacemakers, Inc., St. Paul, MN)

and the client's usual pattern of activity. With conventional insulin therapy of one or two daily injections, the timing of meals and snacks must be consistent from day to day. To prevent hypoglycemia, the client must avoid long periods between meals. Consistency in timing, nutrient content, and caloric level is more important for blood glucose control than the restriction of any specific food item. It is generally more effective to adapt a client's insulin program than to expect major changes in eating habits. Establish a meal plan that is nutritionally adequate and acceptable to the client; then monitor blood glucose levels to integrate insulin therapy.

2. Provide for a normal growth rate in children and the attainment and maintenance of desirable body weight in adults. Periodically record the child's height and weight on a growth chart such as the one developed by the National Center for Health Statistics. Any abnormal change in growth rate warrants an assessment of diabetes control and caloric intake. Adults with IDDM also need periodic assessment of weight and, if necessary, help in achieving and maintaining a desirable body weight.

3. Prevent or delay the development of the long-term cardiovascular, renal, retinal, and neurologic complications associated with diabetes mellitus. Epidemiological evidence suggests that the prevention of hyperglycemia can prevent or mitigate microvascular complications. To attain this goal, clients must be willing and able to monitor their nutrient intake.

Distribution of Nutrients in the Meal Plan. The following percentages of carbohydrate, protein, and fat that make up the meal plan are general recommendations, not rigid requirements. They may be adapted to meet individual eating habits.

Approximately *50%* to *60%* of the total calories in the meal plan should come from *carbohydrates*. There is no need to restrict disproportionately the intake of carbohydrates in the diet as was once common in the management of diabetes. Increased dietary carbohydrate without increased total calories does not increase insulin requirements. Insulin need is more closely related to total caloric intake than to carbohydrate intake, mainly because of the excellent ability of the liver to manufacture glucose from a variety of noncarbohydrate sources.

Research in the mid-1970s demonstrated that increasing the carbohydrate content of the diet actually improved glucose tolerance (Brunzell et al., 1974). In the intestinal wall, in muscle and adipose tissue, and apparently in all tissues involved in glucose utilization and metabolism, a high-carbohydrate diet leads to better metabolism of glucose through enzyme adaptation.

The blood glucose levels produced by various foods are described by the **glycemic index.** This index tells which foods will raise blood glucose levels quickly and which

Nursing Research Note

Tallman V: Effect of venipuncture on glucose, insulin, and free fatty acid levels. *West J Nurs* 1982; 4(1):21–29.

The effect of venipuncture on fasting levels of glucose, insulin, and free fatty acids was studied. The author hypothesized that catecholamine release during stress, such as a venipuncture, might alter these levels.

In a sample of 21 inpatients an intracatheter was inserted into an antecubital vein. Blood was drawn immediately after catheter insertion and again 15 minutes after and 30 minutes after insertion.

The glucose levels indicated no significant differences between any test times. Insulin levels dropped significantly after the first drawing and 15 minutes after catheter insertion. At the 30-minute interval, the insulin levels increased somewhat but not significantly. For the free fatty acid levels, there was a significant drop between the first sample and the sample drawn after 30 minutes.

From these results, the author suggested that fasting insulin levels and free fatty acid levels are affected by venipuncture. It was recommended that when accuracy is essential, these blood tests should be drawn 30 minutes after the venipuncture.

will cause a more moderate rise. Researchers are beginning to learn which foods fall into each category as well as what occurs when foods are eaten separately and when they are eaten as part of a meal.

Many factors affect the glycemic index. The physical form in which food is eaten may affect blood glucose levels. Whole foods, which have a smaller surface area exposed to intestinal enzymes, may be absorbed more slowly than ground foods. Raw foods tend to slow blood glucose response. The meal in which the carbohydrate food is eaten may also be important. Slowly digested carbohydrates eaten in one meal not only cause less blood glucose response after that meal but also lessen the response after the next meal. Finally, carbohydrates taken in small amounts over several hours cause less response than the same amount eaten all at once.

Dietary fiber is another component of food that can affect blood glucose and blood lipid levels. *Dietary fiber* is the term applied to all the constituents derived from the plant cell walls that are not digested by the endogenous secretions of the human digestive tract. Water-insoluble fibers (eg, cellulose, lignin, and many hemicelluloses found in whole grains and wheat bran) seem to have a major effect on gastrointestinal transit time and fecal bulk but less impact on serum glucose and lipid levels. In contrast, water-soluble fibers (eg, pectins; gums; storage polysaccharides; and a few hemicelluloses found in fruits, vegetables, oats, and legumes) have little effect on fecal bulk but affect serum lipid levels and possibly serum glucose levels. The average daily intake of dietary fiber is 10 to 20 g. A recommended level is between 25 and 40 g, or 20 g per every 1000 calories in the daily meal plan. Table 42–4 lists the fiber content of various foods.

Table 42–4	Fiber Content of Various Foods	
Food	**Portion for Approximately One Exchange of Each Food Grouping**	**Approximate Dietary Fiber**
Vegetables	½ to ¾ cup cooked; 1 to 2 cups raw	2 g
Fruits: fresh or canned	½ cup; 1 small fresh	2 g
Breads: whole wheat breads and crackers	1 slice or 1 oz	2 g
Cereals: dry or cooked bran cereals	Varies Varies	3 g 8 g
Starchy vegetables: potatoes, brown rice, bulgur, green peas	½ cup	3 g
Legumes: peas, beans, lentils	½ cup	8 g
Nuts, seeds, peanut butter	1 oz (¼ cup) or 2 tbsp	3 g

SOURCE: Adapted with permission from Franz MJ: *Exchanges for All Occasions: Meeting the Challenge of Diabetes.* Minneapolis: International Diabetes Center, 1983, pp. 44–48.

The recommended level of *protein* intake is *15%* to *20%* of total daily calories. Protein is usually found in combination with fat in foods. The only foods that contain protein without containing fat are nonfat dairy products such as skim milk and vegetable proteins such as beans, peas, and lentils. Therefore, to keep fat within the recommended limits, protein must be kept at reasonable levels as well.

It is recommended that *fat* intake be reduced from the North American average of 40% to 50% of daily calories to approximately *25%* to *30%*. Dietary fat does not have an immediate effect on blood glucose levels but must be considered for two reasons. First, a gram of fat supplies 9 calories, whereas a gram of carbohydrate or protein supplies only 4 calories. Foods containing large amounts of fat will therefore be high in calories, and counting calories to maintain or attain desirable body weight is a major goal for clients with diabetes. Second, the restriction of foods high in fat, especially saturated fat, reduces blood cholesterol and triglyceride levels and decreases the risk of coronary artery disease (CAD). Because people with diabetes have twice the risk of CAD, such restriction is especially important for them.

Saturated fats are found in animal fats, coconut and palm oils, solid shortenings, and dairy foods that contain fat. As noted, these fats raise blood cholesterol levels. Polyunsaturated fats are liquid vegetable oils such as safflower, sunflower, corn, soybean, and cottonseed oils. They have been shown to lower blood cholesterol levels. Monounsaturated fats are neutral fats that neither raise nor lower blood cholesterol levels. They are found in olives, olive and peanut oil, and most nuts.

Cholesterol is manufactured in the body and is obtained in the diet only from animal foods. Although cholesterol is usually found in combination with fat, there are a few foods (eg, eggs and liver) that are high in cholesterol without being high in fat.

The following dietary recommendations help reduce fat intake:

- Eat lean meats and pay careful attention to portion size, with a daily limit of 6 oz of meat, fish, poultry, cheese, and eggs. Use poultry and fish whenever possible, avoiding high-fat meats such as cold cuts, bacon, sausage, frankfurters, and prime cuts such as marbled steaks.

- In place of butter, use margarine with a liquid oil listed as the first ingredient on the label.

- Whenever possible, replace hydrogenated or hardened shortenings with liquid vegetable oils. Hydrogenation changes unsaturated liquid fat into a hardened, saturated fat.

- Use nonfat or low-fat dairy products (eg, skim milk and low-fat cheeses) and avoid products that contain dairy fat. Persons with diabetes, starting with children aged 2, should use skim milk. Plain yogurt can be substituted for sour cream and mayonnaise.

- Restrict foods containing cholesterol, such as eggs and liver.

In summary, it appears the ideal diet is high in carbohydrate with an emphasis on fiber; low in total fat, especially saturated fat; and adequate in protein.

Exchange Lists. The most widely used system for translating the previous information into a method for food selection is the Exchange Lists for Meal Planning. These lists were developed by the American Diabetes Association and the American Dietetic Association in the 1950s and most recently revised in 1976. The exchange system divided food into lists (Table 42–5). Each list contains food items similar in calorie, carbohydrate, protein, and fat content.

Table 42–5 Exchange Lists

One Exchange	Equals	Calories	Carbohydrate (gram)	Protein (gram)	Fat (gram)
Milk	=	80	12	8	—
Vegetable	=	25	5	2	—
Fruit	=	40	10	—	—
Bread	=	70	15	2	—
Meat, lean	=	55	—	7	3
Medium fat	=	75	—	7	5
High fat	=	100	—	7	8
Fat	=	45	—	—	5

SOURCE: Summarized from *Exchange Lists for Meal Planning.* New York: American Diabetes Association and Chicago: American Dietetic Association, 1976, pp. 1–24.

Therefore, any food item on a given list can be exchanged, or substituted, for any other item on the same list.

A meal plan tells how many servings a person may select from each list at each meal and snack. In individualizing such a plan, the best way to start is to take a dietary history to find out what, where, and how much the person would eat if he or she did not have diabetes. Give as much consideration as possible to the person's preferences with respect to types of foods and eating schedules.

Next, determine the client's caloric needs based on desirable body weight and current activity level. It is not necessary to determine the precise caloric need immediately. An estimate can be used as a starting point, and appropriate adjustments made on the basis of experience. The following generalizations are helpful in determining daily caloric levels:

- Children under 12 require an average of 1000 calories plus 100 calories per year of age. Thus, a 4-year-old would require 1400 calories.
- Boys from ages 12 to 15 usually require all of the above plus 200 calories per year of age after 12. Thus, a 14-year-old needs approximately 2600 calories (1000 + 1200 + 400).
- Girls' caloric requirements begin to drop between the ages of 12 and 15.
- A moderately active young man requires approximately 40 calories per kilogram of body weight daily. Thus, a 70-kg (154 lb) man requires approximately 2800 calories/day. A relatively inactive young man may require as few as 30 calories/kg (2100 calories), whereas a young man who habitually engages in heavy activity may require as many as 50 calories/kg (3500 calories).
- A typical young woman requires approximately 30 to 35 calories per kilogram of body weight. Thus, a young woman weighing 58 kg (128 lb) who is moderately active needs approximately 1800 to 2000 calories/day.

- Older individuals usually require fewer calories in relation to body size: 30 to 35 calories/kg (or 15 calories/lb) of desirable body weight for the moderately active; 28 calories/kg (13 calories/lb) of desirable body weight after age 55 or for the sedentary; and 20 calories/kg (10 calories/lb) of desirable body weight for the very obese or very inactive.

Children and teens with diabetes must have adequate caloric intake to grow normally. Because size and activity levels vary considerably in children of the same age, the formulas given here should be used only as guidelines. Too frequently, inadequate calories are prescribed for children and teens with diabetes.

For lean individuals, an initial diet plan that is generous helps emphasize that the main goal is regulation rather than deprivation. Satiety, appetite, and hunger are usually reliable guides to caloric requirements, but body weight is the definitive long-term guide.

After approximating caloric requirements, design a tentative meal plan based on the diet history and discuss use of the exchange lists with the client. The next step is to total the grams of carbohydrate, protein, and fat in the meal plan. The sample breakfast plan in Table 42–6 contains 52 g of carbohydrate, 19 g of protein, and 10 g of fat. To determine the total calories, multiply the grams of carbohydrate by 4, the grams of protein by 4, and the grams of fat by 9. The total calories for this breakfast plan are 374. After the entire day's totals have been calculated, determine the percentages of calories from carbohydrate, protein, and fat by dividing the calories from each nutrient by the total calories.

After the basic meal plan has been designed, consider the following questions:

- Is it nutritionally adequate?
- Are the total calories appropriate?
- Are the proportions of carbohydrate, protein, and fat appropriate?

Table 42–6 Sample Breakfast Meal Plan

Exchange	Number of Servings	Carbohydrate (gram)	Protein (gram)	Fat (gram)
Milk, skim	1	12	8	—
Fruit	1	10	—	—
Bread	2	30	4	—
Meat	1	—	7	5
Fat	1	—	—	5
TOTAL		52	19	10

- Does the meal plan accommodate activity or exercise patterns?
- Has the client had problems with hypoglycemia at certain times during the day that could be prevented by changes in eating habits?
- Does the client have hypertension, abnormal lipid values, or renal disease necessitating further restriction (eg, sodium)?

The best way to monitor the effectiveness of the meal plan is to have the client try it and report problems to the nutritional counselor.

Children's meal plans should be evaluated at least twice a year, because their schedules and activities change frequently, and caloric needs increase or decrease depending on their growth pattern. Adults' meal plans should be evaluated once or twice a year. If weight gain or loss becomes a problem, changes must be made. Continuing education of all clients is essential for long-term adherence to meal planning.

Special Circumstances Affecting the Meal Plan. There is no need to use special or "dietetic" foods. In fact, many so-called dietetic products (ice cream, cookies, cakes, and chocolate candies) are sweetened with sorbitol or fructose and contain as many calories as the products they replace. Clients generally enjoy their food more and spend less when they use regular foods and substitute correctly in their meal plans. Some products with limited calories may be useful, however. Examples are dietetic jams, jellies, soft drinks, and hard candies; fruit canned without sugar; sugarless gums; and artificial sweeteners.

As mentioned, sorbitol and fructose, frequently advertised as being of benefit to people with diabetes, contain the same amount of calories as sucrose (4 calories/g). If used, they must be counted in the meal plan. Saccharin and aspartame (sold as Equal and NutraSweet) are currently available as nonnutritional sweeteners, and when used in moderation they appear safe.

A general rule is: Servings of food that contain 20 calories or less may be considered "free," with a limit of two or three per day. Foods containing more than 20 calories per serving must be included in the meal plan.

Alcohol is a hypoglycemic agent that augments the effects of insulin. The liver is the major organ for alcohol metabolism. Alcohol cannot be converted to glucose or amino acids. However, it can be used as an energy source or converted into fatty acids and triglycerides without requiring insulin.

Clients with diabetes mellitus are more vulnerable to the hypoglycemic effects of alcohol. Hypoglycemia occurs at blood alcohol levels that do not exceed the range of mild intoxication; 35 g of ethanol (2 oz of alcohol) may produce hypoglycemia in a fasting person with IDDM. Fasting depletes hepatic stores of glycogen, making active gluconeogenesis necessary to maintain blood glucose levels. Alcohol inhibits the formation of new glucose from amino acids and other precursors. Larger doses of alcohol may cause a small but transient rise in the blood glucose level, followed a couple of hours later by a fall below the fasting level.

Alcohol is high in calories (7 calories/g) and devoid of nutritional value. Many alcoholic drinks (beer and sweet wines) also contain appreciable amounts of carbohydrate. Even so, most clients with diabetes may have an occasional drink. In normal-weight, insulin-dependent individuals whose diabetes is well controlled, moderate use of carbohydrate-free alcohol (2 oz daily) may be regarded as an "extra," best used with or following a meal. One ounce of alcohol is the equivalent of 1.5 oz of distilled beverage (whiskey, scotch, rye, vodka, gin, cognac, rum, or dry brandy), 12 oz of beer, or 4 oz of dry wine. If alcohol is used daily, calories from alcohol are added to the total daily caloric intake. No food should be omitted, because of the danger of hypoglycemia.

During pregnancy, the diabetic mother must maintain strict control of her blood glucose level to reduce the likelihood of fetal morbidity and mortality. The diet plan must take into account not only the metabolic requirements of the mother but of the developing fetus as well. A total weight gain of 24 to 30 lb is recommended, with the pattern of weight gain more important than the total amount. Pregnancy is not a time for weight reduction.

Caloric requirements can be met by the addition of 300 calories/day to the prepregnancy meal plan. Additional calories should be supplied by 50 g of carbohydrate and 30 g of protein. The diet should contain approximately 1800 to 2500 calories a day. The importance of regular meals and snacks must be emphasized. In particular, the bedtime snack is essential because of the tendency toward nocturnal hypoglycemia and ketosis.

Insulin Administration

Clients must master several concepts and skills in learning insulin self-administration. To ensure that the same insulin is purchased consistently, the client must know the brand name, formulation, purity, concentration, and species source of insulin. This is difficult because there is a wide array of insulins and because insulin is an over-the-counter item in most states. To avoid confusion, advise clients to show their current insulin vials to the pharmacist at the time of purchase.

Insulin vials in use should be stored at room temperature, away from temperature extremes and direct sunlight. Extra vials should be refrigerated. Insulin should be used before the expiration date printed on the label.

Insulin syringes must match the concentration of insulin, or an incorrect dose will result. If injecting U100 insulin, U100 syringes must be used. Low-dose syringes are available for injections of 50 units or less and usually are more economical.

Consistency in the timing of insulin injections is important in maintaining blood glucose control. In conventional therapy, injections are given approximately 30 minutes before meals. Injection times should not vary more than 1 hour from day to day. Intensive therapy permits more flexibility in the timing of injections.

Insulin dosage changes recommended during a health care visit should be given to the client in writing. Written dosage algorithms that guide the client in making dosage changes based on blood glucose results are also helpful.

Insulin is injected in areas of the body containing sufficient subcutaneous tissue (Figure 42–2). An easy guideline for clients to remember is to inject where they can "pinch an inch" of tissue. Recommended sites are the lateral and dorsal surfaces of the upper arm, abdomen, anterior and lateral thighs, and buttocks. A written plan for rotating sites is helpful in selecting sites and encourages the use of several areas of the body for injection. Site rotation plans should be individualized to account for body size and distribution of subcutaneous tissue, the client's preference for sites, and ease of learning.

A written step-by-step outline of the subcutaneous injection technique for single and mixed formulations of insulin is helpful for the individual who has recently learned the technique as well as for the experienced insulin user. Review of these skills and concepts is an important component of periodic health care visits.

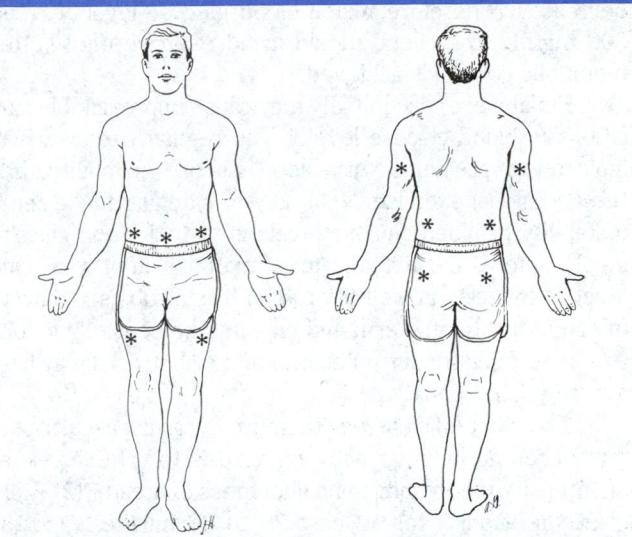

Figure 42–2

Sites for subcutaneous injection of insulin.

SOURCE: Courtesy of Etzwiler DD et al.: *Learning to Live Well With Diabetes.* Minneapolis, MN: International Diabetes Center, 1985.

Exercise

Persons with diabetes experience the same cardiorespiratory, psychological, and weight control benefits that anyone gains from a regular exercise program. In addition, the client with IDDM may benefit from decreased blood glucose levels and improved glucose tolerance. Exercise stimulates glucose uptake in exercising muscles, lowering blood glucose levels and increasing the body's sensitivity to insulin. Thus, regular exercise may decrease the need for injected insulin. Physical training can also help reverse the resistance to insulin that occurs as a result of obesity.

Exercise decreases the levels of very low-density lipoprotein (VLDL) and low-density lipoprotein (LDL). Exercise also is associated with increases in high-density lipoprotein (HDL), which appears to protect against coronary artery disease. Regular exercise also results in lower blood pressure.

To enjoy all the benefits safely, clients with IDDM must take certain precautions before, during, and after exercise. Because exercise adds to the blood glucose-lowering effect of injected insulin, it can increase the likelihood of hypoglycemia. Blood glucose will continue to decrease for up to 24 hours following exercise as muscle and liver glycogen stores are replaced. Food intake may need to be increased before exercising, depending on pre-exercise glucose levels.

Exercise lowers blood glucose levels only when adequate insulin is available. If blood glucose has been chronically higher than approximately 300 mg/dL, especially with mild ketosis, exercise will stress the body and drive blood glucose levels even higher. This occurs because hepatic glucose production increases and peripheral use of glucose decreases. Therefore, when blood glucose levels exceed 300 mg/dL, the client should avoid exercise until better metabolic control is achieved.

Finally, exercise initially may cause unpredictable variations in blood glucose levels. The regular exerciser will have fewer problems with blood glucose instability than the occasional exerciser. The key to safeguarding against instability of blood glucose levels is to test blood glucose levels before, during, and after exercise until a specific level of exercise is well tolerated. It is also wise to avoid injecting insulin into arm and leg sites immediately before exercise. Injecting into the abdomen or buttocks may help avert hypoglycemia.

The most efficient way to improve cardiovascular performance and burn fat with exercise is to (1) exercise at an intensity that results in no shortness of breath, (2) exercise continuously for at least 20 to 30 minutes, and (3) exercise three to five times a week. Aerobic exercise is of low intensity, is of long duration, and uses stored fat as the major energy source. Anaerobic exercise is of short duration (under 2 to 3 minutes), is of high intensity, and uses stored carbohydrate or glycogen as the major energy source. This activity quickly produces exhaustion. Thus, aerobic exercise is best for general fitness and blood glucose control. Aerobic activities require large amounts of oxygen and usually involve movement of the arms and legs, which contain a large part of the body's total muscle mass. Often-recommended aerobic exercises include brisk walking, jogging, swimming, skating, cross-country skiing, bicycling, jumping rope, aerobic dance, and jumping or running in place on a minitrampoline.

Any exercise program should be preceded by a medical evaluation. The program should build gradually in duration and intensity. Each session should consist of:

- *Warm-up period.* Stretching and cardiovascular warm-up for 10 to 12 minutes.
- *Training period.* Aerobic activity for 20 to 30 minutes with heart rate in the target zone (between 70% and 85% of the predicted maximal heart rate, which is approximately 220 minus the client's age).
- *Cool-down period.* Ten to 12 minutes of cardiovascular cool-down, specific muscle-strengthening exercises, and exercises for flexibility and relaxation.

Foot Care

Diabetic foot lesions result from the interplay of peripheral vascular disease and peripheral neuropathy as described in Figure 42–3. The primary cause of diabetic foot ulcers is an insensitive foot. Muscle atrophy causes dorsiflexion of toes and creates new pressure points on the plantar surface of the foot. Minor injury often goes undetected until ulceration and infection develop. Treatment is lengthy and includes antibiotics and the elimination or reduction of weight bearing with bed rest or a weight-bearing cast. Amputation is necessary if these treatment measures fail, but long-term survival following amputation is poor.

From 50% to 70% of the nontraumatic amputations in the United States occur in diabetic clients. Most of these amputations are preventable with proper care (Levin & O'Neal, 1983). Therefore, the prevention of foot lesions is a critical aspect of diabetes education and management. Clients should inspect and cleanse their feet daily and use an unmedicated, unscented lubricating cream to prevent the development of skin fissures. Detailed inspection of the feet should be part of the health care visit. Proper footwear stresses comfort over style. As deformities develop, corrective shoes help reduce stress. Corns, calluses, and nails should be trimmed by a health professional skilled in foot care. The client should avoid chemical abrasives. Minor uninfected injuries can be treated with cleansing, daily dressing changes, and rest. Any deviation from normal healing requires prompt medical attention.

Self Monitoring of Blood and Urine

Clients monitor the effectiveness of nutrition, exercise, and insulin therapy with blood or urine glucose tests. The two types of urine glucose tests are semiquantitative and quantitative. The semiquantitative method tests a small amount of urine with a glucose-sensitive reagent strip or tablet. The result is assumed to reflect the blood glucose level at a specific time. Semiquantitative urine tests correlate poorly with simultaneous blood glucose levels, however. Inaccuracies result from deviations (low and high) from the usual renal threshold for glucose of 160 to 180 mg/dL, the delay between glomerular filtration of urine and collection, and sensitivity and specificity problems with urine test materials.

Despite its disadvantages, however, urine glucose testing is recommended for those who are unable or unwilling to monitor blood glucose levels. Up to four daily preprandial tests are recommended for clients with IDDM. Using fresh second-voided specimens obtained within 30 minutes of emptying the bladder may improve the tests' accuracy.

The success of self blood glucose monitoring (BGM) suggests that it will be the predominant method for self-monitoring of diabetes management in the future. A 1979 report on the initial clinical success with BGM, along with the introduction of convenient testing products, stimulated idespread interest in the method (Tattersall, 1979).

Self BGM is accurate, convenient, and eliminates the disadvantages of urine glucose testing. A drop of capillary blood from a fingertip or earlobe puncture is applied to a glucose-sensitive reagent strip (Figure 42–4). The strip's coloration correlates directly with the blood glucose level and is interpreted visually or by a reflectance meter. Self BGM is recommended for everyone taking insulin. It is mandatory in diabetic pregnancy and intensive therapy, when rigid blood glucose control is necessary.

The frequency of monitoring depends on the type of diabetes, stability of control, degree of control desired, and client preference. Thus, a pregnant diabetic woman may test five to eight times daily, whereas one day of tests

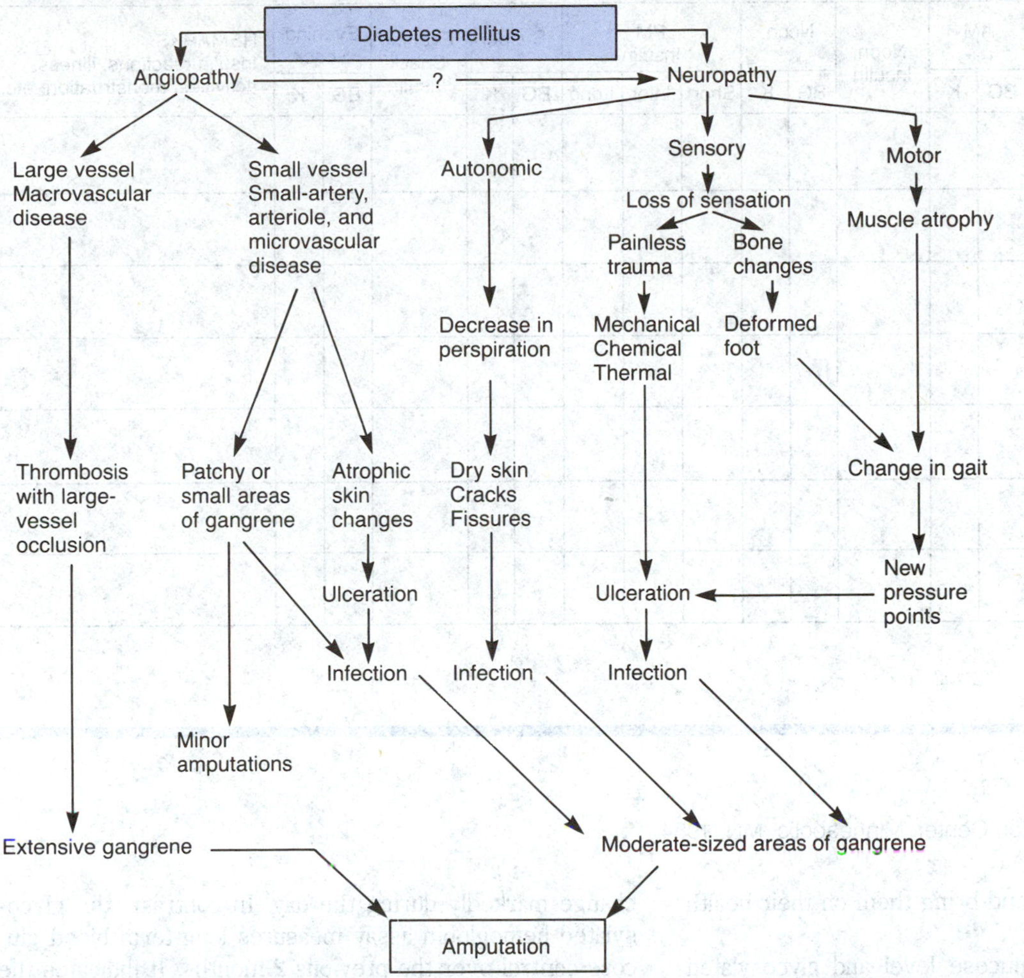

Figure 42–3

Pathogenesis of diabetic foot lesions.
SOURCE: Levin ME: Medical evaluation and treatment. In: *The Diabetic Foot,* 3rd ed. Levin ME, O'Neal LW (editors). St. Louis: Mosby, 1983.

Diabetes mellitus

Angiopathy — ? → Neuropathy

Large vessel Macrovascular disease

Small vessel Small-artery, arteriole, and microvascular disease

Autonomic

Sensory

Motor

Loss of sensation

Muscle atrophy

Painless trauma

Bone changes

Decrease in perspiration

Mechanical Chemical Thermal

Deformed foot

Thrombosis with large-vessel occlusion

Patchy or small areas of gangrene

Atrophic skin changes

Dry skin Cracks Fissures

Change in gait

Ulceration

New pressure points

Ulceration

Infection

Infection

Infection

Minor amputations

Extensive gangrene

Moderate-sized areas of gangrene

Amputation

a week may be sufficient for the older adult with stable diabetes.

Self BGM does not eliminate the need for urine ketone testing. Ketone testing for the nonpregnant client is suggested whenever preprandial blood glucose levels exceed 240 mg/dL or urine glucose tests exceed 0.5%, especially during illness.

Initial and ongoing client education stressing the importance of blood glucose monitoring is essential. Clients should maintain a written record of test results. Figure 42–5 illustrates a common format. Review of the record at each health care visit provides important information on day-to-day control and presents an excellent opportunity for education and support.

Clients should understand whether to test preprandially or postprandially, how frequently to test, what preprandial or postprandial blood or urine glucose targets are, and what action to take if targets are not met. Periodically, the nurse should verify the client's ability to use the testing method. Those using self BGM can compare a capillary blood glucose level with a serum glucose level obtained during the health care visit. The colors of some brands of blood test strips are stable for several days after the reaction if properly stored. Clients can record their visual inter-

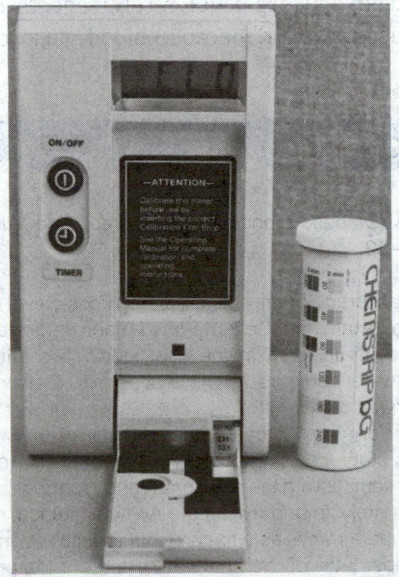

Figure 42–4

One model of a blood glucose monitoring system: The Accu-Chek bG/Chemstrip bG blood glucose monitoring system by Bio-Dynamics.

Month	AM Insulin			AM		Noon Insulin	Noon		PM Insulin			Supper		Evening Snack Insulin	Evening Snack		REMARKS Insulin reactions, illness, activities, menstruation, etc.
Date:	Short	Inter	Long	BG	K		BG	K	Short	Inter	Long	BG	K		BG	K	
8																	
9																	
10																	
11																	
12																	
13																	
14																	

Key: BG = Blood glucose
      K = Ketones

Figure 42–5

Diabetes record book.
SOURCE: International Diabetes Center, Minneapolis, MN, 1984.

pretations on these strips and bring them on their health care visit to verify results.

The random serum glucose level and glycosylated hemoglobin assay are two laboratory determinations commonly used to assess the effect of diabetes therapy. A random serum glucose level rarely reflects overall glycemic status, however, because blood glucose levels can change markedly during the day. In contrast, the glycosylated hemoglobin assay measures long-term blood glucose control over the previous 2 months. It indicates the percentage of hemoglobin attached to glucose (glycosylated). The level of glycosylation depends on the glucose concentration during the 60-day half-life of erythrocytes and hemoglobin. A glycosylated hemoglobin assesses long-

Nursing Research Note

Hilton BA: Diabetic monitoring measures. *Can Nurse* 1982; 73(5):26–32.

The accuracy of urine and blood glucose level testing by nurses was examined. Seventy-one nurses participated in the study; five participated in the pilot study. Two urine testing methods were compared—Clinitest 2 drop method and the Acetest method.

In performing Clinitests, the majority of the nurses followed the steps correctly; however, only 42% correctly compared the sample with the color chart and reported the glucose level accurately. In performing the Acetest method, the majority of the nurses were able to carry out the steps correctly. For both groups, 54% of the sample carried out the procedures correctly, 18% made one mistake, 20% made two, and 6% made three critical errors. Thirty percent of the nurses indicated they would test the first specimen if unable to get a second; 83% of the nurses stated they would use a sterile needle and syringe to withdraw urine from a catheter; 8.5% stated they would disconnect the catheter.

In testing blood using Chemstrip bG, 56% expressed the correct values, 11% expressed the correct range of values, and 32% had either incorrect values or the value ranges were unreliable or undependable. Sixty-three percent did not allow the alcohol to dry on the skin after cleansing. Although the majority was able to carry out the remaining steps with accuracy, 61 had had an inservice program before the Chemstrip test, and this group made fewer errors. Thirty-nine nurses performed the Dextrometer test; the majority was able to follow the steps correctly.

The researcher concluded that nurses are not necessarily able to perform blood glucose and urine glucose testing correctly. Experience did not ensure accuracy. The author recommends inservice education in techniques for blood and urine glucose measurement.

term control but cannot be used to make specific changes in day-to-day therapy. Daily blood or urine glucose test results are used for this purpose.

Self BGM enhances the client's role in diabetes self-management. Self-adjustment of conventional insulin therapy is based on the principles of basic pattern control outlined in Box 42–2. Table 42–7 illustrates how these principles are used.

Box 42–2 Principles of Basic Pattern Control in Conventional Insulin Therapy

Blood glucose levels are affected by meal plan, activity, insulin, and emotional or physical stress. Determine whether stressors or inconsistent activity or meal plans exist before adjusting insulin.

Make insulin adjustments on the basis of blood glucose patterns rather than isolated values.

Assess at least 3 days of blood glucose levels to determine a pattern.

Use the time activity of insulin to determine which insulin is responsible for a blood glucose pattern:

- The prebreakfast short-acting insulin affects the prelunch blood glucose level.
- The prebreakfast intermediate-acting insulin affects the predinner blood glucose level.
- The predinner short-acting insulin affects the bedtime blood glucose level.
- The predinner intermediate-acting insulin affects the prebreakfast blood glucose level the following day.

Increase or decrease insulin 1 to 2 units at a time. Monitor the effect for at least 3 days before making another adjustment.

SOURCE: Adapted with permission from Skyler J et al: Use of insulin in insulin-dependent diabetes mellitus. In: Insulin Update: 1982. Princeton, *Excerpta Medica,* pp. 133–139.

Table 42–7 Application of Basic Pattern-Control Principles

Preprandial targets = 80–120 mg/dL
Snacks: Midmorning, midafternoon, and bedtime

Date	AM Insulin Short	Intermediate	AM Blood Glucose	Noon Blood Glucose	PM Insulin Short	Intermediate	Dinner Blood Glucose	Evening Snack Blood Glucose
9/27	8	17	126	48	4	9	117	99
9/28	8	17	89	60	4	9	96	87
9/29	8	17	102	51	4	9	107	130

Problem: Prelunch hypoglycemia
Recommendation: Decrease prebreakfast short-acting insulin 2 units

Preprandial targets: 80–140 mg/dL
Snacks: Midafternoon and bedtime

Date	AM Insulin Short	Intermediate	AM Blood Glucose	Noon Blood Glucose	PM Insulin Short	Intermediate	Dinner Blood Glucose	Evening Snack Blood Glucose
12/6	10	24	121	89	3	8	176	120
12/7	10	24	107	104	3	8	184	131
12/8	10	24	118	93	3	8	157	109

Problem: Predinner hyperglycemia
Recommendation: Increase prebreakfast intermediate-acting insulin 2 units

Medical and Nursing Approaches to Complications of IDDM

Acute, intermediate, and chronic complications are associated with IDDM. The major complications and their management are discussed in this section.

Acute Complications

Acute complications develop within minutes to days. They include hypoglycemia and diabetic ketoacidosis (DKA).

Hypoglycemia. Hypoglycemia is a serum glucose level below approximately 50 mg/dL accompanied by adrenergic and neurologic symptoms. Normally, catecholamines, glucagon, and GH are released to counteract hypoglycemia. The early symptoms of hypoglycemia, such as palpitations, anxiety, and perspiration, are catecholamine induced. If hypoglycemia persists, cerebral function is impaired, and confusion and irritability result. Severe hypoglycemia produces unconsciousness and seizures.

Because IDDM may impair the usual mechanisms to correct hypoglycemia, this condition should always be treated promptly. Mild symptoms reverse with the ingestion of 10 g of carbohydrate, such as a half cup of fruit juice or nondiet soft drink. If no response occurs within 10 to 15 minutes, treatment is repeated. Overtreatment should be avoided, however, to prevent excessive hyperglycemia. Glucose gel preparations can be administered if the person is uncooperative yet has an intact swallow reflex.

To treat hypoglycemia in an unconscious person in the home setting, administer a glucagon injection. Glucagon produces a transient rise in blood glucose levels, and small, frequent feedings should be started as soon as the person regains consciousness. In the health care setting, severe hypoglycemia is treated with the IV administration of 25 mL of 50% dextrose solution.

Common causes of hypoglycemia include delayed or inadequate food intake, increased activity, and excessive insulin. Snacks and meals scheduled to coincide with the time activity of insulin are important in preventing hypoglycemia. A midmorning snack may be necessary if the client uses prebreakfast short-acting insulin. A midafternoon snack is helpful if the client takes intermediate-acting insulin before breakfast. To prevent nocturnal hypoglycemia, a bedtime snack is essential for everyone taking insulin. Before and during prolonged exercise, extra food is necessary. When hypoglycemia cannot be explained by alterations in food or activity, the client should decrease the insulin taken.

In some individuals, the *Somogyi phenomenon*, or unrecognized hypoglycemia resulting in rebound hyperglycemia, occurs at night. A reduction in insulin or an increase in the bedtime snack is necessary in this case.

Diabetic Ketoacidosis. DKA is a serious but preventable complication of IDDM that can develop within several hours to days. The mortality rate in severe DKA is 5% to 15% and is usually due to the underlying cause (Barrett & DeFronzo, 1984). Infection is the most common precipitating factor.

DKA results from an insulin deficiency combined with increased secretion of counter-regulatory, or anti-insulin, hormones. Insulin deficiency produces hyperglycemia, because the body's uptake of glucose is reduced and gluconeogenesis is increased. Marked hyperglycemia causes an osmotic diuresis, dehydration, and electrolyte depletion. When insulin is deficient, free fatty acids are mobilized from adipose tissue and converted to ketones in the liver. Serum ketone levels rise, causing metabolic acidosis and compensatory hyperventilation. Ketones are excreted in urine; one form, acetone, is volatile and can be detected on the breath. Acidosis produces peripheral vasodilation and hypotension. Levels of glucagon and other counter-regulatory hormones are elevated and contribute to further gluconeogenesis and conversion of free fatty acids to ketones.

Symptoms and signs that precede DKA are hyperglycemia, ketonuria, polyuria, fatigue, and nausea. When vomiting occurs, dehydration and acidosis can develop rapidly. Listlessness; rapid, deep respirations (Kussmaul's breathing); and severe abdominal pain accompany signs of marked dehydration. A serum pH under 7.2 indicates severe acidosis and results in coma and death if untreated.

DKA can be prevented by having the client take measures such as those listed in Box 42–3 to recognize and treat hyperglycemia and ketonuria. If additional insulin is necessary, usually 20% of the total daily dose is given in the form of short-acting insulin.

The first step in treating moderate or severe DKA is fluid replacement. The rapid IV infusion of 3 to 4 L of isotonic or hypotonic saline within several hours restores tissue perfusion. When serum glucose levels fall below 250

Box 42–3 Client Guidelines for Brief Illness

Monitor blood glucose and urine ketone levels every 4 hours. Notify your health care provider if blood glucose levels are elevated or if urine ketones develop.

Never omit insulin. The need for insulin continues or increases during illness.

If you are not able to eat regular food, replace carbohydrates with liquids or soft foods. About 50 g of carbohydrate should be taken every 3 to 4 hours. Water, tea, clear broth, or other clear fluids should be taken frequently.

If nausea, vomiting, or diarrhea occur, take small sips of fluids (1 or 2 tbsp every 15 to 30 minutes) and notify your health care provider.

If illness persists beyond 24 hours, notify your health care provider.

SOURCE: Adapted with permission from Franz M, Joynes J: *Diabetes and Brief Illness.* Minneapolis: International Diabetes Center, 1984, pp. 1–7.

mg/dL, the infusion is changed to 5% dextrose to prevent hypoglycemia.

The second step of therapy is continuous IV infusion or intermittent IM administration of low doses of short-acting insulin. In adults, the dosage generally ranges from 4 to 8 units per hour.

Replacement of potassium may be necessary. Initially, serum potassium may be elevated in DKA, but as ketosis and dehydration are corrected, potassium shifts intracellularly creating hypokalemia. Treatment of the underlying illness that contributed to the development of DKA is also a vital part of therapy.

Intermediate Complications

The intermediate complications of IDDM develop over several months. Children in whom diabetes is poorly controlled are retarded in growth and delayed in development. In the hyperglycemic state, hundreds of calories may be lost in the urine each day. The lack of insulin decreases protein synthesis and reduces levels of substances that control the effect of GH.

The risks during pregnancy for a diabetic mother and her child have decreased significantly because of the emphasis on control of maternal glycemia and improvements in perinatal and neonatal care. Nevertheless, the incidence of congenital anomalies in diabetic pregnancy is four times the rate in nondiabetic pregnancy. The congenital malformations in children born to diabetic mothers occur in organ systems that develop during the first 8 weeks of life. Thus, optimal diabetes control is ideally established before conception.

Maternal complications include a greater risk of hypoglycemia during intensive therapy. It is not yet clear whether diabetic pregnancy in the absence of hypertension accelerates the development of maternal renal and retinal disease.

Long-Term Complications

The long term vascular and neurologic complications of IDDM generally take years to develop and usually become evident in adulthood.

Retinopathy. Diabetes mellitus affects various ocular structures, but its major impact is on the retina. Approximately 5000 new cases of blindness related to diabetes mellitus are reported annually, and nearly 85% of these are due to retinopathy. More than 80% of diabetic clients have some form of retinopathy 15 years after diagnosis. About 2% of persons with diabetes are legally blind from retinopathy (L'Esperance & James, 1983).

Several factors are associated with the development of retinopathy. Its onset is slower in clients diagnosed as diabetic before age 30. Hypertension and lengthy duration of diabetes are predisposing factors. Finally, some evidence suggests that poor metabolic control, particularly mean blood glucose levels exceeding 200 mg/dL, is associated with retinopathy.

Retinal ischemia is important in the etiology of retinopathy. Red blood cell aggregation and capillary basement membrane thickening are two of several processes that diminish oxygen delivery to the retina. Ultimately, damaged vessels leak blood and serum into the retina.

Diabetic retinopathy is divided into two stages, background diabetic retinopathy (BDR) and proliferative diabetic retinopathy (PDR). BDR develops in nearly everyone with diabetes and may progress no further. It is characterized by microaneurysms, flame-shaped (Figure 42–6) and small "dot-and-blot" hemorrhages, and hard exudates that form from serum leakage. Unless the macula is involved, vision is not affected.

Preproliferative diabetic retinopathy (PPDR), an advanced form of BDR, heralds the development of PDR. PDR, the most vision-threatening stage, occurs when new blood vessels form (neovascularization) and hemorrhage into the vitreous. Severe visual loss occurs if hemorrhage occurs near the macula. Eventually, blood from hemorrhages stimulates the development of fibrous membranes, which exert tension on the retina and cause retinal detachment.

Client education about the detection, prevention, and treatment of visual impairment is a key responsibility of the nurse. Advise clients to have an annual examination by an ophthalmologist beginning 5 years after the diagnosis of IDDM. Eye symptoms warrant prompt medical attention. Encourage and promote the client's efforts to achieve metabolic control and emphasize the importance of early diagnosis and aggressive treatment of hypertension and dia-

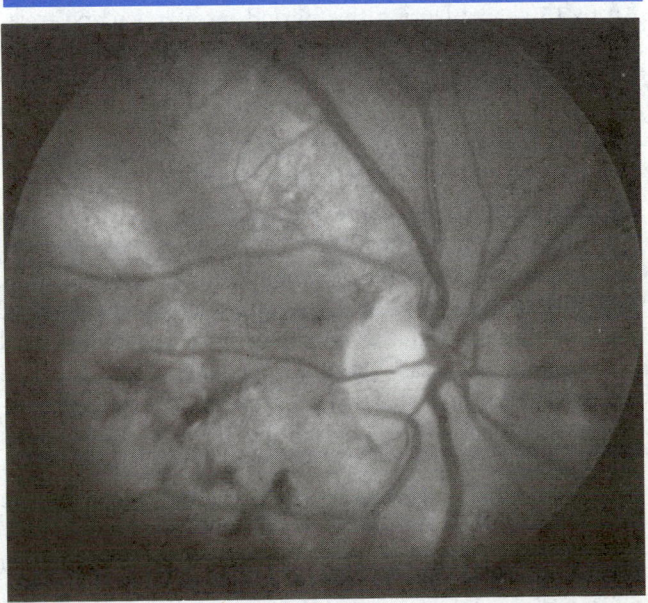

Figure 42–6

Flame-shaped hemorrhages in the retina of a client with diabetes mellitus. (Courtesy of Millard Fillmore Hospital, Buffalo, NY)

betic renal disease. If visual loss occurs, refer the client to rehabilitation services to support adaptation.

Laser photocoagulation, the most effective treatment of PDR, reduces the incidence of severe visual loss by at least 50%. Photocoagulation destroys new blood vessels, leaking blood vessels near the macula, and infarcted areas of the retina. It also produces adhesions that may counterbalance traction from fibrous membranes.

When retinal detachment and massive vitreous hemorrhage develop, vitrectomy restores partial vision in some cases. This procedure removes the blood-filled vitreous and fibrous membranes and replaces them with clear fluid (see Chapter 72).

Nephropathy. Approximately 4000 new cases of diabetic end-stage renal disease occur annually in the United States. Renal failure is the leading cause of death among people with IDDM. Those diagnosed with IDDM before the age of 20 have a 50% chance of developing nephropathy after 20 years.

Diabetic nephropathy includes diffuse and nodular glomerulosclerosis. Diffuse glomerulosclerosis is a generalized thickening of the glomerular basement membrane. Nodular glomerulosclerosis, or Kimmelstiel–Wilson syndrome, is the development of nodules in the mesangium of the kidney and is specific to diabetes mellitus. The diabetic kidney is also prone to atherosclerotic lesions, particularly in the presence of hypertension. Although the cause of diabetic nephropathy is unclear, the evidence suggests that poor metabolic control is an important factor.

The clinical progression of diabetic nephropathy occurs in three stages, each with specific prevention and treatment objectives. The early or asymptomatic stage may last 10 to 15 years. During this period, prevention and treatment of conditions that might impair renal function are important. For example, hypertension and urinary tract infections should be vigorously managed. Repeated use of urethral instrumentation and nephrotoxic agents such as certain drugs and radiologic contrast dyes should be avoided. Metabolic control should be encouraged.

Proteinuria is usually the first sign of renal disease. Its presence signals the beginning of the middle stage, which lasts 2 to 10 years. As renal function deteriorates, diuretic therapy and a low-sodium, protein-modified meal plan become necessary. Insulin requirements may decrease up to 50% as nephropathy progresses to end-stage disease. This final stage generally lasts 1 to 2 years and is characterized by chronic renal failure. Dialysis or transplantation is recommended when the creatinine clearance rate is 10 mL/min and serum creatinine exceeds 6 mg/dL.

Hemodialysis is the most common type of therapy in end-stage renal disease and is preferred for older adults. Approximately 50% survive 3 years, a less favorable outcome than that among nondiabetic clients on dialysis. Continuous ambulatory peritoneal dialysis is an alternative now under evaluation.

Renal transplantation is the preferred treatment for chronic renal failure in selected clients under the age of 60. Compared with hemodialysis, transplantation is associated with more complete rehabilitation, longer survival, better stabilization of retinopathy, and greater improvement of neuropathy (see Unit Five).

Cardiovascular and Peripheral Vascular Disease. Atherosclerosis occurs earlier and more frequently in clients with diabetes mellitus. Coronary artery disease is the most common complication of the total diabetic population. Longitudinal studies, including the Framingham Study, indicate that diabetes is a significant risk factor in the development of heart disease.

Therefore, it is particularly important for diabetic adults to adopt risk reduction strategies recommended for the general population. Meal planning and exercise help the client reduce serum lipid and glucose levels and maintain desirable weight. Hypertension should be treated aggressively to prevent both microvascular and macrovascular disease.

Up to 30% of myocardial infarctions in diabetic individuals are "silent," or painless. This may be due to neuropathy that impedes sensation.

Peripheral vascular disease is the result of both macroangiopathy and microangiopathy. Macroangiopathy, or damage to large and small vessels, is caused by atherosclerotic changes. Microangiopathy involves thickening of the capillary basement membrane. The consequences of microangiopathy are not yet clearly understood but may include increased cell wall permeability. Symptoms and signs of peripheral ischemia include intermittent claudication, cold lower extremities, pain at rest, dependent rubor, diminished or absent pulses, shiny skin with loss of hair, ulcers, infection, and gangrene. Peripheral vascular disease associated with diabetes is often diffuse. Occlusions occur in many segments of vessels, and collateral circulation is involved. The disease usually affects the smaller vessels of both extremities. For these reasons, vascular surgery is difficult.

Glycemic control helps reduce elevated blood lipid levels associated with atherosclerotic changes. Although hyperglycemia alone does not appear to be related to the development of peripheral vascular disease, it should be prevented. Aggressive treatment of hypertension is helpful, and smoking should be discouraged.

Neuropathy. The effects of diabetic neuropathy have been described for over a century and are among the most common, yet puzzling, complications of diabetes mellitus. The causes are unknown but may include a biochemical imbalance of Schwann's cell metabolism and ischemia. Although the central nervous system is not affected, both the peripheral and autonomic nervous systems may be extensively involved. Peripheral sensory polyneuropathy occurs more often in the lower than in the upper extremities and is usually bilateral and symmetrical. One form is characterized by severe pain that is worse at night. Painful neuropathy often subsides spontaneously after several months.

Treatment is limited and directed at the relief of symptoms. Control of hyperglycemia may reverse symptoms and should be attempted. Analgesic, anticonvulsant, and antidepressant drugs have occasionally proven effective.

The less painful, more insidious form of neuropathy is characterized by proprioceptive disturbances and diminished sensation to touch, pain, and temperature. These sensory deficits increase the possibility that injury will occur and go unnoticed. Peripheral motor involvement results in muscle atrophy and weakness in the upper and lower extremities. The loss of muscle function leads to deformities, particularly in the feet.

Mononeuropathies, which involve single nerves, are symmetrical, painful, and abrupt in onset. Paralysis of cranial nerves III and VI (oculomotor and abducens nerves) is the most common form. Recovery occurs spontaneously after several months.

Autonomic neuropathies often exist concurrently with peripheral neuropathies. These conditions may include orthostatic hypotension, neurogenic bladder, delayed gastric emptying, and frequent diarrhea. Impotence, one of the most common manifestations of autonomic dysfunction, affects 50% of diabetic men. Diabetic impotence has both neurologic and vascular causes. Treatment consists of the implantation of a penile prosthesis.

DIABETES MELLITUS TYPE II (NIDDM)

Type II diabetes mellitus (NIDDM) is the second major form of the disease. It accounts for approximately 90% of cases and has been diagnosed in more than 5 million adults in the United States.

Type II differs from Type I diabetes mellitus in several ways. It is usually diagnosed after age 40 and is frequently associated with obesity. It results from faulty pancreatic insulin secretion combined with cellular resistance to the insulin produced. Increased hepatic glucose production is also a factor. Because insulin production is sufficient to sustain life, DKA rarely develops.

As with IDDM, the etiology of NIDDM is unknown. Viral and autoimmune causes are unlikely. There is strong evidence that NIDDM is hereditary, but the HLA system is not involved. A landmark study demonstrated a 93% concordance for NIDDM among identical twins compared with a 50% concordance for IDDM (Tattersall & Pyke, 1972).

Obesity is clearly a risk factor for NIDDM. Insulin resistance is associated with obesity. Many obese persons with NIDDM have abnormally high blood insulin levels. They have a delayed and prolonged release of insulin in response to carbohydrate intake. Insulin secreted in this manner is less efficient in controlling blood glucose levels. The action of insulin depends on the binding of circulating insulin to specific receptors on the cell membrane, followed by intracellular events. Chronically high levels of circulating insulin decrease the number of receptors, resulting in hyperglycemia and, possibly, impairment of intracellular insulin action.

Clinical Manifestations

Unlike the onset of IDDM, the onset of NIDDM is insidious and may go undetected for years. Of the estimated 5 million persons with undiagnosed diabetes in the United States, virtually all have NIDDM. Fatigue, polyuria, polydipsia, delayed healing, chronic infections, and fluctuating vision frequently herald its onset. Occasionally, in long-standing undetected NIDDM, vascular complications are already present at diagnosis.

Therapeutic Measures

The goal of therapy in NIDDM is identical to that in the treatment of IDDM: the restoration of normal blood glucose levels and nutrient metabolism. NIDDM was once regarded as a relatively benign form of the disease. However, as awareness of the morbidity and mortality associated with NIDDM has increased, so have the efforts to improve its detection and management. The three methods of therapy are nutritional management, exercise, and oral hypoglycemic agents or insulin.

Nutritional Management
Sixty to 90% of persons with NIDDM are obese at diagnosis or have a history of obesity. Many produce enough insulin to maintain normal blood glucose levels if they reduce caloric intake, weight, or both. Therefore, the first goal of nutritional management is calorie restriction and increased activity to achieve and maintain a desirable body weight. The calorie-restricted meal plan should be nutritionally adequate.

The second goal is to control hyperglycemia. For some, dietary modification is sufficient to restore normal blood glucose levels. Calorie restriction and weight loss reduce hepatic glucose production, increase the number of insulin receptors, and improve intracellular insulin action.

The third goal of nutritional management is to prevent or treat hypertension, hyperlipidemia, and cardiovascular and renal disease. Often NIDDM coexists with other chronic disease or is diagnosed after the development of a chronic complication. Therefore, nutritional management focuses on treating both diabetes and the related health problem.

Oral Hypoglycemic Agents and Insulin
If properly followed nutritional management fails to correct hyperglycemia, oral hypoglycemic agents or insulin are necessary. The oral hypoglycemic agents, or sulfonylureas, have similar mechanisms of action (Table 42–8). They decrease hepatic glucose production, increase insulin secretion, increase the number of insulin receptors, and enhance intracellular insulin activity. In 1970, results of a long-term study, the University Group Diabetes Program,

Table 42–8	Sulfonylureas (Oral Hypoglycemic Agents)		
Generic Name	**Trade Name**	**Dosage Range (mg/day)**	**Duration of Action (hour)**
Acetohexamide	Dymelor	250–1500	12–18
Chlorpropamide	Diabinese	100–750	60
Glipizide	Glucotrol	5–40	24
Glyburide	DiaBeta, Micronase	2.5–30.0	24
Tolazamide	Tolinase	100–1000	12–24
Tolbutamide	Orinase	500–3000	6–12

SOURCE: Adapted with permission from Rifkin H (editor): *The Physician's Guide to Type II Diabetes (NIDDM): Diagnosis and Treatment.* New York: American Diabetes Association, 1984, p. 41.

suggested that oral agents increased cardiovascular mortality. Those conclusions were challenged, and in 1979 the American Diabetes Association issued a policy statement indicating that restrictions on the use of oral agents are not valid (Whitehouse et al., 1979).

Oral agents are appropriate only for those who secrete insulin. Therefore, they should not be used for IDDM. They are most effective in those recently diagnosed as having NIDDM (1) who are at or above desirable body weight and have never received insulin or (2) whose condition has been controlled with fewer than 40 units of insulin daily.

If hyperglycemia persists despite nutritional and oral agent therapy, insulin is used to supplement the body's supply. In contrast to IDDM, control in NIDDM may be achieved with relatively small doses of intermediate-acting insulin given once daily. The lowest dose of insulin necessary to achieve control should be used; overaggressive insulin therapy may increase hunger and promote weight gain, further increasing insulin resistance.

The use of oral agents in combination with insulin has been attempted, but its value is unproven. Therefore, such therapy should be limited to research.

Specific Nursing Measures

Nutritional Approaches
The steps in creating a meal plan for clients with NIDDM are the same as for those with IDDM. When NIDDM is treated with oral hypoglycemic agents or insulin, the timing of meals is important to prevent hypoglycemia. For those treated with a meal plan alone, the total caloric intake and distribution of nutrients throughout the day are more important than the timing of meals. Snacks are not necessary to prevent hypoglycemia but may help curb the appetite and prevent overeating at meals.

Clients will not follow for long meal plans that are unrealistically low in calories. Plans in the range of 1200 to 1500 calories for women and 1500 to 1800 calories for men promote better adherence and allow gradual weight

loss. Because 1 lb of body fat contains approximately 3500 calories, weight loss is a slow process. A loss of 1 to 2 lb a week is a reasonable goal.

A major problem for those with NIDDM is maintaining weight loss once it has been achieved. A professionally supervised weight control program that emphasizes individual preferences, long-term behavioral changes, and regular exercise is necessary if clients are to achieve and maintain weight goals.

Exercise
Exercise is an important aspect of treatment for clients with NIDDM. Physical activity increases energy expenditure and leads to weight reduction. It also can reduce insulin resistance even before weight loss occurs. Exercise promotes cardiovascular health by decreasing serum triglyceride, LDL, and insulin levels. It also results in increased HDL levels, which may prevent cardiovascular disease. These are important benefits, because those with diabetes mellitus are twice as prone to cardiovascular disease as the general population.

Self Blood Glucose Monitoring
In assessing the effect of NIDDM therapy, self BGM is especially helpful. The renal threshold for glucose increases with age, so it is not uncommon for older adults with NIDDM to obtain negative urine test results when significant hyperglycemia exists. Semiquantitative urine testing has limited value in NIDDM management.

Testing frequency varies widely. Clients treated with meal plans alone or in combination with oral agents may perform self BGM once a week. Those taking insulin generally test once daily or several times on 1 day each week. Although clients with NIDDM are less likely to develop DKA, urine ketone testing is recommended during illness.

Although blood glucose levels tend to fluctuate less in NIDDM than in IDDM, a random serum glucose level may inaccurately reflect overall control. As in IDDM, the glycosylated hemoglobin assay measures chronic blood glucose status better.

Medical and Nursing Approaches to Complications of NIDDM

NIDDM may result in acute and long-term complications. The major complications and their management are discussed in this section.

Acute Complications

Acute complications of NIDDM are hypoglycemia and hyperglycemic hyperosmolar nonketotic coma (HHNK). Hypoglycemia is a complication of sulfonylurea therapy. HHNK can be life threatening.

Hypoglycemia. Hypoglycemia is particularly likely with long-acting agents such as chlorpropamide. The symptoms and signs are the same as those in insulin-induced hypoglycemia. Regular meals and snacks protect against hypoglycemia. For clients whose meal patterns are erratic and who have impaired renal or hepatic function, a short-acting agent is preferred. Clients receiving sulfonylureas, especially chlorpropamide, should understand that alcohol consumption may produce a disulfiram (Antabuse)-like reaction. Disulfiram and alcohol in combination cause nausea, copious vomiting, throbbing headache, sweating, dyspnea, weakness, and confusion. This is a side effect rather than a complication of drug therapy.

Hyperglycemic Hyperosmolar Nonketotic Coma. HHNK coma is most frequently noted in the elderly. It develops in days to weeks. The pathophysiology of HHNK coma is similar to that of DKA except that ketosis is rarely present. The distinguishing clinical features are severe hyperglycemia in excess of 600 mg/dL; absent or minimal ketosis; profound dehydration with hyperosmolality greater than 340 mOsm/kg; and neurologic abnormalities, including seizures. Confusion and excessive thirst are often present. Precipitating factors may include prolonged therapy with hyperglycemia-inducing drugs, acute infection, and excessive fluid loss. Typically, HHNK coma occurs in the infirm who may not recognize or respond to thirst. Health professionals who work with this population should observe fluid intake and output patterns in clients with NIDDM.

Treatment of HHNK coma is similar to that for DKA. The rapid IV infusion of hypotonic saline corrects volume depletion. Low-dose insulin, potassium replacement, and correction of the precipitating factor are other facets of therapy.

Long-Term Complications

Clients with NIDDM are subject to the same long-term vascular and neurologic complications associated with IDDM. The types of diabetes mellitus differ, however, in the likelihood of developing these complications.

Macrovascular complications have a major impact on the health of clients with NIDDM. Coronary artery disease is the major cause of morbidity and mortality in adults, and those over the age of 40 are also at greater risk for diabetic foot problems.

Nephropathy is less likely to develop in NIDDM than in IDDM. Retinopathy, however, may be present at diagnosis. Adults with NIDDM are also more prone to developing cataracts, so annual ophthalmologic examinations for cataracts and retinopathy should begin at diagnosis.

Section II: Reactive Hypoglycemia

Reactive hypoglycemia, a fall in blood glucose concentrations to symptomatic levels several hours after a meal, presumably is a response to factors stimulated by food intake. Most clinicians agree that a history of postprandial symptoms that disappear after food intake, reproduction of these symptoms during testing, and a serum glucose level in the hypoglycemic range during the symptoms are necessary to establish diagnosis.

Clinical Manifestations

Reactive hypoglycemia may occur as part of the "dumping syndrome," but the form that has attracted widespread attention is spontaneous reactive hypoglycemia. Health professionals frequently encounter clients who attribute symptoms such as palpitations, anxiety, depression, weakness, chronic fatigue, and irritability to "hypoglycemia,'" either self-diagnosed or professionally diagnosed. An extensive body of lay health literature focuses on dietary, medicinal, and psychological remedies for hypoglycemia.

The etiology of reactive hypoglycemia is unclear, and there is ample evidence to suggest it is overdiagnosed.

The oral glucose tolerance test (GTT) is the most commonly used diagnostic tool, but substantial doubt exists as to its value in detecting reactive hypoglycemia. Hogan et al. (1983) studied 33 persons with a diagnosis of spontaneous reactive hypoglycemia and noted no relation between hypoglycemia during an oral GTT and symptoms.

Moreover, many normal individuals experience asymptomatic serum glucose levels in the hypoglycemic range during an oral GTT. In a 1982 policy statement on this issue, the American Diabetes Association asserted that there is no evidence to suggest that hypoglycemia causes depression, chronic fatigue, allergies, or behavioral problems (Rizza & Gerich, 1982).

Therapeutic Measures

Nutritional management is the main form of treatment for hypoglycemia, regardless of its cause. The traditional recommendations have included frequent feedings in the form of a low-carbohydrate, high-protein, high-fat diet that avoids simple sugars. Research has demonstrated, however, that a diet high in complex carbohydrates and fiber improves glucose tolerance (Leichter, 1979). Studies of adults with reactive hypoglycemia have shown that carbohydrate restriction impairs glucose tolerance (Anderson & Herman, 1975). High-fat diets also appear to interfere with normal glucose tolerance.

The current nutritional recommendation for clients with reactive hypoglycemia is a diabetic type of diet with 45% to 50% of the calories derived from carbohydrates. Clients should avoid rapidly absorbed sugars such as sucrose. Water-soluble fibers found in fruits and legumes are helpful because they delay gastric emptying by retarding glucose absorption in the gastrointestinal tract. Frequent feedings and moderate alcohol and caffeine consumption also are recommended. Because high-fat diets may interfere with the body's ability to use insulin, reducing dietary fat to improve glucose tolerance and maintain ideal weight is beneficial.

Specific Nursing Measures

Nurses play a significant role in educating the public about reactive hypoglycemia. There is a critical need to disseminate reliable health information substantiated by valid data because there is considerable misinformation about reactive hypoglycemia.

For the client who reports symptoms suggestive of hypoglycemia, recommend a thorough medical evaluation. Whether the diagnosis is confirmed or not, symptoms may persist. The nutritional recommendations outlined earlier represent a healthy approach to relieving symptoms in any case.

Chapter Highlights

Diabetes mellitus is a chronic disease characterized by abnormal carbohydrate, fat, and protein metabolism as well as vascular deterioration. It is the most common disorder of glucose regulation.

Approximately 90% of cases of diabetes mellitus in the United States are Type II, or noninsulin-dependent diabetes mellitus (NIDDM), and less than 10% are Type I, or insulin-dependent diabetes mellitus (IDDM).

The key difference between IDDM and NIDDM is that in IDDM the pancreas is unable to produce sufficient insulin to sustain life.

The goals of therapy for both IDDM and NIDDM are the normalization of blood glucose levels and the restoration of normal carbohydrate, fat, and protein metabolism in an effort to prevent long-term vascular complications.

The major approaches to therapy for clients with diabetes mellitus are insulin or oral hypoglycemic agents, nutritional management, and exercise. Nutritional management is the foundation of therapy for both IDDM and NIDDM.

Conventional insulin therapy consists of one or two daily insulin injections. Intensive therapy includes three or more daily injections or continuous insulin infusion (CSII) by a pump.

The overall goal of nutritional management in both types of diabetes is to normalize blood glucose and blood lipid levels while maintaining good nutrition and health.

The ideal meal plan is high in carbohydrate, with an emphasis on fiber; is low in total fat, especially saturated fat; and contains adequate amounts of protein.

Regular aerobic exercise reduces insulin resistance, increases HDL, reduces LDL, and lowers blood pressure.

Self blood glucose monitoring (BGM) is preferable to urine glucose testing because it is direct, immediate, and accurate.

The glycosylated hemoglobin assay reflects the preceding 2 months of blood glucose control and is valuable in judging the long-term effectiveness of diabetes therapy.

Diabetes education is divided into immediate, in-depth, and continuing stages, each with different goals.

The acute complications of diabetes mellitus include hypoglycemia, diabetic ketoacidosis (DKA), and hyperglycemic hyperosmolar nonketotic (HHNK) coma. The intermediate complications are delayed growth and development in children and fetal morbidity and mortality in diabetic pregnancy. The major chronic complications are retinopathy, nephropathy, coronary artery disease, neuropathy, and peripheral vascular disease.

The most important factor in preventing fetal morbidity and mortality in diabetic pregnancy is maternal blood glucose control.

The stages of retinopathy are background diabetic retinopathy (BDR) and proliferative diabetic retinopathy (PDR). Preproliferative diabetic retinopathy (PPDR) is an advanced form of BDR and heralds the development of PDR.

Hypertension accelerates the progression of diabetic retinopathy and nephropathy.

The two primary pathological conditions leading to diabetic foot problems are peripheral neuropathy and peripheral vascular disease.

Oral hypoglycemic agents increase insulin secretion, reduce hepatic glucose production, increase the number of cellular insulin receptors, and enhance intracellular insulin activity.

Reactive hypoglycemia is a postprandial fall in blood glucose concentrations that results in adrenergic and neurologic symptoms.

Dietary management is the mainstay of therapy for clients with reactive hypoglycemia.

Bibliography

Anderson JE, Herman RH: Effects of carbohydrate restriction on glucose tolerance of normal men and reactive hypoglycemic patients. *Am J Clin Nutrition* 1975; 28(7):748–755.

Barrett E, DeFronzo R: Diabetic ketoacidosis: Diagnosis and treatment. *Hosp Pract* (April) 1984; 19(4):89–104.

Brunzell JD et al: Effect of a fat-free, high carbohydrate diet on diabetic subjects with fasting hyperglycemia. *Diabetes* 1974; 23(2):138–142.

Cahill G, Etzwiler DD, Freinkel N: Blood glucose control in diabetes. *Diabetes* 1976; 25(3):237–239.

Cahill G, Etzwiler DD, Freinkel N: "Control" and diabetes. *New Engl J Med* 1976; 294(18):1004–1005.

Chambers JK: Save your diabetic patient from early kidney damage. *Nurs 83* (May) 1983; 13:58–63.

Dolan–Heitlinger J, Antle M: *Recombinant DNA and Human Insulin: A Source Book.* Indianapolis: Eli Lilly, July 1983.

Etzwiler DD: Education of the diabetic. In: *Clinical Diabetes: Modern Management.* Podolsky S (editor). New York: Appleton–Century–Crofts, 1980.

Forbes K, Stokes SA: Saving the diabetic foot. *Am J Nurs* (July) 1984; 84(7):884–888.

Fredholm N, Vignati L, Brown S: Insulin pumps: The patients' verdict. *Am J Nurs* (Jan) 1984; 84(1):36–38.

Freinkel N: On the etiology of diabetes mellitus. In: *Diabetes Mellitus.* Rifkin H, Raskin P (editors). Bowie, MD: Robert Brady, 1981.

Garcia CA, Ruiz RS: Diabetes and the eye. *Ciba Clin Symp* 1984; 36(4):2–32.

Graham S, Morley M: What 'foot care' really means. *Am J Nurs* (July) 1984; 84(7):889–891.

Hogan M et al: Oral glucose tolerance test compared with a mixed meal in the diagnosis of reactive hypoglycemia. *Mayo Clin Proceedings* 1983; 58(8):491–496.

Keen H, Jarrett RJ: The WHO multinational study of vascular disease in diabetes: Macrovascular disease prevalence. *Diabetes Care* 1979; 2(2):187–195.

Leichter SB: Alimentary hypoglycemia: A new appraisal. *Am J Clin Nutrition* 1979; 32(10):2104–2114.

L'Esperance F, James W: The eye and diabetes mellitus. In: *Diabetes Mellitus: Theory and Practice,* 3rd ed. Ellenberg M, Rifkin H (editors). New Hyde Park, NY: Medical Examination Publishing, 1983.

Levin ME, O'Neal LW (editors): *The Diabetic Foot,* 3rd ed. St. Louis: Mosby, 1983.

McCarthy J: The continuum of diabetic coma. *Am J Nurs* 1985; 85(8):878–882.

National Diabetes Advisory Board: National standards for diabetes patient education programs. *Diabetes Care* 1984; 7(1):31–35.

National Diabetes Advisory Board: *Prevention and Treatment of Five Complications of Diabetes: A Guide for Primary Care Practitioners.* US Department of Health and Human Services, 1983.

National Diabetes Advisory Board: *The Treatment and Control of Diabetes: A National Plan to Reduce Mortality and Morbidity.* US Government Printing Office, Nov 1980.

National Diabetes Data Group, National Institutes of Health: *The Scope and Impact of Diabetes,* Dec 1981.

Rizza R, Gerich J: Statement on hypoglycemia. *Diabetes Care* 1982; 5(1):72–73.

Tattersall RB: Home blood glucose monitoring. *Diabetologia* 1979; 16:71–74.

Tattersall RB, Pyke DA: Diabetes in identical twins. *Lancet* 1972; 2:1120–1125.

West KM: *Epidemiology of Diabetes and Its Vascular Lesions.* New York: Elsevier, 1978.

Whitehouse F et al: Policy statement: The UGDP controversy. *Diabetes* 1979; 28(2):168.

Zinman B, Vranic M: Diabetes and exercise. *Med Clin North Am* 1985; 68(1):145–157.

Suggested Readings

Etzwiler D, Franz MJ, Hollander P, Joynes J: *Learning to Live Well With Diabetes.* Minneapolis: International Diabetes Center, 1985. This comprehensive diabetes manual was written by the staff and consultants of the International Diabetes Center. It is written for clients with diabetes, but health professionals will also find it a valuable reference covering every aspect of diabetes management and education.

Franz MJ: *Exchanges for All Occasions: Meeting the Challenge of Diabetes.* Minneapolis: International Diabetes Center, 1984. Written for both clients and health professionals, this comprehensive book provides guidelines for ethnic foods, traveling, entertaining, illness, exercise, and other situations that affect the basic meal plan. Readers will learn new ways to add variety, flexibility, and interest to meal plans.

National Diabetes Advisory Board. *The Prevention and Treatment of Five Complications of Diabetes: A Guide for Primary Care Practitioners.* US Department of Health and Human Services Publication No. 83–8392, 1983. A basic guide for primary care providers that outlines the detection, prevention, and treatment of DKA; adverse outcomes in pregnancy; retinopathy; foot problems; and renal complications.

Rifkin H (editor): *The Physician's Guide to Type II Diabetes (NIDDM): Diagnosis and Treatment.* New York: American Diabetes Association, 1984. This comprehensive and practical reference on the diagnosis and treatment of Type II diabetes mellitus and its complications is suitable for all health professionals.

The Client With Noninsulin-Dependent Diabetes Mellitus

I. Descriptive Data

Mrs Margaret Smith, a mildly obese 59-year-old female, is seen for an outpatient visit to begin insulin therapy. She is accompanied by her daughter. She appears calm but states: "I'm not looking forward to giving shots. My aunt has taken insulin for many years but doesn't really watch her diabetes. I'm afraid to take insulin shots, but I know I need to feel better."

II. Personal Data

Date and Time:	10:30 AM, July 2, 1986
Name:	Margaret Ann Smith
Social Security Number:	000-00-0000
Address:	122 Elm St., Minneapolis, MN 55416
Telephone:	Office: 000-0000
	Home: 000-0000
Sex:	Female
Marital Status:	Widowed
Age:	59
Birthdate:	6-17-27
Religion:	Protestant
Race:	Caucasian
Occupation:	Executive secretary
Usual Health Care Provider:	Mary Koren, MD

III. Health History

Source of Information:	Client
Reliability of Informant:	Excellent
Chief Concern:	"I'm here to learn how to take insulin."

History of Present Illness:

Mrs Smith has been mildly obese since the birth of her second child over 30 years ago. She was diagnosed with NIDDM 4 years ago and achieved normal preprandial blood glucose levels on a 1500-calorie meal plan following a 12-lb weight loss. Four months ago, she noted a gradual rise in her preprandial blood glucose levels to 180–200 mg/dL despite adherence to her meal plan. Her glycosylated hemoglobin was 6% (N = 3.8 – 5.3%).

She started chlorpropamide 250 mg daily with reduction of her preprandial blood glucose level to 140 mg/dL. Five weeks after beginning oral therapy, she developed cholestatic jaundice. Oral therapy was discontinued, and her preprandial blood glucose levels are now 300–350 mg/dL. She is not ketotic but is experiencing fatigue, polyuria, and polydipsia. She is referred to begin insulin therapy as an outpatient.

Past Health History:

Childhood:	Usual childhood illnesses
Immunizations:	Influenza and pneumonia, 1985
Medical Problems:	Hypertension × 8 years, currently controlled on propranolol 40 mg t.i.d.; osteoarthritis × 4 years; NIDDM × 4 years
Surgeries:	None
Pregnancies:	P2G2, 1951, 1955
Trauma:	None
Transfusions:	None
Allergies:	Sulfa—hives
Current Medications:	Naproxen 250 mg b.i.d., propranolol 40 mg t.i.d.

Case Study written by LeAnn McNeil and Marion J. Franz.

Family History:

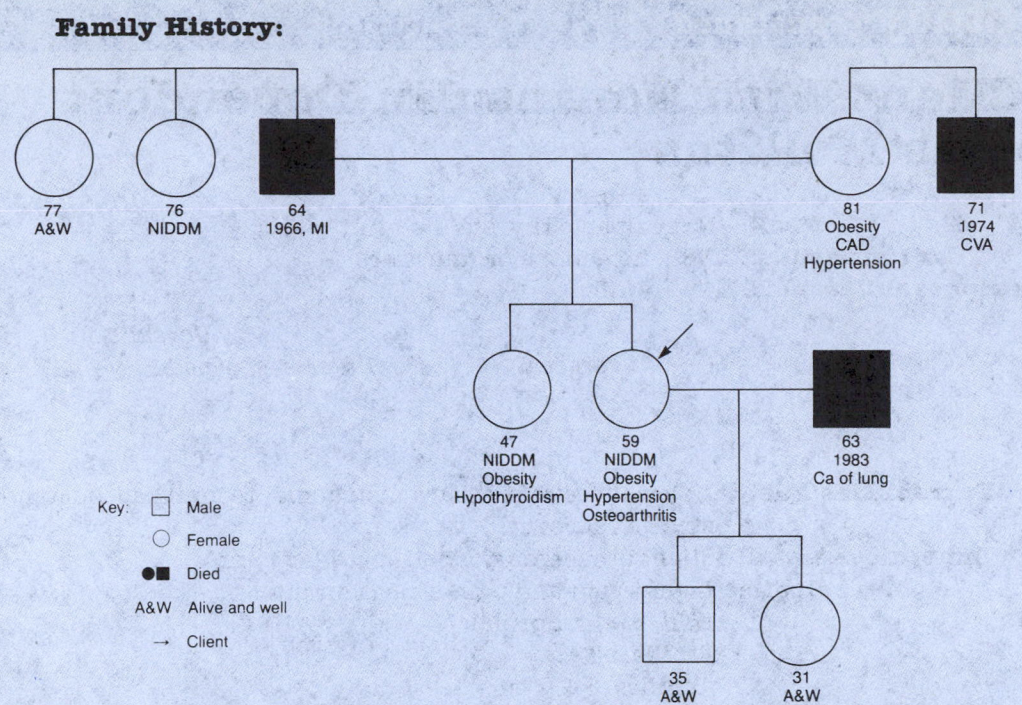

Key:
☐ Male
○ Female
●■ Died
A&W Alive and well
→ Client

(Family tree shows:)
- 77 A&W (female)
- 76 NIDDM (female)
- 64 1966, MI (male, died)
- 81 Obesity CAD Hypertension (female)
- 71 1974 CVA (male, died)
- 47 NIDDM Obesity Hypothyroidism (female)
- 59 NIDDM Obesity Hypertension Osteoarthritis (female, Client)
- 63 1983 Ca of lung (male, died)
- 35 A&W (male)
- 31 A&W (female)

Personal/Social History: Mrs Smith has been employed full time as an executive secretary to the president of a small engineering firm for 13 years. Her husband died 3 years ago within 6 months of a diagnosis of lung cancer. She feels she has finally adjusted to his death. She has retained relationships with several couples with whom she and her husband socialized. Her children and grandchildren live in the Minneapolis area, and she sees them about twice a month. Her hobbies include bridge, gourmet cooking, and gardening. She walks 3 miles a week, does not smoke, and drinks 1–2 glasses of wine a month.

Review of Systems:
General: Increasing fatigue for 3 weeks. Weight stable. No sleep or appetite disturbances.

HEENT: Wears glasses for myopia; last ophthalmology exam 10 months ago was normal; has noted fluctuating distance vision since discontinuing oral therapy; no eye pain or diplopia

Mouth: Constant thirst

Cardiovascular: No chest pain, dyspnea or edema; last blood pressure check 2 months ago normal

Genitourinary: Polyuria every 1–2 hours for 3 weeks; nocturia three times/ night; no dysuria, hematuria, fever, or incontinence

Musculoskeletal: Intermittent minor early morning pain and stiffness both knees; no swelling

Endocrine: Polydipsia for 3 weeks

Neurologic: No pain or paresthesia

Emotional: Anxious about lifestyle adjustment to insulin therapy

IV. Physical Assessment
Height: 5 ft 4 in
Weight: 149 lb
Vital Signs: Temperature 98°F (36.7°C); pulse 82; respirations 18; BP 134/86 rt arm, sitting

Relevant Organ Systems:
Eyes: Snellen with glasses—20/30 OD, 20/40 OS; conjunctivae clear; PERRLA; no retinopathy; visual fields intact

Mouth: Dry mucosa, no ulcerations

(continued)

The Client With Noninsulin-Dependent Diabetes Mellitus

Neck: Nonpalpable thyroid; no bruits
Cardiovascular: NSR, no gallops or murmurs
Peripheral Vascular: 4+ = full

		Femoral	Popliteal	Dorsalis pedis	Posterior tibial
	R	4+	3+	3+	3+
	L	4+	3+	3+	3+

Extremities/Feet: No evidence of pressure or trauma; toenails adequately trimmed straight across
Musculoskeletal: Slight broadening of both patellar joints
Neurologic: Light touch and pain sensation intact
DTR: 3+ = normal
Patellar: 3+
Achilles: 3+

V. Summary Mrs Smith and her daughter met with the nurse and nutritionist to begin instruction for insulin therapy

VI. Nursing Care Plan

Nursing Diagnosis	Client Care Goals	Plan/Nursing Implementation	Expected Outcomes
Nutrition, alteration in: less than body requirements Urinary elimination, alteration in pattern of Knowledge deficit related to: diabetes mellitus, insulin administration, insulin reactions, and self BGM	Client will be able to: select basic meal plan; prepare and administer insulin; self-monitor blood glucose levels regularly; prevent or recognize and treat hypoglycemia; establish ongoing care with health professionals	*Day 1:* 3 h. Nutrition assessment and counseling; revise meal plan for insulin therapy to include three meals with morning, afternoon, and bedtime snacks, 1300–1400 calories with 50% CHO, 20% protein, and 30% fat; review of diabetes as a chronic disease; review self-monitoring of blood glucose and recommend t.i.d.—q.i.d. preprandial testing until satisfactory insulin therapy achieved; discuss prevention, recognition, and treatment of hypoglycemia *Day 2:* 2 h. Client administration of 2 units of regular with 6 units of NPH human insulin; orientation to insulin and syringes; nutrition counseling; establish system for telephone follow-up with nurse and dietitian; review Day 1 content as needed *Day 3:* 1.5 h. Client administration of insulin; instruct in management of minor illness and foot care; nutrition counseling; establish telephone follow-up with nurse and dietitian for insulin, meal plan, and exercise adjustment over next 4 wk; set appointment with nurse, physician, and dietitian in 4 wk; set appointment for in-depth education in 3 to 6 mo to obtain advanced content; review Day 1 and 2 content as needed	Achievement of glycemic control with resolution of symptoms within 4 wk of beginning insulin therapy; mastery of self BGM and insulin administration techniques by Day 3 of program; mastery of basic meal plan concepts within 4 wk of Day 3; mastery of concepts of prevention, treatment, and recognition of hypoglycemia on Day 3; progress toward emotional adaptation within 4 wk of beginning insulin therapy; plan for ongoing health care established on Day 3; plan for obtaining in-depth diabetes education established on Day 3; client and family adapt to chronic illness and adopt healthy behaviors

Chapter 43

Specific Disorders of the Thyroid and Parathyroid Glands

Anne Herrstrom Skelly

Objectives

When you have finished studying this chapter, you should be able to:

Identify disorders commonly associated with the thyroid gland.

Describe the subjective and objective assessment parameters used to obtain information from a client suspected of having thyroid dysfunction.

Explain the laboratory studies that might indicate hyperfunction or hypofunction of the thyroid gland.

Discuss hyperthyroidism—the major subjective and objective findings, treatment approaches, and nursing care.

List the symptoms and signs of thyroid storm and rank the nursing interventions involved.

Discuss hypothyroidism—the major subjective and objective findings, treatment approaches, and nursing care.

List the symptoms and signs of myxedema coma and specify the nursing interventions involved.

Compare the common causes of enlargement of the thyroid (goiter, thyroiditis, and neoplasm) in terms of subjective and objective findings, treatment approaches, and nursing care.

Discuss hyperparathyroidism—the major subjective and objective findings, treatment approaches, and nursing care.

Describe causes of hypercalcemia other than hyperparathyroidism.

Discuss hypoparathyroidism—the major subjective and objective findings, treatment approaches, and nursing care.

Develop a plan of care for the client with tetany.

Anticipate the psychosocial/lifestyle implications of thyroid and parathyroid dysfunction for the client and family and outline specific nursing interventions to address their needs.

Disorders of the thyroid gland may be characterized by either an abnormality in the secretion of thyroid hormone or a change in the size or contour of the gland. An excess of thyroid hormone produces hyperthyroidism; a deficiency produces hypothyroidism. (*Euthyroidism* refers to normal thyroid function.) Disorders associated with changes in size or contour may or may not be accompanied by altered secretion of thyroid hormone; pressure from an enlarged gland may, by itself, produce symptoms. Such disorders include simple goiter (nodular goiter or nontoxic goiter), thyroiditis, and neoplasm.

Similarly, disorders of the parathyroid glands are characterized by abnormalities in the secretion of parathyroid hormone (PTH). Excess PTH produces hyperparathyroidism, whereas a PTH deficiency produces hypoparathyroidism. Changes in the body's PTH levels alter the regulation of calcium and phosphorus.

Specific disorders of the thyroid and parathyroid glands are classified as multifactorial, infectious or inflammatory, or neoplastic in origin. The multifactorial group includes hyperthyroidism, hypothyroidism, simple goiter, hyperparathyroidism, and hypoparathyroidism. Thyroiditis is discussed under infectious and inflammatory disorders. The neoplasms include benign adenomas and carcinomas.

Section I: Disorders of Multifactorial Origin

HYPERTHYROIDISM

Hyperthyroidism is characterized by an increase in secretion and plasma levels of the hormones thyroxine (T_4), triiodothyronine (T_3), or both. Symptomatic hyperthyroidism may also be referred to as *thyrotoxicosis*.

Hyperthyroidism associated with diffuse enlargement of the thyroid (goiter) and exophthalmos (protrusion of the eyeballs) is traditionally known as *Graves' disease*. Some clients with exophthalmos may exhibit no clinical or laboratory signs of hyperthyroidism, however. A synonym for Graves' disease is *diffuse toxic goiter*.

Thyroid storm, which may threaten the client's life, results from a sudden release of thyroid hormone into the bloodstream. Although now rare, thyroid storm may be precipitated in clients with hyperthyroidism by trauma, infection, surgery, or withdrawal from antithyroid drugs (Kaye & Rose, 1983).

The etiology of the various categories of hyperthyroidism is shown in Table 43–1. Primary hyperthyroidism (originating within the thyroid itself) and tertiary hyperthyroidism (from exogenous intake) account for 98% to 99% of all cases (Kaye & Rose, 1983). Secondary hyperthyroidism, resulting from excessive secretion of thyroid-stimulating hormone (TSH), is rare and usually results from a tumor of the adenohypophysis.

Graves' disease, the term often applied to all forms of hyperthyroidism, is classically defined as hyperthyroidism associated with thyromegaly (goiter) and exophthalmos (Figure 43–1). Graves' disease accounts for 40% to 60% of all cases of hyperthyroidism. Its pathophysiology remains unknown, but several lines of research are being followed.

The plasma of 40% to 60% of clients with hyperthyroidism has been found to contain an IgG immunoglobulin that increases the thyroid activity of laboratory animals. The effects of this substance, called long-acting thyroid stimulator (LATS), were found to be similar to those of TSH but with a longer onset of action. The exact function of LATS in Graves' disease remains unclear, because its presence or absence has not been found to correlate with the clinical course of the disease.

Another current theory holds that Graves' disease is caused by thyroid-stimulating immunoglobulins (TSIs), which are produced by lymphocytic tissue in response to thyroid antigens. These immunoglobulins are thought to bind to the TSH receptors in the thyroid cell and to increase the activity of the thyroid. Random mutation of the lymphocytes and genetic disturbances in immunity have been given as reasons for clients' producing these immunoglobulins and developing hyperactivity of the thyroid. A third theory proposes that Graves' disease is essentially an autoimmune disorder produced by an autoantigen and that LATS and TSI are secondary by-products of this process (Saxton et al., 1983).

About 50% of all clients with hyperthyroidism have a positive history of preceding physical or emotional trauma (Kaye & Rose, 1983). The highest incidence of hyperthyroidism is seen in women between the ages of 20 and 40. In Graves' disease, women are affected seven times more frequently than men.

Table 43–1 Etiology of Hyperthyroidism	
Categories of Hyperthyroidism	**Etiology**
Graves' disease	Long-acting thyroid stimulator (LATS) in the plasma causing hyperthyroidism, diffuse thyromegaly, exophthalmos
Nodular hyperthyroidism	Increased production of thyroid hormone by an autonomous thyroid nodule
Chronic thyroiditis	Chronic inflammation of the thyroid causing hyperthyroidism
Factitious and iatrogenic hyperthyroidism	Hyperthyroidism induced by the ingestion of exogenous thyroid hormone
Chorionic thyroid-stimulating hormone (TSH)	Hyperthyroidism and thyromegaly seen in women with choriocarcinoma of the placenta and in men with choriocarcinoma of the testes
Struma ovarii	Hyperthyroidism associated with ovarian carcinoma; the tumor is composed of thyroid tissue and secretes thyroid hormone

Clinical Manifestations

The clinical manifestations of hyperthyroidism are directly related to the amount of excessive circulating hormone and the length of time it has been circulating, the age of the client, and the client's concomitant disorders. Hyperthyroidism affects almost all the systems of the body. The most common subjective and objective findings are summarized in Table 43–2.

In the elderly, thyroid dysfunction is often called the "great imitator" because it may mimic other disorders. A cardiac dysrhythmia, especially atrial fibrillation, that responds poorly to digitalization may be the first sign of thyroid dysfunction in an older adult. Occasionally, paroxysmal supraventricular tachycardia may be seen. Congestive heart failure that seems not to respond to treatment may also be a presenting sign of hyperthyroidism in the elderly as well as in other clients with a history of cardiac disease.

Thyroid Storm

Thyroid storm, or thyrotoxic crisis, is a potentially life-threatening emergency characterized by an increase in all the symptoms and signs of hyperthyroidism. It is a result of a sudden release of thyroid hormone into the bloodstream and may be precipitated by infections, surgery, trauma, radioactive-iodine therapy, aggressive manipulation of the thyroid gland, diabetic ketoacidosis, abrupt withdrawal of antithyroid drugs, or severe stress. With better diagnostic and treatment approaches, thyroid storm now is so rare that it accounts for only 2% of all hospital admissions for hyperthyroidism.

Symptoms and signs of thyroid storm include (Kaye & Rose, 1983):

- Marked restlessness and anxiety
- Rise in temperature to 104°F to 106°F (40°C to 41°C)
- Extreme tachycardia (130 to 160 beats per minute)
- Dehydration
- Nausea and vomiting
- Diarrhea
- Delirium and psychosis

Hyperthyroidism is diagnosed from the clinical signs and symptoms (Table 43–2), elevated plasma levels of T_4, T_3, or both; and elevated radioactive iodine uptake (RAIU). A thyroid scan may help differentiate diffuse toxic goiter from a toxic multinodular goiter. Plasma levels of T_4 are used as a screening tool. When the diagnosis is uncertain, thyroxine-binding globulin (TBG) may be measured to rule out the possibility of abnormalities in the T_4-binding proteins. LATS and TSI are not measured routinely but may be tested more frequently as assay methods become available. Evaluation of TSH levels, though used only occasionally, can be of value in distinguishing primary from secondary hyperthyroidism.

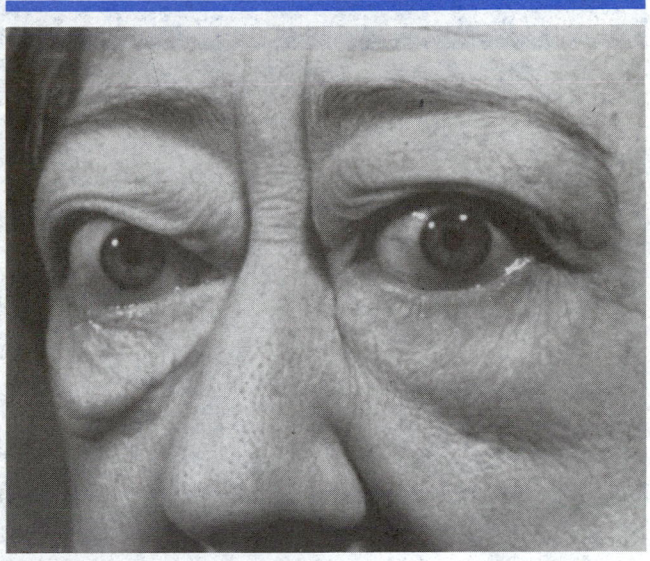

Figure 43–1

Exophthalmos in a client with Graves' disease. (Courtesy of Millard Fillmore Hospital, Buffalo, NY)

These and other tests used in the laboratory evaluation of thyroid disorders are presented in Table 41–2. Other incidental laboratory findings in clients with hyperthyroidism include abnormalities in liver enzymes, decreases in neutrophil count, leukopenia with lymphocytosis, hypercalcemia (in 5% of clients), and hypocholesterolemia.

Therapeutic Measures

The choice of therapy for the treatment of hyperthyroidism depends on the cause of the disorder. Symptomatic therapy involves the oral administration of an adrenergic blocking agent to treat the increased activity of the sympathetic nervous system that accompanies hyperthyroidism. Propranolol is the agent most commonly used to minimize the sympathetic effects. Others include reserpine, guanethidine, and alpha-methyldopa. Definitive measures for the treatment of hyperthyroidism include antithyroid drugs (eg, propylthiouracil or methimazole [Tapazole]), radioactive iodine, and thyroidectomy. See Box 43–1 for a description of antithyroid drugs.

Radioactive Iodine (^{131}I) Therapy

Radioactive iodine is an inexpensive and easily administered therapeutic agent used mainly to treat hyperthyroidism in clients ages 40 and above, although the age limit is not an absolute. Pregnant women should not be given ^{131}I.

The thyroid gland cannot distinguish between normal and radioactive iodine and will absorb both isotopes and store them. Concentrated in the thyroid, ^{131}I will destroy cells that store it by localized irradiation, resulting in a

Table 43-2 Common Findings in Hyperthyroidism

Subjective Findings	Objective Findings
Clients often note:	*Examiners often observe:*
General: Intolerance to heat, fatigue, insomnia, and hyperactivity; increased anxiety, irritability, restlessness, and nervousness; emotional lability	Hair: Fine, silky Nails: Loosening of the nail from the nail bed **(onycholysis)**
Skin: Flushing, sweating	Skin: Smooth, soft, thin, moist; excessive sweating **(hyperhidrosis);** palmar erythema, ankle swelling; a hard, nonpitting swelling over the anterior tibia (pretibial edema)
Eyes: Photosensitivity, diplopia	Eyes: Widened palpebral fissures (stare), **exophthalmos,** lid lag, lid retraction, diminished convergence, increased lacrimation
Neck: Tightness of collars and necklaces	Neck: Thyromegaly with diffuse or symmetrical enlargement; bruits related to increased vascularity; nodules, thyroid tenderness
Cardiovascular system: Palpitations	Cardiovascular system: Increased systolic blood pressure, tachycardia, wide pulse pressures, systolic flow murmurs, dysrhythmias, peripheral vasodilation with bounding pulses and warm, slightly erythematous extremities
Gastrointestinal system: Weight loss, nausea, diarrhea, abdominal pain	Gastrointestinal system: Weight loss, hyperactive bowel sounds
Neurologic system: Muscle weakness	Neurologic system: Fine tremor of tongue, eyelids, and fingers; hyperactive DTRs with a brisk Achilles reflex; sometimes muscle atrophy
Reproductive system: Impotence, decreased libido, infertility (men); **amenorrhea,** hypomenorrhea, decreased libido, infertility (women)	Reproductive system: Male: gynecomastia

SOURCE: Adapted with permission from Kaye D, Rose LF (editors): *Fundamentals of Internal Medicine.* St. Louis: Mosby, 1983.

decrease in T_4 secretion and a reduction in the size of the gland.

Improvement of symptoms may occur 2 to 4 weeks after treatment, with euthyroidism occurring in about 3 months. Occasionally, if the condition does not resolve, a second dose may be administered.

Radioactive iodine is administered on an outpatient basis in the form of an oral "cocktail." When a large dose of ^{131}I is required, the client may need to be hospitalized and placed on radiation safety precautions.

About 10% of ^{131}I-treated clients may develop hypothyroidism in the first year, and about 3% of them may do so every year thereafter. These clients need hormonal replacement. All clients should have periodic medical follow-up and reevaluation after attaining a euthyroid state.

Care of Exophthalmos
Local care of the eyes includes the use of methylcellulose drops (artificial tears) and steroid ophthalmic drops. For severe inflammation of the eyes, oral prednisone may be necessary. Thiazide diuretics can relieve periorbital and lid edema.

In case of rapid progression of proptosis or development of optic neuritis with changes in visual acuity, irradiation of the retro-orbital tissues or surgical orbital decompression may be instituted. In severe cases of exophthalmos, surgery may correct lid retraction and ophthalmoplegia (eye muscle paralysis).

Management of Thyroid Storm
The rare development of thyroid storm poses a serious threat to life. Treatment must be started immediately. The treatment usually includes:

- Propylthiouracil (800 to 1200 mg daily) via a nasogastric tube
- Propranolol (20 to 60 mg q. 4 h PO or 1 to 2 mg IV every 1 to 2 hours)
- Potassium iodide (500 mg q. 6 h or sodium iodide 0.5 g IV q. 8 h)
- Intravenous therapy

- Measures to reduce hyperthermia (eg, cold packs, hypothermia blanket)
- Oxygen
- Corticosteroids in high doses if the client fails to respond to initial treatment in 12 to 24 hours
- Digoxin with cardiac failure
- Additional measures to lower plasma thyroid levels rapidly (eg, plasmapheresis, exchange transfusions, and peritoneal dialysis)

Hyperthyroidism is often cyclic and may be precipitated by either psychological or physiological stress. Recurrence rates are usually in the range of 20% to 30% with any form of therapy except radical thyroidectomy and large doses of ^{131}I. With proper treatment and long-term follow-up, the clinical results are often good, although more as an induced remission than a cure. Hypothyroidism is common in the post-treatment period and may occur several years after a subtotal thyroidectomy or treatment with ^{131}I. Thyroid storm has a poor prognosis and is best prevented by careful preoperative preparation of the client.

Specific Nursing Measures

The nursing care of the client with hyperthyroidism is directed toward ameliorating the symptoms and signs associated with this disorder. Typically, clients with hyperthyroidism are nervous, agitated, slender, often irritable, and subject to emotional lability. They may be hyperactive and restless (because of the increased metabolic rate), have difficulty concentrating for long periods, be intolerant of heat (excessive perspiration), have gastrointestinal problems, and experience sexual dysfunction. In instances of exophthalmos, they may have dryness of the conjunctiva and cornea or visual impairment. These symptoms present a problem not only to the client but also to significant others who are called on to provide support during diagnosis and treatment.

In general, nurses caring for clients with hyperthyroidism should focus on:

- Assessing clients thoroughly
- Maintaining client comfort
- Promoting emotional well-being of client and family
- Monitoring intake and output, diet, and elimination patterns
- Educating clients and their families

Client assessment should include vital signs (temperature, pulse, respirations, and blood pressure) every 4 hours and daily weight. The physician may order a sleeping pulse rate because in hyperthyroidism, the pulse rate often increases during sleep. Especially important is an assessment of the client's mental state, particularly the degree of agitation and restlessness, because increasing restlessness and anxiety may be an early indicator of impending thyroid storm. Also be alert for any symptoms and

Box 43–1 Usual Drug Therapy in Hyperthyroidism (Antithyroid Drugs)

Propylthiouracil 100 to 150 mg q. 8 h., lowered to maintenance doses of 50 mg q. 8 h. after 4 to 8 weeks

or

Methimazole (Tapazole) 10 to 20 mg q. 8 h., lowered to maintenance doses of 5 mg q. 8 h. after 4 to 8 weeks

signs of impending cardiac failure (dyspnea on exertion, shortness of breath, paroxysmal nocturnal dyspnea, dysrhythmias, or rales). Cardiac failure is often a serious complication of hyperthyroidism; it may be seen in the elderly and also in clients with a previous history of cardiac problems.

Clients may require daily baths and frequent linen changes because of profuse perspiration. Give special care to clients who are confined to bed, with attention to bony prominences and other potential areas of skin breakdown. The room temperature should be lowered because of the client's intolerance to heat. Bedding and sleepwear should be lightweight.

In general, clients' activities should be restricted to provide maximum rest and alleviate fatigue. This restriction may further agitate restless, hyperactive clients and provide a challenge for the nurse. To calm such clients, refer them to the occupational therapy department for suitable diversions, alternate the schedule of activity and rest periods, and remove potential sources of stimulation from the environment. Some clients may need to be sedated.

For clients with ocular involvement, elevating the head of the bed may help relieve edema of the periorbital areas. Methylcellulose drops, or artificial tears (0.5% to 1%), alleviate dryness of the eyes and protect against irritation. They should be given as ordered. In clients with severe protrusion of the eyeballs (proptosis), the lids may need to be taped during sleep or a sleeping mask worn to prevent drying of the cornea and conjunctiva. Sunglasses may help minimize the effects of glare. Visual acuity should be assessed and observations made for increasing proptosis and ophthalmoplegia.

Clients with hyperthyroidism are often subject to mood swings, which disturb both client and family. In addition, clients are often irritable, restless, easily upset, and distracted. They often benefit from attempts to create a calm, soothing environment in which the routine and primary caretakers change as little as possible. These clients should be assigned to private rooms. Visitors should be screened or at least educated to avoid disturbing or anxiety-producing topics of conversation. Although it is not always possible in practice, attempt to help the client and significant others see the relation between the client's behavior and physiological state. Because the client may also have some degree of sexual dysfunction, try to provide opportunities to discuss this in a calm, relaxed situation to assure client and family that this, too, is a manifestation of the underlying clinical disorders.

Clients with hyperthyroidism, in spite of an increasing appetite, usually lose some weight because of tissue catabolism resulting from high metabolic rates. They may need 4000 to 5000 calories a day in the form of a high-protein, high-carbohydrate diet. The client should avoid consumption of excessive fiber because of its effect on peristalsis. The amount of caffeine consumed may need regulation to avoid overstimulation. Snacks between meals and at bedtime are beneficial. One of the parameters in assessing the efficacy of a treatment regimen in hyperthyroidism is the maintenance of a stable weight (or weight gain), so weight should be monitored each day or every other day.

Clients with hyperthyroidism often require an increased fluid intake (usually in the range of 4000 mL daily unless there are cardiac or renal contraindications) to overcome excessive fluid loss from increased perspiration due to the high metabolic rate. The increased production of metabolic wastes also requires enough fluid intake to enable their dilution and excretion by the kidneys. This increased fluid intake can be provided in a variety of ways to meet the individual client's needs and tastes. A careful explanation of the purpose of the additional fluid intake may ensure client cooperation.

Clients with hyperthyroidism may also produce stools more often because of the higher rate of peristalsis. This can cause perianal skin breakdown and irritation. Carefully and thoroughly clean the area and apply creams and lubricants as needed.

Client and family education should focus on the basic self-care essential for the client with hyperthyroidism:

- Symptoms and signs of both hyperthyroidism and hypothyroidism—what to report to the doctor and when and the effect of increased thyroid production on the body

- The client's treatment regimen and its purposes—the name, dosage, action, and side-effects of each medication

- Any dietary prescriptions

- The need for regular medical supervision and its purpose—the date and time of the next medical appointment and a telephone number where client and family can call with questions

In addition, because of the emotional and mental changes, explain to the client and significant others the relation between these behaviors and the overproduction of thyroid hormone as well as to reassure them that medical treatment will ameliorate these changes. Emphasize that the treatment for hyperthyroidism often takes a long time to

show an effect. Because subsequent hypothyroidism is also a concern, vigilance is necessary, even after the hyperthyroidism has resolved.

HYPOTHYROIDISM

Hypothyroidism is characterized by a decreased secretion of thyroid hormone. Hypothyroidism may range from a mild state, which is often difficult to diagnose, to myxedema coma. Deficiency of thyroid hormone, which produces the symptoms and signs of hypometabolism, affects almost every system of the body and may be seen in persons of all ages. The major forms of hypothyroidism are cretinism, juvenile hypothyroidism, and myxedema.

Cretinism, or congenital or infantile hypothyroidism, is a state of severe mental and physical retardation resulting from a deficiency of thyroid hormone during the fetal or neonatal period. It is seldom apparent at birth because of the persistent effect of the maternal thyroid hormones. The causes of congenital cretinism include an absent or rudimentary thyroid gland, defects in hormone synthesis, goiter, or atrophy of the thyroid gland. Because approximately 50% of brain growth occurs within the first 6 months of life, early diagnosis and treatment of conditions leading to cretinism are essential to prevent mental and physical retardation.

Juvenile hypothyroidism begins in childhood and is characterized by moderate mental and growth retardation and sexual infantilism. The causes of juvenile hypothyroidism, which may be idiopathic, include atrophy of the gland, defective thyroid function, thyroiditis or thyroidectomy, and pituitary deficiency.

Myxedema, or adult hypothyroidism, is a fairly common disorder that is five times more frequent in women than in men; clients are usually in the 30- to 60-year age range. Symptoms may appear so slowly and insidiously that clients are often unaware of the changes. In severe cases of untreated hypothyroidism, myxedema coma may develop. Myxedema coma is characterized by an intense exaggeration of the symptoms and signs of hypothyroidism, with neurologic impairment leading to loss of consciousness. Myxedema coma occurs in clients of all ages and usually is the result of a precipitating event such as a respiratory tract or other infection; the use of drugs, especially narcotics, tranquilizers, or barbiturates; myocardial infarction or cerebrovascular accident; gastrointestinal bleeding; or exposure to cold. The mortality in myxedema coma has been estimated at 60% to 70%, so prompt recognition of symptoms and early treatment are essential.

The causes of myxedema may be primary (pathology within the thyroid gland itself) or secondary (pituitary insufficiency). Primary thyroid dysfunction is much more common than secondary thyroid dysfunction.

More than 50% of all cases of hypothyroidism are

idiopathic. Primary hypothyroidism may also be iatrogenic (ie, may result from thyroidectomy, treatment of the thyroid by ^{131}I or antithyroid drugs such as propylthiouracil or methimazole) or it may be caused by ingestion of goitrogens (Box 43–2) or by chronic thyroiditis. Autoimmunity has been proposed as a cause of primary hypothyroidism, because autoimmune antibodies have been found in the serum of 70% of clients with the disease (Muthe, 1981). Hashimoto's thyroiditis, another cause of hypothyroidism, is also thought to be an autoimmune disorder.

Secondary hypothyroidism usually follows destruction of the pituitary gland by a tumor (chromophobe adenoma) or by postpartum necrosis (Sheehan's syndrome). These conditions cause a decrease in the secretion of TSH by the anterior pituitary gland, resulting in atrophy of thyroid tissue and deficiencies in circulating T_4 and T_3. Because thyroid hormone is necessary for the function of all the endocrine glands, deficiencies in its secretion may result in a secondary hypofunction of the pituitary, adrenal, and other glands.

Clinical Manifestations

The clinical manifestations of hypothyroidism relate directly to the degree of hormonal deficiency and range from mild, often nonspecific symptoms (eg, fatigue, weight gain, or menstrual irregularities) to full-blown myxedema. Symp-

Box 43–2 Goitrogens (Foods or Drugs Capable of Causing Goiter)

Dietary goitrogens
- Cabbage
- Rutabaga
- Turnip
- Mustard plant
- Soybeans
- Kale

Drug goitrogens
- Propylthiouracil
- Methimazole
- Perchlorate
- Thiocyanate
- Iodides in pharmacological doses
- Lithium salts
- Resorcinol ointments
- Aminoglutethimide

toms may appear slowly and be characterized by a gradual slowing of both mental and physical processes. Table 43–3 lists the most common subjective and objective findings in hypothyroidism.

In the elderly, symptoms of hypothyroidism are easy to overlook because of the gradual slowing of metabolism that accompanies the aging process. The nurse must be alert for subtle symptoms and signs while assessing older clients.

The onset of myxedema coma, which may be gradual, is signaled by a pronounced increase in both the number and magnitude of the findings listed in Table 43–3; there

Table 43–3 Common Findings in Hypothyroidism	
Subjective Findings	**Objective Findings**
Clients often note:	*Examiners often observe:*
Fatigue, lethargy, generalized weakness	Drooping of the eyelid
Intolerance to cold	Thickened facial tissues
Constipation	Dull facial expression
Anorexia, indigestion, flatulence	Lateral third of the eyebrow thinned or absent
Weight gain (10 to 20 lb)	Enlarged tongue
Deepening or hoarseness of the voice	Slow speech
Dyspnea, chest pain	Decreased hearing
Enlargement of the neck	Abdominal distention
Scalp, axillary, and pubic hair loss	Thyromegaly
Dry, coarse skin; brittle nails	Bradycardia
Numbness and tingling of the hands and feet	Decreased body temperature
Changes in memory and mental ability	Cool, coarse, dry skin
Decreased libido and impotence (men)	Nonpitting edema of the lower extremities
Menorrhagia (women)	Delay in relaxation phase of DTRs (pseudomyotonia)
	On x-ray examination, cardiomegaly, pleural and pericardial effusions

is almost always neurologic involvement as well. Prominent clinical manifestations of myxedema coma include:

- Hypothermia, which can be as severe as 74°F (23.3°C) and is a poor prognostic sign; a normal temperature suggests infection
- Hypotension (50% of clients)
- Intestinal ileus or fecal impaction
- Urinary retention
- Seizures (25% of clients)
- Congestive heart failure or pericardial effusion
- Respiratory failure characterized by hypoxia, retention of carbon dioxide, and respiratory acidosis
- A bilateral positive Babinski's sign

Besides myxedema coma, the major complications of hypothyroidism include cardiac involvement, which is a result of advanced coronary artery disease and congestive heart failure; an increased susceptibility to infection; and organic psychoses with paranoid delusions (the so-called myxedema madness). Infertility is another possible complication of hypothyroidism; it usually responds well to treatment.

The diagnosis of hypothyroidism is made from a careful history including family history of goiter or hypothyroidism, drug use (especially propylthiouracil, methimazole, lithium carbonate, iodides, mercaptopurine, oral hypoglycemic agents, and thyroid hormones), and previous thyroid surgery or treatment with ^{131}I. Laboratory findings consistent with hypothyroidism include serum T_4 levels under 3.5 μg/dL and low or low-normal T_3 resin uptake.

When the diagnosis of hypothyroidism has been established, radioimmunoassay of TSH levels will help to distinguish between a primary or secondary cause. Plasma TSH levels are elevated in primary hypothyroidism and depressed in secondary hypothyroidism. Other laboratory abnormalities that may be present in clients with hypothyroidism include macrocytic anemia (also possibly normocytic, normochromic, or hypochromic anemia); basophilia; elevation of serum cholesterol and triglyceride levels; elevations of the creatine kinase (CK), SGOT, and lactic dehydrogenase (LDH) levels; hyperuricemia; and elevated serum carotene levels.

Characteristic ECG abnormalities may be noted: low voltage, sinus bradycardia, and flattened or inverted T waves. Cardiomegaly, pleural effusion, or both may be seen on chest x-ray.

Therapeutic Measures

The main approach to the treatment of hypothyroidism is the correction of the underlying cause. Treatment might involve discontinuation of drugs blocking thyroid synthesis, dietary correction, or administration of thyroid hormones to correct the hormonal deficiency. Thyroid hormone replacement drugs are listed in Box 43–3. Clients receive an initial dose of the drug, which is then adjusted to achieve the optimal effect. The client's hormonal levels are then stabilized by a maintenance dose.

Myxedema coma is a medical emergency. The immediate steps in treating it are:

- Administration of thyroid hormones (500 μg of T_4 or 100 μg of T_3 given stat). Subsequent dosages of T_4 should be 100 μg/day IV and of T_3, 10 to 25 μg IV every 8 to 12 hours.
- Administration of glucocorticoids to cover any adrenal insufficiency; IV hydrocortisone, q.d., which can be decreased to 50 to 75 mg q.d.
- Correction of hypothermia. Blankets are recommended. Aggressive correction is contraindicated, because it diverts the circulatory flow to the periphery and away from the vital organs.
- Maintenance of ventilation.
- Fluid restriction (to less than 1 L/day) if client shows signs of hyponatremia.
- Administration of 50% glucose if client shows signs of hypoglycemia.
- Treatment of any precipitating causes (eg, infection, myocardial infarction, or gastrointestinal bleeding).

The prognosis for hypothyroidism is good; many clients can be treated easily and effectively with replacement therapy. Restoration of the euthyroid state is possible, but relapse may occur if treatment is stopped. Depending on the type of medication used, the effects of the therapy may not be seen for up to 2 weeks, with complete resolution of symptoms taking several months and more. Share this information with the client and family to avoid discouragement.

Specific Nursing Measures

The nursing care of the client with hypothyroidism can be rewarding because of the satisfaction from seeing successful response to treatment. Remember, however, that the euthyroid state is achieved gradually.

Nursing management includes assessment of the client's response to replacement therapy. Positive results are indicated by a decrease in lethargy and fatigue, decrease in

---

Box 43–3   Thyroid Hormone Replacement Drugs

Levothyroxine (Synthroid)

Liothyronine (Cytomel)

Liotrix (Euthroid, Thyrolar)

Thyroglobulin (Proloid)

Thyroid USP (desiccated thyroid)

edema, weight loss, improvement in mentation and speech, increased tolerance to cold, improvement in appetite, resolution of constipation, and normalization of the menstrual cycle. Improvements in the hair, skin, and nails are more gradual. Anemia may not be corrected for 2 to 3 months.

Elderly and cardiac clients should be closely monitored for increased shortness of breath, dyspnea on exertion (DOE), cough, chest pain, or angina. Cardiac status is monitored by checking vital signs regularly and reporting any symptoms and signs of incipient congestive heart fail-

---

Box 43-4 Teaching Material for Clients With Hypothyroidism

Living With Hypothyroidism

You have learned from your physician that you have hypothyroidism. This leaflet will answer questions most often asked by persons who have just learned that they have an underactive thyroid gland as you do. This leaflet and the instructions given by your physician or nurse will give you the information needed to live easily with hypothyroidism.

What is the thyroid?

The thyroid is an endocrine gland that controls the rate of many body functions such as use of oxygen, use of food, and production of heat. The term *endocrine* means the gland makes hormones or body chemicals that travel in the bloodstream to body cells where they do their job.

The thyroid gland is located in the front of the neck and at both sides of the Adam's apple. Thyroid hormone travels from this location to all body cells.

What is hypothyroidism?

Hypothyroidism is a common disorder caused by partial or complete lack of thyroid hormone. Since thyroid hormone affects so many body functions, lack of the hormone causes problems. Complete lack of thyroid hormone for prolonged periods can endanger life. Fortunately, it is easy to supply the lacking thyroid hormone in pill form. Thyroid medication gives the body the hormone needed for normal living.

What are the symptoms of hypothyroidism?

The most common symptoms and signs of hypothyroidism are weakness, sluggishness, dry skin, puffiness of the face, a husky voice, constipation, and feeling cold. You may have noticed some of these symptoms and other signs that your body and mind have slowed down. As the lack of thyroid hormone is supplied by medication, you will notice that these symptoms gradually disappear and you will begin to feel like yourself again.

Infants and children have hypothyroid symptoms similar to those affecting adults. In addition, affected infants may feed slowly, and children may have difficulties in school work.

How is hypothyroidism diagnosed?

Hypothyroidism is diagnosed through examination and laboratory tests. Many symptoms of hypothyroidism are general symptoms of various disorders and are not specific for hypothyroidism. Evaluation includes blood tests that measure the levels of thyroid hormone in your blood. These tests are also done at intervals after diagnosis to check the effectiveness of thyroid medication.

What causes hypothyroidism?

There are many causes of hypothyroidism. The thyroid gland can be destroyed by inflammation, or hypothyroidism may be the result of treatment for an overactive thyroid (hyperthyroidism). Hyperthyroidism is treated with radioactive iodine, surgery, or medication. Often, these treatments cause hypothyroidism, which is easily treated.

Other causes of hypothyroidism include genetic defects and injury to the pituitary gland, which controls the thyroid.

How is hypothyroidism treated?

Treatment is the simple part of hypothyroidism. Your physician will prescribe a tablet to replace the missing thyroid hormone. All you must do is one simple but important thing—YOU MUST TAKE YOUR MEDICATION ON A REGULAR BASIS. Your physician will give you a dose of thyroid hormone that is equal to what a normal thyroid would make. In some cases, your physician will start with small amounts of thyroid hormone and will slowly increase the dose over a period of weeks or months until you have reached a normal level of thyroid hormone. You can help the physician know if the level is reached by reporting how you feel.

If you notice a fast heart rate, nervousness, increased sweating, or heat sensations, report this to your physician. It may indicate that your level of thyroid hormone is too high.

Will hypothyroidism affect my life?

Once you are taking regular medication to replace thyroid hormone, you can live as you did before you had hypothyroidism. The only change is the taking of daily medication. No restrictions of diet or activity are necessary.

Hypothyroidism is almost always a lifelong disease. Thyroid medication cannot be stopped for long periods of time without problems.

After your optimal dose of thyroid medication is determined, your physician may want to check you once or twice a year. If you change physicians, tell your new physician that you are taking thyroid medication. It is wise to carry a medical identification card in your wallet stating that you take thyroid medication.

Important points

1. Your symptoms will disappear slowly. Complete improvement may take several months.
2. You need thyroid medication daily. Set aside a specific time daily to take your thyroid pill. It is helpful to tie this in with a morning routine such as eating breakfast.
3. Living with hypothyroidism is easy when you are an informed partner in your health care.

Medication _____

Dosage _____

SOURCE: Reprinted with permission from Musante–Wake M, Brensinger JF: The nurse's role in hypothyroidism. *Nurs Clin N Am* (September) 1980; 15(3):465–466.

ure, chest pain, increase in angina, or pulse rate over 100. If these occur, discontinue thyroid replacement until the physician is notified.

The client should be kept warm and should be weighed daily to assess fluid loss as an indicator of improvement. Deep breathing and ambulation will improve hypoxia. Lotions and creams will help skin dryness.

The client's drug regimen must be closely monitored, because the hypometabolic state potentiates many drugs, such as digitalis and insulin, requiring a lower dosage. Dosage requirements will change as the client attains the euthyroid state.

Encourage a diet low in calories and high in protein and fiber. Small, frequent portions may be helpful with the anorexic client. Encourage increased fluids if there is no sign of cardiac involvement. Assess the client for constipation and fecal impaction. Stool softeners may be needed. Clients with hypothyroidism have a decreased response to infection. They must be carefully protected, because infection may precipitate myxedema coma.

Health Teaching

Client and family education should stress not only the favorable prognosis for hypothyroidism with treatment but also the need for clients to remain on medication for the rest of their lives. In teaching clients with hypothyroidism, be aware that their slowed mentation and memory may interfere with their ability to learn and retain new information. Therefore, including a family member or significant other in the teaching sessions is helpful for review of the material with clients after the teaching session. Printed information is useful for this purpose. Box 43–4 (on previous page) is an example of material that could be given to clients and their families or friends.

Important teaching areas to cover include:

- The symptoms and signs of both hyperthyroidism and hypothyroidism—what to observe and when to call the physician
- The pathophysiology of hypothyroidism, including the role of thyroid hormone in the body
- The need for lifelong medication and medical follow-up
- Any dietary prescriptions
- The drug regimen, including the name and dosage of medications, their expected action and outcomes, and possible side effects

Hypothyroidism can be especially distressing to a family or significant others because of the changes they see in their loved one (weakness, lethargy, and slowing and dulling of mental abilities). An important nursing role is the psychological support of client and family through the initial diagnosis and treatment period, including reassuring them that most of these observable symptoms and signs will improve and be resolved as treatment progresses.

Another important nursing role in hypothyroidism centers on its prevention, particularly regarding ingestion of goitrogens (see Box 43–2). The pediatric nurse should be thoroughly familiar with the symptoms and signs of hypothyroidism in the infant and child (prolonged jaundice after birth, swollen eyelids, protruding tongue, poor appetite, feeding difficulties, hoarse cry, placidity, lethargy, respiratory difficulties, and resistant constipation), because prompt referral and treatment will allow normal growth and development.

GOITER

An enlargement of the thyroid gland is called a *goiter*. A goiter associated with either hypofunction or hyperfunction of the gland is a toxic goiter, whereas nontoxic goiters are associated with euthyroidism. Goiters are classified into three major categories:

- Diffuse goiters (simple goiter)
- Multinodular goiters
- Uninodular goiters

Toxic nodular goiter accounts for 15% of the cases of hyperthyroidism (Saxton et al., 1983). In toxic nodular goiter, the affected thyroid gland usually has one or more nodules that hyperfunction autonomously without the normal feedback control, resulting in clinical symptoms and signs of hyperthyroidism. Hyperfunction of such nodules suppresses TSH levels and consequently suppresses function of the unaffected thyroid tissue. Hyperfunctioning thyroid nodules, also called "hot nodules," concentrate ^{131}I and thus produce a patchy scintiscan. Figure 41–2 shows a scintiscan of an autonomous hyperfunctioning thyroid nodule before and after TSH stimulation.

A nodule must be at least 0.75 to 1 cm to be palpable. Toxic multinodular goiter occurs more frequently in clients between the ages of 50 and 70, and it is four times more frequent in females than in males.

The causes of nontoxic simple goiter may include iodine deficiency, goitrogens, tissue resistance to thyroid hormone, thyroiditis, or biosynthetic or enzymatic defects. Clients in certain geographic areas, usually away from the seacoast, lack iodine. Insufficiency of iodine in the diet or intrathyroid biosynthetic defects result in a decreased secretion of thyroid hormone. This hypoproduction of hormone results in an increase in TSH secretion by the anterior pituitary gland and a compensatory increase in the size of the thyroid gland. This often returns the thyroid hormone levels to normal but does not resolve the underlying problem. Although iodine deficiency is still common in certain undeveloped areas of the world, it is far less common today in North America because of the prevalence of iodized salt and the use of iodine compounds to preserve foods.

Today, the most common cause of nontoxic goiter is minor intrathyroidal biosynthetic defects (Kaye & Rose, 1983), which appear to occur sporadically and may be acquired or familial. The exact cause of these minor intrathyroidal defects is unknown. Genetic factors are thought to play a role, because 30% to 49% of these clients' relatives show similar goiters or clinical evidence of thyroid disease. Simple goiter may also occur transiently when there is a greater need for thyroid hormone (eg, at the onset of puberty and during pregnancy and lactation). Goitrogens in water, food, and drugs have also contributed to the formation of goiters. Nontoxic diffuse goiters have also been seen in rare cases of tissue resistance to thyroid hormones. Thyroiditis, which is discussed fully in the next section, also causes goiter.

The most common cause of nontoxic multinodular goiter is the long-term changes in the thyroid gland of clients with nontoxic diffuse goiters. These are thought to be degenerative changes that occur in the gland over time.

The causes of nontoxic uninodular goiter include thyroiditis, cysts, hemorrhage, and benign or malignant neoplasms. Thyroiditis and neoplasms are discussed in subsequent sections.

Clinical Manifestations

The major clinical manifestation of goiter is a visibly enlarged, palpable gland. The enlargement may be diffuse or nodular. Thyroid nodules have been detected in up to 4% of the general population and in 15% to 20% of individuals on autopsy.

The client may be completely asymptomatic or may complain of dysphagia, wheezing, or respiratory distress resulting from compression of structures in the neck or upper chest. A prominent bulge in the neck presents cosmetic problems for many clients.

The diagnosis of simple goiter is made after taking a careful history (investigating place of residence; ingestion of goitrogens; familial history of goiter, thyroid disease, or both; and high-stress states), a physical examination, and laboratory testing. Generally, serum T_4 and T_3 levels and RAIU levels are within normal ranges.

If nodules are present, percutaneous needle or open biopsy may be needed to rule out a malignancy. Ultrasonography can differentiate among solid, cystic, and mixed solid and cystic nodules of the thyroid. Figure 43–2 shows an ultrasound of a thyroid cyst. RAIU combined with thyroid scintiscan will yield the number and functional activity of any thyroid nodules present (Williams, 1981). Figure 41–2 shows a thyroid scintiscan illustrating "hot" (functioning) and "cold" (nonfunctioning) nodules and diffuse thyroid enlargement.

Simple goiters either resolve spontaneously or increase to a point where the client has symptoms of compression. In persons over age 50, long-standing multinodular goiters are likely to become toxic. The incidence of malignancy in these clients has not been established. Simple goiter can be prevented with a dietary intake of 100 to 200 ng of iodine daily. The dosage may be increased to the upper limits during puberty, pregnancy, lactation, or periods of stress. This amount is included in a gram or two of iodized salt. In some geographic areas, iodinated oil has been used as a prophylactic measure for goiter.

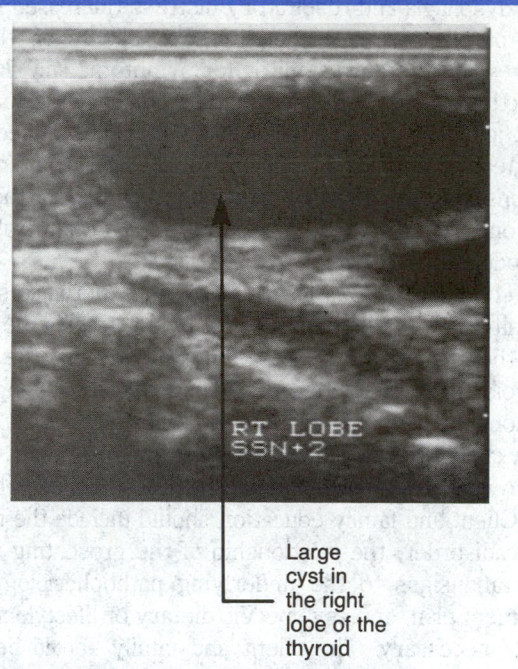

Large cyst in the right lobe of the thyroid

Figure 43–2

Ultrasound exam showing a cyst in the right lobe of the thyroid. (Courtesy of Health Care Plan, Buffalo, NY)

Therapeutic Measures

The most common approach to the treatment of goiter is to suppress the further enlargement of the thyroid gland and to reduce it to normal size. Depending on the cause of the goiter, this may be accomplished by nutritional measures; by medical measures; or, in some cases by surgery.

Levothyroxine (0.2 mg per day) is used to suppress TSH and thyroid hormone production. It should reduce the goiter to normal size in 2 to 6 months. Iodine therapy (Lugol's solution or saturated solution of potassium iodide [SSKI]) is indicated only when iodine deficiency has been established; iodine prophylaxis in other instances may induce hypothyroidism. Medications that promote the formation of goiters (eg, propylthiouracil, methimazole, tolbutamide, and iodine preparations) should be avoided.

Surgery is indicated only to assist in establishing the diagnosis and to rule out potential malignancies. A subtotal thyroidectomy may also be done to reduce the mass of a very large gland in a symptomatic client. Surgery may be followed by medical suppression, because hyperplasia and regrowth of thyroid tissue may occur.

Specific Nursing Measures

Nursing intervention in the care of the client with goiter should focus on client assessment, maintaining client comfort, and client and family education. Client assessment includes reporting and recording symptoms of compression: dysphagia and respiratory distress (increased shortness of breath and wheezing). For clients on thyroid suppression therapy, monitor for symptoms and signs of hyperthyroidism (increased anxiety, tachycardia, palpitations, and diarrhea). These findings should be immediately reported to the physician. Also carefully monitor the client's response to treatment by assessing changes in the size and consistency of the thyroid gland and carefully watching for nodules.

The client with a large goiter can experience significant alterations in comfort. Assist by positioning the client with the head of the bed elevated; by advising the client to avoid tight, restrictive neckwear; and by making sure the consistency of the client's food facilitates swallowing. For a client with significant **dysphagia,** mealtime should not be rushed. Frequent, small feedings may be helpful.

Client and family education should include the nature of the disorder, the relationship of the presenting symptoms and signs to the underlying pathophysiology, the treatment plan, and any specific dietary or lifestyle adjustments necessary. The client and family should be fully familiar not only with the therapeutic regimen but also the overall goals of the treatment plan. Clients should be warned to avoid dietary goitrogens of the sorts listed in Box 43–2.

The nurse's role in the prevention of goiter centers on teaching the necessity of including iodine in the diet. Such teaching is of special importance in geographic areas where goiter is endemic. The early recognition and prompt referral of clients with goiter or thyroid nodules is also an important nursing function. Generally, the smaller a goiter is, the more amenable it is to treatment. Because of the possibility of thyroid carcinoma, the earlier a thyroid nodule is evaluated, the better the prognosis if it is malignant.

HYPERPARATHYROIDISM

Hyperparathyroidism is characterized by a hypersecretion of parathyroid hormone, which brings about an increase in circulating plasma levels of calcium and a decrease in circulating plasma levels of phosphorus. Although one of the major clinical manifestations of hyperparathyroidism is hypercalcemia, it is important to remember that hypercalcemia has several different causes (Box 43–5). Hyperparathyroidism affects women twice as often as men and is more common in persons over age 40. It rarely occurs in childhood.

Hyperparathyroidism can be classified as primary or secondary according to its cause. Primary hyperparathyroidism originates within the gland itself and in about 90% of all cases is caused by a single benign adenoma of one gland. In 8% to 10% of all cases, primary hypertrophy and hyperplasia of all four glands are involved, and in 2% of all cases, carcinoma of one gland is the cause of the primary hyperactivity of the parathyroid glands. Secondary hyperparathyroidism is almost always associated with hyperplasia of all four parathyroid glands and is a compensatory mechanism to combat the hypocalcemia arising from chronic renal disease, rickets, osteomalacia, and acromegaly.

Box 43–5 Causes of Hypercalcemia

- Increased gastrointestinal calcium absorption:
  Vitamin D intoxication
  Sarcoidosis
  Tuberculosis

- Increased calcium resorption from bone:
  Primary hyperparathyroidism
  Malignancy with bone metastases
  Malignancy without bone metastases
    Ectopic parathyroid hormone (PTH) secretion
    Prostaglandin E production
    Synthesis of a vitamin D-like substance
  Multiple myeloma, leukemia, and lymphomas
  Chronic immobilization
  Hyperthyroidism
  Vitamin A intoxication

- Increased renal tubular calcium reabsorption:
  Therapy with thiazide diuretics

- Unclear mechanism:
  Milk-alkali syndrome
  Adrenal insufficiency
  Renal disease
    Chronic hemodialysis
    Renal transplantation
    Polyuric phase of acute renal failure

SOURCE: Reprinted with permission from Jubiz W: *Endocrinology: A Logical Approach for Clinicians.* New York: McGraw–Hill, 1979, p. 201.

Clinical Manifestations

The clinical symptoms and signs of hyperparathyroidism are related to involvement of the skeletal system, renal system, and hypercalcemia. Certain clients may also have asymptomatic hypercalcemia.

Skeletal symptoms and signs include bone and joint pain; pathological fractures of the spine, long bones, and ribs, which may lead to progressive kyphosis; bone cysts; giant-cell tumors of the jaw; hypermotility of the joints; and systemic decalcification of the skeletal system. Urinary tract manifestations include polydipsia and polyuria, "sand" or "gravel" in the urine, calcium phosphate or oxalate renal calculi, nephrocalcinosis, decreased glomerular filtration rate; decreased urine concentration, and secondary renal infection and obstruction that may lead to progressive renal failure and uremia.

Symptoms of hypercalcemia include anorexia, nausea, vomiting, and polydipsia. In addition, the client may have constipation, anemia, weight loss, and asthenia.

Other clinical manifestations of hyperparathyroidism include hypertension, hypotonia, paresthesia, easy fatigability, and depression of the reflexes. Clients may initially have peptic ulcers and pancreatitis (sometimes recurrent). Changes in the psyche include changes in mentation and personality, depression, apathy, mood swings, and even confusion and coma. Changes in the toenails and fingernails include increased thickening and ridging. Calcium deposits may be observed in the cornea (**band keratopathy**) and, in secondary hyperparathyroidism, in the soft tissues around the joints.

According to Muthe (1981), when renal calculi are the main pathological condition, bone changes tend not to occur. Conversely, when bone changes are the major symptom, renal calculi tend not to occur. One of the primary concerns in hyperparathyroidism is progressive renal damage from calcium deposits. This may result in hypertension and lead to death from uremia or congestive heart failure. Early detection and intervention are important, because renal lesions tend to progress, whereas bone lesions heal completely. Figure 43–3 depicts symptoms of hyperparathyroidism and hypercalcemia.

Hyperparathyroid crisis, although rare, may occur after a parathyroidectomy. The crisis is probably precipitated by the release of excessive amounts of PTH into the circulation during surgery. The symptoms and signs are those of acute hypercalcemia and include anorexia, nausea, vomiting, abdominal pain, weakness, polydipsia, dyspnea, and coma. Hyperparathyroid crisis is potentially life threatening and therefore should be reported immediately to the physician. Prompt intervention and careful observations are needed to restore the balance of calcium and phosphorus in the body.

The most common diagnostic tests used in the evaluation of hyperparathyroidism include measurements of serum and urinary levels of calcium and phosphorus, radioimmunoassays of PTH, assessment of serum alkaline phosphatase, and x-ray examination. In primary hyperparathyroidism, the serum calcium level is usually elevated; serum phosphorus level is low or normal; and urinary levels of calcium and phosphorus are elevated (hypercalciuria and hyperphosphaturia), respectively. The serum alkaline phosphate levels are elevated when clinical bone disease is present (approximately 25% of all cases). Elevated serum levels of PTH are also found. The ECG may show shortening of the Q–T interval.

X-ray examination may reveal the following findings if the skeletal system is involved (Muthe, 1981):

- Subperiosteal resorption of the bone (increased in the radial aspects of digits)
- Diffuse dimineralization and decalcification of the bones
- Bone cysts
- Loss of lamina dura of the teeth
- **Chondrocalcinosis** (calcification of the articular cartilage)
- Calculi in the urinary tract and nephrocalcinosis
- In secondary hyperparathyroidism, soft-tissue calcifications in the regions around the joints and in the blood vessels

Therapeutic Measures

The only treatment indicated for overt primary hyperparathyroidism is parathyroidectomy. Pharmacologic measures may be used to treat hypercalcemia, and medical

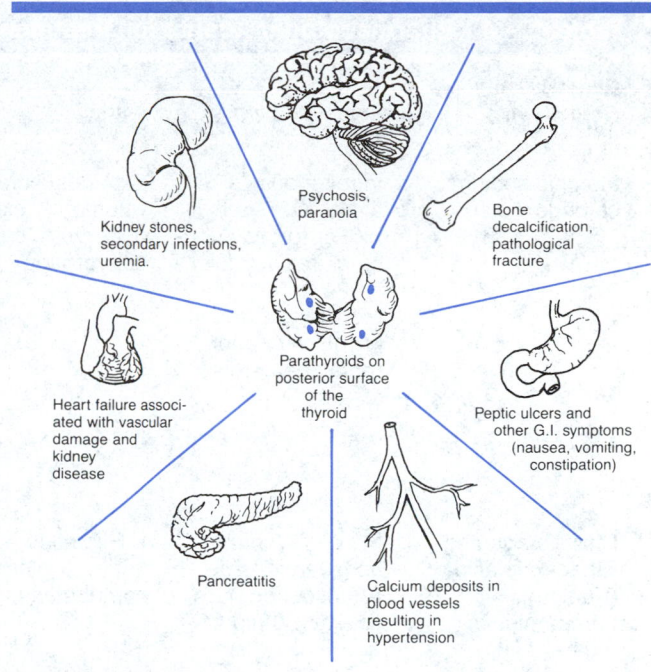

Figure 43–3

Symptoms of hyperparathyroidism and hypercalcemia.
SOURCE: Adapted from Muthe NC: *Endocrinology: A Nursing Approach.* Boston: Little, Brown, 1981.

measures to treat the mild hyperparathyroidism usually found by routine screening procedures. Table 43–4 summarizes the pharmacologic agents used in hypercalcemia. Medical measures in hyperparathyroidism are summarized in Box 43–6.

The surgical treatment of choice is subtotal parathyroidectomy. Sufficient residual tissue is left to preserve function (three glands and a portion of the fourth are resected). The goal of surgery is to remove all affected parathyroid tissue. Surgical intervention is especially indicated in clients with renal and bone involvement, pancreatitis, peptic ulcer, or possible malignancy.

Generally, the prognosis for clients with hyperparathyroidism is good if it is identified and treated surgically early in the course of the disease. In cases that are identified and treated later, the bone lesions generally will heal, but the renal involvement has been found to progress.

Specific Nursing Measures

Nursing approaches to the care of the client with hyperparathyroidism should address the potential for renal calculi, ulcers, pancreatitis, constipation, bone fractures, hypertension, depression, confusion, and changes in cognition.

Potential for Renal Calculi

The nurse should institute a strict, accurate intake and output record for all clients with hyperparathyroidism. In

Table 43-4 Pharmacologic Agents for Treatment of Hypercalcemia

Generic Name (Trade Name)	Administration	Action	Side Effects	Nursing Implications
Isotonic sodium chloride	Intravenous a. 1 L q. 4–6 h b. For forced diuresis: 6 L/q. 24 h (contraindicated in clients with poor renal and cardiac status)	Expands extracellular fluid volume; ↑ excess excretion of calcium; combats dehydration	Circulatory overload	Assess client closely for signs of circulatory overload and renal failure: • Keep strict, accurate I&O record (may be ordered hourly) • Record daily weight • Monitor serum electrolytes
Diuretic agents: Ethacrynic acid (Edecrin) Furosemide (Lasix)	PO q. 1–2 h; may be given in large IV doses: eg, furosemide 80 mg q. 1–2 h	↑ Excretion of calcium into urine; ↓ plasma calcium; contributes to forced diuresis	Also ↑ loss of Na, K, and Mg	As above
Phosphorus (Neutra-Phos, Neutra-Phos-K, Phos Tabs, Fleet's Phospho-Soda) (In-Phos, Hyper-Phos-K)	PO IV	↑ Serum phosphorus levels (to correct hypophosphatemia) and ↓ serum calcium levels by: a. ↑ Deposition of calcium in bone b. ↓ Absorption of calcium by GI tract	Precipitation of calcium-phosphate salts into soft tissues; hypocalcemia	Monitor serum electrolytes; report and record promptly all side effects
Mithramycin	IV as a single injection or as a 6–8-h continuous infusion	Inhibits bone resorption in areas where resorption is actively occurring; effects usually visible within 48 h	Thrombocytopenia; necrosis of the liver with ↑ LDH and SGOT and ↓ clotting factors; ↑ BUN; nausea and vomiting (Hoffmann & Newly, 1980); hypocalcemia	Monitor electrolytes (especially serum Ca); observe for signs of bleeding and report immediately; support during nausea and vomiting
Calcitonin-salmon (Calcimar)	IM or SC	Decreases rate of bone resorption; increases renal clearance of calcium and phosphorus; very expensive; found to be less effective in managing hyperparathyroidism than mithramycin and phosphorus	Fairly safe; clients may have mild nausea; local inflammatory reactions at injection site may occur	Monitor serum electrolytes; report and record promptly any untoward reactions

the absence of cardiac or renal contraindications, the daily fluid intake should be increased to approximately 3000 to 4000 mL to help prevent the formation of renal calculi. The urine may be strained for sediment, and the client should be carefully assessed for symptoms of urinary-tract infections and the presence of hematuria, which may occur asymptomatically. The diet should be low in calcium, and dairy products should be limited. A diet high in acid ash is recommended to acidify the urine and prevent the precipitation of calcium salts. Foods high in acid ash include cranberries, prunes, tomatoes, corn, asparagus, grapes, meats, poultry, fish, eggs, and cereal.

Potential for the Development of Ulcers, Pancreatitis, and Constipation

Be alert to the symptoms and signs of pancreatitis (epigastric and right-upper-quadrant pain, increased flatulence, nausea, vomiting, prostration) and peptic ulcers (epigastric pain that occurs an hour or two after meals or that awakens the client in the night, hematemesis, and

Box 43–6 Medical Measures for Treatment of Hyperparathyroidism

For mild hyperparathyroidism (relatively asymptomatic clients):
• Fluids are increased.
• Immobilization is avoided.
• Diuretics are given.
• If renal function is good, phosphorus is prescribed.
• If client is postmenopausal, estrogen is prescribed.

For hypercalcemic crisis (acute):
• IV fluids are increased to facilitate excretion of Ca.
• Phosphorus, calcitonin, mithramycin, sodium chloride, and/ or prednisone may be prescribed.

For hypercalcemia (subacute):
• Force fluids—3000 to 4000 mL/day (unless contraindicated by cardiac status)—to combat dehydration arising from severe nausea and vomiting and to prevent renal calculi by diluting calcium concentration.
• Keep accurate I&O record.
• Limit dietary calcium intake, especially of dairy products.
• Maintain an acid urine to prevent renal calculi and incidence of urinary tract infections (alkaline urine enhances precipitation of Ca salts); provide foods high in acid ash (eg, cranberries, prunes, tomatoes, corn, asparagus, grapes, meat, poultry, fish, eggs, and cereals).
• Hypercalcemia may be treated by peritoneal dialysis or hemodialysis, especially in hypercalcemic clients with severe kidney damage.

melena). Report and record them immediately. Ambulation should be encouraged unless contraindicated. Fluids should be encouraged and fiber added to the diet. Stool softeners may also be needed.

Potential for Fractures of the Bone
Hyperparathyroid clients with skeletal involvement should be assisted with ambulation because of the danger of pathological fractures. Bear in mind that safety is a prime concern and institute the proper procedures (keep the bed in the low position at all times with siderails up and assist with ambulation).

Potential for Changes in Cognitive Processes and for Depression
Because confusion, depression, paranoia and other mental problems are seen in clients with hyperparathyroidism, report any of these changes and support and reassure both client and significant others. Helpful interventions include organizing the environment to provide rest, a sense of security, and a minimum of disturbances as well as activities to promote interest and involvement.

Potential for Hypertension
Because the hypertension in hyperparathyroidism places an additional work load on the heart, carefully assess the client for any signs of cardiac damage or failure. Check vital signs periodically and report any abnormalities. Clients

receiving digitalis should be carefully monitored because hypercalcemia has been known to increase the toxicity of digitalis (Muthe, 1981).

HYPOPARATHYROIDISM

Hypoparathyroidism results from a deficiency in the secretion of PTH hormone or a decrease in the effectiveness of its action. It is characterized by the presence of low serum calcium levels, high serum phosphorus levels, normal levels of alkaline phosphatase, and negative urinary calcium. The most prominent feature of hypoparathyroidism is hypocalcemia. In its most severe form, it is called hypocalcemic tetany. This deficiency of calcium has the potential to affect the function of many bodily systems including the neuromuscular, cardiovascular, integumentary, and gastrointestinal systems. In addition, hypocalcemia may cause changes in the basal ganglia, cerebellum, and eyes (Muthe, 1981).

Remember there are other causes of hypocalcemia that do not involve PTH deficiencies. These include severe renal insufficiency, dietary inadequacies or malabsorption syndromes, insufficiency of vitamin D, and chronic diarrhea. Also remember the relation between vitamin D and calcium; adequate vitamin D is necessary for the proper absorption and utilization of calcium by the body.

Hypoparathyroidism may have iatrogenic or idiopathic causes. The iatrogenic causes of hypoparathyroidism include damage to the parathyroid glands from thyroid surgery; surgery for tumor of the parathyroid; or, rarely, irradiation of the neck or administration of large doses of iodine for cancer of the thyroid. Accidental removal of healthy parathyroid tissue, formation of scar tissue, injury, or compromise of blood supply to the parathyroid glands can result in either a temporary or permanent loss of function (Muthe, 1981).

Idiopathic hypoparathyroidism is thought to arise from either genetic predisposition or an autoimmune failure. Hypoparathyroidism is often seen in association with pernicious anemia and thyroiditis, both of which have an autoimmune component. Hypoparathyroidism is also seen in association with candidiasis and Addison's disease. The incidence of idiopathic hypoparathyroidism is higher in children than in adults.

Clinical Manifestations

Symptoms of hypoparathyroidism can appear suddenly or slowly. Hypoparathyroidism can be precipitated by infection, pregnancy, menses, surgery, or other physiological stresses to the body. Symptoms of acute hypoparathyroidism include muscle cramping, increased irritability, dyspnea, photophobia, diplopia, dysuria, abdominal cramping, nausea, vomiting, and diarrhea or constipation. Symptoms and signs of chronic hypoparathyroidism appear gradually and are often vague. They include increased lethargy, per-

Nursing Research Note

Long J, West G: The Olympic Trach-Button as an interim airway following tracheostomy tube removal. *Respiratory Care* 1981; 26(12):1269–1271.

This was a prospective study of 163 clients over 12 months who were in the process of tracheostomy tube removal and met criteria for Olympic Trach-Button placement. The study confirmed that the button did not cause problems or have important deficiencies. The device functioned well and was especially important for 15 subjects who had to have their tracheostomy tubes reinserted because of disease exacerbation. Without the button, those tracheostomies would have healed over, and new tracheostomies would have been necessary.

sonality changes (depression, agitation, psychosis, delirium), changes in mentation, anxiety, and blurring of vision.

Signs of hypoparathyroidism include convulsions, **carpopedal spasm,** wheezing, respiratory stridor, positive **Chvostek's sign** (twitching of the facial muscles when facial nerve is percussed), positive **Trousseau's sign** (carpopedal spasm with inability to open the hand when a blood pressure cuff is placed on the arm, elevated over the systolic reading, and left in place for 2 to 3 minutes), cataracts, thinness and brittleness of the nails, dryness and scaliness of the skin, increased incidence of candidiasis, loss of eyebrows and patchy alopecia of the scalp, and hyperactivity of the deep-tendon reflexes (secondary to increased neuromuscular excitability). In addition, if the hypoparathyroidism has occurred in childhood, abnormalities of the teeth may be noted.

The major clinical manifestations of acute hypocalcemic tetany include increasing anxiety, tingling in the hands and circumoral area, painful muscle spasms, facial spasms and grimaces, palpitations, and sometimes convulsions. A positive Chvostek's and Trousseau's sign may be present. Acute tetany may be associated with vocal cord paralysis

and may lead to respiratory obstruction. In this instance, the presence of stridor should alert the nurse to the need for possible emergency intervention (tracheostomy). Severe hypocalcemia may also precipitate heart failure. A positive Chvostek's sign may be seen in 10% of the normal population. Also, a positive Chvostek's and Trousseau's sign may be elicited in conditions other than hypocalcemia (eg, alkalotic states associated with primary aldosteronism and hyperventilation).

The diagnosis of hypoparathyroidism is based primarily on laboratory tests, supportive x-ray findings (calcifications in the basal ganglia and increased density of the long bones), and supportive changes in the eyes (early formation of cataracts) and ECG (prolongation of the Q–T interval). In addition, the ECG may show a generalized dysrhythmia that disappears with treatment if the etiology is hypocalcemia. Specific laboratory findings suggestive of hypoparathyroidism include low serum calcium levels, elevated serum phosphorus levels, normal serum levels of both alkaline phosphatase and magnesium, normal creatinine clearance, low or absent urinary calcium, and low or absent levels of serum PTH (by radioimmunoassay).

Therapeutic Measures

The therapeutic approach to both acute and chronic hypoparathyroidism employs both medical and dietary measures. Although treatment of acute hypothyroidism is usually fairly straightforward with good results, long-term treatment is often tedious and expensive for the client and family. Because no effective preparation of PTH is available, periodic assays of serum levels of calcium and phosphorus are required to provide an indicator of possible

Box 43–7   Medical Measures in Chronic Hypoparathyroidism

After the acute phase, the goal of medical treatment is to maintain a normal serum calcium level by means of drugs and diet.

Pharmacologic agents:
• Oral calcium salts
• Dihydrotachysterol
• Calciferol

High-calcium, low-phosphorus diet:
• Increase in milk and milk products (caution: may be restricted because of phosphorus levels)
• Egg yolk (may also be restricted because of high phosphorus levels)
• Green, leafy vegetables (turnip and dandelion greens; spinach avoided because of its oxalate content)

Box 43–8   Treatment of Acute Tetany

Patent airway

Calcium chloride 5 to 10 mL of a 10% solution IV given slowly

or

Calcium gluconate 10 to 20 mL of a 10% solution IV

Either calcium chloride or calcium gluconate may be added to 1 L of 5% D/W or N/S and given by slow IV drip

Oral calcium salts:
• Calcium gluconate
• Calcium lactate powder
• Calcium chloride
• Calcium carbonate (Os-Cal)

Calciferol (ergocalciferol, vitamin D_2) or dihydrotachysterol (an active metabolite of vitamin D)

Parathyroid hormone injection (for short-term use if absolutely necessary)

Phenytoin and phenobarbital (as adjunctive treatment)

Aluminum hydroxide gel (to lower serum phosphorus levels)

Table 43–5 Pharmacologic Agents for Treatment of Hypocalcemia

Generic Name (Trade Name)	Administration	Action	Side Effects	Nursing Implications
Calcium chloride ($CaCl_2$)	PO or IV (cannot be given IM); IV should be given slowly; 1 mL/min	Elevates serum calcium levels	PO irritating to the gastric mucosa; IV irritating to veins; may ↑ CHF and cause peripheral vasodilation	When given orally should be given with milk or meals; assess client at regular intervals for hypotension secondary to peripheral vasodilation; monitor pulse for irregularities in rate and rhythm; to enhance the effectiveness of calcium salts, teach client to use rebreathing bag; this ↑ acidosis, which results in an increase in the amount of ionized calcium in the serum
Calcium gluconate	PO, IM, IV	Drug of choice given IV in acute tetany	Give slowly as with $CaCl_2$; not irritating to the gastric mucosa	
Vitamin D (calciferol)	50,000 to 250,000 units per day	Promotes calcium absorption and excretion of phosphorus in large doses	Overdose can produce vitamin D toxicity associated with hypercalcemia	Monitor serum calcium levels
Dihydrotachysterol	PO	May be given instead of vitamin D; has similar action; faster	Same as for vitamin D	Monitor serum calcium and phosphorus levels closely; client should be aware of the need for frequent follow-up; use care in giving calcium salts in clients on digoxin, because calcium potentiates the toxic effects of digoxin
Parathyroid hormone (bovine PTH)	SC, IV 3–5 × q.d. (maximum duration of use: 1 week)	Promotes mobilization of calcium from bone; increases absorption of calcium from small bowel	Made from bovine parathyroid glands; sites of degradation and specific side effects unclear	Rarely used, even in acute tetany; giving calcium and vitamin D is much safer

overtreatment or undertreatment. Medical measures used in the treatment of chronic hypoparathyroidism are listed in Box 43–7. Pharmacological agents used in the treatment of hypocalcemia are summarized in Table 43–5. Treatment measures for acute tetany are given in Box 43–8.

Specific Nursing Measures

The nursing management of clients with hypoparathyroidism considers both acute and chronic situations. During the acute hypocalcemic state (tetany), the nurse should:

- Observe the client closely for symptoms and signs of laryngeal stridor and/or respiratory obstruction and report them immediately to the physician.
- Keep a tracheotomy tray and endotracheal setup at the bedside along with IV equipment.
- Institute seizure precautions (padded siderails, no pillow) and monitor the client closely for seizures.
- Make sure that anticonvulsive agents are readily available.
- Review and report serum calcium and phosphorus levels.

For the client with chronic hypoparathyroidism, important nursing responsibilities include client and family education regarding diet, goals of the medication regimen, and the need for frequent follow-up evaluation. In addition, because clients with chronic hypoparathyroidism often have symptoms involving both the integumentary and gastrointestinal systems, specific nursing measures should be directed toward these problems (eg, using lotions and emollients for dryness of the skin, increasing fiber and milk in the diet, and encouraging fluid intake to prevent constipation).

Disorders of the thyroid and parathyroids pose complex problems for clients and significant others. Acute dysfunction may be a threat to life; chronic dysfunction usually requires lifelong treatment and follow-up. Effective nursing interventions can do much to help the client and family not only to adjust to the disorder and its impact on their lives but also to improve the quality of their lives.

Section II: Infectious and Inflammatory Disorders

THYROIDITIS

Thyroiditis is an inflammation of the thyroid gland. The three major forms of this disorder are acute suppurative thyroiditis, subacute thyroiditis (also known as de Quervain's thyroiditis), and lymphadenoid goiter (or Hashimoto's thyroiditis). Thyroiditis can be acute, subacute, or chronic.

Acute Suppurative Thyroiditis

Acute suppurative thyroiditis, or bacterial thyroiditis, is usually triggered by staphylococci, pneumococci, or streptococci, which are transmitted to the thyroid from another site of infection in the body. This is a fairly rare disorder that is differentiated from primary pathology of the lymphatic system. The incidence is greatest in women between the ages of 50 and 60 (Kaye & Rose, 1983).

Subacute Thyroiditis

Subacute thyroiditis is thought to arise from an immune response to a viral infection because it often appears several weeks after a client has had a viral infection. This also is a fairly uncommon disorder seen three to four times more frequently in women between the ages of 25 and 50 years.

Hashimoto's Thyroiditis

Hashimoto's thyroiditis is thought to arise from an autoimmune response of the body. The incidence of this particular form of thyroiditis has been increasing over the past few years (Muthe, 1980). Kaye and Rose (1983) report that it now accounts for 90% of the cases of nontoxic diffuse goiter seen in children and 50% of those seen in adults. The incidence is greater in women between the ages of 20 and 50 than in men, and it tends to run in families; a positive family history is seen in 70% of diagnosed clients. Interestingly, the family histories of these clients also show a high incidence of Graves' disease. Hashimoto's thyroiditis can also be seen in clients with other diagnosed autoimmune diseases, such as rheumatoid arthritis, systemic lupus erythematosus, and Sjögren's syndrome.

Clinical Manifestations

The clinical symptoms and signs of acute suppurative thyroiditis, usually abrupt in onset, include:

- Fever
- Either localized or diffuse swelling over the thyroid with tenderness over the thyroid on palpation
- Pain radiating to the ears
- Localized erythema and increased warmth over the thyroid
- Dysphagia

The clinical symptoms and signs of subacute thyroiditis usually appear several weeks after a viral illness (eg, upper respiratory infection, influenza, mumps) and may begin as a persistent sore throat or earache. On palpation, the thyroid is found to be diffusely enlarged and mildly to moderately tender. Infrequently, a localized area of tenderness or a single nontender nodule may be identified. Kaye and Rose (1983) report that 10% to 20% of clients with subacute thyroiditis may have systemic symptoms and signs of hyperthyroidism (fever, tachycardia, severe dysphagia, chills, sweats, and headache). This is thought to result from the sudden release of large amounts of thyroid hormone from the inflamed cells.

In Hashimoto's thyroiditis there is usually a small to medium-sized goiter, especially nontender, with a firm, rubbery consistency on palpation. This goiter enlarges slowly, becoming firmer and more nodular. The enlargement occurs insidiously. Occasionally, a larger goiter compresses the trachea and esophagus, producing localized lymphadenopathy and hoarseness from involvement of the vocal cords.

The diagnosis of acute suppurative thyroiditis is made from a careful history and physical examination. Thyroid function studies are usually normal. If a thyroid scan is done, the suppurative area may show decreased function.

In mild cases of subacute thyroiditis, all laboratory studies may be within normal limits. In clients with moderate to severe inflammation, the following laboratory abnormalities may be seen (Kaye & Rose, 1983):

- Elevated sedimentation rate, mild leukocytosis, and mild anemia.

- Depression of the RAIU, except in localized disorders, in which instance the scan may show decreased uptake in the involved area.

- Early in the disease, increased levels of thyroid hormone and decreased ^{131}I uptake. This is followed in 2 to 4 weeks by a period of transient hypothyroidism characterized by a low level of serum T_4 or low-normal T_4 levels with continued suppression of ^{131}I. In this instance, the return of the ^{131}I uptake to normal ranges usually correlates with recovery.

- Low titers of thyroid antibodies in 50% to 60% of clients.

The diagnosis of Hashimoto's thyroiditis is also based on a careful history and physical examination, particularly the finding of a firm, diffusely enlarged goiter. Laboratory studies show:

- Normal T_4 and T_3 levels.
- Increased or normal RAIU levels.
- High titers of thyroid antibodies. In 30% to 50% of clients with Hashimoto's thyroiditis, however, the antibody tests are negative or very low.

In all forms of thyroiditis, a needle biopsy will provide a histologic diagnosis. Kaye & Rose (1983) report that differentiation among the various forms of thyroiditis based on clinical and laboratory tests without biopsy is accurate in only 70% to 80% of clients.

Therapeutic Measures

The therapeutic measures for thyroiditis depend on the clinical etiology. Approaches range from the use of antibiotics, to symptomatic support, to the use of thyroid hormone to reduce the size of the gland. Corticosteroids may be used in subacute and Hashimoto's thyroiditis to reduce the size of the gland. In rare instances, surgery may be needed to drain an abscess or reduce a large goiter.

Any of the complications of an acute infection may occur in clients with suppurative thyroiditis. Generally, subacute thyroiditis is a self-limiting disease that resolves in 1 or 2 months. The subacute form is often characterized by remissions and exacerbations; clients may have an initial transitory hyperthyroidism. Therapy is generally nonspecific. The prognosis for recovery is usually excellent. In Hashimoto's thyroiditis, permanent destruction of the thyroid cells may result in hypothyroidism in certain clients. Although the prognosis for clients with Hashimoto's thyroiditis is good, this condition has been associated with the later development of carcinoma and lymphoma of the thyroid.

Specific Nursing Measures

The nursing management of the client with thyroiditis largely depends on the type of thyroiditis involved. For the client with acute suppurative thyroiditis, the care is the same as for any client with an acute infection (eg, increased fluids and fever management). For the client with subacute or Hashimoto's thyroiditis, the nursing care depends on specific client problems and might include administration of analgesics, thyroid medications to reduce the size of the gland, or corticosteroids. The client may need preparation for surgery.

Section III: Neoplastic Disorders

BENIGN ADENOMAS OF THE THYROID

Adenomas are classified according to their histologic characteristics. The most common adenomas are papillary, follicular, and Hürthle cell.

These neoplasms usually are well encapsulated, mobile, and noninvasive; they grow slowly. The rest of the uninvolved thyroid remains normal. Follicular adenomas may retain their ability to produce thyroid hormone, and hyperthyroidism may occur when a large adenoma is present (greater than 3 cm). Clients with benign adenomas are usually clinically euthyroid, however.

CARCINOMAS OF THE THYROID

Carcinoma or malignancy of the thyroid is rare, accounting for fewer than 1% of all malignancies. The incidence is two times greater in women than in men. The average age at diagnosis is 45.

Thyroid cancer can be of four distinct types: papillary, follicular, medullary, and anaplastic carcinoma. These cancer types vary in their degree of malignancy. It is also possible to have metastatic malignancies in the thyroid from other parts of the body. Thyroid carcinoma has been postulated to result from excessive long-standing stimulation by pituitary TSH, seen especially in clients with thyroiditis and certain types of goiter. High levels of TSH have been

reported in clients with thyroid cancer (Muthe, 1981). Persons who received x-ray to the head, neck, or upper mediastinum in infancy or childhood are at risk for thyroid carcinoma later in life.

Clinical Manifestations

Thyroid carcinoma usually presents as a painless, hard, fixed, irregular nodule on the thyroid. The client is usually clinically euthyroid and essentially asymptomatic at onset. As the tumor progresses, the client may experience pressure symptoms such as hoarseness, dyspnea, or vocal cord paralysis. Progression is usually slow, although some types grow rapidly. Metastasis does not often occur; if present, it is usually to the adjacent lymphatic structures, the lungs, or the bones. Certain factors suggest the possibility that a nodule may be carcinoma:

- Age of client is under 40
- Solitary nodule, rapidly progressive
- History of therapeutic radiation to the head, neck, or upper mediastinum (as seen in childhood treatment of enlarged tonsils, acne vulgaris, or treatment of disorders of the thymus)
- Development of secondary symptoms of hoarseness, paralysis of the vocal cords, or enlargement of the lymph glands

- No change or an increase in the size of the nodule after treatment with a 12-week course of thyroid hormone
- Nonfunctioning or "cold nodule" on thyroid scan

Table 43–6 differentiates among the various forms of carcinoma according to incidence, distinguishing characteristics, and prognosis.

A major diagnostic test in the evaluation of neoplasms of the thyroid is the thyroid scan, which is used to differentiate between "hot" (functioning) and "cold" (nonfunc-tioning) nodules. Although this test is frequently used, its results are not definitive because the most common cause of cold nodules is not neoplasm but benign thyroid lesions (cysts, goiter, or benign adenomas). In addition, only one out of every five "cold nodules" on scan is malignant.

The use of needle biopsy in diagnosis is controversial. Some practitioners consider it valuable in diagnosing thyroiditis and identifying carcinoma. Others cite specific problems with the technique; eg, the needle may miss questionable tissue or may not remove sufficient specimen for a thorough pathological analysis, and the technique may

Table 43–6 Classification of Carcinoma of the Thyroid

Type	Incidence	Distinguishing Characteristics	Prognosis
Papillary carcinoma	↑ In clients under the age of 40; more common in women under 40; accounts for 50% of all cases of carcinoma of thyroid and for 75% of carcinoma of thyroid seen in children	Slow growing; ↑ incidence in young adults with past history of irradiation to face, neck, or chest; may metastasize to regional lymph nodes; distant metastases are rare; tumor will not concentrate radioactive iodine or respond to suppression therapy	Excellent with early recognition and treatment; in papillary and follicular carcinoma, survival may exceed 80% at 10 years after diagnosis
Follicular carcinoma	Accounts for 25% of all thyroid carcinomas; ↑ in clients between 40 and 60 years of age; more common in women	More malignant than papillary carcinoma; has a tendency for hematogenous spread resulting in metastases to lung, liver, and bone; tumor will take up and concentrate radioactive iodine; rarely, tumor will also synthesize thyroid hormone, so thyrotoxicosis may occur if lesion is very large	Good
Medullary carcinoma	Accounts for 5%–10% of all thyroid carcinoma; may be caused by an autosomal dominant gene; ↑ in clients between age of 40 and 60; 56% of clients are women	Degree of malignancy lies between follicular and anaplastic types; tumor secretes calcitonin, which can be used to identify clients, follow the results of treatment, and screen family members; spreads by lymphatic channels to adjacent lymph nodes; may metastasize to lung and liver; does not concentrate radioactive iodine; may be associated with hyperparathyroidism, pheochromocytoma, and mucosal neuromas; may also produce certain ectopic hormones such as ACTH, prostaglandins, and serotonin	Poor
Anaplastic carcinoma	Accounts for 10% of all thyroid malignancies; ↑ over the age of 50; slightly more common in women	Rapidly growing tumor with metastasis throughout body; may present as a neck mass that is painful and tender; early involvement of adjacent structures may cause dysphagia, hoarseness, respiratory obstruction, and deviation of the trachea; mass usually hard and fixed; metastases to brain, liver, and lung; tumor does not concentrate radioactive iodine	Very poor; 75% of all clients die within 3 to 6 months

spread the malignancy to uninvolved tissue. Opponents of needle biopsy recommend surgical excision of the node with pathological examination. The use of thyroid echograms in the evaluation of cystic thyroid nodules is still under evaluation.

All thyroid function laboratory tests are usually normal unless thyroiditis or a hyperfunctioning nodule is present. Serum thyroglobulin levels may be elevated in clients with thyroid carcinomas and have been found to correlate with the presence of metastases. Return to normal values following thyroidectomy has suggested to researchers that thyroglobulin levels may be of value in the initial evaluation of all clients with thyroid nodules. Elevations of serum

thyrocalcitonin are found in medullary thyroid carcinoma, especially in the familial form. Figure 43–4 summarizes the recommended approaches to the evaluation of clients with thyroid nodules.

Therapeutic Measures

The approach to treatment of thyroid neoplasms depends on their cause. The main concern is the diagnosis of a client with a single thyroid nodule. For clients with thyroid carcinoma, the approach to treatment must consider the type of tumor, presence of metastases, client's age, and the ability of the tumor to take up radioactive iodine.

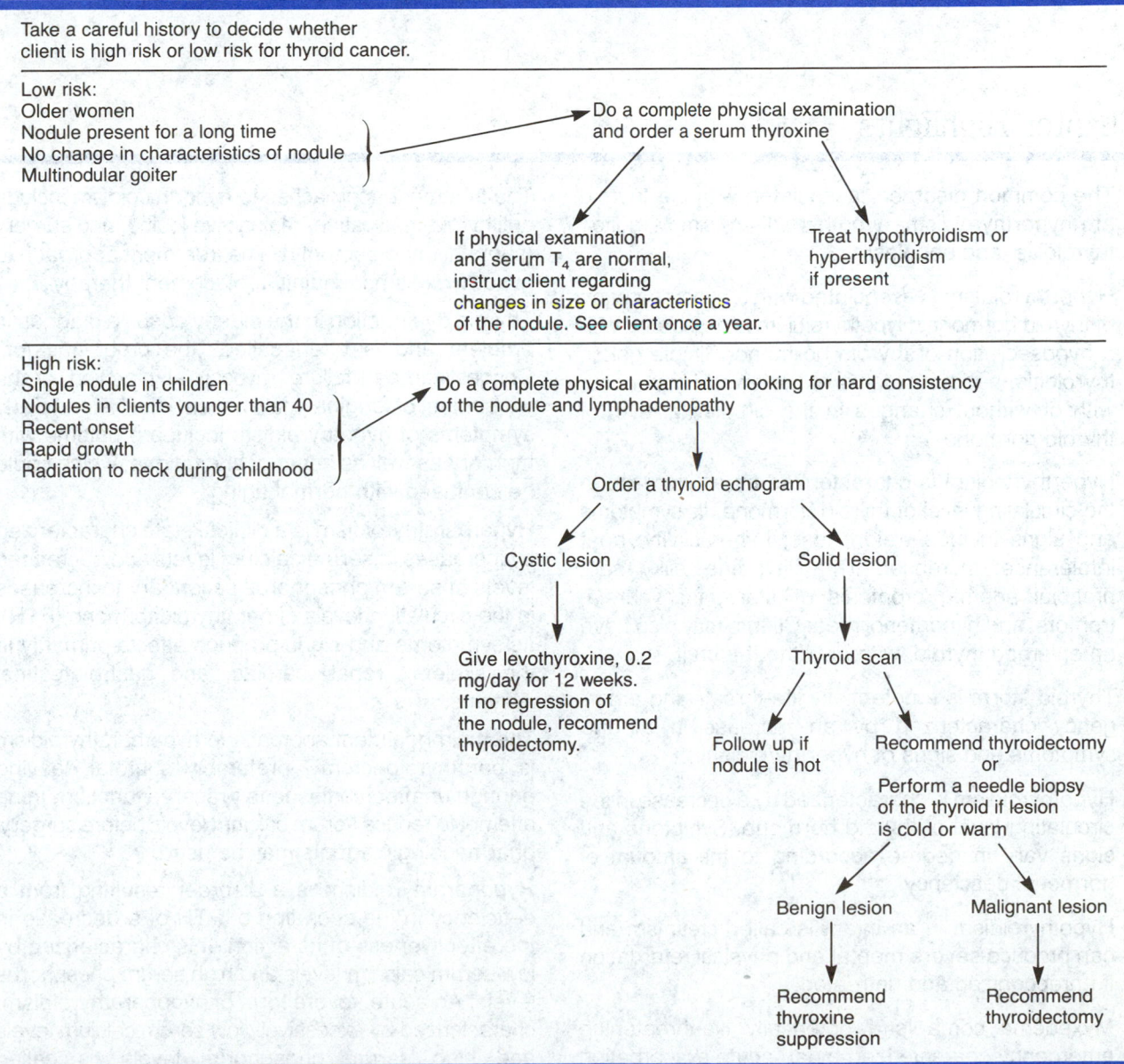

Figure 43–4

Recommended diagnostic, medical, and surgical approaches to the evaluation of clients with thyroid nodules.
SOURCE: Jubiz W: *Endocrinology: A Logical Approach for Clinicians.* New York: McGraw–Hill, 1979.

For benign nodules in clients at low risk for thyroid carcinoma, thyroid suppression may be started with re-evaluations at 3-month intervals. If after 6 months, there is evidence of further growth of the nodule, the client may be referred for surgical excision.

For clients at low risk for thyroid carcinoma who are clinically euthyroid and asymptomatic, close observation for changes in the size or characteristics of the nodule may be all that is indicated. For clients with thyroid cysts, thyroid suppression is started with aspiration of the cysts at 1- to 3-month intervals (Kaye & Rose, 1983). Surgical excision is usually performed if the cyst recurs after the third aspiration.

Surgical approaches in thyroid carcinoma may include total thyroidectomy with or without radical neck dissection or removal of the affected lobe and isthmus. Hypoparathy-roidism and vocal cord paralysis can occur following approaches involving radical neck dissection.

Thyroid-suppressive therapy may be used in papillary tumors or postoperatively to keep T_4 in a normal range and to suppress TSH. Radioactive iodine has been used with follicular tumors and in treatment of functioning metastases.

Specific Nursing Measures

The nursing care of the client with neoplasms of the thyroid involves the same considerations as care of the client following thyroid surgery (Chapter 45). If the client has a diagnosis of carcinoma, the nurse should recognize its implications for both the client and family.

Chapter Highlights

The common disorders associated with the thyroid are hyperthyroidism, hypothyroidism, simple goiter, thyroiditis, and neoplasms.

Hyperthyroidism is associated with a hypersecretion of thyroid hormone. Hypothyroidism is associated with a hyposecretion of thyroid hormone. Simple goiter, thyroiditis, and neoplasms of the thyroid may occur with or without changes in the circulating level of thyroid hormone.

Hyperthyroidism is characterized by an increase in the circulating level of thyroid hormone. Its symptoms and signs include weight loss; hyperactivity; heat intolerance; increased irritability; fine, silky hair; pretibial edema; proptosis or stare; tachycardia; tremors; and hypomenorrhea. Clients may also have an enlarged thyroid, with or without a bruit.

Thyroid storm is a potentially life-threatening emergency characterized by an increase in all the symptoms and signs of hyperthyroidism.

Hypothyroidism is characterized by a decrease in the circulating level of thyroid hormone. Symptons and signs vary in degree according to the amount of hormonal deficiency.

Hypothyroidism in an infant is called cretinism and can produce severe mental and physical retardation if unrecognized and untreated.

Myxedema coma is a potentially life-threatening emergency characterized by an acute exacerbation of all the symptoms and signs of hypothyroidism.

The treatment approaches to hyperthyroidism include antithyroid medication, radioactive iodine, and surgery (subtotal thyroidectomy). The treatment approach to hypothyroidism is mainly replacement therapy.

Thyroid dysfunction in the elderly poses a diagnostic problem and is often called "the great imitator." Congestive heart failure, myocardial infarction, or the worsening of angina may be an initial sign. Early symptoms of hypothyroidism include problems with memory as well as lethargy and fatigue, which could be confused with normal aging.

Hyperparathyroidism is a clinical state characterized by increases in serum calcium levels and decreased levels of serum phosphorus secondary to increases in the circulating levels of parathyroidhormone (PTH). Its symptoms and signs produce effects primarily in the skeletal, renal, cardiac, and gastrointestinal systems.

The main treatment approach to hyperparathyroidism is parathyroidectomy, preferably subtotal, leaving enough unaffected tissue to preserve function. In an attempt to reduce serum calcium levels before surgery, pharmacologic agents may be used.

Hypoparathyroidism is a disorder resulting from a deficiency in the secretion of PTH or a decrease in the effectiveness of its action. It is characterized by low serum calcium levels and high serum phosphorus levels. An acute severe form of hypoparathyroidism, characterized by excessively low serum calcium levels and high serum phosphorus levels, is called hypocalcemic tetany and is potentially life-threatening.

Hypoparathyroidism is most often secondary to thyroid disease. Symptoms and signs of acute hypoparathyroidism include muscle cramping, nausea, vomiting, abdominal cramping, increasing lethargy, and personality changes. Tetany is characterized by increasing anxiety, respiratory obstruction, painful muscle spasms, tingling in the hands and circumoral area, palpitations, and possible convulsions.

The main treatment approaches to hypoparathyroidism are pharmacological and dietary. The overall goal is to maintain the serum calcium levels and prevent further complications.

Three possible causes of enlargement of the thyroid gland are goiter, thyroiditis, and neoplasm (both benign and malignant).

Bibliography

Bates B: *A Guide to the Physical Examination,* 3rd ed. Philadelphia: Lippincott, 1983.

Evangeslistic JT, Thorpe CJ: Thyroid storm: A nursing crisis. *Heart Lung* 1983; 12:184–193.

Grimes J, Iannopollo E: *Health Assessment in Nursing Practice.* Monterey, CA: Wadsworth, 1982.

Hahn AB et al: *Pharmacology in Nursing,* 15th ed. St. Louis: Mosby, 1982.

Hoffmann JJ, Newly TB: Hypercalcemia in primary hyperparathyroidism. *Nurs Clin North Am* 1980; 15(3):469–480.

Honigman RE: Deciphering diagnostic studies: Thyroid function tests. *Nurs 82* (April) 1982; 12:68–71.

Jenkins EH: Living with thyrotoxicosis. *Am J Nurs* 1980; 80:956–958.

Jubiz W: *Endocrinology: A Logical Approach for Clinicians.* New York: McGraw–Hill, 1979.

Kaye D, Rose LF (editors): *Fundamentals of Internal Medicine.* St. Louis: Mosby, 1983.

Musante–Wake M, Brensinger JF: The nurse's role in hypothyroidism. *Nurs Clin North Am* 1980; 15(3):453–467.

Muthe NC: *Endocrinology: A Nursing Approach.* Boston: Little, Brown, 1981.

Saxton DF et al: *The Addison–Wesley Manual of Nursing Practice.* Menlo Park, CA: Addison–Wesley, 1983.

Sharkey PL, Myer DA: Hyperthyroidism. *Critical Care Update* 1981; 8(5):12–15, 17–19, 22–24.

Wartofsky L: Guidelines for the treatment of hyperthyroidism. *Am Fam Physician* (July) 1984; 30:199–210.

Williams RH (editor): *Textbook of Endocrinology,* 6th ed. Philadelphia: Saunders, 1981.

The Client With Hyperthyroidism

I. Descriptive Data	Mrs Janine Figoerella, age 42, was referred to the endocrine clinic of the university teaching hospital by an occupational health nurse at her place of employment. This is her first visit to the facility, and she is somewhat anxious.
II. Personal Data	
Date and Time:	March 16, 1986, 11:30 AM
Full Name:	Janine A. Figoerella
Address:	14 Deurtt Ave., Detroit, MI
Telephone:	Home: 000-0000
	Work: 000-0000, ext 714
Sex:	Female
Age:	42
Birthdate:	6-8-43
Marital Status:	Married
Race:	Caucasian
Culture:	Italian—American
Religion:	Catholic
Occupation:	Secretary
Usual Health Care Provider:	Leonard Hyzy, MD, who retired from his practice several years ago; she has not found another care provider, nor had need of one until now.
III. Health History	
Source of Information:	Client
Reliability of Informant:	Reliable
Chief Concern:	"Nervousness and insomnia for 6 months, increasing in severity."
History of Present Illness:	Client states that for the past 6 months she has experienced increasing nervousness and anxiety with frequent verbal outbursts and crying spells. She also has had a difficult time getting to sleep. States family and associates have commented on her irritability and weight loss (17 lb despite an enormous appetite and abundant food intake) as well as her eyes, which she describes as "looking like they're popping out of my head." She first began to notice the changed appearance of her eyes 3 to 4 months ago and feels they are definitely becoming more prominent. She also feels her neck has increased in size. No headache, changes in visual acuity, diplopia, seizures, or blackouts. No sore throat, swollen glands, neck pain. Feels home and work environments are not unusually stressful; family and peer relationships generally good but strained by her outbursts and anxiety. She does not have polyuria, polydipsia, abdominal or epigastric pain, nausea, or change in character of stool.
	This is the first occurrence of these symptoms for this client. She has no history of major health problems and takes no medications. She has never been treated for mental health problems.
Past Health History:	
Childhood:	Rheumatic fever, pertussis
Immunizations:	Basic series complete; tetanus booster, 1980
Medical Problems:	Pneumonia 1968, not hospitalized; recurrent low back pain since fall on ice in 1974
Surgeries:	T&A, 1950; tubal ligation, 1979

Case Study written by Anne Herrstrom Skelly.

Transfusions:	None
Special Diagnostic Procedures:	X-ray of the lumbo-sacral spine, 1974; no pathology
Trauma:	Fall on ice, winter 1974 c̄ injury to L-S spine
Allergies:	None
Medications:	Sominex, ṫ to ṫ q. H.S. for sleeplessness; takes no other medications
Family History:	Father, age 73, S/P MI, ASHD
	Mother, died age 51, automobile accident
	No siblings
	Husband, age 48, A&W
	Daughters, ages 18 & 20, A&W
	MGF, Ca bowel, maternal aunt, thyroid disorder. No known family history of CVA, ↑ BP, TBC, DM
Personal/Social History:	The client resides with her husband of 20 years and two teenage daughters, ages 20 and 18. She has been employed as a secretary in the office of a nearby developmental center for 7 years and expresses enthusiasm for her job and a liking for the developmentally disabled children she comes in contact with. Usual daily schedule: arises at 6:30 AM; works from 8 AM to 4 PM; arrives home around 4:45 PM; fixes dinner and spends evening at home, usually doing household chores. One night a week she bowls with team from developmental center. On weekend, attends church and on Sunday, usually has father and in-laws over to house for dinner and visiting. Occasionally, on weekend will go out with husband for dinner and a movie. Feels she no longer enjoys herself because of her "nerves."
	She is a high school graduate and has a 2-year degree from Bryant and Stratton Business Institute. She worked as a secretary for a produce firm for 13 years before taking her current position. She has never traveled outside of North America.
Habits:	She eats three to six meals daily to combat weight loss; enjoys bowling and uses her exercise bicycle about three times a week; has never used drugs; has an occasional mixed drink on weekends; smokes one pack of cigarettes per day × 22 years (22 pack years); has no desire to quit, although her husband and children have been urging her to.
	Has had difficulty getting to sleep at night for 6 to 7 months; sleeps 3 to 5 hours with much tossing and turning; does not have nightmares or early morning wakening; has "lost interest in sex" since "trouble with nerves"; intercourse one to two times monthly, usually without orgasm.
	She and her husband are practicing Roman Catholics and attend mass regularly. They have no major financial concerns. She feels she has good support systems. Her symptoms are worrisome to her; she feels she must be having a nervous breakdown because of her inability to control her emotions. She also verbalizes fear of a brain tumor.
Review of Systems:	
General Health:	Extremely fatigued; states, "I just know there's something terrible wrong with me."
Skin:	Has noted increased perspiration; hair has become finer
Eyes:	See HPI
Neck:	See HPI

(continued)

The Client With Hyperthyroidism

Chest:	No DOE, no PND, occasional smoker's cough
Heart:	No chest pain; recently has had several episodes of palpitations
Gastrointestinal:	Increased frequency of stool (two to three times daily), brown in color, soft
Gynecologic:	LMP 3-1-86, 31-day cycle; flow used to be heavy and continue for 3 to 5 days; for past 5 months, has had a very light flow that lasts only 1 to 2 days
Neurologic:	Has noted tremors of her fingers, which she never had before

IV. Physical Assessment

Height:	5 ft 7 in
Weight:	108 lb (weight 6 months ago 125 lb)
Vital Signs:	BP 160/70 supine rt arm; seated 162/68; apical rate 104 and regular; T, 99.8°F (37.6°C); R, 22
Relevant Organ Systems:	
Skin/Hair:	Bodily skin very smooth with increased warmth; scalp hair fine and silky; skin feels moist to touch; ō lesions; ō excoriations
Eyes:	Eyebrows silky and fine; conjunctivae pink; sclerae white; PERRLA c̄ mild degree of difficulty with convergence; bilateral proptosis, symmetrical; ⊕ lid-lag; fundi: disk margins flat and distinct; A-V ratio 2:3, ō H or E, OU
Neck:	Carotids 2 + and equal s̄ bruits; ō lymphadenopathy; thyroid, soft, diffusely enlarged, no bruits, nontender, ō nodules
Heart:	Rate 104 and regular with soft grade I–II/VI early systolic murmur heard best at apex to LSB; ō gallops
Lungs:	Clear to A & P, ō rales, rhonchi, or wheezes
Extremities:	1 +, nonpitting edema noted bilaterally in pretibial areas, ⊖ Homans' sign; ō erythema; ō warmth; all pulses 2 + and symmetrical
Neurologic:	
Mental Status:	Demonstrates difficulty concentrating on tasks, decreased attention span
Motor-sensory:	Fine tremors of fingers and tongue
Cranial Nerves II–XII:	Intact
Cerebellum:	Intact
Reflexes:	

V. Diagnostic Data	Mrs Figoerella was admitted to the hospital and scheduled to have a series of tests. The results are as follows:
ECG:	Tachycardia; normal sinus rhythm
Chest X-ray:	wnl
T$_4$:	13 μg/dL (norm: 4 to 12 μg/dL)
T$_3$ Uptake:	Increased, indicating hyperfunctioning
RAIU Thyroid Scan:	Shows increased uptake by gland with an early peak

  Mrs Figoerella was diagnosed as having hyperthyroidism (Graves' disease).

VI. Nursing Care Plan

Nursing Diagnosis	Client Care Goals	Plan/Nursing Implementation	Expected Outcomes
Comfort, alteration in, related to heat intolerance, diaphoresis, and exophthalmos	Maintain client comfort; prevent skin and eye complications	*If diaphoretic:* Change bed linen frequently; provide linen and sleepwear light in weight; frequent sponge baths; attention to bony prominences; observe for signs of skin breakdown and treat immediately; keep room temperature cool *For exophthalmos:* Elevate head of bed to relieve periorbital edema; methylcellulose drops (0.5% to 1%) to alleviate dryness of conjunctiva and cornea as ordered; for severe proptosis, lids may be taped shut during sleep or sleep mask provided; room lighting should be lowered; minimize glare; provide sunglasses if light is bright or client goes outdoors in sunlight	Will experience comfort and relief from diaphoresis and proptotic symptoms; no signs of skin breakdown
Sleep pattern disturbance, related to insomnia and hyperactivity	Obtain sufficient rest to reduce fatigue	Restrict activities to provide for maximum rest and to alleviate fatigue; explain limitations and rationale to client and family; manipulate environment to decrease excessive stimulation (room temperature, lighting, numbers of visitors, radio, television); schedule rest periods between periods of activity; refer to occupational therapy or recreational therapy for diversion; provide sedation as ordered	Client will not be excessively fatigued; will sleep restfully
Nutrition, alterations in, related to polyphagia and weight loss	Maintain adequate nutritional status	Weight daily or q. 2 days; diet up to 4000 to 5000 calories per day; diet high in protein and carbohydrate; low in fiber; restrict caffeine; provide snacks between meals and at bedtime; frequently assess visual acuity and measurements of EOMs	Client's weight will remain stable
Coping, ineffective individual	Maintain minimal exposure to internal and external stressors	Create as calm an environment as possible; decrease external stimuli; provide consistency in caretakers; establish a routine with as little change as possible; provide private room if needed; visitors should be screened and family education provided to avoid topics that will produce anxiety in the client; provide an opportunity for client and family to discuss their concerns and fears; provide client and family education regarding the physiological and psychological changes in the client; provide support and reassurance to client and family	Client will experience minimal anxiety
Elimination, alterations in, related to fluid loss and increased metabolic rate	Maintain adequate fluid–electrolyte balance	Increase fluid intake to 4000 mL/day (unless there are cardiac or renal contraindications); monitor intake and output; explain to client and family the need for additional fluids; monitor serum electrolytes and urine values	Client will not experience any deficits in fluid volume: No signs of dehydration; specific gravity of urine will remain in normal range; serum electrolytes will remain in normal range

(continued)

The Client With Hyperthyroidism

VI. Nursing Care Plan (continued)

Nursing Diagnosis	Client Care Goals	Plan/Nursing Implementation	Expected Outcomes
Injury: potential for, related to infection, stress, surgery	Prevent severe thyroid storm or crisis	Assess client regularly for indications of thyroid storm: Marked restlessness and anxiety; fever (104°F to 106°F); extreme tachycardia (130 to 160 beats per minute); dehydration; nausea and vomiting; diarrhea; delirium and psychosis; report these immediately to physician; educate client and family about these symptoms and signs	Symptoms and signs of thyroid crisis will be recognized and treated immediately; severe thyroid storm or crisis will be prevented
Knowledge deficit, related to hyperthyroidism	Explain the disease and its treatment clearly and accurately	Review hyperthyroidism with client and family or significant others including: Symptoms and signs of both hyperthyroidism and hypothyroidism; effects of increased thyroxine production in the body; the treatment regimen and its purposes; name, dosage, action, and side effect of each medication; dietary management; need for regular medical supervision and its purpose; date and time of next medical appointment; what to report to the physician; telephone number where client or family can call with questions	Client and family will understand hyperthyroidism and its management

Chapter 44

Specific Disorders of the Pituitary and Adrenal Glands

Anne Herrstrom Skelly

Objectives

When you have finished studying this chapter, you should be able to:

Identify the common disorders of the pituitary and adrenal glands.

Describe the clinical manifestations of disorders of the pituitary and adrenal glands.

Identify therapeutic measures specific to disorders of the pituitary and adrenal glands.

Specify the common drugs used in treating adrenal and pituitary disorders and discuss their potential side effects.

Explain the specific nursing interventions for clients with problems of the pituitary and adrenal glands.

Anticipate the temporary or permanent lifestyle modifications frequently necessary for clients with problems involving the pituitary and adrenal glands.

Discuss the psychosocial/lifestyle implications of pituitary and adrenal dysfunction for the client and significant others and outline specific nursing interventions to address their needs.

Because of the complex actions of the pituitary and adrenal glands, as well as their interaction with each other and with other bodily systems, their dysfunctions have a variety of causes and clinical manifestations. The nursing process will assist the nurse in understanding and caring for clients with disorders of the pituitary and adrenal glands.

Section I: Disorders of Multifactorial Origin

Among the pituitary disorders of multifactorial origin are pituitary dwarfism, panhypopituitarism (Simmonds' disease), diabetes insipidus, and the syndrome of inappropriate antidiuretic hormone (SIADH). Adrenal disorders in this category are Cushing's syndrome and Addison's disease.

PITUITARY DISORDERS
Pituitary Dwarfism

The causes of excessively short stature in children include growth hormone deficiency of unknown origin, craniopharyngiomas that directly invade the pituitary, nonre-

sponsiveness of peripheral tissues to growth hormone (GH) (seen in African pygmies and Turner's syndrome), and systemic diseases associated with shortness of stature (eg, chronic renal insufficiency, congenital cyanotic heart disease, and juvenile hypothyroidism).

Deficiency or undersecretion of GH that can cause dwarfism is usually *not* apparent at birth, because growth during fetal life is not dependent on GH. Deficiency is suspected when there is an abnormality in growth later in childhood (ages 2 to 4 years). The usual presentation is excessively short stature. The actual frequency of dwarfism due to a deficiency of GH is not known, yet deficiency of endocrine hormones is thought to be the least common cause of dwarfism (Muthe, 1981). Many instances of undiagnosed conditions of short stature are thought to result from mild deficiencies of GH. Deficiencies of GH resulting in pituitary dwarfism are also thought to result from an undersecretion of GH releasing factor or from an oversecretion by the hypothalamus of the growth hormone inhibitor, somatostatin.

Thirty-three percent of clients with pituitary dwarfism have nonsecreting pituitary tumors and craniopharyngiomas. A high percentage of the other cases are idiopathic. These individuals have no identifiable pathology (sella turcica is normal); familial genetic traits and birth injury are thought to be implicated (Muthe, 1981). Boys seem to be affected twice as frequently as girls.

Clinical Manifestations

There may be a positive family history of dwarfism. The client's general health is usually good, although some may be subject to hypoglycemia and diabetes insipidus. The client may experience a deficiency of other pituitary hormones as well.

The client's height is three to four standard deviations below the mean for chronological age. The mental development is usually normal, but facial and body proportions are childish: the face is often pudgy and doll-like with fine wrinkling of the skin; the body, though small, is normally formed. Sexual maturity may or may not be normal. Figure 44–1 shows a 6-year-old girl with hyposomatotropic dwarfism before and after treatment.

Therapeutic Measures

The treatment of pituitary dwarfism with human growth hormone is initiated in childhood. Early recognition and referral are important. Many children who are adequately treated develop into normal-sized adults.

Specific Nursing Measures

Nursing interventions in an adult with pituitary dwarfism should address emotional support and health education. Provide opportunities for the client to express thoughts and feelings about body appearance and sexual functioning.

Dwarfism poses many problems for clients. Besides having to deal with threats to body image and self-esteem, their size forces them to face a series of adjustments in the activities of daily life. Clothes must be tailor-made; normal-sized furniture is often uncomfortable, fairly inaccessible, and often hazardous. Equipment designed for use by adults of average height may be uncomfortable or even unusable for the dwarf. Medications and dosages of contrast media must often be calculated according to body size (as in pediatrics). Because of their small proportions, many of these clients are treated as children and may respond accordingly in their behavior.

Teach clients receiving therapy for a deficiency of other hormones the name of the drug, dosage, action, and possible side effects. Clients should also be familiar with the symptoms of overdosage and underdosage of these hormones. Teach them what symptoms to report to the physician and encourage them to carry an identification card or bracelet.

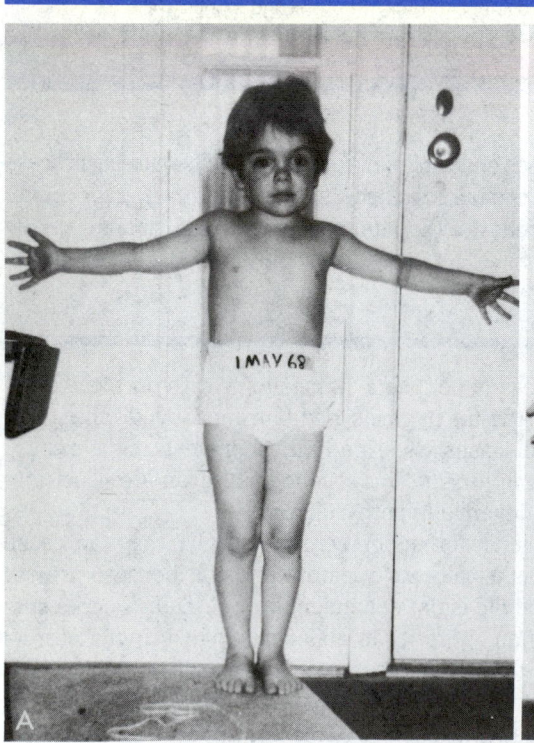
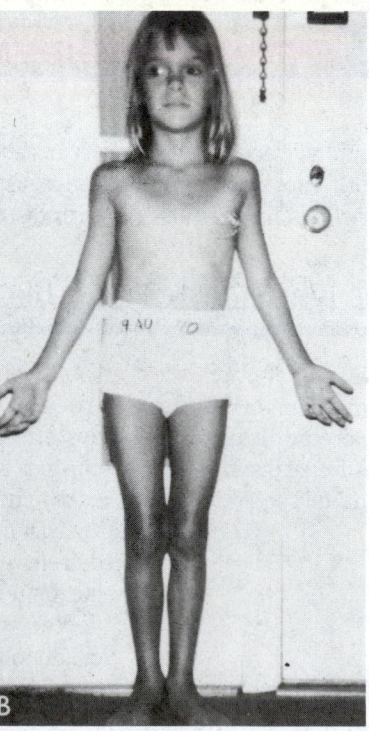

Figure 44–1

A. A six-year-old girl with hyposomatotropic dwarfism secondary to a craniopharyngioma. **B.** After treatment for 2 years.

SOURCE: Williams R: *Textbook of Endocrinology*, 6th ed. Philadelphia: Saunders, 1981, p. 98.

Panhypopituitarism

Panhypopituitarism (Simmond's disease) is characterized by a deficiency of all the hormones of the anterior pituitary. For this to occur, 75% to 90% of the pituitary must be destroyed (Muthe, 1981). Total deficiency of all adenohypophyseal hormones without replacement is fatal.

Primary tumors of the pituitary (craniopharyngioma, adenoma of the chromophobe cells, and eosinophilic adenomas) are one cause of panhypopituitarism. These nonsecreting tumors destroy healthy secreting cells as they enlarge, resulting in hyposecretion of the anterior pituitary hormones. Other etiologies include Sheehan's syndrome (thrombosis of the hypophyseal vessels sometimes associated with postpartum shock); vascular abnormalities (aneurysms, sickle cell anemia, cavernous sinus thrombosis); metastatic tumors; infiltrative and granulomatous disease; hypothalamic dysfunction (causing secondary hypopituitarism); infectious processes; and iatrogenic factors, including surgical and radiological ablative procedures.

Sheehan's syndrome remains the major cause of non-neoplastic spontaneous hypopituitarism in women. In cases of Simmond's disease arising from tumor, infarct, or infection, usually some hormonal function is preserved, and the resulting symptoms are not as severe. In surgical hypophysectomy, the total loss of hormonal production results in deficiencies of gonadotropins, somatotropin, thyrotropin, corticotropin, and prolactin (the latter only in postpartum necrosis of the pituitary). As the amount of destruction of the pituitary increases, the clinical signs of these deficiencies appear.

Clinical Manifestations

The clinical manifestations of panhypopituitarism are related to the multiple hormonal deficiencies and present a wide range of subjective and objective findings. The lack of stimulation by the anterior pituitary causes atrophy in the thyroid, adrenals, and gonads, which results in an undersecretion of their hormones as well.

Findings of panhypopituitarism obtained during the health history may include symptoms of hypothyroidism (intolerance to cold; subnormal body temperature; and changes in the texture of the skin, hair, and nails). Symptoms of gonadal deficiency such as changes in libido, impotence, atrophy of the penis and testes occur in men and menstrual irregularities, infertility, and atrophy of the breasts occur in women.

Symptoms of adrenal insufficiency can also occur—hypoglycemia, weakness, weight loss, hypotension, and changes in skin pigmentation. Clients may note personality changes (eg, lethargy and apathy) and may also suffer nausea, vomiting, and epigastric distress. If an enlarging neoplasm is the cause of the panhypopituitarism, the client may enter the health care system with symptoms of diabetes insipidus (extreme polyuria and polydipsia) or with headache, visual changes, or anorexia.

Objective findings in clients with panhypopituitarism may include retardation of growth and development if the condition occurs before epiphyseal closure. There are often indications of general wasting of muscle and weight loss; osteoporosis is possible. The skin may appear waxy or yellowish; in some instances, it may be dry and wrinkled, giving the impression of aging. The amount of body hair is decreased. The client may also have hypotension, a slow pulse, and symptoms of postural hypotension as well as hypoglycemia from decreased secretion of somatotropin and adrenocortical hormones. Atrophy of the prostate may be found in men and atrophy of the ovaries and uterus in women.

The diagnosis of panhypopituitarism is based on history and physical findings and largely on laboratory studies. Laboratory tests used in the evaluation of anterior pituitary function are discussed in detail in Chapter 41.

Therapeutic Measures

Hypopituitarism is treated with surgery or radiation if the etiology is tumor, and hormones are replaced as necessary no matter what the etiology. Because the tropic hormones are not readily available (except for adrenocorticotropic hormone, ACTH), the target-gland hormones are usually administered (cortisol, thyroid hormone, testosterone, estrogen). With replacement therapy, prognosis for a normal life span is good. In cases of tumor-caused hypopituitarism, the prognosis also depends on the type of tumor and its response to treatment.

Specific Nursing Measures

The nursing care of clients with panhypopituitarism is the same as that for clients experiencing any of the single hormonal deficiencies (eg, hypothyroidism and adrenal insufficiency) and is discussed under these specific disorders. The psychosocial implications of panhypopituitarism for the client are also similar to those discussed under the specific disorders but magnified by the involvement of multiple hormones. Some general points to consider include:

- Encouraging adequate diet and hydration because clients with Simmonds' disease are often anorexic. Also a high-calorie, high-vitamin diet may be necessary for treating debilitation.
- Preventing complications of bed rest, especially if the client is emaciated and immobile for long periods.
- Encouraging ambulation and exercise as tolerated to promote circulation and improve the sense of well-being.

Diabetes Insipidus

Diabetes insipidus is a disorder of the posterior pituitary characterized by the excretion of excessively large amounts of hypotonic urine. Diabetes insipidus can be further classified into two clinical entities based on etiology:

- Pituitary diabetes insipidus, characterized by defective secretion of antidiuretic hormone (ADH)

• Nephrogenic diabetes insipidus, a congenital familial disorder characterized by the failure of significant urinary concentration in association with the secretion of greater than normal amounts of ADH

The result of both these disorders is the production of excessively large amounts of hypotonic urine. This leads to increased thirst, the body's compensating mechanism to prevent dehydration.

Pituitary diabetes insipidus is idiopathic in about 50% of clients. The idiopathic form is known as primary diabetes insipidus and has been associated with familial and congenital factors as well as with subclinical encephalitis. Secondary diabetes insipidus is pituitary diabetes insipidus arising from a variety of causes: hypophysectomy, tumors (metastatic carcinoma of the breast, craniopharyngioma), trauma (basilar skull fractures), vascular lesions (hemorrhage and aneurysms), infections (syphilis, encephalitis, meningitis), histiocytosis, and granulomatous disease (sarcoidosis, tuberculosis).

Nephrogenic diabetes insipidus arises from a tubular defect in the kidney, which results in failure of the kidney to respond to ADH. This is a rare hereditary condition, present at birth. The diagnosis is based on the finding of a hypotonic urine in an infant along with dehydration, vomiting, and fever.

If there has been a temporary injury to the hypothalamus, the client may experience a transient episode of polydipsia and polyuria, which can be followed by either complete recovery or permanent diabetes insipidus. The danger in this situation occurs when the client is unable to drink enough fluids to prevent dehydration and/or unable to communicate an increasing sense of thirst. These clients require careful monitoring of their intake and output and blood pressure as indicators of the need for further fluid replacement.

Clinical Manifestations

The two primary clinical manifestations of diabetes insipidus are persistent polyuria and polydipsia. Polyuria may amount to 5 to 20 L/day depending on the degree of pathology; an output of 4 to 5 L is the most common (Muthe, 1981). The urine has an abnormally low specific gravity (1.001 to 1.005) with no other abnormalities. The client may have headache, visual disturbances, muscular weakness, myalgia, anorexia, and weight loss. Symptoms of electrolyte imbalance may be seen. Persistent polydipsia and polyuria can interfere with sleep, causing fatigue, lethargy, and irritability. If the fluid intake is not sufficient to compensate for the amount lost through the urine, profound dehydration and shock may ensue.

Diabetes insipidus is not a life-threatening disorder unless severe electrolyte imbalances occur. These imbalances are not usually seen in individuals who can compensate for the excessive fluid losses by an increased fluid intake.

Diabetes insipidus is diagnosed by routine screening tests such as specific gravity of urine, plasma sodium levels, osmolality tests, and water deprivation and water-loading tests. The diagnosis is confirmed if a deficiency of ADH is demonstrated and the client's kidneys are shown to respond normally to ADH. In response to a water deprivation challenge, clients with diabetes insipidus will demonstrate an inability to increase the specific gravity and osmolality of the urine. These tests, their indications for use, expected outcomes, and abnormal findings are discussed in detail in Chapter 41. The differential diagnosis involves other causes of polyuria. A brain scan, skull x-rays, visual fields testing, and a full neurologic examination may be done to rule out the presence of a tumor.

Therapeutic Measures

The major therapeutic measure used in diabetes insipidus is replacement therapy. Even though a client may be able to compensate for the excessive loss of fluids by drinking large quantities of liquids, this is often impractical and may involve major adjustments in lifestyle. Administration of exogenous vasopressin (ADH) helps to reestablish a normal fluid balance and relieves the symptoms of polyuria and polydipsia. The drugs used to treat diabetes insipidus are explained in Table 44–1.

Specific Nursing Measures

The nursing care of clients with diabetes insipidus involves:

• Measuring intake and output (q. 1 h in certain clients) as a baseline for treatment and as an indicator for fluid replacement
• Monitoring specific gravity of urine
• Measuring blood pressure and weight before and after treatment is begun
• Encouraging increased oral fluid intake:
  - Assess client's fluid preference. (Clients with diabetes insipidus often prefer ice water for reasons not well understood.)
  - Keep liquids readily accessible to the client
• Restricting salt and protein to help reduce urinary output
• Observing the client for symptoms and signs of dehydration and electrolyte imbalance (eg, intense thirst, weight loss, dryness of the oral mucosa, loss of normal skin turgor)
  - Look for any signs of skin breakdown due to poor skin turgor
  - Prevent skin breakdown by turning and repositioning q. 2 h, ambulation, skin lotion, and gentle massage

After replacement treatment has been started, be alert for symptoms and signs of water intoxication secondary to overmedication with vasopressin (change in level of consciousness, confusion, headache, and weight gain). If these symptoms appear, the medication should be stopped, fluids restricted, and the physician notified immediately. Also be alert for diarrhea resulting from increased peristalsis and

Table 44–1 Pharmacologic Agents Used in the Treatment of Diabetes Insipidus

Generic and Trade Name	Usual Dosage	Action	Side Effects
ADH or vasopressin (Pitressin in aqueous solution)	Parenteral: SC, IV or IM; 5–10 units (0.25–0.5 mL) b.i.d. or t.i.d. p.r.n. for short-term treatment	Increases renal absorption of water	Vasoconstriction, smooth muscle contraction (↑ BP, uterine cramping, ↑ peristalsis)
ADH or vasopressin (Pitressin tannate in oil)	IM: 2.5–5 units q. 36–72 h (based on return of symptoms); warm solution and thoroughly shake before administering IM	Increases renal absorption of water	Vasoconstriction, smooth muscle contraction
Lypressin (Diapid)	Intranasally: 1 or 2 sprays in each nostril q.i.d.	Increases renal reabsorption of water	Vasoconstriction, smooth muscle contraction, irritation of nasal mucosa
Desmopressin acetate (DDAVP)	Intranasally: 0.1–0.2 mL daily in single or divided doses	Increases renal reabsorption of water	Vasoconstriction, smooth muscle contraction, irritation of nasal mucosa
Chlorpropramide (Diabinese)	Oral; 200–500 mg q.d.	Stimulates ADH release from the pituitary; increases vasopressin action in the kidney	Hypoglycemia
Clofibrate (Atromid-S)	Oral; 500 mg q.i.d.	Stimulates ADH release from the pituitary; increases vasopressin action in the kidney	Nausea, weakness, muscle cramps

chest pain, especially in elderly clients with a history of coronary artery disease.

Before discharge, the client and family should be familiar with the disorder and the need for careful recording of intake, output, and daily weights. Clients should carry an identification card and wear a Medic-Alert bracelet or tag, as should all clients with pituitary dysfunction requiring medication. Clients who are to receive vasopressin parenterally should be skilled in the technique of self-injection; know how to prepare and store the medication, the purpose of the medication, and potential side effects. Clients receiving vasopressin by nasal spray should have practiced the correct administration before discharge from the hospital.

Teach the client and family the symptoms and signs of overdosage and underdosage of medications and when to report these to the physician. Overdosage is indicated by water intoxication; underdosage is indicated by dehydration. The interaction of other medications (epinephrine and heparin) and alcohol and vasopressin should be discussed as well as the importance of regular medical evaluation.

Syndrome of Inappropriate Antidiuretic Hormone

The syndrome of inappropriate antidiuretic hormone, or SIADH, is a condition characterized by autonomous release of ADH without regard to plasma osmolality. The body is unable to dilute the urine appropriately, so fluid is retained,

which expands the extracellular fluid compartment and leads to hyponatremia. SIADH can be caused by release of the hormone from a secreting tumor or from the posterior pituitary from a variety of causes. These etiological factors are outlined in Box 44–1 on the next page.

Clinical Manifestations
Clients with SIADH may gain body weight because of fluid retention. They may also be confused, lethargic, weak, and have convulsions due to their hyponatremia. Clinically, serum sodium levels are below 135 mEq/L, whereas the urinary sodium concentrations are elevated. SIADH is diagnosed by laboratory evaluation of serum and urine sodium and chloride levels and of serum and urine osmolality levels. These tests are discussed further in Chapter 41.

Therapeutic Measures
Treatment of SIADH is directed toward its underlying cause. The client may be placed on water restriction. The hyponatremia is usually not treated unless the client has severe symptoms.

Specific Nursing Measures
Nursing care of the client with SIADH involves:

- Assessing for symptoms and signs related to water intoxication and hyponatremia
- Measuring and recording intake and output, blood pressure, and weight

Box 44–1 **Etiology of Syndrome of Inappropriate Antidiuretic Hormone (SIADH)**

Central nervous system: Head injury, CVA, brain tumor/abscess, encephalitis, meningitis, Guillain-Barré syndrome, acute intermittent porphyria, seizure disorders, lupus cerebritis, schizophrenia

Intrathoracic causes: Pneumonia, lung abscess, aspergillosis, tuberculosis, cystic fibrosis, positive-pressure respirator (causes sudden release of ADH)

Tumors: Oat cell carcinoma of the lung, adenocarcinoma of duodenum and pancreas, thymoma, Hodgkin's disease, lymphosarcoma, Ewing's tumor, carcinoma of the ureter

Exogenous drugs:
• Drugs that increase release of ADH (nicotine, clofibrate, vincristine)
• Drugs that potentiate ADH (chlorpropramide, thiazide diuretics)
• Drugs that increase renal reabsorption of water (vasopressin, oxytocin)

Other: Surgery, Addison's disease, hypopituitarism, myxedema, emotional stress, idiopathic disorders

SOURCE: Adapted from Kaye D, Rose LF: *Fundamentals of Internal Medicine.* St. Louis: Mosby, 1983, p. 914. Solomon BL: The hypothalamus and pituitary gland: An overview. *Nurs Clin North Am* 1980; 15(3):449.

• Assisting clients in managing thirst because clients are often on fluid restrictions:
  - Assess fluid preferences
  - Use ice chips rather than water
  - Relieve dryness of mucosa through care of mouth
  - Space fluids over 8-hour time periods
• Teaching regarding nature of disorder, treatment plan, and procedures

ADRENAL DISORDERS

Cushing's Syndrome

Cushing's syndrome arises from an excess of cortisol circulating in the plasma. Common synonyms for this condition are glucocorticoid excess syndrome and hypercortisolism.

The etiology of Cushing's syndrome may fall into one of three categories, which have in common the oversecretion of cortisol by the adrenal cortex:

• Primary Cushing's syndrome
• Secondary Cushing's syndrome or Cushing's disease
• Tertiary Cushing's syndrome

Primary Cushing's syndrome, also called adrenal Cushing's syndrome, usually results from autonomous secretion of glucocorticoid from a unilateral adrenal neoplasm. About half of these tumors are malignant.

Secondary Cushing's syndrome, also called pituitary-dependent Cushing's syndrome or Cushing's disease, is

the most common. It is due to an excess secretion of ACTH that leads to bilateral adrenal hyperplasia.

Tertiary or ectopic Cushing's syndrome arises from the autonomous production of ACTH by at least 25 different extrapituitary malignancies, including carcinoma of the lung and of several organs in the gastrointestinal tract. It is characterized by markedly increased ACTH levels and bilateral hyperplasia of the adrenal glands (Kaye & Rose, 1983).

Cushing's syndrome can also be iatrogenic (ie, occurring in clients who have been given cortisol or ACTH over a period of time). Whatever the etiology, the result of hyperfunction of the adrenal cortex in Cushing's syndrome is an excess of plasma cortisol that produces certain characteristic effects, as described in Table 44–2.

Clinical Manifestations

Hypertension results from the retention of sodium and water. Retained water expands the extracellular fluid volume and increases sensitivity of the vasculature to circulating catecholamines.

Central or truncal obesity, along with a characteristic moon face and buffalo hump, occurs because of deposition

Table 44–2 **Common Findings in Cushing's Syndrome**

Subjective Findings	Objective Findings
Clients often note:	*Examiners often observe:*
Red, full face	Plethoric moon face
Change in body shape	Truncal obesity with muscle wasting of extremities
Muscle weakness and fatigability	Supraclavicular fat pads
	Pendulous fat pad in chest and abdomen
	Buffalo hump in interscapular area
Skin and hair changes	Loss of skin thickness
Easy bruisability	Skin pigmentation
	Multiple ecchymoses
	Purple abdominal striae
	Acne and hirsutism in women
Susceptibility to infection and bone fractures	Osteoporosis
	Hypertension
Menstrual changes (oligomenorrhea, amenorrhea)	Hypokalemia
Irritability, emotional lability, depression, confusion, sleeplessness	Diabetes mellitus (usually in clients with a family predisposition)
Glucose intolerance	

of body fat in the abdominal wall, facial, and interscapular areas. The face of the client with Cushing's syndrome is often round and plethoric (Figure 44–2). Because of a loss of muscle mass resulting from the increased breakdown of protein, the extremities may appear thin, and there may be proximal muscle weakness, especially of the pelvic girdle. Muscle weakness, as well as potential cardiac dysfunction, may be related to hypokalemia resulting from urinary excretion of potassium.

Cutaneous **striae** may be present on the abdomen, breast, perineum, and buttocks. The striae are wide and pinkish purple (Figure 44–3). The skin becomes thinner and more prone to trauma because of the breakdown of collagen. Clients with Cushing's syndrome are also prone to ecchymosis. If the etiology of Cushing's syndrome is pituitary dysfunction, hyperpigmentation of the skin may be present because of increased plasma levels of ACTH. Hyperpigmentation is not found when Cushing's syndrome is of adrenal origin; therefore, it provides a valuable diagnostic sign to rule out the possibility of an adrenal tumor. Acne, hirsutism, **oligomenorrhea,** and amennorhea may be secondary effects of the overproduction of androgen (Sanford, 1980).

Oversecretion of cortisol can also increase susceptibility to fractures from osteoporosis (especially of the spine) because of cortisol-stimulated calcium resorption from the bone. Glucose intolerance (hyperglycemia) may develop secondary to the anti-insulin effect of cortisol. Diabetes mellitus may develop in individuals with a predisposition.

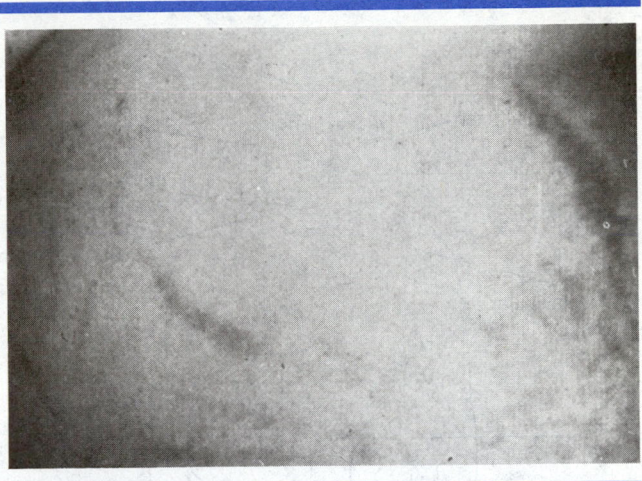

Figure 44–3

Cushing's syndrome: Client with abdominal striae.
SOURCE: Jubiz W: *Endocrinology: A Logical Approach for Clinicians.* New York: McGraw-Hill, 1979, frontispiece.

In addition, there may be emotional symptoms (eg, depression, increased anxiety, euphoria, and frank psychosis). There are increased susceptibility to infection and potential for masking of infection. These symptoms and signs create a typical "cushingoid" presentation (Figure 44–4). The disorder not only causes problems of altered body image and self-esteem but also poses serious potential health concerns.

One of the most important diagnostic findings in the evaluation of Cushing's syndrome is the persistent elevation of serum cortisol levels with loss of the normal diurnal variation. All signs and symptoms are related to this pathophysiological change. Other tests commonly used in the evaluation of this disorder include serum aldosterone and ACTH levels, urinary tests (17-hydroxycorticosteroids [17-OHCS], 17-ketosteroids, aldosterone, and free cortisol) and special tests (dexamethasone suppression test, ACTH stimulation test, and metyrapone test). The routine screening tests and other methods used in the evaluation of adrenal dysfunction are discussed in Chapter 41.

Therapeutic Measures

The treatment of Cushing's syndrome and disease depends on the etiology. If a tumor is involved, treatment also depends on whether the lesion is benign or malignant. Therapeutic modalities used in the treatment of Cushing's disease are surgical measures, pharmacologic agents, and medical measures such as radiation and diet therapy.

Surgery is the most common modality. Transsphenoidal microsurgery, transfrontal craniotomy, and unilateral or bilateral adrenalectomy are possible approaches to treatment of Cushing's syndrome, depending on the location of the tumor. Surgical procedures used in the care of individuals with endocrine disorders are discussed in Chapter 45.

The use of pharmacologic agents is restricted to situations in which there is an inoperable tumor and radiation

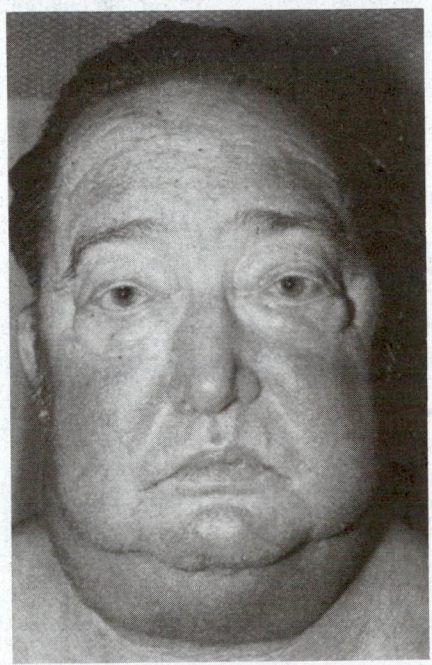

Figure 44–2

Cushing's syndrome: Client with plethoric face.
SOURCE: Jubiz W: *Endocrinology: A Logical Approach for Clinicians.* New York: McGraw-Hill, 1979, frontispiece.

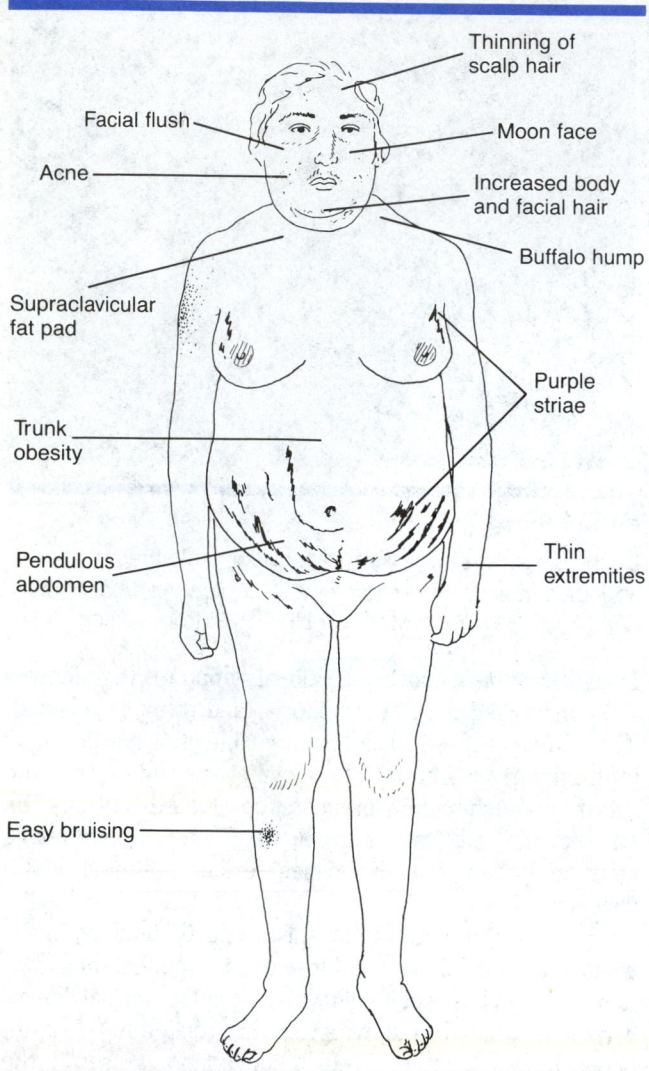

Thinning of scalp hair

Facial flush

Moon face

Acne

Increased body and facial hair

Buffalo hump

Supraclavicular fat pad

Purple striae

Trunk obesity

Pendulous abdomen

Thin extremities

Easy bruising

Figure 44–4

A client with typical cushingoid findings.

has been unsuccessful. Their use generally has been only of short-term value.

When surgery is performed, replacement hormonal therapy is often mandated. It is the responsibility of the nurse to be familiar with the therapeutic use of steroids and their long-term effects and to teach these to the client and family. Table 44–3 summarizes the common side effects of long-term glucocorticoid therapy.

Specific Nursing Measures

The nursing management of Cushing's syndrome focuses on psychological support for the client and family or friends, relief of symptoms, protection of the client from possible complications related to the increased production of cortisol, and client and family education. Psychological support for clients with Cushing's syndrome is especially important because the alterations in body image may affect their self-

esteem and their ability to cope with their present life situation. In addition, clients with Cushing's syndrome often have rapid mood changes, which are of concern to both them and their significant others. Provide for a climate of acceptance; create opportunities for both the client and family to express and discuss their questions, feelings, and concerns; and educate the client and family about the nature of the disorder, its clinical course, and the goals of the medical treatment and nursing care plans.

To help relieve the symptoms of Cushing's syndrome:

- Encourage proper diet and fluid intake (eg, low calorie, high protein, high potassium, low sodium) to help correct the metabolic imbalances.
- Monitor vital signs regularly and report any significant elevations in blood pressure immediately.
- Obtain daily weight on the same scale to monitor rate of fluid retention and loss.

Table 44–3 Common Side Effects of Long-Term Glucocorticoid Therapy

Side Effects	Physiological Basis
Retention of sodium; loss of potassium with resulting fluid retention and ↑ BP	Associated mineralocorticoid effect
Increased susceptibility to infection	Suppression of immune system
Muscle weakness, muscle breakdown	↑ Protein catabolism by glucocorticoids
Glucose intolerance, hyperglycemia	↑ Gluconeogenesis by glucocorticoids
Increased deposition of fat in trunk	↑ Lipid synthesis by glucocorticoids
Growth suppression	↓ Of growth hormone action by glucocorticoids
Emotional changes, possible psychosis	Not understood
Osteoporosis, ↑ incidence of fractures	Changes in calcium metabolism leading to ↑ resorption of bone
Gastritis; gastric, peptic ulcers	Direct irritation or protein-wasting effects of protein
Glaucoma	Interference with aqueous outflow in eye; ↑ intraocular pressure
Cataracts	Not understood
Pancreatitis	Possible effect of glucocorticoids on lipid metabolism

SOURCE: Adapted from Clark JB, Queener SF, Karb VB: *Pharmacological Basis of Nursing Practice.* St. Louis: Mosby, 1982, p. 440.

• Promote physical and emotional rest; provide emotional support during mood changes, offer explanations as needed, and provide opportunities for verbalization of feelings regarding changes in body appearance and the long-term implications of the disorder.

To help prevent complications related to the increased production of cortisol:

• Check urine periodically for glucose and acetone to screen for the presence of diabetes mellitus.
• Assess the client carefully for infection, remembering that one of the effects of increased cortisol production is the suppression of the immune system and masking of infections; attempt to create as safe an environment as possible for the client by preventing exposure to infection and by recognizing that mild symptoms may actually represent a more severe situation.
• Provide protection from injury and trauma because clients' muscle weakness and tendency toward osteoporosis make them susceptible.

Client teaching should include the nature of the disorder, prognosis, goals of the medical (or surgical) treatment plan, and goals of the nursing care plan. If clients are to receive medications, they and their families should be familiar with their purpose, action, dosage, administration, and side effects. Box 44–2 lists the important nursing implications of long-term glucocorticoid therapy. Actively attempt to create a climate in which both the client and family feel free to discuss the implications of the disorder and its effects on their lives. Consider making a public health nursing referral to evaluate the client's home environment for possible safety factors, assist the family in obtaining adaptive equipment if needed, and monitor the client's progress. Box 44–3 provides a general teaching plan for clients on glucocorticoid therapy.

The outlook for Cushing's syndrome clients is brighter now than in the past. The use of transsphenoidal microsurgery to resect pituitary tumors has been one of the major advances in the surgical approach to treatment. The increased use of physical assessment skills by nurses has contributed to the early recognition of possible cushingoid clients, and earlier diagnosis and treatment have improved the outcome for both clients and their families.

Addison's Disease

Adrenocortical insufficiency may be primary (Addison's disease) or secondary. The primary type arises from pathology occurring within the gland itself; the secondary type arises from pathology of the pituitary or hypothalamus or is iatrogenic. Primary adrenal insufficiency is characterized by insufficient production of all three adrenal hormones. The physiological manifestations are those of deficiency of the glucocorticoids and mineralocorticoids. (The adrenals are only a secondary source of the sex hormones,

---

Box 44–2   Nursing Implications of Long-Term Glucocorticoid Therapy

If the course of steroid therapy lasts less than 7 to 10 days, side effects are unlikely.

Monitor the client's weight and blood pressure at frequent intervals.

Check the client's urine regularly for the presence of glucose and acetone.
• For clients who require insulin therapy to treat hyperglycemia, the dosage of insulin varies with the dose of steroids.
• Individuals with diabetes mellitus who require steroid therapy will need adjustment of the regular insulin dosage.

Assess clients carefully for symptoms and signs of gastric irritation that might indicate an ulcer (dyspepsia, epigastric burning, increased flatulence, hematemesis, coffee-ground emesis, and melena). Ulcers may also develop in clients who receive steroids parenterally.
• Steroids should be taken with meals if possible.
• Physician may prescribe the use of cimetidine (Tagamet) and antacids up to four to six times daily while client is receiving steroids.
• Client may benefit from more frequent, small meals.
• All foods and liquids the client feels contribute to gastric symptoms should be carefully noted and excluded from the diet (eg, coffee, tomato products, alcohol). Aspirin is also contraindicated unless specifically ordered by the physician.

Assess clients, especially postmenopausal females, carefully for symptoms and signs of osteoporosis.
• Client should be taught to report any persistent musculoskeletal pain.
• Client should be advised to avoid strenuous physical activities (eg, contact sports, heavy lifting, and strenuous physical labor).
• Care should be taken in the lifting and transfer of any immobilized client on long-term glucocorticoid therapy to reduce the chance of spontaneous fracture.

Advise clients to consult an ophthalmologist every 3 to 6 months to screen for possible glaucoma and early cataract formation.

Clients with a history of tuberculosis or positive tuberculin reactors who are receiving long-term steroid therapy may also receive antituberculosis medications while they are receiving steroids.

Pregnant women should not take steroids unless they are receiving replacement therapy or are in a potentially life-threatening situation. In this case, close monitoring by the endocrinologist and obstetrician is essential.

The complete return of adrenal function after long-term glucocorticoid therapy may take up to 1 year. The client requires careful assessment during this period and may need corticosteroid treatment if stress or infection occurs or if surgery is to be performed.

SOURCE: Adapted from Clark JB, Queener SF, Karb VB: *Pharmacological Basis of Nursing Practice*. St. Louis: Mosby, 1982, pp. 446–447.

so deficiencies of adrenally produced hormones tend to be compensated for by normal ovarian or testicular function.)

It is important to remember that a major difference between primary and secondary causes of adrenal hypofunction is that secondary failure is not usually associated

---

Box 44–3 Teaching Plan for a Client on Glucocorticoid Therapy

A comprehensive teaching plan for any client on glucocorticoids, especially long-term therapy, should cover the following points:

Purpose of therapy (eg, replacement of deficient hormones or treatment of a specific disorder).

Medication: Name, action, dosage, administration, desired effect, side effects.

Importance of taking the medications regularly and of informing the physician immediately when unable to do so. Some clients with adrenal insufficiency may not be able to tolerate taking steroids orally; they must be taught to administer steroids parenterally.

What symptoms and signs to report immediately to the physician:
- Any side effects of the medication (most will resolve when steroid therapy is stopped).
- Any symptoms and signs of infection: Fever, chills, cough, sore throat. (Clients should be encouraged to avoid all other persons who have symptoms and signs of an infection.)
- Any episodes of increased stress (fatigue, infection, emotional upset) that may call for increased dosages of steroids.

Importance of wearing a Medic-Alert tag and carrying a card identifying the client, the diagnosis, and medications. Clients receiving steroid therapy should inform all health care providers.

Rationale for tapering off glucocorticoid therapy and/or rationale for alternative-day treatment. Client should be advised against abruptly stopping the medication.

Importance of diet as a treatment. Diet should include foods high in protein and potassium and low in sodium and carbohydrates. Dietary consultation with nutritionist is often beneficial.

SOURCE: Adapted from Clark JB, Queener SF, Karb VB: *Pharmacological Basis of Nursing Practice.* St. Louis: Mosby, 1982, pp. 446–447.

---

with a marked deficiency of aldosterone. Another differentiating feature is that hyperpigmentation of the skin is only seen in primary adrenal insufficiency. Increased serum levels of ACTH, which is structurally similar to melanocyte-stimulating hormone (MSH), are thought to cause the increased skin tone found in scars, areolae, and skin folds of clients with Addison's disease. Figure 44–5 shows this hyperpigmentation.

Clinical Manifestations

The signs and symptoms of Addison's disease relate directly to the effect of reduced circulating levels of glucocorticoids and mineralocorticoids. Symptoms may appear slowly or as an acute crisis precipitated by stress.

The addisonian client loses sodium in the urine as the distal renal tubules lose the ability to exchange sodium for potassium. This causes hypovolemia and hypotension, which result in decreased renal perfusion and elevated BUN levels as well as hyperkalemia from the retention of potassium. The deficiency of plasma cortisol inhibits the secretion of certain gastrointestinal enzymes; hence, clients with

Addison's disease may experience diarrhea, vomiting, anorexia, and abdominal pain, all of which further decrease fluid levels and thus aggravate the hypovolemia and hypotension. Generalized weakness, decreased physical endurance, changes in mental acuity, and weight loss are consistently seen in clients with Addison's disease.

Hypoglycemia occurs in about 50% of the clients diagnosed with adrenal insufficiency. Deficiencies in circulating cortisol cause a decrease in gluconeogenesis by the liver and increased uptake of glucose by the tissues.

Adrenal Crisis. Some clients with adrenal insufficiency who experience sudden physical or emotional stress or who do not follow their medication regimen may develop an acute and sometimes fatal state of circulatory collapse. Known as adrenal crisis or addisonian crisis, this is characterized by:

- Severe hypotension (the most prominent feature)
- Confusion progressing to coma
- Nausea and vomiting
- Abdominal cramping and diarrhea
- Cyanosis and fever

The symptoms and signs of adrenal crisis are simply the exaggerated symptoms and signs of the disorder. Adrenal crisis is an emergency that requires immediate medical and nursing intervention.

Adrenal crisis can also occur following pituitary or adrenal surgery or after trauma to or hemorrhage into the adrenal cortices. Adrenal hemorrhage can occur with overwhelming septicemia (Waterhouse–Friderichsen syndrome) as a sequela of a meningococcal infection.

Tests used in establishing the diagnosis of adrenal

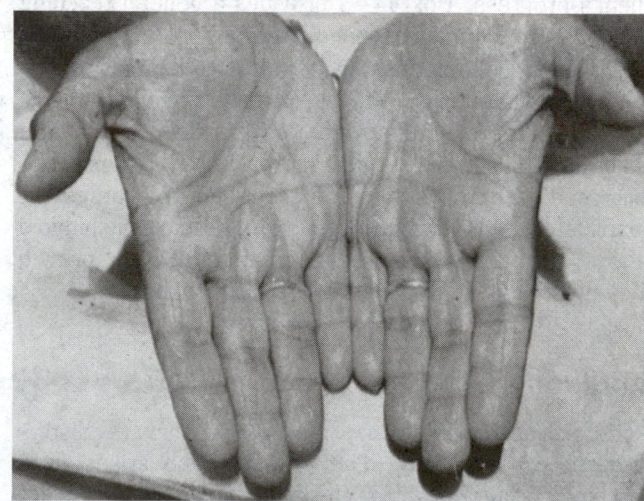

Figure 44–5

Client with Addison's disease showing hyperpigmentation of the palmar creases.
SOURCE: Jubiz W: *Endocrinology: A Logical Approach for Clinicians.* New York: McGraw-Hill, 1979, frontispiece.

hypofunction and their implications are discussed in detail in Chapter 41. Briefly, serum cortisol and metyrapone tests are used for screening. For more definitive results, serum ACTH is measured, or the ACTH stimulation test is used.

Serum cortisol values tend to be low in primary adrenal insufficiency; in secondary adrenal insufficiency, they may be in the low-normal range. The metyrapone test is the procedure of choice in nonacute conditions. When administered to the client, metyrapone should inhibit cortisol synthesis and thus result in a fall in circulating cortisol levels. This should cause an increase in the synthesis of ACTH and a rise in the serum levels of the cortisone precursor 11-deoxycortisol. If this occurs, the pituitary–adrenal feedback loop is assumed to be intact. An impairment of response could indicate primary adrenal insufficiency (failure of adrenals to respond to ACTH) and/or secondary adrenal insufficiency (inability of the pituitary–hypothalamic axis to secrete ACTH).

Although serum cortisol levels tend to be low in both primary and secondary adrenal insufficiency, the operation of the pituitary–adrenal feedback loop causes serum ACTH levels to be low when pituitary malfunction is causing adrenal insufficiency but high in primary adrenal insufficiency. Hence, serum ACTH permits the diagnostician to distinguish between primary and secondary adrenal insufficiency. The study of urinary 17-OHCS has also been used to quantitate the response of the adrenals. The ACTH stimulation test is used to demonstrate primary adrenal insufficiency. It studies the response of the adrenal gland (ie, production of cortisol) after an exogenous administration of ACTH. In primary adrenal insufficiency, the gland does not respond even to repeated administrations of ACTH. In secondary adrenal insufficiency, even though the response to the original ACTH challenge may be subnormal, it will return to normal with repeated administrations. There are various modifications of the test. A graph depicting plasma cortisol response to exogenous ACTH is shown in Figure 44–6.

Therapeutic Measures

Replacement therapy is the usual treatment for adrenal insufficiency. During periods of physical or emotional stress, shock, or surgery, addisonian clients need careful moni-

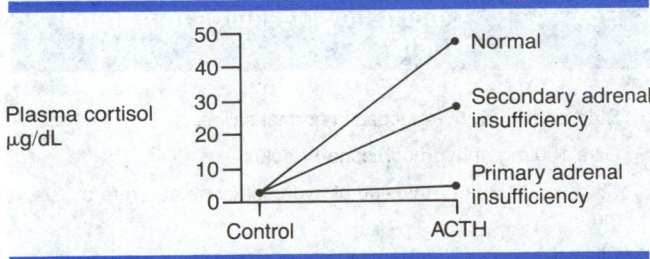

Figure 44–6

Plasma cortisol responses to exogenous ACTH in normal subjects and clients with adrenal insufficiency.

> **Box 44–4   Sample Steroid Therapy Schedule for Clients With Addison's Disease Undergoing any Major Surgery**
>
> Before and during surgery:
>
> Night before surgery: 50 mg cortisone acetate IM (as protection in case of difficulty with infusion)
>
> For first 24 hours and during surgery: Continuous infusion of IV hydrocortisone at 10 mg/h
>
> Day after surgery:
>
> Hydrocortisone 100 mg bolus (to increase circulating cortisone levels)
>
> Daily dose *decreased* as follows (dose may be oral if tolerated): 75 mg/day for 2 days; 60 mg/day for 2 days; 50 mg/day for 2 days; then daily replacement dose of 30 mg

toring of glucocorticoid administration and fluid balance. Box 44–4 presents a sample steroid schedule for addisonian clients undergoing any major surgery. A summary of the pharmacologic agents used in Addison's disease is in Table 44–4.

Specific Nursing Measures

Nurses are actively involved in both the chronic and acute care of clients with adrenal insufficiency. For clients with chronic disease:

- Assess blood pressure, apical–radial pulse, and respirations because addisonian clients are subject to hypotension, especially orthostatic hypotension due to sodium depletion.
- Monitor body weight. Weight loss with adrenal insufficiency is related to gastrointestinal disturbance. Clients should be encouraged to eat a well-balanced high-protein, high-calorie diet with meals at regular intervals and snacks as required. Advise the client that fasting might precipitate adrenal crisis.
- Assess clients for generalized weakness and malaise. The hyperkalemia, hyponatremia, and loss of the normal diurnal variation in cortisol that accompany Addison's disease may give rise to increased muscular cramping and cardiac dysrhythmias. Clients should be counseled to plan several rest periods during the day to avoid fatigue.
- Assess clients for possible hypoglycemic symptoms (weakness, diaphoresis, lightheadedness, abdominal cramps). Addisonian clients are highly susceptible to hypoglycemia.
- Assess clients' mental status and ability to tolerate physical activity, because this is affected by depletion of the adrenal hormones.
- Assess clients for symptoms and signs of infection. Counsel clients to call their physician at the first sign

Table 44–4   Pharmacologic Agents Used in Addison's Disease

Generic and Trade Name	Usual Dosage	Action	Side Effects
Hydrocortisone*	Usual oral dose: 20 mg in AM, 10 mg in PM	Short-acting corticosteroid with mineralocorticoid activity	Overdosage produces symptoms of Cushing's disease; abrupt withdrawal produces symptoms of adrenal insufficiency
Prednisone/prednisolone	Usual oral dose: 7.5 mg daily in divided doses	Increases glucocorticoid activity; decreases mineralocorticoid activity; four to five times more potent than hydrocortisone	Same as hydrocortisone. Overdosage may cause GI irritation; use with caution in clients with liver disease
Methylprednisolone (Medrol)	Dosage must be individualized according to client response	Further increases glucocorticoid activity; decreases mineralocorticoid activity	Overdosage produces cortisol effects on protein, fat, and carbohydrate metabolism; does not significantly affect sodium retention
Fludrocortisone acetate (Florinef)	Usual oral dose: 0.1 mg daily or three times per week	Marked increase in glucocorticoid activity and marked increase in mineralocorticoid activity	Symptoms of mineralocorticoid overdosage: Increased retention of Na and water; increased potassium loss

*Client may need double or triple maintenance dose of hydrocortisone during crisis situations or stress. Some physicians cover these clients by adding prednisone (10–15 mg per day) to maintenance hydrocortisone, to be discontinued after stress is relieved.

of infection. Infection places the body under stress and can precipitate adrenal crisis.

- Screen clients with a tuberculin skin test such as the Mantoux test and/or a chest x-ray before the initiation of steroid therapy. Clients on corticosteroid therapy are considered at high risk for acquiring tuberculosis.
- Teach clients and their significant others the nature of the disorder, its prognosis, and the need for lifelong regular medical treatment and supervision.
- Teach the importance of wearing a Medic-Alert tag and carrying an emergency kit with a syringe filled with 100 mg of hydrocortisone and instructions for use.
- Teach clients and significant others to recognize the symptoms and signs of impending adrenal crisis and of steroid overdosage.
- Teach the importance of maintaining a proper diet to avoid precipitating adrenal crisis.
- Teach the importance of rest periods to avoid fatigue and the need to change position slowly if experiencing vertigo or syncope due to postural hypotension.

The nurse may also be called on to care for clients in adrenal or addisonian crisis. This is an emergency requiring prompt intervention and careful assessment. The immediate goal of medical treatment is to reverse the symptoms of acute deficiency of the adrenal steroids (ie, severe hypotension, vasomotor collapse, and hyperkalemia). The emergency treatment is summarized in Box 44–5.

Nurses caring for a client in an adrenal crisis should:

- Monitor blood pressure, apical–radial pulse, respirations, and temperature q. 15 min during the acute phase.
- Administer intravenous fluids and IV and IM medications as ordered.
- Measure fluid intake and output every hour or as ordered.
- Be alert for symptoms and signs of worsening crisis.
- Administer oxygen or plasma as ordered.
- Support the client and family or friends; provide an environment free from additional physical or emotional stressors.
- Attempt to discover what factors (eg, emotional upset, infection, or missed medication dose) might have precipitated the crisis.

Box 44–5   Emergency Measures in Adrenal Crisis

Start an IV with 5% glucose in normal saline.

Give 100 mg of hydrocortisone IV bolus.

Start continuous IV infusion of hydrocortisone at a rate of 10 mg/h.

Clinical course will determine further dosages.

In addition, antibiotics may be ordered to combat any concurrent infection.

Section II: Neoplastic and Obstructive Disorders

Neoplastic and obstructive disorders of the pituitary include gigantism, acromegaly, and Cushing's disease. Adrenal disorders in this category are aldosteronism and pheochromocytoma.

PITUITARY DISORDERS

Gigantism and Acromegaly

Increased secretion of somatotropin by the anterior pituitary results in gigantism (before puberty) or acromegaly (after puberty). The term *acromegaly* refers to enlargement of the acral parts—head, hands, and feet. The crucial factor is the time onset of the disorder. If the hypersecretion of growth hormone occurs during the individual's growth period before the epiphyses of the long bones have closed, gigantism will occur. Acromegaly occurs after epiphyseal closure.

Acromegaly usually starts between the ages of 20 and 50. Physical changes depend on the amount of hormone oversecretion and the age at which the disorder begins. Acromegaly usually develops slowly and insidiously. Younger adults may be more physically affected than older adults (Muthe, 1981). The disorder is characterized by coarsening of the facial features, enlargement of the extremities, and a high incidence of impaired glucose metabolism. Individuals may also experience impaired vision.

Gigantism starts in infancy or childhood and is characterized by continuous growth of the body until epiphyseal closure occurs. Gigantism in adults is defined as a height over 80 in. In children, it is defined as three standard deviations above the mean for the child's age as measured on a growth curve (Degroot et al., 1979). Pituitary giants may be as tall as 8 ft (240 cm) and may weigh more than 300 lb (135 kg) (Kaye & Rose, 1983). Individuals with gigantism may develop some associated acromegalic features—very large hands and feet—in adult life (Muthe, 1981).

Both acromegaly and gigantism are traceable to an autonomous hypersecretion of somatotropin caused by an anterior pituitary tumor, usually an eosinophilic adenoma (DeGroot et al., 1979). Eosinophilic adenomas are usually benign; however, they secrete excessive amounts of somatotropin and prolactin, which may create pressure in the brain, causing visual symptoms and headache. Eosinophilic adenoma is the most common cause found in clients on autopsy. Hyperplasia of the somatotropin-producing cells and primary pituitary carcinoma are rare.

Clinical Manifestations of Gigantism

Clients with gigantism usually live about 20 years. They are subject to a general debilitation, which is progressive, and are likely to die as the result of pituitary failure leading to adrenal cortical insufficiency.

Objective findings include:

- Extremely large size
- Enlargement of the heart, liver, spleen, kidneys, pancreas, thyroid, parathyroids, adrenals, soft tissues, and peripheral nerves
- Increased metabolic rate
- Incomplete or slow development of secondary sex characteristics
- Glucose intolerance with resulting hyperglycemia and diabetes mellitus
- Possible excess secretion of other anterior pituitary hormones (prolactin, MSH, ACTH, TSH)

Advanced signs include extreme muscular weakness and crippling osteoarthritis, which may be associated with a severe kyphosis.

The symptoms of gigantism are usually attributable to the effects of compression of the adjacent tissues by the tumor or by metabolic changes. Symptoms include headache, which may be mild to severe and may be persistent; **bitemporal hemianopia** and other visual field defects (eg, changes in color perception and diplopia) because of pressure in the optic chiasm; and seizures and stroke due to increased intracranial pressure.

Clinical Manifestations of Acromegaly

Clients with acromegaly do not grow especially tall because onset occurs after puberty. However, the hypersecretion of somatotropin stimulates all tissues of the body—including the soft tissues, organs, and bones—to grow wider and thicker. The term *acromegaly* refers to abnormal enlargement of the extremities. The bones formed by intramembranous ossification continue to grow, leading to enlargement of the skull (especially the forehead), jaw, and supraorbital ridges.

The course of the disease varies among individuals: it may be slowly progressive, or it may cause death only a few years after onset. In some instances, progressive increases in the size of the tumor may result in generalized hypopituitarism.

Symptoms and signs are referable to the pituitary tumor or the excess GH circulating in the plasma. Figure 44–7 is a schematic representation of the symptoms and signs of acromegaly.

During the health history, clients may reveal a variety of symptoms. They may report mild to severe persistent headache. Visual changes can include diplopia, changes in visual acuity and color perception, and loss of a field of vision. Clients may note an increase in hat, glove, ring, or shoe size over the past year or a change in facial appearance. Clients may complain of paresthesia or arthralgia. Hyperhidrosis (excess sweating) may occur, which can be associated with a disagreeable odor during an active phase of the disorder. Clients may report symptoms related to

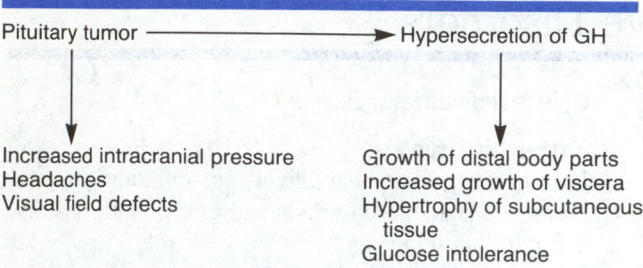

Figure 44–7

Symptoms and signs of acromegaly.

either hypersecretion or deficiency of the other anterior pituitary hormones (eg, in late stages, clients may have loss of libido or amenorrhea). Because of the diabetogenic effect of GH, symptoms of diabetes mellitus—polydipsia, polyuria, polyphagia, and weight loss—appear. The voice may become deeper as a result of hypertrophy of the larynx.

Objective findings include the characteristic changes in facial appearance: the mandible lengthens, thickens, and protrudes **(prognathism);** spaces between the teeth and overbite may develop; the forehead becomes more prominent; the orbital ridge thickens; the soft tissues of the nose, tongue, ears, and lips become enlarged. The skin appears rough and leathery. The pores become increasingly visible as the amount of connective tissue increases. The amount of body hair and skin pigmentation may increase. The hands and the feet become enlarged; fingers assume a spadelike configuration. Thoracic circumference increases secondary to changes in the costal cartilages. Kyphosis often develops.

In addition to these visible external findings, the disorder produces internal changes such as visceromegaly of the heart, liver, kidneys, spleen, and pancreas; enlargement of the thyroid, parathyroid, and adrenal glands; and joint pathology. Degenerative changes, similar to and easily confused with those of osteoarthritis and other arthritic syndromes, appear as bony overgrowth destroys the joints. The client may also exhibit signs of carpal tunnel syndrome—pain and paresthesia along the course of the median nerve—occurring when overgrown fibrotic tissue entraps and compresses the median nerve. Osteoporosis due to loss of calcium may develop in the vertebrae. Hypertension is common, although the exact mechanism is unknown.

The diagnostic measures used to evaluate anterior pituitary dysfunction are discussed in Chapter 41. In general, the history and the physical findings form the basis for the diagnosis of gigantism and/or acromegaly. The laboratory measures simply confirm the diagnosis. Some changes may be noted on x-ray (eg, the sella turcica in 90% of clients with acromegaly will be enlarged). Changes in glucose tolerance are found in about 40% of clients.

Clients should be carefully evaluated for any visual field defects. Although the typical presentation is bitemporal hemianopia, other changes in vision may be present as well.

Therapeutic Measures

Because the usual cause of gigantism or acromegaly is a tumor of the anterior pituitary, the main therapeutic measure is destruction of the tumor by either surgery or radiation. The two major surgical approaches to pituitary tumors are transfrontal craniotomy (transcranial subfrontal hypophysectomy) and transsphenoidal hypophysectomy. These two procedures, their indications, and nursing care are discussed in Chapter 45. Transsphenoidal hypophysectomy is the treatment of choice for a client with active acromegaly. It generally produces improvement or cure in 90% of clients (Jubiz, 1979). Somatotropin levels will drop a few minutes after resection of the tumor; over a period of months, soft tissues regress, and the client loses weight and feels less arthritic pain (Muthe, 1981).

Irradiation of the tumor either externally or internally can be used to control the activity of the disease. Conventional high-voltage irradiation has been found to be successful in more than half of the clients treated (Kaye & Rose, 1983). Its two major disadvantages are the limitation in radioactivity that can be delivered, which should not exceed 5500R, and its slow action (ie, plasma GH levels take at least 6 months to become normal). High-energy particle radiation, delivered by a cyclotron, requires expert techniques and is applicable only in situations where the tumor is confined to the sella turcica (Kaye & Rose, 1983). Implantation of yttrium and/or other radionuclides has been reported to be successful and is used in Europe. Complications secondary to this procedure include meningitis and rhinorrhea (Jubiz, 1979).

The use of medications in the treatment of gigantism and acromegaly is still being researched. Research centers on agents that will block the release of GH from the tumor. Currently under investigation for clients with acromegaly is a dopaminergic agent, bromocriptine, which has been useful in clients who have received conventional radiotherapy and are waiting for the effects to appear (Kaye & Rose, 1983). A GH release-inhibitor hormone in the hypothalamus has been identified and has been found to act on the anterior pituitary to decrease the output of somatotropin. Its possibilities for therapeutic use are still being evaluated. The use of serotonin receptor antagonists to suppress GH levels in clients with acromegaly is also under investigation.

Specific Nursing Measures

Nursing care of the client with acromegaly and gigantism varies with the client's symptoms. Because early recognition and treatment can help reduce the extent of pathological change, the importance of a thorough history and careful physical assessment cannot be overemphasized. Height, body weight, and length of extremities should be carefully observed and recorded, then compared to growth tables. Any abnormal results in a child or an adult should be reported to the physician for further evaluation. These baseline data also serve as a check on progress after treatment is begun.

Monitor clients for weight loss and for constipation or anorexia, which are common with pituitary dysfunction. Clients may require a high-fiber, high-calorie diet to meet hypermetabolic requirements. Those who are anorexic need smaller, more frequent meals and should be weighed daily. Carefully measure intake and output. Monitor clients for symptoms and signs of diabetes mellitus.

If clients become weaker or increasingly lethargic, help them plan daily activities to alternate periods of rest and activity. Also encourage a slower pace of activities and help with personal care as needed.

One of the nurse's most important functions is to teach clients about their condition and to allow for client questions. Clients should be made aware of the significance of taking periodic body measurements and accurately recording the results. Because diabetes mellitus is so often a complication of both gigantism and acromegaly, the client should be instructed in its symptoms and signs and taught how to check the urine for glucose. The importance of periodic fasting blood-sugar levels should also be discussed.

Clients should be familiar with the symptoms and signs of recurring or expanding tumor. In particular, they should be instructed to report immediately any changes in vision, any increase in severity or frequency of headaches, or any increasing lethargy or weakness.

Because adrenocortical insufficiency can develop in clients with gigantism or acromegaly, they should be familiar with its symptoms and signs. Instruct clients to call the physician immediately if any of these occur or if they have an infection or are undergoing emotional stress.

Clients receiving medications should be familiar with names, dosages, actions, and side effects. Teach clients the symptoms and signs of overdosage and underdosage and when and what to report to the physician. If there are any special instructions regarding sick days, clients should receive a written copy of these "sick-day rules" and should become thoroughly familiar with them. Sick-day rules are simply instructions for clients to use if they become ill. The instructions are another tool to promote self-care and independence. In addition, clients should be encouraged to wear a Medic-Alert tag or carry a wallet card describing the condition and their medications.

Provide opportunities for clients to discuss their feelings and ask questions about the changes in their physical appearance. The child with gigantism or the adult with acromegaly needs to know not only the reason for the changes in physical appearance but what might occur in the future. The physical changes seen in gigantism and acromegaly often cause suffering. Clients must deal with a major change in body image that may threaten their self-esteem.

Provide opportunity for clients to express their feelings about changes in libido, impotence, or the consequences of amenorrhea. Often, nurses, because of their interactions with clients and families over time, are in a position to help clients verbalize and explore their feelings about what is happening to them. Changes in sexual ability and loss of fertility are important concerns to clients and their significant others; these problems should be considered as important as any others in formulating the nursing care plan.

The importance and purpose of ongoing medical supervision and evaluation should be discussed with both client and significant others. They all should be aware of the diagnosis, the symptoms and signs of the condition, and the objectives of the treatment plan.

Cushing's Disease

Hypersecretion of ACTH by the anterior pituitary results in increased stimulation to the adrenal cortex. This causes excessive secretion of glucocorticoids by the adrenal cortex, which in turn produces the characteristic cushingoid features: moon face, truncal obesity, decreased glucose tolerance, supraclavicular fat pads, abdominal striae, abnormal skin pigmentation, and pendulous fat pad in chest and abdomen. This condition is known as Cushing's disease, or pituitary-dependent or secondary Cushing's syndrome, and is characterized by excessive secretion of ACTH, hyperplasia of both adrenal glands, and overproduction of cortisol (Jubiz, 1979). If the excessive secretion of glucocorticoids is due to a primary adrenal disorder, as explained earlier in this chapter, the condition is known as Cushing's syndrome.

Clinical Manifestations
The clinical manifestations and diagnostic procedures for all clients with a cushingoid presentation are the same. Refer to the discussion of Cushing's syndrome earlier in this chapter.

Therapeutic and Specific Nursing Measures
The treatment of choice in pituitary-dependent Cushing's disease is destruction of the tumor. The medical measures, surgical measures, and specific nursing measures are the same as those discussed for clients with acromegaly.

ADRENAL DISORDERS

Aldosteronism

Primary aldosteronism, or Conn's syndrome, a condition caused by excessive production of aldosterone by the adrenal cortex, is characterized by hypertension, excessive urinary loss of potassium, and retention of sodium. Primary aldosteronism is thought to be the cause of hypertension in 1% to 2% of all clients with diagnosed hypertension. This is one form of hypertension that is completely curable. Primary aldosteronism originates from one of three sources (Kaye & Rose, 1983): a single adrenocortical tumor (generally a benign adenoma), bilateral hyperplasia of the adrenal cortices, and tumor of the juxtaglomerular (JG) cells of the kidney, which produce renin autonomously. (A secondary form of aldosteronism occurs when increased renal secretion of renin leads to the increased production of aldosterone. The increased renin secretion results from other pathological processes in the body, such as heart failure, nephrosis, and cirrhosis. The production of aldosterone it triggers in turn initiates a cycle of pathologic changes, resulting in increased fluid retention, further compromising cardiac and hepatic function.)

Clinical Manifestations

The major clinical manifestations of primary aldosteronism are hypertension, excessive urinary loss of potassium resulting in hypokalemia, and retention of sodium (hypernatremia). The hypertension in clients with primary aldosteronism is usually a moderate elevation of the diastolic blood pressure. The client may complain of headaches. On physical examination, early hypertensive retinopathy and cardiomegaly may be noted.

The symptoms attributable to hypokalemia range from mild fatigue to profound weakness. The client may complain of paresthesia, loss of stamina, muscular weakness, and intermittent periods of paralysis. If hypokalemic alkalosis occurs, resulting in tetany, physical examination may elicit positive Trousseau's and Chvostek's signs (see Figure 5–4 in Chapter 5).

Because of the increased reabsorption of sodium and water, hypernatremia and hypervolemia occur. Generally, edema is not present. The hematocrit may appear abnormally low as a result of the hemodilution. In addition to these major clinical signs, the client with primary aldosteronism may also have severe polydipsia, polyuria, and nocturia resulting from the renal tubules' inability to respond to ADH.

Primary aldosteronism should be suspected in all clients with hypertension, particularly the young. The finding of hypertension, hypokalemia (below 3.5 mEq/L), and excessive mineralocorticoid production (ie, increased serum aldosterone levels) suggest the diagnosis. These findings become more significant if an excessive excretion of urinary potassium is found along with increased serum levels of sodium (hypernatremia) and decreased excretion of urinary sodium.

A spironolactone test may be used in conjunction with determination of serum potassium levels. Spironolactone is an aldosterone antagonist and, when given orally for 3 to 4 days, will stop the urinary excretion of potassium and restore serum levels to normal. Serum potassium levels have been shown to drop again 5 to 7 days after the drug is stopped. Other tests employed in the evaluation of clients with primary aldosteronism are discussed in detail in Chapter 41.

To localize an aldosterone-producing adenoma before surgery, various techniques may be used. Noninvasive procedures such as nuclear scanning with [131]I-19-iodocholesterol, computerized tomography (CT) scanning, and ultrasonography may be employed as well as invasive procedures such as arteriography and retrograde adrenal venography.

Therapeutic Measures

The two forms of therapy utilized in primary aldosteronism are surgery and drug therapy. Surgery is indicated when there is a unilateral aldosterone-producing tumor. In cases of hyperplasia, a subtotal or total adrenalectomy may be performed. Postoperatively, the return of normal aldosterone secretion by the remaining adrenal tissue may take several months. Following resection of the tumor, the blood pressure will return to normal in most clients, but in one-third it may only be lowered slightly (Kaye & Rose, 1981).

Spironolactone, an aldosterone antagonist, may be given orally over short periods if surgery is contraindicated. Triamterene may also be used. The action and side effects of spironolactone and triamterene are summarized in Table 44–5.

Specific Nursing Measures

The nursing care of clients with primary aldosteronism should include daily weights and measurement of intake and output to assess degree of fluid retention and loss, as well as frequent assessment of blood pressure, pulse, and respiratory rate. Symptoms and signs of increased blood pressure (eg, headaches, changes in visual acuity, and hypertensive retinal changes) should also be noted. Observe

Table 44–5 Pharmacologic Agents Used in Primary Aldosteronism

Generic and Trade Name	Usual Dosage	Action	Side Effects
Spironolactone (Aldactone)	25 mg–200 mg g.d. PO in divided doses	Potassium-sparing diuretic; blocks action of aldosterone on Na-K exchange pump	Should not be used in clients with renal dysfunction; may cause potentially dangerous increases in serum K levels; may cause menstrual irregularities, hirsutism, gynecomastia
Triamterene (Dyrenium)	100 mg b.i.d. PO, after meals	Potassium-sparing diuretic, action similar to that of spironolactone but not a steroid	Triamterene may cause blood dyscrasias; both drugs may cause GI symptoms, skin rashes, "drug fever"

for symptoms and signs of cardiac decompensation and congestive heart failure (eg, increasing shortness of breath, jugular venous distention, rales at lung bases, orthopnea, and paroxysmal nocturnal dyspnea) and irregularities in heart rate and rhythm.

Assess the client for symptoms and signs of hypokalemia, muscle weakness, cramping, fatigue, and skin breakdown. Also evaluate the client for paresthesia and tetany (related to low serum calcium levels resulting from hypokalemic alkalosis). Provide for adequate rest because the client may have nocturia and may need a daytime nap to make up for lost sleep. The diet should be high in protein, low in sodium, and high in potassium. Calories may be restricted if weight reduction is desired. The preoperative and postoperative nursing care of clients undergoing adrenal surgery is discussed in Chapter 45.

Instruct clients with primary aldosteronism on the nature of the disorder (pathophysiology, symptoms and signs, and prognosis); the goals of the medical, surgical, and nursing treatment plan; and how those goals are to be implemented. If they are to be placed on medication, clients should be familiar with its purpose, action, dosage, administration, and side effects. They should know the essentials of their diet and should recognize the need for regular medical evaluation. Postsurgically, clients should be aware that normal endocrine function may take several months to return and that they may need medication during this period. Other clients may not require medications postsurgically or may require lifelong treatment.

Teach clients who are able to take their own blood pressure and pulse regularly, to interpret the findings, and when to report them to the physician. If clients are unable to monitor themselves, family members or friends should be taught to do so.

Pheochromocytoma

Pheochromocytomas are tumors composed of chromaffin cells. The tumors may be found in the adrenal medulla or, less frequently, in the sympathetic ganglia of the abdomen, bladder, or chest. Pheochromocytomas are usually benign and characteristically produce both catecholamines (epinephrine and norepinephrine), although some tumors may release only one of the catecholamines. Hypersecretion of epinephrine elevates the blood pressure by increasing the strength of contraction of the heart, resulting in an increase in cardiac output. Norepinephrine causes arteriolar vasoconstriction, increasing the peripheral vascular resistance to blood flow. Both of these effects result in the marked elevation of both diastolic and systolic blood pressures, which is characteristic of pheochromocytoma. Although clients find its symptoms frightening, pheochromocytoma has a good prognosis.

Pheochromocytomas are thought to occur more often than clinically recognized because they are difficult to diagnose. Pheochromocytomas may be present for varying amounts of time before symptoms occur. Tumors that produce primarily epinephrine are often associated with profuse diaphoresis, palpitations, tremor, anxiety, heat intolerance, and pallor followed by flushing. Tumors that produce primarily norepinephrine are associated with fewer symptoms; the symptoms are similar to those in clients with essential hypertension, hence the difficulty in diagnosis.

Most pheochromocytomas are benign, unilateral adrenal tumors; 10% are bilateral or multiple; 10% are extraadrenal; and 10% are malignant. Men and women are equally affected; the peak incidence is in the fourth and fifth decades of life, although they have occurred in very elderly clients and in newborns. Pheochromocytomas can also be found in association with certain familial neurocutaneous disorders (neurofibromatosis, hemangioblastoma), with hyperparathyroidism, and with thyroid medullary carcinoma (Blacklow, 1983).

Both epinephrine- and norepinephrine-producing tumors may secrete catecholamines paroxysmally, episodically, or continuously. The most severe symptoms are usually seen in clients with the paroxysmally functioning tumors because of the rapid and marked changes in serum catecholamine levels. About 40% of clients with pheochromocytoma have paroxysmal hypertension, whereas the remainder experience either sustained or labile elevations in the blood pressure (Petersdorf et al., 1983).

The paroxysmal attacks vary in frequency, severity, and duration. Both the onset and resolution tend to be abrupt, with the average attack lasting a few minutes to a few hours. In many clients, these attacks may occur without warning, whereas others may be able to identify a prodrome of dermal paresthesia and increasing anxiety. Paroxysmal attacks are also precipitated by emotional changes (eg, laughing, sexual activity, and pain), postural changes (especially flexion or bending of the body), and/or physical exertion. Attacks may increase in frequency and duration over time. These attacks may result in pulmonary edema, cerebral hemorrhage, or ventricular fibrillation and hence may be fatal.

Clinical Manifestations

Symptoms of pheochromocytoma include headache, diaphoresis, and intense palpitations. The client may also complain of extreme anxiety, tinnitus, excessive weakness and tremor, blurred vision, vertigo, dyspnea, and anginal chest pain. After the attack, the client may report a feeling of complete prostration.

Signs of pheochromocytoma include marked elevation of the diastolic and systolic blood pressure (which may rise as high as 200 to 300/150 to 175 mm Hg), often with excessive diaphoresis, anxiety, dilation of the pupils, and tachycardia. Orthostatic hypotension due to contraction of the blood volume and hypertensive retinopathy may occur in clients with persistently functioning tumors. Hyperglycemia and glycosuria are also frequently associated with pheochromocytoma because of catecholamine inhibition of insulin and elevation of plasma glucose levels (Blacklow, 1983).

Pheochromocytoma should always be suspected in hypertensive clients who have symptoms and signs of sympathetic hyperactivity, although fewer than 1% of all hypertension is from pheochromocytoma. The diagnosis of pheochromocytoma is based on the demonstration of excessive catecholamine levels in the serum and urine. In clients with pheochromocytoma, elevated levels of epinephrine; norepinephrine; and their metabolites, metanephrine, normetanephrine, and vanillylmandelic acid, will be present in the urine.

In the past, pharmacologic tests such as the histamine test and phentolamine blocking test were used in the diagnosis of pheochromocytoma. These have largely been replaced by the more reliable and safer urinary assays, which are discussed in Chapter 41.

After excessive catecholamine secretion has been determined, studies are done to confirm the diagnosis and localize the tumor. Common methods are CT scans of the adrenal glands or radiological studies such as the intravenous pyelogram with nephrotomograms, abdominal arteriograms, and selective venography.

Therapeutic Measures

The definitive treatment for pheochromocytoma is surgical excision of the tumor. In the 10% of clients who are not surgical candidates (because of malignant pheochromocytoma with metastases or serious medical problems), control of symptoms is attempted with the use of alpha-adrenergic blocking agents such as phentolamine and phenoxybenzamine hydrochloride. Beta-adrenergic blocking agents may be used in clients with cardiac dysrhythmias or those not responsive to treatment with alpha-adrenergic agents. Clients with pheochromocytoma who are receiving beta-blocking agents should also be receiving alpha blockers to prevent the severe hypertension that can result from unopposed alpha stimulation (Camunas, 1983). Both alpha- and beta-blocking agents should be used with caution because clients can be exquisitely sensitive to them.

The surgical approach to pheochromocytoma is discussed in detail in Chapter 45. The client may have either a midline or transverse upper abdominal incision. The abdominal incision is preferred because it allows complete visualization of both adrenals as well as the extraadrenal sites. The induction of anesthesia and the incision and manipulation of the tumor can precipitate severe hypotension, myocardial infarction, intracerebral hemorrhage, cardiac failure, or hyperthermia (Camunas, 1983).

Specific Nursing Measures

The preoperative and postoperative nursing care for clients with pheochromocytoma is discussed in Chapter 45. In almost 10% of all clients with this tumor, precise localization of the tumor may not be possible before surgery, creating even more anxiety for the client. Hence, it is important to adopt a confident, supportive approach while ensuring that the client and family have an opportunity to discuss their fears and concerns.

Discharge planning should stress the need for lifelong medical supervision. In pheochromocytoma, there is a 10% to 13% chance of recurrence of the tumor, which may be malignant (Camunas, 1983).

The need for lifelong replacement therapy must be emphasized if a bilateral adrenalectomy has been performed or if the remaining tissue is nonfunctioning. Positive aspects of this disorder that can be stressed in client education are that it is a curable cause of hypertension and has a good prognosis.

Disorders of the pituitary and adrenal glands pose many problems and concerns for clients and their significant others. Because of the nature of these disorders—the visible physical changes, the mental and emotional involvement, the often disabling reduction in energy levels and ability to withstand stress—clients and families require considerable nursing support as well as excellent client education. They also need an opportunity to discuss freely their feelings and concerns about their disorder and its meaning for them. Because nurses can make important contributions to the recovery of clients in these areas, technical aspects of nursing care should not be allowed to surpass them.

Chapter Highlights

Pituitary dwarfism is usually not apparent at birth but is suspected when an abnormality in growth is noted later in childhood. It is associated with a deficiency or undersecretion of growth hormone, or somatotropin.

Panhypopituitarism is characterized by deficiency of all the hormones of the anterior pituitary. Total deficiency of these hormones without replacement is fatal.

Diabetes insipidus is a disorder of water metabolism characterized by the excretion of excessively large amounts of hypotonic urine. It may be pituitary or nephrogenic in origin.

The syndrome of inappropriate antidiuretic hormone (SIADH) is characterized by autonomous release of ADH without regard to plasma osmolality. The body is unable to dilute the urine appropriately. The consequences are fluid retention, expansion of the extracellular fluid compartment, and hyponatremia.

Cushing's syndrome, also known as hypercortisolism, is characterized by an excessive level of cortisol in the plasma.

Addison's disease, or primary adrenal insufficiency, is characterized by a deficiency of all three types of adrenal hormones. However, only the effects of deficiencies of the glucocorticoids and mineralocorticoids are usually seen.

Gigantism, defined as a height over 80 in in an adult, is characterized by an increased secretion of somatotropin before puberty. If the excessive secretion of somatotropin occurs after puberty (ie, epiphyseal closure), the condition is called acromegaly.

Cushing's disease is a disorder characterized by hypersecretion of ACTH, resulting in increased stimulation to the adrenal cortex and excessive secretion of glucocorticoids.

Primary aldosteronism, or Conn's syndrome, is caused by excessive production of the adrenocortical mineralocorticoids, particularly aldosterone. Clients with primary aldosteronism often have hypertension, excessive loss of potassium through the urine, hypokalemia, and sodium retention.

Pheochromocytoma is characterized by excessive secretion of the catecholamines (epinephrine and norepinephrine), which produces systolic and diastolic hypertension, profuse diaphoresis, and anxiety.

Pituitary and adrenal disorders, because of their visible physical effects, may cause clients great mental and emotional anguish. Clients often also have a disabling reduction in energy levels and ability to withstand stress. These conditions cause many problems and concerns for clients and their significant others.

Bibliography

Aveson J: Human oddities: Naturally different. *Nurs Mirror* 1980; 150(7):30–32.

Barber LR, Burton JR, Qieve PD (editors): *Principles of Ambulatory Medicine.* Baltimore: Williams & Wilkins, 1982.

Bentley PJ: *Endocrine Pharmacology: Physiologic Basis and Therapeutic Applications.* New York: Cambridge University Press, 1980.

Blacklow D: *MacBryde's Signs and Symptoms,* 6th ed. Philadelphia: Lippincott, 1983.

Burnett J: Congenital adrenocortical hyperplasia: Nursing interactions. *Am J Nurs* 1980; 80:1309–1311.

Camunas C: Pheochromocytoma. *Am J Nurs* 1983; 83(6):887–891.

Clark JB, Queener SF, Karb VB: *Pharmacological Basis of Nursing Practice.* St. Louis: Mosby, 1982.

DeGroot L et al: *Endocrinology.* New York: Grune & Stratton, 1979.

Jubiz W: *Endocrinology: A Logical Approach for Clinicians.* New York: McGraw-Hill, 1979.

Kaye D, Rose LF (editors): *Fundamentals of Internal Medicine.* St. Louis: Mosby, 1983.

Malseed RT: *Pharmacology: Drug Therapy and Nursing Considerations.* Philadelphia: Lippincott, 1982.

Mondal BK: Acromegaly: A change in size. *Nurs Mirror* 1981; 153(81):38–39.

Muthe NC: *Endocrinology: A Nursing Approach.* Boston: Little, Brown, 1981.

Petersdorf RG et al (editors): *Harrison's Principles of Internal Medicine,* 10th ed. New York: McGraw–Hill, 1983.

Sanford SJ: Dysfunction of the adrenal gland: Physiologic considerations and nursing problems. *Nurs Clin North Am* 1980; 15(3):481–498.

Saxton DF et al: *The Addison–Wesley Manual of Nursing Practice.* Menlo Park, CA: Addison–Wesley, 1983.

Solomon BL: The hypothalamus and the pituitary gland: An overview. *Nurs Clin North Am* 1980; 15(3):435–451.

Williams R (editor): *Textbooks of Endocrinology,* 6th ed. Philadelphia: Saunders, 1981.

The Client With Addison's Disease

I. Descriptive Data

Mr Walter Warren is a 54-year-old white male who has his first appointment at the outpatient clinic at a large, urban hospital because of generalized weakness and weight loss.

II. Personal Data

Date and Time:	March 14, 1986, 9:30 AM
Full Name:	Walter A. Warren
Address:	13 Sloan Ave., Buffalo, NY
Telephone:	Home: 000-0000
	Work: 000-0000
Sex:	Male
Age:	54
Birthdate:	11-7-31
Race:	Caucasian
Culture:	Scotch–Irish
Marital Status:	Married
Occupation:	Steelworker
Religion:	Catholic
Usual Health Care Provider:	No regular medical care; has received episodic care at the emergency department of a local hospital; last physical examination in 1972 for insurance company

III. Health History

Source of Information:	Client
Reliability of Informant:	Reliable
Chief Concern:	Weight loss, easy fatigability, and anorexia × 2–3 months, increasing in severity

History of Present Illness: Client states that for the past 2–3 months he has experienced a progressive decrease in his appetite, resulting in a weight loss of 23 lb, generalized weakness, and decrease of physical endurance causing him to miss at least 1 day of work per week; he also has a slight feeling of nausea, occasionally accompanied by abdominal cramping. The nausea and cramping seem unrelated to the ingestion of food and are not relieved by antacids. He has experienced these periods of nausea approximately 1–3× daily for a period of 25–35 minutes. The abdominal cramps are mild, lasting a few minutes and recurring 1–5× daily; they felt like "gas pains" to him although they were unrelieved by the passage of flatus or by eructation; BMs are regular (one daily) and stools are dark brown. Has no epigastric pain, fever, chills, emesis, hematemesis, or melena; no history of peptic ulcer disease, food intolerance, or esophageal, gallbladder, or pancreatic problems.

For the past week, he has experienced transient episodes of palpitations, occurring at rest and with exertion. Episodes last 1½ minutes and resolve. His family became concerned about this development and "forced him" to make this appointment. He denies any accompanying chest pain, SOB, cough, PND, or DOE. He has no past history of cardiac or vascular disease.

Past Health History:

Childhood:	Rheumatic fever, mumps
Immunizations:	Td booster, 1981
Medical Problems:	None
Surgeries:	T&A, 1933; appendectomy, 1950; rt menisectomy, S/P trauma, 1981

Case Study written by Anne Herrstrom Skelly.

Transfusions:	None
Special Diagnostic Procedures:	None
Trauma:	Fell off catwalk at work in 1981, with resulting tear to cartilage of rt knee
Allergies:	Sulfa (generalized rash)
Medications:	Maalox, 1 tbsp p.r.n. nausea
	Acetaminophen, 300 mg, q. 4 h. p.r.n. pain
	Multivitamins, $\frac{.}{1}$ q.d.
	Vitamins, C and E, $\frac{.}{1}$ q.d.
Family History:	Father, age 75, A&W, DJD
	Mother, died age 42, cause unknown
	Brother, age 58, A&W, hypothyroidism
	Sisters, ages 56 and 51, A&W, eldest c̄ ↑ BP, DJD
	Sister, died age 3, pneumonia
	Wife, age 55, A&W
	Daughters, ages 25 and 28, A&W
	PGF, pernicious anemia; maternal aunt, Ca breast; PGM, Parkinson's disease; MGM, CVA; No ⊕ FHx, DM, TBC, MI
Personal/Social History:	Client resides with wife of 29 years who is in good health. They own their own home and have no major financial problems. Two married daughters, both in good health, reside nearby. Usual daily schedule: arises at 5 AM; works 5 days a week at steel plant, where he has been employed for the past 34 years. Concerned about possibility of plant closing because of depressed economic times. Returns home usually at 4 PM and spends rest of day working in garden or "tinkering with automobiles." On weekend, routine includes shopping with wife, entertaining grandchildren (ages 3 and 6½ years) and working on home remodeling projects. Lately, has been unable to do any of these activities because of increasing weakness and lack of stamina.
	Mr Warren is a high school graduate and a World War II veteran. He was stationed in the South Pacific. Since the war, he has not traveled outside the United States except for an occasional trip across the border to Canada and a trip to Bermuda for 1 week in 1980.
Habits:	Used to eat three substantial meals a day; now only able to eat two small meals; enjoyed walking and bowling 1–2× weekly before onset of symptoms. Has never smoked; drinks one to two beers on weekends; used to sleep 6–7 hours a night; at present needs 9–10 hours, with an occasional daytime nap; has also noted some decrease in libido for past 2–3 months; is very concerned about his diminished strength and stamina.
Review of Systems:	
General Health:	"Felt I was in pretty good health, until a few months ago; now everything is going downhill."
Genitourinary:	Some mild difficulty starting urinary stream, no nocturia, no dysuria, no hematuria, no frequency, no penile discharge
Neurologic:	Lightheadedness on rapid position change without vertigo; no syncope, no blackouts, no headaches
Psychological:	Feels more irritable; "can't seem to think as clearly."
IV. Physical Assessment	
Height:	5 ft 9 in
Weight:	170 lb (weight 11-85 was 193 lb)
Vital Signs:	BP supine rt arm 138/72; seated rm arm 120/60; temperature 98.8°F (37°C); resting P. 72; R. 20

(continued)

The Client With Addison's Disease

Relevant Organ Systems:

Skin: Bronzing of skin with increased pigmentation in skin folds and creases, areolae, and in RLQ surgical scar

Eyes: EOMs intact s̄ nystagmus, fundi benign

Mouth: Pigmentation in buccal mucosa

Neck: No jugular venous distention; thyroid not enlarged; no lymphadenopathy; carotids 2+ and = without bruits

Heart: Rate 72 and regular with 2–3 ectopic beats per minute, no gallops or murmurs

Lungs: Clear to A&P, without rales, rhonchi, wheezes

Abdomen: RLQ surgical scar, bowel sounds normoactive, no bruits; soft, s̄ masses, nontender; no organomegaly; inguinal nodes not palpable; no CVA tenderness

Extremities: Rt patellar scar; well healed

Neurologic: Grossly intact, Romberg ⊖; reflexes, wnl

V. Diagnostic Data

Mr Warren was admitted to the hospital and had the following diagnostic work-up:

ECG: Unusually tall, thin T waves with 1–2 PVCs/30 sec

Chest x-ray: wnl

CBC: wnl

Sodium: 132 mEq/L (normal 135–145 mEq/L)

Potassium: 6.1 mg/L (normal 3.5–5.5 mEq/L)

Glucose: 75 mg/dL, random nonfasting specimen

Serum cortisol levels (at 8 AM): 6 μg/dL (normal 5–25 μg/dL)

Metyrapone test: Failure of adrenals to respond to ACTH challenge

Urine 17-hydroxycorticosteroids and 17-ketosteroids: Markedly decreased

On the basis of his history, physical examination, and diagnostic study findings, Addison's disease was diagnosed.

VI. Nursing Care Plan

Nursing Diagnosis	Client Care Goal	Plan/Nursing Implementation	Expected Outcome
Injury, potential for, related to orthostatic hypotension and hypoglycemia	Remain free from injury	Counsel client to change positions slowly and rest in a supported position until symptoms abate if experiencing orthostatic hypotension (dizziness and lightheadedness in fast positional changes); monitor BP and pulse frequently in supine and seated positions, watching for a drop in the diastolic pressure accompanied by a rise in the pulse rate; instruct severely symptomatic clients to call for assistance before changing positions (call bell nearby, siderails up); encourage client not to skip or postpone meals because of possibility of hypoglycemia; observe client for symptoms and signs of hypoglycemia (weakness, diaphoresis, lightheadedness, abdominal cramps); instruct client to take medications as ordered and plan several rest periods during the day to avoid fatigue	Client free of symptoms secondary to orthostatic hypotension and hypoglycemia

Nursing Diagnosis	Client Care Goal	Plan/Nursing Implementation	Expected Outcome
Nutrition, alteration in, related to anorexia	Maintain adequate nutritional status and normal weight range	Monitor body weight; encourage client to eat a high protein, high carbohydrate diet: Potassium and sodium intake depend on individual status (eg, serum levels and type of medication taken); may need small, more frequent feedings; snacks should be provided and encouraged; keep accurate record of daily caloric intake and fluid intake and output; assess food preferences and desires and factors that might interfere with digestion (dentures); monitor laboratory parameters (glucose, BUN, hemoglobin, hematocrit, sodium, and potassium levels) and report any changes to the physician; counsel the client and the family that fasting may precipitate adrenal crisis; administer antiemetics or antacids (if client is on corticosteroids), as ordered; promote adequate hydration but may want to limit fluids 1 h before meals to prevent early satiety	Client will maintain adequate nutrition, hydration, and electrolyte balance; weight will remain within normal limits
Cardiac output, alteration in, related to possible dysrhythmia	Maintain normal potassium levels; remain free from dysrhythmia	Monitor apical heart rate and rhythm, BP, and respirations frequently (at least q. 4 h); assess client for complaints of palpitations, SOB, ↑ DOE, and muscle cramping; monitor serum potassium and sodium levels and report immediately any fluctuations from normal; place client on a cardiac monitor if ordered (Note: depressed T waves are an indication of hypokalemia; tall peaked T waves, an indication of hyperkalemia); if client is receiving steroids, observe for symptoms and signs of hypokalemia; ie, dysrhythmias, muscle weakness, and hypotonicity	Client free of symptoms of dysrhythmias secondary to hyperkalemia or hypokalemia
Sleep pattern disturbance	Obtain sufficient rest and sleep to perform ADL without undue fatigue	Assess client carefully for physical and mental activity tolerance and adjust daily schedule accordingly; plan frequent rest periods during the day; instruct client about relation of energy deficit, medication regimen, and increased emotional and physical stress; medication should be taken as ordered to maintain the normal diurnal variation of the hormone	Client will adjust lifestyle to accommodate to changes in body function
Knowledge deficit, related to Addison's disease	Understand diagnosis, treatment, and symptoms and signs of potential complications	Instruct client and family regarding nature of the disorder, treatment goals, prognosis, and need for lifelong medication and supervision: Instruct client and significant others regarding the symptoms and signs of adrenal crisis and steroid overdosage; client and family should be encouraged to call the physician at the first sign of adrenal crisis, infection, or increased physical or emotional stress; client should carry a Medic-Alert tag or card; instruct	Client will be knowledgeable about his disorder and independent in self-care; client and significant others will feel confident about symptoms and signs signaling a need for physician intervention

(continued)

1399

The Client With Addison's Disease

VI. Nursing Care Plan (continued)

Nursing Diagnosis	Client Care Goal	Plan/Nursing Implementation	Expected Outcome
		client and family about specific dietary requirements and the need for rest periods to prevent excessive fatigue; the mental slowing and emotional instability from decreased cortisol secretion are often a concern to both client and family; provide opportunities for discussion of these concerns, with appropriate feedback about the origin of these changes and the role of medication in relieving them	

Surgical Approaches to Endocrine System Dysfunction

Anne Herrstrom Skelly

Objectives

When you have finished studying this chapter, you should be able to:

Identify the nursing implications of hypophysectomy, including preoperative preparation, postoperative care, and discharge planning.

Anticipate the physiological and psychosocial/lifestyle implications of hypophysectomy for the client and family or significant others.

Identify the nursing implications of adrenalectomy, including preoperative preparation, postoperative care, and discharge planning.

Anticipate the physiological and psychosocial/lifestyle implications of adrenalectomy for the client and family.

Identify the nursing implications of thyroidectomy, including preoperative preparation, postoperative care, and discharge planning.

Anticipate the physiological and psychosocial/lifestyle implications of thyroidectomy for the client and family or significant others.

Identify the nursing implications of parathyroidectomy, including preoperative preparation, postoperative care, and discharge planning.

Anticipate the physiological and psychosocial/lifestyle implications of parathyroidectomy for the client and family.

The primary objectives of surgical therapy in endocrine disorders are to control the abnormal hormonal levels, to relieve the symptoms produced by enlargement of the affected gland, and to rule out possible malignancies of the gland. The major endocrine surgeries are hypophysectomy, adrenalectomy, thyroidectomy, and parathyroidectomy. Hypophysectomy and adrenalectomy also are treatment approaches for clients with cancer of the breast, ovary, and prostate.

Endocrine surgery may have profound physiological and psychosocial/lifestyle implications for the client and family. Many clients require lifelong medication and medical supervision and are at risk for problems related to underdoses or overdoses of these medications. Clients may also have difficulty withstanding stress and infection, necessitating major adjustments in lifestyle.

Section I: Surgical Approaches to Disorders Affecting the Pituitary Gland

Microsurgery has virtually replaced other approaches to pituitary surgery. Nursing care in this section is focused on clients undergoing hypophysectomy employing microsurgical techniques.

HYPOPHYSECTOMY

Hypophysectomy, the surgical removal of the pituitary gland, may involve the resection of a small tumor or the complete removal of the gland. The major indications for hypophysectomy are a primary neoplasm of the pituitary gland (adenoma) and the need to retard the growth and spread of such endocrine-dependent malignancies as cancer of the breast, ovary, and prostate. In the last instance, hypophysectomy does not cure the disease but simply removes the source of the gonadotropic hormones that support the neoplasm. This may provide a remission for several months. Hypophysectomy also can be used to relieve pain in these malignancies.

Surgical Procedure

Pituitary ablation has been achieved by external radiation therapy or by using a radioactive implant; by surgical destruction using stereotactic cryosurgery (freezing); or by surgical excision via a transfrontal craniotomy. Currently, transsphenoidal microsurgery is the most common surgical approach. Whether radiation, surgery, or drugs are used depends on the type and amount of hormonal dysfunction, the size of the tumor, and whether it extends outside the sella turcica.

Transfrontal Craniotomy

A transfrontal craniotomy is indicated when the tumor extends beyond the pituitary fossa and is impinging on the optic chiasm, because this procedure provides the best view of the operative field. For a detailed discussion of the various procedures involved in performing a transfrontal craniotomy, refer to Chapter 39.

Transsphenoidal Hypophysectomy

If the tumor does not extend beyond the sella turcica, the surgeon may use a transsphenoidal approach, employing an operating microscope and televised radiofluoroscopy. Because it causes minimal damage to healthy tissue, the transsphenoidal approach has become the procedure of choice.

During a transsphenoidal hypophysectomy, the client receives general anesthesia while in a sitting position facing the surgeon. The sella turcica is entered by way of the sphenoidal sinus cavity. The initial incision is a horizontal one made in the gingivae over the maxillary bone, so there is no external incision. Following the intrasellar procedure, the surgeon often patches the opening in the dura mater with fascia lata reinforced with muscle tissue or fat from the thigh. The floor of the sella turcica may be reconstructed with cartilage from the nasal septum.

Following surgery, the nasal cavities are usually packed for 48 to 72 hours with petrolatum gauze impregnated with an antibiotic ointment. A gauze sling may be placed under the nasal cavities to absorb secretions. A dry dressing is placed over the thigh wound.

Implications for the Client

Because of the proximity of the optic nerves, optic chiasm, carotid arteries, cavernous sinus, and hypothalamus to the operative area, the surgery involves some risk. The optic nerves or optic chiasm can be injured directly or can be damaged by compromise to their vascular supply. Postoperative visual problems can also result from compression by a hematoma. Prompt detection of visual deterioration is esential so that reoperation can be performed while there is still a chance to reverse the damage. The carotid arteries and cavernous sinus lie lateral to the sella turcica and are vulnerable to injury should the surgeon stray off the midline.

Postoperative diabetes insipidus is not uncommon but is less likely following removal of a microadenoma. A deficiency of ADH is the result of mainpulation or sectioning of the pituitary stalk or damage to the hypothalamus.

Transient CSF leaks can occur following removal of the nasal packings. Most leaks respond to conservative measures aimed at keeping the ICP low. Damage to the dental pulp and injury to the nerves or blood supply to the anterior maxillary teeth have also been reported.

Psychosocial/lifestyle implications for the client will depend on the reasons for the surgery and the final outcome. Clients with acromegaly can expect cessation of further growth and a significant reduction in soft tissue swelling. In the months following surgery a remarkable improvement in facial appearance occurs. Clients with prolactinomas can expect return of menses as well as fertility.

The lifelong hormonal replacement imposed by total hypophysectomy is a considerable financial burden. Some clients may be angry and resentful about their dependence on medication. Others may fear being caught in a situation in which their medications are unavailable.

Physiological and psychosocial/lifestyle implications of transsphenoidal hypophysectomy are summarized in Table 45-1.

Nursing Implications

Preoperative Care

The preoperative preparation of the client for a transsphenoidal hypophysectomy is similar to that for a transfrontal craniotomy, except the removal of scalp hair is not required. It is important to establish a supportive relationship with the client and significant others, because they may be extremely anxious. In addition to the client teaching for a craniotomy, it is important to stress the importance of avoiding activities that increase intracranial pressure (ICP) in the immediate postoperative period (eg, coughing, sneezing, nose blowing, straining with urination or defecation, bending over, or lifting). The client and family should understand the need for lifetime hormonal replacement following hypophysectomy. Clients should be informed that in the immediate postoperative period, they will receive IV fluids and nutrients. The nurse will fre-

Table 45–1 Transsphenoidal Hypophysectomy: Implications for the Client

Physiological Implications	Psychosocial/Lifestyle Implications
Although this is an intracranial procedure, manipulation is usually confined to the sella turcica and the area immediately above it. Cerebral edema and seizures are unlikely	Following hypophysectomy the lifelong dependency on hormonal replacement requires lifestyle modification and may be cause for anxiety.
In the client with metastatic disease, relief of bone pain is achieved and further metastases may be arrested or slowed	For the client with metastatic disease, lifestyle is greatly enhanced by relief of pain and freedom from potent analgesics.
In clients with acromegaly further bony growth will be arrested and a substantial reduction in soft tissue swelling can be expected	For the client with acromegaly, surgery has a positive effect because the gradual but often remarkable improvement in appearance enhances body image; relief of associated symptoms allows for a more normal lifestyle.
Surgical risks are related to the proximity of the optic nerves and chiasm, the carotid arteries, cavernous sinuses, and hypothalamus	For the client with visual impairment there may be no significant improvement; occasionally vision may be further impaired, requiring significant alterations in lifestyle
Visual deterioration or loss can result from direct injury to the optic chiasm, optic nerves, or from compromise to their blood supply	Sexual dysfunction associated with pituitary dysfunction may cause considerable stress, altered body image, and lowered self-esteem
Injury to the hypothalamus may occur with radical excision of large suprasella lesions	
Operative mortality secondary to carotid artery damage is rare	
Rhinorrhea may be transient and frequently responds to measures aimed at keeping ICP low	
Diabetes insipidus may occur	

A corticosteroid preparation is given 1 day before surgery and on the day of surgery to avoid adrenal insufficiency secondary to the removal of the source of ACTH. An in-dwelling catheter may be inserted to enable frequent, accurate determination of postoperative urinary output, which is important in determining the need for ADH replacement. Before surgery, an IV cannula is inserted, and an infusion is started.

Closely monitor clients with diagnosed pituitary tumors for symptoms and signs of pituitary apoplexy, which include severe headache, changes in level of consciousness (LOC), diplopia, loss of vision, and shock. Pituitary apoplexy occurs when there is spontaneous hemorrhage into the tumor secondary to rupture of the blood vessels or rapid enlargement of the adenoma with resulting infarction. It is an emergency requiring immediate intervention.

Postoperative Care

The postoperative care of a client with a transfrontal craniotomy is similar to that for other clients with craniotomies discussed in Chapter 39. In particular, observe the client closely for:

- Symptoms and signs of increased ICP: increased blood pressure; decreased pulse rate; change in pupil size, equality, and reaction to light; and changes in the client's LOC, mental, or neurologic status
- Signs of adrenal insufficiency
- Signs of hypothyroidism (which may develop over several weeks)
- Symptoms and signs of meningitis (elevated temperature, headache, motor restlessness, photophobia, and nuchal rigidity)
- Symptoms and signs of fluid imbalance, which may indicate transient or permanent diabetes insipidus

Following transsphenoidal hypophysectomy, observe the client closely for leaking of cerebrospinal fluid (CSF) through the nares. This can be differentiated from the normal nasal secretions by special CSF testing materials or a test strip for glucose. Glucose is found only in CSF, not in nasal secretions. Report positive glucose test results to the physician. Place the client on bed rest with the head of the bed elevated to 30° to decrease pressure on the sella turcica.

Most clients recover rapidly from transsphenoidal surgery and are allowed out of bed within 24 hours. Fluids are taken orally the evening of surgery, and the diet is increased as tolerated.

Because of the nasal packs, the client is forced to breathe through the mouth and may report a temporary loss of smell. Oral hygiene—rinsing the mouth with saline or clear water—is important to keep the oral mucosa moist. Brushing the teeth is usually contraindicated because of possible tension on the suture line. The nasal packs are usually removed in 48 to 72 hours. The client may be placed on prophylactic antibiotic therapy in either the pre-

quently check their temperature, blood pressure, pulse, and respirations. Clients also should be told that their eyes may be ecchymotic and that a nasal drip pad will be used for drainage from the nose.

operative or postoperative period because of the increased danger of infection using the transsphenoidal approach.

Headache may be a problem in the postoperative period and should be reported to the physician immediately because of the danger of meningitis. Headache is usually treated with non-narcotic analgesics or codeine. Because codeine tends to be constipating, carefully monitor the client's bowel status to prevent straining at stool and increased ICP. If analgesics are used, carefully assess the client's LOC and do a neurologic evaluation to monitor the client's progress.

A major complication in the postoperative period is hypopituitarism, which may develop into addisonian crisis and transient or permanent diabetes insipidus. Therefore, observe the client closely for symptoms and signs of addisonian crisis (weakness, lethargy, fever, nausea, hypotension, and dizziness) and diabetes insipidus (fluid and electrolyte imbalances). In the immediate postoperative period, carefully measure the intake and output of all clients as a guide to fluid balance; check the specific gravity of urine after each voiding.

The usual medication regimen is to administer a cortisone preparation preoperatively and continue it intravenously until the client can tolerate an oral dose. This dose is gradually adjusted until a maintenance level is achieved, and a replacement dose of cortisone is continued for the rest of the client's life. In addition, the client may require

replacement of thyroid and sex hormones (testosterone and estrogen). A few clients may require ADH to control polyuria. After a total ablation of the pituitary gland, menstruation ceases, and the client becomes infertile.

For men, testosterone may relieve changes in libido and impotence secondary to the surgery. Estrogen may be prescribed for women to relieve atrophy of the vaginal mucosa. Human pituitary gonadotropins have been successful in treating infertility in posthypophysectomy clients, especially women. Be sensitive to the effect of this type of surgery on reproductive capacity and functioning and provide ample opportunity for clients to express their thoughts and feelings. Appropriate referral for counseling has also proven beneficial for both the client and sexual partner.

Discharge Planning

Two important nursing responsibilities in the discharge of clients following hypophysectomy are instructions regarding (1) medications (cortisone, thyroxine, sex hormones, and ADH), including their purpose and side effects, and (2) the importance of regular follow-up care. The client should also know the proper administration of these hormones, the symptoms and signs of hormonal imbalance, and circumstances under which the physician should be contacted.

Section II: Surgical Approaches to Disorders Affecting the Adrenal Glands

Surgery of the adrenal glands is done for adrenal tumors or to control metastasis in clients with malignancy of the breast or prostate. Adrenalectomy is the major surgery to be discussed in this section.

ADRENALECTOMY

An adrenalectomy is the surgical removal or resection of one or both of the adrenal glands. A bilateral adrenalectomy involves the removal of both adrenal glands, and a unilateral adrenalectomy is the removal of one adrenal gland. In a subtotal adrenalectomy, a part of an adrenal gland is excised.

The major goal of adrenalectomy is to reduce the excessive secretion of the adrenal hormones. The procedure is indicated when there is hyperfunction secondary to a tumor or hyperplasia of the gland, in pheochromocytoma, and in advanced cases of cancer of the breast and prostate. These malignancies are known to be affected by the hormones of the endocrine system; estrogen has an effect on breast carcinomas and testosterone, on carcinomas of the prostate. In certain clients, these hormones are still present after endocrine suppression and have been found to arise from the adrenal cortex. In premenopausal women with cancer of the breast who are to have adren-

alectomy; an oophorectomy is performed first. In men with cancer of the prostate who are to undergo adrenalectomy, an orchiectomy is performed first.

Surgical Procedure

The two major surgical approaches to adrenalectomy are the transabdominal and lateral approaches. A posterior or transthoracic approach has also been used in certain circumstances.

The transabdominal approach uses a bilateral subcostal or midline incision, which requires preoperative preparation of the entire abdomen and lower thorax from the nipple line to the symphysis pubis. The surgeon opens the abdominal wall and explores the peritoneal cavity. The wound is closed in the same manner as in a routine laparotomy.

The lateral approach involves an incision under the twelfth rib in the rear flank area. This incision is similar to that made for a nephrectomy and is used in clients who are obese or at risk for wound dehiscence. The lateral approach is also useful in clients with large adrenal tumors where the posterior approach cannot be used. The eleventh and twelfth ribs may be resected during the procedure to better expose the upper pole of the kidney. The wound is closed by a sequential replacement of the tissue layers—eg, muscle, fascia, subcutaneous tissue, and skin (Gruendemann & Meeker, 1983).

Implications for the Client

Physiological and psychosocial/lifestyle implications of adrenalectomy include loss of adrenocorticol hormones with lifelong replacement therapy. Implications are covered in Table 45–2.

Nursing Implications

Preoperative Care

Preoperative nursing care focuses on stabilization of the client. In a client with Cushing's syndrome, this involves controlling such problems as hypertension, decreased resistance to stress and infection, emotional lability, edema, hyperglycemia, and hypokalemia. In a client with a pheochromocytoma, nursing care involves managing paroxysmal labile hypertension, severe headache, visual disturbances, excessive sweating, and palpitations.

In addition to general preoperative care discussed in Chapter 14, the nurse should consider the following points in planning preoperative care for clients facing adrenalectomy. The environment should be organized to provide maximum physical and emotional rest for the client. Be aware of the effect of hyperadrenocorticolism on the emotions and provide support and reassurance to the client and family during periods when the client is emotionally labile. Monitor the client for any symptoms and signs of infection, and report these promptly to the physician.

Check the client's blood pressure and vital signs at regular intervals, especially if the client has a pheochromocytoma. Report any marked elevations of the blood pressure to the physician. Clients who are hypertensive before surgery may be placed on phentolamine (Regitine), phenoxybenzamine hydrochloride (Dibenzyline), or both to attempt to reduce the vasomotor tone and lower the blood pressure. The client also may be following a salt-restricted diet to control hypertension. In this instance, check body weight and edema at least daily as assessment criteria.

Check serum electrolytes and urinary glucose and acetone levels at regular intervals to screen for hypokalemia and hyperglycemia. All fluid and electrolyte imbalances must be recognized and corrected in the preoperative period because of the profound physiological changes in the postoperative period. Measure the client's intake and output and weigh the client daily to assess the degree of fluid retention. The potassium-depleted client may receive a solution of potassium chloride. If the client is anemic, transfusion with whole blood or packed cells may be ordered.

Diet in the preoperative period centers on three important factors: hypertension, hyperglycemia, and hypokalemia. In addition, the client with excessive hyperadrenocorticolism may have protein depletion (hypoproteinemia) reflected by a low serum albumin level (LeMaitre & Finnegan, 1980). In general, diet control involves a high-protein diet for protein depletion, reduced carbohydrates and calories for hyperglycemia, restrictions of salt intake for hypertension and fluid retention, and increased potassium intake for hypokalemia. An ulcer also requires special dietary planning.

In the immediate preoperative period, an in-dwelling catheter is usually inserted, as well as a nasogastric (NG) tube to reduce vomiting and abdominal distention postoperatively. Corticosteroids are administered preoperatively as well as during surgery to prevent adrenal insufficiency in the postoperative period. Intravenous fluids are usually

Table 45–2 Adrenalectomy: Implications for the Client	
Physiological Implications	**Psychosocial/Lifestyle Implications**
Loss of adrenocortical hormones, which are essential to life, in proportion to the amount of tissue removed; causes profound physiological changes, especially in the postoperative period	Great effect on psychological status and lifestyle from the loss of adreno-cortical hormones
	Possible need to arrange life and activities to avoid emotional crises, infections, overfatigue, and extremes of temperature
Lifelong glucocorticoid and mineralocorticoid replacement after bilateral adrenalectomy	Possible occupational change to avoid stress, because stress may precipitate an adrenal crisis if the hormonal output is not sufficient to meet the needs of the moment
In unilateral adrenalectomy, cortisol administration during and after surgery, with gradual adjustment of the dosage until remaining adrenal function is adequate	Lifetime medical supervision
	Dependency on medication and the need to know medication regimen, including the name of the drug, dose, frequency, and side effects
In immediate postoperative period, possible acute adrenal insufficiency or addisonian crisis precipitated by stress	Need to watch for the symptoms and signs of medication overdose or hyperadrenocorticolism (edema, weakness, hirsutism, and hypertension) and underdose, or adrenal insufficiency (headache, weakness, malaise, nausea, vomiting, and hypotension)

started and infused slowly to allow prompt administration of corticosteroids and vasopressors if needed.

Because both the transabdominal and lateral approaches involve incisions close to the diaphragm, the client's postoperative respirations tend to be shallow, and coughing is extremely uncomfortable. Therefore, one of the most important preoperative responsibilities of the nurse is to teach clients what to expect and how best to breathe deeply and cough postoperatively (using a pillow to support the incision).

Client teaching before adrenalectomy also should include:

- What to expect in the immediate postoperative period. (The client will be in the recovery room or intensive care unit until stable, and vital signs will be monitored regularly.)
- The importance of coughing, deep breathing, and early ambulation for prevention of complications.
- The nature of the procedure, its indication, and its expected outcome, including the need for lifelong medication and medical supervision.

Postoperative Care

The greatest postoperative concern after adrenalectomy is adrenal insufficiency. Also important are possible hypotension caused by the rapid withdrawal of mineralocorticoids, electrolyte imbalances, and infection resulting from suppression of the immune system. The surgical hazards associated with adrenalectomy include possible injury to the spleen, duodenum, and common bile duct, as well as hemorrhage (LeMaitre & Finnegan, 1980).

Postoperative nursing care of the client following adrenalectomy includes frequent monitoring of the vital

---

Nursing Research Note

Kosel K, Gibb–Matas P, Seaborne L, Westerberg J: Total pancreatectomy and islet cell autotransplantation. *Am J Nurs* 1982; 82: 568–571.

Care of 10 clients who underwent total pancreatectomy and islet cell transplantation was discussed. Care required skilled nursing personnel and support of many health care professionals. Client education was of primary importance and dealt primarily with preoperative teaching, diabetic counseling, and postdischarge education. It was also necessary for nurses to assess each client's ability to cope with anxiety, discomfort, and the use of narcotics. Postoperative care of these clients also presented challenges.

With progress in surgery, protocols and nursing care plans must be continually revised to meet the special needs of clients undergoing extensive surgical procedures. Nurses must always be alert to finding improved ways to assess, teach, and evaluate client progress.

---

signs, including LOC and especially blood pressure, for at least the first 48 hours after surgery. Blood pressure is monitored every 15 minutes in the immediate postoperative period until it is stabilized. The client may also have central venous pressure monitoring. Report any unexplained or significant fall in blood pressure to the physician, because it may indicate impending adrenal insufficiency. Any complaints of chest pain should also be reported immediately, because they may indicate cardiac involvement or a pulmonary embolus.

Monitor blood chemistry reports and fluid balance regularly until they are stabilized. Serum sodium, potassium, and glucose levels are obtained and possibly, urine sodium levels. Carefully record intake and output, and promptly report any imbalances. In the acute postoperative phase, the client's urinary output is measured hourly. Be alert for symptoms and signs of renal shutdown, such as oliguria, anuria, and increasing BUN and creatinine levels.

Monitor the client for symptoms and signs of addisonian crisis. Early signs of adrenal insufficiency may be subtle, including restlessness, dehydration, and tachycardia. Later signs preceding overt shock are increased weakness, hypotension, increased temperature, and vomiting. Addisonian crisis is an emergency and requires prompt intervention with increased corticosteroids, hypertonic saline solutions, or both. In rare cases, peripheral vasoconstrictors are used.

The client should may remain on bedrest for 2 to 3 days until the vital signs are stabilized. To prevent complications of immobility, change the client's position and encourage coughing and deep breathing exercises done every 2 hours. An NG tube prevents postoperative vomiting and minimizes abdominal distention. After the NG tube is removed, the client progresses to a clear liquid diet and then to a diet as tolerated.

Administration of corticosteroids is continued by IV infusion until the client is able to tolerate oral doses of cortisol. In some instances, IM injections of desoxycorticosterone may be administered but are usually replaced by oral cortisol when the client can tolerate it. Be alert for symptoms and signs of hyperadrenocorticolism and adrenal insufficiency and report them promptly. When the IV corticosteroids have been discontinued, the IV may be kept open until the client is completely stable. This precaution provides a quick route for the administration of corticosteroids or a vasopressor as needed.

Special Postoperative Considerations With Pheochromocytomas. If an adrenalectomy was done because of pheochromocytoma, there are important nursing considerations other than the usual postoperative care. Because of the possibility of extreme fluctuations in the blood pressure in the immediate postoperative period, monitor blood pressure every 15 minutes until it is stabilized. Clients with a pheochromocytoma may require a longer period for their blood pressure to become stabilized than other postadrenalectomy clients. Be alert for any sudden elevations of blood pressure in the early postoperative period, which may occur because of the release of epinephrine and norepinephrine from the tumor as it was being excised. Phentolamine or another adrenergic blocking agent may be used intravenously if the blood pressure rises excessively.

Severe hypotension may also develop postoperatively in these clients. If untreated, this can lead to shock. Metaraminol bitartrate (Aramine) and norepinephrine bitartrate (Levophed), usually given via IV infusion, may be used to stabilize the blood pressure. The dosage of these vasopressors is titrated to the client's blood pressure. Therefore, accuracy is essential in measuring the blood pressure, as well as in regulating the flow rate of the infusion. The physician prescribes the rate of flow.

Advise all clients with pheochromocytomas to change positions slowly to avoid symptoms of orthostatic hypotension. They are on bed rest for several days until the vital signs are stabilized. When the head of the bed is elevated, check the blood pressure to assess the result of position change. Blood pressure is also closely monitored when the client is first allowed out of bed. If a significant drop occurs, the client is placed back on bed rest in a supine position. Elastic stockings may be ordered to prevent pooling of blood in the extremities.

Discharge Planning

Clients who have had a bilateral adrenalectomy should understand the significance of the procedure and the fact that hormonal replacement therapy is required for the rest of their lives. They must remain under close medical supervision and should know the indications of adrenal crisis and how it can be precipitated by infection or severe stress. Clients also should be aware of the symptoms and signs of corticosteroid overdose (edema, weakness, hypertension, and hirsutism) and the need to report them to the physician. Those who had hyperadrenocorticolism before surgery should know that these symptoms will slowly subside. Because cortisone tends to mask the symptoms of infection, and adrenalectomy clients are more susceptible to infection, they should be instructed in the subtle signs of illness and encouraged to keep their resistance up and avoid infection whenever possible. They should report early signs of infection immediately to the physician because of the danger of adrenal crisis.

Clients who have a subtotal adrenalectomy should be given the same instructions. They may not need lifelong hormonal replacement but will require careful observation for several months to determine when the remaining adrenal tissue can meet the body's demand. In the meantime, these clients are also at risk for potential adrenal crisis and should be advised to avoid infection, stress, overfatigue, and extremes of temperature. Help clients understand the symptoms and signs of adrenal insufficiency and hyperad-

renocorticolism and the importance of reporting them to the physician.

One of the most important nursing responsibilities in discharge planning is to emphasize the need for continued medical care. Emergency medical tags or bracelets will protect clients in emergency situations when they may be unable to communicate. Counsel clients about resuming activities slowly. The proper amount of hormonal replacement may take several months to achieve, and clients should expect frequent dosage readjustments. Many clients who begin corticosteroid therapy will experience a transient insomnia for the first 2 to 3 weeks, but it usually is resolved without treatment. Tell clients who have had an adrenalectomy because of a pheochromocytoma that their blood pressure may not stabilize within an acceptable range for up to 3 months.

Although corticosteroid therapy has been discussed in relation to adrenal and pituitary surgery, it is important to remember that any surgical client could be receiving corticosteroids for a variety of reasons. Box 45–1 reviews the important nursing considerations for any surgical client receiving corticosteroids.

Box 45–1 Influence of Corticosteroids on Any Surgical Client

The nurse caring for any surgical client receiving corticosteroids should be aware of several important facts. Corticosteroids may be given as replacement therapy (in Addison's disease, hypopituitarism, bilateral adrenalectomy), as well as therapeutically for collagen diseases (rheumatoid arthritis, lupus erythematosus, scleroderma, and periarteritis nodosa). They are also used selectively to treat asthma, iritis, and thrombocytopenic purpura (Moroney, 1982). Clients who have received corticosteroid therapy for long periods usually experience a medically induced adrenal insufficiency because of the suppression of pituitary ACTH. The return of normal pituitary and adrenal function following prolonged therapy may take up to 1 year, and during this period the client must be protected by corticosteroids, especially if surgery is necessary (Muthe, 1981).

Surgical candidates receiving corticosteroid therapy should have the dosage of their steroids increased before and during surgery to meet the increased demands of the anesthetic and surgical procedure. If this is not done, acute adrenal insufficiency may result.

Possible complications of corticosteroid therapy for the surgical client are:

- Exacerbation of peptic ulcer (eg, increased bleeding)
- Reactivation of latent tuberculosis
- Cardiac failure
- Increased incidence of fulminating infections

In addition, the client may develop other side effects of corticosteroid therapy such as osteoporosis, hirsutism, psychosis, and acne (Moroney, 1982).

Section III: Surgical Approaches to Disorders Affecting the Thyroid Gland

Surgical removal of all or part of the thyroid gland may be indicated in clients with hyperthyroidism, goiter, thyroid nodules, or carcinoma of the thyroid. Thyroidectomy is the major surgery to be discussed in this section.

THYROIDECTOMY

Thyroidectomy, the surgical removal of the thyroid gland, may involve a complete removal of the gland or the removal of a lobe (thyroid lobectomy) or portion (subtotal thyroidectomy). Occasionally, clients with enlarged goiters have tissue extension into the substernal or intrathoracic area, and a substernal or intrathoracic thyroidectomy is performed. A thyroglossal duct cystectomy is performed to prevent recurrent cyst formation and infections in clients with a diagnosed cyst of the thyroglossal duct. The thyroglossal duct is an embryological structure that, when present in adults, forms a cystic pouch attached to the hyoid bone in the pretracheal area (Gruendemann & Meeker, 1983). The clinical indications for thyroidectomy are hyperthyroidism (Graves' disease), simple goiter, thyroid nodules, and papillary carcinoma of the thyroid gland.

If surgery is required in Graves' disease, its objective is to remove enough of the thyroid gland to normalize the plasma levels of circulating hormone but to leave enough of the gland to secrete sufficient amounts of T_4 and T_3. Thyroidectomy is also indicated in clients with Graves' disease who, because of sensitivity, are unable to take antithyroid medications as well as in clients for whom the use of radioactive iodine is contraindicated. When there is inflammation of the thyroid gland, or thyroiditis, surgery is only indicated to relieve symptoms of obstruction of the trachea or if malignancy is suspected (LeMaitre & Finnegan, 1980).

Goiter, a condition characterized by an increased amount of thyroid tissue as a means of producing more thyroid hormone, is not characterized by excessive hormone production or inflammation. The objective of surgery in clients with goiter is to relieve esophageal or tracheal obstruction or to improve cosmetic appearance (Gruendemann & Meeker, 1983).

Thyroid nodules can be discrete or multiple and can be benign or malignant. The objective of surgery for clients with these nodules is to rule out possible malignancy.

In cases of goiter, thyroid nodules, or hyperthyroidism, a subtotal thyroidectomy is performed. This involves resection of about five-sixths of the thyroid gland. The remainder of the gland is usually sufficient to provide the necessary thyroid hormones, so replacement may not be needed (Muthe, 1981). Most cancer of the thyroid, however, is treated with a total thyroidectomy, so the client will require lifelong replacement with thyroid hormone. In cases of papillary carcinoma of the thyroid, a total or nearly total thyroidectomy is usually performed. If a primary tumor has been isolated in one lobe, a neck dissection on the involved side may also be indicated because of the proximity of the thyroid to the regional lymph nodes, the primary route for metastasis (LeMaitre & Finnegan, 1980). The mortality rate from thyroid surgical procedures is low; approximately 90% of adult clients will be cured (Muthe, 1981).

Surgical Procedure

Important factors in the surgical approach to the thyroid are the vascularity of the thyroid, the proximity of the parathyroid glands to the thyroid (see Figure 45–1), the relation of the trachea and larynx to the thyroid gland, and the proximity of the recurrent laryngeal nerve to the thyroid. Figure 45–2 shows the surgical site for removal of

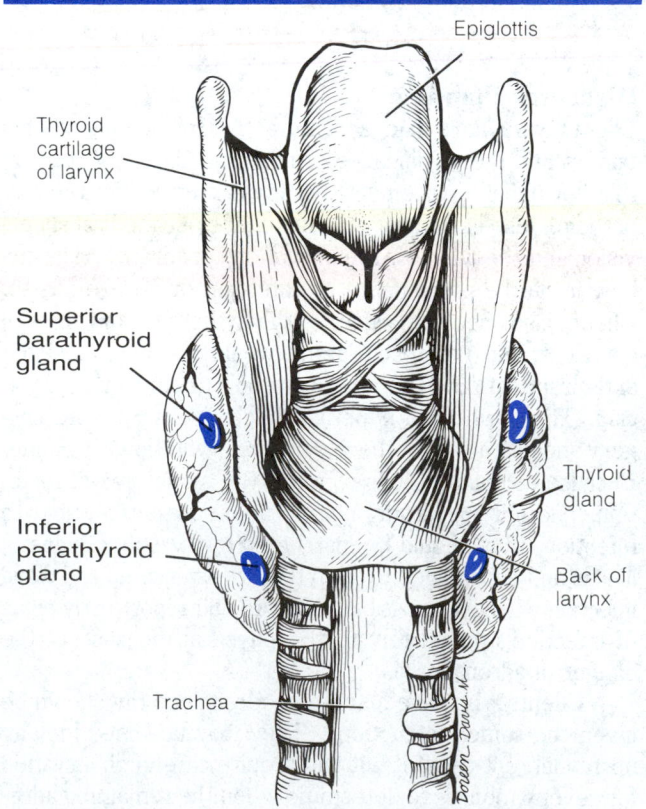

Figure 45–1

Thyroid and parathyroid glands.
SOURCE: Spence AP, Mason EB: *Human Anatomy and Physiology,* 2nd ed. Menlo Park, CA: Benjamin/Cummings, 1983, p. 440.

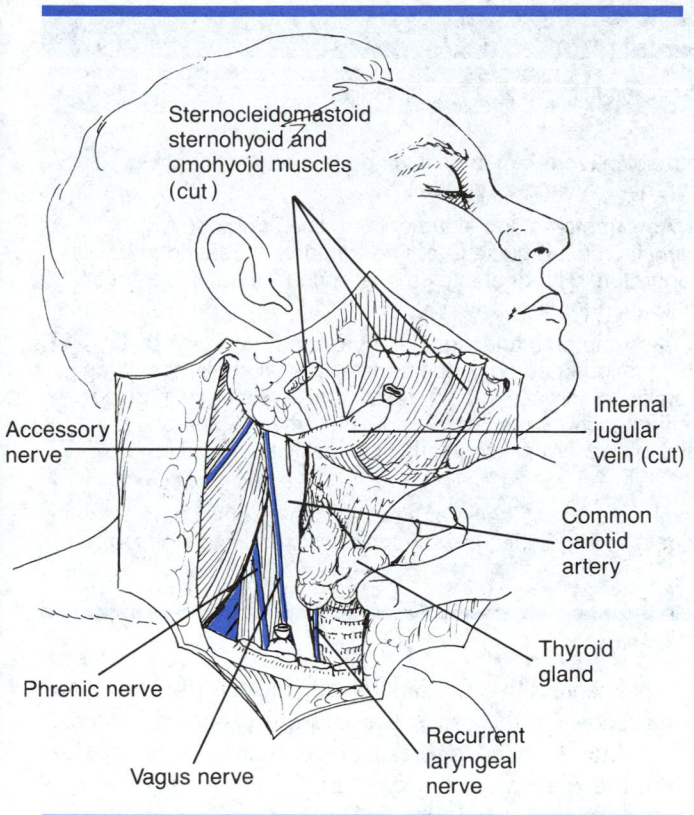

Figure 45–2

Surgical site for removal of the thyroid gland.

the thyroid gland. Note the relative position of the structures mentioned.

In a thyroidectomy, a curvilinear incision is made parallel to the lower crease in the neck, one finger's breadth above the supraclavicular notch. The incision ends laterally at the insertions of the sternocleidomastoid muscles on the clavicle. The gland is then exposed, and the blood supply to the area to be resected is divided. The nerves to the vocal cords are identified and left intact. The thyroid tissue is resected, and the incision is then closed (LeMaitre & Finnegan, 1980). A Penrose drain may be used, or the wound may be allowed to drain laterally through the lateral aspect of the incision and sternocleidomastoid muscles. Fine silk sutures are used to approximate the skin edges. A gauze dressing is applied and fastened with a thyroid collar dressing (Figure 45–3).

Surgical complications include hemorrhage from the superior thyroid arteries; damage to the parathyroid glands because of their proximity to the thyroid; damage to the trachea during surgery, resulting in the aspiration of blood or the postoperative formation of a tracheocutaneous fistula; perforation of the esophagus; and damage to one or both of the recurrent laryngeal nerves, resulting in hoarseness or total aphonia.

Implications for the Client

Among the physiological and psychosocial/lifestyle implications of thyroidectomy are lifelong thyroxine therapy. Implications for the client are discussed in Table 45–3.

Nursing Implications

Preoperative Care

Preoperative preparation of the thyroidectomy client depends to a degree on the clinical indications for the surgery. For example, the emotional care for the client who is to undergo thyroidectomy for an undiagnosed mass in the neck must include the possibility of carcinoma. Clients having a thyroidectomy for Graves' disease require a different approach because of their emotional lability secondary to the oversecretion of thyroxine.

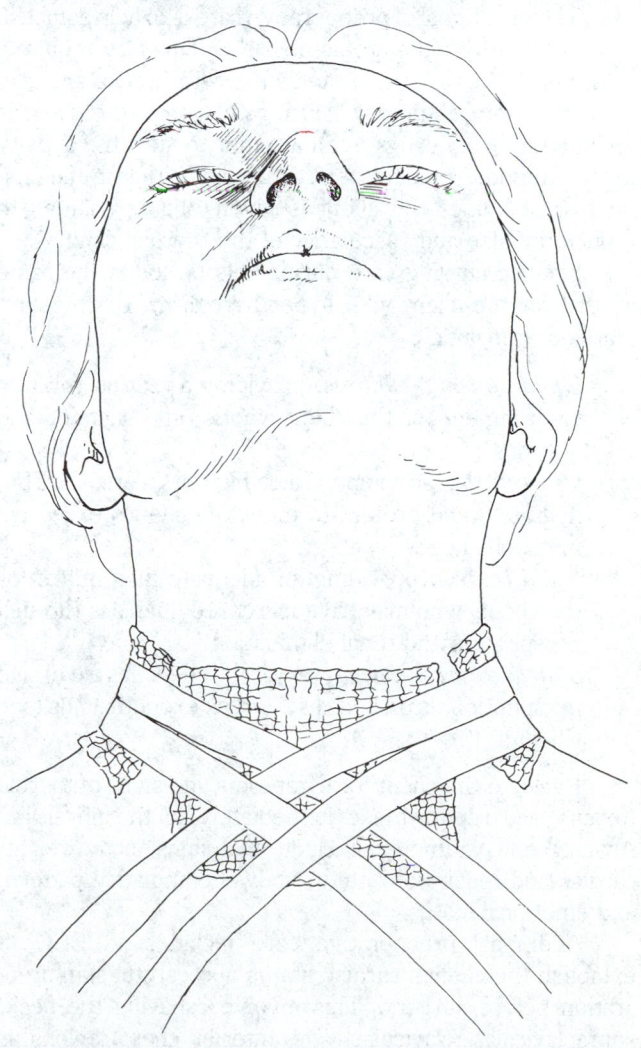

Figure 45–3

Thyroid collar dressing.

Table 45–3 Thyroidectomy: Implications for the Client

Physiological Implications	Psychosocial/Lifestyle Implications
Lifelong thyroxine therapy after total thyroidectomy and possibly after subtotal thyroidectomy Immediate postoperative risk for hemorrhage; respiratory complications; tetany from hypocalcemia caused by inadvertent removal of, or injury to, the parathyroid glands; injury to the recurrent laryngeal nerve; and (rarely) thyroid crisis or storm (may develop rapidly in the first 24 hours)	Need to know the medication regimen, including the name of the drug, indications, dose, frequency, and side effects Need to watch for the symptoms and signs of thyroxine overdose (hyperthyroidism), including increased pulse rate, fine tremors, increased appetite, increased temperature with heat intolerance, amenorrhea, exophthalmos, and the development of fine silky hair Need to watch for the symptoms and signs of thyroxine underdose (hypothyroidism), including fatigue, lethargy, coarseness of scalp hair, nonpitting edema of the extremities, increase in body temperature, increase in pulse and respirations, changes in mentation (decline in memory or pseudopsychosis), reduced libido, menstrual irregularities, sensitivity to cold, and weight gain Visible thyroidectomy scar on the neck for several months until complete healing takes place; in some clients, a disfiguring scar requiring clothing modification

The major goal of preoperative care is to help establish as near a euthyroid state as possible. This may require a treatment period lasting between several weeks and 2 to 3 months before surgery. During this time, the client is given antithyroid drugs in an attempt to slow the activity of the thyroid. Ten days before surgery, either in the hospital or at home, the client is given Lugol's solution to reduce the size and vascularity of the thyroid gland.

Specific nursing care during this period is the same as that for the client with hyperthyroidism. Briefly summarized, it includes:

- *Environmental controls:* providing a restful, relaxing environment for the client who is often agitated and nervous
- *Diet control:* providing a diet high in calories, carbohydrates, and protein to meet the client's excessive metabolic needs
- *Fluid control:* providing an adequate fluid intake for the client, who may have increased fluid loss through perspiration and renal elimination
- *Skin and eye care:* necessary if the client has excessive perspiration, is on bed rest, or has exophthalmos (see Chapter 43)

Evaluate the client for symptoms and signs of thyroid toxicity and report these immediately to the physician. Assessment parameters include vital signs, body weight, cardiac and respiratory status, bowel elimination pattern, and emotional status.

Additional preoperative care includes an ECG to establish the client's cardiac status and careful skin preparation before surgery. This involves shaving the neck, supraclavicular, clavicular, and anterior chest regions as well as the face in a man. The client's blood is typed and crossmatched for 2 units of blood before surgery (LeMaitre & Finnegan, 1980).

Preoperative teaching should include the nature and indication for the procedure and the expected outcome, including the need for lifelong medication and supervision. Tell the client what to expect in the immediate postoperative period (ie, vital signs will be checked frequently, there will be a dressing on the neck, the neck must be kept relaxed and in good alignment avoiding flexion and hyperextension, head movements should be minimized, the throat may be sore for a few days, and medication will be available for discomfort). Give the client an opportunity to express and discuss any fears and anxieties regarding the surgery and its physiological and cosmetic results.

Postoperative Care

Assemble the following equipment at the bedside for use as needed in the postoperative period:

- Emergency tracheotomy tray
- Oxygen equipment
- Suction machine and cannulas

In addition, a humidifier, IV equipment, and ampules of calcium chloride or calcium gluconate should be available. Tubes for the collection of specimens for serum calcium levels should be readily accessible.

Following thyroidectomy, closely observe the client for the first 48 postoperative hours because adverse symptoms may develop quickly and can pose a threat to life. The major complications that may occur in the postoperative period are hemorrhage, respiratory distress, damage to the recurrent laryngeal nerve, hypocalcemia and resultant tetany, and thyroid storm or crisis (Muthe, 1981).

Important observations in the postoperative period include vital signs, which are initially checked every 15 minutes until stabilized. Respiration is carefully monitored with special attention to cyanosis or signs of respiratory

Chapter 45

Surgical Approaches to Endocrine System Dysfunction 1411

distress. Check the client's temperature rectally for the first day or two. Immediately report all fluctuations in vital signs to the physician. In addition, evaluate the client's level of consciousness, including restlessness, apprehension, or anxiety. Assess the client for persistent or increasing weakness of the voice or hoarseness. (Some hoarseness should be expected in the immediate postoperative period, but it should not persist more than 3 days.)

Maintain the client in a semi-Fowler's position immediately after surgery to encourage venous drainage from the neck. The head and neck should be in good alignment and may be supported by a small pillow. Flexion and hyperextension of the neck are contraindicated, and the client should keep head movements to a minimum. Place sandbags or small pillows at the sides of the head to aid immobilization. Muscle tension and spasm often develop in the cervical area as a consequence of this immobilization and can be relieved by massage. As clients progress, teach them to assist in the movement of the head and neck by supporting the head at the sides and in the occipital area. After the skin clips or skin sutures have been removed, the surgeon may order gradual active and passive exercises of the neck.

Once the vital signs have stabilized, the client is allowed out of bed, usually on the first postoperative day. Early ambulation is necessary to prevent stasis in the pulmonary and circulatory systems. During ambulation, remind the client to hold the head in good alignment and to walk erect (the tendency is to flex the neck to minimize tension on the suture line).

Encourage coughing and deep breathing. Coughing may be painful for clients; support and encourage them during this activity. Discourage excessive coughing, however, because it increases throat discomfort and places tension on the suture line. In the early postoperative period, suction may be used to assist the client in clearing the upper airways of excessive mucus secretions. Persistent throat soreness should be reported to the physician, and a room humidifier or medication may be ordered.

Intravenous fluids are usually given until the client can tolerate oral liquids. Liquids are started after nausea subsides and continued until the client can tolerate a soft diet (usually in 2 to 3 days when there is less pain with swallowing). An adequate oral fluid intake will obviate the need for further IV therapy, provide hydration for the client, and maintain renal function.

Usually no medications other than analgesics are ordered in the postoperative period. Meperidine hydrochloride (Demerol) or morphine are given in the first 48 hours to relieve discomfort and apprehension; administer the drug as ordered after careful client evaluation. Postthyroidectomy clients often experience a sense of compression in the neck until the edema subsides. This can be frightening and may make them apprehensive and restless. Careful evaluation of the client before the administration of an analgesic is important to determine the cause of the discomfort.

Postoperative Complications

Hemorrhage. Signs that should alert the nurse to the possibility of hemorrhage include a drop in blood pressure accompanied by a rapid, thready pulse. The nurse may notice either excessive blood on the dressing or behind the neck as well as swelling of the tissues around the dressing. If bleeding is suspected, peel back the outer layers of the dressing carefully and observe the amount of oozing. For clients in the dorsal recumbent position, remember that evidence of bleeding should be assessed laterally and posteriorly to the neck as well as anteriorly. The client may have increased "tightness" of the dressing and difficulty breathing. Wound hemorrhage in a client following thyroidectomy can cause respiratory obstruction by compressing the tissues. Therefore, closely observe the client for cyanosis and asphyxia, which may develop quickly.

If hemorrhage is suspected, the surgeon should be notified immediately and the client placed in the semi-Fowler's position. The dressing may be loosened to promote drainage. An emergency tracheotomy tray, sterile dressings, and oxygen equipment should be brought to the bedside. If the surgeon is not available immediately, the nurse may be instructed to remove the neck skin sutures or clips and separate the skin edges with a Kelly clamp to allow drainage of the accumulated blood. Cover this with a thick sterile dressing until the surgeon arrives (LeMaitre & Finnegan, 1980).

Respiratory Distress. Respiratory distress in the client following thyroidectomy can be caused by hemorrhage, edema of the glottis, or pressure on the trachea from edema. The nurse may note respiratory stridor, "crowing respirations," signs of dyspnea and cyanosis, and the use of the accessory muscles of respiration. The client should be placed in a high Fowler's position and given humidified oxygen by mask. Notify the physician immediately, even for early signs of respiratory distress. Swift nursing interventions are needed to prevent anoxia and cardiac arrest. A tracheotomy tray and endotracheal setup should be at the bedside to use if severe obstruction occurs.

Injury to the Recurrent Laryngeal Nerve. Recurrent laryngeal nerve injury and the resultant loss of voice are usually caused by resection of one or both of the nerves, edema, or trauma. Check the client's voice immediately after surgery by asking the client to repeat a few words; excessive talking is not required. Hoarseness or aphonia immediately after surgery is most likely caused by surgical injury to the recurrent laryngeal nerve. If the quality of the client's voice is good in the immediate postoperative period but then becomes hoarse, it is usually a temporary condition caused by edema (LeMaitre & Finnegan, 1980) or pressure from hemorrhage. Also be aware of the possibility of paralysis of the vocal cords, which can result in closing of the glottis and respiratory obstruction. Nursing interventions include careful observation and early reporting of symptoms and signs.

Hypocalcemic Tetany. Hypocalcemic tetany can be caused by (1) accidental removal of the parathyroid glands during thyroidectomy, (2) injury to the parathyroid glands, or (3) edema of the parathyroid glands. The tetany can occur within the first 24 to 48 hours after surgery as well as up to 6 or 7 days later. The client will have increasing nervousness, tingling in the hands and circumoral areas, painful muscle spasms, and facial spasms and grimaces. Palpitations may also occur.

The nurse may be able to elicit positive Chvostek's and Trousseau's signs. To elicit Chvostek's sign, percuss the facial nerve against the bone just anterior to the ear. Contraction of the facial muscle in the immediate area is considered a positive sign and indicative of neuromuscular irritability (impending tetany). A negative Chvostek's sign (no contraction) is considered normal. To elicit Trousseau's sign, place a blood pressure cuff on the arm, inflate it over the systolic pressure, and leave it on for 1 to 4 minutes. Observe the position and movements of the hand. In a positive Trousseau's sign, which again indicates neuromuscular irritability, the hand will assume a characteristic clawlike position, and contractions (carpopedal spasms) may be seen (see Figure 5–4 in Chapter 5). If either of these signs is elicited, the physician should be informed immediately and plasma calcium and phosphorus levels determined. Treatment is often initiated on the basis of these signs even before the laboratory results have been obtained.

Emergency treatment of hypocalcemic tetany consists of IV administration of 1 g of 10% solution of calcium gluconate. When therapy with calcium is ineffective, it may be followed by the oral administration of calcium or parathyroid hormone (PTH). Keep a tourniquet, a 10-mL syringe, and a 10% solution of calcium gluconate at the bedside (Muthe, 1981).

Thyroid Storm or Crisis. Thyroid storm or crisis is a potentially fatal complication of thyroid surgery rarely seen today because of extensive preoperative preparation of the client and ligation of the blood vessels before the thyroid tissue is handled during surgery. Thyroid storm is caused by a sudden surge of thyroid hormone into the circulation, usually because of excessive manipulation of a toxic gland during the surgical process. The symptoms and signs are the same as those seen in severe hyperthyroidism, including high fever, extreme agitation and restlessness, and extreme tachycardia. The nurse who observes any of these signs should contact the physician immediately because this is an emergency requiring prompt medical intervention. Treatment includes IV sodium iodide, oxygen, steroids, and sedatives. Assemble emergency equipment at the bedside while awaiting the physician's arrival.

Discharge Planning

Because clients are returning home much sooner after surgery than they did in the past, the nurse has a more limited time for client instruction. Some postthyroidectomy clients may be discharged on their third or fourth postoperative day. It is helpful if discharge instructions are written as well as verbal so the client and significant others have something to refer to at home.

Discharge instructions for the client include the importance of returning to the physician for further evaluation and follow-up care. This involves evaluation for any recurrent hyperthyroidism or hypothyroidism, as well as for any signs of hypoparathyroidism. The client should understand the medication regimen, its purposes, and its side effects. Explain any restrictions on activity and diet.

Neck exercises are usually prescribed, and the client should be able to redemonstrate the exercises to the nurse to ensure that they are being performed correctly. Also, the client may be instructed to use a moisturizing cream or emollient on the suture line to prevent contraction of the scar and improve the cosmetic effect.

Clients should know the symptoms and signs of hyperthyroidism, hypothyroidism, and hypoparathyroidism. They should understand the importance of calling their health care provider if any of these symptoms or signs occurs.

Section IV: Surgical Approaches to Disorders Affecting the Parathyroid Glands

Surgery of the parathyroid glands may be indicated for clients with adenoma, hyperplasia, or malignancy of the parathyroids. Parathyroidectomy is the surgery to be discussed in this section.

PARATHYROIDECTOMY

Parathyroidectomy is the surgical removal of all or a portion of the parathyroid glands. The major clinical indications for parathyroidectomy are a single or multiple adenoma of the parathyroid glands and primary hyperplasia of the glands, which produce hyperparathyroidism. About 1% of the adenomas of the parathyroid gland are malignant. Hyperparathyroidism resulting from either adenomas or hyperplasia of the parathyroid glands results in abnormally high levels of calcium in the blood, which affects the central nervous system, renal system, and skeleton. The only treatment for this situation is surgical, which has as its goal the restoration of normal serum calcium levels and the prevention of further complications.

Surgical Procedure

The procedure for parathyroidectomy is similar to that for thyroidectomy except that surgical removal of the parathyroid glands can be more difficult because of their minute size, variability in number, and variability in location (some parathyroid tissue may be found in the mediastinum). The goal of surgery is to remove the required amount of tissue while leaving enough to maintain sufficient PTH levels.

In hyperplasia of the parathyroid glands, which usually affects all four glands, the surgeon may remove three glands and do a subtotal resection of the fourth. One-half of a parathyroid gland is usually enough to maintain a normal level of circulating PTH. In clients with an adenoma, the gland with the adenoma is removed and sent for a frozen section. The other glands are then inspected and biopsied. Depending on the results of this assessment and the frozen section, the glands may be left in place, or a neck dissection may be performed.

Surgical hazards to these clients are similar to those for clients undergoing thyroidectomy, as discussed in the preceding section. In particular, the client is at risk for either temporary or permanent hypoparathyroidism if the glands have been traumatized or resected. Acute hypocalcemia may be seen postoperatively on the first to fourth days.

The prognosis with surgical treatment of hyperparathyroidism is good if the condition is identified early. When the diagnosis is made later, bone lesions usually respond well, but kidney lesions tend to progress (Muthe, 1981).

Implications for the Client

Physiological and psychosocial/lifestyle implications of parathyroidectomy include possible temporary or permanent hypoparathyroidism. Implications for the client are discussed in Table 45–4.

Nursing Implications

Preoperative Care

The preoperative nursing care of the client with hyperparathyroidism is directed toward the management and stabilization of the symptoms and signs of hypercalcemia. These include weight loss, severe dehydration, nausea and vom-

iting, bone pain, polydipsia, and polyuria (LeMaitre & Finnegan, 1980).

The client may be in a weakened condition and have bone pain with pathological fractures. A client with hypercalcemia or bone pain should be on bed rest and be protected from falls. Monitor blood pressure, pulse, and cardiac status carefully. Gastrointestinal symptoms should be evaluated, especially those related to ulcers (hematemesis, melena, and epigastric pain 1 to 2 hours after eating) and acute pancreatitis (vomiting, intense epigastric pain, fever, and chills), which are more common in clients with hyperparathyroidism. Changes in LOC or mentation—especially the development of confusion, excessive sleep, depression, or paranoia—should be closely evaluated.

Assessment of the client's renal function is important in both preoperative and postoperative nursing care, because preexisting renal damage from hypercalcemia may compromise renal function. Urine may be strained for calculi, and the client could be placed on an acid-ash diet to acidify the urine and prevent calculus formation. (Calcium calculi are soluble in a high-acid urine and not as soluble in an alkaline urine.) Monitor intake and output. Fluids can be pushed up to 4000 mL/day to prevent calculus formation, cardiac status permitting. Observe the client for symptoms and signs of urinary tract infection and renal failure.

The client may be placed on a low-calcium diet. If the client is constipated, stool softeners are ordered and additional fiber included in the diet.

Preoperatively, IV phosphate may be ordered to block the absorption of calcium from the gastrointestinal tract. Calcitonin also can be used in some instances to lower the serum calcium levels.

The preoperative preparation of the surgical site is the same as that described for thyroidectomy. Assemble the same equipment as that discussed for the client with thyroidectomy.

Client teaching in the preoperative period should include discussion of the nature of the procedure, its indication, and expected outcome. The client should know what to expect in the immediate postoperative period: vital signs will be checked frequently, there will be a dressing on the

Table 45–4 Parathyroidectomy: Implications for the Client

Physiological Implications	Psychosocial/Lifestyle Implications
Possible temporary or permanent hypoparathyroidism after surgery	Possible need for lifelong medical supervision
Immediate postoperative risk of hypocalcemia and tetany, hemorrhage, respiratory distress, recurrent laryngeal nerve injury, and hyperparathyroid crisis	Possible postoperative medication for months (especially if bone disease is present)
Impeded recovery because of preexisting damage to the central nervous system, heart, skeleton, or kidney	Need to understand the medication regimen, including the name of the drug, dose, frequency, route of administration, and side effects
	Need for client and family to understand any dietary restrictions and the essentials of meal planning

neck, the head may be immobilized by sandbags, the neck will be kept relaxed and in good alignment, head movements will be kept at a minimum, the throat may be sore for a few days, and medication will be available for discomfort. Provide an opportunity for the client to express and discuss any fears and anxieties related to the surgery.

Postoperative Care

The postoperative care of the client with a parathyroidectomy is essentially the same as the postoperative care of the client with a thyroidectomy. Of primary concern is the observation of the client for any symptoms and signs of tetany, including tingling and paresthesia circumorally and in the extremities, tremors, and positive Chvostek's and Trousseau's signs. Any of these symptoms and signs should be reported to the physician immediately. Suction equipment, a tracheotomy set, an endoctracheal tube, and oxygen equipment should be available at the bedside because

tetany requires immediate intervention and treatment. To monitor for hypocalcemia, serum calcium levels are usually evaluated every 12 hours and are expected to return to normal ranges within 24 to 48 hours postoperatively (LeMaitre & Finnegan, 1980).

Be alert for respiratory distress, hemorrhage, and damage to the recurrent laryngeal nerve. Any evidence of these complications also should be reported immediately to the physician.

Discharge Planning

Discharge planning for the client following a parathyroidectomy is similar to that discussed for clients who have had a thyroidectomy, except the client will be evaluated for any evidence of recurrent hyperparathyroidism or the development of hypoparathyroidism. The client needs to be aware of the symptoms and signs of these two clinical situations.

Chapter Highlights

The primary objectives of surgical therapy in endocrine disorders are controlling abnormal hormonal levels, relieving symptoms produced by enlargement of the gland, and ruling out possible malignancies.

Endocrine surgery may have profound physiological and psychosocial/lifestyle implications for the client and significant others. Many clients require lifelong medication and medical supervision.

Hypophysectomy, the surgical removal or resection of the pituitary gland, is performed primarily for a neoplasm of the pituitary or when an endocrine-dependent malignancy is present.

The two major procedures used in hypophysectomy are transfrontal craniotomy and transsphenoidal hypophysectomy. Hypophysectomy can be a threatening and anxiety-provoking surgery for clients and their significant others.

Postoperatively, the client with hypophysectomy requires lifelong hormonal replacement and medical supervision.

Adrenalectomy is the surgical removal or resection of one or both adrenal glands. It may be bilateral, unilateral, or subtotal. It can be performed using a transabdominal or lateral approach.

The clinical indications for adrenalectomy are hyperfunction secondary to a tumor or hyperplasia of the glands, pheochromocytoma, or advanced cancer of the breast and prostate.

Postoperatively, monitor the adrenalectomy client for symptoms and signs of adrenal insufficiency,

hypotension (caused by the rapid withdrawal of mineralocorticoids), electrolyte imbalances, and infection (from suppression of the immune system).

Thyroidectomy, the surgical removal of the thyroid gland, may involve the complete removal of the gland, resection of a lobe, or resection of a portion of the gland.

The clinical indications for thyroidectomy include hyperthyroidism, simple goiter, thyroid nodules, and papillary carcinoma of the thyroid gland.

The major goal of nursing care in the preoperative period is to establish as near a euthyroid state as possible.

Postoperatively, closely monitor the client for symptoms and signs of hemorrhage, respiratory distress, damage to the recurrent laryngeal nerve, hypocalcemia and resultant tetany, and thyroid crisis or storm.

Parathyroidectomy is the surgical removal of all or a portion of the parathyroid glands.

The major clinical indications for parathyroidectomy are a single or multiple adenoma of the parathyroid glands or primary hyperplasia of the glands.

The preoperative management of the client with hyperparathyroidism is directed toward management and stabilization of hypercalcemia.

Postoperatively, closely monitor the client for symptoms and signs of tetany as well as respiratory distress, hemorrhage, and damage to the recurrent laryngeal nerve.

Bibliography

Arnold J: Nursing care study: Giving the necessary support. *Nurs Mirror* 1983; 156(2):47–48.

Camunas C: Transsphenoidal hypophysectomy. *Am J Nurs* 1980; 80:1820–1823.

Eitel DM: Nursing care for hypophysectomy. *AORN J* 1981; 33:256–260.

Entwhistle K: Nursing care study: Thyroidectomy: A strangling feeling. *Nurs Mirror* 1981; 152(16):35–36.

Fode NC, Laus ER, Northartt RC: Pituitary tumors and hypertension: Implications for neurosurgical nurses. *J Neurosurg Nurs* 1983; 15(1):33–35.

Gruendemann BJ, Meeker MH: *Alexander's Care of the Patient in Surgery,* 7th ed. St. Louis: Mosby, 1983.

Kloegman S, Sagor G: Nursing care study: A lump in the throat. *Nurs Mirror* 1983; 156(4):54–56.

Lee KJ, Goodrich I, Pensak M: Pituitary surgery: Current status including transsphenoidal surgery. *Am J Otolaryngol* 1984; 5:138–150.

LeMaitre GD, Finnegan JA: *The Patient in Surgery: A Guide for Nurses,* 4th ed. Philadelphia: Saunders, 1980.

Mauldin BC: The hypophysectomy patient in the OR. *AORN J* 1981; 33:253–255.

Moroney J: *Surgery for Nurses,* 15th ed. New York: Churchill Livingstone, 1982.

Muthe NC: *Endocrinology: A Nursing Approach.* Boston: Little, Brown, 1981.

Paterson AG, Velster DJ: Adrenalectomy for advanced breast cancer: A reappraisal. *Anticancer Res* 1983; 3(2):151–153.

Suggested Readings

Kruger LB: Complications of transsphenoidal surgery. *J Neurosurg Nurs* (June) 1985; 17:179–183. Transsphenoidal surgery is discussed, including anatomical and physiological considerations, indications for surgery, the operative procedure, and surgical complications. The nurse's role in client assessment and care management is also presented.

Propst CL: Nursing care of a patient undergoing transsphenoidal hypophysectomy. *J Neurosurg Nurs* (Dec) 1983; 15:332–338. Assessment of the needs of a client with a pituitary tumor and implementation of a preoperative and postoperative plan of care are the focus of this article. Discharge instructions are also emphasized.

Volner JS: Endocrine dysfunction associated with pituitary adenomas and pituitary surgery. *J Neurosurg Nurs* (Dec) 1983; 15:325–331. The author reviews the anatomy and physiology of the pituitary and its hormones. Symptoms associated with pituitary adenoma are thoroughly discussed. Postoperative nursing care with adenoma removal and total hypophysectomy is presented.

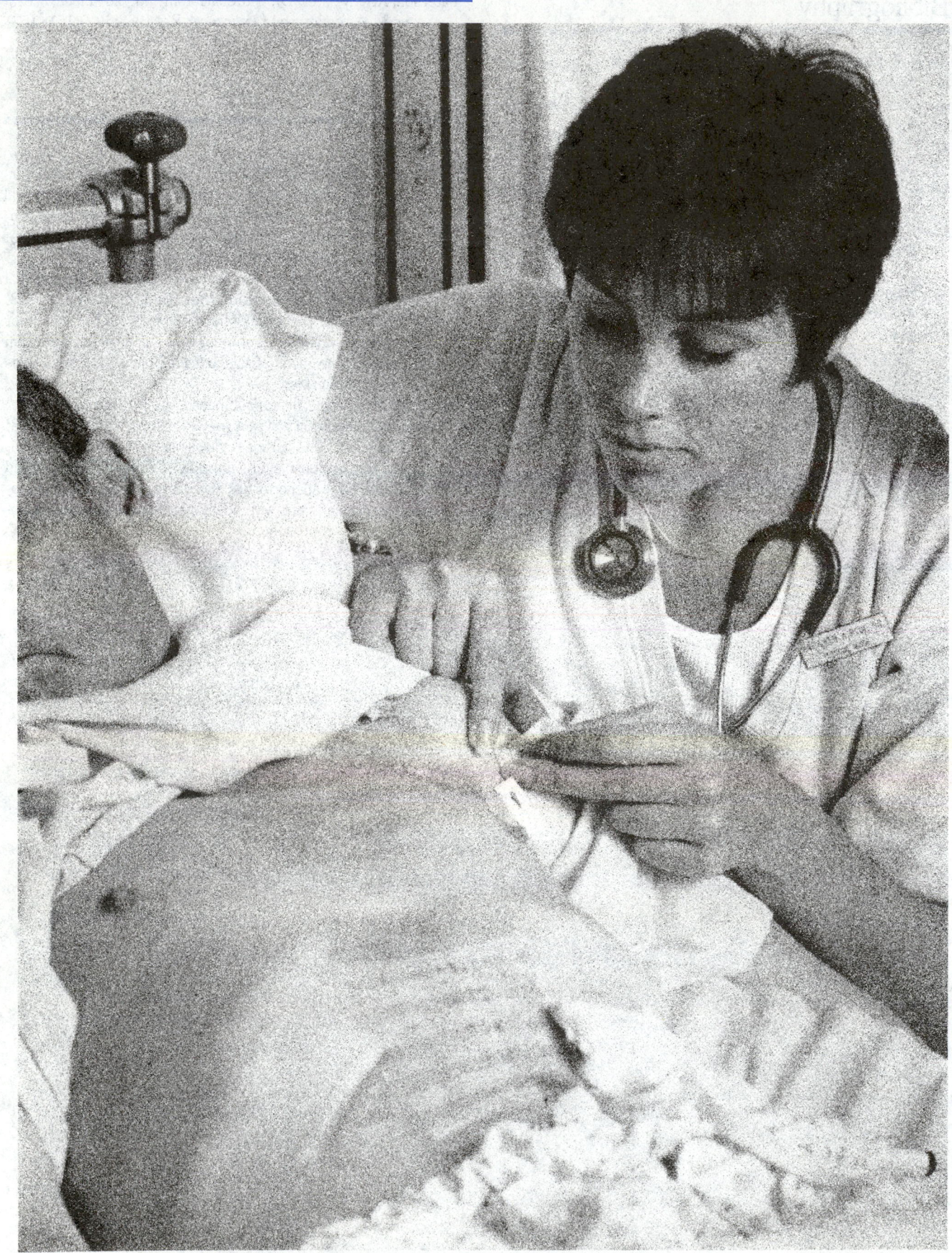

The Client With Gastrointestinal System Dysfunction

Chapter 46

The Gastrointestinal System in Health and Illness

Nancy Nuwer Konstantinides

Objectives

When you have finished studying this chapter, you should be able to:

Cite the major anatomical structures of the gastrointestinal tract.

Describe the normal physiology and regulatory processes of the gastrointestinal system.

Identify the pathophysiological consequences of altered regulatory processes of the gastrointestinal tract.

Recognize the impact of gastrointestinal pathophysiology on other body systems.

Anticipate the psychosocial/lifestyle influences and effects of gastrointestinal pathophysiology.

The gastrointestinal system plays an essential role in maintaining homeostasis by assimilating ingested nutrients and eliminating wastes. Food enters the system through the mouth and esophagus. It then undergoes successive digestive processes as it is passed through the stomach, small and large intestines, being broken down to its elemental components (nutrients, fluid, and electrolytes). Solid wastes that accumulate in the course of the digestive process are excreted through the anorectum. (Waste fluids are further broken down by the kidneys and excreted as urine; this process is discussed in Unit Five.) The liver and gallblad-

der, which play an important role in digestion, are discussed in Unit Nine.

Because all bodily functions are ultimately dependent on the nutritional status of the body's individual cells, any dysfunction of the gastrointestinal system necessarily affects all other systems to some degree. No wonder, then, that individuals with disorders of this system make up a large part of the client population in any health care facility and are commonly seen by nurses practicing in outpatient settings and in the community.

Section I: Structural and Functional Interrelationships

The gastrointestinal (GI) tract or alimentary canal is essentially a tube through which food is conveyed as it undergoes the process of digestion, that is, conversion into substances the body can use. The canal extends from the mouth through the anorectum (Figure 46–1). The pan-

creas and the biliary tract, which are considered auxiliary GI structures, are adjacent to the stomach and duodenum, to which they are connected by the pancreatic duct and the common bile duct respectively. These abdominal organs, known collectively as the viscera, are covered by a serous

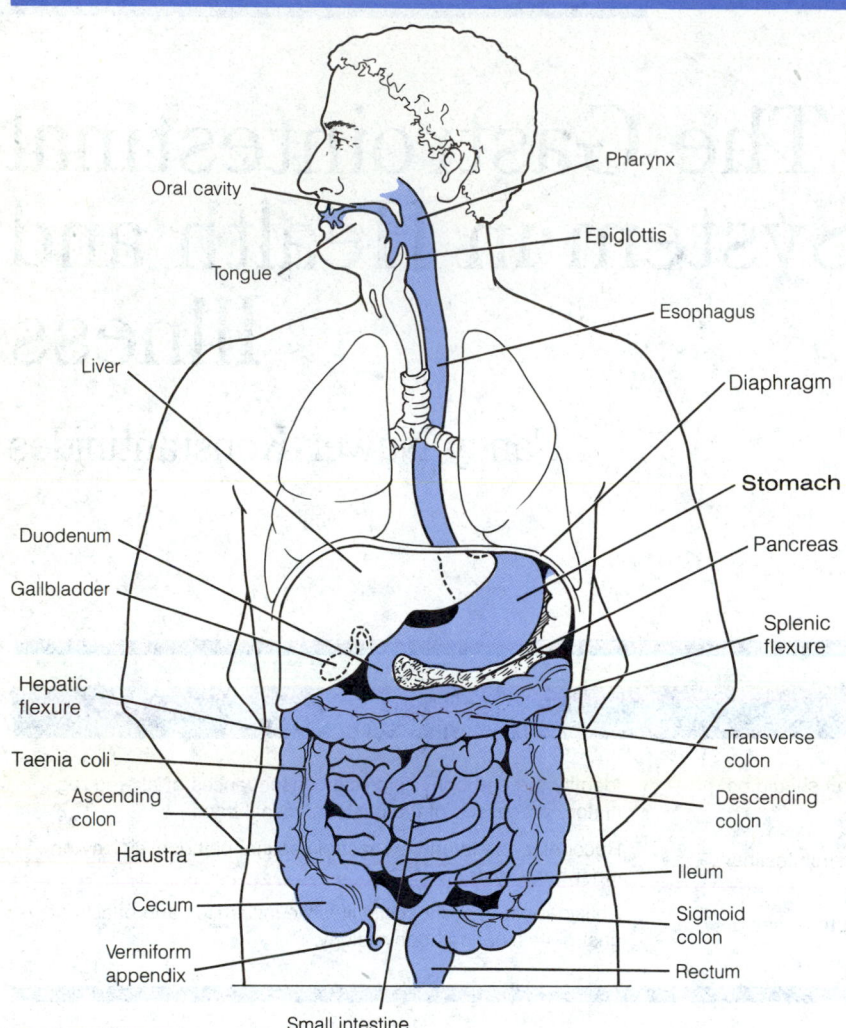

Figure 46–1

The gastrointestinal tract.

SOURCE: Spence AP, Mason EB: *Human Anatomy and Physiology*, 2nd ed. Menlo Park, CA: Benjamin/Cummings, 1983.

membrane called the peritoneum, which also lines the abdominal cavity.

STRUCTURE OF THE MOUTH

Food enters the alimentary canal via the mouth, or buccal cavity. Besides providing a portal of entry for nutrients and fluids, the mouth contains receptors for taste sensations. The initial preparation of food for the digestive process takes place in the mouth during **mastication** (chewing), when the food is ground into a pulp and mixed with saliva.

The roof of the mouth consists of the hard and soft palates; its sides are the insides of the cheeks. The floor of the mouth contains the tongue as well as muscles and three pairs of salivary glands: the sublingual, the submaxillary, and the parotid glands. The parotid glands are the largest. These structures are covered with mucous membrane which, in the case of the tongue, is modified into numerous small projections called *papillae,* some of which contain the taste buds.

The mouth also contains the teeth. Generally, an adult with healthy teeth will have 28 teeth plus two pairs of adult molars, or "wisdom teeth" (unless any or all of these have been removed, which is frequently the case). See Figure 46–2. Congenital absence of one or two teeth is fairly common and follows a familial pattern (Crowley, 1983).

STRUCTURE OF THE ESOPHAGUS

The sole function of the esophagus is to provide for the transit of food and fluid from pharynx to stomach. Food that was initially lubricated by saliva in the mouth is further lubricated by mucus secreted by esophageal glands. The esophagus is located behind the trachea and passes through the diaphragm to connect with the stomach. This opening in the diaphragm is called the esophageal hiatus.

The esophagus is a tubular structure approximately 22 cm (8.8 in) long and 2.5 cm (1 in) in diameter in the adult. It is muscular yet readily distensible and is easily displaced by other structures. The upper portion of the

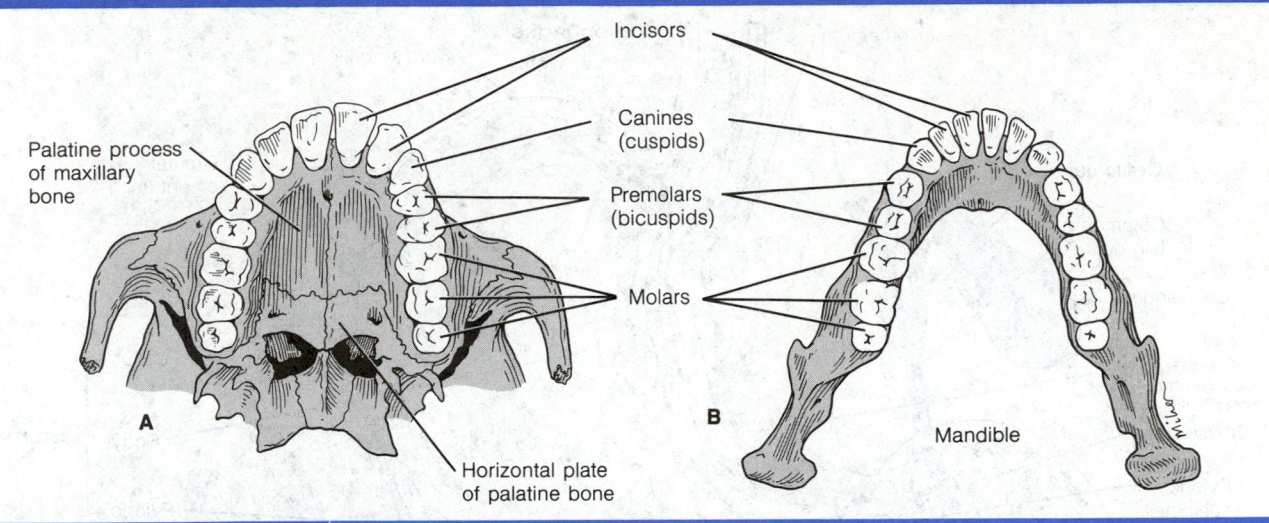

Figure 46–2

Permanent teeth in **A**, the upper jaw, and **B**, the lower jaw.
SOURCE: Spence AP, Mason EB: *Human Anatomy and Physiology,* 2nd ed. Menlo Park, CA: Benjamin/Cummings, 1983.

esophagus is composed primarily of striated muscle and the lower portion of smooth muscle. Food passes from the esophagus into the stomach at the *esophageal–gastric junction.* The *lower esophageal sphincter* controls the passage of the food bolus into the stomach. Once the bolus has passed into the stomach, the lower esophageal sphincter closes to prevent **reflux** (backward flow) of gastric contents.

STRUCTURE OF THE STOMACH

The major functions of the stomach include secretion, storage, emptying, and mixing. It has a reservoir capacity of approximately 1 L. As volume in the stomach increases, a feedback mechanism involving baroreceptors (nerve endings sensitive to pressure) is thought to help deter further consumption of food by decreasing appetite. While in the stomach, the food bolus is mixed with gastric juices and churned by the stomach's musculature. The food bolus is now referred to as **chyme,** which is gradually released into the small intestine through the duodenum.

The stomach is essentially a hollow pouch of muscular tissue that lies primarily in the upper left quadrant of the abdomen (Figure 46–3). Its major regions include the fundus (the uppermost portion), the body, and the antrum (distal portion). At each end of the stomach is a sphincter—the lower esophageal sphincter at its entrance and the pyloric sphincter where the stomach is joined with the duodenum. Blood is supplied to the stomach primarily by the celiac artery and is drained to the liver via the portal vein.

The mucosa lining the stomach has complex secretory functions and a correspondingly complex cellular structure. The principal cell types are:

- Mucous cells
- Parietal cells, which secrete hydrochloric acid and intrinsic factor
- Chief cells, which secrete digestive enzymes

Secretion by the gastric mucosa is influenced by the vagus nerve. The lining of the stomach has a mucosal barrier to prevent autodigestion by enzymes and gastric acids.

The stomach musculature is highly motile; its churning of the chyme facilitates digestion. Gastric motility is controlled by the autonomic nervous system; parasympathetic stimuli increase gastric motility, and sympathetic stimuli decrease it, via the vagus nerve.

STRUCTURE OF THE SMALL INTESTINE

The small intestine (small bowel) consists of the duodenum, the jejunum, and the ileum. Digestive enzymes in the small intestine break down food into its component nutrients (fats, proteins, and carbohydrates). The presence of bile, secreted into the duodenum through the common bile duct at the *ampulla of Vater,* is necessary for the efficient digestion of fat (see Chapter 51). Digestive enzymes synthesized in the pancreas also reach the small bowel via the ampulla of Vater. Certain hormones are also produced in the small intestine.

The duodenum, or proximal portion of the small intestine, begins at the gastric pylorus and extends for about 25 cm (10 in) to the *ligament of Treitz,* where it joins the jejunum. The duodenal mucosa contains both hormone-secreting cells and cells that secrete mucus, which is necessary to protect the walls of the duodenum from digestive enzymes and chyme.

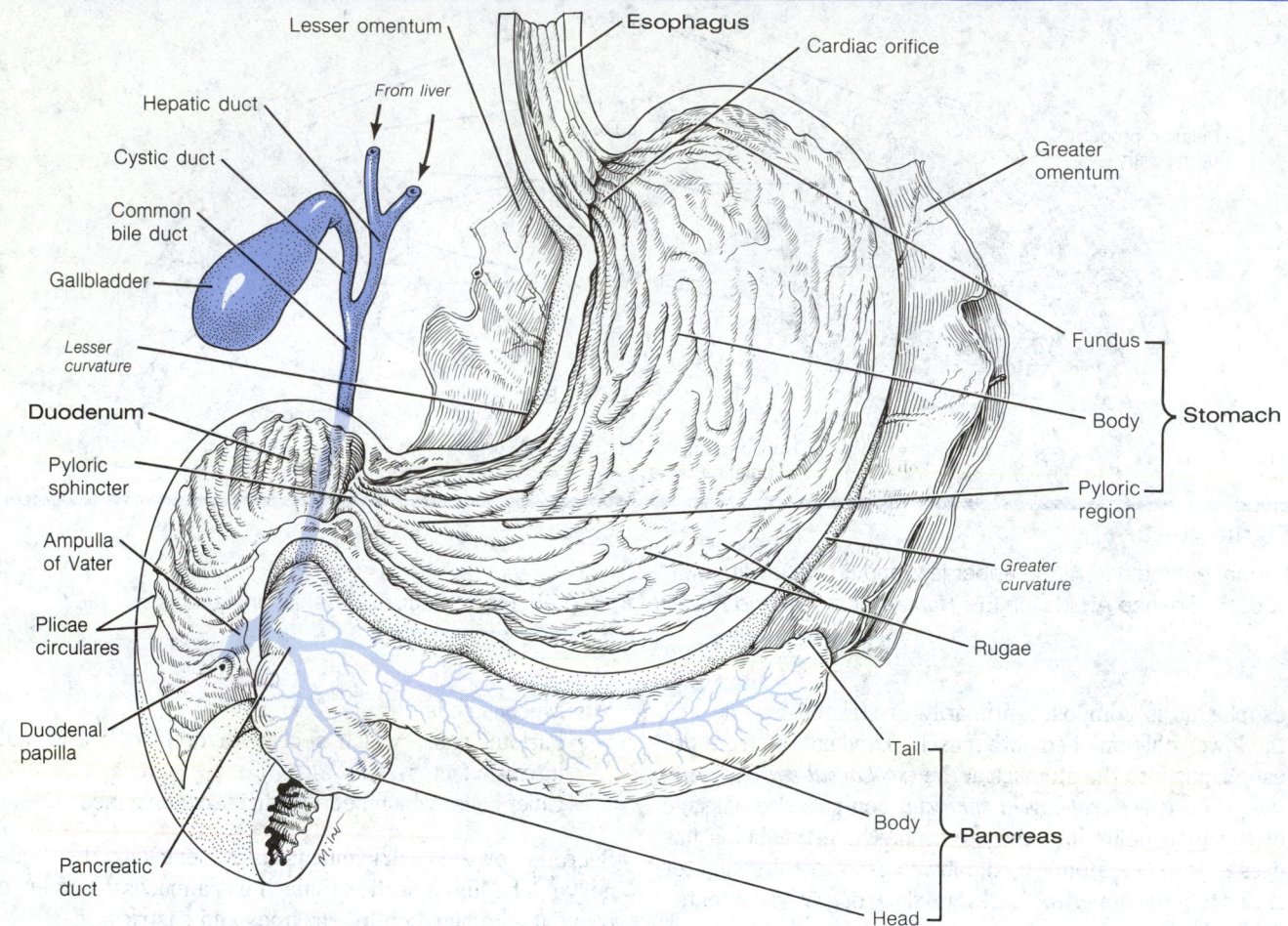

Figure 46-3

The stomach, duodenum, and pancreas.

SOURCE: Spence AP, Mason EB: *Human Anatomy and Physiology*, 2nd ed. Menlo Park, CA: Benjamin/Cummings, 1983.

The length of the small intestine varies, averaging about 6 m (18 to 21 feet) in the adult (Spence and Mason, 1983). The small bowel is lined with intestinal villi, finger-like projections that contain capillaries and lymphatics. Figure 46-4 illustrates the complex morphology of an intestinal villus—one of 4 to 5 million such structures in the small bowel of the average adult. This configuration of the intestinal mucosa vastly increases the surface area where absorption of nutrients can take place. The small bowel has a complex arterial blood supply, the superior mesenteric artery being one of the main arteries. Venous drainage ultimately leads to the portal vein and thereby into the liver.

Chyme passes into the colon, or large intestine, through the *ileocecal valve* at the distal portion of the ileus. Like the lower esophageal sphincter, this sphincter valve not only allows passage of chyme to the next portion of the alimentary canal but helps prevent the contents of the colon from flowing back into the small intestine.

STRUCTURE OF THE LARGE INTESTINE

The large intestine, or colon, has three major functions: absorption of fluid and electrolytes, synthesis of vitamin K by intestinal bacteria, and storage of fecal material until it is eliminated. The odor of the stool is affected by the presence of bacteria in the intestinal tract.

The colon begins at the ileocecal valve. Its various segments are the cecum, ascending colon, transverse colon, descending colon, and sigmoid colon (Figure 46-5). The colon is approximately 1.5 m long (4 to 5 feet) and is larger in diameter than the small intestine. The appendix, a small,

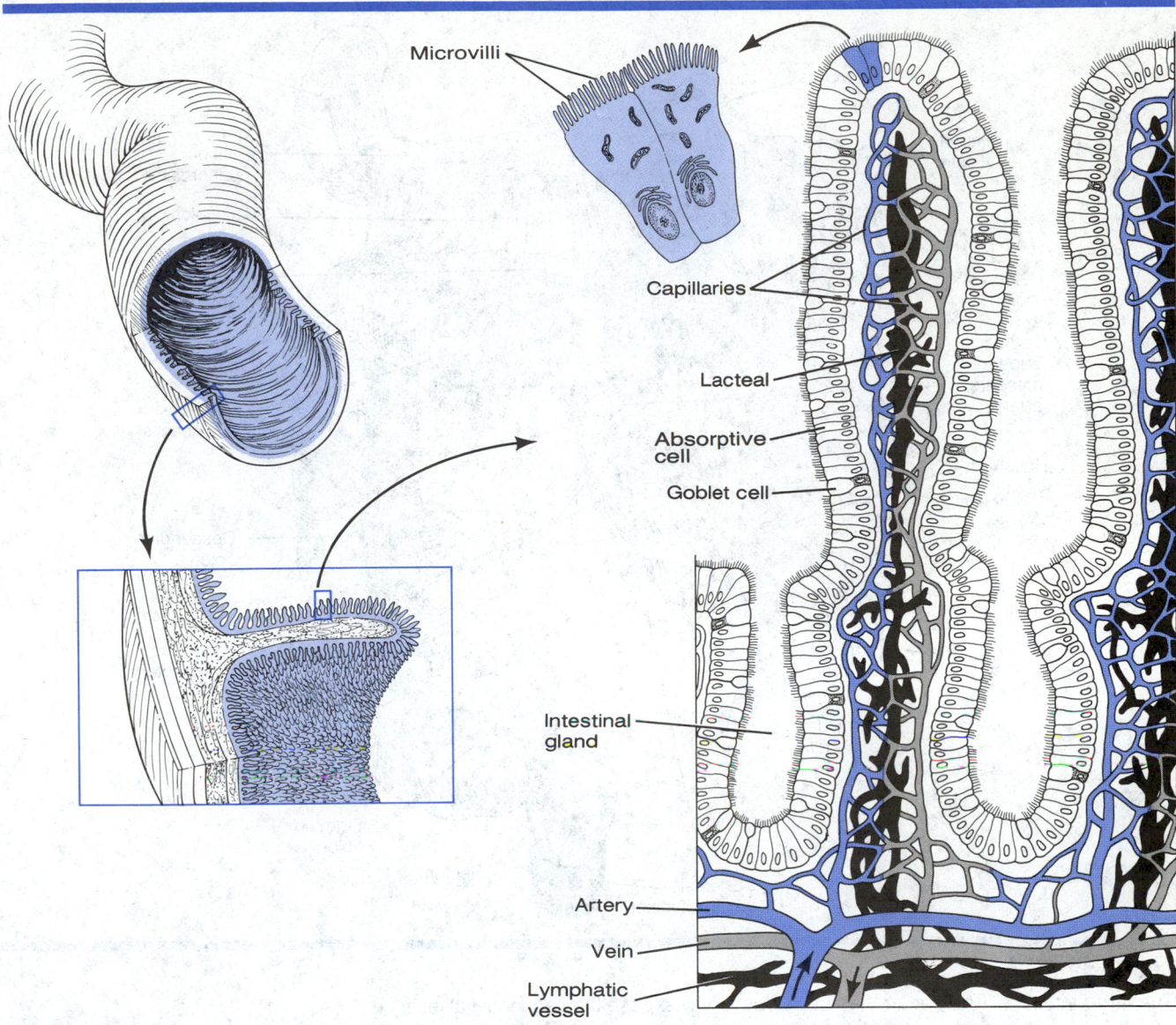

Microvilli

Capillaries

Lacteal

Absorptive cell

Goblet cell

Intestinal gland

Artery

Vein

Lymphatic vessel

Figure 46–4

An intestinal villus.

SOURCE: Spence AP, Mason EB: *Human Anatomy and Physiology,* 2nd ed. Menlo Park, CA: Benjamin/Cummings, 1983.

narrow pouch, projects from the cecum. The superior and inferior mesenteric arteries supply blood to the colon; it is drained by the superior and inferior mesenteric veins.

STRUCTURE OF THE ANORECTUM

Solid waste (feces) leaves the body via the anorectum (the rectum and the anus). The combined structures are about 17 cm (6.5 in) long, the distal 5 cm (2 in) comprising the anal canal. The anus contains both an internal sphincter, under involuntary control, and an external sphincter, which is under voluntary control. Under normal conditions, fecal material is approximately 75% water and 25% solids, including roughage, dead bacteria, fat, protein, and inorganic matter. Its normal brown color is caused by bilirubin derivatives; therefore, absence of brown coloration (**acholic**, or clay-colored, stools) is indicative of biliary dysfunction (see Unit Nine).

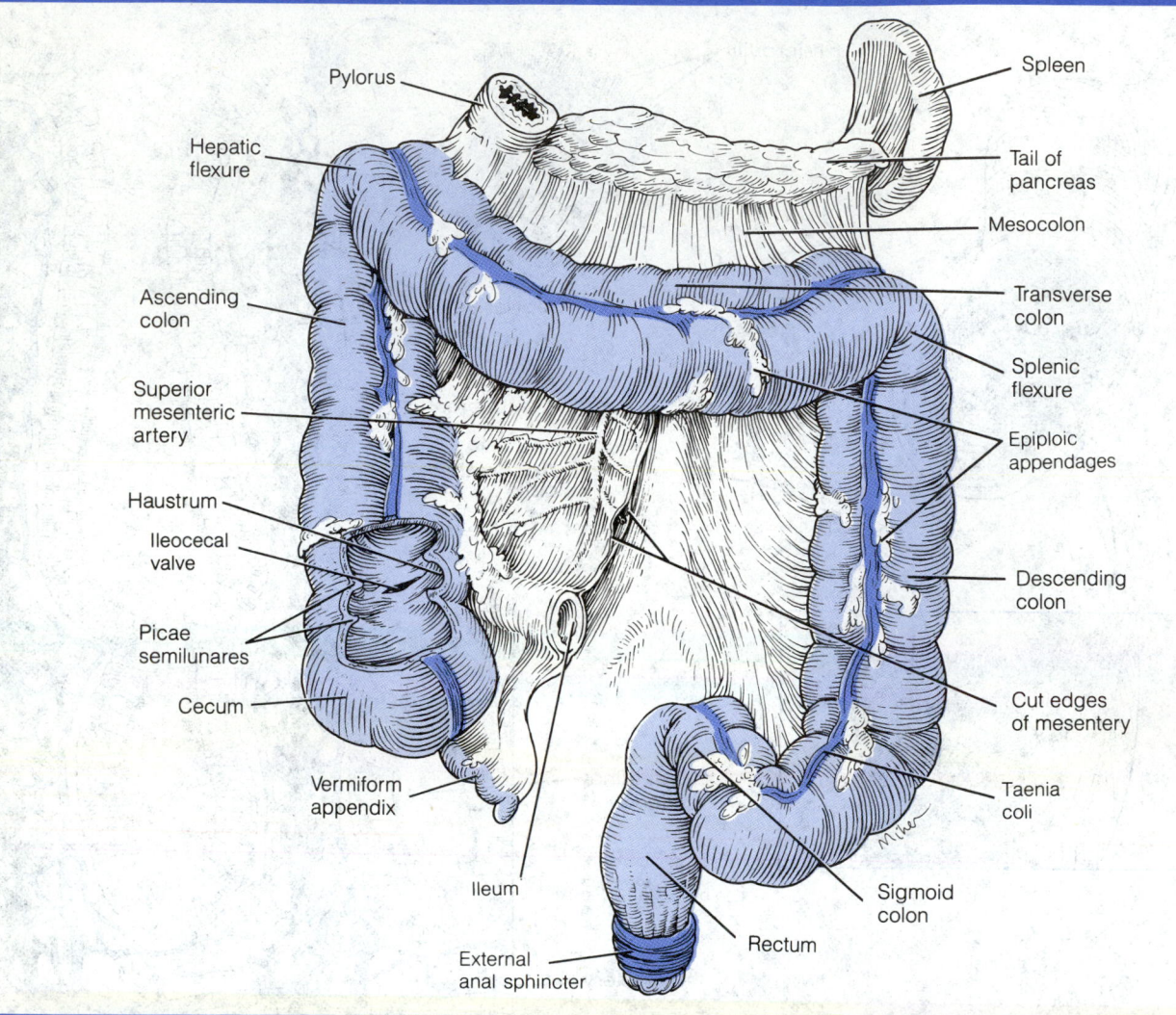

Figure 46–5

The large intestine. The cecum has been opened to expose the ileocecal valve.
SOURCE: Spence AP, Mason EB: *Human Anatomy and Physiology*, 2nd ed. Menlo Park, CA: Benjamin/Cummings, 1983.

THE PANCREAS

The pancreas, one of the accessory organs of the gastrointestinal system, has both exocrine and endocrine functions. Its endocrine functions, which include the production and secretion of insulin by the islets of Langerhans, are discussed in Unit Seven. Its exocrine functions involve secretion of ions (electrolytes), water, and digestive enzymes in response to stimulation by the autonomic nervous system and several hormones synthesized in the GI system.

The electrolytes released by the pancreas consist mainly of sodium, potassium, bicarbonate, and chloride. The principal purpose of these ions is to adjust the pH of the duodenal contents to a level suitable for the activity of the pancreatic enzymes. Enzymes secreted by the pancreas include proteases, protein-digesting enzymes; amylases, which break down carbohydrates; lipases, which act on fats; and peptidases, which further break down protein. Sympathetic stimuli decrease the rate of secretions, whereas parasympathetic stimuli increase the secretory rate of the pancreas.

The pancreas lies close to the stomach and duodenum (see Figure 46–1). It is composed of three main segments: the head, which lies close to the duodenum; the body, which lies posterior to the stomach; and the tail, which extends toward the spleen. Its total length in the adult is approximately 14 cm (5.5 in). The main pancreatic duct (the duct of Wirsung) empties into the duodenum at the ampulla of Vater, together with the common bile duct.

REGULATORY PROCESSES OF THE GASTROINTESTINAL SYSTEM

Swallowing

Before food and fluids can be processed in the alimentary canal, they must be swallowed. The initial phase of the swallowing sequence, which normally occurs after solid materials have been masticated and lubricated by saliva, is voluntary. Once a bolus of food touches the oropharynx, swallowing becomes a reflex controlled by cranial nerves V, IX, X, and XII. The sequence is depicted in Figure 46–6. As food is forced into the oropharynx, the epiglottis closes over the larynx to prevent aspiration; the soft palate closes off the nasal pharynx; and the tongue rises against the roof of the mouth to prevent food from reentering and to push it farther along the pharynx. The upper esophageal sphincter then relaxes, and food moves into the esophagus, where peristalsis and the force of gravity combine to propel the bolus of food toward the stomach.

Secretory Functions

All major structures of the gastrointestinal system produce secretions of some kind—mucoid, digestive, or hormonal. The secretions protect the gastrointestinal mucosa and facilitate digestion and absorption. Secretory activity is initiated in response to neuronal stimulation (primarily from the autonomic nervous system) as well as hormonal and mechanical stimuli.

The Oral Cavity

Most oral secretions are produced by the three pairs of salivary glands. In the normal adult, these glands secrete 1000 to 1500 mL of saliva per day (Spence and Mason, p. 635). Saliva is released in response to psychic stimuli (for example, a television commercial featuring a favorite "fast food"), olfactory stimuli (for example, the smell of bread warm from the oven), and/or mechanical stimuli (such as the touch of food on the tongue). Besides acting as a lubricant to facilitate swallowing, saliva helps dissolve dry particles of food. Saliva contains ptyalin, an enzyme that breaks down starches (complex carbohydrates). Clients with conditions that reduce the flow of saliva or dry out the mouth (for example, certain medications or mouth breathing related to respiratory obstruction) may have a difficult time chewing and swallowing food.

The Esophagus

Most esophageal secretions are mucoid. They facilitate passage of the food bolus by lubricating it and also protect

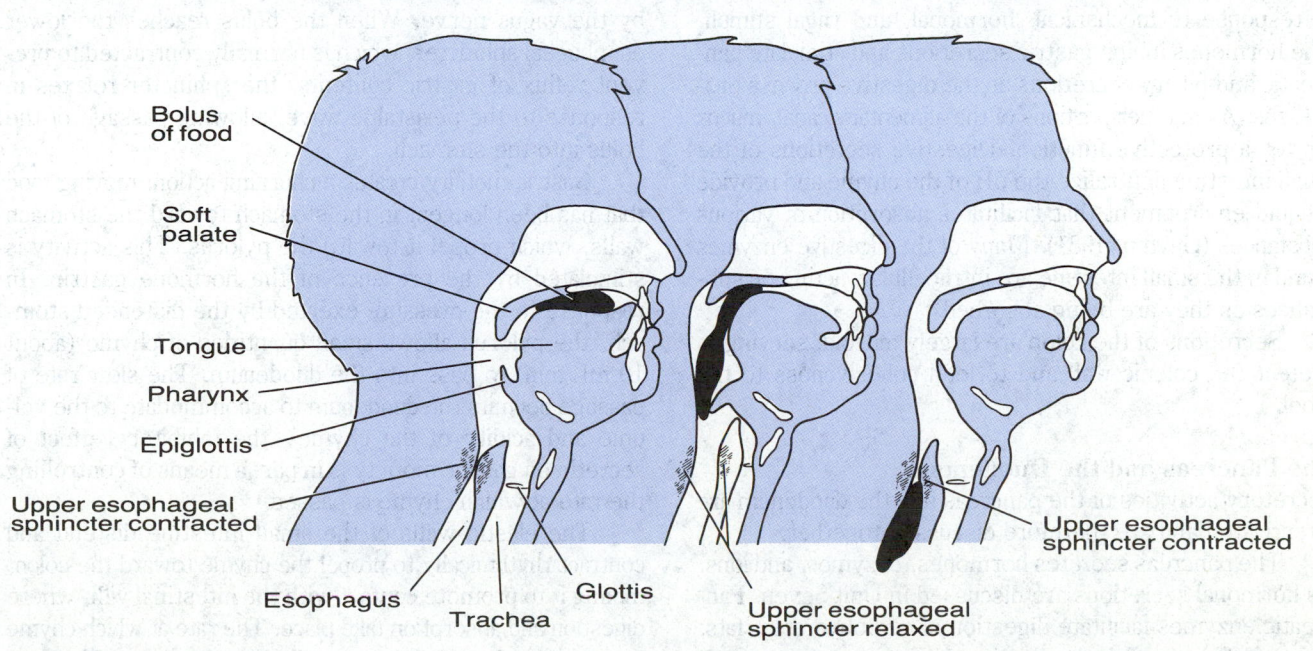

Figure 46–6

The swallowing mechanism.
SOURCE: Spence AP, Mason EB: *Human Anatomy and Physiology,* 2nd ed. Menlo Park, CA: Benjamin/Cummings, 1983.

the esophageal wall by reducing the abrasiveness of swallowed material.

The Stomach

The stomach produces up to 3 L of secretions per day. Some are digestive, some hormonal, and some mucoid. *Pepsinogen,* a proteolytic enzyme, is formed when hydrochloric acid produced by the parietal cells combines with pepsin released by the chief cells. Hydrochloric acid is released in response to a hormone, *gastrin,* which is released into the bloodstream when cells in the lower portion of the stomach are chemically and/or mechanically stimulated by the presence of food. Hydrochloric acid also creates an acidic environment in the stomach. Parasympathetic neuronal pathways—especially the vagus nerve—are also involved in regulating gastric secretions.

Another important gastric secretion is intrinsic factor. This mucoprotein secreted by the parietal cells plays an essential role in the absorption of vitamin B_{12}. Intrinsic factor combines with vitamin B_{12} and is carried through the small intestine. Absorption occurs primarily at the terminal ileum.

Mucoid secretions coat the mucosal wall of the stomach, preventing autodigestion by digestive enzymes and hydrochloric acid. Mucus also coats food particles, facilitating their passage, and is capable of buffering small amounts of acids or alkalis (Guyton, 1981).

The Intestines

The wall of the small intestine secretes up to 2 L of fluid per day, including mucus, digestive juices, and hormones in response to mechanical, hormonal, and vagal stimuli. The hormones inhibit gastric secretions and stimulate pancreatic and biliary secretions as the digestive process progresses. As in other portions of the alimentary canal, mucus serves a protective function. Digestive secretions of the small intestine neutralize the pH of the chyme and provide a liquid environment that facilitates absorption of various substances (Guyton, 1981). Many of the digestive enzymes found in the small intestine are intracellular, acting on substances as they are being absorbed.

Secretions of the colon are largely mucoid, serving to protect the colonic wall and to lend cohesiveness to the stool.

The Pancreas and the Duodenum

Secretory activities of the pancreas and the duodenum are interrelated and are therefore discussed together.

The pancreas secretes hormones, enzymes, and ions. Its hormonal secretions are discussed in Unit Seven. Pancreatic enzymes facilitate digestion of carbohydrates, fats, and proteins, as already discussed. Ionic secretions regulate intestinal pH. Inactive forms of the digestive enzymes are also secreted by the pancreas in response to vagal stimulation.

Bicarbonate ion is necessary to neutralize acidic gas-

tric juices when they enter the intestine, thus providing a pH in which pancreatic enzymes can function. This neutralizing action also prevents damage to the intestinal wall. Release of large quantities of bicarbonate by the pancreas is stimulated by *secretin,* a hormone released by the duodenal mucosa in response to the presence of hydrochloric acid. Secretin is absorbed by the bloodstream and reabsorbed by the pancreas.

Some proteolytic enzymes are released by the pancreas in inactive form and are activated only upon entering the duodenum. Without this mechanism, the pancreas could be consumed by its own enzymes. Release of some of these inactive enzymes occurs in response to stimulation of the pancreas by *cholecystokinin,* a hormone produced and released by the duodenum when products of protein digestion are present. Other inactive pancreatic enzymes are released in response to vagal stimulation. See Box 46–1 for a summary of representative activities of the GI hormones.

Motility

The alimentary canal is motile, that is, able to move spontaneously without conscious control. Its motility serves both in mixing and in propulsion of food along the digestive tract.

Once a bolus has been moved into the esophagus by swallowing, it is propelled toward the lower esophageal sphincter by peristalsis, a wave of contraction that passes along the alimentary tract for varying distances and with varying force. In the esophagus, peristalsis is controlled by the vagus nerve. When the bolus reaches the lower esophageal sphincter, which is normally contracted to prevent reflux of gastric contents, the sphincter relaxes in response to the peristaltic wave, allowing passage of the bolus into the stomach.

Gastric motility creates a churning action, moving food that has been longest in the stomach toward the stomach walls, which propel it toward the pylorus. This activity is stimulated by the presence of the hormone gastrin. In response to the pressure exerted by the distended stomach, the pylorus allows small quantities of chyme (about 10 mL/min) to pass into the duodenum. The slow rate of passage permits the duodenum to accommodate to the volume and acidity of the chyme—the inhibitory effect of secretin on gastric motility is in part a means of controlling the rate at which chyme is passed.

The elastic walls of the small intestine distend and contract rhythmically to propel the chyme toward the colon, mixing it to promote contact with the intestinal villi, where digestion and absorption take place. The rate at which chyme passes into the colon is controlled by the ileocecal valve, which also prevents fecal material from flowing back into the ileum.

The mixing contractions of the colon are called *haustrations.* These movements bring the chyme into contact with the intestinal wall to promote absorption. Mass movements (mass peristalsis) are strong periodic contractions that move feces into the rectum several times a day.

Digestion

Digestion is the process by which ingested substances are broken down in the GI tract and converted into absorbable forms. Digestion has both mechanical and chemical aspects. Mastication (chewing) and gastric and intestinal mixing of chyme are mechanical activities. The activity of enzymes and other secretions are chemical activities. Table 46–1 summarizes the principal enzymes involved in the digestion of carbohydrates, proteins, and lipids.

Carbohydrates

Digestion of carbohydrates begins in the mouth, where food is chewed and ptyalin begins the breakdown of starches (complex carbohydrates) into simple sugars. As chyme enters the duodenum, pancreatic amylase continues the breakdown of carbohydrates. The wall of the small intestine contains enzymes that further break down carbohydrates into monosaccharides, which are absorbed into the bloodstream.

Fats (Lipids)

Digestion of fats is a complex process that begins in the small intestine, where fats are emulsified by bile salts. Once emulsified, the fat can be broken down by the pancreatic enzyme *lipase*. For example, triglycerides are broken down into monoglycerides, free fatty acids, and glycerol. The monoglycerides and free fatty acids then combine with bile salts, which transport them to the intestinal wall for absorption into the lymphatics. Dietary cholesterol is broken down by pancreatic enzymes; bile salts transport cholesterol to the intestinal wall for absorption into the bloodstream.

Proteins

Digestion of proteins is also a complex process that begins in the stomach, where pepsinogen breaks down the protein into a simpler form. In the small intestine, pancreatic enzymes such as trypsin and chymotrypsin further break down proteins—some of them into amino acids. Intracellular enzymes in the intestinal wall complete the digestion of protein.

Absorption

Absorption occurs in the intestinal tract by means of two mechanisms that are basic to all cellular function: diffusion and active transport. *Diffusion* is movement along an electrochemical gradient from areas of high concentration or charge to areas of lower concentration. *Active transport* is generally *against* a gradient and requires the expenditure of energy as well as the presence of a carrier. Water is absorbed into the bowel by diffusion. Sodium is absorbed

---

Box 46–1　Representative Activities of the Gastrointestinal Hormones

Gastrin: Stimulates gastric secretion, particularly the secretion of hydrochloric acid

Secretin: Inhibits gastric acid secretion when the stomach is actively secreting and the mechanisms that cause gastrin release are strongly stimulated. Stimulates the release of a watery fluid that contains bicarbonate from the pancreas. Stimulates the secretion of bile.

Cholecystokinin: Inhibits gastric acid secretion when the stomach is actively secreting and the mechanisms that cause gastrin release are strongly stimulated. Stimulates the release of enzymes from the pancreas. Stimulates the contraction of the gallbladder.

Gastric inhibitory peptide: Inhibits gastric acid secretion when the stomach is actively secreting and the mechanisms that cause gastrin release are strongly stimulated.

---

by active transport. Sodium absorption is important since the bowel secretes 20 to 30 g/day, reabsorbing all of this plus 4 to 5 g of the dietary intake (Guyton, 1981).

Nutrients and other substances are absorbed at various sites. Concentrated solutions of glucose can be absorbed through the buccal mucosa. The gastric mucosa has minimal absorptive properties—except for absorption of alcohol. The small intestine—the principal site of absorption—absorbs water, nutrients, electrolytes, and vitamins. Major nutrients absorbed by the duodenum include iron, calcium, fat, carbohydrates, and some amino acids. The jejunum absorbs carbohydrates and amino acids. The distal ileum reabsorbs bile salts (see Chapter 51), and the terminal ileum absorbs vitamin B_{12} combined with intrinsic factor.

Both the small and large intestines absorb water and electrolytes; 8.0 to 8.5 L per day are absorbed by the small intestine, and 0.5 to 1.0 L are absorbed by the colon. Under normal circumstances, only 50 to 200 mL of water are lost daily in the feces.

Elimination

Once digestion has taken place and water, nutrients, and electrolytes have been absorbed, solid waste, or feces, is expelled through the anorectum. Fecal matter is first propelled into the rectum by strong contractions of the colon that occur several times a day. A reflex contraction stimulated by these mass movements relaxes the internal sphincter, creating an urge to defecate. Under normal conditions, the external sphincter of the adult is under conscious control, allowing the individual to determine the time and place of defecation. If the urge to defecate is ignored, it subsides until the next mass movement. If sphincter control is lost—for example, due to disease or in cases of sudden, intense fear or stress—stool can ooze involuntarily out of the rectum.

Table 46–1 Principal Enzymes Involved in the Digestion of Carbohydrates, Proteins, and Lipids*

Enzyme	Source	Action
Carbohydrates		
Salivary amylase	Salivary glands	Splits starch into the disaccharides maltose and isomaltose
Pancreatic amylase	Pancreas	Splits starch into the disaccharides maltose and isomaltose
Disaccharidases	Intestinal epithelium	Split disaccharides into monosaccharides
Maltase		Splits maltose into glucose
Isomaltase		Splits isomaltose into glucose
Sucrase		Splits sucrose into glucose and fructose
Lactase		Splits lactose into glucose and galactose
Proteins		
Pepsin (pepsinogen)	Chief cells of stomach	Splits proteins into smaller peptide chains of amino acids
Trypsin (trypsinogen)	Pancreas	Splits proteins and peptides into smaller peptides
Chymotrypsin (chymotrypsinogen)	Pancreas	Splits proteins and peptides into smaller peptides
Carboxypeptidase (procarboxypeptidase)	Pancreas	Frees terminal amino acid from the carboxyl (acid) end of an amino acid chain
Aminopeptidases	Intestinal epithelium	Free terminal amino acid from the amino end of an amino acid chain
Tetrapeptidases	Intestinal epithelium	Split final amino acid from tetrapeptides, producing tripeptides and free amino acids
Tripeptidases	Intestinal epithelium	Split tripeptides into dipeptides and free amino acids
Dipeptidases	Intestinal epithelium	Split dipeptides into free amino acids
Lipids		
Pancreatic lipase	Pancreas	Splits triacylglycerols mainly into monoacylglycerols and free fatty acids
Epithelial cell lipase	Intestinal epithelium	Splits monoacylglycerols into glycerol and fatty acids
Cholesterol esterase	Pancreas	Splits cholesterol esters into free cholesterol and free fatty acids

*Substances in parentheses are precursors of active enzymes.

Section II: Pathophysiological Influences and Effects

Pathophysiology of the GI tract can be associated with many conditions, as well as psychosocial factors and disturbances of related organ systems. A general overview of functional alterations is presented here; pathophysiological and psychosocial factors related to specific disorders are discussed in Chapters 48 and 49.

ALTERATIONS IN SWALLOWING

Swallowing is primarily a reflex mechanism. Alterations in swallowing include difficulty in swallowing (**dysphagia**) and backward propulsion of food or gases into the esoph-

agus or through the mouth (reflux, eructation, regurgitation, and vomiting).

Dysphagia

Difficulty in swallowing may be related to mechanical neuromuscular, or psychological factors. Physical abnormalities, obstruction, or inflammatory responses may cause dysphagia. Interruption of the continuity of the tongue, oropharynx, and esophagus may also be implicated. Difficulty in chewing—because of poor dentition, inadequate dentures, or pain in the temporomandibular joint (TMJ), may affect the ability to swallow, since food may not be sufficiently mixed with saliva or sufficiently masticated. Injury or paralysis of the cranial nerves and fibrotic disorders may affect the swallowing reflex. In clients under anesthesia or in coma, the gag reflex is suppressed or absent. Various emotional states, such as anxiety, may affect the voluntary phase of the swallowing process.

Dysphagia has several consequences, such as malnutrition and pain. The client may avoid foods that worsen the problem. Clients with advanced Parkinson's disease, for example, may have to avoid solid foods because neurological impairment interferes with propulsion of solids into the esophagus. Clients who have had a cerebrovascular accident (stroke) may have difficulty swallowing liquids if the oropharyngeal muscles have been paralyzed.

Dysphagia may be associated with pain that the client describes as "heartburn," indigestion, or chest pain. Pain can be severe, causing the client to alter eating habits—for example, to eat only soft foods—or to seek relief by taking antacids.

Backward Flow of Food

Malfunction of the lower esophageal sphincter may cause gastric juices to flow back into the lower esophagus (*gastric reflux*). These highly acid juices may irritate or erode the esophageal mucosa. Belching (**eructation**) is usually associated with swallowing of air—for example, by eating too rapidly or talking while eating. If retained, the swallowed air may cause discomfort associated with distention or may be expelled as "gas" (*flatulence*). *Regurgitation* is reflux of partially digested food into the mouth. It usually causes a sour taste and may occur in association with eructation.

Vomiting is the release of gastric contents through the mouth. It is related to a number of conditions and may be preceded by nausea. The vomiting mechanism is triggered by neurological stimuli. Vomiting causes a loss of gastrointestinal fluids and electrolytes that can be life threatening if excessive. In clients whose gag reflex has been altered by anesthesia or disease, vomitus may be aspirated into the bronchi, causing *aspiration pneumonia* or even respiratory arrest. Forceful vomiting can tear or rupture the esophagus—a severe complication.

CHANGES IN SECRETORY FUNCTION

The mucoid, digestive, and hormonal secretions of the GI tract protect the integrity of the gastrointestinal wall, promote the passage of food or chyme, and facilitate digestion and absorption. Secretory changes may involve either an increase or a decrease and may be related to many different conditions, including:

- Inflammatory disorders (eg, in clients with inflammatory bowel disease, secretion of mucus into the feces is increased)

- Infections (eg, exocrine secretions of the pancreas are reduced in clients with pancreatitis)
- Degenerative disorders (eg, in clients who are malnourished, secretion of lactase and other enzymes may be diminished)
- Neoplastic disorders (eg, in Zollinger–Ellison syndrome associated with pancreatic neoplasms, secretion of gastric acids is increased)
- Neurohormonal disorders (eg, disturbances of the vagus nerve are associated with an increase in gastric acid secretions)
- Mechanical insult as with trauma or surgical excision (eg, production of intrinsic factor—and thus absorption of vitamin B_{12}—is decreased after a gastrectomy)
- Psychosocial conditions (eg, autonomic nervous responses to fear or anxiety inhibit salivary, gastric, and pancreatic secretion)

Because secretory activity of the GI system is so complex and so critical to its functioning, changes in secretory activity may have numerous and far-reaching consequences. A decrease in mucus secretion or alterations in buffering ability (eg, release of bicarbonate ions by the pancreas) can interfere with protective mechanisms, leading to irritation, erosion, and ulceration. Alteration in secretions can also lead to digestion of tissues by their own secretions (**autodigestion**), especially in the stomach and pancreas. Reduced secretion of saliva in the oral cavity can cause dysphagia; elsewhere in the GI tract, a decrease in mucus can interfere with propulsion of chyme through the alimentary canal.

Digestion and absorption may be seriously affected by alterations in secretory activity, leading to serious sequelae. For example, if production of intrinsic factor is impaired or absent, vitamin B_{12} cannot be absorbed. Since vitamin B_{12} is essential to synthesis of erythropoietin, and to the production of red blood cells, malabsorption leads to pernicious anemia.

Absorption of nutrients depends on unimpaired secretion of various hormones and enzymes. For example, pancreatic lipase is necessary for digestion and absorption of both fats and fat-soluble vitamins A, D, E, and K. Conversely, an excess of hydrochloric acid or bile salts may be associated with diarrhea and loss of fluids and electrolytes.

Malnutrition can both cause and result from abnormalities of GI secretions. It causes the intestinal villi to atrophy, diminishing absorption and thus further impairing the client's nutrition. It impairs production of enzymes, which are composed of amino acids. Other sequelae of malabsorption related to malnutrition include loss of muscle mass, changes in skin and hair, impaired wound healing, alterations of immune function, and increase in surgical complications. These and other effects of malnutrition are discussed in Chapter 8.

CHANGES IN MOTILITY

Alterations in motility may be associated with many conditions of mechanical, neurohormonal, or inflammatory origin. Motility may be increased (*hypermotility*) or decreased (*hypomotility*). Mechanical conditions associated with altered motility (usually hypomotility) include ileus (intestinal obstruction) and surgical resection. Neurohormonal conditions include endocrine disorders and reactions to pharmacologic agents. Parasitic infection is one of many inflammatory conditions that alter motility—usually by increasing it.

Hypermotility

Gastrointestinal hypermotility has numerous effects. *Dumping syndrome,* rapid emptying of gastric contents accompanied by tachycardia, palpitations, syncope, diaphoresis, cramping, and bloating, is related to changes in the osmolality, acidity, and volume of chyme entering the duodenum. Hypermotility is often associated with pain and discomfort. Moreover, when chyme moves too rapidly through the intestinal tract, digestion and absorption can not be completed. Diarrhea may result, and fluids and electrolytes may be lost, leading to systemic imbalances.

Hypomotility

Hypomotility also adversely affects homeostasis. Slowing of peristalsis can cause chyme to reflux. Gastric retention related to hypomotility can cause feelings of fullness, nausea, and emesis. Intestinal hypomotility promotes bacterial overgrowth, leading to flatulence and, eventually, to hypermotility related to inflammation. Hypomotility of the colon may lead to constipation and fecal impaction.

CHANGES IN DIGESTION

Digestion and absorption are closely linked. Most nutrients cannot be absorbed until digestive enzymes have broken them down to elemental form. Normal digestion depends on availability of food in the GI tract, availability of digestive enzymes, and unimpaired enzymatic function. If no nutrients are available in the GI tract—for example, in a client who is NPO or one whose nutritional intake is from intravenous sources—digestion slows. Enzyme availability may be impaired by disorders affecting the tissues or organs where the enzymes are synthesized—for example, the pancreas or the intestinal mucosa. Alterations of enzyme activity may be related to:

- Mechanical disturbances (eg, surgical resection or bypass procedures, or obstruction of the pancreatic ducts, as in cystic fibrosis)
- Inflammatory disturbances (eg, pancreatitis)

- Malnutrition
- Disturbances of secretion (eg, pancreatic enzymes may be inactivated if greatly increased secretion of gastric acids lowers duodenal pH)

Alterations in production of bile associated with disorders of the liver and gallbladder may also affect digestion, specifically of lipids.

When enzyme activity is altered, carbohydrates, fats, and/or protein are inadequately digested. If digestion is inadequate, absorption may be impaired or absent. Inadequate absorption may lead to malnutrition which may further impair digestion. Altered digestion and absorption of fat may lead to fatty stools (**steatorrhea**), described as stools that are frequent, frothy, foul, and floating. Acholic (clay colored) stools are related to altered secretion of bile.

CHANGES IN ABSORPTION

Most gastrointestinal absorption takes place in the small bowel, where fluids, electrolytes, and elemental nutrients diffuse or are actively transported via the intestinal lumen to the bloodstream and the lymphatic circulation. Malabsorption is frequently related to maldigestion (see previous section); however, other conditions may be involved, including mechanical insult, neurohormonal disorders, and/or inflammation. Mechanical causes include surgical resection of the intestine, intestinal bypass, proximal ileostomy, and fistula tracts. The consequences of malabsorption include nutrient deficiencies and fluid and electrolyte imbalances. Malabsorption of fats may lead to steatorrhea.

CHANGES IN ELIMINATION

Elimination is the process by which waste products are excreted from the GI tract. Although television commercials and popular opinion promote the virtues of "regularity" (at least one bowel movement per day at the same time), not everyone is regular. In assessing "irregularity," the important determination is whether bowel habits of the individual have *changed*, and in what manner. A change in bowel habits is one of the classic "seven warning signals" of cancer.

Alterations in elimination may include diarrhea, constipation, and bloody stools. Difficult or painful elimination may also occur.

Diarrhea

Diarrhea—loose, watery stools—may be related to many conditions, including hypermotility, inflammation, secretory disturbances, malnutrition, and malabsorption/maldigestion. It may cause loss of fluids and electrolytes and incapacitation of the client due to urgency and frequency. Diarrhea can also be associated with fecal incontinence.

Constipation

Constipation—passage of hard, dry stools—may be related to hypomotility, dehydration, voluntary postponement of defecation, or immobility. Some drugs (eg, opiates) promote constipation, as do diets low in fiber. Constipation may cause abdominal discomfort, painful defecation, and general irritability. Prolonged constipation may cause hemorrhoids (distended anal veins) to form. Laxatives, enemas, or suppositories may be needed to induce defecation, and impacted stool may have to be removed manually.

Blood in the Stool

Detection of blood in the stool has important implications, and may signal such disorders as ulcers, hemorrhoids, anal fissures, diverticulitis, inflammatory disorders, and malignancy. Stools may appear tarry (**melena**), or frank red blood may be present. Melena is usually associated with bleeding of the upper GI tract; the natural red color is lost during passage through the bowel. Frank red blood is usually seen in disorders involving the distal colon or the anorectum (eg, hemorrhoids).

Anemia is frequently associated with loss of blood in the stools. Severe cases of gastrointestinal hemorrhage may lead to shock or even death. Detection of blood in the stools indicates the need for thorough testing to determine its origin; these tests are discussed in Chapter 47. Hidden blood in the stool, (melena or occult blood), or frank blood can each signal cancer and should be investigated without delay, especially in clients over 35 years of age.

Painful or Difficult Defecation

Pain or difficulty in defecating is usually related to an abnormality of the anorectum, most commonly anal fissures or hemorrhoids. Both present a potential for blood loss. Hemorrhoids may become strangulated (constricted), although this is uncommon. Fissures may develop into fistulas opening into the skin or, in the female, into the vagina. Rectal fistulas are often associated with Crohn's disease (regional ileitis). Painful defecation may cause the client to try to avoid defecation, worsening any existing constipation.

Section III: Related System Influences and Effects

Since body systems are not disparate entities but are part of a functioning organism, disorders affecting any system will affect all to some extent. The GI tract is no exception.

THE NEUROLOGIC SYSTEM

Because neurologic regulation plays an important part in GI function, any disorder that affects the initiation or transmission of neuronal stimuli, either locally or systemically, affects gastrointestinal homeostasis.

Dysphagia

Swallowing, being essentially a reflex, is especially susceptible to conditions affecting the cranial nerves. Among conditions in which dysphagia is a potential complication are Parkinson's disease, cerebrovascular accident, multiple sclerosis, and amyotrophic lateral sclerosis (Lou Gehrig's disease). The client with dysphagia may require alternative sources of nutrients, either intravenous supplementation or total parenteral nutrition.

Alterations in Motility or Secretory Activity

Alterations in neurological stimulation may alter motility, secretory activity, or both. Autonomic neuropathy may lead to gastric paresis, correctable by use of gastric stimulants.

Intracranial surgery or severe brain injury may be associated with hypersecretion of gastric acids and thus with gastric hemorrhage, perforation, or ulcer formation.

Intestinal motility may be reduced in conditions affecting neurological stimulation; for example, autonomic neuropathy may lead to hypomotility, proliferation of intestinal bacteria, flatulence, and cramping. Neuropathy may also affect digestion, absorption, and intestinal secretion.

Alterations in Elimination

Conditions associated with spinal cord injury, such as paraplegia and quadriplegia, may affect bowel regulation and sphincter control. Incontinence and/or constipation may develop. Defecation may be regulated by use of laxatives, enemas, suppositories, or digital stimulation on a regular schedule. If these methods are ineffective, manual removal of impacted stool may be required. Nurses play an important role in facilitating elimination in clients with spinal cord injuries and in teaching them bowel function control.

THE RESPIRATORY SYSTEM

Alimentary structures lie close to the bronchi, lungs, and diaphragm. Any protrusion from the abdominal cavity (for example, hiatal hernia, gastric distention, ascites, a neoplasm, or a pseudocyst) can impinge on the movements of the diaphragm or otherwise create pressure on respiratory structures, decreasing vital capacity. Such pressure may create respiratory difficulties ranging from mild dyspnea to severe obstruction. Partially because of proximity, pancreatitis can lead to left pleural effusion and atelectasis because lymph drainage from the pleural space is impaired. Pneumonia and adult respiratory distress syndrome are major complications of pancreatitis.

Several disorders are related to respiratory sequelae. Cystic fibrosis affects the lungs as well as the pancreas since oversecretion of mucus obstructs both organs. Peptic ulcer disease has been associated with chronic obstructive pulmonary disease (COPD), especially when steroids are used to improve ventilatory status. The exact mechanism of the relationship is not clear, although it is thought that increased PCO_2 levels may increase gastric acid secretion. Malignant tumors of the GI tract may raise levels of the neurotransmitter serotonin. Increases in serotonin may be associated with bronchoconstriction and wheezing.

THE CARDIOVASCULAR SYSTEM

To perform their functions, the structures of the GI system require an adequate supply of oxygenated arterial blood. Capillaries and lymphatics must function efficiently to provide for absorption of nutrients and their transport to the tissues. If arterial circulation is impaired, ischemic damage to GI structures can occur; for example, thrombosis of the mesenteric artery may be associated with intestinal ischemia so extensive that massive resection of the bowel is necessary. Gastrointestinal disorders can affect the oxygenation of tissues to the extent that the client develops shock syndrome—for example, in pancreatitis or massive GI hemorrhage. Impairment of lymphatic drainage may interfere with the body's utilization of absorbed fats, especially if the thoracic duct has been affected.

Anemia

Gastrointestinal bleeding on any scale can lead to anemia; the volume of blood lost varies with the site of hemorrhage and type of lesion present. Clients receiving anticoagulant therapy or having disorders of coagulation are especially at risk of GI bleeding—as are clients receiving chemotherapy. (These conditions are discussed in relevant chapters throughout this text.) Anemia also may be related to inadequate nutritional intake, especially of iron, folic acid, or vitamin B_{12}. The importance of intrinsic factor to absorption of vitamin B_{12}, and thus to red blood cell synthesis, has already been discussed. If the site where these nutrients are absorbed is surgically removed, eg, by resection of the small bowel, deficiencies may occur.

THE HEPATIC–BILIARY SYSTEM

The hepatic–biliary system is intimately interrelated with the gastrointestinal system and is usually considered an accessory to it. This system is discussed in Unit Nine. Disorders affecting either system frequently affect both in varying degrees. For example, several GI disorders lead to liver disease; gallstones (**cholelithiasis**) are a potential complication of Crohn's disease. Hepatic lesions can develop in relation to ulcerative colitis or as a complication of jejunoileal bypass surgery.

Any disorder affecting the liver is likely to affect the GI system. Nutrients absorbed by the intestine are transported to the liver for processing; the liver also detoxifies many ingested substances. Normal production and secretion of bile by the liver and gallbladder are necessary to the digestion and absorption of fats and fat-soluble vitamins (A, D, E, and K). Hepatic failure promotes portal hypertension and consequent backup of venous blood into accessory vessels. Eventually, clients develop hemorrhoids and esophageal varices. These clients are prone to gastrointestinal bleeding which is exacerbated by the clotting abnormalities associated with hepatic dysfunction.

Ascites—accumulation of serous fluid in the peritoneal cavity—is related to hepatic disease but affects all abdominal organs. Hepatic failure has also been associated with peptic ulcer disease, although the mechanism is not clearly understood. Infectious hepatitis, another disorder originating in the hepatic–biliary system, is associated with such gastrointestinal manifestations as anorexia, nausea, vomiting, and diarrhea.

THE URINARY SYSTEM

Since gastrointestinal structures are closely adjacent to structures of the genitourinary tract, a large neoplasm in either system may impinge upon the other. Disorders of the GI system can affect the urinary system, as when large amounts of fluid are lost through diarrhea. The kidneys, which play a major role in fluid homeostasis, compensate by concentrating the urine. If synthesis or absorption of vitamin K by the intestine is impaired, hematuria may occur. Renal calculi (**nephrolithiasis**) are a potential complication of Crohn's disease and ileal bypass surgery.

Conversely, urinary disorders can cause or compound GI disorders. Clients with chronic renal failure may develop pancreatitis, peptic ulcer disease, and other gastrointestinal complications. Renal failure may also be associated with anorexia, nausea, oral ulcerations, and an unpleasant taste in the mouth—major deterrents to optimal nutrition. The dietary restrictions and absorption problems related to renal failure make maintaining adequate nutrition difficult or even impossible.

THE ENDOCRINE SYSTEM

Like the nervous system, the endocrine system is intimately involved with gastrointestinal function and with utilization of absorbed nutrients. Thyroid deficiency may affect GI motility; enlargement of the thyroid gland may feel like a lump in the throat to the client, inducing dysphagia. Hyperparathyroidism is associated with development of peptic ulcer disease and pancreatitis. Tumors of the islets of Langerhans can stimulate increased secretion of gastric acids, leading to ulcer formation and diarrhea.

Pancreatic disorders can have both endocrine and exocrine sequelae. As pancreatitis progresses, disturbances of endocrine function can lead to diabetes mellitus. As diabetes progresses (whether or not related to pancreatitis), autonomic neuropathy can affect GI motility. Impaired motility leads to both gastric and intestinal stasis, which, in turn, leads to proliferation of bacterial flora resulting in diarrhea and flatulence. Many diabetics alternate between constipation and diarrhea because of hypomotility.

MULTISYSTEMIC EFFECTS

Musculoskeletal and integumentary effects of Crohn's disease include arthralgias and dermatitis. Inadequate absorption of nutrients can have various integumentary manifestations and can affect other organ systems as well. **Icterus** (jaundice), pruritus, and spider angiomas are associated with hepatic cirrhosis. The serotonin secreted by some malignant tumors can cause flushing. Anti-inflammatory agents used in treating arthralgias may erode the gastric mucosa.

Multisystem stressors such as infection, trauma, burns, and surgery also affect gastrointestinal function, sometimes severely. Ileus is a not uncommon sequela to surgery. Stress ulcers can develop in response to acute or chronic stress, for example, burns, surgery.

Section IV: Psychosocial/Lifestyle Influences and Effects

Think of the many common expressions linking emotional states to the gastrointestinal organs. Having "butterflies in the stomach" means being nervous or apprehensive; bravery or courage "takes guts."

The psychosocial influences and effects related to alimentary function may be associated with factors such as age, culture and lifestyle, occupation, and environment. For nurses committed to the holistic view of human health, an overview of these factors will be helpful in assisting clients to preserve or recover optimum GI function.

SEX AND AGE

Certain GI dysfunctions and their related treatments may affect one sex more than the other. For example, abdominal perineal resections may be associated with impotence in males. Peptic ulcer affects more men than women, although that seems to be changing. Conversely, ulcerative colitis has been more common in women than in men.

Constipation is frequently associated with elderly persons. Although the problem does occur more often among the elderly, it is associated with both degenerative diseases and decreases in some neuronal and hormonal function as people age. Many older people reduce their activity level, whether because of long-term illnesses or, in some cases, because they live in inner cities where they are afraid to leave their homes. Older persons may reduce their consumption of fiber, in some cases because of inadequate dentition or poorly fitting dentures. Mastication may be impaired, leading to digestive difficulties or poor absorption of nutrients. The elderly may also have an inadequate fluid intake. Any of these conditions may lead to constipation and use and eventual overuse of laxatives.

Nurses working with the elderly have many opportunities to help their clients avoid or cope with these problems. Nurses can teach their elderly clients how minor changes in diet, such as eating whole grains, breads and cereals, and fresh fruit, and increasing their fluid intake and activity level can improve overall health as well as alleviate problems of elimination. Encouraging clients to engage in social contact or recreational activities suitable to their physical condition may also direct attention away from concerns about bodily function.

PSYCHOEMOTIONAL FACTORS

A number of disorders of the GI system—notably peptic ulcer, "irritable bowel syndrome," and ulcerative colitis—have traditionally been considered wholly or partially psychogenic. The popularization of such concepts as "anal retentive" or "ulcer personality" has reinforced this view. It is true that mental and emotional states can influence GI function. Fear, anger, anxiety, and other emotional states may increase or decrease intestinal motility. Secretion of hydrochloric acid may increase in states of anger or hostility; secretin production may decrease in clients who are depressed or withdrawn.

The knowledge that some GI disorders are linked to psychosomatic mechanisms, that is, to the physiological effects of mental states, has sometimes led the general public, and even health professionals, to conclude that such disorders are "all in the client's mind." In recent years, biophysiological research has continually unearthed new information that underscores that mind and body are not merely linked: they are essentially one. Unconscious mechanisms such as sphincter control and secretory activity have become better understood, and their link to such previously unknown factors as neurotransmission has been at least partially elucidated.

Accumulating knowledge indicates that GI illnesses

thought to be "psychological" in origin are related less to "neuroses" than to differences in the amount of stress to which individuals are subjected and the vastly different ways in which each individual copes with stress. Persons who "swallow their anger" but who are continually exposed to situations that make them angry may develop peptic ulcers. Those who divert the anger into physical activity may avoid such illnesses. The nurse who helps clients identify their coping patterns and change maladaptive patterns to health-promoting ones is providing a great service.

BODY IMAGE RELATED TO FOOD INTAKE AND ELIMINATION

Various GI diseases and their treatments have profound psychosocial implications, particularly for body image. Disorders or treatments that alter the route of either ingestion or elimination require tremendous adjustments on the part of clients and significant others.

Although a number of conditions may require temporary alteration in the manner of food intake—for example, intestinal obstruction or major surgery—disorders that require long-term nutritional support present the most problems of coping. For clients who have cancers of the head and neck requiring resections that are often mutilating, ingestion of food and fluids via the oral route may have to be bypassed permanently. Considering how much cultural and social life revolves around food—the "coffee break," the "after-theater snack," the wedding receptions and bar and bas mitzvahs—it is not surprising that clients who undergo such profound changes have difficulty in adjusting.

Clients for whom tube feeding and parenteral nutrition require tubes visible to others usually undergo disturbances of body image. Alterations in elimination patterns may be even more distressing. Treatment of some disorders, including cancer of the bowel, inflammatory bowel disease, or trauma to the bowel, require that elimination of waste be diverted to a stoma, a surgically constructed outlet. Having one's feces evacuate through an opening on the abdomen into a collecting bag requires major adjustments in both personal habits and body image. Many clients hesitate or refuse to touch or even look at their stomas for some time after surgery. Since the client may have little control over the passage of feces or flatulence, he or she may fear that others will hear these normally private functions or smell an odor. A client may fear rejection by a spouse or interference with sexual relations. A client whose sexual preferences center on the affected structures may experience severe adjustment problems related to sexuality.

The nurse can be of great help to such clients during the early postoperative period and when they resume their usual activities. Specific suggestions may be found in the following chapter and in discussions of specific disorders.

Nursing Research Note

Trainor M: Acceptance of ostomy and the visitor role in a self-help group for ostomy patients. *Nurs Res* 1982; 31:102–106.

The helper therapy principle states that helpers benefit most from their helper role. This research examines that principle in studying ostomates who volunteer as visitors to other ostomates. The visitor and nonvisitor subjects of this study were members of the United Ostomy Association. It was hypothesized that visitors would have greater acceptance of their own disability than nonvisitor ostomy clients. The researcher also speculated that there was a relation between time since surgery and acceptance; that is, the longer the time since the ostomy surgery, the more likely was acceptance.

According to the results, visitors were most often men, were more educated, and had their ostomy for a longer period of time than nonvisitor ostomy clients. Acceptance of the disability was greatest in the visitor group. Acceptance was not significantly related to length of time since surgery. However, it was demonstrated that as time since surgery increased, the more likely the individual was to serve as a visitor. Age was not a significant factor in determining who would serve as a visitor, but younger individuals were more likely to be visitors.

The study concluded that acceptance of an ostomy is greatest among visitors. Age, sex, length of time, and type of surgery did not affect acceptance significantly.

Nurses can play an essential role in assisting clients to accept their disabilities. Referrals to self-help groups may prove beneficial. The nurse can also serve as a link between clients to enhance coping and acceptance of surgery.

CULTURE AND LIFESTYLE

The cultural beliefs and lifestyles of clients will affect gastrointestinal status and their attitude toward it and will affect whether they consider themselves well or ill when dysfunction occurs. In some cultures feces are considered toxins, and frequent bowel movements are considered necessary to health. If the client believes that having a bowel movement every day is a fundamental aspect of being healthy, not having had a movement for 24 hours past the usual time will make that client feel ill. The nurse who fails to take such beliefs into account may completely misinterpret the significance of this change to the client. The belief that elimination is a dirty or shameful activity will influence the client's adjustment to alterations in elimination, perhaps increasing the client's embarrassment and leading to isolation and withdrawal.

Eating habits can affect both gastrointestinal function and nutrition. Diets low in fiber have been associated with cancer of the colon; cultures in which many whole grains and fresh fruits and vegetables are consumed have a low incidence of colon cancer. Diets high in fiber promote rapid transit of food and chyme through the alimentary canal. It is thought that intestinal stasis associated with diets low in fiber leads to prolonged contact of carcinogens with the intestinal mucosa.

Cigarette smoking has been linked to development of some gastrointestinal cancers, for example, cancer of the esophagus. Smoking of pipes and cigars and use of chewing tobacco has been correlated with cancers of the oral cavity. Excessive consumption of alcohol affects bowel function and can contribute to the development of gastritis and pancreatitis. Insufficient activity and low fiber diet are often associated with constipation.

OCCUPATION AND ENVIRONMENT

Occupational and economic effects of gastrointestinal illnesses are similar to those of any illness that may require expensive and prolonged treatment. Occupational stress has been associated with the development of gastrointestinal disorders, especially peptic ulcer. Air traffic controllers, who work under continual tension, have a high incidence of this disorder.

Environmental sanitation, especially sanitation of food and water supplies, is strongly linked to infectious GI disorders. Water supplies may be contaminated by sewage or by swimmers who defecate or urinate in ponds and lakes. Rural drinking water, which may come from individual wells, is especially vulnerable to contamination by seepage. Consumption of contaminated water may lead to gastroenteritis.

Intestinal parasites may be spread by contaminated food (eg, trichinosis may be spread by contaminated pork that is insufficiently cooked). Infectious diseases may be spread by food handlers who are ill or who do not use proper handwashing techniques. Nurses can do much to encourage clients and the public to practice sanitation.

Chapter Highlights

The gastrointestinal system plays an essential role in maintaining homeostasis by assimilating food products and providing for elimination.

Alteration in gastrointestinal function disrupts this homeostatic balance.

Alteration in swallowing may result from mechanical, neuromuscular, or psychological causes, leading to changes in dietary intake.

Secretory function may be disrupted by inflammatory, degenerative, neoplastic, neurohormonal, and mechanical causes leading to alterations in gastrointestinal wall integrity, digestion, and absorption.

Gastrointestinal motility may be disrupted by mechanical, neurohormonal, and inflammatory causes, interfering with digestion and absorption.

Digestion and absorption may be disrupted by mechanical, inflammatory, or neurohormonal causes, leading to malnutrition.

Alterations in elimination include change in stool character and painful or difficult defecation.

Malnutrition can be caused by alterations of gastrointestinal structure and function or can lead to pathophysiological changes.

Gastrointestinal disorders can result from psychosocial influences and can lead to psychosocial problems, especially when the normal route of ingestion and/or elimination is altered.

Normal gastrointestinal function is highly dependent on nervous innervation and vascular supply. Pathophysiology results from alterations.

The physical proximity of the gastrointestinal tract to other body systems (eg, genitourinary, respiratory) makes these systems especially vulnerable when space occupying disorders (eg, tumors, cysts, ascites) occur in the GI tract.

Gastrointestinal function is often disturbed by multisystem stressors, resulting in potential stasis or stress ulcers.

Bibliography

Anderson L et al: *Nutrition in Health and Disease.* Philadelphia: Lippincott, 1982.
Bailey FE, Walker ML: Socioeconomic factors and their effects on the nutrition and dietary habits of the black aged. *Gerontol Nurs* 1982; 8:203–207.
Coleman V: Hidden connections. *Nurs Mirror* 1982; 155:29–30.

Crowley LV: *Introduction to Human Disease.* Monterey, CA: Wadsworth, 1983.
Drossman DA et al: The prevalence of irregular bowel patterns in healthy young adults. *Gastroenterology* 1981; 80:1139.
Drossman DA: The physician and patient. Pages 3–20 in: *Gastrointestinal Disease.* Sleisinger MH, Fordtran JS (editors). Philadelphia: Saunders, 1983.
Edwards GK: Is there a correlation between occupational stress and physical disease and mental symptoms in upper level management? *Occup Health Nurs* 1982; 38:18–28.

Guyton AC: *Textbook of Medical Physiology*. 6th ed. Philadelphia: Saunders, 1981.

Spence AP, Mason EB: *Human Anatomy and Physiology*. 2nd ed. Menlo Park, CA: Benjamin/Cummings, 1983.

Warneka P: Stress and psychological problems of patients undergoing APR. *J Enterostom Ther* 1981; 8:14–15.

Wilson HS, Kneisl CR: *Psychiatric Nursing*. Menlo Park, CA: Addison-Wesley, 1983.

Wolf S: The psyche and the stomach. *Gastroenterology* 1981; 80:605–614.

Suggested Readings

Howland RJ: The digestive system. *Nursing* (Oxford) 1982; 2:86–88. A structural approach to the anatomy and physiology of digestion with reference to pathophysiology.

Moog F: The lining of the small intestine. *Sci Am* 1981; 245:154–158. An in-depth discussion of digestion and absorption in the small intestine.

Chapter 47

The Nursing Process for Clients With Gastrointestinal System Dysfunction

Patricia Brown

Objectives

When you have finished studying this chapter, you should be able to:

Specify the major components of a health history to be obtained for clients with gastrointestinal system disorders.

Determine specific physical assessment approaches in evaluating clients with dysfunction of the gastrointestinal system.

Identify diagnostic tests commonly performed to determine the presence and/or progress of gastrointestinal disease.

Describe the relationship between alterations in diagnostic test results specific to clients with gastrointestinal disorders and the progress of gastrointestinal disease.

Explain nursing implications, including preprocedure and post-procedure care, for clients undergoing diagnostic tests specific to assessment of dysfunction of the gastrointestinal system.

Anticipate common nursing diagnoses for clients with gastrointestinal disorders.

Identify appropriate client care goals and plans of care for clients with gastrointestinal dysfunction.

Specify nursing skills necessary for comprehensive care of clients with gastrointestinal problems.

Discuss desired outcomes of care for clients with disorders of the gastrointestinal system.

Clients with disorders of the gastrointestinal (GI) system turn to nurses for help in many situations. Some of these encounters will be professional, some personal. They may occur on the medical/surgical unit, at a health maintenance organization, or in the client's home where, for example, a visiting nurse helps a client learn self-care after an ileostomy.

The "client" may be a neighbor worried about blood she found in her stool that morning or a traveler seeking help at an immediate care facility because of severe diarrhea. No matter how casual the encounter, the nursing process is employed. Assessment may be a few brief questions; intervention may consist of advice on where to seek professional care; evaluation may be a quick phone call to ask, "Did you have those tests yet?" Regardless of the simplicity or complexity of each phase, the principles learned by studying this chapter will assist in helping the client.

Section I: Nursing Assessment: Establishing the Data Base

A comprehensive assessment, including a careful health history, is essential regardless of the organ system involved. If the symptoms for which the client sought care suggest a gastrointestinal disorder, or if the existence of a GI disorder has already been established, the assessment should concentrate on data specific to that system. Observations should focus on alterations in swallowing, secretion, motility, digestion, absorption, and elimination, including both objective signs and subjective symptoms reported by the client.

Be sure to obtain psychosocial as well as physiological data. Disorders of the GI system can both affect, and be affected by, psychosocial factors.

SUBJECTIVE DATA

A detailed health history provides a major source of data for the nurse. Remember, though, that limited, spontaneous assessments continually take place in the course of day-to-day nursing care, and much valuable data can be obtained through apparently casual questions. Subjective data elicited from clients with gastrointestinal disorders should include nutritional assessment and assessments of the function of the alimentary canal.

Nutritional Assessment

Detailed discussion of nutritional assessment pertaining to states of overnutrition and undernutrition may be found in Chapters 8 and 9. Thorough assessment of the client's nutritional state is imperative in evaluating possible origins and potential consequences of gastrointestinal dysfunction. Often, a nutritional problem will precipitate a GI problem, herald its presence, or result from its occurrence. A food intolerance, for example, may be related to malabsorption or may be a cause of diarrhea. Furthermore, malnutrition is associated with many GI disorders. Protein-calorie malnutrition is especially prevalent among clients with gastrointestinal cancer.

Diet History
The diet history includes a thorough assessment of what the client eats, as well as recent changes in intake, food tolerance, energy level, and weight. Are there foods the client cannot tolerate? Have bowel or bladder habits changed recently? How? Greater frequency? Less? What about the client's energy level? Diet content can best be assessed by asking the client to describe a typical day's meals and snacks. Remember that overweight clients, in particular, may be sensitive about what they eat, and a more comprehensive description may be forthcoming once trust and rapport have been established. Nonhospitalized clients may

be asked to keep a daily record of food intake on forms the nurse provides. Once client and nurse have determined what is actually eaten, servings per food group can be calculated and problems identified.

Ask the client about indigestion (**dyspepsia**), constipation, and diarrhea, since these conditions may be related to poor nutrition. Be sure that the client describes exactly what he or she means by constipation, since individuals who assign great importance to regularity may consider any variation from a daily movement as constipation. Note any food intolerances and whether they are of recent manifestation.

Has the client gained or lost weight recently? The thin person being assessed may be a "fat person in disguise" who has recently lost weight with a fad diet; the client who appears fat may be a "yo-yo" dieter who was thin last year. Some clients of apparently normal weight are bulimic; extreme thinness may signal anorexia nervosa. (These problems are discussed in Chapter 9.) Rapid weight loss or gain may be associated with malnutrition. Does the client seem lethargic or energetic? A low energy level may signal malnutrition.

Sociocultural Influences
What is the client's attitude toward food? Everyone has food preferences and prejudices related to psychological makeup, cultural and family background, and finances. Knowing these is helpful to the nurse, both in assessing the client's condition and in making realistic plans for care. The immediate environment also affects what and how people eat. A client used to eating at home, in the company of friends and family, may find that eating alone from a tray in the tense atmosphere of a hospital promotes anorexia (loss of appetite).

Are there ethnic foods to which the client is especially attached? What about religious restrictions on diet? Southeast Asians may prefer rice to potatoes; Italians, pasta. Remember, though, not to generalize—not to assume on the basis of a name or appearance that the client eats (or does not eat) particular foods. Ask each individual what his or her preferences are.

Dietary Considerations With the Elderly
Older adults should be carefully evaluated for signs of malnutrition. Many psychosocial problems that are especially likely to affect the elderly predispose them to nutritional deficits. In addition to problems such as loneliness or lack of money, older people often become indifferent to food because taste sensation diminishes with age; the number of taste buds declines, and those remaining may atrophy (Tichy & Chong, 1981). Deficiencies in protein, calcium, iron, and vitamins A and C are especially prevalent (Kohrs, 1983). Fiber may be missing from the diet. Medications,

both prescribed and OTC, may alter intestinal absorption, especially antibiotics and laxatives.

The Upper Gastrointestinal Tract

Since the mouth, esophagus, and stomach function in swallowing and digestion, assessment should focus on alterations of these functions.

The Mouth and Esophagus

Has the client experienced **aphagia** (inability to swallow) or dysphagia (difficulty in swallowing)? What about difficulty in eating in general? Has the client noticed any oral lesions? Discolorations, vesicles, ulcerations, or growths? Does the client use tobacco or alcohol? Use of these substances often promotes development of leukoplakia—small, elevated, patchy white lesions that may precede oral cancer.

Routine assessment should include noting any reports of bleeding, inflammation, infection, ulceration, or spread of disease already present. Specific therapy may be needed to maintain oral hygiene or to prevent spread of infection. Does the disease process interfere with the client's ability to eat or speak? Alternative methods of eating (ie, tube feeding) or communicating may have to be devised. Box 47–1 gives history-taking suggestions for assessment of the oral cavity.

The Stomach

Has the client experienced nausea or vomiting? Heartburn? Indigestion? Excessive eructation? In older adults, motility of the gut decreases, and fewer digestive enzymes are secreted, often leading to heartburn or indigestion (Tichy & Chong, 1981). If disease is already present, ask the client about any changes in the number, severity, or pattern of symptoms, since this information can be useful in evaluating therapies and nursing care plans.

Nausea and Vomiting. If the client reports vomiting, note the odor, color, consistency, and quantity of vomitus. Has the client noticed **hematemesis** (bloody vomitus)? Digested or undigested food in the vomitus? A fecal odor? A fecal odor may indicate reflux of bowel contents due to intestinal obstruction. A coffee-ground appearance of the vomitus may indicate the presence of partially digested blood. These observations help clarify the course of the client's problem and assist in assessing potential problems related to nutritional and fluid–electrolyte status.

Encourage the client to determine whether symptoms are related to eating any particular food. How long after a meal do symptoms begin? How long do they last? Does eating make symptoms worse or does it alleviate them (as it may, for example, in peptic ulcer)?

Try also to determine whether symptoms are related to emotional states or social situations. Is the client having marital difficulties or conflicts with adolescent children? Meals fraught with tension and discord can cause digestive

---

Box 47–1   History-Taking Suggestions: The Oral Cavity

Ask the client about any past or present:

- Severe or persistent pain in mouth or throat
- Recurrent infections, especially streptococcal
- Serious or disabling tooth, gum, or jaw problems
- Chronic hoarseness or laryngitis
- Change in voice
- Pain while chewing
- Difficulty swallowing (dysphagia)
- Impairment of speech (dysphasia)
- Tendency to breathe by mouth
- Sore tongue
- Bloody saliva
- Impaired sense of taste
- Lesions in mouth
- Tonsillectomy or adenoidectomy
- Oral surgery
- Orthodontia work

Also ask about the client's general dental health. Are all the natural teeth present? Any dentures? Partial plates? Any sores or areas of irritation under the dentures? Any problem with toothache or sore, swollen, or bleeding gums? What is the client's daily dental hygiene regimen? How often does the client see a dentist? When was the last appointment?

The following is an example of a write-up history for the mouth that could be found under a review of systems:

Mouth—no hx lesions, dysphagia, or hoarseness; frequent sore throats × 2 years; two documented strep throats—6/80, 11/85; has all natural teeth; annual dental exams; brushes and flosses daily; no hx bleeding gums or frequent dental caries; does not smoke a pipe, cigar, or cigarettes; does not chew tobacco.

Adapted with permission from: Malkiewitz J: What assessing the mouth can tell you. *RN* (May) 1982; p. 66. Copyright 1982 Medical Economics Company Inc., Oradell, NJ.

---

upsets or even long-term dysfunction. Are special stresses arising at work? Perhaps anxiety-producing meetings are regularly scheduled just after lunch. Individuals vary in their response to stress and anxiety, but emotional changes can precipitate diarrhea, constipation, nausea, vomiting, indigestion, or other symptoms. In older adults, loneliness, grief, depression, or financial worries can precipitate or worsen gastrointestinal disease.

Medications and Vitamins. Does the client take prescribed or over-the-counter drugs to relieve gastrointestinal symptoms—for example, antacids, antiemetics, or antiflatulents? How often? How well do they work? It is a good idea to use brand names when asking about these products, because clients are often unaware of the generic names of the preparations they are taking. What about vitamins? Vitamin E, for example, may cause nausea if not taken with meals. Fat-soluble vitamins should be ingested with foods to be effectively absorbed; many clients are not aware of this, and asking about vitamins provides opportunity for health teaching. Ask also about aspirin and anti-inflammatory medications, especially in clients of middle age or older, who may be receiving treatment for arthritis. These medications may irritate the gastric mucosa.

Pain. When asking clients about abdominal pain, remember that visceral pain (pain in specific organs) such as that from the stomach, intestine, or pancreas is poorly localized and may be referred to other parts of the body. The point where the client feels the pain, therefore, may not be the point where the pain originates. Also, because visceral pain is so diffuse, the client may have difficulty describing it. Use open-ended approaches to help clients describe their pain: "Tell me about your pain." If the client finds it hard to describe the quality of the pain, suggest terms such as stabbing, aching, or dull. Remember that in older adults and in persons with some degenerative diseases that affect the nerve endings (for example, diabetes), responsiveness to internal sensations like abdominal distention may have diminished. These clients may not be fully aware of their pain and thus may not report it accurately.

Pain receptors in the visceral organs are most responsive to stretch stimuli. Pain related to distention (from gas, organ enlargement, or neoplasia) may thus be more severe than pain associated with other conditions. Pain in the GI tract tends to increase with peristaltic activity and to decrease with elimination, such as by vomiting or defecation. Visceral pain is often intensified with movement that increases pressure. Peritoneal irritation (that is, irritation of the mucous membrane that contains the viscera) is often intensified by movement alone. Pain related to the effect of gastric acid on the gastric mucosa is often associated with a low pH (high acidity) and may therefore be intensified when the stomach is empty.

The Lower Gastrointestinal Tract

Since the functions of the small intestine, the colon, and the anorectum involve motility, absorption, and elimination, questions should focus on alterations in these functions.

Alterations in Bowel Function

Some clients find discussion of bowel function embarrassing and may consider some symptoms undignified or shameful. Asking questions in a matter-of-fact way may help. A surprising number of adults still resort to euphemisms ("number 2") when discussing bowel function. Encourage clients to use any forms of expression that put them more at ease.

Ask the client about anorectal conditions such as hemorrhoids, anal bleeding, or pruritus. Have there been any episodes of fecal incontinence? Although fecal incontinence may have a benign etiology, it may also be a sign

of colorectal cancer. Since the association of rectal bleeding with cancer has been so well publicized, the client may need realistic reassurance that other causes are possible or even likely.

Ask the client to describe the odor, color, consistency, and frequency of bowel movements. Have there been any recent changes? Changes in the regularity of bowel movements may be indicative of disease or may be related to therapy. As with nausea or indigestion, try to determine whether dietary or emotional factors are related to any changes. Does the client take laxatives or use enemas to facilitate bowel movements? What kind? How often? Does the client eat fresh fruits and vegetables? Whole grains? Bran? Or "fast foods" and highly refined foods lacking in fiber?

Intestinal obstruction will prevent the passage of stool and flatus, causing the abdomen to become distended. Obstruction may be related to tumors, strictures, hernias, intussusceptions, or adhesions (fibrous scar tissue). Post-operative clients are especially susceptible to obstruction related to paralytic ileus (intestinal paralysis); therefore, they are checked frequently to determine whether they are passing flatus or stool and whether abdominal distention is present.

Color and Consistency of the Stool

Ask the client about any changes in the color and consistency of the stool. The following findings are especially significant:

- Melena (black, tarry stools), which indicates digested blood from upper GI hemorrhage
- Bloody stools (frank, red blood), which indicate lower GI or anorectal bleeding
- Yellow or green stools, often signifying infectious processes
- Steatorrhea (fatty, foul-smelling, greasy, floating stools), signifying maldigestion or malabsorption
- Loose, frequent stools (diarrhea)
- Hard, infrequent stools (constipation)

Such findings warrant further investigation, in many cases by diagnostic or laboratory tests.

Pain

Pain is usually present if the bowel is hyperactive or tensely distended. Does the client experience pain or tenderness with defecation? Additional questions pertaining to pain are similar to those already discussed under lower GI, subjective data.

OBJECTIVE DATA

Objective data are obtained by thorough physical assessment of the oral, abdominal, perianal, and rectal areas. Nutritional status should also be evaluated. Basic procedures of the physical assessment are described in detail in

Chapter 7. Only those parameters specifically relating to gastrointestinal dysfunction will be mentioned here.

Physical Assessment

Nutritional Assessment

Objective data relating to nutrition include both clinical observations and the taking of anthropometric measurements—height, weight, body frame, midarm circumference, skinfold measurement, and arm muscle circumference. These measurements and standard parameters for them are presented in Chapter 8.

Clients who are likely to be malnourished should be weighed daily—for example, those who are NPO for prolonged periods and clients with anorexia, malabsorptive disorders, or long-standing diarrhea. In such clients, the body may begin to break down its own fat and protein stores, leading to negative nitrogen balance, weight loss, and debilitation.

Compare each client's weight to the ideal height and weight standards in Table 8–6 and also, in the case of hospitalized clients, to weight on admission.

Assessment of the Oral Cavity

Assessment of the oral cavity also includes assessments related to respiratory status; these are discussed in Unit Three and in Chapter 7. The normal mouth is depicted in Figure 47–1. While assessing for signs related to gastrointestinal status, routinely note any signs pertaining to disorders of other systems. Inspection and palpation will also yield signs of the client's need for oral hygiene, which often presents a problem in GI disease.

Diseases of the oral cavity include inflammatory and infectious processes, degenerative processes, and abnormal growths. Congenital abnormalities may also be seen in older clients; today these are frequently corrected surgically in childhood. If the presence of disease was established prior to the examination, assess for amelioration or spread of the disease. Note any changes in coloration, odor, or discharge. Also note whether any condition that interferes with eating is present.

Comprehensive assessment includes the teeth, gums, tongue, cheeks, and palate. Note any evidence of neoplasms or lesions, inflammation, discoloration, exudate, swelling, or difficulty in swallowing. Note that sublingual

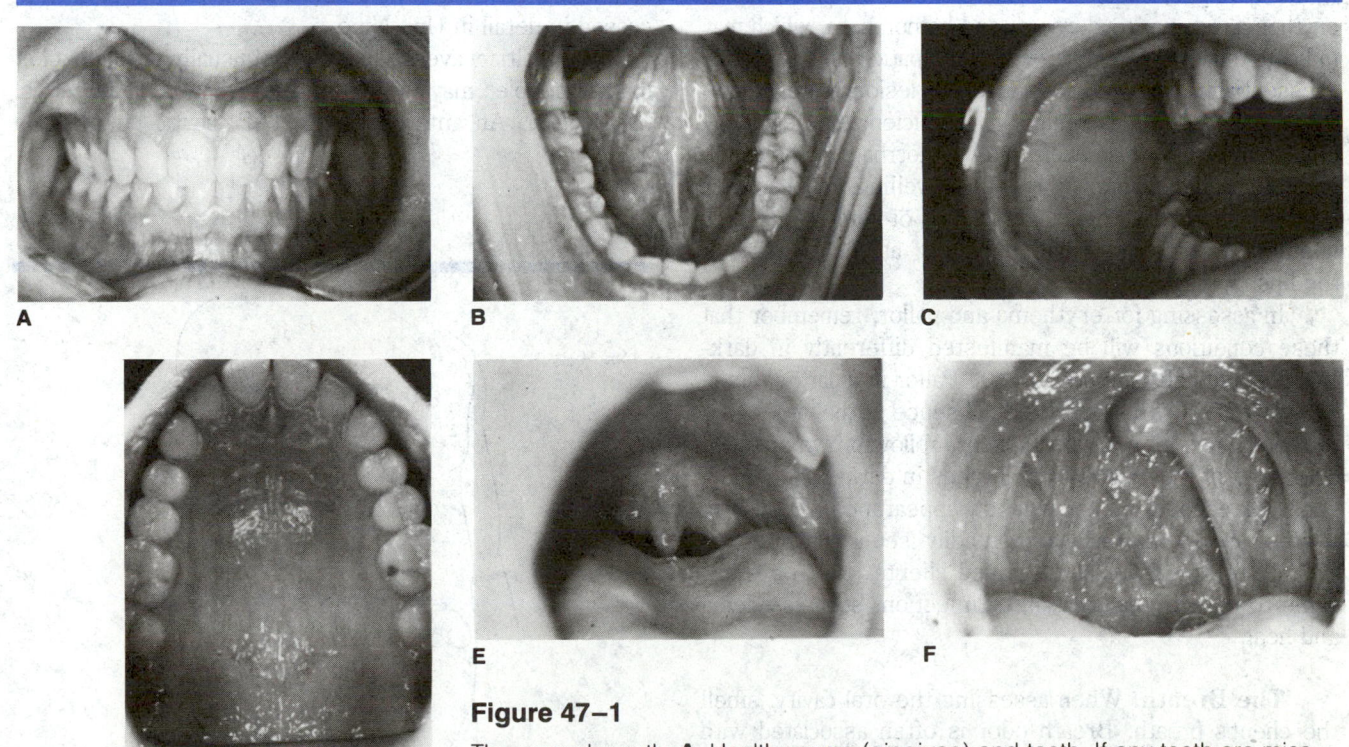

A   B   C
D   E   F

Figure 47–1

The normal mouth. **A.** Healthy gums (gingivae) and teeth. If any teeth are missing, record their location. **B.** The sublingual area, which contains salivary ducts, should always be moist. **C.** Be sure to inspect the buccal mucosa on both sides. **D.** The hard palate is a good place to spot signs of jaundice. Normally, it is pink. **E.** The uvula and soft palate should rise above this position when the client says "A-a-a-h." **F.** The oropharynx should be pink and free of drainage.

spider nevi are normally present in about 50% of older adults and are not pathological (Tichy & Chong, 1981).

Dentition. Inspect the teeth (dentition) for caries, which can be painful and may interfere with eating, ultimately affecting nutritional status. Palpate the teeth to determine whether any are painful to touch or loosened from their sockets. Assess for absence or misalignment of teeth. If teeth appear to be missing, ask the client whether they have been extracted. Congenital absence of one or two teeth, often familial, is a fairly common finding (Crowley, 1983).

If the upper (maxillary) and lower (mandibular) dentition do not meet properly—a condition called malocclusion—the client may not be able to chew food properly. Malocclusion may also lead to pain in the temporomandibular joint (TMJ pain) or in some cases to headaches. Referral to an orthodontist may be indicated. Diseases that affect the jaw such as trauma or arthralgias may impede movement of the mouth or may cause anorexia related to fear of pain with eating.

The Gingivae and the Oral Mucosa. The gingivae (gums), tongue, cheek, and palate should be examined for erythema, edema, tenderness, and hemorrhage, which may indicate inflammation or infection. Palpation for neoplasms is essential in assessing for cancerous lesions. Oral inflammation may also indicate nutritional deficiencies. Deficiency of vitamin C may cause edema and hemorrhage of the gums, and folic acid deficiency may cause swelling, redness, and tenderness of the tongue. Deficiency of some B complex vitamins is associated with cracking at the corners of the lips.

In assessing for erythema and pallor, remember that these conditions will be manifested differently in dark-skinned and light-skinned clients. Pallor in a dark-skinned person is usually discernible by absence of the underlying red tones that are normally present. Yellow-brown or ashen coloration of the mucous membranes in dark-skinned persons corresponds to the whitish appearance of pallor in whites. Erythema, which is readily seen in whites, is difficult to detect in dark-skinned clients. Rely on other signs to detect inflammation or infection, such as edema and heat.

The Breath. When assessing the oral cavity, smell the client's breath. Breath odor is often associated with disease. In diabetic ketoacidosis, for example, the breath has a fruity or acetone odor. A foul odor may indicate extensive caries, infection, or cancer. Clients with esophageal disorders may also have foul breath; if an esophageal lesion inhibits the passage of ingested food, the action of bacteria on accumulated food creates rancidity. However, a foul odor may simply be related to poor oral hygiene.

Assessment of the Abdomen

An abdominal assessment, although providing data specific to the gastrointestinal system, is commonly performed in caring for clients with many different disorders. The usual techniques of inspection, palpation, percussion, and auscultation are employed, but in assessing the abdomen, the usual order of examination is changed. Because percussion and palpation may alter the bowel sounds, auscultation is performed first. Inspection always continues throughout the physical assessment.

Inspect the abdomen for contour and symmetry. Masses or enlarged organs will produce bulging and/or asymmetry. In clients with umbilical hernia, the umbilicus may be displaced or may bulge outward (Figure 47–2). Asymmetry of the upper abdomen may be related to disorders of the stomach, pancreas, or transverse colon; asymmetry of the lower abdomen can occur with disorders of the ascending and descending colon (Grimes & Iannopollo, 1982).

Distention or asymmetry of the abdomen may be from ascites (fluid in the abdominal cavity), or it may be related to excessive flatus. These conditions must be distinguished from distention related to urinary retention, which is primarily seen in the suprapubic area. In clients with ascites, the abdomen is tense and distended. The skin is tightly stretched, usually shiny, and the flanks bulge. Ascites is commonly associated with hepatic disorders. It is discussed in detail in Unit Nine.

Peristaltic waves, which are not usually visible except in thin people, may be observable in cases of intestinal obstruction. An anteroposterior (AP) aortic pulsation in

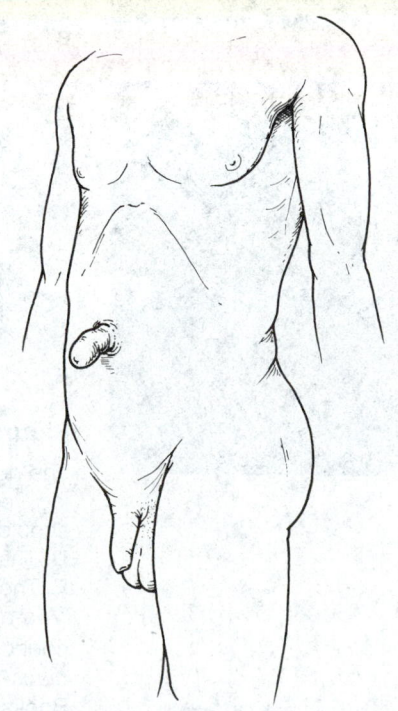

Figure 47–2

Umbilical hernia.

the midepigastric area is normal in thin clients. When the pulsation is lateral as well as AP, it may be related to aortic aneurysm. Note, however, that the abdominal wall becomes progressively thinner and more flaccid with age, so peristaltic waves and aortic pulsations will be more apparent in older adults, even under normal circumstances (Tichy & Chong, 1981). Peristalsis can best be visualized by directing a light obliquely over the abdomen while keeping your eyes at abdominal level.

Carefully inspect the abdominal skin, being especially alert for special kinds of changes. Multiple small nodules may herald gastric carcinoma. Localized ecchymoses in the flank may indicate abdominal or peritoneal hemorrhage.

Place the diaphragm of the stethoscope lightly on the abdomen to auscultate for bowel sounds. Bowel motility is likely to be altered in clients with GI disorders, for example, in cases of diarrhea, intestinal obstruction, and paralytic ileus. The high-pitched tinkling sound associated with intestinal obstruction is caused by peristalsis occurring in a bowel that is tensely distended with air. Peristalsis increases above the point of developing obstruction, causing **borborygmi** (hyperactive bowel sounds). Hyperperistalsis, and therefore borborygmi, also occur in gastroenteritis and intestinal hemorrhage. In older adults, louder bowel sounds may occur normally (Tichy & Chong, 1981). Besides auscultating for bowel sounds, assess for arterial bruits with the bell of the stethoscope (see Chapter 7). Aortic bruits may be heard with abdominal aortic aneurysm.

By percussing the abdomen, the presence of masses, ascites, and visceral enlargement can be determined. Any of these conditions may indicate abdominal pathology. The loud, musical drumlike quality of tympany should predominate in the abdomen, especially over the stomach and intestines. Remember that a stomach full of food or a colon filled with feces may simulate dullness that could be mistaken for visceral enlargement. A nurse should be able to percuss for gastric dilation, a common symptom of gastrointestinal lesions. A nurse may also percuss to detect ascites. This procedure is discussed in Chapter 52.

Palpation is used in detecting or evaluating masses and inflammatory processes in the abdomen. It is not uncommon to mistake feces for a mass—or a mass for feces. If a neoplasm or an inflammatory process is present, the client will usually feel pain on palpation. Responses vary, however, and the type of response may provide valuable clues for diagnosis.

Peritoneal inflammation is usually associated with pain more constant than that of visceral disorders. Peritoneal pain does not change when pressure is applied. Visceral pain, which may be intermittent, may diminish with pressure. Ask the client whether there is less pain when mild pressure is placed on the area involved. A "yes" may indicate that the pain originates in the viscera. Also, ask whether it hurts the client to move. This may indicate peritoneal involvement. Since palpation may cause additional pain for a client who is already uncomfortable, be sure to explain that these procedures are necessary to determine the origin of the client's discomfort.

Inflammation of the peritoneum—eg, in appendicitis, pancreatitis, or diverticulitis—often causes muscle rigidity (guarding) and rebound tenderness (pain occurring upon release of pressure). To assess for rebound tenderness, press the tips of the approximated fingers gently into the abdomen and quickly release them. The client will experience pain in the affected region as the peritoneum is released. *Note that assessing for rebound tenderness should be reserved for experienced examiners. Palpation of the abdomen, if not carefully and properly performed, can cause appendiceal rupture or other dangerous and even life-threatening iatrogenic sequelae.* The pancreas is not normally palpable. If malignancy or inflammation is present, this organ can be detected in the midabdomen above the umbilicus.

Assessment of the Perianal and Rectal Areas

This examination may be especially embarrassing for the client. Make sure that privacy and respect for the client are maintained.

Observe and palpate the perianal area for masses, inflammation, excoriation, ulceration, fissures, and bleeding. If the client has diarrhea, the need for skin care and hygiene may be apparent. Check for the presence of hemorrhoids. Thrombosed external hemorrhoids or prolapsed internal hemorrhoids may appear as painful bluish, shiny, ovoid masses.

To perform the rectal exam, ask the client to lie on his or her left side with the hips and knees flexed. Relax the external sphincter by applying some pressure to the anus; then insert a lubricated, gloved finger into the anal canal, pointing toward the umbilicus (Figure 47–3). Assess for tenderness and/or the presence of nodules or masses. The presence of hard stool may signify fecal impaction, which may have to be removed. Figures 47–3C, D show rectal palpation of the prostate in the male and the cervix in the female.

Examine any stool remaining on the examining finger when it is withdrawn. Are color and consistency normal? Determining whether frank or occult blood is present is especially important. Frank blood is apparent upon inspection, whereas occult blood may be apparent only with testing, either on the nursing unit (Hemoccult test) or in the laboratory.

Diagnostic Studies

Many alterations in gastrointestinal function can be objectively assessed through analysis of laboratory data and diagnostic studies. Specific findings will usually be associated with particular pathological conditions. The nurse should understand how various findings relate to the client's gastrointestinal health status, and which findings indicate the presence of disease processes. By understanding diagnostic studies, the nurse will be able to prepare clients physically and psychologically for the tests. Understanding

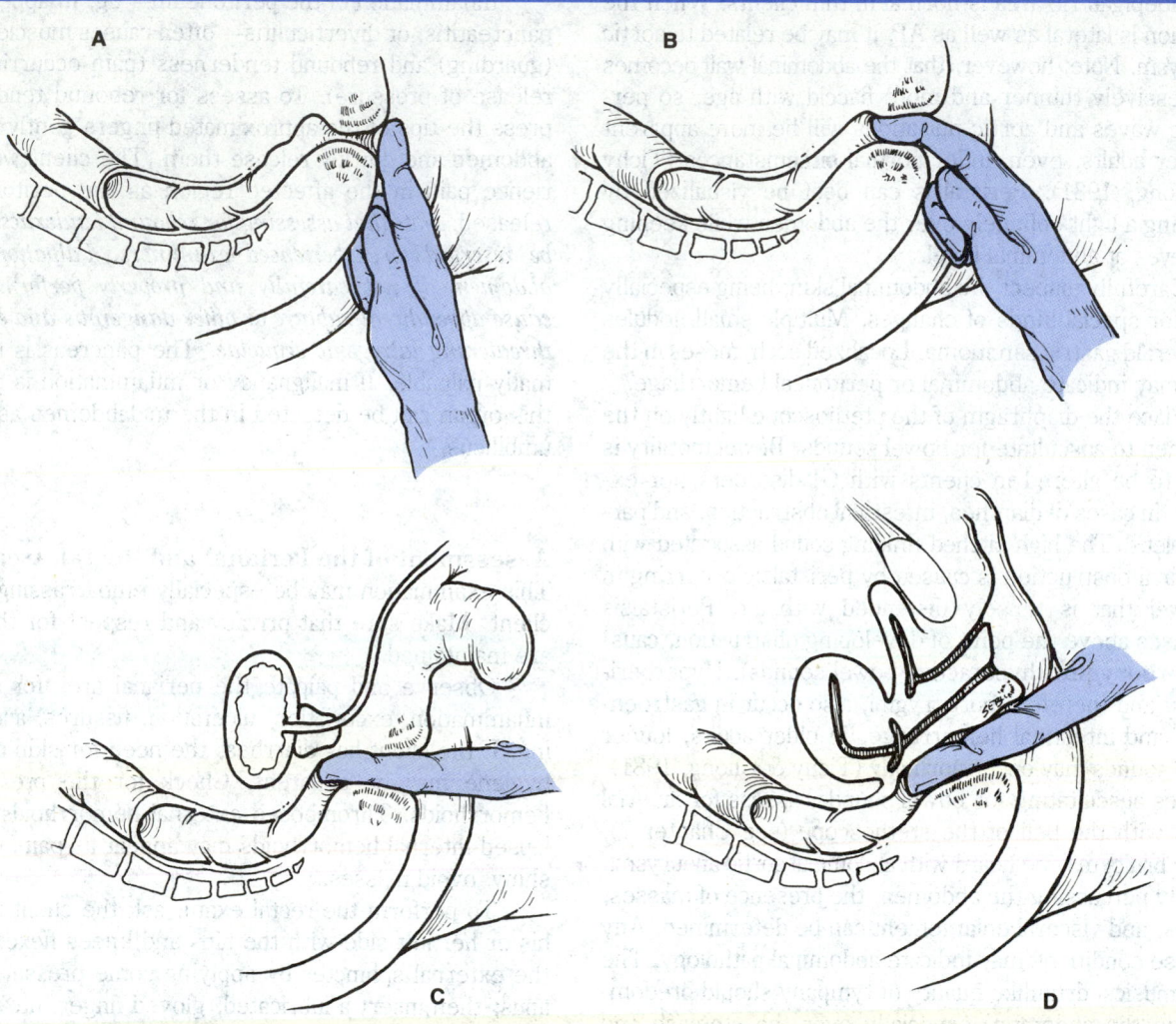

Figure 47–3

Examination of the rectum: **A.** Light digital pressure against the anus causing relaxation. **B.** Gloved, lubricated index finger slowly introduced in direction of the umbilicus. **C.** The finger is rotated to palpate the male prostate. **D.** The cervix in the female.

how certain diagnostic procedures are done will also help in reinforcing the physician's explanation when legal consent must be obtained.

Laboratory tests commonly used in evaluating the GI system are summarized in Table 47–1. Many of these tests are used in evaluating other systems as well; only findings relevant to GI status are given here. Since gastrointestinal status can significantly alter nutritional status, tests used to assess for the presence of malnutrition are included. Only tests associated with the function of the mouth, esophagus, stomach, intestines, and some pancreatic functions are given here; tests used to evaluate hepatic–biliary status are listed in Unit Nine.

Hematologic Studies

Various categories of disorders are associated with specific alterations in blood values. In hemorrhagic disorders—for

example, bleeding peptic ulcer—blood components will be altered. Hemoglobin (Hb), the primary component of the red blood cell (RBC), will be reduced, since there will be fewer RBCs in circulation. Hematocrit (Hct), the percentage of RBCs in a given volume of blood, will also be decreased. In inflammatory and infectious disorders—for example, appendicitis—the production of white blood cells will increase in the client with a normal immune response, and the leukocyte (WBC) count will therefore rise.

Pancreatic Enzyme Levels

Enzymes produced by the pancreas (amylase, lipase) may escape into tissues and into the bloodstream when acute pancreatic disease is present. With chronic pancreatic disease, amylase levels may be decreased. With these enzymes unavailable to digest fats, steatorrhea occurs.

Table 47-1 Laboratory Tests Common to the Gastrointestinal System

Laboratory Test	Normal Expected Value	Disease State	Expected Abnormal Finding
Hemoglobin	Male: 14–18 g/dL Female: 12–16 g/dL	GI bleeding	Decreased
Hematocrit	Male: 40%–54% Female: 37%–47%	GI bleeding	Decreased
Red blood cell count	Male: 4.5–6.2 million/μL Female: 4.0–5.5 million/μL	GI bleeding	Decreased
White blood cell count	4500–11,000/μL	Inflammatory and infectious processes, such as appendicitis, peritonitis, pancreatitis, diverticulitis; also GI cancer	Increased
Serum amylase	60–150 Somogyi μ/dL	Cancer of head of pancreas, acute pancreatitis Chronic pancreatitis	Increased Decreased
Serum lipase	Below 1.5 units/mL	Acute pancreatitis, obstruction of the pancreatic duct	Increased
Serum glucose (fasting blood sugar)	65–100 mg/100 mL	Pancreatic cancer, pancreatitis, pancreatic insufficiency	Increased
Urine glucose	15 mg/100 mL Negative for sugar when testing fractional urines	Pancreatitis	Increased
Serum bilirubin	Total 0.3–1.4 mg/dL Direct 0.1–0.4 mg/dL	Obstructive jaundice due to cancer of the head of the pancreas	Increased Increased
Serum sodium (Na^+)	135–145 mEq/L	Vomiting, gastric suction Diarrhea	Increased Decreased
Serum potassium (K^+)	3.6–5.0 mEq/L	Vomiting, gastric suction Diarrhea	Decreased Decreased
Serum bicarbonate (HCO_3)	21–28 mEq/L	Vomiting, gastric suction Diarrhea	Increased Decreased
Serum chloride (Cl^-)	95–108 mEq/L	Vomiting, gastric suction Diarrhea	Decreased Variable
Serum carotene	40–200 μg/dL (mcg/dL) 0.74–3.72 μmol/L (SI units)	Malabsorption syndrome, pancreatic insufficiency, cystic fibrosis (intestinal), protein malnutrition	Decreased
Serum carcinoembryonic antigen (CEA)	less than 2.5 ng/mL	GI tract and pancreatic cancer, pancreatitis and ulcerative colitis	Increased
Serum albumin	3.5–5.5 g/dL	Malnutrition	Decreased
Serum total iron-binding capacity (TIBC)	250–450 μg/dL	Malnutrition	Decreased
Serum transferrin	22–46 μg/dL	Malnutrition	Decreased
Urine examination: Creatinine	Male: 20–26 mg/kg per 24 h Female: 14–22 mg/kg per 24 h	Malnutrition	Decreased

(continued)

Table 47–1 Laboratory Tests Common to the Gastrointestinal System (continued)

Laboratory Test	Normal Expected Value	Disease State	Expected Abnormal Finding
Urea nitrogen	6–17 g/24 h	Malnutrition	Decreased
Ketones	0.3–2 mg/dL	Malnutrition	Increased
Stool examination:			
Blood	None	Upper GI bleeding	Black stools, occult blood (+)
		Lower GI bleeding	Visible red blood
Fat	1–7 g/24 h	Pancreatic and malabsorptive disorders	Increased
Urobilinogen	40–250 mg/24 h	Obstructive jaundice, such as found with cancer of the head of the pancreas	Decreased
Ova and parasites	None present	Parasitic infection	Parasites present
Culture	Normal flora	Infectious intestinal disorders	Abnormal flora

Adapted with permission from Byrne et al: *Laboratory Tests: Implications for Nursing Care*. 2nd ed. Menlo Park, CA: Addison-Wesley, 1986.

Glucose Levels

Disorders of the pancreas alter insulin production. Since insulin is required for metabolism of glucose, insufficiency or unavailability of insulin will precipitate hyperglycemia—elevation of blood sugar levels. Glucose will also appear in the urine (**glycosuria**) as the body tries to eliminate the excess.

Bilirubin Levels

Cancer of the head of the pancreas may obstruct the common bile duct, precipitating obstructive jaundice. Serum bilirubin will rise, as will levels of bilirubin in the urine. Levels of bilirubin in the stools will decrease, since flow of bile to the gut has been reduced; stools will be acholic, lacking the bile pigments. These findings may also be associated with a number of hepatic–biliary disorders as well.

Serum Electrolytes

Serum electrolytes are an important gauge of GI status. Vomiting, diarrhea, malabsorption, and gastric or intestinal suctioning are especially likely to disturb homeostatic balance by depleting the body of electrolytes and fluids. If fluid loss is sufficient to produce dehydration, the hematocrit level will also decrease. Loss of secretions produced by the pancreas, hepatic–biliary system, or lower bowel may promote metabolic acidosis, since these secretions are alkaline. Diarrhea, mechanical suction, or the presence of a fistula may cause loss of these substances. Conversely, loss of the acidic secretions of the upper GI tract through vomiting or suction may precipitate metabolic alkalosis. (Fluid–electrolyte balance and metabolic acidosis and alkalosis are discussed in Chapter 5.)

Vitamin Levels

Deficiency of vitamin K, which is vital to coagulation of the blood, may be related to malabsorption, diarrhea, ulcerative colitis, intestinal obstruction, or malnutrition. Hepatic–biliary dysfunction may also affect levels of this vitamin. Serum levels of carotene, a precursor of vitamin A, will be depressed in clients with malabsorption syndromes and other GI disorders. Carotene, which is found in green and yellow fruits and vegetables (especially carrots and sweet potatoes), is absorbed from the intestine. If absorption is depressed, serum carotene levels will be low despite ample carotene in the diet.

Carcinoembryonic Antigen Levels

Tests for carcinoembryonic antigen (CEA) are performed as an adjunct to other tests in diagnosing GI cancer and monitoring treatment. CEA is a nonspecific test (Kee, 1983).

Blood and Urine Studies Related to Malnutrition

Malnutrition, often associated with GI disorders, depletes protein stores and creates a negative nitrogen balance in the body. Tests that will show evidence of protein depletion include:

- Serum albumin. Albumin, the smallest of the protein molecules, contributes the majority of total protein value.
- Total iron-binding capacity. Measures the amount of iron-transporting protein in the serum.
- Urinary nitrogen and creatinine (a nitrogen-containing compound).
- Serum transferrin. A transporter of protein and a sensitive indicator of visceral protein stores.

Transferrin levels may be calculated from the total iron-binding capacity. They may also be measured independently, but this technique is not yet widely available.

Protein depletion will also be evidenced by a diminished immune response, since production of lymphocytes and antibodies depends on the presence of protein. The client will show delayed response to common skin test antigens, although this delayed reactivity is not specific to malnutrition-related immunocompetence. The protein-depleted client will also be susceptible to infection and slow to heal, although this, again, is not a condition specific to malnutrition.

Urine ketones will be increased as the body attempts to provide necessary energy by breaking down lipid tissue. Assessment of urinary ketone levels can be easily performed in the course of daily nursing care.

Fecal Abnormalities

Examination of the feces is important in identifying bleeding disorders, malabsorptive and digestive diseases, biliary obstruction, and parasitic and bacterial infections. In infectious processes, the stool must be examined to determine the causative organism. If intestinal infection is suspected, three separate specimens should be collected and tested before the possibility of disease can be ruled out. Sterile containers should be used, and the specimen should be delivered immediately to a laboratory and refrigerated (Byrne et al., 1986).

Routine Radiographic Studies

Abnormalities of the mouth, such as the presence of a mass, dental caries, or abnormal dentition, can be detected by x-rays. An abdominal x-ray (flat plate) can reveal masses in the stomach, intestine, or pancreas, obstruction of the small bowel, trauma to abdominal tissue, and ascites.

Nursing Implications. Testing may be done on an inpatient or outpatient basis. Clients having oral x-rays are usually not restricted in any way. Those having abdominal studies may be asked to fast for 8 hours before the test. Radiographic studies should not be done during the first trimester of pregnancy except in cases of extreme urgency when delay in diagnosis would be dangerous to client and/or fetus. Explain to clients what precautions will be taken to prevent excessive radiation.

Fluoroscopic Barium Studies

Fluoroscopy—visualization with motion—requires use of a contrast agent that can be visualized as it passes through or outlines GI structures. Barium sulfate is the agent used.

Upper GI Series. Fluoroscopic examination of the upper GI tract (esophagus, stomach, duodenum, and other portions of the small bowel) is called an upper GI series. The client must swallow barium sulfate (a chalky white substance, sometimes flavored) or another contrast medium. Films are taken sequentially as this material moves through the upper GI tract (Figure 47–4A); the process may also be monitored on a screen similar to a TV screen.

The upper GI series is performed routinely to rule out gastritis; peptic ulcer; neoplasia or strictures of the esophagus, stomach, or duodenum; hiatal hernia; gastric polyps; gastric or duodenal diverticula; or foreign bodies in the tract. A variation of the procedure, known as hypo-

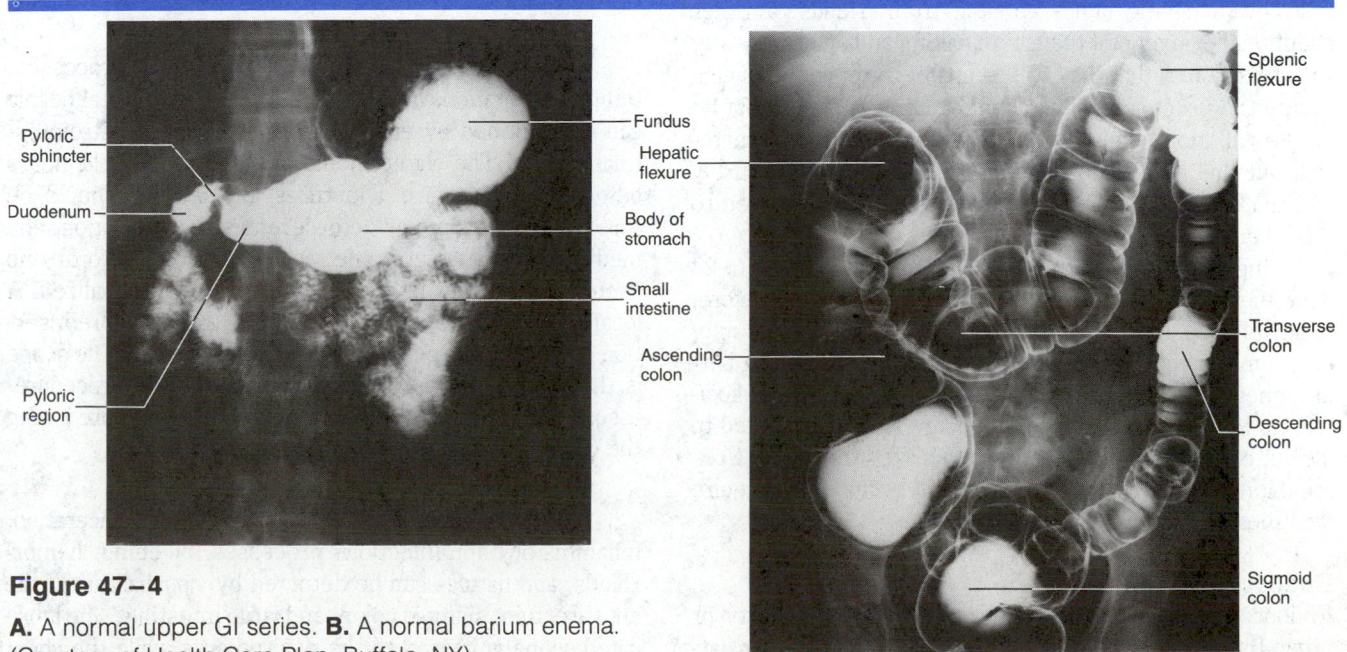

Figure 47–4

A. A normal upper GI series. **B.** A normal barium enema. (Courtesy of Health Care Plan, Buffalo, NY)

tonic duodenography, involves administration of glucagon, atropine, or propantheline bromide (Pro-Banthine) to slow down small-intestinal peristalsis. It may be used if the client has hyperperistalsis, duodenal spasticity, or a space-occupying lesion such as a tumor of the head of the pancreas (Kee, 1983).

A *long GI series* is used to rule out Crohn's disease, parasitic infection, diverticulitis, or malabsorption. In a long series, the regular test is performed first; the client then swallows additional contrast medium, and more x-rays are taken. A GI series may last from 1 to 6 hours, depending on what part of the alimentary canal is being assessed.

Nursing Implications. The client should be NPO for 8 to 12 hours before testing to ensure that the GI tract will be empty. The client should also be advised not to smoke, since smoking stimulates motility. If a long GI series is planned, the client may have to fast for 10 to 12 hours prior to the test. Mouth care is important after upper GI testing to remove the taste of barium.

After the procedure, a laxative should be prescribed and administered. Tell the client to expect light-colored stools for several days. Constipation and fecal impaction may occur, requiring treatment.

Lower GI Series. To visualize the lower gastrointestinal tract, barium sulfate is instilled into the colon by means of a rectal tube (barium enema) (Figure 47–4B). Air may be instilled in addition (double-contrast study). The client must retain the enema while x-ray films are taken. Polyps, tumors, lesions, colitis, diverticulitis, and fistulae can be identified in this way.

Nursing Implications. Many clients dread this test, often having heard about it from friends or other clients. They expect it to be both painful and embarrassing. Clients may fear that they will be unable to retain the enema during the procedure. The client can be reassured that he or she will most likely be able to retain the contrast material, but that many people are unable to control it entirely and that x-ray personnel are professionals accustomed to this eventuality, should it occur.

The client should be on a clear liquid diet for 18 to 24 hours before testing and NPO from supper the night before. A bowel prep—cleansing of the bowel with laxatives and/or enemas—may be required. Immediately after the barium enema, the client should attempt to defecate. A laxative and/or enema after the procedure is recommended to facilitate passage of barium from the intestinal tract. Constipation and fecal impaction may occur and require treatment.

Endoscopy

Endoscopy involves the visualization of a body cavity or organ by means of an endoscope—an instrument consisting of a combination of lenses and a light source at the end of a long, slender tube. With the development of fiberop-

tics, a flexible tube can be employed, since light traveling along these optic fibers can travel around a curve. Earlier endoscopes had to employ straight tubes and complex systems of mirrors.

Various forms of endoscopy derive their names from the area viewed. In the case of gastrointestinal endoscopy, these include:

- Esophagoscopy (the esophagus)
- Gastroscopy (the stomach)
- Esophagogastroscopy (the esophagus and stomach)
- Duodenoscopy (the duodenum)
- Esophagogastroduodenoscopy (the esophagus, stomach, and duodenum)
- Proctoscopy (the anus and rectum), from the Greek *proktos,* for anus
- Sigmoidoscopy (the sigmoid colon)
- Proctosigmoidoscopy (the anus, rectum, and sigmoid colon)
- Colonoscopy (the large intestine)

Nursing Implications. Endoscopy may be performed in a hospital or clinic. Written consent must be obtained. The procedure must be explained to the client, the client's records must be consulted to ensure that preparation requirements (NPO status, bowel prep, sedation if any) have been met, baseline vital signs must be recorded, and the safety and privacy of the client must be ensured.

Draping the client helps alleviate embarrassment. Procedures of the lower tract may produce discomfort and flatus; instruct the client to breathe deeply and slowly to promote relaxation. After endoscopy, whether of the upper or lower GI tract, the client should rest. Vital signs must be taken. Perforation is a rare complication associated with pain, abdominal distention, and hemorrhage (Kee, 1983).

Upper GI Endoscopy. Inflammatory processes, tumors, ulceration, hemorrhage, cancer, and hiatal hernia can be identified by endoscopy of the upper gastrointestinal organs. The client should be NPO for 8 to 12 hours before the procedure. Dentures and jewelry should be removed. Sedation may be ordered as premedication, and medication such as atropine may be prescribed to dry up secretions so that the mucosa may be clearly visualized. A local anesthetic may be applied to the throat before insertion of the endoscope to diminish the gag reflex. The scope is then passed to the desired area. After the procedure, assess the client for return of the gag reflex before giving the client fluids or food.

Lower GI Endoscopy. Polyps, tumors, ulceration, inflammatory and infectious processes, bleeding, hemorrhoids, and fistulas can be detected by visualization of the anus, rectum, sigmoid colon, and large intestine. The lubricated scope is passed to the desired area while the client assumes a knee-chest position (with a rigid scope) or side-lying position (with a flexible scope). The client should have light meals for 1 to 2 days and an 8-hour fast immediately prior to the procedure. A bowel prep involves the use of laxatives the night before the procedure and saline enemas the day of the test. Intravenous meperidine and/ or diazepam may be given to promote comfort and relaxation. Atropine may be given to limit GI tract secretions. After the procedure, the client should be assessed for unusual pain, bleeding, or shock, which could indicate perforation of the bowel.

Ultrasonography

Ultrasonography, also called ultrasound, sonography, or echography, involves the use of sound waves to visualize body structures. It is considered a noninvasive technique with no known harmful effects. To produce the image, a transducer is passed over the body area to be assessed; it emits sound waves and receives echoes "bounced" off body structures. These echoes are converted to electrical impulses, which may be viewed on a screen or photographed. In assessing the GI system, ultrasonography may be used to visualize the abdominal aorta to detect aneurysms and to detect tumors, cysts, and inflammation of the pancreas. NPO restrictions should be observed for 8 to 12 hours prior to ultrasonography. Advise the client that the abdomen will be smeared with thick lubricant to facilitate movement of the transducer and that the procedure is painless, although the client will have to remain still for the duration of the examination.

Computerized Tomography

In computerized tomography scanning (CT or CAT scanning) a narrow x-ray beam is directed at the body from various angles. Esophageal disease, intra-abdominal masses, and organ enlargement can be detected by CT scan, which produces less radiation than standard radiography. Contrast medium is often administered intravenously to enhance visualization.

The client remains alone in a room with his or her body inside a scanner. The test takes about 1½ hours; the client may be asked to take and hold several deep breaths during this time.

Nursing Implications. Since contrast medium may be used, question the client about allergy to iodine (including fish and seafood, since the client may not realize that these foods contain iodine). Explain the procedure, and tell the client that a warm, flushed sensation, accompanied by temporary nausea, may occur if contrast medium is injected. Showing the client a picture of the scanner may help, since the size of CT scan equipment is often frightening. Obtain written consent.

Esophageal Manometry
(Esophageal Motility Study)

Esophageal manometry provides an estimate of esophageal motility by measuring pressure under different conditions: the resting esophageal sphincter, the sphincter

relaxation response, and esophageal peristalsis. Water-filled catheters, connected to transducers, are passed via the nose or mouth through the esophagus and into the stomach. The catheters are gradually withdrawn, 1 cm at a time, as pressure measurements are taken along the esophagus. Electrodes sensitive to pH can be attached to measure esophageal acidity. This increasingly common test is thought beneficial in diagnosing achalasia (failure of the esophageal sphincter to relax during swallowing) and other esophageal disorders in clients with chest pain and dysphagia (Meshkinpour et al., 1982).

Nursing Implications. The client should be NPO from the previous night. Explain that a local anesthetic will be applied topically to the throat to prevent gagging and discomfort. The client should also know that swallowing will be required during the test. Written consent should be obtained.

Schilling Test

The Schilling test, which determines the client's ability to absorb vitamin B_{12}, is commonly used to diagnose pernicious anemia. It is also used to diagnose malabsorption syndrome. Adequate uptake of vitamin B_{12} requires the secretion of intrinsic factor by the stomach and normal absorptive capacity of the terminal ileum (see Chapter 46). For this test, radioactive B_{12} is administered orally, along with an IM injection of B_{12}. A 24-hour urine sample is collected. A finding of subnormal urinary levels of B_{12} indicates that secretion of intrinsic factor or absorption of vitamin B_{12} is abnormal. The abnormality may be due to malabsorption, renal dysfunction, or lack of intrinsic factor (pernicious anemia). A further test is then done in which intrinsic factor is administered. If excretion remains subnormal, pernicious anemia is ruled out, and malabsorption or renal disease is implicated.

Nursing Implications. The client should be NPO for 8 to 12 hours before the test. Written consent should be obtained. Explain that nonradioactive B_{12} is administered parenterally before the radioactive B_{12} is administered orally. The parenteral dose saturates the liver and protein-binding sites so that the oral dose is absorbed and excreted. The urine is collected in a clean container that need not be refrigerated. The client should be cautioned, however, that all urine must be voided or poured into the container, or the test results will not be accurate.

Xylose Absorption Test

Xylose is an easily absorbed monosaccharide that requires no digestion. In the xylose absorption test, used to diagnose intestinal malabsorption, the client first fasts for 10 to 12 hours. After voiding, an oral dose of D-xylose is given with water. Urine is collected for 5 hours and tested for the presence of sugar. In malabsorption disorders such as sprue and Crohn's disease, little D-xylose is excreted, since little is absorbed (Given & Simmons, 1984).

Lactose Tolerance Test

In evaluating a client for lactose deficiency, a lactose tolerance test may be done. This involves drawing a fasting blood sample, after which lactose is given by mouth. Over a period of 2 hours, further blood samples are drawn and tested for blood glucose. Elevated glucose levels in conjunction with the onset of intestinal symptoms signify a positive test. False positive and false negative results can occur, however, because the test is affected by glucose metabolism and gastric emptying time. A breath test for hydrogen before and after the ingestion of lactose is a more sensitive test for lactose deficiency. Unabsorbed lactose is converted to hydrogen by intestinal bacteria, resulting in an elevation of breath hydrogen.

Bernstein Test (Esophageal Acid Perfusion Test)

The Bernstein test is used to determine the presence of esophagitis or an ulcerated esophageal lesion. A nasogastric tube is passed into the stomach after the client has fasted. First saline and then a mixture of saline and hydrochloric acid is instilled into the lower esophagus. If the client feels pain when the acid is instilled, the result is positive (Given & Simmons, 1984).

Nursing Implications. The client should be kept in a sitting position during the test. Explain the procedure and keep the client comfortable.

Biopsy and Cytologic Examination

Specimens of tissue for biopsy or cell scrapings for cytologic examination may be obtained during endoscopic examinations, during surgery, or when gastric tubes are inserted. Special instruments (biopsy forceps, cytology brushes) are used by the physician. The specimens obtained are microscopically examined for changes in cellular morphology, as occurs, for example, in malignancy.

Nursing Implications. Written consent is necessary. Special postprocedure observation of the client for signs of hemorrhage is indicated. For *biopsy of the small bowel,* a specimen is obtained by passing a tube through the oral cavity. The client should be NPO for 8 hours prior to the procedure, and dentures should be removed. Since hemorrhage is a potential complication of this procedure, vital signs should be taken prior to, during, and afterward. The procedure takes about an hour and may be used in diagnosis of malabsorption disease such as nontropical (celiac) and tropical sprue (Beck, 1981b).

Secretion Analysis

Gastric Analysis. Gastric analysis (analysis of gastric secretions) is important in the diagnosis of peptic ulcer, Zollinger–Ellison syndrome, and achlorhydria (absence of hydrochloric acid in the stomach), which is associated with gastric cancer. The client is kept NPO for 8 hours preceding the test, and medications that can affect gastric secretions are withheld for 24 hours. A nasogastric tube is passed, and stomach contents are intermittently or continuously aspirated for 1 to 2 hours. If secretions are scant, medications are given to stimulate more. Secretions must be measured and sent to the laboratory for analysis. Limited secretion of gastric juices occurs with gastric ulcer. Achlorhydria suggests gastric cancer. Mildly elevated secretion of gastric juices suggests peptic ulcer, and greatly elevated gastric acid secretion may signify Zollinger–Ellison syndrome.

Tubeless Gastric Analysis. With this technique, the client is given a gastric stimulant. One hour later, a resin dye is given by mouth. Two hours later, urine is examined for dye. Presence of dye indicates that free hydrochloric acid is present in the stomach—a normal condition. Absence of dye indicates achlorhydria and the possibility of gastric cancer (Kee, 1983).

Pancreatic Secretion Analysis. If pancreatic disease is present, depressed or elevated levels of pancreatic enzymes will be noted in reflux tests that stimulate the pancreas. A duodenal aspiration (duodenal drainage test) involves the administration of secretin or another pancreatic stimulant. A nasogastric tube is first passed into the stomach, where contents are aspirated and then discarded. The client is positioned on the right side to facilitate passage of the tube into the duodenum near the ampulla of Vater. A control specimen of duodenal contents is obtained, and a stimulant is then administered. Duodenal contents are then aspirated and tested for bicarbonate, amylase, trypsin, lipase, blood, mucus, cholesterol, and malignant cells. Elevated levels of enzymes and bicarbonate are expected. Abnormally high elevations may occur with alcoholism and hepatic cirrhosis. Depressed levels are associated with pancreatic cancer, collagen diseases, and diabetes, and after Billroth I and II surgeries (see Chapter 50) (Given & Simmons, 1984).

Section II: Nursing Diagnosis

Once subjective and objective data have been collected during the nursing assessment, client needs will begin to emerge as the information gathered is analyzed and synthesized. Pieces of data from various sources may coalesce into a holistic view of the client's individual situation that highlights specific problems the client and nurse may approach together. Nursing diagnoses commonly seen with GI dysfunction are listed in Box 47–2.

Note that the listings in Box 47–2 are general. True nursing diagnoses will expand upon these general categories to specify the etiology involved and will relate to the condition of the individual client. For example, *alteration in nutrition, less than body requirements* may be related to anorexia in one client, dysphagia in another, and vomiting in a third. Unless the etiology is identified in making the diagnosis, the nurse will not be able to help the client address the problem.

ALTERATION IN BOWEL ELIMINATION

Diarrhea

Diarrhea, passage of frequent, loose, unformed stools, is a frequent occurrence in gastrointestinal disorders. Diarrhea may be associated with:

- Inflammatory or infectious disease of the intestines (eg, infectious enteritis)
- Partial obstruction of the intestines (eg, diverticular disease or neoplasia)
- Disorders of intestinal secretion (pancreatic disease; Zollinger–Ellison syndrome; obstructive jaundice; and short small bowel, often related to surgical resection)
- Disorders of digestion (subtotal or total gastrectomy, lactose intolerance)
- Disorders of absorption (sprue, intestinal resection, colectomy, ulcerative colitis, regional enteritis)

Other physiological conditions may be related to diarrhea as well, and stress may also be a precipitating factor.

The client with diarrhea may be fatigued or exhausted by the almost constant defecation. Moreover, the rapid and frequent passage of chyme limits the absorption of fluid and nutrients and can promote fluid/electrolyte loss, weight loss, and malnutrition.

Frequent passage of acidic stools may cause the perianal area to become excoriated and painful. In some cases, diarrhea may be associated with painful cramps related to severe intestinal spasm. Fecal incontinence may develop, adding to the client's discomfort and embarrassment.

Constipation

Constipation, the passage of dry, hard, infrequent stools, may be precipitated by a number of conditions. The physiological basis of constipation is discussed in the preceding chapter. Briefly, constipation may be related to reduced motility or to obstruction, or it may be secondary to lesions that cause painful defecation (eg, hemorrhoids or fissures) that induce the client to ignore the urge to defecate. Paralytic ileus is another possible cause, particularly in postsurgical clients. Any of these conditions prolongs the transit

> ### Box 47–2 Nursing Diagnoses Commonly Related to Gastrointestinal Dysfunction
>
> **Diagnoses directly related to gastrointestinal dysfunction**
> *Bowel elimination, alteration in: constipation*
> *Bowel elimination, alteration in: diarrhea*
> *Comfort, alteration in: pain*
> *Skin integrity, impairment of: potential*
> *Nutrition, alteration in: less than body requirements*
> *Fluid volume deficit: potential*
>
> **Additional potential nursing diagnoses**
> *Knowledge deficit*
> *Self-care deficit*
> *Self-concept, disturbance in: body image, role performance*
> *Sexual dysfunction*
> *Nutrition, alteration in: potential for more than body requirements*
> *Skin integrity, impairment of: actual*
> *Fluid volume deficit: actual*
> *Anxiety*

time of the stool, with reabsorption of much of its fluid content, causing stools that are hard, dry, and difficult to pass. Constipation usually follows diagnostic studies in which barium is used. Stress, inactivity, or long periods of NPO status and/or diet restrictions that limit residue also contribute to constipation.

The constipated client feels bloated and uncomfortable. Appetite may be diminished, confounding the problem, since adequate bulk and fluid are needed to promote elimination. Straining related to constipation may promote the formation of hemorrhoids.

ALTERATION IN COMFORT: PAIN

Clients with GI disorders will experience various types of pain: pain associated with pressure exerted by neoplasms, pain related to gaseous distention, and incisional pain with GI surgery. Pain may also be related to excessive secretion of gastric acids. Some clients will express pain more readily than others, demonstrating anxiety and restlessness, whereas others appear more stoic. (Pain and individual reactions to it are discussed in Chapter 5.)

Pain can interfere with recovery by discouraging the client from coughing and deep breathing or moving about and becoming independent. The inactivity may actually worsen the client's discomfort, for example, discomfort related to postoperative gaseous distention. Pain associated with defecation, if hemorrhoids are present, may contribute to constipation.

POTENTIAL IMPAIRMENT OF SKIN INTEGRITY

Impairment of skin integrity can be related to various conditions. The presence of GI secretions on the skin can promote excoriation. Diarrhea can promote rectal excoriation. Secretions from draining wounds and fistulas can excoriate the chest or abdominal area. (A fistula is an abnormal opening between body cavities or between the body and the environment.)

Tubes passed through the client's nose into the GI tract can cause irritation and breakdown of the nasal mucosa. Finally, tubes surgically inserted into the GI tract, such as a gastrostomy tube (from the stomach through the abdominal wall) can cause excoriation at the site of insertion by friction from the tube and/or leakage of secretions from it.

Excoriated skin will appear red and edematous and may weep fluid. The client will describe the associated pain as soreness or burning.

ALTERATION IN NUTRITION: LESS THAN BODY REQUIREMENTS

Disorders affecting the alimentary tract alter swallowing, digestion, and absorption. Singly or in combination, alterations in these functions can leave the client moderately or severely malnourished. Neoplasms or strictures of the mouth or esophagus can prevent normal ingestion of foods or fluids. Pancreatic and gastric disorders alter digestive processes; disorders of the bowel alter both digestion and absorption. Moreover, during the course of diagnosis and treatment, the client with GI disease may be subjected to long periods when food and/or fluids are restricted or prohibited. Thus, the client's nutritional state is impaired at a time when the metabolic needs imposed by the body's defense mechanisms, or by the disease itself, as in cancer, actually increase nutritive requirements.

Anorexia, nausea, and/or vomiting are common in GI disease, although these symptoms are also associated with dysfunction of other systems. If ingestion of food is associated with pain or discomfort, the client may be afraid to eat. Secretions and/or odors, such as those from diarrhea or wound drainage, may contribute to a less-than-appetizing atmosphere. Anorexia may also be directly associated with the disease process itself, especially in clients with cancer.

Fatigue is common, especially if vomiting is violent. Large amounts of fluid and electrolytes may be lost in the vomitus and imbalances may occur. Problems associated with deficiencies of particular nutrients may also develop.

POTENTIAL FLUID VOLUME DEFICIT

Diarrhea, anorexia, nausea and vomiting, and long periods of NPO status can contribute to fluid volume deficits (dehydration). Disease states that interfere with normal eating and/or later digestion and absorption can also contribute to this problem. Further loss of fluid may occur through hemorrhage, drainage of wounds or fistulas, gastrointestinal suctioning, and extensive use of laxatives and enemas.

The client who is dehydrated will have dry skin and mucous membranes, poor skin turgor, and will be thirsty. When fluid is lost, body electrolytes will also be lost. Table 47–2 shows the pH and electrolyte content of various gastrointestinal fluids; it is estimated that the GI tract normally secretes a total of about 8500 mL per day (Given & Simmons, 1984). Electrolyte and acid–base disturbances are explained in Chapter 5.

NURSING DIAGNOSES RELATED TO PSYCHOSOCIAL STATUS

Many treatments associated with gastrointestinal disorders may temporarily or permanently alter the client's lifestyle. Clients and their families may have to learn new ways of living, and the nurse may diagnose a knowledge deficit related to the prescribed regimen.

For example, a client with diverticulitis may not know which foods are suitable for the high-residue diet that has been prescribed. The client with a colostomy (an artificial opening from the large intestine to the abdominal wall to provide for fecal elimination) must learn how to care for it and how to cope psychologically with this new method of elimination. (Colostomy is discussed at length in Chapter 50.)

Table 47–2 Milliequivalents (mEq) of Electrolytes per Liter of Gastrointestinal Fluid and pH					
Fluid	pH	Na$^+$	K$^+$	Cl$^-$	HCO$_3^-$
Saliva	6.0–7.0	20–80	16–23	24–44	20–60
Gastric juice	1.0–3.5	20–100	4–12	52–124	0
Bile	7.8	120–200	3–12	80–120	30–50
Pancreatic juice	8.0–8.3	120–150	2–7	54–95	70–110
Intestinal juice	7.5–8.9	80–130	11–21	48–116	20–30

SOURCE: Given BA, Simmons SJ: *Gastroenterology in Clinical Nursing*, 4th ed. St. Louis: Mosby, 1984, p. 72.

Pain, weakness, and poor self-image may interfere with the client's self-care activities, including eating, bathing, dressing, and eliminating wastes. Alterations in body image accompany many treatments, most notably surgical construction of an ostomy. Other disturbances in self-concept may be related to role changes, if, for example, a family breadwinner is immobilized or permanently disabled by disease or treatment, or if the marital partner who has assumed the major responsibility for child care can no longer do so. Sexual dysfunction, while not directly related to gastrointestinal disease, may occur, for example, in a client who has a colostomy and avoids sexual contact because of feelings of disgust or shame.

Section III: Planning and Implementation

Once nursing diagnoses specific to the individual client have been determined, enlist the client's participation in establishing goals of care. Sometimes priorities are obvious, being dictated by the diagnosis—eg, control of vomiting or diarrhea. At other times, priorities may be matters for discussion; the client's priorities may not be the nurse's, and vice versa. Clients to whom independence is extremely important may place considerable emphasis on caring for themselves as soon and as completely as possible. Clients in pain usually give first priority to pain relief and may need a careful, concerned explanation if this goal must be superseded.

Client care goals related to nursing diagnoses commonly encountered in gastrointestinal illness, together with appropriate planning and intervention, are summarized in Table 47–3, a sample nursing care plan. Note that nursing interventions should not alter the client's medical regimen. However, observations made in the course of nursing care, or problems encountered by the client in carrying out a prescribed regimen, should be brought to the physician's attention by the nurse in the role of client advocate.

PREVENTING AND MANAGING CONSTIPATION

Constipation may be related to a disease process or to dietary alterations, such as limited fluid or residue. The nurse cannot alter the disease process, except to ensure that prescribed therapy is implemented. The nurse can, however, encourage the client to consume high-residue foods and to increase fluid intake. Also encourage the client to move about as much as possible, since inactivity is associated with reduced motility.

If these measures are ineffective, laxatives and/or enemas may be prescribed. Commonly prescribed stimulant laxatives are listed in Table 47–4. Categories of laxatives with their disadvantages and actions are shown in Table 47–5. Enemas may be tap water or soap suds or may be the prepackaged (Fleet type) variety. If long-term constipation has led to fecal impaction—the presence of accumulated hard, dry stools that will not pass—oil retention enemas or manual removal of the stool may be necessary. Ensure privacy and make the client as comfortable as possible, allowing adequate time for the client to defe-cate. Many persons find it difficult to defecate while using a bedpan. Using a low fracture pan may be helpful.

PREVENTING AND MANAGING DIARRHEA

Diarrhea may be related to a disease state or to psychosocial factors. In either case, food should be withheld at first. Eating can gradually resume as the diarrhea diminishes. Foods low in fiber should be provided at first, since these will be less stimulating to the intestines. Provide a nonstressful environment, since stress may precipitate or worsen diarrhea. Antidiarrheal medications may be prescribed; these are listed in Table 47–6. Antispasmodics may also be helpful. Medications relieve only symptoms, however, and the underlying disorder must be diagnosed. Skin in the rectal area should be carefully observed for signs of breakdown. Try to ensure privacy, since the client may be embarrassed by foul odors. Finally, output from diarrhea should be carefully measured and charted as part of fluid balance assessment. Maintenance of fluid intake is essential, and clients should understand its importance so they do not become dehydrated.

PROMOTING COMFORT: PAIN RELIEF

Many GI disorders exert pressure on body structures or promote gastrointestinal distention. Careful implementation of the therapeutic regimen will assist in alleviating these conditions. Analgesics may be ordered for symptomatic relief. Stress-reducing drugs such as tranquilizers may be helpful, since stress is often a precipitating factor in GI disease and the pain associated with it.

Nursing responsibilities include discerning the source of the pain and taking measures to diminish it by administering prescribed medications, providing distraction, and promoting relaxation. If pain is related to excessive flatus, encourage the client to ambulate. An antiflatulent such as simethicone may be required. A *Harris flush* (also called colonic irrigation) may be ordered. This procedure is similar to an enema but is done to relieve discomfort related to excessive flatus. Consult a nursing fundamentals text for details of the procedure.

(continued on p. 22)

Table 47–3   Sample Nursing Care Plan for Clients With Gastrointestinal Dysfunction

Nursing Diagnosis	Client Care Goals	Plan/Nursing Implementation	Expected Outcomes
Bowel elimination, alteration in: constipation	Maintain normal bowel elimination; reduce or eliminate constipation	Encourage the client to * "establish a consistent pattern of food intake and elimination; eat breakfast or at least take a hot beverage upon arising; eat foods providing roughage; eat foods such as prunes that contain natural laxatives"; drink more than 1500 mL of fluids each day; establish a pattern of regular exercise; use psyllium instead of laxatives	Client incorporates health teaching into lifestyle that results in daily soft bowel movements that easily pass without straining; should constipation occur, as it often does with traveling and change in usual diet or activity levels, client feels confident to manage problem
Bowel elimination, alteration in: diarrhea	Manage diarrhea effectively	Encourage client to limit intake to liquids initially, gradually adding solids as tolerated; avoid milk and milk products, foods with extremes of temperature, and concentrated sweets, since these may promote diarrhea; eat foods containing pectin, such as bananas and applesauce, since these are naturally acting substances that will limit intestinal activity; eat low-fiber foods initially to avoid stimulating the bowel; clients who tend to have loose stools secondary to life stresses may benefit from regular use of psyllium; relaxation and stress reduction approaches are often helpful	Client incorporates health teaching into lifestyle; bowel elimination is normal: stools are formed, not liquid, and are passed with normal frequency
Comfort, alteration in: pain	Reduce or eliminate pain; explain pain prevention and pain management approaches	Determine the source of pain and eliminate it if possible; provide distraction for the client, ie, reading, television, visitors; encourage relaxation: deep-breathing, yoga, etc.; in cases where pain is associated with flatus, encourage the client to avoid: • Foods that produce gas • Carbonated beverages • Air swallowing • High-fat meals • Reclining immediately after meals • Eating rapidly Administer antiflatulents as ordered; when pain is associated with excessive	Client understands measures to reduce pain and incorporates them in daily activities; should pain occur, client feels confident to manage pain; knows when to consult care provider

Nursing Diagnosis	Client Care Goals	Plan/Nursing Implementation	Expected Outcomes
		gastric acid secretion, administer prescribed ant-acids; antacids that contain simethicone help in reducing flatulence; if there are no contraindications, have client assume the knee-chest position, which aids in passing flatus	
Skin integrity, impairment of: potential	Remain free from skin breakdown	Keep skin clean and dry; assess skin for signs of breakdown, especially areas most susceptible to breakdown; apply lubricant to areas prone to irritation and skin protectants to areas prone to excoriation; use collection bags when excessive drainage is present	Skin integrity is normal: skin shows no signs of breakdown and is smooth, soft, of normal color and moisture, and is not edematous
Fluid volume deficit, potential	Remain free from dehydration	Assess the client for signs of dehydration; keep accurate weight and intake and output records; encourage oral fluid replacement for lost fluids; careful monitoring of IV infusions and laboratory electrolyte values	Excessive loss of fluid is prevented (eg, diarrhea); fluid and electrolyte balance is within normal limits
Nutrition, alteration in: less than body requirements	Maintain normal nutritional intake; describe nutritional management and home care required	When alteration in nutrition is from diarrhea, nursing care plan associated with the problem of diarrhea should be followed; when alteration in nutrition is from client's continual NPO status, make sure meals are provided as soon as possible, once NPO status is no longer in effect; when alteration in nutrition is related to anorexia: • Determine and provide food preferences for the client • Provide small, frequent feedings • Provide a relaxed atmosphere, free of foul odors and secretions When alteration in nutrition is related to nausea and vomiting, encourage the client to: • Eat and drink slowly • Eat small, frequent meals to avoid overdistention of abdomen	Client does not become malnourished; client incorporates teaching regarding nausea and vomiting into daily activities; client is well prepared to manage home tube feedings, special diets, or dietary supplements

(continued)

Table 47–3 Sample Nursing Care Plan for Clients With Gastrointestinal Dysfunction (continued)

Nursing Diagnosis	Client Care Goals	Plan/Nursing Implementation	Expected Outcomes
		• Drink fluids between rather than with meals • Eat dry toast or crackers when feeling nauseous • Avoid poorly tolerated foods • Stay quiet for at least an hour after meals • Relax, take deep breaths, and swallow when feeling nauseous Administer prescribed antiemetics as necessary; if the client is taking oral supplements, offer cold feedings with varied flavors; when tube feedings are given, proper technique should be followed, and mouth care should be provided, since the mouth may become extremely dry	

*Under Plan/Nursing Implementation column, content on constipation and diarrhea from Suitor & Hunter, *Nutrition: Principles and Application in Health Promotion.* Philadelphia: Lippincott, 1980, p. 267.

Table 47–4 Oral Stimulant Laxatives

Generic Name	Trade Name	Therapeutic Effect (Hours)	Stool Consistency	Remarks
Bisacodyl	Dulcolax	6	Soft	Not to be taken within 1 hour after ingestion of milk or antacids to prevent premature dissolving of enteric coating and gastrointestinal irritation
Castor oil	Neoloid emulsion, Castor oil	2–6	Watery	Chilling, mixing with fruit juice or carbonated drinks increases palatability
Cascara sagrada	Cascara sagrada	6–8	Soft, formed	Gives a yellowish brown color to acid urine; reddish color to alkaline urine
Danthron	Dorbane, Modane	6–8	Soft, semifluid	Gives a pink color to alkaline urine; do not give to nursing mother; drug is excreted in milk
Phenolphthalein	Ex-Lax Feen-A-Mint Phenolax	4–8	Semifluid	Gives pink color to alkaline urine or feces; action may persist for 3 to 4 days; may cause skin eruptions as dermatitis
Senna	X-prep, Senokot	6–12	Soft	Crude senna may cause urine discoloration like cascara

SOURCE: Hahn AB, Barkin RL, Oestreich SJK: *Pharmacology in Nursing,* 15th ed. St. Louis: Mosby, 1982, p. 514.
Table by permission of the author of the chapter, "Drugs Acting on the Gastrointestinal Tract," Robert L. Barkin.

Table 47–5   Traditional Laxatives

	No Prescription Required					Prescription Required
	Irritant/ Stimulant Type	Osmotic/ Saline Type	Stool Softener/ Surfactant or Wetting Agent Type	High-Fiber and Bulk-Forming Type	Lubricant/ Emollient Type	Lactulase Syrup
Disadvantages with repeated frequent (long-term) administration	Watery stools, griping	Watery stools, cramps	Unreliable results, may contribute to liver toxicity	Obstruction of narrowed lumen, some difficulty in chewing and swallowing	Anal leakage, lipid pneumonia	Early, transient flatulence and cramps; nausea has been reported
Increases rate of transit in small bowel	Yes	Yes	Yes	Yes	Unknown	Possibly
Causes net secretion of water and electrolytes in small bowel	Yes	Yes	Yes	Yes	No	No
Inhibits absorption in small bowel	Yes	Yes	Yes	Yes	Yes	Not reported
Increases mucosal permeability in small bowel	Yes	Not studied	Yes	Not reported	Not reported	No
Causes mucosal damage in small bowel	Yes	Not studied	Yes	Not reported	Not reported	No
Acts only in colon (not small bowel)	No	No	No	No	Yes	Yes
Indicated for long-term treatment	No	No	No	Probably	No	Yes
Examples of type	Anthraquinone and isatin derivatives, phenolphthalein, castor oil	Magnesium salts, MOM, sodium phosphate, magnesium citrate	DSS, DCS	Methylcellulose, sodium CMC, psyllium seed, agar, plantago	Mineral oil	Chronulac
Physical or chemical property responsible for action	Mucosal surface irritation to stimulate or increase intestinal motor function or activity	Hyperosmolar ingredients trap water in intestinal lumen; hypertonicity of colon increases liquid in colon	Changes surface tension of fecal mass, provides increased penetration of colonic water; penetrates and softens fecal mass by wetting agents	Absorbs water on surface, increases soft fecal mass, adds bulk and moisture to feces causing distention and elimination	Coats over fecal mass, passes with ease, lubricates gastrointestinal tract and softens feces	Colon-specific increase in stool water content and stool softening by increase in osmotic pressure and colon acidification

SOURCE: Hahn AB, Barkin RL, Oestreich SJK: *Pharmacology in Nursing,* 15th ed. St. Louis: Mosby, 1982, p. 510. Table by permission of the author of the chapter, "Drugs Acting on the Gastrointestinal Tract," Robert L. Barkin.

Table 47–6 Drugs Used in Diarrhea Treatment

Official or Nonproprietary Name	Trade Name or Synonym	Dosage	Comments
Locally Acting Antidiarrheal Drugs			
Aluminum hydroxide gel USP	Amphojel	30 mL	Adsorbent
Activated attapulgite	Claysorb	2–5 g	Adsorbent
Activated charcoal USP	—	10 g	Adsorbent
Bismuth subcarbonate	—	500 mg–4 g	Adsorbent
Bismuth subgallate	—	500 mg–2 g	Adsorbent-protective
Bismuth subnitrate USP	—	300 mg–2 g	Adsorbent
Bismuth subsalicylate	—	600 mg–2 g	Adsorbent-protective
Calcium carbonate, precipitated USP	Precipitated chalk	1–2 g	Adsorbent
Carboxymethylcellulose sodium USP	—	1–6 g	Hydrophilic-adsorbent
Kaolin USP	—	2–5 g	Adsorbent
Kaolin mixture with pectin	Kaopectate	30 mL	Adsorbent-hydrophilic
Pectin USP	—	50–300 mg	Hydrophilic-adsorbent
Psyllium hydrophilic mucilloid	Metamucil	4–10 g	Hydrophilic-absorbent
Polycarbophil	—	1–1.5 g	Hydrophilic-absorbent
Zinc phenolsulfonate	—	10–60 mg	Astringent
Systemically Active Drugs			
Antiperistaltic opiates			
Opium, powdered USP	—	20–60 mg	—
Opium, tincture USP	Laudanum	0.6–1.5 mL	—
Paregoric USP	Camphorated tincture of opium	5–10 mL	—
Antiperistaltic opioid derivatives			
Diphenoxylate HCl USP	In Lomotil	5 mg	—
Loperamide	Imodium	2 mg	—
Belladonna alkaloids and synthetic antispasmodics			

SOURCE: Rodman MJ, Smith DW: *Clinical Pharmacology in Nursing.* Philadelphia: Lippincott, 1984, p. 858.

If pain is related to excessive secretion of gastric acid, antacids or acid antagonists may be ordered. Antacids are listed in Table 47–7. Cimetidine (Tagamet), an acid antagonist in common use, inhibits gastric secretion and can be administered orally, IM, or IV. The average dose is 300 mg four times a day (Hahn, Barkin & Oestreich, 1982).

MAINTAINING AND IMPROVING SKIN INTEGRITY

Clients who have diarrhea, ostomies, draining wounds or fistulas, or various kinds of tubes inserted are susceptible to skin breakdown and should be carefully monitored for

Table 47–7   Common Antacid Preparations

Preparation*	Dosage
Aluminum carbonate gel, basic (Basaljel)	As antacid: two capsules or tablets, or 10 mL regular suspension (diluted in juice or water), or 5 mL of extra-strength suspension as needed every 2 hours; not more than 12 doses daily To prevent phosphate stones (urinary phosphate stones are reduced by binding; the phosphate is decreased in the urine): two to six capsules or tablets, 10 to 30 mL suspension, or 5 to 15 mL extra-strength suspension taken 1 hour after meals and at bedtime; both suspensions diluted in juice or water
Aluminum hydroxide gel (ALternaGEL, Alu-Cap, Alu-Tab, Amphojel, Dialume)	600 mg three or four times daily between meals and at bedtime
Aluminum phosphate gel (Phosphaljel)	15 to 30 mL undiluted every 2 hours between meals and at bedtime
Calcium carbonate (Alka-2, Amitone, Chooz, Dicarbosil, Tums, others); chewable tablets range from 330- to 650-mg strengths	0.5 to 2 g as needed
Dihydroxyaluminum aminoacetate (Robalate)	Two to four tablets chewed well with water four times daily between meals and at bedtime
Dihydroxyaluminum sodium carbonate (DASC) (Rolaids)	One or two tablets chewed as needed; repeat hourly if symptoms return
Magaldrate (Riopan); available in tablets (chewable and swallow) and suspension (a distinct chemical entity, hydroxymagnesium aluminate, equivalent to approximately an average of 33% magnesium oxide and 21% aluminum oxide)	400 to 800 mg between meals and at bedtime
Magnesium carbonate powder	0.5 to 2 g between meals with a half glass of water
Magnesium hydroxide (milk of magnesia—MOM, various manufacturers); available in tablets and liquid	As antacid: adults, 5 to 15 mL four times daily; children, 2.5 to 5 mL with water As laxative: adults, 30 to 60 mL with water once daily; children, 7.5 to 30 mL
Magnesium oxide (various); available in tablets, capsules, and powder	250 to 1500 mg administered with water or milk four times daily
Magnesium trisilicate (various); available in tablets and powder	1 to 4 g four times daily with water
Sodium bicarbonate (Soda mint, Bell-ans, various); available as tablets and powders ranging from 325 to 650 mg	0.3 to 2 g one to four times daily

*Other ingredients found as single entities and in combination are: bismuth aluminate, bismuth subcarbonate, defatted skim milk, glycine, ipecac, mineral oil, simethicone bismuth subnitrate, sorbitol, and others. Effervescent tablets and powders contain acetaminophen, citric acid, flavoring, potassium bicarbonate, sodium bicarbonate, sodium citrate, and tartaric acid. Simethicone is a gastric defoaming additive breaking or coalescing gas bubbles. Several antacid combinations have added this agent for acute gas-related symptoms.
SOURCE: Hahn AB, Barkin RL, Oestreich SJK: *Pharmacology in Nursing,* 15th ed. St. Louis: Mosby, 1982, p. 500.
Table by permission of the author of the chapter, "Drugs Acting on the Gastrointestinal Tract," Robert L. Barkin.

this problem. Meticulous skin care is essential. The skin should be kept clean and dry. If a tube has been inserted through the client's nose, apply a water soluble lubricant to the nostrils to prevent irritation and tape the tube to the nose to prevent pulling. A skin protectant such as tincture of benzoin or karaya gum may be used on areas prone to excoriation or breakdown; antacids (eg, Maalox) may be used for this purpose. If wounds or fistulas are draining copiously, collection bags may be applied to prevent continual contact between secretions and skin.

IMPROVING NUTRITIONAL STATUS

If the client has been NPO, make sure an appetizing meal is provided as soon as the client is able to eat. If diarrhea is involved, handle the problem as discussed in the section pertaining to diarrhea. Specific nursing interventions for malnutrition related to anorexia include:

- Determining the client's food preferences and making every effort to provide meals that include them
- Making mealtime a peaceful, appetizing experience
- Keeping the client comfortable and removing unappetizing secretions and odors from the environment
- Providing small, frequent feedings to stimulate appetite

If the client is experiencing nausea and vomiting, determine whether any environmental factors precipitate or worsen the symptoms and try to eliminate them. Oral hygiene may be indicated as well. Antiemetics may also be necessary (Table 47–8).

In all cases of altered nutrition, careful intake and output measurements should be kept and used as guidelines in determining nutritional needs. Weigh the client daily.

The client may require nutritional support through oral nutritional supplements, gastric or enteral tube feedings, feedings through surgically inserted tubes, or total parenteral nutrition (TPN).

Oral Supplementation

Oral supplements, usually high in protein and carbohydrate, are offered between meals. Standard prepackaged formulas can be used for most clients. Defined or specialty formulas are available for clients with malabsorption or maldigestion syndromes. The supplements should be served cold, in small amounts throughout the day. Flavors can be varied to maintain appetite.

Tube Feedings

Standard formulas for tube feeding are available. A sampling of these preparations is provided in Table 47–9. Tube feedings may be administered through a gastric tube or through a small-caliber, weighted tube passed to the duodenum or the proximal jejunum (Gramse, 1983). Tubes for feeding may also be surgically inserted into the esophagus (esophagostomy), stomach (gastrostomy), duodenum (duodenostomy), or jejunum (jejunostomy).

Tube feedings into the stomach are usually tolerated well because the stomach has a reservoir capacity, increasing tolerance to volume of feedings. The risk of aspiration is minimized when the esophageal gastric junction is bypassed with a gastrostomy tube. Esophagostomy and nasogastric tubes prevent complete closure of the esophageal–gastric junction, thereby increasing the risk of aspiration.

Many commercial formulas are available for tube feedings. In the past, formulas were compounded by pureeing baby foods or table foods in a blender. This method is impractical, time consuming, vulnerable to contamination, and does not allow for good control of nutritional intake. Table 47–10 outlines many available formulas, most requiring

Nursing Research Note

Kagawa–Busby K, Heitkemper M, Hansen B, Hanson R, Vanderburg V: Effects of diet temperature on tolerance of enteral feedings. *Nurs Res* 1980; 29:276–280.

The effect of temperature of enteral feedings on tolerance of such formulas was studied. Ensure formula was instilled via a nasogastric tube at 50 mL/h at three temperatures: cold (8 to 11° C), room temperature (23 to 26° C), and warm (36 to 39° C). The formula was marked with a blue dye to act as a stool marker to estimate transit time through the gastrointestinal tract.

The results suggest that there is no statistically significant relation between formula temperature and gastric motility as determined by amplitude and frequency of gastric contractions as well as time taken for digestion. Three of the six sample subjects experienced abdominal cramping and diarrhea 6 to 9 hours following infusion of the cold formula. However, two of the three were premenstrual and normally had diarrhea at the beginning of the menstrual cycle.

According to this study, temperature does not seem to be a factor in symptomatic tolerance of enteral formulas. Nevertheless, the nurse must assess enteral feeding tolerance for each client. Because three subjects experienced symptoms after cold feedings, the nurse must be alert to this possibility.

no preparation. The dietitian is important in formula selection for tube feedings and in prescribing the appropriate amount to meet individual needs. Most formulas contain all the necessary nutrients, but some are incomplete and must be supplemented; balanced nutritional intake is essential. Lactose intolerance, a frequent problem, is avoided by using lactose-free formulas for tube feedings.

Feedings may be given intermittently or continuously. The intermittent approach involves administration of formula 5 to 6 times daily given over 30 minutes. This is the most practical and best tolerated method of administering feedings. Giving the formula too rapidly causes cramping, bloating, nausea, vomiting, and diarrhea. Continuous feeding over 24 hours ties the client down, impairing mobility. Feeding pumps are usually used for continuous feeding to control the infusion rate.

When tube feeding is initiated, the client should be allowed 3 to 4 days to acclimate to the feedings, especially if the gastrointestinal tract has been without feedings for 7 days or more. The placement of the tubing should be checked prior to each feeding. Formulas should be started at low concentration and a slow rate, advancing slowly to full strength and full volume. The feeding should be administered with the head of the bed elevated to prevent aspiration. This method will minimize gastrointestinal complaints and facilitate good nutritional support.

Nursing care with tube feedings entails careful monitoring for complications. Clients who receive tube feedings may experience diarrhea, nausea, abdominal distention, or asphyxia. Increasing the strength and amount of the formula gradually and ensuring that the head of the bed is elevated 30° should prevent these difficulties. Antidi-

Table 47−8 Centrally Acting Antiemetic Agents

Official or Nonproprietary Name	Trade Name	Dosage*
Benzquinamide HCl	Emete-con	50 mg IM; 25 mg IV
Buclizine HCl	Bucladin-S	50 mg
Cesamet	Nabilone	2 mg
Chlorcyclizine HCl USP	Diparalene; Perazil	50 mg
Chlorpromazine HCl USP	Thorazine	10−25 mg
Cyclizine HCl USP	Marezine	50 mg
Dimenhydrinate USP	Dramamine	50 mg
Diphenhydramine USP	Benadryl	25−50 mg
Diphenidol HCl	Vontrol	25−50 mg
Doxylamine succinate	In Bendectin	20−40 mg
Droperidol	Inapsine	1.25−5 mg IV
Fluphenazine HCl USP	Permitil; Prolixin	1.25 mg IM
Haloperidol USP	Haldol	1−5 mg
Haloperidol lactate USP	Haldol lactate	1−5 mg IM
Meclizine HCl USP	Bonine; Antivert	25−50 mg
Metoclopramide HCl	Reglan	1−2 mg/kg IV
Perphenazine USP	Trilafon	4−8 mg
Prochlorperazine edisylate USP	Compazine edisylate	5−10 mg IM
Prochlorperazine maleate USP	Compazine	5−10 mg
Promazine HCl USP	Sparine	25−50 mg
Promethazine HCl USP	Phenergan, Remsed	25−50 mg
Scopolamine HBr USP	Hyoscine	0.5−1.0 mg
Thiethylperazine maleate	Torecan	10−20 mg
Triflupromazine HCl USP	Vesprin	10−20 mg
Trimethobenzamide HCl USP	Tigan	250 mg

*Oral except where indicated.
SOURCE: Rodman MJ, Smith DW: *Clinical Pharmacology in Nursing.* Philadelphia: Lippincott, 1984, p. 866.

arrheal medications may be necessary. If diarrhea persists, a different formula may be tried.

To prevent abdominal distention, check the client for residual formula in the stomach before and several hours after a feeding; withhold feeding if more than 150 mL of residual formula is found. A large residual volume implies slow gastric emptying and may require an altered approach to the feeding regimen.

Table 47−11 lists common problems associated with tube feedings as well as measures to correct them. In addition, electrolyte imbalance, alterations in glucose levels, and deficiency of fatty acids may occur; laboratory studies should be monitored for changes in these values (Hoppe, 1980).

Specific nursing techniques for insertion, use, and removal of apparatus used for tube feedings may be found in nursing fundamentals texts. Care associated with TPN is described in Chapter 8.

Clients whose nutritional status is compromised are especially prone to infection. Since they are highly susceptible to infectious disease, special precautions should be taken to avoid exposure. Be alert to symptoms of infection.

MAINTAINING NORMAL FLUID VOLUME

Assess the client for signs of dehydration. Keep careful intake/output records and encourage the client to consume all food and fluids provided. Give careful consideration to fluid preferences. Weigh the client daily.

Table 47–9   Standard Formulas for Tube Feeding

Ingredient	Measure	Weight (g)	kcal	Protein (g)	Fat (g)	Carbo-hydrate (g)	Iron (mg)	Vitamin C (mg)
Standard Hospital Tube Feeding								
Milk, whole	2 c	488	318	17	17	24	0.2	4.0
Milk, instant, nonfat, dry	1 c	70	250	24	0	35	0.4	5.0
Corn syrup	4¾ T	97.4	280	0	0	71	1.3	0
Egg, powdered, pasteurized*	4 T	30	163	13	12	1	2.3	0
Salt	1 t	5.5	—	—	—	—	—	—
Vitamin preparation	5 mL	—	—	—	—	—	—	—
Total	—	—	1011	54	29	131	4.2	9.0
Standard Blenderized Tube Feeding								
Milk, evaporated	1½ c	428	517	26.4	29.8	36.6	0.4	4.5
Farina, cooked, enriched	1 c	245	108	3.2	0.2	21.3	12.3	0
Egg, powdered, pasteurized*	6 T	45	243	18.5	18.0	1.5	3.3	0
Liver, pureed	1 jar	100	94	14.0	3.1	2.4	6.8	27.4
Orange juice, fresh	½ c	123	49	0.7	0.2	11.0	0.2	64.0
Carrots, cooked	½ c	77	22	0.6	0.2	4.8	0.5	1.5
Total	—	—	1033	63.4	51.5	77.6	23.5	97.4

Note: Nutrient compositions are adapted from USDA Home and Garden Bulletin No. 72. Enough water is added to the total ingredients to make 1000 mL of solution.

*To avoid salmonella contamination, do not use fresh raw eggs. One egg is equivalent to 15 g of powdered egg. Cooked egg custard, salmonella-free frozen eggs, or egg yolks processed for infant feeding may also be used.

SOURCE: Hui YH: *Human Nutrition and Diet Therapy.* Monterey, CA: Wadsworth, 1983, pp. 503, 504.

IMPROVING PSYCHOSOCIAL STATUS

Alterations related to specific disorders are discussed in the sections pertaining to those disorders. Such issues as body image, self-concept, and coping are discussed in Unit One.

Section IV: Evaluation

Evaluation will focus on the goals determined with and for the individual client. If goals are being met, implementation of existing plans is continued. If not, nurse and client must together reevaluate both physiological and psychosocial status to see whether problems were identified correctly. As the client recovers, new goals may be formulated in light of the client's improved status.

Chapter Highlights

A nutritional assessment is always indicated in caring for clients with gastrointestinal disorders.

Nursing assessments to determine the presence of peristalsis include assessments for abdominal distention, presence of bowel sounds, and the passage of stool or flatus.

Clients with gastrointestinal system disorders often

(continued)

Table 47–10   Commercially Available Formulas for Tube Feeding

Classification	Product Names	kcal/mL	mOsm/kg water	Advantages	Disadvantages
Blenderized	Compleat B	1	405	Nutritionally complete* High residue makes them ideal for elderly or those who have altered bowel function	High viscosity makes administration difficult through small-bore tubes Most contain lactose Not for oral consumption Relatively expensive
	Compleat Modified	1	300		
	Vitaneed	1	375		
Milk-based	Carnation Instant Breakfast	1	615–650	Palatable Good for clients who have increased protein and calorie requirements	High lactose content High osmolality
	Meritene	1	505–690		
	Sustacal Powder	1	644		
	Sustagen	1.7	1110		
Lactose-free	Ensure	1	450	Nutritionally complete* Relatively inexpensive Free-flowing consistency May be used orally	Protein quality not as high as blenderized or milk-based formulas
	Isocal	1	300		
	Osmolite HN	1	310		
	Nutri-Aid	1	300		
	Osmolite	1	300		
	Portagen	1	354		
	Renu	1	300		
	Sustacal Liquid	1	625		
	Travasorb	1	450		
High density lactose-free	Ensure Plus	1.5	600	Nutritionally complete* Relatively inexpensive Free-flowing consistency Ideal for fluid-restricted clients	Protein quality not as high as blenderized or milk-based formulas Must be diluted and advanced slowly
	Isocal HCN	2	740		
	Magnacal	2	590		
	Sustacal HC	1.5	650		
Chemically defined	Citrotein	0.66	500	Require minimal digestion Lactose-free Low viscosity so easily administered through small bore tubes	High osmolality Some are relatively unpalatable Relatively expensive Some contain minimal amounts of long-chain fats
	Criticare HN	1	650		
	Isotein HN	1.2	300		
	Precision Isotonic	1	300		
	Precision HN	1	500		
	Precision LR	1	525–545		
	Travasorb HN	1	560		
	Travasorb MCT	1 to 2	300–500		
	Travasorb Std	1	560		
	Vital HN	1	460		
Free amino acid	Vivonex HN	1	810		
	Vivonex Std	1	550		
Specialty formulas	Amin-Aid	1.9	1095	May be given by tube or mouth Require minimal digestion	High osmolality High carbohydrate Some are nutritionally incomplete Very expensive Formulas designed for trauma do not meet currently accepted standards for nutritional requirements for increased stress
	Hepatic-Aid	1.6	1158		
	Travasorb Hepatic	1.1	690		
	Travasorb Renal	1.35	590		
	Trauma-Aid	1	800		
	Trauma-Cal	1.5	550		

(continued)

Table 47–10 Commercially Available Formulas for Tube Feeding (continued)

Classification	Product Names	kcal/mL	mOsm/kg water	Advantages	Disadvantages
Modules	*Carbohydrate*			Flexible—may be combined to yield specific formula	Takes longer to prepare
	Moducal	4 kcal/g	(powder)		May alter taste and/or texture if added to food
		2 cal/mL	725	May be added to food	
	Polycose	4 kcal/g	(powder)		
		2 kcal/mL	850		
	Sumacal	4 kcal/g	(powder)		
	Fat				
	Lipomul	6 kcal/mL	Not applicable for fats		
	MCT (medium chain triglyceride)	7.7 kcal/mL			
	Microlipid	4.5 kcal/mL			
	Protein				
	Casec	4 kcal/g	24 g protein/30 mL		
	Promix	4 kcal/g	24 g protein/30 mL		
	Propac	4 kcal/g	23 g protein/30 mL		

*Nutritionally complete when given in appropriate volumes.

SOURCE: Konstantinides NN, Shrouts E: Tube feeding: Managing the basics. *Am J Nurs* 1983; 83:1316.

Chapter Highlights (continued)

experience symptoms of anorexia, nausea and vomiting, diarrhea, and constipation.

In assessing clients with gastrointestinal disorders, the functions of swallowing, secretion, motility, digestion, absorption, and elimination need to be determined.

Dietary influences include psychological, social, cultural, and economic factors.

The nurse should ensure the privacy of clients with gastrointestinal disorders, since they may experience embarrassment due to symptoms associated with their disease.

Elderly clients are especially prone to malnutrition and constipation.

Nutritional support is often indicated for clients with gastrointestinal disorders.

Nutritional support includes supplementary oral feedings, gastric and enteral feedings, feedings through surgically inserted tubes, and hyperalimentation.

The client with a gastrointestinal disorder may experience changes in self-concept, such as body image and role performance.

Fatigue is often experienced by clients subjected to the numerous and often lengthy diagnostic procedures associated with gastrointestinal disease.

The client with a gastrointestinal disorder is especially prone to fluid and electrolyte and acid–base imbalances related to the excessive fluid losses that often accompany gastrointestinal disease.

Bibliography

Arnold C: Why that liquid formula diet may not work (and what to do about it). *RN* (Nov) 1981; 35–39.

Baker JP et al: Nutritional assessment: A comparison of clinical judgment and objective measurements. *N Engl J Med* 1982; 306:969–972.

Beck ML: Preparing your patient psychologically for an esophagogastroduodenoscopy. (a). *Nurs 81* (Jan) 1981; 11:28–30.

Table 47–11   Common Problems of Tube Feedings

Factors to Assess to Determine How Client Is Tolerating the Feeding	Possible Causes of Problems	Corrective Measures
Gastrointestinal function		
Vomiting	Feeding too soon after intubation	Allow client time to relax and rest after tube is inserted
	Improper location of tip of feeding tube	Repositioning of tube by qualified health professional
	Rapid rate of infusion	Administer slowly
	Excessive volume: (1) Air (2) Formula	Be sure tube feeding container does not run dry before feeding is completed Check with physician regarding number and size of feedings
	Position of client	Position on right side for ½ hr following feeding—reverse Trendelenburg or semi-Fowler's
(Applies to both vomiting and diarrhea)	Food infection or poisoning Anxiety	Check sanitation of formula and equipment Explain procedures; provide reassurance and other needed types of support; provide privacy
Diarrhea	Rapid rate of infusion High osmolality of formula or high concentration of formula	Administer slowly—very slowly if formula is cold Adapt client to formula gradually
	Lactose intolerance	Contact physician regarding change of formula
Constipation	High content of milk in formula Lack of fiber Inadequate fluid intake	Contact physician regarding: (1) Change in formula (2) Laxatives (3) Increasing fluid
Fluid and electrolyte balance		
Dehydration	Rapid infusion of carbohydrate → hyperglycemia → osmotic diuresis → dehydration	Administer slowly; exogeneous insulin sometimes needed
	Excess protein and electrolytes in formula Inadequate fluid intake	Change formula and/or increase fluid according to physician's orders
Edema	Excessive sodium in formula	Check with physician about change in formula
Nutritional adequacy		
Undernutrition (gradual weight loss)	Inadequate number of calories to meet energy requirements	Check to see if client is receiving prescribed amount of formula; estimate client's caloric intake Check with physician regarding increasing the volume, concentration, or number of feedings given
Overnutrition (gradual gain of undesirable weight)	Excessive caloric intake	Check with physician regarding decreasing the volume, concentration, or number of feedings given
Undernutrition (inadequate intake of protein and/or micronutrients leading to biochemical or clinical signs of deficiency)	Amount of standard formula needed to maintain weight is too low to meet requirements for essential nutrients	Check with physician regarding providing appropriate nutrient supplements

SOURCE: Suitor CW, Hunter MF: *Nutrition: Principles and Applications in Health Promotion.* Philadelphia: Lippincott, 1980, p. 371.

Beck ML: Two intestinal tests: one oral, one anal. (b). *Nurs 81* (July) 1981; 11:20–22.

Bryne CJ, Saxton DF, Pelikan PK, Nugent PM: *Laboratory Tests: Implications for Nursing Care.* 2nd ed. Menlo Park, CA: Addison-Wesley, 1986.

Crowley LV: *Introduction to Human Disease.* Monterey, CA: Wadsworth, 1983.

Given BA, Simmons SJ: *Gastroenterology in Clinical Nursing,* 4th ed. St. Louis: Mosby, 1984.

Gramse CA: A review of tube feeding techniques. *Nurs 83* (Feb) 1983; 13:32B–32P.

Grimes J, Iannopollo E: *Health Assessment in Nursing Practice.* Belmont, CA: Wadsworth, 1982.

Hahn AB, Barkin RL, Oestreich SJK: *Pharmacology in Nursing.* St. Louis: Mosby, 1982.

Hoppe M: The new tube feeding sets, or your patients are what you feed them. *Nurs 80* (March) 1980; 10:79–85.

Hui YH: *Human Nutrition and Diet Therapy.* Monterey, CA: Wadsworth, 1983.

Kee JL: *Laboratory and Diagnostic Tests with Nursing Implications.* Norwalk, CT: Appleton-Century-Crofts, 1983.

Kohrs MB: New perspectives on nutritional counseling for the elderly. *Contemporary Nutrition* (March) 1983; 8(3).

Konstantinides NN, Shrouts E: Tube feeding: Managing the basics. *Am J Nurs* 1983; 83:1312–1320.

Meshkinpour H et al: Esophageal manometry: A benefit and cost analysis. *Dig Dis Sci* 1982; 27:772–775.

Moghissi K, Boore JRP: *Parenteral and Enteral Nutrition for Nurses.* Rockville, MD: Aspen Systems, 1983.

Rodman MJ, Smith DW: *Clinical Pharmacology in Nursing.* 2nd ed. Philadelphia: Lippincott, 1984.

Stiklorius C: Beginning this month: GI studies. *RN* (March) 1982; 64–65.

Stiklorius C: Preparing for two uncomfortable tests: Gastric analysis and liver biopsy. *RN* (Sept) 1982; 64.

Suitor CW, Hunter MF: *Nutrition: Principles and Application in Health Promotion.* Philadelphia: Lippincott, 1980.

Tichy AM, Chong D: When assessing the aged don't be fooled by these false alarms. *RN* (Sept) 1981; 58–62.

Veninga KS: An easy recipe for assessing your patient's nutrition. *Nurs 82* (Nov) 1982; 12:57–59.

Suggested Readings

Bayer LM, Scholl DE, Ford EG: Tube feeding at home. *Am J Nurs* 1983; 83:1321–1325. This article discusses preparation and administration of tube feedings in the home.

Konstantinides NN, Shronts E: Tube feeding: Managing the basics. *Am J Nurs* 1983; 83:1312–1320. This article provides extensive current data on nutritional assessment and administration of tube feedings.

Salmond SW: How to assess the nutritional status of acutely ill patients. *Am J Nurs* 1980; 80:922–924. This article discusses protein calorie malnutrition and how to recognize the nutritionally deficient client.

Taylor Sr K: Meeting the challenge of fistulas and draining wounds. *Nurs 80* 1980; 10:45–51. Nursing interventions to control the odor, drainage, and skin breakdown associated with draining abdominal wounds and fistulas are discussed. A framework of individualized, comprehensive, total client care is presented.

Resources

SELF-HELP GROUPS AND OTHER ORGANIZATIONS

American Celiac Society
45 Gifford Ave
Jersey City, NJ 07304
Phone: (201) 432-1207

> The members of this organization are individuals with gluten-sensitive enteropathy and health care professionals (including dieticians and nutritionists) who coordinate and distribute information on celiac sprue, support research into the disorder, and help members locate sources of gluten-free specialty foods. The organization also conducts educational conferences for clients and health care professionals. They publish the American Celiac Society Newsletter.

American Digestive Disease Society
420 Lexington Ave.
New York, NY 10017
Phone: (212) 687-3088

> This voluntary health organization distributes information on digestive disorders and makes referrals to specialists in digestive disorders to special clinics for the management of pain and emotional stress associated with digestive diseases and delivers special programs on nutrition education.

National Foundation for Ileitis and Colitis, Inc.
295 Madison Ave.
New York, NY 10017
Phone: (212) 685-3440

> This nonprofit foundation provides information on inflammatory bowel diseases to the public and to professionals and funds-related research. Clients and family members can also obtain referrals to government-sponsored services for persons with ileitis and colitis.

United Ostomy Association, Inc.
2001 W. Beverly Blvd.
Los Angeles, CA 90057
Phone: (213) 413-5510

> Most members in this organization are ostomates. It provides client mutual-support groups as well as educational programs in ostomy care and management, and assistance in developing and locating ostomy equipment and supplies. It publishes the *Ostomy Quarterly.*

In Canada:

Canadian Foundation for Ileitis and Colitis
212 King St, West, Suite 102
Toronto, Ontario
Canada M5H 1K5
Phone: (416) 593-2740

This foundation for clients with inflammatory bowel disease has 25 chapters in most Canadian provinces and publishes a quarterly, *The Journal*. Specific addresses can be obtained from the headquarters listed here.

HOT LINES

Gutline (American Digestive Disease Society)
Phone: (301) 652-9293, Tues & Thurs, 7:30–9:00 PM, Eastern Time

HEALTH EDUCATION MATERIAL

From:

Patient Information Library
Krames Communications
312 90th St.
Daly City, CA 94015-2621
Phone: (415) 994-8800
Pamphlets
Abdominal Sonogram, 1984. $.35
Appendectomy, 1984. $.35
Barium Enema, 1984. $.35
Oral Cholecystogram, 1981. $.35
Upper GI Series, 1984. $.35
Lower GI Endoscopy, 1983. $.35
Upper GI Endoscopy, 1983. $.35

Booklets
Irritable Bowel Syndrome, 1984. $.70
A Guide to Understanding Colon Surgery, 1984. $.85
The Hemorrhoid Book, 1984. $.85
The Hernia Book, 1984. $.90

From:

Stuart Pharmaceuticals
Division of ICI Americas, Inc.
Wilmington, DE 19897
The following pamphlets for clients with peptic ulcer disease are available free:
Hyperacidity
Did You Say Ulcer?
Straight Talk About Your Ulcer

From:

National Foundation for Ileitis and Colitis, Inc.
295 Madison Ave.
New York, NY 10017
The following pamphlets (appropriate for professionals and clients) on Crohn's disease and ulcerative colitis are available:
Questions and Answers About Diet and Nutrition in Ileitis and Colitis
Questions and Answers About the Complications of Ileitis and Colitis
Questions and Answers About Emotional Factors in Ileitis and Colitis
Questions and Answers About Ileitis and Colitis

From:

American Cancer Society, Inc.
National Headquarters
777 Third Ave.
New York, NY 10017

The following educational materials, available free, provide information on the epidemiology, diagnosis, and treatment of the topic discussed.
Beazley RM, Cohn I: *Pancreatic Cancer*. Professional Education Publication 82-50M-No. 3386-PE, 1982.
Facts on Stomach and Esophageal Cancer. Professional Education Publication, 1978.
Colorectal Cancer—Go For Early Detection. 83-1MM-No. 2051-LE, 1983.

From:

U.S. Department of Health and Human Services
Public Health Service
National Institutes of Health
Bethesda, MD 20014
Cancer of the Colon and Rectum. NIH Pub. No. 83-1552, January 1983.
NCI Research Report: Cancer of the Colon and Rectum. NIH Pub. No. 82-95, September 1982.
Cancer of the Pancreas. NIH Pub. No. 82-1560, May 1982.
Cancer of the Stomach. NIH Pub. No. 83-1554, August 1983.

From:

Hoescht–Roussel Pharmaceuticals, Inc.
Rte. 202-206 North
Somerville, NJ 08876 (Advertising)
What You Should Know About Hemorrhoids and Fissures, 1982. This short pamphlet is intended as an information brochure for clients.

All the following are available free from:
Blistex, Inc.
1800 Swift Dr.
Oak Brook, IL 60521
Attn: Richard K. Green
Executive Vice-President
Canker and Mouth Sores, What You Should Know. A fact sheet discussing the etiology and treatment of mouth sores.
Your Lips' Health and Beauty: A Guide From the Lip Care Experts at Blistex. A fact sheet specific to lip disorders and their care.
Mini-Teaching Guide on Lip Care. Discusses special problems associated with the lips and special care required.

From:

General Mills
Attn: Gloria T. Florey
PO Box 1112, Dept 65
Minneapolis, MN 55440
A monthly newsletter, *Contemporary Nutrition*, is available to food and health professionals.

PROFESSIONAL ORGANIZATIONS

International Association for Enterostomal Therapy, Inc.
505 N. Tustin Ave, Suite 282
Santa Ana, CA 92705
Phone: (714) 972-1720

The membership in this organization is limited to enterostomal therapists and other interested individuals who hold licenses in medicine or nursing. Its goal is to provide care and rehabilitation to persons with abdominal stomas, fistulas, draining wounds, pressure sores, and incontinence. Dues: $65.

Society of Gastrointestinal Assistants
211 E. 43rd St

New York, NY 10017
Phone: (212) 867-4663

This association of RNs, LPNs, LVNs, and physicians develops educational programs in digestive diseases, promotes optimal client digestive diseases. Dues: $40.

Chapter 48

Specific Disorders of the Mouth and Esophagus

Patricia Brown

Objectives

When you have finished studying this chapter, you should be able to:

Identify risk factors associated with disorders of the mouth and esophagus.

Initiate client assessments specific to disorders of the mouth and esophagus.

Discuss the role of the nurse in prevention of disorders of the mouth and esophagus.

Describe therapeutic measures, including any medical and surgical treatments, associated with disorders of the mouth and esophagus.

Specify appropriate nursing care for clients with disorders of the mouth and esophagus.

Anticipate psychosocial/lifestyle implications for clients with disorders of the mouth and esophagus.

List oral hygiene measures appropriate for clients with disorders of the mouth.

Plan the dietary modifications most often indicated for clients with disorders of the mouth and esophagus.

The primary significance of disorders of the mouth and esophagus is that they can significantly alter nutritional status by interfering with ingestion, digestion, and/or absorption. Moreover, many of these disorders are associated with considerable symptomatic discomfort and temporary or permanent alteration in body image. Complications related to these disorders, such as aspiration or infection, can compromise other body systems and affect the overall health status of the individual.

Section I: Disorders of Multifactorial Origin

Disorders of multifactorial origin that affect the mouth and esophagus develop during the natural life span of the individual. Some are related to environmental factors, some to lifestyle. Some are preventable, some are not. Teaching preventive measures to clients and the general public is a major nursing responsibility. Once disorders have occurred, dietary instruction and nutritional support may be indicated.

Since these disorders are frequently associated with dysphagia, the client may have to make dietary adjustments to alleviate or compensate for this difficulty. For example, liquid or soft foods may be easier to swallow; small, frequent feedings may be easier to ingest. Oral hygiene measures may prevent the onset or spread of infection and promote the client's personal comfort.

The nurse's support and encouragement will help clients make dietary changes that involve a change from their usual lifestyle, for example, avoiding refined carbohydrates. Referring the client to a dietitian for counseling may be advisable. Some clients with oral and/or esophageal disorders may be undernourished so that providing a well-balanced diet with nutritional supplementation and nutritional support as needed will be an important nursing responsibility.

DENTAL CARIES

Dental caries, or tooth decay, is the principal cause of tooth loss up to the fourth decade of life (Petersdorf, 1983). Dental caries involves demineralization (decalcification) of tooth enamel and dentin, the main tissue of the tooth (Figure 48–1). Caries can cause pain. The disorder may also interfere with eating, promote halitosis, cause cosmetic changes that embarrass the individual, and lead to loss of teeth. Treatment of dental caries consumes large amounts of money and time.

Caries formation is believed to result from interaction of certain foods (notably refined sugars) and oral bacteria (notably *Streptococcus mutans*) (Schachtele, 1980). Intake of carbohydrates leads to formation of *dental plaque,* a soft, spongy, tenacious material composed of bacteria, protein, and carbohydrate. Bacterial action on ingested carbohydrates produces acids that are destructive to the teeth. Frequent ingestion of carbohydrates, therefore, is of particular significance in the development of dental caries, and numerous studies have linked increased consumption of sugar and sugar-sweetened foods to an increased prevalence of caries.

Clinical Manifestations

The client with caries may not perceive pain until considerable damage has been done to the teeth. Darkening and erosion of the dental surface may be noted on inspection. Accurate assessment of damage to the teeth usually requires x-rays. Once a carious lesion has become extensive, pulpitis (inflammation of the dental pulp) may occur. At this point, the client may notice pain when ingesting cold foods and fluids. Abscesses and more extensive infections may then occur; these are discussed later in this chapter.

Therapeutic Measures

Dental caries is preventable. Meticulous oral hygiene, including brushing and flossing, is recommended. Stannuous fluoride, which interferes with bacterial activity on teeth, may be used, either by means of fluoridated water supplies or individual application. Since some religious groups and other groups concerned with chemical additives in water have raised questions about the advisability of fluoridating community water supplies, recent emphasis has been on individual application. Fluoride may be applied topically in sprays, gels, and/or toothpaste, or may be taken in capsules or tablets.

Dietary modification has also been recommended. It is generally believed that the incidence of caries may be reduced by:

- Decreasing the frequency of carbohydrate consumption, particularly refined carbohydrates such as those in candy; soft drinks; ice cream; and most cakes, pies, and other baked goods
- Reducing the time sugars remain in contact with the teeth (eg, by prompt brushing or at least rinsing the mouth after eating)

Approaches still being evaluated include combating causative bacteria by topical application of iodine or by introducing nonvirulent bacteria that might inhibit the activity of cariogenic species. Immunization has also been suggested.

Specific Nursing Measures

Prevention is the key factor in management of dental caries. A nurse has many opportunities to teach and encourage preventive measures during interactions with clients,

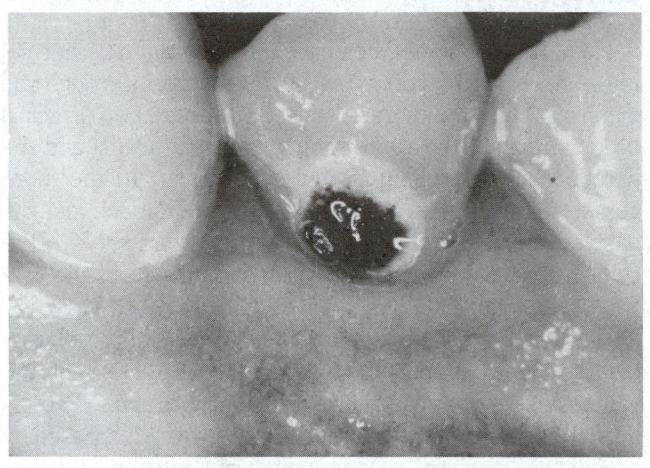

A

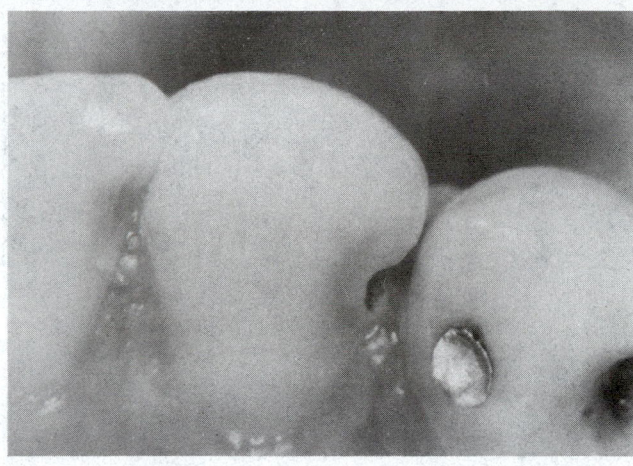

B

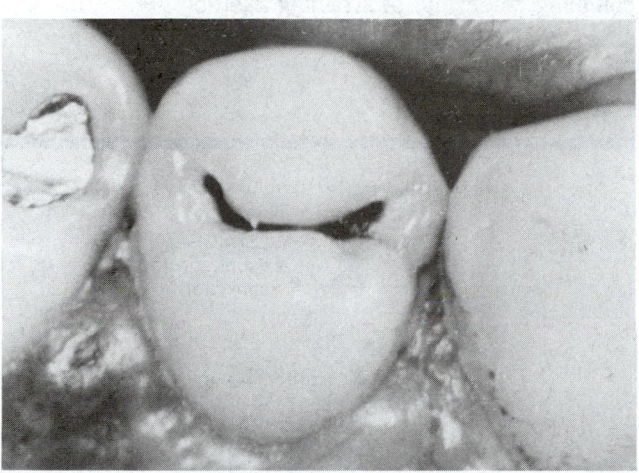

C

Figure 48-1

A. Gumline caries, premolar. **B.** Interproximal caries, lateral incisor and cuspid. **C.** Occlusal caries (chewing surface), premolar. (Courtesy of Gerald Wieczkowski, Jr., DDS, School of Dentistry, State University of New York at Buffalo)

especially during routine physical examinations. Because the etiology of dental caries has been identified rather recently, many adults may not be aware of the role of bacterial action. Has the client been shown how to brush properly? To floss? To use a soft brush? Does the client know what plaque is? A demonstration, using dye, may be revealing, especially to someone whose oral hygiene practices are relatively good.

Changing one's diet is not easy, especially given the American predilection for sugary snacks. Some clients may find it difficult to brush or floss after meals, especially while at work or traveling. Recent studies show that good control can be achieved by thorough brushing and flossing once a day combined with rinsing after meals. Does the client know how to use a Water Pik™ to best advantage? Does the client see a dentist twice a year? All these areas offer opportunities for health teaching.

For clients who are unable to perform their own oral hygiene measures, the nurse will have to do so. It is important to continue brushing and flossing, even if the client is comatose.

MALOCCLUSION

Malocclusion refers to imperfect alignment of teeth that affects how they meet during chewing (the "bite"). Various types have been identified (eg, overbite, underbite, crossbite), and most are discovered and corrected in childhood.

Malocclusion related to abnormal development of the teeth and jaws usually becomes evident in childhood when the permanent teeth erupt. Sometimes malocclusion occurs in adults after oral trauma or with extraction or loss of carious teeth. With improved techniques of correction, more adults are undergoing therapy.

Clinical Manifestations

Malocclusion can cause difficulty in chewing, temporomandibular joint (TMJ) pain, and bone loss. Malocclusion often coexists with TMJ disorders, although the relationship remains unclear. Severe malocclusion may also affect facial appearance as well as the appearance of the teeth (Figure 48–2).

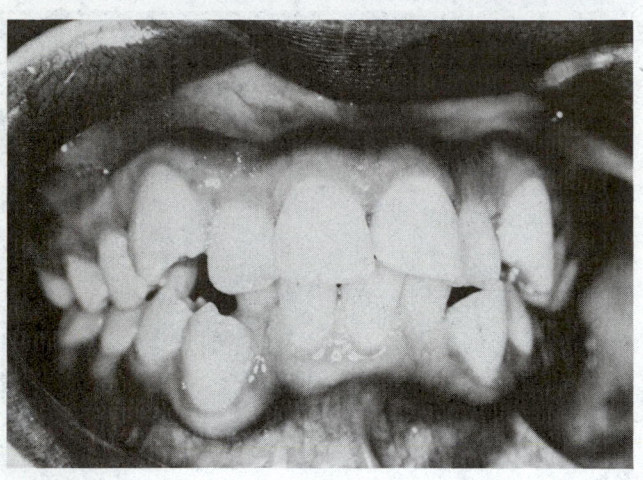

Figure 48–2

Malocclusion. (Courtesy of Sebastian G. Ciancio, DDS, School of Dentistry, State University of New York at Buffalo)

Therapeutic Measures

Teeth may be brought into alignment by bands and/or wires that exert pressure (braces). The process is long because it relies on changes in the underlying bone that occur over time in response to pressure. Sometimes teeth must be extracted to make room for the remaining teeth. Sometimes oral (maxillofacial) surgery is employed; for example, wedges of bone may be removed or inserted to correct the shape of the dental arch. Because correction of malocclusion is a long, usually expensive process, a great deal of commitment is required from the client. Oral hygiene is both crucial and time consuming while the client is wearing braces.

Specific Nursing Measures

Ask the client about pain or difficulty in chewing. Improper chewing can affect digestion; pain may cause the client to avoid eating, promoting malnutrition. Nutritional assessment may be required, and nutritional support may have to be provided.

The client with braces may require instruction regarding their care and reinforcement of the importance of meticulous mouth care. These appliances readily harbor microorganisms. Removable appliances (such as retainers) should be washed daily with soap and water and kept clean. Since braces are so conspicuous and generally associated with adolescence, the adult client may be embarrassed about wearing them and concerned about body image. The late adolescent client may experience intense embarrassment at a time when issues of body image assume great importance.

HIATAL HERNIA

A hiatal hernia (sometimes called a diaphragmatic hernia) is the herniation (protrusion) of the stomach through the diaphragm into the thoracic cavity. There are two principal types of hiatal hernia, the sliding or direct hernia and the paraesophageal (rolling or indirect) hernia. In the more common sliding type, the fundus of the stomach and the gastroesophageal junction ride into the thorax. With the rolling type, a part of the stomach separate from the gastroesophageal junction is involved (Figure 48–3A, B).

A hiatal hernia may be related to weakening of gastroesophageal supports, longitudinal contraction of the esophagus, or increased intra-abdominal pressure (Petersdorf, 1983). Intra-abdominal pressure may be increased by pregnancy, obesity, ascites, physical exertion, trauma, coughing, sneezing, or straining at stool.

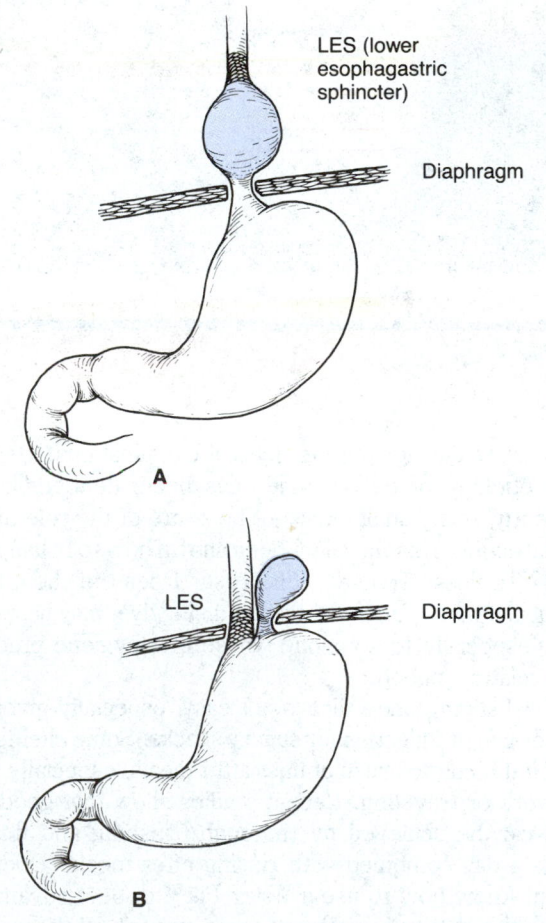

Figure 48–3

Hiatal hernias. **A.** Sliding (direct); **B.** Paraesophageal (indirect or rolling).

Hiatal hernia is more common in women, and in both sexes incidence increases with age. Petersdorf (1983) reports that prevalence in persons ages 50 to 59 is approximately 60%.

Clinical Manifestations

Hiatal hernias may be asymptomatic. In cases of sliding hiatal hernia, reflux of gastric contents into the esophagus may be related to incompetence of the lower esophageal sphincter. Reflux produces burning substernal discomfort ("heartburn") and acid regurgitation. Eructation and flatulence may also occur as the client swallows air to reverse the reflux. Reflux and regurgitation may be associated with aspiration, promoting inflammation and/or infection of the respiratory tract.

Continual reflux of gastric contents may cause esophagitis and damage to esophageal tissue. Resulting fibrosis and scarring may cause strictures and decreased esophageal motility, so the client finds it difficult to swallow. Any conditions that increase intra-abdominal pressure may aggravate symptoms, as may the recumbent position.

Rolling hernias may incarcerate (become trapped) as the protruding stomach is caught above the diaphragm. Resultant impairment of circulation may cause ulceration of tissue; total ischemia may cause tissue necrosis.

A feeling of fullness after eating is a common symptom of either type of hiatal hernia. Diagnosis is made on the basis of symptoms and diagnostic testing, including radiography, fluoroscopy, endoscopy, and tests of esophageal motility and pH.

Therapeutic Measures

Antacids are prescribed to reduce acidity and alleviate discomfort. Spicy foods and irritants such as caffeine are eliminated from the diet. The client is advised to eat slowly and to eat smaller, more frequent meals. Smoking, which stimulates gastric secretion, should be discouraged. Avoiding the recumbent position for at least 30 minutes after meals may be helpful, and preventive measures for conditions that increase intra-abdominal pressure (eg, straining at stool, obesity) are instituted (eg, increased fiber to prevent constipation, weight loss program). Drinking water after meals may help, as may sleeping on the right side (Given & Simmons, 1984). If these measures fail to control esophagitis and other serious symptoms, surgical repair may be indicated.

Specific Nursing Measures

Relief of symptoms is a high priority. Explain to the client and family the importance of eating small, frequent, non-irritating meals; remaining upright after meals; and avoiding increased intra-abdominal pressure. Try to help the client determine what seems to precipitate symptoms. Heavy meals? Spicy foods such as chili, pizza, ethnic specialties? Acid foods, such as peppers, tomatoes, citrus fruits? Caffeine, which is found in coffee, tea, cola drinks, and chocolate? Are symptoms worse at night when the client is lying down? Is the client swallowing air while eating, while talking or because some life situation is making the client nervous or apprehensive? Once these factors have been identified, nurse and client can work out a plan for avoiding them.

Administer antacids as ordered, and explain how they should be used. (See Table 47–7 Common Antacid Preparations.) Assess for respiratory complications and for esophagitis, which is discussed later in this chapter.

ESOPHAGEAL ACHALASIA

Esophageal achalasia (also called *esophageal cardiospasm* or *esophageal aperistalsis*) is a disorder of motility. The esophageal sphincter does not relax properly, and esophageal peristalsis is abnormal.

This neuromuscular disorder, which is related to defective innervation of the esophagus, occurs in all age groups and both sexes. It may occur as a primary disorder or may be secondary to other disorders, especially esophageal neoplasia (Sandler, Borzymski, & Orlando, 1982). Primary achalasia is more prevalent.

Clinical Manifestations

Common symptoms of esophageal achalasia include dysphagia, chest pain, and regurgitation with eating and/or drinking. Halitosis may occur because of a food bolus that will not pass. Aspiration and subsequent respiratory complications may accompany regurgitation. Symptoms may be potentiated by emotional disturbances, upper respiratory tract infections, excessive consumption of spicy and/or cold foods or fluids, hurried eating, or pregnancy (Given & Simmons, 1984). Chronic dysphagia and difficulty in eating may promote malnutrition and weight loss. Achalasia is a long-term, progressive disease; symptoms increase in frequency and severity if the condition is not treated. Chest x-ray, fluoroscopy, and esophageal manometry (see Chapter 47) are useful in diagnosis.

Therapeutic Measures

Measures to relieve symptoms and prevent complications of esophageal achalasia include changes in diet and eating habits. Soft, pureed, or liquid foods are given as tolerated. Ingesting and chewing food slowly may be helpful, as may arching the back and flexing the chin across the sternum while swallowing (Given & Simmons, 1984). Medications have generally been found ineffective in treating achalasia.

Balloon dilation of the esophagus, shown in Figure 48–4, has proven successful in providing at least temporary relief in 85% of clients (Petersdorf, 1983). This pro-

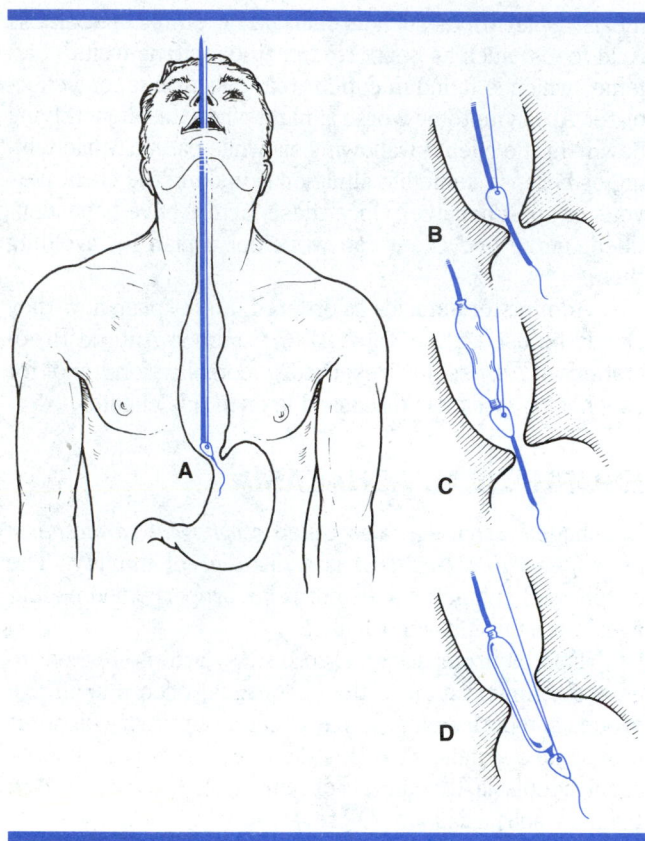

Figure 48–4

Balloon dilation of the esophagus.

cedure, which is done under fluoroscopic monitoring, may be uncomfortable for the client. Hemorrhage and perforation are potential complications. Signs of perforation are elevated pulse rate, chest pain, elevated temperature, and subcutaneous emphysema. Relief provided by balloon dilation may be temporary, and the procedure may have to be repeated periodically.

Surgical myotomy to open the esophageal sphincter may be performed if other therapies are not successful.

Specific Nursing Measures

Nursing measures used in dysphagia are discussed in Chapter 47. The client with esophageal achalasia may experience pronounced discomfort. If regurgitation occurs, a bland diet,

maintaining the sitting position after meals, and elevating the head of the bed at night may alleviate symptoms. For clients being treated at home, the nurse may explain how to use pillows to elevate the upper body. Explain dietary changes and the importance of eating slowly. Careful nutritional assessment is mandatory.

ESOPHAGEAL DIVERTICULA

A diverticulum is an outpouching of a mucosal wall through a defect in the mucosa (Figure 48–5A). Esophageal diverticuli can occur at any point in the esophageal wall, obstructing the passage of food and creating accumulations of food in the diverticular pouch. Dysphagia is common, and large esophageal diverticuli can cause total esophageal stricture.

Esophageal diverticuli may be related to inherent weakness of the esophageal wall, motility disorders such as achalasia, adhesions, or dilation of the esophageal glands which produce mucus. Diverticuli can also occur in the upper area of the stomach, just below where it joins the esophagus (Figure 48–5B).

Clinical Manifestations

In addition to dysphagia, regurgitation may be noted, especially with recumbency. Retention of food and saliva in diverticular pouches can promote halitosis due to decomposition of the food. Nutritional problems can occur, since passage of food is impeded. Barium studies are useful in diagnosis.

Therapeutic Measures

Surgery is the treatment of choice for symptomatic diverticuli (diverticulectomy). Myotomy may be performed to relieve tenseness of the esophageal musculature. Medical therapy is principally dietary; soft, pureed, or liquid foods may be prescribed. If obstruction is severe, the client may need intensive nutritional support.

Specific Nursing Measures

Nutritional assessment is especially important, since oral ingestion may be drastically reduced. Malnutritive states will require correction. Advise the client to eat small meals and to remain upright after eating. Mouth care promotes comfort and alleviates halitosis.

Section II: Inflammatory and Infectious Disorders

Inflammation of the mouth and esophagus, whether or not accompanied by infection, may be related to internal or external irritation or to invasion by foreign organisms (bacteria, viruses, or fungi).

Some of these disorders (eg, periodontitis) are common in the adult population. Others tend to recur in certain individuals, eg, stomatitis. Many may be prevented by oral hygiene. Oral or esophageal inflammation or infection may affect nutritional status by interfering with ingestion. These disorders may induce degeneration of tissue and consequent dysfunction of tissues or organs. Infection may spread to other body areas or to other individuals.

The nurse can be instrumental in teaching clients and the general public how to cope with these disorders and how to prevent their occurrence through oral hygiene and improved diet. Preventing spread of infectious disorders is a crucial nursing responsibility.

PERIODONTAL DISEASE

Periodontal disease, or *periodontitis,* is a chronic inflammatory process that affects the soft tissues and bones that surround and support the teeth. In its advanced stages, periodontal disease promotes degeneration of tissue and separation of teeth from their supports (Figure 48–6A). Gingivitis (inflammation of the gingivae), characterized by red, edematous, bleeding gums, commonly accompanies periodontal disease, which affects over 75% of the US adult population to some extent (DePaola, Alvares, & Etzel, 1982) (Figure 48–6B).

The major etiologic factor in periodontal disease is thought to be plaque. Poor oral hygiene can contribute to excessive plaque formation with subsequent development of periodontitis, and inadequate nutrition may accelerate the process or decrease an individual's resistance to it. Pregnant women, persons with Down's syndrome, and diabetics are especially susceptible to periodontal disease, whereas the use of oral contraceptives and phenytoin (Dilantin) promote development of gingivitis (Petersdorf, 1983). Increased levels of prostaglandins have been found in inflamed gingival tissue, and it is thought that prostaglandins may be at least partially responsible for the bone resorption that accompanies periodontal disease (Petersdorf, 1983).

Gingival hyperplasia, where the gingiva proliferate and may actually cover the teeth, is an untoward side effect of treatment with phenytoin (Dilantin), nifedipine (Procardia), or cyclosporine. The hyperplasia appears to be plaque related (Figure 48–7).

Clinical Manifestations

The client with periodontal disease will have symptoms of gingivitis: reddened, swollen gums that bleed easily with minimal trauma, such as from brushing the teeth. Pyorrhea (discharge of pus) may occur if the disease is advanced. Gums may recede, and teeth may loosen.

The client with gingival hyperplasia has difficulty chewing. Body image problems often occur because of the unsightly appearance of the gingival overgrowth.

Therapeutic Measures

Periodontal disease is more easily prevented than treated. Regular brushing, flossing, and dental examinations are

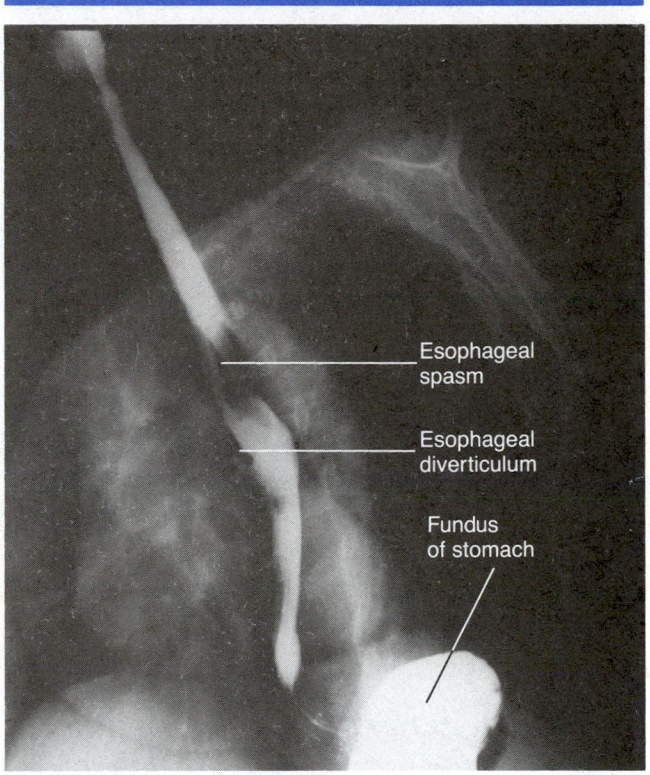

A

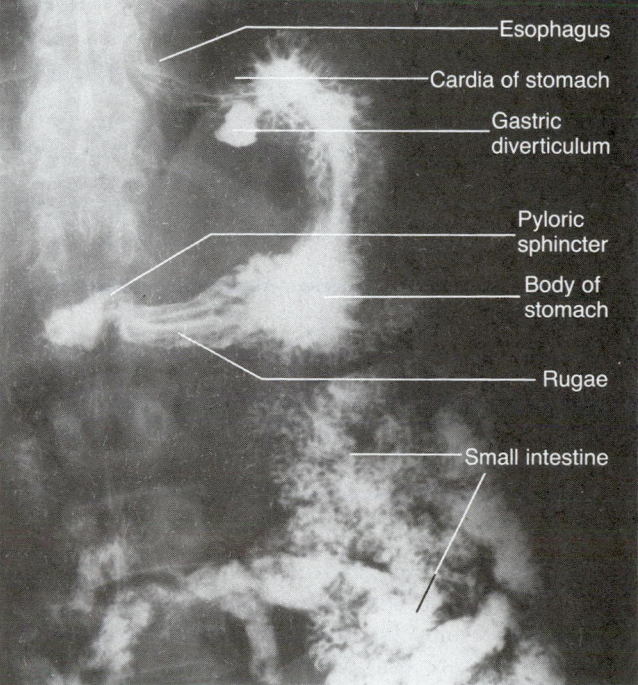

B

Figure 48–5

A. X-ray of an esophageal diverticulum visualized on a barium swallow. **B.** X-ray of a gastric diverticulum located on the lesser curvature of the stomach, just below the cardia (the upper orifice of the stomach connecting with the esophagus). (Courtesy of Health Care Plan, Buffalo, NY)

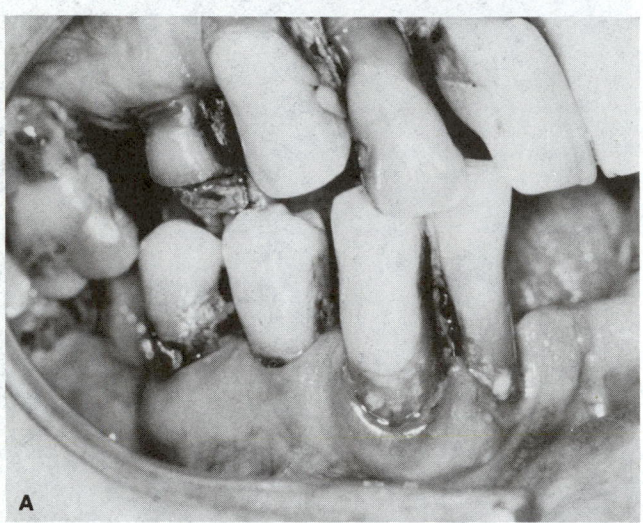

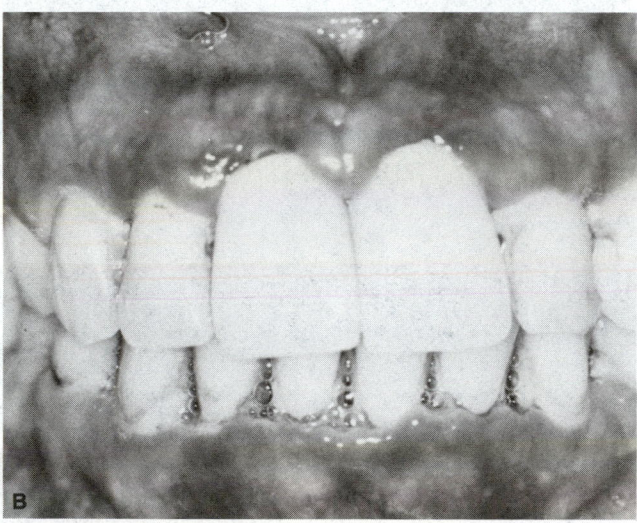

Figure 48-6

A. Severe periodontal disease. **B.** Gingivitis related to plaque formation; gums bleed easily. (Courtesy Sebastian G. Ciancio, DDS, School of Dentistry, State University of New York at Buffalo)

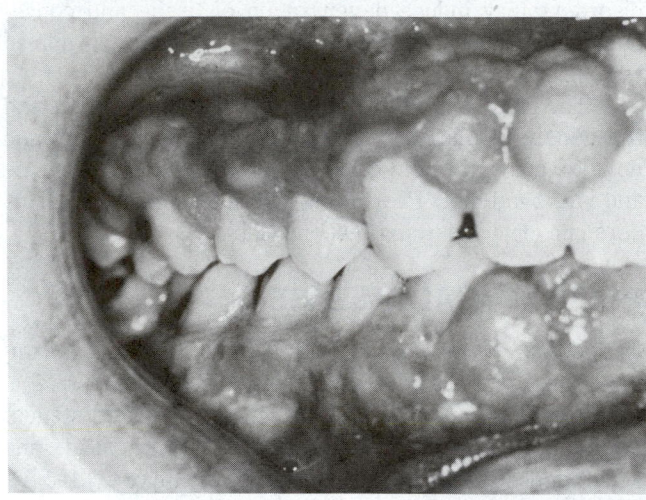

Figure 48-7

Gingival hyperplasia in a client taking phenytoin. (Courtesy of Sebastian G. Ciancio, DDS, School of Dentistry, State University of New York at Buffalo)

Specific Nursing Measures

Since prevention is so important in control of periodontal disease, nurses can help all clients by teaching oral hygiene and dietary measures. If evidence of periodontal disease is seen during a routine examination, refer the client to a dentist or periodontist. Teach clients who are treated with phenytoin, nifedipine, or cyclosporine that regular brushing and flossing can minimize the amount of gingival hyperplasia (Figure 48-8).

PULPAL INFECTION

Infection of the pulp of a tooth may culminate in formation of an abscess, the most common oral infection (Rose, Hendler, & Amsterdam, 1982). Abscesses that involve the apices of teeth (*periapicular abscess*) or the alveoli—the bony tooth sockets—(*alveolar* or *dentoalveolar abscess*) occur most often. Abscess formation is usually related to death of a tooth's nerve or degeneration of its pulp.

Nerve death or pulpal degeneration is usually related to invasion by caries with resultant pulpitis. Abscesses also occur in relation to physical or chemical trauma. The client with suppression of the bone marrow related to chemotherapy or radiotherapy is also susceptible to periodontal infection and abscess formation.

Clinical Manifestations

Sensitivity of the affected teeth is an early sign of abscess formation. Later, moderate to severe pain may predomi-

mandatory. Conventional treatment involves control of plaque through rigorous oral hygiene techniques, including scaling and planing the teeth to remove pockets where plaque and bacteria can collect. Dietary counseling may be necessary; the diet should include at least the recommended dietary allowances (RDAs) for basic nutrients, with emphasis on calcium and phosphorus balance. Infection may have to be controlled with antibiotics. If teeth are lost because of periodontal disease, the client may have to wear dentures. In severe advanced cases, however, the supporting bone may be so badly affected that denture wear becomes difficult.

nate. Oral inspection may reveal one or more decayed teeth. Edema and tenderness may be seen in the cheek or at the chin opposite the abscess. Elevated temperature and other signs of systemic infection may occur.

Therapeutic Measures

The infection must first be localized and then removed, usually by a dental specialist at an office or clinic. The diseased pulp may be removed (root canal therapy), or the tooth may be extracted and the abscess drained. Antibiotics are generally given, usually penicillin, since most oral bacteria are sensitive to it (Rose et al., 1982). Prophylactic antibiotic medication is particularly indicated for clients with a history of rheumatic heart disease or valvular disease, since subacute bacterial endocarditis is frequently associated with tooth extraction in these individuals (Petersdorf, 1983).

Preventing spread of bacteria present in the purulent abscess drainage is critical. Drainage secretion precautions must be taken; that is, gowns and gloves must be worn when in contact with infected material. Careful handwashing is important, and affected secretions and materials should be double-bagged.

Specific Nursing Measures

Relief of symptoms is a primary goal for client and nurse. If pain is severe, analgesics should be given as ordered; distraction and promotion of relaxation may be sufficient for less severe pain. Applying hot compresses to the cheek or chin proximal to the abscess relieves pain and speeds removal of toxic products from the infected area by promoting vasodilation. If teeth are painful or sensitive, the client may have difficulty eating; softer foods or a liquid diet may be required. Extremely hot or cold fluids should be avoided, since they may increase discomfort.

The client undergoing root canal therapy or tooth extraction should be encouraged to take analgesics as prescribed and to apply warm compresses. Rinsing with warm saline solution helps remove debris and can promote comfort.

Any gauze applied to the oral cavity for pressure and/or collection of blood and debris should be sterile. Gauze should remain in the mouth for the period prescribed by the dentist or endodontist. Observe for excessive blood loss. Advise the client to continue taking antibiotics for the entire period prescribed to ensure that all infection has been eradicated.

Infection control measures described under therapeutic measures should be instituted.

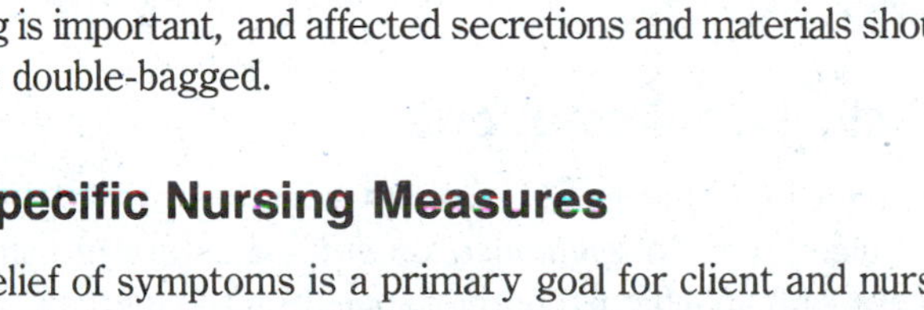

Figure 48–8

Meticulous oral hygiene can reduce dental plaque formation, minimizing gingival hyperplasia in clients taking phenytoin and other drugs.

SOURCE: Reproduced from Ciancio SG, Bourgault PC: *Clinical Pharmacology for Dental Professionals*. 2nd ed. Littleton, MA: PSG Publishing, 1984, p. 195.

Nursing Research Note

Sime AM, Libera MB: Sensation information, self-instruction, and responses to dental surgery. *Res Nurs Health* 1985; 8:41–47.

Clients undergoing gingivectomy were randomly assigned to one of four information groups—sensation, self-instruction, combined sensation and self-instruction, or a control group. They were also separated according to their level of state or trait anxiety. The time seated in the dental chair for the procedure was the period of evaluation. High state anxiety was viewed as a transitory state, whereas high trait anxiety, based on a dental anxiety scale specific to dental care, was viewed as relatively stable over time.

High state anxiety subjects showed the most favorable responses to treatment and benefited from each treatment condition. High state anxiety subjects reported less tension and distress during surgery after receiving sensation information and less tension after receiving self-instruction information. Neither low state anxiety subjects nor high trait anxiety subjects benefited from any of the treatment strategies.

This research suggests a need to explore treatment strategies most effective for individual clients in specific threatening situations.

PAROTITIS

Inflammation of the parotid glands, or parotitis, is both inflammatory and infectious. Aside from parotitis related to mumps, which occurs most frequently in children, this disorder occurs most often in the elderly and in debilitated clients (Petersdorf, 1983).

Parotitis may be related to poor oral hygiene or may be associated with dryness of the mouth **(xerostomia)** promoted by general anesthesia or medications that dry oral secretions. *Epidemic viral parotitis* (mumps) occasionally occurs in adults; more information about mumps may be found in a pediatric nursing text. Mumps occurring in an adult can cause serious problems, including sterility in men.

Sialolithiasis (formation of salivary calculi) may cause parotitis if a stone lodges in the parotid gland. Pain and edema may be associated with eating if the parotid gland is obstructed by a calculus. This condition may be diagnosed by palpation or by x-ray; surgical removal (sialolithotomy) may be required.

Therapeutic Measures

Antibiotic therapy may be combined with hydration, oral hygiene techniques, and massage of the involved gland. Increased hydration facilitates drainage of infected contents. Stimulating salivary secretion, for example, with hard candy, may also promote drainage.

Specific Nursing Measures

The nurse can play an important part in preventing parotitis by maintaining oral hygiene after anesthesia and surgery. Regular brushing and flossing should be carried out, and the lips, tongue, and mucous membranes should be kept moist by rinsing or swabbing. If the client cannot do this, the nurse will have to. A family member can also be taught the importance of maintaining good oral hygiene for the client. If parotitis is present, the client's oral secretions must be aseptically managed. Warm compresses and nursing comfort measures are helpful. Adequate rest and nutrition promote body defenses and healing. Nursing measures to alleviate xerostomia are discussed in Section III.

STOMATITIS

Stomatitis is a general term referring to inflammation of the mouth. Various oral structures may be involved, including the lips, the tongue (glossitis), the gingivae (gingivitis), the mucous membranes, and/or the palate, depending on the origin of the problem and its extent. Stomatitis may involve ulceration and degeneration of tissue.

Stomatitis may be primary or may be a symptom of another disease. Chickenpox, melanoma, infectious mononucleosis, syphilis, leukemia, lymphosarcoma, and nutritional deficiency disorders are a few of the disorders with which stomatitis may be associated. Stomatitis is also common with chemotherapy and/or irradiation of the head and neck. Stomatitis induced by chemotherapy peaks within 7 days of initiation of treatment and lasts about 2 weeks (Beck, 1979). Stomatitis induced by radiotherapy develops 1 to 2 weeks after treatment is initiated. Some symptoms of radiologically induced stomatitis may persist for long periods after treatment. For example, taste sensation may be lost for as long as 6 months, and excessive dryness of the mouth (xerostomia) may be permanent (Lane & Forgay, 1981).

Aphthous stomatitis (aphthous ulcers, canker sores) have an undetermined etiology, although a microbial origin has been suggested. Physical and/or emotional stresses are thought to induce changes in body chemistry that promote development of these lesions. Physical stresses may include spicy foods, bruising, or poorly fitting oral appli-

ances (for example, orthodontic braces). Emotional stresses may be related to virtually any life change event. Canker sores are more common in women and may appear during menses.

Infection with the herpes simplex (type I) virus may cause *acute herpetic gingivostomatitis,* commonly known as a cold sore or fever blister. This lesion is often seen after stress or at the start of menses.

Bacterial infection of the gingivae, mucous membranes, pharynx, and tonsils may cause *necrotizing ulcerative gingivitis* (trench mouth, Vincent's stomatitis). This form of stomatitis occurs frequently in debilitated clients, especially those with nutritional deficiencies.

The Candida species of fungus can cause *thrush,* also known as oral candidiasis or oral moniliasis. Debilitated clients are especially susceptible, as are those receiving steroids or antibiotics, which may alter the oral pH and the composition of oral flora.

Poor oral hygiene, immunosuppression, and bone marrow suppression can contribute to stomatitis of any etiology. Moreover, oral trauma can provide an easy portal of entry for causative organisms.

Clinical Manifestations

Stomatitis may be characterized by bleeding, painful gums, and ulceration. In *aphthous stomatitis,* clusters of painful ulcers with an inflamed border appear on the mucosa. The lesions heal within 1 to 2 weeks but can cause scarring and may recur.

In *herpes simplex infection,* the lip and oral mucosa are generally affected. Painful vesicles that contain a clear yellow fluid form, rupture, and develop a crust that may ulcerate. Gingivitis and a foul odor may be noted in the oral cavity. A systemic response including elevated temperature and lymphadenopathy may occur. Fever blisters are less common in adults than in children. Uncomplicated lesions heal within 10 to 14 days.

Trench mouth is characterized by gingivitis, foul breath, and a bad taste in the mouth. Systemic symptoms such as fever and cervical lymphadenopathy may occur in severe cases.

Thrush causes white patches in the mouth that reveal a raw, bleeding surface when rubbed. Lesions may occur anywhere in the mouth.

Diagnosis of infectious stomatitis is determined by inspection and smear or culture of lesions.

Therapeutic Measures

Regardless of which type of stomatitis the client has, symptoms must be relieved, infection must be eliminated, and its spread prevented.

In bacterial infections, antibiotic therapy may decrease the severity of ulcerations; antibiotics should be used cautiously, however, since they disrupt normal oral flora and may render the client susceptible to invasion by virulent microbes (Lane & Forgay, 1981). Although topical or systemic steroid therapy can relieve symptoms, it is generally not advisable, since steroids may promote development of candidiasis (Daeffler, 1981). Nystatin (Mycostatin) may help control candidiasis. A nystatin suspension may be used as a mouthwash or as flavored ice pops, or vaginal suppositories may be used as lozenges. A new form of treatment for oral candidiasis, clotrimazole (Mycelex) lozenges, has demonstrated a high rate of effectiveness in cancer clients.

Specific Nursing Measures

Local anesthetics, such as lidocaine 2% used as a rinse, may be prescribed prior to meals, since eating may be painful and difficult. A bland liquid or soft diet is indicated and spicy or hot foods should be avoided. The client may be better able to ingest food through straws or syringes.

Local discomfort may be relieved by rinsing with warm saline or bicarbonate of soda solution (1 teaspoon to a glass of warm water) (Bennett, 1979). The teeth and oral cavity should be cleansed every 4 hours with a 1:4 solution of hydrogen peroxide and normal saline applied with an Asepto syringe and a soft cloth or toothbrush. Warm saline may be used as a rinse. Normal brushing and flossing and commercial mouthwashes may be too irritating. Water soluble lubricants help alleviate discomfort from dryness and cracking. Ice chips and cool fluids are also helpful. A 1:1 mixture of cough syrup with diphenhydramine hydrochloride, such as Benylin syrup, and Kaotin-pectate used as a mouthwash has also been suggested for pain relief (Nursing Update, 1983). A case study for the client with stomatitis is presented at the end of this chapter.

ESOPHAGITIS

Inflammation of the esophagus (esophagitis) is a nonspecific disorder characterized by erythema, edema, deterioration, and possible ulceration of the esophageal wall. Destruction of tissue can lead to fibrosis, and scarring of esophageal tissue may lead to loss of function.

Reflux of acidic gastric contents or bile into the esophagus causes *reflux esophagitis,* the most common form of this disorder. Malfunction of the esophageal sphincter, as in hiatal hernia, is a frequent etiologic factor. Other conditions associated with esophagitis include bacterial invasion, chemical irritation (for example, from dust or pollutants), and physical irritation related to smoking. Irritation

may also be related to ingestion of alcohol, spices, or very hot or very cold liquids. Trauma may also promote esophagitis.

Clinical Manifestations

Clients with esophagitis describe burning pain in the area of the sternum; pain may radiate to the neck, jaws, arms, and back. Pain is often related to the recumbent position and/or increased intra-abdominal pressure. Eructation with or without regurgitation of bitter acidic fluid is common. Dysphagia related to edema and lack of esophageal muscle tone may occur, especially at the beginning of meals. The client may notice discomfort in relation to particular substances such as citrus fruits, alcohol, salicylates, coffee, spices, and high-residue foods. Bleeding may occur and will usually be most evident in the stools, since blood is likely to be swallowed.

Therapeutic Measures

Conservative therapy seeks to eliminate the cause. Antacids may be used between meals and at bedtime to reduce acidity and limit trauma related to it. Cimetidine (Tagamet) may be prescribed for gastric reflux and cholestryamine (Questran) for biliary reflux (Kanin, 1980). A bland, low-residue diet will be prescribed to be given in small, frequent feedings. Elevating the upper body at night with pillows or elevating the head of the bed with blocks helps prevent reflux related to the recumbent position.

If strictures related to fibrosis have developed, balloon dilation may be performed periodically (see discussion of esophageal achalasia). Surgical treatment may be necessary if symptoms persist, including vagotomy with antrectomy or pyloroplasty, and myotomy; these procedures are defined and described in Chapter 50.

Specific Nursing Measures

Nursing care focuses on assisting the client with relief of symptoms. Help the client identify and eliminate offensive foods and medications (see previous section). Teach the rationale for remaining upright after meals and elevating the upper body at night. Assistance with weight reduction may be indicated, since obesity increases intra-abdominal pressure. The client should be instructed about prescribed medications and possible side effects and taught to monitor the stool for signs of bleeding.

Section III: Neoplastic and Obstructive Disorders

Tumors of the mouth and esophagus may be benign or malignant. Esophageal cancer is especially virulent. Oral and esophageal cancers occur more frequently in men, especially after the fifth decade of life. Smoking and excessive use of alcohol are major etiologic factors.

Cancers of the oral cavity and esophagus and the treatments related to them may cause severe disfigurement and consequent disturbances of body image. Furthermore, these cancers can seriously compromise nutritional status by interfering with ingestion. Malnutrition is a common sequela. Oral and esophageal cancers are associated with significant morbidity and mortality, especially when the diagnosis is made late in the course of the disease.

GENERAL NURSING IMPLICATIONS

Clients with oral or esophageal cancer require a great deal of psychological support to cope with their disease effectively. Any diagnosis of cancer is frightening, but oral cancers can be especially disfiguring and disruptive to the client's daily life. The nurse will need solid rapport with client and family to help them through difficult times. Esophageal cancer, especially, is associated with a grave prognosis; the 5-year survival rate is only 5% (Crowley, 1983). Client and significant others may need help with grieving, in coping with body image alterations, and in adapting to alternative methods of feeding.

Oral cancers can be detected early, and nurses, who frequently assess the mouth during routine physical examinations or in the course of nursing care, can help significantly by being familiar with early signs of these lesions. Explain to tobacco users and heavy users of alcohol that these practices greatly increase their risk of oral cancer. Encourage them to stop or at least reduce smoking and alcohol use, and to seek frequent physical examinations. Teach early warning signs and self-examination for oral cancer. Figure 48–9 shows a step-by-step approach to a complete oral self-examination for cancer.

In taking the health history, focus on risk factors. Does the client smoke? Chew tobacco? Consume alcoholic beverages? How often? How much? ("Excessive use" is generally defined as more than 2 oz of alcohol per day.) Is dysphagia a recurring problem? Achalasia may accompany cancer of the esophagus. Investigate any lumps, sores, tenderness, or pain. Ask the client how long these have persisted.

To examine the mouth, the following supplies are needed: a tongue blade, gauze, finger cots, mirrors, adequate lighting, and familiarity with early signs of oral cancer. Carefully palpate the oral cavity, including glands and lymph nodes. Pay particular attention to any sores, growths, or lumps, noting size, tenderness, consistency, and fixation. Any client with a history of oral cancer should be checked periodically for recurrence.

Nutritional assessment is of special importance for clients with oral or esophageal cancers, since they frequently experience problems of ingestion, anorexia, and malnutrition. Clients undergoing radiation or chemotherapy may have special problems such as stomatitis or pharyngitis.

How is the client coping with body image changes associated with the disease or with treatment? Is the client withdrawing from social contact? How are family members reacting to any disfigurement? Does the client seem able to adapt to alternative methods of feeding? Coping abilities

of client and family must be continually assessed and strengthened, especially if the prognosis is grave or death is impending.

CANCER OF THE ORAL CAVITY

Most cancers of the oral cavity are squamous cell carcinomas. Adenocarcinomas may arise from the mucous and salivary glands, and basal cell carcinoma, malignant melanoma, sarcoma, and lymphoma may also occur. Areas affected, in order of frequency, are the lips, tongue, buccal mucosa, gingivae, floor of the mouth, and the tonsils. (Cancer of the tongue and the tonsils—both of which affect respiratory status—are discussed in Unit Three.) Approximately 29,000 new cases of oral cancers and over 9000 deaths related to this disorder in the United States were projected for 1985 (1985 Cancer Facts and Figures, 1985). Males, especially those over 40, are more frequently affected.

Heavy use of alcohol and/or tobacco (smoking, chewing tobacco) are identified risk factors; it is thought that irritation by these substances leads to mucosal changes in the mouth. Other factors apparently related to development of oral cancer are chronic irritation from appliances in the mouth (braces, dentures) and poor oral hygiene. Persons with *Plummer–Vinson syndrome* (an iron-deficiency syndrome) are considered at risk, as are those with syphilitic glossitis and those who have had x-rays or radiation therapy of the head and neck. Exposure to intense sunlight has been implicated in development of cancer of the lip (Petersdorf, 1983).

Clinical Manifestations

The client may describe sores that do not heal, swelling, difficulty in chewing, dysphagia, difficulty in talking or moving the tongue, and/or drooling. In its late stages, cancer of the salivary gland may be a painful mass associated with neurological signs such as paresis or paralysis. Pain from cancer anywhere in the mouth may radiate to the face or ear. Lesions may be white, gray, dark brown, or black, and may bleed. An inflammatory response, with erythema and edema, may be seen upon inspection.

Early, primary lesions include:

- Leukoplakia (white, nodular patches on the oral mucosa that do not rub off)
- Speckled leukoplakia (white nodular patches interspersed with erythematous areas)
- Erythroplakia (persistent velvety red patches on the oral mucosa) (Kennett, 1980)

These early lesions are usually benign but are considered premalignant.

Enlargement of cervical lymph nodes may occur as cancer metastasizes, and underlying bone and muscle may

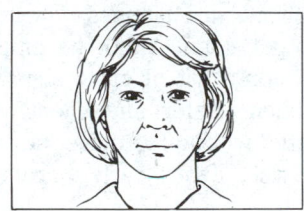

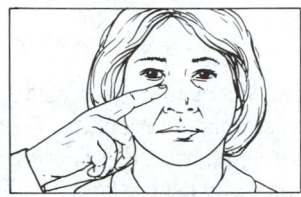

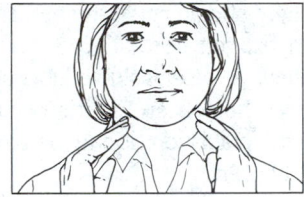

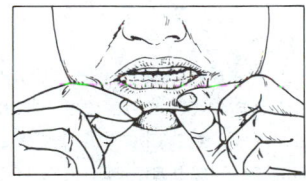

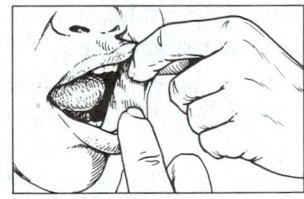

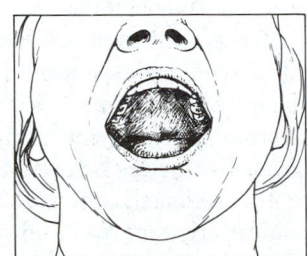

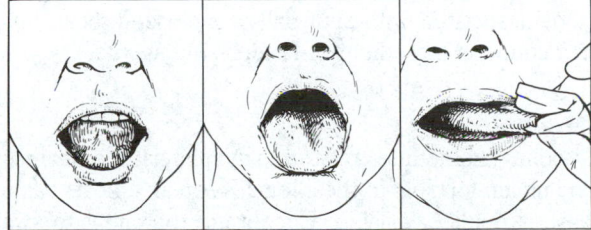

A mirror and adequate lighting are necessary for the self-exam.

Step 1   Symmetry
Look at your face and neck. The right and left sides are normally symmetrical; this means they have the same shape. Any differences in shape, such as a lump or swelling on one side, should be noted.

If similar lumps, bumps or other features are found at the same place on both sides of the face, neck or inside the mouth, they are probably normal.

Step 2   Face
Inspect the skin of the face, neck and lips. Look for changes in skin color, lumps or sores. If glasses are worn, remove them and look closely at the area around the eyes and the bridge of the nose. Replace glasses.

Step 3   Neck
With your fingers press along the sides and front of the neck to detect any lumps or tenderness. (As in Step 1, use symmetry to help identify normal features.)

Any dentures or partial plates should be removed at this point

Step 4   Lips
Pull the lower lip down to view any possible sores or color changes. With your fingers feel for any lump which may not be seen. Repeat procedure for upper lip.

Step 5   Cheek
Use your fingers to expose the left inner cheek surface to observe any white, red or dark patches. Place your thumb on the inside of your cheek and your index finger on the outside. Gently squeeze your cheek between your fingers; check for any lumps or areas of tenderness. Repeat procedure for right cheek.

Step 6   Roof of the Mouth
Tilt the head back and open the mouth wide to observe any color differences or lumps.

Step 7   Floor of Mouth and Tongue
Place the tip of the tongue to the roof of the mouth. Inspect the floor of the mouth and under-surface of the tongue for any color changes or sores. Examine the floor of the mouth by gently pressing with your finger to detect any abnormal lump or swelling.

Extend the tongue and inspect the top surface.

Using a gauze compress or a tissue, gently but firmly grasp the tongue and pull it forward to view the sides. Any swelling or color changes should be noted.

Figure 48–9

Oral self-exam for cancer. (Courtesy of National Cancer Institute)

Box 48–1 Early Signs of Oral Cancer

Oral mucous membranes
    White patches (leukoplakia)
    Red patches (erythroplakia)
    Ulcers
    Masses
    Areas of pigmentation (brownish or black)

Lips
    Fissures
    Ulcers
    Patches of leukoplakia
    Areas of pigmentation

Floor of mouth (under the tongue)
    Leukoplakia
    Masses
    Areas of ulceration

Tongue
    Masses or lesions
    Areas of pigmentation

Asymmetry of the head, face, jaws, or neck

become involved. Prognosis varies, depending on the site of the lesion and its extent. The overall 5-year US survival rate for oral cancer is 40%; survival is highest for cancer of the lip, since these lesions are usually noticed early (1985 Cancer Facts and Figures, 1985).

Diagnosis and ongoing assessment employ physical examination, biopsy, cytology, and radiography.

Therapeutic Measures

Early detection is crucial. Many precancerous lesions are discovered by dentists in routine checkups. Radiation therapy and surgery are the preferred conventional treatments, although chemotherapy is sometimes indicated. Both the primary lesion and any affected lymph nodes are irradiated, and radioactive implants may also be used. Among the surgical approaches are such radical procedures as glossectomy (removal of the tongue), radical neck dissection, and maxillectomy (removal of all or part of the maxilla). These surgeries are discussed in Unit Three in relation to cancers affecting the respiratory system.

Nutritional status must be maintained—a formidable problem because of pain, dysphagia, and the effects of radical surgery. Soft or liquid foods of moderate temperature may be given at frequent intervals, or tube feedings or total parenteral nutrition may be required.

Measures to control pain will be necessary, especially in late stages of the disease. Bacterial infection of lesions must be scrupulously avoided.

Specific Nursing Measures

The facial disfigurement and lifestyle changes that can result from oral cancer and its subsequent treatment can be overwhelming to clients and families. Therefore, the importance of early detection cannot be emphasized enough. See Box 48–1 for a list of early signs to watch for on routine inspection. Refer any client with these signs for a diagnostic workup. Advise alcohol and tobacco users of their risk. Teach early warning signs and oral self-examination.

Mouth Care

Clients with oral cancer may have halitosis, a foul taste in the mouth, xerostomia, or drooling. Frequent mouth care should be encouraged, with the nurse assisting as necessary. In addition to brushing and flossing to the extent possible, the client should rinse the mouth with saline solution or dilute hydrogen peroxide. Other antiseptic rinses may be prescribed. A water-soluble lubricant may be applied to dry or cracked lips. If stomatitis occurs, for example, in association with irradiation, it may be treated as described earlier in this chapter.

Xerostomia

Excessive dryness of the mouth (xerostomia) may be related to salivary gland dysfunction; fever; administration of atropine, antihistamines, tricyclic antidepressants, or phenothiazines; or surgery or irradiation of the salivary glands. Xerostomia related to radiation may be permanent. Measures to increase moisture in the mouth are indicated. Fluids should be encouraged, irritating foods should be avoided, and lubricants such as mineral oil may alleviate symptoms.

The client may wish to suck on hard candies to stimulate saliva production. Although this may be helpful, sugar-free candies should be used as dental caries may develop. Lemon-flavored candies are especially helpful since their acidity helps stimulate salivation.

Papase, a proteolytic enzyme derived from papaya juice, may be given 10 minutes before meals to help break up thickened oral secretions (Larsen, 1982). This agent is available without prescription. Note, however, that papaya is a common allergen. (Ask the client about allergic reactions associated with artificially tenderized meats; papain is a common ingredient of tenderizing agents.)

Drooling

Drooling, sometimes related to dysphagia, is embarrassing and uncomfortable to the client. Keep an emesis basin and tissues readily available. Encourage the client to swallow frequently if possible. Suctioning may be necessary. Anticholinergics, belladonna derivatives, or atropine may be prescribed.

Nutritional Needs

Continual assessment of nutritional status has already been stressed, as has the use of soft or liquid foods and frequent small feedings. Encourage the client to participate actively in meeting nutritional needs; involvement in all activities of daily living is psychologically beneficial. Teach family or significant others how to assist the client with feedings. Both client and family will have problems of adjustment to contend with in addition to the disease itself.

Pain and Discomfort

The importance of alleviating pain and discomfort with analgesic therapy and nursing comfort measures cannot be overemphasized. Pain related to cancer is discussed in Chapter 12; a general discussion of pain may be found in Chapter 5.

CANCER OF THE ESOPHAGUS

Cancer of the esophagus is relatively uncommon in the United States; over 9000 new cases and over 8500 deaths were predicted for 1985 (1985 Cancer Facts and Figures, 1985). Esophageal cancer is common, however, in other parts of the world such as Japan, China, Iran, the Soviet Union, and South Africa. This fact should be considered when examining emigrants from these areas. Males are affected more often than females, and the incidence of esophageal cancer has risen significantly for both male and female American blacks. The disease is most common in individuals ages 50 to 70.

Esophageal tumors include squamous cell carcinomas, adenocarcinomas, and, less frequently, melanomas and sarcomas. Metastasis is common.

Tobacco use and excessive alcohol consumption are risk factors already mentioned. Other predisposing conditions include (Boyce, 1982):

- Ingestion of lye
- Tylosis (hereditary palmar–plantar hyperkeratosis)
- Achalasia
- Barrett's esophagus (in which normal squamous cell epithelium is replaced by columnar cells)
- Plummer–Vinson syndrome (esophageal web formation associated with iron deficiency anemia in premenopausal women)

Clinical Manifestations

Symptoms are not usually apparent until esophageal cancer is advanced, accounting for the high mortality rate associated with late-stage detection. The client will experience progressive dysphagia as the tumor obstructs the esoph-

agus. Clients often describe burning or tightness with swallowing, especially with hot liquids. Pain, anorexia, and weight loss may occur, and hoarseness, coughing, regurgitation, and aspiration may be present. By the time esophageal cancer is diagnosed, regional lymph nodes are usually involved, although the involved nodes may not be clinically palpable. Malnutrition, GI hemorrhage, and aspiration pneumonitis are major causes of death in clients with esophageal cancer.

Diagnosis is made by barium swallow, endoscopy, computed tomography (CT) scanning, biopsy, and cytology.

Therapeutic Measures

If tumor growth and/or evidence of metastasis is minimal, an attempt may be made to remove the tumor surgically (*esophagectomy*), although morbidity and mortality are high. If the tumor is inoperable, radiotherapy may be used. Irradiation has been found to relieve symptoms as well as surgery, but it can induce edema that obstructs the esophagus. Chemotherapy has not proved effective (Boyce, 1982).

Esophageal dilation may be performed in combination with radiotherapy to relieve dysphagia and allow more normal eating (Bachrach, Boyce, & Jackson, 1981). An anesthetic spray or gargle may be used during the procedure, or meperidine or diazepam may be used for preprocedure sedation. Esophageal dilation is discussed in Section I under esophageal achalasia. Symptomatic relief may indirectly improve compromised nutritional status, but malnutrition may persist despite dilation, and nutritional support may be necessary. Prosthetic devices may be inserted into the esophagus to bypass the tumor, especially in the presence of esophagopulmonary fistulas and associated aspiration of food into the respiratory tract. The esophagus is dilated with the client under sedation, and the device is inserted under fluoroscopic monitoring. Pain control will be necessary, and use of narcotics may be indicated.

Specific Nursing Measures

Emotional support is of high priority. Clients must cope with a grave prognosis or certain expectation of death, as well as many lifestyle changes including alternative methods of feeding. Both client and family will need the nurse's support. Comfort measures and nutritional support as discussed in Chapter 47 will be necessary. Soft or liquid foods must be provided if the client is able to ingest food orally, and foods should be made as appetizing as possible to counteract anorexia. The nurse is in a key position to assess the client's ability to tolerate foods and should continually determine, along with the client, what kinds of food will be best tolerated.

Section IV: Traumatic Disorders

Trauma to the mouth and esophagus may be related to irritation, accident, or assault. It may involve any part of the upper GI tract, including the lips, cheeks, gingivae, palate, tongue, teeth, or salivary glands.

Traumatic oral/esophageal disorders are especially serious if they interfere with ingestion. They may also be painful and disfiguring, especially if they involve the mouth. Esophageal trauma may be associated with respiratory complications. Prevention of infection and other complications is an important nursing responsibility. Pain relief may be required. Throughout the ordeal of treatment and recovery, the client will need emotional support.

GENERAL NURSING IMPLICATIONS

Often the nurse in the emergency room is the first health professional to see the client with trauma. The importance of accurate assessment cannot be overstressed. Any trauma to the head may be accompanied by trauma to the oral cavity, and this area should therefore not be overlooked. Any trauma to the chest or abdomen may include esophageal trauma, so this should also be considered.

Try to find out from the client or whoever accompanied him or her what actually caused the injury: A blow? From what sort of instrument? A cut? From a sharp or jagged object? Determining whether the wound is contaminated is especially important, since aggressive therapy may be needed to prevent infection. Are there signs of hemorrhage? Ecchymosis? Pain? Numbness? Loss of function? What is the client's immunization status?

Comfort measures will be needed, as well as emotional support. Prescribed analgesics should be freely offered; only the client can judge the extent of perceived pain. The mouth should be cleansed of dried blood, tooth fragments, and other debris. Cold compresses may be applied to the oral cavity to avert formation of excessive edema, a natural consequence of the inflammatory process. After 24 hours, warm compresses may help relieve edema.

If the injury interferes with eating, alternative means of feeding may be required, and pertinent observations about food tolerance will have to be made. Nutritional assessment is indicated.

TRAUMA TO THE ORAL CAVITY AND ESOPHAGUS

The mouth may be injured in vehicular accidents, falls, fights, or accidents related to employment or recreation. Although esophageal trauma may also have these causes, it is more often caused by ingestion of foreign bodies or burns, especially chemical burns. Suicide attempts may involve ingestion of sharp objects or caustic substances. One source reports that 74% of esophageal perforations

are iatrogenic, usually associated with esophagoscopy or dilation (Keszler & Buzna, 1981). Penetrating wounds may be caused by stabbing or gunshot, and crushing injuries may cause stricture or obstruction.

Clinical Manifestations

Oral trauma may consist of puncture wounds, lacerations, or abrasions accompanied by hemorrhage, edema, erythema, and/or pain. With any deep trauma to the cheek, trauma to the parotid gland should be suspected. Injury to the teeth may cause fracture or avulsion; sensitivity to touch and temperature is a sign of dental fracture. Loosened teeth may be painful and movable. An avulsed tooth is completely out of its socket. Edema and debris in the mouth may cause obstruction of the airway.

If the esophagus has been penetrated, the client will experience retrosternal chest pain and fever. Invasion of the respiratory tract by esophageal hemorrhage will result in bloody sputum. Mediastinitis (inflammation of the mediastinum) may occur.

Oral/esophageal trauma with accompanying inflammation may lead to fibrosis of the involved tissue with scarring and loss of function. Difficulty in chewing or swallowing may occur at the time of injury or later.

Any client with trauma to the chest or thoracic cavity should be assessed for possible esophageal injury by x-ray or by cautious passage of an indwelling aspirating tube. Additional symptoms of esophageal trauma include dyspnea, cyanosis, upper abdominal pain, hypotension, and subcutaneous emphysema in the cervical or anterior thoracic regions.

Therapeutic Measures

Trauma to the oral cavity requires meticulous cleansing and care of the wound to prevent infection. Suctioning of blood and debris may be necessary. Insertion of an airway may be necessary to maintain a patent breathing passage. Lacerations may have to be sutured. Injuries to the parotid gland may also be sutured, and a Penrose drain may be inserted to drain saliva until healing has occurred. Dislodged teeth may be successfully reimplanted if they have been out of their socket less than 2 hours. The dislodged tooth must be held in place in the mouth until dental treatment is begun. Dislodged teeth may also be kept alive for up to 12 hours if immersed in cold milk (Johnson, 1983).

Minor esophageal perforations that can heal spontaneously may respond to medical treatment. The client is kept NPO and fed by means of a gastrostomy or by total parenteral nutrition, and tubes are inserted in the chest to drain accumulated fluids that may extravasate from the esophagus. The client may be kept in Fowler's position, and antibiotic therapy may be employed. Larger perforations should be repaired by surgical suturing. If treatment is delayed too long after the injury, surgery may not be possible.

Foreign bodies are removed by fiberoptic endoscopy; a magnet may be attached to the endoscope to remove metallic objects. Perforation is a possible complication of this procedure. Proteolytic enzymes may sometimes be employed to dissolve dislodged food particles.

Chemical burns of the oral cavity and esophagus should be immediately rinsed with large volumes of water. Steroids may be given to reduce inflammation, and prophylactic antibiotic therapy is generally employed. Fluids may be given as tolerated, but tube feeding and intravenous fluid replacement are often necessary. Stricture and obstruc-

tion may be associated with scarring; peroral dilation may be necessary.

Prophylactic antibiotic therapy and tetanus immunization may be given if the wound is contaminated.

Specific Nursing Measures

Nursing measures will focus on supporting the client and family, preventing infection and complications, promoting comfort, promoting healing, and maintaining nutritional status. Careful assessment of the extent of injury and potential for complication is imperative. The client should be involved in care as much as possible. These and other components of nursing care of the client with oral/esophageal trauma are discussed at the beginning of this section.

Chapter Highlights

Clients with disorders of the mouth and esophagus are especially susceptible to malnutrition.

Clients with disorders of the mouth and esophagus often require dietary alterations with soft or liquid foods, given in small amounts frequently.

The nurse can play an important role in prevention of disorders of the mouth and esophagus through teaching clients about associated risk factors.

Cancers of the oral cavity can easily be detected in the early stages during a routine nursing assessment.

In disorders of the mouth, such as stomatitis, nursing comfort measures are of high priority.

Good oral hygiene is imperative in prevention of disorders of the oral cavity.

Esophageal cancer, although relatively uncommon in the United States, has a high mortality rate.

Bibliography

Bachrach N, Boyce HW, Jackson D: Problems in swallowing and esophageal carcinoma. *Heart Lung* 1981; 10:525–531.

Beck S: Impact of a systematic oral care protocol on stomatitis after chemotherapy. *Cancer Nurs* (June) 1979; 2:185–199.

Bennett J: Oral care of cancer patients undergoing head and neck irradiation. *Dental Hygiene* (May) 1979; 53:209–212.

Boyce HW: Approaches to management of cancer of the esophagus. *Hosp Pract* (Nov) 1982; 109–124.

1985 Cancer Facts and Figures. New York: American Cancer Society, 1985.

Ciancio SG, Bourgault PC: *Clinical Pharmacology for Dental Professionals* 2nd ed. Littleton Mass. PSG Pub. Co, 1984.

Crowley LV: *Introduction to Human Disease.* Monterey, CA: Wadsworth, 1983.

Daeffler R: Oral hygiene measures for patients with cancer III. *Cancer Nurs* (Feb) 1981; 4:29–35.

Dealing with Emergencies, Nursing Photobook. Springhouse, PA: Intermed Communications, 1981.

DePaola DP, Alvares O, Etzel KA: Nutrition and periodontal disease. *Contemporary Nutrition* (Dec) 1982; 7:12.

Given BA, Simmons SJ: *Gastroenterology in Clinical Nursing,* 4th ed. St. Louis: Mosby, 1984.

Giving Emergency Care Completely. Springhouse, PA: Intermed Communications, 1980.

Johnson R: Milk is a natural. (Letter.) *Nurs 83* (Aug) 1983; 13:66.

Kanin J: Chronic esophagitis. *Consultant* (April) 20(4): 1980; p. 153.

Kennett S: Recognizing premalignant conditions in the mouth. *Consultant* (Jan) 1980; 32–44.

Keszler P, Buzna E: Surgical and conservative management of esophageal perforation. *Chest* 1981; 80:158–162.

Lane B, Forgay M: Upgrading your oral hygiene protocol for the patient with cancer. *Canadian Nurs* (Dec) 1981; 27–29.

Larsen G: Rehabilitation of the patient with head and neck cancer. *Am J Nurs* 1982; 82:119–122.

Nursing update: Nursing implications of cancer chemotherapy. *Nurs 83* (Aug) 1983; 13:64a.

Petersdorf RG et al: *Harrison's Principles of Internal Medicine.* New York: McGraw-Hill, 1983.

Rose L, Hendler BH, Amsterdam JT: Temporomandibular disorders and odontic infections. *Consultant* (Dec) 1982; 22(12): 110–136.

Sandler RS, Bozymski EM, Orlando RC: Failure of clinical criteria to distinguish between primary achalasia and achalasia secondary to tumor. *Dig Dis Sci* (March) 1982; 27:209–212.

Schachtele CF: Bacteria, diet and the prevention of dental caries Part I. *Contemporary Nutrition* (July) 1980; 5:7.

Suggested Readings

DePaola DP, Alvares O, Etzel KR: Nutrition and periodontal disease. *Contemporary Nutrition* (Dec) 1982; 7:12. This article discusses the factors associated with periodontal disease. Nutritional influences are highlighted.

Lane B, Forgay M: Upgrading your oral hygiene protocol for the client with cancer. *Can Nurse* (Dec) 1981; 77:27–29. Provides an extensive overview of mouth care, concentrating on the treatment of stomatitis associated with chemotherapy and radiotherapy.

Schachtele CF: Bacteria, diet and the prevention of dental caries: Parts I & II. *Contemporary Nutrition* (July–Aug) 1980; 5:7–8. These articles provide an overview of factors associated with dental caries.

The Client With Stomatitis

I. Brief Descriptive Data	Mary Ann Vanner, a 33-year-old, single, white schoolteacher, belongs to the local HMO. Recently, she was treated for acute sinusitis with ampicillin; the condition has now cleared up. However, she subsequently developed a sore mouth with white patches on the mucous membranes that bleed easily.

II. Personal Data

Date and Time:	Sept 30, 1986; 11 AM
Full Name:	Mary Ann Vanner
Social Security Number:	000-00-0000
Address:	46 Winchester Rd., Whitestone, NY
Telephone:	Home: 000-0000
	Work: 000-0000
Sex:	Female
Age:	33
Birthdate:	6-10-53
Marital Status:	Single
Race:	Caucasian
Religion:	Catholic
Occupation:	Schoolteacher
Usual Health Care Provider:	James Santasiero, MD
	Celestine Springate, RN, NP

III. Health History

Source of Information:	Client
Reliability of Informant:	Reliable
Chief Concern:	"My mouth is sore with some white material. It has also been bleeding."
History of Present Illness:	Three days after starting to take ampicillin for sinusitis, Ms Vanner noticed white spots in her mouth, especially on the insides of her cheeks. Soon after, bleeding was noted with even mild irritation of the mouth (as in brushing and eating), and the white patches rubbed off easily. The soreness in her mouth has progressed in severity.
	She is not a smoker and does not eat highly spiced foods. Recent routine dental examination was normal. She has never had oral surgery or any diseases of the head and neck. Approximately 10 years ago, she developed a yeast infection in the vagina secondary to treatment with penicillin for streptococcal pharyngitis.
Past Health History:	
Childhood:	Usual childhood diseases: measles, mumps, chickenpox
Immunizations:	Has had all routine immunizations; does not remember dates
Medical Problems:	Acute sinusitis occasionally, usually during winter months; no other medical problems
Surgeries:	None
Transfusions:	None
Special Diagnostic Procedures:	Routine chest x-rays
Pregnancies:	None
Trauma:	Fracture left wrist, 1981, fall on ice
Allergies:	None

(continued)

Case Study written by Patricia Brown

The Client With Stomatitis

Family History:

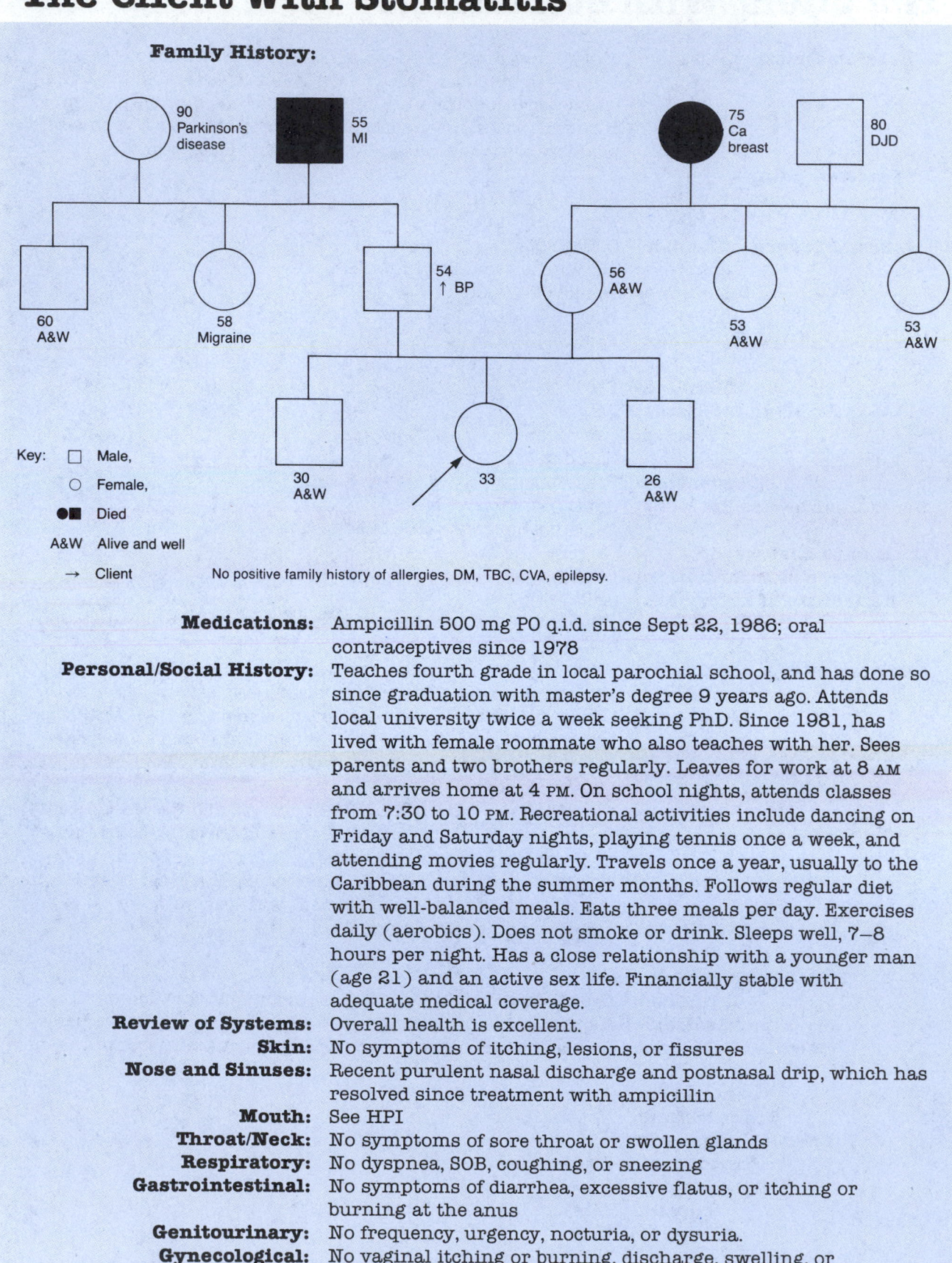

Key:
☐ Male,
○ Female,
■● Died
A&W Alive and well
→ Client

No positive family history of allergies, DM, TBC, CVA, epilepsy.

Medications:	Ampicillin 500 mg PO q.i.d. since Sept 22, 1986; oral contraceptives since 1978
Personal/Social History:	Teaches fourth grade in local parochial school, and has done so since graduation with master's degree 9 years ago. Attends local university twice a week seeking PhD. Since 1981, has lived with female roommate who also teaches with her. Sees parents and two brothers regularly. Leaves for work at 8 AM and arrives home at 4 PM. On school nights, attends classes from 7:30 to 10 PM. Recreational activities include dancing on Friday and Saturday nights, playing tennis once a week, and attending movies regularly. Travels once a year, usually to the Caribbean during the summer months. Follows regular diet with well-balanced meals. Eats three meals per day. Exercises daily (aerobics). Does not smoke or drink. Sleeps well, 7–8 hours per night. Has a close relationship with a younger man (age 21) and an active sex life. Financially stable with adequate medical coverage.
Review of Systems:	Overall health is excellent.
Skin:	No symptoms of itching, lesions, or fissures
Nose and Sinuses:	Recent purulent nasal discharge and postnasal drip, which has resolved since treatment with ampicillin
Mouth:	See HPI
Throat/Neck:	No symptoms of sore throat or swollen glands
Respiratory:	No dyspnea, SOB, coughing, or sneezing
Gastrointestinal:	No symptoms of diarrhea, excessive flatus, or itching or burning at the anus
Genitourinary:	No frequency, urgency, nocturia, or dysuria.
Gynecological:	No vaginal itching or burning, discharge, swelling, or discomfort with intercourse

IV. Physical Assessment

Height:	5 ft 5 in
Weight:	130 lb
Vital Signs:	BP 130/70; pulse 76; respirations 18; oral temperature 98.8°F (37°C)

Relevant Organ Systems:

Skin:	Without lesions
Mouth:	White patches with white, curdlike discharge noted, especially on buccal mucosa; tongue and palate also involved; with palpation, white patches rub off easily and reveal raw surface with bleeding; pain noted with palpation
Neck:	Without nodes
Gynecological:	No erythema at urethra or introitus; vaginal mucosa without lesions; no vaginal discharge

V. Diagnostic Data

A wet prep with KOH and culture were taken of the oral discharge; *Candida albicans* was identified.

VI. Medical Regimen

Diet:	Soft, bland foods recommended until symptoms disappear
Medications:	Nystatin (Mycostatin) oral suspension 400,000 U q.i.d.
Treatments:	Oral hygiene q.4h with a soft toothbrush and warm saline rinses (1 tsp salt to a glass of warm water); use rinses p.r.n. for discomfort; return to HMO if oral symptoms do not disappear or if pain, itching, burning, or lesions are noted on the skin or at the anus or vagina or if discomfort is noted with defecation, urination, or intercourse

VII. Nursing Care Plan

Nursing Diagnosis	Client Care Goals	Plan/Nursing Implementation	Expected Outcomes
Oral mucous membrane, alterations in: related to fungal infection	Reduce or eliminate pain; restore tissue integrity; describe cause of infection	Explain that antibiotics sometimes cause an overgrowth of fungus; explain rationale for soft bland foods; explain bland diet; explain rationale for and use of medication (nystatin should be swished in the mouth and held there as long as possible before swallowing); discuss preparation and use of mouthwash	Client is able to manage medication regimen; client follows diet closely, avoids further irritation of oral mucous membranes, and practices prescribed oral hygiene
Comfort, alteration in: potential for, related to possible candidiasis of other body areas such as the skin, vagina, and GI tract	Monitor symptoms and signs of candida infection in other body areas	Teach client signs and symptoms of candida infection of other body areas; suggest yogurt to normalize vaginal flora after antibiotic therapy	If infection occurs, client will contact care provider to report symptoms

Chapter 49

Specific Disorders of the Stomach, Intestines, and Pancreas

Patricia Brown

Objectives

When you have finished studying this chapter, you should be able to:

Identify the etiology and risk factors associated with disorders of the stomach, small and large intestines, and pancreas.

Explain the role of the nurse in primary prevention of disorders of the stomach, intestines, and pancreas.

List therapeutic measures, including any medical and surgical treatments, associated with disorders of the stomach, intestines, and pancreas.

Describe specific nursing care for clients with disorders of the stomach, intestines, and pancreas.

Anticipate the psychosocial/lifestyle impact of disorders of the stomach, intestines, and pancreas on clients and their significant others.

Discuss the crucial role of nutritional assessment and support in caring for clients with disorders of the stomach, intestines, and pancreas.

Plan diet regimens appropriate for clients with disorders of the stomach, intestines, and pancreas.

Apply the nursing process in all phases of care for the client with disorders of the stomach, intestines, and pancreas.

Dysfunction of the stomach, small and large intestines, and pancreas can adversely affect an individual's lifestyle and nutritional status. The problem may go almost unnoticed until acute, life-threatening complications—hemorrhage, for example—cause the client to seek professional health care.

Nurses may care for clients with problems of these organs in the home, occupational settings, clinics, or hospitals. Dietary and lifestyle factors are frequently implicated. Nurses are often in a position to identify risk factors as well as counsel the client about preventive approaches. Early detection is another crucial part of the nurse's function, especially when clinical symptoms have not yet become apparent.

Section I: Disorders of Multifactorial Origin

Disorders of multifactorial origin primarily affect the stomach and intestines; disorders that affect the pancreas generally have a more specific etiology. Multifactorial disorders develop and manifest themselves during an individual's life span, although some may be familial or hereditary. They often are related to the individual's reaction with the environment, and many are related to dietary intake.

General Nursing Implications

Symptoms and signs of gastrointestinal (GI) disorders of multifactorial causation may be detected while taking the health history or in the course of a routine physical examination. In the early stages, these disorders may have no acute manifestations; symptoms are often vague. Careful attention to the history may offer clues to the presence of undetected disorders. Pay particular attention to the client's eating habits and to any clues relating symptoms to the timing of meals. For example, does epigastric discomfort occur just before a meal, when the client is hungry? Just after a meal? An hour later? Also, ask the client about life events that may be causing stress.

During the physical assessment, be alert to abdominal pain or tenderness. Does the rectal examination seem to cause undue discomfort? Inspect and palpate for hemorrhoids and/or fissures.

Once the client's disorder has been diagnosed, follow-up assessments will monitor the client's progress and the effectiveness of therapy. Are symptoms becoming less severe? Is the client more comfortable? Ongoing nutritional assessment will also be required since GI disorders may seriously alter nutritional status.

Diet counseling is a major component of therapy. Counseling should be individualized because different clients are adversely affected by different foods. If a special regimen such as a high-residue or low-residue diet is prescribed, the client will need counseling about which foods to choose and how to prepare them. A dietitian may plan the actual diet, but the nurse, who sees the client regularly, often has more opportunities for both formal and impromptu counseling.

If medications are prescribed, the nurse is generally responsible for explaining why, how, and when to take them and what side effects or toxic reactions should be anticipated.

LACTOSE INTOLERANCE

Lactose intolerance, also known as *lactase deficiency*, is characterized by an inability to digest lactose, a disaccharide found in milk and milk products. In normal persons, the enzyme lactase, found in the small intestine, hydrolyzes lactose so it can be digested and absorbed. This enzyme is absent or insufficiently active in persons with lactose intolerance.

Insufficient activity of lactase may be primary or may be related to an underlying disorder of the small intestine, for example, celiac sprue, Crohn's disease (regional enteritis), or tropical sprue. Primary lactase deficiency occurs in from 5% to 10% of the adult white population and in 60% to 80% of American blacks, African Bantus, and Orientals (Greenberger, 1981). It is less common among persons of Oriental descent who are born in the United States than among Orientals who have emigrated (Hui, 1983). Primary lactase deficiency may appear to evolve developmentally, with lactase activity decreasing with age, but

in rare cases it is present from birth. In some persons in whom the disorder is not severe, it may be first identified when consumption of milk or dairy products increases, for example, during pregnancy.

Clinical Manifestations

If lactase is deficient, ingested lactose remains unabsorbed in the intestine, where it absorbs water and precipitates abdominal distention, painful cramping, excessive flatulence, borborygmi, and diarrhea. These symptoms may occur within 15 minutes to 4 hours of ingesting milk or milk-based products such as ice cream or soft cheeses. The severity of symptoms depends on the degree of lactase deficiency.

Lactose intolerance may go undiagnosed in mild cases, although a meticulous diet history may reveal the presence of symptoms. Diagnosis may be made by a lactose tolerance test (see Chapter 47), or the client's breath may be tested for the presence of hydrogen. (Intestinal bacteria convert unabsorbed lactose to hydrogen.)

Therapeutic Measures

Treatment for lactose intolerance primarily focuses on eliminating enough lactose from the diet to prevent symptoms. Major sources of lactose are milk and cream, ice cream, and soft cheeses, but breads, cakes, pancakes, margarine, and various commercially prepared and processed foods also contain lactose. The extent of dietary restriction will depend on how sensitive to lactose the individual client is.

Lactose in beverages is often better tolerated if the beverage is sweetened (Gudmond-Hoyer & Simony, 1977) or if the food containing lactose is taken as part of a meal (Bayless & Paige, 1978). Furthermore, some clients are better able to tolerate dry cheeses and fermented milk products such as cultured buttermilk, yogurt, and sour cream (Suitor & Hunter, 1980). A lowfat milk with 70% of the lactose removed (LactAid) is available commercially, and LactAid enzyme may be purchased and used to treat milk and other foods before they are eaten.

Clients with severe, long-standing lactose intolerance may develop dehydration, nutritional deficiencies, and fluid/electrolyte disturbances that require treatment.

Specific Nursing Measures

Clients with lactose intolerance generally do not require hospitalization. The nurse is often the first health care provider to detect this disorder and, together with the dietitian, the one most involved in care. It may be helpful to provide the client with a list of permitted and prohibited foods (see Table 49–1). LactAid products are not available in all areas; information may be obtained from the manufacturer (SugarLo Company, PO Box 111, Pleasantville, NJ 08232).

Table 49–1	Lactose-Restricted Diet
Food Group	**Foods to Avoid**
Beverages	Milk or milk drinks including whole, skim, and chocolate milk
Bread and equivalents	All bread products, muffins, biscuits, and pancakes containing milk or lactose
Cereals	Instant Cream of Wheat, dry cereals containing lactose or milk
Eggs	Eggs or omelets prepared with cream, milk, or milk products
Fats	Margarine or salad dressings with added milk or milk products; spreads or dips containing sour cream, cream cheese, whipping cream
Fruits, fruit juices	Fruit drinks containing lactose
Vegetables, vegetable juices	Any prepared with milk or cheese
Meat, fish, poultry, cheese	All creamed or breaded food; cold cuts, weiners, or other meat with added lactose; all cheese products
Potatoes and equivalents	Any prepared with milk, cheese, or butter; commercial potato products
Soups	Commercial and homemade soups prepared with cream, milk, or milk products
Desserts	Any desserts containing milk or milk products; commercial desserts or mixes, ice cream, sherbet
Sweets	Cream or chocolate candies; any commercial or homemade candies containing milk, lactose, or molasses
Miscellaneous	Cocoa mixes, cream sauce, nonfat dry milk, milk chocolate

PEPTIC ULCER DISEASE

Peptic ulcer disease has various forms: chronic erosion of the stomach (gastric ulcer), chronic erosion of the duodenum (duodenal ulcer), and acute erosion of the stomach or duodenum (stress ulcer). Duodenal ulceration is most common, affecting up to 10% of the US population, especially men, who are affected 6 to 10 times as frequently as women. Most clients are aged 30 to 50, whereas clients with gastric ulcers tend to be slightly older (40 to 60).

Essentially, peptic ulceration is related to erosion of the gastric or duodenal mucosa by acidic digestive juices (Figure 49–1). In severe and chronic ulcer disease, erosion may penetrate muscle tissue and even the serosa, allowing acidic juices to enter the abdominal cavity.

Although the etiologic pattern of peptic ulcer is not fully understood, it is known to involve intricate interrelationships between (1) secretion of digestive juices and (2) the condition and function of the gastric and/or duodenal mucosa. Individuals who have type O blood and who lack group AB antigens in the saliva are at risk for development of gastric ulcer or duodenal ulcer (Hui, 1983).

With *gastric ulcer,* malfunction of the pyloric valve with subsequent reflux of bile into the stomach, is thought to play a role in ulceration. Chronic inflammation of the stomach (gastritis) is often a causative factor, predisposing the mucosa to breakdown. Smoking has also been implicated in development of gastric ulcer, as have various medications, including steroids, salicylates, indomethacin, phenylbutazone, and reserpine.

Duodenal ulcer disease occurs as a result of excessive gastric acid secretion, as a consequence of an increase in the number of acid-secreting (parietal) cells in the gastric mucosa. In conjunction with more rapid gastric emptying, duodenal contents become more acid, causing ulceration.

Various disorders have been linked with development of duodenal ulcers, including hepatic and pancreatic disorders, endocrine disorders, and Zollinger–Ellison syndrome, which is discussed below. Some studies show an association between duodenal ulcer and ingestion of caffeine, alcohol, and certain medications (salicylates, steroids, indomethacin, phenylbutazone, and reserpine). An increased incidence of duodenal ulcer disease has been noted in cigarette smokers, who respond less well to therapy and have a higher mortality with the disease. (Petersdorf, 1983). The role of psychological factors such as longstanding psychic conflict, anxiety, and stress in ulcer disease remains controversial.

In Zollinger–Ellison syndrome, gastrin-secreting tumors (gastrinomas) are present in the pancreas and other organs. The elevated levels of circulating gastrin lead to excessive secretion of gastric acid and subsequently to ulceration, usually duodenal.

Stress ulcers occur in up to 90% of clients with severe trauma, burns, infection, and shock (Petersdorf, 1983). The two basic types of stress ulcers, Cushing's ulcer and ischemic ulcer, may affect either the stomach or the duodenum (Greenberger, 1981). *Cushing's ulcer* is characterized by marked hypersecretion of gastric juices related to profound stimulation of the vagus nerve. It commonly occurs

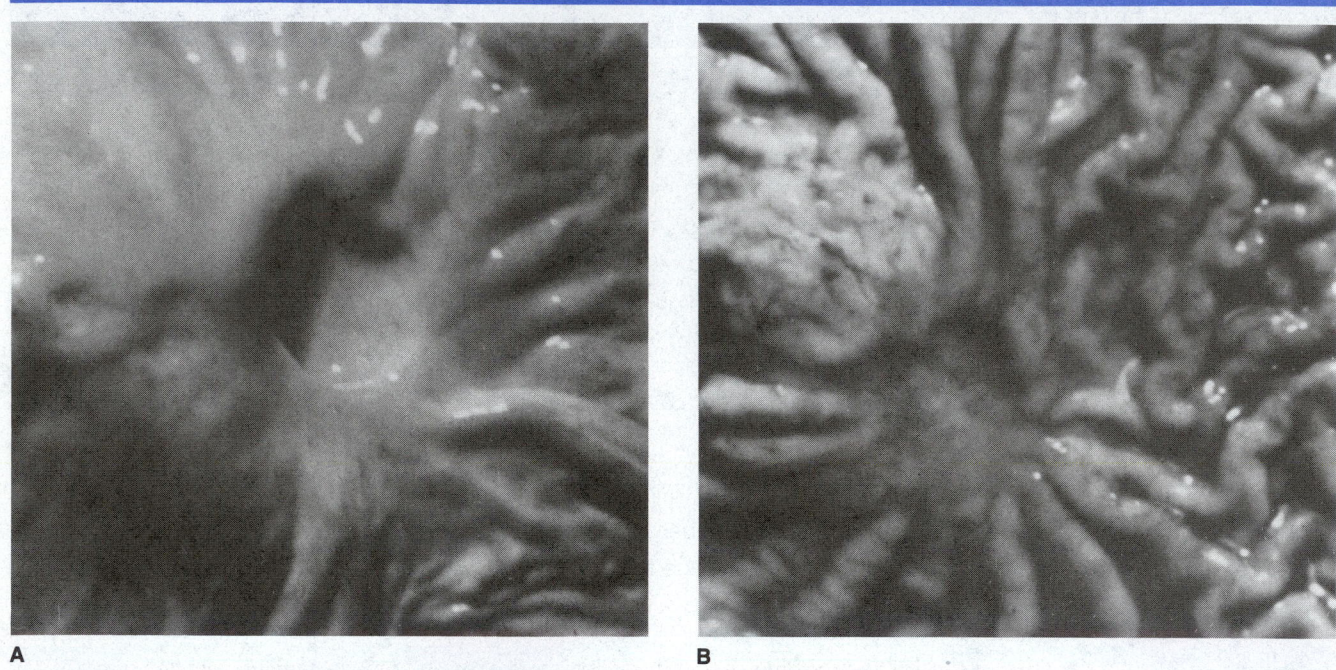

A   **B**

Figure 49–1

A. Gastric ulcer. **B.** Healed gastric ulcer. (Courtesy Millard Fillmore Hospital, Buffalo, NY)

in clients with severe brain injury or those who have undergone neurosurgery. *Ischemic ulcer* is related to ischemia of unknown cause that renders the gastroduodenal mucosa more susceptible to the action of gastric acids.

Clinical Manifestations

The client with chronic ulcer disease may describe symptoms of "burning" postprandial epigastric pain. The pain of gastric ulcer tends to occur sooner after meals than the pain of duodenal ulcer. Pain may radiate to the back and thorax and may be intensified by stress, tension, fatigue, or exposure to cold (Given & Simmons, 1984). Eating or taking an antacid may relieve symptoms, especially with duodenal ulcer.

Chronic peptic ulcer disease should be suspected whenever a client describes epigastric pain that is relieved by eating or by taking antacids. Diagnosis can be confirmed by an upper GI series, but if a gastric lesion is suspected, endoscopy is usually performed to rule out the possibility of gastric carcinoma. If Zollinger–Ellison syndrome is suspected, serum gastrin levels may be elevated; elevated levels suggest the presence of the disorder.

Complications, which occur in up to 25% of clients with peptic ulcer disease, include hemorrhage, GI obstruction, perforation, or intractable ulcer (an ulcer that responds poorly to treatment and frequently recurs). Elderly clients are at higher risk of complications and mortality (Permutt & Cello, 1982).

Hemorrhage, possibly severe, may occur if the ero-

sion is deep enough to alter the continuity of blood vessels. Hemorrhage may be heralded by hematemesis or melena, depending on its severity. (A full discussion of gastrointestinal bleeding is provided later in this section.)

Gastrointestinal obstruction may be related to fibrotic occlusion secondary to tissue damage and scarring. Abdominal distention, nausea, and vomiting will persist until the obstruction is relieved.

If ulceration is severe enough to penetrate the intestinal lining, gastric or duodenal contents spill into the peritoneum, causing inflammation. Peritonitis (inflammation of the peritoneum) is a serious, life-threatening condition. If the pancreas is affected by spillage, pancreatitis may occur. Both conditions are discussed in the section on infectious and inflammatory disorders.

Stress ulcers, which develop from 2 to 10 days after the precipitating insult, are not generally associated with any symptoms except bleeding. Bleeding may be scant, or severe hemorrhage may occur. With severe hemorrhage, a mortality rate of over 50% has been reported (Given & Simmons, 1984). Bleeding may be manifested by melena, hematemesis or, if the client has a nasogastric tube, blood may appear in the drainage.

Therapeutic Measures

Therapy in cases of peptic ulcer disease focuses on relieving symptoms, preventing complications, and healing the lesion. Healing may be accomplished in 4 to 6 weeks, but ulcers may recur in a new location.

Pharmacologic Therapy

The primary drug therapy for peptic ulcer is administration of oral antacid agents, usually taken 1 to 3 hours postprandially and at bedtime. Drugs that inhibit histamine-stimulated gastric acid secretion (H_2 receptor antagonists such as cimetidine) may be prescribed with meals and at bedtime. Sometimes anticholinergic agents are used to decrease gastric acid secretion. Medications are usually given orally, but if the client has severe complications and is NPO, antacids may be given via nasogastric tube, and H_2 receptor antagonists may be given intravenously.

Prophylactic administration of antacids and H_2 receptor antagonists may be successful in clients who are likely to develop stress ulcers (for example, burn clients). Antacids may be given as often as every 30 to 60 minutes through a nasogastric tube, if the client is NPO. If stress ulceration occurs, it is treated similarly to chronic ulceration.

If ulceration is due to Zollinger–Ellison syndrome, surgery must ultimately be performed to remove gastrinomas, although the measures described above may be used temporarily.

Dietary Therapy

Modification of diet is a cornerstone of peptic ulcer therapy; however, the traditional "ulcer diet" with a high proportion of milk and cream is no longer used. The dietary regimen will depend on the stage of the disease and other factors. Smaller, more frequent meals may be given to prevent exacerbation of symptoms related to an empty stomach. A semibland diet may be prescribed, and the client may be advised to avoid fruits and spicy foods, but this must be decided on an individual basis with the client's condition and preferences in mind. Foods that promote symptoms in that particular client should be eliminated. Frequent offenders include coffee (with or without caffeine), alcohol, and foods containing caffeine, such as chocolate and some soft drinks. Some researchers report that a diet high in fiber appears to prevent recurrence of healed duodenal ulcers (Rydning et al., 1982).

Surgical Treatment

Some clients with peptic ulcer disease will require surgery, especially when persistent hemorrhage, perforation, obstruction, or intractable ulcer are present. Surgical therapies for duodenal ulceration include various combinations of vagotomy (severing of the vagus nerve), pyloroplasty, and resection of portions of the stomach and/or duodenum. Surgical procedures used in gastric ulceration include various forms of resection and anastomosis, for example, antrectomy with gastroduodenal anastomosis (Billroth I). These procedures are discussed in Chapter 50.

Specific Nursing Measures

Assessment, especially of food intolerances, is a major nursing responsibility in caring for clients with diagnosed peptic ulcer disease. When caring for surgical clients, burned

clients, and those with severe trauma, be alert for signs of bleeding that may signal the development of stress ulcers (eg, black tarry stools). In all clients with peptic ulcer disease, evaluate client comfort and response to therapy on an ongoing basis. Because complications such as hemorrhage or peritonitis can be life threatening, continual assessment of stools, emesis or GI drainage, peristalsis, and pain level are essential.

Once a plan of care has been developed, help clients integrate it into their particular lifestyle. Explain medication and diet regimens and warn the client about side effects and possible toxicity. Clients should avoid coffee, cola, cigarettes, aspirin, and other irritating drugs. New health care providers should be informed about the client's history of ulcer disease. The client must be instructed about the course of the disease and the nature and signs of possible complications. For example, hematemesis or black tarry stools (melena) should be reported immediately, because they signal the recurrence of bleeding.

Because psychosocial stresses can worsen the disease, the nurse, client, and significant others should work together to reduce stresses in the client's environment. Stress reduction techniques such as relaxation breathing can help the client cope (see Chapter 4). For hospitalized clients, reduction of stresses associated with the hospital setting is mandatory.

INTESTINAL DIVERTICULAR DISEASE

Diverticulosis is the asymptomatic presence of herniations or outpouchings of the intestinal mucosa (**diverticuli**). Fecal material may become entrapped within one or more diverticula; the resulting inflammation, which causes symptoms, is called diverticulitis. Diverticulosis may affect either the small or the large intestine. A congenital form (Meckel's diverticulum of the ileum) exists, but most cases of diverticulosis are acquired. Diverticuli of the large intestine are shown in Figure 49–2.

The incidence of diverticulosis increases with age; two-thirds of individuals 85 years or older in the United States are believed to have the disorder. In younger age groups, it is predominantly a disease of males and in older age groups, of females (Greenberger, 1981).

One suggested etiology is increased pressure on the lumen of the intestine that produces herniation at weak areas, for example, where blood vessels penetrate the intestinal wall. Other suggested etiological factors include atrophy or weakness of the bowel musculature related to aging, obesity, chronic constipation and straining at stool, and abnormalities of intestinal motility.

The role of diet in the formation of diverticuli has recently received considerable attention. Incidence of the disorder is higher in cultures where highly processed foods low in fiber form a significant part of the diet; it is lower among populations who consume large amounts of fiber. It is known that the presence of fiber (roughage) speeds the transit of the stool; conversely, the stool remains longer

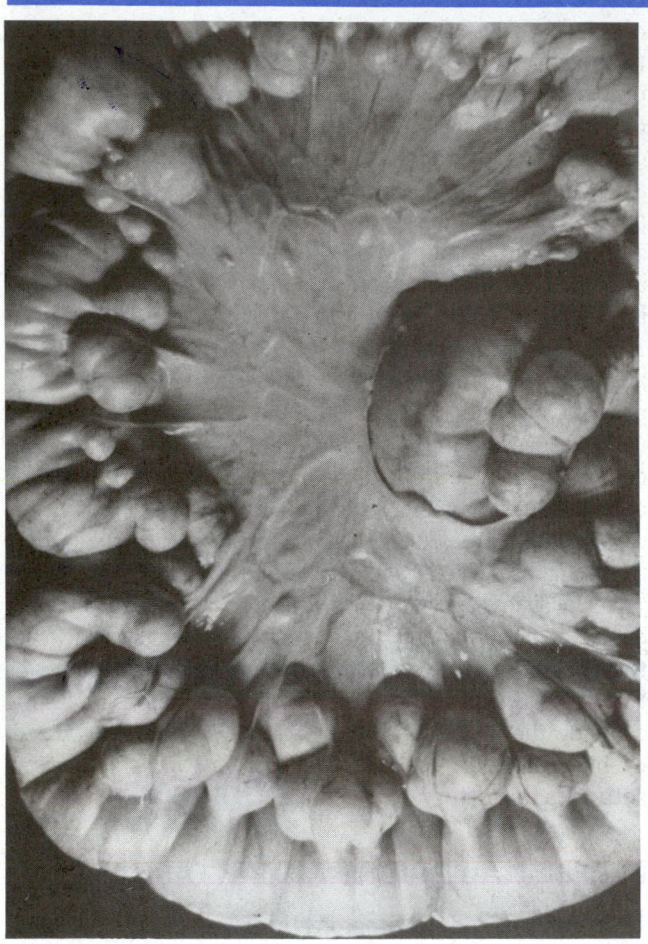

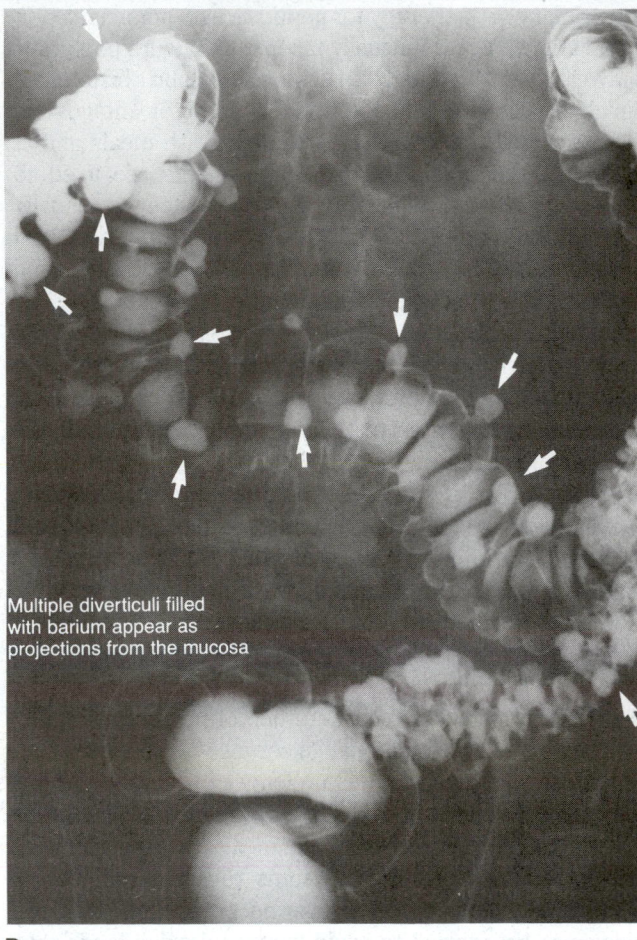

Multiple diverticuli filled
with barium appear as
projections from the mucosa

Figure 49–2

A. Diverticuli of the large intestine. **B.** Multiple diverticuli of the large intestine as seen on barium enema. The diverticuli filled with barium appear as projections from the mucosa (arrows). (A, Photo by James A. Pierotti, Millard Fillmore Hospital. B, Courtesy of Health Care Plan, Buffalo, NY)

in the intestine if fiber is inadequate. More water is reabsorbed from the stool, leaving harder, drier feces and promoting constipation. Accumulation of a hard mass of dry stool (a **fecalith**) in a diverticular sac may cause it to become inflamed.

Clinical Manifestations

Diverticulosis is usually asymptomatic, although constipation, vague abdominal pain and cramping, and abdominal distention may occur. Usually, the diagnosis is made incidentally during diagnostic evaluation for a different problem.

If diverticulitis occurs, however, the client may report episodic, dull midabdominal or lower-abdominal pain that can radiate to the back. Change in bowel habits, excessive flatulence, bloating, and fever may also occur (Given & Simmons, 1984). Acute symptoms typically follow ingestion of a large meal, alcohol, or a large quantity of roughage. Rectal bleeding may also be noted.

In severe cases of diverticulitis, inflammation may lead

to perforation and thus to peritonitis. Edema or fibrosis associated with diverticular inflammation may cause intestinal obstruction. Fistulae may form between the intestine and the urinary bladder, ureter, vagina, abdominal wall, or perineum. These complications increase morbidity and the risk of mortality.

Diagnosis may be confirmed by barium studies, although these are contraindicated in acute diverticulitis, since they may cause further irritation and even perforation. The WBC and ESR may be elevated, reflecting the inflammatory process. Endoscopy may be used to differentiate diverticular disease from carcinoma, but, like barium studies, this procedure is contraindicated in acute diverticulitis.

Therapeutic Measures

Treatment of diverticular disease depends on whether inflammation (diverticulitis) is present. If it is not, therapy focuses on avoiding increases of intraluminal pressure, which could precipitate diverticulitis. Bulk laxatives such as psyllium and a high-fiber diet are used to prevent constipation and straining at stool.

Diverticulitis can be managed by nonsurgical means in 90% of clients (Given & Simmons, 1984). Treatment is aimed at allowing the colon to rest so the inflamed diverticula can heal. Depending on the severity of symptoms, the client may be treated at home or in the hospital. If hemorrhage, perforation, or obstruction are present, hospitalization is necessary. The client may be NPO, or a low-residue diet may be ordered. A nasogastric tube may be passed to decompress the intestinal tract. Clients who are NPO may be given intravenous supplementation or, if NPO status is prolonged, total parenteral nutrition (TPN). Antibiotics may be prescribed. Although analgesics are sometimes ordered, caution is indicated since symptoms of complications may be masked.

Acute attacks of diverticulitis generally subside within a week. In 10% of cases, diseased portions of the colon may be resected, especially if therapy is ineffective or if episodes of inflammation continually recur. A temporary colostomy may be indicated.

Specific Nursing Measures

The nursing care plan should focus on promoting comfort, maintaining adequate nutrition, evaluating treatment outcomes, and monitoring for complications. Clients may be apprehensive about the treatment regimen or may fear that cancer is present, especially if rectal bleeding has occurred. Once the results of tests and diagnostic studies are known, the nurse can reassure the client and reinforce explanations of the findings.

If NPO status and/or intravenous therapy is ordered, the nursing responsibilities associated with these therapies must be carried out. Once food is permitted, a low-residue diet may be ordered. The regimen must be explained to the client and preparations for home care made.

INTESTINAL HERNIA

Protrusion of a portion of the intestine through the abdominal wall is called an intestinal (abdominal) hernia. Although the condition may be congenital, it is usually acquired as a result of conditions that increase intra-abdominal pressure and/or cause the abdominal wall to weaken. Increased pressure may be associated with obesity, pregnancy, coughing or sneezing, lifting, constipation, or straining at stool. Weakening of the abdominal wall may be associated with disease or with aging.

Various types of intestinal hernias are given names according to their location: umbilical hernia (at the umbilicus), inguinal hernia (at the inguinal ring), and femoral hernia (at the femoral ring). An intestinal hernia may also occur at the site of an abdominal incision (incisional or ventral hernia) (Figure 49–3). Inguinal hernias are the most common, usually occurring in males.

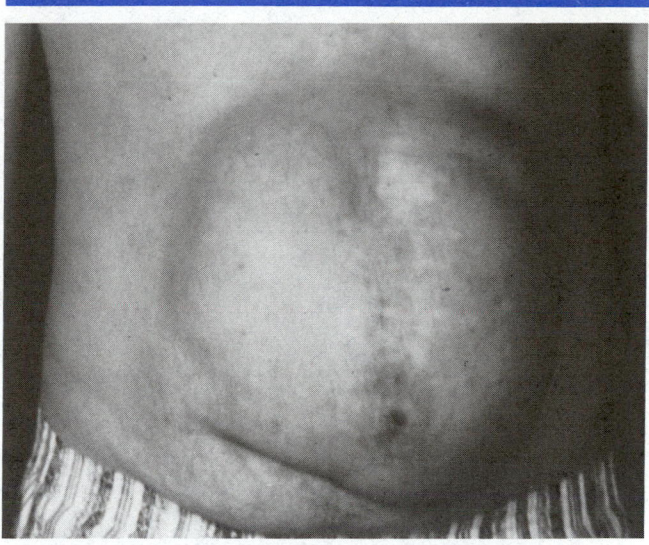

Figure 49–3

Ventral incisional hernia. (Courtesy Millard Fillmore Hospital, Buffalo, NY)

Clinical Manifestations

An abdominal bulge may be seen on physical examination. Palpation discloses a soft, tender mass. The client may notice that the hernia increases in size during straining or exertion and may feel tenderness at the site.

Major complications of hernia include strangulation and incarceration. In strangulation, the margins of the defect constrict the protruding loop of bowel so severely that blood flow is obstructed, leading to tissue necrosis and/or infection. If a hernia cannot be pushed back into the abdominal cavity (reduced), the condition is called incarceration. Both conditions may be associated with severe pain, nausea, vomiting, and fever. An incarcerated hernia may cause symptoms typical of intestinal obstruction. Figure 49–4A shows the herniation of a loop of intestine through the abdominal wall. Figure 49–4B shows the appearance of the herniated bowel during surgical repair.

Therapeutic Measures

The client with a hernia is generally advised to avoid any activities that increase abdominal pressure. Stool softeners, psyllium, and a high-residue diet may be prescribed to prevent constipation and straining at stool, which could aggravate the condition. The client is usually told to avoid straining and stretching and to use proper body mechanics. A truss (firm support) may be prescribed; it should be worn as much as possible, especially when the client is ambulating. Temporary reduction of the hernia by pushing it manually back through the abdominal wall may make the client more comfortable and avert strangulation and incarceration. Permanent reduction can be accomplished only

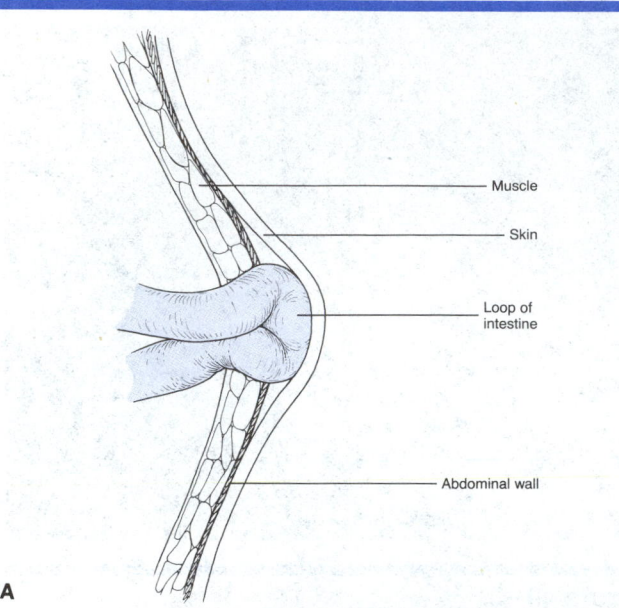

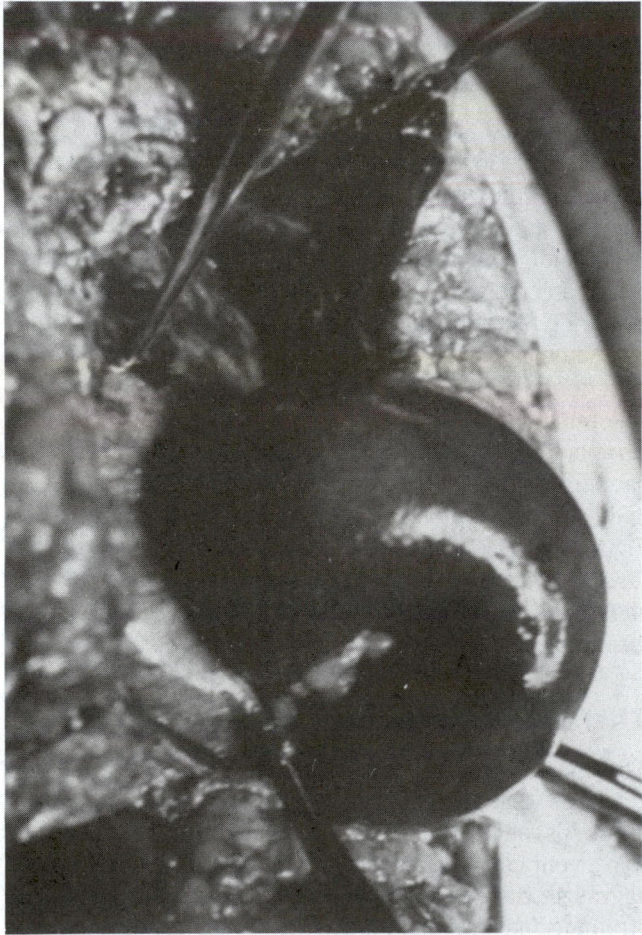

Figure 49–4

A. Herniation of a loop of intestine through the abdominal wall. **B.** Appearance of the herniated bowel during surgical repair. (Courtesy Millard Fillmore Hospital, Buffalo, NY)

by surgery (herniorrhaphy), which is described in Chapter 50. Hernias may recur after surgical repair, so the client will need to learn proper body mechanics and other preventive measures.

Specific Nursing Measures

Observe the client for complications. Instruct the client about the importance of a high-fiber diet with adequate fluids and the avoidance of straining and stretching. Many persons are unaware of proper body mechanics, which the nurse can teach. Clients should also avoid weight gain and should give up smoking to eliminate the continual problem of smoker's cough.

IRRITABLE BOWEL SYNDROME

Irritable bowel syndrome, the most common functional intestinal disorder, is a disturbance of motility that cannot be attributed to an organic cause. The disorder is variously (and inappropriately) referred to as irritable colon, functional diarrhea, spastic colitis, and mucous colitis. It affects women more often than men and is often first seen when clients are in their twenties or thirties.

Various etiologies have been suggested, including emotional turmoil and food intolerance. Some recent research has suggested that the disorder is related to elevated levels of the hormones gastrin and cholecystokinin, which may excessively stimulate an unusually sensitive GI tract (Legerton, 1981). Increased symptoms have been noted following cholecystectomy, possibly in relation to increased levels of cholecystokinin postoperatively.

Clinical Manifestations

Symptoms of irritable bowel syndrome generally fall into one of three basic patterns (Legerton, 1981):

- Alternating constipation and diarrhea, with or without abdominal pain
- Constipation associated with abdominal pain
- Persistent, usually painless, diarrhea

Symptoms are generally chronic and may be triggered or worsened by stress. Because the intestine is irritated and unusually sensitive, excessive mucus may appear in the stools. Diarrhea, when present, generally occurs in the morning and in clusters. Tests of the stool for signs indicating a known organic cause—blood, pus, excessive fat, parasites, or ova—are usually negative.

The symptoms of irritable bowel syndrome closely resemble those of lactose intolerance, and this diagnosis must be ruled out before a definitive diagnosis can be established. Clients with irritable bowel syndrome are usually advised to have routine examinations to detect any organic disease that might develop, but irritable bowel syndrome has not been associated with inflammatory bowel disease or cancer.

Therapeutic Measures

Since no organic cause is known, treatment of irritable bowel syndrome is primarily symptomatic. The client can be helped but probably not cured. Treatment generally occurs outside the hospital.

If constipation is present, a high-fiber diet, adequate fluid intake, and increased activity are indicated. Bulk laxatives may be prescribed. For treatment of diarrhea, anti-motility drugs may be indicated, such as anticholinergics (tincture of belladonna), diphenoxylate hydrochloride (Lomotil), or opiates (paregoric). The client should avoid foods that aggravate symptoms.

The persistent bowel symptoms associated with irritable bowel syndrome can seriously affect the client's lifestyle. Clients frequently suffer from depression (manifested by fatigue, insomnia, and lethargy) and may require psychological counseling or medication. Because symptoms of irritable bowel syndrome are often stress related, the caregiver should discuss this aspect of the disorder with the client. Stress reduction techniques may be helpful.

Specific Nursing Measures

The client with irritable bowel syndrome needs a great deal of psychological support. Not only are the symptoms unpleasant, inconvenient, and often painful, but the absence of a clear organic etiology for the disorder may lead some caregivers to dismiss the client as "neurotic" and not deserving of serious attention.

The nurse can help the client determine which foods seem to promote or aggravate symptoms. Client, nurse, and dietitian together may plan a dietary regimen appropriate to the client's culture and lifestyle. The relation of stress to the client's symptoms can be explored with a view toward eliminating stressful situations where feasible. The nurse may also teach techniques for stress reduction (see Chapter 4).

HEMORRHOIDS AND FISSURES

Hemorrhoids and fissures are common acquired disorders of the anorectal area. Hemorrhoids are excessively distended veins in the anal area. They may be internal (generally remaining within the anal area and covered with mucous membrane) or external (prolapsing through the anal canal). Fissures are cracks in the skin at the anus. Both conditions are associated with increased pressure in the anal area related, for example, to chronic constipation and straining, obesity, or pregnancy.

Clinical Manifestations

Both hemorrhoids and fissures can be detected on physical examination. External hemorrhoids appear as a cluster of red, blue, or pink tissue at the anal area; internal hemor-

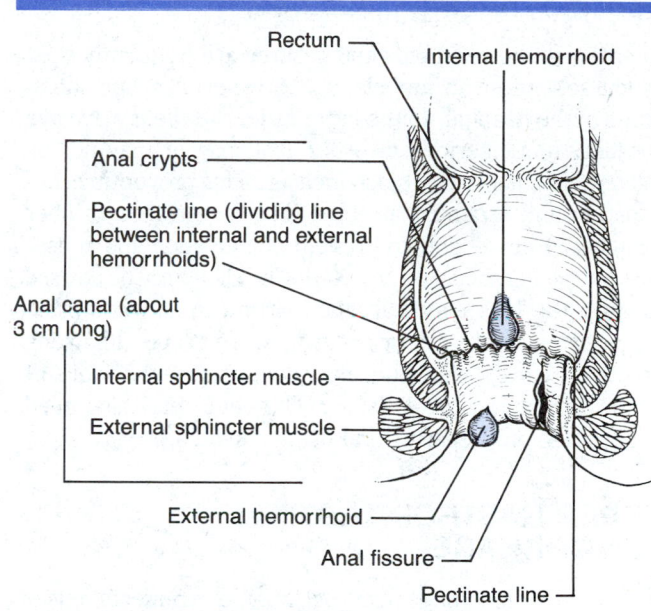

Figure 49–5

Anorectal structures with external and internal hemorrhoids and anal fissure.

rhoids may be palpated on digital examination. Fissures are generally apparent on inspection and may be inflamed (Figure 49–5). A fissure causes extreme pain when a digital rectal examination is performed.

The client with hemorrhoids or fissures will generally describe symptoms of pain and bleeding, especially in association with defecation. Pruritus may also occur, especially with external hemorrhoids. Hemorrhoids may become thrombosed, and both hemorrhoids and fissures may become infected, with or without abscess formation. Bleeding may also occur.

Therapeutic Measures

Treatment is generally aimed at decreasing pressure in the perineum and relieving pain and/or itching. If symptoms are acute, a low-residue diet may be prescribed to prevent further irritation and allow the lesion to heal. Generally, however, a high-residue diet, stool softeners, and bulk laxatives are prescribed to prevent constipation and straining.

Symptoms can often be relieved by limiting activity, applying moist heat (sitz baths), and applying local anesthetic agents (usually containing benzocaine), or anti-inflammatory creams (usually containing steroids). Good hygiene is important in preventing infection.

Fissures generally heal spontaneously. Hemorrhoids can be alleviated, but acute symptoms may recur. Hemorrhoidectomy may be required if complications occur or if symptoms are especially troublesome. This procedure is discussed in Chapter 50.

Specific Nursing Measures

Clients with hemorrhoids and fissures are frequently seen by nurses, often in ambulatory care settings but sometimes in the hospital. In the latter case, the client may have another, more serious disorder that may or may not be related. The nurse can teach measures for preventing constipation and straining at stool. The importance of fiber (roughage) in the diet to prevent constipation and consequent straining should be stressed. The client may be advised to keep the legs elevated when sitting to alleviate pressure related to obesity or pregnancy. Teach good hygiene practices: careful cleansing after defecation and use of soft white, unscented toilet tissue. The client may also need information on preparing and using a sitz bath.

UPPER GASTROINTESTINAL HEMORRHAGE

Upper GI hemorrhage may occur as a manifestation or complication of a number of disorders of the upper gastrointestinal tract. Hemorrhage can significantly compromise a client's physiological and psychological status and can increase the morbidity and mortality associated with the primary disease process.

The most common causes of upper GI bleeding are peptic ulcer disease, erosive gastritis, and esophageal varices (Petersdorf, 1983) (Figure 49–6). (Care of the client with bleeding esophageal varices is discussed in Unit Nine.) Other primary disorders associated with upper GI hemorrhage include esophagitis; esophageal, gastric, and

intestinal cancer; and trauma. Mallory–Weiss syndrome (esophageal laceration secondary to vomiting and retching) and blood dyscrasias that alter coagulation are also associated with upper GI bleeding.

Clinical Manifestations

Upper gastrointestinal hemorrhage may be accompanied by hematemesis, melena, hematochezia, and/or occult blood in the stools. Hematemesis (bloody vomitus) may appear red, dark red, brown, or black, depending on how long blood and gastric acids have been in contact. Ordinarily, the longer the contact, the darker the vomited blood. The characteristic "coffee-ground" appearance of the emesis occurs when blood clots have undergone digestion. If blood is not vomited, digestive changes that occur during its passage through the GI tract will promote a characteristic black tarry appearance of the stool (melena).

If a large amount of blood is present in the intestine, however, intestinal motility increases, and blood that originates high in the GI tract will be bright red when it is passed from the rectum (**hematochezia**). Generally, however, hematochezia signifies bleeding from the small or large intestine, or the rectum.

In many cases, bleeding will be less obvious. Hidden (occult) blood in the stool can be identified only by specific testing (eg, Hematest or guaiac testing). Note that stool tests will be positive for up to 3 weeks after a bleeding episode.

Hemorrhage may be acute or long term. Long-term (chronic) blood loss may go undetected until stools are tested for occult blood, often in the course of routine examination, or signs of iron-deficiency anemia appear (weakness, fatigue, lethargy, pallor).

Acute hemorrhage and major blood loss often appear without warning and may be life threatening. It may appear as hematemesis, melena, or hematochezia. If the client has a nasogastric tube to suction, blood will be apparent in the aspirated drainage.

Rapid, acute blood loss of less than 500 mL is rarely associated with systemic signs in adults, except in the elderly and in clients who are anemic. With losses greater than 500 mL, however, the client will experience orthostatic hypotension, syncope, nausea, thirst, and diaphoresis. As blood loss approaches 40% of total blood volume, hypovolemic shock may follow, with pallor; cool, clammy skin; hypotension; and tachycardia (Petersdorf, 1983). A large quantity of blood in the GI tract may cause nausea, abdominal distention, cramping, diarrhea, and borborygmi.

Laboratory studies will reflect hemorrhage and altered hemodynamics. Hemoglobin (Hb) and hematocrit (Hct) readings will eventually reflect a decrease in the number of circulating erythrocytes, although blood loss may not be accurately reflected for up to 36 hours (Greenberger, 1981). Initially, Hb and Hct readings remain normal. An elevated blood urea nitrogen (BUN) level in the presence of a nor-

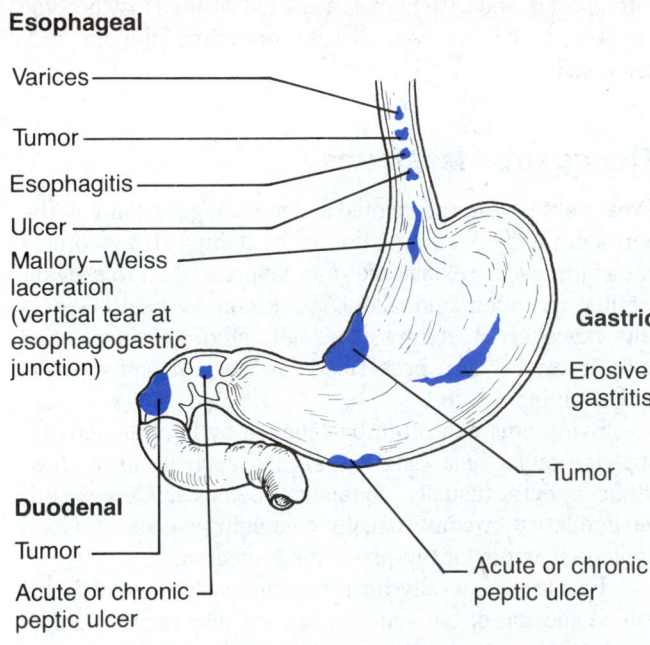

Esophageal

Varices

Tumor

Esophagitis

Ulcer

Mallory–Weiss laceration (vertical tear at esophagogastric junction)

Gastric

Erosive gastritis

Tumor

Duodenal

Tumor

Acute or chronic peptic ulcer

Acute or chronic peptic ulcer

Figure 49–6

Common causes of upper GI bleeding.

mal serum creatinine level suggests upper GI blood loss in excess of 1000 mL. The BUN level is elevated as a consequence of digestion and absorption of blood protein from the GI tract (Greenberger, 1981).

Various assessments may be used to estimate blood loss. In the *tilt test,* pulse and blood pressure are measured first while the client lies flat and again after the client has sat for 1 minute (Lamphier & Lamphier, 1981). Losses of less than 500 mL generally cause a rise in pulse rate of 20 to 25 beats per minute. Blood losses greater than 500 mL generally cause more significant increase in the pulse rate and a drop in systolic pressure. A client who experiences hypotension and tachycardia while supine has probably lost at least 50% of total blood volume. *Leg raising* while the client is in the reclining position will cause the pulse rate to decrease and the blood pressure to increase if volume depletion is significant (Lamphier & Lamphier, 1981).

Therapeutic Measures

Unless anemia is severe, the client with chronic blood loss may be treated as an outpatient. The primary source of the blood loss must be identified and any iron-deficiency anemia corrected. A client with acute, severe hemorrhage is critically ill and must be hospitalized. Treatment priorities include controlling the hemorrhage, preventing shock, and determining the cause of the hemorrhage. A careful history obtained from the client or a reliable significant other helps identify factors that could precipitate hemorrhage (eg, heavy use of alcohol or aspirin, anticoagulant therapy, history of ulcer disease). Endoscopy, angiography, and barium studies may also be used in diagnosing the primary condition.

Immediate intravenous fluid replacement is generally initiated. Normal saline and plasma expanders are generally infused until the client's blood has been typed and crossmatched and whole blood is available for transfusion. Packed red cells may be prescribed to prevent circulatory overload if the client has heart disease or congestive heart failure. Fresh frozen plasma or fresh whole blood is generally not necessary unless many transfusions of stored blood have been administered. In this case, coagulation factors, often lost in stored blood, must be replaced from fresh whole blood or plasma.

Strict intake/output measurement is initiated, and an indwelling catheter may be inserted to facilitate frequent assessment of blood volume status as reflected in urinary output. A central venous pressure (CVP) line or Swan–Ganz catheter may also be inserted so circulatory volume can be continually assessed. Nasogastric intubation may be necessary so accumulated blood and clots can be aspirated and blood loss measured. Iced saline lavage may also be initiated; the cooled solution promotes vasoconstriction and helps stop hemorrhage.

Pharmacologic therapy is generally initiated as soon as possible to stop or prevent bleeding. Antacids are generally ordered and instilled via the nasogastric tube. Intravenous cimetidine (Tagamet) is also generally prescribed.

Among the specific procedures that may be implemented to control hemorrhage are selective angiography combined with vasopressin infusion or embolization, or endoscopy with electrocoagulation or laser therapy. In the first case, selective angiography localizes the hemorrhage. Vasopressin may be infused to promote vasoconstriction, or natural or synthesized clots may be injected into the bleeding vessel (embolization). Endoscopy may also be used where the bleeding vessel is cauterized by electrocautery or by a laser beam.

Surgery to control hemorrhage may be indicated when hemorrhage requires more than 6 to 8 units of blood, when hemorrhage remains uncontrolled for more than 24 to 48 hours, or when blood transfusion fails to restore circulatory volume (Lamphier & Lamphier, 1981). If the source of hemorrhage is unknown, exploratory laparotomy is indicated; if the cause is known, the appropriate procedure is performed.

Specific Nursing Measures

The client with upper GI hemorrhage challenges all the nurse's assessment and intervention skills. Keen observation can be instrumental in detecting signs of anemia in a client with slow, chronic bleeding. Precise assessment is critical in monitoring the client's status during an episode of acute bleeding accompanied by shock and deterioration. Quick thinking and quick action are required.

Intake/output records must be meticulously maintained and transfusions administered safely. If posttransfusion Hct readings are ordered, keep current with the results. Hydration and circulatory status must be frequently assessed: output may be measured every half hour, as may vital signs; urinary specific gravity may be monitored, and skin should be assessed for pallor and turgor.

If the client has a nasogastric tube to suction, its patency must be closely monitored and the tube irrigated (if permitted) as often as necessary to ensure that clots do not obstruct the flow of drainage. If iced saline lavage is to be performed, the procedure described in Box 49–1 should be followed. Antacids or other medications instilled via the nasogastric tube should be followed with water, and suction should be halted temporarily so that the medication can be absorbed and is not washed out.

The client's physiological and psychological comfort deserves careful attention. If hemorrhage has been severe, the client may be covered with blood and should be washed, provided with a clean gown, and otherwise made comfortable. Losing large amounts of blood is frightening as well as dangerous, and the nurse should take time to reassure the client and family and to explain briefly what is being done to control the hemorrhage. Family members should be permitted to be at the bedside if at all possible, since the presence of familiar persons may help calm the client.

Positioning is important, especially for clients in shock. The recumbent position with legs elevated is generally recommended. The client may be in pain; prescribed analgesics and nursing comfort measures are indicated.

LOWER GASTROINTESTINAL HEMORRHAGE

Gastrointestinal bleeding distal to the duodenum—ie, from the jejunum, ileum, colon, or rectum—is characterized as lower GI hemorrhage. It may be mild, moderate, or severe. Hemorrhage may be a chronic manifestation of a disease process or may appear spontaneously and be life threatening.

Lower GI hemorrhage may be precipitated by a number of disorders discussed in this section, including hemorrhoids and fissures, rectal fistula, proctitis, cancer of the bowel, polyps, infectious diarrhea, inflammatory bowel disease, ischemic colitis, intestinal diverticular disease, trauma, colonic angiodysplasia (distended colonic vasculature, a degenerative process associated with aging), or radiation-induced bowel disease. The most common cause is diverticular disease.

Clinical Manifestations

Acute, severe lower GI hemorrhage is usually characterized by hematochezia, but melena may herald the condition if constipation or obstruction is present. The client may have abdominal pain, cramping, distention, and/or diarrhea. *Chronic,* slow blood loss generally presents as iron-deficiency anemia and occult blood in the stool.

Like upper GI hemorrhage, bleeding in the lower tract may be accompanied by hypovolemic shock and alteration in laboratory values, depending on the severity of blood loss. Refer to the discussion of upper GI hemorrhage for clinical manifestations of blood loss and means of estimating its severity. In some cases, lower GI hemorrhage may be associated with intestinal perforation and peritonitis.

Therapeutic Measures

Treatment is designed to stop bleeding, prevent shock, and determine the underlying cause of the hemorrhage. Sigmoidoscopy and/or colonoscopy is often performed, although the usual bowel preparation is omitted if the client is actively bleeding. Angiography with vasopressin infusion or embolization may be performed to control severe bleeding (see discussion under upper GI hemorrhage). Barium studies may be performed once active bleeding has ceased, if no diagnosis has been established.

The gastrointestinal tract is generally allowed to rest, and the client is generally kept NPO and hydrated intravenously. Nasogastric intubation may be used for decompression, but iced saline lavage is not indicated. Fluid/electrolyte balance must be carefully monitored, and an indwelling catheter may be inserted to facilitate input/output measurement and urine studies. Fluid and/or blood replacement is provided as indicated (see discussion under upper GI tract). Prophylactic antacids and cimetidine may be prescribed to prevent stress ulceration.

After an acute episode of upper GI bleeding, or in cases of chronic hemorrhage, a low-residue diet is generally indicated. Iron-deficiency anemia, if present, will require treatment.

Surgery may be required if hemorrhage remains uncontrolled and/or severe, or if it recurs.

Specific Nursing Measures

Supportive therapy will be required, including efficient, accurate, and safe assessment and implementation. Measures used are similar to those discussed under upper GI hemorrhage.

Section II: Inflammatory and Infectious Disorders

Inflammatory and/or infectious disorders of the stomach, intestine, and pancreas may be related to internal or external irritation, diet, or proliferation of pathogenic bacteria. These disorders are fairly common in the adult population and therefore pose a significant health problem.

Significant interference with the lifestyle of the individual may be associated with symptoms such as persistent pain with eating, intolerance to certain foods, and diarrhea. Furthermore, some complications of these disorders, such as hemorrhage, sepsis, and malnutrition, may be life threatening. Clients with infectious or inflammatory GI disorders are often cared for in the community, although a client whose physiological status is seriously altered may be hospitalized.

PERITONITIS

Peritonitis, an inflammation of the peritoneum, is a potentially life-threatening complication of disorders of the abdominal organs. It is associated with significant morbidity and mortality and is the most common cause of death following abdominal surgery (Given & Simmons, 1984).

Various disorders can lead to peritonitis, including perforated peptic ulcer, ruptured appendix, gangrene of the bowel, perforated diverticulum, trauma, and, as already mentioned, abdominal surgery (Figure 49–7). Drainage from a perforated or infected area, as well as the introduction of foreign matter (eg, talc in surgical gloves), can chemically or mechanically irritate the peritoneal cavity,

stimulating the inflammatory process and fostering the proliferation of pathogenic bacteria.

Clinical Manifestations

The onset of peritonitis is sometimes slow and progressive but more often is acute. The vascular hyperemia integral to the inflammatory process causes accumulation of fluid in the abdominal cavity, and thereby abdominal distention and rigidity, pain, anorexia, nausea, and vomiting. The client will often describe pain as severe and report that it intensifies with movement. Muscle guarding is generally noted, and the client may obtain some relief by flexing the knees while recumbent.

Fever and tachycardia will be present, and rebound tenderness will be apparent on palpation. On auscultation, bowel sounds may be diminished or absent, as paralytic ileus may develop. Respiratory function may be seriously compromised, since abdominal distention can inhibit full

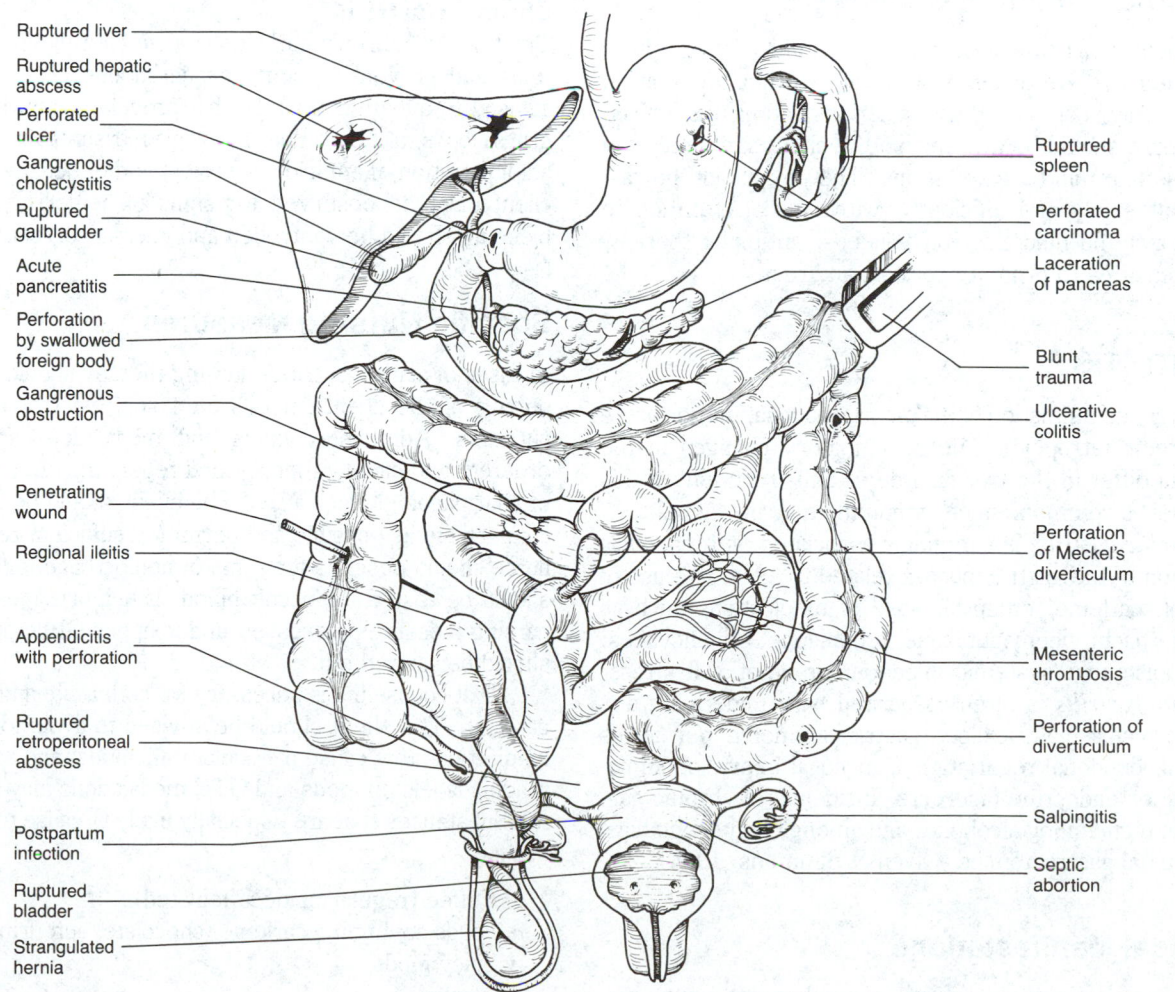

Figure 49–7

Causes of peritonitis.

expansion of the diaphragm. Respirations may become shallow, and hypoxia with signs of tachycardia, restlessness, and cyanosis may occur. Hemodynamics can be seriously affected, leading to shock.

Therapeutic Measures

Septic peritonitis is life threatening and requires prompt and rigorous treatment. The source of irritation must be identified and removed (eg, by appendectomy, gastrectomy, etc.). An exploratory laparotomy will be performed if life-threatening symptoms persist and the source has not been identified. Supportive treatment involves careful monitoring of fluid intake and output; observation for shock; maintenance of circulating fluid volume with intravenous fluids; correction of nutritional, electrolyte, and acid–base imbalances; and administration of antibiotics. Pain relief is also indicated, but analgesics must be used cautiously to prevent masking of diagnostic clues. To alleviate nausea and vomiting, antiemetics are often prescribed.

Specific Nursing Measures

The client with acute peritonitis is generally frightened and apprehensive. He or she may have been healthy, only to be suddenly hospitalized with a serious and painful illness. The nurse should be available so the client and family can express fears and ask questions. Therapy should be carried out safely and efficiently, with special attention to nutritional and fluid/electrolyte needs, antibiotic therapy, and measures to promote comfort and rest.

GASTRITIS

Gastritis, inflammation of the gastric mucosa, may be acute or chronic (atrophic). The inflammatory changes in the mucosa differ in the two disorders. Self-treatment of this disorder is common, since symptoms may be vague.

Acute gastritis is commonly associated with chemical irritation of the gastric mucosa related to excessive use of alcohol, caffeine, or spices; use of medications such as indomethacin, phenylbutazone, prednisone, or salicylates; food poisoning; systemic infection; or emotional stress. *Chronic gastritis* is often associated with underlying disorders such as gastric ulcer, gastric carcinoma, pernicious anemia, duodenal regurgitation, mucosal injury, or immunologic or endocrine disorders. Incidence of chronic gastritis is high among alcoholics and among clients who have had partial gastrectomies (Given & Simmons, 1984).

Clinical Manifestations

Chronic gastritis is sometimes asymptomatic; acute gastritis is always symptomatic. Symptoms of either disorder include epigastric discomfort, bloating, anorexia, nausea, vomiting, abdominal cramping, diarrhea, and eructation.

Hemorrhage may occur and can present as hematemesis, melena, or occult blood in the stool. Iron-deficiency anemia can result from long-term blood loss. Diagnosis is generally based on history, gastroscopy, and biopsy.

Therapeutic Measures

Acute Gastritis

The client with acute gastritis is treated symptomatically. The stomach is permitted to rest and heal while the client is kept NPO and is nourished intravenously until symptoms dissipate. Nasogastric suctioning may be necessary, and, if the client is bleeding, iced saline lavage may be used. A full discussion of treatment and nursing care for upper GI hemorrhage was presented earlier in this chapter.

Antacids are generally administered, by mouth or by nasogastric tube. Antiemetics may also be prescribed, as may anticholinergics or analgesics. As the inflammation subsides and symptoms diminish, the client gradually returns to a normal diet, although any particularly offensive foods are eliminated.

Chronic Gastritis

Treatment of chronic gastritis is aimed at relieving symptoms and preventing acute exacerbations. The client is advised to avoid substances that provoke symptoms (eg, drugs, foods, alcohol). Pharmacologic measures may include administration of antacids, steroids, and/or sedatives. The client must be observed for signs of hemorrhage. Any bleeding should be controlled and anemia corrected.

Specific Nursing Measures

In cases of acute gastritis, nursing therapy should be supportive of the client's needs for fluids, electrolytes, and nutrients. Administer fluids and medications safely as ordered, and closely monitor and report the effectiveness of pharmacologic measures. The client should be made as comfortable as possible and permitted sufficient rest. The nurse should observe for signs of hemorrhage, and stools should be tested for occult blood. If hemorrhage occurs, nursing measures discussed under upper GI hemorrhage should be carried out.

Diet counseling is necessary for both acute and chronic gastritis. The client should be advised to avoid foods and medications that cause particular difficulties, and advice on reading labels on foods and OTC medications may be helpful. Substances that are especially likely to cause problems include:

- Coffee (regular or decaffeinated)
- Foods containing caffeine (chocolate, soft drinks, tea)
- Spicy foods
- Alcohol
- Salicylates (ie, aspirin and aspirin-containing preparations)
- Ibuprofen (Motrin, Rufen, Advil, Nuprin)

- Indomethacin (Indocin)
- Phenylbutazone (Butazolidin, Azolid)
- Steroids

PANCREATITIS

Inflammation of the pancreas, or pancreatitis, may occur in either acute or chronic form. Both forms may be relapsing and, in both cases, inflammation may cause extensive pancreatic tissue changes and/or damage. In some cases tissue regeneration and healing occurs. In others, pancreatic damage may be permanent.

Any disorder that interferes with the flow of biliary or pancreatic secretions or renders secretions more viscous, may precipitate stasis and/or reflux of secretions into the pancreas, leading to inflammation. Autodigestion of pancreatic cells by pancreatic enzymes has also been suggested as a cause of inflammation, degeneration, and, in severe cases, necrosis. Pancreatitis may accompany:

- Excessive use of alcohol
- Excessive use of certain medications:
    thiazide diuretics
    steroids
    acetaminophen
    oral contraceptives
- Biliary tract disease
- Abdominal surgery
- Trauma
- Penetrating duodenal ulcer
- Metabolic disorders
- Infection

The exact mechanism by which these factors are associated with pancreatitis is unclear.

Clinical Manifestations

Both acute and chronic pancreatitis are associated with similar symptoms: anorexia, nausea, vomiting, and upper abdominal pain. The pain is generally steady and may radiate to the upper back. The pain is so severe and intractable, even in chronic pancreatitis, that the client may be unable to eat or to work and may even become addicted to narcotics (Kosel et al., 1982). Fever is common.

On examination, abdominal rigidity and muscle guarding will be noted, and bowel sounds may be diminished. If the common bile duct is obstructed, jaundice occurs. The client is usually unable to tolerate fatty foods, and diarrhea and steatorrhea commonly occur, because enzymes capable of hydrolyzing lipids are absent or deficient. If symptoms persist, the client may lose weight and develop nutritional deficiencies. Fluid shift related to the inflammatory process may precipitate dehydration, pleural effusion and hypoxia, ascites, peritonitis, and/or shock. Hemorrhage related to tissue damage may also occur.

Blood studies reveal leukocytosis (related to inflammation and/or infection) and elevated glucose levels (related to pancreatic cellular damage or to stress). In the absence of lipolytic enzymes, calcium may be used to digest accumulated fats in the pancreas, leading to hypocalcemia. Clinical manifestations of altered glucose metabolism and calcium imbalance may be present. Chronic pancreatitis can precipitate diabetes. Ultrasound and CT scanning may be useful in diagnosis.

Therapeutic Measures

Therapeutic goals include identifying and, if possible, eliminating the cause, relieving symptoms, and preventing complications. Surgery may be necessary to correct the primary disorder. Symptomatic relief measures include nasogastric intubation to rest and decompress the GI tract, analgesics, antiemetics, and anticholinergics (to reduce pancreatic and ductal spasm). Intravenous fluids and electrolytes and parenteral hyperalimentation are administered as necessary to maintain fluid/electrolyte and nutritional balance.

The client is initially NPO. As symptoms subside and clinical and laboratory data improve, a low-fat diet is prescribed. In chronic cases, degeneration may lead to impaired enzyme production (pancreatic insufficiency). Oral administrations of pancreatic enzymes (eg, pancrelipase, pancreatin) may be necessary in such cases.

If glucose metabolism has been seriously altered, insulin may be administered to control hyperglycemia. In severe cases of pancreatitis, the pancreas may be surgically drained or totally or partially resected (pancreatectomy). If pancreatectomy is performed, the client may have to take pancreatic enzymes indefinitely. Surgical treatment is discussed in Chapter 50.

In rare cases, acute pancreatitis follows a fulminant course, causing death within a short time. In most cases, however, progressive healing occurs, and the client recovers after a difficult course.

Specific Nursing Measures

In acute pancreatitis, the nurse is responsible for assessing the client's symptoms and evaluating the effectiveness of therapy, monitoring for complications, promoting normal fluid/electrolyte and nutritional status, and fostering the client's comfort. Nursing assessments include monitoring the urine for glucose and acetone and observing the client for hypoglycemic or hyperglycemic reactions. Since serum calcium levels may be subnormal, observe for clinical signs of hypocalcemia. Nutritional status warrants special attention, and ongoing nutritional assessment and support are indicated.

The client recovering from acute pancreatitis or suffering from the chronic form is generally required to follow a low-fat diet. Although the diet itself is usually provided by the dietitian, the nurse should ensure that the client understands the regimen in terms of the individual's lifestyle and culture. Informing the client about the proper administration of any prescribed medications as well as side effects and toxic reactions is part of discharge planning.

APPENDICITIS

Appendicitis is acute inflammation of the vermiform appendix, thought to be related to ulceration at the area. It may occur as a single attack or as repeated episodes. Appendicitis occurs most often in the second and third decades of life (Petersdorf, 1983).

Several etiologic factors have been suggested for appendicitis, including viral infection and obstruction of the lumen of the appendix. Obstruction may be related to a primary inflammatory process associated with edema, development of fecaliths, the presence of foreign bodies or worms, or an infectious process with enlargement of lymphatic tissue.

Clinical Manifestations

Ulceration and inflammation at the appendix commonly cause anorexia, nausea, vomiting, bowel changes, and pain that begins as diffuse midabdominal pain and eventually localizes at McBurney's point in the right lower quadrant of the abdomen (Figure 49–8). An elevated temperature and leukocytosis are generally noted. Physical examination will reveal rebound tenderness, shallow respirations, and guarding. Pain will also be noted on rectal or vaginal examination.

Infection, with or without abscess formation, may occur, as may necrosis and gangrene. Rupture of the inflamed appendix with perforation of the intestinal wall and consequent peritonitis is a serious potential complication. A fistula may develop between the appendix and the urinary bladder, small intestine, sigmoid colon, or cecum. In some cases, inflammation and infection heal spontaneously, although adhesions may develop and cause obstruction at some later date.

Early diagnosis of appendicitis is important to limit possibly life-threatening complications such as perforation and peritonitis. Diagnosis may be delayed in the elderly, since older persons are less likely to develop a temperature, or in the pregnant client, in whom symptoms may be mistaken for a side effect of pregnancy. Hospitalization and observation are generally indicated when any suspicion of appendicitis exists.

Therapeutic Measures

The client with acute appendicitis requires prompt, effective treatment to eliminate inflammation and infection and to prevent complications. To rest the bowel, NPO status is instituted and the client is given fluids intravenously. A nasogastric tube is passed to decompress the GI tract. Enemas and cathartics must be avoided, since they may irritate an already inflamed area and promote perforation. Antibiotics, an important component of treatment, are gen-

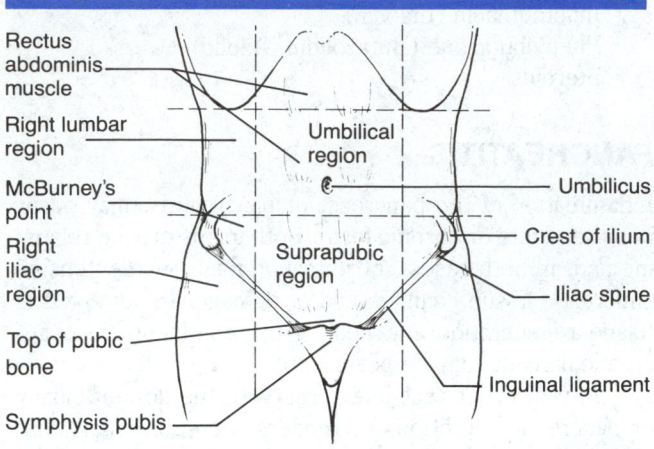

Figure 49–8
McBurney's point.

erally administered intravenously. Analgesics may be given, but caution is indicated, since they may mask symptoms. Surgery (appendectomy) is generally performed as soon as possible. This operation is discussed in Chapter 50.

Specific Nursing Measures

Accurate nursing assessments are crucial to the client's well-being. Any increase in abdominal pain and rigidity may herald life-threatening perforation and/or peritonitis and must be reported promptly. The nurse is responsible for the timely and accurate administration of antibiotics, for monitoring fluid/electrolyte balance, and for administering intravenous solutions. Nursing comfort measures are especially important if analgesics are withheld or kept to a minimum. Explaining that pain medication may mask crucial symptoms may help the client in coping with pain. Keep the client and family informed about tests and treatments. The client will probably require surgery, so preoperative preparation should begin promptly.

INFLAMMATORY BOWEL DISEASE

Although the term "inflammatory bowel disease" could be applied to any inflammatory disorder of the small intestine or colon, it is generally used to designate two conditions: ulcerative colitis and Crohn's disease (regional enteritis, regional ileitis, granulomatous colitis). Both are chronic, recurrent diseases that pose significant health problems.

Ulcerative colitis, the more common, primarily affects the superficial mucosal layers of large areas of the colon. It should not be confused with other forms of colitis (Box 49–2). Crohn's disease affects all layers of the ileum and/or the colon and frequently causes patchy lesions interspersed with normal tissue. Both disorders occur equally in both sexes and occur more commonly in Caucasians, especially those of Jewish origin (Petersdorf, 1983).

Box 49−2 Other Forms of Colitis

Hemorrhagic colitis: Mucosal bleeding, seen in response to the administration of some antibiotics, may be noted after treatment of an upper respiratory tract infection with penicillin or derivatives.

Pseudomembranous colitis: Necrosis and tissue destruction, often seen in response to antibiotics, may be from an overgrowth of bacteria in the intestinal tract; associated with abdominal pain, cramping, fever, diarrhea, and leukocytosis.

Ischemic colitis: Colonic ischemia, as a result of vascular degeneration with aging; generally a short-term problem (2 to 4 weeks); associated with pain and bloody diarrhea.

Various factors have been implicated in the etiology of inflammatory bowel disease. Its familial tendency suggests a hereditary component. Infection, immune factors, and psychosocial factors have been proposed.

Clinical Manifestations

Ulcerative Colitis

The inflammation associated with ulcerative colitis destroys tissue, causing ulceration and necrosis that in turn, precipitate abdominal pain and diarrhea. The stool may contain blood and/or mucus, or may be watery. Symptoms may occur as an isolated attack, may be intermittent or recurrent, or may be continuous. In severe or prolonged episodes, fever, leukocytosis, infection, fluid/electrolyte imbalance, and malnutrition may occur. Fissures, hemorrhage, and formation of abscesses or fistulas can occur as complications. Scarring associated with healing of tissue may obstruct the bowel at a later time. Toxic megacolon (severe dilation of the colon) is a serious complication that can predispose the client to perforation and peritonitis.

Crohn's Disease (Regional Enteritis)

The client with Crohn's disease will experience symptoms similar to those of ulcerative colitis, but the course of the disease is generally more slowly progressive. Fever, abdominal pain, and diarrhea frequently occur, as well as anorexia, nausea, and vomiting. Malabsorption and steatorrhea as well as fluid/electrolyte and nutritional disturbances may also be encountered. Potential complications include intestinal perforation, obstruction, infection, fistula formation (Figure 49–9), fissures, and hemorrhage, although bleeding is generally less severe than with ulcerative colitis.

Chronic, frequent, and/or prolonged episodes of inflammatory bowel disease subject the client to serious, long-standing nutritional imbalances and to weight loss. These clients often appear thin, even emaciated. The chronic aspect of the disease, and the symptoms associated with it, may make the client anxious and/or depressed. The client's lifestyle is greatly altered, especially if bowel resec-

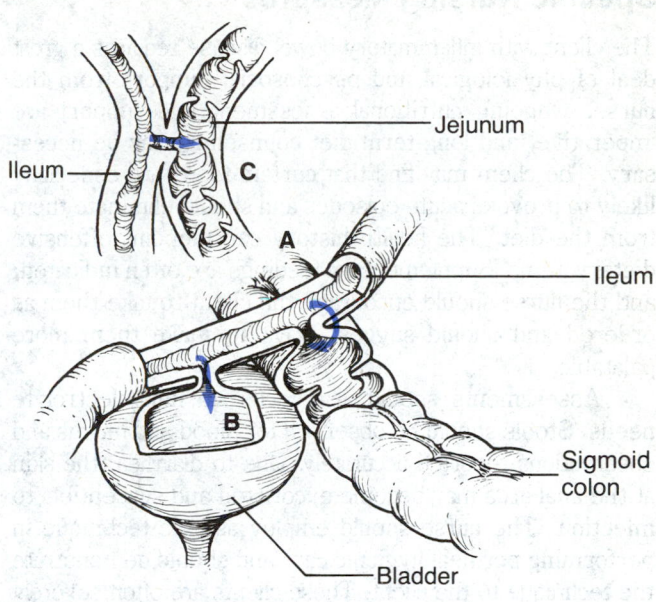

Figure 49–9

Fistula formation in Crohn's disease. **A.** Ileosigmoid fistula. **B.** Internal fistula between ileum and bladder. **C.** Ileojejunal fistula.

tion becomes necessary. Diagnosis is confirmed through the use of barium studies, endoscopy, biopsy, and stool analysis.

Therapeutic Measures

Treatment for ulcerative colitis and Crohn's disease is essentially the same. If symptoms are severe, if complications occur, or if nutritional status is greatly impaired, the client must be hospitalized. In acute episodes, the intestinal tract is allowed to rest. The client is kept NPO and nourished intravenously until symptoms subside. If the client's intake is restricted for a long period, TPN may be indicated to replace nutritional losses. Gradually, a low-residue diet is introduced, as tolerated. Any anemia precipitated by blood loss is corrected.

Pharmacologic measures may include use of anti-inflammatory agents, steroids, anticholinergics, and antispasmodics to control diarrhea, and antibiotics (especially sulfasalazine) to prevent or control infection. Psychological counseling may assist the client in coping with stresses associated with chronic illness. Although ulcerative colitis often subsides (at least temporarily) with treatment, Crohn's disease may persist and may progressively worsen.

In severe, intractable cases of inflammatory bowel disease, surgical intervention may be necessary. The diseased portion of the bowel is resected, and a temporary or permanent ileostomy may be required. Surgery is curative in ulcerative colitis. With Crohn's disease, the recurrence rate is high. These procedures are discussed in Chapter 50.

Specific Nursing Measures

The client with inflammatory bowel disease requires a great deal of physiological and psychosocial support from the nurse. Ongoing nutritional assessment and support are imperative, and long-term diet counseling may be necessary. The client may find that certain foods are especially likely to provoke acute episodes and should eliminate them from the diet. The health history can pinpoint offensive dietary items. Supplementary feedings are often indicated, and the nurse should encourage the client to take them as ordered and should suggest ways to make them more palatable.

Assessments should also focus on fluid/electrolyte needs. Stools should be observed for blood and mucus and observations reported accurately. Due to diarrhea, the skin at the anal area may become excoriated and susceptible to infection. The nurse should employ aseptic technique in performing perineal hygienic care and should demonstrate the technique to the client. These clients are often severely stressed both physiologically and psychologically. Talking over their problems and reactions with them is an integral part of nursing care. Care of the client with an ostomy is discussed in Chapter 50.

SPRUE

Sprue is a disorder of malabsorption. *Tropical sprue* is found primarily in tropical regions but may be seen in returning visitors. *Nontropical sprue* (celiac disease, celiac sprue, gluten-induced enteropathy) is more pervasive.

The etiology of tropical sprue, though not well understood, is thought to be related to nutritional deficiencies and microorganisms endemic to tropical islands. Symptoms are related to changes that occur in the villi of the intestinal tract. Nontropical sprue, which varies in severity, affects women more often than men and also causes intestinal mucosal changes with markedly flattened villi. Consequently, the extensive absorptive capacity of the small intestine is lost. Sensitivity to gluten is thought to be involved, although an immunologic factor has also been implicated.

Clinical Manifestations

Symptoms of tropical and nontropical sprue are similar; anorexia, diarrhea, weight loss, abdominal distention, malabsorption, steatorrhea, nutritional deficiencies, undernutrition, and anemia are common. In nontropical sprue, symptoms are precipitated by ingestion of gluten. The disorder may be associated with extraintestinal manifestations, many of which may have an immunological basis: bone disorders, diabetes, thyroid disorders, interstitial lung diseases, primary biliary cirrhosis, and pericarditis (Faizallah et al., 1982).

Diagnosis is based on tests for absorption abnormalities and on biopsy. In the case of tropical sprue, questions about recent travel asked during the health history may yield a valuable diagnostic clue.

Therapeutic Measures

Tropical sprue is treated with a 2- to 4-week course of antibiotics, usually sulfonamides or tetracycline. Nontropical sprue responds well to a gluten-free diet. Corticosteroids and TPN are also sometimes necessary.

Specific Nursing Measures

The major nursing responsibility is instructing clients with nontropical sprue to avoid gluten-containing foods. Wheat, buckwheat, rye, barley, malt, and oats are gluten-containing grains and are found in many common food stuffs. Important facts about gluten-free diets are listed in Box 49–3. Mucosal changes will return to normal in a majority of clients who carefully follow the diet. Since many of these clients are malnourished by the time they are diagnosed, a nutritionist can be helpful in planning a high-calorie, high-protein, high-vitamin, and mineral diet that is also gluten free.

For the hospitalized client who may be fatigued and dehydrated, the nurse should ensure that fluid and electrolyte and nutritional losses are monitored and replaced as needed. Maintaining an environment conducive to rest is also important.

INFECTIOUS GASTROENTERITIS

Inflammation and infection of the GI tract, causing diarrhea among other symptoms, is usually related to invasion or overgrowth of microbes. Serious morbidity can be associated with these infections (especially among the elderly or malnourished), but most clients can be treated on an outpatient basis. Viral gastroenteritis (also known as infectious diarrhea) is the second leading cause of illness in the United States (Petersdorf, 1983).

Infections are commonly associated with situations in which bacteria, viruses, or parasites gain entry into the GI tract and then proliferate. Infectious gastroenteritis may follow ingestion of contaminated food or water, an upper respiratory infection, or oral/anal or anal/genital contact. Factors that decrease the acidity of gastrointestinal fluids (eg, gastric ulcer, gastric surgery), depress motility, or diminish or destroy normal flora (eg, antibiotic therapy) increase the client's risk of GI infection. Infectious gastroenteritis caused by food poisoning is discussed in detail in Chapter 11.

Clinical Manifestations

The client with gastroenteritis may experience vomiting, diarrhea, abdominal cramping, respiratory symptoms, otitis media, and pharyngitis. Malabsorption often characterizes the infection, and steatorrhea may appear. Temporary lactose intolerance may also develop. These symptoms combine to make the client fatigued and susceptible to fluid/electrolyte imbalance, nutritional deficiencies, and weight loss. Symptoms generally persist for a week or more.

Diagnosis is generally based on symptoms and stool culture. Biopsy of the small bowel may be necessary to diagnose some infections.

Therapeutic Measures

Treatment is generally supportive. The client is rehydrated as necessary; oral electrolyte-glucose mixtures are available for this purpose. In serious fluid imbalance, hospitalization with intravenous replacement may be necessary. A low-residue diet is generally prescribed until symptoms dissipate. Pharmacologic therapy commonly includes bismuth subsalicylate (Pepto-Bismol) administered at half-hourly intervals for 4 hours. In some cases, antibiotics are prescribed.

Specific Nursing Measures

Nursing care is also supportive. Encourage the client to comply with the low-residue diet, emphasizing the need for fluids. Advise the client to rest and to resume activities as symptoms permit. Assess for dehydration and explain to the client how to do so. Explain the medication regimen. Since many of these disorders can be spread through the fecal–oral route, advise the client to follow enteric precautions and explain how to do so.

PILONIDAL CYST

A pilonidal cyst is a foreign body reaction to ingrown hair that develops in the upper end of the cleft between the buttocks in the sacrococcygeal region. Affected clients usually have a deep intergluteal cleft and heavy hair growth in the area. Obesity and jobs that require considerable sitting contribute to the friction, warmth, and moisture that exacerbate the problem.

There are often several openings (sinus tracts) to the skin. The client may only become aware of the cyst when purulent drainage occurs through the sinus tracts from secondary infection in the area. Pain, localized erythema, and swelling may accompany the drainage.

In the past, pilonidal cysts were believed to be of embryological origin. Currently, foreign body reaction with secondary infection is thought to be the predominant etiology.

Therapeutic Measures

Initial treatment involves probing the sinus tracts under local anesthesia with removal of all hair and debris. The wound is packed open and is kept packed until healing takes place. If the cyst recurs, surgical excision of the sinus tract is required. Primary closure is attempted. If the excision is too wide, the wound is packed and allowed to heal by granulation.

Specific Nursing Measures

Since most clients are discharged early, nursing care mainly involves teaching client and family about protection of the surgical site from trauma and from contamination by urine and feces. For promoting comfort and relieving strain on the surgical area, the side-lying position with the upper leg supported by pillows is often the most comfortable.

RECTAL ABSCESS

A localized infection of the perirectal area (rectal abscess) may be caused by chronic inflammation and eventual infection of hair follicles, contamination of rectal fissures, or thrombosed hemorrhoids.

Clinical Manifestations

The primary manifestation of rectal abscess is pain, especially with defecation. The abscess may be apparent with inspection and can generally be felt with palpation. An abscess high in the rectum generally produces additional symptoms of pain and malaise. Pelvic discomfort may be present. Fistulas may form between the abscess and other body areas, especially the bladder and vagina.

Therapeutic Measures

Analgesics and sitz baths may relieve symptoms. Antibiotics may be prescribed. Incision and drainage are usually necessary and are discussed in Chapter 50.

Specific Nursing Measures

Nursing care is supportive and is aimed at relieving symptoms. The client should be assisted with the use of the sitz bath, and aseptic hygienic practices should be stressed.

Section III: Neoplastic and Obstructive Disorders

Neoplasia of the stomach, intestine, and pancreas may be benign or malignant; in either case, the client may experience significant morbidity with altered digestion, absorption, and elimination. Nutritional deficiencies and weight loss are common. The mortality associated with late detection of these cancers is high. Treatment of neoplastic and obstructive GI disorders may necessitate extensive changes in the client's lifestyle. Serious threats to self-concept and body image—for example, if a colostomy is necessary—may occur.

Early detection, which may be crucial to survival, may depend on the nurse's observations. Once the disorder has been diagnosed, the client will need ongoing physiological and psychosocial support.

General Nursing Implications

The nurse is often in a position to detect presymptomatic signs or early symptoms of neoplastic and obstructive disorders of the stomach, intestine, and pancreas. Whether taking a history, performing a physical examination, or providing routine care, the nurse should be alert for:

- Any history of continuing anorexia, nausea, and/or vomiting
- Weight loss without dieting
- Epigastric or abdominal pain that persists
- Changes in bowel habits
- Blood in the stool or black tarry stools in a client who does not take iron or Pepto-Bismol

These changes may be significant and should be reported promptly for further investigation. In performing an abdominal or rectal examination, the nurse should pay particular attention to any asymmetry, distention, masses, or areas of tenderness.

Once a neoplastic or obstructive disorder has been diagnosed, ongoing assessment is crucial to the client's care. Since digestion, absorption, and elimination may be impaired, serious nutritional deficiencies and fluid/electrolyte imbalances may occur. As therapy is instituted, the nurse is responsible for careful monitoring of the client's symptoms and response to therapy.

Ongoing psychosocial assessment will also be required. How does the client feel about the illness? The diagnosis? Hospitalization? Prospective surgery? How are client and family coping, especially if the prognosis is grave or death is impending?

INTESTINAL OBSTRUCTION

Obstruction of the small or large intestine, with inhibition of the passage of intestinal contents, may occur as an acute or chronic problem. Adhesions or hernias cause a majority of small bowel obstructions. These may be a consequence of previous intestinal surgery, trauma, pelvic surgery, or appendectomy.

Obstruction of the large intestine is commonly related to cancer, diverticulitis, volvulus (twisting of the bowel), or intussusception (invagination of the bowel) (Figure 49–10). Paralytic (adynamic) ileus may also be considered a form of intestinal obstruction. Paralytic ileus occurs to some degree after any peritoneal insult (for example, abdominal surgery). Usually, it persists for 2 or 3 days and gradually subsides without treatment.

Clinical Manifestations

Symptoms are precipitated when fluid (gastric, pancreatic, or biliary secretions or saliva), gas, and ingested substances accumulate proximal to the site of obstruction. The client generally has abdominal pain and distention and may vomit. If the obstruction is near the lower end of the intestinal tract, vomiting can occur late and may have a foul, fecal odor caused by bacterial overgrowth in the intestinal tract. The client will probably report being unable to pass stools or flatus. In partial obstruction, diarrhea may be noted. **Singultus** (hiccups) is common.

Borborygmi may be noted on physical examination, except in cases of ileus or peritoneal irritation, in which bowel sounds are diminished or absent. Peristaltic rushes (periodic loud bursts of sounds) are common. Low-grade fever may also be present.

Fluid/electrolyte and acid/base imbalances are common, since fluid shift and absorption in the intestines are abnormal, and output losses may be extreme. Nutritional deficiencies and weight loss also occur. Complications include peritonitis and strangulation (impaired blood supply) and/or incarceration (impaired blood supply and necrosis) of the bowel, which may also promote infection and/or sepsis.

Therapeutic Measures

Supportive treatment is given while the primary cause of the obstruction is sought. The client is kept NPO, and fluid/electrolyte and nutritional needs are met with intravenous fluids and TPN as necessary. A nasogastric or intestinal (Cantor, Miller–Abbot) tube to suction decompresses the intestinal tract and alleviates nausea and vomiting.

Intake and output are carefully measured, and an indwelling catheter may be inserted to facilitate this process. Replacement of fluid losses is imperative. Antibiotics may be prescribed to prevent infection. Analgesics are ordered for pain relief but must be used with caution, since they can mask diagnostic symptoms. Surgery (exploratory laparotomy) is performed as soon as possible to identify and/or treat the primary disorder. Surgical treatments are discussed in Chapter 50.

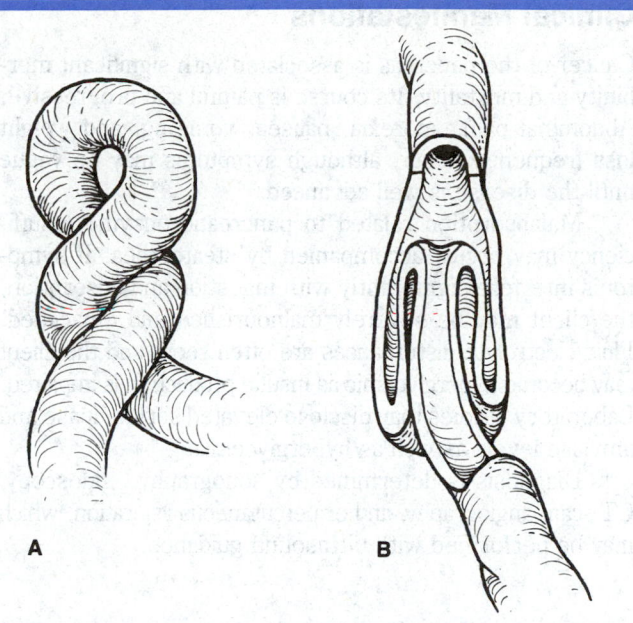

Figure 49–10

A. Volvulus, twisting of the bowel. **B.** Intussusception, small bowel telescopes into itself.

Specific Nursing Measures

The client with intestinal obstruction requires efficient, accurate measurement and recording of intake and output. Intestinal-tract drainage should be carefully described as well. Skin turgor, urine specific gravity, and the client's thirst should be assessed frequently to determine hydration status. Abdominal girth is measured to monitor distention.

Explain why NPO status is necessary and provide mouth care frequently to make the client more comfortable. If analgesics are being withheld for diagnostic reasons, explain why this is being done. Ensure the patency of the nasogastric or intestinal tube and irrigate it as necessary (unless this is contraindicated).

If the client has an intestinal tube, the nurse should realize that it is intended to advance along the intestinal tract to provide for decompression as distally as possible. Often the physician will order that the tube be advanced a few inches at a time by the nurse. Passage of the tube is facilitated by assisting the client into the right-sided semi-Fowler's position.

Throughout the course of care, be available to provide psychological support when needed and encourage the client and family to express any fears about the diagnosis, which may be uncertain.

POLYPS

A **polyp** is a projection of the mucosal surface of the lumen of an organ. Polyps may occur in the stomach or intestine and may be single or multiple, benign or malignant (poly-poid carcinoma). The most common form is the adenomatous polyp (adenoma), which may originate in the benign form and then undergo malignant changes (Petersdorf, 1983).

Familial colonic polyposis, which generally appears in childhood or adolescence, is a hereditary disorder characterized by numerous polyps. It has a 100% association with cancer of the colon by age 40 (Petersdorf, 1983). Gardner's syndrome, also characterized by numerous lesions and a high association with cancer, appears later in life. Polyps are generally diagnosed by digital examination, endoscopy, and biopsy.

Clinical Manifestations

Polyps may produce hemorrhage, diarrhea, and, if large, signs and symptoms of intestinal obstruction. Polyps may, however, be asymptomatic.

Therapeutic Measures

Once identified, polyps are generally removed by colonoscopy, sigmoidoscopy, or gastroscopy as an outpatient procedure or during hospitalization. A low-fiber diet is generally prescribed prior to polypectomy to inhibit inflammation and bleeding. In diagnosed Gardner's syndrome and familial colonic polyposis, prophylactic colectomy, with or without formation of a colostomy, is generally indicated. These procedures are discussed in Chapter 50.

Specific Nursing Measures

Nursing care of the client with a GI polyp is primarily supportive. Explain any treatment such as polypectomy and support the client physiologically and psychosocially throughout the experience. Counsel the client about the relationship of polyps to the incidence of cancer, stressing the importance of routine checkups and prompt reporting of symptoms.

CANCER OF THE STOMACH

Malignant tumors of the stomach affect males more often than females and usually appear after the fourth decade of life. The incidence of gastric cancer has steadily declined in the United States in recent years; nevertheless, it was estimated that 24,700 new cases and 14,300 deaths from gastric cancer would occur in 1985 (1985 Cancer Facts and Figures, 1985). Thus stomach cancer is still a major potentially lethal health problem, especially if detected late in its course.

Although now relatively uncommon in the United States (except in Hawaii), cancer of the stomach is a common problem in Japan, Central and South America, Mexico, Malaysia, and parts of eastern Europe (Austria). Immigrants from these regions and also their first-generation descendants also have an increased incidence of this disease.

Dietary factors have been implicated in the etiology of gastric cancer, notably a diet high in starches, smoked foods, and preservatives. Cancer of the stomach has also been associated with achlorhydria, group A blood type, chronic (atrophic) gastritis, adenomatous polyps, pernicious anemia, and surgical repair of peptic ulcer (Petersdorf, 1983).

Clinical Manifestations

Unfortunately, symptoms are generally slowly progressive and appear late in the course of the disease. The client may report anorexia, nausea, vomiting, weight loss, bloating, and epigastric discomfort. A mass may be noted on palpation, and occult blood may be present in the stool. Anemia may occur as a very late manifestation. Diagnosis is made on the basis of barium studies, gastroscopy, biopsy, and gastric analysis.

Therapeutic Measures

Gastric cancer is treated by surgery (gastrectomy), chemotherapy, and in some cases, radiation. Nutritional support and fluid/electrolyte maintenance are generally indicated. The client with severe symptoms may have to be NPO, and nasogastric intubation may be used to decompress the digestive tract.

If the client is permitted to eat, small, frequent feedings are helpful. Antiemetics may be ordered for nausea, and analgesics for pain. Any anemia is treated as well. Metastasis, if it occurs, affects the liver, bones, and lungs.

Specific Nursing Measures

Consult Chapter 12 for a detailed discussion of cancer nursing. The client with cancer of the stomach requires consistent nutritional assessment and support. Nursing measures to promote the client's nutritional status are indicated. Often, the client will require TPN to maintain nutritional and fluid/electrolyte needs.

Pain control requires the nurse to use comfort measures and to administer analgesics as necessary. Careful assessment of pain is indicated, and any signs or suspicions of metastasis should be noted.

CANCER OF THE PANCREAS

Cancer of the pancreas is the fourth most common cause of cancer-related death in the United States, occurring more commonly in men (Petersdorf, 1983). It generally appears in the sixth or seventh decade of life. The head of the pancreas is most commonly affected.

The etiology of pancreatic cancer remains unclear. Increased incidence, however, has been associated with diabetes, smoking, and pancreatitis.

Clinical Manifestations

Cancer of the pancreas is associated with significant morbidity and mortality. Its course is painful and progressive. Abdominal pain, anorexia, nausea, vomiting, and weight loss frequently occur, although symptoms may be vague until the disease is well advanced.

Malabsorption related to pancreatic enzyme insufficiency may occur, accompanied by steatorrhea. If symptoms interfere significantly with ingestion and absorption, the client may be severely malnourished and emaciated. Fluid/electrolyte disturbances are often seen, and the client may become hyperglycemic as insulin production is impaired. Laboratory studies may disclose elevated serum lipase and amylase levels as well as hyperglycemia.

Diagnosis is determined by sonography, endoscopy, CT scan, angiography, and/or percutaneous aspiration, which may be performed with ultrasound guidance.

Therapeutic Measures

The client with cancer of the pancreas requires supportive treatment to help alleviate symptoms. The client may be more comfortable if kept NPO with nasogastric intubation to decompress the bowel. Nutritional support, often with hyperalimentation, is imperative. Antiemetics and analgesics are indicated.

Most pancreatic tumors are inoperable, but in some cases resection of the pancreas and duodenum (pancreatic–duodenal resection) is performed. A *Whipple procedure,* involving removal of the head of the pancreas, a portion of the stomach, the duodenum, and the common bile duct, is an alternative. After pancreatic surgery, replacement of insulin and pancreatic enzymes is necessary. Surgical treatment is discussed in Chapter 50.

Radiation and chemotherapy may also be used. In general, survival rates are poor, and the disease is often fatal within a year of onset of symptoms.

Specific Nursing Measures

The client with cancer of the pancreas requires tremendous physiological and psychological support from the nurse. Monitor nutritional and fluid/electrolyte status continuously. Check fractional urines q.i.d. to detect glucose abnormalities. Nursing measures to promote nutrition and comfort are of high priority. Monitor all symptoms and evaluate the effectiveness of any measures to control them. The client receiving radiation treatment or chemotherapy requires specialized care as discussed in Chapter 12.

Throughout the course of the client's illness, be available to answer questions from the client and significant others. Both client and family need opportunities to express their feelings about the symptoms of the disease and its grave prognosis.

CANCER OF THE COLON AND RECTUM

Primary neoplasms of the intestinal tract usually affect the large intestine or rectum. Cancer of the small intestine is rare. Excluding skin cancer, the incidence of colorectal cancer is second only to cancer of the lung. Male and female incidence is equal. Colorectal cancer most often appears in the fifth to seventh decades of life.

Dietary factors have been implicated in colorectal cancer. Low-fiber diets, which promote slow stool transit time and stasis of bowel contents, are thought to be related to possible carcinogenic changes in the GI tract. A high intake of fats and meats may also be related. An increased risk for colorectal cancer is associated with familial colonic polyposis, Gardner's syndrome, and inflammatory bowel diseases.

Clinical Manifestations

Clients frequently describe changes in bowel habits, black tarry stools, or bleeding from the rectum. Pain may also be present. Unfortunately, the client may not report these symptoms as soon as they are detected.

As the disease progresses, bleeding may increase, and symptoms of obstruction may occur as the neoplasm grows. Anemia can develop as a consequence of bleeding. Location and occurrence of major symptoms associated with colorectal cancer are summarized in Table 49–2.

Early detection is possible. The American Cancer Society recommends that digital examination, stool guaiac testing, and proctosigmoidoscopy be performed as noted in Box 49–4. Barium studies and biopsy are also useful in diagnosis.

Box 49–4   Recommended Protocol for Early Detection of Colorectal Cancer

The American Cancer Society (1985) recommends the following tests:

Digital rectal examination: once every year for a client over 40 years of age

Stool guaiac test: once each year for the client over 50 years of age; can be done by the client at home

Proctosigmoidoscopy: following two negative annual examinations, once every 3 to 5 years for the client over age 50

Clients who are at higher risk (eg, personal history of polyps or family history of cancer of the colon or rectum) should receive more frequent, thorough examinations beginning at an earlier age

---

Therapeutic Measures

A combination of surgery, chemotherapy, and radiation therapy may be used for treatment. Surgery generally involves resection of the malignant area, and a temporary or permanent colostomy may be necessary. Surgeries commonly performed for cancers of the large intestine are highlighted in Table 49–3 and are fully discussed in Chapter 50.

Prior to surgery, the bowel is thoroughly cleansed with enemas, laxatives, and/or irrigations to prevent operative contamination. Antibiotics are also generally prescribed preoperatively to decrease bacterial flora in the GI tract. Symptoms are relieved with analgesics, and nutri-

---

Table 49–2   Location and Occurrence of Major Symptoms of Cancer of Large Intestine

Symptom	Right Colon	Left Colon	Rectum
Abdominal mass	Right lower quadrant: 69%	Left lower quadrant: 29%	
Pain	Vague, dull, uncharacteristic (aggravated by walking): 89%	Gas pain, cramps: 82%	Late feature: 65%
Blood in stool	Dark or mahogany red mixed in stool: 30%	Bright red, coating surface of stool: 49%	Bright red, coating surface of stool: 80%
Flow of stool	No alteration	Decrease in caliber of stools, tendency toward constipation	Sense of incomplete evacuation; tenesmus
Weight loss (>5 kg)	50%	35%	7%
Obstruction	Acute: 7%	Causes progressive abdominal distention, pain, vomiting, and constipation: 16%	7%
Changes in bowel habits	54%	69%	71%

SOURCE: Given BA, Simmons SJ: *Gastroenterology in Clinical Nursing*. St. Louis: Mosby, 1984, p. 366.

Table 49–3 Surgeries for Cancer of Large Intestine Identifying Scope of Resections	
Location of Lesions	**Procedure**
Cecum and ascending colon	Right colectomy: remove terminal ileum, cecum, ascending colon, and right half of transverse colon
Proximal and midtransverse colon	Right colectomy extended to include transverse colon; anastomose ileum to descending colon
Splenic flexure, descending or sigmoid colon	Left colectomy: remove distal transverse, entire descending, and sigmoid colon; anastomose transverse colon to upper rectum
Sigmoid colon	Sigmoid resection
Upper rectum	Anterior colon resection
Lower rectum and midrectum	Miles' operation: combined abdominal–perineal resection with sigmoid or descending colon removed and colostomy

SOURCE: Given BA, Simmons SJ: *Gastroenterology in Clinical Nursing.* St. Louis: Mosby, 1984, p. 369.

tional and fluid/electrolyte imbalances and anemia are corrected as necessary. A low-residue diet is generally indicated prior to surgery. The prognosis for survival is good with early detection and treatment, but the outlook is more grave if metastasis has occurred.

Specific Nursing Measures

Since early diagnosis is so crucial to the outcome of colorectal cancer, the nurse alert to early signs and symptoms may literally save a client's life. Encourage clients to have periodic examinations as recommended by the American Cancer Society.

Once a diagnosis has been established, physiological and psychological support and nutritional assessment and support are ongoing nursing responsibilities. The client's weight must be monitored and stools observed for signs of bleeding. Nursing comfort measures and analgesics promote comfort and relief from pain.

If the client is to receive chemotherapy or radiation therapy, be prepared to support the client throughout the experience and to provide symptomatic relief as necessary. If a colostomy is performed, the client will need teaching about colostomy care and assistance in adjusting to a new body image (see Chapter 50). Since a diagnosis of cancer is so frightening to many clients, the nurse should encourage verbalization of feelings by client and family. If the client is expected to die, the nurse can work with the client and family as they go through the grieving process.

Section IV: Traumatic Disorders

Traumatic disorders of the stomach, intestines, and pancreas account for a fairly significant percentage of all disorders of these organs. Abdominal trauma may occur as a consequence of fights or falls, motor vehicle accidents, sports injuries, or assault by gun or knife. Trauma may be localized or may involve a large area and a number of abdominal organs.

Trauma to these organs may be difficult to determine and may go undetected, with serious consequences for the client. If the alimentary tract is traumatized, the normal processes of digestion, absorption, and elimination may be impaired, with consequent serious alterations in nutrition, fluid/electrolyte status, and elimination. Complications of trauma to these organs may include hemorrhage, shock, infection, peritonitis, and obstruction, any of which may be life threatening.

TRAUMA TO THE STOMACH, INTESTINES, AND PANCREAS

The stomach, intestines, and pancreas are often traumatized when abdominal injuries are sustained. Major or minor contusions, lacerations, and perforations are frequently encountered. Often, internal injury may be present without overt signs of trauma. These injuries may be fatal if left undiagnosed and untreated.

Trauma to these organs may be blunt or penetrating. Blunt trauma is frequently related to motor vehicle accidents, falls, and fights. Vehicular seatbelts may cause blunt abdominal trauma if worn incorrectly or if an accident is severe. Penetrating wounds are frequently caused by bullets, knives, or stones. Trauma from gunshot wounds is usually more extensive than wounds caused by other penetrating objects, because of the high velocity of the bullet.

Clinical Manifestations

Blunt abdominal trauma may or may not be associated with external injury. When external bruises, lacerations, and contusions are present, however, they frequently correlate with the site of internal involvement. Although external trauma is apparent with penetrating wounds, it may not accurately reflect the extent of internal injury. The angle of entry of a penetrating object may be helpful in localizing internal damage.

Trauma to internal organs will cause enlargement and tenderness on palpation. *Palpation must be performed with utmost care if there is any likelihood of internal trauma. Assessment for rebound tenderness should be done only by a skilled examiner employing all precautions against further injury.* Abdominal distention, inhibition of respirations, and guarding may also be noted.

Crepitation (subcutaneous emphysema) may be noted as crackling sounds as the fingertips palpate an area where extravasation of air has occurred (eg, from an injured colon or diaphragm). Bowel sounds may be diminished or absent if intestinal trauma or irritation has occurred. If an organ has ruptured, causing fluids to leak into the abdominal cavity, peritonitis will result.

Hemorrhage may accompany trauma. Injury to the stomach or intestine may cause bleeding into the GI tract, evidenced by hematemesis or, in severe bleeding, hematochezia. If a nasogastric tube is in place, drainage will contain blood. Frequently, blood from damaged organs seeps into the peritoneal cavity. Cullen's sign (ecchymosis at the umbilicus) and Turner's sign (ecchymosis at the flank) indicate retroperitoneal bleeding and internal injury.

To check for intra-abdominal injury, paracentesis or abdominal lavage may be performed. In lavage, the preferred procedure, a catheter is inserted into the peritoneal cavity through a short umbilical incision, and a small sample of fluid is aspirated and inspected for blood. The presence of blood confirms internal injury and indicates the need for surgery. If the sample of fluid shows no gross evidence of blood, irrigation fluid is instilled through the catheter and allowed to drain. Drainage is inspected for gross signs of blood and is also sent to the laboratory for analysis.

Perforation, peritonitis, and sepsis may follow intestinal trauma. Trauma to the rectum may also have occurred and should be evaluated. Complications of pancreatic trauma may include formation of abscesses or fistulae, enzyme insufficiency and malabsorption (with steatorrhea), and hyperglycemia related to abnormal insulin production or secretion.

Therapeutic Measures

The client with suspected or apparent internal injury is immobilized and made comfortable. Any open wounds should be protected and cleansed. Protruding objects should be left in place. An IV is generally started immediately to provide a route of administration for fluids, blood, and medications.

When internal injury is apparent, an exploratory laparotomy is performed to determine the extent of injuries and to repair damaged organs. Tears or lacerations are generally repaired by suturing. Severely traumatized tissues or organs may have to be removed. In cases of stomach injury, temporary gastrostomy may be necessary, regardless of the extent of surgical repair. If intestinal injury has occurred, the client may require a temporary or permanent colostomy. These surgical procedures are discussed in Chapter 50.

Supportive care includes analgesics, fluid/electrolyte and/or blood replacement, and treatment for shock. Antibiotics are given to prevent or control infection, and tetanus prophylaxis is also administered. The client gradually resumes normal activity as tolerated.

Specific Nursing Measures

The client with trauma to the stomach, intestine, or pancreas may be cared for in the community, the hospital, or an emergency facility. In an emergency situation, the nurse may give care at the scene of the accident as a bystander. Wherever the trauma occurs, the nurse must be knowledgeable about care and possible consequences.

In caring for the client with abdominal trauma, the nurse must be alert to:

- Signs and symptoms that will localize the injury
- The extent and seriousness of the injury
- Early signs of complications

The nurse should obtain a history to determine the exact cause of the injury and the presence of any preexisting disease. It is especially important to determine whether the wound is dirty (contaminated), since aggressive therapy is needed to prevent infection of a contaminated wound. A medication and immunization history should also be obtained. If the client is unable to provide the necessary information, another reliable source should be sought. An accurate description of the location and nature of pain is especially important.

Since abdominal trauma may be associated with trauma to other body areas—especially the respiratory and urinary tracts—the function of all body systems should be evaluated and monitored. Once therapy is instituted, the nurse is responsible for ongoing assessment of the client's symptoms and the effects of therapy. Moreover, the nurse should assess the client's psychological status, since injured clients are often anxious and fearful.

Use sterile technique in caring for any open wounds. Blood and debris should be removed, but any protruding objects (eg, a knife) should be left in place initially, since removal could cause hemorrhage. During the process of wound healing, carefully evaluate the area for any signs of infection, with each dressing change. These should be reported promptly to the physician.

The nurse must pay particular attention to maintaining fluid/electrolyte balance and measuring intake and output frequently and precisely. If the client is permitted to eat, observe how food is tolerated. With intestinal trauma, bowel status must be monitored. Administer medications as ordered and explain the rationale for their use to the client.

In the course of nursing care, the nurse should involve the client and family to the greatest extent possible. Trauma to the body, mild or severe, is accompanied by trauma to the spirit. Answer questions and provide information as necessary, encouraging expression of feelings.

Chapter Highlights

Disorders of the stomach, small and large intestines, and pancreas can significantly alter the nutritional status of a client through interference with the digestion and absorption of nutrients.

Clients with disorders of the stomach, intestines, and pancreas frequently have signs and symptoms of bleeding and/or obstruction, each requiring prompt and efficient medical and nursing care.

The change in elimination status and bowel regimen that may accompany disorders of the intestine can have significant impact on the self-esteem, body image, and lifestyle of an affected client.

Some disorders of the stomach, intestines, and pancreas may be prevented through dietary discretion.

The nurse can play an important role in the prevention of disorders of the stomach, intestines, and pancreas through health teaching about associated risk factors.

The nurse can promote the early detection of disorders of the stomach, intestines, and pancreas through teaching clients to observe and report such symptoms as bleeding, stool changes, and epigastric discomfort.

Early detection of cancers of the stomach, intestines, and pancreas is imperative, since survival rates increase with early treatment.

Bibliography

Bayless TM, Paige DM: Lactose tolerance by lactose malabsorbing Indians. *Gastroenterology* 1978; 74:153.

Bordley DR et al: Early clinical signs identify low-risk patients with upper-GI hemorrhage. *JAMA* (June 14) 1985; 253(22): 3282–3285.

Faizallah R et al: Adult celiac disease and recurrent pericarditis. *Dig Dis Sci* 1982; 27:728–730.

Gilman CJ: Improving survival in patients with rectal cancer. *Am Fam Physician* (Jan) 1984; 29:165–169.

Given BA, Simmons SJ: *Gastroenterology in Clinical Nursing.* St. Louis: Mosby, 1984.

Greenberger NJ: *Gastrointestinal Disorders.* Chicago: Yearbook Medical Publishers, 1981.

Gudmond-Hoyer E, Simony K: Individual sensitivity to lactose in lactose malabsorption. *Amer J Digestive Dis* 1977; 22:177.

Hill SC: Fecal occult blood: Efficacy of testing measures. *Nurse Pract* (Sept/Oct) 1980; 5:15–21.

Hui YH: *Human Nutrition and Diet Therapy.* Monterey CA: Wadsworth, 1983.

Infectious diarrhea? What's the cause? *Patient Care* (May 15) 1983; 79–115.

Jones VA et al: Food intolerance: A major factor in the pathogenesis of irritable bowel syndrome. *Lancet* (Nov 20) 1982; 1115–1117.

Kodner IJ, Fry RD: Inflammatory bowel disease. *Clin Symp* 1982; 34(1):3–32.

Kosel K et al: Total pancreatectomy and islet cell autotransplantation. *Am J Nurs* 1982; 82:568–571.

Kraft SC: What you can do about rectal polyps. *Consultant* (April) 1981; 219–222.

Lamphier TA: Small-bowel obstruction: Think of it early. *Consultant* (Jan) 1981; 165–172.

Lamphier TA, Lamphier RA: Upper GI hemorrhage: Emergency evaluation and management. *Am J Nurs* 1981; 81:1814–1816.

Legerton CW: Current thinking on irritable bowel syndrome. *Consultant* (June) 1981; 25–29.

Lewicki LJ, Lesson MJ: The multisystem impact on physiologic processes of inflammatory bowel disease. *Nurs Clin North Am* 1984; 19(1):71–80.

Myer SA: Overview of inflammatory bowel disease. *Nurs Clin North Am* 1984; 19(1):3–9.

Nostrant TT, Wilson JAP: How good is screening for colorectal cancer? *Postgrad Med* (June) 1983; 73:131–139.

Permutt RP, Cello JP: Duodenal ulcer disease in the hospitalized elderly patient. *Dig Dis Sci* (Jan) 1982; 27:1–6.

Petersdorf RG et al: *Harrison's Principles of Internal Medicine.* New York: McGraw-Hill, 1983.

Petlin AM, Carolan JM: Getting your patient through a lower GI bleed. *RN* (Feb) 1982; 42–45.

Rydning A et al: Prophylactic effect of dietary fibre in duodenal ulcer disease. *Lancet* (Oct 2) 1982; 736–738.

Segal HL: Clues to cancer of the digestive system. *Consultant* (Dec) 1981; 101–103.

Simmons MA: Using the nursing process in treating inflammatory bowel disease. *Nurs Clin North Am* 1984; 19(1):11–25.

Simplifying diagnosis of malabsorption. *Patient Care* (Oct 15) 1981; 128–178.

Smith CW Jr: The irritable bowel syndrome. *Female Patient* 1985; 10:81–90.

Soballe PW: Peritoneal lavage in blunt abdominal trauma. *Am Fam Physician* (March) 1984; 29:193–198.

Stotts NA, Fitzgerald KA, Williams KR: Care of the patient critically ill with inflammatory bowel disease. *Nurs Clin North Am* 1984; 19(1):61–70.

Suitor CW, Hunter MF: *Nutrition: Principles and Application in Health Promotion.* Philadelphia: Lippincott, 1980.

Thomson NA: Convert your assessment into a lifesaving care plan for the patient with abdominal trauma. *Nurs 83* (July) 1983; 13:26–33.

Whitehead WE et al: Learned illness behavior in patients with irritable bowel syndrome and peptic ulcer. *Dig Dis Sci* (March) 1982; 27:202–208.

1985 Cancer Facts and Figures. New York: American Cancer Society, 1985.

Suggested Readings

Burkhart C: Upper gastrointestinal hemorrhage: The clinical picture. *Am J Nurs* 1981; 81:1817–1820. This case study of a client with acute GI bleeding accurately portrays the experience of the client and presents nursing care appropriate to the situation.

Hartwig MS: Sticking to a gluten-free diet. *Am J Nurs* 1983; 83:1308–1310. A detailed discussion of a gluten-free diet, with suggestions to ensure the client's compliance.

Supporting the patient with Crohn's disease: Nursing grand rounds. *Nurs 83* (Nov) 1983; 13:46–51. A case study of a client with Crohn's disease, with detailed discussion of the nursing care required.

The Client With Bowel Obstruction and Possible Malignancy

I. Brief Descriptive Data	Mr John Jones, a 50-year-old engineer, has been admitted to the surgical unit from the emergency room. He has been experiencing persistent symptoms of anorexia, nausea, vomiting, and tenderness in the abdomen for the last 24 hours. His wife accompanies him.

II. Personal Data

Date and Time:	Jan 26, 1986
Full Name:	John Henry Jones
Social Security Number:	000-00-0000
Address:	42 Scott St, Martysville, Maine
Telephone:	Home: 000-0000
	Business: 000-0000
Sex:	Male
Age:	50
Birthdate:	8-18-35
Marital Status:	Married
Race:	Black
Religion:	Catholic
Occupation:	Electrical engineer
Usual Health Care Provider:	Jane O'Donnell, MD

III. Health History

Source of Information:	Client and wife
Reliability of Informant:	Reliable
Chief Concern:	"I started to vomit yesterday, and my stomach feels full and sore."
History of Present Illness:	Twenty-four hours prior to admission, Mr Jones noted the onset of anorexia and nausea. Soon after, he began vomiting dark green liquid and undigested food. He limited his intake to toast and tea but continued to vomit. He has been unable to sleep, although he feels exhausted from all the discomfort and vomiting. At the urging of his wife, he came to the emergency room for examination.

In January 1983, he had a colon resection for a small benign tumor of the descending colon. He has experienced no problems with his bowels since the surgery until now. He has not had a BM or passed gas in 3 days. Prior to this, stools have been well formed, brown, and were passed easily without straining. He has noted no black tarry stools nor blood in the stool. Annual checkups since the surgery have all been normal.

He eats a well-balanced diet including fruits, vegetables, and bran cereal. Since his surgery, he has avoided fatty foods, quit smoking, and maintained a regular exercise program. He takes no medications. Family history is positive for malignancy of breast, prostate, colon. Brother with benign colon polyp.

Past Health History:	
Childhood:	Usual childhood diseases
Immunizations:	Last Td 1978
Medical Problems:	None
Surgeries:	Colon resection 1/83, benign tumor descending colon
Transfusions:	None

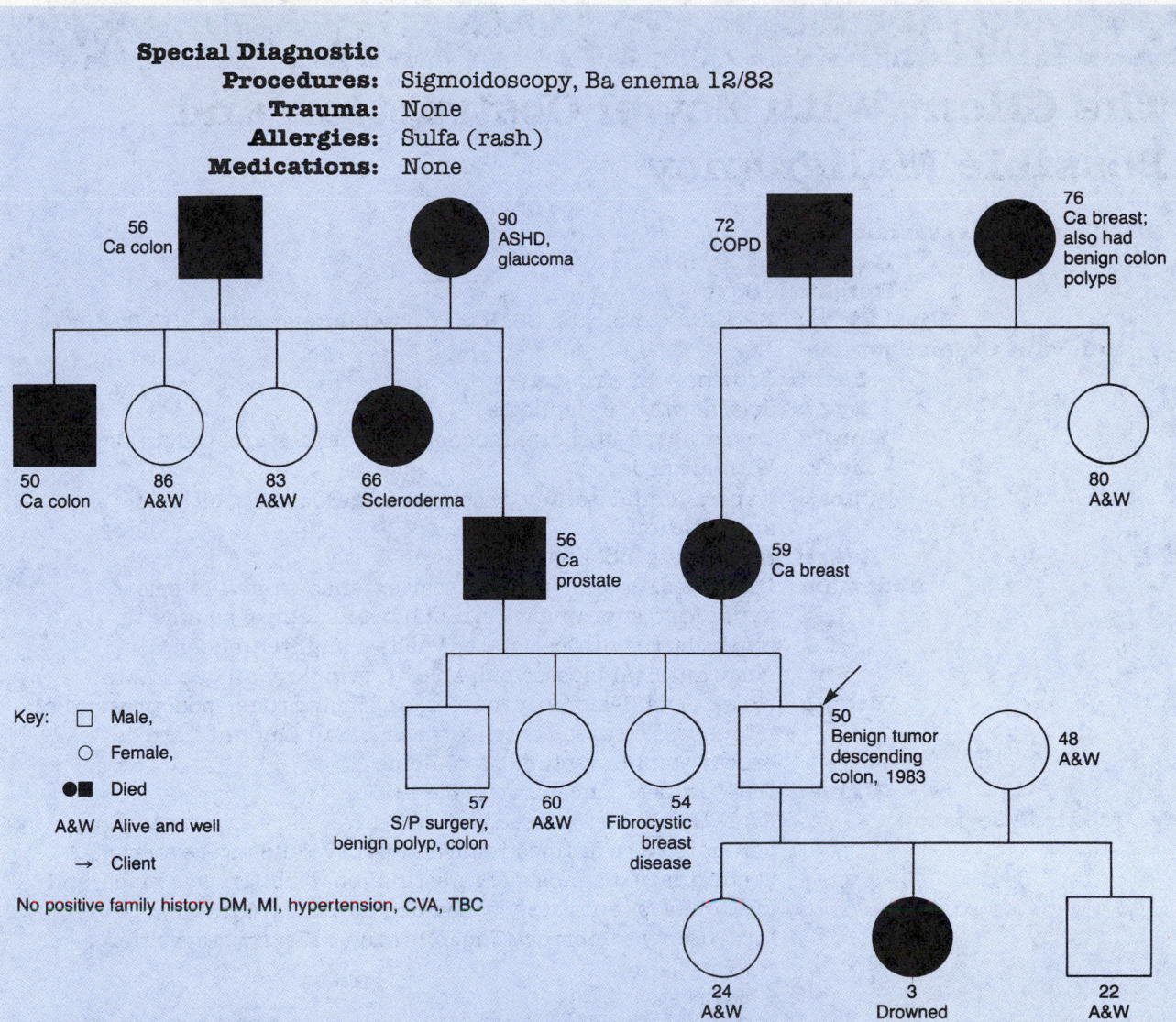

Special Diagnostic
Procedures: Sigmoidoscopy, Ba enema 12/82
Trauma: None
Allergies: Sulfa (rash)
Medications: None

Key:
- □ Male,
- ○ Female,
- ●■ Died
- A&W Alive and well
- → Client

No positive family history DM, MI, hypertension, CVA, TBC

Personal/Social History: Has worked as electrical engineer for past 25 years. Lives with wife in home they own. Daughter and son both in graduate school out of town, return home for holidays. He maintains a good relationship with them. Leaves for work at 7:45 AM and returns home at 5:30 PM. Recreation includes health club activities 2 evenings per week and playing cards 1 evening per week. Eats three meals per day (states they are well balanced with fresh fruit and vegetables). Sleeps well (7 to 8 hours per night), except for recent problem. Financially stable with adequate medical coverage. States he is generally relaxed and not a highly anxious person, although now he is worried about the possibility that cancer is causing his problem.

Review of Systems: States overall health is excellent, energy level good, weight stable

Chest: No cough; no SOB; no history of pneumonia, TBC, or chest trauma

Heart: No chest pain, no palpitations, no DOE, no PND; ECGs always wnl; no history of murmur, dysrhythmia

Gastrointestinal: See HPI

Genitourinary: No nocturia, dysuria, hematuria, polyuria, hesitancy, urgency, frequency, or problems with urinary stream; no history of UTI, renal calculi; able to maintain erection; no pain with intercourse or problem with ejaculation

(continued)

The Client With Bowel Obstruction and Possible Malignancy

IV. Physical Assessment

Height:	5 ft 9 in
Weight:	180 lb
Vital Signs:	BP 120/80; apical P 86; R 20; rectal temperature, 100°F (38°C)

Relevant Organ Systems:

Skin:	Brown; poor skin turgor
Eyes:	Sclerae without jaundice
Mouth:	Dry, cracked lips; oral mucous membranes and tongue dry
Neck:	Without nodes
Chest:	Expansion-bilaterally; resonant to percussion, clear to auscultation
Heart:	Apical rate, 86, regular; S_1 S_2 nl; ō ⓜ
Abdomen:	Distended, midline vertical scar extends from 2 in below xyphoid to suprapubic region; ō bruits; bowel sounds hyperactive with peristaltic rushes; slightly tender all quadrants; no masses palpable; ↑ tympany all quadrants
Rectal:	No external lesions or masses; sphincter tone good; prostate nl; no masses or areas of tenderness; small amount hard dark brown stool in rectum; stool heme ⊖
Urine:	Dark amber, concentrated; SG 1.033.

V. Medical Regimen

An N/G tube was passed and 300 mL of dark green gastric contents were drained immediately; IV fluids were started. A preliminary diagnosis of intestinal obstruction was made, and Mr Jones is tentatively scheduled for an exploratory laparotomy tomorrow. The following orders were written:

- NPO
- Bed rest
- IV 5% dextrose in 0.33 normal saline at 150 mL/hr
- NG to low Gomco suction, irrigate p.r.n.
- Intake and output
- Monitor specific gravity of urine q.8h.
- Prochlorperazine (Compazine), 10 mg q.6h. p.r.n. for nausea
- Ampicillin, 500 mg q.6h. IV

VI. Nursing Care Plan

Nursing Diagnosis	Client Care Goals	Plan/Nursing Implementation	Expected Outcomes
Fluid volume deficit, actual: related to excessive losses	Maintain normal fluid balance	Administer IVs as ordered; monitor for signs of normal hydration and dehydration (thirst, check skin turgor, check mouth and lips for dryness); monitor urine SG; strict intake and output; determine if balanced and report inconsistencies	Clients hydration status should show improvement as therapy is instituted; skin turgor should be normal; mouth should be moist; urine SG should be normal; and I&O should be balanced
Oral mucous membranes, alterations in: related to dehydration	Reduce or eliminate dryness of mouth and lips	Allow client to suck on gauze pad moistened with water or use ice chips, as	Condition of client's mouth will improve; lips and mouth will be

Nursing Diagnosis	Client Care Goals	Plan/Nursing Implementation	Expected Outcomes
		permitted; provide materials for frequent mouth rinse; lubricate lips with sterile jelly or use Chapstick; continue mouth care with attention to flossing and brushing of teeth; instruct client and wife in mouth care	moist and not cracked and dry; wife will demonstrate involvement in husband's care
Nutrition, alteration in: less than body requirements, related to disruption of normal GI function	Maintain nutritional status	Alleviate nausea and vomiting through use of nasogastric tube; maintain patency with irrigation p.r.n.; give prochlorperazine as needed; provide fluid and electrolyte replacement as ordered; observe for symptoms and signs of electrolyte imbalance; monitor laboratory values; report problems to MD promptly; monitor client's weight daily	Electrolyte status remains normal; nutritional assessment reveals no weight loss
Self-care deficit: related to weakness and bed rest	Reduce or eliminate discomfort; promote hygiene	Assist client p.r.n. with use of bedpan, urinal; keep within easy reach; provide materials and water for hygiene; assist p.r.n.; should client and wife desire, teach wife management of urinal and bedpan and where to save urine for I&O	Client will be clean, with all needs for hygiene and elimination met; urine will be measured and discarded promptly
Bowel elimination, alteration in: related to probable obstruction	Maintain bowel elimination status	Monitor bowel elimination status frequently; check frequently for bowel sounds, change in abdominal distention, passage of stool or flatus; report any improvement or deterioration of bowel status promptly	Client's elimination status improves (passes stool or flatus, bowel sounds normal) or remains status quo
Anxiety; related to uncertainty of diagnosis	Express fears of malignancy, colostomy because of strong positive family history of cancer	Encourage client to verbalize fears and feelings; keep client and wife informed about his status; encourage family to ask questions and verbalize their feelings as well; encourage family to visit and participate in care; if any possibility of colostomy exists, urge the surgeon to discuss this fully with client and spouse; remain with client after this discussion to clarify any questions	Client appears calmer; expresses his fears more readily; does not manifest signs of severe anxiety

Chapter 50

Surgical Approaches to Gastrointestinal Dysfunction

Nancy Nuwer Konstantinides

Objectives

When you have finished studying this chapter, you should be able to:

List the indications for surgical intervention with gastrointestinal and pancreatic disorders.

Describe common surgical procedures used in gastrointestinal and pancreatic disorders.

Explain the physiological implications of these surgical treatments.

Anticipate the psychosocial/lifestyle implications of these surgical interventions.

Outline the pertinent nursing interventions in caring for clients with surgery of the gastrointestinal tract and pancreas.

The earlier chapters in this unit have identified the crucial role of the gastrointestinal system in the maintenance of life and health. When medical management cannot control gastrointestinal dysfunction or prevent gastrointestinal complications, surgical treatment becomes necessary. Surgery may also be needed to ensure the integrity and effective functioning of the other body systems that depend on the supply of nutrients provided by a healthy GI tract.

Clients undergoing surgical treatment of the gastrointestinal system often experience lengthy hospitalizations, altered body image, the need to adjust to a different way of taking in food or eliminating waste products, and embarrassment over the public nature of what are usually, at least in the case of elimination, private functions. The nurse who cares for these clients must be sensitive as well as skilled.

This chapter discusses surgical approaches to dysfunction of the esophagus, stomach, small and large intestine, anorectum, and pancreas as well as surgical treatment for persons with life-threatening obesity. Surgery of the mouth and oral cavity has been covered in Chapter 21; jaw wiring is discussed in Chapter 19.

Section I: Surgical Approaches to Disorders Affecting the Esophagus

Surgery is performed on the esophagus to treat such disorders as achalasia, strictures, esophageal diverticuli, neoplasms, reflux esophagitis, and hiatal hernia.

ESOPHAGOMYOTOMY

When a client has difficulty eating because of achalasia and medical treatment has not relieved symptoms, an esophagomyotomy can be performed.

Surgical Procedure

The surgeon makes either an abdominal or a thoracic incision and cuts the lower esophageal muscle longitudinally to facilitate passage of food into the stomach.

Implications for the Client

Physiological Implications

Esophagomyotomy relieves the discomfort of achalasia,

1523

but reflux esophagitis may develop. The irritation produced by reflux esophagitis can cause esophageal stenosis, requiring further surgery.

Psychosocial/Lifestyle Implications

To the extent that the process of eating is returned to normal, the psychosocial implications are limited to dealing with the presence of a scar and the experience of surgery.

Nursing Implications

Client teaching for prevention of reflux esophagitis is an important nursing responsibility. The approaches described in Box 50–1 will help to prevent reflux irritation.

ESOPHAGECTOMY

The entire esophagus or sections of it may be excised because of strictures, esophageal rupture, damage from caustics, or neoplasm. With esophageal neoplasms, surgical excision is performed for curative or palliative reasons. (See Chapter 48 for discussion of esophageal cancer.)

Surgical Procedures

The extent of the resection in an esophagectomy varies, as does the structure to which the remaining esophagus is surgically attached (anastomosed).

Esophagostomy

With a ruptured lower esophagus or other condition that cannot be repaired, the upper esophagus may be diverted to the skin to form an esophagostomy, which will drain saliva and any swallowed liquids or foods. When the damage is to the upper esophagus, a feeding esophagostomy may be constructed.

Box 50–1 Approaches for Prevention of Reflux Esophagitis

Avoid bending over or lying down soon after eating.

Elevate the head of the bed on blocks if reflux tends to occur when lying down.

Eat small, more frequent meals to avoid overdistention of the stomach.

Use liquid antacids one-half hour after meals and at bedtime.

Avoid increased intra-abdominal pressure by:

1. Maintaining normal weight
2. Wearing nonconstricting clothing
3. Stopping smoking to decrease coughing

Esophagogastrostomy

The lower portion of the esophagus is excised and the remaining portion sutured to the stomach, which may have to be pulled into the thoracic cavity to reach the anastomosis site.

Colonic Interposition

When a significant portion of the esophagus is removed, it may be desirable to construct a conduit for passage of swallowed food and liquid using a portion of the colon or the small bowel. A colonic interposition is usually a second-stage procedure performed after a client has sufficiently recovered from an esophagectomy. The amount and section of the colon used varies, depending primarily on blood supply.

With a large esophageal resection, either the left, transverse, or right colon is excised. A portion of the ileum is removed when the right colon is used for interposition. The blood supply of the resected portion is kept intact, and the portion is brought into position for anastomosis to the remaining esophagus and the anterior wall of the stomach. The unresected bowel is anastomosed to bowel, as indicated by the extent and portion excised.

Implications for the Client

Physiological Implications

The physiological implications of esophagectomy depend in part on the extent to which an internal food conduit is restored, as well as the extent to which other structures (stomach, small or large intestine) are disturbed or put to new uses. Creation of an artificial opening to the exterior (a stoma) will change the physical nature of feeding. It will also produce a situation in which normally internal secretions can come in contact with the skin, with the possibility of irritation and skin breakdown.

Psychosocial/Lifestyle Implications

The psychosocial/lifestyle implications of a partial or complete esophagectomy depend in part on the reason for performing it. If the surgery is a life-saving procedure following trauma, the implications will not be the same as if surgery is made necessary by a suicide attempt or because of an esophageal carcinoma.

The diagnosis of malignancy carries the unknowns of a potentially terminal diagnosis as well as the temporary or permanent problems of inability to ingest food and liquids in the usual way. If esophageal damage was secondary to swallowing a caustic substance in a suicide attempt, the life problems that contributed to the self-destructive behavior remain after the surgical intervention. Referral to a mental health professional is essential with these clients as they begin to realize how their lives have been permanently changed by the esophageal damage. Depression and suicidal tendencies may be the aftermath of such insight.

Table 50–1 Esophagectomy: Implications for the Client

Physiological Implications	Psychosocial/Lifestyle Implications
Chewing helps maintain oral health and stimulates gastric secretions; clients who are able may chew food and then expectorate it; this may also have a psychological benefit.	Inability to swallow normal saliva and nasopharyngeal secretions causes drooling, need for expectoration and an acceptable way to manage accumulated secretions.
Wiping of accumulated saliva from lips or frequent licking of lips causes dryness and cracking; moisturizing agents are important.	Inability to eat normally may interfere with family and social relationships as well as with the client's body image.
Frequent oral care helps to maintain integrity of mucous membranes and prevent infection.	Client may be facing a terminal diagnosis and all that it involves.
If an N/G tube is present, frequent nasal and oral care are essential.	If esophagectomy was secondary to a suicide attempt, early referral to a mental health professional is essential to deal with the depression that may follow realization of what has occurred. The underlying problems that led to the suicide attempt also have to be addressed.
If a gastrostomy stoma is present, good skin care is essential to prevent irritation and breakdown.	

With the excision of the esophagus, either complete or partial, and the formation of an exterior stoma, the client must learn an array of new, often embarrassing, and sometimes frightening procedures. Family members may also need education and support. See Table 50–1 for a summary of physiological and psychosocial implications.

Nursing Implications

Preoperative Care
Preoperative nursing care for esophageal surgery is the same as for any major surgery, with one exception. If there is a possibility that the esophagus is not to be restored to its normal state, the client may be extremely anxious about the quality of postoperative life.

Postoperative Care
Nursing care following an esophagectomy will vary with the approach and with the extent of excision. If the lower esophagus is removed and a stoma created to drain the upper esophagus, a drainage bag will be needed to collect the swallowed material. Skin integrity around the stoma must be maintained. Nursing care for a feeding esophagostomy requires the same care for skin integrity, but in addition requires learning a new method of taking nourishment. (Feeding formulas and procedures are discussed in Chapter 47.)

Following a partial esophagectomy that includes an anastomosis to the stomach, small intestine, or portion of the colon to make an intact conduit for food, a nasogastric tube is usually used to prevent postoperative gastric retention. It is important to prevent any manipulation of the anastomosis. The nasogastric tube should be taped securely in place and should not be repositioned; a rupture of the esophageal anastomosis can be devastating. The nurse should observe the client to make sure the tube is clear of obstructions and draining properly. If the tube is not clear, irrigation may be necessary but should be done very gently to prevent pressure on the suture line.

If the esophagectomy is performed through the thorax, the client will require a chest tube to drain the pleural space. Nursing responsibilities with chest tubes are discussed in Chapter 18.

Nursing care following a colonic interposition includes maintaining gastric suction to prevent distention, maintaining chest tube drainage, and maintaining adequate respiration. Tube feedings into the stomach or small bowel may be required temporarily to maintain good nutritional status.

HIATAL HERNIA REPAIR

Hiatal hernia repair is more common than other types of esophageal surgery. If the esophageal–gastric junction bulges into the thoracic cavity (herniates), perhaps because of increased abdominal pressure, gastric secretions can reflux into the esophagus, producing irritation (heartburn). When medical treatment is unsuccessful in controlling the symptoms, surgical repair may be indicated. Definite indications for surgical repair include obstructive stricture and hemorrhage.

Surgical Procedure

One relatively common surgical approach to the repair of a hiatal hernia is *Nissen fundoplication* (Figure 50–1). The surgeon wraps the fundus of the stomach around the lower esophagus and sutures the fundus to itself. The fundus prevents the esophageal–gastric junction from slipping into the thoracic cavity so the symptoms of heartburn and pressure will not recur.

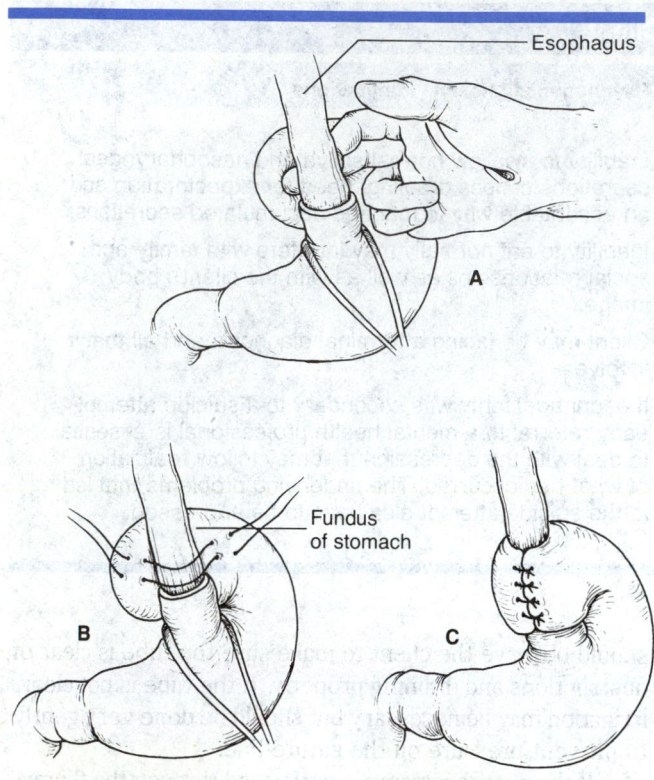

Figure 50–1

Nissen fundoplication.

Implications for the Client

Physiological Implications

Because the incision for hiatal hernia repair is so close to the diaphragm, coughing and deep breathing become uncomfortable, and belching may be impaired. Possible complications of surgical repair include those common to all major surgery (hemorrhage, infection, and pulmonary embolus) and those specific to esophageal surgery (dysphagia or difficulty in eating and swallowing, esophageal obstruction, esophageal perforation, and formation of a fistula).

Psychosocial/Lifestyle Implications

The psychosocial implications of hiatal hernia repair are generally limited to the effect of the incision on body image and the experience of major surgery. There may also be a reluctance to breathe deeply enough to ventilate the lungs properly because of pain or the fear of pain. The physiological and psychosocial/lifestyle implications are summarized in Table 50–2.

Nursing care specific to hiatal hernia repair includes maintaining respiratory status, maintaining gastric suction, and promoting appropriate nutritional intake when the client can begin to eat. Appropriate pain control measures may enhance the ability to aerate the lungs adequately. Clients should not be allowed to smoke for several days and should be encouraged to quit altogether. The nurse should instruct the client in ways of preventing the recurrence of reflux (see Box 50–1).

The client should begin a liquid diet when able to take in fluids. Gas-producing fluids such as carbonated beverages should be avoided because belching may be impaired and gas discomfort may develop. Transient dysphagia may be experienced as a result of edema around the lower esophagus. The client advances to eating solids according to tolerance.

Table 50–2 Hiatal Hernia Repair: Implications for the Client	
Physiological Implications	**Psychosocial/Lifestyle Implications**
Proximity of incision to diaphragm makes coughing and deep breathing uncomfortable.	Abdominal incision may affect body image.
Eructation may be impaired postoperatively.	To prevent recurrence, tight clothing should be avoided, smoking stopped, normal weight maintained, and emotional stress reduced.
Postoperative complications include: hemorrhage, infection, pulmonary embolus, dysphagia, esophageal obstruction, perforation, fistula formation.	Measures to avoid flatulence include eating slowly to avoid excessive air swallowing; avoiding carbonated beverages; and eliminating foods such as beans, broccoli, and cabbage from the diet.

Section II: Surgical Approaches to Gastric Disorders

Surgery for disorders of the stomach is indicated primarily for ulcer disease, tumor, morbid obesity, and conditions requiring a surgically implanted gastric tube for drainage or feeding. Surgical approaches to morbid obesity are discussed in Section III.

GASTRIC RESECTION

A partial or total gastrectomy is indicated primarily for ulcer disease or tumor. When the medical management of an ulcer is unsuccessful at controlling the symptoms and preventing complications, surgery is necessary. A gastric resection may be performed for hemorrhage, perforation, or obstruction resulting from ulcer disease. Gastric tumors are resected for cure or palliation.

Surgical Procedures

The specific surgical procedure performed for ulcer disease or tumor varies with the area and extent of involvement.

Vagotomy

A vagotomy, severing of the vagus nerve, is performed most commonly to decrease gastric acid secretion in duodenal ulcer disease. The type of vagotomy depends on where the nerve is severed—truncal, proximal, or selective.

Pyloroplasty

A pyloroplasty, enlarging the pyloric sphincter, is often performed with a vagotomy to control peptic ulcer disease. A pyloroplasty increases the rate of gastric emptying.

Subtotal Gastrectomy

A portion of the stomach, usually the lower portion, is removed. A vagotomy is performed along with a subtotal gastrectomy to control peptic ulcer disease. A subtotal gastrectomy may also be performed for gastritis, tumor, or gastric outlet obstruction.

Billroth I (Gastroduodenostomy)

Following the resection of the lower stomach, as with a subtotal gastrectomy, the remaining stomach is sutured end-to-end to the duodenum in a Billroth I procedure (Figure 50–2). This is performed primarily for ulcer disease.

Billroth II (Gastrojejunostomy)

Another option for an anastomosis following a subtotal gastrectomy is the Billroth II procedure, where the stomach stump is sutured end-to-side to an opening along the jejunum (Figure 50–3). A blind loop or afferent loop (portion of bowel ending in a dead end) is created that includes the duodenum. This decreases stimulation to the duodenum without interrupting the normal secretion of pancreatic juices into the small bowel.

Total Gastrectomy

The entire stomach may be removed as treatment for tumor or Zollinger–Ellison disease (see Chapter 49), although a subtotal gastrectomy is preferred for localized gastric neoplasms in order to maintain some gastric function. With a total gastrectomy, the esophagus is sutured either to the duodenum or the jejunum. A portion of colon or jejunum may be interpositioned between the esophagus and remaining small bowel to reconstruct the continuity of the gastrointestinal tract.

Implications for the Client

Physiological Implications

Severing the vagus nerve may decrease gastric motility, and the result of gastric retention may be bloating, pain, and vomiting. However, vagotomy may also result in abrupt emptying of stomach contents into the intestine (dumping syndrome), which produces vasomotor symptoms (flushing, palpitations, lightheadedness, tachycardia, diaphoresis, and postural hypotension) and may produce diarrhea. The cause of the dumping syndrome is thought to be related to the rapid entrance of hypertonic chyme from the stomach into the small bowel, causing fluid to be drawn into the bowel lumen. Plasma volume drops, and the intestine becomes distended, causing cramping and an urge to defecate.

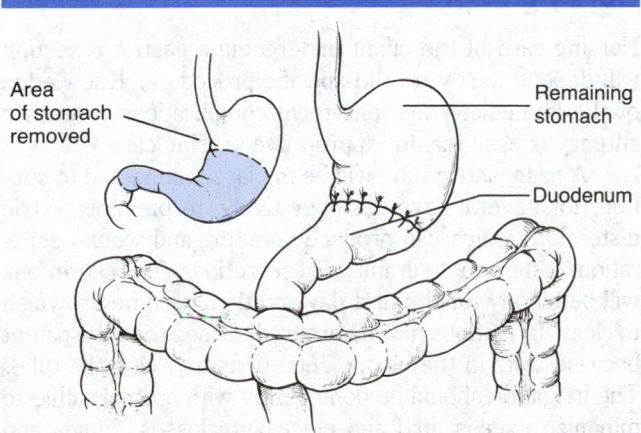

Figure 50–2

Billroth I procedure.

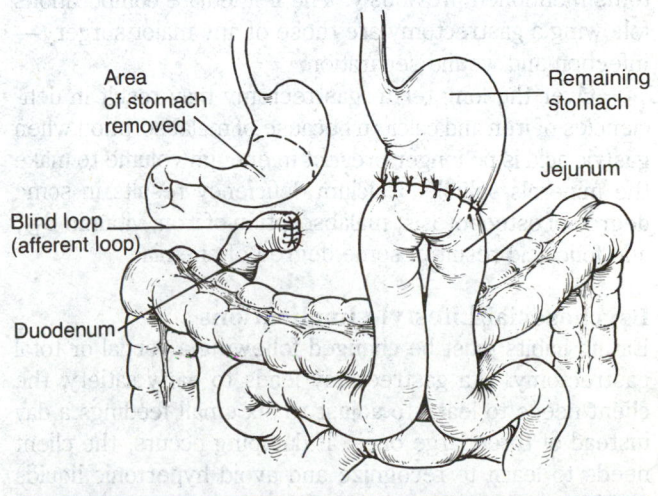

Figure 50–3

Billroth II procedure.

Table 50–3 Gastric Resection: Implications for the Client

Physiological Implications	Psychosocial/Lifestyle Implications
Vagotomy may decrease gastric motility, causing bloating, pain, and vomiting.	Partial gastrectomy may lead to early satiety, necessitating a change in eating habits to six small feedings per day.
Vagotomy may increase gastric emptying, causing diarrhea and symptoms of dumping syndrome.	Client should learn to recognize and avoid hypertonic liquids and high carbohydrate foods to decrease dumping syndrome.
Vagotomy may be associated with dysphagia, cholelithiasis, and recurrent ulcer.	If vitamin B_{12} absorption is greatly impaired, the client may need to plan for regular B_{12} injections for life.
Achlorhydria following gastric resection and vagotomy may be associated with risk of gastric cancer.	Client may have to learn strategies for coping with dumping syndrome and diarrhea.
Alkaline intestinal secretions may reflux into the stomach, causing gastritis.	Lifestyle may be altered by the development of osteoporosis.
Gastric surgery may result in dumping syndrome.	Chronic anemia may cause fatigue, affecting home life and work.
Gastrointestinal symptoms of dumping syndrome include bloating, cramping, diarrhea, nausea, and vomiting.	
Vasomotor symptoms of dumping syndrome include flushing, palpitations, lightheadedness, tachycardia, diaphoresis, and postural hypotension.	
Long-term complications following gastrectomy may include: 1. Iron and calcium deficiency because these minerals require gastric acid to increase solubility 2. Bone disease—osteoporosis 3. Anemia from maldigestion and malabsorption of iron, vitamin B_{12}, and folic acid 4. Weight loss and malnutrition	

Gastric resection with vagotomy results in achlorhydria, which is associated with some risk of gastric cancer in the future. Also, alkaline intestinal secretions may reflux into the stomach, causing gastritis. Gastrectomy may result in the dumping syndrome even when the vagus nerve remains intact, with resultant bloating, cramping, diarrhea, nausea, and vomiting as well as the vasomotor symptoms mentioned previously. The immediate complications following a gastrectomy are those of any major surgery— infection and wound separation.

Over the long term, gastrectomy may result in deficiencies of iron and calcium because of malabsorption when gastric acid is no longer present in enough volume to make the minerals soluble. Calcium deficiency results in some degree of osteoporosis; malabsorption of iron, vitamin B_{12}, and folic acid result in some degree of anemia.

Psychosocial/Lifestyle Implications

Eating habits must be changed following a partial or total gastrectomy. If a gastrectomy leads to early satiety, the client needs to learn to adjust to six small feedings a day instead of three large ones. If dumping occurs, the client needs to learn to recognize and avoid hypertonic liquids and high carbohydrate foods. If chronic anemia occurs or vitamin B_{12} absorption is greatly impaired, the client may have to adjust to a lifelong course of vitamin B_{12} injections

and may have to learn strategies to deal with chronic fatigue at work and at home. Also, the client may have to develop strategies for avoiding or coping with chronic diarrhea. The physiologic and psychosocial impact of a gastrectomy is outlined in Table 50–3. The primary nursing responsibilities include preventing complications, promoting comfort, and maintaining adequate nutrition.

Nursing Implications

Nursing care of the client undergoing a gastric resection will depend partly on the specific procedure. Knowledge of the immediate and long-term complications of gastric surgery is essential for appropriate nursing care.

A nasogastric tube will be in place, connected to suction, for several days postoperatively, to prevent gastric distention (which can produce vomiting and wound separation) and promote drainage of secretions. The secretions will be bloody for the first day and then become brownish to clear. Irrigations may be ordered to keep the tube patent because clots in the bloody secretions may clog the tube. The irrigation should be done gently with normal saline to minimize excess fluid and electrolyte losses. Fluids and electrolytes are given intravenously to replace the gastric losses.

The incision line should be inspected for signs of infection, hemorrhage, and wound separation (**dehiscence**). Sterile technique should be used when changing the dressing; the first dressing change may be performed by the surgeon. Some remove the original dressing 3 days postoperatively and leave it off. Dressings saturated with fresh blood should be replaced rather than reinforced, since blood can harbor organisms that can infect the site.

The nurse should promote client comfort following gastric surgery. Elevating the head of the bed will facilitate breathing as well as lessen the strain on the suture line. Holding a pillow over the incision may lessen the pain of deep breathing, coughing, and moving. Oral and nasal care can also promote comfort when a nasogastric tube is present. Unless contraindicated, the tape that holds the nasogastric tube in place should be reinforced or replaced when necessary. It is important to avoid changing the tube position when changing the tape to avoid pressure on the internal suture line. The nares should be cleansed if crusted secretions build up around the tube.

The client's nutritional status may be maintained with parenteral nutrition for several days postoperatively (the average is 4 days). Bowel motility will not return until several days after surgery because of the minor degree of postoperative paralytic ileus that normally occurs after abdominal surgery. The nurse should listen for bowel sounds and ask the client if any flatus has been passed. A decrease in nasogastric secretions usually accompanies the return of bowel motility. Oral fluids may be initiated; ice chips are generally well tolerated. The oral intake should be minimal with gastric suction to prevent excess fluid and electrolyte losses. When the nasogastric tube is no longer required, clear liquids can be initiated. The diet is slowly advanced to solid food. To avoid the dumping syndrome, caused by rapid flow of chyme into the small intestine, high carbohydrate foods and fluids should not be given. With a partial gastrectomy, the client may need six small feedings a day to prevent distention while promoting good nutritional intake. Early satiety with large meals can cause undernutrition. Nutrition is important following a gastrectomy since clients are vulnerable to malnutrition and weight loss.

GASTROSTOMY

A gastrostomy is an opening into the stomach. Generally, a tube is inserted into the opening, externalizing the gastrostomy for drainage or feedings. A gastrostomy for drainage is used with longstanding or progressive obstruction of the gastric outlet or intestine. This method is used, for example, as palliation when metastatic carcinoma causes bowel obstruction. A gastrostomy in this setting should relieve frequent and persistent vomiting. Gastric drainage is enhanced by gravity or by suction.

A gastrostomy can also be used for feeding in conditions where oral feeding is contraindicated for relatively long periods of time but the gastrointestinal tract is functioning. Examples are some head and neck carcinomas, esophageal rupture or massive resection, conditions with impaired swallowing such as advanced multiple sclerosis, or amyotrophic lateral sclerosis (ALS).

Surgical Procedure

The gastrostomy tube is placed in the stomach through an incision in the abdominal wall. The tube is secured within the stomach as well as at the exit site to avoid slippage. Generally, a large bore tube is used, such as a polyvinylchloride nasogastric tube or a rubber tube (eg, Foley catheter). Where general anesthesia is contraindicated, a technique has been devised to insert a gastrostomy tube percutaneously using local anesthesia.

Another surgically inserted feeding tube similar to the gastrostomy is the esophagostomy (also referred to as a cervical esophagostomy). The esophagostomy tube is inserted in the neck area, threaded through the esophagus, with the end of the tube placed into the stomach. A large bore tube such as the polyvinylchloride nasogastric tube or a rubber tube is usually used. This esophagostomy is used for feeding purposes. See Chapter 47 for specific information about tube feedings.

Implications for the Client

Physiological and psychosocial/lifestyle implications of gastrostomy on client and family are discussed in Table 50–4.

Nursing Implications

Nursing care includes site care to maintain skin integrity, prevent infection, and maintain tube patency. The gastrostomy site should be observed daily for drainage and the area cleansed with the appropriate solution, usually hydrogen peroxide, povidone-iodine, or alcohol. A dressing should be placed over the site to prevent contamination. The tube should be securely taped to the skin to prevent stress on sutures or accidental tube dislodgement.

A surgically inserted gastrostomy tube has a psychosocial impact on the client. The presence of a tube, especially when exposed to others, affects the client's body image. The inability to eat in the normal oral way will greatly affect a client who places much value on oral consumption—tasting the food, chewing, swallowing. Altered eating methods may affect the social practices of mealtime, leaving the client feeling isolated. If long-term feedings are required, the client will have to learn how to administer them at home and how to obtain the necessary supplies. The client and family members will require time to adjust to the altered eating style. The nurse can help by suggesting strategies to keep the client integrated into the family group. When insurance does not cover these expenses, the client may feel guilt about the financial burden to the family.

Table 50–4 Gastrostomy: Implications for the Client	
Physiological Implications	**Psychosocial/Lifestyle Implications**
Skin irritation and breakdown around the gastrostomy tube from gastric secretions are prevented by close observation and thorough cleansing of the skin.	External feeding tubes may affect the client's body image.
Tube dislodgement is prevented by careful taping of the tube and vigilance during dressing, feeding, and activities of daily living.	Usual interaction with family and friends at mealtime may be altered.
Diarrhea may be prevented through use of lactose-free formulas.	Inability to taste and chew food may be upsetting to the client.
Cramping, bloating, nausea, vomiting, and diarrhea are prevented by slow administration of the feeding.	Social situations where food and drink are served may be uncomfortable for the client as well as for all others present.
Reflux of the feeding into the esophagus or backflow into the gastrostomy tube is prevented by having the client remain upright for one-half to 1 hour after eating.	

Section III: Surgical Approaches to Morbid Obesity

Surgical intervention for obesity is indicated for individuals who persistently weigh twice their ideal weight with no endocrine causes for the obesity. Such obesity is called *morbid* because it is severe enough to impair activities of daily living as well as to place a tremendous strain on the body. Surgical alternatives are considered when diet, behavior modification, and medications have been unsuccessful in adequately reducing weight. The primary surgical interventions used to control morbid obesity include gastrointestinal bypass, gastroplasty, and jejunoileal bypass. Most of the desired weight loss occurs within the first year following the procedure.

Surgical Procedures

Gastrointestinal Bypass

In a gastrointestinal bypass, the surgeon partitions the stomach to create a pouch with approximately one tenth the capacity of the stomach. The pouch is anastomosed to the jejunum, thus bypassing the lower stomach and the duodenum (Figure 50–4). This procedure has resulted in many medical problems.

Gastroplasty

Gastroplasty, also referred to as gastric stapling or gastric partitioning, was instituted as an alternative to the gastrointestinal bypass. The advantage of this procedure is that it causes less disruption of the gastrointestinal tract, allowing for normal digestion and absorption. Gastroplasty involves the creation of a small pouch by stapling the stomach together, using the upper portion of the stomach (Figure 50–5). The capacity of this pouch begins at approximately 50 mL, although stretching eventually increases it. A small channel is formed by removing several staples

from the stapling device before stapling. This channel allows food to pass from the pouch into the remaining stomach, thus maintaining the continuity of the gastrointestinal tract.

Jejunoileal Bypass

The jejunoileal bypass is performed to reduce intestinal absorption by bypassing most of the small intestine, thus promoting weight loss by malabsorption of nutrients. The surgical procedure involves the resection of the jejunum 14 in from its origin and suturing the end nearest to the

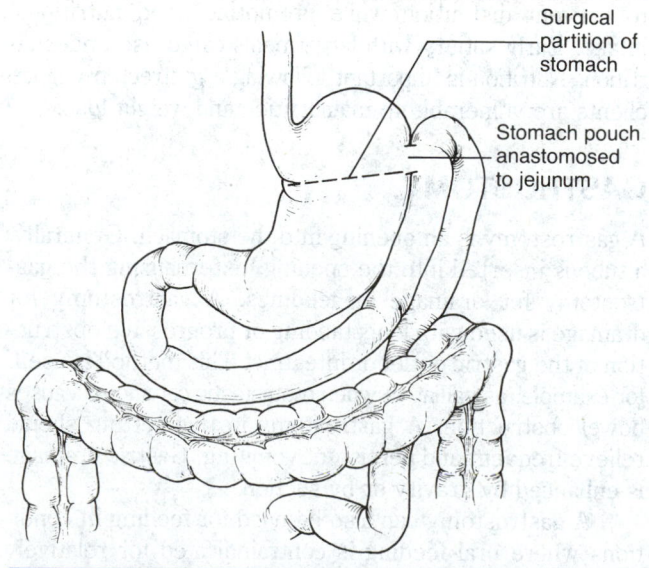

Figure 50–4

Gastrointestinal bypass.

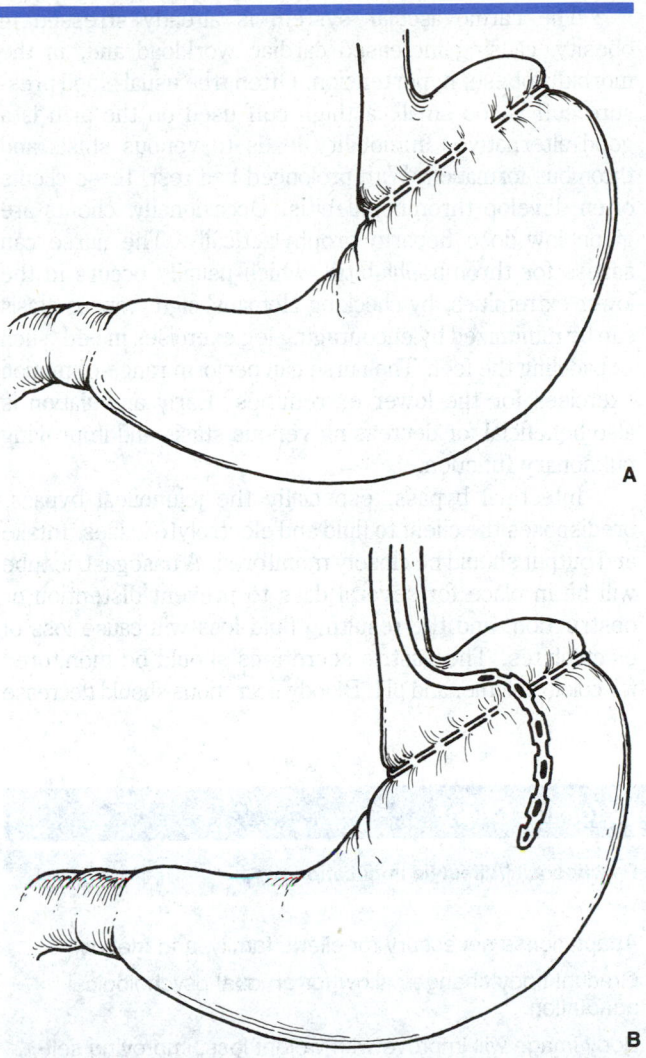

Figure 50–5

Gastroplasty. **A.** A double row of staples form the partition. Defect in the staple line where staples have been removed forms small funnel-shaped, uniformly calibrated opening to distal stomach. **B.** Nasogastric tube ensures postoperative drainage of both proximal pouch and distal portion.

stomach to the terminal ileum 4 in from the ileocecal valve (Figure 50–6). Maintaining the integrity of the ileocecal valve reduces diarrhea because this valve controls movement of contents from the small intestine into the large intestine. Postoperative complications of jejunoileal bypass include wound infections and thromboembolism.

Implications for the Client

Physiological Implications

Any bypass surgery disrupts gastrointestinal integrity and results in maldigestion and malabsorption. With the gastrointestinal bypass, there is malabsorption of iron, calcium, and vitamin B_{12}, with the possibility of anemia and osteoporosis. Therefore, appropriate replacement is essential.

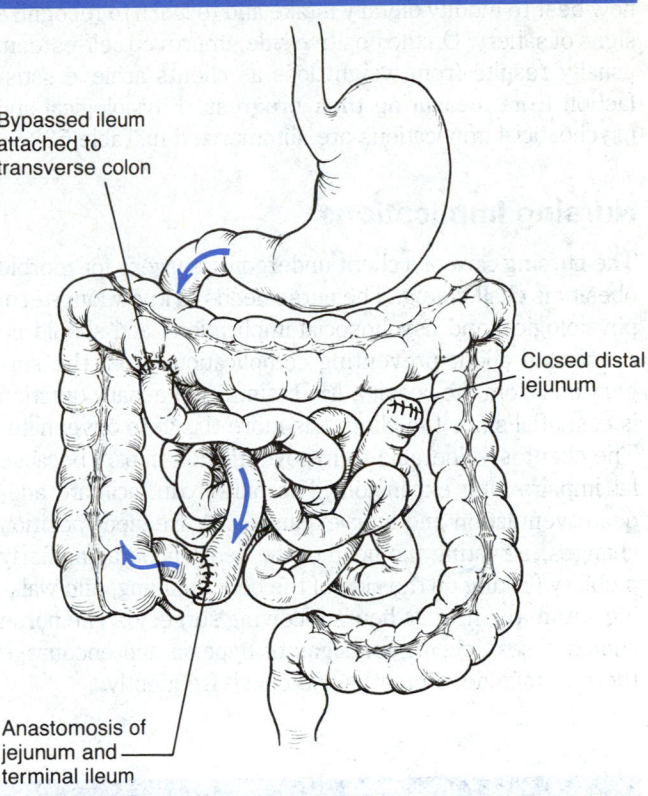

Bypassed ileum attached to transverse colon

Closed distal jejunum

Anastomosis of jejunum and terminal ileum

Figure 50–6

Jejunoileal bypass.

A life-threatening risk is that the pouch created by a gastrointestinal bypass can rupture, spilling food into the peritoneal cavity. Over time, food will stretch it, although excessive stretching weakens the pouch. The channel created in gastroplasty tolerates liquids better than solid foods.

All clients experience diarrhea after a jejunoileal bypass, but the frequency and volume are variable. Liver damage can occur following small bowel bypass, possibly as a result of accumulation of hepatotoxins or release of unknown toxic substances from the bypassed bowel. Hypokalemia may develop secondary to diarrhea. Malabsorption of calcium and magnesium produces deficiency unless appropriately replaced. Renal calculi and gallstones can occur secondary to the malabsorption of calcium. A migratory polyarthritis may develop and is thought to be caused by circulating immune complexes. Reversal or modification of the procedure may be necessary to manage some of these complications effectively.

Psychosocial/Lifestyle Implications

All clients who have a bypass or gastroplasty for morbid obesity must adapt psychologically. Not only the client but also family members and friends must adapt to the changes. On the negative side, the client may have expected magical results from the surgery and be upset and depressed when it alters the capacity to eat but not the desire; it may be frustrating wanting to splurge or binge on food while being physically unable to do so. The client will need to learn how best to modify dietary intake and to learn to recognize signs of satiety. On the positive side, improved self-esteem usually results from weight loss as clients achieve satisfaction from measuring their progress. Physiological and psychosocial implications are summarized in Table 50–5.

Nursing Implications

The nursing care of a client undergoing surgery for morbid obesity is challenging. The nurse needs to know long-term physiological and psychosocial implications and should be concerned about preventing complications from the surgery and from the obesity. Maintaining pulmonary function is essential since the client has more tissue to oxygenate. The client is vulnerable to hypoventilation in part because fat impairs lung expansion. The nurse can facilitate adequate ventilation and lung expansion by frequent position changes, elevating the head of the bed, encouraging early mobility (sitting on the side of the bed, standing, and walking within the first 24 hours following surgery). The nurse should assess clients for signs of hypoxia and encourage them to take deep breaths and cough frequently.

The cardiovascular system is already stressed in obesity, causing increased cardiac workload and, in the morbidly obese, hypertension. Often, the usual blood pressure cuff is too small; a thigh cuff used on the arm is a good alternative. Immobility leads to venous stasis and thrombus formation. With prolonged bed rest, these clients often develop thrombophlebitis. Occasionally, clients are given low-dose heparin prophylactically. The nurse can assess for thrombophlebitis, which usually occurs in the lower extremities, by checking Homans' sign. Venous stasis can be minimized by encouraging leg exercises in bed, such as paddling the feet. The nurse can perform range-of-motion exercises for the lower extremities. Early ambulation is also beneficial for decreasing venous stasis and improving pulmonary function.

Intestinal bypass, especially the jejunoileal bypass, predisposes the client to fluid and electrolyte losses. Intake and output should be closely monitored. A nasogastric tube will be in place for several days to prevent distention or obstruction, and the resulting fluid loss will cause loss of electrolytes. The gastric secretions should be monitored for color, volume, and pH. Bloody secretions should decrease

---

Table 50–5 Surgery for Morbid Obesity: Implications for the Client

Physiological Implications	Psychosocial/Lifestyle Implications
Bowel integrity is disrupted with bypass surgery, causing maldigestion and malabsorption. Gastrointestinal bypass: • Results in malabsorption of iron and vitamin B_{12}, leading to anemia • Results in decreased stimulation of the pancreas since the duodenum is bypassed The pouch created with gastrointestinal bypass and gastroplasty can stretch, rupture, or become obstructed. The channel created in the gastroplasty tolerates liquids best. Jejunoileal bypass: • Results in malnutrition from malabsorption of vitamins, minerals, and amino acids • Results in electrolyte imbalance, worsened with diarrhea, especially loss of potassium, magnesium, and calcium • Can result in liver damage • Can cause bacterial enteritis in the bypassed bowel • Can result in gallstones, renal stones, and migratory polyarthritis	Adaptation is necessary for client, family, and friends. Gradual body changes allow for gradual psychological adaptation. Body image will improve with weight loss, improving self-concept. Progress in weight loss may give client hope and a sense of pride, increasing self-esteem. Client may experience some frustration in the adjustments because of side effects and limit in ability to splurge because of early satiety from gastrointestinal bypass and gastroplasty. Client may not alter need for oral gratification or improve willpower. Client must adapt to long-term medical follow-up. Client must alter or buy clothes, which may be a financial burden. Client can usually live and work normally. Client must realize that a reversal or modification of the procedure may be necessary. Client must modify dietary intake for life; clients having gastroplasty must drink liquids for 8 to 12 weeks. Clients having gastroplasty and gastrointestinal bypass must eat slowly and chew food well. All must respond to signs of satiety, because the pouch or anastomosis will rupture with excessive stretching, leading to hemorrhage, peritonitis, shock, and possibly death.

by the second postoperative day. The nurse should check tube patency, irrigating it if ordered. Complaints of abdominal pain and distention may indicate a nasogastric tube obstruction and should be promptly reported.

Diarrhea also promotes fluid and electrolyte losses, particularly of potassium, magnesium, and calcium. The nurse must closely monitor for electrolyte losses even after the nasogastric tube has been removed. Potassium loss will cause neuromuscular weakness and dysrhythmias. Clients may require supplementary potassium. Encourage clients to eat foods high in potassium such as oranges, apricots, bananas, baked potatoes, milk and milk products, percolated or instant coffee, tea, or prune juice.

The nurse should maintain skin integrity in obese clients. Dampness in skin folds may promote excoriation and fungal infections. Diarrhea may cause anal irritation and skin breakdown. Local application of ointments or sitz baths may be soothing.

Wound management of the obese can be difficult, because their wounds heal poorly. Abdominal wounds are particularly vulnerable to separation or dehiscence, and infection may result. The wound site should be handled aseptically and observed for signs of edema, redness, drainage, or separation. A drainage suction device may be used to facilitate removal of secretions from around the wound.

Maintenance of nutrition is essential. Most clients will start sipping liquids within 3 to 4 days of surgery. The diet is slowly advanced to full liquids; however, gastroplasty requires a liquid intake for several months. The transition to food can be frustrating for all clients. Certain foods such as cabbage will worsen bloating, flatulence, and diarrhea; these foods should be discouraged. All clients need to make dietary modifications. Emphasis should be placed on balanced nutritional intake. Working with a dietitian is helpful.

The nurse plays a crucial role in helping clients, their family, and friends adapt to lifestyle changes as well. Help the client identify strategies of dealing with the inability to splurge or binge on food, and with the frustration experienced as a result, by meeting the need for oral gratification in other ways. Also instruct the client not only to respond to signs of satiety by stopping eating but how to recognize those signs.

Make clear what the risks are: a rupture of the pouch or the anastomosis that spills food into the peritoneal cavity is life threatening, and stretching the pouch excessively not only weakens it but is in opposition to the reason for performing the operation in the first place. See Chapter 9 for a more complete discussion of strategies for coping with eating problems.

Section IV: Surgical Approaches to Disorders of the Intestines

The many indications for surgical treatment of intestinal disorders include inflammatory bowel disease; bowel obstruction from tumor, adhesions, or hernia; vascular insults; trauma; neoplasia; polyps; and conditions requiring diversion of the fecal stream. The most common surgical interventions for these disorders are the feeding jejunostomy, appendectomy, herniorrhaphy, polypectomy, and bowel resection (including colostomy, ileostomy, and abdominal–perineal resections).

FEEDING JEJUNOSTOMY

A feeding jejunostomy is an adjunct to major abdominal surgical procedures of the esophagus, stomach, duodenum, pancreas, or biliary tract, or is used in the presence of an enterocutaneous fistula when feeding into the esophagus, stomach, or duodenum is undesirable. A feeding jejunostomy is usually contraindicated with inflammatory bowel disease, obstruction of the bowel, or when bowel rest is indicated.

Surgical Procedure

A feeding jejunostomy is established by inserting a feeding tube or catheter through an abdominal incision into the jejunum. The feeding catheter is usually inserted through

a needle (a narrow catheter is preferred), which is tunneled through the jejunum wall, then into the jejunum. The surgeon withdraws the needle and sutures the catheter in place at the point where it enters the jejunum and at the abdominal wall.

Implications for the Client

Physiological Implications
Because the jejunum does not have the reservoir capacity of the stomach, it is sensitive to the volume of the feedings. The jejunum is also sensitive to osmolality; an isotonic formula is preferred. Normal digestion and absorption are disrupted because the jejunostomy bypasses the stomach and duodenum. As a result, partially digested formulas are usually given. Intolerance to the strength and volume of the formula leads to nausea, cramping, bloating, tachycardia, palpitations, and diaphoresis.

Psychosocial/Lifestyle Implications
Occasionally, a feeding jejunostomy is required for long periods. These clients in particular feel the psychosocial impact of this alternative feeding route. They are denied the pleasure of chewing, swallowing, and tasting, and may feel isolated from the rest of the family at mealtime. Their body image is affected by the presence of the tube and

their lifestyle affected by the need to feed slowly. Home jejunostomy feedings require education of both client and family, including a method for obtaining supplies. Because this may initially be disruptive to a client and family, the nurse has an important role in helping them to adapt.

Nursing Implications

Nursing care includes flushing the catheter to keep it open; small-caliber catheters are especially vulnerable to clogging. The catheter should be well anchored to the abdominal wall to prevent its being dislodged; feeding into a dislodged catheter could deliver formula into the peritoneal cavity.

Site care is similar to that of any postoperative drainage tube. The nurse should cleanse the area daily (usually with hydrogen peroxide, povidone-iodine, or alcohol), inspect the tube site for infection, and cover it with a sterile dressing. An antimicrobial ointment may be applied to the site.

Feedings should be initiated at dilute strengths and low volumes to avoid problems such as discomfort or diarrhea, and should be administered with an enteral infusion pump to control the rate. Feedings administered continuously are best tolerated. The best formula for a feeding jejunostomy is partially predigested, low in viscosity (to avoid clogging the catheter), and isotonic. Refer to Chapter 47 for a complete discussion of tube feedings.

APPENDECTOMY

An appendectomy is the surgical removal of the appendix, a small, pouchlike structure attached to the cecum. An appendectomy may be performed in the presence of infection (appendicitis), to allay symptoms and prevent perforation (ruptured appendix), or as a prophylactic measure in clients having other abdominal surgery.

The appendix becomes inflamed in response to an obstruction in its narrow lumen, most frequently caused by feces or vegetable fibers. As a result, bacteria multiply within the appendix and cause inflammation, usually accompanied by pain, nausea, vomiting, fever, and elevated white blood cell count. As the inflammation continues, the peritoneum becomes irritated, which increases the pain.

To verify that pain is from appendicitis, look for rebound tenderness (pain following the release of deep pressure) in the right lower quadrant at McBurney's point. With pain from peritoneal irritation, clients will tighten their abdominal muscles (guarding) with palpation and feel more comfortable with the knees drawn up to the chest. Caution clients with suspected appendicitis to avoid cathartics because the stimulation may worsen the symptoms or cause the appendix to rupture.

Surgical Procedure

The surgical procedure is relatively simple. The appendix is excised from the cecum through an abdominal incision.

Because a major complication of appendicitis is a rupture with peritonitis, the inflamed appendix must be handled carefully during surgery.

Implications for the Client

Physiological Implications
The appendix is not known to have an important physiological role, and its removal produces no known physiological consequence, aside from the possible complications of the surgery itself. Abdominal adhesions in later years may be secondary to a ruptured appendix or to the appendectomy.

Psychosocial/Lifestyle Implications
An appendectomy has few psychosocial implications; the scar is small and inconspicuous, except for those with major wound infections. It may be hard for some young adults to accept that activities must be limited for several weeks until the wound has healed completely. Older clients may find that it takes longer for them to resume their normal lifestyle.

Nursing Implications

The postoperative course of an uncomplicated appendectomy includes a hospital stay of 3 to 4 days. A nasogastric tube is necessary only for complications. Incisional care is similar to that for other postoperative wounds. If there was excessive preoperative vomiting, fluids and electrolytes are monitored and replaced parenterally if needed.

POLYPECTOMY

A polypectomy is the surgical removal of a polyp. A polyp is a general term used for a tumor or growth usually on a stalk. Polyps can occur in various places, including the colon and rectum. Intestinal polyps usually extend inward into the lumen of the bowel and can cause bleeding or intestinal obstruction. Most colon and rectal polyps are benign, but some have malignant potential (eg, villous adenoma). A polypectomy is performed when polyps cause symptoms (such as bleeding) or when there is concern that the polyp may be premalignant.

Surgical Procedure

The safest and therefore the most common method for removing colon and rectal polyps is to snare them through an endoscope, either a flexible colonoscope or a rigid sigmoidoscope. This may be an outpatient procedure. The surgeon can also approach the lesion through an abdominal incision when the polyp cannot be reached or appears to be malignant.

The polyp is located and confirmed by x-ray, endoscopy, or both. The surgeon advances the endoscope to the area of the polyp, inserts a wire snare into one of the lumens of the endoscope, places the snare around the polyp stalk, and tightens it. Using cautery diathermy (burning electrical current), the surgeon excises the polyp at the stalk with minimal bleeding. The polyp is usually retrieved by the endoscope biopsy snare and sent for complete histological analysis to determine the presence or absence of cancer. The client is sedated for the procedure; general anesthesia is usually not required.

Implications for the Client

Physiological Implications
Most clients having polyp removal are over 50 years of age. With the rigid sigmoidoscope, the endoscopy procedure is done in the knee–chest position on a sigmoidoscopy table. Many clients find the position (and the procedure) uncomfortable and may become dizzy, nauseated, or feel faint during endoscopy. Postprocedure care involves evaluating vital signs and checking for rectal bleeding. Clients who are going home immediately after the procedure should be checked to be sure they can ambulate safely and are not feeling dizzy or faint. Regular follow-up is important, including colonoscopy or sigmoidoscopy every 2 to 3 years to detect recurrence.

Psychosocial/Lifestyle Implications
Psychosocial implications include the fear that the lesion is malignant or premalignant. Clients may feel anxious about the intrusion into their privacy caused by the procedure.

Nursing Implications

Preoperative Care
The bowel is prepared for a polypectomy by restricting oral intake and using cathartics, enemas, and possibly antibiotics to clear normal colon flora. Prepare the client for the fact that the procedure may be somewhat painful and embarrassing. Provide the client with the opportunity to discuss any fear of malignancy.

Postoperative Care
Preprocedure sedation wears off in several hours. The client should be observed for a day or two for signs of hemorrhage. Slight bleeding from the rectum is not uncommon. The client who is returning home shortly after the procedure should be prepared for the possibility of some mild bleeding.

BOWEL RESECTION

A bowel resection is the surgical excision of any portion of the small or large intestine or rectum. There are numerous indications for a bowel resection, including trauma, ischemic injury, obstruction, fistula, neoplasm, inflammation, and conditions that benefit from temporary or permanent fecal diversion (eg, rectovaginal fistula). The most common indications are obstruction, carcinoma, and inflammatory bowel disease.

Although cancer can involve any portion of the intestines, the sigmoid colon and the rectum are most frequently involved. Surgical excision is usually indicated. Preservation of the continuity of the intestinal tract is desirable but not always possible with resection of intestinal carcinoma. Many surgical excisions of cancer of the rectum or sigmoid colon include the construction of a stoma (an opening) for fecal elimination through the abdominal wall (Table 50–6).

Inflammatory bowel disease, including chronic ulcerative colitis and Crohn's disease (regional enteritis), often requires surgical intervention when medical management is unsuccessful or complications develop such as obstruction, hemorrhage, abscess, or fistula formation. Crohn's disease can affect the entire intestinal wall, leading to fistula and abscess formation. The extent of intestinal wall involvement may make medical and surgical management difficult. Ulcerative colitis generally affects only the mucosal layer of the colon; therefore, spontaneous fistulas are much less common. The presence of ulcerative colitis increases the risk of colon cancer, which develops after 7 to 10 years. Therefore, surgical excision of the entire colon is desirable.

In the past, for clients with ulcerative colitis, the rectum was sometimes left in place and the ileum pulled down and anastomosed to the rectum, avoiding an ileostomy. However, the incidence of recurrence of ulcerative colitis in the retained rectum was high, often requiring more surgery leading to ileostomy. New surgical techniques use the client's rectum and anus and prevent ileostomy. See discussion of ileal-anal reservoir below.

Diverticulitis may be treated with surgical excision. A temporary diverting colostomy may be necessary to allow time for healing of excised areas.

Surgical Procedures

A number of different surgical procedures fall under the heading of bowel resections. They are explained below.

Small Bowel Resection
The resection of the small bowel is indicated primarily for Crohn's disease, ischemic damage, and obstruction. The area and extent of resection are variable. The small bowel can be anastomosed to another portion of the small bowel (ileoileostomy), to the colon (ileocolostomy), or to the anorectum. The small bowel may be used to form an ileostomy (ostomy of the ileum).

Colectomy
A colectomy is the surgical excision of the colon. Removal of the right half of the colon (right hemicolectomy) or the left half (left hemicolectomy) can be done, leaving the rectum in place. The entire colon can be excised (total colectomy) with or without removal of the rectum. An external ostomy stoma may be constructed as a result of partial or total colectomy, or the colon may be anastomosed to another portion of the colon or to the rectum.

Table 50–6   Types of Ostomies

Type	Indication	Usual Location of Stoma	Consistency of Stool
Conventional ileostomy (Brooke ileostomy)	Ulcerative colitis; fecal diversion; temporary bowel rest; Crohn's disease; familial polyposis	Right lower quadrant	Liquid to pastelike
Continent ileostomy	Ulcerative colitis; familial polyposis	Right lower quadrant	Liquid to pastelike
Ascending colostomy	Fecal diversion	Right upper or lower quadrant	Liquid to semiformed
Transverse colostomy, single barrel	Fecal diversion; trauma; unresectable obstructing carcinoma	Right lower quadrant	Liquid to semiformed
Transverse colostomy: • Double barrel • Loop	Fecal diversion; trauma; unresectable obstructing carcinoma	Proximal in right lower quadrant Distal on left side	Liquid to semiformed
Descending colostomy	Colorectal cancer; diverticulitis	Left lower quadrant	Semiformed to solid
Sigmoid colostomy	Colorectal cancer; fecal diversion	Left lower quadrant	Semiformed to solid

Proctectomy

A proctectomy is the surgical excision of the rectum. With cancer of the lower and middle third of the rectum, a subtotal rectal resection can be performed. The rectal remnant (Hartmann's pouch) is closed and a colostomy constructed, or the left colon is stapled to the rectal remnant.

Total Proctocolectomy

The surgical excision of the entire colon and rectum, total proctocolectomy, is indicated for ulcerative colitis and multiple polyposis. The total removal of the colon and rectum makes an ileostomy necessary.

Ileostomy

An ileostomy involves bringing the ileum (usually the terminal ileum) onto the abdominal surface to form a stoma. An ileostomy is done either as a temporary measure (eg, for bowel rest) or as a permanent measure (eg, in ulcerative colitis with a total proctocolectomy). Types of ileostomies include conventional ileostomy, loop ileostomy, and continent ileostomy. The conventional ileostomy is constructed by pulling the proximal end of the ileum through the abdominal wall and turning it over itself to form a cuffed stoma (Figure 50–7). A properly constructed ileostomy has a 1-in protrusion to decrease complications of peristomal skin irritation. Fecal contents drain from the stoma into a collection pouch, which is worn continuously. The distal end of the remaining intestine may be sutured to form a blind loop, or it may be removed entirely.

The loop ileostomy involves pulling the intact ileum through the abdominal wall, placing a rod underneath the resulting loop to support it above the abdominal cavity, and making an opening on the top of the loop to permit fecal passage into a collection pouch. This procedure is used when a temporary ileostomy is necessary to promote healing of an anastomosis of the ileum to the anus.

A continent ileostomy involves the construction of an internal reservoir pouch for stool to control stool output. With the continent ileostomy, wearing an external collection device is unnecessary, which makes this form of ostomy preferable for psychosocial and sexual reasons. Contraindications include short bowel syndrome, Crohn's disease,

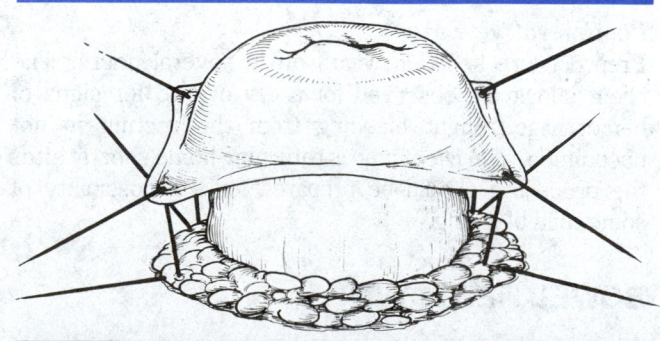

Figure 50–7

Ileostomy stoma construction (conventional). The end ileostomy is gradually everted so that a 3-cm spout is obtained. Note the subcuticular placement of the mucocutaneous sutures, to avoid ileal mucosal implants in the skin. Further sutures are placed between the four quadrant sutures and tied down.

obesity, high-dose steroids, and psychological instability that would render the person unable to perform necessary intubations.

The ileal reservoir pouch for the continent ileostomy is constructed by suturing ileal loops together with a nipple valve to maintain continence of feces and gas (Figure 50–8). The pouch capacity is around 100 to 600 mL, expanding to a larger volume with time. Although the client does not need to wear a collection pouch, mucus will be produced, and an absorbent dressing should be worn over the stoma. The stoma (which is usually even with the abdominal wall) needs to be intubated with a catheter two to four times daily to remove feces.

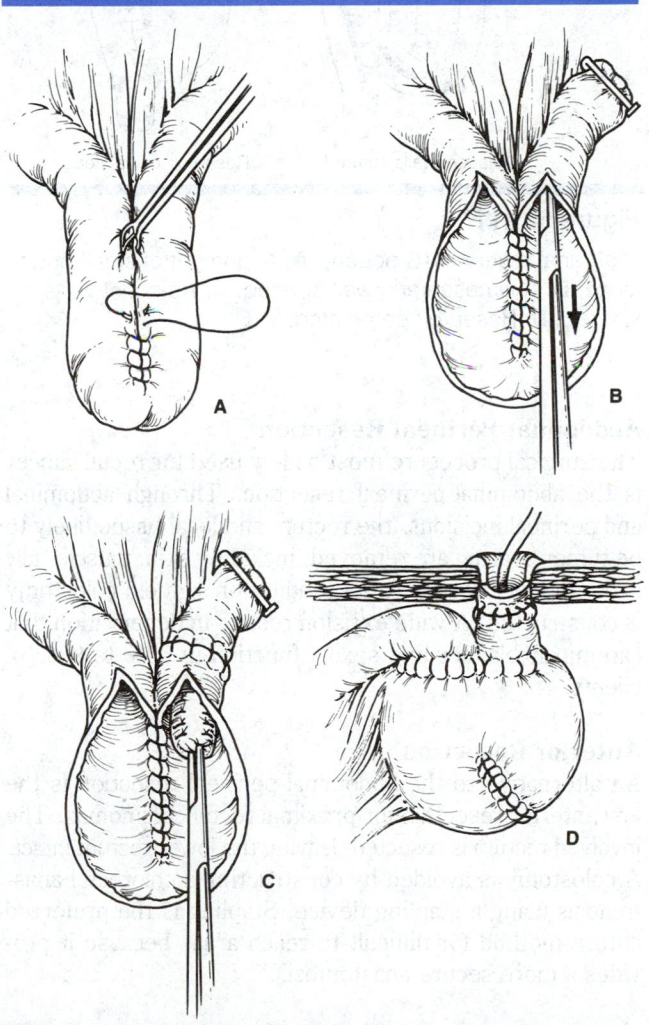

Figure 50–8

Construction of a continent ileostomy (Kock pouch). **A.** Surgeon loops ileum back on itself so that it is 15 cm on each side. **B.** Loop is sutured at its center along the anti-mesenteric border where the two segments touch. **C.** A long U-shaped incision is made around the 30-cm loop, close to suture line. **D.** Ileum opens up into a cuplike shape.

Cecostomy

This rarely performed procedure is an opening into the cecum, usually placed temporarily for decompression prior to a colectomy or an ileal-rectal anastomosis. The cecostomy usually has a tube in place for drainage.

Colostomy

A colostomy is a surgical opening of some portion of the colon onto the abdominal surface. The colostomy is constructed with either the proximal end of the remaining bowel or with a loop of colon. The loop colostomy is generally a temporary measure performed on the transverse colon. The loop may be kept intact with both proximal and distal openings together, or the loop may be severed to form two stomas (a double-barrel colostomy). The double-barrel colostomy prevents fecal passage into the distal bowel. Consistency of stool changes in the colon; therefore, the more distal the colostomy, the more formed the stool (Figure 50–9).

Mucous Fistula

A mucous fistula is a stoma constructed from a dormant portion of bowel following a bowel resection. This is an option when it is desirable to avoid a blind pouch, or when it is necessary to delay reanastomosis. In this procedure, a colostomy or ileostomy is constructed leaving the rectum intact; the proximal end of the rectum is brought up to the abdominal wall for drainage, thus forming the mucous fistula. This procedure prevents intraperitoneal leakage from

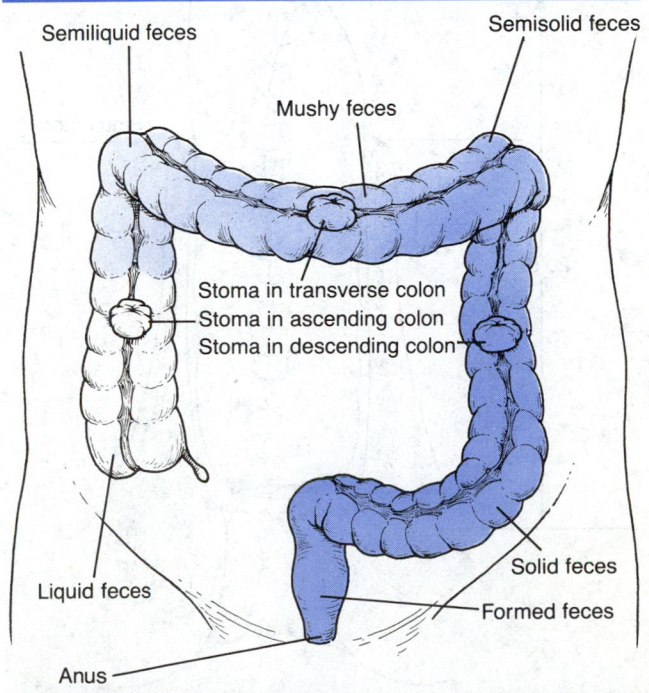

Figure 50–9

Stoma site and fecal consistency.

the rectal suture line where healing may be impaired, eg, after radiation therapy.

Ileal-Anal Reservoir

This procedure is optimal for multiple polyposis and ulcerative colitis because it preserves the rectal sphincter. Because no permanent stoma is needed, this procedure avoids the dramatic change in body image associated with wearing a collection pouch. The ileal-anal reservoir requires an intact anus and functional rectum. The entire colon is resected and rectal mucosa is stripped away, leaving the rectal muscles and anus. A reservoir is constructed with two or three loops of the terminal ileum and stapled to the anus. A J pouch is formed with two loops of terminal ileum (Figure 50–10), or an S-shaped pouch with three loops (Figure 50–11). As a result, the continuity of the intestine is maintained, and a permanent stoma is avoided. The reservoir acts to slow the passage of stool, although the client will experience diarrhea three to eight times per day. To promote healing of the reservoir and suture line, a temporary loop ileostomy is usually constructed for fecal drainage for about 3 months to allow time for healing the anal anastomosis.

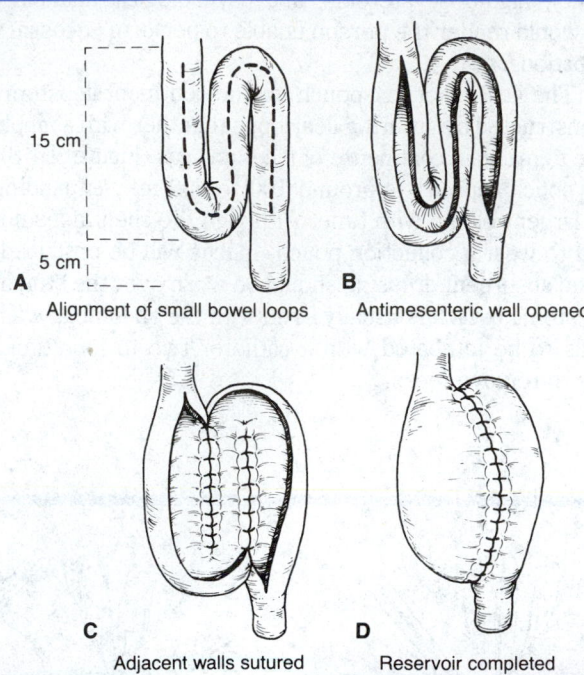

Figure 50–11

Ileal–anal reservoir (S pouch). **A.** Alignment of small bowel loops. **B.** Antimesenteric wall opened. **C.** Adjacent walls sutured. **D.** Reservoir completed.

Abdominal-Perineal Resection

The surgical procedure most widely used for rectal cancer is the abdominal-perineal resection. Through abdominal and perineal incisions, the rectum and local tissue likely to be tumor bearing are removed, including skin, muscle, fat, and lymphoid tissue. A descending or sigmoid colostomy is constructed. A wide excision results in denervation that can impair bladder and sexual function in 50% to 95% of clients.

Anterior Resection

An alternative to the abdominal-perineal resection is the low anterior resection for proximal rectal carcinomas. The involved rectum is resected, leaving the lower rectum intact. A colostomy is avoided by constructing a colorectal anastomosis using a stapling device. Stapling is the preferred suture method for difficult-to-reach areas because it provides a more secure anastomosis.

Implications for the Client

Physiological Implications

The physiological implications of bowel resection depend on the location and length of resection, the presence or absence of the ileocecal valve, the length of the bypassed bowel, and whether intestinal continuity is maintained. Resection of the small bowel will alter digestion and absorption of fluid and nutrients. If a long portion of the

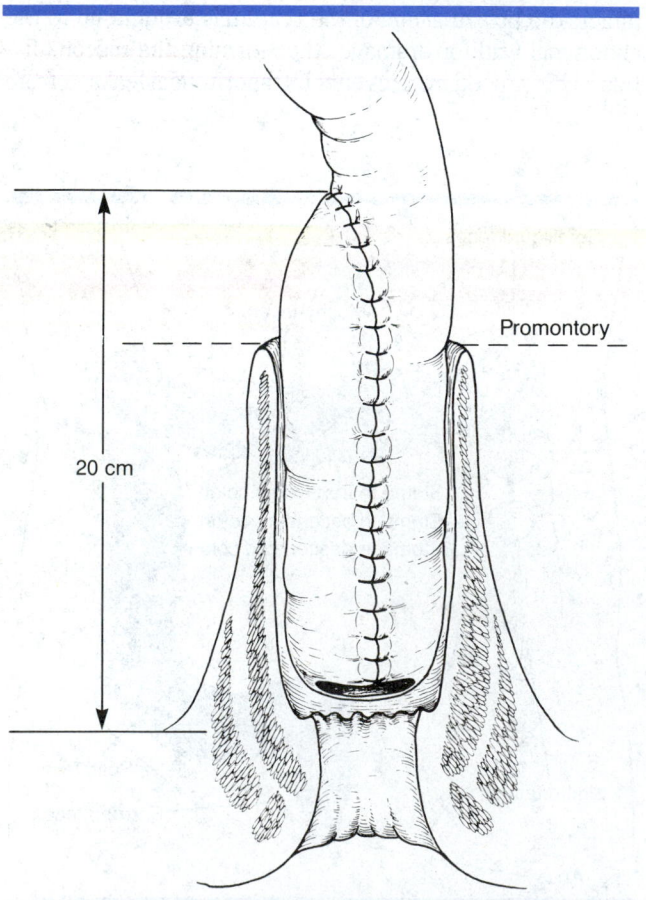

Figure 50–10

Ileal–anal reservoir (J pouch).

small bowel is removed or bypassed, malabsorption and diarrhea ensue (short bowel syndrome).

Resection or bypass of the ileocecal valve has specific implications because this valve controls the passage of stool into the colon and prevents backflow of feces into the small bowel. Resection or bypass of the ileocecal valve may result in diarrhea. When the terminal ileum is resected, vitamin B_{12} absorption is impaired, causing anemia.

Finally, when the entire colon is resected, excessive fluid loss may occur with frequent stooling. With time, fluid loss is decreased as the small intestine increases its absorption of fluid and electrolytes. With resection of the upper rectum and lower colon, it is ideal, if possible, to connect the remaining bowel to the remaining rectum to maintain intestinal continuity.

With ostomies, an inappropriate placement or inadequate stomal protrusion can make appliance management difficult. The stoma must be placed on a flat surface of the abdomen away from the incision line, other stomas, bony prominences, scars, indentations, skin folds, inguinal creases, and the umbilicus. A too-wide stoma can cause hernia or prolapse, whereas one that is too narrow can result in stenosis or obstruction. Other complications include skin irritation, stomal edema, stomal necrosis, and stomal recession.

Pregnancy and obesity can both cause problems. Pregnancy may lead to obstruction or prolapse, although both are uncommon. Obesity may interfere with the initial construction of the stoma, may contribute to decreased blood supply to the stoma or to a retracted stoma.

In an ileostomy, complications include fluid and electrolyte loss, malabsorption of vitamins (B_{12}) and minerals (zinc, sodium, and magnesium), and obstruction from food blockage or adhesions. In a continent ileostomy, further complications are possible, including incontinence, difficult intubation, perforation by catheter, and inflammation of the reservoir from bacterial overgrowth (pouchitis).

In an abdominal-perineal resection, the perineal wound is likely to require drains, and healing may be delayed.

For an ileal-anal reservoir, a two-stage procedure may be required, with a temporary ileostomy. This procedure results in persistent diarrhea, and it may take 6 to 12 months before adequate bowel function is established. Drugs or bulking agents may be needed for control. The reservoir may become inflamed or may have to be intubated to promote drainage. Other complications include excessive as well as persistent diarrhea, anastomotic leak, and incontinence.

Psychosocial/Lifestyle Implications

Psychosocial adjustment to a bowel resection when intestinal continuity has been maintained is directly related to the disease process necessitating resection (eg, benign polyp, malignancy) and quality of postoperative recovery from this major abdominal surgical procedure. In addition to these factors, psychosocial and lifestyle adjustment to an ostomy involve learning to live with a stoma on the

abdomen where intestinal contents are discharged in various states from liquid to solid.

With a stoma, clients often fear withdrawal of friends and family, loss of job or social status, inability to perform sexually, and rejection by the sexual partner. They may worry about being unable to have children or, in the case of a woman, how a pregnancy might interfere with bowel function and stomal viability. Clients may be frustrated at their inability to be completely independent—especially while becoming comfortable with the ostomy equipment, skin care, and problems caused by foods previously enjoyed. Concern over flatulence and fecal odors may contribute to social isolation.

Ostomy clients can live a completely normal life. They need to be helped to manage their ostomy in a caring, supportive, and practical manner. Because each client is unique and each lifestyle different, the nurse should understand as much as possible about the client's lifestyle—diet, exercise, bathroom facilities, travel, sexual preferences, work situation, and support systems. Then instruction can be individualized to meet the client's unique needs. Tables 50–7, 50–8, and 50–9 discuss physiological and psychosocial/lifestyle implications of ostomies, abdominal-perineal resection, and ileal-anal reservoir for the client.

Nursing Implications

Appropriate and adequate nursing care for a client undergoing a bowel resection depends on the specific surgical procedure, extent of reconstruction, and the likely pathophysiological consequences. The nurse must obtain from the surgeon the details of the resection and must apply that information to a solid knowledge of gastrointestinal physiology to plan appropriate care.

Preoperative Care

Preoperative management includes both physical and psychological preparation. The client will be restricted to oral fluids only for 2 to 3 days to control fecal accumulation. Cathartics, enemas, and/or suppositories are given to empty the intestines of feces, to minimize fecal contamination of the operative site. Antibiotics are often ordered to reduce bacterial flora, especially in the colon. Systemic broad-spectrum antibiotics may be used immediately preoperatively and continued postoperatively to control infection.

Clients may enter the hospital with fluid and electrolyte imbalances that need to be corrected before surgery. Anemia may also need correction (by iron or blood administration) to improve oxygen transport. Nutritional status of all clients should be assessed preoperatively since malnutrition leads to postoperative complications. (Debilitated clients may need several weeks of parenteral nutrition to improve nutritional status.)

For clients who will have an ostomy performed, the enterostomal therapist (usually a nurse) plays a crucial role in the client's physical and psychological care both preoperatively and postoperatively. The client's nurse should work

Table 50–7 Ostomy: Implications for the Client

Physiological Implications	Psychosocial/Lifestyle Implications
Inappropriate stoma placement can lead to difficult appliance management.	Adjustment is difficult when the client has unrealistic expectations, eg, ostomy will solve all problems or perceives it as only temporary.
Too wide a stoma opening can lead to hernia or prolapse; stoma too small can lead to stenosis or obstruction.	Client should be able to resume previous activities including recreation, social life, and work.
Stoma that does not protrude enough makes successful pouching difficult.	Procedure involves a complex psychosocial adjustment. May initially feel frustrated, discouraged, isolated, or depressed. May feel they have lost control and become dependent.
Obesity may interfere with constructing the stoma and may contribute to decreased blood supply to the stoma or to a flush or retracted stoma.	Client may have many fears, including rejection by significant others; loss of job; loss of role and status; interference with sexual relations; fear others will notice appliance under clothes, hear gas passing, and smell foul odors.
Pregnancy may lead to obstruction or prolapse, although this is uncommon.	
Colostomy may require irrigations if client desires.	Continent ileostomy requires intubation for drainage two to four times daily. A public restroom may be necessary for drainage.
Complications of an ileostomy include fluid loss (usual output 500 to 1500 mL/day); electrolyte, vitamin, and mineral loss (especially sodium, magnesium, zinc, and vitamin B_{12}); obstruction from food blockage or adhesions.	Body image and self-esteem alterations occur because of body changes and loss of sphincter control.
Complications of an ileostomy and of a colostomy include skin irritation, stomal edema, stomal necrosis, and stomal recession or prolapse.	Client may be concerned about ability to bear children.
	When learning physical skills, client may initially feel a lack of confidence and frustration.
Continent ileostomy advantages include no appliance necessary, little potential for skin excoriation.	Clothing preferences do not have to change.
Continent ileostomy must be emptied by inserting a catheter two to four times daily; fewer problems with gas, noise.	Dietary changes may be necessary, including need to increase fluid intake to prevent dehydration and avoiding foods that increase gas and odor of feces, eg, baked beans, onions, eggs, fish.
Complications of continent ileostomy include incontinence, difficult intubation, fistula, abscess, obstruction, perforation by catheter; may have malabsorption of fat, iron, folate, and vitamin B_{12}; fluid and electrolyte imbalance; pouchitis—inflammation due to bacterial overgrowth.	Client may want to meet others with ostomy for support.

Table 50–8 Abdominal-Perineal Resection: Implications for the Client*

Physiological Implications	Psychosocial/Lifestyle Implications
Perineal wound healing may be prolonged with complications such as infection, wound separation, and hemorrhage. This wound may require drains.	Psychological reactions are related to having cancer, fear of recurrence, and adjustment to mutilating nature of surgery.
Denervation in the perineal resection may lead to bladder and sexual dysfunction.	Body image is affected by having an ostomy and having had perineal resection with closure of anus.
The abdominal wound has the potential complications of infection, hemorrhage, and wound separation.	Oversewing of anus may impact homosexual relations. Client may fear rejection of lover.

*See also Table 50–7, Ostomy: Implications.

with the enterostomal therapist in the preoperative psychological preparation. The client's knowledge and perception of life with an ostomy should be assessed and any misconceptions corrected. The client should be taught the basics of gastrointestinal physiology, how the ostomy will alter the normal physiology, and what strategies are available to compensate for the changes. The client's anxieties should be addressed and support system and coping mech-

Table 50–9 Ileal-Anal Reservoir: Implications for the Client

Physiological Implications	Psychosocial/Lifestyle Implications
A sphincter-preserving surgery with no ostomy required and no appliance. This procedure may fail with recurrent disease to rectal stump, necessitating an ileostomy. May require a two-stage procedure with a temporary ileostomy. Diarrhea will persist and can be excessive. May be necessary to intubate anus with catheter to drain. May take 6 to 12 months until adequate bowel function is established. May need to use drugs or bulk agents for adequate control. Complications include excessive diarrhea, anastomotic leak, incontinence, urgency, pouchitis. Perineal skin protection is important.	Client can avoid having an ostomy. Procedure may fail if disease recurs in rectal stump. Client must learn self-intubation of anus with S pouch. Client may have to deal with incontinence or soiling, especially at night. Client will require regular follow-up with sigmoidoscopy and biopsies to detect recurrence or malignant changes associated with ulcerative colitis.

anisms evaluated. This knowledge will help in understanding and planning for postoperative reactions. Clients and their families must be encouraged to share their feelings and concerns. Good preoperative rapport with client and family will facilitate postoperative adjustment.

The enterostomal therapist can also arrange for the client to meet someone who already has had an ostomy—an ostomate. Discussion with a well-adjusted ostomate can relieve anxiety and helps both client and family to feel they are not alone. The ostomate often continues the relationship with client and family and may play an important role in facilitating postoperative adjustment and return to home and society.

Postoperative Care

Postoperative nursing goals include preventing complications, promoting wound healing, monitoring bowel function, promoting comfort, and maintaining adequate nutritional status. The principal goals of ostomy care include facilitating self-care and psychosocial adaptation, maintaining peristomal skin integrity, and promoting appropriate bowel elimination. Specific care needs for the client with a conventional ileostomy, continent ileostomy, or colostomy are discussed later in this section.

Preventing Complications. Decompression of the bowel will help to prevent complications. The bowel may be decompressed with a nasogastric tube, an intestinal tube, a cecostomy tube, a rectal tube, or a tube placed into the continent ileostomy reservoir. The principles of nasogastric tube management are discussed in Chapter 47 and in nursing fundamentals textbooks. A long intestinal tube, similar to a nasogastric tube, can be advanced into the small bowel (usually by a mercury bolus attached to the tube), where it decompresses the small bowel generally by attachment to low suction.

The cecostomy tube, rectal tube, and continent ileostomy tubes are relatively short tubes with wide lumens. Stool can plug these tubes, which may require periodic gentle irrigation to maintain patency. The continent ileostomy drainage tube is left in place for 2 weeks to promote healing.

The nurse should monitor drainage from all tubes carefully for amount, consistency, and characteristics. This information should be recorded every 2 hours.

Promoting Wound Healing. The nurse's role in wound management following bowel resection begins with observing the incision line for infection, hemorrhage, or separation. Sterile technique must be observed in changing dressings. Drainage tubes may be placed into the wound or along the incision to promote drainage of fluids, which

Nursing Research Note

Gloeckner MR: Perceptions of sexual attractiveness following ostomy surgery. *Res Nurs Health* 1984; 7:87–92.

This research evaluated feelings of sexual attractiveness in four groups of ostomy clients: those with colostomies, ileal conduits, ileostomies, and the Kock pouch.

The results suggest that in the first postoperative year, feelings of sexual attractiveness are lower than feelings preoperatively. After the first year, feelings of sexual attractiveness increased. Clients with Crohn's disease and ulcerative colitis had increased feelings of sexual attractiveness in subsequent postoperative years, surpassing preoperative feelings.

These findings may assist nurses in educating clients undergoing ostomy surgery regarding changes in body function and body image. Nurses should openly discuss issues of sexuality with the client and sexual partner, encouraging verbalization of feelings and sharing of perceptions, concerns, and fears between partners.

may otherwise impair healing. Drainage tubes may drain by internal pressure or by externally applied suction. Portable vacuum collection devices are frequently used when drainage is expected. These collection devices should be emptied regularly and the drainage characteristics and amount recorded.

The stoma should be observed for normal pink or red color, indicating adequate blood supply. The skin around the stoma (peristomal skin) should be protected by a skin barrier such as karaya gum (a protective resin) or a pectin wafer product (eg, stomadhesive, Hollihesive) soon after surgery before stool output begins. The stoma should be covered with a transparent collection pouch to protect the skin, to protect the incision from contamination by drainage from the stoma, to allow observation of the stoma and assessment of bowel function, and to decrease odor and increase client acceptance.

Perineal wound management presents a challenge to the nurse. When the entire rectum is removed, an empty space remains, which will eventually fill with granulation tissue. To promote drainage and healing, the perineal wound may be left open with gauze dressings packed inside, may be partially closed with a drainage tube in place, or may be completely closed. Nursing care will differ for each approach. The perineal wound is also uncomfortable for clients, making positioning and sitting difficult. Pain management is essential.

Monitoring Bowel Function. The nurse should continually monitor the client's bowel function following bowel resection. For several days, bowel motility will be minimal. Observe for return of bowel activity by auscultating for bowel sounds, asking clients if they have passed flatus, and monitoring any ostomy output. With an ostomy, stool output is expected within 4 to 7 days after surgery.

Maintaining Adequate Nutritional Status. Maintaining nutritional status in the postoperative period is another important nursing responsibility. When oral intake is delayed for up to a week or longer, parenteral nutrition is indicated. The parenteral solution should be tailored to the client's specific nutritional requirements, as determined by the dietitian or parenteral nutrition pharmacist, if one is available. Parenteral nutrition includes carbohydrates, amino acids, vitamins, trace elements, and electrolytes. Intravenous fat is supplied by a separate solution. Parenteral nutrition is best administered through a central venous catheter into the superior vena cava or right atrium. The rate of the infusion is controlled by an infusion pump to prevent fluctuation of blood sugar levels. The nurse must handle the parenteral nutrition and delivery system carefully to prevent inadvertent contamination. The client should be maintained on parenteral nutrition until oral intake reaches more than half of the required intake for 3 consecutive days. (Parenteral nutrition is discussed in greater detail in Chapter 8.) Specific nutritional considerations are discussed in the following section.

Ostomy Care

Care of the Conventional Ileostomy. The conventional ileostomy will drain serosanguineous fluid within 24 hours of surgery. Stool output begins with the return of bowel function in 3 to 5 days. The drainage is involuntary and frequent, especially at first. The stool is liquid, and may approach 1500 mL per day, but as the body adapts to the ileostomy, the drainage becomes pasty and about 500 mL per day. Because feces contain enzymes that are irritating to the skin, skin protection is critical. The ileostomy appliance (drainage device) used postoperatively should be disposable, drainable, adhesive backed, and odorproof. A skin barrier must be used as well. When the postoperative stomal swelling subsides, the client and enterostomal therapist can discuss appliance alternatives. There are two basic types, disposable and reusable. The many criteria to be considered in appropriate appliance selection include stoma construction, character of the peristomal skin, cost, client preference, and the client's manual dexterity.

Appliances without a skin barrier will require the addition of a skin protector prior to application. The peristomal skin should be cleansed with mild soap and water when the appliance is changed. The frequency of change depends on the type of appliance and the construction of the stoma. The appliance is easiest to change when output is minimal, generally early in the morning. All equipment necessary for change should be organized and ready. The new appliance should be prepared before the old one is removed. The collection pouch should be drained as soon as it is one third full of gas and/or stool. The nurse should measure the output. Care should be taken when handling the pouch so client acceptance is enhanced. For example, a facial expression while changing the pouch may say more to the client than words ever could.

With a new ileostomy, introduction of food into the diet should be gradual. Clients will slowly learn which foods cause increased drainage, odor, or gas. Cabbage and onions are common odor offenders. Yogurt may be eaten to control odor. When there is considerable air in the pouch, it should be emptied to prevent leakage. There are a number of deodorizers on the market, which can be swallowed or put into the bag. Blockage of the ileostomy should be avoided as far as possible by diet manipulation. Chewing food well, avoiding high-fiber foods, and adequate hydration will help to keep the ileostomy patent.

Clients and a family member, if possible, need to learn ileostomy care prior to discharge. Teaching must include emotional support and discussion of client concerns; skin care; equipment care; emptying, preparing, and applying the appliance; where to obtain supplies; odor management; and dietary modifications. The client should be encouraged to resume all previous activities.

Care of the Continent Ileostomy. For several weeks postoperatively, the ostomy is intubated continuously with a catheter set at low suction. This prevents distention of the new pouch and therefore promotes healing. After 2 to 3 weeks, the ostomy is periodically and gently intubated with a soft catheter to drain the contents of the pouch. The frequency of intubation can be decreased as the pouch capacity increases. Fibrous food is avoided to prevent blockage. The client can drink grape juice as a mild laxative to keep stool liquid. Skin integrity is maintained with daily cleansing, and the stoma is kept covered with an absorbent dressing between emptying. The nurse teaches the client proper intubation and how to detect signs of obstruction.

Care of the Colostomy. The most common colostomy is the sigmoid or descending colostomy. Transverse loop colostomy is less common and presents more difficulties in maintaining skin integrity and proper appliance fit. The sigmoid colostomy will usually drain formed stool on a relatively regular schedule, making care easier than ostomies with frequent, liquid drainage. Many clients prefer a closed and odorproof pouch and are willing to use irrigations to maintain regularity. If irrigations are not desired or are inappropriate, a drainable pouch is indicated. Skin barriers are optional, but a correctly fitting appliance is essential to prevent breakdown of peristomal skin.

Colostomy irrigations (Figure 50–12) may give the client some control over elimination. The procedure takes approximately 1 hour, and it is usually performed in the bathroom. The client fills a container with 500 to 1000 mL of warm, not hot, tap water; hangs the container at shoulder level; and flushes water through the tubing to remove the air. A cone tip is attached to the irrigating tubing and lubricated. The colostomy appliance is removed, and the belted irrigating sleeve is applied. The cone tip is inserted gently into the stoma. This device fits snugly into the stoma and prevents backflow. The water is infused slowly over 3 to 5 minutes to prevent cramping and distention. The client then removes the cone, and fecal material drains directly through the irrigating sleeve into the toilet. When drainage is complete, the client cleans and dries the peristomal skin. The appropriate appliance is applied with or without skin barrier.

The client should be adequately prepared for discharge. Time is needed to recover from surgery and develop confidence in colostomy management. Teach the client site care; emptying, preparing, and applying the pouch; equipment care; proper irrigations; and dietary modifications. Provide emotional support. Discharge planning should include what supplies are necessary, where to obtain them, and where to obtain home help. Referral to a home health agency may be needed.

Psychosocial Support With an Ostomy. The psychological reaction to having an ostomy varies. An effect on body image and self-esteem is expected. Clients experience many fears—realistic and unrealistic. The nurse can support clients by helping them to express their feelings

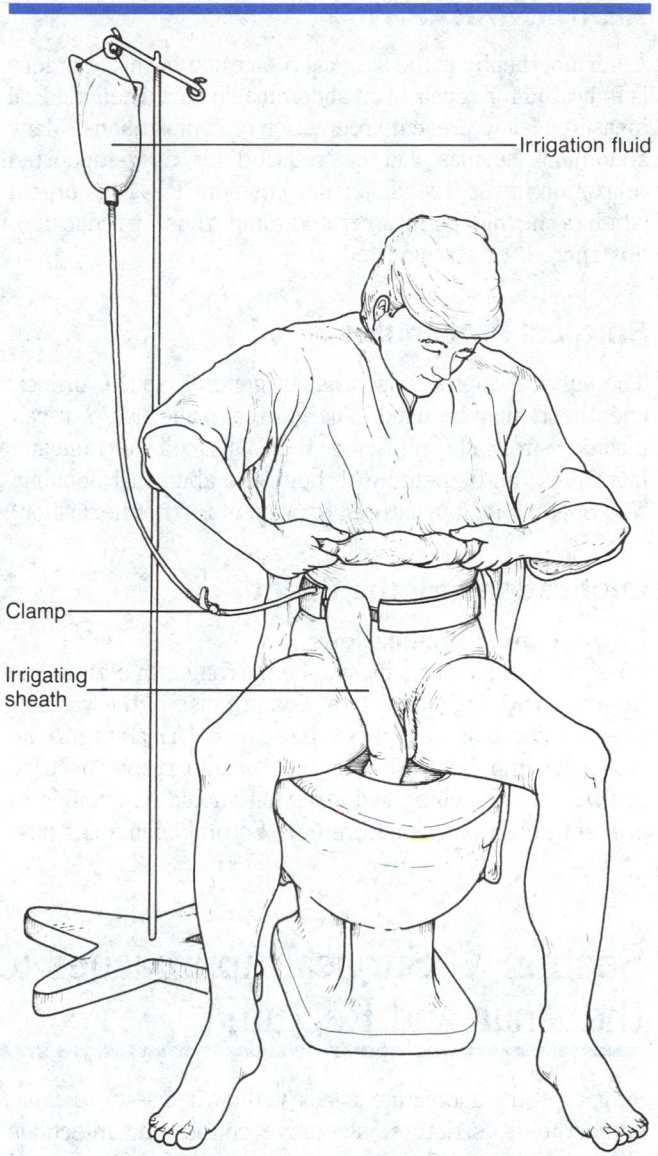

Irrigation fluid

Clamp

Irrigating
sheath

Figure 50–12

Client position for colostomy irrigation.

and anxieties. Many clients worry about the impact of an ostomy in social interactions. Some fear that the stoma will be obvious to others, and many fear it will interfere with sexual relations. If appropriate to the client's situation, the significant other should be included in discussions regarding resumption of normal activities, including sexual relations. There are times when ostomy surgery, or any surgery, may cause a person to feel less desirable sexually or may cause the partner to view the loved one in that way. Helping clients accept the alteration as a minor change in bodily appearance or function that has not decreased their worth as a person will assist them most when working out their own relationships with loved ones. If nurses can help clients to feel good about themselves, then clients will be better prepared to face the world outside.

HERNIORRHAPHY

A herniorrhaphy is the surgical repair of a hernia. Surgery is indicated for repair of an abdominal hernia when medical measures fail to prevent progression or complications. Many abdominal hernias can be reduced by drug-supported relaxation in the Trendelenburg position. Repair is urgent when a hernia is incarcerated (and thus, irreducible), obstructed, or strangulated.

Surgical Procedures

The surgical approach is variable; general, spinal, or local anesthesia may be used. The general principles of repair include surgically replacing the displaced peritoneum, intestines, and omentum through the abnormal opening. The opening is then sutured to prevent further herniation.

Implications for the Client

Physiological Implications

Possible complications include hemorrhage, infection, and (for men with inguinal hernia) compromise of the vas deferens or the blood supply to the testes. Urination may be somewhat impaired with an inguinal herniorrhaphy because of the pain. Coughing and straining should be avoided to prevent strain on the suture line. Scrotal edema is a possible postoperative complication. A scrotal support with an ice bag will help to reduce edema and pain.

Psychosocial/Lifestyle Implications

Physical and sexual activity should be limited for several weeks and heavy lifting avoided for up to 6 weeks. Recurrent herniation may require a change in employment or in a lifestyle that includes heavy lifting.

Nursing Implications

Nursing care following a hernia repair depends on the surgical approach and anesthesia. General measures include promoting comfort, preventing straining, assessing urinary status, and observing the incision for signs of infection or hemorrhage and the scrotum for edema. The client may ambulate soon after surgery, which will facilitate voiding. There are no special dietary modifications except to avoid constipating foods and to increase bulk and fiber. The nurse should explain physical limitations to the client, paying close attention to activities of daily living which need modification to prevent straining. Postoperative discomfort from inguinal hernias may be decreased with the use of a scrotal support. Some hernia repairs are performed on an outpatient basis, limiting the time the nurse has for teaching and postoperative observation.

Section V: Surgical Approaches to Disorders of the Anus and Rectum

Surgery of the anorectum is indicated for neoplasm, trauma, hemorrhoids, stricture, ulcerative colitis, and infectious disease (inflamed fissure, rectal abscess and fistula, and warts). A discussion of proctectomy is included under bowel resection in the preceding section.

HEMORRHOIDECTOMY

A hemorrhoidectomy is the surgical excision of a hemorrhoid. Surgery is indicated when medical measures, such as dietary modification, are unsuccessful in controlling progression or complications such as bulging of internal hemorrhoids into the anal canal, strangulation, pain, bleeding, thrombosis, itch, and fecal incontinence.

Surgical Procedure

The surgical approach to hemorrhoids, which is designed to remove or reduce the affected tissue, is frequently performed on an outpatient basis. Several methods are used, including rubber band ligation, sclerotherapy, and excision. Rubber band ligation, a quick and simple procedure, is performed only on internal hemorrhoids (Figure 50–13) because it is too painful for the external hemorrhoids, which have more sensory nerves. The internal hemorrhoid is isolated, and using special equipment, a rubber band is slipped over the base of the hemorrhoid. This will cause the hemorrhoid to shrink from ischemia and slough off or to scar and atrophy. Postprocedural rectal fullness makes it preferable to ligate only one or two hemorrhoids at one time, allowing 4 to 6 weeks for complete healing. Sclerotherapy (injection of a sclerosing agent) is a less common technique used to control internal hemorrhoids. In this procedure, the hemorrhoid is isolated and injected with a sclerosing agent designed to reduce swelling by atrophy of the involved tissue. Surgical excision, referred to as a closed hemorrhoidectomy, is the preferred procedure for external hemorrhoids where thrombosis has occurred. Anesthesia is local, spinal, or general. The involved tissue is surgically excised with the area sutured closed.

Implications for the Client

The physiological, psychosocial, and lifestyle implications are discussed in Table 50–10. Complications of hemorrhoidectomy are also briefly outlined in the table.

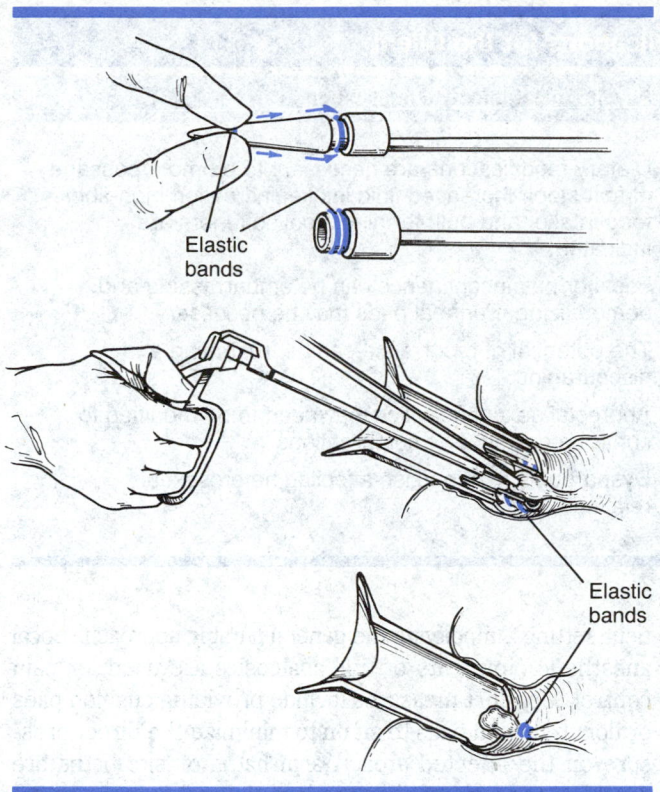

Figure 50–13
Rubber band ligation of hemorrhoids.

Nursing Implications

Nursing care following hemorrhoidectomy includes promoting comfort, promoting elimination, and observing for complications. Comfort measures include mild oral analgesics and local moist heat. Sitz baths or warm tub baths soothe the inflamed tissue and cleanse the area. Slight bleeding may occur for the first day, but excessive bleeding is of concern. Some clients prefer wearing a protective perineal pad to prevent soiling of clothes and bedding. The nurse should instruct the client in dietary modifications to prevent constipation. Increased intake of fluids and high-

fiber foods are helpful. Bulk-forming stool softeners such as psyllium mucilloid (Metamucil) can promote normal stooling. Clients should be advised that the first bowel movement may be uncomfortable—some describe the feeling as "passing glass." Clients should be encouraged to avoid straining during a bowel movement.

SURGERY FOR ANORECTAL INFECTION

Surgery may be indicated for infectious disorders of the anorectum. Infections can result from traumatic fissures (cracks or ulcers) or infected anal glands. An infected anal gland can progress to form an acute abscess, which can progress further to form a fistula (sinus tract). Disorders that predispose to the development of anorectal infection include Crohn's disease, trauma, radiation therapy, and cancer. Surgical intervention for anorectal infections is generally indicated when medical management does not control the unpleasant symptoms.

Surgical Procedures

A wide variety of surgical procedures may be used. Selection of a procedure depends upon the extent of the anorectal infection.

- Incision and drainage involve a surgically created opening that allows for passage of secretions. Removing purulent secretions promotes internal healing and decreases discomfort from pressure. This procedure is often preferred for fistulas and abscesses.
- Fistulotomy is the incision and drainage of a fistula. This may be preferred to an excision, which may leave a gaping wound.
- Fistulectomy is the surgical excision of the involved tissues around a fistula. This creates a wound that requires meticulous care to prevent reinfection.
- Fissurectomy is the surgical excision of a fissure. Since a fissure can be more superficial than a fistula, the

Table 50–10 Hemorrhoidectomy: Implications for the Client	
Physiological Implications	**Psychosocial/Lifestyle Implications**
Complications include infection, hemorrhage, stricture, difficult defecation, and stool incontinence.	Dietary modification is necessary to promote regular bowel movements and avoid constipation. Increased fluid intake and high-fiber foods are helpful.
Hemorrhoids can recur.	
Client should avoid straining and constipation.	With immediate postoperative fecal or blood oozing, soiling of clothing can be embarrassing. The need to wear protective pads can also be humiliating to some.
If taking anticoagulants or aspirin, the client must be closely observed for bleeding.	Weight reduction is advised for the obese client.
	Regular exercise also helps to maintain normal bowel function.

Table 50–11 Surgery for Anorectal Infections: Implications for the Client	
Physiological Implications	**Psychosocial/Lifestyle Implications**
Complications include wound infection, hemorrhage, stricture, difficult defecation, fecal impaction, fecal incontinence, and urinary retention.	Dietary modifications are necessary to promote passage of soft stool. Increased fluid intake, increased high-fiber food intake, and bulk-forming stool softeners are indicated.
Anorectal infections have a high rate of recurrence.	
Crohn's disease, trauma, radiation therapy, and cancer can predispose to recurrence.	Fecal or pus incontinence can be embarrassing and demoralizing. Perineal pads may be necessary.
Lesions can extend into the vagina, causing drainage and dyspareunia.	The potential of recurrence can be frustrating and discouraging.
With prior radiation therapy, healing will be impaired, possibly necessitating a diverting colostomy to prevent fecal contamination.	Anorectal sexual activities may need to be modified to control recurrence or complications.
	Dyspareunia may persist, affecting heterosexual relations.

area of excision is not as large. If the excised area becomes reinfected, a fistula or abscess can result.

- Sphincterotomy is an opening or excision to enlarge the sphincter to prevent further tearing and promote healing of an anal fissure.

Implications for the Client

See Table 50–11 for physiological and psychosocial/lifestyle implications of surgery for anorectal infections.

Nursing Implications

The nursing care following surgery for anorectal infections includes promoting comfort, promoting wound healing, promoting elimination, and preventing complications. Anorectal procedures may be performed in outpatient or inpatient settings, modifying the general nursing approach. Local anesthetic ointments or oral analgesics are used for pain control. Comfort measures include providing cushion pads or donut-shaped pads to sit on to minimize the direct pressure on the affected area. Warm baths or sitz baths are soothing and promote cleansing of the incision; the warm water may also promote the drainage of purulent secretions.

Wound management varies. Open wounds may be packed with sterile gauze. Gauze soaked in solutions designed to draw out purulent secretions or with bacteriostatic action may be packed or applied to the lesion. Close attention to wound management is essential, since anorectal infections tend to recur.

Proper elimination is promoted by ingestion of high-fiber foods, increasing fluid intake, and administering bulk-forming stool softeners. Defecation should be encouraged to prevent fecal impaction.

Section VI: Surgical Approaches to Disorders of the Pancreas

Surgical treatment for disorders of the pancreas is indicated for trauma, neoplasm, inflammation, and obstruction (eg, calculi). A client with pancreatitis may need surgery for such complications as hemorrhage or pseudocyst or when gallstones cause pain or clinical deterioration because of obstruction. The client with pancreatic pseudocyst may need surgery for obstruction, infection, hemorrhage, rupture, or uncontrolled pain. Surgical treatment of pancreatic carcinoma is indicated with localized disease or as a palliative measure.

Surgical Procedures

Drainage of Pancreatic Pseudocyst

The pseudocyst can be drained internally into adjacent structures such as the stomach, duodenum, or jejunum—

the preferred method. However, placing a drainage tube into an external collection device is sometimes necessary. Percutaneous drainage of the pseudocyst can be effective while avoiding risks associated with general surgery. Draining the pseudocyst relieves compression of nearby structures and promotes healing.

Resection of the Tail of the Pancreas

The resection of the pancreatic tail is indicated to remove disease localized in the distal portion of the organ. With local adenocarcinoma, the tail of the pancreas and the spleen are removed. The spleen is removed because the proximity of this highly vascular organ increases the risk of metastasis. Tail resection is also indicated for chronic calcified pancreatitis.

Pancreaticojejunostomy

With chronic recurrent calcific pancreatitis, a pancreaticojejunostomy is indicated. This measure is effective when the pancreatic duct is obstructed in the proximal portion of the pancreas. The pancreatic duct and the jejunum are split longitudinally, placed side to side, and sutured together. This drains the pancreatic secretions directly into the jejunum.

Partial Pancreatectomy

When the body and tail of the pancreas are severely diseased with chronic pancreatitis, they can be removed in a partial pancreatectomy. This procedure may also be employed when previous surgical procedures have failed to control the pain of chronic pancreatitis.

Radical Distal Pancreatectomy

The radical distal pancreatectomy involves the resection of 95% of the pancreas. All but part of the head of the pancreas and the spleen are included in the resection. This procedure is performed when the entire pancreas is involved with chronic pancreatitis.

Total Pancreatectomy

A total pancreatectomy is indicated in some resectable carcinomas, hyperinsulinism, traumatic injury, selected cases of chronic pancreatitis, and in acute fulminant pancreatitis with total pancreatic necrosis.

Pancreatoduodenectomy (Whipple Procedure)

The pancreatoduodenectomy, also referred to as the Whipple procedure, is among the most extensive resections for pancreatic disease. The Whipple procedure is indicated for carcinoma of the head of the pancreas, ampulla of Vater, lower common duct, or duodenum. The procedure involves the resection of the right side of the pancreas, distal stomach, duodenum, gallbladder, and (if indicated) the spleen (Figure 50–14A). Reconstruction is necessary, suturing the common duct, pancreas, and stomach to the jejunum as illustrated in Figure 50–14B. For unresectable carcinomas, palliative measures can be taken to divert biliary and pancreatic secretions.

Implications for the Client

Physiological and psychosocial/lifestyle implications of pancreatic surgery are discussed in Table 50–12.

Nursing Implications

Nursing care of the client undergoing pancreatic surgery depends on the procedure performed. The primary nursing responsibilities include preventing complications, promoting comfort, and maintaining fluid/electrolyte and nutritional status.

Following pancreatic surgery, the client should be monitored closely for pulmonary complications. Proximity of the surgery to the chest cavity makes clients vulnerable

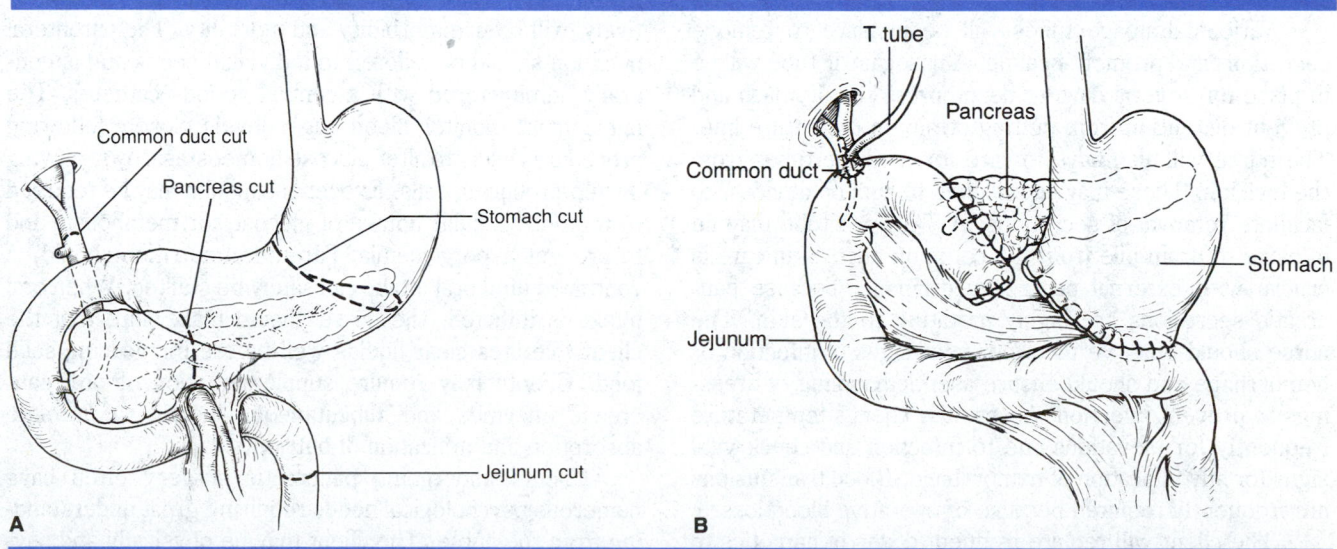

Figure 50–14

Whipple procedure. **A.** Margins of excision. The extent of the resection is indicated. Note that approximately 65% of the stomach is removed. The common duct is divided above its junction with the cystic duct. The jejunum is divided approximately 5 cm distal to the ligament of Treitz. The pancreas is divided at its neck, where it crosses the superior mesenteric and portal veins. **B.** Reconstruction. Completed reconstruction of the digestive tract. Note the end-to-side pancreatojejunostomy is proximal to other anastomoses. The anterior wall of the jejunum has been approximated to the anterior surface of the pancreas with interrupted fine silk sutures. End-to-side hepaticojejunostomy has been constructed using a T-tube to splint the anastomosis. A gastrojejunostomy has been performed distal to the hepaticojejunostomy.

Table 50–12   Pancreatic Surgery: Implications for the Client

Physiological Implications	Psychosocial/Lifestyle Implications
Incidence of postoperative complications is increased with prior narcotic or alcohol abuse, diabetes, poor nutritional status, and fluid and electrolyte imbalance.	Failure of pain control following surgery can be discouraging and frustrating.
Endocrine effects of pancreatic resection include disturbed glucose homeostasis from altered insulin and glucagon production.	Narcotic addiction can result from attempts to control pain of pancreatitis.
Exocrine effects of pancreatic resection lead to malabsorption from maldigestion, steatorrhea, diarrhea, and coagulation problems from impaired absorption of vitamin K.	Dietary modifications may be indicated for extensive excisions and reconstruction (eg, to prevent dumping syndrome following a Whipple procedure).
Postoperative complications include infection, sepsis, hemorrhage, fistula formation, and necrosis to adjacent structures from leakage of pancreatic enzymes.	Abdominal incision may affect body image.
Resection of the distal stomach as part of the Whipple procedure leads to dumping syndrome.	Clients with pancreatic carcinoma are facing a generally fatal diagnosis. Client and family need time to adjust and assistance with planning approaches to maximize the time the client has left.
Procedure may fail to control pain of chronic pancreatitis.	
Proximity to chest increases risk of pulmonary complications postoperatively.	

to pulmonary complications. Pneumonia, atelectasis, and pleural effusion may follow pancreatic surgery. The nurse must encourage clients to aerate their lungs fully by deep breathing. Coughing will facilitate removal of secretions. Pulmonary toilet may be indicated. Frequent measures to improve ventilation are essential to prevent pulmonary insufficiency.

Various drainage tubes will be in place to remove secretions and promote healing. A nasogastric tube will be in place for several days to decompress the stomach and prevent distention from putting strain on the suture line. The nurse will also have to care for drainage tubes from the incision. These may be attached to suction devices, to facilitate removal of secretions. A T-shaped tube may be in place to drain bile from the common duct. Skin care is crucial with external pancreatic drainage, because pancreatic secretions are highly irritating to the skin. The nurse should observe the wound for signs of infection or hemorrhage and should ensure aseptic handling of dressings to prevent infection. Assess the client's temperature frequently for elevations due to infection and check vital signs for any indication of hemorrhage. Blood transfusions are frequently required because of operative blood loss.

The client will require frequent doses of narcotics to control pain following pancreatic surgery. Adequate pain control facilitates cooperation with efforts to cough and deep breathe and to change position. However, doses large enough to cause sedation may result in respiratory depression, further increasing the chance of pulmonary complications.

Following pancreatic surgery, fluid and electrolyte balance must be restored. The specific requirements will vary from individual to individual. Close monitoring of fluid status and laboratory values will assist the nurse in fluid and electrolyte management.

Maintenance of nutritional status is essential in pancreatic surgery. Often, these clients show poor nutritional status, either because of chronic disease or alcohol abuse. Preoperative parenteral nutrition, continued postoperatively, will reduce morbidity and mortality. The parenteral nutrition should be tailored to individual needs and is generally administered with a central venous catheter. The nurse must monitor blood sugar levels closely following procedures likely to alter glucose homeostasis by removing insulin-producing cells. Exogenous insulin may be required to promote cellular uptake of glucose for metabolism and to prevent hyperglycemia. Parenteral nutrition should be continued until oral intake can safely be started. When oral intake is initiated, the nurse should make sure that the client tolerates clear liquids well before introducing solid food. Clients may require supplementation of oral pancreatic enzymes and subcutaneous insulin to promote absorption and utilization of nutrients.

Clients undergoing pancreatic surgery often have numerous psychological needs requiring great understanding from the nurse. The client may be physically and psychologically worn down from chronic disease and unrelenting pain. The client may be facing a terminal diagnosis. There may be a long history of drug or alcohol abuse with all the accompanying personal and family difficulties. These problems, compounded by the discomfort of surgery, require a consistent and caring approach that can pose a challenge for the nurse.

Chapter Highlights

Normal gastrointestinal function is disturbed by surgically altering the continuity of the gastrointestinal tract, requiring compensatory measures.

With esophageal surgery, manipulation of the nasogastric tube should be avoided to prevent disruption of the surgical site.

Complications of surgery on the gastrointestinal system include infection, sepsis, hemorrhage, wound separation, and paralytic ileus.

Respiratory effort may be impaired when gastrointestinal surgery close to the thoracic cavity affects abdominal muscles used in breathing and coughing or produces incisional pain on breathing or coughing.

Drainage via a nasogastric tube is frequently used with gastrointestinal surgery to decompress the stomach, intestine, or both.

Parenteral nutrition is often provided before and after gastrointestinal surgery to maintain nutritional status through the period of intestinal paralysis that follows gastrointestinal surgery.

Safe and effective tube feeding requires appropriate administration and adequate client monitoring.

When surgery results in drainage of gastrointestinal fluids, careful replacement of fluids and electrolytes is essential.

Preoperative evaluation for stoma placement is essential to assure a proper fit of a drainage appliance.

Psychosocial adjustment to an ostomy includes knowledge of the altered physiology, psychological comfort in managing the ostomy, and a realistic understanding of the impact on lifestyle.

Pancreatic surgery can affect both exocrine and endocrine functions of the pancreas.

Supportive family and friends greatly affect the client's coping abilities, adjustment to, and recovery from gastrointestinal surgery.

Bibliography

Boehmer VW, Turk MF: Caring for the gastroplasty patient. *AORN J* 1981; 34:1036–1042.

Broadwell DC, Jackson BS: *Principles of Ostomy Care*. St. Louis: Mosby, 1982.

Fazio VW, Turnbull RB: Ulcerative colitis and Crohn's disease of the colon. *Med Clin North Am* 1980; 64:1135–1159.

Gloeckner MR: Perceptions of sexual attractiveness following ostomy surgery. *Res Nurs Health* 1984; 7:87–92.

Goldberg SM, Gordon PH, Nivatvongs S: *Essentials of Anorectal Surgery*. Philadelphia: Lippincott, 1980.

Kosel K et al: Total pancreatectomy and islet cell autotransplantation. *Am J Nurs* 1982; 82:568–571.

Maingot R: *Abdominal Operations*. Vol 1 and 2. New York: Appleton-Century-Crofts, 1980.

Miller BK: Jejunoileal bypass: A drastic weight control measure. *Am J Nurs* 1981; 81:564–568.

Mojzisik CM, Martin EW: Gastric partitioning: The latest surgical means to control morbid obesity. *Am J Nurs* 1981; 81:569–572.

Parks AG, Nicholls RJ, Belliveau P: Proctocolectomy with ileal reservoir and anal anastomosis. *Br J Surg* 1980; 67:533–538.

Patterson RS, Andrassy RJ: Needle-catheter jejunostomy. *Am J Nurs* 1983; 83:1325–1326.

Patras AZ: The operation's over, but the danger's not. *Nurs 82* 1982; 12:50–56.

Rucker RD Jr et al: Searching for the best weight reduction operation. *Surgery* 1984; 96:624–631.

Sabiston DC: *Textbook of Surgery*. Philadelphia: Saunders, 1981.

Saxton DF et al: *Manual of Nursing Practice*. Menlo Park, CA: Addison-Wesley, 1983.

Sleisinger MH, Fordtran JS: *Gastrointestinal Disease*. Philadelphia: Saunders, 1983.

Stout K: The surgical treatment of morbid obesity. *Nurs Clin North Am* 1982; 17:245–250.

Utsunomiya J et al: Total colectomy, mucosal proctectomy and ileal anal anastomosis. *Am Society of Colon and Rectal Surg* 1980; 23:459–466.

Weakley FL: Cancers of the rectum. *Surg Clin North Am* 1983; 63:129–135.

Wilpizeski MD: Helping the ostomate return to a normal life. *Nurs 81* 1981; 11:62–66.

Suggested Readings

Everett WG: Hemorrhoidectomy without tears—or not too many. *Nurs Times* 1982; 78:526. Brief description of the surgical technique of hemorrhoidectomy. Nursing care related to site care, reinstitution of bowel movements, and psychological support is addressed.

Fazio VW: Regional enteritis (Crohn's disease): Indications for surgery and operative strategy. *Surg Clin North Am* 1983; 63:27–48. An in-depth update on types of Crohn's disease, indications for surgery, preoperative preparation, and surgical procedures.

Goligher JC: Alternatives to conventional ileostomy in the surgical treatment of ulcerative colitis. *J Enterostom Ther* 1983; 10:79–83. A description of alternative surgical procedures to avoid the complications of total proctocolectomy in ulcerative colitis.

Groszek DM: Promoting wound healing in the obese patient. *AORN J* 1982; 35:1132–1138. This article describes the role of the respiratory, cardiovascular, and hepatic systems in wound healing in the obese. Wound complications are discussed with nursing interventions.

Kobza L: Impact of ostomy upon the spouse. *J Enterostom Ther* 1983; 10:54–57. A report of a study based on interviews of spouses of persons with an ostomy. Results support the need to include the spouse in rehabilitation.

Schumann D: Wound healing in your abdominal surgery patient. *Nurs 80* 1980; 10:34–40. A nursing discussion of abdominal wounds addressing high-risk clients; factors interfering with wound healing; and nursing measures to minimize vomiting, distention, and pain. Nutritional effects, respiratory function, and dressing change technique are also discussed.

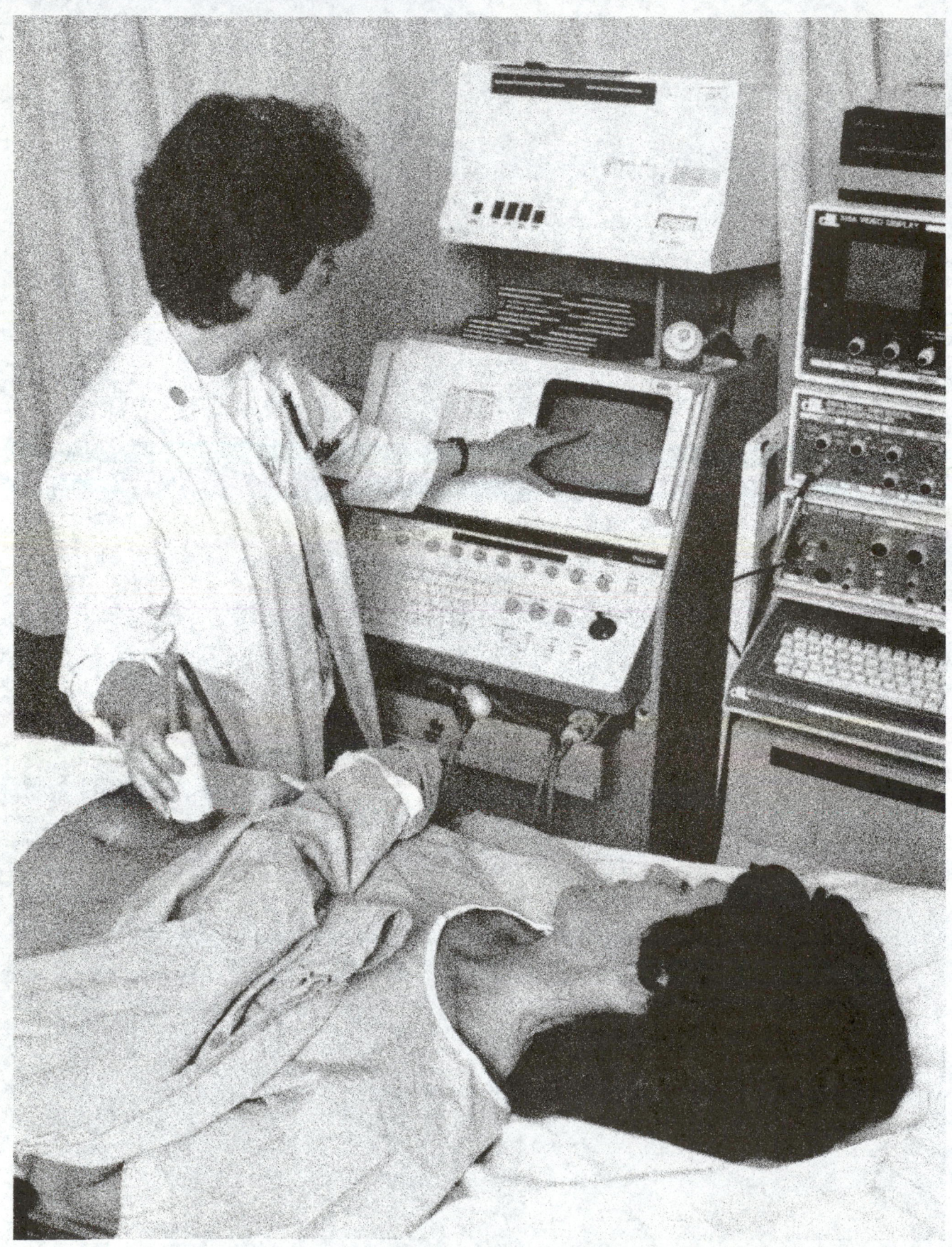

The Client With Hepatic–Biliary System Dysfunction

Chapter 51

The Hepatic–Biliary System in Health and Illness

Jane Hokanson Hawks

Objectives

When you have finished studying this chapter, you should be able to:

Describe the gross anatomy of the liver and gallbladder and their relationship to other abdominal organs.

Discuss the regulatory functions of the liver.

Describe the structure of the liver lobule in relation to physiological function.

List the regulatory functions of the gallbladder and describe their interrelationship with liver function.

Explain pathophysiological influences and effects related to organ enlargement and atrophy, impairment of tissue perfusion and gas exchange, increased susceptibility to infection, impaired bilirubin excretion and detoxification capacity, alterations in fluid volume and nutrition-related functions, biliary infection, and ammonia toxicity.

Analyze interrelationships between hepatic–biliary dysfunction and dysfunction of the integumentary, cardiovascular, and neurological systems.

Identify common psychosocial/lifestyle influences on hepatic–biliary function and describe their effects.

The liver and gallbladder perform several regulatory functions essential to maintenance of homeostasis. The liver synthesizes a number of substances, including coagulation factors, that are vital to life. The gallbladder plays an important role in the digestive process, in particular, the digestion of fats. Although the human body can survive loss of the gallbladder—for example, by surgical removal—survival without a liver is not possible.

Section I: Structural and Functional Interrelationships

The hepatic and biliary systems are both structurally and functionally interrelated. The liver, the largest of the internal organs, performs the following functions:

- Storage and filtration of the blood—a vascular function
- Production of bile—a regulatory function
- Removal of bilirubin from the body—an excretory function
- Metabolism of carbohydrates, fats, and proteins—a metabolic function
- Storage of vitamins A, D, B_{12}, and iron
- Synthesis of coagulation factors

- Detoxification of chemicals

The principal function of the gallbladder is to store and release bile, the nature and properties of which are discussed later in this chapter.

STRUCTURE OF THE LIVER

The normal liver of an adult weighs about 1500 g. The wedge-shaped organ lies in the upper right quadrant of the abdominal cavity, where it is protected by the rib cage. The superior surface underlies the diaphragm. The posterior and inferior surfaces together are generally referred to as the *visceral surface*. The right visceral surface is in contact with portions of the colon, the kidneys, the adrenal glands, and the duodenum; the left visceral surface is bordered by the stomach and spleen. Figure 51–1A depicts the anterior view of the liver with supporting ligaments. Figure 51–1B shows the superior surface of the liver.

The liver is divided into two major regions, the right and left lobes, separated by fissures on the inferior surface of the liver. On the posterior and inferior surfaces of the right lobe are two smaller lobes, the caudate and quadrate lobes. The gallbladder and the inferior vena cava lie in two shallow fossae that parallel the fissures. Veins, arteries, nerves, and lymphatic vessels enter and leave the liver through a space between the caudate and quadrate lobes.

Except for the so-called *bare area,* which rests against the diaphragm, the liver is covered by visceral peritoneum, a thin layer of connective tissue that extends into each lobe to divide the liver into 50,000 to 100,000 liver lobules. These tiny structures, a few millimeters in length and 1 to 2 mm in diameter, are the functional units of the liver.

The Functional Liver Lobule

Each liver lobule (Figure 51–2) is composed of platelike "spokes" of hepatic cells that radiate from a "hub" or central vein that passes through the connective tissue between lobules. The central veins are branches of the portal vein that, together with the portal artery, furnish the blood supply of the liver. (See following section.) Bile is manufactured in the hepatic plates, each of which is generally two cells thick. Tiny bile canaliculi, or bile channels, lying between the hepatic plates carry the bile to bile ducts. Like tributaries forming ever larger streams, the bile ducts merge to form larger ducts. Eventually, they form two hepatic ducts, one from the right lobe and one from the left. These in turn join to form a single hepatic duct that merges with the cystic duct to form the common bile duct. Bile manufactured by the liver, together with bile stored and later secreted by the gallbladder, leaves the hepatic–biliary system via the common bile duct.

The septa between lobules contain venules and arterioles, both of which drain into the hepatic sinusoids, where

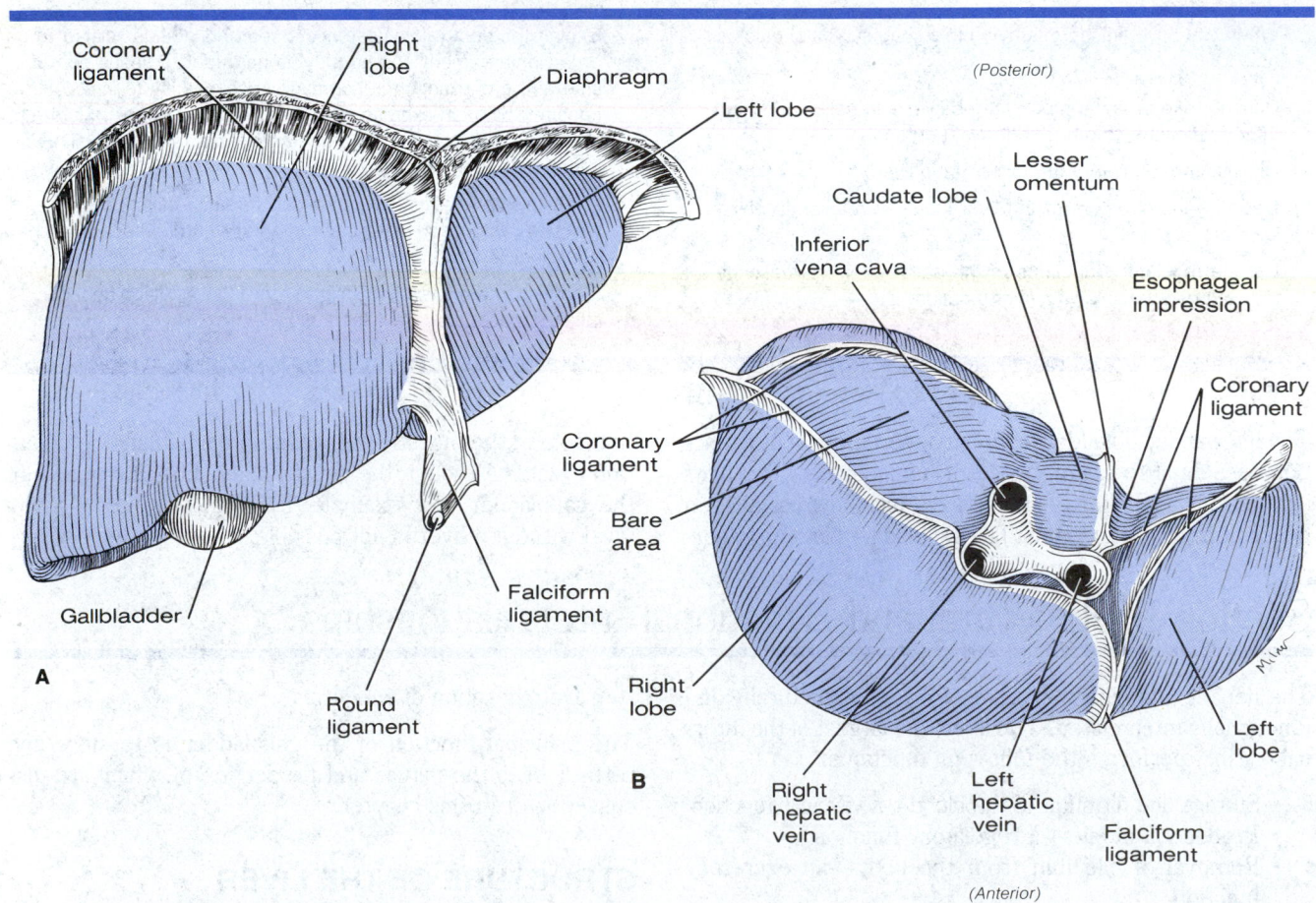

Figure 51–1

A. Anterior view of the liver and its supporting ligaments. **B.** Superior (diaphragmatic) surface of the liver.

SOURCE: Spence AP, Mason EB: *Human Anatomy and Physiology,* 2nd ed. Menlo Park, CA: Benjamin/Cummings, 1983.

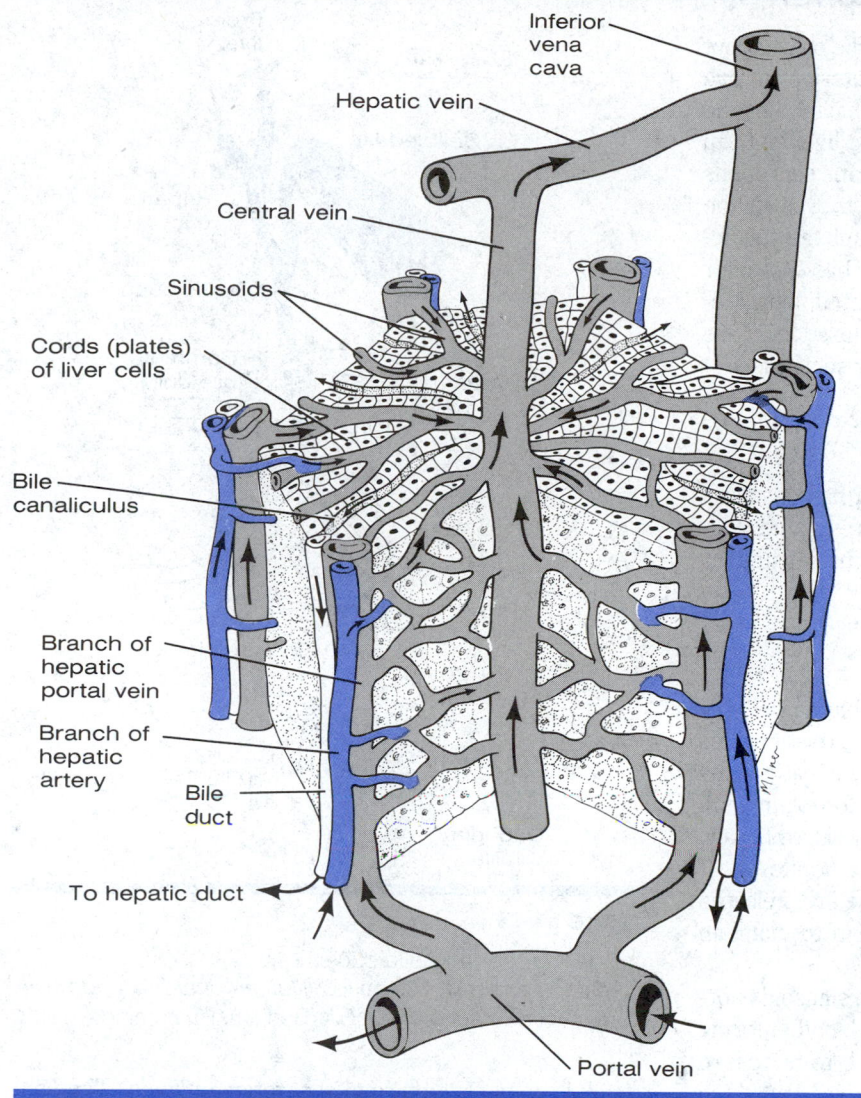

Inferior vena cava

Hepatic vein

Central vein

Sinusoids

Cords (plates) of liver cells

Bile canaliculus

Branch of hepatic portal vein

Branch of hepatic artery

Bile duct

To hepatic duct

Portal vein

Figure 51–2

Microscopic anatomy of a liver lobule. The arrows show the direction of the flow of blood and bile.

SOURCE: Spence AP, Mason EB: *Human Anatomy and Physiology*, 2nd ed. Menlo Park, CA: Benjamin/Cummings, 1983.

venous and arterial blood mingle. This mingling is related to the detoxifying and metabolic functions of the hepatic system. Plasma, including proteins, can diffuse out of the blood. For example, nutritive or toxic substances carried from the intestine in the blood diffuse through the epithelial lining of the sinusoids into the hepatic cells, where they are metabolized, stored, or altered. The sinusoids are also lined by Kupffer cells, phagocytic cells that remove bacteria and other foreign substances from blood that passes through the liver (Spence & Mason, 1983).

Hepatic Circulation

The liver is richly supplied with both arterial and venous blood. Each minute approximately 1100 mL arrives from the hepatic portal vein and 400 mL from the hepatic artery to mix in the sinusoids before returning to the heart via the inferior vena cava. Portal venous blood coming from the intestines has a low concentration of oxygen but a high

concentration of substances absorbed by the intestine during digestion. Blood coming from the hepatic artery is high in oxygen but low in nutrients. The pressure of blood in the portal and hepatic veins is low, allowing easy diffusion of nutrients and other substances along the concentration gradient. Oxygen-rich blood from the hepatic artery maintains the integrity of the liver; if perfusion is absent or diminished, necrosis of hepatic cells will occur (Spence & Mason, 1983).

Arterial and venous vessels, bile ducts, and lymphatic vessels travel together through the liver in so-called *portal tracts*. The direction of flow is from the portal tracts through the sinusoids and into the central veins of the liver lobules. Thus, oxygen and nutrient supply is richest in the hepatic cells nearest the portal tracts and poorest near the central veins. The cells adjacent to the central veins, due to their relatively poor nutritional state, are more susceptible to damage from circulatory disturbances (eg, shock or heart failure) and more vulnerable to toxins than the outermost cells (Crowley, 1983).

STRUCTURE OF THE GALLBLADDER

The gallbladder is a pear-shaped, hollow, saclike organ about 7 to 10 cm long that lies in a fossa on the inferior surface of the liver (Figure 51–1). The *cystic duct,* which drains the gallbladder, joins with the hepatic duct of the liver to form the *common bile duct* (Figure 51–3). Pancreatic secretions also enter this duct via the pancreatic duct. Bile in the common bile duct enters the duodenum through the sphincter of Oddi. When this sphincter is relaxed, bile can enter the duodenum; when the sphincter is contracted, bile manufactured by the liver is stored in the gallbladder. The function of bile is discussed in the following section.

FUNCTIONS OF THE LIVER

As already mentioned, the hepatic system has vascular, secretory, and metabolic functions. It stores some vitamins and iron, detoxifies chemicals, and forms substances necessary for the coagulation of blood.

Vascular Functions

The liver is capable of storing a considerable quantity of blood, the amount depending on the pressure relationships in the arteries and veins. If pressure in the hepatic veins increases by a few millimeters of mercury, for example in the presence of congestive heart failure, cirrhosis, or hepatic congestion, as much as 300 to 400 mL may be stored. If hemorrhage occurs anywhere in the body, the liver releases this stored blood into the circulatory system to maintain circulatory volume (Guyton, 1981).

The phagocytic Kupffer cells lining the sinusoids normally remove 99%–100% of bacteria from blood entering the liver. Kupffer cells multiply in response to increased levels of foreign particles in the blood. Since blood entering the liver through the portal vein contains intestinal bacteria, the Kupffer cells play an important role in the body's defense against infection. Any condition that damages these cells or inhibits their replication increases the body's susceptibility to infection.

Secretory Functions

The hepatic cells of each liver lobule continually secrete small amounts of bile, a thick, greenish yellow, slightly alkaline fluid. When first secreted from the liver through the canaliculi, bile is composed of water, bile salts, bilirubin, cholesterol, fatty acids, and lecithin as well as sodium, potassium, calcium, chloride, and bicarbonate ions.

Bile is concentrated in the gallbladder, which contracts during digestion to squirt it into the duodenum, where it functions as a kind of "biological detergent" to emulsify fat particles (Crowley, 1983). The bile salts decrease the surface tension of fat particles so the agitation of the intestinal tract can break them into small globules easily acted upon by digestive enzymes. Lecithin acts similarly. Fat is digested much more slowly if bile is not present.

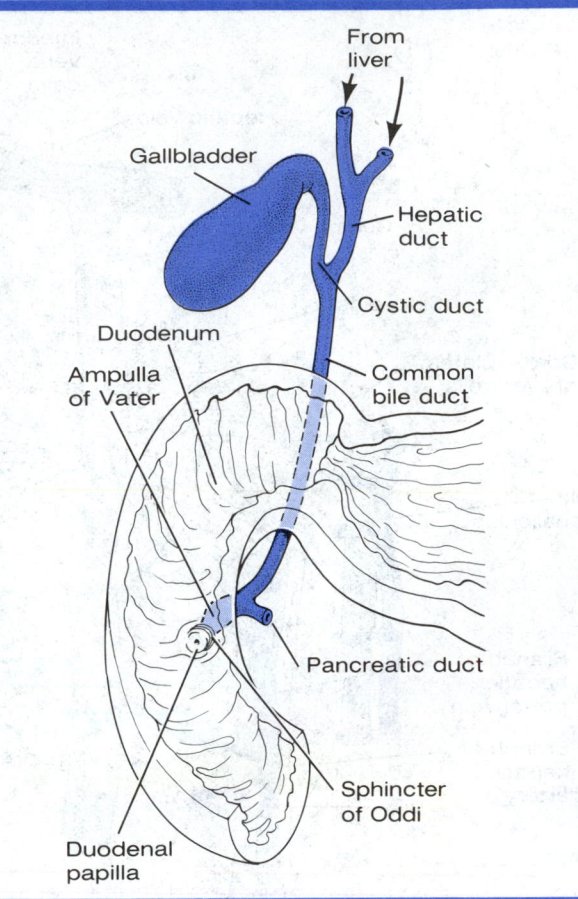

Figure 51–3

The gallbladder and bile ducts.
SOURCE: Spence AP, Mason EB: *Human Anatomy and Physiology,* 2nd ed. Menlo Park, CA: Benjamin/Cummings, 1983.

Bile salts also improve absorption of lipids. The salts combine with fatty acids and monoglycerides to form small complexes called micelles. The ion charges provided by the bile salts enhance diffusion of the micelles across the intestinal mucosa into the bloodstream (Guyton, 1981).

If absorption of fats is diminished because of absence of bile, vitamins A, D, E, and K, which are fat-soluble, cannot be absorbed.

Bile salts are "recycled" from 15 to 20 times in a process known as enterohepatic circulation (Guyton, 1981). From 90%–95% of bile salts secreted are reabsorbed in the distal ileum and carried in the portal vein back to the hepatic cells, which reabsorb and then resecrete them.

Excretory Functions

Bilirubin (bile pigment), a major waste product of hemoglobin metabolism, is excreted by the liver. Normally, erythrocytes have a life span of about 120 days. They are then broken down by the reticuloendothelial cells, and the iron (heme) from the worn-out red cells is conserved for reuse in the synthesis of fresh hemoglobin. The remaining iron-free pigment is free (unconjugated) bilirubin, which is continually present in the bloodstream in small quantities. As blood passes through the liver, unconjugated bilirubin is removed. It is then combined (conjugated) with other substances and excreted via the bile ducts. (A small amount of conjugated bilirubin returns to the blood.)

Conjugated bilirubin is more soluble and less toxic than unconjugated bilirubin. In the intestines, conjugated bilirubin is converted into a highly soluble substance called *urobilinogen,* which is excreted primarily in the feces in an oxidized form known as *stercobilin.* Some 5% of urobilinogen is absorbed into the bloodstream and excreted via the kidneys in an oxidized form called *urobilin.* Since stercobilin gives feces their brownish color, acholic (clay-colored) stools are a classic sign of biliary tract abnormalities.

Metabolic Functions

Carbohydrate Metabolism
The liver plays a major role in carbohydrate metabolism. One aspect of this role is a glucose buffer function that contributes to maintenance of normal blood sugar levels. The liver can remove excess glucose from the blood, store it as glycogen, and reconvert and release it as glucose in response to hypoglycemia. If blood glucose concentrations fall and glycogen is not available, the liver can convert proteins or amino acids to glucose—a process known as glyconeogenesis. The liver is also capable of converting galactose to glucose.

Fat (Lipid) Metabolism
Synthesis of fat from carbohydrates and proteins occurs primarily in the liver. The lipoprotein produced in this process is transported in the bloodstream to the body's adipose tissue for storage. The liver is also capable of rapid metabolism of ingested fat in response to energy requirements. The liver can also synthesize lipoproteins, cholesterol, and other phospholipids.

Protein Metabolism
Before amino acids can be converted into carbohydrates or fat or used to supply caloric needs, a process known as *deamination* (liberation of ammonia) must occur. The liver is the principal site of deamination and the only site where ammonia is detoxified by conversion into urea. In addition, nearly all the plasma proteins are synthesized in the liver, as are several nonessential amino acids.

Storage Functions

Vitamin Storage
The liver is capable of storing up to a four-months' supply of vitamins B_{12} and D and up to a ten-year supply of vitamin A for release as needed. Because of this storage capacity, excessive ingestion of vitamins A or D can have toxic effects on liver function.

Iron Storage
Except for the iron stored in hemoglobin, most of the body's iron is stored in the liver as *ferritin.* Stored iron is released when blood levels of iron fall, a process known as *iron buffering* (Guyton, 1981).

Synthesis of Coagulation Factors

Prothrombin and factors VII, IX, and X, necessary for effective blood coagulation, are synthesized in the liver. Vitamin K is necessary to promote synthesis of these clotting factors, but if bile secretion is inadequate, absorption of this fat-soluble vitamin cannot occur. The liver also synthesizes fibrinogen, another clotting factor.

Detoxification

Many chemicals are detoxified in the liver, including such medications as barbiturates, antidiuretic hormone (ADH), amphetamines, aldosterone, and estrogen. If these substances were not detoxified, they could be fatally toxic to body tissues or organs or could have other adverse effects such as, for example, feminization of males or masculinization of females.

FUNCTIONS OF THE GALLBLADDER

The major regulatory processes of the biliary system involve concentration and storage of bile and regulation of bile secretion.

Concentration and Storage of Bile

The hepatic cells can produce from 600 mL to 1000 mL of bile in 24 hours—over ten times the 50 mL to 75 mL storage capacity of the gallbladder. The mucosa of the gallbladder concentrates bile by absorbing water and electrolytes. This leaves a solution of bile salts, cholesterol, lecithin, and bilirubin that is five to ten times as concentrated as bile secreted by the liver.

Regulation of Bile Secretion

When ingested fat enters the small intestine, a hormone called cholecystokinin is released from the intestinal mucosa. The cholecystokinin travels to the gallbladder via the bloodstream, initiating contraction of the smooth muscle in the wall of the gallbladder and relaxation of the sphincter of Oddi. Vagal stimulation also contributes to contraction of the gallbladder. While the hormone secretin, produced by the jejunal and duodenal mucosa, weakly stimulates bile secretion by the liver, peristalsis stimulated by food further relaxes the sphincter of Oddi. These factors combine to produce squirting of bile into the duodenum with each gallbladder contraction and peristaltic wave. The gallbladder empties poorly in the absence of ingested fat but empties completely within an hour if fat is present. Approximately 94% of the bile salts released into the duodenum are reabsorbed and returned to the liver via the bloodstream (Figure 51–4).

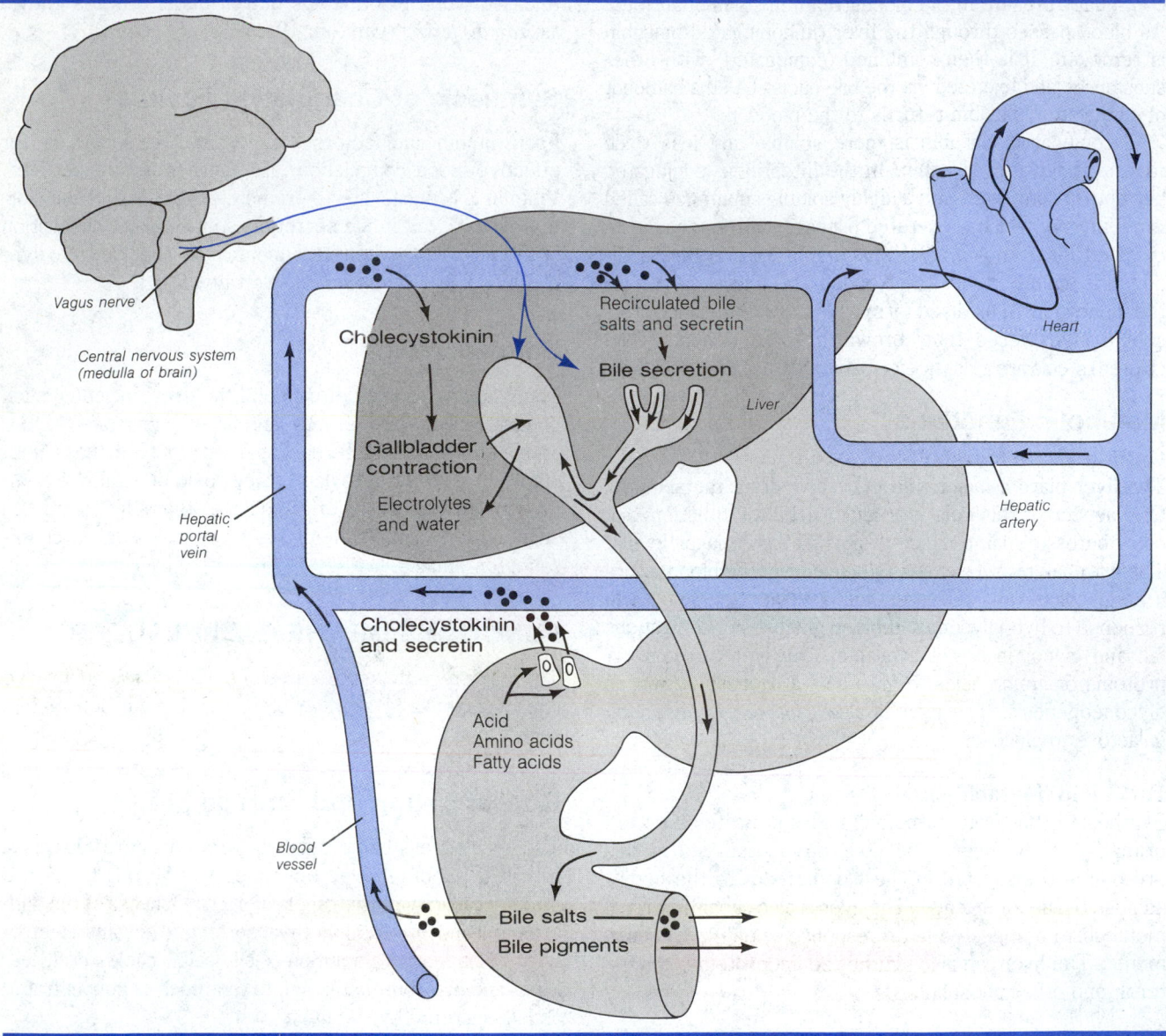

Figure 51–4

Regulatory pathways for bile secretion and bile release from the gallbladder. (Neural regulation is shown in color.)
SOURCE: Spence AP, Mason EB: *Human Anatomy and Physiology,* 2nd ed. Menlo Park, CA: Benjamin/Cummings,1983.

Section II: Pathophysiological Influences and Effects

Pathophysiological changes commonly seen in hepatic or biliary dysfunction are discussed in this chapter. Special influences and effects related to specific illnesses are presented in Chapter 53.

ENLARGEMENT OF THE LIVER

Under normal circumstances, the liver is capable of regeneration once an acute condition (eg, drug toxicity, abscess, or inflammation) has been alleviated. If the pathogenic influence persists, however, regeneration will be of fibrotic origin.

When dead or diseased cells are replaced by fibrous tissue, the liver becomes enlarged (**hepatomegaly**) (Figure 51–5). Fibrotic scar tissue may impede emptying of blood from the hepatic veins, causing the liver lobules to become engorged. This engorgement leads to further enlargement. Pressure exerted on abdominal nerves by the enlarged liver or displacement of other abdominal organs may cause discomfort or pain. Hepatomegaly may also be related to invasion and multiplication of neoplastic cells.

ATROPHY OF THE LIVER

Although the liver may be enlarged during the early stages of hepatic pathology, it eventually atrophies if the pathogenic influence is not removed. In the alcoholic client, for example, continued ingestion of alcohol combined with malnutrition cause scar tissue to replace the dead cells. In time, the scar tissue shrinks, and the liver becomes smaller than normal. Adjacent organs tend to encroach on the space formerly occupied by the liver. (For this reason, a liver from a donor smaller than the recipient is best for transplant purposes.)

PORTAL HYPERTENSION

As hepatic tissue becomes increasingly fibrotic, the portal venules become compressed. This compression increases back-pressure as portal venous blood volume rises. Portal hypertension results, with pressures in the portal vein as high as 20 mm Hg. This contributes to the development of **ascites,** the accumulation of protein-rich serum in the peritoneal cavity.

Collateral pathways develop between the portal and systemic circulation in areas where tributaries of portal and systemic veins are in close approximation. The most common collateral pathways are shown in Figure 51–6. As portal pressure increases, all collateral pathways between the portal and systemic circulation enlarge.

Collateral vessels in the lower esophagus dilate because they are not anatomically structured to carry the extra blood shunted via the azygous system. These dilated veins, called esophageal varices, may rupture causing massive hemorrhage. Hemorrhoids (rectal varices) can result from the increased pressure in hemorrhoidal veins. Splenomegaly can develop secondary to engorgement of the splenic veins.

When esophageal varices hemorrhage, treatment is complicated by abnormalities in blood coagulation related to impaired hepatic function. As bile production becomes impaired, absorption of vitamin K is also impaired. Insufficiency or lack of vitamin K leads to decreased production of prothrombin and coagulation factors VII, IX, and X. Insufficiency of clotting factors, in turn, is related to increased clotting times. This pathogenic sequence may be signaled by ecchymoses all over the body, bleeding of the gums, or blood in the stool.

IMPAIRMENT OF GAS EXCHANGE

Although the vascular dehydration seen in hepatic failure may mask erythrocytopenia, red blood cell deficiency does occur in relation to several factors. For instance, the impaired liver cannot store sufficient vitamin B_{12} and iron for erythrocyte synthesis. In alcohol-related pathologic states, ingestion of large quantities of alcohol inhibits renal synthesis of erythropoietin; the blood contains a higher proportion of immature erythrocytes and fewer mature red

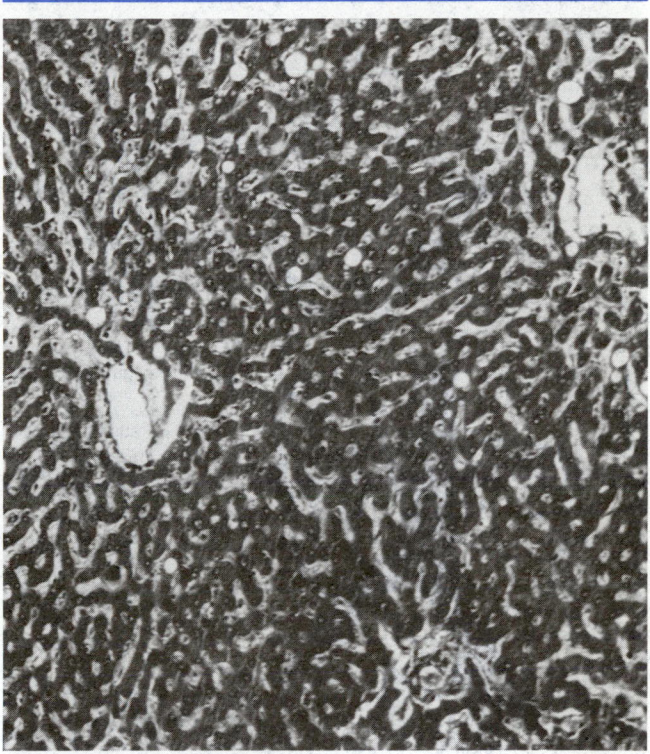

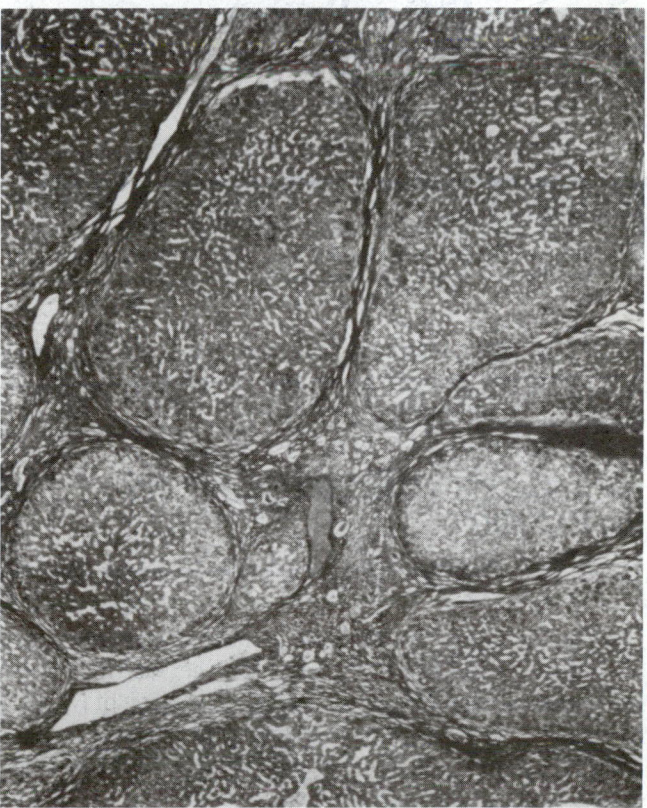

Figure 51–5

Top. Photomicrograph showing cellular structure of normal liver. **Bottom.** Photomicrograph of cirrhotic liver illustrating nodules of liver cells circumscribed by scar tissue. SOURCE: Crowley LV: *Introduction to Human Disease.* Belmont, CA: Wadsworth, 1983.

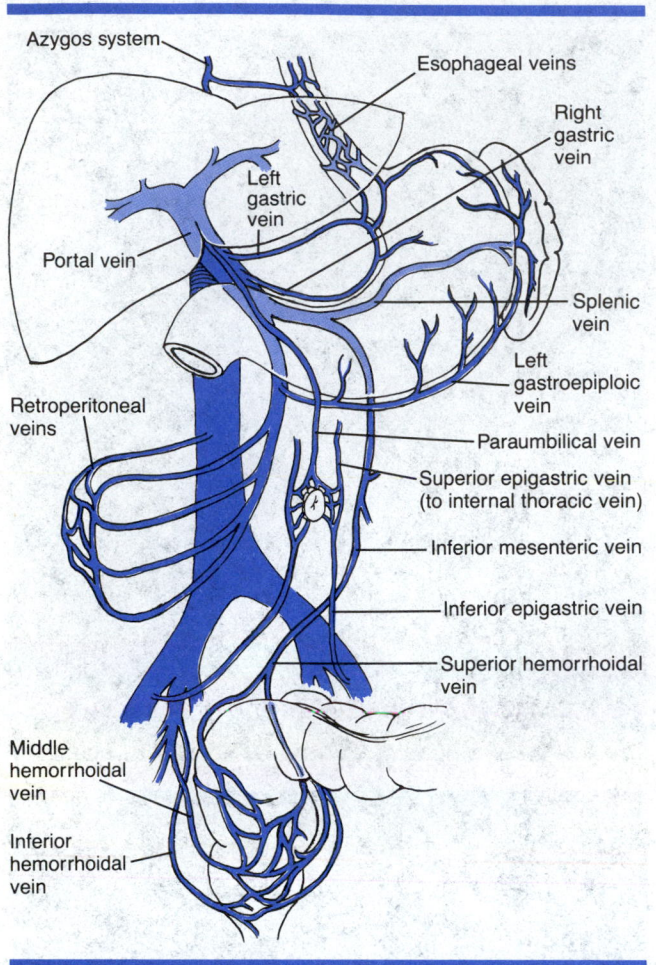

Figure 51–6

Common collateral pathways in portal hypertension.

cells. This deficit may be manifested as dyspnea, increased cardiac output, cardiomegaly, and clubbing of the fingers (Schearman and Finlayson, 1982).

INCREASED SUSCEPTIBILITY TO INFECTION

Injury to the liver is accompanied by damage to or destruction of the Kupffer cells. Phagocytosis is impaired. Microorganisms enter the general circulation and may form abscesses in the liver tissue itself. Whereas the normal liver accounts for 25% of the body's production of lymphocytes, the diseased liver is incapable of lymphocyte production (Guyton, 1981). Lymphocytopenia increases the body's susceptibility to infection.

IMPAIRMENT OF BILIRUBIN EXCRETION

In a compromised liver, absorption and conjugation of bilirubin are impaired. Increased levels of unconjugated bilirubin in the blood and body fluids lead to jaundice, or icterus. The skin becomes yellowish and pruritic, renal

excretion of unconjugated bilirubin causes the urine to become mahogany colored, and the stools are clay colored (acholic) due to the absence of stercobilin.

Not all cases of jaundice are related to impairment of bilirubin conjugation. For example, if the common bile duct is obstructed by gallstones (**choledocolithiasis**) or a neoplasm, bilirubin that has been conjugated by the liver cannot be excreted into the duodenum. Levels of bilirubin rise, and the symptoms of jaundice occur. Icterus may also be related to **cholecystitis** (inflammation of the gallbladder) or to spasms of the sphincter of Oddi, often associated with cholelithiasis. These conditions are discussed in Chapter 53.

Overproduction of bilirubin related to hemolytic states is another cause of jaundice. For example, reaction to a blood transfusion can induce a hemolytic state. The production of unconjugated bilirubin exceeds the conjugating capacity of the liver, and levels of circulating unconjugated bilirubin rise.

In newborn infants, a deficiency of glucuronyl transferase, the enzyme necessary for bilirubin conjugation, may lead to development of jaundice. This type of jaundice may usually be corrected by exposing the infant to ultraviolet light therapy.

Some hereditary disorders are also associated with jaundice, for example, Gilbert's disease or Dubin–Johnson syndrome. Gilbert's disease is associated with deficiency of glucuronyl transferase; Dubin–Johnson syndrome is associated with impaired hepatic excretion of bilirubin.

Principal causes of jaundice are summarized in Box 51–1.

BILIARY INFECTIONS

In the presence of inflammation or obstruction, the gallbladder may become swollen by accumulated mucus secretions or purulent drainage. Staphylococcal, streptococcal, or enteric organisms may infect the gallbladder, or it may become gangrenous.

AMMONIA TOXICITY

As the functional capacity of the liver diminishes, the ability to convert ammonia to urea for excretion by the kidney is impaired. Moreover, the collateral circulation caused by portal hypertension allows ammonia formed in the intestines to bypass the liver and enter the general circulation. The combined effect of these phenomena is ammonia toxicity. This toxicity manifests itself in hepatic encephalopathy, an altered mental state that begins with confusion and progresses to combative states and ultimately to hepatic coma. Another characteristic symptom of ammonia toxicity is **asterixis** ("liver flap"), a flapping tremor of the hand.

ALTERATION IN NUTRITION-RELATED FUNCTIONS

Injury to hepatic cells compromises bile production and interferes with other nutrition-related hepatic functions such as synthesis of glycogen. The decrease in appetite that often occurs in liver disease is followed by weight loss, subnormal body temperature, fatigue, and the metabolism of body fat and muscle to meet caloric requirements. Impairment of bile secretion leads to fat intolerance and decreased fat absorption. The use of muscle mass as an energy source combined with decreased capacity for urea formation lead to a negative nitrogen balance. The limbs become emaciated while the abdomen swells with ascites. Skin breakdown is common. Inability to metabolize the amino acid methionine adequately produces **fetor hepaticus**, a sweet breath odor resembling acetone or old wine.

Deficiencies of folic acid and the B complex vitamins often occur in clients with alcoholic liver disease. Alcohol increases the demand for B vitamins, impairs absorption of folate and the B vitamins, and generally contributes to an inadequate consumption of all nutrients. Folic acid deficiency is manifested by a macrocytic anemia, glossitis, and diarrhea. Lesions of the oral mucosa and tongue, fissures at the corners of the mouth (**cheilosis**), and peripheral neuropathies result from lack of B complex vitamins.

Diminished fat absorption leads to deficiencies of the fat-soluble vitamins A, D, E, and K. Night blindness is associated with deficiency of vitamin A. Osteoporosis may occur in relation to vitamin D deficiency, putting the client at risk for fractures. Vitamin E deficiency can cause impaired red blood cell survival in adults. Coagulation disorders associated with vitamin K deficiency have already been discussed.

ALTERATIONS IN FLUID VOLUME

Among the substances synthesized by the normal liver is the plasma protein albumin, which is necessary for maintaining the colloidal osmotic pressure of the plasma. If plasma albumin is insufficient or absent the normal colloidal osmotic pressure of the blood is not maintained. Plasma seeps into the interstitial spaces, causing peripheral and dependent edema. Pulmonary edema may lead to right-sided conges-

---

Box 51–1   Principal Causes of Jaundice

- Impaired bilirubin conjugation
- Obstruction of the common bile duct (choledocolithiasis, neoplasia)
- Cholecystitis
- Spasms of the sphincter of Oddi
- Overproduction of bilirubin related to hemolysis
- In newborns, deficiency of glucuronyl transferase
- Inherited disorders (eg, Gilbert's disease, Dubin–Johnson syndrome)

---

tive heart failure. Ascites may be related to hypoalbuminemia and failure of the liver to detoxify aldosterone, as well as to portal hypertension. Accumulations exceeding 2 L may lead to problems often also associated with pregnancy: difficulty breathing from pressure on the diaphragm, decreased appetite, feeling of fullness, constipation, flatulence, and umbilical hernia. The weight and bulk of the fluid may also restrict activity.

IMPAIRMENT OF DETOXIFICATION

The diminished detoxification capacity of the compromised liver may compound the problems related to hypoalbuminemia. Increased levels of circulating aldosterone and ADH increase retention of sodium and water, respectively, further complicating the client's edema. Intravascular dehydration—lack of plasma in the blood vessels—related to the hypoalbuminuria may mask erythrocytopenia, because the dilution state of the blood has been altered.

Alteration in detoxification may also induce other problems related to excessive levels of hormones, chemicals, or drugs. Changes associated with an excess of estrogen may occur: loss of axillary, pubic, and body hair; soft skin; and gynecomastia and testicular atrophy in males. Decreased libido, impotence, spider angiomas, and palmar erythema are also associated with increased estrogen levels. Alcohol, antibiotics, psychotropic drugs, and some antihypertensive medications may also accumulate in toxic levels when liver function is impaired.

Section III: Related System Influences and Effects

Since the hepatic–biliary system performs multiple functions related to several other body systems, impairment of hepatic–biliary function can affect these systems to varying degrees.

INTEGUMENTARY SYSTEM

Yellowing of the skin is characteristic of jaundice. **Pruritus** (itching) associated with jaundice may become so severe

that clients scratch until they bleed. The break in skin integrity increases the client's susceptibility to infection. (Pruritus and the itch-scratch cycle are discussed in Unit 13.)

Xanthomas and **xanthelasmas** may occur in clients with biliary problems in whom serum cholesterol levels are high. These foamy cholesterol-filled cells may appear anywhere on the body but are commonly seen on the hands and around the eyes.

Edema and poor nutritional status also may make the skin highly susceptible to breakdown. Decubitus ulcers may form within hours in clients who are not frequently repositioned.

White nails, where 80% of the proximal nail bed is white leaving a distal band of normal pink, are often associated with cirrhosis. In hepatolenticular degeneration (Wilson's disease), the lunulae (half-moons in nail beds) are colored light blue instead of the normal white.

carrying capacity from erythrocytopenia may lead to increased cardiac output as the heart labors to deliver oxygen to starved tissues. Increased portal vein pressure related to hepatic fibrosis increases pressures within adjacent vessels and thereby leads to esophageal varices, splenomegaly, and periumbilical dilation. Hemorrhage of esophageal varices may further reduce the erythrocyte count. Increased clotting time because of deficiency in coagulation factors may produce hemorrhage and hypovolemic shock.

CARDIOVASCULAR SYSTEM

Fluid overload or congestive heart failure may occur in response to excessive levels of aldosterone and ADH. (See section on impairment of detoxification.) Reduced oxygen-

NEUROLOGIC SYSTEM

Ammonia toxicity is related to alteration in mental states ranging from confusion to hepatic coma. The client who is confused or combative has a high potential for injury.

Section IV: Psychosocial/Lifestyle Influences and Effects

Like all body systems, the hepatic–biliary system both influences and is influenced by psychosocial factors. Factors having a generalized effect are discussed in this section; factors related to specific disorders or therapies are discussed in subsequent chapters.

may inadvertently prescribe medications that interact unfavorably for the client. Self-medication with over-the-counter remedies—especially laxatives—may compound the overdosage. Overuse of laxatives is taxing to the liver and kidneys.

SEX AND AGE

Cholelithiasis (gallstones) occurs in women four to five times as often as it does in men. This increased incidence is thought to be related to the action of the female hormones estrogen and progesterone, which increase the cholesterol saturation of bile. The higher the cholesterol saturation, the greater the risk that gallstones will form. Pregnant women and those taking contraceptive pills are at even higher risk of developing cholelithiasis, especially those who have had several pregnancies or who have been on oral contraceptives for several years.

Cholelithiasis is more common in persons over 40 years of age. It can occur at any age, however, especially in association with risk factors such as high fat intake, obesity or diabetes, multiple pregnancies, or an oral contraceptive regimen.

Young adults and elderly individuals are at greater risk of contracting viral hepatitis. This increased risk may be associated with poor nutrition or with crowded or unsanitary living conditions.

Elderly persons are susceptible to problems of drug toxicity, in part because renal and hepatic function declines with age. At age 70, renal and hepatic efficiency may be half what it was at age 20, yet prescription of medications for elderly clients often do not reflect this fact. A drug may be prescribed at twice the dosage actually needed; if the client misunderstands dosage instructions or increases the dosage in the supposition that "more is better," severe toxic reactions can occur. The elderly often have multiple health problems. Several different health care providers

ALCOHOL AND DRUG ABUSE

Abuse of alcohol is a factor in many, though by no means all, conditions that damage the liver. Drug abuse, especially of injected substances, is associated with a high risk of contracting hepatitis. Cultural and psychological aspects of alcohol and drug abuse are discussed in Chapter 10.

LACK OF SANITATION

Drinking water or water used in preparation of foods such as fresh fruit or salad greens may become contaminated by secretions or fecal material from persons with viral (type A or type B) hepatitis (see Chapter 53). Shellfish caught in waters contaminated by untreated or inadequately treated sewage may also transmit the virus of hepatitis A. Sanitation is an important factor in control of hepatitis. Nurses, especially those working in community settings, can help inform their clients of the importance of washing hands before handling food and after using toilet facilities.

DIETARY HABITS

High-fat diets can contribute to the development of cirrhosis of the liver as well as to gallbladder disease. Biliary diseases are more common in cultures where food is prepared mostly by frying or large amounts of fat are used in cooking. Conversely, the incidence of gallbladder disease is low in African and South American countries where fat consumption is low. Due in part to the popularity of fast food chains and fried snack products, the American diet is currently high in fat. A high intake of alcohol and associated malnutrition also contribute to the development of hepatic and biliary disease. (Alcohol abuse is discussed in Chapter 10, and nutrition is discussed in Chapters 8 and 9.)

ECONOMIC FACTORS

Although malnutrition is usually associated with poverty, a high income does not ensure a balanced diet. Reliance on fast foods and snack foods and consumption of a fat-laden diet occur in all socioeconomic classes. Poor sanitation and high alcohol consumption may also occur at any income level.

OCCUPATION AND AVOCATION

Exposure to all types of hepatitis is a special risk of health care professionals, who may be exposed to virus-contaminated blood or secretions. Laboratory and operating room personnel and those who work in hemodialysis units risk contamination through exposure to body fluids. Nurses administering intravenous therapy or disposing of secretions may be exposed to hepatitis if strict asepsis and isolation principles are not followed. Dentists may be exposed to the hepatitis virus in the saliva of a hepatitis carrier or a person with active disease.

Exposure to toxic chemicals may be related to occupation, leisure-time hobbies, or a pharmaceutical regimen. Halothane and chloroform, to which operating room personnel are exposed, are hepatotoxic. Carbon tetrachloride, used in dry cleaning and in various industrial processes, is hepatotoxic, as are toluene and other chemicals used in paint thinners and other compounds used by both professionals and hobbyists. Gold, used in the jewelry trade and in fabrication of some electronic components, is also hepatotoxic. Among the medications that may have a toxic effect on the liver are a number of antibiotics (including erythromycin, oxacillin, and clindamycin), some psychotropic medications, and oral contraceptives. (A more extensive list of hepatotoxic substances appears in Chapter 52.) Highly stressful occupations or those that require a great deal of socialization may contribute to alcohol abuse.

In taking the health history, the nurse who is alert to these psychosocial factors can identify clients who appear to be at risk and refer them for detection of early pathological conditions affecting the hepatic–biliary system.

Chapter Highlights

The liver is essential to life and functions as a regulator for many homeostatic systems.

Principal functions of the liver include (1) storage and filtration of blood, (2) secretion of bile, (3) conjugation and excretion of bilirubin, (4) metabolism of carbohydrates, fats, and proteins, (5) storage of vitamins and iron, (6) synthesis of coagulation factors and lymph, and (7) detoxification of ingested substances.

The basic functional unit of the liver is the liver lobule, of which there are 50,000 to 100,000 in the adult liver.

The principal function of the gallbladder is concentration and storage of bile.

Fibrotic enlargement of the liver is characteristic of most liver disorders; eventually, scarring may result in atrophy in late stages of liver disease.

Increased back-pressure in the portal venous system related to hypertrophy and fibrosis of the liver is the principal cause of periumbilical dilation, esophageal varices, and ascites, and may be related to splenomegaly and hemorrhoids.

Erythrocyte production decreases when the liver is compromised, owing to inadequate storage of vitamin B_{12} and iron (heme).

The client with impaired hepatic function is at risk for hemorrhage related to diminished production of clotting factors due in part to deficient absorption of vitamin K.

Destruction of phagocytic Kupffer cells and impairment of lymph production in a diseased liver increases the client's susceptibility to infection.

Jaundice associated with liver disease is related to impairment of bilirubin conjugation and excretion.

Inability of the compromised liver to convert ammonia to urea for excretion leads to ammonia toxicity, a condition that causes impairment of mentation sometimes leading to coma, as well as asterixis.

Hypoalbuminemia and impaired detoxification of ADH and aldosterone can lead to development of ascites and peripheral edema as well as vascular dehydration, which may mask erythrocytopenia by altering blood viscosity.

Lifestyle factors contributing to hepatic disease include alcohol abuse and work-related exposure to hepatotoxic substances.

Women are more susceptible to cholelithiasis than men, especially those who have had multiple pregnancies and those taking oral contraceptives; obesity, diabetes, high fat intake, and age over 40 are additional risk factors.

Bibliography

Crowley LV: *Introduction to Human Disease.* Monterey, CA: Wadsworth, 1983.

Groer ME, Shekleton ME: *Basic Pathology: A Conceptual Approach,* 2nd ed. St. Louis, MO: Mosby, 1983.

Guyton, AC: *Textbook of Medical Physiology,* 6th ed. Philadelphia: Saunders, 1981.

Petersdorf RG et al (editor): *Harrison's Principles of Internal Medicine,* 10th ed. New York: McGraw-Hill, 1983.

Ramsey JM: *Basic Pathophysiology: Modern Stress and the Disease Process.* Menlo Park, CA: Addison-Wesley, 1982.

Schearman DJC, Finlayson, ADC: *Diseases of the Gastrointestinal Tract and Liver.* London: Churchill Livingstone, 1982.

Sherlock S: *Diseases of the Liver and Biliary System,* 6th ed. Oxford: Blackwell, 1981.

Spence AP, Mason EB: *Human Anatomy and Physiology,* 2nd ed. Menlo Park, CA: Benjamin/Cummings, 1983.

Vick RL: *Contemporary Medical Physiology.* Menlo Park, CA: Addison-Wesley, 1984.

Suggested Readings

Fredette SL: When the liver fails. *Am J Nurs* 1984; 1:64–67. Brief discussion of underlying pathophysiology that is essential for writing effective nursing diagnoses.

Pierce L: Anatomy and physiology of the liver. *Nurs Clin North Am* 1977; 12:257–272. One of several *Nursing Clinics* articles on hepatic disease. Excellent review of anatomy and physiology in relation to clinical assessment. A classic.

Taylor DL: Gallstones: Physiology, signs, and symptoms. *Nurs 83* 1983; 13(6):44. Brief, well-illustrated discussion explains physiology of gallstone formation and reviews diagnostic signs.

Taylor DL: Jaundice: Physiology, signs and symptoms. *Nurs 83* 1983; 13(8):52–54. Brief, well-illustrated description of hemolytic, obstructive, and hepatocellular jaundice, including diagnostic signs.

Chapter 52

The Nursing Process for Clients With Hepatic–Biliary System Dysfunction

Jane Hokanson Hawks

Objectives

When you have finished studying this chapter, you should be able to:

Discuss the complete assessment of a client with hepatic–biliary dysfunction.

Identify the nursing implications of appropriate laboratory tests and diagnostic studies for clients with hepatic–biliary disease.

Specify nursing diagnoses for the client with hepatic–biliary dysfunction.

Plan nursing care for clients with hepatic–biliary dysfunction.

Formulate expected outcomes to evaluate the effectiveness of nursing interventions for clients with problems of the hepatic–biliary system.

The nursing process for clients with hepatic and biliary dysfunction encompasses a wide range of assessments and interventions. Nursing responsibilities generally applicable to hepatic and biliary disorders are discussed in this chapter. Nursing measures applicable to specific disorders and surgical approaches are discussed in Chapters 53 and 54.

Section I: Nursing Assessment: Establishing the Data Base

SUBJECTIVE DATA

In assessing a client's health status, the health history furnishes valuable clues to past and present problems, as well as to risk factors that can indicate where future problems may develop. Usually the client is the chief source of information, but significant others may be able to contribute useful data. The health history as it pertains to overall health assessment is discussed in Chapter 7. This chapter discusses data related specifically to the hepatic and biliary systems.

The client should be questioned about any recent loss of weight, change in appetite, or changes in bowel patterns. What color are the client's stools? What color is the urine? Clay-colored stools or mahogany-colored urine suggest obstruction of the common, hepatic, or cystic duct or an abnormality of bilirubin excretion. Was a change in color

of stool or urine accompanied by yellowing of the sclera or the skin? Did pruritus occur when these changes were noticed? Associating these symptoms may help the client remember when they began.

Has the client lost weight or lost interest in food? A positive reply might suggest development of hepatitis or hepatic cancer, depending on other symptoms and signs elicited during the assessment.

What does the client usually eat? High fat intake might suggest cholelithiasis. Does the client bruise easily or bleed for a long time after a minor cut? Decreased absorption of vitamin K—possibly associated with hyperbilirubinemia—can affect blood coagulation.

Edema of the ankles, difficulty breathing, and collection of fluid in the abdomen could indicate right-sided heart failure, hypoalbuminemia, portal hypertension, or inadequate detoxification of antidiuretic hormone (ADH) and

1567

Box 52–1	Drugs and Chemicals Capable of Causing Hepatic–Biliary Dysfunction

Drugs:

*Acetaminophen (Tylenol, Datril)	Methimazole (Tapazole)
	Methotrexate
Acetohexamide (Dymelor)	Methyldopa (Aldomet, Aldoril)
Allopurinol (Zyloprim)	
Aminosalicylic acid (PAS)	Monoamine oxidase inhibitors
Androgens and anabolic steroids	Nitrofurantoin (Furadantin, Macrodantin)
*Azathioprine (Imuran)	
Chlorpromazine (Thorazine)	Oral contraceptives
	Oxacillin (Prostaphilin)
Chlorpropamide (Diabinese)	*Phenacetin
Clindamycin (Cleocin)	Phenazopyridine (Pyridium)
Erythromycin estolate (Ilosone)	Phenylbutazone (Butazolidin)
Ethionamide (Trecator SC)	Phenytoin (Dilantin)
	Propoxyphene (Darvon)
Gold salts	*Rifampin
Imipramine (Tofranil)	Sulfonamides
*Isoniazid (INH)	Tetracyclines

Inhalation Anesthetics

Halothane (Fluothane)	Methoxyflurane (Penthrane)

Industrial Inhalants

*Arsenic	*Yellow phosphorus
*Carbon tetrachloride	

*Hepatotoxins (dose related)

aldosterone. The client may not remember when such changes began, but asking when clothing became tight around the waist or shoes no longer fit might jog the memory.

Has the client had frequent infections? Increased incidence of infection may be related to destruction of Kupffer cells. Has the client been exposed to hepatitis or mononucleosis? Has the client had any recent blood transfusions? A positive answer may be correlated with other evidence suggesting hepatitis. Impotence or loss of libido may be related to impaired estrogen detoxification. Questioning about this sensitive subject might best be postponed until rapport has been established with the client. Tactful questioning of the client's sexual partner may elicit data suggesting sexual dysfunction.

Determining whether alcohol abuse might be related

to liver dysfunction also requires discretion and tact. One should not presuppose that the client is an alcohol abuser, even if the suspected disorder is commonly associated with consumption of alcohol. The client who does have an alcohol problem may be reluctant to answer, may evade questions, or may deny any drinking problems. Sometimes significant others will verify unexplained changes in behavior that may suggest alcohol abuse. Psychosocial changes related to alcohol abuse are discussed at length in Chapter 10.

Specific, nonjudgmental questions are most likely to yield useful data about drinking habits:

- What do you like to drink?
- How often do you drink? Every day? Several times a day? A week? A month? Such specifics are more useful than generalities such as "rarely" or "often."
- How much do you drink? One drink? Three or four?
- How many shots do you put in a highball? Do you order drinks "up" or with ice? Does wine with dinner mean a glass or a carafe? By "a few beers" do you mean a couple of cans? A six-pack?

Remember that alcohol in any form (wine, beer, or hard liquor) has the same effect. A 12 oz bottle of beer, a 4 oz glass of wine, and a 1 oz shot of Scotch contain the same amount of alcohol. Chapter 10 contains a chart of comparative alcohol content of various drinks that may be helpful in estimating the client's consumption.

Other questions related to drinking habits might be:

- When you drink, how much do you consume in 24 hours?
- What is the most you've drunk in 24 hours?
- Do you drink in the morning? At or after work? With friends? Alone?
- Have you ever blacked out?
- Does drinking make you sick or does it make you feel better? Gastritis related to alcoholism will be alleviated by a drink (Hawks, 1983).

Remember not to concentrate on alcohol while ignoring other clues. What is the client's occupation? Does it involve exposure to solvents, dry-cleaning solutions, anesthetic agents, or other hepatotoxic substances? Does the client have hobbies such as furniture refinishing that might have hepatotoxic side effects? A list of common substances causing hepatic damage is presented in Box 52–1.

OBJECTIVE DATA
Physical Assessment

Physical assessment of the client with hepatic–biliary dysfunction involves careful inspection of the skin, nails, and hair. Physical findings that suggest cirrhosis include:

- Ascites (Figure 52–1)
- Ankle edema
- Muscle wasting

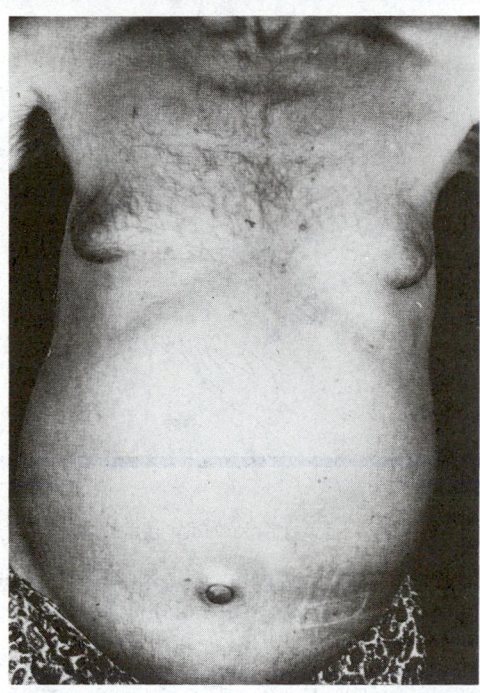

Figure 52–1

Ascites and gynecomastia.

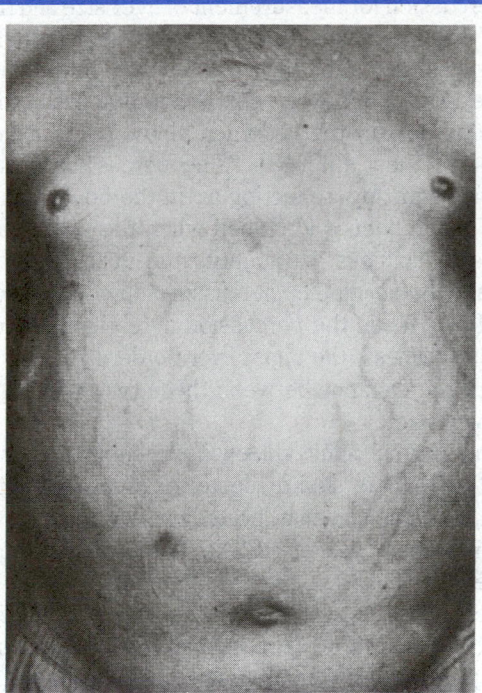

Figure 52–2

Dilated periumbilical veins.

- Dilated periumbilical veins (caput medusae) (Figure 52–2)
- Ecchymoses
- Spider angiomas (Figure 52–3)
- Loss of body hair
- **Gynecomastia** (breast enlargement in males) (Figure 52–1)
- **Jaundice** (yellow coloration to skin and sclerae)
- Clubbing of the fingers

If the client is in a late stage of liver dysfunction, asterixis related to ammonia toxicity will be observed—the hands rapidly clench and unclench. Inflating a blood pressure cuff on the arm will worsen the tremor. Asterixis may also be seen in clients with cancer of the liver. In clients with hepatitis, however, only ecchymoses and jaundice will be apparent unless the condition is long standing. Bruising and jaundice may sometimes accompany hepatic abscess; however, diminished appetite may be the only sign of this disorder. As mentioned previously, jaundice may also be secondary to an obstructive condition or an abnormality affecting bilirubin conjugation.

The abdomen should be auscultated before it is palpated. Diminished bowel sounds are common in clients with ascites. At the same time, auscultation of the lungs may elicit evidence of rales or rhonchi related to pulmonary edema. Listen for hepatic bruits, which may be heard with hepatic carcinoma.

Hepatomegaly and splenomegaly can be present in clients with hepatitis, cholecystitis, hepatic abscess, mononucleosis, cirrhosis, or cancer of the liver. *Because of the*

danger of damaging or rupturing these organs, the inexperienced nurse should not palpate the liver or spleen. If enlargement is severe, these organs may be felt by very light palpation of the abdomen. Swollen lymph nodes may be palpable in the neck or in the groin with an infectious disorder such as mononucleosis. Techniques for detecting peripheral neuropathies as seen in chronic alcoholism are described in Chapter 7 under neurologic assessment.

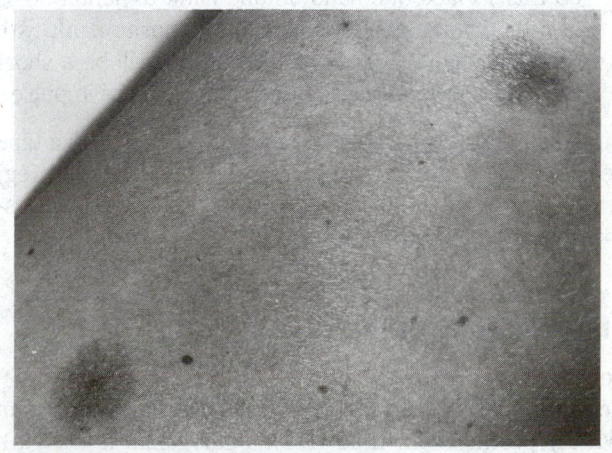

Figure 52–3

Spider angioma on the skin of a client with cirrhosis.
SOURCE: Binnick SA: *Skin Diseases: Diagnosis and Management in Clinical Practice.* Baltimore, MD: Williams & Wilkins, 1982.

Percussion for measurement of liver size and the usual area of splenic dullness helps determine whether either organ is enlarged. The normal liver span at the midclavicular line (MCL) is 6 to 12 cm. When percussing the liver size, begin low in the abdomen below the umbilicus and percuss up the right MCL. The percussion note heard initially is tympany, reflecting air in the bowel. The lower border of the liver is identified when the percussion note changes to dullness. To identify the upper liver border, begin above the nipple, percussing downward along the right MCL. When the percussion note changes from resonance to dullness, the upper liver border has been located. Measure the distance between these two points to determine liver size.

The normal adult spleen lies behind the ninth and eleventh ribs, at or slightly posterior to the left midaxillary line (MAL). The spleen is located by percussing downward in the intercostal spaces (ICS) at the left MAL, beginning in the eighth left ICS. The percussion note should change from resonance to splenic dullness at about the tenth left ICS. A large area of dullness may indicate feces in the splenic flexure of the colon, a full stomach, or splenomegaly. Note that clients who have had organ transplants may have undergone splenectomy.

Three assessment techniques can be used to determine whether fluid is present in the abdomen.

1. With the client supine, both flanks may be percussed for dullness, which indicates the presence of fluid.

2. When the client assumes a side-lying position, fluid will fall toward the side on which the client is lying, where it may be percussed for dullness.

3. The presence of a fluid wave may be determined as follows: Have the client lie flat and place his or her hand, ulnar side down, along the abdominal midline and apply pressure to anchor the fat in the mesentery. (If the client is too ill to participate, an assistant can do this.) Place one hand on one flank to detect signs of a fluid wave while tapping the opposite flank with the other hand (Figure 52–4). There will be a short time lag between the tap and receipt of the impulse.

Abdominal girth should be measured daily with a tape measure. Measurements taken at the same location (eg, at the level of the umbilicus) assist in evaluating progression and/or treatment of ascites.

Diagnostic Studies

Hematologic Studies

Blood samples for determination of white blood cell count (WBC), prothrombin time (PT), hemoglobin level (Hb), and hematocrit (Hct) may be drawn at any time. Hemoglobin and hematocrit values are unaffected by early stages of hepatic disease but may drop if there is hemorrhage from esophageal varices and in response to malnourishment. Prothrombin time will increase with vitamin K deficiency, for example, in cirrhosis, hepatitis, cholecystitis, choleli-

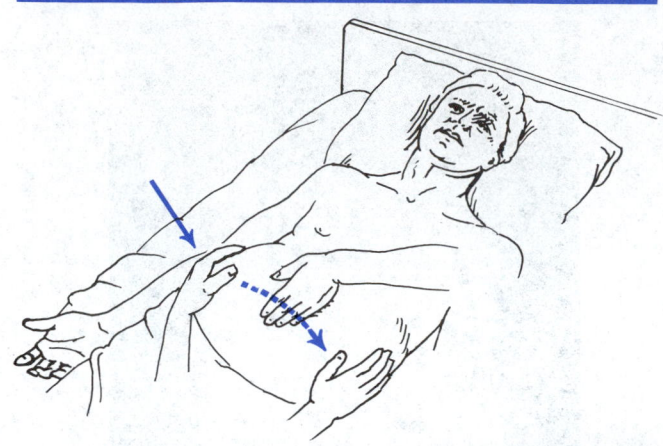

Figure 52–4

Assessing for ascites by checking for a fluid wave.

thiasis, mononucleosis, or cancer of the liver. Leukocyte levels increase in clients with mononucleosis, hepatitis, and abscesses.

Serum Enzyme Studies

Elevated serum enzyme levels occur when hepatic cells are damaged and enzymes are released into the blood. Values that are likely to be elevated with liver or gallbladder disease include:

- Lactic dehydrogenase (LDH)
- Serum glutamic oxaloacetic transaminase (SGOT); also called aspartate aminotransferase (AST)
- Serum glutamic pyruvic transaminase (SGPT); also called alanine aminotransferase (ALT)

Nursing Research Note

Keck J, Swerhun P: Hepatitis B: An occupational risk. *Can Nurse* 1980; 76(11):33–35.

This case study describes how one hospital dealt with a case of hepatitis B found in a nurse employee during the preemployment physical. The individual was permitted to return to work after 4 weeks when values from liver function tests had improved, but the serum was still positive for HBsAg. He was restricted from serving meals and from performing venipunctures and other treatments. The nurse also attended a course in cardiopulmonary resuscitation (CPR).

The author offers suggestions for preventing cross-infection among staff members having CPR training. All staff members must have HBsAg and HBsAb levels drawn within 3 months of starting the course. Results must be available before training begins. A history must be obtained to rule out acute or chronic medical conditions. No staff member should participate who has a positive blood test for HBsAg, an upper respiratory infection, herpes simplex, or a dermatological lesion. Plastic protectors must be placed over the mannequin's mouth. The mannequin head must be disassembled after each use and washed with soap and water plus 0.5% sodium hypochlorite solution. The mannequin must be closely inspected for cracks and tears. Inservice education of CPR instructors on preventing cross-infection is essential.

- Alkaline phosphatase
- Gamma-glutamyl transpeptidase (GGT)

LDH, SGOT, and SGPT values are significantly increased in obstructive jaundice and mononucleosis; they are also markedly elevated in acute and toxic hepatitis, cirrhosis, and hepatic neoplasia. Alkaline phosphatase levels, important in measuring biliary obstruction, are extremely elevated in obstructive jaundice, significantly elevated in cancer of the liver and mononucleosis, and slightly elevated in hepatitis (viral or toxic) and cirrhosis. Elevation of gamma-glutamyl transpeptidase is the most accurate enzymatic indicator of hepatic disease. Enzyme levels will rise as the disease progresses, peaking at the time of maximum cell death, and then begin to fall.

Serum Lipid Values

Changes in serum lipid values are related to the type of disorder. Serum lipids are elevated in obstructive disorders of the biliary system such as cholelithiasis or neoplasia. They are decreased in disorders causing destruction of hepatic cells, for example, in cirrhosis or hepatitis.

Bilirubin Values

Studies of bilirubin values are important in determining the cause of jaundice and hyperbilirubinemia. Direct or conjugated bilirubin levels will be elevated if biliary ducts are obstructed and conjugated bilirubin cannot be excreted. Indirect or unconjugated bilirubin levels will be high if parenchymal (liver lobule) cells have been damaged.

Elevated levels of urobilinogen in the urine indicate parenchymal liver disease such as cirrhosis, toxic or infectious hepatitis, or infectious mononucleosis—or they may indicate cholelithiasis. By impairing excretion of bilirubin in the stool, these conditions lead to increased excretion by the kidneys. Urine that contains bilirubin develops a yellow foam when shaken. Fecal levels of urobilinogen are decreased if the bile ducts are obstructed, but this test is rarely performed because of the difficulty in obtaining accurate values.

Blood Ammonia Values

Blood ammonia levels rise when cirrhosis is present because the disease impairs conversion of ammonia to urea for renal excretion. Bleeding esophageal varices exacerbate ammonia toxicity, since the ammonia produced by the action of intestinal bacteria on the protein in blood adds rapidly to already elevated serum ammonia levels. Hepatic coma can result.

Other Laboratory Test Values

Changes in serum protein levels are common in hepatic and biliary disorders. Serum albumin levels drop (hypoalbuminemia) and gamma globulin levels rise when parenchymal cell damage occurs. Serum antigen-antibody levels are helpful in evaluating hepatitis. For example, hepatitis B surface antigen (HBsAg) is present in the blood of persons who have hepatitis B and also in those who are carriers of the disease. Clients with hepatitis B surface antibody (anti-HBs) in their blood have immunity to hepatitis B.

Laboratory tests commonly used in diagnosis of hepatic and biliary disorders are summarized in Tables 52–1 and 52–2.

Ultrasound

The general principles of ultrasonography are described in Chapter 7. For some clients, especially those for whom oral cholecystography or intravenous cholangiography are contraindicated, ultrasound offers a noninvasive alternative. This technique is being used with increasing frequency to investigate ambiguous findings obtained by other techniques. It is useful in differentiating benign cysts and tumors from malignancies. Liver abscesses and dilation of intrahepatic ducts can be identified by ultrasound, as can gallstones, biliary tumors, and tumors of the extrahepatic ducts (Figure 52–5). In a client with jaundice, dilation of the extrahepatic ducts suggests extrahepatic obstruction. If the ducts appear normal, jaundice is likely to be related to an extrahepatic or prehepatic condition (Pagana and Pagana, 1982). Hepatic icterus is related to abnormalities of bilirubin conjugation or excretion. Extrahepatic icterus is related to obstruction of the hepatic, common, or cystic bile ducts. Prehepatic icterus is associated with an abnormality that takes effect before circulating bilirubin reaches the liver—for example, hemolysis or neonatal icterus.

Nursing Implications. To ensure that the gallbladder is at maximum size for the test, the client must be kept NPO after midnight on the day of testing. Were the client to eat, contraction and emptying of the gallbladder would reduce its size, making it more difficult to visualize. NPO orders are not necessary for visualization of the liver. If barium contrast studies have been performed prior to the ultrasonography, a laxative will be ordered to cleanse the bowel of residual contrast medium.

In explaining the procedure to the client, the nurse can offer reassurance that the study is not painful. The client should be prepared for the copious amount of lubricant that will be applied to the skin to enhance transmission of the sound waves. The rationale for any NPO order should be explained. The procedure will take about 20 minutes.

Liver Scan

Radionuclide scanning techniques are briefly reviewed in Chapter 7. A radionuclide is administered intravenously. Thirty minutes later a detecting device is passed over the client's abdomen to record the distribution of radioactive particles in the liver. Although this technique exposes the client to far less radiation than x-rays, it can only demonstrate filling defects greater than 2 cm in diameter. It is contraindicated for pregnant clients and those who might have difficulty lying still during the scan, which takes about one hour.

Table 52–1 Laboratory Tests Common to the Hepatic–Biliary System

Laboratory Tests	Normal Expected Value	Disease State	Expected Abnormal Findings
Hemoglobin	M 14–18 g/dL F 12–16 g/dL	Prolonged hepatitis or cirrhosis; carcinoma of liver	Decreased
Hematocrit	M 40%–54% F 37%–47%	Prolonged hepatitis or cirrhosis; carcinoma of liver	Decreased
Prothrombin time	11–15 sec	Cirrhosis, hepatitis, cholelithiasis, cholecystitis, carcinoma or abscess of liver	Prolonged. Extent of prolonged time indicates severity of dysfunction fairly well.
Alkaline phosphatase	25–85 IU 1.5–4.5 Bodansky units/dL	Biliary obstruction	Elevated
LDH	60–100 Wacker units 15–60 IU/L 200–450 U/mL	Cirrhosis, hepatitis, abscess, carcinoma of liver, mononucleosis	Elevated
SGOT or AST SGPT or ALT	12–30 U/L 5–30 U/L	Cirrhosis, hepatitis, abscess, carcinoma of liver, mononucleosis	Elevated
Gamma-glutamyl transpeptidase (GGT)	4–60 U/L	Hepatitis	Elevated
Cholesterol	120–260 mg/dL	Biliary obstruction Liver cell damage	Elevated Decreased
Triglycerides	20–190 mg/dL	Biliary obstruction Liver cell damage	Elevated Decreased
WBC count	4500–11,000 cells/mm³	Hepatitis, abscess, cirrhosis	Normal early, then elevated
Bilirubin total indirect (unconjugated) direct (conjugated)	0.3–1.4 mg/dL 0.2–0.8 mg/dL 0.1–0.4 mg/dL	Jaundice Hemolysis; hepatic damage Biliary obstruction	Elevated Elevated Elevated
Urine bilirubin	None	Occurs only when serum direct or conjugated bilirubin is increased	Elevated
Urine urobilinogen	0.5–4.0 Ehrlich units/24 h	Biliary obstruction	Decreased or absent
Stool urobilinogen	40–250 mg/24 h	Biliary obstruction	Decreased or absent
Serum ammonia	70–200 µg/dL whole blood; 56–150 µg/dL plasma	Cirrhosis, hepatitis, abscess, or carcinoma of liver	Elevated
Albumin	3.5–5.5 g/dL	Cirrhosis, hepatitis, carcinoma of liver	Decreased
Gamma globulin	700–1800 mg/dL	Cirrhosis, hepatitis, carcinoma of liver	Elevated
Dye clearance studies Bromsulphalein (BSP)	Less than 5% in blood after 45 minutes	Cirrhosis, hepatitis, carcinoma of liver, biliary obstruction	Dye retained if liver damage

Nursing Implications. No special preparation is required for this study. The nurse should explain the procedure and explain that small amounts of radioactive substances are used. Some clients are apprehensive about the amount of time required for the scan, and it is helpful to explain that the scanning device does not emit radiation but rather records radiation emanating from the injected radioisotope. Pregnant health care providers should not be assigned to the client for at least 24 hours after the radionuclide injection.

Dye Clearance Studies

For this procedure, the client fasts for 12 hours prior to the test. Dye is injected intravenously (about 5 mg/kg of

Table 52–2 Immunologic Antigen–Antibody Tests for Viral Hepatitis A and B

Antigen/Antibody Tests	Comments
anti-HAV (antibody to hepatitis A virus)	Early antibody is of IgM class; convalescent antibody of IgG class; clients with anti-HAV in serum are immune to reinfection.
HBsAg (hepatitis B surface antigen)	Specific for hepatitis B infection; appears about 4 weeks after exposure to hepatitis B; originally called Australian antigen
anti-HB$_s$ (antibody to hepatitis B surface antigen)	Its presence in the blood indicates immunity to hepatitis B.
HB$_c$Ag (hepatitis B core antigen)	The core of the Dane particle; core antigen is difficult to identify.
anti-HB$_c$ (antibody to hepatitis B core antigen	In the absence of Hb$_s$Ag and anti-Hb$_s$, a high titer of anti-HB$_c$ reflects ongoing viral replication.
HB$_e$Ag (hepatitis B "e" antigen)	Found in HB$_s$Ag positive serum only; an indicator of relative infectivity of the client with hepatitis B; persistent positives may be associated with chronic hepatitis.
anti-HB$_e$ (antibody to hepatitis B "e" antigen)	Its presence is associated with a lower degree of infectivity.

HAV (hepatitis A virus): RNA virus, present in serum and stool.
HBV (hepatitis B virus—Dane particle): DNA virus, present in serum, saliva, semen, breast milk.

body weight). Blood is drawn 45 minutes after the injection and inspected for the presence of dye. Normally, less than 5% of the dye will be found in the serum; the presence of a greater proportion of the dye indicates liver cell damage—the impaired cells cannot absorb the dye from the blood. If hepatic damage is known to exist, lower dosages of dye are administered. Either indocyanine green (ICG) or Bromsulphalein (BSP) is used for this study.

Oral Cholecystography

An oral cholecystogram, or "gallbladder series," provides visualization of the gallbladder following oral ingestion of a radiopaque iodinated dye. Figure 52–6 shows a normal cholecystogram. In the first test of the series, gallstones when present may be visualized as dark shadows in a dye-filled gallbladder. Satisfactory visualization of the gallbladder can be obtained only if the gallbladder has concentrated

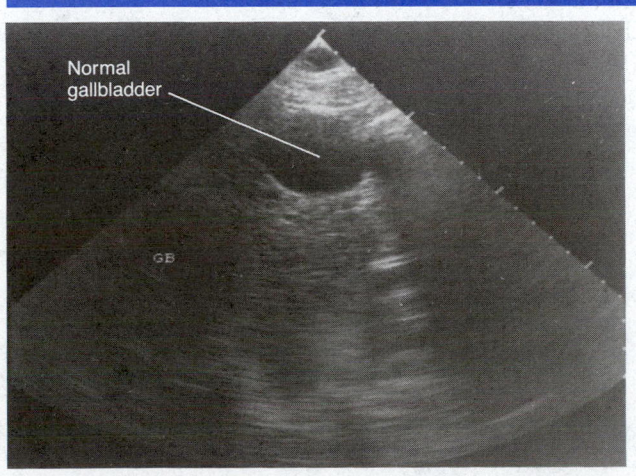
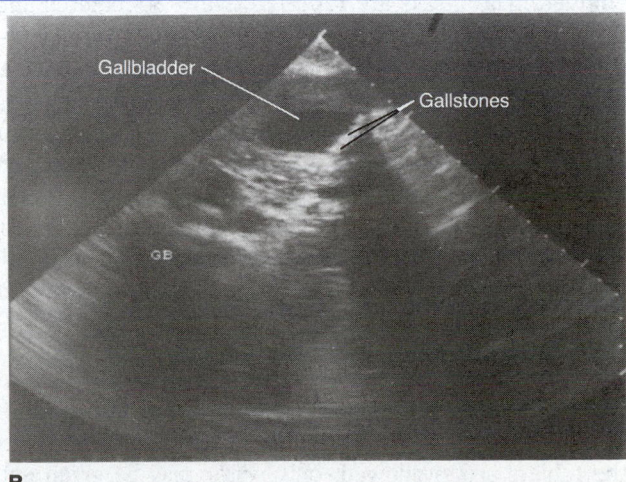

Figure 52–5

A. Ultrasound of a normal gallbladder. **B.** Ultrasound of a gallbladder containing gallstones. Courtesy of Health Care Plan, Buffalo, NY.

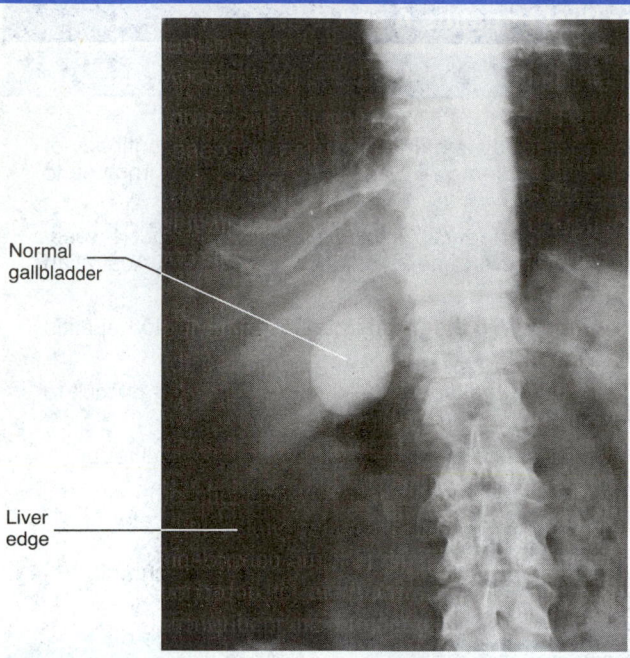

Normal gallbladder

Liver edge

Figure 52–6

A normal oral cholecystogram. The gallbladder is filled with contrast dye. Courtesy of Health Care Plan, Buffalo, NY.

the dye. Adequate concentration depends on correct dosage of the dye, adequate absorption of the dye from the gastrointestinal tract (ie, no nausea or vomiting), and absence of food in the digestive tract (ie, NPO after midnight). If nonvisualization occurs, the test is repeated the next day with a doubled dosage of dye. Hepatocellular dysfunction, cystic duct obstruction, or inflammation of the biliary mucosa will prevent visualization.

In the second phase of the series, the client is given a fatty meal immediately following the first phase, and x-rays are taken to determine how well the gallbladder empties. The x-rays are repeated every 30 minutes until the dye is gone and the gallbladder can no longer be visualized. This may take one to five hours but usually takes no more than three.

Oral cholecystography is contraindicated for pregnant women, clients too ill to swallow the dye tablets or to eat a meal, and persons allergic to iodine. Ultrasonography may soon replace oral cholecystography because it is less invasive, more accurate in diagnosing cholelithiasis, and can be used with pregnant clients and those who cannot take the oral contrast agent.

Nursing Implications. The client will have to swallow seven or eight tablets of absorbable iodine dye (Telepaque, for example) the evening prior to the test. Once the tablets are swallowed, only water may be given until midnight; after midnight the client is kept NPO. Nursing implications include:

- Verifying that no iodine allergy exists. The client should be questioned about seafood allergies, since not all clients are aware of what foods contain iodine.

- Ascertaining that the client is given a low-fat meal on the evening before the test.
- Verifying that serum bilirubin is less than 1.8 mg/dL (so that visualization will be possible).
- Explaining the procedure to the client.
- Administering the tablets at five-minute intervals.
- Observing for adverse effects of the dye. (Anaphylactic reactions have occurred.)
- Maintaining NPO status.

Intravenous Cholangiography

Intravenous cholangiography allows visualization of the hepatic and common bile ducts in addition to the gallbladder and cystic duct. It is used for clients with acute inflammatory disorders, those with proven gallstones, and those who are NPO or unable to tolerate the orally ingested dye used in cholecystography. It is contraindicated for clients with serum bilirubin levels higher than 3.5 mg/dL, for those allergic to iodine, and for pregnant clients. While supine, the client is given an intravenous infusion of iodinated contrast medium. X-rays are then taken at intervals for up to eight hours.

Nursing Implications. No special diet is required for this procedure. Usually, bisacodyl (Dulcolax) is ordered to be given on the morning of the examination. In explaining the procedure to the client, mention that it is normal to feel heat with the administration of the contrast medium. Verifying that the client is not allergic to iodine is an important precaution. The nurse is also responsible for administering the cathartic, verifying bilirubin level, and maintaining NPO status. The client should be kept as comfortable as possible; for example, oral hygiene may be administered during the intervals between films.

Intraoperative Cholangiography

Cholangiography may be performed during a surgical procedure to ascertain that all calculi have been removed from the common bile duct, reducing the probability of complications or follow-up surgery. Dye is injected to enhance visualization.

T-Tube Cholangiography

A T-tube cholangiogram may be taken seven to ten days following a cholecystectomy. The T-tube is placed during surgery. Later, dye is injected via the T-tube so the common bile duct may be visualized and its patency ascertained.

Endoscopic Retrograde Cholangiopancreatography

The icteric client with bilirubin levels above 3.5 mg/dL cannot be evaluated by oral cholecystography or intravenous cholangiography. Endoscopic retrograde cholangiopancreatography (ERCP) and percutaneous hepatic cholangiography (PTHC—see following section) are alternative techniques for these clients. ERCP studies allow visualization of the bile ducts as well as benign masses, cysts, and malignant neoplasms.

A type of fiberoptic endoscope (a duodenoscope) is inserted into the duodenum via the esophagus. Intravenously administered secretin immobilizes the duodenum, facilitating visualization of the ampulla of Vater. Contrast material combined with a broad-spectrum antibiotic are administered through a small cannula inserted into the ampulla, and films are taken periodically for approximately an hour. The antibiotic is given to prevent gram-negative sepsis that may occur if bacteria are forced into the bloodstream by the pressure of the dye injection. Perforation of the esophagus, stomach, or duodenum is another possible complication of ERCP, so this procedure is not used for combative clients (Pagana and Pagana, 1982).

Nursing Implications. A consent form is necessary for this procedure. In teaching the client about the procedure, explain that an impulse to gag will be felt when the tube is passed. The client is kept NPO after midnight. Meperidine and atropine are administered intramuscularly before the client is taken to the radiology department. Emotional support should be given as needed. After the procedure, the client's pulse, temperature, and blood pressure are monitored for signs of shock that may arise from perforation or hemorrhage and for signs of septicemia. Pancreatitis may occur in response to the pressure exerted on the pancreatic duct during the procedure; therefore, a serum amylase test should be performed on the day following an ERCP.

Percutaneous Transhepatic Cholangiography

Like ERCP, percutaneous (through the skin) transhepatic cholangiography (PTHC) is used for icteric clients with serum bilirubin levels above 3.5 mg/dL. During this procedure, a combination of contrast medium and antibiotic is injected into the intrahepatic bile duct to visualize the biliary system. The area below the right costal margin is locally anesthetized, and a spinal needle is inserted directly into the liver guided by fluoroscopy. When bile appears through the needle, it is withdrawn by syringe. Radiopaque dye is then injected directly into the biliary tree. Fluoroscopy is used to determine filling of the biliary tract.

The client is intravenously sedated during the procedure, which takes about one hour. If obstruction is found, a catheter may be left in place for drainage of bile. A PTHC is contraindicated for clients who have prolonged clotting times or iodine allergy, for clients who have had recent gastrointestinal contrast studies or are unlikely to tolerate surgery, and for combative clients. Bile peritonitis, hemorrhage, and septicemia are possible complications.

Nursing Implications. A consent form is required for this procedure, and coagulation studies as well as information regarding possible iodine allergy must be verified. The client is kept NPO after midnight. A laxative may be prescribed if gastrointestinal studies using barium have been recently administered. An intravenous infusion is started for venous access, and the client is premedicated with meperidine and atropine before leaving the unit. After the procedure, the client is kept NPO and in bed for 12 to 24 hours or, if very ill, until the condition improves. Vital signs must be monitored as for a postsurgical client. A sterile closed system must be maintained if a catheter has been left in place.

Liver Biopsy

The purpose of a liver biopsy is to obtain a sample of tissue for histologic examination. Prior to the procedure, a liver scan may be done to determine the precise location of the liver, and a coagulation profile must be obtained so the risk of hemorrhage can be calculated. The client's blood is typed and crossmatched in case a transfusion is needed.

For the study, the client is assisted into a supine or left lateral position. The skin is aseptically cleansed and anesthetized, and a small incision is made to allow insertion of a specialized needle into the liver. A small core of hepatic tissue is then withdrawn and sent for microscopic evaluation (Figure 52–7).

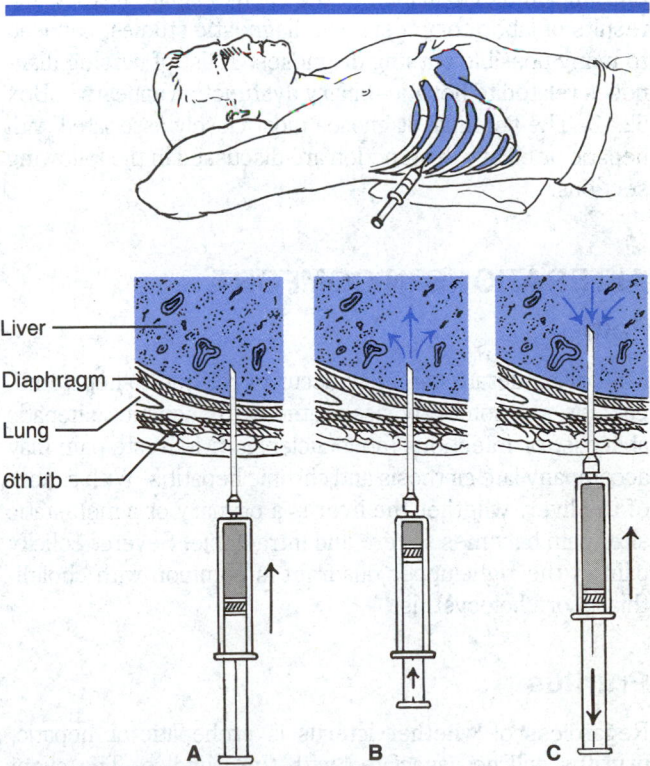

Figure 52–7

Liver biopsy procedure. **A.** Have the client hold his/her breath at the end of expiration to bring the liver and diaphragm to the highest position; the physician then inserts the biopsy needle into the liver. **B.** Approximately 1 mL of saline is injected to clear the needle of blood and tissue. **C.** The needle is pushed farther into the liver. Liver tissue is aspirated, the needle withdrawn, and pressure applied to the injection site. The liver specimen is expelled into formalin to preserve it for analysis.

Nursing Implications. This procedure requires a consent form. The client is kept NPO after midnight. Nursing responsibilities include:

- Checking coagulation studies and consent form.
- Maintaining NPO status.
- Recording pre-procedure vital signs.
- Providing emotional support for the client; this procedure can be frightening and uncomfortable.
- Explaining the procedure to the client, emphasizing the importance of lying still.
- Immediately prior to needle insertion asking the client to inhale deeply, exhale completely, and hold the breath at the end of expiration. This immobilizes the chest wall and keeps the diaphragm at its upper level during the procedure (which takes 5 to 10 seconds).

- Applying pressure to the biopsy site after needle removal.
- Turning client onto right side with a pillow under the costal margin to maintain pressure to the site.
- Assisting the physician as indicated.
- Monitoring post-procedure vital signs (q. 15 min. x4, q. 30 min. x4, then q4h), and administering comfort measures after the procedure.

The client should remain immobile on the right side for several hours and be closely observed for signs of hemorrhage, extravasation of fluid from the biopsy site, peritonitis, and pain. Pain in the right upper quadrant and right shoulder area is common. The client should be reassured about this while being encouraged to report any change in pain level. Analgesics, if given, must be nonhepatotoxic and must not affect clotting.

Section II: Nursing Diagnosis

Assessment of the client with hepatic or biliary dysfunction, including evaluation of the client's health history and results of laboratory tests and diagnostic studies, can lead to many possible nursing diagnoses. A list of nursing diagnoses related to hepatic–biliary dysfunction appears in Box 52–2. The potential diagnoses most closely associated with hepatic or biliary dysfunction are discussed in the following sections.

ALTERATIONS IN COMFORT

Pain

Mild or moderate pain may occur in relation to hepatomegaly or splenomegaly associated with hepatitis, hepatic abscess, or infectious mononucleosis. Moderate pain may accompany late cirrhosis and chronic hepatitis. With cancer of the liver, whether the liver is a primary or a metastatic site, pain becomes severe and intractable. Severe, colicky pain in the right upper quadrant is common with cholelithiasis or cholecystitis.

Pruritus

Regardless of whether icterus is prehepatic or hepatic, pruritus will be associated with the jaundice. The client may scratch the skin until it bleeds. The condition may be intensified by damp clothing or bedding caused by perspiration or by poor ventilation.

POTENTIAL FOR IMPAIRMENT OF SKIN INTEGRITY

If pruritus is severe and the client scratches frequently, skin integrity may be broken. In cirrhosis and cancer of

the liver, edema and negative nitrogen balance cause the skin to be susceptible to breakdown. If the client is not turned every hour or two, decubitus ulcers can form within 12 to 24 hours.

SEXUAL DYSFUNCTION AND DISTURBANCES IN SELF-CONCEPT

Disturbances in self-concept may be related to body image alteration and role performance. Softening of the skin, loss of body hair, or gynecomastia may be related to impaired estrogen detoxification. In men, these feminizing changes disturb the client's sense of masculinity. Ascites and icterus further affect self image. Complications associated with severe disease such as cancer or cirrhosis—for example, ascites and pleural effusion—may necessitate the client's changing occupation or retiring. Loss of occupational role can severely damage self-esteem.

Sexual dysfunction may also accompany impairment of estrogen detoxification. Loss of libido may occur in both sexes, and male clients may become impotent. The client may be hesitant to discuss these matters with health care professionals.

ALTERATION IN THOUGHT PROCESSES

Ammonia toxicity is related to the inability of the compromised hepatic cells to convert ammonia to urea for excretion in the urine. The ammonia interferes with brain metabolism, leading to alterations of mentation ranging from slight confusion to coma. Initially, clients may be somewhat confused or disoriented—unable, for example, to remember their names or where they are. Asterixis may also be apparent. Clients may then progress through lethargy to combativeness and abusiveness before lapsing into coma.

Gastrointestinal hemorrhage further increases serum ammonia levels owing to bacterial action on blood in the gut. Wernicke-Korsakoff syndrome, characterized by confusion, disorientation, and amnesia with confabulation, is sometimes seen in alcoholics. The syndrome is thought to be related to thiamine deficiency.

ALTERATION IN NUTRITION

Hepatic dysfunction is associated with impaired metabolism of proteins, fats, carbohydrates, and vitamins. Weight loss, fatigue, negative nitrogen balance, vitamin B deficiency, and deficiencies of fat-soluble vitamins A, D, E, and K are common. The client should consume a balanced diet high in carbohydrates, vitamins, and (unless ammonia toxicity is present) proteins. Abdominal pressure from ascites may cause a constant feeling of fullness as well as flatulence or constipation. These conditions may also diminish appetite, further depleting nutritional status.

In cholelithiasis or cholestasis, a low-fat diet should be consumed because fat metabolism is reduced by disturbances in biliary function. Deficiency of vitamin K may also accompany these disorders.

IMPAIRMENT OF GAS EXCHANGE

Several conditions related to hepatic and biliary disease impair exchange of oxygen and carbon dioxide. Retention of sodium and water is associated with pleural effusion and ascites. Ascites exerts pressure on the diaphragm, interfering with inspiration. Inadequate oxygenation of body tissue related to erythrocytopenia also impairs gas exchange.

ALTERATIONS IN FLUID VOLUME

Alterations in fluid volume may be either deficits or overloads. For example, when the compromised liver can no longer detoxify ADH and aldosterone, retention of sodium and water contributes to circulatory congestion and hypertension. Conversely, fluid volume deficit can be related to hemorrhage of esophageal varices (leading to shock) or to overuse of diuretics. If plasma colloidal osmotic pressure is reduced because of hypoalbuminemia, fluid extravasation into the interstitial space will cause edema despite intravascular dehydration. In this instance, diuretics alone will be ineffective in reducing edema and will, moreover, worsen dehydration.

> ### Box 52–2 Nursing Diagnoses Commonly Related to Hepatic–Biliary Dysfunction
>
> **Diagnoses Directly Related to Hepatic–Biliary Dysfunction**
>
> *Comfort, alteration in,* related to pain
>
> *Comfort, alteration in,* related to pruritus
>
> *Self concept, disturbance in,* related to body image or role performance
>
> *Sexual dysfunction*
>
> *Skin integrity, impairment of, potential*
>
> *Thought processes, alterations in*
>
> *Nutrition, alterations in: less than body requirements*
>
> *Gas exchange, impaired*
>
> *Fluid volume, alterations in*
>
> *Tissue perfusion, alterations in, gastrointestinal*
>
> **Additional Potential Nursing Diagnoses**
>
> *Urinary elimination, alteration in patterns of,* related to increase (diuretics) or decrease (owing to impaired detoxification of ADH and aldosterone)
>
> *Self-care deficit* related to severe hepatic dysfunction or hepatic coma
>
> *Knowledge deficit* related to surgical procedures, diet, lifestyle changes
>
> *Grieving, anticipatory*
>
> *Bowel elimination, alteration in*
>
> *Sensory perceptual alterations* related to ammonia toxicity or peripheral neuropathy
>
> *Injury, potential for,* related to ammonia toxicity, bleeding tendency

ALTERATIONS IN TISSUE PERFUSION

Increased cardiac output associated with hypertension is related to fluid volume alterations discussed above. Erythrocytopenia can lead to increased cardiac output as the heart attempts to compensate for tissue oxygen needs.

Section III: Planning and Implementation

Nursing diagnoses and related planning, implementation, and evaluation for the client with dysfunction of the hepatic–biliary system are presented in a sample nursing care plan (Table 52–3). They are also discussed in this section and the following one in terms of objectives of care.

Table 52–3   Sample Nursing Care Plan for Clients With Hepatic–Biliary Dysfunction

Nursing Diagnosis	Client Care Goals	Plan/Nursing Implementation	Expected Outcome
Comfort, alteration in, related to pruritus.	Maintain comfort. Reduce or eliminate jaundice and pruritus. State cause of pruritus.	Be sure itching is not related to allergy; rest; good diet; ventilation; cotton clothing; change wet sheets; distraction; no alkaline soaps; infrequent baths; whirlpools; emollients; keep nails short; have client wear gloves to decrease breaking skin integrity from scratching; diphenhydramine as ordered; teach about pruritus.	Performs ADL without scratching; rests comfortably without scratching; relief from itching; describes cause of pruritus.
Comfort, alteration in, related to pain.	Ambulate without undue discomfort; rest comfortably.	Avoid hepatotoxic drugs; use those broken down and excreted by kidney; Brompton's cocktail or morphine infusion drip for intractable cancer pain; meperidine, nitroglycerin, or phenobarbital for cholelithiasis pain; nursing comfort measures.	Performs ADL without undue pain; rests comfortably without severe pain; relief from pain.
Skin integrity, impairment of: potential.	Maintain skin integrity. Understand need for eating diet high in protein.	Teach about and provide high protein diet; relieve itching; turn every one to two hours; relieve pressure on edematous areas with positioning; prevent infection with good skin care.	Normal skin integrity; evidence client is eating high protein diet.
Self-concept, disturbance in: related to altered body image and sexual dysfunction.	Accept body image changes.	Instruct about causes of body changes; allow client to ventilate feelings; encourage family support.	Describes causes of body changes; discusses feelings openly.
Thought processes, alteration in.	Maintain satisfactory thought processes.	Assess for change in mental status; have client write name daily, pump BP cuff to note severity of asterixis; safety measures; potassium to improve cerebral metabolism of ammonia; tap water enemas to decrease blood in intestines from bleeding varices; assess for fetor hepaticus; prevent swallowing of blood from esophageal varices; rest; neomycin to decrease intestinal bacteria; lactulose to increase diffusability and excretion of ammonia.	Writes name daily without changes; states name, place, date correctly; absence of asterixis.
Nutrition, alteration in: less than body requirements.	Ingest a well-balanced diet.	High potassium diet; low salt diet; increased carbohydrate and protein diet; increase appetite: oral hygiene, antiemetics, fresh air; decrease fat intake; correct vitamin deficiencies.	Client will consume a well-balanced diet; a correction of nutritional deficiencies will be observed. Evidence of increased food intake; client lists foods high in potassium and low in salt.
Gas exchange, impaired.	Maintain adequate O_2/CO_2 exchange with minimal breathing difficulties.	Careful positioning, diuretics, and albumin to reduce edema and decrease pressure of ascites on diaphragm; O_2 as needed; assist with paracentesis; increased iron	Client will perform ADL without use of O_2; client will not have bluish tint to lips; normal hemoglobin values; increased energy

Nursing Diagnosis	Client Care Goals	Plan/Nursing Implementation	Expected Outcome
		intake; blood transfusions, vitamin K as ordered.	shown by resuming knitting, reading, or other activities of interest.
Fluid volume, alteration in.	Maintain normal fluid volume balance; minimal edema.	Daily weights; assess skin turgor; careful recording of I and O; use of aldosterone antagonists as ordered to decrease sodium and water retention; careful administration of diuretics and albumin.	Good skin turgor; decreased circumference of extremities; I and O measurement that indicates correction of fluid volume alteration.
Tissue perfusion, alteration in.	Maintain adequate tissue perfusion.	Correct RBC value with transfusion, iron, vitamins K and B_{12}; care related to edema and portal hypertension as above.	Blood pressure of no more than 140/80; hemoglobin values within normal limits; prothrombin time within normal limits.

PROMOTING COMFORT

For the client with hepatic—biliary dysfunction, alterations in comfort are likely to be associated with pain or pruritus.

Pain Relief

Mild to moderate pain associated with various disorders may be controlled with nonnarcotic, nonaspirin analgesics. Aspirin should not be administered because of its anticoagulant properties. Clients with hepatic dysfunction are likely to have coagulation abnormalities related to poor absorption of vitamin K. Drugs causing hepatic damage should also be avoided (see Box 52–1); the drugs of choice are those excreted by the kidneys.

For the severe, intractable pain associated with cancer of the liver, Brompton's cocktail may be prescribed because it relieves pain without clouding the mind. Brompton's cocktail is an elixir of morphine, cocaine, alcohol, chloroform water, flavoring syrup, and a phenothiazine antiemetic. In England, heroin is substituted for morphine. Effective alterations in Brompton's cocktail used experimentally in North America include methadone as a substitute for morphine and a dextroamphetamine as a substitute for cocaine.

For pain associated with cholelithiasis, meperidine is usually the drug of choice. Morphine is rarely administered, since most physicians believe it exacerbates spasms of the sphincter of Oddi, increasing pain. Nitroglycerin or phenobarbital may promote comfort by relaxing smooth muscle.

Nursing measures such as giving a backrub, assisting the client in changing position, providing distraction, and offering emotional support may supplement analgesic medication.

Pruritus Relief

The pruritus associated with icterus can be extremely upsetting to the client. It is important to rule out any pos-

sibility that the condition is related to an allergy. Measures to alleviate itching include dry clothing and bedding, emollients, a well-balanced diet, and distraction. Alkaline soaps should be avoided, and baths are given only every two or three days, if possible. Whirlpool baths are preferred. Diphenhydramine hydrochloride (Benadryl) is often prescribed for clients with jaundice because of its sedative and antipruritic effects; this drug is excreted by the kidney and thus is not hepatotoxic. Nursing care of the client with pruritus is discussed in Unit 13.

MAINTAINING AND IMPROVING SKIN INTEGRITY

Several nursing interventions are crucial to maintenance of skin integrity. Relieving pruritus should receive high priority. Frequent turning and repositioning to relieve pressure on edematous areas prevents formation of decubitus ulcers. A low-sodium diet, fluid restriction, and diuretic therapy may be prescribed to induce diuresis and lessen peripheral and abdominal edema. Care of the client with ascites and edema will be further discussed in later sections, but it is important to remember that decubitus ulcers can form in 12 to 24 hours if turning and repositioning are not done conscientiously every 1 or 2 hours.

Preventing infection presents a challenge, because the client's reticuloendothelial system is severely compromised. Careful handwashing is essential. It is recommended that sterile technique be maintained during dressing changes for surgical wounds and at catheter sites.

Nutritional measures may be used to promote healing and improvement of skin integrity. See the discussion under Improvement of Nutritional Intake.

IMPROVING SELF-CONCEPT AND SEXUAL FUNCTION

Jaundice that accompanies cholelithiasis is often reversible. Bodily changes associated with hepatic disorders often are not. A client may react to perceived unattractiveness by hiding under the bed covers, refusing to leave the room, avoiding other clients, or keeping the curtains drawn around the bed. Remarks such as "I look like I'm six months pregnant" or "I look like a banana" are clues to diminished self-esteem.

Helping the client toward an improved self-image is not easy, but the nurse who has gained the client's confidence can promote acceptance of body changes. Explaining the conditions underlying icterus, ascites, gynecomastia, decreased libido, impotence, and other body changes to client and significant others is usually helpful. Giving the client opportunity to express feelings is essential. Suggestions about clothing colors that tone down yellow skin or clothing styles that disguise a protruding abdomen are appreciated by the client both for their practical value and as expressions of the nurse's acceptance and concern. Clients who must be isolated because of hepatitis often feel rejected; care givers should be encouraged to visit the client often. Touching the client is especially helpful.

Advanced hepatic disease is frequently accompanied by physical and libidinal changes in sexual function. Counseling may be needed to help client and sexual partner adjust to these changes.

MAINTAINING AND IMPROVING THOUGHT PROCESSES

Evaluating the client's mental status, promoting safety, and monitoring for decreasing ammonia toxicity are nursing responsibilities. Mentation may be monitored by assessing the client's orientation to person, place, and time. One convenient technique for detecting changes in ammonia toxicity levels is having the client write his or her name daily and comparing the signatures. Severity of asterixis may be evaluated by pumping up a blood pressure cuff on the client's arm; the more rapidly the hand clenches and unclenches, the higher the serum level of ammonia. The client's breath should be assessed for fetor hepaticus, which is similar to the odor of acetone or old wine.

As the person who administers most medications, the nurse must be alert to the possibility that a hepatotoxic drug or dosage has been inadvertently prescribed. (See Box 52–1.) Detoxification capacity declines in older individuals, even under normal conditions; this impairment will be worsened in hepatic disease.

Safety measures such as padded siderails or restraints may be necessary to protect clients who are confused or combative as a result of hepatic encephalopathy. The client must be reminded not to get out of bed unassisted. Activities of daily living should be supervised, as should smoking.

REDUCING AMMONIA LEVELS

Various therapeutic measures may be prescribed to decrease serum ammonia levels. Intravenous administration of glucose may provide protein-conserving carbohydrates. Rest

can decrease release of ammonia associated with muscle contraction.

Pharmacologic measures may also be employed. Potassium is sometimes given to improve cerebral metabolism of ammonia. Antibiotics such as neomycin may be administered orally or by enema to reduce the number of ammonia-synthesizing bacteria in the gut. Since neomycin is poorly absorbed from the intestine, its bactericidal action in the intestine is prolonged; however, this antibiotic may cause ototoxicity or nephrotoxicity if administered for more than six days (Malseed, 1982).

Lactulose (Cephulac, Duphalac) may be given orally or by nasogastric tube. This drug acts by acidifying the colon so ammonia couples with hydrogen ions and is excreted in the feces. Improvement may be seen within 24 hours, with serum ammonia levels being reduced by 25%–50% in most clients. Diarrhea is common with lactulose therapy, so electrolyte levels must be monitored. In some cases, hemodialysis may be necessary to reduce serum ammonia levels.

The nurse should routinely check stools for occult blood and monitor vital signs for changes that might indicate gastrointestinal hemorrhage. Bacterial action on blood in the gut may cause ammonia levels to rise. If esophageal varices are bleeding, tap water enemas may be ordered to cleanse the intestines of all contents, including protein-rich blood.

IMPROVING NUTRITIONAL INTAKE

Unless ammonia toxicity is present, the client with hepatic dysfunction should receive a diet high in protein to promote hepatic healing and prevent loss of muscle mass. The diet should be low in salt and high in vitamins, carbohydrates, and calories. If ammonia toxicity is present, low-protein, potassium-rich foods should be provided. The client with biliary dysfunction should reduce the quantity of fats consumed.

Promoting a well-balanced diet with a client who often has no appetite is a challenge. Appetite may be improved by providing oral hygiene and fresh air, minimizing movement, and administering prescribed antiemetics. The nurse can work with the dietitian in providing appetizing meals, perhaps in small frequent feedings supplemented by nourishing snacks. Protein supplements may be used if not contraindicated by ammonia toxicity. It is helpful if the mealtime environment is pleasant and free of unpleasant odors. Food preferences elicited in the nursing history should be considered. Explaining the rationale for the diet may encourage the client to eat more.

If the client is unable to eat enough to meet caloric needs, feeding via nasogastric tube or total parenteral nutrition may be prescribed.

IMPROVING GAS EXCHANGE

Several measures may be prescribed to improve oxygenation. If dyspnea occurs at rest or upon exertion, oxygen therapy may be initiated. Oral iron supplements or a transfusion of packed red cells may be given to improve hemoglobin and hematocrit levels. Intramuscular injections of vitamin K_1 (AquaMEPHYTON) improve clotting. Diuretic therapy or administration of albumin may be prescribed to reduce pleural effusion, which hinders gas exchange, or to decrease ascites, which exerts pressure on the diaphragm.

The nurse may be called upon to assist with paracentesis (Figure 52–8) to remove ascitic fluid from the abdomen. The client is assisted to a sitting position. The abdomen is cleansed with an antiseptic solution and draped. Local anesthesia is administered, and a trochar is inserted and tubing attached. Fluid drains via gravity into a sterile container. Up to 2 L of fluid may be removed; removal of a larger quantity may lead to shock. The nurse documents the amount and color of ascitic fluid removed before sending a sample of the fluid for laboratory evaluation. Paracentesis may be repeated periodically as fluid reaccumulates.

Ascites may also be controlled by a LeVeen or Denver shunt procedure; these are discussed in Chapter 54.

RESTORING NORMAL FLUID VOLUME

Edema related to hepatic dysfunction is misleading because vascular dehydration frequently accompanies it. (See Chapter 51.) Diuretic therapy alone can worsen dehydration. Diuretics should not be overused and should be given in conjunction with albumin. Aldosterone antagonists are the diuretics of choice since edema is related to inadequate detoxification of aldosterone. Intake-output records should be maintained and electrolyte values and skin turgor assessed. The client should be weighed and girth measured daily to assess fluid volume status; weight loss should not exceed half a pound (0.23 kg) a day. Greater losses may result in a shift of fluids into the abdominal cavity, may promote electrolyte imbalance, and may precipitate hepatic encephalopathy.

In the client with ascites, accumulated fluid may stretch the skin so tightly that it tears. The client should be urged to avoid restrictive clothing, take good care of the skin, and change positions frequently. Place a pillow under the costal margin for support if the client is lying on his or her side.

Support hose should be worn and the limbs elevated frequently to minimize peripheral edema. When seated clients should be warned to support their legs, not to cross them or let them dangle.

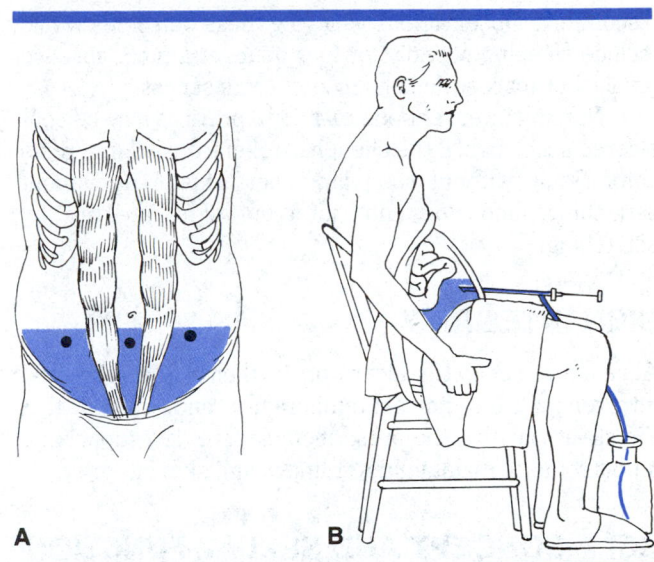

Figure 52–8

Paracentesis in a client with ascites. **A.** The preferred sites for trocar insertion are indicated to avoid injury to the deep inferior epigastric vessels. **B.** Assist the client to a comfortable seated position with the chest and abdomen draped. In this position the intestines will float away from the paracentesis site.

A fluid deficit may occur, for example, during episodes of variceal hemorrhage. Lost blood must be replaced and vital signs closely monitored. Nursing care for the client with variceal bleeding is discussed in Chapter 53.

IMPROVING TISSUE PERFUSION

Tissue perfusion may be improved by correcting anemia; iron supplements, vitamins B_{12} and K, and blood transfusions may be administered. When hemoglobin and hematocrit values are restored to normal levels, the heart pumps blood throughout the body more efficiently. Ecchymoses and gingival hemorrhage may indicate vitamin K deficiency. If the client has coagulation disorders, injections—especially intramuscular injections—should be avoided whenever possible, and pressure should be applied after any injection is given. Decreasing fluid overload, if present, will improve cardiac output.

Section IV: Evaluation

Expected outcomes for the client with hepatic–biliary dysfunction are presented in the sample nursing care plan (Table 52–3). The discussion below supplements the data in the table. If data collected do not substantiate these expected outcomes, nursing plans must be revised.

COMFORT

Nursing interventions related to pain are successful when the client is resting comfortably without severe pain and can perform activities of daily living (ADL) without undue discomfort. Observations verifying these outcomes would include sleeping soundly for four hours at a time, absence of facial grimaces, and absence of restlessness.

Nursing interventions related to pruritus may be considered successful if the client has relief from itching, rests comfortably without scratching, performs ADL without scratching, and does not interrupt skin integrity by scratching.

SKIN INTEGRITY

Absence of decubitus ulcers or erythema at surgical and intravenous sites, normal temperature, and evidence that the client is eating the prescribed diet are data supporting an outcome of maintaining or improving skin integrity.

SELF-CONCEPT AND SEXUAL FUNCTION

When a client can discuss the causes of body changes and openly discuss feelings about sexual dysfunction, body image, and role changes, nursing interventions have helped attain the expected outcomes. Additional mental health counseling may be needed before this goal can be attained.

THOUGHT PROCESSES

Orientation to person, place, and time, absence of asterixis, and the ability to write one's name the same way on sequential days are evidence that supports maintenance of thought processes. If asterixis develops or changes in handwriting are noted, the nurse may need to modify plans and interventions.

NUTRITION

Expected outcomes for improving nutritional status and knowledge of nutrition include the ability to list foods high in protein and potassium and low in salt and fats, evidence of increasing intake of well-balanced foods, and signs that nutritional deficiencies are being corrected. This will be a slow process, but if a client is eating half the food on the tray instead of nothing, improvement has been shown. Consulting with the client to make a list of favorite foods and seeing that those foods are served may improve consumption. Cultural and ethnic preferences should be considered in planning the diet.

GAS EXCHANGE

One expected outcome might be the client's ability to ambulate without oxygen supplementation. Another is return of the hemoglobin level to normal. Others might be absence of dyspnea on exertion; absence of cyanosis; or increased energy shown by knitting, working a crossword puzzle, or writing a letter. If these data can be observed, the nursing plan may be considered successful.

FLUID VOLUME

Expected outcomes related to fluid volume include good skin turgor, decreased circumference of edematous extremities or abdominal girth, and intake and output measurements indicative of correction of a fluid volume alteration. Correction of fluid volume alterations may take a long time, and several plans and revisions may be required.

TISSUE PERFUSION

A blood pressure no greater than 140/80 mm Hg and normal hemoglobin and prothrombin time are indications of adequate tissue perfusion. Hemoglobin and hematocrit values and blood pressure readings may be deceiving if vascular dehydration is present.

Chapter Highlights

When interviewing the client to assess for hepatic or biliary dysfunction, ask about bowel habits, yellowing or itching of the skin, swelling of the ankles, diet patterns, drinking habits, and exposure to hepatitis or toxic chemicals.

In the client with liver dysfunction, hemoglobin, hematocrit, albumin, and serum lipid values are below normal; prothrombin time, LDH, SGOT, SGPT, GGT, WBC, indirect bilirubin, serum ammonia, and gamma globulin levels are elevated.

In the client with biliary dysfunction, hemoglobin, hematocrit, and urinary and fecal urobilinogen values are below normal; prothrombin time, alkaline phosphatase, serum lipids, and direct bilirubin values are elevated.

Diagnostic studies used for clients with known or suspected hepatic or biliary dysfunction include ultrasound, radionuclide scanning, dye clearance studies, oral cholecystography, intravenous cholangiography, endoscopic retrograde cholangiopancreatography (ERCP), percutaneous transhepatic cholangiography (PTHC), and T-tube and operative cholangiography.

For the client with alteration in comfort related to pruritus, promoting comfort includes ruling out allergy, encouraging rest and a well-balanced diet, providing ventilation and dry clothing and linen, avoiding frequent baths and alkaline soaps, applying emollients, and keeping fingernails short.

Nursing measures related to relief of pain for the client with hepatic–biliary dysfunction include administering analgesics appropriate to the source and severity of pain, avoiding hepatotoxic analgesics, and providing nursing comfort measures.

Nursing measures related to maintenance of skin integrity include providing a high-protein diet (unless ammonia toxicity is present), relieving pruritus, repositioning and turning the client with edema every one to two hours, and providing good skin care.

Helping the client with hepatic or biliary disease maintain satisfactory mentation involves assessing for changes in mental status; instituting safety measures; providing a low-protein diet; preventing aspiration of blood from variceal hemorrhage; giving tap water or neomycin enemas; and administering potassium, neomycin, or lactulose as prescribed.

Nursing measures to overcome nutritional deficiencies include encouraging intake of a well-balanced diet high in potassium, vitamins, carbohydrates, and proteins (if appropriate), and low in sodium.

Promoting adequate O_2/CO_2 exchange in the client with hepatic or biliary dysfunction involves proper positioning for adequate expansion of the diaphragm; administering diuretics and albumin to correct edema; assisting with paracentesis; and administering iron, vitamin K, and blood transfusions as ordered.

Nursing measures to promote normalizing of fluid volume include administering albumin and diuretics, weighing the client and measuring abdominal girth daily, recording intake and output, and monitoring skin turgor and possible hemorrhage of esophageal varices.

Nursing measures to promote adequate tissue perfusion in clients with hepatic and biliary disorders include correction of fluid overload by administering diuretics as ordered and correcting low hemoglobin and hematocrit values by administering iron, vitamins K and B_{12}, and transfusions of packed red cells as prescribed.

Bibliography

Byrne CJ et al: *Laboratory Tests: Implications for Nursing Care.* Menlo Park, CA: Addison-Wesley, 1981.

Hawks JEH: Alcoholism: An overview. *Plast Surg Nurs* 1983; 3:49–52.

Malseed RT: *Pharmacology: Drug Therapy and Nursing Considerations.* Philadelphia: Lippincott, 1982.

Pagana KD, Pagana TJ: *Diagnostic Testing and Nursing Implications.* St. Louis, MO: Mosby, 1982.

Thompson JM, Bowers AC: *Clinical Manual of Health Assessment.* St. Louis, MO: Mosby, 1980.

Suggested Readings

Gannon RB, Pickett K: Jaundice. *Am J Nurs* 1983; 83(3):404–407. Comprehensive discussion of jaundice—its causes and phases—and nursing care. Discussion of assessment thoroughly covers laboratory tests and physiological basis for pathological changes.

Gever LN: Lactulose: A crucial element in treating hepatic encephalopathy. *Nurs 82* 1982; 12(8):76–78. Concise description of what lactulose is, why it is given, how it is administered, and what side effects it causes.

Goldenberg DA: Management of bleeding esophageal varices. *Crit Care Q* 1982; 5(2):33–46. In-depth discussion of treatments. Contains diagrams, photographs, and 47 references.

King DE: How to give your portal hypertension patients a fighting chance. *RN,* July 1983: 31–37. Full coverage of causes and effects of portal hypertension, assessment techniques, preoperative history taking and data evaluation, surgical procedures, and signs and symptoms of postoperative complications.

Resources

ORGANIZATIONS AND SELF-HELP GROUPS

American Digestive Disease Society
(Includes gallbladder disease; see Resources in Chapter 47.)

American Liver Foundation
30 Sunrise Terrace
Cedar Grove, NJ 07009
Phone: (201) 857-2626
This volunteer-run agency funds research education and training programs for the public and professionals and programs for detecting and treating liver disease.

For clients with cancer refer to the resources list at the end of Chapter 12.

For clients exposed to hepatotoxic substances refer to the resources list at the end of Chapter 13.

For alcoholic clients refer to the resources list at the end of Chapter 10.

HEALTH EDUCATION MATERIALS

Krames Communications
312 90th St.
Daly City, CA 94015
   This organization provides the following client education materials:

The Gall Bladder Book, in English or Spanish, $ .90

Abdominal Sonogram, in English or Spanish, $ .35

Oral Cholecystogram, in English or Spanish, $ .35

Chapter 53

Specific Disorders of the Hepatic–Biliary System

Jane Hokanson Hawks

Objectives

When you have finished studying this chapter, you should be able to:

Describe nursing interventions for clients with congenital disorders of the hepatic–biliary system.

Identify nursing, medical, and pharmacological measures for clients with cirrhosis.

Compare and contrast type A; type B; type non-A, non-B; toxic; drug-induced; and chronic active forms of hepatitis.

Describe the etiology and treatment of hepatic abscess.

Discuss risk factors, signs and symptoms, and pharmacological and nursing management of cholecystitis and cholelithiasis.

Explain the circumstances associated with carcinoma of the hepatic–biliary system and interventions for these clients.

Identify types of hepatic–biliary system trauma and nursing care for the traumatized client.

Specific disorders of the hepatic–biliary system include some life-threatening illnesses with long-term implications, for example, cirrhosis. Viral hepatitis, a disease with increasing incidence, has assumed considerable importance in recent years, and health care providers may themselves be at increased risk of contracting this disease. Disorders of the hepatic–biliary system may be generally classified as congenital, multifactorial in origin, infectious, neoplastic and obstructive, and traumatic.

Section I: Congenital Disorders

Congenital disorders of the hepatic and biliary system are present from birth, although they may not be visibly apparent or symptomatic until adulthood. The disorders to be discussed in this section include Gilbert's syndrome, Dubin–Johnson syndrome, Rotor's syndrome, and hepatolenticular degeneration (Wilson's disease). All are transferred by genetic inheritance.

Persons with congenital disorders are seen rarely in adult health nursing; most persons with uncorrectable disorders do not survive to adulthood. As corrective techniques and health care measures improve, however, more such persons are living beyond childhood. They may seek medical care when symptoms of their disorder first appear or when exacerbations occur.

GILBERT'S SYNDROME

Gilbert's syndrome is a familial disorder characterized by a deficiency of glucuronyl transferase, an enzyme necessary for conjugation of bilirubin. (See Chapter 51.) Due to the enzyme insufficiency, serum levels of unconjugated bilirubin rise, with consequent hyperbilirubinemia and icterus

(Sherlock, 1981). No pathologic changes occur in the liver with this disorder, so liver function studies will yield normal results except for the elevated bilirubin levels. There is no hemolysis or obstruction.

DUBIN–JOHNSON SYNDROME

Dubin–Johnson syndrome is chronic idiopathic icterus characterized by exacerbations and remissions. A brown, coarsely granular pigment is found in the hepatic cells.

ROTOR'S SYNDROME

Rotor's syndrome is a genetically transferred chronic conjugated hyperbilirubinemia. Pigmentation of the hepatic cells does not occur with this disorder.

HEPATOLENTICULAR DEGENERATION

Hepatolenticular degeneration, also known as Wilson's disease, is a rare (1 in 200,000) disorder of varied symptoms related to a disturbance of copper metabolism. It is transmitted by autosomal recessive inheritance.

Although normal amounts of copper are consumed, excess copper is retained in the liver, perhaps due to inability to excrete it in the bile. The normal liver stores between 18 and 45 μg of copper per gram of dry weight. When hepatic concentration of copper reaches 500 to 2000 μg per gram, necrosis of hepatic cells begins. Copper is released into the serum and deposited in other tissues, particularly the brain, cornea, and kidneys. This process takes years.

Clinical Manifestations

Clinical manifestations usually begin to appear between ages 6 and 20 but may appear as late as age 40. A variety

of symptoms and signs may occur, including hemolytic anemia, neurologic disease, psychiatric disorders, renal disease, and skeletal abnormalities, in addition to the usual symptoms and signs of hepatic dysfunction. The characteristic diagnostic indications of hepatolenticular degeneration are signs of basal ganglion disease accompanied by the **Kayser–Fleischer** ring, a rusty-brown corneal accumulation of copper. These signs are not apparent in the early stages of the disease, however.

The course of the disease varies among individuals. An asymptomatic period may follow the acute hepatic stage. Once the neurologic stage begins, the disease is progressive; if not treated, Wilson's disease is usually fatal. Yet in 40% of affected persons, liver disease is not recognized until the client has entered the neurologic stage. Wilson's disease should be considered as a possible diagnosis in any person over 30 who has chronic hepatitis.

Therapeutic Measures

Wilson's disease is treated by administering sulfurated potash to prevent further accumulation of copper and administering the copper-chelating agent D-penicillamine to mobilize copper from body tissues and increase renal excretion. Potash is generally taken for 6 to 12 months; chelation therapy is continued for life.

Specific Nursing Measures

In addition to assessment for hepatic and neurologic symptoms, nursing care involves client and family education, emotional support, and encouragement of genetic counseling.

Section II: Disorders of Multifactorial Origin

Disorders of multifactorial origin are those for which no single, specific etiologic agent has been identified. For the hepatic–biliary system, cirrhosis is the major disease process of multifactorial origin.

CIRRHOSIS

Cirrhosis is a chronic process in which the normal configuration of liver lobules is disrupted. (See Figures 51–5A and B.) Cell death occurs, and regeneration is associated with scarring. Nodular cells formed during regeneration distort the morphology of the liver and obstruct hepatic flow of blood and lymph. Eventually, cirrhosis leads to hepatic failure and portal hypertension.

Cirrhosis may be classified as: (1) Laennec's cirrhosis,

(2) biliary cirrhosis, or (3) postnecrotic cirrhosis. Laennec's cirrhosis is usually caused by chronic alcohol abuse. Biliary cirrhosis is related to prolonged obstructive jaundice or to an infection that ascends from the gallbladder to the small bile ducts by way of the hepatic duct. Postnecrotic cirrhosis is related to formation of scar tissue following hepatitis or hepatic abscess.

Clinical Manifestations

Cirrhosis is often but not invariably preceded by fatty infiltration of the liver (**steatosis**). Either fatty liver or cirrhosis may be related to nutritional disorders, biliary obstruction, hepatotoxicity, iron storage disorders, and ethanol ingestion (Groer and Shekleton, 1983). Histologic

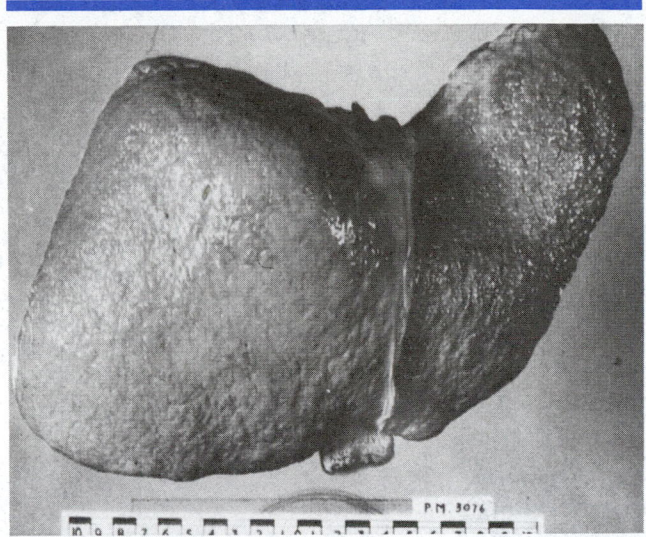

Figure 53–1

Cirrhotic liver with hobnail appearance.

examination of the liver reveals fatty infiltration, cellular necrosis, and disruption of the lobes. Gross inspection reveals a "hobnail" appearance; the hepatic surface is often stippled and nodular, somewhat like a football (Figure 53–1). Other pathophysiological changes are consistent with those discussed in Chapter 51.

Portal hypertension results in compensatory development of collateral blood vessels in the esophagus. These vessels, called esophageal varices, dilate as portal hypertension increases. Because such vessels are inadequate to accommodate the increased blood flow, hemorrhage may occur.

The client has a characteristic appearance. The skin is orange-yellow, the eyes are sunken, and the facial bones are prominent. The limbs are emaciated, whereas the abdomen is enlarged due to ascites.

Therapeutic Measures

Therapeutic measures employed in treatment of cirrhosis generally include those discussed in Chapter 52, including analgesic, antiemetic, and diuretic therapies; nutritional interventions; and treatments directed at controlling variceal hemorrhage and ascites. Pharmacological therapies commonly employed in cirrhosis are listed in Box 53–1.

Esophageal variceal hemorrhage may be controlled temporarily by administering infusions of vasopressin (Pitressin) to promote diffuse arterial vasoconstriction and to lower portal pressure by constricting the splanchnic arterial bed. The infusion may be given systemically or via the superior mesenteric artery. Either method provides only temporary control and is associated with complications, including systemic arterial hypertension and coronary vasoconstriction possibly leading to myocardial infarction.

If vasopressin administration is unsuccessful, gastric lavage with ice-cold saline, use of the Minnesota tube or Sengstaken–Blakemore tube, or portal-systemic shunting may be implemented to control bleeding temporarily. A Sengstaken–Blakemore tube has three lumens: one suctions gastric contents, one inflates a gastric balloon, and one inflates an esophageal balloon (Figure 53–2A). The Minnesota tube has a fourth lumen used to aspirate esophageal contents (Figure 53–2B). Shunts are discussed in Chapter 54.

Injection sclerotherapy, an alternative long-term control measure, may be performed as a bedside procedure with the client sedated with diazepam (Valium) or meperidine hydrochloride (Demerol). Sclerosing solutions are injected directly into the bleeding varices by means of fiberoptic endoscopy. Various solutions are used; an example is 5% sodium morrhuate, alone or with bovine thrombin. Complications include chest pain, transient fever, ulceration of the injection sites, and formation of strictures. Most are self-resolving; strictures may be treated by dilatation. Perforation, a major complication, is rare, since the instruments used are flexible. If perforation does occur, it is treated by keeping the client NPO, suctioning gastric contents, and administering antibiotic therapy; surgery is seldom required.

Specific Nursing Measures

Nursing care for the client with cirrhosis generally requires interventions for all the nursing diagnoses identified in Chapter 52. It is important to emphasize that clients with cirrhosis must abstain from alcohol. They are plagued with jaundice and associated pruritus, ammonia toxicity, ascites, edema, and hemorrhagic tendencies, especially in the gastrointestinal tract. Laboratory test findings will be consistent with the discussion in the previous chapter. Because cirrhosis is a chronic condition, most nursing interventions will be related to the client's comfort. Teaching clients and the public about the affects of alcohol may have preventive benefits. A case study of a client with cirrhosis is presented at the end of this chapter.

Nursing measures for clients with esophageal hemorrhage include explaining treatments to the client and assessing frequently to determine whether hemorrhage

Box 53–1	**Pharmacological Agents Commonly Used in Treatment of Cirrhosis**
Albumin	Lactulose
Aldosterone antagonist diuretics	Neomycin
Anticholinergics	Potassium
Antiemetics	Propranolol (Inderal)
Diphenhydramine (Benadryl)	Vitamin K
Emollients	

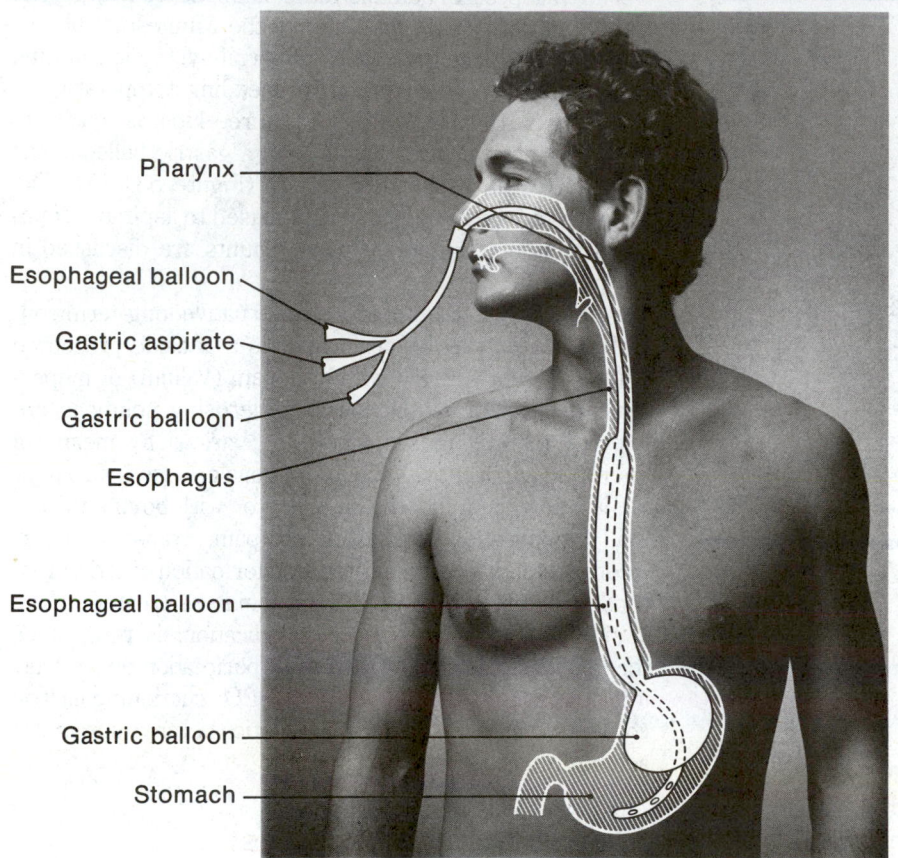

Pharynx

Esophageal balloon

Gastric aspirate

Gastric balloon

Esophagus

Esophageal balloon

Gastric balloon

Stomach

A

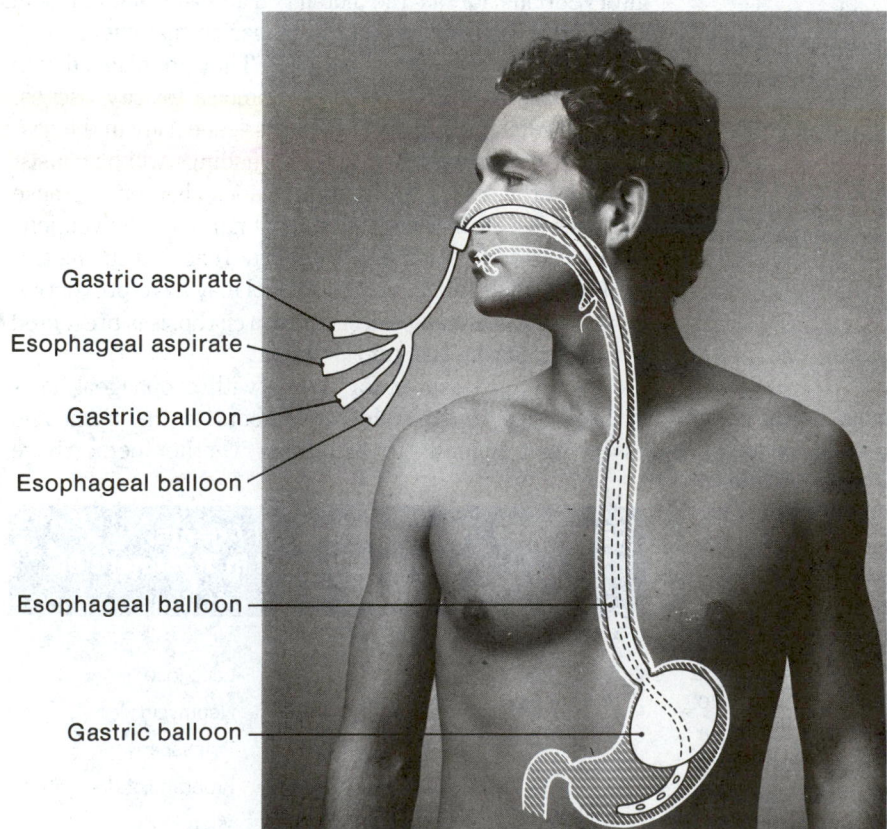

Gastric aspirate

Esophageal aspirate

Gastric balloon

Esophageal balloon

Esophageal balloon

Gastric balloon

B

Figure 53–2

A. Triple-lumen esophageal-naso-gastric (Sengstaken–Blakemore) tube. **B.** Four-lumen (Minnesota sump) tube.

SOURCE: Swearingen PL: *The Addison-Wesley Photo-Atlas of Nursing Procedures.* Menlo Park, CA: Addison-Wesley, 1984, p. 228.

has ceased. As with any hemorrhage, the nurse is responsible for monitoring blood replacement therapy. Bleeding esophageal varices create a crisis for client and family. Timely explanations of ongoing interventions and anticipated results will help the client cope with panic and fear of death. Providing nursing care in a decisive, supportive manner helps the client regain control and to participate in the therapy. To provide optimum crisis care, the nurse should assess the family support structure and provide information and support to significant others as well as the client.

Section III: Infectious and Inflammatory Disorders

Infectious and inflammatory disorders of the hepatic–biliary system can involve the liver or the gallbladder. Hepatic infection may be associated with inflammation of hepatic cells, hyperplasia of Kupffer cells, bile stasis, or tissue necrosis. Biliary infections may be associated with dilation of the gallbladder, which will be filled with bile, pus, and blood. Infectious and inflammatory disorders discussed in this section include hepatic abscess, cholecystitis, and five types of hepatitis: viral hepatitis (type A; B; and non-A, non-B), toxic or drug induced hepatitis, and chronic active hepatitis. About 50% of persons with hepatic–biliary dysfunction have one of the infectious disorders.

VIRAL HEPATITIS

Hepatitis is an inflammation of the liver. The viral forms of hepatitis may be classified as type A, type B, or non-A, non-B. The viruses responsible for hepatitis A and B have been identified; the virus or viruses responsible for non-A, non-B hepatitis are not yet known (Table 53–1). Hepatitis A and B are characterized by three stages: prodromal, icteric, and recovery. (Non-A, non-B hepatitis is often not associated with icterus.) The prodromal (preicteric) stage lasts 1 to 3 weeks; the icteric or jaundiced stage lasts 6 to 8 weeks, and the recovery stage may last from 3 to 4 months. The three types of viral hepatitis are discussed separately.

Hepatitis A (Infectious Hepatitis)

Hepatitis A, an infectious hepatitis associated with brief incubation (3 to 5 weeks) and low mortality (1% or less), is known to be caused by an RNA virus. Outbreaks of hepatitis A have occurred in institutional settings in association with poor sanitation and a large population. The virus is found in blood, feces, saliva, and urine of infected individuals, and transmission is usually by the fecal–oral route. Raw shellfish from polluted waters may also carry the virus. The type A virus may be transmitted from person to person or by way of contaminated water or food. Young adults (15 to 29 years), middle-aged adults, and persons living in crowded conditions appear more susceptible to the type A virus. Washing hands after bowel movements

Table 53–1   Comparison of Types of Viral Hepatitis

	Hepatitis A	Hepatitis B	Non-A, Non-B Hepatitis
Cause	Type A virus	Type B virus	Unidentified virus
Incubation period	3–5 weeks	5–25 weeks	2–23 weeks
Carrier	No	Yes	Yes
Chronicity	No	Yes	Yes
Type of virus	RNA	DNA	Unknown
Transmission	Feces, blood	Blood and body fluids (semen; vaginal, oral, and nasal secretions; breast milk, CSF)	Blood
Symptoms	May have none. Flulike, headache, fatigue, anorexia, fever, dark urine, jaundice, hepatomegaly, aversion to cigarettes	More severe than hepatitis A. Fever, rash, arthralgia, headache, aversion to cigarettes, hepatomegaly, dark urine, jaundice, fatigue, anorexia	Similar to hepatitis B. Often no jaundice
Prevention	Immune serum globulin after exposure	Hepatitis B immune globulin after exposure; hepatitis B vaccine before exposure	None

and before eating, and environmental sanitation are the most effective means of preventing the spread of hepatitis A.

Clinical Manifestations

Flulike symptoms may occur in the preicteric stage, including headache, fatigue, malaise, anorexia, pruritus, weakness, fever, and aversion to cigarettes. Sometimes, however, the client is asymptomatic. At the end of the preicteric stage, the urine appears mahogany-colored and the stools are acholic. During the second (icteric) stage, the urine remains dark, the stools light. The skin usually appears jaundiced, and the liver and spleen are swollen and tender. Laboratory studies will show elevated white blood count (WBC), SGOT, SGPT, alkaline phosphatase, and indirect bilirubin levels. Serum protein and lipid values will be slightly below normal.

Therapeutic Measures

Therapeutic measures are directed at relieving symptoms. Vitamin K may be prescribed if coagulation abnormalities are found. Frequent high-calorie meals, intravenous fluids, and restricted physical activity may be prescribed.

Anyone who comes in contact with hepatitis A should receive intramuscular administrations of immune serum globulin (ISG) or gamma globulin within 1 week. Gamma globulin or ISG provides immunity for 6 to 8 weeks. The usual dosage is 0.02 mL/kg of body weight. Smaller dosages are sometimes administered prophylactically every 2 to 3 months to persons at high risk—for example, health care personnel who work with many clients with hepatitis.

Specific Nursing Measures

Persons with hepatitis A may often be cared for at home. Hospitalized clients will require interventions for alterations in comfort (pruritus and pain), nutritional intake, and

---

fluid volume; impairment of skin integrity and O_2/CO_2 exchange; and disturbances in self-concept. (See Chapter 51.) In addition to these measures, the client with hepatitis A is placed in enteric isolation. The nurse must wear gloves when in contact with fecal matter, bedpan, or linens soiled with stool. Persons giving care in the home should also wear gloves if contact with feces is possible. Gowns should be worn in any situation where gross soiling occurs. Careful attention to handwashing is essential for clients and for those giving care.

Discharge planning for hospitalized clients includes encouraging the client to get ample rest, ingest a well-balanced diet, drink at least 3000 mL of fluid per day, and avoid alcohol and OTC medications for at least 6 months. These clients should be told they will have a lifetime immunity to hepatitis A virus. There is no chronic carrier state with hepatitis A. The client will not progress to chronic hepatitis or cirrhosis.

Hepatitis B (Serum Hepatitis)

The hepatitis B virus, a DNA virus, usually causes a more serious form of the disease. The incubation period for hepatitis B (also called serum hepatitis or long-incubation hepatitis) is long—5 to 25 weeks, and the mortality rate is 1% to 10% (Gurevich, 1983). Incidence of hepatitis B is higher in populations of individuals who have received blood transfusions, in recreational drug users who may share infected needles or syringes, and in homosexuals. All ages are affected, but young adults appear most susceptible.

The serum from clients with hepatitis B contains three distinct structures—spherical particles, Dane particles, and filamentous forms (Figure 53–3). Spherical particles and filamentous forms consist of hepatitis B surface antigen (HBsAg) only. The Dane particle has an outer coat containing HBsAg and an inner core called hepatitis B core antigen (HBcAg).

The virus may be found in blood, saliva, tears, nasal secretions, breast milk, semen, and vaginal secretions of infected individuals and in blood-sucking insects that have ingested the virus from infected persons. The disease may be contracted via the parenteral route (eg, during blood transfusion, by injection, or during hemodialysis), by intimate contact with carriers or persons acutely ill with the disease, from contaminated instruments, or by transmission from mother to infant. Hepatitis B carriers may be asymptomatic.

Less than 1 mL of blood is required to transmit infection. Health care personnel who have any break in skin integrity can readily contract the disease from contaminated secretions. Tattooing and ear piercing have been associated with hepatitis B.

Clinical Manifestations

Hepatitis B is characterized by many of the same symptoms as hepatitis A, but in more virulent form. Clients who recover sometimes develop chronic hepatitis. Develop-

---

Nursing Research Note

James AM, Skolnick RB, Habel L, Agee B: A survey of hepatitis B vaccination programs for hospital employees. *Am J Infect Control* 1985; 13(1):32–34.

A survey of county hospitals in Los Angeles determined community practice regarding hepatitis B virus screening and immunization of employees. Only 33% of the hospitals had an immunization policy, and 73% of these planned to screen their employees. The hepatitis B virus vaccine became available in June 1982, and policies were left to the discretion of the individual hospitals because risks varied among hospitals.

The vaccine continues to be controversial because of the cost of the screening and the vaccination serum itself. Nurses who work in high-risk areas where exposure to hepatitis B virus is prevalent should read the literature about its efficacy. Nurses should also inquire about their hospital's policies regarding hepatitis immunization.

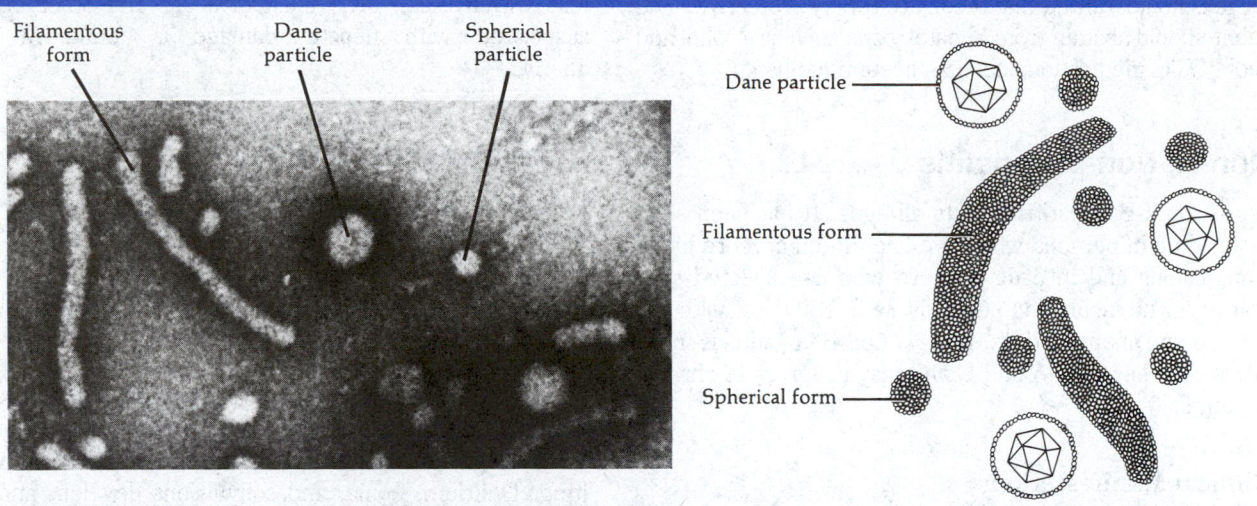

Figure 53–3

Left. Electron micrograph showing the three distinct types of hepatitis B particles. **Right.** Diagram of each particle.
SOURCE: Tortora GJ, Funke BR, Case CL: *Microbiology: An Introduction,* 2nd ed. Menlo Park, CA: Benjamin/Cummings, 1986.

ment of a subclinical carrier state is also possible with hepatitis B. General malaise, arthralgia, rash, pruritus, gastrointestinal symptoms, and hepatomegaly are common in the prodromal stage. Severe nausea and vomiting accompany jaundice in the icteric stage. Common laboratory findings include elevated WBC, SGOT, and SGPT levels as well as elevated alkaline phosphatase and indirect serum bilirubin. The presence of hepatitis B surface antigen (HBsAg) is diagnostic of the disease.

Therapeutic Measures
Medical measures for treatment of hepatitis B may include the intravenous administration of fluids and electrolytes, since the anorexia associated with the disease may cause dehydration and electrolyte imbalance. Vitamin K is given to most clients, and various measures for relief of symptoms may be prescribed such as antihistamines for pruritus and antiemetics for nausea and vomiting.

Preventive Measures
Persons at high risk for exposure to hepatitis B include health care professionals working in dialysis units, emergency rooms, and operating rooms. Also at increased risk are intravenous therapy nurses, oral surgeons, dental hygienists, and medical technologists. All nurses are at some risk by being in health care environments.

Passive immunoprophylaxis is available against hepatitis B via hyperimmune globulin or hepatitis B immune globulin (HBIG). For example, with a needle stick injury, passive immunoprophylaxis may be given with HBIG. HBIG must be given as soon as possible after exposure, preferably within seven days. The recommended prophylactic dose of HBIG is two IM injections—0.06 mL/kg of body weight, given 30 days apart.

Until recently, no safe active vaccine was available against hepatitis B. Now there is a live vaccine, which enables recipients to develop antibodies against the disease. It is given in 3 IM dosages (initial dose, second dose one month later, third dose 6 months after initial dose) in the deltoid muscle. Gluteal IM administration should not be used because of erratic absorption of vaccine. It is known to be effective for up to 5 years and perhaps much longer. There seem to be no major risks from hepatitis B vaccine. The question has been raised whether AIDS can be contracted from the vaccine because the vaccine is made from the plasma of human hepatitis B carriers, who may be gay men. To date there are no known cases of AIDS resulting from hepatitis B vaccine.

Specific Nursing Measures
Rest, frequent high-calorie meals, and at least 3000 mL of fluid per day are important to recovery. Hepatotoxic medications must be avoided. Whether the client is hospitalized or at home, care givers should avoid direct contact with any of the client's bodily fluids. Gloves should be worn when handling the client's eating utensils, soiled tissues, linens, wash cloths, bath towels, and underwear. The nurse should be particularly careful when giving injections, drawing blood, or removing intravenous tubing to avoid needlestick injuries or direct contact with the client's serum. For protection of other health care workers and housekeeping personnel, extreme care must be observed in disposal of needles and IV equipment.

Discharge teaching includes cautioning clients not to donate blood, informing them that they will have lifetime immunity to hepatitis B following recovery, and encouraging them to get adequate rest. Clients must be cautioned not to engage in sexual relations until serum liver function tests return to normal (which could be as long as 3 to 4 months) because semen and vaginal secretions will infect others. If sexual contact does occur, clients should use protective barrier measures such as condoms, although there is no guarantee that these are totally protective. The client should abstain from hepatotoxins such as alcohol and avoid OTC medications such as acetaminophen.

Non-A, Non-B Hepatitis

Non-A, non-B hepatitis affects all ages. It has been seen most often in persons who have had fifteen or more blood transfusions and in drug abusers who use injected substances. The incubation period is 14 to 160 days, with the mean being about 50 days. Non-A, non-B hepatitis is more lethal than hepatitis A and B and may progress to chronic hepatitis.

Clinical Manifestations
As with other types of hepatitis, there are inflammation of hepatic cells, hypertrophy of Kupffer cells, and bile stasis. During the prodromal phase, the client experiences malaise, anorexia, headache, and lassitude and is febrile. Later, hepatomegaly, liver tenderness, and arthralgia occur. The client is often without icterus.

Therapeutic and Specific Nursing Measures
Adequate hydration, nutrition, and rest are essential for recovery. The client with non-A, non-B hepatitis is usually hospitalized because of the need for intravenous fluid replacement, tube feedings or total parenteral nutrition, relief from pruritus, and rest. Vitamin K is prescribed to correct coagulation abnormalities.

Extreme care must be taken with needle punctures to avoid hemorrhage or spread of the disease. Blood isolation precautions are observed, but enteric isolation is not necessary, since the disease is blood borne. Other nursing activities are similar to those already described.

Since blood transfusions are associated with risk of contracting non-A, non-B hepatitis, nurses may wish to suggest to clients planning to have elective surgery that they donate their own blood for use if transfusions are necessary.

TOXIC AND DRUG-INDUCED HEPATITIS

Certain agents, including carbon tetrachloride, yellow phosphorus, and acetaminophen (in large doses) are hepatotoxins. When ingested or inhaled they cause necrosis of hepatic cells. Hepatitis related to these substances is called toxic hepatitis.

Varying patterns of hepatic dysfunction are seen in response to use of other drugs and anesthetic agents. For example, halothane, methyldopa, and isoniazid can produce a reaction indistinguishable from viral hepatitis. Chlorpromazine, erythromycin estolate, and methimazole can cause intrahepatic cholestasis with jaundice. Phenylbutazone and the sulfonamides can produce granulo-

mas within the liver. (A list of drugs and other agents associated with hepatic damage is found in Box 52–1).

Clinical Manifestations

Both drug-induced and toxic hepatitis are manifested by inflammation of hepatic cells, hyperplasia of Kupffer cells, and bile stasis; however, toxic hepatitis is associated with acute cellular necrosis. The onset of both forms is similar to that of viral hepatitis, from which they must be quickly distinguished if detoxification is to be initiated to save the client's life. Anorexia, jaundice, and hepatomegaly are common. In *toxic hepatitis*, the illness may progress rapidly, with rising fever, subdermal hemorrhage, and severe vomiting. Delirium, coma, and convulsions develop, and the client dies within a few days. If the toxin is promptly identified and exposure is discontinued, however, the client may recover quite rapidly. Cirrhosis sometimes develops after recovery.

Drug-induced hepatitis may develop after repeated exposures have sensitized the client to a drug. For this reason, any medication that causes pruritus or other symptoms of sensitivity should be immediately withdrawn and the sensitivity noted on the client's record. Chills, fever, rash, pruritus, arthralgia, and nausea are early signs of drug-induced hepatitis. Icterus, hepatomegaly, and hepatic tenderness follow. The urine is dark. Symptoms may subside once the drug is withdrawn, but drug-induced hepatitis may be fatal, and postnecrotic cirrhosis also may develop. The anesthetic agent halothane has been linked to episodes of drug-induced hepatitis; therefore, anesthetics should be rotated for clients undergoing repeated surgical procedures.

Therapeutic and Specific Nursing Measures

Treatment is directed at removal of the toxin or sensitizing agent, if known. There are no antidotes.

Early diagnosis is important. The health history taken by the nurse yields data indicative of toxic or drug-induced hepatitis. Attention should focus on occupational history, possible exposure to hepatotoxins during hobby activities (for example, furniture refinishing), and medication history, including OTC medications and self-prescribed vitamin therapy. (Large doses of vitamins A and D may be hepatotoxic.) Once the disease has been diagnosed, nursing care focuses on comfort measures and replacement of blood, fluids, and electrolytes.

CHRONIC ACTIVE HEPATITIS

Chronic active hepatitis, or chronic active liver disease (CALD), is related to active inflammation with associated hepatic necrosis. Usually the person has had hepatitis B or non-A, non-B hepatitis before development of the chronic condition. CALD is usually fatal within a few years. Remission may occur, but the client usually develops cirrhosis.

Clinical Manifestations

The client is fatigued, icteric, anorexic, anemic, and has a low-grade fever. Arthralgia and abdominal pain are common, and women may be amenorrheal. There is speculation that CALD may be related to interaction with the immune system because IgG, IgM, and IgA values are elevated. Antinuclear antibodies are also found in the serum of persons with CALD.

Therapeutic and Specific Nursing Measures

Rest and adequate nutrition are required, and steroids may be prescribed to lessen the intensity of the immune reaction. Other nursing care is as described in Chapter 52.

HEPATIC ABSCESS

Hepatic (or liver) abscess is an invasion of the liver by microorganisms producing a localized collection of pus in a cavity formed by destruction of tissue. Hepatic abscess may be caused by fungi, several types of bacteria, or even protozoa. An infection anywhere in the body can lead to formation of a hepatic abscess, but gastrointestinal infections are especially likely to do so.

Usually, microorganisms that invade the liver are destroyed by the phagocytic Kupffer cells, but occasionally a few survive. The lobular structure of the liver tends to keep the infection small and circumscribed, but several lobules may be affected. As the microorganisms multiply, the toxins they produce destroy hepatic cells. Concurrently, the body's defense system acts to destroy the invading organisms, and the cavity becomes filled with a mixture of leukocytes, microorganisms, and dead and necrotic hepatic cells.

Clinical Manifestations

The client will have a high fever, a painfully enlarged liver, anemia, elevated WBC level, and icterus. As the temperature rises, the client has alternating episodes of chills and diaphoresis; toxic shock can occur within hours. If identified soon enough, the infective agent can be controlled with antimicrobial therapy. Sometimes, septicemia cannot be reversed, and the client dies.

Therapeutic Measures

Nonaspirin analgesics, intravenous fluid therapy, and parenteral antimicrobial agents may be prescribed. Occasion-

ally, surgical intervention may be indicated to drain large abscessed areas or to resect an abscessed portion of the liver. This is done rarely, however, because coagulation abnormalities associated with liver dysfunction increase the risk of severe hemorrhage. The most common surgical intervention is percutaneous drainage. This may be done intermittently, or continuous catheter drainage may be employed.

Specific Nursing Measures

Continual assessment is a crucial part of nursing care. Has the client had an infection within the last 6 months? Is the client diabetic? In diabetics, infections that have apparently resolved sometimes lodge in the liver.

Hourly monitoring of temperature and vital signs may be required to determine whether the client is becoming septic or whether antimicrobial therapy is taking effect. Hepatic abscess is accompanied by pain and fever, so supportive care with comfort measures is necessary. If surgical intervention is indicated or drainage initiated, the nurse will teach the client about the procedure, provide reassurance, and assess for hemorrhage.

CHOLECYSTITIS

Cholecystitis is an inflammation of the gallbladder. It may be either acute or chronic. An acute inflammation may begin in the mucosal layer as a primary infection. More often it is superimposed on a chronic infection initially related to cholelithiasis. The gallbladder becomes dilated and filled with bile, pus, and blood. Common infective organisms include staphylococci, streptococci, and enteric organisms.

Clinical Manifestations

Major symptoms of cholecystitis are intense pain, tenderness, and rigidity in the right upper quadrant of the abdomen associated with nausea, vomiting, and the usual signs of inflammation. Jaundice may be present if there is an obstruction. If the gallbladder is filled with frankly purulent matter, the condition is called empyema of the gallbladder. Although chronic cholecystitis may be related to an acute attack, it is almost always associated with cholelithiasis.

Therapeutic and Specific Measures

The gallbladder is usually resected after acute inflammation has been relieved by medical intervention. Surgical removal of the gallbladder (cholecystectomy) is discussed in Chapter 54. Because cholecystitis and cholelithiasis are closely associated, medical and nursing measures are discussed in the following section on obstructive disorders.

Section IV: Neoplastic and Obstructive Disorders

Although hepatic and biliary neoplasia and cholelithiasis may both be classified as obstructive, the two types of obstruction have little in common. Nursing measures will therefore be discussed for each disease process.

CANCER OF THE GALLBLADDER

Cancer of the gallbladder is rare. Malignant tumors are usually columnar cell carcinomas that cause symptoms of inflammation and obstruction (Groer and Shekleton, 1983). In part because of its rarity, biliary carcinoma may be overlooked or confused with cholelithiasis.

CANCER OF THE LIVER

Most cases of hepatic cancer in the United States involve metastatic lesions. Primary carcinoma of the liver is rare in the United States and Canada but common in Asia and Africa. The frequency of primary hepatic cancer in parts of the Third World is thought to be related to the large number of hepatitis B virus carriers in these populations. Chronic carriers are at increased risk of developing liver cancer.

Primary malignant neoplasia of the liver generally is an adenocarcinoma (see Chapter 12) arising from hepatic cells or bile ducts. The larger right lobe is more frequently involved than the left. The lesion develops most frequently in persons aged 60 to 79, with males having 6 to 10 times the incidence of females. The highest incidence is in Orientals (Baldanado and Stahl, 1982). In addition to hepatitis B, factors associated with primary hepatic carcinoma are cirrhosis, intestinal parasites, hemochromatosis, and schistosomiasis (liver flukes).

Metastatic carcinomas are seen in over 50% of end-stage cancers. Often the tumors will enlarge the liver to seven times its normal size.

Clinical Manifestations

Signs and symptoms are not pathognomonic of cancer; instead, symptoms are related to the extent of hepatocellular damage and functional failure of the liver. Initially, the client may lose weight; later, increase in weight may be associated with ascites and fluid retention. Other manifestations are cachexia, anemia, abdominal fullness and pain, fever, hemorrhage, obstructive icterus, splenomegaly, and hepatomegaly. Liver function test results will show abnormalities.

Therapeutic Measures

Nonmetastatic solitary localized tumors are surgically resected. Because of the liver's capacity for regeneration, as much as 90% of liver tissue has been successfully removed. Chemotherapy is usually instituted to promote regression of the tumor and prolong client survival. Methotrexate, 5-fluorouracil, or other agents may be administered systemically or by intrahepatic arterial line. Arterial lines are being used with increasing frequency because the drug reaches the tumor at full strength, yet partial detoxification within the hepatic cells minimizes systemic side effects. Radiation therapy may also be employed.

Severe, intractable pain frequently is associated with hepatic carcinoma; morphine drip or Brompton's cocktail may be prescribed. A low-sodium diet, tube feedings, or total parenteral nutrition may be necessary, as well as measures to alleviate other manifestations of hepatic dysfunction (for example, paracentesis; see Chapter 52). Pharmacological agents commonly used in treating hepatic carcinoma are listed in Box 53–2.

Specific Nursing Measures

Nursing care is consistent with general care of the client with hepatic dysfunction as discussed in Chapter 52 and cancer as discussed in Chapter 12. If an intrahepatic arterial line is in place, the nurse must assess for placement of the line, occlusion, and hemorrhage. Continuity of the line must be maintained to avoid contamination or development of an air embolus. Clients are usually kept in bed while the line is in place.

Precautions related to chemotherapy and radiation exposure are discussed in Chapter 12.

CHOLELITHIASIS

Cholelithiasis, the formation of gallstones, can lead to obstruction of the bile ducts associated with obstructive

---

Box 53–2   Pharmacological Agents Commonly Used in Treatment of Hepatic Carcinoma

Chemotherapeutic agents:
  Doxorubicin HCL (Adriamycin)
  Methotrexate
  5-fluorouracil

Aldosterone antagonist diuretics

Antiemetics

Diphenhydramine (Benadryl)

Emollients

Potassium

Brompton's cocktail

Morphine drip

icterus and severe colicky pain. An estimated 20 million Americans have cholelithiasis, and almost 1 million new cases are diagnosed each year.

Several predisposing factors are related to development of cholelithiasis:

- Women are affected four times as frequently as men.
- Persons over 40 are affected more often than younger persons.
- Women taking oral contraceptives are twice as likely as other women to develop gallstones.
- Cholelithiasis occurs more often in multigravidas than in childless women.
- High fat intake and cholesterol saturation of bile predispose a person to cholelithiasis.
- Obesity and diabetes are associated with increased risk of gallstone formation.
- Persons who have had extensive bowel resection (as for Crohn's disease) have a threefold to fivefold higher incidence of cholelithiasis, possibly because recirculation of bile salts is interrupted (Thorpe and Caprini, 1980).

The physiological basis for these risk factors is discussed in Chapter 51.

Cholesterol saturation of bile appears to be a major factor in development of gallstones. The underlying cause may be dysfunction of the hepatic cells where bile is synthesized. Bile salts precipitate from supersaturated bile, forming nuclei for accretion of layers of cholesterol, calcium, and bilirubin to form calculi within the gallbladder.

Gallstones are classified as either cholesterol or pigment stones. Cholesterol stones are usually of mixed composition and contain more than 70% cholesterol plus calcium salts, bile pigments, fatty acids, and proteins. There is a high incidence of cholesterol stones in North America. Pigment stones are primarily calcium and bilirubin and contain less than 10% cholesterol. Pigment stones are less common in North America but have a high prevalence in Japan.

Clinical Manifestations

Calculi formed in the gallbladder may move into the cystic duct, the common bile duct, or even into the liver via the hepatic ducts. Calculus obstruction of the pancreatic duct may cause pancreatitis.

The most common symptom of cholelithiasis is colicky pain believed to be related to spasms of the sphincter of Oddi. Pain may also be related to obstruction and distention of a bile duct. Usually, the pain is felt in the epigastrium or the right upper quadrant of the abdomen, but it may radiate up the back between the scapulae to the right shoulder or around the abdomen to the back, making it difficult for the client to assume a comfortable position. Biliary colic may occur at varying intervals following meals or may awaken the client from sleep. Usually, symptoms occur at pro-

gressively shorter intervals after ingestion of almost any food. Occasionally, however, a single pain episode will never be repeated.

In addition to the characteristic pain, nausea and vomiting are common, as is elevated temperature. Distention of the bile ducts stimulates the vomiting center. If the common bile duct is obstructed by a calculus, greenish-yellow jaundice develops. Pruritus often develops before the jaundice is visible in the sclerae. Icterus is accompanied by acholic stools and dark, frothy urine. Ecchymoses may be evident.

Laboratory and diagnostic studies assist in confirming the diagnosis. WBC levels, direct bilirubin levels, prothrombin time, and alkaline phosphatase and serum lipid levels will be elevated. Urine urobilinogen levels will decrease, but bilirubin will be found in the urine. Cholecystography, cholangiography, or endoscopic retrograde cholangiopancreatography (ERCP) may be ordered. These diagnostic studies are described in Chapter 52.

Therapeutic Measures

If symptoms are mild, a low-fat diet may be sufficient to control them. The diet should be high in proteins and carbohydrates. Depending on the client's nutritional status, intravenous glucose and protein supplementation may be indicated. A nutritious diet promotes healing and helps prevent hepatic damage. Vitamin K may be required if coagulation abnormalities are demonstrated.

If the client's serum cholesterol and triglyceride levels are markedly elevated, antilipemic agents may be prescribed. One such agent, cholestyramine (Questran), combines with bile so it is excreted and lipids are not absorbed; this drug may cause constipation. Because cholestyramine may impair absorption of other medications, they should be given 1 hour before cholestyramine. Clofibrate (Atromid-S) and niacin have also been used to reduce serum lipid levels but are associated with severe side effects.

Medications that dissolve gallstones have been used experimentally. One such agent, chenodeoxycholic acid or chenodiol has been in clinical use in many countries for some time. It is effective only for calculi formed of cholesterol; gallstones containing large amounts of calcium do not respond (Hofmann, 1982). The treatment is currently expensive, involving a 2-year regimen for dissolution of the calculi and maintenance therapy thereafter. Chenodiol has recently been approved for use in the United States for clients who have radiolucent pure-cholesterol stones.

Side effects may include diarrhea, hepatotoxicity, and an elevation in serum cholesterol levels. Because chenodiol may affect fetal growth and development, it should not be given to women capable of conception unless they have adequate contraceptive protection. Persons with chronic liver disorders or biliary obstruction should not receive chenodiol because of possible hepatotoxicity.

Pharmacological agents used in treating cholelithiasis and cholecystitis are listed in Box 53–3.

Box 53–3 Pharmacological Agents Used in Treatment of Cholelithiasis and Cholecystitis

Nonaspirin analgesics	Vitamin K
Meperidine	Cholestyramine
Phenobarbital	Chenodiol
Nitroglycerin	

Box 53–4 High-Fat Foods to Be Avoided by Clients With Cholelithiasis

Cream and artificial creamers

Whole milk

Rich rolls, doughnuts, pancakes, and waffles (especially with added butter)

Pastries

Ice cream

Cookies, cakes, and pies

Fried foods

Mayonnaise

Avocados

Cheese (except low-fat cottage cheese or ricotta)

Cream soups and sauces

Peanut butter

Nuts

Chocolate

High-fat snack foods such as potato chips

Butter, margarine, and cooking oils

Bacon, sausage, and other fatty meats

If gallbladder function is impaired or if the bile ducts are obstructed, surgical intervention is required. Surgical approaches to biliary obstruction are discussed in Chapter 54.

Specific Nursing Measures

In addition to comfort measures and administering analgesics and other prescribed medications, the nurse can consult with the dietitian and the client to work out a palatable low-fat diet. The client may find a list of foods useful (Box 53–4). Additional nursing measures generally applicable to biliary disease are discussed in Chapter 52. A case study of a client with cholelithiasis is presented at the end of Chapter 54.

Section V: Traumatic Disorders

Characteristics and care of clients with gallbladder trauma vary considerably from those for hepatic trauma. Principles applicable to each type of disorder will be discussed separately below.

TRAUMA TO THE GALLBLADDER

Acute acalculous cholecystitis—cholecystitis not related to biliary calculi—may occur in clients who have sustained abdominal trauma, for example, in an automobile accident. The condition is related to necrosis of biliary tissue resulting from the original insult. The gallbladder is full of bile so viscous (the consistency of crankcase oil) that it cannot drain. Usually, the cholecystitis is not apparent while the client is NPO and has a nasogastric tube in place. If fever, an elevated WBC level, abdominal pain, and postprandial emesis develop in a posttrauma client, acute acalculous cholecystitis should be suspected.

Generally, a cholecystectomy is performed. Nursing care for the client with a cholecystectomy is discussed in Chapter 54.

TRAUMA TO THE LIVER

Trauma to the liver may be penetrating or blunt. Penetrating trauma is usually from gunshot wounds or stab-

bings; blunt injuries are caused by motor vehicle accidents, falls, or assaults. Blunt trauma is more serious, since it can fracture the liver capsule. Parenchymal cell damage may occur with or without disruption of the capsule. Other complications of hepatic trauma include hepatic hematoma, hemorrhage into the biliary passages, and intraperitoneal hemorrhage.

Therapeutic Measures

Surgical intervention is usually necessary for debridement of the wound and control of hemorrhage. Intravenous fluid administration, blood expanders, blood replacement, and other measures to control shock may be prescribed. Antibiotic therapy is used to prevent or control infection. Vitamin K supplementation may be ordered postoperatively to correct coagulation abnormalities related to impaired hepatic function.

Specific Nursing Measures

Nursing responsibilities include assessing the client for signs of hemorrhage and shock prior to surgery and for symptoms of hemorrhage, infection, renal failure, and pulmonary embolism after surgery. Aggressive treatment of shock will be necessary preoperatively and postoperatively. Other postsurgical nursing responsibilities include administration of antibiotics, intravenous fluids, blood, albumin, glucose, and vitamin K as ordered. Additional interventions are those related to good preoperative and postoperative care (Chapter 14) as well as emotional support for client and significant others. Psychosocial interventions for trauma and other emergencies are discussed in Chapter 13.

Chapter Highlights

Nursing interventions for clients with congenital disorders of the hepatic–biliary system include promoting comfort, encouraging genetic counseling, providing emotional support, and educating the client and significant others.

Care for the client with cirrhosis includes general care discussed in Chapter 52, especially promoting comfort; maintaining skin integrity, tissue perfusion, and thought processes; improving nutritional intake; and correcting fluid volume alterations.

Hemorrhage of esophageal varices may be controlled with vasopressin therapy, gastric lavage with iced saline, placement of a Sengstaken–Blakemore or Minnesota tube for temporary control, and injection sclerotherapy or portal-systemic shunting for long-term control.

Hepatitis A, also known as short-incubation or infectious hepatitis, is associated with a lower mortality rate than other forms, is transmitted via the fecal–oral route, and provides lifetime immunity for persons who have had the disease.

Hepatitis B, also known as long-incubation or serum hepatitis, is transmitted via all bodily fluids with the possible exception of feces; it can progress to chronic hepatitis or to a subclinical carrier state.

Prophylactic administrations of immune serum globulin (ISG) for hepatitis A and hepatitis B immune globulin (HBIG) for hepatitis B are given within one week of exposure. Hepatitis B vaccine is available for persons continually exposed to this disease and to high-risk individuals such as dialysis clients.

Non-A, non-B hepatitis, seen in persons with multiple transfusions and in abusers of parenterally administered drugs, is more lethal than hepatitis A and B.

Toxic hepatitis, caused by drugs or chemicals that induce cell necrosis, and drug-induced hepatitis, caused by drugs that sensitize the liver, can be completely reversed if the sensitizing or toxic agent is removed; in many cases the agent cannot be identified in time. The health history can help identify possible sources of toxicity.

Chronic active hepatitis, seen in persons who have previously had hepatitis B or non-A, non-B hepatitis, is believed to involve an immune interaction because IgG, IgM, and IgA values are elevated.

Hepatic abscesses, often in adjoining liver lobules, are pockets of necrotic cells, infectious microorganisms, and leukocytes.

Metastatic cancer of the liver is 25 times as common as primary liver cancer. Hepatic carcinoma is associated with weight loss, ascites, cachexia, anemia, abdominal fullness and pain, fever, hemorrhage, obstructive icterus, splenomegaly, and hepatomegaly.

Cholecystitis is inflammation of the gallbladder frequently associated with cholelithiasis and characterized by intense pain, tenderness, and rigidity in the right upper quadrant of the abdomen.

Bibliography

Baldanado AA, Stahl DA: *Cancer Nursing: A Holistic Multidisciplinary Approach,* 2nd. ed Garden City, NY: Medical Examination Publishing, 1982.

Crowley LV: *Introduction to Human Disease.* Monterey, CA: Wadsworth, 1983.

Dong B et al: Viral hepatitis. *Nurse Pract* (March) 1984; 9:27–32.

Epstein M: Renal complications of liver disease. *Clin Symp* 1985; 37(5):3–32.

Gallbladder trouble after trauma. *Emerg Med* 1980; 12:98.

Groer ME, Shekleton ME: *Basic Pathophysiology: A Conceptual Approach,* 2nd ed. St. Louis, MO: Mosby, 1983.

Hofmann AF: Gallstone-dissolving drugs: New approach to an old disease. *Drug Therapy,* February 1982:57–71.

Keith JS: Hepatic failure: Etiologies, manifestations, and management. *Crit Care Nurs* 1985; 5(1):60–86.

Kirkman-Liff B, Dandoy S: Hepatitis B: What price exposure? *Am J Nurs* (August) 1984; 84:988–990.

Malseed RT: *Pharmacology: Drug Therapy and Nursing Considerations.* Philadelphia, PA: Lippincott, 1982.

Mar DD: New hepatitis B vaccine: A breakthrough in hepatitis prevention. *Am J Nurs* 1982; 82:306.

Schoenfield LJ: Gallstones and other biliary diseases. *Clin Symp* 1982; 34(4):2–32.

Sherlock S: *Diseases of the Liver and Biliary System,* 6th ed. Oxford, Blackwell, 1981.

Suggested Readings

Gurevich I: Viral hepatitis. *Am J Nurs* 1983; 83:571–586. Presents a thorough overview of types A, B, and non-A, non-B hepatitis, including excellent discussion of precautions for health care providers.

Halberstam MJ: Doctor, I feel queasy after eating . . . *Ladies Home Journal* 1980; 97–174. Presents a client's view of the pain associated with gallbladder disease.

Newell J: Portal systemic encephalopathy. *Nurse Pract* (July) 1984; 9:26–37. The pathogenesis, clinical manifestations, disease stages, diagnosis, and treatment of portal systemic encephalopathy are discussed. Client and family education for self-management is emphasized.

Thorpe CJ, Caprini JA: Gallbladder disease: Current trends and treatments. *Am J Nurs* 1980; 80:2181–2185. Risk factors, signs and symptoms, diagnostic studies, and medical interventions for gallbladder dysfunction are discussed.

Wimpsett J: Trace your patient's liver dysfunction. *Nurs '84*, 1984, 14(8):56–57. This very short narrative is supplemented with a detailed diagram of pathophysiological changes and related client symptoms.

The Client With Cirrhosis

I. Brief Descriptive Data	Mr John Smith, age 55, has been admitted to the hospital with a diagnosis of prehepatic coma secondary to Laennec's cirrhosis. His skin and sclerae are slightly jaundiced, and he complains of itching skin. Ascites, peripheral edema, multiple bruises, confusion, and drowsiness are apparent.

II. Personal Data

Date and Time:	Sept. 25, 1986; 7:00 PM
Full Name:	John Adam Smith
Social Security Number:	000-00-0000
Address:	Box 28956, Branston, Colo
Telephone:	Work: 000-0000
	Home: 000-0000
Sex:	Male
Marital Status:	Married
Age:	55
Birthdate:	5-1-31
Religion:	Protestant
Race:	Caucasian
Occupation:	Carpenter
Usual Health Care Provider:	Joe Adams, MD

III. Health History

Source of Information:	Client and wife
Reliability of Informant:	Client confused at times; wife is reliable but apathetic
Chief Concern:	Itching, confusion, and drowsiness off and on
History of Present Illness:	Has been admitted several times during the past ten years for problems associated with cirrhosis—ascites and peripheral and pulmonary edema. Bleeding esophageal varices, 1981. LeVeen shunt placed, 1982. Was also hospitalized in 1960, 1966, for alcohol-related automobile accidents. Sustained fx rt femur, 1960; mild concussion, 1966.

Current main concern of client is itching skin and being "tired" much of the time; no fatigue pattern identified. Wife identifies recent confusion and forgetfulness as most significant concern. Ten days ago wife noted husband's increased episodes of confusion and decreased appetite. No vomiting, but has been nauseated on occasion late in afternoon; bowel movements twice a day—some stools are tarry, black, while others are lighter in color; flatulence has increased and caused some cramping discomfort; epigastric discomfort accompanies nausea at times. Still ingests alcohol—one to two beers per evening prior to dinner; continues to drink 5–6 cups caffeinated coffee per day; stays on low roughage diet. Concerned about loss of job because of worsening condition and financial difficulties.

Past Health History:	
Childhood:	Childhood diseases—measles, mumps, chickenpox
Immunizations:	Polio, 1961; Td, 1982; influenza and pneumonia, 1982
Medical Problems:	Hepatitis B, 1948; cirrhosis, 1978; congestive heart failure, 1980; esophageal variceal hemorrhage, 1981
Surgeries:	Appendectomy, 1961; paracentesis, 1980, 1981; LeVeen shunt, 1982
Blood Transfusions:	1974, 1976, 1978, 1981, 1982

(continued)

Case Study written by Jane Hokanson Hawks.

The Client With Cirrhosis

Trauma: Auto accidents, 1960 (fx femur); 1966 (mild concussion); minor auto accidents, 1971, 1974, 1977

Allergies: None

Medications: Furosemide, 40 mg PO b.i.d.

Family History: Propranolol, 20 mg PO t.i.d.

Spironolactone, 25 mg PO t.i.d.

Family genogram:

- 72 Colon cancer (male, died)
- 62 Cirrhosis (male, died)
- 78 Hypertension, heart disease (female)
- 73 Breast cancer 10 years ago (female)
- 5 Accident (male, died)
- 58 Heart disease, hypertension (male)
- 50 A & W (female)
- 55 Cirrhosis 8 years (male, Client — arrow)
- 52 A & W (female)
- 35 A & W (female)
- 33 A & W (female)
- 31 A & W (male)

Key:
- □ Male
- ○ Female
- ●■ Died
- A&W Alive and well
- → Client

Personal and Social History: Currently works about 20 hours per week as a carpenter; condition has prohibited more than that for last 5 years; children are all away from home and doing well; wife works full time as secretary for local attorney; very little exercise as tolerates it poorly; likes to build wagon wheel lamps and tables in spare time; 3-pack-a-day smoker × 30 years; quit 3 years ago; wife is supportive; children call often.

Review of Systems: General health has begun to deteriorate over past 2 years.

Skin: Frequent itching

Mouth: States, "Gums bleed when brushing"

Respiratory: Has shortness of breath on exertion

Gastrointestinal: See HPI

Urinary: Voids approximately 10 times per day, nocturia × 2 at night; denies dysuria, urgency, hesitancy

Genital: Unable to achieve erection for two years; both client and wife find this upsetting

Endocrine: Denies polydipsia, polyphagia

Psychological: Believes he will get well; becomes frustrated when unable to remember things

IV: Physical Assessment

Height: 6 ft, 0 in

Weight: 200 lb

Vital Signs: BP 160/95; pulse 105; respirations 28; temperature 98.2°F (36.8°C). Tall, ill-appearing, obviously jaundiced, somewhat confused 55-yr-old w/m

Relevant Organ Systems:

Skin: Orange—yellow discoloration, spider angiomas on anterior chest; no breaks in skin integrity; bruises noted on all extremities

Eyes: Sclerae yellow

Breasts: Mild gynecomastia

Chest: Dyspnea noted in supine position; DOE; rales both lower lobes posteriorly

Heart: PMI palpable 5th left ICS, 2 cm lateral to MCL; apical rate 98, regular

Abdomen: Obvious ascites, dilated periumbilical veins; decreased bowel sounds, no bruits; liver edge palpable 5 cm below rt costal margin; liver 15 cm by percussion at rt MCL; fluid wave present; spleen not palpable

Genitourinary: Thinning pubic hair; urine very dark yellow and frothy

Extremities: 3+ ankle edema bilaterally; limbs emaciated except for areas of edema

Neurologic: Confused at times; some decreased sensation in toes and hands (unable to distinguish hot and cold)

V. Diagnostic Data   Results of laboratory data include hypokalemia, prolonged prothrombin time, decreased plasma albumin, and increased bilirubin and serum ammonia levels.

VI. Medical Regimen

Diet: 500 mg Na, 15 g protein, 1500 mL fluid restriction

Treatments: Tap water enema

Medications: Neomycin, 20 g PO q.i.d.
Spironolactone (Aldactone), 25 mg PO t.i.d.
Diphenhydramine (Benadryl), 50 mg PO h.s. p.r.n. for itching
Vitamin K (AquaMEPHYTON), 2 mg IM, MWF
Furosemide (Lasix) 40 mg PO b.i.d.
Propranol HCL (Inderal), 20 mg PO t.i.d.
Potassium, 20 mEq PO t.i.d.

VII. Nursing Care Plan

Nursing Diagnosis	Client Care Goals	Plan/Nursing Implementation	Expected Outcome
Comfort, alteration in: related to pruritus	Reduce or eliminate pruritus; increase comfort; sleep throughout the night	Rest, good diet, ventilation, cotton clothing, change wet sheets, distraction, no alkaline soaps, infrequent baths, whirlpool, emollients, keep nails short, diphenhydramine 50 mg p.r.n., have client wear gloves	Performs ADL without scratching; rests comfortably; relief of itching
Skin integrity, impairment of: potential	Change position frequently; take in well-balanced diet; understand effects of prolonged pressure on skin integrity	Well-balanced diet (low protein, low Na because of diagnosis); relieve itching; frequent turning, use of air or water mattresses, and position change to relieve pressure on edematous areas; keep skin clean, dry; keep sheets wrinkle-free; teach about effect of pressure on skin	Normal skin integrity; avoids staying in same position more than 1 hour; client and family understand mechanism of skin breakdown
Thought processes, alteration in	Regain satisfactory thought processes	Have him write name daily, check extent of asterixis by pumping BP cuff, potassium	Writes name daily without changes; oriented to date, time, place; client and

(continued)

The Client With Cirrhosis

VII. Nursing Care Plan *(continued)*

Nursing Diagnosis	Client Care Goals	Plan/Nursing Implementation	Expected Outcome
		20 mEq t.i.d.; tap water enema, assess for fetor hepaticus, rest; Sengstaken–Blakemore or Minnesota tube if esophageal varices bleed; may assist with ice lavage; neomycin sulfate 1 g q.i.d., 15 g protein, ↓ Na diet; fluid restriction	family aware of dietary restrictions and adhere to them; absence of asterixis
Fluid volume, alteration in: related to ascites and portal hypertension	Improve fluid volume balance	Potassium 20 mEq t.i.d., Furosemide 40 mg b.i.d., 500 mg Na diet, spironolactone 25 mg t.i.d.; intake input and output; monitor esophageal varices, daily weight, abdominal girths; assess patency of LeVeen shunt; measure circumference of extremities; 1500 mL of fluid restriction	Good skin turgor, decreased abdominal girth and circumference of extremities, increased output in comparison to intake
Fluid volume, alteration in: related to potential for hemorrhage	Decrease bruising, possibility of other bleeding problems	Vitamin K 2 mg IM, MWF; monitor prothrombin time and observe for bleeding; check stool hemoccults; explain that caffeine, alcohol are irritants to the GI tract and can cause gastritis and ulcer disease	Prothrombin time within normal limits; absence of bleeding or further bruising; avoids GI irritants such as caffeine, alcohol
Knowledge deficit related to effect of alcohol use and other hepatotoxins	Understand effects of alcohol use on body; describe other common substances that can cause hepatic damage	Explain that cirrhosis and portal hypertension are related to history of alcohol use; also explain need to avoid substances that may further damage the liver (drugs, chemicals)	Abstinence from alcohol and other hepatotoxins; does not use over-the-counter drugs without checking with care provider
Sexual dysfunction	Understand how cirrhosis leads to hormonal imbalances, causing impotence	Explain hormonal imbalances that accompany cirrhosis to client and wife; discuss alternative approaches to meeting sexual needs if couple is interested	Both partners understand effects of cirrhosis on sexual function and can talk about the situation with each other

Chapter 54

Surgical Approaches to Hepatic–Biliary System Dysfunction

Jane Hokanson Hawks

Objectives

When you have finished studying this chapter, you should be able to:

Explain the procedure and identify rationale for insertion of a LeVeen shunt.

Specify nursing and client implications associated with the insertion of a LeVeen shunt.

Identify rationale for a liver resection and the nursing and client implications.

Describe the procedure and indications for insertion of an hepatic arterial line.

Discuss client implications and nursing care related to placement of an hepatic artery line.

Describe the procedure and list the altered states for which liver transplantation would be considered.

Enumerate physiological, psychosocial, and lifestyle client implications associated with liver transplantation.

Explain the preoperative and postoperative nursing care for a client undergoing liver transplantation.

Compare and contrast the indications for cholecystostomy, cholecystectomy, and choledochostomy.

Describe and compare the procedures for cholecystostomy, cholecystectomy, and choledochostomy.

Specify nursing and client implications for cholecystostomy, cholecystectomy, and choledochostomy.

Surgical procedures involving the hepatic–biliary system have serious implications related to the compromised status of the client. Impaired synthesis of coagulation factors, often associated with poor absorption of vitamin K in the absence of bile, renders the client susceptible to hemorrhage. Moreover, impaired hepatic function is generally associated with metabolic imbalances. For these reasons, the client undergoing any surgical treatment for hepatic or biliary disease must be closely observed to avert and treat complications. A solid understanding of normal physiology is mandatory for making these assessments.

Section I: Surgical Approaches to Disorders Affecting the Liver

LEVEEN SHUNT

Before the LeVeen peritoneal–jugular shunt came into use in the mid-1970s, treatment for ascites was limited to a medical regimen (low-salt diet, decreased fluid intake, and diuretic therapy) or treatments involving paracentesis and creation of portacaval shunts. Extracellular fluid volume could be reduced by medical measures, but hyponatremia, hypovolemia, oliguria, and azotemia were common side effects. Portacaval shunt procedures were associated with high operative mortality and encephalopathy. Valuable plasma proteins were lost in abdominal paracentesis. The LeVeen shunt and similar procedures such as the Denver shunt minimize these risks and side effects.

Principles of the LeVeen and Denver Shunts

The LeVeen shunt provides a route for reinfusion of ascitic fluid into the venous system. It operates according to a simple principle of physics: Matter flows along a pressure gradient from areas of high pressure to low. When properly positioned, the shunt runs from the abdominal cavity through the peritoneum and under the subcutaneous tissue into the superior vena cava. Figure 54–1 illustrates a shunt in place, showing its main components—a perforated peritoneal tube, a valve consisting of a one-way diaphragm supported by rubber struts, and a venous catheter.

The valve remains open only so long as pressure in the peritoneal cavity is at least 3 cm H_2O higher than pressure in the superior vena cava. At this pressure, the valve struts flex, moving the diaphragm away from the tube to allow ascitic fluid to pass into the venous catheter. Figure 54–1C illustrates the valve and the open and closed positions of the diaphragm.

During inspiration, pressure in the intraperitoneal cavity usually rises to about 5 cm H_2O higher than pressure in the vena cava, and ascitic fluid moves along the pressure gradient from the abdomen into the venous circulation. On expiration, the pressure drops, and the valve closes.

The diaphragm flattens on inspiration as the lungs fill with air, increasing the pressure within the peritoneal cavity. By practicing breathing exercises, the client can learn to raise intraperitoneal pressure sufficiently to allow fluid to flow through the shunt.

Several safety features are built into the shunt design. The valve prevents blood from flowing into the venous catheter and causing thrombotic obstruction. The valve is

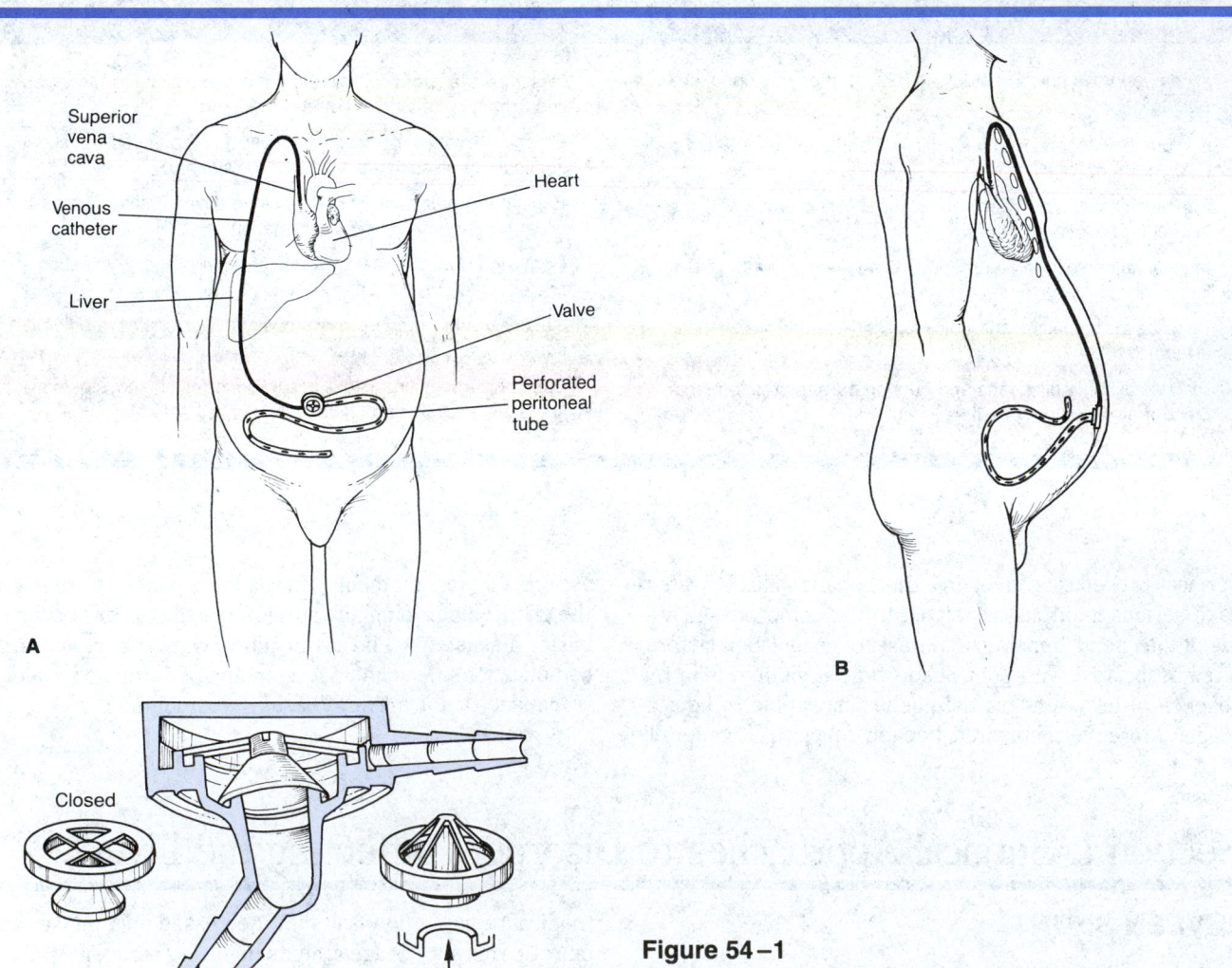

Figure 54–1

A. Anterior view of LeVeen shunt. **B.** Lateral view of LeVeen shunt. **C.** Valve of LeVeen shunt.

designed to remain closed unless intraperitoneal pressure is at least 3 cm H_2O higher than vena caval pressure; thus, if the client's vascular system is overloaded, the valve remains closed, avoiding further overload.

A modified version of the LeVeen shunt is the *Denver shunt*. With the Denver shunt, an internal bulb is positioned so it can be felt externally and pumped to increase intraperitoneal pressure and force fluid into the vena cava. The Denver shunt may be used for clients who are unable to practice breathing exercises to enhance fluid movement. It is the preferred shunt for treatment of ascites related to a malignancy.

Surgical Procedure

The LeVeen shunt may be placed under general anesthesia or with the client sedated and the incision areas locally anesthetized. The shunt valve may be placed in either the upper left or right quadrant of the peritoneal cavity through a transverse incision 2 to 3 cm below the costal margin. The peritoneal tube is inserted through the small abdominal incision surrounded by purse-string sutures, which are then drawn closed. A ligature is then used to guide the venous catheter from the abdomen through a subcutaneous tunnel to an incision in the neck. There the catheter is inserted into the inferior vena cava and sutured into place. The incisions are irrigated with an antibiotic solution before closure.

Implications for the Client

Physiological Implications
Hemodilution usually occurs during the first postoperative week because the shunt pumps large amounts of ascitic fluid into the general circulation. A drop in the hematocrit of as much as 10% to 15% may be expected, and a transfusion of packed red cells may be needed to bring the hematocrit to normal. Cardiac overload and congestive heart failure as well as renal overload are possible complications. The client with a shunt is susceptible to wound infection and septicemia. Other possible complications include extravasation of ascitic fluid from the incision sites, sub-cutaneous or gastrointestinal hemorrhage, and occlusion of the shunt.

Psychosocial/Lifestyle Implications
To increase the success of the LeVeen shunt in reducing ascites, the client must participate in a regimen that includes abstaining from alcohol, following a low-salt diet, and practicing breathing exercises. Some clients will be unwilling to make these lifestyle changes, perhaps believing that "I'm going to die soon anyway, so I might as well eat what I like."

Positive changes following the LeVeen shunt procedure include reduction of ascites with consequent improvement in appearance; relief of dyspnea; and ability to resume activities of daily living, self-care, and possibly employment. The client may also resume sexual activity once he or she recovers from the surgery, assuming sexual function was normal before the operation. If decrease in libido or physical changes related to impaired endocrine detoxification have already occurred, sexual function will probably not improve significantly. The LeVeen procedure itself has no detrimental effect on sexual activity.

Client implications of the LeVeen procedure are summarized in Table 54–1.

Nursing Implications

Preoperative Care
The client's weight must be checked and recorded daily before breakfast. Comparison of daily weights will identify any fluid gain and will provide a baseline for measuring fluid loss after the procedure. Measure abdominal girth at the umbilical level daily for the same reasons. Accurate intake–output records are also necessary to establish a baseline for determining fluid loss after surgery. Prophylactic antibiotic therapy is started 24 hours before surgery.

Several laboratory values must be obtained before surgery:

- If possible, 24-hour urine collections should be done for 2 or 3 days to test for electrolyte imbalances.
- Ascitic fluid should be drawn on 2 or 3 consecutive days for chemical analysis.

Table 54–1 LeVeen Shunt: Implications for the Client	
Physiological Implications	**Psychosocial/Lifestyle Implications**
Hemodilution results in decreased hematocrit	Abstention from alcohol
Cardiac overload and congestive heart failure are possible	Low-salt diet
	Breathing exercises
Renal overload	Resumption of ADL and self-care as ascites is gradually reduced
Septicemia, wound infection can occur	
Hemorrhage	Improved appearance

- Liver function tests and bilirubin, BUN, creatinine, protein, and electrolyte studies are required.
- A complete blood count (CBC) must be done and prothrombin time obtained.

If CBC values show anemia, the client should receive a transfusion of packed red cells to bring hematocrit levels up to normal before surgery. Vitamin K is indicated if prothrombin times are too long. Monitor creatinine and BUN values closely, because medical treatment of ascites can induce hepatorenal syndrome resulting in renal failure or death.

Postoperative Care

Several preoperative measures are continued postoperatively. Weigh the client immediately after the operation and then daily. Measure and record abdominal girth daily. Urine output is recorded hourly.

Furosemide may be administered immediately after surgery and again if urine output falls or peripheral edema is evident. Hematocrit values are monitored every 4 hours during the first postoperative day so the extent of hemodilution can be evaluated. A transfusion of packed red cells may be ordered. A vein is kept open for quick access if complications arise. To prevent fluid overload, a minidrip tubing setup is preferred, although infusion pumps may also be used. The amount infused should not exceed 125 mL per 8 hours.

After the first 24 hours, the nurse tightly applies an abdominal binder to promote removal of fluid. Intake–output records, prophylactic antibiotic therapy, and 24-hour urine collections are also continued. Ascitic fluid for analysis is drawn once daily for 2 days and then weekly.

The nurse can begin teaching the client how to inhale against resistance to facilitate the flow of ascitic fluid through the shunt. Having the client use a blow bottle will make instruction easier. The client begins eating a regular low-salt diet. If signs of ammonia toxicity are present, the diet may also be low in protein. Potassium supplementation may be ordered if hypokalemia develops.

Monitoring for complications is a continuing responsibility. Possible complications include cardiac or renal overload, shunt occlusion, disseminated intravascular coagulation (DIC), hemorrhage, infection, and extravasation of ascitic fluid from the incisions.

Discharge planning includes dietary instruction, which may reinforce the dietitian's teaching or may originate with the nurse. Clients should demonstrate ability to do the breathing exercises and must be shown how to maintain records of daily weights and temperatures. Reassure clients that daily living activities, including sexual relations, can be resumed as tolerated.

PORTAL–SYSTEMIC AND PORTACAVAL SHUNTS

The purpose of shunt procedures is to decompress esophageal varices and maintain optimal portal perfusion. If var-

iceal hemorrhage continues despite attempts to control it by medical means, the client may be a candidate for a portal–systemic or portacaval shunt—not the ideal solution for problems associated with portal hypertension but an option nonetheless. A portacaval shunt permits blood to flow directly into the inferior vena cava so it no longer needs to circumvent the scarred hepatic cells by way of the collateral circulation. (See Chapter 51.) A portal–systemic shunt (such as splenorenal shunt) connects the splenic vein to the renal vein also bypassing the scarred hepatic cells. Since pressure in the portal system is reduced, dilation of the esophageal varices is also reduced, decreasing the risk of hemorrhage.

Clients with portal hypertension are poor surgical risks; however, continued episodes of variceal hemorrhage are associated with an equal or higher mortality rate than the surgery. Nonalcoholic clients respond more favorably than alcoholic clients, and better results are obtained if the procedure is elective rather than an emergency.

Surgical Procedure

Various types of shunting procedures may be performed, depending on the pathological condition. Shunts are classified according to their influence on portal hemodynamics as:

- End-to-side portacaval shunts, by which all portal blood is diverted around the liver and hepatic perfusion is interrupted
- Side-to-side portacaval, mesocaval, and splenorenal shunts, by which only a portion of portal blood flow is diverted but hepatic venous perfusion is interrupted
- Distal splenorenal shunts, by which partial perfusion of the liver is maintained

Schematic illustrations of some shunt procedures are presented in Figure 54–2. Indications for various shunt procedures and their advantages and limitations are compared in Table 54–2.

Implications for the Client

Physiological Implications

The most common complication is hepatic encephalopathy related to impaired detoxification of ammonia, drugs, and toxins after the hepatic circulation has been surgically rerouted. Diminution of metabolic functions of the liver—for example, synthesis of coagulation factors and albumin—and depletion of glycogen stores lead to hypocoagulability of the blood, ascites, and hypoglycemia. Hypovolemia may develop in association with hemorrhage or diuretic therapy. Ascitic pressure on the diaphragm, guarding related to incisional pain, or encephalopathy may cause hypoventilation leading to hypoxemia. Peripheral edema may increase following a mesocaval shunt, in which venous drainage of the lower body is reduced. Nutritional defi-

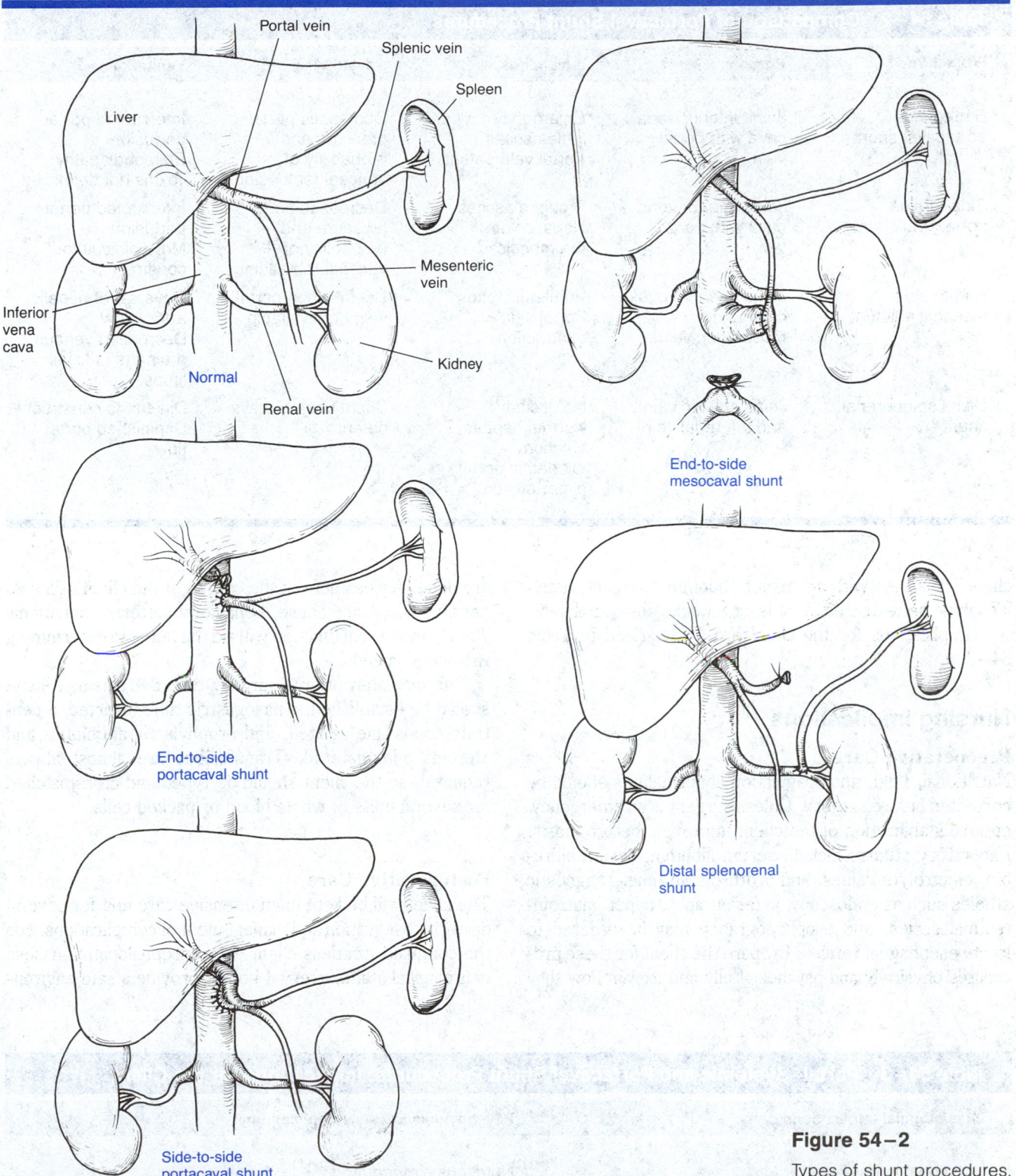

Liver

Portal vein

Splenic vein

Spleen

Mesenteric vein

Inferior vena cava

Kidney

Normal

Renal vein

End-to-side portacaval shunt

Side-to-side portacaval shunt

End-to-side mesocaval shunt

Distal splenorenal shunt

Figure 54–2

Types of shunt procedures.

ciencies related to a history of malnutrition can lead to delayed healing and skin breakdown.

Psychosocial/Lifestyle Implications

Consumption of alcohol must be eliminated and a nutritionally sound diet encouraged. Memory loss, confusion, and lethargy should be expected postoperatively, related to encephalopathy and temporary decrease in hepatic function. These changes may be frightening and upsetting to client and family. Advanced hepatic disease is frequently accompanied by physical and libidinal changes in sexual function, and counseling may be necessary to help the

Table 54–2 Comparison of Portacaval Shunt Procedures

Procedure	Purpose	Indications	Advantages	Limitations
End-to-side portacaval shunt	Joins inferior vena cava with portal vein	Emergency Little ascites Portal vein patent	Decreases portal pressure and probability of variceal rebleeding	Interrupted portal perfusion Encephalopathy Toxins not detoxified
Side-to-side portacaval shunt	Joins inferior vena cava with portal vein	Problem ascites Hepatic vein thrombosis	Decreases portal pressure and probability of variceal rebleeding	Interrupted portal perfusion More difficult to construct
End-to-side mesocaval shunt	Joins inferior vena cava and mesenteric veins	Problem ascites Portal vein obstruction	Useful when portal vein not available	Reversal of hepatic artery flow Decreased venous drainage of lower limbs
Distal splenorenal shunt	Joins splenic vein and left renal vein	No ascites Normal hepatic function Idiopathic portal hypertension	Shunt usually stays patent	Difficult to construct Diminished portal flow

client adjust. As with any major abdominal surgery, activities must be restricted for at least 6 weeks postoperatively.

Implications for the client are summarized in Table 54–3.

Nursing Implications

Preoperative Care

Nutritional, fluid, and coagulation abnormalities should be corrected before surgery. Unless surgery is an emergency, optimal stabilization of the client improves the prognosis. Laboratory studies include serum albumin, serum bilirubin, electrolyte values, and prothrombin time. Diagnostic studies such as endoscopy, arteriography, upper gastrointestinal series, and esophagography may be ordered to locate esophageal varices. Prepare the client for these procedures physically and psychologically and explain how they

are done. Assessment of the course of the client's illness, possible substance abuse, behavioral patterns, nutritional status, and sexual function will aid the nurse in determining the client's needs.

Immediately prior to surgery, effective plasma volume should be established, a nasogastric tube inserted, a central venous line started, and prophylactic antibiotics and steroids administered. Transfusions are almost always required, so the client should be typed and crossmatched for several units of whole blood or packed cells.

Postoperative Care

The client will be kept in an intensive care unit for several days for observation and management of complications. For the confused, restless client with encephalopathy, assess neurological status every 4 hours, provide a safe environ-

Table 54–3 Portal–Systemic and Portacaval Shunt Procedures: Implications for the Client

Physiological Implications	Psychosocial/Lifestyle Implications
Nutritional imbalances	Nutritious diet required
Decreased oxygenation	Abstention from alcohol
Peripheral edema	Memory loss, confusion should be explained to client and significant others and necessary support given
Decreased fluid volume	
Increased clotting time	Altered sexual function
Confusion, lethargy associated with hepatic encephalopathy	Limitation of activity as for any abdominal surgery

ment, reorient often to reality, see that protein intake has been restricted, and administer neomycin and lactulose as prescribed. Care for the client with alteration in thought processes is discussed in detail in Chapter 52.

If injections cannot be avoided, small-gauge needles should be used. Vitamin K administration may be ordered to decrease the risk of hemorrhage. Both stools and secretions from the nasogastric tube should be regularly tested for indications of internal hemorrhage; platelets may have to be administered. Blood glucose levels should be monitored and 10% dextrose given if hypoglycemia occurs. Total parenteral nutrition with amino acid solution (Travasol) and 25% dextrose with added vitamins, minerals, and trace elements may be used to maintain blood glucose levels and to correct nutritional deficiencies. A low-sodium diet or intravenous infusions may be prescribed to minimize peripheral edema and ascites formation. More detailed discussion of these possible complications may be found in Chapter 52.

LIVER RESECTION

A liver resection, or lobectomy, is a serious operation performed only when a lesion—usually a neoplasm—can be totally excised. Resection is not indicated for metastasized malignancies. Occasionally, a large hepatic abscess may be resected if antimicrobial therapy and percutaneous drainage have been unsuccessful in eradicating an infection.

A client can survive with only 10% of the liver functioning; complete destruction or removal of the liver is not compatible with life. The liver has unique regenerative capacities. Some sources have reported regeneration within 6 months of a successful resection of 90% of liver tissue. Resection is most successful, however, when less tissue is removed. If as little as 20% of hepatic tissue is resected, regeneration takes place within months.

Surgical Procedure

Liver resections involve considerable risk of massive hemorrhage followed, within minutes, by death. To reduce this risk, hypothermia is commonly employed to slow down metabolism and restrict circulation.

For a right lobectomy, a large thoracoabdominal incision is required to expose the right lobe. Hemorrhage and pulmonary complications commonly accompany this type of incision. A large abdominal incision is made for a left lobectomy; evisceration is a possible additional complication of this approach.

Once the liver has been exposed, all large vessels are ligated or cauterized to prevent severe hemorrhage before the tissue is removed. Once the resection is completed, control of hemorrhage remains a primary concern. Occasionally, an incompletely ligated vessel may hemorrhage after the incision is closed. If the client's vital signs suggest shock or hemorrhage, a return to the operating room may be indicated.

Implications for the Client

Physiological Implications

Because of the homeostatic functions of the liver, meticulous postoperative care will be needed to prevent complications and correct metabolic abnormalities. The client should be made aware of the seriousness of the surgery. Prepare the client for the monitoring and supportive instrumentation that will be in place following the surgery and for the possibly frightening and disorienting atmosphere of the intensive care unit.

Common complications include cardiopulmonary failure, shock, liver dysfunction, and hemorrhage. Metabolism of carbohydrates, proteins, and fats may be impaired. Hypoglycemia is common, requiring close monitoring of blood glucose levels and administration of intravenous glucose. Drugs that are toxic to the liver must be avoided. (A list of hepatotoxic medications is in Chapter 52.)

Pain is a major problem for the client for the first 3 to 7 postoperative days. Its control is more challenging because of medication restrictions related to hepatotoxicity. Coughing and deep breathing may be so painful that pneumonia develops or other pulmonary problems, such as pneumothorax or collapse of a lung, occur because of accumulated secretions. A chest tube may have to be inserted to reexpand the lung. (Pulmonary complications and related nursing care are discussed in Unit Three).

Psychosocial/Lifestyle Implications

The importance of good nutrition cannot be emphasized enough. Usually, a lobectomy is performed to remove a tumor; the client with a diagnosis of cancer requires a great deal of support and encouragement. (See Chapter 12.) As with any abdominal surgery, activities are limited for at least 6 weeks after surgery. The client cannot return to work, lift heavy objects, or perform activities such as vacuuming during this recovery period. Lobectomy has no direct effect on sexual activity. Once the incision has healed and pain is minimal or absent, the client will be able to engage in whatever sexual activities were customary for him or her prior to surgery.

Client implications of liver resection are summarized in Table 54–4.

Nursing Implications

Preoperative Care

The nurse is the key person in helping the client meet physical and emotional needs. Abnormalities related to nutrition, fluid and electrolyte levels, and coagulation must be corrected before surgery. Several laboratory and diagnostic studies will need to be done. The nurse prepares the client for these procedures and explains why and how they are done. Usually, a bowel preparation procedure of cathartics, enemas, and intestinal antibiotics is begun 2 days before surgery.

Table 54–4 Liver Resection: Implications for the Client	
Physiological Implications	**Psychosocial/Lifestyle Implications**
Hemorrhage leading to shock	Emotional support needed
Pneumonia; other pulmonary complications	Good nutrition required
Cardiac complications	Must avoid alcohol and hepatotoxins
Hypoglycemia	Activities limited postsurgically as for any abdominal operation
Susceptibility to hepatotoxins	With diagnosis of malignancy, client and family require guidance, explanation, and support; coping strategies should be planned
Pain	
Rapid regeneration of hepatic tissue	

Postoperative Care

Postoperative care includes measures appropriate for any abdominal or thoracic procedure. Constant attention is needed to correct metabolic abnormalities and prevent complications, especially during the first 72 postoperative hours. Clients are often assigned to the intensive care unit during the immediate postoperative period. The family and significant others may require the support of the nurse as they cope with the critical diagnosis and serious surgery. Discharge planning is consistent with that for any abdominal or thoracic procedure; see relevant chapters for detailed discussion. The nurse should emphasize the importance of avoiding alcohol and hepatotoxins.

INSTALLATION OF HEPATIC ARTERIAL LINE

As discussed in Chapter 53, the hepatic arterial line provides a route for administering chemotherapeutic agents directly to the liver without dilution in the bloodstream. Systemic side effects are minimized by hepatic detoxification.

Surgical Procedure

The client is kept NPO and sedated prior to this procedure. An intraarterial catheter is inserted under fluoroscopic guidance via one of three routes:

- Through the antecubital fossa into the brachial artery, then to the subclavian artery, into the aorta, and finally into the hepatic artery
- From the groin area via the femoral artery and aorta into the hepatic artery
- Through the abdomen into the hepatic artery

Once the catheter has been inserted properly, it is sutured into place. X-rays are used to verify placement of the catheter; these are often repeated daily while the catheter is in place.

Insertion via the abdomen or the antecubital fossa has the advantage of allowing the client more freedom of movement. If the catheter is inserted into the groin, bed rest

is mandatory. Chemotherapeutic agents are administered, usually over a period of 5 days, and the catheter is removed when the chemotherapy has been completed.

Implications for the Client

Physiological Implications

Because the catheter is inserted via the arteries, hemorrhage and occlusion are possible complications. Vital signs and circulatory status must be monitored frequently. If continuity of the tubing is interrupted, hemorrhage, air embolism, or infection can occur. If the catheter is displaced, chemotherapeutic agents, most of which are toxic or caustic, might be misdirected.

Psychosocial/Lifestyle Implications

Mobility and independence are reduced when a hepatic artery line is in place because the area where the catheter exits must be immobilized. (See Nursing Implications.)

Administration of chemotherapy carries all the implications associated with cancer, and the client will need the best possible emotional support. Nursing considerations related to the psychosocial effects of cancer are discussed in Chapter 12.

Physiological and psychosocial/lifestyle implications of this procedure are summarized in Table 54–5.

Nursing Implications

Preoperative Care

Preoperatively, the nurse instructs the client and significant others about the procedure, offers support as for any surgical procedure, and reviews the results of coagulation studies. If bleeding times are prolonged, vitamin K therapy may be prescribed for several days prior to the procedure.

Postoperative Care

Postoperative nursing care includes maintaining the patency of the line and monitoring for complications. A pressurized infusion containing heparin, usually in 5% dextrose and water, is continued while the line is in place. (Pressure is necessary to keep the solution running and to prevent

Table 54–5 Installation of Hepatic Arterial Line: Implications for the Client	
Physiological Implications	**Psychosocial/Lifestyle Implications**
Chemotherapy administered directly to tumor Fewer systemic side effects of chemotherapy Complications include hemorrhage, catheter displacement, infection, air embolism, decreased arterial circulation	Restricted mobility and independence while line is in place Side effects of chemotherapy Client and significant others require emotional support with diagnosis of cancer

thrombosis.) Secure all tubing connections and be sure there is no tension on the tubing. Death from hemorrhage can ensue in minutes if the tubing becomes disconnected. As a precaution, a hemostat should be kept near the client at all times, and client and family should be taught how to clamp the tubing.

If the catheter exits at the antecubital fossa, the client's arm and shoulder must be immobilized in a sling to prevent dislodgement of the catheter. An arm board, which permits shoulder movement, does not provide sufficient immobilization. If the line exits at the groin, bed rest with the leg straight out at all times is necessary. Check pedal or radial pulses, depending on the catheter site every 1 to 2 hours to ascertain that circulation is adequate in the immobilized limb. Vital signs are taken every 2 to 4 hours to monitor for possible hemorrhage or development of an infection.

Two common chemotherapeutic agents, doxorubicin (Adriamycin) and 5-fluorouracil, are associated with severe side effects requiring nursing interventions for comfort, alleviation of vomiting, and emotional support.

LIVER TRANSPLANTATION

Liver transplantation is a relatively new technique that may be considered for persons with liver dysfunction who are free of infection, malignancy, severe atherosclerosis, or cardiopulmonary disease. Although infants with potentially fatal hepatic and biliary disorders are prime candidates, clients with cirrhosis or chronic hepatitis are also potential candidates.

Surgical Procedure

To be usable for transplantation, a liver must be obtained from a donor who is brain dead but free of disease. Also, the donor's blood pressure and volume must be maintained at levels sufficient to sustain a 3-hour operation for removal of the liver. Ideally, the donor is smaller in size than the intended recipient because a liver in late stages of disease is smaller than a normal liver.

Two transplantation techniques are possible: (1) The diseased liver can be removed and a donor liver placed in the same area of the right upper quadrant of the abdomen. (2) The diseased liver is left in place and the donor liver

placed in the groin or pelvis. Both techniques require reconstruction of the biliary drainage system. Immunosuppressive therapy is usually instituted prior to surgery and continued after revascularization and total hemostasis have been achieved.

Implications for the Client

Physiological Implications

Once the transplant has been completed, the client's condition will begin to improve. Ascites will diminish and liver function will return to normal—provided the complications of rejection, infection, or occlusion of vessels do not arise. Intensive monitoring is required for several days to 2 weeks after transplantation surgery. Mechanical ventilation must be provided, and ECG and arterial monitoring is required. Laboratory values are assessed frequently.

Immunosuppressive drugs such as prednisone have side effects that affect the client's appearance. Cushing's syndrome (moon face, thinning of skin and hair, fluid retention, buffalo hump) and osteoporosis are some of the characteristics associated with long-term corticosteroid therapy.

Cyclosporine, a new drug isolated from soil fungus, has been used for prophylaxis of organ rejection in kidney, liver, and heart transplants. It seems to suppress only that part of the immune system that rejects foreign tissue. It has no effect on the body's ability to fight infection. Cyclosporine is given orally or IV and works well only in conjunction with corticosteroids.

Psychosocial/Lifestyle Implications

Liver transplantation is an extremely serious operation with grave risks, performed only in clients who are critically ill to begin with. The experience is emotionally draining for client and family. Significant others will be anxious about the client's condition, especially in the early postsurgical period when visits must be strictly limited.

After hospital discharge, transplant recipients must continue to limit exposure to crowds and sick persons because immunosuppressive therapy significantly decreases resistance to infection. They should avoid shopping malls, theaters, and large restaurants, particularly at the height of the cold and flu season.

Immunosuppressants must be taken daily; rejection can occur after one dose of drugs has been omitted. For this reason, if the client is nauseated and the medication cannot be taken by mouth, it should be administered intravenously by a health professional or intramuscularly by the client or significant other. Signs of impending rejection are shown in Table 54–6.

Alterations in body image related to immunosuppressive therapy are difficult to cope with. Clients may be disturbed by the idea that a portion of their body once belonged to someone else. The possibility of rejection poses a constant threat accompanied by fear of death. A renal transplant recipient whose kidney is rejected can resume dialysis. The liver transplant recipient has no such alternative if rejection cannot be reversed.

Client implications related to liver transplantation are summarized in Table 54–7.

Nursing Implications

Preoperative Care
Transplant candidates must undergo rigorous physiological tests, including liver function studies, coagulation studies,

and hemoglobin and electrolyte profiles. They are also given psychological tests and interviewed to determine if they are capable of coping with the stress of the surgery, possible rejection, and the concept of having a part of someone else's body. The nurse can offer support during this testing phase and explain the need for the tests to the client and significant others.

The nurse is also the key person in providing information about the surgical procedure, the mechanisms of rejection, and postoperative monitoring and medications. The nurse also helps prepare the client and significant others for the lifestyle changes that will occur once the surgery is successfully completed.

Postoperative Care
Intensive postoperative nursing care is required for the transplant recipient. This is best provided in a transplant unit, where nurses are accustomed to caring for transplant clients and have specialized knowledge of the unique problems associated with transplantation. Mechanical ventilation and constant ECG and arterial pressure monitoring

---

Table 54–6   Signs of Organ Rejection in Liver Transplant Recipients

Sign	Related Comments
Elevated lymphocyte level	Sensitized lymphocytes destroy cells of transplanted organ
Decreased hepatic vascular perfusion	Can be detected by dye clearance studies discussed in previous chapter
Elevated temperature	Part of inflammatory process of rejection
Abnormal liver function tests, for example, SGOT, SGPT, indirect bilirubin	Client would have icterus, mahogany-colored urine, acholic stools
Enlargement and tenderness of liver	
Hypertension	
Tachycardia	
Altered results of liver scan	

Table 54–7   Liver Transplantation: Implications for the Client

Physiological Implications	Psychosocial/Lifestyle Implications
Improved condition	Experience is emotionally draining for client and significant others
Rejection of transplant	
Infection	Client alone during critical hours; requires support, encouragement, and human contact
Occlusion of vessels	Immunosuppressive drug regimen must be meticulously followed without interruption
Cushing's syndrome and other side effects associated with steroid therapy	Alterations in body image
	Fear of organ rejection and death
	Exposure to crowds must be limited.

will be required for the first 48 to 72 hours. Signs of rejection are monitored through liver function tests such as the SGOT, bilirubin studies, liver scans, and cholangiography. Coagulation studies, electrolyte levels, and hemoglobin profiles are also watched closely.

Bed rest for 24 to 48 hours is important. Intravenous fluids, antibiotics, and immunosuppressive drugs are administered by the nurse. The nurse must also be alert for signs of rejection such as an elevated temperature, swollen and tender liver, and abnormalities of coagulation or liver function. If signs of rejection occur, dosages of immunosuppressants are increased.

Considering the many responsibilities of physical care, the nurse may find little time to attend to the client's need for human interaction, especially in the early postsurgical hours when the client is alone and separated from family and familiar stimuli. These considerations are discussed in some of the annotated readings listed at the end of this chapter.

Family members must be kept informed of the client's condition. Their need for encouragement and support often can best be met by nurses who are caring for their loved one. As the client's condition improves, visiting time can be extended. Client and significant others will need to know what medications will be prescribed, what their purpose is, and how important it is to follow instructions conscientiously. In most units, clients take their medications and keep logs of important information such as temperature, before they are discharged. These practices assist the nurse in evaluating the client's comprehension and enhance the client's chances for success as an outpatient.

The importance of never missing a single dose of immunosuppressive agents must be stressed repeatedly. Discharge teaching should include instructions for obtaining an intravenous or intramuscular administration of the immunosuppressant if nausea or vomiting prevent taking of oral medication. Since a health care provider may not be immediately available, the nurse should teach the client and a family member how to give an intramuscular injection. The technique of giving an injection can be practiced with sterile saline prior to discharge.

Discharge planning should also include the importance of avoiding crowds and fatigue and information about a special diet, if one has been prescribed.

PERCUTANEOUS DRAINAGE OF ABSCESSES

Until recently, surgical incision and drainage was the standard procedure for drainage of pyogenic hepatic abscesses that did not respond to antibiotic therapy. Percutaneous drainage with either intermittent or continuous catheterization is now more common and successful.

Surgical Procedure

Preparation of the client and insertion of the stylet are similar to liver biopsy. (See Chapter 52.) Once the stylet is withdrawn, purulent material can be drained from the abscess. The drained material is cultured, and appropriate antibiotic therapy is initiated. The drainage procedure may be repeated again in 5 to 10 days as needed until the client becomes afebrile. The combination of percutaneous drainage and antibiotic therapy usually clears up the abscess with minimal risk. Although continuous catheterization may be used, it restricts the client's mobility and provides an avenue for reinfection.

Implications for the Client

Percutaneous drainage presents little risk for the client. The principal drawbacks are temporary discomfort when the stylet enters the liver and the inconveniences of intravenous antibiotic therapy. Pain diminishes as the abscess is resolved. Analgesic medications are restricted because of the risk of hepatotoxicity. Hemorrhage is a possible complication.

Nursing Implications

Nursing care is similar to that for the client who has had a liver biopsy, including monitoring of vital signs, assessments, and comfort measures. (See Chapter 52.) Additional measures include monitoring temperature to determine whether the infection is clearing and administering antibiotic therapy.

Section II: Surgical Approaches to Disorders Affecting the Gallbladder

CHOLECYSTOSTOMY

A **cholecystostomy** is the surgical formation of an opening in the gallbladder. A cholecystostomy is performed to relieve acute or chronic cholecystitis in clients who would be at great risk if cholecystectomy were performed.

Surgical Procedure

Under general anesthesia, the gallbladder is incised, and calculi, bile, and purulent material are removed. A drainage tube is sutured into place.

Implications for the Client

Physiological Implications

The client will be relieved of pain and infection. Hemorrhage is the most common complication. As with any major surgery, pneumonia can develop if the client does not cough and deep breathe sufficiently. Fat absorption may be impaired, possibly leading to deficiency of fat-soluble vitamins.

Psychosocial/Lifestyle Implications

Restrictions on activity and mandated changes in diet may be difficult for the client to adjust to. Other psychosocial considerations are those associated with any major surgical procedure. (See Chapter 14.)

Implications related to cholecystostomy are summarized in Table 54–8.

Nursing Implications

Preoperative Care

Preoperative care is similar to that for any surgical procedure, including instructing the client in coughing and deep breathing.

Postoperative Care

A major nursing responsibility in the postoperative period is connecting the drainage apparatus and ensuring its patency, sterility, and preventing dislodgment. The client will require intravenous therapy, and vitamin K may be prescribed if clotting abnormalities occur. Administration of medications and nursing measures for relief of pain, nausea, and vomiting will be required.

Pneumonia is a common complication. Assist the client with turning, coughing, and deep breathing by helping the client splint the incision and administering analgesics.

Discharge instructions should include information about required medications (vitamins, anticholinergics, antispasmodics), low-fat diet, skin care, and aseptic technique for dressing changes around the drainage tube. The client should also know signs and symptoms of potential complications such as infection or dislodgement of the drainage tube, which generally remains in place until the client is well enough to tolerate a cholecystectomy.

CHOLECYSTECTOMY AND CHOLEDOCHOSTOMY

A **cholecystectomy** is a resection of the gallbladder. A **choledochostomy** involves incision of the common bile duct for removal of biliary calculi and the insertion of a T-tube. These operations are performed on some clients who have acute or chronic cholelithiasis and cholecystitis.

The client with acute cholecystitis usually requires cholecystectomy. The optimal timing of the surgery remains controversial. When perforation or empyema is suspected, immediate surgery is indicated. Delayed surgical intervention is prudent in clients with a questionable diagnosis or in clients who are poor surgical risks. The latter group may be managed with cholecystostomy and gallbladder drainage, with elective cholecystectomy at a later date.

Cholelithiasis is *not* an automatic indication for surgical intervention. If the gallstones cause no symptoms ("silent" gallstones), cholecystectomy is usually not recommended. Small gallstones are associated with greater risk than large gallstones because small stones are more likely to move into the bile ducts, causing obstruction.

Surgical Procedure

For a cholecystectomy, the most common approach is through a right subcostal incision. The gallbladder is dissected from the liver after ligation of the cystic duct and related vasculature.

For a choledochostomy, an incision is made into the common bile duct, and calculi as well as any purulent material are removed. A T-tube is inserted (Figure 54–3) to allow drainage of bile and to maintain the patency of the common duct during the postsurgical period, when edema develops at the operative site. The arms of the T are inserted into the hepatic duct (leading from the liver) and the common bile duct (leading into the duodenum). The tail of the T exits from a stab wound in the abdomen and is attached to a drainage collection system. Drainage of 200 to 500 mL of bile during the first 24 hours is considered normal; the amount of drainage then diminishes. A T-tube cholangiogram is usually performed 7 days postoperatively (see Chapter 52). If findings are normal, the T-tube is removed and the client discharged the following day.

Table 54–8 Cholecystostomy: Implications for the Client	
Physiological Implications	**Psychosocial/Lifestyle Implications**
Relieves pain	Fat in diet restricted
Relieves infection	Activity limited
Client may have problems related to deficiency of bile: coagulation problems, inadequate absorption and digestion of fats and fat-soluble vitamins	Client usually too ill to work or perform all ADL
Pneumonia and hemorrhage are possible complications	Drainage tube in place until client is well enough to tolerate surgical removal of gallbladder

Implications for the Client

Physiological Implications
Although the client may experience considerable pain for several days after surgery, cholecystectomy and choledochostomy ultimately remove the source of pain and inflammation. Pneumonia is the most common complication related to this surgery; because of the subcostal location of the incision, coughing and deep breathing are painful.

With the gallbladder removed, lipid digestion relies solely on bile produced by the liver. Gone are the concentrating and storage regulation formerly provided by the gallbladder. (See Chapter 51.) Fats are not digested completely because bile reaches the duodenum in unconcentrated form. Flatulence is common. Fat intake must be limited for 4 to 6 weeks after surgery.

Psychosocial/Lifestyle Implications
The client may find it difficult to restrict fat intake if he or she has been accustomed to a high-fat diet. Activities, especially lifting, vacuuming, and related activities, are restricted for at least 8 weeks. Most clients can return to their jobs after 8 weeks.

Implications of these procedures are summarized in Table 54–9.

Nursing Implications

Preoperative Care
In addition to the usual preoperative concerns, the nurse has several further responsibilities for the client undergoing cholecystectomy and choledochostomy. Vitamin K will be prescribed if clotting abnormalities are found. A prolonged prothrombin time or positive results of reagent strip tests (Hemastix) performed on emesis should alert the nurse to coagulation problems. Intravenous infusions are started 24 to 48 hours before surgery to hydrate the client, correct electrolyte imbalances, and increase hepatic glycogen stores.

Relieving the client's pain is another nursing goal. Meperidine (Demerol) may be used, although some physicians prefer to prescribe nitroglycerin or phenobarbital. Nitroglycerin, given sublingually, relieves pain by relaxing smooth muscle. Phenobarbital sedates the client and also relaxes smooth muscle. Morphine is not used because it is

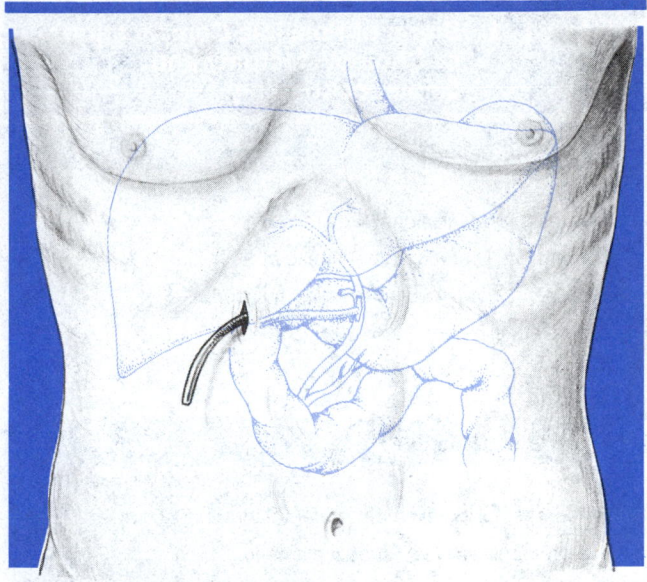

Figure 54–3

T-tube placement.

believed to increase spasms at the sphincter of Oddi. Nursing comfort measures such as repositioning, providing distraction, and removing noxious stimuli from the environment to reduce nausea may also be employed.

A nasogastric tube and suction are often prescribed to relieve abdominal distention and remove gastric juices that stimulate the secretion of cholecystokinin. Antiemetics are also prescribed.

In addition to the teaching accompanying any major surgical procedure (see Chapter 14), preoperative teaching includes explanation of the nature and function of the T-tube. The client should expect to be given intravenous infusions for several days following the operation, until oral ingestion of food and fluid can be tolerated. Because of the location of the incision, teaching the client how to splint the incision during coughing and deep breathing is especially important.

The client is placed on NPO status at midnight. (Often these clients are already NPO because a nasogastric tube has been inserted.)

Table 54–9 Cholecystectomy and Choledochostomy: Implications for the Client	
Physiological Implications	**Psychosocial/Lifestyle Implications**
Relieves pain	Low-fat diet
Relieves inflammation	Heavy lifting, some ADL restricted
Fat absorption impaired	May have T-tube in place when discharged
Complications may include pneumonia, hemorrhage, or thrombosis	

Box 54–1 Signs of Possible Complications of Cholecystectomy and Choledochostomy

Signs of Infection

Redness ⎱
Warmth ⎬ at incisional area, site of drainage tube, or site of previous intravenous infusions
Swelling ⎰

Temperature higher than 100°F (37.7°C)

Purulent drainage at T-tube site

Signs of Obstruction

Tenderness or pain in right upper quadrant of abdomen

Bile drainage around T-tube if clamped

Nausea and vomiting

Acholic (clay-colored) stools

Jaundice

Mahogany-colored urine

Signs of Tube Dislodgement

Decreased drainage

Evidence that tube has shifted position

Postoperative Care

As with any abdominal surgery, the goal is to prevent complications. Taking vital signs and assessing for hemorrhage are important responsibilities. Pneumonia is a common complication of gallbladder surgery. Encourage the client to take ten deep breaths per hour and to cough. The nurse assists the client in splinting the incision to reduce pain when coughing.

Care of the T-Tube. Care of the T-tube is primarily the responsibility of the nurse. The tube must remain attached to the drainage collection bag, it must not be kinked, and the contents of the bag should be measured at least once during each shift. During the initial 24-hour post-surgical period, drainage of 200 to 500 mL is normal. When a few days have elapsed, such amounts may indicate obstruction of the common bile duct.

Placement of the T-tube is important. Its purpose is to form a passage so bile can drain out under pressure. Make sure the tube is not kinked. It should be taped on the abdomen slightly below the T-tube wound site. Taping it too low creates too much drainage. Taping it too high prevents free drainage and allows fluid to flow back into the common bile duct.

Once the client resumes eating, the T-tube may be clamped to aid digestion. It is usually removed 7 to 10 days following surgery. Some clients are discharged with a T-tube in place to drain excess bile or to remove small stones that could lodge in the common bile duct.

Assessing for Complications. The nurse must assess for complications unique to the biliary tract. The appearance of icterus may indicate injury to the ducts or obstruction of a duct by a calculus. Acholic stools may also be related to duct injury or obstruction. Excessive T-tube drainage several days after surgery might suggest obstruction of the common bile duct. Excessive loss of bile may necessitate recycling the client's bile by straining it and adding it to juice for oral ingestion. Fever and abdominal pain may be symptoms of infection, whether wound infection or bile peritonitis. These symptoms may also be related to pancreatitis from trauma to the pancreas during surgery. Hemorrhage is a possible complication related to decreased absorption of vitamin K and decreased synthesis of prothrombin.

Discharge Planning. General discharge teaching is similar to that for any abdominal surgery. Special points to emphasize include avoiding fatigue, lifting, and excessive exercise during the first 8 weeks. Fat intake should be limited.

Clients who are to be sent home with a T-tube in place should be instructed in its care. Remind the client to be sure the tube is not kinked or obstructed, to tape it securely, and to place it correctly. Although a daily shower provides adequate cleansing of the T-tube site, additional cleansing with an antiseptic solution helps prevent infection. A dry, sterile dressing is placed over the wound and tube and then taped into place. It should be changed daily and more often if it becomes soiled or wet. Povidone–iodine ointment may be applied to the wound site. Zinc oxide may be applied where the tube exits and on nearby skin to prevent skin irritation from bile.

Being discharged with a T-tube may cause considerable anxiety. Drawing a picture of the biliary system with the T-tube in place, explaining the function of the tube, and teaching the client how to unclamp the tube and measure drainage may alleviate fears. Sometimes the tube is kept clamped at all times. Clients should also be prepared for the possibility of a repeat cholangiogram after discharge.

Tell the client to consult a health care provider regarding signs of possible complications, such as infection, obstruction, or dislodgement of the tube. A list of signs is provided in Box 54–1. Before the client is discharged, measure the length of the T-tube from the wound site to the connecting tube. The client who uses this measurement as a baseline will be able to tell whether the tube has moved or been dislodged.

Chapter Highlights

The LeVeen shunt works on the principle of diffusion along a pressure gradient to reinfuse ascitic fluid into the venous system by way of a pressure-sensitive valve.

Possible complications associated with insertion of a LeVeen shunt are hemodilution, cardiac or renal overload, and infection.

Nursing care for the client with a LeVeen shunt includes careful monitoring of intake-output, abdominal girth, weight, electrolyte levels, and hematocrit.

Portal–systemic or portacaval shunts are used as a last resort for controlling portal hypertension and variceal hemorrhage, but the rate of survival is not much better than for clients treated medically.

A liver resection, or lobectomy, is done only if the lesion, an abscess or tumor, can be totally excised.

Prior to any hepatic or biliary surgery, coagulation abnormalities, fluid and electrolyte balance, and cardiopulmonary abnormalities must be corrected.

Postoperative nursing care of the client with a liver resection includes carrying out prescribed interventions for correction of metabolic imbalances, assessing for complications as for any abdominal or thoracic surgery, keeping significant others informed, and providing encouragement and emotional support for client and family.

The hepatic arterial line provides for administration of chemotherapeutic agents directly to a hepatic lesion, reducing systemic side effects by means of hepatic detoxification.

Nursing care for the client with a hepatic arterial line involves maintaining the patency of the line, immobilizing the site of entry, checking pulses in the affected areas, providing nursing comfort measures, and supporting client and significant others through the stresses related to a diagnosis of cancer.

The client who receives a liver transplant will require lifelong immunosuppression, but symptoms related to liver dysfunction will be alleviated once the immediate postoperative hazards associated with acute rejection, infection, and hemorrhage are overcome.

Liver transplant recipients are best cared for in a transplant unit where mechanical ventilation and continual ECG and arterial pressure monitoring can be provided. The client will require intravenous fluid administration and careful monitoring of homeostatic functions.

The nurse must teach client and family about medications, daily records, and signs of transplant rejection and verify their comprehension before the client with a liver transplant can be discharged.

During a cholecystostomy, the gallbladder is opened, and calculi, bile, and purulent matter are removed. A bile drainage tube is usually inserted.

During a cholecystectomy, the gallbladder is excised. This procedure is often done in conjunction with a choledochostomy, in which the common and hepatic bile ducts are explored and obstructions are removed.

A T-tube is often inserted into the common bile duct after gallbladder surgery to allow bile to drain and to maintain ductal patency in the presence of edema.

Preoperative nursing care for the client having gallbladder surgery involves (1) administering measures to correct coagulation, fluid, and electrolyte abnormalities; (2) relieving pain; (3) reducing nausea and vomiting; and (4) providing preoperative teaching, especially regarding coughing and deep breathing.

Postoperative care for the client with gallbladder surgery includes (1) preventing complications including hemorrhage, thrombus formation, abdominal distention, and especially pneumonia; (2) promoting relief from pain and nausea; (3) caring for the T-tube apparatus; and (4) providing discharge teaching.

Bibliography

Cooperman AM (editor): Liver, spleen, and pancreas. *Surg Clin North Am* (Feb) 1981; 61:1.

Klopp A: Shunting malignant ascites. *Am J Nurs* 1984; 84:212–213.

McDermott WV Jr: *Surgery of the Liver and Portal Circulation.* Philadelphia: Lea & Febiger, 1974.

Matolo NM (editor): Biliary tract disease. *Surg Clin North Am* (Aug) 1981; 61:4.

Munoz E et al: Surgonomics: The cost of cholecystectomy. *Surgery* 1984; 96:642–647.

Petersdorf RG et al: *Harrison's Principles of Internal Medicine,* 10th ed. New York: McGraw-Hill, 1983.

Taylor PD: Liver transplantation. *Am J Nurs* 1981; 81:1672–1673.

Thorpe CJ, Caprini JA: Gallbladder disease: Current trends and treatments. *Am J Nurs* 1980; 80:2181–2185.

Suggested Readings

Clark M, Shapiro D: Master transplanter. *Newsweek* 1982; 99:58. Brief overview of life of Dr Thomas Starzl, the first surgeon to transplant a liver.

Garvey EC, Manganaro M: Nursing implications of hepatic artery infusion. *Cancer Nurs* 1982; 5:51–55. Discusses nursing care; examines small study of procedure.

Jackson BS, Carlisle PM: How post-op complications can burgeon into crisis. *RN* (Jan) 1981; 44:26–32. Discusses complications of cholecystectomy from a nursing perspective.

Klopfenstein ML: Hepatic artery cannulation. *AORN J* 1981; 34:956–964. Describes procedure from an operating room perspective.

The Client With Cholelithiasis

I. Brief Descriptive Data	Mrs June Jones, 44 years old, mother of six children, has been admitted to the hospital with a diagnosis of cholelithiasis. She is mildly icteric, obese, and has nausea and vomiting.

II. Personal Data

Date and Time:	May 15, 1986; 10 a.m.
Full Name:	June Ellen Jones
Social Security Number:	000-00-0000
Address:	1400 Star Rd, Middletown, Iowa
Telephone:	Home: 000-0000
	Work: 000-0000
Sex:	Female
Age:	44
Birthdate:	2-24-42
Marital Status:	Married
Race:	Caucasian
Religion:	Catholic
Occupation:	Part-time accountant
Usual Health Care Provider:	Evan Hanson, MD

III. Health History

Source of Information:	Client
Reliability of Informant:	Reliable
Chief Concern:	Pain in the right upper abdomen with nausea and occasional vomiting after meals.
History of Present Illness:	Two weeks before admission, Mrs Jones developed right upper quadrant abdominal pain that radiated around to the back and was associated with nausea and vomiting after meals. Two days before admission she noticed that her urine was very dark and her stools lighter in color. She had also been more flatulent in the past months. She enjoys fried foods, dairy products, pastries, and chocolate although they have recently caused her some abdominal discomfort after eating. Adheres to a modified low-salt diet because of mild hypertension diagnosed in 1975. Doesn't smoke; usual alcohol intake is 1 to 2 glasses of wine on the weekend. Had 6 full-term pregnancies; kept at least 5 extra pounds after each one; has always had a tendency to be slightly overweight. Takes no medications.

Past Health History:

Childhood:	Usual childhood diseases—measles, mumps, chickenpox
Immunizations:	Polio, 1961; Td, 1978 (dog bite)
Medical Problems:	1975, slightly hypertensive, controlled on modified low-salt diet
Surgeries:	Tonsillectomy, 1948; appendectomy, 1975
Blood Transfusions:	None
Pregnancies:	Para 6, gravida 7, miscarriage 1; all children delivered vaginally; all children weighed under 9 pounds at birth.
Allergies:	Penicillin (hives)
Medications:	None; does not use oral contraceptives
Personal and Social History:	Busy household with active, intelligent children; she has college degree and works 3 days a week for accounting firm; husband has college degree and is corporate executive for Northern Gas Company; enjoys traveling and sailing during the summer.

(continued)

Case Study written by Jane Hokanson Hawks.

The Client With Cholelithiasis

Active lifestyle but doesn't exercise regularly; never smoked; consumes 1 to 2 alcoholic beverages per week; satisfactory sex life; Catholic; rhythm method for birth control; financially stable; close to parents and siblings; husband has no living family.

Top generation (left family):
- 74 A & W
- 67 Hypertension 20 years
- 13 Accident
- 70 Stroke two years ago

Top generation (right family):
- 65 Hypertension; obesity
- 67 Heart attack; obesity
- 62 A & W
- 60 Breast cancer 5 years ago

Middle generation:
- 21 Killed Viet Nam
- 40 A & W
- 36 A & W
- 38 A & W
- 44 A & W (Client)
- 46 A & W

Bottom generation:
- 20 A & W
- 18 A & W
- 15 A & W
- 14 A & W
- 12 A & W
- 7 A & W
- Miscarriage

Key:
- □ Male
- ○ Female
- ●■ Died
- A&W Alive and well
- → Client

Review of Systems: Overall health is generally good except for obesity and slight hypertension, which has been controlled with low-salt diet.

Skin: Some episodes of intense itching in last 48 hours

Cardiovascular: History of hypertension since 1975; BP remains within normal limits on low-salt diet; has never taken BP medication

Gastrointestinal: See HPI

Hematopoietic: States, "I've bruised easily lately."

IV. Physical Assessment

Height: 5 ft 7 in

Weight: 192 lb

Vital Signs: BP 140/90; pulse 84; respirations 20; temperature 100°F (38°C) Overweight, fair-skinned, articulate 44-yr-old w/fe in NAD

Relevant Organ Systems:

Skin: Slightly jaundiced; several bruises 1 to 2 cm in diameter on both lower legs, rt arm

Eyes: Sclerae icteric

Abdomen: Obese; appendectomy scar RLQ; 2 to 4 bowel sounds per minute; soft, tender-to-deep palpation RUQ; no hepatomegaly or splenomegaly; increased tympany throughout

Urinary: Urine dark and frothy

V. Diagnostic Data Laboratory results showed elevated direct bilirubin, alkaline phosphatase, and slightly elevated SGOT and LDH levels. Absence of urine urobilinogen. Because of the high bilirubin values, the oral cholecystogram and intravenous cholangiogram were not helpful in visualizing the gallbladder. An ultrasound of the gallbladder permitted a diagnosis of gallstones to be made. An endoscopic retrograde cholangiopancreatography (ERCP) confirmed the diagnosis and ruled out the presence of a tumor. A cholecystectomy and common bile duct exploration are scheduled.

VI. Preoperative Regimen

Diet: Low-fat, 2 g Na
NPO night before surgery and if nauseated

Medications: Cholestyramine (Questran), 6 g PO q.i.d.
Vitamin K (AquaMEPHYTON), 2 mg IM MWF
IV D5W with 20 mEq of KCl 125 cc/hr
Meperidine (Demerol), 75 to 100 mg IM q. 3 to 4 h. p.r.n. pain
Diphenhydramine (Benadryl), 50 mg PO or IM q. 6 h. p.r.n. for itching

Treatments: Nasogastric tube to low intermittent suction evening before surgery

VII. Nursing Care Plan

Nursing Diagnosis	Client Care Goals	Plan/Nursing Implementation	Expected Outcome
Comfort, alteration in: related to pruritus	Remain comfortable; sleep through the night; tolerate pruritus once cause understood	Ventilation, cotton clothing, no alkaline soaps, whirlpool, emollients; Diphenhydramine 50 mg PO or IM q. 6 h.; teach about bilirubin as cause of pruritus	Relief from itching; incorporate information into daily self-care activities
Fluid volume, alteration in: related to potential for hemorrhage	Remain free from hemorrhage with no further bruising; understand reason for bruising	Vitamin K 2 mg IM MWF; monitor prothrombin time and observe for bleeding; teach about vitamin K and resultant bruising	Prothrombin time within normal limits; absence of further bruising; careful to avoid unnecessary trauma
Nutrition, alteration in: less than body requirements related to nausea and vomiting	Maintain nutritional status	IV fluids; nasogastric tube to low intermittent suction to relieve distention; remove noxious stimuli; administer antiemetics as ordered; mouth care	Relief from nausea and vomiting; fluid and electrolyte balance maintained
Anxiety related to planned surgery	Understand surgical procedure and related treatment; will discuss questions and feelings about upcoming surgery	Teach about surgery; teach about risk factors that contribute to gallstone development; allow to ventilate feelings and ask questions	Minimal anxiety in anticipation of surgery
Knowledge deficit related to preoperative, intraoperative, and postoperative procedures	Understand pre, intra, and postop procedures and explain rationale for each	Explain that client will have IV before and after surgery until tolerating foods again; explain purpose of T-tube; explain reason for deep breathing, coughing, and turning; have client demonstrate coughing with pillow splint; explain what is done during surgical procedure and in recovery room; explain postoperative management in detail regarding: 1. Prevention of complications such as hemorrhage, pneumonia, thrombus formation, abdominal distention 2. Relief of pain 3. Maintaining patency of T-tube	Client and family will be comfortable with each phase of surgical care and participate actively in prevention of postop complications

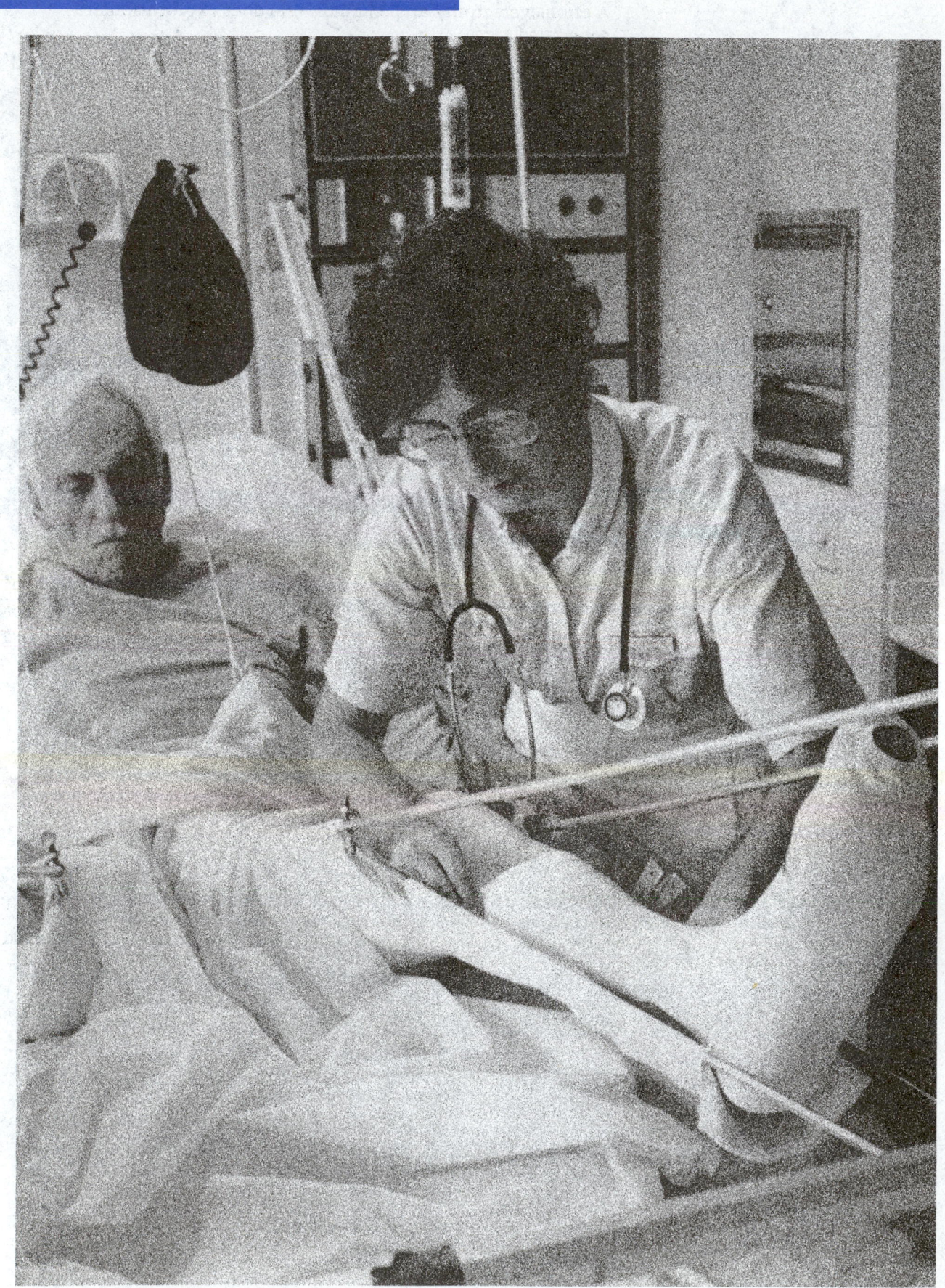

The Client With Musculoskeletal System Dysfunction

Chapter 55

The Musculoskeletal System in Health and Illness

Linda Heim McCausland

The musculoskeletal system is composed of many anatomical structures that work together to produce movement, support, and protection of the body and its parts. These structures include the bones and joints of the skeletal system; the skeletal muscles; and the tendons, ligaments, and other elements that connect muscle to bone or bone to bone.

Section I: Structural and Functional Interrelationships

STRUCTURE AND FUNCTION OF BONES

The human skeletal system has several functions that are reflected in the structure of the bones. The skeleton as a whole provides a framework for supporting the other body tissues. Individual bones may protect vital organs and soft tissues or serve as levers that are moved by attached muscles. Bones are also responsible for hematopoiesis, or production of blood cells, and serve as storage sites for minerals such as calcium and phosphorus. Bones differ from one another in form and in tissue type.

The Form and Parts of a Bone

Bones are classified into four major groups according to shape:

- Long bones, consisting of two knobs connected by a shaft, are the major bones of the limbs.
- Short bones make up the wrist and ankles.
- Flat bones form the ribs and sternum, as well as much of the braincase.
- Irregular bones include the vertebrae and some of the bones of the face and pelvic girdle.

A less common type, called a sesamoid bone, develops within a tendon; the most prominent example of a sesamoid bone is the patella.

The parts of a long bone, such as the femur, are shown in Figure 55–1. The knobby ends of the bone are called epiphyses or heads. The proximal epiphysis is the end closer to the trunk; the distal epiphysis is farther from the trunk. The epiphyses are covered with articular or hyaline cartilage, which is resilient and provides padding for the opposing joint surfaces. The shaft of the bone is known as the diaphysis. Periosteum, a dense white fibrous membrane, covers the diaphysis, providing a surface for the attachment of tendons and ligaments. The inner layer of the periosteum, richly supplied with blood vessels and nerves, contains bone-forming cells called osteoblasts,

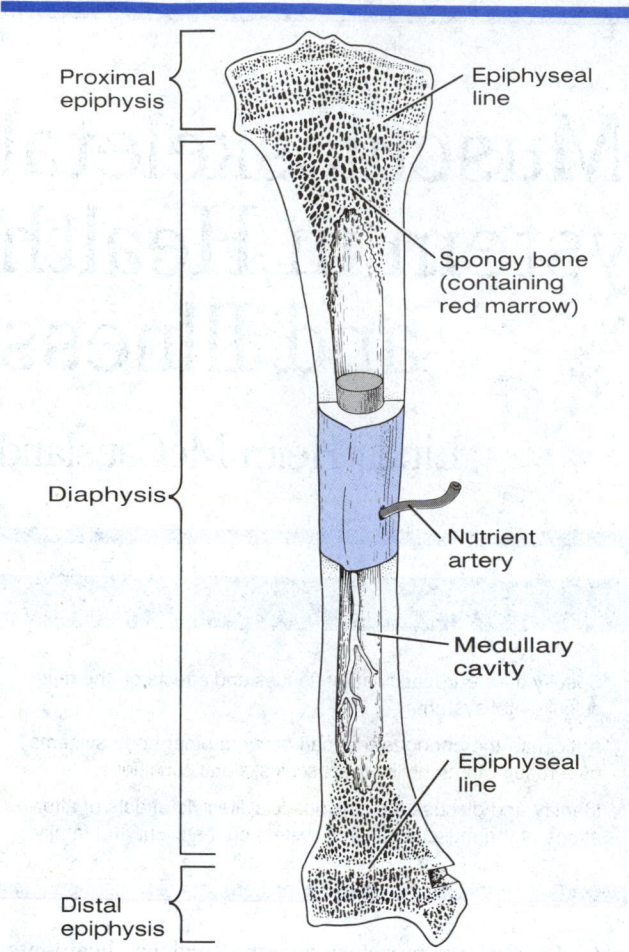

Figure 55–1

Structure of a long bone.

SOURCE: Spence AP, Mason EB: *Human Anatomy and Physiology,* 2nd ed. Menlo Park, CA: Benjamin/Cummings, 1983.

necessary for repair and for increase in growing bone diameter. Between the epiphysis and diaphysis of growing bones is the epiphyseal plate, responsible for growth in length. When growth stops, the epiphyseal plate is replaced by bone. Inside the shaft of a long bone is the medullary canal or cavity, which is filled with yellow bone marrow. The canal is lined with a layer of osteoblasts.

The Structure of Bone Tissue

Bone is a connective tissue and thus is composed of an acellular matrix and cells. The matrix of bone is a network of collagen fibers impregnated with mineral salts, primarily calcium carbonate and calcium phosphate. This combination of fibers and minerals provides bone with its great strength and hardness. The bone cells, called *osteocytes,* are found in spaces within the matrix.

Bone tissue can be either spongy (cancellous) or compact (dense). Spongy bone is porous, resembles a sponge, and contains red bone marrow in its spaces. Short, flat and irregular bones and the epiphyses of long bones are mostly

made of spongy bone. Compact bone, which is much less porous than spongy bone, forms the shafts of long bone as well as a protective layer (cortex) over spongy bone. A microscopic view shows the structural differences in the two types of tissue (Figure 55–2). Spongy bone has an irregular, open-spaced framework made up of thin plates of bone called trabeculae, separated by spaces that contain red marrow in some bones. Osteocytes are found in the spaces; they receive their blood supply from vessels of the periosteum that penetrate the spongy bone. The compact bone of an adult has a concentric structure not present in spongy bone.

Concentric cylindrical layers, or lamellae, of calcified matrix surround a central channel called a haversian canal. The haversian canals run longitudinally through the bone and contain small blood vessels, lymphatics, and nerve fibers. Spaces between the lamellae, known as lacunae, contain the osteocytes. Tiny canals, or canaliculi, connecting the haversian canal and the lacunae bring nourishment and oxygen to the osteocytes and remove wastes. This entire structure—haversian canal, lamellae, lacunae, osteocytes, and canaliculi—is known as a haversian system and is illustrated in Figure 55–3. In compact bone, several haversian systems are adjacent to each other and closely fitted together. Nerve fibers and blood vessels from the periosteum connect with those in the haversian canals and medullary cavity.

Bone Growth and Turnover

Bones grow in length at the epiphyseal plates. In a growing long bone cartilage, cells proliferate rapidly in the epiphyseal plates and are gradually replaced by bone cells through a process called **ossification.** In this manner, the shafts of the long bones continue to increase in length until a person is about 20 to 25 years old, when the epiphyses close and ossification is complete. A process called *remodeling*—selective bone resorption and formation that maintains the epiphyses at a relatively constant size—occurs as the bone increases in length.

Bones grow in circumference as bone-forming *osteoblasts* deposit new layers of bone tissue around the outside. At the same time, bone-destroying cells called *osteoclasts* dissolve away bone cells on the inner aspect of the bone, increasing the size of the medullary cavity.

Bone is a dynamic structure that is continuously remodeled by bone cell activity. Old bone is removed and new bone is formed through the processes of *resorption* (eating away) and *deposition,* performed by osteoclasts and osteoblasts respectively. The replacement of bone tissue through resorption and deposition is called *turnover.* The process of resorption may be more active in the elderly, the inactive, and in some disease states. In the normally active adult, the two processes are generally balanced.

Bone formation and remodeling occur in response to the stresses exerted on the bone. During prolonged periods of bed rest, the forces applied to bones are changed, and the bones may become fragile and lose structural mass.

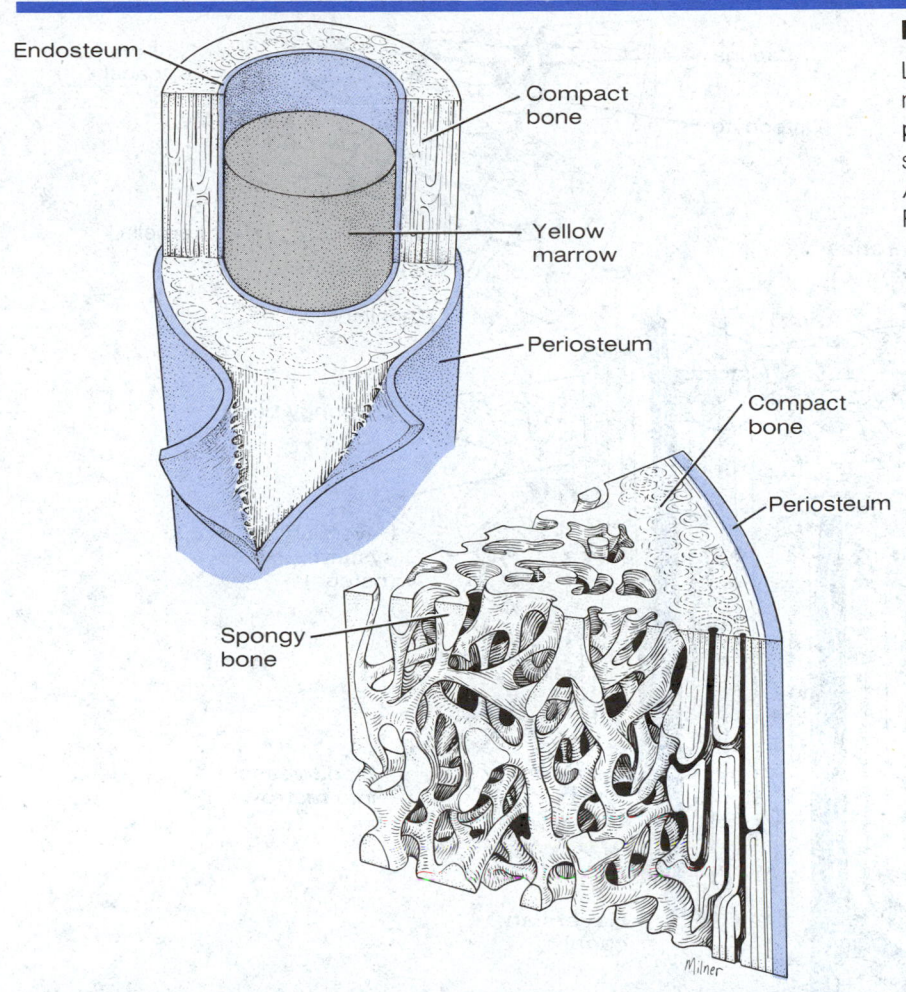

Endosteum

Compact bone

Yellow marrow

Periosteum

Compact bone

Periosteum

Spongy bone

Milner

Figure 55–2

Longitudinal section and inset of higher magnification showing spongy and compact bone.
SOURCE: Spence AP, Mason EB: *Human Anatomy and Physiology,* 2nd ed. Menlo Park, CA: Benjamin/Cummings, 1983.

Healing of Disrupted Bone Tissue

A break in the continuity of bone tissue is called a **fracture.** Fracture healing occurs by formation of new bone tissue and can be described in four stages, as diagrammed in Figure 55–4.

1. *Procallus (hematoma) formation.* Bleeding occurs at the broken ends of the bone just as it does in other injured tissues. The bleeding, which is from damaged vessels in the bone, the bone marrow, the periosteum, and surrounding soft tissues, forms a hematoma at the fracture site. Initial healing actually begins with the formation of a hematoma called a procallus. The hematoma becomes a fibrin network. New capillaries form, fibroblasts invade the clot, and granulation tissue is formed. Dead cells and tissue debris are removed by phagocytosis.

2. *Callus formation.* The fibroblasts differentiate into cells, which lay down a new matrix for bone formation. A collar of soft fibrocartilaginous tissue known as callus surrounds the fracture site, bridging the gap. The callus is much wider than the bone's diameter and extends above and below the fracture line.

3. *Ossification.* Mineral salts are deposited in the new matrix, and the callus eventually becomes bone. The fracture ends are firmly bound together but are not yet strong enough for weight bearing.

4. *Consolidation and remodeling.* The callus is remodeled by osteoclastic and osteoblastic activity according to the stresses placed on the bone by muscles and weight bearing. The excess callus is eventually absorbed and the bone assumes a more normal shape.

The rate of healing depends on several factors, such as the person's age and the type and location of the fracture. A child's bone heals much faster than an adult's bone. Favorable conditions for healing include good circulation, adequate nutrition, absence of infection, and proximity and immobility of the fracture ends. In some cases fracture healing can take a year or longer.

STRUCTURE AND FUNCTION OF JOINTS

Bones are bound together at joints, which allow the bones varying degrees of mobility. Together with the muscles, ligaments and tendons, the movable joints provide stabilization and permit motion of the body parts. The many

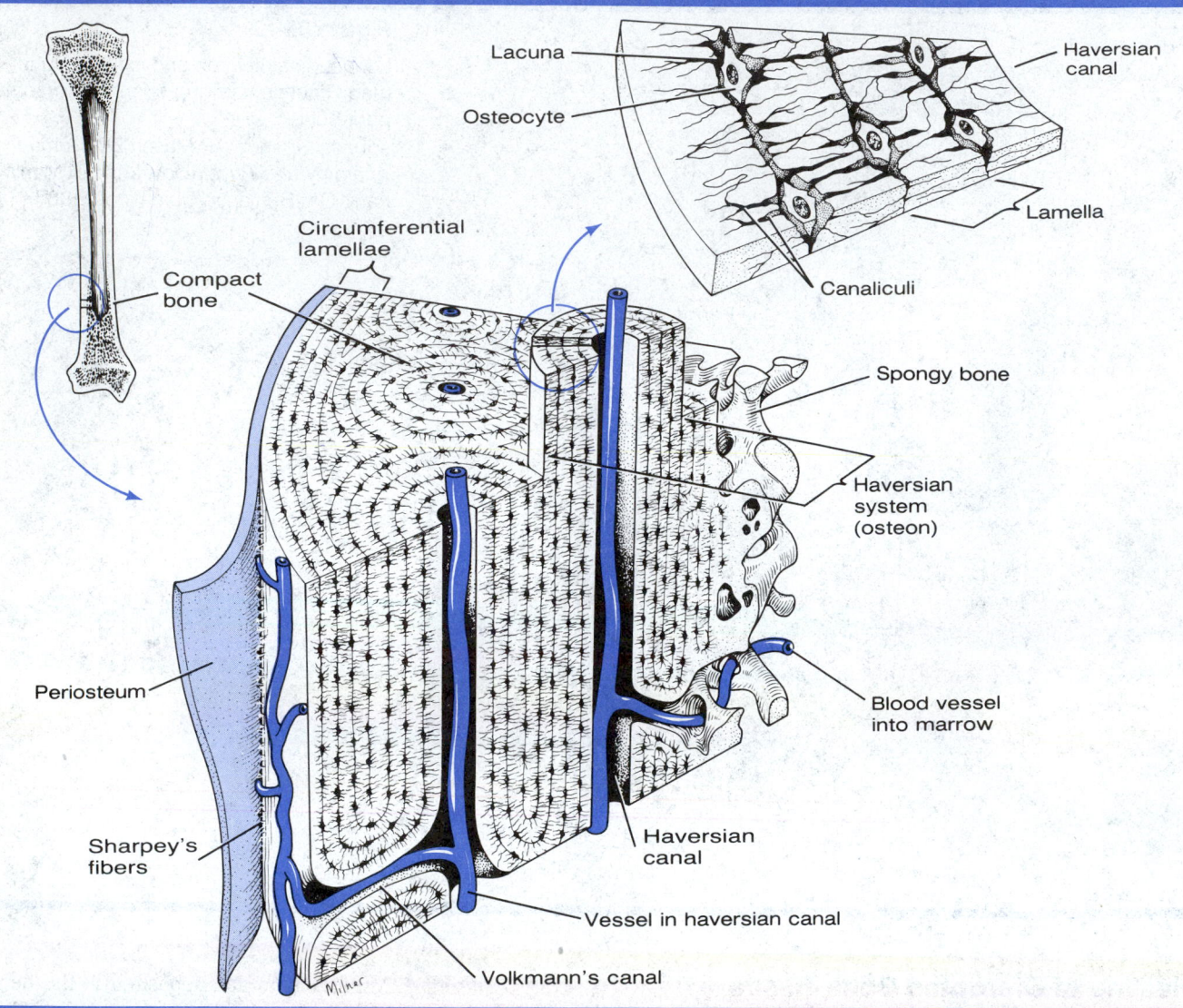

Figure 55–3

Magnified haversian system as seen in compact bone tissue. The periosteum has been pulled back to show a blood vessel entering the haversian system through a Volkmann's canal.

SOURCE: Spence AP, Mason EB: *Human Anatomy and Physiology,* 2nd ed. Menlo Park, CA: Benjamin/Cummings, 1983.

joints of the body allow for a variety of movements that can be coordinated into agile or skilled activities. Consult Chapter 7 for a review of the normal range of joint motion.

The joints of the body are classified into three types:

- *Synarthroses,* or immovable joints, such as those in the sutures of the skull
- *Amphiarthroses,* slightly movable joints, such as the symphysis pubis
- *Diarthroses,* or freely movable joints, such as those in the knee and hip

The structure of the diarthroses will be discussed because changes in this type of joint most often affect health. A diarthrotic joint (Figure 55–5) has a *synovial cavity* and is, therefore, also known as a synovial joint. The

cavity is surrounded by a *joint capsule* of strong fibroelastic tissue, which is attached to the periosteum of the articulating bones. The capsule allows movement while resisting dislocation. The inner surface of the joint cavity is lined with *synovial membrane,* which secretes *synovial fluid.* The cartilage-covered bone ends and the synovial fluid reduce friction as joint surfaces rub against each other. The amount of synovial fluid is small but is enough to lubricate the joint and provide nourishment for the articular cartilage. The synovial membrane can also secrete antibodies to protect the joint from disease.

Some diarthrotic joints have *articular discs (menisci)* made of fibrocartilage (Figure 55–5B), which lie between the articulating bone surfaces and act as shock absorbers. In the knee, these are known as *semilunar* cartilages. Many

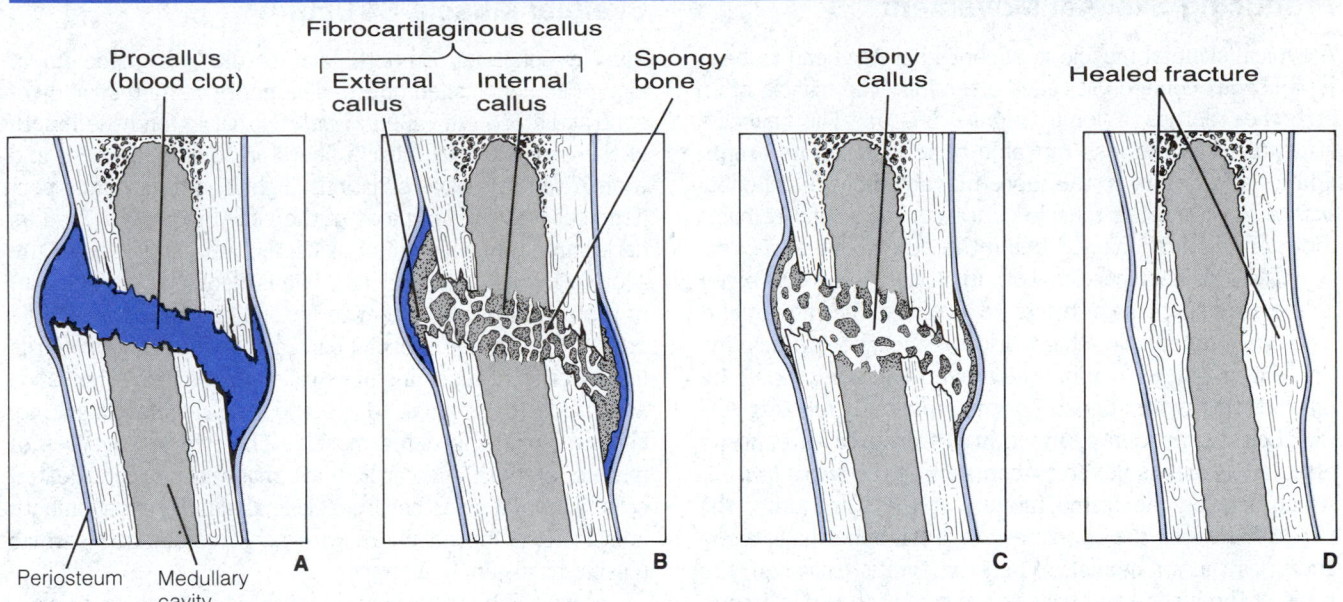

Figure 55–4

Healing of a fracture. **A.** Initial repair begins with formation of a blood clot called a procallus. **B.** Connective tissue invades the procallus, replacing it with a fibrocartilaginous callus. **C.** The fibrous callus is eventually replaced by bone that develops from cells of the periosteum. **D.** Healed fracture.
SOURCE: Spence AP, Mason EB: *Human Anatomy and Physiology,* 2nd ed. Menlo Park, CA: Benjamin/Cummings, 1983.

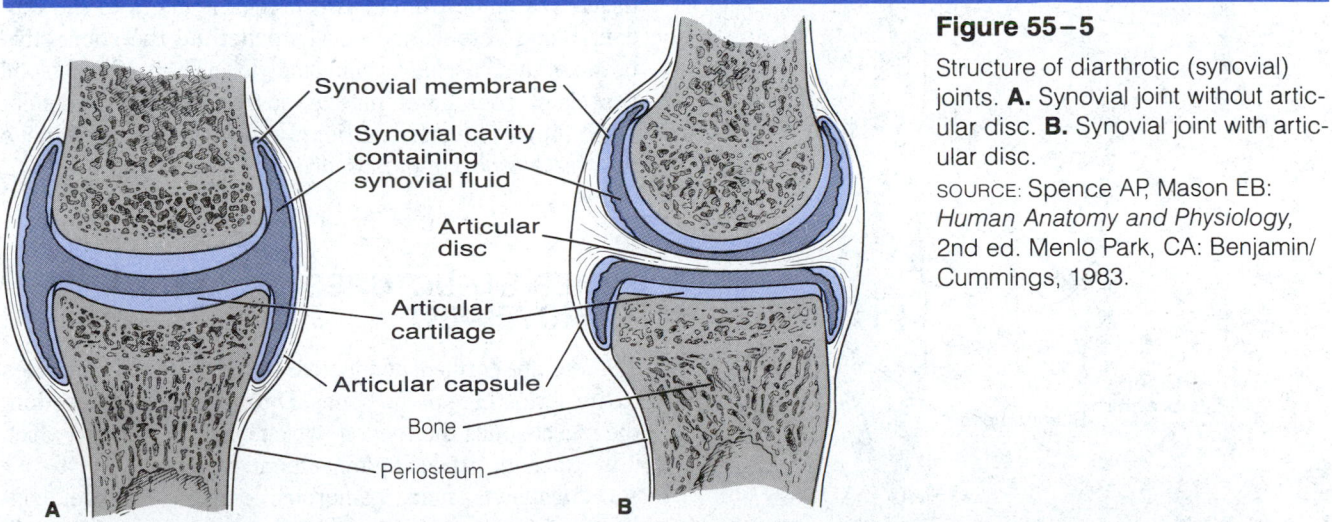

Figure 55–5

Structure of diarthrotic (synovial) joints. **A.** Synovial joint without articular disc. **B.** Synovial joint with articular disc.

SOURCE: Spence AP, Mason EB: *Human Anatomy and Physiology,* 2nd ed. Menlo Park, CA: Benjamin/ Cummings, 1983.

diarthrotic joints have ligaments inside and outside the joint capsules to bind the bones together and give additional stability.

STRUCTURE AND FUNCTION OF SKELETAL MUSCLES

Contraction of skeletal muscle is responsible for moving the bones of the skeleton. The bone serves as a lever, the joint serves as a fulcrum upon which the bone pivots, and the muscle provides the force that moves the lever. A second function of skeletal muscles is maintenance of body posture. There is a residual amount of contraction in the muscles, known as *muscle tone,* which serves to keep the body erect and ready for action. A third function is heat production. When a person is cold, small rapid contractions of skeletal muscle, called shivering, produce body heat.

Producing Skeletal Movement

A typical skeletal muscle is anchored at each end to bone by a fibrous connection called a tendon. The muscle often stretches across a joint (Figure 55–6). The muscle's attachment to the less movable bone is called its *origin,* and its attachment to the more movable bone is called its *insertion.* When the muscle contracts, one bone remains more or less stationary, forcing the other bone to move.

Most skeletal muscles work in groups. The *prime mover* is the muscle that contracts to produce the movement. *Synergists* are muscles that work together with prime movers to assist in performing the movement. *Antagonists* are muscles that work opposite prime movers by relaxing during their contraction or by acting to produce an opposite effect. The arm is flexed by contracting the *biceps brachii,* which acts as the prime mover; at the same time, the *triceps brachii* on the opposite side of the humerus relaxes, acting as the antagonist. When the arm is extended, the roles of the biceps and triceps are reversed. An **isotonic contraction** occurs when a muscle shortens during contraction. An **isometric contraction** occurs when a muscle becomes tense while remaining the same length.

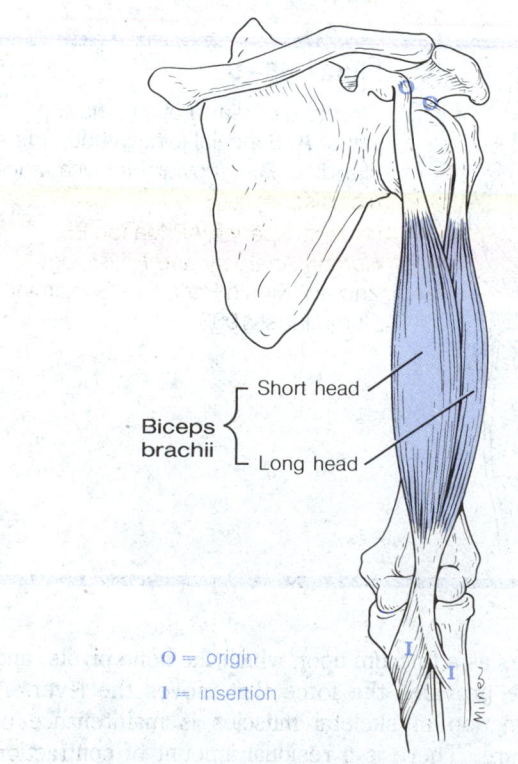

Figure 55–6

The biceps brachii muscle—a typical skeletal muscle, showing origin and insertion.

SOURCE: Spence AP, Mason EB: *Human Anatomy and Physiology,* 2nd ed. Menlo Park, CA: Benjamin/Cummings, 1983.

Skeletal Muscle Structure

Muscle—skeletal, smooth, and cardiac—is made up of elongated cells called fibers. The fibers contain strands of contractile protein called *myofibrils* that extend the length of the cell. Skeletal muscle fibers are multinucleated, and their myofibrils have striations: light and dark bands perpendicular to the long axis of the cell (Figure 55–7). The dark bands (anisotropic or A bands) are composed of the protein myosin and the light bands (isotropic or I bands) of the protein actin. A dense fibrous line called the Z line crosses the center of each I band and divides the myofibrils into a series of repeating units called *sarcomeres.* The bands are visible to the unaided eye and give skeletal muscle its alternate name, striated muscle. The two other types of muscle, smooth and cardiac, are made up of uninucleated cells. They differ further from skeletal muscle in that smooth muscle has tapered fibers with no striations and cardiac muscle has branched fibers.

Muscle fibers are bound together by connective tissue into small bundles called fascicles, visible to the unaided eye. Fascicles are bound into larger bundles, which collectively form the muscle. The entire muscle is enclosed by a connective tissue covering called the epimysium, which is continuous with the connective tissue surrounding the fascicles and fibers. The epimysium is also continuous with the tendon or other connective tissue attachment of muscle to bone. Thus, there is a continuous network of connective tissue extending from individual muscle fibers to the tendon. Blood vessels and nerves penetrate the connective tissue of the muscle, reaching individual fibers. Small blood vessels surround each muscle, so muscle has an excellent blood supply to furnish nutrients and oxygen and to remove the waste products of muscular activity.

OTHER STRUCTURES RELATED TO MOVEMENT

Tendons are cords of connective tissue that attach muscles to the periosteum of the bones. During muscle contraction, the muscle pulls the tendon, which pulls the bone to which it is attached, producing movement.

Ligaments, made of fibrous connective tissue, connect bones to one another. They have the ability to stretch while providing stability. The knee joint, for example, is stabilized by ligaments, such as the anterior and posterior cruciate ligaments, which bind the femur to the tibia within the joint capsule, and by the medial and lateral collateral ligaments outside the joint capsule (Figure 55–8).

A *bursa* is a fluid-filled sac that facilitates motion of structures that move against each other. It can be found between skin and bone, muscle and bone, tendons and bone, ligaments and bone, and between muscles. The bursae function as padding between structures to reduce the friction caused by moving parts.

Connective tissue, in the broad sense of the term,

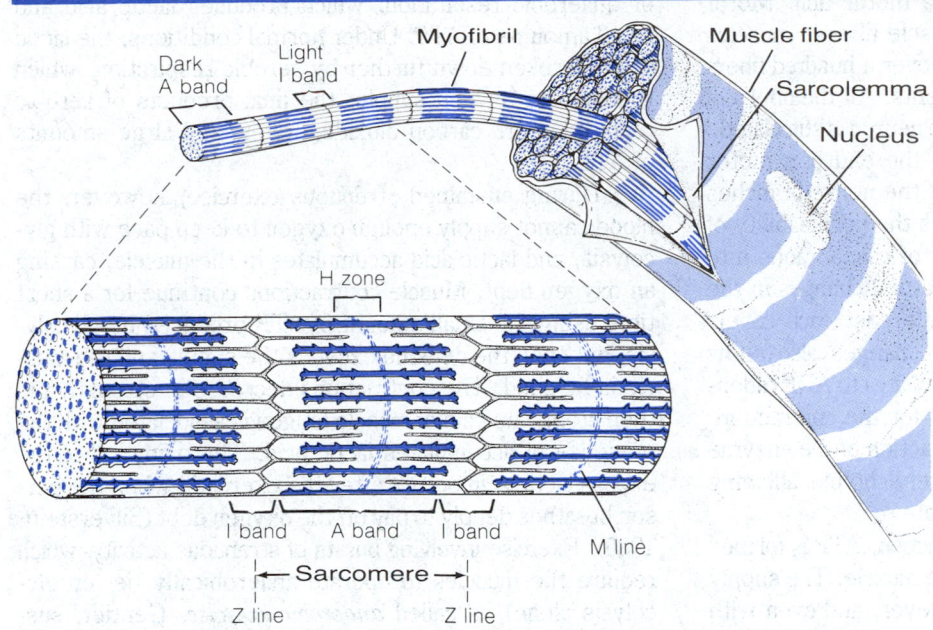

Dark A band
Light I band
Myofibril
Muscle fiber
Sarcolemma
Nucleus
H zone
I band
A band
I band
M line
Sarcomere
Z line
Z line

Figure 55–7

Striated muscle. Microscopic anatomy of an individual skeletal muscle fiber (cell). Note the striated (striped) appearance of the muscle fiber and the myofibrils.

SOURCE: Spence AP, Mason EB: *Human Anatomy and Physiology,* 2nd ed. Menlo Park, CA: Benjamin/Cummings, 1983.

includes all tissues made up of cells in a matrix: bone, cartilage, blood, and lymph, for example. The term is used in a more limited sense, however, when discussing diseases of the connective tissues. In this sense, connective tissue means the binding and covering tissues of the body, including tendons, ligaments, muscle fascia, and the deep layers of the skin. This kind of connective tissue (sometimes called "connective tissue proper") is essential in holding together all the components of the musculoskeletal system.

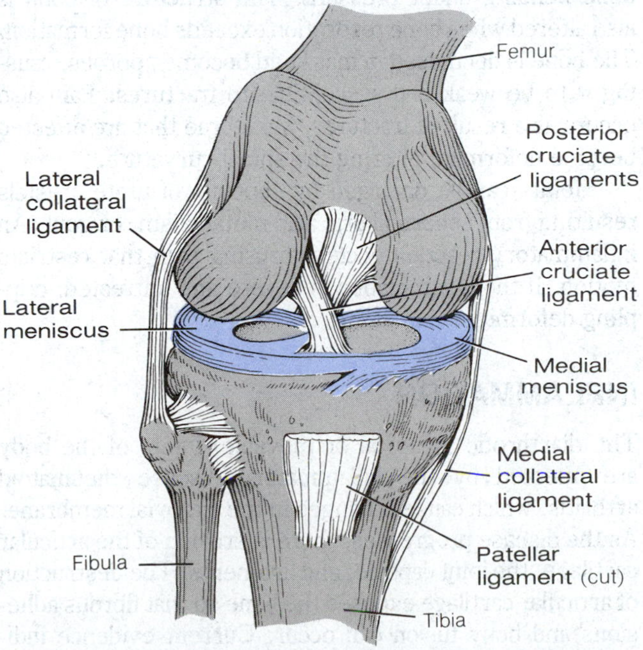

REGULATORY PROCESSES

Regulation of the Calcium Content of Bone

The calcium in bone contributes to the bone structure. The bone itself serves as a reservoir for calcium-requiring physiological processes. The exchange of calcium between the bones and the circulatory system is under hormonal regulation.

Two endocrine hormones affect the amount of calcium stored in the bones: parathormone (PTH) and calcitonin. The parathyroid gland secretes parathormone in response to a lowered serum calcium level. Parathormone stimulates resorptive (bone-destroying) activity to release calcium from the bone, increases calcium and phosphate absorption from the gastrointestinal tract, and increases calcium reabsorption in the kidney. The thyroid gland secretes calcitonin when the serum calcium level is high. Calcitonin inhibits bone resorption, decreasing the calcium blood level. Vitamin D is also important in calcium metabolism because it stimulates calcium absorption by the intestine.

Skeletal Muscle Contraction

Skeletal muscle contraction begins with the stimulus of a muscle fiber by a motor neuron. Every motor neuron ends in many fine branches, each branch connecting with an individual muscle fiber. A group of muscle fibers activated

Femur
Posterior cruciate ligaments
Anterior cruciate ligament
Lateral collateral ligament
Lateral meniscus
Medial meniscus
Medial collateral ligament
Patellar ligament (cut)
Fibula
Tibia

Figure 55–8

Ligaments of the right knee joint. (The femur is flexed slightly to allow the ligaments to be seen.)

SOURCE: Spence AP, Mason EB: *Human Anatomy and Physiology,* 2nd ed. Menlo Park, CA: Benjamin/Cummings, 1983.

by a single motor neuron is called a motor unit. Motor units range in size from a single muscle fiber in muscles controlling fine, skilled movements to over a hundred fibers in muscles involved in gross movements. All the fibers of a motor unit contract together when the neuron is stimulated.

When a nerve impulse reaches the end of a motor neuron, small vesicles in the ends of the nerve branches release acetylcholine, which increases the permeability of the muscle cell and causes an influx of calcium ions into the cell. The calcium ions cause structural changes in the myofilaments that allow them to slide past each other, causing contraction. The structural changes also allow breakdown of ATP (adenosine triphosphate) to ADP (adenosine diphosphate) to provide energy for the contraction. The muscle relaxes as a result of the action of the enzyme cholinesterase, which breaks down acetylcholine, allowing the muscle to return to its resting state.

At the beginning of muscle contraction, ATP is formed from creatine phosphate stored in the muscle. The supply of creatine phosphate is limited, however, and even with mild muscle activity, additional ATP must be formed from ADP. The energy for forming this additional ATP is supplied by respiration—the breakdown of fats and carbohydrates by the cell. The first step in respiration is glycolysis,

or anaerobic respiration, which produces lactic acid and small amounts of ATP. Under normal conditions, the lactic acid is broken down further by aerobic respiration, which requires an oxygen supply; the final products of aerobic respiration are carbon dioxide, water, and large amounts of ATP.

During sustained strenuous exercise, however, the blood cannot supply enough oxygen to keep pace with glycolysis, and lactic acid accumulates in the muscle, causing an oxygen debt. Muscle contractions continue for a short time using the small amount of ATP produced by glycolysis, but soon the demand exceeds the supply and the muscle is fatigued. The contractions decrease in strength and then stop. The pain of muscle fatigue is associated with the presence of accumulated lactic acid. The oxidation of the excess lactic acid occurs after the exercise, when the person breathes deeply to pay off the oxygen debt (Silverstein, 1980). Exercise involving bursts of strenuous activity, which require the muscles to operate anaerobically (ie, on glycolysis alone), is called *anaerobic exercise*. Gentler, sustained exercise that stimulates rapid aerobic respiration without outstripping the oxygen supply is called *aerobic exercise*.

Section II: Pathophysiological Influences and Effects

The primary function of the musculoskeletal system is to provide body movement. When disease or trauma alters the system, the individual's mobility and relations are usually affected, which may profoundly affect a person's lifestyle. Movement is often still possible, but not without pain or difficulty. This section introduces the pathophysiological alterations that can occur in the musculoskeletal system: metabolic alterations, inflammation, degenerative changes, infection, neoplasm, and trauma. Specific disorders involving these alterations will be discussed in later chapters of this unit.

The alterations covered here occur in disorders usually seen in adults. There are also many congenital disorders affecting the musculoskeletal system, but since these are first encountered in childhood, they will not be covered in this unit. Nurses often see adult clients with paralysis, deformities, and other effects of childhood musculoskeletal disorders. For a full discussion of congenital conditions, consult a pediatric nursing textbook.

METABOLIC ALTERATIONS

The structure of bone may be disrupted by inadequate calcium content. Since calcium gives bone its hardness, a deficiency causes bones to be soft and deformed. Pain is caused by stresses on the bone from weight bearing or when a considerable pull is exerted by muscles: nerve end-

ings in the periosteum are stimulated by the weakened bone bending under pressure. The structure of bone is also altered when bone resorption exceeds bone formation. The bone is decreased in mass and becomes porous, causing it to be weak and susceptible to fractures. Pain also occurs as a result of fractures. Vertebrae that are affected become deformed, altering the spinal curvature.

Joints can be damaged by deposits of urate crystals resulting from abnormal uric acid metabolism, or gout. An inflammatory reaction occurs, causing pain that restricts motion. If the inflammation is severe and untreated, crippling deformities may occur.

INFLAMMATION

The diarthrotic (synovial or movable) joints of the body are affected by the inflammatory disease rheumatoid arthritis, which causes changes in the synovial membrane. As the disease progresses, there is erosion of the articular cartilage, the joint capsule, and ligaments. The destruction of articular cartilage exposes the bone so that fibrous adhesions and bony fusion can occur. Current evidence indicates that immune reactions are involved in the changes in the joint (Porth, 1983). Other tissues of the body are also affected by the disease. The effects of the disease include pain, limited joint mobility, and joint deformity.

Inflammation may occur in other musculoskeletal

structures from excessive or repeated strain as well as bacterial invasion. Restricted motion and pain usually result. Other connective tissues of the body may be affected by inflammation, resulting in changes in other organs as well as changes in the musculoskeletal system. Many of these connective tissue disorders are believed to be associated with immune processes. The specific conditions will be discussed in Chapter 57.

DEGENERATIVE CHANGES

The joint is the musculoskeletal structure most frequently influenced by degenerative disease. Changes are most often associated with aging, obesity, trauma, and inflammatory conditions. The degenerative process is a wearing out of the joint surfaces. The articular cartilage softens, thins, and ulcerates, and the joint surface becomes rough. There may be a narrowing of the joint space, swelling of adjacent soft tissue, and formation of bone cysts (Koerner & Dickinson, 1983). The normal smooth-gliding joint action is diminished. The periosteum becomes irritated by friction, stimulating the growth of bone spurs at the joint margins (Silverstein, 1980). The effects of this destruction include joint pain, stiffness, and joint deformity, which result in slight to moderate limitation of movement.

The intervertebral disks are also affected by degeneration. The water content of the disks decreases with age, causing them to become thinner. The surrounding fibers (ligaments) also change with age, so the disk becomes unstable. These changes cause decreased height and painless restriction of spinal movement. Sometimes the condition becomes more severe, with pressure on nerves causing pain and neurologic deficits.

Somewhat akin to degeneration is the process of **atrophy,** or wasting away. Muscle and bone can atrophy as a result of disuse. The normal strain on muscles and bones contributes to their development and to the maintenance of their size, shape, strength, and composition. Through disuse, muscle cells become reduced in size and weakened, the muscle mass becomes more fibrous, and bone cells become demineralized. Inactivity can also lead to joint **contracture.** The muscle fibers become shortened and fixed, and the joint's range of motion becomes limited. These conditions are reversible if the person resumes normal activity. Contractures can progress to an irreversible state without treatment, however. Ligaments can also lose their ability to maintain joint stability.

INFECTION

Bone can become infected by pathogens entering the bone by way of the circulation or through open wounds, including surgical incisions. The proliferation of bacteria causes pressure, bone destruction, and eventual bone necrosis. The resulting pain usually limits mobility. Some infections become chronic, with perpetual draining abscesses.

Nursing Research Note

Lambert VA: Study of factors associated with psychological well-being in rheumatoid arthritic women. *Image* (Spring) 1985; 17:50–53.

This research identified and described factors associated with well-being in women afflicted with rheumatoid arthritis. Social support, severity of the illness, and demographic characteristics were examined in relation to each other and to the level of psychological well-being. The study sample consisted of 92 women ranging in age from 21 to 80 years with a mean age of 55 years. Data were collected by a structured interview.

Under the category of severity of the illness, pain was the single significant predictor of psychological well-being (ie, psychological well-being decreases as joint pain and difficulty in carrying out tasks increase). Dependence on others was significantly correlated with difficulty in performing tasks.

Clients with rheumatoid arthritis need to understand pain prevention and joint preservation approaches to optimize their quality of life. Nurses have a responsibility to provide this kind of information to clients. Because many older women with rheumatoid arthritis have limited support systems, nurses can assist clients in locating support services.

Other musculoskeletal structures, such as joints and bursae, can be infected by pathogens entering from penetrating wounds or via the circulation. Pain and restricted motion are common.

NEOPLASIA

Neoplastic growths in the musculoskeletal system can be benign or malignant. Benign tumors grow slowly or not at all and usually are encapsulated. They may cause mild pain, tenderness, and sometimes an abnormal prominence on the bone. Malignant tumors grow rapidly, causing intermittent to persistent pain (especially at night), tiredness, limited movement, swelling, and spontaneous fractures. Other effects may occur as a result of a tumor pressing on other structures, eg, nerves, blood vessels, or organs.

Malignant lesions may be from growths originating in musculoskeletal tissue (primary) or to metastatic lesions (secondary). The most common are bone lesions due to metastasis, generally from the lung, breast, intestine, thyroid, kidney, and prostate. Since the malignant cells can spread via the circulation, and the bones have a rich blood supply, the cells easily migrate to the bone. This is especially true for bones with large amounts of red marrow such as the spine, pelvis, and ribs. Cellular activity in the tumor may be osteolytic (bone destroying) or osteoblastic, forming abnormal new cells. Malignancy of the bone marrow was discussed in the chapter on blood forming organs (Chapter 29).

Malignant neoplasms of the bone, muscle, and cartilage are called sarcomas. The prefixes of the tumor names indicate the tissue in which the tumors are present, for example, osteogenic sarcoma (bone), rhabdomyosarcoma (muscle), and chondrosarcoma (cartilage). See Chapters 2 and 12 for a further discussion of tumor classification.

The effects of neoplastic growths can range from treatable conditions with no residual problems to death from tumor growth or resulting complications. Depending on the specific neoplasm, the client may experience a temporary limitation in mobility (due, for example, to surgery for tumor removal) or permanent limitation due to mutilating surgical excision, such as amputation of a limb.

TRAUMA

Trauma to a bone can cause a fracture. A person with a fracture has limited mobility, if not from instability or deformity then from the pain movement would cause. Soft tissue adjacent to a fracture, such as blood vessels, nerves, muscles, and adjacent organs may be damaged from the actual traumatic event or from the sharp edges of the bro-

ken bone. If the skin has been broken because of the fracture, the opening becomes a potential site for infection. The wound and the generous blood supply of the bone provide an excellent medium for bacterial growth. Muscle spasm at the fracture site can pull on the segments of the bone, holding the bone in an angulated position or causing side-by-side displacement of the bone fragments. A displaced segment of bone must be repositioned so the bone can heal in proper alignment.

Skeletal muscle can be injured by trauma. Fortunately, skeletal muscle fibers can regenerate, but when the damage is extensive, the fibers are replaced by scar tissue (Silverstein, 1980). Trauma to the musculoskeletal structures supporting the joints is common. Muscle fibers may be injured due to overuse, overstretching, forcible twisting, and other abnormal movements. The fibers may be torn, or stretched too far, and joint surfaces may dislocate, that is, separate partially or completely. Associated blood vessels and nerves may be damaged in the process. Pain and limited motion are the result.

Section III: Related System Influences and Effects

PROBLEMS RELATED TO IMMOBILIZATION

Musculoskeletal disease can lead to immobilization; immobilization is also a method of treatment for many musculoskeletal conditions. Immobilization affects every system in the body to some extent, including the musculoskeletal system itself. Although immobility may help some musculoskeletal conditions heal, it may give rise to others. The effects of immobility on the body systems are summarized in Table 55–1.

NEUROLOGIC AND VASCULAR PROBLEMS

Neurologic and vascular problems can cause or contribute to musculoskeletal disorders. Since muscle functioning is the result of the combined effect of muscle fibers and motor nerves, damage to or interference with the nerves can

impair muscle functioning. Decreased functioning can cause muscles to atrophy, and paralysis can occur. Likewise, disruption of the vascular supply to bones or muscles can limit the nutrients and oxygen supplied to the cells and interfere with removal of cellular waste products. Prolonged interruption of circulation leads to necrosis of the tissues ordinarily supplied by the vessels.

Musculoskeletal disorders can also give rise to neurologic or vascular problems, which may in turn cause further musculoskeletal damage. Pressure from bandages, traction equipment, casts, tumor growth, and poor positioning are a few problems that can hinder nerve and blood vessel functioning. Trauma to muscles causes edema and hemorrhage in soft tissues, increasing the pressure within a confined space. Pressure on nerves and blood vessels in the area can become so great as to produce irreversible necrosis of the muscle tissue. An ugly, crippling, permanent contracture of the limb may occur, as well as loss of motor and sensory functioning.

Section IV: Psychosocial/Lifestyle Influences and Effects

Age, sex, nutritional status, occupation, lifestyle, and emotional status can contribute to the development or exacerbation of a musculoskeletal problem, or make one person more susceptible to a given problem than another. Musculoskeletal dysfunction, in turn, has far-reaching psychosocial implications. By altering mobility, comfort, and appearance, it can affect the client's emotional status, social and sexual functioning, occupation, and lifestyle. This sec-

tion will consider how psychosocial influences contribute to musculoskeletal alterations and how musculoskeletal alterations affect the psychosocial aspects of a client's life.

AGE AND SEX

The aged person is more prone to injuries because of vision problems, loss of balance, and falls. With osteoporosis,

Table 55-1	Summary of Effects of Immobility on the Body System
System	**Results**
Musculoskeletal	Demineralization of bone; decreased muscle mass and strength; joint stiffness; contractures; instability
Cardiovascular	Orthostatic hypotension; increased thrombus formation; increased workload on the heart
Respiratory	Decreased respiratory efficiency due to: decreased respiratory muscle movement, decreased movement of respiratory secretions, change in CO_2 and O_2 exchange; hypostatic pneumonia
Gastrointestinal	Anorexia; change in bowel habits, eg, constipation
Urinary (especially from prolonged supine position)	Stasis of urine in kidney pelvis; formation of renal calculi; urinary retention; urinary tract infection
Integumentary	Abrasions; decubitus ulcer formation
Psychological	Loneliness; boredom; depression; sensory deprivation

which is common in postmenopausal women, fractures are more likely. Men also have a moderate decrease in bone density and muscle mass as they age because of a reduction in testosterone secretion.

DIETARY HABITS

Nutritional intake can affect the functioning of the musculoskeletal system in several ways. Nutritional excesses leading to obesity can cause stress fractures and excessive wear on joints. Vitamin deficiencies can cause bones to be deformed during growth, affect the turnover of bone in adulthood, and cause bones to be thin and porous. Vitamin D is especially important because it enhances the absorption of calcium and phosphorus from the intestinal tract. Musculoskeletal effects of vitamin deficiency diseases are uncommon in developed countries because an ordinary diet is usually adequate to prevent these symptoms. However, people with poor eating habits, such as alcoholics, occasionally develop vitamin deficiency diseases. Alcoholics tend to skip meals because their hunger is satisfied by the alcohol, so their nutrient intake is often inadequate. Also, foods they do eat may not be absorbed well because of inflammation and changes in the gastrointestinal tract. Vegetarian diets that exclude all animal foods including dairy products and eggs require careful planning to ensure there are enough nutrients to prevent deficiency states.

Mineral deficiencies can also cause problems. Calcium imbalances affect the muscular and skeletal systems, because calcium is essential for bone growth and turnover and for muscle contraction. A calcium deficit can result in increased neuromuscular excitability and bone demineralization, whereas calcium excess can cause muscular weakness. Low-calcium intake is often a contributing cause of osteoporosis, a disease involving bone demineralization that is common

in the elderly. Bone demineralization can also occur from a deficiency of phosphorus.

OCCUPATION AND RECREATION

A person's occupation can contribute to alterations in the musculoskeletal system, especially alterations resulting from trauma. Constant stress on joints, as from the use of a jackhammer, for example, can cause arthritic changes. Jobs involving heavy lifting and working with machinery have a high risk of traumatic injuries, including injuries to bones, joints, and muscles. People who work on assembly lines with dangerous machinery are susceptible to hand injuries. Today employee health and safety measures are reducing the incidence of such accidents in many countries.

Some musculoskeletal conditions require long-term or permanent changes in a client's way of life. Clients with an amputation, for example, may need to change their occupations. Various musculoskeletal disorders can reduce the number of hours clients can stay on their feet on the job.

The current interest in physical fitness has prompted many people to become active in athletic endeavors. While more and more people are becoming aware of the conditioning and training necessary to participate in physical activities, numerous injuries still occur.

Sport injuries are of two kinds, those that are acute and those that result from overuse. Acute injuries occur most often in contact sports and include breaks, strains, sprains, and dislocations. Overuse injuries are usually a result of repetitive motions common to a particular sport or of a sudden change in the sport, such as increasing the distance run, using different equipment, or playing on a different surface. The most common overuse injuries are inflammation of tendons and stress fractures. Ankle and foot injuries, dislocated hips, strains, and sprains of the back and neck have been seen in breakdancers. Engaging in high-risk sports such as race car driving increases the potential for personal injury.

With musculoskeletal disorders, clients may have to abandon recreational activities because they can no longer perform them or because the activities will cause further damage. Roles within the family may change; for example, a housewife may go out to work while her husband assumes the child-rearing responsibilities. Occasionally, it is necessary to modify a client's home, such as lowering the kitchen cupboards and work spaces. All these changes require a period of adjustment for all persons affected.

ECONOMIC FACTORS

Lengthy hospitalization, numerous surgical procedures, and the need for appliances and adaptive devices may add up to an enormous expense for the client and family. Those injured on the job frequently receive worker's compensation, but many injuries are not job related. Persons with health insurance coverage may have all or most of their medical expenses covered, but they usually are not compensated for income lost from not working.

ROLES AND RELATIONSHIPS

Conditions of the musculoskeletal system particularly affect a person's emotions because these conditions usually affect independence and mobility. A person who is temporarily or permanently dependent on others for assistance with activities of daily living may have feelings of powerlessness, loss of security, and a decrease in self-esteem. Being placed in a cast or in traction increases feelings of powerlessness. The chronic nature of many musculoskeletal problems may make clients wonder if they are becoming a burden on their families. They may no longer feel needed or useful to others because of their limitations. Some elderly people fear that they will be judged incapable of caring for themselves and be sent to a nursing home.

The nurse will see orthopedic clients in various phases of the *grieving process* (see Chapter 16). The grief may be for a lost body part or lost function, or even for lost loved ones who were killed in the same accident in which the client was injured. Other clients are uncertain about the outcome of their conditions and may have fears of deformity, disfigurement, or paralysis.

Body image may be altered as a result of a deformity or from devices used in treating the condition. Client self-perception will include anything connected to the body, such as a traction apparatus, cast, crutches, or even the bed. Confinement to a bed or room for an extended period of time may cause sensory deprivation, resulting in such manifestations as boredom, anxiety, and confusion. (See Chapter 4 for a discussion of body image, sensory deprivation and overload.)

With all this change, grief, fear, and doubt, changes in behavior are not surprising. Clients may seem unreasonable, demanding, frustrated, or depressed. They may realize a new source of power in voicing their anger. Musculoskeletal pain exacerbates clients' emotional reactions, making them feel even worse.

SEXUAL EXPRESSION

Some treatments for musculoskeletal conditions may provide obstacles to sexual activity. Examples are casts, traction, and long confinement in the hospital. The client's feeling of freedom to engage in sexual activity may be affected by fear of causing pain or of disrupting a healing injury or surgical repair.

The individual's sexual self-concept may be altered by changes in role or body image or by feelings of dependence and inadequacy. Sexual dysfunction may be related to feelings of depression and anxiety. The partner's perception of the client as a sexual being may be altered, affecting their sexual relationship. The couple may need to find new approaches for intercourse or other methods of sexual satisfaction.

Chapter Highlights

Normal development and functioning of muscles and bones requires the usual physical stresses and strains of daily activities.

Alterations in anatomy and physiology of the musculoskeletal system can result in limited motion, pain, and deformity.

Bone structure can be disrupted by vitamin and mineral deficiencies, altered bone metabolism, infection, tumors, and trauma.

Muscular structure and function can be altered by degenerative changes, inactivity, trauma, and abnormal calcium levels.

Joints can be damaged by degenerative changes, inactivity, infection, inflammation, and trauma.

Musculoskeletal conditions can result in long-term problems requiring lengthy medical treatment and adaptation to changes.

The emotional status of a client with limited mobility may be affected because of loss of independence and self-esteem, changes in body image, and alterations in sexual functioning.

Irreparable damage can occur to muscle and bone tissues when there is interference with their nerve or blood supply.

Immobilization for treatment of musculoskeletal conditions can have adverse effects on all body systems.

Bibliography

Crelin ES: Development of the musculoskeletal system. *Clin Symp* 1981; 33(1): 2–36.

Garrick JG: The sports medicine patient. *Nurs Clin North Am* 1981; 16:759–766.

Koerner ME, Dickinson GR: Adult arthritis: A look at some of its forms. *Am J Nurs* 1983; 83:254–262.

Porth C: *Pathophysiology: Concepts of Altered Health States.* Philadelphia: Lippincott, 1983.

Price SA, Wilson LM: *Pathophysiology: Clinical Concepts of Disease Processes,* 2nd ed. New York: McGraw-Hill, 1982.

Rosse C, Clawson DK: *The Musculoskeletal System in Health and Disease.* New York: Harper & Row, 1980.

Silverstein A: *Human Anatomy and Physiology.* New York: Wiley, 1980.

Spence AP, Mason EB: *Human Anatomy and Physiology,* 2nd ed. Menlo Park, CA: Benjamin/Cummings, 1983.

Suggested Readings

Hilt NE, Cogburn SB: *Manual of Orthopedics.* St. Louis: Mosby, 1980. Written by nurses, this book covers many aspects of orthopedic care, including anatomy, physiology, assessment, and interventions.

Krause MV, Mahan LK: *Food, Nutrition, and Diet Therapy,* 7th ed. Philadelphia: Saunders, 1984. A book on basic nutrition and specific therapy for nutritional care in disease.

Lentz M: Selected aspects of deconditioning secondary to immobilization. *Nurs Clin North Am* 1981; 16:729–737. Covers the effects of immobilization on the cardiovascular and musculoskeletal systems, with relevant nursing interventions.

Turner P: Caring for emotional needs of orthopedic trauma patients. *AORN J* 1982; 36:566–570. Identifies many emotional problems of orthopedic clients and gives suggested nursing care.

Chapter 56

The Nursing Process for Clients With Musculoskeletal System Dysfunction

Linda Heim McCausland

Objectives

When you have finished studying this chapter, you should be able to:

Describe the essential subjective data to be obtained on clients with musculoskeletal problems.

Discuss specific areas to examine when gathering objective data on clients with musculoskeletal conditions.

Identify diagnostic tests specific for clients with musculoskeletal dysfunction.

Specify nursing diagnoses common to clients with orthopedic problems.

Anticipate general nursing interventions for clients with musculoskeletal dysfunction.

Formulate general criteria for evaluating the effectiveness of nursing interventions for clients with orthopedic problems.

Orthopedics is the branch of medicine that studies and treats conditions of the bones, muscles, joints, and associated structures. An orthopedic nurse is one whose practice is primarily concerned with orthopedic clients. Almost all nurses, however, deal with at least some clients who have orthopedic problems, whether in the emergency department, surgical suite, intensive care units, ambulatory care settings, nursing homes, or medical and surgical units. This chapter discusses application of the nursing process to clients with musculoskeletal disorders in general. The following chapters treat aspects of nursing specific to clients with particular musculoskeletal conditions.

Section I: Nursing Assessment: Establishing the Data Base

The nursing assessment of the orthopedic client requires special emphasis on the musculoskeletal, neurologic, and vascular systems. The general techniques for assessing these systems are covered in Chapter 7. Assessment of musculoskeletal trauma in emergency situations is covered in Chapter 13. In emergencies, nurses must deal first with life-threatening conditions such as hemorrhage and breathing difficulties; broken bones can usually wait until more urgent problems are treated. Assessing the emergency client for spinal injury is also important before attempting assessment of range of joint motion.

SUBJECTIVE DATA

Clients can provide important information about what they are experiencing as a result of their condition.

Pain

Pain, sometimes severe, is a common manifestation of musculoskeletal problems. Ask clients to describe their pain thoroughly, including location, intensity, quality, duration, radiation, precipitating factors, and successful relief measures. Ask the client to point to the location where it hurts most; point tenderness (a highly localized sensitivity to touch) may be the site of a fracture in a trauma client. Some clients ache all over and need to indicate each of the areas involved. Knowing the quality of pain may help pinpoint a specific problem, but the client may need help in describing the pain. A burning pain under a cast may indicate pressure sore formation or skin irritation, whereas pain radiating down a leg may indicate pressure on spinal nerves. All these data are helpful in making a nursing diagnosis and may also aid the physician with the medical diagnosis.

Some orthopedic clients experience pain so severe they cannot tolerate moving or being touched. Others have learned to live with chronic pain for so long that they may require less postoperative analgesia than usual. Pay attention to descriptions of pain that seem unusual or excessive for the client's condition. Such complaints warrant a thorough assessment. The pain may indicate a new or undiagnosed condition; eg, pain in the calf several days postoperatively may be the result of a complication such as thrombophlebitis.

Paresthesia

The client may describe abnormal sensations, or paresthesia, such as tingling, numbness, and diminished or absent sensation. The affected area should be defined as precisely as possible. Paresthesia is an indication of a neurologic problem and requires an in-depth assessment by the nurse. Neurologic assessment is covered in the discussion of objective data.

Changes in Activities of Daily Living and Mobility

The nurse can obtain additional subjective data by asking the client how the problem affects activities of daily living (ADL) and mobility. Changes in normal activities may be from pain alone or from additional causes such as fatigue, weakness, stiffness, or decreased mobility of a particular body part. One client may report an inability to sleep at night because of leg pain, whereas another may say pain begins after walking as far as the bus stop. A client may have made adjustments to maintain independence ("I have to ride the elevator for just one floor now") or abandoned certain activities ("I can't serve a tennis ball any more because my shoulder hurts so much"). Encouraging clients to discuss their view of the situation helps to bring insights and misconceptions to the surface. Clients might also reveal feelings such as fear of dependence or of being a burden, or worries about being unable to support or care for a family.

Assistive Devices

The nurse should ask the client about any assistive devices used to help maintain independence. The client may use aids for walking, eating, dressing, bathing, toileting, or all of these. Some people are creative and adaptive in finding new ways to meet their daily needs.

History of the Injury

Subjective data are particularly helpful in the case of injury when the client can describe the traumatic event and the action taken. The health care team will want to know:

- What was the client doing when the injury occurred?
- How long ago did the injury happen?
- What caused the injury?
- What position was the limb in at the time of injury?
- Did the client hear a crack or pop when the injury occurred?
- What initial symptoms (bleeding, deformity, bone protrusion, change in sensation, bruises, swelling, pain) did the client notice?
- What action (elevating the limb, applying ice, applying heat, continuing to use the limb, immobilizing the limb) did the client or someone else take in response to the injury?
- Were alcohol or drugs involved in the accident?
- Was any medication given?

This information can help the health care team determine what tissues and structures were injured as well as anticipate potential problems. If the client is unconscious or unable to supply the information because of shock, pain, or emotional distress, the health team needs to obtain a description of the accident from someone who accompanied the client to the hospital. It is important to ask people who bring in trauma clients to stay until someone can question them.

OBJECTIVE DATA

Physical Assessment

Objective data include the results of physical assessment and of laboratory and other diagnostic tests. In assessing clients with musculoskeletal disorders, the nurse considers vital signs, posture, muscle strength and tone, ability to ambulate, and neurologic status.

Vital Signs
An assessment of the vital signs is of particular importance in musculoskeletal trauma. Be alert to signs of shock. A

temperature elevation may accompany inflammation and is common with an infection such as osteomyelitis (infection of the bone). Observing respiration is essential when injury occurs to the face, neck, or chest. Clients with spinal or chest deformities may also have abnormal respirations.

Inflammation and Swelling

Inflammation results from injury to tissues caused by physical trauma or by chemicals, bacteria, or foreign substances. Swelling occurs as inflammatory exudate forms to defend the tissues from the injury. Edema (usually resulting from circulatory problems) may also be present. Inspection and palpation are used when assessing clients for swelling and inflammation and comparing one extremity to the other for size, warmth, and erythema (redness). A joint will appear swollen when there is an increase in synovial fluid or when blood or purulent material is present in the joint capsule. This swelling is known as **effusion.** Effusion in the knee is detected by displacing the fluid with an upward stroke along the medial side of the knee and then pressing on the lateral side. The fluid will return and form a bulge (the bulge sign). Be gentle when assessing inflamed areas because they are usually tender. It is best to start palpating at a distance from the obvious tender area and work toward it, letting clients know when and where they will be touched and reassuring them that the touch will be gentle. Describe the amount of any swelling, and take note of how the injury was first treated. The latter is important for determining the significance of the amount of swelling. For example, after the same initial damage, an extremity that was iced and elevated after injury will have less swelling than one that was held in a dependent position while being soaked in warm water.

Skin Integrity

Injury or disease processes may cause changes in the skin. Discoloration results when trauma to soft tissues causes **ecchymosis** (bruising). The skin may be broken or torn as a result of injury. Describe any lesions completely; include the location, length, depth, and appearance of the involved tissue. If there is any drainage, describe the amount, color, type, and odor.

Rashes are common in connective tissue disorders. Look for changes in the skin such as discoloration, dryness, scaliness, and lesions. Terminology used to describe rashes is covered in Chapter 7. Areas to observe are the face (including the eyes and mucous membranes), trunk, and extremities. Also assess the hair and nails because alopecia (hair loss) and nail changes can accompany some types of arthritis. Discoloration, usually redness, may occur in the palms, over joints, and at the distal ends of toes and fingers. Normal pigmentation may also be altered. Observe for thickening or thinning of the skin. Thin skin is especially susceptible to skin tears. Nodules characteristic of some arthritic conditions may be noted when palpating and observing the skin.

Nursing Research Note

Southwick JR, Callahan DJ: A study of blood-drainage patterns on synthetic cast materials. *Orthop Nurs* (March-April) 1985; 4:72–75.

This study investigated blood drainage in five types of fiberglass casting materials and one type of plaster of Paris. The fiberglass cast material did not absorb blood. The blood was drained to the outside of the cast or was absorbed into the casting pad. With plaster of Paris, however, blood was absorbed into the plaster material.

The authors stated that, with fiberglass casts, wound drainage will be found on bed linen or on the cast pad. Clients must be alerted to the possibility of bleeding and what to expect. This visible drainage is a method for assessing client status and wound status postoperatively.

Other skin changes may be the result of treatment such as immobilization, casts, and traction. The nurse must therefore assess the skin condition of clients receiving such treatment. Pressure sores can occur readily at any point of pressure. Assess the skin around cast edges frequently and any areas touched by the traction apparatus. If the client cannot be turned, take advantage of any opportunity to view normally hidden areas. For example, check the skin of the heels and sacrum when the client is raised for back care.

Deformities

Assess joints for deformities by observation and palpation. Compare joints in one extremity with those in the corresponding extremity, checking for symmetry, position, and changes in alignment. See Box 56–1 for the major points in general joint assessment.

When there is a joint dislocation, the normal shape of the joint is lost. There may be an abnormal bulge or mass in the joint area (as when the patella is displaced to the side, for example), or the two extremities may differ in length. Leg length discrepancy can be ascertained by measuring from the anterosuperior iliac spine to the medial malleolus when the client is lying down, as shown in Figure 56–1.

Another type of deformity to be assessed is a deviation in the angle of the limbs. A *valgus* deformity is one in which the part of the body distal to the joint is angled away from the midline of the body; for example, genu valgum is the term for knock-knees. A *varus* deformity is one in which the part of the body distal to the joint is angled toward the midline of the body; eg, *genu varum* is the name for bowlegs. These deformities are illustrated in Figure 56–2. The same adjectives, *valgus* and *varus,* are used to describe foot deformities; when the heel is turned outward, the term is *talipes valgus;* turned inward, *talipes varus.*

Box 56–1 General Joint Assessment

Examine all joints in sequence from head to toe.

Examine painful joint last so less pain and fewer muscle spasms are induced.

Compare joints from one side to the other for symmetry.

Note size and contour of joints.

Observe for joint deformity, swelling, contractures, subluxation (partial dislocation), ankylosis (fixation).

Inspect color of overlying skin.

Palpate for temperature.

Touch gently to locate areas of tenderness in surrounding skin, muscles, bursae, and ligaments.

Palpate synovial membrane. Normally, the membrane is about the thickness of paper; the abnormal membrane feels boggy or doughy. Test for bulge sign.

Evaluate range of motion (ROM), active and passive.

Palpate for crepitation (a grating sound) on motion.

Assess muscle strength.

Observe for muscle atrophy.

Assess the spine for abnormal curvature (Figure 56–3). A lateral curve is known as **scoliosis.** An increased convex curve of the thoracic spine (hunchback) is called **kyphosis,** whereas an increased concave curve of the lumbar spine (swayback) is known as **lordosis.** With a deformity, the client may shift another body part in the opposite direction to compensate for the imbalance; eg, the pelvis may tilt to compensate when one leg is shorter than the other. Look for these compensatory changes.

Abnormal bone growths, unnatural bone position, or a bone discontinuity can be observed. Suspicious areas should be palpated for tenderness or irregularity. When a part of the bone has moved out of its original alignment, it is said to be angulated. Angulation could be the result of abnormal development, a current injury, or an old fracture that healed in improper alignment. Bony fragments protruding from an open wound are an obvious deformity.

Consider the effects of any deformities when assessing the client's posture, gait, range of joint motion, and other functional abilities.

Range of Motion

Normal range of joint motion is described in Chapter 7. Range of motion (ROM) is measured with an instrument called a goniometer (Figure 56–4). Placing the arms of the goniometer parallel to the axis of the bones that form

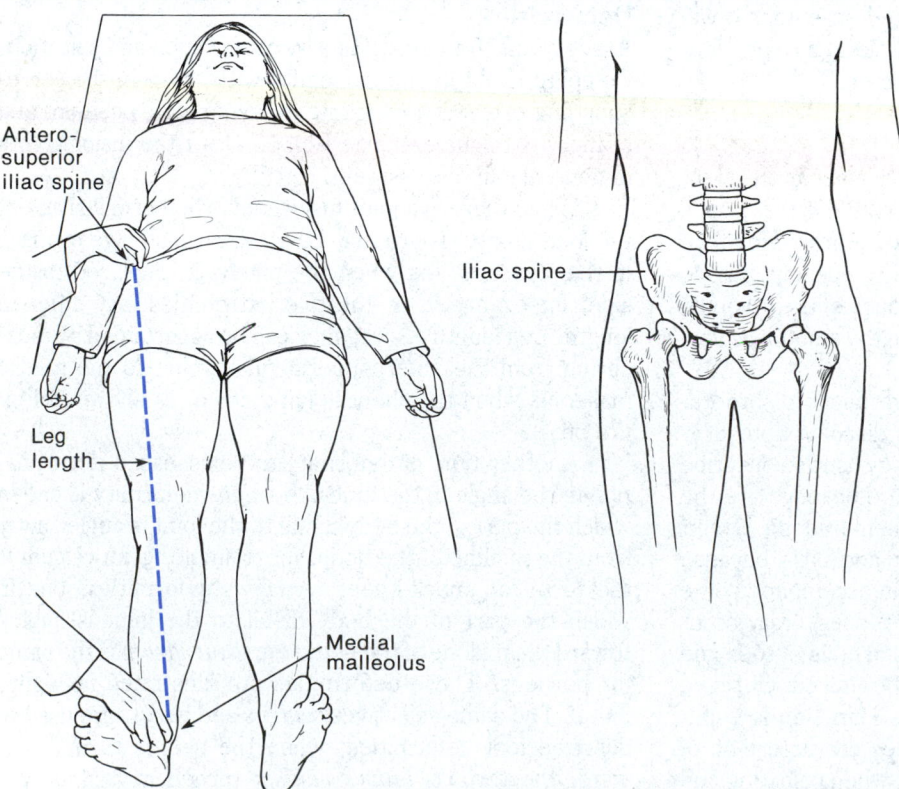

Figure 56–1

Measurement of leg length with client supine.

Antero-superior iliac spine

Iliac spine

Leg length

Medial malleolus

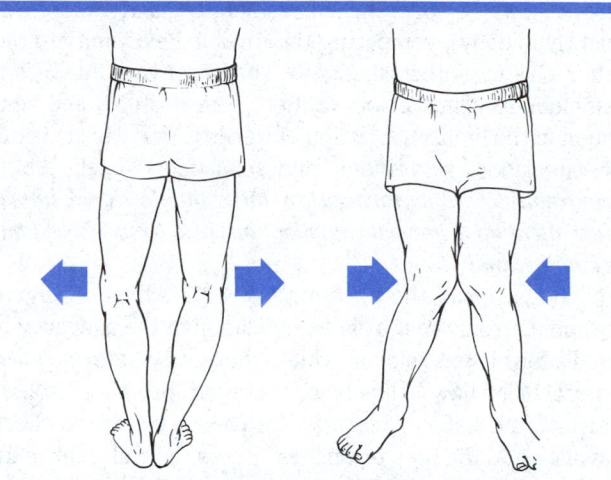

Figure 56–2

Left: Genu varum (bowlegs). **Right:** Genu valgum (knock-knees).

the joint, the examiner measures the angle for the typical positions of the joint. The elbow's normal flexion, for example, is 160°, whereas its normal extension is 0° (Rodts, 1983). To determine what is normal for a client, compare a joint with an apparently abnormal ROM to the corresponding joint in the other extremity. Elderly people are likely to have some normal decrease in ROM, so it would be incorrect to use the average range as the standard for them.

Ask the client to do ROM actively during evaluation. If the client is unable to move the extremity because of

paralysis, determine ROM through passive movement. Do not move a joint beyond the point of comfort, and do not assess ROM in an acutely inflamed joint because it will be tender.

During the assessment of ROM, note joint stiffness, instability, and deformity. A grating sensation may be heard or felt during movement when there is a rough surface on the articular cartilage or when broken bone ends rub together. This grating is known as bony **crepitation**. A limitation of motion may be due to a *contracture* (permanent muscle shortening). The nurse who detects early signs of limitation of movement can implement measures to improve the ROM and prevent further limitations.

Posture

Observe the client's standing posture for abnormalities. Posture can be affected by deformities, anomalies, muscle weakness, trauma, and pain. Clients may hold themselves in positions that relieve or decrease pain. Observe the symmetry of the body parts. Deformities of the spinal column may affect posture, causing exaggeration of any of the normal spinal curves. Posture is also an indication of energy and muscle tone. Normally posture is erect but not as rigid as a soldier standing at attention.

Muscle Strength, Size, and Tone

Muscle strength, size, and tone help diagnose disease conditions and also give the nurse information about the amount of assistance a client may need when ambulating and participating in activities. The examiner tests muscle strength by asking the client to resist movements or to move against resistance applied by the examiner. Strength is graded on a scale of 0 to 5 (see Box 56–2).

Observe and palpate muscles bilaterally to check their size and any asymmetry. If there seems to be a discrepancy in size, measure the limb circumferences with a tape measure to see if there are significant differences.

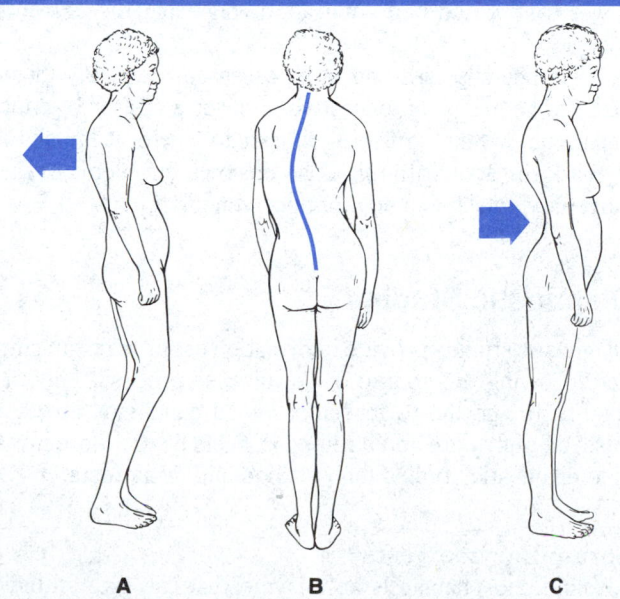

Figure 56–3

Abnormal spinal curves. **A.** Kyphosis. **B.** Scoliosis. **C.** Lordosis.

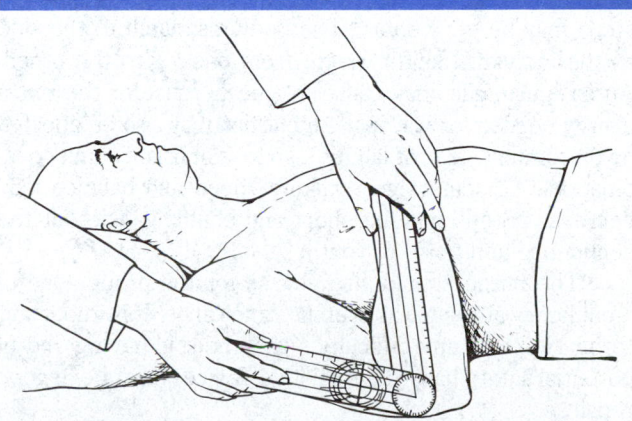

Figure 56–4

Use of a goniometer to measure the range of motion of a joint.

Box 56–2   Grading Muscle Strength

Grade 0: no evidence of contractility

Grade 1: trace of contractility

Grade 2: active movement with gravity eliminated

Grade 3: active movement against gravity

Grade 4: complete motion against gravity and some resistance

Grade 5: normal, complete motion against gravity and full resistance

---

Muscle tone is assessed by moving the extremities passively. While the client is relaxed, the examiner moves the extremity through the range of motion, noting resistance to movement. A muscle with diminished tone is described as *flaccid*. When the muscle is tight and tense from involuntary contraction, it is said to be *spastic*.

Function of the muscles depends on proper function of the nervous system. Muscle abnormalities noted during the assessment may be due to disorders of the nervous system, which are discussed in Unit Six. Specific disorders of the muscles are covered in Chapter 57.

Ability to Ambulate

To assess ability to ambulate, ask the client to get up to walk across the room, turn around, and come back. Note whether the client has any difficulty getting up from the chair or bed. Normally when a person walks, the feet are about 2 to 4 in apart, and the body shifts from side to side about 1 in (Larson & Gould, 1978). Posture is erect, with toes pointed straight ahead and shoulders in a straight line; the arms swing back and forth at the person's side, and movement is smooth with good balance.

There can be a variety of irregularities in walking. A limp can occur from abnormalities of leg length, joint motion, muscle strength, or other causes. The gait may appear stiff, unsteady, or wide-based; the feet may drag, or the steps may be very short. The body may lurch to the side as the individual shifts weight from one leg to the other. An irregular gait may cause fatigue because of the extra energy needed for walking. Ambulation may also be affected by discomfort, fear of falling, and loss of balance and coordination. As adults age, walking speed and balance may decrease. Steps may be short and shuffling, without the confidence and poise of youth.

The nurse should also assess for the proper use of ambulatory aids such as crutches and canes. It is important to be aware of any difficulties the client is having and of potential safety hazards. Assistive devices must be in good repair.

Neurovascular Status

Assessment of neurovascular status in the extremities is important for clients with traumatic injuries, surgery, casts,

and traction. Perform the assessment regularly (more frequently initially), comparing the involved extremity to the other one to detect changes. The acronym CMTS is a reminder to check color, motion, temperature, and sensation in the limb. A variation of this is CMS, which stands for circulation, movement, and sensation (Distel, 1982). *Abnormalities in neurovascular status should receive immediate attention to prevent complications and irreversible damage to the limb.*

The color of the extremity or of the toes or fingers extending from the cast is an indication of the adequacy of circulation. If the color is white, there may be inadequate arterial blood flow; if it is blue, there may be venous stasis. Perform the *test for blanching* (or capillary refill) to check circulation to the toes or fingers. Press the nail firmly until it turns white, then release the pressure quickly; the normal pink coloring should return in 3 to 5 seconds. If the color is slow to return, there may be reduced arterial blood flow to the extremity.

Interference with the nerves supplying the extremity can cause a decrease in motion and change in sensation. To check motion, ask the client to move (flex, extend, abduct, and adduct) all the toes or fingers of the involved extremity within the limitation imposed by pain (or cast). Observe for diminished or absent motion. Assess all toes or fingers of the extremity for changes in sensation because some digits are innervated by one nerve and some by another. Test sensation by pricking the toe or finger with an object such as the end of a straightened paper clip. The client should describe the sensation, such as numbness, tingling, burning, dull pain, or no sensation.

Temperature is assessed by feeling the extremity and comparing to the other one. Take into consideration that a wet cast or ice bag application can make the extremity cold.

Peripheral pulses should be assessed, especially those distal to an injury, an operative area, or a cast or traction apparatus. When a pulse is difficult to locate, it is helpful to mark the spot with ink. Also observe for edema of the extremity, which is a sign of poor venous return.

Diagnostic Studies

Diagnostic studies provide information useful in diagnosing and following the course of the disease process. Laboratory tests specific to musculoskeletal conditions are discussed briefly here and outlined in Table 56–1. More invasive diagnostic studies follow blood and urine tests.

Serum Enzyme Tests

Alkaline phosphatase is an enzyme that can give an indication of new or active bone formation, because osteoblasts secrete large quantities of this enzyme when they are actively depositing bony matrix. Extreme elevations are common with Paget's disease of the bone, metastatic tumors to

Table 56–1	Laboratory Tests Common to the Musculoskeletal System		
Laboratory Test	**Normal Expected Value**	**Musculoskeletal Dysfunction**	**Expected Abnormal Findings**
Alkaline phosphatase	1.5–4.5 U/dL (Bodansky units) 4–13 U/dL (King-Armstrong units) 0.8–2.3 U/mL (Bessey-Lowry-Brock units)	Paget's disease Metastatic cancer to the bone Osteogenic sarcoma Healing fractures Osteomalacia Rickets Hyperparathyroidism	↑ ↑ ↑ ↑ ↑ ↑ ↑
Antinuclear antibodies (ANA)	Negative	Rheumatoid arthritis Sjögren's syndrome Polymyositis Scleroderma Systemic lupus erythematosus Dermatomyositis Felty's syndrome Periarteritis nodosa Chronic discoid lupus	May be positive ↓ ↓ ↓ ↓ ↓ ↓ ↓ ↓
Calcium (Ca^{++})	8.5–10.5 mg/dL or 4.3–5.3 mEq/L	Hyperparathyroidism Metastatic cancer to the bone Multiple myeloma Prolonged immobilization Healing fractures Hypoparathyroidism Osteomalacia Rickets	↑ ↑ ↑ ↑ ↑ ↓ ↓ ↓
Creatine phosphoki-nase (CPK) or creatine kinase (CK)	5–25 U/mL 10–135 U/L ⎫ in women 5–35 U/mL 20–170 U/L ⎫ in men	Skeletal muscle disease Strenuous exercise Polymyositis Following IM injections	↑ ↑ ↑ ↑
Erythrocyte sedimenta-tion rate (ESR, sed. rate)	0–20 mm/h Wintrobe ⎫ in women 0–9 mm/h Wintrobe Westergren ⎫ in men (Increased in elderly)	Inflammatory diseases Collagen diseases Multiple myeloma Sarcoma Rheumatoid arthritis	↑ ↑ ↑ ↑ ↑
Serum glutamic-oxa-loacetic transaminase (SGOT, GOT)	3–21 IU/L 8–40 U/mL	Dermatomyositis Muscle damage Muscular dystrophy	↑ ↑ ↑
Human lymphocyte antigen B27 (HLA-B27)	Positive or negative	Ankylosing spondylitis Reiter's syndrome Psoriatic arthritis Enteropathic arthritis Juvenile rheumatoid arthritis	May be positive ↓ ↓ ↓ ↓
Lactic dehydrogenase (LDH)	80–120 Wacker units 71–207 IU/L 150–450 Wroblewski units	Muscular dystrophy Dermatomyositis Skeletal muscle malignancy	↑ ↑ ↑
Lupus erythematosus cell preparation (LE prep)	Negative	Systemic lupus erythematosus Chronic discoid lupus Rheumatoid arthritis Periarteritis nodosa Sjögren's syndrome Dermatomyositis	May be positive ↓ ↓ ↓ ↓ ↓
Phosphorus (PO$_4$$^{--}$)	3.0–4.5 mg/dL 1.8–2.6 mEq/L	Osteoporosis Healing fractures Hypoparathyroidism	↑ ↑ ↑

(continued)

Table 56−1 Laboratory Tests Common to the Musculoskeletal System (continued)			
Laboratory Test	**Normal Expected Value**	**Musculoskeletal Dysfunction**	**Expected Abnormal Findings**
Rheumatoid factor (RF, latex fixation)	Negative	Rheumatoid arthritis Some chronic inflammatory diseases	Titer of 1:40− 1:160 Lower titers
Uric acid	2.0−6.6 mg/dL, women 2.1−7.5 mg/dL, men	Gout Multiple myeloma Arthritis Hyperparathyroidism	↑ ↑ ↑ ↑
Urine calcium	1+ to 2+ turbidity with Sulkowitch test	Hyperparathyroidism Osteolytic bone disease Osteoporosis Hypoparathyroidism Osteomalacia	↑ ↑ ↑ ↓ ↓

bone, and osteogenic sarcoma. (This enzyme is also elevated in liver disease.)

Blood tests performed to detect presence of muscle disease measure levels of enzymes released when muscle tissue is destroyed or injured. These enzymes are creatine phosphokinase (CPK) or creatine kinase (CK), lactic dehydrogenase (LDH), and serum glutamic-oxaloacetic transaminase (SGOT), also known as aspartate aminotransferase (AST). The same tests indicate cardiac muscle destruction in the client with a myocardial infarction.

Serum Tests for Antibodies and Antigens

Antinuclear antibodies (ANA) are autoantibodies, produced against components of one's own cell nuclei. They are often present in clients with inflammatory connective tissue diseases, such as systemic lupus erythematosus or rheumatoid arthritis. The antibodies are detected by immunofluorescence, which is used as a screening test for clients with symptoms of such conditions. When ANA is present, the fluorescent dye used as a stain reacts within the antibodies and shows up under ultraviolet light (a positive result). The dye forms certain patterns that have been associated with disease. ANA results may also be positive with advancing age, but otherwise the test should be negative in the absence of connective tissue disease. After the presence of ANA is established, specific tests are done to identify particular antibodies such as anti-DNA (specific for systemic lupus erythematosus) and anti-RNA (specific in mixed connective tissue disease and systemic lupus erythematosus).

The test for the rheumatoid factor (RF) is specific for rheumatoid arthritis. The test, also called latex fixation, is frequently negative in the early stages of the disease but is usually positive in advanced rheumatoid arthritis. RF is also present in some chronic inflammatory diseases, including connective tissue disorders, but the titers are lower.

The test for the presence of human lymphocyte antigen B27 (HLA-B27) is used to help diagnose or rule out ankylosing spondylitis and Reiter's syndrome. This antigen is present in 90% of those with these diseases (Tilkian, Conover, & Tilkian, 1983). The antigen can also be found on tissue cells of those without these diseases, however, so its presence is not sufficient for a diagnosis.

Serum Calcium and Phosphorus

The level of calcium in the blood is used to detect bone disease and parathyroid gland disorder. A test for calcium is usually ordered along with serum phosphorus level because their concentrations are interrelated. Generally, when one level is elevated, the other is lowered. Conditions that increase bone resorption (osteoclastic activity) such as hyperparathyroidism, invasive bone disease, bone atrophy, osteoporosis, and osteomalacia cause an increase in the level of serum calcium.

Serum Uric Acid

Serum uric acid is elevated during an acute episode of gout but may be normal during remission. The serum uric acid level is also used as an indication of kidney function.

LE Cell Preparation

The LE prep (lupus erythematosus cell preparation) is useful in diagnosing systemic lupus erythematosus (SLE). It is positive in 90% of untreated SLE; however, false positive and false negative results do occur. Since negative results do not eliminate the diagnosis of SLE, and since results may be positive in other diseases, this test is not used as much today as it has been in the past. The anti-DNA test is more specific for diagnosing SLE.

Erythrocyte Sedimentation Rate

The erythrocyte sedimentation rate (ESR or sed. rate) is a test in which the settling of red blood cells in uncoagulated blood is timed. It is not a specific test for any particular disease, but elevations occur during inflammatory conditions and tissue necrosis. Changes in the ESR give an indication of improvement or worsening of the condition.

Urine Calcium

The amount of calcium excreted in the urine is a reflection of the level of serum calcium.

Synovial Fluid Analysis

Synovial fluid may be analyzed to detect inflammatory joint conditions, arthritis, and joint infection. The fluid is removed from an involved joint by aspiration (arthrocentesis). The procedure is done with aseptic technique, including skin preparation, local anesthetic, and use of a sterile needle and syringe. Normal joint fluid is clear and straw colored, with high viscosity and a white blood cell count (WBC) of less than $200/\mu L$. In disease conditions, the fluid may appear cloudy, turbid, green, gray, or red, with decreased viscosity and an elevated WBC. The fluid may be used for a mucin clot test: A drop of synovial fluid normally forms a firm clot when added to an acetic acid solution, but in some inflammatory conditions, the clot will be soft and friable. When joint infection is suspected, Gram's stain and culture of the fluid are done to detect the causative organism.

X-rays

Examination by x-ray helps diagnose bone and joint problems; it also allows following of the progress of a condition and its response to treatment. Abnormalities of bones that can be detected by x-ray include fractures, changes in density, and changes of position. X-rays also show joint changes such as erosion of joint margins, joint space narrowing, bone spurs, loose bodies, and dislocation. Specific injuries to soft tissues such as tendons and ligaments do not show on x-rays, but soft tissue swelling may be obvious. There is no special preparation for x-rays, but the client should be instructed to remain still when asked. When a fracture is suspected, clients should be moved cautiously to and from the x-ray department as well as on and off the cart and x-ray table to prevent further injury. It is essential to splint an extremity before the client is moved.

Special x-rays requiring injection of radiopaque substances are sometimes used for further study. Question the client before the procedure to determine any allergy to radiopaque dyes or iodine (because many dyes contain iodine). An *arthrogram* is an x-ray of a joint following the injection of radiopaque dye; the injection requires sterile technique. The internal structure of the injected joint can be visualized on the x-ray because the dye outlines the intracapsular joint space. Changes in the joint structure, such as injury to the ligaments and meniscal tears, show on the x-ray as patterns taken by the dye.

A *myelogram* is an x-ray and fluoroscopic exam of the spinal cord and subarachnoid space following the injection of a contrast medium, which is introduced by way of a lumbar puncture (see Chapter 36). Abnormalities such as a herniated disk can be localized when filling defects are seen on the x-ray. When Pantopaque medium is used, the postprocedural care is like that following a lumbar puncture. A newer medium, metrizamide (Amipaque), is being used for lumbar myelography. It provides the advantages of better visualization and use of a smaller needle. The medium does not need to be withdrawn. When Amipaque is used, the postprocedural care includes prevention of nausea, vomiting, headache, and seizures. The head of the bed must be elevated 30–40° for 8 hours, followed by flat bed rest with bathroom privileges for the next 16 hours. Oral fluids are encouraged. Phenothiazines, MAO inhibitors, and tricyclic antidepressants should be withheld 48 hours prior to the myelogram to decrease the possibility of seizure activity. Phenothiazines must also be avoided for 24 hours after the procedure (Branson, 1982).

Bone Scan

A bone scan provides a picture of radioactivity in bones after intravenous injection of a radioactive isotope, usually technetium 99. The radioactive substance accumulates in areas of increased osteoblastic activity, which then show up as dark spots on the screen. Since some malignant bone tumors have accelerated osteoblastic activity, the bone scan is useful in diagnosing these tumors. A bone scan may be done when bone metastasis from other tumor sites is suspected. A bone scan can detect lesions at an earlier stage of disease than a routine x-ray. Tell clients that the injection may be a little uncomfortable and that they must remain still during the scan itself.

Arthroscopy

Arthroscopy is the examination of a joint through a special fiberoptic endoscope called an arthroscope (Figure 56–5). The knee is the joint most commonly examined by this means. The instrument has lenses and a light source permitting photography and surgical procedures through it. The procedure is done in the operating room using aseptic technique, usually with the use of a local anesthetic, although a general anesthetic may be given. A tourniquet helps to reduce blood flow to the area. A cannula is inserted into the joint, through which the scope is introduced, and normal saline is instilled to provide a viewing medium. The technique can be used for biopsy of the synovium or cartilage, as well as removal of loose bodies from the joint. After the procedure, a compression dressing, such as an Ace bandage, is applied. The client may be allowed to bear weight, avoiding excessive use for a few days, or may be directed to avoid use for 24 hours, depending on the surgeon's preference and the nature of the procedure. Teach the client to observe for signs of infection. The procedure is frequently done on an outpatient basis (Farrell, 1982).

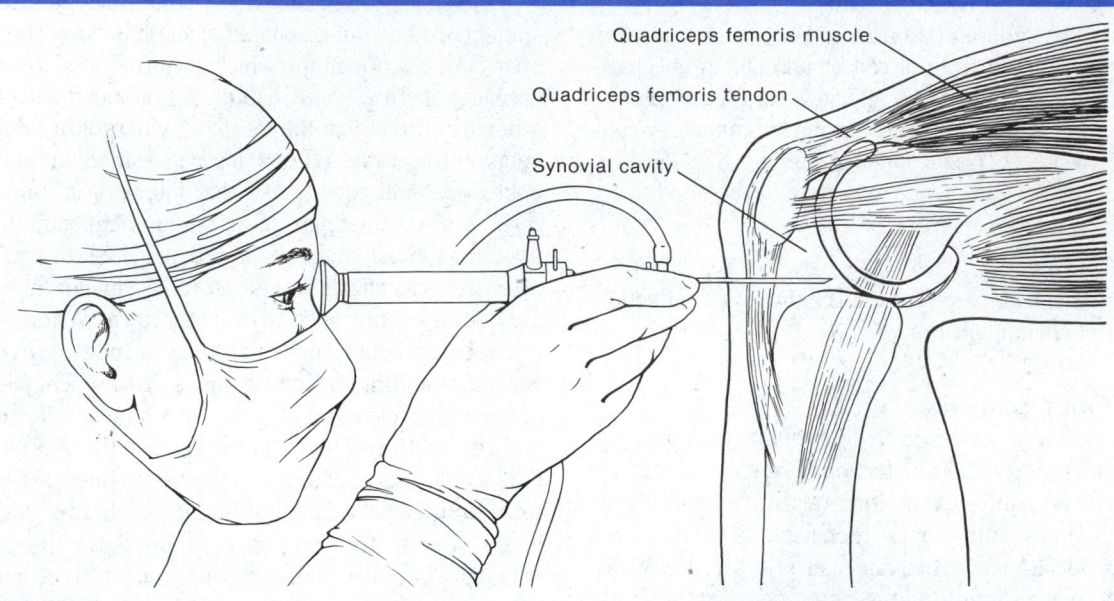

Quadriceps femoris muscle

Quadriceps femoris tendon

Synovial cavity

Figure 56–5

Use of an arthroscope to view interior of the knee.

Electromyogram

The **electromyogram** (EMG) is a test to measure the electric currents produced by muscles, at rest and during contraction. Small needle electrodes are inserted into the muscles being tested and then connected by wires to an electromyograph machine. The results are recorded, displayed on a screen, and heard on a speaker. Changes in muscle electrical activity may be helpful in diagnosing neuromuscular disease. The test is particularly useful in differentiating muscular disease from neurologic disease. There is no special preparation before the test. Inform the client that small needles will be inserted into skin and muscle, causing some discomfort but that there is no danger of electrical shock.

Biopsy

A biopsy is the removal of tissue for the purpose of microscopic examination; it may be done to confirm diagnosis or to follow the course of a disease or the effectiveness of treatment. Specimens may be obtained by means of a special needle or punch, excision of a piece of tissue during open incision, or aspiration of fluid. When a lesion is suspected, the location is approximated by means of examination and diagnostic tests. When a needle biopsy is done on an internal lesion, there is no certainty that the sampled area contains cells from the lesion. Therefore, an open incision in which the lesion is visualized may be the method of choice in some biopsies. Needle or punch biopsies can be done at the client's bedside, in the physician's office, or in surgery. The incisional biopsy is an operative procedure done under general or local anesthesia.

Various biopsies may be performed on the musculoskeletal system. Bone may be obtained by open or needle biopsy to diagnose or follow a bone disease or lesion. Skin, obtained by a punch biopsy, is examined to diagnose some of the connective tissue disorders. Muscle biopsies are usually operative procedures done to evaluate muscle disease. Synovial membrane can be biopsied by means of an arthroscopy, a needle biopsy, or an open incision. Synovial membrane analysis is useful in diagnosing different types of arthritis. Buccal mucosa may be biopsied to help diagnose Sjögren's syndrome, and the temporal artery may be biopsied to diagnose temporal arteritis.

Section II: Nursing Diagnosis

Several nursing diagnoses evolve from the nursing assessment of clients with musculoskeletal problems. (See Box 56–3 for nursing diagnoses commonly related to the client with musculoskeletal dysfunction.) The most notable diagnosis is *impaired physical mobility*. A nursing care plan for this diagnosis is covered in general in Table 56–2. Most of the common diagnoses presented in the table are potential problems. Therefore the nursing interventions are primarily preventive measures. This care plan should be individualized to specific client conditions.

Alteration in bowel elimination: constipation is another common nursing diagnosis. Since this problem is frequently associated with immobility, the nursing care plan to deal with it is covered within Table 56–2 under "potential for constipation." *Ineffective breathing pattern* is a possible nursing diagnosis because of immobility. The nursing care plan for this potential problem is covered in Table 56–2 under "potential for hypostatic pneumonia."

Sexual dysfunction may result from obstacles created by such forms of treatment as casts, traction, and prolonged hospitalization. Pain, deformity, altered body image, and role change can lead to sexual dysfunction. A general nursing care plan for this diagnosis is presented in Table 56–3. Care also should be individualized to the client and specific problem. *Disturbance in self-concept:* body image is covered more thoroughly in Chapter 4.

Alteration in comfort: pain is a common nursing diagnosis for this system. Pain is discussed in Chapter 5. *Impairment of skin integrity: potential* is also a risk area for musculoskeletal conditions. The care plan for this potential problem is covered within Table 56–2 under "potential for skin breakdown" and also is covered in Chapter 78.

Altered peripheral tissue perfusion can occur in musculoskeletal problems when casts, traction, and bandages are applied, when surgery is done, or when trauma occurs. Clients who have limited mobility and pain may find they cannot participate in their usual interests and therefore will need to learn new diversional activities.

Some clients with musculoskeletal conditions will experience a *self-care deficit* because of pain, deformity, loss of strength, and limited mobility. Because this is common for those with rheumatoid arthritis, it will be covered specifically for that condition in Chapter 59.

Box 56–3	Nursing Diagnoses Commonly Related to Musculoskeletal Dysfunction

Diagnoses Directly Related to Musculoskeletal Dysfunction

Mobility, impaired physical

Tissue perfusion, alteration in

Skin integrity, impairment of, potential

Comfort, alteration in, related to pain

Sexual dysfunction, potential

Self-care deficit

Breathing pattern, ineffective

Bowel elimination, alteration in, related to constipation

Self-concept, disturbance in, related to body image

Additional Potential Nursing Diagnoses

Coping, ineffective individual

Coping, ineffective family: compromised

Sleep pattern disturbance

Injury, potential for, related to trauma

Diversional activity, deficit

Section III: Planning and Implementation

Several general nursing interventions are common to many musculoskeletal problems.

PROMOTING REST

Rest is particularly useful in treating inflammatory conditions of the joints, especially during the acute phase, because it helps relieve pain and prevent further destruction of joint tissues. Rest is also helpful after musculoskeletal trauma because it helps minimize pain and swelling and promotes healing of injured tissues. A fractured bone is rested by use of a splint, cast, or traction after the bone is placed in good alignment. Rest is also used to relieve muscle spasms.

Rest may be prescribed for the whole body (bed rest) or for local areas by use of splints or casts. Bed rest may be helpful during joint inflammation and is necessary with traction. Because prolonged bed rest can result in many complications, specific nursing measures are necessary to

prevent their occurrence (see Table 56–2). Splinting joints provides stability, relieves pain caused by movement, and maintains the joint in a functional position. Rest may also be achieved by restricting weight bearing on an injured extremity, thus resting it.

A balance between rest and activity is desired so that function can be maintained while additional disability is prevented. Clients with arthritis need extra rest periods and extra hours of sleep at night. They need to be taught the importance of planning for this additional rest to control fatigue and restore energy.

In addition to physical rest, emotional rest is necessary in inflammatory disease because exacerbations can occur during emotional upset. Nurses can teach clients relaxation techniques and encourage clients to minimize negative life stresses and to respond with humor to stresses that cannot be avoided.

(continued on p. 1654)

Table 56–2 Sample Nursing Care Plan for Clients With Impaired Physical Mobility

Nursing Diagnosis	Client Care Goals	Plan/Nursing Implementation	Expected Outcome
Mobility, impaired physical, related to: 1. Potential for muscle atrophy	Actively exercises the involved muscles within the limits of prescribed therapy; understands the causes of muscle wasting and the benefits of active exercise	Assess muscle size, strength, symmetry; ambulate as much as possible; encourage participation in ADL; teach isometric exercises when isotonics are not possible; active ROM, at least b.i.d.; teach how active exercise prevents muscle wasting	Muscle symmetry, size, strength equal to those of uninvolved extremity; ambulates and participates in ADL with minimal assistance; describes reason for active exercise
2. Potential for joint contracture	ROM exercises of the involved joints within the limits of prescribed therapy; understands the causes of joint contracture and the benefits of exercises and correct alignment; maintains proper body alignment when sitting or lying	Assess the client's ROM; ROM at least b.i.d.; position in correct body alignment; change position frequently; use assistive devices that maintain position, such as hand cones, footboard; encourage participation in ADL; teach ROM exercises, correct positioning; teach how mobility prevents contractures; rest in a functional position, ie, avoid hip rotation, wrist drop, footdrop	Retains normal range of joint motion; describes reasons for exercises and correct alignment
3. Potential for bone demineralization (osteoporosis)	Changes position frequently; carries out daily weight-bearing exercises and activities; understands the effects of immobility on the bone; eats a well-balanced diet	Encourage weight bearing as much as possible including standing, sitting, ambulation; encourage resistive exercises; encourage participation in ADL; teach how mobility helps prevent bone demineralization; implement frequent position changes; encourage eating a well-balanced diet with adequate intake of calcium, vitamin D, and protein	Performs weight-bearing exercises regularly; describes the reasons for activity, weight bearing, and balanced diet; shows no evidence of bone pain or porous bones (on x-ray)
4. Potential for skin breakdown	Changes position frequently; takes in a well-balanced diet and 2000–3000 mL of fluids per day; understands the effects of prolonged pressure on skin integrity; observes own skin for pressure sores where possible	Encourage position changes q.1 h; assess and teach client to assess skin for signs of potential skin breakdown: redness, edema, pain; keep skin clean, dry, and lubricated; check every 4–8 h; keep sheets wrinkle free; use special devices to decrease pressure such as air or water mattresses; teach client to shift weight periodically; encourage a well-balanced diet with at least 2000–3000 mL of fluids per day; teach how prolonged pressure causes decubitus ulcer formation.	Avoids staying in the same position for more than 1 h; skin shows no signs of breakdown; describes how skin breaks down from prolonged pressure
5. Potential for urinary calculi	Takes in 3000 mL of fluids per 24 h; understands the relationship of immobility and stone formation; changes position frequently and ambulates when able	Encourage fluid intake of 3000 mL per 24 h; I & O; ambulate as much as possible; change position frequently; especially use an upright position periodically; teach that mobility helps decrease stone formation; observe for signs of stone formation such as hematuria, flank pain, dysuria; check urine pH daily; check serum Ca^{++} values	Shows no signs of urinary calculi formation; ambulates and changes position regularly; describes reason for activity and increased fluid intake; fluid intake is 3000 mL per 24 h; urine pH remains slightly acidic
6. Potential for urinary retention and/or incontinence	Empties bladder adequately, voluntarily; understands the relationship between	Note voiding pattern (frequency, amount); assess for signs of urinary retention, such as inability to void, abdominal distention; I & O; use a	No signs of bladder distention or incontinence; describes how activity aids voiding

Nursing Diagnosis	Client Care Goals	Plan/Nursing Implementation	Expected Outcome
	decreased activity, decreased muscle tone, and difficulty voiding; changes position frequently	sitting (or standing) position to void; provide privacy; encourage activity and ambulation as much as possible; teach that mobility aids the ability to void normally; use methods to facilitate voiding, such as running water within hearing distance	
7. Potential for constipation	Ambulates and exercises regularly; understands the causes of constipation; takes in 3000 mL of fluids per 24 h; includes roughage in diet	Question client regarding a BM daily; I & O; ambulate as much as possible; encourage fluids, at least 3000 mL per 24 h; encourage foods containing fiber; use a sitting position for BM; provide privacy; consult with physician as needed for orders for laxatives, stool softeners; teach relationship between mobility, fluids, fiber, and constipation	Maintains usual bowel pattern; describes how constipation is related to immobility
8. Potential for hypostatic pneumonia	Practices coughing and deep-breathing exercises (C & DB); ambulates and changes position frequently; understands the effects of immobility on respiratory system	Assess rate, depth, rhythm of respirations q. 4 h; assess the chest for abnormal breath sounds; assess skin color for hypoxia; teach and encourage C & DB exercises q. 2 h; encourage ambulation as much as possible; encourage frequent position changes, especially upright; observe for obstructions to respirations, such as a tight cast or bandage; teach about the relationship between immobility and respiratory problems	Shows no signs of respiratory problems; explains how inactivity affects the respiratory system; performs C & DB exercises q. 2 h
9. Potential for orthostatic hypotension	Safely ambulates or assumes upright position regularly; understands the relationship between immobility and postural hypotension	Encourage regular exercise and ambulation; encourage the upright position; have client wear elastic stockings; teach and encourage client to get up slowly; check BP while dangling, before standing, and q. 4 h; observe for light-headedness when upright; teach the relationship between hypotension and immobility	Blood pressure remains stable when upright; explains the cause of postural hypotension and the reason for rising slowly; engages in regular activity including ambulation
10. Potential for thrombus formation	Exercises the extremities actively; understands the tendency for clot formation during inactivity; increases fluid intake to at least 3000 mL per 24 h	Observe for signs of thrombus formation, such as tenderness, edema; check Homan's sign; have client wear elastic stockings; encourage active leg exercises regularly, such as pedaling the feet, drawing imaginary circles with the toes; avoid positioning with acute angle flexion of the knees, such as using the knee gatch on the bed or pillows under the knees; change position q. 2 h; encourage fluid intake of at least 3000 mL per 24 h; avoid trauma to the limb; avoid positioning with one limb leaning on the other, causing pressure; teach about the relationship between immobility and blood clot formation	No signs of thrombus formation; explains the relationship between thrombus formation and immobility; carries out active leg exercises at least q. 2 h

(continued)

Table 56–2 Sample Nursing Care Plan for Clients With Impaired Physical Mobility (continued)

Nursing Diagnosis	Client Care Goals	Plan/Nursing Implementation	Expected Outcome
11. Potential for changes in the mental status	Expresses feelings about condition and situation; uses all senses; remains oriented; maintains independence as much as possible; interacts with others regularly; participates in activities as able	Encourage participation in ADL; encourage independence; exercise and ambulate frequently; change position frequently; encourage client to be out of room, socializing with others; encourage visitors and phone calls; orient or reorient as necessary (calendar, clock, familiar objects); encourage participation in usual hobbies and activities, when possible; provide opportunities for decision making; encourage expression of feelings; allow client to vent feelings about immobility, role change, restrictions; assess for changes in emotional reactions, orientation, motivation, body image, and self-concept; provide a change of scenery or encourage family to do so; use sensory stimuli such as touch, radio, TV	Shows proper orientation to person, place and time; demonstrates normal psychosocial status, as indicated by family; displays emotional reactions that are appropriate to the circumstances; maintains maximum independence; actively participates in interactions and activities; shares feelings and frustrations
12. Change in ability to ambulate	Exercises the muscles to be used in ambulation; uses any ambulatory aids correctly; understands safety measures for ambulation; adjusts home environment to facilitate ambulation, as needed	Teach exercises appropriate for ambulation: (1) isometrics of the quadriceps, abdominal, and gluteal muscles (2) doing pushups when prone (3) lifting buttocks off bed while sitting by pushing down on bed with hands. Teach use of trapeze appropriate for client, ie, bending knees and raising back and buttocks off the bed; shifting weight periodically, without holding breath when lifting; try the upright position a few times before ambulation for those who have been flat; use sturdy shoes when ambulating; get help when ambulating the first time and as needed; dangle feet first; teach transfer activities, eg, lock wheelchair wheels, elevate head of bed; teach correct use of ambulatory aids (physical therapist may do this but nurse should be familiar with methods to aid ambulation on the unit); make sure ambulatory aids are correct height, size; teach client to keep head up, looking forward (not down) when walking; assess balance; provide a safety belt for client's waist, for nurse to hold when walking; remove clutter, loose rugs, wet spots on floor, other items that may cause falls; also teach client and family; observe that client is using proper gait for aids used; make sure client can ambulate well enough to maneuver up and down stairs and in and out of bed before discharge; have someone assess client's home environment for safety and possible nec-	Ambulates with minimal assistance; describes safety measures necessary for ambulation; correctly uses ambulatory aids; participates in appropriate exercises; uses trapeze as taught; accidents or injuries do not occur in either hospital or home environment

Nursing Diagnosis	Client Care Goals	Plan/Nursing Implementation	Expected Outcome
		essary alterations to assist ambulation; have family member make necessary adjustments before discharge	
13. Change in ability to perform ADL	Participates in ADL, as able; learns new ways to perform ADL when necessary and able; adjusts to changes in ADL abilities	Assess ability to perform ADL; assess need for assistive devices; encourage participation in ADL; give reinforcement (acknowledgment, reward) for good performance and effort; place objects client will use nearby to facilitate self-help; teach alternative methods for achieving ADL; consult with physician, OT, PT for additional intervention as needed; consult for financial aid through social services, when needed for assistive devices, etc.; encourage family involvement when client will need assistance at home; encourage resourcefulness and creativity when trying adaptive techniques (buying a tool for every activity is not necessary); allow expression of feelings, eg, of discouragement or anger; give encouragement as needed and encourage family to do so	Functioning with as much independence as is possible; able to cope with necessary adjustments in performing ADL; client and family creatively adapt usual life activities to client's impairment in mobility

Table 56–3 Sample Nursing Care Plan for Orthopedic Clients With Potential Sexual Dysfunction

Nursing Diagnosis	Client Care Goals	Plan/Nursing Implementation	Expected Outcome
Sexual dysfunction related to: • Musculoskeletal discomforts • Prolonged hospitalization • Restrictions in motion	Understands alternative forms of sexual activity; adjusts sexual activity to avoid musculoskeletal discomfort; adjusts sexual activity to hospital environment; adjusts sexual activity to limitations imposed by condition or treatment; accepts changes imposed by musculoskeletal problem	Assess for affects of musculoskeletal pain, prolonged hospitalization, restricted motion, and change in role on sexuality; include effects on both client and significant other; teach that other forms of sexual activity are possible such as alternative positions, masturbation; encourage any type of sexual activity that is appealing and gratifying without causing discomfort or disrupting treatment; encourage client to discuss problem with partner so they can work out something mutually gratifying	States that sexual satisfaction is achieved without causing discomfort; describes alternative forms of sexual activity; expresses feelings about the sexual adjustment necessitated by musculoskeletal problems
• Changes in role and body image		Encourage verbalization of sexual concerns by both client and partner; teach client which positions are prohibited, eg, acute hip flexion after total hip replacement; encourage partner to express love and affection, as appropriate; provide opportunities for decision making and self-care (to increase feelings of independence, when role is changed)	

MAINTAINING PROPER POSITION AND BODY ALIGNMENT

Positioning the client is a nursing measure to prevent complications as well as a therapeutic measure to aid healing in proper alignment. Correct body posture and methods of positioning are covered in fundamental nursing textbooks. The nurse should be familiar with proper posture for lying, standing, and sitting. Important points relevant for musculoskeletal conditions will be emphasized here.

A firm mattress is especially important for the client confined to bed for an extended period of time, for those having back problems, and for those with heavy casts requiring support. A trapeze on the bed is useful to allow clients to shift their body weight periodically.

The client with an injured extremity or who has had surgery on an extremity will usually have the extremity elevated on pillows; the foot of the bed may be elevated in addition. When elevated, the entire length of a cast or splint should be supported to avoid strain on the unsupported area. When the client is lying on one side, the uppermost limb should be supported with pillows along its entire length to avoid adduction. Particular attention should be given to avoid pressure over nerves and bony prominences.

The normal curves of the back should be supported with small pads when the client is supine. Use of only a small pillow under the neck helps prevent neck flexion contracture. Trochanter rolls are used to prevent external hip rotation when supine. The prone position should be included in the positioning schedule when the client's condition allows.

A client with an inflamed or painful extremity will hold it in the most comfortable position. In most cases, that position involves flexion of a joint. Without exercise and changes in position, a contracture will develop. When joints are acutely inflamed or painful, a splint may be applied to rest the joint in a *functional position* (one that would be most useful if the joint became frozen in that position). Make sure splints fit properly, are removed periodically for skin care, and are reapplied. When handling painful extremities, the least distressing method is to support the limb above and below the affected area, handling it gently.

MAINTAINING COMFORT

Pain and discomfort should be assessed thoroughly before attempting nursing interventions. Because some orthopedic problems are chronic, dependence can occur with prolonged drug use. Comfort measures and relaxation approaches should be attempted and not abandoned because they were not effective initially.

The comfort measures learned in nursing fundamentals courses should be tried. Change the client's position and give a back rub or massage, where not contraindicated. Handle a painful limb gently or allow clients to move their own limbs, even if it takes time. Encourage resting the

painful limb. Sometimes elevating the limb relieves discomfort but lowering it increases the pain. Application of heat or cold, whichever is appropriate, may provide analgesia. When the weight of covers causes discomfort, a foot cradle or footboard may be helpful. Check for dressings that might be too tight, causing pain. Crumbs in a cast can be removed by a portable vacuum.

These measures should supplement the use of analgesics to relieve discomfort. Transcutaneous electrical nerve stimulation (TENS) or biofeedback may also be helpful (see Chapter 5).

APPLYING HEAT OR COLD

The use of either hot or cold applications provides temporary relief of pain and increased range of motion of joints. It used to be common to apply heat only to arthritic joints, but cold has also been found to be helpful for many people. Alternating application of heat and cold can be effective in some. Physicians suggest using whatever works for the arthritic client. Contraindications for heat or cold include poor circulation, decreased temperature sensation, and hypersensitivity to heat or cold. Use is limited in those who are not alert enough to note abnormal sensations from the heat or cold, including those who are sedated.

Heat specifically causes vasodilation, thereby increasing blood flow. It relaxes muscles, relieves morning stiffness, and provides analgesia. Heat is not used on acutely inflamed joints but is useful in subacute or chronic joint problems (Simpson, 1983). Many forms of heat, including dry and moist heat, are used for arthritic conditions. *Moist heat* is more penetrating and can be applied by a shower; by foot, hand, or tub baths; and by hot packs or compresses. *Dry heat* can be administered at higher temperatures than moist heat. Methods of dry heat include diathermy (electromagnetic waves) and ultrasound (high frequency sound waves), usually administered by a physical therapist. Heating pads, lamps, and hot water bottles also provide dry heat. Paraffin baths provide heat as the client dips the affected hand into melted paraffin. The hand is then wrapped in a towel or blanket for about 20 to 30 minutes to hold the heat (Larson & Gould, 1978).

Heat is often applied before exercise and massage. The exposure should last about 15 to 30 minutes, depending upon the method used. Prolonged use of heat causes vasoconstriction. The need for safety measures in applying heat cannot be overemphasized. The area should be checked frequently (every 5 minutes, at least) for redness, tissue damage, and discomfort. Clients should be instructed to get attention immediately if the application feels too hot. Clients should be taught not to adjust the heat source themselves.

Cold applications cause vasoconstriction, decreasing blood flow and helping to decrease or prevent swelling after injury. Pain may be relieved because cold raises the pain threshold. In some people, stiffness is relieved by cold. Cold is more useful in those with acute pain or acutely inflamed joints. It can be applied by cold compresses, ice bags, or a cold bath. Ice is applied to traumatic injuries for the first 24 hours after the accident to decrease fluid accumulation, control bleeding by vasoconstriction, and decrease pain. Prolonged use of cold, however, causes vasodilation. Therefore, cold is applied for 15 to 30 minutes, removed for 10 to 15 minutes, and then reapplied in a cyclical pattern. In between, dry the skin and check for untoward signs such as paleness, cyanosis, mottling, and secondary vasodilation. At times, ice is applied continuously to reduce swelling. If continuous cold is ordered, check the client frequently (every 5 minutes, at least) for undesired effects.

MAINTAINING SKIN INTEGRITY

Prolonged bed rest or wearing a cast, splint, or traction device may cause skin breakdown. Basic nursing care for prevention is covered in Table 56–2 under "potential for skin breakdown." Clients with deformity and inability to perform ADL will need special attention to hygiene if unable to help themselves. Some clients are reluctant to ask for assistance with bathing because they do not want to be dependent on others. Be tactful in assessing the need for assistance with skin care, and intervene appropriately.

PROMOTING EXERCISE AND AMBULATION

The benefits of exercise include increased circulation, maintenance of joint mobility, improvement in joint mobility, preservation of muscle strength, and improved muscle strength. ROM exercises, whether active or passive, help prevent contractures.

Isometric or muscle-setting exercises are done when a muscle contracts without movement, thereby maintaining strength, increasing tone, and aiding circulation. The client should be taught to contract or tighten the muscle, holding it until the count of 10, then relax. This should be done 10 to 15 times every 3 to 4 hours when awake. To instruct clients in isometric quadriceps exercises, tell them to try pushing the back of the knee against the mattress while sitting in bed. If this is done properly, the thigh muscle tightens and the heel raises off the mattress. Encourage clients to try it on the unaffected leg first to demonstrate the method. Quadriceps atrophy begins in 1 week if the muscle is not exercised (Farrell, 1982). Isometrics should be done on quadriceps, gluteal, and abdominal muscles to prepare the client for ambulation.

Isotonic exercises are done with uninvolved extremities. When the client will be using crutches, the arms can be strengthened by push-ups when prone, lifting the buttocks off the bed by pushing the palms against the mattress while sitting, weight lifting, and use of the trapeze. Commercial weights may be used, but objects such as sandbags or books can also serve as weights for lifting.

Exercises beneficial to arthritics include ROM and isometrics. Acutely inflamed joints are not exercised. Studies have shown that rest and splinting of inflamed joints cause minimal or no permanent joint mobility loss. Arthritic clients should not use isotonic or weight-lifting exercises that stress affected joints. They should also limit the number of repetitions of each movement (Simpson & Dickinson, 1983).

All clients should be encouraged to move all unrestricted body parts. Participation in ADL provides some exercise and should be encouraged. Those with a cast or splint should exercise the joints above and below the appliance, unless contraindicated. Clients with an arm cast tend to hold their shoulder in one position. For them, the sling should be removed and ROM exercises performed to keep the shoulder free. See the nursing care plan in Table 56–2 for nursing interventions to prevent muscle atrophy or joint contracture and to prepare for ambulation.

Physical therapists usually are consulted to help the client with ambulation. They also measure and fit the client for ambulatory aids such as crutches, canes, walkers, and wheelchairs. However, physical therapists are not readily available in most ambulatory care settings or emergency departments, where a majority of musculoskeletal injuries are treated. Therefore nurses should familiarize themselves with this information, in case they are called upon to measure crutches and teach crutch-walking. In most inpatient settings, an appropriate gait is taught and practiced in physical therapy. Nurses are responsible for assisting the client on the unit during ambulation, so they must be familiar with proper crutch posture and crutch-walking gaits. Proper posture includes: head held high, feet under the pelvis, crutches about 10 inches in front and slightly to the sides of the feet, and weight carried on the wrists and palms, not the axilla. If the weight rests on the axilla, the radial nerve may be injured, causing paralysis of the elbow and wrist extensor muscles. When the client is standing upright with shoulders relaxed, the axillary bar should be one to two fingers below the axilla. Both client and nurse should be aware of the amount of weight bearing allowed on the affected leg or legs: full, partial, or none.

Measuring a client for crutches can be done in bed or standing, with the shoes on. Measure from the axillary fold to a point 6 to 8 in lateral to the heel. Another method is to subtract 16 in from the height. The hand bar should be placed so that the elbow has 30° flexion (see Figure 56–6) when resting. The elbow extends when a step is taken. The crutches should be assessed for safety. Bolts should be tightened; rubber tips should not be worn down. A pad may or may not be used on the axillary bar. The client should wear low-heeled shoes with nonskid bottoms.

The most common crutch-walking gait is the three-point gait. The crutches are moved forward first, then the involved leg, and then the uninvolved leg. This gait is used when partial or no weight bearing is allowed on the involved leg. The two-point gait is used when some weight bearing is allowed on both feet. The client advances one crutch and the opposite leg simultaneously, then the other crutch and remaining leg together. The four-point gait is also used when some weight bearing is allowed on both feet. One

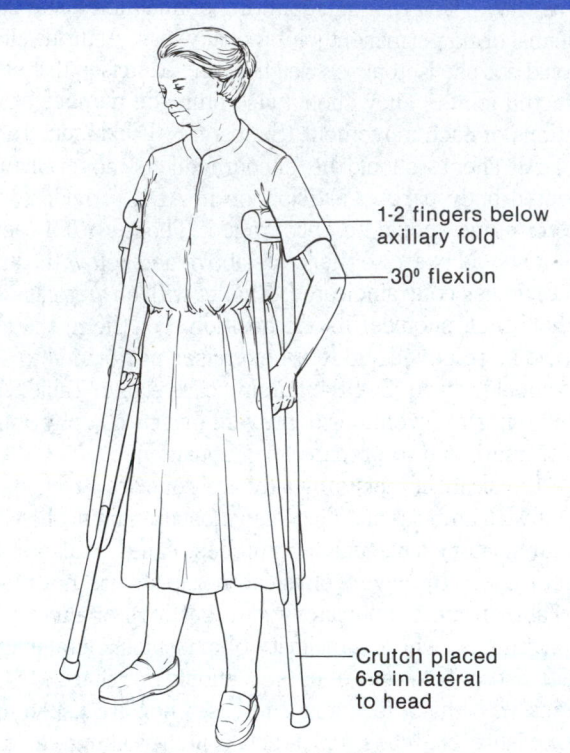

1-2 fingers below axillary fold

30° flexion

Crutch placed 6-8 in lateral to head

Figure 56–6

Correctly fitted crutches.

A walker is often used by elderly people because it provides greater support and a feeling of security. It is useful for clients with an unsteady gait and when partial weight bearing is necessary. The client can pick up and move the walker or push it forward. Walkers come in different sizes or can be adjusted. They are the correct height when the client's elbows are flexed 15° to 30° while holding the handles. Walkers are not very useful on stairs unless the tread is very deep, so the client may require assistance when navigating stairs.

Safety precautions are necessary with all types of aids to ambulation. At home, the family should remove clutter and loose rugs. Clients should wear sturdy shoes. Finally, clients should be assisted until they are ambulating well without help. It is important to plan ahead by instituting an exercise program to prepare the client for ambulation. Ambulation should begin with plenty of time available for practice before the client is discharged.

USING ASSISTIVE DEVICES

Many self-help devices are sold to aid the disabled client in maintaining independence. It is not always necessary to purchase these items; many suitable devices can be made at home. Many clients and their family members are creative in improvising to meet their needs.

Various modified eating utensils are available, some with built-up handles, others with long handles, and some with handles at a different angle than is usual (Figure 56–7).

Clients who cannot reach their feet adequately can use elastic shoelaces and various long-handled appliances such as shoehorns and stocking holders (Figure 56–8). Those who cannot raise their arms can use reachers and long-handled combs. The use of Velcro fasteners, rather than buttons, aids those with difficulty in fine motor skills. In the bathroom, an elevated toilet seat, handrails, a shower chair, nonskid mats, and a long-handled bath sponge can be helpful.

The occupational therapy (OT) department can assist the client in developing self-care abilities and make recommendations for easier, safer methods to do many tasks. In some facilities, the nurse can make referrals to OT; in others, the nurse must consult with the physician.

When a client normally uses special devices for self-care at home, encourage continued use when hospitalized. Any methods that keep clients independent should be encouraged, even if doing a task themselves takes longer or creates a mess. A nursing care plan for encouraging self-care is provided in Table 56–2 under "change in ability to perform ADL."

PROVIDING DIVERSIONAL ACTIVITY

Clients who are bedridden or confined to the hospital for a long time may become restless, depressed, and even disoriented. They may become preoccupied with their illness unless they have activities to hold their interest. Find-

crutch is advanced, then the opposite leg, then the remaining crutch, and finally, the other leg. This gait is harder to learn but provides more stability because three "points" are always on the floor.

The nurse can assist the client to gain confidence in walking on crutches by having the client wear a belt that the nurse can grasp as needed to keep the client from falling. The nurse should walk slightly behind and to the affected side. For crutch-walking on stairs, the affected leg should move together with the crutches. When the stairs have a railing, the client can put both crutches under the arm opposite the railing while the near hand holds the rail. When climbing, the client advances the unaffected leg first, then the crutches (while standing on the unaffected leg, as the affected leg dangles). When descending, the client moves the crutches first, and the unaffected leg last. Going down the stairs with crutches is particularly frightening; clients should practice with supervision until they gain skill in this maneuver.

A cane is used to lessen weight bearing on a hip or knee. It provides a wider than normal base of support and aids balance. The client should hold the cane on the side opposite the involved leg, taking part of the weight off the sore leg. Canes with three (tripod) or four (quad) legs are also available and provide added stability. A properly fitted cane allows slight (15° to 30°) flexion of the elbow when it is being held and extension of the elbow during weight bearing.

ing diversional activity that interests a bed-fast client may be a challenge. The nurse can suggest that the client and family members list activities that interest the client and think of ways those interests can be pursued in bed, eg, hobbies, crafts, reading, TV, and visitors. Sometimes the client's bed can be moved to a day room to encourage socializing. A nursing care plan to encourage activity is provided in Table 56–2 under "potential for changes in the mental status."

IMPROVING NUTRITIONAL STATUS

Nutrition for the client with a musculoskeletal problem includes a well-balanced diet and maintenance of recommended body weight. The diet, in general, should contain adequate vitamin D, calcium, and protein for maintenance of the musculoskeletal system. The client who is confined to bed or is inactive should eat plenty of roughage to prevent constipation. The arthritic client who is obese should be placed on a weight reduction diet to further remove stress from the joints.

PREPARING FOR SURGERY

The preparation of the orthopedic client is like that of other clients going to surgery (see Chapter 14) with a few special considerations. Additional laboratory tests may be done including erythrocyte sedimentation rate, serum calcium, phosphorus, and alkaline phosphatase. Coagulation studies and typing and crossmatching of blood are usually done because bones are highly vascular, and hemorrhage is possible.

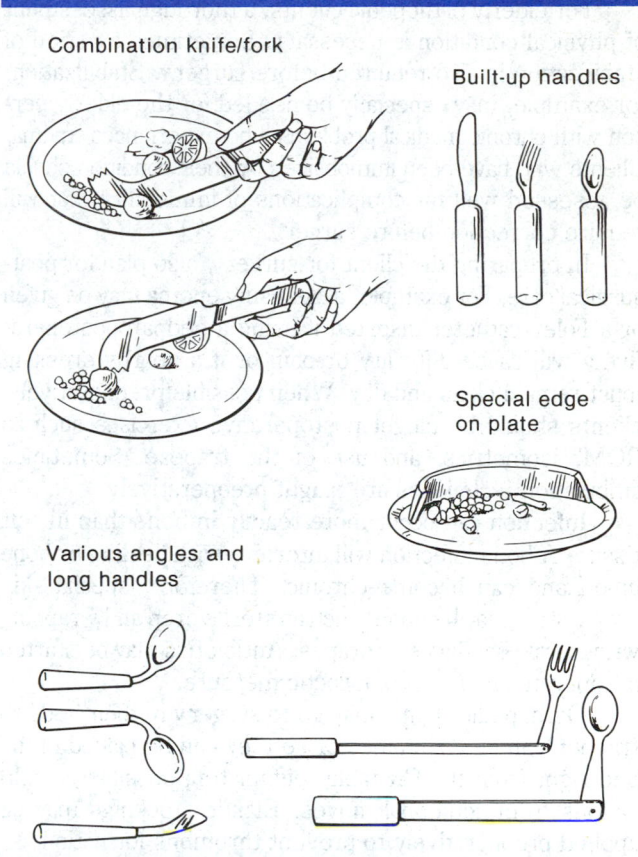

Figure 56–7

Assistive aids for eating.

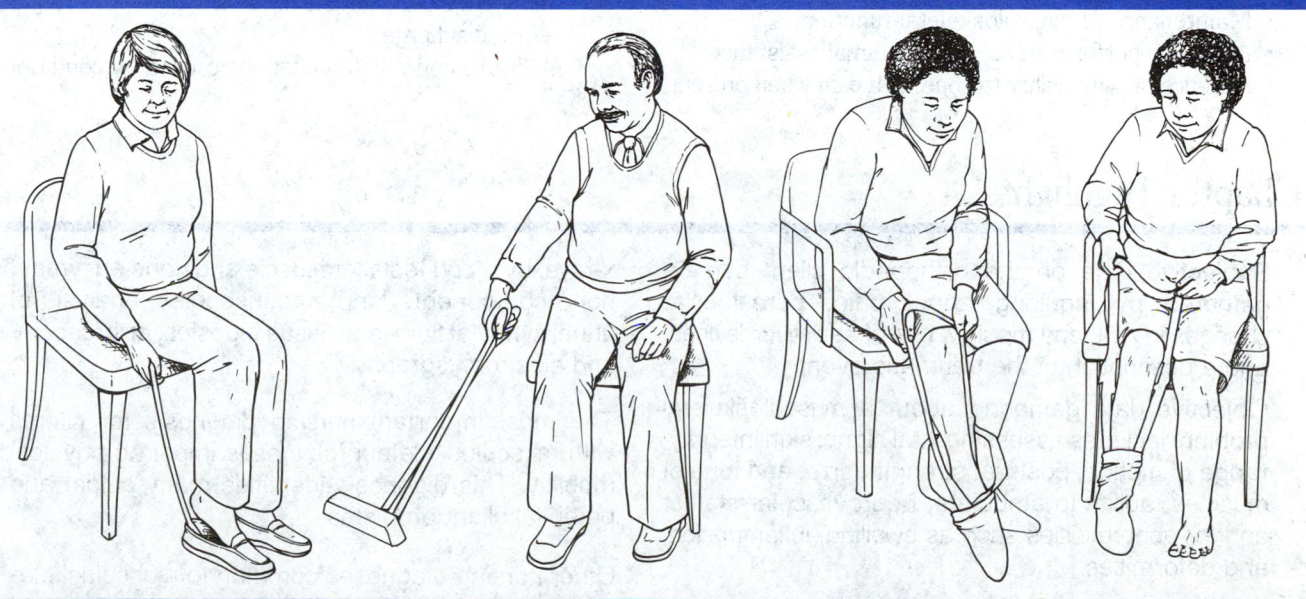

Figure 56–8

Long-handled assistive devices.

For elderly orthopedic clients, a thorough assessment of physical condition is necessary. Sometimes a period of stabilization is also required before surgery. Stabilization, for example, may especially be needed for the elderly person with chronic medical problems who experiences trauma. Clients who have been immobilized by their condition should be assessed well for complications of immobility that will require correction before surgery.

In preparing the client for surgery, also plan for postsurgical care. For example, a cleansing enema may be given or a Foley catheter inserted if using a bedpan postoperatively will cause difficulty or pain or if a nearby dressing must remain clean and dry. When possible preoperatively, clients should be taught postoperative exercises such as ROM, isometrics, and use of the trapeze. Sometimes ambulation techniques are taught preoperatively.

Infection can occur more readily in bone than in soft tissue. A bone infection will interfere with healing or bone union and can become chronic. Therefore, special skin preparation may be done, such as sterile prep and wrapping with sterile bandages or drapes. Antibiotics may be started preoperatively as a prophylactic measure.

Orthopedic clients may go to surgery in their beds so traction can be maintained or so they can be placed in the bed right from the OR table, eliminating possible complications from additional moves. Elastic stockings may be applied preoperatively to prevent thrombus formation.

Psychological preparation for orthopedic surgery depends on the client's condition, age, and mental state. A complete assessment of the client's mental state provides the nurse with clues to appropriate interventions. For example, for an elderly client, a broken hip may bring fear of final loss of independence and autonomy. For these clients, the need to mourn should be recognized. For those whose condition requires repeated surgeries, the nurse should plan to help the client deal with depression, frustration, or apathy. An example is the client with peripheral vascular disease who faces amputation and repeated stump revision and who feels angry and hopeless.

For clients who have high hopes of improvement in their condition or relief from pain, the nurse may be able to concentrate on instruction in the techniques that may be needed postoperatively. Even the hopeful client may have misconceptions, however, and the instruction period provides an opportunity for the nurse to discover those and correct them. For those who face orthopedic surgery, common fears are of pain, loss of body parts, and in some cases the possibility of paralysis.

In addition to psychological preparation for surgery, the nurse may plan for postoperative psychological support. For clients who go into surgery directly after trauma, the nurse may have to plan for postoperative psychological assistance in facing a sudden and permanent change in lifestyle or a long and unexpected confinement.

Section IV: Evaluation

Criteria for evaluation are normally specific to each condition. Some general criteria for musculoskeletal problems are:

- Maintenance of musculoskeletal function
- Ability to perform ADL, with minimal assistance
- Absence of pain; ability to cope with pain when present

- Absence of complications of immobility
- Absence of deformity; if deformity unavoidable, position is functional
- Knowledge of condition and ability to do care required before discharge
- Ability to cope with limitations caused by condition

Chapter Highlights

Subjective data on the orthopedic client can be gathered by inquiring about pain, paresthesia, changes in ADL and mobility, use of assistive devices, and a description of the traumatic event.

Objective data gathering about a musculoskeletal problem includes assessing vital signs; skin integrity; range of motion; posture; strength, size, and tone of muscles; ability to ambulate; neurovascular status; and for abnormalities such as swelling, inflammation, and deformities.

In addition to other routine diagnostic tests, the musculoskeletal system can be assessed by specific

x-rays; by blood tests for muscle and bone enzymes, bone components, and autoantibodies; analysis of urine, synovial fluid, and tissue biopsies; arthroscopy and electromyography.

The most important nursing diagnosis for clients with musculoskeletal problems is impaired physical mobility. This diagnosis identifies many actual and potential client problems.

Other nursing diagnoses common to musculoskeletal clients include pain, altered body image, altered peripheral tissue perfusion, possible sexual dysfunction, and deficits in diversional activity and self-care.

Nursing measures common to musculoskeletal problems include rest, positioning in correct alignment, comfort measures, hot or cold applications, good skin care, exercise, ambulation, introducing assistive devices, diversional activity, nutritional support, and preparation for surgery.

The effectiveness of nursing interventions is evaluated by determining if musculoskeletal function and ADL are maintained and if pain, deformity, and complications of immobility are absent. Clients should understand their condition and be able to give or obtain necessary care and cope with any limitations.

Bibliography

Baird SE: Development of a nursing assessment tool to diagnose altered body image in immobilized patients. *Ortho Nurs* 1985; 4(1): 47–54.

Bates B: *A Guide to Physical Examination,* 3rd ed. Philadelphia: Lippincott, 1983.

Branson KA: Patient management following Amipaque myelography. *Ortho Nurs* 1982; 1(6):38–40.

Distel N: A nursing quality assurance investigation of orthopedic patient care. *QRB* 1983; 8:20–22.

Farrell J: Arthroscopy. *Nurs 82* (May) 1982; 12:73–75.

Farrell J: *Illustrated Guide to Orthopedic Nursing,* 2nd ed. Philadelphia: Lippincott, 1982.

Fischbach F: *A Manual of Laboratory Diagnostic Tests,* 2nd ed. Philadelphia: Lippincott, 1984.

Johnson LL: Diagnostic and surgical arthroscopy. *Clin Symp* 1982; 34(3):2–32.

King PA: Foot problems and assessment. *Geriatr Nurs* (Sept/ Oct) 1980; 182–186.

Larson CB, Gould M: *Orthopedic Nursing,* 9th ed. St. Louis: Mosby, 1978.

Rodts MF: An orthopedic assessment you can do in fifteen minutes. *Nurs 83* (May) 1983; 13:65–73.

Self-help devices: When hand function is compromised. *Patient Care* (April 30) 1984; 48–99.

Shannon ML: Five fallacies of pressure sores. *Nurs 84* (Oct) 1984; 14:34–41.

Simpson CF: Heat, cold, or both? *Am J Nurs* 1983; 83:270–273.

Simpson CF, Dickinson GR: Exercise. *Am J Nurs* 1983; 83:273–274.

Tilkian SM, Conover MB, Tilkian AG: *Clinical Implications of Laboratory Tests,* 3rd ed. St. Louis: Mosby, 1983.

Treseler KM: *Clinical Laboratory Tests: Significance and Implications for Nursing.* Englewood Cliffs, NJ: Prentice-Hall, 1982.

Tucker JB, Marron JT: The qualification/disqualification process in athletics. *Am Fam Physician* (Feb) 1984; 29:149–154.

Vanderbeck KA: Getting the facts: a guide to orthopaedic assessment. *Ortho Nurs* 1984; 3(5):31–34.

Wells R, Trostle K: Creative hairwashing techniques for immobilized patients. *Nurs 84* (Jan) 1984; 14:47–51.

Suggested Readings

Cohen S, Viellion B: Patient assessment: Examining joints of the upper and lower extremities. *Am J Nurs* 1981; 81:763–786.

A programmed instruction unit covering joint assessment, with elaborate illustration of range of motion.

Dickinson GR, Gorman TK: Adult arthritis: The assessment. *Am J Nurs* 1983; 83:262–265. This article covers general subjective and objective data collection for arthritis. It is part of a continuing education unit.

Dunn BH: Components of musculoskeletal examination. *Ortho Nurs* 1982; 1(6):33–36. Provides a good overview of musculoskeletal assessment for nurses.

Farrell J: Orthopedic pain: What does it mean? *Am J Nurs* 1984; 84:466–469. This article offers guidelines for evaluating and managing pain in selected orthopedic conditions. Total knee replacement, total hip replacement, fractured femur, and fractured tibia are discussed.

Taylor SL: Lower back pain assessment: Part I—History-taking. *Ortho Nurs* 1983; 2:4, 11–16. Part II—Defining range of motion. 2:5, 39–44. Part III—The physical examination. 2:6, 21–27. This series of articles is written for nurse practitioners. It covers terminology and thorough explanations accompanied by illustrations to assess low back pain systematically.

Wassel A: Nursing assessment of injuries to the lower extremity. *Nurs Clin North Am* 1981; 16:739–748. This article gives thorough explanations of types of lower extremity musculoskeletal injuries, including signs, symptoms, treatment, and rehabilitation.

Resources

SELF-HELP GROUPS AND OTHER ORGANIZATIONS

American Alliance for Health, Physical
Education, Recreation, and Dance
Promotions Unit
1201 Sixteenth St. NW
Washington, DC 20036
Phone: (202) 833-5554
This voluntary educational organization answers questions about recreation and fitness opportunities for the handicapped.

American College of Sports Medicine
1440 Monroe St.
Madison, WI 53706
Phone: (608) 262-3632
An informational resource for questions about sports medicine which also provides referrals to sports medicine specialists.

American Lupus Society
23751 Madison St.
Torrance, CA 90505
Phone: (213) 373-1335
> Volunteer workers promote public awareness of lupus, obtain funds for client care, and sponsor programs where clients and their families can meet to exchange information and offer mutual support.

Arthritis Foundation (National Headquarters)
1212 Avenue of the Americas
New York, NY 10036
> This foundation funds research and provides information to the public and profession for education and training. Local chapters throughout the United States support clinics, home care programs, rehabilitation services, and mobile consultations units for clients with arthritis.

Arthritis Information Clearing House
PO Box 34427, Dept N 79
Bethesda, MD 20034
Phone: (301) 881-9411
PO Box 9782
Arlington, VA 22209
Phone: (703) 558-8250

Muscular Dystrophy Association
810 Seventh Ave.
New York, NY 10019
Phone: (212) 586-0808
> This voluntary health agency provides comprehensive free client care programs in local chapters throughout the country to persons with muscular dystrophy and related disorders, free loan of medical equipment and appliances, group recreation programs, and personal counseling by trained volunteers.

National Amputation Foundation
12-45 150th St.
Whitestone, NY 11357
Phone: (212) 767-0596
> This membership organization of both civilian and veteran amputees offers information and support, a program of social rehabilitation, and referrals to centers throughout the country for the manufacture of prosthetic devices and training in their use (they maintain a prosthetic device center in New York City). Their "Amp-to-Amp" program offers person-to-person counseling.

National Lupus Foundation
5430 Van Nuys Blvd., Suite 206
Van Nuys, CA 91401
Phone: (213) 885-8787
> This non-profit organization run by volunteers raises funds to support research and distribute literature to the public and professionals.

United Scleroderma Foundation, Inc
PO Box 350
Watsonville, CA 95077-0350
Phone: (408) 728-2202

HOT LINES

Arthritis Medical Center
Phone: (800) 327-3027
> Sponsored by Arthritis Medical Center. A physician will answer telephone questions; printed literature is also available.

Medical Advice for Jogging Related Problems
Phone: (202) 785-8050
> Sponsored by the National Jogging Association. Advice is given to members for problems related to jogging.

HEALTH EDUCATION MATERIAL

Patient Information Library
Krames Communications
312 90th St.
Daly City, CA 94015-2621

Osteoarthritis, 1983, $.75
Cast Care, 1984, $.90
Arthroscopy, 1984, $.80
Back to Backs: A Guide to Preventing Back Injury, 1984, $.95
Your Back Is Always Working, 1984, $.90
Fitness, $.90
Slips, Trips and Falls, 1984, $.90
A Guide to Hand Safety, 1984, $.90
Back Owners Manual: A Guide to the Care of the Low Back, 1984, $.90
Neck Owners Manual: A Guide to the Care and Treatment of Common Neck Problems, 1984, $.90
Knee Owners Manual: A Guide to the Care and Treatment of the Problem Knee, 1984, $.90
Shoulder Owners Manual: A Guide to the Care and Treatment of Common Shoulder Problems, 1984, $.90
Foot Owners Manual: A Guide to Good Foot Care, 1984, $.90
Hand and Wrist Owners Manual: Treatment of Hand and Wrist Injuries, 1983, $.90
Ankle Owners Manual: A Guide to Common Ankle Injuries, 1984, $.75
Physical Therapy: Improving Movement and Function, 1984, $.75
Running: Putting Together a Safe Running Program, 1984, $.75
The Foot Book: A Guide to Podiatric Care, $.95
Back Exercises for a Healthy Back, 1985, $.75

NURSING ORGANIZATION

National Association of Orthopedic Nurses
Box 56
Pitman, NY 08071
Phone: (609) 582-0111
> Members of this organization are nurses involved in the care of orthopedic clients. The association's goals are to enhance personal and professional growth through continuing education and the promotion of research. Dues are $35.

Chapter 57

Specific Disorders of Connective Tissue and Muscles

Rita A. Colicchia
SueAnn Wooster Ames

Objectives

When you have finished studying this chapter, you should be able to:

Describe the clinical manifestations and significance of disorders of connective tissue and muscle.

Identify therapeutic measures specific to disorders of connective tissue and muscles.

Specify the common drugs used in muscle and connective tissue disorders and discuss their potential side effects.

Formulate specific nursing interventions for clients with disorders of connective tissue and muscles.

Anticipate the temporary or permanent lifestyle modifications frequently necessary for clients with problems involving muscles and connective tissue.

Explain necessary health teaching for clients with specific disorders of connective tissue and muscles.

Injury to connective tissue and muscle may arise from congenital or acquired disease or from trauma. Diseases and traumatic injuries that primarily affect the joints are discussed in Chapter 59; this chapter deals with injury to muscles and connective tissues surrounding the joints or in other parts of the body. Many of the diseases affecting the musculoskeletal system are systemic disorders with widespread and often serious effects. The discussion of nursing care in this chapter will focus on the muscular and connective tissue manifestations of these disorders; treatment of other symptoms is covered more fully in other chapters of this text.

Section I: Congenital Disorders

Congenital disorders of connective tissue are structural connective tissue defects present at birth. Most of these disorders are transmitted by a single autosomal dominant gene. Although there are many congenital connective tissue disorders, most are rare; this section will present two of the better known ones; Marfan's syndrome and Ehlers–Danlos syndrome. The obvious manifestations of these disorders may not appear until the second decade of life or later (Petersdorf et al., 1983).

Both syndromes are serious and require the diversified services of many health care professionals. Clients and their families are burdened by financial, psychological, and social problems that the health care team must deal with straightforwardly. Assistance and counseling for parents of affected children are covered in textbooks of pediatric nursing. The discussion in this book will be limited to the problems of adults.

It is important for an affected person to have genetic counseling before having children. Although the physician and genetic counselor may be the main sources of information, the client may ask the nurse to repeat or explain what they have said. Therefore, the nurse should have a basic knowledge of human genetics when caring for clients with these syndromes. Health care providers should gather careful family histories detailing the patterns of disease transmission so families can see the degree of risk with each pregnancy.

The nurse is in a unique position to support parents and clients with a congenital connective tissue disorder. It is important to listen carefully and to help them develop realistic goals. Many decisions regarding therapy require informed reflection, since occasionally the risks outweigh the benefits. In these cases, the nurse can be available to explain, to reassure, and to support. The nurse can also be an excellent source for referrals to community agencies and groups that may be of assistance. The March of Dimes Birth Defects Foundation has an international directory for genetic services (see Resources, end of Chapter 56).

MARFAN'S SYNDROME

Marfan's syndrome is a relatively rare generalized disorder of connective tissue inherited as an autosomal dominant trait. Abraham Lincoln had Marfan's syndrome. New mutations of the disease have been attributed to sperm from fathers of advanced age. The classic triad of Marfan's syndrome involves the cardiovascular, visual, and skeletal systems, although there is wide variability in clinical manifestations. The average age of death is between age 40 and 50, but some people have survived into their 70s.

Clinical Manifestations

The major *cardiovascular* complication involves the aorta. Marfan's syndrome causes degeneration of the elastic fibers of the aortic media, which can lead to dissecting aneurysm. Aortic regurgitation may occur producing a diastolic murmur. Mitral valve prolapse, thickening of the coronary arteries, conduction system abnormalities, and aortic coarctation have also been associated with Marfan's syndrome.

 Echocardiogram is useful in following aortic and mitral valve abnormalities. Clients with valve involvement are at risk for endocarditis. These clients should have antibiotic prophylaxis for any dental work causing bleeding or for any other invasive procedures, to prevent bacteremia, which can lead to endocarditis.

 Ocular problems are a result of defective supporting tissue of the lens, which can cause bilateral subluxation or total dislocation of the lens. The dislocation is usually upward, but slit lamp examination must be done to detect more subtle variations. Complications such as reduced visual acuity, uveitis, glaucoma, cataracts, retinal detachment, and myopia may also occur.

 The most obvious *skeletal* manifestations are extreme height and long extremities. People with Marfan's syndrome are usually much taller than other members of their families and have excessively long arms and legs in relation to their bodies. The measurement from fingertip to fingertip with the arms outstretched is greater than the body height. The fingers are extremely long, a condition known as *arachnodactyly,* or "spider fingers." The sternum may bulge outward (*pectus carinatum,* or pigeon breast), or it may be depressed (*pectus excavatum,* or funnel breast). See Figure 57–1. If the chest deformities are extreme, the echocardiogram becomes unreliable.

 Kyphoscoliosis may be quite severe because of the

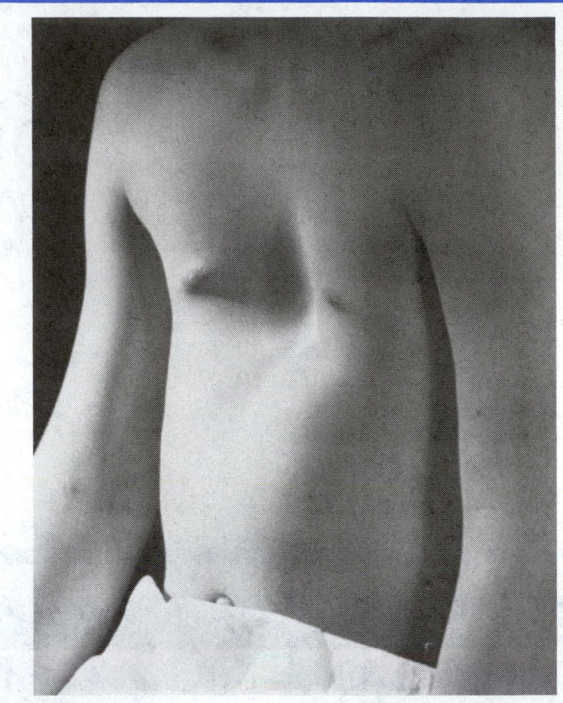

Figure 57–1

Pectus excavatum, or funnel breast, as seen in Marfan's syndrome. (Photo courtesy Millard Fillmore Hospital)

weakness of the ligaments and other supporting connective tissues. Other skeletal manifestations include a long and narrow skull, with a high, arched palate, and flat feet. Joints and ligaments are hyperextensible leading to recurrent dislocations of the knees and hips.

Therapeutic Measures

Therapeutic approaches in Marfan's syndrome are directed toward the specific manifestations. Yearly ophthalmological examinations aid in early detection of retinal detachment and lens dislocation (see Unit Twelve).

 Since cardiovascular problems are the major cause of mortality, most of the diagnostic and treatment efforts are directed to the heart and aorta. Echocardiograms are done yearly, unless the diameter of the aorta exceeds the upper limits by 50%, in which case echocardiogram is performed every 6 months. Drugs such as propranolol (Inderal), which decrease myocardial contractility and thus diminish stress on the aorta, have been used in an attempt to delay aortic complications. Left-sided strain and congestive heart failure are strong indications for surgery, since digitalis preparations may increase aortic enlargement.

 The risk of cardiovascular surgery is greater for clients with Marfan's syndrome because sutures may not hold well due to the abnormal connective tissue. Nevertheless, prophylactic aortic repair is being done with less than 10% mortality (Krupp & Chatton, 1981). Aortic valve prostheses have also been implanted successfully, although prolonged anticoagulation therapy places the client at risk for hemorrhage.

Kyphoscoliosis is the most deforming and disabling skeletal manifestation of Marfan's syndrome. Clients should be examined twice a year so therapy can be initiated quickly if this condition develops. Mechanical bracing, physical therapy, and in severe cases, spinal fusion are used to correct or retard the deformity (Figure 57–2).

As can be easily seen from Figure 57–2, the thoracic cavity in clients with kyphoscoliosis can be so reduced that cardiac and respiratory function are compromised. These clients are particularly susceptible to upper respiratory infections and should be treated aggressively if an infection occurs.

Prepubertal females are often given estrogen and prepubertal males are given androgens to decrease height and also decrease the incidence of kyphoscoliosis. The sex hormones not only cause early epiphyseal closure but also bring about the physical and psychosocial changes of puberty, which can create numerous other stresses for a young person already having body image problems. Clients with Marfan's syndrome should have genetic counseling because their children will have a 50% chance of having the syndrome. Pregnancy in a Marfan's client with aortic changes may be hazardous because the cardiovascular overload and increased intra-abdominal pressure may contribute to aortic rupture.

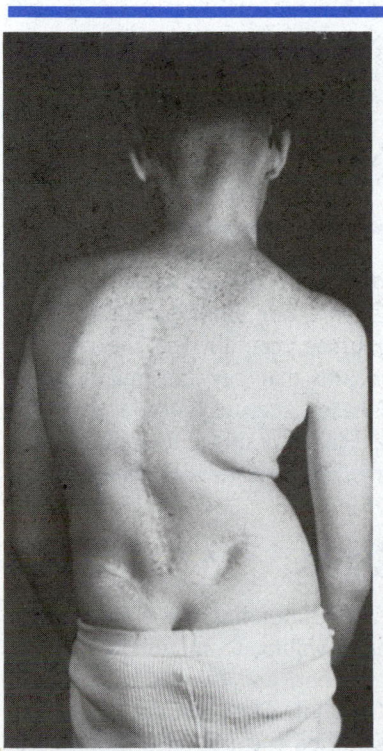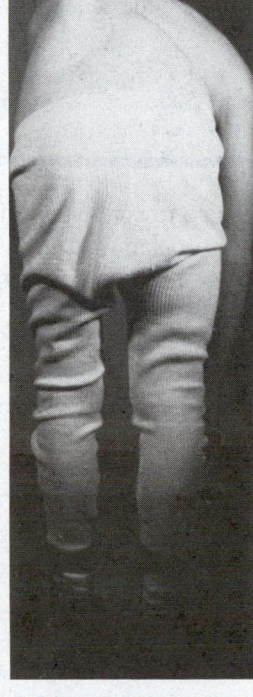

Figure 57–2

Left: Young man with kyphoscoliosis standing up straight.
Right: Same young man bending forward (scars are from spinal fusion). (Courtesy Millard Fillmore Hospital)

Specific Nursing Measures

The health history is extremely important in clients with congenital disorders such as Marfan's syndrome. Particular attention should be paid to the client's coping abilities in terms of living with a chronic disease that involves numerous changes in body image. Assessing the client's financial resources is important because the complications of Marfan's syndrome can be quite costly.

Thorough assessment of the eyes, the cardiovascular system, and the musculoskeletal system are extremely important.

- Eyes. Look for tremor of the iris as it is moved horizontally. This is an indication of subluxation of the lens. The client may also have myopia (nearsightedness) and blue sclera (due to the presence of thin sclerae through which the vessel-rich choroid can be seen).
- Cardiovascular. Listen for the early diastolic murmur of aortic regurgitation. This consists of a high-pitched blowing sound, heard best with the diaphragm of the stethoscope over the second right or third left intercostal space. Increased pulse pressure and water-hammer pulse may also be evident. Occasionally, a midsystolic click indicative of mitral valve prolapse may be auscultated.
- Skeletal. Observe for increased height compared with family proportions and a very thin build, arachnodactyly, pigeon or funnel breast, hyperextensibility of the joints, and kyphoscoliosis.

Nursing intervention is basically that of psychological support, education, and symptomatic care. The nurse should be prepared to discuss the nature and course of the disease with the client. Explain the importance of genetic and pregnancy counseling. Encourage the client to have echocardiograms and ophthalmological exams once a year and orthopedic exams twice a year, to detect problems in their early stages. The client should understand the need to avoid trauma and invasive surgical procedures (when the risks outweigh the benefits). Explain the need for prophylactic antibiotic therapy before any dental or urinary procedures, to prevent endocarditis.

EHLERS–DANLOS SYNDROME

Ehlers–Danlos syndrome is a rare genetic disorder of connective tissue that affects the skin, joints, and hematopoietic systems. It is usually transmitted by an autosomal dominant gene, but it may also be transmitted by an autosomal recessive or an X-linked recessive gene.

Clinical Manifestations

The major manifestations of Ehlers–Danlos syndrome are fragile and increased elasticity of skin, hyperextensible joints, and fragility of blood vessel walls. Researchers have divided the syndrome into eight distinct types, according to severity, systems involved, and manner of transmission.

The client's *skin* is very smooth and hyperextensible; ie, it can be pulled away from the body but returns to its original shape. Fragility and bruising are often evident. Minor cuts cause gaping "fish mouth" wounds with little bleeding. Even the slightest trauma may cause purpura or hematomas that calcify and resemble tumors. These pseudotumors occur particularly over pressure points such as knees and elbows.

The *joints* are so hyperextensible in Ehlers–Danlos that many people with this syndrome have become circus personalities with names like the Indian Rubber Man or the Human Pretzel. Dislocations, effusions, and hemarthrosis of the hip, patella, and shoulders may occur. Kyphoscoliosis, flat feet, and hyperextensible knees are often present. Thoracic deformities are not as common but do sometimes occur, as does a forward slipping of the lower lumbar vertebrae (spondylolisthesis).

The client may have episodes of bleeding, including spontaneous epistaxis; bleeding into the joints (hemarthrosis); blood in the sputum (hemoptysis); dark, tarry stools (melena), indicating bleeding in the digestive tract; and bleeding gums. It is not known whether the abnormal bleeding is from weakness in blood vessel walls or abnormal interactions of platelets with collagen.

Abnormalities of the *heart and blood vessels* occur only in one severe type of the syndrome. These include mitral valve prolapse, right bundle branch block, and other conduction abnormalities. Rarely is there any aortic disorder. However, the client with this type of Ehlers–Danlos syndrome has friable arteries, so any invasive angiography should be done cautiously.

Other manifestations of Ehlers–Danlos syndrome can include spontaneous bowel rupture or pneumothorax following surgeries, premature births due to early membrane rupture, and diaphragmatic hernias or diverticuli. In rare instances, a client may have glaucoma, retinal detachment, or corneal abnormalities. People with this condition are highly mobile and often make good acrobats or ballet dancers. Management of their problems includes use of salicylates, joint protection, and joint conditioning exercises.

Specific Nursing Measures

Care for Ehlers–Danlos clients consists of symptomatic treatment and support, since no specific treatment exists. The main concern is to protect the client's skin and joints from cuts, bruises, and dislocations. The nurse should inquire about bleeding gums, melena, hemoptysis, and nosebleed. Be alert to inadequate wound healing or wound dehiscence after any surgical procedure. Postsurgical assessment of the lungs for pneumothorax is important.

As with any chronic condition, the nurse needs to teach clients and their families about the nature and course of the disease. Genetic counseling should be referred to an expert because it is complicated by the varying modes of transmission of the syndrome. A client with Ehlers–Danlos syndrome who becomes pregnant is at risk for exacerbation of joint problems, increased bruisability, abdominal hernia, and varicosities. Serious complications may arise with cesarean section because sutures do not hold well and wound dehiscence may result.

Section II: Inflammatory Disorders

BURSITIS AND TENDINITIS

Many pathological conditions involve inflammation of connective tissue. Most inflammatory conditions covered in this chapter are related to alterations in the immune system and are discussed in the next section. This section deals only with bursitis and tendinitis, inflammatory conditions not usually associated with immunological disorders.

Bursitis is an inflammation of the synovial membrane lining a bursa; *tendinitis* is an inflammation of a tendon. These inflammations may result from trauma, or they may be secondary to disease. Although both conditions are usually acute, they can become chronic and quite disabling with repeated injury or inadequate care.

Bursitis and tendinitis develop from prolonged overuse of a particular muscle group that can eventually damage a bursa or tendon. Overuse may be due to repetitive work movements or to a sports activity. Since the vascular supply of tendons is poor, their healing is limited, and inflammation can become chronic, resulting in tissue damage and persistent pain. Often a person with a chronic condition is unable to continue performing the movements that led to the problem and must seek other employment. Calcium deposits in tendons or bursae may also be the cause of inflammation. Tendon sheaths may become inflamed secondarily to systemic diseases such as gout, rheumatoid arthritis, or scleroderma. Since bursitis and tendinitis have similar causes, symptoms, and treatments, they will be discussed together.

Clinical Manifestations

The major symptom of bursitis/tendinitis is pain, often so severe that the client is unwilling to move the affected part. Swelling may be present, and this alone may keep the client from moving the joint. The pain may awaken the client at night, especially when turning onto the affected area during sleep. Any of the body's many bursae and tendons can become inflamed, but some joint areas are more commonly affected than others and will be discussed here. Note, however, that acute pain and erythema in joint areas may also be due to infection, gout, or rheumatoid arthritis.

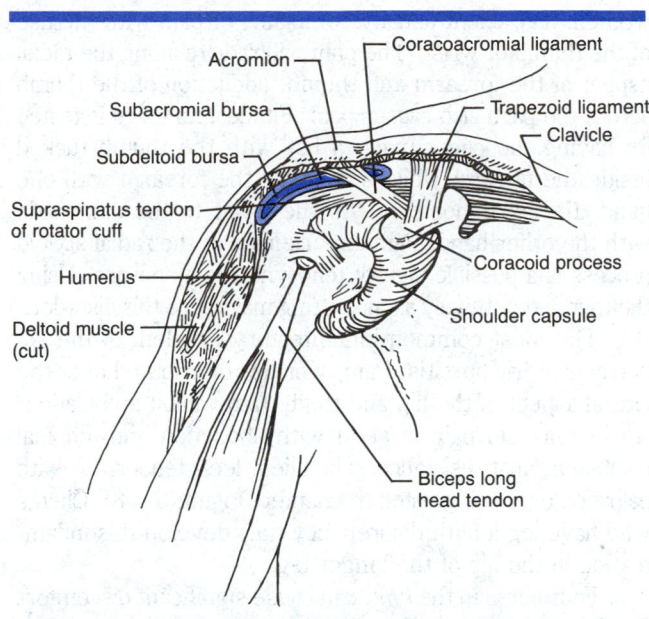

Figure 57–3

Location of subacromial and subdeltoid sections of the bursa and supraspinatus tendon.

Bursitis and tendinitis of the *shoulder* involve the subacromial and subdeltoid bursa (which are different sections of the same large bursa) and the tendon of the supraspinatus muscle. Figure 57–3 shows the location of the

involved structures. The onset of bursitis or tendinitis in the shoulder usually follows activities involving repetitive movements of the whole arm, such as sanding, painting, sawing, or repeated lifting. Pain in the deltoid area increases when the client lies on the shoulder or actively abducts the arm. A classic sign of bursitis or tendinitis of the shoulder is the "painful arc" between 80° and 120° of active arm abduction as shown in Figure 57–4; the client is unable to support the weight of the arm at these angles. Further abduction causes no pain, and the examiner can perform passive range of motion (ROM). If passive ROM causes pain, suspect capsulitis, or inflammation of the joint capsule, rather than a periarticular disorder.

Inflammations of the *elbow* region most often involve the olecranon bursa and the medial and lateral epicondyles (Figures 57–5 and 57–6). Tennis elbow is generally lateral epicondylitis, and pitcher's elbow is medial epicondylitis. These inflammations cause pain that radiates from the elbow down to the forearm. The client may drop heavy objects because of a feeling of decreased strength, although no real loss of strength actually occurs. Palpation of the involved epicondyle causes pain. There is no loss of motion of the joint. Activities involving lower arm movement, such as tennis or hammering, may precipitate an attack. Olecranon bursitis usually is caused by leaning or falling on the elbow. There may not be severe pain, but swelling is often extensive and alarming to the client (Figure 57–7).

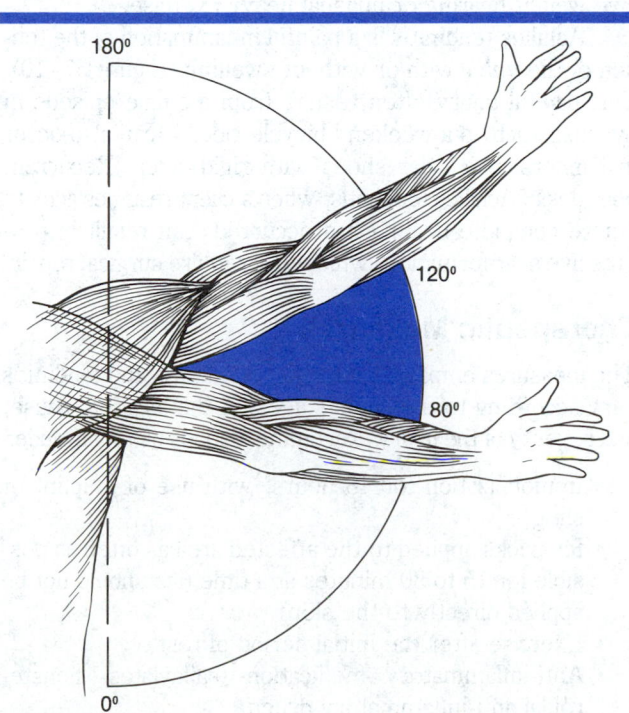

Figure 57–4

The painful arc in tendinitis and bursitis of the shoulder.

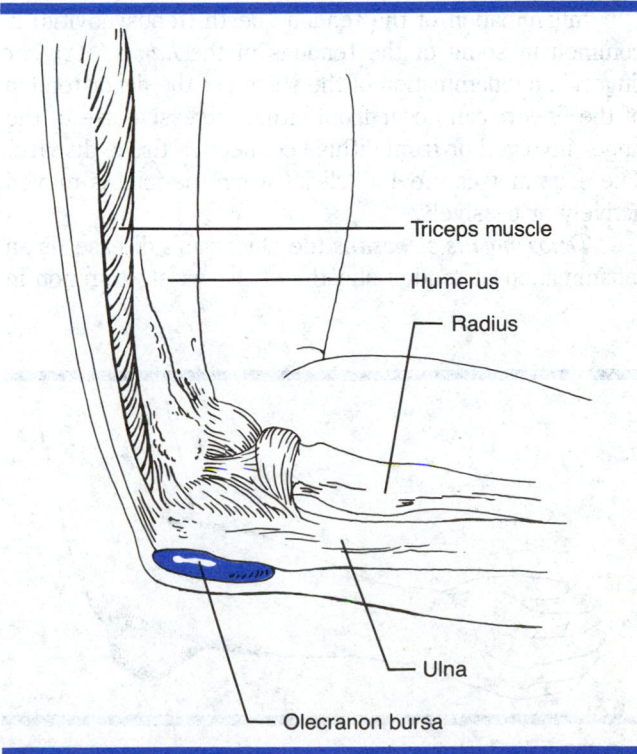

Figure 57–5

Olecranon bursa.

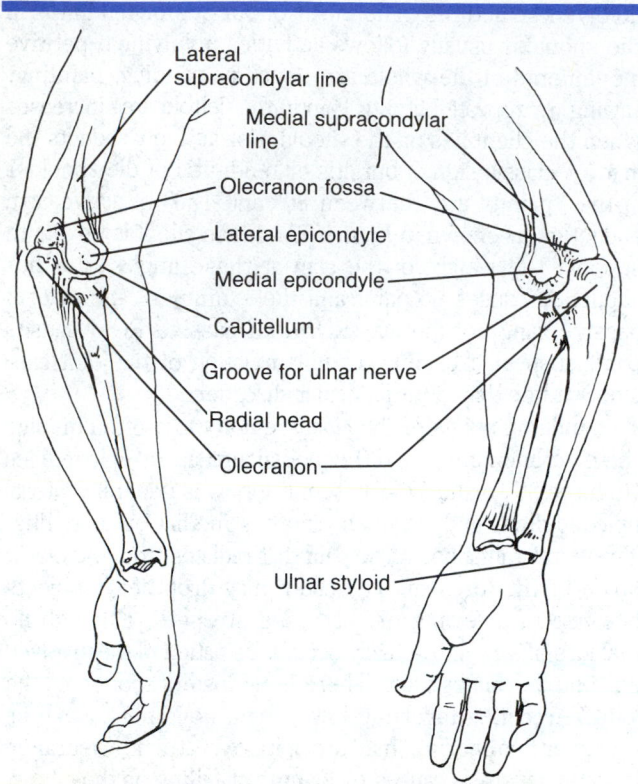

Figure 57–6

Left: Lateral epicondyle of the elbow. **Right:** Medial epicondyle of the elbow.

Inflammation of the tendon sheath (tenosynovitis) is common in some of the tendons of the *hand*. "Trigger finger," an inflammation of the sheath of the flexor tendon of the finger, can occur from either excessive use of the finger involved or from diffuse connective tissue disease. The examiner can feel a "click" when the joint is moved actively or passively.

Tenosynovitis stenosans (de Quervain's disease) is an inflammation of tendon sheaths of the wrists common in

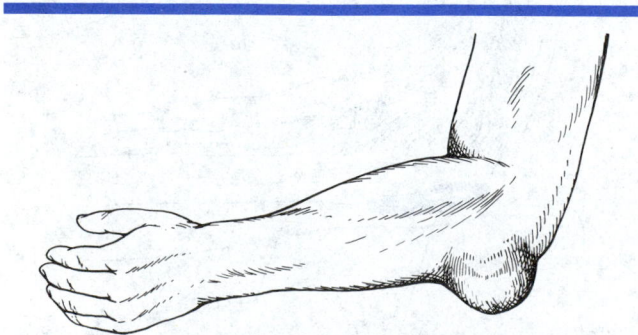

Figure 57–7

Localized swelling of the olecranon bursa.

women. The client usually complains of pain with the use of the thumb or wrist. The pain will radiate along the radial aspect of the forearm and thumb; adduction of the thumb across the palm also causes pain. Finklestein's sign is tested by having the client make a fist with the thumb tucked inside the fingers; while stabilizing the forearm with one hand, the examiner deviates the wrist to the ulnar side with the other hand. Pain experienced at the radial styloid process is a possible sign of tenosynovitis stenosans. Using the thumb repetitively as in knitting may cause this disorder.

The most common inflammatory problem of the *hip* is trochanteric bursitis. Pain, which is distributed over the lateral aspect of the hip and thigh, may inhibit ambulation. An increase in pain is seen with abduction and internal rotation against resistance. The client feels tenderness with palpation over the greater trochanter (Figure 57–8). Clients who have leg length discrepancy may develop this inflammation in the hip of the longer leg.

Four bursa in the *knee* can cause significant discomfort for the client when inflamed:

- Prepatellar bursa
- Superficial infrapatellar bursa
- Deep infrapatellar bursa
- Pes anserine bursa (see Figure 57–9)

Prepatellar bursitis (housemaid's knee) results from the combined action of excessive kneeling and leaning forward as in washing floors or gardening. Superficial infrapatellar bursitis (clergyman's knee) can result from excessive kneeling in a prayerful position. Deep infrapatellar bursitis and pes anserine bursitis are secondary to excessive weight bearing or unusual heavy exercise.

Achilles tendinitis is a painful inflammation of the tendon of the *ankle* with or without swelling (Figure 57–10). This painful injury often results from a single episode of overuse such as a weekend bicycle ride. It can also occur in runners who wear shoes with rigid soles. Recurrent episodes of Achilles tendinitis, when a client resumes activity before complete healing has occurred, can result in progressive scar formation, which may require surgical repair.

Therapeutic Measures

The measures employed for relief of bursitis and tendinitis vary according to the client's age and the location, cause, and severity of the injury. Recommendations usually include:

- Immobilization for 48 hours, with use of a splint or sling
- Ice packs applied to the affected area as often as possible for 15 to 30 minutes at a time (ice should not be applied directly to the skin)
- Exercise after the initial period of rest
- Anti-inflammatory medication (salicylates, nonsteroidal anti-inflammatory drugs)
- Occasionally, local corticosteroid injections into the inflamed bursa or tendon area

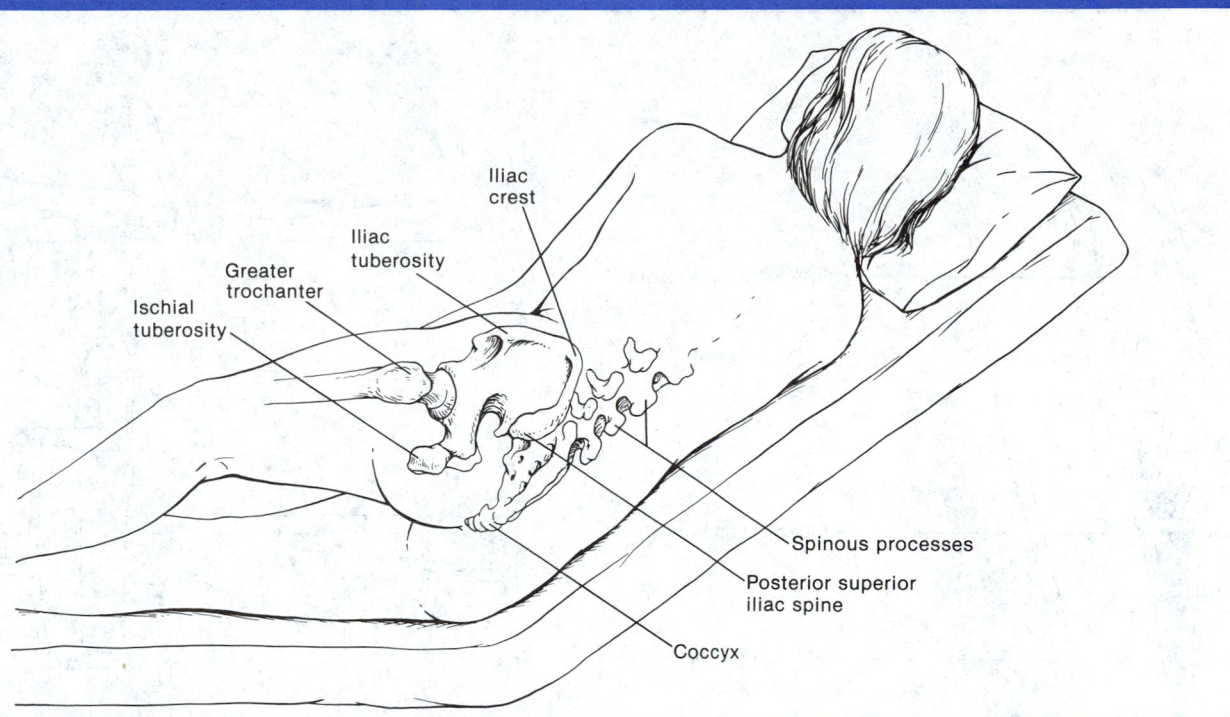

Figure 57–8

Greater trochanter.

Exercise is crucial in the rehabilitation process, and active movement is started early. For example, in bursitis of any bursa of the knee, quadriceps-setting exercise is begun as soon as pain allows (Figure 57–11). When pain and tenderness have completely subsided, range of motion and full quadriceps activity are initiated. Physical therapists are often involved in designing exercises for clients, according to their individual needs. Occupational therapists may also participate if the nature of the problem involves a modification or change in job.

Fluid may be aspirated from the bursal space to relieve the symptoms. Fluid obtained should be cultured and inspected microscopically. Heat therapy by means of hot packs, ultrasound, or diathermy is used following cold therapy with some clients. *X-rays* of joints are usually normal, but in some instances calcium deposits can be identified as the precipitating factor. *Arthrography* is indicated in specific types of shoulder trauma to rule out any disruption of the joint capsule. *Surgery* is rarely used for bursitis or tendinitis unless rupture of the tendon occurs.

Specific Nursing Measures

Nurses are most likely to encounter clients with bursitis or tendinitis in ambulatory care or in emergency rooms. Goals of nursing care are to relieve the client's pain, maintain maximum mobility, and prevent joint contracture.

Assessment of pain and range of motion is important both initially and after treatment to measure the effectiveness

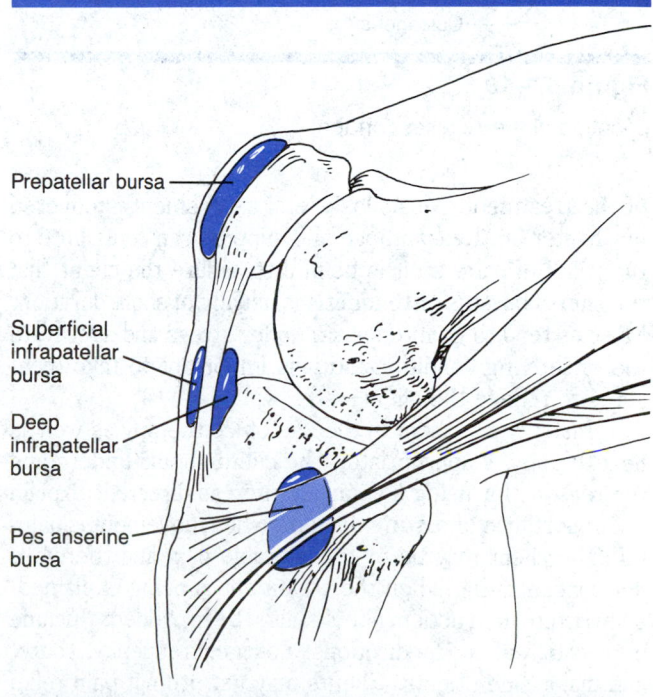

Figure 57–9

Clinically significant bursae of the knee.

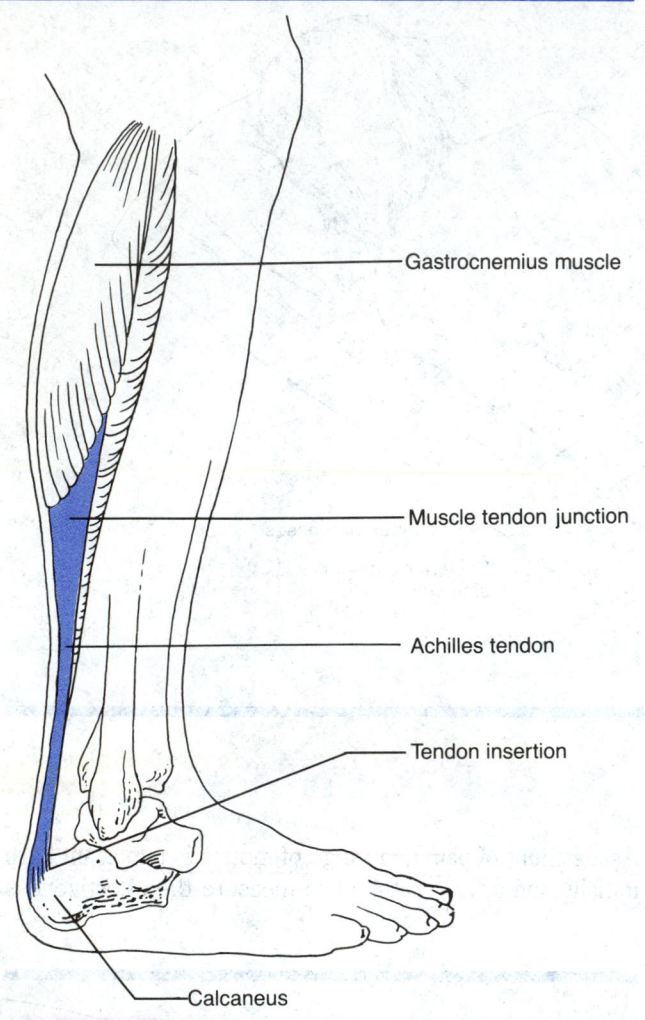

Figure 57–10

Location of the Achilles tendon.

- Gastrocnemius muscle
- Muscle tendon junction
- Achilles tendon
- Tendon insertion
- Calcaneus

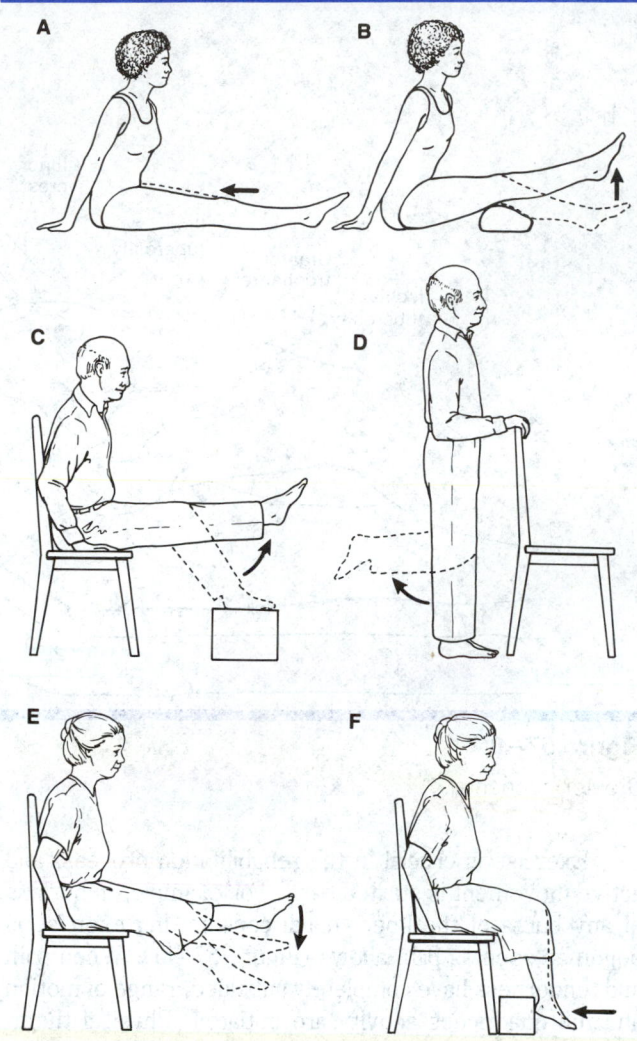

Figure 57–11

Exercises for rehabilitation of the knee. **A.** Isometric quadriceps exercise. **B,C.** Isotonic quadriceps exercises. **D.** Gravity-resisted isotonic flexion exercise. **E.** Gravity-assisted isotonic flexion exercise. **F.** Isometric flexion exercise.

of the treatment. Musculoskeletal assessment is covered in Chapter 56. Reassurance and support can contribute to the relief of pain, so it is helpful to assure the client that the pain of bursitis or tendinitis is usually of short duration. Muscles tend to go into spasm under stress and aggravate the underlying condition, so it is important to take measures to relieve the client's stress.

Instruct the client in the use of ice therapy as well as heat therapy, if appropriate. The client should understand the reasons for using a splint or sling as directed; explain the importance of resting the joint while movement is painful. The client may be in considerable pain and therefore not concentrating when the treatment is being explained, so written instruction should also be provided. Include information about medications: dosage, frequency, route, and major side effects. Clients may get prompt pain relief from medications and be tempted to use the affected area too soon. Caution them to refrain from early resumption of activity to avoid reinjury.

Teach exercises for rehabilitation of the affected area. Some simple shoulder exercises are illustrated in Figure 57–12. The first, the gravity-assisted pendulum exercise, can usually be initiated very early. As pain allows, the arc of the pendulum swing should increase. Figures B and C illustrate walking the fingers up the wall in two positions. Figure D demonstrates the use of a pulley to raise the affected arm as high as possible, and Figure E shows the client using a towel to simulate the motion of drying the back with alternating arm movements. Provide a good deal of encouragement because exercises will be uncomfortable at first. If physical therapy is needed, be sure the client has an appointment with the therapist and understands the importance of keeping it.

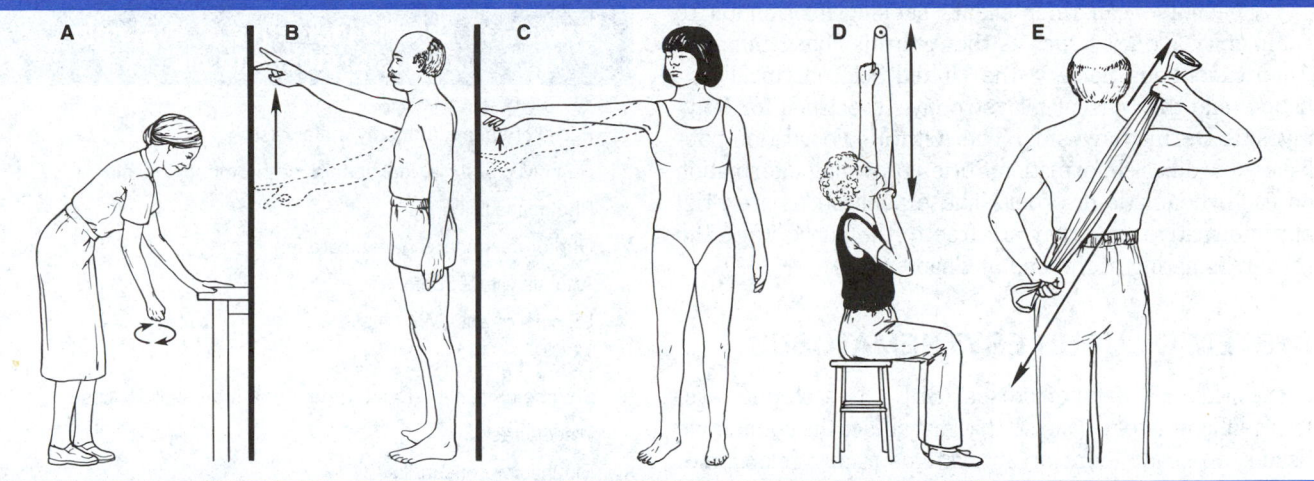

Figure 57–12

Exercises for rehabilitation of the shoulder. **A.** Gravity-assisted pendulum swing. **B, C.** Wall-walking exercises in two positions. **D.** Use of pulley to raise arm. **E.** Drying-of-back motion to exercise shoulder.

Section III: Immunologic Disorders

The disorders to be covered in this section (systemic lupus erythematosus, scleroderma, dermatomyositis, polymyositis, and amyloidosis) are believed to be caused by an autoimmune mechanism—that is, the body makes antibodies against its own tissues. In many autoimmune diseases, viruses are thought to be the initiating factor.

Autoimmune disorders are classified as organ specific or generalized. The connective tissue diseases are generalized autoimmune disorders, usually involving a progressive degradation of collagen in connective tissues throughout the body. Rheumatoid arthritis is included in these autoimmune disorders but will be discussed in Chapter 59 because joint involvement is the major problem.

There are serious consequences for those with autoimmune disorders of the connective tissues. Significant morbidity or even death may occur, but with the current emphasis on early diagnosis and treatment people are surviving and learning to live with these chronic illnesses. Although remissions occur, these disorders may leave their mark in the form of distorted self-image; permanent tissue damage; and psychological, economic, family, and social problems. Successful therapy for clients with autoimmune disease requires the services of various health professionals: physicians, nurses, physical therapists, occupational therapists, psychologists, social workers, and dietitians.

Familiarity with each disorder will prepare the nurse to be alert for manifestations signaling potential problems and to teach the client about them. Assessment skills to evaluate all body systems are essential because autoimmune disorders are systemic with different presentations in each individual. The nurse should also be familiar with the medications used for these disorders: their purpose, action, side effects, dosage, and contraindications. Since clients may be taking a combination of drugs, it may be difficult for them to figure out a workable dosing schedule; the nurse should help clients incorporate their medications into their daily routines. Comfort measures are another important aspect of nursing care during acute phases or exacerbations of autoimmune disorders. Proper positioning; use of splints; and small comfort measures such as back rubs, smoothing wrinkled sheets, and keeping noise and light down can all contribute to the client's well being.

The nurse will explain to clients how they can try to prevent exacerbations of specific manifestations of their disease and how to cope with them when they do occur. Preventive measures may include avoiding stress, cold, sun, or certain drugs, depending on the disease and its manifestations in the individual client. Exacerbations may cause extreme fatigue, so the client must learn to balance the proper amounts of rest and exercise.

People with immunological disorders are usually afraid of developing new and more severe manifestations, and often worry about dying. Their bodies seem to be rebelling against them, and though in the prime of life, they may feel totally defeated. The nurse must understand their fear and discouragement and become a source of information, encouragement, and support. Try to assist clients to adjust their lifestyles to their limitations rather than fighting them. Listening to the client is important, and being available when the client wants to talk is the best therapy the nurse can offer. Encourage clients to join or help form a group of people with the same illness. Seeing someone else cope with problems they thought were insurmountable sometimes gives new impetus to their lives.

The nurse can refer clients seeking information to community agencies such as the Arthritis Foundation, the American Lupus Society, the United Scleroderma Foundation, and the Muscular Dystrophy Association for Polymyositis/Dermatomyositis. The Arthritis Foundation publishes a Medical Information Series providing information on each rheumatic disorder. These publications are brief but informative, and they are free to the public. (See the resources listing at the end of Chapter 56.)

SYSTEMIC LUPUS ERYTHEMATOSUS

Systemic lupus erythematosus (SLE), is a chronic systemic inflammatory disease that may affect the connective tissue of one or more organ systems at any given time. Joints, skin, blood, heart, lungs, and glomeruli can be involved, although usually not all are involved in the same individual. Occasionally, the disease is fulminating and rapidly fatal. For the most part, however, SLE follows an irregular course with exacerbations and remissions. Women of childbearing age are most often affected.

Of the many theories regarding the etiology of SLE, none is proved. All researchers are confident that the immune system is somehow involved. The role of slow or latent viruses, genetic factors, hormones, and drugs are all being investigated. It is postulated that SLE may not be a single disease entity but several closely related disorders with different genetic, immunologic, and pathogenic causes. The hallmark of SLE is the presence of antinuclear antibodies (ANA) in the serum. ANA forms immune complexes with specific antigens, and these complexes penetrate the cell membrane, causing diffuse damage in various organ systems. The complement system is also implicated in the tissue damage. Further discussion of these processes can be found in Chapter 2.

The diagnosis of SLE is established by the presence of at least four of the clinical criteria listed in Box 57–1. The presence of ANA or other abnormal laboratory results is not diagnostic unless accompanied by clinical symptoms. (This is true of all immunologic disorders of the muscle-connective tissue system.) Absence of ANA does not rule out a diagnosis of SLE. A negative ANA decreases the likelihood of this diagnosis, however.

Clinical Manifestations

The *joints* are the most common areas of involvement in SLE, and many clients are misdiagnosed as having rheumatoid arthritis. In the arthritis of lupus, the affected joints often appear normal, although they can be hot, swollen, and tender as in typical rheumatoid arthritis. The most commonly affected joints are the proximal interphalangeal (PIP) joints, knees, wrists, and metacarpophalangeal (MCP) joints. Most people also complain of morning stiffness. Deformities and bone erosions are rare, but aseptic necrosis of the hip sometimes occurs because of high steroid

---

Box 57–1 Criteria Indicative of Systemic Lupus Erythematosus

Facial erythema (butterfly malar rash)

Hemolytic anemia, leukopenia, or thrombocytopenia

Photosensitivity

Oral or nasopharyngeal ulceration

Arthritis without deformity

LE cells or anti-DNA

ANA

Profuse proteinuria (>3.5 g/day) or urinary cellular casts

Discoid rash

Pleuritis or pericarditis

Psychosis, convulsions, or neurologic deficits

SOURCE: Rodnan GP, Schumacher HR (editors): *Primer on the Rheumatic Diseases* 8th ed. Atlanta: Arthritis Foundation, 1983.

---

dosage. Infectious arthritis of one or more joints may appear because of the client's decreased resistance to infection.

The *skin* is the second most common area of involvement. Malar (cheekbone area) rash in butterfly distribution (Figure 57–13) is a classic sign of SLE although not frequently seen. In clients with skin involvement, exposure to sunlight often brings on the skin eruptions. Patchy alopecia, oral or nasal ulcers, and Raynaud's phenomenon may also be present. (Raynaud's phenomenon is described in the discussion of progressive systemic sclerosis later in this section.)

The pleura and pericardium may be involved. Clients may experience pleuritic-type chest pain, and a pleural friction rub may be heard on auscultation, with pleural effusion visible on x-ray. Pericarditis may be present, as evidenced by a pericardial friction rub on auscultation, pericardial effusion on x-ray, and ECG changes.

Kidney involvement occurs in approximately 50% of clients and is one of the most serious manifestations of SLE, since it can lead to renal failure and death. The first signs of renal damage are proteinuria, hematuria, and cellular casts. Monitor the client's blood pressure closely because an increase in blood pressure may herald renal involvement.

Central nervous system manifestations sometimes occur and are varied. Seizures, psychosis, emotional lability, cranial nerve abnormalities, migraine headaches, and major motor weakness may occur. Psychological changes must be evaluated carefully however, because they may be from high-dose steroid therapy rather than SLE. The highest SLE mortality rates are in clients with central nervous system and/or renal involvement.

SLE can affect *blood elements*. Possible hematologic problems include hemolytic anemia, leukopenia, lympho-

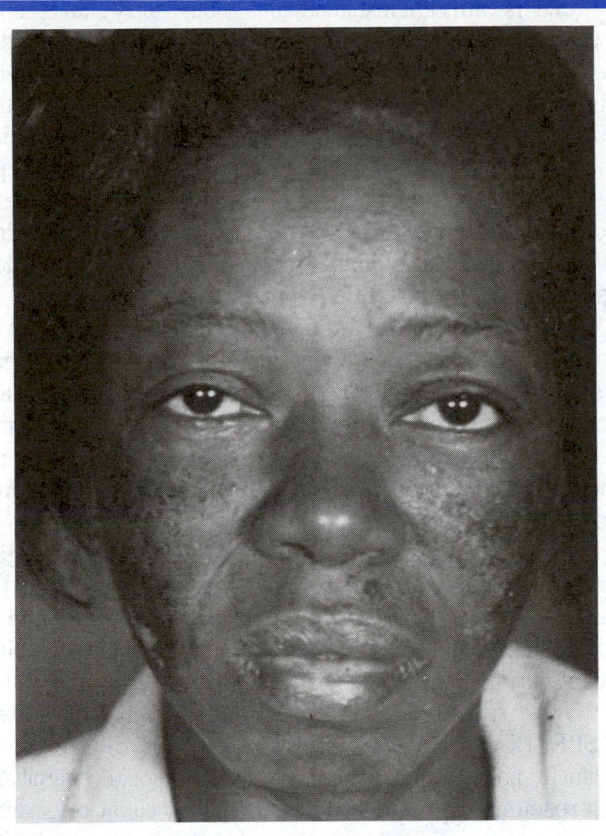

Figure 57–13
Butterfly rash of systemic lupus erythematosus in malar (cheek) region. (Photo courtesy Millard Fillmore Hospital)

penia, and thrombocytopenia; these can occur even in the absence of drug therapy.

Other common clinical manifestations are fever, malaise, arthralgia, myalgia, lymphadenopathy, anorexia, weight loss, nausea and vomiting, and abdominal pain. Extreme fatigue may be an early symptom of SLE.

Menstrual abnormalities are not uncommon in the early stages of SLE. Pregnant clients usually do well with careful management if they have no active renal disease. An exacerbation of the disease may occur in the last trimester or in the postpartum period. It is best for a client to become pregnant while in remission and taking no medications. Miscarriages, premature births, and stillbirths do occur.

Therapeutic Measures

The goal of treatment is to control symptoms and suppress the disease activity as much as possible. Specific measures vary depending on the clinical manifestations in each client. Although there is no known cure for SLE, proper treatment may decrease the number of exacerbations and prolong life. Much of the treatment is supportive and educational and is described under Specific Nursing Measures.

Various drugs are used, separately or in combination,

to treat the symptoms of SLE. *Salicylates* are used for arthralgia, arthritis, myalgia, and fever. If skin problems are also present, *antimalarials* may be used. These are administered in low doses because of the chance of causing retinopathy. Clients taking antimalarial drugs should have ophthalmological exams every 6 months. Clients with skin manifestations are advised to avoid the sun and to use sunscreens when exposure is unavoidable.

Corticosteroids, when indicated, usually have a dramatic effect. They are never used prophylactically, however, because they do not prevent serious manifestations. Indications for corticosteroid therapy are CNS or renal involvement, pericarditis, pleurisy, severe myositis, hemolytic anemia, clotting problems, leukopenia, and thrombocytopenia. Corticosteroids are often given every other day so symptoms of persistent SLE activity can be detected on the off day. Alternate-day therapy can also preserve or restore the hypothalamic–pituitary–adrenal axis and causes fewer side effects than daily doses.

With severe nephritis, cytotoxic agents are sometimes used in addition to corticosteroids. These drugs are used with extreme caution because of their serious side effects of marrow toxicity, hemorrhage, alopecia, and sterility. The full effects of long-term use of these drugs are still unknown.

Although plasmapheresis has been used in some cases, it has no proven effect on the symptoms of SLE. Dialysis and renal transplantation have been used in renal failure with some success (Decker, 1982). A low-sodium, low-protein diet is prescribed for renal failure.

Specific Nursing Measures

Assessment for Complications
Nurses may see clients with SLE in both inpatient and ambulatory care settings. Discovering early symptoms and signs of exacerbations and complications is important in prolonging the life of clients with SLE. Table 57–1 lists assessment priorities in identifying complications. Carefully monitor all diagnostic study reports to remain well informed about the client's progress.

Client Education
The nurse can instruct clients and their families about preventing exacerbations. Discuss medications with them: dosage, actions, side effects, and scheduling. Clients can buy their medications in bulk to save money, and they may want to shop around for the best buy. Clients should not change the dosage of the drugs they are taking without consulting the physician and should continue to take their medications even when they are feeling well. Clients taking steroids should wear a medical alert bracelet because they may need an increased dosage in case of a major accident or surgery. Clients should know that drugs such as birth control pills, antibiotics, hydralazine, procainamide, and tetanus toxoid may trigger or exacerbate symptoms. Advise

Table 57–1	Assessment for Complications of Systemic Lupus Erythematosus
System Involved	**Subjective and Objective Findings**
Cardiopulmonary	Chest pains, tachypnea, dyspnea, orthopnea, tachycardia
Renal	Increased weight, decreased urinary output, edema, hematuria, proteinuria, cellular casts, elevated BP
Gastrointestinal	Nausea and vomiting, diarrhea, pain, distention, decreased or absent bowel sounds
Neurologic	Diplopia, ptosis, nystagmus, ataxia, seizures, personality change, paranoid or psychotic behavior
Hematopoetic	Malaise, weakness, fever, chills, petechiae, epistaxis, hematemesis, positive stool for occult blood

clients to avoid over-the-counter drugs and hair dyes or cosmetics, except those approved by their physician.

Suggest that clients try to avoid stress-producing people and situations. Clients and their families may undertake a stress management program of their own using some of the suggestions and exercises described in Chapter 4. Stress management groups may also be beneficial. Clients should rest periodically throughout the day; midmorning and midafternoon naps are advisable in addition to a full 8 hours of sleep at night. Clients should try to adjust their activities so a low level of activity follows a high level and should discontinue any activity before becoming tired. Because clients with SLE are susceptible to viral and bacterial infections, they should avoid crowds and people with infections and colds during seasons when upper respiratory infections are common. Clients who develop an infection should be evaluated by their health care provider.

Box 57–2	The CREST Syndrome of Scleroderma

C • Calcinosis (subcutaneous calcifications)

R • Raynaud's phenomenon

E • Esophageal hypomotility

S • Sclerodactyly

T • Telangiectasia

SOURCE: Rodnan GP, Schumacher HR (editors): *Primer on the Rheumatic Diseases*, 8th ed. Atlanta: Arthritis Foundation, 1983.

Clients with skin manifestations should apply skin cream as directed. If exposure to the sun causes exacerbations, clients should wear protective clothing and broad-brimmed hats or use sunscreens. If oral ulcers are present, clients should eat soft foods and take meticulous care of their mouths. Clients with Raynaud's phenomenon should keep their hands warm; they should wear gloves in cold weather and when putting their hands into a freezer. They should also try to avoid air-conditioned rooms because in some cases this can precipitate a Raynaud's attack.

Teach clients with troublesome arthritis ROM exercises and methods for applying ice and heat (see Chapter 56). Also demonstrate proper body alignment and postural techniques to preserve function and decrease deformities. Stress the importance of regular health care even when feeling well for early detection of exacerbations or complications.

Encourage clients to maintain a positive self-image through careful attention to dressing and grooming. If makeup is used, it should be hypoallergenic. Maintaining independence and usual role routines is usually possible except during acute exacerbations.

The Arthritis Foundation publishes helpful literature on SLE. Discussion groups of people with SLE have been helpful for both clients and families. Nurses should be familiar with resources in their own local areas for client referral.

PROGRESSIVE SYSTEMIC SCLEROSIS

Progressive systemic sclerosis, also called PSS or *scleroderma*, is a connective tissue disorder. It causes fibrous changes in the skin, synovium, and small arteries of the digits, as well as in various internal organs, most notably the esophagus, intestines, heart, lungs, kidney, and thyroid. The disease occurs in various forms, ranging from a skin condition (localized scleroderma) to the CREST variant of PSS (Box 57–2), which is thought to be a more benign type, to involvement of visceral organs (systemic scleroderma). Some clients with the CREST syndrome have subsequently developed visceral and more extensive cutaneous lesions of PSS.

In all forms of the disease, there is vascular injury at the level of small arteries and capillaries, and the resulting decrease in circulation is the cause of the tissue changes. What precipitates the vascular damage is unknown, although investigations show that immunologic mechanisms may be involved. Collagen also increases, which causes fibrosis of the affected organ.

There is no laboratory test to diagnose PSS. Autoantibodies occur in this disorder, and the ESR may be elevated. Skin biopsies are not diagnostic, but a recent technique shows some promising results. In this technique, a thin layer of immersion oil is placed on the nail fold, which is then observed with an ophthalmoscope set at +20 or +40 diopters. In PSS, dilated capillary loops

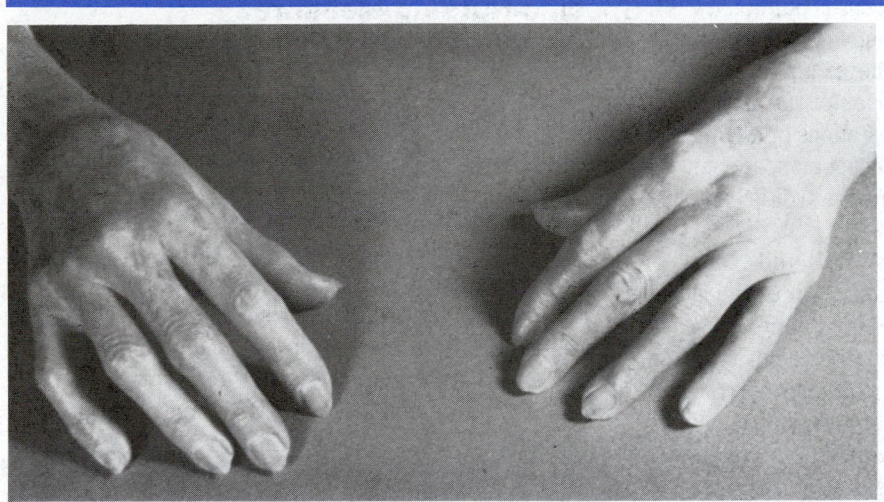

Figure 57–14
Tapering of the fingers with tightness of the overlying skin as seen in scleroderma. (Photo courtesy Millard Fillmore Hospital.)

can be observed (Phillips, 1981). At this time, however, diagnosis is based on clinical manifestations.

Clinical Manifestations

The most frequent presentation in PSS is the clinical triad of *skin changes, Raynaud's phenomenon,* and *esophageal hypomotility.* However, other organs must be continually monitored for involvement.

The most typical changes in PSS occur in the skin. (Scleroderma means "hard skin.") Typically, skin changes begin with swelling of the hands and gradual thickening, tightening, and hardening of the skin of the fingers (sclerodactyly) (Figure 57–14). The fingers become tapered and eventually even clawlike. Ulcers may develop on fingertips and over knuckles as the skin becomes taut. Sometimes the skin changes progress proximally at a slow rate, eventually affecting the face. The skin of the face becomes tight and shiny with a loss of normal wrinkles and skin folds. The nose may become beaked, and sometimes radial furrowing is seen around the mouth (Figure 57–15). The person cannot open the mouth completely. In extreme cases, the face becomes expressionless.

Most clients with PSS have *Raynaud's phenomenon,* and this is often the first symptom to appear. With Raynaud's there is diminished blood flow to the digits secondary to vasoconstriction of the digital arteries, triggered by cold, vasoconstricting drugs, or emotional states. The initial sign is digital pallor. The digits then become blue as a result of cyanosis and later become red secondary to erythema on rewarming.

The client may have pain and stiffness in both small and large peripheral joints. Occasionally, a client develops arthritis and synovial effusion. Contractures and atrophy of the fingers may eventually occur.

Hypomotility of the *esophagus* occurs in a majority of clients with PSS. There is gastroesophageal reflux, with

resulting heartburn and stricture. The client may have difficulty swallowing. Esophageal dilation is sometimes needed, and the client's nutrition may be impaired. Gastrointestinal involvement can progress to the intestine and colon, with development of hypomotility of the small intestine and wide-mouth diverticuli.

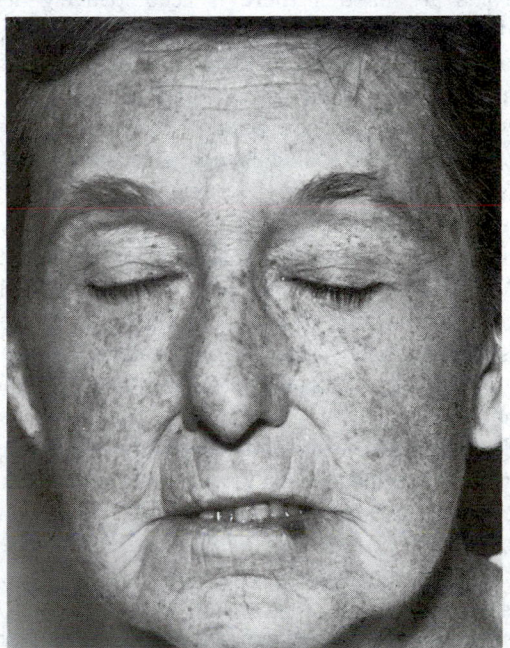

Figure 57–15
Taut facial skin, beaked nose radial furrowing around the mouth, and telangiectasias as seen in scleroderma.
SOURCE: Binnick SA: *Skin Diseases: Diagnosis and Management in Clinical Practice,* Baltimore, MD: Williams & Wilkins, 1982.

The systemic disease can also cause cardiopulmonary problems. Dyspnea may develop because of pulmonary hypertension and interstitial fibrosis. The examiner may hear fine dry rales or crackles at the bases of the lungs, and spirometry is often abnormal. Manifestations involving the heart are primarily the result of lung complications. Dysrhythmias, conduction disturbances, pericarditis, and pericardial effusions sometimes occur.

The *kidneys* are sometimes seriously affected, with malignant hypertension rapidly producing renal failure. Renal failure is the leading cause of death in PSS. Clients with affected kidneys have high renin levels and proteinuria.

Hematologic problems, in addition to a mild normochromic, normocytic anemia, include vitamin B_{12}/folic acid deficiency anemia, which may occur secondarily to bacterial overgrowth because of atony of the small intestine. There also may be some GI bleeding and resultant iron deficiency.

Other manifestations include thyroid involvement, which may cause Hashimoto's thyroiditis or even produce hypothyroidism. Biliary cirrhosis, trigeminal sensory neuropathy or other cranial nerve neuropathies, and Sjögren's syndrome are possible.

Therapeutic Measures

Treatment of PSS is symptomatic, and much of it will be described under nursing measures. Drugs such as corticosteroids are used if there is accompanying disabling myositis or severe mixed connective tissue disease. Uncontrolled studies have shown some improvement with D-penicillamine, which reduces skin thickening, but this is not generally accepted treatment. Some researchers have advocated colchicine to inhibit collagen accumulation but its effects remain questionable. Immunosuppressive agents are also being studied.

If skin ulcers develop, soaks and debridement along with topical antibiotics may be necessary. Physical therapy for the hands is important to prevent contractures. For clients with Raynaud's phenomenon, biofeedback is sometimes useful for controlling temperature in the hands and feet.

Some clients with esophageal dysmotility require intermittent esophageal dilation. In cases of malabsorption by the small intestine, absorption often improves with the use of tetracycline, which destroys the bacterial overgrowth that occurs with hypomotility.

Hypertension is treated aggressively with drugs to prevent irreversible renal damage. Propranolol, clonidine, and minoxidil, drugs that block the renin-angiotensin pathway, are most often used. Dialysis may be necessary with progressive renal failure.

Arthritis responds to NSAIDs, and the dry eyes (sicca syndrome) of Sjögren's syndrome are helped by artificial tears. A client with dry mouth (xerostomia) should have frequent dental exams because this condition predisposes people to severe dental caries.

Specific Nursing Measures

Assess the client's skin and joints and cardiovascular, pulmonary, and gastrointestinal status. Evaluate the eyes and mouth for adequate lacrimal and salivary gland secretion. Monitor blood pressure closely and review laboratory results. Venipuncture in the antecubital area may be difficult because of skin changes. Avoid finger sticks because of the client's compromised circulation; the earlobe may afford the best site if only a capillary tube of blood is needed.

Explain the nature and course of PSS to client and family and help them become knowledgeable about signs of more serious involvement. Teach them about prescribed medications and demonstrate ROM exercises to prevent joint contracture. Encourage the liberal use of skin lotions to decrease dryness.

Advise clients with Raynaud's phenomenon to avoid cold, ergotamine, and amphetamines. They should wear gloves and socks in winter and whenever their hands and feet are exposed to cold. Smoking should be avoided since nicotine causes pronounced peripheral vasoconstriction, which markedly aggravates Raynaud's.

Clients with esophageal dysmotility should eat small, frequent meals; chew their food thoroughly; and follow meals with water. They should avoid any foods that cause them particular problems. Antacids after meals and at bedtime help to relieve gastric irritation. Raising the head of the bed on blocks will decrease nocturnal esophageal reflux.

The face and hands often undergo considerable change in scleroderma, which alters the client's appearance and manual dexterity. The facial skin becomes taut, the nose may become beaked, and telangiectasias may appear on the face. Tapering of the fingers with tightness of the overlying skin occurs, and flexion contractures may be present.

The nurse who has established a relationship of trust with clients may be able to help them express their thoughts and fears. These clients are dealing with a diagnosis with a varied prognosis that causes significant body image changes. The possible loss of hand function may be more stressful than the facial changes to many clients because of potential loss of independence. The mental health clinical nurse specialist can be of considerable assistance to these clients and also to the nursing staff caring for them.

DERMATOMYOSITIS AND POLYMYOSITIS

Dermatomyositis and polymyositis are closely related disorders involving degenerative and inflammatory changes in connective tissues. Dermatomyositis involves skeletal muscle and skin; polymyositis, skeletal muscle alone. The rate of onset and progression of symptoms are varied. There is evidence that these disorders may be caused by a viral infection or by an autoimmune response. Sometimes a malignancy is the precipitating cause. In this case, the tumor probably initiates an immunologic reaction directed against an antigen common to both the tumor and the muscle tissue.

Clinical Manifestations

The most outstanding symptom of dermatomyositis and polymyositis is extreme muscle weakness. Clients experience weakness in the proximal limb muscles making it difficult for them to raise their arms, go up and down stairs, or get out of a bathtub or a chair. They may be unable to raise their heads from the pillow or to squat. Often the client feels no pain, but the muscles may be tender to palpation. Occasionally, there is aching pain in the buttocks, thighs, and calves. The pharyngeal and laryngeal muscles may be affected, resulting in dysphagia and dysphonia (difficulty in speaking or hoarseness). Raynaud's phenomenon and arthritis may also be present.

Occasionally, cardiac abnormalities such as dysrythmias occur. With severe cardiac involvement, there may be necrosis of the myocardial fibers resulting in death. Cough and dyspnea may be an indication of interstitial pneumonitis and fibrosis.

The skin lesions in dermatomyositis consist of diffuse erythema of the face, neck, and anterior chest and a purple-hued maculopapular rash that occurs periorbitally and on the nose, cheeks, forehead, and fingernails (heliotrope eruption) (Figure 57–16A). Pruritus and periorbital and perioral edema may also be present. Papules on the knuckles (Gottron's papules) occur in about 50% of clients (Figure 57–16B).

Laboratory findings include elevated muscle enzymes including SGOT, SGPT, CK, and aldolase (see Chapter 56). Positive ANA, rheumatoid factor, and elevated ESR are common. The EMG reveals inflammation, and muscle biopsy findings show tissue changes such as muscle necrosis and regeneration. The muscle biopsy should be taken from muscle that is involved but not atrophied. The diagnosis is based on the clinical picture, along with an abnormal EMG, elevated muscle enzymes, and a positive muscle biopsy. Evaluation of muscle enzymes is helpful in monitoring the client's response to treatment.

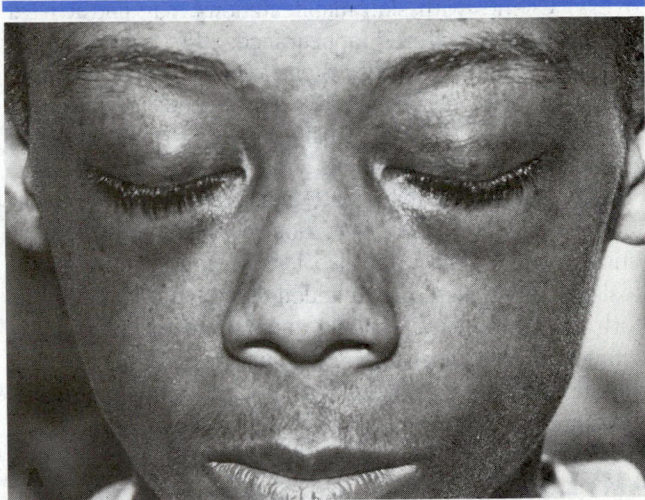
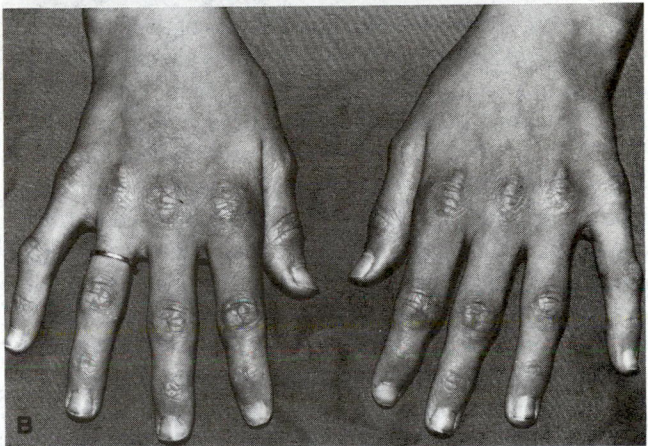

Figure 57–16

A. Periorbital rash and edema of dermatomyositis.
B. Papules on the knuckles (Gottron's papules) in dermatomyositis.
SOURCE: Binnick SA: *Skin Diseases: Diagnosis and Management in Clinical Practice.* Baltimore, MD: Williams & Wilkins, 1982.

Therapeutic Measures

Corticosteroids are the cornerstone of therapy, and their effects can be determined by monitoring the muscle enzyme levels. Decreasing or discontinuing the steroid too soon may cause an exacerbation that may be difficult to control. If clients respond poorly to steroids, immunosuppressive drugs such as azathioprine may be added to the regimen.

Clients who do not respond to corticosteroids should have a workup for a malignancy. If a malignancy is found and treated, the muscle weakness should resolve.

Specific Nursing Measures

Clients with dermatomyositis or polymyositis present a challenge for the nurse because their severe muscle weakness and inability to move against gravity make them almost immobile. In the initial phase, clients will need complete care and meticulous attention to prevention of the complications of immobility.

The dysphagia resulting from pharyngeal weakness can cause numerous problems such as choking and aspiration pneumonia. Anyone offering food or fluids to the client should be fully aware of the client's difficulty in swallowing and offer oral medications, fluids, and food slowly with the client in a comfortable upright position. A gastrostomy tube or hyperalimentation is sometimes necessary.

Continuous assessment of the client is important to monitor response to corticosteroids. Muscle weakness can be evaluated by the client's ability to move the limbs against resistance. Assessment of the skin, lungs, and cardiovascular system are important nursing responsibilities.

In helping clients and families with the psychosocial problems that inevitably arise from such a disabling condition, reinforce the fact that most clients make a full recovery. Clients with skin manifestations may find it hard to accept their altered appearance; the nurse should encourage them to express their feelings and assist them to look as good as possible. Gently encourage independence even if it is in the smallest task. Praise for small accomplishments is essential.

Teaching the family gentle massage and ROM activities is beneficial to the client, not only to prevent complications of immobility but also for the touching involved. Resistive exercises can be added as enzyme levels drop. Both client and family should understand the medication regimen prior to discharge. Community health nursing visits to the home may be helpful as well as referral to relevant community agencies.

AMYLOIDOSIS

Amyloidosis is characterized by deposits of the fibrous protein *amyloid* in connective tissue. The disorder may be diffuse, involving major organs, or it may be limited, with little effect on a person's life. Diffuse (or generalized) amyloidosis is progressive and usually leads to death in 1 to 4 years, although clients sometimes live as long as 10 years. The major cause of death is renal failure, but sudden death can occur from cardiac dysrhythmias. There are six recognized types of amyloidosis, some involving other disorders such as multiple myeloma and Mediterranean fever. (For further information on classification of amyloidosis, see the selected readings at the end of the chapter.)

The etiology of amyloidosis, like that of most connective tissue diseases, is unknown, but it appears to involve the immune system. People with amyloidosis have marked depression of T-lymphocytes, with normal or hyperactive B-lymphocytes. Other immunologic abnormalities may also be involved. One classification of amyloidosis is familial, and the mode of inheritance seems to be autosomal dominant. The exception is Mediterranean fever, which has an autosomal recessive mode of transmission.

Clinical Manifestations

The clinical manifestations of amyloidosis are varied and depend upon the site of amyloid deposition.

If the *kidneys* are affected, there is mild proteinuria with few RBCs. Hypertension is rare unless there has been long-standing illness. Renal involvement eventually leads to azotemia and death.

The *liver* is commonly affected, and liver function may be abnormal in later stages of the disease. Elevated serum alkaline phosphatase and Bromsulphalein excretion (BSP) are most indicative of liver amyloid (Cohen, 1980). Hepatosplenomegaly may also develop.

If the *heart* is involved, the client may have congestive heart failure, cardiomegaly, and dysrhythmias. ECGs and angiograms are abnormal. People with amyloidosis may be hypersensitive to digitalis, so it should be used with caution.

When the *skin* is affected, characteristic, slightly raised waxy papules cluster in the axillary, anal, and inguinal folds as well as on the face, neck, and ears or in the mucosal area of the tongue. These papules are seldom pruritic and sometimes can only be detected on biopsy. Gentle rubbing of the skin may produce purpura.

The *gastrointestinal tract* is often involved; clients may have obstruction, ulceration, malabsorption, hemorrhage, and diarrhea. Infiltration of the tongue with amyloid may lead to macroglossia. Even if not enlarged, the tongue may be stiff and firm to the touch.

If the *central nervous system* is affected, clients may experience peripheral neuropathy, the inability to sweat, hoarseness, and sphincter incompetence. Adie's pupil, which is a sluggish pupillary reaction to both light and accommodation, may develop.

Clients may have *joint* symptoms, since amyloid can affect the articular cartilage and synovial membrane. Amyloidosis often resembles rheumatoid arthritis because it causes symmetrical inflammation of the small joints, morning stiffness, nodules, and fatigue. Bilateral carpal tunnel syndrome is common. Amyloidosis clients with these joint problems are often later diagnosed as having multiple myeloma.

The *lungs* may be affected because amyloid often blocks ducts of the sinuses and the air passages of the respiratory tract. *Blood* disorders may include fibrinogenopenia, increased fibrinolysis, and clotting deficiencies.

Because of the variable course and presentation of amyloidosis, it can be years before a client is correctly diagnosed. The care provider should suspect amyloidosis in clients with chronic infections or inflammatory disease or when unexplained proteinuria, hepatomegaly, or splenomegaly suddenly appear. The specific diagnosis of amyloidosis is made by biopsy specimen from the rectum, skin, gums, kidney, or lung; the rectal biopsy is the most common. Laboratory abnormalities include proteinuria, elevated ESR, and a decrease or increase in serum immunoglobulins (IgG, IgA, IgM).

Therapeutic and Specific Nursing Measures

Treatments for amyloidosis are entirely symptomatic. Renal transplants have been successful in a few people with kidney involvement. Colchicine has been shown to prevent acute attacks of Mediterranean fever and is thought to inhibit amyloid deposition.

Specific nursing measures depend on the client's clinical manifestations. Because the most frequent cause of death is renal failure or cardiac dysrhythmias, carefully assess output, presence of proteinuria, and vital signs. Check the apical rate and rhythm as part of the vital signs. In addition to the renal and cardiovascular systems, the respiratory, gastrointestinal, musculoskeletal, neurologic systems, and skin are evaluated for progression of the disease.

Often it takes years and much client and family frustration before the diagnosis of amyloidosis is made. By then, the symptoms can be advanced. Clients with amyloidosis have survived up to 10 years, although death usually occurs several years following diagnosis.

Support for the client and family is essential. Sometimes it is almost easier for them to deal with the facts of the disease, even though the prognosis is poor, than to suffer through years of not knowing what is wrong.

Section IV: Traumatic Disorders

SPRAINS AND STRAINS

Traumatic injuries to the soft tissues surrounding joints—muscle, ligaments, and tendons—are called sprains and strains. The injury may arise from blunt trauma to the muscle or joint; excessive exercise; or twisting, stretching, or forcible extension of a joint. Surgery is seldom needed unless complete rupture occurs, but the pain of such an injury can be severely limiting. Serious sprains or strains can be more debilitating than fractures or internal knee derangement.

A *sprain,* an injury to a ligament, is the result of forcing a joint beyond its normal ROM. The ligament may be stretched or actually torn. Often a blunt blow to the joint can sprain it. Sprains usually occur during sports activities or falls. A *strain* is an injury to a muscle and/or tendon at any location from origin to insertion. Strains are associated with excessive stretching of a muscle or muscle unit; they usually do not occur because of a blow or direct trauma. Poor conditioning, improper warm-up before activity, muscle fatigue or weakness, and strength imbalance can all contribute to muscle strain. Precipitating events include lifting improperly, sudden straining motions, and falls. Intermittent joggers and weekend sports buffs often have strains; well-conditioned athletes are usually spared. Strains have a high incidence of recurrence.

Clinical Manifestations

A *sprain* causes pain, swelling, local hemorrhage, spasm of the muscle that moves the joint, and disability (Table 57–2). The pain occurs with passive movement of the joint, and there is intense pain over the involved ligament itself. Sprains are graded according to damage to the ligaments and the resultant joint instability.

Ankle sprains, the most common, occur when inversion of the foot tears a ligament, usually the anterior talofibular ligament. *Knee sprains* cause swelling, hemarthrosis, significant decrease in the range of motion, and joint laxity. The injured person is usually unable to bear weight. Often the person hears a "pop" when the injury occurs and later describes the knee as feeling as if it is going to "give way." The medial collateral ligament is most commonly involved.

Strains cause pain, swelling, muscle spasm, and hemorrhage into the muscle (Table 57–3). Discoloration and weakness may also be present. Pain increases with active

Table 57–2	Grading and Treatment of Sprains	
Degree of Injury	**Treatment**
First degree: tenderness and swelling over the ligament; the joint is stable	PRICE, NSAIDs
Second degree: partial ligament disruption with some joint instability in addition to tenderness and swelling	PRICE, immobilization, NSAIDS, x-rays to determine need for further treatment
Third degree: complete tearing of the ligament with loss of joint stability on the side of the ligament rupture	

flexion or passive stretching, which helps in differentiating strains from sprains. Strains are graded according to loss of muscle strength.

Therapeutic and Specific Nursing Measures

Treatment is basically the same for strains and sprains. The nurse should take a thorough history to determine the

Table 57–3	Grading and Treatment of Strains	
Degree of Injury	**Treatment**
First degree: local pain, tenderness, swelling with pain on active flexion or passive stretching; no loss of strength or motion	PRICE, NSAIDs
Second degree: partial disruption resulting in some loss of strength	PRICE, NSAIDs, splinting
Third degree: complete disruption with a functionless muscle-tendon unit	Surgical repair

---

Box 57–3   PRICE Treatment for Sprains and Strains

P • Protection

R • Rest

I • Ice

C • Compression

E • Elevation

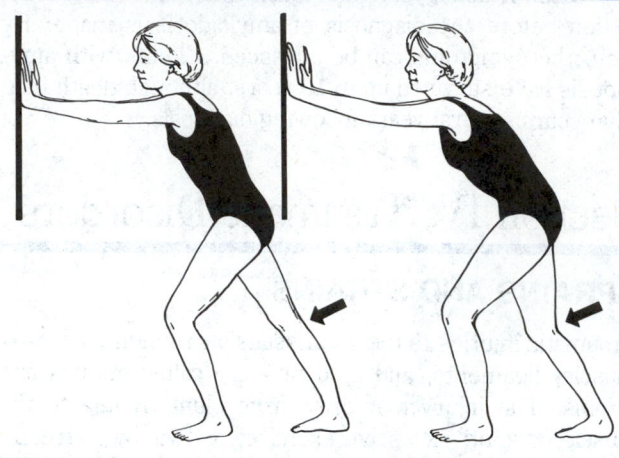

Figure 57–17

Achilles tendon stretch.

---

nature and cause of the injury as well as any significant health problems that may influence the treatment. When a suspected strain or sprain occurs, the PRICE treatment is initiated (Box 57–3). Cold compresses should immediately be applied to minimize swelling and to decrease spasm and pain. The extremity is then wrapped with an elastic bandage, which is soaked first in cold water to aid the cooling process, and elevated above heart level to limit the amount of dependent edema and swelling. The PRICE regimen is usually continued for the first week after injury, although there is some controversy about whether cold or heat is used after the first 24 hours. Cold is usually recommended for 5 to 7 days because of its anti-inflammatory and analgesic effect. Then wet heat is encouraged to aid in relaxation of muscles and to promote blood flow to the

---

Box 57–4   Nonsteroidal Anti-Inflammatory Drugs (NSAIDs) for the Treatment of Sprains and Strains

Indomethacin (Indocin)

Ibuprofen (Motrin)

Tolmetin sodium (Tolectin)

Sulindac (Clinoril)

---

area. Sometimes heat is used immediately after the first 24 hours of injury.

With a second or third degree sprain, an x-ray is always taken to rule out a fracture (Table 57–2). Clients with sprains are usually immobilized for 1 week. When all pain on motion has ceased, clients can begin active ROM and muscle-strengthening exercises. Nonsteroidal anti-inflammatory drugs is the treatment of choice (Box 57–4).

The PRICE regimen and NSAIDs are also appropriate for management of a strain (Table 57–3). Emphasis is placed on prevention of recurrence through the use of muscle-strengthening and stretching exercises. The importance of doing warm-up exercises before engaging in strenuous activity is stressed. For example, recurrent ankle sprains are often associated with tight Achilles tendons. Daily slow stretching of the Achilles tendon can effectively reduce the incidence of ankle sprain (Figure 57–17). Should complete muscle rupture occur, surgical intervention is needed. Many professional athletes elect to have surgery even for partial rupture because this promotes faster healing.

Chapter Highlights

Congenital disorders of connective tissue and muscle are genetically transferred as single gene defects of the autosomal dominant type. Therefore, thorough family histories must be taken, and genetic counseling is of great importance.

Clinical manifestations of Marfan's syndrome include lens subluxation, aortic anomalies, skeletal abnormalities—especially archnodactyly and excessively long arms and legs in relation to the trunk.

Ehlers–Danlos clients have hyperextensible joints and

fragile, hyperextensible skin, along with bleeding disorders.

Nursing interventions for clients with congenital disorders are essentially psychological support, client education, and symptomatic care.

Pain is the most important symptom in evaluating bursitis and tendinitis. Therefore, a careful pain assessment is an important part of the data base.

The most common sites for bursitis and tendinitis are the shoulders, elbows, hands, hips, knees, and ankles.

Therapeutic measures for bursitis and/or tendinitis consist of rest, ice, exercises, analgesics, and anti-inflammatory drugs, and local injections of corticosteroids.

Medications used in immunologic disorders are toxic. Therefore, the nurse, client, and family should be familiar with symptoms and signs of toxicity.

Systemic lupus erythematosus is now thought to be a number of closely related, but separate illnesses that have different immunologic, genetic, and pathogenic causes.

Clinical manifestations of immunologic disorders of muscles and connective tissue may include arthritis, myositis, integumentary changes, gastrointestinal changes, nephritis, CNS disturbances, and cardiopulmonary abnormalities. Fever, malaise, anorexia, and weight loss may also be among the primary symptoms.

Therapeutic goals for clients with immunologic disorders are to control symptoms and suppress the disease activity. Various medications such as salicylates, NSAIDs, antimalarials, corticosteroids, and immunosuppressives are used.

Serious sprains and strains can be more debilitating than fractures and have a high incidence of recurrence. Therefore, education for prevention is the primary nursing concern.

General therapeutic measures for sprains and strains include protection, rest, ice, compression with Ace bandages, elevation, and immobilization to minimize pain, decrease edema, and prevent further injury.

Bibliography

Birrer RB: *Sports Medicine for the Primary Care Physician.* New York: Appleton-Century-Crofts, 1984.

Brody DM: Running injuries. *Clin Symp* 1980; 32(4):2–36.

Decker JL: The management of systemic lupus erythematosus. *Arthritis Rheum* 1982; 7:891–894.

Garrett WE: Sprains and strains in athletes. *Postgrad Med* 1983; 73(3):200–209.

Hoffman GS: Tendinitis and bursitis. *Am Fam Physician* 1981; 23(6):103–110.

Krupp MA, Chatton MJ: *Current Medical Diagnosis and Treatment.* Los Altos, CA: Lange, 1981.

Lewis KS: Systemic lupus erythematosus: The great masquerader. *Nurs Prac* 1984; 9:13–22.

Lynch HT, Fain P, Marrero K: *International Directory of Genetic Services,* 6th ed. White Plains, NY: March of Dimes Birth Defects Foundation, 1980.

Petersdorf RG et al: *Harrison's Principles of Internal Medicine,* 10th ed. New York: McGraw-Hill, 1983.

Phillips RM, Wasner CK: Scleroderma: Current understanding of pathogenesis and management. *Postgrad Med* (Sept) 1981; 70:153–168.

Pyeritz RE, McKusick VA: Current concepts: The Marfan syndrome—diagnosis and management. *New Engl J Med* 1979; 14:772–777.

Rodnan GP, Schumacher HR (editors): *Primer on the Rheumatic Diseases,* 8th ed. Atlanta: Arthritis Foundation, 1983.

Roy S, Irvin R: *Sports Medicine.* Englewood Cliffs, NJ: Prentice-Hall, 1983.

Sheon RP et al: The hypermobility syndrome. *Postgrad Med* 1982; 71(6):199–209.

Simkin PA: Tendinitis and bursitis of the shoulder. *Postgrad Med* 1983; 73(5):177–190.

Suggested Readings

Dunwoody CJ, Pais MB, Wandel CR: Introduction to muscular skeletal disorders. In: *Nurse's Reference Library: Diseases.* Horsham, PA: Intermed Communications, 1981. Good general source for concise descriptions of musculoskeletal disorders. Diagnosis, treatment, and nursing interventions are all discussed in a relevant manner. Written for nurses, the chapter is a valuable resource for quick reference.

Hart D: Disseminated connective tissue diseases. *Nurs Mirror, Clinical Forum* (Nov) 1981. This article gives the reader a concise overview of the more common connective tissue disorders. Other articles in this Clinical Forum will also be of interest to the student who is dealing with clients who have rheumatic diseases.

Pigg JS: Nursing care of the hospitalized patient with rheumatic disease. In: *Rehabilitation and Management of Rheumatic Conditions.* Ehrlick GE (editor). Baltimore: Williams & Wilkins, 1980. This chapter is valuable for nurses who care for the hospitalized client with a rheumatic disease. Nursing implications and interventions related to common problems of clients with rheumatic disorders are thoroughly discussed. A section on common rheumatic drugs and their implications is also included.

Proceedings of the conference on current perspectives on the immunology of systemic lupus erythematosus. *Arthritis Rheum* 1982; 7:721–910. Entire issue is devoted to SLE. It contains detailed articles explaining current investigations into the pathogenesis, immunologic manifestations, and management of this disease.

The Client With Systemic Lupus Erythematosus

I. Brief Descriptive Data	Mrs Kathleen Oates, age 35, comes into the physician's office with a complaint of fatigue, migratory joint pain with swelling, and a rash over both cheeks.

II. Personal Data

Date:	June 10, 1986
Insurance:	Blue Cross/Blue Shield 50/51
Full Name:	Kathleen Elizabeth Oates
Social Security Number:	000-00-0000
Address:	12 Stone Ln., Orchard Park, Fla
Sex:	Female
Age:	35
Birthdate:	9-1-50
Marital Status:	Married
Occupation:	Elementary school teacher
Race/Culture:	Caucasian
Usual Health Care Provider:	Sharon Evert, MD

III. Health History

Source of Information:	Client
Reliability of Informant:	Excellent historian
Chief Concern:	Rash over both cheeks that began after working in the garden. Also fatigue and occasional joint pains.
History of Present Illness:	About 10 years ago, when living out of town, Mrs Oates experienced pain and swelling of both knees. She sought help at a hospital outpatient department and was diagnosed as having rheumatoid arthritis. She was placed on aspirin with only slight relief of symptoms. Over the years, she has experienced intermittent, mild arthralgia in the ankles, shoulders, knees, hands, and wrists, which she has learned to live with. However, during the last 3 months she has experienced progressive worsening of pain, swelling, and fatigue and has developed daily morning stiffness on arising lasting approximately 3 hours. Last week while in the sun, she developed a rash over her cheeks and has come to her physician for evaluation. She denies Raynaud's symptoms, psoriasis, or other skin problems. Her only medication is Bufferin 650 mg t.i.d. She expresses concern about her recently developed symptoms and desires more information about her condition.
Past Health History:	
Childhood:	Measles, mumps, chickenpox
Immunizations:	Last Td, 1978
Medical Problems:	None
Surgeries:	T&A, 1955
Transfusions:	None
Special Diagnostic Procedures:	None
Pregnancies:	None
Trauma:	Fracture of right tibia, 1962 (fall from bicycle)
Allergies:	None known
Medications:	Bufferin 650 mg t.i.d.; multiple vitamin $\frac{-}{i}$ q.d.; various OTC preparations p.r.n. episodic sinus congestion

Case Study written by Rita A. Colicchia and Carolyn Czech Montgomery.

Family History:	Father, age 60, A&W; emphysema, DJD
	Mother, age 59, A&W; hypertension, RA
	Brother, age 41, A&W
	Brother, age 37, A&W; mixed connective tissue disease
	Spouse, age 39, A&W
	No known significant health problems in other blood relatives.
Personal/Social History:	Mrs Oates and her husband live on a 40-acre farm, which they recently purchased. They share a hobby of training horses for show and maintain the property themselves. Client spends her school vacation time working on a garden and redecorating their home. Drives her own car into nearby community, 7 miles away, for work, purchasing groceries, and needed services. She has a master's degree in education. Enjoys teaching first grade, September through June. They are financially comfortable with two incomes.
Habits:	Eats three balanced meals a day and has no difficulty maintaining weight. Exercises daily by working with horses but this has become increasingly difficult over the past several months. Does not smoke. Rare alcohol intake—notices flushing of face with alcohol. Denies other drug use. Sleeps 8 to 9 hours per night, bedtime at 10 or 11 PM, arises at 6 AM.
Sexual Functioning:	Sexually active without problems; they plan to have no children; husband had a vasectomy for birth control.
Coping Patterns:	Husband is very supportive; she relies on him and her own inner strength when symptoms are immobilizing; her brothers and neighbors help with the horses as needed; also has several close, supportive women friends.
Review of Systems:	
Skin:	See HPI
Nose:	Chronic nasal rhinitis and postnasal drip
Heart:	Occasional palpitations since 1980; denies knowledge of precipitating or aggravating factors
Gyn:	Menses, regular 30-day cycle; recently having heavy 3-day flow followed by 3 days of spotting; moderate dysmenorrhea.
Musculoskeletal:	See HPI
Psychological:	Gets depressed because of fatigue and recent difficulties accomplishing tasks at home.

IV. Physical Assessment

Weight:	123 lb
Height:	5 ft 4 in.
Vital Signs:	Temp 97°F(36°C); P-64; R, 16; BP 130/70
Relevant Organ Systems:	
Skin:	Flat, erythematous rash over malar area and bridge of nose; no digital ulcers or alopecia noted
ENT:	wnl without mucosal ulcers; adequate saliva
Lungs:	Normal resonance with percussion; clear to auscultation A&P
Heart:	PMI slightly medial to MCL at 5th LICS; 64/min, regular; no rubs, murmurs, or gallops
Abdomen:	Bowel sounds wnl; no masses or tenderness; liver, spleen, kidneys not enlarged
Musculoskeletal:	Generalized symmetrical synovitis, especially of the hands and wrists; 2+ swelling with tenderness, heat, and limited motion of hands; decreased grip strength noted bilaterally; slight decrease of ROM both wrists; no atrophy or deformities visualized
Neurologic:	Gait, coordination, sensation, and deep tendon reflexes all wnl

(continued)

The Client With Systemic Lupus Erythematosus

V. Diagnostic Data
- Erythrocyte sedimentation rate (ESR), 38 mm/h
- VDRL, reactive
- Antinuclear antibody (ANA), positive, 1:80
- Hct, 36%
- Platelets adequate
- Complement C_4, decreased, 8.0 (16.0–45.0 mg/dL, normal)
- Urinalysis within normal limits

VI. Summary

After evaluating Mrs Oates, her diagnosis was established as systemic lupus erythematosus (SLE). The treatment regimen was as follows:
- Increased periods of rest
- Ice therapy to inflamed joints and elastic bandages to wrists
- Medications: Prednisone 5 mg q.d., Hydroxychloroquine (Plaquenil) 200 mg q.d., Aspirin 325 mg q.i.d., Hydrocortisone cream 1% to malar rash b.i.d.

VII. Nursing Care Plan

Nursing Diagnosis	Client Care Goals	Plan/Nursing Implementation	Expected Outcomes
Mobility, impaired physical: related to painful joints	Reduce or eliminate joint pain	Instruct client to take medications as prescribed to maintain proper blood levels; teach proper method to apply ice: cover skin with cloth; keep ice packs on for 20 min q.i.d.; instruct regarding proper application of elastic bandages	Absence of joint pain, swelling and stiffness; client performs ROM exercises b.i.d. independently; performs ADL without evidence of fatigue
Skin integrity, impairment of: related to erythematous rash	Reduce or eliminate facial rash	Instruct to apply hydrocortisone 1% sparingly as prescribed by physician; avoid the sun; wash with hypoallergenic soap and use hypo-allergenic makeup if makeup must be worn	Malar rash will resolve without complications
Self-concept, disturbance in: body image, related to having a chronic illness	Discuss feelings openly; describe feeling less anxious; participate in treatment and care	Explore the causes of the anxiety and sense of helplessness by open discussion and effective listening; help client to recognize her strengths; help her view herself as a total person and not just to focus on her limitations; encourage expression of feelings; involve husband and/or close friends in plan of care if acceptable to client	The client expresses feelings and thoughts about body image; there are no signs of anxiety; client shows increased interest in participation in treatment and self-care; husband and/or close friends remain supportive and loving

Nursing Diagnosis	Client Care Goals	Plan/Nursing Implementation	Expected Outcomes
Knowledge deficit, related to nature and cause of SLE and actions of newly prescribed medications	Discuss the disease process and proper use of new medications	Teach client and family about the use of corticosteroids; (they should only be taken with food so as to decrease GI upset); client should know never to discontinue the drug on her own; advise client to wear medical alert bracelet that says she is taking corticosteriods; observe for the side effects of corticosteroids, ie, moon faces, flushing, acne, buffalo hump, headaches, etc; since on hydroxychloroquine, client should have oph-thalmological exams every 6 months; teach client and husband about SLE; provide pamphlets, refer to the Lupus Foundation; explain need to avoid drugs such as sulfa, birth-control pills, and OTC medications; client should avoid becoming pregnant, which is currently not a consideration but could change in the future	Client can describe the nature, cause, and progression of SLE; client takes medi-cations with food, can relate side effect of medications; client wears medical alert bracelet; client understands need to check with primary care provider before taking any new medication by prescription or OTC, and before discontinuing any current medication

Chapter 58

Specific Disorders of the Bones

Linda Heim McCausland

Conditions affecting the bones usually interfere with a person's mobility, comfort, and independence and sometimes require prolonged treatment and rehabilitation. The disorder may leave the client with a deformity, which may cause numerous physiological and psychosocial consequences. Some conditions affecting bone can be life threatening, particularly those caused by malignancy. This chapter will cover the specific disorders that affect bones in adults; these can be classified as disorders from metabolic alteration, infection, neoplasm, or trauma.

Section I: Metabolic Disorders

Metabolic disorders affecting bone interfere with bone formation, weakening the bone. The metabolic disorders *osteoporosis, osteomalacia,* and hyperparathyroidism all cause demineralization and loss of bone mass. The first two disorders are discussed in this section; hyperparathyroidism, an endocrine disorder, is covered in Unit Seven. *Paget's disease of the bone,* also discussed in this section, involves deposition of weak bone and has symptoms similar to those caused by bone loss.

Manifestations of metabolic bone disorders are pain (especially in the spine and legs), bone tenderness, and weakness; all these problems can make ambulation difficult. If allowed to progress, metabolic bone disorders eventually cause skeletal deformities, such as abnormal spinal curvature or bone enlargement, and may lead to pathological fractures. Clients with these disorders may also experience anorexia and weight loss.

Because the onset of metabolic disorders is insidious, clients with metabolic bone disorders may not be hospitalized until their condition is severe or a fracture occurs. If ambulatory care nurses and community health nurses are aware of the conditions contributing to these diseases, they may be able to detect them in their early stages and encourage clients to seek medical intervention. They can also intervene for those at risk by teaching about the benefits of a nutritionally balanced diet, regular exercise, and good body mechanics.

General Nursing Implications

Nursing intervention for clients with metabolic bone disorders includes measures to prevent deformities and fractures. The client needs to be turned frequently but must be handled gently to prevent fractures. When a brace or corset is prescribed, teach the client to apply it properly and encourage its use. With an explanation that the device provides support and prevents deformity, the client may be more willing to adapt to its use.

Clients with metabolic bone disorders need extra rest but must also avoid the hazards of immobility. The nurse can teach exercises for preventing joint contracture and muscle atrophy and can instruct the client in the use of correct body mechanics. Encourage safety measures because an injury could cause fractures; advise the client, for example, not to walk on snow or ice and to avoid sudden bending and lifting. Also suggest ways of preventing strain and fatigue, such as wearing good supportive shoes, sleeping on a firm mattress, maintaining recommended body weight, planning for rest periods, and using ambulatory aids. Clients may need help with food selections to comply with the prescribed diet, and the nurse may want to refer them for nutrition education. Interventions involving rest, exercise, ambulation, and positioning are discussed more fully in Chapter 56.

OSTEOPOROSIS

Osteoporosis is a condition in which the rate of bone resorption exceeds the rate of bone formation, reducing bone mass. An osteoporotic hand and wrist is compared to a normal one in Figures 58–1A and B. Osteoporotic bones become porous, brittle, and subject to fracture from minimal trauma or normal stress. Bones most often affected are the vertebrae, ribs, and wrist and hip bones.

All people lose some bone as they grow older, beginning at about age 30, but when bone mass is less than normal for someone's age, the person is considered to have osteoporosis. Several factors contribute to excessive bone loss. Osteoporosis is much more common in postmenopausal women than in men and appears to be related to the *diminished levels of estrogen* occurring after menopause, whether natural or surgically induced. *Immobility* or lack of exercise is also associated with increased bone resorption. The bones need the usual stress of weight bearing and activity to continue normal bone turnover; otherwise, demineralization occurs. Elderly people who become less

active with age are subject to *disuse osteoporosis.* Astronauts in space experience osteoporosis related to *lack of gravity,* despite the exercises they perform.

Osteoporosis is sometimes associated with *inadequate nutrition,* such as deficiencies in calcium and vitamin D, and excess phosphorus. High-protein diets for weight reduction may increase bone resorption because the increased acid resulting from increased nitrogen is buffered by calcium taken from the bones. Osteoporotic changes occur secondarily to several endocrine problems such as Cushing's disease, hyperthyroidism, hyperparathyroidism, diabetes mellitus, and acromegaly. Medications associated with osteoporotic changes are corticosteroids, when used for long periods, and heparin.

Clinical Manifestations

Osteoporotic changes may go on a long time before they are noticed; Lukert (1982) states that 50% of women past 65 years of age have asymptomatic osteoporosis. Initial symptoms include weakness, unsteady gait, stiffness, and poor appetite. The symptom that brings the client to the physician is commonly back pain, usually in the lower thoracic or lumbar region. The onset of the pain may be sudden or insidious. Changes in the spine cause loss of height, rounded back (kyphosis), and pressure on nerves. Spinal deformity may also decrease the size of the thorax, causing changes in respiratory function. Other areas that are often painful are the hips, pelvis, and legs. Elderly people often experience pathological fractures in weight bearing or other stress-bearing areas such as the hips, wrists, and vertebrae due to osteoporosis; in fact, over two-thirds of clients with hip fractures are found to have osteoporosis.

The serum calcium, phosphorus, and alkaline phosphatase levels of osteoporotic clients are usually normal. On x-ray, the affected bones appear thin, porous, and radiolucent; fractures may also be obvious.

Therapeutic Measures

The best strategy for osteoporosis is prevention through regular activity, exercise, and an adequate calcium intake throughout life. Women over 35, who do not have sufficient calcium in their diets, should probably begin oral calcium supplements. Exercise reduces the rate of normal bone loss. If osteoporosis does develop, treatment is prescribed according to the contributing factors. Exercise and a well-balanced diet with foods from the four food groups are recommended for anyone with osteoporosis; calcium and vitamin D supplements are prescribed for clients with dietary deficiencies.

The use of estrogen is controversial. Studies have shown that estrogens retard the rate of bone loss, but the long-term benefits have been questioned. There is also an

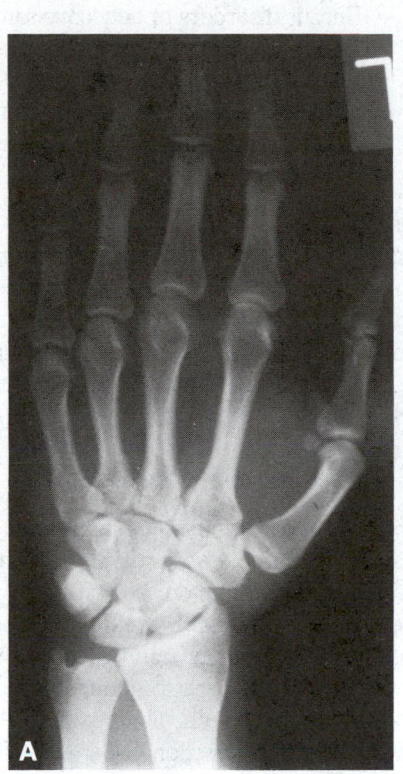
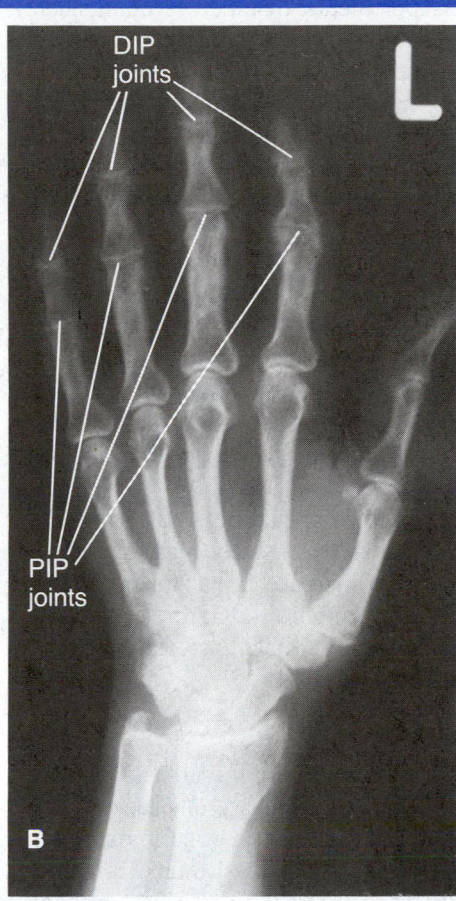

Figure 58–1

A. X-ray of a normal hand. **B.** X-ray of a hand with osteoporotic changes and degenerative joint disease. Note the loss of bone matrix in the phalanges and the joint space narrowing, especially the DIP joints. (Courtesy of Health Care Plan, Buffalo, NY)

increased risk of endometrial carcinoma when estrogens are used to treat a postmenopausal woman with an intact uterus. Lindsay (1982) suggests giving progestogen (synthetic progesterone) once a month or every 3 months to a woman with a uterus who is taking estrogen to help decrease the incidence of endometrial shedding. The combined estrogen–progesterone regimen will cause the woman to have cyclical uterine bleeding. The side effects of this hormone combination are the same as those for birth control pills; including phlebitis and emboli. A woman taking these hormones needs an annual gynecological examination. The question of whether there is greater risk from endometrial cancer or from the significant morbidity and disability that may accompany osteoporosis remains unanswered. Women may have to answer that question for themselves in terms of their own quality of life.

Sodium fluoride stimulates osteoblastic activity, and when given with calcium, bone mass increases. Studies are underway to determine the best therapeutic use of fluoride in osteoporosis.

Specific Nursing Measures

Osteoporosis is one of the hazards of immobility, so a nurse caring for any client requiring prolonged immobilization or bed rest must be concerned with its prevention. A sample nursing care plan for preventing disuse osteoporosis is given in Chapter 56. Since the nursing measures for prevention of osteoporosis are similar to those for its treatment, this section will discuss them together.

Nutrition

Proper nutrition is essential for both prevention and treatment of osteoporosis. The recommended dietary ratio of calcium to phosphorus is 1:1. The American diet, however, has much larger percentages of phosphorus than calcium. Those over 45 years of age consume about half the recommended dietary allowance (RDA) of calcium (Gorrie, 1982). High phosphate intake stimulates parathyroid activity and thus increases bone resorption. A dietary history is helpful in assessing deficient intake; the client may need dietary changes or supplements to meet recommended allowances. In general, a diet adequate in vitamin D, calcium, and protein, will provide the nutrients necessary for bone formation. The nutritional management for osteoporosis is summarized in Table 58–1.

Milk products usually are recommended for increasing calcium intake, but some elderly clients do not tolerate milk because of discomfort from intestinal lactase deficiency. For these people, the nurse should recommend cottage cheese, aged or extra sharp cheddar cheese, and green leafy vegetables. Also make suggestions for preparing vegetables such as collards, kale, and turnip greens because some people may have never tried them. Clients can take preparations of lactase with milk products to prevent the cramping and diarrhea of lactase deficiency (Wolanin & Phillips, 1981).

People with osteoporosis should not consume high-protein diets because a diet excessively high in protein (more than 100 g/day) may increase urinary excretion of calcium. Since many high-protein foods are also high in phosphorus, decreasing protein intake also aids in maintaining a lower phosphorus intake.

Exercise

The nurse and client should plan a program of exercises in which movement and weight bearing are emphasized. All clients who are able should engage in regular exercise, such as walking 30 to 60 minutes at least 3 times a week. Other beneficial exercises are bicycling, stationary cycling, and aerobic dancing. The client should avoid activities that would add pressure to or jar weight-bearing joints and vertebrae, such as jogging.

Other measures the nurse can discuss with the client include safety precautions; good posture and body mechanics; a firm mattress (or a bedboard under a sagging mattress) to provide adequate support to the spine; and corsets for back support. A client with acute back pain should have a few days of bed rest on a supportive mattress, with ice applied intermittently to reduce muscle spasm.

OSTEOMALACIA

Osteomalacia is an adult form of *rickets,* a disease in which bone tissue fails to calcify and becomes soft and flexible. Instead of affecting bone growth, as rickets does in a child, osteomalacia affects the turnover of bone because bone growth is completed in the adult.

Osteomalacia results from vitamin D deficiency, which depresses calcium absorption, causing bone demineralization. Vitamin D deficiency occurs with:

- Inadequate dietary intake of vitamin D
- Deficient vitamin D synthesis in the skin because of lack of exposure to sunlight
- Malabsorption of vitamin D or calcium from the intestine (as occurs in any intestinal disorder associated with steatorrhea)

- Chronic renal failure interfering with metabolism of vitamin D
- Hepatic disorders or anticonvulsant therapy that impairs absorption and conversion of vitamin D
- Gastrectomy, which contributes to diminished intake or defective absorption of vitamin D secondary to the rapid passage of stomach contents past the duodenum

In osteomalacia, normal bone is replaced with osteoid tissue, which is structurally weak and subject to deformity and fracture with stress. Osteomalacia, although not common in North America, does occur in the housebound elderly, in women who have little sun exposure and who undergo repeated pregnancies and prolonged lactation, and in over 50% of clients with chronic renal failure.

Clinical Manifestations

In addition to the changes mentioned earlier, clients with osteomalacia have severe muscle weakness, nagging pain resulting from strain on the soft bone, and decreased height because of kyphosis. Softening of bone also leads to angulation of the sternum and deformities of the pelvis and femoral necks. On x-ray, diminished bone density and bone deformities are seen, along with pseudofractures (bands of decalcification perpendicular or oblique to the bone surface). Laboratory findings include decreased serum calcium and phosphorus levels and elevated alkaline phosphatase levels. The diagnosis of osteomalacia can be confirmed by bone biopsy.

Therapeutic and Specific Nursing Measures

Osteomalacia caused by dietary deficiency can be prevented by supplying the adult with adequate vitamin D (5 μg daily with an additional 5 μg daily during pregnancy and lactation), calcium (800 mg daily with an additional 400 mg daily in pregnancy and lactation), and phosphorus. See Table 58–1 for nutritional management in osteomalacia. The nurse should determine the reason for dietary deficiency so that the cause can be treated: Is it due to poor eating habits, lack of knowledge of a balanced diet, or lack of available foods? Does the client use antacids? Many clients ingest large amounts of antacids containing aluminum hydroxide, which interfere with phosphorus absorption. Explain that antacid use can lead to phosphorus deficiency. The client may need help in planning and selecting a balanced diet based on financial resources, food preferences, and the availability of foods.

If osteomalacia develops, it is treated with high doses of vitamin D: 25 to 125 μg daily, increasing to 1250 μg daily if malabsorption is evident. Calcium and phosphorus supplements may also be given. When a client is taking such large doses of vitamin D for an extended time, serum and urine calcium levels should be monitored for hyper-

Table 58-1 Nutritional Management in Osteoporosis and Osteomalacia

Nutrient	Recommendation in Osteoporosis	Recommendation in Osteomalacia	Sources
Calcium	↑ to 1500 mg q.d.	At least 800 mg q.d.; add 400 mg more in pregnancy and lactation	Dairy products; collards; kale; turnip, dandelion, and mustard greens; canned sardines and salmon eaten with bones; oysters
Vitamin D	Maintain usual level if frequent sun exposure; if house-bound, increase intake	↑ intake	Exposure to sunlight, fortified milk and cereals, eggs, butter, fish liver oils
Phosphorus	↓ intake	800 mg q.d.; add 400 mg more in pregnancy and lactation; ↓ use of antacids containing aluminum hydroxide, which interfere with phosphorus absorption	Beef, poultry, fish, soft drinks
Protein	Avoid excessive intake	Avoid excessive intake	Meat, poultry, fish, dairy products, eggs, cheese, grains, beans, peas, nuts

calcemia and hypercalciuria. Signs of vitamin D toxicity are excessive calcification of bones and soft tissues and symptoms of hypercalcemia such as malaise, headache, anorexia, nausea, vomiting, weakness, constipation, polyuria, and polydipsia (Krause & Mahan, 1984).

Encourage clients to expose their skin to sunlight so they can synthesize their own vitamin D. (Precautions against overexposure to the sun are discussed in Unit Thirteen.) A client with osteomalacia will also benefit from a firm mattress and a brace or corset for support.

PAGET'S DISEASE OF THE BONE

Paget's disease (osteitis deformans) of the bone is mentioned here because it has some similarities to metabolic bone diseases, although it does not cause a decrease in bone mass or demineralization of bone. In the early stages of Paget's disease, increased osteoclastic resorption of bone occurs. As the disease progresses, normal bone is replaced by immature woven bone, the haversian system disappears, and bone architecture becomes highly disorganized. These changes lead to a mosaic structure that is weak and fractures easily. The bone remodeling leads to swelling and deformity of bones; for example, the long bones become thicker and bow. The number of affected bones ranges from one to many; commonly involved are the vertebrae, pelvis, long bones, and skull.

The cause of Paget's disease is unknown, although a viral etiology is suspected. The disease is uncommon before the age of 40 but incidence increases steadily with each subsequent decade. Often there is a positive family history. Osteogenic sarcoma is a rare but usually fatal complication of Paget's disease.

Clinical Manifestations

Some clients are asymptomatic; others have pain and aching. Manifestations vary with the location of the lesion and the extent of the condition. Enlargement of the skull may cause facial pain, headaches, and need for a larger hat size. Hearing loss may occur secondary to direct involvement of the ossicles of the inner ear or to compression of cranial nerve VIII, the vestibulocochlear nerve. Long bones such as the femur or tibia may appear swollen, deformed, or bent, and the skin over the affected bone will be warm due to increased vascularity (Figure 58-2). There may be changes in gait. The serum alkaline phosphatase level is extremely elevated, an indication of the increased bone activity. On microscopic exam, the bone lesion shows the characteristic mosaic pattern. X-rays show opaque and radiolucent areas.

Therapeutic and Specific Nursing Measures

Most clients require no treatment because the disease is localized and causes no symptoms. Otherwise, treatment is supportive and symptomatic, with emphasis on good body mechanics. Ambulatory aids may be necessary for a

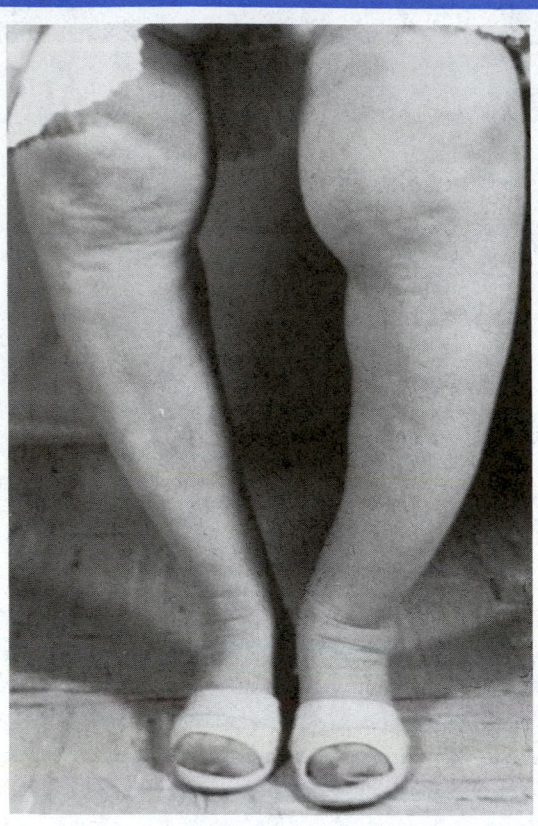

Figure 58–2

Paget's disease of the long bones of the leg. (Courtesy of Millard Fillmore Hospital, Buffalo, NY)

Table 58–2	Pharmacological Approaches to Paget's Disease
Drug	**Action**
Aspirin and nonsteroidal anti-inflammatory agents	Analgesia
Steroids	Suppress the disease, but only in large doses, so are not recommended
Sodium fluoride	Decreases symptoms, but may lead to poorly mineralized bone
Salmon, porcine and human calcitonin	Inhibits bone resorption, decreases serum alkaline phosphatase levels; given subcutaneously
Cytotoxic drugs, eg, mithramycin	Inhibits bone resorption, decreases serum alkaline phosphatase levels; given intravenously
Etidronate disodium (EHDP)	Inhibits bone resorption, decreases serum alkaline phosphatase levels; can be taken orally

client with an altered gait. Analgesics or nonsteroidal anti-inflammatory agents are given for pain. A person with an extremely high rate of bone turnover may be given drugs to suppress bone activity—eg, calcitonin, mithramycin, or etidronate disodium (see Table 58–2).

The general nursing implications covered earlier apply to clients with Paget's disease of the bone. The nurse must explain the importance of good body mechanics. Emotional support is essential, because this is a chronic condition with no definitive treatment, and the client may become discouraged and frustrated.

If the client is inactive, hypercalcemia may occur. A hypercalcemic client needs a low calcium diet and high fluid intake to help prevent urinary calculi. The client should drink about 3 to 4 L/day, unless this high intake is contraindicated for other reasons. Fluids to offer, in keeping with the low calcium requirement, are water, tea, coffee, and cranberry or prune juice.

Section II: Infectious Disorders

OSTEOMYELITIS

Infections of the bone, bone marrow, and surrounding soft tissues by *pyogenic* (pus-forming) bacteria are called *osteomyelitis*. Such infections, which usually involve the long bones, can be acute or can progress to a chronic state; in either case, they cause bone destruction, limited mobility, and severe pain.

The organism most often responsible for osteomyelitis is *Staphylococcus aureus;* hemolytic *Streptococcus* is the second most common; *Neisseria gonorrhoeae, Hemophilus influenzae,* and *Salmonella* may also infect bones. The bacteria enter the bone by way of the bloodstream (bacteremia), by extension of a local soft tissue infection, or from open wounds.

Osteomyelitis can be divided into three types: acute infectious, acute localized, and chronic. In *acute infectious* osteomyelitis, also known as *hematogenous,* the infection enters the bone from another site in the body. This type of bone infection is most common in children, usually affecting the metaphysis (the area in the shaft next to the epiphyseal plate) of long bones. However, it can occur in adults as a more localized infection, especially of the vertebrae. There is often a history of mild, local trauma, which causes decreased resistance in the bone. A systemic infection already present in the body (eg, from tonsillitis, otitis media, upper respiratory infection, impetigo, or a tooth infection) may then move via the bloodstream into the area of decreased resistance. The ends of long bones are usually affected because they are highly vascularized, with sluggish circulation. *Acute localized* osteomyelitis, also known as *exogenous,* occurs when there is direct invasion of bacteria from open fractures, septic surgery, or penetrating wounds. The infection usually remains localized. *Chronic* osteomyelitis is a dreaded condition that can follow the other types because of inadequate or ineffective treatment during the acute phase. It is characterized by remissions and exacerbations; the client may be asymptomatic during the remission phase, but pain and inflammation occur during exacerbation as the body tries to rid itself of necrosed bone fragments, called *sequestra.* Sinuses form, drain purulent material, heal over, and form again.

After bacteria enter the bone, they multiply and destroy cells, and macrophages enter to kill the bacteria. The collection of debris and resulting edema cause a rise in pressure in the rigid bone structure. When the pressure reaches arteriolar pressure, blood (and the antibiotics it carries) cannot enter the area. Eventually, the pus leaks out of the bone and the pressure elevates the periosteum (Figure 58–3), stripping the bone of its surrounding blood vessels and causing necrosis. The pocket between the periosteum and the bone surface is called a subperiosteal abscess; sequestra are found beneath such abscesses. The bone lays down new bone cells over the sequestrum in an attempt to heal itself, forming a new bone covering called an *involucrum.* The involucrum encloses the bacteria in the bone, interferes with normal phagocytosis, and acts as a barrier to antibiotics, thus causing a chronic condition. Sinus tracts may form between the sequestra and the skin or into an adjacent joint, draining the purulent material contained in the abscess.

Infections of the bone are extremely difficult to irradicate. An acute infection can progress into a chronic one involving many hospitalizations and prolonged disability. An infection that is present when a fracture is trying to heal will result in poor healing, nonunion, or malunion. If an infection occurs involving a prosthesis used for joint replacement, the prosthesis frequently must be removed, leaving the client with a significant disability.

Clinical Manifestations

Acute osteomyelitis is characterized by an abrupt onset of severe pain in the involved extremity. Edema, redness,

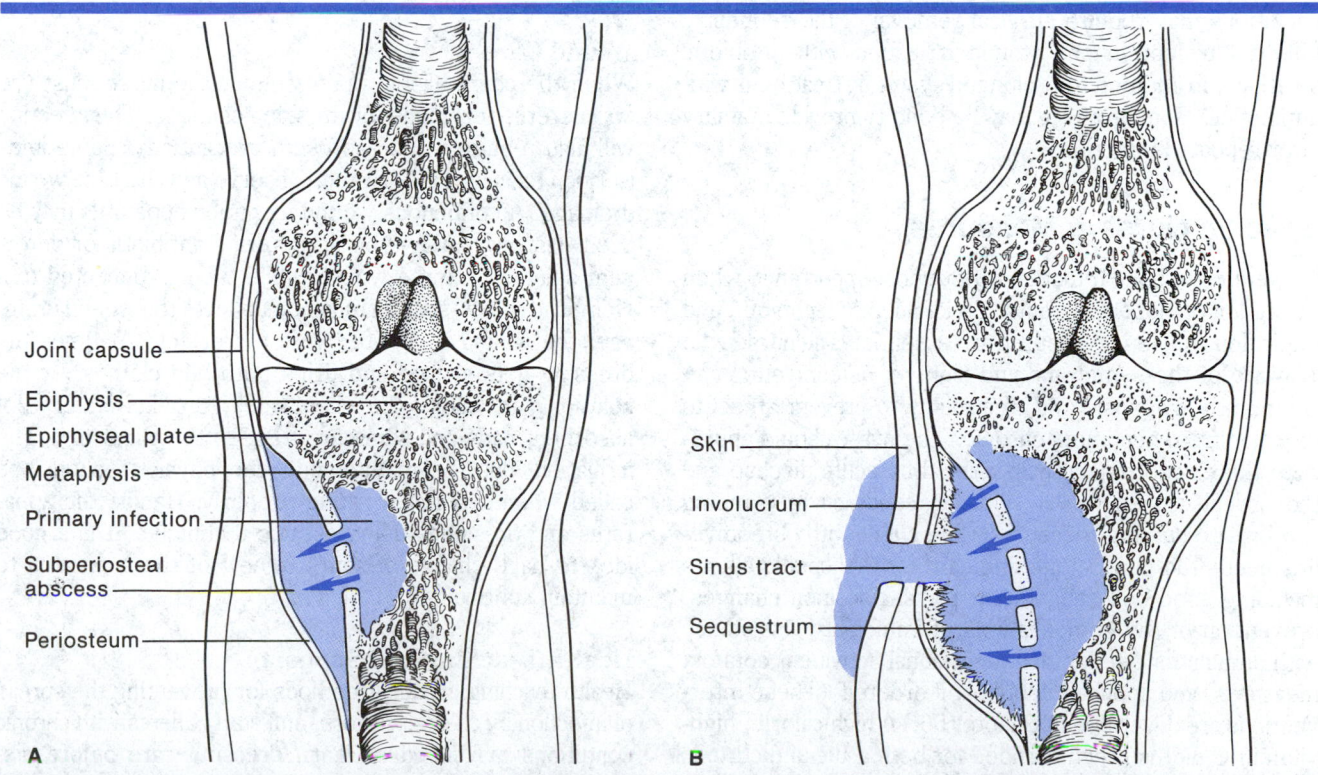

Figure 58–3

Bone lesion in osteomyelitis. **A.** Pus leaks out from the infection site, lifting the periosteum and its blood vessels away from the bone. **B.** The fragments of dead bone are called sequestra. The new bone layer is called the involucrum. Sinus tracts form between the sequestra and the skin.

and heat occur locally. Clients may have muscle spasms and hold the extremity in flexion, resisting any attempts to touch it. Other manifestations include fever, chills, diaphoresis, malaise, headache, and nausea. The white blood cell (WBC) count is very high, and the erythrocyte sedimentation rate (ESR) is elevated. X-rays are negative until about 2 weeks after the onset, when the bone will have areas of density and radiolucency.

In the chronic phase, an exacerbation may be characterized by low grade fever, pain, and persistent drainage from a sinus tract. A *sinogram,* an x-ray in which dye is injected into the open sinus, reveals the course of the sinus tract.

Therapeutic Measures

Since it is essential to begin antibiotic therapy before the infection becomes isolated, multiple antibiotics are given as soon as blood or wound culture specimens are obtained. When the culture results are available, inappropriate antibiotics are discontinued, and others, specific to the causative organism, are begun. Antibiotics are continued for several weeks. In acute infectious osteomyelitis, abscesses are incised and drained if the response to the antibiotics is slow. In acute localized osteomyelitis, I&D (incision and drainage) allows removal of any hardware (metal used for bone repair) as well as drainage of the wound. Chronic conditions may require surgical removal of the sequestra followed by continuous wound irrigation with antibiotic solutions, in addition to prolonged systemic treatment with antibiotics. Bone grafting may be done to provide stability after repeated infections.

Specific Nursing Measures

Prevention of bone infection is of utmost importance when caring for orthopedic clients. Strict aseptic technique and meticulous hygiene measures are essential. The nurse who is aware of the symptoms and signs of osteomyelitis can aid in early diagnosis and treatment, to prevent an acute infection from becoming chronic. The nurse should appreciate the extraordinary pain caused by acute disease and the ordeal caused by the chronic condition in planning appropriate nursing measures. The client with osteomyelitis needs the general nursing care for orthopedic clients including good body alignment, regular position changes, prevention of the complications of immobility, assistance with ambulation, sedentary diversional activities, comfort measures, and application of heat if ordered. (These interventions are described in Chapter 56.) A high-calorie, high-vitamin C diet is recommended for both acute and chronic osteomyelitis, and a vitamin C supplement may be helpful in promoting healing. Encourage generous intake of fluids, particularly when fever is present. Vital signs should be taken every 4 hours when the client's temperature is elevated; antipyretics may be needed.

Pain Relief and Immobilization

Dealing with the client's pain may be a challenge. When moving the client, give analgesics first, get help, and support the limb well so that the joints above and below the painful area are stabilized. All movements should be gentle and smooth, to prevent pathological fractures as well as pain. Sometimes, just touching the bed causes the client pain, so it is a good idea to post signs warning others to avoid bumping or touching the bed. Treatment will involve some method of immobilizing the limb, such as a splint, cast, or traction. (Specific nursing measures for clients in casts or traction are covered in the discussion of fractures.) The extremity should be maintained in a functional anatomic position. The extremity is often elevated. Do not allow continued flexion of the limb; prevent footdrop by means of a splint. A bed cradle may be useful for keeping sheets off the painful limb.

Antibiotics and Hydration

The client will be receiving antibiotics intravenously, and the nurse must see that these are given on time to assure sustained blood levels. It is essential that the client receive proper hydration if IVs are interrupted to give antibiotics; intake and output should be measured. Since antibiotics are given in high dosages and for prolonged periods, the nurse must watch for side effects of the medications. (See Chapter 11 for specific side effects of antibiotic therapy.)

Wound Care

When the client has an open wound, the nurse must use strict sterile technique for dressing changes. The infection will also require wound and skin precautions. Sometimes isolation technique is indicated. Observe and chart the wound drainage. A continuous wound irrigation apparatus may be used. Usually, an IV-type setup drips antibiotic or detergent solution into the wound while tubing connected to a Hemovac or low-suction machine collects the wound drainage; the wound is covered with a dressing. At times the dressing gets soaked and drips onto bed clothes, or the solution runs along the client's leg; provide waterproof absorbent pads and skin care to keep the client dry. The irrigation must be maintained—the physician should be called when it is not working properly. Handle the apparatus and dressings using aseptic technique. It is a good idea to have change-of-shifts review of the apparatus to maintain continuity.

Health Teaching and Support

Health teaching includes methods for preventing the spread of infection by clients, visitors, and staff. Clients with chronic conditions may need to learn dressing care before discharge. Caution them to avoid weight bearing until instructed, to prevent fracture. Clients should also know about the drugs they will be taking at home: their action, correct dosage, and possible side effects.

Clients with chronic disease require emotional support. They may be faced with intermittent pain, an unsightly limb because of scars from draining wounds, and foul-smelling drainage. They may fear loss of the limb. These problems require nursing interventions appropriate for body image changes (see Chapter 4). Allow clients to verbalize their feelings and help correct any misconceptions.

Encourage continuing medical supervision. The nurse may want to make a referral to a community health nurse to be certain that the client is managing wound care properly at home. In addition, the nurse can assess the client's mental status and overall adjustment to the disease.

Section III: Neoplastic Disorders

Tumors of the bone can be of three types: benign, primary malignant, and secondary malignant (metastatic). A benign bone tumor originates in bone tissue, as does a primary malignant tumor. A secondary malignant bone tumor occurs as a result of metastasis from primary lesions elsewhere in the body, eg, from the breast, lung, prostate, intestine, thyroid, or kidney; this is the most common type of bone tumor in adults. The most common primary malignant bone tumor in adults is multiple myeloma, which will be covered in Chapter 29 with disorders of blood-forming organs. This section will discuss the second most common primary malignant bone tumor, osteogenic sarcoma, and the most common benign bone tumor, the giant cell tumor. Giant cell tumors can become malignant if not completely removed.

Bone tumors cause pain, sometimes severe, and interfere with mobility. They may cause permanent limitation and disfigurement if amputation of a limb is necessary. These tumors frequently occur in young people and pose a threat to body image and self-concept, which are extremely important in the adolescent and young adult years.

Clients with malignant bone tumors have a poor prognosis, but early detection of such a tumor may promote early treatment and prevent metastasis. The nurse should be aware of the symptoms and signs of bone cancer (described under the specific diseases) and encourage the client to seek medical attention without delay.

OSTEOGENIC SARCOMA

Osteogenic sarcoma, also known as osteosarcoma, is the most common malignant primary neoplasm of bone, occurring primarily in young people 10 to 25 years old. It also can occur later in life secondarily to Paget's disease of the bone, chronic osteomyelitis, or previous bone irradiation. The areas affected most often are the ends of long bones (especially around the knee) including the distal femur, proximal tibia, and proximal humerus. The etiology of this disease is unknown, and the prognosis is generally poor.

The lesions of osteogenic sarcoma may vary in appearance. Osteolytic osteogenic sarcomas dissolve the bone and invade adjacent soft tissues. Osteoblastic osteogenic sarcomas form new bone. The bone may become weak and fracture, particularly when the tumor grows slowly. The tumor may metastasize, most often to the lung, resulting in a poorer prognosis.

Clinical Manifestations

Clients usually have pain at night, sometimes intermittently. They may experience sudden onset of pain, perhaps after minor trauma. As with other bone tumors, clients are likely to have a local swelling or mass and may walk with a limp. In addition, the client with osteogenic sarcoma may complain of fatigue.

The lesion is visible on x-ray; a bone scan shows increased activity at the tumor site. Serum alkaline phosphatase is elevated in 50% of clients. When initial alkaline phosphatase levels are very high, the course is often rapidly fatal. Analysis of a biopsy of the lesion will confirm the diagnosis. Candidates for limb salvaging procedures should have needle biopsy under fluoroscopy. An open bone biopsy may disrupt the tumor, making limb salvage difficult.

Therapeutic Measures

The tumor must be removed or destroyed. The location of the tumor dictates the extent of the surgery. The most satisfactory surgical procedure is amputation, but in some cases the tumor and the area around it can be removed without amputation. Limb salvaging procedures have been made possible by advances in chemotherapy and endoprosthetics. Clients must have achieved most of their bone growth to be candidates for these procedures. Therefore amputation remains the procedure of choice in younger children. The client may be given chemotherapy preoperatively and postoperatively. See Box 58–1 for pharmacological measures in osteogenic sarcoma.

Box 58–1 Pharmacological Measures in Osteogenic Sarcoma

Analgesics

Antiemetics

Chemotherapeutic agents:
- Cyclophosphamide (Cytoxan)
- Doxorubicin hydrochloride (Adriamycin)
- Methotrexate sodium (Folex, Mexate)
- Vincristine sulfate (Oncovin)

Specific Nursing Measures

Most of the nursing interventions appropriate for bone tumor clients are discussed elsewhere in this text. Measures for preventing deformity, assisting with ambulation, providing comfort, and changing position are included in Chapter 56. Routine preoperative and postoperative care are covered in Chapter 14. Nursing care related to surgical procedures such as amputation and internal fixation will be covered in Chapter 60. Measures to deal with the specific problems of cancer, radiation therapy, chemotherapy, and surgery for cancer clients are covered in Chapter 12, as are measures used to encourage nutrition for those receiving radiation therapy and chemotherapy.

Help with emotional problems is likely to be as important as any other nursing intervention. Dealing with changes in body image and self-concept is discussed in Chapters 4 and 56. The client, who may be young, may be grieving over loss of a limb or impending death. Encourage expression of feelings, and accept expressions of anger and frustration. The entire family will need emotional support. A referral to a mental health or religious counselor may be helpful.

GIANT CELL TUMORS

A giant cell tumor is usually a benign tumor of the bone, although there are some malignant types. A previously benign tumor may undergo malignant transformation. Giant cell tumor occurs most often in the 20- to 25-year age range and is commonly found at the end of long bones, especially around the knee (distal femur and proximal tibia) and the distal radius. It is made up of large numbers of multinucleate giant cells or osteoclasts; its cause is unknown. Giant cell tumors tend to recur, and the chances of malignancy increase if they are not completely removed.

Clinical Manifestations

The clinical manifestations of giant cell tumor are pain, tenderness, a local mass or swelling, and sometimes a limp. Occasionally, a pathological fracture occurs. The lesion will be visible on x-ray (Figure 58–4).

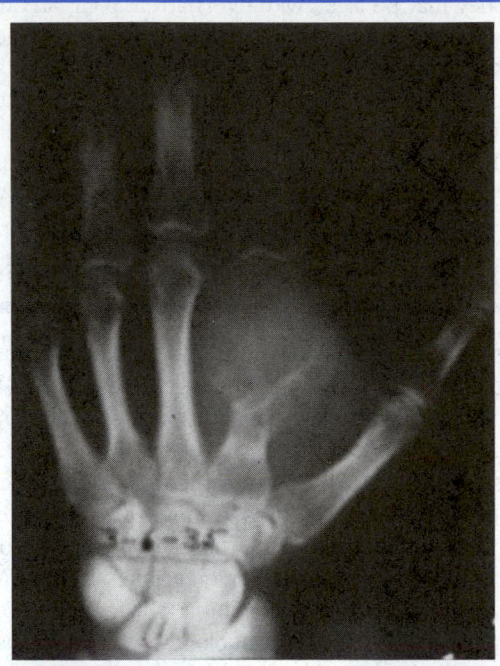

Figure 58–4

Giant cell tumor of the index finger. (Courtesy of Millard Fillmore Hospital, Buffalo, NY)

Therapeutic and Specific Nursing Measures

The tumor is surgically removed along with normal bone around it, and bone grafting may be done to fill in the cavity. Newer methods believed to decrease recurrence of the tumor are cryotherapy after tumor excision or cryotherapy and filling in the cavity with the bone cement methyl methacrylate (Connolly, 1981). Depending upon the extent of the tumor and its recurrence, amputation may be necessary. Radiation therapy is used for difficult-to-remove lesions, such as those in the pelvis, sacrum, or spine. Nursing measures are those referred to in the discussion of osteogenic sarcoma.

Section IV: Traumatic Disorders

Traumatic conditions affecting the bones include fractures and amputations. Since amputations are treated surgically, they will be covered in Chapter 60.

FRACTURES

A **fracture** is a break in the continuity of a bone. Fractures can cause disruption of more than the bone, however; surrounding soft tissues and adjacent organs can be damaged either from the injury itself or from sharp bone fragments.

For example, fractured ribs may puncture the lung, or a fractured pelvis may injure the bladder. Nerves or blood vessels may be damaged or severed. Therefore, management of fractures includes thorough assessment for related problems. Fractures interfere with bodily movements such as ambulation and ADL and may also be painful. If untreated, fractures may heal in deformed positions, affecting the future use of the part, or they may not heal at all. Many complications can occur as a result of fractures, including complications resulting from treatments such as casts, traction, and immobilization. The nurse must quickly identify any signs and symptoms of complications and seek prompt, appropriate treatment. The nursing care of clients with fractures is mainly concerned with measures to prevent complications and deformities.

Types of Fractures

Many terms are used to describe types of fractures. A fracture in which the skin over the injury remains intact, so there is no connection between the bone and the skin surface, is known as a *closed* fracture (formerly called a simple fracture). An *open* fracture (formerly known as compound) is one in which the skin surface over the injury is broken and the surface wound connects with the fracture. The open wound may have been caused by the fracture fragments piercing the skin or by a force from outside the body, such as a bullet which pierced the skin, hit the bone, and caused the fracture. Fracture fragments that break through the skin may protrude from the wound or they may move back inside; in the latter case, the examiner does not know whether the wound communicates with the fracture. A person who administers first aid should note whether the bone protruded. An open fracture is more complicated than a closed one because of the potential for infection. The fracture can be described further by indicating the area of bone involved. Long bones are divided into thirds: proximal, middle, and distal. Thus, one might describe a fracture as a closed fracture of the distal femur. Various kinds of fractures are diagrammed and described in Table 58–3.

Fractures occur when a bone is unable to absorb or transmit a stress placed upon it. The stress can occur from a direct force such as a blow, falling, or crushing, or from an indirect force like twisting or extreme muscle contraction. As already discussed, minimal stress can break a weakened bone (pathological fracture). A *stress fracture* can occur in normal bone that is subjected to repeated stresses, such as strenuous activity. Jogging can cause stress fractures, for example, in experienced as well as inexperienced joggers.

Clinical Manifestations

The manifestations of a fracture depend upon its type and location and on the other tissues involved. A history of the traumatic event may suggest the possibility of a fracture. Severe pain usually occurs immediately, and there may be *point tenderness* at the fracture site. There may be obvious *deformity*: The limb may be bent, shortened, or twisted, or the contour of bones in the skull may be changed. Protrusion of bone fragments through an open wound is an obvious sign of fracture.

Swelling may be caused by bleeding into the tissues and accumulated serous fluid at the site of injury. *Ecchymosis* may also occur due to bleeding, but this usually takes a few days to be apparent. Involuntary and painful *muscle spasm* may occur around the site of injury; spasm is sometimes caused by attempts to move the limb. Spasm also occurs with the loss of normal tension on the muscle from the fracture. The examiner may hear or feel *crepitation,* a grating caused by bone fragments rubbing together; do *not* try to elicit this sign, however, because movement of sharp bone fragments may cause further damage to surrounding tissues. The limb may display abnormal motion; for example, a long bone fractured along the shaft may bend at the point of fracture, where it would normally be rigid. There may be loss of function due to displacement of bone fragments, muscle spasms, instability, or pain; injury to a nerve may cause *paralysis*. A final manifestation of fracture is *shock,* which may occur as a result of hemorrhage or extensive traumatic damage. X-rays confirm the diagnosis and provide the physician with information about the type of fracture and the displacement of fragments.

Occasionally, a client may have an impacted fracture or one without displacement of fragments and will be able to use the limb. The only symptoms may be pain with direct pressure and some swelling. When medical care is finally obtained, an x-ray will reveal the fracture line.

Therapeutic Measures

Some specific types of fractures and their treatment are covered in other units in this textbook. Fractures of the jaw, nose, and ribs are covered in Unit Three. Fractures of the vertebrae, including halo traction, are covered in Unit Six. The general objectives of fracture management are:

- Realigning the bone fragments, a process called *reduction.*
- Maintaining the alignment by *immobilization.*
- *Restoring function* to the part.

Reduction of a fracture can be accomplished in three ways. *Closed reduction* is the manipulation of the bone fragments until the bone is realigned. Some manual traction and rotation of the limb may be necessary. This type of reduction is done on closed fractures with or without a local or general anesthetic. Sedation may also be used. The realigned bone is then immobilized by application of a cast or splint. *Open reduction* is a surgical procedure in which the fracture fragments can be directly visualized to place them back into alignment. The bone is immobilized by use of nails, rods, plates, screws, or pins, which hold the bone fragments together, a procedure known as *open reduction internal fixation* (ORIF). These surgical approaches will be covered in Chapter 60.

The third type of reduction is *traction.* **Traction** is pulling force applied to the limb to overcome muscle spasm and realign the fracture. The traction pull maintains the bone in alignment, so traction is also a means of immobilization. X-rays are taken after application of traction to

Table 58–3 Types of Fractures		
Type	**Description**	**Illustration**
Closed (simple)	The skin over the fracture remains intact.	
Open (compound)	The skin surface over the fracture is broken, and the surface wound connects with the fracture.	
Comminuted	The bone is broken into three or more fragments.	
Transverse	The break runs straight across the bone, ie, perpendicular to the bone's long axis.	

Type	Description	Illustration
Oblique	The break runs at an angle, or slanted, across the bone.	
Spiral	The break coils around the bone. This usually occurs from torsion (twisting) of the limb such as occurs in a skiing accident when the foot is stuck in one position while the leg continues to turn.	
Impacted	The fracture fragments are pushed into each other (telescoped). This can occur when a person falls straight down, landing on the feet.	
Greenstick	The fracture does not go all the way through the bone; rather it splinters on one side. This occurs in children because their bones are soft, much like the flexible green limb of a tree, which does not break through completely when one tries to snap it in two. These fractures heal rapidly.	
Pathological	The fracture occurs at a point in the bone weakened by disease, such as with tumors or osteoporosis. The break may occur from only a small force or normal activity such as sneezing or twisting.	
Avulsion	A fragment of bone connected to a ligament breaks off from the rest of the bone.	

(continued)

Table 58-3 Types of Fractures (continued)

Type	Description	Illustration
Extracapsular	The fracture is close to a joint but remains outside the joint capsule.	
Intracapsular	The fracture is within the joint capsule.	

determine that alignment is appropriate and that the pieces are not too far apart. In addition to fracture management, traction may be used to correct deformities, to reduce muscle spasms, and to rest injured or diseased joints.

Immobilization is essential after the fracture fragments are realigned. If the fragments are not immobilized, hematoma and callus formation will be disrupted and the bone will heal slowly or in poor alignment. Splints, casts, traction, and internal and external fixation tools are used for immobilization. Internal fixation was described in the discussion of open reduction. External fixation also requires surgery but uses an external device for immobilizing the fracture fragments. During surgery, pins are inserted into the bone above and below the fracture; these extend through the skin and are clamped to an external framework. This surgical procedure will be described in more detail in Chapter 60. The use of casts and traction will be covered in detail in a later section of this chapter.

Restoration of function is accomplished by preventing complications during immobility and by rehabilitation methods that prepare the client for mobility and maintain muscle strength, tone, and range of joint motion. The physical therapist is often involved in planning an exercise and ambulation program with the client.

The Use of Casts in Fracture Management

Casts are used to immobilize fracture fragments after they have been reduced. Casts can also be used to correct deformity; to rest weak, injured, or diseased parts; and to immobilize parts after such surgeries as joint fusion or reconstruction. Some common types of casts are described and illustrated in Table 58-4. The pressure points are also shown.

Applying the Cast. The most common casting material is mesh bandage impregnated with *plaster of paris,* a powder made from gypsum. The bandage is supplied in various-sized rolls or strips (splints). When the rolls or splints are immersed in water, a chemical reaction takes place between the water and the powder, giving off heat and forming crystals. The crystals interlock and produce a strong, firm cast as the material dries. When wet, the bandage can be molded to fit the contour of the body part. The strength of the cast depends on the number of layers of plaster bandage applied.

Casts can be applied in the physician's office, the emergency room, a special cast room, or the operating room. The plaster is messy, so the person applying the cast wears an apron and rubber gloves and covers the

Table 58–4	Types of Casts	
Type	**Description**	**Illustration and Pressure Points**
Short arm cast	Extends from below the elbow to the palm or fingers. The thumb may or may not be included in the cast, depending on the location and type of fracture. Used for fractures of the distal forearm, wrist, carpals, or metacarpals.	Radial and ulnar styloids
Long arm cast	Extends from above the elbow to the palm or wrist. Used for fracture of the distal humerus, forearm, or carpals.	Radial and ulnar styloids Olecranon Epicondyles
Hanging long arm cast	Cast hangs from a special sling attached to the cast and looped around the client's neck. As it hangs, the weight of the cast provides traction to realign a fracture of the humerus. This combines the principles of casting and traction. The cast must remain hanging, unencumbered to maintain the traction force; ie, the cast should not be supported or rested on anything.	Neck and shoulders Olecranon Radial and ulnar styloids Epicondyles

(continued)

Table 58–4   Types of Casts (continued)

Type	Description	Illustration and Pressure Points
Short leg cast	Extends from below the knee to the toes. Used for fractures of the ankle or foot.	Shin bone — Medial and lateral malleoli — Achilles tendon — Heel
Long leg cast	Extends from above the knee to the toes. Used for fractures of the femoral condyles, tibia, fibula, or ankle.	Knee — Fibular head — Shin bone — Medial and lateral malleoli — Achilles tendon — Heel
Cylinder cast	Extends from the ankle to the thigh. Used for injuries to the knee and stable fractures of the distal femur and proximal tibia.	Fibular head — Knee — Shin bone

Type	Description	Illustration and Pressure Points
Body cast	Covers the trunk; it may include the upper chest or start below the axillae. A window is cut over the abdomen to prevent pressure on the internal organs. Used for fractures or dislocation of the spine, for scoliosis, or after spinal surgery.	Iliac crests
Hip spica cast	A *spica cast* is applied with a figure-eight turn of the plaster rolls between the body and an appendage. There are shoulder spica and thumb spica casts, but the hip spica cast is the one most often referred to as a spica cast. The hip spica may include the trunk and both legs (double spica), one leg (single spica), or a one-and-a-half spica, which extends to the toes of one leg and the knee of the other. A window is cut over the abdomen, and an opening is left in the groin area. Used for fractures of the femoral shaft, the upper femur, or the hip and for hip dislocations. It is also used for immobilization of the hip after special reconstructive surgery or joint fusion.	Fibular head, Iliac crests, Shin, Abductor bar, Achilles tendon, Heel, Malleoli
Cast brace	A device used to immobilize a fracture while permitting joint mobility. It is most frequently used to treat fractures of the femoral shaft after a few weeks of skeletal traction. A snug thigh cast of plaster is applied from the high upper thigh to above the knee joint. Another cast is applied to the lower leg; it may be a walking cast or a cylinder cast. The two casts are connected by two hinges at the knee joint. Sometimes the thigh area includes a minispica cast around the pelvis. Allows early ambulation and weight bearing, which facilitate healing and shorten the rehabilitation period. (Recall that the stresses placed on a bone stimulate bone formation.) The hinges can be locked for walking and unlocked for exercising the knee. Problems with this type of appliance include pressure sores at the edges of the thigh cast, swelling of the knee, and difficulty sitting on the bedpan or commode. The extremity should be elevated when the client is not walking.	Cast edges, Shin, Achilles tendon, Malleoli, Heel

client's clothing. The client may need analgesics before the cast is applied, and the client should be helped to relax. Clients should be told that the cast will be heavy and will give off heat for 10 to 30 minutes while drying because of the chemical reaction. Frequently, the nurse holds the limb in position as the cast is applied.

First, the skin over which the cast will be placed is inspected well to note any redness, abrasions, open areas, or bruises. These areas may require special care before casting and evaluation after, through a cast window and during cast change, to see that the skin is not breaking down. The skin is cleansed and dried. After the fracture is reduced, the limb is usually covered with tubular stockinette. The stockinette, which is long enough to extend beyond both ends of the cast, is rolled up and applied smoothly, to prevent wrinkles. Next, rolls of sheet wadding, a feltlike material, are wrapped around the limb. Sheet wadding can be molded to the shape of the limb; it is layered to provide a comfortable padding and wrapped sufficiently over bony prominences to prevent pressure. A roll of plaster bandage is placed in tepid water until it is evenly soaked, and excess water is squeezed out. Tepid water is used because hot water (along with the heat of the chemical reaction) may cause burns on the client's skin, whereas cold water may cause delayed drying time. The plaster bandage is wrapped over the sheet wadding in smooth layers and molded to the shape of the limb. The person holding the limb must use the flat palms of the hands rather than fingertips, which can cause indentations in the cast and thus pressure areas on the extremity. The ends of the stockinette are folded over the edges of the cast and fastened in place with a final wrap of plaster. The cast is *set* in a few minutes but is still subject to indentations. It may take 24 to 48 hours or longer to dry completely, depending upon its thickness and the humidity and temperature of the air. The finished cast is placed on pillows, and the extremity is x-rayed to make sure the bone is aligned.

Pressure points must be avoided in the application of any immobilizing device. With cast application, bony prominences such as the head of the fibula, the malleoli of the ankle, or the epicondyle of the distal humerus are protected by padding. However, the proper molding of the cast around bony prominences following the normal contour of the extremity is more important in preventing pressure areas than is the application of excessive padding.

Pressure areas can form under the cast at any time because of muscle spasms causing continued friction over joints, toys or other objects dropped down the cast, or rolling up of the padding material under the cast.

Alternative Cast Materials. Materials other than plaster of Paris have been used for casts recently—eg, fiberglass and plastic. Casts made of these materials are lighter and more porous than plaster casts, yet they are strong. They are also easier to clean and do not deteriorate when wet, as a plaster cast does. The client may be allowed

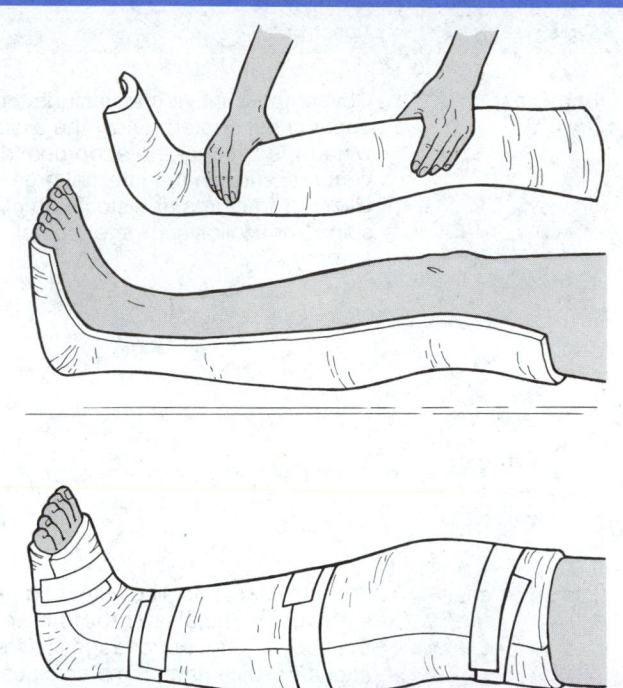

Figure 58–5

A bivalved cast.

SOURCE: Kozier B, Erb G: *Techniques in Clinical Nursing: A Nursing Process Approach*, 2nd ed. Menlo Park, CA: Addison–Wesley, 1986.

to immerse a cast made from such materials in water, as long as the cast and skin are thoroughly dried afterward to prevent skin maceration. A blow dryer set on medium is used for drying after immersion, which may take up to a few hours. The material used for padding under the cast is made of a synthetic that dries quickly.

Fiberglass and plastic casts become hard and strong in about 15 minutes or less. One type, called a light-cured fiberglass cast, is applied from a roll and then exposed to ultraviolet light for a few minutes until it hardens. Other lightweight materials are softened in hot water or immersed in cool water before application and then are molded to the extremity. These newer casting materials are more expensive than plaster, so they are not used on clients who require frequent cast changes. They also are inappropriate for an injury where bleeding may occur because the drainage will not be absorbed as it would be with plaster.

Cast Alterations. Occasionally, alterations are made in casts. A cast *window* may be formed by cutting out a small section of the cast. A cast cutter is used to cut a rectangular area in the cast, the plaster is removed, and the sheet wadding is cut to expose an area of skin that requires observation or care. There may be a wound requiring dressings, a pressure area causing discomfort, or stitches may need to be removed. The plaster square that is cut out should be saved because it is frequently put back to prevent the limb from swelling into the opening. The window plug may be taped in place with adhesive or wrapped with an elastic bandage. When wound care is given through the window, it is important to avoid getting the cast wet.

In another cast alteration, known as *bivalving,* the cast is split by the cast cutter along both the entire lateral and medial cast surfaces. This may be done to relieve edema or to change the cast into a half-shell splint. The splint is formed by removing the upper (or lower) half, allowing the limb to rest in the other half. A half-shell splint allows access to the joints and limb, but still provides support. The removed half of the cast is saved, and it is put back in place when the client is turned. The two shells are fastened together with straps, adhesive, or elastic bandaging (Figure 58–5).

A *walking heel* may be applied to a leg cast to allow weight bearing. If a client wonders why he or she does not have a walking cast, explain that this is only used when the type of fracture and position of the limb allows walking before healing is complete. Sometimes a walking heel is added later, when sufficient callus formation occurs, to allow weight bearing. The client must wait until the plaster dries before trying to walk on it. An alternative to the heel is a cast shoe worn over the cast (Figure 58–6).

Removing the Cast. When the fracture is healed, the cast is split with an electric cast cutter, which has a blade that oscillates rather than cuts (Figure 58–7). The vibrating blade is raised quickly as it breaks through the plaster (or synthetic cast) so it does not cut through the padding underneath. The cutter is noisy, and the client may feel some pressure and heat. All this can be frightening; the client will need reassurance that the cutter will not go through to the skin. After the cast is split, the cut edges are spread apart with tools, and the sheet wadding is cut with bandage scissors.

The Use of Traction in Fracture Management

Traction is applied by ropes, pulleys, weights, and an apparatus that connects them to the body part. The traction is adjusted to hold the fracture fragments in the proper alignment while healing takes place. When a force pulls in one direction, it is necessary to have a counterforce pulling in the opposite direction to keep the client from being pulled off the bed. In most cases, the countertraction is the client's body weight and the position of the bed (eg, the foot of the bed may be elevated). It is important to note the position of the client and the bed when traction is set up and to maintain these; otherwise the traction pull may be changed, altering the bone alignment.

Placing a person in traction means confinement to bed and usually a lengthy hospitalization (unless this is a temporary measure, eg, until a cast is applied). The bed should

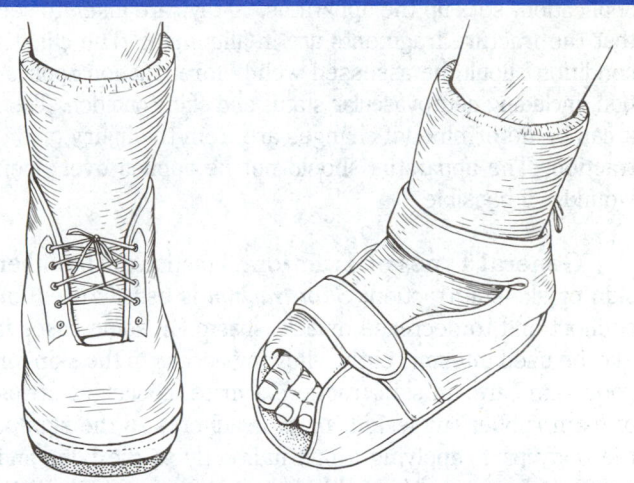

Figure 58–6

Cast shoe.

have a firm mattress, bedboard (if there are springs on the bed), and an overhead trapeze. An overbed frame is frequently necessary to connect traction equipment. An alternating air mattress or egg-crate-type foam rubber on the mattress is helpful in preventing pressure sores. A water mattress may be used as long as the limb remains in alignment on it. The physician, or someone trained in traction

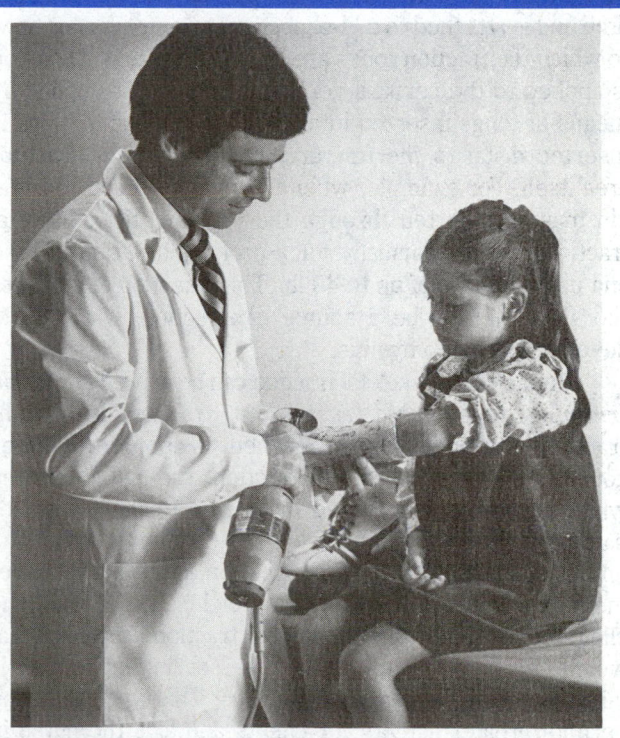

Figure 58–7

Cast cutter. (Photo courtesy of Stryker Corporation, Kalamazoo, MI)

application, sets up the apparatus. X-rays are taken to see that the fracture fragments are in alignment. The client's condition should be assessed well before traction application, including neurovascular status and skin condition. Then it can be determined if changes are from the injury or the traction. The apparatus should not be applied over open wounds, if possible.

General Types of Traction. Traction can be either skin or skeletal traction. *Skin traction* is usually used for comfort and to decrease muscle spasm. In some cases it may be used intermittently, allowing access to the skin for good skin care. In skin traction, a material such as strips of foam rubber, moleskin, or tape adheres to the skin of the body part, applying a pull indirectly to the bone and muscle. The material is held in place by wrapping the limb with elastic bandaging. Skin traction can also be applied by use of a halter around the head for cervical traction or a pelvic belt for traction of the lower vertebrae. In the case of Buck's extension (described later), a foam boot is used and fastened with Velcro straps. Skin traction is used for a shorter length of time than skeletal traction (up to 4 weeks) and uses small weights. The skeleton is capable of tolerating more weight than the skin.

Skeletal traction is applied directly to the bone. It is used for long-term alignment of fracture fragments. Under local or general anesthesia, a pin or wire is inserted aseptically through the skin and bone so traction weights can be applied to it. The pin extends through both sides of the limb and is attached to a U-shaped metal spreader, or bow, to which the traction ropes are tied. When skeletal traction is applied to the cervical vertebrae, the pull is applied by means of tongs inserted into the skull. The pin or wire is inserted distal to the fracture, not through the fracture area itself. For example, when the femur is fractured, the pin may be inserted through the proximal tibia. Skeletal traction is applied usually for a prolonged period of time and uses weights of up to 40 lb. The insertion of pins into the skeleton may be a source of infection, which could develop into osteomyelitis.

Both skin and skeletal traction can be applied as *straight (running)* or *balanced (suspension)* traction. In straight traction, the body weight and bed position are used as countertraction. In balanced traction, the pull is exerted while the limb is supported by use of a sling, splint, or hammock, and weights provide the countertraction. The limb is suspended rather than lying on the bed, and movement is permitted because the weights move when the client moves, maintaining constant traction. Any slack that would otherwise occur in the ropes during movement is taken up by the suspension apparatus. This type of traction permits greater activity for clients and aids the nurse in giving care because clients can be moved slightly to relieve pressure on the back. They can raise to use the bedpan and receive back care without changing the pull of the traction.

Specific Traction Devices. Some specific types of traction are described below. Readers wanting more information should consult orthopedic nursing textbooks.

Buck's extension is an example of straight skin traction (Figure 58–8A–C). It is applied to the lower leg:

- To relieve muscle spasm
- For preoperative immobilization of a fractured hip or femur
- For maintaining alignment after hip surgery
- To reduce hip or knee contractures
- To rest a diseased hip or knee

It can be used on one or both legs. Frequently, the nurse applies Buck's extension. Various types of apparatus are used to apply this type of traction. When adhesive tapes are used, the nurse may shave and cleanse the leg and coat it with protective skin spray such as tincture of benzoin. Opinions differ about the advisability of shaving and use of tincture of benzoin because shaving may cause skin abrasion, and benzoin is not as useful for protecting against infection or beneficial for adherence as was once believed (Farrell, 1982). Nonadhesive strips require skin care and assessment but not shaving. The nurse places the tape or strip along the medial and lateral aspects of the calf (and sometimes the thigh also), leaving space at the bottom for inserting the spreader or footplate used for attaching the traction rope. Folded or rolled stockinette can be placed just above the malleoli to keep the tapes off the ankles. Elastic bandaging is wrapped *smoothly* over the tapes, from above the ankle to the knee, to secure them. Particular care is taken to avoid pressure over the fibular head (the lateral side of the calf below the knees), to prevent pressure on the peroneal nerve. The traction rope and weight are applied to the spreader or footplate; the spreader should be wide enough to keep the tapes off the malleoli. A boot-type of apparatus with Velcro straps may be used instead of tapes and bandages (Figure 58–8D). The weights for this type of traction should not exceed 8 to 10 lb; otherwise, the skin will break down. A pillow may be placed under the lower leg with the heel extending over the end of it. The foot of the bed may be elevated to provide countertraction. The physician should let the nurse know if the traction can be removed for skin care; however, the adhesive-tape type is not removed. Problems that can occur from this type of traction are skin breakdown or neurovascular damage from the apparatus being too tight (eg, peroneal nerve palsy), allergy to the materials, pressure sores on the heels, or slipping of the traction apparatus so traction is not maintained.

Russell's traction is a type of skin traction (Figure 58–9) applied to treat fractures of the shaft of the femur and to correct knee and hip deformities. It can also be used bilaterally to treat back pain. The lower leg is wrapped as in Buck's extension to provide horizontal pull. In addition, a sling is placed under the knee to provide vertical lift. The back of the knee is padded with thick felt or foam

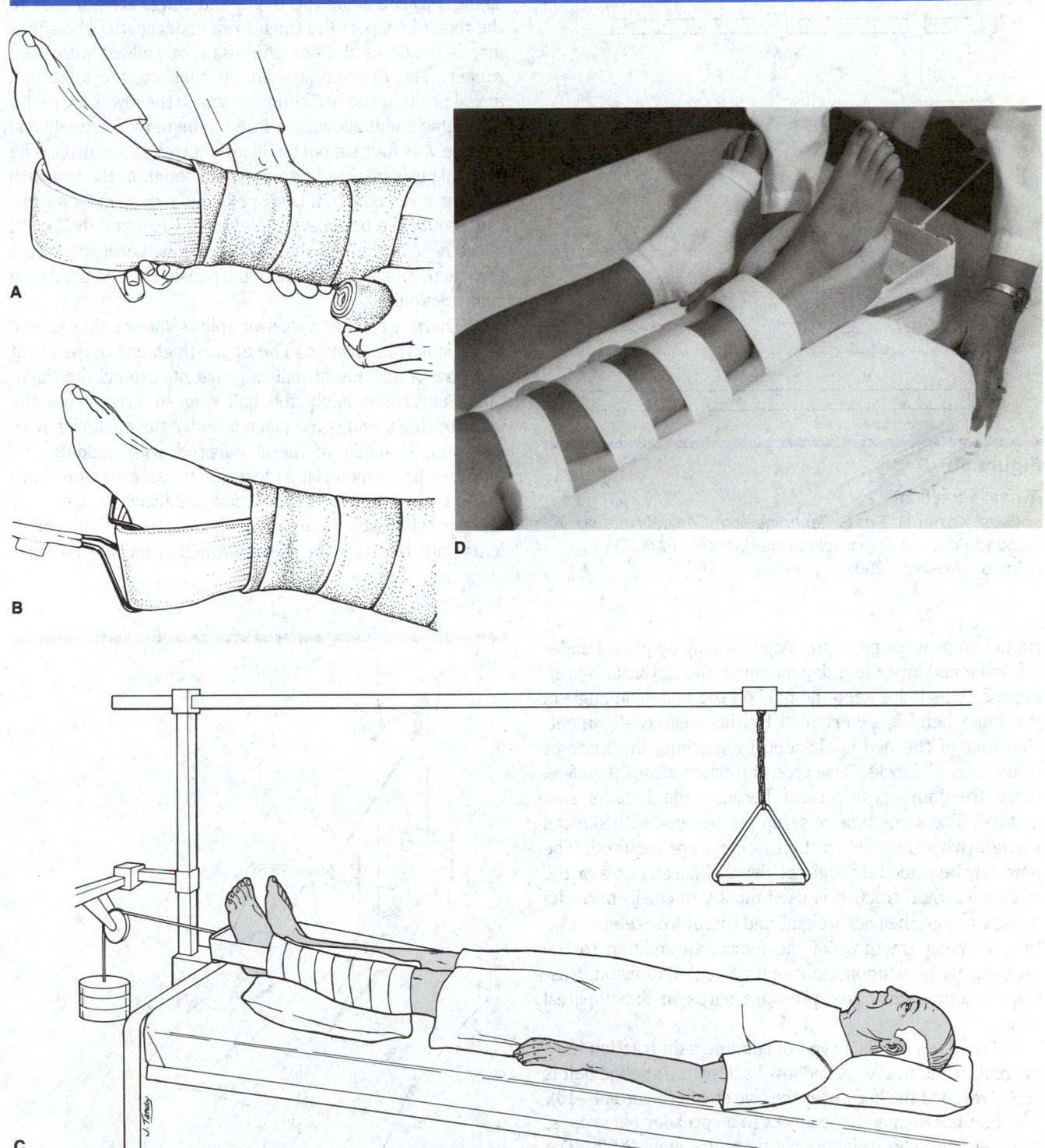

Figure 58–8

Applying Buck's extension. **A.** The leg is supported while being wrapped. The strips are placed along the medial and lateral aspects of the calf. Elastic bandage is applied smoothly and evenly from above the ankle to the knee. **B.** The spreader keeps the strips away from the malleoli. **C.** Buck's extension traction in place. **D.** A Buck's boot for extension traction.

SOURCE: **C,** Kozier B, Erb G: *Techniques in Clinical Nursing: A Nursing Process Approach,* 2nd ed. Menlo Park, CA: Addison–Wesley, 1986; **D,** Swearingen, PL: *Addison–Wesley Photo-Atlas of Nursing Procedures*. Menlo Park, CA: Addison–Wesley, 1984.

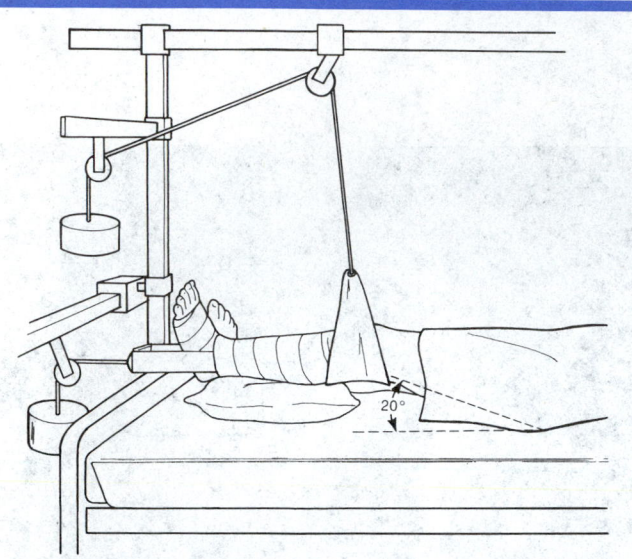

Figure 58-9

Russell's traction.
SOURCE: Kozier B, Erb G: *Techniques in Clinical Nursing: A Nursing Process Approach,* 2nd ed. Menlo Park, CA: Addison-Wesley, 1986.

rubber to prevent pressure. A pillow may be placed under the knee and lower leg, depending on the physician's preference. This helps keep the heel off the bed. The angle of the knee bend is determined by the desired alignment. The foot of the bed is elevated by gatching the knee or using "shock" blocks. This type of traction allows the client more freedom of movement because the limb is suspended. The same type of setup can be used with skeletal traction when heavier traction weights are required. The pins may be placed through the distal fibula and tibia or the calcaneus. Skin traction is used mostly in children; adults usually require heavier weight, and therefore skeletal traction, to treat fractures of the femur. In addition to the problem areas mentioned above for Buck's extension, Russell's traction can cause pressure sores in the popliteal area.

Pelvic traction is a type of running skin traction used to treat pelvic fractures and low back pain. A pelvic belt is applied around the body over the iliac crests (Figure 58-10). The belt has straps that connect to a spreader bar, ropes, and weights. The weights may be up to about 20 lb. The foot of the bed is elevated or knees gatched. Problems occurring from this type of traction include pressure sores on the iliac crests, sore elbows from shifting in bed, and slipping of the pelvic belt due to improper fit or application. If the head of the bed is elevated too high, the client may slip down in bed, negating the traction.

The *Thomas* or *Harris splint* and *Pearson attachment* are used when balanced skeletal traction is applied to treat fractures of the shaft of the femur (Figure 58-11). The

splint is placed along the thigh, and slings are attached to the rods to support the thigh from underneath. The slings may be made of cloth or sheepskin or padded with foam rubber. The Pearson attachment supports the knee in a flexed position and has slings on which the lower leg rests. This attachment allows the knee to be moved actively and passively. A foot support is used to prevent footdrop. The skeletal pin is inserted into the distal femur or the proximal tibia and connected to a U-shaped bow, ropes, and a weight. The foot of the bed may be elevated. Changing the height of the head of the bed should not be done because it alters the traction. A similar form of suspension can be used with skin traction.

There are other types of splints for traction known by various trade names. The upper-thigh end of the splint may have a full ring or half ring that fits around the thigh. Some physicians apply the half ring so it is across the anterior thigh, and some place it under the posterior side. The ring is made of metal covered with padding and moisture-proof material or leather. It can cause pressure in the groin and skin irritation, and is difficult to keep clean and dry with use of the bedpan and bathing. Other problems with this type of skeletal traction include infection

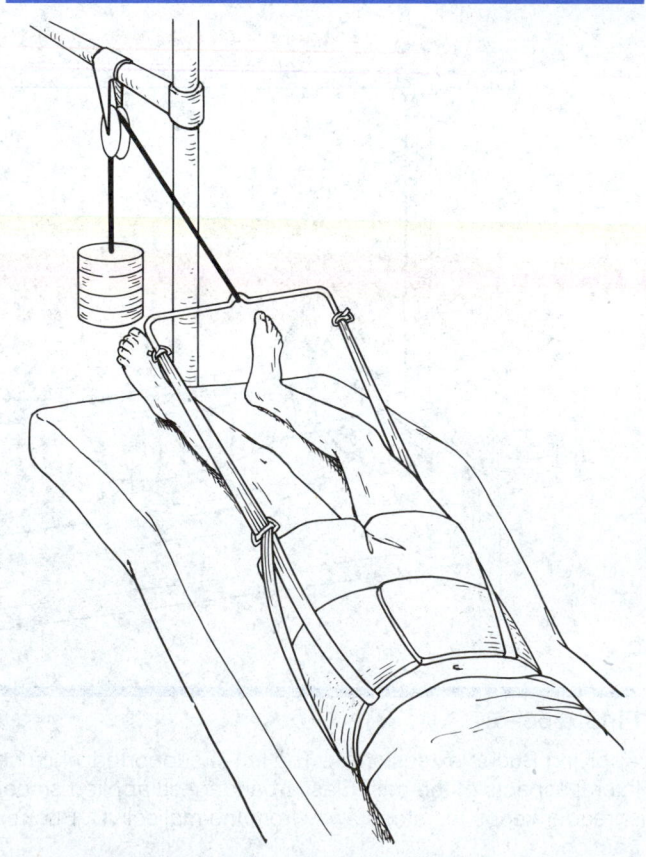

Figure 58-10

Pelvic girdle traction.

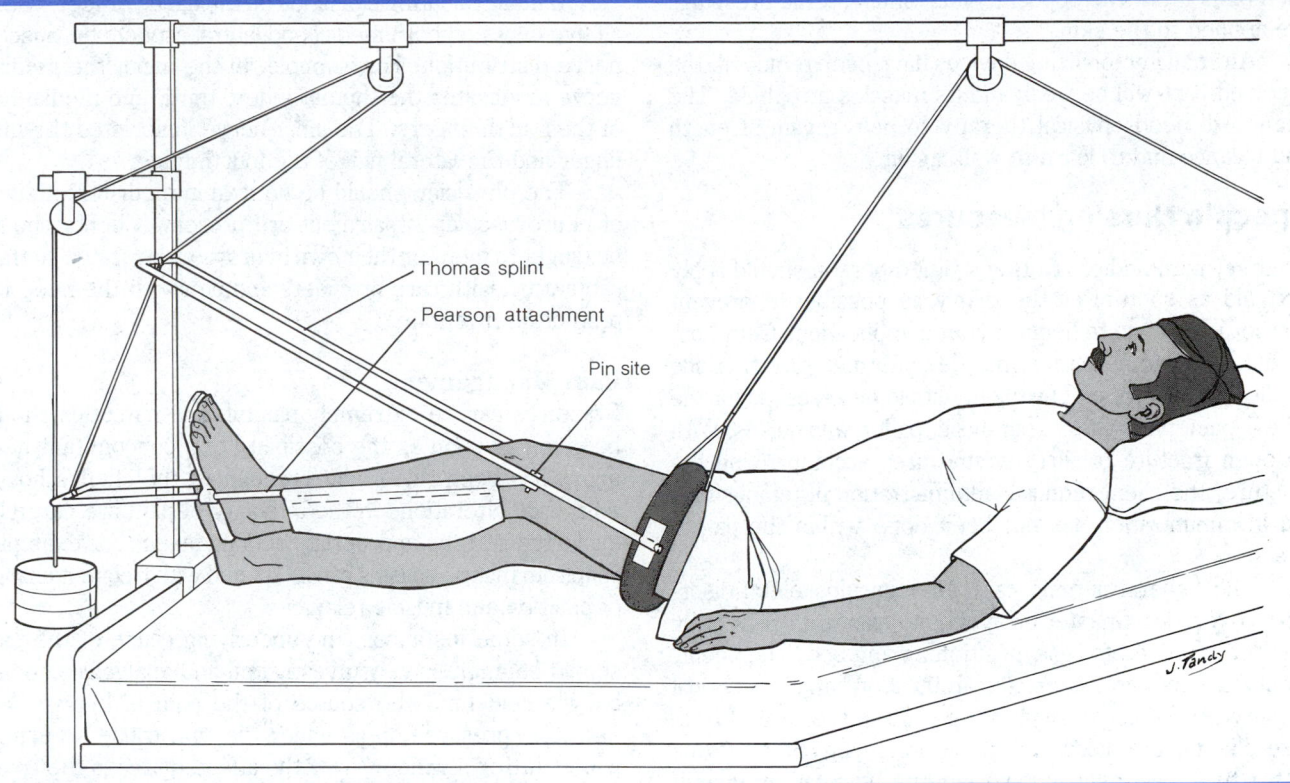

Thomas splint

Pearson attachment

Pin site

Figure 58–11

Thomas splint and Pearson attachment.

SOURCE: Kozier B, Erb G: *Techniques in Clinical Nursing: A Nursing Process Approach,* 2nd ed. Menlo Park, CA: Addison-Wesley, 1986.

from insertion of skeletal pins and pressure sores in the ischial area and the areas of skin that touch edges of the slings.

Crutchfield tongs are used for skeletal traction to treat fractures and dislocations of the cervical vertebrae (Figure 58–12). The pins are inserted about a half inch into the skull after the area is shaved, scrubbed, and anesthetized, and tongs are attached to ropes and weights. The weight may be as much as 35 lb. The head of the bed may be kept elevated slightly by physician's order. Frequently, a special turning bed such as the Roto Rest kinetic treatment table, Circo-electric bed, or Stryker frame is used. This type of apparatus and treatment are used on clients with neurological problems (see Unit Six).

Halo traction may also be used for cervical fractures. The traction headpiece is attached to a vest, maintaining head and neck immobilization. This allows early ambulation of the client (see Chapter 37).

Removing the Client From Traction. When the client is removed from traction, a cast or surgical fixation device may be needed. Skeletal wires are removed after the surrounding skin and exposed wires have been scrubbed with antiseptic solution. The physician depresses the skin around the wire, cuts the wire beneath the skin surface,

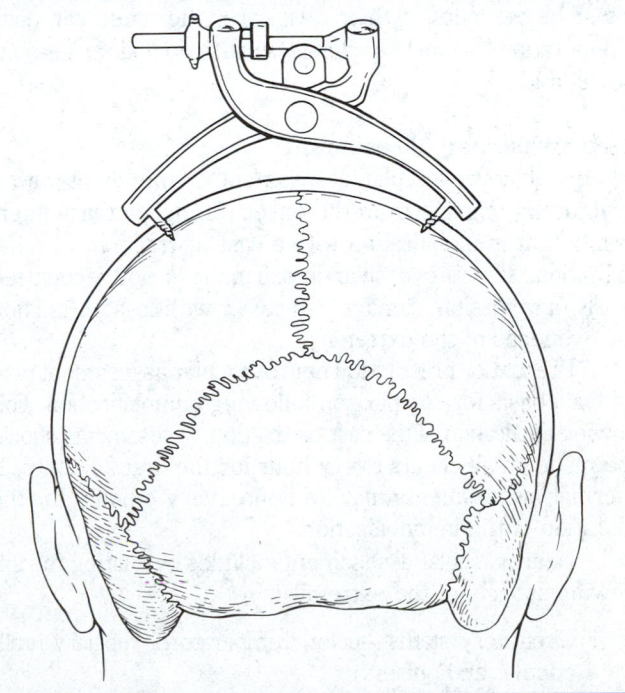

Figure 58–12

Crutchfield tongs.

then pulls it out the opposite side. Small sterile dressings are applied to the skin.

After all immobilizing devices have been removed, the involved part will be weak and its muscles atrophied. The client will need physical therapy to help regain strength and balance and to learn to walk again.

Specific Nursing Measures

A nurse, paramedic, or other trained person should apply first aid as soon after the injury as possible to prevent further injury and to help prevent complications from fractures. First aid measures include splinting, elevation, ice application, and rest. The client should be assessed for the 5 Ps—pain, paresthesia, paralysis, pallor, and pulses. With an open fracture or dirty wound area accompanying the fracture, the client requires administration of tetanus toxoid if immunization has not been done within the past 5 years.

The general nursing care for musculoskeletal disorders covered in Chapter 56 applies to fractures, especially measures related to rest, positioning and body alignment, comfort, skin care, exercise, ambulation, and diversional activity. Additional measures, specific to the care of fracture clients, are discussed in the following. Some forms of fracture treatment involve lengthy hospitalization and/or limited mobility after the client is discharged. Clients undergoing such treatment need considerable emotional support and encouragement to participate in the activities necessary for rehabilitation. A nurse who feels sorry for clients and does not encourage the exercises necessary to maintain strength may delay return of mobility. Clients must be partners in their own care; the nurse can elicit cooperation by teaching clients what to do and the reasons for doing it.

Neurovascular Assessment

Frequent neurovascular assessment of the client with a fracture is ongoing from the onset through surgical intervention or immobilization with a cast or traction, to rehabilitation. If neurovascular impairment is not recognized early, irreversible damage can result with loss of function or even loss of the extremity.

Precast or pretraction neurovascular assessment provides a basis for comparison following immobilization. Following application of the cast or traction, assessments should be made on all clients every hour for the first 24 hours. If normal, assessments may be done every 4 hours for the duration of the immobilization.

Neurovascular assessment includes evaluating the following aspects of the extremity:

- Circulatory status—color, temperature, capillary refill, edema, and pulse(s)
- Neurologic status—sensation, mobility, presence of numbness and tingling

When evaluating sensation on the hands or feet, check all five digits on both medial and lateral aspects because of nerve distribution. For example, in the hand, the median nerve innervates the thumb, index, third, and medial half of the fourth fingers. The ulnar nerve innervates the fifth finger and the lateral half of the fourth finger.

The physician should be notified immediately if signs of neurovascular impairment are present. Clients should be taught to monitor their own neurovascular status so they can alert health care providers and family to the need for prompt intervention.

Pain Management

Fractures can be extremely painful, and narcotics should be given as soon as the possibility of a concomitant head injury has been ruled out. Throughout the client's hospitalization, alterations in the intensity of pain are carefully evaluated and the appropriate actions taken. For example, pain from muscle spasms can be treated with frequent change of position and muscle relaxants.

In some instances, the underlying cause of the pain should be aggressively investigated and analgesics should be withheld until the source of the pain is known. For example, pressure areas under the cast cause a burning pain. Cutting a window over the affected area is the treatment of choice. Ischemic pain, such as occurs with impaired neurovascular status or compartment syndrome, is managed by bivalving the cast to relieve pressure.

Avoiding Hazards of Immobility

All measures to prevent the hazards of immobility are essential. Encourage the client to exercise all uninvolved extremities every 4 hours while awake. Joints not confined by a cast or traction need ROM, and the client should do isometric exercises to maintain muscle strength in unaffected extremities. (Refer to the exercises in Chapter 55.) The physician should prescribe specific exercises for the affected limb. Encourage self-care, and place articles and the call bell where they can be reached. Clients will need help with ADL, especially when their hand or arm is confined in a cast or traction. Diversional activities are necessary. Remember that casts and traction also affect the client's body image and sexual needs (see Chapter 56).

The client with a leg cast or with traction will be able to maneuver in bed better with use of an overhead *trapeze*. Clients will need instructions on how to use the trapeze, eg, bend the good leg to help lift, pull the body upward, and avoid breath-holding while lifting. When holding the breath to lift, a person performs the Valsalva maneuver, which increases the intrathoracic pressure, decreasing blood flow to the heart. When the person exhales, the intrathoracic pressure decreases, causing a sudden surge of blood to the heart. A client with heart problems may not be able to compensate for the sudden increase of blood flow.

Skin areas susceptible to pressure should be assessed hourly for 48 to 72 hours after a cast or traction is first applied. Care to obvious pressure areas should begin before any problems are noted. Elbow and heel protectors are useful in preventing soreness to these areas, which are easily irritated from shifting the body weight around in bed.

Nutrition

Metabolic needs are greatly increased following trauma. Extensive fracture healing may require an intake of 3000 to 4000 calories per day. Additional fiber and fluids help prevent constipation caused by immobility. The client whose intake is inadequate may receive vitamin and protein supplements. Increased calcium is usually discouraged because calcium is mobilized from the bones during immobility (disuse osteoporosis), and excesses can cause urinary calculi. Therefore, the client's fluid intake should be at least 3000 mL per day, if not contraindicated.

Caring for a Client With a Cast

Drying the Cast. A finished cast is placed on pillows, both to elevate the extremity and to avoid placing the cast on a hard surface, which could flatten it as it dries. Pillows should provide support along the entire length of the cast, except a leg cast should be positioned so the heel hangs over the edge to prevent pressure on the heel. It is best to use pillows *without* plastic or rubber covering because airtight pillows trap the heat and may cause burns to the skin (Farrell, 1982). If plastic-covered pillows must be used, place several layers of toweling or a bath blanket between the cast and pillow to allow the heat to dissipate.

The nurse may need extra help to move a client with a fresh cast into a bed while supporting the cast. Be sure to handle the wet cast with the palms, not the fingertips. Plaster that got on the surrounding skin during cast application should be removed with plain water. Turn the client to expose all surfaces of the cast while it is drying. If the client feels cool or chilled during the drying, cover uncasted areas of the body for warmth. Occasionally, lights or cast dryers are used to help dry the cast quicker. Take care to place the lamp far enough away from the cast (15 in) and to prevent intense heating. Cast dryers can cause uneven drying with a dry outside and an unstable interior. When the cast is completely dry, it is hard and odorless. Weight bearing is not allowed until then (if it is a weight-bearing cast). When the cast is dry, the client may be turned to any comfortable position because the fracture fragments are immobilized by the cast.

Edema. Ice bags may be applied to the fracture site intermittently (on for 20 to 30 minutes, off 10 to 15 minutes, as described in Chapter 56) for the first 24 to 48 hours. Place the ice bags along the sides of the cast rather than on top. The ice bags should be only about half full so

they are not heavy enough to cause indentation. Swelling under the cast may impair circulation. Therefore, it is important to elevate the cast higher than the heart, if possible, unless compartment syndrome exists. Occasionally, a change in position will relieve pressure from the cast.

Skin Care. Skin care along the cast edges includes washing and drying every day, being careful not to get the cast wet. The skin can be massaged with alcohol but not with lotion, which tends to soften the skin and may cause maceration. Run the fingers under the cast edge to remove plaster crumbs, which may irritate the client's skin. A portable vacuum cleaner may also be helpful. Also inspect the skin for signs of breakdown. Care of the skin can also be taught to both client and family.

Clients in a cast or traction should use a fracture bedpan. Sometimes people are afraid to use such a small bedpan, thinking they will overfill it, as indeed they do occasionally if the foot of the bed is elevated. Disposable underpads and good skin care after bedpan use are important. Those unfamiliar with the fracture bedpan tend to insert it backwards so the client is sitting in the deepest part. The shallow, flat end of the pan should be pointed toward the head of the bed.

Cast Care. The nurse should inspect the cast for fit and for softened areas, which would tend to cause changes in alignment of the fracture fragments. Initial swelling that has subsided may cause the cast to be too loose. If the cast does not have a stockinette finished edge, the edges can be finished by placing "petals" along them after the swelling and pain subsides. This is done by cutting strips of adhesive tape, rounding one end, and tucking the other end under the cast smoothly so it adheres to the sheet wadding inside the cast, being careful not to roll the tape edges. The free end of the tape is brought over the cast edge and secured to the outside cast surface. The petals should overlap to cover the entire cast edge; they help keep it from breaking down and prevent skin irritation from rough edges. Casts can be protected from soiling in the perineal region by tucking waterproof material under the cast and fastening it to the outside with adhesive. A dirty cast can be cleaned a little with scouring cleanser and a slightly moistened cloth. A cast should not be painted or varnished, because it must remain porous so evaporation can take place.

Infection and Drainage. The nurse should assess the cast for unusual odors, which can be an indication of infection under the cast. This means sniffing right next to the cast. Hot spots along the cast may also be an indication of infection. Drainage coming through the cast is a sign of infection or bleeding underneath. Expect bleeding to occur through the cast for the first few days after surgery. Most nurses circle the drainage area with ink and label the date

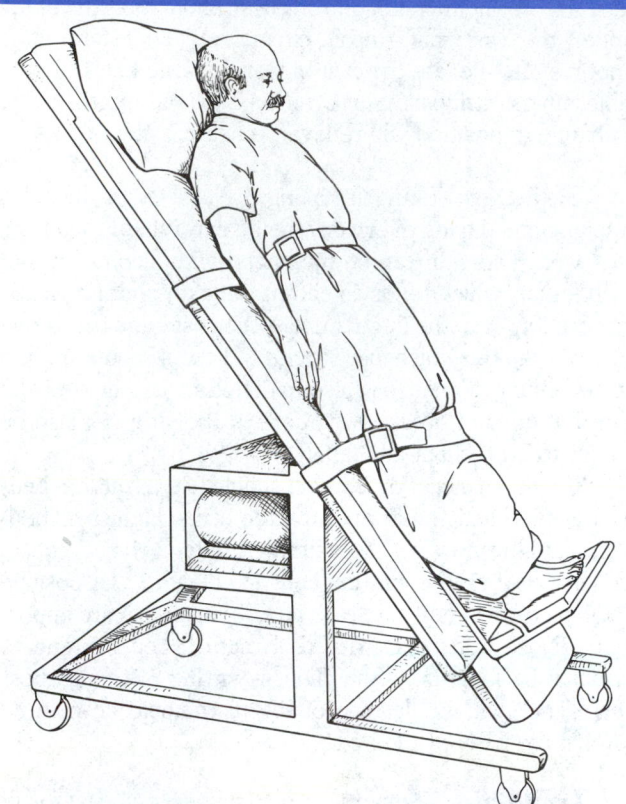

Figure 58–13

A tilt table is used to aid the client in gradually adjusting to the upright position.

and time on the cast; later checks will show if the area extends. However, some think visible drainage is a poor indication of amount of drainage, and some physicians do not want anything drawn on a client's cast. Excessive drainage should be reported. Remember to check the undersurface of the cast, as drainage will flow downward.

Specific Types of Casts. The client with an *arm cast* usually wears a sling to support the arm when not lying down. Refer to a fundamental nursing text for correct application of a sling. The hand should not hang off the end of the sling, and it should be higher than the elbow. If the physician permits, the client should remove the sling at least four times a day and put the arm, and especially the shoulder, through ROM exercises. If the client does not use a sling, the arm should be kept elevated unless the cast is specifically meant to hang (eg, to provide traction for a fractured humerus). A hanging arm cast should not rest on pillows, and the client must sit upright to provide proper alignment of fracture fragments. Areas to assess for pressure with arm casts include bones of the wrist and elbow.

The client with a *leg cast* will need to learn to use some type of ambulatory aid to get around. Warn clients

that their toes may swell when the cast is lowered, and encourage them to elevate the extremity when sitting or lying back supine. The cast may be heavy, and extra help may be needed to move the leg when getting in and out of bed. When up in a wheelchair, the client's leg should be elevated and tied to the footrest along with a supporting pillow so it does not fall. Areas to assess for pressure with a leg cast include the head of the fibula on the lateral surface of the leg, which is near the peroneal nerve; the anterior tibia; the kneecap; the heel; and both sides of the ankle.

The client in a *hip spica cast* is usually confined to the cast for several months. Clients need to be turned regularly and require assistance for this in addition to helping themselves with the overhead trapeze. Clients usually turn onto the unaffected side while the nurse supports the cast. When on their sides, position clients with pillows between the legs and against the back. While the cast is still wet, the client must be turned frequently from supine to prone because this cast takes a few days to dry. It is important to support the wet cast as the client rolls and to place pillows for supporting the cast. If the cast has an abductor bar between the legs, the bar should not be grasped to move the client. If the client begins to ambulate with the cast, it is done gradually, first trying the upright position by use of a tilt table (Figure 58–13). The cast requires sitting in a reclining-type position, which hinders client participation in personal care.

Health Education and Support. A list of points to cover when teaching the client about cast care is provided in Table 58–5. The client should be taught not to tamper with or alter the cast and not to scratch under it with any object. The client will experience frequent itching under the cast, and the temptation to poke something under the cast for scratching will be great. If scratching occurs, the skin underneath can become injured or irritated, causing sores under the cast. Forcing air under the cast with a bulb syringe or a hair dryer on cool setting may be helpful for soothing an itch.

Wearing a cast can be frustrating because it is heavy and clumsy and restricts independence. The client needs encouragement to try new methods of performing tasks to remain independent or to accept temporary dependence on others.

Care After Cast Removal. When the cast is removed, the casted extremity will appear thin and flabby, and the skin will be scaly and may be foul smelling. The nurse should prepare the client for this ahead of time. The limb will also be weak and may be painful to use; balance may be unstable. The scaly skin requires gentle cleansing followed by application of oil or lanolin; the skin is tender and should not be scrubbed. Some physicians recommend soaking the limb to remove the scales. The weak limb should be supported when moved. The limb will swell when held in a dependent position; instruct clients to continue

Table 58–5 Instructions for Clients Being Discharged in a Cast

1. Check the color, temperature, movement, and sensation of all toes or fingers exposed from the cast at least twice a day (more often for a new cast).

2. Elevate the limb (toes higher than the knee; hand higher than the elbow). For an arm cast, wear a sling when not lying down.

3. Do not alter the cast in any way (except adhesive tape petals can be applied over sharp edges).

4. Keep the cast clean and dry. Plastic over the cast will help when going out in bad weather. The cast can be cleaned a little by using a slightly damp cloth and scouring cleanser. Avoid soaking.

5. Wash the skin along the cast edges and dry well every day. Skin can be massaged with alcohol, but do not use lotion at cast edges.

6. Inspect the skin along cast edges every day; run fingers under the edges to remove cast crumbs.

7. Inspect the cast for drainage, odors, cracked or softened areas, and hot spots.

8. Do not scratch under the cast or poke any objects under the cast.

9. Exercise the joints above and below the cast at least four times a day, if permitted by your physician.

10. Notify your physician if:
    - You have a fever.
    - The cast is loose, cracked, or softened.
    - There is a foul odor from the cast.
    - There is drainage coming through the cast.
    - Swelling does not go down when the cast is elevated.
    - Fingers or toes are changed compared to those on the other limb, for example, cold, numb, no feeling, pale, or unable to move.
    - There is pain or burning under the cast.
    - The skin around the cast edges becomes broken and sore.

11. Continue to see your physician for scheduled appointments.

the nurse should study it, know what it is supposed to look like, and keep everything the same, even the placement of pillows. It may be a good idea to take a picture of the bed and hang it at the bedside for reference. The traction should never be altered without the physician's order. Instructions from the physician should be clear about how much movement is allowed, for example, in raising and lowering the head of the bed, or in turning, and to which side. If the traction can be removed temporarily, as is sometimes done, that should be made clear in the physician's orders. The nurse should instruct the client about the positions allowed, especially if there are electric controls on the bed.

Assess the traction apparatus at least once every shift. Weights should hang freely without touching or resting on anything. The traction would not be maintained if, for example, the client slid toward the foot of the bed so the weight sat on the floor. The footplate or spreader should not touch the foot of the bed or frame. The rope should be examined to see that it is not frayed, that the knots are secure, that it is not rubbing against the overbed frame, and that it is resting in the groove of the pulley. Sometimes the rope gets caught at the edge of the wheel in the pulley, changing the traction pull. The ends of the rope can be taped to the rope to prevent knots from slipping. The weights should be fastened securely and hung so they are not jarred or hit by traffic going by.

Making a Traction Bed. It is usually easier to make the bed from top to bottom when the client is in traction and cannot be turned. The nurse must get sufficient help. The client assists by lifting with the trapeze; an assistant can help lift the client as allowed. The dirty linens are removed as the clean ones are pulled into place; top linens are not tucked under the mattress. While the helper is available, give back care. Observe the back and sacral area for pressure sores. If the client cannot be lifted enough for good skin observation and care, depress the mattress with a hand to make more room. Back care may be necessary every few hours. Use the same method to administer the bedpan. It is important to get extra help when lifting the client and giving care so as not to cause the client needless pain and to keep the pull of the traction constant.

Exercise. Isometric exercises can be done to the involved extremity in many kinds of traction but it is best to check with the physician to see if exercises are permitted because they are contraindicated for some people.

Pin Care. The care of skin around skeletal pins (Figure 58–14), known as *pin care*, varies according to physician preference. Frequently, the physician places a sterile gauze pad around the pin, with an iodine or antibiotic ointment applied to the site. Some physicians do not apply any dressing. Some want the skin cleansed around the pin to remove the drainage that accumulates; others do not.

to elevate the extremity and reassure them that with activity and exercise, the tendency for swelling will subside. The physician will prescribe exercises and instruct the client in the amount of activity or weight bearing allowed. A physical therapist may assist in the rehabilitation program.

Caring for the Client in Traction

Maintaining the Traction. The traction pull should be in alignment with the axis of the long bones. During the first week of traction, the physician may make traction adjustments as the muscle spasms decrease and the bone position changes. After the traction apparatus is set up,

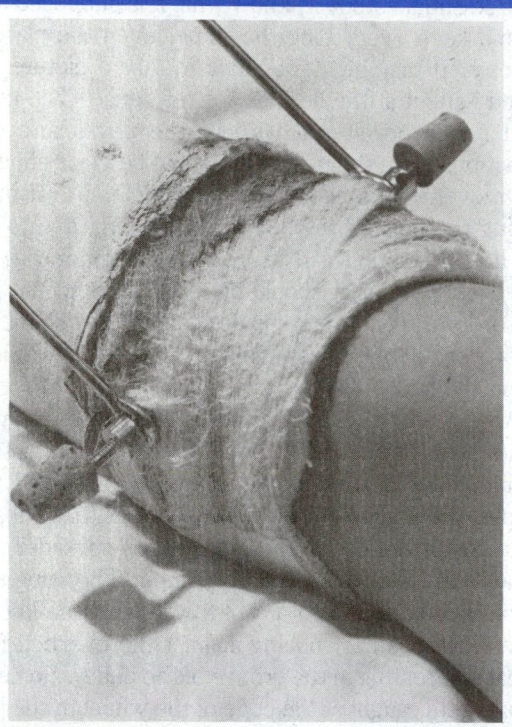

Figure 58–14

Skeletal traction: A pin through the bone with covering the ends.

SOURCE: Swearingen PL: *Addison–Wesley Photo-Atlas of Nursing Procedures.* Menlo Park, CA: Addison–Wesley, 1984

Therefore, the physician must order pin care, and it should not be done otherwise. One method is to clean around the pin with half-strength hydrogen peroxide solution on a cotton swab, then apply a gauze pad with povidone–iodine (Betadine) ointment, using aseptic technique. Cut a slit in the pad with sterile scissors so the pad can be placed around the pin, or use drain sponges with a slit already made in them. Inspect the skin around the pin at least once a day, and check the pin to see that it is not loose or slipping to one side. Bring any changes to the physician's attention. Indications of infection include redness, tenderness, and purulent drainage. Cover the pin ends with cork (the rubber stoppers from venipuncture tubes also work well) to keep from getting scratched or catching the linens.

Care After Traction Removal. Confinement in traction can be a source of emotional stress, as was discussed in Chapter 55. The client may be afraid to move, so the nurse should provide clear explanations of the amount of movement and activity allowed, with assurance that the traction apparatus will maintain the bone in alignment.

When clients are removed from traction and begin ambulation, they must slowly acclimate to the upright position. This can be done with a few sessions on a tilt table or by slow elevation to a seated position and eventually to

the upright position, with each attempt progressing as far as tolerated. The nurse observes the client for signs of orthostatic hypotension such as pallor, a lowering of blood pressure, faintness, or dizziness with position change. Explain to clients that the limb will be weak and unsteady at first, and encourage them to follow the physician's instructions concerning the amount of weight bearing and activities permitted. The criteria to evaluate the effectiveness of nursing interventions in fracture care are listed in Box 58–2.

Complications of Fractures

Infection as a complication of fracture healing was described earlier in this chapter under osteomyelitis. The *complications resulting from immobility* are also possible with fracture treatment. Prevention and treatment of these complications are covered in Chapter 56. This section discusses other complications that can arise during healing of fractures.

Problems of Bone Union

Delayed union of the fracture occurs when the bone does not unite in the usual amount of time. This delay can have various causes, including infection, inadequate reduction or immobilization, poor circulation to the bone, and metabolic disturbances that affect the protein and vitamins available for healing. *Nonunion* is the failure of healing so firm union does not take place. The causes of nonunion include those listed for delayed union, as well as separation of the bone fragments so that callus cannot span the gap,

---

Box 58–2 Criteria to Evaluate the Effectiveness of Nursing Interventions in Fracture Care

The client with a fracture will:

Demonstrate good body alignment and good posture

State that pain is relieved

Describe and comply with the prescribed restrictions in activity

Demonstrate recommended exercises and ambulation techniques correctly

Adjust to the temporary body image changes

Cope with the limitations imposed by the injury and treatment

Describe symptoms and signs of complications that can occur from fractures and their treatment

Display no signs of infection, deformity, skin breakdown or other hazards of immobility

Display no signs of complications such as those from neurovascular impairment or fat embolism

Effectively and safely use ambulatory aids

Describe and correctly demonstrate care required after discharge

massive loss of bone from the injury, or soft tissue between the fracture fragments. Delayed union and nonunion are treated by discovering and correcting the underlying problems.

For nonunion, surgical revision of the fracture ends or bone grafting may be helpful. A new method of treatment that is proving effective is electrical stimulation to promote bone formation (Bassett, Mitchell, & Gaston, 1981). One method uses noninvasive equipment that can be placed over the skin or cast surface (Figure 58–15). The client takes the equipment home and uses it about 10 to 12 hours a day, usually during sleep. The treatment may be continued about 3 to 8 months. Another method uses a semi-invasive technique in which insulated electrodes are inserted percutaneously into the medullary canal of the fracture, utilizing image-intensified fluoroscopy to determine placement. The electrodes are connected to a battery pack outside the cast. The client must avoid weight bearing to prevent pulling out the electrodes and should be seen by the physician once a month. The electrodes are removed after 12 weeks of treatment (Connolly, 1981).

Malunion is a complication in which union occurs in a deformed or angulated position. This can occur from inadequate reduction and immobilization. If the condition is severe, it may be treated by remanipulating the bone or by surgical intervention.

Compartment Syndrome

Compartment syndrome occurs when swelling or pressure develops within a confined space, or compartment, in an extremity. A compartment is a normally occurring area in which a muscle group is enclosed in tough fascial tissue. Small openings allow blood vessels and nerves to enter and exit the compartment. Little room remains for swelling. Tight bandages and casts may cause pressure from outside the compartment, or inflammation and resulting edema or hemorrhage may cause pressure from within, compromising circulation in the extremity. *Ischemia* (lack of blood supply) of the muscle occurs if enough pressure builds up, and ischemia leads quickly to nerve damage. The first symptom of compartment syndrome is pain that increases in severity, especially with passive stretching, and is unrelieved by narcotics. Other symptoms and signs include paralysis, paresthesias, decreased or absent pulses, and tense skin over the limb. Farrell (1982) states that irreversible damage begins in muscles and nerves after 6 hours of ischemia, and the extremity becomes useless in 24 to 48 hours. Ischemic muscle tissues are replaced by fibrotic tissue, forming contractures. For example, Volkmann's contracture (Figure 58–16) can occur with injuries in the elbow region. The hand and forearm become permanently disabled, and motor and sensory function are lost.

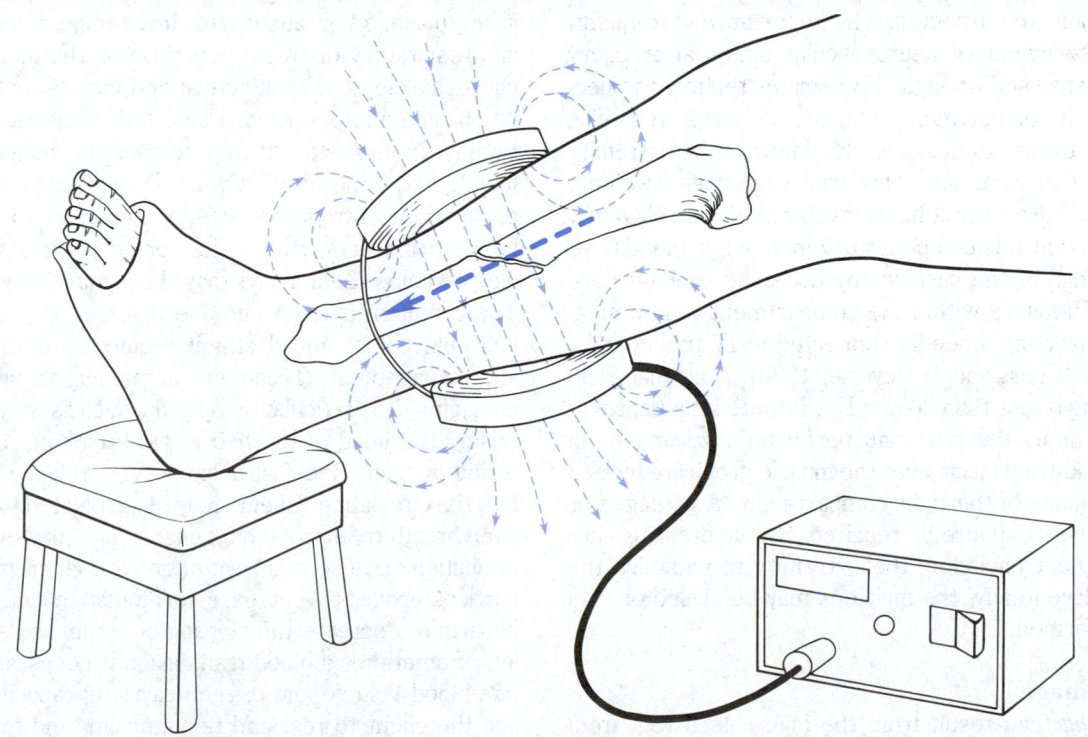

Figure 58–15

Electrical stimulation to promote bone formation.

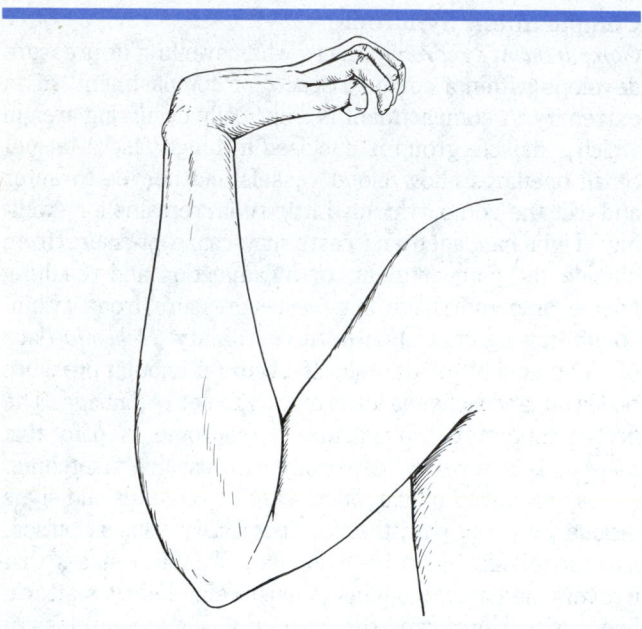

Figure 58–16

Volkmann's contracture.

Preventive measures for compartment syndrome include elevation of an injured extremity and intermittent ice application; frequent, regular neurovascular assessment for early detection; avoiding tight dressings, splints, or casts and IV infiltration; and listening to the client's complaints and seeking prompt medical attention when complications are suspected. The importance of frequent, regular assessment of neurovascular status after injury cannot be stressed enough. Immediate treatment is necessary when compartment syndrome is suspected. The heart may attempt to increase blood flow to the extremity in response to ischemia. This will exacerbate swelling. Keeping the extremity at heart level, rather than elevated, may circumvent this compensatory increase in blood flow. The front half of the cast or any occlusive bandages are removed. Pressure within the compartment can be measured by inserting a needle connected to IV tubing and a manometer (Crossland & Deyerle, 1980). A normal pressure reading is less than 20 mm Hg. If there is no improvement in 1 hour, the physician performs a *fasciotomy*, in which the skin and fascia over the muscle group are incised to allow release of the tight compartment. A damaged or bleeding vessel can also be repaired. Sterile dressings are applied without encircling the extremity to minimize the pressure. Eventually, the incisions may be closed or skin grafts performed.

Nerve Damage

Nerve damage can result from the injury itself (eg, from sharp bone fragments) or from the treatment. The peroneal nerve runs along the lateral side of the lower leg below the head of the fibula where it is superficial and can easily be affected by pressure from a cast or traction apparatus. Damage to this nerve can result in footdrop. Peroneal nerve function can be checked by asking the client to dorsiflex the ankle and to extend the toes. Sensory function is checked by pricking the lateral side of the great toe and the medial side of the second toe. The damage may be permanent but is sometimes temporary. Wristdrop can occur from injury to the radial nerve. To test for motor function, the client is asked to hyperextend the wrist or thumb. To test the sensory status, prick the skin in the web between the thumb and index finger. When nerve damage is impending or suspected, treatment includes splitting the cast or adjusting the traction apparatus.

Fat Embolism

Fat embolism can occur as a complication of fractures or surgery of the long bones, from multiple trauma, or from other conditions unrelated to trauma. The cause of fat embolism is not completely understood but is probably at least partly related to a release of bone marrow fat into the circulation, a change in the fat composition in the circulation after trauma, or both. Apley and Solomon (1982) state that circulating fat globules occur in most adults with closed fractures of long bones, but only a small portion of these people develop problems.

Measures to prevent fat embolism are prompt immobilization of fractures and avoidance of manipulation of the fracture fragments. Signs and symptoms usually occur 12 to 72 hours after surgery or injury and include steadily rising pulse, respiratory rate, and temperature; cyanosis and respiratory distress; petechiae on the upper anterior chest, axillae, and conjunctiva; and mental confusion, agitation, and apprehension. Frequently, a change in sensorium is the first sign. It may be a subtle change such as a feeling that something is wrong. Diagnostic tests show low oxygen concentration in arterial blood and sometimes fat in the urine or sputum. The serum lipase level may be elevated, and chest x-rays may show pulmonary infiltrates. The condition is a serious one that can progress to convulsions, coma, and death; it requires prompt diagnosis and management. Treatment is supportive and includes managing the particular symptoms, such as treating shock, raising the head of the bed to aid breathing, or administering oxygen. Bed rest helps prevent release of more fat into the circulation. Clients may be instructed to cough and deep breath to improve oxygenation and may even require intubation and use of a respirator. The client may receive corticosteroids to decrease inflammation and edema or heparin to decrease the clotting of serum lipids and platelets. Sometimes a blood transfusion is necessary to maintain blood volume and oxygen-carrying capacity. Encourage the client to rest and remain calm, and provide both client and family with emotional support during this crisis.

Pulmonary embolism, also a complication of fractures due to immobility, is discussed in Chapter 14.

Avascular Necrosis

Avascular necrosis, also known as *aseptic necrosis,* occurs when a bone is deprived of its blood supply, causing bone death. This is a common complication of fractures, especially fractures of the femoral neck. Vessels within the joint capsule that supply the head of the femur may be damaged from the trauma; without the normal blood supply, the bone becomes osteoporotic and necrotic. Avascular necrosis can also occur with joint dislocation; high-dosage, long-term steroid therapy; and other conditions. The client experiences pain and limited movement. Treatment is usually surgical removal of the femoral head and replacement with a hip prosthesis (see Chapter 60).

Cast Syndrome

Cast syndrome, a complication of body casts, is caused by compression of part of the duodenum by the superior mesenteric artery, resulting in obstruction. The signs and symptoms of cast syndrome include prolonged nausea and vomiting, abdominal distention (seen through a cast window cut over the abdomen), and vague abdominal pain. The condition can be fatal if allowed to progress. Treatment includes gastrointestinal decompression, maintaining NPO, fluid and electrolyte replacement, and removal of the cast (Farrell, 1982).

Chapter Highlights

Metabolic disorders of the bone include hyperparathyroidism, osteoporosis, and osteomalacia. These conditions may result in bone pain, weakness, deformities, and pathological fractures.

Paget's disease of the bone leads to swelling and deformity of bone with weakness and potential for fracture.

Osteomyelitis is an acute or chronic infection of the bone and surrounding tissues, causing pain, bone destruction, and limited mobility.

Prevention of bone infection is of utmost importance because an acute infection may progress into a chronic one. Signs and symptoms of infection include heat, odor, drainage, redness, swelling, pain, and fever.

The more common bone neoplasms are giant cell tumor (benign) and osteogenic sarcoma (malignant). These conditions interfere with mobility and comfort.

Signs and symptoms of bone cancer include pain, tenderness, local swelling, a mass, and walking with a limp. Medical attention should be sought without delay upon detection.

Bone tumors must be surgically removed or destroyed by chemotherapy or radiotherapy.

A fracture is a break in the continuity of a bone. It causes pain, swelling, limited movement, and possibly damage to surrounding tissues and organs.

Fractures can occur from a fall; a blow; crushing; twisting; muscle contraction; stress on the bone; and bone disease.

A fracture heals best when the bone fragments are realigned in close proximity, immobilized to maintain alignment and when circulation is good, infection is absent, and nutrition is adequate.

Methods used to immobilize a realigned fracture include casts, splints, internal fixation, external fixation, and traction.

Assessment of a limb with a fracture includes checking for pain, pallor, paresthesia, paralysis, and pulselessness. Abnormalities noted must be brought to the physician's attention immediately.

To prevent changing the contour of a wet cast, it must be handled with flat palms and placed on pillows to support its entire length. Casted extremities should be elevated above heart level when possible.

Traction equipment must remain in the position set by the physician to maintain the alignment and immobilization of the bone fragments.

Traction should be assessed at least every shift to evaluate alignment and maintain the intended pull. The ropes should be in the pulley grooves, and weights should be hanging freely.

General nursing interventions for clients with bone disorders include measures to prevent the hazards of immobility; comfort measures such as analgesics and position changes; exercising unaffected extremities; encouraging self-care; providing diversional activities; giving emotional support; encouraging a nutritionally balanced diet; and assisting with the use of ambulatory aids and ADL.

Any complaint of a client treated with a cast or traction should be investigated fully and promptly to avoid complications.

Nerves and skin can deteriorate from pressure of casts, splints, and traction apparatus. Areas to assess for pressure include: area over the fibular heads; both

(continued)

Chapter Highlights *(continued)*

malleoli; anterior tibia; heels; knees; radial and ulnar styloids; elbows; epicondyles of the elbow; iliac crests; and skin touching the edges of casts and traction equipment.

Complications of fractures include delayed union, nonunion, malunion, infection, the hazards of immobility, compartment syndrome, nerve damage, fat embolism, pulmonary embolism, avascular necrosis, and cast syndrome.

Lengthy hospitalization and recovery period may be an emotional and financial burden for clients with fractures and for their families.

Before discharge, the nurse teaches the client about cast care; wound care; signs and symptoms of complications; ambulation restrictions; good body mechanics; and necessary rest, exercise, nutrition, and follow-up care.

Bibliography

Apley AG, Solomon L: *Apley's System of Orthopaedics and Fractures,* 6th ed. London: Butterworth, 1982.

Bassett CAL, Mitchell SN, Gaston SR: Treatment of ununited tibial diaphyseal fractures with pulsing electromagnetic fields. *J Bone Joint Surg* 1981; 63:511–523.

Burg ME: Compartment syndrome. *CCQ* 1983; 6(1):27–32.

Connolly JF (ed): *DePalma's the Management of Fractures and Dislocations: An Atlas,* 3rd ed. Philadelphia: Saunders, 1981.

Crossland S, Deyerle W: Compartmental syndrome. *Nurs 80* 1980; 10(11):51–53.

Farrell J: *Illustrated Guide to Orthopedic Nursing,* 2nd ed. Philadelphia: Lippincott, 1982.

Geier KA, Hesser K: Electrical bone stimulation for treatment of nonunion. *Ortho Nurs* 1985; 4(2): 41–49.

Gorrie TM: Postmenopausal osteoporosis. *JOGN Nurs* 1982; 11:214–219.

Kaplan FS: Osteoporosis. *Clin Symp* 1983; 35(5):2–32.

Krause MB, Mahan LK: *Food, Nutrition, and Diet Therapy,* 7th ed. Philadelphia: Saunders, 1984.

Lane JM, Vigorita VJ: Osteoporosis. *Ortho Clin North Am* 1984; 15(4): 711–728.

Lindsay R: The role of sex hormones and synthetic steroids in prevention of post-menopausal osteoporosis. *Clin Invest Med* 1982; 5(2/3):189–194.

Lukert BP: Osteoporosis: A review and update. *Arch Phys Med Rehabil* 1982; 63:480–487.

Merkow RL, Lane JM: Current concepts of Paget's disease of bone. *Ortho Clin North Am* 1984; 15(4): 747–763.

Mirra JM: *Bone Tumors: Diagnosis and Treatment.* Philadelphia: Lippincott, 1980.

Mourad L: *Nursing Care of Adults With Orthopedic Conditions.* New York: Wiley, 1980.

Powell M: *Orthopaedic Nursing and Rehabilitation,* 8th ed. London: Churchill Livingstone, 1982.

Richards M: Osteoporosis. *Geriatr Nurs* 1982; 3(2):98–102.

Searls K et al: External fixation: General principles of patient management. *CCQ* 1983; 6(1):45–54.

Southwick JR, Callahan DJ: A study of blood drainage patterns on synthetic cast materials. *Ortho Nurs* 1985; 4(2): 72–75.

Sproles KJ: Nursing care of skeletal pins: A closer look. *Ortho Nurs* 1985; 4(1): 11–19.

Winick M: *Nutrition in Health and Disease.* New York: Wiley, 1980.

Wolanin MO, Phillips LRF: *Confusion: Prevention and Care.* St. Louis: Mosby, 1981.

Suggested Readings

Brunner NA: *Orthopedic Nursing,* 4th ed. St. Louis: Mosby, 1983. A programmed learning text covering nursing care of orthopedic clients. Includes surgical and nonsurgical care.

Kuska BM: Acute onset of compartment syndrome. *JEN* 1982; 8(2):75–79. The etiology and treatment of compartment syndrome are described as well as an explanation of how to measure compartmental pressure.

Lane PL, Lee MM: New synthetic casts: What nurses need to know. *Ortho Nurs* 1982; 1(6):13–20. An excellent article on the use and care of various types of synthetic casts.

Milazzo V: An exercise class for patients in traction. *Am J Nurs* 1981; 81:1842–1844. An account of what a group of nurses did to decrease boredom and prepare clients in traction for crutch walking. A list of sample exercises is provided.

Notelovitz M, Ware M: *Stand Tall: The Informed Women's Guide to Preventing Osteoporosis.* Gainesville, FL: Triad Publishing, 1982. From the public library, the book gives an overview of osteoporosis including treatment and prevention.

Southmayd W, Hoffman M: *Sports Health: The Complete Book of Athletic Injuries.* New York: Quick Fox, 1981. From the public library, this book describes the causes, symptoms, treatment, and prevention of recurrence of sports injuries.

Trigueiro M: Pin site care protocol. *Can Nurse* 1983; 79(8):24–26. A detailed report of pin site care, suggesting an alternative method for care.

Chapter 59

Specific Disorders of the Joints

Carolyn Czech Montgomery
Rita A. Colicchia
SueAnn Wooster Ames

Objectives

When you have finished studying this chapter, you should be able to:

Discuss joint problems of multifactorial origin, including ankylosing spondylitis, Reiter's syndrome, psoriatic arthritis, gout and pseudogout, low back pain, scoliosis, Charcot joints, and carpal tunnel syndrome.

Identify the clinical manifestations and treatments for degenerative joint disease.

Describe the articular and extra-articular manifestations of rheumatoid arthritis (RA) and the various approaches to treatment of this disease.

Compare RA with Felty's syndrome in regard to symptoms and signs, clinical manifestations, and treatment.

Explain the nursing interventions for Sjögren's syndrome and shoulder–hand syndrome.

Recognize the circumstances leading to infectious disorders of the joints, describing the kinds of pathogens involved, their differential diagnosis, and treatment measures.

Describe the various kinds of benign tumors of the joints and specific nursing interventions for these disorders.

Discuss the clinical manifestations and therapeutic measures for synovial sarcoma and clear cell sarcoma.

Specify the nurse's role in the therapeutic and preventive care of traumatic disorders of the joints.

A joint is the point of articulation between two bones. Because of their location and constant use, joints are susceptible to stress, injury, and inflammation. This chapter discusses the major disorders affecting the joints.

Section I: Disorders of Multifactorial Origin

Joint problems of multifactorial origin include a wide variety of conditions, including ankylosing spondylitis, Reiter's syndrome, psoriatic arthritis, gout and pseudogout, low back pain (low back strain and intervertebral disk disease), scoliosis, Charcot joints, and carpal tunnel syndrome.

Joint disorders of multifactorial origin usually affect people in the prime of life. The disruption of normal life activities can be monumental, and families and job security can disintegrate unless clients seek proper medical attention and counseling. Although only gout can be cured, the other disorders can be controlled to varying degrees so that in most instances the client can maintain a fairly normal lifestyle.

ANKYLOSING SPONDYLITIS

Ankylosing spondylitis (Marie-Strümpell disease) is an inflammatory disease of the ligamentous insertion site into the bone (primarily the bones of the spine). Although in the past it was considered a variant of rheumatoid arthritis (RA), new evidence disputes this assertion and classifies ankylosing spondylitis as a prototype of a group of disorders listed as seronegative spondyloarthropathies. These disorders are characterized by the absence of the rheumatoid factor in the blood, the lack of rheumatoid nodules, and the presence of HLA-B27 histocompatibility antigen in the blood. Although the illness is more severe in men, women are affected equally often—a fact only recently discovered.

Although ankylosing spondylitis was thought to be rare, recent studies have shown it has a 1% incidence in the general population. The etiology is unknown, but theories focus on heredity, an immune response, the *Klebsiella* bacteria, and other infectious agents.

Clinical Manifestations

Articular symptoms and signs of ankylosing spondylitis include the gradual onset of back pain and morning stiffness. The client has a history of pain for 3 months or more that typically improves with exercise. Clients affected are usually under age 40 and have a strong history of relatives who are positive for HLA-B27. Physical examination of the spine reveals sacroiliac tenderness, decreased spinal mobility, and muscle spasm.

All too often, people do not seek medical help until there is already deformity of the spine and contractures of the hips. Deformities can be prevented with proper client education and physical therapy, although some degree of spinal mobility loss will still occur. Because of the similarity of symptoms, ankylosing spondylitis and intervertebral disk disease must be carefully differentiated. Table 59–1 shows their differences and similarities. Intervertebral disk disease is discussed later in the section on low back pain.

Peripheral joint involvement is possible, exhibiting pain, swelling, and effusion. Hip and shoulder symptoms may be most apparent. Table 59–2 shows the differentiating characteristics of ankylosing spondylitis and RA, a disease discussed later in this chapter.

Extra-articular symptoms and signs of ankylosing spondylitis include fatigue, fever, and weight loss. Conjunctivitis or iritis may occur, and both are more frequent in clients with peripheral joint involvement. The limited spinal mobility decreases thoracic excursion, predisposing the client to respiratory difficulties. Cardiovascular problems such as aortic incompetence, cardiomegaly, and conduction defects may occur. Neurologic problems may be seen in later stages with an insidious onset of leg or buttock pain; sensory, motor, bowel, and bladder impairment; or a combination.

A diagnosis of ankylosing spondylitis is made by x-ray determination of bilateral sacroiliitis of the sacroiliac joints. Vertebral squaring, or a "Bamboo spine," also may be seen in some clients (Figure 59–1). Although HLA-B27 antigen is usually present, it is not diagnostic. There are no specific abnormalities in laboratory test results, but an elevated ESR and a mild anemia may be present.

Therapeutic Measures

The majority of individuals with ankylosing spondylitis today have a good prognosis, but client education is important to ensure compliance with prescribed regimens. Although chronic discomfort and decreased spinal mobility may occur, total ankylosis occurs in only a few people.

The cornerstone of management is physical therapy, and constant effort is required to promote extension of the spine and maintain normal posture in sleeping, standing, sitting, and walking. A warm shower before exercise helps the client perform extension exercises. The client should change positions frequently and avoid bending over for long periods of time. Deep breathing exercises are essential, and swimming is one of the best general exercises a client with ankylosing spondylitis can perform.

The following exercises from Cohen and Killian (1982) can also be helpful:

- *Vertebral push-ups.* The client stands in a corner with arms fully extended and hands on an adjacent wall. The client falls forward as far as possible and then returns to the starting position.

- *Rocking chair maneuver.* The client lies prone on the

Table 59–1 **Differentiating Characteristics of Ankylosing Spondylitis and Intervertebral Disk Disease**

Characteristic	Ankylosing Spondylitis	Intervertebral Disk Disease
Morning stiffness	Present	Absent
Amelioration of discomfort with rest	Absent	Present
Amelioration of discomfort with activity	Present	Absent
Onset	Insidious	Rapid
Neurologic deficits	Absent	Present
Radiation of pain to legs	Infrequent, usually not below knees	Frequent
ESR	Elevated	Normal
HLA-B27	Present in 90% of cases	Present in 7% of cases
Sacroiliitis	Present, but may be radiographically absent early in disease	Absent

SOURCE: Reprinted with permission from Cohen LM, Killian PJ: Spondyloarthropathies: The spondylitis associated disorders. *Postgrad Med* (Nov) 1982; 72:128.

Table 59–2 **Differentiating Characteristics of Ankylosing Spondylitis and Rheumatoid Arthritis**

Characteristic	Ankylosing Spondylitis	Rheumatoid Arthritis
Age	20 to 40	20 to 60s
Sex	Predominantly men	Predominantly women
Race	Predominantly white	Similar distribution among whites and blacks
Familial association	Strong	Weak
Arthritis	Oligoarticular, asymmetric	Polyarticular, symmetric
Joint erosions	Uncommon	Common
Sacroiliitis	Present	Absent
Eye involvement	Iritis	Episcleritis/scleritis
Rheumatoid nodules	Absent	Present
ESR	Elevated	Elevated
HLA-B27	Present in 90% of cases	Present in 7% of cases
Rheumatoid factor	Absent	Present in 80% of cases

SOURCE: Reprinted with permission from Cohen LM, Killian PJ: Spondyloarthropathies: The spondylitis associated disorders. *Postgrad Med* (Nov) 1982; 72:129.

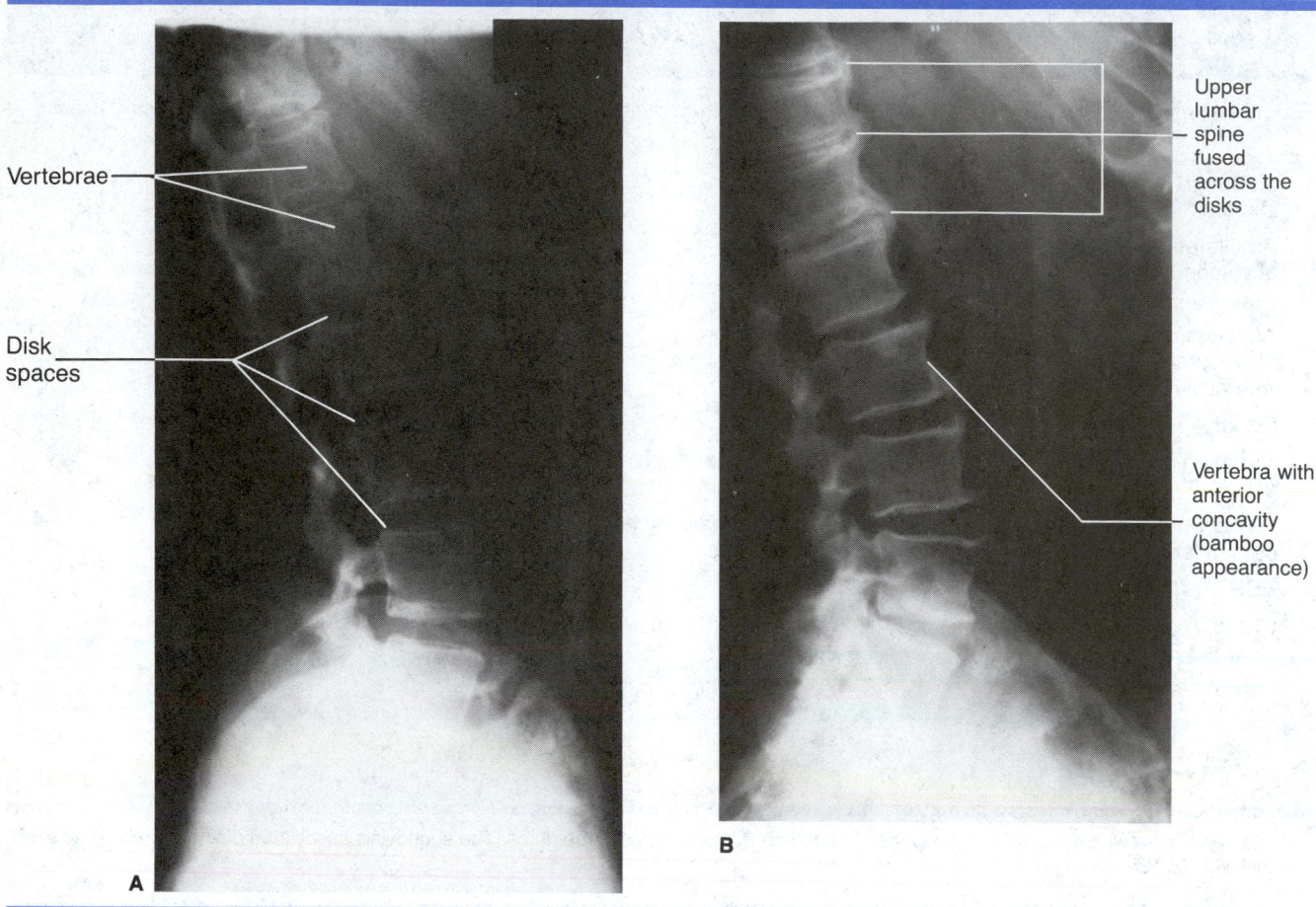

Vertebrae

Disk spaces

Upper lumbar spine fused across the disks

Vertebra with anterior concavity (bamboo appearance)

A

B

Figure 59–1

A. Normal lumbar spine. Vertebrae normal in size, shape, and density. Disk spaces between vertebrae are normal.
B. Ankylosing spondylitis. Note the fusion across the disk spaces in the upper lumbar area. Also note the anterior concavity of the vertebrae enhancing their resemblance to bamboo. (Courtesy of Health Care Plan, Buffalo, NY)

floor, raises the head and legs, and arches the back. This is held for 5 seconds and then repeated.

Indomethacin (Indocin) is usually the drug of choice for treatment of ankylosing spondylitis. Other nonsteroidal anti-inflammatory drugs (NSAIDs) or aspirin can also be used.

Total hip replacement may benefit clients with severe hip involvement. Occasionally, flexion deformities of the spine are surgically corrected by vertebral wedge resection and refusion.

Offspring of people with HLA-B27 antigen should seek genetic counseling.

Specific Nursing Measures

Assess the joint range of motion, thoracic excursion, and degree of client discomfort. Instruct the client and family or significant other in proper positioning, encourage frequent position change, and discourage heavy lifting. The client should maintain proper posture in all positions. Advise the client to sleep on a firm mattress with no pillow, if possible. Assist the client with vertebral push-ups and the rocking chair maneuver when indicated. Instruct the client in deep breathing, chest expansion, and back exercises. The client should be urged to discontinue smoking because of possible future lung involvement.

Administer medications as prescribed. Be sure to give them with food or antacids to decrease the chance of gastrointestinal disturbances. Indomethacin is known to cause headaches and elevate blood pressure in some people, so monitor clients closely for these signs. Explain the action and side effects of any drugs taken to both client and significant others. Applications of heat, cold, or massage may also be prescribed for pain relief.

REITER'S SYNDROME

Reiter's syndrome is an asymmetric arthritis occurring with urethritis and conjunctivitis. As in ankylosing spondylitis, there is an association with the histocompatibility antigen HLA-B27. The triad of symptoms may follow dysentery or a sexually transmitted disease. *Shigella, Salmonella,* and *Chlamydia* are a few of the agents thought to be involved. Males between the ages of 20 and 40 are most commonly affected.

Clinical Manifestations

In Reiter's syndrome, an acute onset of arthritis affects two or more joints and may recur. The knees, ankles, and small joints of the feet are most frequently affected. Large effusions may be present. A "sausage toe" is a typical lesion resulting from inflammation of the interphalangeal joints and the flexor tendon sheath. The joints are warm, erythematous, and painful. Urethritis may be manifested after an episode of diarrhea. Prostatitis, seminal vesiculitis, and cystitis also may occur. Women may have asymptomatic cervicitis and urethritis.

Conjunctivitis may be so mild that it escapes notice by the client. The discharge is sterile and subsides quickly. Uveitis, however, can occur later in the disease and cause debility. Mucocutaneous lesions on the glans penis, mouth, palms, and soles may be seen. Oral ulcers are painless and usually not clinically noticed because they disappear in a few days.

Clients with Reiter's syndrome and a positive HLA-B27 may develop ankylosing spondylitis. It is not known, however, whether a person who is positive for HLA-B27 and develops Reiter's syndrome is more likely to develop ankylosing spondylitis than a healthy person who is positive for HLA-B27. Cardiovascular involvement may include first-degree heart block, complete heart block, S-T segment changes, palpitations, transient murmurs, pericardial friction rub, and aortic regurgitation.

There is no absolute diagnostic test for Reiter's syndrome, so a detailed history and physical examination are used to make the diagnosis. X-rays show nothing in early illness, but progression of the disease brings narrowing of the joint space, erosive changes, and possibly calcaneal spurs.

The ESR may be elevated, and a mild leukocytosis may be present. The HLA-B27 antigen is found in a majority of clients. Synovial fluid examination shows an increase in white blood cells and is helpful in ruling out infectious joint disease. The rheumatoid factor is negative.

Therapeutic Measures

Tetracycline 500 mg q.i.d. for 14 days is the treatment of choice for nonspecific urethritis. The arthritis is treated with indomethacin or phenylbutazone. Nonsteroidal anti-inflammatory drugs (NSAIDs) or salicylates may also effectively treat some clients. When more aggressive treatment is needed, immunosuppressive drugs are used. Physical therapy is essential to prevent flexion contractures.

Specific Nursing Measures

When taking a history of a client with monoarticular or asymmetrical arthritis, ask about urethritis, inflammation of the glans penis, eye disease, and mouth ulcers. Inquiring about bowel function is also important because diarrhea may precipitate Reiter's syndrome. Include back pain and stiffness in a review of systems.

Instruct the client in physical therapy activities, and put joints through range-of-motion (ROM) exercises where indicated. Finally, explain the side effects of medications, and help clients schedule medications around food.

PSORIATIC ARTHRITIS

Psoriasis is often associated with inflammatory arthritis and a negative rheumatoid factor. The psoriatic skin lesions usually precede the arthritis, and in most cases there is correlation between joint flares and skin flares. Clients with psoriasis are most likely to develop joint problems, although many people with psoriasis never have joint symptoms at all. Also, some clients with psoriatic arthritis have very mild psoriatic skin lesions or no lesions. Heredity is the most specific factor in the development of psoriatic arthritis. Environmental factors also may influence this illness, but the exact etiology is unknown.

Clinical Manifestations

The manifestations of psoriatic arthritis vary from client to client. Some have distal joint involvement, whereas others have widespread deformity, ankylosis, and joint destruction. The disease can be symmetrical or asymmetrical, and some clients have spondylitis, sacroiliitis, eye problems, or a combination. Nodules are not present with psoriatic arthritis. Some people have both psoriatic arthritis and RA at the same time.

Silver-white scaly patches are seen on the elbows, legs, scalp, and back. Nails are pitted (20 pits or more per nail), and arthritis is more common with nail changes than with skin lesions. Onycholysis is very common.

Joint symptoms usually begin with the acute onset of pain and swelling of distal interphalangeal (DIP) joints. A goutlike symptom in the great toe often gives a "sausage" appearance to the joint, but the disability is usually not as great as with RA. Spondylitis is often found in families with a strong background of psoriatic arthritis. Upon x-ray examination, some people show marked articular destruction with resorption of bone. A shortening of the middle phalanx of the DIP joints of fingers and toes has a characteristic cuplike appearance, and sometimes an entire phalanx is destroyed. Extra-articular symptoms include some conjunctivitis, episcleritis or uveitis, and no rheumatoid nodules.

Laboratory studies reveal some anemia, an elevated ESR, a negative rheumatoid factor, positive antinuclear antibodies (ANA), and an elevated uric acid level. Diagnosis is made by considering nails, peripheral arthritis, and spinal involvement. Nail and skin changes in psoriatic arthritis may be hard to differentiate from those in Reiter's syndrome.

Therapeutic Measures

Therapeutic measures for psoriatic arthritis are aimed at both the arthritis and the psoriasis. The treatment of psoriasis is covered in Chapter 79, and the treatment of RA is covered later in this chapter. The only pharmacological treatment measure for RA that is not applicable to psoriatic arthritis is gold (chrysotherapy). Gold can cause pruritus and dermatitis, which aggravate the psoriasis.

Specific Nursing Measures

See Section III in this chapter for a discussion of the specific nursing measures for RA. Nursing measures for psoriasis are covered in Chapter 79.

GOUT

Gout is a disease that produces joint inflammation because of the deposition of uric acid crystals (monosodium urate crystals) in the articular tissue. Deposition occurs either because of an increased production of uric acid or a decrease in uric acid excretion. Gout can be classified as either primary or secondary. In primary gout, an unknown metabolic defect is responsible for increased serum uric acid. Men are most often affected, and the disease seems to run in families.

The reason for the increase in serum uric acid in secondary gout is either an excessive turnover of cells, as in leukemia, Hodgkin's disease, or myeloma, to name a few, or impaired excretion of uric acid by the kidney because of chronic kidney failure or the effects of drugs on the kidney, especially diuretics. Some other problems that may precipitate attacks of secondary gout are alcohol, starvation, psoriasis, and sarcoidosis.

Clinical Manifestations

Kelley (1981) describes the following four stages of gout.

Asymptomatic Hyperuricemia
In the first stage of gout, the uric acid level is elevated, but there are no arthritis symptoms, tophi (nodules that contain monosodium urate crystals), or calculi. About 5% of these clients will develop gouty arthritis. In men, hyperuricemia is defined as a uric acid level of 7.0 mg/100 mL or greater, and in women as 6.0 mg/100 mL or greater. A value greater than 7.0 mg/100 mL increases the risk of renal calculi or gout attacks. Gout usually occurs after 20 to 30 years of sustained hyperuricemia. However, some people will have renal colic before their first episode of arthritis.

Acute Gouty Arthritis
The primary manifestation of the acute gouty arthritis stage is an extremely painful arthritis, usually monoarticular, beginning at night. Later the joint is so swollen, red, and tender that the client cannot even tolerate the pressure of bedclothes. There can be polyarthritis and fever. The attacks are of short duration, and intervals are completely free from pain. Ninety percent of individuals experience their acute attack in the great toe (podagra—involvement of the first metatarsophalangeal joint) (Figure 59–2). The acute attack can be caused by minor trauma, surgery, or excessive alcohol consumption.

Intercritical Gout
After an acute attack of gout, 7% of clients will never have a second episode. Most, however, will have another attack within 1 year, although the interval may be as long as 10 years. The second attack is polyarticular and more severe, lasts longer, and may occur with fever.

Chronic Tophaceous Gout
If untreated, individuals progress to chronic polyarticular disease and develop tophi. These are difficult to differentiate from rheumatoid nodules on physical examination. Tophi occur in cartilage, synovial membrane, and soft tissue. If they ulcerate, a white, chalky, pasty material containing uric acid crystals is found (Figure 59–3).

Other manifestations of gout include renal dysfunction (which occurs in 90% of clients with a history of gouty arthritis) and albuminuria (a possible initial manifestation). Renal calculi occur in 10% to 25% of clients with gout, sometimes before joint symptoms appear. Obesity, elevated triglyceride levels, and hypertension may also accompany gout.

Initially, there are no x-ray abnormalities, but later bone erosions with an overhanging margin may be seen. This helps differentiate gout from RA.

Diagnosis is made by using a polarized light microscope to visualize uric acid crystals within the white blood

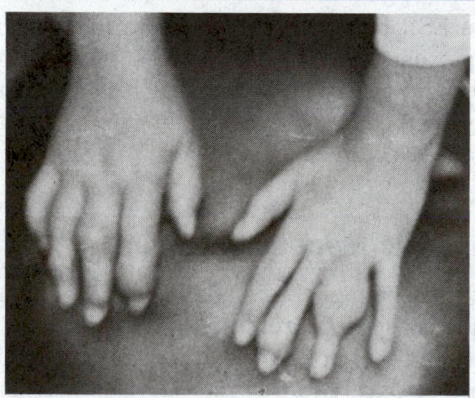

Figure 59–2

Tophaceous gout of the hands. (Courtesy of Ralph Argen MD, Buffalo, NY)

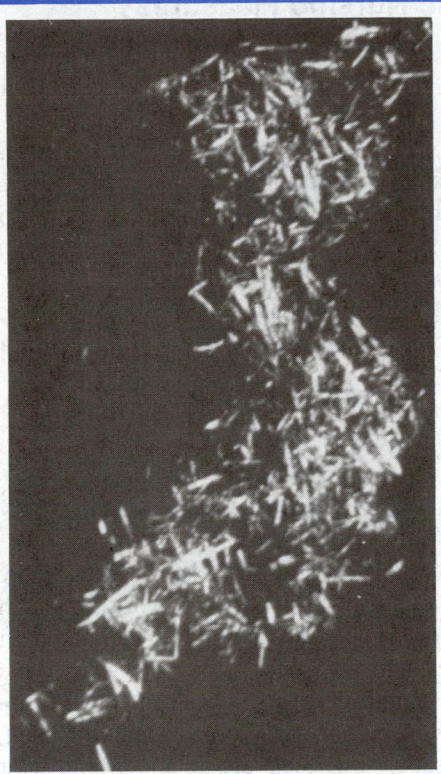

Figure 59–3

Uric acid crystals as seen in aspirate or tissue sections of tophaceous deposits. (Courtesy of Millard Fillmore Hospital, Buffalo, NY)

cells found in synovial fluid from the inflamed joints. It is important to culture synovial fluid to rule out infection. A presumptive diagnosis can be made if the client has hyperuricemia, classical clinical features, and a dramatic response to colchicine.

Therapeutic Measures

Acute attacks of gout respond to rest and NSAIDs such as naproxen (Naprosyn) and indomethacin (Indocin). Colchicine can also be given orally; however, since the higher doses needed cause abdominal cramps and diarrhea, it is not usually used. Colchicine is also available for IV use but is used rarely because it is an irritant and causes severe pain and necrosis if it infiltrates. The drug should be diluted in normal saline and infused in no less than 5 minutes. Other side effects are bone marrow depression, seizures, alopecia, hepatocellular failure, mental depression, ascending paralysis, respiratory depression, and death. Toxic effects are greater in those clients with hepatic, bone marrow, and renal disease.

According to Kelley (1981), indomethacin is the treatment of choice in clients with an established diagnosis of gouty arthritis. If a single joint is involved, aspiration and intra-articular injection of steroids are beneficial. The acute symptoms usually resolve in a few days.

The long-term management of gout includes measures to lower serum uric acid levels; these should be initiated after the acute attack subsides for clients who continue to be hyperuricemic. Small doses of colchicine (1 to 2 mg q.d.) may be used prophylactically. In addition, antihyperuricemic agents are often used to lower serum uric acid levels to less than 7.0 mg/100 mL. These either increase the renal excretion of uric acid or decrease uric acid production.

Drugs that increase the renal excretion of uric acid include sulfinpyrazone (Anturane) and probenecid (Benemid). Their long-term use promotes resorption of tissue deposits and tophi. Aspirin should not be given with these drugs since it blocks the uricosuric effect. These agents can precipitate an acute gouty attack because they mobilize tissue deposits of uric acid. Therefore, they are used only after the full resolution of a gouty attack. They are often used in combination with prophylactic colchicine or NSAIDs to prevent future episodes of gout. These drugs also can precipitate renal calculi, so it is important to maintain adequate fluid intake.

Allopurinol (Zyloprim) decreases uric acid production. The usual dose is 300 mg q.d., although it is used in a lower dose if there is renal dysfunction. Significant side effects include gastrointestinal distress, skin rashes, fever, alopecia, bone marrow suppression, hepatitis, jaundice, and vasculitis.

Other measures that may improve the client's symptoms are weight reduction, joint rest, joint protection, heat or cold therapy, and a decreased purine diet. Diet restriction is usually limited to alcohol and glandular meats. Strict purine restriction is unrealistic since most foods contain purines.

Specific Nursing Measures

Assess joints frequently for erythema, tenderness, tophi, and swelling. Bed cradles are used in the hospital so bedclothes will not press on painful joints, and clients at home can improvise similar protective devices. Resting the affected joint is important, and nonpainful joints should be put through frequent ROM exercises. As the acute symptoms subside, the affected joint should also be exercised. Apply heat or ice as ordered.

Maintain fluid intake at 2 to 3 L per day to decrease the chance of renal calculi. Clients should understand the rationale for increased fluids, which is even more important for those taking uricosuric medications. Monitor intake and output carefully. If a renal calculus is suspected, urine must be strained in an attempt to trap the calculus for laboratory evaluation. For the hospitalized client, the nurse should monitor all laboratory reports for uric acid and albuminuria. Also, be alert for gout attacks 24 to 96 hours after any surgical procedure on a client with gout.

Client education includes instructing the client and significant others in the use of heat and cold for joint symptoms and the importance of increased oral fluids. Because many clients with gout are overweight, a condition that stresses the joints, weight reduction is important. Teach clients with gout to avoid rich foods, which are high in purines and contribute to elevated triglyceride levels and obesity. Other purine-rich foods are organ meats (eg, liver and sweetbreads), alcohol, and fried foods. Base-forming foods, such as milk, cream, vegetables (except corn and lentils), fruits (except cranberries, plums, and prunes), molasses, carbonated beverages, and baking soda and baking powder, may be helpful. They will alkalinize the pH of urine.

The client should understand the action of all medications taken. Provide written instructions that include the amount, dose, frequency, route of administration, and potential side effects. Tell the client taking probenecid or sulfinpyrazone to avoid aspirin.

PSEUDOGOUT

Pseudogout, or calcium pyrophosphate crystal deposition (CPPD), is an inflammatory arthritis caused by the deposition of calcium pyrophosphate dihydrate crystals in the joint. X-ray findings of articular cartilage calcification usually accompany it. It is equally distributed in both sexes and generally occurs in people over age 50. Many clients with pseudogout have other disorders such as diabetes, hypothyroidism, and gout, to name a few.

The arthritis in pseudogout is probably brought on by a release of crystals from the cartilage into the joint cavity. This results in the activation of vasoactive and chemotactic factors. The mechanism for initial deposition into the cartilage is unknown.

Clinical Manifestations

In pseudogout, arthritis occurs in the knee and other large joints. The joint is erythematous, swollen, warm, and painful. Like gout, pseudogout is usually monoarticular, but involvement of other joints can follow in succession. Attacks are often precipitated by trauma, surgery, or medical illness. Attacks are rapid and reach their peak in 12 to 36 hours. Episodes are intermittent, usually involve the same joint, and last about 1 to 2 weeks. Joints are normal between attacks.

Diagnosis is made by microscopic inspection of joint fluid for calcium pyrophosphate dihydrate crystals, as well as by x-ray evidence of cartilage calcification. As in gout and all monoarticular arthritis, bacterial cultures and smears should be done on the aspirated synovial fluid.

Therapeutic Measures

Acute attacks of pseudogout are treated with nonsteroidal anti-inflammatory drugs. Sometimes intermittent intra-articular steroid injections are used. However, the deposition of calcium pyrophosphate dihydrate crystals cannot be reversed or prevented (Petersdorf et al., 1983).

Specific Nursing Measures

Nursing measures for pseudogout include careful joint assessment, ice or heat therapy as prescribed, and monitoring for symptoms and signs of systemic illness and side effects of medications. The nurse assists the physician with intra-articular steroid injections. Ask clients about allergies before the injection because lidocaine (Xylocaine) is often given along with the steroid. A sterile container is needed for the joint fluid specimen.

Client education for home care includes instruction in heat or ice therapy, ROM exercises, and the nature and side effects of drugs. If the client is overweight, a weight reduction diet promotes the long-term health of the knees, the major weight-bearing joints.

LOW BACK PAIN

Low back pain is a term that includes many different types of problems. A client could have a mild strain or a malignant tumor when first consulting a physician about this condition. Low back pain is one of the major causes of disability in North America and is, therefore, of extreme importance. Two common disorders causing low back pain will be discussed: low back strain and intervertebral disk disease.

Erect posture and a sedentary lifestyle predispose people to low back pain. Certain stressors that put unequal pressure on the spine also contribute: congenital anomalies, leg length discrepancy, asymmetrical development of the spine, weak abdominal muscles, and acquired injuries. Obesity also contributes to low back pain.

Clinical Manifestations

Low back strain is the most common cause of low back pain. There is usually a history of injury, most often a minor injury followed by an immediate or delayed pain in the lower back. Pain can radiate down into the buttocks and even down the back of the leg (sciatic type of pain). Any motion of the spine causes pain, but coughing and sneezing do not aggravate it. Clients often assume distorted positions to be comfortable.

Many lifestyle characteristics predispose people to low back pain, so they may be easily injured when a minor trauma occurs. Lack of exercise, weak abdominal muscles, and obesity all contribute to the problem. Additional influencing factors include improper reaching, lifting, or bending; sitting too long in overstuffed, nonsupportive chairs; lying on soft, lumpy mattresses; or riding in a car for long periods in low bucket seats. History taking should include information about these aspects of the client's life. People who carry a large wallet or credit card case in a rear pants pocket cause asymmetrical pressure on the lower back when sitting, which also contributes to low back pain.

Physical examination reveals tenderness and spasm of the paravertebral muscles. The ROM of the lower lumbar spine decreases, and tender areas may be palpated at the posterosuperior iliac spines. There may be a discrepancy in leg length.

The straight leg raising test to differentiate low back strain from herniated disk is done with the client supine. Raise the leg on the affected side straight up until pain is experienced, then lower the leg slightly and dorsiflex the foot, which stretches the sciatic nerve (Figure 59–4). If pain occurs in the back or along the sciatic nerve distribution with dorsiflexion of the foot, herniated disk is suspected. In low back strain, there is no pain on dorsiflexion of the foot and no sensory, motor, or reflex changes noted in the legs.

With intervertebral disk disease, there is severe low back pain with radiation into the buttocks, legs, and feet, usually on one side. Coughing, sneezing, bending, and riding in a car will increase the pain. Disk disease is common in elderly people, because compression fractures of the vertebrae increase from osteoporosis. Being on steroids compounds the problem.

Physical examination usually reveals sensorimotor loss and, later, weakness and muscle atrophy. The straight leg raising test induces a sciatic type of pain rather than back pain. The most common location is the disk between L4-L5 or L5-S1. Pain is relieved with rest and increased with motion. Disk disease can also affect the cervical area, C5-C6 or C6-C7. Usually, a chronic aching pain radiates to the shoulders and into the neck or goes down to the arm and into the hand. The hands and fingers may be numb.

Diagnosis of a herniated disk can be determined by history and physical examination. A computerized tomography (CT) scan confirms the diagnosis and can be used to monitor treatment. Both nucleated disks and lateral spinal stenosis can be seen on a CT scan.

Diagnosis of low back pain should include a full blood count; ESR; a biochemical profile including serum calcium, phosphate, alkaline phosphatase, and serum protein levels; and electrophoresis. Men should have a serum acid phosphatase drawn and a thorough rectal examination to rule out cancer of the prostate. Spine x-rays are not taken routinely but should be ordered if physical examination suggests even a remote possibility of ruptured disk.

Myelograms are only necessary if surgery is being considered. A CT scan is ordered if spine x-ray results are within normal limits but the client's condition does not improve with treatment.

Therapeutic Measures

Low back strain is usually self-limiting. Bed rest, analgesics, muscle relaxants, heat or ice therapy, and flexion exercises can relieve the initial spasm. After severe pain subsides, abdominal muscle strengthening exercises and back exercises can prevent recurrences. Lumbar girdle support also can be helpful to younger clients.

The conservative treatment of intervertebral disk disease involves bed rest, sometimes for as long as 1 to 3

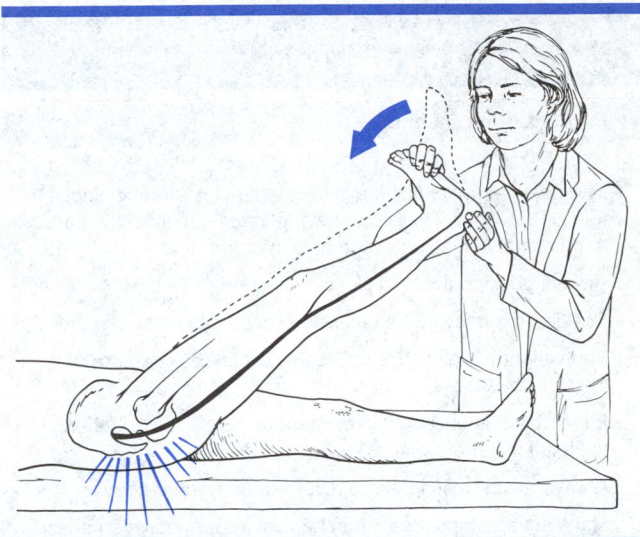

Figure 59–4

Straight leg raising exam in which dorsiflexion of the foot produces sciatic pain.

months. Traction, lumbar corset support, analgesics, physical therapy, and exercises are all potentially helpful approaches to treatment. Epidural injections with steroids can sometimes help clients who are not responsive to other measures. Transcutaneous electrical nerve stimulation (TENS) also helps relieve pain in some clients. Because not everyone responds, clients are advised to rent the unit for 2 weeks and use it at home before purchasing it.

Chemonucleolysis, a procedure with some risk, may be considered for clients who do not do well with other treatment. The enzyme chymopapain is injected into the disk to shrink it, thereby relieving pressure. The other option is surgical intervention; laminectomy is the most common procedure. Both chemonucleolysis and laminectomy are discussed in Chapter 60.

Specific Nursing Measures

The primary function of the nurse in the management of low back disorders is prevention. Therefore, the main thrust is toward client education, which includes instruction about proper lifting technique, muscle-strengthening exercises, and posture (Box 59–1).

Most people lift incorrectly, using a straight back and flexed knees. This technique throws people off balance, and they either fall or incorrectly straighten their legs and flex their back to avoid falling, straining the lumbar area (Owen, 1980).

In addition to poor lifting techniques, weak lumbar muscles, weak abdominal muscles, prolonged sitting, poor posture, and obesity all contribute to back insults. Therefore, the strengthening of abdominal and lumbar muscle groups, along with proper lifting techniques, proper posture, and weight reduction, reduces the risks of back injuries. All exercises should be done gently and slowly to build

Box 59–1 Approaches to the Prevention of Low Back Pain

Proper Lifting Technique

The best height for lifting a load is when it is already placed 2 feet off the floor. Therefore, having loads consistently placed at this level in the workplace aids in proper lifting.

Always position the load close to the body.

Position the body so that muscle groups can work together.

The weight to be lifted is excessive if it is 35% or more of the lifter's body weight.

If the object is bulky (30 in or more to a side) do not attempt to lift it if it is more than 20 lb.

Always avoid twisting; try to pivot with the entire body.

Make several trips; use a mechanical apparatus when possible; and do not hesitate to ask for help if needed.

Do not bend over at right angles.

Make sure no obstacles are in the way and that the feet are secure.

Exercises

Flexed-knee sit-ups to strengthen the abdomen

Bent-knee leg lifts to strengthen the abdomen

Knee–chest leg lifts to stretch the lower back and tighten the abdomen

Back flattening to stretch the lower back and tighten the abdomen

Posture

Sleep on the back or side with a small pillow. Keep the knees flexed while in bed. A small pillow under the knees may help, but a pillow should be used cautiously if there are joint problems with the knees, since flexion contracture of the knees can occur quickly.

Sleep on a supportive mattress.

Use a straight-back chair when sitting.

Do not cross the legs or sit with the legs straight out on a footstool.

Wear flat-heeled shoes.

When standing, use a small stool to rest one leg at a time; shift the weight from one leg to the other when standing for long periods.

up endurance. In addition, exercises should always be done with the knees flexed.

Teach clients about the side effects of medication; for example, muscle relaxants may cause some drowsiness, and NSAIDs may exacerbate ulcer problems. Explain the proper and discriminate use of analgesics, because back pain can be a long-term problem. If the client is hospitalized, explain procedures and therapies before they are

encountered to allay anxiety. Before myelography, ask the client about allergies; the radiopaque dye contains iodine, and people who are allergic to seafood are usually allergic to the dye. Explain that myelography is an uncomfortable procedure and that sedation will be given beforehand. Following myelography, the client must remain supine for 6 to 9 hours to prevent headache and must drink adequate fluid. Postprocedure care includes monitoring vital signs and assessing neurologic function.

Help the obese client formulate a nutritional and realistic diet. Refer the client to an accessible weight reduction program or begin one.

Offer supportive care for emotional ramifications of back injuries. In addition to the costs from lost wages, medical expenses, and insurance premiums, the costs to the client and family or significant others can be great in psychological trauma.

Explain to the client with a back injury that complete bed rest is essential initially, and that the more activity, the longer it will take to improve. Apply heat and cold therapy safely and instruct the client in home use. Take advantage of massage and other comfort measures to help relieve pain. Finally, perform ROM exercises, and instruct the client in active ROM if other joints are involved.

SCOLIOSIS

Scoliosis is a lateral curvature of the spine, most commonly in the thoracic area with convexity to the right and compensatory convex curves to the left in the cervical and lumbar areas. Scoliosis can be functional (a result of poor posture or leg length discrepancy) or structural (a result of deformity of the vertebral bodies, paralysis, congenital malformations, or idiopathic causes). Idiopathic causes are the most common and appear when the growth spurt begins in adolescence.

Clinical Manifestations

Symptoms of backache, fatigue, and dyspnea occur only after scoliosis is well established. Screening and early referral of children during their elementary school years are essential to prevent long-term problems. Untreated scoliosis can result in pulmonary insufficiency from decreased lung capacity, back pain, degenerative arthritis of the spine, intervertebral disk disease, and sciatica.

The older adult client, most often female, may exhibit kyphosis, a postural curvature of the spine that is due to aging, disk degeneration, atrophy of spinal muscles, osteoporosis, or vertebral collapse. Adults with kyphosis have a rounded back and possibly weakness and generalized fatigue. Kyphosis rarely produces local tenderness except in severe osteoporosis with compression fractures.

Therapeutic Measures

Early treatment of scoliosis consists of exercises, bracing, surgery, or a combination of these. If the client is untreated in adolescence, problems that develop in adulthood can only be treated symptomatically. These clients have severely compromised lung capacity, and any upper respiratory tract infection must be treated aggressively to prevent pooling of secretions, pneumonia, and atelectasis.

Specific Nursing Measures

Clients with scoliosis often have body image problems related to the deformity. They have trouble finding clothes that fit properly and difficulty finding comfortable positions in which to sit or lie. When the older adult with severe kyphosis or scoliosis is hospitalized for any problem, careful attention to positioning is essential (eg, on x-ray tables, operating room tables, and carts, as well as for gynecologic examinations); improper positioning is not only extremely uncomfortable for the client, but it can precipitate a vertebral fracture, especially in a client with osteoporosis.

School nurses are in an ideal position to monitor adolescents for scoliosis with yearly screening. If scoliosis is detected early, exercises and bracing usually can correct the problem. Some adolescents will require surgical intervention, however. With vigilance on the part of school nurses and active programs to instruct parents about signs of scoliosis, adults with scoliosis will be a problem of the past.

To prevent abnormal spinal curvature in older women, usually resulting from osteoporosis, regular exercise and calcium supplements are important. Some sources suggest that women begin calcium supplementation as early as age 35 to prevent the numerous complications of osteoporosis, one of which is vertebral collapse.

CHARCOT JOINTS

Charcot joints, also called *neurologic joints,* develop in clients with a variety of neurologic problems that affect proprioception, deep pain sensation, or both. These disorders include tabes dorsalis (a manifestation of late syphilis), diabetic neuropathy, and syringomyelia. Because of the neurologic loss, the supporting structures of the joint relax; thus, the joint undergoes abnormal trauma and stress during regular motion.

Degeneration of cartilage, recurrent fractures, and marked proliferation of adjacent bone become evident with time. The joints affected depend on the illness. Tabes dorsalis usually affects the knees, hips, ankles, and lumbar spine. Diabetic neuropathy more often affects the tarsometatarsal, metatarsophalangeal, and tarsal joints. Syringomyelia affects the shoulders, elbows, and cervical spine.

Clinical Manifestations

The joint enlarges because of bone overgrowth and effusion. The affected client experiences only mild discomfort in relation to the actual structural abnormalities found on

x-ray examination. A sudden onset of severe pain usually indicates an intra-articular fracture.

Physical examination reveals instability and hypermobility of the joint with effusion and crepitation as the disease progresses. X-ray examination shows cartilage degeneration, loose bodies, and marginal osteophytes that are larger and more disorganized than in degenerative disease. Callous formation is also common, and callous breakdown can cause large ulcers that are difficult to heal.

Therapeutic Measures

The goal of treatment for Charcot joints is to provide stability and relieve pain; treating the underlying neurologic problem does not help the joint problem. External supports are helpful but must be used carefully, because clients will not be aware of abrasions or tender spots caused by braces. Therefore, supports must be inspected frequently and adjusted meticulously. Arthrodesis may provide stability, but frequently the bones do not unite.

Specific Nursing Measures

Assess the joint for ROM, swelling, pain, and muscle strength. Evaluate sensory perception in the extremities. Monitor the client's pain level, and medicate as ordered. Clients should understand that joint rest is important even when there is no pain, because stressful activity on joints can cause fractures.

Client education regarding proper foot care is important to prevent infections and traumatic lesions. Also instruct the client and significant others about safety precautions in the home, such as eliminating loose throw rugs, clutter on stairs, and electric cords in frequently traveled areas. Clients should learn to avoid walking on wet floors and must be extremely careful on icy surfaces in winter.

Instruct the client in the use of crutches or walkers, and demonstrate proper fitting and gait procedures (see Chapter 58). Help the client understand that damage can occur without noticeable discomfort, so regular physician follow-up for monitoring of the illness is advisable.

CARPAL TUNNEL SYNDROME

Carpal tunnel syndrome is an entrapment neuropathy resulting from pressure on the median nerve as it passes through the space formed by the bones of the wrist and the transverse carpal ligament (Figure 59–5). A variety of problems can cause entrapment of the median nerve, including tenosynovitis, trauma, rheumatoid arthritis, gout, pseudogout, acromegaly, edema of pregnancy, and premenstrual edema. Carpal tunnel syndrome, which is much more common in women than men because women's carpal tunnels are smaller, occurs most often in the age range of 40 to 50 years. The dominant hand is affected most often, but the condition can be bilateral. Median nerve paralysis can occur if the nerve entrapment is not treated.

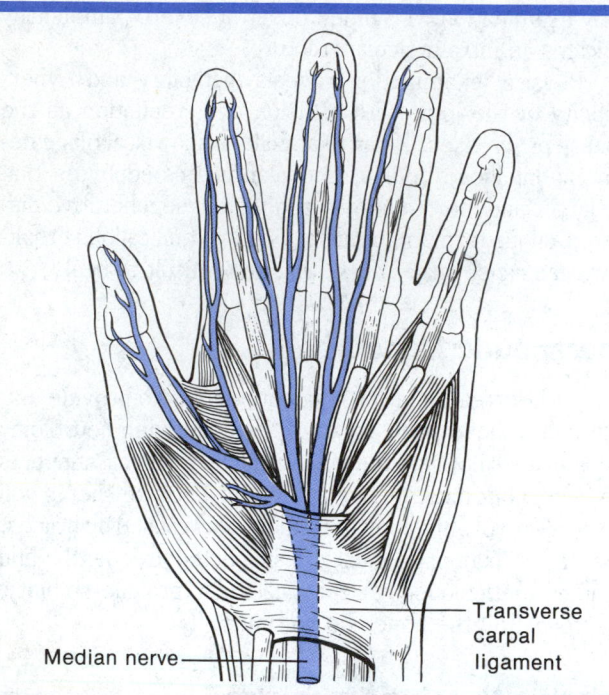

Figure 59–5

Carpal tunnel: anatomic relation of median nerve.

Median nerve

Transverse
carpal
ligament

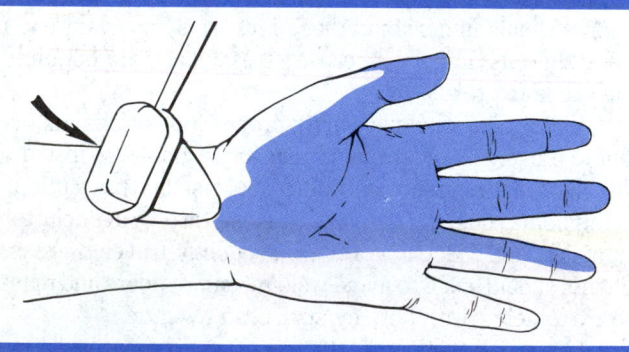

Figure 59–6

Tinel's sign.

Clinical Manifestations

Paresthesia occurs in the areas supplied by the median nerve: the thumb, the index and middle fingers, and the adjacent side of the ring finger. Pain may radiate up the arm and is worse at night. Some fine motor movements may be difficult. There may be atrophy of the thenar eminence (fleshy entrance at the base of the thumb) as time progresses, and abduction of the thumb weakens. A positive Tinel's sign is elicited by light percussion over the median nerve on the flexor surface of the wrist. Normally, there is no response, but in carpal tunnel syndrome the percussion elicits a tingling sensation in the 3½ digits innervated by the median nerve (Figure 59–6). Electromyography can confirm the diagnosis.

Therapeutic Measures

Diuretics and a low-salt diet may be helpful if edema is a factor in carpal tunnel syndrome. Splinting of the wrist at night as well as during the day helps avoid flexion. Local injections of steroids may provide relief for some clients. Surgical release of the transverse carpal ligament may be necessary (see Chapter 60).

Specific Nursing Measures

Explain the nature of carpal tunnel syndrome to the client, and encourage the use of a low-salt diet. Discuss the rationale for diuretic therapy and frequent follow-up with the care provider when diuretics are given on a long-term basis. Check the potassium levels of clients on diuretic therapy every 3 months.

Instruct the client to inspect the skin of the wrist frequently when using the splint. The hands should not be overused, and rest is essential when symptoms are present. The client can remove the splint several times a day to expose the skin and do gentle ROM exercises.

Section II: Degenerative Disorders

DEGENERATIVE JOINT DISEASE

Degenerative joint disease (DJD), also known as *osteoarthritis,* is the only disease to be discussed in this section. One of the most common joint problems seen in clinical practice, it is primarily a disorder of the articular cartilage. Aging seems to be the most important factor in the development of DJD.

In DJD, the bony tissue near the cartilage becomes more dense, and overgrowth (osteophytes or spurs) occurs near the joint edges. The joint space eventually becomes severely narrowed, and ultimately bone rests on bone, resulting in a deformed joint (Figure 59–7).

Degenerative joint disease may be classified as primary or secondary. Primary DJD occurs in the older age group without evidence of predisposing abnormality. It is essentially a wear-and-tear phenomenon. Secondary DJD results from previous joint damage and may begin at any age. Clinical findings are similar in primary and secondary DJD.

Clinical Manifestations

The onset of pain in DJD is gradual. Local pain in the affected joint or joints is usually worse after activity and relieved with rest. There may be a history of some morning stiffness, but this usually lasts for only a brief period.

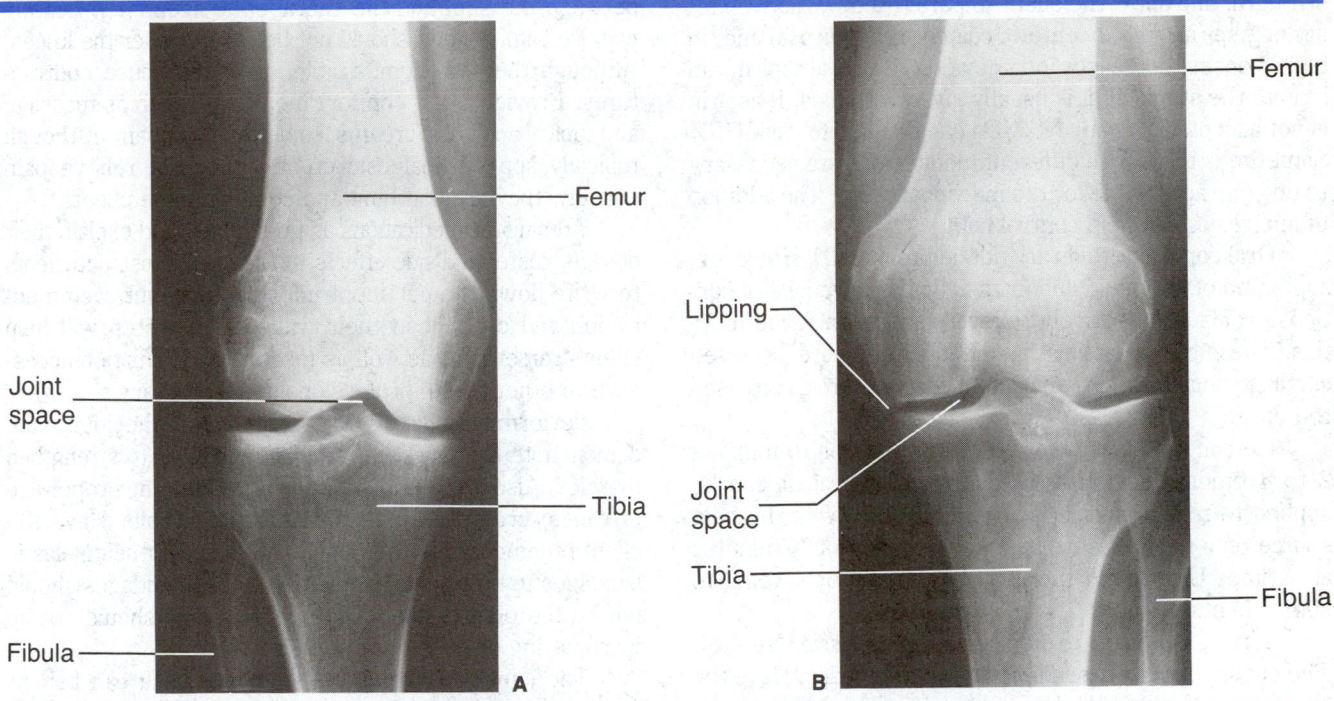

Figure 59-7

A. X-ray of a normal right knee. Note the joint space. **B.** X-ray of the left knee in a client with DJD. Note the joint space narrowing, sharpened articular margins, and the marginal osteophyte formation (lipping). (Courtesy of Health Care Plan, Buffalo, NY)

Because DJD is not a systemic disorder, fatigue is mild and not incapacitating. As time goes by, the joint becomes restricted in motion, and surrounding muscles may atrophy. Pieces of cartilage that break off can irritate the synovial lining, and inflammation and swelling may occur.

Joints most affected by DJD are distal interphalangeal (DIP) joints, proximal interphalangeal (PIP) joints, carpometacarpal joint of the thumb, cervical and lumbar spines, metatarsophalangeal (MTP) joint of the big toe, acromioclavicular joints, knees, hips, and temporomandibular joints. Although DJD is usually asymmetrical, generalized DJD may occur; it mimics a more systemic arthritis when numerous joints are affected at once.

Physical assessment may reveal crepitation on movement of the joint, limited range of motion, and atrophy of surrounding muscles. Bony overgrowths may be seen on the DIP joints of the fingers (Heberden's nodes) (Figure 59-8) and the PIP joints of the fingers (Bouchard's nodes).

X-rays of various joints involved confirm the diagnosis of DJD. Although cartilage itself cannot be seen on x-ray film, DJD involves a narrowing of joint space. There may also be osteophytes and bone cysts as the disease progresses, along with joint deformity. If erosive, inflammatory arthritis is present, the x-ray film may show erosions of the bones that may be difficult to distinguish from RA.

Laboratory analysis of the blood is not diagnostic in DJD, but various tests can rule out the other types of arthritis, which may occur simultaneously. If a joint is aspirated, culture and analysis of the fluid are mandatory to rule out infection. Joint fluid in DJD usually appears normal.

Therapeutic Measures

The goal of treatment in clients with DJD is to relieve pain, decrease swelling, increase joint function, improve muscle

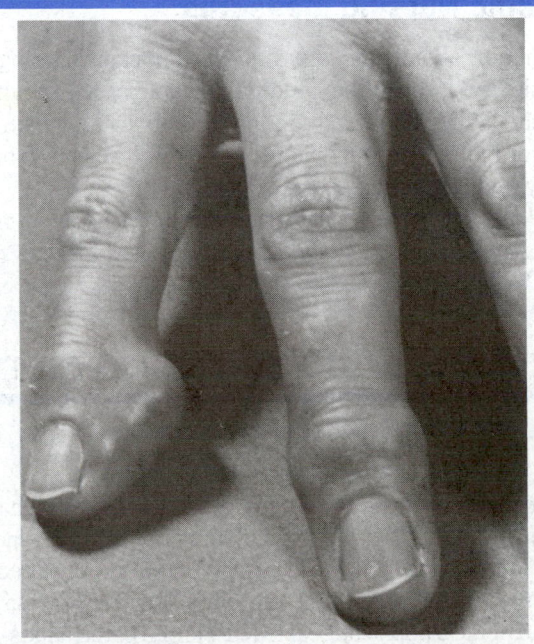

Figure 59-8

Heberden's nodes as seen in DJD. (Courtesy of Millard Fillmore Hospital, Buffalo, NY)

strength, and allow the client to pursue a more active life-style. Aspirin, usually enteric coated, relieves pain and, in higher doses, decreases inflammation. Because aspirin can irritate the stomach, it is usually given with food. If aspirin is not acceptable, many NSAIDs can be used to treat DJD. Sometimes trials with different medications are necessary to find one acceptable for the individual client. The addition of analgesics can help control pain.

Oral corticosteroids are not helpful in DJD. However, aspiration of joint fluid and intra-articular injections of corticosteroids do effectively relieve pain and increase function. These injections must be infrequent because increased cartilage degeneration can occur if corticosteroids are used too often.

Ice can be applied to relieve swelling for 10 minutes 2 to 4 times a day. If the client prefers heat, it can be applied to reduce muscle spasm but always with the heat source on a medium setting for a maximum of 20 minutes at a time. Ultrasound therapy also has brought relief to some clients.

Various isometric exercises improve muscle strength. The quadriceps exercise improves knee function. Have the sitting client extend the leg and hold for 6 seconds; repeat 5 times. While watching television, the client can do this each time a commercial comes on—a handy way to remember to do the exercise. Elastic bandages, canes, and walkers also can protect the joint from stress.

When clients do not respond to conservative treatment, surgery and possibly total joint replacement can be an option (see Chapter 60). Joint replacement of a hip or knee is most common, but prosthetic implants are possible for other joints as well.

Specific Nursing Measures

Instruction about pain relief is an important nursing responsibility. Explain the need for rest and paced activities. The client should understand that activity causing pain that lasts for hours is too strenuous. Instruct the client to begin slowly and add activities gradually.

Administer ice or heat therapy—whichever is most effective—and instruct the client in its use. Place a towel between the skin and the therapeutic agent (eg, heating pad, ice bag). Pillows should not be placed under the knees. Although they are comfortable, they can cause contractures. Provide other comfort measures, such as massage and topical analgesic creams, to help relieve pain. Although topically applied analgesic creams may not relieve pain entirely, they are soothing and comfort some clients.

Administer medications as prescribed, and explain their dosage, route, and side effects to the client. Instruct clients to write down the pertinent information about each medication and carry it in their wallets. This step will help clients remember, as well as make the information accessible to other health professionals, if necessary.

Perform passive ROM exercises on the joint, and demonstrate the types of isometric exercises to strengthen muscles. Also provide instruction regarding the proper use of canes, crutches, and walkers, if applicable. Have the client redemonstrate their use. Tell the client using elastic bandages to wrap toward the heart. The bandages should not be too tight or too loose and generally should not be worn during sleep.

The joints of the hips, knees, and back can benefit from weight reduction, because stress from added weight can cause more rapid cartilage breakdown. If the client is overweight, help plan a realistic weight loss program. Urge clients of normal weight to be conscientious about maintaining that weight level. Instruct the client about safety measures to be taken at home to prevent injury, especially from falls.

Elderly clients with DJD face additional problems. Some have other disease processes with which to cope. Also, their support groups may be more limited, because spouses and friends may be deceased, and children may live far away or be involved in their own lives. Older persons may also be at a disadvantage financially, because their incomes may be fixed and they cannot afford needed medications. These clients need a great deal of emotional support to relieve anxiety and decrease muscle tension, which may contribute to their pain. Suggestions of support groups, referral to specific agencies, or arranging for community health nursing visits are possible approaches nurses should pursue.

Section III: Immunologic Disorders

RHEUMATOID ARTHRITIS

Rheumatoid arthritis (RA) is a systemic disease characterized primarily by chronic inflammation of the synovial lining of the joints. Joints are usually symmetrically affected. The most commonly involved joints are the wrists, PIP joints, metacarpophalangeal (MCP) joints of the hands, and MTP joints of the feet. Extra-articular involvement of RA includes muscle atrophy; anemia; osteoporosis; and skin, ocular, vascular, pulmonary, and cardiac symptoms. The course of the illness is variable, with a few or every joint in the body invaded. The long-term results are also unpredictable in regard to remission and exacerbation. Although classified in the 1983 *Primer on the Rheumatic Diseases* as a diffuse connective tissue disorder, RA is discussed in the chapter on joints because its major manifestation is joint inflammation. Women develop RA three times more often than men.

The etiology of RA is unknown. Whatever the cause, it releases various chemical mediators of inflammation (antigen–antibody complexes) into the joint. These chemicals cause synovial lining proliferation and cell lysis, a destructive process that eventually heals in a way that leaves a particular kind of scar tissue called *pannus*. Pannus generally tightens as other scar tissue does and pulls on structures already weakened by the destructive process. This results in flexion contractures and fibrosis, with possible calcifications.

Clinical Manifestations

Articular Manifestations

Swollen joints develop, especially the PIPs, MCPs, MTPs, and wrists, in bilateral symmetrical distribution; monoarticular involvement is also possible. The swelling is caused by proliferation of the synovial membrane that produces increased synovial fluid. Joint symptoms usually are insidious over weeks to months. Morning stiffness lasting from 30 minutes to several hours is characteristic of RA because of the synovial congestion, increased synovial fluid, and capsule thickening.

Deformities may occur later in the course of the disease because of soft tissue weakness and joint destruction. Ulnar deviation of the fingers is most common in RA (Figure 59–9). Swan-neck deformity of the fingers occurs when there is hyperextension of the PIP joints in conjunction with flexion of the DIP joints. Similarly, a boutonnière deformity of the fingers results from a flexion deformity of the PIP joints and extension of the DIP joints. Carpal tunnel syndrome with paresthesia of the thumb and the second, third, and radial aspects of the fourth digit may occur secondary to synovitis of the wrist, which compresses the median nerve beneath the transverse carpal ligament.

Extra-articular Manifestations

Fatigue, weakness, anorexia, and weight loss may be present because of the systemic effect of the inflammatory process. Anemia, which is associated with a chronic arthritis, also may develop.

Rheumatoid nodules—firm rounded or oval nodules that occur in subcutaneous or deeper connective tissue—may be present over the extensor surface of the elbows (Figure 59–10) or Achilles tendons. These benign lesions are uncomfortable, mainly because they have been produced by friction and pressure.

Vasculitis of the coronary, cranial, and mesenteric vessels has been reported, as well as vasculitis of small peripheral vessels. Myocardial infarction, neuropathy, skin necrosis, and leg ulcers may also result. Pericarditis appears more often in males and is unrelated to the duration of the disease. The course of the pericarditis varies from mild and self-limiting to cardiac tamponade and death.

Lung involvement includes pleurisy with or without effusion, pulmonary fibrosis, and rheumatoid nodules of the lung. Clients exposed to dust (eg, coal miners) can develop

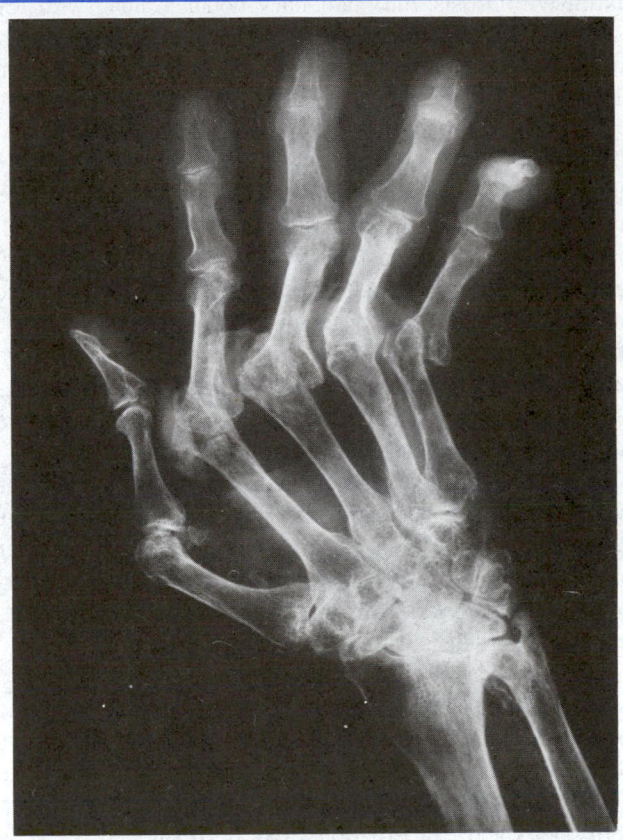

Figure 59–9

X-ray of a hand of a client with rheumatoid arthritis. Note the ulnar deviation of the fingers and the enlarged DIP joint in the ring finger.
SOURCE: Spence AP, Mason EB: *Human Anatomy and Physiology,* 2nd ed. Menlo Park, CA: Benjamin/Cummings, 1983.

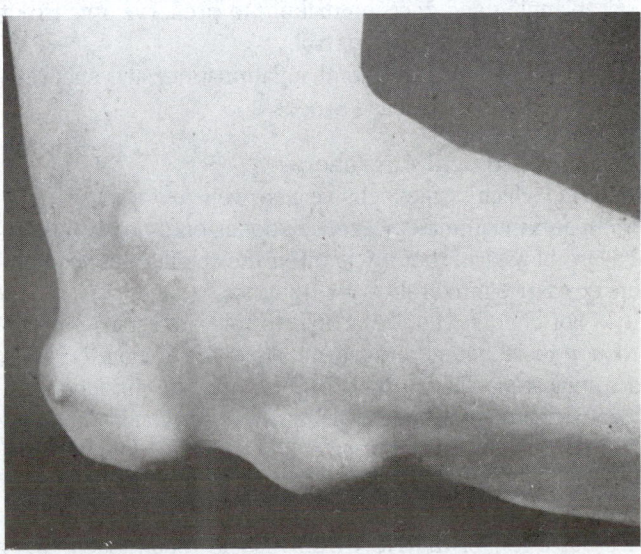

Figure 59–10

Rheumatoid nodules of the elbow. (Courtesy of Millard Fillmore Hospital, Buffalo, NY)

extensive fibrosis and pulmonary nodules along with RA (called Caplan's syndrome).

Dry eyes, corneal and conjunctival lesions, episcleritis, and scleritis also may occur in conjunction with RA.

Diagnosis

Diagnostic study data to be gathered include blood work, synovial fluid analysis, and x-rays. The ESR is elevated, parallel to the disease activity. There may be a normocytic, monochromic, or hypochromic anemia. The rheumatoid factor is present in 70% of adults with RA but is not specific for the disease. Complement levels are depressed. Five to ten percent of clients with RA have false positive tests for syphilis. Antinuclear antibody (ANA) test results are positive in 25% of cases, with a diffuse pattern.

Synovial fluid analysis can help establish the diagnosis when polymorphonuclear leukocytosis is present. X-rays early in RA show soft tissue swelling and periarticular osteoporosis. As the disease progresses, joint space narrowing and bony erosions are seen. In late RA, malalignment and ankylosis can be visualized.

Diagnosis of RA is made over time, as the disease settles into a bilateral, symmetrical, polyarticular arthritis usually by the end of 1 to 2 years. At that point, laboratory tests help confirm the diagnosis, and x-ray changes are usually present. The disease's natural progression varies; remissions and exacerbations may be related to the type of onset, age of the client, and the presence of the rheumatoid factor in high titers.

Therapeutic Measures

In spite of the variable course of RA, client care plans should include the following goals:

- Involve the client and family in all aspects of therapy planning and decision making to preserve a sense of personal value and control.
- Decrease pain and joint inflammation, and suppress the systemic disease process.

Pharmacological Approaches

Aspirin, which is inexpensive and well tolerated, is used as an anti-inflammatory agent in doses of 2.4 to 4.0 g/day. Failure of aspirin therapy is often the result of noncompliance, gastric intolerance, or tinnitus.

For clients who are unable to tolerate aspirin or who require more potent anti-inflammatory medication, NSAIDs are indicated. These work by blocking the production of local inflammatory mediators such as prostaglandins and kinins, thereby reducing pain and inflammation and promoting joint mobility. Ibuprofen (Motrin), indomethacin (Indocin), naproxen (Naprosyn), and tolmetin (Tolectin) are but a few of the NSAIDs available today. Each has a similar action, but clients are unique in their response to them. At least a 2-week trial of each drug is recommended before discontinuation because clients may initially do well

on a drug, and then the effect may dissipate; in this case, another NSAID should be tried. Because the main side effect of all NSAIDs is gastrointestinal distress, all clients should take them with food or milk, and they should be given cautiously to people with ulcers. Analgesics can be used in conjunction with anti-inflammatory agents when necessary. These include acetaminophen (Tylenol), propoxyphene hydrochloride (Darvon), and codeine.

Gold is used as a suppressive agent in RA to potentiate remission. Gold therapy is presently available in either injectable or oral forms. Both are equally effective. Injectable gold is available as sodium thiomalate (Myochrysine) and aurothioglucose (Solganol). Initially 10 mg of gold is given IM to detect any hypersensitivity. If no reaction occurs, the client will receive 50 mg IM once a week until improvement or a total of 1 g is reached. Injections will be continued indefinitely at varying time intervals if there is significant improvement, but will be discontinued when no improvement is evident or hypersensitivity develops. Toxic effects of injectable gold include mild skin rash, proteinuria, exfoliative dermatitis (a rare complication), mouth ulcers, and aplastic anemia.

Oral gold, auranofin (Ridaura), is similar in action to injectable gold, but smaller doses are effective. The usual dose of auranofin is 3 mg twice a day. As with injectable gold, there is a time factor involved (3 to 6 months) before efficacy can be determined. Diarrhea is the most common side effect, but this may be controlled by decreasing the dosage. Both oral and injectable gold must be monitored closely with blood and urine samples. Prescriptions for auranofin should be written for one month at a time to maintain client–physician contact for adequate monitoring.

Penicillamine (Depen, Cuprimine) is similar to gold in its action and percentage of remission produced, but it has the benefit of being an oral agent. The medication is given in increasing increments monthly. Toxicity to penicillamine may be as high as 50%, and clients should be monitored for proteinuria or bone marrow depression. A common benign side effect of the drug is a blunting of taste sensation, which usually disappears as the client continues taking the medication. Chemically related to penicillin, this drug usually should not be administered to individuals with a known penicillin allergy.

Steroids are seldom used to treat RA except in a severe exacerbation or for intra-articular injections. Cytotoxic agents are used in rare cases for immunosuppression. They are effective but dangerous because of their toxicity.

Methotrexate, however, is one immunosuppressive that has been effective in the treatment of RA. Studies have shown that 70% of clients tested improve significantly in a short period of time on both oral and injectable forms. Therapy usually involves giving 5–15 mg once a week. This type of pulse dose decreases the incidence of cirrhosis, which can occur with daily dosing. Methotrexate should only be used for clients who have been refractory to conventional therapy.

Activity, Rest, and Exercise

Exercise is always indicated for clients with RA to strengthen and preserve muscle groups affecting the involved joints. The client should never approach exercise too aggressively, however. If pain is present for longer than 2 hours after exercise, the client has done too much and should decrease the amount of activity at the next session. During acute exacerbations, performing passive ROM exercises twice a day is optimal therapy. When the disease course is stable, exercise is best done in divided doses three to four times per day. Water exercises are excellent for arthritics, because the buoyancy allows easier joint movement.

Heat and cold therapy raise the client's pain threshold and help decrease muscle spasms. It is useful to use heat or cold in conjunction with exercise to increase joint range of motion and decrease stiffness. Contraindications to heat include poor circulation, decreased sensation, skin infection, heat hypersensitivity, and decreased alertness. Contraindications to cold include vasculitis, Raynaud's phenomenon, cryoglobulinemia (the presence of an abnormal protein in the blood that forms gels at low temperatures), and paroxysmal cold hemoglobinuria (a rare disorder associated with blood in the urine on exposure to cold).

Cold is often more effective for acute pain, whereas heat works better for subacute chronic pain. An easy method of applying cold therapy to a joint is to use a bag of frozen peas. The bag retains its temperature while molding to the involved joint. Methods of heat application include paraffin baths, diathermy, ultrasonography, hydrotherapy, saunas, or showers. Determining factors for this treatment include client preference, ease of use, and cost.

Rest is a necessary therapy for clients with both acute and chronic RA. In acute stages of the illness, the client may have to maintain bed rest for 1 to 2 weeks to allow joint rest and muscle relaxation. Too much rest can result in contracture and permanent damage to the joint, however. Encourage clients with chronic stable RA to alternate activity with rest, allowing 1 to 2 hours of rest during the day and 10 to 12 hours of sleep each night.

Surgical Approaches

Fusions performed in wrists or ankles may increase stability and decrease pain, although joint function is lost. Surgical implants or repair work can increase joint function. Implant procedures generally give good results. Total joint replacements are most effective in the hip, although finger, shoulder, and knee replacements also can be done. Early synovectomy is not beneficial in RA; long-term results show no lasting positive outcome (see Chapter 60).

Specific Nursing Measures

Monitor the client's vital signs, level of pain, and other joint symptoms and signs. Continuously evaluate the client for new joint involvement and extra-articular manifestations of RA by assessing all joints, the chest and heart,

Nursing Research Note

Burckhardt C: The impact of arthritis on quality of life. *Nurs Res* 1985; 34(1):11–16.

The quality of life experienced by individuals with arthritis was investigated. The results suggest that positive self-esteem, belief in internal control over health, positive perceptions regarding support, and low negative attitudes toward the illness contributed to a higher quality of life. The severity of the arthritis and subsequent impairment indirectly affected the quality of life through the mediator variables of self-esteem and internal control over health.

Because self-esteem, a sense of personal control over health, supportive relationships, and a low negative attitude toward the illness result in higher levels of perceived quality of life, nursing care should be aimed toward enhancing these variables. Education, and client and family involvement in decision-making and care requirements are possible approaches.

the eyes, and skin. Follow laboratory results, especially ESR, rheumatoid factor, and x-rays. Monitor the client's weight, and encourage a balanced diet. There is no diet therapy in the treatment of RA except for ensuring good nutrition and ideal weight to decrease stress on joints.

Prepare the client thoroughly for all procedures. Administer medications as ordered, explain their side effects, and evaluate the client's response to the drugs. Watch for gastrointestinal distress when aspirin or NSAIDs are used. Observe for proteinuria, skin rash, and bone marrow depression with gold or penicillamine therapy.

Medicate the client for pain before each exercise session when necessary, and evaluate results. Apply heat or cold therapy, especially after exercise sessions. Encourage the client to manage activities of daily living, and provide enough time to accomplish tasks. Schedule periods of activity alternating with periods of rest. Apply splints as indicated.

Evaluate the client for problems with self-esteem, body image, and depression. Referral to mental health professionals can help clients who are having problems coping with a disease that will markedly alter their lives. Social workers can help clients who face a change in occupation. Inform the client and family about the Arthritis Foundation and its activities, particularly the client support groups and education classes.

Discharge planning involves careful instruction regarding all therapeutic measures to be used at home (eg, exercises and heat or cold treatments). Both client and family or significant others should know all medications to be used and their potential side effects. Emphasize the importance of frequent follow-up visits with the health care provider.

FELTY'S SYNDROME

Felty's syndrome is a variant of RA with splenomegaly and leukopenia. Some clients with RA develop a superimposed infection that leads to either leukopenia or splenomegaly, so this possibility must be ruled out before making a definite diagnosis of Felty's syndrome. Two-thirds of clients with Felty's syndrome are female, usually between the ages of 50 and 70 years.

As with RA, the etiology of Felty's syndrome is unknown. The leukopenia and splenomegaly usually occur 10 years or more after the arthritis appears. The true incidence is thought to be less than 1% of clients who have RA. Felty's syndrome appears to occur more often in clients with severe articular disease than in those with milder forms.

Clinical Manifestations

Articular Manifestations

Refer to the preceding discussion on articular manifestations of RA.

Extra-articular Manifestations

The extra-articular manifestations of Felty's syndrome include splenomegaly and leukopenia, as well as possible anemia and thrombocytopenia. Weight loss may be striking and unexplained, often for several months before the diagnosis is reached. The client has a history of recurrent gram-positive infections that respond to antibiotic therapy. Frequent leg ulcerations may occur.

Mild liver function abnormalities occur in 25% of clients. Other laboratory findings include a positive rheumatoid factor, which is present in 98% of clients. There may be low serum complement levels. One-third of clients have a positive lupus erythematosus (LE) cell test, and two-thirds have positive ANA test results. X-ray examination findings are as described in the section on RA.

A diagnosis of Felty's syndrome is made by the presence of the triad of characteristics: RA, splenomegaly, and leukopenia.

Therapeutic Measures

Refer to the preceding section on RA for therapeutic approaches to the management of joint problems. Splenectomy is indicated in clients with recurrent or serious infection. Hematologic improvement will result, as well as decreased synovitis and leg ulcers. Gold or penicillamine therapy can increase the severity of leukopenia while suppressing the arthritis component of this syndrome.

Specific Nursing Measures

Explain the nature of the illness to the client and significant others. They will need support in coping with this chronic and sometimes debilitating syndrome.

Maintain a clean environment to prevent client exposure to pathogens. For example, use proper handwashing techniques before contact with the client, as well as aseptic technique when changing dressings. Carefully inspect and care for all skin areas.

Administer medications as ordered. See the discussion of RA for the drugs usually administered and their side effects.

SJÖGREN'S SYNDROME

Sjögren's syndrome (SS) is a chronic inflammatory disorder characterized by a sicca syndrome—decreased lacrimal gland secretions, which causes dry eyes (keratoconjunctivitis), and decreased salivary gland secretions, which causes a dry mouth (xerostomia)—that occurs along with a connective tissue disease. Originally, SS was most commonly associated with RA, but now it is also linked to systemic lupus erythematosus, progressive systemic sclerosis, polyarteritis nodosa, and polymyositis. There is even a form of SS that is a distinct process in itself with no associated disorder. Sjögren's syndrome is more prevalent in women, with an average age of onset of 50 years.

The etiology of SS is unknown. As with other immune disorders, 50% of SS clients appear to have an autoimmune response of the body—on the exocrine organs in this instance.

Clinical Manifestations

A slowly developing dryness of the eye occurs that clients often describe as a sensation of a foreign body in the eye or as a sandy or gritty feeling. The client may experience a burning sensation, decreased tearing, and redness of the eye. Thick, ropy strands of discharge may be present at the inner canthus, especially in the morning. Little or no saliva present in the mouth leads to lip cracking; dental caries; and ulcerations of the mouth, tongue, and lips. The client may also have difficulty in chewing, swallowing, and phonation. Nasal dryness results in epistaxis or abnormalities of taste and smell. Lower respiratory tract involvement can cause chronic bronchitis, tenacious sputum, and a dry mouth.

Dyspareunia or a burning sensation in the perineal region may occur because of vaginal dryness. Generalized skin dryness is common. One half of SS clients may develop parotid or submandibular salivary gland enlargement. This is symmetrical and may occur with fever, tenderness, and erythema.

Laboratory studies of SS clients who also have RA show mild anemia, increased serum immunoglobulin levels, and lowered serum complement levels. Schirmer's test can roughly evaluate lacrimal secretions; normal result is the wetting of 15 mm or more of the standard filter strip in 5 minutes. Biomicroscopy of the eye, which involves the use of a microscope with a slit lamp, can indicate the presence of superficial erosions when the bulbar conjunctiva or cornea is stained with rose bengal dye.

Diagnosis of SS is made when keratoconjunctivitis, xerostomia, and a connective tissue disease are present. When xerostomia and keratoconjunctivitis alone occur, sicca syndrome is the diagnosis.

Therapeutic Measures

Therapeutic measures for SS largely treat its symptoms. Artificial tears (0.5% methylcellulose) help decrease ocular symptoms and prevent local complications. Increasing fluid intake is the primary treatment for xerostomia, although artificial lubricants and sugar-free lozenges may also relieve symptoms. Careful brushing and dental flossing of the teeth are mandatory to maintain oral health. Saline soaks can relieve nasal dryness, and water-soluble lubricants applied at the introitus and into the vagina help prevent dyspareunia. Eucerin cream or any other nonalcohol-based moisturizer is recommended for dry skin therapy.

Specific Nursing Measures

Explain the nature and management of the illness to the client and significant others. Maintain a fresh container of water and other fluids within reach for the hospitalized client to drink. Teach proper oral care. Monitor the client's eyes frequently for infection and other eye symptoms. Explain the importance of avoiding oil-based lubricants for the nose or vagina to avoid lipid pneumonia or vaginitis. Teach the client proper skin care: Little or no soap should be used, and the skin should be lubricated frequently.

SHOULDER–HAND SYNDROME

Shoulder–hand syndrome is the most common form of reflex sympathetic dystrophy. The client has impaired mobility of the shoulder accompanied by erythema, pain, swelling, osteoporosis, and immobility in the ipsilateral (same side) hand or wrist. There may be bilateral shoulder–hand involvement and, rarely, elbow involvement.

Shoulder–hand syndrome is thought to be secondary to overactivity of the sympathetic nervous system. Pain fibers carry impulses to the spinal cord, where a cycle of reflexes may lead to local sympathetic nervous system overload resulting in inappropriate and prolonged arterial vasoconstriction. Shoulder–hand syndrome may be precipitated by myocardial infarction, cerebrovascular accident, cervical disk disease, or trauma. The cause is unknown in other clients.

Clinical Manifestations

Shoulder–hand syndrome begins with a gradual or acute onset of stiffness and weakness in the upper extremity, followed by swelling, vasomotor changes, hyperesthesia, and disability. Microscopic evidence of synovitis is seen in the affected joint. These symptoms remain for 3 to 6 months, when vasomotor signs decrease and atrophy and contracture develop. The prognosis is unclear, but a majority of clients are free from pain within 2 years.

X-rays show patchy osteoporosis in the head of the humerus, wrist, and phalanges. No other diagnostic studies are indicated.

Early diagnosis is difficult, because the shoulder–hand syndrome simulates RA. Presentation of the clinical manifestations with patchy osteoporotic x-ray changes aids in diagnosis.

Therapeutic Measures

Early in the course of this syndrome, heat, exercise, and reassurance are necessary and effective treatments. Salicylates provide symptomatic relief, and high-dose steroid therapy (prednisone, 60 to 80 mg/day) for 2 to 3 weeks with a slow tapering of the dose assists in the resolution of symptoms. A cervical sympathetic block is done in clients with severe, unrelenting symptoms.

Specific Nursing Measures

If shoulder–hand syndrome occurs along with myocardial infarction or other disease processes, nursing care is directed to the client's total health care needs. Specific care for shoulder–hand syndrome involves pain assessment, administration of medication as ordered, and careful monitoring for side effects, especially because the client may be taking a variety of drugs for multiple problems. Have the client do gentle shoulder, elbow, and wrist exercises to maintain mobility and prevent contracture. Heat or cold applications may be helpful to relieve pain.

Section IV: Infectious Disorder

INFECTIOUS ARTHRITIS

Infectious arthritis is the inflammation of a joint resulting from an invading organism that attacks the synovium and synovial fluid. Viral, bacterial, and fungal infections all predispose susceptible people to arthritic involvement. Pathogens present in the host circulate freely in the bloodstream and become trapped in the richly perfused synovial membrane, leading to the inflammatory and subsequent degenerative changes. Infectious arthritis is an opportunistic disease that takes advantage of people who are immu-

nocompromised by chronic illness or medication, or who already have joint destruction from an immune disorder such as RA. Diabetics, clients receiving steroids, and the elderly are prime candidates for such joint involvement. Swift diagnosis and treatment can prevent serious degenerative changes.

Clients with infectious arthritis undergo repeated arthrocentesis, which is stressful for people afraid of needles and medical procedures. Clients may require hospitalization for the duration of therapy, which ranges from 2 to 4 weeks in acute disease to as long as 1 year in subacute or chronic infections. Financial difficulties may result for clients and their families through the loss of a wage earner's salary and added hospitalization expenses.

The nurse should be available to both the client and significant others for psychological support, physical care, health education, and monitoring of the client's response to therapy. The control of pain and protection of the involved joint or joints are priorities of nursing management. The nurse who is familiar with the pathophysiology of the infections and the differences between the various invading organisms will know when aggressive therapy is needed to prevent destruction versus when the disease is self-limiting and will lead to little or no residual damage.

Bacterial Arthritis

Bacterial infections most commonly affect clients who are unable to resist invading organisms. The old, young, and those who have compromised defense mechanisms because of chronic illness or immunosuppressive drugs are especially susceptible. A primary bacterial source of infection, such as pneumonia, endocarditis, or a simple urinary tract infection, is prerequisite for the arthritis.

Gram-positive cocci such as staphylococci, gram-positive rods, mycobacteria, and *Treponema* present a clinical picture of similar arthritic and systemic components. Onset of the arthritis is usually abrupt, and the client has a single hot, erythematous, swollen joint, usually the knee. X-rays demonstrate soft tissue swelling soon after onset. After several weeks of disease activity, osteomyelitis may be visualized. In general, the client feels ill and is febrile with shaking chills. Leukocytosis is present in 50% of cases.

Gonococcal infections, the most common cause of bacterial arthritis, are the exceptions to the rule. This gram-negative coccus usually affects young, healthy, sexually active adults (women more often than men). People who develop gonococcal arthritis usually experience fever at its onset, with migratory polyarthralgias and polyarthritis. Tenosynovitis is common in the upper extremities, especially in the wrists and small joints of the fingers. A generalized rash occurs two-thirds of the time and may involve maculopapular, pustular, vesicular, or bullous lesions. Of clients with gonococcal arthritis, 30% to 50% have a purulent joint effusion; the rest have a sterile effusion.

Tuberculosis (TBC) arthritis, caused by the bacillus *Mycobacterium tuberculosis,* was common in the past and still must be considered in a differential diagnosis for infectious arthritis. Its onset is insidious, usually monoarticular, and primarily affecting the hips or knees. The client may not have concurrent active TBC but has a positive tuberculin skin test and usually shows evidence of previous TBC on chest x-ray. Tubercle bacilli will be present in the synovial fluid.

Viral Arthritis

Arthritis of viral origin is an interesting subunit of infectious arthritis. Its transmission, like that of any other infec-

tious agent, is through the bloodstream. The viral arthritic process may have all the signs of a much more harmful process, such as RA, but will resolve of its own accord. Viral arthritis is a self-limiting infection in which the potential for joint damage is minimal. The viral illnesses most commonly responsible for secondary arthralgias include rubella, mumps, herpes, mononucleosis, and hepatitis A or B. Viral arthritis also can be acquired after immunization with live rubella virus.

Fungal Arthritis

Four fungal diseases are most commonly associated with the development of fungal arthritis: coccidioidomycosis, sporotrichosis, blastomycosis, and candidiasis. In general, arthralgias occur with the primary infection from the fungi without residual joint damage. However, joint destruction is possible when the organism disseminates into a secondary arthritis. Treatment of fungal arthritis is the same for all fungal organisms.

Therapeutic Measures

The invading organism in infectious arthritis should be identified as quickly as possible to prevent joint destruction. Isolating the organism will guide in the selection of antibiotics and the level of aggressiveness needed to control the infection. Pathogens are identified through the aspiration of synovial fluid, synovial fluid cultures, and synovial biopsy. Appropriate antimicrobial medications are then instituted. For example, isoniazid or rifampin may be given for TBC arthritis, and amphotericin B may be used to treat fungal arthritis.

Depending on the severity of the arthritis, the client may be kept in bed and given aspirin or an NSAID in addition to the antimicrobial agent. The client with a viral arthritis will be on aspirin or NSAIDs alone, because there are currently no effective antiviral agents.

A key diagnostic and therapeutic point with gonococcal arthritis compared with other kinds of bacterial arthritis is the rapid resolution of symptoms upon the administration of penicillin or other appropriate antibiotic therapy. Within 24 to 48 hours, the joint effusion begins resolving, making routine aspirations unnecessary. This rapid recovery after drug therapy initiation helps provide a diagnosis in cases where the bacterium *Neisseria gonorrhoeae* has not been isolated from either the involved joint or the genitourinary tract.

Other therapeutic measures for infectious arthritis include surgical excision of the affected synovium in instances where destruction of the joint cartilage, tendons, or both appears imminent.

Specific Nursing Measures

In taking the client's history, the nurse should realize that it is a key to diagnosis. Has the client recently had a viral illness (eg, rubella, mumps, or hepatitis)? Has the client had a urinary tract infection, pneumonia, or other bacterial infection? Has the client received any recent immunizations? Question the client about sexual activity and whether the partner has any known infection. Ask about dysuria and urgency or frequency related to urination because gonorrhea may cause urinary symptoms. Since fungal infections are often endemic to certain areas of the country, ask about recent travel. Is the client taking immunosuppressants? Does the client have a history of TBC or positive tuberculin test? Has the client had any recent invasive diagnostic studies or treatments (eg, hyperalimentation, venipuncture, or cystoscopy)? Also investigate thoroughly the onset of the arthritis using the seven dimensions discussed in Chapter 7.

To protect the intra- and extra-articular structure from future damage and reduce the client's discomfort, immobilize the involved joint during the acute arthritic stage. Because the client is usually on complete bed rest, active and passive ROM exercises for uninvolved joints are essential. Apply warm compresses to the involved joint.

Assess the involved joint frequently for drainage and any change in condition. Use sterile technique with any dressing changes. Administer antimicrobials, anti-inflammatory agents, and analgesics as ordered, and observe the client carefully for side effects.

For the client receiving parenteral fluids, measure intake and output accurately. Promote cooling for the client with fever by frequent sponging, encouraging fluids, and using a hypothermia blanket, if necessary. Monitor laboratory test results daily, especially the results of culture and sensitivity tests. Assist with joint aspirations or synovial biopsy using proper aseptic technique.

The education of the client and family or friends for home care should include instruction about ROM exercises to maintain joint mobility; dressing change techniques and wound care, if appropriate; and the names, dosages, actions, and potential side effects of all medications to be taken at home. The client and others involved should be aware of symptoms and signs of repeated infection (eg, increased pain, fever, swelling, redness, and drainage). They must take care to avoid any trauma to the joint.

Section V: Neoplastic Disorders

BENIGN TUMORS OF THE JOINT

The discussion of tumors of the joints and surrounding structures will be limited to the benign and malignant lesions generally included in a differential diagnosis for arthritis. The use of the term *benign tumor* is a misnomer in some cases. The client with a lesion of this type may experience years of intermittent minor problems with the involved joint. There may be a history of discomfort and an unstable joint. Because the symptoms of a benign tumor can remain innocuous for long periods, joint damage may result. No matter what the extent of damage, joint surgery is required for therapy; in cases of recurrence, surgery must be repeated. Nurses should recognize and deal with the frustrations of a client subjected to repeated hospitalizations and therapies for a "benign" disorder.

Lipoma

A lipoma of a joint is a lobulated fatty mass similar in appearance to lipomas that occur in other parts of the body. Lipomas develop most frequently in an elbow or knee joint of a client who has osteoarthritis.

Clinical Manifestations
The client seeks medical attention when the involved joint begins locking or when pain, decreased motion, or an effusion occurs. Effusion aspirate is clear, and x-rays are nondiagnostic.

Therapeutic Measures
Arthroscopy or surgical removal of the lesion is the recommended therapy. These procedures have an excellent prognosis.

Hemangioma

Hemangiomas are rare vascular tumors often associated with arteriovenous malformations or skin vascular disease. They affect a young age group (often teenage females who have been symptomatic since childhood). The knee is usually the involved joint.

Clinical Manifestations
There is a history of episodic and unilateral doughy joint swelling; pain; limitation of motion; and locking, buckling, or both. Aspirations of the knee repeatedly produce serosanguineous fluid in the absence of trauma. X-rays early in the course of a hemangioma may appear normal, whereas enlarged epiphyses, joint narrowing, and enlargement of the intercondylar notch later may be visualized.

Therapeutic Measures
Surgical removal yields good results in the treatment of a localized hemangioma. Because of the vascular nature of this tumor, however, a diffuse form may involve the entire joint capsule and make a resection impossible. Radiation therapy is attempted in these clients and produces mixed results.

Synovial Chondromatosis

Synovial chondromatosis is a condition of unknown etiology in which numerous cartilaginous nodules form. These nodules involve the joint, bursae, and sometimes the tendon sheaths of a knee, hip, elbow, shoulder, or ankle. It is a self-limiting affliction that most frequently affects young and middle-aged males.

Clinical Manifestations

Synovial chondromatosis is a slowly progressing ailment, and many years pass before the client seeks evaluation for the problem. As in other previously described tumors, presenting symptoms usually consist of swelling, pain, stiffness, limitation of motion, and joint locking. Particularly with synovial chondromatosis, the client experiences joint crepitation or a grating sensation from the multiple intrasynovial nodules. X-ray findings may demonstrate calcified free-floating bodies in the synovium.

Therapeutic Measures

Excision of the involved synovium and removal of all loose bodies is the treatment of choice. Surgical therapy has a good prognosis, although the condition may recur if removal is incomplete.

Pigmented Villonodular Synovitis

Pigmented villonodular synovitis is a condition of unknown etiology in which the synovial lining cells have a marked proliferation that results in the appearance of innumerable villi and folds. The formation of these fingerlike projections can affect not only the synovial lining of a joint but also the tendon sheath, bursa, and bone. Unilateral involvement of the knee, hip, ankle, or elbow joint of young adults is most common.

Clinical Manifestations

There are two forms of pigmented villonodular synovitis: localized and diffuse. The diffuse type causes pain and mild, episodic joint swelling over a period of months to years. Occasionally, the client may note an acutely painful, warm, swollen joint with limited motion. Repeated aspirations of joint fluid yield dark serosanguineous fluid in the absence of trauma.

The localized type of pigmented villonodular synovitis occurs in either the medial or lateral knee compartment as a solitary nodule. It, too, may begin with episodic pain and mild swelling and can be misdiagnosed as a torn meniscus. Serosanguineous fluid is rarely aspirated with this type of lesion.

X-rays may show a soft tissue density, but arteriograms are more useful because of the vascularity of these tumors. Most often, however, arthroscopic examination enables the condition to be diagnosed.

Therapeutic Measures

Surgical resection is the treatment for both types of pigmented villonodular synovitis. The localized form is cured with simple excision. With the diffuse type, lesions may recur if synovectomy is incomplete. Clients who have knee involvement also can experience a recurrence of the condition.

Specific Nursing Measures for Benign Tumors of the Joint

During the diagnostic phase of benign tumors, the health history is important. The nurse should concentrate on any significant joint trauma. Ask the client if there is any past history of arthritis. Obtain a detailed description of swelling, pain, limitation of motion, or joint instability.

Instruct the client in the use of a cane or crutches in cases of severe joint instability. Apply warm soaks to the area for relief of mild pain, and instruct the client and family or friends in the use of heat. Prepare the client for surgery through physical preparation, instruction about the prevention of postoperative complications such as thrombophlebitis, and attention to psychological needs.

Postoperative care includes checking for wound drainage or signs of infection, changing sterile dressings as necessary, and splinting the involved area. Assess the client's level of discomfort, and give pain medication as ordered. To prepare the client for discharge, provide instruction in the care of the surgical site and restrictions on activities, as well as on follow-up appointments with the physician and physical therapist.

MALIGNANT TUMORS OF THE JOINT

Malignant tumors of the joint are rare. However, whenever a client has a slow-growing monoarticular mass, a malignancy should be suspected.

Synovial Sarcoma

The highly malignant synovial sarcoma, which is fortunately rare, is the most common primary tumor of the joint. It can appear at any age, although it seems to predominate in young adults. The growth generally appears on a lower extremity, but synovial sarcomas have been known to develop in an upper extremity, the neck, or chest.

Clinical Manifestations

The client usually appears with a slow-growing mass that may have been present for months to years, depending on how deeply seated it is in tissue. Pain may be present, or the client may have a vague sensation of discomfort over the involved area. There also may be localized swelling. Tumor involvement of the neck may produce hoarseness, dysphagia, or dyspnea.

The average survival time from presentation to death

is about 7 years; the 10-year survival rate is approximately 30%. Survival rates are highest in the very old and very young, as well as in clients with tumors less than 0.5 cm in diameter.

Therapeutic Measures
Ideally, the goal of therapy for synovial sarcoma is to eliminate the tumor and preserve a functional limb. Preoperative chemotherapy and radiation therapy may be undertaken to decrease the size of the tumor. An open wedge biopsy of the tumor is performed. If the biopsy is positive, the surgeon performs wide resection with radical lymph node dissection. Chemotherapy and radiation therapy are continued postoperatively, and the client is kept on a high-protein diet.

Clear Cell Sarcoma

Clear cell sarcoma is a rare tumor that involves tendons rather than joint spaces. It can occur in any age group and usually is found on parts of the foot such as the heel, toes, or ankle. Because of this lesion's location, it is very difficult to remove entirely; thus, it is an ultimately deadly lesion because of recurrence and metastasis.

Clinical Manifestations
The tumor appears as a slowly progressing, painless growth during a period of months to years. Diagnosis is made by biopsy.

Therapeutic Measures
Preoperative and postoperative chemotherapy and radiation therapy are employed, along with radical resection of the tumor-infested area.

Specific Nursing Measures for Malignant Tumors of the Joint

Supportive nursing care is essential for clients who face a diagnosis of cancer, possible amputation of a limb, and side effects from chemotherapy and radiation therapy. Encourage both client and family or significant others to verbalize their thoughts and fears. Include the family or friends in client care activities and education whenever possible.

Help the client select foods that are appetizing in addition to being high in calories and vitamins, and provide snacks between meals. Administer medications as ordered, including antibiotics, analgesics, antiemetics, and antidiarrheals. Promote physical activities as much as possible, balancing them with periods of rest.

Postoperative care includes checking dressings frequently for bleeding, drainage, or a foul odor. Monitor vital signs every 4 hours, especially temperature. Provide optimal nutrition, and record intake and output. See Chapter 60 for postoperative care of the client following amputation. Finally, help the client set realistic goals for recovery.

Section VI: Traumatic Disorders

Permanent structural changes may occur in a joint as a result of cartilage and capsular tears, detachment of menisci, hemorrhagic effusions, articular fractures, or repetitive trauma. Because of the realignment of involved bone, bursa, and tendons, a mechanical deterioration of articular cartilage results in DJD.

Acute traumatic arthritis may result from unexpected force, such as sports or automobile accidents. Repetitive trauma is an internal occurrence—a chronic injury resulting from repeated smaller stresses to a joint through vibrations, blows, abnormal strain, or position. This type of injury is related to occupation and lifestyle, eg, the stress placed on the MTP joints of a ballerina or the knees of a jogger. Over time, repetitive trauma may realign the joint and lead to the same result as an acute injury.

The client with traumatic arthritis must make lifestyle changes. The football player who has developed DJD of the knees as a result of multiple tackles may need to wear special equipment or stop playing. The factory worker exposed to repeated vibratory trauma may need a different job assignment. As obvious as these solutions are, they may not be popular with the client, and the decision to make a lifestyle change must come from the client. The responsibility of the care provider is to give the client accurate information about the alternatives available.

The nurse plays an important role in the therapeutic and preventive care of traumatic disorders. As the first person on the scene of an accident, the nurse may be able to prevent any residual damage by protecting the limb by splinting, elevating the area, applying ice, and not allowing weight on the area. At the workplace, the nurse can evaluate jobs for injury and health risks. It may be possible to identify tasks that expose employees to repetitive trauma; employees then can rotate through these jobs rather than be assigned permanently to potentially harmful tasks.

JOINT EFFUSIONS

Joint effusions can occur as a result of simple trauma or secondary fractures, internal derangements, or severe sprains. Within 24 hours after a blow to the joint, synovial fluid accumulates. If blood vessels in the synovium are broken, a hemarthrosis also occurs. The knee is most commonly affected by this injury.

Clinical Manifestations

In simple cases of traumatic synovitis, joint swelling with mild pain occurs. Aspiration of the joint produces clear fluid with elevated protein content and decreased viscosity.

Hemarthrosis, which usually develops from 15 minutes to 2 hours after the trauma, is usually more painful than a clear effusion and is accompanied by low-grade fever. Aspiration of the joint produces bloody fluid. Diagnosis of traumatic synovitis is primarily by physical examination, but x-ray examination is done to rule out fracture.

Therapeutic Measures

Apply ice initially for 30 minutes q.i.d. to reduce swelling and relieve pain. After the first 24 hours, apply moist heat to the area for 30 minutes q.i.d. Repeated joint aspirations are necessary if fluid reaccumulates. Compression dressings applied to the joint, along with bed rest or limited weight bearing, may be necessary, depending on the severity of the injury.

Specific Nursing Measures

Assist the physician with joint aspirations. Apply compression dressings and cold and heat therapy. Instruct the client in the application of cold and heat as well. Emphasize the need to protect the joint while pain is present to prevent reinjury. Teach the use of crutches, if necessary.

DISLOCATION AND SUBLUXATION

When a joint's articulating surfaces are completely displaced because of trauma, it is termed a dislocation. Partial displacement of the articulating surfaces results in a subluxation. Both subluxations and dislocations can damage soft tissues, nerves, or blood vessels if not attended to promptly. The joints most often affected are shoulders, wrists, elbows, fingers, hips, knees, and ankles.

Clinical Manifestations

After injury, the joint appears deformed; it is tender, and motion is limited. The involved extremity is shortened.

Joint pain may be intense, especially if articular surface fractures are present. With immediate treatment, there is good prognosis. However, bone necrosis can result if reduction of the subluxation or dislocation is delayed.

The diagnosis is made through physical examination and client history. X-rays are taken to evaluate joint displacement and to determine whether fractures are present.

Therapeutic Measures

The longer the delay in correcting a joint displacement, the more difficult the procedure becomes because of edema and muscle spasms. Two types of procedures can correct this injury. Closed reduction is manual traction done under local or general anesthesia. Narcotics may be given for analgesia, and tranquilizers are administered for their antispasmodic effect. Open reduction is done where wire fixation of the joint or repair of torn ligaments is necessary. A splint, cast, or traction is used for 3 to 6 weeks after reduction.

Specific Nursing Measures

At the accident site, the nurse should splint the joint as is—even if crooked—to prevent further damage. Apply ice to decrease pain and swelling.

The hospitalized client requires immediate orthopedic examination. Observe the area distal to the injury for evidence of vascular damage (pallor, absent pulse, or abnormal coolness) and nerve damage (paresthesia or paralysis).

After reduction, monitor respirations and keep a ventilating bag and airway at the bedside, since the narcotics and tranquilizers administered can depress respirations. Check the dressing or cast for pressure that may impair blood flow. Instruct the client regarding gradual mobilization of the joint when the dressing or cast is removed.

Chapter Highlights

Ankylosing spondylitis is a seronegative spondyloarthropathy characterized by the lack of rheumatoid nodules, absence of rheumatoid factor in the blood, and the presence of serum HLA-B27 antigen. The ligamentous insertions into the bone, primarily the spine, are the areas which become inflamed as a result of this disorder.

Reiter's syndrome presents as a triad of asymmetrical arthritis, urethritis, and conjunctivitis. It is thought to occur following a diarrheal infection or after a sexually transmitted infection, although there is an association with serum HLA-B27 antigen.

Psoriatic arthritis presents as a seronegative inflammatory arthritis, caused by either hereditary or environmental factors. It is a variable condition that involves only a subsection of clients who have psoriasis. Therapeutic measures are aimed at controlling both the arthritis and the psoriasis.

Gout is a disease which produces joint inflammation as a result of deposition of uric acid crystals in the articular cartilage.

Pseudogout is an inflammatory arthritis caused by the deposition of calcium pyrophosphate dihydrate crystals in a large joint, such as the knee. Attacks may be precipitated by trauma, surgery, or medical illness.

Low back pain can have a multiplicity of causes including congenital anomalies, leg length discrepancies, asymmetrical development of the spine, weak abdominal muscles, acquired injuries, sedentary lifestyle, and/or obesity.

Low back strain is the most common cause of low back pain. It is a self-limiting condition treated with bed rest, analgesia, muscle relaxants, heat or ice, and flexion exercises.

The nurse's main role in the management of back disorders is prevention. Clients should be taught proper lifting techniques, muscle strengthening exercises, and the importance of proper posture.

Screening for and treatment of scoliosis is important in early adolescence, because untreated, it can lead to decreased lung capacity, back pain, degenerative arthritis of the spine, intervertebral disk disease, and sciatica.

Carpal tunnel syndrome is an entrapment of the median nerve due to tenosynovitis, trauma, rheumatoid arthritis, gout, pseudogout, acromegaly, edema of pregnancy, or premenstrual edema. Paresthesia of the thumb, index, middle, and medial side of the ring finger occur.

Degenerative joint disease (DJD) is primarily a disorder of articular cartilage resulting from "wear and tear" (primary) or traumatic causes (secondary). The pain of DJD is gradual in onset, most severe after activity, and relieved with rest.

The treatment goals of DJD are to relieve pain, decrease swelling, increase joint function, and allow the client to lead a more active lifestyle. Aspirin or NSAIDs, heat or ice, exercise, and possibly surgery can help to relieve the discomfort and achieve treatment goals.

Rheumatoid arthritis (RA) is a systemic disease characterized primarily by chronic inflammation of the synovial lining of joints. Symmetrical swelling of joints occurs most commonly in the MCPs, PIPs, MTPs, and wrists.

Because of the systemic nature of RA, clients should temper activity with periods of rest to avoid fatigue.

Exercise is indicated for clients with RA to strengthen and preserve muscle groups around involved joints.

Felty's syndrome is a variant of RA with splenomegaly and leukopenia. Along with the standard therapeutic measures for RA, splenectomy may be necessary.

Sjögren's syndrome is a chronic inflammatory disorder characterized by decreased lacrimal gland and salivary gland secretions. Treatment for Sjögren's syndrome is mainly symptomatic.

Shoulder–hand syndrome is the most common form of reflex sympathetic dystrophy. It is thought to be secondary to overactivity of the sympathetic nervous system precipitated by myocardial infarction, a cerebrovascular accident, cervical disk disease, or trauma.

Infectious arthritis can occur due to bacterial, viral, or fungal invasion of the richly perfused joint synovium and synovial fluid. The invading organism must be identified early in the course of the arthritis so that appropriate therapy can be initiated. Joint destruction occurs swiftly with fungal and certain bacterial infections, whereas viral arthritis is a self-limiting illness.

Benign tumors of the joint include lipomas, hemangiomas, synovial chondromatosis, and pigmented villonodular synovitis. These tumors, while noncancerous, may cause pain, limitation of motion, and joint instability. Treatment is surgical removal.

Malignant tumors of the joint are rare, slow-growing, monoarticular masses. Synovial and clear cell sarcomas are the two most common forms. Treatment includes supportive care, chemotherapy, radiation, and possible limb amputation.

Traumatic arthritis may occur from a sudden, unexpected force, or from repeated trauma. Joint effusions, dislocations, and subluxations occur as a result of acute trauma. If not attended to promptly, long-term damage occurs to the joint and its surrounding soft tissue.

Bibliography

Burckhardt CS: The impact of arthritis on quality of life. *Nurs Res* 1985; 34(1):11–16.

Carette S et al: The natural disease course of ankylosing spondylitis. *Arthritis Rheum* 1983; 26(2):186–189.

Chaffman M, Brogden RN, Heel RC: Auranofin—A preliminary review of its pharmacological properties and therapeutic use in rheumatoid arthritis. *Drugs* 1984; 27:378–424.

Cohen LM, Killian PJ: The spondyloarthropathies: The spondylitis associated disorders. *Postgrad Med* 1982; 72(5):127–136.

Delany P: Neurologic complications of systemic lupus erythematosus. *Am Fam Physician* July 1983; 28(1):191–193.

Garber E, Bluestone R: Evaluating arthritis in the elderly. *Consultant,* July 1980; 20(7):97–106.

Harris CJ: Rheumatoid arthritis and the pregnant woman. *Am J Nurs* 1985; 85(4):414–417.

Hawley, DH (editor): Symposium on arthritis and related rheumatic diseases. *Nurs Clin North Am* Dec 1984; 19(4): 565–725.

Kay MMB, Golphin J, Makinodan T: *Aging, Immunity and Arthritic Disease.* New York: Raven Press, 1980.

Kelley WN et al: *Textbook of Rheumatology.* Philadelphia: Saunders, 1981.

Koerner ME, Dickerson GR: Adult arthritis. *Am J Nurs* 1983; 83(2):255–277.

Laborde JM, Powers MJ: Life satisfaction, health control orientation, and illness related factors in persons with osteoarthritis. *Res Nurs Health* 1985; 8(2):183–190.

Lambert VA: Study of factors associated with psychological well-being in rheumatoid arthritic women. *Image* Spring 1985; 17(2):50–53.

Lorig KR: Arthritis self-management: A patient education program. *Rehabil Nurs* 1982; 7(4):16–19.

Meenan RF et al: The arthritis impact measurement scales: Further investigation of a health status measure. *Arthritis Rheum* 1982; 25(9):1048–1053.

Owen BD: How to avoid that aching back. *Am J Nurs* 1980; 80(5):894–897.

Petersdorf RG et al: *Harrison's Principles of Internal Medicine,* 10th ed. New York: McGraw-Hill, 1983.

Phillips KF: The use of gold therapy with rheumatoid arthritis. *Ortho Nurs,* July/Aug 1983; 2(4):31–34.

Platz CM: Rheumatoid arthritis: Guidelines for office management. *Postgrad Med* 1981; 70(3):143–149.

Rodnan GO, Schumacher HR, Zvaifler NJ: *Primer on the Rheumatic Diseases.* Atlanta: Arthritis Foundation, 1983.

Simpson CF: Heat, cold or both. *Am J Nurs,* Feb 1983, pp 270–273.

Steinberg FU: *Care of the Geriatric Patient.* St. Louis: Mosby, 1983.

Strodthoff C: Pathophysiology of rheumatoid arthritis. *Nurse Pract* 1982; 7(June):34–35.

Waxman J: Localized rheumatologic diseases. *Postgrad Med* 1983; 75(2):189–196.

Weinblatt ME, Coblyn JS, Fox DA et al: Efficacy of low dose methotrexate in rheumatoid arthritis. *N Engl J Med* 1985; 312:818–822.

Suggested Readings

Dickinson GR: A home care program for patients with rheumatoid arthritis. *Nurs Clin North Am* 1982; 25(9):1048–1053. The author discusses characteristics of RA and assessment of the client with RA. Detailed home care plans are developed based on the characteristics of the disease and thorough client assessment. Specific instructions for clients are given regarding splints, joint protection, application of heat and cold, exercises, and energy conservation.

Owen BD, Damron CF: Personal characteristics and back injury among hospital nursing personnel. *Res Nurs Health* 1984; 7:305–313. This research study used a sample of 64 female nursing personnel, 32 with back injuries and 32 with no back problems. Demographic, physical characteristics, and lifestyle data were looked at with some interesting results!

The Client With Rheumatoid Arthritis

I. Descriptive Data

Mr David Watts, a 45-year-old black male who has had rheumatoid arthritis (RA) for 5 years, was seen by his primary physician at the HMO 1 month ago for a pruritic, generalized skin rash and given a tentative diagnosis of "gold reaction." He comes to the HMO's Rheumatology Department today for further evaluation and recommendations.

II. Personal Data

Date:	Oct 2, 1986
ID Number:	00000-00-0
Full Name:	David Ernest Watts
Address:	35 Beach St., Hanover, NY 14002
Telephone:	Home: 000-0000
	Work: None
Sex:	Male
Marital Status:	Married
Age:	45
Birthdate:	12-12-40
Religion:	Baha'i
Race/Culture:	Black
Occupation:	Presently on disability. Formerly employed as a millwright.
Primary Health Care Provider:	Paul Marine, MD

III. Health History

Source of Information: Client and medical records

Reliability of Informant: Client is reliable but reticent to reveal information unless specifically questioned

Chief Concern: "My wrists, hands, knees, and feet are swollen and hurt all the time. The pain even wakes me up when I try to roll over at night."

History of Present Illness: Mr Watts joined the HMO in 1979. Shortly thereafter, he developed migratory joint pains, which involved his hands, his wrists, shoulders, knees, and metatarsals of his feet. These acute problems were unifocal and resolved following application of moist heat, rest, and nonsteroidal anti-inflammatory (NSAID) therapy. Laboratory studies were within normal limits. X-rays of the hands showed soft-tissue swelling.

In March 1980, Mr Watts developed a symmetrical painful swelling of his MCPs, PIPs, wrists, knees, and metatarsals. He experienced morning stiffness, which would gradually lessen by afternoon, lost 20 lb in 6 weeks, and complained of anorexia and chronic fatigue. A rheumatoid factor was positive with a titer of 1:1640. An ANA was positive with a diffuse pattern and a titer of 1:20. ESR was 60 mm/h. At this point, he was diagnosed as having RA.

His symptoms became progressively worse as he continued to work. Finally, he took a disability leave from his job with a local car manufacturer, per his physician's advice. ASA and NSAIDs were not sufficient to control Mr Watts's inflammation and arthralgias, and he was given intermittent oral steroids to control symptoms. Since this therapy is not recommended long-term, gold therapy was initiated 12/83. A considerable

(continued)

The Client With Rheumatoid Arthritis

improvement in his condition was noted by the spring of 1984, and he was maintained on gold salts (Myochrysine) 50 mg IM q.4 weeks, sulindac 200 mg b.i.d., and acetaminophen p.r.n.

Five weeks ago, a maculopapular, pruritic rash started on the client's anterior and posterior thorax, arms, and legs. It was determined that the gold injections were the probable cause, and the drug was discontinued. With questioning, Mr Watts admits to morning stiffness lasting approximately 3 hours. He has increased pain and swelling of his MCPs, PIPs, wrists, and knees. He is currently taking sulindac 200 mg b.i.d., ASA gr X q.4 h, and diphenhydramine 25 mg t.i.d. p.r.n. for pruritus (has not needed any for past 1 week). He appears discouraged with this present setback and voices fear that he will never be as well again as he was with the gold injections.

Past Health History:
Childhood: Mumps, measles, chickenpox
Immunizations: Tetanus toxoid, 1979; unsure of other immunizations
Medical Problems: No other problems but RA
Surgeries: Tonsillectomy, 1946; appendectomy, 1958
Transfusions: None
Special Diagnostic Procedures: None
Trauma: Fracture right radius age 10 with no sequelae
Medications: Diphenhydramine (Benadryl), 25 mg PO t.i.d. p.r.n.
Sulindac (Clinoril), 200 mg b.i.d.
ASA gr X q.4 h p.r.n.

Family History:

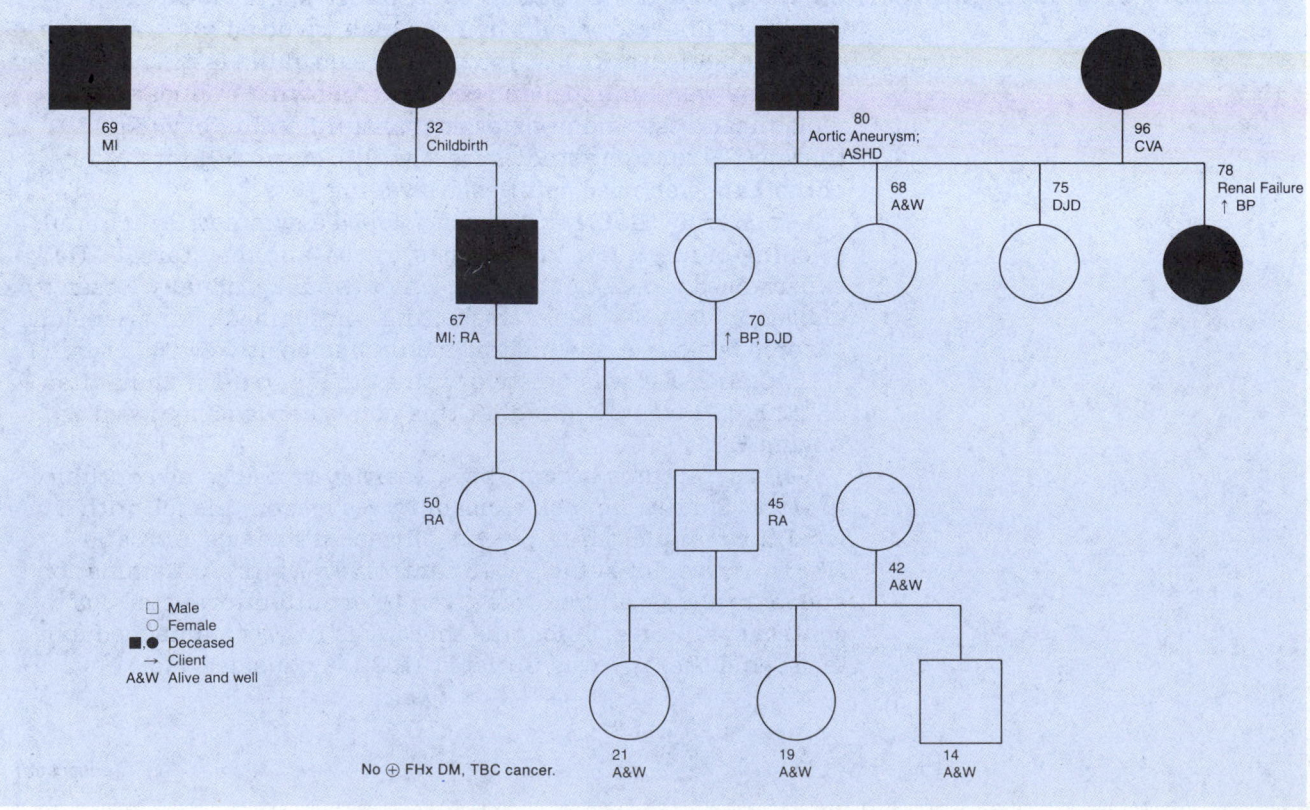

- □ Male
- ○ Female
- ■,● Deceased
- → Client
- A&W Alive and well

No ⊕ FHx DM, TBC cancer.

Personal/Social History:	Lives with spouse and children in a modest split-level home, which they own. Mr Watts spends his time on a woodworking hobby that he hopes to turn into a full-time business. At present, he sells his wood name plates, sconces, and wall hangings at craft shows and fairs to supplement his family's income. Drives his own car. Son and Mr Watts care for outside home maintenance.
	High school graduate. Worked as a millwright for 22 years before taking disability leave. There are no current financial problems because he had good personal disability coverage.
Habits:	Eats three balanced meals a day. Loses weight whenever RA is in severe exacerbation. Has not felt capable of exercising regularly. Most of exercise comes from walking when RA is in remission. Smokes 1½ packs of cigarettes a day for 28 years. Has rare ETOH intake. Attempts to sleep 7 hours a night, but pain has been waking him; he then watches late night television for distraction. He will rest for 1 to 2 hours in the afternoon if arthritis is in exacerbation.
Sexual Functioning:	Sexually active with wife without difficulties.
Coping Pattern:	Tends to ignore or deny the chronicity of RA; alters medications on his own and misses appointments with the physician when he feels well. Wife and children are supportive to client; family is close-knit; outside support systems limited.
Review of Systems:	States overall health is good, but fatigue is a chronic problem that interferes with activities.
Skin:	Rash has resolved; no current pruritus.
Eyes:	Requires glasses for reading but otherwise has good vision.
Mouth:	Has noted dry mouth and lack of saliva, which makes swallowing difficult periodically.
Lungs:	No cough, dyspnea, or pain with deep breath.
Vascular:	Notes numbness and blanching of fingers with cold weather, followed by erythema of involved areas with warming.

IV. Physical Assessment

Weight:	148 lb
Height:	6 ft 2 in.
Vital Signs:	T. 98°F(36.7°C); P. 88; R. 20; BP 120/76
Relevant Organ Systems:	
Skin:	Brown, warm to touch, without lesions or nodules
Lungs:	Normal resonance with percussion; clear to auscultation A & P
Heart:	PMI at 5th LICS, medial to MCL; apical pulse 88/min, regular; no rub, ⓜ, or gallop
Vascular:	2+ brachial, radial, femoral, popliteal, DP, and PT pulses
Musculoskeletal:	
Hands:	Bony enlargement of MCPs, PIPs with swelling, erythema; areas warm to touch, tender, with "boggy" texture on palpation; ulnar drift and interthenar wasting noted; grip strength decreased; 2 cm ganglion cyst on dorsum of left hand
Wrists:	1+ effusion of right wrist; bilaterally tender radial styloids; limitation of motion noted bilaterally
Shoulders:	45° lateral abduction of right arm with tenderness
Knees:	3+ effusion of right knee; 1+ effusion of left; crepitation palpable with ROM; "doughy" texture to joints on palpation Posture and balance are within normal limits. Client limps, favoring right leg.

V. Diagnostic Data

- Bilateral x-rays of hands and knees show joint space narrowing and bony erosions.
- CBC: WBC 5.9, RBC 4.8, Hgb 13.4, Hct 39.8%, MCV 84, MCHC 33.8

(continued)

The Client With Rheumatoid Arthritis

- Urinalysis: Color: yellow; clarity: clear; specific gravity: 1.013; protein, glucose, ketones, blood: negative; 0–2 WBCs, 0–1 epithelial cells
- Erythrocyte sedimentation rate (ESR): 68 mm/h
- ANA positive—1:40 titer with diffuse pattern
- Rheumatoid factor—1:640
- Serum complement—within normal limits

VI. Summary

After evaluating Mr Watts, his rheumatologist concurred with the diagnosis of gold toxicity rash and decided to change to penicillamine. Penicillamine 250 mg $\frac{-}{1}$ q.d. for 2 weeks and then b.i.d. after that time was prescribed. Mr Watts was advised of the toxic effects of the medication and told to return for a follow-up appointment in 1 month.

VII. Nursing Care Plan

Nursing Diagnosis	Client Care Goals	Plan/Nursing Implementation	Expected Outcomes
Mobility, impaired physical, related to increased pain and stiffness	Reduce or eliminate pain and diminish joint stiffness and swelling	Suggest keeping a time chart for medications; stress importance of maintaining a blood level for medications; encourage to alternate rest with periods of light activity	Will take NSAIDs and acetaminophen on a regular schedule; will begin penicillamine as directed; will avoid activities that cause further joint pain/stiffness or swelling
Activity intolerance, related to current flare-up of arthritis	Decrease fatigue	Plan with client a realistic rest schedule (eg, 2 hours midmorning and midafternoon) until acute flare-up resolves	Client will moderate activities and maintain a specific rest schedule to decrease fatigue
Self-concept, disturbance in: related to altered role performance	Share feelings and frustrations	Allow time at appointment sessions for client to discuss feelings, share frustrations; organize a group session of clients who have RA to allow mutual support	Acceptance of present physical situation; improved coping ability
Noncompliance, when acute phase is over	Understand importance of following medication regimen and activity modifications	Instruct in pathophysiology of RA and in the importance of long-term management, including compliance with medication regimen, proper joint rest, and follow-up care	Client will continue medication as instructed; client will plan rest and activity periods carefully; client will keep follow-up appointments
Knowledge deficit related to current drug therapy	Recognize signs of adverse drug reactions	Instruct in benign and serious side effects of penicillamine (pruritic rash, abnormal taste sensation, renal damage)	Will competently manage penicillamine therapy and will contact physician if a problem occurs
Knowledge deficit related to complications of RA	Explain need for joint exercise to prevent contracture	Instruct client in ROM exercises to be done when joint is not acutely inflamed; explain contracture formation; refer to physical therapy if available	Client will demonstrate more joint ROM and express confidence in managing his condition

Nursing Diagnosis	Client Care Goals	Plan/Nursing Implementation	Expected Outcomes
Nutrition, alteration in: less than body requirements	Discuss proper nutrition and importance of keeping up nutritional status when exacerbations of RA occur	Discuss food likes and dislikes with client and offer suggestions for adding more calories to diet	Maintains present weight during acute flare-ups; gains 5 to 10 lb when feeling good

Chapter 60

Surgical Approaches to Musculoskeletal System Dysfunction

Linda Heim McCausland

Objectives

When you have finished studying this chapter, you should be able to:

List the indications for surgical intervention of musculoskeletal disorders.

Describe surgical procedures for musculoskeletal disorders.

Discuss the physiological implications of surgical treatment of disorders of the musculoskeletal system.

Anticipate the psychosocial/lifestyle implications of surgical treatment of musculoskeletal disorders.

Identify nursing interventions appropriate for clients undergoing surgical treatment of musculoskeletal disorders.

This chapter discusses the surgical procedures used in musculoskeletal disorders and the nursing measures appropriate to each procedure. The disorders themselves are discussed in Chapters 57, 58, and 59 of this unit. General preoperative preparation for orthopedic surgery clients is discussed in Chapter 56, as are general nursing interventions for orthopedic conditions.

INTERNAL FIXATION OF FRACTURES

Internal fixation immobilizes reduced fractures by means of nails, rods, plates, screws, pins, or even unabsorbable sutures. The metals being used today, such as Vitallium and stainless steel, are less likely to cause a foreign body reaction than those used in the past. Occasionally an individual does develop a tissue reaction, however, due to sensitivity to metals in the alloys.

Internal fixation is used to maintain reduction when closed treatment is unsuccessful, impossible, or contraindicated. For example, it is useful for fractures that are prone to nonunion, such as fractures of the femoral neck, and for those that will be pulled apart by the action of muscles, such as transverse fractures of the patella (Apley & Solomon, 1982). For a client with multiple fractures, treatment by surgical fixation of one fracture may allow closed treatment of another fracture.

Connolly (1981) states that fixation of severely comminuted (crushed) fractures is usually inadequate, so another form of treatment is recommended, eg, a cast or traction. Internal fixation may be used to treat pathological fractures, such as those caused by malignancy or osteoporosis, if the metal device can be secured to the bone adequately; however, with a pathological process affecting the bone, that may be difficult. Acrylic cement may be helpful in these cases in holding the metal securely to the bone. Open fractures should not be treated with internal fixation devices because incidence of complications such as wound or bone infection is higher for open fractures than closed ones.

Surgical fixation of fractures is a good treatment method for elderly clients, because it preserves the range of joint motion and often permits earlier mobility than treatment by traction alone, thus avoiding the hazards of immobility. Internal fixation is also used to hold a bone together when reconstructive bone surgery is done; an example of such surgery is osteotomy, discussed later in this chapter.

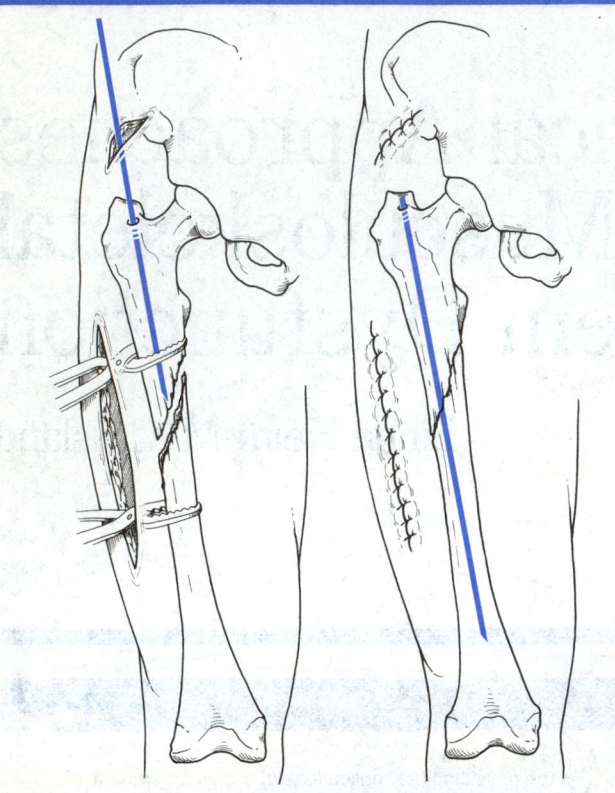

Figure 60-1

Intramedullary rod insertion. An incision is made at the top of the trochanter to insert the rod. Another incision is made over the fracture so the rod can be manipulated across the fracture line.

Surgical Procedure

An intramedullary (IM) rod, nail, or pin is used to treat a fracture of the shaft of a long bone. The procedure is done under general anesthesia. For a fracture in the shaft of the femur (Figure 60-1), an incision is made on the lateral aspect of the thigh over the fracture site so that the bone and rod can be manipulated under direct visualization. Another, smaller incision is made near the top of the trochanter to insert the rod, or to allow manipulation when the rod is inserted through the lower incision. The rod is inserted through the medullary canal (either upward from the fracture site or downward through the top of the trochanter) so the rod crosses the fracture site, joining the proximal and distal portions of the femur. A compression dressing is applied to the surgical site. The patient may be placed in balanced suspension traction or in a cast-brace postoperatively, or no supplemental immobilization may be used at all.

A similar procedure known as closed nailing uses image intensified fluoroscopy. An incision is made at the end of the long bone, and the rod is inserted through the medullary canal, across the fracture site. An incision over the fracture site is not required, because fluoroscopy replaces direct viewing. Closed nailing is more difficult to perform,

and malrotation is common (Apley & Solomon, 1982). However, there is less morbidity associated with closed nailing. It may be the best option for debilitated clients. According to Connolly (1981), the rod used for internal fixation should be removed when the fracture is completely obliterated, which should be at least one year after the fixation.

Some other fixation devices are shown in Figure 60-2. Metal plates are used on fractures of the shaft of long bones. They are held in place by screws made of the same metal as the plate (Figure 60-2A). The plate must be strong and securely fixed with at least two screws penetrating the bone cortex on both sides of the bone, above and below the fracture. Fractures that have small fragments of bone may be repaired with other hardware, such as screws (Figure 60-2B) or wires (Figure 60-2C). Combinations of devices are also used. Fixation devices are inserted through an incision over the area of fracture. A temporary posterior splint, firm on one side and soft on the other, may be applied in the operating room and left in place until swelling subsides. Then a cast may be applied. The follow-up treatment, including immobilization, depends upon the type and

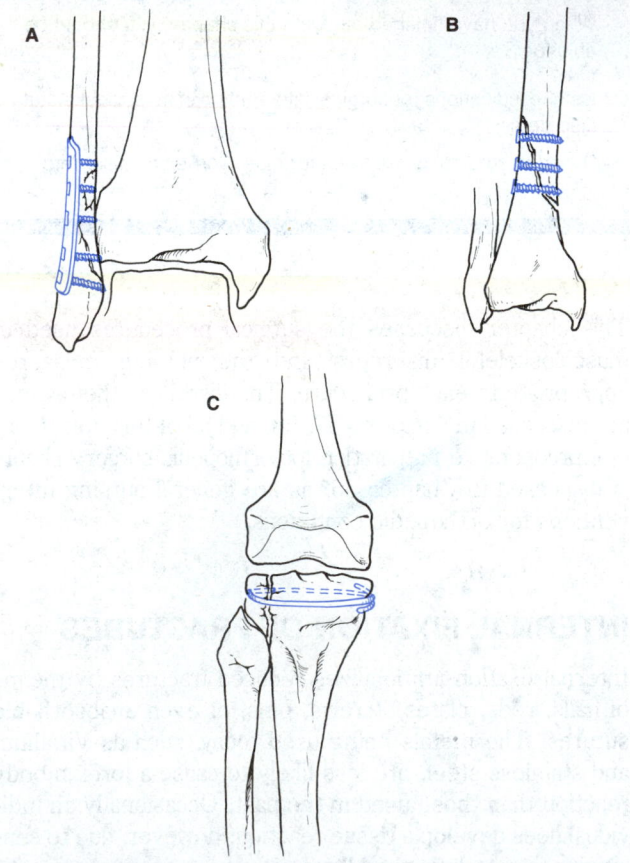

Figure 60-2

Internal fixation devices. **A.** Plate and screws holding together a comminuted fracture of the distal fibula.
B. Screws used to hold an oblique fracture of the tibia.
C. Wire used to secure a fragment of the tibial plateau.

location of the fracture, as well as the procedure. The hardware may be removed after complete healing, according to the physician's preference and the client's response to it; if it is not causing a problem, it may be retained.

Implications for the Client

Physiological Implications
Internal fixation devices keep the fragments in alignment so bone healing can occur in situations where it otherwise might not. Other physiological advantages to the client arise from the early mobility this treatment sometimes provides (eg, intramedullary rod fixation of the femur may provide earlier mobility than treatment by traction only). Thus, the client's chances of experiencing the hazards of immobility are decreased.

Bone infection is a potential complication of surgical intervention, since the procedure creates an opening through which pathogens can enter. During surgical manipulation of the tissues, nerves and blood vessels can be damaged, causing complications. A metal plate may break unless it is protected from stress while the fracture unites. Some metal devices may loosen or migrate, causing pain and instability.

Psychosocial/Lifestyle Implications
Early mobility has a positive effect: The client is able to be more independent earlier than with other procedures, and may be discharged sooner. Some internal fixation procedures require use of traction or cast postoperatively, however. The psychosocial effects of casts and traction are discussed in detail in Chapter 58. The implications of internal fixation procedures for the client are summarized in Table 60–1.

Nursing Implications

Preoperative Care
The preoperative preparation for internal fixation is the same as for other orthopedic surgical clients. Sometimes clients are taken directly from the emergency room to the operating room with little time to prepare them for what to expect. Such a client may need postoperative instruc-

tions on topics that normally would be taught preoperatively, such as exercises, coughing, and deep breathing.

Postoperative Care
Postoperative positioning in correct body alignment is important for maintaining the integrity of the fixation device. After an intramedullary rod is inserted, traction may be used to keep the limb from rotating until the client regains muscle control. Otherwise, sandbags may be placed along the sides of the limb to prevent external rotation. Care of the client in traction or a cast is covered in Chapter 58.

The affected limb is elevated postoperatively. The nurse checks the dressing or cast for bleeding and assesses the client's neurovascular status regularly to detect signs of complications. Dressing changes require sterile technique. Care will be needed to prevent the hazards of immobility. Provide analgesics and comfort measures to relieve pain. All these nursing measures are discussed in more detail in Chapter 58. Isometric exercises help maintain muscle strength and stimulate callus formation. For an intramedullary rod, the isometrics press the bone fragments together and help prevent them from pulling apart.

After surgical fixation of a lower extremity, clients must stay in bed until they can move the limb well. When they are allowed out of bed, the physician specifies how much, if any, weight bearing is allowed. The client must use crutches until bony union is evident on x-ray.

Before discharge, teach the client the signs and symptoms of infection, how much weight bearing is allowed, wound care, and cast care and ambulation techniques when these are appropriate. Encourage follow-up visits with the physician. A sample discharge handout is shown in Box 60–1. It is general enough to be used for postoperative clients after other surgical orthopedic procedures. Also, for a client in a cast, refer to the teaching described in Table 58–5.

EXTERNAL FIXATION OF FRACTURES

External fixation is a method of holding fracture fragments in alignment so healing can take place. Pins inserted into

Table 60–1 Internal Fixation: Implications for the Client

Physiological Implications	Psychosocial/Lifestyle Implications
Alignment maintained so bone healing can occur.	When used on fracture of femoral shaft, allows earlier mobility than treatment by traction would.
Earlier mobility than with traction alone may decrease the chances of immobility hazards.	Casts, splints, or traction may be used after internal fixation, causing alterations in independence.
Temporary pain and local swelling occurs.	May require the use of an ambulatory aid.
Potential complications: wound infection, bone infection, vascular or nerve injury, metal plate may break, device may loosen or migrate.	

Box 60–1 General Discharge Handout for Postoperative Orthopedic Clients

1. Elevate the limb (toes higher than the knee; hand higher than the elbow). For arm surgery, wear a sling when not lying down.

2. Your surgical wound should be cared for as follows: _____ _____

3. Exercise your arms and legs as instructed: _____ _____

4. The amount of activity you are allowed with your involved limb is _____ _____

5. Activities not allowed (check those appropriate):
   _____ Tub bath
   _____ Shower
   _____ Driving
   _____ Sexual intercourse
   _____ _____

6. Continue to use (walker, crutches, cane) as taught until instructed otherwise by your physician.

7. Notify the physician if:
   • You have a fever
   • The area of your incision appears reddened, swollen, hot, or has a foul odor
   • You have any drainage from the incision
   • You have numbness or loss of feeling in your leg or arm
   • You are unable to move your fingers or toes
   • You have severe pain at the incisional area

8. Continue to see the physician for scheduled appointments.

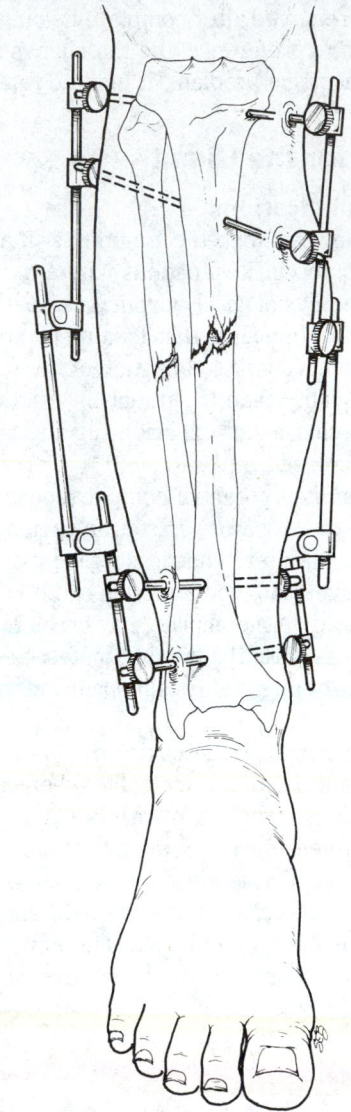

Figure 60–3

External fixation devices.

---

the bone above and below the fracture are attached to an external metal framework, which exerts pressure on the pins to stabilize the fragments in the proper position (Figure 60–3).

External fixation is used for complicated fractures that are difficult to repair by the usual methods of casts, traction, or internal fixation. Such fractures include open fractures with extensive soft tissue damage; comminuted fractures; fractures in which part of the bone is lost (eg, from a bullet wound); infected fractures; fractures complicated with burns; and severe open fractures, possibly with neurovascular damage, which might otherwise result in amputation of the limb. External fixators are most commonly applied to fractures of the leg but are also used on fractures of the forearm and pelvis.

Surgical Procedure

External fixators are applied under general anesthesia in the operating room. Small incisions are made over the pin insertion sites. Pins are inserted through the tissues and bone above and below the fracture site. The usual number of pins is 4 to 6, although as many as 12 may be necessary. The physician then connects the pins to external clamps and rods and manipulates them until the bone fragments are in alignment and confirmed by x-ray.

Implications for the Client

Physiological Implications

When there is an open wound over a fracture site, an external framework allows observation and care of the wound. In contrast, a cast would require a cast window to allow wound care. While providing stabilization of the fracture, external fixation allows movement of unaffected joints and muscles and may permit earlier ambulation than traction. There is a decreased risk of fat embolism because the bone fragments are stabilized (Hay & Karas, 1981). When part of the bone is missing, the fixator maintains the gap between fracture fragments, so that bone healing occurs between them and the limb does not shorten (Hay & Karas, 1981).

The limb will be painful for a few days after surgery because of manipulation of the extremity. Thereafter, the client is usually fairly comfortable, requiring only oral analgesics. Local swelling will be present after surgery. Temporary or permanent neurovascular damage may occur from surgical manipulation or from the injury itself. The insertion of pins into the bone provides a potential site for infection.

Psychosocial/Lifestyle Implications

The appearance of an external fixation device is rather shocking to anyone who has never seen one. The device is also heavy and makes movement awkward. The client will need to adjust to these psychological and physical problems. If the alternative treatment is amputation of the limb, the client will probably find the device tolerable.

Clients who need an external fixator may be taken to surgery immediately after being injured, so there is little or no opportunity to prepare them for the appearance of the device. Client and family will require explanations of the purpose of the apparatus. Body image will surely be affected by this abnormal addition; the client may be reluctant to look at the limb and may worry about the reactions of others.

Injuries requiring treatment by external fixation may also require a long hospitalization and adjustment to some type of ambulatory aid. Getting clients involved in wound and pin care gives them something to do and trains them for the care they must continue after discharge. Clothing may need to be adjusted to accommodate the device.

The implications of an external fixation device are summarized in Table 60–2.

Nursing Implications

Preoperative Care

Preoperatively, the nurse should describe the appearance and function of the external fixation device to the client and family. A picture of such a device or seeing another client with one is more helpful than a verbal description. Since this type of treatment has been uncommon in the past, most people have never seen the apparatus. Explain to the client that the device holds the bone together to permit healing while allowing care of the open wound. Clients should understand that they must not adjust the apparatus in any way, since that would alter the bone alignment. Preoperative preparation is the same as for any surgical orthopedic client (see Chapter 56).

Postoperative Care

Postoperatively, the limb is elevated to reduce swelling. This is frequently done by means of balanced suspension traction, applied by tying traction ropes directly to the fixator. Traction care is covered in Chapter 58. If traction is not used, elevate the limb on pillows or by raising the foot of the bed. Move the limb by grasping the frame rather than the limb itself. The sharp pin ends can be covered with cork, Vacutainer plugs, or the plastic ends that come with some pins. Assess the client's neurovascular status regularly, and provide comfort measures as necessary to relieve pain. Antibiotics are given to prevent infection.

Exercise and Ambulation. Help the client maintain joint mobility by doing range of motion (ROM) exercises at least twice a day and maintain strength by doing frequent isometric exercises, as allowed. When clients are ambulating, the physician should specify whether they can bear weight on the affected leg. The physical therapist can prepare clients for ambulation and teach them the use of ambulatory aids, usually crutches. Encourage clients to move slowly and smoothly because the heavy, awkward fixator may affect balance and coordination. It is important for someone to help clients get in and out of bed and move around until they can manage safely on their own.

Wound and Pin Care. Wound care is a challenge with the external framework in the way. The fixator is not

---

Table 60–2 External Fixation: Implications for the Client	
Physiological Implications	**Psychosocial/Lifestyle Implications**
Provides stability of fracture fragments.	Alters body image.
Allows visualization and care of open wound.	Device is heavy and awkward.
Allows movement of unaffected joints and muscles.	Hospitalization and/or recuperation may be lengthy.
Allows earlier ambulation in many cases.	Client must learn use of ambulatory aid.
Decreases risk of fat embolism.	Client or family member needs to learn to give wound and pin care for home care.
Prevents bone shortening by maintaining distraction when a part of the bone is missing.	The type of clothing that can be worn with the device may require adjustment after discharge.
Pain is usually minimal after a few days postoperatively.	The device may interfere with return to work.
Local swelling occurs immediately postoperatively.	
Potential complications: wound infection, bone infection, nerve or vascular damage.	

sterile, but wound care requires *strict* aseptic technique. Sterile gloves and/or sterile forceps are necessary, and the nurse must avoid touching them on the framework. The dressings may be maneuvered into place by use of sterile instruments or sterile tongue blades. These dressing changes take longer than others.

Daily pin site care is necessary to prevent infection. The type of pin care should be specified by the physician. Serous fluid will normally drain around the pin sites and form crusts. The fluid forms as a result of the soft tissues sliding over the pins. Pin site care requires cleansing of each site with a separate sterile cotton-tipped applicator to remove the crusts. Crust removal is important because crusts can harbor bacteria when left in place. Usually, hydrogen peroxide is used for cleansing, followed by normal saline. Observe the skin for redness, pain, tenderness, odor, or skin tension. An antibacterial agent such as iodophor ointment or foam may be applied, or antibiotic ointments are sometimes used. Sterile technique requires the use of many sterile cotton-tipped applicators, one per site. Sterile dressings are sometimes applied.

As soon as clients are able, they should be involved in pin site and wound care. Involvement in care helps pass the time and trains clients for their care after discharge. The nurse can teach sterile technique and observe until clients perform satisfactorily. Teach clients to notify the physician of any abnormal signs or symptoms, or if a pin becomes loose. Loose pins contribute to destabilization of the fracture, and it may enhance development of infection by irritation of soft tissue. Clients can keep the fixator clean by wiping it with a clean damp cloth.

Sometimes the external rods are removed and a cast is applied over the pins, incorporating them into the cast. Then the nurse needs to teach the client cast care (see Chapter 58) before discharge. Wearing clothing over the device may take simple tailoring so that sleeves or pantlegs can be snapped over the fixator. Velcro fasteners are helpful.

To help clients adjust to changes in body image, encourage expression of feelings about the wound and external fixator, and involve them in their own care. Encourage them to discuss their situation and their feelings about it. The fixator may interfere with the client's return to work. A referral to a social worker may be necessary if prolonged hospitalization or recuperation causes worries about financial matters.

HIP PINNING

Hip pinning (or nailing) is a type of internal fixation procedure used for repair of fractures of the proximal femur. Hip fractures are most common in the elderly; the average age of occurrence is 73. Seventy percent of hip fractures occur in women (Connolly, 1981). Characteristics of the elderly that probably contribute to falls and hip fracture include poor vision; slowed reflexes; problems with balance; weak muscles; postural hypotension; and weak, fragile bones from osteoporosis. Hip fractures may occur from

falls, a twisting motion, direct trauma, or stress on diseased bone. Common sites of fracture are illustrated in Figure 60–4.

Assessment of the client with a hip fracture usually reveals a leg that is shortened, externally rotated, and abducted. The client experiences pain, especially when attempting to move the extremity, and may resist anyone touching it. The skin over the hip may be ecchymotic and swollen.

In some hip fractures, the bone fragments are not displaced, and these fractures can be treated conservatively with rest. For most hip fractures, however, surgery is the treatment of choice.

Surgical Procedure

Many procedures and fixation devices are used to treat fractured hips. The procedure is determined by the type and location of the fracture. The surgeon selects the device that will best secure the fracture fragments in place and provide a functioning joint. A brief description of some of these procedures follows; some of the devices are illustrated in Figure 60–5.

A fracture of the femoral neck in which the fracture is incomplete or the fragments are not displaced may be

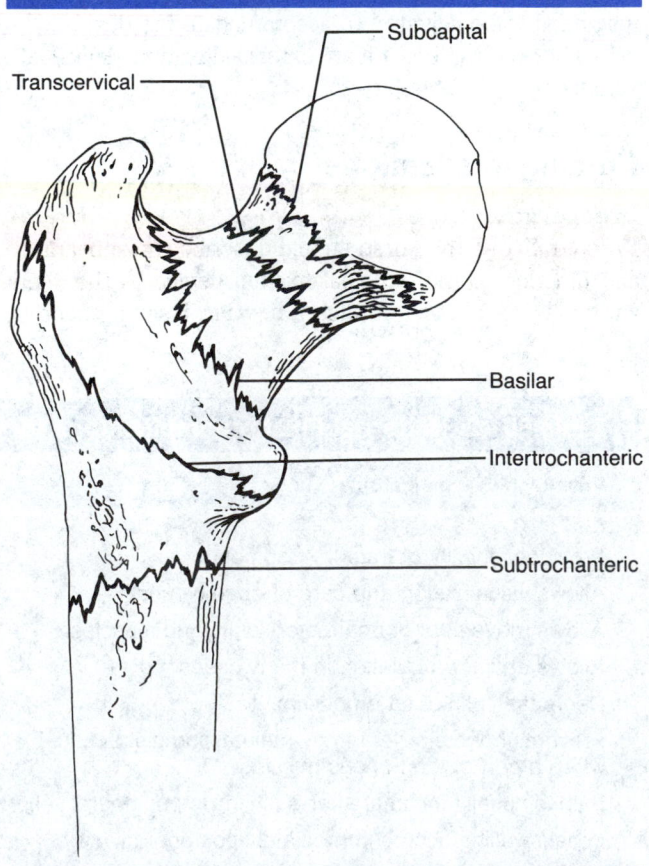

Figure 60–4

Common sites of hip fractures.

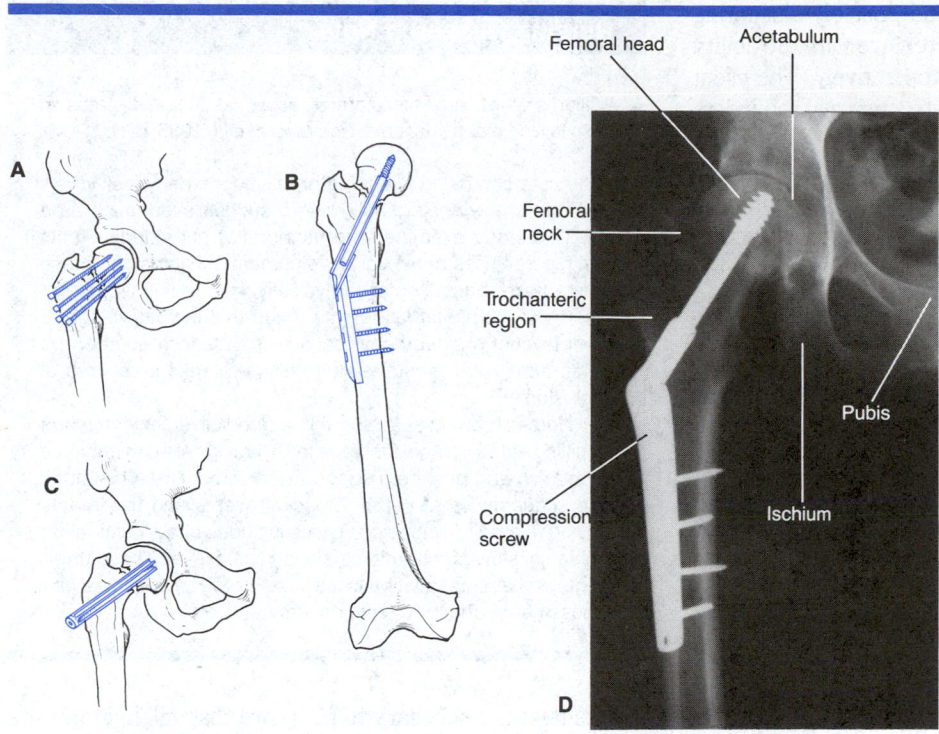

Femoral head

Acetabulum

Femoral neck

Trochanteric region

Compression screw

Pubis

Ischium

D

A

B

C

Figure 60–5

Types of internal fixation devices for fractured hips. **A.** Knowles pin. **B.** Compression screw. **C.** Nail. **D.** A compression screw used to treat a fracture of the right femoral neck (Courtesy of Health Care Plan, Buffalo, NY).

fixed by pins, such as Knowles pins (Figure 60–5A). Under general anesthesia, the incision is made on the lateral thigh just below the greater trochanter. The pins are inserted using fluoroscopy to guide the placement.

A device known as a compression screw (Figure 60–5B) has been used recently to treat some femoral neck and intertrochanteric fractures. The device has two components: a screw with large threads that grasp the head of the femur from within and a side plate that is screwed to the shaft of the femur. The side plate has a barrel, through which the screw is inserted. The two pieces slide closer together as bone resorption occurs at the fracture site. Under general anesthesia, the fracture is reduced, and an incision is made over the trochanteric region after x-rays demonstrate that satisfactory reduction has been accomplished. Instruments are used to ream out a hole in the bone from below the greater trochanter, up through the neck of the femur and into the femoral head. The compression screw is inserted, the barrel of the plate is fitted over the screw, and the side of the plate is fastened with screws to the femoral shaft. Compression is applied to pull the pin and plate together. The compression is helpful in preventing nonunion by decreasing the gap between fracture fragments. The sliding quality prevents the screw from penetrating through the femoral head (Connolly, 1981).

Another device for fractures of the femoral neck consists solely of a nail that traverses the fracture site to hold the fracture fragments in alignment (Figure 60–5C). The nail may be triflanged, rather than round, to prevent rotation of the bone around the nail. Other devices for hip fractures combine pins or nails with side plates.

Implications for the Client

Since hip pinning is a type of internal fixation, the implications summarized in Table 60–1 apply here.

Physiological Implications

The advantage of hip pinning, as opposed to fracture treatment by traction or cast, is earlier mobility. In most cases, the client gets out of bed within 1 or 2 days after surgery. The disadvantages are the same as those for other internal fixation procedures. In addition, interruption of blood supply to the head of the femur, from either the traumatic event or the surgery, may cause aseptic (avascular) necrosis. Then, further surgery may be necessary (see the following section, covering hip prosthesis).

Other physiological effects of surgery include pain, local swelling, ecchymosis, and possible hemorrhage and shock. Full weight bearing is not allowed until sufficient healing occurs, which may take as long as 5 months.

Psychosocial/Lifestyle Implications

Fear of dying as a result of hip fracture is common. Many people remember an elderly friend or relative who died during hospitalization following a hip fracture. Indeed, 30% of hip fracture clients die within 1 year after the injury, sometimes from pulmonary embolism, myocardial infarction, or pneumonia but mostly from old age (Connolly, 1981).

Confusion is common in the elderly client who is hospitalized. Contributing factors include pain, shock, a strange environment, medications, and fluid and electrolyte imbalances. A confused client may try to get out of bed, especially at night, jeopardizing safety and possibly disrupting the surgical repair. Confusion may interfere with the ability to participate in physical therapy postoperatively. The client who is forgetful may need frequent instruction and reminders about contraindicated positions and activities.

The client may also fear loss of independence because of loss of function. A temporary or permanent change in lifestyle may be necessary. Some people cannot return to their former level of independence and require a change in living accommodations, such as moving in with a relative, temporary or permanent residence in a nursing home, or the assistance of a homemaker or home aide. The client and family should begin planning for discharge soon after admission so hospitalization is not prolonged.

Any of these fears or actual consequences may cause the client to be depressed. On the other hand, the early mobility allowed by hip pinning should have a positive effect on the client's mental status since it increases independence and reduces the sense of helplessness. The specific implications of a fractured hip and surgical hip repair are summarized in Table 60–3.

Nursing Implications

Preoperative Care

Since hip fracture clients are usually elderly, their condition may be complicated by the chronic diseases that accompany old age. The client's condition must be stabilized before surgery is attempted; as with any preoperative client, fluid and electrolyte balance and nutritional status should be optimal. An elderly client is particularly susceptible to the hazards of immobility, and the longer stabilization is delayed, the longer the client is immobile. Surgery should be done within 48 hours of injury if the client is medically stable.

On admission, the nurse and several assistants transfer the client gently to the bed. An egg crate or air mattress should be applied to the bed first. A thorough preoperative

assessment is necessary to plan care that will help get the client in optimal condition for surgery. Include assessment for other injuries. Buck's extension or Russell's traction may be applied to reduce pain and muscle spasm, or the client may be allowed to assume a position of comfort without traction. The nurse should not attempt to align the leg as long as the neurovascular status is satisfactory (Farrell, 1982). Turning the client should be done with pillows between the legs.

In addition to the usual preoperative preparation (see Chapter 56), a type and crossmatch is done to have blood available for surgery. The nurse may start an intravenous infusion to give preoperative antibiotics. Prepare the client to expect the following postoperatively: an IV, Hemovac, antibiotics, a dressing in the trochanteric region, and anal-

Table 60–3 Hip Pinning: Implications for the Client*	
Physiological Implications	**Psychosocial/Lifestyle Implications**
Client's medical condition must be stabilized before surgery is performed.	Client may fear dying as a result of hip fracture.
Surgery should be performed as soon as condition is stable to prevent hazards of immobility.	Elderly client may become confused, jeopardizing safety, surgical repair, and interfering with cooperation in therapy.
Aseptic necrosis may occur if the blood supply to the femoral head is damaged.	Elderly clients who are forgetful require clear instructions and reminders about contraindications.
Procedure usually causes pain, local swelling, ecchymosis.	Former level of independence may be decreased temporarily or permanently.
Hemorrhage and shock may occur.	Client may require a change in living accommodations.
Full weight bearing is not permitted until healing occurs (possibly as long as 5 months).	Client may be depressed.
	Early mobility may have a positive effect on the client.

*See Table 60–1 for implications of internal fixation.

gesics for pain. Explain the positions that will be allowed, exercises that will need to be done, and use of the trapeze.

Postoperative Care

The postoperative care may be specific according to the physician's preference. In general, the nurse assesses the client's neurovascular status and the condition of the dressing each time vital signs are taken. Observe the part of the dressing under the client carefully, since drainage will flow downward and may be missed from a side view. A Hemovac is usually used for a few days postoperatively and should be kept collapsed. Measure the drainage each shift; the amount should decrease with time. An IV is usually used to give intravenous antibiotics. Provide comfort measures and analgesics after a thorough assessment of the client's pain. Good skin care and observation of common pressure areas are important.

Coughing, deep breathing, and incentive spirometry are necessary to prevent respiratory problems. The client wears elastic stockings; remove these at least twice a day to give skin care and to observe the heels for signs of breakdown. Range of motion exercises are necessary for all uninvolved joints, and the client should do isometric exercises to maintain strength in the quadriceps, abdominal, and gluteal muscles (see Chapter 56).

A fracture bedpan prevents unnecessary flexion of the operative hip and pain. Incontinence of urine or stool may soil the nearby dressing, requiring prompt dressing change to prevent wound contamination. To prevent constipation, encourage adequate intake of fluids and roughage; exercise, stool softeners, and laxatives may also be helpful. The client is often able to tolerate regular foods the day after surgery. Nutritional management for those with fractures is covered in Chapter 58.

Positioning and Turning. Physicians' postoperative orders vary mostly in regard to positioning the client. Some physicians use traction (Buck's or Russell's) or a cast to reduce muscle spasm and maintain alignment. Turn the client only as ordered. In general, the client can and should be turned every 2 hours. The doctor may have a preference for which direction the client may be turned (toward the operative or unoperative side). Whenever the client is moved, avoid extreme positions and movements such as acute angle flexion of the operative hip. Adduction and external rotation should also be avoided. Tell the client to keep toes pointing toward the ceiling while resting in bed. Trochanter rolls or covered sandbags placed beside the leg are helpful in preventing rotation, but avoid pressure on the upper lateral calf to prevent peroneal nerve injury. Place pillows between the client's legs to maintain abduction. Whenever the client is turned, assistance will be needed to support the uppermost leg in abduction. Be sure pillows have been placed between the client's legs to prevent a strain on the operative area.

With pinning, the risk of displacement of the surgical device is less than with a hip prosthesis (see next section),

but gentle handling and proper positioning are still necessary. Assess frequently for maintenance of good body alignment. Do back care and skin observation when the client is in the side-lying position.

Ambulation. When clients are allowed out of bed, the nurse should know specifically how to get them up and what positions are allowed. Most clients are allowed out of bed the first or second day after surgery, with no weight bearing on the operative leg. The nurse should assess how well the client will follow directions. If the ability to follow directions is questionable, it is better to lift the client into the chair. The chair should be firm, not low, and should have armrests. It should be placed parallel to and touching the bed, positioned so the client can move toward the strong (unoperative) side. The client should wear firm, nonskid shoes, and the chair and bed wheels should be locked. Give clear instructions, with the assurance that the staff will be there to assist at all times.

To get up, the client turns to the side, swivels into a sitting position, dangles until stable, stands with weight on the unoperative leg only, pivots, and eases into the chair by grasping the armrests. All this is done with the assistance of the nurse, using good body mechanics. The physician should specify if the leg should remain elevated when the client is in the chair. The first time out of bed should be only about 15 to 20 minutes, unless the client wants to be up longer. While up, personal hygiene, hair care, and oral care can be done, or the client can eat a meal, as long as there is no discomfort. Prolonged sitting in a chair should be avoided to prevent pelvic vein thrombosis (Connolly, 1981). The client returns to bed by reversing the order of the actions used to get up.

Walking begins according to the client's readiness and the physician's preference. A physical therapist instructs the client in the use of a walker, usually without weight bearing on the operative leg. The walker and no weight bearing are necessary until the fracture is healed—about 4 months.

Safety Measures. The nurse should evaluate the client's mental status for planning interventions according to the level of orientation. When the client is confused, interventions to maintain safety are necessary. Siderails should be up, and a small light may be left on in the room at night. Use restraints only as a last resort. Interventions to control pain and maintain hydration may help combat some of the causes of confusion; in addition, the nurse should evaluate the effects of the medications the client is taking. It will be necessary to repeat instructions and supervise the client's activities at times. Providing orientation and encouraging family visits may help the client's mental status. Encouraging independence and participation in self-care is helpful for the client who is depressed because of feelings of helplessness.

Discharge. Consult the family when preparing the client for discharge. The home should be made safe for use of a walker, eg, by removing throw rugs, clutter, and electric cords from traffic areas. Families will need to obtain a walker and perhaps an elevated toilet seat. The client should use a firm chair with armrests. The client and family may be referred to social services to plan for help in the home or to plan discharge to a specialized facility when necessary. Encourage follow-up visits to the physician, who will use x-rays to evaluate healing and to detect signs of complications, such as avascular necrosis.

HIP PROSTHESIS

Insertion of a hip prosthesis is a surgical procedure used to treat certain hip fractures. A metal device consisting of a ball-shaped head attached to an intramedullary rod is used to replace the head and neck of the femur (Figure 60–6). The material covered in the previous section on hip pinning is pertinent here also and will not be repeated. This discussion will deal only with the differences in the treatment and care for the client with a hip prosthesis.

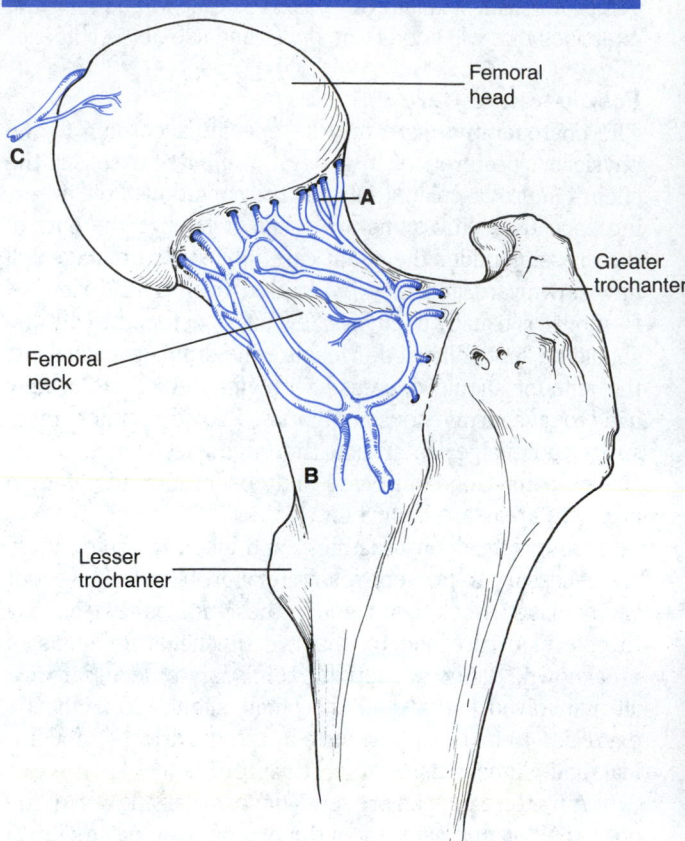

Figure 60–7

Blood supply to the femoral head. **A,** posterior superior retinacular vessels. **B,** posterior inferior retinacular vessels. **C,** the artery of the ligamentum teres.

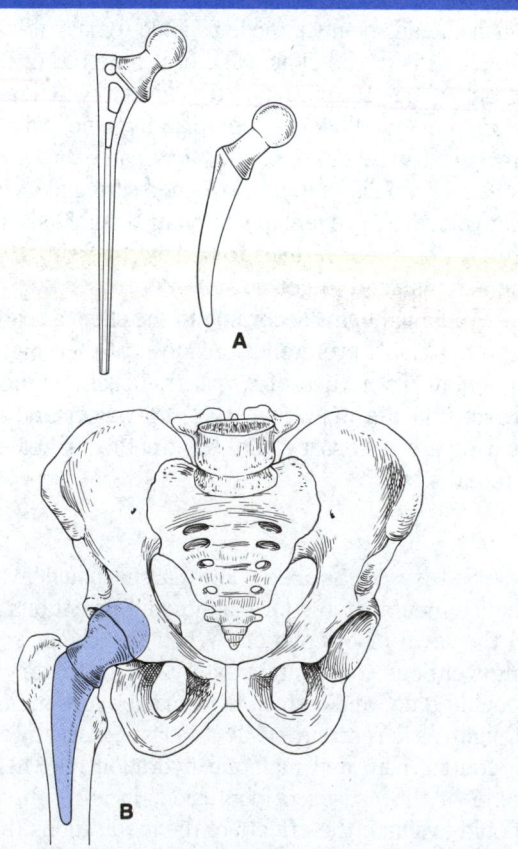

Figure 60–6

Hip prostheses. **A.** *Left,* an Austin-Moore prosthesis. *Right,* a cemented prosthesis. **B.** A hip prosthesis in place. The ball fits into the acetabulum; the stem is inserted into the femoral medullary canal.

Use of a hip prosthesis is indicated for hip fractures that are prone to development of avascular necrosis (see Chapter 58). Figure 60–7 shows the blood supply to the femoral head. The vessels in the femoral neck are vulnerable to injury when the femoral neck is fractured, especially when there is displacement of the fragments. Disruption of the vessels interferes with healing and may cause avascular necrosis. Connolly (1981) states that a hip prosthesis is the most effective treatment for people over 70 years old who have femoral neck fractures with displacement. A hip prosthesis may also be used for comminuted femoral neck fractures and other fractures that are difficult to reduce.

Surgical Procedure

The hip prosthesis is inserted under general anesthesia. An incision is made in the trochanteric region. The femoral head is removed, and the femoral neck is reshaped to receive the prosthesis. The medullary canal is reamed to remove the cancellous bone so the canal can accommodate the prosthesis rod or stem. The surgeon determines the correct size of the prosthesis so the prosthesis head is the same size as the femoral head. The Austin Moore (AM) prosthesis, a metal self-locking device in use for several years, has holes in the stem through which bone consolidation occurs, locking the device in place. Newer devices, such as the Cathcart prosthesis, are designed to be cemented into the medullary canal providing a stronger bond. The ellipsoid head of the Cathcart prosthesis allows synovial fluid to perfuse the acetabulum (Connolly, 1981) and provides less incidence of erosion of the prosthesis through the acetabular cartilage.

Implications for the Client

The implications of hip pinning summarized in Table 60–3 apply here as well.

Physiological Implications

A hip prosthesis provides a functioning hip joint without the risk of avascular necrosis that may exist with other types of hip fracture repair. Another advantage is earlier weight bearing, since there is no fracture to heal. The chief disadvantage of this type of surgery is increased chance for dislocation of the hip postoperatively. The postoperative positioning of the client is important in preventing dislocation.

Other potential problems are loosening of the prosthesis in the medullary canal and erosion of the prosthesis head through the acetabular cartilage. The newer-shaped prostheses, which can be cemented in place, reduce the chances of these complications (Connolly, 1981).

Psychosocial/Lifestyle Implications

The positions allowed postoperatively may restrict the movements of the client and interfere with comfort. Nursing measures are helpful in relieving discomfort. The earlier weight bearing allowed with a prosthesis should make using a walker easier than it would be with a hip pinning. Table 60–4 lists those implications that are different for hip prosthesis clients.

Nursing Implications

The nursing care for clients with hip pinning, described in the previous section, is pertinent here also. The positioning of the client is important to prevent hip dislocation and strain on the incisional area. The approach of the incision into the joint capsule dictates postoperative positioning, which the surgeon specifies. As with hip pinning, avoid acute flexion and adduction of the hip. To maintain the operative leg in an abducted position, use a wedge-shaped abductor pillow or a splint (Figure 60–8). The pillow fastens with Velcro straps. It is important to prevent circulatory problems from tight straps and to prevent decubitus ulcers from pressure of the appliance. The straps should not be placed over the upper fibula where the peroneal nerve lies. Remove the appliance to provide skin care and

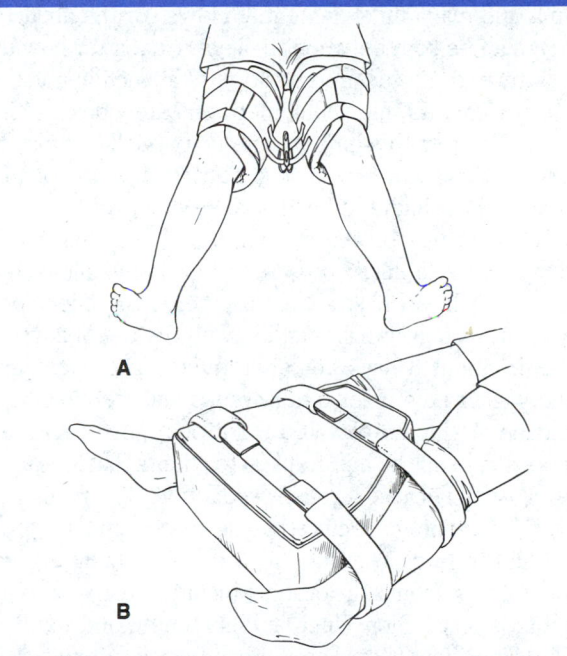

Figure 60–8

Abductor splint (**A**) and pillow (**B**).

Table 60–4 Hip Prosthesis: Implications for the Client*	
Physiological Implications	**Psychosocial/Lifestyle Implications**
Provides a functioning hip joint without the chance of avascular necrosis.	Postoperative positioning may be restrictive.
Earlier weight bearing is allowed than with hip pinning.	Use of walker may be easier than with hip pinning because weight bearing is allowed earlier.
Chances of hip dislocation require adherence to specific preventive positioning orders.	
Complications are loosening of the prosthesis and erosion of the prosthetic head through the acetabular cartilage.	

*See Table 60–3 for implications of hip pinning.

to observe the skin condition while the client keeps the leg in the required alignment. The length of time the abduction device is used depends upon the physician's preference and the client's progress. Some physicians use ordinary pillows or sandbags to position the leg in abduction instead of the abduction devices.

The client is allowed to turn only with physician's orders because some physicians prefer the supine position only. When clients are not allowed to turn, the nurse teaches them to use the trapeze to help lift themselves for linen changes and frequent back care. Lifting the client in this way is much easier and safer with extra assistance. The operative leg must be kept in the desired alignment while lifting.

If the client is allowed to turn to a side-lying position, the specific side is ordered by the surgeon. Generally, the client turns onto the operative hip, since the bed can splint the limb and maintain alignment. Pillows (or the abductor device) must be kept between the legs. No matter how the client is turned, the desired position of abduction must be maintained, and the hip should not be acutely flexed. Elevation of the operative limb on one or two pillows may be ordered; otherwise it should be kept flat. The surgeon may also specify how high the head may be elevated.

The client may be allowed out of bed 1 to 3 days after surgery to sit in a chair; no weight bearing is allowed on the operative leg. Physical therapy helps the client progress to ambulation; weight bearing with the use of a walker may begin about 3 days postoperatively. The client may find the walker helpful for 6 to 8 weeks and then begins to use a cane. Using an elevated toilet seat postoperatively prevents strain on the hip. Explain to clients that legs must not be crossed because it causes adduction. The reason for all these positioning specifications is to prevent the prosthetic head from dislocating out of the acetabulum. Signs and symptoms of hip dislocation include sharp pain and abnormal limb position, such as shortening and external rotation. The client should notify the physician immediately if these things happen; the client may have to return to surgery for treatment.

SYNOVECTOMY

Synovectomy is a surgical procedure in which the synovial membrane is removed from a joint to relieve pain.

The client with rheumatoid arthritis with a painful, swollen joint that responds poorly to intra-articular steroids is a candidate for synovectomy. The procedure should be done before the cartilage and bone are eroded by the disease; once that has happened, the client requires arthroplasty. Synovectomy is most often done on the knee but is also a common procedure for the fingers, wrist, and elbow.

Surgical Procedure

Synovectomy is usually done under general anesthesia. A tourniquet may be used on the extremity to decrease bleeding. The joint capsule is opened, and the synovial tissue is removed carefully to prevent damage to nerves and blood vessels. The capsule is repaired, and a bulky soft pressure dressing is applied after wound closure. The dressing remains for a few days postoperatively.

Implications for the Client

Physiological Implications

Removal of the inflamed synovium provides relief of pain in the majority of clients. Synovectomy also preserves joint functioning, although some motion may be lost. After knee synovectomy, 50% to 75% of clients have relief of pain, although they may lose some joint motion, especially flexion. The synovium regrows and may develop the disease, but usually in a milder form. This procedure may be a palliative measure, and arthroplasty may be done later as the condition progresses.

The surgical procedure will cause localized pain, edema, and decreased ROM postoperatively. Range of motion exercises and ambulation are begun early, with weight bearing as soon as it is tolerated.

Psychosocial/Lifestyle Implications

The client should benefit psychologically from the relief of pain. Postoperatively, there is some inconvenience with the bulky dressing and limited use of the joint. Depending upon the joint affected, the client may need help with ADL, but only temporarily until strength and ROM are regained. Recurrence of the disease in the joint may be depressing and discouraging to the client. The implications of synovectomy are summarized in Table 60–5.

Nursing Implications

Assess the client's neurovascular status, dressing, and vital signs regularly. Elevate the extremity. The client will begin exercises a few days postoperatively. Ambulation and amount of weight bearing are specified by the surgeon. Otherwise, routine postoperative nursing care is necessary.

OSTEOTOMY

An osteotomy is a surgical procedure in which a bone is cut so it can be realigned. A wedge of bone may be removed or inserted, or the bone may be rotated to adjust the weight-bearing alignment or to decrease pain. The procedure actually causes a fracture of the bone.

Osteotomy is performed when a deformity in a limb interferes with joint function, causing pain and difficulty with movement. The deformity may be caused when a fracture heals in poor alignment. Other causes of deformity are congenital conditions and bone diseases, such as rickets. An osteotomy may also be helpful in altering alignment to change the weight-bearing surface in an arthritic joint. This may help relieve joint pain.

The procedure is done most often on the femur for

Table 60-5 Synovectomy: Implications for the Client	
Physiological Implications	**Psychosocial/Lifestyle Implications**
Provides relief of pain.	Relief of pain allows psychological rest.
Preserves joint function; some joint motion may be lost.	Temporary inconvenience of bulky dressing and decreased use of the involved extremity. May require assistance with ADL.
The synovium regrows and can develop rheumatoid synovitis.	Recurrence of the disease may be discouraging.
Exercises will be necessary to regain strength and function.	
Temporary swelling and pain occur from the surgical procedure.	
Potential complications: wound infection, joint infection, nerve or blood vessel damage.	

correcting malposition of the head of the femur in the acetabulum (Mourad, 1980).

Surgical Procedure

Osteotomy is done under general anesthesia. The bone is cut, repositioned, and held in place with some type of internal fixation device. The angle of the limb is measured and calculated carefully by the surgeon to provide the desired alignment. The fresh cut bone surfaces must be brought together firmly to facilitate bony union. One example of an osteotomy is illustrated in Figure 60-9. A cast is frequently applied to maintain alignment.

Implications for the Client

The implications of osteotomy are generally the same as those for a client with internal fixation (see Table 60-1).

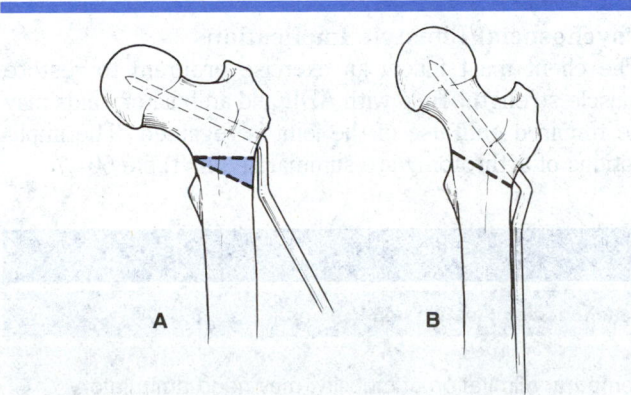

Figure 60-9
Osteotomy with the use of a blade plate to hold the bone together. **A.** The wedge shaped section is removed to realign the bone. **B.** The two cut surfaces are brought together and held in place by an internal fixation device.

Physiological Implications
Osteotomy provides the client with a functioning limb and relief of pain. When the procedure is done on an osteoarthritic hip, it may delay the progression of the arthritis (Powell, 1982).

The client must avoid weight bearing until the union is complete. Client progress and the location of the osteotomy influence when weight bearing can begin and the amount of weight allowed. Possible complications include overcorrection or undercorrection of the deformity and the complications of internal fixation, such as infection.

Psychosocial/Lifestyle Implications
Undergoing an elective procedure in hopes of improving comfort and functioning may cause considerable ambivalence. Clients may wonder if they are doing the right thing by having surgery instead of trying to live with the disability. They may fear complications and further disability.

Postoperatively, the client should experience the psychological benefits of pain relief if the surgery is a success. There may also be an improvement in appearance if a deformity is less noticeable or a limp is absent. Clients will have to adjust to the immobility of a cast or internal fixation device until union is complete. Additional implications of osteotomy are summarized in Table 60-6.

Nursing Implications

Preoperative Care
Preoperatively, the nurse should encourage clients to express their concerns about undergoing the procedure and plan appropriate interventions. Nursing care is the same as that given to a client with a fracture who has had internal fixation. The care of a client in a cast, described in Chapter 58, is pertinent here.

Postoperative Care
Postoperatively, the nurse should expect a large amount of bleeding through the cast from the surgical area for about

Table 60–6 Osteotomy: Implications for the Client*	
Physiological Implications	**Psychosocial/Lifestyle Implications**
May provide relief of pain.	May provide relief of pain, improving quality of life.
May improve functioning of the limb.	In some cases, provides improved appearance of a limb.
May delay progression of the osteoarthritic process in the involved joint.	Difficulty with ambulation (eg, limping) may be less noticeable.
Weight bearing is not allowed until union is complete.	
The site of the procedure and the progress of the client influence when and how much weight bearing is allowed.	
The deformity may be overcorrected or undercorrected.	

*See Table 60–1 for implications of internal fixation.

2 days (Farrell, 1982). Therefore, vital signs are checked every 4 hours for signs of shock.

Teach isometric and ROM exercises and encourage the client to do them regularly to maintain muscle strength and joint ROM. Also encourage isotonic exercises to prepare for ambulation (see Chapter 56). Physical therapy will be ordered to prepare the client for ambulation and to teach the use of ambulatory aids. The length of time the client must spend in a cast, on crutches, and without weight bearing are all determined by the surgeon.

ARTHROTOMY

An arthrotomy is a surgical opening into a joint to visualize the intra-articular structures for diagnosis or to perform surgical procedures. Arthrotomy is not used often as a diagnostic procedure since arthroscopy is now so widely used (see Chapter 56). The knee is the joint on which arthrotomy is most often performed.

Arthrotomy is used to drain an abscess or hematoma in a joint, to remove loose bodies or damaged structures, to inspect the joint structures, to take biopsies, and to perform a synovectomy.

Surgical Procedure

Arthrotomy is done under general anesthesia. The joint capsule is opened and irrigated with sterile normal saline.

The joint structures can be seen directly and the desired procedure performed. After the joint capsule is closed, pressure dressing is usually applied.

Implications for the Client

Physiological Implications
Depending upon the procedure done, the surgery may improve functioning of the joint and relieve discomfort. The arthrotomy will cause temporary weakness of the joint and pain in the area. The client should rest the joint for a few days afterward and then engage in movement, the amount and kind depending upon the procedure done. The surgeon will prescribe specific exercises to strengthen the joint. Since vessels may bleed into the joint, a compression dressing is used. An opening into a joint provides a portal for microorganisms, so antibiotics are frequently given postoperatively to prevent joint infection. Arthroscopy is being used more today to perform operative joint procedures as well as diagnosis. Its advantages over arthrotomy are a decrease in morbidity and a faster return to normal activity.

Psychosocial/Lifestyle Implications
The client must follow an exercise program to restore muscle strength. Help with ADL and ambulatory aids may be required until use of the joint is regained. The implications of arthrotomy are summarized in Table 60–7.

Table 60–7 Arthrotomy: Implications for the Client	
Physiological Implications	**Psychosocial/Lifestyle Implications**
May provide improved joint functioning and relief of discomfort.	Temporary limitation of mobility; may need ambulatory aids and help with ADL.
The joint will be weak temporarily, requiring exercises to strengthen it later.	Improved joint functioning and decreased discomfort may improve quality of client's life.
Potential complications: bleeding into the joint, nerve or blood vessel damage, wound infection, joint infection.	

Nursing Implications

Preoperative Care

The preoperative preparation is the same as for other orthopedic conditions (see Chapter 56).

Postoperative Care

Postoperatively, the nurse should observe the dressing for bleeding and check neurovascular status along with vital signs. The extremity should be elevated on pillows. Mild analgesics and comfort measures are necessary to relieve pain. The amount of joint movement, exercises to be done, and the amount of weight bearing to be allowed will be ordered by the surgeon. Straight-leg raises and quadriceps setting exercises, for example, are done when surgery is performed on the knee. The client may need to use ambulatory aids.

ARTHRODESIS

Arthrodesis is the surgical fusion of a joint to provide stability or relief of pain. Joint movement is no longer possible after bony union takes place.

Arthrodesis is indicated when joint movement causes severe pain or instability, and other measures have failed to relieve it. Such a condition may result from joint disease, such as tuberculosis or arthritis; fractures with nonunion; congenital defects; muscle imbalance from neuromuscular disease; or may follow failure of total joint replacements.

If the joint can be fused in a functional position, it may be more useful to the person than before. That is, a fixed position may allow use of an extremity that otherwise would be impossible because movement is so painful or the joint is unstable. For example, fusion of an arthritic's wrist may provide pain-free, functional movement of the hand. Hip fusion may be done on a severely painful hip of a young person who works in a standing position or does heavy work, provided the knee, other hip, and spine are normal. (These joints must be normal because more stress is placed on them after fusion.) Although a slight limp may result, the client can be comfortable and may be able to walk and run (Apley & Solomon, 1982). Other joints on which arthrodesis is performed include the spine, ankle, knee, interphalangeal joints, and shoulder.

Surgical Procedure

Arthrodesis is done under general anesthesia. The articular cartilage is removed from both joint surfaces; the bone surfaces are fashioned to form an approximate fit. Then pieces of bone graft are packed into the remaining small spaces to promote bony union. Usually, the bone ends are held together firmly by internal fixation devices such as staples, an intramedullary rod, pins, or plates and screws. The best positioning of the united joint depends upon the needs of the individual; for example, a fused knee with slight flexion may be good for sitting, but a straight knee is better for walking or standing. A cast is frequently applied to immobilize the joint until union is complete. A person with hip fusion will have a hip spica cast, whereas a knee fusion requires a long leg cast.

One such surgical procedure is triple arthrodesis in which three bones of the ankle are fused to treat instability of the foot. The three affected joints are the talocalcaneal, talonavicular, and calcaneocuboid joints (Figure 60–10). The fusion does not affect the flexion and extension of the ankle, but eliminates eversion and inversion. The client wears a short leg cast.

Implications for the Client

Physiological Implications

The benefits of arthrodesis are relief of pain and instability. If pain is caused by joint movement, fusion of the joint should eliminate the pain. In some areas, stability may be more important than movement if the movement is faulty.

The implications of internal fixation, summarized in Table 60–1, are pertinent here also. The operation will cause pain and swelling in the operative area, requiring analgesia and elevation. Weight bearing is not allowed until union has occurred. A complication of arthrodesis is nonunion at the site of attempted fusion.

Psychosocial/Lifestyle Implications

Obviously, an immovable joint is an inconvenience. A fused knee, for example, interferes with using stairs and tying one's shoes. However, the client should weigh the possible inconveniences against the benefits before deciding about surgery. A pain-free, stable joint is likely to improve quality of life, and clients can learn how to cope with limited movement. For example, the client with a fused knee can maneuver on stairs by swinging the involved leg out to the side or forward and using a handrail.

The client will have the added adjustment to immobility of a cast and ambulatory aids until bony union is complete. The effects of a cast are discussed in Chapter

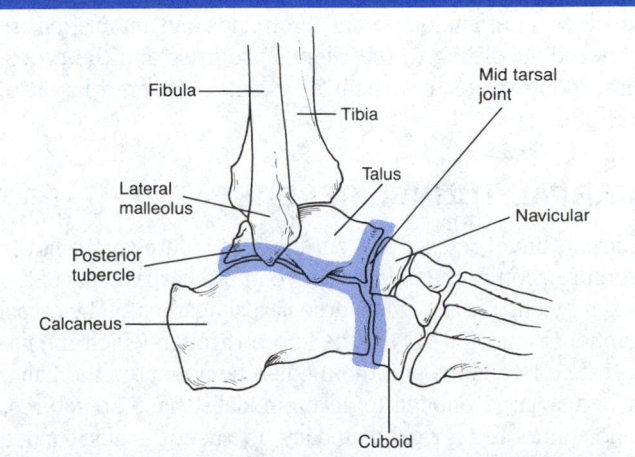

Figure 60–10

Triple arthrodesis. (Shaded portion is site of arthrodesis.)

Table 60–8 Arthrodesis: Implications for the Client*	
Physiological Implications	**Psychosocial/Lifestyle Implications**
Provides relief of pain.	A pain-free, stable joint should improve the quality of life.
Joint is fused into one position, providing joint stability.	The postoperative cast and restricted weight bearing may limit general mobility.
Weight bearing is not allowed until bony union occurs.	A stiff joint may cause a limp or alter the client's ability to move or sit.
	Body image may be altered because of limited movement; however, the stability may improve body image.

*See Table 60–1 for implications of internal fixation.

58. Depending on the procedure done, the client may have a permanent limp or inability to sit properly. This may affect lifestyle and alter body image. However, a client's body image is sometimes improved by pain relief and new stability. The implications of arthrodesis are summarized in Table 60–8.

Nursing Implications

Preoperative Care
Preoperatively, the nurse should assess the client's understanding of the procedure. Since the intended result is an immobile joint, it is particularly important that the client be aware of the outcome and that any misconceptions be clarified before surgery. Other preoperative care is like that for any orthopedic surgical client (see Chapter 56).

Postoperative Care
Postoperatively, check the client's vital signs frequently along with neurovascular status. Any problems with circulation should be reported immediately so the cast can be cut and spread. The extremity should be elevated and ice bags applied intermittently for 24 to 48 hours. There may be a moderate to large amount of bloody drainage on the cast the first few days postoperatively. No weight bearing is allowed until union occurs. Exercises and ambulation are ordered according to the client's progress and the procedure done. Care of a client in a cast is covered in Chapter 58.

CARPAL TUNNEL RELEASE

Carpal tunnel release is a surgical procedure that relieves compression of the median nerve in the carpal canal of the wrist by cutting the transverse carpal ligament. The carpal tunnel (Figure 60–11) is the space through which the finger flexor tendons and the median nerve enter the hand; it is just large enough to accommodate these structures. The tunnel has a rigid boundary because it is surrounded by carpal bones on three sides and on the fourth side by the transverse carpal ligament, which is not very elastic. Any condition causing enough pressure in the tunnel space

to compress the median nerve is known as carpal tunnel syndrome (see Chapter 59). Such conditions include trauma, bony deformity, thickening of the ligaments or tendon sheaths, thickened synovium in rheumatoid arthritis, soft tissue masses such as a ganglion, and edema such as that of pregnancy.

Carpal tunnel release is performed when carpal tunnel syndrome has not responded to conservative therapy, such as rest, splinting, and cortisone injection.

Surgical Procedure

Carpal tunnel release may be done under general or regional anesthesia or axillary block. A pneumatic tourniquet may be used on the arm to decrease bleeding. The tourniquet

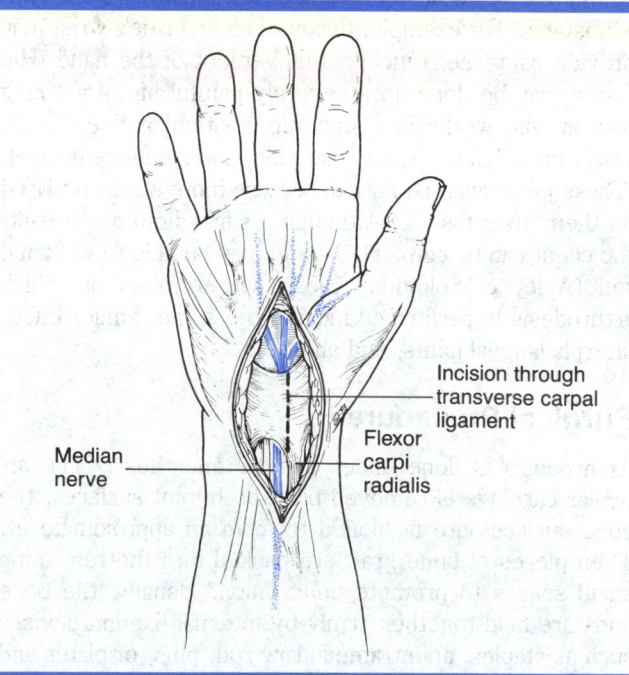

Median nerve

Incision through transverse carpal ligament

Flexor carpi radialis

Figure 60–11

Carpal tunnel release. The transverse carpal ligament is divided to relieve pressure on the median nerve.

looks like a blood pressure cuff attached to a gauge. When inflated properly, it prevents venous oozing without totally obstructing the arterial blood supply (Gruendemann & Meeker, 1983). An incision is made from the proximal palm across the wrist. The transverse carpal ligament is divided longitudinally along its entire length. A segment of the ligament may be removed. A splint-type dressing is applied with an elastic bandage for pressure.

Implications for the Client

Physiological Implications
Sensation usually returns to normal slowly, but occasionally there is some permanent neurological deficit (Apley & Solomon, 1982). The client may have experienced so much pain preoperatively that the postoperative pain is less. The splint remains in place for 1 week and then is removed. Active exercises and normal activity help restore function.

Psychosocial/Lifestyle Implications
Clients should experience relief of chronic pain. They may be able to sleep through the night and resume activities that previously caused discomfort, such as sewing and holding a newspaper to read. Wearing a splint for a week may be an inconvenience, especially when the procedure is done on the dominant hand. The client will need assistance with ADL in the hospital and after discharge until the splint is removed. The implications of carpal tunnel release are summarized in Table 60–9.

Nursing Implications

Preoperative Care
Preoperative care is like that for other orthopedic conditions.

Postoperative Care
Postoperatively, the nurse must assess the neurovascular status of the hand as described in Chapter 56. The hand is elevated on pillows or hung by stockinette from an IV pole. Clients having an axillary block anesthetic may return to the room without having regained full control of their arm. It is fairly common for the bulky splinted hand to hit the client in the face during transfer into the bed. Therefore, the nurse should control the movement of the arm until the client is settled. Analgesics and comfort measures are necessary to relieve pain. Antibiotics are given postoperatively to prevent infection.

Care of the client with a cast, which was discussed in Chapter 58, is pertinent here even though a splint is used rather than a cast. The arm should be elevated in a sling when the client is ambulating. Encourage the client to resume normal use of the hand once the splint is removed. Heavy lifting may be contraindicated for several months.

TOTAL HIP REPLACEMENT

Total hip replacement is a type of joint repair in which both hip surfaces are replaced with artificial prostheses (Figure 60–12). The head and neck of the femur are replaced with a metal femoral component, usually made from stainless steel or Vitallium. The acetabular surface is replaced with a cup-shaped component usually made from high density polyethylene, although sometimes made of metal. The metal-on-plastic articulation creates less friction than metal-on-metal. Both pieces are secured by a bone cement, methyl methacrylate.

The total hip replacement is for those who have damage to both surfaces of the joint resulting in severe pain and poor functioning. Conditions producing such damage include osteoarthritis, rheumatoid arthritis, trauma to the hip, congenital deformities, and aseptic necrosis of the femoral head with damage to the acetabular cartilage.

The long-term effectiveness of methyl methacrylate for arthroplasty (joint repair) is not known. Its use in this country was approved by the FDA in 1969. Many surgeons have hesitated to perform joint replacement surgeries on young people since the long-term effects are not yet known. Some resort to osteotomy or arthrodesis on clients under 55 years of age. Others believe clients of any age are acceptable candidates for joint replacement, even those under 40, provided they are well informed and willing to

Table 60–9 Carpal Tunnel Release: Implications for the Client	
Physiological Implications	**Psychosocial/Lifestyle Implications**
Provides relief of pain and paresthesia.	Relief of chronic pain should provide a psychological lift.
Prevents paralysis of median nerve.	Activities previously curtailed due to pain may be resumed.
Active use is encouraged to restore function when splint is removed.	Use of operative hand will be temporarily restricted by the splint.
Temporary swelling and pain occur from the surgical procedure.	Will need assistance with ADL.
Potential complications: wound infection, nerve or blood vessel damage.	

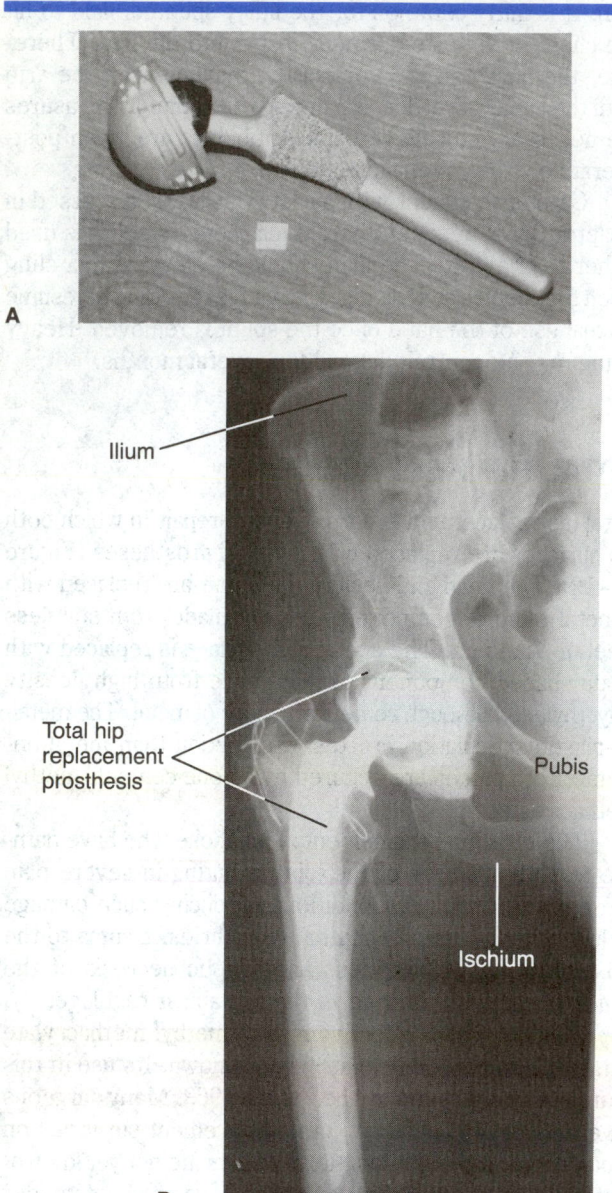

A

Ilium

Total hip
replacement
prosthesis

Pubis

Ischium

B

Figure 60–12

Total hip replacement prosthesis. **A.** A standard total hip
prosthesis with plastic acetabular component and metal
femoral head and neck component. **B.** X-ray of a client with
a total hip replacement. (Courtesy Health Care Plan, Buffalo, NY)

accept the unknown. The procedure is contraindicated in
those who have an active infection or those with inadequate bone to support one of the artificial joint components.

An alternative to the cement is a porous coated prosthesis that permits bony ingrowth into the pores of the
metal, which provides an interlocking bond. This newer
method avoids the failure of the cement. Full weight bearing is not allowed for 12 weeks to 6 months to allow proper
tissue growth and immobilization of the prosthesis in the
bone (Doheny, 1985).

Surgical Procedure

Hip replacement is done under spinal or general anesthesia. The diseased joint surfaces are removed. The acetabulum is reamed out to fit the cup prosthesis, and holes
are drilled or cut into the acetabulum so the cement holds
the cup securely. The cup is fixed in place with methyl
methacrylate. The head and neck of the femur are removed,
the medullary canal is reamed, and the cancellous bone is
removed. The intramedullary stem is cemented into place.
Then the components are put together to reduce the joint.
The prostheses come in a variety of sizes and shapes. The
surgeon selects the type and size that will give the client
the best fit and function and positions the parts carefully
to create as normal a joint as possible.

A suction-type drainage, such as a Hemovac, is inserted
to remove drainage and prevent hematoma formation. The
surgical approach to the hip may require removing the greater
trochanter with its muscles still attached and replacing it
after the prosthesis is inserted. It is reattached with strong
wire so the muscles attached to it do not pull away.

To decrease the chance of wound infection during hip
replacement surgery, special precautions are used in the
operating room. The number of personnel in the room or
moving in and out is limited. A clean air or laminar air flow
room may be used to reduce the amount of particles and
contaminants in the air. Gowns and drapes made of imper-
vious materials may be used; surgeons may double glove.
Antibiotic solutions are used to irrigate the wound.

The amount of blood lost during this procedure is
watched closely and transfusions given as needed. Large
amounts of IV fluids (typically 2000 to 3000 mL) may be
given during surgery to increase the blood volume. This
is done so that the blood pressure is maintained when the
methyl methacrylate is inserted because the substance
causes hypotension (Farrell, 1982). A Foley catheter may
be inserted to observe urine output. Clients may be placed
directly into their bed from the OR table so they will be in
the desired postoperative position and not require further
transfer.

Implications for the Client

Physiological Implications

The results of total hip replacement are usually dramatic.
After 6 months, most clients have little or no pain and can
walk with minimal or no limp. Compared with surgeries
done in the past, this procedure allows early ambulation,
about 2 to 5 days postoperatively. An exercise routine is
necessary to regain function and strength in the operative leg.

Nerves and blood vessels may be damaged during surgical manipulation. Temporary edema occurs in the operative area. The client can lose a great deal of blood, so the
hemoglobin and hematocrit values are evaluated regularly.

Three potential complications may occur. The cement
may fail and loosen the prosthesis, possibly from trauma

or infection. When this happens, pain occurs, and another operation may be necessary.

A second potential problem is wound infection, a dreaded condition that may necessitate removing the prosthesis. The foreign material placed in the body may restrict the body's defense mechanisms, increasing the chances of infection; that is the reason for all the precautions described in the previous section. A wound infection is treated with IV antibiotics, continuous antibiotic wound irrigation, and possibly wound debridement. If the prosthesis must be removed, the client is left with a shortened leg and unstable hip. Surprisingly, the client can still walk, although with an altered gait, using crutches and an elevated shoe. If the infection can be resolved, another joint replacement may be attempted, or surgery can be done to fuse the hip joint (arthrodesis). About 1% to 6% of total hip replacement clients develop wound infections (Mourad, 1980). Infection of the hip can occur from bacterial infection elsewhere in the body, which localizes in the hip. Therefore, the client may be instructed that prophylactic antibiotics are necessary when procedures such as cystoscopy or dental surgery are done in the future or if a bacterial infection develops.

A third potential complication is dislocation of the hip in which the ball moves out of the socket. This happens rarely, but can occur because of laxity of the hip muscles or improper positioning of the leg after surgery. The client will experience sudden pain, may be unable to move the leg or bear weight, and the leg will be shortened. The treatment is traction or a hip spica cast, or surgery may be necessary. This is why proper postoperative positioning is so important.

Psychosocial/Lifestyle Implications

After successful surgery the client has little pain and improved use of the hip. Clients may have had so much pain before surgery that the postoperative pain seems minor. Indeed, they may find the results unbelievable after the suffering they have experienced. Clients may be able to resume activities that were impossible or too painful before the surgery. Depending on their progress and occupation, clients may return to work in about 4 to 6 months.

Some precautions will be necessary, such as maintaining optimal weight and avoiding movements that could cause hip dislocation, such as acute angle hip flexion or extreme extension. The client should learn to be cautious to prevent a fall or other trauma.

Some clients who have total hip replacement may have severe arthritis in other joints, and they may therefore not experience as much improvement in mobility as those with only one damaged joint. They may also be planning to have surgery on another joint in the near future. The implications of hip replacement are summarized in Table 60-10.

Nursing Implications

Preoperative Care
In addition to providing the usual preoperative care for orthopedic surgery (see Chapter 56), teach the client about the specific restrictions and exercises to be followed postoperatively. The surgeon should explain the risks of the surgery, and the nurse should encourage the client to ask questions and express feelings or fears about the procedure. In some hospitals, the physical therapist assesses

Table 60-10 Total Hip Replacement: Implications for the Client	
Physiological Implications	**Psychosocial/Lifestyle Implications**
Provides relief of pain.	A pain-free, functioning hip should improve quality of life.
Provides a functioning hip.	May be able to resume activities previously impossible due to pain.
Nerves and blood vessels may be damaged during surgical manipulation.	Positioning restrictions may be an inconvenience.
Blood loss may be extensive and requires replacement.	The recovery period may be lengthy.
Specific exercises are necessary to regain strength and function.	Use of ambulatory aids is necessary for an extended period of time.
Temporary local swelling and pain occur from the surgical procedure.	Having someone to assist at home is necessary after discharge.
Early ambulation is allowed.	Caution is required to prevent falls.
Complications in the hip itself: wound infection, hip dislocation, loosening or breaking of the prosthesis.	May return to work in 4-6 months, depending on occupation and progress.
	Should not become overweight.
	Habits need to be adapted to prevent dislocation (eg, use caution when sitting and standing; avoid soft, low chairs; avoid leg crossing).

the client preoperatively and teaches some exercises needed for recuperation. An overhead frame and trapeze are placed on the client's bed to teach how to lift.

The client's blood is crossmatched. The nurse may scrub the client's hip and thigh area twice a day with antibacterial soap, and antibiotics may be started prophylactically before surgery, either orally or IV. Clients may start wearing elastic stockings before going to surgery and may go to the operating room in their bed.

Postoperative Care

Postoperatively, the nursing interventions covered in Chapter 56 will be necessary, such as neurovascular assessment, good body alignment, comfort measures, exercises, ambulation, skin care, and preventing the hazards of immobility. Complications to watch for and try to prevent are shock, wound infection, thrombophlebitis, pulmonary emboli, and fat emboli.

Positioning, Lifting, and Turning. The position of the client postoperatively is important to prevent hip dislocation. Required positions vary, depending on the surgical approach as well as the surgeon's preference. The postoperative orders should be clear, and the nurse and client should follow them exactly. The operative hip must be kept in abduction. An abductor pillow or splint (Figure 60–8) may be used, or traction may be applied. Buck's traction, or sometimes Russell's traction (see Chapter 58), may be used to reduce muscle spasm and maintain abduction. The traction may be used continuously for a few days and then applied only at bedtime or discontinued. Rotation of the hip is not generally allowed; the hip should remain in neutral alignment unless specified (some surgeons order slight external rotation). The hip should not be flexed to less than a 90° angle. If elevation of the head of the bed is allowed, it should be only 30° to 45°. Some surgeons allow head elevation only for short periods; the client should be flat some of the time to prevent hip flexion contracture.

The client maintains bed rest for about 2 to 5 days. If turning is not permitted, the staff performs back care and top-to-bottom linen changes by lifting the client straight up in bed. The client lifts with the trapeze and at least three staff members should assist with lifting, one doing the back care. If turning is allowed, orders should specify to which side, because some surgeons prefer turning onto the operative side only. Never turn the client without placing pillows or an abductor splint between the legs. Check a confused client frequently to see that the desired position is maintained.

Monitoring Vital Signs and Drainage. Check the vital signs, the neurovascular status, and the dressing routinely, being careful to observe the part of the dressing under the client. A Hemovac will be in place for about 2 days; keep it deflated and empty it every shift, using aseptic technique to prevent wound infection. Measure and record the nature of the drainage accurately.

Medications. The client is on intravenous broad-spectrum antibiotics for about 2 days postoperatively and then receives oral forms. The IV is discontinued after the switch to oral antibiotics. Postoperative prophylactic anticoagulants are sometimes ordered to prevent formation of emboli, and the client may wear elastic stockings on one or both legs. Clients who are on steroids for rheumatoid arthritis will need to have increased doses during surgery and for a few days afterward. Their adrenal glands cannot produce the increased amounts necessary during this stressful period. Intravenous doses may begin preoperatively, when the client is NPO, and continue until the oral dose is resumed.

Comfort Measures. Analgesics and comfort measures are necessary to relieve pain for the first few days. Pain is mostly from muscle spasms and decreases daily. The client returns to a normal diet according to tolerance and should take plenty of fluids. A Foley catheter may be in place; the client uses a fracture bedpan. It may be difficult for clients to void in the restricted position, so the nurse should watch for urinary retention and bladder distention.

Skin Care and Exercise. Heel protectors and possibly an air mattress are used to protect the skin. The operative thigh is often edematous and tends to develop blisters under the tape; be very careful when changing the dressing. The client's heels, elbows, and sacral region should be observed frequently for signs of breakdown. Heels can be elevated off the bed by means of padding under the calf or with leg troughs.

The client should exercise all unaffected extremities routinely. Isometric exercises and plantar flexion and dorsiflexion on both legs can be done. Incentive spirometry with coughing and deep breathing exercises are also important.

Ambulation and Discharge. Ambulation begins according to the surgeon's preference and the client's progress. Various routines are used; for example, the physical therapist or the nurse may assist the client out of bed for the first time or a tilt table may be used to help the client into the upright position at first. However it is done, hip flexion should be kept to a minimum. The chair used for sitting should be firm and not low, and it should have arms. Physical therapy may begin anywhere from the second to the sixth day postoperatively. The client progresses from parallel bars to crutches or a walker, then to a cane. The amount of weight bearing allowed varies. The physical therapist teaches exercises used for strengthening muscles and gives the client a regimen to follow. The client learns to go up and down stairs and how to put shoes and socks on without acutely flexing the hip. An elevated toilet seat is used for the same reason.

When preparing clients for discharge, instruct them about all restricted activities, such as those listed in Box

Box 60–2 General Guidelines for the Client With Total Hip Replacement After Discharge

Bend the hip only to a 90° angle (right angle), *not less*!

Use a firm chair with arms; seat should be high enough so your hips are not lower than your knees.

*Keep your knees about 12–18 in apart when sitting.

*Do not use a rocking chair; soft, low seats; anything that creates a hammocklike effect.

*Use an elevated toilet seat.

Do not sit for more than 30 minutes at a time. Get up and take a few steps at least every half hour when sitting.

*Do not cross your legs when sitting, standing, or lying.

If allowed to lie on your side, keep a pillow between your legs.

Have someone help with bathing and dressing (eg, putting on your socks) or use special devices.

*Women should avoid high heels.

Use a reacher to pick up objects from the floor or get someone to do it for you. Do not squat or bend way over.

Continue to exercise as instructed by the physical therapist.

Sexual activity may be resumed as long as restricted positions are avoided, such as bending your hip less than a 90° angle and crossing your operative leg beyond your body's midline.

Do not drive a car until your physician permits.

Continue to use whatever aids (walker, crutches, cane) you have learned until instructed otherwise.

Inform your physician if you have a fever; severe pain; redness, swelling, or drainage from your incision; or inability to use your leg.

Keep appointments with your physician for follow-up.

Your physician will instruct you if and when changes in these activities can be made.

*Recommended as lifetime habits.

60–2. A printed sheet with prescribed exercises for reference is given to the client. The nurse also explains the importance of wearing the elastic stockings for another 6 weeks. The occupational therapist may teach clients how to dress without flexing the hip more than 90°. Explain the need for prophylactic antibiotics during future surgical procedures. Clients should have someone at home to assist them after discharge. The length of hospitalization is about 2 to 3 weeks.

TOTAL KNEE REPLACEMENT

Total knee replacement is a type of arthroplasty in which the diseased articulating surfaces of the knee are replaced by artificial components. There are two general types of knee prostheses, condylar and hinged (Figure 60–13). The condylar type consists of a metal femoral component and a high density polyethylene tibial component. They are con-

cave and convex to fit together. The hinged type is a metal prosthesis with components that fit into the distal femoral shaft and proximal tibial shaft; the two components are connected by a hinge. The hinged type is used mostly for unstable knees with faulty supporting ligaments. Both types are usually cemented into place with methyl methacrylate.

Total knee replacement is usually used for a client whose knee is painful as a result of degenerative joint disease when conservative treatment or other surgeries have been unsuccessful in relieving pain. The client may have knee instability and difficulty conducting activities of daily living. Joint destruction may be from rheumatoid arthritis or osteoarthritis. The contraindications for total knee replacement are the same as those for total hip replacement. In addition, obesity and poor motivation are a hindrance to optimum functioning of the new knee.

Surgical Procedure

Knee replacement can be done under general or spinal anesthesia. The conditions in the operating room are the same as those described for total hip replacement. A pneumatic tourniquet is used around the thigh to diminish bleeding. The bone ends are exposed and shaped to fit the prosthesis, which the surgeon has selected to meet the needs of the individual client. The fit and movement are tested, the pieces are cemented into place, and a Hemovac is inserted.

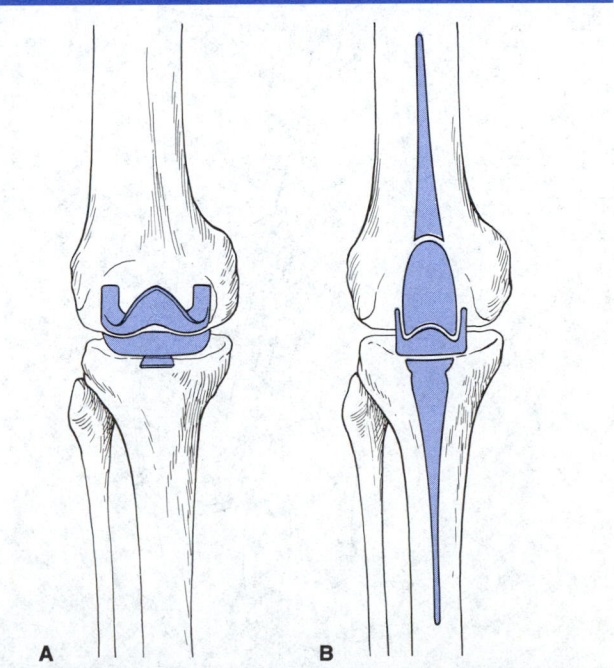

Figure 60–13

Total knee replacement prostheses. **A.** Condylar type with metal femoral component and plastic tibial component. **B.** Hinged type with hinge connecting femoral and tibial components.

After a dressing is applied, the knee is positioned in extension by use of a plaster cast, splint, or knee immobilizer (Figure 60–14). The immobilizer has heavy metal stays to prevent flexion.

Implications for the Client

Physiological Implications
The joint replacement should provide pain-free motion and stability. The overall success of total knee replacements is not the same as that of total hip replacements because its stability depends on the integrity of the knee ligaments. Since the knee normally has a variety of movements, and the hinge-type prosthesis lacks rotation, strain can loosen that type of prosthesis or damage the surrounding bone. If the prosthesis fails, another joint replacement may be attempted, or fusion (arthrodesis) of the knee may be necessary. Arthrodesis of the knee is crippling.

The progress of the knee replacement client depends on the individual's abilities and tolerance for physical therapy and activity. These clients usually have more pain and require a longer rehabilitation period than hip replacement clients.

Potential complications include nerve and blood vessel damage, blood loss, and wound infection, which have been

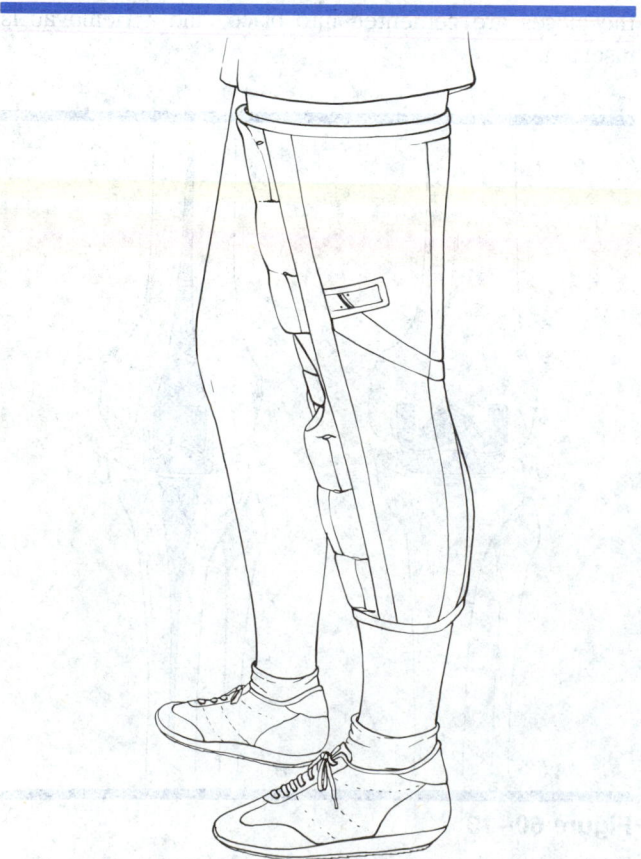

Figure 60–14

Knee immobilizer.

described in the earlier discussion of total hip replacement. The use of a thigh tourniquet in surgery may increase the chances of pulmonary emboli.

Psychosocial/Lifestyle Implications
With successful surgery, clients will have relief of pain and a functional knee. They should be able to carry out normal activities of daily living and feel more secure with a stable knee. Normal activities should not damage the prosthesis, but the client should be careful to avoid falling. Clients may be concerned about how discolored and swollen the leg appears, but this is normal at first.

Rehabilitation takes a long time and requires motivation and hard work on the client's part. Ambulatory aids may be needed for several months. The implications of total knee replacement are summarized in Table 60–11.

Nursing Implications

Preoperative Care
The preoperative preparation is like that described for total hip replacement.

Postoperative Care
The postoperative care is also the same except that there are different restrictions on positioning; traction is not used; and ambulation follows a different course. This section will describe these differences.

The client remains on bed rest for about 1 to 2 days postoperatively, with the operative leg in extension and elevated on pillows. The head of the bed may be elevated to the level of comfort. Care of the client in a cast is described in Chapter 58. If the client is wearing a knee immobilizer, the nurse should check to see that it is neither too tight nor so loose that it slips downward when the client is ambulating. Depending on the procedure done and the surgeon's preference, the immobilizer may be removed from the second to the tenth day postoperatively, may be replaced at bedtime, and/or used for ambulation only. The client may get out of bed to a chair on the first to second postoperative day. The client stands on the unoperative leg, placing limited weight or no weight (as specified by the surgeon) on the operative leg. When the client is in the chair, the leg must be elevated on pillows at first; eventually, clients will be able to bend their knees and lower their legs.

Exercises may begin 1 to 2 days postoperatively to increase strength and function. Straight leg raising and quadriceps setting exercises are important so the client can begin ambulating when the muscles are strong enough to control leg movement. Passive knee flexion and extension exercises progress to active. Clients' ability to exercise depends on their condition before surgery. They need encouragement and reinforcement when exercising because it is difficult and may be exhausting. In physical therapy, they progress from standing between parallel bars to walking with a walker or crutches and learn to climb and descend stairs. Discharge from the hospital occurs about 2 weeks

Table 60–11 Total Knee Replacement: Implications for the Client

Physiological Implications	Psychosocial/Lifestyle Implications
Should provide relief of pain and a functioning, stable knee.	A pain-free, functioning knee may improve quality of life.
Nerves and blood vessels may be damaged from surgery and cast or immobilizer.	May be able to resume activities previously impossible due to pain and instability.
Specific exercises are necessary to regain strength and function.	The recovery period may be lengthy.
Temporary local swelling and pain occur from the surgical procedure.	Use of ambulatory aids is necessary for an extended period of time.
Continuous passive motion decreases pain and swelling, promotes early joint flexibility, and prevents adhesions.	Progress is individualized according to abilities and tolerance.
Complications in the knee itself are possible, such as: wound infection, loosening or breaking of the prosthesis, ligament instability, damage to the surrounding bone.	Wearing a cast or immobilizer may be a temporary inconvenience.
	Caution is required to prevent falls.
	The client may be concerned by the swollen and discolored appearance of the leg.
	Should not become overweight.

after surgery. Clients will walk with crutches or a walker for about 2 more months. They may progress to a cane and eventually walk unassisted. After discharge, clients must follow a prescribed exercise regimen and may increase their activity as tolerated; progress varies from one client to another.

More recently, continuous passive motion (CPM) has been used postoperatively on clients with total knee replacement. Knee movement is provided by a stationary, electrically powered machine or by a dynamic apparatus of suspended ropes and pulleys. The advantages of this treatment include: greater range of motion, faster relief of postoperative pain, earlier discharge, greater muscle strength maintenance, reduced incidence of adhesions, and stronger fixation of the prosthesis due to stimulation of healing. Mobility is restricted since the client must remain supine the greater portion of the day; therefore, the complications of immobility must be prevented (Strang & Johns, 1984).

OTHER JOINT REPLACEMENT

Other joints for which replacement surgery is done include the shoulder, elbow, wrist, fingers, ankle, and toes. These surgeries will be presented together, briefly. The procedures are not as common or as advanced as the hip and knee arthroplasties.

In general, the indication for an arthroplasty is a painful, poorly functioning joint. The condition may be the result of rheumatoid, traumatic, or osteoarthritis. In addition, instability, tumors, and pathological fractures in the joint area may be treated by joint replacement.

Surgical Procedure

Joint replacements may be done under general or regional anesthesia. Pneumatic tourniquets are used where appro-

priate, and diseased articular tissues are removed. Many different types of prostheses are used; some of them are shown in Figure 60–15. For example, a shoulder prosthesis may be a two-part prosthesis with polyethylene glenoid and metal humeral shaft components, cemented into place by methyl methacrylate (Figure 60–15A). A hinged-type prosthesis may be used for the elbow (Figure 60–15B); a two-part carpal–radial prosthesis may be used in the wrist (Figure 60–15C). Bones of the wrist may also be replaced by Silastic implants, a biologically inert, flexible silicone material. In the hand, metacarpophalangeal and proximal interphalangeal (PIP) joints may be replaced by Silastic implants (Figure 60–15D); adjacent tendons or ligaments may be repaired to improve stability also. A two-part polyethylene–metal prosthesis may be used in the ankle. Prostheses used in the toes are similar to those used in the fingers. A splint or other immobilization device is applied when the procedure is finished.

Implications for the Client

As with the hip and knee replacement, these surgeries may provide pain-free, stable, functioning joints, and may even improve appearance (eg, that of the hands). Potential complications are like those of other arthroplasties, including loosening or breaking of the prosthesis, infection, dislocation, fracture of the bone around the prosthesis, and recurrence of pain. Weak muscles may limit the joint's stability and motion.

Nursing Implications

Preoperative preparation and postoperative care are like that described for total hip replacement, except that the positioning and immobilization will be different in each case.

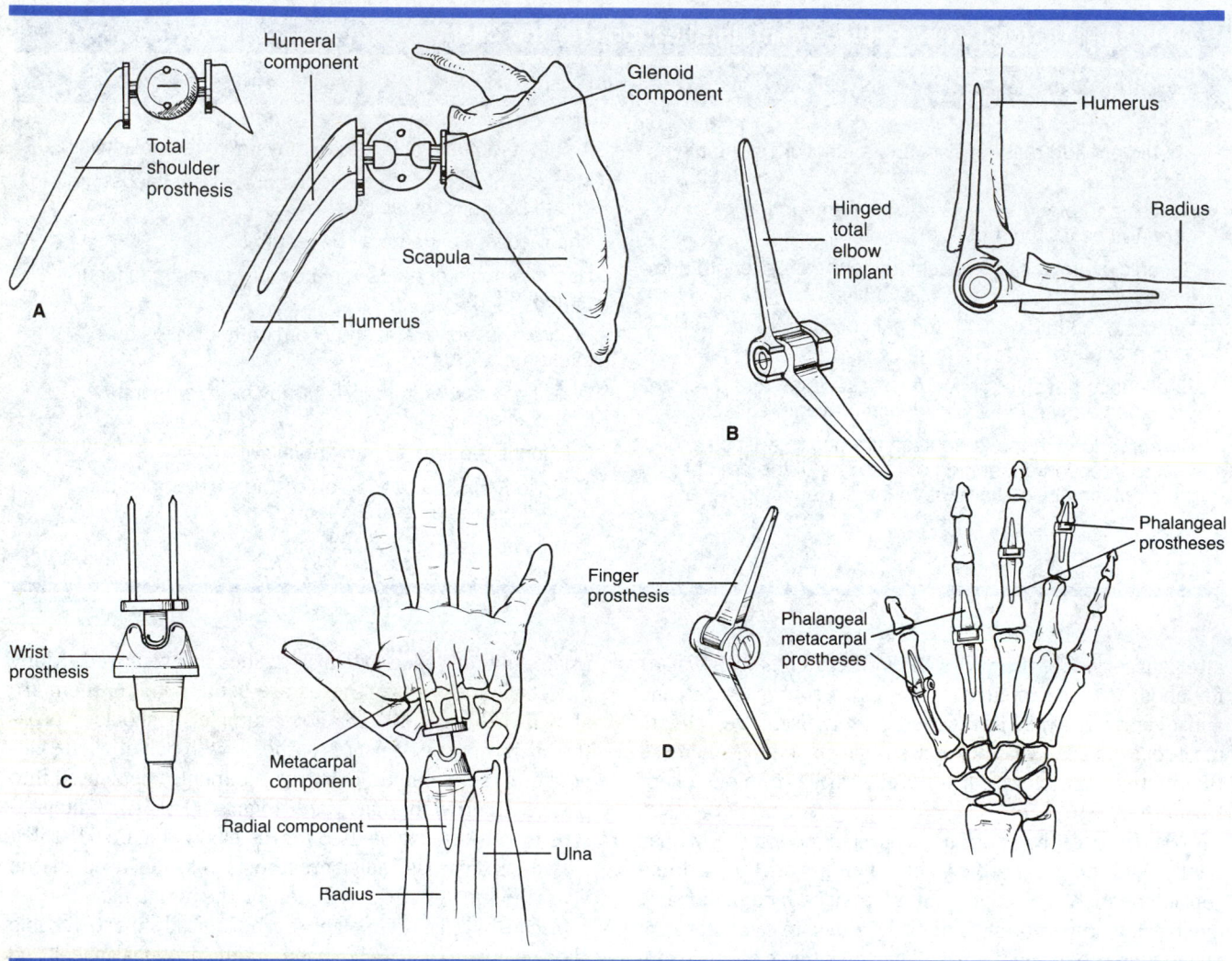

Figure 60-15

Other types of joint replacements. **A.** Shoulder. **B.** Elbow. **C.** Wrist. **D.** Fingers.

After surgery, the extremity should be elevated, and ice bags may be applied intermittently for the first 24 to 48 hours. Frequent neurovascular assessment is important. A Hemovac may be used following shoulder replacement. The client should wear a sling for ambulation after upper extremity surgery. Joints not confined to a splint should be exercised frequently. After the involved joint is no longer immobilized, the client follows a specific exercise program for rehabilitation.

TENDON SURGERY

Various surgical procedures are performed for injury or deformity of tendons (eg, those of the knee, shoulder, hand, and foot). Tendon surgery is indicated for laceration or rupture of a tendon and for an avulsion fracture, in which a tendon tears away still attached to a fragment of the bone. Traumatic damage to a tendon causes loss of function and pain. Other indications for tendon surgery are recurrent dislocation and deformity from congenital or neuromuscular conditions.

Surgical Procedure

Tendon surgery may be done under regional or general anesthesia. A pneumatic tourniquet may be used, if appropriate, to create a bloodless field. Various methods of surgical restoration are used. A tendon may be transplanted, ie, repositioned to alter motion; or it may be lengthened or divided to achieve the desired result. A tendon that is torn or ruptured may be sutured back together or reinserted into the bone. Tendons can also be transferred from elsewhere in the body, possibly to restore movement to a paralytic limb. An avulsion fracture may need open reduction and internal fixation. An immobilization device such as a cast, knee or shoulder immobilizer, or a splint is applied to the joint.

Implications for the Client

Physiological Implications

The client may regain normal functioning and stability with successful surgery. Immobilization will be necessary for about 3 to 8 weeks, depending on the tendon involved. As with any orthopedic operative procedure, blood vessels or nerves can be damaged, and temporary local swelling and pain will occur. Ambulatory aids are necessary after surgery on the lower extremity. The client will need to undertake an extensive exercise program to regain the strength and function of the affected limb. Specific complications are instability, recurrent weakness, problems with motion, or failure of the tendon transfer.

Psychosocial/Lifestyle Implications

Regaining functioning will allow clients to return to their usual activities. Clients with repair of a congenital deformity may be capable of new movements, and they will have to work to strengthen their muscles to achieve the best functioning. Clients with upper extremity surgery will need temporary assistance with ADL because of immobility. The implications of tendon surgery are summarized in Table 60–12.

Nursing Implications

Preoperative Care

The preoperative care is like that for other orthopedic clients (see Chapter 56). The client should be taught the exercises necessary for recovery, such as straight leg raising and quadriceps setting exercises for patellar tendon surgery.

Postoperative Care

Routine postoperative care is necessary, as well as checking neurovascular status frequently, elevating the extremity, and applying ice intermittently for 24 to 48 hours. Observe the dressing or cast when checking vital signs;

cast care is described in Chapter 58. Postoperative pain may be severe and require analgesics and comfort measures. The client with upper extremity surgery will need assistance with ADL and should have the bedside stand placed within reach of the unaffected arm.

The surgeon should specify limitations in weight bearing and use of the limb. A physical therapy program will help restore functioning and teach the use of ambulatory aids. The allowed movement, required exercises, and ambulatory aids will be determined by the specific procedure. The client should have a good understanding of all these when discharged from the hospital.

MENISCECTOMY

A meniscectomy is a surgical procedure in which a torn or damaged meniscus (semilunar cartilage) is removed from the knee joint. The torn part alone or the entire meniscus may be removed.

Meniscectomy is indicated when a meniscus is torn so it causes symptoms such as pain, tenderness, limited motion, mild effusion, and possibly locking. The knee locks when the torn cartilage locates between the femur and tibia and interferes with motion. When locked, it can be flexed but not extended. A torn meniscus commonly occurs from a twisting motion of the knee as in athletic injuries (Figure 60–16). Ligaments of the knee are often injured at the same time.

The medial meniscus is torn most often. A torn meniscus will not heal and must be removed if it is causing difficulty. Surgery is not always necessary, but it is performed if conservative treatment is not successful.

Surgical Procedure

Meniscectomy is done by either open or closed surgery. Open surgery involves the arthrotomy procedure covered

Table 60–12 Tendon Surgery: Implications for the Client	
Physiological Implications	**Psychosocial/Lifestyle Implications**
May provide normal functioning and stability.	Regaining function allows return to previous activity level.
Temporary local swelling and pain occur from the procedure.	For a congenital condition, new movement may be possible allowing greater independence.
An extensive exercise program may be necessary to regain strength and function.	Assistance with ADL is necessary for those with upper extremity surgery.
Ambulatory aids will be necessary for lower extremity surgery.	The necessary exercise program may require a great deal of work.
Potential complications: joint instability, recurrent weakness, movement difficulty, failure of the surgery, nerve or blood vessel damage, and wound infection.	Wearing a cast or immobilizer will be a temporary inconvenience.
	Learning the use of ambulatory aids is necessary for lower extremity surgery.

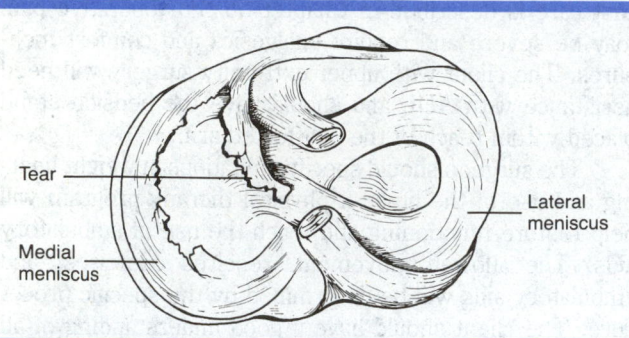

Figure 60–16

A cross-section of a knee joint showing a torn meniscus. This type is called a bucket handle tear. A torn meniscus is a common athletic injury.

earlier in this chapter. A pressure dressing is usually applied, and some physicians use a posterior splint. Closed surgery is done through an arthroscope, which was described in Chapter 56. The torn meniscus or part is cut into tiny particles that are removed by irrigating the joint.

Implications for the Client

Table 60–7 summarized the implications of arthrotomy (open meniscectomy).

Physiological Implications

Removal of the meniscus produces mild rotatory instability of the knee. The client must do strengthening exercises for the knee muscles to overcome the instability. The procedure removes the pain and locking, providing a functional joint. Partial regeneration of the meniscus may occur. Antibiotics are given to prevent infection.

Psychosocial/Lifestyle Implications

The fear of having an undependable knee should be removed. The closed procedure allows much faster recovery; the client can ambulate on crutches the evening of surgery, as opposed to 2 or 3 days later for open meniscectomy.

The general implications of meniscectomy for the client are summarized in Table 60–13.

Nursing Implications

Preoperative Care

Preoperatively, the care is like that for other orthopedic surgery clients. The nurse should teach quadriceps setting and straight leg raising exercises preoperatively.

Postoperative Care

Postoperatively, the nurse assesses vital signs, neurovascular status, and the dressing frequently. The leg is elevated, and ice may be applied intermittently for about 24 hours. All other joints should be exercised. A physical therapy program is necessary to help the client strengthen the muscles. Exercise begins with quadriceps setting and straight leg raising, progressing to crutch walking. The progress depends on how well muscle strength is regained. After arthroscopic surgery, the client may use crutches for about 10 days. With open meniscectomy, crutches may be used for about 6 weeks.

BUNIONECTOMY

Bunionectomy is a surgical procedure done to remove a **bunion**, a bony prominence and bursa on the medial side of the first metatarsal head of the great toe. A bunion is commonly associated with an abnormal position of the great toe known as hallux valgus, in which there is lateral displacement of the great toe at the metatarsophalangeal joint (Figure 60–17). Various procedures are done to remove the bunion and repair the abnormal position.

The indication for bunionectomy is pain unrelieved by conservative measures, which may become severely disabling. Bunions are more common in women than men; they are usually bilateral; and they may be caused by congenital deformity. The influence of footwear as a cause of bunions is disputed; however, improperly fitted shoes do contribute to the worsening of hallux valgus when the deformity exists (Apley & Solomon, 1982).

Surgical Procedure

Various surgical procedures are used for this condition depending on what type of abnormality is present. All procedures remove the bony overgrowth and bursa (bunion-

Table 60–13 Meniscectomy: Implications for the Client*	
Physiological Implications	**Psychosocial/Lifestyle Implications**
Provides relief of pain, eliminates locking.	Diminishes the fear of the knee locking.
Produces mild rotatory instability of the knee.	The closed procedure allows faster recovery than the open procedure.
Exercises strengthen the muscles to overcome this.	
Partial regeneration of the meniscus may occur.	

*See Table 60–7 for Implications of Arthrotomy

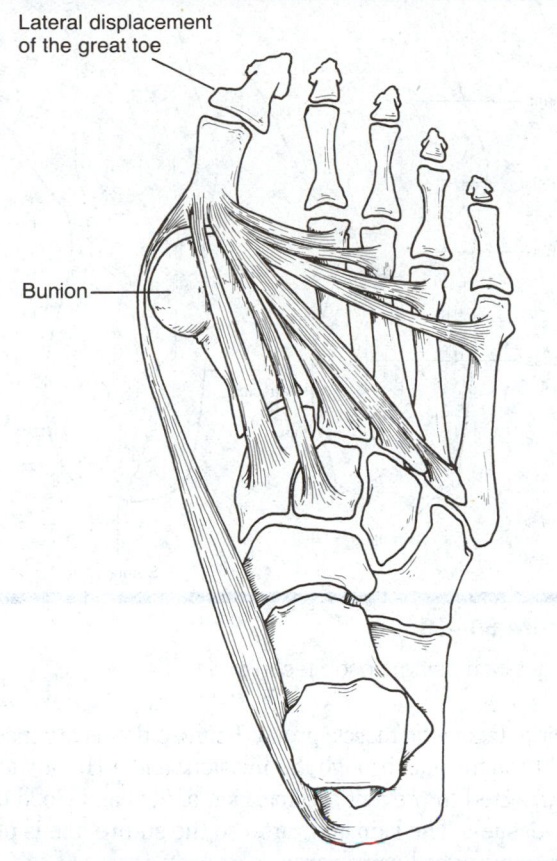

Figure 60–17

Bunion and hallux valgus.

ectomy). Additional repairs to realign the great toe include osteotomy of the first metatarsal, removing the proximal portion of the first phalanx, tendon transplants, or any combination of these. Wire may be inserted to maintain bone alignment during healing of the osteotomy; the wire protrudes from the end of the great toe and is eventually removed. A compression dressing, short leg cast, or a cast just on the foot may be applied.

Implications for the Client

Physiological Implications

The procedure provides relief of pain and alleviates disability. Mobility will be limited at first, depending upon the procedure done. Temporary swelling and pain occur; the pain requires analgesics and comfort measures. Antibiotics are given to prevent infection.

Psychosocial/Lifestyle Implications

The relief of chronic pain should improve the client's quality of life. The procedure will also improve the appearance of the foot; although this is not in itself a reason for doing the surgery, it is certainly an additional benefit. The client will need to use ambulatory aids such as crutches until healing occurs. The client implications of bunionectomy are summarized in Table 60–14.

Nursing Implications

Routine preoperative and postoperative orthopedic care are necessary. The nurse checks neurovascular status, vital signs, and cast or dressing frequently. The operative foot is elevated. Comfort measures and analgesics are given to relieve pain. Cast care is described in Chapter 58. The amount of weight bearing allowed depends upon the procedure done, so the postoperative orders should be specific. Some clients are allowed to walk on their heel at first and progress to weight bearing as tolerated. After osteotomy, on the other hand, the client may not bear weight for 3 to 6 weeks. Physical therapy teaches clients the use of ambulatory aids.

AMPUTATION

An amputation is the removal of all or part of a limb because of disease or injury. An amputation can also occur traumatically as the result of an accident, requiring surgery to care for the resulting wound.

Most lower extremity amputations are necessary due to peripheral vascular diseases (PVD), such as diabetes mellitus and arteriosclerosis. Upper extremity amputations are rarely done for peripheral vascular disease, but they may be necessary as a result of trauma, such as that occurring in explosions or crushing injuries. Other indications include:

- Infection, such as osteomyelitis or gas gangrene
- Tumor, such as osteosarcoma
- Thermal injury, such as frostbite or burns
- Congenital deformity

Table 60–14 Bunionectomy: Implications for the Client	
Physiological Implications	**Psychosocial/Lifestyle Implications**
Provides relief of pain; alleviates disability.	Relief of chronic pain should improve quality of client's life.
Temporary local swelling and pain occur from the procedure.	Appearance of the foot is improved.
Potential complications: nerve or blood vessel damage, wound infection.	Ambulatory aids will be necessary temporarily.

Limbs that seriously interfere with functioning or are extremely painful and have not responded to other treatment may require amputation also.

Surgical Procedure

The choice of the specific site of the amputation involves several factors. The remaining tissues must have an adequate blood supply for healing of the wound. The surgeon tries to save as much of the limb as possible, while providing for the best fit and function of a prosthesis. The higher the level of the amputation, the greater the energy expenditure for ambulation with a prosthesis. There are standard limb lengths that are optimal for use of a prosthesis. However, prosthetists today are able to fashion prostheses for almost any site. Some common amputation sites are:

- Transmetatarsal: part of the foot is removed; does not usually require a prosthesis
- Ankle: foot is removed at the ankle
- Below the knee (BK): 10 to 14 cm of the tibia should be preserved; allows for a more natural gait than at or above the knee, because knee is preserved
- At the knee (knee disarticulation): lower leg is removed at the knee joint
- Above the knee (AK): leg is removed about 6 cm above the knee joint
- Below the elbow: lower arm is removed to about 14 cm below the elbow
- Above the elbow: lower arm is removed; all possible length is preserved down to 5 cm above the distal end of the humerus

The surgical procedure is usually done under general anesthesia. A tourniquet may be used to create a bloodless field.

There are two types of amputation—open (guillotine) and closed (flap). The open technique leaves the wound edges open; the skin, muscle, and bone are all cut at the same level (similar to the way a guillotine would cut). The open wound is necessary when infection is present so purulent material can drain. The main blood vessels are tied off, and a bulky soft compression dressing is applied. Skin traction may be utilized to prevent skin and muscle retraction, which would interfere with fitting a prosthesis. Four traction strips of adhesive or rubber are applied above the dressing and attached to 5 lb of traction weight (see skin traction in Chapter 58). The infection is treated with systemic antibiotics and wound irrigations. When the infection has cleared, the wound may be surgically closed or allowed to heal by granulation.

In the closed technique, the bone is cut 2 in shorter than the skin and muscles so the tissues can cover the end of the bone (Figure 60–18). Major vessels are tied off with ligatures. The muscles may be sutured to the bone or to

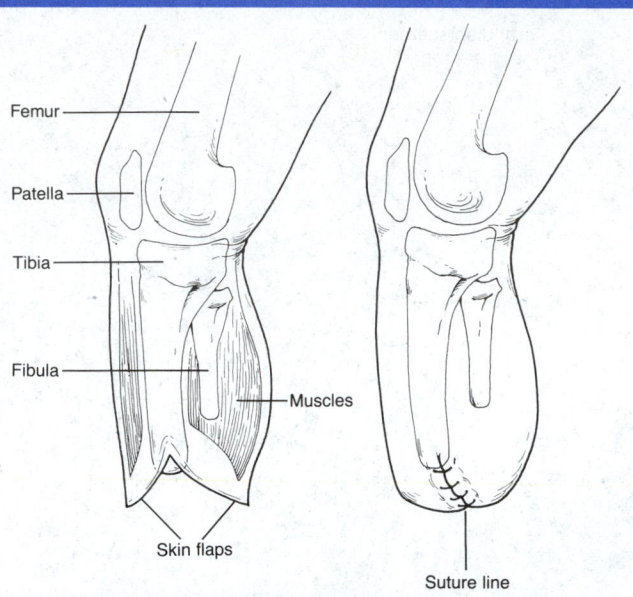

Figure 60–18

Amputation using closed technique.

their antagonistic muscle group. Penrose drains are inserted and brought out through the incision, and a Hemovac may be inserted to prevent accumulation of fluid and blood under the tissues. The skin is sutured so the suture line is placed in a nonweight-bearing area.

The surgeon decides whether to use an early or a delayed prosthesis fitting. If a delayed prosthesis fitting is used (the conventional method), the stump is covered with fluffy absorbent dressing followed by a compression bandage. Elastic bandage is used to decrease swelling and to begin shaping the stump for the future prosthesis.

If the surgeon chooses the early fitting (also called immediate postoperative fitting or rigid dressing), the stump is covered with an absorbent dressing and padding followed by a plaster cast. For a lower extremity amputation, a suspension strap is attached to the cast so it can be connected to a waist belt. A temporary prosthesis, made of a pylon tube and prosthetic foot, is attached to the cast either immediately or a few weeks after surgery (Figure 60–19). Another method employs an air splint over the dressing to provide compression for controlling edema. The client can ambulate while wearing the splint, which is covered with a metal cylinder.

Implications for the Client

Physiological Implications

Undergoing an amputation may relieve pain that was not relieved by other measures. The surgery may eliminate persistent wounds or ulcerations with inadequate circulation. Sometimes amputation is a lifesaving measure (eg, when a tumor may metastasize or an infection is life threatening). In other cases, it removes a limb that has been useless or even a bother.

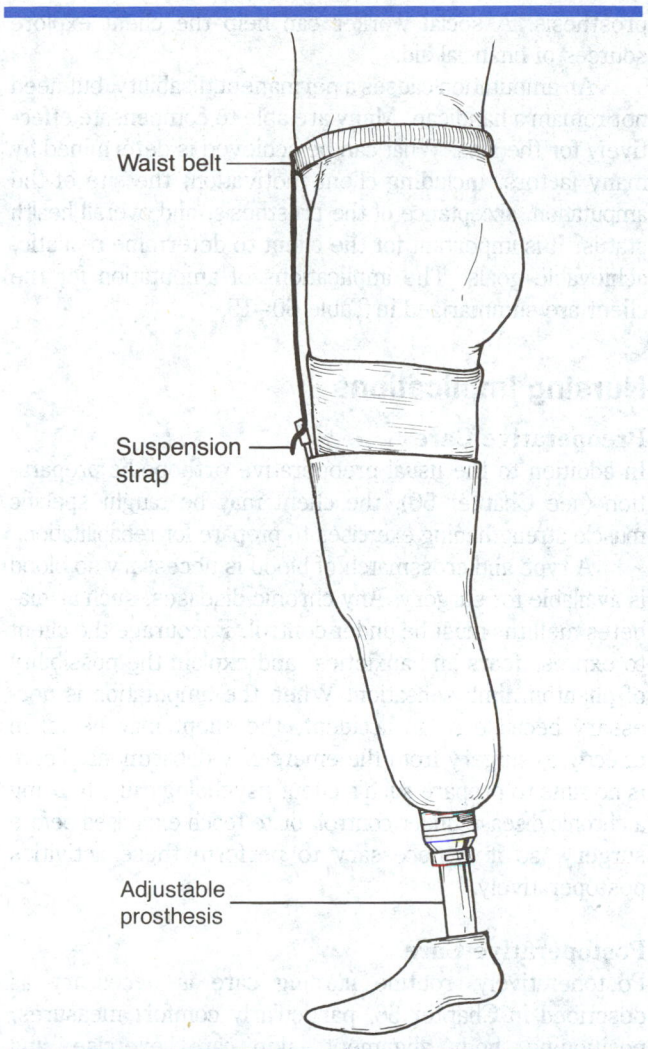

Waist belt

Suspension
strap

Adjustable
prosthesis

Figure 60–19

Immediate postoperative prosthetic fitting (rigid dressing).

Hemorrhage can occur as a result of failure of the ligatures used to tie off vessels in the limb. Severe hemorrhage is rare, requiring emergency treatment to stop the bleeding and restore the blood volume. Upper extremity amputation usually produces severe pain in the stump. The pain following lower extremity amputation is considered mild by comparison; however, Crowther (1982) states that health care workers usually underestimate the client's pain and discomfort.

After the amputation, it may seem to the client as if the missing limb is still there. This feeling, known as phantom limb sensation, may occur briefly or may continue for years; there are instances of reported phantom limb sensation for as long as 20 years after amputation. Exactly why this experience happens is not completely known. It may happen because cut nerve endings that formerly innervated the limb have been stimulated or because the remaining neurons in the stump continue to send impulses to the same area of the brain as before.

Phantom limb sensation eventually disappears. It may

diminish by a process known as telescoping, in which the limb actually seems to be receding or shrinking toward the stump. The thumb, index finger, and great toe are usually the final parts to "disappear." Phantoms of the upper extremity seem to last longer than phantoms of the lower extremity.

Not to be confused with phantom limb sensation is another event called phantom limb pain. Clients have described this pain by using words such as *acute, crushing, grinding,* and *burning.* Fortunately, painful phantoms are relatively rare and occur in only 1% to 2% of all amputations. Why painful phantoms occur is also not clear. Phantom limb pain may result from inflammation or regrowth (neuroma formation) of the cut nerve endings and may occur soon after the amputation or not until many years later. Persistent pain has been treated by nerve block, anti-inflammatory drugs, neuroma excision, electrical nerve stimulation, and psychotherapy. Carpamezapine (Tegretol), an anticonvulsant and analgesic drug, and amitriptyline (Elavil), an antidepressant drug, have also been used. All approaches to treatment of persistent phantom limb pain have met with limited success.

Another physiological reaction, edema of the stump, can be prevented by wrapping the stump with elastic bandage or by use of the rigid postoperative dressing. Complications of skin healing can occur on the end of the stump as a result of pressure, poor circulation, or wound infections. Limited weight-bearing and postoperative antibiotics are used to prevent these complications. Joint contracture is another complication, which can interfere with use of a prosthesis. There is a natural tendency for clients to assume a position of comfort, which frequently involves flexion of a joint. Unfortunately, these positions, while comfortable, may lead to joint contractures. Position changes and exercises are necessary to prevent contracture formation.

The early, or immediate, postoperative prosthesis fitting provides advantages over delayed fitting but is not appropriate for everyone. Clients who may have difficulty with healing postoperatively (eg, those with peripheral vascular disease or infection), are not candidates for the rigid dressing. Skin healing cannot be observed with this fitting, because the cast is kept in place for about 10 days. Some surgeons use Penrose drains and then remove them through a temporary window cut in the cast; others use no drains. The rigid dressing helps prevent edema formation and shapes the stump for the prosthesis. Ambulation can begin earlier with this dressing, but weight bearing is usually just touch down weight bearing, and is strictly limited for about 2 to 3 weeks while wound healing takes place. The permanent prosthesis fitting can also take place earlier than with the delayed fitting, around 3 to 4 weeks postoperatively. The chance of phantom limb pain is less, and there is probably some psychological value to having a prosthesis (even though a crude one) already in place when the client returns from the operating room. A possible complication is skin or wound breakdown from early ambulation and weight bearing.

For the delayed prosthetic fitting, it is necessary to shape the stump by use of elastic bandages so a prosthesis can be applied. A temporary prosthesis may be fitted and applied 2 to 3 weeks postoperatively, or the client may wait for the permanent fitting. The stump shrinks as healing occurs, and the permanent prosthesis fitting is done when shrinkage and shaping is optimal, usually 2 to 3 months after surgery. Ambulation can begin without a prosthesis, but progress is obviously limited.

With both early and delayed fitting, an extensive physical therapy program is necessary to strengthen the muscles used for ambulation and to learn to use the prosthesis. Not everyone with an amputation is a candidate for a prosthesis. Those who are confused, debilitated, elderly, or have a chronic disease or infection may not be able to use a prosthesis and must either learn to ambulate without one or use a wheelchair. A prosthesis for the lower extremity can provide a nearly normal gait; upper extremity prostheses are more limited because they cannot reproduce the fine motor movements of the hand.

Psychosocial/Lifestyle Implications

Religious beliefs may influence a client's decision and feelings about amputation. Some religions oppose amputation; others permit it but require burial of the amputated part. The nurse should try to find out whether the client wants the limb to be buried and help to make the necessary arrangements with the family.

A client may have many psychological reactions to amputation, ranging from grief for the loss to a sense of relief at being rid of a painful or bothersome part. Body image will be altered as the client learns to accept the loss of the limb and the presence of the prosthesis. A person who has had time to prepare for an amputation may adjust more easily than one with a traumatic amputation. Phantom limb sensations will affect the client's emotional well being. The nurse should mention these sensations and explain that they are not abnormal, since the client may avoid mentioning them for fear of appearing "crazy." Clients may have feelings of uselessness, helplessness, and uncertainty about future abilities and may worry about what others think of their abilities or appearance.

Rehabilitation is a long and arduous process that requires strong motivation and hard work. There will be permanent changes in lifestyle; the client will have to abandon some previous activities and learn how to do others in a new way. Clients may not be able to return to their previous occupation, depending upon the nature of the work and the degree of rehabilitation. Although a new occupation may be necessary, a self-supporting life is often a realistic goal. Someone whose dominant hand has been amputated will need to learn to do things with the other hand. For some, limited mobility will mean increased dependence on others; eg, an elderly client may need help getting out of bed into a wheelchair.

Economic problems may arise because of the lengthy hospitalization and rehabilitation period and the cost of a prosthesis. A social worker can help the client explore sources of financial aid.

An amputation causes a permanent disability, but need not remain a handicap. Many are able to compensate effectively for the loss. What can be achieved is determined by many factors, including client motivation, the site of the amputation, acceptance of the prosthesis, and overall health status. It is important for the client to determine realistic, achievable goals. The implications of amputation for the client are summarized in Table 60–15.

Nursing Implications

Preoperative Care

In addition to the usual preoperative orthopedic preparation (see Chapter 56), the client may be taught specific muscle strengthening exercises to prepare for rehabilitation.

A type and crossmatch of blood is necessary so blood is available for surgery. Any chronic diseases, such as diabetes mellitus must be under control. Encourage the client to express fears and anxieties, and explain the possibility of phantom limb sensation. When the amputation is necessary because of an accident, the client may be taken directly to surgery from the emergency department. There is no time to prepare such a client psychologically, to bring a chronic disease under control, or to teach exercises before surgery, so it is necessary to perform these activities postoperatively.

Postoperative Care

Postoperatively, routine nursing care is necessary as described in Chapter 56, particularly comfort measures, positioning, body alignment, skin care, exercise, and ambulation. The dressing is checked frequently along with the vital signs, to detect any sign of hemorrhage. A large tourniquet is kept at the bedside; if hemorrhage occurs, the nurse applies the tourniquet and notifies the physician immediately. Drainage from the dressing is to be expected because Penrose drains are used; however, bright red drainage is a sign of fresh bleeding. The client should do coughing, deep breathing, and incentive spirometry every 1 to 2 hours. Antibiotics are given to prevent infection. Nursing measures to prevent urinary retention, constipation, and skin problems are described in Chapter 56. The diet is advanced as tolerated. Range of motion exercises are necessary for all joints.

Positioning. Assist the client to change position every 2 hours, avoiding positions that would encourage contracture formation. For the client with a lower extremity amputation, the foot of the bed may be elevated for 24 to 48 hours to decrease stump edema. Thereafter, continuous elevation of the legs is avoided to prevent hip flexion contracture. No pillow is allowed under the operative leg or between the legs; a flexion or abduction contracture would interfere with use of a prosthesis. A firm mattress is necessary to prevent hip flexion. The client should assume

Table 60–15 Amputation: Implications for the Client

Physiological Implications	Psychosocial/Lifestyle Implications
May provide relief of pain.	May provide relief of chronic pain, or freedom from a useless limb, improving quality of life.
May prevent metastasis of a tumor or arrest a life-threatening infection.	A permanent handicap occurs that requires changes in many areas of the client's life.
Should eliminate persistent ulceration of extremity.	The grieving process may occur over loss of a limb.
Temporary local pain and edema occur in the stump.	Body image is altered.
A compression dressing is necessary to shape the stump for delayed prosthesis fitting.	May require abandoning previous activities and learning new ways of doing things.
The advantages of early over delayed prosthetic fitting are that the early fitting controls edema, shapes the stump, allows earlier ambulation and permanent prosthesis fitting, and decreases phantom limb pain.	Change in occupation may be necessary.
	May become dependent on others.
An extensive physical therapy program is necessary to build strength and learn prosthesis use.	Lengthy hospitalization and rehabilitation may cause financial problems.
Upper extremity prostheses cannot reproduce fine motor movements of the hand.	Fear and anxiety about self-worth and being a burden may occur.
Ambulatory aids may be necessary for lower extremity amputee.	Adjustment after a traumatic amputation may be more difficult than a planned amputation.
Potential complications: hemorrhage and shock, phantom limb pain, joint contracture, wound infection, and skin breakdown on stump.	Persistent phantom limb pain may be discouraging.
	Motivation and hard work are necessary for rehabilitation.

the prone position for 30 minutes 3 to 4 times a day. For part of the time the client is supine, the bed should be completely flat. Trochanter rolls can be used to prevent rotation of the leg. Discourage continuous knee flexion when the client is in bed or sitting in a chair. The client should begin isometric exercises of the quadriceps, gluteal, and abdominal muscles on the first or second postoperative day and perform them 4 to 5 times a day to maintain strength. The care for a client in skin traction (for an open amputation) is described in Chapter 58.

Stump Conditioning and Bandaging. With the delayed fitting amputation, the client carries out stump conditioning exercises by pushing the stump against an object, beginning with a towel or soft pillow and progressing to harder surfaces. The amputation stump is further prepared for the prosthesis by molding it into a conical shape with elastic bandaging. The nurse begins doing this the first or second postoperative week and should eventually teach the client how to do it. The elastic bandage is wrapped so the greatest compression is at the distal end of the stump, with decreasing compression as the bandage ascends the limb. The bandaging should be rewrapped about five times a day to maintain the compression and checked frequently to note slipping or tightening of the bandages.

The AK amputation stump is wrapped so the bandage is anchored around the hips in figure-eight turns (Figure 60–20). Oblique turns are used on the limb rather than circular turns, which could be constricting. The bandaging should be smooth, so no skin is exposed and the edges of

the bandage do not flap. It should not be so tight as to cause pain or discomfort or interfere with circulation. The BK amputation stump is wrapped using the same principles, with figure-eight turns about the knee (Figure 60–21).

An elastic stump shrinker may be used instead of the bandage. Two sets of bandages should be available, so one can be washed and dried daily as the other is worn. The bandage should be laid flat to dry, to prevent stretching.

The rigid dressing must remain in place on an amputation stump using immediate postoperative fitting. If it falls off, the nurse should wrap the stump with elastic bandages immediately and call the physician to replace the dressing; otherwise, the stump will swell and lose its desired shape.

Rehabilitation After Leg Amputation. The client with a leg amputation will be out of bed in 1 or 2 days postoperatively. The client can stand on the unaffected leg to transfer to a chair. The physical therapist will teach exercises and ambulation technique, which the nurse can reinforce when the client is back on the unit. When a temporary prosthesis is first used for ambulation, only limited weight bearing is allowed. The client progresses from parallel bars to crutches or a walker, then to a cane, and finally to no aids. The rate of progress varies with the individual. An AK amputee eventually uses a prosthesis with a knee joint that locks when weight is applied. The physical therapist is responsible for gait training and teaching the client how to maneuver on stairs.

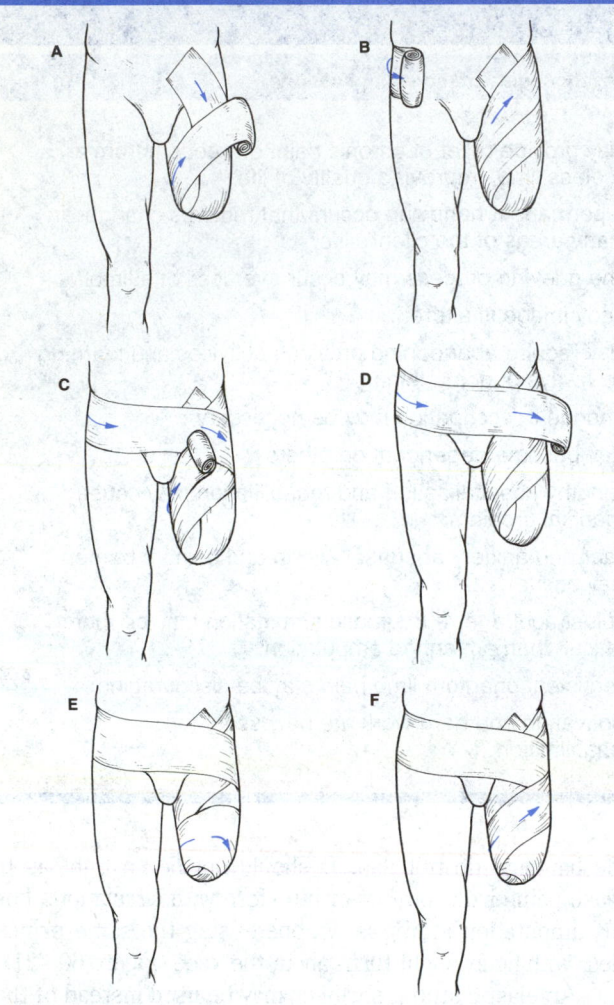

Figure 60–20

Wrapping an AK amputation stump. Four- to six-inch elastic bandage is used. Oblique turns are used rather than circular turns. The bandage is anchored around the hip with a figure-eight turn.

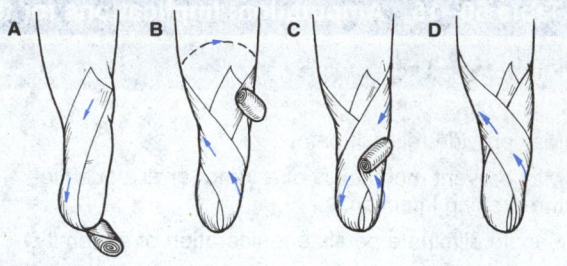

Figure 60–21

Wrapping a BK amputation stump. Four-inch elastic bandage and figure-eight turns about the knee are used.

Research is currently focused on developing methods of computer-assisted mobility.

Fitting and Care of the Prosthesis. A prosthetist measures and fits the client for the prosthesis. Prostheses are made of wood, metal, and plastic. Some prostheses are held on by a belt around the waist; some stay in place by suction (air is forced out as the stump is placed in the socket).

The prosthetist teaches the client how to care for the appliance. A prosthesis is an expensive item and requires conscientious care. The socket should be cleaned daily with mild soap and water and dried thoroughly; the hinges should be lubricated; mechanical parts should not get wet. The client should not alter the prosthesis in any way. The prosthetist should be seen immediately when problems occur with the prosthesis, and a yearly checkup may be recommended.

Rehabilitation After Arm Amputation. People usually experience more pain with arm amputation than with leg amputation, so comfort measures are especially important for a client who has lost an arm. The client wears a sling when out of bed. Range of motion exercises are necessary to prevent contracture; physical therapists teach arm exercises. The client will need to have someone wrap the arm because it is impossible to wrap with one hand.

Use of the arm prosthesis is difficult. Skilled use requires long training with the physical therapist and a great deal of practice; the fine movements of the hand are never replaced. One type of prosthesis for the arm is made with a split hook, which opens voluntarily by means of control cables activated by arm or shoulder movement. Other devices work by electrical power. A cosmetic prosthesis provides less function but is more pleasing to the eye. There have been many improvements in prostheses in recent years, and improvements should continue.

Stump Care With a Prosthesis. The nurse teaches the client stump care so the limb can be maintained in optimal condition. Clients should inspect the stump thoroughly before and after using the prosthesis. They may need a mirror to see all areas of the stump. If there are irritated or sore areas, the prosthesis should not be worn, and the physician should check the stump to avoid development of a more serious problem. The client should wash the skin with mild soap and water, rinse it thoroughly, and dry it well. If a stump sock is worn, it should be washed daily. The client should have enough stump socks to wear a clean, dry sock every day. Stump socks should be discarded if they develop rough spots or holes; they should not be mended because mending causes rough areas. Tell the client that the stump may shrink and require refitting.

Body Image and Sexual Functioning. Nursing care appropriate for body image disturbances is discussed in Chapter 4. A visit from an amputee who has adjusted well to a similar amputation and prosthesis may help the client. Clients may find it hard to use the word "stump" at first, so the nurse can encourage discussion about their "limb" or "leg." A client may become discouraged with the amount of work necessary to learn new skills, especially a client with an arm amputation. Help clients to set realistic goals and to progress steadily toward self-care. Accomplishments should be praised by the health team. Encourage the family to do the same.

Although an amputation should not seriously affect a person's ability to engage in sexual activity, clients may perceive themselves as less attractive or may worry about what their partner thinks or feels. Some changes may be necessary because of the presence of the prosthesis, or because the person no longer has a limb that was once used for sexual activity. A client who has lost a hand will need to use the other one for touching. Assess for potential difficulties and encourage the client and sexual partner to discuss their feelings. The nursing care plan in Chapter 56 includes a section on sexual dysfunction related to musculoskeletal problems.

Preparation for Discharge. Clients may be discharged from the hospital as soon as the wound heals and they can do the prescribed exercises, wrap the stump correctly, and ambulate as directed. Training with the prosthesis is not usually done on an inpatient basis. Urge the client to continue follow-up visits to the physician, prosthetist, and physical therapist and teach care specific to the underlying condition, such as PVD or diabetes mellitus, before client discharge. A referral to a community health nurse may be helpful, to reinforce teaching and assess progress. The client may also be referred to a social worker, to help with financial problems, and to the local Office of Vocational Rehabilitation, which can provide occupational assistance.

LAMINECTOMY

Laminectomy, the removal of one or more vertebral bony arches (laminae), may be done when the severe back and leg pain of a herniated intervertebral disk has not responded to conservative treatment (see Chapter 59). The portion of the protruding disk (nucleus pulposus) that is pressing on the nerve root is removed through the opening provided by the laminectomy (Figure 60–22). This procedure is called a diskectomy (also discectomy). When assessment shows progressive neurological impairment, prompt surgery, without attempts at conservative treatment, is necessary to prevent permanent neurological deficit.

Laminectomy is also indicated to relieve compression of the spinal cord caused by injury or disease, to do surgery on the spinal nerves, and to remove tumors of the spinal cord. The procedure is most common in the lumbar region but may also be necessary in the cervical or thoracic spine. Spinal fusion may be done at the same time if the spine is unstable as a result of either the laminectomy or the underlying condition.

Surgical Procedure

Laminectomy is usually performed under general anesthesia with the client in the side-lying or prone position.

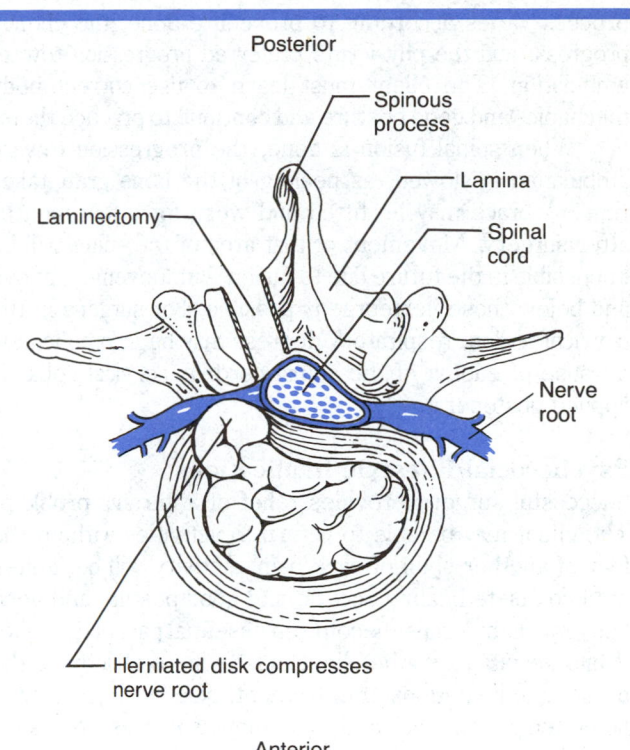

Figure 60–22

Laminectomy for removal of a herniated disk.

Occasionally, a spinal or local anesthetic is given. Other positions such as knee-chest or sitting may be used. An anterior approach (eg, through the abdomen) is used for some spinal surgeries, but the posterior approach to the spine is most common.

For the diskectomy, part of the lamina of one or more vertebrae is removed. The nerve root and dural sac are retracted to expose the disk space, and the herniated fragments of the disk are removed. If spinal fusion is done, bone is usually obtained from the iliac crest. A dressing is applied after wound closure.

Implications for the Client

Physiological Implications

Local pain and some neurologic manifestations may occur in the legs as a result of surgical manipulation and edema at the operative site, eg, tingling, numbness, or temporary anesthesia may occur in the area supplied by peripheral nerves. Therefore, the condition may not seem to be improved immediately after surgery. The success of the diskectomy varies. Spengler (1982) states that a wide range (46% to 90%) of diskectomies are claimed to have excellent results. However, the symptoms may recur, the disk material can reform, or disk fragments may have been missed in surgery (Wilkinson, 1983). Injury to the nerves is possible and may result in permanent neurologic deficits.

After successful surgery, the client will have improvement in ambulation and relief of pain. The rehabilitation process varies according to procedure done, the client's progress, and the physician's preferred progression toward ambulation. The client must learn to use correct body mechanics and good posture and continue to practice them.

When spinal fusion is done, the progression toward ambulation is slowed, as healing of the bone graft takes time. A brace may be fitted and worn for a few months after surgery. Movement of that area of the spine will be impossible in the future due to fusion, but movement above and below those vertebrae is possible. For surgery in the cervical region, respiratory distress may be a complication because of edema of the spinal cord. A cervical collar is applied postoperatively.

Psychosocial/Lifestyle Implications

Successful surgery provides relief of a chronic problem. The client may be able to return to activities without the fear of another spell of back pain. Activity will be limited until complete healing occurs, and good posture and good body mechanics must become an essential part of daily life. While hospitalized, the client must adhere strictly to the prescribed limitations of movement. Needed objects must be placed within reach and adjustment is necessary to such activities as eating while lying on the side. When pain recurs, clients often feel discouraged and frustrated. Back problems are a common cause of disability and may force a person to stop working or change occupation. Other people may imply that the client is a malingerer, causing problems in the client's social relationships. The implications of laminectomy are summarized in Table 60–16.

Nursing Implications

Preoperative Care

Routine preoperative orthopedic care is necessary (see Chapter 56). In addition, the nurse teaches the client how to logroll (described under "Positioning and Turning") and how to get out of bed postoperatively (described under "Ambulation"). Assess the client's neurovascular and comfort status for comparisons to postoperative condition. Many clients fear that paralysis could occur as a complication of back surgery. Encourage clients to verbalize their apprehension and correct any misconceptions. Explain that swelling from surgery may cause the pain and numbness experienced before surgery to remain for some time afterward. The nurse should collect several pillows before surgery for positioning the client afterward.

Postoperative Care

Routine postoperative care includes interventions described in Chapter 56 such as comfort measures, neurovascular assessment, and prevention of the hazards of immobility. When moving the client back into bed from the recovery room cart, at least four people should lift the client gently, keeping the spine in good alignment. The bed should have a firm mattress.

The client's neurovascular status must be assessed with vital signs and any loss of sensation or deterioration in ability to move reported promptly to the physician. The nurse should stress respiratory status assessment in the client with cervical spine surgery. Observe the dressing for signs of hemorrhage or leaking cerebral spinal fluid, either of which should be reported to the physician.

The physician may order elastic stockings. Clients should move their arms, dorsiflex and plantarflex their feet, and cough and deep breathe every 2 hours. Use comfort measures and analgesics to relieve pain. If the client is discouraged because the preoperative symptoms are still present, explain that edema may be responsible.

The nurse should observe for difficulty with voiding because position limitations may be a hindrance. Use a

Table 60–16 Laminectomy: Implications for the Client	
Physiological Implications	**Psychosocial/Lifestyle Implications**
Successful surgery provides relief of pain and improves ambulation.	Chronic pain and disability may be relieved, improving the quality of life.
Local pain and edema occur as a result of surgical manipulation.	Temporary limitation in activity and positioning is necessary.
Neurological manifestations may occur immediately postoperatively due to operative area edema.	Good body mechanics and posture are a lifelong necessity.
Nerve damage can occur, causing permanent neurological deficits.	Recurrence of symptoms is discouraging.
Diskectomy is not always successful in relieving the symptoms; symptoms may recur.	Failed surgery may result in disability or a change in occupation.
A complication of cervical spine surgery is respiratory distress.	Recurrence of condition may cause others to think client is malingering.
Spinal fusion eliminates movement in the involved vertebrae; the recuperation period is lengthy.	A lengthy disability period may cause discouragement and financial problems.

fracture bedpan, and roll, rather than lift, the client onto it.

The diet is advanced as tolerated; foods to prevent constipation are encouraged. Initially, the client will have to eat in the side-lying position. Clients should be positioned on the side that allows them to use the dominant hand to feed themselves.

Positioning and Turning. Positioning varies with the physician's preference and the surgical procedure done. When the spinal fusion client is supine, the bed is completely flat. For diskectomy, the physician may prefer to have the client's legs elevated on pillows along their entire length or in a position with knees and hips flexed. Either of these positions relaxes the back muscles and provides comfort. The head of the bed may be elevated with physician's order only; it is usually elevated after cervical vertebrae surgery. When elevated, the client should be positioned in the bed so bending occurs at the hips, not somewhere along the back; it is important not to slouch. A sign above the client's bed indicating which positions are allowed or forbidden is helpful.

Turn the client every 2 to 3 hours. At first, two nurses are needed for turning since perfect body alignment needs to be maintained. Eventually, clients can turn themselves without help. The method for turning, known as *logrolling*, involves turning the client all at one time, without twisting the spine. The client is moved to one side of the bed, a pillow is placed between the legs, and the arms are crossed over the chest. The nurse places one hand on the client's far shoulder and one on the hip and rolls the client toward her/him while another nurse supports the back in alignment. Place pillows at the client's back for support, a pillow under the head, another between the knees, and one in front of the chest to support the arm. The uppermost knee should be flexed for balance. The client will eventually be able to turn unassisted by logrolling, after healing has begun.

A doubled-thickness drawsheet can also be used as a turning sheet for logrolling. Back rubs should be given and the skin inspected with each position change. Avoid rubbing the operative area. Place the call light near the bed so the client can avoid excessive reaching, which may strain the back.

Ambulation. Progressive ambulation usually begins with dangling, possibly the evening of surgery. Some surgeons prefer to be present when the client dangles for the first time. Two methods are used. In the first, the head of the bed is elevated, and the nurse brings the client's legs over the edge of the bed, swiveling the client's body at the same time without twisting the spine. In the second method, the client begins in the side-lying position, then pushes the upper body into the upright position using one or two hands as nurses move the legs over the edge of the bed and support the back. Observe for postural hypotension, especially if the client has been supine for several days. Getting out of bed is done in the same manner and

may begin from 1 to 5 days postoperatively, or in the case of spinal fusion, perhaps 2 weeks postoperatively. Some clients are allowed only to walk, not stand in one spot. The nurse should encourage good posture when walking. If the client is allowed to sit in a chair, the chair should be firm, with a straight back. Encourage good sitting posture, with the feet flat on the floor. In some cases, sitting is not allowed for several weeks.

Discharge. The length of hospitalization varies, but is typically about 1 to 2 weeks. Before discharge, the physician informs the client about restricted activities, such as driving and sexual activity. The restrictions usually apply for about 4 to 6 weeks postoperatively. The nurse should teach the client good posture and principles of body mechanics. The client's return to work depends on the type of activity the job requires. The prolonged absence from work (which often begins before surgery, when the client is undergoing conservative treatment) may create financial problems. A social worker may help find financial assistance.

CHEMONUCLEOLYSIS

Chemonucleolysis is the surgical procedure in which the enzyme chymopapain is injected into the central portion of a herniated intervertebral disk to shrink it. Pain caused by pressure of the disk on the nerve root is relieved as the disk shrinks.

Chemonucleolysis is indicated when acute leg pain due to a herniated lumbar disk does not respond to conservative treatment (see Chapter 59). A myelogram or computerized tomography (CT) scan shows that the intervertebral disk is herniated.

The procedure is an alternative to laminectomy, which is a major operation. Chemonucleolysis is contraindicated for those with an allergy to chymopapain, which is found in papaya and used in meat tenderizer. An allergy to radiopaque dye is also a contraindication. In addition, people who are experiencing bowel or bladder dysfunction or rapid changes of neurological functioning should not have this procedure but rather prompt disk surgery (Musolf, 1983).

Serious neurologic problems have recently been reported following chemonucleolysis with chymopapain, including paraplegia, cerebral hemorrhage, and transverse myelitis. It is currently recommended that chemonucleolysis be limited to the one disk producing the client's symptoms (Smith, 1984).

Surgical Procedure

Chemonucleolysis is done under general or local anesthesia with the client in a side-lying position. Local anesthesia is recommended and is associated with fewer complications. Spinal needles are inserted into the affected disk and their placement checked by means of fluoroscopy. Radiopaque dye is injected to confirm the diagnosis and the location of the problem disk. A test dose of chymopapain is injected into the disk through the spinal needle, and the client is observed for about 10 to 20 minutes for an allergic reaction. If no reaction is noted, the full dose is injected slowly. A small dressing is applied over the site.

Implications for the Client

Physiological Implications

The procedure is effective in about 70% of cases, providing relief of pain (Spengler, 1982). A few clients experience immediate relief of pain, but others may experience severe back spasms, especially when they move (Musolf, 1983). Analgesics, muscle relaxants, and rest are used to treat the spasms, which can persist for several days or weeks. Leg pain present before the procedure may be present for several days after the injection. Some stiffness, soreness, and edema may occur at the injection site (Musolf, 1983). As with lumbar puncture, a spinal headache can occur (see Chapter 36). Anaphylactic reaction occurs in 0.5% to 1% of clients from allergic reaction to the chymopapain (Gunby, 1983). This is a life-threatening situation requiring immediate treatment with epinephrine and measures to prevent or treat cardiac arrest. (Refer to Chapters 5 and 13.)

The client remains on bed rest for 1 to 2 days postoperatively. Activity and ambulation progress as tolerated.

Psychosocial/Lifestyle Implications

The advantage of this type of surgery is that it provides relief of pain without major surgery. Therefore, the hospitalization is shortened and the return to usual activities is more rapid than after laminectomy, the actual speed depending upon the demands of the client's lifestyle. The implications of chemonucleolysis are summarized in Table 60–17.

Nursing Implications

Preoperative Care

Preoperative care for chemonucleolysis is the usual care given for all operative procedures. Ask the client about allergies to radiopaque dyes, chymopapain, and meat tenderizer. Clients should be aware that the procedure is not without risk.

Postoperative Care

Postoperatively, the nurse checks vital signs routinely and assesses neurovascular status every 2 to 4 hours, reporting any abnormality to the physician. Watch closely for signs of anaphylactic reaction during the first 24 hours. Signs and symptoms include respiratory distress, hypotension, urticaria, pruritus, gastrointestinal discomfort, and eventual cardiac arrest. Suspected reaction requires emergency intervention with epinephrine injection, airway maintenance, and resuscitation. A slow-drip IV is maintained for 24 hours to keep a vein open, should emergency treatment be required.

The client maintains bed rest for 24 to 48 hours postoperatively; any comfortable position can be assumed. The nurse encourages coughing, deep breathing, and extremity movements every 2 hours and provides comfort measures and analgesics as needed. Foods and fluids are resumed as tolerated.

The client is usually discharged about 3 days postoperatively, when able to ambulate comfortably. The physician may prescribe specific exercises. Teach the client principles of good posture and body mechanics so back strain can be avoided.

BONE GRAFTING

A bone graft is a transplant of bone from another site, whether from the same individual (autograft) or another (allograft or homograft). The bone graft provides a matrix on which new bone can be layed; it also introduces viable bone-forming cells and small vessels (Connolly, 1981). Autografts have the best chance of survival and of being incorporated into the bone.

Bone grafts are done to stimulate osteogenesis in nonunion or delayed union of fractures, to fill bone cavities or replace missing bone, and to provide stability to fractures

Table 60–17 Chemonucleolysis: Implications for the Client	
Physiological Implications	**Psychosocial/Lifestyle Implications**
Successful surgery provides relief of pain.	Pain is relieved without major surgery.
A spinal headache may occur temporarily.	Requires shorter hospitalization and recovery than laminectomy.
Back spasms may occur temporarily.	
Anaphylactic reaction may occur from chymopapain or radiopaque dye.	
Leg pain experienced before procedure may persist for several days after injection.	
Stiffness, soreness, and edema may occur at injection site.	

or fused joints. Grafting may be used in combination with other procedures or treatments, eg, with open reduction internal fixation of a fracture or with electrical bone growth stimulation in delayed union.

Surgical Procedure

Bone grafting is done under general anesthesia. Preparation of two surgical sites is necessary when bone is being used from elsewhere in the body. Common donor sites are the iliac crest, tibia, fibula, rib, and radius. The recipient site is prepared, eg, by making a trough across a nonunited fracture site. One or more pieces of bone are cut, sawed, or scraped from the donor site and placed in the prepared recipient site. The fragments are placed in a cavity, packed about a fracture, or otherwise incorporated into the new location (Figure 60–23). Immediate transfer of the bone without prolonged exposure to the air maximizes the viability and effectiveness of the graft (Connolly, 1981). Cadaver bone from a bone bank is another source of grafting material. Some type of immobilization is used after wound closure, usually a cast.

Experimental work is being done with induction osteogenesis (or osteoinduction), a method of stimulating new bone growth using powdered demineralized bone derived from a cadaver or the client's own body. A paste is made of the powder for insertion into the recipient site. This process has been used primarily for craniofacial bones (eg, to fill gaps or augment bony contour) and for construction of new bone in soft tissue (King, 1982).

Implications for the Client

See the implications for internal fixation (Table 60–1) and arthrodesis (Table 60–8), where appropriate.

Physiological Implications

For the client whose fracture has not healed, a bone graft provides a stimulus for bone healing. A bone graft also provides a framework for bone growth when part of the bone is missing.

The donor site provides an additional location for pain,

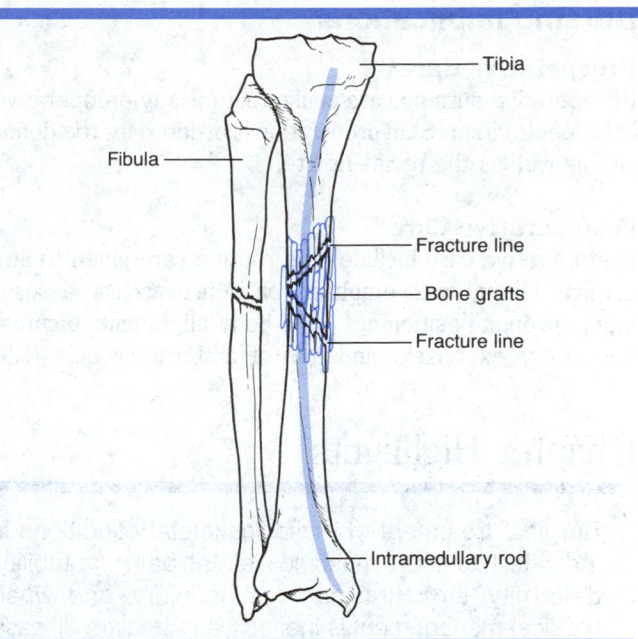

Figure 60–23

Bone grafting. Slabs of cancellous bone packed around a fracture site.

soreness, and complications such as infection. The amount of weight bearing allowed postoperatively and the progression toward ambulation depend on the location of the graft and other circumstances. For example, no movement is allowed when joint fusion (arthrodesis) is done. Some grafts are used on fractures for which weight bearing casts are eventually applied. The weight bearing helps revascularize the graft.

Psychosocial/Lifestyle Implications

The client who has a lengthy recuperation period, during which the fracture has not healed, may be discouraged. A bone graft provides hope that a bone that has failed to heal will eventually do so. With a successful bone graft, the client should be able to abandon ambulatory aids and return to usual activities. The implications of bone grafting are summarized in Table 60–18.

Table 60–18 Bone Grafting: Implications for the Client*	
Physiological Implications	**Psychosocial/Lifestyle Implications**
Provides a stimulus for bone healing for delayed union or nonunion of fractures.	Provides hope that fracture healing will occur.
Provides a framework for bone growth.	May speed the ending of a prolonged recovery period for delayed or nonunion of a fracture.
Two surgical wounds occur when autografts are used, increasing the chances of pain and complications.	
Weight bearing and ambulation depend on circumstances and location of the graft.	

*See Tables 60–1 and 60–8 for implications of internal fixation and arthrodesis.

Nursing Implications

Preoperative Care

Preoperative nursing care is like that for any preoperative orthopedic client. Skin preparation is ordered for the donor site as well as the recipient site.

Postoperative Care

Postoperative care includes the routine care given to any surgical client, with emphasis on neurovascular assessment, proper positioning, good body alignment, comfort measures, exercises, and use of ambulatory aids (see

Chapter 56). The care of a client with a cast is described in Chapter 58, and care following internal fixation and arthrodesis are explained earlier in this chapter.

The nurse should assess the dressing over the donor site as well as that over the other surgical area. Positioning the client comfortably may be difficult when there are two operative sites. Exercises required and progression toward ambulation will be specific to the procedure done. Therefore, the physician should give precise postoperative instructions about required, permitted, and restricted activities for the client and nurse to follow.

Chapter Highlights

Surgical treatment of musculoskeletal conditions is indicated to treat musculoskeletal pain, instability, deformity, structural damage or injury, and when medical management is ineffective in treating disease or injury.

In general, the physiological results of musculoskeletal surgeries are relief of pain, improved functioning, and repair of deformity or injury. The client temporarily experiences local pain, swelling, and limited weight bearing and mobility while recuperating from musculoskeletal surgery.

Potential complications of musculoskeletal surgery include nerve or blood vessel disruption, wound infection, bone or joint infection, hemorrhage, shock, phlebitis, pulmonary or fat embolism, and loosening or breaking of hardware.

Abnormalities noted upon neurovascular assessment must be brought to the attention of the surgeon immediately.

The nurse should position the client in required or permitted positions during the postoperative period and avoid positions that are contraindicated.

Exercises are necessary preoperatively and postoperatively to maintain and regain strength and function.

An important nursing function is preventing the hazards of immobility.

Pain management includes use of analgesics, position changes, and other comfort measures.

Care of the wound requires aseptic dressing changes and observing for signs of infection.

The client will need some assistance with ADL postoperatively especially when mobility is limited.

Client practice of exercises and correct use of ambulatory aids is encouraged and reinforced by the nurse. The nurse should be familiar with the amount of weight bearing allowed and monitor the client.

The surgical treatment may alter the body image because of disfigurement, impaired musculoskeletal functioning, and the use of orthopedic appliances or ambulatory aids.

Lengthy hospitalization and recovery required in most musculoskeletal surgery may be an emotional and financial burden.

Before discharge, the nurse teaches the client about positioning and ambulation restrictions, exercises, signs and symptoms of complications, and wound care.

Bibliography

Agee BL, Herman C: Cervical logrolling on a standard hospital bed. *Am J Nurs* 1984; 84(3):315–318.

Apley AG, Solomon L: *Apley's System of Orthopaedics and Fractures*, 6th ed. London: Butterworth, 1982.

Bartell L: Bunionectomies. *Ortho Nurs* 1985; 4(1): 21–28.

Blake SA: Noncemented femoral prosthesis: Intraoperative focus. *Ortho Nurs* 1985; 4(1):40–42.

Connolly JF (ed): *DePalma's The Management of Fractures and Dislocations: An Atlas*, 3rd ed. Philadelphia: Saunders, 1981.

Crowther HT: New perspectives on nursing lower limb amputees. *J Adv Nurs* 1982; 7:453–460.

Doheny MO: Porous coated femoral prosthesis: Concepts and care considerations. *Ortho Nurs* 1985; 4(1):43–45.

Farrell J: *Illustrated Guide to Orthopedic Nursing*. 2nd ed. Philadelphia: Lippincott, 1982.

Gruendemann BJ, Meeker MH: *Alexander's Care of the Patient in Surgery*, 7th ed. St. Louis: Mosby, 1983.

Gunby P: What is intradiscal therapy anyway? *JAMA* 1983; 249:1121–1123.

Hay BK, Karas CB: External fixation: Option for fractures. *AORN J* 1981; 34:417–426.

King JP: Bones: How to grow new ones. *AORN J* 1982; 35:968–975.

Kostuik JP: *Amputation Surgery and Rehabilitation*. New York: Churchill Livingstone, 1981.

Mourad L: *Nursing Care of Adults With Orthopedic Conditions*. New York: Wiley, 1980.

Musolf JM: Chemonucleolysis: A new approach for patients with herniated intervertebral disks. *Am J Nurs* 1983; 83:882–885.

Powell M: *Orthopaedic Nursing and Rehabilitation*, 8th ed. Edinburgh: Churchill Livingstone, 1982.

Robinson JE, Mar LO: A nail-safe method. *Am J Nurs* 1985; 85(2):158–161.

Smith WS: Letter to doctors and pharmacists dated July 19, 1984, regarding the neurological complications following use of chymopapain. Smith Laboratories, Inc, 1984.

Spengler DM: *Low Back Pain: Assessment and Management*. New York: Grune & Stratton, 1982.

Strang EL, Johns JL: Nursing care of the patient treated with continuous passive motion following total knee arthroplasty. *Ortho Nurs* 1984; 3(6):27–32.

Walsh CR, Wirth CR: Total knee arthroplasty: Biomechanical and nursing considerations. *Ortho Nurs* 1985; 4(1):29–34, 70.

Wilkinson HA: *The Failed Back Syndrome*. Philadelphia: Harper & Row, 1983.

Wright V: *Bone and Joint Disease in the Elderly*. Edinburgh: Churchill Livingstone, 1983.

Suggested Readings

Brown SL: Avoiding postoperative pitfalls with hip fracture patients. *RN* 1982; 45(5)48–54. Describes the postoperative care of clients with pinning. Has several illustrations of fixation devices.

Gallagher LL: Shoulder arthroplasty. *Nurs 80* 1980; 10(7):46–49. The nursing care of the client with shoulder arthroplasty is described with illustrations of the anatomy and the prostheses involved.

Kryschyshen PL, Fischer DA: External fixation for complicated fractures. *Am J Nurs* 1980; 80:256–259. Summarizes the use of external fixation and the nursing care necessary. Has several good photographs to visualize the devices.

McWilliams N: *Manual of Orthopedic Surgery for Nurses*. Bowie, MD: Brady, 1982. A textbook for nurses working with orthopedic clients in the operating room. Provides good pictures of hardware and operating room instruments used for specific procedures.

Miller BK, Gregory M: Carpal tunnel syndrome. *AORN J* 1983; 38:525–532. Describes the syndrome, operative care, and preoperative and postoperative nursing care as well.

Voluz JM: Surgical implants. *AORN J* 1983; 37:1341–1352. A review of a variety of devices used for internal fixation and joint replacement. General nursing measures in the operating room and postoperatively are presented.

Walters J: Coping with a leg amputation. *Am J Nurs* 1981; 81:1349–1352. This article describes four phases in the adjustment process and nursing interventions helpful in assisting clients to cope with amputation.

The Client With a Fractured Hip

I. Descriptive Data

Mrs Joan Williams, age 62, was admitted on Jan 18 to the hospital with a tentative diagnosis of right fractured hip. She was placed on bed rest with 5# Buck's traction to the right leg.

II. Personal Data

Date and Time:	2 PM, Jan 18, 1986
Insurance No.:	NY00000
Full Name:	Joan Marie Williams
Address:	124 Mayne Rd., Hampton, NY 14222
Telephone:	Home: 000-0000
	Work: None
Sex:	Female
Age:	62
Birthdate:	8-2-23
Marital Status:	Widowed
Race/Culture:	Caucasian
Religion:	Jewish
Occupation:	Housewife
Usual Health Care Provider:	William Katz, MD

III. Health History

Source of Information:	Client
Reliability of Informant:	Reliable, good recall
Chief Concern:	"Fell and hurt my hip," "Can't move my leg"
History of Present Illness:	

Mrs Williams slipped on the ice on her steps when returning from the mailbox on Jan 18. She experienced pain in right hip area and found it difficult to get up. After she lay there about 5 minutes, a neighbor saw her and was able to carry her into the house and call an ambulance. She was admitted to the hospital with a tentative diagnosis of a right hip fracture.

Other musculoskeletal system history: denies weakness, myalgia, or muscle cramps. Has osteoarthritis, which primarily affects her hands. Notes intermittent stiffness and swelling of DIP and PIP joints of both hands, especially in the right thumb. Takes Ecotrin 650 mg t.i.d. regularly and applies ice p.r.n., which relieves the discomfort.

Expresses concern that she will not be able to return to her home and resume her independence.

Past Health History:	
Childhood:	Childhood diseases—measles, mumps
Immunizations:	Smallpox vaccination; unsure of others
Medical Problems:	Osteoarthritis; mild hypertension since 1978—well controlled with salt restriction and diuretics
Surgeries:	Appendectomy, 1960; cholecystectomy, 1966
Blood Transfusions:	None
Special Diagnostic Procedures:	Gallbladder x-rays, 1966; mammogram, 1979, negative
Pregnancies:	One in 1943, full-term male; no complications
Trauma:	None
Allergies:	None
Medications:	Ecotrin, 650 mg t.i.d.; Dyazide, $\frac{1}{1}$ b.i.d.
Family History:	Father, died age 71, heart disease, hypertension
	Mother, died age 76, CVA
	Sister, age 59, A&W, hypertension, osteoarthritis

Case Study written by Linda Heim McCausland.

Brother, age 58, A&W, osteoarthritis
Husband, died age 60 (in 1983), MI
Son, age 40, A&W
Maternal uncle, Ca lung
No other significant health problems in blood relatives

Personal/Social History: Lives alone in rural area; owns own home, a small, three-bedroom house, one floor. Intent upon keeping her home and remaining independent. Husband's pension is adequate; does not worry too much about money. Spends average day doing household tasks, gardening, reading, watching TV. Drives her own car. Necessary services, shopping, temple are within 5 miles. Enjoys crocheting, bingo, women's group at temple.

Elementary school education; worked as a clerk in a clothing store until pregnancy. Husband was a mechanic.

Habits: Eats three balanced meals a day, likes sweets but has to avoid them to keep weight down; exercises more in the summer doing yard work, taking walks; weight gain of about 10 lb in winter due to inactivity; alcohol intake, a glass of wine each evening; denies other drug use; never smoked; averages 7 hours of sleep a night; bedtime at 11:30 PM, arises 6:30 AM, occasional nap in evening after dinner.

Son and family visit often and help with chores; very close to her sister, phones daily, visits once a week. States that her strong religious beliefs helped her cope with her husband's death 3 years ago.

Review of Systems: States overall health is good; arthritis is only bothersome when it interferes with her ability to work with her hands

Skin: Complains of dryness on legs, feet, hands from colder weather—has increased with aging; applies lanolin-type lotion b.i.d. with improvement; denies other skin problems

Eyes: Vision good with corrective lenses for reading and for distance (bifocals)

Ears: States hearing is less acute but is not a problem for her

Breasts/Axillae: Had pain in left breast in 1979, mammogram was negative, pain subsided in a few weeks; denies current problems; regularly examines breasts since then

Gastrointestinal: Occasional constipation in the winter when less active, takes psyllium with relief

Gynecological: Menopause at 49, uneventful; sees gynecologist yearly for exam; not sexually active since husband's death

Psychological: Gets depressed at times when she thinks about her late husband; less frequent depression noted as time goes by; supportive family

IV. Physical Assessment

Weight: 140 lb, goes down to 130 lb in summer
Height: 5 ft 6 in
Vital Signs: Temp 98.8°F(37°C); P-88; R-22; BP 148/88
Relevant Organ Systems:
Skin: Pink, warm, decreased elasticity; has dryness of lower legs and both feet; skin on feet is slightly scaly
Cardiovascular: PMI at 5 LICS, slightly medial to MCL, apical rate 86, regular
Musculoskeletal: Right leg appears shorter than left, externally rotated, abducted; unable to move it without severe pain in the right hip region; ecchymotic area 10 × 8 cm over right trochanteric region, with slight swelling present in hip and upper thigh; dorsalis pedis and posterior tibial pulses = bilaterally; unable to locate popliteal pulses; color, motion, temperature, and sensation

(continued)

The Client With a Fractured Hip

(CMTS) of toes of both feet normal; no peripheral edema other than that in right hip area.

Bony enlargement noted in DIP joints in both hands; some limitation of flexion and extension of the fingers and thumbs; no other deformities, tenderness, or swelling noted; ROM good in other joints; muscle strength and tone intact.

Examination of right leg motion and strength deferred; unable to evaluate gait, posture, or balance.

Psychological: Alert, oriented to person, place, time; good recent and remote memory

V. Diagnostic Data
VI. Summary An x-ray of the right hip revealed an intertrochanteric fracture. Mrs Williams was scheduled for a hip pinning 2 days after admission. She was typed and crossmatched for 2 units of blood to have available for surgery. Her CBC, electrolytes, urinalysis, and ECG were within normal limits. Preoperative teaching was done. Family members were present frequently and were supportive.

On Jan 20, a hip pinning was done using a compression screw. General anesthesia was used, and 1 unit of whole blood was given during surgery. A Hemovac drain was inserted. She tolerated the procedure well, progressed satisfactorily in the recovery room, and was returned to her room.

VII. Postoperative Orders
- Vital signs and neurovascular checks q.15 min, until stable, then q.30 min × 4, then q.2h × 2, then q.4h
- IV of 5% dextrose/0.45 normal saline at 125 mL/h until taking fluids well PO; then decrease to 80 mL/h
- Advance diet as tolerated
- I&O; empty Hemovac q. shift
- Bed rest; may turn to either side with pillow between legs

Medications: Meperidine (Demerol), 50 mg IM q.3h p.r.n. pain
Trimethobenzamide HCl (Tigan), 200 mg IM q.6h p.r.n. nausea or vomiting
Cefazolin (Kefzol), 1 g q.6h, IV piggyback
Dyazide, 1 cap b.i.d., resume first day postop

VIII. Nursing Care Plan

Nursing Diagnosis	Client Care Goals	Plan/Nursing Implementation	Expected Outcomes
Comfort, alteration in: related to surgical incision and arthritis	Relieve pain; rest comfortably for 3–4 h periods; participate in diversional activity	Assess pain q.3h; meperidine, 50 mg IM q.3h p.r.n. and evaluate effect; change position q.2h and p.r.n.; back rub, diversional activity; ice to hands for arthritic discomfort; handle right leg gently; teach to request analgesic before pain is severe	Requests analgesics before pain gets severe; able to rest comfortably and participate in ADL with comfort
Fluid volume deficit, potential: related to postoperative hemorrhage	Prevent hemorrhage and shock	Assess VS frequently until stable, then q.4h; check dressing and Hemovac q.2h; I&O	Reports any bloody drainage on dressing; no signs of bleeding or shock

Nursing Diagnosis	Client Care Goals	Plan/Nursing Implementation	Expected Outcomes
Gas exchange, impaired: related to anesthesia and inactivity	Prevent respiratory problems	Explain causes of respiratory problems; assess respirations and auscultate chest q.4h; C&DB q.2h; incentive spirometer; encourage fluid intake of 3000 mL/day; assist with position change at least q.2h	Practices C&DB exercises; changes position frequently; drinks 3000 mL fluids/day; no sign of respiratory problems; understands effects of inactivity on respiratory system
Injury: potential for disruption of surgical repair	Promote fracture healing	Avoid extreme positions (no acute angle hip flexion, adduction, external rotation); position trochanter rolls or sandbags to keep good alignment; support operative leg when turning; when out of bed, no weight bearing on right leg; pivot into chair; firm, high chair; teach her about desired and restricted positions	Uncomplicated fracture healing; explains and practices desired positioning; understands position restrictions
Skin integrity, impairment of: potential, related to inactivity	Prevent areas of skin breakdown	Assess common pressure areas (heels, sacrum, ankles, elbows) q.4h; air mattress; heel protectors; turn q.2h with pillow between legs; check CMTS with VS; back care and massage when turned; balanced diet; 3000 mL fluids/24 h; keep skin clean, dry, lubricated; teach about effects of pressure on skin; apply lanolin to feet and lower legs b.i.d.	Understands effects of prolonged pressure on skin integrity; avoids staying in same position for more than 2 h; no signs of skin breakdown; understands importance of diet and fluids and maintains good intake
Skin integrity, impairment of: potential, related to wound infection in the surgical incision	Prevent wound infection	Assess dressing or incision, and temperature q.4h; check Hemovac drainage; empty q.8h, keep deflated; aseptic technique for dressing changes; change wet or soiled dressings frequently; Cefazolin 1 g IV q.6h; teach signs and symptoms for wound infection	Understands and reports any signs or symptoms of infection
Mobility, impaired physical: related to potential for contractures and muscle atrophy	Prevent contractures and muscle atrophy	ROM to all uninvolved joints b.i.d.; isometric abdominal, gluteal, quadriceps exercises q.i.d.; encourage self-care; teach exercises; position in good alignment; teach benefits of exercise and good alignment	Exercises (ROM) uninvolved joints; does isometric exercises; maintains proper body alignment; participates in ADL; understands benefits of exercise and correct alignment; normal ROM and muscle strength

(continued)

The Client With a Fractured Hip

VIII. Nursing Care Plan *(continued)*

Nursing Diagnosis	Client Care Goals	Plan/Nursing Implementation	Expected Outcomes
Mobility, impaired physical: related to potential for thrombus formation	Prevent thrombus formation	Elastic stockings, remove b.i.d. to give foot care, observe skin and reapply; dorsiflex and plantarflex ankles; assess for calf pain, check Homans' sign; teach how inactivity leads to clot formation	Exercises extremities regularly; understands how clot formation occurs from inactivity; no signs of thrombus formation
Urinary elimination, alteration in pattern: related to potential for urinary retention because of unnatural position on bedpan	Prevent urinary retention	Assess for inability to void or distended abdomen; use fracture bedpan; elevate head of bed 45°; provide privacy; encourage 3000 mL fluid q.d.; I&O; encourage use of commode or toilet when able to be out of bed; use measures to help voiding, (eg, running water within hearing distance)	Empties bladder completely; takes in 3000 mL fluids q.d.; uses commode or toilet when able to be out of bed; no distention; output approximately equal to intake
Bowel elimination, alteration in: potential for constipation related to inactivity	Prevent constipation	Assess daily for BM; encourage foods with fiber, fruit juices; encourage position changes and activity; 3000 mL fluid q.d.; teach measures to prevent constipation	Takes in 3000 mL fluids/day; understands causes of constipation; includes fiber in diet; changes position frequently and increases activity daily; daily BM
Self-concept, disturbance in: potential depression related to dependence on others	Express feelings about her condition; participate in activities as able	Encourage involvement in discharge plans; encourage independence in ADL; encourage her to ventilate feelings	Periods of depression decrease as she recuperates; helps with ADL as much as possible; able to return to own home eventually and care for self
Knowledge deficit related to care necessary after discharge	Feel comfortable and secure with home care	Discuss discharge plans with her and family; encourage self-care; teach wound care; encourage correct use of walker and getting in and out of bed; teach how to modify home for safe use of walker; encourage follow-up visit with physician	Learns to use walker correctly; understands safety measures for use of walker; adjusts home environment to facilitate independence in ADL; describes safety measures for ambulation

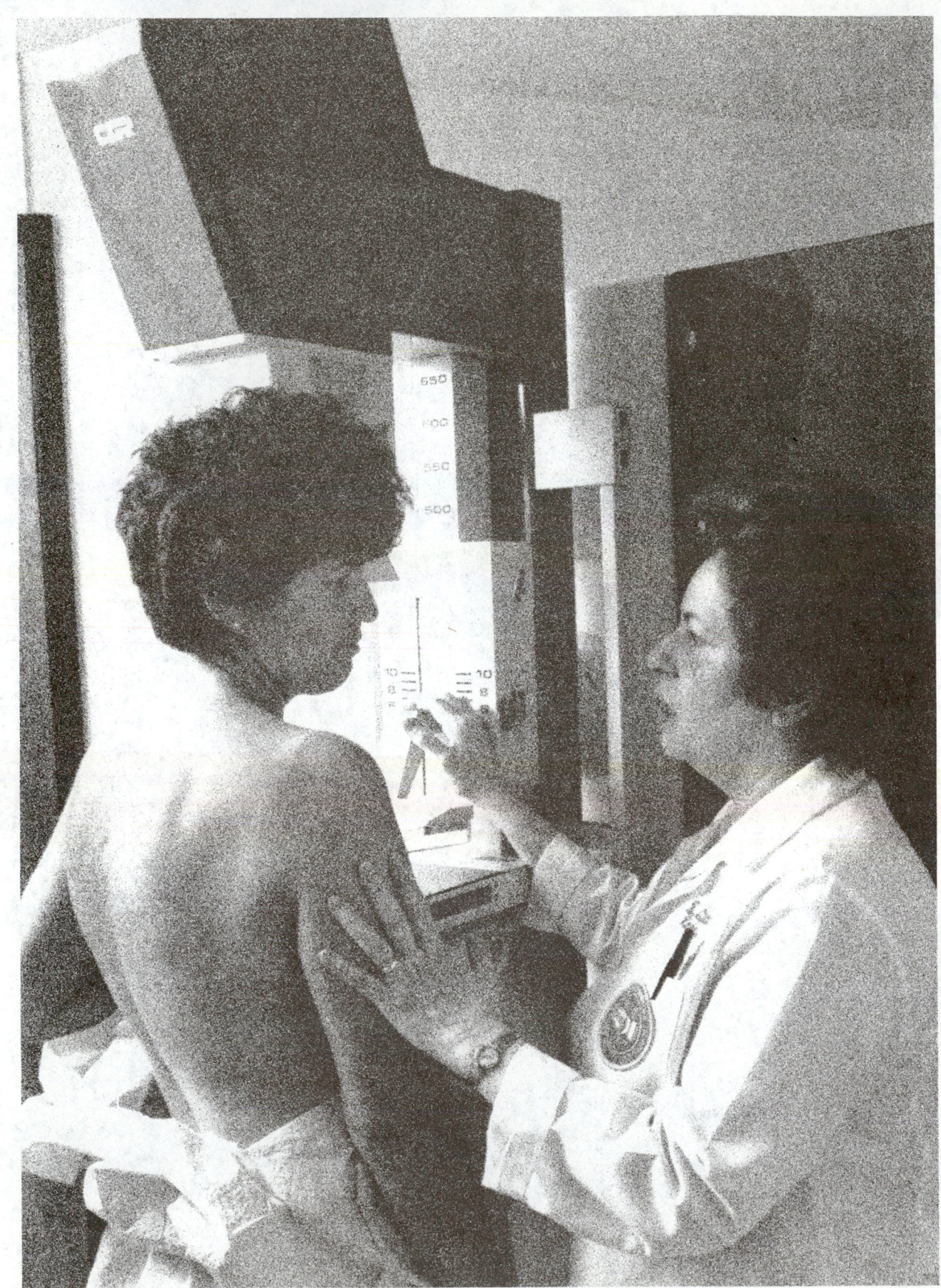

The Client With Reproductive System Dysfunction

Chapter 61

The Female Reproductive System in Health and Illness

Mary Lyn Field

Objectives

When you have finished reading this chapter, you should be able to:

Describe the structures of the external and internal female genitalia and explain their function and changes from birth to menopause.

Trace changes in hormone secretion and their effects in females from birth to menopause.

Describe the four phases of sexual response in women.

Identify the variations in bleeding in women and the major causes and characteristics of pelvic pain.

Discuss the interrelatedness of the female reproductive system with the musculoskeletal, integumentary, urinary, gastrointestinal, and endocrine systems.

Explain the psychosocial influences on the well-being and dysfunction of the female reproductive system in adolescence, young and middle adulthood, and menopause.

Although the structures of the female reproductive system are localized, the system's functions depend on and affect many other structures and systems. The female reproductive system operates in a feedback relation to the neurological and endocrine systems, and the hormones involved affect many other parts of the body. A clear understanding of hormonal actions and neuroendocrine function related to the menstrual cycle will aid assessment and management of many problems of the female reproductive system.

Both the normal variations and the dysfunctions of the female reproductive system may produce great anxiety because of the relation of the system to women's sexual identity, social roles, and body image. Because most nurses are women and most physicians are men, many female clients look to nurses for support and advice about physiological and psychosocial functions of the female reproductive system. Many women are more comfortable discussing reproductive system problems with women than men. Thus, female nurses are in a position to be effective in counseling, teaching, and managing the problems of clients with gynecologic concerns. The nurse who can integrate a knowledge of anatomy and physiology with an understanding of the emotional and social experiences and needs of a female client can offer competent, caring, and comprehensive health services.

Section I: Structural and Functional Interrelationships

STRUCTURE AND FUNCTION OF THE FEMALE REPRODUCTIVE SYSTEM

The female external genitalia provide protection, enhance sexual arousal and pleasure, and are the site of urination.

The internal genitalia are the sites of major biological events in a woman's life, including **menarche** (the onset of menstruation), premenstrual changes, pregnancy, and **menopause** (the cessation of the menstrual cycle).

External Genitalia

The term *vulva* refers to the female external genitalia. Refer to Figure 61–1 in the following discussion of the vulva's specific structures.

Mons Pubis

At the top of the external genitalia is the mons pubis, or mons veneris (see Figure 61–1). This rounded pad of fatty tissue is covered with pubic hair and contains sebaceous and sweat glands. The amount of fat and hair is controlled by such factors as nutrition, steroids, and genetics. The mons pubis becomes fuller in adolescence, and pubic hair appears in the area around 11 or 12 years of age. In menopause, there is a loss of fatty deposits, so the mons pubis becomes less prominent, and the pubic hair thins and decreases. In many women, the hairline forming the superior border of the mons pubis forms a transverse line across the lower abdomen, whereas in others the line extends toward the umbilicus along the linea alba. The mons pubis has three functions: protecting the pelvic bones, making coitus more comfortable; distinguishing the female by its rounded contour; and enhancing arousal. Stimulation of the mons pubis causes orgasm for some.

Clitoris

The clitoris, from the Greek word for key, is considered the most erotically sensitive part of the female genital tract. The clitoris is visible between the folds of the labia minora at the anterior juncture (see Figure 61–1). It is about 5 to 6 mm in length and 6 to 8 mm in diameter. The external portions are the body and glans. The body has two small erectile corpora cavernosa (cavernous bodies) covered by

a dense fibrous membrane. The glans consists of a mucous membrane with an enormous number of free nerve endings; this makes the clitoris a sensitive area of the body requiring, in some women, only light stimulation to bring on orgasm. Innervation of the clitoris is through the terminal branch of the pudendal nerve. The prepuce, or hood, of the clitoris overlying the glans is also erotically very sensitive because of its abundance of free nerve endings. The clitoris produces **smegma,** a substance that has an odor often considered erotically stimulating. There is little change in clitoral response in menopause.

Labia Majora

The labia majora originate in the mons pubis and end in the perineum, uniting to form the posterior commissure (see Figure 61–1). Labia means "lips," and the labia majora are two rounded mounds of tissue that form the lateral boundaries of the vulva. They are homologous to the scrotum of the male. The labia majora contain fatty tissue, sweat glands, hair, blood vessels, lymphatic vessels, and nerves.

The labia majora function mainly as a protective covering for the genitals, but they also serve as a source of erotic pleasure. Pregnancy causes the labia to lose tone, producing a loose appearance. At menopause, the labia atrophy and appear less prominent. There are many normal variations in the appearance of the labia from woman to woman, throughout life.

Because the labia majora have much loose connective tissue, the structure is especially susceptible to edema. The lymphatic drainage of the labia majora is shared with other structures of the vulva. Therefore, labial congestion

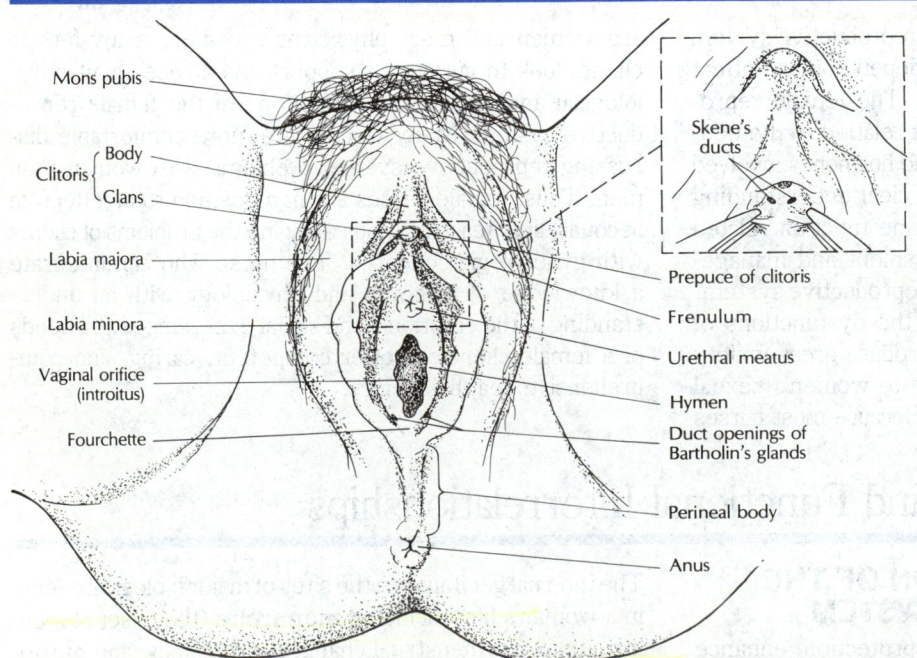

Figure 61–1

Female external genitals, longitudinal view.

SOURCE: Olds SB, London ML, Ladewig PA: *Maternal–Newborn Nursing: A Family-Centered Approach*, 2nd ed. Menlo Park, CA: Addison–Wesley, 1984, p. 71.

Mons pubis

Clitoris { Body / Glans

Labia majora

Labia minora

Vaginal orifice (introitus)

Fourchette

Skene's ducts

Prepuce of clitoris

Frenulum

Urethral meatus

Hymen

Duct openings of Bartholin's glands

Perineal body

Anus

or swelling can be a clue to malignancies in a number of other areas.

The nerves supplying the labia majora are primarily of central nervous system origin. Innervation to the anterior third is from the first lumbar segment, and to the posterior two-thirds from the sacral segment. The area is extremely sensitive to touch, pressure, pain, and temperature. The internal and external pudendal arteries constitute the arterial blood supply. An extensive venous network is in connection with the veins of the clitoris, labia minora, and perineum.

Labia Minora

The labia minora are two thin longitudinal folds of tissue lying inside the labia majora (see Figure 61–1). Their surface is shiny and has no hair follicles. They divide anteriorly to form the prepuce of the clitoris and just below this to form the frenulum (lower fold) of the clitoris. Posteriorly, the labia merge to form the fourchette, the fold of skin immediately posterior to the vaginal orifice that is often traumatized during childbirth.

The tissue of the labia minora is erectile. Because of many tactile nerve endings, a vaginal discharge is potentially irritating. The skin becomes engorged and red during sexual excitement, and the labia distend. By a rich supply of sebaceous glands, the labia minora lubricate the vulvar skin. The labia minora also provide bactericidal secretions and heighten sexual arousal and pleasure. After menopause, the labia minora atrophy, losing fat tissue and becoming flatter as the labia majora do, although to a lesser degree.

Urethral Meatus

The urethral meatus, or external urethral opening, usually is about 2 to 3 cm inferior to the clitoris but may be located at other nearby points where it is more difficult to see. The meatus is slightly elevated and has depressed areas on each side. The opening may be stellate or crescent shaped. The urethral meatus forms the opening through which urine flows (see Figure 61–1).

Paraurethral Glands

The paraurethral glands (Skene's ducts) are located bilaterally and open into the posterior wall of the urethra (see Figure 61–1). Skene's ducts are correlates of the male prostate gland and do not appear to have a specific function in the female. They are susceptible to gonococcal infection, however.

Vestibule, Introitus, and Hymen

The vestibule, visible upon separation of the labia majora, is the elliptical space bordered by the labia minora laterally, the urethra and clitoris superiorly, and the fourchette inferiorly. The vaginal introitus (the opening into the vagina) sits within the vestibule. The hymen (also called the hymenal ring) is an irregular membranous fold of epithelium and fibrous tissue that surrounds and covers the vaginal intro-

itus to varying degrees (see Figure 61–1). The strength and size of the hymen vary among individuals and in the individual at different times. If the hymen is thick, surgery may be necessary to perforate it to allow intercourse, pelvic examination, and menstrual flow. The hymen can be broken through strenuous physical activity, masturbation, or the use of tampons. It may remain intact, however, even in parous women.

Bartholin's Glands

Just inside the middle to lower vaginal introitus are Bartholin's glands, whose ducts appear as two small papular elevations just at the base of the vestibule and external to the hymenal ring (see Figure 61–1). Research has disproved the idea that the Bartholin's glands provide lubrication during intercourse (Olds et al., 1984; Tyler & Woodall, 1982). These glands are thought to secrete mucus that keeps the vaginal mucosa moist.

Perineum

The term *perineum* is often misused to refer to the vulva or external genitalia. The perineum actually includes the skin and tissues between the vaginal introitus and the anal orifice (see Figure 61–1). These structures are all highly vascular, which explains the bleeding that occurs with an episiotomy.

The muscles of the perineum include the ischiocavernous muscles, which curve around the clitoris, extending from the ischium to the base of the clitoris; the bulbocavernous muscles, which envelop the vestibule and surround the lower third of the vagina; the transverse muscle of the perineum and levator ani muscle, which extend from the perineal body and unite behind the vaginal openings; and the rectus abdominis muscle, which is attached to the suspensory ligament and then attaches to the clitoral body. These muscles collectively anchor and protect the pelvic viscera and external genitalia and provide the sphincter activity of the urethra, vagina, and rectum. The contractions of these muscles serve as a major stimulus of orgasm.

Embryonic Development

The female external genitalia are differentiated from the male genitalia in the eighth week of embryonic development. In the female, the absence of testosterone, not the production of female hormones, determines the formation of female external genitalia. If the developing fetus is exposed to testosterone produced by the male testis or by an exogenous source, the external genitalia become masculine (Johnson & Everitt, 1980).

From similar original structures, the two sexes develop different anatomies secondary to the presence or absence of testosterone. The genital tubercle becomes the corpora cavernosa and glans of the penis in the male and the corpora cavernosa and glans of the clitoris in the female. In the female, the urethral folds remain separate and form the labia minora instead of fusing as they do in the male. Labioscrotal swellings become the labia majora in the female, whereas in the male, these swellings fuse and become the scrotum. What is embryonically the urogenital slit becomes the lower vagina and urethra.

Internal Genitalia

The internal organs both respond to hormonal stimulation and secrete hormones, profoundly affecting biopsychosocial responses such as premenstrual stress reactions and postnatal feelings of well-being. Illnesses involving the genital system produce great anxiety for most women, and the structures of the internal genitalia are the sites of the most common health problems related to the female reproductive system, such as dysmenorrhea and vaginitis.

Vagina

The vagina, or birth canal, is like a tunnel, tube, or passageway open at its anterior end and extending inward to the center of the pelvis. This musculomembranous structure accommodates menstrual discharge, the penis in coitus, and the fetal head during delivery.

The vaginal vault is the upper part of the vagina. The cervix of the uterus projects into the upper part of the anterior wall of the vagina, making the anterior wall shorter than the posterior wall by 2.5 cm. The cervix creates a distinct section of the vagina similar to that created by indenting a balloon to make a recess or hollow area (Figure 61–2). The four arches that result from the projection of the cervix into the vaginal vault are called the vaginal fornices. The anterior vaginal fornix is short, the lateral ones are deeper, and the posterior fornix is deepest. The uterus can be palpated above the anterior and posterior fornices.

Semen collects in the posterior fornix with coitus when the woman is supine.

The lining of the vagina is noncornified stratified squamous epithelium that proliferates under estrogenic stimulation. The rugae vaginales are transverse ridges of mucous membrane in the posterior and anterior vaginal walls. The lateral walls are smoother. The surface appears this way from menarche to menopause. After stretching from pregnancies and decreased estrogenic stimulation with menopause, the rugae vaginales smooth out and the lining becomes thinner and drier, or atrophic.

In the past, the vagina was described as a relatively insensitive structure. The pudendal nerve innervates the lower third, and there are no special nerve endings. This explains why vaginal sensations during coitus and sexual excitement are minimal, as well as why pain during the second stage of labor is manageable. There is interesting new evidence, however, about vaginal sensation. Research has revealed a dime-sized area just above the anterior surface of the vaginal wall about one-third to one-half the way into the vagina—the Gräfenberg spot, or G spot (Figure 61–3). This also has been described as the female counterpart of the male prostate gland (Belzer, 1981). Women and their partners report that when the Gräfenberg spot is stimulated, varying amounts of a fluid unlike urine are expelled (Bullough et al., 1984). Whatever its source, the ejaculate seems to be expelled by some women in response to clitoral stimulation. Because of methodological problems, no definitive study has yet proven that the ejaculate is different from urine or vaginal secretions (Heath, 1984).

The vagina is acidic from menarche to menopause, and its surface is moist from fluid secreted by the vaginal

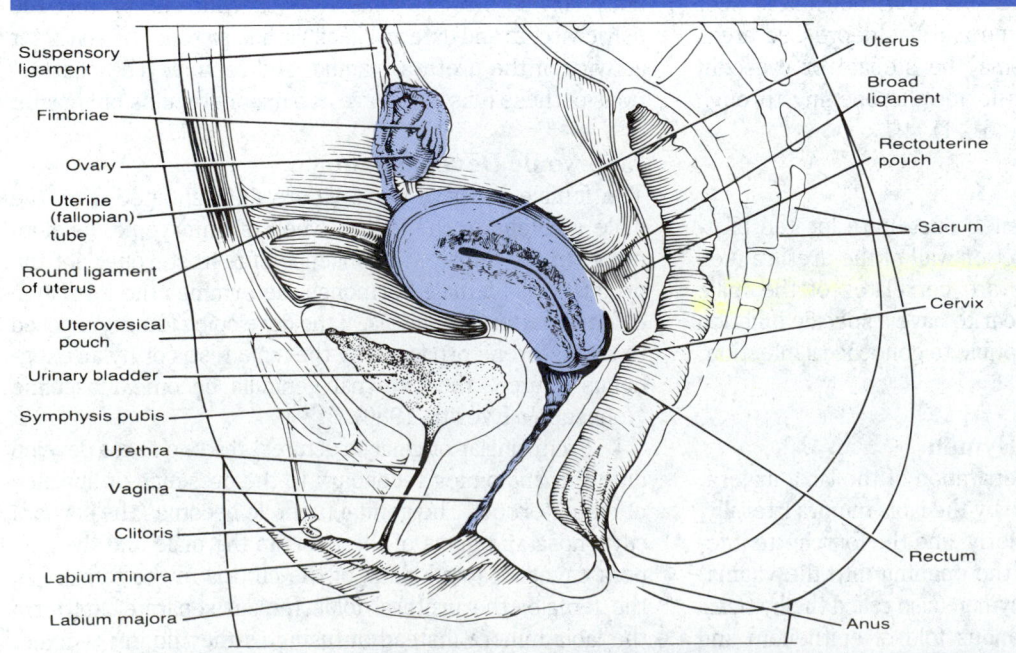

Figure 61–2

Median view of the female pelvis.

SOURCE: Spence AP, Mason EB: *Human Anatomy and Physiology*, 2nd ed. Menlo Park, CA: Benjamin/Cummings, 1983, p. 742.

Suspensory ligament
Fimbriae
Ovary
Uterine (fallopian) tube
Round ligament of uterus
Uterovesical pouch
Urinary bladder
Symphysis pubis
Urethra
Vagina
Clitoris
Labium minora
Labium majora

Uterus
Broad ligament
Rectouterine pouch
Sacrum
Cervix
Rectum
Anus

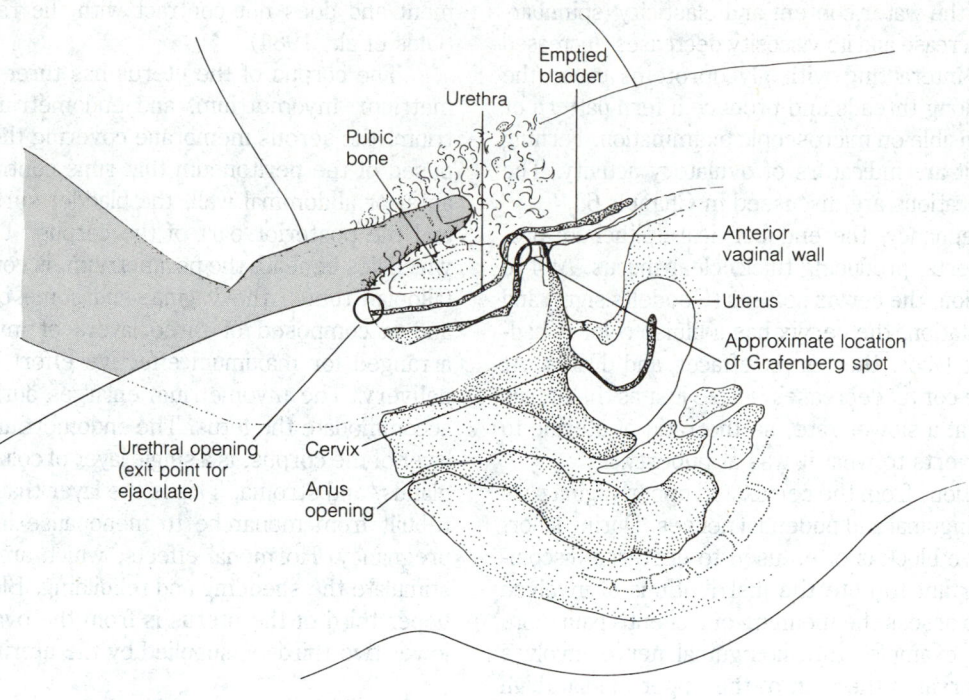

Figure 61–3

Locating the Gräfenberg spot. Two fingers are usually employed, and it is often necessary to press deeply into the anterior wall of the vagina to reach the spot.

SOURCE: Crooks R, Bauer K: *Our Sexuality*. Menlo Park, CA: Benjamin/Cummings, 1983, p. 183.

epithelium. Döderlein's bacilli, which produce lactic acid, and the vaginal contents exist symbiotically. Ovarian hormones regulate the glycogen content and the sloughing and renewal of vaginal epithelial cells. The interaction of the bacilli with this process by enzymatic breakdown of glycogen to lactic acid maintains the acidity of the vagina. Douching interrupts this natural protective process and can make the vagina more susceptible to infection.

The vascular supply of the vagina is different for each segment. Branches of uterine arteries supply the upper third; bladder arteries, the middle third; and internal pudendal and rectal arteries, the lower third. Lymphatic drainage follows a direct pattern and should be included in the assessment of vaginal infections. Drainage from the upper third is into the external and internal iliac nodes; from the middle third, into the hypogastric nodes; and from the lower third, into the inguinal nodes. Nodes in the rectovaginal septum collect drainage from the posterior wall.

Muscular and ligamentous support of the vagina is provided by the levator ani muscle and the transverse cervical, pubocervical, and sacrocervical ligaments at the level of the upper vagina. The urogenital diaphragm supports the middle vaginal portion and the perineal body, the lower segment. The levator ani is the principal muscle that closes the vagina.

Cervix

The cervix of the uterus, as the last structure of the female anatomy visible on external examination, provides much information about menstruation, the presence of infection, pregnancy, and the stages of labor (see Figure 61–2). Its absence indicates past surgery or a congenital condition. The cervix is highly elastic, which is obvious from the fact that it accommodates the fetal skull at birth. The many folds in its surface increase its potential surface area, as does its 10% muscle composition.

The openings of the cervix are the external os at the vaginal end and the internal os at the uterine end; the area between the two is the cervical canal. The cervix is partly vaginal and partly supravaginal. The vaginal cervix appears pink, whereas the supravaginal cervix is redder. Squamous stratified epithelium covers the vaginal cervix, and tall columnar ciliated cells with mucus-secreting glands line the supravaginal cervix. These two linings meet at the squamocolumnar junction, the area from which cells are taken in a Papanicolaou (Pap) test to screen for cervical cancer.

Mucus-secreting cells in the cervical canal produce mucus, which provides lubrication and acts as a bacteriostatic agent. A plug of mucus protects the fetus during pregnancy. The character of cervical mucus is affected by the level of estrogen. Cervical mucus is primarily water. Near ovulation, the water content and elasticity (spinnbarkeit) of mucus increase and its viscosity decreases. Increased salt and water interacting with glycoproteins cause the mucus to form long threads and produce a fern pattern or crystallization visible on microscopic examination. Ferning and spinnbarkeit are indicators of ovulatory activity. The diagnostic implications are discussed in Chapter 63.

During pregnancy, the endocervical epithelium proliferates and everts, producing thick, clear mucus. At 4 to 6 weeks' gestation, the cervix softens (Goodell's sign), and at 8 weeks' gestation, the cervix has a bluish color (Chadwick's sign). At labor, the cervix effaces and dilates. At menopause, the cervix decreases in size just as the uterus does, although at a slower rate, so the ratio of uterine to cervical size reverts to what it was at puberty.

Pain sensations from the cervix and upper vagina pass through the ilioinguinal and pudendal nerves. During labor, a pudendal nerve block is often used to decrease discomfort. It is important to note the distributions of involved spinal nerves to assess the meaning of a client's pain more accurately. For example, the ilioinguinal nerve involves L-1, which innervates the skin of the upper medial thigh and external genitalia as well as the muscles of the lower abdominal wall. The pudendal nerve involves the spinal nerves S-2 through S-4, which innervate the skin of the perineum and the external genitalia. Thus, pain in these areas may reflect pathological conditions in the area of the cervix (Spence & Mason, 1983).

Uterus

The uterus, or womb, is an organ with great significance in health and culture. As a symbol of reproductive ability, it is described in myths and endowed with symbolic meanings. Uterine changes occur at each developmental stage of a woman's life. The shedding of the lining signifies menarche and the possibility of reproductive capability, and the cessation of the shedding signifies menopause. The uterus endows a woman with the capacity to reproduce and sometimes it is the source of discomfort or disease as well.

The uterus is located at the center of the pelvic cavity between the base of the bladder and the rectum and above the vagina (Figure 61–2). The anterior surface is somewhat flat, whereas the posterior surface is convex. It is wider than it is deep anteroposteriorly. The uterus is held in position by the broad and round ligaments in the upper area; the cardinal, pubocervical, and uterosacral ligaments hold it in place in the middle area and at the pelvic floor inferiorly.

The uterus actually consists of two unequal parts. The corpus, or body, forms the upper two-thirds and consists mainly of myometrium. This pear-shaped portion is larger during the reproductive years. The portion of the corpus above where the fallopian tubes attach is the fundus. The neck or cervix (discussed previously) forms the lower part. The isthmus, the slight constriction or narrow part, constitutes the division of the cervix and the corpus.

In pregnancy, the isthmus becomes the lower uterine segment and does not contract with the rest of the uterus (Olds et al., 1984).

The corpus of the uterus has three layers: the perimetrium, myometrium, and endometrium. The perimetrium, the serous membrane covering the uterus, is composed of the peritoneum that runs continuously over the anterior abdominal wall, the bladder surface, the fundus, and the posterior part of the corpus. The myometrium, which lies beneath the perimetrium, is continuous with the fallopian tubes, the vagina, and some ovarian ligaments and is composed of three layers of involuntary muscle arranged for maximum effective effort during labor and delivery. The myometrium enlarges during pregnancy to accommodate the fetus. The endometrium, the innermost layer of the corpus, is a single layer of columnar epithelium, glands, and stroma. This is the layer that is shed and then rebuilt from menarche to menopause in the absence of pregnancy. Hormonal effects, which are discussed later, stimulate the shedding and rebuilding. Blood supply to the upper third of the uterus is from the ovarian artery. The lower two-thirds is supplied by the uterine artery.

Fallopian Tubes

From the sides of the uterus arise the fallopian, or uterine, tubes, which extend almost to the side walls of the pelvis (Figure 61–4). They curve posteriorly and then medially toward the ovaries. Each tube is situated in the superior border of the broad ligament. The tubes are 8 to 13.5 cm long and are moveable, not rigid. The fallopian tubes form a passageway that connects the peritoneal cavity with the

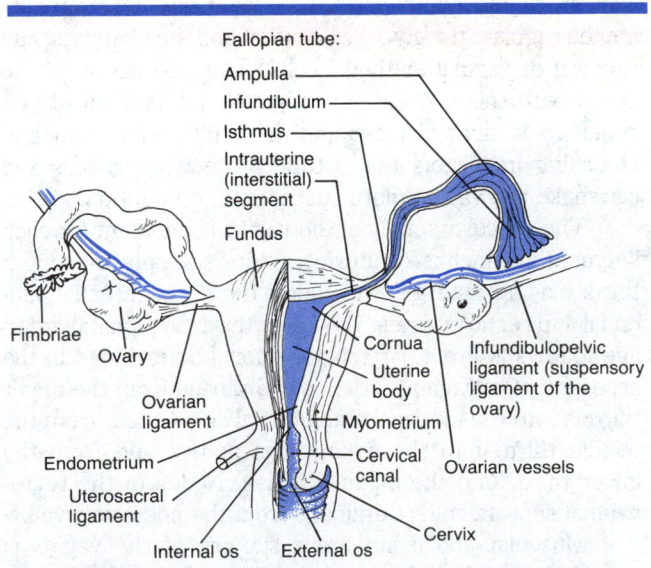

Figure 61–4

The fallopian tubes (oviducts or uterine tubes) and ovaries.
SOURCE: Adapted from Olds SB, London ML, Ladewig PA: *Maternal–Newborn Nursing: A Family-Centered Approach*, 2nd ed. Menlo Park, CA: Addison–Wesley, 1984, p. 82.

external environment via the uterus and vagina, creating the potential for the spread of infection between these areas. The tubes enable transport of the ovum from the ovary to the uterus and provide a favorable, nourishing environment for fertilization.

The fallopian tubes have a four-layered wall: peritoneal (serous), subserous, muscular, and mucous layers. The blood and nerve supply is in the subserous layer. Muscular layer activity gives the tubes a peristaltic movement that helps transport the ovum from the fallopian tube to the uterus. These muscle movements may be spastic in an anxious woman, affecting her fertility by decreasing the chances of effective ovum transport. The mucous layer is composed of ciliated and nonciliated columnar epithelium. The nonciliated cells secrete a fluid that nourishes the ovum, and the ciliated cells move, forming currents that, with the peristaltic action of the tube, help move the ovum toward the uterus.

Depending on the section of the tube, its size or diameter varies from 1 to 4 mm. The uterine opening into the tube is about the size of a hairbrush bristle; the rest of the tube size varies but is approximately the size of a strand of spaghetti. At its funnel-shaped distal end, the infundibulum, the tube fans out to a trumpetlike shape. Around the small orifice of the infundibulum are fimbriae (folds of tissue). The largest fimbria attaches to the ovary, keeping the tube close to the ovarian surface. The fimbriae are mobile, moving the ovum into the tube and then the uterus.

More proximal to the uterus is the ampulla, which has a wide lumen and distensible wall. The meeting of ovum and sperm often occurs here. An infection with subsequent scarring in the tubes can block the passage to the uterus, resulting in infertility or an ectopic pregnancy. The isthmus of the tube is closer to the uterus. This portion is straight and narrow and has a muscular wall. This is the point where tubal ligation is done.

The fallopian tubes are rich in blood supply and innervated by sympathetic and parasympathetic motor and sensory nerves. Women experience pain from the tubes in the area of the iliac fossa.

Ovaries

The ovaries, almond-shaped organs positioned on each side of the uterus, are approximately 1.5 to 3.0 mm wide, 2 to 5 cm long, and 1 to 1.5 cm thick (see Figure 61-4). The ovaries' size increases at adolescence and decreases during menopause.

Each ovary is supported by the mesovarium, which attaches it to the broad ligaments; the ovarian ligament, which connects it to the uterus; and the suspensory ligament, which attaches it to the lateral pelvic wall. An ovary is composed of the medulla (the inner portion, which contains nerves and lymph vessels) and the cortex (the functional outer portion, which contains follicles and ova). Germinal epithelium covers each ovary. A thin protective layer of fibers, the tunica albuginea, is just below it. The peri-

toneum does not cover the ovary; this allows the release of ova but also permits the spread of neoplastic cells.

The ovary usually releases one ovum each month (ovulation). At birth, the ovary contains about 1 million oocytes (developing ova) and at puberty, about 30,000. The functional unit of the ovary is the follicle, which, under the influence of follicle-stimulating hormone (FSH) from the pituitary gland, progresses from a primary follicle, to a growing follicle, and, finally to a graafian follicle. The maturing follicle secretes estrogen, which enhances its growth and maturation. Eventually, luteinizing hormone (LH) from the pituitary gland acts on the follicle, and ovulation occurs with an accompanying reduction of estrogen production and a continuation of progesterone secretion. This process is described more fully in the later discussion of the menstrual cycle.

The follicle's complex structure changes as it matures and again with ovulation. This structure consists of a surrounding theca folliculi that contains an inner rim of secretory cells and an outer rim of connective tissue. The theca surrounding the ovum also contains granulosa cells separated from the theca by a thin layer of membrane. The theca cells produce estrogen, and the granulosa cells secrete progesterone. The zona pellucida separates the ovum from the granulosa cells. As the follicle matures, the granulosa cells proliferate and fluid accumulates. The follicle then bulges and ruptures at ovulation, releasing the ovum and its corona radiata, or collection of surrounding granulosa cells. The remaining granulosa cells fill the collapsed follicle and form the corpus luteum, or yellow body, which retrogresses if pregnancy does not occur. If pregnancy does occur, the corpus luteum enlarges and remains throughout gestation, secreting progesterone.

The surface of the ovary, once tense, shiny, and elastic, becomes scarred and pitted by the development of fibrous tissue known as the corpus albicans; this replaces the area where the corpus luteum was absorbed when it retrogressed in the absence of pregnancy. This process, repeated with each menstrual cycle, results in an ovary progressively more scarred and pitted with age (Figure 61-5).

Embryonic Development

Primitive gonads begin to develop in the growing fetus at about 5 weeks. During the seventh and eighth weeks, the primitive gonads develop into either ovaries or testes. Testosterone secreted by the fetal testes stimulates the mesonephric ducts to develop into the male genital tract. The fetal testes also secrete müllerian regression factor, a hormone that causes degeneration of the müllerian duct preventing the development of the female genital tract.

Pelvis

The female bony pelvis has many functions. It supports the upper torso, protects the organs of the lower pelvis, and forms an axis through which the fetus passes at deliv-

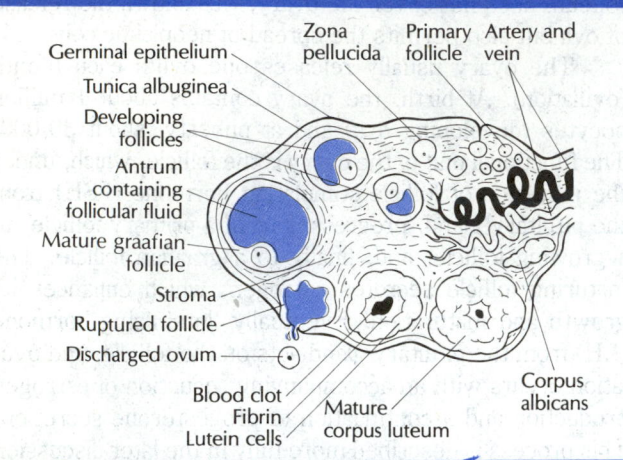

Figure 61–5

Various stages of development of the ovarian follicles.
SOURCE: Olds SB, London ML, Ladewig PA: *Maternal–Newborn Nursing: A Family-Centered Approach*, 2nd ed.
Menlo Park, CA: Addison–Wesley, 1984, p. 98.

ery. Viewed from the top, the pelvis is like a basin open at its base. It is formed by the ischial, iliac, and pubic bones on the sides, with connection in the front by a cartilage "joint," the symphysis pubis. The two iliac bones are joined by a cartilage "joint" with the sacrum and coccyx. The spines of the ilium are what people sit on. The pelvic outlet is formed by the ischial spines and the tip of the coccyx.

Breasts

The female breast is a cutaneous gland that is an accessory of the reproductive system. It is cone shaped and has a "tail" of breast tissue extending into the axilla. The breasts are usually in an approximately symmetrical position on the sides of the chest between the second and sixth ribs and between the sternal edge and the midaxillary line.

The breast is a tightly woven, complex structure composed of a glandular and ductal network, fat, connective tissue, fasciae, blood vessels, nerves, and lymph (Figure 61–6). One breast may be larger than the other, and the weight of each varies from about 150 to 200 g. In the center of the breast are the nipple and the areola, which are pigmented more darkly with puberty, pregnancy, and exogenous estrogen use. The nipple varies from 0.5 to 1.3 cm in diameter. Its erectile tissue responds to sexual excitement, cold, friction, pregnancy, and menses by becoming more rigid and prominent. The surface of the areola is irregular and papillary because of the presence of Montgomery's tubercles, which secrete a liquid that protects the breasts during infant suckling.

The glandular portion of the breast can be visualized as a series of lobes radiating from the nipple, extending anteriorly to posteriorly, separated by adipose tissue. The lobes consist of lobules formed by alveoli, clusters of sac-like structures that are the termination of collecting ducts whose anterior ends store milk during lactation. The epithelium of the alveoli secretes the components of milk. Progesterone, along with estrogen, is responsible for alveolar and lobular development. The growth of the ductal epithelium is regulated by estrogenic hormones (Tyler & Woodall, 1982).

The veins of the breast connect with the superior vena cava and are part of a low-pressure system susceptible to change in intra-abdominal pressure. These veins form a pathway for metastasis of neoplastic cells from the breast to the lungs, pelvis, vertebrae, or skull. Lymph flows mainly toward the axilla, then travels medially, and finally empties into the jugular and subclavian veins—a short route that makes it easy for cancer cells to metastasize into the general circulation (Figure 61–7).

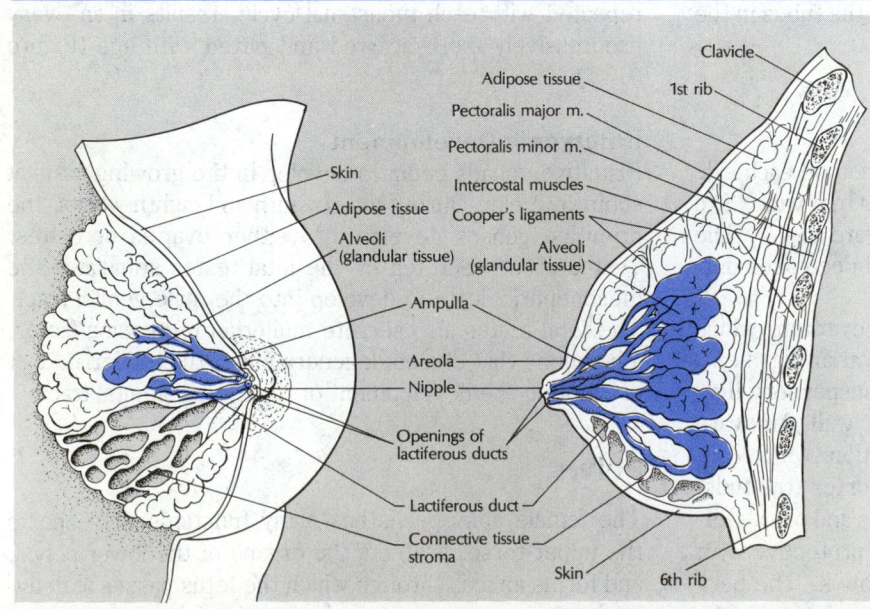

Figure 61–6

Anatomy of the breast. **Left.** Anterior view of partially dissected left breast. **Right.** Sagittal view. (Modified from Spence AP, Mason EB: *Human Anatomy and Physiology*, 2nd ed. Menlo Park, CA: Benjamin/Cummings, 1983, p. 747.)
SOURCE: Olds SB, London ML, Ladewig PA: *Maternal–Newborn Nursing: A Family-Centered Approach*, 2nd ed. Menlo Park, CA: Addison–Wesley, 1984, p. 84.

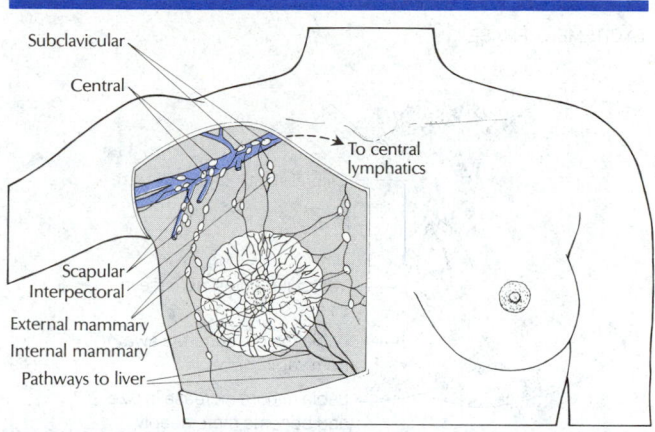

Figure 61–7

Lymphatic drainage of the breast.
SOURCE: Olds SB, London ML, Ladewig PA: *Maternal–Newborn Nursing: A Family-Centered Approach*, 2nd ed. Menlo Park, CA: Addison–Wesley, 1984, p. 85.

Breast development occurs in stages beginning in the neonatal period. At 8 or 9 years of age, the nipples become elevated, followed by an increase in the size of the areolae. About the time of menarche, the breasts develop a cone shape and increase in size.

In early pregnancy, the breasts increase in size and nodularity, with subsequent increases in venous prominence and an increase in pigmentation and erectility. Breast symptoms of pregnancy begin about the third or fourth week of gestation and continue until 5 to 7 days after delivery. At delivery, the anterior pituitary gland secretes increased amounts of prolactin with a concomitant decrease in estrogen and progesterone. Prolactin stimulates the alveolar cells of the breast to produce milk. For the first 2 to 4 days after delivery as lactation is being established, a yellowish creamy fluid called colostrum is secreted. Colostrum is thicker and richer in vitamins, minerals, proteins, and immunoglobulins than milk produced later.

In early menopause, women often experience uncomfortable breast sensations such as fullness and tenderness because of fluctuations in estrogen levels. Later in menopause, hormone levels stabilize. Overall estrogen levels decrease during menopause, resulting in a decrease of fat tissue in the breast and the replacement of fat tissue by fibrous cords.

Female Sexual Response

Female sexual responses, like those of the male, are determined by both psychological and tactile stimuli of either the genital organs or other areas of the body. Both sympathetic and parasympathetic autonomic nerves carry the motor impulses that result in the responses to stimulation. The phases of sexual response—excitement, plateau, orgasm, and resolution—are depicted in Figures 61–8 and 61–9. Although the phases of sexual response are named

the same for both men and women, the durations vary. Male sexual response is discussed in Chapter 62.

The excitement phase can be initiated by many different types of stimuli, including sight, sound, touch, or smell, and its intensity may increase rapidly. The first physical sign of response in women is vaginal lubrication, equivalent to a sweating reaction, which may occur in 10 to 30 seconds. Vasocongestion around and in the vagina causes a transudate to pass through the tissue of the vaginal walls. Other reactions during the excitement phase are: vasocongestion of the labia minora and majora, increase in size of the glans of the clitoris and elongation of the shaft, upward and backward movement of the cervix and uterus, erection of the breast nipples, and increase in alveolar size. The breasts and the labia minora may also become flushed.

If adequate stimulation continues and distraction does not interfere, the plateau phase follows the excitement phase. In this intensification of the excitement phase, the outer third of the vagina becomes engorged, decreasing the opening and forming the orgasmic platform; the labia minora's color deepens to a bright red; the clitoris retracts; and heart rate and blood pressure increase (Hogan, 1980).

The orgasm phase is characterized by rhythmic contractions of muscles, including those of the clitoris, vagina, and uterus. Muscle tension is released, and blood vessels become engorged. Vaginal contractions occur at 0.8-second intervals and vary from 3 to 15 contractions per orgasm (Hogan, 1980). Stimulation of the clitoris results in the same orgasmic changes as those caused by stimulation of the vagina. Women's descriptions of orgasm vary from a slight pleasurable movement sensation to intense throbbing. During orgasm, the respiratory rate increases to as high as 40 respirations per minute and the heart rate to 180 beats per minute. Blood pressure becomes elevated as well.

The resolution phase is characterized by a return to the preexcitement phase. The clitoris returns to normal as swelling disappears. The labia also return to normal size, and in 3 to 4 minutes the vagina loses its distention (Fogel & Woods, 1981).

Biologic causes of sexual dysfunction are less common than psychosocial causes. They include drug effects; neurological disease; surgical, malignant, or degenerative changes in the pelvic structures; infection; and trauma. Psychosocial causes might include cognitive, developmental, intrapsychic, or interpersonal causes.

REGULATORY FUNCTIONS OF THE FEMALE REPRODUCTIVE SYSTEM

Traditionally, many of a woman's life changes have followed the changes in biologic function from puberty to menopause. The interaction of hormones, body changes, and the female psyche will be discussed later. This section discusses the neuroendocrine changes occurring at three major points in female development: (1) in puberty and menarche, (2) in menopause, and (3) during pregnancy.

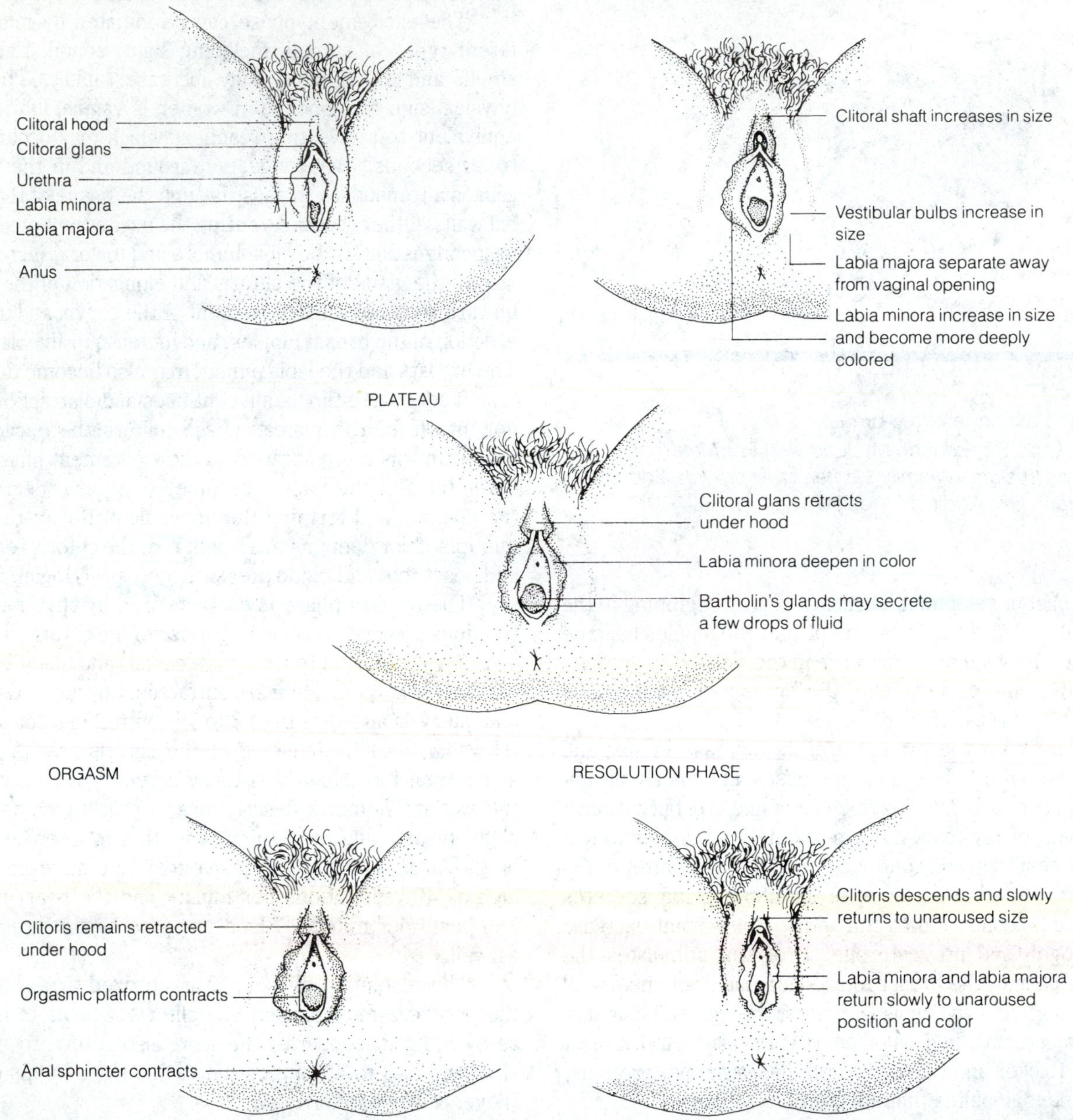

UNAROUSED STATE

Clitoral hood
Clitoral glans
Urethra
Labia minora
Labia majora

Anus

EXCITEMENT PHASE

Clitoral shaft increases in size

Vestibular bulbs increase in size

Labia majora separate away from vaginal opening

Labia minora increase in size and become more deeply colored

PLATEAU

Clitoral glans retracts under hood

Labia minora deepen in color

Bartholin's glands may secrete a few drops of fluid

ORGASM

Clitoris remains retracted under hood

Orgasmic platform contracts

Anal sphincter contracts

RESOLUTION PHASE

Clitoris descends and slowly returns to unaroused size

Labia minora and labia majora return slowly to unaroused position and color

Figure 61–8

Female external genitalia during the sexual response cycle.
SOURCE: Crooks R, Bauer K: *Our Sexuality*. Menlo Park, CA: Benjamin/Cummings, 1983, p. 175.

Regulation of the phases of female development is an interactional process occurring along the hypothalamic–pituitary–gonadal axis. The anterior pituitary gland is controlled by secretions from the anterior hypothalamus, which is under the feedback control of hormones secreted by the ovaries. Gonadotropins are substances produced by the anterior pituitary gland and placenta that have an affinity for acting on the ovaries and control their function. Three hierarchies of hormones in the female endocrine system are part of the axis just described: (1) luteinizing hormone releasing factor (LRF), secreted by the hypothalamus; (2)

FSH and LH, secreted by the anterior pituitary gland in response to stimulation by LRF; and (3) estrogen and progesterone, secreted by the ovaries in response to FSH and LH (Figure 61–10).

Puberty and Menarche

The regulatory mechanisms in the timing of the onset of puberty are not yet fully understood. Research has shown that the onset of puberty is related not only to maturity of

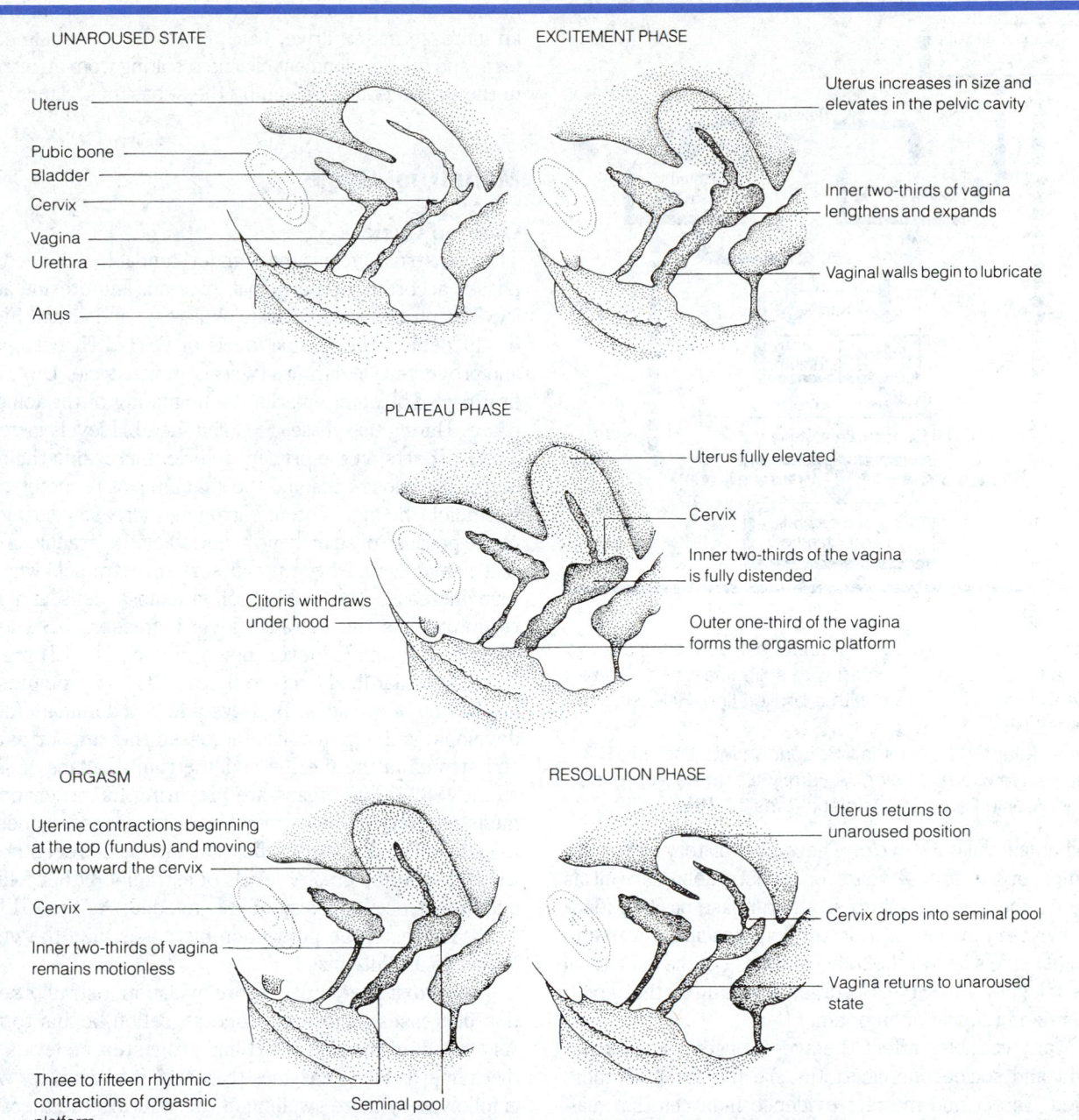

Figure 61–9

Changes of the vagina and uterus during the sexual response cycle.
SOURCE: Crooks R, Bauer K: *Our Sexuality*. Menlo Park, CA: Benjamin/Cummings, 1983, p. 174.

the hypothalamic–pituitary–gonadal axis but also to genetics, the environment, body fat, and other endocrine phenomena.

The hypothalamus seems to become less sensitive to estrogen as it matures. The immature hypothalamus inhibits the secretion of LRF and, in turn, the secretion of FSH and LH, which are necessary for the development and release of an ovum. As the hypothalamus matures, the low levels of circulating estrogen no longer inhibit the secretion of LRF, so LRF is secreted and stimulates the pituitary gland to produce FSH and LH.

Prior to menarche, LH and FSH are secreted at higher levels during sleep. The LH stimulates the ovary to synthesize estrogen precursors, and FSH and LH levels are as high during the day as they are at night. Menarche occurs in response to these higher levels of FSH and LH that ultimately cause follicular growth and development in the ovary. Levels of estrogen also increase, which causes the endometrium of the uterus to proliferate. A cyclic pattern emerges, with feedback to LRF in the hypothalamus resulting in cyclic menstrual bleeding that is caused by sloughing of the endometrium.

At first, uterine bleeding may occur without ovulation,

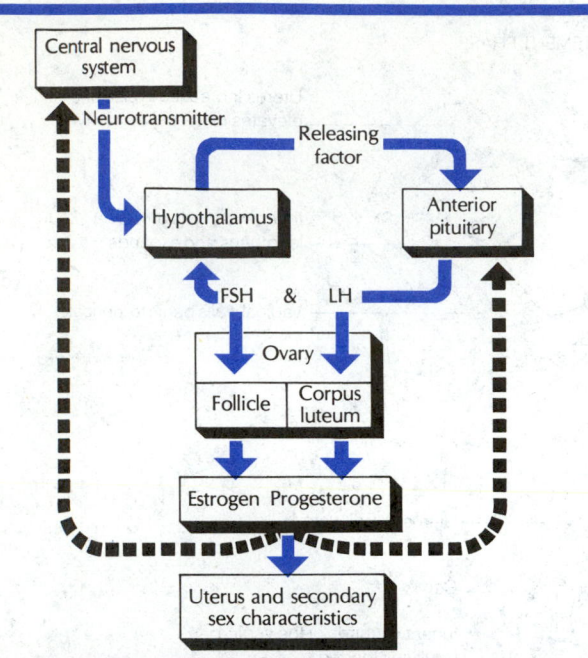

Figure 61–10

The hypothalamic–pituitary–gonadal axis in the female. Positive feedback is illustrated with solid lines, and negative feedback is illustrated with a broken line. Releasing factor is LRF.

SOURCE: Adapted from Olds SB, London ML, Ladewig PA: *Maternal–Newborn Nursing: A Family-Centered Approach*, 2nd ed. Menlo Park, CA: Addison–Wesley, 1983, p. 92.

called an anovulatory cycle. These anovulatory cycles are common in the first 2 years of menstruation as well as later. As the system matures, a two-phase positive feedback system develops within the hypothalamus; a rise in estrogen levels late in the follicular phase of the menstrual cycle triggers an FSH-LH surge, resulting in the development and release of an ovum.

Many variables affect the age of onset of menarche. Weight and socioeconomic status are the variables most studied. Direct and indirect evidence indicates that malnutrition is associated with later age of menarche. The age of menarche in the United States has decreased by about 3 years in the last 80 years or so, which is associated with an increase in size at birth and improved diet. In many countries, age at menarche has been found to be associated negatively with socioeconomic status. Differences in age in other countries range from a few months to 2 years. In developed countries, the mean age at menarche is about 13 years.

The effects of increased estrogen levels during puberty include the development of the ductal part of the breasts; the growth of the external genitalia; and the development of a female body configuration, including fat definition at the hips and thighs. The increased estrogen levels also stimulate sebaceous gland secretions that may result in acne. Testosterone, which is present in small amounts in women, is produced by the interstitial cells and stroma

in the ovary. Testosterone is thought to be responsible for an increase in sex drive, hair growth in a masculine pattern, and the development of acne resulting from an increase in the production of sebum by the sebaceous glands.

Menstrual Cycle

Ovarian Cycle

The menstrual cycle is most understandable if divided into phases according to hormonal, ovarian, and uterine activity. The phases are follicular, ovulatory, and luteal. Figure 61–11 depicts the plasma levels of FSH, LH, estrogens, and progesterone during a typical ovarian cycle. Day 1, the first day of bleeding, marks the beginning of the follicular phase. During this phase, FSH and then LH levels increase. The FSH acts on the primary follicle, increasing the number of granulosa cells and their number of receptor cells. Estradiol, the most potent estrogen, increases during this phase because of an enzyme acquired by the granulosa cells that converts androgen precursors to estradiol, which in turn increases the number of granulosa cells and FSH receptors. As the estradiol level increases, FSH levels begin to fall, and LH levels begin to rise. The LH present in the follicular fluid binds to theca cells and promotes the production of estradiol. By Days 5 to 7, a dominant follicle develops, and estradiol has increased the number of cells and stroma in the uterine endometrium (Emans & Goldstein, 1982). The organs are preparing for pregnancy or menstruation. As the estradiol level increases, so does the LH level. The dominant follicle has increased receptors for LH and secretes greater levels of estradiol. Other follicles undergo atresia, and less FSH is needed. As the LH level rises, progesterone production increases, and the granulosa cells are luteinized.

Approximately 1 day before ovulation, estradiol secretion decreases as progesterone secretion begins to rise. As a result of the rise in LH and progesterone levels, the theca interna forms enzymes that cause it to dissolve, which is followed by more swelling of the wall. As the theca and granulosa cells are luteinized, new blood vessels grow into the follicle wall, prostaglandins are secreted into the follicular tissues, and more plasma seeps into the follicle. This results in more swelling, as well as rupture and release of the ovum. This is what is referred to as **ovulation**.

The luteal phase of the cycle involves an increase in the size of the granulosa cells and an accumulation of lutein to form the corpus luteum. The corpus luteum is highly vascular and secretes progesterone and estrogen. About 8 days after ovulation, it is functionally at its peak. Unless pregnancy occurs, at 10 to 12 days after ovulation, the corpus luteum begins to regress, possibly in response to estrogen. As the corpus luteum regresses, the secretion of estrogen and progesterone decreases. High levels of estrogen and progesterone have been suppressing FSH and LH secretions by the anterior pituitary gland. When the corpus luteum degenerates, therefore, the decreased

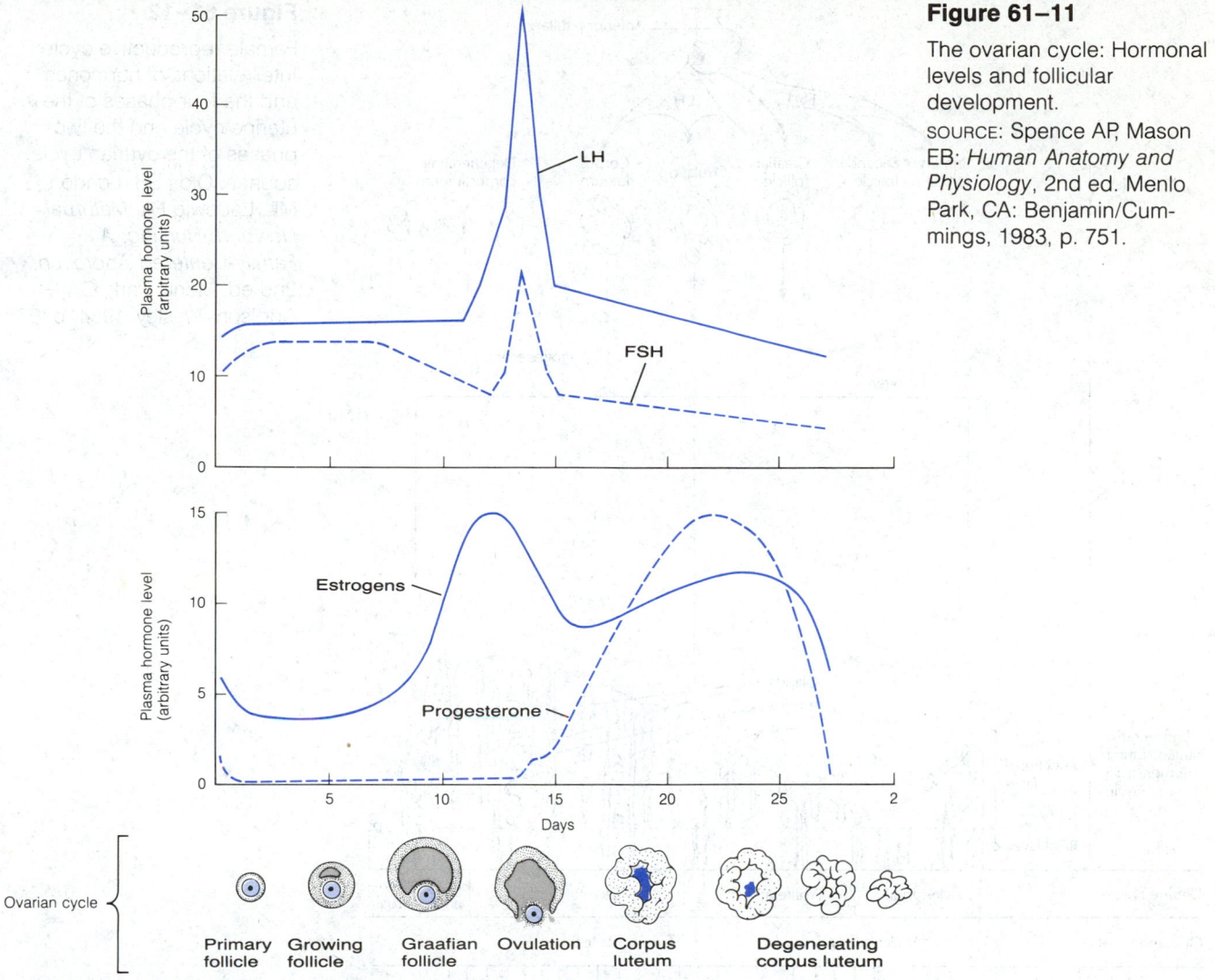

Figure 61–11

The ovarian cycle: Hormonal levels and follicular development.
SOURCE: Spence AP, Mason EB: *Human Anatomy and Physiology*, 2nd ed. Menlo Park, CA: Benjamin/Cummings, 1983, p. 751.

levels of estrogen and progesterone cause the pituitary gland to again produce FSH and LH.

Uterine Cycle

The uterine cycle has two phases: the proliferative and secretory phases. The proliferative phase coincides with the follicular phase of the ovarian cycle just described. Under the influence of estrogen, the endometrium proliferates and increases in thickness. During this phase, there is tortuosity of the endometrial glands, lengthening of the endometrium itself, and mitotic activity in the epithelial cell lining of the endometrial glands. The length of this phase is variable.

The secretory phase coincides with the luteal phase of the ovarian cycle and occurs in response to increasing levels of progesterone, which cause swelling and secretory development of the endometrium. The glands become tortuous and secrete endometrial fluid. In the stromal cells, cytoplasm, liquid, and glycogen increase greatly. The blood supply increases as well, and the endometrium doubles in thickness. Should an ovum implant in the endometrium, it

is now adequately prepared to nourish the development into an embryo. Figure 61–12 depicts the relation between the endometrial and ovarian cycles, the hormones being secreted, and the corresponding days of the menstrual cycle.

Menopause

The depletion of follicles caused by their monthly release from the ovaries over the years results in low levels of estrogen and progesterone. Without estrogen and progesterone feedback to the hypothalamus, releasing factors continue to stimulate pituitary gland secretion of FSH and LH (Olds et al., 1984; Tyler & Woodall, 1982). When the ovaries become unable to respond to the FSH and LH, ovarian activity diminishes.

Menopause generally occurs at about age 50 (see the discussion in Section IV for variations). The ovarian and menstrual cycles gradually become irregular, and many menstrual cycles are anovulatory. The period of premenopausal changes is called the **climacteric**.

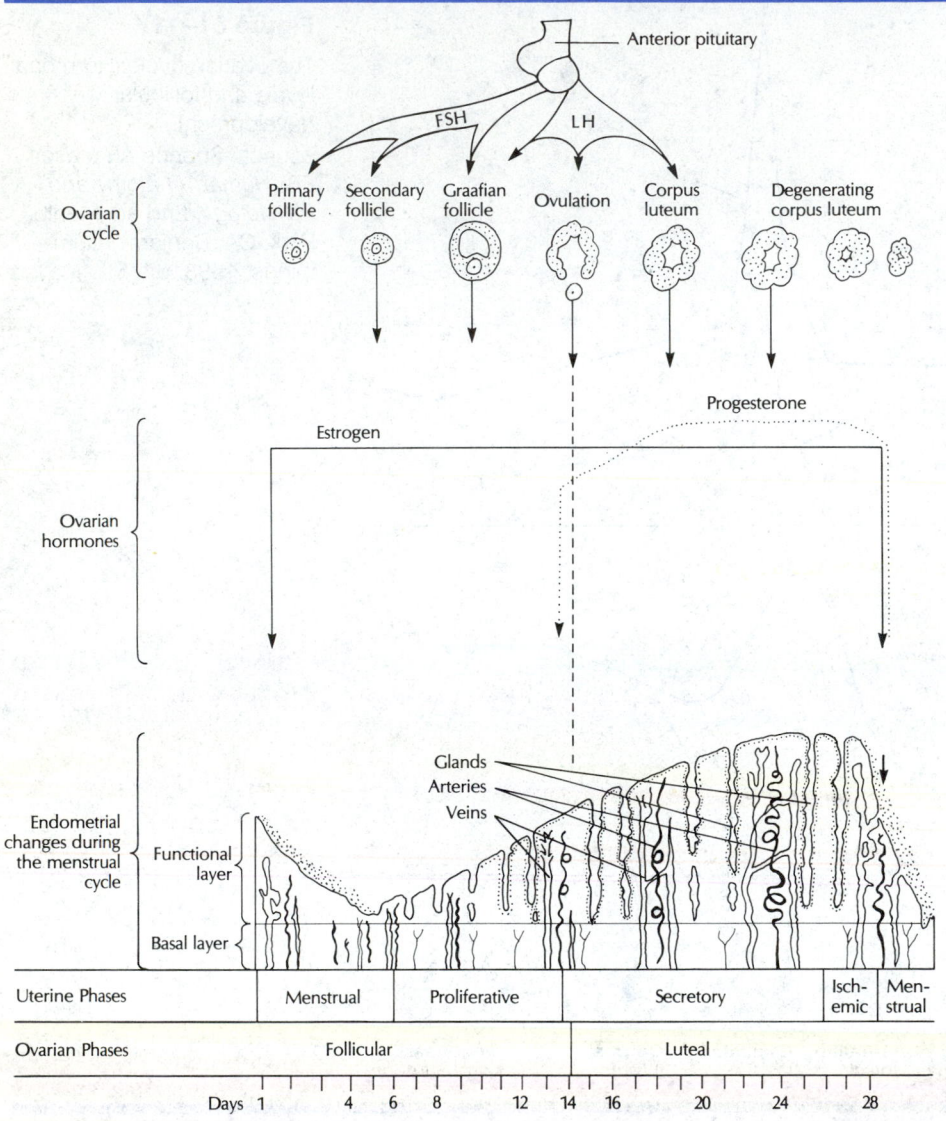

Figure 61–12

Female reproductive cycle: Interrelations of hormones and the four phases of the uterine cycle and the two phases of the ovarian cycle. SOURCE: Olds SB, London ML, Ladewig PA: *Maternal–Newborn Nursing: A Family-Centered Approach*, 2nd ed. Menlo Park, CA: Addison–Wesley, 1984, p. 97.

Vasomotor instability in the form of hot flashes is a common premenopausal symptom. Although estrogen replacement therapy seems to alleviate vasomotor instability, it is not clear whether decreased estrogen levels are the etiological basis for the instability. Many other physical changes that occur during menopause, however, are the result of decreased estrogen. Among these are atrophy of skin, subcutaneous tissue, and mucous membranes, along with osteoporosis or excessive calcium loss. (These physical changes can be slowed with estrogen replacement therapy.) Many of these changes may make sexual activity uncomfortable. The vagina may become drier and more rigid, and in many women, the vulva also becomes dry and pruritic. Atrophic vaginitis and vasomotor instability are the two most common reasons for estrogen replacement therapy.

Pregnancy and Fetal Development

The corpus luteum is the source of most progesterone during the first 10 weeks of pregnancy. At some time between the 7th and 12th week, the placenta assumes this function. Human chorionic gonadotropin (HCG), a glycoprotein similar to LH, is secreted by the trophoblast (a stage in the early development of the embryo) early in pregnancy. It stimulates the corpus luteum to secrete estrogen and progesterone during early pregnancy and then falls to a lower level as placental hormone production increases. FSH, important in the establishment of menstruation and follicular growth, is not inhibited by the steroids from the corpus luteum.

Three types of estrogen are elevated during pregnancy: estrone, estradiol, and estriol. Many of the precursors of these forms of estrogen come from the fetus. The effects of estrogen during pregnancy, mainly in the form of estriol, include enlargement of the uterus, the breasts and their ductal structure, and the external female genitalia. Various pelvic ligaments relax so the sacroiliac joints become limber, facilitating delivery of the fetus.

The placenta also secretes large quantities of progesterone; this causes decidual cells to develop in the endometrium, playing a role in the early nutrition of the embryo. Progesterone also decreases contraction of the gravid uterus, preventing spontaneous abortion, and prepares the breasts for lactation.

Section II: Pathophysiological Influences and Effects

Variation in bleeding and pelvic pain are the two most common pathophysiological changes related to the female reproductive system. Women's visits to health care providers are often related to problems with menstrual cycles. Clients may notice either that they do not bleed, bleed irregularly, bleed too little, or bleed too much. Chapter 64 discusses bleeding variations and **dysmenorrhea** (painful menstruation) in detail.

AMENORRHEA

Amenorrhea, the absence of menses, can be primary or secondary. The less common primary amenorrhea is a condition in which the woman has never menstruated. Causes include congenital obstruction, testicular feminization, and adrenal or ovarian tumors. Secondary amenorrhea is the cessation of menses for over 6 months after menarche. In most women, this is caused by the lack of the LH surge at midcycle (Ellis & Beckmann, 1983). Common causes include severe illness, major life changes or high anxiety, and changes in exercise and dietary habits. The use of phenothiazines, reserpine, or oral contraceptives also may induce secondary amenorrhea (Fogel & Woods, 1981). Amenorrhea after discontinuing oral contraceptive use usually does not last more than 6 months (Goroll, May, & Mulley, 1981). Other less common causes of secondary amenorrhea include pituitary tumors, ovarian cysts, uncontrolled diabetes, hyperthyroidism and hypothyroidism, and Cushing's syndrome.

Secondary amenorrhea also occurs in pregnancy and menopause. A pregnancy test and detailed history confirm or rule out pregnancy. The age of the woman, the mother's age at menopause, and lack of other diagnostic clues confirm imminent menopause; 1 year of amenorrhea confirms menopause.

VARIATIONS IN CYCLE LENGTH

Variations in cycle length include bleeding at intervals of 18 to 21 days or less, uterine bleeding at times other than the normal menstrual flow, or bleeding at intervals greater than 35 days. Increased frequency of menstrual periods is caused by a shortening of either the follicular or luteal phases of the menstrual cycle. Increased frequency is more common during premenopause and just after menarche. Intermenstrual bleeding may occur with cervicitis, malignancy, or at the time of ovulation. Bleeding at intervals greater than 35 days occurs because there is a prolonged proliferative phase of the menstrual cycle, the cause of which is often unclear. A disruption of the hypothalamic–

pituitary–ovarian axis occurs. Possible causes include obesity, malnutrition, emotional factors, ovarian disease, and systemic disease (Ellis & Beckmann, 1983). In addition to causing anxiety about possible pregnancy or pathologies, bleeding at longer intervals decreases fertility and increases the risk of endometrial cancer.

VARIATIONS IN AMOUNT OR DURATION OF BLEEDING

Variations in the amount or duration of bleeding include excessive or prolonged menstrual flow and bleeding at times other than the usual menstrual period and at irregular intervals. Excessive menstrual flow may occur because of ectopic pregnancy or spontaneous abortion. In cycles in which ovulation occurs, other causes of a heavy flow include fibroids, adenomyosis, and erosion into an endometrial vessel by an intrauterine device (IUD) (Fogel & Woods, 1981). Hypothyroidism and blood dyscrasias are possible systemic causes. Medications that can be responsible are anticoagulants, diuretics, anticholinergics, and phenothiazines. Anovulation (absence of ovulation) leads to excessive endometrial buildup followed by heavy bleeding and, usually, prolonged menses. Progesterone deficiency is the basis for the process.

When no local or systemic causes can be found for abnormal increases in the frequency or amount of flow, the term *dysfunctional uterine bleeding* (DUB) is applied. DUB is usually from a dysfunction of the hypothalamic–pituitary–ovarian axis and occurs either early or late in the reproductive years, and is often associated with anovulatory cycles. When it occurs in adolescence, DUB is from immaturity of the axis. Infertility is associated with DUB in teenagers.

In ovarian failure in the perimenopausal years, either little progesterone is secreted or the endometrium becomes so proliferated that sloughing occurs. If progesterone production returns or the endometrium "reaches its limit," bleeding is outside the usual pattern, prolonged, and heavy. Hormone therapy or curettage are indicated, according to the client's age (Fogel & Woods, 1981).

In the postmenopausal woman, any bleeding must be considered serious until proven otherwise. The incidence of malignancy in women with postmenopausal bleeding is high (Ellis & Beckmann, 1983).

PELVIC PAIN

Although a common problem of women, pain in the pelvic area is often hard to diagnose. At times, the pain's origin is never found even though the pain is definitely present. It is particularly difficult for women to localize pelvic pain. Pain can originate from cutaneous and muscle fibers or from visceral innervations. The former is experienced as acute pain; is more easily localized; and is more likely to arise from the labia, vagina, and abdominal wall. Visceral pain is more likely to be burning, aching, or chronic; is often referred pain; and is likely to originate in the uterus, tubes, ovaries, or bladder (Fogel & Woods, 1981). Pelvic pain is further discussed and illustrated in Chapter 63.

Pain is an individual perception; pain is what the client says it is. The frustrated health care provider can inadvertently contribute to the client's pain by contributing to her anxiety through asking her to localize a pain that she is not experiencing as localized. Because pelvic pain often involves a woman's feelings about her femininity or sexual behaviors, it is an anxiety-producing phenomenon.

Section III: Related System Influences and Effects

A number of related systems, such as the musculoskeletal, integumentary, urinary, gastrointestinal, and endocrine systems, affect and are affected by the female reproductive system.

MUSCULOSKELETAL SYSTEM

Postmenopausal women are at risk of osteoporosis (a decrease in bone density), which is thought to be caused by an increased rate of bone resorption as estrogen levels decline. The rate of decline in skeletal mass is much more rapid in women than in men, and 25% of women over 60 have spinal compression fractures (Goroll et al., 1981). Estrogen therapy seems to slow the development of osteoporosis.

Bone formation is thought to be increased by the administration of calcium (1 g daily) to women over 40. Prevention of osteoporosis consists of ensuring the optimal development of maximum bone mass in young people by supplementing calcium and vitamin D where insufficient. One gram of calcium (increased to 1200 mg for pregnant women) and 400 units of vitamin D are recommended for young people.

INTEGUMENTARY SYSTEM

The turgor, elasticity, and color of skin are all affected by ovarian function. Decrease in estrogen causes skin to dry and lose its elasticity. Hormonally induced pigmentary changes occur in pregnancy, oral contraceptive administration, menopause, and in the presence of ovarian tumors. Skin changes are discussed in detail in Chapter 77.

URINARY SYSTEM

Estrogen decline in menopause may result in urethral atrophy, leading to a distal urethritis and stricture formation.

This may result in some bladder obstruction and symptoms of urinary frequency and dysuria. Incontinence is so inconvenient for some women that they withdraw socially and become depressed. Other causes of incontinence include oversedation, confusion, and psychological regression, but in these cases it is usually temporary. Fixed incontinence may be caused by neurological damage, pelvic relaxation secondary to obstetric trauma, and urethral narrowing.

GASTROINTESTINAL SYSTEM

Older women may develop a rectocele—a prolapse of the posterior vaginal wall and rectum into the vaginal canal—from past obstetric trauma resulting in muscle weakness. Constipation may be a side effect of this weakness. Constipation and even bowel obstruction also may occur as uterine fibroids exert pressure on the intestines.

ENDOCRINE SYSTEM

Periods missed because of psychological or environmental factors are the result of an effect on the hypothalamus. Increased adrenal function is thought to increase estrogen precursors, which give feedback signals to the hypothalamus, decreasing the output of LRF and, subsequently, FSH and LH. (This process was described earlier.)

The impact of emotional stress on the menstrual cycle is a prime example of how the body and mind work together. Among incidents leading to missed menses are examinations in school, marital discord, change of job or residence, chronic anxiety, and fear of pregnancy (Fogel & Woods, 1981). Endocrine system influences and effects have been discussed earlier in this chapter. Because the reproductive and endocrine systems relate so closely, it is impossible to discuss the structure and function of the female reproductive system without discussing hormonal function as well.

Section IV: Psychosocial/Lifestyle Influences and Effects

The well-being and dysfunction of the female reproductive system are determined by both biological and psychological

factors. Thus, not only anatomic and physiologic details but also the psychosocial/lifestyle factors affecting women should be an important part of the data used to plan for and give nursing care to women.

DEVELOPMENTAL INFLUENCES

Females mature from 2 to 2½ years faster than males. They become taller than males at age 7, but by adulthood males are 6% taller and 20% heavier. In general, though, females grow up faster, enter puberty sooner, and then cease to grow earlier than males. The onset of adolescence, or puberty, marks a major change in the life cycle of female children. Puberty is more easily identified in girls than in boys because of menarche. The sequence of physical changes in adolescence is much the same for all girls, although the age of onset varies among individuals and cultures.

The internal changes in the uterus, vagina, and ovaries are considered primary sex characteristics, whereas the growth of the breasts, the appearance of pubic and axillary hair, hip development, and skeletal growth are secondary sex characteristics. These changes are caused by an increased production of estrogen by the ovaries, which increases the ratio of estrogens to androgens (male sex hormones). Adrenocorticotropic hormone (ACTH) from the pituitary gland stimulates the adrenal glands to produce androgens. Androgens are responsible for pubic and axillary hair development and clitoral enlargement, and they may be related to increased sex drive. Puberty is also associated with a rapid growth rate in females. Estrogens cause the epiphyses and shafts of the long bones to unite, so female growth stops earlier than male growth.

Menarche is a biologic marker that affects the adolescent's self-image, sexual identity, and societal and cultural expectations. These, in turn, affect the adolescent's accomplishment of developmental tasks. Menstruation is the dramatic confirmation to the adolescent girl that she is indeed female. It signals her ability to conceive and mother a child and clearly demarcates her from her male peers and even her nonmenstruating female peers.

In many cultures, including North America, the family and society impose restrictions on females at menstruation. Menstruation is sometimes regarded as a curse and associated with evil and contamination, or a sickness. In some cultures, the menstruating woman is not allowed to be in the same room with men, serve food, have intercourse, participate in religious ceremonies, or look at infants, chickens, or sprouting beans (because these might get sick and die).

The restrictions and societal attitudes toward menstruation create the potential for ambivalence. The adolescent girl sees menstruation as positive—marking womanhood and reproductive capacity. She also receives contradictory messages about contamination and temporary restrictions on activities such as swimming and bathing. Irregular menses and dysmenorrhea may stimulate questions about the normalcy of adolescent ''femaleness'' and the ability to reproduce. Responses to dysmenorrhea are

likely to be affected by attitudes about menstruation formed at its onset. The extent to which the adolescent girl is restricted and the meanings her mother attributes to menstruation may contribute to the later acceptance or resentment of menstruation as a part of sexuality and normal body function.

After puberty, the female adolescent receives clear messages about her sexual identity. In addition to receiving messages from the social milieu that she is female, her sexual identity is obvious when she looks at her body. Many adolescent girls, however, have ambivalent feelings about their genitalia. They experience biologic urges and a biologic readiness, but sexual activity is usually socially prohibited or at least parentally prohibited. Although the adolescent female may have sexual feelings, she has difficulty expressing these without guilt. Her genital development is the visual reminder of these conflicts.

Reproductive system disorders during adolescence can affect many aspects of sexual function throughout life. For example, pelvic inflammatory disease (PID) from an untreated sexually transmitted disease (STD) such as gonorrhea results in a higher risk of ectopic pregnancy and infertility because of scarring of the fallopian tubes. For the young adolescent who desires pregnancy later in life, the possibility of these disorders and the pain of PID are traumatic. For the adolescent who is experimenting with sexual activity while experiencing a new body image, the occurrence of an STD threatens the development of a positive view of sexuality, especially if it is painful and necessitates public acknowledgment of sexual activity.

For a North American woman with a life expectancy of about 75 years, young and middle adulthood is the period from the end of adolescence to menopause. Many women make major life transitions by making choices regarding work, social supports, marriage, and children. To many women, sexual and reproductive concerns are paramount in the 20s and 30s. Biologic events associated with aging—for example, loss of reproductive function—make biologic reproductive boundaries obvious.

The stage after middle adulthood is menopause, a term that can refer to the perimenopausal years, which include premenopause (the period leading up to menopause), the menopause itself, and postmenopause (the years that follow the cessation of menses). In the United States, the average age for menopause is 51, although it may begin as early as 35 and as late as 60 (Fogel & Woods, 1981).

By the year 2000, it is projected that 1 in every 14 people will be a woman 65 years of age or older (Porcino, 1983). How a woman lives in this period is determined to a great extent by the choices she has made up to this point. Her childbearing years will most likely be over by age 50, and the decision to have or not have children will then have its impact. The option to marry will still be available, but choices about this issue are likely to have been made by this time and thus will have their impact as well.

A positive view of old age comes from the belief that the individual psyche can achieve mastery over negative biologic and societal influences. The task of this part of the life cycle is to maintain integrity and avoid despair, accepting death as a part of a life in which some hopes have been realized and some potential fulfilled.

BODY IMAGE

In adolescence, a profound change in body image occurs because of the development of primary and secondary sex characteristics, skeletal growth, and menarche. Only in the fetal and infant periods do people experience as rapid physical changes. Because body image is essential to overall self-image, the rate of maturation and actual physical appearance of the female adolescent have great psychological impact. Concerns about body image and physical characteristics are central to adolescents. They spend an inordinate amount of time examining physical changes as they occur. Being different or having undesirable physical characteristics puts the adolescent at risk of ridicule.

The early adolescent period is associated with a disturbance of self-esteem in many adolescents, especially females. One-half of the early adolescent girls in some studies reported distress and dissatisfaction with some aspect of their physical development or appearance (Seigel, 1982). Attractiveness is important in adolescence. Adolescents attribute more socially desirable personality traits to those who are physically attractive, and social acceptance depends heavily on physical attractiveness.

The resolution of body image problems in adolescence is important if a girl is to develop into a woman who accepts her body and its natural female processes. Developing other abilities while valuing her unique physical attributes contributes to the adolescent's successful movement from issues of identity to issues of intimacy.

Later, during young and middle adulthood, physical characteristics remain essentially stable. Major body image changes are likely to occur during pregnancy when the effects of reproductive system alterations are experienced in all body systems.

How women encounter menopause varies. Attitudes toward aging and involvement in adult roles strongly determine a woman's adjustment in older age. The importance she places on changes in body image and cessation of her reproductive capacity is influenced by previous experiences and cultural attitudes. For the woman whose self-esteem is broader than physical beauty alone or who does not believe that youth equals physical beauty, the effects of body changes may be slight. Some cultures even value the cessation of menses.

Menopausal symptoms associated with decreased estrogen production by the ovaries can be unsettling. About 80% of women have at least some symptoms. Vasomotor instability is a common symptom, although it is not absolutely clear that it is caused by hormonal changes. Hot flashes, flushes, and episodes of perspiration occur; many women find these uncomfortable and seek medical care. Breasts that begin to sag and the growth of facial hair are

two other body changes that may threaten a woman's feminine body image. Although it is important to recognize negative feelings about body image that may occur during menopause, it is also important to recognize that women who have adequate support systems and who view themselves as competent people with the potential for continued growth may not have negative feelings about their physical appearance.

SEXUAL EXPRESSION

The progression of sexual behavior seems similar for most adolescents. Most proceed in order from holding hands to being held, kissing, necking, light petting, heavy petting, and coitus. Sexual activity of urban girls aged 14 and over is increasing. In 1971, an estimated 30% of the girls in a study sample had been sexually active; in 1976, the figure had risen to 43% and in 1979, to 50%. The major increase was among white adolescents who had never married. The average age at the time of first intercourse was found to be 16.4 for white adolescents and 15.5 for black adolescents (Zelnick & Kantner, 1980).

Some basic differences in male and female sexuality have been noted. Girls are known to masturbate less than boys. Females rarely have orgasm during their first coital experience, in contrast to males. Fear of pregnancy is a potential major deterrent to the female's experience of pleasure with intercourse.

The contraction of an STD is a major risk of coitus in adolescents, and the risk increases for the adolescent who engages in intercourse impulsively or who is uncomfortable discussing the risk or possibility of venereal disease with a partner. Also, the use of oral contraceptives instead of condoms increases the risk of STD contraction for two possible reasons: oral contraceptives provide no physical barrier and result in extrusion of the squamocolumnar junction of the cervix, making it more susceptible to invasion by foreign organisms such as those that cause STDs (such as *Herpesvirus hominis*). Another explanation for the high incidence of STDs in adolescence is the fact that a person who begins sexual activity in adolescence is more likely to have several partners, increasing the risk of exposure. Lack of knowledge, which results in an unknowing transmission of infections, is another contributing factor. Chapter 64 discusses STDs in women of all ages.

Developmental causes of sexual dysfunction can have long-term effects. Although societal attitudes and public education are changing, it is not uncommon for adults to know little about their anatomy and how it relates to the sexual response cycle. Parental attitudes about sex may hinder the development of a healthy sexual outlook in children. An example of potentially harmful teaching is telling young girls that sex is dirty, giving negative labels to their genitals, and punishing them for touching or showing the genital area. Adolescent girls get strong messages to repress sexual impulses and are treated with anxiety and suspiciousness regarding pregnancy. Thus, sex becomes "dangerous" as well as "forbidden." The image of the woman as a sexual object who provides pleasure through passive reception of male sexual advances—an image passed on by society—can influence womens' ability to get pleasure from sexual activity.

Sexual dysfunction can be caused or exacerbated by many interpersonal variables. Anxiety about performance, difficulty with self-esteem and trust, and feelings about the sexual partner strongly influence sexual function. Poor communication as a result of negative self-perception, attitudes, or both is a frequent source of unsatisfactory sexual experiences. A woman is more likely to be stimulated pleasurably if she lets her partner know what works for her, but many women are not skilled at asking directly for what they want. One approach to treating sexual dysfunction in women is to have them describe the phase in which the dysfunction occurs—in interest or libido, in the excitement phase, in the orgasmic phase, or during coitus. This helps the woman client to be specific about what goes wrong during any sexual interaction.

Sexual activity does not necessarily decrease for older women. Many are not sexually active because they have outlived their partners, but some continue to be sexually active with new partners. The older woman might also satisfy sexual needs through masturbation.

DIETARY HABITS

Good nutrition is particularly important for females during adolescence, pregnancy and lactation, middle age, contraceptive use, and menopause. Greater amounts of calories, protein, iron, iodine, niacin, and riboflavin are recommended during adolescence than during most other ages. During adolescence, energy requirements increase as do the rates of protein deposition, nitrogen retention, iron utilization, and calcium absorption and retention.

Dietary changes of adolescent girls are related to their relationships with their parents and peers. As they rebel against parental values and eat more meals away from home, their nutrition is at risk. Many calories come from snacks because it is common for teenagers to snack rather than eat a meal. Other problems of adolescent eating behavior were discussed in Chapter 9.

Oral contraceptives seem to affect nutritional status by altering the metabolic need for several nutrients. Carbohydrate metabolism is altered because estrogen causes increased insulin secretion, increased secretion of growth hormone (GH), and elevated serum glucose levels. Glucose tolerance tests are abnormal in 10% to 11% of women who have taken oral contraceptives for a year (Fogel & Woods, 1981). Serum levels of cholesterol, triglycerides, cholesterol, phospholipids, and lecithin are also elevated. The nutrients thought to be needed in increased amounts by women taking oral contraceptives include vitamins B_6, B_{12}, and C and folic acid. Heavy blood loss during a menstrual period can cause anemia. This is particularly true for women with IUDs. Oral iron supplements can easily correct this condition.

The complex nutritional needs of pregnant and lactating women are discussed in nutrition and obstetric texts. In general, the pregnant woman needs to increase intake of calories, protein, iron, calcium, vitamin A, and the B-complex vitamins. Only iron supplementation is routinely recommended; in most cases, an adjusted diet is expected to provide sufficient intake of the other nutrients. Excessive consumption of vitamins that cross the placental barrier can cause fetal abnormalities or fetal toxicity.

In middle age, the main nutritional problem is a decreasing need for calories; if not respected, this leads to obesity. Women are more prone to obesity than men. Obesity increases a woman's vulnerability to cancers of the breast and endometrium, degenerative joint disease, and cardiovascular disorders. A reduction of caloric intake and an increase in exercise to coincide with a decreased metabolic rate can help combat the problem (see Chapter 9). After menopause, it is essential that women have adequate dietary calcium and supplement their calcium intake.

OCCUPATION AND AVOCATION

Increasing numbers of women over age 16 are joining the labor force in North America. The ability to delay childbearing has contributed to this trend. The effect of working on women's health is under study, but not many conclusions have been drawn. In general, women employed outside the home have neither more nor fewer physical complaints than those who work at home; this could be because sick women do not seek employment, or if they do look for jobs, they are not hired. Women in blue-collar jobs who have preschool children have been found to have high levels of anxiety.

The exposure of pregnant women to toxic and stressful agents in the workplace can be dangerous. Infertility and fetal damage have been associated with exposure to halogenated hydrocarbons, carbon monoxide, benzene, and radiation. Health workers such as nurses are also exposed to hazardous substances in health care environments, especially in operating rooms (see Chapter 14).

Some employers believe that, because of hormonal variations in menstruation and menopause, women's emotions are too labile for them to be reliable and to perform consistently. This attitude places women under more stress than men in similar jobs and hampers women's efforts to achieve their full potential. Recent publicity about premenstrual syndrome (PMS) has drawn added attention to the impact of hormonal variations on women. It is important that studies be done on the impact of the information about PMS on employers' hiring, firing, and promotional practices. Studies also are needed on the actual impact of variations in estrogen and progesterone levels on behavior and performance. The emotional well-being of working women who have negative effects during menses and menopause could be greatly improved by the informed sensitivity and unbiased attitudes of family, friends, and employers.

Chapter Highlights

The female external genitalia include the mons pubis, clitoris, labia majora and minora, urethral meatus, vestibule, introitus, hymen, and perineum.

The female internal genitalia include the vagina, cervix, uterus, fallopian tubes and ovaries.

The breasts are accessory glands of the reproductive system.

The development of the male and female reproductive systems is parallel; differentiation depends on secretion of testosterone by the male fetus.

The female reproductive system is structurally and functionally responsive to the hormonal variations that occur at specific times in a woman's life. The three major developmental points are puberty and menarche, pregnancy, and menopause.

The hormonal variations responsible for structural changes and for events such as menarche and menopause are controlled by the hypothalamic–pituitary–ovarian axis. Its secretions are affected in a complex way by factors such as emotions and surgery.

The timing of the onset of puberty is not fully understood, but menarche begins in response to a cyclic pattern of hormonal secretion involving the hypothalamus, estrogen, LRF, FSH, LH, the pituitary gland, the ovaries, and the uterine endometrium.

The menstrual cycle can be divided into phases according to hormonal, ovarian, and endometrial activity. The ovarian cycle, in turn, can be divided into follicular, ovulatory, and luteal phases. The endometrial cycle has proliferative and secretory phases.

Menopause generally occurs about age 50. Some changes and symptoms during this period can be allowed or alleviated by estrogen replacement therapy.

Both female and male sexual response involves four phases: excitement, plateau, orgasm, and resolution. Causes of sexual dysfunction can be biologic or, more commonly, psychosocial.

Variations in bleeding include primary and secondary amenorrhea, variations in menstrual cycle length, and variations in the amount and duration of bleeding.

Systems affected by the female reproductive system include the musculoskeletal, urinary, gastrointestinal, and endocrine systems.

Each major biologic alteration in the female reproductive system affects social roles, interpersonal relationships, and body image.

Sex role formation begins at birth and is as dependent on social influences as it is on anatomic characteristics. Parental and social expectations of females are different from those for males. This profoundly affects women's interactions and self-esteem.

Female nutritional needs change throughout the life cycle. Especially critical times are adolescence, pregnancy and lactation, middle age, and menopause. Contraceptive use imposes special dietary requirements as well.

Bibliography

Belzer E: Orgasmic expulsions of women: A review and heuristic inquiry. *J Sex Res* 1981; 17:1–12.

Bullough B, David M, Whipple B, et al: Subjective reports of female orgasmic expulsion of fluid. *Nurse Pract* 1984; 8:55–58.

Crooks R, Baur K: *Our Sexuality.* Menlo Park, CA: Benjamin–Cummings, 1983.

Durant R, Jay MS, Linder CW, et al: Influence of psychosocial factors on adolescent compliance with oral contraceptives. *J Adolesc Health Care* 1984; 5(1):1–6.

Ellis JW, Beckmann CRB: *A Clinical Manual of Gynecology.* Norwalk, CT: Appleton–Century–Crofts, 1983.

Emans SJH, Goldstein DP: *Pediatric and Adolescent Gynecology.* Boston: Little, Brown, 1982.

Fogel CI, Woods NF: *Health Care of Women: A Nursing Perspective.* St. Louis: Mosby, 1981.

Gelein JL: Aged women and health. *Nurs Clin North Am* 1982; 17:179.

Goroll AH, May LA, Mulley AG: *Primary Care Medicine.* Philadelphia: Lippincott, 1981.

Guyton AC: *Textbook of Medical Physiology.* Philadelphia: Saunders, 1981.

Heath D: An investigation into the origins of a copious vaginal discharge during intercourse. *J Sex Res* 1984; 20:194–209.

Hogan RM: *Human Sexuality: A Nursing Perspective.* Norwalk, CT: Appleton–Century–Crofts, 1980.

Johnson MH, Everitt BJ: *Essential Reproduction.* Boston: Blackwell, 1980.

Kastner LS: Ecological factors predicting adolescent contraceptive use: Implications for intervention. *J Adolesc Health Care* 1984; 5:79–86.

Lauver DR: Irregular bleeding in women: Causes and nursing intervention. *Am J Nurs* 1983; 83:396–401.

Masters WH, Johnson VE: *Human Sexual Response.* Boston: Little, Brown, 1966.

Olds SB, London ML, Ladewig PA: *Maternal Newborn Nursing: A Family Centered Approach,* 2nd ed. Menlo Park, CA: Addison–Wesley, 1984.

Porcino J: *Growing Older, Getting Better: A Handbook for Women in the Second Half of Life.* Reading, MA: Addison–Wesley, 1983.

Seigel O: Personality development in adolescence. In: *Handbook of Developmental Psychology.* Wolman BB et al (editors). Englewood Cliffs, NJ: Prentice–Hall, 1982.

Shephard DL: Sex differentiation and the development of sex roles. In: *Handbook of Developmental Psychology.* Wolman BB et al (editors). Englewood Cliffs, NJ: Prentice–Hall, 1982.

Spence AP, Mason EB: *Human Anatomy and Physiology.* Menlo Park, CA: Benjamin–Cummings, 1983.

Turner BF: Sex-related differences in aging. In: *Handbook of Developmental Psychology.* Wolman BB et al (editors). Englewood Cliffs, NJ: Prentice–Hall, 1982.

Tyler SL, Woodall GM: *Female Health and Gynecology Across the Life Span.* Bowie, MD: Brady, 1982.

Zelnick M, Kantner J: Sexual activity, contraceptive use and pregnancy among metropolitan area teenagers. *Fam Plann Perspect* 1980; 12:230–237.

Suggested Readings

Crooks R, Baur K: *Our Sexuality,* 2nd ed. Menlo Park, CA: Benjamin–Cummings, 1983. This practical, readable text presents a broad perspective on the basic biology, psychology, and sociology of sexuality. Discussions are enhanced by personal reports of clients from the authors' files and simple, clear illustrations.

Moses AE, Hawkins RO: *Counseling Lesbian Women and Gay Men: A Life-Issues Approach.* St. Louis: Mosby, 1982. This brief text is aimed at members of the helping profession. It examines general issues faced by gays, special counseling issues, and past and current attitudes toward gays in this culture.

Woods NF (editor): *Human Sexuality in Health and Illness,* 3rd ed. St. Louis: Mosby, 1984. This thorough but concise text presents a multidimensional perspective on sexuality in both health and illness. It includes chapters about sexuality throughout the life cycle, sexual dysfunction, sexual assault, and drug effects on human sexual behavior; case examples; guidelines for nursing interventions; and current literature reviews.

Chapter 62

The Male Reproductive System in Health and Illness

Elizabeth Scheidt Farren

Objectives

When you have finished studying this chapter, you should be able to:

Describe the external and internal structures that make up the male reproductive system and discuss their function.

Compare the parallels between the male and female reproductive systems.

Discuss the anatomy and physiology of the male sexual response.

Explain the regulatory processes of the male reproductive system.

List endocrine dysfunctions of the male reproductive system and discuss their implications.

Define infertility and identify its possible causes and implications.

Define sexual dysfunction and discuss its causes and implications.

Describe the impact of diseases of other systems on the male reproductive system.

Identify the impact of drugs on fertility and sexual response.

Discuss psychosocial influences on male sexuality across the life span.

The purpose of any reproductive system is propagation of the species. In human beings, the reproductive organs are also a means for obtaining sexual satisfaction and pleasure. The male reproductive system has three general functions: the regulation of male characteristics, **spermatogenesis** (the formation of sperm), and the performance of the male sexual act. In accomplishing these primary tasks, the reproductive system has significant effects on growth, cellular metabolism, general well-being, and other body systems. The reproductive system is of the utmost importance to the continuation of the species; although failure within the system usually does not have life-threatening effects on the individual, it can result in serious physical and emotional alterations in well-being.

Section I: Structural and Functional Interrelationships

Organs of the male reproductive system play complementary roles in the system's functions. The external organs serve primarily to protect the testes and to propel sperm and urine from the body. For the internal structures, the principal functions are spermatogenesis and testosterone production.

STRUCTURE AND FUNCTION OF THE MALE REPRODUCTIVE SYSTEM

The external male genitalia consist of the penis and scrotum. The internal organs include the testes, a ductal system, and accessory glands.

External Genitalia

The penis and scrotum are designed to deposit sperm in the vagina, accomplish urination, contain and protect the testes, and function in sexual activities.

Penis

The penis is a pendulous soft-tissue structure attached to the anterior and lateral walls of the pubic arch by muscle and suspensory ligaments (Figure 62–1). It is composed of three longitudinal columns of erectile tissue: a central column containing the urethra and two encompassing columns that provide the organ's main structural support. The erectile tissue is overlayed with subcutaneous tissue, a fibrous sheath, and skin that is slightly more pigmented than other body skin. The lateral columns, the corpora

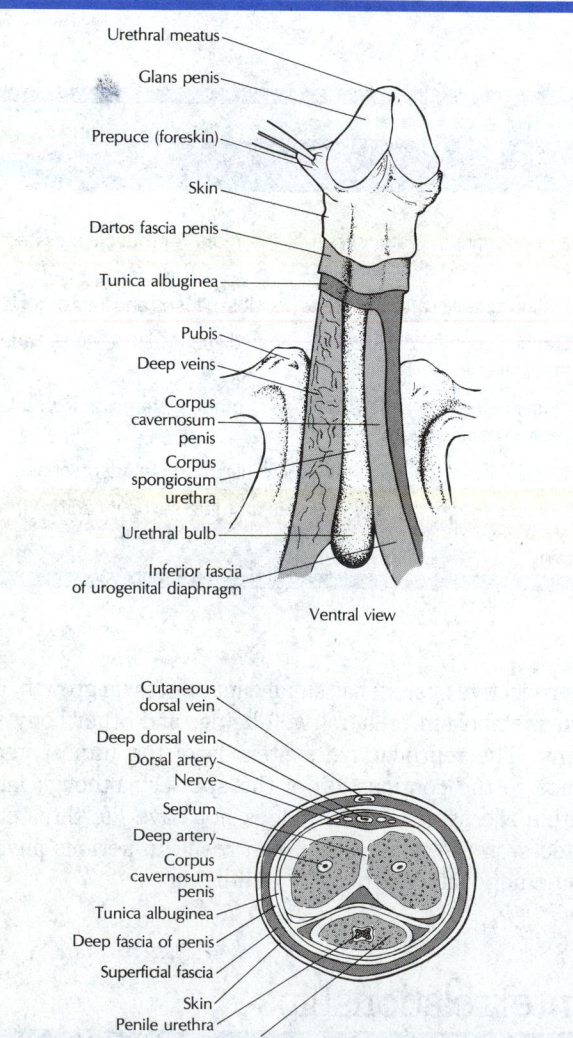

Urethral meatus
Glans penis
Prepuce (foreskin)
Skin
Dartos fascia penis
Tunica albuginea
Pubis
Deep veins
Corpus cavernosum penis
Corpus spongiosum urethra
Urethral bulb
Inferior fascia of urogenital diaphragm

Ventral view

Cutaneous dorsal vein
Deep dorsal vein
Dorsal artery
Nerve
Septum
Deep artery
Corpus cavernosum penis
Tunica albuginea
Deep fascia of penis
Superficial fascia
Skin
Penile urethra
Corpus spongiosum urethra

Cross section

Figure 62–1

Anatomy of the penis.
SOURCE: Olds SB, London ML, Ladewig PA: *Maternal–Newborn Nursing: A Family-Centered Approach.* Menlo Park, CA: Addison–Wesley, 1984, p. 60.

cavernosa penis, are divided by trabecula (connective, elastic, and smooth muscle fibers) into cavernous spaces that become blood-filled sinuses during erection. The central column, the corpus spongiosum urethra, is also divided, but the spaces are smaller and the walls thinner owing to its support of the penile urethra. At the distal end, the corpus spongiosum urethra expands and becomes the glans penis, which surrounds the urethral meatus. The skin covering the penis is continuous from the base of the penis at the pubic arch to the glans penis, where it folds inward and backward upon itself and is called the prepuce, or foreskin. Usually, only the base of the penis is covered with hair.

Blood supply to the penis is via pudendal arteries that form a complex network terminating in the cavernous spaces. The diameter and valves of the arteries are supplied with autonomic parasympathetic fibers from sacral cord segments S-2, S-3, and S-4, which on tactile stimulation cause the arteries to dilate and the cavernous spaces to fill with blood. The pressure of the filled spaces compresses the veins supplying the penis, resulting in the retention of blood within the organ. The penis thus becomes firm and erect, or tumescent.

Cerebral centers also influence erection and have been located in various loci of the limbic cortex. These centers are vulnerable to psychic stimuli, which may enhance or detract from sexual performance and pleasure. Sympathetic fibers from the lumbar portion of the spinal cord control visceral functions such as the emission of semen and rhythmic muscle contractions. When stimulation ceases, detumescence occurs: the arteries constrict, blood is allowed to leave the sinuses, and the organ returns to a flaccid state.

The penis is a functional part of the urinary system that transports the urethra to its external oriface, the meatus. It is also a crucial part of the reproductive system, serving to deposit sperm in the female vagina, as well as an organ of considerable psychic importance in conveying sensations of sexual pleasure and well-being.

Scrotum

The scrotum, a thin-walled sac continuous with the abdominal wall, hangs suspended from the perineal region posterior to the penis. The scrotal wall is composed of deeply pigmented skin and a complex of fascial connective tissue and smooth muscle fibers called the tunica dartos.

The scrotum keeps the testes at a lower temperature than the abdominal cavity would, which is more conducive to sperm viability. The fibers of the tunica dartos layer contract readily with temperature or tactile stimulation. This action draws the scrotum and its contents protectively up toward the body and gives the structure a wrinkled appearance. These soft linear folds are called rugae. At warm temperatures, the scrotum is smooth and pendulous. The surface of the scrotum is supplied with sebaceous glands and is sparsely covered with hair.

The interior of the scrotum is divided by tunica dartos fibers into two compartments, each of which contains a testis, an epididymis, and a ductule system that passes through the inguinal canal. The scrotum is innervated by sacral (S-3) and lumbar fibers and is sensitive to pressure, pain, and temperature. Consequently, it can perform its protective function while serving as an organ of sexual pleasure. In later life, the scrotum stays more relaxed and pendulous.

Breasts

The male breasts do not serve a functional reproductive purpose but are a site of sexual pleasure and arousal for some men. They are structurally the same as the female breasts but are only rudimentary in the well state. The male breasts consist of glandular tissue sensitive to hormonal stimulation, fibrous tissue, and fat. Their blood supply is from thoracic arteries. Lymphatics run along the lower border of the pectoralis major to the axilla. The breasts receive their innervation from cutaneous nerves of the thorax. Each breast has a nipple composed of deeply pigmented skin and erectile breast tissue capable of response to mechanical stimulation. Unlike the female pattern, male breasts change little if at all during puberty.

Internal Genitalia

The function of the testes are to produce sperm and testosterone. The ductal system conveys sperm, and the series of accessory glands secretes a medium for sperm nourishment and transport (Figure 62–2).

Testes

The testes are two small, oval organs that develop within the abdominal cavity of the fetus. Under the influence of testosterone, the testes descend into separate compartments of the scrotum at 24 to 35 weeks of gestation. The peritoneum actually precedes the testes into the scrotum by an invagination process called the processus vaginalis, which forms the tunica vaginalis, the outer covering of the testes. Beneath the tunica vaginalis is the tunica albuginea, and fibroelastic connective tissue containing some smooth muscle cells. The tunica albuginea sends fibrous septa into the body of the testes, dividing it into many wedge-shaped lobes (Figure 62–3).

Within each of the 200 to 300 lobes of the testis are seminiferous tubules tightly coiled into position. Here the

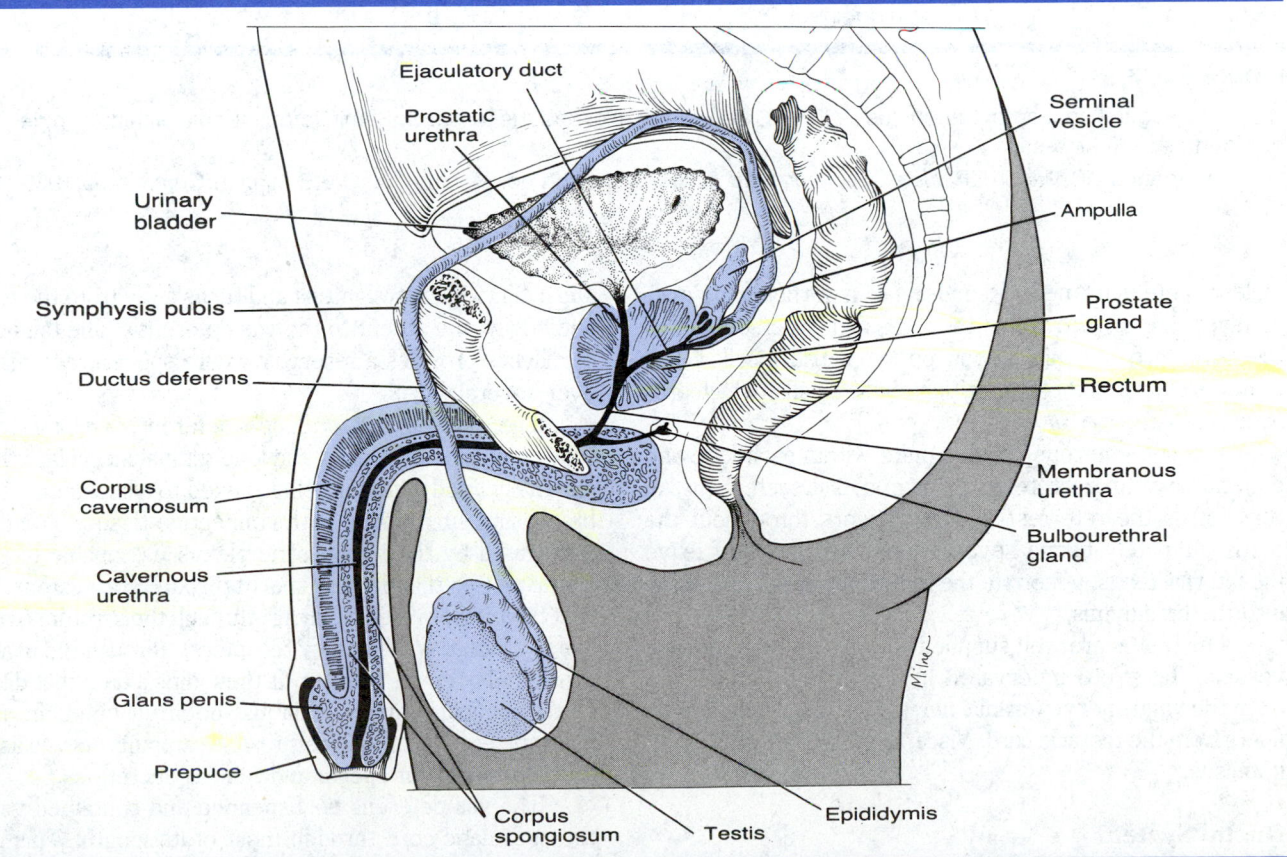

Figure 62–2

Sagittal section of the male pelvis with a portion of the left pubic bone attached to illustrate the path of the left ductus deferens.

SOURCE: Spence AP, Mason EB: *Human Anatomy and Physiology*, 2nd ed. Menlo Park, CA: Benjamin/Cummings, 1983, p. 735.

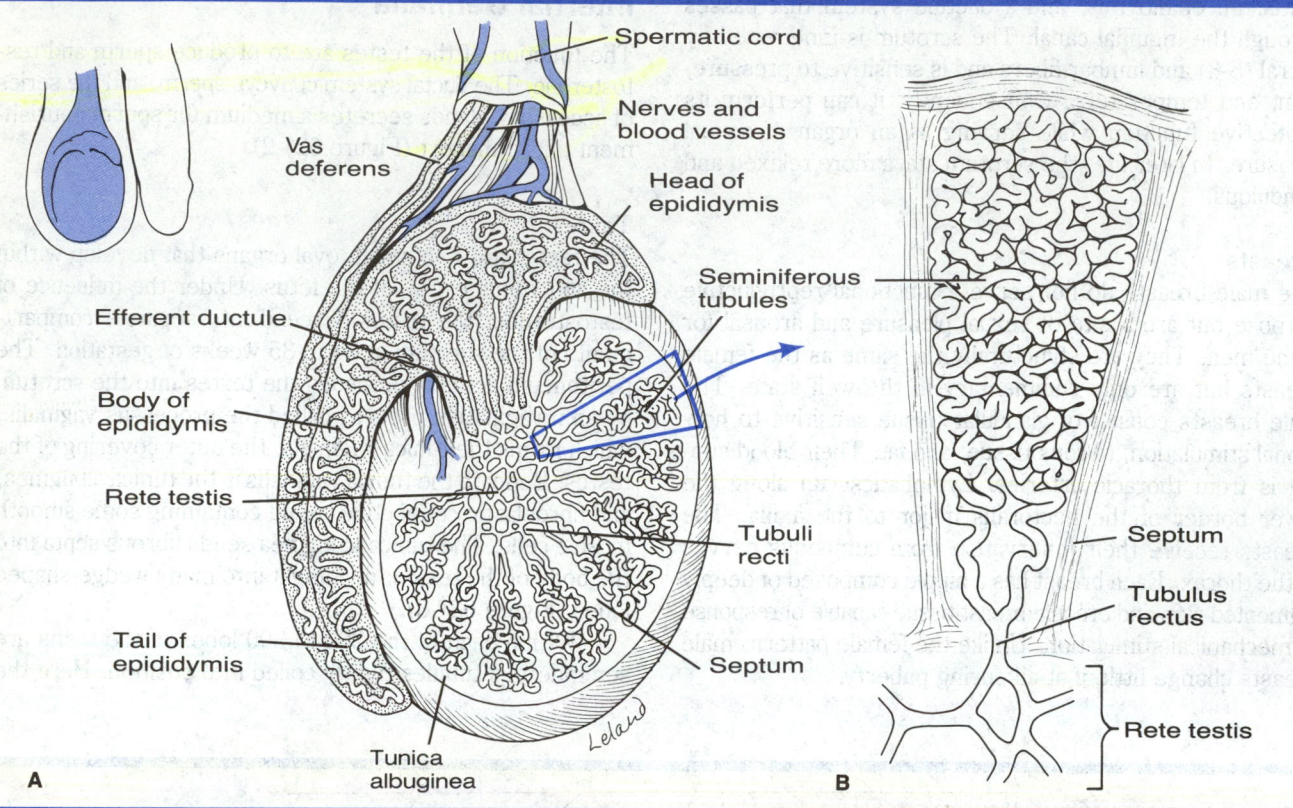

Figure 62–3

Testis. **A.** Sagittal section of the ductus deferens, the epididymis, and the testis. **B.** Seminiferous tubule within a single compartment of the testis.

SOURCE: Spence AP, Mason EB: *Human Anatomy and Physiology,* 2nd ed. Menlo Park, CA: Benjamin/Cummings, 1983, p. 732.

male gamete is formed and undergoes a portion of its maturation process. Also within the lobes and dispersed around the seminiferous tubules are supportive nutritive cells called Sertoli's cells and the interstitial Leydig's cells, which produce testosterone.

The seminiferous tubules unite within each lobe and generally within each testis to form a duct system that in turn forms the rete testis. This network throughout the testis ultimately forms several common ducts that leave the internal testis, penetrate the tunica albuginea, and empty into the epididymis.

The testes are well supplied with blood and lymphatic vessels. They are innervated by parasympathetic fibers from the vagus nerve (cranial nerve X) and by sympathetic fibers from the thoracic cord. Visceral fibers transmit afferent impulses.

Ductal System

The epididymis is the first part of an efferent ductal system leading from each testis through the inguinal canal and finally opening into the prostatic portion of the urethra. The epididymis consists of a continuous tube that is coiled and forms a head (attached to the top of the testis), a body (which descends along the posterior aspect of the testis),

and a tail (which straightens and turns away from the testis and begins the ascent to the vas deferens). The tail of the epididymis provides a reservoir where spermatozoa mature over several days.

The vas deferens, or ductus deferens, is a long simple tube composed of circular and longitudinal muscular layers, internally lined with epithelium, fixed to a basement membrane, and surrounded with connective tissue. The duct, innervated by the hypogastric plexus, is capable of peristaltic motion that propels sperm through the system. The duct travels from the epididymis through the scrotum (where it is innervated with sensory receptors), through the inguinal canal, and over the bladder. It then joins a duct that dilates at its terminal to an ampulla just before it opens into the prostatic portion of the urethra. The ampulla serves as the main reservoir for sperm and tubular secretions.

The vas deferens is suspended and contained within the spermatic cord through most of its length. This connective tissue structure suspends the testis, epididymis, and vas deferens as well as the complex of blood vessels, lymphatics, and nerves that supplies these structures. It extends from the tail of the epididymis to the abdominal inguinal ring and is enclosed by the cremaster muscle and layers of fascia coming from the abdominal wall.

Accessory Glands

Seminal vesicles, the urethral and bulbourethral glands, and the prostate gland make up the male accessory glands. Two seminal vesicles—lobulated glands lined with secretory epithelium—lie posterior to the bladder at the base of the prostate. They secrete a thick, nutritive, alkaline fluid that mixes with sperm on ejaculation. The fluid contains fructose and proteins, which are essential to sperm mobility and metabolism. The seminal vesicles each have a duct that joins the vas deferens to form an ejaculatory duct about 1 in long, where sperm from the vas deferens and nutritive fluid from the seminal vesicles mix and are discharged into the prostatic portion of the urethra.

The urethra is a shared pathway for urine and semen and the final link from the testes to the exterior. This tubelike organ extends from the internal urethral orifice at the bladder to the tip of the glans penis, where it emerges, forming an external meatus. The urethra is lined with a large number of small glands (Littre's glands) along its surface, which produce and contribute mucus. The urethra has an internal sphincter that forms a smooth muscle valve at the outlet of the bladder and responds to parasympathetic and sympathetic stimulation. The external urethral sphincter lies at the point where the urethra penetrates the urogenital diaphragm and is composed of the skeletal muscle; hence, it is under voluntary control. Each portion of the urethra is named for the structures it passes through. Thus, there is the prostatic urethra, the penile urethra, and the membranous urethra (which passes through the urogenital diaphragm).

The bulbourethral glands are two pea-sized glands located on either side of the urethra and opening into it. They produce a lubricating alkaline mucus that is expressed into the urethra during ejaculation, reducing its usually acidic state and creating a more hospitable environment for sperm.

The prostate gland is a spherical body that surrounds a portion of the urethra and lies adjacent and inferior to the neck of the urinary bladder. A capsule of muscle fibers encases this lobulated gland, which contains 30 to 60 branched, ducted segments opening ultimately into the ejaculatory ducts, which in turn open into the prostatic urethra. The gland secretes a thin, milky, slightly acidic fluid containing few nutrients, some minerals, and fibrinolysin. Under both endocrine and neural control, the prostate gland is subject to hyperplasia, which is most common in older men but occurs in men of all ages.

Embryonic Development

An individual's sex is genetically determined at the moment of fertilization, but the reproductive system is undifferentiated to male or female until the eighth week of development. The male and female systems remain similar in structure and function throughout life. In each, the gonads arise from the urogenital ridge of the embryo. In the female, they become the ovaries, and in the male, they become the testes because of testosterone stimulation.

External genitalia also have a common beginning. A genital tubercle arising in the fourth week of gestation swells and lengthens with a urethral groove on its ventral surface; this is called a phallus in both males and females. Labioscrotal swellings arise, and urogenital folds develop about the same time. The phallus elongates under the influence of testosterone, forming the penis. The urogenital folds fuse and form the urethra. In the female, or in a male lacking testosterone, the phallus remains small and becomes the clitoris; the urogenital folds remain open, forming the labia minora. The labioscrotal swellings become the scrotum in the male and the labia majora in the female. A more complete discussion can be found in Chapter 61. See also Figure 61–3.

It is testosterone, then, that differentiates embryological tissue to form male reproductive organs regardless of genetic sex. Injection of testosterone into gravid animals during organogenesis will cause development of male sexual organs, even in female embryos. Conversely, removal of the testes in the male fetus permits development of female organs in that genetic male. The essential testosterone is actually produced by the male embryo in the second month of gestation. Its production is the response of the interstitial cells of the male testes to the message of human chorionic gonadotropin (HCG) produced by the placenta.

Interference with this sequence results in incomplete or inappropriate sexual organ development. Teratogenic influences such as certain drugs or viral invasions during organogenesis also result in structural and functional problems for the system. Some of these effects are amenable to medical or surgical treatment later in life, but some are irreparable and result in lifelong consequences to the individual.

Male Gamete

The male gamete is the sperm, which is produced under the influence of gonadotropic hormones in all the seminiferous tubules of the testis beginning at sexual maturation and continuing throughout life. The gamete's function is to contribute one-half of the genetic material to a new life.

Both the sperm and their source organ originate from a primordial germ cell that differentiates and appears in the embryo early in gestation in the region of the reproductive system. As these germ cells multiply by mitotic division, some organize to form the seminiferous tubules, and some differentiate to form spermatogonia. Spermatogonia proliferate by mitosis and grow, but otherwise they remain relatively inactive throughout fetal development, infancy, and childhood. At sexual maturity, spermatogenesis begins; this process is illustrated in Figure 62–4.

The first phase of spermatogenesis, mitotic division of spermatogonia, results in increased numbers of spermatogonia, some of which grow, undergo morphological changes, and become primary spermatocytes. The others continue to divide and replenish the reservoir of sperma-

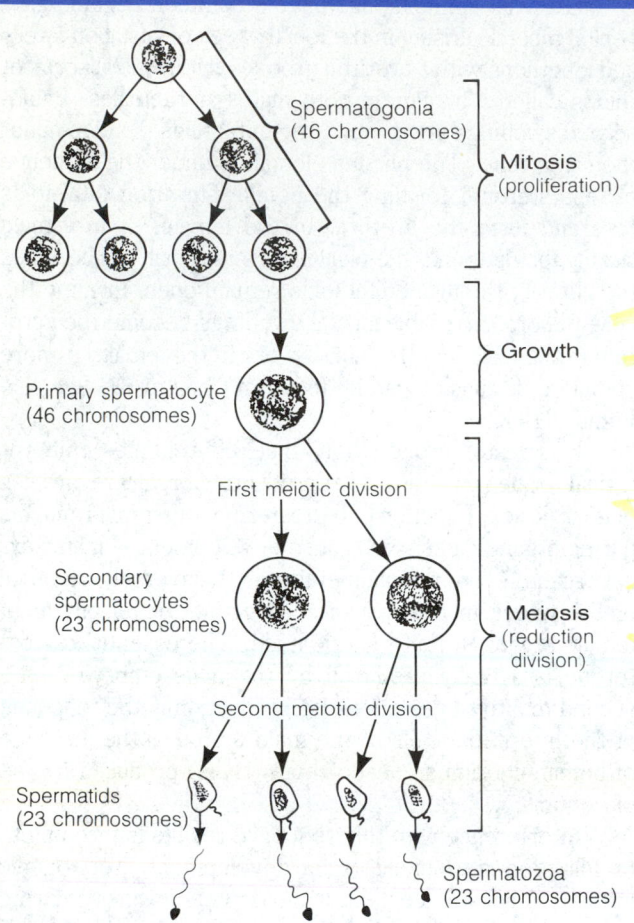

Figure 62-4

The process of spermatogenesis.

SOURCE: Spence AP, Mason EB: *Human Anatomy and Physiology*, 2nd ed. Menlo Park, CA: Benjamin/Cummings, 1983, p. 739.

togonia. All offspring retain 46 chromosomes, including an X and a Y sex chromosome.

In the second phase, the first meiotic division occurs. Each primary spermatocyte produces two cells called secondary spermatocytes and containing one-half the genetic material of somatic cells (23 chromosomes, including either an X or a Y sex chromosome). A second meiotic division occurs, resulting in a total of four daughter cells, called spermatids, from each original primary spermatocyte.

The final phase of spermatogenesis is a differentiation process that takes place with the spermatids attached to the Sertoli's cells within the testes, where they are finally transformed to sperm, or spermatozoa. When first formed, the spermatids have the usual features of epithelioid cells. Through their interaction with Sertoli's cells, however, most of the cytoplasm disappears, and the spermatid lengthens into the recognizable structure of the sperm. There is a head, neck, body, and tail, each with a highly specialized function.

The oval head contains the nucleus and, thus, the genetic message. A structure called the acrosome sits like a helmet on the head of the sperm and contains digestive enzymes used to penetrate the surrounding investment of the ovum. The neck is the site of the centrioles, and mitochondria are arranged in the body. Extending out from the body is a long tail containing large quantities of adenosine triphosphate (ATP) necessary to sustain the continued movement of the tail as it propels the sperm through the female reproductive tract once it is deposited at the mouth of the cervix.

Sperm released from Sertoli's cells are still functionally immature; they are immobile and incapable of accomplishing fertilization. During a 2-week passage from the testes to the vas deferens sperm undergo maturation and capacitation; that is, they become capable of penetrating the investment of the ovum and fusing with its yolk.

Sperm are transported through the system in a seminal plasma, or **semen**, which is the collective product of the male accessory sex glands. Each accessory gland contributes an exocrine secretion to the seminal plasma, which provides the correct environment for sperm at each portion of passage: Seminal vesicles, bulbourethral glands, and urethral glands secrete a mucoid, alkaline fluid, whereas the prostate gland secretes a slightly acidic, milky fluid. The combined products result in a hospitable seminal plasma pH. Although exquisitely sensitive to elevated temperatures, sperm can survive freezing indefinitely and be viable upon their return to normal temperatures.

Viable sperm require a pH of 7.2 to 7.8, sufficient nutrients, and protection during transport to and through the female reproductive tract. The accessory glands contribute over 60 substances, including fructose for metabolism, cholesterol for insulation, zinc for antibacterial activity, and prostaglandins for the enhancement of transport. Substances similar to fibrinogen and fibrinolysin make possible the initial coagulation of the seminal fluid within the ducts. This lasts for 15 to 20 minutes following ejaculation; then the ejaculate liquifies, permitting the sperm to ascend the female tract for fertilization.

The average sperm density in semen in a recent investigation was found to be 80 million sperm per milliliter of semen (Lipshultz & Howards, 1983). This is not necessarily the level needed for initiating pregnancy, however. Fertility always depends on male–female compatibility, including quantity and quality of sperm, quality of the ova, and a conducive physiological environment. It is generally accepted that sperm count diminishes with age and frequency of ejaculation. Viable sperm may be stored up to 6 weeks in the male tract but will survive usually no more than 48 hours in the inhospitable female tract (Lipshultz & Howards, 1983). The presence of supportive and nutritive substances, the proper pH, and the density of sperm directly affect fertility.

Male Sexual Response

As a physiological event, the male sexual response is designed to prepare the male for reproductive union with the female. It consists of two distinct components: a genital vasocongestive reaction (which produces penile erection) and reflex clonic muscular contractions (which result in orgasm). The two components involve different anatomic structures and are innervated by different parts of the nervous system. This distinction becomes important in recognizing and treating sexual dysfunctions.

The male sexual response cycle parallels the female's in its four phases: excitement, plateau, orgasm, and resolution. The erectile component of the sexual response transforms the flaccid penis into a firm phallus that makes insertion into the vagina possible (Figure 62–5A). The response is initiated in the excitement phase with local stimulation of the genitals, psychic stimulation such as erotic thoughts or viewing a desirable partner, or a combination of these experiences. Parasympathetic fibers control the

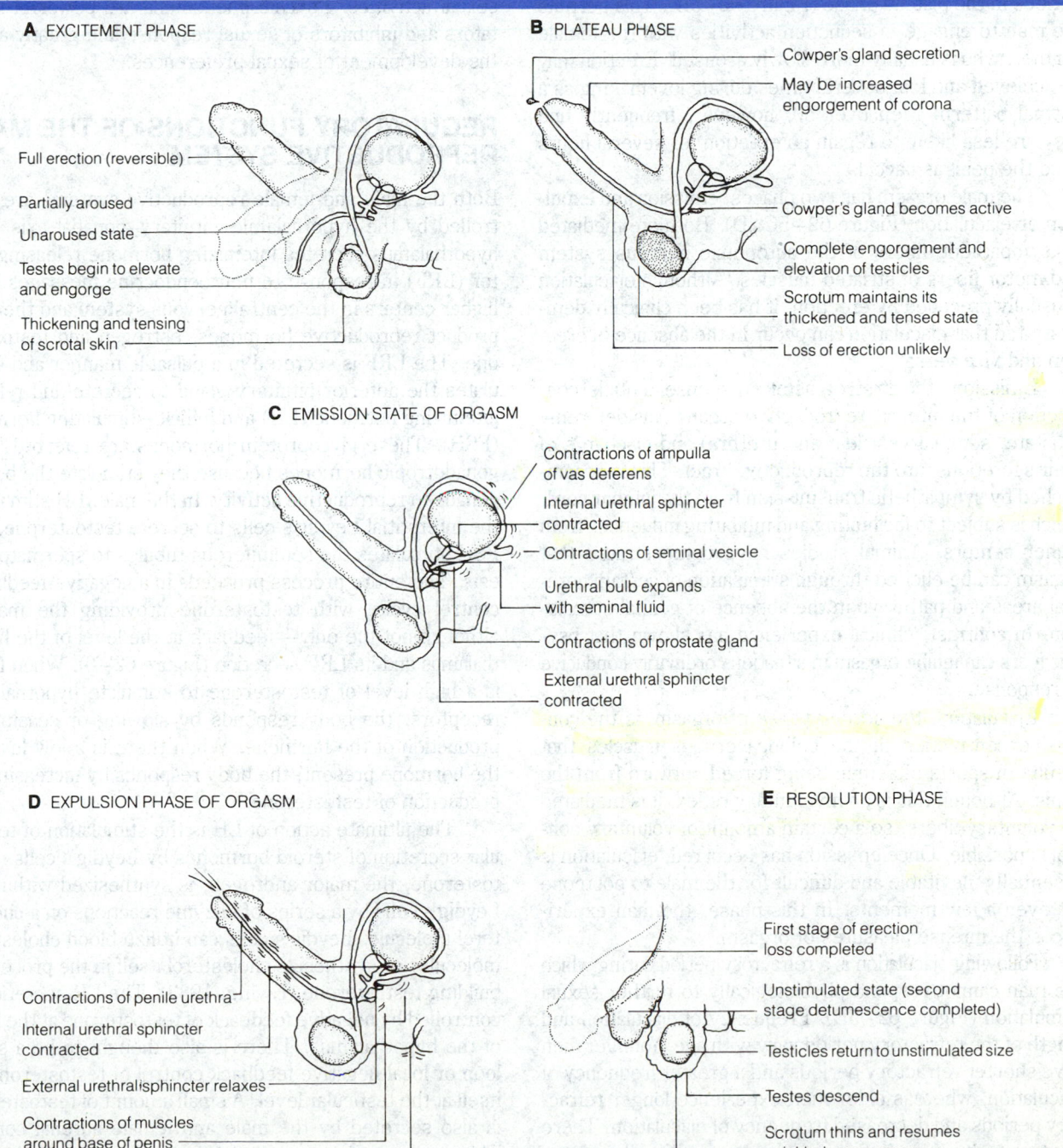

A EXCITEMENT PHASE

Full erection (reversible)
Partially aroused
Unaroused state
Testes begin to elevate and engorge
Thickening and tensing of scrotal skin

B PLATEAU PHASE

Cowper's gland secretion
May be increased engorgement of corona
Cowper's gland becomes active
Complete engorgement and elevation of testicles
Scrotum maintains its thickened and tensed state
Loss of erection unlikely

C EMISSION STATE OF ORGASM

Contractions of ampulla of vas deferens
Internal urethral sphincter contracted
Contractions of seminal vesicle
Urethral bulb expands with seminal fluid
Contractions of prostate gland
External urethral sphincter contracted

D EXPULSION PHASE OF ORGASM

Contractions of penile urethra
Internal urethral sphincter contracted
External urethral sphincter relaxes
Contractions of muscles around base of penis
Contractions of rectal sphincter

E RESOLUTION PHASE

First stage of erection loss completed
Unstimulated state (second stage detumescence completed)
Testicles return to unstimulated size
Testes descend
Scrotum thins and resumes wrinkled appearance

Figure 62–5

Male sexual anatomy during the sexual response cycle.

SOURCE: Crooks R, Bauer K: *Our Sexuality.* Menlo Park, CA: Benjamin/Cummings, 1983, p. 176.

diameter and valves of penile blood vessels; these fibers permit the engorgement of sinuses to produce erection and then the emptying of these vessels and loss of erection. These parasympathetic fibers are the same sacral fibers that innervate the rectum and the detrusor muscle of the bladder. Consequently, diseases, injuries, and surgeries that affect these fibers also affect bowel and bladder function and possibly erectile function.

Once attained, erection can be maintained for long periods in the plateau phase (Figure 62–5B). This permits the man to engage in seduction activities with the female partner, who is usually more slowly aroused. Erection may be achieved and lost several times during lovemaking as a normal pattern. Men over 50, however, frequently find they are less likely to regain an erection for several hours once the penis is flaccid.

The male orgasm has two phases, emission and expulsion or ejaculation (Figure 62–5C, D). Both are mediated by sympathetic fibers of the autonomic nervous system and motor fibers of striated muscles. Although ejaculation is usually preceded by erection, it has been clinically demonstrated that ejaculation can occur in the absence of erection and vice versa.

Emission, the first orgasmic response, entails contraction of the internal reproductive organs (vas deferens, prostate, seminal vesicles, and urethra) and discharge of their secretions into the reproductive tract. This is accomplished by sympathetic transmission from the lumbar cord, which is subject to facilitating and inhibiting influences from higher centers. Animal studies have demonstrated that orgasm can be elicited through stimulation of certain cerebral areas and pathways in the absence of genital stimulation. In contrast, clinical experience has shown that psychic fears can inhibit orgasm in situations ordinarily conducive to response.

Ejaculation, the second phase of orgasm, is the convulsive contraction of the bulbocavernous muscles that results in spurts of semen being forced outward from the penis. Although this is an involuntary reflex, it is mediated by voluntary fibers, so a certain amount of voluntary control is possible. Once emission has occurred, ejaculation is essentially inevitable and difficult for the male to postpone for even a few moments. In this phase, the man experiences the intense pleasures of orgasm.

Following ejaculation is a refractory period during which the man cannot respond physiologically to further sexual stimulation (Figure 62–5E). Frequency of ejaculation and length of the refractory period vary with age. Younger men have shorter refractory periods and a greater frequency of ejaculation, whereas older men experience longer refractory periods and decreased frequency of ejaculation. There is no such alteration in the capacity for erection, however, and older men can continue to enjoy sexual play with simply a decrease in the frequency of ejaculation. The psychic component to the sexual response is at least equal to the physiological response.

Each developing person has certain sexual experiences that profoundly affect orientation to sexuality and pleasure. Cultural factors create a wide range of interpretations, values, and judgments that influence individual sexuality. Such interpretations can enhance or diminish the sexual experience and lead to patterns of seeking or avoiding certain sexual activities throughout life. Even chance experiences, such as a perfect first experience, rape, or incest, can radically change an individual's appreciation of sexual activities. Psychic phenomena are powerful facilitators and inhibitors of sexual response and greatly affect the development of sexual preferences.

REGULATORY FUNCTIONS OF THE MALE REPRODUCTIVE SYSTEM

Both the male and female reproductive systems are controlled by the hypothalamic–pituitary–gonadal axis. The hypothalamus secretes luteinizing hormone releasing factor (LRF) in response to neuroendocrine messages from higher centers in the central nervous system and the end-product reproductive hormones, estrogen and testosterone. The LRF is secreted in a pulsatile manner and stimulates the anterior pituitary gland to secrete and release luteinizing hormone (LH) and follicle-stimulating hormone (FSH). These glycoprotein hormones are referred to as gonadotropic hormones because they stimulate the body's gonads to reproductive activity. In the male, LH stimulates the interstitial Leydig's cells to secrete testosterone, and FSH stimulates the seminiferous tubules to spermatogenesis. The entire process proceeds in a negative-feedback-control cycle, with testosterone providing the main—although not the only—feedback at the level of the hypothalamus and its LRF secretion (Figure 62–6). When there is a high level of testosterone to stimulate hypothalamic receptors, the body responds by slowing or ceasing its production of the hormone. When there is a low level of the hormone present, the body responds by increasing its production of testosterone.

The ultimate action of LH is the stimulation of testicular secretion of steroid hormones by Leydig's cells. Testosterone, the major androgen, is synthesized within the Leydig's cells by a series of enzyme reactions on a cholesterol molecule. Leydig's cells can utilize blood cholesterol molecules or synthesize cholesterol itself in the process of building testosterone (Ewing, 1983). The LH secretion is controlled by negative feedback of testosterone at the level of the hypothalamus. There is also thought to be a short loop or local negative feedback control of testosterone by itself at the testicular level. A small amount of testosterone is also secreted by the male and female adrenal cortex. This secretion is controlled by adrenocorticotropic hormone (ACTH) and does not appear to exert negative feedback effects on the pituitary gland. Under normal conditions, this testosterone is insufficient to stimulate masculinization.

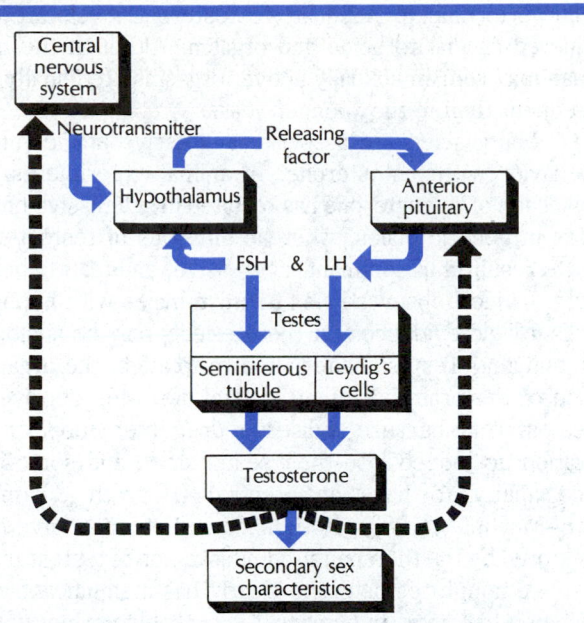

Figure 62–6

The hypothalamic–pituitary–gonadal axis in the male. Positive feedback is illustrated with solid lines, and negative feedback is illustrated with a broken line.

SOURCE: Adapted from Olds SB, London ML, Ladewig PA: *Maternal–Newborn Nursing: A Family-Centered Approach.* Menlo Park, CA: Addison–Wesley, 1984, p. 92.

Reproductive Effects of Testosterone

Testosterone is responsible for the differentiation of the male reproductive tract from the time of the hormone's secretion by the fetal testes at 8 weeks' gestation. It stimulates maturation of internal structures and, finally, the descent of the testes to the scrotum at 24 to 35 weeks. These endocrine-directed morphological changes are irreversible, although failure of testosterone at any time after puberty results in some regression of the reproductive glands.

Puberty is a time in the life cycle when the body matures to become capable of reproduction. All body structures and substances necessary for reproduction have been present since birth but have existed in an immature state. In males usually between the ages of 11 and 13, the level of testosterone begins to rise in response to LH and FSH. The exact cause for this change in previous levels of hormones is not yet known. As gonadotropin levels rise, the testosterone secretion increases many times, and the ducts and accessory glands of the reproductive tract enlarge and become active. Testosterone is necessary for the concentration and secretion of fructose by the seminal vesicles for the nourishment of sperm (Mawhinney, 1983). Spermatogenesis initiation and maturation depend on adequate levels of testosterone, along with FSH. After puberty, testosterone influences the length and width of the penis, scrotal rugae, and genital pigmentation.

Testosterone also directly mediates secondary sex characteristics in the male during and after puberty. Many of these effects are logical consequences of testosterone's metabolic effects and include the appearance and distribution of pubic and axillary hair, lengthening and thickening of the vocal cords, increased activity of sebaceous glands, broadening of the shoulders, and general increase in muscle mass. The maintenance of all these effects requires continued adequate levels of testosterone.

General Effects of Testosterone

Testosterone is an anabolic hormone capable of placing the body into positive nitrogen balance (a state in which less nitrogen leaves the body than was consumed in the form of protein and so can be retained for tissue building). Being a steroid hormone, testosterone enters its target cells and increases cell nuclear activity. Within a few minutes, the amount of RNA increases, followed by an increase in the quantity of cell protein. In many target tissues, the actual number of cells increases within a few days. This action of testosterone is responsible for the more heavily muscled body and thicker skin of the postpubertal male.

Testosterone is converted by various target tissues to several other compounds, including dehydrotestosterone (DHT) and estrogen. It is metabolized in the liver to 17-ketosteroids and excreted in the urine. If liver function is compromised and testosterone is not metabolized, signs of elevated testosterone levels may appear, such as exaggerated secondary sex characteristics. The amount of testosterone is assessed through plasma analysis to determine whether its source is testicular or adrenal. Minimal levels of testosterone in the adult male are below 300 ng/dL (Melman & Leiter, 1983). Analyzing the by-products of testosterone in the urine is not considered useful, because this method cannot discriminate between testicular and adrenal testosterone.

Testosterone has profound metabolic effects, many of which are easily observable at puberty. It can increase the metabolic rate up to 15%. It improves calcium absorption and retention, as well as increases the deposition of calcium salts in bones. Bones grow in thickness, and their matrix density increases. This results in an initial spurt of height, but testosterone also ultimately causes the epiphyses to unite, limiting longitudinal growth. Skeletal muscle increases in quantity and density, and the vocal cords thicken and lengthen. Epithelial cells respond with proliferation, thickening, and coarsening; body hair increases, especially in pubic and axillary areas. All these effects result in the heavier, more densely muscled, deeper voiced, and hairier male of the species.

Puberty, when testosterone effects are at peak level, creates the familiar pattern of the adolescent male with a voracious appetite, burgeoning height, and alto-to-soprano voice who is trying to get accustomed to his rapidly changing body and new psychic drives. Male adulthood is physiologically calmer; maintenance levels of testosterone gradually decrease with time but never cease abruptly as ovarian secretions in the female do. Indeed, spermatogenesis and testosterone secretion continue with aging and decline only slightly. Even this slight reduction in testosterone secretion, however, results in a moderate decrease in muscle mass, bone density, and skin thickness, as well as a change in vocal timbre. Although every man's general appearance changes with age, the extent of the change varies with the individual. A decrease in muscle mass is evident in large muscles responsible for postural changes as well as in small muscles, such as those that contribute to facial contours. The skin loses its elasticity, hair growth slows, subcutaneous fat deposits regress, and the characteristic appearance of the older man becomes established. Calcium is lost from bone and not redeposited at the former rate, resulting in a more brittle skeleton.

Diminishing testosterone levels are directly related to all these changes, but they are probably not the only responsible factor. For example, testosterone increases the deposition of calcium in bones but so does weight-bearing stress. The older man has traditionally engaged in less physical activity, such as running and lifting; therefore, the weight-bearing stress on the skeleton is lessened. This fact, along with the diminished testosterone levels, is probably a more complete explanation of skeletal fragility.

The reduction of testosterone production—whether from age or disease state—also affects sexual responses and performance. Adequate testosterone levels are considered crucial to libido and orgasm. Although the older man may remain sexually active, orgasms are usually less frequent than in the younger years.

Many scientists associate aggressive and dominant behavior with testosterone. In animal experiments, the blockade of testosterone has resulted in submissive behaviors in genetic males, whereas infusions of testosterone have resulted in dominant, aggressive, and mating behaviors. Clinical observations of human males with hypogonadism yield evidence that these effects may be analogous in humans. Testosterone is known to affect the organization of the brain beginning in fetal life. Men deprived of testosterone because of disease, drug interaction, or castration do indeed lose their sexual drive and sometimes the ability to have an erection (Horwith & Imperato–McGinley, 1983). Both libido and potency have been restored by the therapeutic administration of testosterone.

Although testosterone clearly has a significant influence on behavior, in humans it is probably not possible to separate psychosocial factors from biological factors in sexual behavior. Although testosterone can affect the sexual drive and its intensity, it can be assumed that testosterone does not affect how sexual desire is expressed through behavior toward the self and others (Vick, 1984). Behavior is influenced by individuals' psychosocial experiences and choices as they interact with others throughout life.

Section II: Pathophysiological Influences and Effects

The reproductive system, like all the body's systems, is vulnerable to deterioration, infection, and neoplasia. Immune responses and chemical exposures can cause a variety of problems. Congenital defects, although not life threatening, can greatly restrict adequate function. Although influences on the system are many and varied, alterations in function caused by any of these mechanisms result in three basic problems: gonadal endocrine disturbances, infertility, and sexual dysfunction. These problems will be considered here, and specific disease conditions, their etiologies, and their treatment will be discussed in Chapters 67 and 68.

GONADAL ENDOCRINE DISTURBANCES

The adrenal gland and peripheral tissues produce some testosterone, but the amount is insufficient to affect any of the reproductive functions. The testes are the main source of testosterone; consequently, any disease process affecting the testes profoundly affects the reproductive endocrine status. Problems occur with either overproduction or underproduction of the hormone.

Hypogonadal Endocrine Responses

Hypogonadal endocrine responses occur primarily because of a developmental or destructive lesion of the testes. They occur secondarily by failure in the production of the gonadotropins or their releasing factors.

In primary hypogonadal response, an injury may be present at birth; in this case, puberty will not occur. Primary hypogonadism can also be acquired at any time later in life. Certain genetic abnormalities, such as Klinefelter's syndrome (usually an XXY or XXYY chromosome complement), do not support the development of testicular tissue. Acquired conditions resulting in testicular tissue damage can cause either complete or partial failure of function. For example, the testes are especially sensitive to high temperatures, and exposure to high environmental temperatures or fevers secondary to any illness may compromise testosterone production and spermatogenesis. Failure of the testes to descend from the abdomen (cryptorchidism) where the temperature is higher results in testicular atrophy that is usually irreversible beyond puberty. Many infectious diseases, especially viral diseases, also can cause testicular failure. Examples include mumps, tuberculosis, leprosy, gonorrhea, brucellosis, and syphilis.

Neoplastic diseases of the testes may result in either underproduction or overproduction of hormone, usually the latter. This can affect both sperm and testosterone production. The treatment of testicular neoplasms can result in diminished androgen levels and *oligospermia* (diminished number of sperm in the semen) or *azoospermia* (absence or failure of formation of sperm in the semen). Radiation damage from x-rays usually does not occur at therapeutic levels, but 20 rads can damage sperm. Eighty rads can result in oligospermia for as long as 5 years or in complete testicular atrophy. The chemotherapeutic drug cyclophosphamide (Cytoxan) may cause oligospermia or azoospermia from which approximately 50% of clients recover in 3 years (Griffin & Wilson, 1983). Many therapeutic or recreational drugs affect plasma levels of testosterone. Antiandrogens (eg, cyproterone acetate) oppose the action of testosterone, and other drugs suppress its production. Chronic marijuana use, for example, has been correlated with decreased plasma testosterone levels, oligospermia, and impotence.

Secondary hypogonadism, the result of insufficient gonadotropins, can result from pathological conditions of the pituitary gland or lack of releasing hormones from the hypothalamus. The absence of gonadotropins in the blood confirms this etiology. These conditions can be successfully treated with gonadotropin replacement therapy.

When testicular failure occurs congenitally or any time before the normal onset of puberty, puberty does not occur. In this case, the adolescent growth spurt does not take place; the infant genital morphology persists; body hair remains fine and does not increase on the face, axilla, and pubic areas; and the voice does not deepen. Although the growth spurt does not occur, total height may increase because the epiphyses do not unite. A lack of the signs of puberty past ages 15 to 17 should alert the clinician to a possible pathological condition.

In younger adults, testicular failure or removal results in some regression of the secondary sex characteristics, such as beard growth, skin texture, voice timbre, and genital pigmentation. The accessory glands often get smaller, especially the prostate gland. Sperm count and motility decrease, and fertility is compromised. Libido will most likely diminish, and **gynecomastia** (enlarged feminine-appearing breasts) may appear. In the older male, some of these regressive changes may not be noticeable because of expected developmental changes.

Hypergonadal Endocrine Responses

Primary hypergonadism is caused by an androgen-producing testicular tumor, usually a trophoblastic tumor or tumors of Leydig's or Sertoli's cells. These pathological changes usually result in palpable testicular masses and are most common in an undescended testis (occurring in 1 in 2000 undescended testes as opposed to 1 in 100,000 descended testes). Lymphoma, leukemia, and carcinomas of other tis-

sues sometimes produce secondary tumors in the testis (Griffin & Wilson, 1983).

Secondary hypergonadism, the result of increased levels of gonadotropins, may be familial, pituitary, or hypothalamic in origin. Tumors in the region of the third ventricle are commonly the cause. Results of the hypersecretion are the same as for hypersecretion of primary origin, but the treatment differs.

Regardless of its cause, the overproduction of testosterone has various consequences depending on the client's age. In the prepubertal male, the signs of puberty may appear with the onset of disease rather than at the expected age of 12 to 15. The growth spurt will occur, but without treatment, the continued high levels of testosterone will prematurely close the epiphyses and limit total height. In the adult male, few somatic changes are observable with testosterone excess. Some clinicians believe that high levels are associated with behavioral changes, including increased libido and aggression. Often, however, the only demonstrable sign is the palpable testicular mass in the case of testicular disease.

The prostate gland is especially sensitive to androgen stimulation. In cases of androgen excess, the gland can become greatly enlarged, even to pathological proportions. The gland is also sensitive to estrogen stimulation and responds with similar enlargement. This hypertrophic response can have severe consequences for the urinary tract because of the prostate's anatomic position. The hypertrophy of prostatic tissue can actually obstruct the urethra, leading to the inability to void and the eventual destruction of kidney tissue. It also can signal a premalignant state.

INFERTILITY

Infertility is a diagnosis that can be applied to an individual but is most appropriately applied to a couple attempting conception. In primary infertility, there is failure to achieve pregnancy after 1 year of unprotected intercourse. Review of data by Lipshultz and Howards (1983) found that of couples attempting a first pregnancy, 15% fail to conceive within a year. In 30% of all cases significant male pathology exists, and in 20% of cases both male and female pathology exists. Thus, in 50% of infertile couples, the male is at least in part the cause of the failure to conceive.

Factors Affecting Fertility

Sperm can meet ovum for conception only if there is viable, mature, and motile sperm with an unimpeded route from the testes to the fallopian tubes. Many factors can compromise the production of viable sperm. Any infectious, neoplastic, or immunologic disease that affects testicular tissue can diminish or eliminate spermatogenesis. Many chemicals can cause oligospermia, including sulfasalazine (Azulfidine), cimetidine (Tagamet), and nitrofurantoin (Furadantin). Caffeine, nicotine, alcohol, and especially marijuana use—particularly long-standing and frequent use—are correlated with oligospermia. Endocrine failures previously discussed also can result in oligospermia or immature or immotile sperm.

The transport of sperm through the male reproductive tract for deposit in the female is an equally important aspect of fertility. Patent ducts and conducive seminal secretions are required, so the congenital absence of any portion of a duct or accessory gland results in infertility. The most common acquired pathological condition that impedes the passage of sperm is scarring adhesions in the duct tissue secondary to infection such as syphilis, gonorrhea, or tuberculosis. Structural weaknesses such as hydrocele and varicocele also can impede sperm. Obstruction along the ductile system, which can be caused by an enlarged prostate gland, can impair fertility. Finally, the surgical removal of a portion of the vas deferens, or vasectomy, results in infertility.

For fertilization to occur, the production and subsequent passage of sperm through the system must be followed by emission and ejaculation of the sperm into the female reproductive tract. Erection is usually the first stage of the male sexual act, although emission and ejaculation can occur without it. Many disease states, drugs, and psychosexual factors can interfere with erection and will be discussed later.

Because emission and ejaculation are controlled by the autonomic nervous system, any disease state or drug that alters autonomic response will also affect ejaculation. For example, spinal cord lesions caused by trauma or a demyelinating disease such as multiple sclerosis can impair or prevent ejaculation. Drugs affecting the autonomic nervous system also affect sexual response. Phentolamine (Regitine) and prazosin hydrochloride (Minipress), for example, are alpha-adrenergic blockers that can impair ejaculation, leading to infertility.

An ejaculatory problem with an anatomic cause is *retrograde ejaculation,* in which emission occurs but seminal plasma is ejaculated backward into the bladder rather than forward through the urethra to the external orifice. Diabetes, chronic alcoholism, prostatic surgery, and uremia are other common causes of ejaculatory problems. Drugs that depress the central nervous system, such as sedatives, narcotics, and barbiturates, also affect the sex centers of the brain and can impair ejaculation.

Situational Infertility

Many cases of infertility are situational to the couple. The woman's reproductive tract and the man's sperm may or may not be compatible. For example, the contour of a particular female's reproductive tract may slightly prolong the time required for the ascent of sperm. If her partner also has a borderline low sperm count, their pairing may result in infertility. Quite possibly, either partner paired with another person might conceive without difficulty. Some

women have an immune response to certain sperm and actually form antibodies that destroy them.

Certain numbers of sperm must exist to achieve conception, but attempts at defining sperm count adequacy have been difficult for many reasons. Normal values should be based on cross-sectional sampling, but most research comes from limited populations such as couples with complaints of infertility, vasectomy candidates, or restricted age groups. Lipshultz and Howards (1983), have offered minimal standards of adequacy below which the initiation of pregnancy becomes statistically difficult. On at least two occasions, a 1.5- to 5-mL sample of seminal ejaculate must contain more than 20 million sperm per milliliter; furthermore, 60% of the sample must have mobility, and more than 60% must have structural integrity.

The frequency of ejaculation is another situational factor that affects sperm quality. Sperm lose motility and viability with prolonged storage, whereas frequent ejaculation can force sperm through the duct system with inadequate time for maturation. The most effective frequency of intercourse for adequate sperm is every 48 hours.

The timing of intercourse is the simplest situational cause of infertility but also the most frequent. Many couples do not understand the significance of the menstrual cycle nor the life expectancy of sperm, which is approximately 2 days in cervical mucus and only hours in the vagina. They also may not understand the importance of position during intercourse. Depositing of sperm deep in the female reproductive tract at the cervical os can compensate for low sperm counts by improving sperm survival. In some positions, sperm are not as likely to be placed at the cervical os. The female superior position, for example, permits gravity to work against the deposition of sperm at the cervical os; for some couples, this simple fact can affect fertility.

The diagnosis of infertility first requires a relevant psychosocial, sexual, and medical history of the male partner. Concomitant evaluation of the female partner and the couple's sexual patterns and behavior are also essential. The diagnosis of infertility is further discussed in Chapters 63 and 66.

SEXUAL DYSFUNCTIONS

A sexual dysfunction is a physical impairment of the sexual response. In the male, this includes problems with erection, emission, ejaculation, sexual desire, genital muscle spasm, and dyspareunia (painful sexual intercourse). The cause of these dysfunctions may be physical or psychosocial, but the altered response is a physical impairment.

Impotence

To the male, the most devastating sexual dysfunction is probably **impotence,** an impairment of erectile function. Primary impotence is a severe and chronic disorder in men who have never had normal erectile function. It is relatively rare and associated with significant pathological conditions. In contrast, secondary impotence is not associated with significant pathological conditions and occurs in men who previously had normal erectile function. Most men experience occasional episodes of impotence at some time in their sexual lives, and this is not considered abnormal. Erectile difficulties can occur in men of all ages, socioeconomic groups, and races. Impotence may be from physical or psychological factors, but the basic mechanism is impairment of the erectile reflex. The vascular reflex cycle fails to pump sufficient blood to the penile sinuses to make the penis firm and erect.

Physical causes are related to the vascular and neural mechanisms that accomplish erection. Generalized physical factors include debilitation, stress, and fatigue. Specific conditions, which are discussed later in this chapter, include diabetes, multiple sclerosis, cord injuries, surgical trauma, hepatic pathology, and low testosterone levels. The abuse of substances such as caffeine, alcohol, marijuana, and narcotics can profoundly affect potency, as was discussed earlier. Drugs used to treat other conditions may also affect potency.

Psychological causes of impotence are at least as numerous as its physical causes. They may be serious psychiatric disturbances such as depression but more often are attributable to less serious and more immediate factors such as fear of performance failure or moral conflict over a particular sexual experience. The lack of trust between partners often inhibits the sexual response. Young men often fear premature ejaculation, whereas older men may fear impotence itself. Erectile function is impaired as soon as the man experiences anxiety, because the reflex response requires that the situation be supportive and that conscious thoughts not inhibit the reflex sequence. A more accurate understanding of normal developmental erectile responses across the lifespan would relieve many men of considerable discomfort and self-doubt, which sometimes leads to impaired response.

Impotence can occur episodically or be total (at all times with all partners). Men of all ages, races, and cultures invest a great deal of self-esteem in the erectile response, and its failure is uniformly devastating. Depression, anxiety, and loss of self-esteem are almost always associated with the problem of impotence.

Other Sexual Dysfunctions

Impairments of emission and ejaculation include retrograde ejaculation (discussed earlier), **premature ejaculation** (the inability to exert any voluntary control over the timing of the ejaculatory reflex), and failure to reach orgasm. Of these, premature ejaculation is the most common. Physical causes of these problems include (1) impairments in the nerve pathways from trauma or disease and (2) inadequate amounts of neurotransmitters, because of drugs or disease, to effect these responses under autonomic control. The many psychological causes of premature ejaculation are often those described earlier as contributing to impotence. Knowledge deficit also can contribute to premature ejaculation; the man may not be aware of his partner's needs and responses.

Sexual desire may be compromised by inadequate levels of testosterone to stimulate the sex centers of the brain or by lesions of the brain in these areas. Depression is a potent and common cause of this problem.

Dyspareunia, or pain on sexual response, can result from penile anatomic problems such as phimosis (an abnormally tight prepuce) or Peyronie's disease (a hardening of the corpora cavernosa). It can also occur secondary to local infections (such as herpes, scabies, and gonorrhea) or disease within the reproductive system (such as prostatitis, urethritis, or epididymitis).

Any sexual dysfunction significantly affects the well-being of the man experiencing the problem and his relationship with sexual partners. The problems are seldom irreversible, but their diagnosis and treatment depend on a meticulous history and examination by a skilled health care professional. Some medical conditions inevitably lead to impairments in the sexual response, but these often can be managed carefully to control or retard the progression of symptoms.

Section III: Related System Influences and Effects

Many disease conditions outside the reproductive system affect sexuality, sexual response, fertility, and the reproductive system in general. When assessing any individual with a disease, it is important to evaluate the psychological impact the disease may have on reproductive and sexual status. The nurse can gain such information by careful interviews with the client and by researching the pathophysiological mechanisms of the disease in the literature to understand the potential for altered response.

Every health care professional must respond to the client's concern for reproductive status and help a client express these concerns. This can be done by taking a routine but detailed sexual history, along with a history of other systems. If the nurse conveys to the client that reproductive concerns are a legitimate part of the health history, the client will feel more comfortable expressing them. Thus, although the client may be in treatment for diabetes, for example, sexual concerns are a proper and important focus of care.

Any disease that affects neurologic, pulmonary, or cardiovascular function generally will affect the reproductive system through diminished ability to respond to stimuli and compromised tissue integrity. Some conditions have direct effects, a few of which will be discussed here.

Arteriosclerosis in penile arteries impairs the vascular mechanism leading to erection. Neurological damage from disease (multiple sclerosis, myasthenia gravis, or Parkinson's disease) or trauma (such as spinal cord injuries) interrupts the autonomic control of the sexual response. Dysfunction in the central nervous system, such as endogenous depression, tumors, and epilepsy, can cause sexual dysfunctions from these higher centers. Renal dialysis clients and those with severe liver disease are commonly impotent. Although these conditions are currently considered irreversible, they often can be managed to control or retard the progression of symptoms. Careful attention to glucose control in the diabetic client, for example, can retard neuropathy and arteriosclerosis. Exercise, diet, and the cessation of smoking theoretically will slow the progression of arteriosclerosis.

Drug-induced sexual dysfunction, which has been discussed throughout this chapter, is irreversible while the use of the drug continues. When the drug is being used to treat a disease condition, an alternative drug might treat the disease satisfactorily but have fewer effects on the reproductive system. Some drugs that adversely affect male sexuality are drugs to treat hypertension, drugs that affect mental and emotional function, and the cholinergic-blocking drugs that are used in the treatment of Parkinson's disease and peptic ulcer.

It is essential to appreciate the interrelation of all the body's systems and to be alert to potential adverse interactions. On the other hand, organic causes for sexual dysfunction should not be assumed simply because a disease is present. Self-esteem and hope for the future are an important part of the assessment of the whole client. The presence of diabetes, for example, suggests a possible organic cause for impotence. The fear, depression, and anguish associated with a chronic disease, however, may be equally destructive factors. Any approach to treatment of a sexual dysfunction depends on a clear determination of the organic or psychic cause.

Sometimes it is possible to anticipate and prepare the client for a reproductive dysfunction. For example, when chemotherapy is initiated to treat a cancer and it is expected that fertility will be affected, the client could be offered the option of freezing and banking his sperm to be used at a later time. In this way, he could still plan to have his own family even though he would be infertile after treatment.

When results of a pathological condition are severe and irreversible, some further options remain. Reconstructive plastic surgery of the genitals is achieving acceptable results. Penile implants to achieve erection are available and, for many men, provide satisfying and acceptable results (refer to Chapter 68).

Trauma and diseases of the musculoskeletal system can pose a special problem to the reproductive system. Pain, immobility, or disfigurement may make it difficult to find a comfortable position for sexual response. Counseling and guidance to choose a position and comfortable support in a position often can greatly improve a dysfunctional situation.

Section IV: Psychosocial/Lifestyle Influences and Effects

Sexuality is the psychosocial expression of the reproductive system. The biological developmental changes covered in the previous discussion have a powerful effect on sexuality. Sexual identity and gender identity, however, are outcomes of culture, religion, and life experiences.

Gender identity is that part of the self-concept that recognizes maleness and femaleness and composes an acceptable profile of a male or a female for the self. Although this identity includes sexuality, it also encompasses all the learned cultural expressions of what males and females do. In North American society, these definitions are changing. Fifty years ago, few people would have disagreed with the idea that adult males work to support families and adult females care for those families in the home. Today such a statement would not necessarily be accurate. There is no confusion about biological gender, but the role identity of the genders is taking on new definitions. Sexual identity is that part of the self-concept that defines the expression of reproductive drives unique to the individual. This aspect of self-concept is also totally affected by cultural and life experiences.

General wellness affects the reproductive system as it does all body systems. Nutritional status, amount of energy, and general sense of well-being affect sexual response, reproductive status, and sexuality. Libido, or sexual drive, can be altered by psychosocial factors such as rejection or acceptance by peers, as well as by general wellness and energy levels.

DEVELOPMENTAL INFLUENCES

Both gender and sexual identity begin developing in infants. Biological factors heavily influence early development, but cultural experiences and observations are also significant. Gender and sexual identity are influenced profoundly by role modeling of significant adults, which explains why sexual and gender behaviors differ among cultures. Margaret Mead (1935) described societies in which females wielded the real power and initiative, and men learned dances and demonstrated ritual charm. She described a culture in which males and females behaved in a gentle, loving manner and one in which both sexes behaved with equal fierceness and aggressiveness. These behaviors were modeled in those cultures and thus accepted by the majority of their members.

Sigmund Freud believed that most of the self-concept is formed before age 6. Learning and behavior theorists disagree with such a strict limitation but recognize the significance of learning in the early years. For this reason, experiences of urogenital dysfunction and painful or privacy-violating experiences can affect an individual throughout life. Associations can form between the fear-ridden, painful episode and the individual's own use of the reproductive system. Physiological risks to the system in the early years are primarily those of genetic and congenital anomalies. Except for these occurrences, trauma (to the system or the child in general) poses the biggest problem.

Cultural impact on the male reproductive system includes the interpretations that adults make to the child concerning the use and meaning of the genitals in that culture. The child also observes the adults' behavior in regard to privacy, respect, and the use of genitals and forms personal attitudes and behaviors from these experiences. The 2-year-old who is told that his "wee-wee is dirty" may have difficulty later in learning to handle or let sexual partners handle his genitals for pleasurable purposes.

Many cultures have rites of initiation into manhood that simultaneously recognize the initiate's developing manhood and define the norms and expectations of that culture for its members. Following the rite, the initiation of a public sexual image is acceptable, and sexual identity may be broadcast to others. For example, in many North American Indian communities, adolescents are presented at special ceremonial gatherings and allowed to dance a ritual dance. From that time, the community considers them eligible for choosing or being chosen as partners. In North America, the appearance of junior high or high school students at school dances or the use of cosmetics in public may signal their readiness for dating.

Urogenital dysfunctions at this point in the life cycle may provoke extreme anxiety because the young male has not had time to develop familiarity with his reproductive performance or confidence in it. Questions of fertility are usually of less concern to the adolescent than those of potency, although childhood diseases do pose a threat to fertility at and following puberty.

After biological maturity, changes in reproductive status are minor. Throughout adult life, however, psychosocial influences may provoke a wide range of sexual behaviors and habits. With established sexual activity, the male becomes vulnerable to sexually transmitted diseases (STDs), which pose a risk not only to the reproductive system but to many other body systems as well. Hydrocele and cancer are also problems of adulthood.

Pressures and stresses felt in adult life directly influence the sexual response and the energy available for sexual activity. Simple fatigue, such as that experienced by a man working two jobs or engaged in highly competitive and demanding employment, may be sufficient to impair sexual response. Life crises such as job change, death in the family, marriage, separation, and divorce are stressful experiences. People's sexual needs and responses vary greatly during times of stress and include the following patterns: (1) diminished sexual desire; (2) the immediate formation of a new, dependent relationship; and (3) multiple sexual encounters (Svechin–Greatrex, 1983).

In later years, subtle changes in sexual performance may cause the man to believe he is too old for sexual activity. Although this is not physiologically true, cultural expectations may strongly prejudice his attitudes. The most common disease conditions in this age group include hydrocele and prostate problems, which do affect both reproductive status and sexual response. These problems are discussed in Chapter 67.

Religious and cultural factors also strongly affect the frequency of sexual activity and the number and variety of partners. Religious and cultural convictions that limit the number and choices of partners can have a protective effect; research has shown an increased incidence of reproductive system diseases among people with a number of partners (Nass, Libby, & Fisher, 1981). Some religions prohibit the practice of homosexuality, a lifestyle that increases the risk of hepatitis B and acquired immune deficiency syndrome (AIDS), two diseases much less common in heterosexual populations.

DIETARY HABITS

The effect of nutrition on the male reproductive system is primarily on general well-being and tissue integrity. Throughout history, various foods and drinks have been believed to be aphrodisiacs. There is no evidence that any nutritional preparation has a major effect on the reproductive system. Nevertheless, good nutrition is essential for sexual energy and tissue health, just as it is essential to the well-being of other body systems.

OCCUPATION AND AVOCATION

Some occupations can pose a hazard to the male reproductive system. Jobs that require prolonged sitting or standing are associated with an increased incidence of prostate problems. Jobs that require heavy lifting increase the risk of hernia, hydrocele, and varicocele.

Environmental hazards may exist on the job or elsewhere. Society is only beginning to learn of the risks of disease from exposure to toxic chemicals and waste from a variety of agents. Such exposure may have adverse effects on fertility by causing low sperm count or low motility of existing sperm, or it may even cause chromosomal damage to sperm. A few of these substances are (Mann & Lutewak–Mann, 1981):

- Organochlorine compounds (dichlorodiphenyltrichloroethane or DDT, some defoliants, and components of plastic) are easily absorbed through the skin and can damage DNA in the germ cell.
- Dibromochloropropane, a soil fumigant, has antispermatogenic properties. Its inhalation or oral adminis-

tration causes severe degenerative changes in the testes.

- Dibromopropanol (a clothing flame retardant, Tris-BP) is a proven carcinogen to which the scrotum is particularly susceptible.
- Organophosphorus (including many insecticides) inhibits cholinesterase, transiently affecting autonomic response but possibly also affecting spermatogenesis.
- Paraquat (a herbicide used extensively on marijuana) has mutagenic and antifertility properties.

The list of hazardous substances continues to grow as dysfunctions are identified and epidemiologically associated with environmental exposure.

Some occupations pose the risk of trauma to the male reproductive system. Many farm accidents, especially with bailers and mechanized pickers, involve trauma to the external organs of reproduction. Truck drivers who sit over motors may experience heat injuries to the testes or infertility problems because of the heat. Men who manufacture or use hazardous substances are also at risk.

Even recreational activities can pose hazards. Hot tubs and spas have been implicated in heat-induced infertility problems that are usually temporary. Tight-fitting clothing holds the scrotum close to the body, creating temperatures that may be too high for adequate testicular function.

Chapter Highlights

The purpose of any reproductive system is the continuation of the species and providing a means of sexual pleasure and satisfaction.

The external organs of the male reproductive system are the penis and scrotum; the internal organs are the testes, epididymis, vas deferens, and several accessory glands.

The male gamete is the sperm, which is produced by the testes and released into the ductal system, where it is nourished and transported by seminal plasma, or semen. Mature sperm are motile, have 23 chromosomes, and are vulnerable to heat but able to remain viable after freezing.

The male sexual response is governed by the central nervous system and affected by the autonomic nervous system and the circulatory system. Both physical and psychic stimuli can elicit or inhibit the sexual response. In the male, the sexual response changes in frequency and duration but persists throughout the lifespan.

The endocrine reproductive cycle in the male is governed by the hypothalamus, which acts upon the anterior pituitary gland, which acts upon the gonads. A negative feedback cycle fine-tunes the system.

Testosterone, the primary male hormone, is directly responsible for differentiation of the male genitals, maturation of the internal sex organs, maturation of sperm, and secondary sex characteristics.

General metabolic effects of testosterone include deposition of calcium salts in bone, increase of muscle mass, closure of epiphyses, and increased metabolic rate.

Hypogonadal endocrine responses result in the failure of testosterone-dependent processes such as

maintenance of secondary sex characteristics and spermatogenesis.

Hypergonadal endocrine disturbances result in increased testosterone secretion and, consequently, exaggerated testosterone effects such as early puberty and enlarged gonads.

Infertility is the inability to conceive. In the man, it can result from (1) injury to the gonads from such causes as high temperatures or exposure to toxic substances or (2) the absence of any part of the reproductive system.

Sexual dysfunctions are physical impairments of the sexual response. They can result from injury to the genitals or exposure to drugs or diseases that affect autonomic or cardiovascular function.

Any disease or drug that affects the autonomic nervous system, respiratory system, or cardiovascular system can impair the sexual response. General well-being compromised by disease in any system is also likely to affect the sexual response. Some drugs and toxic chemicals also can impair fertility.

Sexuality is the psychosocial expression of the reproductive system.

Gender identity is the self-image of maleness or femaleness constructed by the individual, whereas sexual identity is that part of the self-concept that defines the unique expression of reproductive drives.

Chronological age is responsible for some biological changes in the reproductive system, as well as some changes in sexuality and sexual behavior. There is a definite biological change in the male at puberty, but only a moderate and gradual biological change with aging following middle age.

Bibliography

Aman RP: A critical review of methods for evaluation of spermatogenesis from seminal characteristics. *J Androl* 1981; 2:37.

Ewing L: Leydig cell. In: *Infertility in the Male.* Lipshultz L, Howards SS (editors). New York: Churchill Livingstone, 1983.

Griffin E, Wilson J: Disorders of the testes. In: *Harrison's Principles of Internal Medicine,* 10th ed. Petersdorf RG, Davis R, Martin J, Wilson J (editors). New York: McGraw–Hill, 1983.

Horwith M, Imperato–McGinley J: The medical evaluation of disorders of sexual desire in males and females. In: *The Evaluation of Sexual Disorders.* Kaplan HS (editor). New York: Brunner/Mazel, 1983.

Huckins C: Development of the testes and establishment of spermatogenesis. In: *Infertility in the Male.* Lipshultz L, Howards SS (editors). New York: Churchill Livingstone, 1983.

Lipshultz L, Howards S (editors): *Infertility in the Male.* New York: Churchill Livingstone, 1983.

Mann T, Lutewak–Mann C: *Male Reproductive Function and Semen.* New York: Springer–Verlag, 1981.

Mawhinney M: Male accessory organs and androgen action. In: *Infertility in the Male.* Lipshultz L, Howards SS (editors). New York: Churchill Livingstone, 1983.

Mead M: *Sex and Temperament in Three Primitive Societies.* New York: Morrow, 1935.

Melman A, Leiter E: Urologic evaluation of impotence. In: *The Evaluation of Sexual Disorders.* Kaplan HS (editor). New York: Brunner/Mazel, 1983.

Nass GD, Libby L, Fisher M: *Sexual Choices: An Introduction to Human Sexuality.* Monterey, CA: Wadsworth, 1981.

Svechin–Greatrex TE: Separation and divorce: Crisis and development. In: *Treatment Interventions in Human Sexuality.* Nadelson C, Marcotte D (editors). New York: Plenum, 1983.

Vick RL: *Contemporary Medical Physiology.* Menlo Park, CA: Addison–Wesley, 1984.

Suggested Readings

Fromer MJ: *Ethical Issues in Sexuality and Reproduction.* St. Louis: Mosby, 1983. Written by a nurse, this book explores ethical issues relating to sexuality and reproduction. Topics such as counseling clients with sexual dysfunctions, abortion, artificial insemination, and many other important concerns to the nurse are discussed.

Kaplan HS: *The New Sex Therapy.* New York: Brunner/Mazel, 1974. In this classic, the first of Kaplan's five books on sexual disorders, the sexual response is thoroughly discussed across the life span.

Kolodny RC, Masters W, Johnson V, & Briggs M: *Textbook of Human Sexuality for Nurses.* St. Louis: Little, Brown, 1979. This work is written for nurses in collaboration with a nurse who worked with Masters and Johnson for many years. It has an excellent section on handicapped clients and sexuality.

Nadelson C, Marcotte D (editors): *Treatment Intervention in Human Sexuality.* New York: Plenum, 1983. This comprehensive text uses sociology, psychology, and medicine to explore sexual dysfunctions.

Chapter 63

The Nursing Process for Clients With Female Reproductive System Dysfunction

Carolyn Fritz McCain

Objectives

When you have finished studying this chapter, you should be able to:

Specify the components of the client health history that are necessary for the evaluation of female reproductive system dysfunction.

Discuss the three typical symptoms related to female reproductive system dysfunction.

Determine specific physical assessment approaches in evaluating clients with dysfunction of the female reproductive system.

Identify the diagnostic studies commonly performed to detect the presence or the progress of female reproductive system dysfunction.

Apply nursing methods to promote comfort in clients with female reproductive system dysfunction and pain.

Identify the nursing interventions that can assist clients with knowledge deficits related to early warning symptoms of cancer, ovulation and sexual function, and sexually transmitted diseases (STDs).

State the relation between adequate nutrition and menstrual function.

Formulate nursing interventions that promote perineal skin cleanliness and integrity.

The nursing process for females with reproductive system dysfunction includes both general and specialized assessment skills and interventions. This chapter discusses the planning of individualized client care related to disorders of the breast and female reproductive system dysfunction. Nursing measures that apply to specific female reproductive system disorders and surgical approaches are discussed in Chapters 64 and 65.

Section I: Nursing Assessment: Establishing the Data Base

The assessment of the female reproductive system can be the most difficult part of a history and physical examination. The examiner and the client may experience anxiety or embarrassment while collecting data about sexuality and sexual function. Women with reproductive system dysfunction often require increased time and understanding during assessment because of the highly emotional nature of gynecologic problems. Women are often reluctant to seek medical attention until the symptoms are advanced. This may be because of difficulty in acknowledging the existence of the problem, anxiety, embarrassment, or false hope that the symptoms will disappear.

SUBJECTIVE DATA

The nurse is often the health team member who must elicit primary assessment data and review previous nursing and medical treatment records. Variations in lifestyles and the definitions of acceptable behavior necessitate that the interviewer be nonjudgmental. Phrase questions about social or sexual habits so the client will not feel threatened or defensive.

When collecting data about the client's chief concern, recognize that many reproductive system problems are multifaceted. Disorders of other body systems, such as the urinary and gastrointestinal systems, may produce concerns similar to those caused by gynecologic problems. Furthermore, the woman's own interpretation of the meaning of pain influences her ability to describe it. For example, pelvic pain—one of the most common female complaints—is often difficult to describe. The pain site the client identifies may be a referred site instead of its source. Thus, the examiner must gather information and examine all body systems suggested by the symptoms; finding and treating only one presenting symptom may not be enough.

A detailed health history is essential in assessing the client's gynecologic well-being. Question the client about any changes from her usual pattern of reproductive system function. Examine her current lifestyle, recent significant changes, and stress level. Explore the client's medical and surgical history to determine whether previous illnesses or treatments and her current problem are related.

Asking specific questions helps determine the usual characteristics of the presenting symptoms. Information on the onset and frequency of the symptoms is important, because the timing of the symptoms often suggests their cause. If a symptom is not continuous, question what seems to make it worse or better. Associated signs or symptoms, such as odor or pruritus, should be investigated. The effect the problem has on activities of daily living and self-prescribed treatments needs to be determined. The typical triad of symptoms related to the female reproductive system includes pain, vaginal discharge, and bleeding.

Pain

Pain may be associated with genital lesions or discharge, inflammatory disease, congestion, muscle spasm, obstruction, and irritation. Pain caused by pathological conditions must be differentiated from pain from functional or benign causes. The intense pain from rupture, ischemia, or perforation usually is of sudden onset and can be localized, whereas pain that has a more insidious onset is often the result of infection, congestion, or obstruction.

The timing of the pain's onset in relation to previous normal function is also important. For example, spasmodic primary dysmenorrhea begins with cramping on the first day of flow and is rarely associated with physical abnormalities or pathological conditions. Secondary dysmenorrhea, in contrast, is the onset of painful menses after a previously established pattern of relatively comfortable periods. The cause of secondary dysmenorrhea often is traced to organic problems, frequently endometriosis.

The pain's location may suggest a pathological condi-

tion or functional discomfort (Figure 63–1). Abdominal pain from infection is often bilateral and may involve the entire abdomen. Pelvic congestion or uterine tumors need to be ruled out as a cause of midabdominal or lower back pain. Dysmenorrhea may be of congestive origin and involves a dull, aching pain that often begins before menses and is associated with premenstrual syndrome (PMS). Unilateral lower quadrant pain may suggest an ectopic pregnancy, **mittelschmerz** (ovulatory pain), or an ovarian cyst. Breast pain may indicate neoplasms, cysts, or inflammation.

Dyspareunia (pain associated with intercourse) may have a physiological or psychogenic cause. Vulvar or vaginal infections or a rigid hymen can cause pain upon immediate penetration, whereas pain associated with deep penile penetration can be caused by endometriosis, tumors, or pelvic inflammatory disease (PID). A client may experience dyspareunia from decreased vaginal lubrication because of normal low estrogen levels, such as during the postpartum, lactation, and climacteric–menopausal periods.

Vaginal Discharge

The second symptom of the triad is vaginal discharge and its accompanying distress. Most often a troublesome discharge is caused by infection or irritation, and occasionally a contraceptive agent or disease process is the underlying cause.

Consider the possibility of a sexually transmitted disease (STD) in clients of all socioeconomic classes. Clues to this possibility are often found in the client's motive for seeking care. Gonorrhea may be characterized by a yellow purulent discharge, dysuria, and lower abdominal pain. Painless sores on the genitals or mouth may indicate syphilis. In comparison, herpes simplex infections may cause exquisitely painful genital lesions.

A detailed history assists in the determination of the cause, which may be multifactorial and influenced by stress, hygiene, lifestyle, and lowered nutritional status or resistance to disease. Ask the client when the symptoms began and the character and color of the discharge. Copious, frothy discharge is characteristic of *Trichomonas vaginalis*. *T. vaginalis* and *Hemophilus vaginalis* are also associated with a foul-smelling discharge. Collect data concerning associated symptoms such as pruritus, burning, or tingling. Pruritus of the vulva with a discharge resembling cottage cheese indicates *Candida albicans* infection.

Look beyond the initial cause of vaginal discharge to rule out multifactorial contributors such as systemic disease, frequent douching, or the concurrent use of medications. Unless these are addressed, the treatment is not likely to be effective, and the problem will recur.

Bleeding

The third common symptom in the gynecologic triad is unusual bleeding or the lack of bleeding. This includes

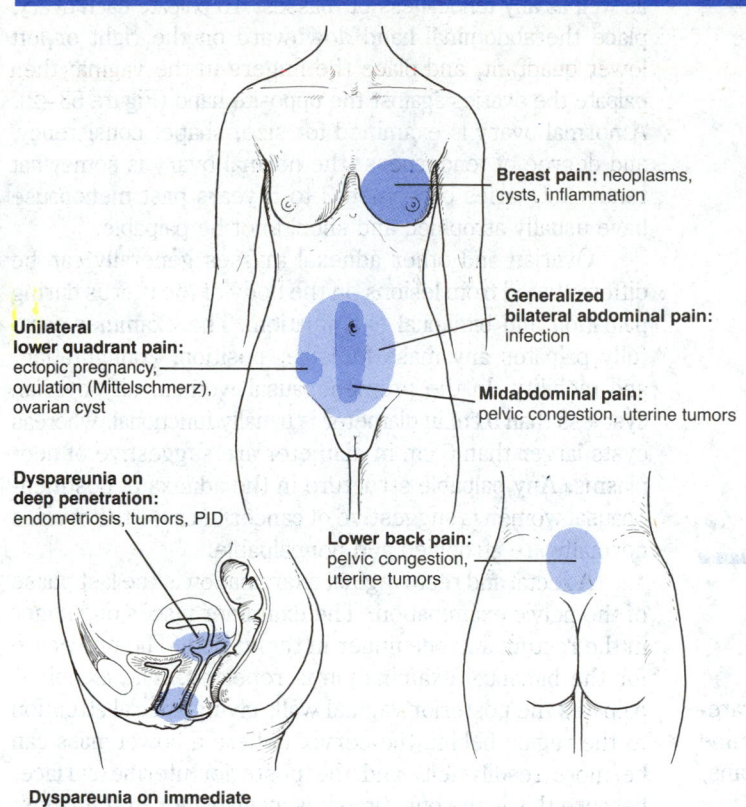

Figure 63-1

Location of pain in the female reproductive system.

Breast pain: neoplasms, cysts, inflammation

Generalized bilateral abdominal pain: infection

Unilateral lower quadrant pain: ectopic pregnancy, ovulation (Mittelschmerz), ovarian cyst

Midabdominal pain: pelvic congestion, uterine tumors

Dyspareunia on deep penetration: endometriosis, tumors, PID

Lower back pain: pelvic congestion, uterine tumors

Dyspareunia on immediate penetration: vulvar or vaginal infections, low estrogen levels, rigid hymen

amenorrhea, changes in the normal menstrual cycle, and spotting between periods. The client's menstrual history is essential in assessing her chief concern. Besides obtaining information about the age of menarche, elicit information about the frequency and duration of the menses. A description of the amount of flow is highly subjective among women. Therefore, try to obtain an accurate picture of how much blood is lost and the character of the bleeding. Ask the client how many pads or tampons she uses during her menstrual period as a whole, as well as on specific days. For example, are panty liners sufficient, or must she use maxipads or superabsorbent tampons? Also determine whether there have been any changes from the client's usual pattern and character of menstruation, including pain.

OBJECTIVE DATA

Physical Assessment

After the history has been completed, the client is prepared for the physical assessment. It is recommended that women over 20, as well as younger sexually active clients, have an annual pelvic examination. Ask the client to empty her bladder and undress before the examination. Drape her adequately to protect her modesty, and allow eye con-

tact with the examiner. Placing a mirror so that the client is able to observe her own cervix facilitates teaching. Explain in advance each step of the physical examination.

The examination begins with a general inspection to determine the development of secondary sex characteristics and to detect a chronically ill appearance. Examination of the breasts usually follows the examination of the heart and lungs. Inspect the breasts for size, shape and symmetry, the appearance of the skin, and the presence of any masses or dimpling. Inspect the nipples for size and shape, as well as redness, ulcerations, and discharge. A uniform palpation pattern of the breast is necessary to note tenderness or nodules. The examiner should describe any nodules palpated by their location, size, shape, consistency, mobility, and tenderness. This is a good time to teach the client how to perform breast self-examination (BSE) or, if she already does BSE, to review the proper procedure (refer to Chapter 7).

After the breast examination, the examiner generally inspects, auscultates, and palpates the abdomen. In the gynecologic examination, the health care provider is alert for symptomatic and asymptomatic abdominopelvic masses. A mass associated with severe pain, fever, or hemorrhage demands immediate action. Laboratory testing of the white blood cell (WBC) count, differential WBC count, and sedi-

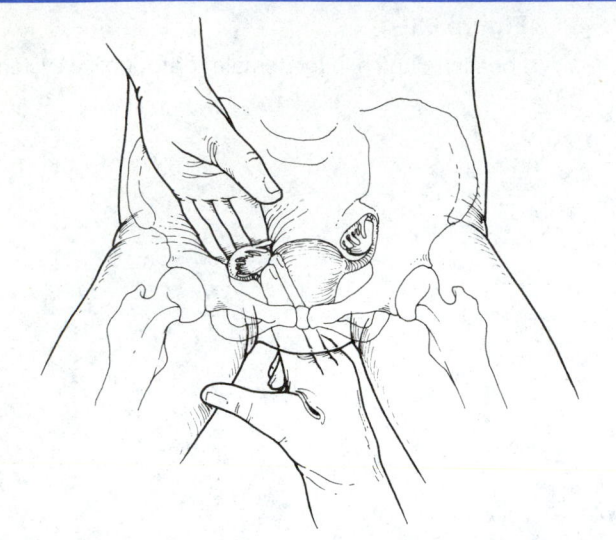

Figure 63-2

Bimanual abdominovaginal palpation of the adnexa.

mentation rate may also be helpful in the diagnosis. A careful history and physical examination can usually determine whether the mass originates in the reproductive organs, bowel, or urinary tract.

As the examination progresses, the client assumes the lithotomy position. Inspect the external genitalia for normal development and signs of inflammation, swelling, ulceration, discharge, or nodules. In older women or those who have had difficult deliveries, it is important to assess perineal support. Ask these women to strain downward, and note any bulging of the vaginal walls, which indicates weakening.

Internal examination of the vagina and cervix is next (see Chapter 7 for description and illustrations). Examination is accomplished by the use of a speculum of the appropriate size and shape, which should be warmed and lubricated with warm water. Other lubricants should be avoided if cytological studies are planned (see the section on diagnostic studies). Inspect the cervix and its os for color, position, ulcerations, nodules, masses, discharge, and bleeding. During pregnancy, the color of the cervix changes to bluish purple as a result of increased vascular congestion (Chadwick's sign). Conditions that produce inflammation and ulcerations of the cervix include herpes simplex type II. Slowly withdrawing the speculum allows inspection of the vaginal tissues for lesions or inflammation.

After withdrawing the speculum, proceed with a bimanual examination, which was described and illustrated in Chapter 7. Two gloved lubricated fingers of one hand are inserted into the client's vagina while the other hand simultaneously palpates the abdomen. This allows examination of the uterus and the adnexa (adjacent structures, including ovaries, fallopian tubes, and uterine ligaments). Note the size, shape, consistency, and mobility of the uterus,

as well as any tenderness or masses. To palpate each ovary, place the abdominal hand downward on the right or left lower quadrant, and place the fingers in the vagina; then palpate the ovaries against the opposite hand (Figure 63-2). A normal ovary is examined for size, shape, consistency, and degree of tenderness (the normal ovary is somewhat tender). Ovaries of women 3 to 5 years past menopause have usually atrophied and should not be palpable.

Ovarian and other adnexal masses generally can be differentiated from lesions on the body of the uterus during palpation and bimanual examination. The examiner carefully palpates any mass for size, position, configuration, and mobility. In the premenopausal woman, any ovarian cyst less than 5 cm in diameter is usually functional, whereas cysts larger than 6 cm in diameter are suggestive of neoplasms. Any palpable structure in the adnexa of postmenopausal women is suggestive of cancer because the ovaries normally are atrophied and nonpalpable.

A rectal and rectovaginal examination is the last phase of the pelvic examination. The examiner places one finger in the rectum and one finger in the vagina. The procedure for the bimanual examination is repeated. The examiner palpates the posterior vaginal wall, giving special attention to the region behind the cervix (where a bowel mass can be more readily felt) and the posterior uterine surface, because this is the only time it is available for examination. The rectal examination makes it easier to detect abnormalities of the deeper structures and the posterior surfaces of the reproductive organs (see Figure 63-3).

Following the pelvic examination, a gentle wiping of the perineal area removes secretions and lubricant. The client may need some assistance in removing both feet from the stirrups at the same time to reduce strain on the perineal muscles. Some clients experience orthostatic hypotension if they sit up too quickly, so the examiner should evaluate the client for signs of dizziness before letting her get off the examining table using a stool. Allow

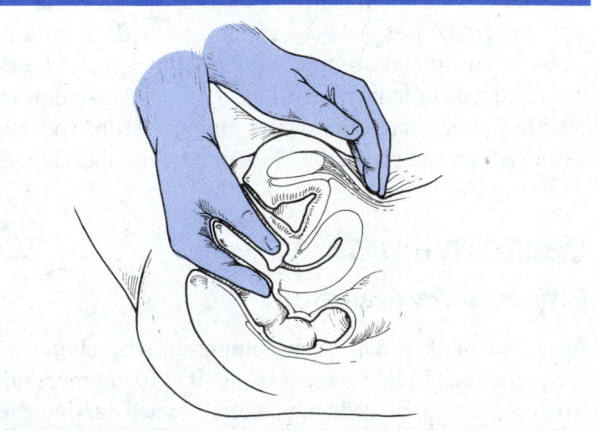

Figure 63-3

Bidigital rectovaginal examination.

adequate time for dressing, and be available to answer questions or interpret collected data.

Diagnostic Studies

Diagnostic studies relevant to the female reproductive system are discussed in this section. Laboratory tests are summarized in Table 63–1.

Papanicolaou and Other Cytologic Tests

The *Papanicolaou* (Pap) *test* has been used since the 1950s to screen for cervical cancer. Most gynecologists recommend that women receive the test annually, and women over 40 and those at high risk may be advised to have semiannual exams. This relatively painless cytologic test can detect precancerous and cancerous cells among the cells shed from the cervix. Occasionally, adenocarcinoma

cells of the endocervix or the endometrial lining of the uterus also will be discovered. Atypical cells discovered in the cytologic screening may be from cervicitis.

The Pap test takes just a few minutes after the woman is in the lithotomy position. After the cervix is visualized through the speculum, a wooden spatula is used to scrape the cervix and endocervix (Figure 63–4A). The specimens are immediately transferred to glass slides and either sprayed or immersed in a fixative solution (Figure 63–4B). If the smear is allowed to dry on the slide before the fixative has been applied, accurate diagnosis will be impossible. A pathologist examines and interprets the smears, and the test results are usually received in 2 to 3 days.

The accepted (Papanicolaou's) classification of the cytologic findings is:

- Class 1: Absence of atypical or abnormal cells
- Class 2: Atypical cytology but no evidence of malignancy

Table 63–1   Laboratory Tests Common to the Female Reproductive System

Laboratory Test	Normal Expected Value	Disease State	Expected Abnormal Findings
Hemoglobin	12–16 g/dL	Anemia, severe hemorrhage	Decreased
Hematocrit	37%–47%	Anemia, severe hemorrhage	Decreased
Prothrombin time	11–15 s	Disseminated intravascular coagulation (DIC)	Increased
Lactic dehydrogenase (LDH)	80–120 Wacker u	Extensive malignancy	Increased
White blood cell count	4500–11,000 µL	Acute infection, hemorrhage, surgery	Increased
	Neutrophils: 60%–70%	Bacterial infection, inflammatory disease, stress	Increased
	Eosinophils: 1%–4% Basophils: 0.0%–1.0% Lymphocytes: 25%–40%	Allergic or parasitic disorder Blood dyscrasia Viral infection	Increased
	Monocytes: 2%–6%	Severe infection	
Estrogen (serum)	Premenopausal: 4–60 ng/dL Postmenopausal: < 3–14 ng/dL	Masculinizing tumor, corpus luteum cyst, Stein–Leventhal syndrome	Increased
		Turner's syndrome, menopause, hypopituitarism, anovulatory bleeding	Decreased
Prolactin	Female: 0–23 ng/mL Male: 0–20 ng/mL	Galactorrhea, pituitary tumor, hypothyroidism	Increased
Testosterone	Total: 30–120 ng/dL	Polycystic ovary, ovarian tumor	Increased
	Free: 0.3–1.9 ng/dL	Female hirsutism, polycystic ovary, virilization	Increased
VDRL	Nonreactive (no flocculation)	Syphilis	Reactive (flocculation)
FTA–ABS test	Nonreactive	Syphilis	Reactive
TPI test	Negative	Syphilis	Positive

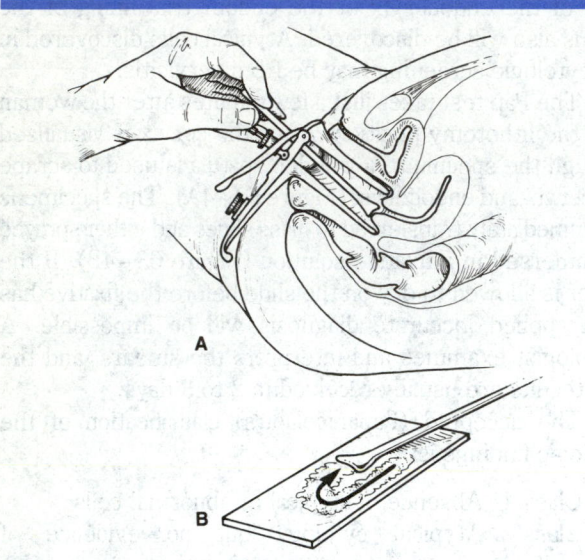

Figure 63-4

The Papanicolaou (Pap) test. **A.** The curve of the wooden spatula allows it to scrape the cervix and the endocervix simultaneously. **B.** Transferring the specimen to a glass slide.

- Class 3: Cytology suggestive of, but not conclusive for, malignancy
- Class 4: Cytology strongly suggestive of malignancy
- Class 5: Cytology conclusive for malignancy

A finding of abnormal cytology, with the exception of Class 5, does not necessarily mean a diagnosis of cancer. Additional studies should be ordered to confirm the test results. These commonly include colposcopy, biopsy and conization, and dilatation and curettage (D and C).

The nurse should schedule the Pap test between the client's menstrual periods. Advise the client to avoid douching, vaginal medications or deodorants, and sexual intercourse for at least 24 hours before the test. Douching will wash away cellular deposits, and vaginal medications or deodorants may cause irritation and confound the cytology. Semen also can confound the cytology.

At the time of the examination, give the client assistance and support as needed. Relaxation techniques, including deep breathing and concentrating on a visual focus point, may be valuable to the apprehensive client. Explain all procedures to the client prior to their performance.

When informing a client that her specimen showed atypical cells, emphasize that only Class 5 is conclusive for malignancy. Provide support and honest answers to the client's questions, and encourage her to return to the clinic for follow-up testing to validate the test results.

Cytologic examinations can also detect viral, fungal, and parasitic disorders and evaluate the client's endocrine status. The vaginal mucosa cells respond cyclically to the monthly fluctuation of steroid hormones, and cell scrapings of the lateral vaginal walls permit easy study of these fluctuations.

Schiller's Iodine Test

Schiller's iodine test is an outpatient procedure to identify unhealthy cervical epithelium. A positive test is only suggestive of neoplasms. To perform the test, the client is placed in a lithotomy position, and the cervix is visualized through a speculum. The entire surface of the cervix is painted with Schiller's iodine solution (1 part aqueous iodine, 2 parts potassium iodide, and 300 parts water).

Normal cervical cells contain glycogen, which reacts with the iodine solution to stain the cells a mahogany brown. Thus, brown staining over the entire squamous epithelial surface of the cervix is interpreted as a negative test result. A positive test, the absence of staining in some sites, indicates that immature cells are present; this is suggestive of neoplasms. Because cancer depletes the epithelial cells' store of glycogen, they cannot react to the stain. Any sites that appear pale in comparison to the surrounding cervical tissue should be biopsied, even though the majority of these sites will be noncancerous.

Vulvar Staining (Collins' Test)

Skin changes of the vulva can be stained and identified for biopsy by a procedure similar to Schiller's test. In Collins' test, a 1% solution of toluidine blue O is painted over the entire vulva. After the skin has dried briefly, it is washed with 1% acetic acid, which removes the blue stain from normal cells. Any areas that retain the dark blue stain are considered positive and should be biopsied.

Colposcopy and Colpomicroscopy

The colposcope and colpomicroscope provide three-dimensional magnification (from 10 to 20 times and up to 400 times, respectively) of the cervical epithelium. Colposcopy is also suited for inspection of the vagina and vulvar epithelium. Either stained or unstained cells may be visualized.

The examiner visualizes the cervix with a speculum and cleans secretions from it. A cotton swab moistens the cervix with saline to allow better visualization of vascular patterns and the squamocolumnar junction. The cervix may be painted with 3% acetic acid, which acts as a mucolytic agent to draw moisture from the tissue and accentuate important morphological features. The colposcope provides intense illumination and magnification to visualize tissue areas under question. A biopsy is still required, however, for accurate diagnosis of questionable sites.

Colposcopy is recommended for any women suspected of having diethylstilbestrol (DES) changes (such as daughters of women who took DES) and for clients with precancerous and malignant lesions to localize the exact site for biopsy. A combination of cytology and colposcopy is recommended.

Cervical Biopsy

A biopsy is the examination of choice to remove cervical tissue for cytologic study. The type and extent of the biopsy vary. If a lesion is clearly visible with a colposcope, a punch biopsy may be used to extract a small column of tissue. Cervical specimens preferably include a portion of the squamocolumnar junction (the area of most cervical malignancies). Cervical punch biopsy can be done as an office procedure without anesthesia, because the cervix has few pain receptors. The biopsy specimen need not cause excessive bleeding; light cauterization with a silver nitrate stick usually is sufficient to control light bleeding.

When no lesions are visible or the Pap test is suggestive of malignancy, a conization (inverted cone biopsy) of the cervix is advisable (see Chapter 65). This requires anesthesia and operating room capabilities. All biopsy specimens are immediately placed in a formalin solution for transport to the cytology laboratory.

The client should be scheduled for the biopsy during the middle of the menstrual cycle, when the cervix is the least vascular. Explain the procedure to the client, paying attention to the physical sensations she might expect. Because cervical biopsy is performed to evaluate areas that could be cancerous, most women are anxious and need time to explore feelings and fears. The use of relaxation techniques often facilitates comfort and expedites the procedure.

Advise the client to rest for 24 hours after the procedure and to avoid any heavy lifting. Although some oozing is considered normal, the client should report any excessive bleeding (more than a regular menstrual period flow). The client should avoid douching and sexual intercourse until the biopsy site has healed completely.

Endometrial Biopsy and Aspiration

Both endometrial biopsy and aspiration are techniques to obtain cells directly from the uterine lining of women at risk for cancer of the endometrium. Endometrial biopsy is also of significant value in assessing functional menstrual disturbances (especially anovulatory bleeding) and infertility. The biopsy should be performed during the immediate premenstrual period to serve as an index of progesterone influence and ovulation. Biopsies done in the last half of the menstrual cycle (approximately Days 21 and 22) can evaluate corpus luteum function and the presence or absence of a secretory endometrium.

An endometrial biopsy is often performed as an office procedure using a small amount of intrauterine anesthesia. After the cervix has been dilated, a curet is passed through the cervix and pressed firmly against the uterine wall, and a portion of the endometrium is withdrawn by either the cuplike end of the curet or by suction. A specimen that contains malignant cells confirms the diagnosis of endometrial cancer. A negative test result does not rule out the diagnosis, however; it only provides evidence that there are no malignant cells in the limited site of the biopsy, and

carcinoma may be present in other areas of the endometrium. Women with symptoms suggestive of endometrial cancer need a diagnostic curettage for accurate diagnosis.

A disposable unit often used to obtain cytologic specimens from the entire uterine cavity is the Gravlee Jet Washer. The client is prepped, and the cervix is dilated as for the endometrial biopsy. A perforated cannula is inserted into the uterine cavity, and a rubber plug is placed at the cervical os to create an airtight system. A saline-filled reservoir and an empty syringe are attached to the end of the cannula. Pulling the plunger of the syringe causes a negative pressure to build up in the uterus, which draws the saline from the reservoir into the uterine cavity and irrigates the entire cavity. This process dislodges cells and small tissue fragments and collects them in the syringe. When the syringe is full, the cannula is removed. An important advantage of this system is the negative pressure created in the uterus. This prevents potentially malignant cells, forced from their implantation site in the uterus, from being pushed into the fallopian tubes.

Culdocentesis

Culdocentesis, or aspiration through the vaginal cul-de-sac, determines the presence or absence of free blood or pus (from a ruptured ectopic pregnancy or infection) in the pelvic cavity. Usually, no anesthesia is required for the insertion of the aspirating needle through the upper portion of the vagina. The amount of information obtained from this procedure is limited, and a negative aspirate is inconclusive.

Culdoscopy

Culdoscopy, a method of pelvic endoscopy, is the simplest procedure for direct visualization of the pelvic cavity, organs, and ligaments in women who may not require surgical intervention. Culdoscopy is highly accurate and useful in women with suspected ectopic pregnancy, primary ovarian disorders and infertility, unexplained pelvic pain, and pelvic masses of undetermined nature.

The knee-chest position is essential to provide the best view of the pelvis during the procedure. The majority of culdoscopies are done with only local anesthesia in the vaginal cul-de-sac. The culdoscope, a tubular instrument with a lamp and lens near its tip, is inserted through the cul-de-sac into the pelvic cavity (Figure 63–5). Inspection combined with abdominal palpation provides a detailed view of the pelvic contents. The examination site heals easily without sutures, but the client is advised not to douche or have intercourse for approximately 2 weeks after the procedure.

Laparoscopy

A second method of pelvic endoscopy is laparoscopy (pelvic peritoneoscopy), which is discussed in detail in Chapter 65. It is frequently used as a diagnostic procedure when minor surgery is anticipated. In addition to the indications

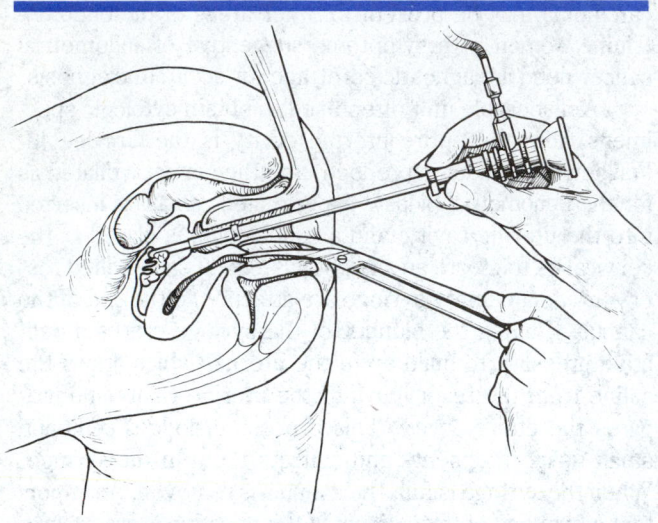

Figure 63–5

Culdoscopy. The culdoscope is inserted through the cul-de-sac. Note that the client is in the knee–chest position for this procedure.

previously listed for culdoscopy, laparoscopy provides a route for procedures such as tubal sterilization, ovarian biopsy, cyst or graafian follicle aspiration (to retrieve ova for in vitro fertilization), and lysis of adhesions around the fallopian tubes.

Hysteroscopy

Hysteroscopy permits an endoscopic view of the interior of the uterus. The hysteroscope uses a lens with fiberoptic lighting in conjunction with an aqueous solution or carbon dioxide to distend the uterus. The examiner inserts the hysteroscope through the cervix following pericervical anesthesia. Because of the necessity for a medium to distend the uterus and the opportunity for cells to be pushed through the fallopian tubes, hysteroscopy is contraindicated in clients with suspected cancer of the cervix or endometrium, as well as pelvic or upper genital tract infection. Since pregnancy is also a contraindication for the procedure, it is best performed 5 days after menses has ceased.

The use of hysteroscopy today is limited. Hysteroscopy may become a potential intrauterine route for tubal sterilization. The technique is now used as a complement to other diagnostic tests for infertility and unexplained bleeding.

Methylene Blue Test

The location of a vaginal fistula is facilitated by the instillation of methylene blue into the client's bladder. Dye that appears in the vagina indicates a vesicovaginal fistula. Dye would not appear in the vagina if the woman had a ureterovaginal fistula or a rectovaginal fistula. A test with negative results is followed by the IV injection of indigo carmine. This dye appears in the vagina of clients with

a ureterovaginal fistula. An intravenous pyelogram (IVP) and cystoscopy may also be performed to determine the location and number of fistulas.

Infertility Studies

Infertility is the failure to conceive after a year or more of regular, unprotected intercourse or the inability to carry pregnancies to live birth. Infertility differs from sterility, which implies a permanent incapacity to conceive. The diagnosis or potential diagnosis of infertility is a crisis for a woman and her partner.

The woman typically seeks treatment for infertility. Because the problem is complex and multifactorial, however, the health care provider should see both partners to obtain a more complete history and data collection. It is important to listen to the couple's separate and joint concerns. The period when the couple admits their infertility to themselves and outsiders is particularly stressful. The initial work-up and probing of the couple's intimate life threaten their maleness and femaleness and can affect their personal relationship. Having both partners available facilitates their ability to process information given to them and makes the treatment a joint concern.

Unless the couple has extenuating circumstances such as advanced maternal age, the infertility work-up is generally not begun until 1 year without conception. The initial investigation consists of a thorough medical, sexual, and social history of each partner. A physical examination and routine laboratory tests are performed for both man and woman to determine their general state of health.

The woman's infertility work-up includes a detailed history of menstruation, previous pregnancies, use of birth control techniques, and any STDs. The man's history includes questions about any previous impregnations, history of STDs, and his ability to achieve and maintain an erection and produce an ejaculate. Because infertility can be multifactorial, finding one cause in one partner does not exclude the possibility of other causes in the same partner or other partner.

To explore such sensitive areas, nurses must develop an effective interpersonal relationship with these clients. This requires an adequate working knowledge of the meaning of the diagnoses, tests, and treatments. Nurses must have worked through personal feelings about the meaning of infertility and the interventions used to treat the problem. They also should be appropriately empathic and able to allow clients to express their feelings.

Many tests employed in the infertility work-up are unpleasant and potentially embarrassing to clients. For example, clinics often are unable to provide adequate privacy and comfort in which couples can obtain semen specimens or have intercourse before a postcoital cervical mucus test. The nurse can assist by providing adequate time and space for couples to collect specimens. Health care providers also must treat the situation discreetly to protect the couple's privacy.

Basal Body Temperature Charting. A basal body temperature chart is a simple graph used as a part of infertility studies to indicate ovulatory function. Immediately upon awakening each morning, the woman takes her temperature with a basal body thermometer. This thermometer is similar to a standard oral thermometer, except the markings between degrees are easier to read. The client must take her temperature before getting out of bed to determine the body temperature at total rest. The client records the temperature on a graph that plots the degrees Farenheit for each day of the menstrual cycle. The client should keep the chart for four or more menstrual cycles to be able to identify recurring patterns. She should indicate on the chart the days when intercourse occurred and any reasons for an elevated temperature, such as fever. The charts are useful in planning optimal times for intercourse and future infertility testing (Figure 63–6).

The normal temperature chart shows a biphasic curve for each menstrual cycle. Normally, the basal body temperature is lower in the preovulatory phase. In the second phase, progesterone affects the temperature curve by causing a sustained increase of 0.4°F or more from the point of ovulation until menses begins. An irregular, low, monophasic pattern indicates anovulation with absent or inadequate progesterone production. A graph that shows a biphasic pattern with a sustained temperature elevation through the first missed period suggests pregnancy.

Keeping the basal body temperature chart can be stressful to the couple, because it calls specific attention to their infertility every day and removes spontaneity from intercourse. The couple may feel as though the chart dictates when they may express desire for each other and when they should have coitus.

Fern Test (Cervical Mucous Arborization Test). The fern test is a second simple way to assess whether a woman ovulates. The test is based on physiological evidence that the amount of sodium chloride, other electrolytes, and various proteins in cervical secretions depends on ovarian hormone production. Cervical mucus under the influence of increasing estrogen production has a high concentration of sodium chloride shortly before ovulation, so it forms crystal patterns when drying. The characteristic fern pattern, which actually resembles fern fronds, is seen in dried cervical mucus only when there is adequate estrogen (Figure 63–7A). Ovulation and the secretion of progesterone inhibits or completely abolishes this pattern even though estrogen is still being produced. During pregnancy, when there is continuous progesterone influence, this pattern also does not occur. The cervical mucus of a menopausal woman will not show ferning because of the absence of sufficient estrogen (Figure 63–7B).

The fern test is easily performed by the health care provider. The client is prepared for a pelvic examination, and her cervix is exposed with a speculum and gently swabbed clean. A sample of endocervical mucus is obtained and smeared on a glass slide. If the sample is spread too thinly or blood is present in the specimen, ferning will not occur. The slide is allowed to air-dry completely for at least 10 minutes before it is read under a microscope.

A positive fern test indicates a predominant estrogen state. The fern test also can help determine ovulation if the cervical mucous smear is inspected twice during the menstrual cycle, once during the preovulatory stage and later after the last date on which ovulation could have occurred in a menstrual cycle. If ovulation has occurred, an amorphous pattern will be present, indicating progesterone production by the corpus luteum.

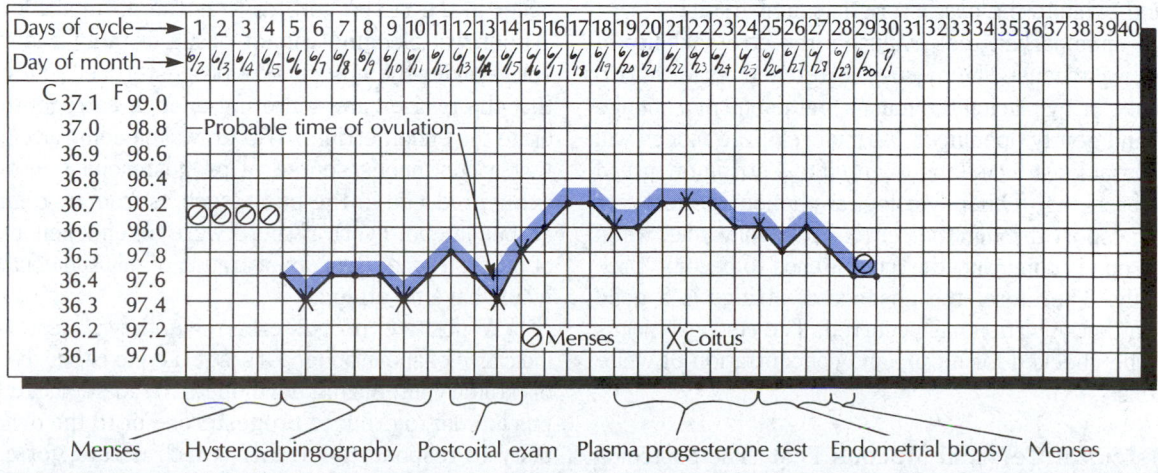

Figure 63–6

Basal body temperature chart with different types of testing and the time in the cycle that each would be performed.
SOURCE: Olds SB, London ML, Ladewig PA: *Maternal–Newborn Nursing: A Family-Centered Approach.* Menlo Park, CA: Addison–Wesley, 1984, p. 115.

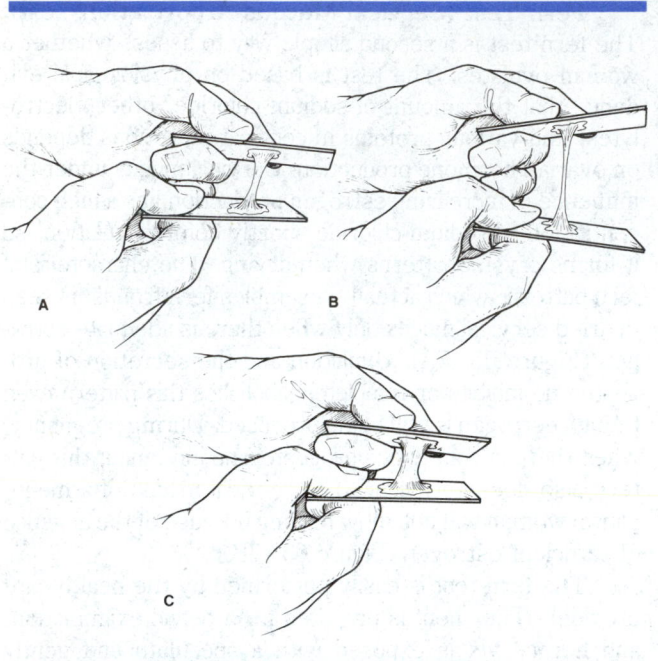

Figure 63–7
Spinnbarkeit test. **A.** Beginning of cycle. Mucus is sparse and viscid. **B.** Midcycle. Mucus is copious, resembles raw egg—white, clear, stretchy, slippery; spinnbarkeit is present. **C.** End of cycle. Mucus becomes thick and cloudy white or yellow with no spinnbarkeit.

Spinnbarkeit Test. The quantity and quality of the cervical mucus respond to the effects of estrogen and progesterone in other ways as well. At the beginning of the menstrual cycle, the mucus is scant and viscid. By midcycle, the mucus is copious, clear, slippery, and stretchy. The watery midcycle mucus has been compared to raw egg white and exhibits the characteristic spinnbarkeit.

The spinnbarkeit test evaluates the stretchability of endocervical mucus. The mucus is stretched between two glass slides or by placing the mucus on the end of a sponge forceps and gently opening it. At midcycle, the mucus will stretch for at least 5 cm (about 2 in) into a string or thread without breaking. This physiological phenomenon assists sperm transport through the cervix. After midcycle, when progesterone is dominant, the mucus tends to become thick and cloudy. Therefore, the absence of strings is a good indication that ovulation has occurred. The cervical mucus also can be checked for its pH and concentration of white blood cells.

Postcoital Cervical Mucous Test. The postcoital cervical mucous test (Sims' test or P–K test) provides both male and female reproductive system assessment data. The couple is advised to abstain from intercourse for 48 hours before the test. The test usually is scheduled on or within 24 hours of the day on which other tests (such as

the basal body temperature test) predict that ovulation should occur. The couple ideally has intercourse 4 to 8 hours (some authorities recommend as few as 2 hours or as many as 8 hours) before the woman is to be examined, and she must not tub bathe or douche after intercourse.

The woman is prepared for a pelvic examination, with the cervix exposed using a nonlubricated speculum. Samples of the endocervical mucus and secretions from the vaginal pool are examined separately under a microscope. Sperm in the cervical mucus indicates that the coital technique is adequate. If the mucus shows midcycle changes, the pH and quality of the mucus will facilitate sperm transport. A cervical mucous sperm count should show 5 to 20 sperm per high-powered field. Normally, 4 hours after intercourse 50% of the sperm will still be active. At 12 hours after intercourse, the number of active sperm normally drops to 25%.

If the cervical mucus is scanty, thick, or contains a large number of leukocytes or epithelial cells, the postcervical mucous test will invariably be abnormal. A single abnormal test result is not conclusive. It may indicate poor coital technique, low sperm count, inadequate seminal fluid, poor cervical mucous quality, or a test scheduled on the wrong day of the menstrual cycle. If the sperm are all immotile, the cervix may have been examined too late after intercourse.

Progesterone Withdrawal Test. The progesterone (progestin) withdrawal test provides data about the endometrial lining of the uterus and the ability of the ovaries to secrete estrogen. The test aids in the diagnosis of anovulation as a cause for amenorrhea.

After a negative pregnancy test, the client takes 10 to 20 mg of short-term progestin orally every day for 5 days. If there has been previous estrogen stimulation, withdrawal bleeding (the sloughing of endometrium) will occur in the next 2 to 5 days as the hormonal levels fall. Withdrawal bleeding cannot occur from an endometrium solely under the influence of progesterone, so it indicates that the ovaries are secreting enough estrogen to proliferate the endometrium. Withdrawal bleeding also indicates that a continuous source of progesterone is not already being produced in the body (such as from a pregnancy or corpus luteum cyst); if there were an endogenous source of progesterone, the administration of this additional amount would have no effect.

A positive progesterone withdrawal test is highly indicative of anovulation. This is related to either the absence of pituitary luteinizing hormone (LH) to stimulate the corpus luteum to produce progesterone or to the ovary's inability to respond to the LH (which occurs, for example, with encapsulated ovaries in Stein–Leventhal syndrome).

Estrogen–Progesterone Withdrawal Test. The investigation for the cause of amenorrhea in the client who does not have withdrawal bleeding following the progesterone withdrawal test continues with an estrogen–progesterone (E–P) withdrawal test. The woman is given 0.02 to 0.05 mg of ethinyl estradiol orally for 21 days followed by 10 to 20 mg of progestin given orally for 7 days. If the E–P withdrawal test is positive (withdrawal bleeding occurs), the client does have an endometrium, but it has not been adequately primed by endogenous estrogen.

Pregnancy Tests

Pregnancy tests are all based on the detection of human chorionic gonadotropin (HCG) in blood or urine. They are included in this text because of their use in ruling out or confirming pregnancy, as well as in aiding in the diagnosis of retained placental tissue, hydatidiform mole, and choriocarcinoma. Furthermore, because many drugs and interventions for preventive or tertiary treatment are teratogenic (causing birth defects in the fetus), the health care provider must be assured that the client is not pregnant.

Biological tests that employ laboratory animals for pregnancy testing have been abandoned in favor of immunologic tests that use a latex particle preparation sensitized to HCG. This is combined with an antiserum and a sample of the client's first voiding of the day, and the mixture is observed for clumping of the latex particles (positive result). Other pregnancy tests produce color changes if results are positive. The most accurate immunologic test results are usually available in 2 to 3 hours, but commercially available tests can provide fairly accurate results in 2 minutes. These tests can detect or rule out HCG reliably in urine specimens of women 10 to 14 days after their first missed period. Some can even detect positive samples 4 to 5 days after a missed period.

The most accurate tests for the presence of HCG in serum are radioimmunoassay and radioreceptorassay. Both use radioactive iodine and are capable of detecting small amounts of HCG in the blood. These tests approach 100% accuracy within the first days after a missed period.

Pituitary Gonadotropin Determination

Determination of the quantitative levels of follicle-stimulating hormone (FSH) and prolactin help in the differential diagnosis of reproductive tract disorders. Most of these tests are now done by radioimmunoassay. The FSH and LH levels are important in the evaluation of subfertile women. Determination of the level of prolactin helps in the investigation of women with galactorrhea (breast discharge) with or without amenorrhea.

Steroid Hormone Determination

In the diagnosis of female reproductive system disorders, the ability to determine the levels of the steroid hormones estrogen and progesterone is extremely important. The client's 24-hour urine sample can be screened for estradiol and pregnanediol (urinary by-products of estrogen and progesterone). The radioimmunoassay technique can detect both plasma estrogen and progesterone at any given time in the menstrual cycle. Progesterone levels can be indicative of ovulation and pregnancy, whereas falling serial levels of progesterone in pregnancy may indicate impending abortion.

Adrenal disorders can affect ovarian function, and the ovaries are capable of producing both adrenal steroids and androgens. Therefore, a simple measurement of the steroid compounds (estrogens, progesterone, androgens, and the corticoids) in urine samples is not always indicative of the organ in which they were produced. Although this can lead to difficulties in the interpretation of test values, most disorders with grossly abnormal organ function have characteristic patterns of steroid hormone excretion.

A measurement of androgen and adrenal corticoid metabolites is obtained from 24-hour urinary 17-ketosteroid determination. An abnormal increase in either androgen or cortisol production will elevate the 17-ketosteroid level.

Chromosomal Analysis

The nuclear sex chromatin pattern is most commonly determined by the study of oral or buccal smears (when analyzing people after birth) or by the study of fetal cells in amniotic fluid obtained by amniocentesis (aspiration of the fluid surrounding the fetus, which is obtained by introducing a needle through the maternal abdominal wall and the uterus). Vaginal smears may also be used but are generally less satisfactory. Chromosomal analysis is indicated for the differential diagnosis of clients with primary amenorrhea and ambiguous external genitalia as well as to rule out rare gonadal tumors.

Rubin's Test

The use of Rubin's test (tubal insufflation) to determine the patency of the fallopian tubes has largely been replaced by hysterosalpingography (see the next section). Rubin's test, however, can be performed in a clinic and does not expose the client to radiation or the dye used for x-ray studies. Unfortunately, it is associated with frequent false-positive readings.

For Rubin's test, carbon dioxide is passed under pressure through a cannula that goes through the cervix into the uterus (Figure 63–8). If the fallopian tubes are patent, the examiner using a stethoscope can hear gas pushing into the abdomen. The pressure changes from 80 to 120 mm Hg in the uterus to 50 to 70 mm Hg as the gas passes through the fallopian tubes. Uterine pressure that builds to 200 mm Hg indicates blocked fallopian tubes. Following the test, women experience abdominal pain and acute shoulder or scapular pain, caused by the gas exerting pressure under the diaphragm and creating pressure on the phrenic nerve. The characteristic shoulder pain (abrupt in onset and sharp but transient) from the free carbon dioxide that rises in the abdomen when the client sits up is the only valid end point that signifies a positive test. The pain

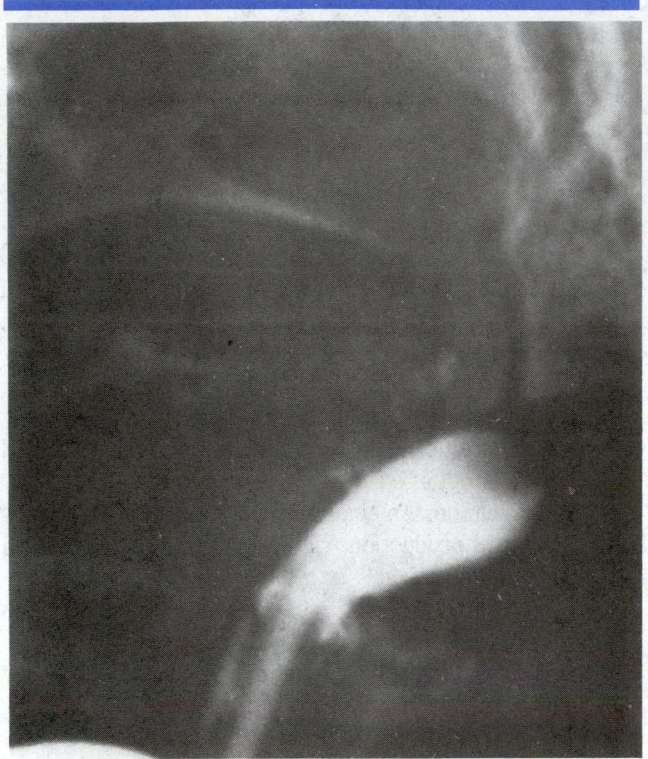

Figure 63-8

Hysterosalpingogram showing an abnormally shaped (uni-cornuate) uterus. (Courtesy of Health Care Plan, West Seneca, NY)

usually subsides in 24 hours and can be relieved by position change.

Hysterosalpingography

Hysterosalpingography is an x-ray examination following the injection of a contrast substance to highlight the interior of the cervix, uterus, and fallopian tubes. The test is useful in the evaluation of tubal anatomy and patency and the detection of uterine abnormalities (fibroids, tumors, or fistulas) in infertility work-ups. Despite the relative simplicity of the test, there is a significant incidence of false-positive and false-negative interpretations. Therefore, the findings should be confirmed by laparoscopy to provide an accurate diagnosis. Nevertheless, the wealth of information that the hysterosalpingogram provides about the interior of the uterus and fallopian tubes makes it a valuable preoperative study.

This examination should be scheduled for the second to fourth day after the end of the client's normal menstrual flow. Scheduling is important to prevent the accidental flushing of a fertilized ovum from the fallopian tube or the exposure of a fetus to radiation. Unlike Rubin's test, this procedure must be performed in a radiology department.

There are no diet restrictions before the examination. The client is usually prepared with a cathartic the evening before the test followed by an enema the morning of the

examination to reduce distortion of the x-rays by gas shadows. If the test is an outpatient procedure, the nurse should check that the client has prepared herself as ordered.

The client signs a consent form before the procedure. The nurse confirms the date of her last menstrual period and records it in the progress notes. The woman may be premedicated to promote comfort and decrease apprehension. The nurse should inform her that she may experience some nausea and vomiting, abdominal cramping, or faintness. Explain that although these are all normal, the client should inform the examiner of any severe, continuous cramping. Listen attentively to the client's concerns, and encourage her to ask questions before and after the procedure.

The client assumes the lithotomy position, and her cervix is exposed by a speculum. A few milliliters of radiopaque dye or an oil-based medium is injected through a cannula into the uterine cavity by the radiologist. Usually, only two to three x-rays are taken to show the path and distribution of the contrast medium. If the fallopian tubes are patent, the dye enters the peritoneal cavity within 10 to 15 minutes.

The phrenic nerve may be irritated by the dye and cause shoulder pain following the procedure. The dye also may drain from the cervix, so the woman should be given a perineal pad to wear for several hours following the test to prevent soiling her clothes. Inform her that she may have some bloody discharge, but if it continues for 4 days or more, she should contact her physician. The client also should contact her physician to report any signs of infection, such as lower quadrant pain, fever, malodorous discharge, and tachycardia.

Additional X-ray Studies in Gynecologic Diagnosis

The following x-ray studies are frequently used to evaluate many gynecologic disorders. An x-ray film of the abdomen that shows the kidneys, ureters, and bladder area (KUB) may show pelvic masses, calcified tumors or fibroids, dermoid cysts, or bone changes characteristic of metastatic cancer. In the routine work-up for gynecologic cancers, an IVP, barium enema, and chest film are taken to determine the extent of any metastasis or the degree of displacement or obstruction of organs caused by the disorder.

Ultrasonography

The use of ultrasonography as a diagnostic technique is becoming routine in most obstetrics and gynecology clinics. It involves no exposure to ionizing radiation and is considered safe for use during pregnancy. A photograph can be taken of the oscilloscope screen for entry into the client's permanent record. Measurement techniques are available to aid in the evaluation of the images on the screen.

In gynecologic practice, the pelvis and abdomen are scanned in a linear fashion to outline and define soft tissue masses and differentiate tumor types, ascites, and encapsulated fluid. Ultrasonography also can locate escaped intrauterine devices (IUDs) and monitor progress or tumor regression following medical treatment. The technique is especially useful in obese clients when bimanual examinations are not satisfactory to make a differential diagnosis. Ultrasonography is further discussed in Chapter 7.

Tests to Identify Pathogens

Wet Prep. A sample of the secretions in the vaginal pool (those that collect in the vagina when the client is on her back) can be obtained at the beginning of an examination that uses a nonlubricated speculum. The wet prep (simple fresh or wet smear), a standard vaginal test, is useful in the diagnosis of trichomonal or candidal vaginitis as well as nonspecific vaginitis or cervicitis. The test also can evaluate atrophic vaginitis. Curdy white plaques seen on the vaginal wall should be scraped and examined to rule out candidal vaginitis.

To perform this test, the specimen is placed on a glass slide, and a drop of saline and a coverglass are applied. The slide is examined under the microscope using both low and high power to confirm or rule out the presence of pathogens.

Other cellular components may be seen in the examination. Epithelial cells (large, nucleated, irregular, distinctly outlined cells) are usually abundant. White blood cells (round, regular, grainy, multinucleated cells) are almost always present in small amounts. Scant red blood cells may be seen even in the absence of menses. Cellular debris, clothing, fibers, and sperm also may be observed in the prep.

Potassium Hydroxide Preparation. Preparation of a vaginal smear with potassium hydroxide (KOH) greatly facilitates the diagnosis of candidal vaginitis. If possible, the specimen is obtained from the white patchy areas on the vaginal walls. If the vaginal patches are unavailable, the specimen is obtained from the erythematous area on the labia or vulva. The specimen is placed on a glass slide and combined with one drop of 10% to 20% KOH solution; this dissolves cellular debris, leaving the stained hyphae (threads or filaments) and yeast forms visible. Because it is often difficult to get a good specimen, even a single spore confirms the diagnosis.

Gram's Stain. Gram's stains are used to identify certain bacterial pathogens, including *Hemophilus vaginalis*. The specimen for the smear is obtained from the lesion or vaginal discharge. Gram's stains may not be useful in the diagnosis of gonococci in vaginal or cervical secretions because of confusion from the large number of other cells in the specimen.

Tzanck Test. The Tzanck test is used to detect genital herpesvirus type II. Scrapings from the base of a lesion

are placed on a slide and fixed with methyl alcohol for 10 minutes. The smear then is stained with Giemsa or Wright's solution and examined under a microscope. Findings typical of *herpesvirus* are giant multinucleated cells or acidophilic intranuclear inclusion bodies.

Vaginal and Cervical Cultures. Vaginal cultures are indicated to identify the pathogenic organism and determine the appropriate antibiotic therapy. Culture media are available for growing *Trichomonas,* but a culture is rarely necessary, because the differential diagnosis is readily made by examination of a wet prep. An inexpensive, accurate culture method uses Nickerson's medium to grow *Candida* in 1 to 5 days in slanted tubes. This method is especially helpful, because the identification of candidal vaginitis by wet prep alone is often difficult. When a nonspecific bacterial vaginitis is suspected, routine bacteriologic cultures and antibiotic-sensitivity studies are ordered. Viral culture mediums are available for suspected herpetic infections of the vagina, vulva, or cervix.

One of the most important cultures in gynecologic practice is the culture to detect *Neisseria gonorrhoeae.* A culture is essential for confirming the diagnosis of gonococcal infection in women, because a large number of clients that harbor the organism are asymptomatic. Collecting the specimen for an endocervical culture is discussed and illustrated in Chapter 11. Specimens also can be obtained from the urethra, rectum, and oropharynx. The swab is then rolled in a Z pattern on a medium that is selective for the growth of gonococcus and inhibits the growth of the usual vaginal and rectal contaminants. The Z pattern is then cross-streaked with a sterile wire loop to help isolate the *N. gonorrhoeae* colonies. Finally, the inoculated plates are incubated in a carbon dioxide–rich atmosphere.

Urinalysis: Culture and Sensitivity. Whenever dysuria accompanies vaginitis, a clean-catch or catheterized urine sample should be sent for analysis and culture. Often, the same organism is involved when urinary tract infections occur at the same time as vaginitis, so the results of a urine culture and sensitivity study may assist in the diagnosis and treatment of the gynecologic problem.

Instruct the client in the proper technique for obtaining a clean-catch urine sample (see Chapter 11).

Dark-Field Examination for Syphilis. A dark-field examination of the clear serum from the surface of the ulcerated lesions aids in the identification of *Treponema pallidum* in primary or secondary syphilis. The spirochete cannot be seen under direct light because it is translucent, and it cannot be stained with the usual dyes. The dark-field method of microscopic examination reflects light through the organism instead of directly onto it. A positive test identifies the spirochetes moving back and forth. If the client has applied alcohol to the lesion or used systemic or local antibiotics, the surface spirochetes will be killed, and the test will yield a false-negative result. If this is suspected, the dark-field examination should be repeated later.

Serologic Tests

Serologic tests analyze blood specimens for antigen–antibody reactions, the body's natural defenses to foreign organisms. This form of diagnostic testing is of benefit only after an infection has become well established. Gynecologic uses of serologic testing include evaluation for syphilis and rubella, as well as blood typing and screening for ABO and Rh incompatibilities. Serum titers also can be used to detect antibodies against the herpesvirus type II. A single titer is not as revealing as serial titers, which can detect the rise in antibodies with exposure to disease.

Venereal Disease Research Laboratory Test.
The Venereal Disease Research Laboratory (VDRL) test is a nontreponemal antigen test used to detect, confirm, and follow cases of syphilis. This test is not absolutely specific or sensitive for syphilis, because both false-positive and false-negative results are possible, but it is economical and highly indicative. Some acute and chronic conditions that cause false-positive results are tuberculosis, infectious mononucleosis, recent smallpox vaccination, rheumatoid arthritis, subacute bacterial endocarditis, and hepatitis.

The results of the VDRL test are read qualitatively. The normal range is nonreactive, and other results may be weakly reactive or reactive. If any reactivity is reported, the result should also be indicated quantitatively as the number of geometric dilutions required until the serum is no longer reactive. A titer of 1:8 or greater indicates syphilis. A titer above 1:32 can indicate the secondary stage of syphilis.

Any trauma to blood vessels that leads to hemolysis can interfere with the test. The blood should be drawn before meals, because any increase in chyle in the serum also can interfere with the test. (Chyle is absorbed from the intestine during digestion.) The client also should avoid alcohol for 24 hours before the test, because it will decrease the sensitivity of the test (Bryne, et al., 1981).

The results of a positive test vary with the stage of syphilis. During the first week after a chancre appears, the test is usually negative because the antibodies have not had enough time to increase sufficiently. The serologic test is usually first positive 1 to 3 weeks after the chancre appears. If the primary syphilis is treated, the serologic titers almost always return to nonreactive levels within 6 months. During the secondary stage of syphilis, the titers are very high and remain high several months after treatment. It may take up to 2 years for the serology tests to become nonreactive. In the tertiary stage of syphilis, the titers are often low and unaffected by treatment. Clients with tertiary syphilis are usually seropositive for life, and the VDRL test cannot effectively detect this latent stage.

Fluorescent Treponemal Antibody Absorption Test.
Another test used in the diagnosis of syphilis is the fluorescent treponemal antibody absorption (FTA–ABS) test. It is most useful in differential diagnosis when there is a diagnostic problem, as in a false-positive reaction to the VDRL test, and is considered the most reliable test to pick up specific antibodies in all syphilitic stages. Once positive, the test is reactive for life; therefore, even treated clients yield positive test results. A reactive FTA–ABS test, then, indicates the presence of FTA–ABS antibodies, but it cannot determine the syphilitic stage or distinguish between syphilis and other conditions caused by the treponema. A nonreactive result means there are no treponemal antibodies. If a client is suspected to be in the very early stages of syphilis (eg, has a chancre) other studies are necessary. A borderline reaction is considered inconclusive. Regardless of results, a repeat test is usually performed before the diagnosis is confirmed.

Treponema Pallidum Immobilization Test.
The *Treponema pallidum* immobilization (TPI) test uses live antibodies and must be performed at the Centers for Disease Control in Atlanta. This is the most sensitive and specific serologic test, but it is expensive, time consuming, and difficult to perform. It has few false-positive results and is used to confirm neurosyphilis.

Breast Screening

Mammography.
Mammography is a soft tissue x-ray study of the breast that is helpful as a screening tool for women at higher-than-normal risk of developing breast cancer. Mammograms are used to detect differences in the density of the breast tissue and are especially helpful in the evaluation of breasts with poorly defined masses, multiple masses or nodules, nipple changes or discharge, skin changes, and pain. Mammography can detect many cancers that are not palpable by physical examination, but some cancers appear benign on mammography. Thus, mammography should not take the place of biopsy when there is a single, dominant lump in the breast.

Mammography usually requires two low-dose x-ray views of each breast: (1) a view of the side and (2) a view from above, with the breast supported on a platform while the client is seated. Mammograms of small breasts are not as effective, because there is not sufficient breast tissue to compress in the x-ray views.

The National Cancer Institute recommends that mammograms not be used in the routine screening of women younger than 35 years but should be provided for any woman with a suspected neoplasm or at high risk for breast cancer. The American College of Radiologists and the American Cancer Society suggest that women between the ages of 35 and 40 have a baseline mammogram and annual mammograms after age 50.

The breasts of premenopausal women have a low fat content and a high percentage of glandular tissue, which increases their overall density. This makes the mammogram much less accurate in the discovery and diagnosis of breast masses. The breasts of postmenopausal women, in contrast, have a much higher fat content, which increases the accuracy of the diagnosis. In young women's breasts, there is little difference in density between normal glandular tissue and neoplasms, whereas in older women, the fatty tissue appears lighter on the mammogram than neoplasms. Cancer and cysts may have the same density, but cysts usually have smooth borders, and neoplasms often have starburst margins.

Immediately before the mammogram, ascertain whether the client is pregnant or suspects she may be pregnant. If there is any question of pregnancy, the client should reschedule the test after the pregnancy is completed. Be sure to document the client's answer to questions about pregnancy in the progress notes. During pregnancy, the breasts are more sensitive and engorged. This tends to make x-ray interpretation more difficult. Mammograms are rarely done on pregnant women because, although shielding of the abdomen is possible, it is impossible to stop the radiation from internal scattering. Biopsy of a suspicious lump is preferred.

As with other nursing interventions, explain or reinforce the purpose and procedure of the test to the client. Explain that mammography is essentially painless but that the woman may experience some discomfort when the breast is compressed during the x-ray. Provide a cover gown and adequate privacy for the client to undress. The actual test takes approximately 15 minutes; ask the client to wait until the x-rays have been developed in case a view needs to be repeated. There are no dietary restrictions prior to the mammogram. Ask the woman not to use creams, powders, or deodorant on the breasts or underarm areas before the x-rays; these products contain aluminum chlorhydrate and may show up as white on x-rays, mimicking calcium clusters.

The client needs appropriate support and time to express her concerns about the mammogram and the presence of any lumps. Address any questions she may have, or refer them to a physician. Communicate the client's concerns in the progress notes, notify the client's physician about them, or both. It is important to have a physician speak to the client to interpret the films as soon as possible after the test.

Since this is a time when the client is anxious about the health of her breasts, it is an excellent time to teach or reinforce techniques for regular monthly BSE. Assess the client's prior knowledge of breast examinations, and ask the client to demonstrate the technique to be sure she understands.

Xeromammography. The xeromammogram uses a much lower dose of radiation than the low-dose mammogram to provide a xerogram of the soft breast tissue. (A xeromammogram is illustrated in Chapter 64.) A special selenium-coated plate is placed under the breast exposed to the x-rays, and the xerogram is photoelectrically recorded on paper without the use of film. This procedure has gradually begun to replace conventional low-dose mammograms, because it is often more accurate, and the bas-relief, high-contrast effect of the picture is easier to read. Xeromammography has the same indications as low-dose mammography.

Thermography. Once thought to be a boon for the routine screening of clients for breast disease, thermography has dropped from favor because it requires expensive equipment and is difficult to interpret accurately. A thermogram is a picture of the surface temperature of the skin that does not employ ionizing radiation. Infrared photography detects the circulation pattern of different areas of the breasts. Areas of increased blood supply (eg, around tumors) produce more heat than normal breast tissue. Thermography can accurately detect large cancers but often fails to detect small or deep neoplasms.

Breast Aspiration and Biopsy. Aspiration and biopsy of suspicious breast nodules are integral parts of the diagnosis of breast masses. Aspiration cytology is useful to help determine whether nodules are benign fibrocystic nodes or solid tumors that might be malignant. If there are any associated changes in the skin, such as dimpling or fixation, the nodule should be incised or excised instead of aspirated.

Fluid aspirated from benign cysts varies from clear to green or dark brown. The color is unimportant unless it appears bloody, which suggests cancer. The fluid is most always thin. If no fluid is returned by aspiration of the nodule, the lesion is solid and should be biopsied. (See Chapter 65 for further discussion of breast aspiration and biopsy.)

Section II: Nursing Diagnosis

Assessment of the client with dysfunction of the female reproductive system can lead to a variety of nursing diagnoses (Box 63–1). The potential diagnoses most closely associated with the female reproductive system are discussed in the following sections.

ALTERATION IN COMFORT

Dysfunction of the female reproductive system can produce mild to severe pain. The client may experience dysmenorrhea and mittelschmerz as a steady, dull aching with a bearing-down sensation in the lower abdomen or as colicky cramps of varying intensity. More severe pain may be associated with endometriosis. Pain associated with spontaneous abortion is similar to labor as the uterus contracts to expel the products of conception. Severe lower abdominal pain and acute abdomen are symptoms of a ruptured tubal ectopic pregnancy. Torsion (twisting) of ovarian cysts, uterine myomas, or the anatomic supports of the adnexa, which are primarily membranous and vascular tissues, causes severe pain. The weight of heavy tumors causes stretching of these tumors into a pedicle that is predisposed to torsion. Even without stretching, torsion of a normal tube and ovary can occur. Acute or chronic PID characteristically produces pain on movement of the uterus and adnexa during jarring or pelvic examination. Pain associated with vaginitis and vaginal discharge or genital lesions can be severe and is exacerbated when urine comes in contact with the lesions during normal voiding.

GRIEVING

Women who experience reproductive system dysfunction often progress through traditional stages of grief because of an actual, perceived, or anticipated loss. (The stages of the grief process are described in Chapter 16.) The loss of reproductive ability caused by hysterectomy, severe pelvic disease, sterilization, or aging produces a characteristic grief reaction in women. Infertility causes not only the woman, but her partner as well, to grieve for the perceived loss of their biological children. Grief is also associated with the surgical removal of a breast. The diagnosis of cancer in any of the reproductive organs and its association with death cause anticipatory grief. Not all women experience the grief reaction with the same intensity; its intensity depends on the importance the woman places on her femaleness and its corresponding evidence of bodily function and beauty.

KNOWLEDGE DEFICIT

Cancer Early Warning Symptoms

The unremitting education of women regarding the early warning symptoms of cancer and the necessity of self-examination and early treatment has begun to make a difference in 5-year survival statistics (from time of diagnosis). Nurses still need to study why more women do not participate in these programs, however. For example, cancer of the breast is a leading cause of cancer death in both black and white women, and women themselves detect over 90% of breast cancers. Nevertheless, difficulty acknowledging the presence of a mass and the false hope that it will go away keep many women who discover a breast lump from seeking medical care.

Early detection by regular monthly BSE and early treatment of a malignant mass dramatically increase the survival rates. Early cancer of the cervix and uterus may be asymptomatic. Initial symptoms include irregular vaginal bleeding and foul-smelling discharge. Pain is not a symptom until late in the disease. Regular pelvic examinations with annual cytologic smears can detect early atypical cells and allow less radical treatment.

Ovulation and Sexual Function

Many misconceptions about the menstrual cycle exist and are propagated. Many young women are unaware of the time of ovulation and may misunderstand the optimal fertile period with respect to planned parenting or contraception. Sexual intercourse may be painful or nonorgasmic because the woman's understanding of her partner's and her own body function may limit her ability to express herself in a sexual relationship.

Sexually Transmitted Diseases

Sexually transmitted diseases are epidemic in the United States. Gonorrhea and syphilis have long been recognized as social problems, but recently other STDs have received media attention. Herpes simplex type II infection, chlamydiosis, trichomoniasis, and condylomata acuminata (venereal warts) are other diseases that can be sexually transmitted. Because women are afraid and ashamed of STDs, they often try to ignore the symptoms until they are severe or until the disease is discovered during a routine examination. Consequently, their partners may become infected and further spread the disease. These diseases have serious consequences. For example, a disease such as gonorrhea, if untreated, can cause chronic PID and sterility.

ALTERATION IN NUTRITION: LESS THAN BODY REQUIREMENTS

Health care providers are seeing an increasing number of young women with menstrual irregularities. Low percentages of body fat have been associated with amenorrhea and anovulation. With the social emphasis on physical fitness, many young women are participating in prolonged, strenuous exercise such as long-distance running. Studies have documented the return of normal ovulation in long-distance runners when they decreased their amount of running time and increased their percentage of body fat. Additionally, society equates beauty with thinness, which may lead some compulsive young women to develop anorexia nervosa or bulimia (see Chapter 9). Unfortunately, menstrual function does not return quickly after treatment for anorexia, and in some instances, menstruation may never return.

SELF-CARE DEFICIT RELATED TO PERINEAL HYGIENE

Because of the proximity of the female urethral, vaginal, and rectal openings, the gynecologic client may be seen for vaginal infections precipitated by incorrect perineal wiping techniques. *Escherichia coli,* a bacterial organism from the colon, causes vaginitis. Infections attributed to postero-anterior perineal wiping usually are labeled nonspecific vaginitis.

DISTURBANCE IN SELF-CONCEPT

A disturbance in self-concept may be initiated by a negative change in body image, role, or personal identity. Contributing factors that relate to female reproductive system dysfunction include loss of body parts or body function because of pathological conditions or maturational processes. Infertility, mastectomy, sexual dysfunction, and menopause often lead to a disturbance in the client's self-concept. The diagnosis of an STD can create feelings of worthlessness and punishment for perceived wrong-doing. The negative change in self-concept parallels lowered self-esteem, and situations such as pain and chronic or terminal illness can emphasize this disturbance.

Nursing Research Note

Ruby EB, Estok P: Intensity of jogging: Its relationship to selected physical and psychosocial variables in women. *West Nurs Res* 1983; 5(4): 325–335.

The authors examined the physical and psychosocial health benefits and risks associated with jogging. The sample consisted of 319 female joggers who had been participants in either a 6.2 mile run or a marathon. The sample was stratified according to the intensity of the jogging. Low-intensity joggers ran 1 to 10 miles weekly, moderate-intensity joggers ran 11 to 40 miles weekly, and high-intensity joggers ran 41 to 112 miles weekly.

A variety of physical symptoms were associated with jogging. One-fourth (25%) of the subjects noted change in appetite, weight loss, muscle soreness, bowel habit alteration, knee and foot pain, and increased libido. Less than 5% had difficulty with torn ligaments, infertility, hematuria, chest pain, heart palpitations, prolapsed uterus, dizziness, or feeling blue. High-intensity runners reported a greater incidence of appetite changes, stress fractures, missed or scant menses, hematuria, and hip problems.

Psychosocially, the majority of the runners reported higher levels of self-esteem and improved interpersonal relationships. High-intensity runners reported more problems with interpersonal relationships; as the intensity of running increased so did the number of problems. Anxiety levels were lower among high-intensity runners.

Educating female joggers about physical and psychological benefits and risks of running is a nursing responsibility. Moderation and a healthy outlook toward the degree of involvement must be incorporated. Education should focus on potential injuries, proper training, and equipment to minimize injury and enhance the benefits.

SEXUAL DYSFUNCTION RELATED TO LOSS OF A BODY PART OR BODY FUNCTION

Pathophysiological, psychological, or situational factors can negatively affect a client's sexual health or function. For example, a woman may perceive her sexual experience as unrewarding or inadequate following a mastectomy or hysterectomy. Vulvar lesions may cause painful coitus. The pressure that infertility places on a couple often causes the sexual relationship to be unsatisfying.

IMPAIRMENT OF SKIN INTEGRITY

Excessive vaginal discharge facilitates the growth of organisms that thrive in a warm, moist environment. Irritation of the vulva with redness, edema, and general malaise often follows. Lesions of the vulva from *Candida albicans* or herpes simplex virus may be associated with intense itching and lead to further skin breakdown attributed to scratching and secondary infections. Mechanical irritation from tight or nonabsorbent clothing and chemical irritants such as deodorants and douches also can cause skin alterations.

Section III: Planning and Implementation

A sample nursing care plan with nursing diagnoses and related client care goals, interventions, and expected outcomes for the female client with reproductive system dysfunction is presented in Table 63–2 and discussed in this section.

PROMOTING COMFORT

The client often can tolerate mild to moderate discomfort associated with common gynecologic disorders such as ovulatory and menstrual pain after being assured that her physiology is normal. Accurate information about the character and length of time the client should feel the pain is also helpful.

Pain is best tolerated when the client can stay in control of the situation. The client can learn relaxation techniques such as controlled breathing, massage, and concentrating on a focal point prior to the anticipated discomfort and use them when needed. A support person can provide reassurance and distraction to help relieve even severe pain after surgery. Dry or wet heat can aid in muscle relaxation and promote healing by increasing circulation to the area. The client should be encouraged to change positions and be made more comfortable with pillows or blankets to decrease pressure or muscle tension.

The nurse may also administer prescribed analgesics to the client, and the choice and dosage of the drug should be appropriate for the severity of the pain. Partially because of its antiprostaglandin effect, aspirin has long been used as an analgesic for dysmenorrhea. Some of the newer pain preparations that contain ibuprofen (Advil, Nuprin) also have this characteristic. Narcotics are prescribed for severe pain associated with a number of gynecologic disorders. Topical anesthetics may be used by clients with vulvar lesions.

WORKING THROUGH GRIEF

Grief can occur without death or terminal illness; the loss of any significant object, function, or relationship can precipitate the grief response. Women might equate mastectomies and hysterectomies with disfigurement and decreased femininity. The loss may be intensified by the lost opportunity for breast feeding, lessened sexual arousal, or the inability to reproduce and menstruate. The loss of "normal" reproductive function and biological children plague infertile couples, who must grieve for the children they never had. Even women who undergo voluntary sterilization experience grief over the permanent prevention of future conceptions.

When working with clients experiencing a grief reaction, be available for supportive listening. Acknowledge the woman's loss and assess her grief stage. Some clients may be in a state of denial and hear only information with which they are capable of dealing. By acknowledging the client's grief and being available, the nurse provides the woman the opportunity to express her feelings.

The client also needs permission to express negative feelings, and discussing these difficult feelings promotes the normal progression of the grief response. Explain the anticipated stages of grief and convey that these feelings are normal and do not progress in a linear fashion. The client should understand that certain circumstances may trigger a return to a previously "completed" stage of grief. Local support groups or community volunteers should be investigated. Time should be allocated during follow-up physical examinations to assess the appropriateness of the client's present stage of grief and the effect it is having on her activities of daily living.

PROMOTING LEARNING
Cancer Early Warning Symptoms

The major early warning symptoms of cancer are discussed in Chapter 12. The following symptoms relate specifically to female reproductive system dysfunction:

- Unusual bleeding or discharge
- A thickening or lump in the breast or elsewhere
- A change in bowel or bladder habits (because of the proximity of the reproductive organs)

Women must develop an awareness of their own bodies to be able to detect subtle changes that could indicate an early malignancy. Female clients should routinely receive information and demonstration of self-examination procedures such as BSE, which is thoroughly discussed and illustrated in Chapter 7. The mass media also help reinforce such teaching. Women should be encouraged to have annual physical examinations and cytologic screening.

Ovulation and Sexual Function

The routine gynecologic examination should include an assessment of the client's understanding of her menstrual cycle. She may be encouraged to keep a daily record of her cycle to assist in determining the time and duration of bleeding. A review of this record is especially helpful to young women as they gain an understanding of their body functions, including an awareness of probable fertile periods. In infertility investigations, a recording of the basal body temperature may accompany the daily record. Be sure that the client understands the principles of the study and the documentation techniques.

In caring for clients with sexual dysfunction, be supportive and nonjudgmental when hearing the chief concern. Some clients may be relieved to know that their

Table 63–2   Sample Nursing Care Plan for a Client With Female Reproductive System Dysfunction

Nursing Diagnosis	Client Care Goals	Plan/Nursing Implementation	Expected Outcome
Alteration in comfort, related to pain	Ability to state physiologic explanation of pain and two nonpharmacologic methods of pain relief, use nonpharmacologic methods, attain pain relief without excess drowsiness or decrease in activities of daily living, avoid pain on voiding or ambulation, sleep and rest comfortably	Explain normal physiology of affected reproductive system component; explain physiological reason for pain (if known); teach relaxation techniques; use comfort measures (ie, heat and massage); teach musculature support; encourage use of support person; provide environment conducive to rest and sleep; administer pain medications p.r.n. if appropriate	Client describes physiology of her pain (if known); states at least two nonpharmacologic methods of pain relief; attempts nonpharmacologic methods of pain relief; performs normal activities of daily living without pain or excess drowsiness; ambulates without pain; voids without pain; sleeps and rests without disturbance from pain
Grieving	Ability to describe the meaning of loss, proceed appropriately through stages of grief, express negative feelings, communicate with significant others, continue to perform activities of daily living	Acknowledge loss to client; be available to listen; explain what to expect in normal grief stages; give permission to express negative feelings; encourage client to express meaning of loss; encourage client to perform activities of daily living; provide contact for support group; provide follow-up assessment of grief stage	Client verbalizes meaning of loss; is in appropriate stage of grief; performs previously expected activities of daily living
Knowledge deficit, related to early cancer warning symptoms	Ability to state warning symptoms of gynecologic cancer and accurately perform monthly BSE; annual Pap test	Teach cancer warning symptoms and BSE; use return demonstration; encourage client to return for cytologic examination	Client states gynecologic cancer warning symptoms; demonstrates correct technique for breast self-examination; performs examinations at regular monthly intervals; returns annually for Pap test
Knowledge deficit, related to ovulation and sexual function	Ability to understand normal menstrual cycle physiology, determine approximate time of ovulation, conceive only when desired, have no pain during intercourse, follow medical orders about sexual relations, experience satisfaction with sexual function	Establish nonjudgmental, supportive relationship; explain normal menstrual cycle physiology; teach techniques for approximating time of ovulation; teach contraceptive methods and help with decision making; provide information on coital techniques to decrease discomfort; provide information on nongenital methods of mutual satisfaction; administer prescribed medications; encourage discussion of feelings with partner	Client states menstrual physiology; indicates approximate time she ovulates; has no unplanned pregnancies or pain with intercourse; states satisfaction with sexual function
Knowledge deficit, related to STDs	Ability to understand symptoms of, mode of, transmission of, and means of protection from, STDs; not experience recurrence of STD after teaching;	Establish nonjudgmental, supportive relationship; teach symptoms and transmission of STDs; teach means of protection from STDs; encourage compliance with complete treatment	Client states symptoms of major STDs, mode of transmission, and means of protection; completes total treatment; has no recurrence of STD after treatment

(continued)

Table 63–2 Sample Nursing Care Plan for a Client With Female Reproductive System Dysfunction (continued)

Nursing Diagnosis	Client Care Goals	Plan/Nursing Implementation	Expected Outcome
	accept and comply with complete course of STD treatment if appropriate		
Alteration in nutrition: Less than body requirements	Ability to state the four basic food groups and obtain adequate food to meet minimum daily requirements; consumption of balanced diet daily; increase in amount of body fat; ability to describe causative factors (if known); normal menstrual function	Teach importance of four basic food groups; refer to supplemental food source services if appropriate; discuss methods of food preparation to increase attractiveness and palatability; divide total daily required calories into smaller frequent meals; refer client to psychotherapy if appropriate; encourage social contact when eating; allow client to choose from menu	Client states four basic food groups; has adequate food supplies available; chooses appropriate foods from menu; consumes at least minimum daily requirements; increases percentage of body fat; resumes normal menstrual function; states causative factor of decreased food consumption
Self-care deficit, related to perineal hygiene	Understanding of the importance of correct perineal wiping (in an anterior-to-posterior direction); cleanliness of perineum	Teach and reinforce correct wiping techniques; teach mode of fecal contamination and relationship to infection; provide ample supplies to encourage correct perineal wiping	Client states importance of correct wiping and states or demonstrates correct wiping technique; maintains clean perineum
Disturbance in self-concept	Ability to develop positive body image, discuss meaning of loss, increase control of own life, perform appropriate activities of daily living	Establish trusting relationship; be an active listener; reinforce positive feelings; clarify misconceptions; promote social interaction; provide anticipatory guidance	Client states improvement of body image; discusses meaning of loss with nurse and significant others; is able to make decisions more easily; performs all previously established activities of daily living
Sexual dysfunction related to loss of body part or body function	Demonstration of movement toward acceptance of loss; ability to discuss meaning of loss; resumption of sexual relations	Establish trusting relationship; encourage discussion of meaning of loss; encourage sharing of concerns with partner; role play through fear of rejection; encourage discussion of strengths of relationship; give permission for resumption of sexual relations	Client views and discusses loss with less discomfort; discusses meaning of loss to self and relationship; states sexual relations have resumed
Impairment of skin integrity	Ability to state cause of skin lesions or pruritus; external genitalia free of edema, redness, irritation, and itching; maintenance of perineal hygiene; avoidance of alkaline soaps, douches, and genital deodorants; completion of prescribed treatment; ability to rest and sleep comfortably	Explain cause of skin breakdown; teach use of sitz baths, heat lamps, and frequent change of pads; provide adequate supplies to maintain hygiene; reinforce necessity of completion of full course of treatment; provide environment conducive to rest and sleep; provide distraction if client has pruritus; encourage client to keep nails short and clean; demonstrate proper method of perineal wiping; encourage use of nonrestrictive, natural-fiber undergarments to allow ventilation	Client states cause of lesions and/or pruritus; has external genitalia without lesions, edema, redness, or itching; maintains perineal hygiene; does not use excessive alkaline soaps, douches, or deodorants; completes total treatment; is able to rest and sleep without disturbance from perineal pain or itching

problem is not unique and that treatment is often successful. The nurse must be comfortable conversing with both members of the couple about intimate details of their sexual lives and may need to interpret medical terminology in terms the couple can understand.

Sexually Transmitted Diseases

The ability to discuss sexuality comfortably is mandatory for the health care provider counseling clients about STDs. The client may feel embarrassed to seek information or treatment about any one of the STDs, so the nurse must convey respect, privacy, and concern to encourage the client to seek or continue with the prescribed treatment. The nurse should advise the client about:

- The meaning of STD
- Early symptoms of STDs
- The mode of disease transmission
- The course of the disease
- The means of disease prevention
- Medical follow-up of sexual partners
- Required reporting of the disease, if applicable

Sexually transmitted diseases are discussed in Chapter 64.

IMPROVING NUTRITIONAL INTAKE

Health care providers must have insight into why a client consumes amounts inadequate to meet nutritional requirements. The possibility of pathological conditions should be eliminated through medical screening. If no such condition exists and adequate food is available, the client may need to seek psychological counseling. Women with inadequate body fat levels to support normal menstrual function should be counseled about a balanced daily diet and appropriate caloric requirements. The nurse may suggest alternative meal plans that might work better in the client's lifestyle. Support and encouragement need to be given through follow-up counseling. Social programs should be explored to assist women who do not have the means to purchase adequate foods. These can provide low-cost foods and preparation guides to maximize the client's food-value intake. (See also Chapter 9.)

IMPROVING PERINEAL HYGIENE

The nurse should advise clients on the correct technique to wipe the perineum: from front to back, disposing of the tissue after a single wipe. This technique prevents inadvertent contamination of the urethra and vagina by rectal flora. During foreplay and intercourse, the client should take care to avoid cross-contamination from the rectal area to the vagina. Intercourse can encourage the development of cystitis by friction and the spread of vaginal bacteria to the urethra. Voiding immediately after intercourse can prevent bacteria from ascending into the urethra.

IMPROVING SELF-CONCEPT

The nurse must develop a trusting relationship with the client, who will then begin to express feelings about the way she views herself. The nurse should be an active listener to facilitate further conversation, provide accurate information, clarify misconceptions, and supply positive feedback. Help the client gain control over her body through adequate rest and relaxation, increased mobility, self-awareness, self-examination of her body, viewing and accepting perceived disfigurement, and identifying stressors and coping mechanisms. Provide health teaching related to the client's specific needs. Through careful guidance, the client can accept her altered body image and lifestyle. Her self-concept will improve as she finds she is gaining control of her life.

IMPROVING SEXUAL FUNCTION

After assessing the cause of the client's sexual dysfunction, use active listening to determine how the dysfunction affects the client. The client's acceptance of sexual dysfunction from the loss of a body part or function is aided by progression through the appropriate stages of grieving (see Chapter 16 and "Working Through Grief" in this chapter). Normal sexual function also depends on a positive self-concept (see the previous section about improvement of self-concept). Upon medical approval, couples need to be given permission to participate in sexual relations, and any restrictions of activity should be fully explained to both

---

Nursing Research Note

Muhlenkamp A, Waller M, Bourne A: Attitudes towards women in menopause: A vignette approach. *Nurs Res* 1983; 32(1):20–23.

Female subjects were studied regarding their attitudes toward menopause. The vignettes consisted of three types of illustrations: a female during climacteric, a nonclimateric female, and a middle-aged male.

There was no difference in semantic ratings of the male at midlife and the climacteric female or between a male at midlife and a nonclimateric female. The subjects ranked females in the vignettes lower than themselves in the semantic differential ratings. There was no difference between male and female vignette characters on semantic ratings. Subjects ranked themselves higher than males in semantic differential ratings. Subjects' levels of self-esteem did not affect the ratings of the vignettes or the rating of themselves.

This study indicates that women see menopause as a normal process and not a disease. There was not a negative attitude once associated with the term *change of life.* Nurses can foster this positive attitude by teaching about normal physiological processes during the middle years. Nurses can also correct misinformation and misunderstanding about menopause.

partners. Encourage clients and their partners to express their concerns about sexual activities and provide them with suggestions to minimize potential difficulties, including ways to project acceptance of the partner and preserve modesty. The client may appreciate information on the use of vaginal lubricants, position changes to prevent pressure discomfort, and nongenital methods of mutual satisfaction.

Women with genital lesions or pathogenic discharge should be advised not to engage in sexual intercourse until they have completed the full course of the treatment. If this is unacceptable to the couple, the male should use a condom.

IMPROVING SKIN INTEGRITY

The improvement of skin integrity depends on the prevention of further skin breakdown. In female reproductive disorders, the genital skin is often compromised because of the continually warm, moist environment. Normal skin integrity requires cleanliness of the perineum, but some vaginal discharge is normal and nonoffensive. Some women have difficulty accepting this physiological phenomenon, however, and routinely use strong alkaline soaps, douches, and deodorants to keep themselves "clean." This assists in the destruction of normal flora, predisposing the client to further skin breakdown.

The client with pruritus should be informed about its causes. Since moist clothing may aggravate pruritus, the client should attempt to stay as clean and dry as possible by frequently changing perineal pads. Distraction can prevent total concentration on the itching, and fingernails should be kept short if the client is inclined to scratch the area. Control of the offending organism by appropriate medication resolves the itching.

In health teaching, recommend undergarments that provide ventilation through natural fibers. Nonrestrictive clothing prevents chafing. Women with heavy vaginal discharge should use and frequently change pads or tampons.

Women being treated for a vaginal infection should complete the total treatment even after the initial symptoms subside. If vaginal tablets or suppositories are prescribed, the woman should remain recumbent for approximately 30 minutes after application to allow for some absorption and dispersal of medication in the upper vaginal area. She should expect some drainage of the medication, which is best coped with by wearing a perineal pad. (Tampons should be avoided because they absorb too much of the medication.) The client should continue treatment even if she begins to menstruate, and she should avoid intercourse until treatment has been completed. If the vaginal irritation is an allergic response, the offending substance must be removed. If the external genitalia are swollen and uncomfortable, sitz baths with warm water can promote comfort and speed healing by increasing circulation to the area. Air drying and exposing the area to a heat lamp also can provide relief.

Section IV: Evaluation

ALTERATION IN COMFORT

Client care goals have been met if the woman is able to perform activities of daily living without pain or excessive drowsiness and if she is able to rest and sleep without disturbance from pain. Unfortunately, gynecologic pain is often cyclical during the reproductive years. Women who suffer from cyclical pain are often best managed with a combination of reproductive physiology teaching, reassurance, comfort and relaxation techniques, and pharmacologic interventions. Nursing interventions are considered effective if the client can state the physiology of her pain, attempts nonpharmacologic pain relief, and appropriately uses pain medications.

GRIEVING

The woman is evaluated as having an appropriate grief response if she is able to perform previously expected activities of daily living. Nursing interventions are considered successful if the client is able to verbalize the meaning of her loss and feels permitted to express the magnitude of her feelings. Warning symptoms of pathological grief include prolonged denial, inappropriate cheerfulness or hostility, agitated depression, continuing isolation, and excessive or disproportionate grieving in relation to the degree of the loss. Individuals most likely to develop these symptoms are those with a history of depression and with poor interpersonal relationships.

KNOWLEDGE DEFICIT

Client education is considered effective if the woman can successfully demonstrate BSE and states that she performs BSE on a monthly basis. The client should also be able to state correctly the warning symptoms of gynecologic cancer. Perhaps more importantly, client education is considered effective if the woman has achieved some control over her own body and is able to seek prompt health care at the onset of her suspicions.

Successful client teaching will enable the woman to describe her menstrual cycle physiology and to utilize this information to promote or prevent conception. The client should feel comfortable enough with the health care provider to be able to discuss coital problems and methods for noncoital sexual satisfaction. Following appropriate therapy, the client should be able to state that she has no pain with intercourse and is satisfied with her sexual function.

Compliance with the total medical treatment of the STD and prevention of recurrence of STDs are data supporting goal achievement. The client needs to feel comfortable discussing sexual concerns with the health care provider if the teaching is to be effective. Goal criteria that must be achieved to prevent a future STD include knowledge of signs and symptoms of STDs, the modes of transmission, and the means of protection.

ALTERATION IN NUTRITION: LESS THAN BODY REQUIREMENTS

Expected outcomes for a female client whose reproductive function is inhibited due to failure to meet minimum nutritional requirements include the ability to state the recommended daily amounts of each of the basic food groups, to choose appropriate foods, and to show an increase in body weight and fat. The client should receive support from the nurse and significant others. The nurse may refer the client to a support group or for psychotherapy.

The resumption of normal menstrual function is not expected immediately upon compliance with the above criteria. The client should understand that the initiation of menstruation may be delayed for some time.

SELF-CARE DEFICIT: PERINEAL HYGIENE

Following effective teaching, the client should be able to state the correct method of wiping the perineum and its importance. Her perineum will remain clean, and there will be no occurrence of urinary or vaginal infection secondary to fecal contamination.

SELF-CONCEPT

Expected outcomes of nursing support and guidance should lead to an improvement of the client's self-image. An effective interpersonal relationship between the nurse and the client should permit her to verbalize feelings of loss and negative thoughts. Anticipatory guidance should assist the woman to clarify misconceptions and perform activities of daily living.

SEXUAL DYSFUNCTION: LOSS OF BODY PART OR FUNCTION

From a respectful and supportive nurse–client relationship, the client is able to verbalize feelings about the meaning of the loss. With increased acceptance of the loss and anticipatory guidance about methods to enhance the sexual relationship, the woman is able to resume a satisfactory sexual life.

SKIN INTEGRITY

Absence of lesions and genitalia discomfort are results of successfully met client care goals. The woman is able to state the correct method of perineal hygiene and refrains from irritants that may alter normal vaginal pH. She also completes the total medically prescribed treatment and is able to rest and sleep without disturbance from perineal discomfort.

Chapter Highlights

When interviewing clients with female reproductive system dysfunction, it is important to assume a supportive and nonjudgmental attitude and to allot sufficient time.

Reproductive system disorders may be multifaceted and produce complaints similar to disorders of other body systems.

Female reproductive system disorders are commonly related to pain, vaginal discharge, and bleeding. They can often be diagnosed from a complete history and information on the timing, character, and location of the symptoms. The physical examination confirms the diagnosis in many cases.

Sensitive support from the nurse will help female clients cope with the wide variety of invasive and noninvasive laboratory and diagnostic studies used in gynecology.

Nursing interventions to promote comfort and alleviate pain in gynecologic disorders include teaching relaxation and control techniques and administering prescribed analgesics.

The loss of menstrual function, as in menopause, can produce a normal grief reaction. Surgical loss of reproductive ability or a breast also can produce grief. Help these clients to express their feelings and provide information about the grief process.

The nurse should instruct clients about the early warning symptoms of gynecologic cancer and self-examination procedures to promote early detection.

The client's knowledge deficit related to ovulation, sexual function, or STDs can be overcome by supportive, nonjudgmental, and informative nursing consultation and advice.

(continued)

Chapter Highlights *(continued)*

Teaching the female client with an inadequate percentage of body fat about good nutrition, and providing her with support and proper food choices, will help promote the return of her menstrual function. Proper perineal hygiene is necessary to prevent urinary and vaginal contamination from fecal material.

Careful nursing guidance can help the client accept altered body image and lifestyle, improve her self-concept, and can improve her sexual function.

The improvement of skin integrity depends on the prevention of further skin breakdown. Health teaching is important to promote normal vaginal flora, control pruritus, and help clients understand and follow treatment regimens for vaginal infections.

Bibliography

Byrne JC et al: *Laboratory Tests: Implications for Nursing Care,* 2nd ed. Menlo Park, CA: Addison–Wesley, 1986.

Cancer Facts and Figures: 1985: New York: American Cancer Society, 1985.

Carpenito LJ: *Nursing Diagnosis: Application to Clinical Practice.* Philadelphia: Lippincott, 1983.

Fischbach F: *A Manual of Laboratory Diagnostic Tests,* 2nd ed. Philadelphia: Lippincott, 1984.

Fogel CI, Woods NF: *Health Care of Women: A Nursing Perspective.* St. Louis: Mosby, 1981.

Frank DI: Counseling the infertile couple. *J Psychosoc Nurs* 1984; 22(5):17–23.

Green TH: *Gynecology: Essentials of Clinical Practice,* 3rd ed. Boston: Little, Brown, 1977.

Jensen MD, Bobak IM: *Maternity and Gynecologic Care: The Nurse and the Family.* St. Louis: Mosby, 1985.

Martin LL: *Health Care of Women.* Philadelphia: Lippincott, 1978.

Peckman BM, Shapiro SS: *Signs and Symptoms in Gynecology.* Philadelphia: Lippincott, 1983.

Sawatzky M: Tasks of infertile couples. *J Gyn Nurs* 1981; 10:132–133.

Suggested Readings

Bell R (editor): *Changing Bodies, Changing Lives: A Book for Teens on Sex and Relationships.* New York: Random House, 1980. This book for the lay population grew out of *Our Bodies, Ourselves: A Book by and for Women.* It can serve as a reference for nurses helping teens and parents with sexual health education. The book, which includes sections about body changes, the development of sexual awareness, and emotional and physical health care in adolescence, is illustrated by relevant diagrams and photographs.

Boston Women's Health Book Collective: *The New Our Bodies, Ourselves: A Book by and for Women.* New York: Simon & Schuster, 1985. This excellent book is based on the premise that women need to learn about their bodies in order to be in control of their lives. It covers all topics pertinent to women's health care.

Carpenito LJ: Alterations in comfort. In: *Nursing Diagnosis: Application to Clinical Practice.* Philadelphia: Lippincott, 1983. This excellent presentation includes etiological factors, assessment criteria, nursing goals and principles, and the rationale of nursing care. The section includes discussions on acute pain and chronic pain appropriate to the care of the gynecologic client.

Menning BE: *Infertility: A Guide for the Childless Couple.* Englewood Cliffs, NJ: Prentice–Hall, 1977. Although this book is a number of years old, it is a comprehensive summary of infertility physiology, psychology, and treatment, appropriate for laypersons as well as health care professionals. Ms. Menning is also the founder and director of RESOLVE, INC. (See resources list.)

Woods NF: Infertility. In: *Health Care of Women: A Nursing Perspective.* Fogel CI, Woods NF (editors). St. Louis: Mosby, 1981. This comprehensive discussion of the etiology of male and female infertility includes sociocultural perspectives and provides an excellent summary of the health assessment of the infertile couple from the initial contact through analysis of test results. The discussion also includes current treatment and the meaning of infertility as a life crisis.

Resources

SELF-HELP GROUPS AND OTHER ORGANIZATIONS

American Fertility Society
1608 Thirteenth Avenue South
Birmingham, AL 35205
Phone: (205) 933–7222

An organization of health care professionals interested in infertility that responds to written requests for referral to infertility specialists in local communities.

Association for Voluntary Sterilization
708 Third Avenue
New York, NY 10017
Phone: (212) 986–3880

This association can refer clients considering tubal ligation or vasectomy to specialists and treatment centers for consultation. It also offers information and sponsors educational programs.

DES–Action
PO Box 1977
Plainview, NY 11803
Phone: (516) 433-7070

This organization is for women who took the hormone

DES during pregnancy and their daughters. It conducts workshops, training courses, and seminars and publishes a newsletter. Also provides referrals to physicians who are specialists in DES exposure and to "rap" groups.

ENCORE (Contact a local YWCA)

This is a national YWCA program for postoperative breast cancer clients. It includes floor and pool exercises and group discussions.

HELP
PO Box 100
Palo Alto, CA 94302
Phone: (415) 321–5134

This organization provides information about herpes genitalis and advice on coping with it.

Janus Information Facility/Gender Clinic
University of Texas Medical Branch
Galveston, TX 77550
Phone: (713) 765–3924

Clients who are considering a sex change operation or who have questions about transsexualism can obtain information from this facility. Requests for information must be accompanied by a contribution of at least $5.00 to cover handling and postage.

National Gay Task Force
80 Fifth Ave., Suite 1601
New York, NY 10011

Offers information and support to gay persons or to those interested in personal and social issues affecting same-sex intimate relationships.

National Woman's Health Network
224 Seventh St., SE
Washington, DC 20003

This feminist health advocacy and resource group offers addresses of local women's health services and is concerned with women's health issues such as maternal and child health during pregnancy and birth, conception control, abortion, breast cancer, and toxic shock syndrome.

Reach to Recovery
American Cancer Society, Inc.
777 Third Ave.
New York, NY
Phone: (212) 371-2900

An American Cancer Society visitor program that offers support for women who have breast cancer. Volunteers who have breast cancer demonstrate exercises and provide information and a temporary breast form.

RESOLVE, INC.
PO Box 474
Belmont, MA 02178
Phone: (617) 484-2424

This national organization provides support, counseling, and referral services for infertile couples through trained telephone counselors. Referrals to artificial insemination and adoption facilities are also offered.

Sex Information and Education Council of the United States (SIECUS)
Suite 304

5010 Wisconsin Ave., N. W.
Washington, DC 20016
Phone: (202) 686–2523

This organization maintains an information clearinghouse on all aspects of human sexuality and will help clients locate information.

HOT LINES

Genetic and Teratogen Hot Line
Phone: (212) 270-2072 from 10 AM to 4 PM weekdays

Genetic counselors from the State University of New York Downstate Medical Center respond to calls about infectious, environmental, and genetic hazards. This hot line also provides information to expectant parents who may want to know the effects of a specific drug on the unborn fetus.

VD National Hot Line
Phone: (800) 227-8922 (nationwide, except CA) from 8 AM to 8 PM weekdays and from 10 AM to 6 PM weekends. In California call (800) 982–5883.

This toll-free number offered by the American Social Health Organization provides confidential answers about venereal disease and the locations of over 5000 free or low-cost treatment services in the continental United States.

HEALTH INFORMATION MATERIAL

From: National Cancer Institute
Bethesda, MD 20205

The Breast Cancer Digest is an excellent 212-page book for professionals. It covers the psychosocial as well as the physiological aspects of breast cancer with a comprehensive guide to audiovisual materials and professional and client educational materials.

Teaching Breast Self-Examination: A Guide for Nurses is a brochure and a pocket-sized card of the basic points to be covered in BSE instruction.

SPECIALTY ORGANIZATIONS

American Association of Sex Educators, Counselors and Therapists
One East Wacker Dr.
Chicago, IL 60601

This organization is involved in sex education, research, and therapy and certifies qualified sex educators and counselors. Provides client referrals.

Nurses Association of the American College
of Obstetricians and Gynecologists (NAACOG)
600 Maryland Ave., SW, Suite 22 East
Washington, DC 20024
Phone: (202) 638-0026

The goals of this organization are to stimulate interest in and promote high standards in gynecologic, obstetric, and neonatal nursing. Membership comprises RNs and allied health workers with primary job responsibilities in these specialty areas. Dues, $60.

Chapter 64

Specific Disorders of the Female Reproductive System

Diane Wind Wardell

Objectives

When you have finished studying this chapter, you should be able to:

List congenital disorders of the female reproductive system and describe the general nursing implications in caring for these clients.

Identify the treatment measures for primary dysmenorrhea and infertility.

Help the client explore changing sexual and reproductive roles in the presence of amenorrhea, alterations in cyclic bleeding, dysfunctional uterine bleeding, endometriosis, and premenstrual syndrome.

Discuss the clinical manifestations and treatment measures

for disorders of pelvic relaxation, including uterine prolapse, cystocele, and rectocele.

Explain the risks and nursing measures involved in the various treatments for menopausal symptoms.

Instruct clients in measures to prevent or reduce the risk of infectious vaginitis or sexually transmitted diseases.

Explain the circumstances associated with neoplastic disorders of the female reproductive tract and interventions for these disorders.

Describe the causes of the most common traumatic disorders of the female reproductive tract and the nursing measures associated with these lacerations, hematomas, and fistulas.

Conditions that affect the female reproductive system include congenital, multifactorial, degenerative, infectious and inflammatory, and neoplastic disorders as well as traumatic disorders from surgery, irradiation, and injury. This chapter will discuss the etiology, significance, clinical manifestations, therapeutic measures, and specific nursing measures for these disorders.

Section I: Congenital Disorders

Congenital disorders affecting the female reproductive system involve some abnormal process in the embryonic development of the fetus at the time of sexual differentiation. Because they affect internal structures, some congenital disorders may not manifest themselves until menarche or when they delay or prohibit menarche. Problems manifested at birth are treated in childhood.

A congenital disorder usually is identified when the client has difficulty with menstruation or fertility. The disorder alters the client's body image because of a conflict between reality and what she anticipates as normal in the reproductive system. The more severe the disorder, the greater its potential to alter body image.

General Nursing Implications

The nurse in the primary care setting is responsible for planning care, teaching the client about the therapeutic regimen, and providing necessary support to enable the client to accept the diagnosis. The nurse informs the client about testing procedures that may be required, such as ultrasonography and laparoscopy, and develops a care plan specific to the client's needs and diagnosis, including referring the client to other resources. The plan may require that the client merely be observed, not treated, over time. The nurse schedules follow-up examinations and stresses the importance of following the therapeutic regimen, and refers the client to appropriate community resources (see Chapter 63, Resources). Finally, the nurse's acceptance of the individual client influences how the client perceives herself in relation to other women.

MÜLLERIAN APLASIA

Müllerian aplasia is the anatomic condition in which the vagina ends in a blind pouch with either no uterus or a rudimentary uterus that does not function. The defect occurs during the development of the reproductive system in the eighth week of embryonic development (see Chapter 61). Müllerian aplasia usually occurs sporadically but may affect members of the same family.

Clinical Manifestations and Therapeutic Measures

The client usually seeks medical attention because of amenorrhea. The normal karyotype of 46XX is present, and the secondary sex characteristics of breast development and growth of pubic and axillary hair usually develop normally. The external genitalia are also normal. The client is infertile but has normal female development. There is no treatment for müllerian aplasia.

Specific Nursing Measures

The nursing measures for müllerian aplasia are similar to those for the infertile woman, which include helping the client accept herself as a woman even though she lacks reproductive capacity. The nurse should discuss the possible implications of infertility for the client and provide emotional support by allowing her to vent feelings of anger and disappointment. The client may feel distressed that a life goal of bearing children is unattainable.

VAGINAL ATRESIA

Vaginal atresia results in the complete absence of the vagina from failure of the vagina to canalize. The client may have a small vaginal pouch and often has a normal uterus, ovaries, and fallopian tubes. The atresia is caused by the fusion of müllerian ducts in the ninth week of embryonic development (see Chapter 61).

Clinical Manifestations

The client does not have a menstrual flow but has cyclic cramping abdominal pain because of the accumulation of blood and mucus from the menses. Chromosomal study reveals a 46XX karyotype, the normal female karyotype. The secondary sex characteristics are present as well.

Therapeutic Measures

Vaginal atresia is treated by the construction of an artificial vagina. Various surgical techniques are used. There are different surgical techniques of vaginoplasty (repair of the vagina), depending on the deformity. Reconstruction is best carried out before 18 months of age but may be performed when the client is older. There is no reason to delay surgery until puberty.

Specific Nursing Measures

Overall preoperative and postoperative nursing management is discussed in Chapter 65. In addition, the nurse instructs the client about the use of vaginal dilators or regular coitus to keep the vagina patent. The nurse also provides emotional support for the client.

TRANSVERSE VAGINAL SEPTUM

Transverse vaginal septum is one of the most common vaginal anomalies. There may be a complete obstruction of the vagina that obscures the cervix from view or a partial obstruction with a small opening. The embryonic origin of this disorder is not clearly understood. It may be caused by the failure of the vagina to canalize.

Clinical Manifestations

The client has a history of cyclic abdominal cramping because of the accumulation of blood and mucus from the menses. A pelvic mass also may develop because of the accumulation of the menses. An imperforate hymen manifests itself by a bulging, bluish membrane in the vagina within three menstrual cycles when there is a high septum, or within about six menstrual cycles if there is room in the vagina for the menses to accumulate. A partial obstruction results in painful coitus or dyspareunia.

Therapeutic Measures

Therapeutic measures involve surgical excision of the membrane. Fertility is maintained, sexual intercourse becomes possible, and dyspareunia is relieved, depending on the location of the membrane before excision.

Specific Nursing Measures

Preoperative and postoperative nursing care is discussed in Chapter 65. The client may be embarrassed about her condition, so the nurse should demonstrate acceptance of the client to put her at ease.

INCOMPLETE MÜLLERIAN FUSION

Incomplete müllerian fusion results in an abnormal shape and division of the uterus. The uterus that results may be unicornuate, arcuate, septate, bicornuate, didelphate, or have other variations (Figure 64–1). This condition results from embryonic failure of the müllerian ducts during the ninth to twelfth week of gestation. The bicornuate and didelphate are the most common disorders.

Clinical Manifestations

Clinical manifestations of incomplete müllerian fusion are infertility, recurrent abortion and prematurity, abnormal fetal position and presentation, and abnormal placental implantation. Many of these clients have normal reproductive capacity, however, and those who do not may have conditions other than the shape of the uterus that adversely affect reproductive capacity.

Therapeutic Measures

Other causes of reproductive failure must be ruled out. Then the uterus may be surgically excised in an attempt to improve fertility.

Specific Nursing Measures

Preoperative and postoperative nursing care of the client having uterine surgery is discussed in Chapter 65. Specific nursing care centers around the reproductive capacity of the client. For example, referral for infertility counseling or to self-help groups such as RESOLVE, Inc. (see resources at the end of Chapter 63) may be necessary, and adoption or other arrangements may be initiated if the client and her partner decide they want children.

DIETHYLSTILBESTROL-EXPOSED CLIENTS

The in-utero exposure of female offspring to diethylstilbestrol (DES) may cause various reproductive tract abnormalities. In the 1950s and 1960s, DES was used to prevent abortion and was given to pregnant women with diabetes, toxemia, premature labor, and other conditions. In 1971, a link between vaginal and cervical cancer and DES exposure in utero was found.

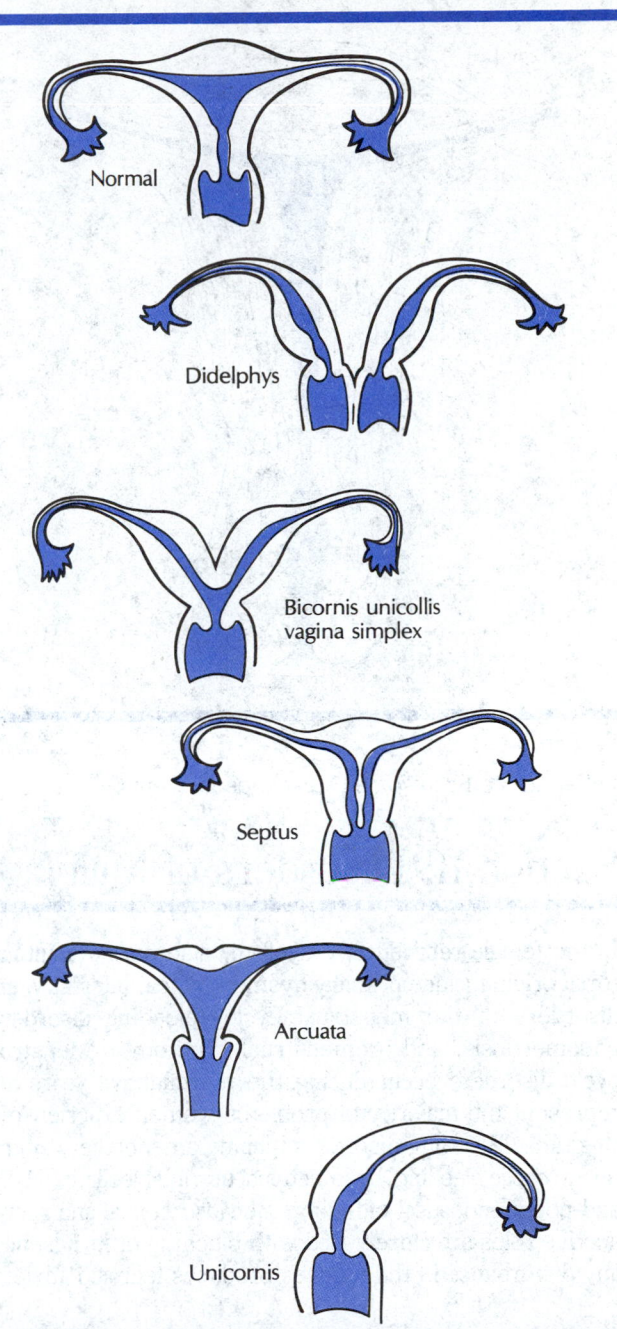

Figure 64–1

Congenital malformations of the uterus.
SOURCE: Olds SB, London ML, Ladewig PA: *Maternal–Newborn Nursing: A Family-Centered Approach.* Menlo Park, CA: Addison–Wesley, 1984.

Clinical Manifestations

The clinical manifestations of in-utero DES exposure depend on when the exposure occurred and may include epithelial changes, a cock's comb–appearing cervix or a cervix with clefts or pseudopolyps, and inelastic fornices. There may be changes in the uterus. The typical T-shaped uterus

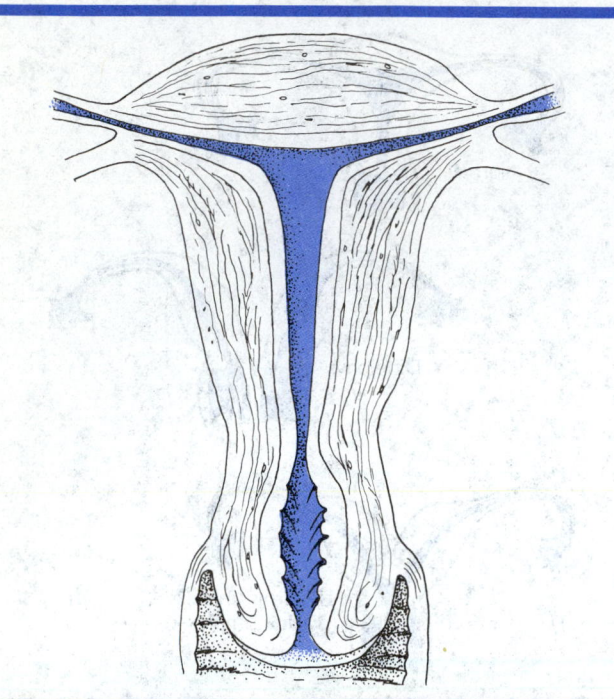

Figure 64–2

T-shaped uterus in some DES-exposed clients.

found in DES-exposed clients (Figure 64–2) may predispose them to infertility and spontaneous abortion.

Therapeutic Measures

In past years, clients exposed to DES in utero underwent the administration of progesterone, skinning of the cervix, or other aggressive procedures such as surgical excision, cauterization, cryotherapy, or laser evaporation of abnormal tissue. Currently, the plan of care includes routine Papanicolau (Pap) tests and careful pelvic examinations yearly. If there is a change in the Pap test or the appearance of the vaginal mucosa, the client is followed more closely.

Specific Nursing Measures

Nursing care involves screening for clients who have been exposed to DES. The client may deny her risk, so the nurse is also responsible for informing the client about the necessity of routine follow-up examinations. The nurse provides emotional support through therapeutic communication skills. Nursing care for the client who develops cancer is described in the later section on neoplastic disorders.

Section II: Disorders of Multifactorial Origin

In the female reproductive system, disorders of multifactorial origin include primary dysmenorrhea, infertility, and disorders of the menstrual cycle (bleeding disorders, endometriosis, and premenstrual syndrome). Menstrual cycle disorders occur during the reproductive years and represent the majority of problems women experience at this time. Bleeding disorders include amenorrhea, alteration in cyclic bleeding, dysfunctional uterine bleeding (DUB), and postmenopausal bleeding. Because sexual and reproductive roles are closely tied with bleeding or its absence, any disturbance in the menses produces fear and anxiety.

PRIMARY DYSMENORRHEA

Dysmenorrhea is painful menses. Primary dysmenorrhea occurs when there is painful menses in the absence of a pelvic pathological condition. In secondary dysmenorrhea, the pain's cause is some pathological condition such as endometriosis, pelvic inflammatory disease (PID), or congenital abnormalities of the reproductive tract. The causes of secondary dysmenorrhea are discussed elsewhere in this chapter, so this section will cover only primary dysmenorrhea.

Primary dysmenorrhea is caused by an excess of prostaglandin, which is formed in the endometrium following ovulation and reaches a peak at menstruation. The increased prostaglandins are thought to result in three conditions: (1) an increase in uterine contractions, (2) ischemia

from the decrease of uterine blood flow, and (3) a lowering of the pain threshold of the nerves in the uterus.

Clinical Manifestations

The onset of symptoms in primary dysmenorrhea is usually within 12 months of menarche. Lower abdominal cramps in waves radiate to the lower back, upper thighs, or both. The pain is most intense during the first 3 days of the menstrual cycle and usually subsides within the first 24 to 48 hours. The accompanying symptoms may include headache, nausea and vomiting, and diarrhea. It is most common in women up to 25 years of age.

Therapeutic Measures

The most frequent treatment for primary dysmenorrhea is the use of nonsteroidal anti-inflammatory drugs (NSAIDs). Aspirin, although an NSAID, has little effect on painful menstruation, and not all NSAIDs are recommended for dysmenorrhea. Some specific NSAIDs that help reduce dysmenorrhea are ibuprofen (Motrin, Advil, and Nuprin), mefenamic acid (Ponstel), and naproxen sodium (Anaprox). These medications are given when the dysmenorrhea occurs and do not need to be given before the onset of menstruation.

Another treatment is the use of oral contraceptives if the client desires birth control. Oral contraceptives decrease the amount of prostaglandins in the menstrual flow. Because of the side effects associated with their use, oral contraceptives should be given only when the client desires birth control. Primary dysmenorrhea often markedly decreases after pregnancy.

Relief from pain usually occurs after several months of treatment. If NSAIDs, oral contraceptives, or pregnancy fail to provide relief, the client should be reexamined for other causes of pain.

Specific Nursing Measures

The nurse can review the client's menstrual history for the onset of dysmenorrhea and its association with menses to help determine the cause of the dysmenorrhea. A review of the client's attitude toward menstruation helps determine whether the symptoms have a psychological base. The nurse can also explore the client's pain threshold.

When primary dysmenorrhea is treated with NSAIDs, the nurse should discuss the possibility of gastrointestinal upset and headache. Less common side effects include peripheral edema, reversible alteration of liver enzymes, urticaria, angioneurotic edema, and bronchospasms in clients with asthma. The side effects of oral contraceptives vary, depending on the type of agent used. The more serious side effects include gallbladder disease, hepatic adenoma, thrombophlebitis, myocardial infarction, stroke or hypertension, and migraine headaches. Caution the client to contact her health care provider if these side effects occur.

Instruct the client that the medication may not relieve the discomfort for several months. Physical exercise, including swimming and the pelvic rock exercise (Figure 64–3), may help decrease the pain. Other measures for relieving discomfort include the use of heat in the form of tub baths, showers, or heating pads as well as increased sleep during menstruation. Instructions in personal hygiene

may help alleviate some misconceptions about how the body functions during the menstrual cycle. Finally, good nutrition can impart a sense of well-being.

INFERTILITY

Infertility is the inability to conceive after 1 year of coitus without contraception. Primary infertility is present when a woman has never conceived, and secondary infertility occurs when a woman who has previously conceived is not able to conceive again after 1 year of unprotected intercourse.

Infertility is usually caused by one or a combination of three conditions: the failure of the woman to ovulate, inadequate sperm production, and structural abnormalities. Fertility problems have been attributed equally to women and men, with other factors such as improper timing during the ovulatory cycle and position during intercourse attributed to the couple. Causes of male infertility are discussed in Chapter 62.

Clinical Manifestations

Infertility is manifested by the inability to become pregnant. When the woman does not ovulate, the typical signs of ovulatory cycles—premenstrual breast tenderness, a feeling that menstruation is about to occur, and uterine cramps during menstruation—are absent. There is a monophasic shift in the basal body temperature chart, compared with the normal biphasic shift.

Abnormalities of the female reproductive tract that cause infertility include congenital disorders mentioned in Section I. Occlusion of the fallopian tubes is an abnormality caused primarily by infectious processes or previous surgery that may have caused peritubal adhesions.

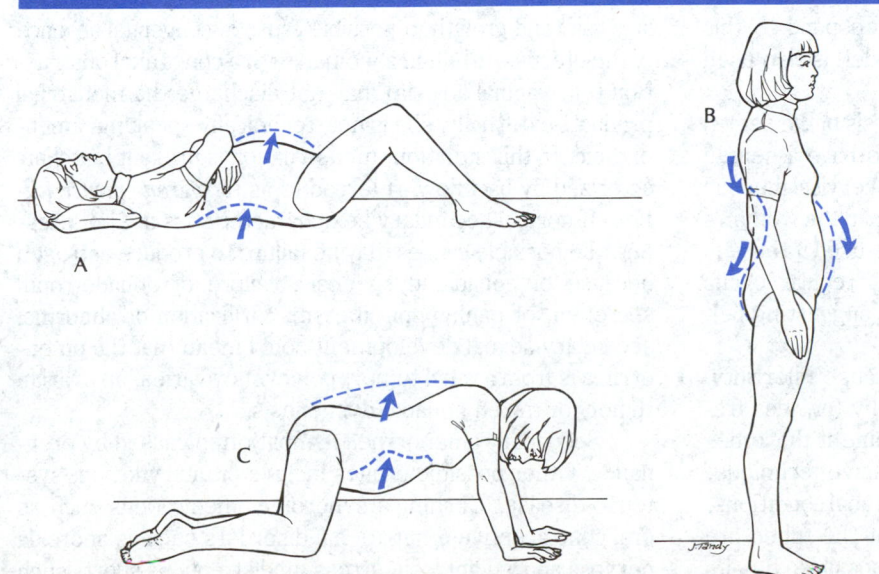

Figure 64–3

The pelvic rock can be performed: **A.** While lying supine. **B.** Standing. **C.** Or on hands and knees. The buttocks and the abdominal muscles should be tightened at the same time while the buttocks are tucked under. This causes the pelvis to rock or tilt forward.
SOURCE: Olds SB, London ML, Ladewig PA: *Maternal–Newborn Nursing: A Family-Centered Approach.* Menlo Park, CA: Addison–Wesley, 1984.

Therapeutic Measures

The most important therapeutic measure in treating infertility is a thorough history and physical examination of the couple (see Chapters 63 and 66). History taking for the woman should include such factors as menstrual and contraceptive history, the nature of previous pregnancies, coital frequency, and the presence or absence of dyspareunia and dysmenorrhea. Other factors to consider are the client's surgical history, infections of the reproductive system, and changes in physical findings. The physical examination emphasizes the thyroid gland, breasts, changes in body habits, secondary sex characteristics, and patterns of hair distribution. The abdomen should be assessed for masses and tenderness, and a thorough internal examination is completed.

The treatment of infertility depends on its cause or causes. If the female does not ovulate, treatment will include hormonal evaluation by measuring follicle-stimulating hormone (FSH), luteinizing hormone (LH), and prolactin levels. These tests help determine whether the lack of ovulation is caused by the hypothalamus, pituitary gland, ovaries, or other conditions. An endometrial biopsy is performed if the client has a history of irregular bleeding to determine hormonal and cyclic changes in the endometrium. If hirsutism and obesity are present, the possibility of androgen excess is also explored by measuring urinary DHA (dehydroandosterone, an androgen occurring in normal human urine) and plasma stenedione and testosterone levels.

The medical management of the anovulatory client includes the use of drugs such as clomiphene citrate (Clomid) to stimulate ovulation. This is given daily on the fifth to the ninth day after a normal or progestin-stimulated menses. Most pregnancies with the use of this drug occur within the first 3 months of treatment. If ovulation does not occur, human chorionic gonadotropin (HCG) is added on the thirteenth day. Human menopausal gonadotropin (HMG) therapy may be used for clients who do not respond to this treatment. Bromocriptine mesylate (Parlodel) is also used for some clients.

Male infertility is diagnosed by an analysis of the semen at various intervals. If the man refuses to have a semen analysis, the woman can undergo the coital cervical mucous test. This should demonstrate viable sperm in the woman's cervical mucus. Donor insemination can be used if there is male infertility, provided the woman has regular cyclic menses and no history or physical findings suggesting pelvic pathology.

When fallopian tube abnormalities cause infertility, various tests such as hysterosalpingography (or, less frequently, Rubin's test) are used to determine if the tubes are patent. Laparoscopy, although an invasive technique, gives the most accurate information about tubal conditions. Pregnancy may occur after these tests if the tubes are patent. Tubal reconstructive surgery is possible, but its success is variable. See Chapter 65 for a description of laparoscopy and tubal surgery, as well as Chapter 63 for a complete description of tests to detect infertility.

Specific Nursing Measures

The female client may be more comfortable discussing her sexual history with the nurse, who then can guide her on the correct positions and timing of sexual intercourse during the ovulatory phases of the menstrual cycle. The initial visit usually includes instructions in charting the basal body temperature, which the nurse can provide (see Chapter 63). Reinforce the instructions pertaining to the other tests performed.

When surgery is performed, the client will be eager to find out if she has a favorable condition for conception to occur. Preoperative and postoperative care is reviewed in Chapter 65.

The client may feel guilty if she is responsible for the inability to reproduce. She may experience lifestyle changes if she and her partner desired a family and the diagnosis concludes that she is infertile. Feelings of hostility toward others who have children or those who question when she is going to have children are normal. The nurse should refer her to the national organization RESOLVE (see Chapter 63) for support, counseling, and referral both during the diagnostic process and afterward.

AMENORRHEA

Amenorrhea, the absence of menstruation, may be classified as primary amenorrhea (in which there has been no bleeding) or secondary amenorrhea (bleeding absent in a previously normal menstruating female).

The causes of primary amenorrhea are categorized according to the client's physical development. If she has normal secondary development of breasts, pubic and axillary hair, and growth, a possible cause is congenital absence of the uterus. Although a woman with a congenital obstruction (eg, vaginal atresia) may not discharge the menstrual products externally, she is not, technically speaking, amenorrheic. In this situation, menstruation is present but characterized by backflow, referred to as *retrograde menstruation*. If normal secondary sex characteristics are not present, the possible causes may be failure to produce estrogen because of gonadal dysgenesis, failure of gonadotropin secretion, or panhypopituitarism. Virilization or abnormal secondary sexual development could mean that the amenorrhea is from a renal tumor, polycystic ovaries, an ovarian tumor, or mixed gonadal dysgenesis.

Secondary amenorrhea is most often caused by pregnancy. Other possible causes include pituitary lesion, systemic disease, Cushing's syndrome, medications such as oral contraceptives, nutritional disorders such as anorexia nervosa and weight loss, stress, and strenuous sports such as long distance running or ballet that decrease body fat.

Clinical Manifestations

In primary amenorrhea, menstruation is absent after the age of 18. In secondary amenorrhea, menstruation is absent for more than 6 consecutive months after normal cycles have been established. The clinical manifestations correlate with the cause.

Therapeutic Measures

For the client with primary amenorrhea, history taking and a physical examination are completed. This is followed by progesterone and estrogen–progesterone withdrawal tests, which demonstrate normal pituitary, ovarian, and uterine function if bleeding occurs. If no withdrawal bleeding occurs, a combined estrogen–progesterone preparation is given cyclically to approximate the normal menstrual cycle. Appropriate treatment depends on the cause of the amenorrhea. In many cases, infertility is diagnosed.

In secondary amenorrhea, pregnancy is first ruled out by physical examination and pregnancy testing (see Chapter 63). Treatment depends on the cause of the amenorrhea. Infertility testing may be necessary.

Specific Nursing Measures

The amenorrheic client may feel that her childbearing potential is threatened. If infertility is identified, the client may need to alter her image of herself as a woman in the childbearing role. When amenorrhea has emotional causes, the nurse can be an effective therapeutic listener. When amenorrhea is caused by weight loss, the nurse can provide dietary counseling to maintain adequate weight for menses to recur. Other more specific nursing measures in anorexia nervosa are discussed in Chapter 9.

ALTERATION IN CYCLIC BLEEDING

Cyclic bleeding is usually related to the ovulatory pattern. Variations on the bleeding pattern involve the amount, duration, interval, or irregularity of the menses. A short, scant pattern of menstruation usually signifies normal frequent ovulation. Excessive menstrual flow that occurs only once may be from spontaneous abortion or ectopic pregnancy. A more frequent cause could be an intrauterine device (IUD), fibroids, or adenomyosis. Other causes include systemic diseases, blood dyscrasias, hypothyroidism, medications, and chronic iron-deficiency anemia.

Clinical Manifestations

A scant menses or excess menstruation are the most common cyclic bleeding alterations. If there is heavy menstruation, anemia can occur as a result of the excess bleeding.

Therapeutic Measures

Conservative treatment for alterations in cyclic bleeding consists of hormonal therapy given in the later part of the

---

Box 64–1 A Self Checklist for Women With Signs and Symptoms of PMS

1. Lessening frequency of headaches, cravings and/or fatigue by keeping the blood sugar level up:
   a. Eating at least 45 grams of protein daily
   b. Eating six meals daily, not more calories but more frequent meals
   c. Eating fruits for snacks, not sweets
   d. Decreasing fluid retention
2. Lessening or controlling depression/irritability by:
   a. Getting 7-8 hours of sleep nightly
   b. Exercising the equivalent of 2 miles of walking daily
   c. Getting with a support group/person to express your feelings
   d. Increasing Vitamin B_6 foods in diet (corn, liver, wheat, yeast, tomatoes, unsalted sunflower seeds, peanuts) or 200 milligrams of Vitamin B_6 daily prior to menses
   e. Increasing foods high in Magnesium in diet (whole grain, dried beans, seafood)
   f. Decreasing stress (exercise, meditation, yoga, relaxation, stop talk—keep mind from unnecessary worries—assertiveness training)
   g. Decreasing fluid retention (no salt at table, 1 lemon in water daily, no more than 1 carbonated beverage a day. Rule of S's—avoid salt, soup, sauces, etc.)
3. Decreasing swelling/bloating, breast tenderness by decreasing fluid retention through:
   a. Using no salt at the table
   b. Eating frozen, not canned foods
   c. Avoiding salty foods (pickles, potato chips, pork, Rule of S's)
   d. Using natural diuretics (1 lemon or tbsp. 100% lemon juice in 8 oz water daily, caffeine, if acceptable.
4. Other measures commonly recommended follow:
   a. Avoiding nutritional irritants by:
      1. Avoiding coffee, chocolate (if one finds these to worsen the symptoms)
      2. Decreasing use of refined sugar by using sweeteners, honey, fruits instead of sweets for snacks
   b. Attaining or maintaining recommended body weight
   c. Using primrose oil capsule for breast tenderness

SOURCE: Kirkpatrick MK, Grady TR: PMS: A self-help checklist. *Occupational Health Nurs* 1985 (February); 33:92.

---

cycle. If fibroids are the cause of the excess bleeding and childbearing is desired, a myomectomy (removal of the fibroids only) can be done. For clients who do not desire children and who have pain associated with fibroids, a hysterectomy can be performed. A discussion of surgical techniques is in Chapter 65.

Specific Nursing Measures

Nursing measures include reinforcement of the idea that the client's short, scant cycles are normal and do not signify disease. The client with heavy menstrual bleeding may become fearful for her life, and support by the nurse is important. Encourage good nutrition, including foods high in iron. Stress the importance of taking medications. If the client takes oral iron preparations, instruct her to take them with meals to decrease gastric irritation; warn her that iron may cause black stools. Preoperative and postoperative care of the hysterectomy client is discussed in Chapter 65.

DYSFUNCTIONAL UTERINE BLEEDING

Dysfunctional uterine bleeding is caused by a hormonal imbalance in the hypothalamic–pituitary–ovarian axis, without an organic pathological condition of the organs of reproduction themselves. The menstrual cycles are usually anovulatory, which interferes with the usual menstrual pattern. The bleeding may be caused by excessive growth of the vascular tissue of the endometrium; this tissue breaks down sporadically, leaving the vascular channels exposed. The diagnosis of DUB is made after the following conditions are found not to be the cause: pregnancy, malignancy, myomas, cervical erosion, polyps, vaginal infection or trauma, ovarian dysfunction, systemic disease, medication, and emotional disturbance.

Clinical Manifestations

Characteristic abnormal patterns of bleeding are **menorrhagia** (excessive profuse menstrual flow), **metrorrhagia** (bleeding between menstrual periods), prolonged menstrual flow, and **oligomenorrhea** (markedly diminished menstrual flow). The interval between menstrual periods and the length of the menstrual period may also be shortened or increased. The client with anovulatory DUB is usually an adolescent or a woman in her 50s.

Therapeutic Measures

There is no single method for treating DUB. The physician tries various measures and closely observes the client for the appropriate response. Pharmacologic measures include the administration of estrogens, progesterones, androgens, and ergot derivatives; ovulation induction; and antiprostaglandin therapy.

Specific Nursing Measures

Any bleeding can concern the client. Because multiple treatments are used for DUB, the client may become concerned about the number of procedures being used. Provide support and instruct the client to keep a record of her bleeding to determine the effectiveness of each treatment.

POSTMENOPAUSAL BLEEDING

Malignancy occurs in 30% to 40% of clients with postmenopausal bleeding, and any bleeding that occurs after menopause is considered to be a sign of malignancy and should be evaluated. If a malignancy exists or there are recurrent episodes of bleeding, the treatment is hysterectomy (see Chapter 65).

Estrogen replacement therapy (ERT) also causes postmenopausal bleeding. When estrogens are needed in the postmenopausal period, a combination of estrogen and progesterone decreases the risk of unopposed estrogens. Unopposed estrogens can lead to endometrial hyperplasia, a precursor to carcinoma. (See the discussion of ERT in the section on menopause.)

ENDOMETRIOSIS

Endometriosis is the presence of functioning endometrial tissue outside the uterus. The common sites of endometriosis are shown in Figure 64–4. The cause of the disease is not known. It is speculated that endometrial tissue refluxes from the uterus into the pelvic cavity at menstruation or that the condition is congenital. The incidence of the disease is not known because it can be present without any symptoms. Some research studies have identified endometriosis in 5% to 50% of gynecologic surgery clients (Duenhoelter, 1983). Endometriosis is usually found in women who have delayed childbearing.

When the endometrial tissue invades the myometrium, the condition is known as adenomyosis. Adenomyosis is usually found in women over 35. Symptoms include excessive and prolonged menses and dysmenorrhea. If symptoms are severe, the treatment is hysterectomy.

Clinical Manifestations

Endometriosis can only be diagnosed by histological identification of endometrial tissue and glands in a lesion that

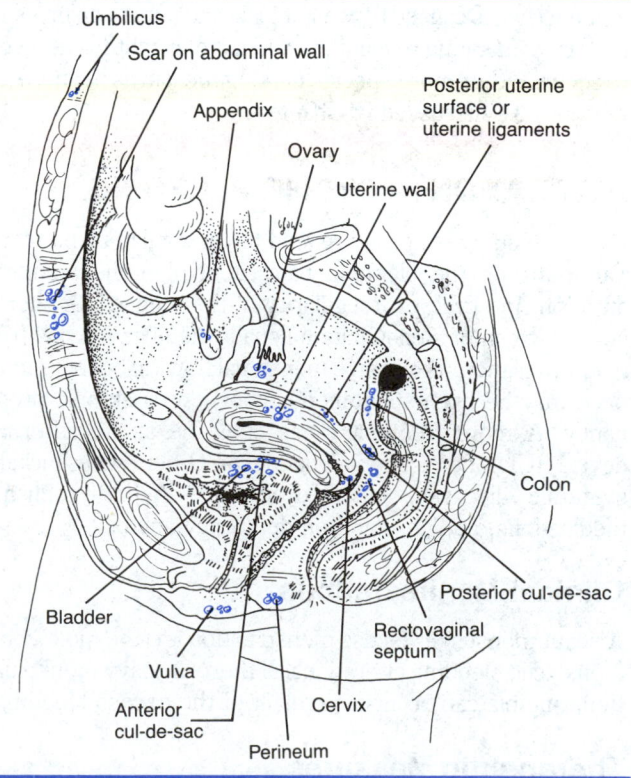

Figure 64–4

Possible sites of endometriosis.

is seen via laparoscopy or laparotomy or in a biopsy specimen of the lesion. The lesions have a bluish "powderburn" gross appearance, and their size can vary from microscopic to larger than 10 cm in diameter.

The symptoms are based on the location of the lesions. The most common symptoms are dysmenorrhea, deep dyspareunia, and sacral backache. The client may also have infertility and menstrual abnormalities. Pain develops gradually and increases in intensity over time. The location of the pain depends on where the lesions are located. The extent of the endometriosis and the severity of the pain and symptomatology are not necessarily related.

Therapeutic Measures

Treatment is highly individualized and depends on the symptoms and the client's desire for childbearing. The medical management of choice includes the use of the anti-gonadotropin, danazol (Danocrine), a synthetic androgen, which is prescribed for a 6- to 9-month period. Danazol is effective and safe but expensive. Danazol is usually given in doses of 600 mg daily for the first month, beginning a few days after menses has begun. The dosage is reduced to 200 mg daily as long as the client remains amenorrheic. The possible side effects of danazol include weight gain, acne, decrease in breast size, oily skin, and deepening of the voice. High-dose birth control pills may also be used to shrink endometrial tissue. High-dose progesterones are no longer recommended by the Food and Drug Administration (FDA). Pregnancy is encouraged because it may cause the disease process to regress and because of the increased risk of infertility as the disease progresses.

Surgical treatment includes total hysterectomy and bilateral salpingo-oophorectomy (TAH-BSO) if no further childbearing is desired. An option is to leave part of an ovary intact for hormonal production if there are no apparent lesions on it. If childbearing is desired, conservative surgery that involves the removal of active implants by excision, as well as lysis of adhesions, is carried out.

Specific Nursing Measures

Preoperative and postoperative nursing measures for TAH-BSO are discussed in Chapter 65. Because endometriosis often results in infertility, the client will need the nurse's emotional support. If pain has been a major factor, the client may be relieved to find its cause. The encouragement not to delay childbearing may necessitate a different family-planning schedule for the client and her partner. Provide support and be an effective listener as the client discusses these concerns and possible changes in plans.

PREMENSTRUAL SYNDROME

Premenstrual syndrome (PMS) is a collection of symptoms that occur in the luteal phase of the menstrual cycle and alter the client's normal physiological and emotional states.

They are not present once the menstrual period is over. According to different studies, the incidence of the syndrome varies from 5% to 95%. The onset of PMS is from 2 weeks to a few days before menses.

No specific cause is known. The peak time for the occurrence of PMS is ages 30 to 40. Environmental stress may play a role in the development of PMS, as may expectations about the menstrual cycle's being a time of distress.

Clinical Manifestations

The symptoms must recur for at least 3 cycles before a diagnosis of PMS is made. The list of PMS symptoms can be divided into physical and psychological. The physical symptoms include edema of the legs and fingers, a bloated feeling in the abdomen, weight gain, breast tenderness, headaches and dizziness, heart palpitations, excessive thirst and appetite, excessive sleeping, constipation, back pain, craving for sweets, and acne. The psychological symptoms include sadness, depression, crying easily, tenseness, anxiety, irritability, restlessness, mood swings, increased or decreased sexual desire, and feelings of irrationality. The symptoms vary with individuals; however, they increase in severity just prior to the onset of menstruation and subside as the menstrual flow starts.

Therapeutic Measures

There is no standardized treatment for PMS. Diuretics can relieve edema, and anxiolytic agents (or minor tranquilizers) can treat symptoms on a short-term basis. Vitamin B_6 also may bring some relief. Bromocriptine mesylate (Parlodel), a prolactin-suppressing drug, may help in the management of breast tenderness, edema, and weight gain. Progesterone may be used to counter estrogen's sodium-sparing actions and may provide a calming effect; however, progesterone works sporadically and can actually worsen symptoms. In some instances, some experts think that psychological counseling is helpful in returning the feeling of bodily control to the client.

Specific Nursing Measures

Nursing measures depend on PMS symptoms and the treatment the physician prescribes. The nurse can direct the client to keep a diary of her symptoms to help better understand them and thus increase her feeling of control over herself. Help the client realize that PMS is a disorder and that individualized treatment is necessary. It is also helpful to include the client's family or significant other in the management of PMS. (See Box 64–1.)

Proper nutrition is important in relieving some of the symptoms, so nutritional counseling should include instructions to consume foods high in vitamin B_6 and magnesium. The dietary sources of vitamin B_6 are pork, glandular meats, cereal bran and germ, milk, egg yolks, oatmeal, and legumes. Dietary sources of magnesium include nuts, legumes, cereal, grains, dark green vegetables, and seafood. Explain that an excess of vitamin B_6 causes headache, dizziness, and nausea. The diet should not contain refined sugars, caffeine, or red meat. Smoking is also discouraged. Exercise should be encouraged.

Section III: Degenerative Disorders

Degenerative disorders of the female reproductive system include pelvic relaxational prolapse (uterine prolapse, cystocele, and rectocele). Pelvic relaxation involves the muscles responsible for support of the uterus, bladder, and rectum; these include the endopelvic fascia, the uterosacral and cardinal ligaments, and the levator ani muscles. Pelvic relaxation is caused by traumatic stretching from childbearing and occupational and unusual athletic activities, heredity, and menopause. Other causes include obesity, asthma and other chronic lung conditions, chronic constipation with straining, and excessive traction on the cervix during a dilatation and curettage (D and C) or traction on the umbilical cord during obstetrical delivery to hasten delivery of the placenta. Approximately 50% of all women who have borne a child have some degree of vaginal and uterine prolapse. However, only about 10% to 20% of those with pelvic support dysfunction experience symptoms severe enough to warrant surgery (Kase and Weingold, 1983).

Menopause is also discussed in this section. Although menopause is a natural state, not a disorder, it is included here because it creates uncomfortable symptoms that may require treatment.

GENERAL NURSING IMPLICATIONS

An essential role of the nurse in degenerative disorders involves health teaching to prevent or reduce the severity of pelvic relaxation and to facilitate the client's understanding of menopause as a natural phenomenon. Physical care is another essential component because many clients with degenerative conditions may undergo surgery or pharmacologic treatment.

UTERINE PROLAPSE

Prolapse of the uterus may result in the descent of the cervix to the vaginal introitus (first-degree prolapse), protrusion of the cervix through the introitus (second-degree prolapse), or prolapse of the entire uterus through the introitus (third-degree prolapse or procidentia). Figure 64–5 depicts the types of uterine prolapse.

Clinical Manifestations

The general symptoms of uterine prolapse may include sacral backache, a feeling of the "insides falling out," a feeling of "sitting on a ball," and a bearing-down sensation. There may be bleeding if the cervix is exposed, as well as cervical erosion caused by congestion and trauma.

Therapeutic Measures

Preventive measures include performing Kegel exercises in the postpartum period. Lacerations of the perineum and episiotomies should be sutured carefully with good approx-

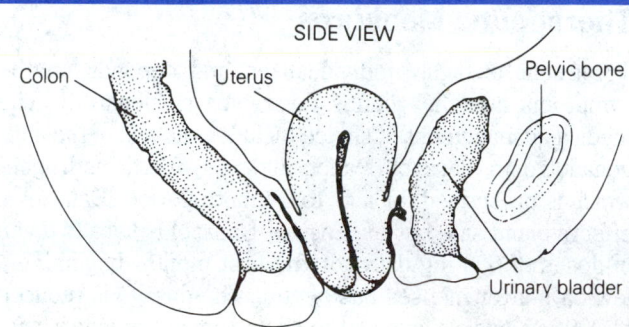

First-degree (cervix comes down to vagina)

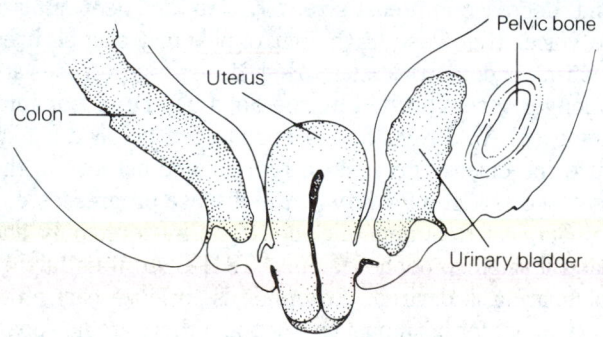

Second-degree (cervix protrudes through vagina)

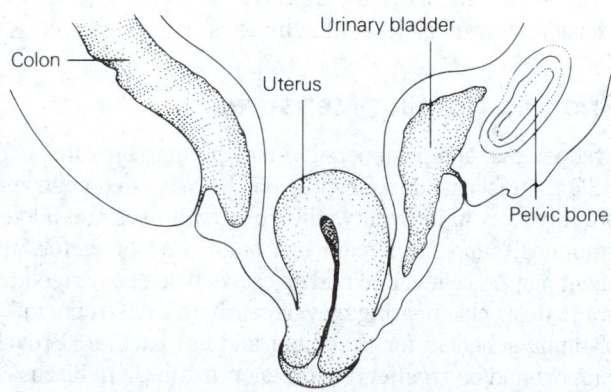

Third-degree — total procidentia (uterus protrudes below vagina)

Figure 64–5

Prolapse of uterus and vagina.
SOURCE: Saxton DF, Pelikan PK, Nugent PM, Hyland PA: *The Addison–Wesley Manual of Nursing Practice.* Menlo Park, CA: Addison–Wesley, 1983.

imation of the structures. Unnecessary traction should not be applied to the cervix and uterus during obstetrical or surgical procedures.

Treatment involves the use of exercises to help strengthen the muscle floor. Surgery, usually hysterectomy, is performed when there are significant symptoms such as pain and bleeding and when a second-degree or third-degree prolapse is present (see Chapter 65). Pessaries, instruments placed in the vagina to support the uterus, may be used by clients who refuse surgery or are not suitable candidates for surgery. Pessaries are discussed and illustrated in Figure 64–6.

Specific Nursing Measures

Preoperative and postoperative care for the client having a hysterectomy is discussed in Chapter 65. If surgery is not indicated, instruct the client in how to perform pelvic tilt and Kegel exercises to tighten the pubococcygeal muscle, improving support to the pelvic organs. Nurses caring for female clients should teach them to perform Kegel exercises to avoid or decrease the severity of uterine prolapse. The exercise can be taught to all women of childbearing age before pregnancy. Instructions for Kegel and other related exercises are given in Box 64–2.

Explain the care of the pessary if one has been inserted. The device must be removed and cleaned with mild soap and water about every 6 weeks, and regular douching may

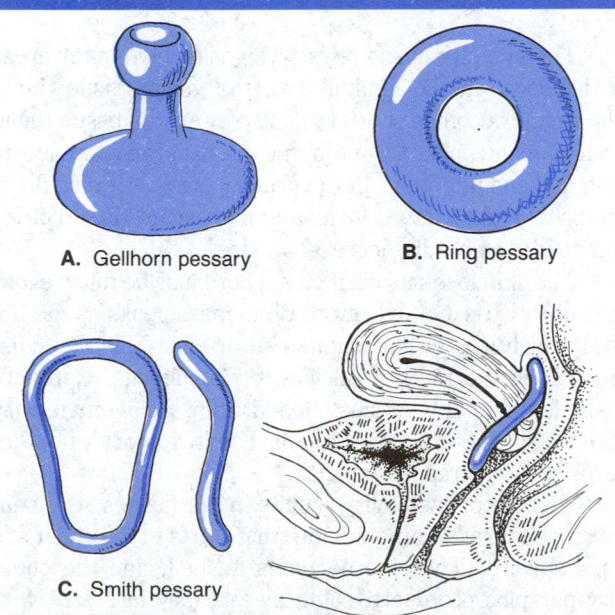

A. Gellhorn pessary **B.** Ring pessary

C. Smith pessary

Figure 64–6

Vaginal pessaries. The Gellhorn **(A)** and ring **(B)** pessaries are most commonly used to relieve urinary prolapse. They are made of a rigid material (usually hard rubber or plastic). Smith's pessary **(C)** is a flexible ring placed around the cervix. It is most commonly used to correct a backward displacement (retroversion) of the uterus.

> **Box 64–2 Exercises for Pelvic Relaxation and Stress Incontinence**
>
> Do all exercises slowly on a firm surface several times daily.
>
> 1. *Kegel exercise*
>   a. When lying on your back, tighten the pelvic floor muscles as hard as you can, holding for the count of 5 seconds, then release. As you learn to do this, it can be done many times daily, while sitting or standing. Repeat at least 10 times in a row.
>   b. When you are urinating, do exercise 1a, using the muscles to stop the flow of urine. Hold for 5 seconds, then relax. Practice this each time you use the toilet.
>   c. Lie on your back with a pillow under your knees. Cross your ankles. Squeeze your buttocks together drawing in the anus, as if to prevent a bowel movement. Grip your knees together. Hold for 5 seconds, then relax. Remember to breath normally. Repeat at least 10 times.
>
> 2. *Pelvic tilt*
>   a. Lie on your back with your knees partly bent and feet flat on the floor. Pull in your abdomen and tighten your buttocks, so the small of your back presses against the floor. Remember to breathe normally. Hold for 5 seconds and relax. Repeat 10 times.
>   b. Repeat exercise 2a while on your hands and knees, using the abdomen and buttock muscles to make your lower back flatten out. Hold 5 seconds and relax. Repeat 10 times.
>   c. Practice pelvic tilts standing with your back against a wall. Pelvic tilts strengthen the abdomen and are the basis for many postural exercises.
>
> 3. *Partial curl-up*. Lie on your back with your knees bent and feet on the floor. Have your arms at your sides, just off the floor. Do a pelvic tilt (exercise 2) and then lift your head and shoulders off the floor. Slowly lie back down. You do not have to do a full sit-up to get the benefits of this exercise. Full sit-ups are not recommended for people who may have back problems. Repeat 5 to 20 times.
>
> 4. Tighten your stomach muscles while sitting and standing. Hold for count of 10, breathing normally. Repeat 5 times.

be necessary. The nurse should also discuss measures that help decrease the risk of infection, using proper hygiene as described in Chapter 63. Clients with pessaries are at increased risk for infection due to trauma from the pessary itself and the long-term presence of material foreign to the body. Instruct the client to notify her health care provider if she experiences pain, changes in the urinary pattern, unusual vaginal discharge or if the pessary is expelled.

CYSTOCELE

A *cystocele* is the herniation of the posterior aspects of the bladder into the vagina through the cervicopubic fascia of the anterior vagina. A *urethrocele* is a herniation of the urethra into the vagina. Both conditions are caused by the same general conditions as uterine prolapse, usually childbearing, obesity, or chronic lung conditions.

Clinical Manifestations

The most common manifestation is urinary stress incontinence. A cystocele may cause an increased incidence of bladder infections because of congestion in the base of the bladder as well as a herniation in the anterior wall of the vagina from the weakened supports.

Therapeutic Measures

Conservative management for stress incontinence includes the Kegel exercises. Alpha-adrenergic receptor stimulants may increase the tone of the bladder and the urethral smooth muscle. Estrogens in small doses may be prescribed for postmenopausal clients. Urinary tract infections should be treated promptly (see also Chapter 33).

Surgical management for cystocele includes anterior colporrhaphy (described in Chapter 65). Other procedures such as uterine suspension, Kelly's plication and the Marshall–Marchetti operation that attempt to support the pelvic structures have low success rates.

Specific Nursing Measures

The nurse should explain the Kegel exercises and review the importance of taking prescribed medications. Be aware of the embarrassment the client may feel if she has stress incontinence or if she must wear pads or plastic protective underpants. Garments that fit well will prevent leaking. Encourage the client to void frequently. Preoperative and postoperative care for anterior colporrhaphy is described in Chapter 65.

RECTOCELE

Rectocele results when the rectovaginal fascia weakens and the rectum herniates into the posterior vaginal wall. An *enterocele* is the herniation of the intestine into the vagina. They are both caused by the same conditions as uterine prolapse and cystocele.

Clinical Manifestations

The general symptoms of a rectocele resemble those of uterine prolapse and cystocele. Specific manifestations include rectal fullness and incomplete evacuation of stool. At times, the client may need to reduce the posterior wall of the vagina manually to evacuate her stool.

Therapeutic Measures

Because rectoceles are present in all parous women to some extent, it is necessary to treat only those with symptoms. Perineal exercises such as Kegel exercises can help premenopausal clients and those without major symptoms. Stool softeners will help prevent constipation and reduce the instances of incomplete evacuation of stool. The sur-

gical technique for repair of a rectocele, posterior colporrhaphy, is described in Chapter 65.

Specific Nursing Measures

The nursing measures for clients with rectoceles are the same as those for clients with cystoceles, except rectocele clients are not prone to bladder infections. Chapter 65 describes client care for posterior colporrhaphy.

MENOPAUSE

Menopause is the cessation of ovarian activity with a concurrent cessation of the menses and a decrease in the ovarian hormones estrogen and progesterone. In the premenopausal state, the menses become irregular, and the flow may decrease. This occurs at different ages between 35 and 60 years; the average age is 51. Menopause is also discussed in Chapter 61.

Clinical Manifestations

The clinical manifestations of menopause result in part from the loss of estrogen and in part from aging. The process of menopause occurs over a period of time as the ovaries gradually decrease in size and function. This period of time is referred to as the *premenopause* and usually lasts for a few months, or sometimes for a few years. Most women experience these as mild changes and adapt with minimal disruption to their usual lifestyle during this premenopausal period.

The symptoms and physical signs involve many areas of the body. In the genital area, the vulval tissue thins. The vagina becomes shorter and narrower; the tissue thins, leading to atrophic vaginitis and perhaps an increase in irritation and infection. In the urinary tract, atrophic distal urethritis and stricture formation may occur. The ovaries and uterus markedly decrease in size.

The skin loses its elasticity. There may be muscle loss with fibrotic tissue formation. Bone mass peaks at age 35, after which it is either maintained or lost. This depends, in part, on the ratio of calcium to phosphorus. Osteoporosis, found mainly in small boned, thin, fair women, may result from the loss of estrogen. Family history of osteoporosis also increases the risk.

Vasomotor instability results in hot flashes, the sensation of overwhelming warmth that starts in the chest and rises upward. The skin becomes flushed, and the client may perspire profusely. Night sweats may interfere with sleep. Hot flashes stop when the body becomes adjusted to the new estrogen levels. Vasomotor symptoms may also include dizziness and numbness and tingling in the fingers and toes.

Psychological symptoms may include irritability and depression. The cause of depression has not been pinpointed, but if it occurs, it is probably due to a combination of factors. Some of the physiologic factors are biochemical and are related to aging and changes in hormone production. Others may be related to psychosocial factors. Menopause heralds the loss of youth and childbearing potential. Many other factors occur in addition to cessation of menstruation. For many women, children have grown up and left home, and anxiety about job security and life accomplishments increases.

Therapeutic Measures

Conservative treatments of menopausal symptoms include vitamins and herbs. Estrogen replacement therapy (ERT) also is used, but it poses greater risks for the client. Bellargal tablets (a combination of phenobarbital, ergotamine tartrate, and belladonna) have also been used for hot flashes. Because the drug contains a barbiturate, it produces a sedative effect and may be addictive.

Always obtain a thorough history of clients who seek medical attention for their symptoms to rule out the possibility that the symptoms are caused by disease processes such as genital carcinoma (in which ERT is contraindicated) rather than menopause. In addition, the history helps to determine clients who would be at increased risk from ERT. The data also alert health care providers to clients with emotional disorders; ERT should not be used to treat depression and irritability.

Vitamin therapy includes the use of calcium supplements and a decrease in the consumption of phosphorus found in foods such as breads, cereal, and soft drinks. Because older persons have a decreased ability to absorb calcium from the intestine in the presence of a high phosphorus level, the maintenance of the calcium–phosphorus ratio will help prevent bone loss.

Herbs and vitamins may alleviate vasomotor instability. Ginseng is thought to normalize the metabolic rate. Vitamin E may promote energy and a feeling of well-being; it also may alleviate leg cramps and relieve hot flashes by decreasing FSH. The vitamin B complex also may aid in the control of hot flashes (Fogel & Woods, 1981; Jensen & Bobak, 1985).

Estrogen replacement therapy is indicated for osteoporosis; severe vasomotor instability; and, in local application, for atrophic vaginitis. It is contraindicated in diseases of the liver, gallbladder, and pancreas; sickle-cell disease; and tumors of the uterus. It also may be contraindicated with thromboembolic disease, pulmonary embolism, hypertension, myocardial infarction, and tumors of the breast. The major risk of ERT is an apparent increase in the incidence of endometrial cancer with prolonged ERT. The lowest effective dose of estrogen should be used for only short periods—a few months or, at most, only a year—when the physical discomforts associated with menopause are at their peak. The estrogens used for ERT are ethinyl estradiol (0.02–0.05 mg), estradiol (Estrace, 1–2 mg), or conjugated estrogens (eg, Premarin, 0.3–1.25 mg). It is recommended that ERT be given on a cyclic schedule of 3 weeks on and 1 week off (Rodman & Smith, 1984). An increased incidence of blood clotting episodes has been seen in women who are on ERT for longer periods or who take larger doses. Vitamins B and C may be depleted in clients on ERT.

Specific Nursing Measures

It is important to stress the normalcy of menopause. Most women do not have difficulty with the climacteric (the time when menstrual cycles become further apart and blood flow decreases in amount). If serious effects are present, however, either vitamin therapy or ERT may be considered. The nurse can instruct the client in keeping a diary of her menstrual pattern.

Educate the client on the types of food to avoid, such as those high in phosphorus (see Box 24–1 in Chapter 24). Encourage a diet rich in calcium and vitamins E and B. Calcium can be found in cheese, milk, sesame seeds, and seaweed. Vitamin E is found in vegetable oils, wheat germ, soybeans, peanuts, and spinach; this vitamin takes from 2 to 4 weeks to begin decreasing FSH and effectively preventing hot flashes. Vitamin B is found in wheat germ, yogurt, whole grains, brewer's yeast, liver, and milk. The client should avoid a high protein diet.

Discuss the risks of ERT with the client. Prepare the client for the possibility of side effects with low-dose ERT such as breast tenderness, occasional gastrointestinal upset, and spotting. Inform the client that bleeding is normal when estrogens are withdrawn. Reassure the client that bleeding does not indicate a renewal of menstruation nor the possibility of becoming pregnant in postmenopausal women.

Section IV: Infectious and Inflammatory Disorders

Infectious and inflammatory disorders of the female reproductive system can be limited to the vaginal tract alone, to one or more reproductive organs, or result in disease affecting many systems in the body. The common vaginal infections and sexually transmitted diseases (STDs) will be discussed here, as well as the more encompassing disorders of PID and toxic shock syndrome. Parasitic infestations that may be sexually transmitted are discussed in Chapter 79.

Infectious vaginitis is one of the most frequent reasons clients seek medical attention. A number of different agents can produce signs and symptoms of infectious vaginitis. After the causative agent has been identified, treatment is directed toward eliminating the infection. This section will discuss the most common types of infectious vaginitis and their treatment.

Sexually transmitted diseases include syphilis, herpes genitalis, gonorrhea, and those that are discussed here as types of infectious vaginitis (*Candida albicans, Gardnerella vaginalis,* and *Trichomonas vaginalis* infections as well as chlamydial vaginitis).

GENERAL NURSING IMPLICATIONS

General nursing measures for infectious and inflammatory disorders include following the principles of good hygiene, which are discussed in Chapter 63. Possible reactions of the client include emotional shock, anger, guilt, fear, and decrease in self-esteem. Being an active listener and providing the client with support and health information are central nursing roles. All sexual partners need to be treated to prevent STD infection of others. Inform the client that syphilis and gonorrhea must be reported to the local public health department, which, in turn, reports cases to the Centers for Disease Control (see Chapter 11). The client can personally notify her sexual partners, or the public health department will assist her in notifying contacts.

YEAST INFECTIONS

The most common type of yeast infection is that from the overgrowth of *Candida albicans.* Yeast infections are most common in diabetic and pregnant women because of their high blood glucose level. The overgrowth of *Candida albicans* also can occur with the use of broad-spectrum antibiotics, which decrease the normal vaginal flora.

Clinical Manifestations

The vaginal discharge is thick, white, and cheesy. There is also perineal pruritus, and severe infections may cause dysuria from vulval, perineal, and periurethral excoriation. Diagnosis is made by microscopic evaluation of the discharge using saline or potassium hydroxide for slide preparation or by culture of the discharge (see Chapter 63).

Therapeutic Measures

Therapeutic measures for yeast infections include the insertion of miconazole nitrate (Monistat) or clotrimazole (Lotrimin) suppositories or cream into the vagina nightly for 5 to 7 days. These pharmacologic agents treat the infection effectively. Consider suggesting treatment of the partner, because the yeast may be present on the prepuce, the folds of skin on the penis, and the scrotum.

Specific Nursing Measures

Instruct the client to avoid a high-carbohydrate diet. Test the client for possible diabetes because the organism thrives in a high-carbohydrate environment. It also grows in warm, moist environments. Advise the client to take off her bathing suit after it becomes wet and to avoid tight jeans and nylon underwear.

GARDNERELLA VAGINALIS INFECTIONS

The hemophilus bacterium *Gardnerella vaginalis* can cause vaginal infection. The bacteria can be transmitted sexually but can also exist normally in the vagina in small amounts without causing symptoms. When vaginal acidity is decreased, the bacteria will overgrow.

Clinical Manifestations

The vaginal discharge is profuse and has a pronounced fishy odor. Microscopic examination shows characteristic epithelial cells covered with bacteria, referred to as *clue cells,* as well as a large number of leukocytes. A general bacterial culture can also confirm the presence of *Gardnerella vaginalis.*

Therapeutic Measures

Therapeutic measures include tetracycline (500 mg q.i.d. for 10 days) or metronidazole (Flagyl) (500 mg t.i.d. for 5 to 7 days). If the client is allergic to these pharmacologic agents, erythromycin or ampicillin may be used. Treatment of the client's sexual partner will prevent reinfection. Screen clients for pregnancy because it will contraindicate some of the drugs used. Ampicillin should be used to treat pregnant women.

Specific Nursing Measures

Tell the client to avoid sexual contact until the treatment has been completed. Institute general nursing measures as discussed in Chapter 63.

TRICHOMONAS VAGINALIS INFECTIONS

Trichomonas vaginalis infections are caused by the protozoan of that name. This one-celled parasite is transmitted sexually and possibly by contact with objects contaminated by vaginal or urethral discharge from an infected person.

Clinical Manifestations

A *Trichomonas vaginalis* infection has symptoms that include a profuse thin, foamy, yellow-green discharge with an unpleasant odor. The vagina or cervix may have a strawberry color from small petechiae. The protozoan can be easily identified by microscopic examination using a saline preparation (see Chapter 63).

Therapeutic Measures

Treatment by metronidazole, either 250 mg t.i.d. for 7 days or 2 g in a single dose, effectively eradicates the infection if the sexual partner is also treated. If not, the client will become reinfected. Pregnant clients should not take metronidazole.

Specific Nursing Measures

Specific nursing measures include the identification of pregnancy because pregnant women should not be treated with metronidazole. Instead, a povidone-iodine gel can help decrease the discharge; however, it does not eradicate the infection. Because the organism can live in moist environments outside the body for up to 6 hours, clients should be cautioned against sharing towels or other personal items with others.

CHLAMYDIAL VAGINITIS INFECTIONS

Chlamydial vaginitis is caused by some of the organisms in the genus *Chlamydia*. Chlamydia are also a major cause of nongonococcal urethritis (NGU) (discussed in Chapter 67). It is the most prevalent STD in the United States.

Clinical Manifestations

The vaginal discharge is thin, white, and bubbly, with little odor. The diagnosis is made by culture using a special medium or by excluding other possible causes.

Therapeutic Measures

Treatment for chlamydial vaginitis involves either tetracycline (500 mg a day for 7 days) or erythromycin (250 mg t.i.d. for 7 days). Sexual partners also should be treated.

Specific Nursing Measures

General nursing measures to decrease the risk of infection should be implemented. The client should avoid intercourse or condoms should be used until the treatment has been completed.

SYPHILIS

The incidence of syphilis increased 17% in women from 1977 to 1980 (Miles, 1984), although the incidence of syphilis, in general, is decreasing in the 1980s. Syphilis affects 12 out of 100,000 people. As the rate for women increases, the incidence of congenital syphilis also increases. The disease can be found in newborns, who contract it from the mother after the third month of gestation.

Clinical Manifestations

The causative agent, the spirochete *Treponema pallidum,* is detected by dark-field examination of the lesion (chancre) during the first stage of the disease after the incubation period of 10 to 90 days. The routine serologic test for syphilis is the VDRL test (see Chapter 63), which is positive after about 3 months of exposure.

Different stages of syphilis have different symptoms. As the organism incubates, there are no symptoms. The

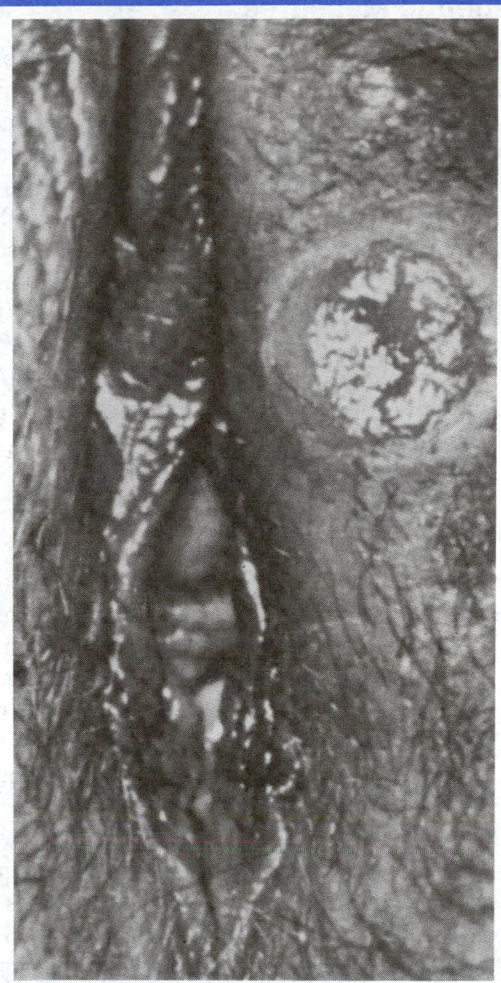

Figure 64–7

Syphilitic chancre on the labia.
SOURCE: Crooks R, Bauer K: *Our Sexuality,* 2nd ed. Menlo Park, CA: Benjamin/Cummings, 1983.

primary stage involves the formation of a lesion, a chancre, which appears after the 10- to 90-day incubation period. There is usually only one chancre, which begins as an indurated papule; the surface then erodes, forming a painless ulcer (Figure 64–7). If treatment is not begun at this time, the ulcer will heal in about 3 to 9 weeks. The regional lymph nodes also may be enlarged at this time.

The female client with secondary syphilis has systemic symptoms such as malaise, headache, and fever. The characteristic vulval lesions, condylomata lata, are raised, flat, moist, and gray. They may be ulcerated and indurated. Lesions also can be found in the mouth and pharynx, under the breasts, and in the axillae. There usually is painless inguinal adenopathy.

The third stage of the disease is not discussed here because its chief manifestations involve areas other than the reproductive system. Third-stage syphilis is discussed in Chapter 37.

Therapeutic Measures

The treatment for syphilis in the primary and secondary stages is the administration of penicillin G benzathine (2.4 million units IM in a single dose). Probenecid (Benemid) is given 30 minutes before the injection. Probenecid delays excretion of penicillin resulting in higher plasma levels for longer periods. Aqueous penicillin G procaine (600,000 units IM daily for 8 days) also may be administered. Clients allergic to penicillin may be given tetracycline hydrochloride (500 mg PO q.i.d. for 15 days). If a pregnant client has a penicillin allergy, erythromycin (500 mg PO q.i.d. for 15 days) should be given instead of tetracycline. Erythromycin is also given to those allergic to both penicillin and tetracycline.

Specific Nursing Measures

The specific nursing measures for syphilis depend on the stage of the disease. The nurse should identify pregnancy in the client so the appropriate therapy can be given. Also identify clients allergic to penicillin. Warn the client that the administration of high doses of penicillin can create soreness at the injection site.

Tell the client who is being treated during the secondary stage that a post-treatment reaction may occur approximately 4 hours after treatment. This reaction, the *Jarisch–Herxheimer reaction,* results from the sudden massive destruction of spirochetes by antibiotics. It is characterized by chills, elevated temperature, general body aches, headache, malaise, and increased skin lesions. The reaction usually peaks in about 8 hours and lasts for about 16 hours. If this reaction occurs, clients are less likely to be made anxious by it if it is explained to them and they anticipate its possibility. Offer the client symptomatic relief and reassurance during this uncomfortable period. Treatment should not be discontinued unless the symptoms are severe or threaten to be fatal, or if laryngitis, auditory neuritis, or labyrinthitis is present since these may signify the possibility of irreversible damage.

Encourage the client to contact the sexual partner or partners so that they can receive effective therapy. The client should return for repeat serologic tests 3, 6, and 12 months after treatment.

HERPES GENITALIS

Infections with herpes simplex viruses (HSVs, or *Herpesvirus hominis*) are common STDs. Herpes simplex type II is the one found most often in the genital area. Herpes simplex type I also can be found there but is more often associated with infections of the mouth, such as cold sores. Herpes genitalis is not a reportable disease, although its incidence seems to be increasing. The infection is found most often in the age group of 15 to 30 years.

There is no known cure for herpes genitalis. The inactive form lies dormant in the spinal root ganglia. The virus causes serious complications to the newborn who contracts it during delivery or after the membranes rupture. HSV has been linked to cancer of the cervix and vulva.

Clinical Manifestations

The primary course of herpes genitalis is more severe than its recurrences. In the primary form of the disease, vesicles rupture and cause a painful ulcer; this form also has systemic effects such as fever, malaise, and inguinal node enlargement. These symptoms occur approximately 2 to 7 days after incubation. The ulcers have a yellowish gray color with a surrounding raised edge and are usually present on the medial aspects of the labia minora and the clitoris, vagina, urethra, and cervix (Figure 64–8). They can last from 4 to 6 weeks. Secondary infections can recur from every few weeks to once or twice a year. These ulcers do not last as long, and there is no associated lymphadenopathy. The recurrences occur more often in men than women. The disease may be transmitted to others when lesions are present.

Diagnosis of herpes genitalis is made by microbiological smear by touch preparation on a slide; multinucleated giant cells are usually found. The Pap test also may be used.

Therapeutic Measures

Although there is no known cure, acyclovir (Zovirax) can be used to help reduce the duration of the first attack of the disease and to reduce pain and itching. It does not eliminate latent infection, so there are recurrences, but it may reduce the risk of recurrences and, thus, the transmission of the disease.

Alcohol and other drying agents can be used to dry

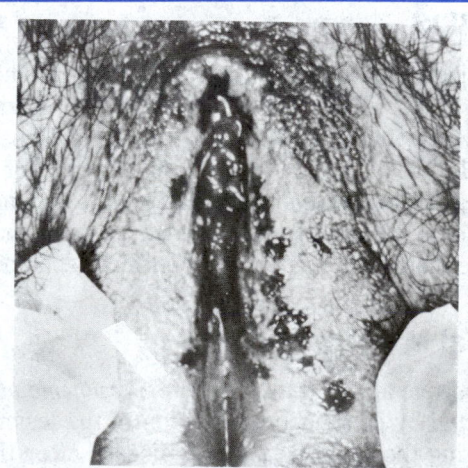

Figure 64–8

Genital herpes blisters on the labia.
SOURCE: Crooks R, Bauer K: *Our Sexuality,* 2nd ed. Menlo Park, CA: Benjamin/Cummings, 1983.

lesions on the vulva. The client may need sedation during the first week of the disease when the lesions are the most painful. Hospitalization may be necessary if extensive lesions prevent normal voiding.

Specific Nursing Measures

The diagnosis of herpes genitalis can cause severe emotional trauma when the client realizes there is no cure. She may have difficulty notifying her sexual partner or partners, feel violated, and experience guilt feelings for contracting an STD. The nurse must recognize the client's fear and anxiety.

During the painful primary stage, evaluate the client's need for pain medication and inform her that recurrences of the disease will not be as incapacitating. Instruct clients to refrain from intercourse when lesions are present. Close follow-up during pregnancy is necessary because of the risk of the unborn child's contracting a highly fatal neonatal infection or congenital deformities.

GONORRHEA

One of the most common STDs is caused by *Neisseria gonorrhoeae,* a gram-negative diplococcus. Approximately 1 million cases are reported each year, and a total of 3 million are suspected because of underreporting of the disease. The organism has become increasingly resistant to penicillin (see Chapter 67).

Clinical Manifestations

It is estimated that between 50% and 75% of women with gonorrhea are asymptomatic or have mild symptoms, including transient vaginal discharge, dysuria, low abdominal discomfort, or a change in menstrual patterns (Miles, 1984). The endocervix is the primary site of infection in women. The infection can spread up the reproductive system and cause PID as it spreads into the fallopian tubes, possibly during menstruation. It also can spread downward, leading to a urethral infection that causes dysuria, discharge, and urinary frequency. Gonorrhea can also be present in Bartholin's glands, causing infection with signs of labial pain and edema. A disseminated gonococcal infection causes symptoms of fever; skin lesions that begin as maculae and progress to vesicles and hemorrhagic pustules; and joint pain with or without swelling, erythema, and heat.

Diagnosis in the woman is made by culturing the endocervix, rectum, and pharynx, depending on the type of sexual involvement. If oral sex has occurred, a culture of the pharynx also is obtained.

Therapeutic Measures

The key to the treatment of gonorrhea is effective antibiotic administration. The following guidelines are based on the recommendations of the Centers for Disease Control (CDC) (1982).

In uncomplicated cases of gonorrhea in adults, treatment is a single dose of aqueous penicillin G procaine (4.8 million units IM) divided and given in two sites and probenecid (1.0 g PO). Because it requires only one dose, this method is useful if a client is not perceived to be reliable. Disadvantages are that many gonococci are resistant to penicillin, the client may be allergic to either penicillin or procaine, and the injection is painful. Often chlamydial infections coexist with the gonococcus, and penicillin will not eradicate them.

Other treatment options are tetracycline hydrochloride (500 mg PO q.i.d. for 7 days) or doxycycline (100 mg PO b.i.d. for 7 days). These drugs are well absorbed, raise both urine and urethral drug levels, and are effective against coexisting chlamydial infections. Disadvantages are that strict compliance to the drug regimen is needed, some gonococci are resistant to tetracyclines, and tetracyclines are not effective in treating anorectal infections.

Clients may also be treated with one dose of amoxicillin (3.0 g PO) or ampicillin (3.5 g). Usually, 1.0 g probenecid is given with these drugs to interfere with renal tubule excretion of the penicillins and therefore increase serum levels. These drugs will not treat coexisting chlamydial infections and are not effective against anorectal or pharyngeal infections. The problem of possible organism resistance also exists.

Spectinomycin hydrochloride (Trobicin; 2.0 g IM) is used if the organism is penicillin resistant or if the client is allergic to penicillin. Again, 1.0 g of probenecid is usually administered by mouth as well. Some strains may be resistant to spectinomycin hydrochloride and it, too, is ineffective against coexisting chlamydial and pharyngeal infections.

The CDC recommends that all PPNG (penicillinase-producing *Neisseria gonorrhoeae;* those that are resistant to all forms of penicillin) strains be tested for spectinomycin resistance. In these instances, clients should be treated with cefoxitin sodium (Mefoxin) or cefotaximine (Claforan) in combination with probenecid.

Treatment of pharyngeal gonorrhea is the same. Anorectal gonorrhea is treated with aqueous penicillin G procaine or spectinomycin (2.0 g IM). Treatment for disseminated gonorrhea is aqueous crystalline penicillin G (10 million units IM per day until improvement is seen); then amoxicillin (500 mg PO) or ampicillin (500 mg PO) is given q.i.d. for at least 7 days. Other treatment regimens may also be followed.

Specific Nursing Measures

Educate the client about the disease, methods of transmission, disease process, and management. Clients with no symptoms may have trouble understanding that they have a serious infection. Teach good hand-washing techniques to prevent the infection's spread to the conjunctiva. Give instructions for taking oral medication if necessary, and warn the client not to share her medication with her partner.

A repeat culture is necessary 2 weeks after pharmacologic treatment has begun to determine whether the infection was cured or if it is caused by a penicillinase-producing strain. Until a negative culture has been obtained, tell the client to avoid sexual relations. Emotional support includes allowing the client to discuss concerns about the treatment plan as well as personal concerns.

PELVIC INFLAMMATORY DISEASE

Acute pelvic inflammatory disease (PID) is an infection of the uterus and fallopian tubes that can extend into the pelvic cavity and involve the broad ligament, adjacent blood vessels, and lymphatics. Salpingitis, or inflammation of the fallopian tube, is the most common clinical finding.

Complications of PID are numerous. The disease leads to infertility in 10% of women who have had it once. Chances of infertility increase to 25% after two episodes and to 50% after three or more episodes. PID also can lead to ectopic pregnancy. Recurrent infections are another risk. Chronic abdominal pain is present in about 15% of the cases and may be a result of pelvic adhesions.

The most frequent cause of PID is infection by *Neisseria gonorrhoeae,* the causative organism for gonorrhea. Other sexually transmitted infecting organisms are *Chlamydia trachomatis* and genital mycoplasmas. PID also can be caused by organisms that are not sexually transmitted, such as aerobic and anaerobic bacteria, which are in the normal flora of the cervix and vagina.

The risk of PID increases with the number of sexual partners as well as in clients with IUDs. The disease occurs more often in younger sexually active females, with the highest rate (1.5% to 2.0%) in clients 15 to 19 years old.

Clinical Manifestations

The clinical manifestations of PID vary from mild to severe. As has been discussed, salpingitis is the most common finding. The most common symptom, abdominal pain, is usually present only for a short time if it results from salpingitis. There may be an increase in vaginal discharge, as well as metrorrhagia and menorrhagia from endometritis. Less than half the clients have a fever. Nausea and vomiting occur when the bowel serosa and muscularis are involved.

Diagnosis is based on the history of contact with an infected partner and the physical examination, which usually demonstrates tenderness of the lower abdominal area, cervix, uterus, and adnexa. The sedimentation rate and white blood cell (WBC) count may be elevated. A Gram's stain of the cervical secretions may reveal *Neisseria gonorrhoeae.* The cervical secretion is also cultured to detect *N. gonorrhoeae* and *Chlamydia trachomatis.* If examination of the male partner reveals a gonococcal infection, PID is suggested in the female. Ultrasonography may help diag-

nose pelvic abscesses. Laparoscopy can be used to obtain a culture of the infecting organism from the fallopian tubes.

Therapeutic Measures

Treatment for the milder forms of PID include bed rest at home in a semi-Fowler's position to promote drainage. In 1982, the Centers for Disease Control recommended the following medications: cefoxitin (2.0 g IM), amoxicillin (3.0 g PO), ampicillin (3.5 g PO), or aqueous penicillin G procaine (4.8 million units IM), each with probenecid (1 g PO). Each of these medications is followed by doxycycline (100 mg PO b.i.d. for 10 to 14 days) or tetracycline hydrochloride (500 mg PO q.i.d. for 10 to 14 days).

If the case of PID is more severe or outpatient treatment fails, inpatient treatment is needed. Analgesics are given for pain. Decreased fluid intake is corrected, and electrolyte balance is restored intravenously. Bed rest and a semi-Fowler's position are used. There is no standard antibiotic regimen. However, intravenous doxycycline may be given, followed by an oral dose; clindamycin given intravenously plus gentamicin or tobramycin given intravenously also may be used. Clindamycin or doxycycline is then used as an oral medication.

Specific Nursing Measures

Bed rest is maintained as previously described. Depending on the organism, the nurse may ask the client to notify her sexual partner or partners for treatment. Give supportive care by being accepting of the client and providing time for discussion of client concerns. Give pain medication as ordered for relief of abdominal pain. Monitor fluid intake if the client is receiving fluids intravenously or vomiting. Explain the treatment regimen to the client, along with the possible side effects of the medication. A case study of a client with PID follows this chapter.

TOXIC SHOCK SYNDROME

In one study, most cases (97%) of toxic shock syndrome (TSS) coincided with tampon use during the menstrual cycle (Cibulka, 1984). This infection suddenly causes various symptoms. It can occur without tampon use in association with infected wounds, deep abscesses, lacerations, and insect bites. The causative agent is usually toxin secreted by strains of *Staphylococcus aureus,* but the mechanisms are not clearly understood. In cases involving tampon use, there seems to be a correlation between the chemical fibers used in superabsorbent tampons and the incidence of TSS. In a recent study (Mills et al., 1985), the production of the toxin associated with TSS was controlled (in the laboratory) by the concentration of magnesium; the lower the concentration of magnesium, the higher the concentration of the toxin. Fibers that bind the magnesium in the vagina were demonstrated to increase strikingly the amount of toxin produced. The incidence of TSS in the United States is 6.2 cases per 100,000 menstruating women per year.

Clinical Manifestations

The toxin can affect almost any body system. The symptoms include a rapid onset of fever of 102°F (38.9°C) or higher, nausea and vomiting, and a diffuse rash followed by desquamation of the skin of the palms and soles about 1 to 2 weeks after the disease's onset. Hypotension with a systolic blood pressure less than 90 mm Hg is also a symptom.

Three or more of the following organ systems or structures must be involved for the disease to be considered TSS:

- The gastrointestinal system, with vomiting and diarrhea at the onset of the illness
- The musculoskeletal system, with severe myalgia and a creatine phosphokinase (CPK) level at more than twice normal
- The mucous membranes, with hyperemia
- The kidneys with impaired renal function and elevated blood urea nitrogen or CPK levels at least twice the upper limit of normal
- The hepatic system, with serum glutamic-oxaloacetic transaminase (SGOT) or serum glutamic-pyruvic transaminase (SGPT) at twice the upper limit of normal
- The hematologic system, with thrombocytopenia
- The central nervous system, with confusion, alterations in consciousness, and possible combative behavior

A differential diagnosis of TSS requires that negative results be obtained from blood and cerebrospinal fluid cultures. Serologic tests for Rocky Mountain spotted fever, leptospirosis, and measles also must be negative.

Therapeutic Measures

The tampon should be removed and the client placed in isolation. Treatment for TSS includes bed rest and antibiotic therapy with beta-lactamase–resistant antibiotics such as nafcillin and gentamicin. As soon as possible, obtain cultures from the nasopharynx, blood, urine, stool, and open sores. Intravenous infusion can prevent shock from hypotension and electrolyte loss. If the infusion does not prevent hypotension, a vasopressor drug may be used. Oxygen may be needed if the client shows signs of respiratory distress.

Specific Nursing Measures

Administer antibiotics and assess the client's temperature frequently; a hypothermia blanket may be needed. Nausea and vomiting may necessitate a nasogastric tube. Administer medication for nausea and vomiting as ordered. Because of prolonged bed rest, assess the client's skin frequently and help eliminate areas of pressure. Provide passive ROM and turn the client frequently. Encourage coughing and deep breathing.

Monitor fluid intake and output for signs of circulatory overload (headache, flushed skin, a rapid pulse, venous distention, coughing, and shortness of breath). Also monitor arterial blood gases for signs of adult respiratory distress syndrome (see Chapter 20).

If TSS affects the central nervous system, the client may become confused and combative. If necessary, protect her with soft restraints, and frequently orient her to time, person, place, and events. Prevent sensory overload by ensuring a quiet environment. Support the client's family or significant others by explaining procedures and answering questions. Clients who have had TSS should know that they are at risk for TSS in the future and should probably avoid tampon use.

Section V: Neoplastic Disorders

The malignant disorders discussed in this section are cancer of the uterus (both endometrial cancer and cervical cancer), ovarian cancer, vulval cancer, and cancer of the breast. Fallopian tube cancer is very rare and will not be discussed here. The benign disorders discussed include uterine leiomyomas, benign ovarian tumors, and benign breast disease.

GENERAL NURSING IMPLICATIONS

Carcinomas of the reproductive system, including the breast, account for more than 40% of all female cancers and are the most common cause of cancer deaths in the female client. The incidence and deaths from cancer of the reproductive system are compared by site in Table 64–1. Early

Table 64–1	Cancer Incidence and Deaths: Female Reproductive System	
Site	**Incidence**	**Deaths**
Breast	119,000	38,400
Cervix	15,000	6800
Endometrium	37,000	2900
Ovary	18,500	11,600
Other	4400	1100

SOURCE: American Cancer Society: *1985 Cancer Facts and Figures.* New York: American Cancer Society, 1985.

detection increases the rate of cure and survival. The results of early detection screening can be seen in the 70% decrease in uterine cancer during the past 40 years. The decrease in deaths is primarily attributable to the Pap test. The survival rate in breast cancer is almost 100% if the cancer is treated before it has become invasive (American Cancer Society, 1985). This means that a crucial nursing role is the prevention and early detection of reproductive system cancers.

A neoplasm of the reproductive system can in some instances, mean an end to a woman's reproductive years or pose a threat to personal, family, and career goals. Caring for these clients requires a combination of technical and psychosocial skills. Specific nursing measures for both malignant and benign neoplasia are discussed in this section. General therapeutic measures for cancer have been discussed in Chapter 12 and specific surgical treatments for both benign and malignant neoplasia in Chapter 65.

ENDOMETRIAL CANCER

Endometrial cancer affects mostly mature women between the ages of 50 and 64. Although it can occur in younger women, it is rare before the age of 40 (Quilligan, 1983). The conditions that put women at risk for the development of endometrial cancer are obesity, history of infertility, failure of ovulation, hypertension, and diabetes in a postmenopausal woman. Other conditions include late menopause and the prolonged use of ERT. (See Table 64–1 for incidence and mortality.)

Clinical Manifestations

Endometrial hyperplasia is present before the development of cancer; this may result from unopposed estrogen. The major symptom of endometrial cancer is some form of abnormal bleeding. Any vaginal bleeding in a postmenopausal client should be evaluated. A D and C is performed to assess the uterine lining for signs of endometrial hyperplasia or carcinoma. The Pap test, although highly effective in detecting early cervical cancer, is only 50% effective in detecting endometrial cancer. An endometrial biopsy at menopause is a more accurate method of detection.

Therapeutic Measures

Surgery combined with radiation therapy is usually the treatment of choice for endometrial cancer depending on the stage of the disease and the individual health characteristics of the client. Staging for endometrial cancer is defined in Box 64–3. Stage Ia tumors are treated surgically without irradiation. In Stage II and more extensive carcinomas, the TAH-BSO (discussed in Chapter 65) is performed along with lymph node dissection. Preoperative radiation therapy either by radium implants or external irradiation is used in endometrial cancers of Stage Ib and greater when clients are capable of undergoing surgery. In

those clients with inoperable tumors (usually stages III and IV) and those with postoperative recurrences, treatment includes external and/or intracavitary irradiation.

Clients with tumors that are positive estrogen and progesterone receptors usually respond to hormonal therapy. Progestins or megestrol acetate may be used in premenopausal clients who do not choose to have a TAH-BSO because they wish to preserve childbearing potential. For clients with advanced disease (extended outside the uterus) or recurrent disease, hydroxyprogesterone caproate (Delalutin) may be effective. Tamoxifen citrate (Nolvadex) may be effective in clients whose disease has progressed after therapy with progestins.

There is no specific combination of chemotherapy agents used in advanced disease. Combinations of vincristine, dactinomycin and cyclophosphamide, or dacarbazine and doxorubicin, have been shown to be somewhat effective.

Specific Nursing Measures

Nursing measures for endometrial cancer clients are discussed in Chapters 12 and 65. These chapters discuss surgical approaches and care of the client receiving radiation, respectively.

CERVICAL CANCER

There are two types of cervical cancer. The most common type, squamous cell carcinoma, is believed to be viral in origin and almost never occurs in virgins. The other type, adenocarcinoma, may be present in virgins as well as nonvirgins. Cervical cancer begins as a change in the epithelial covering of the cervix and eventually involves the epithelial layer. This change can be considered premalignant and is called cervical intraepithelial neoplasia (CIN); at this stage, there is no metastasis of the cells. The Pap test is highly

---

Box 64–3   Staging of Endometrial Cancer

Stage I: Carcinoma confined to the corpus

Subdivision according to size of uterus:
Ia: Uterine cavity sounds to 8 cm or less
Ib: Uterine cavity sounds to more than 8 cm

Subdivision according to histology:
G1: Highly differentiated adenomatous carcinomas
G2: Differentiated adenomatous carcinomas with partly solid areas
G3: Predominantly solid or entirely undifferentiated carcinomas

Stage II: Carcinoma has involved corpus and cervix

Stage III: Carcinoma has extended outside uterus but not outside true pelvis

Stage IV: Carcinoma has extended outside true pelvis or has obviously involved mucosa of bladder or rectum. Bullous edema as such does not permit allotment of a case to stage IV

effective in detecting these early changes. Invasive carcinoma extends beyond the surface, involves the body of the cervix, and from there can spread to the lymphatic system and extend to surrounding structures such as the vagina, bladder, and rectum. Incidence and mortality are listed in Table 64–1.

Clinical Manifestations

The client is symptom-free in the early stages, although early changes in cellular structure can be diagnosed by the Pap test. Therefore, regular examination of the cervix, vagina, and vulva are necessary along with a complete pelvic examination. A lesion can be visualized by colposcopy or more in-depth evaluation of the cells can be accomplished by a cone biopsy if the lesion extends into the endocervical canal. Staging of cervical cancer is defined in Box 64–4.

Therapeutic Measures

Treatment depends on the extent of the disease, the state of the client's general health, her age, and whether or not she wishes to have her reproductive potential preserved. The treatment of premalignant lesions can consist of cryotherapy, electrocautery, laser therapy, or conization. Hysterectomy is performed for carcinoma in situ. Stage 0 (carcinoma in situ) and stage I and Ia carcinoma can also

---

Box 64–4 Staging of Cervical Cancer

Stage 0: Carcinoma in situ, intraepithelial carcinoma

Stage 1: Carcinoma strictly confined to the cervix (extension to the corpus should be disregarded)
  Ia: Microinvasive carcinoma (early stromal invasion)
  Ib: All other cases of stage I; occult cancer should be marked "occ"

Stage II: Carcinoma extends beyond the cervix, but not to the pelvic wall; the carcinoma involves the vagina, but not as far as the lower third
  IIa: No obvious parametrial involvement
  IIb: Obvious parametrial involvement

Stage III: Carcinoma extends to the pelvic wall; on rectal examination, there is no cancer-free space between the tumor and the pelvic wall; the tumor involves the lower third of the vagina; all cases with a hydronephrosis or nonfunctioning kidney are included
  IIIa: No extension to the pelvic wall
  IIIb: Extension to the pelvic wall and/or hydronephrosis or nonfunctioning kidney

Stage IV: Carcinoma extends beyond true pelvis or has clinically involved the mucosa of the bladder or rectum; a bullous edema as such does not permit a case to be allotted to stage IV
  IVa: Spread of the growth to adjacent organs
  IVb: Spread to distant organs

---

be conservatively managed by cervical conization, transvaginal roentgentherapy, and laser treatment. Clients who are conservatively managed should be closely evaluated at least yearly for further appearances of cancer. Either surgery or radiation is used for stages Ia and IIa cancer of the cervix.

The surgery for stage Ia involves a TAH, or a TAH with removal of the upper vagina, depending on the tumor depth. For stages Ib and IIa, radical abdominal hysterectomy and bilateral pelvic lymphadenectomy are performed. Irradiation is used alone for stages IIb and III. In stage IV, pelvic exenteration, although rarely used, may be performed.

Radiotherapy is effective in the treatment of cervical cancer and is often used in combination with surgery. In early stages, intracavitary applications of radium are used. In the operating room, vaginal cylinders are placed in the lateral vaginal fonices. Once the client returns to her room, the applicators are loaded with the radioactive material. The dose and time are calculated by a computer; the usual insertion length is 48 to 72 hours. During this period of time, the client remains on bed rest with a catheter and a low residue diet.

In advanced tumors (stages III and IV), external radiation is beneficial in reducing the symptoms. External and internal radiation may be used together. Interstitial radiation, the direct insertion of radioactive needles into the tumor, is another treatment modality.

Chemotherapeutic agents that have been used with some success include methotrexate, cyclophosphamide, and combinations of hydroxyurea or doxorubicin and radiotherapy. Combination chemotherapy is used for late and recurring carcinomas and includes such drugs as bleomycin, mitomycin C, and cisplatin. A description of surgical techniques is found in Chapter 65, and chemotherapy and radiation therapy are discussed in Chapter 12.

Specific Nursing Measures

See Chapter 65 for a discussion of preoperative and postoperative nursing care for the various procedures. Chapter 12 discusses chemotherapy, radiation therapy, and general nursing care of the cancer client.

OVARIAN CANCER

Ovarian cancer is more difficult than endometrial cancer to detect in its early stages, and therefore the disease has often spread by the time it is detected. The survival rate is only about 30% (Dugan, 1985). Ovarian cancer occurs in all age groups but is more common in women 40 to 65 years old. By 55 years, it is the fourth most common cause of cancer deaths in women. (See Table 64–4 for incidence and mortality rates.)

Ovarian malignancies are caused by 19 different cell types with 27 subtypes, based on the histologic examination of the lesion. Because of this wide range of cell types,

---

Box 64–5 Staging of Ovarian Cancer

Stage I: Tumor limited to ovaries
  Ia: Limited to one ovary; no ascites
  Ib: Limited to both ovaries; no ascites
  Ic: Limited to one or both ovaries with ascites or positive peritoneal washings

Stage II: Tumor of one or both ovaries with pelvic extension
  Ia: Extension and/or metastases to uterus and/or tubes only
  IIb: Extension to other pelvic tissues
  IIc: As in IIa and IIb with ascites or positive peritoneal washings

Stage III: Tumor of one or both ovaries with intraperitoneal abdominal metastases; involvement of retroperitoneal lymph nodes or extension to small bowel or omentum within pelvis

Stage IV: Tumor of one or both ovaries with distant metastases outside of peritoneal cavity

---

ovarian cancers differ in their characteristics and potential for metastasis.

Clients at high risk are those with ovarian imbalance as demonstrated by infertility, nulliparity, and early menopause. There is also a correlation between a diet high in animal fat and an increased incidence of ovarian cancer.

Clinical Manifestations

Most ovarian cancers are not diagnosed until the lesion has metastasized outside the pelvis. The client may have an increase in abdominal girth from the growth of the tumor, ascites, or both. Any adnexal mass after menopause should be evaluated by laparoscopy or laparotomy. Other symptoms that should be evaluated are an adnexal mass 6 cm in diameter or greater in a woman of any age, a mass less than 6 cm in diameter that persists through one menstrual cycle, and any solid mass that cannot be diagnosed as a uterine leiomyoma. Staging of ovarian cancer is defined in Box 64–5.

Therapeutic Measures

Evaluation of the tumor determines what type of surgery is indicated in premenopausal clients. If the cancer is a dysgerminoma (derived from the germ cells of the embryonic gonad), only the affected ovary need be removed. In postmenopausal clients, a TAH–BSO is performed. The omentum and lymph nodes may also be removed if there is evidence of metastasis.

Radiation is best accomplished by external abdominal and pelvic irradiation using cobalt or supervoltages. Chemotherapeutic agents are thought to be responsible for remissions in some instances. The chemotherapeutic agents used include alkylating agents, cisplatin, doxorubicin, and various combinations of these agents.

Specific Nursing Measures

Nursing measures for surgical care of the client are discussed in Chapter 65. Care of the client with cancer is discussed in Chapter 12.

VULVAL CANCER

Cancer of the vulva is usually found in elderly women, with the highest incidence between ages 70 and 80. It is the fifth most common female reproductive cancer and the fourth most common pelvic reproductive cancer. Those most at risk have had chronic vulvitis treated by various methods without biopsy. The disease progresses from a dysplasia through intraepithelial neoplasia to invasive cancer. The premalignant dysplasia and epithelial involvement may be present for 10 years or longer, and the invasive lesion may extend locally for a time before it metastasizes. As with other cancers, the earlier the disease is recognized and treated, the better the client's chances for recovery. Thus biopsy should be performed on all lesions suggestive of cancer.

Clinical Manifestations

The most common symptom of vulval cancer is vulval pruritus. There may also be a history of chronic vulvitis (chronic inflammation of the vulva). A neoplasm should be suspected in any woman with a chronic irritation that fails to heal with treatment, or when an ulceration develops. A raised, grayish white hypertrophic patch on the vulva, referred to as **leukoplakia,** may precede invasive cancer in up to 50% of cases (Kase & Weingold, 1983). Fewer than 10%, however, become malignant. Staging for carcinoma of the vulva is defined in Box 64–6.

Therapeutic Measures

The treatment for vulval cancer is surgical removal of the vulva (vulvectomy) and the superficial inguinal lymph nodes. Radiation therapy is not performed because of the high probability that it will cause extensive tissue necrosis. Chapter 65 describes the vulvectomy procedure.

Box 64–6 Staging of Vulval Cancer

Stage I: Tumor 2 cm or less confined to vulva; no suspicious lymph nodes

Stage II: Tumor over 2 cm confined to vulva; no suspicious lymph nodes

Stage III: Tumor extending beyond vulva (urethra, vagina, perineum, anus); no suspicious lymph nodes. Tumor of any size confined to vulva with grossly positive nodes

Stage IV: Tumor of any size extending to upper urethra or bladder, rectum, or bone with fixed or ulcerated lymph nodes or distant metastases

Specific Nursing Measures

The elderly woman may hesitate to have a vulvectomy because of embarrassment. She will need the nurse's support during both diagnosis and treatment. Chapter 65 reviews the nursing care of the vulvectomy client.

BREAST CANCER

Breast cancer is the most common cause of cancer deaths in women, although it is anticipated that the lung cancer death rate for women will surpass the breast cancer death rate by 1986 (American Cancer Society, 1985).

About one out of every 11 women in the United States will develop breast cancer. Its incidence has been rising over the last 15 years, but so has the survival rate. (See Table 64–1 for incidence and mortality.) As a woman ages, her risk of developing breast cancer increases. Breast cancer is most often found in women over the age of 50, but the incidence has increased in women aged 20 to 30. A personal history of breast cancer and a family history of the disease—especially if it occurs before menopause and is bilateral—increase the risk. Women who have never had children or delayed pregnancy until after the age of 30 are also at an increased risk. The onset of menses and menopause influence the risk of developing breast cancer: If menses occurs before the age of 14 and menopause occurs later than age 55, the risk of breast cancer development is higher. Some nutritional factors also have been linked to the development of breast cancer, including being overweight by more than 40% and consuming a diet high in fat.

Breast cancer usually develops in the epithelial breast tissue. The most common sites are the ducts (90%) and the lobules (5%), with the remaining 5% being other types, including Paget's disease of the nipple and inflammatory carcinoma (USDHHS, 1984). The epithelial cells undergo hyperplasia, which may or may not gradually progress to carcinoma in situ and then to invasive carcinoma. The most common type is invasive ductal carcinoma, which often spreads to the axillary nodes. About half the tumors develop in the upper outer quadrant of the breast (Figure 64–9).

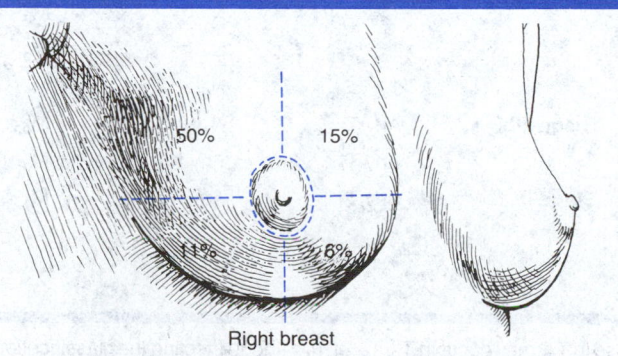

50%   15%
11%   6%

Right breast

Figure 64–9

Location of breast cancer. About half of all breast cancers develop in the upper outer quadrant of the breast.

Breast cancer can be detected by breast self-examination (BSE), mammography, thermography, ultrasonography, computerized tomography (CT), and nuclear magnetic resonance (NMR) imaging. At this time, mammography (discussed and illustrated in Chapter 63) is the most widely used method for detecting small tumors and distinguishing between benign and cancerous conditions. The most definitive method of diagnosis of cancer is biopsy of the tumor. The best hope for recovery from breast cancer lies in early treatment.

Clinical Manifestations

The early clinical manifestations of breast cancer may be the appearance of a lump upon palpation, routine mammography screening, or other technique. Most excised breast lumps (70%) are benign (Sheehan, 1984).

A unilateral increase in breast size may signify a breast tumor. A change in the shape of the breast also can be a warning sign. The most important change in shape is dimpling of the skin, which can be from the retraction of a fibrous strand from an underlying tumor.

Nipple changes include retraction, ulceration, scaliness, or discharge. Any pain or tenderness of the nipple may also be a sign of breast disease. Blood-stained discharge from the nipple may be a sign of a duct papilloma.

Edema of the skin, which may be caused by lymphatic drainage failure, gives the breast a *peau d'orange* ("orange peel") appearance. Lesser degrees of edema may be palpable as an increase in the thickness of the skin. Other skin changes may include the appearance of prominent subcutaneous veins and, with advanced tumors, infiltration by direct extension of the tumor.

Pain is not a frequent symptom in cancer of the breast, and severe pain is usually a symptom of inflammation. When cancer is present, the client usually perceives the pain as a pricking sensation. Clinical manifestations of the metastasis of breast cancer most often occur in the chest wall and lymph nodes. Advanced disease involves metastasis to the bone, lung, liver, and brain.

Therapeutic Measures

The treatment of breast cancer is based on the recognition that breast cancer is not strictly a localized disease, but is instead a systemic one. Both localized and systemic treatments are used. The treatment for breast cancer depends on the stage of the disease (Box 64–7) among other factors. Today the decision about the type of treatment considers the woman's desire for preservation of the breast. Even when surgery is required to remove the breast, later reconstruction can provide a breast mound that enables the client to look normal in clothes and eliminates the need for a breast prosthesis. Diagnostic and surgical methods of treatment are reviewed in Chapter 65.

Several radiotherapeutic techniques are used to treat breast disease. In the early stage of the disease, simple

Box 64–7 Staging of Breast Cancer

Primary tumor (T)

T_x: Tumor cannot be assessed.

T_0: No evidence of primary tumor.

T_{1s}: Paget's disease of the nipple with no demonstrable tumor. *Note:* Paget's disease with a demonstrable tumor is classified according to the size of the tumor.

T_1*: Tumor 2 cm or less in greatest dimension.

    T_{1a}: No fixation to underlying pectoral fascia or muscle.

    T_{1b}: Fixation to underlying pectoral fascia and/or muscle.

        I: 0.5 cm

        II: 0.6 to 1.0 cm

        III: 1.0 cm

T_2*: Tumor more than 2 cm but not more than 5 cm in its greatest dimension.

    T_{2a}: No fixation to underlying pectoral fascia or muscle.

    T_{2b}: Fixation to underlying pectoral fascia and/or muscle.

T_3*: Tumor more than 5 cm in its greatest dimension.

    T_{3a}: No fixation to underlying pectoral fascia or muscle.

    T_{3b}: Fixation to underlying pectoral fascia and/or muscle.

T_4: Tumor of any size with direct extension to chest wall or skin. *Note:* chest wall includes ribs, intercostal muscles, and serratus anterior muscle, but not pectoral muscle.

    T_{4a}: Fixation to chest wall.

    T_{4b}: Edema (including peau d'orange), ulceration of the skin of the breast, or satellite skin nodules confined to the same breast.

    T_{4c}: Both of the above.

Lymph nodes (N)—definitions for clinical diagnostic stage.

N_x: Regional lymph nodes cannot be assessed clinically.

N_0: Homolateral axillary lymph nodes not considered to contain growth.

N_1: Movable homolateral axillary nodes considered to contain growth.

N_2: Homolateral axillary lymph nodes considered to contain growth and fixed to one another or to other structures.

N_3: Homolateral supraclavicular or infraclavicular nodes considered to contain growth or edema of the arm.[†]

Lymph nodes (N)—definitions for surgical evaluative and postsurgical treatment—pathologic.

N_x: Regional lymph nodes cannot be assessed (not removed for study or previously removed).

N_0: No evidence of homolateral axillary lymph node metastasis.

N_1: Metastasis to movable homolateral axillary nodes not fixed to one another or to other structure.

N_{1a}: Micrometastasis 0.2 cm in lymph node(s).

N_{1b}: Gross metastasis in lymph node(s).

    I: Metastasis more than 0.2 cm, but less than 2.0 cm in one to three lymph nodes.

    II: Metastasis more than 0.2 cm, but less than 2.0 cm in four or more lymph nodes.

    III: Extension of metastasis beyond the lymph node capsule (less than 2.0 cm in dimension).

    IV: Metastasis in lymph node 2.0 cm or more in dimension.

N_2: Metastasis to homolateral axillary lymph nodes which are fixed to one another or to other structures.

N_3: Metastasis to homolateral supraclavicular or infraclavicular lymph node(s).

Distant metastases (M)—all time periods.

M_x: Not assessed.

M_0: No (known) distant metastasis.

M_1: Distant metastasis present.

Clinical or pathologic stage grouping

Stage T_{1s}: In situ.

Stage X: Cannot stage (unstageable).

Stage I	T_{1ai}	N_0	M_0
	T_{1aii}	N_0	M_0
	T_{1aiii}	N_0	M_0
	T_{1bi}	N_0	M_0
	T_{1bii}	N_0	M_0
	T_{1biii}	N_0	M_0
Stage II	T_0	$N_{1a \text{ or } 1b}$	M_0
	$T_{1a \text{ or } 1b}$	$N_{1a \text{ or } 1b}$	M_0
	$T_{2a \text{ or } 2b}$	N_0	M_0
	$T_{2a \text{ or } 2b}$	$N_{1a \text{ or } 1b}$	M_0
Stage IIIa	T_0	N_2	M_0
	$T_{1a \text{ or } 1b}$	N_2	M_0
	$T_{2a \text{ or } 2b}$	N_2	M_0
	$T_{3a \text{ or } 3b}$	N_0	M_0
	$T_{3a \text{ or } 3b}$	N_1	M_0
	$T_{3a \text{ or } 3b}$	N_2	M_0
Stage IIIb	Any T	N_3	M_0
	Any T_4	Any N	M_0
Stage IV	Any T	Any N	M_1

*Dimpling of the skin, nipple retraction, or any other skin changes except those in T_{4b} may occur in T_1, T_2, or T_3 without affecting the classification.

Note: cases of inflammatory carcinoma should be reported separately.

[†]Edema of the arm may be caused by lymphatic obstruction and lymph nodes may not then be palpable.

SOURCE: US Department of Health and Human Services: *The Breast Cancer Digest.* NIH Publication No. 84–1691. Bethesda, MD: National Cancer Institute, 1984, pp. 202–203.

excision of the tumor and sampling of the axillary nodes are followed by a course of radiation therapy, the dose and length of treatment depending on the axillary node involvement. A "booster" dose of radiation may supplement the external radiation; this is accomplished by an implant of radioactive material or by an electron beam from a linear accelerator. Iridium is typically implanted in breast tissue. Small tubes are threaded through the breast tissue, usually under local anesthesia, and then filled with seeds of the radioactive material. The tubes are left in place for approximately 50 to 60 hours and deliver approximately 2000 rads to the surrounding tissue. Figure 64–10 shows an iridium implant. Radiation therapy also can be used in the advanced stage of breast cancer, when metastasis has occurred. It then is often used with other methods of treatment, which are combined to decrease symptoms and provide remission of the disease.

The medical management of breast cancer also includes the use of hormonal therapy, chemotherapy, and immune system stimulants such as bacillus Calmette–Guerin (BCG) or Levamisole, used in combination. These methods are most often used in advanced breast disease, when surgery and radiation have been unable to destroy the cancer growths, but they also can be used to prevent metastasis, which may occur from a few months to 30 years later. The mean interval for recurrence is 3 years.

Hormonal therapy can be valuable in the treatment of breast cancer. Estrogen receptor protein (ERP) in the tumor is measured to determine whether the tumor is estrogen-rich, which most often occurs in the postmenopausal period. The rate of response to hormonal therapy

of ERP-positive tumors is 50% to 60%, and of ERP-negative tumors, less than 10%. When both the progesterone receptor protein (PRP) and the ERP are positive, the response to hormonal therapy increases to 77% (USDHHS, 1984).

The goal of the various methods of hormonal therapy is to reduce the amount of estrogen produced in the body. This can be accomplished surgically by oophorectomy or adrenalectomy. Adrenalectomy can be replaced by hypophysectomy or the use of aminoglutethimide to inhibit adrenal steroid synthesis (these procedures are discussed in Unit Seven). The antiestrogen used is tamoxifen citrate (usually 20 mg PO per day for at least 6 weeks) to assess the level of effectiveness. Diethylstilbestrol (5 to 10 mg t.i.d. for at least 6 weeks) is given to women with metastatic disease, who are postmenopausal for at least 5 years, to assess the level of effectiveness and then is continued until relapse occurs.

Various chemotherapeutic agents used to treat breast cancer are effective in combination rather than as single agents. A universally effective regimen has not been demonstrated, so various drug combinations are used, depending on such factors as the stage of the disease, the client's age, and the type of tumor. The most common chemotherapeutic agents include cyclophosphamide, methotrexate, fluorouracil, and doxorubicin.

Specific Nursing Measures

Specific nursing measures are reviewed in Chapter 65 for the various surgical diagnostic and therapeutic procedures for breast cancer, as well as for reconstructive surgery. Specific nursing measures related to chemotherapy and radiation therapy are reviewed in Chapter 12.

It is important to remember that the client may have many decisions to make after the diagnosis of breast cancer. Her coping mechanisms may be overwhelmed at this time, so she will need the nurse to provide support in the decision-making process and to explain alternative types of treatment. The type of treatment depends on such factors as the stage of the disease, the type of disease, the age of the woman, and her feelings about breast preservation. The nurse can anticipate questions clients have regarding the treatment process and provide information. It is also important to assess the support systems available to the client. The family or significant others will also need the support of the nurse during this critical time.

UTERINE LEIOMYOMAS

A uterine leiomyoma is a benign tumor, known to many clients as a fibroid, that is composed of smooth muscle cells and some connective tissue. It compresses the normal uterine muscular tissue as it grows and may involve the submucosa layer or be intramural in origin (Figure 64–11 on next page). They are the most common uterine tumor mass.

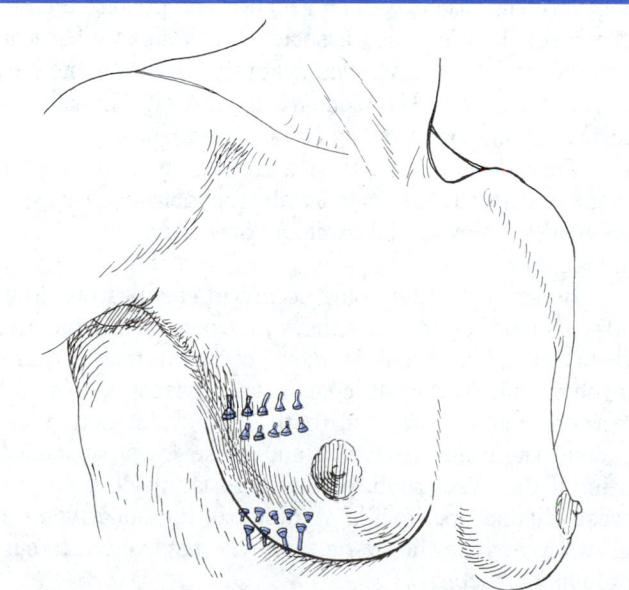

Figure 64–10

The iridium implant provides a concentrated "booster" dose of radiation to the area where the cancer was located.

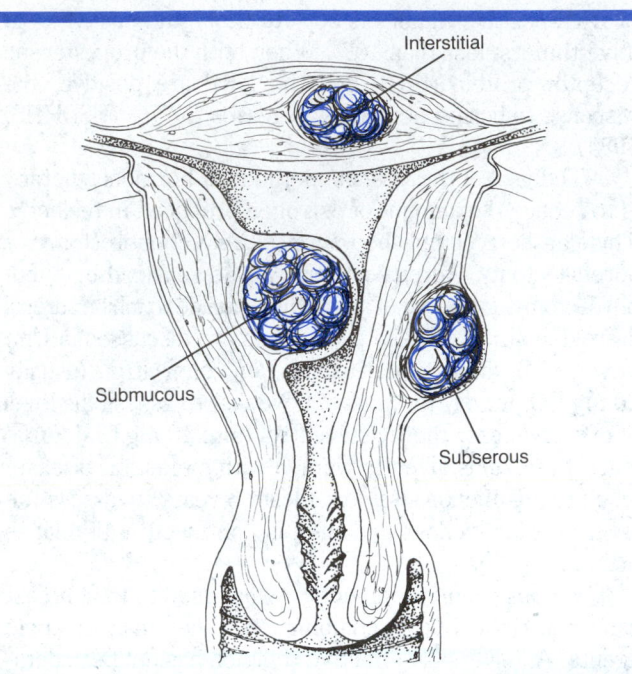

Figure 64–11

Uterine leiomyomas.

Clinical Manifestations

The clinical manifestations of uterine leiomyomas include an enlarged, irregular uterus. The client may experience prolonged and heavy or painful menstruation. Depending on the location or size of the tumor or on the number of tumors, the client may also experience other symptoms such as a feeling of heaviness in the lower abdomen or pelvic region, constipation, frequency of urination, or varicosities of the lower extremities or vulva. There may be no symptoms, however, and the tumor may be found on pelvic examination.

Therapeutic Measures

The treatment of the leiomyomatous uterus depends on the client's symptoms and desire for future childbearing. The client with no symptoms is informed of the fact that she has a benign tumor that does not require treatment. She is instructed to report any changes in her bleeding pattern, such as prolonged or heavy menses.

Myomectomy (removal of the tumor) is performed if the leiomyoma interferes with maintaining a pregnancy. A total hysterectomy is performed when heavy and prolonged menstruation results in anemia. A hysterectomy is also performed if the tumor results in a uterus larger than one of a 12-week gestation or when the woman cannot carry out activities of daily living because of excess bleeding. After menopause, the tumor will decrease in size;

however, if the uterus continues to enlarge, a TAH–BSO is performed.

Specific Nursing Measures

Before the pelvic examination, have the client void so the bladder is not confused with a tumor. Pregnancy testing also should be performed if there is a possibility of conception. The preoperative and postoperative nursing care for the hysterectomy client is reviewed in Chapter 65.

BENIGN OVARIAN NEOPLASMS

More neoplasms arise from the ovary than from any other reproductive organ, and the ovary is the most frequent site of a pelvic mass in the female reproductive tract. Most of the benign neoplasms manifest themselves during the reproductive years. They include functional cysts such as follicle cysts, corpus luteum cysts, theca lutein cysts, and polycystic ovaries. Benign neoplasms of the ovaries also include tumors derived from the germinal epithelium such as the serous cystadenoma, pseudomucinous cystadenoma, benign cystic teratoma (dermoid cyst), ovarian fibroma, and the Brenner tumor. These tumors appear in different age groups. This discussion will include only the common tumors.

Clinical Manifestations

Follicle cysts are usually small and may rupture upon pelvic examination. They usually disappear spontaneously during the menstrual cycle either by absorption or rupture.

Corpus luteum cysts are less common. The client has delayed menstruation with an irregular and prolonged onset of menses. Pain is usually associated with the cyst because of intraluminal bleeding. The cyst may rupture on its own or regress slowly. Ultrasonography can differentiate the corpus luteum cyst from an ectopic pregnancy.

Theca lutein cysts, the least common of the ovarian cysts, are usually associated with trophoblastic disease of pregnancy. They are bilateral and may reach 20 to 25 cm in diameter.

Benign cystic teratoma occurs in clients from 20 to 30 years old; they may be either cystic or solid in structure. Unilateral involvement is more common than bilateral involvement. The cysts contain fatty, viscoid sebaceous material, matted hair, and teeth. The cystic tumors are pedunculated and may twist and cause lower abdominal pain. If the cysts rupture, the material inside them can cause chemical peritonitis. A tumor of the solid type can grow larger than the cystic type and may adhere to surrounding structures.

Ovarian fibromas have no unique symptomatology. They may produce estrogen and are usually unilateral and pedunculated (thus, they may undergo torsion). Ascites usually accompanies the larger lesions.

Therapeutic Measures

Follicle cysts are managed conservatively and observed over a number of menstrual cycles. Gonadotrophic suppression may cause regression of the cyst. If it enlarges beyond 6 cm in diameter, laparoscopy is performed, at which time the cyst may be aspirated.

Corpus luteum cysts must be differentiated from ectopic pregnancy by ultrasonography or laparoscopy. They may regress slowly, or rupture and cause intraperitoneal bleeding and require surgical intervention. The preservation of ovarian tissue is the goal of treatment.

Theca lutein cysts usually completely regress after evacuation of the trophoblastic tissue. They should not be removed or drained.

If clients with a benign cystic teratoma or ovarian fibroma desire preservation of fertility, management involves preserving as much of the ovary as possible. Hemorrhage, torsion, rupture, or infection may necessitate removal of the ovary and fallopian tube, however.

Specific Nursing Measures

If the client has a cyst that will be observed over the menstrual cycle, instruct the client to note any symptoms and to return for follow-up care. If the client will undergo surgery, she and her family or significant other may find the potential diagnosis of cancer traumatizing. Nursing care with the diagnosis of cancer is reviewed in Chapter 12, and the nursing care of the surgical client undergoing oophorectomy or other ovarian surgery is discussed in Chapter 65.

BENIGN BREAST DISEASE

Benign breast disease includes the majority of breast masses that develop in women. These include fibrocystic disease, also referred to as *cystic hyperplasia* and *chronic mastitis;* fibroadenomas; and intraductal papillomas. The reactions of a woman who palpates a breast lump may be fear of cancer, denial of the possible significance of the lump, and anxiety. The diagnosis of benign breast disease involves evaluation to rule out cancer.

Clinical Manifestations

Fibrocystic disease usually first occurs at the median age of 30. A painful and tender mass decreases and increases in size in relation to the menstrual cycle, becoming larger and more painful as menses approaches. The mass is characteristically firm, mobile, and regular in shape and is usually found in the upper outer quadrant of the breast. Aspiration of the mass usually produces a gray-green fluid. The

disease usually regresses after menopause as the ovarian hormones decrease.

Fibroadenomas are usually found in the younger client but may occur between the ages of 15 and 60. Fibroadenomas are usually painless and do not change in size in relation to the menstrual cycle. They are mobile, spherical, firm, and usually 2.0 to 2.5 cm in diameter when discovered. The chance of another fibroadenoma occurring is about 10% to 20% (Schwartz, 1982).

Intraductal papilloma occurs most often in women between the ages of 35 and 45 years. The primary symptom is a serous or serosanguineous nipple discharge. There is usually no palpable mass. The location of the discharge from the nipple can be used to determine which duct is involved. During excision of the duct, the papilloma is usually found to be less than 0.5 cm in diameter and within 1 cm of the areolar margin.

Therapeutic Measures

A mass reported to have cyclic changes is first followed over a menstrual cycle to verify these changes. The primary surgical measure used in fibrocystic disease is aspiration biopsy for diagnosis, which is discussed in Chapter 65. Surgical excision or incision is necessary to rule out cancer when the cyst fails to produce fluid when aspirated, the fluid is bloody, the cyst rapidly refills with fluid, or a combination of these signs occurs. The medical treatment of fibrocystic disease includes the promotion of a diet low in fat and substances with methylxanthine such as chocolate, coffee, tea, and cola products. The daily use of vitamin E (600 units) also may help decrease the symptoms.

Fibroadenomas are treated by surgical excision (see Chapter 65). Removal of surrounding tissue is not usually necessary, because the mass is usually easily demarcated from surrounding breast tissue.

Intraductal papillomas are surgically treated by excision of the involved duct by wedge resection (see Chapter 65). A limited ductal excision of the involved duct will preserve enough tissue so that a woman can breast-feed if she desires.

Specific Nursing Measures

The nurse has an important role in providing the client with necessary support during the diagnostic procedures by explaining the procedures and their implications. The role of the nurse in care of the client having a biopsy and further surgical management is discussed in Chapter 65. The client diagnosed as having benign breast disease may still feel apprehensive about changes in her body image caused by scarring from the surgical procedure. She may worry about the effects of radiation exposure to her breasts in mammography. Provide the opportunity for the client to discuss her fears and concerns to aid adjustment.

Section VI: Traumatic Disorders

This section discusses lacerations, hematomas, and fistulas as well as trauma that may result from sexual assault or domestic violence. Although rape is a violent sexual act against either a woman, a man, or a child, the discussion in this section is focused on adolescent and adult females.

LACERATIONS, HEMATOMAS, AND FISTULAS

Traumatic disorders of the female reproductive tract occur either by direct injury to the vulva, vagina, or breasts, or as the result of surgery or irradiation. Trauma to the vulva, although rare, may result in a laceration or in hematoma formation. Trauma to the vagina usually results from an intercourse injury or the insertion of foreign bodies into the vagina. Trauma from surgery or irradiation can result in fistula formation.

The majority of fistulas (95%) are the result of surgery to the bladder or the reproductive tract (Pauerstein, 1982). Fistulas between the bladder and vagina are known as vesicovaginal fistulas. There are also ureterovaginal, urethrovaginal, rectovaginal, perineal–vaginal, vesicouterine, and vesicocervical fistulas (Figure 64–12).

Clinical Manifestations

Symptoms of vulval or vaginal trauma include pain, possible bleeding, and the presence of lacerations or hematomas. The client with a fistula has involuntary leakage of urine or involuntary leakage of stool from the vagina. When the fistula is located between the bladder or ureter and the vagina, there is involuntary leakage of urine from the vagina. Urine may leak intermittently if the urethra is involved. When the fistula is between the rectum and vagina, there is leakage of stool from the vagina.

Therapeutic Measures

To repair minor lacerations of the vulva or vagina, a local anesthetic can be used before suturing; this is usually an outpatient procedure. Extensive lacerations should be repaired in the operating room with adequate anesthesia.

Hematomas of the vulva may need to be drained, depending on the size, type, and location of the vessel involved. If the hematoma is small or of moderate size and is not expanding, close observation is all that is necessary.

Fistulas are surgically managed; techniques depend on their extent and site. A vaginal approach is often used to repair postoperative vesicovaginal fistulas. Surgeons may use the abdominal approach if tumors and radiation therapy caused the fistulas. With very large fistulas, urinary or fecal diversion may be necessary.

Specific Nursing Measures

If direct injury caused the trauma, nursing care involves observation of the laceration and hematoma. Ice can reduce pain and edema with a hematoma. The client will need emotional support during the emergency situation. This can be accomplished by staying with the client, answering her questions, and reassuring her. If surgery is needed for repair, the client should receive preoperative and postoperative care individualized to her specific needs.

The client with a fistula will need long-term physical care and help in adjusting to her changed body image. The lack of control over body functions can cause her to feel helpless. Therefore, the nurse is a needed source for venting feelings and frustrations.

RAPE

A woman is raped in the United States approximately every 6 minutes (Braen, 1982), and most of these occur during the hours between 10 PM and 2 AM. The assailant is usually known to the woman. The rape may occur anywhere: in her home, work place, or other familiar area as well as in streets and alleys.

It should never be assumed that the rape victim somehow provoked the incident. Many victims blame themselves even though they did nothing to provoke the attack and most likely could have done nothing to prevent it. The effects of the victimization often can lead to emotional and psychological problems that can persist for years.

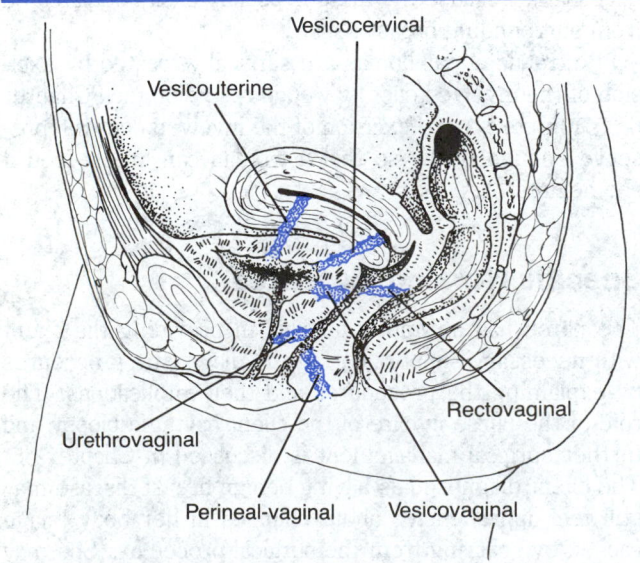

Figure 64–12

Fistulas that may develop in the female reproductive system.

Clinical Manifestations

There may be external evidence of trauma to the breasts, thighs, buttocks, and back. Other injuries may include fractures of the eye orbits, fractured mandible, human bites of the hands and breasts, long bone fractures, broken ribs, trauma to the abdomen, and lacerations and contusions of the skin.

Trauma to the perineal area and vagina occurs in about 8% of rape victims (Braen, 1982). These include lacerations and contusions of the vulva, introitus, or vagina. Lacerations of the cervix can occur when foreign objects are inserted into the vagina during the assault.

The oral cavity and rectum may also have been traumatized. The mouth may show evidence of bruises, a torn frenulum, or other signs of trauma. The anal area should be inspected for bruising, bleeding, and lacerations.

Therapeutic Measures

The victim of rape usually is seen in the emergency room of the hospital, and if extensive trauma exists, she may be admitted to the general unit. On arrival to the hospital, the rape victim often is both psychologically and physically traumatized. She has experienced a loss of control, self-esteem, and security.

Because rape is a violent crime certain steps should be taken to ensure the client's legal rights. The client has the right to refuse examination and may choose to receive only the physical and psychological care necessary. The emergency care of the rape victim is outlined in Table 64–2. The rape kit may be used as a standard emergency department procedure in obtaining specimens for legal action. An example of this kit is described in Table 64–3. When transferring evidence from one authority to another,

Table 64–2 Emergency Assessment and Nursing Intervention With the Sexual Assault Victim

Component	Nursing Interventions
Written consent for examination, lab tests, photographs, and release of information to appropriate legal authorities	Explain reasons for securing the victim's informed consent. Explain that victim has a right to refuse all or part of the examination, treatment, or release of information, and support victim's decision. Although reporting the attack to appropriate authorities should be encouraged, the victim should not be coerced.
History: Age, marital status, parity, menstrual history, date of last menstrual period, current methods of contraception, last coitus prior to assault	Explain that this information is gathered as part of the *routine* examination of sexual assault victims.
	Reassure the victim that staff are not being accusatory, but are gathering this essential information for the victim's protection in the event of future legal action.
	Explain that it is important to ascertain the risk of pregnancy from the assault or from prior intercourse.
Change of clothing, bathing, douching, voiding or defecation since the attack	If the client has not done so, advise not to douche, bathe, wash, change clothes, void, or defecate prior to the examination as this may interfere with the collection of evidence.* Clothing should be placed into a paper (not plastic) bag and labeled appropriately.
Ingestion of fluids, use of mouthwash, or brushing teeth since the assault	If oral penetration occurred, client should be advised not to drink fluids, brush teeth, or use mouthwash until oral swabbings and cultures have been obtained.
Use of drugs or alcohol (general habits as well as use within past 24 hours)	These questions should be asked in a straightforward, nonaccusatory manner. This information is needed as part of the chain of legal evidence. It may be used in court to confirm or disaffirm the victim's credibility.
Description of assault—the circumstances, including who (if known or a description), when, where, and what (penetration, ejaculation, use of contraceptive, extragenital acts, threats of violence, etc.)	The victim should be asked to recount the attack as she recalls it. The nurse should convey to the client an awareness that this may be emotionally distressful for the victim, explaining that it is necessary to establish the sequence of events.
	Use of universality may lessen the victim's embarrassment or anguish (eg, the nurse may offer, "Some attackers force their victims to engage in anal intercourse. Did this happen to you?" or, "Most women who have been sexually assaulted feel embarrassed and wonder whether they did anything to provoke the attack. How are *you* feeling?"
	Be aware of and sensitive to the victim's nonverbal behaviors, acknowledging them appropriately and reassuring the victim that her reactions are "normal."

(continued)

Table 64–2 Emergency Assessment and Nursing Intervention With the Sexual Assault Victim (continued)

Component	Nursing Interventions
	"Why?" questions should be avoided as they may reinforce feelings of self-blame and may sound accusatory.
Physical examination	The physical examination should be performed by a qualified gynecologist who has experience in examining sexual assault victims. A nurse or sexual assault crisis counselor should stay with the victim during the examination to offer explanations, reassurance, and emotional support.
	The victim's privacy should be protected with the utmost sensitivity and care.
	The client should not be asked to undress until just prior to the start of the examination to preserve her feelings of control.
General appearance: Inspection for bruises, lacerations, abrasions, etc. Photographs may be taken with victim's consent	Explain reasons for inspection. Protect victim's privacy. The nurse should maintain an objective yet sensitive and supportive manner.
Genito-rectal examination: Inspection of external genitalia, perineum, vagina, cervix, and rectum	Client preparation for each portion of the examination is imperative. Explanations of what is being done and why should be given.
Aspiration, swabbing, or washings of vagina (and mouth or rectum if indicated) for motile sperm, acid phosphatase, and blood group antigens	The absence of motile sperm does not rule out that penetration occurred since the assailant may not have ejaculated, may be oligospermic or aspermic, or may have used a condom.
	The acid phosphatase level may validate the time interval since penetration occurred.
Pap smear	Routine
Bimanual examination	Assist client to relax during examination with verbal reassurance, deep breathing, and distraction techniques.
Fingernail scrapings, pubic hair combings, clippings of matted pubic or other hair	Explain to client that these are obtained to test for foreign skin cells, blood, semen, and clothing fibers to aid in identifying assailant.
Urinalysis for drug screen, motile sperm, and pregnancy test	Laboratory evidence should be collected, labeled, and recorded in accordance with the emergency facility's written protocol.
Blood samples for alcohol and drug screen, and VDRL	
Treatment: Care of physical injuries (lacerations, etc.). Antibiotic prophylaxis may be administered (for venereal disease possibility)	Explanations of all procedures should be given and the victim's consent obtained.
Prevention of pregnancy with estrogens (especially in a client whose history places her at risk) may be warranted	Caution client about side effects of estrogens (nausea, vomiting, breakthrough bleeding).
Follow-up gonorrhea culture at 7 days and 6 weeks postassault	
Follow-up serology for VDRL at 6 weeks postassault	
Follow-up pregnancy test if indicated	
Emotional support and referral for follow-up care	Provide facilities and supplies for client to wash, bathe or shower, and change clothing.
	Encourage client to contact a supportive friend or relative.
	Contact local rape crisis center (with client's consent), and inform client of services offered such as individual crisis counseling, support groups, literature, legal assistance, etc.

Component	Nursing Interventions
	Encourage client to seek follow-up care. Reassure client that fears, depression, and other emotional symptoms may persist for months. Prepare victim for possibility of a delayed reaction to the assault. Nightmares, sleep difficulties, and fear of being alone are common sequelae.
	Provide client with a *written* list of names, addresses, and telephone numbers of community agencies that provide services for victims of sexual assault.
	Discharge client in the care of a family member or friend or a volunteer from rape crisis service.
	Provide victim with written instructions for follow-up physical care, and the name and telephone of an emergency department nurse the victim can contact if she has additional questions at a later date.
	Telephone the victim in 3 or 4 days to check how she is doing and offer continued support.

*Sexual assault victims often feel dirty and want to wash or bathe as soon as possible. Those who have been forced to engage in oral sex may feel nauseated or may even vomit (any vomitus should be saved for analysis, as should urine or stool).

SOURCE: Prepared by Janis P. Bellack, MN, RN.

Table 64–3 Rape Kit for Standard Emergency Department

Test	Kit Contents	Test	Kit Contents
1. Clothing collection	Standard paper clothing bags	8. Vaginal washing (if no specimen is visible in the vagina)	10 cc of saline (also use aspiration pipette and bulb from test 6 if these weren't used to aspirate vaginal contents)
2. Urine for pregnancy test and drug screen	Two urine containers		
3. Fingernail scrapings	Fingernail file (or broken wooden stick from a swab), envelope or red-topped blood tube	9. Pap smear	Cervical scraper (wooden), two clean slides, pap smear fixative
4. Pubic hair trimming (if semen is detected)	Forceps, scissors, envelope	10. Gonorrhea culture	Thayer-Martin plates or Transgrow media from laboratory, cotton-tipped swabs
5. Pubic hair combing	Plastic comb, large paper towel to comb hair into envelope to put comb and folded towel into	11. Saliva for secretor status	Three cotton-tipped swabs and a red-topped test tube
6. Aspiration of vaginal contents	Vaginal speculum, aspiration pipette (available from lab) and bulb for pipette, red-topped test tube and stopper	12. Blood samples	Three red-topped test tubes, tourniquet, *nonalcohol* swab to prep the skin, syringe and needle
7. Swab of vagina	Two glass slides (one frosted at one end), two cotton-tipped swabs, red-topped test tube, and stopper, pencil for marking slide	*Other contents*	Appropriate laboratory forms, rape examination forms, labels for samples, camera and film (optional)

SOURCE: Braen GR: Rape and sexual assault of the adolescent and adult female. *Top Emer Med* 1982; 3(1):56.

it is important that the procedure be signed and witnessed. This includes transferring samples from one person to another. All samples should be properly labeled with client's name, number, date, time of collection, site, and collector's name.

The prevention of venereal disease is important. The client is most frequently exposed to gonorrhea during the attack. Therefore, an endocervical culture is obtained, and the client is offered immediate antibiotic therapy as if she had been exposed to a known case of gonorrhea. Antibiotic treatment for gonorrhea was discussed earlier in this chapter. It is estimated that only one out of every 1000 rape victims develops syphilis (Warner & Braen, 1982). A serologic test for syphilis, the VDRL, is performed to rule out preexisting disease and repeated in 6 weeks if the initial test is negative. See Section IV for treatment of venereal disease.

Pregnancy as a result of rape develops in about 1% of clients (Warner & Braen, 1982). A careful gynecologic history is obtained to determine the risk for pregnancy. A radioimmunoassay for HCG may be performed to ensure that pregnancy did not exist before the attack. Before giving any medication for the prevention of pregnancy, the client's written consent should be received and the possibility of pregnancy ruled out. The medications used are diethylstilbestrol (25 mg orally twice a day for 5 days), conjugated estrogens (30 mg orally once daily for 5 days), or ethyl estradiol (5 mg orally once daily for 5 days). The client may choose to wait and have suction curettage abortion or menstrual extraction once pregnancy has occurred, rather than to take preventive hormonal treatment.

Psychological help for the rape victim in the emergency room begins with the staff. The client should be placed in an area with privacy and treated with sensitivity, understanding, and careful consideration. Support after discharge can be given by woman antirape groups, which might be available in the community. Short- or long-term counseling may be desired or needed by the client and her family.

Specific Nursing Measures

The nurse's attitude of acceptance and support of the client during the various procedures is of primary importance. The response of the client may include fear, shock, hysterical behavior, and anger. Her usual coping methods may be overwhelmed. It is not uncommon for the initial reactions of the client also to include denial or behaving in a very controlled and rational manner. With support, the client can then begin to express her feelings about the rape. It is only after this rapport is developed that the interview and physical examination should begin.

A detailed history of the rape is obtained, including such questions as time, date, place; use of force, threats of force; and type of assault and frequency. A gynecologic

and medical history are also obtained. The client's activities after the rape, such as douching, bathing, urination, and ingestion of alcohol or medication, are explored.

After the treatment of physical injuries and the collection of specimens (if the client consents), the nurse can assist the client in performing treatments that may provide a sense of cleanliness and possibly prevent disease. These may include such things as a cleansing douche, mouthwash, antiscabies shampoo, a shower, and a change of clothing.

The support systems and coping mechanisms of the client should be assessed. Family, friends, and significant others may need to be contacted. Referral to community resources should be made and instructions for follow-up care provided.

The rape victim needs to know what reactions to the rape may occur later. Somatic symptoms such as disrupted sleep patterns and nightmares, loss of appetite, fatigue, soreness, aches, and genital or urologic problems, may occur even when physical injuries are absent. The feeling of fear continues long into recovery; fear of being alone is very common. Feelings of guilt may occur, but the client should be made aware that she is not responsible for the assault. Depression may also occur once the client attempts to resolve the issues surrounding the rape; psychological assistance is especially helpful at this point. There may be withdrawal from sexual relationships because of the client's loss of self-respect and also because sexual relationships may reawaken the unpleasant memories associated with the sexual assault. The need for comfort and closeness, however, is heightened. For the elderly, there may be a loss of independence that might not be regained. The elderly woman may also worry more about what others might think and need reassurance of her value as a person.

DOMESTIC VIOLENCE

The battered woman is a victim of domestic violence. This violence involves both psychological and physiological trauma. It is estimated that approximately 2 million women in the United States are battered annually (Schechter, 1982). In 1970 there supposedly were few women who were actually victims of violence such as beatings or rape in the home, and as late as 1974 the term "battered women" was not a part of the vocabulary.

The woman who is battered does not have a specific psychological profile. She is as varied as any random group of women. The reason a woman is battered is not completely known and is not merely due to psychopathology on the part of either victim or assailant. It may be due in part to society's emphasis on male dominance and control, not genetics. The battering is seen as purposeful behavior with the intention of bringing about control.

The woman who is the victim of domestic violence is likely to be pregnant, and during pregnancy the batterings escalate. The social factors associated with battering are inadequate income, unemployment, youth, urban residence, and minority group status.

Clinical Manifestations

Injuries are inflicted both verbally and physically. The verbal abuse attacks the woman's sense of self-worth. Verbal abuse also includes threats about possible violent acts and what the partner will do to punish the victim if she leaves.

The physical injuries are caused by slapping, pushing, punching, kicking, or inflicted by weapons such as belts, knives, and razors. Hot liquids and hot utensils are also used and cause burns and scalds. The injuries are more likely to be on the face, breasts, chest, and abdomen. Some attackers strategically direct the assault to areas of the body that are not exposed when clothed. Marital rape may also occur after a beating.

It is important to realize that many victims of domestic violence do not seek help after repeated beatings. The reasons for this are varied—the woman lives with her victimizer, the man betrays her trust and love and also asserts that the beatings are her fault, or her failed relationship with her partner raises doubts about her capabilities.

In addition to physical injuries, the battered woman is often physically and psychologically drained. She fears leaving the partner because she believes she is incapable of surviving by herself in the world. She fears that her partner is fragile and that her leaving may cause his self-destruction. At the same time she may feel as if she can no longer cope, value her children's well-being, and fear that her partner may kill her.

The characteristics that will aid in the identification of victims of domestic violence include (Goldberg & Carey, 1982):

- Repeated emergency department visits for minor injuries
- History of being "accident prone"
- Soft-tissue injuries
- Injuries on areas of the body normally covered by clothing
- Implausible explanations for injuries
- Simplistic or vague explanations for injuries
- Psychosomatic complaints
- Depression
- Pain—especially chronic
- Substance abuse in client or spouse
- Suicidal gestures or attempts
- Psychiatric history in client or spouse
- Previous marriage counseling
- History of prior physical abuse
- History of observing someone else being abused
- History of sexual abuse

> ## Box 64–8 Questions to Determine Domestic Violence
>
> The following questions should be directed to clients believed to be victims of domestic violence.
>
> 1. Have you ever been in a relationship in which you were hurt in any way? Are you in one now?
> 2. How does your partner act when he has been drinking? Is there any verbal or physical abuse?
> 3. Have there been times in your relationship that you have had physical fights?
> 4. How is your partner with the children? Does he lose his temper?
> 5. You seem to have some special concern about your partner. Can you tell me more about this? Are you afraid? Has he ever hurt you?
> 6. Do your verbal fights also include physical contact?
> 7. Many women tell me that they argue with their partners and later on state that they have also been beaten. Could this be happening to you? Are you being beaten?
> 8. Sometimes when men are overprotective and jealous as you describe, they can react strongly and use physical force. Is this happening to you?
> 9. I noticed you have a number of bruises. Can you tell me how they happened?

Adapted from Goldberg W, Carey AL: Domestic violence victims in the emergency setting. *Top Emer Med* 1982; 3(1):67.

The presence of these characteristics should alert the nurse to ask the questions provided in Box 64–8.

Therapeutic and Specific Nursing Measures

Once the battered woman has been identified it is important to diagnose and treat her physical injuries. An evaluation of the client's strengths and weaknesses needs to be performed. After this evaluation, it can be determined what actions clients can take on their own behalf. Information about alternatives to remaining with a battering partner can be given. These may include a women's shelter, legal action, and other community resources.

The referral to other agencies should occur at the initial visit because many of the clients do not return for follow-up care. Adequate referral is needed to prevent the client from returning to a potentially lethal environment. A mental health consultant or psychiatric nurse specialist can provide support, counseling, and follow-up care.

It is important to acknowledge the client's problems may seem overwhelming to her. A nonjudgmental attitude is very important in obtaining factual information. The client can be reassured that there are alternatives to a situation in which she is battered.

Chapter Highlights

A congenital disorder of the female reproductive system is usually identified when the client is having difficulty with menstruation or fertility.

The more severe the congenital disorder of the female reproductive system, the greater its potential to alter body image. These disorders include müllerian aplasia, vaginal atresia, transverse vaginal septum, and incomplete müllerian fusion.

The in-utero exposure of female offspring to DES may cause various reproductive tract abnormalities.

Any disturbance in reproductive bleeding may produce fear and anxiety.

The symptoms of PMS vary with individuals. The symptoms increase in severity just before menstruation and subside as the menstrual flow starts.

Pelvic relaxation—uterine prolapse, cystocele, and rectocele—is caused by traumatic stretching from childbearing and occupational and unusual athletic activities, heredity, and menopause.

Perineal exercises, such as Kegel exercises, can be beneficial in preventing or reducing the severity of pelvic relaxation problems.

The clinical manifestations of menopause are caused in part by the loss of estrogen and in part by aging.

It is important to emphasize the normalcy of menopause when caring for the client.

Infectious vaginitis is one of the most frequent reasons women seek medical attention.

All sexual partners must be treated to prevent the infection of others when an STD is diagnosed.

Pelvic inflammatory disease leads to infertility in 10% of women who have had the disease once.

Most cases of toxic shock syndrome coincide with tampon use during the menstrual cycle.

The decrease in deaths related to cervical cancer is primarily attributable to the Pap test.

The best hope for recovery from breast cancer lies in early treatment.

Most breast masses in women are from benign breast disease, including fibrocystic disease, fibroadenomas, and intraductal papillomas. The diagnosis of benign breast disease involves evaluation to rule out cancer.

Lacerations, contusions, and hematomas of the reproductive organs can be the results of accidents, rape, or domestic violence.

The majority of fistulas are the result of surgery to the bladder or the reproductive tract. They may also result from irradiation.

Bibliography

American Cancer Society: *1985 Cancer Facts and Figures*. New York: American Cancer Society, 1985.

Braen GR: Rape and sexual assault of the adolescent and adult female. *Top Emer Med* 1982; 3(1):55–63.

Centers for Disease Control: Sexually transmitted disease treatment guidelines. *MMWR* 1982; 31:Suppl to No. 25.

Cibulka NJ: Toxic shock syndrome and other tampon related risks. *JOGN Nurs* 1983; 12(2):94–99.

Coates A: Current status of chemotherapy of breast cancer. *Drugs* 1984; 2:93–98.

Couch RB et al: Genital herpes: An epidemic disease. *Heart Lung* 1983; 12:320–324.

Cramer D et al: Dietary animal fat in relation to ovarian cancer risk. *Obstet Gynecol* 1984; 63:833–838.

Del Regato J, Spjut H, Cox JD: *Ackerman and Del Regato's Cancer Diagnosis, Treatment, and Prognosis*, 6th ed. St. Louis: Mosby, 1985.

De Vita VT, Hellman S, Rosenberg S: *Cancer Principles and Practice of Oncology*, Vol I, 2nd ed. Philadelphia: Lippincott, 1985.

Duenhoelter JH: *Greenhill's Office Gynecology*, 10th ed. Chicago: Year Book Medical Publishers, 1983.

Dugan KK: The bleak outlook on ovarian cancer. *Am J Nurs* 1985; 85(2):144–147.

Finkelhor D et al (editors): *The Dark Side of Families*. Beverly Hills, CA: Sage Publications, 1983.

Fogel CI, Woods NF: *Health Care of Women: A Nursing Perspective*. St. Louis: Mosby, 1981.

Goldberg W, Carey AL: Domestic violence victims in the emergency setting. *Top Emer Med* 1982; 3(4):65–76.

Harris J, Hellman S, Silen W: *Conservative Management of Breast Cancer: New Surgical and Radiotherapeutic Techniques*. Philadelphia: Lippincott, 1983.

Hassey M, Bloom LS, Burgess SL: Radiation alternative to mastectomy. *Am J Nurs* 1983; 83:1567–1569.

Jensen MD, Bobak IM: *Maternity and Gynecologic Care: The Nurse and the Family*, 3rd ed. St. Louis: Mosby, 1985.

Kase N, Weingold A (editors): *Principles and Practice of Clinical Gynecology*. New York: Wiley, 1983.

Kirkpatrick MK, Grady TR: PMS: A self-help checklist. *Occup Health Nurs* 1985 (February); 33:90–92.

Lauerson NH: Recognition and treatment of PMS. *Nurs Pract* 1985 (March); 10:11–12.

McNall LK: *Contemporary Obstetric and Gynecologic Nursing*. St. Louis: Mosby, 1980.

Miles PA: Sexually transmitted diseases. *JOGN Nurs* 1984; 13(Suppl):102s–124s.

Mills JT et al: Control of toxic-shock-syndrome toxin-1 (TSST-1) by magnesium ion. *J Inf Dis* 1985; 151:1158–1161.

Parsons CA (editor): *Diagnosis of Breast Disease: Imaging, Clinical Features and Pathology.* London: Chapman and Hall, 1983.

Pauerstein CJ (editor): *Gynecologic Disorders: Differential Diagnosis and Therapy.* New York: Grune & Stratton, 1982.

Peckham BM, Shapiro SS: *Signs and Symptoms in Gynecology.* Philadelphia: Lippincott, 1983.

Pitkin R, Zlatnik F (editors): *The Yearbook of Obstetrics and Gynecology.* Chicago: Year Book Medical Publishers, 1984.

Quilligan EJ (editor): *Current Therapy in Obstetrics and Gynecology,* 2nd ed. Philadelphia: Saunders, 1983.

Rilvin ME, Morrison JC, Bates GW (editors): *Manual of Clinical Problems in Obstetrics and Gynecology.* Boston: Little, Brown, 1982.

Rodman MJ, Smith DW: *Clinical Pharmacology in Nursing.* Philadelphia: Lippincott, 1984.

Savage EW: Carcinoma of the female reproductive system. *Fam Community Health* 1982; 5:1–12.

Schechter S: *Woman and Male Violence.* Boston: South End Press, 1982.

Schwartz GF: Benign neoplasms and "inflammations" of the breast. *Clinical Obstet Gynecol* 1982; 25:373–385.

Senie RT, Rosen PP, Kinne DW: Epidemiologic factors associated with breast cancer. *Cancer Nurs* (Oct) 1983; 5:367–371.

Shafer M et al: Self-concept in the diethylstilbestrol daughter. *Obstet Gynecol* 1984; 63:815–819.

Sheahan SL: Management of breast lumps. *Nurse Pract* 1984; 2(2):19–22.

US Department of Health and Human Services: *The Breast Cancer Digest.* NIH Publication No. 84-1691. Bethesda, MD: National Cancer Institute, 1984.

Warner CG, Braen GR: *Management of the Physically and Emotionally Abused: Emergency Assessment, Intervention and Counseling.* Norwalk, CT: Appleton–Century–Crofts, 1982.

Weingourt R: Never to be alone: Existential therapy with battered women. *J Psychosoc Nurs* 1985; 23(3):24–29.

Wilhelm–Hass E: Premenstrual syndrome: Its nature, evaluation, and management. *JOGN Nurs* 1984; 13(4):223–229.

Suggested Readings

Bernhard LA: Endometriosis. *JOGN Nurs* 1982; 11(5):300–304. This article discusses the pathology, symptoms, and medical and surgical management of endometriosis. It also includes a nursing care plan developed for the client with this disorder.

Britton J: *To Live Each Moment: One Woman's Struggle Against Cancer.* Downers Grove, IL: InterVarsity Press, 1984. A woman's experience when she discovered she had breast cancer is described.

Hassey M, Bloom LS, Burgess SL: Radiation alternative to mastectomy. *Am J Nurs* 1983; 83:1567–1569. This article reviews the breast cancer management by excision of the mass and radiation therapy.

Knobf MK: Breast cancer: The treatment revolution. *Am J Nurs* 1984; 84:1110–1117. The first part in a continuing education series reviews current trends in the treatment of breast cancer.

Lauver D: Irregular bleeding in women: Causes and nursing interventions. *Am J Nurs* 1983; 83:396–401. This article reviews how to develop the data base for providing care to clients with irregular bleeding. It explores the causes of irregular bleeding, its treatment, and nursing care.

Miles PA: Sexually transmitted diseases. *JOGN Nurs* 1984; 13(Suppl):102s–124s. A comprehensive review of STDs using a home-study approach.

Parker M: Psychological problems in the treatment of gynecological malignancy. *Nurs Times* 1983; 79(10):56–57. The ways in which reassurance and encouragement can support the client with a malignancy are explored.

Perley NZ, Bills BJ: Herpes genitalis and the childbearing cycle. *MCN* 1983; 8:213–217. This article reviews the clinical course of herpes genitalis and discusses the effect of herpes on pregnancy and the newborn. It also gives recommendations about the nurse's role in counseling dysmenorrheic women.

Whettam J: Update on toxic shock: How to spot it and treat it. *RN* 1984; 47(2):55–56,58,60. A review of the course of TSS includes the nursing care involved.

Wilhelm–Hass E: Premenstrual syndrome: Its nature, evaluation, and management. *JOGN Nurs* 1984; 13(4):223–229. The nature and incidence of PMS are reviewed, and a nursing protocol is presented.

The Client With Pelvic Inflammatory Disease

I. Descriptive Data	Sally Jones, age 25, has been admitted to the hospital with a tentative diagnosis of acute pelvic inflammatory disease. She is complaining of chills and abdominal pain. She is bent over and grasping her abdomen.

II. Personal Data

Date and Time:	Sept 2, 1986; 11 AM
Full Name:	Sally Ann Jones
Social Security Number:	000-00-0000
Address:	1456 East La., Pittsburgh, PA
Telephone:	Work: 000-0000
	Home: 000-0000
Sex:	Female
Marital Status:	Single
Age:	25
Birthdate:	10-4-61
Religion:	None
Race:	Caucasian
Occupation:	Secretary
Usual Health Care Provider:	Susan Smith, MD

III. Health History

Source of Information:	Client
Reliability of Informant:	Reliable
Chief Concern:	Lower abdominal pain and chills
History of Present Illness:	This is Sally's first hospitalization. Two days ago she developed lower abdominal pain, which was initially relieved by two extra-strength acetaminophen tablets. Gradually, the pain became more severe and any movement made it worse. She also developed chills and a low-grade fever.

Her last menstrual period was 8-24-86; she has a 26- to 30-day cycle and a moderate flow for 5–6 days; menarche age 13. Last Pap 2-86—normal. She has never been pregnant; contraceptive method is spermicidal foam. Her last period was normal; she has noted no vaginal discharge and has no pain with intercourse; most recent intercourse was 14 days ago. Her sexual partner had no sores or discharge from the penis as far as she could tell. No polyuria, frequency, urgency, nocturia, or hematuria. Has noted a mild dysuria for about 5 days, but not with every voiding. Has never had an UTI. Bowel movements are normal, brown, soft; has a BM daily without difficulty.

Her past health has been excellent. She was treated once in 1983 for gonorrhea with 1 million units of penicillin G procaine after a positive culture was obtained from the cervix.

Past Health History:	
Childhood Diseases:	Mumps and chickenpox
Immunizations:	Polio, 1970; DPT, 1973; smallpox, 1963
Medical Problems:	Gonorrhea, 1983
Surgeries:	T & A, 1969
Blood Transfusions:	None
Trauma:	Fractured rt humerus, 1968 (fell out of a tree)
Allergies:	None
Medications:	Extra-strength acetaminophen for headache once or twice a month

Case Study written by Diane Wind Wardell.

Family History:

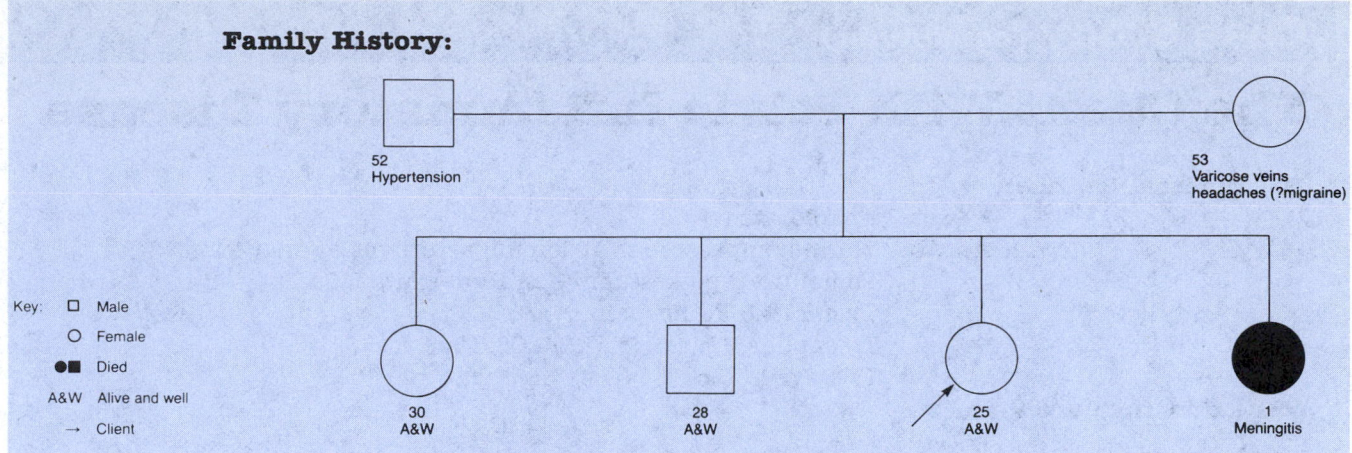

Key:
☐ Male
○ Female
●■ Died
A&W Alive and well
→ Client

52 Hypertension			53 Varicose veins headaches (?migraine)
30 A&W	28 A&W	25 A&W	1 Meningitis

Personal/Social History: Currently works 40 hours a week as a secretary in a computer firm; lives in an apartment near her parents; dates sporadically and does not identify any significant relationship with a particular male friend; last date 2 weeks ago was with a new partner; is active in social events in apartment complex; enjoys swimming, bicycling, and boating; skis in winter months; visits parents and siblings every Sunday at parents' home; maintains a good relationship with the family.

Smokes ½ PPD × 5 years; does not drink alcohol. Diet is well balanced; eats primarily vegetables but also eats chicken and fish.

Review of Systems: General health has been good until 2 days ago. Usual weight 115 lb, no recent weight change, fatigued

Skin: Has not noted any rashes or sores

Respiratory: No symptoms of respiratory difficulty

Gastrointestinal: No symptoms of food intolerance; no nausea, vomiting, or diarrhea

Hematopoietic: Denies easy bruising or excessive bleeding

Psychological: Rarely moody or depressed; occasionally has mild mood swings prior to menses

IV. Physical Assessment

Height: 5 ft 6 in

Weight: 112 lb

Vital Signs: BP 110/64; pulse 98; respirations 26; temperature 103°F

PE: Attractive, neatly dressed, 25-yr-old female; face flushed

Relevant Organ Systems:

Skin: Warm to touch, face flushed

Breasts: Firm, symmetrical; no masses; no nipple discharge

Chest: Breath sounds vesicular without rales or wheezes

Heart: PMI palpable 5th left ICS, 7 cm from MSL, apical rate 98, regular. No murmurs.

Abdomen: Flat, no scars; bowel sounds hypoactive; kidneys, spleen not palpable; liver 7 cm at right MCL; tenderness in suprapubic area with light palpation

Genitalia: Vulva reddened; cervix, pus from nulliparous os; no cervical lesions; uterus anterior, midline; tender to gentle palpation; adnexa tender bilaterally; vagina: rugae apparent, no lesions

V. Diagnostic Data Results of laboratory tests include increased white blood cell count, an increase in polymorphonuclear leukocytes and bandforms on the differential peripheral blood smear, and an increased erythrocyte sedimentation rate. The cervix, urethra, anus, and throat were all cultured. Gram's stain of exudate from the cervix showed gram-negative diplococci (*Neisseria gonorrhoeae*).

(continued)

The Client With Pelvic Inflammatory Disease

VI. Medical Regimen

Diet: As tolerated
Treatments: Warm compresses to abdomen; semi-Fowler's position
Penicillin G potassium 20 million units IV daily
Tylenol #3 PO for pain
Tylenol qr V p.r.n. for T > 100.8°F
IV D5W, 100 cc/h

VII. Nursing Care Plan

Nursing Diagnosis	Client Care Goals	Plan/Nursing Implementation	Expected Outcome
Comfort, alteration in: pain	Client will experience a decrease in pain each day during hospitalization	Heat to abdomen to increase circulation; therapeutic touch; comfort measures such as back rub, bed rest in semi-Fowler's position, warm tea/liquids; medicate as ordered for pain	Client will be pain free by discharge without medication
Injury: potential for	Client will have decreased signs of infection	Monitor vital signs q. 4 h for increased temperature; monitor laboratory values for increased leukocytes; maintain semi-Fowler's position to decrease chance of abscess formation; administer antibiotic therapy as ordered; monitor vaginal discharge for amount, odor, color, consistency; check IV site for signs of infection (phlebitis) and infiltration: eg, swelling, redness, coolness, or excess warmth; maintain ordered IV flow rate; reinforce need for handwashing to prevent infection of eyes	Client will be at decreased risk of recurrent disease; client's fertility will be maintained; no further signs of infection or discharge
Self-concept, disturbance in: related to body image change	Client will verbalize feelings and fears regarding illness	Check frequently for signs of distress: crying, silence, others; spend time with client discussing concerns; use therapeutic techniques in communicating such as: open-ended questions, reflection; inform client of availability to talk if she desires	Client will express positive self-concept at discharge
Knowledge deficit: related to understanding of disease process	Will discuss disease pathology and implications for self	Assess level of knowledge; review female anatomy; discuss causative organism; explain how organism spreads; review course of disease; instruct that treatment of sexual partner is necessary; discuss need for follow-up evaluation after discharge; instruct that intercourse must be avoided until negative cultures are obtained from partner as well as self	Will verbalize knowledge of disease pathology and implications for self

Chapter 65

Surgical Approaches to Female Reproductive System Dysfunction

Sandra E. Seff
Diane Wind Wardell

Objectives

When you have finished studying this chapter, you should be able to:

Discuss the indications for surgical approaches to female reproductive system disorders.

Provide a brief description of the surgical procedures used in treating dysfunction of the female reproductive systems.

Recognize the implications that the surgical procedures of the

female reproductive system have on the physiological function of the client.

Describe the impact that the surgical procedures of the female reproductive system have on the psychosocial adaptation and lifestyle of the client.

Discuss the nursing implications of caring for these clients in the preoperative and postoperative periods.

Female reproductive surgeries include operative procedures of the breasts, uterus, cervix, ovaries, fallopian tubes, vagina, and vulva, as well as their supporting structures. These procedures may be done for diagnostic, therapeutic, cosmetic, or sterilization purposes.

The nurse who cares for a woman undergoing reproductive surgery must be sensitive to the psychological impact the procedure may have. The loss of sexual organs or reproductive capacity can result in disturbances of body image and feelings of loss and grief. The degree to which the woman's emotional well-being is affected depends on the type of surgery, her knowledge of reproductive function, her self-concept, her lifestyle, and her support system.

Most women adjust to the physiological consequences of their surgery without serious psychological disruption, but many have difficulty coping with the emotions these operations can engender. For example, a woman who places a high value on her physical attractiveness and relates to others primarily through her sexuality may be devastated by the removal of a breast or a scar from a large abdominal incision. Likewise, a woman whose self-esteem depends on her reproductive ability may experience depression after any operation that alters her reproductive capacity.

Often reproductive surgery is required during the perimenopausal years, a time when many women confront the fear of aging, physical changes, and changes in lifestyle. Surgery becomes an additional stress that can accentuate feelings of sexual inadequacy and loss of physical attractiveness. When surgery is for the treatment of cancer, the fears of death, uncontrollable pain, and disfigurement become paramount.

The nurse must recognize the emotional adjustments associated with reproductive surgery. The nurse's role includes assisting the client in recognizing her fears and anxieties so she will be able to discuss them in a nonthreatening nurse–client relationship. Ideally, the nurse initiates this process preoperatively to allow the client sufficient time to begin resolving her feelings before the physical stress of surgery. The client's physical recovery is influenced by her age, health status, emotional well-being, and extent of her disease. To provide optimum nursing care, the nurse must understand the interrelation of these factors.

Some clients have advanced gynecologic disease because they have failed to seek early medical care. Often these delays are caused by failure to recognize the symptoms as pathological and by the embarrassment many women experience from a gynecologic examination. Older women often find it disconcerting when their physician of many years retires, and they may not feel comfortable establishing a new relationship with a physician. Furthermore, all women fear sexual disfigurement and may fail to have early symptoms evaluated to avoid confronting the possibility of surgery. Clients can be informed about new surgical technologies that result in less tissue destruction and disfigurement. It is hoped that these delays can be reduced by sensitive health care personnel and accurate health education.

Much of reproductive surgery is performed in middle-aged and elderly women, so chronic illness such as cardiopulmonary disease, hypertension, or diabetes mellitus can become a complicating factor. Osteoporosis in postmenopausal clients predisposes them to fractures if nurses do not carefully position them for gynecologic procedures, especially those that require the lithotomy position.

Society's emphasis on thinness can lead to poor dietary habits and nutritional anemias. Problems arise when these anemias become superimposed on the lowered hemoglobin values associated with women in the reproductive age group. This situation becomes clinically important because certain types of gynecologic diseases are associated with bleeding, and many gynecologic surgeries result in significant blood loss.

The obese client presents a unique set of problems. Some women fail to have routine examinations because they fear their physicians will scold them for gaining weight. Marked obesity can make adequate physical assessment of the pelvic organs difficult. Obviously, these situations can hinder early diagnosis of disease states and result in treatment delays. Obese clients also are at an increased risk for anesthetic and postoperative complications.

Gynecologic nursing thus requires a broad knowledge base. The ability to give postoperative care is not enough. Sensitivity to the psychological issues associated with reproductive surgery, an understanding of the medical conditions that can be unique to these clients, and an assessment of the client's knowledge of reproductive and sexual function are also essential.

Section I: Surgical Approaches to Disorders Affecting the Female Reproductive Organs

CERVICAL DILATATION AND UTERINE CURETTAGE

Cervical dilatation and uterine curettage (D and C), the most frequent gynecologic surgery, can be done for diagnostic or therapeutic purposes. The indications for the procedure include dysfunctional uterine bleeding (DUB) (to determine the histologic composition of the endometrium); infertility (to determine the presence of ovulation); and the need to diagnose endometrial cancer or tuberculosis, remove uterine polyps, and remove early products of conception (to eliminate hemorrhage or other complications when a spontaneous incomplete abortion has occurred or when an elective abortion is desired). A D and C is also performed prior to other gynecologic surgeries to ensure that intrauterine pathology does not exist.

Surgical Procedure

The D and C can be performed under local anesthesia with mild sedation or under general anesthesia. The choice of anesthesia depends on the client's age, health state, ability to cooperate, the indication for the procedure, and the facility in which the D and C is done.

The client assumes a lithotomy position. The physician uses a uterine probe to determine the length and direction of the uterine cavity. Next, dilators that gently stretch the muscles and fibers of the cervix gradually enlarge the cervical canal and internal os. After this dilatation has been completed, the uterine cavity undergoes systematic curettage (scraping). Specimens obtained from the cervical canal and uterine cavity are sent to the laboratory for histologic examination.

Implications for the Client

Physiological Implications
Complications of the D and C include perforation of the uterus and cervical laceration, which lead to hemorrhage. Occasionally, vasovagal effects also occur at the time of cervical dilatation. Physical discomfort is generally mild and limited to uterine cramping. Bleeding resembling a menstrual cycle for 5 to 7 days postoperatively is usual.

Psychosocial/Lifestyle Implications
A D and C may follow the loss of a desired pregnancy, and the client may manifest her grief by crying and expressing sadness. When the D and C terminates an unwanted or unplanned pregnancy, feelings of grief and guilt may occur. The client may not have anticipated these feelings and may find them initially difficult to express. Usual activities, including intercourse, may be resumed in 2 to 3 weeks. Table 65–1 summarizes the client implications of a D and C.

Nursing Implications

Preoperative Care
The D and C often is conducted in an outpatient setting, so the nurse should provide the client clear instructions

Table 65–1	Cervical Dilatation and Uterine Curettage: Implications for the Client	
Physiological Implications	**Psychosocial/Lifestyle Implications**
Perforation of the uterus or cervical laceration, leading to hemorrhage	Grief after loss of desired pregnancy
Occasional vasovagal effects at the time of cervical dilatation	Guilt and grief after termination of unwanted pregnancy
Uterine cramping	Normal activities, including intercourse, may be resumed in 2–3 weeks
Bleeding for 5–7 days	

for preliminary preparation. Specific information regarding dietary restrictions, arrival time, and arrangements for postoperative transportation will facilitate a successful outcome.

When the client arrives for surgery, ascertain that she has complied with the preoperative instructions and has signed the operative permit. The nurse may make a brief health assessment to establish changes in the client's health status since the previous examination. Obtain vital signs, and report significant deviations from normal to the surgeon. After explaining the procedure, orient the client to the surgical surroundings. The woman should empty her bladder and then change into the appropriate gown for the procedure.

Escort the client to the operating room, assist her onto the table, and begin preparation for the D and C. When assisting the client into the lithotomy position, be sure to support her legs at the popliteal areas and ankles. Positioning both legs simultaneously prevents muscle strain. If resistance is encountered because of pain or immobility, stop and notify the surgeon.

When the D and C is performed as an inpatient procedure, the preoperative preparation is similar. A mild sedative may be given prior to the procedure.

Postoperative Care

The client will remain in a recovery area until fully reacted (approximately 1 hour). Monitor the vital signs every 15 minutes until stable. A falling blood pressure with a rapid pulse should alert the nurse to the possibility of hemorrhage from a cervical laceration or uterine perforation.

Assess the client's perineal pad frequently. Vaginal bleeding should not be heavier than that of a normal menstrual period. A woman in a dorsal recumbent position can have significant undetected bleeding, because gravity allows the blood to flow in the direction of her buttocks and sacrum. Therefore, check not only the perineal pad but also the area under the buttocks.

Discomfort is generally mild. The client may experi-

ence uterine cramping, which is readily alleviated with mild analgesics and rest. Pain not relieved by these measures must be brought to the physician's attention.

When the D and C is associated with the loss of a wanted pregnancy, the nurse must be sensitive to the client's perceived loss and allow her to express her grief (see Chapter 16). Statements such as, "You can always have another baby," or, "It wasn't really a baby yet," are inappropriate. The nurse also should help the client express grief and guilt over the termination of an unwanted or unplanned pregnancy.

Discharge instructions should include information on when the pathology report will be available, the recommended method of contraception, when the client may resume normal activities, and the time of her next appointment. Remind the client that signs or symptoms such as fever, heavy bleeding, or severe uterine cramping require emergency care.

LAPAROSCOPY

Within the last decade, laparoscopy (pelvic peritoneoscopy) has become widely used to visualize the pelvic cavity. Laparoscopy enables the surgeon to perform many diagnostic and therapeutic procedures that otherwise would require major abdominal surgery. The technique is often preferable to traditional laparotomy, which requires an abdominal incision, because laparoscopy requires less operative time, less hospital confinement, less discomfort, less cost, and less time lost from normal activities.

The diagnostic uses include exploration of the pelvic cavity and reproductive organs, tissue biopsy, aspiration of pelvic cysts, and the evaluation of infertility. It is usually combined with a diagnostic D and C. The therapeutic uses are for surgery on pelvic adhesions, tubal sterilization, removal of an intrauterine device (IUD), aspiration of pelvic cysts, aspiration of ova (for in vitro fertilization), and the removal of an early ectopic pregnancy.

Surgical Procedure

Laparoscopy is usually done under general anesthesia, but it also can be performed under local anesthesia with mild sedation. After the client is anesthetized, she is placed in a dorsal lithotomy position. Both the abdomen and the perineum are cleaned and draped so the surgeon can perform an emergency laparotomy at any time during the procedure if it becomes necessary. The bladder is emptied by a straight catheter, and a D and C is performed. A forceps is placed on the cervix to allow manual manipulation of the uterus during the laparoscopy.

Next, the client is placed in a 10° to 15° Trendelenburg's position to cause the intestines to fall away from the pelvic cavity. A **pneumoperitoneum** is created by filling the abdominal cavity with carbon dioxide or dinitrogen monoxide (nitrous oxide) through a needle inserted below the umbilicus. This lifts the abdominal wall from the pelvic viscera to provide better visualization. When sufficient insufflation is achieved, the surgeon introduces a trochar and cannula into the peritoneal cavity through a small (3- to 4-cm) infraumbilical incision. Once in place, the trochar is removed, and the laparoscope is inserted. This instrument enables the surgeon to visualize the pelvic organs and perform the necessary surgery (Figure 65–1). A second probe may be inserted through a suprapubic incision. This alternate procedure allows for additional instrumentation and is thought to increase visualization. Upon completion of the procedure, the laparoscope is removed, the abdomen is deflated, and the skin wound is closed with the appropriate sutures and covered with a small dressing or plastic bandage.

Implications for the Client

Physiological Implications
Complications from a laparoscopy are rare but can be life threatening. Peritonitis, necrosis of the bowel, catastrophic hemorrhage, and cardiopulmonary impairment have occurred. Abdominal discomfort from the incision is mild, but the residual gas can irritate the phrenic nerve and cause referred sudden intermittent sharp shoulder pain. The pain diminishes in a few days as the gas is absorbed. Because women undergoing a laparoscopic procedure are usually healthy and in the reproductive age group, major complications can be devastating.

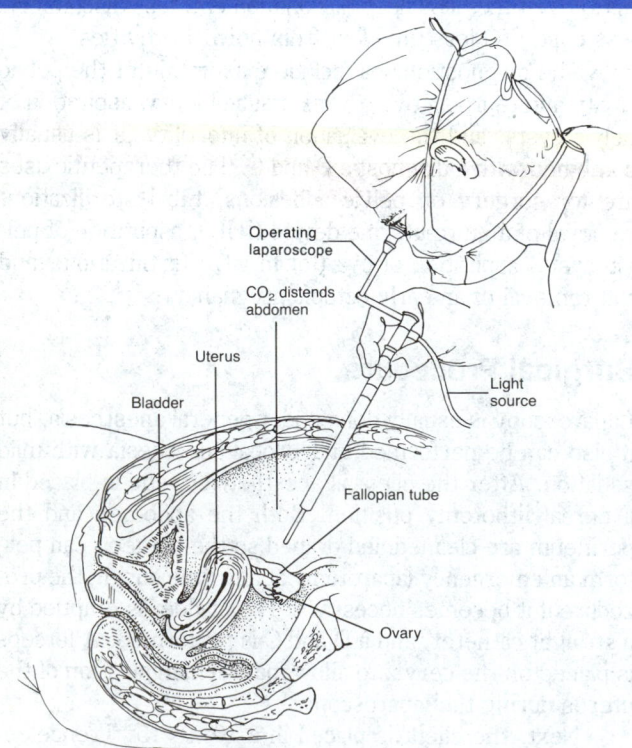

Figure 65–1

Laparoscopy. The laparoscope is inserted through a small infraumbilical incision. Gas distends the abdominal wall lifting it away from the pelvic organs.

Table 65–2	**Laparoscopy: Implications for the Client**
Physiological Implications	**Psychosocial/Lifestyle Implications**
Rare complications of peritonitis, necrosis of the bowel, catastrophic hemorrhage, cardiopulmonary impairment	Same-day surgery reduces lifestyle limitations
Mild abdominal discomfort	Minimal restrictions on activity
Referred sudden intermittent sharp shoulder pain from pneumoperitoneum for a few days	Avoid tub bathing until incision heals
	Change own dressing (plastic bandage)

Psychosocial/Lifestyle Implications
Clients may be admitted and discharged the same day. There are minimal limitations on strenuous activity from the first 5 to 7 days postoperatively. The client will be responsible for changing her own dressing, usually a plastic bandage. Subcuticular sutures are usually used; they are absorbed and thus do not need to be removed. Nonabsorbable sutures are removed approximately 1 week later. Tub bathing should be avoided until the incision has healed. Physiological and psychosocial/lifestyle implications for the client undergoing laparoscopy are listed in Table 65–2.

Nursing Implications

Preoperative Care
Preoperative nursing care is similar to that for a D and C. Discussing postoperative discomforts at this time might help to minimize the client's anxiety.

Postoperative Care
Postoperative nursing care is similar to that for a D and C but also includes assessment of the infraumbilical incision for drainage or hematoma formation. Mild analgesics may be helpful in the first few postoperative days to alleviate the shoulder pain caused by residual gas from the pneumoperitoneum. Only oral analgesics are necessary if the client's anxiety has been reduced by preoperative preparation. Discharge instructions in addition to these are similar to those given for a D and C. Because clients are often discharged the same day of the surgery, provide instructions on wound care and dressing changes.

CERVICAL CRYOSURGERY

In gynecology, cryosurgery frequently is used to destroy areas of cervical dysplasia or chronic cervicitis. It is also used to remove small vulval lesions. Cervical cryosurgery has basically replaced cervical cauterization as a surgical treatment. Laser treatment for treating cervical dysplasia or chronic cervicitis is also available. Because it requires special equipment and skills, it is not as readily available as cryosurgery. The discussion in this section can also be applied to cervical laser surgery.

Surgical Procedure

Cryosurgery is an ambulatory procedure often performed in the physician's office. It requires no anesthesia and is almost painless. The freezing agent is applied with a cryoprobe applied directly to the involved tissue (Figure 65–2). Total treatment time is about 2 minutes.

Implications for the Client

Physiological Implications

The client should expect a profuse watery discharge from the treated area and possible spotting after cryosurgery. Necrotic tissue sloughs in about 10 days and complete healing may take 2 to 3 months. A possible complication is cervical stenosis requiring dilation.

Psychosocial/Lifestyle Implications

The client should avoid intercourse for 2 weeks postoperatively. A follow-up visit to the physician or other health care provider in 2 weeks is routine. Regular cytologic exams are necessary to monitor the condition of the cervix. The client implications of cryosurgery are found in Table 65–3.

Table 65–3 Cervical Cryosurgery: Implications for the Client	
Physiological Implications	**Psychosocial/Lifestyle Implications**
Profuse watery discharge	No intercourse for 2 weeks
Possible spotting	Return visit to health care provider in 2 weeks
Complication of cervical stenosis requiring dilation	Regular cytologic exams (Pap smear)

Nursing Implications

Preoperative Care

Preoperative nursing care is similar to that for other outpatient gynecologic procedures. Nursing care has been described under D and C.

Postoperative Care

After cryosurgery is completed, instruct the client to avoid intercourse for 2 weeks and to expect a profuse watery discharge and possible spotting. Stress the importance of returning to the health care provider regularly for cytologic follow-up examinations, because dysplasia can recur in other areas of the cervix.

CERVICAL CONIZATION

Conization is the surgical removal of a cone-shaped piece of tissue from the uterine cervix for diagnostic or therapeutic purposes. In past years, many women who were found to have abnormal cervical cytology underwent this procedure. Conization now has been replaced by the less traumatic cryosurgery and laser techniques. Surgical conization is still indicated, however, when the pathological lesion cannot be visualized via the colposcope or when cervical dysplasia persists despite repeated conservative therapies.

Surgical Procedure

Under either general or regional anesthesia, an electrical instrument or a surgical knife is inserted into the external os and rotated to cut and remove an inverted cone of tissue (Figure 65–3). The area is then coagulated. The biopsy specimen is placed immediately in a formalin solution and transported to the cytology laboratory. The os may or may not be packed with gauze.

Implications for the Client

Physiological Implications

Complications of conization include hemorrhage and, in some instances, infertility because of the removal of mucus-

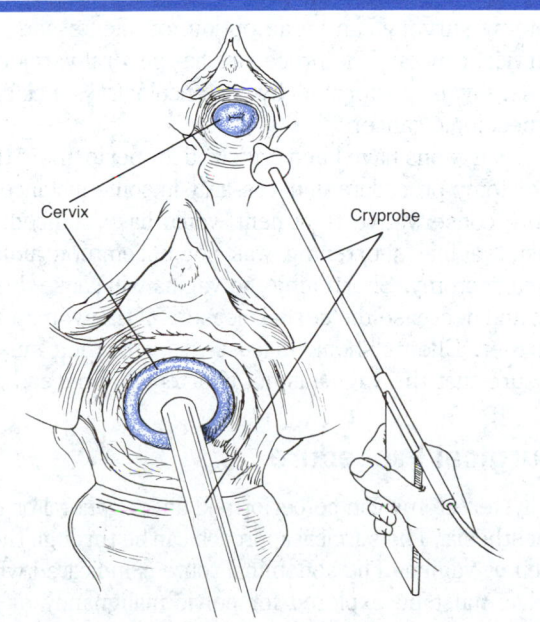

Figure 65–2

Cervical cryotherapy.

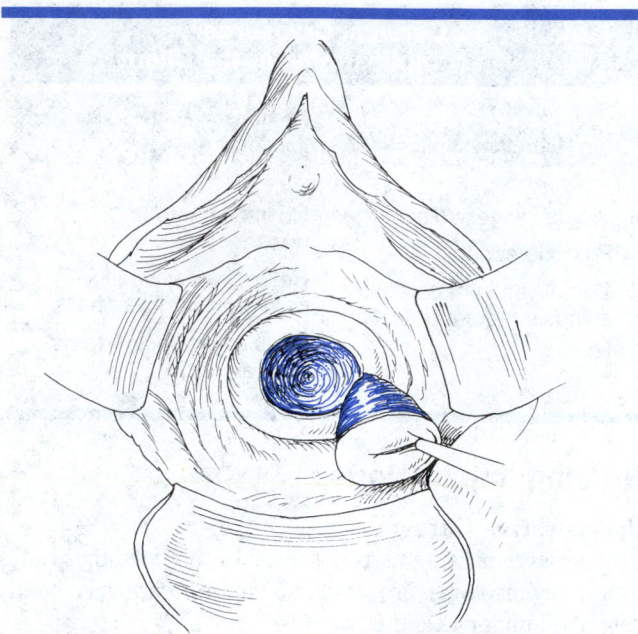

Figure 65–3

Cervical conization. A cone-shaped piece of tissue has been removed from the cervix.

producing glands and the formation of scar tissue. Some discharge is normal. A pack may be in place.

Psychosocial/Lifestyle Implications

The client should abstain from intercourse for at least 3 weeks after surgery, rest for 24 hours, and avoid heavy lifting for 2 to 3 weeks. The client will need regular cytologic examinations. Table 65–4 summarizes the client implications of conization.

Nursing Implications

Preoperative Care

Explain the conization procedure to the client, including physical sensations. Fear of cancer also should be discussed.

Table 65–4	**Cervical Conization: Implications for the Client**	
Physiological Implications	**Psychosocial/Lifestyle Implications**
Possible hemorrhage	No intercourse, douching, or tampon use for at least 3 weeks
Possible infertility	
Some discharge	Rest for 24 hours
Cervical packing possible	No heavy lifting for 2–3 weeks
	Need for regular cytologic examinations

Postoperative Care

Postoperative nursing care is similar to that for a D and C. Later hemorrhage can be a significant complication, so discharge instructions must be directed toward preventing this problem. Advise the client to abstain from coitus, douching, or the use of tampons for at least 3 weeks. The client should report immediately to the physician any bleeding heavier than a normal menstrual period or associated with the passage of clots. Remind the client of the need for regular cytologic examinations.

HYSTERECTOMY

A hysterectomy is the surgical removal of the uterus. The indications for this operation include large leiomyomas, adenomyosis, malignancy, uterine prolapse, severe pelvic infection, endometriosis, and DUB that is unresponsive to conservative measures.

When the uterine body and cervix are removed, the procedure is called a *total hysterectomy.* Occasionally, the physician may find it necessary to remove only the uterine body and leave the cervix in place. This procedure, called a *subtotal hysterectomy,* is seldom performed today unless surgical complications or the client's debilitated state require rapid surgery. After surgery, these clients still have a cervix, so they will continue to need regular Pap tests for cytologic screening and remain at risk for cervical cancer. When the uterine body, cervix, both ovaries, and both fallopian tubes are removed, the procedure is called a *total abdominal hysterectomy with bilateral salpingo-oophorectomy* (TAH-BSO). Removal of the uterine body, cervix, connective tissue, the upper third of the vagina, and pelvic lymph nodes is called a *radical hysterectomy.* The ovaries and fallopian tubes may also be removed. Radical hysterectomy surgery can be an option for clients with stage I cervical cancer. The procedure has several variations and generally is performed by an oncologist specializing in gynecologic cancer.

Surgeons have been criticized for performing the hysterectomy procedure unnecessarily in some instances when more conservative treatment would have sufficed. In the past, vaginal shortening was not uncommon along with hysterectomy. Shortening the vagina will cause dyspareunia and decrease the sexual pleasure of the woman and her partner. Clients should discuss this with their surgeon to ensure that the vagina is not shortened unnecessarily.

Surgical Procedure

A hysterectomy can be performed under general or regional anesthesia. The surgical approach can be through the abdomen or vagina. The abdominal route is indicated when the pelvis must be explored for pelvic malignancy or severe infection and when the uterus is too large to remove vaginally. The surgical incision for the abdominal approach may be vertical or transverse. Vertical midline incisions are quicker to perform and easier to extend if complications occur; some women feel these incisions produce less discomfort. The scar is more obvious and the incision is weaker than the transverse incision, however. The transverse incision is more difficult to perform and may not allow adequate exposure. Its strength and less obvious scar are its major advantages.

The vaginal approach is indicated for prolapse of the uterus and cancer in situ of the cervix. This route allows more rapid recovery because there are less restriction of mobility, less postoperative discomfort and no abdominal incision. Its major disadvantages are the limited exposure of the surgical site and the increased risk of infection.

Implications for the Client

Physiological Implications

Complications of all four types of hysterectomy include hemorrhage, infection, and thromboembolic disease. Clients undergoing the abdominal approach may have more postoperative pain than those with the vaginal approach. In a radical hysterectomy, wound drains are inserted during surgery and removed 4 to 5 days postoperatively. These clients also are at risk for hypokalemia and hypoalbuminemia.

The clients who have a subtotal or total hysterectomy will no longer have menstrual periods and will be sterile. (In rare instances, when sufficient endometrial tissues remain after subtotal hysterectomy, menstruation may be possible in the premenopausal woman.) Hormone replacement is not necessary, however, because the ovaries have been left intact. This is also true of clients after a radical hysterectomy when the ovaries are left intact. Premenopausal clients may notice some of the same premenstrual symptoms they had prior to the surgery. They should document when the premenstrual symptoms occur; the cyclical nature of the symptoms will establish that they are benign. Because both ovaries are removed in a TAH-BSO and sometimes in a radical hysterectomy, premenopausal clients will experience a sudden climacteric. Hormone replacement with estrogen and progesterone is usually required to minimize the menopausal symptoms.

The client having a radical hysterectomy may be left with a hypotonic bladder with decreased sensation and high bladder capacity. The cause of this dysfunction is thought to be nerve damage, resulting from interference in autonomic innervation to the bladder. Disruption in the innervation to the rectum may also prevent complete expulsion of feces.

Psychosocial/Lifestyle Implications

Clients are sterile after all forms of hysterectomy. Dyspareunia is possible whenever the procedure involves vaginal shortening and in subtotal hysterectomy if cervical discharge is a problem. Body image problems are possible with all surgeries.

Clients having both ovaries removed may possibly need hormonal replacement depending on the age of the client

Nursing Research Note

Schilling J, Molen M: Physical fitness and its relationship to postoperative recovery in abdominal hysterectomy patients. *Heart Lung* 1984; 13(6):639–644.

The relation between preoperative level of physical fitness and recovery from abdominal hysterectomy was examined. It was postulated that clients with higher levels of preoperative physical fitness would have fewer circulatory and pulmonary complications, shorter hospital stays, more favorable physical conditions immediately after surgery, and a greater capacity to perform activities postoperatively than clients with lower levels of physical fitness.

Physical fitness was measured by the postexercise heart rate response to the Canadian Home Fitness Test and a questionnaire that assessed amount and type of physical activity 2 weeks before surgery. Postoperative recovery was measured by length of hospital stay, presence of circulatory and respiratory complications, clients' self-evaluation, and ability to perform specified routine activities. Nineteen white females composed the sample.

The relation between physical fitness and the number of pulmonary and circulatory complications was not significant. A significant relation was found between higher levels of physical fitness and shorter lengths of hospital stay. A significant relation existed between indicators of physical fitness and clients' self-evaluation of physical condition. The relation between physical fitness and physical capacity to perform activities independently was not significant. The researchers believed that the small sample size may have altered results. Preoperative assessment of level of physical fitness by nurses may designate clients at risk for complications, longer hospital stays, and a more complicated recovery.

and the reason for the surgery. Clients with disrupted innervation to the bladder or rectum after radical hysterectomy will need to employ Crede's maneuver to facilitate bladder emptying at 2- to 3-hour intervals and use mild laxatives on a regular basis to promote complete emptying of the rectum. Implications for the hysterectomy client are summarized in Table 65–5.

Nursing Implications

Preoperative Care

The routine preoperative preparation common to other abdominal surgery (see Chapter 50) is also indicated for a hysterectomy. In addition, the physician may order an antiseptic vaginal douche the evening before surgery. A Foley catheter may be inserted prior to the client's going to the operating room. If the hysterectomy is performed through the vagina, the client will be given prophylactic antibiotics before the operation.

Although the client should have been informed by the physician of the exact nature of the hysterectomy procedure and its implications, it is a nursing responsibility to make sure the client understands the procedure. Inform the client of implications discussed earlier.

Table 65–5 Hysterectomy: Implications for the Client

Type of Surgery	Organs Removed	Physiological Implications	Psychosocial/Lifestyle Implications
Subtotal hysterectomy	Uterine body	Possible hemorrhage, infection, thromboembolic disease; cessation of menses in premenopausal women; sterility; possible continuation of cyclic premenstrual symptoms; continued cervical cancer screening	Sterility; possible body image problems
Total hysterectomy	Uterine body; uterine cervix	More postoperative pain with abdominal approach than vaginal approach; possible hemorrhage, infection, thromboembolic disease; cessation of menses in premenopausal women; sterility; possible continuation of cyclic premenstrual symptoms	Sterility; possible dyspareunia if vaginal shortening was part of the procedure; possible body image problems
Total abdominal hysterectomy with bilateral salpingo-oophorectomy (TAH-BSO)	Uterine body; uterine cervix; fallopian tubes; ovaries	More postoperative pain because of abdominal approach; possible hemorrhage, infection, thromboembolic disease; sudden climacteric in premenopausal clients; sterility	Sterility; possible dyspareunia if vaginal shortening was part of the procedure; possible body image problems; possible need for hormonal replacement
Radical hysterectomy	Uterine body; uterine cervix; supportive structures; pelvic lymph nodes; may also include ovaries and fallopian tubes	More postoperative pain because of abdominal approach; possible hemorrhage, infection, thromboembolic disease; risk of hypokalemia and hypoalbuminemia; wound drains inserted at time of surgery and remaining for 4 to 5 days; cessation of menses in premenopausal women; sterility; possible continuation of cyclic premenstrual symptoms; sudden climacteric if ovaries removed in premenopausal women; possible disrupted innervation to bladder and rectum	Sterility; possible dyspareunia if vaginal shortening was part of the procedure; possible body image problems; nerve damage to bladder requiring that client be discharged with Foley catheter or cystotomy tube; need to use Credé's maneuver to empty the bladder completely when urinary drainage apparatus is removed (see Chapter 33); need for laxatives for adequate bowel function

Postoperative Care

The postoperative nursing care for the hysterectomy client is determined by her previous health status, the indications for surgery, and the surgical approach. In general, nursing interventions involve the promotion of healing through adequate nutrition, the alleviation of discomfort, the prevention of complications, and the promotion of a positive self-concept.

Initially, hydration is maintained and electrolytes are replaced by supplements and IV fluid therapy. Monitor these fluids to make sure they infuse at a rate conducive to the client's present health state.

Clients with abdominal hysterectomies are NPO for 24 hours or until nausea subsides and bowel sounds return. They are then placed on a diet that progresses from clear liquids to solid food. Vaginal hysterectomy clients can consume food earlier, because there has been less bowel manipulation. When clients are able to select their own menus, assist them in choosing foods rich in nutrients that promote tissue healing. Flatulence, a common problem in gynecologic surgery, can be relieved by simethicone (Gas-X, Mylicon), a rectal tube, the left lateral Sims' position, and increased physical activity.

The amount of postoperative discomfort varies according to the placement of the surgical incision, the surgical approach, the amount of tissue manipulation, and the client's level of anxiety. Anxiety can be reduced if the nurse informs clients that pain is a normal response to surgery and that medication is available. As a rule, clients with vaginal hysterectomies experience less discomfort and are mobile sooner than those who have had abdominal procedures. Clients with transverse abdominal incisions may have more discomfort than those with midline incisions. For pain control, narcotics are ordered every 4 to 6 hours if appropriate during the first 48 hours. The nurse should administer these drugs, assess their effectiveness, and observe clients for side effects. Nursing comfort measures include proper positioning and splinting of the incisional area with movement.

Hemorrhage can occur with any type of hysterectomy but is more frequent with the vaginal approach. Monitor vital signs every 15 minutes until stable. Any fall in blood pressure associated with unusual postoperative pain should alert the nurse to the possibility of occult hemorrhage. Observe perineal pads for bright red blood; a small amount of serosanguineous discharge is expected. Clients with vaginal procedures may have vaginal packings for the first 24 hours to put mild pressure on the suture line and control postoperative oozing. The abdominal dressing should remain dry, and the nurse should report significant discharge or bleeding.

In gynecologic surgery, the most common sites of postoperative infection are the lungs, incision site, urinary tract, and pelvic cavity. As with other types of major surgery, the risk of infection depends on the client's health status, the indication for surgery, the anesthesia, and the surgical technique.

Pulmonary atelectasis, bronchitis, and pneumonia are complications that can be minimized by nursing intervention. Encourage mobility and pulmonary exercises. Incentive spirometry should be used for clients at increased risk for pulmonary infection because of obesity, smoking, or chronic lung disorders. Clients who have been instructed in these measures preoperatively will be better prepared to participate in preventing complications.

Wound infections, abscesses, or cellulitis can occur at both abdominal and vaginal incision sites. Infections of the vaginal cuff (the closed-off portion of the upper vagina after removal of the cervix) are more common, because the nonsterile environment encourages growth of pathogens. Be alert for foul-smelling discharge on the client's dressing or perineal pad. Again, a small amount of serosanguineous drainage is expected. Report temperature elevations to the surgeon. Therapy consists of systemic antibiotics.

Because of its proximity to the reproductive organs, the urinary system is susceptible to trauma and infection. Clients return to the unit with indwelling urethral catheters, which the nurse must evaluate for patency. Urinary drainage should be assessed for hematuria. Catheter care requires sterile technique. In the absence of complications, the catheter is removed in 12 to 24 hours. Some clients have difficulty voiding after catheter removal because of the edema and discomfort from surgery. Check for frequent small voiding as a clue to residual urine. Distention of the bladder requires repeat catheterization. Once adequate voiding has been established, remind clients to wipe from front to back to prevent fecal contamination of the urethra and vagina. Avoid bacterial concentration in the bladder by encouraging fluids that flush the urinary tract.

Peritonitis is a severe complication of gynecologic surgery. Predisposing factors include preexisting infection, intestinal trauma, obesity, and excessive tissue oozing. Abdominal pain, rigid abdomen, nausea, vomiting, and fever

are classic signs the nurse should recognize.

Thromboembolic disease includes conditions of vascular clotting and their sequelae. Pulmonary embolus suggested by fever, tachycardia, dyspnea, and pleuritic chest pain is a serious form of this disorder. Manipulation and trauma of the pelvic vessels predispose the gynecologic client to this problem, and a prior history of thromboembolic disease, pelvic malignancy, and obesity accentuates the risk. Exercises while in bed, early postoperative ambulation, and the use of antiembolic stockings are thought to minimize these complications. Encourage women to avoid positions that obstruct venous return from the lower extremities.

OOPHORECTOMY

Oophorectomy is the surgical removal of one or both ovaries. The indications include ovarian malignancy, unresolved benign ovarian neoplasm, tubo-ovarian abscess, and the need for prophylaxis in perimenopausal and menopausal clients having hysterectomies.

Surgical Procedure

An oophorectomy can be done under general or regional anesthesia. The surgeon usually uses a laparotomy incision to allow adequate exposure to explore the abdominal cavity. This is essential when malignancy is suspected, because metastasis to the diaphragm can occur. When malignancy is confirmed, the surgeon removes the ovaries, uterus, and fallopian tubes.

Implications for the Client

Physiological Implications

If malignancy is found during oophorectomy, the fallopian tubes and uterus may be removed with the ovaries. The premenopausal client having both ovaries removed will experience a sudden climacteric and sterility. The use of hormonal replacement therapy depends on the client's age and the indication for surgery. If only one ovary is removed, the remaining one usually can meet physiological needs. Complications of oophorectomy are similar to those of abdominal hysterectomy.

Psychosocial/Lifestyle Implications

Because bilateral oophorectomy causes sterility, the client faces the loss of her reproductive capability. She may also have to cope with the diagnosis of cancer. Client implications for oophorectomy are listed in Table 65–6.

Nursing Implications

Preoperative and postoperative nursing care are similar to that for abdominal hysterectomy clients. Complications are also similar to those that may be expected with abdominal hysterectomy.

Table 65–6	Oophorectomy: Implications for the Client	
Physiological Implications	**Psychosocial/Lifestyle Implications**
If malignancy is found, possible removal of fallopian tubes and uterus	In bilateral procedure, sterility and possible need for hormonal replacement in premenopausal women
In bilateral procedure, sudden climacteric and sterility	Possible body image change
In unilateral procedure, ability of remaining ovary to meet physiological needs	Fears associated with malignancy
Complications similar to abdominal hysterectomy (see Table 65–5)	See also Table 65–5

SALPINGOPLASTY

Salpingoplasty (tuboplasty) is the surgical repair or reconstruction of the fallopian tubes to treat infertility. The most common reason for infertility in women is the inability of the ovum to reach the fallopian tube or to be propelled through the tube to be fertilized by the sperm. These problems usually result from peritubular adhesions or tubal occlusion in association with pelvic surgery, pelvic inflammatory disease (PID), endometriosis, previous sterilization, or ectopic pregnancy.

Surgical Procedure

The specific tubal pathology determines the surgical approach and procedure employed. Most salpingoplasties are done under regional or general anesthesia. Recent advances in microsurgery have made these procedures more common.

Salpingolysis, the release of peritubular adhesions, can be accomplished by either an abdominal laparotomy or by a laparoscopy. The surgical approach depends on the extent of the adhesions.

Fimbriaplasty is the repair of a partial fimbrial occlusion, whereas a *salpingostomy* repairs a complete fimbrial occlusion. Because these conditions are associated with peritubular adhesions, salpingolysis may be performed at the same time.

When the fallopian tubes have been separated by surgical sterilization or closed by infection, anastomosis of the tubes can reestablish tubal patency in some cases. The type of procedure the surgeon uses depends on the pathological condition or the previous method of sterilization. An end-to-end anastomosis reunites the two ends of the severed or damaged tube, and a tubouterine anastomosis reconnects the tube to the cornua of the uterus (the horn-

shaped portion of the upper uterine body). These procedures require laparotomy incisions.

Implications for the Client

Physiological Implications

Complications from salpingoplasty are rare. Infection, wound disruption, and hemorrhage have been reported. The long-term complications include peritubular adhesions, fibrosis, and tubal occlusion. These long-term problems increase the risk of ectopic pregnancy. The reestablishment of fertility and a resulting full-term pregnancy is the ideal outcome of salpingoplasty. Because of current microsurgical techniques, this goal can be accomplished in approximately 60% of the clients suitable for surgery (Gomel, 1983).

Psychosocial/Lifestyle Implications

Salpingoplasty may fail to restore fertility. The client who has had unrealistic expectations for the surgical outcome will then need to adjust to the loss of reproductive potential. Since great hope is placed on the success of the procedure, couples can be emotionally distressed by a poor outcome. Unresolved feelings of guilt and failure may lead to sexual dysfunction and marital disruption. Client implications of salpingoplasty are summarized in Table 65–7.

Nursing Implications

Preoperative and postoperative nursing care of clients having salpingoplasty depends on the surgical approach. The care of laparoscopy clients having abdominal gynecologic surgery is discussed earlier in this chapter. Unique to salpingoplasty is the preoperative and postoperative administration of dexamethasone (Decadron), a synthetic corticosteroid thought to diminish the initial inflammatory response to surgery and thereby reduce the possibility of a failed procedure. Because this drug also can mask infection, it is used in conjunction with prophylactic antibiotics.

Table 65–7	Salpingoplasty: Implications for the Client	
Physiological Implications	**Psychosocial/Lifestyle Implications**
Complications of infection, hemorrhage, peritubular adhesions, fibrosis, tubal occlusion	Possible failure to restore fertility resulting in possible sexual dysfunction and marital disruption
Higher risk for ectopic pregnancy	
Tubal patency and possibly fertility restored	
Term pregnancy in 60% of procedures	

VULVECTOMY

Vulvectomy involves excision of the external genitalia. The indications for this surgery include premalignant vulvar lesions, cancer in situ, or invasive carcinoma.

Surgical Procedure

Both simple and radical vulvectomy are performed under general anesthesia. Simple vulvectomy usually involves the clitoris, labia majora, labia minora, and tissues between them (Figure 65–4). With invasive carcinoma, a radical vulvectomy may be performed to remove the entire vulva, lymphatics, subcutaneous fat, and skin portions from the abdomen and groin (Figure 65–5).

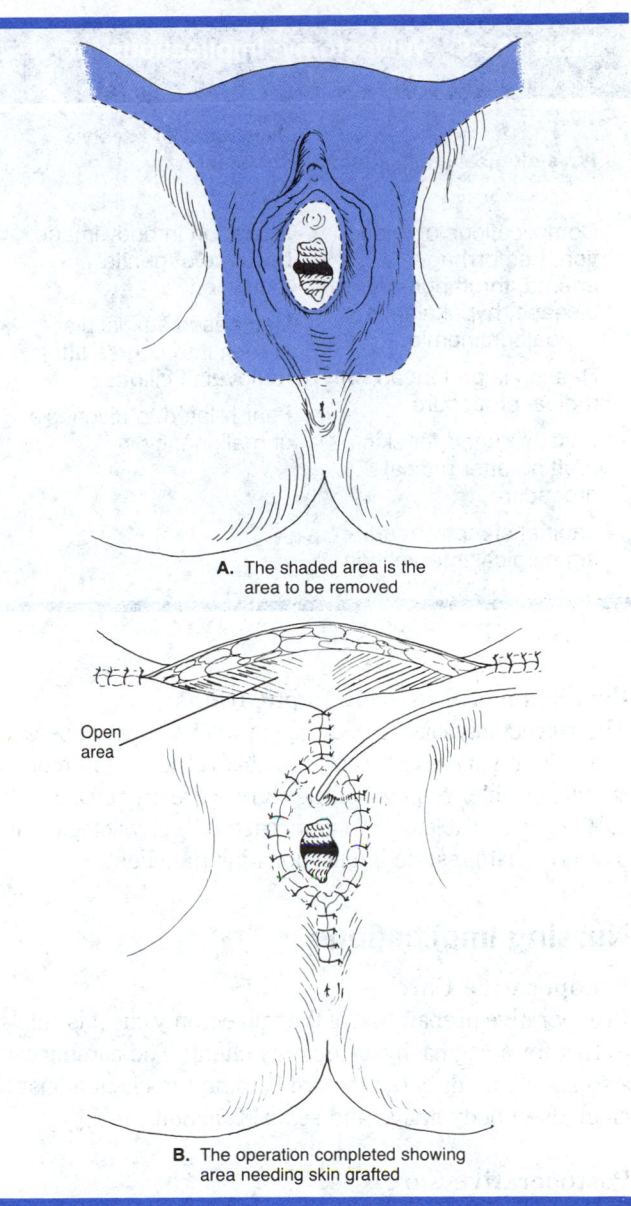

A. The shaded area is the area to be removed

B. The operation completed showing area needing skin grafted

Figure 65–5

Radical vulvectomy. **A.** The shaded area is the area to be removed. **B.** The operation completed, showing area needing skin grafted.

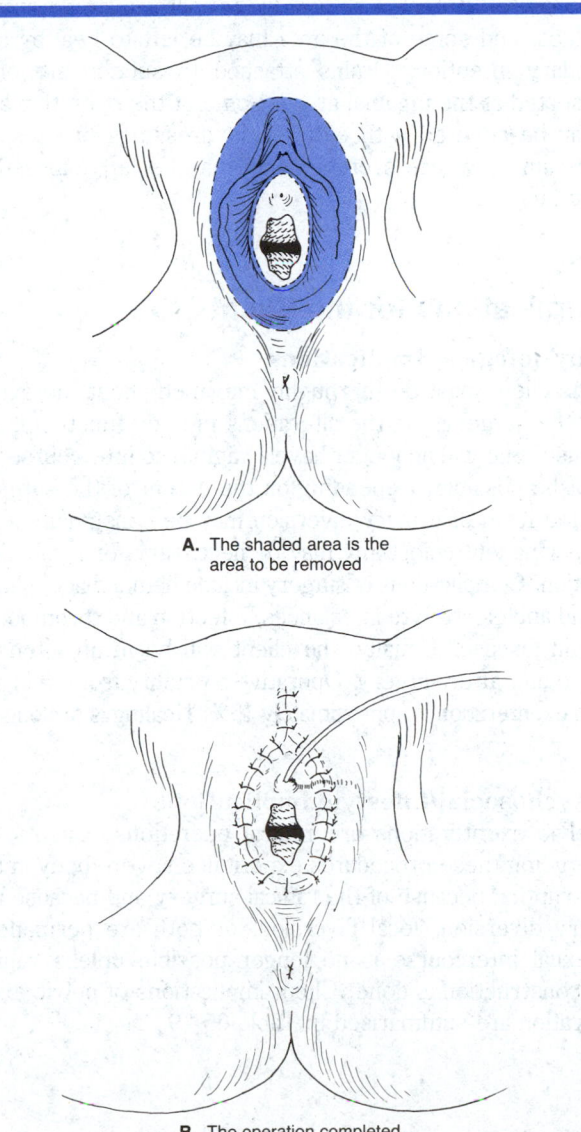

A. The shaded area is the area to be removed

B. The operation completed

Figure 65–4

Simple vulvectomy.

Implications for the Client

Physiological Implications

Postoperative complications of vulvectomy include infection, hemorrhage, edema, and thromboembolic disease. Radical vulvectomy clients are at increased risk of infection because of prolonged healing, extensive tissue destruction and because they are usually of advanced age. Skin grafting may be necessary after the removal of large amounts of tissue. Hypokalemia and hypoalbuminemia can result from extensive tissue destruction and fluid loss. Vaginal stenosis from scar formation can occur and requires surgical intervention.

Table 65–8 Vulvectomy: Implications for the Client	
Physiological Implications	**Psychosocial/Lifestyle Implications**
Complications of infection, hemorrhage, edema, thromboembolic disease, hypokalemia, hypoalbuminemia	Alteration in body image because of genital mutilation
Healing is prolonged with radical procedure	Decreased sexual pleasure in intercourse after removal of clitoris
Possible need for skin grafting after radical procedure	Fear related to diagnosis of malignancy
Vaginal stenosis requiring surgical intervention	

Psychosocial/Lifestyle Implications

The vulvectomy client's body image will be impaired because of mutilation of the external genitalia. Although intercourse is still possible, removal of the clitoris greatly reduces sexual pleasure. Table 65–8 summarizes the physiological and psychosocial/lifestyle implications for the client.

Nursing Implications

Preoperative Care

Preoperative preparation of the vulvectomy client is similar to that for a vaginal hysterectomy client. The nursing care also should be directed toward helping the client adjust to changes in body image and sexual function.

Postoperative Care

Prevention of infection, hemorrhage, and edema are primary postoperative nursing concerns with the simple vulvectomy. These complications can be prevented by pressure bandages, the use of sterile technique in dressing changes, and the use of wound drains. Prophylactic antibiotics initiated prior to the surgery are continued for 48 hours postoperatively to prevent infection. Poor healing with wound dehiscence can result from poor circulation and infection. Sitz baths are controversial; although they provide generalized heat, they also may contribute to infection. Heat lamps promote circulation and thus the supply of oxygen at the wound site. In many instances, healing occurs by secondary intention—a long and uncomfortable process that requires meticulous attention to preventing infection. The nursing care for clients with skin grafts is described in Chapter 80.

Fluid and electrolyte management is essential in these clients to prevent hypokalemia and hypoalbuminemia. Older clients may require wedge pressure monitoring by a Swan–Ganz catheter to regulate fluid replacement.

PELVIC EXENTERATION

Total pelvic exenteration is the removal of the entire female reproductive tract, along with both urinary and fecal diversion. Modifications of this procedure involve removal of the reproductive organs with only urinary diversion or removal of the reproductive organs with only fecal diversion. This surgery is performed on clients with invasive cancer of the uterine cervix.

Surgical Procedure

The surgical procedure is similar to that for radical vulvectomy. Procedures for urinary and fecal diversion may also be performed (see Chapters 34 and 50). Deep pelvic node and groin node excision are likely to be part of the surgical procedure. It may not be possible to approximate the wound edges, and some of the area may be left to heal by secondary intention. Drains attached to suction are often inserted at the inguinal areas. Some of the operative area may be covered with either light dressings or pressure dressings, whereas other parts may be left exposed to the air.

Implications for the Client

Physiological Implications

The client must be thoroughly informed about the extent of the surgery and the alterations in body function it will cause. She will no longer have a vagina, so intercourse will not be possible. Depending on the extent of the surgery, some form of urinary diversion may be constructed, and a permanent colostomy may be necessary for fecal elimination. Complications of surgery include hemorrhage, shock, fluid and electrolyte imbalances, infection and thromboembolic disease. Usually, the client will be in an intensive care unit after surgery. Operative mortality from total pelvic exenteration is approximately 15%. Healing is prolonged.

Psychosocial/Lifestyle Implications

Pelvic exenterations are radical operations. Clients undergoing these procedures experience severe body image disruption because of the radical surgery and because urinary diversion, fecal diversion, or both are permanent. Sexual intercourse is no longer possible unless vaginal reconstruction is done. Client implications of pelvic exenteration are summarized in Table 65–9.

Nursing Implications

Preoperative Care

Preoperative nursing for pelvic exenteration is similar to the care of clients undergoing vulvectomy (discussed ear-

Table 65-9	Pelvic Exenteration: Implications for the Client
Physiological Implications	**Psychosocial/Lifestyle Implications**
Removal of vagina	Severe disruption of body image
Prolonged healing	
Possible fecal and urinary diversion	Sexual intercourse no longer possible unless vagina is reconstructed
Complications of hemorrhage, shock, fluid and electrolyte imbalances, infection, thromboembolic disease	Need to adapt to both urinary and fecal diversion (see Chapters 34 and 50)
Stay in intensive care unit	
High mortality rate (15%)	

lier in this chapter) and those having urinary and fecal diversion (as discussed in Chapters 34 and 50, respectively). The nurse must devote considerable time toward allowing these clients to verbalize their anger and fears.

Postoperative Care

The long surgical procedure and a fluctuating blood volume predispose pelvic exenteration clients to hemorrhage and shock. Clients need to be monitored carefully so corrective measures can be taken immediately. In the surgical intensive care unit, fluid maintenance and electrolyte balance are major concerns. Because of the radical surgery, infection is a major cause of death. The postoperative care for bladder and fecal diversion are discussed in Chapters 34 and 50. These clients may also be receiving chemotherapy or radiation (see Chapter 12).

Section II: Surgical Approaches to Tubal Sterilization

The term *sterilization* encompasses a variety of surgical procedures that are performed to terminate a person's ability to bear children. Sterilization is considered a permanent form of contraception. This section will discuss methods of tubal sterilization, which involves the surgical alteration of the fallopian tubes to prevent the union of the ovum and sperm.

Surgical Procedure

Tubal sterilization can be performed under local or general anesthesia. It is usually an outpatient procedure. The surgical approach (entry into the pelvic cavity) can be by laparoscopy, as previously described; by minilaparotomy; or through the vagina. The tubal occlusion can be accomplished by dissection, ligation (Figure 65-6), electrocautery, a polymeric silicone (Silastic) ring, a metal clip, or a combination of any of these methods.

Laparoscopy can be used in most types of tubal occlusion procedures. This surgical operation has been discussed previously in this chapter. Tubal sterilization by minilaparotomy is performed through a small transverse suprapubic incision. In the postpartum client, the surgeon often uses a small infraumbilical incision because the fallopian tubes are elevated at this time. Postpartum tubal sterilization has the greatest incidence of unintended recannulation because the pelvic organs are highly vascular immediately after childbirth.

Tubal sterilization also can be performed transvaginally through an incision in the anterior vaginal wall. This approach is seldom performed now because of its high infection rate and the ease of laparoscopy.

Implications for the Client

Physiological Implications

Sterility because of occlusion of the fallopian tubes is the major implication. Complications from tubal sterilization are few. Perforation of the urinary bladder is the major problem that can occur with the suprapubic approach. The vaginal approach carries a greater risk of infection. The

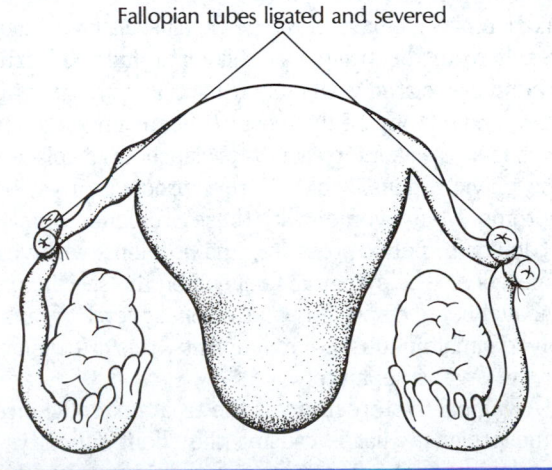

Fallopian tubes ligated and severed

Figure 65-6

Pomeroy method of tubal ligation. Both fallopian tubes are ligated and severed, which interrupts continuity of the tube.

SOURCE: Olds SB, London ML, Ladewig PA: *Maternal-Newborn Nursing: A Family-Centered Approach.* Menlo Park, CA: Addison-Wesley, 1984, p. 128.

possibility of mistaking another structure for the fallopian tube is a risk with all methods of tubal occlusion, as is recannulation, which allows pregnancy.

Psychosocial/Lifestyle Implications

Tubal sterilization causes permanent sterility, so women should be certain that they will desire no future pregnancies. Some surgeons recommend that young women seeking sterilization undergo procedures such as the Silastic ring that cause the least amount of tubal destruction, in case they wish to have the operation reversed in the future. Clients should also be aware that the tubes can recannulate and cause unplanned pregnancy. Clients who desire no future pregnancies feel relieved that they no longer need to use temporary contraceptive methods. Clients who change their minds later experience anxiety over whether fertility can be reestablished. Table 65–10 summarizes the physiological, psychosocial, and lifestyle implications of tubal sterilization.

Nursing Implications

Preoperative Care

The preoperative nursing care for clients undergoing tubal sterilization is similar to that for other gynecologic procedures such as D and C. The nurse must inform clients of the permanence of the procedure and avoid terms such as

| Table 65–10   Tubal Sterilization: Implications for the Client ||
Physiological Implications	Psychosocial/Lifestyle Implications
Sterility because of occlusion of fallopian tubes	Sterility
With suprapubic approach, possible perforation of the bladder	Possible unplanned pregnancy from tube recannulation
With vaginal approach, greater risk of infection	Anxiety over surgical reestablishment of fertility if pregnancy is desired in the future
Possible recannulation	

tubes tied and *tubal*. Many women erroneously think that reversal of the procedure merely involves "untying" the tubes. Also inform clients that although it is rare, the tubes can recannulate and cause unplanned pregnancy.

Postoperative Care

Postoperative care focuses on the relief of discomfort and the prevention of infection. Postoperative nursing care depends on the surgical approach. Care was described earlier in the section on laparoscopy.

Section III: Surgical Approaches to Relaxation of the Pelvic Musculature

Relaxation or weakness of the pelvic musculature is thought to result from the trauma of childbirth and the hormone reduction associated with menopause. The uterus, vagina, bladder, and rectum are the most frequently involved organs. The muscle relaxation causes prolapse or displacement of the pelvic organs, which in turn produces a variety of symptoms. Many women with these problems complain of low back pain, pelvic pressure, and problems with voiding or defecation. The symptoms depend on the specific organs that have been displaced, and often several organs are involved simultaneously. For simplicity, this discussion will treat the organs separately.

A vaginal hysterectomy is the treatment of choice for uterine prolapse that is causing the client difficulty. The surgical procedure and nursing care were discussed earlier in this chapter and will not be repeated here. When the primary symptom is urinary stress incontinence, a variety of surgical procedures to suspend the uterus and associated structures (uterine suspension, Marshall–Marchetti, Kelly's plication) may be employed. It should be noted that these procedures have a low rate of success. Stress incontinence is discussed in Chapters 33 and 34.

ANTERIOR COLPORRHAPHY

Cystocele and urethrocele are the indications for anterior colporrhaphy. Anterior colporrhaphy repairs the weakness of the anterior vaginal wall.

Surgical Procedure

When a cystocele occurs without stress incontinence, a simple anterior colporrhaphy corrects the vaginal weakness and returns the bladder to its anatomic position. This operation is performed under general or regional anesthesia. The client is placed in a lithotomy position, and the surgeon makes an incision into the anterior vaginal wall. The bladder is mobilized, and the fascia between the bladder and vagina is tightened with sutures. Excess vaginal tissue is then removed, and the vaginal wall is closed. If stress incontinence was a problem, the surgeon can modify this procedure with added sutures to draw the suburethral ligaments under the urethra and restore the vesicourethral angle. Anterior colporrhaphy is often performed in conjunction with posterior colporrhaphy, vaginal hysterectomy, or both.

Implications for the Client

Physiological Implications

Anterior colporrhaphy relieves stress incontinence and reduces the incidence of bladder infection. Serious complications, including hemorrhage, are rare. Postoperative urinary tract infections, voiding difficulties, and dyspareunia can occur, however. In addition, 10% of clients have a recurrence of the cystocele.

Psychosocial/Lifestyle Implications

This procedure relieves stress incontinence and its accompanying embarrassment to the client. Dyspareunia may make sexual intercourse difficult for some clients. See Table 65–11 for a summary of implications for the client of anterior colporrhaphy.

Nursing Implications

Preoperative Care

Preoperative care is similar to care for clients undergoing vaginal hysterectomy. Vaginal hysterectomy was discussed earlier in this chapter.

Postoperative Care

After surgery, the client returns to the unit with vaginal packing, which is removed in 24 to 48 hours. Because packing can mask overt signs of bleeding, monitor vital signs frequently. Instruct the client to report dizziness or light-headedness, symptoms indicating acute blood loss.

Voiding is difficult because of urethral narrowing, edema, and postoperative discomfort. Urinary drainage is accomplished by a Foley catheter or suprapubic cystostomy tube. Foley catheters are removed in 2 to 4 days. If the client has small frequent voidings, suspect urinary retention. Residual urine volumes greater than 100 mL usually necessitate the reinsertion of the Foley catheter. When the suprapubic drainage system is used, the tube is clamped for voiding. Residual urine can be directly measured after each voiding by unclamping the cystostomy tube.

POSTERIOR COLPORRHAPHY

Rectocele or enterocele are the indications for posterior colporrhaphy. Posterior colporrhaphy repairs the posterior vaginal wall.

Surgical Procedure

Like the anterior repair, posterior colporrhaphy is done under general or regional anesthesia. The surgeon makes an incision into the posterior vaginal wall, separates the rectocele from the wall, and obliterates it by tightening the fascial layer between the rectum and vagina. The excess vaginal tissue is removed, and the incision is repaired. This procedure is often performed along with an anterior colporrhaphy, vaginal hysterectomy, or both.

Table 65–11 Anterior Colporrhaphy: Implications for the Client	
Physiological Implications	**Psychosocial/Lifestyle Implications**
Relief of stress incontinence	Reduction in embarrassment from incontinence
Reduction in number of bladder infections	Decreased sexual pleasure from dyspareunia in some instances
Possible complications of urinary tract infection, voiding difficulties, dyspareunia, hemorrhage	
Recurrence of cystocele in 10% of clients	

Implications for the Client

Physiological Implications

A posterior colporrhaphy resolves symptoms of the rectocele, although complete rectal strength will take at least 6 weeks to return because of slower healing of the fibrous tissue and fascia. Complications can include bleeding, infection, and dyspareunia. These clients also may have urinary retention because of the surgical manipulation and the discomfort associated with bearing down.

Psychosocial/Lifestyle Implications

The client must consume a high-fiber diet to prevent constipation and weakening of the musculature. Stool softeners and laxatives also may be needed. Dyspareunia may sometimes occur and can cause problems with sexual intercourse. The client implications of posterior colporrhaphy are summarized in Table 65–12.

Table 65–12 Posterior Colporrhaphy: Implications for the Client	
Physiological Implications	**Psychosocial/Lifestyle Implications**
Resolution of symptoms of rectocele	High-fiber diet to prevent constipation and musculature weakening
Delay in return of complete rectal strength for at least 6 weeks	Possible need for stool softeners and laxatives
Possible bleeding, infection, dyspareunia, urinary retention	Decreased sexual pleasure from dyspareunia possible in some instances

Nursing Implications

Preoperative Care

Preoperative nursing care of posterior colporrhaphy clients is similar to that of clients undergoing other vaginal surgeries. Some physicians order preoperative barium enemas to rule out other causes of excessive straining for defecation.

Postoperative Care

Assess postoperative clients for bleeding and infection. If operative oozing was excessive, it may be necessary to place a drain in the incision; this reduces the possibility of infection by lessening the risk of hematoma formation. An in-dwelling Foley catheter will initially resolve the problem of urinary retention. Sitz baths are helpful in promoting healing and relieving discomfort. Stool softeners are used to prevent straining.

The nurse must assess the client's dietary habits and instruct her to include foods that contain bulk and fiber. A high-residue diet is thought to facilitate defecation, preventing recurrence of the rectocele.

Section IV: Surgical Approaches to Disorders of the Breast

The surgical approaches to disorders of the breast presented here include breast biopsy, mastectomy (breast removal), breast reconstruction, and breast augmentation and reduction mammoplasty. All these surgical procedures result in a changed body image, so the impact of the procedure depends on the woman's perception of the breasts' significance in her self-image and the value she places on the breasts in determining femininity and sexuality. The nurse who is with the client before surgery, when she first sees her changed body, and during the recovery period can offer support, information, and comprehensive care.

BREAST BIOPSY

Breast biopsy is the removal of material from a breast mass or the removal of the mass itself for histologic study of the cells to determine whether cancer is present. Any breast mass should be evaluated for the possible diagnosis of cancer. Biopsy can differentiate whether a fibrocystic lesion is (1) a simple cyst or cysts caused by a change in the cells lining the ducts and the secretion of fluid or (2) a premalignant condition that is caused by hyperplasia of the cells. Biopsy also can identify fibroadenomas and intraductal papillomas. A histologic examination is performed on the discharge, and a biopsy is performed on the duct involved. If no mass is present with nipple discharge, as in mammary duct ectasia, diagnosis is made by histologic examination of the discharge.

Surgical Procedure

The breast biopsy is performed by aspiration of the fluid or tissue from the tumor, incisional removal of a portion of the tumor, or excision of the whole tumor (Figure 65–7). Fluid aspiration requires no anesthesia. The lump is first located by palpation or diagnostic techniques such as mammography or ultrasonography. A large-bore needle is used to aspirate the contents from the tumor, and the contents are then placed on a slide for Papanicolaou evaluation. When an incisional or excisional biopsy is performed, a local anes-

thetic is usually used. The tumor cells are then histologically evaluated using the frozen section technique.

Implications for the Client

Physiological Implications

During the aspiration biopsy, the client feels minimal discomfort as the needle is inserted into the tumor. During

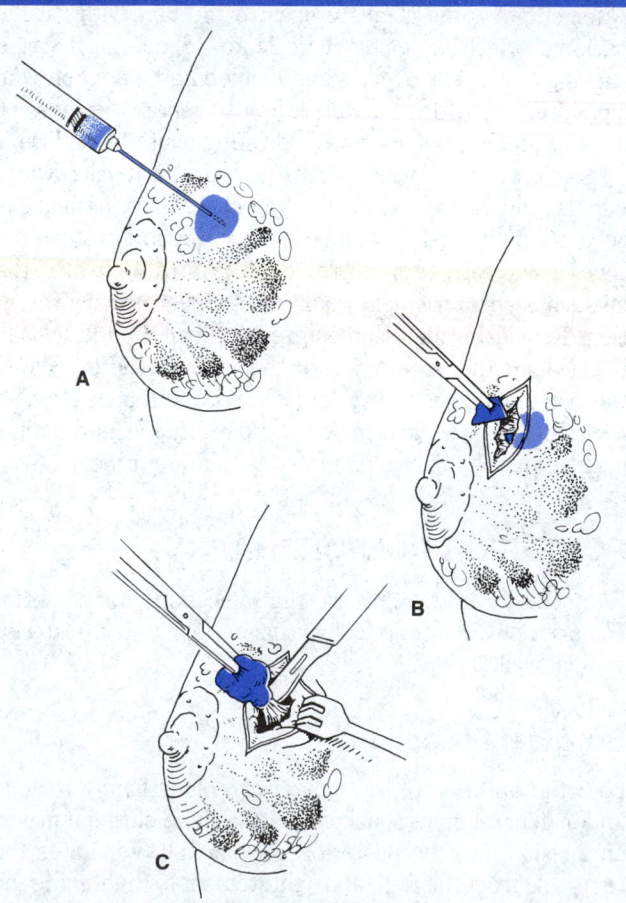

Figure 65–7

Types of breast biopsies. **A.** Aspiration biopsy. **B.** Incisional biopsy. **C.** Excisional biopsy.

Nursing Research Note

Scott D: Anxiety, critical thinking, and information processing during and after breast biopsy. *Nurs Res* 1983; 32(1):24–28.

Critical thinking ability, anxiety, and information processing were examined in a group of women 18 through 60 years of age undergoing breast biopsy for the purpose of diagnosing a carcinoma. The sample was tested during hospitalization and retested again 6 to 8 weeks after biopsy when results were known.

The findings suggest that critical thinking abilities are reduced during hospitalization compared with 6 to 8 weeks postbiopsy. Anxiety levels during hospitalization before a benign test result were extremely high. The anxiety was reduced 6 to 8 weeks after hospitalization. The anxiety level was correlated with difficulty in the reasoning process and decision-making abilities. Information processing was not significantly reduced in the hospitalized group, but information processing declined somewhat with high anxiety levels.

Because anxiety diminishes critical thinking abilities and impairs information processing, nurses must pay special attention to clients and monitor health teaching. These clients also need intense nursing support to cope with immediate stressors.

an incisional or excisional biopsy performed under local anesthetic, the client may feel pulling and probing but should not feel pain. A mild analgesic may be needed for incisional pain following the procedure, and a support bra is worn day and night through the first week. Biopsy rarely leads to complications or wound-healing problems. The breast usually continues to function if the client is in her reproductive years.

Psychosocial/Lifestyle Implications

Before the biopsy, most clients are anxious about the possible diagnosis of cancer, anticipated pain, possible change in body image because of disfigurement, and invasion of their bodies. Anxiety may continue even after the diagnosis of a benign tumor because of breast changes such as the scar and the absence of breast tissue, which alter the body image. A diagnosis of cancer and discussion of options for treatment are emotionally difficult and require support (see Chapter 12).

Good nutrition is a preventive measure for fibrocystic disease and a possible preventive measure for breast cancer as well. With the diagnosis of fibrocystic disease, remind the client to eliminate substances with methylxanthine such as coffee, tea, and chocolate from her diet. Reducing fat and increasing fiber in the diet may help prevent breast cancer (see Table 12–2). Emphasize the importance of monthly breast self-examination (BSE). Client implications of breast biopsy are summarized in Table 65–13.

Nursing Implications

Preoperative Care

Preoperative instructions to the breast biopsy client vary according to the type of anesthesia used and the type of biopsy performed. Needle aspiration of a potential cyst is usually performed in a primary care setting, whereas excisional and incisional biopsy procedures may be performed in the hospital. Give instructions on dietary restrictions to the client undergoing general anesthesia. Tell all clients about arrival time, preoperative laboratory work, and the need for transportation postoperatively. Information about the sensations to expect during the biopsy is also important. Provide emotional support by listening to the client's fears and providing information on the procedure. Tell the client when the results of the histological test will be available.

Postoperative Care

Immediate postoperative nursing care includes assessment of the site for bleeding and monitoring of vital signs. Ice applied to the incisional area may decrease swelling. A supportive bra may provide comfort and should be worn at night. Mild analgesics may relieve incisional pain.

Provide emotional support for the client and significant others. Discharge teaching will include information on nutrition, incisional care, and scheduling of a return visit to the health care provider for removal of sutures if appropriate. Teach or review monthly BSE procedures.

MASTECTOMY

A mastectomy, or removal of the breast, is the most common surgical procedure performed when a malignant tumor is found. The mastectomy procedure is controversial; many women are demanding more conservative and less destructive surgery for breast cancer, a move supported by many cancer authorities. This section discusses the various types of mastectomies and the more limited surgical procedures for breast cancer. The type of surgery

Table 65–13	Breast Biopsy: Implications for the Client	
Physiological Implications	**Psychosocial/Lifestyle Implications**
Sensations of pulling or probing during the procedure	Anxiety
	Fear of cancer
Mild postoperative discomfort	Alterations in body image because of scar and absence of breast tissue
	Need for emotional support
	Decisions about type of treatment if cancer is diagnosed
	Dietary changes: elimination of methylxanthine substances, increase in fiber, decrease in fats
	Monthly BSE

depends on the staging of the tumor and the client's preferences. The smaller the tumor in the absence of metastasis, the greater the survival rate and the number of alternatives for treatment. When the cancer involves the muscle or interpectoral node, more muscle and tissue must be removed.

Radiation therapy, hormonal therapy, and chemotherapy have all been discussed in the section on breast cancer in Chapter 64. This discussion is limited to surgical treatment of breast cancer and assumes that the client has discussed the various therapeutic approaches, as well as their risks and benefits, with the health care team.

Surgical Procedure

In the United States, the standard surgical procedure for treatment of breast cancer has been the *modified radical mastectomy*. This aggressive procedure removes the involved breast tissue as well as the nipple and areola, surrounding skin, lymph nodes of the axillary region, and possibly the smaller pectoral muscle. The greater pectoral muscle is left intact. Figure 65–8A illustrates the procedure and

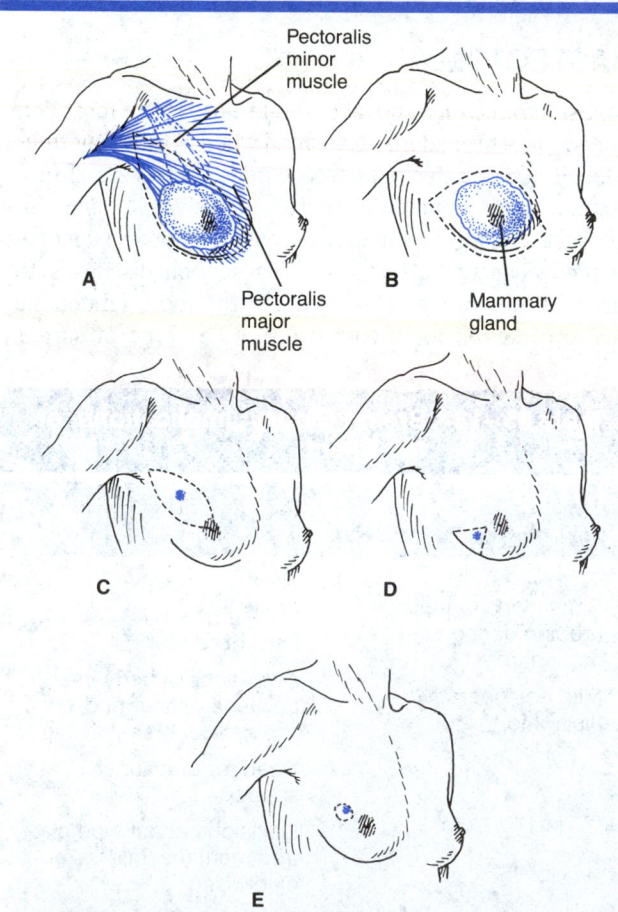

Pectoralis minor muscle

Pectoralis major muscle

Mammary gland

A B C D E

Figure 65–8

Mastectomy procedures. **A.** Modified radical mastectomy with drainage tube in place. **B.** Simple or total mastectomy. **C.** Quadrantectomy. **D.** Partial mastectomy (segmental resection). **E.** Lumpectomy (tylectomy).

placement of the drainage tube. If the lymph nodes are found to be cancerous, chemotherapy may be recommended. A simple mastectomy, or total mastectomy, involves removal of the breast only and is indicated for Paget's disease of the nipple and other localized cancers. Lymph nodes and the pectoral muscles are left intact (Figure 65–8B). It is also used as a palliative measure when a large tumor has metastasized and may cause ulceration and draining.

In the *quadrantectomy,* the excision includes the entire quadrant of the breast containing the tumor, the fascia covering the greater pectoral muscle, and the entire smaller pectoral muscle (Figure 65–8C). *Partial mastectomy* (also called segmental resection) involves an excision of the tumor and a 2- to 3-cm wedge of tissue surrounding it (Figure 65–8D). A portion of the overlying skin and the underlying fascia are also excised. Both procedures usually include nodal dissection to determine the need for chemotherapy. *Lumpectomy* or tylectomy is similar to excisional biopsy, discussed earlier; it removes the tumor and the near surrounding tissue but leaves the skin and fascia intact. Axillary lymph nodes may or may not be removed through a separate incision. Lumpectomy is also illustrated in Figure 65–8E.

The *Halsted radical mastectomy,* a more extensive and destructive surgical dissection, removes the breast, nipple and areola, axillary nodes, and both pectoral muscles. Variations of this procedure have also included removal of part of the rib cage to excise the internal mammary lymph nodes as well as removal of the supraclavicular lymph nodes. The Halsted procedure is rarely used today.

Implications for the Client

Physiological Implications

Radical and simple mastectomy procedures remove all the functional breast tissue. The removal of muscle and lymphatics, along with subsequent scarring, causes the physiological alterations the client experiences. With the modified radical and Halsted radical mastectomies, alterations caused by the removal of the breast and lymphatics—and the removal of all the muscles of the chest wall in the case of the Halsted procedure—may decrease movement of the affected arm in the immediate postoperative period. The client may find ambulation difficult if a large breast was removed, because there will be an imbalance in gait. This imbalance also may cause a stooping shoulder.

Complications of radical mastectomies include hemorrhage, which requires surgery to control, and nerve injury. Other complications are wound infection and necrosis of the scar, which along with obstructed flow can lead to lymphedema, in which the arm becomes swollen, painful, and edematous. The drainage of fluid from the operative site via a suction catheter aids wound healing. Complications are more common and movement of the affected arm more limited after a radical mastectomy because it is a more extensive procedure. Nerve injury, lymphedema, and limited movement of the arm on the operated side usually do not occur with partial mastectomy or quadrantectomy. Client implications from lumpectomy are the same as from breast biopsy.

Radiation therapy may be given if appropriate as described in Chapter 12. Radiation may be used following surgery if lymph nodes are positive for cancer. When a simple mastectomy is performed for advanced breast cancer, the wound may not heal as readily as it would if the cancer were not as advanced, and infection is more common.

Psychosocial/Lifestyle Implications

The woman faced with removal of a breast must confront the fear of death, her relationships with others, and her sexuality. Female sexuality is a key point in the recovery of the postmastectomy client. Some clients recover from the surgery and find their sexuality improved, whereas others never fully recover psychologically and sexually. Less extensive procedures such as quadrantectomy and partial mastectomy, although they do not involve removal of an entire breast, can still leave the breast markedly disfigured. Lumpectomy leaves only a visible incisional scar. Some clients find it difficult if not impossible to look at a disfigured breast or extensive scar. Clients may experience depression, anxiety, altered body image, and sexual dysfunction. Phantom breast sensations (feelings that the removed breast is still present) also may occur.

The client's emotional makeup, relationships, age, and other factors influence her recovery. A woman with previous depression, low self-esteem, and ineffective coping mechanisms will have more difficulty with full recovery than a woman with a sense of self-worth and strong coping skills. A woman with good relationships with her partner will often recover with less difficulty than one who lacks a support system or has a poor relationship with a partner. Because the younger client is more likely to have more of her self-worth invested in her body image she may have a more difficult postoperative adjustment. If the client sees cancer as a punishment for sexual pleasure, her postoperative adjustment also may become difficult.

The mastectomy client may need to wear a breast prosthesis. She also will need to protect the affected arm from injury and infection thereafter (see the section on postoperative care). Client implications of mastectomy are summarized in Table 65–14.

Nursing Implications

Preoperative Care

The nurse is in a position to offer both instruction and emotional support before the mastectomy. Contact with a caring professional will enable the client to express her concerns and fears and discuss anticipated body image and sexual changes. She may need to review her choice for treatment and discuss the alternatives (see also Chapter 64).

Preoperative teaching includes the need for deep

Table 65–14	**Mastectomy: Implications for the Client**
Physiological Implications	**Psychosocial/Lifestyle Implications**
Loss of functional breast tissue	Anxiety because of fear of death
Decreased movement of the affected extremity	Need to confront relationships and sexuality
Possible instability in gait and drooping shoulder after removal of a large breast	Maladaption to body image change manifested by inability to look at the scar, depression, anxiety, sexual dysfunction
Pain depends on extent of surgery	
Complications of hemorrhage, nerve damage, infection, necrosis of the scar, lymphedema	Phantom breast sensations possible
	Need for support system
	Breast prosthesis
Possible radiation therapy	Need to protect the affected arm from injury

breathing exercises because of a restrictive dressing that may decrease chest expansion. Emphasize the need to move the affected extremity after surgery to increase circulation, decrease edema, and reduce arm and shoulder stiffness and numbness. Explain that a suction apparatus will be placed in the wound, discuss its purpose, and inform the client that removal can be anticipated about 3 days after a modified radical mastectomy.

Postoperative Care

In the postoperative period, emotional support is an important aspect of nursing care of a mastectomy client. Physical care includes making the client comfortable and avoiding complications, providing exercise instruction, preventing infection and lymphedema, and teaching about breast prostheses.

Emotional Support. Emotional support by the nurse and other members of the health care team is of paramount importance in the postoperative period. The nurse can describe the incision to the client who cannot initially look at it, share the experience of looking at the incision with her, and let her express her fears concerning her body image changes. The services of an American Cancer Society Reach to Recovery volunteer, a woman who has had a mastectomy, also can assist the client in adjusting to her surgery and her new body image. In this program, knowledgeable and well-adjusted breast cancer clients visit new clients to demonstrate how they are coping with their illness and the effects of their surgery. Emotional support and an exercise program are offered by the ENCORE program of the YWCA. Clients participate in floor and swimming pool exercise sessions and group discussions. Both programs are in the resources list in Chapter 63. Other general resources for the cancer client are listed in Chapter 12.

The client should be consulted about her involvement in physical care and treatment to reduce her feelings of vulnerability. Help the client identify support systems and discuss her usual coping mechanisms.

Both the client and her partner can view the wound postoperatively if they wish. Affection can be encouraged by hand-holding and touch. Concerns about returning to sexual relations should be discussed before the client is discharged. Discussing potential sexual problems or the partner's response to the woman's loss of her breast may be difficult for the client. During hospitalization, she may be more concerned initially about physical care. Clients' feelings about their disease and its treatment are not easily resolved, and it may take months to years for them to work out their feelings. During this period, the woman may avoid sexual intimacy because she fears her partner's reaction to her changed body.

The partner may also experience a wide range of emotions, such as fear that sexual overtures will be rebuffed or that lovemaking that included the breast may have somehow caused the cancer. The partner may fear that facial expressions may betray his or her difficulty in coping with the client's changed appearance. Although some partners may be physically repelled by a missing or disfigured breast, most adjust quickly. A partner's facial expression of concern, sadness, or anxiety may stem from distress about what the surgical procedure represents—a threat to life. When the client interprets such facial expressions as rejection, her worst fears may be validated.

Describing the scar and showing illustrations of the mastectomy incision will help the partner and the client know what to expect when first seeing the operative area. It is helpful for clients to know that in a national survey, the National Cancer Institute (1981) found that 81% of the men surveyed reported that they would feel compassion for a partner and be supportive of her after a mastectomy. Box 65–1 has guidelines for initiating a discussion on sexuality with a client and her partner.

Physical Care. Pain is controlled by analgesics, depending on the severity of the surgical procedure and the client's pain tolerance. The client can also be made more comfortable with proper positioning. Check the dressing and the bedclothes beneath the client for bleeding. Also check the affected arm for warmth, color, edema, and feeling. Care of the suction catheter includes accurate measurement of output, the possible application of povidone-iodine (Betadine) ointment around the site, and daily sterile dressing changes. Tell the client that the suction catheter is usually removed in about 3 days and may cause only mild discomfort. Assist the client out of bed on the day following surgery if not before. After the effects of anesthesia have disappeared, diet can be as tolerated.

Box 65–1 Guidelines for Initiating a Discussion on Sexuality

Be comfortable with the topic of sexuality. The client and her partner should not be embarrassed or slighted because their needs surpass the nurse's limits. A nurse who feels uncomfortable in helping a couple with sexual concerns is responsible for consulting another health care professional who feels comfortable in this area.

Designate one nurse on a unit to discuss the feelings, beliefs, and attitudes pertaining to breast cancer, the surgery, and sexuality with a given client and her mate. In this way, the psychosexual aspects of the woman's care are included in the care plan, but the client and her partner will not be bombarded with a host of well-intentioned nurses.

Arrange for the discussion to take place in a relaxed and quiet area.

Include the client's partner in the discussion. Other family members may be included if the client desires or it is seen by the nurse to be of therapeutic value.

Initiate the discussion by starting with less threatening items, such as instructions on breast forms or range-of-motion exercises. Essentially, the more physical or external topics provide a basis for delving into the emotional aspects of the surgery.

Exhibit a caring, supportive, nonjudgmental attitude throughout the discussion. Any signs of disgust or horror will only lower the client's opinion of herself.

Be certain that the words used in discussion are not only familiar but also are interpreted similarly by all involved. This is not to say that either party has to use words that may seem unnatural. However, the nurse needs to become desensitized to words that the client population commonly uses when describing sexual relations and that the nurse finds offensive. It has been suggested that the nurse can get used to hearing such words by repeating them aloud while alone in a secluded place.

Keep in mind the client's cultural and religious beliefs as well as the effects of other medicines and/or illnesses upon her level of sexual functioning.

Do not force the client and her mate to divulge their concerns about sexuality. However, they need to know that a concerned individual is there to listen and guide them when they are ready.

Do not overwhelm or rush the couple during the discussion period. Instead, it is important that the nurse keep pace with the needs and interests of the couple.

Do not assume that all breast cancer clients have or want a sexual partner or that the sexual partner is male.

SOURCE: Adapted from *The Breast Cancer Digest* US Department of Health and Human Services: NIH Publication No. 84–1691. Bethesda, MD: National Cancer Institute, 1984, p. 149.

Exercise Instruction. The client should begin exercising the extremity immediately after surgery with encouragement to move the fingers. Range-of-motion (ROM) exercises are crucial to maintain joint mobility, maintain circulation, and reduce edema. Mobility is essential in resuming everyday activities, such as fastening a bra, pulling up a zipper, grooming, cooking, and engaging in sports. Assisted ROM exercises for the involved shoulder may be started as soon as the client returns to her room. Exercise is progressive and follows a routine format: sets of ten performed three times daily. Clients who have had a modified radical mastectomy should be encouraged to undertake self-care activities by the next day; these include washing the face and upper body, applying cosmetics, and combing or brushing their hair using the involved arm.

Some clients, especially those who have had a Halsted radical mastectomy, may be unable to lift the involved arm without assistance. Help the client lift her arm rather than taking over self-care activities for her. When the client is able to lift the involved arm without help, she is ready for a more complex exercise such as that illustrated in Figure 65–9.

Assistive devices will also help maintain joint flexibility and can be adapted for home use during the later recovery period. They include using a rope end pulley, "climbing

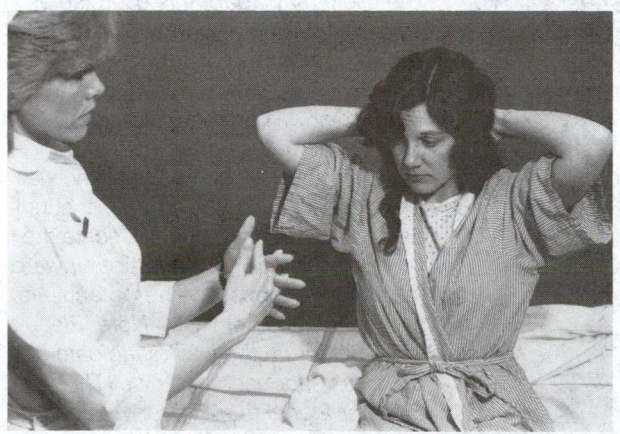

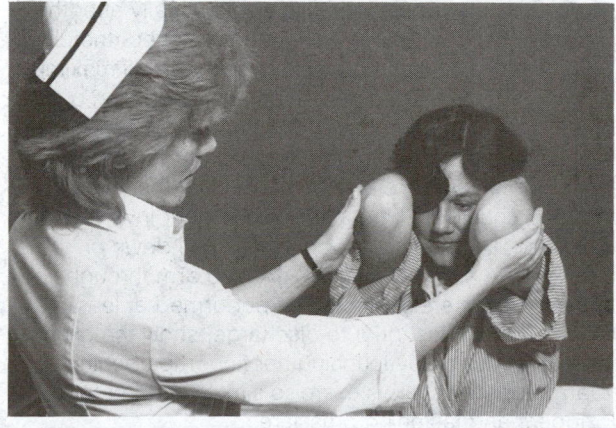

Figure 65–9

Exercise after mastectomy. **Top.** When the client is able to lift her involved arm actively without assistance, instruct her to clasp her hands behind her head (as shown). **Bottom.** She should then attempt to touch her elbows together, or to bring them as close together as possible. This movement will flex, externally rotate, and adduct the involved shoulder.

SOURCE: Swearingen PL: *Photo-Atlas of Nursing Procedures.* Menlo Park, CA: Addison–Wesley, 1984.

a wall," and pulling down on a rope held behind the back (Figure 65–10).

The client should perform more exercises as she can tolerate them. In planning exercises, consider the amount of discomfort the client experiences. Usually, the more muscles that are cut and the more tissue removed, the greater the discomfort. Clients are often apprehensive and worry that exercises may delay healing or disrupt the sutures. Explaining the purposes of the exercises, the resilience of the body, and the strength of the sutures, as well as assuring the client that she will not be required to perform exercises beyond her level of tolerance, will all help reduce the client's apprehension.

Prevention of Infection and Lymphedema. Removal of the axillary nodes and lymphatic channels predisposes the client to infection and lymphatic obstruction. To prevent these complications, it is important not to take the blood pressure and blood samples on the involved side. Medications should not be injected into the affected arm. Heavy objects, including purses, should not be carried on the affected side. Instruct the client to use a protective glove when doing chores, avoiding injuries and exposure to strong detergents and chemicals. Any breaks in the skin should be promptly treated. The client should apply lanolin-based hand cream daily or more often if necessary. Instruct the client to report pain, redness, increased swelling, or hardness to her health care provider.

A collateral lymphatic drainage system usually develops within 3 to 4 weeks postoperatively. In the interim, elevating the involved arm so the elbow is higher than the shoulder and the hand is higher than the elbow helps prevent or reduce edema. Massaging the arm from the hand toward the shoulder is another useful technique. Women who exercise, elevate, and massage the involved arm for at least 3 months after surgery are less likely to have severe lymphedema. Severe lymphedema that occurs many months, or sometimes even years, after surgery should always be promptly assessed for infection and related treatment if appropriate. The client may wear a supportive elastic sleeve similar to an antiembolic stocking to reduce lymphedema. This should be applied in the morning before the client sits or stands. Lymphedema is much less frequent after modified radical mastectomies than after Halsted radical mastectomies.

Breast Prostheses. Most women who have had a mastectomy are concerned about restoring their normal appearance as soon as possible. A temporary breast prosthesis is usually provided by a Reach-to-Recovery volunteer before the client is discharged from the hospital. This lightweight, soft prosthesis is used while the incisional area is healing and until tenderness and edema dissipate in about 6 weeks. By that time, most clients are ready to be fitted for a more natural-looking prosthesis.

Commercial breast forms are available in a wide variety of sizes and shapes and are sold in most large depart-

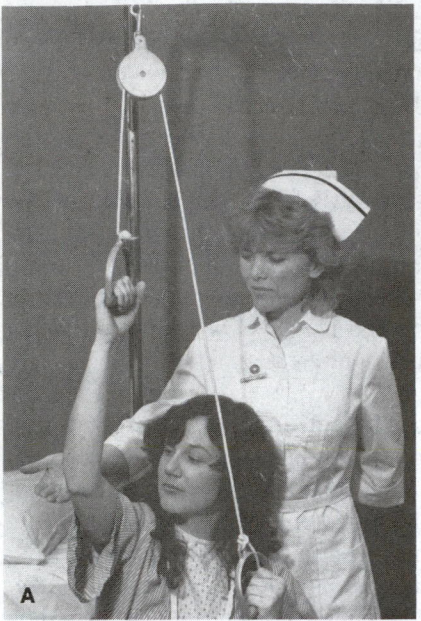

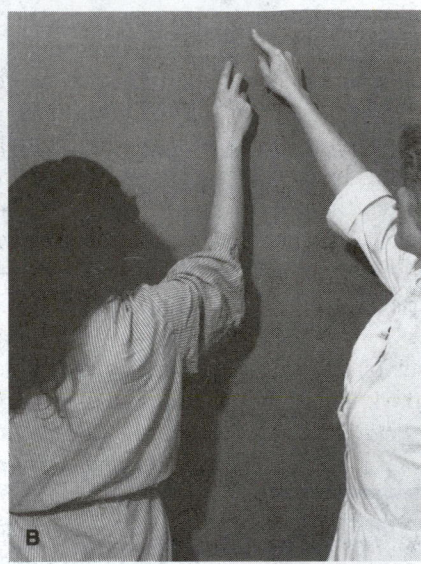

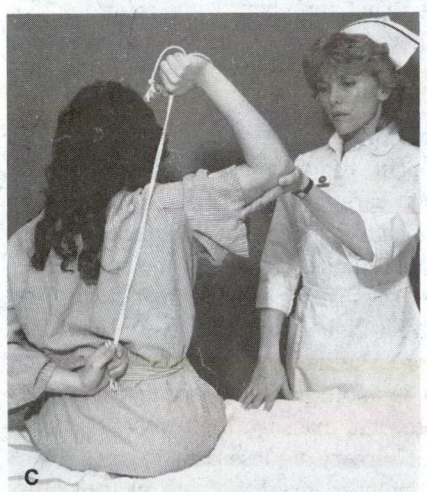

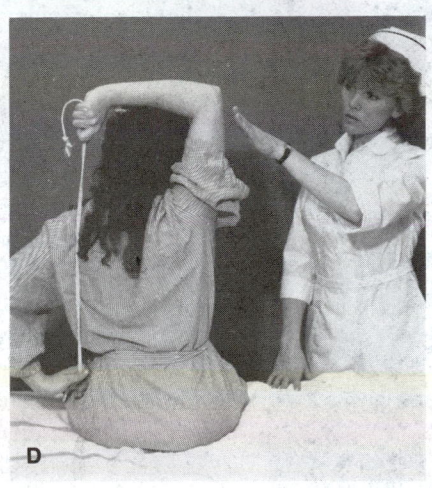

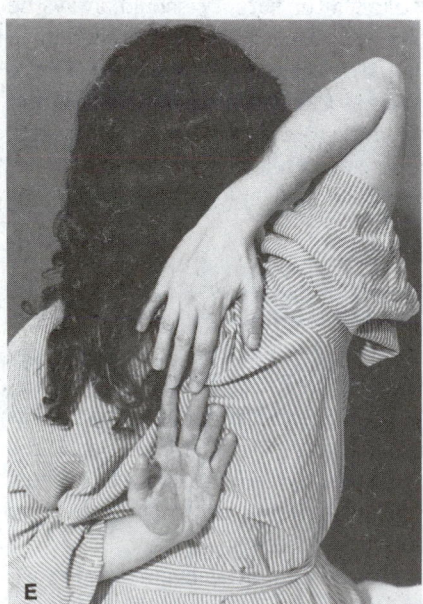

Figure 65–10

A. The client can also use assistive devices to achieve shoulder flexion. With physician approval, assemble a rope and pulley system onto an overhead trapeze bar. The client should grasp the hand grips and begin the exercise with the involved arm in the lower position. Instruct her to pull down gently with the hand of the uninvolved arm, allowing the involved arm to be raised gradually (as shown). Explain to the client that some discomfort and a sensation of stretching the incision is normal, but that to achieve maximum shoulder range, she should flex the shoulder as much as possible. *Note: The client may adapt this exercise at home by placing a rope over a stable shower curtain rod or over a wall hook.* **B.** Teach the client how to "climb a wall," which will promote shoulder flexion without the use of an assistive device. The client should face the wall and position her involved arm at shoulder level. Gradually, she will scale the wall by "walking" her fingertips upward (as shown). Encourage her to achieve maximum shoulder ROM. *Note: Place a tape marker on the wall to indicate her progress after each exercise. This will give her a goal to strive for with each new attempt.* **C.** Around the second postoperative week, usually after the sutures have been removed, the client can begin exercises that will maximize external rotation and abduction of the shoulder. A 75-cm (30-in) rope can be used to assist the client in achieving maximum range. Instruct her to grasp the rope, holding the lower end in her uninvolved hand in the back at the level of her waistline. The top of the rope should be held in the hand of her involved arm at about the level of her head. **D.** She should very gently pull down on the rope with the hand of her uninvolved arm, guiding the involved arm through abduction and external rotation. This exercise should be performed at least three times daily in sets of ten each. **E.** Just prior to discharge, show the client how to achieve maximum shoulder flexion by touching her fingertips behind her back with the involved arm uppermost. This exercise simulates the range required for zipping back zippers and fastening brassieres.

SOURCE: Swearingen PL: *Photo-Atlas of Nursing Procedures*. Menlo Park, CA: Addison–Wesley, 1984.

ment stores (where specially trained fitters help the client select an appropriate prosthesis), surgical supply stores, and some pharmacies, or by mail order. Like natural breasts, the weight and consistency of prostheses vary; they may be filled with foam rubber, chemical gel, water, ceramic particles, or silicone gel. Silicone prostheses are the heaviest and most expensive (from $100 to $200). Their advantage is that their weight provides better balance and reduces problems such as muscle strain caused by asymmetry. Some forms are available with a modified nipple; nipple prostheses can be purchased to augment prostheses without nipples or can be used by women who have had reconstructive surgery that did not replace the nipple. In some locations, it is possible to purchase a custom-designed prosthesis made from a mold of the breast before surgery; these cost about $400.

Reach-to-Recovery volunteers and fitters in department stores can often recommend bras that fit comfortably and can be adapted to suit each woman's individual needs. Specially designed clothing is also available in department stores and by mail order.

Insurance companies may fully or partially reimburse clients for prostheses and specially designed or altered bras. This information is usually supplied by Reach-to-Recovery volunteers or is available through the American Cancer Society. In many instances, clients will need a physician's prescription and receipts to take the medical deduction from federal income tax.

BREAST RECONSTRUCTION

Breast reconstruction is performed on clients who have had a mastectomy. It does not fully restore the normal appearance of the breast but creates a breast mound, which helps the woman look normal in clothes and eliminates dependence on a prosthesis. The chief indication for the procedure is the client's decision to have a breast reconstructed. There is no medical need to replace the lost breast; however, for many women, the psychological benefit of a restored self-image is sufficient justification for undergoing the procedure. Any woman who has had a breast removed may elect to have breast reconstruction. Reconstruction requires further consideration or might be contraindicated where the client needs extensive skin grafting or extensive irradiation or when the client has unrealistic expectations for the reconstructed breast.

Surgical Procedure

Breast reconstruction surgery is performed under general anesthesia either after the mastectomy has healed, which takes a minimum of 3 months, or at the same time as the mastectomy. Immediate reconstruction may have poorer cosmetic results because of the effects of radiation therapy or chemotherapy, and it increases the risk of complications such as fibrous capsular contracture (discussed later in this section).

The breast reconstruction procedure depends on the type of mastectomy and the type of deformity. When the muscle is not damaged, the reconstruction can be accomplished by the placement of a silicone gel implant beneath the pectoral and serratus muscles. Another type of simple breast reconstruction is accomplished by using an expander implant. This implant is placed submuscularly as is the silicone gel implant. The essential difference is that the expander implant has a built-in filler port that allows it to be injected with sterile normal saline. The injections are repeated several days to a week apart until the implant has expanded beyond the desired size. After the implant has been in place for several weeks or months, it is replaced with a permanent silicone gel implant of appropriate size. Overstretching the skin and muscle by overfilling the expander implant creates a more normal drape, with a more natural appearance, over the smaller implant. These procedures are used when muscle and skin are adequate. Figure 65–11 shows the good results that are possible with this procedure.

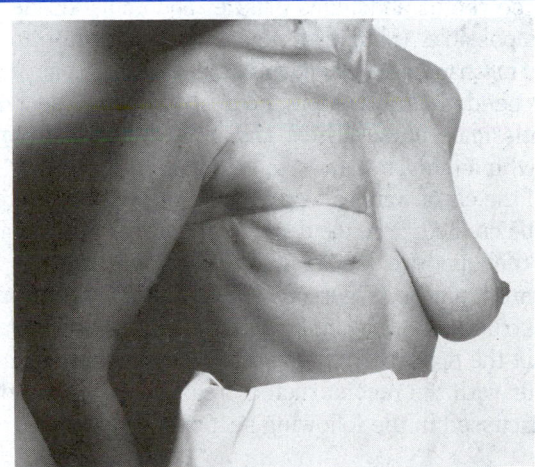
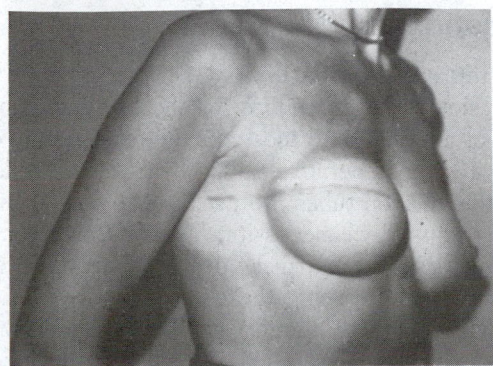

Figure 65–11

Pre- and postoperative views of a client who underwent breast reconstruction with an expander implant on the right. A later breast reduction on the left brought the breasts into better symmetry.

SOURCE: Woods JE: Current state of the art in breast reconstruction. *Plas Surg Nurs* 1984; 4:86.

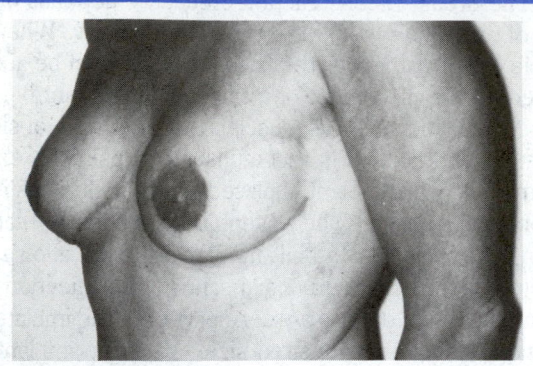

Figure 65–12
Reconstructed nipple and areola using perineal skin and sharing the nipple from the opposite breast.
SOURCE: Woods JE: Current state of the art in breast reconstruction. *Plas Surg Nurs* 1984; 4:86.

When soft tissue, muscle, and skin are inadequate for placement of an implant alone, reconstruction using grafts from the rectus abdominis muscle, abdominal tissue, and skin is possible. (Skin grafting and tissue transfer are discussed in Chapter 80.) If enough tissue is present, an implant is not needed. Another procedure combines a section of the latissimus dorsi muscle and overlying skin from the back with an implant.

If the client wants a nipple on the reconstructed breast, it can be created, once the desired contour has been attained, from the opposite nipple, inner thigh, buttock, or labia majora or minora (Figure 65–12). At the time of breast reconstruction, it may be necessary to decrease, enlarge, or uplift the opposite breast to achieve symmetry and match contour with the reconstructed breast. These procedures are discussed in the following section.

Implications for the Client

Physiological Implications

The physiological implications for the breast reconstruction client are similar to those for the mastectomy client. There will be postoperative pain. A hematoma may develop even when suction tubes are used in the wound. If hemorrhage occurs, it will necessitate a return to surgery. The restrictive dressing may make deep breathing and coughing difficult, predisposing the client to atelectasis. If an abdominal lipectomy ("tummy tuck") was also performed, bed rest may be necessary for several days; this increases the risk of thrombophlebitis and pulmonary embolism. Infection from the incision is another risk. A hypertrophic scar or keloid may develop. The most common problem is fibrous capsular contracture, the formation of a fibrous capsule around the implant; this contracts, makes the breast round and hard, and may displace it upward.

The implant does not increase the risk of cancer. It will not hinder the detection of cancer unless the cancer is underneath the implant. Most recurrences of cancer are in the skin or just beneath the pectoral muscle.

Psychosocial/Lifestyle Implications

The client's satisfaction from the surgery is high if preoperative expectations are reasonable. Improved self-concept and body image following the surgery may manifest themselves in increased self-confidence and a more positive attitude.

Activities of daily living can be resumed after discharge. However, the client should not wear a bra for the first 3 months, and should avoid heavy lifting, strenuous exercise, contact sports, sleeping on the abdomen, and any activity that puts pressure on the reconstructed breast for 6 weeks. To decrease the risk of fibrous capsular contraction, the client should perform breast massage as illustrated and described in Figure 65–13. This also keeps the implant mobile and stretches the surrounding tissue to help achieve a more natural appearance; this, in turn, positively affects the client's self-image.

Because reconstructive surgery is similar to mastectomy, the client again may encounter her fears of death from cancer. She may feel guilty about having elective surgery. Complications that arise may represent to the client a return of the cancer and increase her anxiety. Abnormal adjustment to breast reconstruction may include the feeling that it will "cure" the cancer and neglect of the breast because the care reminds the client that she has cancer.

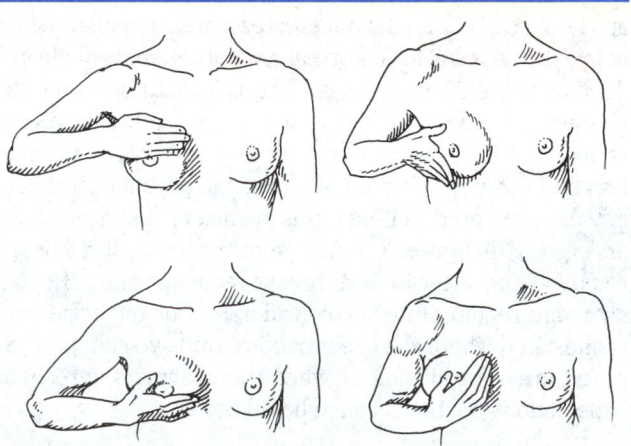

Figure 65–13
Postoperative breast massage technique to help the breast soften and become more natural in contour. Gently press the breast mound with the palm of the hand on each side for a count of five. Move from superior to lateral, to inferior, and to medial aspects, and repeat the sequence five times. Perform the exercise at least three times daily or more often as directed for 3 to 6 months postoperatively.

Table 65–15	Breast Reconstruction: Implications for the Client
Physiological Implications	**Psychosocial/Lifestyle Implications**
When on bed rest, increased risk for thrombophlebitis and pulmonary embolism Complications of hematoma, atelectasis, infection, hypertrophic scar or keloid, fibrous capsule around the implant, hemorrhage	Improved self-concept and body image No bra for first 3 months Restriction of activities that put pressure on the new breast for 6 weeks Need to perform breast massage Renewed fears about the diagnosis of cancer Monthly BSE

This is an especially important time for the client to continue monthly BSE. Client implications of breast reconstruction are summarized in Table 65–15. See Chapter 80 for client implications of skin grafting and free tissue transfer.

Nursing Implications

Preoperative Care
The nurse's function before surgery is to develop a rapport with the breast reconstruction client to provide support. Clients commonly experience fears about the diagnosis of cancer, along with guilt and anxiety. Review the client's expectations (eg, the client must understand that reconstruction is not a replacement for the lost breast but merely a breast mound). Preoperative teaching should include techniques of manual breast massage as well as information on what to expect postoperatively (wound suction, dressings, and the need for frequent deep breathing and turning).

Postoperative Care
Emotional support must be continued in the postoperative period. Physical care includes management of the dressing and incision and observation for complications. Pain can be controlled by analgesics. Review the manual massage procedure, and have the client gently demonstrate massage before discharge with the surgeon's approval. Teach and review BSE as well. If the reconstruction involved grafting, the client will have an extended period of bed rest.

BREAST AUGMENTATION AND REDUCTION MAMMOPLASTY

Breast augmentation mammoplasty is the surgical method of increasing the breast size. The client requests the surgery to improve her body image. The physician elects not to perform the augmentation if the client has unrealistic expectations of the surgery. Breast augmentation also may be used as a reconstructive procedure after mastectomy.

Breast reduction mammoplasty is performed when the breasts have hypertrophied, are very large, or are asymmetrical. Large breasts may cause back pain and shoulder discomfort from bra straps. Both breast augmentation and reduction give women important opportunities to make choices about their bodies.

Surgical Procedure

The breast augmentation procedure is similar to breast reconstruction following mastectomy. The surgeon makes an inframammary or periareolar incision, and places a silicone sac (usually filled with either silicone gel or saline solution) in a subpectoral or subcutaneous submuscular pocket. Figure 65–14 illustrates the results that can be achieved with breast augmentation.

The reduction procedure is more involved. Excess tissue and skin are removed, and the nipple is transplanted to its proper position on the reconstructed breast. Figure 65–15 illustrates hypertrophy of the breasts, and the postoperative result after reduction mammoplasty. General anesthesia is used for both procedures.

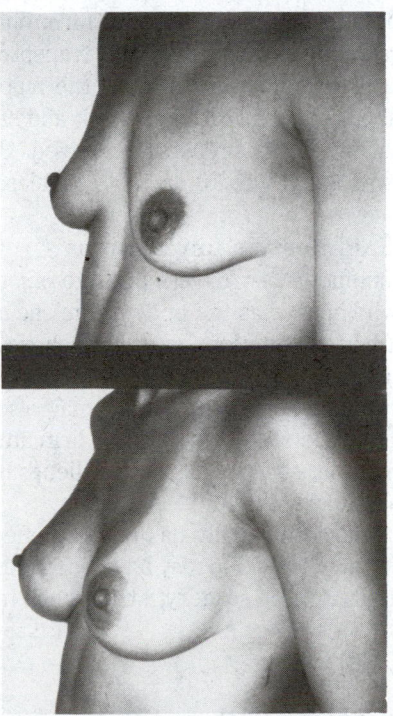

Figure 65–14

Breast augmentation. **Top.** Preoperative. **Bottom.** Postoperative (Courtesy of Dr. Muldowney).

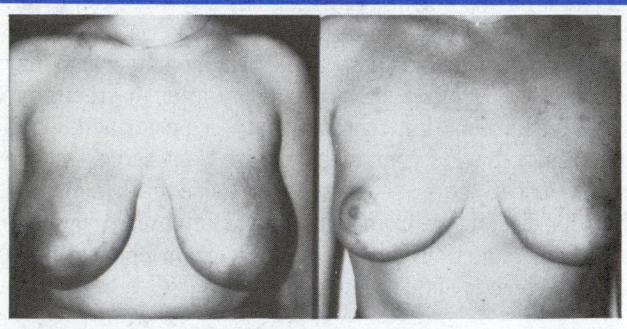

Figure 65–15
Breast reduction. **Left.** Preoperative. **Right.** Postoperative
(Courtesy of Dr. Muldowney).

Implications for the Client

Physiological Implications
Breast augmentation carries the risk of fibrous capsular contraction. Other complications, such as hematoma and infection, are rare. The Food and Drug Administration (FDA) has questioned the safety of the implants and is considering requiring manufacturers to carry out long-term studies proving that silicone does not seep into the body.

After reduction mammoplasty, biological function of the breast is lost and breast feeding is not possible. The complications of the procedure are the same as for breast reconstruction, including infection, hematoma, and hypertrophy of the scar. Complications are rare, however. The reestablishment of circulation to the transplanted nipple may cause a black scab to form over the nipple, but this falls off in about a week. Previous back and shoulder discomfort from the heavy breasts is relieved. Pain is common during the initial 7 to 10 days of convalescence.

Psychosocial/Lifestyle Implications
Breast augmentation may have a positive emotional effect on a client who finally has the body image she has wanted. However, if her expectations were unrealistic, such as to save a failing relationship or restore her sexuality, she may be disappointed in the results. She may also be disappointed if the breasts are too large or firm after augmentation. In any case, surgery alters the client's body image, necessitating an adjustment.

Breast reduction usually has positive effects. Before surgery, unwanted attention may have been focused on the client's bust size. After surgery, she may be more willing to socialize.

Table 65–16	Breast Augmentation and Reduction Mammoplasty: Implications for the Client
Physiological Implications	**Psychosocial/Lifestyle Implications**
Possible fibrous capsular contracture after breast augmentation	Positive body image change
Complications of hematoma, infection, hypertrophy of the scar	Satisfaction with procedure influenced by expectations
Possibility of silicone seepage into the body with breast augmentation	Improved social interaction
Relief of backache after breast reduction (no excess weight of large breasts)	Monthly BSE
Loss of breast function after breast reduction	Need to wear a support bra by day and an Ace bandage at night for about the first 2 weeks after breast augmentation
Pain for 7–10 days	

The breast reduction or augmentation client must continue monthly BSE. She will wear a support bra during the day and an Ace bandage at night for the first 2 postoperative weeks. Physiological and psychosocial implications for the client after breast reduction and augmentation are summarized in Table 65–16.

Nursing Implications

Preoperative Care
The nursing implications in the preoperative period are similar to those for breast reconstruction clients. The nurse should support the client's decision for breast size change and be available to discuss possible guilt and anxiety over the procedure.

Postoperative Care
Postoperative nursing implications also are similar to those for breast reconstruction clients. Manual massage should be performed to prevent fibrous capsular contracture. If fibrous capsular contracture occurs, it is treated by the plastic surgeon with manual rupture or surgery to release the fibrotic tissue. Discharge teaching involves wound care, signs of infection, and the techniques and importance of monthly BSE.

Chapter Highlights

Female reproductive surgeries include operative procedures of the breasts, uterus, cervix, ovaries, fallopian tubes, vagina, and vulva, as well as their supporting structures. Surgery can be done for diagnostic, therapeutic, cosmetic, or sterilization purposes.

Body image disturbances and feelings of loss and grief are potential problems for many gynecologic surgery clients.

An assessment of the client's knowledge of reproductive and sexual function is essential to the nursing process.

Infection, hemorrhage, and thromboembolic disease are the major complications of gynecologic surgery.

Many of these procedures can be done on an outpatient basis.

Major gynecologic surgeries are often preceded by laparoscopy, D and C, or both.

Surgical approaches to disorders affecting the female reproductive organs include cryosurgery, conization, hysterectomy, oophorectomy, salpingoplasty (tuboplasty), vulvectomy, pelvic exenteration, anterior colporrhaphy, and posterior colporrhaphy.

Tubal sterilization can be performed by laparoscopy, minilaparotomy, or via the vagina.

Surgical approaches to disorders of the breast include breast biopsy, mastectomy (breast removal), breast reconstruction, and breast augmentation and reduction mammoplasty.

The nurse's role in caring for clients with breast surgery involves providing support, information, and comprehensive care, depending on the type of surgery and the reason for it.

Breast biopsy, mastectomy, and breast reconstruction often involve the diagnosis of cancer, which necessitates additional nursing support and information. Monthly BSE becomes especially important for these clients.

Breast reconstruction, augmentation mammoplasty, and reduction mammoplasty are performed at the client's request to improve her body image. The procedures usually have positive effects.

Bibliography

Aitken DR, Minton JP: Complications associated with mastectomy. *Surg Clin North Am* 1983; 63(6):1331–1349.

Benson R: *Current Obstetric and Gynecologic Diagnosis and Treatment,* 5th ed. Los Altos, CA: Lange, 1984.

Dinner MI, Dowden RV: Breast reconstruction: State of the art. *Cancer* 1984; 53:809–814.

Fogel CI, Woods NF: *Health Care of Women: A Nursing Perspective.* St. Louis: Mosby, 1981.

Goldberg P, Stolzman M, Goldberg H: Psychological considerations in breast reconstruction. *Ann Plast Surg* 1984; 13:39–42.

Gomel V: *Microsurgery in Female Infertility.* Boston: Little, Brown, 1983.

Jones H, Rock J: *Reparative and Constructive Surgery of the Female Generative Tract.* Baltimore: Williams & Wilkins, 1983.

Lierman LM: Support for mastectomy. *AORN J* 1984; 39:1150–1157.

Masterson BJ: *Manual of Gynecologic Surgery.* New York: Springer–Verlag, 1979.

Pfeiffer CH, Mulliken JB: *Caring for the Patient With Breast Cancer: An Interdisciplinary/Multidisciplinary Approach.* Reston, VA: Reston, 1984.

Reynolds M: *Gynaecological Nursing.* Boston: Blackwell, 1984.

Ridley JH: *Gynecologic Surgery. Errors, Safeguard, Salvage,* 2nd ed. Baltimore: Williams & Wilkins, 1981.

Rutledge DN: Nurses' knowledge of breast reconstruction: A catalyst for earlier treatment of breast cancer? *Cancer Nurs* 1982; 5:469–473.

Schwartz GF: Benign neoplasms and "inflammations" of the breast. *Clin Obstet Gynecol* 1982; 25:373–385.

Sheahan SL: Management of breast lumps. *Nurse Pract* 1984; 9:19–22.

Weatherley–White RC: *Plastic Surgery of the Breast.* New York: Harper & Row, 1980.

Woods JE: Current state of the art in breast reconstruction. *Plast Surg Nurs* 1984; 4:85–88.

Suggested Readings

Northouse LL: Coping with the mastectomy crisis. *Top Clin Nurs* 1982; 4(2):57–65. This is a comprehensive review of the use of the nursing process in the care of a mastectomy client.

Paritzky JF, Overby BA: Preoperative teaching on a gynecologic unit. *JOGN Nurs* 1982; 11(6):384–386. A discussion of preoperative preparation for any client about to undergo gynecologic surgery, with a focus on the nurse's teaching role.

Stanfill PH: The psychosocial implications of hysterectomy. *JOGN Nurs* 1982; 11(5):318–322. This article discusses the fears and anxieties of women having hysterectomy and the body image adaptations necessitated by different types of hysterectomies.

Weisenthal M: Reach-to-Recovery Program of the American Cancer Society. *Cancer* 1984; 53:825–827. The components of American Cancer Society's Reach-to-Recovery Program are discussed. Provides the nurse with a quick guide to the wide variety of services this program offers.

Chapter 66

The Nursing Process for Clients With Male Reproductive System Dysfunction

Phyllis Foster Healy

Objectives

When you have finished studying this chapter, you should be able to:

Gather appropriate subjective data concerning male sexual function.

Identify the components of a physical examination of the male reproductive system.

Interpret the significance of selected laboratory and diagnostic tests that relate to reproductive function.

Anticipate common problems affecting the male reproductive system.

Develop interventions to help the male client resolve reproductive tract problems.

Nurses caring for the male client who is experiencing a disorder of the reproductive system undoubtedly find their physiological as well as psychosocial nursing skills challenged. Intruding on what is usually an extremely personal and private area of a client's life makes the need for trust and confidentiality, important in any nurse–client interaction, central to the care plan.

Section I: Nursing Assessment: Establishing the Data Base

Female nurses, especially those who are inexperienced, often feel uncomfortable in assessing the reproductive systems of male clients. Parts of the health history and physical examination of the male reproductive system may be better conducted by a male nurse, an experienced female nurse, a nurse practitioner, or a male physician. The nurse can, however, form the necessary nonjudgmental attitude through careful guidance and introspection about personal values and sexuality.

SUBJECTIVE DATA

A thorough history of the male client's past and present psychosocial and physical health related to sexual function is a critical part of the nursing data base. In gathering this history, consider the following and then proceed. Is the data asked for appropriate? What is the client's comfort level? What is the comfort level of the history taker? Is the interviewer truly nonjudgmental and genuinely accepting? Has the nurse overcome personal taboos related to the discussion of sexuality? Can the nurse demonstrate an acceptance of alternative sexual practices? Is there sincerity?

The health history should include questions about sexuality and reproduction. Because the male urinary tract and reproductive system share common pathways, questions related to urinary history should also be included (see Chapter 32). Before beginning the history, clarify terms with the client to avoid misunderstandings over the meanings of words.

The male sexual and reproductive history should include the following questions:

- What is the client's sexual preference?
- Does he have a significant relationship or available partner?
- Does this client have one or a number of partners? Are these partners heterosexual, homosexual, or both?
- What is the client's level of knowledge related to reproductive and sexual function?
- What religious and cultural values are significant to this client?
- What is the client's role and gender identity?
- Is the client married?
- Is the client experiencing impotence or infertility?
- Does the client use recreational or therapeutic drugs known to affect sexual and reproductive function?
- Has the client had any known exposure to sexually transmitted diseases (STDs)?
- What is the client's overall health status? Pay particular attention to any condition that might affect sexual function, such as diabetes, endocrine disorders, renal failure, cardiac problems, neurological problems, or psychological problems.
- Is the client aware of any lumps or lesions in the genital area?
- Has the client experienced any trauma to the genital region?

The pertinent urinary history includes questions about urethral discharge, burning on urination, frequency, difficulty starting and stopping the urinary stream, a decrease in the urinary stream, the presence of nocturia, the presence of blood in the urine, and any problem with urinary incontinence.

Questions concerning health practices should cover the following areas. Does the client or partner use one or more birth control methods? Does the client practice testicular self-examination (TSE)? Does the client wear tight synthetic underwear or an athletic supporter? These can increase the temperature of the testes, contribute to decreased sperm production, and also can create a warm, moist environment where fungi thrive (Siemans & Brandzel, 1982).

OBJECTIVE DATA

The data gathered in the history are augmented and clarified through both the physical examination and diagnostic studies.

Physical Assessment

The physical assessment of the male reproductive system includes inspection and palpation. In the inspection, note the general shape and condition of the genitals, including skin condition and any discharge. Palpation detects inflammation, tenderness, and alterations in shape and contour.

The physical examination is a critically important aspect of the nursing assessment, since it provides data related to the development of secondary sexual characteristics, and can reveal the presence of infections, cancer, or asymmetry that may indicate a neoplasm or other disorder.

Inspection

For inspection of the male genitalia, the client should stand facing the examiner. General observation includes assessment for the presence of secondary sex characteristics (pubic hair and appropriate testicular and penile development), which should be present in the normally developed adult man. The testes are generally symmetrical, although the left testis is slightly lower than the right.

Further inspection includes observing the condition of the integument, noting whether the skin is intact and whether there are any lesions or ulcers. Common lesions on the penis include the chancre and condylomata acuminata, or venereal warts. Chancres, usually caused by syphilis, are painless, reddened, rounded, eroded ulcers with induration at their bases. Venereal warts have a cauliflower, wartlike, pedunculated, reddened, moist appearance. Carcinoma of the penis is rare in North America but is a significant worldwide health problem. It most often occurs in uncircumcised men as a nodule or ulcer on the glans penis or the inner aspect of the prepuce. Because the prepuce may cover this type of lesion, the client should retract the prepuce, if possible, for inspection (Figure 66–1A). These lesions are usually painless. As with any other potential

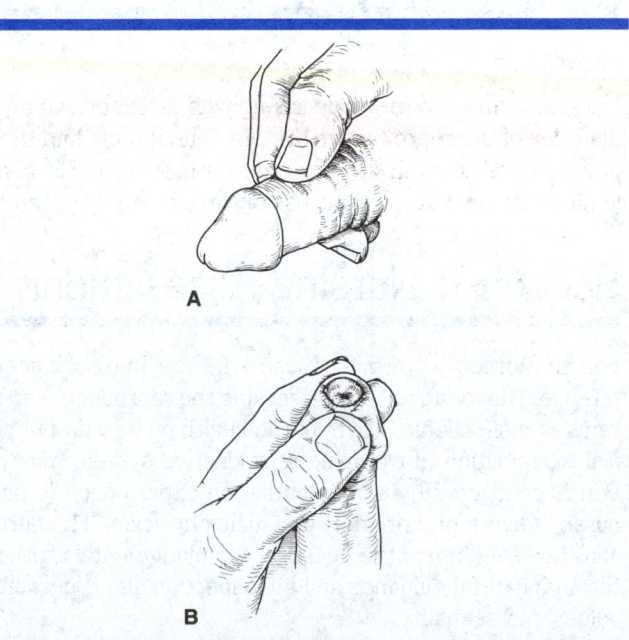

A

B

Figure 66–1

Inspecting the glans, meatus, and distal urethra. **A.** Retraction of prepuce and examination of glans, subpreputial area, and meatus. **B.** Separation and inspection of the meatus.

cancer, any sore that does not heal must be investigated further.

When the prepuce is retracted, inspect the glans for leukoplakia (white patches that could be precancerous) and smegma (a cheeselike secretion of sebaceous glands that builds up if hygiene is poor). Determine if the prepuce is retractable and easily returned. In phimosis the prepuce cannot be retracted; in paraphimosis, the retracted prepuce cannot be returned.

To inspect the distal end of the urethra, ask the client to squeeze the penis between his fingers near the head (Figure 66–1B). If discharge is present, obtain a smear and gonococcal culture. Note the location of the urethral opening, which should be central. An opening on the inferior surface is known as hypospadias. Some degree of hypospadias is common, but more pronounced conditions are usually corrected in childhood. Epispadias, a urethral opening on the anterior part of the penis, is less common. In this abnormality's mildest form, the urethral opening is found on the front of the glans. Epispadias is more severe if it is found further along the dorsum of the penis. In its most serious form, the condition is associated with exstrophy of the bladder. Surgery is necessary to correct epispadias.

Next, inspect the scrotum. For good visualization, ask the client to hold the penis up and to the side so it is out of the way. Remember to inspect both the anterior and posterior surfaces of the scrotum, noting its contour and symmetry; the left testis will be slightly lower. Check for lesions, nodules, or edema. Scrotal size changes, depending on muscle tone. The dartos muscle contracts when cold and relaxes when warm. Also, because muscle tone decreases with age, the scrotum may become more pendulous.

The groin is closely observed for swellings or bulges that could indicate an inguinal hernia. Make this observation with the client at rest and as he bears down.

Palpation

Wear gloves during palpation only if lesions or an infection is present. Palpate the penis for any signs of inflammation, tenderness, and changes in size and contour. Hard, painless plaques under the skin on the dorsal surface of the penile shaft indicate Peyronie's disease and may be accompanied by complaints of dyspareunia and crooked erections.

The testes are most easily palpated if the skin is warm and relaxed. Gently roll the testes between the thumb and fingers (Figure 66–2). Normally, they are smooth, mobile, bilaterally consistent in size, and somewhat sensitive to pressure. In the majority of men, the epididymis can be palpated behind and lateral to the testis. The spermatic cord and vas deferens are identified by following them from the epididymis up to the inguinal ring and bilaterally palpating each between the thumb and forefinger. Report nodules, inflammation, tenderness, or swelling of the epididymis, spermatic cords, and vas deferens.

If any swelling or irregularities are noted in the scrotum, the scrotum is transilluminated. The room is darkened and a flashlight placed behind the scrotum. Normally, a red glow is present as the light shines through serous fluid (tissues and blood will not transilluminate). Any hard, irregular masses that do not transilluminate should be reported. Since cancer of the testes is a serious health problem in men from ages 15 to 40, any irregularities should be considered suggestive of problems and be referred.

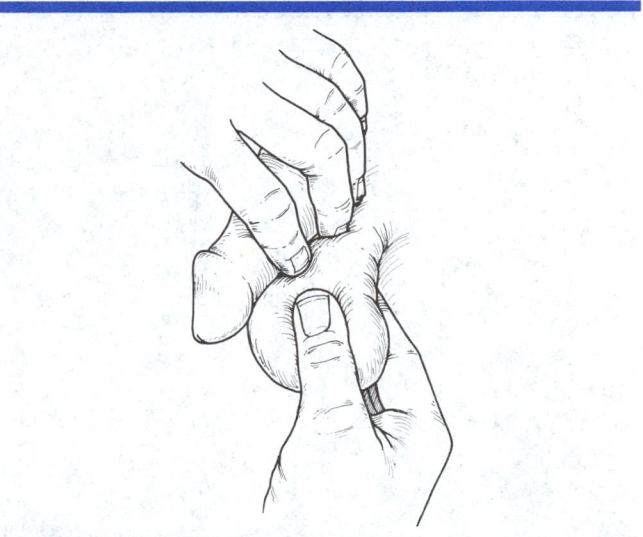

Figure 66–2

Palpating the testis and epididymis.

Early detection and treatment are critical for the client with testicular cancer. All adolescent males should be taught TSE and perform it monthly. (TSE is described and illustrated in Chapter 7.) In a study of male college students, Haggerty (1984) reported that only 8% practiced TSE and only 42% had ever heard of it. Judging from these results, nurses have an important educational function to perform. Tell clients to examine themselves after a warm shower, when scrotal muscles are relaxed. They should hold their scrotums in their hands and palpate for hardenings or lumps by gently rolling the testes between the thumb and forefingers. Any lumps, hardenings, or lack of symmetry should be promptly reported.

Thorough assessment of the male reproductive system also includes palpation of the prostate. Techniques for this examination vary according to the client's health status. The ambulatory client is best examined while standing. He should bend at the waist, turn his toes in, and rest his upper body across an examining table. In this way, the gluteal muscles relax, the buttocks flatten, and the rectum and anus become more accessible (Figure 66–3). A client unable to tolerate this position is placed on his left side, his right knee flexed and his buttocks close to the edge of the table.

The examiner uses a gloved, lubricated index finger to palpate the posterior prostate, which protrudes about 1 cm into the anterior rectal wall. The lateral lobes and median sulcus can be identified. The size, shape, consistency, and

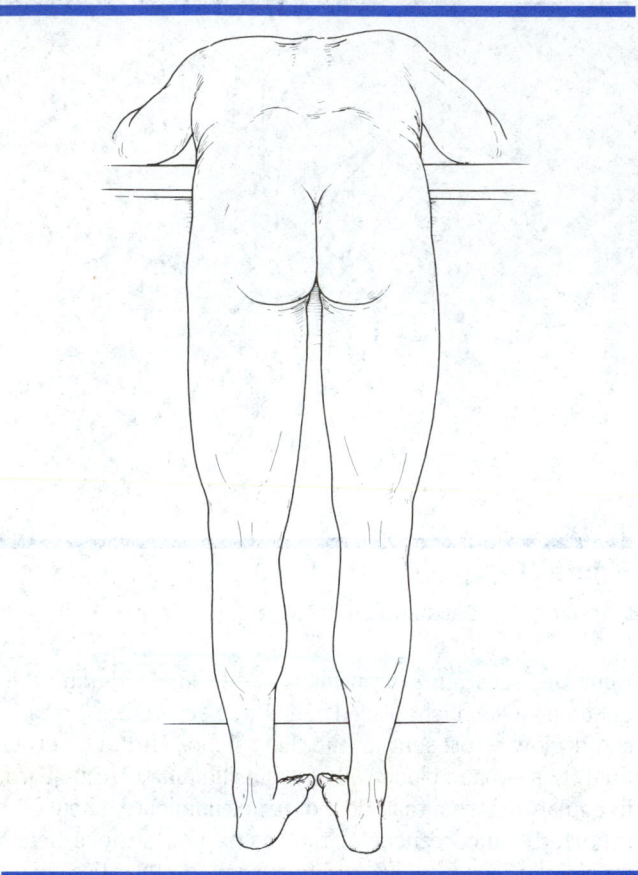

Figure 66-3

Client position for examination of prostate.

symmetry should be noted. In a client with benign prostatic hyperplasia, the prostate may be soft, smooth, and symmetrically enlarged, protruding more than 1 cm into the rectal wall. The enlargement may obliterate the median **sulcus** (a midline groove that separates the two lobes). Tenderness, edema, and bogginess may indicate prostatitis. If this condition is suspected, the prostate can be massaged to force discharge into the urethra for culture. Any irregular, hard, fixed nodules might indicate cancer of the prostate. Because cancer of the prostate frequently begins in the posterior lobe and is easily palpable on rectal examinations, this procedure is recommended annually for all males over age 40.

During palpation, the examiner also should feel for the presence of an inguinal hernia. To palpate for an indirect hernia, have the client slightly bend his knee on the same side. The examiner's little or index finger then follows the inguinal canal inward as far as it goes. At that point, the client is asked to bear down. A bulging mass indicates a hernia. This same examination is then done on the opposite side. The examiner should use the left hand on the left side and the right hand on the right side. A direct hernia is palpated by asking the client to bear down while two fingers are placed bilaterally over the inguinal rings. A bulge indicates a direct inguinal hernia. Palpating for a hernia is illustrated in Chapter 7.

Diagnostic Studies

A variety of diagnostic studies assists in the assessment and diagnosis of problems with the male reproductive system. These are discussed in this section and the laboratory tests are summarized in Table 66–1.

Serologic Tests

Serologic tests for the male reproductive system are described in Chapter 63. They include the Venereal Disease Research Laboratory (VDRL) test, fluorescent treponemal antibody absorption (FTA–ABS) test, and *treponema pallidum* immobilization (TPI) test.

Serum Acid Phosphatase Test

Serum acid phosphatase levels are studied to detect prostatic cancer. Acid phosphatase is an enzyme found in many body tissues, including the kidney, red blood cells, platelets, liver, spleen, and bone. The major concentration is in the prostate, where it is 100 times more concentrated than in other tissues.

The normal values for serum acid phosphatase are 0 to 1.1 Bodansky units/mL, 1 to 4 King–Armstrong units/mL, and 0.13 to 0.63 Bessey–Lowry units/mL, depending on the method of measurement. An increase in acid phosphatase levels indicates the metastasis or extension of a tumor, and a decrease in acid phosphatase levels indicates a response to treatment. Prostatic massage will cause a false elevation of acid phosphatase levels; to avoid this, the test should be performed before a rectal examination or at least 24 hours afterward. A false increase also can occur if the client has received clofibrate (Atromid-S), which decreases low-density lipoproteins and may be taken by the man who needs more than dietary control to lower his serum cholesterol and triglyceride levels. The ingestion of fluorides, oxalates, or phosphates may cause a false decrease. After the specimen is drawn, it must be sent to the laboratory immediately.

Serum Human Chorionic Gonadotropin Test

The presence of human chorionic gonadotropin (HCG) in the serum may indicate testicular choriocarcinomas or other testicular tumors. Radioimmunoassay to measure HCG levels is invaluable for the early detection of testicular tumors. In one study, HCG was increased in 7.7% of clients with seminoma, 60% of clients with embryonal testicular cancer, and 100% of clients with choriocarcinoma (Javadpour, 1980). With effective treatment, the HCG levels decrease to normal.

Alpha-Fetoprotein Test

Another testicular tumor marker is alpha-fetoprotein (AFP), which is also measured by radioimmunoassay. AFP is produced in the liver, yolk sac, and gastrointestinal tract of the fetus and is the major circulating protein. The normal level for males and nonpregnant females, less than 25 ng/mL, increases in 70% of clients with embryonal testicular

Table 66–1 Diagnostic Tests Common to the Male Reproductive System

Laboratory Test	Normal Expected Value	Disease State	Expected Abnormal Findings
Serum acid phosphatase	0–1.1 Bodansky units/mL; 1–4 King–Armstrong units/mL; 0.13–0.63 Bessey–Lowry units/mL	Prostatic cancer	Elevated
Human chorionic gonadotropin (HCG) (radioimmunoassay)	3 m/μ/mL	Testicular cancer, especially that caused by choriocarcinoma	Elevated
Alpha-fetoprotein (AFP) (radioimmunoassay)	< 25 ng/mL	Embryonal testicular cancer	Elevated
Testosterone analysis	Male: 406–954 ng/dL	Hypogonadism	Decreased
24-h urine test for 17-ketosteroids	8–25 mg/25 h	Testicular cancer Hypogonadism	Elevated Decreased
Semen analysis	Motility: 60%–70% moving forward Appearance: 70% normal in shape and motility Density: more than 20 million/mL Volume: 2–6 mL	Infertility	Decreased; with sperm count below 20 million, endocrine testing and testicular biopsy are performed

cancer. AFP levels should decrease with effective treatment. AFP is measured before and after orchiectomy (removal of the testis). Elevated AFP levels after orchiectomy suggest metastasis.

Testosterone Analysis
In a client with fertility problems, serum or plasma testosterone levels are determined. Abnormally low levels may be found in infertility. In males, the normal level is 406 to 954 ng/dL.

Complete Blood Count
To gather baseline data on health status, a complete blood count is conducted for the male experiencing a problem with the reproductive system. Anemia could contribute to problems with potency or fertility. Leukocytosis could indicate an infectious process.

Blood Chemistry Analysis
Blood chemistry analysis is used to screen for general physical problems. Clients with renal problems often have problems with sexual performance, so serum creatinine levels are determined to check for renal function. Glucose tolerance and thyroid function may be tested if endocrine dysfunction is suspected to be a contributing cause of infertility.

Urinalysis
Urinalysis is a screen for any abnormalities. Urine cultures check for urinary tract infections; a colony count greater than 100,000 indicates infection. A 24-hour urine test for

17-ketosteroids (a metabolite of androgen) may be performed (refer to Chapter 41). Testicular cancer causes an increase in 17-ketosteroids, whereas in hypogonadism, 17-ketosteroids levels are decreased. Normal levels are 8 to 25 mg/24 h.

Semen Analysis
Semen analysis, a part of fertility testing, identifies abnormalities in one of the following areas:

- *Sperm motility*. Normally, at least 60% to 70% of sperm are moving forward.
- *Morphology and quality of sperm*. More than 70% should be motile and normal in appearance.
- *Volume/density*. There should be at least 20 million sperm per mL of ejaculate. Ejaculatory volume should be between 2 and 6 mL.

Before the semen analysis, the client should be sexually abstinent for at least 48 hours. Abstinence should not be longer than 5 days, however, because the quality and motility of the sperm will decrease. Heat and cold will destroy the sperm, and the specimen must be delivered to the laboratory within 2 hours; thus, the client should masturbate in the physician's office while wearing a condom to collect the specimen. Some male clients are uncomfortable with the request to masturbate to obtain semen because of religious beliefs or personal reasons (Orthodox Judaism and Roman Catholicism have sanctions against masturbation). These clients can be instructed to collect semen in a condom during sexual intercourse and to take the specimen to the laboratory immediately. Even this method may be unsatisfactory for persons who believe that the sole purpose of ejaculation is reproduction. The semen analysis is performed at least twice. If the sperm count is less than 20 million/mL, endocrine testing and testicular biopsy are indicated (Pagana & Pagana, 1982).

Gonococcal Culture

If gonorrhea is suspected, a urethral gonococcal culture is usually obtained. (See Chapter 11 for discussion and illustration of urethral culture.) Both a culture and Gram's stain can be performed, but a culture is particularly important because of gonococcal resistance to antibiotics (Harrison, 1984).

Lymphagiography

Clients with testicular, prostatic, or penile cancer may have lymphangiography performed. See Chapter 28 for a discussion of this procedure.

Biopsy of the Prostate or Testis

To detect cancer, a prostatic biopsy may be performed. First, a cystoscopy is performed, and the area of the biopsy is identified by rectal examination. A needle is then inserted into the perineal skin, and prostatic tissue is aspirated. Usually, a biopsy is performed on more than one area. A small dressing is placed on the site of needle insertion using aseptic technique (Lerner & Khan, 1982).

A testicular biopsy may be performed to check for a testicular abnormality if no sperm are obtained on semen analysis. This biopsy is done bilaterally; an incision is first made into the scrotal skin, and separate incisions are then made into each testis. Testicular biopsy specimens should not be placed in a preservative because it will alter cellular structure and kill live sperm making the results inaccurate. Afterward a dressing is applied, and a scrotal support is used to prevent scrotal edema. The client may feel mild pain (Lerner & Khan, 1982).

Other Diagnostic Studies

A variety of other tests can be used to evaluate the condition of the male urinary tract in the diagnosis of reproductive abnormalities. Kidney, ureter, bladder (KUB) films can be taken to determine the presence of structural abnormalities or radiopaque calculi. An intravenous pyelogram (IVP) with postvoiding films may be ordered to check for obstruction and for a filling defect in the bladder that indicates marked benign prostatic hypertrophy. A cystoscopy may be performed to visualize the prostate as well as the bladder. A computerized tomography (CT) scan may be used to evaluate testicular and prostatic cancer by measuring tissue density. Further details on these procedures are provided in Chapter 31.

Section II: Nursing Diagnosis

The primary nursing diagnoses for disorders of the male reproductive system are sexual dysfunction and alteration in the urinary elimination pattern. These and other related nursing diagnoses are in Box 66–1.

SEXUAL DYSFUNCTION

The many possible causes of sexual dysfunction are premature ejaculation, impotence, infertility, STDs, knowledge deficit, fear, anxiety, grief, altered body image, altered self-concept, role change, or a number of altered physiological states. To determine when a diagnosis of sexual dysfunction is appropriate, look for some of the following characteristics:

- Expression of sexual problems or lack of sexual satisfaction
- Physical alterations that indicate a potential or actual dysfunction
- Significant role changes
- Feelings of shame or guilt
- A violation of cultural or religious sexual taboos
- A loss of privacy
- A loss of power or control
- Ingestion of recreational or therapeutic drugs that affect sexual function

---

Box 66–1 Nursing Diagnoses Commonly Related to Dysfunction of the Male Reproductive System

Diagnoses Directly Related to Male Reproductive System Dysfunction

Sexual dysfunction, related to premature ejaculation, impotence, infection, altered cardiovascular function, or infertility

Urinary elimination, alteration in pattern of, related to incontinence, urinary tract obstruction, or retention

Fluid volume deficit, actual or potential

Knowledge deficit

Self-concepts, disturbance in, body image, self-esteem, or role performance

Additional Potential Nursing Diagnoses

Anxiety

Coping, ineffective individual and family

Skin integrity, impairment of

ALTERATION IN URINARY ELIMINATION PATTERN

Causes of an alteration in the pattern of urinary elimination include incontinence after prostatectomy, dysuria and urethral discharge secondary to infection, urinary tract obstruction and retention as a result of benign prostatic hyperplasia, or catheter insertion because of urinary retention or as a postoperative procedure. To determine when the diagnosis of alteration in patterns of urinary elimination is appropriate, look for defining characteristics such as nocturia, hesitancy, incontinence, urinary retention, and the presence of an in-dwelling catheter.

Section III: Planning and Implementation

As with any client having a health problem, planning and goal setting for the male client with reproductive system dysfunction must include a mutual identification of goals and client involvement in all aspects of planning. This is especially important when dealing with the personal, private concerns of the male reproductive system. Frequently, it may be necessary, with the client's consent, to include the sexual partner in the plan of care. The precise plan depends on the client's problem and particular needs for resolution, so a thorough assessment to determine the exact nature of the problem is necessary. A sample nursing care plan appears in Table 66–2.

Table 66–2 Sample Nursing Care Plan for a Client With Dysfunction of the Male Reproductive System

Nursing Diagnoses	Client Care Goals	Plan/Nursing Implementation	Expected Outcome
Sexual dysfunction, related to premature ejaculation and impotence	Client and partner satisfaction with sexual function; improved ability to perform sexually; development of alternate means to achieve satisfaction	Assess client for possible cause; provide client opportunity to ventilate feelings and frustrations; provide information on possible causative factors of secondary impotence; help client modify lifestyle to decrease contributory factors; refer client for diagnostic work-up of possible physiological causes; refer client for sex counseling or therapy; instruct client in use of techniques to improve sexual communication, satisfaction, and function (general body touching, genital touching, position change with woman on top, more frequent ejaculations, smaller orgasms, stop-start and squeeze techniques, oral genital stimulation); refer for penile implant if desired and appropriate	Client has increased perception of sexual satisfaction; improved ability to function sexually; satisfactory use of alternative means to achieve satisfaction; improved self-esteem; improved communication with partner; decrease in anxiety and other stressors
Sexual dysfunction, related to infection	Awareness of cause of treatment of infection; ability to identify and inform contacts if infection is from an STD; compliance with medical regimen; demonstration of good sexual hygiene	Identify infection's cause; identify and inform contacts; administer antibiotics as prescribed; teach client how to prevent future infections and about appropriate use of medications; teach client appropriate sexual hygiene	Client is free of infection, refrains from sexual contact with infected partners, demonstrates appropriate hygiene practices; partners are treated for infection
Sexual dysfunction, related to altered cardiovascular function	Decrease in cardiac work load during sexual activity; freedom from discomfort during sexual activity	Instruct client about less exerting positions (woman on top or side-lying position); about prophylactic use of pain-relieving medication (eg, nitroglycerin to relieve angina or analgesics for joint pain); about alternative means of sexual satisfaction	Client verbalizes a perception of sexual satisfaction; is free of excessive fatigue and discomfort

(continued)

Table 66–2 Sample Nursing Care Plan for a Client With Dysfunction of the Male Reproductive System (continued)

Nursing Diagnoses	Client Care Goals	Plan/Nursing Implementation	Expected Outcome
Sexual dysfunction, related to infertility	Identification of correctable contributing factors; ventilation of feelings of inadequacy and frustration; open discussion of problem by client and partner; exploration of acceptable alternatives; relief from problem where possible	Provide opportunity for client to ventilate feelings; encourage open communication with partner; assist with diagnostic work-up; identify possible correctable contributing factors; refer client for counseling or medical-surgical correction as needed; explore acceptable alternatives with couple	Client demonstrates adaptive coping with problem; accepts childless lifestyle or finds a suitable alternative, such as adoption; identifies cause of infertility and corrects it where possible
Alteration in pattern of urinary elimination, related to urinary tract obstruction and retention	Freedom from urinary retention, obstruction, and urinary tract infection	Have client stand to void and use other measures to induce voiding; maintain patency of urinary catheter; force fluids to 3000 mL/24 h; maintain closed system; practice strict asepsis; provide catheter care at least every 24 h or more often as needed	Bladder is undistended; urinary output is at least 1200 mL/24 h; catheter is patent; urine is clear and free of infection
Alteration in pattern of urinary elimination, related to incontinence	Urinary continence; freedom from problems of incontinence (wetness, odor, skin breakdown)	Teach exercises to strengthen pelvic floor; limit caffeine, alcohol, and diuretics, if possible; develop fluid intake and voiding schedule; use protective pads; change incontinent client's clothes and linen immediately; use external drainage device; bathe perineal area; use protective ointments	Client is continent, clean, and dry; client and immediate environment are odor-free

ACHIEVING SATISFACTORY SEXUAL FUNCTION

The overall goal for a client experiencing sexual dysfunction is the achievement of a satisfactory level of sexual function. When this level has been achieved will vary according to a client's values and cultural and religious beliefs.

Establishing Effective Communication

To intervene effectively, the nurse must have an open, caring approach to the client to build a rapport that encourages discussion of the client's concerns. The inexperienced professional nurse is most likely to be in the role of history taker and screener. If any significant problems are uncovered, the inexperienced nurse might refer the client to someone more experienced with sexual counseling.

Any problems of sexual dysfunction require open communication between the sexual partners. Teaching effective communication techniques to the partners can be most helpful. Techniques include active listening, clarifying and paraphrasing, and the use of "I" messages. Touch is an important means of nonverbal communication and can provide positive sexual stimulation.

Active listening is sometimes described as listening with a third ear; the person intently focuses on what the other is saying. This intent listening is communicated nonverbally by facial expressions and nodding and verbally by asking for examples or by encouraging the speaker to continue by using such phrases as "I see" and "Go on."

Seeking clarification by asking, "Are you saying that. . . ?" conveys that the partner is listening and clears possible misconceptions. In paraphrasing, the listener summarizes the other's messages, as in the following example: Speaker: "I wish I didn't always have to be the one to begin the lovemaking." Listener: "Oh, I see you think I should be more forward."

In an "I" message, a person accepts responsibility for his or her own needs or feelings by using such statements as "I need," "I feel," "I want," or "I like." These messages communicate the person's needs and are preferable to statements that tend to blame someone else, such as, "You make me feel. . . ." Partners also should avoid *why* questions that ask for an explanation of behavior. Many people are unaware of their motivation; others may be aware of it, but do not wish to share it. Why questions tend to make them feel defensive and may close off, rather than open up, communication between the couple.

Treating Sexual Dysfunction Related to Premature Ejaculation

Premature ejaculation concerns many male clients and their partners because it can interfere with sexual satisfaction for both. The nurse can teach clients techniques to help delay ejaculation. For example, the male's lying on his back in a relaxed, passive position decreases the muscular tension that occurs with the male on top, which often contributes to premature ejaculation. Ejaculating more frequently also may help delay ejaculation; the response slows after the first orgasm, so having a second one will delay ejaculation. Having smaller orgasms can lead to sustained muscle control and increased ejaculatory control (Crooks & Baur, 1983). Improved verbal communication also can aid in delaying ejaculation because the man can inform the partner when to stop stimulation.

Two other techniques can prevent premature ejaculation. In the stop–start technique, the penis is stimulated until there is a feeling of ensuing orgasm; then the stimulation is suddenly stopped. These steps are repeated to increase the threshold of excitability. With the squeeze technique, the partner squeezes the head of the penis using the thumb and first two fingers for 3 to 4 seconds just before orgasm. This stops the urge to ejaculate.

Treating Sexual Dysfunction Related to Impotence

As discussed in Chapter 62, impotence can be primary (the client has never attempted or achieved an erection) or secondary (the client had previously achieved erections). Secondary impotence is most common, and most men experience it at least occasionally. Crooks and Baur (1983) and many others note that anxiety is a major cause of erectile difficulty, so an important intervention is to reduce the pressure for performance. A trusted partner can greatly help reduce performance pressure. Daily stress often contributes to impotence problems. Helping the client learn stress-reducing techniques (see Chapter 4) and relieving boredom and fatigue often improve secondary impotence. The client also should reduce or curtail the use of recreational drugs known to contribute to secondary impotence. As with premature ejaculation, honest communication and trust between partners is essential.

It is important to rule out a physiological cause of the impotence. This can be done by measuring nocturnal penile tumescence in a sleep laboratory or at home using a portable device. Most men normally have erections during sleep, and absence of sleep erections indicates a physiological cause of impotence.

Clients with erectile dysfunction may find alternate means of sexual satisfaction useful. Techniques include general body touching, manual genital stimulation, use of sexual aids such as vibrators, and oral–genital stimulation. These techniques can reduce the pressure on the man with psychogenic impotence, and intercourse can then be attempted. If erectile difficulties still occur, the client should revert to one of the other techniques.

Sexual and psychological counseling also can be useful for the impotent client. Counseling may help the client with psychogenic impotence uncover the source of the problem. The client may need emotional support to deal with the decreased self-esteem and altered body image that impotence can cause. A penile implant (see Chapter 68) may help the client with inorganic impotence and is also sometimes used for psychogenic impotence if other forms of therapy are not successful.

Treating Sexual Dysfunction Related to Infection

Infection is another cause of sexual dysfunction. The overall goal of nursing care is to relieve symptoms of the infection and prevent its spread to others. To prevent the infection's spread, the client must understand its cause and mode of transmission. He must understand the need for appropriate antibiotic treatment and for identifying and treating sexual contacts if the infection is an STD. Clients should understand that they must take the full course of antibiotic therapy and not resume sexual activity without protection until both they and any partners have been treated. Wearing a condom will provide a barrier to the spread of infection for those who resume sexual activity before treatment is completed. Infection control by the nurse includes proper hand-washing techniques, the use

Nursing Research Note

Ewald BM, Roberts CG: Contraceptive behavior in college-age males related to Fishbein model. *ANS* 1985; 7(3):63–69.

Beliefs, attitudes, and intention to use condoms as a contraceptive method were studied in male college students aged 18 to 20. Fishbein's Belief-Attitude-Intention Behavior (BAIB) model was used as a theoretical framework. The BAIB model shows specific behavior is a function of intention to perform that behavior. The intention to perform is seen as a function of an attitude toward a behavior and the person's perception of what significant others think about a behavior. The attitude is a function of belief about the consequences of a behavior and personal evaluation of these consequences. The model attempts to predict and understand particular behaviors.

Positive beliefs about condom use were significantly correlated with positive attitudes about condom use. Attitudes about condom use were also related to intention to use condoms. The result indicated that intention to use condoms was positively associated with use in the past month during the study. Therefore, this study supports the Fishbein model in that positive beliefs and attitudes combined with intention to use were positively associated with utilization of this birth control method.

The Fishbein model indicates that beliefs result in particular behaviors. Altering beliefs may alter behaviors. Therefore, teaching birth control use may be more effective if it is aimed at altering beliefs rather than behaviors.

of sterile technique with dressing changes, and the timely administration of antibiotics.

Treating Sexual Dysfunction Related to Altered Cardiovascular Function

Clients with altered cardiovascular function often need to reduce the work load of the heart and the chance of pain during sexual activity. They can achieve this goal through position changes; both the female-superior and side-lying positions are less exerting for the male. The appropriate use of medications is also important. For example, taking a nitroglycerin tablet before intercourse can relieve anginal pain. If needed or desired, the client can employ alternative means of sexual satisfaction. (See also Chapter 24.)

Treating Sexual Dysfunction Related to Infertility

Clients often perceive infertility as a blow to their self-esteem and sense of male identity. The overall nursing goal is to assist the client in identifying possible correctable contributing factors and in coping effectively with the problem. Implementation includes identifying possible contributing factors such as retrograde ejaculation (ejaculation into the bladder), varicocele (varicosities in the testis), low sperm count from wearing tight pants or briefs, the use of drugs, and any problems with the partner.

The nurse should allow the client to ventilate his feelings of frustration and failure, as well as encourage open communication between partners. The infertile couple may choose to accept being childless or may choose such alternatives as adoption, artificial insemination, in vitro fertilization, or surrogate parenting.

PROMOTING URINARY FUNCTION

The overall goal for the client with an alteration in the pattern of urinary elimination is the achievement of continent, pain-free, nonobstructed urinary flow.

Treating Urinary Tract Obstruction and Retention

For the client with simple urinary retention, such as that often experienced after surgery, measures to induce voiding may be helpful. For the male client, standing to void often solves the problem. Hearing running water and placing the hand in water also may help relax the sphincter.

A client with prostatic hyperplasia may develop acute urinary retention or chronic retention. An in-dwelling catheter is usually inserted when a client has acute retention. Urinary drainage systems should be closed to prevent infectious organisms from ascending. The catheter should be free of dependent loops, and the collection bag should be kept below the level of the bladder to prevent backflow.

To maintain the normal penile–scrotal angle, prevent urethral pressure, and prevent trauma, tape the catheter to the upper thigh or abdomen. Strict asepsis is needed to prevent urinary tract infections from in-dwelling catheters. (See the suggestions in the section on nosocomial infection in Chapter 11.) Wash the penis with soap and water, retracting the prepuce if the client is uncircumcised. Remove crusts around the catheter with hydrogen peroxide. In many institutions, catheter care also includes wiping around the urinary meatus with an antiseptic and then applying an antibacterial ointment. Whether these measures are helpful is controversial. Unless otherwise contraindicated, force fluids to 3000 mL/24 h to flush the urinary tract and prevent stasis.

Treating Incontinence

Exercises to strengthen the pelvic area and urinary sphincter can help the client with incontinence. These exercises include alternately tightening and releasing the pelvic muscles and starting and stopping urination. (See the discussion of Kegel exercises in Box 64–1.) The intake of diuretics and substances such as alcohol and caffeine make incontinence more difficult to control and should be reduced if possible. The client should have easy access to a bathroom or urinal so he can relieve himself when the urge is present. The elderly or disabled male may require assistance because of impaired mobility, but it is important that the client's privacy be maintained.

Clients with incontinence may wear protective pads, which may be an asset when the incontinence is contributing to social isolation. Protective pads must be used with caution and with the client's consent, because they may cause the client to feel as though he is being treated like a child. A client who is incontinent should have his clothes and linens changed immediately. His skin should be protected with a nonwater-soluble protective ointment such as vitamin A and D or Desitin ointments.

For the incontinent male client, external condom drainage may be an appropriate solution but should not be used until other attempts have been made to control incontinence. If external drainage is used, the nurse should continue to assess changes in the client's condition. Too often this external drainage device is left on when frequent offering of the urinal could achieve the same purpose. Successful use of the urinal can increase the client's sense of dignity and independence. The penile skin is prone to irritation, so the nurse should apply tincture of benzoin or another protective solution before the condom is applied. Institutional policies vary, but usually the condom should be removed every 24 hours, the area washed with soap and water and checked for excoriation, and a new condom applied. If the penile skin is excoriated, the condom should not be reapplied. Also check to see if the condom twists at the tip of the penis, obstructing urinary drainage. The condom is apt to leak, so check frequently to be sure the client is dry. A leaking condom should be changed.

Section IV: Evaluation

Evaluation of the client with sexual dysfunction depends on its cause. Successful outcomes include the perception of increased sexual satisfaction, relief from infection, the improvement or acceptance of infertility, and a decrease in fatigue or pain during intercourse (for the client with a physical disability). The nurse should determine the level of the client's awareness of his sexual function and sexual health problems.

Successful outcomes for the client with an alteration in pattern of urinary elimination include the client's remaining clean, dry, and free of incontinence. The perineal skin should be free of breakdown. The client should be free of urinary retention problems either by voiding without difficulty or by having a freely flowing urinary drainage system.

Chapter Highlights

When interviewing the male client to assess for reproductive system dysfunction, nurses must maintain an open, accepting approach and have insight into their own and the client's feelings about the sensitive data being gathered.

The health history should include information about the client's sexual preference and practices, exposure to STDs, the presence of lumps or lesions, problems with the urinary stream, and general health practices.

The physical examination of the male reproductive system begins with observation of the secondary sex characteristics and inspection of the external genitalia. Next, the nurse palpates the penis, testes, scrotum, prostate, and inguinal canal.

Laboratory tests to detect male reproductive system problems include serologic tests; tests to determine levels of serum acid phosphatase, serum HCG, AFP, and testosterone; complete blood count; blood chemistry analysis; urine testing; semen analysis; and gonococcal culture.

Among the diagnostic studies performed on the male reproductive system are lymphangiography and biopsy of the prostate or testis.

Two common nursing diagnoses in clients with male reproductive system dysfunction are sexual dysfunction and alteration in urinary elimination pattern.

For the client with sexual dysfunction, nursing interventions to promote satisfactory sexual function begin with establishing effective communication between nurse and client and between the client and sexual partner.

Other nursing interventions for clients with sexual dysfunction depend on the type of dysfunction: premature ejaculation, impotence, altered cardiovascular function, or infertility. Nursing actions involve identifying the problem's cause and encouraging the expression of feelings, lifestyle modification, referrals, and increased partner communication.

Nursing measures for the client with a reproductive system infection include teaching sexual hygiene, identifying and treating the client's sexual contacts, and administering medication.

Nursing interventions for clients with urinary tract obstruction and retention include helping the client induce voiding, forcing fluids, and providing correct catheter care.

Helping the client control incontinence includes teaching pelvic strengthening exercises, limiting diuretics, and providing easy access to a bathroom.

Nursing evaluation of the client with sexual dysfunction includes assessment of the degree of sexual satisfaction, relief from infection, improvement or acceptance of infertility, and amount of fatigue or pain during intercourse.

The nurse evaluating the client with an alteration in the urinary elimination pattern should watch for signs of incontinence and impairment of perineal skin integrity. The client should void without difficulty or have a freely flowing urinary drainage system.

Bibliography

Byrne JC et al: *Laboratory Tests: Implications for Nursing Care,* 2nd ed. Menlo Park, CA: Addison–Wesley, 1986.

Crooks R, Baur K: *Our Sexuality,* 2nd ed. Menlo Park, CA: Benjamin–Cummings, 1983.

Fishbach F: *A Manual of Laboratory Diagnostic Tests,* 2nd ed. Philadelphia: Lippincott, 1984.

Haggerty BJ: Prevention and differential of scrotal cancer. *Nurse Pract* 1984; 8(10):45–52.

Harrison WO: Gonococcal urethritis. *Urol Clin North Am* 1984; 11(1):45–54.

Javadpour N: Germ cell tumor of the testes. *CA* 1980; 30:242–255.

Kneisl CR, Wilson HS: *Handbook of Psychosocial Nursing Care.* Menlo Park, CA: Addison–Wesley, 1984.

Lerner J, Khan Z: *Mosby's Manual of Urologic Nursing.* St. Louis: Mosby, 1982.

McConnell EA, Zimmerman MF: *Care of Patients With Urologic Problems.* Philadelphia: Lippincott, 1983.

Malasanos L et al: *Health Assessment,* 3rd ed. St. Louis: Mosby, 1985.

Pagana KD, Pagana TJ: *Diagnostic Testing and Nursing Implications.* St. Louis: Mosby, 1982.

Pearson JC et al: Radioimmunoassay of serum acid phosphatase after prostatic massage. *Urology* 1983; 21:37–41.

Roseman D, Ansell JS, Chapman WH: Sexually transmitted diseases and carcinogenesis. *Urol Clin North Am* 1984; 11(1):27–44.

Siemens S, Brandzel RC: *Sexuality: Nursing Assessment and Intervention.* Philadelphia: Lippincott, 1982.

Suggested Readings

Carpenito LJ: *Nursing Diagnosis: Applications to Clinical Practice.* Philadelphia: Lippincott, 1983. The student wanting further help with the nursing process in reproductive system dysfunction will find this book useful.

Crooks R, Baur K: *Our Sexuality,* 2nd ed. Menlo Park, CA: Benjamin–Cummings, 1983. This is a very good book for those who need more information on sexual function, sexual problems, and social issues related to sexuality.

Hogan R: *Human Sexuality: A Nursing Perspective.* New York: Appleton–Century–Crofts, 1980. This comprehensive book discusses all aspects of sexuality. It includes strong chapters on culture and religion as they relate to sexuality, as well as chapters on a variety of health deviations and sexuality.

Lerner J, Khan Z: *Mosby's Manual of Urologic Nursing.* St. Louis: Mosby, 1982. This book will be particularly helpful in the preparation of nursing care plans.

Siemens S, Brandzel RC: *Sexuality: Nursing Assessment and Intervention.* Philadelphia: Lippincott, 1982. Information on sexual assessment, body image and sexuality, sex roles and sexuality, and sociosexual problems are contained in this book.

Resources

(See also the resources list in Chapter 63; for resources on acquired immune deficiency syndrome [AIDS], see the resources list in Chapter 28.)

SELF-HELP GROUPS AND OTHER ORGANIZATIONS

Impotents Anonymous
5119 Bradley Blvd.
Chevy Chase, MD 20815

This organization, founded in 1981, offers information about the causes of impotence, treatments available, and emotional support. Meetings are held once or twice a month, and no dues or fees are collected. An associated organization, I-Anon (modeled after Al-Anon) gives impotent men's partners the chance to share their concerns and to benefit from the experience of others. Both organizations guarantee anonymity.

Chapter 67

Specific Disorders of the Male Reproductive System

Phyllis Foster Healy

Common disorders of the male reproductive system include congenital disorders; disorders of multifactorial origin; and infectious, neoplastic, and traumatic disorders. Included in this chapter's discussion are clinical manifestations of these disorders, their therapeutic measures, and the nursing measures specific to clients with these conditions. Male clients with reproductive system disorders often undergo changes in body image and sexual dysfunction. Therefore, emotional support is among the most important nursing interventions.

Section I: Congenital Disorders

Most significant congenital disorders of the male reproductive system are corrected during childhood. Failure to treat them early can seriously affect a person's psychosocial development, contributing not only to possible physiological dysfunction but also to severe body image problems. Two examples are hypospadias (the condition in which the urethra opens on the underside of the penis or the perineum) and epispadias (the absence of the upper wall of the urethra). Complete information on these problems can be found in a pediatrics textbook. Cryptorchidism, which contributes to infertility and greatly increases the risk of testicular cancer in the adult male, is discussed in this chapter.

CRYPTORCHIDISM

Cryptorchidism, failure of one or both testes to descend into the scrotum, is the most common disorder of prenatal sex differentiation in males. The testes usually descend by 24 to 35 weeks' gestation. Not surprisingly, the incidence of cryptorchidism is higher in premature male neonates (30%) than in full-term males (3.4%). At least half of these undescended testes descends into the scrotum by 1 month, and by 1 year the incidence of cryptorchidism is 0.7% to 0.8% (Zelikovsky, 1983).

Clinical Manifestations

Cryptorchidism is diagnosed by the absence on palpation of one or both testes in the scrotum. The testes may involuntarily retract out of the scrotum as a result of the *cremasteric reflex* activated by exposure to cold, touch, excitement, and physical activity. This is not true cryptorchidism; these testes usually fully descend by puberty and present no health problems for the client during adulthood.

Cryptorchidism causes concern because of its common complications. An atrophic scrotum on the affected side causes concern about appearance. Up to 90% of infants with cryptorchidism have inguinal hernias and are prone to torsion of the spermatic cord (Zelikovsky, 1983). Fibrotic changes have been reported in the seminiferous tubules in infants as young as 18 months. Ultimately, these changes can affect spermatogenesis and cause infertility, probably because of the higher temperature in the abdomen. A significant increase in testicular cancer—35 to 48 times greater—is also associated with cryptorchidism (Zelikovsky, 1983). This risk applies to both the affected testis and the contralateral one.

Therapeutic Measures

The general therapeutic measure in cryptorchidism is to bring the testis down early. If the testes have not descended by the third month after birth, they are unlikely to descend and treatment is instituted as soon as possible. Boys may be treated with human chorionic gonadotropin (HCG) (3000 to 5000 mg IM for 3 to 5 days) to encourage the testes' descent. The usual treatment, however, is surgical fixation of the testes in the scrotum (orchiopexy).

Specific Nursing Measures

Most cryptorchidism is treated in infancy. The nurse's role with the adult client is to obtain an accurate history to determine whether the client had the condition as an infant and, if so, when and how it was repaired. It is important to determine whether the client developed any complication of cryptorchidism. The infertile client needs emotional support and information on the cause of infertility. All adolescent males should be taught testicular self-examination (TSE), but it is especially important for clients with cryptorchidism because of the increased incidence of testicular cancer in these clients. See Chapter 7 for more information on TSE.

Section II: Disorders of Multifactorial Origin

Disorders of multifactorial origin have a variety of contributory factors; their exact cause varies with each client. These disorders may affect both the client's body image (by changing the appearance of the genitals) and urinary and sexual function.

General Nursing Implications

Disorders of multifactorial origin often alter the client's body image, so psychological support is a particularly important nursing intervention. Because deficient hygiene may contribute to problems such as phimosis or paraphimosis, health education is also an important part of nursing care for these clients.

PHIMOSIS

Phimosis, which is seen in the uncircumcised male, is the inability to retract the prepuce over the glans penis (see Figure 67–1). Phimosis most often is secondary to infection that has resulted from poor hygiene. The infection leads to scarring and fibrosis, which in turn lead to more infection and further scarring.

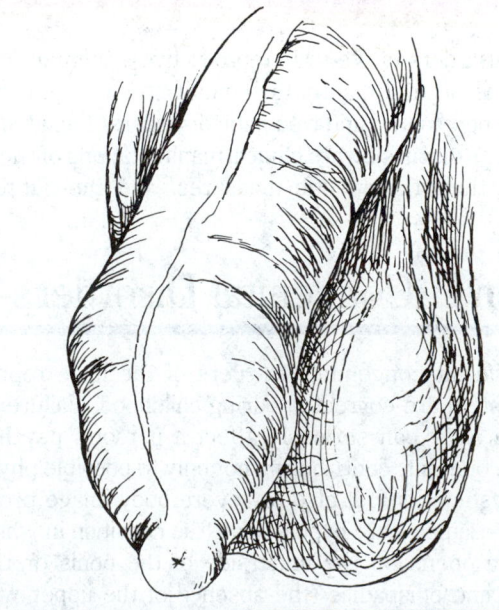

Figure 67–1

Phimosis. Note pinpoint opening of prepuce.

Clinical Manifestations

The clinical manifestations of phimosis include scarring; the inability to retract the prepuce; and signs of infection such as swelling, warmth, and exudate under the prepuce. Penile constriction and urethral obstruction are possible complications.

Therapeutic Measures

The administration of antibiotics and warm soaks to the penis relieves the infection. Creating a dorsal slit in the prepuce relieves any constriction or urethral obstruction the phimosis is causing. After the infection is resolved, a circumcision is performed.

Specific Nursing Measures

Preventive health teaching about basic hygiene is particularly important to prevent infection and resultant phimosis. The uncircumcised client should retract the prepuce daily and wash the penile shaft with soap and water; this removes the smegma from the penis and prevents infection. Instruct the client with phimosis to administer warm soaks and give him information on the proper administration of antibiotics. The client facing circumcision needs information about the procedure as well as emotional support. See Chapter 68 for more information on circumcision.

PARAPHIMOSIS

Paraphimosis is the inability of the uncircumcised retracted prepuce to be returned easily. Like phimosis, it is usually the result of recurrent chronic infections.

Clinical Manifestations

Because the retracted prepuce forms a constrictive ring around the penis, the penis becomes edematous and the foreskin becomes even more difficult, if not impossible, to return. Bluish discoloration of the penis results from obstruction of the blood supply; gangrene is possible (see Figure 67–2).

Therapeutic Measures

Manual reduction of the paraphimosis is the initial treatment measure. The glans penis is squeezed for 5 minutes in an attempt to decrease penile size. The penis is then pushed back while the prepuce is pulled forward. If this is unsuccessful, a surgical dorsal slit into the constricting ring relieves the pressure. Any infection is treated prior to a circumcision, which prevents the recurrence of paraphimosis.

Specific Nursing Measures

The most important nursing intervention for the client with paraphimosis is providing information and emotional sup-

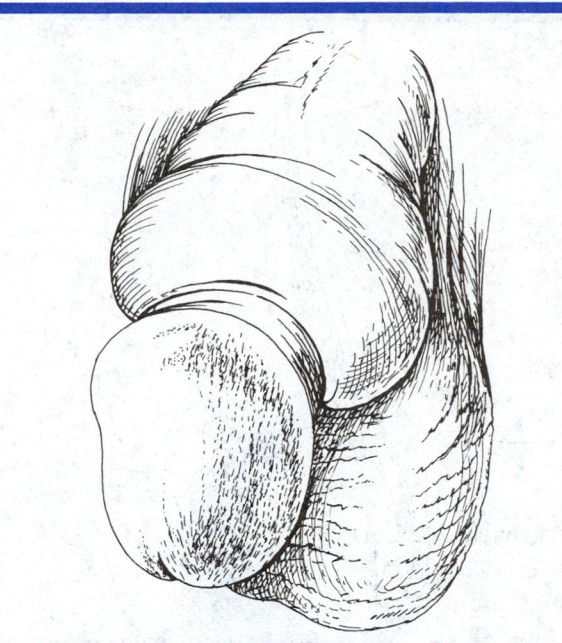

Figure 67–2

Paraphimosis. Retracted prepuce has become a constricting band around the penis.

port because the constriction of circulation to the penis causes severe anxiety. As in the case of the client with phimosis, it is important to prevent infection with basic hygiene. Nursing measures for circumcision are discussed in Chapter 68.

HYDROCELE

A hydrocele is accumulation of fluid in the tunica vaginalis testis (Figure 67–3). Hydrocele is frequently a congenital anomaly associated with an inguinal hernia. It can also occur after injury or irradiation to the scrotum.

Clinical Manifestations and Therapeutic Measures

A hydrocele usually appears as a transilluminating painless, oblong, soft mass in the scrotum. If the hydrocele is neither large nor causing discomfort, treatment is not required. Treatment is indicated, however, if physical or emotional discomfort occur because of the hydrocele's appearance or if circulation to the testis is impaired by pressure from the hydrocele. At times, it is important to reduce the size of the hydrocele so the testes can be examined carefully because a hydrocele can occur as a complication of testicular cancer.

Conservative treatment involves aspiration of the fluid. Hydroceles tend to recur, and the fluid may need to be reaspirated every 6 to 20 weeks. If this treatment is not adequate, surgical excision (hydrocelectomy) may be necessary. Chapter 68 discusses hydrocelectomy.

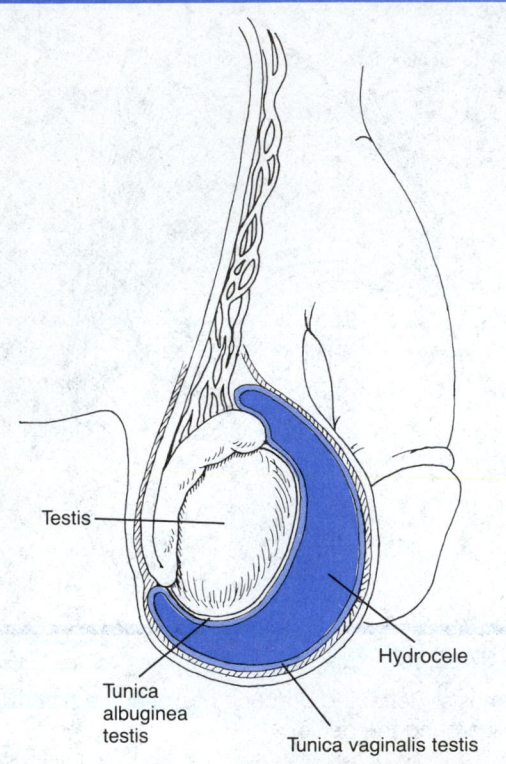

Figure 67–3

Hydrocele.

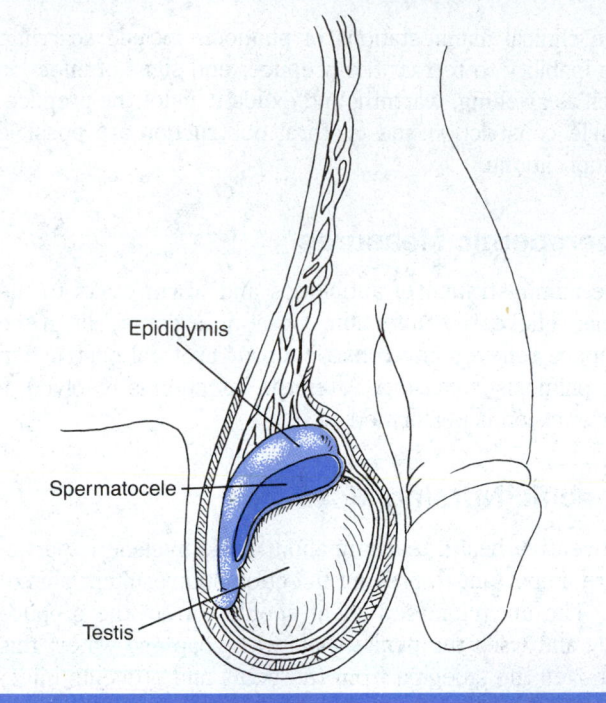

Figure 67–4

Spermatocele of the epididymis.

Specific Nursing Measures

Be sure the client understands the reason for aspirating the hydrocele, and explain that reaspiration may be necessary. A scrotal support may decrease discomfort caused by the weight of the hydrocele. Provide emotional support as needed for the client's altered body image or concern over the cause or effect of the hydrocele. Nursing measures for the client having hydrocelectomy are discussed in Chapter 68.

SPERMATOCELE

A spermatocele is a cyst of the epididymis or rete testis that contains dead sperm (Figure 67–4). Spermatoceles occur at the upper pole of the testis adjacent to the epididymis.

Clinical Manifestations and Therapeutic Measures

The mass is usually small, asymptomatic, and painless. If the mass becomes large, it may be mistaken for a hydrocele. If a spermatocele is firm, it should be distinguished from a tumor; unlike a tumor, a spermatocele is freely moving and will transilluminate. On aspiration, a white opaque liquid with dead sperm cells is observed. Usually no treatment is needed. A large spermatocele requires spermatocelectomy, however (see Chapter 68).

Specific Nursing Measures

Provide information and emotional support to the client as needed. Nursing measures for the spermatocelectomy client are discussed in Chapter 68.

VARICOCELE

A varicocele is a varicosity in the pampiniform plexus (a complex of veins from the testis and the epididymis that constitutes part of the spermatic cord). A varicocele usually results from incompetent vein valves (Figure 67–5). It is far more common on the left side, where the veins drain at a right angle. According to Belker (1981), 8% to 22% of all men have varicoceles; more significantly, 21% to 30% of men seen in infertility clinics have this condition. Varicoceles probably contribute to infertility by increasing scrotal temperature. Because even small varicoceles can contribute to infertility, accurate diagnosis is of the utmost importance.

Clinical Manifestations

To detect a varicocele, the client stands and performs Valsalva's maneuver (see Chapter 74). If there is a varicocele, the examiner will feel a rush of blood in the scrotum and will hear it with the Doppler stethoscope. The client may complain of an aching, pulling feeling in the scrotum. Semen analysis may show decreased sperm production, more immature sperm, and decreased sperm motility. The

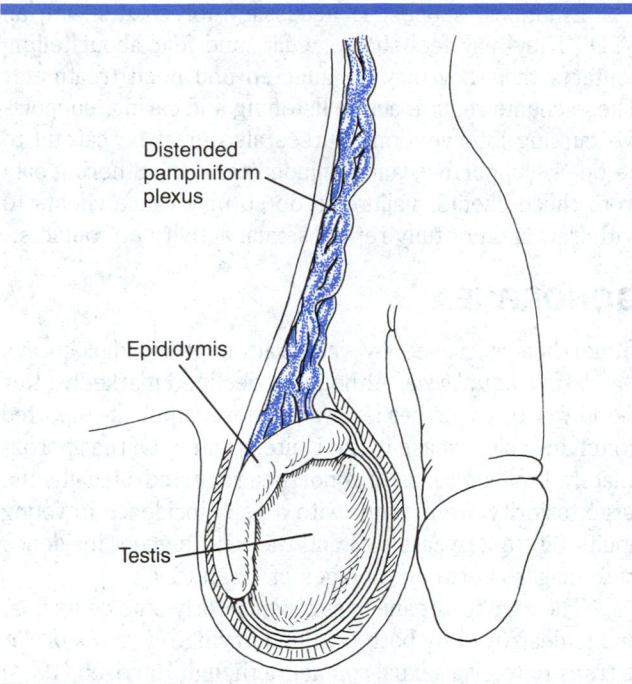

Figure 67–5
Varicocele.

swelling formed by the varicocele feels like a "bag of worms" and appears bluish through the skin of the scrotum.

Therapeutic Measures

Varicoceles usually are not treated unless the client has a problem with infertility or discomfort. The semen quality improves in most clients after varicocelectomy. Chapter 68 describes this surgical procedure and its nursing management.

Specific Nursing Measures

Inform the client about the relationship between varicoceles and infertility. Make the client comfortable so he can ventilate feelings and anxiety. Give information and support the client so that he can make an informed decision about surgery. Be sure he is not inadvertently raising his intrascrotal temperature by wearing tight pants or under-

wear. A scrotal support may help the client bothered by a heavy, pulling feeling.

PRIAPISM

Priapism is a state of constant erection not associated with sexual desire. It is caused by congestion or sludging of blood in the corpora cavernosa penis with obstruction to the outflow of blood, often secondary to leukemia, sickle-cell disease, or spinal cord injury. Priapism also can result from tardive dyskinesia, a complication of the prolonged use of high doses of phenothiazines. Priapism can cause urinary retention.

Clinical Manifestations

The persistent erection of priapism is usually painful. There is marked turgor of the corpora cavernosa although the glans penis and the corpus spongiosum are flaccid. If the erection has been prolonged, the penis may be discolored because of ischemia. If it causes urinary retention, priapism becomes a urologic emergency by posing a threat to the renal parenchyma from backflow of urine.

Therapeutic Measures

The client is usually sedated with meperidine (Demerol), which has the side benefit of reducing blood pressure and thus reducing circulatory congestion in the penis. Warm enemas may cause venous dilation and thus allow the congested blood to flow out. A urethral catheter is inserted, and saline or heparin irrigations may be used. If these measures are not successful, it may be necessary to create a surgical fistula to shunt blood from the corpora cavernosa to the corpus spongiosum. The cause of the priapism also should be investigated and treated.

Specific Nursing Measures

Provide information to the client on the possible cause of priapism and keep him informed about possible treatments. Give analgesics as needed, and evaluate the client for relief of pain. Provide emotional support to the client because this experience may frighten and embarrass him. Other nursing measures are determined by the treatment measures employed.

Section III: Infectious Disorders

Sexually transmitted diseases (STDs) are among the most common infectious disorders of the male reproductive system. Males, especially adolescents and young adults, seem to have an increased incidence of STDs; this may be because of contact with anonymous sexual partners or because men with STDs seek medical care more quickly than women.

The external male genitalia are more easily inspected than the female's and the client himself is able to see lesions or discharges.

Gonorrhea is the most-reported infectious disease in the United States, and chlamydial infections are even more prevalent. The incidence of syphilis is markedly increased in homosexuals. STDs are more common in blacks than in whites and are more common in whites than in Orientals. The incidence of STDs is also higher among single, divorced, and separated individuals as well as among homosexuals and heterosexuals with multiple partners.

Men may be carriers of organisms that cause infectious vaginitis in women. Although they may not have symptoms of a disease, they should be treated to avoid reinfecting their partner or infecting a new partner. See the discussion of infectious vaginitis in Chapter 64. Scabies and pelvic lice are also sexually transmitted. These infestations are discussed in Chapter 79. Acquired immune deficiency syndrome (AIDS) is discussed in Chapter 29.

General Nursing Implications

Health teaching is the key to preventing the spread of STDs. Because of the age groups at risk, the nurse must provide this information early—at the same time as basic sex education. The nurse needs great skill in educating adolescents without leading them to believe that sex is dirty or shameful. The need for imparting this information is clear in light of the psychological and physical discomfort, risk of sterility, and risk to unborn children from STDs.

Teaching should include the fact that the spread of STDs can be prevented if sexual activity is limited to one or a few known partners. The use of condoms may help prevent the spread of some STDs. Information should include the mode of transmission of these diseases and the fact that contacts usually must be identified and treated. The nurse's suggestion to limit partners or use condoms may appear to the client as an attempt to judge and moralize. Nurses must recognize their role as information givers while remembering that the choice belongs to the client. If a nurse is to continue to be an effective caregiver, he or she must accept the client's choice in a nonjudgmental manner.

Treatment for infectious diseases of the male reproductive system almost always involves antibiotics. Before administering an antibiotic, be sure to check for allergies. The client who is given penicillin parenterally should be observed for 30 minutes for a possible anaphylactic reaction. Note the motivation and ability to comply of the client who is to be given antibiotics orally. The client needs to understand that he should take the doses on schedule and must complete the full course even if the symptoms go away. Be aware that clients taking broad-spectrum antibiotics such as ampicillin and amoxicillin are at risk of developing superinfections. An empty stomach increases absorption of these drugs, so the client should be instructed to take them 1 hour before or 2 hours after meals. The client receiving any of the tetracyclines should be instructed not to take them with milk products, antacids, or iron preparations because they will not be absorbed. Children under 8 years old and pregnant women should not take tetracycline because it delays bone growth and stains secondary teeth. Tetracycline can also cause superinfections and photosensitivity upon exposure to sunlight.

Emotional support is necessary for clients with an STD. They may feel shame, guilt, and fear about telling contacts that they may be infected and need treatment. These clients require active listening and caring, supportive nursing intervention. Nurses also must be careful to be open, supportive, and nonjudgmental in gathering data from these clients. Failure to do so may cause clients to withdraw and not fully report sexual activity or contacts.

GONORRHEA

Gonorrhea is caused by the gram-negative diplococcus *Neisseria gonorrhoeae*. Although it declined markedly after World War II, gonorrhea is now the most commonly reported communicable disease in the United States. Of the approximately 1 million cases of gonorrhea reported annually, the large majority are in men, with a peak incidence in young adults (20 to 24 years old) and the next highest incidence in teenagers between the ages of 15 and 19.

The aerobic organism survives poorly outside its host and is destroyed by both heat and drying. *N. gonorrhoeae* is transmitted via sexual contact, although Harrison (1984) notes rare reports of viable organisms' being recovered from toilet seats after 18 hours and from wet towels between 10 and 24 hours after contact. The organism has become increasingly resistant to penicillin since the 1950s. A strain referred to as PPNG (penicillinase-producing *Neisseria gonorrhoeae*) was first identified in 1976 on US military bases and cities in the Philippines. Since then, this strain has been identified in approximately 30 countries in North America, Europe, Asia, Africa, and the Pacific islands. It was imported from Southeast Asia and West Africa, where PPNG is most common (Krieger, 1984).

Clinical Manifestations

In men, the gonococcus usually causes gonococcal urethritis or, depending on the client's sexual practices, rectal inflammation and pharyngitis. Usually, the incubation period is 3 to 10 days. Harrison (1984) reports that the PPNG strain can cause symptoms and a positive culture 12 hours after contact.

Manifestations of gonorrhea in men include dysuria and a white or yellowish green cloudy urethral or rectal discharge. These symptoms range from severe to minimal. A client can also be asymptomatic and spread the organism without knowing it. Without treatment, the inflammation subsides within 2 to 4 weeks, and the individual may become a carrier.

Diagnosis is based on Gram's stain and a culture of the urethral discharge to identify penicillin-resistant gonococci. The PPNG strain is often also resistant to other antibiotics, such as tetracycline.

Therapeutic Measures

The key to the treatment of gonorrhea is effective antibiotic administration. Treatment guidelines based on the recommendations of the Centers for Disease Control (CDC) are provided in Chapter 64. All clients treated for gonorrhea should have follow-up cultures performed 4 to 7 days after treatment is completed. It is recommended that throat, urethral, and rectal cultures also be performed. All sexual partners must be identified, examined, cultured, and treated. Ineffective treatment can result in epididymitis; genital abscesses; and proctitis and pharyngitis in clients practicing oral-genital, ano-genital, or ano-oral sex.

Specific Nursing Measures

Prevention is the key in the nursing management of the client at risk of developing gonorrhea. Education of adolescent and young adult men about the risk of developing gonorrhea as well as other STDs must be emphasized and imparted in a straightforward, matter-of-fact, nonjudgmental way. Give the facts, and allow clients to form their own value judgments based on these facts.

Information given to the young client should include facts about the incidence, risk, and transmission modes of gonorrhea. The client should understand that all contacts must be identified and treated. He also must understand the risk of the infection and possible subsequent sterility in female partners. Using a condom during intercourse and limiting sexual contacts to one or a few known sexual partners can help prevent the transmission of the disease. Other important information includes making sure the client realizes that he can become reinfected if he has contact with an untreated partner. The client being treated for gonorrhea should refrain from intercourse until the follow-up cultures are negative. A client who has had intercourse with a high-risk individual should begin an antibiotic regimen.

Before administering antibiotics, check for any drug allergies. It is particularly important to determine the client's ability and willingness to comply with the planned drug regimen; clients known to be unreliable are best treated with a single injection. Explain the importance of returning for a follow-up culture, and make an appointment for the client. Finally, the client should be able to express any feelings of anxiety, shame, or guilt. If telling a partner presents particular difficulty, the nurse can help by being a supportive listener as the client works through this problem.

NONGONOCOCCAL URETHRITIS

The client with nongonococcal urethritis (NGU) has symptoms of urethral inflammation, but the gonococcus is not present on culture. There are many causes, but the most common are *Chlamydia trachomatis* and *Ureaplasma urealyticum*. This disease can occur at any age, and its incidence is increasing. Clinics treating STDs report that over half of the urethritis seen is NGU (Bowie, 1984). The greatest incidence is in the young adult age group (20 to 24 years). The incubation period varies between 1 and 5 weeks.

Clinical Manifestations

The manifestations of NGU are similar to those of gonococcal urethritis but often less acute. Dysuria and a thin, watery discharge are early symptoms. Later, the discharge may be thick, white, and creamy. For definitive diagnosis, the urethra should be milked and a Gram's stain and culture performed. Nongonococcal urethritis is more difficult to treat than gonococcal urethritis; penicillin is not effective, and the discharge is slow to clear. Between 30% and 40% of cases recur within 6 weeks (Bowie, 1984). The diagnosis and treatment may be further confounded because a client can have NGU and gonorrhea at the same time.

Therapeutic Measures

Tetracycline hydrochloride (500 mg q.i.d. for 7 days) effectively eradicates *Chlamydia trachomatis*. Doxycycline (100 mg PO b.i.d. a day) is more effective against *Ureaplasma urealyticum* and will also treat gonorrhea. For the client unable to take tetracycline hydrochloride, treatment with erythromycin (500 mg PO q.i.d. for 7 days) is recommended.

Specific Nursing Measures

Prevention of NGU is difficult, because the causative organisms are prevalent, the affected individuals are frequently asymptomatic, and the organisms commonly are resistant to the prescribed drugs. As with other STDs, the nurse can teach the client that having one or a limited number of known partners will help control the disease's spread. The use of condoms or spermicides also may be helpful.

The client should be taught to avoid alcohol during the treatment phase. He should not resume intercourse for 4 weeks after treatment because recurrence is common; if he does resume intercourse during this time, the client should be sure to use a condom. It is important that the client comply with the treatment regimen because untreated cases usually have complications, the major one being epididymitis. Partners need to be identified and treated.

EPIDIDYMITIS

Inflammation of the epididymis, or epididymitis, is the major complication of NGU. When it occurs in a man under 35 years of age, epididymitis is usually caused by the gonococcus or *Chlamydia trachomatis*. In clients who practice anal intercourse, it may be caused by the *Escherichia coli*. The likely cause in those over age 35 and in preadolescent males is either a coliform or pseudomonas bacteria; rather than being sexually transmitted, the infection is usually caused by urinary tract disease.

Clinical Manifestations

One-sided scrotal pain, redness, and swelling are typical of epididymitis (Figure 67–6). Diagnosis is based on a urine

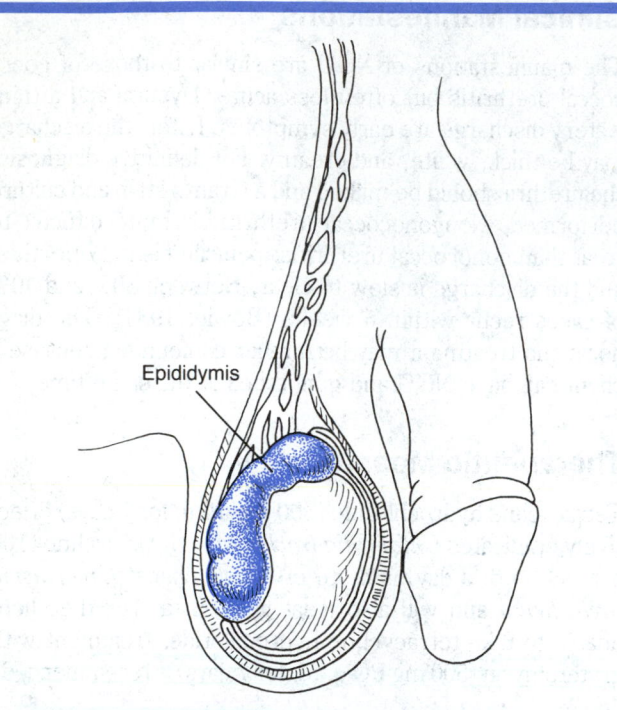

Figure 67–6

Epididymitis. Note swelling of the epididymis and the scrotum.

and urethral culture. Testicular tumor, spermatic cord torsion, and abscess should be ruled out. Epididymitis can lead to abscess formation.

Therapeutic Measures

A culture is performed; until the results are obtained, a broad-spectrum antibiotic from the aminoglycosides or cephalosporins is used. One of the following drugs is usually recommended to treat epididymitis: tetracycline hydrochloride (500 mg PO q.i.d. for 10 days), doxycycline (100 mg PO b.i.d. for 10 days), or amoxicillin (500 mg t.i.d. for 10 days). Erythromycin also may be used. If the epididymitis is not sexually transmitted, its cause should be determined. When epididymitis has been sexually transmitted, the partner is also treated.

The client's activity is limited to either bed rest or bed rest with bathroom privileges. Ice applied to the scrotum for the first 24 hours and scrotal elevation may reduce inflammation. An anti-inflammatory agent such as indomethacin (Indocin) may be given, and analgesia is necessary.

Specific Nursing Measures

The exquisite pain caused by epididymitis makes pain relief a priority in the early period. Assess the client frequently for pain and the effectiveness of the analgesic. The client probably will take an oral analgesic such as oxycodone with acetaminophen (Percocet) every 4 hours; be sure the medication is administered on time and is given before the pain

cycle begins so the client is spared intermittent painful episodes.

Inform the client that bed rest will reduce metabolic demands and aid in healing. The scrotum should be elevated to decrease dependent edema; this is best achieved by the use of the Bellevue bridge (Figure 67–7). When the client is out of bed, he should wear an athletic supporter. Further nursing interventions include monitoring the client's temperature every 4 hours and forcing fluids to maintain hydration and keep the temperature down.

PROSTATITIS

Prostatitis, inflammation of the prostate gland, is the most common complication of STDs. Acute bacterial prostatitis is usually not sexually transmitted. It is caused by *Escherichia coli*, *Klebsiella pneumoniae*, *Proteus mirabilis*, or *Pseudomonas aeruginosa*. Chronic nonbacterial prostatitis is more common in 30- to 45-year-olds and is thought to be caused by the sexually transmitted organisms *Chlamydia trachomatis*, *Ureaplasma urealyticum*, and *Trichomonas vaginalis*.

Clinical Manifestations

The symptoms of prostatitis include dysuria, suprapubic and perineal pain, urethral discomfort, rectal fullness, nocturia, urgency and frequency of urination, and blood in the ejaculate. With acute bacterial prostatitis, the client has severe symptoms of a systemic and prostatic infection. On rectal examination, the prostate feels enlarged, tender, and boggy. Massage should not be attempted because it can cause septicemia. Chronic nonbacterial prostatitis is difficult to treat because the cause is uncertain. The symptoms

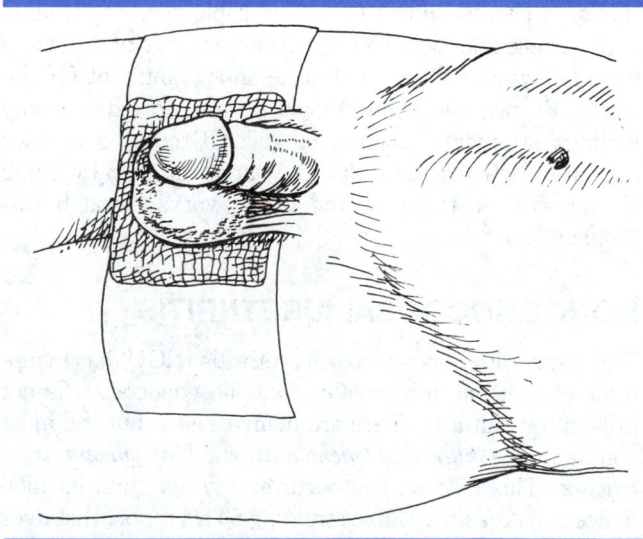

Figure 67–7

Elevating the scrotum with a Bellevue bridge. The bridge is built of gauze lying on top of tape.

of chronic nonbacterial prostatitis are generally similar but subacute.

Therapeutic Measures

Acute prostatitis is usually treated with tobramycin given intramuscularly until the client is afebrile. The dose is based on body weight and is usually 3 to 5 mg/kg. Afebrile clients usually receive a drug such as trimethoprim or sulfamethoxazole orally for 30 days. If the infection becomes chronic, treatment is more difficult.

Specific Nursing Measures

If the cause of the prostatitis is sexual transmission, identify and treat contacts. Explain to the client the mode of transmission and possible preventive measures. Be sure the antibiotics are administered in a timely manner, and closely monitor the renal function of clients taking tobramycin. Alcohol, caffeine, and spicy foods aggravate prostatitis, so instruct the client to avoid them.

LYMPHOGRANULOMA VENEREUM

Lymphogranuloma venereum is an STD caused by several subtypes of *Chlamydia trachomatis*. It can be acute or chronic and cause a wide range of generalized symptoms and transitory perineal lesions. Although a worldwide disease, it is more common in tropical and subtropical areas.

Clinical Manifestations and Therapeutic Measures

The lesions appear 1 to 2 months after exposure. They are vesicular or papular and heal rapidly, so the client may not notice them. Days to weeks after the lesions appear, symptoms of lymphadenitis occur. Inguinal lymph nodes are painful, palpable and matted, and necrotic, purulent fistulas form. At this point, chills and fever, headache, joint pain, nausea, and vomiting also may occur. A skin rash may also be present. Late changes that occur with lymphogranuloma venereum include rectal strictures and elephantiasis of the external genitals. Lymphogranuloma venereum is usually treated with tetracycline hydrochloride (500 mg PO q.i.d. for 2 weeks).

Specific Nursing Measures

Assist the client with identification of contacts so they can be treated. Explain the mode of transmission, and be sure the client understands the need to have the full range of antibiotic treatment. Instruct the client that washing with soap and water after sexual exposure may be a successful preventive measure.

SYPHILIS

Syphilis is caused by the spirochete *Treponema pallidum*. The incidence of syphilis has dropped sharply recently (the total number of cases dropped 30% from 1982 through 1985). The CDC attributes the declining syphilis rate to a major change in sexual behavior in homosexual men because of fear of AIDS. Gay men have accounted for more than half of the syphilis cases in the United States. Changes in sexual activity, away from anonymous sex and toward monogamous relationships, have reduced the risk of STDs in homosexual men.

Clinical Manifestations

The incubation period of primary syphilis is 10 to 90 days, with an average of 21 days. *Treponema pallidum* thrives in a warm, moist environment. The chancre (the painless lesion of syphilis) is a papule that progresses to a reddened, indurated, painless ulcer (Figure 67–8A). The chancre may last from 2 to 8 weeks, when regional lymphadenopathy may also occur.

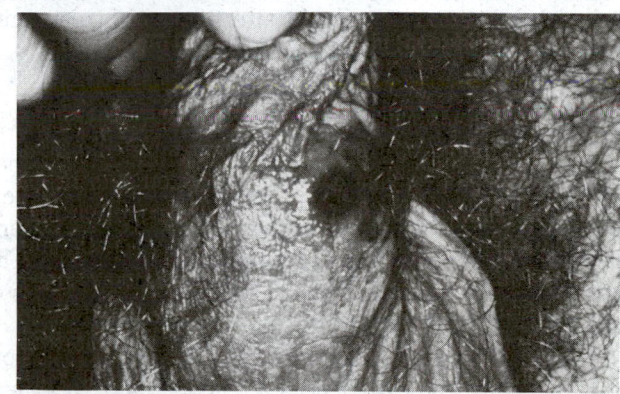

A

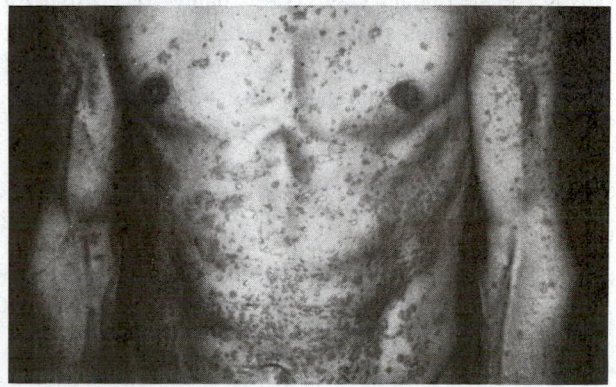

B

Figure 67–8

Characteristic lesions associated with syphilis at various stages of development. **A.** Chancre of primary stage on a male. **B.** Skin rash of secondary stage.

SOURCE: Centers for Disease Control, Public Health Service, U.S. Department of Health and Human Services, Atlanta, Georgia.

Diagnosis is hindered by the fact that the chancre may appear on the rectum, lips, tongue, or pharynx rather than on the more typical place, the penis. Drusin (1984) reports that misdiagnosis is common; the chancre is often mistaken for cancer of the rectum, tongue, and penis. (The VDRL test and other laboratory tests to detect syphilis are discussed in Chapter 63.)

Secondary syphilis occurs when the organism enters the bloodstream. On the average, this occurs about 6 to 8 weeks after the infection begins. The client has a generalized maculopapular rash, fever, aches, sore throat, hair loss, and lymphadenopathy (Figure 67–8B). In blacks, the rash appears annular with a clear center (Drusin, 1984).

Between 4 and 12 weeks after the initial infection, syphilis becomes latent. If untreated, it manifests itself as tertiary syphilis about 18 to 20 years after the initial infection. Tertiary syphilis often involves the neurological and cardiovascular systems.

Therapeutic Measures

For treatment of syphilis see therapeutic measures for syphilis in Chapter 64. Follow-up examinations should be scheduled 3, 6, and 12 months after the initial treatment.

Specific Nursing Measures

The basic preventive measures that apply for other types of STDs also apply to syphilis. These include limiting intercourse to one or a limited number of known partners and using a condom to help prevent the disease's spread. The nurse should assist the client in identifying all contacts of the last 3 months, who will require treatment.

Provide comfort measures and physiological support for the client who experiences a reaction after treatment during the secondary stage (see Chapter 64). Finally, the client with syphilis should understand that he is at risk of developing the disease any time he is exposed to the organism; there is no immunity to syphilis.

CHANCROID

One cause of genital ulcer is the chancroid caused by *Hemophilus ducreyi*. This STD is more common in tropical areas, with less than 1000 cases reported in the United States each year.

Clinical Manifestations

Chancroids are tender, and their bases may be covered with an exudate. Lymph nodes may be tender and swollen. The incubation period is 1 to 14 days. This condition must be distinguished from syphilis; the chancroid lesions appear similar, but the treatment is different. The organism can be isolated and identified by culture.

Therapeutic Measures

Treatment is either with erythromycin (500 mg q.i.d.) or trimethoprim/sulfamethoxazole DS (160/800 mg PO b.i.d. for at least 10 days or until the ulcer heals). Apply sterile soaks to the ulcers to remove necrotic material. As with other STDs, the client's partner or partners also need to be treated.

Specific Nursing Measures

Nursing measures for chancroid are similar to those for other STDs. They include advising the client how to prevent transmission, assisting him in identifying contacts and emphasizing the importance of following the treatment regimen.

CONDYLOMATA ACUMINATA

Condylomata acuminata (venereal warts) are considered a "minor" STD. According to Margolis (1984), however, they account for 1 million office visits per year and can undergo carcinogenic changes.

Clinical Manifestations

Clients may have warts on the shaft of the penis; on the scrotum; and, in homosexuals, in the anorectal area. The practitioner should examine the client for other STDs and distinguish these warts from the condylomata lata of syphilis. The warts also should be biopsied to check for cancer. The incubation period is 1 to 2 months.

Therapeutic Measures

The area where the warts occur must be kept dry to prevent their spread. One common treatment is the topical application of 10% to 25% podophyllin solution in tincture of benzoin (four weekly applications). It is important to avoid normal tissue to prevent irritation and scarring. Normal tissue should be protected with petrolatum jelly or other protective covering and the solution removed in 1 to 4 hours. Other treatments include cryotherapy, electrosurgery, and surgical excision. The removal of warts in the urethral meatus may cause stricture formation.

Specific Nursing Measures

The nurse must support the client as he undergoes the treatment regimen. Be sure the client is fully informed about the possible treatment options.

MOLLUSCUM CONTAGIOSUM

Molluscum contagiosum occurs worldwide in adults and children and is spread by direct skin contact, often sexually transmitted in adolescents and young adults. It is caused by a poxvirus whose incubation period is 2 to 7 weeks.

Clinical Manifestations

The lesions are firm, rounded, translucent papules that contain encapsulated bodies of caseous material. Lesions appear on the genitals, thighs, and abdomen in no particular pattern. The lesions spontaneously regress in 9 to 12 months.

Therapeutic Measures

The purpose of treatment is to prevent self-infection, to stop the spread, and to improve appearance. The lesions are surgically treated by curettage, or podophyllin, phenol, or silver nitrate caustic substances can be used. Cryotherapy with liquid nitrogen also may be performed.

Specific Nursing Measures

Explain the treatment to the client, and provide support through the therapeutic regimen. These clients often have multiple sex partners, so all partners should be identified and treated.

HERPES GENITALIS

Sexually transmitted herpes simplex infections are on the rise. The exact incidence and prevalence are not known because herpes genitalis is a nonreportable disease, and some individuals are asymptomatic. Herpes genitalis seems to rank after gonorrhea and chlamydia infections as a leading STD. The majority of genital infections are caused by *Herpesvirus hominis* type II, although at least 15% are caused by *Herpesvirus hominis* type I; the virus that causes cold sores (a reflection of the increase in oral-genital sex). Herpes genitalis can be transmitted via a genital or oral-genital route. The incubation period is 2 to 10 days.

Clinical Manifestations

Generally, herpes genitalis is less severe in men than women. The first episode is the worst and may last about 3 weeks. The client usually has multiple bilateral painful pustules or ulcerative lesions on the penis, genital area, groin, or rectum (Figure 67–9). The lymph nodes are tender, and generalized symptoms of malaise and fever may appear. As some vesicles form pustules, ulcerate, crust, and heal, new vesicles appear. During the period of open lesions, the virus sheds from the lesions, and the infection can be spread to sexual contacts. Half the males infected with *Herpesvirus hominis* complain of dysuria, and the virus can be isolated from the urethra. In fact, herpes simplex without external lesions can cause NGU. The herpesvirus may be simultaneously present in other areas of the body. Mertz

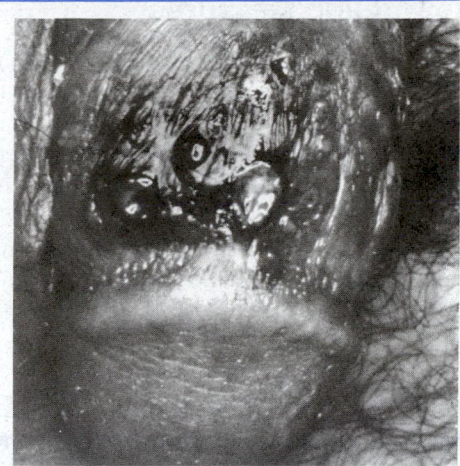

Figure 67–9

Genital herpes blisters on the penis.
SOURCE: Centers for Disease Control, Public Health Service, U.S. Department of Health and Human Services, Atlanta, Georgia.

and Corey (1984) report that 10% of clients with primary herpes genitalis have pharyngitis and lesions on their buttocks and fingers.

The herpesvirus lies dormant in the spinal root ganglia and can reactivate at any time. The exact cause of recurrence is not known, but it is believed that emotional stress or tight clothing that increases warmth in the genital area may be factors. Recurrent infections are usually not as severe as the first infection, but they occur more often in men than women. There are fewer systemic manifestations, the lesions cover a smaller area, and usually they heal more quickly. Urethritis does not usually recur. Fifty percent of clients have a prodromal period with an itching, tingling sensation before the lesions break out (Mertz & Corey, 1984).

The disease can cause neurologic complications such as aseptic meningitis and sacral radiculopathy, an inflammation of the roots of the sacral nerves. It also can cause proctitis and prostatitis.

Therapeutic Measures

There is no cure for herpes genitalis, and researchers are seeking a cure or a vaccine. The major breakthrough so far has been the drug acyclovir (Zovirax), a nucleoside analogue. A topical ointment containing 5% acyclovir used early during the primary outbreak shortens healing time and viral shedding and reduces the severity of pain and itching (Mertz & Corey, 1984). An intravenous form of the drug is available for immunosuppressed clients. FDA approval has been sought for the oral form. Clinical trials indicate that oral acyclovir is the first medication to offer hope for decreasing the pain and discomfort in clients with recurrent infections (Reichman, 1984).

Specific Nursing Measures

Herpes genitalis is prevented by avoiding intimate contact with an individual with active lesions. Condoms do not necessarily provide protection. Teach the client to avoid touching other parts of his body because autoinoculation is possible and to keep the blisters clean and dry. The client needs to know that acyclovir treatment must be started early in the outbreak. He should cover all lesions with the ointment every 3 hours six times a day for 7 days (Centers for Disease Control, 1982).

Section IV: Neoplastic Disorders

A neoplasm in the male reproductive tract often causes obstruction signaled by impaired urinary output. Benign prostatic hyperplasia (BPH) is a common health problem for men over 50 years old, and prostatic cancer is a major cause of cancer death in this age group. Testicular cancer, although rare, affects men at the prime of their lives. Early detection can significantly affect the outcome and survival rates of these cancerous conditions. Any sore that does not heal; asymmetry in the scrotum or prostate; or an unusual lump or hardening in the testes, penis, or prostate may indicate a neoplasm.

General Nursing Implications

Because early detection can significantly affect the outcome and survival rates for clients with neoplastic disorders, nurses play an important role in prevention and early detection through health education. The client with an obstructive or neoplastic disorder needs complete information at all times. The diagnostic process will probably provoke anxiety and fears of disfigurement and sexual dysfunction. Thus, emotional support for the client and his family or significant other is a crucial part of all nursing interventions. If sexual dysfunction becomes a problem, the client should be referred for counseling and possible surgical penile implant, if indicated.

BENIGN PROSTATIC HYPERPLASIA

Benign prostatic hyperplasia (BPH) is caused by an increased production of prostatic cells (Figure 67–10). The term *hypertrophy*—an increase in the size of the cells—is commonly misapplied to BPH. The prostate gland increases in size because the number of prostatic cells (not their size) increases. BPH is the most common neoplastic growth in men; at least 50% of men over age 50 have some degree of hyperplasia. The progressive increase in size of the prostate gland can obstruct urine flow and lead to urinary tract infections, hydronephrosis, and the eventual destruction of renal parenchyma.

Exactly why prostatic hyperplasia occurs is not known. It may be related to aging or an unexplained hormonal mechanism.

Herpes genitalis causes psychological pain and suffering in addition to physical discomfort. The client may feel stigmatized and ashamed. He will have to avoid sexual contact during active outbreaks and faces having to tell his partner the reason. A client with herpes genitalis should tell future sexual partners about the condition. These clients need complete information and emotional support as they work through the changed self-concept the diagnosis generates.

Clinical Manifestations

Early in BPH, the increasing obstruction causes compensatory hypertrophy of the detrusor muscle of the bladder wall (see Figure 67–10) to overcome urethral resistance. The symptoms at this point may depend on the compensatory ability of the bladder, but ultimately diverticula may form in the bladder wall and lead to residual urinary stasis and urinary tract infection. Later, when the bladder can no longer undergo hypertrophy, signs of decompensation include acute urinary retention, bilateral hydroureter and hydronephrosis, and infection because of urinary stasis. Typical symptoms of BPH include hesitancy, frequency, nocturia, urgency, decreased urinary stream, and difficulty

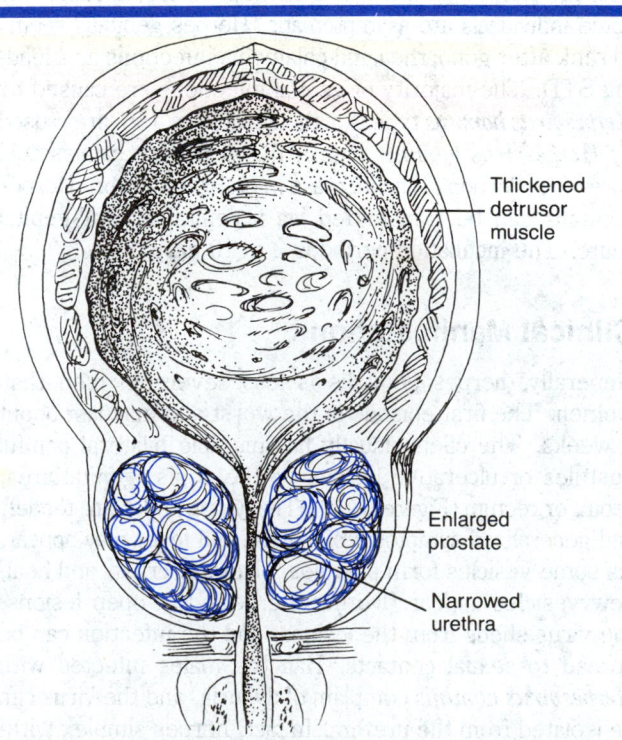

Thickened detrusor muscle

Enlarged prostate

Narrowed urethra

Figure 67–10

Benign prostatic hyperplasia.

starting the stream. Sexual function, sexual frequency, and quality of erection may decline.

Therapeutic Measures

A drug history is first obtained. Any of the following drugs can cause urinary symptoms: parasympatholytics, bronchodilators, antispasmodics, antihistamines, muscle relaxants, tranquilizers, and ganglionic blocking agents. Discontinuing the drug may correct the problem. An infection must be treated before any manipulative procedure such as cystoscopy is performed because these procedures carry a high risk of sepsis.

The client with acute urinary retention has a small Foley catheter inserted to relieve pain, prevent the loss of bladder tone from distention, and prevent further hydronephrosis. Usually, once decompression has been performed, the client is treated surgically by prostatectomy (see Chapter 68). The client who is not a good surgical candidate will have a small in-dwelling catheter that remains in place. The urine is usually kept acidic to decrease the chance of infection by giving methenamine mandelate (Mandelamine) q.i.d. or vitamin C (500 mg q.i.d.). Antibiotics are administered only if the client develops epididymitis. Complications of long-term catheterization include stricture, recurring epididymitis, and periurethral abscess. If these occur, a suprapubic catheter is indicated.

Specific Nursing Measures

Nursing interventions for BPH clients include keeping the client well informed and preparing him for catheterization and surgery. Maintain continuous catheter drainage and perform catheter care every shift using aseptic technique. For further interventions, see Chapter 32 for catheter care and Chapter 68 for care after prostatectomy.

CANCER OF THE PROSTATE

Cancer of the prostate is the second most common cancer and the third most common cause of cancer deaths in the US male population. It represents a significant health problem for men over 50, and its incidence peaks at age 70. Although its cause is not known, a familial tendency suggests the possibility of a genetic basis. The incidence is higher in blacks than whites and in clients who have received androgenic hormones. It is hypothesized that prostatic cancer is caused by hormonal changes, but neither the exact cause nor the relationship between host and tumor factors is clear.

Clinical Manifestations

The early clinical manifestations of prostatic cancer are similar to those of BPH, including obstructive urinary

Nursing Research Note

Scott DW, Oberst MT, Bookbinder MI: Stress-coping response to genitourinary carcinoma in men. *Nurs Res* 1984; 33(6):325–329.

Stress responses were studied in males undergoing periodic evaluation of genitourinary carcinoma. All subjects had previously been diagnosed as having a noninvasive chronic bladder cancer.

The results demonstrated that anxiety levels of the subjects were within normal range for a general outpatient population and lower than in most medical–surgical clients. It was also determined that as anxiety levels increased, critical thinking abilities declined. Educational level and critical thinking abilities were inversely related to anxiety levels postprocedure. Additional stressors and other unresolved problems were found to increase anxiety levels in this sample. Subjects exhibiting higher anxiety levels had lower educational levels, lower critical thinking skills, and were unable to resolve major problems. This group with higher anxiety levels exhibited greater behavioral responses, such as depression and helplessness.

This research suggests that assisting clients to cope effectively with life stressors is an important nursing responsibility. Coping skills can be enhanced through client education, active involvement of both family and client, adequate preparation for discharge, and follow-up.

symptoms and blood in the ejaculate. The obstruction may progress more rapidly than with BPH.

Metastasis is common in prostatic cancer, and the diagnosis is often not made until this stage. Metastatic symptoms include bone pain, low back pain radiating down the legs, weight loss, and anemia. The major site of metastasis is the bone, and other common sites include the lung, liver, and lymph nodes. With metastasis, serum acid phosphatase levels are elevated. Hematuria is a late symptom.

Rectal palpation of the prostate is recommended yearly for all men over 40 years old because this screening examination may detect the tumor in its early stages. Any asymmetry or hard lumps felt through the rectal mucosa could indicate cancer of the prostate. Differentiating between BPH and prostate cancer by rectal examination may be difficult in the early stages, so prostatic biopsy is recommended. A hard, fixed nodule may be palpated in later stages. Cystoscopy, intravenous pyelography, ultrasonography, and computerized tomography (CT) scans also may be performed as part of the diagnostic work-up. Regional lymph nodes are not usually symptomatic. Peripheral edema may occur with massive pelvic lymph node involvement. To check the status of the lymph nodes, lymphangiography and lymph node biopsy may be performed. The course of the disease is influenced by the tumor's growth rate, the tendency to metastasis, and the tumor's response to treatment.

A controversy surrounds the clinical staging classification for prostatic cancer. The two most accepted classifications are the A-B-C-D and the tumor, nodes, and

Box 67-1   Staging of Prostatic Cancer

A-B-C-D system

Stage A or stage I cancer is not clinically apparent but is detected on biopsy after surgery for BPH. Stage A prostatic cancer occurs two to three times more frequently than is actually determined clinically, according to autopsy findings.

Stage B or stage II cancer is confined within the prostatic capsule.

Stage C or stage III cancer is present with clinical evidence of local extension but no distant metastasis.

Stage D or stage IV cancer is present, along with evidence of distant metastasis.

TNM system

T: Tumor extent.

   T_x: The extent of the primary tumor cannot be assessed.

   T_0: No tumor is palpable.

   T_1: An intracapsular tumor is surrounded by a normally palpable prostate.

   T_2: The tumor is confined to the gland but is deforming its contour.

   T_3: The tumor extends beyond the capsule.

   T_4: The tumor is fixed or involves adjacent structures.

N: Node involvement.

   N_x: Metastatic regional lymph node involvement cannot be assessed.

   N_0: No involvement of regional lymph nodes exists.

   N_1: A single node is involved.

   N_2: Multiple nodes are involved.

   N_3: A fixed pelvic wall mass exists with a free space between the mass and the tumor.

   N_4: Juxtaregional nodes are involved.

M: Metastasis.

   M_x: Distant metastasis cannot be assessed.

   M_0: No metastasis has occurred.

   M_1: Distant metastasis has occurred.

metastasis (TNM) systems, although even within these systems, authorities may disagree. The A-B-C-D system is most widely accepted (see Box 67–1).

Therapeutic Measures

The treatment of prostatic cancer is based on the stage. Because there is no universal agreement on staging, however, differences in treatments vary accordingly. Stage A disease may be treated either by surgery or observation, because survival rates for both methods generally match a control group of similar age.

Stage B disease is usually treated with a radical pros-

tatectomy, possible lymph node dissection, and supplemental external beam radiation. Supervoltage radiation may be used without radical surgery. One study, however, demonstrated a significantly increased survival rate for clients after radical prostatectomy (90%) as opposed to radiation therapy (62%) (Schmidt, 1984). Some clinicians treat more advanced stages B and C disease with interstitial radiation therapy using implants of radioactive iodine (^{125}I), radioactive gold (^{198}Au), and radioactive iridium (^{192}Ir). These implants are usually performed in conjunction with pelvic lymphadenectomy.

The most common form of treatment for stage C prostatic cancer is radiation therapy with doses of 6500 to 7000 rads to the prostate and 5000 to 5500 rads to the pelvic lymph nodes. A palliative approach is taken with stage D disease. Treatment usually includes estrogen therapy, bilateral orchiectomy, or both. In most clients, the initial response to estrogen therapy is dramatic, with a disappearance of bony metastasis and bone pain as well as a shrinkage of the prostate. Hormonal failures are usually treated with chemotherapeutic agents. Fluorouracil, cyclophosphamide, cisplatin, doxorubicin, and mitomycin-C alone or in combination are administered to clients with metastatic prostatic cancer.

Specific Nursing Measures

Early detection of prostatic cancer improves the prognosis, so the nurse should teach men over age 40 to have yearly checkups that include rectal examination. Furthermore, because there is a significant correlation between gonococcal infection and later prostatic cancer, the prevention and prompt treatment of gonorrhea may help decrease the incidence of prostatic cancer.

The client with prostatic cancer feels anxious and fearful, and his body image is threatened. Not only does the client view the diagnosis of cancer as life threatening; the location in this case includes a threat to his sexual potency and overall masculinity. All nursing interactions stem from the client's need for clear, accurate information about his condition and for emotional support as he works through this massive disruption in his life. Nursing interventions related to the client facing prostatic surgery are discussed in Chapter 68.

External radiation therapy usually decreases the obstructive symptoms and increases client comfort. Proctitis, diarrhea, and urinary frequency can result, however. The client who undergoes radiation therapy in the genital area faces possible temporary or permanent sterility or impotence. Approximately 30% of these clients have problems with impotence, so for most it is realistic to believe that potency can be maintained. Chromosomal damage is also a risk. The client needs clear information about these risks as well as a good deal of emotional support as he faces these significant life changes. If the client is concerned about fertility, his sperm may be placed in a sperm bank before radiation therapy is begun. For further care of the client receiving radiation therapy, see Chapter 12.

The client receiving antiandrogen therapy (estrogen or orchiectomy) should be evaluated for a regression of symptoms. Tell the client that obstructive symptoms usually decrease, bone pain decreases, and he will gain weight and strength. Usually anemia also improves. X-rays usually show that the metastatic bone lesions are healing. Also inform the client about the side effects of this therapy, including a decreased libido and impotence; feminization, including tender gynecomastia; and edema of the ankles. Teach the client to reduce his salt intake to help control the edema. Furosemide (Lasix) also may be prescribed. These clients have an increased incidence of thromboembolism and of death from this complication. Attempt to prevent this through the use of antiembolic stockings, ambulation, and ankle pushes when in bed. Because the client may be debilitated and in great pain, mobility may be difficult to maintain.

TESTICULAR CANCER

Testicular cancer affects otherwise healthy young men between the ages of 15 and 40, and it is one of the leading causes of cancer death in that age group. Marked advances in diagnosis and treatment have increased the potential for cure, even when metastasis is present. Risk factors associated with testicular cancer include a history of cryptorchidism, a possible genetic predisposition (incidence is much higher in whites than blacks), and carcinoma in situ (malignant changes in the epithelial tissue). Skakkebaek, Berthelson, and Mitter (1982) have noted that invasive cancer occurs within 5 years of the first biopsy that detects carcinoma in situ in 50% of infertile or fertile clients with cryptorchidism.

More than 90% of testicular cancer arises from the germ cell epithelium of the testis. There are two main classifications of these tumors—seminomas and nonseminomas—depending on the tissue type. Nonseminomas are further subdivided into teratomas, embryonic carcinoma, and choriocarcinoma. The type of tumor affects both treatment and prognosis.

Clinical Manifestations

The earliest manifestation of testicular cancer is a smooth, painless lump. It usually does not adhere to the scrotal wall, so scrotal shape is maintained. If the tumor is large, the scrotum is taut and glistening. Often, the client discovers the tumor as a lump or hardening in the testes. The tumor will not transilluminate. More advanced signs include general abdominal and inguinal aching and heaviness. Pain is a late sign. When first seen by the physician, 35% of clients have either lymph node or distant metastasis.

The client with metastasis may have signs and symp-toms of a supraclavicular or abdominal mass from lymphatic spread—abdominal pain, bowel or urinary obstruction, a cough from lung metastasis, and general weight loss and anorexia. Any testicular tumor may cause gynecomastia, especially if the tumor is from choriocarcinoma.

Radioimmunoassay is performed to detect elevated HCG and alpha-fetoprotein levels; their increase depends on the type of tumor. The HCG level is often elevated in clients with embryonal cancer and is always elevated in clients with choriocarcinoma (Javadpour, 1980). Alpha-fetoprotein levels are often elevated in clients with teratoma and embryonal cancer.

Therapeutic Measures

Therapy for testicular cancer is based on the stage of the disease. Staging classifications vary, but there is general agreement on progression (Javadpour, 1980): in stage I or A, the tumor is limited to the testis; in stage II or B, there is metastasis to regional lymph nodes; and in stage III or C, there is metastasis to distant organs.

An orchiectomy with high ligation of the spermatic cord is performed upon the initial discovery of the tumor. The surgery is useful for diagnosis, differentiation of the tumor, and staging. Seminomas, the most common type of testicular tumors, are radiosensitive; postoperative radiation therapy to the lymph drainage areas of the testes is employed to treat this type of tumor. Javadpour (1980) reports that radiation therapy results in a 5-year survival rate of more than 90%. In stage I, supervoltage radiation is given to the inguinal, aortic, and caval lymph areas. In stage II, the mediastinal and supraclavicular lymph nodes are also included. The prophylactic dose is 2000 rads in 2 weeks and the therapeutic dose, 3000 rads in 3 weeks. The survival rates with stage III are between 28% and 55% after radiation therapy (Javadpour, 1980). Stage III disease is treated with chemotherapy (usually cyclophosphamide and cisplatin).

Nonseminomatous tumors with negative tumor markers (HCG and AFP are not elevated) and nodes are treated postoperatively with x-rays and followed with tumor markers for 2 years. Clients who have stage II disease showing either positive nodes or markers are treated with chemotherapy. Those with stage III disease are treated with node dissection and chemotherapy.

Babian (1984) describes the following chemotherapeutic regimen for the treatment of nonseminomatous testicular tumors: vinblastine sulfate (Velban; 0.3 mg/kg in two equally divided doses on Days 1 and 2), cisplatin (100 mg per square meter in 3 to 5 equally divided doses starting on Day 1), and bleomycin (30 units on Day 1 and repeated weekly for a total of 360 units). The vinblastine sulfate and cisplatin regimens are repeated every 3 weeks for four courses. Other agents that have been used to treat nonseminomatous tumors include methotrexate, actinomycin D, chlorambucil, and vincristine sulfate.

Specific Nursing Measures

Early detection and treatment are critical for the client with testicular cancer. Therefore, all adolescent males should be taught TSE and should perform it monthly. Testicular self-examination is discussed and illustrated in Chapter 7.

The client with testicular cancer should be informed that prompt treatment holds the promise of cure. He requires a great deal of emotional support as he faces surgery, radiation, or chemotherapy. Most men maintain sexual function after surgery, although retrograde ejaculation may cause infertility problems. Artificial insemination using the client's sperm is possible if sperm is obtained, frozen, and banked before treatment.

The client receiving chemotherapy faces problems of bone marrow depression leading to anemia, susceptibility to infections, and the potential for hemorrhage. He also may face the disfigurement of alopecia and the discomfort of stomatitis, nausea, and vomiting. Providing long rest periods, protecting the client from infection, and avoiding any trauma that can lead to hemorrhage are important nursing interventions. Antiemetics such as perphenazine (Trilafon) should be given before meals and chemotherapy treatments to help decrease nausea and vomiting. To help relieve stomatitis, the client should avoid spicy foods and have frequent mouth care with a nonalcohol-based mouthwash (commercial mouthwashes contain alcohol). Gargling with an anesthetic mouthwash such as viscous lidocaine (Xylocaine) before meals may help relieve the pain so that the client can eat. The alopecia is temporary, and the client may wish to wear a hairpiece or hat during this time. For further nursing care related to the client receiving radiation therapy or chemotherapy, see Chapter 12.

CANCER OF THE PENIS

Although rare in North America, cancer of the penis is a significant worldwide health problem. Its highest incidence is in men in their 60s and 70s. A contributing causative factor is poor hygiene.

Clinical Manifestations

Lesions considered to be precancerous are leukoplakia and painful velvety red plaques (erythroplasia of Queyrat) on the dorsal aspect of the uncircumcised penis. The most common cancerous lesion is squamous cell carcinoma, which usually is seen as a visible lesion on the glans or prepuce. Penile discharge also may be present.

There is no consensus on the staging of penile carcinoma. Babian (1984) stages clients in the following manner: in stage I, the tumor is confined to the penis; in stage II, there is suggested ilioinguinal regional node metastasis; and in stage III, there is disseminated metastasis.

Therapeutic Measures

The treatment of cancer of the penis depends on the stage and location. In stage I, if the disease is on the prepuce, a circumcision is performed. If the lesion is on the distal shaft, a partial penectomy is performed. Any stage other than stage I requires a total penectomy. Lymphadenectomy is indicated if the nodes are diseased. In a young client with a small lesion, external radiation may be used instead of surgery. A client with inoperable nodes or metastatic disease is treated with systemic chemotherapy (usually bleomycin or methotrexate). The 5-year survival rates for cancer of the penis are not good: stage I has a 65% survival rate; stage II, a 20% rate; and stage III, a 1% survival rate (Babian, 1984).

Specific Nursing Measures

Teaching clients the importance of basic hygiene is important in the prevention of penile cancer. The uncircumcised client must understand that daily retraction of the prepuce and washing the penis are essential. The client and his partner require a great deal of emotional support as they face disfiguring surgery that directly threatens male identity, sexual performance, and fertility.

Section V: Traumatic Disorders

Trauma to the male genitals can have a variety of causes. Some causes include a penetrating or blunt injury, catching the clothing in a power tool, the congestion or impairment of circulation, or a drug reaction.

General Nursing Implications

Trauma to the genitals, like any other trauma, can constitute an emergency. If major blood vessels have been damaged, life-threatening hemorrhage can occur; the client needs treatment for shock. The prompt relief of impaired circulation to the penis may preserve this vital organ. Quick reporting and surgical exploration of scrotal injuries may preserve testicular function.

The client who has suffered a penetrating injury to the genitals should be assessed for the point of entry of the bullet, knife, shrapnel, or other object. Discoloration of the penis or scrotum may indicate trauma, impaired circulation, or both. The nurse should note the presence of hemorrhage.

TRAUMA TO THE PENIS

Trauma to the penis can result from a bullet or stab wound or can be caused by catching the clothing in a power tool. Circulation to the penis can be impaired as a result of strangulation from a twisted condom catheter, a string wrapped around the penis, a tight ring, or a worker's tool. A blunt injury to an erect penis can lead to corporeal or urethral rupture.

Clinical Manifestations and Therapeutic Measures

The clinical manifestations depend on the cause of the trauma. Treatment also depends on the cause of the trauma. Damage from a penetrating missile must be surgically repaired as soon as possible. The management of a strangulation injury includes removal of the object.

Specific Nursing Measures

Teach the client to avoid wrapping anything tight or constricting around the penis and to use power tools carefully. The client with trauma to the penis needs substantial emotional support in dealing with the disfigurement and surgery.

SCROTAL INJURIES

Scrotal injuries are not common, because the scrotum is mobile and the scrotal muscles retract reflexively. Blunt or penetrating objects can injure the scrotum, however.

Clinical Manifestations and Therapeutic Measures

The signs and symptoms of scrotal injuries are determined by the cause. Trauma to the scrotum usually requires surgical exploration and treatment for the particular problem. Prompt surgical intervention minimizes damage to the testes. Nonsurgical intervention includes elevating the scrotum and applying ice. Neither measure preserves the testes, however.

Specific Nursing Measures

Provide the client with specific information about the extent of injury and treatment, and emotional support. Bed rest and scrotal elevation are quite important after a scrotal injury. Whenever the client is ambulatory, the client should wear a scrotal support and should avoid strenuous activity, lifting heavy objects, or climbing stairs for several days after the injury.

Chapter Highlights

Disorders of the male reproductive system can result from congenital anomalies, infectious diseases, neoplasms, or trauma; they also may be of multifactorial origin.

The male client with a reproductive system disorder may undergo an altered body image and sexual dysfunction. Thus, emotional support is a key nursing intervention.

Cryptorchidism, failure of the testes to descend into the scrotum, is the most common disorder of prenatal sex differentiation in males.

Male reproductive system disorders of multifactorial origin include phimosis, paraphimosis, hydrocele, spermatocele, varicocele, and priapism.

The incidence of STDs is increasing and is a major cause of infectious disease of the male reproductive system.

An important nursing role in caring for STD clients is teaching them about the disease's incidence, mode of transmission, preventive measures, and treatments.

Infectious disorders that affect the male reproductive system include gonorrhea, NGU, epididymitis, prostatitis, lymphogranuloma venereum, syphilis, chancroid, condylomata acuminata (venereal warts), molluscum contagiosum, and herpes genitalis.

Neoplasms of the male reproductive system contribute significantly to the overall mortality of male clients.

Benign prostatic hyperplasia is the most common neoplasm in men. Surgery is the most common therapeutic measure.

Early detection of prostatic cancer improves the client's prognosis, so the nurse should encourage yearly rectal examinations for men over age 40.

Testicular self-examination is a simple means of early detection of testicular cancer. This should be taught to all adolescent males and practiced throughout adulthood.

Trauma to the penis or scrotum can constitute an emergency and can result in serious damage to urinary and sexual function.

Bibliography

Alexander RE: Maternal and infant sexually transmitted diseases. *Urol Clin North Am* 1984; 11(1):131–139.

Babian R: Malignant tumors of the urogenital tract. In: *Conn's Current Therapy*. Pakel RE (editor). Philadelphia: Saunders, 1984.

Belker A: The varicocele and male infertility. *Urol Clin North Am* 1981; 8(1):41–45.

Bowie WR: Nongonococcal urethritis in sexually transmitted disease. *Urol Clin North Am* 1984; 11(1).

Centers for Disease Control: Sexually transmitted disease treatment guidelines. *MMWR* 1982; 31:Suppl to No. 25.

Droller MJ: Cancer of the testes: An overview. *Urol Clin North Am* 1980; 7(3):731–733.

Drusin LM: Syphilis: Clinical manifestations, diagnosis and treatment. *Urol Clin North Am* 1984; 11(1):121–130.

Haggerty BJ: Prevention and differential of scrotal cancer. *Nurse Pract* 1983; 8(10):45–52.

Harrison WO: Gonococcal urethritis. *Urol Clin North Am* 1984; 11(1):45–54.

Holmes KK, Bell TA, Berger RE: Epidemiology of sexually transmitted disease. *Urol Clin North Am* 1984; 11(1):3–12.

Ireton RC, Berger RE: Prostatitis and epididymitis. *Urol Clin North Am* 1984; 11(1):83–93.

Javadpour N: Germ cell tumor of the testes. *CA* 1980; 30:242–255.

Krieger JN: Biology of sexually transmitted disease. *Urol Clin North Am* 1984; 11(1):15–25.

Lerner J, Khan Z: *Mosby's Manual of Urologic Nursing*. St. Louis: Mosby, 1982.

Long PP: Prostatic cancer. *Nurs 81* (Dec) 1981; 11:22–23.

Margolis S: Genital warts and molluscum contagiosum. *Urol Clin North Am* 1984; 11(1):163–170.

Martin DC: Malignancy in the cryptorchid testis. *Urol Clin North Am* 1982; 9(3):371–375.

McConnell EA, Zimmerman MF: *Care of Patients With Urologic Problems*. Philadelphia: Lippincott, 1983.

McDougal WS, Persky L: *Traumatic Injuries to the Genitourinary System*. Baltimore: Williams & Wilkins, 1981.

Mertz G, Corey L: Genital herpes simplex virus infections in adults. *Urol Clin North Am* 1984; 11(1):103–117.

Messing E, deKernion JB: Adjuvant therapy for genitourinary cancer. *Surg Clin North Am* 1981; 61(6):1331–1343.

Reichman RC et al: Treatment of recurrent genital herpes simplex infections with oral acyclovir: A controlled trial. *JAMA* 1984; 251:2103–2107.

Ritchie JP, Garnick MB: Changing concepts in the treatment of non-seminatous germ cell tumors of the testes. *J Urol* 1984; 131:1089–1092.

Roseman D et al: Sexually transmitted disease and carcinogenesis. *Urol Clin North Am* 1984; 11(1):27–44.

Schmidt JD: Treatment of localized prostatic carcinoma. *Urol Clin North Am* 1984; 11(2):305–309.

Skakkebaek NE, Berthelson JG, Mitter J: Carcinoma in situ of the undescended testes. *Urol Clin North Am* 1982; 9(3):377–386.

Spirnack PJ, Resnick ML: Disturbed sexual function due to spermatocele. *Med Aspects Hum Sexuality* 1984; 18(1):221–236.

Sullivan LD: Benign prostatic hyperplasia. In: *Conn's Current Treatment*. Pakel, RE (editor). Philadelphia: Saunders, 1984; 534–538.

Zelikovsky G: Cryptorchidism. *Med Aspects Hum Sexuality* (April) 1983; 17(4):135–147.

Suggested Readings

Berger RE (editor): Symposium on sexually transmitted diseases. *Urol Clin North Am* 1984; 11(1). [Entire issue.] An excellent group of articles describes the current status and treatment of STDs.

Campbell CE, Herton JR: VD to STD: Redefining venereal disease. *Am J Nurs* 1981; 81:1629–1635. This review of STDs includes informative charts and illustrations.

Haggerty BJ: Prevention and differential of scrotal cancer. *Nurse Pract* 1983; 8(10):45–52. Testicular cancer and TSE as a means of early detection are described.

Centers for Disease Control: *Questions and Answers on Genital Herpes*. US Department of Health and Human Services, Washington, DC, 1982. Available from the CDC Center for Prevention Services, Atlanta. This brochure is useful in the nurse's health teaching and is suitable for distribution to clients.

Weisner PJ: Magnitude of the problem of sexually transmitted diseases in the United States. 1980 Status Report. Center for Prevention Services, Centers for Disease Control. This article identifies the problem of dealing with STDs in our society.

Chapter 68

Surgical Approaches to Male Reproductive System Dysfunction

Phyllis Foster Healy

When you have finished studying this chapter, you should be able to:

Identify common types of surgery performed on the male reproductive tract.

Delineate the usual indications for surgical intervention in male reproductive problems.

Describe basic surgical procedures performed on the male reproductive tract.

Explain the physiological and psychosocial/lifestyle implications of surgical intervention for male reproductive system disorders.

Discuss the preoperative nursing care for the male facing surgical intervention for a reproductive tract problem.

Develop a postoperative plan of care for the client with each disorder.

Specify nursing interventions to prevent anticipated postoperative complications.

Surgical approaches to disorders of the male reproductive system include operative procedures of the prostate gland, penis, and testes and related structures. Like women, men react to the loss of sexual organs and the ability to reproduce with changes in body image and feelings of loss and grief. The client's physical and emotional recovery from reproductive system surgery is affected by the type of surgery, knowledge level, self-concept, lifestyle, and support systems. The well-informed nurse plays an important role in providing education and emotional support to these clients.

Section I: Surgical Approaches to Disorders Affecting the Prostate Gland

The surgical removal of the prostate gland is called a prostatectomy. Often only the adenomatous (enlarged) tissue is removed, resulting in a subtotal prostatectomy. A complete prostatectomy, in contrast, includes removal of all prostatic tissue, as well as the prostatic capsule. Four general approaches are used for prostatectomy: the transurethral, suprapubic, retropubic, and perineal. Factors such as the client's general physical condition and the specific urologic problem affect the selection of surgical approach.

Radical prostatectomies are performed on clients with cancer of the prostate. They are called radical because in addition to the removal of the prostate gland, the seminal vesicles, bladder neck cuff, and often the pelvic lymph nodes, are also surgically removed. They are performed as a retropubic or perineal prostatectomy. The newer retropubic approach is increasingly preferred because of the increased exposure it allows and because the pelvic lymph glands can be explored and removed at the time of surgery. Because the procedure for radical surgery is extensive, it is generally agreed that the candidate should have at least a 10-year life expectancy, be under 70, and be in good medical condition. Most surgeons agree that clinical stage B prostatic cancer should be treated with radical prostatectomy. Selected clients with stages A and C cancer also may be treated in this fashion. Debate continues on the risks versus advantages of pelvic lymphadenectomy, but for selected clients it will increase life expectancy.

TRANSURETHRAL RESECTION

The transurethral resection (TUR) of the prostate, or transurethral prostatectomy (TURP), is by far the most common type of prostatic surgery. Between 85% and 95% of clients needing prostatectomies are treated with TUR, which involves removal of the prostate gland via the urethra. The major indication for performing a TUR is obstructive benign prostatic hyperplasia that no longer can be managed medically. This approach requires no surgical incision, which makes it particularly useful for the elderly client needing relief of obstructive symptoms, such as from malignant prostatic nodules. Very small cancerous lesions also can be removed transurethrally.

For a successful TUR, most surgeons think the prostate should be small (less than 40 g). A TUR is contraindicated for clients with hip joint problems or prior hip surgery because the procedure requires that the client be in a lithotomy position. If bladder diverticula or large bladder calculi are present, an open surgical procedure (usually a suprapubic prostatectomy) is performed. One major disadvantage of the TUR is that prostatic tissue remains, so hyperplasia can occur again.

Surgical Procedure

After the administration of anesthesia, the client is placed in a lithotomy position. Spinal anesthesia is preferred, but general anesthesia is sometimes used. A cystoscopy is performed, and a resectoscope is then inserted through the cystoscope and used to scrape out the medial lobe of the enlarged prostate (Figure 68–1). Irrigating fluid is constantly infused into the bladder to keep the operative field visible, and full visualization is achieved by the use of a fiberoptic light. A retention catheter is frequently inserted at this time to provide for continuous irrigation and drainage during the postoperative period.

Implications for the Client

The physiological and psychosocial/lifestyle implications of clients undergoing TUR are similar to those for clients undergoing the other three prostatectomy approaches. Following is an overview of all client implications, with an emphasis on TUR.

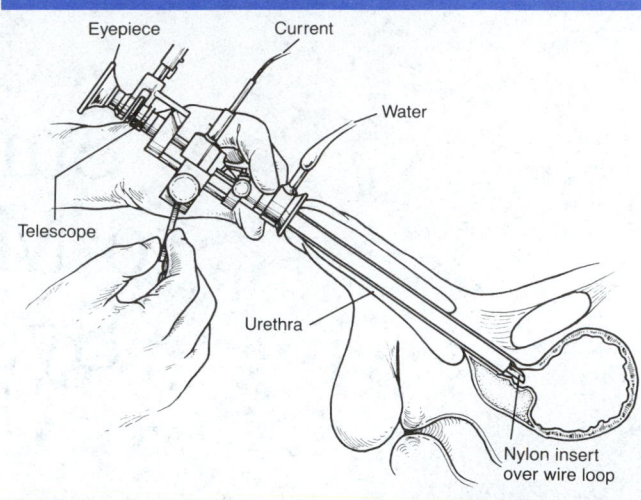

Figure 68–1

Transurethral prostatectomy. The telescope and lamp assist the surgeon in locating and resecting prostatic tissue. A rotating wire loop at the end of the resectoscope connected to a cutting current shaves off the enlarged prostatic tissue, which is then flushed away.

Physiological Implications

After a prostatectomy, **retrograde ejaculation** (backflow of ejaculate into the bladder) occurs as a result of injury to the bladder neck. Although the client is not sterile, he is infertile and his urine appears cloudy after orgasm. Impotence should not be a problem after TUR, but it sometimes occurs. Usually, there is no apparent physical cause for impotence after a TUR. It is believed to be related to a high level of fear and anxiety associated with the surgery. A positive approach, telling the client that he should be able to resume his previous level of sexual functioning, might prevent the condition from developing.

Urinary incontinence can occur after prostatectomy as a result of damage to the urinary sphincter. Usually, the incontinence is temporary and may be brought on by urgency or stress.

Postoperative hemorrhage and clot formation are serious and frequent complications that present risks after any prostatectomy. A TUR may cause a great deal of intraoperative bleeding. Venous bleeding is common in the initial postoperative period, and delayed bleeding may occur during the first 2 to 3 weeks. Dark blood is common in the urine. Bleeding is usually treated by inserting a large retention catheter, inflating the balloon with 30 mL or more of fluid, and then pulling the catheter so the balloon lodges against the bladder neck, applying pressure on the bleeding prostatic fossa (Figure 68–2). Usually, traction is maintained for 4 to 8 hours, depending on the client's condition. A two- or three-way Foley catheter is left in place and connected to gravity drainage.

Surgical opinion about continuous bladder irrigation is divided; this technique mechanically irrigates the bladder, preventing clots from forming and clogging the catheter. Some surgeons routinely use a three-way catheter and con-

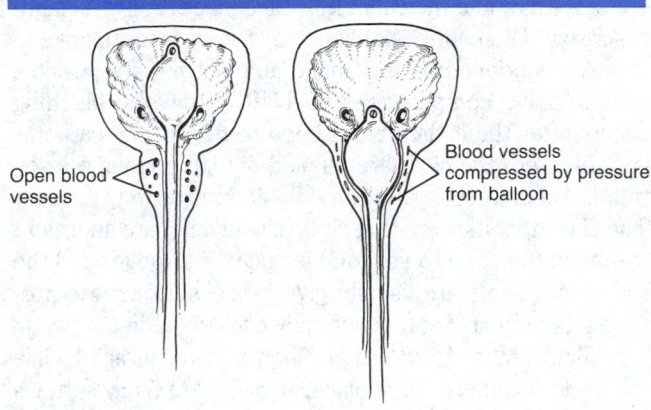

Open blood vessels

Blood vessels compressed by pressure from balloon

Figure 68–2
Traction by in-dwelling catheter after prostatectomy.

tinuously irrigate with a solution such as 1.5% glycine for 24 hours postoperatively. Others do not think continuous bladder irrigation is necessary and do not order it unless the catheter is not draining.

At the end of surgery, clients are usually given 20 to 40 mg of furosemide (Lasix) intravenously to promote diuresis. Some surgeons administer the antifibrinolytic drug epsilon-aminocaproic acid (EACA) to decrease bleeding by inhibiting the action of urokinase in the urine.

Like other surgical clients, the postprostatectomy client is at risk of developing atelectasis, pulmonary embolism, and other respiratory complications. This is particularly true for clients with pre-existing respiratory problems and those whose prostate is removed via an abdominal approach. In addition, the lithotomy position used for TUR clients

makes them particularly vulnerable to postoperative deep vein phlebitis. Postoperatively, the client also is at risk for urinary tract infection, bladder spasms, and urethral stricture. Electrolyte system imbalances may develop, especially hyponatremia from the absorption of irrigating fluid.

Because clients undergoing TUR are usually over 60 years old, they may have other health problems such as cardiovascular insufficiency, pulmonary insufficiency, renal dysfunction, or hepatic dysfunction. TUR should be performed only after such conditions have been assessed and stabilized. Urinary tract infections should also be eradicated before TUR.

Psychosocial/Lifestyle Implications

After prostatectomy, clients' sexual relationships may be a problem because of impotence. Further social isolation may occur because of urinary incontinence. Incontinence usually resolves a few days or weeks after catheter removal, however. Infertility caused by retrograde ejaculation may be a problem for some clients. Clients should avoid strenuous activity for 6 weeks and intercourse for 4 to 6 weeks. The physiological and psychosocial/lifestyle implications of the client undergoing a TUR are summarized in Table 68–1.

Nursing Implications

Preoperative Care

Clients facing any type of prostatectomy have many concerns that the nurse should address. Clark and O'Connell (1984) list clients' major concerns as: Will I be impotent? Will I be less masculine? Will I be sterile? Will I be able to go back to work? Will I lose control of urination?

Table 68–1 Prostatectomy: Implications for the Client	
Physiological Implications	**Psychosocial/Lifestyle Implications**
Retrograde ejaculation	Impaired relationship as a result of impotence
Urinary incontinence (usually temporary)	Social isolation as a result of incontinence
Postoperative hemorrhage and clot formation	Infertility secondary to retrograde ejaculation
Atelectasis, pulmonary embolism, and other respiratory complications	No strenuous activity for 6 weeks
Postoperative deep vein thrombosis, especially if exaggerated lithotomy position required	No intercourse for 4 to 6 weeks
Urinary tract infection	Body image and self-esteem changes with altered sexual functioning
Bladder spasms	
Urethral stricture	
Electrolyte system imbalances (especially hyponatremia)	
Risk of impotence, especially with perineal prostatectomy	
Scrotal and leg lymphedema after radical prostatectomy	
Urinary and fecal incontinence from sphincter damage during perineal prostatectomy	

Providing full information to the preoperative client facing a prostatectomy is a critically important nursing function, not only because the client needs accurate information to help allay his fears but also because the client has a right to this information. The nurse should explain, for example, any activity limitations the client will face postoperatively. Besides giving information, provide the opportunity for the client to verbalize his concerns so his preoperative anxiety can be kept at a manageable level. For example, fears of cancer are common and not unrealistic.

Standard preoperative preparation includes a general preoperative work-up, blood typing and crossmatching, renal function tests (BUN and serum creatinine tests), an intravenous pyelogram, voiding cystograms, and cystometric evaluation. The client with a urinary tract infection should have a culture and sensitivity study done, and specific antibiotic therapy should be started before surgery. Surgery is delayed until the urinary tract infection is under control. Some surgeons administer antibiotics prophylactically, although this use of broad-spectrum antibiotics is controversial. If the client has a urinary catheter in place preoperatively, strict aseptic technique is essential. The maintenance of catheter drainage is an important aspect of nursing care.

A client facing a prostatectomy should come to surgery well hydrated, so encourage drinking of fluids and monitor the client being hydrated with preoperative IV fluids. Because prostatic surgery is usually performed on elderly clients, overhydration must be avoided.

Preoperative preparation also should include a careful history to check for any prior respiratory or vascular problems that may contribute to postoperative complications. Clients should be informed about what tubes and drains to expect postoperatively. After a TUR, a client will have a two- or three-way Foley catheter in place. He also may have continuous bladder irrigation. Tell the client that this may cause him to feel the urge to void, but caution him that bearing down as if to void will contribute to bladder spasms. Bladder spasms will be relieved with antispasmodics.

Elastic bandages are usually placed on the legs preoperatively and are also used intraoperatively and postoperatively. Anticipate the need for antiembolic stockings and take calf measurements preoperatively so stockings will be available as soon as possible postoperatively.

Postoperative Care

The usual nursing care given any client after surgery also applies to the postprostatectomy client. Take vital signs every 15 minutes until they are stable, then progress to every hour and then every 4 hours. Intake and output, level of mobility, and consciousness also should be assessed. Monitor electrolyte, BUN, and creatinine levels.

Generally, ambulation and hourly deep breathing and coughing are performed on the first postoperative day. Frequent turning, toe wiggling, and gentle leg exercises should be done with assistance the night after surgery. Fluids are administered intravenously until the first post-operative day, and the client may take fluids orally the night of surgery. Thereafter, the client may take a diet as tolerated.

As mentioned, hemorrhage and clotting are possible postoperative complications of TUR. If delayed bleeding occurs after the catheter has been removed, the catheter is reinserted, the clots are flushed out, traction is reinstituted, and diuresis is instituted by administering IV fluids. The clues that indicate that clots are forming are an urgent feeling of the need to void and leakage of urine around the catheter. Clients are usually given stool softeners to prevent straining at stool, which may cause bleeding.

Fluid intake of 2 to 3 L/day should be encouraged while the urinary catheter is in place, usually 2 to 5 days after a TUR. If the client has continuous bladder irrigation, the nurse should carefully record intake and output, making sure to account for the irrigating fluid. If the urine is bloody, the catheter stays in longer, and the rate of irrigating fluid should be increased. Restraints may be required because clients confused after surgery may try to get out of bed and pull out their catheters. If clots form in the single-lumen catheter, manual irrigation may be required to remove them.

The 30-mL balloon and traction used after a prostatectomy contribute to the postoperative problem of painful bladder spasms. These spasms are made worse if clotting obstructs the catheter or the client attempts to void around the catheter. The spasms can be recognized by the client's subjective sensation of pain, by palpation of the contracted bladder, and leakage of urine around the catheter. Instruct the client not to attempt to void around the catheter even though he may feel an intense urge to do so. Explain that this urge is caused by the feeling of fullness created by the large balloon and the traction. Maintaining catheter patency will reduce the frequency of spasms. Belladona and opium (B and O) suppositories or other antispasmodics are used to relieve spasms.

The risk of infection increases when an in-dwelling catheter is present. Forcing fluids to prevent stasis of urine is one means to help prevent infection. Strict asepsis and maintaining a closed drainage system are also important. Report any signs of urinary tract infection, such as fever; cloudy, foul-smelling urine; or mucous shreds in the urine. The high risk of infection after prostatectomy usually necessitates the administration of prophylactic antibiotics.

The client may experience urinary incontinence for a few days after catheter removal. Teach the client to do exercises designed to increase sphincter tone, such as Kegel exercises, which are done by tightly squeezing the perineal muscles five to ten times each hour. (Kegel exercises are described in Chapter 64.) Starting and then stopping the urinary stream also helps strengthen the sphincter. Medications such as propantheline bromide (Pro-Banthine) or ephedrine may be used. Propantheline bromide relaxes the bladder, thus decreasing the voiding reflex. Ephedrine increases sphincter tone. The client with incontinence that continues for 6 months after surgery may require external drainage or the insertion of an artificial sphincter. Straining to void and a decrease in the urinary stream could indicate the development of urethral stricture. Observe for these signs and report them to the physician.

Assess the client for signs of hypervolemia and hyponatremia by watching for signs of cerebral edema (changes in level of consciousness, notable confusion, twitching, irritability, convulsions, and coma) within the first 24 hours. The irrigating fluid used for continuous bladder irrigation should be isotonic. A client with water intoxication may be placed on restricted fluids and given sodium.

Positioning during surgery may affect postoperative recovery. Because clients who have had a TUR will have been in the lithotomy position, which predisposes them to deep vein thrombosis and subsequent pulmonary embolism, they may be treated with prophylactic minidoses of 4000 to 5000 units of heparin every 8 to 12 hours.

If elastic bandages or antiembolic stockings have been used, they should be removed each shift and the condition of the underlying skin checked. Early ambulation, hourly coughing and deep breathing, and ankle exercises while in bed also can be helpful preventive measures. Avoid applying pressure on the popliteal and calf areas. The client should not cross his legs, and the bed should not be gatched. Because of the risk of pulmonary embolus, calf massage should be avoided.

Most persons over age 60 still have active sex lives, so postoperative impotence is a serious concern. The impotent client needs time to grieve and verbalize his feelings postoperatively because the impotence will threaten his masculine identity and body image. The client may be a candidate for a penile implant, or alternatives to genital sex can be explored. If impotence presents a problem for the client after a simple prostatectomy, the possible psychosocial sources of this problem should be explored.

Basic instructions that the nurse should give the client upon discharge include:

- No intercourse for 4 to 6 weeks. See the physician before resuming sexual activity.
- No strenuous activity or heavy lifting for at least 6 weeks because activities that increase intra-abdominal pressure may cause bleeding.
- Avoid all driving as well as riding on bumpy roads.
- Take stool softeners as ordered to prevent the straining that occurs with constipation.
- Maintain a daily fluid intake of 2 to 3 L.
- Watch for delayed hemorrhage, and report it immediately to the physician.

SUPRAPUBIC PROSTATECTOMY

In the suprapubic approach, the prostate gland is removed through an incision in the bladder via the lower abdomen. This procedure can relieve the symptoms of obstructive prostatic hypertrophy and is often used when surgical removal of bladder calculi or diverticula is also needed. It also may be used when the prostatic enlargement is too great for TUR.

Surgical Procedure

The suprapubic prostatectomy is sometimes referred to as transvesical prostatectomy because the prostate is approached through a low abdominal suprapubic incision and then through an incision in the bladder (Figures 68–3A and B). The bladder contents are aspirated, the mucosa over the prostate is removed by electrocautery, and the prostatic contents are removed digitally. Both a urethral catheter and suprapubic tube are placed, and a small drain is placed in the lower abdomen (Figure 68–3C).

Implications for the Client

Physiological Implications
The abdominal approach used in suprapubic prostatectomy increases the risk of respiratory complications, especially in vulnerable clients. Urine leaking from the bladder into surrounding tissues can lead to infection. Other physiological implications for the client are similar to those for clients undergoing TUR. Hemorrhage and bladder spasms

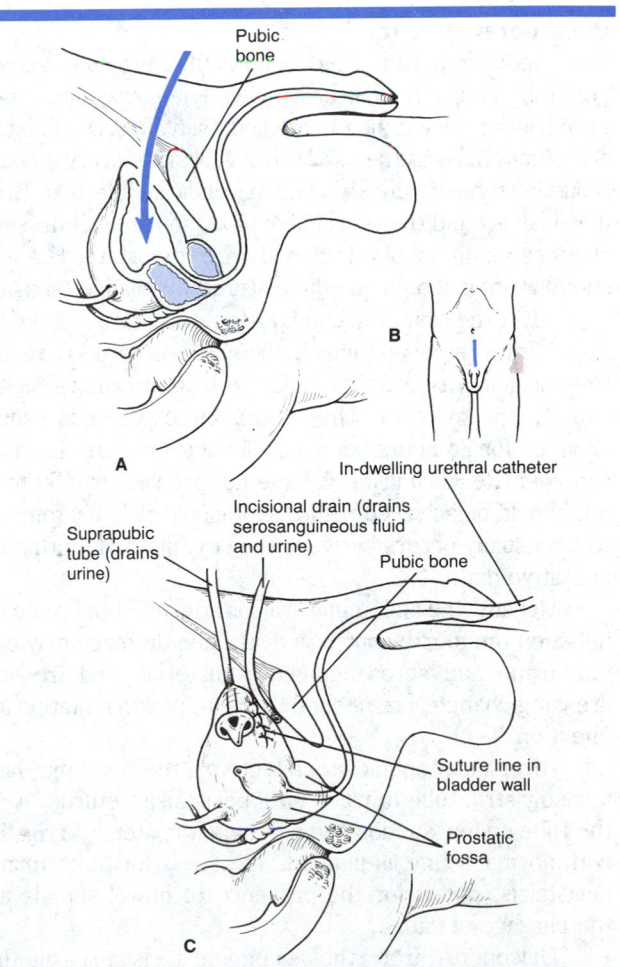

Figure 68–3

Suprapubic prostatectomy. **A.** Side view. **B.** Incision line. **C.** Suture lines and drainage tubes.

are some of the more common postoperative problems. Urinary continence and sexual function usually are unaltered, however. The client is NPO and receives IV fluids until intestinal motility returns in 3 to 5 days.

Psychosocial/Lifestyle Implications

The psychosocial and lifestyle implications for the suprapubic prostatectomy client are similar to those for clients undergoing TUR. A summary of the client implications for suprapubic prostatectomy is found in Table 68–1.

Nursing Implications

Preoperative Care

Preoperative care for the client having a suprapubic prostatectomy is similar to that for a client having a TUR. Major nursing activities include providing information about implications of the procedure, maintaining catheter care, monitoring hydration, and taking a history to assess the risk of postoperative complications.

Postoperative Care

The recovery period after a suprapubic prostatectomy is generally longer than after a TUR. The nurse should perform routine daily catheter care and maintain accurate intake and output measurements. Assess vital signs every 4 hours. A sudden temperature elevation may indicate infection. Urine may leak around the suprapubic tube, so frequent dressing changes using aseptic technique are important. B and O suppositories should be administered for bladder spasms.

After the first or second postoperative day, one of the catheters is removed (usually the Foley catheter) to reduce the possibility of urethral stricture from inflammation and subsequent scarring. The suprapubic catheter is usually clamped for 24 hours before removal to be sure the client can void. Residual urine volume not greater than 50 to 75 mL should be achieved before suprapubic catheter removal, which usually occurs between the seventh and tenth postoperative day.

Usually, the abdominal drain is advanced and removed between the fourth and sixth days. The drainage may contain urine and serosanguineous material, and frequent dressing changes are needed to prevent skin irritation and infection.

After a suprapubic prostatectomy, the client may have a nasogastric tube in place until peristalsis returns. Keep the tube on low suction and maintain its patency, irrigating with normal saline as needed. To assess for the return of peristalsis, check for the presence of bowel sounds and the passage of flatus.

Discomfort from the abdominal incision is another postoperative condition requiring nursing intervention. Narcotic analgesics can relieve incisional pain. Other applicable postoperative nursing interventions are discussed in the section on TUR.

RETROPUBIC PROSTATECTOMY

In the retropubic approach (also called a retrovesical prostatectomy), a low abdominal incision is made, and the prostate gland is entered directly. The retropubic approach, which totally removes all prostatic tissue, is used when the prostate is larger than 100 g (too large for TUR) or when malignant tissue needs to be surgically excised. Because the client is in a supine slight Trendelenburg's position, this approach can be used when the lithotomy position is contraindicated. The procedure's two major advantages over the suprapubic approach are better control of bleeding because of direct access to the surgical site and elimination of the need for a suprapubic catheter postoperatively unless there is extensive bleeding.

Surgical Procedure

This procedure is performed under general anesthesia. The surgeon makes a low abdominal incision without making an opening into the bladder (Figures 68–4A and B),

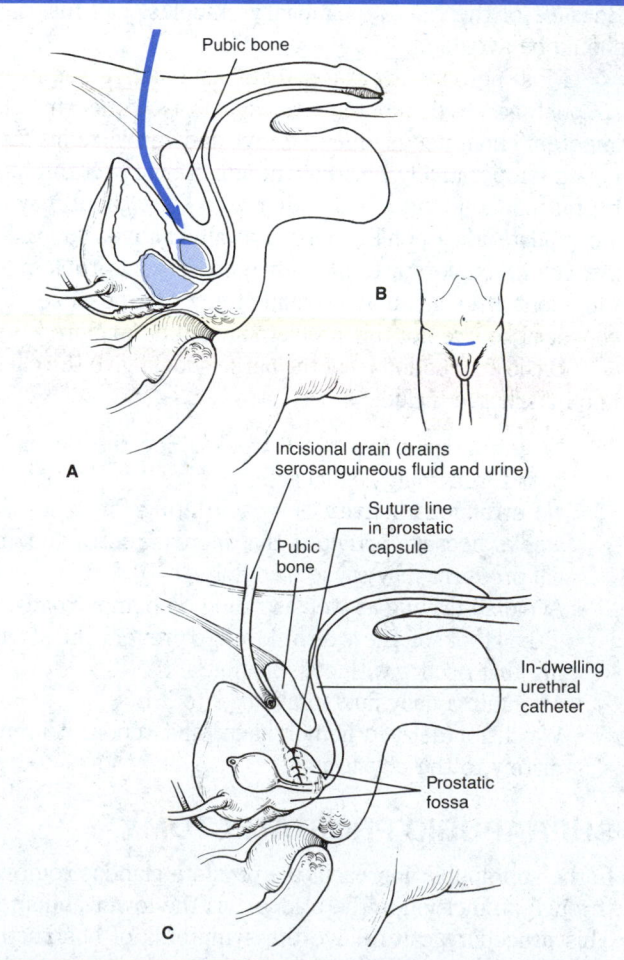

Figure 68–4

Retropubic prostatectomy. **A.** Side view. **B.** Incision line. **C.** Suture lines and drainage tubes.

incises the capsule of the prostate, and in a simple retropubic prostatectomy, removes glandular tissue. One or two drains are placed into the abdominal incision, and an indwelling urethral catheter is also placed (Figure 68–4C).

A radical retropubic prostatectomy involves the total removal of the prostate, ejaculatory ducts, seminal vesicles, and fascia. Frequently, a radical lymphadenectomy is performed prior to the removal of the prostate. Some surgeons think that if metastatic nodes are found, the surgery should not be performed (Veenema & Wechsler, 1984).

Implications for the Client

Physiological Implications
The abdominal approach used in the retropubic prostatectomy increases the risk of respiratory complications, especially in vulnerable clients. Rectal injury may occur during radical retropubic prostatectomy and is usually repaired at the time of surgery. Severe damage can lead to bowel incontinence. The client who has a radical retropubic prostatectomy with lymphadenectomy may have a problem postoperatively with scrotal and leg edema. Almost all clients are impotent after a radical prostatectomy because of damage to the parasympathetic nerves and after lymphadenectomy because of damage to the sympathetic nerves. Thus, the client facing radical surgery should be informed that impotence is likely. For clients who wish to remain sexually active, a penile implant can be inserted later to correct this problem.

The incision causes postoperative discomfort. Retropubic prostatectomy clients have minimal problems with bladder spasm or intraoperative and postoperative hemorrhage, however. See the section on TUR for further physiological implications.

Psychosocial/Lifestyle Implications
Refer to the discussion of TUR. Physiological and psychosocial/lifestyle implications of retropubic prostatectomy are summarized in Table 68–1.

Nursing Implications

Preoperative Care
Clients undergoing radical prostatectomy often have a bowel preparation preoperatively to be sure the bowel is cleared in case of bowel injury. This consists of enemas, the administration of an antibiotic such as neomycin, and a low-residue diet. For other nursing implications of retropubic prostatectomy, refer to the discussion of TUR.

Postoperative Care
After a retropubic prostatectomy, the client has an indwelling catheter in place. Assess its patency and measure intake and output. A major postoperative nursing goal is the prevention of urinary tract infection; thus, the nurse should maintain the integrity and sterility of the drainage system. After a simple prostatectomy, the catheter is usu-

ally removed on the sixth postoperative day. After a radical retropubic prostatectomy, the catheter may have traction applied for 1 week, and the catheter may remain in place for as long as 3 weeks.

The drain inserted around the incision site is usually advanced on Day 6 and removed on Day 7. After a radical retropubic prostatectomy, however, the drains are advanced after 1 week and removed in 10 days if no urine leakage is present.

Like the suprapubic prostatectomy client, the retropubic prostatectomy client may have a nasogastric tube in place until peristalsis returns. Keep the tube on low suction, and maintain its patency by irrigation with normal saline as necessary. IV fluids are required at this time.

Incisional pain can be controlled by narcotic analgesics. The skin is kept dry by a change of abdominal dressing at least twice daily. If scrotal and leg edema occur, the legs and scrotum should be elevated, and the nurse should carefully observe the client for increasing edema. Chronic edema may become a problem after lymphadenectomy, especially if the client has had postoperative pelvic irradiation. Another common serious problem after lymphadenectomy is thromboembolism. Elastic bandages or antiembolic stockings help prevent venous stasis as well as edema. Other postoperative procedures are described in the discussion of TUR.

PERINEAL PROSTATECTOMY

The perineal approach is useful when the prostate is enlarged beyond 40 to 60 g and when the abdominal approach is contraindicated, as it may be in a severely obese client or a client at risk of suffering postoperative respiratory complications. The surgical time is short, so fewer cardiopulmonary complications are associated with perineal prostatectomy. This approach also is used for removal of a prostate with calculi. The perineal approach provides excellent exposure for vesicourethral anastomosis (the connection of the bladder to the urethra). If cancer is suspected, the perineal prostatectomy can be used for open biopsy and frozen section. A simple or radical perineal prostatectomy then can be performed based on the findings from the frozen section.

The perineal approach carries the risk of rectal injury and urinary fistula to the perineum or rectum. Because the lymph nodes are poorly exposed, the perineal procedure is not the best choice if lymph node biopsy or lymph node resection is anticipated. This approach also necessitates placing the client in the lithotomy position, which is a contraindication for some clients.

Surgical Procedure
The perineal prostatectomy is an open surgical procedure in which the prostate is approached through an incision in the perineum between the anus and the scrotum (Figure 68–5). After spinal or general anesthesia has been admin-

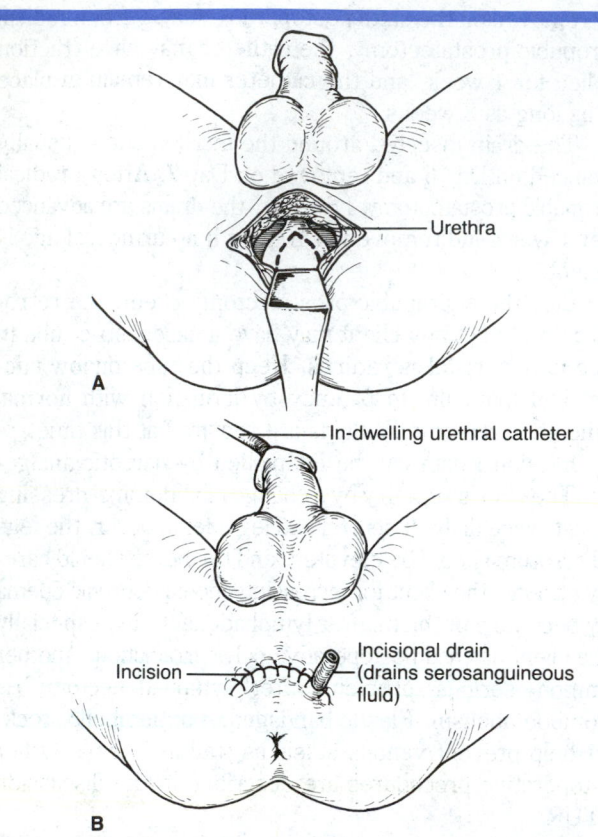

Figure 68–5

Perineal prostatectomy. **A.** Structures are visualized after incision is made. **B.** Suture line and drainage tube.

istered, the client is placed in an exaggerated lithotomy position; the knees are flexed almost to the chest, and the feet point upward. A simple perineal prostatectomy removes the prostate gland by incision of the capsule through the perineum. A radical perineal prostatectomy, in contrast, removes the entire prostate gland with capsule, the vas deferens, the seminal vesicles, and the pelvic lymph nodes. For both types, a drain in the perineal incision and a urethral in-dwelling catheter are placed (see Figure 68–5).

Implications for the Client

Physiological Implications

The exaggerated lithotomy position used for perineal prostatectomy makes these clients, like TUR clients, vulnerable to postoperative deep vein thrombosis. If the surgery includes pelvic lymph node removal, the client will experience increased pelvic congestion, possible pelvic infection, and possible peripheral edema. Impotence from dam-

age to sympathetic or parasympathetic nerves and urinary incontinence from damage to the urinary sphincter are common, and fecal incontinence from nerve damage or rectal sphincter damage usually from an unrepaired laceration also can occur. See the discussion of TUR for other physiological implications of prostatectomy.

Psychosocial/Lifestyle Implications

See the section on TUR for psychosocial/lifestyle implications of prostatectomy. In addition, clients undergoing radical perineal prostatectomy cannot achieve an erection and may need to consider having a penile implant. Urinary and fecal incontinence and altered sexual capacities lead to changes in self-concept. A summary of client implications appears in Table 68–1.

Nursing Implications

Preoperative Care

A bowel preparation before perineal prostatectomy minimizes the chance of postoperative wound infection. The nurse should give the client opportunities to express feelings related to threatened loss of normal sexual function, loss of masculinity, and changes in self-esteem and self-worth. See the discussion of TUR for other aspects of preoperative nursing care.

Postoperative Care

After a perineal prostatectomy, the client usually has a Foley catheter in place for 2 weeks, and a closed drainage system is essential to prevent infection. A drain also will be present in the perineal area. This drain is usually removed on the seventh postoperative day.

Pay strict attention to keeping the incision clean and dry to promote healing and prevent infection, change the dressing at least twice daily, and cleanse the incision with soap and water after each bowel movement. Incisional pain, although mild, may require analgesics. To prevent rectal perforation or fistula development, the client should receive nothing by rectum. This includes no rectal thermometers, enemas, suppositories, rectal tubes, or any other rectal procedure during the postoperative recovery period.

Encourage the client to communicate with his spouse or sexual partner feelings of loss of masculinity and self-esteem. Alternate methods of sexual expression or penile implants may also be discussed.

Urinary incontinence may take longer to resolve than with other prostatic surgeries. Dribbling can be corrected by Kegel exercises and gluteal exercises performed five to ten times per hour. See the section on TUR for additional postoperative nursing measures.

Section II: Surgical Approaches to Disorders Affecting the Penis

CIRCUMCISION

A circumcision, the removal of the prepuce, is often performed in infancy because of religious or cultural reasons.

Routine circumcision is now questioned, and the practice is not as common as it once was. In the adult, a circumcision is usually performed for a problem such as phimosis, paraphimosis, or carcinoma in situ on the prepuce. Adult clients may delay seeking treatment because they fear penile damage or sexual dysfunction as a result of surgery.

Surgical Procedure

An adult circumcision is usually performed under local anesthesia; 1% lidocaine without epinephrine is injected around the circumference of the penis. Any adhesions are released, and the appropriate amount of prepuce is excised and the skin edges are reapproximated. Figure 68–6 illustrates one circumcision technique.

Implications for the Client

Physiological Implications

Hemorrhage and edema are potential postoperative complications. Pain is usually present in the immediate postoperative period but can generally be managed with analgesics. If a wide area of the prepuce is excised (eg, for carcinoma in situ) and the shaft of the penis is denuded, skin grafting may be required. After circumcision, the client with phimosis or paraphimosis will be more comfortable and better able to provide personal hygiene.

Psychosocial/Lifestyle Implications

Sexual intercourse should be avoided until healing is complete. Some clients may continue to fear damage to the penis or impaired sexual function after surgery until they are reassured by the appearance and function of the penis after it has healed.

Clients experience an altered body image and changes in sensation depending on the extent of the surgery. Most clients experience little difficulty in incorporating the body change. Clients who have extensive prepuce removal for

Table 68–2	Circumcision: Implications for the Client	
Physiological Implications	**Psychosocial/Lifestyle Implications**
Hemorrhage	No sexual intercourse until healing complete
Edema	
Pain, usually minimal	Fear of damage to penis or impaired sexual function
Potential skin grafting if large area of prepuce removed	
	Altered body image and changes in sensation
Increased comfort	Fear of cancer progression or extension
Enhanced ability to maintain hygiene	

cancer or who require skin grafting will be faced with adjusting to more extensive changes. The fear of progression or extension of cancer may be a problem for these clients. The implications for the adult client undergoing circumcision are summarized in Table 68–2.

Nursing Implications

Preoperative Care

Circumcision is not minor surgery to the client facing it. The client needs complete information about the circumcision procedure, and the nurse should allow him to verbalize his fears.

Postoperative Care

The client will return from surgery with a pressure dressing of petroleum jelly gauze and a dry sterile dressing on top. Carefully assess for bleeding, a potential postoperative problem. The dressing and wound site must remain clean and dry, so the dressing should be changed after voiding. Carefully observe for and document the first voiding to ensure that the urethra is patent. If the client is discharged with a dressing in place, he should be taught to care for the operative area until it heals.

PARTIAL OR TOTAL PENECTOMY

A partial penectomy is the amputation of the distal penis; total penectomy removes the entire penis. These operations are usually performed for cancer of the penis. The partial penectomy is preferred over the total penectomy, because it allows the client to stand to void and to direct his urinary stream. Normal sexual function is impaired, however. Partial penectomy is performed for cancer on the distal third of the penis. Carcinoma on the proximal shaft or base of the penis necessitates a total penectomy, usually with radical removal of the ilioinguinal lymph nodes and surrounding connective tissue.

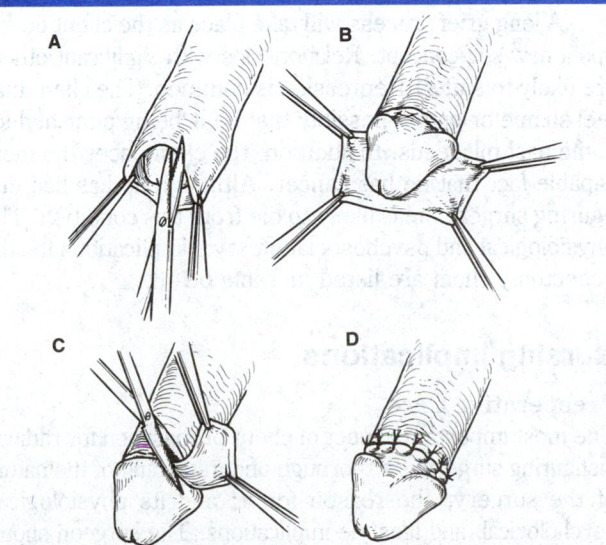

Figure 68–6

Circumcision.

Surgical Procedure

With the client in a lithotomy position, a tourniquet is placed around the penis, and an incision is made at the area where the corpora cavernosa, corpus spongiosum, and urethra are to be amputated. The principle of a partial penectomy is to remove the diseased distal penis and leave a 2 cm tumor-free margin proximal to the tumor. The remaining urethra is split slightly to prevent stricture formation, and the retracted skin is brought down and sutured to form a penile stump with a urethral opening.

In a total radical penectomy, the incision starts at the pubis and extends to the perineum, circling around the penis. The ilioinguinal lymph nodes and connective tissue in the pubic area are excised; the urethra is identified and isolated; the penis is amputated, the urethra is brought out through the perineum, forming a perineal urethrostomy; and the scrotal wound is closed. A drain is placed in the wound, and an in-dwelling catheter is inserted through the urethra (Figure 68–7). To prevent edema and fluid buildup under the scrotal flap, a pressure dressing is placed on the wound.

Implications for the Client

Physiological Implications

Penectomy is disfiguring major surgery. The client is no longer able to have sexual intercourse. He will have to void

Table 68–3	Partial and Total Penectomy: Implications for the Client
Physiological Implications	**Psychosocial/Lifestyle Implications**
Inability to engage in intercourse	Alteration in self-concept and body image
Need to void from penile stump while standing, or to sit to void	Feelings of powerlessness
Infection leading to hemorrhage or tissue sloughing	Grief reaction
Lymphedema	Changed relationships because of altered sexual function
Thrombophlebitis	Depression, shame, or guilt
	Need to deal with possible death

from a penile stump while standing or, in the case of total penectomy, sit to void. Postoperative complications can include infection, which increases the risk of hemorrhage and tissue sloughing. Lymphedema after radical penectomy and thrombophlebitis are other postoperative problems.

Psychosocial/Lifestyle Implications

The psychosocial and lifestyle implications of partial and total penectomy are great. This disfiguring surgery greatly affects the client's self-concept; he is likely to feel emasculated and powerless. Both penile appearance and normal sexual function are altered, and the total penectomy client is further emasculated by the fact that he needs to sit to void.

A long grief process will take place as the client develops a new self-concept. Relationships with significant others are likely to suffer. Depression is common. The client may feel shame or guilt—possibly that he is being punished for some past misdeeds. In addition, the client faces the inescapable fact that he has cancer. Although he has had disfiguring surgery, he is likely to die from this condition. The physiological and psychosocial/lifestyle implications for the penectomy client are listed in Table 68–3.

Nursing Implications

Preoperative Care

The most important aspect of client preparation for radical, disfiguring surgery is a thorough understanding of the nature of the surgery; the reason for it; and its physiological, psychological, and lifestyle implications. The surgeon should clearly explain this information, but it is the nurse's role to confirm that the client understands the implications of the surgery. The nurse should inform and guide the client rather

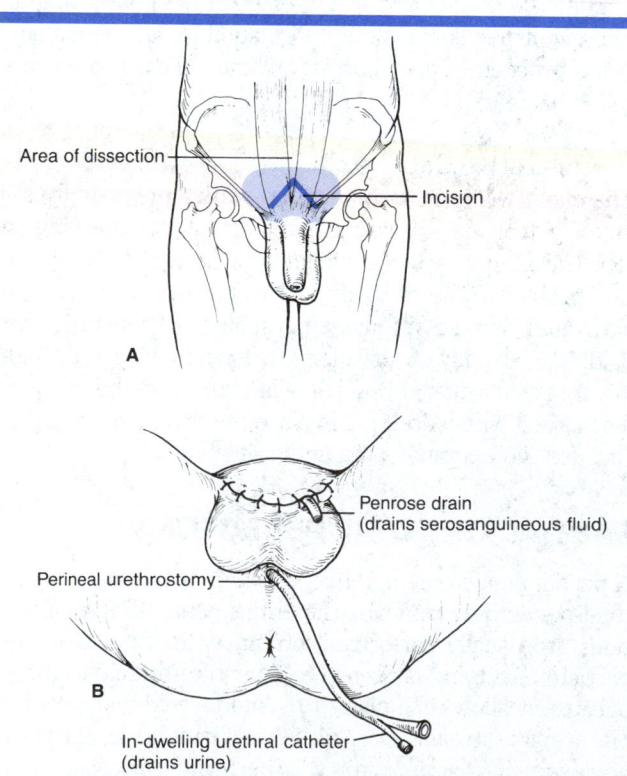

Figure 68–7

Total penectomy. **A.** Area of incision. **B.** Suture line and drainage tubes.

than make decisions for him. Because this client is likely to feel powerless, it is important for him to have as much autonomy as possible to feel some sense of control over his life.

The grieving process over the lost body part and sexual function will no doubt begin during the preoperative period, and the family or significant others should be included as an ongoing support system. The client will need to feel accepted and loved to get through this difficult and trying time. Encourage the client and his sexual partner to communicate openly with each other, and provide time for the family or significant others to express their concerns and grief. The client needs to spend time verbalizing his concerns and doubts about his ability to cope with what lies ahead. Some clients manifest their anxiety by withdrawing and saying little. Be aware that the client's silence may result from feeling overwhelmed rather than from "accepting" the impending surgery. A quiet client actually may have a more difficult time adjusting postoperatively.

Almost all penile cancers are infected. The infection should be resolved using antibiotics before surgery, because a postoperative infection increases the risk of tissue sloughing and hemorrhage. Because of the potential for postoperative hemorrhage, blood typing and crossmatching should be carried out. An extensive preoperative workup also will be done.

Postoperative Care

Be particularly vigilant after this major radical procedure for signs of shock or hemorrhage. Take vital signs every 15 minutes until stable, then every half-hour for 2 hours, then every hour for 4 hours, and finally every 4 hours.

A compression dressing will be in place for 36 to 48 hours after surgery, and drains will be present around the suture line. The surgeon should change the first dressing. The nurse should reinforce it as needed and carry out frequent dressing changes thereafter.

An in-dwelling catheter will be placed in the perineal urethrostomy for about 5 days. Be sure gravity drainage and patency are maintained. Once the catheter is removed, the client will have to sit to void. Sitting, voiding, and then needing to wipe the perineal area (much as women do) makes the client realize how extensive surgery was. The nurse must allow the client total privacy at this extraordinarily difficult time.

A frequent complication after a total penectomy and radical ilioinguinal lymph node dissection is necrosis of the skin covering the wound, occurring between the 4th and 12th postoperative days. The resultant skin sloughing and infection contributes to the development of bleeding, so antibiotics are continued until the incision heals. To prevent lymphedema, the client should be fitted with elastic stockings, and precautions should be taken to avoid injury to the legs. The client should elevate his legs whenever possible.

If the client has had a radical ilioinguinal lymph node dissection, he will be on bed rest for 5 to 7 days after the procedure. Suction catheters are in place for the first 5 to 7 days. Throughout this time, the legs are kept in an elevated position. To prevent thrombophlebitis, the client is treated with either small doses of heparin or warfarin sodium (Coumadin) postoperatively.

The nurse must provide postoperative support as the client grieves the loss of the body part and slowly comes to terms with a new self-image. Psychological adjustment will be difficult and will require the support of everyone around the client. The client's sexual partner and other family members also will require support. Referrals for individual or couple counseling should be made.

PENILE IMPLANT

A penile implant is the insertion of a prosthesis into the corpora cavernosa so the client can achieve an erection and thus improve his sexual performance and satisfaction. An implant is one means of treating impotence. Usually, the client undergoes an extensive physical and psychosocial evaluation before the decision is made to try surgical correction of the impotence. Clients with organic impotence not amenable to endocrine therapy are candidates for this surgery. This group can include diabetics, clients with spinal cord injuries, and those on antihypertensive medications. Some clients with psychogenic impotence who have not been responsive to psychological counseling also can benefit from penile implants.

Surgical Procedure

Two basic types of implantable penile prostheses are the solid-rod (noninflatable) and inflatable types. The solid-rod prosthesis consists of paired semirigid rods easily inserted through a small incision in the suprapubic, scrotal, or perineal area (Figure 68–8) in a 30-minute procedure. After the incision is made, the surgeon measures the corpora

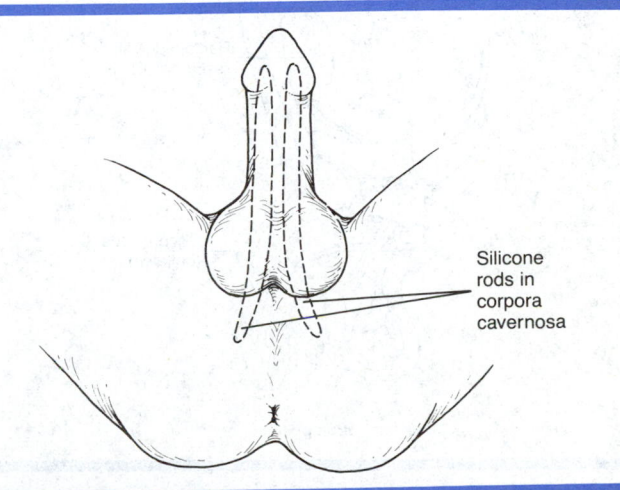

Silicone rods in corpora cavernosa

Figure 68–8

Noninflatable penile prosthesis.

cavernosa after exposing and dilating them and inserts the appropriate-sized prosthesis.

The inflatable prosthesis is usually inserted via an upper scrotal approach, which allows direct access for both cylinder and pump placement. Tunnels are created in the corpora cavernosa on both sides of the penis, and an appropriate-sized cylinder is inserted into each tunnel. The pump used to inflate and deflate the cylinders is implanted in the most dependent portion of the scrotum. The fluid-containing reservoir is placed beneath the rectus muscle in front of the bladder (Figure 68–9).

Implications for the Client

Physiological Implications
The Small–Carrion solid-rod prosthesis is made of semi-rigid Silastic and remains semirigid. The Jonas prosthesis has a malleable core, so some positional shaping of the penis can occur. The Flexi-rod prosthesis has a perineal hinge, so it can be folded into the perineum. This is better for appearance but may require manual manipulation of the penis during intercourse.

Malfunction of solid-rod prostheses is rare, although

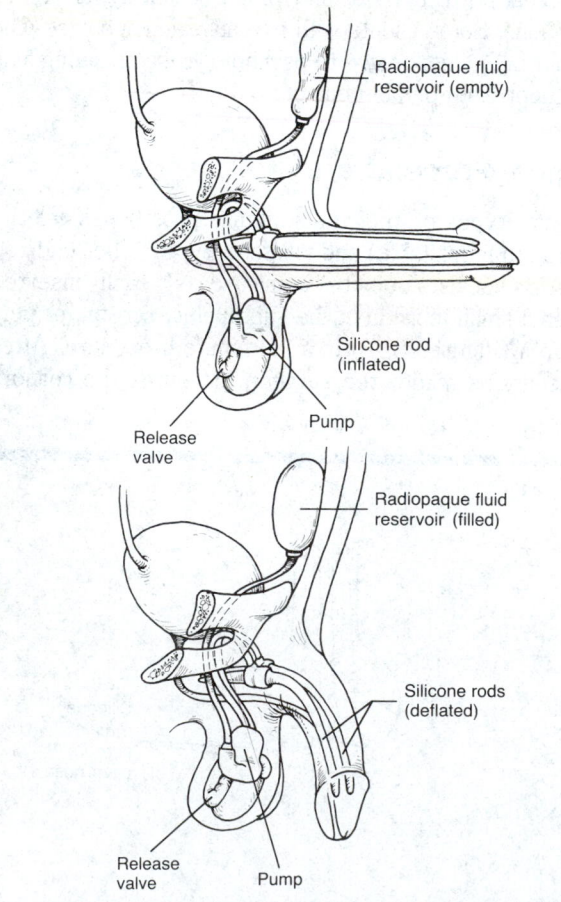

Figure 68–9
Inflatable penile prosthesis.

sexual function is not the same as normal. The penis is neither as large nor as rigid as with a physiological erection. The cylinders can interfere with voiding and are not advised for clients in whom a cystoscopy or TUR may be necessary. Googe and Mook (1983) report added benefits to the insertion of the solid rod: Clients with condom catheters report they can more easily keep the condom in place, and clients who do self-catheterization report that the more rigid penis is easier to catheterize.

The inflatable penile prosthesis, first used in the early 1970s, simulates a normal physiological erection in both size and appearance; in addition, it cannot be detected when deflated. This prosthesis includes two inflatable silicone rods in the corpora cavernosa, a 60-mL inflatable reservoir, and a scrotal pump with a release valve (see Figure 68–9). The client activates the mechanism by squeezing the bulb of the pump through the scrotal skin. This pressure sends the radiopaque fluid from the reservoir into the cylinders, creating an erection. The erection remains until the client presses the release valve at the base of the pump, returning the fluid to the reservoir.

Some advantages to the inflatable prosthesis are that there is no cosmetic change; cystoscopy or a TUR can be performed if necessary; and there is no interference with intercourse, orgasm, or ejaculation. the prosthesis will, however, reduce any partial erection the client may have. Sensation will be normal if normal sensation was present before. Reproduction is possible.

Two problems can develop with inflatable prostheses. The client may have an allergic reaction to the fluid if a leak occurs, or he may be physically unable to activate the pump. Mechanical failure usually occurs from a kink in the tubing. Both this malfunction and a leak can be corrected surgically using a local anesthetic. Client satisfaction is high; 80% of clients select the inflatable device over the solid-rod type (Gregory, 1982).

Postoperative complications of both types of penile prostheses are similar. Scrotal edema generally subsides after 7 to 10 days, and discoloration lasts for approximately 2 weeks.

Psychosocial/Lifestyle Implications
The client with a solid-rod penile prosthesis may find the continually semi-erect penis embarrassing; others find it preferable. In addition, the penis may need to be manipulated manually during intercourse. In general, however, most clients report satisfaction with sexual function. The inflatable penile prosthesis also generally satisfies clients. It improves the client's potency, and he can reproduce if no other problems exist. Mechanical failure can cause embarrassment, however.

The client with a penile prosthesis should avoid strenuous activity for 3 weeks. He should not have intercourse for at least 6 weeks, and even then he may experience some discomfort. Table 68–4 summarizes the implications for the penile implant client.

Table 68–4 Penile Implant: Implications for the Client	
Physiological Implications	**Psychosocial/Lifestyle Implications**
Solid-rod prosthesis Small–Carrion prosthesis: penis always semirigid	Embarrassment from continual erection for some; improved cosmetic appearance for others
Jonas prosthesis: positional shaping of penis possible because of malleable core	Possible need to manipulate penis manually during intercourse
Flexi-rod: perineal hinge allowing for folding into perineum	General satisfaction with sexual function
Sexual function not the same as normal	No strenuous activity for 3 weeks
Less penile rigidity and decreased girth on erection	No intercourse for 6 weeks
Possible interference by cylinders in voiding, cystoscopy, or TUR	
Temporary scrotal edema and discoloration	
Inflatable prosthesis Simulation of normal physiological erection	General satisfaction with improved potency
No change in external appearance	Possible reproduction ability
No interference in cystoscopy or TUR	Embarrassment if mechanical failure occurs
Maintenance of intercourse, orgasm, and ejaculation	No strenuous activity for 3 weeks
Decrease in client's own partial erection	No intercourse for 6 weeks
Possible allergic reaction to fluid	
Need to be able to activate pump	
Temporary scrotal edema and discoloration	

Nursing Implications

Preoperative Care

The nurse's first priority in preoperative care is to be sure the client is well informed about the types of procedures available and that he is given sufficient time to think through his options before making a decision about this elective procedure. When possible, the client's sexual partner should participate in the decision making. The nurse should demonstrate the various devices to the client. The nurse may also administer preoperative prophylactic antibiotic therapy (usually an aminoglycoside or cephalosporin).

Postoperative Care

The antibiotics administered preoperatively are continued during the postoperative period. In addition, postoperative pain is first relieved by a parenteral narcotic, such as 2 mg of hydromorphone hydrochloride (Dilaudid) given intramuscularly every 4 to 6 hours for the first 24 hours. The client's comfort level then can usually be maintained with an oral agent such as oxycodone hydrochloride (Percodan) or oxycodone hydrochloride and acetaminophen (Percocet) (one to two tablets given every 4 hours). The need for analgesics usually decreases about 48 hours after surgery.

Blood loss is generally minimal, but for the first 24 hours, check the dressing every 2 hours and change it as needed. Some surgeons insert a wound drain into the scrotum. With a drain, up to 30 mL of drainage a day is considered within normal limits (Googe & Mook, 1983). Wound drains are usually removed after 24 to 48 hours.

The client returns from the operating room with an in-dwelling catheter, which is usually removed after 24 hours. Carefully check voiding after catheter removal. The client should be ambulating within 24 hours after surgery.

An inflatable prosthesis should not be inflated until the first visit to the surgeon 1 week after surgery. Starting on the second postoperative day, the client should pull the pump to the lowest part of the scrotum by locating the pump between his thumb and index finger and gently pulling it downward. The client is usually discharged on the third postoperative day. He has no dressing and can shower or bathe.

Because some manual skill is involved, provide a prosthetic model on which the client can practice deflation and inflation. Three weeks after surgery the client should start inflating his own prosthesis daily and continue for 6 weeks to create a fibrous tissue sheath around the reservoir (Googe & Mook, 1983). The client inflates the device by squeezing the pump 10 to 15 times with one hand while holding it stationary with the other hand. He deflates the prosthesis by gently pressing a release valve. The valve is difficult to find and occludes the flow if pressed too hard. Thus, it is important for the client to practice using the prosthesis to avoid embarrassment when first attempting intercourse.

Section III: Surgical Approaches to Disorders Affecting the Testes and Related Structures

ORCHIECTOMY

An orchiectomy is the removal of the testis. Simple orchiectomy involves removal of the testis alone, whereas radical orchiectomy involves high ligation of the spermatic cord and may include retroperitoneal lymphadenectomy. A simple orchiectomy is performed for recurrent epididymo-orchitis when more traditional medical treatment has failed. It also is used as palliative treatment for cancer of the prostate. A radical orchiectomy is performed whenever there is cancer of the testis, epididymis, or spermatic cord. Bilateral orchiectomy may be performed for metastatic cancer of the prostate.

Surgical Procedure

In a simple orchiectomy, the surgeon makes a scrotal incision and removes the testis. Scrotal drainage is usually necessary for at least the first 24 hours. If there is an infection, the drain may remain in place for 7 to 10 days.

A radical orchiectomy is also referred to as an inguinal orchiectomy, because the testis is exposed via an inguinal incision. The spermatic cord is also exposed, and the testis and all cord structures are removed. Rubber-shod clamps are placed at cord margins to prevent tumor spill (Stewart, 1982). A wound drain will be in place postoperatively.

Retroperitoneal lymphadenectomy is usually performed with a radical orchiectomy, especially if the testicular tumor is embryonal carcinoma or teratocarcinoma. The client should have no clinical evidence of metastasis. This extensive surgery requires a midline incision from the xiphoid process to the suprapubic area. The surgeon excises all tissue containing nodes.

Implications for the Client

Physiological Implications
If the orchiectomy is unilateral, the client will still produce testosterone and retain his masculine characteristics, including potency and fertility. Potential postoperative complications can include phlebitis and, after radical orchiectomy with retroperitoneal lymphadenectomy, respiratory and vascular problems and injury to major abdominal organs with resultant hemorrhage, fistula formation, or inflammation.

Psychosocial/Lifestyle Implications
Testicular cancer appears in the young adult man just as he may be making career and family plans. He probably fears that the surgery will emasculate him. If the alteration in the scrotum's appearance concerns the client, a gel-like prosthesis can be inserted. In addition, this client will also fear for his life. Implications for the orchiectomy client are summarized in Table 68–5.

Nursing Implications

Preoperative Care
The major preoperative preparation of the client is psychological preparation. The nurse needs to provide emotional support to the client as he verbalizes his concerns about cancer, emasculation, and lifestyle changes.

Postoperative Care
Recovery is rapid for the client who has had an orchiectomy without retroperitoneal lymphadenectomy. A general diet and ambulation are usually started the day of surgery; as with other types of genitourinary surgery, early ambulation usually can avert phlebitis. An ice pack applied to the scrotum for 24 hours after surgery reduces edema and bleeding. Analgesia may at first be accomplished by parenteral narcotics, but usually after the first 24 hours oral analgesics are sufficient.

The extent of the surgery and incision necessitate bed rest for the first 24 to 48 hours after an orchiectomy with retroperitoneal lymphadenectomy. Respiratory and vascular complications are likely to follow, so the nurse should help the client with ankle pushes, turning, deep breathing, and coughing every 2 hours. The extensive abdominal manipulation in this surgery leads to paralytic ileus, and the client will have a nasogastric tube set to suction until bowel sounds return and flatus is passed.

VASECTOMY

A vasectomy is the removal of all or part of the vasa deferentia. Approximately 500,000 elective vasectomies are performed each year in the United States (Kessler, 1982). The wish to be sterile is the major reason clients have vasectomies. The other reason is to prevent epididymitis

Table 68–5 Orchiectomy: Implications for the Client	
Physiological Implications	**Psychosocial/Lifestyle Implications**
Potency and fertility maintained after unilateral orchiectomy	Fear of cancer
Potential for postoperative phlebitis	Fear of emasculation from surgery
After lymphadenectomy, possible respiratory, vascular, and abdominal complications	Possible improvement in appearance with a prosthesis

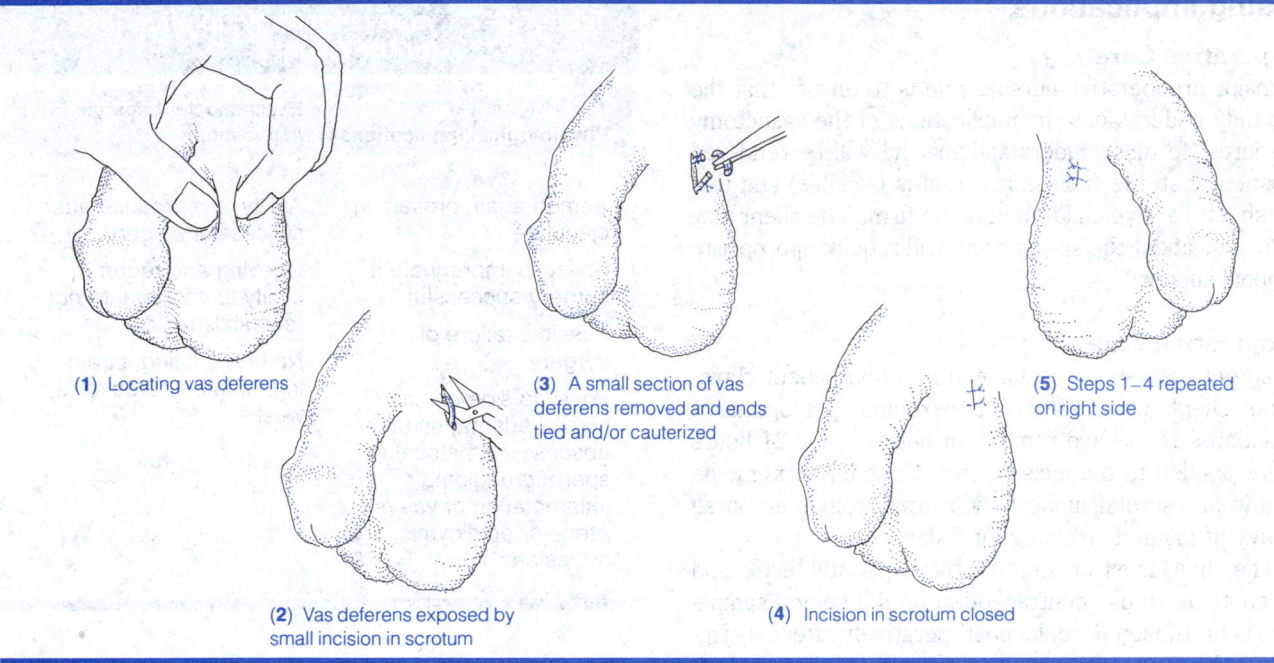

(1) Locating vas deferens

(3) A small section of vas deferens removed and ends tied and/or cauterized

(5) Steps 1–4 repeated on right side

(2) Vas deferens exposed by small incision in scrotum

(4) Incision in scrotum closed

Figure 68–10

Vasectomy. The procedure is demonstrated in steps 1 through 5.
SOURCE: Crook R, Bauer K: *Our Sexuality*. Menlo Park, CA: Benjamin/Cummings, 1983, p. 367.

after a prostatectomy. Anyone about to undergo a vasectomy should fully realize that the procedure may be permanent. The client should not expect that this procedure can be reversed at a later date. He must be an emotionally mature, stable individual who has rationally arrived at the decision not to have more children. Although consent of the marital partner is not generally required, the consensus among surgeons is that in most cases, the partner should be informed (Kessler, 1982).

Surgical Procedure

A vasectomy usually can be performed in an outpatient setting using local anesthesia and a scrotal incision (Figure 68–10). A variety of surgical procedures is used. The success rate is generally high, but each technique has some failures. Some techniques combine both excision and fulguration with electrocautery.

Implications for the Client

Physiological Implications
A vasectomy causes permanent sterility unless it can be reversed. This is not an immediate effect, however, and the client is fertile for at least 6 weeks postoperatively. Minor scrotal edema or more serious problems can occur after a vasectomy. The surgery may fail and the client remains fertile. Scrotal abscess, hematocele, sperm granuloma, inflammation of the vas deferens or epididymis, and adhesions also can occur. Some researchers have reported an increase in autoimmune diseases and atherosclerosis after vasectomy, but these claims have yet to be upheld

by well-controlled studies. Vasectomy is considered a safe, effective, and inexpensive means of birth control (Kessler, 1982).

Psychosocial/Lifestyle Implications
The client's inability to reproduce usually allows him and his partner to relax more fully during intercourse. However, the infertility may create problems if the client wants to reproduce in the future, (such as after a remarriage or the loss of a child). The client should not have intercourse or do heavy lifting or straining for 7 days after surgery. The physiological and psychosocial/lifestyle implications for the vasectomy client are summarized in Table 68–6.

Table 68–6	Vasectomy: Implications for the Client
Physiological Implications	**Psychosocial/Lifestyle Implications**
Permanent infertility	Inability to reproduce
Possible side effects of scrotal edema, scrotal abscess, hematocele, sperm granuloma, inflammation of vas deferens or epididymis, and adhesions	Relaxation of client and partner during intercourse
	Problems from infertility if client's lifestyle changes
Possible failure of surgery	

Nursing Implications

Preoperative Care
The major preoperative nursing role is to ensure that the client fully understands the implications of the vasectomy procedure. He must understand that he will be rendered permanently sterile (unless reversal is possible) and that his wish not to have children must be firm. The client may feel anxious about the surgery and will require appropriate emotional support.

Postoperative Care
This surgery is usually performed in an outpatient clinic, so the client must clearly understand postoperative instructions. He should remain on bed rest for 24 hours with ice applied to the incision site. Once ambulatory, he should wear a scrotal support and refrain from intercourse or heavy lifting and straining for 7 days.

The client must understand that he is still fertile and must continue to use contraception until a semen sample (which is first taken 6 weeks postoperatively after 20 ejaculations) shows no sperm in $20\times$ magnification under high power. If any sperm—even immotile ones—are in the ejaculate, the client is still not sterile (Kessler, 1982).

VASOVASOSTOMY

A vasovasostomy is surgery on the vasa deferentia to reverse the effects of a vasectomy. The high rate of divorce and remarriage in the United States has resulted in an increase in requests for reversal of vasectomy (approximately 2 requests in 1000 vasectomies). The major reason is remarriage; other reasons include loss of children; a change of mind; and less commonly, chronic testicular pain or concern about atherosclerosis (Kessler, 1982).

Surgical Procedure

The repair can be achieved by either a macrosurgical or microsurgical technique, depending on surgical skill, experience, and preference. A scrotal incision is used, scar tissue is excised, and one of several methods of reanastomosis is performed. One study reported a 92% potency and a 49% pregnancy rate using a macrosurgical technique performed in an outpatient operating room (Kessler, 1982).

Implications for the Client

Physiological Implications
The success of vasovasostomy is determined by the presence of semen in the ejaculate. The most common problem with this procedure is the failure to reestablish fertility. Often, although the sperm count is adequate, decreased motility of sperm or other unexplained problems prevent impregnation. Some evidence suggests that after a vasectomy, antibodies are produced against sperm, which affects pregnancy rates after vasovasostomy (Kessler,

Table 68–7 Vasovasostomy: Implications for the Client	
Physiological Implications	**Psychosocial/Lifestyle Implications**
Semen again present in ejaculate	Ability to reproduce after successful surgery
Ability to impregnate if surgery successful	Grieving and regret if ability to impregnate not reestablished
Possible failure of surgery	No heavy lifting, straining, or intercourse for 3 weeks
Possible side effects of scrotal edema, scrotal abscess, hematocele, sperm granuloma, inflammation of vas deferens or epididymis, and adhesions	

1982). Other postoperative complications are the same as those after vasectomy.

Psychosocial/Lifestyle Implications
The renewed ability to reproduce is the main psychosocial and lifestyle implication of a successful vasovasostomy. The client and his partner must wait a considerable time before surgical success can be determined, however. If pregnancy does not occur, the couple must deal with grief and regret. In the immediate postoperative period, heavy lifting, straining, and intercourse are avoided for 3 weeks. Client implications for a vasovasostomy are listed in Table 68–7.

Nursing Implications

Preoperative Care
The nurse should support the client preoperatively as he verbalizes his concern about the outcome of the surgery. Regret over ever having chosen to have a vasectomy is common.

Postoperative Care
The client should wear a scrotal support for 10 days after surgery. Ice packs will be used for the first 24 hours to decrease edema. Discharge instructions include no heavy lifting, straining, or intercourse for 3 weeks. A semen analysis is performed 1 month postoperatively. Sperm may be present but are commonly abnormal in appearance and motility. Motility usually peaks at 6 months. Clients and their partners will need a great deal of emotional support as they wait and hope for a successful outcome, as will those whose surgery is unsuccessful.

VARICOCELECTOMY

A varicocelectomy is the removal of a varicocele in the channels of the spermatic cord. The major indications for the procedure are client discomfort and infertility.

Surgical Procedure

The surgeon makes an inguinal incision. The spermatic cord and veins are identified, and dissection and ligation of the veins are performed.

Implications for the Client

Usually, the client can anticipate improved fertility and relief from pain after removal of the varicoceles. Scrotal edema occurs postoperatively in most cases. Appearance of the scrotum is improved by removal of varicosity. Client implications are listed in Table 68–8.

Nursing Implications

Before surgery, the nurse should be sure the client understands the procedure and provide emotional support. Postoperatively, the client will have an ice pack on the scrotum for the first 24 hours. He should wear a scrotal support after surgery until edema subsides.

SPERMATOCELECTOMY

A spermatocelectomy is the removal of a sperm-filled sack in the scrotum (spermatocele). Because spermatoceles are usually small, they usually do not require surgery. Surgery is indicated only if the client experiences pain or is embarrassed by the scrotum's appearance.

Surgical Procedure

The surgeon makes an anterior scrotal incision. The spermatocele is then dissected.

Implications for the Client

Implications are similar to those for varicocelectomy. Client physiological and psychosocial/lifestyle implications are summarized in Table 68–8.

Nursing Implications

The nurse should be sure the client is fully informed and understands the spermatocelectomy procedure. For the first 24 hours after surgery, he may place an ice pack on the scrotum to prevent or reduce edema. The client should wear a scrotal support and may be placed on anti-inflammatory drugs.

Table 68–8 Varicocelectomy, Spermatocelectomy, and Hydrocelectomy: Implications for the Client	
Physiological Implications	**Psychosocial/Lifestyle Implications**
Possible increased fertility	Possible increased fertility
Relief from pain, discomfort, or feeling of heaviness	Need to wear scrotal support and use ice pack until edema subsides
Scrotal edema	Improved appearance
Scrotal drain likely with hydrocelectomy	Self-care of incision site and dressing

HYDROCELECTOMY

A hydrocelectomy is the removal of a fluid-filled sac in the scrotum (hydrocele). If no underlying pathology is present, hydroceles are usually removed only if they are large enough to be uncomfortable and embarrassing.

Surgical Procedure

A transverse incision is made in the anterior scrotal wall so any prominent vessels are avoided. The hydrocele is brought forward, and the sac is opened so the testis and epididymis can be inspected. The sac is then excised and the testis replaced in the scrotum.

Implications for the Client

Hydrocelectomy relieves the scrotal heaviness and discomfort caused by the added weight of the hydrocele in the scrotum. Scrotal edema may occur in the early postoperative period.

A major benefit of hydrocelectomy is improved appearance. Large hydroceles may have caused the client embarrassment or affected his lifestyle by limiting clothing selection. Participation in sports and other recreational activities may have been uncomfortable because of the added weight. The physiological and psychosocial/lifestyle implications for the client undergoing hydrocelectomy are listed in Table 68–8.

Nursing Implications

The nurse should provide preoperative emotional support to the client, as well as information on the procedure and postoperative implications. A scrotal drain will be in place for 24 to 48 hours postoperatively, and an absorbent dressing and scrotal support will be necessary for several days. Usually, the client will receive an oral anti-inflammatory drug for 1 week postoperatively to prevent edema.

Chapter Highlights

Transurethral resection (TUR) of the prostate is a common surgical procedure performed for benign prostatic hyperplasia. Postoperative hemorrhage, bladder spasms, and deep vein phlebitis are common complications.

Other surgical approaches to prostatectomy include suprapubic, retropubic, and perineal prostatectomies.

Impotence usually results after a perineal prostatectomy, and the client should be aware of this.

Adult circumcision is usually performed for such problems as phimosis, paraphimosis, or carcinoma in situ on the prepuce.

Partial or total penectomy is disfiguring surgery performed for cancer of the penis. The physiological, psychosocial, and lifestyle implications to the client are far-reaching.

Penile implants can be used to correct organic impotence as well as some forms of psychogenic impotence. Clients are usually satisfied with solid-rod and inflatable prostheses.

Radical orchiectomy is usually performed for testicular cancer. Potency and fertility are maintained when surgery is unilateral.

Vasectomy is a safe and effective means of birth control. It should be performed only if the client is sure he does not want more children, however.

Vasovasostomy can reverse vasectomy. The most common reason men desire reversal is remarriage. Pregnancy rates after vasovasostomy are lower than the number of clients who again show sperm in their ejaculate.

Varicocelectomy, the removal of a varicocele, is performed if the client is infertile or having discomfort. The surgery is usually successful in increasing fertility and relieving discomfort.

The removal of a spermatocele or hydrocele by spermatocelectomy or hydrocelectomy, respectively, relieves pain and improves appearance.

Bibliography

Clark N, O'Connell P: Prostatectomy: Answering your patients' unspoken questions. *Nurs 84* (April) 1984; 14:48–51.

Crawford ED, Borden TA: *Genitourinary Cancer Surgery.* Philadelphia: Lea & Febiger, 1982.

Datta PK: The post-prostatectomy patient. *Nurs Times* (Oct 7–13) 1981; 77:1759–1761.

Glenn JF: *Urologic Surgery.* Philadelphia: Lippincott, 1983.

Glenn JF, Werneth, JL: The male genital system. In: *Textbook of Surgery,* 12th ed. Sabiston D (editor). Philadelphia: Saunders, 1981.

Googe MC, Mook TM: The inflatable penile prosthesis: New developments. *Am J Nurs* 1983; 83:1044–1047.

Gregory JG: Impotence: The surgical approach. *Surg Clin North Am* 1982; 62(6):981–998.

Hogan R: *Human Sexuality: A Nursing Perspective.* New York: Appleton–Century–Crofts, 1980.

Kessler R: Vasectomy and vasovasostomy. *Surg Clin North Am* 1982; 62(6):971–980.

Kramer SA: Circumcision. In: *Urologic Surgery.* Glenn JF (editor). Philadelphia: Lippincott, 1983.

LeMaitre GD, Finnegan JA: *The Patient in Surgery: A Guide for Nurses.* Philadelphia: Saunders, 1980.

McConnell EA, Zimmerman MF: *Care of Patients With Urologic Problems.* Philadelphia: Lippincott, 1983.

Molitar P: Transurethral resection. *Nurs Mirror* (Oct 5) 1983; 153:22–27.

Stewart BH: *Operative Urology.* Baltimore: Williams & Wilkins, 1982.

Veenema RJ, Wechsler M: Commentary: Radical retropubic prostatectomy. In: *Current Operative Urology,* 2nd ed. Whitehead ED, Leiter E (editors). New York: Harper & Row, 1984.

Vogel CH: Sex after radical prostatectomy. *Nurs 80* (June) 1980; 10:90–91.

Whitehead ED, Leiter E: *Current Operative Urology,* 2nd ed. New York: Harper & Row, 1984.

Zinike H, Utz DC: Surgical management of prostatic cancer. In: *Principles and Management of Urologic Cancer,* 2nd ed. Javadpour N (editor). Baltimore: Williams & Wilkins, 1983.

Suggested Readings

Clark N, O'Connell P: Prostatectomy: Answering your patients' unspoken questions. *Nurs 84* (April) 1984; 14:48–51. This is a very useful article written in terms the client can understand and includes a reproducible client instruction sheet.

Googe MC, Mook TM: The inflatable penile prosthesis: New developments. *Am J Nurs* 1983; 83:1044–1047. This overview discusses the causes of impotence, the historical development of penile implants, and the current use of the inflatable prosthesis. It also reviews the preoperative and postoperative preparation of the client.

Gregory JG: Impotence: The surgical approach. *Surg Clin North Am* 1982; 62(6):981–998. A thorough discussion includes the causes of impotence, the methods of diagnosis, and nonsurgical and surgical interventions used.

Kessler R: Vasectomy and Vasovasostomy. *Surg Clin North Am* 1982; 62(6):971–980. This article reviews vasectomy and the reasons why reversal is sometimes selected. It discusses the surgical approach and emphasizes the need for careful reasoning before deciding to have a vasectomy.

The Client With Benign Prostatic Hypertrophy

I. Descriptive Data

Mr Charles Egan, age 68, arrives at the emergency department of the local hospital because he has been unable to void for 24 hours and is quite uncomfortable. He is accompanied by his wife. This is the first time Mr Egan has been hospitalized.

II. Personal Data

Date and Time: Nov 19, 1986, 6 AM
Name: Charles Egan
Social Security Number: 000-00-0000
Medicare Number: 000000000
Supplemental BC/BS
Number: 0000000000
Address: 1816 Fulton St, Melton, NH 00040
Telephone: 000-0000
Sex: Male
Age: 68
Birthdate: 10-15-18
Marital Status: Married
Race: Caucasian
Religion: Catholic
Occupation: Retired railroad worker
Usual Health Care
Provider: Stephen Riley, MD

III. Health History

Source of Information: Client
Reliability of Informant: Alert, oriented, and reliable
Chief Concern: "I haven't been able to pass water since yesterday and it sure does hurt."

History of Present Illness: Mr Egan has noticed that over the past 10 years he has had increasing difficulty starting his urinary stream and in stopping it once it starts. His urinary stream has decreased in force, and he usually wakes up twice a night to void. During the past week, he has noticed increased frequency, burning on urination, and nocturia up to five times a night. It has been increasingly difficult for him to start the stream. Yesterday he was totally unable to void; he has not voided since.

He has no history of UTIs, STDs, or any abdominal surgery. He has not noted any lumps, lesions, or bulging in the genital area. He has had no trauma to the perineal area. He has a soft, brown, formed stool every morning without difficulty. His stools have never been black. He takes no medication.

Client is married; his wife of 40 years has been his only sexual partner; sexually active but reports frequency has decreased from weekly to once or twice a month. Last had intercourse 2 weeks ago without difficulty.

Past Health History:
Childhood: No major health problems
Immunizations: Has not had a shot in 30 years
Medical Problems: None
Surgeries: None
Trauma: None
Allergies: None
Medications: None

(continued)

Case Study written by Phyllis Foster Healy.

The Client With Benign Prostatic Hypertrophy

Family History: Father, died age 70 from pancreatic carcinoma
Mother, age 90, A&W; has cataracts
Sisters × 2, ages 64 and 62, A&W
Wife, age 65, A&W
Sons × 3, ages 39, 37, and 34, all A&W
    No ⊕ FHx DM, MI, CVA, hypertension, or malignancy except for his father; states that he comes from a family of "long livers," and that his father was the first and only one to have cancer.

Personal/Social History: Lives with wife on a small farm in New Hampshire. They enjoy a good relationship and are active in the Catholic church and local Grange. In summer, client spends his time caring for a productive vegetable garden and taking care of his two cows, three goats, and ten chickens. At harvest time, he sells his produce at the farmer's market and participates in the county fair. During the winter, he cares for his animals and otherwise busies himself inside or with church activities.
    Completed eighth grade. He reads a lot and is well informed on current events. Retired 4 years ago as a railroad conductor on a commuter train between Boston and New Hampshire. He has not traveled outside New England except for serving with the Marines in the Pacific during World War II.
    He feels the family is financially stable. They own their own farm. He makes extra income on vegetables and eggs, receives a railroad pension, and has $20,000 in savings.

Habits: States he is a meat-and-potatoes man; eats eggs and bacon every morning for breakfast. Walks at least 2 miles every day. Cares for garden and animals. Has never smoked. Drinks one shot of whiskey every night. States, "It warms me up and keeps my motor going."

Review of Systems:
General: Weight stable; no symptoms of fatigue, anorexia, or difficulty sleeping
Eyes: Wears glasses for reading; no eye pain or decreased vision
Ears: States he "doesn't hear the wife as well as he used to"; also has difficulty hearing in a crowded room with many voices in the background
Cardiopulmonary: No chest pain, no cough, no DOE; last chest x-ray 20 or 30 years ago; no TBC exposure; never had a TBC skin test; no PND, no ankle edema; never had an ECG
GI: No food intolerance, no dysphagia, no hx of ulcer disease, no reflux, no abdominal pain
M-S: Occasional low back pain with excessive bending and lifting; relieved by rest and ASA
Psychological: No major worries except about current symptoms; usual coping pattern is to walk or tend the garden if upset

IV. Physical Assessment Client is tanned with well-developed shoulder, abdominal, and leg muscles. Appears younger than stated age and overall health seems to be good.
Height: 5 ft 11 in
Weight: 185 lb
Vital Signs: T: 99°F (32.2°C), P: 84, R: 20
BP: 130/80 (L) arm, sitting

Relevant Organ Systems:

Cardiovascular: Apical rate 84, regular; no murmurs or gallops; pedal pulses 3 + and equal bilaterally

Abdomen: 0 scars, 0 bruits, muscular, nontender; no CVA tenderness; L-S-K not palpable; bladder dull to percussion and palpated to 4 cm below the umbilicus

Genitals: Penis circumcised; no lesions, masses, or discharge; scrotum without masses or lesions; no inguinal or femoral hernias

Rectum: No perianal lesions, no ext hemorrhoids; sphincter tone good; rectal walls without lesions; prostate, enlarged symmetrically, soft, smooth, slightly tender to palpation

V. Summary

Mr Egan was admitted to the hospital as an emergency case. An 18 F Foley catheter was inserted, 1000 mL of urine was drained, and the catheter was clamped. One hour later, the catheter was unclamped, and another 800 mL of urine was drained; the catheter was left open to straight drainage.

Urine was sent to the laboratory for urinalysis and urine culture and sensitivity. Mr Egan was scheduled for an IVP, a voiding cystogram, and cystometric evaluation. Routine blood work, an ECG, and a chest x-ray were done in anticipation of surgery.

Mr Egan was placed on ampicillin to treat a urinary tract infection. Five days after admission, with the UTI under control, Mr Egan was taken to the operating room for a transurethral resection of the prostate gland.

VI. Nursing Care Plan

Nursing Diagnosis	Client Care Goals	Plan/Nursing Implementation	Expected Outcome
Tissue perfusion, potential alteration in: related to postoperative hemorrhage	Client has postoperative course free of hemorrhage and hypovolemic shock	Assess skin temperature, skin color; check vital signs q. 15 min; progress to q. 30 min and to q.1h as they become stable; assess for large amounts of bright red bleeding through and around the catheter; maintain catheter traction; administer stool softeners to prevent straining; instruct client to watch for and report signs of delayed bleeding; in preparing client for home care, instruct him to avoid heavy lifting and riding on bumpy roads	Client's vital signs remain stable; any untoward bleeding is discovered early so hypovolemic shock is prevented; client has a postoperative course free of active hemorrhage and clots
Urinary elimination, alteration in patterns of	Client free of urinary retention and obstruction	Maintain catheter patency by gravity drainage; no dependent loops; maintain continuous bladder irrigation as ordered; teach perineal exercises to decrease dribbling after catheter is removed; force fluids to 3000 mL/day	Catheter patent and free of obstruction
	Client free of urinary tract infection	Administer antibiotics as ordered; maintain sterile closed system; practice strict asepsis; give catheter care q.12h	Urine clear and free of infection
Comfort, alteration in: related to pain	Client relatively pain-free	Maintain continuous bladder irrigation to prevent formation of clots; teach client not to try and void around catheter even	Client free of bladder spasms and comfortable

(continued)

The Client With Benign Prostatic Hypertrophy

VI. Nursing Care Plan *(continued)*

Nursing Diagnosis	Client Care Goals	Plan/Nursing Implementation	Expected Outcome
		though he may have that sensation; administer B and O suppositories for relief of bladder spasms	
Sexual dysfunction	Client to verbalize an understanding of temporary sexual dysfunction	Tell client that usual intercourse may be resumed 6 weeks after surgery but that he should check with his doctor before resuming; explain that impotence is not expected after TUR; encourage nongenital touching to express caring until intercourse can be resumed	Client expresses understanding of need for a temporary restriction on sexual intercourse; client and partner are able to express caring to each other; satisfactory sexual relations reestablished
Tissue perfusion, potential alteration in: related to postoperative phlebitis	Client will be free of signs of phlebitis	Reinforce preoperative teaching of leg and ankle exercises and have client practice them q.1h while awake; have client wear elastic bandages or antiembolic stockings; teach client to avoid pressure on calf or popliteal space by not crossing legs or gatching knee-break of bed; administer low-dose heparin as ordered; ambulate client at least three times a day; encourage significant others to participate in client's care	Client practices exercises, ambulates frequently, and avoids positions that decrease venous return; significant others remind and encourage client when he is reluctant to exercise; client's extremities are free of signs of phlebitis

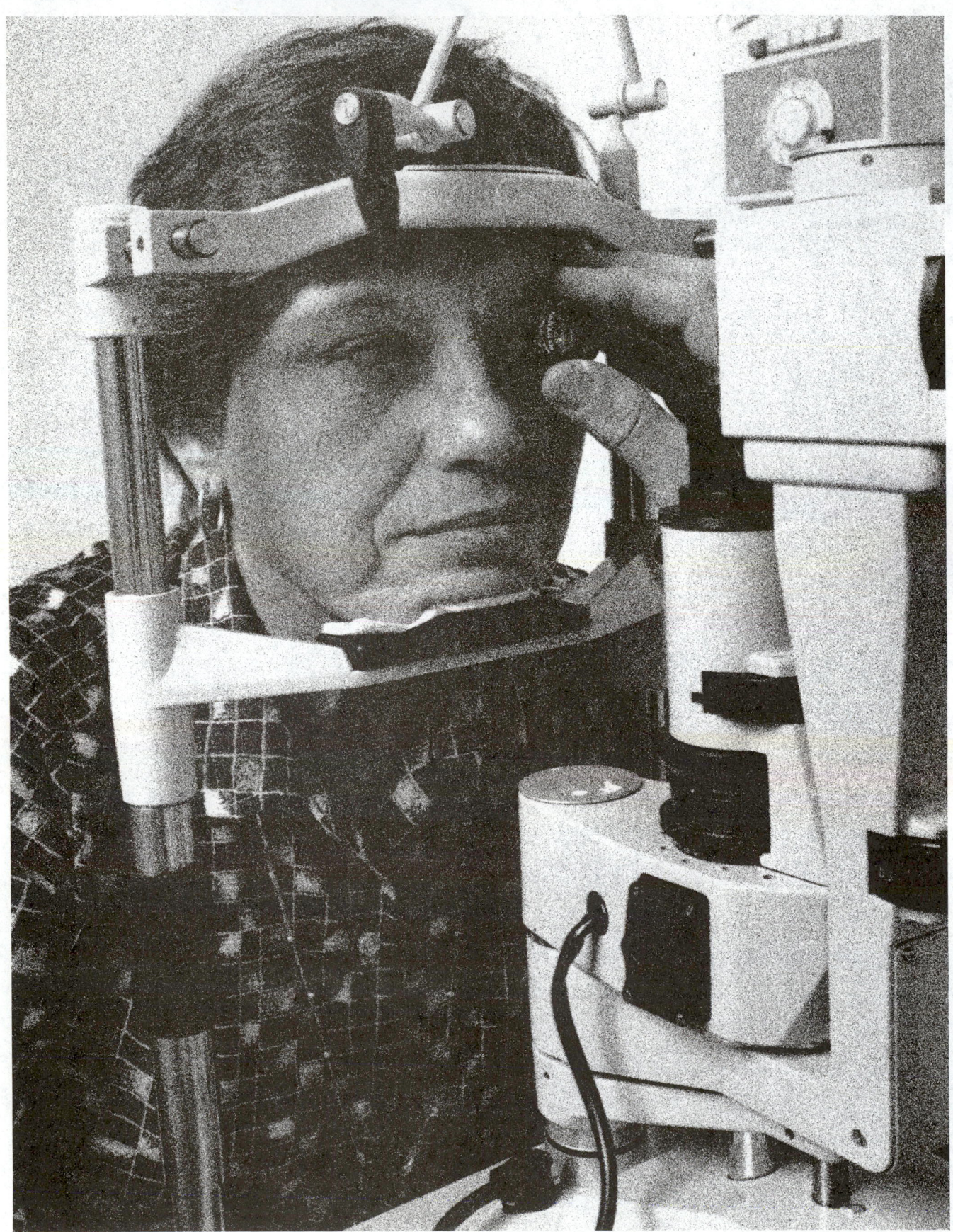

UNIT 12

The Client With Visual and Auditory System Dysfunction

Chapter 69

The Visual System in Health and Illness

Mardy Nord Meadows
Theresa M. Flaherty
Carol Ren Kneisl

Objectives

When you have finished studying this chapter, you should be able to:

Identify the anatomic structures of the eye.

State the functions of the eye structures.

Identify pathophysiological influences that can adversely affect the function of the eye.

Describe alterations in other body systems that can influence the eye's anatomy and role.

Discuss psychosocial influences and their effects on the structure and function of the eye.

The eye, the sole sensory organ for gathering visual data, is a complex anatomic and physiological structure. The data it gathers allow a person to detect changes in the environment and to direct a variety of activities. In addition, visual sensations contribute to feelings of self-worth and self-concept. They provide pleasure and the ability to share human experiences. Mobility, communication, financial security, independence, career, and self-image—in other words, all of life—frequently depend on the normal structure and function of the eyes. Throughout history, the eye has always carried a unique importance and mystique. Various cultures have credited the eyes with supernatural powers. It is often said that the eye is a window or a link to the world, and people without this link may experience many fears and losses.

Section I: Structural and Functional Interrelationships

STRUCTURE AND FUNCTION OF THE EYE

The eye is approximately 1 inch in diameter and nearly spherical with the anterior portion slightly more convex.

The eye can be divided anatomically into the protective structures; the external, middle, and inner layers; and the refracting media. The muscles, nerves, and blood supply of the eye interrelate to the main structures.

Protective Structures

Orbit

Only one-sixth of the eye is exposed; the rest is recessed and protected by the orbits (bony sockets) formed by the cranial bones. Posteriorly, the eye is cushioned by fat pads and connective tissues. In addition to protecting the eye, the orbit provides a pathway for the nerves and blood vessels that supply the eye.

Eyelid

The eyelids protect the eye from external irritation and can prevent about 99% of light from entering. (Note, however, that the eyelids will *not* prevent retinal damage from ultraviolet rays, as when a person lays face up in the sun.) The eyelids' protective function is mediated by three mechanisms: movement of the eyelids (blinking), the screening and sensing action of the cilia (eyelashes), and lubrication of the cornea. The first mechanism, blinking, occurs about 25 times per minute when a person is awake. Blinking is the most important element in the protective action of the eyelids. Opening and closing the eyelids may be voluntary or reflexive. The eyelids are closed by the orbicularis oculi muscle, and the levator palpebrae superioris muscle opens them (Figure 69–1A). Second, the cilia prevent dust and small particles from entering the eye. The third mecha-

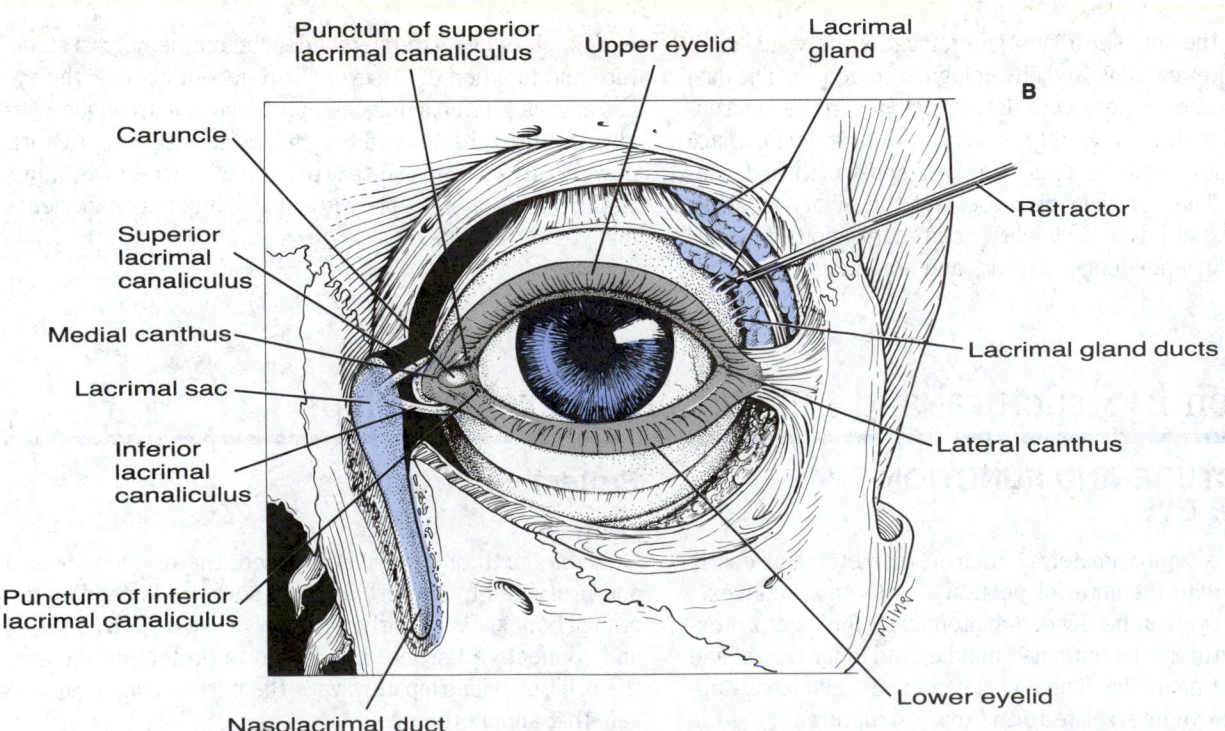

Figure 69–1

Accessory structures of the eye. **A.** Sagittal section. **B.** Anterior view (the lacrimal gland has been retracted to show the ducts).
SOURCE: Spence AP, Mason EB: *Human Anatomy and Physiology,* 2nd ed. Menlo Park, CA: Benjamin/Cummings, 1983.

Superior rectus muscle
Levator palpebrae superioris muscle
Eyebrow
Orbicularis oculi muscle
Superior conjunctival fornix
Palpebral conjunctiva
Bulbar conjunctiva
Palpebral fissure
Eyelashes
Meibomian glands
Tarsal plate
Cornea
Orbicularis oculi muscle
A
Retina
Inferior conjunctival fornix

Punctum of superior lacrimal canaliculus
Upper eyelid
Lacrimal gland
Caruncle
B
Superior lacrimal canaliculus
Retractor
Medial canthus
Lacrimal gland ducts
Lacrimal sac
Inferior lacrimal canaliculus
Lateral canthus
Punctum of inferior lacrimal canaliculus
Nasolacrimal duct
Lower eyelid

nism, the secretions of the meibomian glands (sebaceous glands), supplies moisture to the cornea and conjunctiva and helps prevent the rapid evaporation of the normal tear layer.

The skin of the eyelids, the thinnest in the body, is loose and elastic. This gives the eyelids a great potential for swelling. Fibrous connective tissue in the eyelids (the tarsal plate) maintains their shape. The site at which the eyelids meet is called the canthus. The medial canthus is on the nasal side, and the lateral canthus is on the temporal side. A small protuberance of modified skin in the medial canthus is called the caruncle. These structures are all illustrated in Figure 69–1.

Tears

Tears are secreted by the lacrimal glands. Composed of salts, mucin, and lysozyme (a bactericidal enzyme), tears bathe the anterior surface of the eye, cornea, and conjunctival epithelium. The tears drain into the superior and inferior lacrimal canaliculi (short passages that lead to the lacrimal sac) through the *puncta* (small openings into the lacrimal canaliculi located on the eyelid near the medial canthus), into the lacrimal sac to the nasolacrimal duct, and from there to the nasal cavity (Figure 69–1B). Blinking spreads tears over the surface of the eye.

Tears provide a consistent moistened surface to prevent friction between the eyelids and conjunctiva and inhibit the growth of microorganisms. The mechanical flushing action of tears also rids the eye of cellular debris and foreign bodies. Tears also have a role in the nutrition of the cornea. They provide small amounts of glucose necessary for corneal metabolism and for the maintenance of corneal transparency. The uptake of oxygen through the tear film is also essential for corneal metabolism. Hyposecretion or hypersecretion of tears may cause complaints of dry or wet eyes, respectively.

Conjunctiva

The conjunctiva provides a protective lubricating environment between the eyelid and eyeball when the eye blinks or moves. The conjunctiva is composed of a thin, transparent, avascular mucous membrane that covers the inside surfaces of the eyelids and the anterior surface of the sclera. The area where the conjunctiva lining the eyelid (palpebral conjunctiva) joins the conjunctiva lining the anterior surface of the sclera (bulbar conjunctiva) is called the fornix (see Figure 69–1A).

External Layer

Sclera

The outermost layer of the eye is composed of two structures: the sclera and the cornea. The sclera is the fibrous outer protective coat of the eye (Figure 69–2). It is continuous with the cornea anteriorly and with the dural sheath of the optic nerve posteriorly. Although the sclera is continuous with the cornea and similar to the cornea in tissue

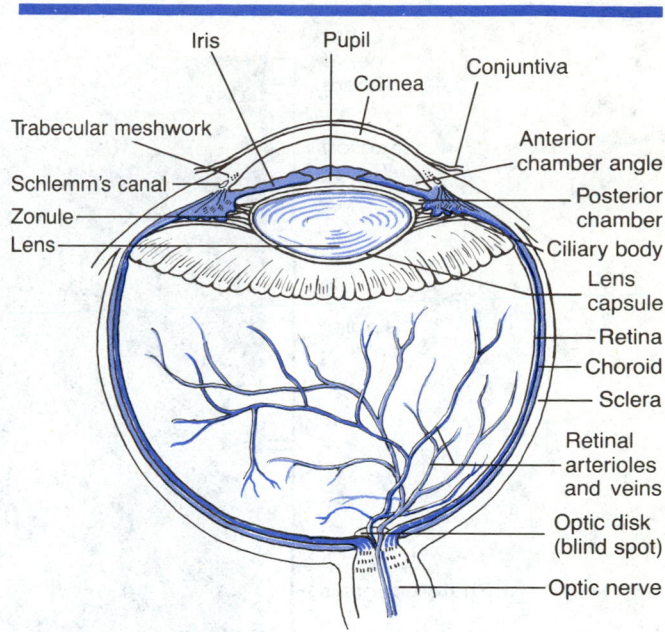

Figure 69–2

Internal structures of the eye.

structure, it is white and opaque (unlike the transparent cornea) because of its continuous state of hydration, which allows the sclera to reflect and scatter light. Because the sclera is composed of dense connective tissue and many collagen fibers, it helps preserve the shape of the eye and protect the more delicate internal structures. The sclera forms five-sixths of the external layer of the eye.

Cornea

The cornea, a transparent avascular tissue, makes up one-sixth of the external layer of the eye and is situated in front of the iris. It functions as a refracting and protective window through which light rays pass en route to the retina. The cornea's greater curvature causes it to protrude from the sclera (see Figure 69–2).

The cornea has five distinct layers: the pavement epithelium, Bowman's membrane, stroma, Descemet's membrane, and endothelium (Figure 69–3). The epithelium, which is continuous with the conjunctiva, serves as a barrier to microorganisms and has an abundance of nerve fibers. Thus, abrasions to the corneal epithelium are very painful and may lead to infection of the deeper layers. Bowman's membrane, which is clear, lies between the epithelium and the stroma. The stroma makes up about 90% of the corneal thickness. This layered structure has cell fibers running the full length of the cornea, which makes corneal splitting, as done in superficial keratoplasty, relatively easy (see Chapter 72). Descemet's membrane, also a clear membrane, lies between the stroma and the endothelium. The endothelium of the cornea is important in the maintenance of corneal dehydration.

The curve of the cornea bends light rays, producing approximately 50% of the focusing power of the eye. Only

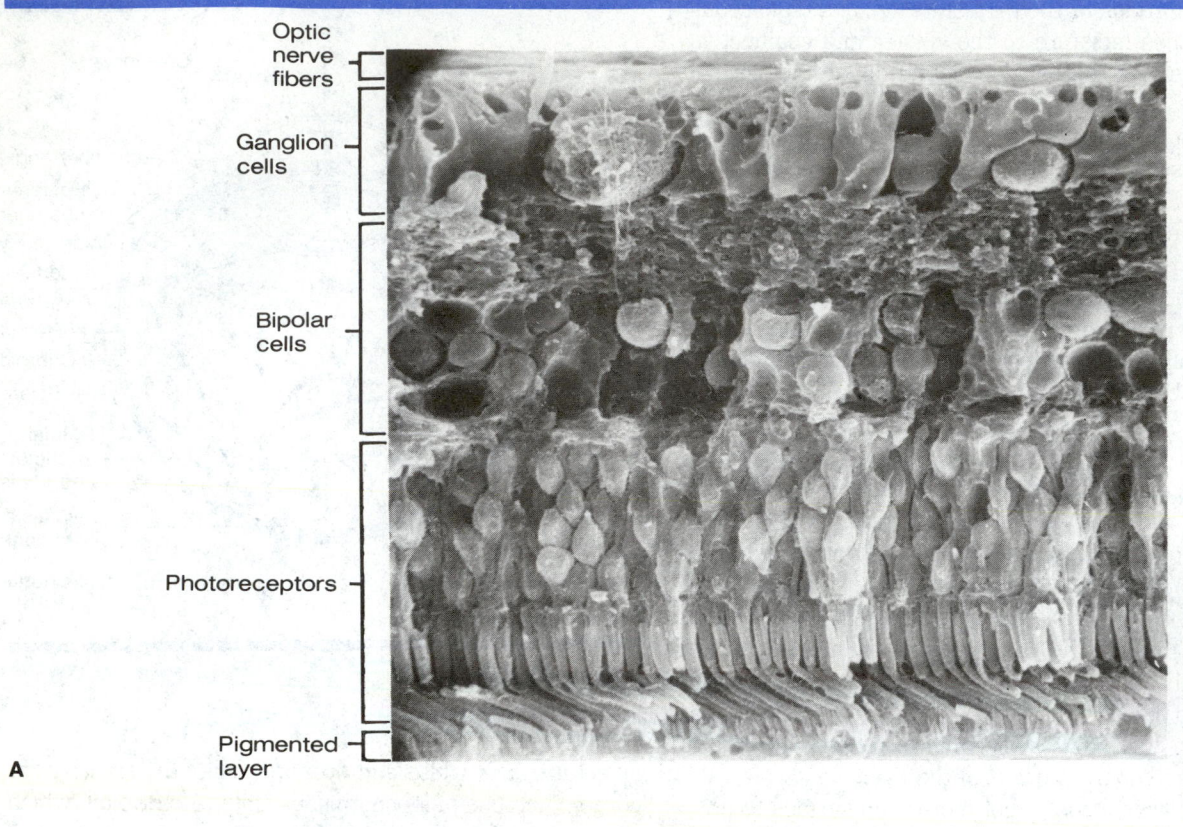

A

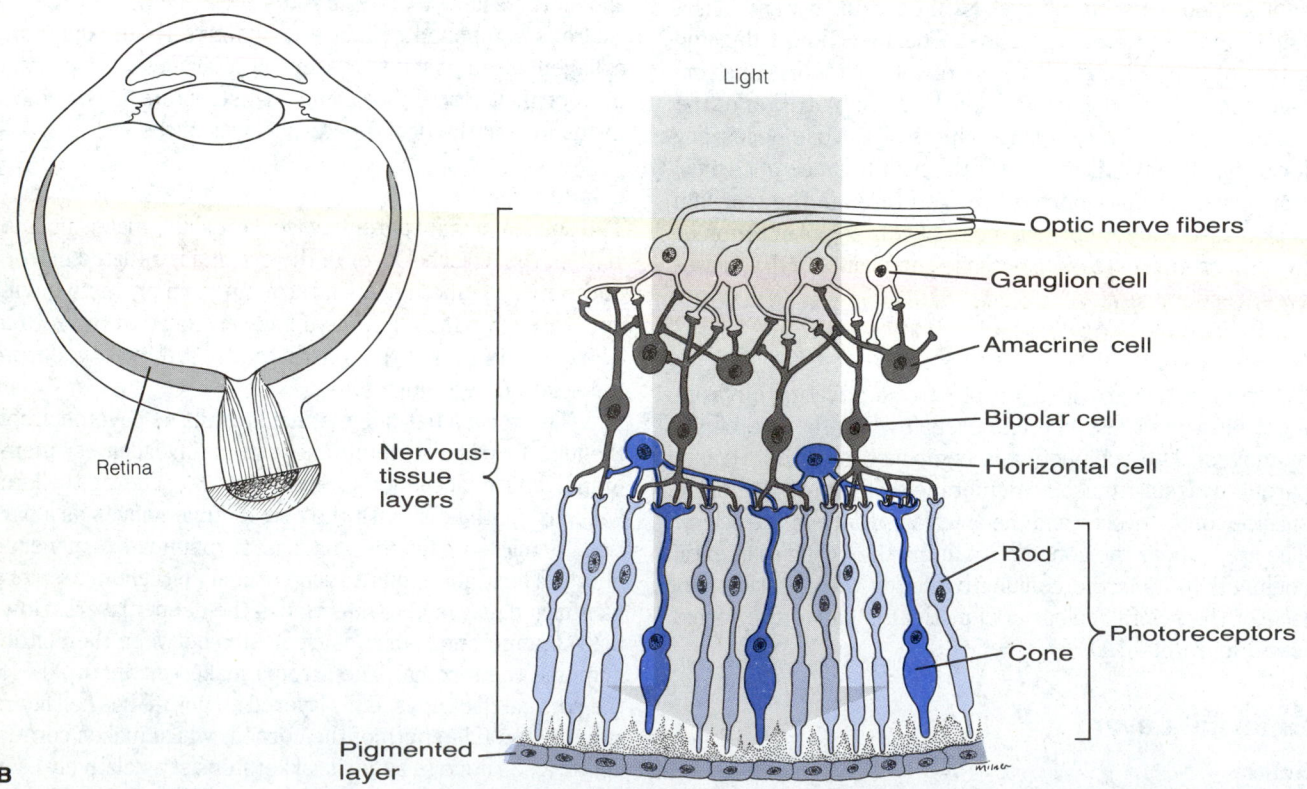

B

Figure 69–3

The structure of the retina. **A.** Scanning electron micrograph (× 1500). **B.** Schematic view.

SOURCE: **A,** Kessel RG, Kardon RH: *Tissues and Organs: A Text-Atlas of Scanning Electron Microscopy*. New York: W.H. Freeman, 1979; **B,** Spence AP, Mason EB: *Human Anatomy and Physiology*, 2nd ed. Menlo Park, CA: Benjamin/Cummings, 1983.

the cornea possesses the regulatory processes necessary to maintain its state of dehydration and hence its transparency. One of these processes involves the normal evaporation of water from the precorneal tear film. This creates a hypertonicity of the film, which elicits an osmotic reaction that draws water from the corneal stroma to the tears. In addition, the endothelial and epithelial layers of the cornea have a sodium-potassium pump that actively draws water from the cornea. Damage to the epithelium, and especially to the endothelium, of the cornea alters the normal dehydration processes and causes an influx of water. Hydration, in turn, causes swelling and alters the uniform structure of the corneal cells. Light reflected by the water makes the cornea appear cloudy.

Middle Layer

Choroid

The middle layer of the eye, the *uveal tract,* is a vascular layer composed of three structures: the choroid, the iris, and the ciliary body and ciliary muscles. The choroid, a layer of tissue that lies between the retina and the sclera, extends from the edge of the optic nerve posteriorly to the ciliary body anteriorly (see Figure 69–2). It is composed largely of blood vessels that supply oxygen and nutrients to the outer portion of the underlying retina. The choroid has highly pigmented cells that absorb light and prevent it from being reflected within the eyeball. Because of the close relationship of the choroid and the retina, choroidal disease almost always affects the retina and may impair central vision.

Iris

The iris is the pigmented circular membrane behind the cornea and in front of the lens that gives the eye its color (see Figure 69–2). It contains a central aperture, the pupil, which regulates the amount of light entering the eye and increases the eye's depth of focus. Sphincter and dilator muscles within the iris regulate these processes by either dilating or constricting the pupil.

The pupil itself is not a structure, but a large hole in the center of the iris. It appears black because light rays entering the eye are absorbed by the choroid and are not reflected. Although changes in the size of the pupil are most often related to how much light enters the eye, drugs and changes in emotional states or attitudes also can affect pupil size.

Ciliary Body and Ciliary Muscles

The ciliary body is anterior to the choroid and extends to the root of the iris (see Figure 69–2). A circular array of tiny spiderweblike fibers, the *zonules,* stretches from the ciliary body to the lens to hold it in place. The ciliary muscles contract and relax the zonular fibers to the lens to put images upon the retina, adjusting focus between far and near objects (**accommodation**). The ciliary body also

manufactures a steady flow of aqueous humor (discussed later in this chapter).

Inner Layer: The Retina

The retina is a thin structure with a neural tissue layer and a pigmented layer covering the inner wall of the posterior portion of the globe, or the inside of the back of the eye (see Figure 69–2). The pigmented layer stores vitamin A, an important precursor to the photosensitive pigment, *rhodopsin*. The neural layer contains more than 125 million photoreceptor cells, called *rods* and *cones* because of their respective shapes (Figure 69–3). Each photoreceptor cell is specialized to perceive various kinds of stimulation by light rays.

Cones are specialized for fine visual discrimination and color perception. They are stimulated by medium and high levels of illumination. (That is why color cannot be detected by moonlight.) Cones are most densely concentrated in the yellow central portion of the retina, or macula. The center of the macula is the fovea centralis. Visual acuity is the greatest in this portion of the retina. Because of the high concentration of cones in the center of the retina, central vision has far better acuity than peripheral vision. Damage to the macular area of the eye affects central vision and causes difficulty in reading, whereas damage to the peripheral portion of the retina affects side vision.

Rods, in contrast, are located peripherally to the fovea centralis. More sensitive to light than cones, rods can be stimulated by dim light. Rods also allow perception of shapes and movement in dim light and aid in peripheral vision.

The prime function of rods and cones is to absorb light. The energy from this absorbed light initiates a chemical reaction within the rhodopsin stored in the rods, causing depolarization of the cells. Depolarization, in turn, stimulates electrical impulses to flow from the rods and cones into the bipolar and ganglionic cellular layers of the retina. Axons from the ganglion cells converge at the back of the eyeball to form the optic nerve (Figure 69–2). The point at which the nerve fibers leave the eye to form the optic nerve is called the *optic disk*. Because it is free of photoreceptors and is light insensitive, the optic disk is called the *blind spot*. The optic nerve dispatches electrical impulses initiated in the retina to the brain for interpretation.

Diverging blood vessels emerge from the optic disk— usually in pairs of an artery and vein—and spread over the retinal surface. Because each person's retina has a unique pattern of branching vessels, retinal identification is being investigated as a means of controlling access to secure installations such as military bases and top-secret nuclear research facilities. Chapter 7 discusses and illustrates retinal visualization through ophthalmoscopy.

Refractive Media

The *refractive media* are the transparent parts of the eye having refractive power, the ability to bend light rays at the surfaces of two transparent media. The eye has four refractive media: the cornea (already discussed), the lens, the aqueous humor, and the vitreous humor. Refraction is discussed in detail in the section, "Regulatory Functions of the Eye."

Lens

The lens, a biconvex, avascular, transparent body about 8 mm in diameter, focuses light rays on the retina (see Figure 69–2). It is composed of a *cortex* and a central *nucleus* and is encased in a supportive elastic *capsule*. As has been described, the lens is held in place behind the pupil by zonular fibers, which focus the lens in **accommodation**. With age, the central nucleus hardens, leading to decreased elasticity of the lens. This decreases the ability of the lens to change shape when the ciliary muscle contracts and thus leads to a decreased refractive power and a decreased ability to focus on near objects.

Accommodation also is altered when the eyeball is either abnormally long (as in nearsightedness, or **myopia**) or abnormally short (as in farsightedness, or **hyperopia**). Visual images are focused in front of or behind the retina, respectively, and the lens lacks adequate strength to focus (accommodate) objects on the retina. Disorders such as myopia and hyperopia are usually easily corrected with glasses or contact lenses.

Vitreous Humor

The vitreous humor is a clear, jellylike fluid that maintains the transparency and form of the eye. The vitreous fills the intraocular space from the retina to the posterior lens. Because the vitreous does not regenerate, its loss in any significant quantity as a result of trauma or surgery may create tension within the eye and distort other ocular structures. The vitreous may also disintegrate with age, allowing pigment or blood cells to become suspended in it and cast shadows (**floaters**) on the retina.

Aqueous Humor

The aqueous humor is a clear watery fluid that serves as a refracting medium, provides nutrients to the lens and cornea, and contributes to the maintenance of intraocular pressure. It is secreted by the ciliary body into the posterior chamber of the eye (the area behind the iris and in front of the lens). Aqueous humor flows through the pupil into the anterior chamber of the eye, a narrow space between the cornea and iris, toward the trabecular meshwork and Schlemm's canal. The *trabecular meshwork* (sometimes called the spaces of Fontana) is a series of small openings or perforations in the connective tissue. Aqueous humor flows through and is filtered by the trabecular meshwork on its way to Schlemm's canal. *Schlemm's canal* is a large outflow channel that leads into the venous circulation. Failure of the aqueous humor to drain through Schlemm's canal causes eventual blindness due to optic nerve damage from increased intraocular pressure (see the discussion of glaucoma in Chapter 71).

Muscles of the Eye

Muscles of the eye that adjust it internally for vision are referred to as intrinsic muscles. They include the ciliary and the sphincter pupillae muscles (circular muscles) and the dilator pupillae muscles (radial muscles), which are all located in the iris. Other muscles originate in the orbit and insert on the outside surface of the eyeball. These extrinsic muscles move the eyeball in various directions; so sensitively is their action adjusted that each fovea centralis normally is directed at the same object. Of the six extrinsic muscles, the four rectus muscles (the superior, inferior, lateral, and medial rectus) are responsible for abducting, adducting, elevating, or depressing the globe. The two oblique muscles' (the inferior and superior oblique) main functions are inward rotation and elevation of the eye. The muscles are illustrated in Figure 69–4. There are six **cardinal directions of gaze**—directions in which the globe can move depending on which muscle is acting predominantly. These are illustrated in Figure 69–5.

Innervation of the Eye

The eye is supplied with motor and sensory nerves. The abducens (cranial nerve VI), trochlear (cranial nerve IV), and oculomotor (cranial nerve III) nerves are the three main motor nerves that innervate the extrinsic muscles of the eye. Cranial nerve III also supplies the intrinsic muscles of the eye. The sympathetic (adrenergic) portion of CN III innervates the dilator pupillae muscle, so stimulation of the sympathetic nervous system will dilate the pupil. Conversely, blockage of the sympathetic nervous system causes pupil constriction. The parasympathetic nervous system (cholinergic portion) innervates the sphincter pupillae and ciliary muscles. Parasympathetic stimulation thus causes pupil constriction and increases accommodation.

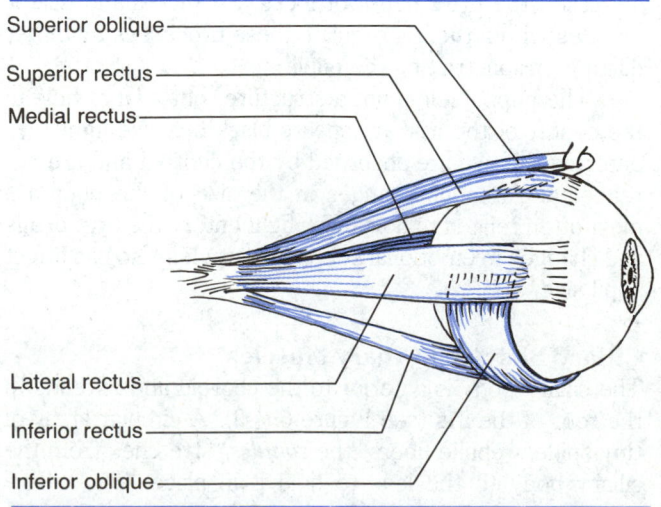

Superior oblique
Superior rectus
Medial rectus
Lateral rectus
Inferior rectus
Inferior oblique

Figure 69–4

The extrinsic muscles of the eye.

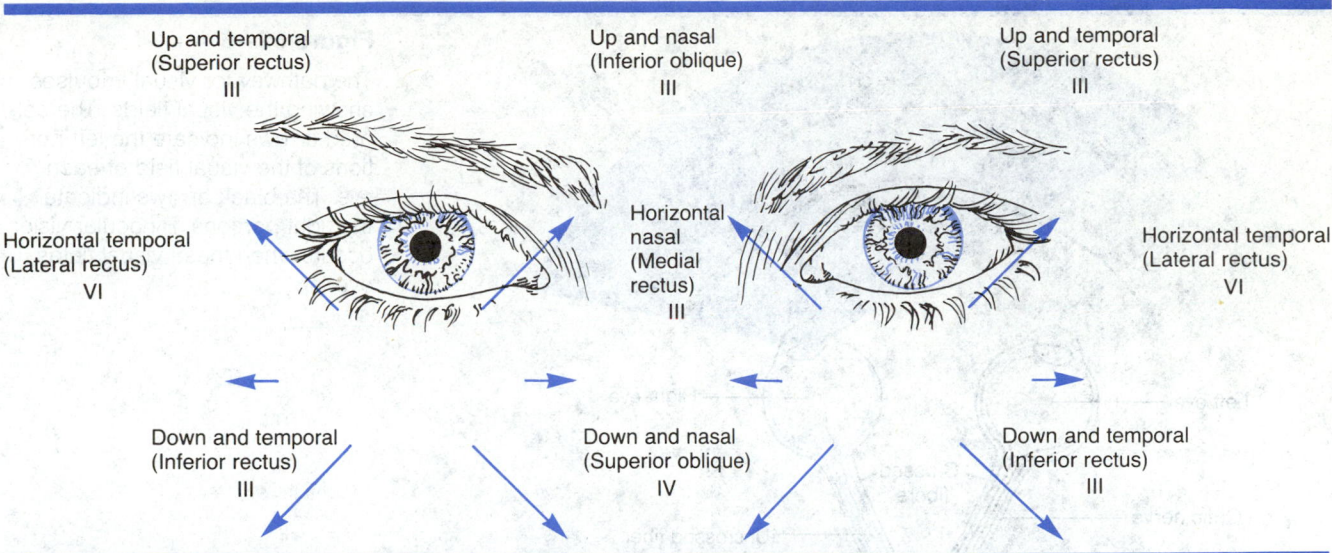

Up and temporal
(Superior rectus)
III

Up and nasal
(Inferior oblique)
III

Up and temporal
(Superior rectus)
III

Horizontal temporal
(Lateral rectus)
VI

Horizontal
nasal
(Medial
rectus)
III

Horizontal temporal
(Lateral rectus)
VI

Down and temporal
(Inferior rectus)
III

Down and nasal
(Superior oblique)
IV

Down and temporal
(Inferior rectus)
III

Figure 69–5

The six cardinal directions of gaze. The muscles that act predominantly are given in parentheses. The cranial nerves responsible for innervation are also listed.

The optic nerve (cranial nerve II), a "trunk" consisting of approximately 1 million axons arising from the retina, is the chief sensory nerve of the eye. It serves as a pathway for vision. The optic nerve emerges from the back of the globe and passes through a circular opening in the sclera to the optic chiasm, the area at the base of the brain just anterior to the pituitary gland where the left and the right optic nerves come together, and where one half of the fibers then cross to the opposite sides of the brain. The fibers then form the left and right optic tracts, which continue to the primary visual cortex, or visual area of the brain, in the occipital lobes. Each optic tract contains fibers from both retinas—the lateral retina of the same side and the medial retina of the opposite side (Figure 69–6). This anatomic structure has diagnostic significance because specific defects in the visual fields help to pinpoint the location of tumors or damage to the retina, optic nerve, or optic pathway. This is further discussed and illustrated in Chapter 37.

Another sensory nerve of the eye is the ophthalmic nerve, a branch of the trigeminal nerve (cranial nerve V). It carries sensations of pain, touch, and temperature to the eye. The facial nerve (cranial nerve VII) innervates the orbicularis muscle, which closes the eyelid.

Blood Supply to the Eye

The eye receives its main blood supply from the ophthalmic artery, a branch of the internal carotid artery. The ophthalmic artery in turn branches into several smaller arteries: the ciliary arteries, the lacrimal arteries, and the muscular artery branches, each supplying blood to specific portions of the eye. The external carotid artery, in addition to the internal carotid artery, contributes to the blood supply of the eye and eyelids.

REGULATORY FUNCTIONS OF THE EYE

For normal binocular vision to occur (see Figure 69–6), the two eyes must simultaneously focus images on the same points of the two retinas. This provides a larger visual field and the ability to perceive depth. A coordinated process of refraction, accommodation, regulation of pupil size, and the meeting of visual lines (convergence) makes normal binocular vision possible.

Refraction

Refraction involves the passage of light rays from a transparent medium (such as air) into a second transparent medium with a different density (such as water) (Figure 69–7A). Refraction bends light rays at the surface of the two media. The light rays entering the eye are bent as they pass through the cornea and the lens on their way to the retina. If an object is 20 ft or more from the viewer, the reflected light rays are nearly parallel to one another and are sufficiently bent to fall on the fovea centralis, where sharpest vision takes place. However, objects closer to the viewer have reflected light rays that are divergent rather than parallel to each other. These divergent light rays must be refracted (bent) more toward each other for them to fall on the fovea centralis. This change in refraction ability is the responsibility of the lens.

Accommodation

The lens, through accommodation, can change shape; it becomes more convex or concave, thereby changing its focusing power. The more a lens curves outward, the more acutely it bends the light rays toward each other. When the eye is focusing on a close object, the reflected light rays are more divergent; thus, the lens curves greatly to

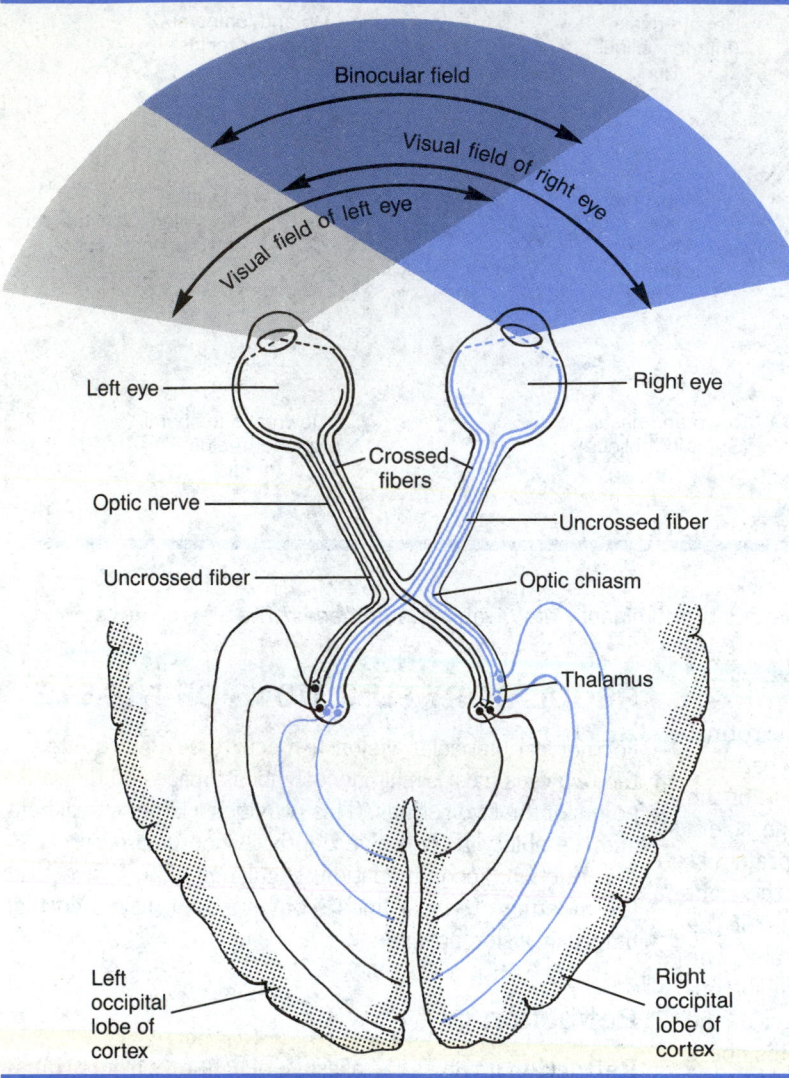

Figure 69–6

The pathway for visual impulses showing the visual fields. The colored arrows indicate the left portions of the visual field of each eye. The black arrows indicate the right portions. Binocular vision occurs when these visual fields overlap.

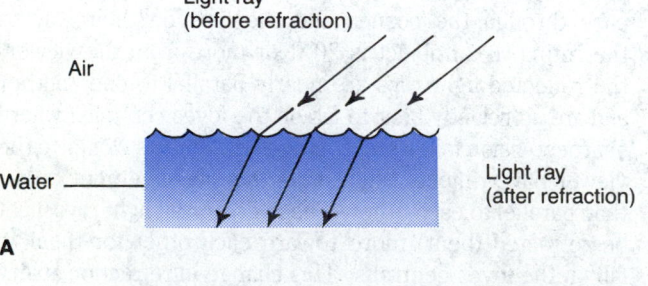

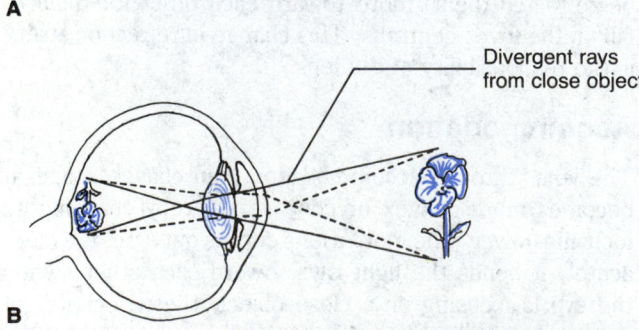

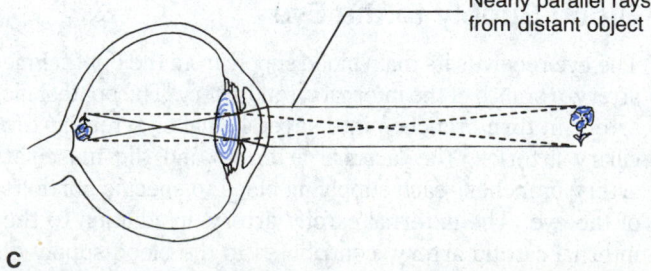

Figure 69–7

Refraction and accommodation. **A.** Refraction bends light rays as they pass from air into water. **B.** Accommodation for near vision. **C.** Accommodation for far vision.

bend the rays toward the fovea centralis. During accommodation, the ciliary muscle contracts and releases the tension on the lens, allowing it (because of its elasticity) to shorten, thicken, and bulge outward. In near vision, the ciliary muscle is contracted, and the lens is bulging (Figure 69–7B). In far vision, the ciliary muscle is relaxed, and the lens is flatter (Figure 69–7C). With aging, the lens loses elasticity and thereby loses some of its ability to accommodate. Any abnormalities related to improper refraction, such as myopia, hyperopia, **astigmatism** (irregularities in the surface of the lens or cornea), or a lens opacity (cataract) may produce blurred or distorted visual images.

Regulation of Pupil Size

The regulation of pupil size is another crucial process in the formation of clear retinal images. The contraction of the circular muscle fibers of the iris causes pupil constriction, which narrows the diameter of the hole through which light rays enter the eye. This prevents light rays from entering the eye through the periphery of the lens. (These rays would not be focused on the retina and would result in blurred vision.)

Convergence

Convergence of the eyes—the medial movement of the two eyeballs so they are both directed toward the object being viewed—also is associated with focusing images on the retina. Convergence allows light rays to fall on and stimulate identical spots on the two retinas, resulting in the perception of a single image. If the extrinsic eye muscles are weak, damaged, or uncoordinated (as in strabismus), light rays from an object fall on different points of the two retinas, and two objects are perceived (**diplopia**).

After an image has been formed on the retina by refraction, accommodation, constriction of the pupil, and convergence, light impulses must be converted into nerve impulses by rods and cones. The light breaks down the photosensitive chemicals in either rods and cones (depending on the degree of illumination), which stimulates electrical impulses to be conducted to the brain for interpretation. The exact mechanism by which this occurs is not clear.

Regulation of Intraocular Pressure

Pressure in the eye is controlled by minute structures in the anterior chamber of the eye (the trabecular meshwork and Schlemm's canal) located at the *anterior chamber angle* between the cornea and the iris. Normally, this is where aqueous humor leaves the eyeball and enters the venous circulation. Essentially, the trabecular meshwork functions as release valves. If the intraocular pressure is too low, outflow decreases; if the pressure is too high, outflow increases. In glaucoma, the fluid fails to flow normally into Schlemm's canal, and the accumulation of fluid causes intraocular pressure to rise. Increased intraocular pressure may cause atrophy of the optic nerve and result in loss of vision.

Section II: Pathophysiological Influences and Effects

Many pathophysiological influences can alter the normal function of the eye. They may cause mild, temporary effects such as blurred vision and itchy eyes, or more severe and permanent afflictions such as blindness.

CONGENITAL ALTERATIONS

Congenital alterations are genetically determined and are present at or before birth. They tend to occur in families and are usually bilateral. **Abiotrophic diseases**, which are not present at birth but manifest themselves later in life, are not true congenital alterations but will be considered as such because they are genetically determined. Abiotrophies include such diseases as corneal dystrophy, retinitis pigmentosa, glaucoma, cataracts, and optic atrophy. All can lead to progressive visual impairment.

Refractive errors, motor anomalies (eg, ptosis and nystagmus), and congenital cataracts interfere with the normal development of sight unless corrected. Congenital metabolic disorders frequently associated with other anomalies also may contribute to a variety of alterations to the eye. The lens, the cornea, or both may be clouded; the nervous system may be affected; **photophobia** (ocular discomfort induced by bright light) may occur; and a number of other alterations may be present. In short, they all impair vision, and they may all be associated with pain, psychological adjustments, and even blindness.

MULTIFACTORIAL ALTERATIONS

Multifactorial alterations are contracted after birth or in utero. They are not genetically inherited, although it is often difficult to determine the mode of acquisition. Syphilis or rubella of the mother, premature birth, infant oxygen intoxication, trauma, and drugs ingested by the mother during pregnancy all have been associated with dysfunctions of the eye and reduced vision.

DEGENERATIVE ALTERATIONS

The aging eye undergoes many normal degenerative processes. The eyelids may wrinkle or droop because of decreased skin elasticity. Senile plaques and infiltrates are occasionally found on the conjunctiva or cornea and produce distorted vision. The lens may lose its transparency and its ability to change shape with ciliary muscle constriction, thereby producing blurred vision and decreased accommodation. Arteriosclerosis of vessels supplying the choroid and retina may result in decreased central vision, night blindness, or complete blindness.

Degenerative alterations also may occur as a secondary phenomenon resulting from other diseases. These may be either monocular or binocular. Inflammations of the cornea, conjunctival disease, and chronic glaucoma may lead to degeneration of the cornea, epithelial tissue, and lens, respectively. These, along with many other degenerative alterations, can affect the eyes with varying degrees of severity.

IMMUNOLOGIC ALTERATIONS

Allergens such as pollen, dust, hay, and cats may cause rapid vascular congestion (edema), itching, tearing, and burning of the eyes. These symptoms are usually temporary and have no residual effects. Inherited allergenic diseases are termed atopic diseases and are antibody mediated.

Nonatopic immunologic (cell-mediated) diseases of the eye include corneal allograft reactions and corneal ulcers formed in response to bacteria. Systemic immunologic diseases such as multiple sclerosis, rheumatoid arthritis, and systemic lupus erythematosus can also adversely affect the eye, causing disorders such as optic neuritis, glaucoma, cataracts, or corneal lesions that in turn cause pain, mental anguish, and loss of vision.

INFECTIOUS ALTERATIONS

Bacterial, viral, or fungal microorganisms can infect the external eye structures (eyelids, lacrimal glands, and conjunctiva) relatively easily and cause swelling, redness, pain, tearing, discharge, and blurred vision. Hordeola (styes) and cysts are common problems associated with infection of the cilia or meibomian glands. The loss of the corneal epithelium, which acts as a barrier to most infections, may result in corneal ulcers that cause pain and impaired vision.

Infectious involvement of the central nervous system may give rise to muscle palsies and optic neuritis.

NEOPLASTIC ALTERATIONS

A wide variety of both benign and malignant tumors occurs in the eye, eyelid, and orbit. These tumors may destroy important structures, interfere with their function and cause mild to severe effects, or both. Intraocular lesions may obstruct vision, interfere with aqueous humor drainage, displace the lens, or cause retinal detachments. Corneal lesions produce decreased vision. Retrobulbar and orbital tumors may displace the eye forward and cause diplopia and exophthalmos. Like any neoplasm, a neoplasm in the eye may invade blood vessels, become dispersed in surrounding tissues, and eventually lead to death.

TRAUMATIC ALTERATIONS

Despite the many protective mechanisms of the eye, the incidence of eye injuries is high. Trauma to the eye is one of the most frightening and rapid assaults the body can experience partly because of the influence the eye has in shaping our self-concept and the great extent to which we depend on normal vision in performing activities of daily living.

Whether the effects of trauma are long or short term depends on the extent and type of injury incurred and which tissues are damaged. Corneal abrasions, burns, and perforations cause pain, scarring, photophobia, and possible infections. Contusions can affect all eye structures and elicit edema, vitreous hemorrhages, retinal detachments, hyphema (blood in the anterior chamber of the eye, usually from trauma), lens dislocation, glaucoma, and optic nerve damage. The effects of these conditions include pain, photophobia, decreased acuity and vision, blindness, ecchymoses (a "black eye"), and body image changes. Penetrating injuries frequently cause ocular infections and may lead to blindness. All eye injuries carry the potential for further injury and increased chances of permanently impaired vision. Prolonged social and economic hardships are two additional effects of severe eye trauma.

Section III: Related System Influences and Effects

Function of the eyes, like that of many structures of the body, is related to the normal function and processes of other body systems. Any alterations in these other systems (especially the nervous and cardiovascular systems) can cause dysfunction of the eyes.

NERVOUS SYSTEM

Central nervous system disorders such as meningitis and encephalitis may alter the function of the optic nerve

or motor nerves or interfere with the visual pathways. Guillain–Barré syndrome may lead to corneal ulceration if facial paralysis results in the inability to close the eyelids. Clients with multiple sclerosis may have blurred vision when paralysis of the extrinsic muscles occurs. Ocular symptoms also occur with cerebral palsy, head trauma, and brain abscess. These alterations may result in a variety of symptoms (eg, the loss of peripheral or central vision or vision loss in one eye) and can affect vision permanently or temporarily.

CARDIOVASCULAR SYSTEM

Blood vessels of the eye are subject to the same changes from diseases such as arteriosclerosis, atherosclerosis, and hypertension as vessels of the same size elsewhere in the body. A decrease in cardiac output, vascular occlusions, and thrombi all may impair blood supply to the eye. Increased intraocular pressure may result from an obstruction to the superior vena cava. Hypertension may potentiate *retinopathy* (noninflammatory degeneration of the retina) or intraocular hemorrhages. It is also possible that hypertension results in increased production of aqueous humor, thus contributing to glaucoma. Again, the conditions may temporarily or permanently impair vision, and a variety of symptoms may occur. Ischemia of the internal carotid artery frequently causes **amaurosis fugax** (a transient loss of vision in one eye). Aneurysms within the blood vessels of the brain or within the circle of Willis may cause pain above the eye, diplopia, and ptosis.

ENDOCRINE SYSTEM

Diabetes mellitus is the most common cause of blindness in young people and in older people who have had diabetes for more than 10 years. Diabetes mellitus often causes retinopathy and, less frequently, the development of cataracts, optic neuropathy, and changes in refractive error.

Hyperthyroidism is frequently accompanied by prominent ocular changes such as exophthalmos because of an increase in the volume of orbital contents and eyelid retraction.

MUSCULOSKELETAL SYSTEM

Most autoimmune diseases, such as systemic lupus erythematosus and rheumatoid arthritis, influence ocular functions. The predominant effects of systemic lupus erythematosus are inflammation of the sclera (scleritis) or conjunctiva, the simultaneous inflammation of the cornea and conjunctiva, and retinal hemorrhage. The eyelids may sometimes be involved in facial lesions. Rheumatoid arthritis may herald scleritis and episcleritis (superficial scleritis) from circulating antigen–antibody complexes. These antigen–antibody complexes cause systemic inflammation and nodule formation in various body structures, including the sclera of the eye.

Just as many systemic diseases affect the function of the eye, so can alterations of the eye affect other body systems. For example, holding the head in a certain position to see, as is sometimes necessary with extraocular muscle dysfunctions, can lead to musculoskeletal problems such as stiffness of the neck or contractures.

HEPATIC–BILIARY SYSTEM

Many other systemic diseases will not affect vision but may alter the eye's appearance. For example, liver diseases such as hepatitis cause icteric (jaundiced) sclera from the excess bilirubin in the blood. Such nonfunctional alterations are important clues in the diagnosis of other disease processes in the body. In this way, the eye serves as a window to the rest of the body.

Section IV: Psychosocial/Lifestyle Influences and Effects

Reduced vision or blindness has both psychosocial influences and effects. Because sight is such an integral part of life, anything that affects the eye will affect the person's human relationships, self-concept, self-confidence, physical integrity and activity, communication, and career and financial security.

The way in which a person reacts to the loss of vision varies with the severity of impairment, the age at which the handicap occurred, the available support systems, and the way in which the person has dealt with other stressors in life. A loss of sight mandates many changes in learned behavior and in activities of daily living. Impaired vision also presents difficulties in meeting basic needs, including security, safety, nutrition, activity, and self-esteem.

In the United States alone, approximately 1.5 million people are visually handicapped and another 1 million are blind. Legal blindness is defined as corrected visual acuity of 20/200 or less or the loss of a total visual field of 20° or less. Rehabilitation methods such as braille reading and writing, white canes, guide dogs, and occupational training have made a notable contribution in meeting the needs and restoring the self-esteem of blind people. Many agencies

also help the newly blind in dealing with emotions and attitudes that might adversely affect their rehabilitation.

DEVELOPMENTAL INFLUENCES

People blind from birth seem to experience increased learning difficulties throughout life, because they have no memory of objects, color, or the environment. In addition, they suffer disturbances in proprioception and in achieving various social and developmental milestones. People who become blind later in life may have difficulty with developmental milestones that occur after sight has been lost.

AGE

With normal aging comes degenerative changes in the eyes' structures and, commonly, a gradual decrease in vision. These degenerative changes that accompany aging and result in impaired vision include presbyopia, dry eyes, glaucoma, macular degeneration, and cataract formation. Reduced vision leads to many psychosocial and behavioral changes in older people. For example, increased anxiety is prevalent among the elderly with impaired vision as their world becomes a confusing place. Visual loss, especially in the elderly, increases susceptibility to illusions, withdrawal, disorientation, and interpersonal isolation. People first experiencing presbyopia sometimes deny it and refuse to get glasses. Feelings of insecurity and isolation intensify for the aged driver with night blindness.

Other emotions experienced by the elderly with visual impairments include boredom, fear, depression, resentment, grief, anger, and lability of affect. Dry eyes (lack of tear secretions) are not only annoying; they also may evoke fear of further damage to the eye, such as ulceration. Artificial tears help correct this problem, but the frequent instillation required is often difficult for older people.

Other ocular changes occur well before old age. Adolescents generally experience mild hyperopia, because accommodative power can no longer counteract the hyperopic error. At about age 50, a further hyperopia tends to develop that is caused by lens changes. Myopia can be manifested early in life, occasionally at birth. It also can occur during periods of rapid growth and may continue to advance through adult life when degenerative changes occur. Thus, age plays a role in progression, and treatment varies accordingly.

CULTURE AND LIFESTYLE

The eyes and things associated with them, such as makeup, glasses, and eye contact, have different significance and implications to various cultures and individuals. Some people think eye makeup brings attention and adds beauty to the eyes, whereas others feel it is unnatural and hides true beauty. Many in this culture equate the use of eye makeup with maturity and sophistication, because it is used mostly by adults. However, eye makeup is a common source of eye infections and allergies, so it should be used with care.

People also vary in their perception of correctional lenses (glasses or contacts). Many stereotypes are associated with glasses or types of glasses. For example, thick, horn-rimmed glasses are frequently associated with studious people. Some people see the need for glasses as an imperfection or a signal that they are getting older. To people of economically deprived countries, glasses may express a form of affluence; many individuals cannot afford glasses, let alone eye examinations. The overall acceptance of glasses in American culture seems to be increasing. This is because of the current fashion trend of designer frames and tinted lenses, as well as the widespread knowledge of the improved vision that glasses permit.

People's attitudes toward eye contact also vary depending on both the individual and the culture. Eye contact signals respect and intimacy to many people, whereas others perceive it as a disrespectful invasion of privacy.

DIETARY HABITS

Poor nutrition adversely affects all body systems. Alterations of the eye may arise from systemic diseases resulting

from poor nutrition or from specific vitamin deficiencies. Vitamin A deficiency is most commonly associated with night blindness. Vitamin A is required for the regeneration of rhodopsin. Thus, a deficiency in vitamin A leads to a delay in darkness adaptation. Vitamin A deficiency also may contribute to a loss of integrity of the epithelial structures. The conjunctiva and cornea may become dry, keratoconjunctivitis (simultaneous inflammation of the cornea and conjunctiva) may occur, and corneal ulcers may develop.

Although no other specific vitamin deficiencies have been conclusively identified as a cause of specific eye conditions, many associations are being researched. Disorders of galactose metabolism are thought to contribute to the development of cataracts. Other associations are vitamin B deficiency with retrobulbar neuropathy and intraocular hemorrhages with clinical scurvy (vitamin C deficiency) (McLaren, 1980). These associations are most common in less developed rice-dependent countries.

ECONOMIC FACTORS

Economic situations may also indirectly affect the function of the eye. Insufficient financial resources of families or societies often contribute to nutritional deficiencies of individuals. In addition, the lack of education and poor sanitation and housing conditions associated with the financially deprived may lead to increased eye infections and a decreased resistance to other diseases. People often avoid health care (eg, routine eye examinations and corrections) because they lack money to pay for the care received, there is a lack of health care facilities, or they are unable to pay for transportation to health care facilities. Some may not know of special provisions in income tax laws for blind people.

Trachoma, a chronic contagious form of conjunctivitis, is directly associated with depressed economic conditions leading to poor personal hygiene, as well as climatic conditions such as dryness and dust. This widespread disease affects approximately 400 million people and blinds approximately 20,000 of them. Immigrants to the United States in the early 1900s were regularly tested for trachoma; if it was diagnosed, they stayed at Ellis Island before being returned to their country of origin.

OCCUPATION AND AVOCATION

Various occupations increase the risk of ocular trauma and irritation, and occupational causes account for approximately 80% of all eye injuries (Voke, 1982). Chemical burns can damage the cornea and conjunctiva, causing pain, ulcers, and possible blindness or permanent visual loss. Chemical or thermal burns also can cause external scars to form, which impair the normal function of the eyelids.

Metal and engineering trades have a higher incidence of corneal abrasions and penetrating injuries, because industrial machines can propel foreign materials into the eyes of nearby personnel. Abrasions are generally painful and may impair vision either temporarily or permanently if infection, scars, or ulcers develop. Foreign material (eg, metal pieces or wood splinters) that penetrates the eye may cause rupture of the globe, inflammatory reactions, or retinal degeneration, all of which impair vision. Because of the risk of significant eye injury while working, safety glasses and other safety precautions, such as the designation of restricted areas and the provision of ocular irrigation fountains, are now mandatory in a number of industrial settings. Contusions to the eye are more prevalent in people whose occupations or leisure activities involve physical contact, such as athletes. The effect of trauma varies according to the extent of the injury; however, vitreous and subconjunctival hemorrhages are the most common. Hemorrhages generally resolve with time or can be surgically corrected, and vision is only temporarily impaired.

Sports injuries, especially those from racket sports (tennis, squash, and racketball), cause an increasing number of eye injuries each year. Hyphema is the most common eye injury. It is usually temporary, and normal vision is restored after the clot is absorbed in approximately 4 to 7 days. However, it may affect vision permanently if glaucoma or retinal detachments develop. Corneal abrasions and lacerations are also possible. Since some of the balls used in racket sports can travel more than 100 mph when hit with force, the loss of an eye to extensive injury also can occur when protective eyewear is not worn. With hockey and lacrosse, blows to the face and eyeball, as well as cuts and lacerations across the front of the eye, are common.

Workers in some occupations incur exposure to radiant energy (ultraviolet light, infrared light, and other electromagnetic waves) at higher levels than normal. These occupations include welding, glassblowing, and any other jobs with prolonged exposure to the ultraviolet rays of the sun. Exposure to radiant energy may cause photophobia, superficial corneal lesions, and cataracts.

Many occupations now require the frequent or lengthy use of video display terminals (VDTs). At the request of labor unions, the National Institute for Occupational Safety and Health (NIOSH) has conducted an investigation to determine the potential health hazards associated with use of VDTs. The study indicates that the potential for visual alterations is practically nil. Visual discomfort (tearing, burning, and itching) and eyestrain are the most common complaints of users. These problems may be reduced by ensuring adequate illumination, reducing reflected glare, and providing frequent rest periods for users. Continued research in the relatively new field of VDT ophthalmic pathology should keep the public abreast of new hazards and the long-term effects of VDTs. At present, NIOSH recommends mandatory preplacement vision testing and periodic vision examinations for VDT operators, primarily to ensure that the operator has the appropriate corrected vision for performing the work task (U.S. Department of Health and Human Services, 1981). Special colored lenses for eyeglass wearers (purple for a green VDT screen and red for an amber screen) are being tested to see if they reduce visual discomfort.

ENVIRONMENTAL FACTORS

Environmental influences may also adversely affect the function of the eye. These effects, which are usually temporary, include conjunctival irritation, tearing, blurred vision, and superficial infections. Smog, the prevalence of toxic chemicals, and water pollution are some of the contributing factors. Prolonged exposure to the sun without sunglasses can lead to photophobia and superficial lesions. Smokers frequently have conjunctival irritation, blurred vision, and difficulty seeing colors accurately. Some nonsmokers, because of high sensitivity, experience the same symptoms by just being in a room with a smoker.

The environment influences and affects blind or visually impaired people differently than it does sighted people. Activities usually taken for granted, such as grocery shopping, driving a car, or walking across a busy street, become more difficult, more dangerous, or impossible for the visually impaired. Many federal, state, and local agencies provide assistance to people with severe visual impairment. These agencies attempt to decrease the environmental barriers and increase the safety of visually impaired people. Talking crosswalk signals and the use of braille in public places (such as elevators) are just two of the many aids instituted by such agencies. See the resources list at the end of Chapter 70 for agencies that provide assistance to the visually impaired.

Chapter Highlights

The eye, the sole means by which people gather visual data, is a crucial sensory organ.

Protection is provided to the eye by the orbit, eyelids, tears, and conjunctiva.

The eyelids protect the eye from external irritation and can prevent about 99% of light from entering.

Tears provide nutrition to the cornea, prevent friction between the eyelids and conjunctiva, and inhibit the growth of microorganisms.

The eye consists of three layers: the sclera and cornea make up the outer layer; the choroid, iris, and ciliary body constitute the middle layer; and the retina is the innermost layer.

(continued)

Chapter Highlights *(continued)*

The cornea is transparent because of its relative state of dehydration and uniform structure.

The choroid's primary function is to supply oxygen and nutrients to the retina.

The ciliary body's main function is to assist with accommodation. It also manufactures aqueous humor.

The retina contains photoreceptors (rods and cones) that, when stimulated, send impulses to the brain via the optic nerve. Cones are specialized for visual acuity and color discrimination, whereas rods are concerned with peripheral vision and vision under dim light.

The center of the retina is called the macula; at the very center of the macula is the fovea centralis where fine vision occurs.

The refractive media consist of four transparent structures: the cornea, lens, vitreous humor, and aqueous humor.

Through accommodation, the lens assists in focusing near or far objects.

The aqueous humor produced in the ciliary body is important in the maintenance of intraocular pressure.

The intrinsic muscles of the eye adjust it internally for vision, whereas the extrinsic muscles move the eyeball in different directions.

The eye is supplied with both sensory and motor nerves.

The eye receives its main blood supply from the ophthalmic artery.

The regulatory process of the eyes that provides binocular vision involves refraction, accommodation, regulation of pupil size, and convergence.

Congenital, multifactorial, degenerative, immunologic, infectious, neoplastic, and traumatic alterations can affect the normal function of the eye. Effects may be mild or severe, and vision may be permanently or temporarily impaired.

Alterations in other body systems often adversely affect the eye.

Loss of vision impoverishes human relationships and affects psychosocial development.

Culture and lifestyle may influence the function of the eye and the normal process of vision.

Bibliography

Collins F: *Handbook of Clinical Ophthalmology.* New York: Masson Publishing USA, 1982.

Dickman R: *A Vision Impairment of the Later Years: Macular Degeneration.* Washington, DC: Public Affairs Committee, 1982.

McLaren DS: *Nutritional Ophthalmology,* 2nd ed. London: Academic Press, 1980.

Moses R: *Adler's Physiology of the Eye.* St. Louis: Mosby, 1981.

Smith JF, Nachazel P: *Ophthalmic Nursing.* Boston: Little Brown, 1980.

Smolin G, O'Connor G: *Ocular Immunology.* Philadelphia: Lea & Febiger, 1981.

Spence AP, Mason EB: *Human Anatomy and Physiology,* 2nd ed. Menlo Park, CA: Benjamin-Cummings, 1983.

US Department of Health and Human Services. *Potential Health Hazards of Video Display Terminals.* Washington, DC: US Government Printing Office, 1981.

Vaughan D, Asbury T: *General Ophthalmology,* 9th ed. Los Altos, CA: Lange, 1980.

Voke, J: Eye hazards in industry. *Occup Health* (Feb) 1982; 34–36.

Suggested Readings

Carroll TJ: *Blindness, What It Is, What It Does, and How To Live With It.* Boston: Little Brown, 1970. Somewhat old, this book still accurately reflects the meaning of blindness for clients and their families and friends. It also discusses the special problems of rehabilitation for the blind.

Hammond RE: *Human Vision.* Raleigh, N.C.: Carolina Biological Supply Co., 1980. This colorful 25-page booklet describes the structure and function of the eye, common disorders, and suggests activities for clients and students such as determining the size of the blind spot, color vision, and after images among others.

National Advisory Eye Council of the National Eye Institute. *Visual Research: A National Plan. 1983–1987.* Washington, DC, National Eye Institute, 1983. This three-volume report details the programs and services provided by the National Eye Institute (NEI) and data on vision research projects being supported by NEI, government agencies, and private organizations.

Wertenbaker L: *The Eye: Window to the World.* Vol in *The Human Body.* Washington, DC: US News Books, 1982. This interesting book discusses the myths, misconceptions, and superstitions related to the eye. Other topics are color vision, visual pathways, and imperfections of the eye.

Chapter 70

The Nursing Process for Clients With Visual System Dysfunction

Theresa M. Flaherty
Mardy Nord Meadows
Carol Ren Kneisl

Objectives

When you have finished studying this chapter, you should be able to:

Determine components of the client's health history necessary for establishing a data base in the assessment of the eyes.

Discuss the objective data to be obtained in establishing a data base for clients with visual impairment.

Identify the instruments commonly used for visualization of the ocular fundus.

Describe the tests performed to determine visual impairments.

Develop nursing diagnoses related to disorders of the eye.

Identify psychosocial adjustments that take place when a person becomes visually impaired.

Anticipate the important elements in nursing planning and implementation related to promoting optimal vision, including providing care, preserving vision, and preventing visual loss.

List the categories of ophthalmic medications and their effects, duration, mechanism of action, indications and contraindications, and side effects.

Discuss the nursing evaluation of clients with visual dysfunction.

Loss of vision, or the threat of it, affects clients physiologically as well as psychosocially. Providing holistic nursing care to clients facing vision loss is a nursing challenge.

This chapter discusses the nursing process as applied to clients with visual system disorders.

Section I: Nursing Assessment: Establishing the Data Base

The nurse must be aware of significant eye symptoms and the potential for their causing permanent visual loss to be able to help clients prevent loss or further deterioration of vision. In addition, eye changes often give clues to the presence or progression of disorders in other systems. The eyes essentially serve as windows to the rest of the body. Assisting in the improvement of a client's eye function can be extremely satisfying, and any information the

nurse can collect in the assessment will accelerate the restoration of vision.

SUBJECTIVE DATA
Assessing the Chief Concern

The nurse begins assessment of a client with a visual disorder by determining the client's perception and feelings

Table 70–1   Common Systemic Drugs With Potential Ocular Side Effects

Drugs	Cataract Formation	Corneal and Lens Effects	Cycloplegia	Decreased Visual Acuity	Diplopia	Disturbed Accommodation	Disturbed Color Vision	Increased Intraocular Pressure	Miosis	Mydriasis	Optic Neuritis	Photophobia	Retinopathy	Visual Loss	Yellow Sclera
Acetazolamide (Diamox)												X			
Amitriptyline (Elavil)			X									X			
Benztropine (Cogentin)										X					
Chlordiazepoxide (Librium)						X									
Chloroquine (Aralen)					X	X						X	X		X
Chlorpromazine (Thorazine)		X										X	X		
Chlorpropamide (Diabinese)						X									
Dexamethasone (Decadron)		X						X							
Diazepam (Valium)						X									
Digoxin (Lanoxin)					X	X	X								
Ethambutol (Myambutol)			X												
Hydrochlorothiazide (Aldactazide, Esidrix)							X								
Hydrocortisone		X						X							
Imipramine (Tofranil)										X					
Insulin		X													
Methotrexate (Mexate)												X			
Methyldopa (Aldomet)										X					
Prednisolone		X						X							
Prednisone	X	X						X							
Promethazine (Phenergan)		X								X		X			
Propantheline (Pro-Banthine)								X		X		X			
Quinidine gluconate (Quinaglute)					X	X	X					X			
Streptomycin											X				
Thioridazine (Mellaril)			X										X		

about the illness—the chief concern. Documentation of the client's primary concern is fundamental in making an accurate diagnosis, so a careful history is essential.

Determine the following in regard to symptoms: time of onset, duration, and whether the symptoms occur when the client is in certain positions or situations. It is important to determine whether the client has had treatment for the complaint and is currently taking medication. Inquire about all medications the client is taking, because many drugs used for conditions unrelated to the eye have potential ocular side effects. These commonly prescribed systemic drugs are listed in Table 70–1. Ask clients when

they last had an eye examination and whether they wear corrective lenses and if so what kind. The nurse also will need to know the answers to such questions as:

- Has a decrease in visual acuity occurred?
- Has the client noted it in one eye or in both eyes?
- What exactly does the client see (or not see)?
- Does the client have pain?

General questions like these provide a starting point in collecting subjective data. The following sections identify specific areas to explore.

Changes in Vision

The client may complain of *halos,* which are rainbow-colored rings encircling bright lights caused by an alteration in the ocular media. An incipient cataract is the most common cause, but rapidly increased intraocular pressure from acute angle-closure glaucoma also may cause halo symptoms.

Photopsia, or the appearance of flashing lights, can disturb the client despite the phenomenon's short duration (less than a fraction of a second). The phenomenon seems to worsen after dark and may be a warning signal of impending retinal detachment.

Floaters, small moving spots seen before the eye because of fine vitreous opacities, are visualized only when the eye is open. They are particularly apparent when viewed against an evenly illuminated bright background (such as a blue sky). Floaters are often due to the aging process; the vitreous degenerates and releases tissue deposits or sloughs off tissue. Floaters also may be due to hemorrhagic diseases (eg, diabetic retinopathy and hypertension) or to retinal tears, where small hemorrhages release red blood cells into the vitreous. Numerous or conspicuous floaters may help locate a retinal hole (indicating a vitreous hemorrhage). Most floaters do not warrant treatment or cannot be treated.

Diplopia, a common visual disorder, can be confused with vertigo because of certain similarities between the two, such as the inability to focus the eyes and a subsequent lack of equilibrium. It is important to determine the time of onset and duration of this symptom, as well as whether it occurs in certain positions or situations. Diplopia involves a weakness or paralysis of one or more of the extraocular muscles, and the visual axes of both eyes are not directed at the same object. Unilateral diplopia can occur with corneal opacity and cataracts by reflecting split light rays. Diplopia is often also seen in myasthenia gravis, thyroid exophthalmos, transient ischemic attacks, and orbital injuries with globe displacement.

Pain and Irritation

Ocular pain takes many forms and necessitates careful investigation to determine its cause. It is often helpful to determine initially whether the pain occurs after extensive use of the eyes. Such pain is often **asthenopia**—ocular discomfort related to an uncorrected refractive error. The term *eyestrain,* commonly used to describe this condition, is actually misleading; strain connotes damage, but prolonged use of the eyes does not damage them.

Pain can range from aches (from accompanying fatigue, frontal sinusitis, or muscle imbalance) and stabbing pain (from penetrating injury or corneal ulceration) to sensations of pressure usually resulting from an abrupt increase in intraocular pressure (from angle-closure glaucoma). Severe pain can occur with inflammations of the iris and ciliary body, scleritis, and herpes zoster ophthalmitis. Other causes of pain include chemical irritants and blepharitis. Severe eye pain always warrants an examination by a physician.

In evaluating the client's pain, consider his or her anxiety level. A fear of blindness (the most dreaded sensory loss) or any alteration in the function of the eye may be paramount in the client's mind, possibly affecting not only the client's response but also the degree of discomfort experienced. Providing reassurance, encouragement, and ongoing explanation are important nursing responsibilities that promote trust. Pain is a private and personal experience, and the nurse should obtain the best description the client can give to understand what it means for the client (see Chapter 5).

Headaches are a common discomfort associated with the eyes; they have numerous possible causes, many of them unrelated to the visual system. Assess the type of headache and its history of onset, relationship to eye use, location, duration, and associated symptoms. A refractive error seldom causes a headache. Should the client experience eye fatigue, the associated headache will probably be frontal, and the results of refraction testing may concur with the complaint. Other eye examinations can rule out an ocular basis for the headache, and a more complete physical assessment then becomes necessary. Headache assessment is discussed more fully in Chapter 37.

Severe deep ocular pain usually indicates an increase in intraocular pressure, as is found in glaucoma. In severe acute congestive glaucoma, the pain may be intense enough to precipitate nausea and vomiting. Untreated, a severe attack of acute glaucoma can cause permanent blindness within a few days.

Acute localized pain aggravated by movement of the eye or eyelid suggests a foreign body or corneal abrasion. Misdirected eyelashes rubbing on the cornea (*trichiasis*), **entropion** (inversion of the eyelid margin), conjunctivitis, and keratitis can cause considerable discomfort and require ophthalmic treatment.

Burning and itching generally do not indicate serious eye disease. The most frequent cause is inflammation of the eyelids or conjunctiva from irritation or infection. Smoke, smog, wind, and allergic reactions from hay fever or eye makeup can precipitate such symptoms. Prolonged use of the eyes (eg, long periods of time sitting at a computer terminal) also can cause mild irritation. Tabor (1981) cited five reasons for eye fatigue after work at a computer terminal: (1) too much or too little light in the computer room, (2) a contrast glare effect from the light or brightly colored background of the monitor screen, (3) contour sharpness deterioration from the phosphors wearing out (the phosphors interact to produce the forms on the screen), (4) the flicker effect (the repetitive bead of light beaming more than 25 times a second), and (5) a poorly designed work station that is not individualized for the computer operator. Another report by the University of Vienna reported color-contingent problems with computer use. Fatigue and changes in color perception were noted after use of video display terminals (VDTs). Extended viewing of a VDT has been noted to cause a color aftervision phenomenon (McCullough effect). Sensitive individuals see an opposite color when looking from the VDT to another object (eg, people who use green screens see red or red-edged objects; people who use amber screens see blue objects; people who use red screens see green objects; and people who use blue screens see amber objects). Long-term ocular effects of computer terminal use are not known.

Dryness of the eyes occurs for many reasons ranging from conditions characterized by hypofunction of the lacrimal glands (Sjögren's syndrome; see Chapter 57) to excessive evaporation of tears (caused by such factors as dry climate and exposure) and mucin deficiency (caused by such conditions as avitaminosis A and chemical burns). As dry spots appear on the corneal and conjunctival epithelium, vision may become slightly impaired, the client may feel burning or smarting, and secondary bacterial infections may occur. Early preventive treatment may reduce these complications.

Epiphora, excessive watering of the eye, is a common condition; it occurs when any portion of the lacrimal system is blocked or when the lower eyelid is displaced due to congenital, traumatic, inflammatory, or degenerative causes.

Lacrimation is the overproduction of tears; apart from emotion, it is caused by local irritation of the conjunctiva, cornea, or iris or by photophobia. Facial nerve paralysis (Bell's palsy) may cause unilateral lacrimation. Abnormal regeneration of the facial nerve fibers and an invasion of the salivary gland secretory fibers into the lacrimal glands (as occurs in Bell's palsy) results in increased tear secretions (crocodile tears) while eating. The origins of emotional, or psychogenic, tearing (crying) are in the hypothalamus. Emotional tearing is always bilateral.

Photophobia, an abnormal intolerance to light, is most often caused by corneal inflammation, iridocyclitis (inflammation of the iris and the ciliary body), and **aphakia** (absence of the lens). The albino population has photophobia because of insufficient pigment for the absorption of excess illumination. Photophobia can sometimes be associated with emotional distress and needs careful assessment. Regardless of its cause, the sudden appearance of severe photophobia may indicate a serious eye condition. The nurse should respond by darkening the room and providing supportive therapy. Some medications may produce photophobia including methotrexate and related antimetabolites, chlorpromazine (Thorazine), amitriptyline hydrochloride (Elavil), quinidine gluconate (Quinaglute), propantheline bromide (Pro-Banthine), promethazine hydrochloride (Phenergan), chloroquine hydrochloride (Aralen), and acetazolamide (Diamox) (see Table 70–1). All mydriatic ophthalmic medications also produce photophobia.

Change in the Eye's Appearance
Red eye is due to congestion of blood in the conjunctival or ciliary blood vessels. The eye displays a diffuse redness, the extent of which depends on the etiology and may alarm the client. Red eye is a cardinal sign of ocular inflammation

and provides a detectable warning signal of many diseases. Conjunctival **injection** (congestion of blood vessels) is uncomfortable but does not compromise visual function. Because a red eye is the most obvious symptom nurses can recognize, they should also give serious attention to accompanying symptoms such as loss of vision, pain, visible loss of transparency of normally clear parts of the eye, irregular pupils, and a definite circular pattern around the cornea. These symptoms may indicate vision-threatening disorders such as acute angle-closure glaucoma, uveitis, and keratitis; or systemic diseases such as Sjögren's syndrome, hyperthyroidism, polycythemia vera, and gout.

Hyphema, or blood in the anterior chamber between the cornea and iris, results from a tear in the ciliary body. Hyphema is easily detected by a penlight. A subconjunctival hemorrhage is a localized, patchy area of bleeding from the rupture of a small blood vessel beneath the conjunctiva. Yellow sclera are commonly associated with jaundice; bilirubin accumulates in the conjunctiva and makes it look yellow. The sclera also may appear yellow from the use of antimalarial drugs (a normal side effect) or from their toxicity. The sclerae of blacks and other dark-skinned people are often yellowish in the normal state. A tumor beneath the sclera (melanocytoma or staphyloma) may cause discoloration (a blue nevus or black elevated mass, respectively). In Wilson's disease, abnormal copper metabolism causes a rust-colored corneal ring, the Kayser–Fleischer ring.

A mucopurulent drainage from the eyes usually indicates a bacterial infection and can arise from blepharitis, conjunctivitis, dacryocystitis, or keratitis. The nurse should note the character and amount of discharge, when it occurs, and whether chronic crusting of the eyelid margins occurs. A specimen for microscopic identification, culture, and sensitivity testing may be required.

Assessing the Client's Health History

Once the nurse has clearly defined the client's chief concern, the client's health history should be assessed. Determine whether the client has ever had a similar or related visual problem and if so, determine the signs and symptoms of that complaint. Determine if the client wears contact lenses or glasses and if so, how old they are and when the last eye examination occurred.

Major illnesses and operations, especially the most recent, should be documented. If the client has recently sustained trauma, note the type and time of injury, as well as any emergency treatment given. Elicit information regarding past trauma to the eye and any permanent damage the eye may have sustained (eg, an irregularly shaped pupil). Diseases such as diabetes mellitus, hypertension, and vascular thrombosis may cause ocular changes and are crucial in the collection of a relevant data base. Also note medications currently taken and allergies to medicines.

History taking should emphasize questions that may

help confirm or negate the tentative diagnosis. Certain signs and symptoms can be expected to accompany a suspected diagnosis, and their absence or presence will further narrow the possibilities.

A family history will document congenital disorders of the eye or glaucoma within the client's blood relatives. A history of other diseases in the family that have ocular complications, such as hypertension and diabetes mellitus, is also significant.

Assessing Lifestyle

Lifestyle considerations are important in gathering subjective data for clients with ocular dysfunctions. Assess nutrition because ocular pathology related to vitamin deficiency has been noted. Avitaminosis A has been associated with corneal ulcers and xerophthalmia (dryness of the conjunctiva and cornea). In avitaminosis C (scurvy), hemorrhages may develop in the eye as well as the skin, mucous membranes, and other parts of the body. Finally, people with poor nutritional habits may develop nutritional amblyopia (dimness of vision). Heavy alcohol intake and heavy smoking have also been associated with dim vision. A proper diet, particularly one with adequate thiamine, helps correct this type of amblyopia.

The client's age is important in determining senile changes and in helping determine treatment. However, loss of vision often is attributed to a natural change of old age when, in fact, a condition exists that can be corrected by medical attention. An astounding example is the fact that clients with cataracts make up the second largest group of blind individuals in the United States (Newell, 1982). Ignorance and fear play a major role in this unfortunate and preventable statistic. The nurse should determine how the client copes with and understands the many changes that occur with aging and provide education and support as needed. Indeed, erroneous beliefs about visual changes prevent many clients from seeking treatment for many treatable degenerative processes such as cataracts and glaucoma (see Box 70–2 later in this chapter).

The client's occupation often provides insight into how well the client functions day to day, as well as insight into possible etiologic factors. The nurse should inquire about whether the client's job involves VDTs, working with small objects, exposure to machinery, or exposure to chemicals, all of which can cause eye fatigue or visual loss. Decreased job performance may be a clue to blurred vision or intrusive symptoms such as headaches. In addition, sports activities can provide additional information on causes of problems (see Chapter 69).

Assessing Social Support Systems

Impaired vision or complete loss of vision can be devastating, causing depression, anxiety, and feelings of helplessness and isolation. Without visual aids, the formerly independent client may abandon hobbies, reading, and writing. Clients cut off from these activities of daily living and from visual stimuli may experience sensory deprivation (see Chapter 4). They may become depressed, may hallucinate, and may even become suicidal. Therefore, the health care team should assess the client's available support systems in an attempt to optimize self-sufficiency.

Determine the client's home situation. Is the client living alone? Are family or friends in the area, and how do they feel about the client's visual loss? How is the client managing activities of daily living? What transportation is available? What is the client's economic status? Can the client resume the former job, or does he or she need to seek another career direction? If the client requires medication such as insulin how will it be administered? Has the client been through a rehabilitation program to relearn mobility with a cane or to learn to use other aids to assist with activities of daily living? These and similar questions help the nurse assess the client's social support systems.

OBJECTIVE DATA

Objective data are gathered through direct and indirect inspection of the eye and through related laboratory tests and diagnostic studies. Use aseptic technique when examining the eye, because microorganisms are easily transmitted from one eye to another and from the hands to the eye. Hands should be washed *before and after* each ophthalmic examination. Instruments should be cleaned appropriately, and some (eg, the tonometer) ideally should be sterilized between uses. When eye medication such as local anesthetics are instilled, make sure the dispenser tip does not touch the client's eye or eyelid.

Physical Assessment of the Eye

Physical examination of the eye consists primarily of inspection with and without specific ocular tools. Before inspecting the eye, examine the client. Note posture that may be compensating for a lack of clear vision. For example, a compensatory head posture, with the chin depressed and tilted to the uninvolved side, can be characteristic of a CN IV nerve palsy, where the superior oblique muscle depresses and causes intorsion of the eye (tilting of the eye toward the midline of the face). A lesion of CN III can cause **ptosis** (a drooping of the upper eyelid), a fixed dilated pupil, and eye abduction and intorsion. Evaluate the expression on the client's face; a wrinkled forehead might indicate eye pain, photophobia, or an attempt to elevate the upper eyelid in ptosis. Squinting may indicate strabismus. Look to see whether there is symmetry between the eyes, noting the presence of ptosis, exophthalmos, keratoconus, or facial nerve paralysis.

Ask the client to remove glasses or contact lenses for the examination. Preexamination medications such as local anesthetic eyedrops are generally not necessary until ton-

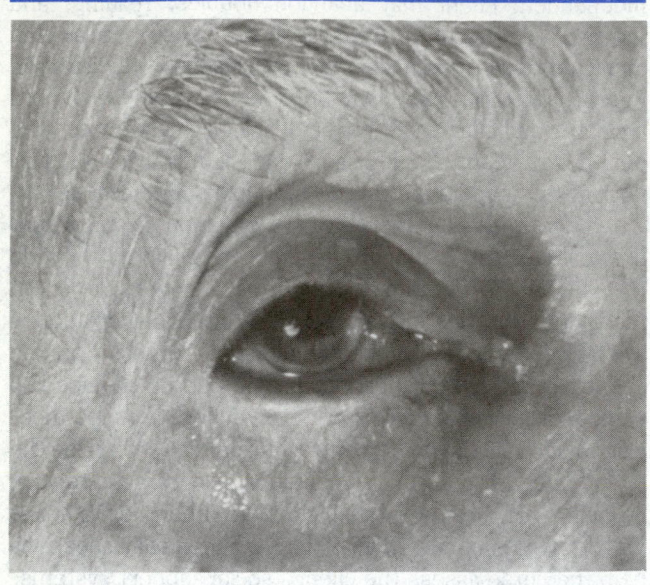

Figure 70-1

Inspecting the external eye. The epiphora of this client is due to ectropion.

ometry is performed. Dilation of the pupils is desirable for examinations and will be discussed later in this chapter.

A systematic approach to the physical inspection is helpful. In good illumination, examine the superficial parts, progressing to the ocular fundus with the use of the ophthalmoscope. Gentleness and reassuring the client are of utmost importance in ocular examinations.

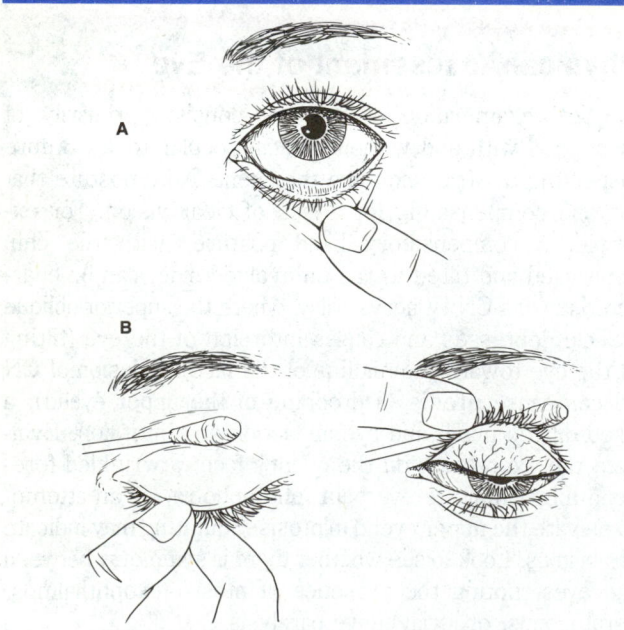

Figure 70-2

A. Everting the lower eyelid. **B.** Everting the upper eyelid.

Check the position of the eyelids, noting ptosis or drooping of the lower lid (**ectropion;** Figure 70-1). The closed eyelids should fit snugly without exposing the cornea. The eyelids are highly elastic, and any degree of swelling should be noted, along with redness and other signs of inflammation. Examine the inward surfaces of the eyelids for foreign bodies, defects, discharge, and other abnormalities. Also examine the eyelashes to determine if they are rubbing on the cornea or crusting because of discharge.

The conjunctivas should be inspected for color; they should be a pale glistening pink. Note conjunctival injection, **chemosis** (edema of the conjunctiva around the cornea), and excessive discharge. Look for evidence of hemorrhage and the presence of foreign bodies. To complete the conjunctival examination, gently evert the eyelids. The lower eyelid is easily everted by pulling down the skin inferiorly (Figure 70-2A). The upper eyelid is somewhat more difficult to evert. A step-by-step procedure is illustrated in Figure 70-2B.

The sclera may change color in disease states. A blue sclera occurs in disorders of the connective tissue; icteric sclera (a yellow sclera) is observed in cases of jaundice, where tissues are stained with bile pigments. The sclera is normally smooth, and the nurse should note inflammation, abnormal growths, or bulging.

Check the cornea for clarity, noting cloudiness or spots. The cornea's surface should be smooth and regular. Examine broken areas by staining the surface of the eyeball with sodium fluorescein, as discussed later in this chapter (see Figure 70-11). Test corneal sensation by touching a wisp of sterile cotton to each corneal surface; decreased sensitivity (a decreased blink response) can indicate CN V lesions or a herpes keratitis. On the other hand, persons who have worn contact lenses for a long period of time may have diminished corneal reflexes without neurological damage.

The diameter and curvature of the cornea are measured using calipers and the keratometer, respectively. Measuring the corneal diameter is useful in determining pathological conditions; a diameter greater than 12 mm can indicate congenital glaucoma, and small corneas (less than 10 mm in diameter) can indicate either hyperopia or angle-closure glaucoma. Corneas are also measured for placement of intraocular lens implants. A keratometer is used to measure the radius of curvature of the anterior surface of the cornea primarily for contact lens selection, but it is also useful in diagnosing keratoconus. An experienced ophthalmic nurse should be able to carry out these procedures without difficulty; however, the ophthalmologist usually makes these assessments. Because of the cornea's rich nerve supply, the client may feel severe pain from seemingly minor irritation. Thus, the nurse should promote comfort as necessary.

The iris may be examined directly. Compare its color in the two eyes; differences can indicate a uveal inflammation, tumor, or retained foreign body. Abnormalities of the iris may distort the shape of the pupil. Note each pupil's shape, size, reaction to light and whether they are equal. The pupil's light reflex is then examined under darkened conditions by shining a penlight from the side of the eyeball inward. The light reflex is a neuromuscular response to light stimulus that constricts the pupil according to the amount of illumination falling on the retina. This response progresses to the optic nerve along the optic tract to the midbrain. The CN III is then stimulated and innervates the sphincter muscle of each iris. For this reason, illumination of one eye constricts the opposite pupil simultaneously (consensual light reflex). An optic tract lesion could be the cause of dissimilar constrictions during unilateral illumination.

A dilated pupil can be caused by dimmed light, acute glaucoma, myopia, the use of sympathomimetic drugs, and old and new eye injuries. A constricted pupil will be seen with bright illumination, iris inflammation, glaucoma with pilocarpine treatment, and morphine and heroin use. Old age also can cause constricted pupils (senile miosis), but pupillary reflexes normally remain intact. Irregularly shaped pupils invariably indicate an abnormality such as iritis, central nervous system syphilis, injury, previous eye surgery, or congenital defects. Sphincter muscle tears can give the pupil border a scalloped appearance, and tears at the base of the iris produce a D-shaped pupil. A normal pupil and some of the alterations in various conditions are illustrated in Figure 70–3.

When the normally transparent avascular lens becomes opaque (cataract), vision is reduced and surgery is often indicated. Cataract formation is often a senile change but can be seen in young people as a congenital defect. Trauma and diabetes also may be associated with the formation of cataracts. Any clouding of the lens and the degree of vision impairment should be documented.

Full movement of the eyeball is regulated by the integrity of CNs III, IV, and VI. The nurse should note deviations of the eyeball and observe for unequal directions of gaze (see Chapter 69). Diplopia often results when only one eye is directed at the intended object of regard (strabismus). Measurement of deviation will be necessary to determine the treatment of choice. Since strabismus is common and can be corrected as early as 6 months of age, consult a pediatric nursing textbook for discussion about appropriate diagnostic tests and corrective treatment.

The retinal area, the *ocular fundus,* is viewed with the ophthalmoscope. The direct ophthalmoscope visualizes the optic disk, the macula, and the retinal vessels. Visualization is monocular, and images are magnified 15 times. Chapter 7 discusses the ophthalmoscopic examination in detail and illustrates the structures of the fundus. If the ocular fundus cannot be easily inspected, the pupil may be dilated with a short-acting anticholinergic such as tropicamide (Mydriacyl 11%) or phenylephrine hydrochloride (Neo-Synephrine). Analyze the client's total systemic status before dilating the pupils, because some mydriatics and other ophthalmic medications can interact with other

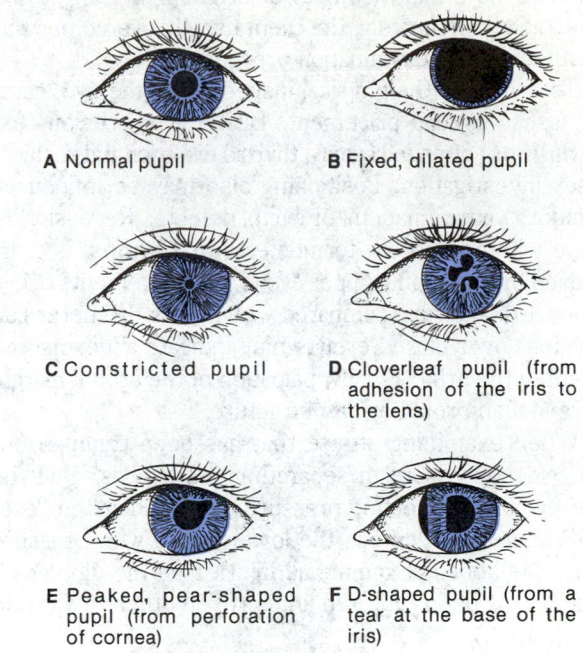

Figure 70–3

Pupil signs.

medications or diseases and produce adverse effects, such as exacerbating glaucoma. (Table 70–4, later in this chapter, lists common ophthalmic medications and their possible interactions with other medications, as well as contraindications for other diseases.) After the eyes have been examined, a miotic such as pilocarpine hydrochloride can be used to reverse the effect of mydriasis. Usually, however, the client wears a pair of sunglasses until dilatation wears off (approximately 4 hours).

Indirect ophthalmoscopy is stereoscopic and has a bright light source emerging through a hole in a mirror to give a total inverted image. It provides a larger field of vision and a better view of the peripheral retina than does direct ophthalmoscopy. The examiner wears the indirect ophthalmoscope on the head and uses a scleral depressor that gently pushes the retina toward the pupil to observe the extreme retinal periphery and ciliary body. Magnification is five times, so small hemorrhages or microaneurysms cannot be seen.

The slit lamp, a biomicroscope used in combination with a hand-held contact lens to flatten the corneal surface, can visualize the anterior part of the eye with great detail. It illuminates the cornea and lens up to 50 times. The light beam itself can be varied from a full circle beam to a narrow slit of light for examining a small section of the cornea or lens.

The direct and indirect ophthalmoscope and slit lamp examinations are always conducted in a darkened room. Explain all tests to the client to obtain accurate responses and reduce anxiety. Most eye examinations take 10 minutes, and the initial moments of bright light can be uncomfortable. Fortunately, the client usually overcomes this discomfort as the examination proceeds.

To complete the physical inspection of the eye, carefully assess eyeball placement. Bilateral protrusion (**exophthalmos**) often indicates a thyroid disorder and requires further investigation. Positioning also may be influenced by tumors, inflammation, or birth defects. Recession of the eye within the orbit, termed **enophthalmos,** is characterized by a drooping upper eyelid. Measurements of eye position are taken and compared with norms. Compression (palpation) over closed eyelids may indicate abnormal tissue within the orbit. Finally, palpation of the orbital margin may reveal an orbital or nasal fracture.

When examining an eye that has been traumatized, never exert pressure in separating the eyelids. Pull the upper eyelid up, exerting pressure only against the "eyebrow" bone, and depress the lower eyelid with pressure on the cheekbone. Examine all injuries on the globe as if the globe has been ruptured until proven otherwise (Stein & Slatt, 1983).

Assessing Refraction

The eye that sees a focused object at a distance of 20 ft is said to be normal (in a state of emmetropia). Farsightedness (hyperopia) is a failure of the light rays to converge at the retina; instead, the rays focus posterior to the retina, and vision consequently is blurred for distant objects and even more blurred for nearer objects. Vision cannot be improved by stepping farther away from the object, but the hyperopic condition can be resolved by the placement of convex lenses to neutralize the abnormal eye focus.

Nearsightedness (myopia) is caused by too strong a lens system for the distance of the retina behind the lens. In other words, the light rays focus before they reach the retina; by the time they do reach the retina, they have spread apart again, causing an unfocused object. Myopics see close objects without difficulty (the image can be brought closer to the eyes to focus the light rays on the retina) but cannot focus on distant objects. A concave lens corrects this refractive error.

Astigmatism is more complex to resolve and involves an irregular cornea or egg-shaped rather than spherical lens. Light rays cannot focus a clean image because of a dissimilarity in the cornea's north–south and east–west curves. A lens with more curvature in one direction than the other can correct astigmatism. These conditions are discussed and illustrated in Chapter 71.

Retinoscopy

Refraction is determined objectively with a retinoscope, an instrument that shines a beam of light through a trial lens. Emerging rays of light from the retina are focused at the examiner's eye. The retinoscope can precisely determine the refractive error and is especially useful in testing

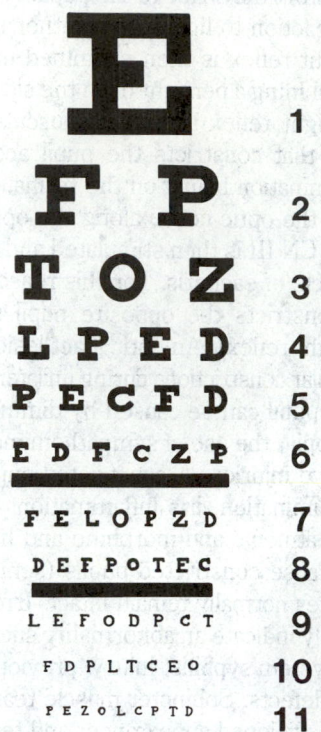

Figure 70–4

Snellen's chart.

young children and people who respond slowly or have difficulty in choosing the best lens.

Snellen's Chart and Pinhole Test

Visual acuity is the degree of detail that the eye can discern in an image; it is determined primarily by the function of the cones at the fovea centralis. The examiner can measure the ability to distinguish shapes or identify symbols to determine myopia, hyperopia, accommodation function, and the presence of clear transparent structures and an intact fovea centralis. If the client normally wears corrective lenses, the following tests should be conducted with and without the lens aid.

Snellen's chart is a group of letters that become smaller from top to bottom (Figure 70–4). The client has one eye occluded with an opaque card while the other eye is tested. At a distance of 20 ft, the client reads the line that he or she sees most clearly and continues to read each line in order of diminishing size until the letters are incorrectly identified. Acuity is recorded as a fraction; the numerator represents the client's distance to the chart, and the denominator represents the distance at which a normal eye can read the line. For example, 20/40 means that at 20 ft the client can correctly read a line that the normal eye is able to read at 40 ft. Legal blindness is defined as visual acuity of 20/200 or less in the better eye with best correction.

The pinhole test is a simple, useful test for determining decreased acuity that is due to retinal disease. With one eye occluded, the client looks at Snellen's chart through a pinhole punched in an opaque card. This prohibits all but the central rays from passing on to the macula. If the client has a refractive error, the pinhole will improve vision. Organic loss of vision, in contrast, cannot improve with a pinhole.

Assessing the Visual Field

The **visual field** is the area within which stimuli produce sight when the eye is looking straight ahead. By performing peripheral and central visual field tests, the nurse can assess the functions of the retina, optic nerve, and optic pathways. The confrontation test is an easy way to determine a decrease in peripheral vision. The examiner sits opposite the client and, with the directly opposite eye closed on both client and examiner, holds up a finger as far to the side as possible and slowly moves the finger inward into the line of vision. The client with normal vision visualizes the finger simultaneously with the examiner with normal vision.

Perimeters are tests for the peripheral field that allow the examiner to make gross estimated interpretations of visual field capacities. The client fixates on a center target point. The examiner moves an object from outside the field into the field on a radial line toward the fixation point, and the client announces when he or she sees the object.

The tangent screen is useful in determining visual field defects closer to the fovea centralis. A black felt screen is used, and test objects from 1 to 50 mm in size are randomly placed on the screen. Blind spots and **scotomata** (areas of depressed vision) can be demonstrated as each eye is individually tested for visualization of the spots (Figure 70–5) (see also Figure 37–1).

Assessing Intraocular Pressure

Normal intraocular pressure is 12 to 20 mm Hg. Tonometry can determine the pressure by measuring the amount of corneal indentation produced by a given weight. Schiotz's tonometer, shown in Figure 70–6, is one instrument that may be used. A topical anesthetic is instilled, and the supine client fixates a spot on the ceiling. The examiner places the tonometer on the apex of the cornea. The attached scale measures the amount of indentation made in the cornea by the weight of the tonometer, thus determining the pressure in the eye. The noncontact (or air-puff) tonometer is rapidly replacing Schiotz's tonometer as a screening tool in vision care facilities. It does not touch the eye. Rather, a puff of pressurized air is directed at the cornea. The deflections of the cornea in response to the puff of pressurized air are measured (Figure 70–7). Caution clients that the release of pressurized air results in an audible sound and a slight but nonpainful fleeting pressure on the cornea. Unprepared clients are often startled by the sound

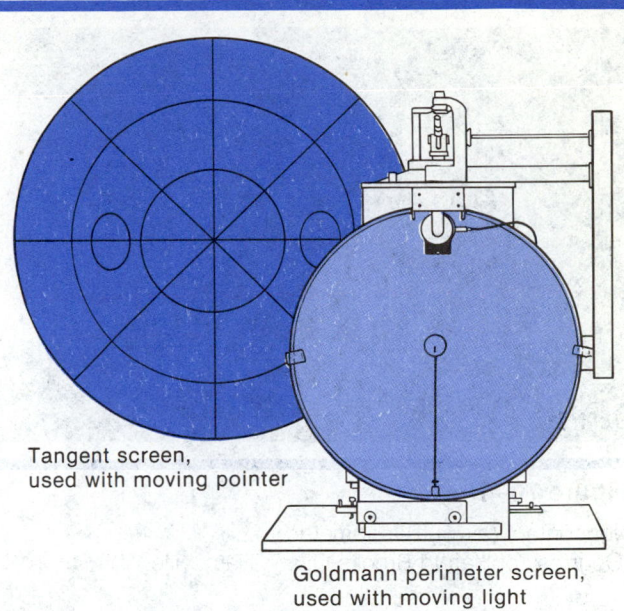

Tangent screen, used with moving pointer

Goldmann perimeter screen, used with moving light

Figure 70–5

Peripheral vision test.

and sensation and become apprehensive over testing of the second eye.

Since the signs and symptoms of glaucoma are insidious and often missed, the nurse should encourage anyone over 40 years old to have regular ophthalmologic examinations, which should always include an intraocular pressure measurement.

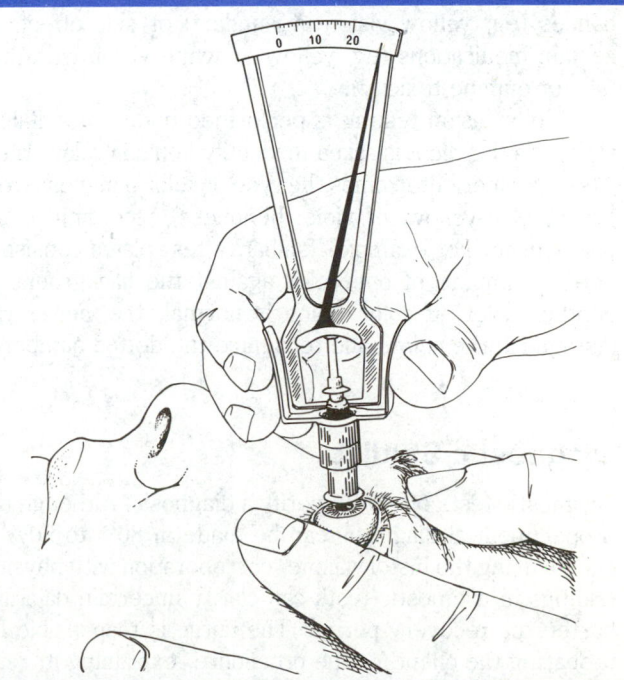

Figure 70–6

Schiotz's tonometer.

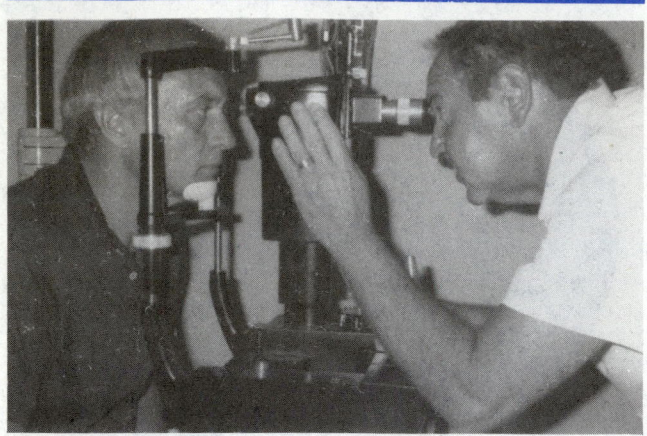

Figure 70-7
Noncontact (air puff) tonometer.
(Courtesy of Harold Brooks OD, Williamsville, NY)

Assessing Color Vision

Color blindness is inherited in 7% of men and 0.5% of women and is known to be an abnormality of the X chromosome. Central retinal degeneration and optic nerve disease also can cause loss of color vision in one eye from decreased cone function. Malnutrition and the ingestion of drugs—for example, digoxin (Lanoxin), quinidine gluconate (Quinaglute), and hydrochlorothiazide (Aldactazide and Esidrix)—can affect color vision bilaterally. Color vision problems also may be associated with systemic disturbances (eg, yellow vision in jaundice) or side effects of certain medications (eg, yellow or white vision with digitalis or quinine toxicity).

Color vision testing is performed under good illumination, as the client is asked to identify items in color plates. The examiner determines the type of color blindness (red-green, blue-yellow, or violet blindness) according to the plates used. For example, Ishihara's test plates consist of dotted numbers of one color against the background of another color. If color vision is normal, the viewer can distinguish the colors and recognize the dotted number.

Diagnostic Studies

Diagnostic tests often can verify a diagnosis. Although the proper medical diagnosis can be made in 80% to 90% of clients using the history alone, corroboration with physical findings in diagnostic tests can clarify uncertain data and hasten the recovery period. The nurse is responsible for preparing the client for the procedure, explaining it, reinforcing the physician's explanation, and offering support throughout the process.

Diagnostic studies help complete the history and physical assessment of the client. All clients admitted to the hospital have complete blood counts and urinalysis done. If the family history includes such disorders as hyperthyroidism or diabetes, the examiner should recognize the potential usefulness of obtaining related blood values, such as determining the glucose level. Intradermal skin and mucous membrane tests of suspected allergens are often done to identify an allergic cause of an eye problem. Skin tests may also be done to determine whether tuberculosis or histoplasmosis are possible sources of an eye infection. Related laboratory studies used to assess eye disorders are discussed in Table 70-2.

Ocular Culture
Nurses may participate in investigations requiring specimens through collection, proper handling, and client education. To obtain a specimen for determination of the organism present in an ocular infection, take a sterile swab and gently brush the conjunctival surface to obtain contact with possible pathogens. Transfer it to the appropriate medium to favor the growth of either aerobic or anaerobic microbes, viruses, or fungi. Do not instill antibiotic drops or ointments until after the specimen has been collected. Culturing the eye is illustrated in Figure 11-9.

Conjunctival Scraping
A conjunctival scraping may assist in the diagnosis of a disease; the histology can be studied under the microscope to identify abnormalities. In this procedure, the eye is topically anesthetized, and a conjunctival scraper (an aluminum rod with flattened ends) is gently brushed over the exposed conjunctiva by an ophthalmologist to obtain a surface scraping. The specimen is spread evenly on glass slides, dried, and sent to the laboratory for staining and examination.

Fluorescein Staining of the Cornea
Breaks in the cornea can be identified by applying a moist paper strip impregnated with sodium fluorescein to the inferior conjunctival cul-de-sac. Tears distribute the dye over the cornea. Irrigating the surface of the cornea will wash away excess dye, leaving only areas in which the corneal epithelium is absent stained green. Fluorescein staining may be combined with a slit lamp examination. A blue filter on the slit lamp highlights the fluorescein-stained cornea.

Gonioscopy
Gonioscopy is a test used to examine the angle of the anterior chamber. The device looks much like a jeweler's loupe and has a contact lens containing a mirror. When it is placed on the eye it facilitates the detection of a narrow angle (Figure 70-8).

Table 70–2   Laboratory Tests Related to Disorders of the Eye

Laboratory Test	Normal Expected Value	Disease State	Expected Abnormal Findings
Red blood cells	M 4.5–6.2 million/μL F 4.0–5.5 million/μL	Anemia (retinal and choroidal hemorrhage, loss of vision from ischemic optic neuropathy with massive hemorrhages)	Decreased
		Polycythemia (reduced flow of blood through the eye, central retinal vein occlusion, optic disk infarction, amaurosis fugax, retinal hemorrhage)	Increased
White blood cells	4500–11,000/μL	Leukemia (dilatation of retinal arteries and veins, microaneurysms, hemorrhages)	Increased
		Infectious process that is due to acute or chronic bacterial infections (eg, iridocyclitis, chorioretinitis, conjunctivitis [gonorrheal], ulcerative keratitis, orbital cellulitis)	Increased
Platelets	150,000–400,000/μL	Thrombocytopenic purpura (retinal and choroidal hemorrhages)	Decreased
Sickle-cell test: Hemoglobin S (Hb S)	Negative Hb S	Sickle-cell anemia (occlusion of small peripheral arterioles of the retina, leading to weakened neovascularization and susceptibility to severe hemorrhage)	Positive Hb S
Blood sugar, fasting	80–120 mg/dL	Diabetes (retinopathy, lens changes [cataract], iris changes with diminished pupillary responses, extraocular muscle palsy)	Increased
Thyroxine (T$_4$)	4.5–11.8 μg/dL	Hyperthyroidism, or Graves' disease (severe exophthalmos can lead to corneal ulcers, fibrosis of extraocular muscles, optic neuropathy)	Increased
Triiodothyronine (T$_3$) uptake	25%–35%	Same as T$_4$ disease state	Increased
Gram's stain	Conjunctiva free of microbes except possibly small quantities of diphtheroids and staphylococci	Isolated organisms causing infectious reaction	Identification of either gram-positive or gram-negative bacteria
Cultures	Same as Gram's stain	Same as Gram's stain disease state	Presence of coliform bacilli and related enteric organisms, *Klebsiella pneumoniae,* pathogenic fungi and viruses, *Hemophilus influenzae, Staphylococcus aureus, Diplococcus pneumoniae, Neisseria gonorrhoeae*

Computed Tomography

Computed tomography (CT) of the orbit is a diagnostic method that can detect abnormalities such as intraocular foreign bodies, orbital disease, and retinoblastoma much more dependably than conventional roentgenography. Contrast dye is injected, and the eyeball is then scanned through 180° in a path from 0.9 to 1.0 cm wide. Tumors can be correctly determined in pictures that are 100 times more accurate than conventional x-ray films.

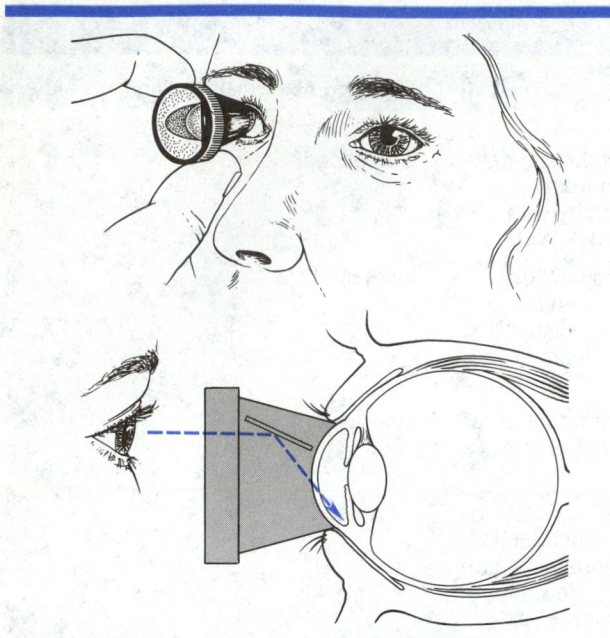

Figure 70–8

Gonioscopy. The mirror inside the lens facilitates detection of a narrowed angle.

Ultrasonography

Ultrasonography plays a useful role in determining pathological conditions of the eye, especially the lens, retina, and choroid. Sound waves with frequencies of 5000 to 20,000 Hz are used in the diagnosis of both intraorbital and orbital tumors. Lesions such as retinal detachment and fibrous tissue proliferation also can be documented easily as reflected vibrations are converted into electric potential and displayed by an oscillograph. In this noninvasive procedure, a probe is simply placed on the eyelid to reflect back to the sound probe and form an echogram. Ultrasonography is a useful adjunct to the ophthalmoscope when opacities deter visualization.

Fluorescein Angiography

Photographs of the ocular fundus, including the retina and retinal blood vessels, may be obtained through fluorescein angiography. This diagnostic test is probably the most frightening to the client because of its invasiveness and discomfort. The nurse can provide explanations and reassure the client as the ophthalmologist performs the procedure.

The fluorescein is injected into the antecubital vein and should appear in the retinal arterioles in 10 seconds. Rapid-sequence photographs are taken through the pre-dilated pupil, and the presence of vascular obstructions, neovascularizations, microaneurysms, abnormal capillary permeability, and defects of the retinal pigment epithelium may be noted. The client needs a complete explanation of the procedure, including warning of the hot sensation experienced when the dye is injected (it lasts about 10 seconds and is similar to stepping into a hot shower) and the potential for an allergic reaction (itching and hives).

Radioactive Phosphorus (^{32}P) Nuclear Studies

Radioactive phosphorus is injected into the antecubital vein when a malignant intraocular tumor is suspected. Approximately 36 to 48 hours later, the ocular area is scanned using a special probe to determine the extent of phosphorus uptake. An elevated reading signals the presence of an intraocular tumor. This can be a difficult test to perform properly; the probe must be as close to the suspected tumor location as possible to obtain an accurate reading. If the tumor is thought to be located in the posterior area, a conjunctival incision may need to be made to place the probe appropriately. Its chief function is to differentiate between a melanoma (which requires enucleation) and a nevus, preventing unnecessary enucleation. Clients need to be prepared for what to expect when this study is performed. Inform clients that ^{32}P has a short life span and quickly passes out of the body. There is no discomfort other than that from the insertion of the IV needle.

Section II: Nursing Diagnosis

Several nursing diagnoses can be considered in the nurse's assessment of a client's response to a visual impairment. Box 70–1 lists nursing diagnoses related to the visual system, and the following sections discuss the most common diagnoses.

VISUAL SENSORY-PERCEPTUAL ALTERATION

The brain receives 90% of its sensory input through sight, so impaired or reduced vision obviously inhibits sensory perception. An infant born blind has no memory of objects, colors, the environment, or spatial relationships, making the learning process exceedingly difficult. Decreased vision or blindness that occurs later in life profoundly alters the client's lifestyle. The client will grieve for the vision loss and must develop new problem-solving abilities to fit altered communication patterns and sensory perception.

KNOWLEDGE DEFICIT

A knowledge deficit may complicate the visually impaired client's sensory deficit or even cause it through unfamiliarity with self-care measures to prevent visual system problems. Furthermore, the client may be unaware of possible rehabilitation or treatments that could correct or improve the visual defect. Erroneous beliefs are common and often interfere with appropriate treatment (see Box 70–2 later in the chapter).

IMPAIRMENT OF COMMUNICATION

The visually handicapped must make substantial adjustments to facilitate communication, or social isolation and its subsequent frustration will be almost inevitable. The client's inability to visualize the body language and facial expressions of speakers can lead to unhappiness and misinterpretation for both sides. In addition, the client may find it difficult to verbalize frustrations and may withdraw rather than deal directly with the impairment.

SELF-CARE DEFICIT

The client with deteriorating vision or sudden visual loss will need new ways of performing activities of daily living, which suddenly acquire new, challenging, or even frightening aspects. Most of these clients become dependent on others to some degree, at least initially. For most mature adults, this loss of independence is devastating, and many feel hopeless.

DISTURBANCE IN SELF-CONCEPT

Visually impaired clients must reevaluate their entire way of life. They may require a complete career change, and the problems in cooking or caring for small children may provoke depression and feelings of hopelessness. The clients' roles within the family or other social support systems often change as they require assistance for activities of daily living. Dependence on spouses or children is particularly difficult for clients to accept, and both parties may misinterpret emotional responses to dependency such as anger, loss of patience, or withdrawal. Lowered self-esteem is common and can cause an inability to function.

INEFFECTIVE CLIENT COPING

As has been said in the previous paragraphs, visual alterations can induce many coping mechanisms, including depression, anger, resentment, fear, anxiety, withdrawal, denial, delusions, and hallucinations. Such adaptive behavior can profoundly affect rehabilitation and the client's ability to meet life's demands. The client will profit from a healthy, honest relationship with the family and friends but may be overcome with grief and other emotions that inhibit normal relationships.

Box 70–1 Nursing Diagnoses Commonly Related to Visual System Dysfunction
Diagnoses Directly Related to Visual System Dysfunction
Sensory-perceptual alteration: visual *Knowledge deficit:* related to visual impairment *Communication, impaired visual* *Self-care deficit:* related to visual impairment *Self-concept, disturbance in:* related to self-esteem and role performance *Coping, ineffective individual* *Coping, ineffective family* *Fear:* related to vision loss
Additional Potential Nursing Diagnoses
Comfort, alteration in: pain *Diversional activity, deficit in* *Home maintenance, impaired management of* *Mobility, impaired physical*

INEFFECTIVE FAMILY COPING

The visually impaired client's family or significant others may exhibit as much shock over the vision loss as the client does. Emotions may range from grief and compassion to feelings of guilt related to the cause of the injury or the preventable nature of the problem. The family or friends may respond in a number of ways. They may interfere in rehabilitation because of inability to accept the client's handicap, or may deal with their feelings by being overprotective of the client. The family may overcompensate for the client's loss by cutting up food and feeding the client, insisting that the client do little activity or household tasks, etc. This can put extreme pressure on the client, increase his or her anxiety, and possibly create feelings of resignation and inescapable dependency and helplessness.

FEAR

Fear of blindness is common in humans and probably develops as early as the first eyeglass fitting. Ignorance about vision can contribute to an unrelenting preoccupation with blindness and the inability to deal with vision problems realistically. Ignorance also hinders communication between client and health care givers and can intensify the client's fears.

Section III: Planning and Implementation

In addition to providing care to clients with visual system dysfunction, nurses have an important role in preserving vision and preventing its loss. Both roles are discussed in this section and in the sample nursing care plan in Table 70–3.

PRESERVING VISION AND PREVENTING LOSS OF VISION

Teaching people how to protect and preserve their eyesight is a critical nursing role that can take place in a wide variety of settings—schools, industry, the ambulatory care setting, the acute care setting, and community groups, among others. Persons without visual dysfunction should learn self-care measures to prevent injury and be able to recognize visual system dysfunction. Clients with a visual disorder should have a basic understanding of the disorder, its progress, how to maintain and enhance eyesight, and how to prevent complications. The general principles to incorporate in health teaching are discussed here.

1. Wash hands carefully to protect client.
2. Remove drainage and crusts from eye and lashes using sterile cotton and saline. Wipe from inner to outer canthus once, then discard.
3. Ask client to tilt face upward and head back.
4. Instruct client to look up.
5. Gently pull down lower lid exposing conjunctiva, taking care not to apply pressure to the eyeball.
6. Prevent contamination of medication, eye dropper, or tube.

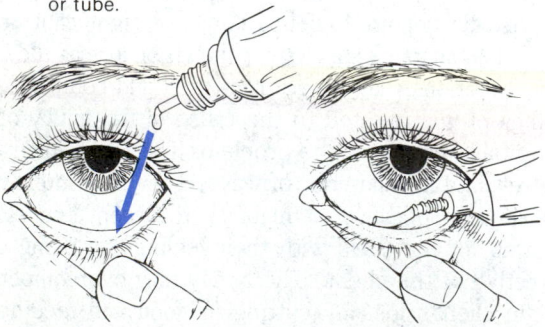

7. Squeeze the prescribed number of drops into the inferior conjunctival cul-de-sac, *not on the eye itself.*
8. Apply pressure at the inner canthus for 1 to 2 minutes, keeping the eyelid open.

7. Squeeze ointment onto the lid margin for ¼ to ½ in. Blinking and body temperature will distribute and melt the ointment.
8. Instruct client to close eyes gently for about 2 minutes.

9. Clean the client's cheek of any excess moisture or ointment.
10. Wash hands carefully to protect self from inadvertent systemic effects from client's medication.
Note: If client is to receive more than one type of eyedrop, instill the least viscous medication first, and wait at least one minute before instilling the second medication.

Figure 70–9

Instilling topical ophthalmic medications.

Regular Eye Examinations

Thorough eye examinations are important at birth; before beginning grammar school; at about 9 years of age; prior to beginning high school, college, or graduate school; and about every 5 years in early adulthood. At about 35 to 40 years of age, when many adults begin to experience vision problems, regular eye examinations every 2 years are recommended. Advise clients who have diabetes, glaucoma, or a family history of these disorders to contact a health care provider for an eye examination more frequently. An eye examination should be done whenever the client experiences any of the following:

- Disturbances of vision such as blurring, loss of peripheral vision, seeing halos around lights, or diplopia
- Pain
- Redness
- Sudden appearance of floaters
- Photophobia
- Persistent watering
- Purulent discharge
- Lesions of the eye or eyelid
- Trauma to the eye or eyelid
- Pupil irregularities

These symptoms and the disorders in which they occur are discussed in Chapter 71.

A number of health care providers are specialists in eye care. The client should know what services each provides to determine the appropriate person to consult. An *optician* grinds and fits corrective lenses and adjusts frames. An *optometrist* assesses refractive errors and eye muscle disturbances; adjusts lenses to changes in refraction and accommodation of the eye; prescribes corrective lenses, low-vision aids, and eye muscle exercises; and performs screening tests for glaucoma and color blindness. An *ophthalmologist* is a physician who specializes in the diagnosis and treatment of disorders of the eye, performs surgery, and prescribes corrective lenses and medication.

Eye Care

Because they are exposed organs, the eyes are especially vulnerable to infection and trauma. Caution clients to keep their hands away from their eyes, faces, and hair to reduce the likelihood of introducing bacteria. If the eyes must be touched, the hands should be washed thoroughly first. Eye makeup is a frequent source of infection and irritation. It should be used by one person only, not shared with others. Old eye makeup should be discarded, since it provides a good culture medium for bacteria.

The same rationale applies to discouraging clients from using someone else's eyedrops or eye ointment: Infection can be spread through contaminated materials. Proper methods for instillation of eyedrops is shown in Figure

Table 70–3   Sample Nursing Care Plan for a Client With Visual System Dysfunction

Nursing Diagnosis	Client Care Goals	Plan/Nursing Implementation	Expected Outcomes
Sensory-perceptual alteration: visual	Understanding of disease course and ability to cope with impaired vision; ability to grieve for visual loss as warranted	Educate client about potential progression of visual impairment, explaining disease process; encourage client to talk about deteriorating vision, coping methods, and attitudes toward blindness; discuss with client rehabilitation options that allow maintenance of independence; encourage participation in support groups	Client effectively copes with visual impairment; client verbalizes anxieties about visual impairment; client demonstrates an independence that allows a satisfactory lifestyle
Knowledge deficit related to visual impairment	Understanding of the limits of visual loss; recognition of available preventive treatment; seeking of treatment/care to restore optimal vision	Educate client about possible cause of visual loss, including clarification of erroneous beliefs (see Box 70–2); educate client about potential disease processes that predispose people to visual disorders; encourage the use of protective goggles and safety masks for industrial or sports activities that may compromise vision; encourage examinations for clients with symptoms of pain, redness, blurring, crossed eyes, persistent floaters, sudden photophobia, persistent watering, or purulent discharge; encourage a complete eye examination with cycloplegic refraction for people beginning grammar school, at 9 years of age, and before beginning high school, college, and graduate school; if client wears corrective lenses, encourage examinations every 5 years and after 35 to 40 years of age, every 2 years	Client recognizes the need to seek medical attention for visual impairment; client recognizes that most blindness is preventable with appropriate early therapy; client takes opportunity to correct refractive errors as demonstrated at eye examination
Communication, potential for impaired visual	Verbalization of frustration at inability to communicate and see others and at not knowing where objects are in unfamiliar surroundings	Encourage client to talk about frustrations and offer reassurance that effective communication is possible; always announce presence and departure; acquaint client with surroundings; use full description when talking about a thing, place, or person's appearance; facilitate communication using touch appropriately without startling the client; address client by name	Client resumes prior communication efficacy and copes with impaired communication in a healthy, realistic manner
Self-care deficit related to visual impairment	Maximization of functional abilities and achievements	Encourage client to dress self, feed self, and ambulate (with degree of assistance necessary); encourage caretaker to consult client if uncertain whether help is needed; educate client about rehabilitation options related to mobility training and braille; reassure client that some dependency is necessary, such as in transportation, reading menus, and selecting clothes	Client resumes prior lifestyle as appropriate; demonstrates ability to care for self; is aware of rehabilitative potential

(continued)

Table 70–3	Sample Nursing Care Plan for a Client With Visual System Dysfunction (continued)		
Nursing Diagnosis	**Client Care Goals**	**Plan/Nursing Implementation**	**Expected Outcomes**
Self-concept, disturbance in related to self-esteem and role performance	Ability to resume employment with acquired skills through career search and analysis of job skills; achievement or maintenance of financial security and independence	Encourage rehabilitation early in adjustment period; educate client about legal blindness tax deductions and state and federal funding for rehabilitation; reassure client that dependency on support groups and significant others is warranted and that qualified professionals can assist client in learning new skills; encourage client to verbalize methods for coping, attitudes toward blindness, and anxiety	Financial security; satisfactory employment; resolution of feelings of loss; ability to cope with reactions and support from significant others
Coping, ineffective client and family	Verbalization of feelings about visual impairment; return to daily functioning as physically and socially active as possible; as much autonomy as possible; maximization of achievements, functional abilities, and use of other senses; orientation to time and place	Provide opportunities to allow client to talk about shock of blindness or impaired vision; suggest counseling or psychotherapy to work out feelings of loss; encourage activities of daily living with visual aids for assistance as necessary; encourage independence as much as possible within a safe environment; emphasize remaining capabilities	Client can cope with impaired vision in a healthy, realistic manner; client demonstrates normal psychosocial status and return to previous functional ability
	Normal relations with family; ability to discuss loss with family member; maintenance of as much client independence as possible; ability to keep anxiety of family to a minimum to ease adjustment to blindness; ability of client to keep perspective regardless of family interference	Encourage client and family to talk about grieving process (allow sufficient time); suggest that client and family seek counseling if developing guilty feelings become obsessive and interfere with client's rehabilitation; educate family about goals of rehabilitation; discourage dependency attitudes such as feeding client and inhibiting activities; encourage family to allow client to perform tasks; educate family to allow client to bump into objects in the rehabilitation period without excessive expressions of sympathy or overreaction; encourage family understanding and patience; educate family about potential of rehabilitated client; dissuade family from promoting unrealistic hopes for cures	Family overcomes grieving and can promote client's rehabilitation; family understands importance of allowing client to learn and develop skills and reason for client's frustrations; family exhibits patience and understanding; family accepts reality of blindness in their loved one and assists positively in rehabilitation
Fear related to vision loss	Realistic understanding of potential blindness; development of rapport with health care givers that can assist in effective coping; ability to effectively perform activities of daily living without preoccupation with potential blindness	Educate client about disease process and expected level of visual functioning; develop client trust to assist in coping with disease process in healthy, effective manner; begin rehabilitative measures in timely manner so client will have confidence in management of activities of daily living; educate client about community groups that can provide support	Client recognizes the ability of unyielding fear to interfere with a healthy outlook on life; client understands the progression of disease without undue surprises; client overcomes fear and learns measures that allow maximum autonomy

70–9. In addition, this practice may be harmful in other ways. One person's eye medication may be contraindicated for another person because of allergies, other health conditions, interaction with other medications, or the nature of the eye disorder causing the symptoms (eg, cycloplegics and mydriatics are contraindicated in glaucoma).

Encourage clients to be alert to work, school, and hobby situations in which the potential for eye injury is high. Encourage them to wear eye protection when working with caustic chemicals or when exposed to dust and dirt, wood, metal, or glass fragments. Caution clients against rubbing their eyes; rubbing can spread infection or, if a foreign body has entered the eye, cause corneal abrasions or lacerations. The nozzle of spray products should be directed away from the eyes. Leisure and recreational activities such as racket sports or games in which sticks or flying objects are used are also potentially dangerous. In addition to helping clients assume responsibility to protect their eyes, nurses as citizen activists can support legislation outlawing the sale of dangerous toys and fireworks and promote the use of shatterproof glass, safety goggles, and protective sports equipment. First aid treatment for eye injuries and foreign bodies in the eye is discussed in Chapter 71.

The client can prevent or reduce eye fatigue by following a few guiding principles:

- Use adequate illumination. The lamp or light should not cast shadows on the work or reading area. Table lamps should be about 24 in high and placed on the nondominant side (eg, to the left for someone who is right handed).
- Rest the eyes often during prolonged use. Looking away to focus on other objects in the distance or closing the eyes helps rest them.
- Individualize the work area that contains a VDT. Screen glare can be avoided by using a tilt table or turntable, adjusting the lighting or the location of the VDT (if possible), applying a nonglare coating to the screen, or purchasing eyeglasses specifically designed to ease eye fatigue from VDT work.

Discourage the practice of using old (and no longer accurate) or secondhand eyeglasses. Although they may improve vision, the refraction correction can be off considerably. Purchasing over-the-counter reading glasses that magnify print may be a very brief solution when reading glasses are lost or broken, but these lenses are not individualized and should not be used for a long period of time. Explore with clients the reasons for using any of these eyeglasses. If clients are unaware that these glasses can cause eye fatigue, the information provided will encourage clients to discontinue their use. If the reason is financial, arrange a social service referral to help clients obtain corrective lenses especially for them.

Discussing eye care provides the nurse with the opportunity to clarify any misconceptions clients may have about eye care, eye health, and visual disorders. Some

Box 70–2 Myths About Visual Impairments and Their Clarification

Myth: *Overuse of the eyes will wear them out; if one eye is not viable, use of the other eye may produce damage from strain.*
Fact: **There is no way either one or both eyes can be worn out.**

Myth: *Reading in dim light harms vision.*
Fact: **Reading in dim light will not damage vision; however, it may cause fatigue and discomfort.**

Myth: *Sitting too close to the television ruins vision.*
Fact: **Sitting close to the television does not harm eyesight.**

Myth: *The eyeball is removed for surgery.*
Fact: **The eyeball remains intact during surgery. Its removal would damage the vessels and nerves at the posterior portion, and replacement would be impossible.**

Myth: *Red eye is an insignificant symptom.*
Fact: **Redness of the eye is the cardinal sign of ocular inflammation and can indicate serious disease (as well as minor disorders).**

Myth: *Glasses that fit incorrectly can worsen vision.*
Fact: **Glasses that are too weak or too strong may cause blurring or discomfort but do not irreparably harm the eyes.**

Myth: *Wearing glasses makes people dependent on them.*
Fact: **After the removal of glasses, an adjustment period may be necessary. However, unnecessary glasses will not harm or further damage the eye.**

Myth: *Exercises can correct refractive errors.*
Fact: **Exercises can strengthen eye muscles but cannot correct a refractive error that is due to an anatomic defect (inadequate length of the eyeball or irregular curvature).**

Myth: *Extra vitamins or megadoses of vitamins A and B will maintain or enhance eye health.*
Fact: **Although vitamin A and B deficiencies may cause problems such as night blindness and impairment or deterioration of the cornea, lens, and retina, an excess intake may cause papilledema and impair vision by damaging the optic nerve.**

Myth: *Eyewashes and other over-the-counter (OTC) preparations to cleanse the eye help promote eye health and prevent infection.*
Fact: **The natural secretions of the eye do a good job of cleaning the eye and should not be removed. The OTC preparations may contain substances to which some people are allergic. Furthermore, using the eyecup provided with these preparations may spread infection from one eye to the other.**

common erroneous beliefs and what the nurse can say to clarify them are discussed in Box 70–2.

Ophthalmic Medications

The drugs prescribed by the ophthalmologist are usually applied to the eye in the form of drops and, more rarely, ointments. The categories of ophthalmologic medications and the effects they produce are listed here:

- **Adrenergics.** These drugs release epinephrine from the sympathetic nerve fibers and produce mydriasis and vasoconstriction of the ocular vessels. Adrenergics may be used in conjunction with miotics when miotics cannot completely control the intraocular pressure of clients with open-angle glaucoma.

- **Anesthetics.** Topical anesthesia with benoxinate hydrochloride (Dorsacaine) or proparacaine hydrochloride (Ophthaine) is most common in cataract surgery, iridectomy, prior to removing foreign bodies and sutures, and prior to performing certain diagnostic procedures such as tonometry and gonioscopy. Anesthetics produce short-acting, rapid anesthesia. Retrobulbar infiltration may be required for some surgical procedures (see Chapter 72).

- **Anticholinergics.** These drugs block the passage of impulses through the parasympathetic nerves, resulting in mydriasis and paralysis of accommodation. They are relatively short acting, lasting only a few hours.

- **Antimicrobials.** These drugs are administered topically, subconjunctivally, or systemically to treat bacterial, fungal, or viral infections by destroying or inhibiting the organism's growth.

- **Beta-adrenergic-blocking agents.** These agents block the release of epinephrine and reduce both normal and increased intraocular pressure. Their exact mechanism of action is not yet clear; they are thought to reduce the production of aqueous humor but in some instances have been observed to increase its outflow.

- **Carbonic anhydrase inhibitors.** These drugs are thought to inhibit the activity of the enzyme carbonic anhydrase, which apparently plays a role in the control of ocular fluid formation. The result is a reduction in intraocular pressure. Carbonic anhydrase inhibitors are generally used on a short-term basis to treat glaucoma.

- **Cholinergics.** The cholinergics are parasympathomimetics that act directly to release acetylcholine from parasympathetic nerve fibers. They produce miosis, contraction of the ciliary muscles, dilation of blood vessels, and increased aqueous humor outflow.

- **Cholinesterase inhibitors.** These newer agents are more potent miotics than the cholinergics. They act indirectly by inhibiting the enzymatic destruction of acetylcholine. The acetylcholine then accumulates and acts on the iris sphincter and ciliary muscles, causing miosis. The short-acting compounds are used more often than long-acting compounds, which may actually decrease fluid outflow and increase intraocular pressure.

- **Corticosteroids.** Corticosteroids dramatically relieve ocular pain and discomfort. By suppressing ocular inflammation, they inhibit redness, swelling, capillary dilation, exudation, cellular infiltration, and collagen deposits.

- **Cycloplegics.** In addition to producing mydriasis, these drugs (usually anticholinergics) paralyze accommodation (cause **cycloplegia**) by blocking the action of acetylcholine on the iris sphincter and ciliary muscles. Cycloplegics are used for refractive purposes and when it is desirable to keep the pupil dilated (eg, for infectious conditions of the iris and ciliary body, in corneal diseases, and after certain operations). They should not be administered to clients with glaucoma.

- **Hyperosmotics.** These agents create a rapid increase in extracellular fluid osmolality, causing fluid to move out of the eye and reducing intraocular pressure. They are used before or during surgery when it is desirable to reduce the intraocular pressure and to treat glaucoma. They may be administered parenterally or orally.

- **Miotics.** These drugs constrict the pupil (cause **miosis**). In addition, they produce accommodation and facilitate increased aqueous humor outflow, thus reducing intraocular pressure. Miotics are commonly used in the treatment of glaucoma. Both cholinergics and cholinesterase inhibitors can produce miosis.

- **Mydriatics.** Dilation of the pupil (**mydriasis**) can be produced by adrenergics and anticholinergics. Their use facilitates thorough examination of the fundus. Because they prevent the outflow of fluid and thus increase intraocular pressure, mydriatics should not be administered to clients with glaucoma. They do not interfere with accommodation and thus do not have a cycloplegic effect.

Most of these drugs are applied topically, although some may be administered orally or parenterally. Topical application, however, does not guarantee that unwanted systemic effects will be avoided. Cholinergic and miotic drugs (those that constrict the pupil) are most likely to cause systemic reactions. Scrupulously adhering to the prescribed dose helps avoid systemic reactions. Applying pressure at the inner canthus for 1 to 2 minutes after administration compresses the lacrimal duct, preventing systemic absorption through the mucous membranes of the nose. Keep the client's eyelids apart for several seconds while applying pressure to allow the drug to act on the surface of the eye. People instilling miotics should wash their hands when finished to prevent systemic absorption from a drug-contaminated finger that comes in contact with the mucous membranes.

Procedures for instilling eyedrops and ointments are discussed in Figure 70–9. Remember that whoever instills the eye medication—nurse, client, family member, or significant other—should begin only after careful handwashing; prevent contamination of the medication, eyedropper, or tube; and be gentle to avoid any injury to the eye.

A diffusional system is sometimes used to provide controlled consistent delivery of a drug for periods of up to a week. The system is a plastic device slightly larger than a contact lens, which is inserted into the conjunctival

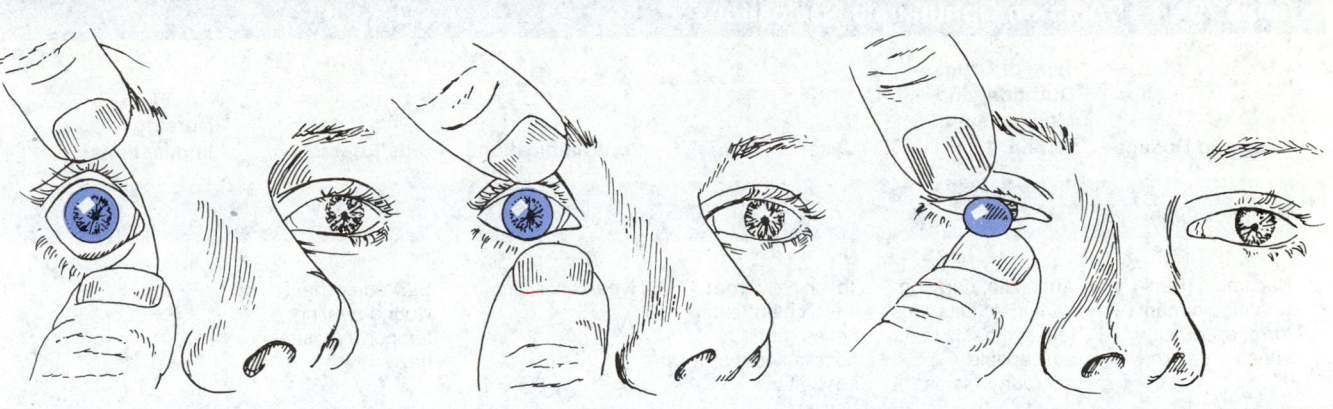

Figure 70–10

Emergency removal of hard contact lenses. **A.** After the eyelids have been separated and the corneal contact lens has been correctly positioned over the cornea, widen the eyelid margins beyond the top and bottom edges of the lens. **B.** Move the lower eyelid margin near the edge of the bottom of the lens; then move the upper eyelid margin near the edge of the top of the lens. Move under the bottom edge of the lens by pressing slightly harder on the lower eyelid while moving it upward. **C.** After the lens has tipped slightly, move the eyelids toward one another and thereby cause the lens to slide out between the eyelids. Reprinted by permission of American Optometric Association.

sac. The drug is contained in a reservoir between two membranes that allow it to diffuse into the eye. A diffusional system frees clients from having to administer multiple doses of eyedrops and is most commonly used for glaucoma, because the intraocular pressure can be controlled more consistently.

As with the administration of any drug, the nurse should make sure that the right drug in the right dose is given to the right client in the right way at the right time. Accidentally administering a mydriatic instead of a miotic to a client with primary angle-closure glaucoma, for example, could precipitate an acute attack and result in blindness. Keeping the medication at the client's bedside helps avoid confusion and lessens the likelihood of contamination.

Many ophthalmic solutions deteriorate rapidly. Check expiration dates and also discard solutions that become cloudy or change color. Table 70–4 discusses some of the most common ophthalmic medications.

APPLYING EYEPATCHES OR EYESHIELDS

Eyepatches are frequently used as protection for an affected eye. They also serve as bandages, to collect drainage, and to provide rest to limit eye movement. A tight pressure patch is occasionally used for corneal abrasions (to promote epithelial attachment) or after an enucleation (to prevent bleeding). Metal-pierced shields are common practice, placed over an eyepatch to provide extra protection, particularly at night. Eyepatches should be securely taped from the middle of the forehead outward to the cheekbone. They should be changed at least twice a day and more often when

drainage is noted. It is important to dispose of the patches as warranted (drainage from infections requires that patches be separated from other refuse). Good hand-washing is essential before and after changing patches, and cross-contamination from one infected eye to another is avoided by cleansing the hands between care of each eye.

PROMOTING ADAPTATION TO VISUAL SENSORY-PERCEPTUAL ALTERATION

Coping with changes in visual sensory perception is a long-term process facilitated by the client's new abilities to function in activities of daily living. Encourage the client to talk about the deteriorating vision and methods of coping. Preconceived attitudes about blindness may hinder the rehabilitative progress and thus should be identified at the onset.

The client care goals for those with sensory-perceptual changes are relearning independence through rehabilitation, education about visual pathology and treatment, and developing the ability to cope with impaired vision in a healthy, realistic manner. Finally, the client must reexamine how to continue to meet basic needs with a visual alteration. Specific suggestions on attaining these goals are discussed below and throughout this section.

The nurse should offer the client consistent encouragement and motivation throughout this difficult adjustment period. Encourage the client to discuss coping methods and evaluate his or her progress so that the health care program can be tailored to meet the most important psychosocial needs.

(continued on p. 2021)

Table 70–4   Common Ophthalmic Medications

Drug and Dosage	Type of Drug, Duration, and Mechanism of Action	Uses	Contraindications	Side Effects	Nursing Implications
Antimicrobials					
Bacitracin (Baciguent); ointment form; application varies greatly	Antibiotic; duration varies; inhibits protein synthesis in susceptible microorganisms	To topically treat infections of external eye and adnexa caused by susceptible bacteria	Hypersensitivity	Slowed corneal wound healing; temporary visual haze	
Chloramphenicol (Chloromycetin, Chloroptic) Neomycin sulfate (Myciguent) Gentamicin sulfate (Garamycin) Tobramycin (Tobrex): 1–2 gtt up to every hour (varies greatly)	Antibiotics; duration varies; inhibits protein synthesis in susceptible microorganisms	Same as for bacitracin	Hypersensitivity	Hypersensitivity; alteration in normal microflora of the ocular tissue; nausea and vomiting; occasional burning and stinging of the eye	Culture and sensitivity tests should be performed initially, and periodically during continued treatment; watch for signs of superinfection; protect drug from light and check expiration dates
Dexamethasone 0.1%, neomycin sulfate, polymyxin B sulfate (Maxitrol): 1–2 gtt up to every hour, also in ointment form 3–4 times daily	Combination steroid/antibiotics; duration varies; suppresses inflammatory response and acts against specific organisms	To treat ocular inflammation when concurrent use of an antimicrobial is judged necessary	Dendritic keratitis vaccinia; varicella; microbacterial infection of the eye; hypersensitivity	Allergic sensitizations; increased intraocular pressure with possible development of glaucoma; optic nerve damage (infrequent)	
Bacitracin zinc, neomycin sulfate, polymyxin B sulfate (Polysporin); ointment form; applied q. 3–4 h	Antibiotic; duration varies; inhibits protein synthesis in susceptible microorganisms	Same as for bacitracin	Hypersensitivity	Possibly retarded corneal healing; overgrowth of nonsusceptible organisms	
Carbonic Anhydrase Inhibitors					
Acetazolamide (Diamox, Hydrazol); tablets: 125–250 mg q.i.d.; sustained-release capsules: 500 mg b.i.d.; IM 500 mg initially, then 250 mg q.4h. May be given IV during an acute attack	Diuretic; 4–6 h; affects carbonic anhydrase in ciliary body, thus reducing secretion of aqueous humor	To treat chronic simple (open-angle) glaucoma, secondary glaucoma; preoperatively in acute angle-closure glaucoma where surgery is delayed to lower intraocular pressure	When sodium and/or potassium blood serum levels are depressed; marked kidney and/or liver disease	Lowered serum potassium; gastric distress; diarrhea; kidney stones; shortness of breath; fatigue; tingling extremities	Give in morning if possible to avoid interference with sleep as a result of diuretic action; monitor intake or output; observe for, and advise client to report signs of hypokalemia: muscle weakness; respiratory distress, heart irregularities, and signs of metabolic acidosis (malaise, headache, weakness, nausea and vomiting, and abdominal pain); IM injections cause intense pain

Drug and Dosage	Type of Drug, Duration, and Mechanism of Action	Uses	Contraindications	Side Effects	Nursing Implications
Corticosteroids					
Prednisolone acetate (Pred Forte) 1.0% and 0.12%: 1–2 gtt q.i.d. up to q.1h	Steroid; duration varies; inhibits edema, fibrin deposition, capillary dilation, phagocytic migration of the acute inflammatory response, capillary proliferation, deposition of collagen, scar formation	To treat inflammatory conditions of anterior segment of eye, allergic conjunctivitis, uveitis, keratitis	Acute superficial herpes simplex, vaccinia, varicella, and most other viral diseases of the cornea and conjunctiva	Increase in intraocular pressure; slow wound healing; increased risk of glaucoma or cataracts; hypersensitivity	Shake gently before using; drug may increase intraocular pressure and mask infection, so warn client to report incidence of slow healing or persistent inflammation; protect drug from light
Hyperosmotic Agents					
Mannitol (Osmitrol): 1–3.2 gm/kg of body weight of 20% solution should be administered 1–1½ h prior to surgery over a 30-min period	Osmotic diuretic; 5–6 h; reduces intraocular pressure by making plasma in the blood system hypertonic relative to aqueous humor	To treat acute (angle-closure) glaucoma; preoperatively and postoperatively when reducing intraocular pressure is indicated	Hypersensitivity; hypotension; inadequate renal function; unstable cardiovascular status; severe dehydration; pregnancy	Diuresis; fluid and electrolyte imbalance; dryness of mouth, thirst; headache; blurred vision; nausea and vomiting; dizziness; tachycardia	Monitor intake, out, and electrolytes; avoid extravasation (observe injection site for signs of inflammation or edema); do not give fluids to allay dryness or thirst, since this counteracts the desired effect; client may suck on small amounts of cracked ice
Miotics					
Carbachol (Isopto Carbachol) 0.75%–3.0%: 1–2 gtt 3–4 times daily	Synthetic cholinergic 4–6 h; constricts pupil	To manage glaucoma	Corneal abrasions; acute iritis	Spasm of ciliary body resulting in reduced accommodation, plus headache and sensitivity	Occlude tear duct; instruct client to avoid squeezing lids together
Physostigmine, eserine 0.25%–0.5%: 1–2 gtt 3–4 times daily	Short-acting cholinesterase inhibitor; 1–24 h; acts on iris sphincter and ciliary muscles to cause pupil constriction	To manage glaucoma	Coronary occlusion; parkinsonism; bradycardia; intestinal obstruction; hypotension; primary angle-closure glaucoma	Allergic reactions (have caused limited use of the drug)	Occlude tear duct; use only clear, colorless solutions; discard solutions that turn pink or red; store in tightly covered, light-resistant containers in a cool place to slow rate of deterioration; inform client that lid-twitching, temporary blurred vision, and difficulty seeing in dim light may occur

(continued)

Table 70–4   Common Ophthalmic Medications (continued)

Drug and Dosage	Type of Drug, Duration, and Mechanism of Action	Uses	Contraindications	Side Effects	Nursing Implications
Pilocarpine hydrochloride 0.5%–4.0%: 1–2 gtt up to 6 times daily	Cholinergic; 4–6 h; most commonly used miotic; constricts pupil; causes ciliary spasm; deepens anterior chamber; causes vasodilation of trabecular meshwork	To manage glaucoma; postoperatively to prevent displacement of vitreous; to reverse the effect of mydriatics	Where constriction is undesirable (eg, acute iritis); interacts with cyclopropane or halogenated hydrocarbons to cause arrhythmias and tachycardia; interacts with tricyclic antidepressants to potentiate cardiac effects	Spasm of ciliary body resulting in reduced accommodation	Preserve in tightly covered, light-resistant containers; may cause blurred vision and difficulty focusing; caution client against driving a motor vehicle or operating machinery until vision is clear; occlude the tear duct for 1–2 min after administration to avoid excessive systemic effects
Timolol maleate (Timoptic) 0.25%–0.5%: 1–2 gtt b.i.d.	Beta-adrenergic-blocking agent; 12–28 h; reduces aqueous humor formation; possibly increases outflow	To manage glaucoma, decrease intraocular pressure and secretion of aqueous humor	Possible increased effect when used with epinephrine or carbonic anhydrase inhibitors; bronchospasm; severe COPD; uncontrolled cardiac failure; increased ocular and systemic effect with propranolol and other oral beta-adrenergic-blocking agents; hazardous increased effect when used with MAO inhibitors	Asthma; increased blood pressure; hypersensitivity reactions; ocular irritations	Occlude tear duct; instruct client on instillation; monitor blood pressure and heart rate (both may decrease with systemic absorption); instruct client not to touch dropper to eye or surrounding tissue
Mydriatics and Cycloplegics					
Atropine sulfate (Isopto Atropine) 0.5% and 1.0% w/ v: 1–2 gtt b.i.d.	Anticholinergic; up to 6 days; relaxes ciliary muscle; dilates pupil; paralyzes accommodation	Preoperative and postoperative use in intraocular surgery; to treat keratitis, iritis, cyclitis; to perform refractive work in children	Primary angle-closure glaucoma	Dryness of the mouth; photophobia	Have client avoid hazardous activities if blurred vision or dizziness occurs; discontinue if eye pain, conjunctival palpitation, rapid pulse, or dizziness occur; occlude tear duct; encourage dark glasses; mydriatic effect can last up to 6 days
Cyclopentolate hydrochloride (Cyclogyl) 0.5%–1.0%; 2.0% solution for darkly pigmented irises: 1–2 gtt q. 10 min	Anticholinergic; less than 24 h; see homatropine hydrobromide for mechanism of action	Whenever mydriasis is required with minimal cycloplegia; refraction; to treat iritis or iridocyclitis	Primary angle-closure glaucoma	Local sensitivity; signs of CNS toxicity (rare)	Encourage wearing of dark glasses for photophobia; medication can burn when instilled; occlude tear duct; have client avoid hazardous activities

Drug and Dosage	Type of Drug, Duration, and Mechanism of Action	Uses	Contraindications	Side Effects	Nursing Implications
Epinephrine hydrochloride (Epifrin) 0.5%–2.0%: 1–2 gtt 1–2 times daily	Adrenergic; 12–72 h; stimulates dilator smooth muscle to dilate pupil	To manage open-angle glaucoma (long duration, no miosis); for early control of glaucoma to decrease morning intraocular pressure	Cardiac history; shallow anterior chamber; primary angle-closure glaucoma; with cyclopropane or halogenated hydrocarbons, can cause arrhythmias and tachycardia; with tricyclic antidepressants or antihistamines, can potentiate cardiac effects of epinephrine	Systemic effect; headache; heart palpitations; allergies; long-term use can cause melanoma deposits in conjunctival cells	Drug causes mydriasis with blurred vision and sensitivity to light; if using with miotic, instill miotic 2–10 min before epinephrine because of limited capacity of conjunctival sac; transient stinging may follow initial administration, and headache is common at first but decreases with continued use; solutions that turn brown should be discarded
Homatropine hydrobromide (Isopto Homatropine) 1.0% and 2.0% w/v: 1–2 gtt q. 10–15 min	Anticholinergic; 6–24 h; blocks responses of sphincter muscle of the iris and accommodative muscle of the ciliary body to cholinergic stimulation; produces pupillary dilation and paralysis of accommodation	Ophthalmic examination; intraocular surgery; to treat keratitis, iritis, cyclitis	Primary angle-closure glaucoma	Local sensitivity	Do not exceed recommended dosage; photophobia can occur so encourage use of dark glasses; occlude tear duct; have client avoid hazardous activities
Tropicamide (Mydriacyl) 0.5%–1.0%: 1–2 gtt every 30 min	Anticholinergic; 30–40 min; blocks normal sphincter tone of iris, causing pupil dilation	To perform diagnostic procedures; to dilate eye to view fundus preoperatively and postoperatively	Primary glaucoma	Muscle rigidity; pallor; nausea and vomiting; cyanosis	Transient stinging may occur, as well as photophobia and blurred vision; encourage use of dark glasses; occlude tear duct

Vision Aids and Environmental Modification

Clients with problems of visual sensory perception can be helped by a variety of vision aids and alterations in the environment.

- Eyeglasses. Glass or plastic lenses in a cosmetically appealing plastic or metal frame can be used to correct refractive errors and are further discussed in Chapter 71.
- Contact lenses. Made of plastic, contact lenses also correct problems of refraction. They are discussed in detail in the following section.
- Cataract glasses. These heavy, thick glasses are used after cataract surgery. Their advantages and disadvantages are discussed in Chapter 72 in the section on cataract surgery.
- Intraocular lens implants. These permanent plastic lenses are inserted into the eye at the time of cataract surgery. They simulate natural vision closely and are discussed and illustrated in Chapter 72.
- Magnifiers. Hand-held magnifiers can be used to enlarge print or for fine detail. Chest-supported and stand magnifiers leave the hands free.
- Monocular telescope. This device, when held to the eye, can be used to read street signs and enhance distant vision.
- Night vision microscope. Worn on the head, this device enables clients to see better in the dark.

- Field-widening devices. For clients with constricted visual fields such devices as press-on prisms for glasses help to widen the peripheral field.

- Enlarged print. Large print books, magazines, and newspapers (eg, *The New York Times*) may be purchased or borrowed from the local library.

- Optical-to-tactile converters. These devices convert vision into tactile sensation. A miniature camera moved along a line of print reproduces the outline of a letter on a tactile screen by adjusting a series of tiny rods.

- Talking books, magazines, and newspapers. Records or tapes of books, magazines (eg, *Newsweek*), and newspapers are available on loan from agencies for the blind or public libraries. Tapes are also available for purchase.

- Braille. Agencies for the blind and correspondence courses will teach a client how to use the braille system of writing and printing by means of tangible points or dots. Specially designed braille watches, household devices, books, magazines, playing cards, and medical aids are available.

- Guide dogs. Especially trained dogs help blind persons become mobile. Month-long training courses teach blind persons how to use this technique and how to care for the dog.

- Magnifying television screens. Additions to a regular television set make TV more accessible.

- Telephone aids. Special dials are available for telephones in both large print and braille.

- Canes. White canes with red tips help to identify the blind person who uses a cane to locate obstacles in the environment. Newly developed laser canes cannot only locate objects, but can also identify changes in the terrain as far away as 20 feet.

New aids are always being developed. The agencies listed in the resources section at the end of this chapter will be able to provide current information.

Contact Lenses

The inventor and artist Leonardo da Vinci first proposed fitting the eye with a lens to correct vision problems. Today more than 20 million people wear contact lenses, plastic disks that float on the tear layer that covers the cornea and are held in place by surface tension. They are preferred by many because of their cosmetic appeal. In some instances (after cataract surgery is one), they provide better vision correction than the more conventional eyeglasses.

Various types of contact lenses are available. Some are especially good for people with astigmatism, while others are safer for people who play sports. Some should not be worn by persons who work near chemical vapors or fumes. Table 70–5 lists the advantages and disadvantages of each

---

Box 70–3 Health Education for Contact Lens Wear

Wash hands carefully before insertion or removal; be sure hands are thoroughly dried if using soft lenses.

Check for lens damage and foreign bodies before insertion.

Never wet contact lenses with saliva.

Clean lenses after each wearing (work over a clean towel).

Keep storage case clean; replace solution on a regular basis; inspect case for damage.

Use only recommended cleaning, soaking, and storage solutions.

Avoid getting eye makeup or hair spray on hands or lenses, and avoid using overhead hair dryers.

Keep nails trimmed to avoid damaging lenses.

Remove lenses before swimming to avoid loss or absorption of irritating chemicals.

Avoid sleeping or napping while wearing contact lenses.

Keep use limitations in mind; do not overwear contact lenses.

Avoid rubbing the eyes when wearing contact lenses or using eyedrops unless recommended by a vision care provider.

Wear safety equipment when necessary on the job or during athletic activities; do not rely on contact lenses for eye protection.

Carry a medical emergency card calling attention to the contact lenses.

Have regular vision care examinations.

---

type and the care they require and illustrates proper insertion and removal.

Contact lenses require time, effort, skill, and proper management on the part of the wearer. Box 70–3 provides a list of dos and don'ts that should reinforce instruction provided to the client.

Emergency removal of contact lenses may also become a nursing responsibility. When clients are comatose or unable to remove contact lenses by themselves, nurses may have to remove them manually. Figures 70–10 (p. 2017) and 70–11 illustrate emergency removal. *Note the caution in Figure 70–11.* Do not attempt to remove contact lenses if the cornea cannot be visualized, the eye is injured, or removal is difficult; contact an ophthalmologist instead.

ENHANCING COMMUNICATION

Clients with impaired vision because of disease or eye-patches will have their anxiety lessened when care providers announce their presence and departure, letting clients know who they are and what they are doing. Remember to address clients directly when speaking to them and provide descriptions of people, places and things. Avoid startling clients by touching them unexpectedly.

It is helpful (and safe practice) to acquaint visually impaired people with their surroundings and how they can obtain help if they need it.

PROMOTING ADAPTATION TO THE HOSPITAL ENVIRONMENT

A trusting rapport can be initiated by taking time to introduce the hospital environment to the visually impaired client upon admission for a medical or surgical procedure. If placed in a two- to four-bed ward, it is helpful to place the visually impaired client closest to the bathroom. The client should be walked around the room (and the bed), holding on to the nurse's elbow, to find his or her bearings. Descriptions such as "The nightstand is just to the right of the head of the bed as you're facing the bed" or "There is an armchair at the foot of the bed" are helpful (and important) information. The nurse should have the client touch the various pieces of furniture to understand the spatial scheme of his room. Location of the nurse's call light and telephone should be within easy reach. The bedside table should be placed on the client's most visual side of the bed. Tissues and paper bags for refuse taped to the raised siderails are convenient for the visually impaired. When assisting the client in unpacking personal belongings, it is advisable to allow the client to place any articles in the drawers to increase awareness of their location and promote independence in retrieving items as needed during the hospital stay.

When meal trays arrive, the client is often able to feed himself or herself provided the location of each food on the plate has been described. A common practice is to refer to each food on the plate by times on the clock (eg, "The potatoes are at 3 o'clock"). Assisting with the opening of condiment packages and milk cartons is helpful. It is best for the nurse to cut up the food, butter the bread, and warn the client of any hot beverages on the tray.

Discourage the newly visually impaired client from getting out of bed at night without assistance. Despite thorough orientations to the geography of the hospital, darkness may invite unsafe conditions and a client with one eyepatch or bilateral patches may have a different perception of his or her surroundings.

IMPROVING SELF-CARE ABILITY

Health care team members should formulate a plan for restoring order in the client's life as early as possible. Evaluate the client's basic personality, and maximize his or her accomplishments. The nurse should encourage as much self-care as possible, such as in dressing, eating, and ambulating. Consulting the client when unsure if assistance is needed avoids impinging on the client's independence. The client should be aware, however, that some dependency is necessary, especially at first, for activities such as home management, transportation, assistance with menu selections, and selection of daily wardrobe. Educate the

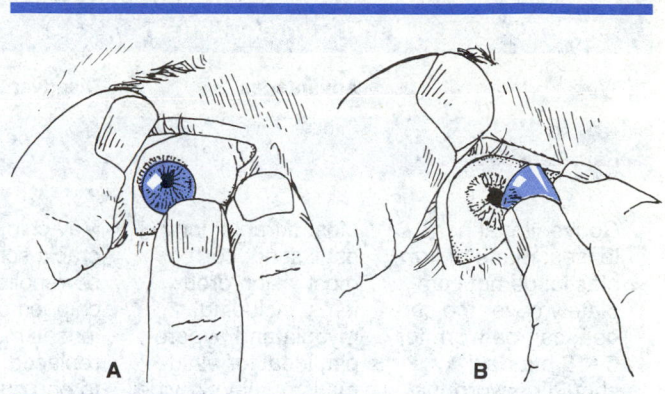

Figure 70–11

Emergency removal of soft contact lenses. 1, with clean hands, pull down the lower lid with the middle finger and place the index fingertip on the lower edge of the lens. **A.** 2, Slide the lens down to the white part of the eye. 3, Compress the lens lightly between the thumb and index finger. 4, Bring thumb and index finger together in a "pinching" motion, causing the lens to double up between fingers, allowing air underneath. **B.** 5, Remove the lens from the eye. **Caution:** Inadequate tearing caused by severe injury or shock may cause the lens to adhere to the eye. If the lens resists removal, flush the eye with normal saline solution, wait several minutes, then follow the above five steps for removal. Reprinted by permission of American Optometric Association.

client about mobility training and learning braille if appropriate to promote as much independence as possible.

IMPROVING SELF-CONCEPT

The client regaining autonomy during the rehabilitation process recognizes his or her self-worth and accomplishments. Thus, early rehabilitation alleviates problems from changed role performance and lowered self-esteem, as well as helps achieve or maintain financial security and independence.

Encourage the client to evaluate career options realistically. Often a different job with the same employer is possible, but newly acquired skills may be necessary. If career changes are necessary, educate the client about public funds available for rehabilitation. Health care team members should reassure the client that dependency on support groups and significant others is warranted in learning new skills. The resources listed at the end of this chapter can lead the client to professionals qualified to teach new skills easily and efficiently.

IMPROVING CLIENT AND FAMILY COPING

The adjustment period to visual loss or blindness is difficult for both client and family or significant other. Both parties need many opportunities to verbalize their reactions to the

Table 70–5	Guide to Contact Lenses			
Type	**Advantages**	**Disadvantages**	**Care**	**Insertion and Removal**
Hard Lenses				
Conventional hard lenses: made of firm plastic; do not completely cover the cornea; can be worn for 8–15 h a day; should be worn for approximately the same number of hours each day	Most durable; longest lasting; correct most vision problems, including myopia and hyperopia; ideal for astigmatism; may provide better vision than soft lenses in some cases; easier to clean and less expensive to maintain, not as fragile as soft lenses	May chip, scratch or crack; scratches can be repolished, but chipped or cracked lenses must be replaced; more likely to pop out or slip off center than soft lenses; longer and more difficult adjustment period (possibly several weeks before worn comfortably); two or three office fittings may be required; wearer may notice lens edge or reflected glare; spectacle blur (blurring of vision with glasses for approximately 1 h after removing lenses); foreign bodies may lodge under lens	Apply cleaning solution on removal to remove mucus and other debris; clean regularly according to the recommended schedule; rinse well and store in soaking/disinfecting solution	Insertion: 1. Wash hands. 2. Inspect each lens for damage. 3. Place lens, cupside up, on tip of index finger. 4. Apply a few drops of wetting solution. 5. Use middle finger of same hand to gently pull down lower eyelid. 6. Lift the upper eyelid with the other hand and look at the lens. Place the lens on the eye, release both eyelids, and close both eyes.
Gas-permeable hard lenses: composition similar to that of conventional hard lens; slightly larger than hard lens	Easier adjustment than with conventional hard lens; can be worn for longer periods; allow oxygen to pass through to the cornea; less irritating than hard lenses; spectacle blur less likely; as durable as other hard lenses; ideal for	Expensive	Some types may require disinfection on a regular basis or need to be stored in a special solution	Removal: 1. Stretch the outer canthus of the lower eyelid. 2. Cup the other hand under the eye. 3. Catch the lens as it falls after blinking.

Type	Advantages	Disadvantages	Care	Insertion and Removal
Hard Lenses				
	astigmatism when conventional hard lenses cannot be tolerated			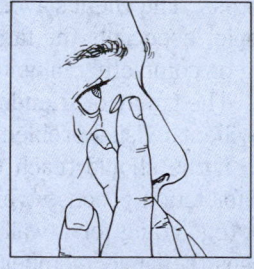
Soft Lenses				
Conventional soft lenses: made of gel-like plastic; cover the cornea and part of the sclera; flexible; can be worn up to 18 h a day	Easy adjustment period; greatest wearing comfort; may be worn part-time; seldom pop out or slip off center; foreign bodies less likely to lodge under lens; lens edge not noticeable and there is less reflected glare; ideal for athletes; can be fitted in one or two office visits	More expensive than hard lenses; harder to clean and require greater care to avoid bacterial and fungal infections; less durable than hard lenses; require more frequent replacement (about 1½ years); vision may not be as sharp as with hard lenses; may absorb cigarette smoke, chemical vapors, and aerosol spray	Clean and rinse lenses after each removal; disinfect after each removal in the recommended way using either a heating unit or a disinfecting solution; alternating the method may damage the lenses; soaking in a special solution to remove protein deposits may also be required; must not be allowed to dry out	Insertion: 1. Wash and dry hands thoroughly. (Wet hands may cause lenses to flatten.) 2. Inspect each lens for damage. 3. Place lens, cup-side up, on tip of index finger. 4. Use middle finger of same hand to gently pull down lower eyelid. 5. Look up exposing white area. 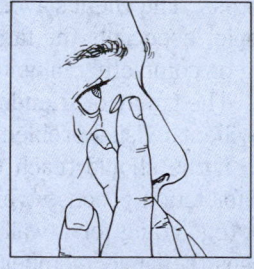 6. Gently place the lens on the white area, remove the finger, and release the lower eyelid. 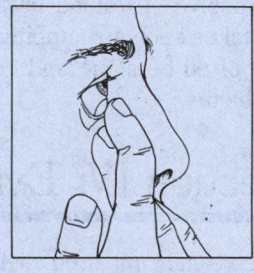

(continued)

Table 70–5	Guide to Contact Lenses (continued)			
Type	**Advantages**	**Disadvantages**	**Care**	**Insertion and Removal**
Soft Lenses				
Extended wear soft lenses: Made of a more flexible gel-like plastic than conventional soft lenses; can be worn for 24 h a day for long periods	Can be worn for extended periods; allow oxygen to penetrate to cornea; ideal for persons who have difficulty in handling lenses; ideal after cataract surgery	More expensive than conventional soft lenses; easily damaged; require more frequent replacement than regular lenses	Require special handling for protein deposits and frequent vision care visits	7. The lens will center itself on blinking. Removal: 1. Look up and slide the lens down off the pupil with the finger. 2. Gently squeeze the lens with thumb and index finger and lift it off the eye.

visual loss, as well as time to work through the grieving process. The client's avoidance of interaction with support people, especially the family or significant other, can prolong or completely inhibit rehabilitation.

The family or friends should understand the causes of the client's visual problem and the goals for rehabilitation. The nurse should teach them how to promote a healthy rehabilitation process while giving the client greater control (eg, going for a walk with the client while the client grasps the family member's elbow or encouraging the client to perform certain tasks independently). Such suggestions allow the family to feel useful and the client to feel normal. Discourage excessive expressions of sympathy and unrealistic hopes for a cure while encouraging the need for patience and understanding. The family should allow themselves to stand back and let the client make small mistakes such as bumping into objects, because the client will often be alone and needs to learn to cope with such problems.

OVERCOMING FEAR

The health care provider should recognize that a client's fear of blindness may not be unrealistic. However, excessive fear or obsession interferes with healthy adjustment to visual impairment and needs to be addressed. Often fearing the unknown is worse than facing the actual situation, and what the client needs is education in dealing with the visual impairment. The client must develop trust in the caregivers to believe in the reality of the disease process. As the client recognizes fear and places it in perspective, he or she can begin to learn rehabilitative measures for managing the activities of daily living. The client also should be made aware of community groups that can provide support during the adjustment period (see the resources list at the end of this chapter).

Section IV: Evaluation

The visually impaired client who is coping effectively demonstrates a good understanding of the disease process and the procedures necessary to promote eye health, as well as shows the ability to verbalize emotions about the visual loss. One of the primary methods of coping is the ability to share fears, anxieties, and frustrations with family and significant others (including health care givers). An effective rehabilitation will enable the client to resume the prior level of communication, be aware of his or her potential, take control of the rehabilitation pace, and derive pleasure in accomplishing autonomous tasks.

The client's family also should accept the reality of the visual loss and provide encouragement while allowing self-sufficiency where possible. A reexamination of client and family roles is necessary initially, but the rehabilitated client eventually will resume normal family responsibilities. The

client should be satisfied with his or her career decision and contribution to the family budget.

The client with a potential for complete visual loss should be able to verbalize the ultimate fear—blindness—and place it in perspective. It should not interfere with daily life. Specific expected outcomes have been included in Table 70–3.

Chapter Highlights

The nurse should clearly establish the chief concern of the visually impaired client in initiating the assessment.

The nurse should determine the time of onset and duration of the symptom, whether the client has been treated in the past for the same symptom, and any medications the client may be taking.

Assessment of the client's lifestyle and social support systems is an important component of subjective data collection.

Physical examination of the eye consists of inspection with and without ocular tools. As the visual examination takes place, the examiner should explain the procedures and regularly reassure the client.

The objective eye examination includes use of the ophthalmoscope, slit lamp, Snellen's chart, retinoscope, pinhole test, perimeter, tonometer, color vision tests, computed tomography, fluorescein angiography, ultrasonography, and laboratory studies.

Nursing diagnoses for clients with impaired vision fall

broadly into the following classifications: visual sensory-perceptual alteration, knowledge deficit, impaired communication, self-care deficit, alteration in self-concept, ineffective coping, alterations in family interactions, and fear.

Teaching people how to protect and preserve their eyesight is a critical nursing role.

In planning and implementing care for the visually impaired client, the nurse must consider job factors, home maintenance, child care, financial security, transportation, self-care deficits, and independence.

Clients and their families should be instructed in the safe and effective administration of ophthalmic medications.

The legally blind individual (one with a visual acuity of 20/200 or less in the better eye with best correction) may have difficulty keeping a job and remaining independent; this client may require assistance from other people, agencies, or devices to maintain an optimal lifestyle.

Bibliography

Chawla HB: *Essential Ophthalmology.* New York: Churchill Livingstone, 1981.

Milder B, Weil B: *The Lacrimal System.* Norwalk, CT: Appleton-Century-Crofts, 1983.

Moses S: "What's the score on sports and eye injuries?" *Can Nurse* (April) 1980; 76:43–45.

Newell FW: *Ophthalmology,* 5th ed. St. Louis: Mosby, 1982.

Osguthorpe NC: If your patient has contact lenses. *Am J Nurs* 1984; 84:1255–1256.

Parr J: *Introduction to Ophthalmology.* New York: Oxford University Press, 1982.

Rooke FCE, Rothwell PJ, Woodhouse DF: *Ophthalmic Nursing.* New York: Churchill Livingstone, 1980.

Saunders WH et al: *Nursing Care of Eye, Ear, Nose and Throat Disorders,* 4th ed. St. Louis: Mosby, 1979.

Smith JF, Nachazel PP: *Ophthalmic Nursing.* Boston: Little, Brown, 1980.

Stein HA, Slatt B: *The Ophthalmic Assistant: Fundamentals and Clinical Practice,* 4th ed. St. Louis: Mosby, 1983.

Tabor M: "Video display terminals: The eyes have it!" *Occup Health Safety* (Sept) 1981; 50:30–39.

Vaughan D, Asbury T: *General Ophthalmology,* 9th ed. Los Altos, CA: Lange, 1980.

Suggested Readings

Belmont O: Some common visual symptoms: What they mean and what to do about them. *Occup Health Nurs* (June) 1981; 29:21–24. Common visual symptoms are described, including blurred vision, papilledema, diplopia, flashing lights, floaters, and halos.

Boyd-Monk H: Practical methods of how to examine the external eye. *Occup Health Nurs* (June) 1981; 29:10–14. This article discusses a systematic approach to the assessment of the eye, describing potential pathological conditions noted on inspection.

Gillin SL: Simple nursing procedures for the occupational health nurse. *Occup Health Nurs* (June) 1981; 29:18–20. This article describes techniques for various ophthalmologic procedures assigned to the nurse, such as corneal staining, eyelid eversion, and eye irrigation.

King RC: Taking a close look at the eye. *RN* (Feb) 1982; 47:49–56. A review of the physical assessment of the eye includes inspection with the ophthalmoscope. The article contains useful illustrations.

Norman S: The pupil check. *Am J Nurs* 1982; 82:588–591. Pupil abnormalities are discussed and illustrated in this article.

Saunders WH et al: *Nursing Care of Eye, Ear, Nose, and Throat Disorders*. St. Louis: Mosby, 1979. This is the most current and complete ophthalmology nursing book. It covers the spectrum of eye disorders and related nursing interventions.

Resources

SELF-HELP GROUPS AND OTHER ORGANIZATIONS

American Foundation for the Blind, Inc.
15 W. 16th St.
New York, NY 10011
Phone: (212) 787–2618

A national research and service agency for the blind. Publishes books, pamphlets, and professional reports including the *Directory of Agencies Serving Blind Persons in the United States*. Sells aids and appliances (kitchen, medical, sewing) for the visually handicapped.

Bold, Inc. (Blind Outdoor Leisure Development)
533 E. Main St.
Aspen, CO 81611
Phone: (303) 925–8922

Over 20 clubs nationwide are dedicated to providing outdoor recreational opportunities for the blind. They promote a more active life through skiing, swimming, rafting, camping, fishing, horseback riding, and golfing.

Eye Bank Association of America
3195 Maplewood Ave.
Winston-Salem, NC 27103

Provides corneas, sclerae, and vitreous humor without charge.

Eye Bank for Sight Restoration, Inc.
210 E. 64th St.
New York, NY 10021

Receives donated eyes for distribution where needed to ophthalmologists.

Hadley School for the Blind
700 Elm St.
Winnetka, IL 60093

Provides tuition-free correspondence courses for the blind including vocational and university-level courses.

Library of Congress
Division for the Blind and Physically Handicapped
Washington, DC 20540
Phone: (202) 882–5500

Provides books in braille and talking book and magazine records and reproducers for these records. Distributes and maintains talking book machines through their 34 regional distributing libraries.

Local and/or state libraries

Supply books, magazines, and newspapers in large print as well as records and games.

National Retinitis Pigmentosa Foundation
8331 Mindale Cir.
Baltimore, MD 21207
Phone: (301) 655-1011

An organization with over 40 chapters that supports research into retinitis pigmentosa and allied retinal degenerative diseases. Educates professionals and the public and trains self-help leaders.

National Society for the Prevention of
Blindness, Inc.
79 Madison Ave.
New York, NY 10016
Phone: (212) 684-3505

Specializes in programs to eliminate preventable blindness through education, research, and prevention services.

New Eyes for the Needy, Inc.
549 Millburn Ave.
Short Hills, NJ 07078
Phone: (201) 376-4903

This nonprofit group of volunteers solicits used metal eyeglass frames and sells them to scrap refineries to raise money to buy prescription eyeglasses or prosthetic eyes for those who cannot afford them.

Recording for the Blind, Inc.
215 E. 58th St.
New York, NY 10022
Phone: (212) 751–0860

A nonprofit organization that provides records or tapes of textbooks and other educational material. Will record books at the specific request of borrowers.

In Canada:
Blind Organization of Ontario with
Self-Help Tactics (BOOST)
100 Richmond St. E., Suite 408
Toronto, Ontario, Canada M4S 1E9
Phone: (416) 364-4639

Helps obtain employment for the blind and works toward improved legislation. Also provides a speakers bureau.

Canadian Council of the Blind
96 Rideout St. S.
London, Ontario, Canada N6L 3X4
Phone: (519) 434-4339

Promotes employment, public education, prevention of blindness, and social bonds between blind and sighted persons.

Canadian National Institute for the Blind
1931 Bayview Ave.
Toronto, Ontario, Canada M4G 4C8
Phone: (416) 486–2636

Offers counseling, education, social service, employment opportunities, and mobility training. Permanent resident accommodations (at a fee) are available.

John Milton Society for the Blind in
    Canada
40 St. Clair Ave. E., Suite 201
Toronto, Ontario, Canada M4T 1M9
Phone: (416) 921-4152
> Founded by Helen Keller and church leaders from major denominations, this organization facilitates the spiritual development of the visually handicapped and assists them in participating in church and community work.

GUIDE DOG SERVICES

There are several centers that provide guide dog services for legally blind persons. Most programs are 4 weeks long and require full-time residence at the training facility where clients are matched and trained with a guide dog. There is no charge for the guide dog or the training program; however, not all training facilities cover travel expenses. Training services are provided by the following organizations:

Guide Dogs for the Blind, Inc.
P.O. Box 1200
San Rafael, CA 94902
Phone: (415) 479-4000
> Training facilities in San Rafael, California.

Guide Dog Foundation for the Blind, Inc.
109-19 72nd Ave.
Forest Hills, NY 11375
Phone: (212) 263-4885
> Training facilities in Long Island, New York.

Guiding Eyes for the Blind
106 E. 41st St.
New York, NY 10017
Phone: (212) 683-5165
> Training facilities in Yorktown Heights, New York.

International Guiding Eyes, Inc.
P.O. Box 18
North Hollywood, CA 91603
Phone: (213) 877-3937
> Training facilities in North Hollywood, California.

Leader Dogs for the Blind
1039 South Rochester Road
Rochester, MI 48063
Phone: (313) 651-9011
> Training facilities in Rochester, Michigan.

Pilot Guide Dog Foundation
33 East Congress Parkway
Chicago, IL 60605
Phone: (312) 922-7081
> Training facilities in Columbus, Ohio.

(The) Seeing Eye, Inc.
P.O. Box 373
Morristown, NJ 07960
Phone: (201) 539-4425
> Training facilities in Morristown, New Jersey.

Guide Dog Users
Box 174, Central Station
Baldwin, NY 11510
Phone: (304) 471-1490
> This is an organization of persons who use guide dogs. Promotes education of its members and the public on guide dog training and supports the development of mobility aids for blind persons.

SPECIALTY ORGANIZATION

American Society of Ophthalmic Registered
    Nurses
P.O. Box 3030
San Francisco, CA 94119
Phone: (415) 921-4700
> Membership in this organization is composed of RNs working full- or part-time in ophthalmic nursing. The goal of the organization is to maintain excellence in client care through education of its members. Dues, $35.

Chapter 71

Specific Disorders of the Visual System

Theresa M. Flaherty
Mardy Nord Meadows

Objectives

When you have finished studying this chapter, you should be able to:

Explain the importance of genetic counseling for clients with retinitis pigmentosa.

Identify what therapeutic measures are available for the treatment of clients with ptosis and strabismus.

Summarize the clinical manifestations and therapeutic and nursing interventions for clients with retinal detachment.

Describe the four kinds of refractive error and how each can be corrected, noting the role of both hard and soft contact lenses.

Discuss the four classifications of glaucoma, their clinical manifestations, and the nurse's role in the prevention of this disorder.

Identify the clinical manifestations and therapeutic and nursing

interventions for the major degenerative disorders affecting the visual system.

Discuss ways in which both clients and health care providers can limit the effects of allergic ocular reactions.

Describe the major infectious disorders of the eye—hordeola, chalazia, blepharitis, conjunctivitis, trachoma, keratitis and corneal ulceration, and uveitis—related to the nurse's role in the prevention of their spread and in providing symptomatic relief.

Explain why psychosocial support of the client plays a major role in nursing care of clients with neoplastic disorders of the eye.

Identify the six specific types of traumatic ocular injuries, their clinical manifestations, and the role of health care providers in their treatment.

Disorders of the visual system that affect adults can be divided into the following categories: congenital, degenerative, immunologic, infectious, neoplastic, and traumatic. In addition, some conditions, such as retinal detachments and glaucoma, can originate from a variety of factors. Common adult eye diseases differ in their clinical manifestations, therapeutic approaches, and nursing measures.

Many disorders of the visual system can be diminished in effect or prevented completely with early detection, prevention of injury, and appropriate treatment. The nurse plays an important role in all aspects of the care and prevention of eye disorders.

Section I: Congenital Disorders

Congenital ocular disorders tend to be abiotrophic and bilateral. Their exact etiologies are frequently unknown, and treatment is often only palliative, not curative. Most

congenital disorders of the visual system are very rare; the more common ones, although still fairly rare, include corneal dystrophy, retinitis pigmentosa, ptosis, and strabismus. Congenital ocular disorders are important because they often impair vision, produce pain, and require many psychological adjustments.

General Nursing Implications

The nurse's role in working with clients with congenital disorders of the visual system includes providing genetic counseling, client education, client assessment, rehabilitative measures, and emotional support. Genetic counseling is of the utmost importance in families with a history of retinitis pigmentosa. The early assessment and treatment of ptosis and strabismus often can avert potential complications and learning disabilities. The nurse may conduct widespread testing and assessment programs for these disorders in preschools or clinics.

The nurse often has a great influence on clients experiencing progressive visual impairment. These individuals often require extensive rehabilitation and ongoing emotional support, both of which are important nursing activities.

CORNEAL DYSTROPHY

Corneal dystrophy encompasses a group of rare hereditary disorders of the cornea characterized by abnormal deposits of substances on the cornea, such as collagen fibers, calcium salts, lipids, or amyloids, and by corneal structural changes such as keratoconus, a usually bilateral conical protrusion of the cornea. Dystrophy disorders occur bilaterally and can affect any of the five layers of the cornea. Corneal dystrophies are slowly progressive diseases that generally do not affect vision unless the entire cornea is involved. The etiology of corneal dystrophy is unknown.

Clinical Manifestations

Corneal dystrophy disorders usually manifest themselves by the second decade. They may remain stable or slowly progress with increasing visual impairment over the years. Lacrimation, photophobia, and irritation of the eye frequently accompany these disorders. Pain may be present if corneal erosion occurs. The cornea appears cloudy because of edema, and the ophthalmologist usually notes epithelial defects of the cornea such as surface irregularities as well as web, dot, or fingerlike opacities.

Therapeutic Measures

If vision is sufficiently impaired to warrant treatment, a penetrating keratoplasty is done (see the section in Chapter 72 on corneal transplants). Blurred vision from corneal edema is frequently treated with hyperosmotic eyedrops and ointment (5% sodium chloride) in an attempt to dehydrate the epithelium and make it clear again.

Specific Nursing Measures

Because of the rarity of corneal dystrophy and the fact that vision is often not impaired until late in the disease, the nurse will have little exposure to these clients. Interaction between the nurse and the affected client usually occurs during routine eye examinations or when the client is admitted to the hospital for a corneal transplant. Thorough explanations of the disease process, emotional support, and reassurance are the mainstays of nursing management for these clients. Nursing care of the client undergoing a corneal transplant is discussed in Chapter 72.

RETINITIS PIGMENTOSA

Retinitis pigmentosa, a hereditary disorder, involves the degeneration and clumping of the retinal pigment. This pigment lines the sensory retina (where the rods and cones lie) and serves a role in the physiological function of the rods and cones essential for vision. Degeneration of the retinal pigment curtails the physiological activity of the sensory retina, and it, too, begins to degenerate. Retinitis pigmentosa is primarily a disease of the rods; the cones are affected only late in the disease. The disorder may be mild or progress to total blindness, depending on the cause and duration of the disease. Other problems, such as deafness and mental retardation, can be associated with retinitis pigmentosa. The primary defect in retinitis pigmentosa is unknown, but investigations to determine its etiology are being carried out.

Transmission patterns of retinitis pigmentosa vary; the trait can be sex linked, autosomal dominant, or autosomal recessive. Sex-linked retinitis pigmentosa seems to be the most disabling and rapidly progressive form. Approximately 55% to 60% of all reported retinitis pigmentosa cases affect males. Overall incidence reports differ; one study showed that 5 per 1000 people are diagnosed as having retinitis pigmentosa. From 20% to 50% of cases are autosomal recessive (Bloome & Garcia, 1982).

Clients with retinitis pigmentosa have a higher incidence of vitreous opacities, glaucoma, cataracts, retinal detachment, and myopia than the normal population.

Clinical Manifestations

The first signs of retinitis pigmentosa are usually seen by age 10. Night blindness is often the initial symptom, progressing to complaints of tunnel vision (even in the daylight) and, finally, total blindness, often by age 30 (Figure 71–1). Some cases remain stable instead of progressing. The final outcome for vision is better if the symptoms develop at an older age.

An ophthalmoscopic examination reveals small, needle-shaped pigment debris in the midperiphery of the retina, a waxy pallor of the optic disk, and attenuated retinal vessels that appear as thin red threads because of their constriction and degeneration from the disease process.

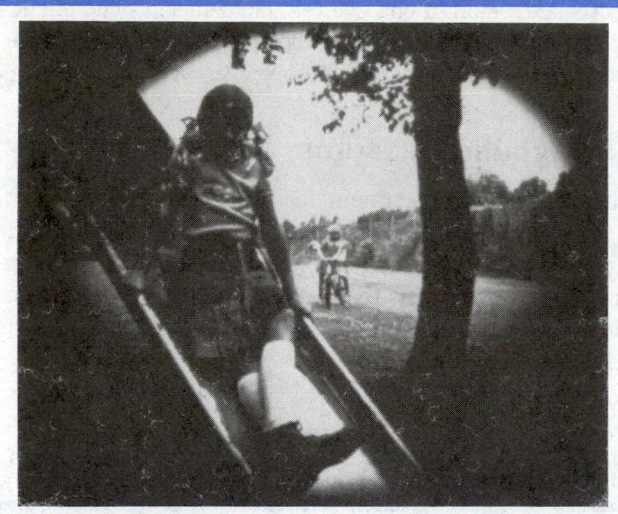

Figure 71–1

Vision changes in retinitis pigmentosa. (Courtesy of National Eye Institute, Bethesda, MD)

Therapeutic Measures

No curative treatment of retinitis pigmentosa exists. The administration of vitamin A has been attempted without significant effects. Treatment should emphasize genetic counseling. Clients with the disease should be told that the chance of having an affected child is one in two and that the child may be more or less affected than they are themselves. The genetic background of the other parent does not influence the evaluation unless the family history also indicates the presence of retinitis pigmentosa. Information should be presented in a statistical way to facilitate the client's understanding of the genetic implications. Avoid advising the client on whether to have a child or not because that is a decision only the client and partner can make. This is obviously an extremely difficult time for a couple wanting their own natural child. Feelings of hopelessness are common, and counseling may be warranted.

Clients with retinitis pigmentosa should be treated for complications (eg, myopia or retinal detachment). Low-vision aids may provide slightly more vision, although most people have difficulty adjusting to them or find them troublesome. Low-vision aids for clients with retinitis pigmentosa include (1) field-widening devices for constricted peripheral fields (eg, Fresnel Press-On prisms applied to the spectacles); (2) hand-held magnifiers; and (3) night vision microscopes, which provide sufficient light amplification to allow the impaired cones to function. Rather than use such devices, many clients opt to deal with their progressing disease by learning early the rehabilitation methods used for the blind. Using a cane, learning braille, or possibly changing to a career that the client will be able to continue as vision deteriorates are a few rehabilitation methods that may be suggested.

Specific Nursing Measures

There is no treatment for retinitis pigmentosa, and it often leads to blindness; therefore, emotional support of the client and family or significant others becomes the most important nursing intervention. Encourage the client to contact the National Retinitis Pigmentosa Foundation for counseling, reassurance, and information regarding testing for carriers and new lines of therapy (see resources section of Chapter 70). Genetic counseling also should be encouraged.

PTOSIS

Ptosis, the drooping of the upper eyelid, allows only partial coverage of the eyeball. It may affect one or both eyes and be constant or intermittent. Ptosis is most often a congenital disorder, although it also can be acquired later in life. Congenital ptosis is transmitted as a dominant characteristic. It results from developmental failure of the levator muscle in the upper eyelid. Acquired ptosis can result from either myogenic factors (eg, myasthenia gravis) or neurogenic factors (eg, paralysis) or trauma.

Clinical Manifestations

Severe ptosis is immediately obvious to even the untrained eye. The lid appears smooth and flat, and the tarsal fold is absent. Mild ptosis becomes more evident when the individual looks upward. If the lid droops enough to cover the pupil, the client's forehead will be wrinkled, or the head will tilt back in an effort to compensate. Amblyopia may also accompany a blocked pupil.

Therapeutic and Specific Nursing Measures

The treatment of choice for congenital ptosis is a surgical procedure that shortens the levator muscle. If ptosis is associated with a systemic disease (acquired), the disease should be treated before surgery for ptosis is attempted. Nursing interventions are based on the client's surgery and are discussed in Chapter 72.

STRABISMUS

Strabismus is a pathological condition characterized by a malalignment of the visual axes. The eyes appear to be crossed, with only one eye looking at the intended object. The malalignment causes separate images to be focused on the two retinas, and the client sees double.

Strabismus can be paralytic or nonparalytic. Paralytic strabismus, which is generally acquired, results from damage to the extraocular muscles or nerves. The affected eye is unable to move in certain directions. Nonparalytic strabismus is usually an inherited anomaly in which there is a defect in the position and fusion ability of the two eyes.

Strabismus affects approximately 3% of children and 1% of the overall population. It has both cosmetic and visual consequences, but prompt care may prevent its crippling effects. Since strabismus affects mostly children and treatment usually occurs before school age, this text will not provide an in-depth discussion. Consult a pediatric nursing or opthalmic text for further information.

Clinical Manifestations

Strabismus is generally easily observed; indicative signs in addition to crossed eyes include squinting, head tilting, closing of one eye to improve vision, and evidence of decreased vision in one eye (eg, clumsiness). The client's symptoms also may include diplopia, blurred vision, decreased visual acuity, and photophobia.

Therapeutic Measures

The objective of treatment for strabismus is good visual acuity, binocular vision, and an acceptable cosmetic appearance. Drugs (long-acting miotics), glasses, orthoptics, and surgery are the common modes of treatment. Surgery is the preferred method for the repair of congenital strabismus.

Section II: Disorders of Multifactorial Origin

Some disorders of the visual system have a range of possible etiologies. For example, retinal detachments can result from inflammation caused by trauma or from degeneration of the retina with age. Refractive errors can be from inheritance, disease, injury, or degeneration. Glaucoma is the third disorder recognized as having many potential causes, including congenital, degenerative, neoplastic, and traumatic causes. The disorders discussed in this section are of particular importance because of their relatively high incidence.

General Nursing Implications

Nurses often see glaucoma and retinal detachment in an acute phase, with surgery expected. Preparation of the client for surgery and subsequent therapies essentially involves promoting comfort and giving emotional support. Clients inevitably have great anxiety; they should recognize the potential for loss of vision in the affected eye while also receiving reassurance.

Nurses often see clients with refractive errors in ambulatory care, school, and occupational health settings. In these cases, the nurses' role includes explanations of procedures and education about the eye.

RETINAL DETACHMENTS

A retinal detachment is possible because the retina is physically attached to the inside of the eye (the choroid) in only two places: at the very back (the optic nerve) and at its front edge (the ciliary body). The remaining retina is held in position by the gentle pressure of the vitreous. A hole or tear can develop in any part of the retina but is most frequent near the front edge, where it is thinnest (Figure 71–2A). A detachment may be spontaneous or follow trauma.

When a tear occurs, vitreous leaks through the retinal hole. Vitreous seeps behind the retina, lifts it from the choroid in a progressive fashion, and enlarges the detachment. Vision becomes compromised as the rods and cones are deprived of their choroidal nutritional supply. Untreated retinal detachment often eventually results in massive fibrosis of the retina and vitreous cavities; this frequently is complicated by uveitis and cataract formation. The eye

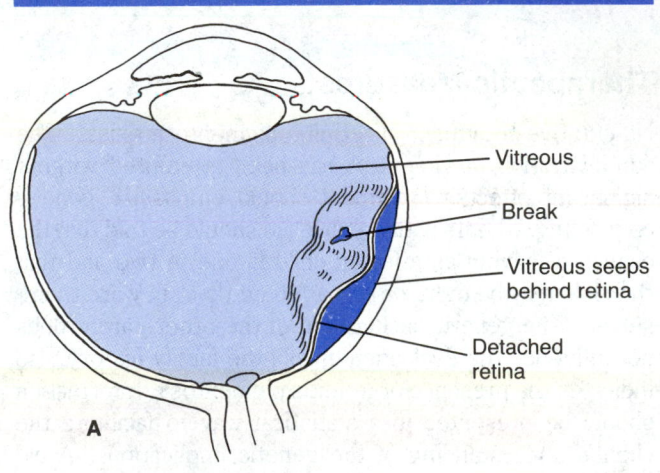
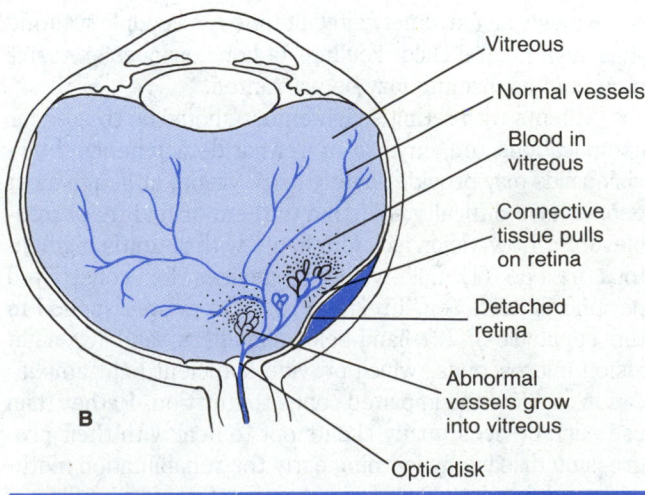

Figure 71–2

A. Retinal detachment. **B.** Traction retinal detachment because of neovascularization in diabetic retinopathy.

may eventually become glaucomatous or atrophic and blinded (Chignell, 1980).

As has been mentioned, retinal detachments may have a variety of causes. Chignell (1980) cites myopia, aphakia, retinal degeneration, trauma, and retinal neovascularization as predisposing factors. Vitreous degenerates in myopia and results in the separation of the vitreous from the retina. The higher the degree of myopia, the greater the risk of retinal detachment (Kaufman et al., 1980). The exact relationship between aphakia and retinal detachment is not known, but the vitreous may detach from the posterior retina in an effort to occupy the former lens space. A contusion or penetrating injury also can cause retinal detachment; in fact, detachment occurs in about 80% of ocular contusions. Racket sports are becoming major culprits in trauma-induced retinal detachments, and safety goggles are finding new clients as athletes recognize this danger. *Neovascularization*, commonly seen in diabetic retinopathy (discussed in Chapter 42), can extend into the vitreous. Traction along these vessels can cause severe vitreous hemorrhage and retinal detachment (Figure 71–2B).

Clinical Manifestations

The symptoms of retinal detachment include a "shadow" or "curtain" spreading across the field of vision (Figure 71–3). The client may notice the sudden appearance of photopsia or floaters in one eye, followed eventually by a loss of a portion of the visual field (see visual field testing in Chapter 70). These floaters are caused by shadows cast by pigment or blood cells freed into the vitreous at the time the retina tears. Vision is at first blurred and becomes progressively worse. Nontraumatic retinal detachments have a strong bilateral tendency.

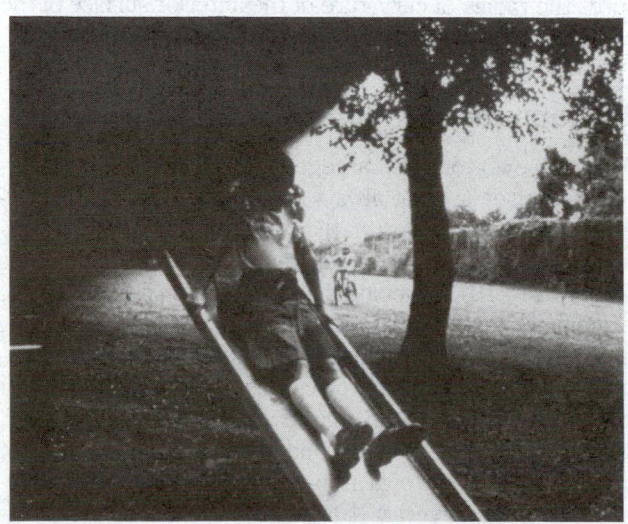

Figure 71–3

What a person with retinal detachment sees. (Courtesy of National Eye Institute, Bethesda, MD)

Therapeutic Measures

The goal of treatment in retinal detachment is to seal holes and prevent their further development. Nonsurgical measures include cryotherapy, diathermy, and photocoagulation. In addition, panretinal photocoagulation, a "scatter treatment" with a wide band of laser spots, is sometimes performed to prevent neovascularization in diabetics. Surgical procedures for the repair of retinal detachments are discussed in Chapter 72, as are cryotherapy, diathermy, and photocoagulation.

Specific Nursing Measures

Orientation of the client to the environment prior to the preoperative application of bilateral eyepatches is essential. Encourage the client to ask for assistance, since he or she will be unable to perform even basic tasks, such as self-feeding. Bilateral eyepatches prevent eye movement and may prevent further detachment.

Retinal surgery is unsuccessful in reattaching the retina about 20% of the time. Eye examinations are frequent after the procedure, and repetitive procedures may still be unsuccessful in 10% of the cases. The nurse needs to understand the added anxiety caused by the long-term nature of the treatment and provide support as needed. Client education in the symptoms of retinal holes and detachment is essential, because delay of repair may result in an uncorrectable injury to vision.

REFRACTIVE ERRORS

As described in Chapter 69, refraction is a deviation of light rays passing from one transparent medium into another of a different density. In regard to the eye, everyone has a degree of refractive error; if symptoms are bothersome enough, the person requires glasses.

Refractive errors include myopia (nearsightedness), hyperopia (farsightedness), astigmatism (asymmetric focus), and presbyopia (lack of focusing power). In myopia, light rays converge anterior to the retina; by the time the rays reach the retina, they have spread apart again, displaying a blurred subject (Figure 71–4A). Close objects are easily focused, but distant objects are not visualized clearly. Hyperopia also is a failure of the light rays to converge at the retina; these rays focus posterior to the retina, and vision is blurred for both near and far objects (Figure 71–5A). Astigmatism can coexist with the myopia or hyperopia and is caused by unequal corneal curvature or a lens irregular in shape (Figure 71–6). **Presbyopia**, a loss of ability to focus clearly on objects close to the eye, develops with age (over 40 years).

Refractive error is the most common visual problem in North America. Almost half of the population of the United States wear glasses. Most children are hyperopic at birth. From this stage to age 3, there is an apparent increase in hyperopia. The eye may increase its axial length

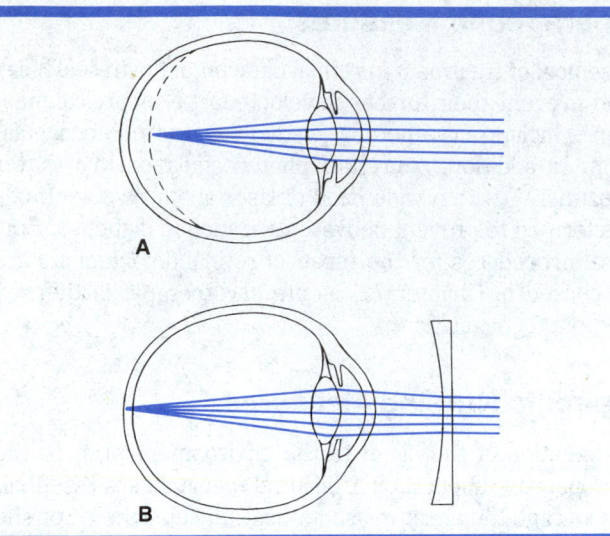

Figure 71–4

Myopia. **A.** In myopia, light rays from distant objects focus in front of the retina. **B.** Most cases of myopia can be corrected by a concave lens, which causes light rays to diverge as they enter the eye.

SOURCE: Spence AP, Mason EB: *Human Anatomy and Physiology,* 2nd ed. Menlo Park, CA: Benjamin/Cummings, 1983.

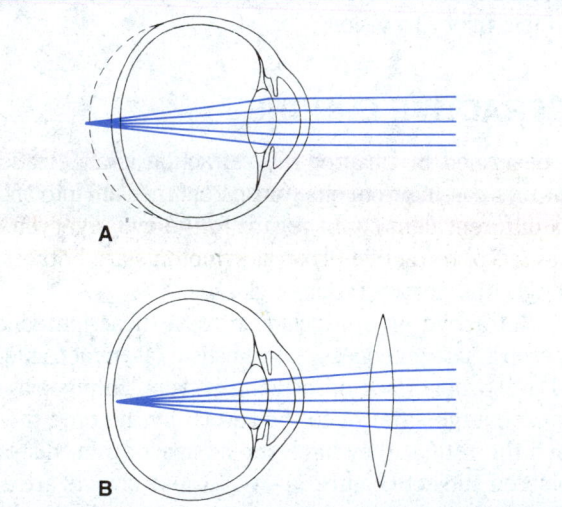

Figure 71–5

Hyperopia. **A.** In hyperopia, light rays from distant objects focus behind the retina. **B.** Most cases of hyperopia can be corrected by a convex lens, which causes light rays to converge as they enter the eye.

SOURCE: Spence AP, Mason EB: *Human Anatomy and Physiology,* 2nd ed. Menlo Park, CA: Benjamin/Cummings, 1983.

from 17 mm at birth to the average adult size of 24 mm by age 8.

An eye's axial length and lens shape are determined genetically. Disease and injury also can cause refractive

errors. For example, orbital and intraocular tumors can cause hyperopia. Uncontrolled diabetes and nuclear sclerosis, a type of senile cataract, can result in myopia. Some antihypertensive drugs, such as hydralazine hydrochloride and chlorthalidone (Hygroton), can induce myopia as well. Astigmatism may be genetic or result from surgical incisions into the cornea, trauma and scarring of the cornea, or growths of the eyelid such as a chalazion (see Section V) pressing on the globe (Newell, 1982). Presbyopia occurs because of an inelastic lens that the ciliary muscle cannot adjust. An inevitable effect of middle age, presbyopia necessitates glasses to change focus from far to near.

Clinical Manifestations

The two main symptoms of refractive error are reduced visual acuity and discomfort related to the use of the eyes. Other symptoms or problems are not likely to be corrected by glasses. The onset of symptoms is generally gradual, and they often are acutely experienced only after intense reading or close work. People often do not realize they have poor eyesight, especially children who experience myopia at an early age (it can start at age 5).

Many people claim headaches are indicative of a refractive error. More often, however, headaches are related to sinusitis or tight neck muscles secondary to tension, and corrective lenses will be of no help. Reduced visual acuity and ocular discomfort may also be symptoms of potentially serious disease processes such as a neurological disorder or systemic problem. This should be considered in the overall plan of care. As described in Chapter 70, visual acuity is subjectively tested with Snellen's chart and the pinhole test. Retinoscopy is an objective measurement of the refractive error.

Keratometry assists in determining a correct contact lens fit. It uses a keratometer, an instrument that measures the radius of curvature of the anterior surface of the central optical portion of the cornea.

Therapeutic Measures

Although everyone has a degree of refractive error, corrective lenses are not always indicated. Some people tolerate slight errors better than the disadvantages of corrective lenses. Myopia is neutralized with concave lenses (Figure 71–4B). Myopic adolescents should have an eye examination every 1 to 2 years to ensure they are wearing the correct lenses; adulthood stabilizes the need for frequent new lenses. Hyperopics require a convex lens for correction (Figure 71–5B); however, if visual acuity is good, muscle balance is normal, and there are no symptoms, correction of hyperopia is probably not necessary, irrespective of its severity (Newell, 1982). Astigmatism may be corrected with cylindrical lenses or hard contact lenses with more curvature in one direction than another. Presbyopia is treated with bifocals, which have a convex portion to correct hyperopia and an adjoining lens for distance

must be handled gently because they tear easily. Extended-wear lenses are soft lenses with a higher percentage of water absorption, allowing constant use for weeks at a time. They are more expensive than soft or hard contact lenses but require minimal maintenance. They are discussed in detail in Chapter 70.

Specific Nursing Measures

Cycloplegic agents are used to block accommodation and dilate the pupil for retinoscopic examination. The nurse should be aware of the client's unusually blurred vision and sensitivity to light from the cycloplegic. Tell the client when making an appointment that dark sunglasses are advised, and that the client should rely on a friend or family member for transportation after the examination (effects can last from 6 hours to 6 days).

The nurse needs to know during the history and physical examination whether a client wears corrective lenses and should assist with the removal of contact lenses when indicated. Particular attention should be paid to the unconscious client who may be wearing contact lenses. If oblique illumination reveals a lens, its removal is warranted to avoid exposure damage or other types of injury. Removal of contact lenses in this situation is discussed and illustrated in Chapter 70. The lenses should be placed in the proper sterile solution and clearly marked with the owner's name and identification of right or left lenses. Promote personal hygiene and daily removal of eye makeup to prevent inflammation, infection, and corneal abrasion.

GLAUCOMA

Glaucoma is a disorder of the eye in which there is sufficiently increased intraocular pressure to cause atrophy of the optic nerve and loss of vision. The increase in intraocular pressure (which is normally between 12 and 20 mm Hg) is caused by an imbalance between the formation and reabsorption of aqueous humor. As Chapter 69 described, aqueous humor is secreted by the ciliary body into the posterior chamber of the eye. It then flows through the pupil into the anterior chamber. The aqueous humor normally drains through the trabecular meshwork (located at the angle of the iris and the cornea) into Schlemm's canal and, finally, into the venous system (Figure 71–7A). Obstruction of the filtration system impairs the outflow mechanism, allowing the aqueous humor no exit. The subsequent accumulation of fluid causes a rise in intraocular pressure. The nerve fibers and blood vessels in the optic disk become compressed and are eventually damaged or destroyed.

Glaucoma is typically bilateral unless it occurs as a result of another disease (secondary glaucoma). However, symptoms in one eye may be more pronounced than in the other eye. Visual impairment varies from blurred vision to complete blindness. Glaucoma is one of the most common causes of blindness in North America. Approximately 2%

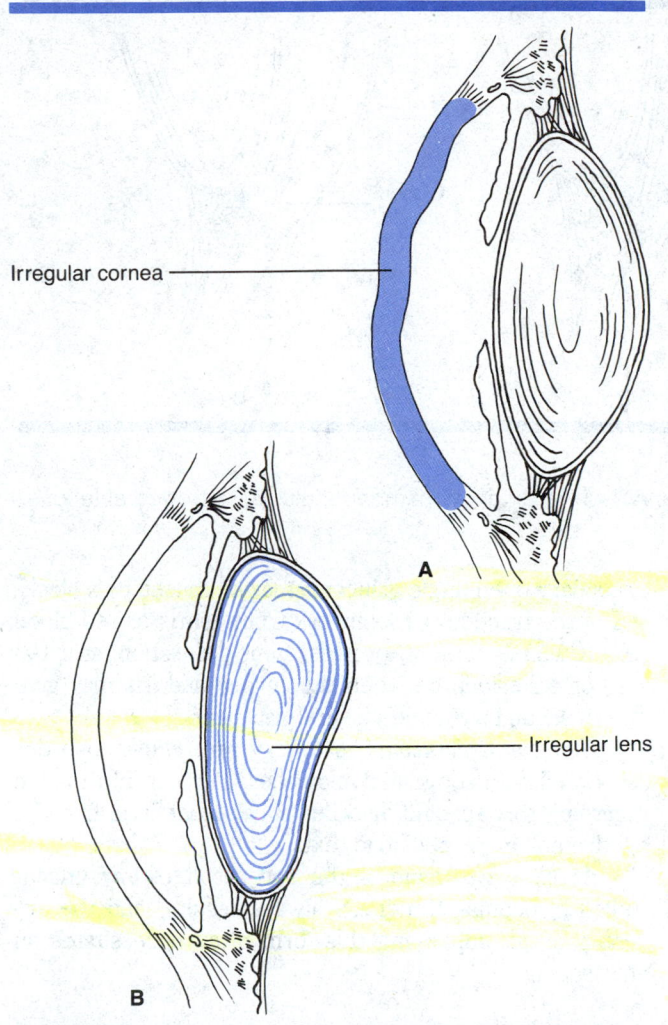

Figure 71–6

Astigmatism from: **A.** An irregular cornea. **B.** An irregular lens.

correction. In this way, two different sets of glasses are not necessary.

Contact lenses, corrective lenses placed directly in front of the cornea, have become exceedingly popular in the last decade. They are substituted for glasses by people who require constant correction for clear vision in myopia or hyperopia, as well as clients who have undergone cataract extraction. Hard lenses, the original contact lenses, are the least expensive, but they require a gradually increased adaptation time to a maximum of 14 hours. Hard lenses are smaller than soft lenses, and some clients cannot tolerate a hard foreign body on their eye. Hard lenses are more likely to cause corneal injury from abrasion; however, hard contacts often provide better vision than the soft variety (eg, for clients with astigmatism).

Soft lenses are desirable because of their shorter adaptation period. They can be useful for athletic activities and are lost less often than hard lenses. However, bacteria tend to adhere more firmly to soft lenses than hard lenses, and clients should sterilize their lenses nightly. Soft lenses

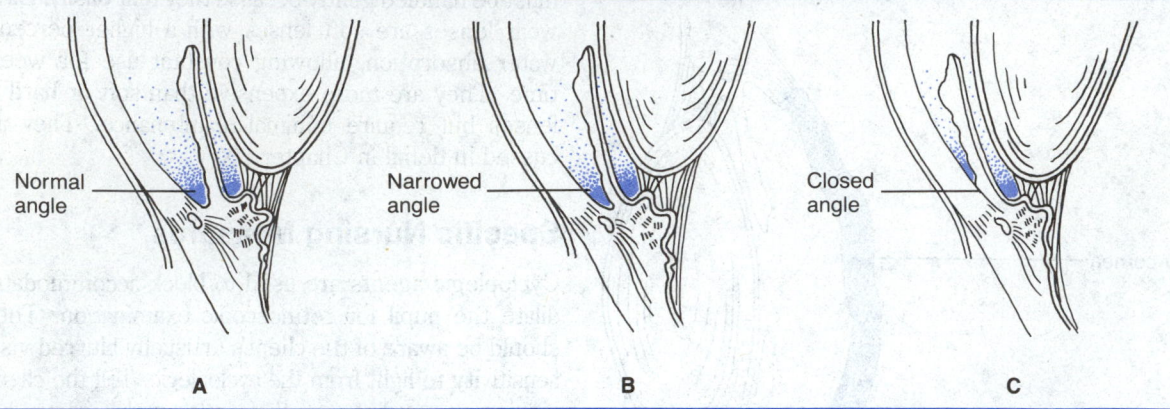

Figure 71–7

The anterior chamber angle in the normal eye and in glaucoma. **A.** Normal anterior chamber angle. **B.** Narrowed anterior chamber angle. **C.** Closed anterior chamber angle.

of all people over 40 years old in the United States have glaucoma, and another 1 million cases have not yet been diagnosed. Glaucoma may be roughly divided into four classifications: (1) primary glaucoma (open-angle and angle-closure glaucoma), (2) secondary glaucoma, (3) congenital glaucoma, and (4) absolute glaucoma.

Primary open-angle glaucoma, often referred to as simple glaucoma, is a chronic disease usually manifested in middle or late life. The most common form of glaucoma, it accounts for approximately 90% of the diagnosed cases. Its onset is gradual, insidious, painless, and usually lacking in any external signs. It results from a progressive narrowing in diameter of the trabecular meshwork openings (rather than from a narrowing or closure of the angle), which creates a resistance to aqueous humor outflow. The production of aqueous humor is then greater than the outflow, resulting in increased intraocular pressure.

Primary angle-closure glaucoma, also called narrow-angle glaucoma, frequently constitutes an ocular emergency. This form of glaucoma may develop into a full-blown attack within 30 to 60 minutes. Attacks are usually acute because of a sudden increase in intraocular pressure resulting from a complete blockage of the filtering angle by the iris. The disorder normally occurs in people who already have a narrow entrance into the filtration angle and a shallow anterior chamber (Figure 71–7B). Dilatation or forward displacement of the pupil causes the iris to push against the trabecular meshwork, thus blocking the exit of aqueous humor (Figure 71–7C). Conditions that would normally dilate the pupils, such as fear and dark adaptation, or medications that cause cycloplegia also may instigate this disorder. It may affect one eye at a time, and the extent of damage varies in relation to the severity and duration of ocular hypertension. Primary glaucoma—both open-angle and angle-closure—has no known basis other than genetic predisposition (Shields, 1982).

Secondary glaucoma results from other diseases of the eye that interfere with the outflow of aqueous humor. It may be of either the open-angle or angle-closure type.

Secondary open-angle glaucoma may be caused by a blockage of the trabecular meshwork from debris or red blood cells (trauma), tumors, or iritis. Lens dislocation, scar tissue, or adhesions between the cornea and iris may give rise to secondary angle-closure glaucoma.

Congenital glaucoma is a very rare ocular disorder associated with congenital anomalies. Further information regarding this specific disorder may be obtained from an ophthalmology or pediatric text.

Absolute glaucoma is the end result of any uncontrolled glaucoma. Blindness always results, and the severe pain accompanying this form often necessitates an enucleation.

Clinical Manifestations

Primary open-angle glaucoma is a slowly progressive disease. Most clients are unaware they have glaucoma (or that they are at risk because of a shallow anterior chamber) unless it has been diagnosed on a routine eye examination, because there are no symptoms until visual impairment occurs. The earliest signs of visual impairment the client may detect include failure to perceive changes in color, blurred vision, premature presbyopia, decreased accommodation, and a persistent aching of the eyes. A decrease in peripheral vision over the years also may occur (Figure 71–8). Examination of the eye will reveal a narrowing of the small vessels on the temporal surface of the optic disk, a cupping appearance of the optic disk, and possible corneal edema. Intraocular pressures are usually elevated, although they may be within the normal range.

Primary angle-closure glaucoma, in contrast, occurs suddenly. The client suffers intense pain and a sudden decrease or loss of vision. Nausea, vomiting, and diaphoresis often accompany an acute attack because of the severe pain. The affected eye usually appears red, and the iris appears dull, gray, and patternless. The pupil is fixed, dilated, and unresponsive to light. The anterior chamber appears shallow upon examination (Figure 71–9). Edema of the

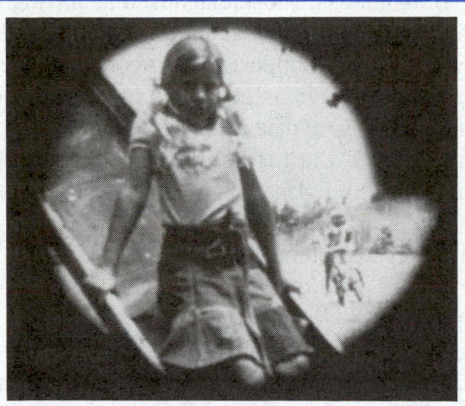

Figure 71–8

What a person with advanced glaucoma sees. (Courtesy of National Eye Institute, Bethesda, MD)

lids, cornea, and conjunctiva also may be present. Intraocular pressure is frequently greater than or equal to 50 or 60 mm Hg. Over 50% of clients with angle-closure glaucoma experience transient subacute attacks. These generally last a few hours and increase in frequency prior to an acute attack. Clients often see halos of blue–violet and yellow–red rings around lights while experiencing a subacute attack.

The clinical manifestations of secondary glaucoma are similar to those of either primary open-angle or primary angle-closure glaucoma, depending on the etiology of the secondary glaucoma.

Therapeutic Measures

Treatment for one type of glaucoma may be contraindicated in another type, so it is imperative to identify the probable etiology before initiating treatment. The specific drugs are discussed in Chapter 70 and the surgeries in Chapter 72.

Primary open-angle glaucoma is a chronic condition that cannot be cured; it can only be controlled to decrease

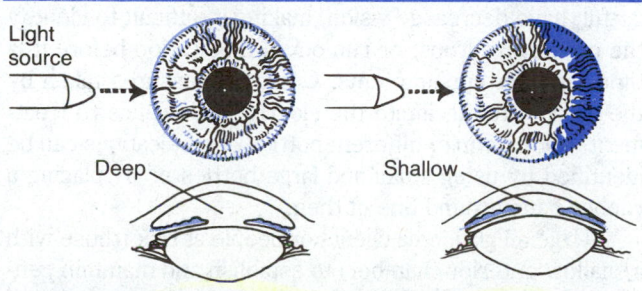

Figure 71–9

Assessing the depth of the anterior chamber. When the anterior chamber is narrow, oblique illumination casts a crescent-shaped shadow on the far portion of the iris, as illustrated.

visual loss. Medical intervention is instituted first, and treatment must be continued for the rest of the individual's life. It can often be controlled for long periods by miotic agents.

Miotic eyedrops, such as pilocarpine (1% to 6%), constrict the pupil and allow opening of the outflow channel (trabecular meshwork and Schlemm's canal) to facilitate aqueous humor drainage, thereby reducing the intraocular pressure. Pilocarpine is usually instilled up to five times a day. Pilocarpine can also be administered through a diffusional system that employs the principle of membrane-controlled drug release, which is similar to the way in which Transderm-Nitro (discussed in Chapter 24) and Transderm-Scop (discussed in Chapter 75) work. Called Ocusert Pilo-20 (or Pilo-40), the system is composed of a disk that contains a core reservoir of pilocarpine surrounded by a synthetic membrane. When placed under the eyelid, the disk delivers 20 to 40 mg of pilocarpine per hour for 7 days. The system's main advantages are that it provides the drug at a constantly controlled rate and eliminates the need for clients to instill eyedrops frequently. Strong, long-acting cholinesterase inhibitors are sometimes used when open-angle glaucoma worsens despite treatment with pilocarpine in an attempt to avoid surgery.

Epinephrine hydrochloride 0.5% to 2% (Epifrin) instilled one to two times a day is often the primary drug used in the initial treatment of open-angle glaucoma. It works by decreasing the secretion of aqueous humor while increasing its outflow, and it produces no miosis. This is an advantage for clients who have cataracts since miotics dim vision by reducing the amount of light that enters the eye. One disadvantage is that the drug's topical administration often causes a temporary stinging sensation.

Timolol maleate (Timoptic) in concentrations of 0.25% to 0.5% is now being widely used in the treatment of open-angle glaucoma although it is not yet recommended in the treatment of angle-closure glaucoma. It lowers the intraocular pressure by decreasing the production of aqueous humor and requires instillation only two times a day. The drug does not cause the dimming of vision that occurs with pilocarpine or the ocular stinging that occurs with epinephrine.

When maximal medical management of open-angle glaucoma is not successful and there is progressive visual field loss, surgery is indicated. Filtering procedures (eg, trabeculectomy or sclerectomy) create a fistula between the anterior chamber and the subconjunctival space. Aqueous humor then passes through the fistula, and the intraocular pressure is reduced. A similar effect can also be obtained by using a laser beam. Laser surgery for both open-angle and angle-closure glaucoma is rapidly becoming the initial surgical procedure of choice because of its ease of performance, low rate of complications, and favorable results (see Chapter 72).

Primary angle-closure glaucoma usually mandates immediate surgical management. Surgery is often curative if the duration of the attack is short and no scars have formed. The surgical procedure of choice is a peripheral iridectomy. A wedge is cut out of the iris, establishing a new outflow channel for the aqueous humor, or a laser iridotomy is performed (refer to Chapter 72). Prophylactic iridectomy or iridotomy is recommended for the other eye to prevent a second acute attack.

An effort is made to decrease the intraocular pressure with medications prior to surgery. Pilocarpine (2% to 4%) instilled every 5 minutes for 30 minutes to 1 hour, then three to four times per hour until surgery, is often required. This pulls the iris away from the trabecular meshwork, allowing aqueous humor outflow. In angle-closure glaucoma, however, treatment with miotics is often only a stopgap measure prior to surgery. Many of the milder miotics by themselves do not provide effective long-term control of intraocular pressure. Sometimes cholinesterase inhibitors such as eserine and neostigmine are used alternately with pilocarpine in an attempt to open the angle. The stronger long-acting cholinesterase inhibitors are not usually administered to clients with angle-closure glaucoma because their powerful and prolonged contracting action can cause a pupillary block by trapping fluid behind the iris, thus pushing it forward and closing the angle.

Hyperosmotic agents (mannitol or oral glycerin), which draw fluid from the eye, are also usually given. Carbonic anhydrase inhibitors such as acetazolamide (Diamox) may also be given intravenously in an attempt to decrease the intraocular pressure quickly. It may be followed by oral doses of 125 to 250 mg four times a day. Pain and nausea must be controlled with narcotics and antiemetics.

Treatment of secondary glaucoma begins by treating the underlying cause. The disorder is then treated the same as open-angle or angle-closure glaucoma, whichever is present.

Marijuana is being used experimentally in some centers where it is available by prescription. Another experimental drug, levobunolol, which is painless when applied topically, is expected to be available in the United States by 1987.

Specific Nursing Measures

Nurses have many roles in the care of clients with glaucoma. However, since glaucoma is a leading cause of blindness in North America, prevention is one of the nurse's most important functions. Mass screening of people over age 40 can be accomplished relatively easily. Temporary or mobile clinics may be set up to perform visual field tests, make tonometry readings, and provide general information regarding the disease. With practice, the nurse should be able to perform tests easily and accurately. Individuals with a family history of glaucoma should be encouraged to have regular tonometry tests well before they reach age 40. Making the public aware of glaucoma and its consequences often encourages people to seek early testing and treatment on their own.

Because of public knowledge that glaucoma is a lead-

ing cause of blindness, those diagnosed as having the disease often are apprehensive about the threat to their sight and require emotional support. It is important to be honest and open with clients in as positive a manner as possible. Discuss information on disease progression and steps that can be taken to prevent further damage. Steps to prevent further damage from glaucoma include:

- Routine eye examinations
- Compliance with the recommended medical regimen
- Prophylactic iridectomy
- Maintenance of general good health
- Avoidance of strenuous activities, which may increase intraocular pressure

Group sessions for individuals having difficulty dealing with their diagnosis of glaucoma often provide encouragement, new ways of coping, and peer support.

Other important functions of the nurse include assisting clients with their regimens of glaucoma therapy and understanding the reasons for possible noncompliance. Some of the most common reasons include avoidance of the side effects of medications, forgetfulness, running out of medications, or the inability to identify the appropriate medications. Instructions regarding the time, amount, side effects, and proper administration of medications also are essential. For example, eyedrops are best placed in the lower fornix while occluding the tear duct to prevent excessive systemic effects. Inform clients of the inconvenience that miotics may cause, eg, increased difficulty seeing in the dark (see Chapter 70). Encourage all glaucoma clients to carry a card stating what medications they are taking and to wear an identification bracelet or necklace in case of an accident. This information not only alerts health care providers that an individual has glaucoma and that the prescribed glaucoma medications should be continued; it also prevents health care providers from using medications that cause pupil dilation (eg, atropine as a preoperative medication), which could precipitate an acute attack of glaucoma.

Many glaucoma clients are elderly and may require additional teaching and support if their regimens are to be followed. Often the elderly live alone; are somewhat forgetful; have decreased vision, making it difficult to identify the proper eyedrops; or run out of medication before it is time for their appointments. Creative measures taken by the nurse often facilitate the elderly's adherence to treatment. For example, different bottles of medications can be identified by using small and large bottles or by placing a rubber band around one of them.

Urge all glaucoma clients or people at risk (those with a shallow anterior chamber) to establish and maintain general health practices. They should avoid constipation, heavy lifting and straining, and activities that increase the intracranial pressure and, hence, the intraocular pressure. Teach clients to wash their hands prior to instilling eye medications, to take care not to touch the eyedropper to the eye, and to clean discharge with normal saline or warm water from the inside corner of the eye outward. In addition, caution clients against rubbing their eyes.

Clients at risk should not use some eye "whiteners" or antihistamines, because they may dilate the pupil and initiate an acute attack. Whiteners such as tetrahydrozoline hydrochloride (Visine) are vasoconstrictors that decrease ocular inflammation and redness.

The nurse also may explain diagnostic procedures to the client and assist the examiner during such procedures. When clients are admitted to the hospital, assess their ability to see and orient them to their surroundings. Administer eyedrops, osmotic agents, narcotics, and antiemetics in a timely manner. Care of the client requiring ocular surgery is discussed in Chapter 72.

Section III: Degenerative Disorders

Degeneration of the visual system is generally associated with old age. Of the population over 65, 80% have one or more chronic ocular conditions with varying degrees of disability. Different parts of the eyeball begin to decline at different ages, and deterioration occurs at different rates. The basic mechanisms underlying the decline and deterioration are not known.

With aging, certain characteristics of the eyeball change. The eyeball appears to shrink because of loss of orbital fat, and poor muscle tone loosens the eyelids. Other changes include reduced visual acuity; decreased power of accommodation to darkness and dim light; loss of peripheral vision, central vision, or both; and difficulty in color discrimination. Presbyopia, the inevitable loss of the ability to focus clearly, develops with age; this accounts for the many elderly adults requiring corrective lenses.

General Nursing Implications

The nurse's primary responsibility to clients with degenerative disorders of the eye is health education. Clients should be taught that blindness is preventable and that regular eye examinations will assist in the appropriate treatment of degenerative disorders. Eyeglasses become increasingly necessary with age, and clients should be urged to be fitted appropriately. They should be assured that cataract extraction, barring other health complications, is safe even for the very old and can improve vision considerably.

Teach elderly clients with decreased vision not to rely on a driver's examination vision test for approval to drive. Snellen's charts are not infallible, and automobile accidents can be avoided if the visually impaired elderly client has ongoing care with an ophthalmologist.

CATARACTS

When the crystalline lens becomes opaque, it is called a cataract. This loss of transparency impairs vision. Many people believe cataracts mean blindness; in reality, however, cataracts develop slowly, and surgical extraction of a cataract can restore vision with little discomfort or risk.

Most cataracts (95%) are thought to be due to the aging process (senile cataracts). The adult lens consists of a peripheral portion (the cortex) and a central portion (the nucleus) encased in a capsule. With age, the nucleus becomes

dense, the cortex can opacify, and the lens becomes hard and unyielding. Furthermore, a gradual reduction in accommodative powers occurs. Cataracts of this degenerative type usually are evident at about age 50, although they may develop much earlier.

Other cataracts may be due to congenital factors (rubella in a pregnant woman during the first trimester can damage the developing lens), heredity, trauma (either a penetrating wound or contusion), inflammation (long-standing uveitis or glaucoma), malignancy, metabolic factors (poorly controlled diabetes mellitus), radiation (prolonged exposure to infrared light), and toxic conditions (long-term corticosteroid use).

Clinical Manifestations

The primary symptom of cataracts is some degree of visual loss. Gradual blurring of vision is the most common complaint (Figure 71–10). Glaring light such as bright sunshine constricts the pupil and makes vision seem worse. Double vision may occur in one eye (monocular diplopia), because

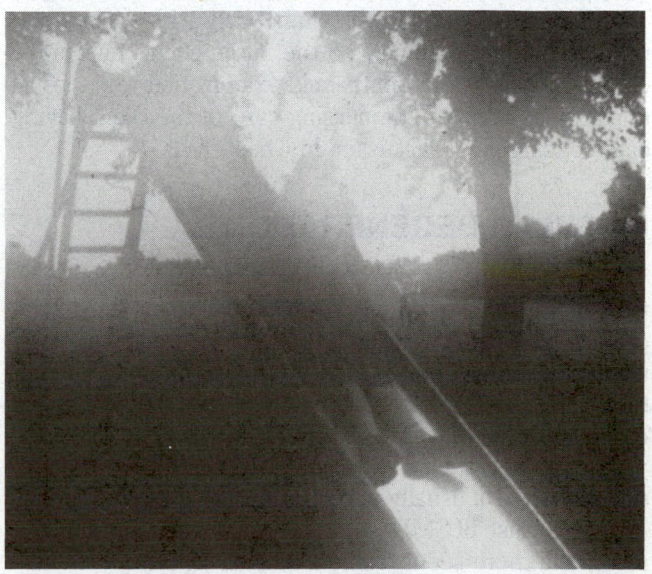

Figure 71–10

What a person with a cataract sees. (Courtesy of National Eye Institute, Bethesda, MD)

the lens opacity splits light bundles, causing two parts of the sensory retina to be stimulated. Senile cataracts are often bilateral, although usually unequal in density. Cataracts cause no pain.

Therapeutic and Specific Nursing Measures

Early stages of cataract development often go unnoticed, because many elderly people believe that old age brings a natural, unpreventable onset of blindness. Ophthalmoscopy, biomicroscopy, or a loupe (a convex magnifying lens) can be used to identify a cataract. Examination is enhanced by mydriasis. Ophthalmoscopy also can indicate how much visual loss a cataract should be causing. If the examiner can see in clearly, the client should be able to see out. In advanced stages, a cataract is visualized as a white discoloration just behind the pupil that is easily observable by oblique illumination.

The only effective treatment of a senile cataract is surgical removal. If the cataract is not removed, the client will eventually become blind. The techniques and management of cataract extraction are discussed in the following chapter. Extraction is usually postponed until vision in the better eye has fallen below 20/50, however, because functional vision is considered more desirable than the clear but distorted vision following cataract extraction. A senile cataract generally progresses slowly and may never attain a state in which extraction is necessary. In the early stages, permanent dilation of the pupil with atropine (three times weekly) may improve vision. Medication to retard or inhibit the formation of cataracts has not proven effective except in the case of diabetic cataracts. In the early stages of a cataract, a change of glasses may be helpful. As the lens becomes more cloudy, however, glasses will not help.

Cataracts can occur simultaneously with other ocular disorders (eg, glaucoma), so the nurse should encourage clients to have a full ophthalmic examination when visual impairment occurs. The nursing care of the client having cataract surgery is discussed in Chapter 72.

MACULAR DEGENERATION

The macula is more vulnerable to disease and degeneration than any other part of the retina. Senile macular degeneration (SMD) is the leading cause of new cases of blindness in the United States, accounting for 14% of the newly blind (Folk, 1982). It has been suggested that the aging of our population will make SMD an epidemic in 25 or 30 years. Degeneration in SMD is bilateral, but the progression in each eye usually occurs at different rates.

The cause of SMD is not known. Most cases are sporadic, and there seems to be a familial tendency. The disease process occurs because of an abnormality at the level of the retinal pigment epithelium and overlying photoreceptors. **Drusen,** yellow deposits, are visualized on ophthalmoscopic examination as mounds on Bruch's mem-

brane (beneath the pigment epithelium). Drusen are thought to represent secretory products from a "tired" retinal pigment epithelium (Folk, 1982). An abnormal fluid transfer then seeps through Bruch's membrane, promoting an elevation or "blistering" of the pigment epithelium and the neurosensory retina. In addition, an abnormal blood vessel from the choroid may grow through the defect in Bruch's membrane and lead to a subretinal hemorrhage, which usually leads to a subretinal scar. Recurrent scarring with decreased nourishment of the macula leads to destruction of the pigment epithelium and photoreceptors, as well as the permanent loss of central acuity. This degeneration of the macula can take years to run its course. Because of the typical client's age (greater than 50 years), arteriosclerotic vascular changes commonly coexist with the degeneration but are not responsible for it.

Clinical Manifestations

Macular degeneration spares peripheral vision. However, the client may experience blurred vision, and a central scotoma is inevitable (Figure 71–11). Visual acuity is distorted. Visualization via ophthalmoscope will show a central retinal detachment and, in advanced cases, fibrosis with surrounding hemorrhage. Fluorescein angiography can help locate leaky vessels.

Therapeutic and Specific Nursing Measures

Laser photocoagulation may help prevent further leakage of fragile vessels and result in transitory visual improvement.

Eventually, an unremitting macular degeneration blinds central vision. Reading is not possible, but the affected client may still have mobility without assistance. The nurse

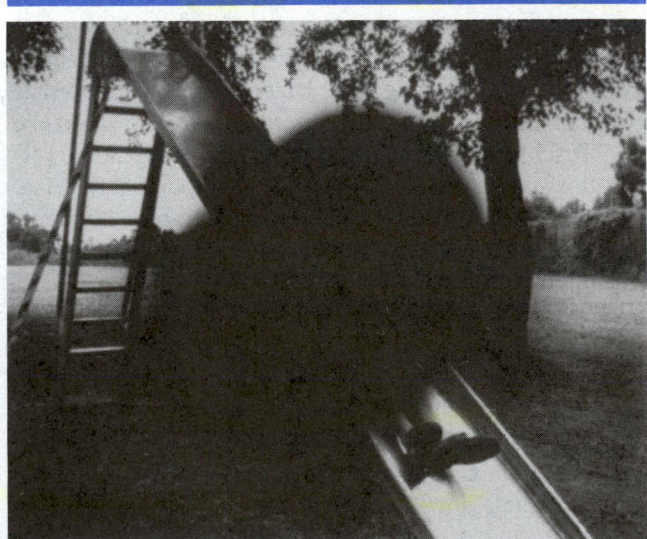

Figure 71–11

What a person with macular degeneration sees. (Courtesy of National Eye Institute, Bethesda, MD)

must remember that the difference between a loss of central vision and the loss of all vision is enormous and should reassure clients that unless other ocular disorders exist, they can perform activities of daily living independently.

Section IV: Immunologic Disorders

Immunologic disorders of the eye may result from the introduction of antigens from the external environment (eg, drugs, bacteria, or pollen) or the internal environment (eg, virally infected cells or transformed cancer cells). Antigens from the internal environment generally cause a systemic activation of the immune system, whereas the response elicited by external antigens is usually limited to the site of contact. The immune reaction of the eye varies in degrees of severity and may be acute or chronic.

The eye is often thought of as a special target of immunologic disease processes. It is not more susceptible to immunologic attacks than other organs of the body, but an attack to the eye is generally more obvious and visible. In an immune response, the eye often appears bloodshot because of the dilation of blood vessels in the conjunctiva. The inflammatory process initiated by the immunologic response may cause the normally transparent media of the eye to become opaque, thus disturbing the images transmitted to the retina. In addition, products of inflammation floating in the vitreous may cast shadows on the retina. Although permanently impaired vision or blindness may result from severe or chronic immune reactions, the most common signs and symptoms associated with immunologic diseases of the eye—burning, itching, and tearing—are temporary and mild.

General Nursing Implications

Nurses play many roles in the prevention, care, and treatment of people with visual and eye disorders. The recognition of immunologic diseases and their prevalence are ways the nurse may become involved with these clients.

Ophthalmic considerations are extremely important in the treatment of immunologic disorders of the eye. Be aware that the corticosteroid therapy frequently used to treat allergic eye conditions not only suppresses inflammation, but also reduces the eye's resistance to invasion by microorganisms (see Table 70–4 in Chapter 70). Client education should include information on proper eye care, the type of eye medications used and how to safely administer them, and the avoidance of specific allergens.

Do not overlook emotional support in working with the allergic client whose symptoms seem minor compared with others. These individuals may become discouraged, despondent, and angry for several reasons; either they are forced to live with their annoying symptoms, or they must make radical changes in their lives (eg, changing jobs or moving) to be successfully treated. The nurse's continued interest and reassurance can help these clients cope with their disorders.

ALLERGIC OCULAR REACTIONS

Allergic ocular reactions are caused by exposure to allergenic materials, which bring about a hypersensitivity response (anaphylaxis).

The conjunctiva and eyelids are the two eye structures most commonly affected. Pollen and other airborne particles are readily introduced into ocular tissue, setting off allergic reactions. Ingested allergens or contact allergens such as makeup, contact lenses, and ophthalmic drugs also can initiate a hypersensitive reaction in the eye. Contact lenses may trap allergens and contribute to allergic reactions. Many allergic reactions can be avoided by limiting exposure to offending agents.

Clinical Manifestations

The client normally experiences itching, tearing, and burning of the eye. Vascular congestion (hyperemia), chemosis, and excessive tearing are the most prevalent signs. Exudate from the eye is clear or whitish if the response is acute and white, thick, and stringy if the allergy is chronic. The conjunctiva frequently appears milky or pink. Corneal edema is rare; if present, however, the client may have pain, photophobia, and blurred vision. Giant papillae (engorged and edematous outgrowths of inflamed conjunctiva) may appear in the tarsal conjunctiva of the upper eyelid of clients who develop an intolerance to their contact lenses.

Therapeutic Measures

The first approach in the treatment of allergies is the avoidance of exposure to the suspected allergen, such as offending foods, animal hair, perfumes, insect sprays, dust, pollen, and irritating fumes (eg, gasoline). If exposure to offending agents cannot be avoided, it should at least be limited. Wearing a mask while cleaning the house to prevent inhalation of dust and wearing goggles to prevent ocular exposure to allergens are two examples of attempts to limit exposure.

Cold compresses provide symptomatic relief of itching and burning, as well as promote vasoconstriction, which diminishes the immune reaction. Sunglasses can help clients with photophobia.

Various pharmacological agents are also used in the treatment of atopic diseases. Topical or subcutaneous epinephrine hydrochloride (Epifrin) provides symptomatic relief of conjunctival chemosis and hyperemia (see Table 70–4 in Chapter 70). Vasoconstricting agents may diminish the loss of fluid and the proliferation of eosinophils from blood vessels. Systemic antihistamines such as diphenhydramine hydrochloride (Benadryl), chlorpheniramine maleate (Chlor-Trimeton), and hydroxyzine hydrochloride (Atarax) may also be beneficial by competing with histamine for receptor sites. Low doses of corticosteroids (eg, prednisolone) may counteract the inflammatory response, although they are generally not warranted in treating atopic ocular diseases. Immunotherapy is another therapeutic measure frequently used in the treatment of clients with allergic reactions.

Specific Nursing Measures

Since most people with ocular allergic reactions are not hospitalized, intervention centers around client education, guidance, and support. Explain to the client and family or friends what allergens to avoid and how to avoid them. Measures that provide symptomatic relief, such as the use of cold compresses, can be encouraged. If the condition worsens or vision becomes impaired, encourage the client to see a physician.

CORNEAL ALLOGRAFT REACTIONS

A corneal allograft is performed in an attempt to replace a diseased cornea with healthy tissue from a donor (see Chapter 72 for a complete discussion). Rejection of the allograft occurs because the body's immune mechanism recognizes the graft as foreign (nonself) and thus initiates pathological changes or destruction of the graft.

Cellular immunity mechanisms are implicated in corneal allograft reactions. The first such mechanism involves the body's recognition of foreign tissue. The second mechanism, a direct consequence of the first, is the body's defensive reaction against the foreign tissue: Antibodies are formed against the allograft, and an antigen–antibody reaction takes place. This reaction produces an inflammatory response, which in turn damages the blood vessels of the cornea and causes ischemia and necrosis of the allograft. Rejection generally starts at the site of maximum vascularization (usually the periphery of the allograft). Trauma or inflammation that dilates the blood vessels may increase the risk of allograft reactions. Interrupted sutures that are left in place too long, producing neovascularization, also increase the probability of allograft reactions.

Allograft reactions occur in about 10% to 15% of the approximately 10,000 corneal grafts performed each year. This low rate of rejection is attributed to (1) the absence of blood vessels and lymphatics in the cornea and (2) the lack of presensitization to tissue-specific antigens in most recipients (Vaughan & Asbury, 1980).

Clinical Manifestations

Corneal allograft reactions may occur as early as 10 days, or as late as many years, after implantation of donor tissue into the recipient eye. The earliest signs are a mild inflammation of the uveal tract, the presence of cells and protein in the anterior chamber, and an accumulation of small keratic (bony) deposits on the endothelium. The donor cornea then becomes edematous and opaque. Clients experience little pain, but their vision is usually blurred.

Therapeutic Measures

The mainstay of treatment for corneal allograft reactions is corticosteroid therapy (see Table 70–4 in Chapter 70). The frequent administration of corticosteroids (often every hour) suppresses the immune system in a number of ways. First, corticosteroids diminish the release of active substances such as histamine. Second, they constrict blood vessels, thereby decreasing vascular permeability. Third, they can reduce the movement of antigen–antibody complexes across cell membranes. Fourth, corticosteroids decrease the number and circulation of lymphocytes. Prednisolone acetate 1% is the topical corticosteroid of choice, since it penetrates the intact corneal epithelium better than prednisolone sodium phosphate. Occasionally, oral corticosteroids are ordered in conjunction with the topical ones. Corticosteroid therapy is continued until the clinical signs abate. Surgical maneuvers to minimize and prevent corneal allograft reaction include (1) using small grafts to reduce the invasion of antibodies, (2) removing interrupted sutures as soon as reparative fibers and blood vessels reach the graft, and (3) using nylon sutures rather than silk.

Specific Nursing Measures

The nursing management of a client experiencing a corneal allograft reaction includes emotional support of client and family or significant others, client education, and ensuring correct management such as proper administration of eyedrops. Emotional support is especially important if the client has had a previous allograft rejection. Client education should include information about the prescribed drugs (ie, the drug name, side effects, and actions). Reinforce the proper method and timing of instillation of eyedrops and maintain the proper schedule of frequent eyedrop instillation, which at times may be inconvenient to the client. Clients should be informed that because grafts are slow to heal, they should be careful to prevent infection and avoid activities that increase intraocular pressure. Encourage follow-up visits to the physician.

Section V: Infectious Disorders

Almost any pathogenic bacteria can cause an ocular infection. Staphylococcus is a constant inhabitant of the anterior portion of the eyeball, and fungi, viruses, spirochetes, pro-tozoa, and parasites are inescapable. The eyeball's intact outer layers provide an effective barrier against infection. However, if microbes have an opportunity to invade the intraocular structures, a serious infection can develop and rapidly spread to adjacent parts of the eye. This is particularly true of streptococcal infections. A great variety of factors are involved in a microorganism's ability to establish a disease process; most important, the infectious agent must be able to penetrate the protective barriers and find a favorable environment for multiplication. Untreated infectious disorders can ultimately lead to blindness.

General Nursing Implications

Most clients with localized infections are not hospitalized; therefore, nursing care consists of teaching the client and family or friends to care for the inflamed or infected eye. Good hygiene should be emphasized. Teach the client how to prevent the spread of the infection and demonstrate consistent clean technique by careful hand-washing and use of individual towels and washcloths (refer to Chapter 70).

HORDEOLA

A hordeolum (stye) is an acute benign abscess of the follicle of an eyelash or accessory gland along the eyelid margins. It may occur in crops as the infection spreads to adjacent hair follicles. The usual cause of a hordeolum is staphylococcal infection. Several hordeola may persistently recur in clients with chronic blepharitis or conjunctivitis or in debilitated people with compromised immune systems.

Clinical Manifestations

A hordeolum is characterized by a localized red, swollen, and acutely tender area. Pain is in direct proportion to the amount of eyelid swelling.

Therapeutic and Specific Nursing Measures

Treatment is usually a topical sulfonamide; however, sensitivity tests are necessary in all chronic and acute cases to ensure the proper choice of antibiotics. Incision and drainage are often indicated when the abscess becomes "pointed" and does not spontaneously drain.

Treatment in acute cases consists of the application of hot, moist compresses for 10 to 15 minutes four times a day. Gentle rubbing away from the eye will mechanically remove infected debris. An antibiotic ointment then may be applied. Urge the client not to squeeze the hordeolum, because the infection could be complicated by the development of cellulitis and can spread along the entire eyelid margin. Advise clients with persistent or recurring hordeola to see their health care provider.

CHALAZIA

A chalazion is a chronic sterile granulomatous inflammation of one of the meibomian glands. Often mistaken for a hor-

deolum, a chalazion is differentiated mainly by the fact that it tends to be on the conjunctival side of the eyelid and does not involve the eyelid margin. The cause of chalazia is unknown, and recurrence may require a biopsy to rule out malignancy.

Clinical Manifestations

Chalazia are characterized by gradual localized swelling of the meibomian gland and inflammation and tenderness not quite as severe as with a hordeolum. Palpation reveals a small swelling at the conjunctival side of the eyelid that feels like a small piece of buckshot. If the chalazion increases in size, astigmatism may develop as the globe is distorted.

Therapeutic and Specific Nursing Measures

Asymptomatic chalazia do not require treatment. Short-term suppuration is treated with a topical antibiotic such as a sulfonamide. If vision is distorted, an excision of the chalazion is indicated. Chronic inflammations may require an incision and curettage. Apply hot, moist compresses to the affected eye q.i.d. for 15 to 20 minutes. A chronic chalazion is annoying and unpleasant for the client, and emotional support is helpful.

BLEPHARITIS

Blepharitis is a chronic scaling inflammation of the eyelid margins. It begins in childhood and frequently continues throughout life, becoming more symptomatic in the sixth and seventh decades (Newell, 1982). There are two types of blepharitis: squamous (seborrheic) and ulcerative (staphylococcal). Both types may be present in an individual. Clients with rosacea and atopic diseases seem to have an increased incidence of blepharitis.

Clinical Manifestations

Squamous blepharitis is associated with scaling of the skin that may cause fine flakes and scales surrounding the lashes and eyebrows. Redness of the eyelid margin, chronic conjunctivitis, and mild keratitis are common. Seborrhea and dandruff are almost always present. Ulcerative blepharitis caused by *Staphylococcus aureus* produces suppurative lesions at the follicles of the lashes, glands of Zeis, and Moll's glands (ciliary glands of the conjunctiva next to the bulbs of the eyelashes). The yellow purulent discharge crusts on the lashes and is difficult to remove. There may be a subsequent loss of lashes (caused by destruction of the hair follicles and the removal of crusts) and distortion of the eyelid margin. These irreversible changes are dangerous to the cornea because of exposure and dysfunction of the lacrimal film.

Therapeutic Measures

Pharmacological management of blepharitis depends on the sensitivity of the offending organism. Local antibiotics such as sulfonamides, gentamicin, erythromycin, and bacitracin are often used in ointment form. Systemic antibiotics may be indicated for severe inflammation. Corticosteroids may decrease the inflammatory effect (see Table 70–4 in Chapter 70). Finally, medicated shampoos and lotions are recommended to control the seborrheic dermatitis.

Specific Nursing Measures

Emphasize the importance of keeping the scalp, eyebrows, and eyelid margins clean. Instruct the client to remove eyelid crusts frequently using cotton and diluted baby shampoo. Crusts are easier to remove when hot, moist compresses are used for 10 to 15 minutes three to four times daily. Stress good hand-washing before and after care of the eyelids, and tell the client to avoid rubbing or touching the eyes. Shampoos containing selenium are easily obtainable, and the nurse should advise the client to use them regularly to control the seborrheic scalp.

CONJUNCTIVITIS

Conjunctivitis is an inflammation of the conjunctiva characterized by hyperemia, cellular infiltration, and exudates. It may be caused by exposure to noxious elements such as bacteria, viruses, fungi, parasites, toxins, allergens, chemicals, and chronic irritation. Conjunctivitis is overwhelmingly the most common cause of an atraumatic red eye. *Pinkeye* is the acute contagious form of conjunctivitis common in children. Chronic conjunctivitis is the most troublesome, particularly in the elderly, since it is recurrent and of long duration. The type of exudate, degree of corneal complication, and severity of infection are influenced to a great extent by the hygiene, nutrition, and general health of the affected individual.

Conjunctivitis is most commonly caused by bacteria (eg, *Staphylococcus aureus,* alpha and beta streptococci, pneumococci, hemophilus organisms, *E coli,* and *Pseudomonas*). Other causative organisms include viruses (eg, herpes viruses) and fungi (eg, *Candida albicans* and *Aspergillus fumigatus*). Endogenous diseases or syndromes that can cause conjunctivitis include Sjögren's syndrome, Reiter's syndrome, and Stevens–Johnson syndrome.

Noninfective causes of conjunctivitis include allergic responses; chemical and irritant responses to acids, alkalies, smoke, and wind; and chronic irritation, such as rubbing, entropion, or contact lens wear.

Clinical Manifestations

Signs of conjunctivitis include hyperemia, tearing, exudation, and pseudoptosis (drooping of the upper eyelid due to increased weight from cellular infiltration). The client complains of a foreign body sensation; a scratching or burning sensation; a sensation of fullness around the eyes; pruritus; and, when the cornea is involved, photophobia. Signs and symptoms of a more serious problem are significant pain, a change in visual acuity, an irregular cornea, and an abnormal pupil size or reaction upon examination. A fluorescein stain should be done to determine the etiology.

A purulent discharge is noted in clients with bacterial conjunctivitis; even if untreated, it may subside within 2 weeks. Viral conjunctivitis is highly contagious and is manifested by a profuse watery discharge and diffuse redness. Fungal and parasitic forms of conjunctivitis are unilateral and often appear as localized inflammatory granulomas; fungal conjunctivitis is uncommon. Toxic or traumatic conjunctivitis also is unilateral. Allergic conjunctivitis may cause considerable swelling, marked pruritus, and a stringy discharge.

Therapeutic Measures

A conjunctival culture should be performed when characteristic clinical manifestations are insufficient to determine the causative organism of conjunctivitis. Bacterial conjunctivitis can be treated with a broad-spectrum antibiotic until a culture and sensitivity test result have been obtained. Treatment of viral conjunctivitis is usually ineffective; it runs its course. Fungal conjunctivitis may respond to nystatin ointment. Topical corticosteroids and vasoconstrictors can relieve the congestion and pruritus associated with allergic conjunctivitis.

Specific Nursing Measures

To prevent the spread of infection, the nurse should instruct the client and family or friends about the importance of good personal hygiene. For example, the use of individual towels and tissues instead of communal towels and handkerchiefs will decrease the spread of the organism. Teach the client and family how to instill eyedrops without touching the eye, and instruct them to instill medication in the unaffected eye first to prevent cross-contamination.

Eyepatches are not used, because enclosure of the drainage would provide optimum conditions for the growth of bacteria and viruses. Irrigations may be ordered (always before instillation of the medication) to remove discharge. Use separate equipment for each eye and wash the hands between treatment of each eye to avoid cross-contamination. Finally, recommend dark glasses for photophobia.

TRACHOMA

Trachoma, a chronic destructive disease of the conjunctiva and cornea, can cause corneal scarring; untreated, it can cause blindness. Trachoma affects 400 million people worldwide and is associated with poor personal and community hygiene, overcrowding, and lack of running water. There is an especially high incidence of trachoma in the

Balkans and Russia. It is also common in the hot arid climates of North Africa and the Middle East, as well as in the Caribbean and Southeast Asia. Immigrants from these countries may carry the disease. Children are more susceptible to trachoma, and mothers may transfer the infection to their children. Trachoma exclusively affects the eye and does not lead to systemic involvement.

The trachoma agent is *Chlamydia trachomatis*. Insects, especially flies and gnats, are believed to play a role in transmission by feeding on the lacrimal secretions of children and people whose eyes have an inadequate lid reflex. Trachoma is a contagious disease transmitted from eye to eye and may be exacerbated by other types of bacterial conjunctivitis.

Clinical Manifestations

The incubation period of trachoma is uncertain, and subclinical infection is the rule. Often signs and symptoms do not become apparent until adulthood. Signs of trachoma often resemble those of a severe conjunctivitis that burns, itches, and waters. There is corneal inflammation and vascularization with severe conjunctival scarring and deformity that may lead to blindness.

Therapeutic and Specific Nursing Measures

Tetracycline, erythromycin, and sulfonamides administered systemically cause striking clinical improvement. Vaccination in an endemic area often gives promising results, and entire communities can be treated prophylactically. Ideally, impoverished areas should have improved waste disposal and fly control to prevent trachoma. Surgical treatment is required for entropion, where the eyelashes chronically rub against the cornea and cause ulcerations, scarring, dehydration, and possible perforation.

Proper nutrition and personal hygiene are paramount in the prevention of trachoma. Emphasize to clients the transmission mode; the importance of good hand-washing; and the need to avoid community towels, linens, and cosmetics.

KERATITIS AND CORNEAL ULCERATION

The outer layer of the cornea, the epithelium, provides an adequate barrier against most microbes into the cornea. If the epithelium is traumatized, however, a variety of organisms can flourish within the stroma and Bowman's membrane, and keratitis (inflammation of the cornea) ensues. Keratitis may be complicated by the formation of a corneal ulcer. Only the epithelial cells and Descemet's membrane are able to regenerate; thus, damage to the cornea usually leaves a permanent scar and may impair vision. The infection also may spread to other ocular structures. Corneal perforation and possible loss of the eye may occur.

Keratitis may be caused by pathogenic bacteria (eg,

Staphylococcus aureus); viruses (eg, herpesvirus); fungi (eg, *Candida albicans*); facial nerve disorders such as Bell's palsy that paralyze the orbicular muscle of the eye (an oval muscle surrounding the eyelid responsible for closing it, wrinkling the forehead, and compressing the lacrimal sac); traumatic insult (eg, from chemicals, excessive ultraviolet exposure, and mechanical means); and exposure (eg, from ptosis or severe ectropion). Despite the formidable corneal barrier, some bacteria are able to penetrate an intact cornea (eg, *Neisseria gonorrhoeae* and *Pseudomonas aeruginosa*). Clients with malnutrition, vitamin A deficiency, diabetes, or decreased resistance are more susceptible to a variety of microorganisms.

Clinical Manifestations

The predominant feature of keratitis is necrosis, often with resultant ulcer formation. Because the cornea has a rich nerve supply, clients may feel severe pain from seemingly minor irritations. Corneal lesions can cause blurred vision, with greater blurring if the lesion is centrally located. Since there are no blood vessels or mucous glands in the cornea, discharges are uncommon, except with a purulent bacterial ulcer. The client often has the sensation of a foreign body in the eye. Photophobia is not uncommon, and the eye may appear reddened (bloodshot).

Therapeutic Measures

It is important to ask the client about a history of trauma, because foreign bodies and erosion are two of the most common corneal disorders. Topical eye medications the client may be taking should be investigated to rule out steroid therapy, which frequently predisposes the recipient to herpetic keratitis.

Culture and smear for Gram's stain are fundamental, as are bacterial identification and sensitivity studies. Broad-spectrum topical antibiotics are used at frequent intervals until diagnosis can be made by the smear. The instillation of atropine sulfate (Isopto Atropine) or scopolamine hydrobromide (Isopto Hyoscine) for pupil dilation keeps the ciliary body and iris at rest, thereby reducing pain. Nystatin or amphotericin B may be beneficial in the treatment of fungal corneal ulcers. Avitaminosis A corneal ulceration resulting from a dietary lack of vitamin A, impaired absorption of vitamin A from the gastrointestinal tract, or impaired utilization of vitamin A by the body is treated with the intravenous administration of 10,000 to 15,000 units of vitamin A daily.

The corneal integrity can be maintained as long as the corneal surface is kept moist by the client's wearing a plastic wrap moisture chamber secured to the surrounding skin with adhesive tape. Another method for keeping the cornea moist is inserting a bandage soft contact lens—a soft contact lens used to treat corneal epithelial erosions secondary to recurrent corneal erosion, corneal dystrophies such as keratoconus, keratitis, alkali burns, and bullous keratopathy. Sometimes taping or suturing of the lids is performed, or a conjunctival flap (see Chapter 72) is used to protect the exposed cornea. Surgical relief of exophthalmos can often cure exposure-induced corneal ulcerations.

Specific Nursing Measures

Hot, moist compresses should be used generously. Eyepatches are not used on infectious or suppurative lesions, however, because they favor bacterial multiplication and prevent the free flow of discharge from the eye. Teach the client proper instillation of eyedrops, including the importance of washing hands before and after and methods of preventing contamination.

UVEITIS

Uveitis, a general term for inflammatory disorders of the uveal tract, encompasses a number of diseases that affect part or all of it. The most frequent form of uveitis is iritis (acute anterior uveitis). Early diagnosis of iritis is important to prevent the formation of posterior **synechiae** (adhesions of the iris to the lens) (Figure 71–12A). In posterior uveitis, the retina is almost always secondarily affected (chorioretinitis). Uveitis is usually unilateral and is principally found in the young and middle age groups.

In addition to inflammation by pathogens, uveitis may also result from a hypersensitivity reaction such as arthritis or ankylosing spondylitis. Microorganisms are rarely identified, and only about one-third of all cases of uveitis have an identifiable cause; the other two-thirds are of unknown etiology.

Clinical Manifestations

Pain, photophobia, and blurred vision are common symptoms of uveitis. Depending on the cause, the onset can be from acute to insidious. Pathogenic invasion may cause a diffusely red eye. Pupils are usually small and irregular as posterior synechiae form (Figure 71–12B).

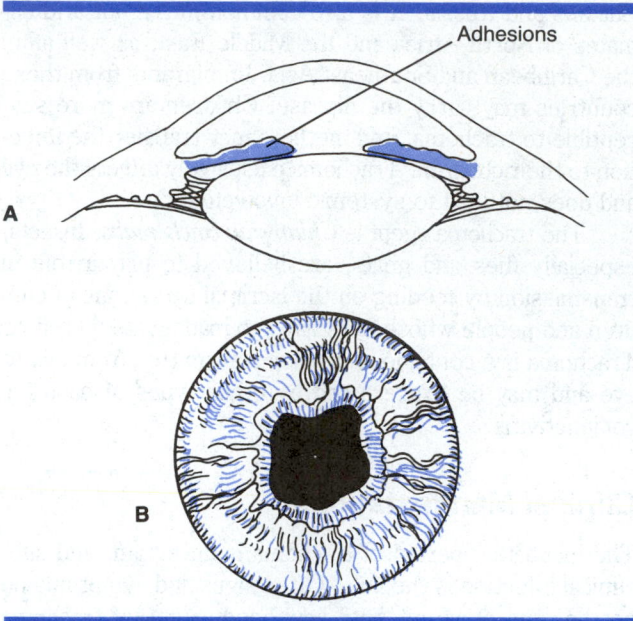

Figure 71–12

Posterior synechiae. **A.** The iris adheres to the lens. **B.** Irregular pupil from posterior synechiae.

Therapeutic and Specific Nursing Measures

Because the tubercle bacillus and *Histoplasma capsulatum* have been known to be causative organisms in uveitis, skin tests may identify the probable cause and consequently aid in treatment. The pupil is kept dilated with atropine sulfate (Isopto Atropine) twice a day to prevent the formation of posterior synechiae (see Table 70–4 in Chapter 70). Steroids are helpful in the treatment of hypersensitivity-caused uveitis. Glaucoma is a common complication, and appropriate measures to decrease intraocular pressure are necessary.

Warm, moist compresses are applied for 10 minutes four times a day; analgesics also promote comfort. Dark glasses are recommended for photophobia.

Section VI: Neoplastic Disorders

Benign and malignant tumors may occur in the eye and surrounding structures. The diagnosis of intraocular and retrobulbar tumors is difficult, and biopsies are necessary to determine cell structure and malignancy. Early diagnosis is crucial in saving vision and in preventing extraocular extension of the tumor and death.

Neoplasms of the eyeball are relatively rare. Of all ocular tumors 85% appear in the choroid; 9%, in the ciliary body (Miller, 1979); and 6%, in the iris.

General Nursing Implications

Clinical manifestations usually do not occur until the late stages of intraocular tumors (unless there is macular involvement), so the nurse usually does not play a role in their early detection. If the client does complain of a change in vision or displacement of the eyeball, the nurse should encourage investigation.

Sometimes a routine ophthalmologic examination reveals the possibility of a tumor. The nurse then can offer emotional support as further studies are required and confirmation of the diagnosis is made. Because enucleation is often the final outcome, the nurse must recognize the client's extremely difficult decision between losing an eyeball and vision or dying. The nurse also should be aware of past experiences the client and family or significant others have had with cancer, because they can highly influence the coping mechanisms used.

CHOROIDAL MELANOMAS

Choroidal melanomas are nonhereditary, unilateral tumors of the middle layer of the eyeball (Figure 71–13). Most choroidal tumors are in the posterior portion of the eye, making biopsy difficult. They usually occur in white men over the age of 50.

The exact cause of choroidal melanomas is unknown. Malignant melanomas are found in 10% of the eyes blind from injury or inflammation, suggesting the possibility that irritation promotes malignancy. In the rare case that a metastatic choroidal melanoma is diagnosed, the probable origin is the breast or lung. The liver is the only organ known to be a site of metastasis from uveal tract melanomas.

Clinical Manifestations

Symptoms of choroidal melanomas often are not exhibited until the late stages of the disease process. A retinal detachment will cause visual distortion with an increase in choroidal volume. The loss of part of the visual field corresponds to the location of the tumor. Generally, the client has no pain unless glaucoma occurs.

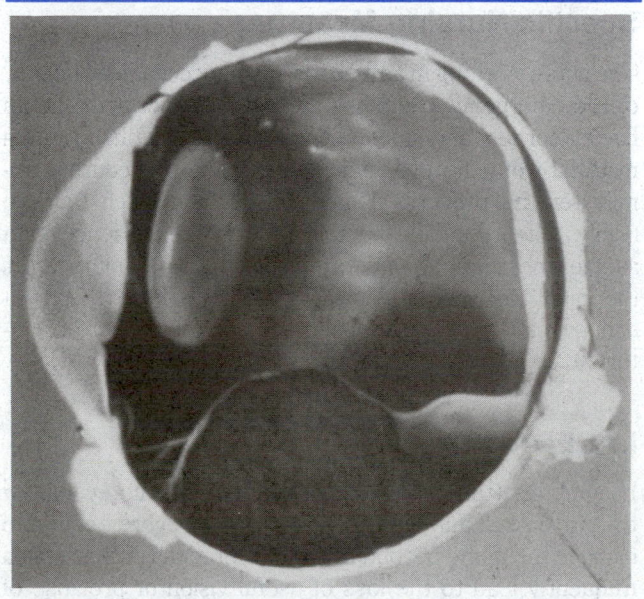

Figure 71–13

Choroidal melanoma. (Courtesy of Millard Fillmore Hospital, Buffalo, NY)

Therapeutic Measures

Once a correct diagnosis has been confirmed by indirect ophthalmoscopy, ultrasonography, fluorescein angiography, or computed tomography (see Chapter 70), appropriate treatment will be instituted. Often a small tumor will not change in size for a long time (months to years). When diagnosis is uncertain, therefore, regular examinations (every 3 to 4 months) are performed to watch for growth, which indicates the necessity for treatment because of the chance of metastasis. Metastatic spread of a uveal melanoma before the primary tumor has become symptomatic is virtually unknown (Zimmerman & McLean, 1980).

A tumor less than 10 mm in diameter is associated with a client mortality of 13%, whereas a tumor greater than 12 mm in diameter has a 70% client mortality. The safest treatment is enucleation, with the age of the client and the size of the tumor being the major determinants. Recently, external proton beam irradiation has been used to treat eyes with tumors. Because this treatment requires the use of a linear accelerator, it is performed in few health care centers. Five- and 10-year survival rates are not as yet known.

Specific Nursing Measures

Clients undergoing external proton beam irradiation are hospitalized prior to this radiation therapy for the insertion of tantalum rings around the tumor. The tantalum rings provide reference markers for radiographic alignment of the proton beam with the tumor. This period of hospitalization affords the nurse the opportunity to provide client education and emotional support prior to irradiation. The client undergoes proton beam irradiation about 2 weeks later. During an 8-day period, the client usually receives five proton beam irradiation treatments. The nurse is unlikely to have contact with the client during the treatment period, and information and support are provided by the personnel at the linear accelerator facility.

The loss of an eyeball can be a devastating experience for a client. With the decision of enucleation to save one's life, the client faces complex ramifications. When the client has reasonably good vision in the other eye and the mortality for the diagnosed neoplasm is low (less than 15%), the choice to enucleate may be easier. Alternatively, some clients may prefer to take a chance with a highly malignant tumor, particularly when the vision in the other eye is compromised.

The client will undoubtedly feel ambivalent about the choice of treatment; thus, psychological support is greatly needed to help the client overcome confusion about the ultimate decision and to be able to cope with and accept the cancer and the treatment approach chosen. Alterations in lifestyle may be necessary, and assisting the client with necessary rehabilitative measures is an important aspect of the nurse's role. The nursing care of the client undergoing enucleation is discussed in Chapter 72.

Section VII: Traumatic Disorders

Ocular trauma is the most common cause of eye disease and represents potential disaster to the eye. It is a major source of blindness in North America. (Untreated eye diseases such as trachoma or glaucoma account for the majority of cases of blindness in the rest of the world.) Approximately 50% of blindness in one eye and 20% of blindness in both eyes is caused by trauma. Because of the size of the eye and its delicate structure, major damage may result from an injury that would be insignificant on another part of the body. In addition, ocular trauma is frequently associated with intracranial injury. Finally, the number of days spent in the hospital recovering from ocular trauma is so high that economic consequences are significant.

General Nursing Implications

The greatest deterrent to ocular trauma is educated awareness of risks and careful avoidance procedures; approximately 50% of serious ocular trauma can be prevented in this way. Nurses play a significant role in both the prevention and treatment of ocular injuries. Encourage safety precautions in both the home and work environments through public education and support of safety legislation.

Prompt care can restore useful vision, whereas improper handling or poor management can destroy the eye. Thus, proper first aid care and avoidance of further damage to the injured eye is extremely important. The nurse must be able to differentiate potentially serious eye injuries from minor ones. Any injury causing decreased vision, bleeding from or within the eyeball, or pain should be promptly referred to a physician.

Emotional support of the client and family or friends is essential. The partial loss of sight and fear of blindness are the most dreaded aftermaths of ocular trauma. Although emotional support is important, it is also important that the nurse be honest with the client and family, because a complete recovery is often not possible.

ABRASIONS

Abrasions are superficial scratches on the eyelid, conjunctiva, or cornea. Abrasions to the eyelid and conjunctiva rarely warrant medical attention, because they heal rapidly without treatment and cause little pain. Corneal abrasions, in contrast, disrupt the corneal epithelium and expose many nerve fibers, causing pain and prompting the client to seek medical treatment. Superficial abrasions normally heal without scarring or visual impairment. Two possible complications of corneal abrasions are delayed healing and recurrent corneal erosion. Infection as a result of an abrasion is rare.

Abrasions of the eye are traditionally found after the removal of foreign bodies and after injuries caused by such objects as paper, fingernails, or twigs of a tree catching the eye. Overwearing of contact lenses can also cause corneal abrasions. Recurrent erosions can occur where regenerated epithelial cells have imperfectly united with Bowman's membrane, so that opening the eyes is sufficient by itself to detach them.

Clinical Manifestations

Clients with corneal abrasions often feel as if they have foreign bodies in their eyes. These abrasions generally cause pain because of the exposure of nerve fibers in the epithelium; excess lacrimation and photophobia are other symptoms. The use of a fluorescein strip aids in the diagnosis of corneal abrasions (see Chapter 70).

Therapeutic Measures

The treatment of corneal abrasions centers around pain relief. Topical anesthetic eyedrops, such as 5% tetracaine, are routinely used. Systemic analgesics are rarely necessary. Continued and frequent instillation of anesthetic eyedrops delays healing and should not be permitted. Antibiotic eyedrops are also used to guard against infection.

A firm patch on the eye prevents movement of the eyelid, thereby promoting healing and relieving pain. The patch should be changed daily during the inspection of the eye. The client should wear the patch until healing occurs (usually within 24 to 72 hours). Rest and avoiding movements of the cheek, which loosen the eyepatch and allow blinking, are recommended.

Specific Nursing Measures

The nurse working in ambulatory care, occupational health, or the emergency room has the most contact with clients having corneal abrasions. These nurses may flush foreign material from the eye, perform staining procedures, administer the prescribed medications, and patch the eye firmly. Clients should be told they may experience pain as the anesthetic wears off, usually 1 to 2 hours after the initial treatment. Also instruct clients how to apply a firm eyepatch in case it loosens or falls off (refer to Chapter 70).

LACERATIONS

Lacerations (tears) to the eye may involve the eyelids or the globe itself and may be superficial or severe enough to damage the globe beyond repair. Lacerations of the cornea frequently lead to the loss of useful vision or prolapse of the iris, ciliary body, lens, or vitreous. The client with a laceration injury is predisposed to intraocular infection, cataract formation, and corneal scarring. Eyelid lacerations may be disfiguring and interfere with the normal flow of tears. Lacerations of either the cornea or eyelid are usually associated with penetration by sharp objects (eg, knives or scissors), explosive injuries, and automobile or bicycle accidents.

Clinical Manifestations

Pain, bleeding, tearing, and shock are common manifestations of eyelid lacerations. They usually are easily visualized by the examiner. Clients with corneal lacerations may have mild to severe pain and symptoms of shock. Tissue prolapse may be evident upon examination. Iris prolapse causes the pupil to look like a teardrop. Other facial trauma often accompanies ocular lacerations.

Therapeutic Measures

The treatment of lacerations depends on the structure injured and whether there is prolapse of tissue. Eyelid lacerations should be repaired as soon as possible, because a delay of 6 to 8 hours significantly increases the risk of infection. The client should be sedated, reassured, and restrained from excessive movement. Eyelid lacerations not near the eyelid margins are sutured in the same way as other skin lacerations. If the laceration occurs at or near an eyelid margin, however, repair becomes increasingly difficult. Inappropriate repair creates a notch in the lid, causing disfigurement and interfering with tear flow.

Corneal lacerations without prolapsed tissue usually require suturing under an operative microscope. The scar must be made as small as possible to afford the least disruption of vision. Cycloplegics and antibiotics are usually indicated. Bilateral patches are usually placed to ensure complete rest of the eyes. Bed rest also may promote healing. Tetanus prophylaxis is indicated in any injury that penetrates the eye. Measures to repair corneal lacerations with prolapsed tissue attempt to replace the prolapsed contents of the eye. If damage is severe and much of the intraocular content has been lost, evisceration or enucleation is indicated.

Small, clean lacerations of the cornea (3 to 4 mm) often seal spontaneously. A rigid eyeshield and antibiotics are generally the only corrective measures taken.

Specific Nursing Measures

Nursing management of clients with ocular lacerations depends on the extent of injury. Eyelid lacerations and corneal lacerations without prolapsed tissue require little nursing intervention other than reassurance and instructions regarding the instillation of medications. If bleeding is present, application of pressure is contraindicated because this can damage the underlying globe.

Corneal lacerations with tissue prolapse generally require hospitalization of the client. Care is discussed more fully in the next section and in the discussion of enucleation in Chapter 72.

FOREIGN BODIES

Foreign bodies in the conjunctiva and cornea are the most common cause of ocular trauma. They generally pose few problems unless laceration and tissue prolapse accompany them. Foreign bodies can also penetrate and perforate the intraocular contents and lodge in almost any structure. Intraocular foreign bodies carry a high risk of impairing sight to some degree. Frequently encountered foreign bodies include dirt, small metallic particles, eyelashes, and glass. Most clients who seek medical attention for known or suspected foreign bodies in their eyes have been hammering, welding, or standing next to an industrial machine that caused particles to blow into their faces and eyes.

Clinical Manifestations

A conjunctival foreign body is usually not painful unless the object is under the upper eyelid. Blinking then moves the particle over the cornea, creating irritation and pain. Corneal foreign bodies cause pain, tearing, and photophobia. The sensation that something is in the eye occurs with both conjunctival and corneal foreign bodies.

Symptoms of intraocular foreign bodies may not be commensurate with the seriousness of the injury. Immediate symptoms may be minimal if the foreign body enters the eye quickly and smoothly. Intraocular foreign bodies usually lodge in the vitreous cavity. Therefore, ophthalmoscopic examination may reveal corneal lacerations, localized areas of conjunctival infection, a hole in the iris, hyphema, or disturbance of the lens. Retinal detachments may occur if the foreign body reaches the posterior portion of the eye.

Therapeutic Measures

Treatment depends on where the foreign body is located. If the object cannot be seen by the naked eye, magnification may be necessary. The client should not rub the eye because this may abrade the corneal tissue or cause the particle to become embedded. Eyes with penetrating injuries should be shielded from pressure. Attempts should not be made to cleanse the area of tears, discharge, and blood or to remove the penetrating object until an ophthalmologist has evaluated the client's condition.

Conjunctival foreign bodies frequently come out spontaneously with blinking. If this does not occur, they can be wiped out gently with a cotton swab moistened with normal saline. If the particle cannot be seen on the exposed conjunctiva, the examiner should evert and inspect the upper eyelid.

Foreign bodies embedded in the cornea must be removed by a physician, preferably an opthalmologist. A local anesthetic, magnification, and the use of a slit lamp facilitate removal. The physician takes care not to penetrate the cornea. Antibiotic ointments (eg, polymyxin B-bacitracin, gentamicin) should be instilled three times a day following removal of the foreign body. Eyepatches may be used if a laceration results.

Ophthalmologic treatment of foreign bodies that have perforated the intraocular contents depends on the type of foreign body and the extent of damage to surrounding tissues. Some inert substances are left in place, whereas organic matter (eg, wood, copper, or iron) is normally removed. Because magnetic material can be removed relatively easily with the aid of a magnet, it creates fewer hazards than does penetration by nonmagnetic foreign bodies. The removal of nonmagnetic particles requires the use of forceps to grasp and remove the objects from the vitreous. Any other damage to the eye must be repaired. Evisceration or enucleation is indicated if trauma and loss of intraocular contents is severe. Any penetrating injury to the eye warrants tetanus prophylaxis as well as the administration of antibiotics and analgesics.

Specific Nursing Measures

The nurse often takes an active role in the care of clients with ocular foreign bodies. Remove conjunctival foreign bodies by using a moist cotton swab or gently irrigating the eye with normal saline. If the foreign particle rests in the upper eyelid, evert the lid using the method discussed in Chapter 70. If corneal or intraocular foreign bodies are suspected, try to ensure that the client will be seen by an ophthalmologist as soon as possible. Meanwhile, shield the eye from pressure; try to provide a quiet, supportive environment; and obtain an order for analgesic medication. The nurse may assist the physician with removal of the foreign body or prepare the client for surgery.

Postoperatively, the nurse provides frequent assessments and should give honest reassurance to the client. Complete postoperative care is discussed in Chapter 72.

ORBITAL FRACTURES

Two types of orbital fracture can occur. The first involves the bony rim of the orbit and is usually detected by x-rays. The second type, a blow-out fracture, involves the disruption of the thin inferior orbital wall, causing the orbital contents to herniate into the maxillary sinus. The inferior rectus muscle often becomes incarcerated in the fracture site. Approximately 15% of orbital fractures are associated with serious eye injury.

Almost all orbital fractures are caused by a direct injury to the eye. Direct injuries usually result from blunt blows to the eye from a golf ball, a piece of equipment, or a motor vehicle accident. Fractures also occur as an extension of fractures in adjacent bones. In a blow-out fracture, pressure from a direct blow pushes the eyeball back and increases the intraocular pressure. This sudden pressure increase causes the inferior orbital wall to fracture next to the air-containing sinuses.

Clinical Manifestations

The client with a blow-out fracture frequently has pain, nausea at the time of injury, and diplopia. Ecchymosis, swelling, and subcutaneous emphysema (if the ethmoid bone is involved) may be present in either type of fracture. Persistent diplopia and enophthalmos are the two complications frequently seen with orbital fractures.

Therapeutic Measures

Surgical reduction of the fracture is undertaken if mobility of the eye is restricted or if endophthalmitis (extensive intraocular infection) is present. This procedure is not emergent and usually can be undertaken 7 to 10 days after the injury takes place to evaluate the indications fully. Simultaneous injury to the globe, however, may require immediate care.

Cold compresses applied during the first 24 hours help minimize swelling and bleeding into the surrounding tissues. Hot packs to speed the absorption of blood may be used after the first 24 hours. Pain medications are prescribed and administered.

Specific Nursing Measures

The nursing management of a client with an orbital fracture involves recognizing such an injury and urging prompt medical attention. The nurse may assist the ophthalmologist in examining the eye and carrying out therapeutic measures. Emotional support and teaching are the two most common and important nursing roles.

BURNS

Burns are tissue injury resulting from exposure to radiant energy, high temperatures, or chemicals. Radiant energy burns usually result from overexposure to ultraviolet rays, which most commonly occurs with the use of sunlamps or with carbon arc lamps used in welding. Overexposure can occur relatively quickly without a protective eye filter. Ultraviolet rays may also be absorbed by the eye when watching the sun or an eclipse, or when tanning in the sun with the face and eyes exposed. Reflections of the sun on snow or water constitute a greater hazard than the sun itself because the ultraviolet light concentrations are higher.

Thermal burns usually involve the eyelids rather than the globe. They usually result from flame, flare such as from a welding torch, or splashes of molten metal or other hot liquids.

Chemical burns occur in both home and work settings when a toxic substance comes in contact with the eye. The substance may be acidic (eg, sulfuric, hydrochloric, nitric, or acetic acid) or alkaline (eg, sodium hydroxide, ammonium hydroxide, lime, or calcium hydroxide). In general, alkali burns penetrate the tissue more quickly and are more serious than acid burns. The extent of damage to the eye depends on the concentration of chemicals, the duration of exposure, and the pH of the solution.

Severe burns to the eye may cause major ocular complications; poor rehabilitative prognosis; and, when bilateral, a life of dependency for the affected individual. Immediate first aid care of the burned eye often limits the amount of damage to the eye. Other organ damage may accompany burns to the eye (eg, extensive burns of the face, body, and upper airways). Care of these burns may supersede or coincide with eye care (see Chapter 15).

Clinical Manifestations

All types of burns may stimulate the free nerve endings in the corneal epithelium and the conjunctiva. When the burn is severe, especially from alkali, there is an immediate rise in intraocular pressure. Radiant energy burns produce no immediate symptoms; they manifest themselves approximately 6 to 12 hours after ultraviolet exposure. The client experiences extreme pain from the development of superficial keratitis. Tearing, photophobia, and congestion of the globe are often present. Severe ultraviolet burns also may burn the macula, causing permanent visual impairment. Photophobia and blurred vision may be present for a week after the accident.

Thermal burns usually cause widespread tissue destruction. Depending on the extent of the burn, pain and shock may be displayed. Corneal sloughing may also be present if damage to the cornea has occurred.

The immediate manifestation of chemical burns is pain. The eye should be copiously flushed for at least 20 minutes with water to remove the foreign substance until the pain subsides. After a chemical burn, the eyelids will be swollen and the conjunctiva reddened. The degree of corneal stromal whitening (marbleization) aids in determining the severity of the burn.

Therapeutic Measures

Radiant energy burns usually cause significant pain and prompt the client to seek medical attention. A topical anesthetic reduces pain and facilitates examination. Mydriatics (eg, homatropine hydrobromide [Isopto Homatropine]) are often used in the initial examination to dilate the pupil (see Table 70–4 in Chapter 70). Visual acuity should always be tested. Patching the eye for 24 hours and applying cold compresses provide symptomatic relief. Recovery usually occurs within 12 to 36 hours without complications.

The treatment of thermal burns is similar to the treatment of skin burns elsewhere, because the eyelid tissue is usually involved. Skin grafts, mucous membrane grafts, or both may be required if eyelid contractures are present.

Chemical burns require the immediate dilution of the chemical, because the extent of damage to the eye depends on the concentration of the contacting solution and the amount of time it is in contact with the eye. Always flush the eye first, then seek medical attention. Copiously flush the eye with water for 20 to 30 minutes. Separate the eyelids well to allow the water to flush the cornea and conjunctiva. Do not try to neutralize the chemical with a buffering solution, because finding the correct solution often delays treatment. Industrial plants and research laboratories must have jet stream irrigating fountains or safety showers. Remove any particulate matter. After irrigation, the eye can be patched and the client sent to an ophthalmologist for examination. Corneal exposure resulting from eyelid edema and retraction or incomplete blinking must be treated quickly by artificial tears or moisture chambers.

The use of steroids for thermal or chemical burns is controversial, and most ophthalmologists avoid it. Instead, they usually order antibiotics to prevent or treat infection. If corneal damage from a chemical burn is severe, corneal transplantation may be undertaken approximately 18 months to 2 years after the accident. The chance of visual improvement with this procedure after severe burn damage is 50% (Pfister, 1983).

Specific Nursing Measures

Nursing intervention with chemical burns to the eye involves immediate irrigation of the eye, as has been discussed. Information regarding the type of chemical involved, its concentration, and the duration of probable exposure should be obtained. The nurse should try to calm the client. Occupational health nurses may be involved in ensuring that all employees follow safety regulations and that all irrigators function properly.

The incidence of ultraviolet burns can be decreased by public awareness. Inform the public formally and informally about the significance of ultraviolet burns and how to avoid them.

CONTUSIONS

An intraocular contusion is a bruising injury in which the exterior of the eye remains intact, but intraocular damage has occurred. This type of trauma most frequently results in a hemorrhage into the anterior chamber (hyphema) or the vitreous or surrounding tissues (ecchymosis). The consequences of such injuries vary and are often not immediately obvious. Contusions of the eyeball may be produced by a severe blow to the eye. The blow is usually blunt and comes from traumatic contact with a tennis ball, fist, golf ball, or baseball.

Clinical Manifestations

A client with an ocular contusion may have a large extravasation of blood under the skin that causes the eye to appear black and blue. Swelling of the surrounding tissues most often accompanies a black eye. Hyphema also may be evident and often can be observed by the naked eye (Figure 71–14). The client may experience impaired vision, pain, and fear. A sudden decrease in vision and complaints of

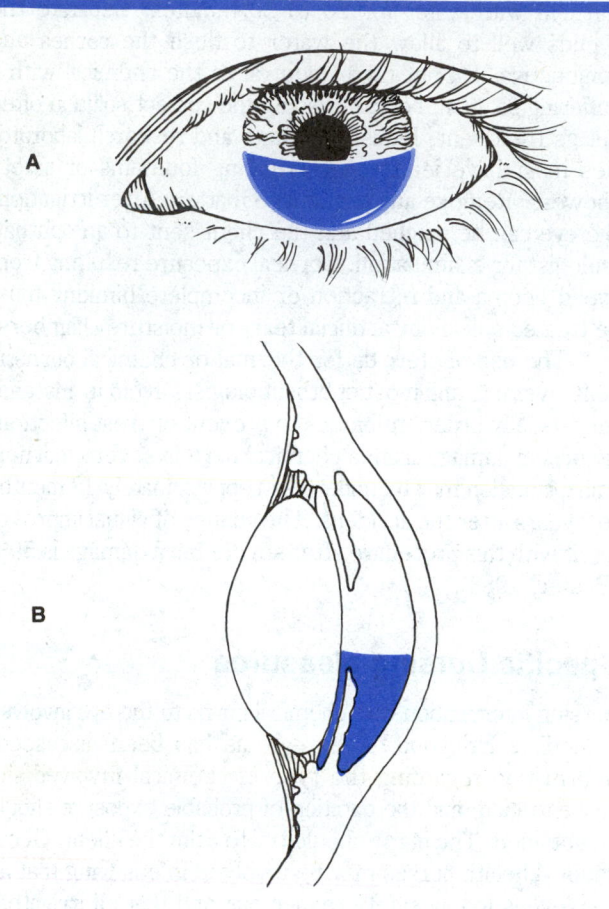

Figure 71–14

Hyphema. **A.** Front view. **B.** Side view.

floaters may indicate a hemorrhage into the vitreous. Intraocular pressure almost always temporarily increases in a contusion of the eyeball.

Other complications that may develop immediately or weeks to months after the injury include lens dislocation, macular edema, retinal detachment, iridodialysis (splitting of the iris resulting in more than one pupil), and rupture of the sclera.

Therapeutic Measures

Most immediate effects of an ocular contusion do not require immediate definitive treatment. Specific treatment depends on the location and extent of damage. Cold compresses and mild analgesics are used to treat ocular contusions. As the blood decomposes and is absorbed, the bruises change color and fade completely in 5 to 7 days.

Clients exhibiting signs of hyphema should have absolute bed rest with bilateral eyepatches to minimize the risks of further bleeding. Diazepam (Valium) may be ordered to decrease anxiety and promote complete rest. Intraocular pressure should be monitored.

Specific Nursing Measures

Clients with hyphema should have the head of the bed elevated. Change the eyepatches daily and provide ongoing emotional support. Since clients have bilateral eyepatches, the nurse must assist with many of the daily living activities, such as feeding and bathing. The nurse also may encourage family members or friends to assist with these tasks and to read to the client. Enforce complete rest using any available measures.

Chapter Highlights

Corneal dystrophies, retinitis pigmentosa, ptosis, and strabismus are the most common congenital eye disorders, although they are all fairly rare.

Treatment for congenital disorders is often only palliative, not curative. The nurse therefore should encourage genetic counseling and provide client education, rehabilitative measures, and emotional support.

Many eye disorders such as retinal detachments, refractive errors, and glaucoma may have a variety of etiologies (be multifactorial in origin). They are important because of their relatively high incidence.

A retinal detachment progressively impairs vision as the retina is pulled from the choroid, depriving the rods and cones of their nutritional supply. It may result from trauma, vitreous traction, or retinal degeneration.

Retinal detachments frequently require surgical intervention. However, cryotherapy, photocoagulation, and diathermy can be used to seal holes, as well as to prevent the proliferation of new vessels in clients with diabetic retinopathy.

Refractive errors occur when light rays fail to converge on the same point on the retina. Myopia (nearsightedness), hyperopia (farsightedness), astigmatism (asymmetric focus), and presbyopia (lack of focusing power) generally cause reduced visual acuity and discomfort but can be easily corrected with glasses or contact lenses.

Glaucoma encompasses a group of ocular disorders that have increased intraocular pressure, usually because of a blockage of the aqueous humor outflow channels. Glaucoma may be primary, secondary, congenital, or absolute.

Miotics, timolol maleate, epinephrine, and diuretics are initially used in the treatment of glaucoma. However, surgical filtering procedures are sometimes required.

Nurses can help prevent the disastrous effects of glaucoma through public education and mass screening of individuals over 40. Assisting clients with their therapy regimen and client education are other important responsibilities of the nurse.

Degenerative disorders such as cataracts and macular degeneration produce such changes as reduced visual acuity, loss of accommodation, loss of peripheral or central vision, and difficulty in color discrimination.

Cataracts develop slowly and cause impaired vision as the lens becomes opaque. Surgical removal of the lens and a corrective lens after surgery correct this disorder.

Antigens introduced from either the internal or external environment can elicit an immune reaction in the eye, causing temporary redness, burning, itching, and tearing.

Corneal allograft reactions, in which the immune system recognizes a corneal allograft as a foreign tissue and rejects it, occur at a low rate.

The invasion of intraocular structures by pathogenic bacteria can cause an ocular infection, which is generally manifested by pain, swelling, redness, and mucopurulent discharge. The administration of appropriate antibiotics is the definitive treatment.

Keratitis, conjunctivitis, and trachoma are the most severe types of ocular infections and may progress to permanent scarring of the eye.

Benign and malignant tumors of the eye are usually not detected until a late stage of the disease. Of all ocular tumors 85% appear in the choroid. Enucleation is often the final outcome of ocular tumors.

Ocular trauma results from the following specific injuries: abrasions, lacerations, foreign bodies in the conjunctiva or cornea, orbital fractures, burns, and contusions of the eyelid or globe. The type and extent of injury determines the amount of visual impairment.

Prompt and appropriate first aid by the nurse may prevent blindness in many cases of ocular trauma. Public education of risks and careful avoidance procedures, as well as support of safety legislation, are further nursing interventions in the prevention of ocular trauma.

Bibliography

Bloome MA, Garcia CA: *Manual of Retinal and Choroidal Dystrophies.* Norwalk, CT: Appleton-Century-Crofts, 1982.

Chawla H: *Essential Ophthalmology.* Edinburg: Churchill Livingstone, 1981.

Chignell AH: *Retinal Detachment Surgery.* New York: Springer-Verlag, 1980.

Dale RT: *Fundamentals of Ocular Motility and Strabismus.* New York: Grune & Stratton, 1982.

Folk J: Senile macular degeneration. *Primary Care* 1982; 9(4):793–799.

Kaufman H et al: The ailing eye: treat, consult, refer? *Patient Care* (April 15) 1980; 14:16–69.

Kilroy J: Care and teaching of patients with glaucoma. *Nurs Clin North Am* 1981; 16(3):393–404.

Miller D: *Ophthalmology.* Boston: Houghton Mifflin Professional Publishers, 1979.

Newell F: *Ophthalmology,* 5th ed. St. Louis: Mosby, 1982.

Pfister R: Chemical injuries of the eye. *Ophthalmology,* 1983; 90(10):1246–1252.

Saunders W et al: *Nursing Care in Eye, Ear, Nose, and Throat Disorders,* 4th ed. St. Louis: Mosby, 1979.

Shields MB: *A Study Guide for Glaucoma.* Baltimore: Williams & Wilkins, 1982.

Smith JJ, Nachazel DD: *Ophthalmic Nursing.* Boston: Little, Brown, 1980.

Theodure FM, Bloomfield SE, Mandine B: *Clinical Allergy and Immunology of the Eye.* Baltimore: Williams & Wilkins, 1983.

Tumulty G, Resker M: Eye trauma. *Am J Nurs* 84:740–745.

Vaughan D, Asbury T: *General Ophthalmology.* Los Altos, CA: Lange Medical Publications, 1980.

Warner GG (editor): *Emergency Care Assessment and Intervention,* 3rd ed. St. Louis: Mosby, 1983.

Zimmerman L, McLean I: A comparison of progress in the management of retinoblastomas and uveal melanomas. In: *Ocular Pathology Update.* Nicholson D, editor. New York: Masson, 1980; pp. 191–210.

Suggested Readings

Ciolini N, Horowitz J: What diabetics need to know about their risk of blindness. *Sightsaving* 1983; 52:2–5. This well-written and well-illustrated article on diabetic retinopathy discusses treatment and research. The journal is published by the National Society to Prevent Blindness.

International Education Committee of the American Academy of Ophthalmology. *The Athlete's Eye.* San Francisco: Academy of Ophthalmology, 1983. The 56-page booklet is written for athletes and those people responsible for their health and safety—coaches, athletic trainers, team physicians, and nurses. Includes color photographs.

Kaufman H et al: The ailing eye: Treat, consult, refer? *Patient Care* (April) 1980; 14:16–69. This article comes from a journal for primary physicians and contains useful current information on examination of the eye, conjunctivitis, iritis, acute glaucoma, corneal abrasion, chemical injury, foreign body, and more.

Kilroy J: Care and teaching of patients with glaucoma. *Nurs Clin North Am* 1981; 16(3):393–404. Up-to-date series on ophthalmologic disorders; takes a nursing perspective.

Warner GG (editor): *Emergency Care Assessment and Intervention,* 3rd ed. St. Louis: Mosby, 1983. Discusses the assessment and treatment of the most common eye injuries seen in the emergency room.

Chapter 72

Surgical Approaches to Visual System Dysfunction

Mardy Nord Meadows
Theresa M. Flaherty

Objectives

When you have finished studying this chapter, you should be able to:

Discuss the nursing implications for the client undergoing general eye surgery.

Discuss the indications for the surgical correction of vitreous opacities or loss, retinal detachments, cataracts, glaucoma, corneal opacities, and ptosis.

Describe the surgical procedure that corrects these conditions.

Explain the indications and surgical procedure for enucleation.

Anticipate physiological and psychosocial/lifestyle client implications related to vitrectomy, retinal detachment surgery, cataract extraction, intraocular lens implantation, iridectomy, sclerectomy and trabeculectomy, corneal transplant, ptosis surgery, and enucleation.

Implement the nursing care required for clients having these surgeries.

Ocular surgery usually offers the client a chance for improved vision, pain relief, and a new outlook on life. Local anesthesia is generally used, and the hospital stay can range from 1 to 7 days. During this time, the client's vision may be significantly limited, because one eye is usually patched. Furthermore, decreased vision in the other eye is common, because many visual dysfunctions (eg, cataracts, myopia, and glaucoma) affect both eyes to varying degrees. Clients therefore depend on health care professionals for their comfort and safety in the hospital environment. Many consider ocular surgery to be frightening because of the importance of vision in daily life as well as the profound fear of blindness and lifestyle changes that accompany it.

GENERAL NURSING IMPLICATIONS IN EYE SURGERY

Many nursing responsibilities and functions in caring for clients having any type of eye surgery are similar. This section briefly discusses the general nursing implications and nursing care during the preoperative, intraoperative, and postoperative phases of eye surgery. General nursing care for clients undergoing eye surgery is listed in Box 72–1. Specific implications of the various types of surgery will be discussed in the sections on specific surgeries throughout the chapter.

Preoperative Care

Upon the clients' admission to the hospital, orient them and their families or friends to their immediate surroundings, the client unit, and personnel. This is particularly important for clients having eye surgery because their vision is frequently already diminished, and one or both eyes may be patched postoperatively. Familiar surroundings may ease the client's anxieties and lessen postoperative disorientation.

The nurse should assess the client's vision, especially in the unoperated eye; because the operated eye will be patched postoperatively, the client will see only with the unoperated eye. The client with poor vision in the unoperated eye or with bilateral eye patches will require stricter

Box 72–1 Nursing Care for General Eye Surgery

Preoperative Phase

Orient the client and family or friends to immediate surroundings, the client unit, and personnel.

Assess the client's vision, ensure the client's safety, and assist with activities of daily living as needed.

Assess the client's level of knowledge and degree of anxiety about the disease state and surgery. Encourage questions and provide answers as well as emotional support.

Preoperative teaching should include:

• Activity and position *restrictions* required postoperatively: coughing; quick, sudden, jarring movements; straining with bowel movements; bending or stooping; nose blowing; lying on operated side; heavy lifting; rubbing, squinting, or tightly closing the eyes; running or jumping; and smoking.
• The time of surgery and appropriate length of the procedure.
• Frequency and effect of eyedrops.
• Dietary restrictions (explain what NPO means and when it is in effect).
• Information regarding eyepatches (types of patches, whether bilateral or unilateral).
• Preoperative sleeping medications to be used.
• Type of anesthetic to be used (local, regional, or general).
• Trimming the eyelashes.
• Effect of preoperative medications; inform client that an IV may be started prior to surgery.

Administer preoperative eye medications in a timely manner.

Instruct or assist the client in cleansing face, shampooing hair, and shaving face (males) as ordered.

Intraoperative Phase

Meet the client upon admission to the operating suite.

Provide support and reassurance to the client during the procedure.

Provide brief explanations of what is happening during the operation, if appropriate.

Enhance the client's ability to rest and relax during the operative procedure.

Carry out the usual tasks of the operating room nurse.

Accompany the client back to the unit or postanesthesia recovery room.

Postoperative Phase

Position the client as ordered (eg, head of the bed elevated 30°; lying supine or on unoperated side).

Postoperative Phase (continued)

Explain to the client the type of, and rationale for, position and activity restrictions.

Ensure the client's safety.

Reorient the client to time and place upon return to room.

Alert the client to the location of the IV, and monitor its infusion.

Check the client's vital signs every 15 to 30 minutes until stable.

Instruct the client to avoid activities that increase the venous pressure and hence increase intraocular pressure. (See the section on the preoperative phase in this box.)

Observe the client for sudden, sharp pain in the unoperated eye because this may signify an increased intraocular pressure, hemorrhage, or other complications. Notify the physician if such pain occurs.

Recognize and deal with nausea, vomiting, and restlessness early. These activities are contraindicated in eye surgery, because they raise the intraocular pressure and place stress on the suture line.

Administer analgesics, antiemetics, and mydriatic eyedrops as ordered.

Encourage the client to flex and extend the extremities to avoid thrombi.

Encourage deep breathing to expand the lungs and keep them free of secretions. Discourage coughing because it increases the intraocular pressure.

Observe aseptic technique for all procedures performed on the operated eye.

Assist the client to the bathroom the first time and thereafter as needed.

Minimize sensory deprivation. For example, encourage the client to listen to music, game shows, or the news; encourage visits from family and friends; make frequent, short visits to clients; suggest that significant others read to clients; and use touch.

Monitor coexisting medical problems, eg, diabetes.

Provide discharge instructions, including:

• Proper administration of eye medications (dosage, effect, and side effects)
• Correct placement of eyepatch or shield
• Signs and symptoms of infection
• Importance of follow-up care
• Use of dark glasses to limit photophobia

safety measures and more assistance with activities of daily living (eg, bathing, eating, and walking).

Before surgery, also assess the client's level of knowledge and degree of anxiety about the disease state and upcoming surgery. Encouraging questions and providing accurate, simple answers often reduces anxiety. Discuss the client's fears and concerns and provide emotional support.

The client should have a thorough understanding of what to expect before, during, and after the surgery. A client information sheet such as the one in Box 72–2 will help reinforce the nurse's preoperative teaching. The

Box 72−2 Client Information Sheet: Ophthalmic Surgery

Preoperative Phase

Become familiar with your surroundings because one or both eyes will be patched after surgery.

Blood and urine samples will be needed, as well as possibly an electrocardiogram (ECG) and chest x-ray.

There will be an order for you to have nothing to eat or drink after midnight the evening before your surgery. (The abbreviation for this is NPO.)

An intravenous line (IV) may be started before or during the surgery to give you fluids, avoid dehydration, and administer necessary medications.

Eyedrops will generally be given. There are many different kinds (eg, antibiotics, anti-inflammatory agents, and pupil dilators) to decrease eye movement and facilitate the surgery.

A tranquilizer will often be administered (either by pills or an injection). This will allow you to relax during the surgery.

Intraoperative Phase

A nurse will meet you upon your entrance to the operating room.

If you will be receiving local anesthesia, it will be important to hold your head still except when asked by the doctor to move.

Anesthetic eyedrops will be given to numb your eye.

Local anesthesia is often given (at the eyelids) to prevent blinking.

Eyelashes may be trimmed.

Sterile drapes will cover the rest of your face during surgery.

Postoperative Phase

You will return to your room after surgery. If you have had general anesthesia, you will go to the postanesthesia room first until you are fully awake.

One or both eyes may be patched for protection and rest, as well as to minimize movement.

If no nausea occurs, eating and drinking are usually allowed the day of surgery.

Postoperative Phase *(continued)*

You will be encouraged to move your legs gently while in bed to prevent the formation of blood clots in your legs.

Breathe deeply to expand your lungs and keep them free of secretions.

If you must cough, keep your mouth open to help decrease pressure inside the head.

Notify the nurse if you are nauseated or if you feel sharp pain or pressure in your eye.

Laxatives may be ordered to avoid straining with bowel movements.

Activity and position restrictions are important and should be followed to prevent complications. Each eye surgery and doctor may have different requirements. Examples are: (1) head of the bed elevated; (2) bed rest; (3) avoiding putting the face down; (4) no lying on operated side to prevent pressure and contamination; (5) no leaning over or stooping (increases the pressure in your eye); and (6) no shaving, hair combing, or tooth brushing.

Be sure to clarify the specific instructions and postoperative restrictions regarding your surgery with your physician and nurse.

Activities that increase blood pressure in the head also increase eye (intraocular) pressure, which is undesirable. Thus, these activities may be restricted for several days to weeks. Examples are straining during bowel movements, heavy lifting, rubbing the eyes, squinting, and tightly closing the eyes.

Eye medications may be ordered, and patches may be changed daily by your physician or nurse. Instructions for taking medications at home will be given to you by the physician, nurse, and pharmacist.

Your family or friends are encouraged to visit and participate in your care as needed or desired.

Television watching and reading may be restricted by the physician.

Avoid eye cosmetics until given permission to use them by your physician.

Your specific surgery will be discussed with you by your physician. If you have any questions, do not hesitate to ask your physician or nurse.

---

required activity and position restrictions should be included in preoperative teaching. Tell the client that he or she probably will be allowed bathroom privileges with assistance the day of surgery and will be able to take short walks and sit in a chair the first postoperative day. Emphasize the need to avoid activities that increase venous pressure and hence intraocular pressure, placing stress on the suture lines. Such activities include coughing; quick, sudden, jarring movements; straining with bowel movements; bending or stooping; nose blowing; lying on the operated side; heavy lifting; rubbing, squinting, or tightly closing the eyes; and running or jumping. The client should be

aware of the rationale for avoiding these activities. Smoking is discouraged both before and after all ocular surgery because a smoker's cough frequently increases the intraocular pressure and stresses the suture lines. In addition, smoke is an irritant to the eye.

Inform the client of the time of surgery and approximately how long the procedure will take. In addition, tell the client that pain medications, antiemetics, and stool softeners will be provided postoperatively as needed. Emphasize the importance of clients informing the nurse about how they are feeling and the potential need for medications.

Immediately prior to surgery, the nurse administers the prescribed medications (narcotics, sedatives, or tranquilizers) to prepare the client for anesthesia. If the client is to have a general anesthetic, IM atropine sulfate is used to decrease secretions. The eye is widely dilated with a mydriatic and cycloplegic eyedrop (eg, phenylephrine hydrochloride 10% [Neosynephrine] or cyclopentolate hydrochloride [Cyclogyl 1%]). In addition, a prophylactic antibiotic eyedrop is often given (eg, gentamicin). The timely administration of preoperative eye medications to ensure adequate dilation of the eye is essential.

Intraoperative Care

The nurse's role in the intraoperative phase is extremely important. Most eye surgeries are carried out under local anesthesia, an anxiety-provoking experience for many clients. Meeting the client upon admission to the operating suite, explaining what is happening to the client, and providing interested and concerned support and reassurance throughout the surgical procedure will help the client feel less isolated. Brief explanations of what is happening often prevent anxiety-producing misinterpretations on the client's part. Remind the client to hold his or her head still during the procedure. Remember, however, not to interfere with the relaxation that preoperative tranquilizers can provide the client; do not talk too much or provide long or unnecessary explanations.

Local and regional anesthesia are given for the client's comfort and to prevent blinking during surgery. A lid speculum helps enlarge the operative field, and traction muscle sutures (Figure 72–1) steady the globe. The operating microscope magnifies the small structures of the eye to 15 to 20 times and provides adequate illumination so delicate surgery can be performed more easily. Foot controls allow

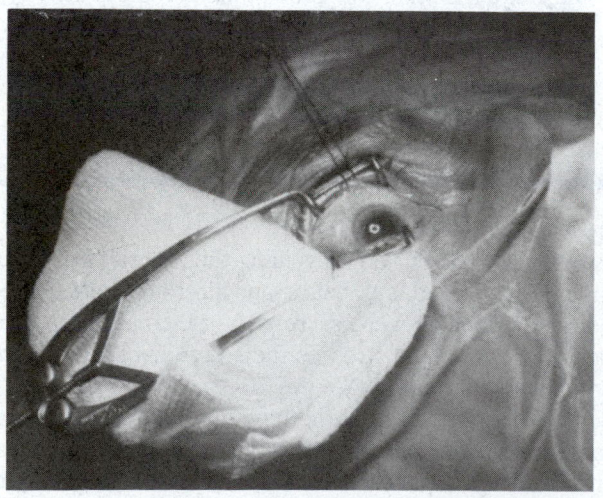

Figure 72–1

The operative ocular field. A lid speculum is in place and the traction muscle sutures steady the globe.

Nursing Research Note

Hill BJ: Sensory information, behavioral instructions and coping with sensory alteration surgery. *Nurs Res* 1982; 31(1):17–21.

An experimental design was used to examine the relation between behavioral instructions, sensory information, and general information and their effect on the coping behavior of postsurgical cataract clients. The combination of behavioral instruction and sensory information decreased the time of the client's first venture from home. Explaining typical sensations to be expected by postsurgical cataract clients improved client outcome. Presurgical behavioral instructions for cataract clients (eg, how to reduce discomfort in the operative eye and appropriate self-care skills) are beneficial and should be instituted by nurses.

the surgeon to manipulate the microscope without disrupting the sterile field.

Accompany the client back to the client unit (or the postanesthesia recovery room if the client has received a general anesthetic).

Postoperative Care

Postoperative nursing care of the client with eye surgery focuses on observing for complications, promoting client comfort, and helping the client return to normal activities of daily living. Monitor vital signs every 15 to 30 minutes until stable. Thereafter, take vital signs according to the client's medical status. Co-existing medical problems such as diabetes also should be monitored by blood sugar, urine sugar, and acetone tests and a clinical assessment of the client.

Position the client with the head of the bed elevated 30° and lying either supine or on the unoperated side unless ordered otherwise. This position helps maintain intraocular pressure and minimizes swelling. Explain position restrictions to the client, and reinforce them as necessary.

Promote safety by keeping the siderails of the bed up until the client is fully awake and oriented, until bilateral patches have been removed, or until they are no longer deemed necessary for the client's protection. Place the call light within the client's reach. Do not allow the client to smoke unsupervised.

Postoperative confusion is frequently a problem with eye clients, especially the elderly. Nurses must reorient the client to time and place and reintroduce themselves upon the clients' return to their rooms and thereafter as necessary.

Postoperative activity varies with each eye surgery, client, and surgeon. Often on the first postoperative day the client is allowed to sit in a chair and take brief walks in the hall with assistance. The nurse should supervise and assist the client with activities after checking specific orders.

Encourage the client to flex and extend the extremities to avoid thrombi, as well as to take deep breaths to expand the lungs and keep them free of secretions. Discourage coughing because it increases the intraocular pressure and places stress on the suture line. Reinforce the importance of avoiding activities that increase intraocular pressure (see the section on preoperative care).

Postoperative pain is often controlled solely by acetaminophen or aspirin, although meperidine hydrochloride (Demerol) administered every 3 to 4 hours may be required for relief of more intense pain. Observe the client for sudden, sharp, or persistent pain in the operated eye because this may be the first sign of a complication such as increased intraocular pressure or hemorrhage. Notify the physician if such pain occurs. Note the amount of lid edema and ecchymosis when administering eye medications or changing the eyepatch. Aseptic technique should always be used.

Antiemetics are given to avoid nausea and emesis, which increases the intraocular pressure. The nurse administers mydriatic and cycloplegic eyedrops two to three times a day (see Table 70–4 in Chapter 70). Prophylactic antibiotic eyedrops and corticosteroids to reduce inflammation might also be ordered. Stool softeners or laxatives help avoid constipation.

Minimize sensory deprivation for clients with impaired vision and limited activity orders. Make frequent short visits to the client, and encourage family and friends to visit. Provide diversional activities such as listening to the radio and television game shows or the news, or suggest that a visitor read to the client.

Prior to discharge, be sure the client, family, or friends can properly and safely administer eye medications. Provide information on the purpose and potential side effects of each medication. The client should understand home care instructions (eg, the correct placement of an eyepatch or shield and the use of dark glasses to limit photophobia) and the necessity of making temporary lifestyle adaptations. As with any surgery, emphasize the importance of follow-up care.

VITRECTOMY

A vitrectomy is a microsurgical procedure in which the preretinal membranes are cut and abnormal vitreous is removed via suction and replaced by a balanced salt solution. This often prevents loss of vision from retinal damage.

A vitrectomy is performed when there is sufficient loss of vitreous or damage to the vitreous to cause a retinal tear or detachment or to block the light rays from the retina. Vitreous hemorrhage and retinal detachment from proliferative diabetic retinopathy are the main indications for a vitrectomy. Other indications include vitreous loss, vitreous opacity, and traction detachments.

Trauma of the globe is caused by such items as BBs, needles, or metal; if the globe is penetrated, vitreous is lost through the wound, and there is potential for retinal detachment. Vitreous loss may also be an iatrogenic (physician-induced) complication occurring during cataract, iris, or corneal surgery.

Hemorrhage, the most likely cause of an opaque vitreous, usually results from trauma or systemic diseases (eg, diabetes or hypertension). When there is hemorrhage without a significant retinal detachment, the physician normally waits 6 months or more for signs of absorption before undertaking surgery. Inflammation of the choroid and retina can also cause opacities of the vitreous because of a secondary cellular invasion of the vitreous fluid.

The formation and invasion of preretinal and vitreous membranes create traction on the retina. This traction pulls on the retina and may cause it to detach from the pigment epithelium. Proliferative diabetic retinopathy, vasculitis, and sickle-cell disease often give rise to retinal traction detachments.

Surgical Procedure

Ultrasonography prior to surgery is often useful in identifying the presence and position of a retinal detachment that is caused by a vitreous abnormality. A local anesthetic is generally used to avoid postoperative nausea, vomiting, and delayed recovery. A general anesthetic or the availability of a general anesthetic may be necessary depending on the complexity of the case, the health of the client, and the client's ability to tolerate the procedure. The pupil should be widely dilated prior to the surgery. The eye is then prepared (lashes trimmed, cleansed, draped, etc.) as for any other surgery. A lid speculum is placed, and the globe is steadied with traction muscle sutures.

The *pars plana vitrectomy* is the most widely used procedure. This approach is made possible by the development of a special surgical instrument that cuts the vitreous, removes the diseased tissue by suction, and replaces the aspirate with a balanced salt solution. A small (3 mm) incision is first made through the conjunctiva and sclera into the vitreous cavity at the pars plana (the flat part of the ciliary body from where the ciliary muscle extends back to and becomes part of the choroid). The retina is visualized with the aid of a fiberoptic light attached to the vitrectomy instrument. The damaged vitreous is aspirated, and a balanced salt solution such as Ringer's solution is simultaneously infused to prevent collapse of the eyeball; the solution eventually is replaced by body fluids. The instrument is then withdrawn, and the incision is sutured closed. Atropine sulfate (Isopto Atropine) 1% and a combination antibiotic-corticosteroidal ointment are instilled in the eye. The eye is then patched, and the client returns to his or her room. The vitrectomy instrument is also useful for removing foreign bodies.

Implications for the Client

Physiological Implications

Approximately 82% of vitrectomy clients show improved visual acuity, and vision is markedly improved if no macular damage has occurred. Diseases such as diabetic retinopathy may cause irrevocable damage to the retina, however, and vitrectomy improves visual acuity in only 50% to 75% of these cases (Little, 1983). Often the vitrectomy client's vision is so poor preoperatively (20/200) that any improvement is gratifying.

Postoperative pain varies from individual to individual; however, it is usually minimal, and acetaminophen (Tylenol) or acetaminophen with codeine usually provides sufficient relief. Patching one or both eyes promotes rest and reduces edema, thereby assisting in pain relief.

Possible complications following a vitrectomy include lens damage, retinal holes, delayed healing of the corneal epithelium, and glaucoma. Lens damage may occur if the tip of the vitrectomy instrument touches the lens during the surgical procedure. Retinal holes may result from the surgeon's inadvertently cutting the retinal tissue, roughly touching the retina with the instrument, or exerting traction on the retina while cutting the fibrous membranes that adhere to the retina. Damage to the corneal epithelium from direct contact with the vitrectomy instrument or a nonwatertight sclerotomy may delay healing of the epithelial tissue. Glaucoma may be induced in the early postoperative phase if intraocular gas, which is sometimes injected into the vitreous to compress the retina, expands. Glaucoma may also be induced if degenerated red blood cells in the vitreous enter the anterior chamber and obstruct the outflow of aqueous humor.

Psychosocial/Lifestyle Implications

A temporary alteration in the client's normal lifestyle and daily activities will be necessary. The client should avoid any activities that increase intracranial pressure, because these also increase intraocular pressure and place undue stress on the suture lines (see Box 72–1). The client should take a 1- to 3-week leave from work—longer if heavy manual labor is required on the job or if complications arise. The client may walk around the house and watch television as tolerated. Adjusting to a quiet lifestyle may be difficult for active and independent persons. Anxiety, fear, and concern are normal reactions of any vitrectomy client, although the intensity of such emotions and the ability to cope with them vary dramatically from person to person. Implications for the client with a vitrectomy are summarized in Table 72–1.

Nursing Implications

Preoperative Care

The general considerations of nursing care cited at the beginning of the chapter and in Box 72–1 apply to the care of clients undergoing vitrectomies. Before caring for the client, be aware of the specific type of vitrectomy performed. Care of a client who has had a simple vitrectomy differs from care after retinal detachment surgery. Nursing care will be more complex if the retina was involved. (See nursing implications in the discussion of retinal detachment surgery.)

Table 72–1 Vitrectomy: Implications for the Client	
Physiological Implications	**Psychosocial/Lifestyle Implications**
Markedly improved vision if no macular damage has occurred	Temporary curtailment of strenuous activities
Minimal postoperative pain	Temporary visual impairment with eyepatch
Potential complications, including lens damage, retinal holes, delayed healing of corneal epithelium, and glaucoma	Return to work in 1–3 wk unless complications arise or manual labor is required
	Anxiety, fear, and concern

Often clients having vitrectomy surgery have such poor visual acuity (20/200) that they are considered legally blind. Therefore, safety precautions are imperative. Clients should be oriented to their surroundings and allowed to unpack their own belongings to avoid frustration; the nurse should avoid rearranging the belongings.

Postoperative Care

One or both eyes will be patched upon the client's return to the room, so reorientation to the surroundings and safety precautions are important. Generally, no specific position must be maintained unless there was retinal involvement. A semi-Fowler's position is recommended if persistent bleeding exists to allow the blood to settle below the visual axis. Most clients are allowed bathroom privileges (with assistance) the day of surgery and slow walks in the hall the first postoperative day.

The hospital stay of a vitrectomy client is from 3 to 7 days.

RETINAL DETACHMENT SURGERY

A retinal detachment involves the separation of the neural layer of the retina from the outer pigment layer. The amount of visual loss depends on the amount of retina that detaches. The aim of surgery is to reattach the retina permanently in its original anatomic position and to return the visual function to as close to normal as possible.

Surgical repair is indicated in most tear-induced retinal detachments, because spontaneous reattachment is extremely unlikely. The retinal hole must always be sealed, and if the retina has detached, scleral buckling (a surgical technique in which the wall of the eye is indented toward the detached retina) is indicated. A vitrectomy may be sufficient treatment for a traction detachment caused by fibrous membranes within the vitreous pulling on the retina when no holes are present.

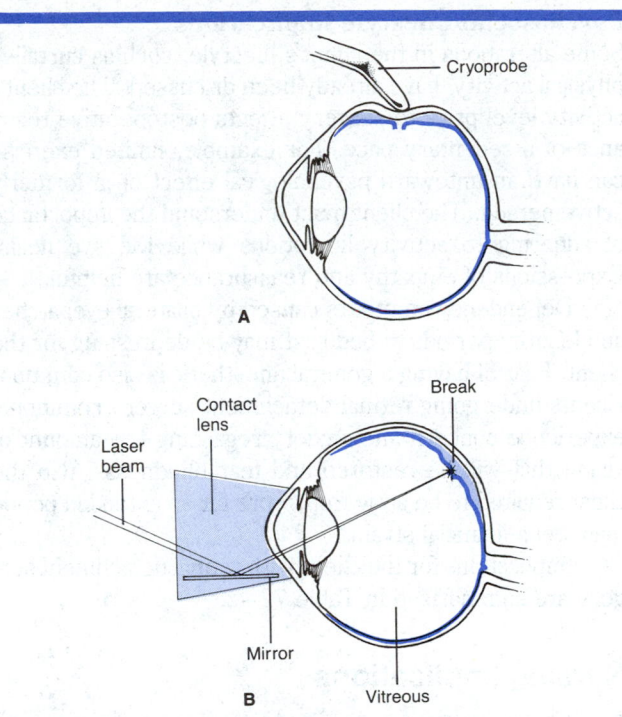

Figure 72-2

Retinal reattachment surgery. **A.** Using a cryoprobe. Scar tissue forms as the frozen area heals, reattaching the retina. **B.** Using a laser. Tiny laser burns weld the retina back together in a process called photocoagulation.

Surgical Procedure

Before the retinal detachment surgical procedure begins, it is essential to determine by ophthalmoscopy or ultrasonography the type of detachment and the location of the retinal hole. This information, in addition to the surgeon's preference, will determine the technique to be used. Mydriatics are instilled prior to surgery.

Sealing of a retinal break by the creation of a chorioretinal adhesion is accomplished by diathermy, cryotherapy, or photocoagulation. These procedures cause a chorioretinal scar to form around the lesion and hence prevent the leakage of vitreous fluid behind the retina. In diathermy, heat is applied directly to the sclera to create an adhesion. This method is being abandoned in favor of cryotherapy and photocoagulation. Cryotherapy involves the use of a supercooled ($-70°C$) metal probe (cryoprobe) applied to the sclera opposite the borders of the retinal hole for a varying period of time (Figure 72-2A). The disruption of the pigment epithelium excites an inflammatory response, which leads to scar formation and retinal reattachment within about 1 week. Photocoagulation employs a bright light (eg, an argon laser or xenon lamp) focused through the refracting media (cornea, lens, vitreous, and aqueous humor) onto the retinal hole (Figure 72-2B). The heat generated by the light induces the retina and underlying retina to coagulate together. This procedure is often

done on an outpatient basis for prophylactic treatment of predisposing peripheral degenerations of the retina. In all three procedures used to create a chorioretinal scar, local anesthetic is administered.

Scleral buckling techniques indent the sclera toward the vitreous by implanting various materials at the retinal break. Implants may be made of absorbable materials such as gelatin or nonabsorbable materials such as silicone rubber.

Absorbable implants are used in uncomplicated cases of retinal detachment to create a temporary buckle. These implants are slowly broken down and absorbed by the host tissues and replaced by a layer of granulation tissue within 3 to 6 months. Absorbable implants are soft, pliable, easy to sterilize, and may be impregnated with antibiotic solutions. These factors, coupled with the fact that absorbable implants are temporary, account for the relatively low rate of infection and erosion. An additional advantage is the swelling of absorbable implants that occurs during the first postoperative days and helps ensure a tighter closure of the retinal break. Absorbable implants cannot be used, however, if the buckle must extend more than 180°.

Nonabsorbable implants are used to create a permanent buckle and are indicated when there is a large break in the retina, multiple breaks, or signs of traction (eg, preretinal proliferation). An encircling element (a silicone rubber band that encircles the eye) is generally used in conjunction with silicone rubber implants and provides permanent relief of vitreous traction (Figure 72-3). The two major disadvantages of permanent implants are pressure necrosis and erosion of the tissue underlying the implant.

The procedures for implanting the absorbable and nonabsorbable implants are similar, and a general anesthetic is usually used. All retinal breaks are identified and sealed with a chorioretinal scar using either cryotherapy or diathermy. The conjunctiva is first excised, and the sclera is then exposed. The implant is placed at the site of the retinal hole. It may be secured on the outside of the sclera (explant) with mattress sutures (see Figure 72-3) or placed within dissected partial-thickness scleral flaps, which are sutured over the implant. If subretinal fluid is to be drained from the eye, a radial incision is made at the selected site

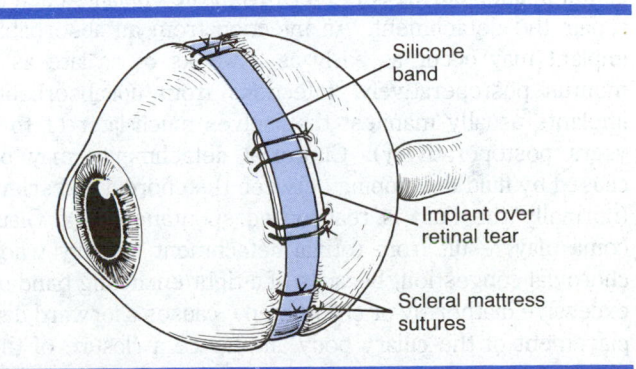

Figure 72-3

Scleral banding for retinal detachment.

to allow the retinal break to rest against the buckle. As soon as subretinal fluid has drained adequately, the buckle sutures are tightened, and the globe is indented. Air may be injected into the vitreous cavity to help reposition the retina against the choroid. The wound is then closed, and a prophylactic antibiotic injection often is given.

Implications for the Client

Physiological Implications

A cautious prognosis should be given to clients requiring retinal detachment surgery because approximately 20% of the initial surgery is unsuccessful, and reoperation still leaves about 10% of clients uncured. The return of central vision is extremely unlikely if the macula has detached. Clients who noticed floaters preoperatively may continue to complain of these postoperatively, since reattaching the retina does not remove the vitreous opacities.

Retinal detachment surgery requires more alterations in physical activity than any other eye surgery. Strict bed rest and the maintenance of specific positions are frequently required both preoperatively and for 1 to 5 days postoperatively. Complications of bed rest (eg, thrombi and atelectasis) must be prevented. Bilateral eyepatches, if ordered, make the client dependent on others for assistance with activities of daily living.

The amount of discomfort in and around the eye varies following surgery. Some lid edema and chemosis are normally present. Chemosis occurs because of the trauma caused by conjunctival incision and the subsequent healing process.

The client is usually discharged from the hospital 3 to 7 days after surgery. An additional 2 weeks of recovery at home is required before sedentary work and activities can be resumed. The client should avoid strenuous activity for about 2 months (Chignell, 1980).

Because general anesthesia is usually used for retina surgery, the client is susceptible to complications such as nausea, vomiting, emboli, pneumonia, and urinary retention. Potential complications related to the surgery itself include infection, choroidal detachment, glaucoma, and vitreous hemorrhage. An infection may develop because of contamination during surgery or from the implants used to repair the detachment. An infection from an absorbable implant may occur as early as 2 weeks or as late as 6 months postoperatively. Infections from nonabsorbable implants usually manifest themselves much later (1 to 8 years postoperatively). Choroidal detachments may be caused by fluid developing between the choroid and sclera (normally the fluid is reabsorbed spontaneously). Glaucoma may result from retinal detachment surgery when choroidal congestion, because of a tight encircling band or excessive diathermy or cryotherapy, causes a forward displacement of the ciliary body and hence a closure of the filtration angle. A vitreous hemorrhage following retinal detachment surgery is usually induced by the trauma of surgery.

Psychosocial/Lifestyle Implications

Some alterations in the client's lifestyle, such as curtailed physical activity, have already been discussed. The client's activity level prior to surgery affects postoperative tolerance of a sedentary pace. For example, limited exercise can have an untoward psychological effect on a formerly active person. The client must understand the importance of adhering to activity limitations while the eye heals. Expressions of empathy and reassurance are helpful.

Dependency on others caused by bilateral eyepatches and lengthy periods of bed rest may be depressing for the client. Fear of having a general anesthetic is also common. Clients undergoing retinal detachment surgery commonly experience concern and anxiety regarding the amount of vision that will be restored and fear blindness. Also the client required to be away from work for an extended period may feel a financial strain.

Implications for the client with retinal detachment surgery are summarized in Table 72–2.

Nursing Implications

Preoperative Care

Clients with a retinal detachment have usually had a sudden loss of sight. They are generally admitted to the hospital soon after the diagnosis has been made and often do not have time to prepare for surgery emotionally or physically.

Table 72–2 Retinal Detachment Surgery: Implications for the Client

Physiological Implications	Psychosocial/Lifestyle Implications
Approximately 80% initial success for surgery; floaters may remain	Need for emotional support
Decreased physical activity	Increased dependency on others while eyes are patched and activity is limited
Potential complications from prolonged bed rest (eg, thrombi and atelectasis)	Concern and anxiety regarding amount of vision restored after surgery
Bilateral eyepatches	Fear of blindness (potential body image changes)
Lid edema and chemosis	Potential sensory deprivation
Possible complications of general anesthesia	Possible adjustment to living with decreased vision
Postoperative complications, including infection, choroidal detachment, glaucoma, and vitreous hemorrhage	Discouragement from potential for recurrence
	Financial strain if out of work for long period

Recognize the intensity of their fear and apprehension. Explanations of the surgical procedure, reassurance, truthful answers to questions, and the provision of realistic hope are nursing interventions that can significantly reduce the client's anxiety.

Upon admission to the hospital, the client is frequently limited to bed rest with bathroom privileges, and bilateral patches are often applied. Bed rest reduces eye movements, decreases the chance of the client's falling and causing further injury to the retina, allows a vitreous hemorrhage to clear, improves the position of the retina, and prevents macular detachment. The client is positioned so that the area of detachment is in the dependent position. Activity and position restrictions vary by surgeon and client. Therefore, the nurse must be familiar with the client's specific orders. Frequent reminders and explanations regarding which positions and activities are permitted encourage client cooperation. Evaluate whether the client needs a sedative to promote relaxation and comfort. For the client confined to bed, safety precautions, attempts to lessen sensory deprivation, and avoidance of potential complications are similar to those described at the beginning of the chapter.

Postoperative Care

Many of the preoperative nursing measures are continued postoperatively. Specific position restrictions depend on the location and extent of the retinal detachment and on whether air was injected into the vitreous to help reposition the retina. If air was injected, position the client so the area of the retina that needs to be repositioned against the choroid is uppermost (Figure 72–4). Gravity then will cause the air bubble to rise and press against the retina. The surgeon should specify the position of the body (prone, supine, or on one side), the position of the head, and the elevation of the head of the bed.

Most clients are allowed bathroom privileges the day of surgery. Short walks in the hall and sitting in a chair for meals is generally permitted the day following surgery, depending on the severity of the case. The client on any degree of bed rest must resume leg exercises and deep breathing postoperatively. Expressions of empathy and reassurance are helpful for the client attempting to limit activity.

Bilateral patches are usually not indicated if the retina is flat at the end of the operation. The nurse should frequently check the dressing of the operated eye for drainage or bleeding but change it only if ordered to do so.

Discharge teaching is similar to that for any eye surgery (see Box 72–1). Emphasize that excessive eyestrain, constipation, straining, lifting heavy objects, contact sports, and stooping should be avoided for at least 6 to 8 weeks postoperatively. Nurses should address psychosocial implications such as fear of reinjury, fear that the repair will not work, or fear of potential blindness prior to discharge. Clients need and appreciate reassurance that these emo-

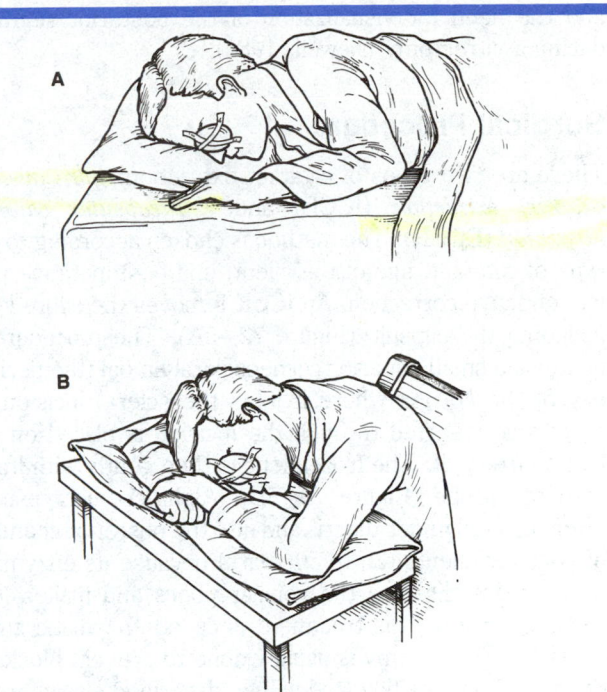

Figure 72–4

Postoperative positioning of client after air injection. Head should be positioned so that air rises and presses retina against choroid. **A.** Position in bed. **B.** Position in chair with tray stand.

tions are common in people having undergone retinal detachment repair.

CATARACT EXTRACTION

As described in Chapter 71, most cataracts (95%) are acquired late in life. Other types may be caused by toxicity (steroids), trauma (contusions), diabetes, and hypocalcemia. The opacities may occur in the lens nucleus, lens cortex, and posterior subcapsule after an ECCE extraction (described below).

Cataract extraction removes the opaque lens, providing clear vision again (with corrective lenses). The procedure can be done with minimal risk in 60 minutes. Cataract extraction is warranted when visual acuity is sufficiently decreased to interfere with the client's occupation, recreational activities, or lifestyle. Age is a consideration; a younger person may have higher demands for eyesight than a sedentary octogenarian.

Extraction is possible for cataracts of any degree of maturity. In the rare hypermature state, the lens may become swollen, burst within the eye, and release lens proteins into the anterior chamber, inducing anterior uveitis or blocking the trabecular meshwork and causing a secondary glaucoma. Other indications for cataract extraction include vision in the better eye of less than 20/50, the need to permit photocoagulation for retinal or choroidal disorders, and the need for visualization of the posterior segment during a vitrectomy (Newell, 1982).

Surgical Procedure

There are two types of cataract extraction: *intracapsular cataract extraction* (ICCE) and *extracapsular cataract extraction* (ECCE). The method is chosen according to the type of cataract, age of the client, and postoperative plan for refractive correction. An ICCE removes the entire lens, including the capsule (Figure 72–5A). The procedure is done via a small superior corneoscleral limbal (the periphery of the cornea where it joins the sclera) incision. A cryoprobe inserted through the incision is placed on the lens to freeze it. The frozen lens is then gently withdrawn with the probe (Figure 72–5B). Alpha-chymotrypsin is often injected under the iris and into the posterior chamber of younger clients (20 to 50 years) because its enzymatic action helps dissolve the zonular fibers and makes lens removal easier. This treatment is called enzymatic zonulolysis. An iridectomy is usually done to prevent blockage of aqueous humor flow and will be described elsewhere in this chapter. The cataract incision is then closed with fine 10-0 nylon suture.

An ECCE removes the anterior capsule, lens nucleus, and lens cortex while retaining the posterior capsule (Figure 72–5C). The same superior corneoscleral limbal incision is made as for the ICCE. First, the lens nucleus is removed; the lens cortex is then removed by irrigation and suction. This type of cataract extraction is common with *intraocular lens* (IOL) *implantation*, because the remaining posterior capsule can provide support for the lens. (Intraocular lens implantation will be described later in this section.) ECCE with IOL is often done on a same-day surgery basis.

A soft cataract involves the lens cortex and is often extracted via phacoemulsification. An ultrasonic needle inserted through a small incision fragments the lens, and the emulsified particles are then aspirated. This procedure is usually reserved for clients under age 50 with no nuclear sclerosis (hardness).

Local anesthesia may be used in any cataract surgery, according to client and physician preference. Local anesthesia blocks the facial nerve, retrobulbar region, and extraocular muscles. A lid speculum provides exposure, and the surgeon usually uses a foot-controlled microscope to improve visualization.

If both eyes have cataracts, surgery is performed on the more opaque cataract first. Surgery on the other eye may be performed approximately 1 month later, assuming the first procedure had no complications.

Implications for the Client

Physiological Implications

The most outstanding feature of a cataract extraction is restored vision with seemingly little discomfort or inconvenience. However, because the client has a refractive error and lacks accommodative power in the aphakic eye, a corrective lens is necessary for adequate visual acuity. Determining whether a client should wear cataract glasses or contact lenses or have IOL placement involves many

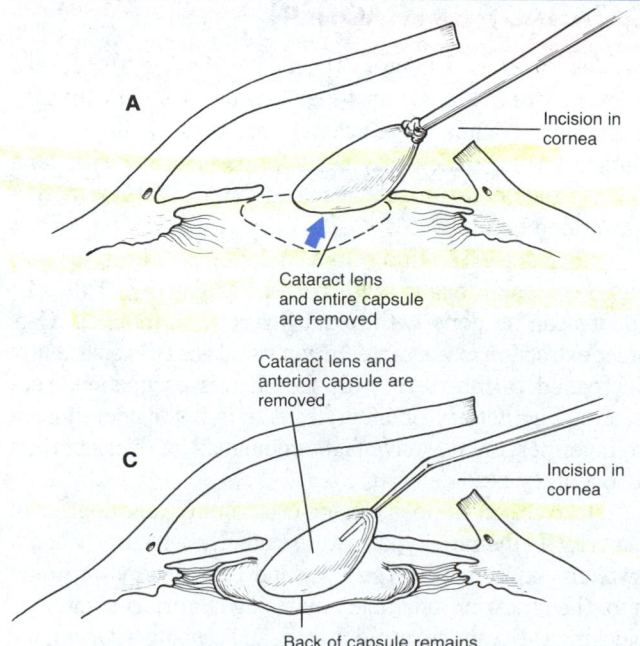

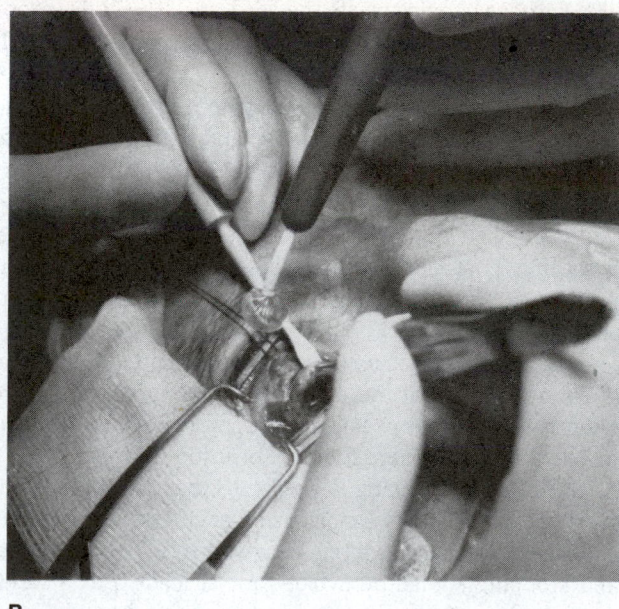

Figure 72–5

Types of cataract extraction. **A.** ICCE. **B.** The cryoprobe is removing the frozen lens in an ICCE. **C.** ECCE.

variables, which will be discussed in the section on psychosocial and lifestyle considerations.

Intraocular lenses are made of poly-methyl methacrylate (a type of plastic) and come in dozens of sizes and shapes. Three types of IOLs are: (1) an anterior chamber lens fixed on the angle of the anterior chamber (Figure 72–6A), (2) a lens fixed to the iris (Figure 72–6B), and (3) a posterior chamber lens held in position either in the capsule of the lens or sutured to the iris (Figure 72–6C). When the type of cataract extraction (ICCE or ECCE) has been determined preoperatively, the appropriate IOL is selected. The power of the IOL is determined according to the client's visual needs. Other lens adjustments consider the eyeball's axial length (measured with A-scan ultrasonography) and the corneal curvature (measured with a keratometer).

Indications and contraindications for IOLs remain controversial because of the possibly serious complications. McCoy (1981) states that IOL implants are contraindicated in clients with only one eye that has potentially good vision; clients with severe myopia; clients whose other eye has had a previous poor operative result; and clients with corneal endothelial dystrophy, glaucoma, or retinal detachment in either eye. The complications associated with any cataract surgery include increased intraocular pressure (from wound leakage) that could cause the anterior chamber to become flatter and shallower; vitreous loss through the wound with accompanying vitreous hemorrhage or retinal holes leading to detachment; and, the most serious, an intraocular infection. The complications of IOL implants can include any of these as well as (1) low-grade immediate postoperative uveitis and inflammation; (2) endo-ophthalmitis caused by fungi; (3) corneal dystrophy from inadvertent continued contact between the cornea and any part of the implant or iris suture; (4) subluxation (dislocation), which is usually caused by a problem with the iris clip of the IOL; and (5) a flat anterior chamber, which is usually caused by a wound leak with or without choroidal detachment (Meltzer & Drews, 1983). The pros and cons of an IOL implant should be discussed with the client, and the current ocular status should be assessed carefully.

After cataract surgery, the eye refraction takes about 3 months to stabilize, and the client will have several ophthalmic examinations in the interim. The client who experiences a shower of floating spots or a progressive dark shadow that may indicate a hemorrhage or retinal detachment should call the ophthalmologist.

Thirty percent of posterior capsules (the structure remaining after ECCE) will ultimately opacify as a result of persistent lens fibers adhering to the capsule or metaplasia of the remaining fibers (Clayman, Jaffe, & Galin, 1983). Repeat surgery or Yag laser treatment can become necessary, so the client should see an ophthalmologist 1 year after surgery and every few years thereafter.

Generally, cataract extraction is relatively safe. A study in 1980 by Krieglstein, Duzanec, and Leydhecker (1980) showed that 81.4% of more than 3500 clients had vision

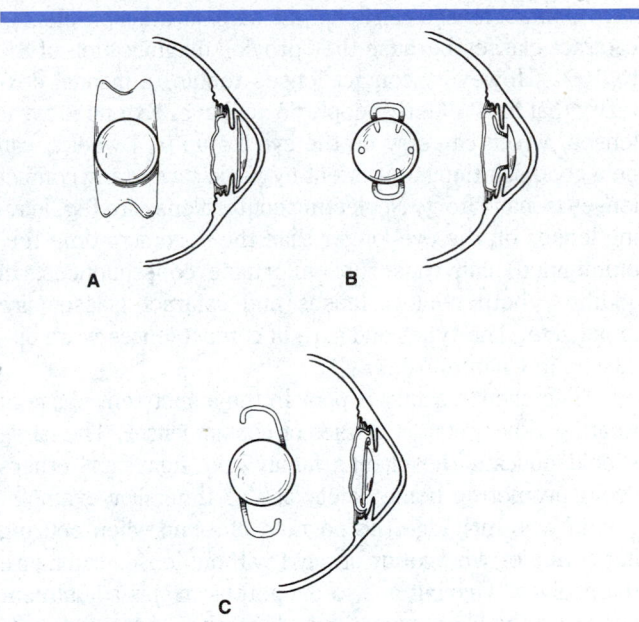

Figure 72–6

Types of intraocular lens implants (IOLs). **A.** Anterior chamber lens. **B.** Iris supported lens. **C.** Posterior chamber lens.

better than or equal to 20/40 after ICCE. Another impressive study showed that 90.5% of 200 clients had better than or equal to 20/40 vision after ECCE with IOL implant (Jaffe, 1979).

Psychosocial/Lifestyle Implications

Clients having same-day surgery avoid hospitalization and return to familiar surroundings shortly after surgery. The postoperative care of the client is assumed by the client and family. Follow-up visits with the eye surgeon are important.

Clients must recognize the lifelong need for corrective lenses after cataract extraction to avoid distorted vision. They can choose among cataract glasses, contact lenses, or IOLs, depending on many factors. Cataract glasses cannot focus both eyes of clients with monocular aphakia. These clients may be fitted with glasses that focus either the operated or unoperated eye (depending on which sees better), but they cannot be fitted to use both eyes together. Only when these clients are fitted with a contact lens—where the correcting lens is closer to the principal planes of the original lens—can they focus objects bilaterally. Cataract glasses magnify objects 25%, which predisposes clients to personal injury during the adjustment process. These glasses also limit side vision, because the aphakic lens allows best acuity only at the central portion. Cataract glasses have the additional disadvantages of being heavy and unattractive. Plastic lenses are lighter than glass lenses, but the magnification problem remains. Also, plastic lenses scratch easily and must be guarded carefully in harsh environments. However, they may be the only alternative for clients who lack the manual dexterity or the ability to provide the special care required by contact lenses.

Contact lenses can solve the magnification problem of cataract glasses because they provide magnification of 8% to 10%. However, contact lenses require a manual dexterity that most elderly people do not have. Extended-wear lenses, which can stay on the eye for up to 4 weeks, can be a good solution. Consistent hygienic care of any contact lenses is mandatory. Neglecting contact lens care (eg, leaving lenses on the eye longer than the maximum time recommended) can cause uncomfortable consequences. In addition, both contact lenses and cataract glasses are expensive. The types and care of contact lenses were discussed in Chapter 70.

The client's acuity is poor in the adjustment phase of wearing either cataract glasses or contact lenses. The nurse should educate the client's family and significant others about promoting home safety at this time. For example, clients who misjudge the position of a cup when pouring hot coffee or who get up at night without lenses can injure themselves. Driving is also dangerous in this adjustment phase, so the client must depend on others for assistance.

Intraocular lenses, when devoid of complications, can release the client from many disadvantages of both cataract glasses and contact lenses. They eliminate the need for removable lenses (except for reading glasses) and provide minimal magnification (0% to 2%).

Fear accompanies any medical or surgical treatment, particularly one that involves vision. Clients may not be informed or may be misinformed about cataract extraction, as well as about their cataract's etiology and surgical outcome. The nurse can relieve their anxiety through education. Table 72–3 summarizes client implications for cataract extraction.

Nursing Implications

Preoperative Care
Educating the client about cataract extraction and its typically successful outcome is only one part of the preoperative care provided by the nurse. As the client enters the hospital, the nurse begins teaching the client and family about what will happen over the next few days. Clarification about what a cataract is and how it will be removed must not be ignored. Same-day surgery clients need additional preoperative instruction. Teach them and their families about the postoperative care the client will require in the home.

Because of the nature of the disease, the client will have no depth perception. Clients with bilateral cataracts often are almost sightless. Thus, the nurse should orient the client to the hospital room and organize possessions within reach of the client's better eye.

Postoperative Care
Postoperatively, the client depends on the nursing staff for assistance in eating, bathing, and ambulating. Bed rest with bathroom privileges is usually allowed the day of surgery, but other activity should be discouraged. Instruct

Table 72–3	Cataract Extraction: Implications for the Client
Physiological Implications	**Psychosocial/Lifestyle Implications**
Restored vision, but aphakic eye	Lifelong need for corrective lenses for refractive error
Choice among cataract glasses, contact lenses, or intraocular lenses (IOLs)	Disadvantages of cataract glasses: weight and physical inconvenience, need for an adjustment process to tolerate a 25% magnification, inability to focus both eyes with monocular aphakia, limited side vision, expensive
Possible complications of IOLs, including corneal endothelium damage, vitreous loss, intraocular infection, postoperative inflammation, and retinal detachment	Contact lenses are a solution to magnification problem; however, conventional contact lenses require manual dexterity, can be expensive, and require scrupulous hygienic care
Three months needed for eye refraction stabilization	
Possible hemorrhage, retinal detachment, or posterior capsule opacification	Need for safety precautions in adjustment phase
Good success rate	Possibility of IOL to relieve client from removable lenses and magnification problems
	Need for education to relieve fear and anxiety

the client to lie on the unoperated side or back. An eyepatch and metal shield will prevent trauma. The head of the bed is usually maintained at 30° to control intraocular pressure and minimize swelling. Clients who find themselves in an unfamiliar environment with monocular vision will appreciate reassurance from the nurse. Pain is nominal, and acetaminophen is usually sufficient to provide relief. Sharp, severe pain is unusual and could indicate a complication, so the doctor should be notified if it occurs.

Reading may begin 24 hours (and light activity 24 to 72 hours) after cataract surgery and should be slowly increased as tolerated. Heavy work is usually not permitted for 4 to 6 weeks. Older people may have heard from friends who had cataract surgery many years ago before new techniques were developed that postoperative activity of any kind is contraindicated. Thus, reassurance and clarification of instructions are necessary before the client is discharged. The client ready for discharge may be required to take eye medication such as atropine sulfate (Isopto Atropine) to prevent posterior synechiae. The client and family or friends need instruction on the correct instillation of eyedrops, as well as on the application of eyepatches and shields. See Box 72–1 for further nursing interventions.

IRIDECTOMY AND IRIDOTOMY

An iridectomy is a simple, effective surgical procedure in which a small portion of the iris is removed. The procedure relieves the blockage of the trabecular meshwork by the periphery of the iris by creating a new channel between the chambers and allowing the iris to fall away from the trabecular meshwork (Figure 72–7). Drainage of aqueous humor via normal pathways is thus reestablished.

An iridectomy is always indicated in an acute attack of angle-closure glaucoma; it is the only hope of permanent cure. Early surgery can maintain stabilization of visual functions and give better long-term results. Prophylactic surgery on the second eye is generally recommended, since a high percentage of second eyes will develop angle-closure glaucoma despite miotic therapy. Surgery on a normal eye (with normal intraocular pressure and without angle-closure glaucoma) before permanent synechiae (adhesions of the iris to the lens and cornea) have formed creates fewer complications and less operative risk than surgery performed during an attack of intraocular hypertension.

Surgical Procedure

Prior to surgical intervention of angle-closure glaucoma, an effort is made to decrease the intraocular pressure with medications. When tensions as near normal as possible have been obtained, an iridectomy is undertaken. Local infiltration (retrobulbar) anesthetics, which paralyze the intraocular and extraocular muscles, along with topical anesthetics, are generally used.

The surgeon makes a small rectangular or triangular flap in the conjunctiva. The anterior chamber is then entered with a 4- to 5-mm incision at the middle of the corneoscleral limbus, preferably in the 11:30 or 1:30 position. Iris prolapse normally occurs spontaneously if the incision is correctly placed. The surgeon grasps the iris with forceps and excises a small peripheral portion. A gentle stroke over

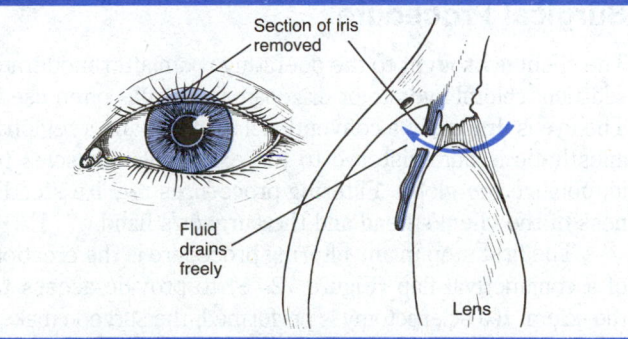

Figure 72–7

Iridectomy and iridotomy.

the cornea will generally reposition the iris. A preplaced suture closes the limbal wound, and a running suture closes the conjunctival wound. Short-acting mydriatic and topical steroids to control inflammation are begun the first postoperative day to counteract the formation of synechiae and are continued until all signs of iritis have ceased.

Laser iridotomies (see Figure 72-7) are increasingly frequent as experience with the procedure grows. They are performed on an outpatient basis using only a drop of topical anesthesia. The laser iridotomy is normally made in the upper quadrant of the middle to peripheral iris. An argon laser is reported to give the best results (Shields, 1982). Low levels of energy are used initially, with the power increasing slowly as necessary. The required number of laser applications for a successful iridotomy varies from individual to individual; the average falls between 60 and 90 applications in a single sitting. Penetration of the iris is manifested by a cloud of pigment entering the anterior chamber from the laser treatment site. Corneal endothelial and epithelial burns at the therapy site are common complications of laser iridotomies. Corneal clouding may result from these burns, but it normally clears within a few days. Retinal burns are another potential complication of laser iridotomies.

Implications for the Client

Physiological Implications

The client is essentially cured of glaucoma and its intense pain after iridectomy if the glaucoma was due solely to a closed angle. No further treatment will be necessary after the eye becomes quiet (lacks inflammation) because angle-closure glaucoma does not involve the trabecular meshwork or Schlemm's canal but only the closure of the outflow angle. Once the angle is reopened (or an iridectomy performed), the other outflow channels will function normally. If trabecular insufficiency because of structural defects and complete or partial blockage of the trabeculum are present, as is sometimes the case with chronic primary angle-closure glaucoma, medical therapy should be resumed.

Although iridectomies are simple procedures, rare complications may occur. Hemorrhage into the anterior chamber is one complication. The blood usually is reabsorbed without intervention, but surgical irrigation may be necessary. Damage to the lens may cause a cataract, requiring possible extraction. Persistent hypertension of the eye warrants medical treatment; sometimes a filtering procedure (eg, trabeculectomy or sclerectomy, which will be discussed in the next section) is required if extensive synechiae have formed. A flat or shallow anterior chamber is associated with a wound leak, and prompt intervention is essential to avoid corneal or lens damage.

Psychosocial/Lifestyle Implications

Essentially no lifestyle changes are required after a successful iridectomy. The client is generally allowed to resume activities of daily living the day after surgery. A single eyepatch may be worn, but this is generally not necessary. No adverse effects follow an iridectomy, because the lid normally covers the superior portion of the cornea where the incision was made. The client is symptom-free, is generally not required to undergo further treatment, experiences no visual changes, and is considered cured of glaucoma.

Implications for the client with an iridectomy or iridotomy are summarized in Table 72–4.

Nursing Implications

General nursing measures for clients undergoing eye surgery are summarized in Box 72–1. The interventions must be modified and adjusted for each individual, because everyone has different needs.

Preoperative Care

Clients with angle-closure glaucoma are usually admitted to the hospital during an acute attack of increased intraocular pressure. They generally suffer excruciating pain in and around the eye and may also be experiencing nausea, vomiting, and blurred vision. Relief of these symptoms is one of the nurse's first responsibilities. Analgesics such as morphine or meperidine hydrochloride (Demerol) are usually administered. Miotics are instilled every 5 to 15 minutes until the pupil constricts. The nurse also might be required to start an IV line for the administration of osmotic agents. Routine hospital admission procedures such as orienting the client to surroundings, obtaining a history, preoperative teaching, and laboratory work, are further nursing responsibilities.

Often the client can focus only on pain relief. Every effort to relieve anxiety and apprehension benefits both the client and health care team. Explaining procedures, answering questions, encouraging verbalization of feelings, and providing support are beneficial. These are important intraoperatively as well, because the client is awake.

Postoperative Care

Orient the postoperative client to time and place upon return to the room. Encourage rest the first day to allow the wound to seal; however, the client may get up to go to the bathroom with assistance. Most clients resume a regular diet the first day.

Other important nursing interventions include the administration of prescribed medications and assessing the client for complications. Severe pain is uncommon and warrants an examination by the physician.

The client is generally discharged the day after surgery. The nurse's discharge teaching should include information on prescribed medications (steroids and mydriatics), signs and symptoms of potential complications (persistent or intense pain, decreased or blurred vision, hyphema) and eye care. It should also emphasize the importance of follow-up care and routine eye examinations.

FILTERING PROCEDURES FOR GLAUCOMA: TRABECULECTOMY AND SCLERECTOMY

Filtering procedures, such as trabeculectomy and sclerectomy, are used in the treatment of open-angle glaucoma when medical management is insufficient. There are many types of filtering procedures; however, they all create a drainage channel from the anterior chamber through the sclera, allowing the aqueous humor to flow into the subconjunctival spaces, where it can be absorbed. Filtering procedures vary primarily according to the method used to create the drainage fistula. Many aspects of the operative procedure and the postoperative care, however, are basically the same. The goals of surgery are to control the intraocular pressure and prevent optic nerve atrophy.

Filtering procedures are indicated in the presence of progressive visual field loss and optic disk changes in association with a persistent elevated intraocular pressure despite maximal medical therapy. High intraocular pressure alone is seldom an indication for surgery.

Surgical Procedure

The client is brought to the operating room after moderate sedation; chloral hydrate or diazepam (Valium) is often used. The eye is draped in a conventional manner, and a regional anesthetic is administered to the extraocular muscles to immobilize the globe. Filtering procedures require steadiness of the client's head and the surgeon's hand.

The first step in any filtering procedure is the creation of a conjunctival flap (Figure 72–8) to provide access to the sclera. If a sclerectomy is performed, the surgeon makes a scleral incision into the anterior chamber behind the insertion of the conjunctival flap. A small hole is then cut or punched through the full thickness of the limbal tissue,

Table 72–4	Iridectomy and Iridotomy: Implications for the Client	
Physiological Implications	**Psychosocial/Lifestyle Implications**
Relief of pain	Minimal lifestyle changes
Cure of glaucoma if increased intraocular pressure was due solely to closed angle	Ability to resume activities of daily living the day after surgery
Rare postoperative complications, including hemorrhage, cataracts, persistent hypertension of the eye, and a flat or shallow anterior chamber	No adverse cosmetic effects
	No visual changes; freedom from glaucoma

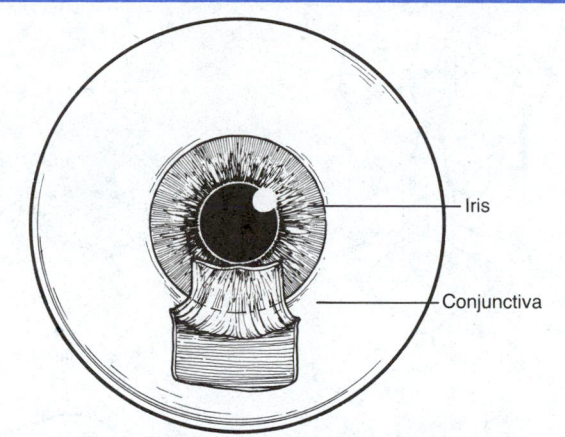

Figure 72–8

Conjunctival flap in trabeculectomy and sclerectomy.

creating a direct opening (fistula) into the anterior chamber, allowing aqueous humor to drain freely.

A trabeculectomy involves a partial-thickness scleral flap, under which lies the fistula to the anterior chamber. This surgical procedure removes a section of the blocked trabecular meshwork. A laser beam technique (trabeculoplasty) achieves the same effect. A peripheral iridectomy usually is then performed in all filtering procedures, and the conjunctiva is sutured to obtain a watertight seal.

As with other glaucoma surgeries, cycloplegics and steroids are prescribed after filtering procedures until all signs of iritis abate. Prolonged iritis following filtering procedures may cause the fistula to scar closed.

Implications for the Client

Physiological Implications
There are relatively few physiological implications for the client having a trabeculectomy or sclerectomy. Control of intraocular pressure should be maintained with the client's own medications upon admission to the hospital. Postoperative pain or discomfort in the operated eye is ordinarily controlled with acetaminophen. Severe or sudden pain often indicates a complication, such as hemorrhage or infection. Clients seldom experience nausea since local anesthetics are generally used.

An eyepatch to maintain cleanliness is often in place for the first day or two after surgery. A metal eyeshield to protect the eye during sleep is recommended for several weeks postoperatively.

Complications of filtering procedures are similar to those of iridectomies and include hyphema from surgical trauma; lens damage from surgical manipulation of the lens or postoperative iritis; and a flat or shallow anterior chamber often associated with hypotonia (reduced tension), detachment, or excessive filtration. In addition, the incidence of choroidal detachment and corneal edema increases, because the eye is opened for the procedure.

Psychosocial/Lifestyle Implications
The success or failure of filtering procedures may determine whether the client will lead a normal life or be required to live with decreased vision or blindness. Thus, the client may experience anxiety. Medical treatment (frequent eyedrops and examinations) is often required postoperatively.

Activity orders following surgery are liberal. Rest is encouraged the day of surgery; thereafter, barring complications, the client may resume normal activities. Other than stopping smoking for 1 week preoperatively and postoperatively, no other lifestyle changes or alterations in personal habits are required.

Table 72–5 lists client implications associated with filtering procedures for glaucoma.

Nursing Implications

Preoperative Care
A client having a filtering procedure for the treatment of glaucoma is usually admitted to the hospital the evening before surgery. The nurse should carry out routine admission procedures according to the institution's and surgeon's protocols. Take time to discuss the client's fears and misgivings and to clear up misconceptions. This often helps relieve the client's and family's anxiety, as well as fosters their cooperation and confidence.

Postoperative Care
Postoperative nursing care of the client having a filtering procedure is similar to care after other eye surgeries (see

Table 72–5	Filtering Procedures for Glaucoma: Implications for the Client	
Physiological Implications	**Psychosocial/Lifestyle Implications**
Postoperative pain and discomfort minimal	Anxiety
Prevention of optic nerve atrophy	Need to conform and adapt to continued medical regimen and follow-up care
Need to control intraocular pressure with medications	
Need for eyepatch and eyeshield at first for cleanliness and protection	Normal activities after 1 day of rest
Postoperative complications, including hyphema, lens damage, flat or shallow anterior chamber, choroidal detachment, and corneal edema	Need to stop smoking for 1 wk preoperatively and postoperatively

Box 72–1). Discharge teaching is consistent with that discussed in the section on iridectomy.

CORNEAL TRANSPLANT

Opacities of the cornea significantly affect visual acuity. A corneal transplant or keratoplasty can restore normal vision by transplanting a donor cornea in place of the excised diseased cornea. This procedure is indicated when inflammation or trauma to the cornea induces the formation of abnormal collagen material (scar tissue) in an otherwise transparent avascular structure. Other conditions that may be helped by keratoplasty include healed lacerations with scarring, chemical burns, corneal degeneration and subsequent corneal thinning, dystrophies, and recurrent infections.

Surgical Procedure

There are two basic types of keratoplasties: lamellar (non-penetrating) and penetrating. In *lamellar keratoplasty,* only the superficial (epithelial and subepithelial) layers are transplanted on the excised superficial opacity. The opacity must be limited to the anterior corneal layers. Lamellar keratoplasty was the first successful corneal transplantation technique from one human to another. Although the number of clear grafts is greater with lamellar keratoplasty than with penetrating keratoplasty, the visual results seldom reach better than 20/40, even in the most favorable cases (Girard, 1981).

Penetrating keratoplasty is indicated for opacification of the deeper layers of the cornea (beneath the two anterior layers). All five corneal layers are replaced, and a cataract extraction may be performed at the same time. Keratoconus is a common reason for performing a penetrating keratoplasty. In this progressive condition, the central cornea develops a noninflammatory conical protrusion that becomes progressively more pronounced, disturbing the eye's focusing system. Other indications for penetrating keratoplasty include other corneal dystrophies and degeneration, trauma, tumors, corneal disease, and bullous keratopathy resulting from previous ocular surgery.

In keratoplasty, either the entire diameter of the cornea or a partial (central or peripheral) section can be replaced. The procedure may combine a penetrating and lamellar keratoplasty.

Prior to surgery, the client is given a miotic such as pilocarpine hydrochloride to flatten and elongate the iris; this extends the iris over the lens and prevents trauma to it. A hyperosmotic agent (eg, intravenous mannitol) may be given preoperatively to decrease intraocular pressure and soften the globe. Keratoplasty is usually performed under a local anesthetic. Using a trephine (cookie-cutter-like instrument), the surgeon cuts the clear cornea from the donor (Figure 72–9A). The opaque cornea is cut from the recipient, and the donor cornea is sutured into place with extremely fine (9-0) silk or 10-0 nylon suture (Figure

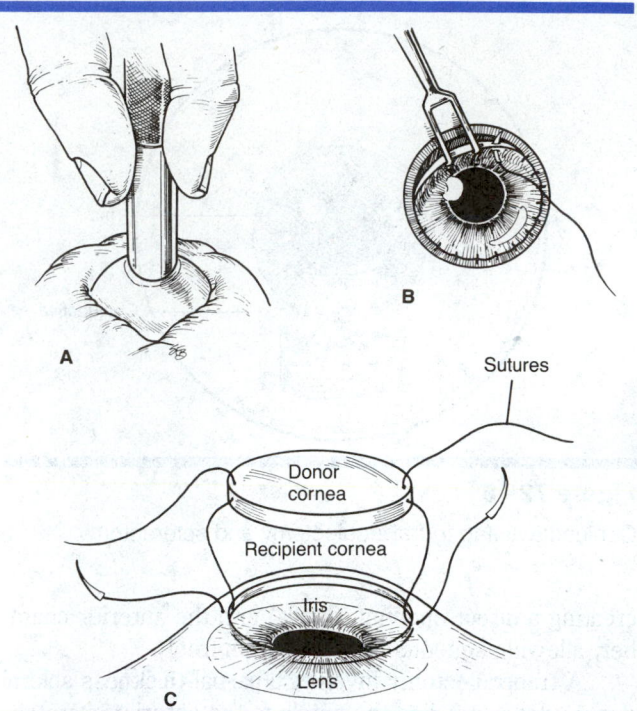

Figure 72–9

Keratoplasty. **A.** Trephination of donor cornea. **B, C.** Suturing donor cornea.

72–9B and 9C). The anterior chamber, if entered, is reformed with a balanced saline solution.

The donor tissue comes from a noninfected human cadaver and should be used ideally within 24 hours if a penetrating keratoplasty is to be done, because of the rapid endothelial death rate. For a lamellar keratoplasty, the cornea can be frozen, dehydrated, or refrigerated for up to 6 months before transplantation. The enucleated eye should come from a donor who died of an acute disease or injury. Some causes of death, such as leukemia, sepsis, central nervous system degenerative diseases, and previous eye disease, render a donor cornea unsuitable for transplantation. After death, the donor's lids should be closed and saline-moistened gauze placed on top. A young donor (25 to 35 years old) is preferable because of the large number of endothelial cells, which optimize transplant success (Box 72–3). People wanting to donate their eyes for keratoplasty should contact an eye bank that is a member of the Eye Bank Association of America or their state's agency for the blind (see list of resources in Chapter 70).

Implications for the Client

Physiological Implications

Because of the absence of blood vessels and lymphatics in the healthy donor tissue, the recipient ideally should not be sensitized to the graft and reject it. However, the rejection rate is approximately 10% to 15%. Rejection is manifested by the donor cornea's becoming opaque from

Box 72–3 Criteria for Donor Material for Corneal Transplants*

I. Cases in which donor tissue may present a health-threatening condition for the recipient or may be contraindicated because of endothelial dysfunction:

- Death from unknown cause
- Creutzfeldt–Jakob disease
- Subacute sclerosing panencephalitis
- Congenital rubella
- Progressive multifocal leukoencephalopathy
- Reye's syndrome
- Subacute encephalitis, cytomegalovirus brain infection
- Septicemia
- Hepatitis
- Rabies
- Intrinsic eye disease (retinoblastoma, conjunctivitis, iritis, glaucoma, corneal disease, malignant tumors of the anterior segment)
- Blast-form leukemia
- Hodgkin's disease
- Lymphosarcoma
- Death from central nervous system diseases of unknown etiology
- Acquired immune deficiency syndrome (AIDS)

II. Cases in which donor tissue may require caution in use:

- Multiple sclerosis
- Parkinson's disease
- Amyotrophic lateral sclerosis
- Jaundice (rule out infectious hepatitis)
- Chronic lymphocytic leukemia
- Diabetes
- Chronic immunosuppression
- Syphilis
- Mechanical respiratory support
- Known or suspected intravenous drug abuse
- Eyes that have had intraocular surgery

III. Age of donor

The lower limit is full-term birth. There is no absolute upper limit. It is recognized, however, that endothelial abnormalities and decreased cell density increase with age.

The interval between donor death and enucleation should be as short as possible (it is generally recommended that enucleation occur within 6 hours of death). Cooling the body and/or placing ice packs over the closed lids is helpful.

IV. Corneal retrieval procedures

The enucleation should be performed by sterile technique, following which the globe should be irrigated with sterile solution and placed in a sterile glass container, which is then put into a shipping container. The contents should be kept cool, but must *not* be frozen.

At the eye bank, the whole eye should be vigorously irrigated with sterile saline and immersed for 5 minutes in Neosporin solution.

The eye bank should report the following information to the surgeon:

1. Gross appearance (eg, clarity, epithelial integrity, foreign objects, opacities, and scleral color) of the eye
2. Microscopic appearance of the eye, including:

- State of the epithelium
- Gross thickness of the stroma
- Presence of folds in deep layers
- Presence of guttata (if possible) or other endothelial abnormalities

V. Methods of preservation of donor material

- The whole eye is placed in a closed, sterile, moist chamber, cooled to 4°C. Eyes so prepared need not necessarily pass through an eye bank.
- The cornea with a rim of sclera is excised, using sterile technique, and placed into a sterile solution consisting of tissue culture medium (TC 199), dextran, and antibiotics (M–K [McCarey–Kaufman] technique).
- Cryopreserved tissue is still available in some eye banks. It requires meticulously careful preserving and thawing.
- Organ-cultured tissue is available in only a few centers and is not generally available to the surgeon.
- Tissue stored in glycerin or frozen at −80°C is useful for lamellar grafts and, rarely, as an emergency patch-graft for a perforation.

VI. Time interval between death and surgery

- Whole or refrigerated eyes may be used up to 96 hours after death of the donor. Surgery is advisable as soon as possible.
- Tissue preserved by the McCarey–Kaufman technique may be used up to 4 days after the death of the donor.
- Cryopreserved tissue may be used up to at least 1 year after the death of the donor.

VII. Responsibility of surgeon and eye bank

The decision to accept a given donor rests with the operating surgeon. The eye bank's responsibility lies in furnishing as full and accurate data as possible to the surgeon, including:

- Age of donor
- Cause of death
- Associated diseases
- Time of death
- Time of enucleation
- Method of preservation
- Results of exam in eye bank

VIII. Miscellaneous

Preoperative cultures are left to the discretion of the individual eye bank.

The surgeon can also take cultures.

Emergency situations may arise where it is necessary to use donor tissue that does not meet all the criteria mentioned above. In such cases the urgency of the situation should be balanced against the overall quality of the donor.

---

*The decision to use a given donor resides with the surgeon.

SOURCE: Eye Bank Association of America, 1983. Reprinted with permission.

endothelial failure, defective healing caused by faulty tissue apposition (poor wound closure), and epithelial defects. Repeated transplants are possible, although corticosteroids often resolve a rejection episode. Corneal allograft reactions were discussed in Chapter 71.

A keratoplasty heals extremely slowly, taking several months to years, because the cornea is avascular. Steroids are used to reduce the inflammatory process, and antibiotics are given postoperatively to avoid infection. Sutures are removed approximately a year or longer after the procedure.

Psychosocial/Lifestyle Implications

Because the keratoplasty heals slowly, the client must remember to curb activities that increase intraocular pressure to avoid stress on the suture line and subsequent leakage of aqueous humor (see Box 72–1). This period of time could be as brief as one month or as long as one year. The client who understands the inherent risks of unsafe care of the eye is often more willing to use protective measures to protect the delicate transplant. The operated eye should be protected from mechanical trauma either by protective glasses (in industrial settings) or a metal eyeshield (at night to avoid rubbing). Good hand-washing and avoidance of touching or rubbing the eyes are also essential to prevent infection.

Rejection of the donor transplant is a major disappointment for the client, especially one who made serious attempts to avoid it. The client may become discouraged and unwilling to undergo another transplant. He or she may withdraw from family and physician, developing mistrust in the health care system and the surgery itself. The client will need extra support at this time and reassurance that another transplant can be performed.

Client implications of keratoplasty are summarized in Table 72–6.

Nursing Implications

Preoperative Care

The keratoplasty is usually done as an emergency, but the client will have expected it and will be excited preoperatively. The nurse helping clients prepare for the procedure can educate them about it, answering questions and clarifying any misconceptions. Emphasize the goals of preventing postoperative trauma to the eye (an eyeshield will be used) and avoiding coughing, bending, or straining. Reassure the client that little pain is experienced postoperatively but that analgesics and tranquilizers will be used as needed. The client's face is cleansed with an antibacterial soap.

Postoperative Care

Antiemetics and cough suppressants may be used postoperatively to avoid stress on the suture line. Promote good general hygiene of the client as needed to prevent infection. Washing the hands before and after care to the

Table 72–6	Corneal Transplant: Implications for the Client	
Physiological Implications	**Psychosocial/Lifestyle Implications**
Rejection rate of 10% to 15%	Activities limited until healing has occurred (from 1 mo to as long as 1 yr)
Months to years of healing; sutures remain in place 1 yr or longer	Need for protection from mechanical trauma and infection in postoperative period
Steroids to reduce inflammation and antibiotics to avoid infection	Fear of graft rejection

eye is especially important in this instance. Assess the client's occupation for potential trauma to the eye. For example, if the client cares for small children, cleans, and cooks, alternatives may be needed to avoid undue stress on the suture line of the cornea. In this case, a family member or friend might provide assistance, and a visiting nurse could provide health care supervision during home visits. See Box 72–1 for further nursing interventions.

SURGERY FOR PTOSIS

Congenital ptosis (dystrophy of the levator palpebrae muscle) can be corrected with surgery. Acquired ptosis due to Horner's syndrome (an interruption of sympathetic nerve supply to Müller's muscle caused by a lesion in the brain stem, upper spinal cord, or peripheral sympathetic chain) also is surgically correctable. Acquired ptosis that results from myasthenia gravis, seen in 95% of myasthenia gravis cases, usually is treated with a drug such as neostigmine, although a skin excision is sometimes done. Traumatic ptosis caused by concussion, surgery (eg, cataract extraction), damage to cranial nerve III (the oculomotor nerve), or direct laceration of the levator palpebrae muscle can be surgically corrected. Correction should be delayed a year after the injury, however, as ptosis can improve, and early intervention may result in overcorrection. Senile ptosis (muscle atony) also can be surgically corrected. Ptosis in children is not in the realm of this discussion, but surgical correction should be done as soon as possible to avoid amblyopic development. Ptosis surgery on adults is usually for cosmetic reasons and will not cure an amblyopic eye.

Surgical Procedure

There are many types of ptosis and at least as many corrective procedures. The preoperative examination is essential for accurate classification of the ptosis type and the proper surgical procedure. Since 50% of the ptosis population suffers from primary levator palpebrae muscle dystrophy (Beard, 1981), the following discussion will describe the associated surgical procedure.

Preoperatively, the degree of levator muscle function is measured using a millimeter ruler to determine the excursion (movement from open to closed lid position) of the eyelid as the client looks downward and then upward. Normal movement measures 15 mm. With a ptotic eyelid that measures approximately 5 to 12 mm, a levator resection is feasible, and this is the most successful procedure in treating ptosis (Beard, 1981).

Local anesthesia is preferred for levator muscle resection, because the client can cooperate and move the unoperated eye for comparison with the operated eye as needed. Either local infiltration or regional block anesthesia is used. The amount of levator muscle to be resected should have been determined during the preoperative examination. An incision is made through the eyelid skin and muscle below the upper tarsal border (Figure 72–10). The levator is exposed and cut away from the skin-muscle lamina, orbital fascia, and upper tarsal border. Excess levator muscle is resected, and the remaining levator muscle is sutured down on the tarsus. Silk (5-0) sutures close the skin wound. Finally, the surgery is concluded by placing a *Frost suture*

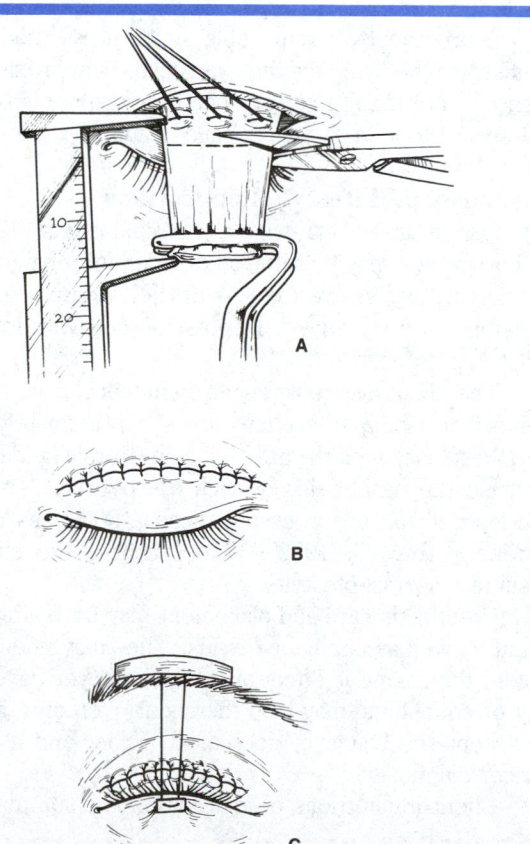

Figure 72–10

Ptosis surgery. **A.** Excess levator muscle is resected. **B.** The skin wound is closed along the lid length where it will be hidden when the lid is open. **C.** A Frost suture in the lower eyelid is taped above the eyebrow.

in the lower eyelid and taping it to the eyebrow to cause lower lid elevation over the cornea for corneal protection (Fox, 1980).

Implications for the Client

Physiological Implications
Swelling or edema may contraindicate the use of the Frost suture. In any event, the cornea must be protected; often all that is needed is a simple eyepatch worn for 1 to 3 days. The Frost suture usually is removed after 2 to 3 days. Swelling generally subsides in 7 to 10 days, although healing can be slow, and the lid can droop for several weeks. The surgeon changes the dressing every day and examines the client to ensure adequate healing and inspect for corneal injury. Artificial tears (0.5% to 1.0% methylcellulose) are used three to four times a day to prevent corneal drying and resultant keratitis.

Postoperative hemorrhage is unlikely, and pressure dressings are neither recommended nor likely to be necessary. Infection is rare because of the eyelid's abundant blood supply. Other possible complications of ptosis surgery include overcorrection or undercorrection of the anomaly. (In undercorrection, the eyelid rests below the desired level.) Both complications may require further surgery. Further complications include uneven positioning of the eyelids, the recurrence of ptosis, ectropion, entropion, loss of eyelashes, poor eyelid contour, and muscle imbalance.

Psychosocial/Lifestyle Implications
The health care team should clearly emphasize to the client before surgery that the greater the ptosis, the poorer the prognosis. Because one goal is cosmetic correction, the client may be extremely disappointed, dismayed, and perhaps angry when the postoperative result is not a perfect eyelid. Sometimes one or two more surgeries may be needed to obtain a satisfactory result. The client must understand the possible necessity of further surgery, although this may cause fear. Excessive activity is contraindicated until the surgeon gives permission.

Implications for the client having surgery for ptosis are summarized in Table 72–7.

Nursing Implications

Preoperative Care
The client may need help accepting the possibility of an unsatisfactory surgical result. Provide empathy and reassurance as needed. The client can also be assured that complications are relatively rare and that success is expected.

Postoperative Care
The client can be observed postoperatively in the hospital for the previously mentioned complications, such as bleeding and discomfort from swelling. High or semi-Fowler's positioning may help prevent edema and provide comfort. Offer analgesics as prescribed. Be aware of whether a Frost

Table 72-7	Surgery for Ptosis: Implications for the Client	
Physiological Implications	**Psychosocial/Lifestyle Implications**
Need to wear eyepatch for 1 to 3 days	Extreme disappointment or anger when surgery fails to give a perfect eyelid
Swelling and slow healing	
Possible corneal dryness	Fear of repeated surgeries to correct postoperative result
Complications, including hemorrhage, infection, overcorrection or undercorrection of anomaly, uneven eyelid positioning, recurrence of ptosis, ectropion, entropion, loss of eyelashes, poor eyelid contour, and muscle imbalance	Excessive postoperative activity contraindicated

suture was used before instilling eyedrops or inspecting the eye. Take care not to disturb the suture.

If the client is discharged the day of surgery, inform the family or significant others of the inevitable eyelid swelling and encourage administration of analgesics as prescribed. Explain that swelling can be minimized with semi-Fowler's positioning.

ENUCLEATION

An enucleation is a complete surgical removal of the eyeball. This procedure is indicated for a blind and painful eye; after trauma that caused irreparable harm; and in cases of infection, **sympathetic ophthalmia** (inflammation of the uveal tract of the uninjured eye), malignancy of the eye (eg, melanoma or retinoblastoma), and absolute glaucoma. When no other treatment is feasible, enucleation is done for palliative as well as lifesaving reasons.

Surgical Procedure

Enucleation is usually performed under general anesthesia. The conjunctiva is opened around the cornea (as close to the corneoscleral limbus as possible), and each of the four rectus muscles are severed from the globe at their insertion. The oblique muscles are then severed from the globe. Finally, the optic nerve is severed from behind the globe, and the globe is removed from the socket. Pressure is applied to stop bleeding. A permanent round plastic or Teflon globe is placed in the empty socket to retain the round shape. The muscles or tissues are sewn over the implant, which allows some movement of it. The conjunctiva is then closed, forming a mucous-membrane-lined socket.

Sometimes only the intraocular contents of the eyeball are removed, and the sclera and cornea are retained in a procedure called an evisceration. For example, panophthalmitis (inflammation of all the structures of the eye) necessitates evisceration or enucleation because an actively suppurative eyeball can give rise to meningitis. Evisceration is seldom done today, however, because of the risk of sympathetic ophthalmia following it.

Implications for the Client

Physiological Implications
An enucleation is usually the end result of a series of attempts to save the eyeball. The client's condition may have already been managed with cryotherapy, radiation therapy, chemotherapy, steroids, and other medications.

Enucleation has relatively few potential complications in comparison with other eye surgeries. Hemorrhage and infection may occur. Infection may be indicated by pain and headache on the side of the enucleation, as well as temperature elevation. Occasionally, infection can result in abscess, thrombosis, or meningitis. To avoid these complications, the client wears a pressure dressing for 2 days to prevent hemorrhage, and may use antibiotics upon discharge.

A prosthesis, a removable artificial eye made by an oculist, can be fitted for the eye socket in approximately 1 month. Until then, a plastic shell (conformer) is placed in the socket to hold its shape while healing.

Psychosocial/Lifestyle Implications
The loss of an eye can have a profound effect on clients. Although they may be relieved of a painful, disfiguring, or blind eye, they grieve the loss of the eye and experience a change in body image. Depression and withdrawal are often experienced.

The client also must adjust to monocular vision. With monocular vision, the client loses approximately 50° of peripheral vision on the affected side (from a field of 180°), because the nasal fields of each eye overlap. Therefore, the loss of one eye does not mean a 50% loss of visual efficiency (Newell, 1982). With practice, the client can resume a normal lifestyle.

Prosthesis care and placement may be trying for the client as well as family or friends. They may need time to accept the cosmetic effect of an artificial eye. Psychotherapy or counseling may help the client overcome grief and to accept the lost eye, decreased vision, and a possible cancer diagnosis.

Client implications of enucleation are summarized in Table 72-8.

Nursing Implications

Preoperative Care
Routine preoperative nursing care is carried out for the client undergoing an enucleation. Emotional support and

Table 72–8 Enucleation: Implications for the Client

Physiological Implications	Psychosocial/Lifestyle Implications
Possible complications (hemorrhage and infection) and need to avoid them by wearing a pressure dressing for 2 days and taking antibiotics	Relief from a painful, disfiguring, or blind eye
	Depression, withdrawal, and the need to grieve
Use of a conformer initially to hold the shape of the socket during healing	Normal lifestyle
	Need to adjust to monocular vision
Use of a prosthesis a month after enucleation	Difficulties in prosthesis adjustment for client and significant others
	Fear of cancer

empathy help relieve some of the anxiety that clients experience.

Chapter Highlights

Clients requiring eye surgery fear vision loss, discomfort, dependence on significant others and health care professionals, and possible lifestyle changes.

The nurse needs to assist the client in verbalizing fears, provide education on procedures and implications, and assist the client in regaining autonomy safely.

The nurse can promote an uneventful postoperative course by providing orientation of time and place to the client with an eyepatch; preventing nausea with antiemetics; encouraging flexing and extending of the extremities to prevent thrombi; promoting deep breathing to expand lungs and prevent secretions; and discouraging coughing, bending, straining with bowel movements, and nose blowing to prevent increased intraocular pressure.

A vitrectomy is indicated when damage to the vitreous or loss of the vitreous from conditions such as diabetic retinoplasty, trauma, and inflammation is severe enough to create a potential for retinal detachment or to block light from the retina.

Retinal holes are sealed using cryotherapy, photocoagulation, or diathermy.

Scleral buckling techniques indent the wall of the eye toward the vitreous in an attempt to reattach the retina to its anatomic position.

Postoperative Care
The postoperative client can move about without restrictions. Observe for bleeding, elevated temperature, and pain. After 48 hours, the instillation of antibiotics may be necessary.

Before discharge, teach the client and family or friends the correct administration of medications and the proper hygienic care of the eye socket. The conformer is a temporary prosthesis and need not be replaced if it falls out. However, the client should learn the care and insertion of a prosthesis. It needs to be removed about twice a month for cleaning. Special polishing, usually done by an optician, is periodically required to remove dried protein secretions.

Prosthesis care should be carried out as follows:

- Wash the hands.
- Pull the lower lid down, and the prosthesis should slip out.
- Wash the prosthesis under running water.
- Reinsert the prosthesis by lifting the upper eyelid against the bony orbit and placing the prosthesis under the lower eyelid while it is pulled down. The prosthesis should slip into place.

Retinal reattachment procedures often require stringent positioning for the immediate postoperative period to keep the retina and choroid in apposition.

Cataract extraction is a relatively risk-free surgical procedure with two techniques: intracapsular or extracapsular cataract extraction.

The aphakic client will have decreased refractive power and no accommodation ability after cataract extraction, so cataract glasses, contact lenses, or an intraocular lens will be necessary for adequate visual acuity.

An iridectomy creates a new channel of aqueous humor drainage by dissecting a small portion of the iris. It essentially cures angle-closure glaucoma and requires few lifestyle changes.

Filtering procedures (trabeculectomy and sclerectomy) create a drainage channel for the aqueous humor in open-angle glaucoma, alleviating intraocular hypertension.

A corneal transplant (keratoplasty) may restore vision by transplanting a donor cornea in place of the excised diseased cornea.

Corneal transplants result in rejection approximately 10% to 15% of the time, and steroids may reverse rejection. Repeated transplants also are possible.

(continued)

Chapter Highlights (continued)

Ptosis surgery for adults is usually for cosmetic reasons and will not cure an amblyopic eye. The client should be prepared for the possibility of a nonperfect eyelid postoperatively, depending on the original defect and possible surgical complications.

Enucleation is the complete surgical removal of the eyeball and is required when other treatment is not feasible or the condition is not treatable.

Bibliography

Beard C: *Ptosis,* 3rd ed. St. Louis: Mosby, 1981.

Boyd-Monk H: Retinal detachment and vitrectomy: Nursing care. *Nurs Clin North Am* 1981; 16(3):383–477.

Chignell A: *Retinal Detachment Surgery.* New York: Springer-Verlag, 1980.

Clayman H, Jaffe N, Galin M: *Intraocular Lens Implantation.* St. Louis: Mosby, 1983.

Fox S: *Surgery of Ptosis.* Baltimore: Williams & Wilkins, 1980.

Girard L: *Corneal Surgery,* Vol. 2. St. Louis: Mosby, 1981.

Jaffe NS: The changing score of intraocular implant lens surgery. *Am J Ophthal* 1979; 88:819–828.

Krieglstein GK, Duzanec Z, Leydhecker W: Cataract surgery: Types and frequencies of complications. Albrecht von Graefes, *Arch Klim Ophthalmology,* 1980; 9–13.

Little H et al: *Diabetic Retinopathy.* New York: Thieme–Stratton, 1983.

McCoy K: Cataracts and intraocular lenses: From cloudy to clear. *Nurs Clin North Am* 1981; 16(3):405–414.

Meltzer D, Drews R: Intraocular lens implantation. In: *Complications in Ophthalmic Surgery.* New York: Churchill Livingstone, 1983.

Morse PH: *Vitreoretinal Disease.* Chicago: Year Book Medical Publishers, 1979.

Newell F: *Ophthalmology,* 5th ed. St. Louis: Mosby, 1982.

Schepens C: *Retinal Detachment and Allied Diseases.* Vol. 1. Philadelphia: Saunders, 1983.

Shields BM: *A Study Guide for Glaucoma.* Baltimore: Williams & Wilkins, 1982.

Smith JF: *Ophthalmologic Nursing.* Boston: Little, Brown, 1980.

Suggested Readings

Boyd-Monk H (editor): *Nurs Clin North Am* 1981; 16(3):383–477. [Entire issue.] This symposium on ophthalmic nursing discusses the treatment, care, and ocular therapeutics of clients with cataracts, glaucoma, and retinal and vitreous abnormalities.

Chignell AH: *Retinal Detachment Surgery.* New York: Springer-Verlag, 1980. This small book is an excellent resource for total explanation of the retinal detachment including examination with excellent color/black/white plates; preoperative and postoperative management and discussion regarding complications.

Fletcher D: An unexpected discovery. *Nurs Mirror* (April 17) 1980; 150:34–35. This article discusses intraocular lenses, including their history, description, indications, and complications. Specific postoperative nursing management is also discussed.

Grabham J: Vitrectomy surgery. *Nurs Times* 1982; 78:2113–2117. The anatomy and physiology of the vitreous; reasons for its removal; and preoperative, intraoperative, and postoperative nursing care are described. The article also includes a definitive list of dos and don'ts for discharged ophthalmic patients.

Schulman J: *Cataracts: The Complete Guide from Diagnosis to Recovery for Patients and Families.* New York: Simon & Shuster, 1984. Printed in large easy-to-read type, this book by an eminent eye specialist explains cataracts and every step of cataract surgery. Written in a conversational tone, the book is directed toward clients and their families.

Smith JF: *Ophthalmologic Nursing.* Boston: Little, Brown, 1980. A comprehensive discussion of preoperative and postoperative nursing care of various eye surgeries also provides a brief description of each surgery.

Today's OR Nurse (March) 1983; 5(1). Marta, M: A guide to the posterior vitrectomy, p. 26+; Whitton, S: Penetrating Keratoplasty: The gift of sight, p. 20+; Zach P, Smirnow I: IOL implantation, p. 13+. These three articles provide a current overview of the various surgical procedures, as well as information on client preparation, nursing implications, and complications. Excellent photographs of instruments and procedures are provided.

The Client With Cataract Extraction and Intraocular Lens Implant

I. Descriptive Data

Mrs Margaret Schwan, an 80-year-old retired librarian, was seen by her ophthalmologist with a complaint of blurred vision and subsequent difficulty reading. She had no complaints of pain other than occasional frontal headaches after long periods of reading.

II. Personal Data

Date and Time:	March 2, 1986; 1 PM
Full Name:	Margaret Louise Schwan
Social Security Number:	000-00-0000
Address:	2323 Lancaster Dr., Oakland, CA
Telephone:	000-0000
Sex:	Female
Age:	80
Birthdate:	8-23-05
Marital Status:	Widowed
Race:	Caucasian
Religion:	Lutheran
Occupation:	Retired librarian
Usual Health Care Provider:	Geraldine Drummond, MD; Michael Laski, RN, NP

III. Health History

Source of Information:	Client
Reliability of Informant:	Very reliable
Chief Complaint:	"For the past six months or so, I've noticed increasing difficulty reading fine print."

History of Present Illness: Mrs Schwan states she has noted a gradual deterioration in visual acuity (left eye more than right) over the last few years interfering with activities of daily living. No diplopia, eye pain, redness, halos, or floaters. She has no history of eye problems except for needing reading glasses since age 50; no eye trauma; no hx of DM, hypertension, cardiovascular disease, renal disease; no ⊕ F hx of eye problems; has occasional headaches behind her eyes relieved by over-the-counter sinus medications; otherwise takes no meds except for acetaminophen for arthritic discomfort and psyllium and an occasional stool softener for constipation.

Past Health History:

Childhood:	Usual childhood illnesses
Immunizations:	Doesn't remember having any; never had dog bite or stitches requiring Td
Medical Problems:	Chronic constipation X 25 years, currently managed with psyllium; osteoarthritis both hands, both hips, left shoulder
Surgeries:	Bunionectomy rt foot, 1974; abd hysterectomy for fibroids, 1960
Pregnancies:	None
Trauma:	None
Allergies:	Sulfa (urticaria)
Medications:	Acetaminophen, gr X AM and PM
	Psyllium 1 tbsp b.i.d.
	Docusate sodium (Colace), 100 mg p.r.n.

(continued)

Case Study written by Mary Nord Meadows and Theresa Flaherty.

The Client With Cataract Extraction and Intraocular Lens Implant

Family History: Father, died age 90, old age
Mother, died age 36, childbirth
Brother, died age 73, MI, also had Type II DM
Sister, age 82, A&W
Husband, died age 70, CVA
   No known positive F hx of TBC, cancer, glaucoma, cataract, or other eye problems

Personal/Social History: Mrs Schwan has been widowed 11 years and lives alone in a one-story apartment; is a former smoker (1 PPD × 20 yr) and is accustomed to a glass of sherry after dinner; active in her church and volunteers 15 hours a week at the public library. She eats simple "convenience" foods, reassuring the interviewer that she gets proper nutrition; has no difficulty sleeping; no longer drives her own car because of her decreasing vision but has several close friends who take her shopping; is able to walk to church and to the library.

Review of Systems: States her overall health is excellent

Eyes: See history of present illness

Ears: Has minor hearing difficulty in rt ear; was tested and told she had some nerve deafness; it does not bother her

Respiratory: No DOE, no cough

Cardiovascular: No chest pain; all past ECGs wnl; no ankle swelling

Gastrointestinal: No nausea, vomiting, change in bowel habits; stools brown; has daily BM with psyllium; eats whole grains and fresh fruits

Gynecological: Was never able to become pregnant, which was a major disappointment in her life; had heavy bleeding with fibroids; no problems since hysterectomy

Musculoskeletal: Often has pain in fingers and hips on damp days and with overuse; joints rarely swell; uses acetaminophen for pain, which controls it well

IV. Physical Assessment

Weight: 152 lb

Height: 5 ft 5 in

Vital Signs: Temperature 36.4°C; pulse 82; respirations 16; BP 130/84, rt arm, seated

Relevant Organ Systems:

Eyes:
- *VA (visual acuity) using Snellen's chart   PH (pinhole)*
OD V (without corrective lenses) 20/80 → 20/80
OS V (without corrective lenses) 20/200 → 20/200
M (manifest: what a client can subjectively achieve when assessing for best acuity)
M = OD no improvement; OS no improvement
- *External exam:*
Lids: Normal, no ptosis, ectropion, or entropion noted
Lashes: Scarce
Lacrimal: Nl; no swelling, erythema, epiphora, or dryness noted
- *EOMs (extraocular movements):* Normal: Full movement OU; orthophoric (no strabismus)
- *Pupils:* Normal size: OD 3 mm → 2 mm (with light); OS 3 mm → 2 mm; round, regular, no defects
- *VFs (visual fields):* Intact to finger confrontation

- *SLE (slit lamp examination):*
  Conjunctiva: White, no injection
  Anterior chamber: Deep without cells or flare (protein)
  Iris: Nl
  Lens: L > R cataract

Frontal	Cross-section	Frontal	Cross-section
OD		OS	
2+ nuclear sclerosis		3+ brunescent (brown) sclerosis	

- *Additional testing of intraocular lens specifications:*
  Keratometry: Curvature = $41.50 - 42.50 \times 90$ diopters
  Ultrasound: Axial length = 23.5 mm
  Power for ametropia calculated to be = +20.50 diopters
    A posterior chamber intraocular lens was chosen, according to above specifications and physician's preference; lens power is to be 21.5 diopters to make client slightly nearsighted without glasses
- *TA (tension applanation):*
  OD = 16 normal intraocular pressure = 8–21; OS = 15
  Dilation with Mydriacyl 1% and Neo-Synephrine 2.5%
- *Fundus, using indirect ophthalmoscope:*
  OD (optic disk, vessels, macula, and periphery): No abnormality
  OS: Hazy view, probably nl optic disk, vessels, macula, and periphery
  Optical media: OD 20/80; OS 20/200

Respiratory: Sinuses, without tenderness; chest, clear to auscultation
Cardiovascular: Apical rate 78, regular; o m; S_1S_2 nl; ECG nl
Musculoskeletal: Heberden's nodes DIP joints of index, middle, and ring fingers both hands
Neurologic: CN II-XII intact; Romberg test negative

V. Diagnosis Bilateral cataracts

VI. Summary Physical examination revealed bilateral cataracts, and surgery was recommended. The ophthalmologist described the cataract extraction procedure and the potential surgical risks to Mrs Schwan. One week later, she was admitted to the hospital for cataract extraction and intraocular lens implant of her left eye, to be followed by extraction of the right cataract at a later date.

VII. Nursing Care Plan

Nursing Diagnosis	Client Care Goal	Plan/Nursing Implementation	Expected Outcome
Sensory-perceptual alteration: visual, with potential for loss of independence in an otherwise active elderly woman	Understands temporary decrease in vision postoperatively; remains independent	Orient client to surroundings and organize possessions within reach of unoperated eye; explain use of an eyepatch postoperatively and the resultant loss of vision in that eye until patch is removed; reassure client that a degree of realistic dependency is necessary during healing process, ie, assistance with transportation, dressing, ambulating; educate about temporary	Cooperation and understanding with regard to visual limitations in postoperative period and contraindicated activities; resumption of previous lifestyle with improved vision

(continued)

The Client With Cataract Extraction and Intraocular Lens Implant

VII. Nursing Care Plan (continued)

Nursing Diagnosis	Client Care Goal	Plan/Nursing Implementation	Expected Outcome
		period postoperatively when there will be less-than-desirable vision in the operative eye; allow client to be active; light reading and TV are OK; instruct client regarding contraindicated activities such as rubbing the eyes, straining at stool, bending over	
Mobility, impaired physical, with potential for increased discomfort from osteoarthritic joints	Experiences minimal arthritic pain; maintains joint flexibility	Maintain activity patterns to retain flexibility of joints; use passive or active range-of-motion exercises; encourage self-care activities such as eating and bathing self; evaluate use of heat or cold for joint discomfort	Arthritis will not be exacerbated by decreased activity; able to resume full activity without limitation
Mobility, impaired physical, with potential for depression	Understands and tolerates the temporary period of inactivity postoperatively	Discuss with client what she is allowed to do, emphasizing activities of daily living; encourage verbalization about frustrations; encourage regular walks in hallways for stimulation; initiate discussion between client and physician regarding resumption of her work and rigorous reading schedule	Will not have change in behavior; remains interested in things around her and does not withdraw; actively plans for discharge and return home
Bowel elimination, alteration in: constipation	Achieves satisfactory nutritional pattern and daily bowel movement	Continue psyllium b.i.d. as is client's regular pattern; encourage 2000–3000 mL of fluids per day; obtain order for a stool softener if client is constipated despite previous measures; evaluate client's normal diet for fibrous foods such as fresh fruits, vegetables, and bran products; encourage regular walks (eg, 20 min walks 2–3 times/day); determine whether a support person is available to share meals and walks	Regular bowel movements without need for straining; states she feels good and has more energy with increase in exercise

Chapter 73

The Auditory System in Health and Illness

Dominica Ann Limburg
Carol Ren Kneisl

Objectives

When you have finished studying this chapter, you should be able to:

Identify the major functions of the auditory and vestibular systems.

Describe anatomic structures in the ear related to the auditory and vestibular systems.

Discuss the functions of the ears in relation to their structure.

Identify pathophysiological influences that can result in structural or functional alterations of the ears.

Identify alterations in other body systems that can affect the ears.

Discuss psychosocial influences that have some relationship to hearing or balance.

The ear may be one of the most overlooked and underrated organs of the body. Some of us pay attention to the outer ear, or at least to how it looks. We notice a misshapen ear or an ear with a particularly attractive earring. We also tend to become aware of our ears when things go awry—when our ears pop or feel stuffed. Otherwise, we seldom think about the auditory system, not even when enjoying a particularly pleasurable piece of music or listening to the sound of waves lapping at the shore, and certainly not as we move and turn our heads as we carry out our daily activities. The auditory system is not only responsible for all the sounds we hear; it also helps us maintain our equilibrium (balance). Along with the eye, the ear is one of the most important sources of information that we have about the world we live in and the space we occupy. The auditory system enables us to receive information about how we affect others and what they think about us. It plays a significant role in the relationships—good or bad—that we have with others.

Section I: Structural and Functional Interrelationships

Although a sensory organ, the ear is also part of the central nervous system. Its two major functions, hearing and the maintenance of equilibrium, interface closely with the central nervous system.

Hearing is a complex mechanism in which the ears receive sound waves, convert them into nerve impulses, and transmit them for interpretation to the central nervous system through the cochlear branch of the vestibulocochlear nerve (also known as the acoustic nerve, cranial nerve VIII, or CN VIII). *Equilibrium*, in contrast, is maintained by the vestibular system of the inner ear, which detects the orientation and movement of the head and transmits this information to the central nervous system via the vestibular branch of CN VIII. Both hearing and equilibrium are discussed later in this section in the discussion of regulatory functions.

Development of the ear begins in the embryo at 3 weeks, and the sensory end organs are completed by 12 weeks. Except for the external ear and the endolymphatic duct, the hearing mechanism (unlike any other organ system) is fully formed and of adult size at birth.

STRUCTURE AND FUNCTION OF THE EAR
External Ear

The external ear consists of two structures: the auricle, or pinna, and the external auditory canal, sometimes called the external acoustic meatus or external auditory meatus.

Auricle
The auricle is the visible funnel-shaped part of the ear that is attached to the skull by muscles and ligaments. In humans these muscles serve no practical function, but lower animals use them to increase their hearing acuity by bending their ears toward sound.

The parts of the auricle are the helix, anthelix, crus of the helix, tragus, lobule, and concha (Figure 73–1). The auricle, with the exception of the lobule, consists of a thin layer of elastic fibrocartilage (more pliable in children than in adults) covered with closely adherent skin. The lobule consists of fatty tissue, which facilitates ear piercing. The auricle is the receptor for the mechanical vibrations of

sounds—it catches sound waves. The helix, anthelix, and the crus of the helix help direct the sound waves through the concha to the external auditory canal.

External Auditory Canal
The external auditory canal (Figure 73–2), which is only about 2.5 cm (1 in) in length, bends downward and forward from the concha to the tympanic membrane (eardrum). The outer third of the canal consists of elastic cartilage, whereas the inner two thirds is bone. Skin lining the canal is continuous with the auricle and tympanic membrane. The thick skin lining the cartilaginous area contains numerous hair follicles, as well as sebaceous and apocrine glands. The hairs help prevent dirt, dust, and foreign bodies from entering the canal. Secretions from the sebaceous and apocrine glands form a yellowish-brown wax, **cerumen,** which serves a number of useful functions. First, it provides a self-cleaning system for the ear; second, it is bacteriostatic because of its acid pH; and third, its enzyme activity prevents drying of the epithelium in the canal (Marshall & Attia, 1983). The bony portion of the canal is lined with thin skin that is extremely sensitive to touch.

At the inner end of the external auditory canal is the *tympanic membrane*, a concave, shiny, pearly gray, translucent membrane that separates the external ear from the middle ear. When sound waves funnel through the canal and reverberate off the sides, they cause the tympanic membrane to vibrate. The anatomical features of the tympanic membrane are more fully described and illustrated in Chapter 7.

Middle Ear

The middle ear, or *tympanic cavity*, is situated within an air-filled cavity of the temporal bone (see Figure 73–2). An opening in the posterior wall, the *tympanic antrum*, connects the middle ear with the mucous-membrane-lined mastoid sinuses of the mastoid portion of the temporal bone. The mastoid portion is located just posterior to the external auditory canal. The middle ear also connects with the nasopharynx through the eustachian tube, which enters the middle ear through an opening in the floor of the temporal bone. This anatomic feature makes it possible for microorganisms to enter the middle ear through the eustachian tube and even to move into the mastoid sinuses through the tympanic antrum, causing infections in either location. Because of the close proximity of the mastoid sinuses to the brain, infections there can spread to the meninges of the brain.

Because it connects the middle ear with the nasopharynx, the eustachian tube equalizes the pressure in the middle ear with atmospheric pressure. Swallowing and yawning open the eustachian tube, and high atmospheric pressure closes it.

Attached to the tympanic membrane is the ossicular chain, or ossicles, a set of three bones—the *malleus* (hammer), *incus* (anvil), and *stapes* (stirrup)—with freely mov-

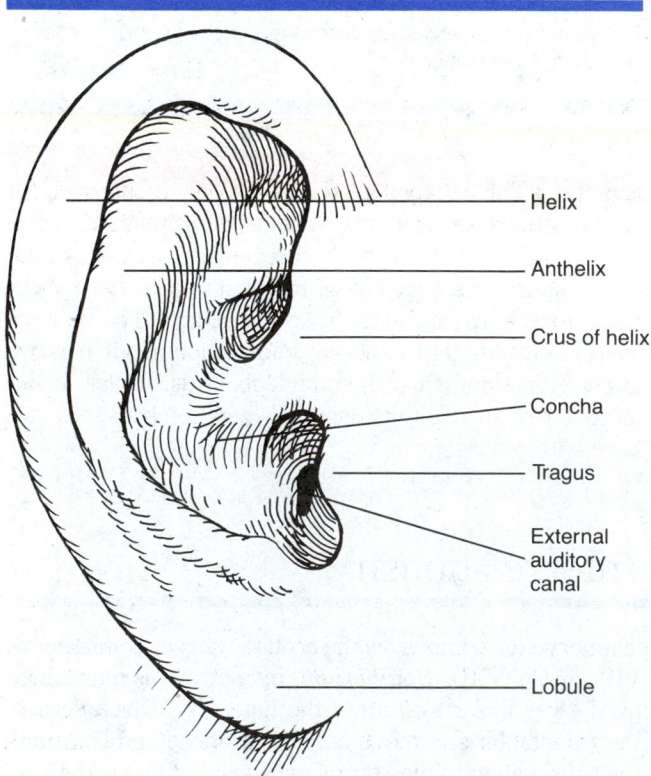

Figure 73–1

Structures of the external ear.

Helix

Anthelix

Crus of helix

Concha

Tragus

External auditory canal

Lobule

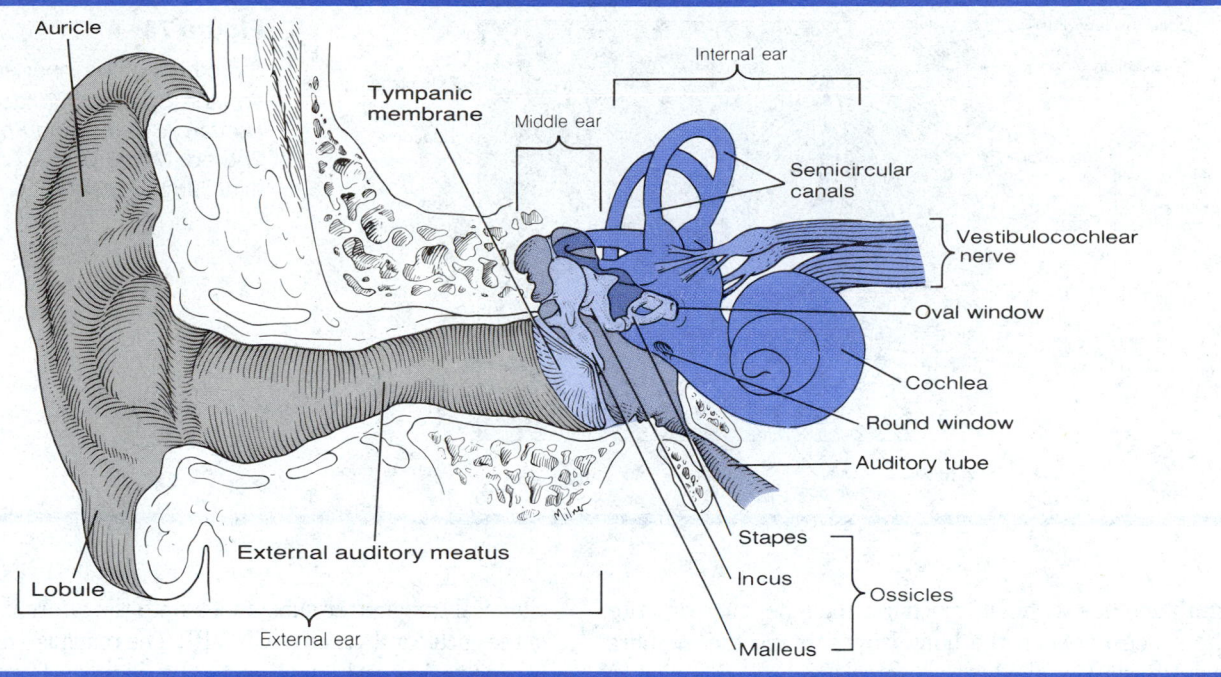

Figure 73–2

The ear.

SOURCE: Spence AP, Mason EB: *Human Anatomy and Physiology,* 2nd ed. Menlo Park, CA: Benjamin/Cummings, 1983.

able synovial joints. The ossicles are the smallest bones in the human body. Figure 73–3 is a close-up view of the ossicles and their relationship to one another. The handle of the malleus is attached to the tympanic membrane. The incus is attached by ligaments to both the malleus and the stapes. The footplate of the stapes fits against the *oval window,* a membrane-covered opening of the temporal bone into the inner ear. These bones act as a chain of levers across the middle ear, transmitting and amplifying vibrations received at the tympanic membrane to the oval window and from there into the inner ear. The middle ear has a second membrane-covered opening into the inner ear called the *round window.*

Inner Ear

In the base of the skull between the sphenoid and occipital bones lies the petrous portion of the temporal bone, the most compact bone in the body. Within this petrous bone lie the inner ear (labyrinth) and the internal auditory meatus, an opening through which the facial nerve (CN VII) and vestibulocochlear nerve (CN VIII) transmit their impulses to the brain.

The inner ear consists of two parts: the bony (osseous) labyrinth and the membranous labyrinth. The bony labyrinth is a series of interconnecting passageways within the petrous portion of the temporal bone. The membranous labyrinth is similar in shape but smaller than the bony lab-

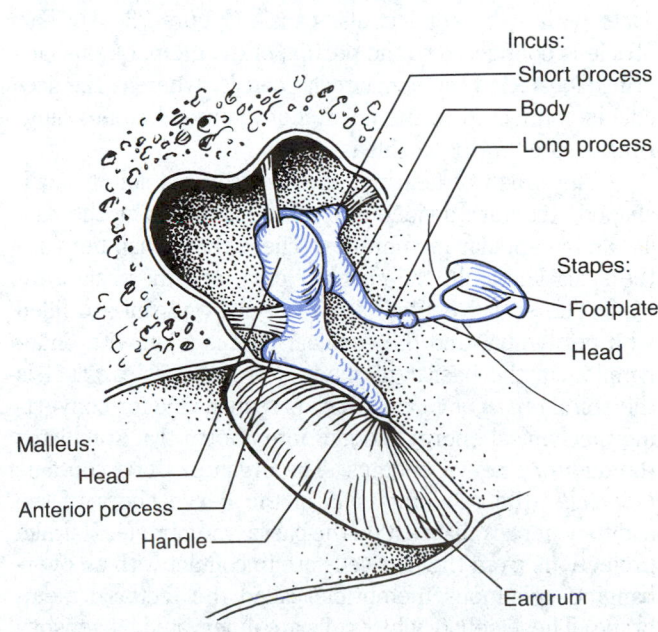

Figure 73–3

The ossicles. The handle of the malleus attaches to the tympanic membrane, through which it receives sound wave vibrations. The vibrations travel through the incus to the stapes and through its footplate to the membrane covering the oval window.

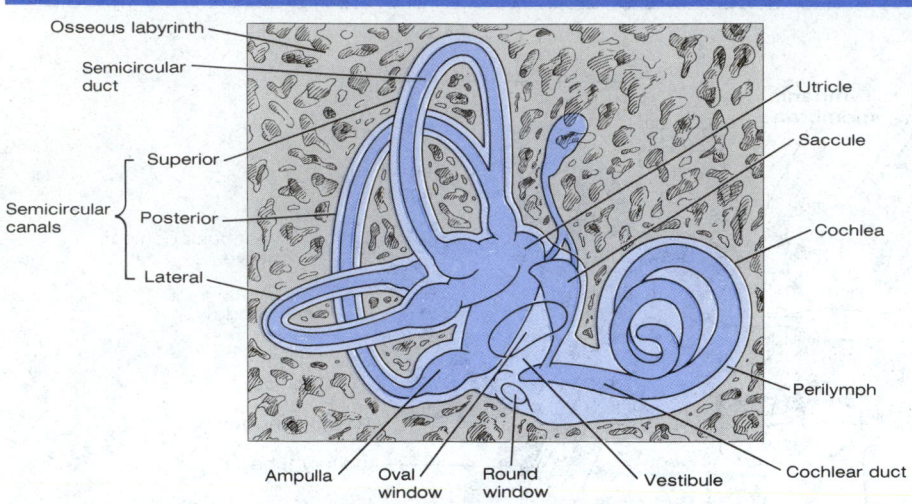

Figure 73–4

Structures of the inner ear.
SOURCE: Spence AP, Mason EB: *Human Anatomy and Physiology*, 2nd ed. Menlo Park, CA: Benjamin/Cummings, 1983.

yrinth and lies within it, much like the inner tube of a tire. The space between the bony labyrinth and the membranous labyrinth is filled with a watery fluid called *perilymph*, which separates them. The membranous labyrinth is filled with a similar fluid called *endolymph*.

The bony labyrinth consists of the cochlea (the anterior part); the vestibule (the central part); and the superior, posterior, and lateral semicircular canals (the posterior part). Correspondingly, the membranous labyrinth consists of the cochlear duct within the cochlea, the utricle and the saccule within the vestibule, and the semicircular ducts within the semicircular canals (Figure 73–4). The utricle is connected to the portion of the membranous labyrinth located in the semicircular canals, whereas the saccule is connected to the portion of the membranous labyrinth located in the cochlea.

The organ of hearing, the *cochlea*, is a spiral, snail-shaped structure divided into three chambers by the basilar and vestibular membranes. These three chambers are the scala vestibuli, the cochlear duct, and the scala tympani. The scala vestibuli and the scala tympani are filled with perilymph, and the cochlear duct is filled with endolymph. On the basilar membrane of the cochlear duct is the spiral *organ of Corti*, which is responsible for converting mechanical energy (sound) into a form that stimulates the auditory nerve endings. The organ of Corti contains *hair cells* (the receptor cells of the nerve fibers of the auditory nerve) that rest on the basilar membrane. Hairlike projections from the hair cells are in contact with an overhanging gelatinous membrane called the tectorial membrane. These sensory hair cells are innervated by sensory fibers from the cochlear division of CN VIII.

When the ossicles vibrate, causing the oval window to move inward, a fluid wave is created in the perilymph. This fluid wave causes the round window to bulge outward into the middle ear and moves the basilar membrane of the cochlear duct, causing the hairlike projections of the hair cells to move against the tectorial membrane and release

chemical transmitter substances onto the afferent endings of the cochlear division of CN VIII. The result is a discharge of electrochemical impulses to the auditory fibers of the cochlear division of CN VIII, which transmits the electrical impulses to the brain.

The vestibule and three bony semicircular canals make up the vestibular system within the ear (refer to Figure 73–4). The *semicircular canals* are arranged at right angles to one another—much like the floor and two adjacent side walls in the corner of a room—and open into the posterior portion of the vestibule. Floating within the semicircular canals are three semicircular ducts. On the end of each duct is an enlargement called an ampulla (see Figure 73–4), which contains a group of receptor hair cells, called cristae, embedded in a gelatinous mass. In response to turning the head, movement of the endolymph bends the hair cells. Consequently, these hair cells fire impulses to the nerve fibers of the vestibular portion of CN VIII.

The saccule and utricle, two enlargements of the membranous labyrinth within the vestibule, contain maculae (similar to cristae) covered with particles of calcium carbonate; these are known as *otoliths*. The otoliths press on the hair cells in response to different positions of the head, sending impulses to the vestibular branch of CN VIII. How equilibrium is maintained is discussed later in this chapter.

Blood and Nerve Supply to the Ear

Blood is supplied to the ear through branches of the internal and external carotid, the maxillary, the superficial temporal, and the occipital arteries. Veins drain into corresponding branches. Lymph from the ear drains into the preauricular, postauricular, occipital, and superficial and deep cervical nodes.

Nerve supply to the ear includes branches of the facial nerve (CN VII), vagus nerve (CN X), trigeminal nerve (CN V), vestibulocochlear nerve (CN VIII), and glossopharyngeal (CN IX) nerve. Stimulation of the vagus nerve accounts for reflex coughing or sneezing during examination of the ears, and stimulation of the trigeminal, facial, and glossopharyngeal nerves accounts for earaches with referred pain from the teeth, tongue, or pharynx. The auditory nerve is the vestibulocochlear nerve (CN VIII), which has two separate divisions—the cochlear and vestibular nerves. The two divisions join to form a common trunk, termed the vestibulocochlear nerve (refer to Figure 73–2). The *cochlear division* innervates the hair cells of the organ of Corti and transmits impulses related to hearing from the organ of Corti to the cortex of the temporal lobe of the brain. The *vestibular division*, which supplies the vestibules and ampullae of the semicircular canals, maintains equilibrium. It transmits impulses to motor areas of the medulla and cerebellum.

REGULATORY FUNCTIONS OF THE EAR

The two primary regulatory functions of the ear are hearing and maintenance of equilibrium. Each of these functions is described here.

Hearing

To hear a sound, the ear must perceive sound waves that travel through the air, pass through the external auditory canal, are transferred to the inner ear, and are transmitted to the brain via the cochlear branch of CN VIII. Thus, hearing is a complex process involving a number of structures and fluids. Box 73–1 describes the steps in this complex process.

Two qualities of sound—pitch and intensity—are important in understanding hearing. *Pitch* is related to the frequency of the sound wave (the number of cycles per second, called hertz, or Hz). Sounds can be high pitched (a soprano voice) or of lower pitch (alto or bass). High-pitched sounds stimulate different portions of the basilar membrane than low-pitched sounds. High-pitched sounds stimulate the basilar membrane near the base of the cochlea; low-pitched sounds stimulate the basilar membrane near the apex of the cochlea.

Intensity is related to the loudness of the sound and is measured in decibels (dB). Each 10-decibel increase in the intensity of sound is actually a tenfold increase in loudness. A ticking watch makes a sound of about 20 dB. A noisy restaurant usually registers at a sound level of about 70 dB. This means that the noisy restaurant is 100,000 times as loud as a ticking watch. Both pitch and intensity are important in interpreting sound.

Equilibrium

The inner ear provides information about the movement and position of the head. The saccule and utricle inform us about position when the head is still, whereas the semicircular canals provide information about changes in position.

Box 73–1   Process of Hearing

Air molecules in the atmosphere are disturbed, which causes them to bump into one another.

The movement of air molecules causes a vibration (sound wave) to form.

The sound wave travels through the air and strikes the auricle, which directs it into the external auditory canal.

The sound wave enters the external auditory canal and strikes the tympanic membrane, causing it to vibrate.

The vibrations are transferred to the ossicles (the malleus, incus, and stapes), which then begin to vibrate, transmitting the sound wave across the middle ear cavity to the oval window and into the inner ear.

The stapes, because of its anatomic design, exerts more than twice as much force on the oval window as is exerted on the malleus at the tympanic membrane. This increases the sound wave by about 3 dB.

Because the tympanic membrane has a much larger surface area than does the oval window (and thus the sound wave is transmitted from a larger to a smaller surface), the sound wave is amplified even further, by about 23 dB.

The amplified sound wave is transmitted to the perilymph, causing it to move in a fluid wave.

After a brief latent period, a reflex called the tympanic or sound attenuation reflex occurs in response to loud sounds. This reflex causes muscular contractions in the middle ear that dampen the vibrations of the ossicles and decrease the transmission of sounds before they reach the cochlea. Because of the latent period, however, this reflex provides little protection against sudden explosive loud sounds.

Pressure waves move the perilymph about; intense pressure waves cause the membrane of the round window to bulge out into the middle ear.

These pressure waves are transferred into the cochlea, where they cause the basilar membrane to move.

Movement of the basilar membrane causes the hairlike projections of the hair cells of the organ of Corti to move.

This movement signals the hair cells to release chemical transmitter substances onto the afferent endings of the cochlear division of CN VIII.

Action potentials are produced and conducted along the cochlear division.

Through synapses in the medulla, midbrain, and thalamus, these impulses are then transmitted to the cerebral cortex, where they are interpreted as sound.

We use this information to coordinate movements and to maintain balance. In these three organs of balance, receptor structures composed of hair cells with hairlike projections in contact with a gelatinous substance are sensitive to stimulation and movement of endolymph caused by changes in position. Displacement of the hairs alters the pattern of nerve impulses transmitted to the medulla and the cerebellum by the vesticular branch of CN VIII.

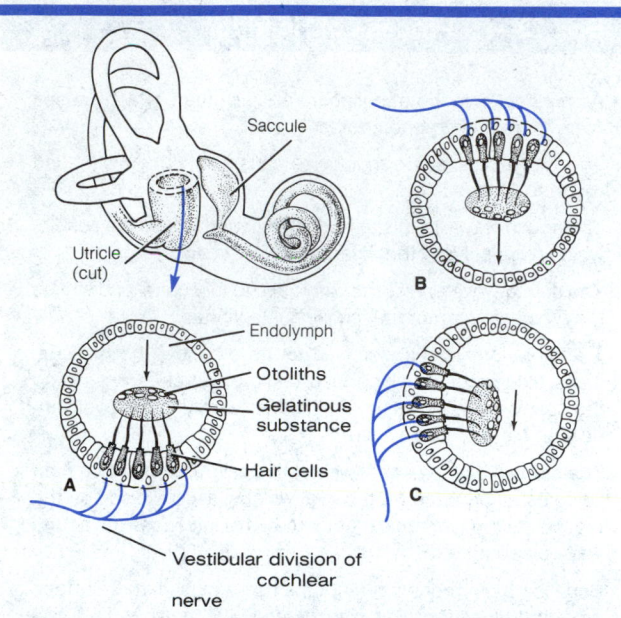

Figure 73–5

Stimulation of the macula within the utricle. The arrows indicate the direction of the force of gravity. **A.** Shows a macula when the head is in an upright position. **B.** Illustrates a macula when the head is inverted. **C.** Shows a macula when the head is in a horizontal position.

SOURCE: Spence AP, Mason EB: *Human Anatomy and Physiology,* 2nd ed. Menlo Park, CA: Benjamin/Cummings, 1983.

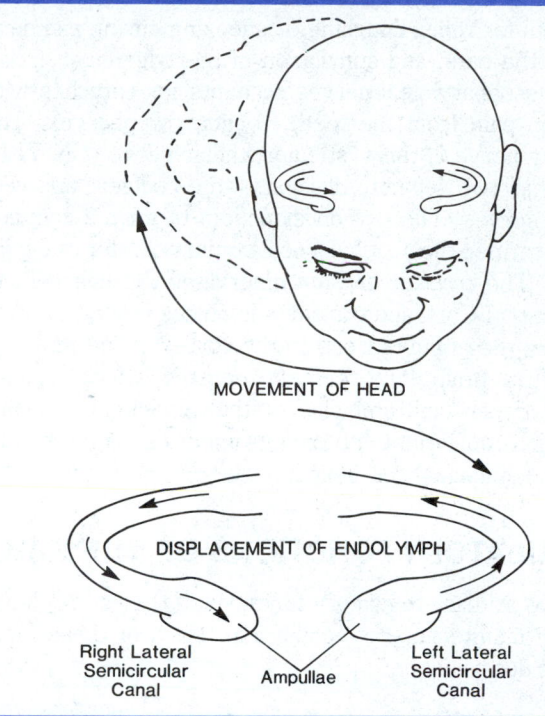

Figure 73–6

Movement of endolymph in relation to the right and left lateral semicircular ducts, which are oriented horizontally. Because the endolymph lags momentarily, movement of the head toward the right increases the pressure on the cupula within the ampulla of the right horizontal duct and reduces the pressure on the cupula in the ampulla of the left horizontal duct. The different nerve messages from the two cristae produce a sensation of turning.

SOURCE: Vick RL: *Contemporary Medical Physiology.* Menlo Park, CA: Addison–Wesley, 1984.

The receptor structure located within the utricle, the macula, and the otoliths that stimulate the hair cells provide information about the position of the head when the head is stationary. Figure 73–5 illustrates how the force of gravity or acceleration causes displacement of hair cells and alters the pattern of nerve impulses transmitted to the brain. Whether the saccule operates in the same way is not yet known.

The semicircular canals provide information about changes in position. The head causes movement of endo-lymph in at least one of the three semicircular canals (Figure 73–6). The receptors in the ampulla, the cristae, help maintain balance during starting, stopping, or turning movements.

Section II: Pathophysiological Influences and Effects

An understanding of pathophysiological influences and their effects on the ear requires a clear knowledge of the concepts of deafness, hearing loss, tinnitus, vertigo, and nystagmus.

A person who is deaf has nonfunctioning auditory systems. A person who has only one deaf ear is not considered deaf; deafness is an absolute lack of response to amplified sound.

A person with a hearing loss, or **hypoacusia,** has a functioning, though defective, auditory system and can respond to amplified sounds. Hearing loss can be classified as *conductive* (or peripheral), *sensorineural* (or perceptive), or *mixed* (or combined). Conductive hearing loss results from defective transmission of acoustic energy (sound) from the auricle to the hair cells of the organ of Corti. Conductive hearing loss generally occurs in the external ear, the middle ear, or both. Modern microsurgical observations have broadened the concept to include the cochlear fluid system in the inner ear (eg, a loss of perilymph fluid would also affect the transmission of energy). Sensorineural hearing loss results from dysfunction occurring anywhere in the neural pathway from the organ of Corti to the auditory cortex of the brain. Sensorineural hearing loss is sometimes referred to as central hearing loss. A combination of conductive and sensorineural hearing loss is called mixed, or combined, hearing loss.

Tinnitus is a sensation of noise such as ringing, buzzing, or hissing in the ear or head. It usually precedes, occurs with, or follows hearing loss. Tinnitus may be subjective (heard by the client) or objective (heard by the examiner).

Vertigo is a sensation of disturbed motion. Clients may feel that the room is twirling while they are stationary or that the room is stationary while they are twirling and falling. Vertigo can result from unequal firing of neurons from the right and left vestibular system in the ear or from other disorders in the central nervous system.

Nystagmus is an abnormal involuntary movement of both eyes either horizontally, vertically, diagonally, or circularly. Nystagmus can be caused by an unequal concentration of endolymph in one side of the semicircular canal or from disorders in the central nervous system.

CONGENITAL ALTERATIONS

Congenital alterations can appear at any time during the life cycle: at birth, immediately after delivery, during childhood, or during adulthood. They may be hereditary or acquired. Congenital hereditary disorders are caused by a genetic defect; they have a familial tendency and are usually associated with other abnormalities. Congenital acquired disorders, in contrast, result from the following:

- Trauma incurred during pregnancy or during delivery
- Syphilis and bacterial or viral infections of the mother during pregnancy
- Certain drugs taken by the mother during pregnancy
- Rh incompatibility
- Prematurity or prolonged anoxia of the infant

Congenital influences can cause structural malformations or missing parts of the ear, which can lead to deafness or conductive, sensorineural, or mixed hearing loss.

DEGENERATIVE ALTERATIONS

Degenerative changes in the ear are similar to those seen in other parts of the body. Loss of elasticity, thinning of the epidermis, and a decrease in secretions from the sebaceous glands result in dryness and pruritus of the external ear and narrowing of the auditory canal. Degenerative changes in the bones and joints of the ossicles can result in conductive hearing loss. Narrowing of blood vessels and the resulting decreased circulation to the inner ear can cause tinnitus, vertigo, or hearing loss. A decrease in the number of hair cells and nerve fibers with aging results in presbycusis, a gradual sensorineural hearing loss.

IMMUNOLOGIC ALTERATIONS

Contact dermatitis evidenced by pruritus and pain in the external ear is caused by an allergic reaction to earrings, hair dyes, cosmetics, or shampoos. Pollens, dusts, and other allergens can increase mucous secretions in the eustachian tube and the middle ear. These sticky secretions

cause malfunctions of the eustachian tube and decreased mobility of the tympanic membrane and ossicles, resulting in conductive hearing loss.

INFECTIOUS ALTERATIONS

Bacteria, yeasts, and fungi are the usual causes of infections of the external ear. These can result in excruciating pain or obstruction of the external auditory canal that leads to mild conductive hearing loss. Upper respiratory tract infections transmitted through the eustachian tube are usually responsible for middle and inner ear infections. These can cause fever, pain, and mild conductive hearing loss.

NEOPLASTIC ALTERATIONS

Neoplastic alterations of the ear, as in other parts of the body, may be benign or malignant. Basal and squamous cell carcinomas as well as melanomas can affect the skin of the external ear. Tumors can affect the middle ear, inner ear, or the auditory and facial nerves as they pass through the internal auditory canal. Middle ear tumors may be accompanied by extreme pain associated with otorrhea (discharge) and conductive hearing loss. Inner ear and nerve involvement can lead to vertigo, tinnitus, sensorineural hearing loss, and facial paralysis.

OBSTRUCTIVE ALTERATIONS

Impacted cerumen, foreign bodies, polyps, or edema can cause obstructions in the auditory system. The amount of cerumen within the ear canal varies from individual to individual; some tend to produce large amounts, which often obstruct the external canal. Foreign bodies include vegetable objects, such as peas or beans; beads; flying insects; or cotton. Attempts to remove such objects often result in trauma and infection, which lead to edema, pain, and temporary conductive hearing loss. Polyps in the external auditory canal may also obstruct the passage of sound waves.

Edema from an upper respiratory tract infection also occurs in the eustachian tube. Obstructions in the eustachian tube prevent air from entering the middle ear, causing an imbalance of pressure on either side of the tympanic membrane. Decreased pressure in the middle ear can disrupt the transmission of sound to the inner ear. Other obstructions resulting from trauma or neoplastic disorders cause pain as well as conductive and sensorineural hearing loss.

TRAUMATIC ALTERATIONS

Frostbite, lacerations, and bruises to the external ear, although painful, usually do not result in hearing loss. Direct blows to the head, however, can result in fractures of the temporal bone, dislocation of ossicles, lacerations in the mucous lining of the middle ear, rupture of the oval window and tympanic membrane, and damage to the auditory nerve. Trauma can lead to vertigo, pain, bleeding from the ear, nausea, vomiting, nystagmus, tinnitus, and conductive and sensorineural hearing losses. Hearing loss also can result from continued exposure to loud noise or sudden but limited exposure to a loud explosive sound.

Section III: Related System Influences and Effects

Disorders of the nervous, respiratory, circulatory, endocrine, and renal systems can affect the ear. Central nervous system disorders such as multiple sclerosis affect the auditory pathways, resulting in hearing loss. Bacterial and viral infections of the upper respiratory system affect the middle ear through the eustachian tube. Decreased circulation or vascular occlusion can result in vertigo; however, more research is needed to show the relationship with hearing losses. Although no definite proof can be found, there appears to be a relationship between hearing loss and hypothyroidism (Goodhill, 1979).

With impairment of the renal system, drugs that are mainly or entirely excreted by the kidneys can accumulate within the bloodstream. Ototoxic drugs (drugs with a noxious effect on CN VIII) may accumulate in the inner ear and cause tinnitus and a gradual sensorineural hearing loss. Acetylsalicylic acid (aspirin) is a drug that is mainly excreted by the kidneys. High doses are administered to obtain anti-inflammatory action in such diseases as arthritis. Acetylsalicylic acid inhibits the biosynthesis and release of prostaglandins, which have a role in the control of renal circulation and thus may impair renal function. The exact cause of ototoxicity of acetylsalicylic acid is unknown, but it is thought to be due to an inhibition of the oxidative enzymes in the cochlea. The hearing loss is usually bilateral but is reversible 7 to 10 days after acetylsalicylic acid use is discontinued. Hemodialysis and renal transplantation are frequently accompanied by sensorineural hearing loss and vestibular lesions. The administration of high doses of drugs may be a factor in this relationship.

Section IV: Psychosocial/Lifestyle Influences and Effects

Impaired hearing has both psychosocial/lifestyle influences and effects: It hinders communication with others, it restricts the ability to be productive, and it interferes with having fun and enjoying life. It reduces feelings of personal security, diminishes the sense of self-worth, and leads to isolation. Thus, impaired hearing strikes at the essence of what it is to be human.

DEVELOPMENTAL INFLUENCES

Problems of hearing affect psychosocial development. Those who do not hear well often find that their ability to communicate verbally is impaired, making it more difficult to resolve the psychosocial tasks successfully at various developmental stages and to meet the challenges of education and job preparation.

Many features of contemporary society lend themselves to disorders of the ear. Our society is mobile, which increases the risk of vehicular accidents, barotrauma during rapid changes of altitude, and aerotitis media related to air travel. Even advancements in medical science are risky (eg, the increased use of ototoxic drugs increases the risk of sensorineural hearing loss). An increase in teenage pregnancies is another factor. Some teenagers may not have medical care available, and others may seek prenatal care only late in their pregnancies, increasing the risk of congenital problems. While postponing prenatal care is a problem regardless of age, it is more common among teenagers.

Psychosocial development, especially in relation to autonomy and independence, is often delayed in hearing-impaired people. Well-meaning family members and friends may be overprotective, thus increasing the person's isolation and dependence on others and decreasing self-confidence. Because hearing-impaired children seldom have the opportunity to meet deaf adults who could function as positive role models, they tend to develop a less positive self-image in relation to hearing adults.

SEX AND AGE

More men than women have hearing impairment. This may be due largely to the fact that men are more likely to have been exposed to harmful levels of noise in the workplace than have women. Now that more women work outside the house, however, there is an increase in their reported instances of hearing problems that can be traced to the work environment. One genetic disorder, otosclerosis, is more common among women.

The instances of hearing loss increase with age (US Public Health Service, 1982); some degree of hearing loss is first noticed around age 50. It is one of the top three chronic conditions among the aging population, occurring in 25% over age 65, in 50% over age 75, and in 90% of the residents in nursing homes (Porcino, 1983).

DIETARY HABITS

Osteomalacia and sensorineural deafness are thought to be associated (Brookes & Morrison, 1981). Deficiencies of vitamin D and ionized calcium are thought to affect the transmission of action potentials generated by the cochlea. Lohle (1982) found a correlation between vitamin A deficiency and auditory thresholds in both animal and human experiments. More research on the role of nutrition in hearing impairment is needed.

ECONOMIC FACTORS

Insufficient family income that results in inadequate shelter, clothing, nutrition, or health care may result in eventual hearing impairment. These factors tend to reduce resistance to infections and to increase exposure to traumatic elements in the environment such as cold, noise, and pollution.

Hearing-impaired people may be forced into early retirement, reducing their income. In addition to its effects on individuals, early retirement under these circumstances also hurts society as a whole because it cannot benefit from the contributions of this segment of the population. Hearing loss can prove to be costly to individuals in other ways as well. For example, although Medicare covers the costs of hearing evaluation and analysis, it does not cover the cost of correcting hearing loss. Medicare specifically excludes hearing aids and related services from reimbursement.

OCCUPATION AND AVOCATION

Hazardous noises in the workplace also cause hearing loss. Industrial workers exposed to the loud sounds of jet engines and heavy machinery, military personnel exposed to gunshots, and entertainers exposed to amplified music are especially vulnerable to noise-induced hearing loss. The Occupational Safety and Health Act (OSHA) of 1971 first established guidelines for acceptable levels of noise exposure and standards for hearing protection and testing in industry. These guidelines were amended in 1983 (see Table 75–2). Noise exposure can be measured more accurately by recently developed individual dosimeters worn by workers. Unfortunately, workers—especially older workers—may be afraid to reveal their hearing loss to employers lest they lose their jobs. They may stay in environments that increase hearing loss.

Hearing loss may cause great stress in people with jobs in which acute hearing is important (eg, musicians, telephone operators, mental health counselors, and secretaries). Hearing loss may require that workers reevaluate their jobs or careers and consider the possibility of making a change.

An increased general interest in physical fitness and conditioning has caused larger numbers of people to participate in sports such as swimming, diving, and racket ball. Ear infections from water sports and trauma to the ear from a ball hit at speeds over 100 mph are possible.

ENVIRONMENT

Community noise is a major problem in contemporary society. Increased noise from vehicular traffic is one aspect of the problem. Another is the growing number of noisy labor-saving devices used in most homes, which exposes residents to levels of noise as hazardous as those in many industrial environments. The tendency of some young people to wear stereo headsets for long periods may also have some damaging effects. Monitoring noise pollution remains a complex problem for study and is discussed further in Chapter 75. Pollution of lakes, rivers, and other waterways can also lead to hearing damage because of infections.

ROLES AND RELATIONSHIPS

Hearing losses create tensions within families and friendships. Because hearing loss is not a visible handicap, many people become impatient with the person whose hearing is impaired. This may result in misunderstandings, irritation, and suspicion on both parts.

Chapter Highlights

The ears are special sensory organs whose major functions are hearing and maintaining equilibrium.

The nurse needs knowledge of the structure and function of the ear to understand the transmission of sound through the ear to the cerebral cortex.

Knowledge of the vestibular system of the inner ear will enable the nurse to understand how the body maintains its sense of equilibrium in coordination with the muscular and ocular systems.

Alterations in the structure and function of the auditory system can lead to deafness, hearing loss, tinnitus, vertigo, and nystagmus.

Deafness is an absolute lack of response to amplified sound. A person who is deaf has bilateral non-functioning auditory systems.

Hearing loss can be classified as conductive, sensorineural, or mixed.

(continued)

Chapter Highlights *(continued)*

Congenital, degenerative, neoplastic, and traumatic alterations can result in sensorineural, conductive, or mixed hearing loss.

Obstructive, immunologic, and infectious alterations usually result in conductive hearing loss.

Disorders of the nervous, respiratory, circulatory, endocrine, and renal systems can adversely affect hearing and equilibrium.

Ototoxic drugs may cause tinnitus and a gradual sensorineural hearing loss.

Hearing loss affects the psychosocial development of an individual. Language and communication skills,

if not developed, can lead to isolation, decreased self-esteem, and dependency.

Contemporary sociocultural changes affecting hearing are increased teenage pregnancies with higher incidences of congenital problems, hearing loss that is due to increased environmental noise, and injuries resulting from an increased interest in physical sports.

Nutritional and economic deficiencies can contribute to increased susceptibility to infections and hearing loss.

Bibliography

Brookes E, Morrison AW: Vitamin D deficiency and deafness. *Brit Med J* (July) 1981; 283: 273–274.

Danino J et al: Tinnitus as a prognostic factor in sudden deafness. *Am J Otolaryngology* 1984; 5(6):394–396.

DeWeese D, Saunders W: *Textbook of Otolaryngology,* 6th ed. St. Louis: Mosby, 1982.

Goodhill V: *Ear Diseases, Deafness and Dizziness.* Hagerstown, MD: Harper & Row, 1979.

Lohle E: The influences of chronic vitamin A deficiency on human and animal ears. *Arch Otorhinolaryngol* 1982; 234(2):167–173.

Marshall K, Attia E: *Disorders of the Ear.* Boston: John Wright-PSG, 1983.

Porcino J: *Growing Older, Getting Better.* Menlo Park, CA: Addison-Wesley, 1983.

US Public Health Service: *Vital and Health Statistics. Hearing Ability of Persons by Sociodemographic and Health Characteristics: United States.* PHHS Pub. No. (PHS) 82–1568. US Government Printing Office, Series 10, No. 140, 1982.

Suggested Readings

Bateman HE, Mason RM: *Applied Anatomy and Physiology of the Speech and Hearing Mechanism.* Springfield, IL: Thomas, 1984. This visually oriented book contains detailed information related to the structure and function of speech and hearing. It is also clinically focused and emphasizes client concerns.

LoGrasso BA: Using words without sound. *Am J Nurs* 1980; 80:2186–2187. In this article, a nurse shares her experience of living, working, and going to school with deaf persons.

Lysons K: *Your Hearing Loss and How to Cope With It.* North Pomfret, VT: David & Charles, 1978. This is an easy-to-read book that deals with the main problems encountered with hearing impairment. The author describes his own feelings about accepting hearing loss; what can be done for rehabilitation; and problems concerning employment, leisure, and family relations. A good book to recommend to clients and their families.

Chapter 74

The Nursing Process for Clients With Auditory System Dysfunction

Dominica Ann Limburg
Carol Ren Kneisl
SueAnn Wooster Ames

Objectives

When you have finished studying this chapter, you should be able to:

Identify specific subjective and objective data essential to establishing a data base for clients with disorders of the ears.

Describe diagnostic studies used for assessing auditory and vestibular functions.

State the essential information the nurse should collect before scheduling a client for radiographic studies.

Discuss nursing diagnoses and their applications to the client with a disorder of the ears.

Describe the planning and implementation of nursing care relative to preventing hearing loss and preserving hearing, maintaining and enhancing communication, and meeting the physiological and psychosocial needs of clients with auditory system dysfunction.

Discuss specific communication skills that the nurse can use when caring for a client with hearing impairment.

Identify specific environmental conditions that enhance the client's hearing during all phases of the nursing process.

Explain the uses, types, limitations, and care of hearing aids.

The nurse plays a significant role in the prevention and early detection of disorders of the ears, as well as in the rehabilitation of clients with these disorders. These activities occur not only in the hospital, but also in schools, industrial environments, and other community settings. To prevent infections in the ears and trauma to the auditory system, the nurse participates in educational programs, teaching proper hygiene of the ears and upper respiratory system. Through auditory screening programs, the nurse engages in the early detection and monitoring of hearing loss. Encouraging and assisting in the monitoring of environmental hazards such as noise pollution and swimming area pollution are also nursing responsibilities. Education about the effectiveness and proper use of protective devices such as earplugs is also part of the nurse's role.

The nurse is frequently the first to recognize hearing impairment through periodic examination of the ears and assessment of hearing. Assessing, diagnosing, and removing impacted cerumen often improves the hearing problem. By learning to communicate with hearing-impaired people, the nurse can help prevent loneliness, depression, and isolation. Educating the client's family members and significant others about aids for communication and safety measures within the home is often necessary. The nurse should encourage family members to include the client in conversations and social gatherings. Family members also need instruction in the care and use of hearing aids.

In the hospital and other health care settings, the nurse cares for the individual both preoperatively and postoperatively. Through accurate assessments, the nurse prevents or identifies complications and begins early interventions. Clients are assisted to return to their previous lifestyles as soon as possible.

Section I: Nursing Assessment: Establishing the Data Base

The nurse should be aware of special considerations in assessing people with disorders affecting the ears. Many have hearing loss, so the nurse should select an environment that enhances hearing. Background noises often affect the ability of the client to hear words correctly. Thus, the room should be quiet, with radios and televisions turned off. Lighting should allow clients to see the nurse's face, because they may be relying on speech reading (watching visible gestures plus lip reading) for communication. A pencil and paper should be available if necessary. If the client uses manual (sign) communication, it might be necessary to use an interpreter.

Attentive listening, using all the senses, is especially important when assessing a hearing-impaired client. Touching, preferably on the arm, is important in gaining the client's attention. Be alert for signs of fatigue; communication is an effort for some hearing-impaired clients, and they hear and understand less when they are tired. Thus, contacts of short duration may yield more information for the nurse.

SUBJECTIVE DATA

The health history should begin with an exploration of the client's chief concern, whether it is pain (otalgia), discharge (otorrhea), tinnitus, vertigo, or a decrease in hearing. Use of the seven dimensions, or the PQRST, of evaluating a symptom will help the nurse gather the pertinent information (see Chapter 7).

Otalgia may be caused by a specific disorder of the ear itself or by referred pain from other diseases of the head and neck. Differentiating between the two in the history is important for accurate care planning. Referred pain to the ear may be associated with temporomandibular joint disorders, malocclusion, or nocturnal teeth grinding (bruxism). Carious teeth; lesions of the mouth, tongue, hypopharynx, or larynx; or calculi in the parotid or submaxillary duct also may cause referred pain to the ear. Otalgia directly related to the ear may be secondary to trauma, infection, allergies, the presence of foreign bodies, impacted cerumen, or benign or malignant growths. Therefore, the history should elicit information about sports activities, particularly swimming and diving. Direct trauma to the ear can be caused by many contact and racket sports. Swimmer's ear (diffuse bacterial external otitis) is a common cause of ear pain. Barotrauma, which results from excessive ear pressure due to rapid or extensive altitude changes, can cause rupture of the tympanic membrane.

The nurse should ask questions about recent infections. For example, the client may have pain from enlarged cervical or auricular lymph nodes secondary to an upper respiratory tract infection that is referred to the ear. However, the client may also have an inflammation of the eustachian tube (eustachian tube salpingitis). The inflammation creates a vacuum in the inner ear with unilateral or bilateral middle ear effusion and retracted tympanic membrane(s), causing discomfort and a feeling that the ear needs to pop or crack.

An allergy history is important to document any seasonal allergies causing ear symptoms and nasal congestion, such as hay fever. Often the symptoms of seasonal allergy are similar to those of a viral upper respiratory tract infection (see Table 19–2 in Chapter 19). Medication allergies are also important, because the client may be using something topically on the auricle for pruritus or discomfort— eg, around a bothersome pierced ear opening—that is causing weeping, flaking, and inflammation rather than curing the problem.

One of the most common trauma and foreign body problems in adults is related to care of the ears. Many people dig in their ears with paper clips and cotton swabs. Clients come to ambulatory care facilities with trauma to the auditory canal or tympanic membrane, or with foreign bodies in their ears, because of improper cleaning with small, sharp objects. Clients might be advised facetiously that nothing smaller than their elbows should enter their ears.

Cerumen is problematic for many clients because it may cause scaling, pruritus, discomfort, and a decrease in hearing. Proper mastication normally takes care of cerumen by moving it to the external ear, where it flakes off unnoticed or is easily washed off. Therefore, a history of dental or jaw problems is significant. Clients with ill-fitting dentures or those who do not wear their dentures at all chew poorly and thus interfere with normal cerumen removal. Clients who work in areas where there is considerable dust and dirt also may build up more cerumen, because the wax, in trapping this foreign material, tends to become harder and thicker. These clients need health education regarding safe ways to loosen and remove cerumen.

Otorrhea is an annoying symptom for many clients. Discharge may accompany external otitis or otitis media, or it may indicate the presence of a foreign body. Question clients about the color, odor, and amount of the discharge. Certain organisms causing otorrhea have characteristic odors (eg, drainage from the ear caused by *Pseudomonas* often smells sweet). (See Table 74–1 for characteristics of otorrhea.)

The nurse should also ask the client about *tinnitus*. This can accompany other symptoms such as otalgia and otorrhea secondary to impacted cerumen, the presence of a foreign body, or inflammation. It may also occur alone, can be extremely annoying and uncomfortable, and can interfere with sleep and normal daily activities. There are two types of tinnitus: ear tinnitus and cranial tinnitus. *Ear tinnitus,* which is caused by disorders of the ear, may be accompanied by hearing loss. *Cranial tinnitus* is associated with cerebrovascular and other intracranial lesions.

Table 74–1	Otorrhea: Color and Usual Cause	
Appearance of Discharge	**Usual Cause**
Yellow	Soft cerumen
Green	Acute external otitis
Serous	Eczematous lesions of auditory canal wall; early acute otitis media; cerebral spinal fluid from fracture of middle cranial fossa
Purulent	Acute or chronic otitis media; tuberculous otitis media; cholesteatoma
Bloody	Trauma to auditory canal walls; rupture of tympanic membrane; fracture of middle cranial fossa

Specific data to be collected include the perceived site of the tinnitus, its loudness and pitch, and its disappearance in the presence of other sounds. Tinnitus may be louder at night or certain times of the day or week. It may vary with the position of the head or body. Low-pitched tinnitus is most often related to disorders of the outer or middle ear, such as infections or trauma. Continuous high-pitched tinnitus often occurs with noise-induced hearing loss. An occupational history elicits noise exposure information. The nurse should explore noise exposure in the home and environment. High-pitched tinnitus is also associated with an ototoxic reaction to drugs such as propranolol, caffeine, salicylates, quinidine, and indomethacin. A drug history is therefore essential and should include all OTC drugs as well as prescription drugs that the client is taking or has taken in the past. The drug history also should include any history of drug allergies or side effects that the client has experienced.

Vertigo is a spinning sensation; either the client feels as if he or she were spinning or as if the room were whirling around the client. It is frequently associated with nystagmus, nausea, and vomiting. Vertigo is the most common symptom of a vestibular disorder. The health history can assist in differentiating between true vertigo and dysequilibrium. Vertigo may accompany diseases of the middle or inner ear; labyrinthitis, Meniere's syndrome, and damage to CN VIII are all possible causes. For these reasons, a thorough history of infections, trauma, and use of ototoxic drugs is essential, as is information on the nature of the spinning, time of day, and aggravating and alleviating factors. *Dysequilibrium* is a nonvestibular symptom of spacial disorientation. It is related to changes in cerebral oxygenation, changes in blood pressure, drugs, visual or emotional disturbances, and various metabolic disorders. Sedatives such as barbiturates can cause dysequilibrium, and antihistamines and diazepam are also implicated. Dysequilibrium is often described as an unsteadiness,

queasiness, faintness, light-headedness, or a blacking-out sensation. It usually is not accompanied by nystagmus.

Careful questioning about any decrease in hearing is critical to the evaluation of the client with ear dysfunction. The client may not report a hearing loss until it is quite extensive. Family members or significant others are usually the first to recognize the loss. The nurse can obtain information relating to impaired hearing through questions such as these:

- Is the hearing loss in one or both ears?
- Was the onset sudden or gradual?
- Is hearing more problematic in particular situations (eg, large groups)?
- Are all sounds or just certain sounds diminished?
- Is there a family history of hearing loss?

For the client with a known hearing loss, information specific to aural rehabilitation should be obtained. For example, does the client communicate manually or use speech reading? Usually, younger clients have been taught these skills, but older clients may need considerable assistance. Does the client use a hearing aid? Is it effective? Often clients have purchased a hearing aid but do not use it. Find out why it is not being used. Many clients are reluctant to accept their hearing disability, so they may reject the use of a hearing aid because it then becomes obvious that they have a hearing impairment. Some may not take the time to adjust to its use, and others may not have the financial resources to purchase a hearing aid and batteries and to provide for repairs. Also, many elderly clients do not have the manual dexterity to use or clean hearing aids.

The nurse can identify any lifestyle changes that have occurred as a result of the hearing impairment by asking about the client's activities during a 24-hour period. The client's role and responsibility in the family may be altered and diminished. An inability to participate in family discussions becomes frustrating for the client. Family members or significant others also become frustrated in trying to communicate and begin to ignore the client when the communication becomes difficult. Communication difficulties can also occur in social groups. The hearing-impaired person finds it difficult to enjoy meetings, parties, or lectures, or even to follow normal dinner table conversation. These difficulties result in client withdrawal from everyday activities and eventually isolation, which can result in depression. The acceptance of the hearing loss helps motivate the client to overcome communication difficulties through rehabilitation programs, the use of a hearing aid, or both.

The nurse should gather additional health history information about health risks. Both smoking and lack of exercise can affect ear disorders. Smoking irritates the mucous membranes in the upper respiratory tract, which can alter the function of the eustachian tube and lead to infections in the middle ear. Nicotine also causes blood vessel constriction. Auditory and vestibular functions rely on good circulation to the structures of the ear. Atherosclerosis and other vascular disorders are related to lack of exercise. A history of other illnesses related to the cardiovascular system may elicit valuable information. For example, clients with diabetes mellitus can experience hearing loss or vertigo because of associated vascular changes.

Eliciting information relating to resources and support systems that the client uses will aid in the planning of care. Support systems may include family, friends, or community groups. The elderly person living alone, however, often has no support system. The nurse also should identify the availability and client use of health services, as well as the availability of emergency contacts. The client's financial status also should be explored. The nurse may identify the need for social work referral for assistance with meeting the costs of rehabilitation programs.

Individuals with hearing loss function effectively in many professions and vocations, but they may experience difficulty in areas of employment that depend on sensory perception for safety, such as some assembly line positions. Through the history, the nurse may identify a need for vocational counseling. Vocational counselors assist clients in job relocation or suggest adaptations in the existing workplace for the hearing-impaired. For example, a client who is gradually developing a noise-induced hearing loss that may be exacerbated by working in a noisy environment may be helped to find a similar position in a quieter environment or to find ways to reduce the noise in the present job.

OBJECTIVE DATA

Objective data related to the ears are obtained from a physical assessment, the assessment of auditory and vestibular functions, laboratory tests, and diagnostic studies. A thorough head and neck examination, the Romberg test, and gait assessment accompany examination of the ears. Since disorders of the ears are often related to problems in other body systems such as the endocrine, renal, or cardiac systems, a comprehensive physical assessment is advisable. However, only specific examination of the ears and related structures will be discussed here. Also see Chapter 7.

Physical Assessment

Vital signs are basic to any physical assessment, including that for auditory dysfunction. Increased temperature alerts the nurse to infection, and blood pressure alterations alert the nurse to any renal or circulatory alterations that may affect auditory function.

Inspection, palpation, and auscultation are used to examine the external ears and mastoid area. Visualization of the external auditory canal and the tympanic membrane requires additional lighting and a speculum.

Examination begins by looking at the position of the auricle. An auricle that is absent, asymmetrical or abnormal in configuration, as well as ears set low, are indications of

Box 74–1   Selected Abnormalities of the Auricle and Around It

Congenital Findings

Microtia: Unusually small auricle

Macrotia: Unusually large auricle

Protrusion of auricle at right angles to the head (lop ear)

Congenital absence of auricle

Nodules

Gouty tophi: Accumulations of uric acid crystals in the helix or anthelix; painless; seen in gout

Keloids: Nodular masses of scar tissue seen on pierced earlobe

Sebaceous cysts: Often seen behind the ear

Darwinian tubercles: Small painless elevations near the upper third of the helix; a congenital variation

Enlarged preauricular or postauricular lymph nodes: More easily palpated than visualized

Lesions

Squamous cell carcinomas: Crusted, ulcerated, or indurated lesions that fail to heal

Warts of viral origin

Trauma-Related Findings

Hematomas: May appear as blue masses on the auricle; should be aspirated to prevent cauliflower ear

Cauliflower ear: Auricle misshapen by fibrosis secondary to trauma

congenital defects. Box 74–1 summarizes selected abnormalities of the auricle and around it. Normally, the position of the ears does not vary or varies slightly from a horizontal line drawn across the inner and outer canthus of the eyes to the tip of the helix. A line drawn from the top to the bottom of the ear should not vary more than 10° from the vertical (Figure 74–1). The anterior and posterior surfaces of the auricle, the external auditory canal, and the mastoid areas are carefully inspected for skin changes, redness, swelling, or evidence of lesions or nodules. Observe clients wearing hearing aids for signs of irritation from ill-fitting molds. Palpation is useful in assessing for tenderness, heat, swelling, deformities, and crepitus. Areas palpated should include the auricles; the mastoid process; and the preauricular, postauricular, occipital, and cervical lymph nodes. Referred pain from the temporomandibular joint may be identified by crepitus in the joint. Palpate the joint by placing a finger in the joint space anterior to the ear while the client opens and closes the jaw or by placing

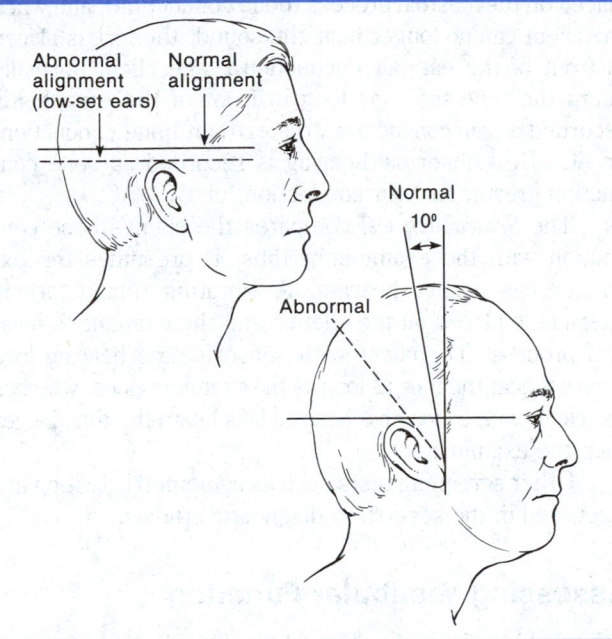

Figure 74–1

Normal and abnormal ear alignment.

Table 74–2 Visible Abnormalities of the Tympanic Membrane	
Appearance of Tympanic Membrane	**Cause**
Areas with white streaks or flecks	Old scarring secondary to healed inflammation
Amber colored	Serous fluid showing through tympanic membrane as amber color; seen with serous otitis media
Air bubbles behind tympanic membrane; air/fluid levels	Serous otitis media with eustachian tube salpingitis
Retracted with accentuated landmarks and distorted or absent light reflex	Eustachian tube obstruction or salpingitis
Bright red and bulging; no luster or light reflex	Acute suppurative otitis media
Blue-black (hematotympanum); no light reflex	Blood in middle ear secondary to trauma
Old perforations (oval holes through which dark shadow can be seen)	Usually secondary to acute otitis media

the finger within the ear and pressing downward while the client opens and closes the jaw. Normally, a click may be heard or felt.

The nurse uses auscultation over the auditory canal to detect objective tinnitus and auscultation over the mastoid area to detect bruits.

The otoscope is used to inspect the auditory canal for cerumen, foreign bodies, inflammation, swelling, bleeding, discharge, lesions, and growths. Removal of the cerumen may be necessary for an unobstructed view and is discussed later in this chapter. The amount, color, odor, and consistency of any otorrhea should be noted at this time.

Skill in the use of the otoscope is necessary for observing the normal landmarks of the tympanic membrane. The use of the otoscope is described and illustrated in Chapter 7. Accentuation of the landmarks suggests a retracted membrane. Inability to visualize any of the landmarks suggests a bulging or thickened membrane. Other abnormalities include changes in color, scarring, increased vascularization (injection), perforations, and discharges. Selected abnormalities and descriptions are found in Table 74–2.

Mobility of the tympanic membrane is tested with a pneumatic otoscope. A rubber squeeze bulb with tube is attached to the otoscope by a connecting tube (Figure 74–2). Squeezing the bulb pushes air into the canal, causing the membrane to move inward. Removing the air causes the membrane to bulge outward. No movement or jerky movement of the tympanic membrane suggests middle ear disease or an obstructed eustachian tube. Tympanometry, discussed in the section on diagnostic studies, is another more accurate assessment of tympanic membrane mobility.

Assessing Auditory Function

Hearing evaluation begins with the initial contact between nurse and client. Nurses should be alert for clues of hearing loss in all client interactions, not just in those related to complaints about the ears. Clues include turning of the head, cupping of the ears, or leaning toward the speaker. Nurses might suspect hearing loss if the client's voice is unusually loud or has a monotonous or unvaried tone, if word endings are omitted, or if certain types of words need to be repeated. Nurses should be alert for hearing loss if

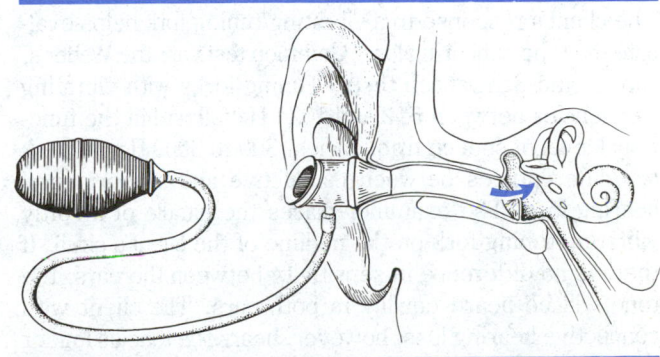

Figure 74–2

Pneumatic otoscopy to detect diminished or absent mobility of the tympanic membrane.

clients do not answer questions when they cannot see the nurse's mouth or if they answer questions inappropriately. Gross hearing screening is performed by the voice, watch tick, and tuning fork tests. More accurate testing requires an audiometer. Hearing tests provide information that assists in the diagnosis of hearing impairment and identifies the client's need for aural rehabilitation.

Voice Test

The voice test provides a gross assessment of the client's ability to hear the whispered or normally spoken word. Each ear is tested separately. The client or examiner masks or occludes one of the client's ears by placing a finger within the ear. This does not prevent all hearing by this ear, so better results are obtained when the occluding finger is rapidly but gently moved back and forth in the ear while the examiner whispers numbers or words to the other ear at a distance of 30 to 60 cm (1 to 2 ft). The examiner then asks the client to repeat numbers that have two equally accented syllables, such as nine-four. To prevent lip reading, the client is asked to look away from the examiner, or the examiner stands behind the client. Normally, softly whispered words are heard bilaterally. If the client cannot hear the whisper, the examiner increases the intensity of the voice to a medium and then a loud whisper, then to a soft, medium, and loud voice.

Watch Tick Test

In performing the watch tick test, the examiner observes the client's ability to hear the ticking of a watch at a distance of 2 to 5 cm (1 to 2 in). Use of the watch tick test is limited, however, because it only tests high-frequency loss. Frequency refers to the number of vibratory cycles per second of sound and is expressed in hertz. A sound perceived as a low tone in pitch has a low frequency, whereas a sound perceived as a high tone in pitch has a high frequency. Hearing is most sensitive in frequencies of 500 to 4000 Hz. Higher frequencies are usually affected first with sensorineural hearing loss. Choose a watch carefully, because many watches today do not have a discernible tick.

Tuning Fork Tests

The client's response to a vibrating tuning fork helps evaluate the type of hearing loss. Common tests are the Weber's, Rinne, and Schwabach tests. Tuning forks with vibrating frequencies between 512 and 1024 Hz fall within the functional level of speech frequencies, 300 to 3000 Hz. *Weber's test* differentiates between conductive and sensorineural hearing loss. The examiner places the handle of a softly vibrating tuning fork on the midline of the client's skull. If there is no difference in sensitivity between the ears, the tone will be heard equally in both ears. The client with conductive hearing loss, however, hears the tone as louder in the poorer ear; the client with sensorineural loss hears the tone as louder in the better ear.

The *Rinne test* also helps evaluate conductive and sensorineural hearing loss. A softly vibrating tuning fork is placed on the mastoid process (bone conduction), and when the client can no longer hear the sound, the fork is placed in front of the ear (air conduction). The client normally hears the tone twice as long in front of the ear; this is recorded as air conduction greater than bone conduction, or AC>BC. Abnormal hearing is recorded as bone conduction greater than air conduction, or BC>AC.

The *Schwabach test* compares the client's bone conduction with the examiner's; thus, it presumes the examiner has normal hearing. A vibrating tuning fork is alternately placed on the client's and the examiner's mastoid process. The client with sensorineural hearing loss does not hear the tone as long as the examiner does, whereas the client with conductive hearing loss hears the tone longer than the examiner.

Other screening tests such as audiometric testing are discussed in the section on diagnostic studies.

Assessing Vestibular Function

Labyrinthine disorders are evaluated by checking for nystagmus, for falling (the Romberg test), or for past pointing. To evaluate past pointing, the client sits facing the nurse with the eyes closed and the arms extended. The nurse touches the client's extended index fingers with his or her own fingers. Maintain this position while the client raises the hands above the head and then attempts to reassume the initial position (touching the fingers). The client's eyes remain closed. Past pointing is interpreted as the client deviating to the right or left of the target fingers and indicates inner ear stimulation or loss of position sense. Checking for nystagmus is discussed later in this chapter, and the Romberg test is discussed in Chapter 7.

Vestibular assessment also include cerebellar testing, including evaluation of gait. Since causes of vertigo are related not only to the vestibular system but also frequently to the central nervous system, an examination of all the cranial nerves is also indicated. Other vestibular studies include electronystagmography (ENG) and the caloric test discussed in the section on diagnostic studies.

Diagnostic Studies

Laboratory and diagnostic studies are used to corroborate historical and physical findings. These studies contribute to an accurate diagnosis or help monitor the results of therapy. Knowledge of the studies aids the nurse in preparing and supporting the client. The hearing-impaired client is usually anxious when hospitalized. To relieve anxiety, the nurse should be sure the client understands the proposed procedure and, if necessary, should support the client during the study.

Culture and Sensitivity

Common microbiological tests related to otologic infections include smears and cultures of secretions plus an antibiotic sensitivity test. Experienced physicians familiar with common infections often make clinical diagnoses without laboratory studies. Cultures are usually indicated when the client has a long history of an infection or does not respond to prescribed therapy.

Sterile cotton-tipped applicators used through a sterile speculum collect specimens from the external ear. For middle ear specimens, it may be necessary to perform needle aspirations through the tympanic membrane (tympanocentesis) or aspirations with a sterile suction tip through a tympanic perforation or small incision in the membrane (myringotomy). Cultures are examined for the presence of bacteria, fungi, or yeasts. Gram's stain is used for a gross differentiation of the bacterial flora. Hansel's stain is used to determine cytological details and for polymorphonuclear leukocytes, eosinophils, and lymphocytes. Such studies assist in the differentiation of allergies and infections. If allergies are suspected, skin testing is done.

Blood and Urine Tests

Serum tests include the fluorescent treponemal antibody absorption (FTA-ABS) test to rule out syphilis. Serum analysis for toxic levels of drugs and hematologic tests rule out leukemia, anemia, polycythemia, or other blood dys-

crasias that produce otologic disturbances. Urinalysis also is used to detect the presence of drugs or other metabolic disturbances. Table 74–3 gives normal and abnormal test values.

Radiographic Studies

Two screening radiographic views of the temporal bone aid in the diagnosis of inflammatory disease and other conditions leading to hearing loss: (1) the Schuller view of the lateral mastoid and (2) the Stenver view of the internal auditory canal, the inner ear, and the petrous pyramid (the densest part of the temporal bone behind the vestibule). Tomography allows visualization of the desired structure while the areas in front of it or behind it are obscured. The tomographic examination of the temporal bone consists of a series of exposures taken 1 or 2 mm apart in different positions. Although total x-ray exposure to the client is an important consideration in using this technique, 30 tomograms expose the client to less radiation than a single routine chest x-ray.

Before exposing a client to radiographic studies, obtain information about allergies (especially to iodine) and the date of the last menstrual period to determine if the client is pregnant.

Table 74–3 Laboratory Studies Related to Disorders of the Ear

Laboratory Test	Normal Expected Value	Disease State	Expected Abnormal Findings
FTA–ABS	Nonreactive	Syphilis	Reactive
White blood cells	4500–11,000 cells/μL	Inflammatory process such as otitis media or furuncles	Increased
Neutrophils	Relative value 54%–75% Absolute value 3000–7500 cells/μL	Increased immune system function (otitis)	Increased
Lymphocytes	Relative value 25%–40% Absolute value 1500–4500 cells/μL	Increased immune system function (otitis)	Increased
Eosinophils	Relative value 1%–4% Absolute value 50–400 cells/μL	Allergies	Increased
Urinalysis	Protein 2–8 mg/100 mL of urine	Kidney disorders	Protein more than 20 mg/ 100 mL of urine
Gram's stain	Middle ear sterile	Otitis media	Presence of gram-negative or gram-positive bacilli or cocci
Cultures	Middle ear, sterile; external ear, certain fungi and bacillus species, diphtheroids, staphylococci	Otitis media, external otitis	Presence of bacteria, *Aspergillus fumigatus, Candida albicans, Pseudomonas aeruginosa, Staphylococcus aureus,* streptococci, coliform bacilli
Antibody susceptibility test	Ability of various antimicrobials to slow or stop growth	Isolated organism from culture	

Audiometric Testing

The *audiometer* is an electronic instrument that generates pure tones of different frequencies and intensities. Audiometric tests differentiate between conductive and sensorineural hearing loss and provide information about the amount and degree of hearing loss. Most audiometric tests are administered by audiologists although nurses in community settings often perform screening (pure tone) audiometry. Audiometric testing should be conducted in a quiet, preferably soundproof, room. The two most common screening tests are pure tone and speech audiometry. *Pure tone audiometry* tests each ear separately for air conduction (via earphones) and bone conduction (via a vibrator placed on the mastoid bone). The examiner varies the intensity (decibels) at tested frequencies of 125, 250, 500, 1000, 2000, 4000, and 8000 Hz. The faintest point at which the client hears the tone is called the *hearing threshold level* (HRT). The audiometer is equipped with a masking noise used when there is a wide difference between the hearing acuity of both ears and the better ear hears the signal intended to test the poorer ear. Thresholds are recorded on a graph called an audiogram. A hearing range of 0 to 20 for the tested frequencies is considered normal. Figure 74–3 shows a normal audiogram.

Speech audiometry tests the client's ability to understand and discriminate sounds. The speech audiometry test is administered via a monitored live microphone or recorded test material. Spondee words (two-syllable words with equal accents, such as hotdog or airplane) are presented. A speech reception test measures how loud speech must be before it is heard. The *speech reception threshold* (SRT) is the minimum intensity required for a client to understand speech. The SRTs are usually consistent with the pure tone averages. The lowest level at which the client correctly repeats 50% of the words is the speech discrimination level and is also recorded on the audiogram.

Speech discrimination testing measures the client's ability to distinguish phonetic elements of speech and thus understand what is heard. Using a live monitored microphone or recorded material at levels above the SRT, the examiner presents lists of single-syllable words, such as day or jam, selected in approximately the same proportion as they occur in spoken English. Clients with normal hearing usually have a discrimination score of 90% to 100%. Less than 90% usually indicates sensorineural hearing loss.

Impedance audiometry helps differentiate ear disorders. The impedance test battery involves three separate evaluations: tympanometry, static impedance, and acoustic reflex tests. Tympanometry measures the mobility of the tympanic membrane as air pressure is varied in the external ear. It works in a way similar to pneumatic otoscopy. The objective is to determine the impedance (resistance) or compliance (flexibility) of the tympanic membrane to sound waves. The test exposes the ear to a constant sound and measures the percentage of sound reflected back from the tympanic membrane with an electroacoustic impedance meter. This measurement is the drum compliance at

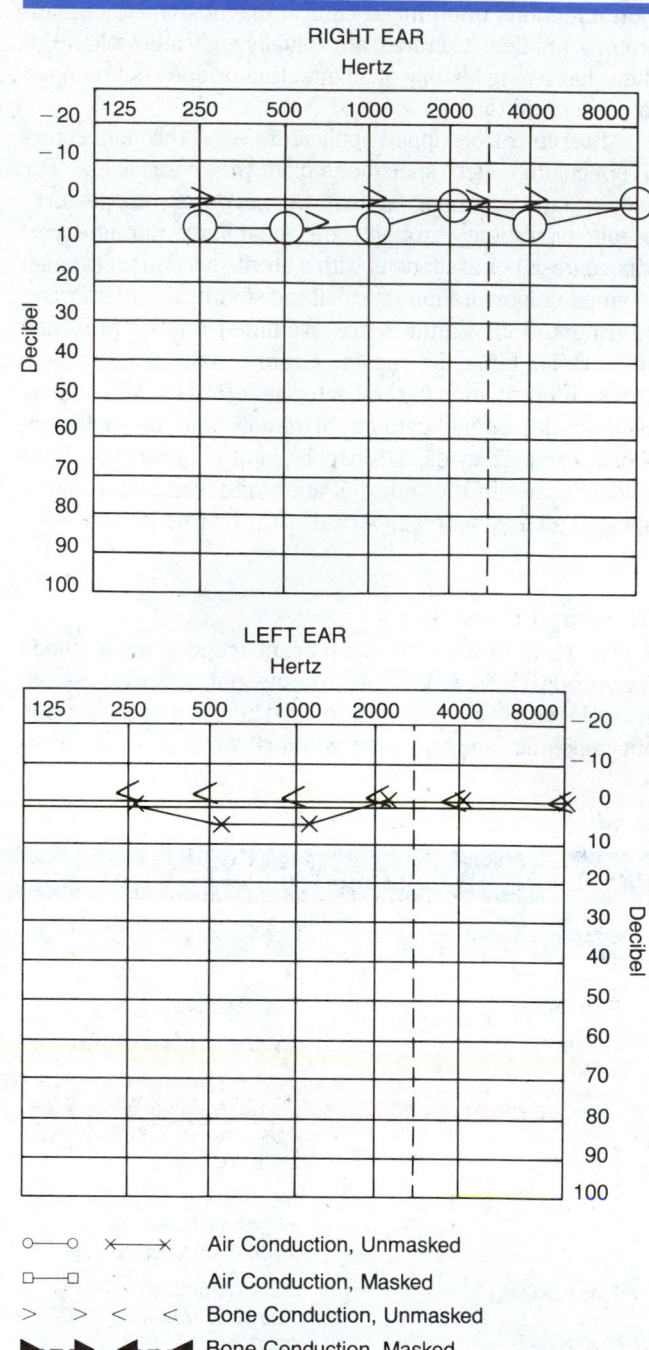

Figure 74–3

Normal audiogram.

a particular pressure. The more rigid the membrane, the less the compliance and the higher the impedance. The test is repeated with varying pressure, and a compliance curve, or tympanogram, is plotted. This curve varies with different ear disorders. The static impedance test measures the compliance of the middle ear at rest. The acoustic reflex test measures the changes in compliance caused by the contraction of the middle ear muscles in response to pure tone signals. In clients with normal hearing, the threshold level for the pure tone signals is usually 95 dB. Absence of the acoustic reflex provides helpful diagnostic information.

Vestibular Tests

Electronystagmography (ENG), a clinical test of vestibular function, evaluates the status of the semicircular canals by measuring their effect on the ocular muscles. The nystagmus is electrically recorded on a graph. The ENG test battery includes a series of ocular, positional, and bithermal caloric tests used to assess clients with symptoms of dysequilibrium, vertigo, and other forms of imbalance. The battery also can be used to monitor vestibular function in clients at high risk for vestibular damage, such as those receiving gentamicin and streptomycin. The results are viewed as a whole, with certain abnormal findings suggestive of peripheral vestibular dysfunctions and others suggestive of CNS disorders (Zarnoch, 1982).

In preparation for the test, advise the client to avoid alcohol, sedatives, tranquilizers, or antivertigo drugs for at least 48 hours prior to the examination; the drowsiness produced by such drugs can reduce or weaken the response. An otoscopic examination and removal of cerumen prior to the examination is necessary, because impacted cerumen

reduces the response. The skin around the eyes is cleansed, removing all makeup and skin oil. The client is placed supine on a table or in a chair with the head elevated 30°. Electrodes are attached to the skin with electrode paste. A ground electrode is attached to the forehead, and electrodes are placed above, below, and at the outer canthus of each eye to record horizontal and vertical nystagmus. The ENG is performed in a dark room and takes approximately 1 hour.

The *bithermal caloric test* compares the nystagmus produced by warm and cold stimulation in each ear. An ear is irrigated with warm (44°C) and then cold (30°C) water with a 5-minute interval between each irrigation. During the procedure, mental alerting tasks such as counting backward from 100 are used to prevent the suppression of responses (Zarnoch, 1982).

A simple caloric test, the *Kobrak caloric test,* stimulates the vestibular labyrinth by directing ice water into the external auditory canal through a Luer-Lok syringe with a 22-gauge needle. Ten to 12 seconds of stimulation will normally induce mild vertigo, nystagmus, and a tendency to fall toward the side of the stimulated ear. Sometimes it also induces vomiting. No response indicates that the labyrinth is nonfunctional.

Section II: Nursing Diagnosis

Nursing diagnoses commonly related to the care of clients with auditory dysfunction, as well as other potentially relevant diagnoses, are listed in Box 74–2. As has been discussed, the nurse should be alert for hearing impairment in all clients, not only those with identified hearing difficulties.

Box 74–2 Nursing Diagnoses Commonly Related to Dysfunction of the Auditory System

Diagnoses Directly Related to Auditory System Dysfunction

Sensory-perceptual alterations, auditory

Sensory-perceptual alterations, kinesthetic

Communication, impaired verbal, related to impaired hearing

Knowledge deficit

Injury, potential for, related to impaired hearing or disturbances in equilibrium

Self-concept, alteration in, related to body image, self-esteem, role performance, personal identity

Additional Potential Nursing Diagnoses

Comfort, alteration in, related to pain

Coping, ineffective individual or family

Sleep pattern disturbance, related to tinnitus

Social isolation, related to problems of hearing

SENSORY-PERCEPTUAL ALTERATION: AUDITORY

Reduced hearing, regardless of its cause, affects all aspects of a client's life and impairs the client's ability to function normally. Tinnitus with or without hearing loss is another disruptive symptom with multiple effects on a person's life (eg, a client with tinnitus may find it extremely difficult to fall asleep and once asleep, may find that sleep is interrupted).

SENSORY-PERCEPTUAL ALTERATION: KINESTHETIC

When the sense of balance is disrupted, the client is also unable to function normally. The client's mobility and equilibrium are disturbed. Vertigo is often accompanied by a number of unpleasant physiological symptoms such as nausea and vomiting.

IMPAIRED VERBAL COMMUNICATION: AUDITORY

Hearing loss may also affect the development of verbal communication. The ears monitor speech, and the client's

Nursing Research Note

Magilvy J: Quality of life of hearing-impaired older women. *Nurs Res* 1985; 34(3):140–143.

Major variables were studied that influence the quality of life perceived by older hearing-impaired women. The study compared the quality of life experienced by women who were deaf before age 19 and those who developed hearing impairments in later life. The variables thought to influence quality of life were health, social support, age, financial adequacy, and social hearing handicap.

The results suggest that women who developed hearing impairments later in life had an overall lower perception of quality of life than the early-onset group. The older group perceived themselves as less healthy, lacking adequate social support, and experiencing greater social handicap. Financial adequacy and age of onset of deafness did not directly influence perceived quality of life in either group.

The findings indicate that quality of life is positively influenced by one's perception of health and by social support networks. Quality of life is negatively affected by perceptions of social handicap. Judging from these findings, nursing intervention with other hearing-impaired clients should focus on health promotion, enhancing social support systems, and facilitating adaptation to the hearing handicap.

voice may be too soft or too loud when this ability is diminished because inflections cannot be heard; the client's voice also may become monotonous. Clients who do not hear themselves talk will be unaware when they have mispronounced words.

KNOWLEDGE DEFICIT

Clients who are unable to understand or hear may have been unable to internalize health teaching or explanations. This puts hearing-impaired clients at a serious disadvantage for being well-informed consumers of health care. Identifying knowledge deficits is crucial in assisting clients in becoming active participants in their own health care, preventing complications, and making rational decisions that affect the quality of life.

POTENTIAL FOR INJURY

Hearing problems predispose clients to accidents and trauma. Clients unable to hear warning signals such as traffic noises, sirens, barking dogs, or shouting people may not be able to prevent injury to themselves or others. Those with vestibular problems may be in grave danger if vertigo occurs while they are driving a car or truck, working with dangerous machinery, crossing a busy street, or doing any of the activities of daily life that people with stable equilibrium take for granted.

ALTERATION IN SELF-CONCEPT

Clients with disturbed auditory function may view themselves negatively. They may misinterpret what others say because they hear it incorrectly, or they may respond with anger to perceived affronts. Sometimes it seems easier to withdraw from relationships with others, and clients soon find that their roles in the family, social, or work group have changed. A heavy reliance on others for communication often leads to increasing dependence on others and decreasing autonomy.

Section III: Planning and Implementation

The role of the nurse working with clients with vestibular dysfunction is discussed in Chapter 75 in the sections on Meniere's syndrome and motion sickness. The role of the nurse working with clients with auditory dysfunction involves the prevention of hearing loss and preservation of hearing, the maintenance and enhancement of communication, and meeting the clients' physiological and psychosocial needs. Table 74–4 gives a sample nursing care plan.

Clients and their families need information about the cause and treatment of the disorder, information about rehabilitative measures and available resources in the community, and encouragement in making the adjustments in their daily lives imposed by hearing impairment. To help clients reach their optimal level of wellness, the nurse may need to encourage them to seek help from various health professionals. The nurse often works collaboratively with the otologist (a physician specializing in disease of the ears) or the otorhinolaryngologist (a physician specializing in diseases of the ear, nose, and throat). Other professionals also provide services necessary for clients with hearing impairments. These include the audiologist (a specialist in

the evaluation and rehabilitation of clients with hearing problems); the speech therapist (a specialist dealing with communication disorders); and others such as the social worker, psychologist, or vocational counselor.

PREVENTING HEARING LOSS AND PRESERVING HEARING

Damage to the structures of the ear, infection, and hearing impairment are often preventable. The crucial role of the nurse in prevention is the education of the client and family regarding routine care of the ear and the prevention of damage from hazardous noise.

Routine Cleaning of the Ear

The external auditory canal is basically a self-cleaning structure. The muscles involved in chewing help work cerumen through the canal to the outer surface, where it can be readily removed with a washcloth in routine washing.

Table 74-4 Sample Nursing Care Plan

Nursing Diagnosis	Client Care Goals	Plan/Nursing Implementation	Expected Outcome
Sensory-perceptual alteration: auditory	Optimal sensory stimulation	Obtain client's attention by touching, or by calling his or her name; speak slowly and clearly, facing client; restate when not understood; talk toward client's best ear; assist client in using hearing aid; control background noises when communicating (eg, radio, television, etc); use hand gestures; use pad and pencil	Client uses assistive devices or speech reading; client uses other senses in communicating
Impaired verbal communication	Optimal pattern of communication	Encourage use of adaptive hearing device; provide a calm, quiet, unhurried atmosphere; encourage communication in whatever manner client is able; provide alternate method of communication; identify areas of speech difficulties; encourage referral to speech pathologist	Improved pattern of communication
Knowledge deficit	Increased knowledge relating to prevention of ear disorders, medical and surgical interventions, use of auditory devices, safety practices, and listening and communication skills	Provide information relating to: proper hygiene of the ears; cause of client's disorder; method of treatment; use and maintenance of hearing aid or other auditory device; safety practices; and listening and communication skills	Client demonstrates proper hygiene of the ear, has decreased anxiety related to surgical interventions; describes appropriate medical treatment used; uses and maintains hearing aid; describes safety measures such as increased use of other senses (eg, visual and tactile); uses listening and communication skills
Potential for injury	Prevention of injury	Clients with hearing loss: Encourage use of other senses and hearing adaptive devices to identify hazards in the environment; provide client with information on adaptive devices and hearing guide dogs if appropriate; tag the hospitalized client's door, bed, and chart to alert other health care personnel to the client's special needs	Risk of potential injury is avoided or decreased
		Clients with vestibular problems: Instruct client to stop activities while experiencing vertigo; provide hospitalized client with call light and bed rails to prevent injury	Client avoids hazardous situations until vertigo has diminished or been relieved
Alteration in self-concept (body image, self-esteem, role performance, and personal identity)	Progression toward a positive self-concept	Encourage client to express feelings; suggest alternative methods of communication; assist client with adaptive devices, hearing aids, etc; encourage seeking help from other health professionals if necessary (eg, audiologist, vocational rehabilitator, etc); support family and assist in adapting; encourage and assist client with family relationships and other social contacts	Client demonstrates positive self-concept by accepting hearing loss; begins learning other methods of communication; begins using assistive hearing devices; reestablishes family and other social contacts; establishes plans for adjusting work situation or seeks alternative plans

Discourage clients from inserting objects such as cotton-tipped swabs, hairpins, safety pins, paper clips, or their own fingers into their ears to clean them. Not only is this likely to be unnecessary, but it is also *dangerous*. Even cotton-tipped swabs are relatively inflexible. A sudden movement of the head because the client has been startled or an accidental push by a person passing by can force the object deeper into the ear canal. This can push the cerumen further in and impair hearing, scratch or irritate the external auditory canal, or puncture the tympanic membrane. In general, it is safest to leave the outer ear alone.

The self-cleaning mechanism of the outer ear may not operate well under certain circumstances. When chewing is impaired, as occurs with a fractured jaw, malocclusion, or ill-fitting or no dentures, cerumen may build up. Cerumen removal by a knowledgeable health care provider may become necessary. The self-cleaning mechanism also may not be operating effectively in other less obvious situations. Consider checking for cerumen buildup in clients who are NPO, on a clear liquid diet, or receiving nourishment through intravenous infusions.

Tell clients to avoid washing their ears with strong soaps or shampoos that can irritate and dry the skin, causing itching. Scratching an irritated ear can result in a secondary infection. Clients who experience dry skin with aging may find this to be a particular problem.

Removing Cerumen

Clients prone to cerumen accumulation (people with a large amount of hair in the outer ear and those who work in dusty or dirty areas) should be taught how to soften and remove cerumen safely. Half-strength hydrogen peroxide solution instilled into the ear with a medicine dropper can help remove cerumen. (Refer to the later section on instilling drops, creams, and ointments.) The hydrogen peroxide should remain in the ear for 5 minutes and be irrigated out with clear water in a medicine dropper or while the client showers. Once a week is usually enough, although clients with a large accumulation may have to treat the problem more often. Commercial ceruminolytic agents such as Debrox (a combination of carbamide peroxide and glycerol) can be purchased OTC. Some people are allergic to OTC ceruminolytics with combined ingredients, however, and the nurse should caution them to avoid their use.

When necessary, a health care provider can remove cerumen in a variety of ways. The nurse can use a specially constructed cotton-tipped ear swab to gently remove accumulated cerumen. Make sure the swab is not inserted too far into the canal and the light is sufficient to be able to see that the cerumen is not being pushed further along the external auditory canal.

Cerumen also may be removed using a curet or suction (Figure 74–4A, B). Both methods require the same precautions spelled out earlier, but suction is safer. Ear irrigation is used least often because it can cause discomfort if the solution is either too warm or too cold. Ear

irrigation should not be used unless the client is known to have an intact tympanic membrane to avoid forcing water or cerumen into the middle ear through a perforation. An otolaryngologist may make an exception, however, to flush out accumulated pus when a client with a perforated tympanic membrane has a severe middle ear infection; in this case, the physician should perform the irrigation. Instructions for ear irrigation can be found in nursing fundamentals textbooks.

Keeping the Ear Dry

Keeping water out of the ear is important, because moisture invites maceration that may result in infection. Thus, clients should try to avoid letting water run into the ears while showering. Using earplugs or Vaseline-impregnated cotton plugs will help. To make a cotton plug, unroll a cotton ball and apply Vaseline to its surface. Roll from one end to the other—Vaseline side out—ending with a cylinder that can be easily molded, cut to the desired length, and inserted into the ear. When swimming, it is best to

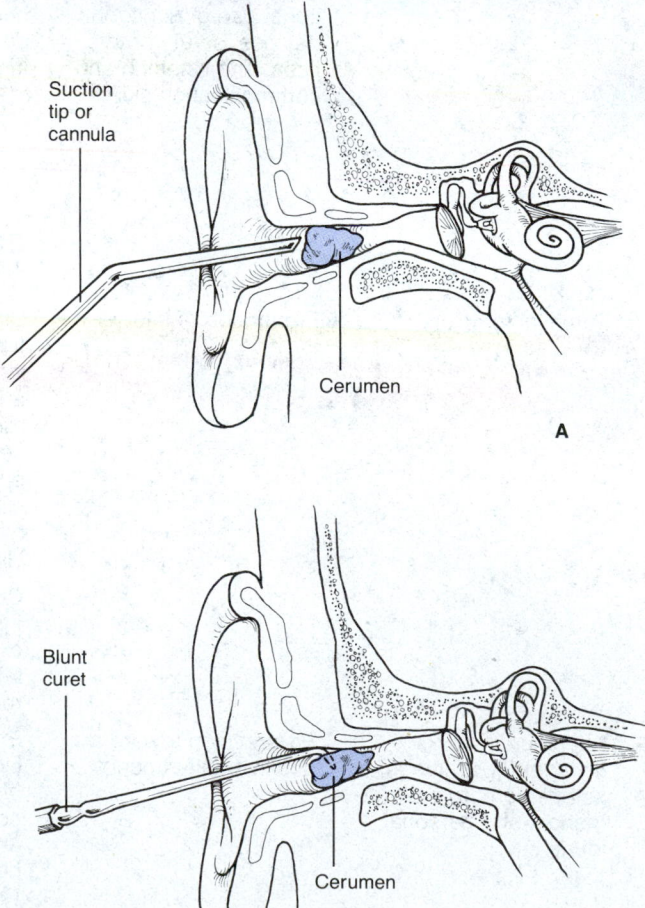

Figure 74–4

A. Removal of cerumen with a curet. **B.** Removal of cerumen using suction.

use earplugs made especially for that purpose. Swimming should be limited to 4 or 5 hours at the most.

The external ear can be dried by using a hair dryer (taking care not to burn the external ear) or instilling a few drops of alcohol into the external auditory canal (being careful not to dry out the skin of the external ear).

Removing Foreign Bodies

Foreign bodies in the ear are a more common problem for children than adults. However, even adults insert foreign bodies into their ears for cleaning purposes and cannot get them out. Flying insects or debris blown into the ear by a strong wind are also common.

Instilling mineral, olive, or vegetable oil or alcohol into the ear will smother an insect and allow it to float out. Irrigation can flush out debris but should not be used if the foreign object is of vegetable origin, because it will tend to absorb the water and swell. Professional help in removing foreign bodies prevents additional damage to the ear.

Equalizing Pressure in the Middle Ear

Changes in altitude and inflammation of the eustachian tube from upper respiratory tract infections or seasonal allergies may cause discomfort when fluid or air is trapped in the middle ear. Clients can use a variety of self-ventilating techniques to help equalize the pressure; yawning, swallowing several times, chewing gum, and opening the mouth about 2 cm and protruding the jaw forward may help. The Valsalva maneuver—holding the nostrils shut and the mouth closed while gently blowing—may be used when the other measures are not helpful. However, clients with congestion from an upper respiratory tract infection should not use this maneuver, because it can force bacteria into the middle ear.

Instilling Drops, Creams, or Ointments

Drops or ointments should be inserted into the external auditory canal when the client is lying on his or her side with the affected ear up. Instruct the client to remain in this position for at least 5 minutes and to insert a cotton ball before assuming a sitting or standing position. This will allow the solution to drain into the cotton ball.

Creams can be carefully applied to the external ear with a cotton swab or cotton ball. Instruct the client to hold the swab close to its cotton-tipped end and to brace the fourth and fifth fingers against the face. This prevents inserting the swab too far and accidentally damaging the tympanic membrane.

Discourage clients from self-treatment with eardrops or oil when they have an earache. This not only delays effective treatment but may allow an infection to progress; keeping the ear canal continuously moist with eardrops or oil also may cause fungal infection.

Earlobe Piercing

Earlobe piercing is a popular cosmetic procedure to facilitate the wearing of earrings. Earlobe piercing should be carried out under aseptic conditions, preferably by a health care provider. Clients who are prone to keloid formation, are diabetic, or have a skin disease should avoid earlobe piercing.

The client must pay meticulous attention to the pierced earlobes while they heal—which can take up to 6 weeks—because the most frequent complication is infection. The earlobes should be cleansed two to three times daily (especially during the first 3 weeks) with half-strength hydrogen peroxide. A mild antiseptic also may be applied at both the front and back of the earlobe. Clients who use alcohol for its antiseptic properties should be aware that it may irritate and dry the skin. The client should turn the ear wire or earring stud during cleaning to maintain patency of the opening. The earring should not be removed until the opening has healed to avoid premature closure.

Another potential problem with ear piercing occurs when people are allergic to the metals or alloys used to make the posts and wires of the earrings. Most people can tolerate 14-karat gold. Those who are sensitive to gold may find surgical stainless steel less irritating.

Preventing Damage From Noise

The problem of noise pollution is increasing in the workplace, the home, and the city streets. Nurses should educate their friends, neighbors, and clients about the damage to the hair cells of the ears that can result from hazardous noise. A review of Table 75–1 shows that some sounds considered normal or innocuous can cause hearing damage if people are exposed to them long and often enough.

Hearing protectors can reduce and even prevent noise trauma; they come in a variety of forms:

- Disposable plugs are almost invisible, because they are placed inside the ear canal.
- Reusable plugs are also placed inside the ear canal. Some come in pairs and are joined by a string.
- Headband plugs can be worn by people who wear glasses or headgear in their work.
- Muffs have foam- or liquid-filled cushions that form a seal around the ear. They are the most effective in blocking out noise but cannot be worn by people who wear glasses or other protective headgear that interferes with their snug fit.

Hearing protectors can be purchased in sporting goods stores, medical supply stores, hearing clinics, and through audiologists; they are usually available in work settings in which noise is a problem. If hearing protectors are not available in such work settings, the client and nurse should bring the problem of noise to the attention of management.

Hearing protectors require relatively little care. Earplugs should be kept clean and stored in a clean case or

Box 74-3 **Guidelines for Protecting Hearing**

Wear hearing protectors at home when working with power tools.

Run appliances one at a time to keep the noise level down, and do not use noisy appliances any more than absolutely necessary.

Be an informed consumer and select the quieter household appliances. Consumer guides often recommend appliances based on their decibel ratings.

Anticipate noise exposure at work, at home, or while engaging in recreational activities. Put on hearing protectors before starting up a motorcycle, a snowmobile, etc.

Avoid sitting close to loud music (either live or recorded).

Be cautious about any noise-making object close to the ears, including stereo headphones worn while jogging or mobile telephones.

Be a citizen activist and help reduce the noise levels in the community.

When caught unprepared by exposure to noise that cannot be controlled (an emergency siren, a malfunctioning automobile horn, a subway train, etc), cover the ears tightly with the hands.

empty wide-mouthed bottle. If they become discolored or hardened, they should be discarded. Headband plugs should be handled carefully, because twisting or bending them may interfere with their performance. Muffs may need periodic cushion replacement and should be stored in a safe place.

Around-the-clock prevention is important in preserving hearing. Box 74-3 lists specific suggestions nurses can make.

MAINTAINING AND ENHANCING COMMUNICATION

The nurse can maintain and enhance communication in a number of ways. A modification of communication style is necessary to account for the special needs of hearing-impaired people. Clients can undertake programs in auditory training, stress reduction, and assertiveness training to enhance their ability to communicate. Environmental modifications and hearing aids also help people hear better. The ultimate aim is to prevent the client's isolation from others.

What the Nurse Can Do

When speaking with someone who is hard of hearing, attract the person's attention first. Gestures and touching are usually helpful ways to signal an intention to communicate verbally. Having attracted the person's attention, stand directly in front of the person and face the light. This gives the person the added advantage of being able to see formed

words and to read lips. Speaking at a calm, relaxed pace lets the client know that the nurse understands and respects his or her limitation without increasing anxiety. The client who is relatively free from stress and anxiety probably will hear better.

Appropriate facial expressions and gestures help the hearing-impaired person comprehend what the nurse is saying more fully. It may be necessary to modify the tone or pitch of the voice so the person can hear better. If the client does not understand what has been said, try rephrasing it. If the nurse does not understand all the client has said, details can be filled in from the context of the communication. Be cautious, however, not to misunderstand without realizing it. A better approach might be to ask the client to repeat or rephrase what has not been understood.

The hospitalized hearing-impaired client should be identified by tags on the door, bed, and call system to alert all hospital staff to the hearing loss. Having a hospital room near the nurses' station helps decrease the client's feeling of isolation and increases the feeling of security. A pad and pencil should be handy in case the client finds it helpful. The nurse should write all important instructions for the client.

What the Client Can Do

Encourage hearing-impaired clients to be assertive in asking others to repeat or rephrase what they have said, to speak louder, to face them directly, to move into the light, or to take any other action that helps clients better understand the verbal communication. Clients may be reluctant to ask others to accommodate them and need to know that most people are willing to be helpful when they understand what is being asked of them, and why. Clients with associated speech problems can anticipate situations in which they may have to repeat themselves or clarify a verbal communication.

When stress is a factor in hearing impairment or anxiety makes communication difficult, stress reduction exercises such as those recommended in Chapter 2 are often helpful. The nurse can teach these exercises to the client and encourage their use.

Some clients may find it necessary to learn speech reading. This helps clients identify spoken words even though they may not hear them. Auditory training is often a helpful adjunct to speech reading. In auditory training programs, people learn to discriminate between sounds and enhance their listening skills. Hearing centers, otologists, audiologists, and the organizations listed at the end of this chapter can direct clients to speech reading and auditory training classes in the local community.

Environmental Considerations for Home and Community

Simple and inexpensive steps to alter the environment are often useful to people who do not hear well. For example, certain materials and furnishings help reduce echoes and muffle irrelevant noises that interfere with a hearing-impaired person's ability to hear. Movable furniture allows hearing-impaired people to sit where they can better hear and see the lips of speakers.

Other less simple and more expensive steps involve communication systems that can be installed in conference rooms, classrooms, theaters, and auditoriums or added to the radio, television, or telephone in the home or at work. These include the following:

- *Audio loops:* Wire loops are installed around the perimeter of a room to permit people with hearing aids or other special equipment to receive amplified sound.

- *Special headsets:* Audio signals from microphones can be transferred into invisible, infrared light that can then be converted back into sound and received through a headset.

- *Amplisound:* The listener is provided with an AM radio receiver with earplugs that transmits sound through a special station located within the building. This can be used with or without a hearing aid.

- *Phonic ear:* Similar to amplisound, the phonic ear is an FM radio broadcasting system.

- *Captioning devices:* Added to a television, these devices will display subtitles or captions at the bottom of the screen. Unfortunately, only a few television programs are currently coded for this service.

- *Telephone communication devices:* Sound amplifiers that can easily be installed on telephones help the hearing-impaired use them. Devices with typewriterlike keyboards help deaf people communicate with Bell System operators with receiving systems in four regional locations (Oakland, Omaha, Boston, and Philadelphia). Toll-free numbers that users of telephone communication devices can call for assistance in placing telephone calls are included in the resources list at the end of this chapter.

- *Sign language interpreters:* People with training in signing at public gatherings and television presentations can be invaluable. Organizations that provide interpreters are listed in the resources list at the end of this chapter.

- *Hearing guide dogs:* Much like seeing eye dogs, these specially trained animals alert the hearing-impaired person who lives alone to the sounds of the doorbell, telephone, alarm clock, and smoke alarm, as well as other sounds in the home or public places. The dogs are trained to protect their masters from danger and to assist them in carrying out daily activities that depend on sound. See the resources list at the end of this chapter.

Hearing Aids

It is estimated that over 1 million Americans wear hearing aids (Hanawalt & Troutman, 1984). A hearing aid receives speech and environmental sounds through a microphone, converts them into electrical signals, strengthens the electrical signals through amplification, and converts the amplified electrical signals back to sound. Hearing aids work by amplifying sound, not merely by intensifying it.

What Hearing Aids Can and Cannot Do

Many hearing aids can now be tailored to the client's specific needs. For example, rather than needing to have all sound made louder, a client with a sensorineural hearing loss may need to have low tones depressed and higher tones enhanced. In contrast, a client with a conductive hearing loss may benefit from amplification alone if it can overcome the blockage or damage that prevents sound from reaching the inner ear. Hearing aids are more likely to be helpful when the hearing loss is conductive rather than sensorineural. In consultation with an otologist and an audiologist, the client can make an informed decision about whether to attempt to use a hearing aid and what kind of hearing aid would be best.

Clients should understand that using a hearing aid does not guarantee perfect hearing and that not everyone is a good candidate. Because hearing aids increase sound, background sounds also are increased. Some people find this distracting and annoying. Also, although speech becomes louder, it may not be clearer. The hearing aid user may be disappointed to find that it may still be difficult to understand what others are saying. To take full advantage of the benefits of a hearing aid and learn to interpret speech more accurately, the hearing aid wearer may need auditory training or to learn speech reading.

Types of Hearing Aids

Tell clients that even though they are believed to be good candidates for hearing aids, the amount or type of hearing loss may limit their choices. Unfortunately, the least obvious hearing aids are also the smallest and are located close to the receiver itself. Their small size and the proximity between hearing aid and receiver limit the amount of amplification that can be achieved; thus, clients with severe hearing loss may not be able to use them. Four common types of hearing aids are discussed below.

- The behind-the-ear (BTE) aid is used most often. It is comfortable and has cosmetic appeal, especially for clients with long or abundant hair to hide it. The hearing aid itself hooks behind the ear and is connected by a short clear plastic tube to an ear mold inserted into the external auditory canal (Figure 74–5A). It is useful for hearing losses in the range of 25 to 80 dB.

- The in-the-ear (ITE) aid is also popular. The one-piece design of this smallest of the hearing aids allows

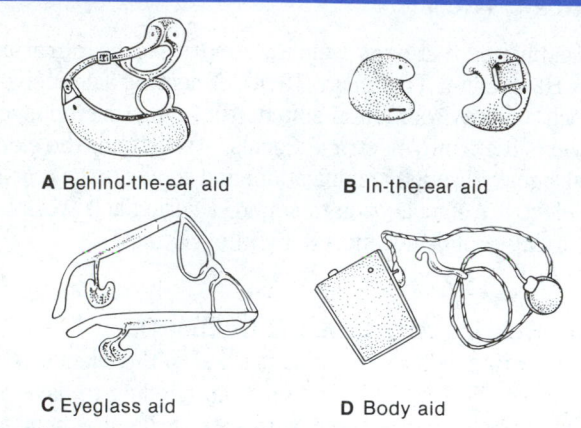

A Behind-the-ear aid   **B** In-the-ear aid

C Eyeglass aid   **D** Body aid

Figure 74–5

Types of hearing aids.

all components—hearing aid, receiver, and battery—to be placed directly into the external auditory canal (Figure 74–5B). It is useful for hearing losses in the range of 25 to 55 dB.

- The eyeglass hearing aid is less popular. The receiver and tubing (which is connected to a microphone that fits in the external auditory canal) are hidden within the eyeglass frame, and the arm of the eyeglass frame conceals the battery (Figure 74–5C). One drawback is that the eyeglass frame must be bulky to conceal the equipment, so style selection is limited. This type of hearing aid is useful for hearing losses in the range of 25 to 70 dB.

- The body aid is used by people with severe hearing loss. Its fitted ear mold attaches to a round receiver, which is connected by wiring to a transmitter that may be clipped to the client's clothing. The transmitter can be readily concealed by clothing, but the round receiver and wire cannot (Figure 74–5D). The body aid is useful for hearing losses in the range of 40 to 110 dB.

Recent research has resulted in the development of a special device to improve hearing. Implanted surgically into the cochlea, the *cochlear implant* is sometimes referred to in the popular literature as an artificial ear or a high-tech hearing aid (see Chapter 76).

Caring for Hearing Aids

Hearing aids are delicate and must be protected from breakage, moisture, and heat. Routine cleaning of a hearing aid, which may be done by client or nurse, involves washing the detached ear mold in warm, soapy water and cleaning the plastic connecting tube, if one exists, with a pipe cleaner. Specific hints for caring for a hearing aid are outlined in Box 74–4. In addition to teaching the client the proper care of a hearing aid, nurses may also find it necessary to care for the hearing aid when the client is unable to do so. If the hearing aid requires more than routine care, a specialist should clean it.

Box 74–4   Hearing Aid Tips

Keep the hearing aid dry and away from high temperatures, such as direct sunlight.

Do not use solvents or lubricants on the hearing aid.

Avoid hair spray (which tends to clog the aid) or use the spray before inserting the ear mold.

When the hearing aid is not in use, turn it off by opening the battery door. This also helps to dry any moisture that seeps in from the skin.

Store the aid in its case or bag.

To clean the aid, detach the ear mold from the battery device and soak the mold in warm, mild soapy water. Rinse with clear water and let it dry thoroughly before reconnecting it. A pipe cleaner may be used to clean the plastic connecting tube. All other cleaning should be done by a specialist.

To change the battery remove the old one(s) and follow the + or − sign indicator in the battery compartment. If batteries are placed wrongly, the compartment door will not close. Batteries usually last from 2 to 4 weeks depending on the amount of usage. Keep spares available and stored in a dry place. Batteries usually come five or six in a wheel-type case. Every hearing aid uses only one type of battery, which can be purchased at local acoustic supply dealers.

SOURCE: Reprinted with permission from Hanawalt A, Troutman K: If your patient has a hearing aid. *Am J Nurs* 1984; 84:900–901.

Inserting a Hearing Aid

The nurse may have to insert a hearing aid when the client is unable to do so, eg, when the client is confused or disoriented, has tremors or mobility problems, does not have the manual dexterity needed, or is comatose or semicomatose. Guidelines for hearing aid insertion are listed in Box 74–5.

Box 74–5   Guidelines for Inserting a Hearing Aid

Turn the hearing aid on to be sure it works. If a squealing or whistling sound (feedback) is heard when turning the hearing aid on high, it is working. If a sound is not heard, the hearing aid may need new batteries. Look in the battery case to see if extra batteries are on hand.

Gently insert the ear mold into the client's ear canal. First, place the ear bore (hole) in the mold into the ear canal. If the client cannot say into which ear the mold should be placed, look to see which ear it will fit if the ear bore is inserted first (ear molds are custom-made).

Once the hearing aid has been inserted, have the client adjust the volume if able. If the nurse must adjust it, use a midrange setting. (The lowest is 1, and the highest is usually 4.)

The tube, if the hearing aid has one, should be placed over the ear and attached to the device that contains the battery. This is a good time to check the tubing to make sure there are no breaks or kinks, because this could distort or interrupt the sound.

If the hearing aid does not seem to be operating properly after insertion, make sure that it has been turned on and inserted properly, that all components are attached, and that the batteries are functional. Also make sure the ear canal or ear mold are not obstructed by cerumen. If the malfunctioning persists, notify the local hearing aid representative, who may be able to supply the client with a loaned hearing aid until repairs have been made. Local chapters of associations listed in the resources listing at the end of this chapter may also loan hearing aids temporarily.

Consumer-Oriented Regulations

Hearing aids may be sold by unqualified people with little or no training. For this reason, it is crucial to encourage clients to seek evaluation by an audiologist and otologist before purchasing a hearing aid. Remind them that not all hearing loss can be helped by a hearing aid, and only an audiologist or otologist should recommend a specific type of aid to be purchased. Make sure that the client also understands the importance of consulting a reputable hearing aid dealer to avoid problems with improperly made ear molds that may not fit or may cause pain.

In 1977, the Federal Trade Commission (FTC) studied the hearing aid industry and ruled that hearing aids may be sold only to people who have had a prior medical evaluation (unless a person 18 years old or older waives this right). Soon after, the Food and Drug Administration established guidelines intended to protect the rights of hearing-impaired people. These may be obtained by writing to the FTC at the address given in the resources list at the end of this chapter.

Section IV: Evaluation

Continual assessment is essential in evaluating the client's achievement of expected outcomes. Outcomes for the most common nursing diagnoses are given in Table 74–4. The nurse should evaluate the client's ability to undertake measures to prevent hearing loss, to conserve hearing, and to maintain and enhance the ability to communicate with others.

Chapter Highlights

Nursing assessment of the ears includes the assessment of auditory and vestibular functions. Otalgia, otorrhea, tinnitus, vertigo, and hearing loss are common presenting symptoms.

The health history for clients with disorders of the auditory system should include exploration of the chief concern; questions about recent infections, allergies, and medications; and questions about ear cleaning.

The nurse should be alert to clinical clues of hearing loss in any client, because clients are often sensitive and do not admit having a loss.

Clients must admit to having a hearing loss before they can accept rehabilitative or adaptive measures.

Families and significant others play an essential role in providing social support for the hearing-impaired client.

Physical assessment of clients with auditory disorders includes inspection, palpation, and auscultation.

Specific tests of hearing loss include the voice, watch tick, and tuning fork tests.

Diagnostic studies for clients with auditory dysfunction include radiographic studies, audiometric testing, and vestibular tests (ENG, including ocular, positional, and bithermal caloric tests).

Hearing loss can have physical, psychological, social, and economic effects on the client.

Nursing diagnoses related to the client with auditory dysfunction include auditory and kinesthetic sensory-perceptual alterations, impairment of verbal communication, knowledge deficit, potential for injury, and alteration in self-concept.

For optimal results in rehabilitation, the family should be included in the rehabilitative process.

The nurse can plan a role in the prevention of auditory dysfunction through education on routine care of the ear and the prevention of damage from hazardous noise.

Assistive devices, aural rehabilitation, stress reduction, assertiveness training, and environmental modifications can enhance communication and prevent isolation and sensory deprivation.

The nurse should ensure that the client understands the uses and limitations of hearing aids, as well as the importance of working only with qualified professionals in the selection and fitting of these aids.

Bibliography

American Council of Otolaryngology—Head and Neck Surgery: *Otologic Referral Criteria for Occupational Hearing Conservation Programs.* Washington, DC: American Council of Otolaryngology, 1981.

Clark JL: Otalgia: Identifying the source. *Postgrad Med* 1981; 70(4):99–103.

Cluff GL: After the hearing test: What then? *Occup Health Saf* (March) 1983; p 14.

Cooper JC: The audiovestibular test battery for vertigo. *Ear Nose Throat J* 1980; 59(9):347–353.

Hanawalt A, Troutman K: If your patient has a hearing aid. *Am J Nurs* 1984; 84:900–901.

Hurvitz J, Carmen R: *Special Devices for Hard of Hearing, Deaf, and Deaf-Blind Persons.* Boston: Little, Brown, 1981.

Koch KH: Hidden handicaps: The deaf and hard of hearing. Some hints. *Nurs Times* 1981; 77(32):19–20.

Rosenblum E: *Fundamentals of Hearing for Health Professionals.* Boston: Little, Brown, 1979.

Ross T: Deafness: Breaking through the sound barrier. *Nurs Mirror* 1981; 152(21):20–23.

Thompson JM, Bowers AC: *Clinical Manual of Health Assessment.* St. Louis: Mosby, 1980.

Zarnoch JM: Hearing disorders: Audiologic manifestations. In: *Speech, Language and Hearing.* Loss N et al. Philadelphia: Saunders, 1982.

Suggested Readings

DeBlase R, Kucler M: Assistive hearing device aids patient-staff communication. *Ger Nurs* 1985; 6(4):223–224. The use of assistive hearing devices (inexpensive, battery-operated amplifiers with headphones) for hearing-impaired clients on medical-surgical and specialty units in a 410-bed general hospital is described.

Franks JR, Bechmann NJ: Rejection of hearing aids: Attitudes of a geriatric sample. *Ear and Hearing* 1985; 6(3):161–166. This article explores the reasons why only 21% of adults 65 and older with hearing impairment use hearing aids.

Holder L: Hearing aids: Handle with care. *Nursing 82* 1982; 12(April):64–65. An illustrated article demonstrating the care of hearing aids.

Oyer HJ, Oyer EJ: Social consequences of hearing loss for the elderly. *Allied Health Behav Sci* 1983; 2(2):123–137. A discussion of the social consequences encountered by older people with sensory and auditory deprivation.

Roseblum E: *Fundamentals of Hearing for Health Professionals.* Boston: Little, Brown, 1979. One of the most complete books on hearing and hearing problems written for nurses and other health professionals.

Sataloff RT, Vassallo LA: Choosing the right hearing aid. *Hosp Prac* 1981; 15:32A–32S. A comprehensive description of hearing aids and the advantages and disadvantages of various types. Problems occurring with the hearing aids are also discussed.

Resources

SELF-HELP GROUPS AND OTHER ORGANIZATIONS

American Academy of Otolaryngology—
Head and Neck Surgery, Inc
1101 Vermont Ave. NW, Suite 302
Washington, DC 20005

This association's members are physicians who specialize in treating people with disorders of the head and neck, especially disorders related to the ear, nose, and throat. The organization provides information and public service pamphlets.

American Athletic Association for the Deaf
3916 Lantern Dr.
Silver Spring, MD 20902
Phone: (301) 942–4042

This is an organization of deaf athletes and individuals interested in promoting competitive sports programs for hearing-impaired persons. They sponsor softball and basketball tournaments throughout the United States. Publish a quarterly bulletin.

American Humane Association
5351 S. Roslyn St.
Englewood, CO 80110
Phone: (303) 779–1400 (voice number)
(303) 287–6230 (TTY number)

Guide dogs trained to alert their masters to sounds such as alarm clocks, doorbells, telephones, or an infant's cry are available free of charge through this organization's Hearing Dog Program. Clients are also instructed in their use.

American Speech, Language, Hearing Association
10801 Rockville Pike
Rockville, MD 20852
Phone: (301) 897-5700

Information on hearing loss, as well as speech and hearing centers in locations across the country, is provided by this organization. Write or call (see Hot Line below) for information packet on cochlear implants, their risks and benefits, and the centers that provide this surgery.

Gallaudet College
Seventh St. and Florida Ave., N. E.
Washington, DC 20001
Phone: (202) 447–0314

This is the world's only liberal arts college for deaf persons.

National Association of the Deaf
814 Thayer Ave.
Silver Spring, MD 20910

This organization provides information on local chapters of interpreters.

Registry of Interpreters for the Deaf
PO Box 1339
Washington, DC 20013

The names of interpreters are also available through this organization.

Self-Help for the Hard of Hearing (SHHH)
PO Box 34889
Bethesda, MD 20033
 Formed for people with hearing problems, their families, and their friends, this organization provides education on hearing loss, remedial aids, and alternative communication skills. It also counsels members on the detection, management, and possible prevention of hearing loss.

Teletypewriters for the Deaf, Inc.
814 Thayer Ave.
Silver Spring, MD 20910
Phone: (301) 588–4605
 This is an organization for deaf individuals who communicate through teletypewriters and for other persons and institutions interested in this form of communication. It encourages the development of networks and the installation of TTYs (teletypewriters) in public facilities, and distributes used equipment to deaf persons at a substantial discount. Publishes a quarterly newsletter and a directory of Teletype terminals currently operated by deaf persons.

In Canada:
Canadian Deaf Sports Association
17512 86th Ave.
Edmonton, Alberta, Canada T5T 0L4
 Promotes athletics for the deaf.

Canadian Speech and Hearing Association
Suite 1202
181 University Ave.
Toronto, Ontario, Canada M5H 3M7
 Provides information on hearing loss and speech difficulties, and referrals to specialty centers throughout Canada.

Purple Cross Deaf Detection and Development Program
B. P. O. Elks of Canada
3420A Hill Ave.
Regina, Sasketchewan, Canada S4S 0W9
 This organization raises funds for programs and research for hearing and speech services in Canada.

HOT LINES

Bell Telephone Company
Phone (800) 342-4181
 Hard-of-hearing people can obtain information on special telephone equipment for the hearing impaired at this number.

Bell Telephone Company
Phone: (800) 855-1155
 People who use special telephone communication devices for the totally deaf can call this number to obtain assistance in placing person-to-person, third-number, collect, and credit card calls.

Hearing Helpline
Phone: (202) 638-7577
 This hot line operated by the Better Hearing Institute answers questions about hearing loss, hearing aids, and hearing aid services.

Kresge Hearing Research Laboratory of the South
Phone: (301) 897-8682
 Call this number collect for information on help for people who can hear at only very high frequencies.

National Association for Hearing and
 Speech Action
Phone: (800) 638-TALK [except Alaska, Hawaii, and Maryland; from these states call collect (301-897-8682)]
 This consumer affiliate of the American Speech, Language, Hearing Association has an active help line.

National Hearing Aid Society Helpline
(Mon–Fri, 9 AM to 5 PM)
Phone: (800) 368-5779 (nationwide)
(292) 472-4222 (Washington, DC; Maryland; and Virginia)
 Call this hot line for hearing aid information, consumer advice on hearing aids, and the names and locations of 2000 member dealers.

White House Hotline for the Hearing-Impaired
Comments Office
Phone: (202) 456–1414 (voice number)
 (202) 456–6313 (TTY number)
Visitors Office
Phone: (202) 456–2200 (voice number)
 (202) 456–2216 (TTY number)
 Two White House offices have installed teletypewriter units so that hearing-impaired citizens can comment on presidential policies or arrange for sign language guided tours of the White House.

HEALTH INFORMATION MATERIAL

From:
 American Academy of Otolaryngology—
 Head and Neck Surgery, Inc
 1101 Vermont Ave. NW, Suite 302
 Washington, DC 20005
 Doctor, What Causes the Noise in My Ears? 1981. Free
 pamphlet.
 Ear Wax, 1984. Free pamphlet.
 Noise, Ears, and Hearing, 1984. Free pamphlet.

From:
 Bureau of Consumer Protection
 Federal Trade Commission
 Pennsylvania Ave. at Sixth St. NW
 Washington, DC 20580
 Write for the September 1978 final report on the hearing aid industry.

From:
 Conference of Executives of American Schools for the Deaf
 5034 Wisconsin Ave., N.W.
 Washington, DC 20016
 Phone: (202) 363–1327
 The April issue of American Annals of the Deaf includes a state-by-state listing of resources and services for the deaf which can be ordered for $6.50.

From:
 Krames Communications
 312 90th St.
 Daly City, CA 94015
 Phone: (415) 994-8800

Dizziness or Vertigo? Understanding Balance Problems, 1984. Booklet, $.75

Ear and Head Noises: Tinnitus, 1983. Brochure, $.35

Hearing Aids: A Guide to Their Wear and Care, 1984. Booklet, $.90

Hearing Conservation: A Guide to Preventing Hearing Loss, 1984. Booklet, $.90

Middle Ear Fluid: Serous Otitis Media, 1984. Brochure, $.35

NURSING ORGANIZATIONS

Otorhinolaryngology Head/Neck Nurses
% Warren Otologic Group
3893 East Market St.
Warren, OH 44484
Phone: (216) 856-4000

Members are RNs who promote continuing education and enhanced quality of patient care in this specialty area, along with a strong sense of professional identity and an open forum for the exchange of ideas, information, and interests in the field. Annual dues are $40.

Chapter 75

Specific Disorders of the Auditory System

Dominica Ann Limburg

Objectives

When you have finished studying this chapter, you should be able to:

Discuss the cause and clinical manifestations of otosclerosis.

Describe the course of Meniere's syndrome, along with nursing interventions for clients in each stage of this condition.

Describe physiological changes occurring in the ears of the elderly and the nurse's role in their detection or prevention.

Discuss good aural hygiene for the prevention of infectious disorders of the ear and distinguish among the specific infectious disorders (external otitis, suppurative otitis media, non-suppurative otitis media, and their various manifestations).

Describe clinical manifestations and nursing interventions for a client with a neoplastic disorder of the ear, including cholesteatoma and acoustic neuroma.

Explain measures to avoid injuries and hearing loss due to trauma.

Disorders affecting the auditory system may be generally classified as congenital disorders; disorders of multifactorial origin; or degenerative, immunologic, infectious, neoplastic, or traumatic disorders. Each type of disorder has characteristic clinical manifestations, therapeutic measures, and nursing implications. In the case of any disorder, hearing impairment must be detected early; a program of aural rehabilitation then can be initiated to prevent client withdrawal and isolation. Emotional support is of primary importance in the nursing care of clients with hearing or vestibular dysfunctions.

Section I: Congenital Disorders

Congenital disorders of the ear may be inherited or acquired. Congenital inherited disorders are caused by a genetic defect and occur at any time during the life cycle, whereas congenital acquired disorders are caused by trauma or toxicity either prenatally, perinatally, or immediately postnatally. Congenital acquired disorders can vary in severity from a mild deformity to the absence of an anatomic part or the total absence of the ear. Congenital disorders are the most common cause of deafness. Any maternal infection or trauma during the prenatal period, especially the first trimester, can cause a congenital disorder resulting in malformation or malfunction.

Congenital malformations are usually identified at birth or shortly thereafter. Abnormalities of the auricle range from a complete absence (anotia) to a variation in its shape and size, such as a small, deformed auricle (microtia) or a large auricle (macrotia). Occasionally, more than one auricle or accessory auricles are present. Other malformations include fissures and enlargement of the lobule or a complete absence of the lobule. Malformations of the auricle can have a psychological effect on the individual. However, they usually do not affect hearing unless they are associated with other defects in the external auditory canal and the middle ear that result in a conductive or sensorineural hearing loss. Deformities of the auricle are often associated with aural atresia (a narrowed or absent external auditory canal) or abnormalities of the middle and inner ear. Congenital deformities of the inner ear are rare but result in deafness.

Congenital anomalies of the middle ear usually involve the ossicles. All or part of the ossicles might be absent, deformed, or fused together resulting in conductive hearing loss. Facial nerve dysfunction is often associated with anomalies of the middle ear; the nerve might be wrapped around the stapes or split in two. Clients may have a flattened cochlea, or a cochlea with only one single coil, or other malformations in the vestibule. Sensorineural hearing loss can be severe at birth or slowly progressive beginning in childhood.

With any congenital malformation, early identification is important. A program of speech training should be started as soon as possible when there is hearing impairment. Surgical cosmetic corrections usually are performed during early childhood to prevent emotional disturbances.

General Nursing Implications

Because nurses maintain close contact with clients, they play a vital role in the prevention and detection of congenital hearing disorders and can refer clients for hearing evaluations early. Nurses also can help prevent congenital disorders by monitoring the medications and radiological studies of pregnant women. Educating women about the causes of congenital disorders also can help prevent them. Nurses also can support hearing-impaired individuals and their families or significant others by providing support and engaging the family's help in the rehabilitation.

OTOSCLEROSIS

Otosclerosis (otospongiosis) is a dystrophy of the temporal bone that begins as a softening of the bone because of resorption and increased vascularity. This spongy bone gradually becomes a dense sclerotic mass. It affects the bony labyrinth of the inner ear and usually invades the ligament around the stapes footplate, causing conductive hearing loss. The progressive involvement of the footplate causes its immobilization, preventing the transmission of sound through the oval window. Occasionally, the lesion invades the cochlea or vestibule of the inner ear and causes sensorineural hearing loss.

Although no definite cause of this bony growth has been established, heredity is a significant factor; 40% to 50% of cases report a family history of otosclerosis. This disease is common in whites but rare in blacks, Orientals, and Native Americans (Jerger & Jerger, 1981). Women have a greater incidence of otosclerosis than men. Puberty, pregnancy, and menopause often exacerbate it, and birth control pills can heighten the effects of the disease (Shambaugh & Glasscock, 1980).

Clinical Manifestations

The onset of otosclerosis usually occurs between 15 and 45 years of age but may occur as late as 70 to 80 years. A slowly progressive, bilateral conductive hearing loss is the primary clinical manifestation. The disease progresses slowly, with periods of inactivity. The client frequently can hear better in a noisy environment, and mild tinnitus often accompanies the hearing loss.

On examination, the external ear and tympanic membrane are normal. Occasionally, the hypervascularity of the sclerotic lesion will be seen on the tympanic membrane as a pink area below the umbo (the slight projection where the malleus attaches). The Rinne test shows that bone conduction is greater than air conduction, whereas Weber's test shows that sound lateralizes to the poorer ear (see Chapter 74). Although otosclerotic changes may not be visible on radiographic studies, these studies are usually ordered to rule out other abnormalities. Audiometric testing shows a progressive conductive hearing loss that over time may progress to a mixed hearing loss. When the disease progresses to the cochlea, mild vertigo may be present.

Therapeutic Measures

Although there is no definitive medical treatment for otosclerosis, sodium fluoride has proven successful in arresting the process for some people. Florical, a combination of calcium carbonate and sodium fluoride sold as a dietary supplement, stops the progression of hearing loss in some clients. Hearing aids combined with a program of rehabilitation usually enable the client to hear. Surgical intervention involving the stapes also usually improves the hearing loss (refer to Chapter 76).

Specific Nursing Measures

Because the onset of otosclerosis usually occurs during the young adult period, affected clients may be anxious about whether the hearing loss will have an effect on their future. Reassure clients that if they use a hearing aid or undergo surgery, career plans usually need not be altered. Instruction in health care for a client with a hearing aid is discussed in Chapter 74, and the nursing care of a stapes surgery client is discussed in Chapter 76. A case study for the client with otosclerosis is presented at the end of this chapter.

Section II: Disorders of Multifactorial Origin

The acquired disorders—motion sickness and Meniere's syndrome (disorders of vestibular function) and psychogenic or nonorganic hearing disorders—are discussed in this section. Their exact etiologies are unknown but are thought to be related to a variety of physical and psychosocial factors. Motion sickness is a common condition, whereas the other two are not, but all have a significant impact on the quality of life.

MOTION SICKNESS

Motion sickness is a temporary disturbance in the functioning of the semicircular canals. Little is known about its exact cause and nature. It happens to some but not all people exposed to repetitive, shifting movement such as riding in a boat, on amusement park rides, or in the back seat of an automobile for long distances. The constantly shifting head position, changes in acceleration, and conflicting vestibular and visual signals are thought to be responsible for motion sickness.

Clinical Manifestations

Symptoms are dizziness and nausea that often progresses to vomiting. Motion sickness may begin soon after the exposure to motion and may not subside until several hours after the stimulation has stopped.

Therapeutic Measures

Some people are helped by taking steps to minimize changes in the visual field. It may help to hold the head in a fixed position and to focus the eyes on a single point. Dancers learn this early in their career; when twirling, spinning, or turning rapidly they keep their eyes fixed on one object and turn their heads rapidly to refocus as quickly as possible on the same object.

Antinauseants such as dimenhydrinate (Dramamine), meclizine hydrochloride (Antivert, Bonine), trimethobenzamide hydrochloride (Tigan), and cyclizine hydrochloride (Marezine) have been used successfully to prevent motion sickness as well as to relieve the symptoms. They may be taken by mouth ½ hour to 1 hour before the anticipated motion begins and then continued until the symptoms subside. If vomiting makes the oral route ineffective, intramuscular administration may be necessary.

Clients who anticipate long trips by air, sea, or car can use a transdermal system (Transderm-Scop), a flat disk with a drug reservoir containing scopolamine applied to intact skin in a hairless area behind the ear. The disk delivers scopolamine at a relatively constant rate to the systemic circulation over a 3-day period. It should be applied approximately 4 hours before the antiemetic effect is needed.

Some clients become too drowsy using Transderm-Scop and discontinue its use.

Specific Nursing Measures

Clients should be taught measures to avoid or reduce motion sickness. Clients taking antinauseants should be cautioned about operating machinery or driving a motor vehicle. Sucking on hard candies will reduce the problems of dry mouth. Whoever applies or removes Transderm-Scop should wash the hands thoroughly with soap and water to prevent scopolamine from coming into direct contact with the eyes. The application site should also be thoroughly washed and dried. Guidelines for applying and removing the Transderm-Scop are given in Box 75–1.

MENIERE'S SYNDROME

Meniere's syndrome (endolymphatic hydrops) is a disorder of the inner ear that results from an increased volume of endolymph with dilation of the membranous labyrinth that can progress to herniation and rupture of the membranous labyrinth. The disease is characterized by exacerbations of three symptoms (vertigo, tinnitus, and sensorineural hearing loss) and remissions until finally a complete remission occurs spontaneously. Meniere's syndrome usually begins between 40 and 60 years of age and is rare in chil-

---

Box 75–1   Guidelines for Applying and Removing the Transderm-Scop System

Apply 4 hours before needed.

Select a hairless area behind one ear, free from cuts or irritations, and wipe the area with a clean dry tissue.

Peel the package open and remove the system.

Remove the clear plastic covering from the round disk without touching the adhesive surface (metallic side) of the disk.

Firmly apply the metallic side with the adhesive surface to the dry skin behind the ear making sure that all edges have good contact with skin.

Do not remove the disk until it will no longer be used. It is good for 3 days but may be removed sooner if desired.

Wash hands with soap and water and dry thoroughly to remove any scopolamine.

Remove and discard the disk after 3 days.

For nausea control longer than 3 days, apply a new system behind the other ear and follow the instructions given above.

Keep the system as dry as possible to prevent it from falling off. Limited contact with water, as in bathing or swimming, is not likely to affect the system.

dren. The incidence of the disorder is unknown, but estimates range from about 0.05% to 0.15% of the population (Jerger & Jerger, 1981).

The exact cause of the increased volume of endolymph—whether excessive production or deficient reabsorption—is unknown. Deficient reabsorption suggests that the defect is in the function of the endolymphatic sac, but other factors also have been suggested, such as viral infections, allergies, endocrine disturbances, and paroxysmal vasomotor dysfunction. The disease seems to be exacerbated by emotional stress.

Clinical Manifestations

A client in the acute phase of Meniere's syndrome is in obvious distress and may be incapacitated and require hospitalization. Symptoms include severe vertigo with nausea and vomiting, tinnitus, and an uncomfortable full feeling in one ear progressing to hearing loss. The vertigo persists from 1 to 12 hours followed by a period of unsteadiness, fluctuating hearing loss, and tinnitus. The client may be anxious, irritable, and depressed. Temperature, pulse, and blood pressure are usually normal.

A period of remission follows the initial acute phase. Future acute attacks can occur at any time from a few weeks to months after the initial attack. Remission between the acute attacks then becomes longer until a complete remission occurs spontaneously. The client is left with varying degrees of hearing impairment, especially for low tones.

Physical examination during the acute attacks reveals nystagmus and ataxia. Tuning fork tests reveal a sensorineural hearing loss, and electronystagmography (ENG) shows hyporeaction. Pure tone audiometry usually indicates a unilateral sensorineural hearing loss. Serial audiograms also illustrate the gradual hearing decline. During remissions, no nystagmus or ataxia is observable; hearing tests can remain abnormal, however, and tinnitus can persist.

Therapeutic Measures

No treatment has been entirely successful in altering the course of Meniere's syndrome, but many drugs are useful for symptomatic relief. Some clients find that vasodilation with histamine phosphate controls the vertigo. Other antivertiginous drugs include dimenhydrinate (Dramamine), meclizine hydrochloride (Antivert, Bonine), and diphenhydramine hydrochloride (Benadryl). Sedatives such as diazepam (Valium) and anticholinergic drugs such as atropine, propantheline bromide (Pro-Banthine), and glycopyrrolate (Robinul) help control nausea, vomiting, and perspiration.

Salt restriction and diuretics such as ammonium chloride may relieve fullness or pressure in the ear. Some clients show an immediate improvement on this regimen and are able to avoid taking high-risk drugs or having sur-

gery. An essentially salt-free diet, called the Fürstenberg diet, is sometimes recommended (see Box 75–2) and may benefit some clients. When allergy appears to be the cause, elimination diets to discover the source of the allergy, followed by desensitization injections, are used. Hearing aids can help with the hearing loss and mask tinnitus for some clients.

Surgical procedures include endolymphatic sac operations to preserve the residual hearing, or destruction of the inner ear to relieve the symptoms. The latter procedure is reserved for clients whose lives are intolerable

---

Box 75–2 Fürstenberg Diet for Meniere's Syndrome

General Guidelines

1. Fluids are unrestricted, but excessive fluid intake is discouraged.
2. Proteins are encouraged.
3. Sodium is restricted.
4. Foods are to be prepared and served without salt.

Specific Guidelines

1. Avoid the following foods at all times:

Bread (salted)	Clams	Meats (salted)
Butter (salted)	Condensed milk	Olives
Carrots	Crackers (salted)	Oysters
Caviar	Endive	Raisins
Cheese	Fish (salted)	Spinach

2. Eat the following foods no more than twice weekly:

Beets	Dates	Peanuts
Buttermilk	Figs	Pumpkin
Cantaloupe	Horseradish	Radishes
Cauliflower	Kohlrabi	Rutabagas
Celery	Limes	Strawberries
Chard	Muskmelon	Turnips
Coconut (dried)	Mustard	Watercress
Currants (dried)	Peaches	

3. Eat the following foods daily:

Bread (unsalted) as desired

Butter (unsalted), candy (except chocolate), cream, honey, jam, jellies, and sugar as desired

Cereals such as farina, oatmeal, puffed rice, puffed wheat, rice

Eggs as desired

Fish as desired

Fowl as desired

Fruits (except those listed above)

Milk as desired

Potato and at least one of the following: corn, cranberries, macaroni, plums, prunes, rice, spaghetti, vegetables (except those listed above)

because of severe attacks of vertigo or who have permanent hearing impairment in the affected ear. These surgical procedures are discussed in Chapter 76.

Specific Nursing Measures

During the acute stage, bed rest with siderails to prevent falling is advisable. Support the client's head with pillows on each side to prevent movement, which usually aggravates the vertigo. The client will need assistance while vomiting. Reassure the client that the acute phase will soon end. Clear liquids as tolerated are encouraged to prevent dehydration, but usually an IV line is started for fluid and drug administration. Watch for signs of any side effects of the drugs administered.

After the acute phase, encourage the client to lead as relaxed a lifestyle as possible, since stress appears to bring on the acute phase. Smoking and alcohol act as vasoconstrictors and can affect the absorption of endolymph. The nurse should encourage programs to reduce stress (see Chapter 2) and to stop smoking.

PSYCHOGENIC OR NONORGANIC HEARING DISORDER

A psychogenic hearing loss has no known organic cause; it is usually precipitated by emotional stress and may be under either involuntary or voluntary control. For example, a person in tremendous conflict (severe psychological stress) may suddenly develop deafness. Known in psychiatric terminology as a conversion disorder (hysterical conversion), this deafness is not under voluntary control; the symptom is symbolic of the client's psychological conflict. The symptom actually helps keep the psychological conflict out of the client's awareness (primary gain). It may enable the client to avoid an unwanted task or to receive support from others because of the disability.

Hearing impairment may also be feigned or exaggerated. In this case, the client has voluntary control over deafness to achieve specific goals, such as avoiding military service or obtaining financial compensation. The purposeful production of false or exaggerated symptoms for these purposes is known as malingering.

A diagnosis of psychogenic hearing loss should not be made until a thorough and comprehensive assessment of the client has determined that a physiological problem does not indeed exist.

Clinical Manifestations

The extent of psychogenic hearing loss varies from client to client, although total hearing loss is likely in conversion disorders. Retests of hearing acuity and audiometric tests may yield inconsistent results, especially if malingering is a factor.

Therapeutic Measures

The treatment for psychogenic hearing loss is determined by the individual client's needs. Many may need psychological counseling.

Specific Nursing Measures

The nurse should maintain a calm, unhurried, understanding attitude. Often health professionals are impatient and annoyed with clients they perceive not to be legitimately ill and thus limit the amount of time they spend with them. Although it may be difficult, it is crucial to strive for a nonjudgmental attitude. The nurse should encourage and support the client who requires psychological counseling.

Section III: Degenerative Disorders

Normal physiological alterations of aging affect the ears, just as they affect other organ systems in the body. Changes in the ear include atrophy of the external auditory canal and a decrease in the elasticity of the auricle, tympanic membrane, and the muscles and ligaments of the ear (Jerger & Jerger, 1981). In the third and fourth decades, the hairs in the wall of the male auditory canal become coarser and longer; when entangled with cerumen, they can cause obstructions. In the female, a decrease in sebaceous gland activity leads to a decrease in sebum production. The number and activity of the ceruminous glands also decrease in the elderly. Although arthritic changes such as calcification of the cartilage and narrowing of the joint spaces can occur in the ossicular joints, studies show these changes do not affect sound transmission (Anderson & Meyerhoff, 1982).

The normal decrease in glandular secretions predisposes the aging population to infections, trauma, and obstruction of the ears. It is estimated that 30% of the elderly have a hearing impairment that affects their communication.

General Nursing Implications

Nurses in the community or long-term care centers are taking a more active role in the care of the elderly. Early detection and prevention of infections, trauma, and obstruction may prevent or restore hearing loss. This, in turn, prevents many social and psychological problems relating to hearing loss.

PRESBYCUSIS

Presbycusis (presbyacusia) is a slowly progressive, bilateral hearing loss due to aging. It is usually more pronounced at frequencies above 2000 Hz.

Presbycusis has been categorized into four different

types: sensory, neural, strial, and cochlear conductive. More than one type of presbycusis is often present in the older adult. *Sensory presbycusis* usually begins in middle age and progresses slowly. Although there is a high tone hearing loss, speech discrimination usually is good. Atrophy of the organ of Corti at its basal end results in loss of outer hair cells and supporting cells, which causes the hearing loss.

Neural presbycusis begins at any age and is due to the loss of cochlea neurons in the auditory pathway. The organ of Corti is usually not affected, so pure tone hearing is relatively normal. However, the loss of neurons leads to poor speech discrimination.

Strial presbycusis, which is slowly progressive, can begin in middle or old age and is often associated with a family history of hearing loss. Pure tone hearing loss is associated with patchy atrophic changes in the stria vascularis (the capillary-containing portion of the membranous labyrinth). Speech discrimination is usually good unless the pure tone loss falls below 50 dB (Anderson & Meyerhoff, 1982).

Cochlear conductive presbycusis begins in middle age and is thought to be related to a stiffening of the basilar membrane. Pure tone and speech discrimination steadily decline on audiometric testing, but no pathological degenerative changes explain the degree of hearing loss.

Hearing loss attributed to degenerative changes can be related to many factors, such as diet, exercise, smoking, noise, metabolism, arteriosclerosis, emotional stress, and heredity. The definitive cause of presbycusis, however, remains unexplained after many studies.

Clinical Manifestations

A gradual progressive hearing loss, the major clinical symptom of presbycusis, is confirmed by hearing acuity tests and audiometry. The rate of progression varies with clients but usually accelerates with age. Some clients complain of tinnitus and dizziness, and families or significant others often notice personality changes in the client such as depression or irritability.

Therapeutic Measures

No effective medical or surgical treatment has been found for presbycusis. Its management consists of aural rehabilitation including hearing aids, psychosocial counseling, and emotional support.

Specific Nursing Measures

Support and reinforce the programs instituted by the audiologist and discourage unproven cures. Safety is a concern whenever dizziness occurs; remind the client to keep safety measures in mind. The nurse's health teaching includes instructing the client and family or significant others about presbycusis and its effect on communication. The family or significant others should be taught how to communicate more effectively with the client and assist with the care of the hearing aid, if necessary. Caregivers should make a special effort to prevent client withdrawal and isolation; the nurse can encourage and even arrange for social contact with community groups or volunteers.

Section IV: Immunologic Disorders

Immunologic factors are possible causes of some of the multifactorial, infectious, and degenerative disorders affecting the ear that are discussed in other sections of this chapter. Immunologic factors associated with allergies of the external ear are essentially dermatologic. Progressive sensorineural hearing loss and vestibular dysfunction in young adults has recently been related to an autoimmune disorder. It is thought that minor trauma such as myringotomy (incision into the pars tensa) may trigger this process. Optimal treatment has not been defined, but steroids and cyclophosphamide are being used (Sataloff, Sataloff, & Vassallo, 1980).

Section V: Infectious Disorders

Infection is the most common disease process of the ear. Infectious disorders of the ear can be bacterial, fungal, or viral. The organism—introduced through the skin of the external ear, through a perforated tympanic membrane, or through the eustachian tube—produces inflammations in susceptible individuals. Infectious disorders can occur in the external, middle, and inner ear. Some infections are mild and heal without treatment, whereas others, if untreated, have serious complications such as mastoiditis (an infection spreading to the bone cells), brain abscess, meningitis, and hearing loss. Still other infections become chronic, resisting treatment.

General Nursing Implications

People often consult nurses about earaches. Some earaches are associated with a self-limited infection, and the knowledgeable nurse can assess the ear and advise people to seek medical care for treatment and prevention of complications when appropriate. Finally, nurses can prevent the spread of some infections through education of the public in aural hygiene measures (discussed in Chapter 74).

EXTERNAL OTITIS

External otitis (otitis externa) is basically an inflammation of the skin. Because of its location, its effect on hearing, and its complications, it is considered to be in the realm of otology even though it overlaps with dermatology.

External otitis can be localized or diffuse. Diffuse otitis is either primarily otological (the skin infection begins in the ear and spreads to surrounding face, neck, and scalp) or primarily dermatological (the infection spreads to the ear from surrounding areas). Primarily dermatological otitis, which includes herpes, warts, seborrheic dermatitis, and eczema, will not be discussed here. When these disorders occur in the ear, they are treated the same way as when they occur in other areas of the skin (see Chapters 77 through 80).

Removal of the normal protective barriers predisposes individuals to external ear infections. Thus, fastidious cleaning of the external auditory canal removes the protective cerumen and allows invading organisms to enter, especially when the skin is traumatized by applicators, pencils, hair clips, or fingernails. Water or moisture retained in the ear after swimming or showering can cause a maceration of the skin. The moisture combines with the keratin, cerumen, and other debris, causing them to swell within the ear. The swelling obstructs the openings of the apocrine and other sebaceous ducts, which decreases the normal protective skin secretions. This process accounts for the greater frequency of infections in hot, humid environments.

The many types of external otitis are categorized according to the causative agent and the clinical course of the infection. A severe life-threatening external otitis, *malignant otitis externa,* occurs in elderly diabetics. It begins in the skin of the external auditory canal and, if not arrested, extends through the soft tissue to the temporal bone and the other bones that form the floor of the cranial cavity— the frontal, sphenoid, ethmoid, and occipital bones.

Furunculosis is a localized external otitis of the hair follicles in the cartilaginous part (outer half) of the external auditory canal (Figure 75–1). It begins as a red papule and develops into a pustule (furuncle), which usually erupts and drains spontaneously. Furuncles are caused by staphylococci, which are usually introduced into the skin by scratching with contaminated fingernails or other objects. Inflammation of multiple follicles is called a carbuncle. Recurrent furuncles occur more frequently in clients with diabetes.

Diffuse bacterial external otitis, commonly called swimmer's ear, affects 5% to 20% of clients seen in health care settings during the summer months. A combination of high temperature, high humidity, and contamination of the skin with gram-negative bacilli causes diffuse bacterial external otitis. Three stages of inflammation can occur;

preinflammatory, acute, and chronic inflammation. In the preinflammatory stage, the cells become macerated because of moisture in the ear. Pruritus with scratching leads to traumatization and infection of the skin, which initiates the acute stage. This stage may be mild, moderate, or severe, depending on the clinical manifestations. Chronic inflammation is recurrent and does not respond to treatment.

Otomycosis, an acute or chronic external otitis, is often found secondary to a bacterial infection, occurring after the extended use of topical corticosteroids and antibiotics. It is caused by fungi, most commonly *Aspergillus niger* and *Candida albicans.* The clinical course, usually occurring in hot weather, runs from a mild to a severe inflammation with frequent recurrences.

Clinical Manifestations

The first symptom of furunculosis is pruritus, which progresses to a persistent, excruciating pain in 24 to 48 hours. The nurse examining a client should be aware that pulling on the auricle, moving the jaw, or inserting a speculum causes extreme pain (see Figure 75–1). Preauricular or postauricular adenopathy may be present. The swelling in the auditory canal may obscure the tympanic membrane. If visible, however, it is normal. With the otoscope, an erythematous swelling is usually visible in the canal. Conductive hearing loss occurs only when the lumen of the canal is completely obstructed. A mild fever may be present until the furuncle erupts. Pain is relieved immediately after the furuncle erupts and drains. The drainage is a whitish-yellow, fetid exudate.

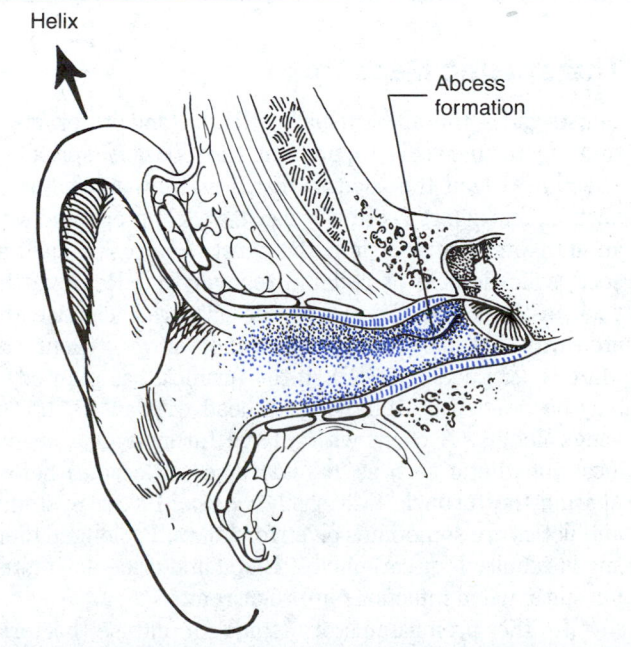

Figure 75–1

External otitis with furunculosis.

During the preinflammatory stage of diffuse bacterial external otitis, the client complains of severe pruritus, and scratch marks may be visible. Slight erythema of the skin in the external auditory canal and a dull (rather than shiny) tympanic membrane are observed during the acute mild stage. Occasionally, a clear odorless discharge may be present. Mild discomfort occurs when pressing on the tragus or pulling the auricle. During the acute moderate stage, the opening of the external auditory canal is partially occluded with seropurulent debris. Periauricular edema causes a moderate amount of pain, and preauricular and postauricular adenopathy may now be present. In the acute severe stage, the pain is so intense that the client is reluctant to move the jaw. Seropurulent bluish-gray or greenish secretions completely obstruct the canal. Severe periauricular edema is present. Cultures usually reveal *Pseudomonas*, and the client usually has a fever.

In chronic diffuse bacterial external otitis, there is a thickening of the skin and edema of the auricle. The skin may appear dry and scaly. A gray-brown or greenish secretion with a fetid odor is present in the canal. Pain is usually not as severe as in the acute stage. The tympanic membrane is thick and dull. Cultures reveal a gram-negative bacillus (usually *Proteus* or *Pseudomonas*) and fungal infections. Fungal infections are discussed in the section on otomycosis.

The client with otomycosis usually seeks care because of severe pain. Often there is a previous history of otomycosis. Otoscopic examination reveals the *Aspergillus niger* as a grayish or bluish membrane with black spots covering the external auditory canal and tympanic membrane. *Candida albicans* appears as a creamy white deposit. Removal of the membrane or deposit leaves a reddened area. A serous or serosanguineous otorrhea may be present.

Therapeutic Measures

Conservative therapy is usually effective and preferable in treating furunculosis to prevent the possible spread of infection. Clean the auditory canal with an applicator or suction, and insert a cotton or gauze wick impregnated with an antibiotic ointment into the canal. Analgesics such as acetylsalicylic acid or codeine relieve pain. Remove the wick in 24 hours; if drainage has occurred, cleanse the area with 70% alcohol and insert another wick (Senturia, Marcus, & Lucenti, 1980). If the furuncle has pointed, it may be drained by removing its head with an 18- or 20-gauge needle. A client with a large furuncle may need a local anesthetic such as 1% lidocaine (Xylocaine) before incising the furuncle (Marshall & Attia, 1983). Systemic antibiotics are sometimes given for 4 days. Prolonged therapy is required for carbuncles. Blood and urine are tested for sugar when infections are recurrent.

In the preinflammatory stage of diffuse bacterial external otitis, treatment consists of irrigating the auditory canal with 3% hypertonic saline to remove debris and carefully drying it with cotton-tipped swabs or a hair dryer. A topical corticosteroid or antibiotic cream is usually effective at this stage.

Avoid irrigation in the acute mild stage. Polymyxin or gentamicin drops or a corticosteroid cream applied to the concha may be helpful.

Treatment for the acute moderate stage is similar to that of the mild stage, except that cultures and sensitivity testing for identification of the organism are obtained. If the auditory canal is obstructed, a gauze impregnated with an antibiotic and corticosteroid is packed into the canal. An oral broad-spectrum antibiotic also is administered. Analgesics and sedatives are necessary to relieve the pain. When the edema in the auditory canal subsides, antibiotic drops may be substituted for the gauze packing. This therapy usually continues for several days.

In the acute severe stage, treatment is similar to that in the moderate stage, except added analgesics are needed to control the pain. Identification of the organism and sensitivity testing are imperative. When the client cannot tolerate oral therapy because of nausea and vomiting, hospitalization becomes necessary for the administration of parenteral antibiotics and parenteral fluids. On rare occasions, an abscess may need to be incised and drained.

The treatment for chronic diffuse bacterial external otitis is similar to the treatment for the mild acute form. The sensitivity of the organism is obtained before antibiotics are administered via a cotton wick impregnated with a mixture of antibiotics and corticosteroid cream packed into the canal. Aluminum acetate packs are applied to the periauricular eczematous areas. Failure of treatment may indicate a secondary fungal infection.

With otomycosis, careful cleaning of the auditory canal with suction or dry wipes is imperative for at least three consecutive days. Many topical antimycotic agents are available for treatment, such as nystatin (Nilstat) and clotrimazole (Lotrimin). Analgesics for pain also may be necessary. Treatment should be continued at least a week after the infection has cleared up.

Specific Nursing Measures

A hot water bottle applied to the ear of the client with furunculosis promotes eruption and drainage. Purulent drainage can cause the spread of the pathogens, however, so take care to prevent this spread by cleaning the discharge with a cotton ear swab. Discourage clients from touching or scratching the ear, because staphylococci in the nares are often transferred to the ear by scratching the nasal mucosa and then the ears. Encourage frequent hand washing with a bactericidal soap. Tell the client to avoid inserting objects into the canal for removal of cerumen, an instruction that can be reinforced by information on the protective value of cerumen. All directions should be explained and written down. Include medication ordered, how it is administered, its side effects, and symptoms of allergic reactions.

Nursing management of the client with diffuse bacterial external otitis consists of cleaning the ear with cotton-tipped swabs and applying creams or drops as indicated. The client should be taught to administer ear drops and apply creams safely (see Chapter 74). Preventive measures are similar to those described for furunculosis. The client should be taught to keep water out of the ear (see Chapter 74) to prevent recurrence or chronicity. People who wear ear molds should pay special attention to cleaning and drying the ears.

Keeping the ear dry is the most important nursing measure for otomycosis. The client should wear earplugs or cotton plugs impregnated with a water-soluble jelly when showering. The nurse can help prevent otomycosis by discouraging self-treatment with ear drops for an earache.

SUPPURATIVE OTITIS MEDIA

Otitis media is an inflammation of the mucoperiosteal lining of the middle ear, including the eustachian tube, middle ear cavity, mastoid antrum, and mastoid air cells. The mucous membrane of the middle ear is continuous with the respiratory mucous membrane of the nasal cavity, sinuses, nasopharynx, eustachian tube, trachea, bronchi, and part of the larynx. Thus, otitis media may affect some or all of these structures. When associated with bacterial infection it is called suppurative otitis media. Inflammation of the middle ear without infection is called serous otitis media and is discussed later in this chapter.

Acute suppurative otitis media (acute purulent otitis media) is a bacterial infection of the middle ear lining. It occurs in people of all ages but especially in children, because their eustachian tubes are shorter and wider than adult eustachian tubes. In children, the condition affects both ears, whereas it usually affects only one ear in adults. *Chronic suppurative otitis media* is a continuous infection in the middle ear that lasts for at least 3 months. Severe cases can lead to an erosion of the ossicles.

The most common cause of acute suppurative otitis media is *Hemophilus influenzae* in children and pneumococci in adults. Beta-hemolytic streptococcus is usually the cause when otitis media occurs as a complication of the common cold. Suppurative otitis media can result from an upper respiratory tract infection, sinusitis, improper nose blowing, and the obstruction of hypertrophied adenoids.

In chronic suppurative otitis media, a permanent central perforation of the tympanic membrane exposes the middle ear lining to bacteria. Exposure of the middle ear lining also seems to make it more susceptible to infection via the eustachian tube.

Clinical Manifestations

Although acute suppurative otitis media is usually a self-limited disease, it runs through characteristic clinical stages depending on the virulence of the bacteria and the sus-

ceptibility of the host. A recent history of upper respiratory tract infection followed by an earache, fever, and sense of fullness in the ear is associated with the first stage. Hyperemic swelling beginning in the eustachian tube and extending to the middle ear causes the signs and symptoms. Hearing is usually normal at this stage. Otoscopy reveals a dull, thickened, injected tympanic membrane.

The second stage occurs 12 to 24 hours later. The formation of an exudate causes occasional vomiting (usually in children) and conductive hearing loss. Otoscopy reveals a bulging, red, lusterless, immobile tympanic membrane with loss of landmarks and cone of light. Superficial tenderness may occur over the mastoid process of the temporal bone. X-rays taken at this time may reveal air cells filled with fluid that appear cloudy; however, the bone cells are intact. Temperature also increases at this stage. If untreated, the tympanic membrane ruptures and expels a purulent discharge. Symptoms subside after the rupture.

A recurrence of pain with fever, deep mastoid tenderness, and an increase in foul purulent discharge indicates mastoiditis. However, this rarely occurs today with antibiotic therapy.

In chronic suppurative otitis media, the mucous membrane, seen through the perforated tympanic membrane, may appear edematous or pale and thin. Conductive hearing loss is present.

Therapeutic Measures

Objectives of therapy are to resolve the infection and prevent its spread into the bone. The absence of fever indicates a viral or mild infection that will resolve spontaneously. When fever is present, antibiotic administration is started and continued for at least 7 to 10 days—even though symptoms subside—to prevent the recurrence of an incompletely resolved infection. Ampicillin, the drug of choice for adults, can be replaced by erythromycin in the case of allergy. The otitis media usually resolves at this stage. Acetaminophen (Tylenol), aspirin, and occasionally codeine are used to relieve the pain. Decongestants may be used with inflammation of the eustachian tube to relieve pressure in the middle ear and eustachian tube.

With fever, extreme pain, and a bulging tympanic membrane, a myringotomy (see Chapter 76) may be performed to release the exudate. Cultures and sensitivity of the exudate should be obtained if the drainage persists. Hearing should be tested after apparent resolution of the infection to be certain there is no residual hearing loss.

Treatment for chronic suppurative otitis media consists of cleaning the external ear with suction or dry wipes. A broad-spectrum antibiotic in boric acid powder is insufflated into the ear once or twice a week until the ear is dry. Exacerbations are treated as they are in acute suppurative otitis media. Surgical closure of the tympanic membrane when the ear is dry improves hearing. If hypertrophied adenoids obstruct the eustachian tube, they are often surgically removed. If mastoiditis occurs, antibiotics and myringotomy are the treatments of choice; mastoidectomy is almost never done today.

Specific Nursing Measures

Care of clients with otitis media focuses on pain management and preventing the spread of the disease. Heat may be used to relieve pain. Cleaning the external ear with dry cotton swabs and placing cotton loosely in the ear prevents the drainage from spreading the infection to surrounding areas. Cold cream can prevent irritation of the skin of the external ear.

Provide the client with written instructions for the recommended treatment. Explain the cause of the disease and the rationale for taking the complete course of medication. Encourage fluids, adequate rest, and the use of earplugs or cotton impregnated with vaseline during showering. When the tympanic membrane is perforated or a myringotomy has been performed, swimming is usually prohibited until the tympanic membrane has healed.

Clients should be aware that forceful nose blowing could force infected pathogens into the middle ear. Clients with an upper respiratory tract infection should not close their nostrils when blowing their noses; sniffing or just wiping the nostrils is safer.

SEROUS OTITIS MEDIA

Serous otitis media (middle ear effusion), a nonsuppurative otitis media, is an accumulation of serous fluid within the middle ear. Acute serous otitis media is a sudden accumulation of fluid. This occurs more frequently in adults, whereas the chronic form, a gradual accumulation, is more commonly found in children. The fluid can remain in the ear for months or years before it is detected.

The incidence of middle ear effusions seems to be increasing. Although it is technically not an infectious disorder, it is discussed here because it is thought to be related to the increased use of antibiotics for treating ear infections, which results in a residual sterile fluid. This condition is also associated with viral respiratory infections, allergies, or obstruction of the eustachian tube. Allergies cause hyperplasia of the secretory cells and increased secretions. An obstruction or dysfunction of the eustachian tube may result from upper respiratory infection, allergy, enlarged adenoidal tissue, trauma, or tumors. The eustachian tube clears secretions and replenishes oxygen to the middle ear mucosa. Thus, obstruction of the eustachian tube causes a negative pressure in the middle ear resulting in removal of fluid from the cells and its accumulation in the middle ear.

Clinical Manifestations

The signs and symptoms of nonsuppurative otitis media are minimal. The most significant sign is poor mobility of the tympanic membrane seen with the pneumatic otoscope or tympanometry. A history of allergies may or may not be present. Adult clients may complain of a feeling of fullness or bubbling and crackling in the ear. Usually, no pain is present. Mouth breathing may occur.

Audiometry detects a conductive hearing loss; if the loss is below 15 dB, however, a Rinne test may not detect it. The tympanic membrane may appear normal, grayish-white, or bluish and may be thickened or retracted. A fluid level or bubbles may be visible through the tympanic membrane (see Figure 75–2). The fluid may be straw colored. If adenoids are causing the condition, they may be visualized in the nasopharynx.

Therapeutic Measures

Although decongestants have been the standard therapy, their efficacy in treating otitis media has not been proven. Often the client is observed for 3 to 4 weeks to allow normal absorption of the fluid with self-ventilating techniques. The client may be referred to an allergist for sensitivity testing and desensitization. Periodic audiometric testing to ascertain hearing loss is necessary.

A Mathes inflator can be used to inflate the eustachian tube. This device provides positive pressure through the nasopharynx while the client swallows, forcing air up the eustachian tube to the middle ear. Tympanocentesis or myringotomy with insertion of ventilating tubes may be performed to remove fluid. These surgical procedures are discussed in Chapter 76. Other surgery includes adenoidectomy or removal of tissue obstructing the lumen of the eustachian tube.

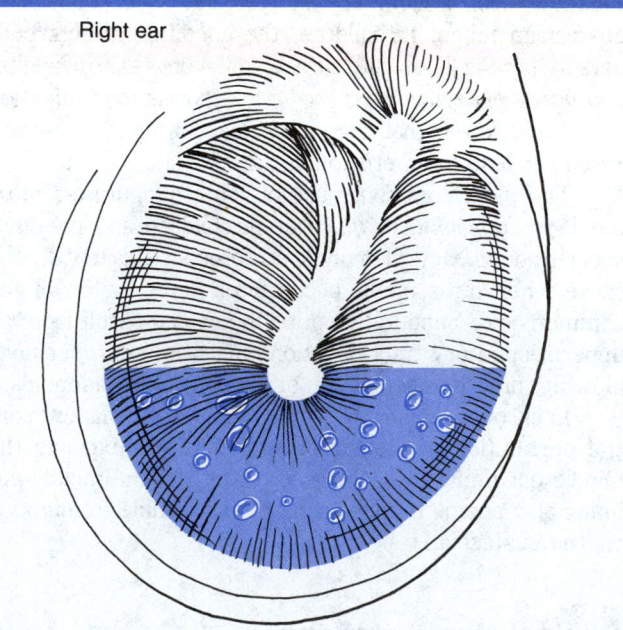

Right ear

Figure 75–2

Fluid level and air bubbles behind the tympanic membrane in serous otitis media.

Specific Nursing Measures

Explain the cause of middle ear effusion to the client. The client should be taught self-ventilating techniques and be encouraged to use them (see Chapter 74). When myringotomy has been performed, take precautions similar to those described previously. Nursing care for a client having a myringotomy is discussed in Chapter 76.

Section VI: Neoplastic Disorders

Neoplastic disorders include benign and malignant disorders of the external, middle, and inner ear. The temporal bone can be invaded by malignant tumors arising in the cranium, parotid glands, salivary glands, nasopharynx, and neck. Metastases from the abdomen or thorax also can infiltrate the temporal bone.

A lack of specific symptoms often results in the spread of the disease before it is recognized. Lesions of the external ear are visible, but tinnitus and a gradual hearing loss may be the only symptoms of middle and inner ear lesions until they are well established. Pain, bleeding, vertigo with nausea, and vomiting occur late in the course of most carcinomas. Chronic otorrhea similar to that occurring with infections should always be explored further.

Neoplastic disorders of the external ear, if not detected early, can result in deformities; thus, they create both psychological and functional problems. Although tumors of the middle and inner ear are rare, they are serious, causing bone erosion, hearing loss, and even death.

General Nursing Implications

Nurses can assist in early detection of neoplastic disorders through cancer-screening programs, hearing testing, and careful inspection of any client with whom they have contact. They can provide emotional support when the diagnosis is made and disfigurement or hearing impairment are imminent. Rehabilitation programs involving nurses are often necessary.

NEOPLASMS OF THE EXTERNAL AND MIDDLE EAR

Neoplastic changes of the external and middle ear may be benign or malignant. Most common benign skin lesions occur in the skin of the auricle and the cartilaginous part of the external auditory canal. These include lipomas, fibromas, sebaceous cysts, warts, and keloids. Keloids, which are more common in the black population, occur where previous trauma has occurred. The lobule is the most common site because of ear piercing. Keloids can grow as large as golf balls. Nodular bony growths (osteophytes, or exostoses) occur in the bony canal. They are usually bilateral and occur more commonly after puberty in males.

Actinic keratosis, a common precancerous lesion, occurs more frequently on the auricle of the elderly. Squamous and basal cell carcinomas are the most common malignant lesions of the external and middle ear. If untreated, basal cell lesions grow and invade local structures such as cartilage and bone. Squamous cell carcinomas slowly invade and metastasize into surrounding tissues. Metastasis to the lymph nodes usually occurs first in the preauricular nodes. Malignant melanoma, which usually originates in a nevus, occurs more frequently in 40- to 50-year-olds.

The exact cause of benign and malignant lesions of the ear is unknown. Excessive exposure to the sun is associated with actinic keratosis and basal cell carcinoma, which are more prevalent in light-skinned individuals. Osteophytes occur in individuals whose auditory canals have been subjected to trauma. These bony growths are associated with frequent swimming in cold water.

Clinical Manifestations

Few symptoms occur with external ear neoplasms. Sebaceous cysts or lipomas feel like smooth, soft, mobile masses under the skin. Exostoses of various sizes are visible in the external auditory canal. The client may complain of the ear feeling blocked, especially when cerumen accumulates behind the bony growth.

Any scaly, translucent lesion should be further investigated. A squamous cell lesion may resemble an external otitis that does not heal. The discharge may be blood tinged, and lymphadenopathy may also be present. When the squamous cell cancer spreads to the bony canal and the middle ear, pain and hearing loss occur. Polyps also may appear in the canal. Paralysis of the facial nerve can become evident in the advanced stages. Biopsy with histological examinations confirms the diagnosis, and radiographic studies show the extent of the lesion.

Therapeutic Measures

Benign tumors are removed surgically if they show signs of growth or secondary infection. Local excision is usually adequate for basal cell carcinomas, whereas radiation and chemotherapy are used to treat lesions that have spread. Squamous cell carcinomas limited to the auricle require radical excision or total auriculectomy, often followed by radiation therapy. Skin grafts may be necessary to aid healing. Auricular prostheses often provide better cosmetic results than auricular reconstruction. Advanced carcinomas may require temporal bone resection with upper neck dissection. Surgical treatment for basal cell and squamous cell carcinomas is discussed in Chapter 80. Head and neck surgery is discussed in Chapter 21 and skin grafting in Chapter 80.

Specific Nursing Measures

Clients with neoplastic disorders require a great deal of emotional support. Try to relieve their anxiety by fully explaining the effects of the neoplasm and all anticipated procedures. Keep the external ear as clean as possible, removing any discharge present to prevent infection.

Many ear surgeries today are performed in outpatient surgical units. Here the nurse is responsible for teaching the client, family member, or significant others whatever care is necessary. Emphasize precautions about infections or getting water into the ear. Rest usually is recommended for the first few days, and the client is told not to touch the ear except to replace a sterile cotton ball within it. In most cases, the nurse will instruct the client to call the next day if no return visit is scheduled. Furthermore, the client, family member or significant others should be instructed to call immediately if there is any change in the client's temperature or if increased pain or bleeding occurs. Long-term follow-up is necessary for clients who need rehabilitation for hearing loss.

CHOLESTEATOMAS

A cholesteatoma is an ingrowth of epidermis (the squamous epithelium) from the external meatus into the middle ear attic. Cholesteatomas are more common during the teenage years and can be primary, secondary, or congenital.

A *primary cholesteatoma,* the most common form, originates as an ingrowth through a perforation in the pars flaccida (Figure 75–3). The cause of primary cholesteatoma is unknown; it is thought to be eustachian tube dysfunction that creates a vacuum within the middle ear, which

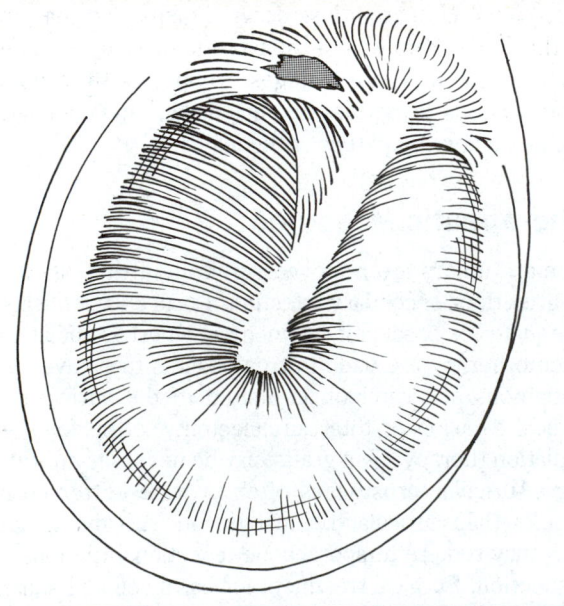

Figure 75–3

Perforation of the pars flaccida.

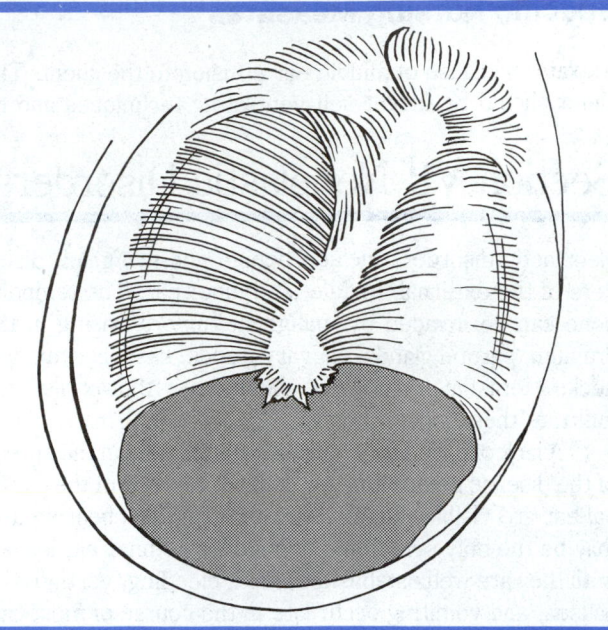

Figure 75–4

Peripheral perforation of the drum.

causes the loosest part of the pars flaccida to invaginate. A *secondary cholesteatoma* is an ingrowth of the annulus fibrosa through a peripheral perforation of the tympanic membrane usually caused by chronic suppurative otitis media (Figure 75–4). A *congenital cholesteatoma,* which is seen in children and young adults, is presumably caused by epidermis congenitally left within the middle ear behind a normal intact tympanic membrane. It is not associated with perforation. Epidermis in the middle ear produces keratin, which accumulates and destroys underlying tissue. As the disease progresses, it may destroy the ossicles and spread to the inner ear (see Figure 75–5). Secondary infection often occurs at the site of the accumulated keratin. A secondary infection occurring in the inner ear is called acute suppurative labyrinthitis; in the mastoid, it is called suppurative mastoiditis.

Clinical Manifestations

An early cholesteatoma may be asymptomatic, and the perforation in the pars flaccida is usually detected during a routine otoscopic examination. The first symptom may be a conductive hearing loss in the affected ear. A painless, fetid otorrhea occurs when a secondary infection is present. As the disease progresses, facial paralysis and vertigo can occur.

Therapeutic Measures

The treatment for a cholesteatoma is surgical removal. All the cholesteatoma must be removed to prevent further growth. If possible, a modified radical mastoidectomy followed by tympanoplasty is performed. Sometimes a radical

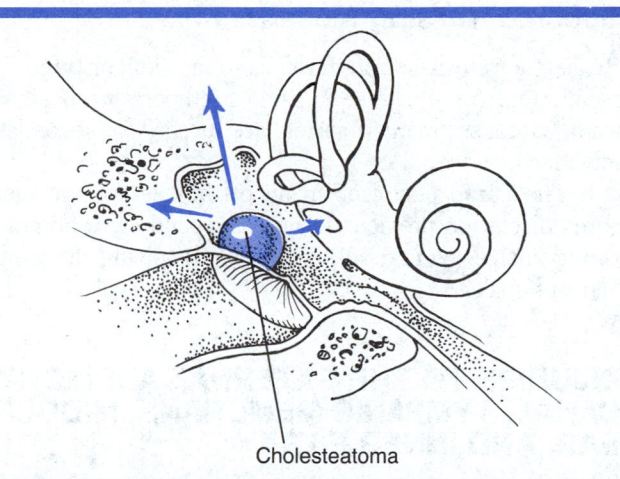

Figure 75–5

Cholesteatoma, which can erode into the inner ear, temporal bone, or epidural space.

mastoidectomy that removes all the mastoid air cells, the ossicles, and the tympanic membrane is necessary. After surgery, periodic lifelong follow-up to detect any new growth is essential (Marshall & Attia, 1983).

Specific Nursing Measures

Refer to the section on mastoidectomy in Chapter 76 for a discussion of the nursing care of a client undergoing surgery for cholesteatoma.

ACOUSTIC NEUROMA

An acoustic neuroma (also called an acoustic neurilemoma or an acoustic schwannoma) is a benign tumor arising from the neurilemmal sheath of the vestibular branch of cranial nerve VIII (the vestibulocochlear nerve) and occurring within the internal auditory canal or in the region of the cerebellopontile angle. As the tumor grows, the cochlear branch of CN VIII becomes involved. The tumor can begin at any age and grows slowly. The specific cause of acoustic neuroma is unknown. A small number of tumors (usually

bilateral) are a feature of von Recklinghausen's disease (see Chapter 37).

Clinical Manifestations

Clinical manifestations usually follow a predicted course as the tumor grows. The most common first symptom is tinnitus, followed by an increasing high-frequency hearing loss with low speech discrimination. As the tumor progresses, symptoms of involvement of the cranial nerves V and VII (trigeminal and facial nerves, respectively) are present; these include an absence of an ipsilateral corneal reflex, facial hypesthesia, trigeminal pain, and loss of taste in the anterior two-thirds of the tongue. As the tumor progresses, nystagmus and ataxia may occur. Cerebellar pressure causing papilledema occurs late in the disease. Diagnostic testing can include the examination of cerebrospinal fluid, which will show an elevation of protein.

Tumors 2 cm in diameter or larger can be detected by a computerized tomography (CT) scan. If the CT scan fails to detect a tumor but symptoms are present, a myelogram may be performed. The response to the electronystagmographic caloric test is reduced or absent.

Therapeutic Measures

The treatment for an acoustic neuroma is its surgical removal (discussed in Chapter 39). However, clients who are not safe candidates for surgery or have an extremely large tumor are treated with steroids. Gamma knife radiation has been successful for removing tumors less than 2 cm (Shambaugh & Glasscock, 1980).

Specific Nursing Measures

The nurse is responsible for preparing the client emotionally and physically for the diagnostic procedures and eventual surgery. Preoperative preparation and postoperative expectations should be discussed with both client and family or significant others. If the tumor affects the client's hearing, a method of communication should be established. Refer to Chapter 39 for surgical management.

Section VII: Traumatic Disorders

Traumatic disorders of the ear can result from injuries to the head, penetrating wounds through the auditory canal, or sudden atmospheric pressure changes. Traumatic conditions that affect auditory and vestibular function also can result from exposure to noise and reactions to certain drugs. Today the prevalence of motor vehicle accidents, industrial and other environmental noises, and exposure to ototoxic drugs account for many traumatic injuries. Because this trauma can result in disfigurement and auditory and vestibular impairment, it leads to physical and emotional problems.

General Nursing Implications

The prevention of traumatic disorders should be of prime importance to nurses, since so many are avoidable. Nurses can encourage safety measures wherever they work. In industrial situations, they can monitor noise levels, work to reduce them, and encourage the use of hearing protectors. Nurses should also be alert for potential ototoxic reactions to drugs. After traumatic injuries have occurred, important nursing measures are: providing meticulous care to prevent secondary infection and residual deformity, administering medications to alleviate pain, providing emotional support especially when hearing loss has occurred, encouraging the client's participation in a program of rehabilitation if one is necessary, and instructing the client in self-care and trauma prevention.

INJURIES TO THE AURICLE

Trauma of the auricle includes contusions, hematomas, abrasions, and lacerations caused by falls, vehicular accidents, blows to the ear, and foreign bodies. The ear's exposed position and the absence of subcutaneous tissue also predispose it to frostbite and burns.

Clinical Manifestations

Conductive hearing loss can be present with any traumatic injury. The client with a contusion and hematoma may complain of pain, numbness, and paresthesia of the auricle. Tenderness, erythema, or ecchymosis may be present. Repeated contusions may cause a thickening of the auricle called cauliflower ear. Lacerations may be small and superficial, be deep into the cartilage, or involve a complete avulsion of the auricle. Burns can cause extensive blistering or destruction of tissue. Frostbite occurs on the upper and outer edges first, and its extent is often not apparent. The frozen area appears waxy and whitish-yellow and feels cold and hard.

Therapeutic Measures

Mild analgesics are usually sufficient for easing pain of contusions and hematomas. Any fluid that accumulates should be aspirated; cotton impregnated with water-soluble jelly should be fitted into the contours of the auricle, and a pressure bandage should be applied for several days to prevent an accumulation of fluid. Antibiotics are recommended if there is evidence of infection.

Abrasions are cleaned thoroughly to remove any foreign matter. After an antibiotic ointment is applied, the wound can be left uncovered.

Surgical lacerations are sutured. When the laceration is contaminated or has been untreated for 24 hours, it may be debrided and treated with antibacterial preparations. Wet dressings with aluminum acetate (Burow's) solution may be used until sloughing occurs, but they should not be tight on the laceration to avoid necrosis of the cartilage. If lacerations are extensive, the auditory canal is packed to prevent stenosis. The packing must be changed frequently to prevent secondary infections. Skin grafts may ultimately be necessary (see Chapter 80). Immediate reattachment of an auricle torn from the head is necessary to be successful; otherwise a prosthesis will have to be used. The treatment of burns is detailed in Chapter 15 and the treatment of frostbite in Chapter 79.

Specific Nursing Measures

Be alert for any associated trauma to the skull or tympanic membrane. Any increase in pain or temperature is significant, because many injuries are prone to secondary infections.

The nurse performs many of the therapeutic measures discussed previously such as wound care, administering analgesics and antibiotics, and applying dressings and wet soaks.

INJURIES TO THE EXTERNAL AUDITORY CANAL, TYMPANIC MEMBRANE, MIDDLE EAR, AND INNER EAR

Abrasions, small lacerations, insect bites, and hematomas can occur in the external auditory canal. The most common serious injury to the ear is perforation of the tympanic membrane. Fractured and displaced ossicles are often associated with a perforated tympanic membrane and fractures of the temporal bone. Fractures involving the temporal bone are the most common fractures of the base of the skull. Temporal bone fractures follow two general pathways: About 80% of the fractures are longitudinal (cross through the middle ear), and 15% are transverse (cross through the internal auditory canal, the optic capsule, or both) (Goodhill, 1979).

A cotton applicator is the most common traumatic tool used by clients, many of whom think that regular cleaning of the external auditory canal is necessary. Injuries are also caused by pencils, paper clips, flying objects, and improper irrigation of the external auditory canal. A blow to the side of the head can cause a longitudinal fracture, whereas a transverse fracture is caused by a blow to the front or back of the head.

Clinical Manifestations

Abrasions, lacerations, or hematomas in the external auditory canal and perforations of the tympanic membrane are usually visible with careful otoscopic examination. Microscopic examinations may be necessary to see small tears in the membrane. Insect bites may cause wheals, vesicles, or ulcerations.

Longitudinal fractures usually cause a perforated tympanic membrane and a bloody discharge in the external auditory canal. Facial paralysis is usually delayed, but conductive hearing loss may be present.

With a transverse fracture, the tympanic membrane is intact, but the examiner can see blood behind the tympanic membrane within the middle ear. Transverse fractures may occur bilaterally. Injury to the inner ear can result from tearing of the membranous labyrinth and rupture of the oval and round windows (Jerger & Jerger, 1981). Vertigo, nystagmus, and sensorineural hearing loss may be present. Any facial paralysis will occur immediately.

Tomography is usually necessary to delineate longitudinal fractures, whereas transverse fractures can be seen on plain films of the skull and mastoid. Serial audiometric testing is necessary to evaluate the hearing loss.

Therapeutic Measures

A topical antiseptic or antibiotic is applied to abrasions, small lacerations, or hematomas in the external auditory canal. If the canal's skin is torn and has an elevated skin flap, an absorbable gelatin sponge (Gelfoam) or a petroleum-jelly-impregnated fabric (Adaptic) inserted into the canal for several days will hold the flap in place.

Foreign objects are removed with curets, suction, or irrigation (see Chapter 74). A few drops of oil or alcohol instilled into the auditory canal will kill an insect and make it float to the top, where it can be easily removed. Water should *not* be used, because it will not kill the insect; in fact, the insect will cling to the canal wall, making it difficult to remove. If the insect has bitten or scratched the canal wall, the instillation of alcohol may be painful. Irrigation is contraindicated if the tympanic membrane cannot be seen or the foreign object is of vegetable origin. Surgery may be necessary to remove an object fixed within the canal.

Small perforations of the tympanic membrane are usually only observed for several days, and sterile cotton is placed in the external auditory canal. If the perforation remains dry after several days without signs of closing, patching with a paper moistened with 10% silver nitrate or a gelatin film promotes healing. Antibiotics prevent infection in the middle ear. When the perforation is large or patching is unsuccessful, surgery (tympanoplasty or myringoplasty) is necessary (see Chapter 76). Surgical exploration and repair of the ossicles may also be necessary.

For temporal bone fractures, the management of intracranial injuries with the establishment of ventilation and maintenance of vital signs takes precedence over the otologic problem. A sterile dressing is applied to the draining ear until the general condition has stabilized. Hearing may fluctuate during the first 6 months after temporal bone fractures, after which exploratory surgery may be necessary. Reconstructive surgery for the tympanic membrane or ossicles can be performed if necessary.

Specific Nursing Measures

The nurse's primary responsibility in caring for clients with injuries to the external auditory canal, tympanic membrane, middle ear, and inner ear may be emotional support and providing knowledge. Emotional distress because of hearing loss or fear of hearing loss, is often the biggest problem in these clients. The removal of foreign bodies and the treatment of minor injuries are accomplished with little discomfort if the nurse reassures the client and explains the procedures.

If possible, elevate the head of the bed for clients with traumatic conditions of the middle or inner ear. Use sterile aseptic technique for all treatment to the ear. Establish a

method of communication with the client until the hearing is improved—during the first 3 weeks after head trauma or gradually over a 6-month period. Instruct clients with perforated tympanic membranes to avoid putting water into their ears and to have regular examinations for evidence of cholesteatoma.

BAROTRAUMA

Barotrauma occurs in clients during takeoff and landing in airplanes or underwater diving. It is caused by a failure of the eustachian tube to open sufficiently, causing an unequal pressure differential between the middle ear and the atmospheric pressure. Barotrauma is more common in clients with upper respiratory tract problems. This problem has increased today with the increased frequency of airplane travel and the popularity of scuba diving.

Clinical Manifestations

Clients with barotrauma usually complain of severe pain, fullness in the ear, and decreased hearing. The tympanic membrane can be retracted. With severe pressure differentials, fluid or blood may accumulate in the middle ear. Rupture of the tympanic membrane can occur (see Figures 75–6A and B). Occasionally, dislocation of the ossicles also may occur.

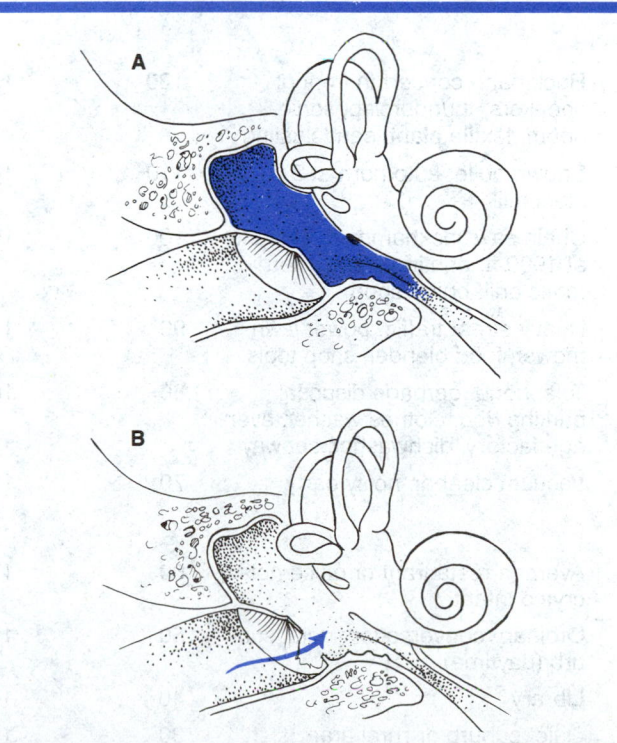

Figure 75–6

A. Barotrauma with blood-filled middle ear from a ruptured blood vessel. **B.** Barotrauma with ruptured tympanic membrane, which provides instantaneous equalization of pressure.

Therapeutic Measures

Analgesics may be required for pain relief, and decongestants may be used to open the eustachian tube. It may be necessary for the otologist to catheterize through the nasopharynx to the eustachian tube to restore the pressure within the middle ear. With severe trauma, a myringotomy can be performed to release the pressure and aspirate any accumulated fluid. Clients with upper respiratory tract infections can take oral decongestants ½ hour before and periodically during flying to prevent barotrauma.

Specific Nursing Measures

Nursing management should concentrate on prevention. For example, instruct clients in self-ventilating techniques (described in Chapter 74) to use when flying. Sucking on hard candy and swallowing will open the eustachian tube.

Discourage clients with upper respiratory tract infections from flying or diving. The client in whom barotrauma has occurred should avoid flying or diving for 2 weeks.

NOISE TRAUMA

Noise-induced hearing loss is a sensorineural hearing loss that develops gradually over months or years from environmental or industrial noise exposure at or above 85 dB. Less intense sounds may cause fatigue or annoyance, but not hearing loss. The degree of hearing loss is proportional to the duration of exposure when the sound level is held constant. Table 75–1 illustrates the effects of common noises of daily life on hearing. The incidence of noise-induced hearing loss is higher in adults than in children, because adults are exposed to more of the conditions that predispose them to noise trauma. Acoustic trauma is an in-

Table 75–1 Effects on Hearing of Common Noises in Daily Life

Sound	Decibel Level	Relative Sound Intensity	Effect
Rocket on launching pad	180	1,000,000,000,000,000,000	Hearing loss inevitable
Jet plane takeoff (close range)	150	1,000,000,000,000,000	Tympanic membrane rupture possible
Gunshot blast	140	100,000,000,000,000	Pain in the ear; possible tympanic membrane rupture; any length of exposure time is dangerous
Rock band concert in front of speakers, thunderclap, sonic boom, textile plant, sandblasting	120	1,000,000,000,000	Immediate danger to hearing
Snowmobile, auto horn at 3 ft, steel mill	110	100,000,000,000	
Chain saw, jackhammer, jet plane at 1000 ft, printing plant, pneumatic drill, boiler shop	100	10,000,000,000	Hearing damage after exposure for 2 hr; with every 5-dB increase, "safe time" cut in half
Heavy street traffic, power lawn mower, food blender, shop tools	90	1,000,000,000	Hearing damage in less than 8 hr
Telephone, garbage disposal, barking dog, clothes washer, average factory, dishwasher, subway	80	100,000,000	Hearing damage after more than 8 hr
Vacuum cleaner, noisy party	70	10,000,000	Critical level at which noise may begin to affect hearing after constant exposure
Average restaurant or office noise, crying infant	60	1,000,000	Intrusive; annoying
Ordinary conversation, quiet suburb (daytime)	50	100,000	
Library	40	10,000	
Quiet suburb or rural area (nighttime)	30	1000	
Rustle of leaves, whispering voices	20	100	
Breathing	10	10	

stantaneous hearing loss from brief exposure to a high-intensity sound at close range, such as gunshots or explosions.

Clinical Manifestations

The client with noise trauma complains of hearing loss, a high-pitched tinnitus, and a feeling of fullness within the ear. Noise-induced hearing loss usually occurs bilaterally, whereas acoustic trauma may be unilateral. Vascular congestion of the tympanic membrane may occur with acute acoustic trauma. High-intensity noise can perforate the tympanic membrane and dislocate or fracture the ossicles.

Therapeutic Measures

No medical or surgical treatment effectively restores the hearing loss after noise trauma. Therefore, prevention is most important. The federal government has determined guidelines for permissible noise exposure, which are given in Table 75–2. The control of noise exposure is the best means of prevention.

If noise trauma has occurred, rest and avoidance of further trauma is recommended. Aural rehabilitation may be necessary. The masking of tinnitus with special hearing aids or biofeedback with masking has been helpful for some clients. Surgery for repair of the tympanic membrane and ossicles may be necessary.

Specific Nursing Measures

The nurse's primary responsibility in dealing with noise trauma lies in prevention. Exposure to noise levels above the federal guideline criteria is hazardous, and nurses should recommend hearing conservation. Nurses can help inform clients about the health hazards of noise. Clients who work in noisy environments, for example, should be made aware of the potential risk to their hearing. Encourage periodic audiometric testing for those at risk, as well as the use of protective devices such as helmets, earplugs, or earmuffs.

OTOTOXICITY

Ototoxicity is a toxic reaction to chemicals and drugs that cause damage to the auditory system, vestibular system, or both. Damage occurs first in the hair cells and is followed by degeneration of the nerve endings and fibers. Cochlear and vestibular damage may occur together or separately. Auditory damage is permanent and may progress even after the drug use has been discontinued. Vestibular damage, in contrast, may be reversed after discontinuing the drug use.

Ototoxic reactions are caused by a variety of substances including aminoglycoside antibiotics, diuretics, arsenic, alcohol, nicotine, lead, carbon monoxide, quinine,

Table 75–2	Federal Guideline Criteria for Permissible Noise Exposure	
Decibels Above Threshold	Duration
90	8 hr
95	4 hr
100	2 hr
105	1 hr
115	15 min

SOURCE: US Department of Labor, Occupational Safety and Health Administration. *Occupational Noise Exposure: Hearing Conservation Amendment, Final Rule* (29 CFR 1910). *Federal Register* 48:9738–9785, US Government Printing Office, 1983.

and aspirin. Vestibular side effects may be caused by drugs such as oral contraceptive agents, sedatives, and tranquilizers, but evidence is lacking to classify them as ototoxic. Factors influencing the occurrence of ototoxicity are impaired kidney function, dehydration, and high drug dosage. Ototoxicity occurs more frequently in infants and the elderly. Congenital hearing loss can result from the administration of ototoxic drugs to pregnant women.

Clinical Manifestations

Signs and symptoms of ototoxicity include bilateral sensorineural hearing loss, tinnitus, vertigo, and ataxia. The onset of hearing loss may be gradual or rapid and may occur while the person is taking the drug or months after the drug use has been discontinued. Table 75–3 shows the characteristic effects of some ototoxic drugs.

Therapeutic Measures

There is no known treatment for vestibular or cochlear damage after it has occurred. Thus, the drug serum levels of clients who are receiving ototoxic drugs should be monitored. Serial audiograms and vestibular function tests also should be performed. Drugs should be discontinued with the first sign of ototoxicity.

Specific Nursing Measures

Nurses are responsible for careful observation of clients receiving ototoxic drugs. They should question clients daily about hearing loss, tinnitus, or dizziness. Clients on long-term treatments with ototoxic drugs should have their intake and output measured. Periodic urinalysis and renal function tests should be performed to make sure renal impairment has not occurred.

Table 75–3 Ototoxic Drugs*

| | Effect | | |
Agent	Cochleotoxic	Vestibulotoxic	Permanent Damage
Antibiotics			
Gentamicin	+	+++	Yes
Kanamycin	+++	+	Yes
Neomycin	++++	+	Yes
Streptomycin	+	++	Yes
Vancomycin	++	+	Yes
Viomycin	++	+++	Yes
Diuretics			
Ethacrynic acid	+	+ or 0	Occasionally
Furosemide	+	+ or 0	Occasionally
Others			
Nitrogen mustard	++	++	Yes
Quinine	+	0	Rarely
Salicylates	+	+	No

*Toxicity is rated on a scale of 0 (none) to ++++ (highest).

SOURCE: Goodhill V: *Ear Disease, Deafness, and Dizziness.* New York: Harper & Row, 1979.

Chapter Highlights

Emotional support is of primary importance to clients with auditory or vestibular dysfunction.

Early identification of hearing impairment is important so a program of aural rehabilitation can be initiated to prevent client withdrawal and isolation.

Congenital disorders are the most common cause of deafness; they can be inherited or acquired. Prevention and detection are the most important nursing implications.

Otosclerosis, which tends to run in families, is a common cause of conductive hearing loss in young adults.

Clients with Meniere's syndrome have extremely uncomfortable paroxysmal attacks of vertigo, tinnitus, and sensorineural hearing loss.

Because there is no effective medical or surgical treatment for presbycusis, nurses should encourage the elderly to seek aural rehabilitation and amplification, along with possible psychological counseling, to prevent depression and isolation and to improve hearing.

Meticulous cleaning of the external ear can remove physiological protective barriers against bacterial, fungal, or viral infections.

External otitis occurs more frequently in warm, humid environments.

A recurrence of pain, fever, and increased otorrhea can indicate a complication of otitis media. Clients should take the complete course of medication for otitis media, even though symptoms have disappeared.

Tinnitus and a gradual hearing loss may be the only early symptoms of neoplasms of the middle and inner ear. Lesions of the external ear, in contrast, are visible.

Clients with perforated tympanic membranes should avoid getting water in their ears and have regular examinations for evidence of cholesteatomas.

Noise-induced hearing loss and barotrauma are increasing problems in our society, but they often can be prevented.

Damage to the auditory system caused by noise and ototoxic drugs is irreversible. Thus, nurses should know the potential side effects and the risk of delayed toxic effect of any drug they administer.

Bibliography

Alpiner J: Psychological and social aspects of aging as related to hearing rehabilitation of elderly clients. In *Aural Rehabilitation for the Elderly*. Henock M (editor). New York: Grune & Stratton, 1979.

Anderson RG, Meyerhoff WL: Otologic manifestations of aging. *Otolaryngologic Clin North Am* 1982; 15(2):353–370.

Goodhill V: *Ear Diseases, Deafness, and Dizziness*. Hagerstown, MD: Harper & Row, 1979.

Jerger S, Jerger J: *Auditory Disorders: A Manual for Clinical Evaluation*. Boston: Little, Brown, 1981.

Marshall K, Attia E: *Disorders of the Ear*. Boston: John Wright-PSG, 1983.

Mawson SR, Ludman H: *Diseases of the Ear: A Textbook of Otology*, 4th ed. Chicago: Year Book, 1979.

Sataloff J, Sataloff RT, Vassallo LA: *Hearing Loss*, 2nd ed. Philadelphia: Lippincott, 1980.

Senturia BH, Marcus MD, Lucenti FE: *Diseases of the External Ear*, 2nd ed. New York: Grune & Stratton, 1980.

Shambaugh GE, Glasscock ME: *Surgery of the Ear*, 3rd ed. Philadelphia: Saunders, 1980.

Suggested Readings

Heller B, Gaynor E: Hearing loss and aural rehabilitation of the elderly. *Top Clin Nurs* 1981; 3(1):21–29. This article focuses on hearing problems of the aged.

Niswander M: Making good "cents" out of hearing conservation. *Occup Health Safety* (March 1983):57–60. A description of the problems experienced by a nurse in establishing an industrial hearing conservation program. The essentials of a good program are discussed.

Rados B: When motion sickness goes along for the ride. *FDA Cons* 1985; 19(2):6–9. This article details the symptoms and causes of motion sickness and offers a number of precautions that help prevent it in susceptible persons. Pharmacologic treatment is also discussed.

Chapter 76

Surgical Approaches to Auditory System Dysfunction

Dominica Ann Limburg

Objectives

When you have finished studying this chapter, you should be able to:

Identify the common surgical procedures of the auditory system.

Describe the rationale for performing surgical procedures of the auditory system.

Anticipate psychosocial effects of hearing loss on client and family.

Describe preoperative nursing assessments relative to auditory procedures.

Implement postoperative nursing interventions for a client who has had auditory surgery.

Discuss postoperative health teaching for clients who have had ear surgery.

Aural surgical procedures are performed to control infections and improve, restore, or maintain auditory function. Prior to the introduction of antibiotics, most surgical procedures were performed to eradicate infections. Today, because the operating microscope permits the surgeon to visualize the tiny structures of the ear more readily, the frequency and number of available surgical procedures for the restoration of hearing have greatly increased. The elimination of infection is still of prime importance, however.

To make an informed decision on whether to risk surgery, the client must be informed of the expected hearing improvement, as well as the risk of sustaining an increased hearing loss. The client should be fully aware of the objectives of the procedure, how it is done, and the preoperative and postoperative care to be expected.

Surgical procedures discussed in this chapter are myringotomy, mastoidectomy, tympanoplasty, and stapedectomy, cochlear implants, and procedures used to treat Meniere's syndrome. Surgical procedures for the removal of acoustic neuromas are discussed in Chapter 39.

Section I: Surgery to Improve, Maintain, or Restore Auditory Function

MYRINGOTOMY

A myringotomy is an incision of the tympanic membrane to release fluid under pressure and to insert ventilating tubes to aerate the middle ear. The drainage of purulent fluid from the middle ear prevents destruction of the ossicles, spread of infection to the mastoid cells, spontaneous rupture of the tympanic membrane, or a combination of these complications. This surgical intervention is usually recommended for the following reasons:

- A severe infection with purulent fluid under tension in the middle ear
- A recurring infection not completely cured with antibiotic therapy
- An accumulation of nonbacterial middle ear effusion

• Occasionally, for diagnostic purposes

Symptoms such as severe pain, fever, mastoid tenderness, and a bulging tympanic membrane are indicative of fluid under pressure in the middle ear.

Surgical Procedure

A myringotomy is usually performed in an ambulatory setting (a physician's office, clinic, or day surgical center). A brief general anesthesia may be necessary for some children and older adults. Generally, a topical agent such as a phenol solution is used to anesthetize the tympanic membrane (Karmody, 1983).

Several inexpensive disposable myringotomy kits are available with instruments and drapes necessary for the procedure. A new sharp myringotomy knife should always be used. A curved posterior inferior incision, a smaller anterior superior radial incision, or a smaller anterior inferior radial incision is made through an aural speculum (Figure 76–1). A radial anterior incision is preferable when inserting a plastic ventilating tube that will remain for a long time (Armstrong, 1983). A culture is then taken to determine the type and sensitivity of the organism present. The culture may be taken from the tip of the myringotomy knife. The fluid and pus are aspirated, and if indicated, a tube is inserted (Figure 76–2). Various types of plastic ventilating tubes are available.

Implications for the Client

Physiological Implications

The client with an acute infection has severe pain, fever, and possibly a mild hearing loss. The escape of pus and fluid immediately relieves the pain. A cotton ball is placed within the external auditory canal to collect the drainage. Antibiotics may be prescribed. If symptoms persist or are

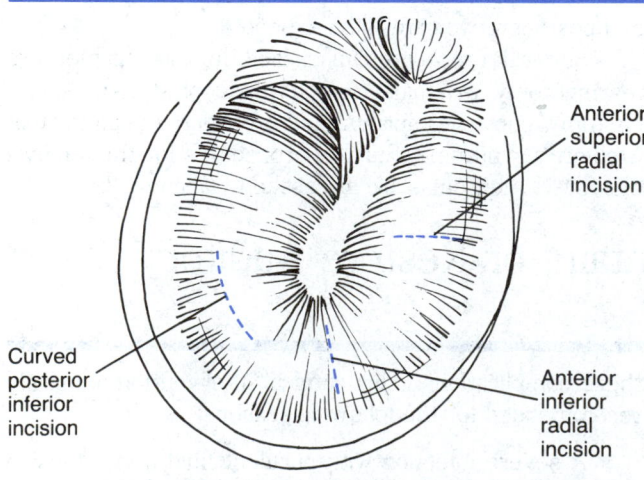

Figure 76–1

Myringotomy incision of tympanic membrane: Location of curved posterior inferior incision, anterior superior radial incision, and anterior inferior radial incision.

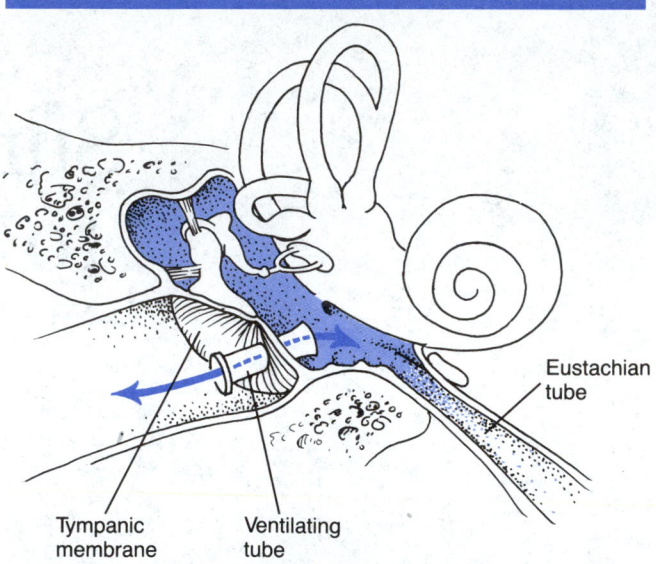

Figure 76–2

Myringotomy to release the exudate in chronic suppurative otitis media.

exacerbated, the client should notify the physician. Ventilating tubes extrude spontaneously after 3 weeks, or the physician may remove them any time after 6 weeks. Occasionally, it may be necessary to reinsert the tube if mechanical drainage is required for a longer time.

To prevent infections of the middle ear, the client should prevent water from entering the ear until the tympanic membrane has healed. Hearing should be tested in 6 to 12 months to detect any reaccumulation of fluid.

Psychosocial/Lifestyle Implications

Clients who have had a middle ear effusion for some time have adapted to diminished hearing. After the insertion of a ventilating tube, therefore, all sounds seem extremely loud. Clients should be warned that traffic sounds on their way home may seem intolerably loud but that they will soon adapt to normal hearing. A myringotomy should have no negative long-term psychosocial or lifestyle effects. Increased hearing, on the contrary, may provide better communication and cognitive skills. The client implications of a myringotomy are summarized in Table 76–1.

Nursing Implications

Preoperative Care

Assesses the client preoperatively, and review the record for drug allergies and physical or psychological limitations that may interfere with the success of the operative procedure. Help alleviate anxiety by listening to the client, answering questions, explaining the procedures, and discussing postsurgical implications. A family member or significant other should participate in any discussions, especially if the client is very young or very old, to provide the support many clients need. A family member or significant other can also help interpret preoperative teaching to a

Table 76–1	Myringotomy: Implications for the Client	
Physiological Implications	**Psychosocial/Lifestyle Implications**
Relief from pain, fever, and possibly mild hearing loss	Marked increase in hearing (possibly uncomfortable at first)
Possible antibiotic use	Improvement in communication and cognitive skills
Need to keep water out of ear until tympanic membrane heals	Unable to engage in water sports until the tympanic membrane heals; must take precautions when showering and performing personal hygiene
Testing for reaccumulation of fluid in 6 to 12 months	

client with hearing loss. Often, though, the nurse must find a method of communicating with the client. Writing all instructions may help the client understand them.

Postoperative Care

Postoperative instructions also should be written so the client can take them home. Health teaching should include:

- Instructions for washing hands before and after touching the ear to prevent the spread of infection
- Instructions for changing and disposing of the cotton ball
- Instructions for taking antibiotics or any other medications prescribed
- Encouragement to keep follow-up appointments
- Instructions for preventing water from entering the ear as long as a ventilating tube is in place or until the tympanic membrane heals

The client should use earplugs when showering and shampooing. The external ear should be cleaned with a washcloth. The client should avoid inserting applicators and going swimming. (These general instructions apply to the care of all clients having surgery of the ear.)

MASTOIDECTOMY

A mastoidectomy is the incision, drainage, and removal of diseased mucosa and bone from the mastoid process of the temporal bone. It may also be done to gain acccess to the middle or inner ear. There are three types of mastoidectomies: the simple (also referred to as complete) mastoidectomy, the radical mastoidectomy, and the modified radical mastoidectomy.

As a result of antibiotic therapy for acute otitis media, simple mastoidectomies are rarely performed today. A modified radical mastoidectomy is indicated for a cholesteatoma and for some carcinomas. The modified radical procedure is followed by a tympanoplasty (described later

in this chapter) to restore hearing. A radical mastoidectomy is performed only when the preservation of hearing is secondary to preventing the spread of disease and is rarely used.

Surgical Procedure

The supine client is placed in a semi-Fowler's position. A general or local anesthesia with preoperative sedation may be used. The advantage of local anesthesia is that the client can be ambulatory the afternoon of surgery and ready to go home the next day. Hair is shaved or clipped to about 3 cm from the periauricular area. Some otologists prefer clipping because they think skin is more prone to infections after shaving. A water-soluble lubricant applied to the hair around the incisional site keeps the rest of the hair away from the operative field.

Two types of incisions, the postauricular and the endaural, may be used for a mastoidectomy. The *postauricular* incision begins at the upper attachment of the auricle to the head and follows the postaural groove to the tip of the mastoid process (Figure 76–3A). The *endaural*

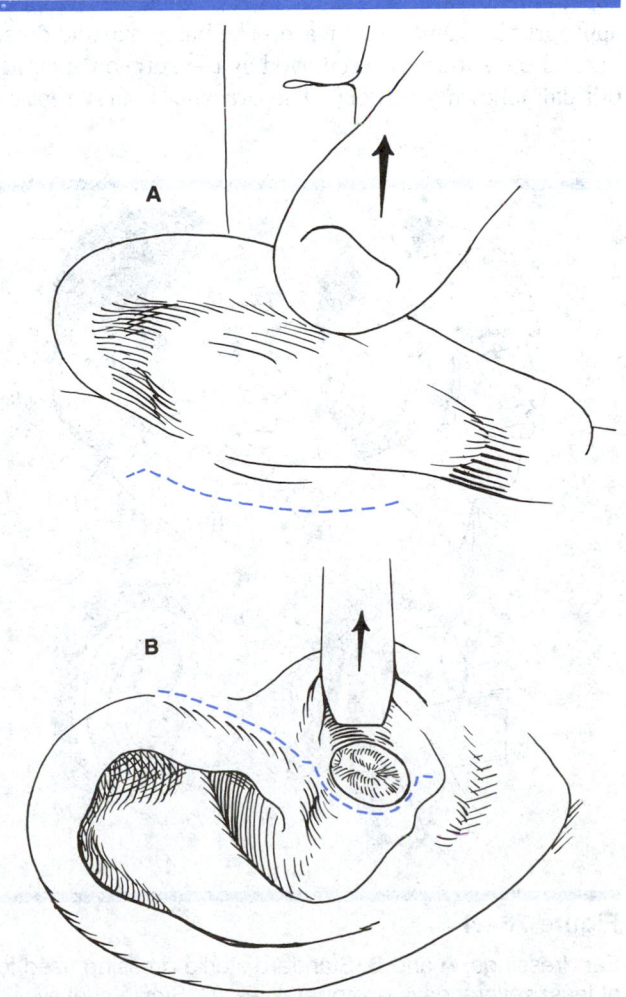

Figure 76–3

A. Postauricular incision. **B.** Endaural incision.

incision begins above the anterior junction of the crus of the helix with the skin of the head and follows the anterior margin of the meatus between the meatus and the tragus (Figure 76–3B). In a simple mastoidectomy, all accessible air cells are dissected, keeping the walls of the mastoid process and external auditory canal intact. In a radical mastoidectomy, all the walls are removed, making one large cavity from the external auditory canal to the mastoid cavity. In a modified radical mastoidectomy, the ossicles and tympanic membrane are kept intact, and the mastoid air cells and posterior canal wall are removed. The skin of the posterior canal wall then is used to line the cavity. A Teflon drain is usually placed through the lower end of the incision. After the operation, a bulky dressing is placed over the ear and held in place with a bandage (Figures 76–4A, B).

Implications for the Client

Physiological Implications
Most clients are ambulatory the evening of the surgery and are discharged in 1 or 2 days. The client may feel dizzy and should seek assistance when getting out of bed. Return appointments are scheduled every week or two until appropriate healing takes place. The bulky mastoid dressing and the sutures are removed by the surgeon about the 6th day following surgery. The dressing is first replaced

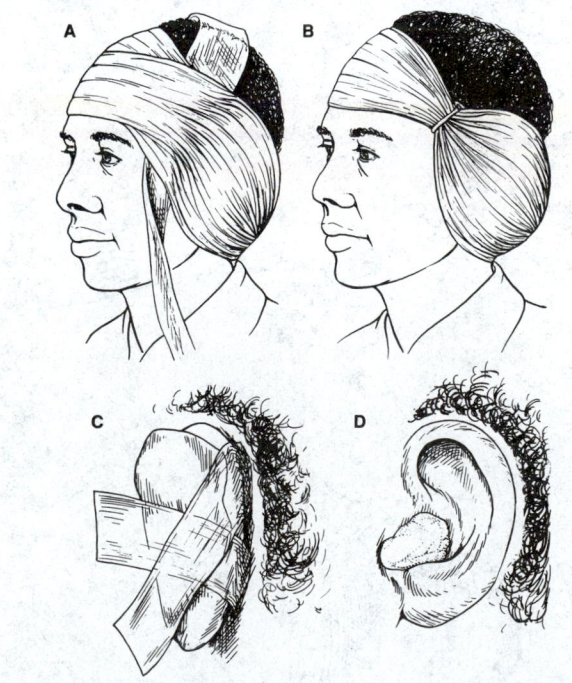

Figure 76–4

Ear dressings. **A** and **B.** Standard sterile dressing used for at least several days postoperatively. **C.** Sterile oval eye patch attached by tape. **D.** Sterile cotton in the concha not taped.

by an eye patch, then by a cotton pledget placed in the outer ear (see Figures 76–4C, D). The client is instructed to change it three times a day as long as drainage is present. Most clients' ears become dry in about 3 or 4 weeks.

Psychosocial/Lifestyle Implications
Following a mastoidectomy the client can resume a normal lifestyle in about 6 weeks. Since most mastoidectomies are followed by tympanoplasty, refer to that section for further lifestyle implications.

Client implications of mastoidectomy are summarized in Table 76–2.

Nursing Implications

Preoperative Care
The client is instructed not to take aspirin or any other medication that may prolong bleeding before the mastoidectomy. Even a small amount of bleeding during aural surgery impairs the surgeon's ability to visualize the tiny structures, so every precaution is used to decrease bleeding.

Postoperative Care
When the client returns from surgery after a mastoidectomy, the head of the bed is elevated at least 30°. Monitor the vital signs and observe for signs of bleeding or drainage. Excessive bleeding should be reported immediately to the physician. Be sure to check the dressing near the back of the head and the bed linens under the head for signs of bleeding. The outer dressing can be reinforced if necessary. Clients may be dizzy in the immediate postoperative period, so siderails are used while the client is in bed.

Because of its location, the facial nerve (CN VII) is vulnerable to injury during all types of surgery involving the middle or inner ear. The nerve enters the petrous

Table 76–2	Mastoidectomy: Implications for the Client	
Physiological Implications	**Psychosocial/Lifestyle Implications**
Precautions to decrease bleeding during surgery	Return to activities in 6 weeks
Discharge in 1 to 2 days and follow-up every week or until healing occurs	See Table 76–3 for implications following tympanoplasty, if performed
Need to change dressing three times a day after bulky dressing removal for 3 to 4 weeks	
Possible dizziness	
Possible facial nerve damage	

portion of the temporal bone through the internal auditory canal, winds around the ossicles, and exits through the mastoid process where it divides into many branches that course through the temporal bone to the lacrimal gland, the tongue, and the salivary glands (Figure 76–5). Watch for signs of facial paralysis, including sagging of the face, drooping of the mouth, drooling, or the inability to close the eyelid on the operative side. As soon as clients can respond, ask them to show their teeth, whistle, and wrinkle their foreheads. Clients who have injury to the nerve are taken back to surgery within 24 hours for decompression and repair of the injured nerve. Edema of the nerve also can cause paralysis, but this paralysis does not appear until several days postoperatively and usually resolves spontaneously.

Nausea and vertigo may be present following surgery, so always assist the client in getting out of bed. Administer medications for nausea, vertigo, and pain relief as ordered. Antibiotics are usually ordered to prevent infections. Encourage oral fluids as tolerated.

Prior to discharge instruct the client to:

- Report any change in drainage, pain, temperature, and weakness of the face.
- Wash hands before and after touching the ear and changing the cotton ball.
- Take medications as ordered. The nurse should write out the side effects of medications for the client.
- Prevent water from entering the ear for about 6 weeks.

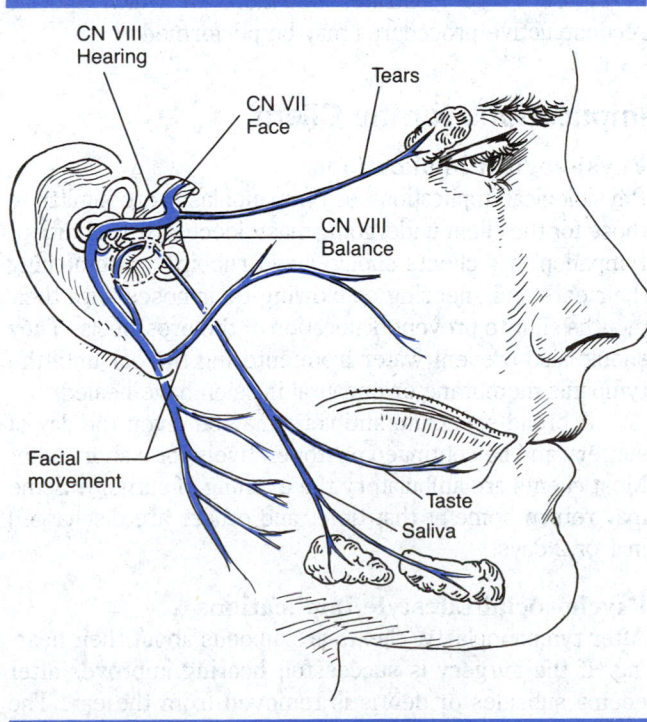

Figure 76–5

Areas affected by facial nerve injury.

TYMPANOPLASTY AND STAPEDECTOMY

Tympanoplasty designates a group of reconstructive procedures for repairing the tympanic membrane and the sound-conducting structures in the middle ear. The procedures may be categorized as:

- Myringoplasty. A reconstructive procedure for the repair of a tympanic membrane perforation.
- Tympanoplasty without mastoidectomy. A surgical procedure used to eradicate disease within the middle ear and reconstruct an impaired sound-conducting apparatus. This procedure can include a myringoplasty.
- Tympanoplasty with mastoidectomy. A surgical procedure used to eradicate disease within the mastoid process and the middle ear and to reconstruct an impaired sound-conducting apparatus. This procedure can include a myringoplasty.

The tympanic membrane and ossicles normally act as a transformer of sound pressure to the oval window. The tympanic membrane also dampens sound pressure, creating a lag in transmitting it to the round window, allowing the stronger pressure to reach the oval window first. With defects in the tympanic membrane or any part of the sound-transmitting apparatus, sound pressure reaches the oval and round windows simultaneously. This equalizes the stronger pressure normally exerted at the oval window, reducing the motility of the endolymph. This, in turn, decreases hair cell stimulation and ultimately decreases hearing. Defects in the sound-transmitting apparatus can be caused by a congenital defect, trauma, otosclerosis, a cholesteatoma, or chronic suppurative otitis media.

The main objective of tympanoplasty is to eliminate the disease and reconstruct or replace the sound-conducting apparatus so hearing can be improved or maintained. A tympanoplasty is contraindicated for clients with an obstructed eustachian tube or sensorineural hearing loss. Without a patent eustachian tube, the air pressure in the middle ear necessary for conduction of sound to the oval window is lacking, which results in sensorineural hearing loss. For clients without sensorineural hearing discrimination, repair of the conductive apparatus is useless. Unless there is an active cholesteatoma, tympanoplasty in children is delayed until the teens because of their greater susceptibility to acute otitis media.

Surgical Procedure

Tympanoplastic surgery is individualized for each client according to the cause and amount of the defect in the sound-conducting apparatus. Surgical procedures are continually being modified and developed. Local anesthesia is generally used; however, for prolonged surgery that includes a mastoidectomy, a general anesthesia may be preferred. Either endaural or postaural incisions are used in tympanoplastic surgery.

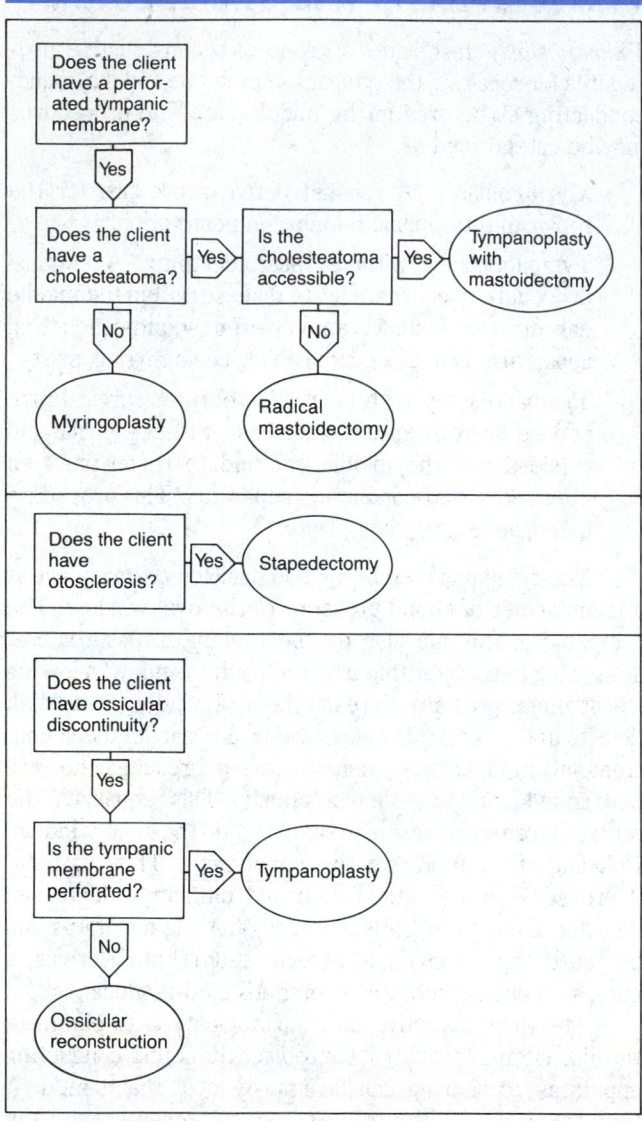

Figure 76–6

Flow chart for tympanoplasty and other reconstructive procedures.

The simplest tympanoplastic procedure is the *myringoplasty,* a reconstruction of the tympanic membrane using a fascia graft taken from the temporal muscle behind the ear. The perforated edges of the tympanic membrane are excised, and the graft, held in place with an absorbable gelatin sponge (Gelfoam), closes the gap. If the handle of the malleus is eroded, the tympanic graft is placed against the long process of the incus. If the incus is eroded, the graft is depressed to establish contact with the head of the stapes. Allograft tympanic membranes with or without attached ossicles also are used successfully for reconstruction.

The most common ossicular discontinuity is at the incudostapedial joint linking the incus and the stapes. The surgeon can reestablish contact between the incus and the stapes by reshaping and repositioning the incus to hold the head of the stapes. The most difficult ossicular defect

to reconstruct is the absence of the handle of the malleus and the arch of the stapes. Plastic or ceramic prostheses are used for partial or total ossicular replacements; however, human bone replacements are desirable, because they are rarely rejected (Hough, 1982). Other surgical procedures depend on whether the ossicles are fixed, whether they are partially or completely eroded, and whether any discontinuity exists in the ossicular chain.

In the past, a stapes that was ankylosed, or fixed, because of otosclerosis was mobilized by removing the otosclerotic lesion around it. This procedure (stapes mobilization) is seldom performed today because the active otosclerotic lesion usually grows back. *Stapedectomy* is the current procedure of choice for an ankylosed stapes caused by otosclerosis. This procedure removes the head, neck, and crus of the stapes. A stainless steel or Teflon piston is inserted into a small hole created in the footplate. A wire loop connects the piston to the incus. This connects the incus to the oval window, bridging the gap between the incus and the inner ear. Some procedures remove the entire footplate and seal the oval window with a plug of fat or Gelfoam connected to a wire looped on the incus. Many other prostheses also are available today.

Some surgeons perform tympanoplasty in stages. During the first stage, they generally perform a modified radical mastoidectomy to remove diseased tissue (eg, a cholesteatoma or otosclerosis) and then reconstruct the tympanic membrane. About 6 months later, they perform the second stage to inspect the cavity for recurrence of the cholesteatoma or otosclerosis and to perform any ossicular reconstruction that may be necessary. The flow chart in Figure 76–6 illustrates situations in which specific reconstructive procedures may be performed.

Implications for the Client

Physiological Implications
Physiological implications of tympanoplasty are similar to those for the client undergoing mastoidectomy. In addition, tympanoplasty clients should avoid rubbing or scratching their ears and sneezing or blowing their noses with their mouths shut to prevent dislocation of the prosthesis. They should also prevent water from entering the ear until the tympanic membrane or endaural incision have healed.

A broad-spectrum antibiotic may be given the day of surgery and be continued postoperatively for a short time. Most clients are ambulatory the evening of surgery. Some may return home at that time, and others are discharged in 1 or 2 days.

Psychosocial/Lifestyle Implications
After tympanoplasty, clients are anxious about their hearing. If the surgery is successful, hearing improves after edema subsides or debris is removed from the ear. The hearing status is best evaluated 4 to 6 weeks postoperatively. Once the hearing status has been established, the client should report any decline.

Table 76-3 Tympanoplasty: Implications for the Client

Physiological Implications	Psychosocial/Lifestyle Implications
Precautions to decrease bleeding during surgery	Hearing improvement after edema reduced and debris absent, if surgery successful
Need to change dressing three times a day after bulky dressing removal for 3 to 4 weeks	Need to report hearing decline
Possible dizziness	After stapedectomy, return to activities in 1 to 3 weeks
Avoidance of rubbing or scratching ear, sneezing or nose blowing with mouth shut, and water in ear until healed	After tympanoplasty with mastoidectomy, return to activities in 6 weeks
Possible broad-spectrum antibiotic administration	Slight clicking or popping heard in wind
Discharge evening of surgery or in 1 to 2 days	Yearly hearing tests
	Possible need for hearing aid

Following stapedectomy and tympanoplasty, most clients can return to work or resume a normal lifestyle, including air travel, in 1 to 3 weeks. A client who has had a tympanoplasty with mastoidectomy, however, may need about 6 weeks to resume a normal lifestyle. In this case, the client also may resume swimming and showering in 6 weeks.

Clients with prostheses may prefer to cover their ears in the wind because of a slight clicking or popping sound they hear as the prosthesis moves. Following surgery for otosclerosis, clients should have yearly hearing tests to detect any recurrence or progression of the lesion. Some clients will need hearing aids for additional hearing improvement. Client implications of tympanoplasty are summarized in Table 76-3.

Nursing Implications

Nursing implications for tympanoplasty are similar to those for mastoidectomy. Postoperatively, the head of the bed is elevated. Monitor the vital signs, observe for signs of bleeding and drainage, and report excessive bleeding to the physician. Outer dressings can be reinforced. If the client is feeling dizzy, the nurse assists in ambulation and uses siderails while the client is in bed. Dizziness may occur for a few hours after a stapedectomy. Be alert for signs of facial paralysis. Loss of taste or facial weakness due to trauma to CN VII should be reported immediately.

Medications administered may include analgesics, sedatives, and antibiotics as ordered. Occasionally, anti-

emetics are administered for nausea. Health teaching should include (1) warnings against nose blowing and keeping the mouth open when sneezing and (2) instructions for changing the cotton ball in the external auditory canals.

COCHLEAR IMPLANTS

A cochlear implant is essentially an electronic inner ear that will enable profoundly deaf adults to hear some sounds such as doorbells and automobile horns. The device picks up sound in the environment, converts it to electrical impulses, and broadcasts it to an implanted receiver, which provides direct electrical stimulation to the nerve fibers of CN VIII in the cochlea.

The House device was approved in late 1984 by the Food and Drug Administration after undergoing clinical trials in more than 400 clients. Other cochlear implant prostheses are being developed and used experimentally.

The cochlear implant is indicated for postlingually deaf adults (those who had learned to talk before losing their hearing) with nonfunctioning hair cells but viable auditory neurons. Controversy surrounds its use in children because they are more prone to middle ear infections, the electrode may enable bacteria to invade the inner ear and nervous system, and scarring might prevent the implementation of a more sophisticated device yet to be developed.

Surgical Procedure

Through a postauricular incision, a mastoidectomy is performed to gain access to the cochlea. An electrode is inserted into the scala tympani to the round window, and an inactive ground wire is placed in the middle ear. Both electrodes are attached to an internal coil embedded in the mastoid cortex (Figure 76-7).

Implications for the Client

Physiological Implications

Physiological implications for clients with cochlear implants are the same as those for clients who have had a mastoidectomy. After the incision has healed, an external coil is placed on the scalp directly over the internal coil. A small microphone placed on a shirt or blouse collar or on the ear picks up sound and carries it to a battery-operated signal processor, about the size of a deck of playing cards and worn on a belt, in a pocket, or attached to a brassiere (Figure 76-7). The processor converts the sound into an electrical signal and transmits it to the external coil and then to the internal coil to activate the electrode in the scala tympani, which stimulates the nerve fibers. Long-term effects of the electrical stimulation are unknown, and research is being conducted to study them (Balkany, 1983).

Psychosocial/Lifestyle Implications

Clients with cochlear prostheses can detect their own voices and learn to detect other sounds in the environment, but

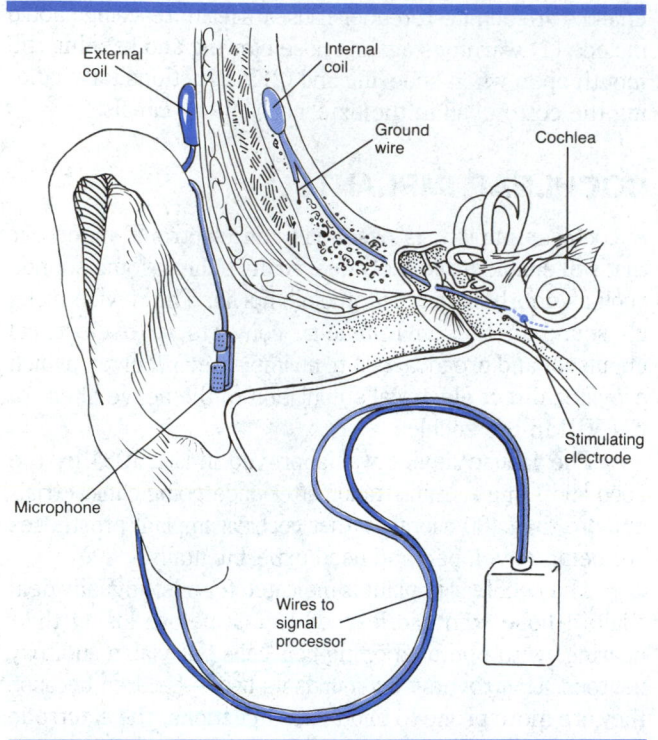

External coil
Internal coil
Ground wire
Cochlea
Stimulating electrode
Microphone
Wires to signal processor

Figure 76–7

Cochlear implant.

Table 76–4 Cochlear Implant: Implications for the Client	
Physiological Implications	**Psychosocial/Lifestyle Implications**
Ability to hear previously unheard sounds	Detection of acoustic cues leading to improved client speech and improved ability to speech read
Possible dizziness	
Long-term effects of electrical stimulation unknown	Detection of environmental sounds promotes safety
Long-term follow-up necessary	Decreased feeling of isolation
Scarring may prevent implantation of other newly developed devices	Increased self-esteem and sense of security
	Background noises may be irritating
	May be uncomfortable with visibility of microphone, wire, external coil, and signal processor

normal hearing is still beyond the scope of cochlear implants. Although the prosthesis does not improve the client's ability to understand speech, it does provide acoustic cues that improve the tone, pace, and stress on words in the client's own speech. The ability to hear environmental sounds promotes safety and decreases feelings of isolation. Clients with implants describe an increased self-esteem and an increased sense of security. Client implications of a cochlear implant are summarized in Table 76–4.

Nursing Implications

Nursing implications for clients with cochlear implants are similar to those for mastoidectomy clients.

Section II: Surgery to Correct Meniere's Syndrome

Clients with continued attacks of Meniere's syndrome—fluctuating sensorineural hearing loss, vertigo, and tinnitus—in spite of medical treatment are candidates for a surgical procedure. Most are desperate for relief of vertigo. Some otologists recommend early surgical intervention to prevent progressive destruction of the inner ear and preserve hearing. Surgical procedures for Meniere's syndrome are classified into two major groups: conservative and destructive. Conservative procedures are performed to reduce vestibular symptoms while preserving hearing. Destructive procedures eliminate vestibular symptoms but cause total hearing loss in the involved ear. Therefore, if there is bilateral involvement, conservative techniques are usually performed on the most severely affected ear.

Surgical Procedure

Ultrasound is a conservative technique for depressing vestibular activity in clients with Meniere's syndrome. An ultrasonic probe inserted through a tympanotomy directs energy at the round window. The effects of ultrasound are not yet well understood.

An endolymphatic subarachnoid shunt is also a conservative technique. After a simple mastoidectomy has been performed, the surgeon opens the endolymphatic sac, creating a shunt between it and the subarachnoid space in the brain. A shunt tube also can be inserted into the endolymphatic sac to drain it into the mastoid cavity. The vestibular branch of CN VIII is usually resected as well.

The most widely used conservative procedure to relieve attacks of vertigo is to section or cut the vestibular nerve through a middle fossa approach (craniotomy approach), described in Chapter 39. This approach preserves hearing and provides permanent relief from vertigo.

Destructive procedures are used only for clients with minimal residual hearing in the involved ear. These procedures can be performed under local or general anesthesia. One of the procedures, labyrinthectomy, can be performed by various techniques. In one technique, the tympanic membrane is flapped over and the promontory between the oval and round windows is opened. The contents of the vestibule are then removed with a suction tip, and the vestibule is packed with Gelfoam soaked in an ototoxic drug such as streptomycin to ensure its complete destruction.

Another labyrinthectomy technique requires a mastoidectomy to expose the horizontal semicircular canal. The surgeon then makes an opening into the canal, through which the membranous labyrinth is removed. A simple mastoidectomy is also performed in the translabyrinthine technique, which is used to open the internal auditory canal. This exposes the superior and inferior vestibular nerves, which are then sectioned to destroy the vestibular end organs. When the major complaint is tinnitus, the cochlear nerve is also sectioned. The labyrinthectomy can also be approached from the middle fossa.

Other techniques and procedures are also performed for Meniere's syndrome. Those described in this chapter are the most common.

Implications for the Client

Physiological Implications

After surgery for Meniere's syndrome, the client remains in the hospital 1 to 3 days unless the subarachnoid space was entered, in which case the client remains a week or more. Although complications with shunt operations are uncommon, there are risks of increased loss of hearing, infection, spinal fluid leakage, and CN VII paralysis. Risks with the middle fossa nerve section, although uncommon, may include all the complications just described, as well as injury to the brain causing speech paralysis and paralysis to the opposite arm or leg.

During the first few days after a labyrinthectomy or nerve section, clients become vertiginous and nauseated when they move their heads. Gradually, accommodation occurs. In about 3 to 4 weeks, the client becomes steady and can walk unassisted.

Some clients may take months to recover their equilibrium fully, and a small percentage who have destructive procedures may experience permanent disequilibrium. Some clients also continually see objects viewed from a distance as jerky. Clients who have destructive procedures will also experience hearing loss in the operative ear.

Table 76-5	Surgical Procedures for Meniere's Syndrome: Implications for the Client	
Physiological Implications	**Psychosocial/Lifestyle Implications**
Hospital stay of 1 to 3 days (longer, if subarachnoid space entered)	Usually can resume work about 4 weeks after discharge
Relief from vertigo and tinnitus	May have to modify lifestyle and continue to attend to safety precautions if unsteadiness or vertigo persist after surgery
Risk of increased hearing loss, infection, spinal fluid leakage, CN VII paralysis, and brain injury	
Vertigo and nausea for 3 to 4 weeks, months, or (rarely) permanently	Depression and frustration if the symptoms are not relieved by surgery
Hearing loss in operative ear with destructive procedures	May need to learn speech reading or undergo auditory training when labyrinthectomy has been performed

Psychosocial/Lifestyle Implications

Depending on the procedure, most clients can resume work about 4 weeks after discharge. If vertigo persists, clients will need to modify their lifestyle accordingly as suggested in the section on Meniere's syndrome in Chapter 75. Depression and frustration are often felt by clients who find little or no relief after undergoing surgery. Clients who have undergone a destructive procedure will have total hearing loss in the operative ear.

Client implications of surgical procedures for Meniere's syndrome are summarized in Table 76-5.

Nursing Implications

See Chapter 75 (Meniere's syndrome) for preoperative nursing care. Postoperative nursing care is similar to that for clients having a mastoidectomy. The hospital stay can be from 1 day to several days or longer if the subarachnoid space was entered. Nursing care after a craniotomy approach is discussed in Chapter 39. The nurse should assist the client until steadiness is regained. Help the client avoid moving quickly or becoming fatigued, which seems to exacerbate the unsteadiness.

Chapter Highlights

Improved hearing obtained by surgical procedures can lead to higher self-esteem and an increased sense of security for clients.

The main objectives of a myringotomy are the release

of fluid under pressure and aeration of the middle ear. This procedure is indicated to prevent the spread of infection to the mastoid cells, prevent destruction

(continued)

Chapter Highlights *(continued)*

of the ossicles, prevent a spontaneous rupture of the tympanic membrane, or a combination.

A mastoidectomy removes infection, bone, or both to gain access to the middle and inner ear.

The main objective of a tympanoplasty is to eliminate disease and reconstruct or replace the sound-conducting apparatus in the middle ear.

The electrical stimulation of auditory neurons with cochlear implants cannot now produce normal hearing but enables clients to detect sounds in the environment.

Surgical procedures are performed to eliminate the vestibular symptoms of Meniere's syndrome and preserve hearing, although some procedures do cause hearing loss.

It is important to check the dressing near the back of the head and the bed linens under the head for signs of bleeding.

The facial nerve, CN VII, is vulnerable to injury during surgery of the middle or inner ear. Check the postoperative client for signs of facial paralysis.

Dizziness or vertigo may be experienced to varying degrees by clients having otologic surgery; the nurse should be sure to assist the client in ambulating and provide safety measures such as bedrails.

An important nursing role is health teaching; postoperative instructions should be written as well as oral since many clients experience some hearing loss.

Bibliography

Armstrong BW: Prolonged middle ear ventilation: The right tube in the right place. *Annals of Otology, Rhinology, Laryngology* 1983; 92:582–586.

Balkany TJ: An overview of the electronic cochlear prosthesis: Clinical and research considerations. *Otolaryngology Clin North Am* 1983; 16:209–215.

Hough JV: Experience in tympanoplasty: Avoiding revisions and complications. *Otolaryngology Clin North Am* 1982; 15:845–860.

Karmody C: *Textbook of Otolaryngology.* Philadelphia: Lee & Febiger, 1983.

Mawson SR, Ludman H: *Diseases of the Ear. A Textbook of Otology,* 4th ed. Chicago: Year Book, 1979.

Shambaugh GE, Glasscock ME: *Surgery of the Ear,* 3rd ed. Philadelphia: Saunders, 1980.

Suggested Readings

Gruendemann BJ, Meeker MK: *Alexander's Care of the Patient in Surgery,* 7th ed. St. Louis: Mosby, 1983, pp. 593–612. Additional information on the necessary instruments and set-ups for surgical procedures used to treat dysfunction of the auditory system.

Loeb GE: The functional replacement of the ear. *Sci Am* 1985; 252(2): 104–111. A highly technical but fascinating account of the development and function of the cochlear implant. Several illustrations and photographs help to explain how the device works.

The Client With Otosclerosis

I. Brief Descriptive Data	Mrs Tina Sharppe, age 32, was admitted to the hospital with a diagnosis of conductive hearing loss due to otosclerosis.
II. Personal Data	
Date and Time:	Oct 9, 1986, 4 PM
Full Name:	Tina Marie Sharppe
Social Security No.:	000-00-0000
Ins. No.:	TX00000
Address:	136 Meadow La., Austin, TX 78758
Telephone:	Home: 000-0000
	Work: 000-0000
Sex:	Female
Age:	34
Birthdate:	1-19-53
Marital Status:	Married
Race/Culture:	Caucasian
Occupation:	Teacher/housewife
Usual Health Care Provider:	Dr Robert Trissen
III. Health History	
Source of Information:	Client
Reliability of Informant:	Reliable
Chief Complaint:	"Can't hear as well as I used to."
History of Present Illness:	Seven years prior to admission, Mrs Sharppe became aware that she was not hearing well in her left ear. Because of a family history of otosclerosis, she had hearing tests, and otosclerosis was diagnosed. At that time, she was told she could get a hearing aid to improve her hearing if she desired. She decided against the hearing aid, but since the birth of her daughter 2 years ago, she has noticed a progression of the hearing loss, especially in the left ear. After having hearing tests, she was encouraged to have a stapedectomy. Mrs Sharppe denies having any earache, tinnitus, or dizziness. She takes no medications except for occasional aspirin for headaches.
Past Health History:	
Childhood:	Childhood diseases—chickenpox, 1959
Immunizations:	DPT, measles, mumps, rubella, polio
Trauma:	Fx rt arm, 1960, age 7
Medical Problems:	None
Surgeries:	None
Pregnancies:	1979, vaginal delivery—male
	1984, vaginal delivery—female
Allergies:	No known allergies to food or medications; no seasonal allergies
Medications:	Aspirin occasionally for headache
Family History:	Father, age 62, A&W, has otosclerosis, wears hearing aid, had two stapedectomies; also has hypertension controlled with medication and diet
	Mother, age 60, A&W, no health problems
	Sister, age 24, A&W
	Husband, age 35, A&W
	Son, age 6; daughter, age 2 (both A&W)
	PGM, otosclerosis; MGM, DM, type II
Personal/Social History:	Mrs Sharppe lives in a small town about 30 mi from the hospital with her husband and two children. Her mother and father live next door. Mother cares for daughter during the day.

(continued)

The Client With Otosclerosis

Mrs Sharppe teaches third grade in the public school, likes her work, and recently returned after a maternity leave. Husband is a physician's assistant. They own their own home.

Educational/Occupational History: Needs nine more credits for master's degree. Goes to classes one night a week. Has worked as an elementary school teacher 8 yr.

Habits: Eats 3 balanced meals a day with snack at night; walks 6 blocks to and from school each day; has never smoked; has an occasional glass of white wine (average of 1/wk); drinks 4 cups of coffee/day; denies drug use; usually arises at 6:30 AM and goes to bed about 11 PM; she and husband belong to gourmet cooking group; also enjoys gardening.

Review of Systems: States overall health is excellent.

Skin: Denies problems

Eyes: Wears contact lenses; last eye exam, 1984

Ears: See history of present illness

Teeth: No problems, last dental visit 4 mo ago

Respiratory: Usually has one cold a year, no cough

Breasts: No pain or lumps, examines breasts once a month

Cardiovascular: Denies problems

Gastrointestinal: No food intolerance, no changes in bowel habits

Gynecological: Menarche, age 13; 28-day cycle, 4-day flow; uses diaphragm for birth control

Endocrine: No excessive thirst, hunger, or urination

IV. Physical Assessment

Weight: 123 lb

Height: 5 ft 4 in

Vital Signs: Temp 98°F, P 76, R 16, BP 118/76

Relevant Organ Systems:

Head: Scalp and skull without masses or lesions; hair—normal distribution, thick, brown

Face: Symmetrical, sinus areas nontender, TMJ freely movable, no crepitation

Eyes: Vision with contacts R 20/20, L 20/30, PERRLA, EOMs intact, fundi benign

Ears: Auricles without lesions; canals patent without excessive cerumen, inflammation, or lesions; both TMs pearly gray, mobile, normal landmarks visible. Hearing (CN VIII): unable to hear whispered voice until repeated louder; unable to hear watch ticking; Rinne, BC>AC bilaterally; Weber, lateralizes to left ear; Schwabach, sound heard longer by client

Nose: Septum midline, nostrils patent, nasal mucosa pink, no discharge

Mouth/Throat: Mucosa pink; teeth in good repair; tonsils present, not enlarged

Neck: Auricular and cervical nodes not palpable

Neurologic: CN I–XII intact except for CN VIII as above; gait normal; Romberg, able to maintain standing position with eyes closed; sensory, pain and light touch intact

V. Diagnostic Data

Laboratory results showed normal CBC, bleeding time, and urinalysis.

VI. Summary

Mrs Sharppe was scheduled for a stapedectomy the next morning under local anesthesia. She progressed well after surgery and was discharged that evening.

The Client With Otosclerosis

VII. Postoperative Orders   Vital signs q. 30 min ×4
Diet as tolerated
Assess ambulatory status ×3 before discharge
Codeine sulfate 60 mg q.6h p.r.n. for pain
Dimenhydrinate (Dramamine) 50 mg q.6h p.r.n. for dizziness

VIII. Nursing Care Plan

Nursing Diagnosis	Client Care Goals	Plan/Nursing Implementation	Expected Outcome
Alteration in comfort related to surgical intervention	Client will remain free from pain and dizziness	Assess client for pain and dizziness; instruct regarding moving head slowly to prevent dizziness; assist client when ambulating if dizzy; explain actions, dose schedule, and potential side effects of medications for home use	Ability to ambulate comfortably without dizziness; client uses analgesics for pain and antivertiginous medication for dizziness safely as needed
Injury: potential for infection related to surgery	Client will remain free of postoperative infection	Instruct client to refrain from touching ear dressing or washing ear; assess for signs of headache or pain	Client competently cares for ear and consults with care provider appropriately
Injury: potential for dislocation of prosthesis	Prosthesis will remain intact	Discuss with client need to keep mouth open when sneezing or coughing and wipe nose instead of blowing	Client sneezing and coughing with mouth open; refraining from nose blowing
Knowledge deficit related to care after discharge	Recovers fully from surgery with improved hearing, without complications	Instruct client to avoid sudden head movements; report unusual symptoms of pain, taste changes, or facial weakness; postpone washing hair for 2 wk; avoid getting water in ear for 4 wk; also instruct to avoid contact with people who have upper respiratory infections and to avoid flying for 4 wk; encourage client to keep follow-up appointments and to have annual hearing tests	Client fully understands postoperative instructions and has uneventful recovery

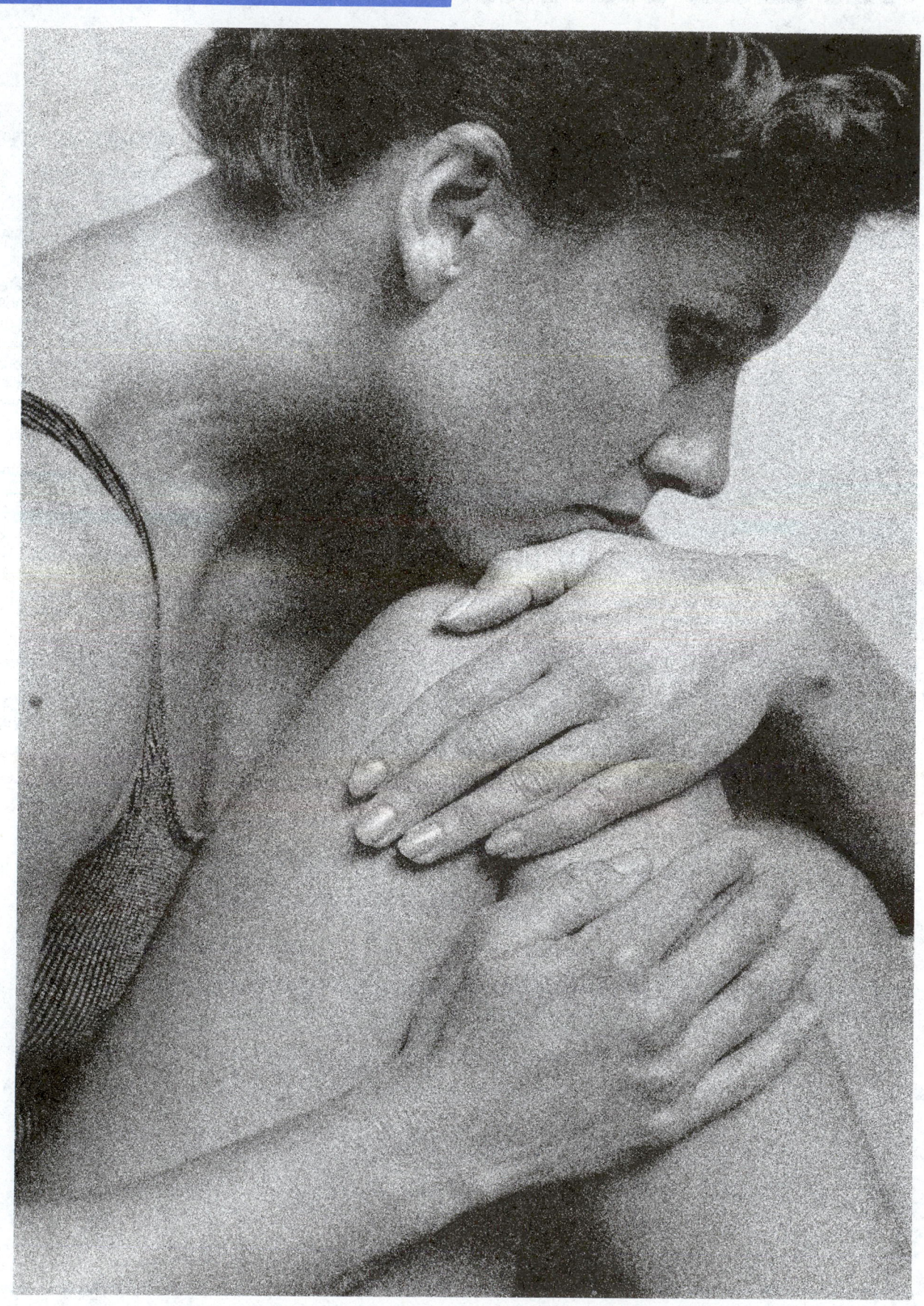

The Client With Integumentary System Dysfunction

UNIT 12

Chapter 77

The Integumentary System in Health and Illness

Carolyn Gorczyca

Objectives

When you have finished studying this chapter, you should be able to:

Identify the basic structures that form the integument.

Discuss the major functions of the integument.

Describe cellular composition, growth patterns, and functions of each layer of skin, the appendages, and melanocytes.

Explain the physiological mechanisms that regulate the activities of the skin.

Identify major factors that influence pathophysiological alterations of the skin.

Describe general cutaneous effects that result from pathophysiology of the skin.

Discuss the interrelations between behavior and skin manifestations.

Correlate phases of growth and development with normal alterations that may occur within the integument at each phase.

Link systemic disorders to their cutaneous manifestations.

Describe how psychosocial factors influence pathogenesis of skin disorders.

The integument, or skin, is the largest organ in the body, covering approximately 3000 sq in. of surface area in an average adult. One square inch of skin contains about 20 yards of blood vessels, 100 oil glands, 65 hairs and muscles, 650 sweat glands, and 78 yards of nerves with 19,500 touch nerve endings, 1300 pain nerve endings, 160 pressure nerve endings, 78 heat nerve endings, and 13 cold nerve endings. In all, there are almost 20 million cells of all kinds in one square inch of skin.

Because the skin is vital to the homeostatic balance of the body, it is essential for physical survival. It provides not only a protective barrier to the outside world, but it also, paradoxically, provides a major means of communicating with others and with the environment through touch and sensation. Therefore, the skin is essential not only for physical survival, but for the development of human behavior as well. Billions of dollars are spent each year to ensure the beauty of the skin and its other components, the hair and the nails. To most persons, physical appearance not only influences how others see them but how they see themselves. The skin is a window to the human body; it also reflects problems in other body systems.

Section I: Structural and Functional Interrelationships

STRUCTURE OF THE INTEGUMENTARY SYSTEM

Two basic layers make up the integument: the epidermis and dermis. A bed of subcutaneous tissue (the hypoder-mis), although technically not considered skin, constitutes the innermost segment. These layers, although structurally different, are continuous with the mucous membranes at body openings of the gastrointestinal and genitourinary tracts. The thickness of skin varies; the thinnest layers

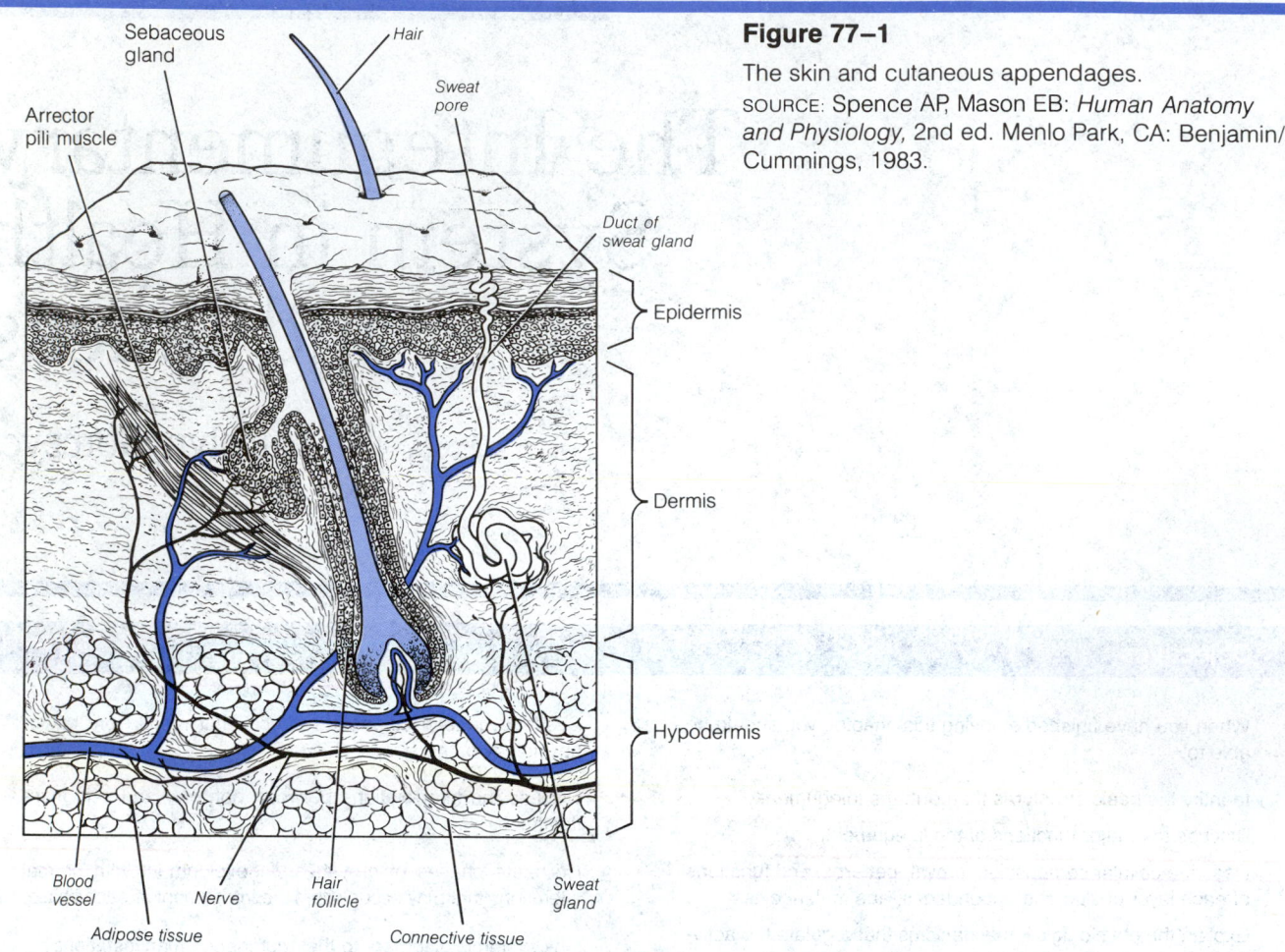

Sebaceous
gland

Hair

Sweat
pore

Arrector
pili muscle

Duct of
sweat gland

Epidermis

Dermis

Hypodermis

Blood
vessel

Nerve

Hair
follicle

Sweat
gland

Adipose tissue

Connective tissue

Figure 77–1

The skin and cutaneous appendages.
SOURCE: Spence AP, Mason EB: *Human Anatomy and Physiology,* 2nd ed. Menlo Park, CA: Benjamin/Cummings, 1983.

are on the eyelids, eardrum, and penis, and the thickest are on the palms of the hands and soles of the feet. Hair, nails, and the sebaceous, eccrine, and apocrine glands are classified as cutaneous appendages. These structures are illustrated in Figure 77–1.

Epidermis

The epidermis, the paper-thin outermost cutaneous layer, is composed of epithelial cells (mostly of the type called *keratinocytes*). There are four major zones, the stratum germinativum (growing layer), stratum granulosum, stratum lucidum, and stratum corneum (horny layer). Keratinocytes, or basal cells, reproduce in the innermost level (stratum germinativum), and each new daughter cell pushes upward on the cell above it. During their migration to the surface, keratinocytes change character; they are flattened, dehydrated, and lose their nuclei. The outermost layer of the epidermis (stratum corneum) consists of dead keratinocytes that eventually are shed. The normal life cycle of epidermal cells lasts about 4 weeks. Any increase

or decrease in the rate of keratinocyte production will alter the character of the skin.

The keratinocyte contains a waterproof, hard protein matter called *keratin* that is produced within the cell. Keratin is also responsible for the formation of hair and nails. Vitamin A is essential to the keratinizing processes and in the maintenance of normal epithelial structures.

The stratum corneum, through its relative imperviousness, protects the internal milieu. In addition, growth of infectious organisms is retarded by the dryness, constant shedding of the outermost layer of the epidermis, and the presence of an acid pH on most areas of the body except for the axilla, groin, and the skin between the fingers and toes (interdigital spaces).

Dermis

The dermis (or corium) is separated from the epidermis by the basement membrane. The dermis is denser than the epidermis and is primarily made up of connective tissue. A combination of fibers, water, and a gelatinous substance (collagen) makes it semisolid. The upper area of the dermis, known as the papillary layer, extends into the epidermis by means of projections or folds called *papillae*. Many of these protrusions contain capillary loops that nourish the epidermis, which has no blood vessels of its own. Curving parallel ridges created by these papillae are responsible for the development of fingerprint and footprint patterns within the epidermal layer of the palms and soles. Besides a network of blood vessels, the dermis also contains hair follicles, the glandular appendages, nerves, and lymphatics. These structures extend into the lower layer of the dermis (also called the *reticulum*).

The elasticity and resilience of the skin result from the presence of collagen, elastin, and reticular fibers in the dermis. Collagen is also important in maintaining durability of cutaneous blood vessels, healing of wounds, and increasing resistance to infection. Its formation requires adequate intake of vitamin C.

Subcutaneous Tissue (Hypodermis)

The hypodermis, also known as subcutaneous tissue or subcutis, is the third layer of the integument. This loose connective tissue is made up primarily of fat cells, but it also contains blood vessels, nerves, lymphatics, and protein fibers. The amount of subcutaneous tissue varies; it is absent from eyelids, penis, scrotum, nipple, areola, and the skin over the anterior surface of the tibia. The abundance and distribution of subcutaneous tissue is determined by sex hormones, heredity, age, diet, and disease states. The subcutis stores energy as fat (adipose tissue), which prevents loss of body heat through insulation and protects internal structures by cushioning mechanical shocks.

Hair

Hair covers most of the body surface except for the palms, soles, lips, nipples, and parts of the external genitalia. The millions of hair follicles, tubelike passages from which the hair grows, are formed during fetal development. They are derived from the epithelial cells in the epidermis and become invaginated in the underlying dermis (Figure 77–2). The external root sheath forms the outermost layer of the follicle, whereas the internal root sheath provides a lining from the bottom of the follicle up to the sebaceous gland. Each hair is a column of keratinized cells that develops at the base of the follicle where the blood vessels within the papillae provide for circulatory and nutritional needs. The root is the part of the hair that forms in the follicle, and the shaft is the dead part of the hair that protrudes through the skin. A cross section of hair shows a central core (medulla) covered by a cortex, which is covered in turn by the cuticle.

The human body has two major types of hair. Vellus hair (referred to as lanugo in newborns) is very fine, short,

lightly colored, and barely visible. It is commonly called "peach fuzz." Terminal hair is long, thick, and pigmented. It occurs on the scalp, arms, legs, axilla, and pubic regions and on the male face and chest. It may be straight, wavy, helical, or spiral. Hair color is proportional to the amount of melanin in the cortex of the hair. Blond, gray, and white hair result from the absence of melanin.

A smooth muscle (the arrector pili) is attached at the base of the follicle. When a stimulus such as cold or fright contracts the muscle, the follicle and hair are brought to an erect position, producing "goose pimples" or "goose flesh."

Hair grows in a cyclic pattern in which each follicle responds independently. A hair may be either in the growth phase (anagen), in transition (catagen), or in the resting phase (telogen). Generally, each strand is shed when new growth begins pushing the old hair upward. Rates of hair regeneration on the various body surfaces differ. The scalp is most active, where 85% to 90% of the hairs may be in the anagen phase for as long as 2 to 6 years.

Hair growth is basically influenced by blood supply and hormones. Normally, a significant change in hair distribution occurs during puberty, when androgen stimulates growth on the axilla and pubic area (and face, chest, and body in men). Black, Indian, and Oriental men normally have far less hair in the pubic and beard areas. Conversely, women of Mediterranean or Middle Eastern (rather than Northern European) ancestry often have more facial hair (for example, on the upper lip). Excesses and losses of hair may occur at various times during the life cycle, in response to normal alterations in hormonal levels. Systemic illness, emotional stresses, drugs, chronic superficial irritation, cutaneous inflammation and infection, temperature extremes, and starvation may also influence hair growth.

Hair is a protection from the elements and from trauma. For example, scalp hair and eyebrows are barriers against sunlight, and nasal hairs and eyelashes filter ambient air. Hair is also an indicator of general health status. Too little or too much hair can have a negative impact on body image.

Nails

Fingernails and toenails are formed from the strata corneum and lucidum (Figure 77–3). They appear as a dense layer of dead flat cells filled with keratin. The stratum germinativum provides an epithelial bed on which the nail plate rests, firmly attached along most of its length by the cuticle or eponychium. Growth is continuous from the nail matrix at the proximal end, also called the *lunula* because of its white crescent moon shape. Normal nails are transparent and durable; the proximity of capillaries accounts for the normal pink coloration. Nails protect the fingers and toes and assist in a variety of utilitarian activities. Nail biting and occupational stresses cause faster growth, thickening, or both. Systemic illnesses may also be reflected in changes

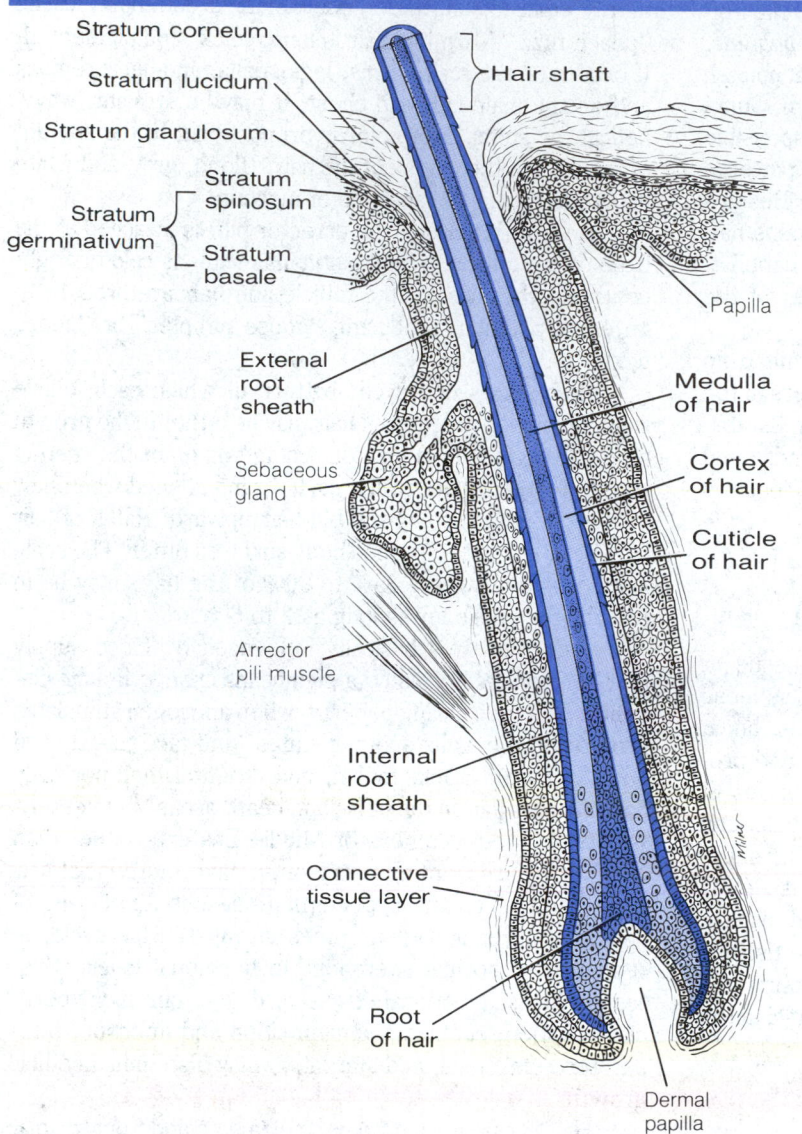

Stratum corneum

Stratum lucidum

Stratum granulosum

Stratum spinosum

Stratum germinativum

Stratum basale

Hair shaft

External root sheath

Sebaceous gland

Arrector pili muscle

Internal root sheath

Connective tissue layer

Root of hair

Papilla

Medulla of hair

Cortex of hair

Cuticle of hair

Dermal papilla

Figure 77–2

Vertical section through a hair follicle.

SOURCE: Spence AP, Mason EB: *Human Anatomy and Physiology*, 2nd ed. Menlo Park, CA: Benjamin/Cummings, 1983.

to the nail or its bed. These are further discussed and illustrated in Chapter 78.

Glandular Appendages

All three kinds of glandular appendages—sebaceous, eccrine, and apocrine glands—are formed from epidermal cells during fetal development and become invaginated in the dermis. They excrete either through a duct that opens directly to the skin surface or into the hair follicle.

The sebaceous (oil) glands are located throughout the entire skin except for the palms of the hands and soles of the feet. They are abundant on the face, scalp, upper chest, and back. The duct of the sebaceous gland joins the hair follicle near the distal end, and the combined structure may be referred to as a *pilosebaceous unit*. The sebaceous gland produces a lipid substance known as **sebum**, which

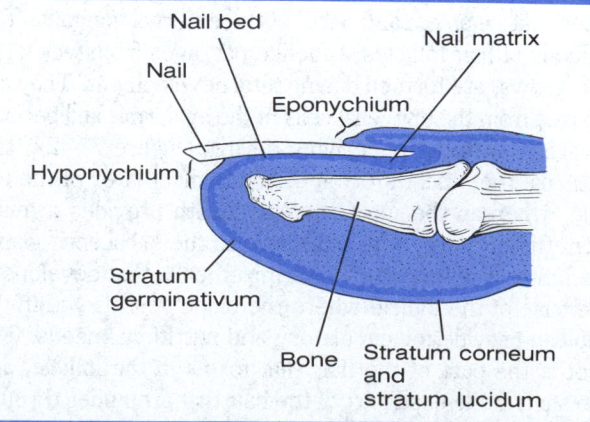

Nail bed

Nail

Nail matrix

Eponychium

Hyponychium

Stratum germinativum

Bone

Stratum corneum and stratum lucidum

Figure 77–3

Structure of a nail.

SOURCE: Spence AP, Mason EB: *Human Anatomy and Physiology*, 2nd ed. Menlo Park, CA: Benjamin/Cummings, 1983.

provides some lubrication of hair and epidermis, has an antibacterial-fungistatic action, and retards evaporation from the skin surface.

Androgens are responsible for the enlargement and functioning of the sebaceous glands. Activation occurs during puberty. Once the glands are functioning, the production of sebum is a continuous process. Sebaceous glands may cause problems such as acne in adolescence and young adulthood.

There are two kinds of sweat glands—eccrine and apocrine glands. Only the eccrine glands participate in heat regulation. Millions of eccrine glands are located over the body with the greatest distribution in the palms of the hands, the soles of the feet, and the forehead.

The apocrine (odoriferous) glands are found most significantly in the axillary, nipple, anal, and pubic areas. Their ducts empty into the upper portion of the hair follicle. These glands do not have a known physiological role in man, although water, salts, and organic matter are secreted. The decomposition of the excreta by bacteria on the skin causes body odor. As with the sebaceous glands, activation occurs during puberty and is hormone dependent. Excretion is a continuous process that is increased by emotional stress.

Skin and Hair Coloring

Melanin is a brown-black pigment that gives color to skin and hair. Melanin-forming cells (melanocytes) are interspersed among the basal cells of the epidermis but are derived from neural rather than epithelial tissue. The amount of pigment production in the melanocytes is regulated by melanocyte-stimulating hormone (MSH) from the anterior pituitary. Dendritic projections on the melanocytes transfer the pigment granules to the keratinocytes. Without melanin, skin looks pink or white depending on the degree of vascularity. The presence of carotene, a precursor of vitamin A found in some vegetables such as carrots, gives a yellow color to the skin.

Because all humans have an equal number of melanocytes, it is the amount, size, and distribution of melanin granules produced that determine skin color. Whites (Caucasians) have the least amount of coloring, with variances in Africans, Asiatics, and Native Americans. Blacks from Africa, New Guinea, and dark-skinned persons from southern India (tropical regions) have a high degree of pigmentation.

The purpose of melanin is to protect living cells from damaging ultraviolet radiation. Cellular damage (sunburn, for example) occurs if the body is unable to defend itself against ultraviolet rays by synthesizing more melanin, which acts as a natural sunscreen. In dark-skinned people, protection is inherent. Those individuals who are capable of increasing melanin production will tan with exposure to the sun (see also Chapter 78 and Table 78–7).

FUNCTION OF THE INTEGUMENTARY SYSTEM

The major biological functions in which the skin and its appendages play a role are protection, thermoregulation, and sensory perception. The skin also has a significant role in metabolic activities.

Protection

The skin is the first line of defense against the external environment. It provides a barrier to a variety of noxious agents (including infectious organisms, parasites, radiant energy, and chemical substances) that could be harmful to internal structures and mechanisms. Because of its great durability, pliability, and adaptability, skin can serve as a buffer against trauma from physical objects and mechanical stressors. The waterproof quality of the outer layer of the skin prevents both excess water absorption and abnormal losses of body fluids. It also aids in maintaining a moist internal environment necessary for metabolism.

Thermoregulation

Blood conducts heat from internal structures to the skin for dissipation. The skin dissipates excess body heat in two ways: by radiation and by evaporative cooling. The intense heat produced during cellular metabolism must be removed from the body's core. Heated blood from the interior flows to the skin, which is cooled by the ambient air, and heat is transferred to the skin cells and from there to the air.

The flow of blood needed to nourish the skin is insignificant compared with the amount needed for thermoregulation. In relatively cool conditions, blood flow to the skin is about 0.4 L (400 mL)/min, but the amount goes as high as 2.8 L/min when maximum vasodilation occurs. To accommodate this great variance, the skin contains a network of blood vessels that can adjust rapidly to increased or decreased demands. Venous plexuses, which are connected to arterioles by arteriovenous anastomoses, hold large volumes of blood during the cooling process (Figure 77–4). When heat must be conserved, or when large quantities of blood are needed elsewhere (as for digestion), the arterioles will constrict to allow only a minimum of blood into the veins. In a cold environment, skin and the adipose tissue in its deeper layers insulate the body's core to retain needed heat.

The nervous system controls thermoregulation by controlling blood flow to the skin. Temperature changes are registered in the hypothalamus, which in turn relays responses requiring vasodilation and activation of the sweat glands (for cooling) or vasoconstriction (for heat retention). These responses are mediated through the sympathetic portion of the autonomic nervous system.

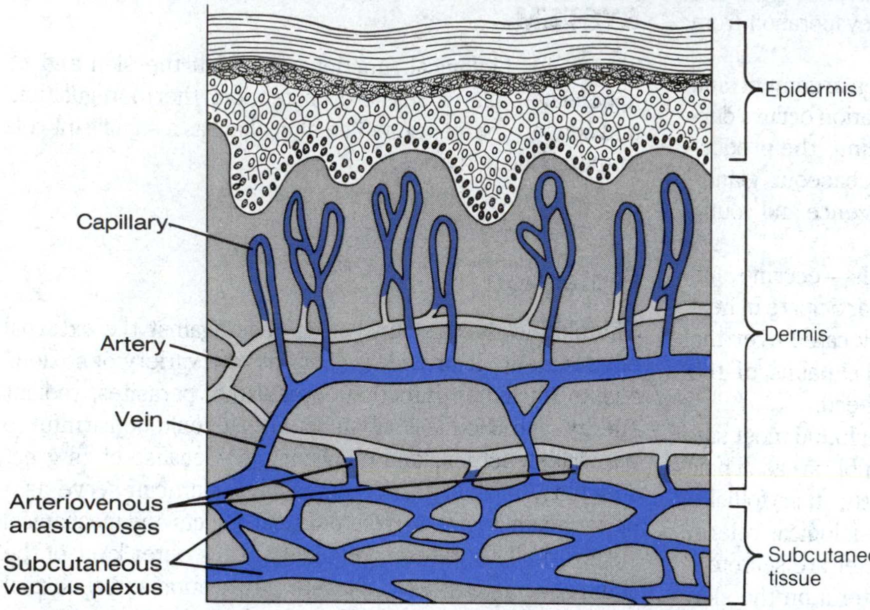

Figure 77–4

Blood vessels of the skin.
SOURCE: Spence AP, Mason
EB: *Human Anatomy and
Physiology*, 2nd ed. Menlo
Park, CA: Benjamin/Cummings, 1983.

Evaporative cooling takes place when the eccrine glands secrete sweat, a hypotonic mixture of water and sodium chloride (salt) with minute amounts of urea, sulfates, and phosphates, into ducts that empty to the surface of the skin. As the sweat evaporates, cooling takes place. Although heat is the primary stimulus for the production of sweat, emotional stress may also trigger increased perspiration.

Sensory Perception

The integument contains several types of receptor cells at various levels in the skin that perceive sensations of pain, pressure, touch, and temperature. Sensory receptors in the skin also play a direct role in the protective function of the skin. For example, the perception of an extreme temperature—dangerously hot or cold—causes an avoidance reaction almost before there is a conscious recognition of the danger. People with sensory receptor deficits (as a result of neurovascular disease, for instance) may fail to perceive the pain of a cut or burn and thus be unable to protect themselves from further damage.

Metabolism

The skin takes part in several metabolic functions. It assists in the regulation of fluids and selected electrolytes by eliminating water and small amounts of sodium chloride through the sweat glands. The amounts excreted are influenced by activity and by ambient temperature. When the kidneys and liver are not working properly, the skin may replace some of their function by excreting nitrogenous wastes and products of metabolism. Also, in the presence of sunlight or ultraviolet radiation, skin begins the process of forming vitamin D (cholecalciferol), a substance needed for absorbing calcium and phosphates from food.

Section II: Pathophysiological Influences and Effects

It is difficult to identify precise pathophysiological influences when studying diseases of the skin (or dermatoses). Few disorders have a single cause; many have several interrelated influences and for some, the cause is still unknown. Generally, the pathophysiology is correlated with one or more of the following factors: genetic and congenital factors, multifactorial or idiopathic causes, immunologic hypersensitivity, infections and infestations, neoplasia, or trauma. These categories are by no means all encompassing; they simply represent the major elements that affect normal structure and function of the skin.

GENETIC AND CONGENITAL FACTORS

Factors such as skin color, thickness, hairiness, and glandular activity are all determined primarily by genetic makeup. Children may be born with "birthmarks." These congenital manifestations include any nonspecific localized skin malformation, usually vascular or pigmented. Mongolian spots (bluish spots in the sacral region), hemangiomas, and certain types of nevi (moles) may be evident. Although precursor cells for pigmented lesions may be present at birth, such lesions are more apt to appear with increasing age (usually after puberty). Freckles constitute an inherited type of alteration in pigmentation, even though they generally appear only as a result of sun exposure. Albinism (hypopigmentation) is caused by a genetic defect that prevents synthesis of melanin and results in the absence of color in the skin and hair. Heredity plays an important role in predisposition to the development of acne and atopic dermatitis (allergic tendency), although other factors are also implicated.

Skin loses water content from natural causes such as aging and low humidity (desert air, eg); however, there are people who tend to have chronic dry flaky skin. A child may be born with a condition called *ichthyosis,* which involves excessive scaling or thickening of the outermost layer of the skin. Such problems may continue into puberty and adulthood.

MULTIFACTORIAL OR IDIOPATHIC CAUSES

Many dermatoses are classified as multifactorial because no outstanding factor can be linked with pathogenesis. A classic example is psoriasis. Although the disorder seems to have a familial tendency, there is no identifiable factor that causes an accelerated rate of cell proliferation. Seborrheic dermatitis (dandruff) is another common condition whose cause is unknown, although it has been associated with constitutional predisposition and with emotional and physical stress. Vitiligo (patches that lack pigment) and chloasma (patches darker than the surrounding skin) involve alterations in skin pigmentation that may be considered idiopathic in origin. Although familial tendency has been correlated with vitiligo, exactly why the skin becomes depigmented remains unknown. Chloasma, on the other hand, has been associated with pregnancy, chronic illness, and Latin American origin.

IMMUNOLOGIC HYPERSENSITIVITY

Immunologic hypersensitivity responses may occur. Normally, there is a balance among the factors that mediate the body's defense against foreign matter. Some individuals, however, have an inborn tendency (atopy) to react adversely to these stimuli. An immediate hypersensitivity response may follow direct contact, inhalation, ingestion, or injection of numerous substances. Common allergens include cosmetics, soaps, perfumes, lotions, sprays, plants, and certain metals. Delayed hypersensitivity is a common reaction with exposure to poison ivy. Skin eruptions and other cutaneous manifestations are common side effects of drugs and are one sign of transfusion incompatibility.

An allergic reaction, localized or general, triggers an inflammatory response. The alterations in the skin include erythema (reddening), rashes, urticaria (hives), and the onset of pruritus (itching) in varying degrees. Anaphylaxis is always possible when an individual has developed an acute sensitivity to any allergen.

The cutaneous manifestations seen in autoimmune disease further illustrate the significance immunity has pathophysiologically. Although the basic reason for the phenomenon is unknown, the body produces antibodies against its own connective tissue. As a result, the skin may atrophy, harden, show changes in vasculature and pigmentation, develop rashes, or become edematous.

Immunity is also linked with the body's defense against cancer. Immune deficiencies have been noted in malignant melanoma, and immunotherapy has been used in an attempt to stimulate the client's antibodies to destroy the abnormal cells.

INFECTIONS AND INFESTATIONS

Infectious agents are responsible for much integumentary pathology. The skin surface supports a normal population of flora, primarily gram-positive bacteria of which staphylococci and diphtheroids are most prominent. Problems occur when pathological organisms gain entry beyond the protective epidermis, perhaps through natural openings such as the hair follicles and the eccrine ducts. More often, organisms invade the body through traumatic breaks in the cutaneous tissue (scratches, lacerations, punctures, bites), through areas damaged by excessive moisture, or by septic administration of parenteral substances. Persons with intertrigo (chafing), an inflammatory dermatosis, may develop infection from normal skin flora. Obese persons are particularly vulnerable because skin folds (axillary, inframammary, inguinal) may become irritated during hot weather. Infection is also involved in acne.

Primary skin infections are commonly caused by bacteria, viruses, and fungi. Secondary infections may occur with stasis dermatitis (where impaired circulation damages skin cells of the feet and ankles), atopic dermatitis, or in decubiti and leg ulcers. Skin damaged by any dermatosis, by diminished circulation, or by a disruption to neurological controls is vulnerable to infection. Nursing care is of particular importance in clients with any such vulnerabilities.

Skin may also become a site for clinical manifestations in systemic infections. Communicable diseases, such as measles, chickenpox, scarlet fever, and Hansen's disease (leprosy) produce classic skin signs and symptoms. Sexually transmitted diseases such as syphilis, genital herpes simplex, and condylomata acuminata (venereal warts) also present characteristic cutaneous lesions.

Infestations involve attacks on the skin by parasitic organisms, which are classified as protozoans, helminthoids (worms), and arthropods. The most common dermatoses involve bites by either of two types of arthropods. Arachnids such as spiders, scorpions, ticks, and mites represent one group; insects such as lice, bedbugs, fleas, flies, mosquitoes, and bees are the other.

NEOPLASIA

Neoplasia in the broadest sense involves the development of new tissues (often called tumors). Increased cellular proliferation is responsible for numerous cutaneous pathological conditions. Friction and chronic pressure are responsible for hyperkeratosis (calluses) in localized areas on the outermost layer of the epidermis. Keloid formation and hypertrophic scarring involve excessive collagen formation after cutaneous injury. People with deeply pigmented skin have a predisposition to develop keloids or hypertrophic scarring, but their occurrence is not limited by skin color. Warts are caused by viral infection, but may also be classified as neoplasia.

Skin cysts are a form of abnormal mass, although most are not technically neoplasia. The growth usually contains some fluid or solid material (or both) and can occur for several reasons. Some are congenital; others arise from obstruction of the pilosebaceous duct. Wens are a form of skin cyst.

Benign or malignant neoplasms may develop from every type of cell in the various layers and structures of the skin, but keratinocytes and melanocytes are the most frequently involved. As with tumors in general, the cause for abnormal cell proliferation is unknown.

Seborrheic keratosis, a hyperplastic epidermal lesion, is a common benign skin condition seen in middle-aged and older adults. Another type of benign tumor is the nevus or mole—a common malformation often considered a birthmark. The nevus is not a simple structure, either in cellular composition or in its cause. Nevi may be vascular or nonvascular, highly pigmented or nonpigmented. A nevus may arise from melanocytes or from epidermal, glandular, connective, or neural tissue. *Junctional nevi* are of most concern because they may develop into malignant melanomas. They are discussed in Chapter 79.

Several epidermal lesions are considered precancerous and require regular examination to detect malignant changes. They include senile keratoses, actinic keratoses, and arsenical keratoses. **Leukoplakia** (white plaques seen on mucous membranes) are also considered precancerous lesions. Long-term exposure to sun; to chemicals such as coal tar, pitch, or creosol; to ionizing radiation (x-rays); to direct contact with or ingestion of arsenic; to chronic irritation; and to smoking has been implicated in cancer. In addition, persons with light-colored hair and skin (Northern European ancestry) have a predisposition to skin cancer. Albinos and individuals with xeroderma pigmentosum (a hereditary disorder that causes photosensitivity) are likely to develop skin cancer if not suitably protected from exposure to sunlight. Epithelial cell lesions may progress into basal cell or squamous cell carcinomas.

TRAUMA

Physical injury to the skin is an ever-present hazard. Superficial lacerations, contusions, abrasions, and punctures occur frequently in accidents at home, in the streets, or at the workplace. Exposure to extremes of temperature can cause injury; extensive burns or frostbite can cause loss of life or a limb. Electrical burns and irradiation damage internal structures even when the skin seems little affected. Everyday mechanical pressures or chronic irritation provokes the development of localized thickening of skin, or **lichenification**. Corns and calluses are good examples of the skin's attempt to adapt to these irritations.

A frequent cause of trauma to the skin is scratching. Scratching is an attempt to alleviate the discomfort of pruritus (itching). The sensation of itching is perceived by nerve endings deep in the epidermis. Many factors can stimulate pruritus: dry skin, insect bites, and topical irritants are examples of external stimuli. Pruritus can also result from chemical mediators released into the skin during inflammation and allergic responses, or from metabolic wastes and irritants exiting through the integument.

Pruritus increases during vasodilation, with tissue anoxia, with venous stasis, and with emotional tension. Vasoconstriction lessens the sensation. Although scratching and rubbing of the irritated areas are defensive actions, too much can traumatize the protective layers of skin. Being unable to relieve an itch is emotionally frustrating. Continual pruritus can disrupt sleep, rest, and socialization. Unbearable pruritus constitutes a dermatological emergency.

Section III: Related System Influences and Effects

Although the skin is not usually thought to be essential to life, without it, death would occur. Like other organ systems, however, the skin depends on proper functioning of the endocrine system, the heart and blood vessels, lungs, kidneys, and gastrointestinal tract. Each person is a multiplicity of cells, every cell functioning uniquely but, most important, working with all the others to maintain life.

ENDOCRINE SYSTEM

At puberty, hormonal changes trigger secretions from the apocrine glands, causing the redistribution of body fat and the development of axillary and pubic hair, and, in men, the development of chest, facial, and body hair. In addition, hormones stimulate secretion by the sebaceous glands, and the apocrine glands. Acne vulgaris, a common disorder in adolescence that may extend into adulthood, is related to the production of sebum, as described in Chapter 79. Although acne is not in itself life threatening, it occurs at a period when boys and girls begin developing roles as men and women. Acne can have a negative effect on body image and self-esteem.

Testosterone decreases growth of hair on the scalp and may be responsible for some forms of alopecia in men. Estrogens, in turn, cause skin to become more vascular. The effects are seen in the premenstrual cycle when retention of fluid causes breast enlargement and edema in ankles and fingers.

For women during the child-bearing years, characteristic changes may occur during pregnancy that cause concern to the client. Pregnancy involves glandular activities that primarily result in the alteration of pigmentation, such as the presence of striae on the body (depressed atrophic stripes), the appearance of chloasma in a characteristic pattern called *pregnancy mask,* color changes to the vulva and nipples, and prominence of freckling and nevi. Pruritus is a fairly common discomfort, possibly resulting from excretion by cutaneous glands. **Hypertrichosis** (excess hair) may occur but in many cases disappears following delivery.

Menopausal changes involve the skin as a target area. Women experience "hot flashes," which entail cutaneous vasodilation and profuse perspiration. Alterations in hair growth and distribution (growth of facial hair) may also cause problems.

Endocrine system disorders such as Addison's disease, Cushing's syndrome, acromegaly, and hyper- and hypopituitarism cause significant changes in skin pigmentation and texture and in the amount and distribution of hair and subcutaneous tissue.

CARDIOVASCULAR AND RESPIRATORY SYSTEMS

Cardiovascular disorders often cause skin changes. For example, clients with peripheral vascular disease fre- quently have changes in the extremities including pallor, dependent rubor, cyanosis, dry scaly skin, cellulitis, ulcerations, and brittle toenail. Gangrene can be a long-term complication of peripheral vascular disease. Clients with chronic obstructive pulmonary disease (COPD) or congestive heart failure will often be cyanotic and have clubbing of the fingers.

Blood dyscrasias often cause skin signs such as petechiae, ecchymosis, and pallor. Alopecia, skin eruptions, and pruritus are seen in some lymphomas.

URINARY SYSTEM

Dysfunction in the urinary system may affect the integument in a number of ways. For example, chronic renal failure may result in pruritus, uremic frost, pallor, or a yellow cast to the skin.

GASTROINTESTINAL AND HEPATIC-BILIARY SYSTEMS

Clients who are malnourished may experience loss of subcutaneous tissue, alopecia, hyperkeratosis, or purpura. Persons who ingest excessively large amounts of vitamin A may have an orange color to the skin; this carotene pigmentation is the result of carotene toxicity. Biliary tract disease often causes jaundice, pruritus, and spider hemangiomas.

MUSCULOSKELETAL SYSTEM

Connective tissue disorders may alter the appearance and function of the integument. For example, systemic lupus erythematosus has a characteristic butterfly-shaped rash on the face and causes small ulcerations of the fingertips. Scleroderma causes a leathery hardening of the skin. A joint disorder—rheumatoid arthritis—often coexists with psoriasis.

Section IV: Psychosocial Influences and Effects

Skin disorders that can be attributed solely to psychological or social causes are rare. However, many conditions show a correlation between emotional stress and the onset of exacerbation of the dermatosis; the skin may become the primary target.

Skin plays a significant role in the communication of feelings. The cutaneous blood vessels are affected by the emotional states of an individual, as are some of the glan- dular appendages. Fear may cause blanching, anger or embarrassment may produce a red face, and anxiety may increase perspiration. Emotions can alter hormone production and circulation, which, in turn, can alter integumentary processes. In addition, emotions can alter behavior (nutrition, cleanliness, substance abuse, willingness to follow instructions, and so on) that can affect the skin.

Some of the more common dermatoses known to be

Nursing Research Note

Randolph GL: Therapeutic and physical touch: Physiological response to stressful stimuli. *Nurs Res* 1984; 33(1):33–35.

Physiological difference between groups reacting to stressful stimuli when treated by either therapeutic touch or physical touch was investigated. Physiological responses measured include skin conduction, muscle tension, and peripheral skin temperatures. Physical touch consisted of placing one's hands on the subject's abdomen and lower back. Therapeutic touch consisted of the practitioner entering a meditative state, concentrating on the subject, and placing hands on the abdomen and back to transfer energy. Sixty healthy college female students were used in the sample. They viewed a stressful film and during the viewing received either therapeutic or physical touch.

There was no significant difference in the psychophysiological measures between the groups. Both groups exhibited significant stress response to the film. Although therapeutic touch has received support in other research, this study failed to demonstrate its effectiveness in reducing stress. Additional research is needed on the effectiveness of therapeutic touch in stress reduction.

influenced by psychological considerations include atopic dermatitis (eczema), alopecia areata, urticaria, and psoriasis. Flare-ups of atopic dermatitis are known to occur with emotional stress. Alopecia areata, in which loss of hair occurs suddenly, often follows a traumatic event, such as the death of a significant person. Psoriasis has a prolonged and unpredictable course. The onset or exacerbation of psoriasis is frequently preceded by some form of stressful or anxiety-producing situation.

The appearance and the health of the skin are directly influenced by an individual's stage of development and nutritional status. Occupational exposures and climatic conditions contribute to problems of the skin. An individual's body image, comfort with sexuality, and with roles and relationships can all be closely intertwined with the appearance of the skin.

SEX AND AGE

The aging process results in multiple effects to the skin for both men and women. Diminished circulation, altered metabolism, reduced immunity, and changes in hormonal activity all cause changes. Generally, there is an overall decrease in tissue mass, which results in a thinner, more transparent skin. Loss of collagen and adipose tissue results in sagging and wrinkling. As total body water decreases, skin becomes dry and scaly. Color changes and keratotic, vascular, and pigmented lesions appear with greater frequency. Increased fragility of blood vessels allows for easy bruising. Sluggish circulation leads to improper nourishment of the living portion of the integument. Finally, for a number of reasons (including all of the above plus, in many

cases, years of chronic irritation), the elderly are predisposed to malignancies of the skin.

DEVELOPMENTAL FACTORS

Tactile stimulation is the first means of communication. The physical closeness of mother and infant and the emotional messages that are relayed by touch through caressing, cuddling, holding, and stroking influence adult life as well as childhood.

Skin disorders that begin in infancy can influence personality development. Infantile forms of eczema can affect mother-child interactions and subsequent tactile communication. Disturbances in intimacy and self-image can be initiated in infancy that form barriers to normal adaptive processes in later life.

DIETARY HABITS

There are no known foods that cause or cure specific skin disorders. At one time, diet was considered relevant in the development of acne. Foods such as chocolate, nuts, cola, whole milk products, fatty meats, and spicy foods were to be avoided. Although these foods do not cause acne, their overconsumption by adolescents remains a general nutritional concern.

Poor nutrition, whether for economic or other reasons, may alter skin integrity. The poor, chronic dieters, or the elderly may not have a well-balanced diet that provides the necessary vitamins, minerals, proteins, and fatty acids. Nutritional deficiencies cause dryness, scaliness, inelasticity, decreased skin and hair pigmentation, edema, pallor, and dermatoses. Also, loss of subcutaneous tissue interferes with the protective and thermoregulatory functions of the skin.

Dietary excesses primarily result in obesity, which has a distinct effect on appearance. Xanthomas, yellow to brown skin deposits that are high in lipid content, are found on the eyelids in persons with hyperlipidemia, a condition associated with cardiovascular disease, or nutritional problems. Xanthomas and hyperlipidemia are discussed in Units Four and Seven. Of major concern is excessive intake of vitamin A, with or without medical supervision, often used to treat skin disorders such as acne. Synthetic derivatives of vitamin A called *retinoids* have been found to be pharmacologically effective in cases of acne, psoriasis, and ichthyosis. Excess vitamin A, however, besides being detrimental to the liver and to bone, causes such problems as dry, fissured skin; rashes; brittle nails; hair loss; and lip inflammation (cheilosis).

CLIMATE

Exposure to excessive sun or humidity can influence the condition of the skin. For example, prickly heat or *miliaria*, a condition that involves blockage of sweat glands, is associated with hot and humid weather, as are cutaneous fungal infections. Premature aging, vitiligo, actinic keratosis, and skin malignancies all increase in body areas that have been exposed to a great deal of sunlight. Persons who live in geographical areas where the sun is strong are at increased risk for these skin disorders.

Sunlight has been considered therapeutic for some skin lesions but is known to aggravate psoriasis, herpes simplex, and atopic dermatitis. Protection must be given to persons with systemic illnesses who may develop photodermatoses. Adverse skin reactions may occur in persons with lupus erythematosis, scleroderma, pellagra, phenylketonuria, hypopituitarism, and albinism.

Some drugs can cause photosensitivity (increased redness on exposure to the sun, which can result in severe sunburn. The most common drugs involved are demeclocycline (Declomycin), doxycycline (Vibramycin), chlorpromazine (Thorazine), hydrochlorothiazide (Hydro-DIURIL), tolbutamide (Orinase), and nalidixic acid (Neg-Gram). Oral contraceptives may also cause photosensitivity.

BODY IMAGE

The American culture sets no age limits on the demand for a youthful appearance. Women have traditionally been the prime victims of the demand, although men are increasingly investing time, energy, and money to ensure a youthful, "fit" appearance. People whose sense of self-worth depends heavily on physical attractiveness often have great difficulty dealing with age-related alterations in appearance. When cosmetics fail to hide the natural changes, elective cosmetic surgery may be used to remove excess skin (sags or wrinkles) or to modify some body change (eg, sagging breasts). Some go to extreme lengths to eliminate the signs of aging, sometimes at great financial cost and occasionally exposing themselves to the traumatizing effects of faulty or unproven procedures.

Skin disorders that cause disfigurement alter the body image as well as one's self-view. The presence of extensive cutaneous lesions, particularly when inflammation or infection is obvious, may arouse fears of contagion in others. Rejection of a person for this reason, or because his or her appearance is repulsive, adds to the emotional stress and feelings of low self-worth the client may feel. In turn, the physiologic problem can be further compounded by the use of cosmetics intended to hide blemishes as the client attempts to present a more attractive appearance.

ECONOMIC FACTORS

The poor may be exposed to skin problems as a result of unsanitary or crowded living conditions, unsafe heating (burns from open fires or unshielded portable heaters), and complications resulting from lack of (or inadequate) treat-

ment. Also, the poor may use community swimming pools where contagion may be a risk. It would be an error to assume that skin disorders have economic boundaries, however. Outbreaks of infections and infestations may occur within any school or community.

The affluent can afford medical services, cosmetics, and plastic or reconstructive surgery, if desired. However, they can also afford vacations in places where the climate guarantees extensive exposure to hot, humid, sunny weather, placing themselves at increased risk.

OCCUPATION AND AVOCATION

Dermatological problems have great significance in occupational health. They are the most frequently reported work-related disorders; 90% are the result of contact with substances causing inflammatory dermatitis. For instance, hand dermatitis is quite common among beauticians, photographers, and furniture refinishers. In addition, folliculitis, acne, pigment changes, neoplasms, ulcerations, and granulomas have been identified as occupationally related. Chronic exposure to sunlight has increased the incidence of skin malignancies in farmers, fishermen, and sailors. Insecticide makers, spray-rig operators, oil refinery workers, and smelter employees who work with arsenic face similar risks. Some of these same substances are used in the pursuit of leisure activities and may cause skin problems. Clients may need to limit, or even to give up, treasured leisure activities.

Some persons may lose jobs as a result of a dermatological condition. Fellow workers may fear "catching" an illness; employers may be reluctant for the employee to have contact with the public. An employer may also be reluctant to retain an employee whose disorder is occupationally induced.

SEXUAL EXPRESSION

The skin plays an important role in how people express their sexuality (through touch), since sexual arousal is facilitated by tactile stimulation of the skin's erogenous zones. In addition, insecurities and uncertainties about sexuality and sexual activity may be amplified by feelings of unattractiveness because of skin lesions. Contact with the skin may trigger unpleasant feelings in either partner. Even the anticipation that unpleasant feelings may be triggered can sometimes be reason enough to avoid sexual activity.

ROLES AND RELATIONSHIPS

One's interpersonal world is also strongly influenced by integumentary problems. For example, fear of being rejected by others may make it difficult to participate in usual socializing activities. Some conditions or symptoms (eg, severe pruritus) may actually interfere with or prevent a person from carrying out usual familial or social roles.

The development of chronic skin disorders whose treatment is exacting and unending may result in depression. Some individuals may withdraw, completely insulate and isolate themselves, or even consider suicide. Finally, fear, anxiety, anger, hostility, guilt, depression, loneliness, and denial may all accompany even a relatively mild skin disorder.

Chapter Highlights

The integument has a vital role in maintaining homeostasis in man.

The integument is composed of three distinct layers of skin, the dermis, epidermis, and hypodermis (or subcutaneous tissue), and contains the cornified (hair and nails) and glandular (sebaceous, eccrine, and apocrine) appendages.

Skin is the first line of defense against noxious agents from the external environment.

Skin is also a key organ in thermoregulation, sensory perception, and metabolism.

Tactile communication is essential to both physiological and psychosocial well-being.

The circulatory, nervous, and endocrine systems act as major regulatory mechanisms of the skin.

General health and emotional state may be reflected in cutaneous manifestations.

The cause-and-effect relationship of skin disorders must be viewed holistically because of the interactions and interrelations between physiological, psychological, socioeconomic, and environmental factors.

In addition to primary disorders of the integument, cutaneous manifestations occur with systemic illness.

Most skin disorders are caused by several interrelated factors; few disorders have a single cause, and for some the cause is still unknown.

Cutaneous effects may involve several alterations in characteristic features, sensations, fluid content, and the appearance of abnormal tissue or growth on the surface of the skin.

The skin is often the primary target when the client is under emotional stress.

Normal alterations in skin and the appendages occur at significant times within the human life cycle.

Climate and occupation influence the condition of the skin.

Alteration in appearance of the skin has significant influence on body image and self-esteem.

Bibliography

Green ML, Harry J: *Nutrition in Contemporary Nursing Practice.* New York: Wiley, 1981.

Groër MW, Shekleton ME: *Basic Pathophysiology: A Conceptual Approach,* 2nd ed. St. Louis: Mosby, 1983.

Guyton AC: *Basic Human Physiology: Normal Functions and Mechanisms of Disease,* 3rd ed. Philadelphia: Saunders, 1981.

Levy BS, Wegman DH: Environmental and occupational hazards. Pages 124–155 in: *Practice of Preventive Health Care.* Scheiderman LJ (ed). Menlo Park, CA: Addison-Wesley, 1981.

Luciano DS, Vander AJ, Sherman JH: *Human Anatomy and Physiology.* New York: McGraw-Hill, 1983.

Muir BL: *Pathophysiology—An Introduction to the Mechanisms of Disease.* New York: Wiley, 1980.

Pillsbury DM, Heston CL: *A Manual of Dermatology,* 2nd ed. Philadelphia: Saunders, 1980.

Sauer GC: *Manual of Skin Diseases,* 4th ed. Philadelphia: Lippincott, 1980.

Spence AP, Mason EB: *Human Anatomy and Physiology,* 2nd ed. Menlo Park, CA: Benjamin/Cummings, 1983.

Wilson HS, Kneisl CR: *Psychiatric Nursing,* 2nd ed. Menlo Park, CA: Addison-Wesley, 1983.

Suggested Readings

Larrabee, WF: The aging face: Why changes occur, how to correct them. *Postgrad Med* (Nov 15) 1984; 76:37–46. The focus of this article is on the aging face and the characteristic anatomic, biomechanical, biochemical, and histologic changes it undergoes. Dermabrasion, chemabrasion, collagen implant, and plastic surgical procedures are discussed. Interesting photographs and illustrations enhance this article.

McAuliffe K, McAuliffe D: I care. *Nurs 84* (April) 1984; 14:58–59. Nursing experiences are offered to indicate the significance of touch in ministering care.

Melamed E: *The Terror of Not Being Young.* New York: Linden Press/Simon & Schuster, 1983. The author relates scientific findings and personally collected data pertinent to the problems of aging as the process affects women in comparison to men and the resulting psychological, social, and economic outcomes. "Buying Youth," one of the chapters, is relevant to this text, because it identifies cosmetic measures to alter the cutaneous effects from aging.

Montagu A: *Touching: The Human Significance of the Skin,* 2nd ed. New York: Harper & Row, 1978. This book represents a scientific study of the skin as a major organ system. The significance of skin to adaptation is highlighted.

Chapter 78

The Nursing Process for Clients With Integumentary System Dysfunction

Carolyn Gorczyca

Objectives

When you have finished studying this chapter, you should be able to:

Apply the nursing process in caring for clients with disorders of the integument.

Collect pertinent subjective data in a dermatological history.

Assess the integument for the major skin signs, color, temperature, texture, turgor, and edema.

Describe primary and secondary types of cutaneous lesions.

Identify relevant nursing diagnoses for clients with disorders of the integument.

Formulate a nursing care plan for a client with a skin problem.

Implement nursing interventions for health problems of the skin.

Identify the specific purposes and nursing implications involved with select modalities of treating skin problems.

Evaluate expected outcomes of nursing interventions.

The many kinds of cutaneous manifestations, the complexity of cause-and-effect relationships, and the interrelatedness of organ systems involved in the development of skin disorders make it imperative that the nurse use a systematic method of assessing, planning, implementing, and evaluating the care to be administered. Because of the great variety in types of nursing care needed for clients with common skin problems, this chapter will primarily examine the nursing process for clients with dermatoses. Burns are discussed in Chapter 15. The components of the nursing process for skin disorders resulting from cold and biophysical injury will be discussed in Chapter 79.

Section I: Nursing Assessment: Establishing the Data Base

The client's problem may be clearly visible when the nurse makes initial contact, but that does not make systematic data-gathering unnecessary. The challenge is for the nurse to provide an atmosphere where the client's concerns may be expressed freely. The nurse's fears about contagion, the possible repulsiveness of the condition, and lack of theoretical understanding of skin disorders may create subtle barriers to verbal communication, perceptions of behavior, and discovery of factors that influence the client's state.

Nurses must realize that how they touch the client and respond to the client's appearance can facilitate or hinder the client–nurse relationship.

SUBJECTIVE DATA

The purpose of the interview is not only to obtain a dermatological history, but to learn the total health picture. The nurse needs to know biographical data, the client's specific and general complaints, how the client sees the lesion or cutaneous manifestations, and how the client thinks the condition came about.

Biographical information should be the starting point. Age, sex, race, occupation, and environment (including climate) may be significant in the assessment of the problem and may expedite the diagnosis. Information about lifestyle, recent travel, economic status, and living conditions within a community will help.

When questioning the client about the actual skin disorder, it is important to elicit the following information:

- The date of onset and duration of the problem
- The initial site of occurrence and progressive involvement of other areas
- Nature of the distribution of the cutaneous signs
- Skin texture, temperature, odor, drainage, and oil and water content
- Any change in cutaneous sensation (numbness, tingling, pruritus)
- Changes in color
- Specific alterations in hair texture, amount, color, distribution, and presence of dandruff
- Specific alterations in nail texture, color, and contour
- Factors that seem to aggravate or alleviate the problem
- Treatment prior to visit

Use terms or phrases that may be easily understood and helpful in facilitating descriptions. Accurate information is beneficial in identifying specific disorders that have characteristic onsets, locations, or symptomatology.

The dermatological history must include an investigation into the following areas:

- Family or personal history involving allergic tendencies (hay fever, asthma, atopic dermatitis)
- Personal history of x-ray treatment for acne
- Family history of skin disorders
- Personal history of childhood diseases (measles, chickenpox, scarlet fever)
- Exposure to external allergens (soaps, deodorants, jewelry, metal, cosmetics, clothing, furs)
- Exposure to internal allergens (foods)
- Current medications, whether prescription drugs or over-the-counter preparations
- Occupational exposure to irritants or toxic substances
- Exposure to environmental factors, such as temperature extremes, excessive sunlight, or high humidity
- Seasonal influence on the condition
- Recent contact with animals, insects, or plants
- Involvement in out-of-door activities
- Menstrual history and sexual contacts
- Dietary and hygienic practices
- Use of public swimming pools, restrooms, gym showers, or other facilities
- Recent travel
- Recent psychosocial stress

Information from client responses in these areas of concern will help to identify etiological factors, appropriate treatment modalities, and preventive measures.

No history will be complete unless the systemic effects and influences are scrutinized. Inquire about:

- General symptoms such as fatigue, anorexia, nausea and vomiting, weakness, weight loss, headache, fever, and chills
- General health with specific focus on each organ system as well as mental health
- Family history of diabetes mellitus
- Alcohol dependency

As the nurse learns more about the effects of the disease, the information about cutaneous manifestations will be obtained through a more dynamic and sophisticated assessment to reveal possible problems with oxygenation, nutrition, metabolism, elimination, immunity, or hormone imbalances.

OBJECTIVE DATA

Physical Assessment

Inspection and palpation are key in the next phase of data gathering. The sun provides the best light in which to view the skin, hair, and nails. Lamps containing 60-watt nonfluorescent bulbs are the recommended alternative. Oblique lighting in a darkened room may be used to determine subtle elevations or depressions. Variations in skin pigmentation may be seen better in subdued light.

Very dark skin may conceal certain skin problems. Nurses must learn to recognize the natural blend of pigmentation in various types of healthy skin and to examine the buccal mucosa, tongue, lips, nail beds, and sclera to supplement skin information. With practice, the nurse will learn to recognize normal variations in pigmentation, such as Mongolian spots, and dermatological problems common to different populations.

The examining room should have a comfortable temperature to prevent both vasodilation and vasoconstriction that might affect the appearance of the skin. A relaxed supportive atmosphere is important to prevent errors such as mistaking an embarrassed blush for erythema.

After proper draping, begin the physical examination by viewing the overall appearance of the client to evaluate general health. Manifestations of systemic involvement should be recorded (such as yellowing that may indicate jaundice), information obtained from vital signs correlated, and any overt signs of toxicity noted. If the client has a history of x-ray treatment for acne, palpate the thyroid.

The examination is then conducted in a set sequence of careful inspection and palpation of all visible components of the integument. Beginning with the hair and scalp, progress from the head and neck to the upper extremities, the trunk, and the lower extremities. Also note the condition of the oral mucous membrane.

Skin

The skin should be assessed for color, temperature, texture, turgor, and the presence of edema. Then note the type, shape, arrangement, and distribution of lesions. It is important to be exact in the observations and to use the correct terms in recording the observations (see Tables 78–1 and 78–2). It will not be possible later to assess the progress of therapy without a clear and exact record of initial condition.

Color. Skin color is affected by pigmentation (melanin, carotene, hemoglobin) and vascularization. Alterations may be localized or general. Depending on the pathogenesis involved, more definite information can often be obtained by looking at the conjunctiva, the palms of the hands, the soles of the feet, the nail beds, and the lips. For example, the pallor of anemia in black clients is more readily visible in the conjunctiva.

Color may be *isochromatic* (uniform) or *versicolored* (a combination of shades). Observations may be documented by notation of the exact colors seen (pallor, rubor, cyanosis).

Temperature. Warmth and coolness of the skin normally reflect adjustments in the circulatory system as it provides for thermoregulation in the body. Touch the skin so relative heat can be sensed by the fingertips. Localized heat may indicate the presence of an inflammatory process, whereas generalized hyperthermia reflects systemic involvement. When the skin feels cold, a question of vascular insufficiency may be considered.

Texture and Turgor. Many factors will influence the constitution and tension of the skin. To assess texture and turgor, gently grasp a small section of skin and evaluate it, then record the findings using the following terms:

- Consistency—May be smooth, rough, scaly, crusty, thin, thick, atrophied, firm, wrinkled, nodular; may show areas of lichenification or ichthyosis
- Accommodation—May be resilient, inelastic, pliable; may show increased or decreased tension
- Moisture and oil—May be dry, oily, moist, or weeping

Edema. Increased fluid content may extend beyond the dermal levels and into the subcutaneous tissue. Edema may be determined by looking and palpating to determine the extent or the degree of involvement. Record the presence and location of edema and use terms such as taut, tight, puffy, indented, or pitting to describe it further. Pitting edema is described according to stages in Chapter 7.

Type of Lesion. The types of primary and secondary skin lesions that appear with disorders of the integu-

ment or disorders associated with systemic diseases are shown in Tables 78–1 and 78–2. The tables describe characteristic features and provide examples of conditions in which the lesions are known to appear. Primary lesions represent the basic cutaneous responses to pathophysiological influences or stressors. Secondary alterations develop from the initial manifestation.

After examining the lesions, record surface conformity, texture, mobility, presence of altered sensation (tenderness, pruritus), and depth of involvement. The skin must also be assessed for vascular lesions such as petechiae, purpura, ecchymoses, and telangiectasis. Any of these signs may aid in diagnosing disorders remote from the skin.

Shape of Lesion. Configurations of individualized lesions should be described whenever feasible. Appropriate terms include round, oval, annular (ring shaped), elongated (tubular), or irregular. The lesions may also have sharp or diffuse (spreading) borders.

Arrangement. The pattern of surface lesions should be recorded because it is of use in making the diagnosis. For example, in herpes simplex, the lesions appear in clusters, whereas in herpes zoster, they are linear and run along the course of a cutaneous nerve. Lesions may appear grouped, confluent (merging together), contiguous (touching or adjoining), disseminated (scattered), or symmetrical. Particular arrangements may be further described as being linear, serpiginous (snakelike), reticular (a network formation), or arcuate (arching).

Distribution. The extensiveness and location of the lesions are significant. The area of involvement should be classified as being isolated, localized, regional, or generalized. The nurse should learn characteristic distributions for common disorders and examine the sites accordingly. Certain problems may involve normally exposed skin, pressure points, or common sites on the body. Conditions such as psoriasis, scabies, acne, and seborrheic dermatitis have classic distribution patterns; these are discussed in Chapter 79.

Hair and Nails

Hair should be examined for color and for dullness or sheen. The nurse should feel the hair to determine whether it is dry or oily, rough or soft, fine or coarse. A strand should be checked for brittleness or pliability. The distribution and amount should be evaluated in terms of the age and sex of the patient. Gains or losses should be identified as being localized or general.

The general appearance of the nails can show physiological changes or disruptions and sometimes emotional stress, as when the nails have been bitten.

The shape of nails may be altered from a normal convexity to a spoonlike or concave appearance, or clubbing

Table 78–1   Primary Skin Lesions

Lesions	Characteristics	Examples	Illustrations
Macule	Small; circumscribed; less than 1 cm in diameter; flat; nonpalpable; brown, red, purple, white, or tan	Ephelis (freckling); purpura; rubeola; rubella; scarlet fever; lentigo; Mongolian and cafe-au-lait spots	
Papule	Circumscribed; elevated; less than 1 cm in diameter; palpable; firm; red, brown, pink, tan, or bluish-red	Mole; acne; pimple; angioma; wart; pityriasis rosea; actinic and seborrheic keratosis	
Vesicle	Superficial; circumscribed; less than 1 cm in diameter; elevated; filled with clear fluid	Blister; chicken pox; smallpox; herpes; poison ivy; contact and atopic dermatitis; insect bites	
Bulla	Similar to vesicle but larger than 1 cm in diameter	Blister with second-degree burn; pemphigus vulgaris; drug eruptions	
Pustule	Similar to vesicle and bullae but filled with pus; white or yellowish-cream	Acne; furuncle; variola; miliaria; impetigo; folliculitis	See vesicle (above)
Wheal	Flat-topped; elevated; variable diameter; irregular shape	Urticaria; insect bites; poison ivy	
Nodule	Circumscribed; elevated; 1–2 cm in diameter; firm; deeper in dermis than papule	Tophi; Heberden's nodes; erythema nodosum; ganglion; dermatofibroma; acne	
Tumor	Elevated; solid; greater than 2 cm in diameter; may or may not be clearly demarcated; may or may not vary from skin color	Epithelioma; fibroma; lipoma; cavernous hemangioma; melanoma	
Patch	Flat; larger than 1 cm in diameter; irregular in shape	Vitiligo	
Plaque	Elevated; flat-topped; firm; rough; over 1 cm in diameter; may be coalesced papules	Psoriasis; seborrheic warts; discoid lupus erythematosus	
Cyst	Elevated, encapsulated mass in dermis or subcutaneous layer; fluid, semifluid, or solid content; may or may not appear raised	Epidermoid; sebaceous	

Table 78–2 Secondary Skin Lesions

Lesions	Characteristics	Examples	Illustrations
Crust	Slightly elevated areas of dried blood, pus, serum; size varies; color may be straw, tan, honey, brown, red, or black	Impetigo; eczema; scab on abrasion or laceration	
Scale	Irregular; dry or oily; thick or thin; flaky exfoliation; varied size; white, tan, or silver	Dandruff; psoriasis; exfoliative dermatitis	
Lichenification	Rough, thickened, hardened epidermis; increased skin markings due to chronic rubbing or irritation; not as clearly demarcated as a plaque	Chronic dermatitis	
Excoriation	Loss of epidermis; exposed dermis	Scratches; linear abrasions	
Fissure	Linear crack or break exposing dermis; small; deep; red	Athlete's foot; dishpan hands; cheilosis	
Erosion	Depressed; moist; glistening break in superficial epidermis; circumscribed; red; follows rupture of vesicle or bulla; larger than fissure	Smallpox; chicken pox; diaper dermatitis	
Ulcer	Depressed; involves total epidermis and all or part of dermis, may involve subcutaneous tissue; concave; varies in size; exudative; red or reddish-blue	Decubiti; stasis ulcers; third-degree burns; chancre	
Scar (cicatrix)	Thin line to thick irregular fibrous tissue; pink, red, or white	Healed wound or surgical incision	
Atrophy	Thin; shiny; translucent; paper-like; skin furrows obliterated	Striae; arterial insufficiency; aging skin	

may occur. Transverse furrows, called Beau's line, may appear as a result of a variety of cutaneous or systemic problems. Onycholysis, separation of the nail plate from the bed, is a common disturbance. Some examples of clinical nail findings are discussed and illustrated in Table 78–3.

The transparency of the plate may be impaired (stained or discolored). This transparent quality makes the nail bed ideal for assessing capillary filling and, ultimately, the adequacy of circulation to the distal portions of the extremities.

The substance of the nail should be observed for bulk (thinness or thickness), smoothness, irregularities or pitting of the surface, and for flexibility or brittleness.

Diagnostic Studies

Direct Examination

The use of a magnified hand lens is helpful in examining small lesions. A Wood's lamp may be used to determine the presence of fungal infections, which show a characteristic yellow–green fluorescence under black light. This ultraviolet long-wave light is also useful in identifying some bacterial infections and aids in the delineation of pigment disorders.

Skin Testing

Skin tests are used to determine hypersensitivity and immune responses by the administration of allergens or antigens on the surface or into the dermis. The three types include patch, scratch, and intracutaneous tests.

Patch testing provides an accurate means for assessing contact sensitivity. One or more suspected allergens is placed on a hairless area of the body (often the skin of the forearm), one allergen per patch, and covered with an adhesive tape or patch-test dressing for 48 to 72 hours. During this time, the site must be kept dry. A positive reaction is shown by the appearance of redness, papules, vesicles, or edema.

Allergens may be introduced into the body through a superficial abrasion or intradermal injection. In the *scratch* test, a needle or special tool is used to scratch the skin. Scratches, 1 cm long and 2.5 cm apart, are made in rows on the client's forearm or back. Within 30 to 40 minutes after introduction of the allergen, the area is assessed for erythema, edema, or both.

Intradermal tests are usually performed to evaluate immunity from prior exposure or sensitization. Several antigens that may have relevance to the integumentary system include tuberculin, blastomycin, and coccidioidin. After inoculation with a tuberculin syringe into the layers of the skin, the reading takes place within 48 to 72 hours. Positive reactions will show signs of induration, or erythema, or both.

Microscopic Examination

The microscopic study of tissue or a culture allows a more decisive diagnosis to be reached. Bacteria, yeast, fungus, spirochetes, parasites, and many viruses can be recog-

nized under a microscope. (For some viruses, an electron microscope is needed.)

Specimens for microscope study are obtained through several means. Scales, crusts, and exudate can be taken by gentle scraping. Smears can be taken of weeping lesions and are useful in diagnosing bullous diseases and vesicular eruptions. Gram's stains, potassium hydroxide (KOH) test, dark-field examinations, immunofluorescence, and various other preparations and methods may be used to facilitate microscopic visualization.

Biopsy

Skin biopsy is a valuable tool in diagnosis. Several methods of acquiring histologic samples are available. A *punch biopsy* usually provides sufficient tissue for examination and is a simple procedure to perform. The physician selects the

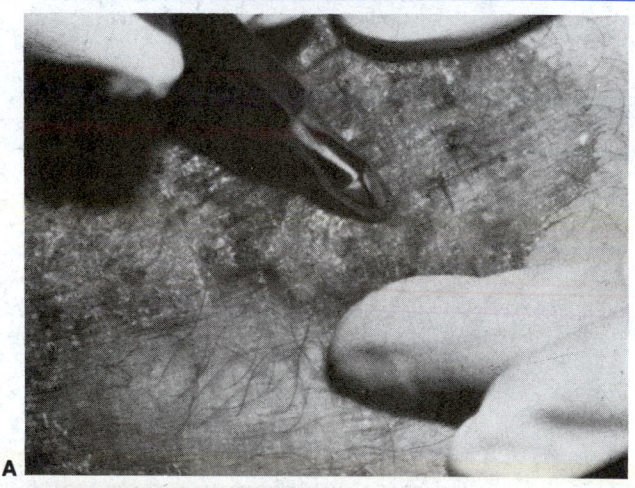

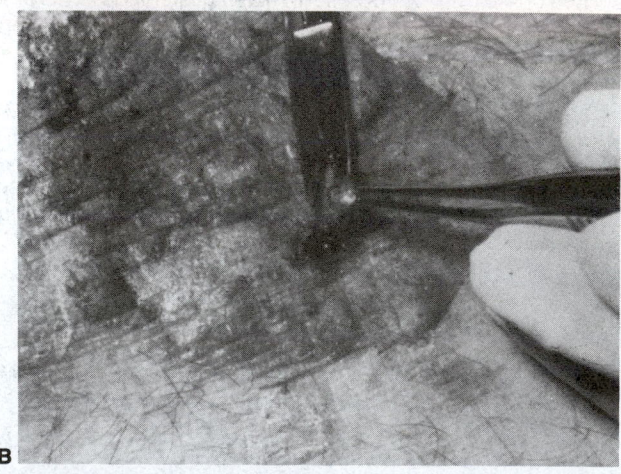

Figure 78–1

Punch biopsy of the skin. **A.** Incising the skin by exerting pressure and rotating the punch. The usual diameter of the cutting edge is 3 or 4 mm. **B.** Cutting the specimen with a curved scissors.

SOURCE: Binnick SA: *Skin Diseases: Diagnosis & Management*. Baltimore, MD: Williams & Wilkins, 1982.

Table 78–3 Clinical Nail Findings

Illustrations	Description	Causes
Onychorrhexis	Brittle nail; frayed and torn borders; steplike appearance at cut edges	Malnutrition; iron or calcium deficiency; thyrotoxicosis; chemical or occupational damage; aging; radiation
Onychauxis	Thickened and hypertrophied nail plate with irregular keratin layers	Trauma; fungal infections; familial; aging
Onycholysis	Separation of nail plate at its free edge from nail bed	Thyrotoxicosis; fungal infections; eczema; psoriasis
Clubbing	Convex, parrot-beak nails; nail angled dorsalward	Pulmonary disease (bronchiectasis, lung abscess, cavitary tuberculosis, emphysema, lung neoplasm); cardiovascular disease (congenital heart disease, subacute bacterial endocarditis, secondary polycythemia)
Spooning	Spoon- or saucer-shaped nails; may be thin	Hypochromic anemias; iron deficiency; Raynaud's syndrome; more rarely in rheumatic fever, lichen planus, syphilis
Splinter hemorrhages	Linear red streaks in the nail bed, run from free margin proximally for several millimeters	Subacute bacterial endocarditis; trichinosis; hypertension; mitral stenosis; occupational damage
Square, wide plates	Square, wide nail plates, more wide than long	Acromegaly; cretinism
Long, narrow plates	Long, narrow nail plates	Eunuchoidism; hypopituitarism; Marfan's syndrome
Beau's line	Transverse furrow in nail plate; eventually grows out with nail	Any severe illness

(continued)

Table 78–3	Clinical Nail Findings (continued)	
Illustrations	**Description**	**Causes**
Mees' line	Transverse white band; eventually grows out with the nail; indicates lesser injury than with Beau's line	Generalized illness; infectious fevers; poisoning (arsenic, thallium, fluoride); chemotherapy
Terry's nails	Proximal 80% is white; distal margin is normal pink	Hepatic cirrhosis
Lindsay's nails (half-and-half nails)	Proximal 40% to 80% is white; distal portion is red, pink, or brown; sharp demarcation between colors	Renal disease
Muehrcke's lines	Paired, narrow bands of pallor; parallel to the lunulae; in the nail beds, not the nail plate	Hypoalbuminemia
Red half-moons	Red rather than white lunulae	Cardiac failure
Blue half-moons	Azure blue rather than white lunulae	Wilson's disease
Partial leukonychia	Irregular white areas in the nail plates	Common; not diagnostically significant

area that is expected to be most informative, cleanses it gently, and administers a local anesthetic. A skin punch instrument specific for this type of biopsy can provide a 2 to 8 mm sample of tissue when it is pressed firmly into the lesion (Figure 78–1, p. 2166). Wound care following the biopsy may involve no more than a simple dressing, although suturing or application of adhesive strips may be necessary if a large sample is taken. Use of caustics or Gelfoam is not usually required.

A *shave biopsy* involves using a scalpel to remove the elevated part of a lesion. A biopsy sample may have to be scooped out from a flat or depressed area. A pedunculated

lesion may be clipped off with scissors, as may a small fold of skin where the cosmetic appearance will not be disturbed. The use of pressure, caustics, or light electrosurgery may be necessary to stop bleeding after any of the above procedures.

Certain lesions warrant surgical excision because histologic study requires an ample amount of tissue for investigation. A wide and deep resection that needs to be performed under general anesthesia entails admission to the hospital either as an outpatient or inpatient. Postoperative care is contingent on the extent of the excision or the site involved and is discussed in Chapter 80.

Laboratory Testing

Diagnostic assessment of a client with a dermatological problem may involve limited laboratory tests. Routine blood cell count and differentials, urinalysis, and chemical analysis may be required, usually when hospitalization is necessary. A wide variety of systemic disorders have cutaneous manifestations. Refer to the appropriate systems chapter for a more detailed explanation.

A common test is culture of the skin exudate. Measurement of immunoglobulins may have some relevance to primary skin disorders because clients with allergic tendencies may show elevations in IgE levels.

Other diagnostic studies may be necessary if metastases are suspected from invasive primary skin lesions. Chest x-rays, liver function studies, and a gastrointestinal work-up are some of the diagnostic measures the physician may order.

Section II: Nursing Diagnosis

Most clients with dermatoses are treated in ambulatory care settings, either in physicians' offices or in dermatology clinics. The nurse in a hospital or extended care facility is usually caring for clients with numerous problems in addition to the dermatological one. Therefore, the care plan may contain several nursing diagnoses that reflect major concerns for actual or potential life-threatening disturbances before a focus on a skin disorder is identified.

Several nursing diagnoses are relevant to the integumentary system and should be considered during client assessment. A list of nursing diagnoses related to integumentary dysfunction appears in Box 78–1. The diagnoses are discussed in the following section.

Box 78–1 Nursing Diagnoses Commonly Related to Dysfunction of the Integumentary System

Diagnoses Directly Related to Integumentary Dysfunction

Skin integrity, impairment of: actual or potential

Injury, potential for trauma

Comfort, alteration in

Sleep pattern disturbance

Self-concept, disturbance in, related to body image disturbances

Additional Potential Nursing Diagnosis

Fluid volume deficit, actual or potential

Self-concept, disturbance in, related to self-esteem or role performance

Knowledge deficit

Self-care deficit, related to bathing/hygiene

Home maintenance management, impaired

Section III: Planning and Implementation

Planning and implementation of care for a client with a cutaneous disorder focus on these specific areas: provision of care (general hygiene, skin and wound care, comfort and emotional support); protection (from further injury, secondary infection, heat losses, fluid and electrolyte imbalances); and teaching self-care and health maintenance. A sample nursing care plan for a client with integumentary system dysfunction is presented in Table 78–4.

CARE OF THE SKIN

Personal hygiene is important not only for the lesion but for all parts of the body that may influence the healing process. Keeping the skin and its appendages healthy requires proper cleansing with soaps that do not cause drying or irritation. Intertriginous areas (where skin contacts skin) should be dried, particularly in the obese or where skin folds may prove problematic. Incontinent clients must be cared for quickly and efficiently. If the skin is dry (because of climate, disease, aging, or other reasons), it may be necessary to limit bathing and lubricate the skin. Body odors should be eliminated primarily by washing with soap and water, with sparing use of deodorants, antiperspirants, and perfumes. Therapeutic soaps, shampoos, powders, lotions, or selective agents may be required for any dermatologic problems.

Table 78–4	Sample Nursing Care Plan for a Client With a Dermatologic Problem		
Nursing Diagnosis	**Client Care Goal**	**Plan/Nursing Implementation**	**Expected Outcome**
Impaired skin integrity: related to weeping vesicular lesions	Improvement of skin integrity	Apply open wet dressings to affected areas using aluminum acetate q4h; apply 1% hydrocortisone cream lightly after soaks; expose area to air as much as possible	Skin integrity will improve with decrease in or absence of redness, vesicle drainage; decrease in discomfort; reduction in or stabilization of altered skin integrity
Potential for injury related to infection	Prevention of injury or infection	Instruct client in daily hygiene of skin, nails, hair; observe for purulent drainage, increased redness, edema, tenderness; monitor temperature b.i.d.; instruct client in handwashing, avoidance of scratching, bumping, coarse clothing against affected area, temperature extremes	Absence of complications will be noted by no alterations in color, temperature, sensation, and fluid content; temperature within normal limits; no signs of malaise or fatigue; no signs of excoriations, bleeding, bruising
Knowledge deficit	Understanding of skin disorder	Discuss substances responsible for hypersensitivity reaction; instruct client to avoid use of those substances	Client demonstrates knowledge of problems such as contact dermatitis by identifying allergens responsible for reaction; indicating methods to eliminate allergens
Comfort, alteration in: related to pruritus	Relief of pruritus; increase in comfort; prevention of further symptoms	Instruct client to bathe in warm water containing bath oils (such as Alpha Keri); dry skin thoroughly; wear only minimal clothing over area; wear absorbent cotton clothing if possible; avoid extremes of physical activity; keep room at cool temperature, nonhumid; cut and clean nails; avoid rubbing and scratching; administer ordered antipruritic drugs; apply topical medications as ordered	Client demonstrates a calm, relaxed appearance and normal posture; sleeps comfortably and for long intervals; experiences decreased discomfort; skin has decreased dryness, no excessive moisture; client demonstrates understanding by avoiding scratching and avoiding situations or stimulation that increase itching
	Reduction of stress level	Discuss physical and emotional factors that may trigger itch–scratch cycle; request family to bring in books, craft material; encourage listening to radio, watching TV	Client involved in diversional activity
Alteration in self-concept: disfigurement; related to visible skin eruptions	Decrease in self-consciousness	Spend additional time with client; provide a specific time and place to discuss feelings; listen carefully; use touch appropriately; discuss implications of feelings and methods of coping; explore ways to facilitate coping; encourage client to socialize with client/family/significant others	Client demonstrates adjustment by expressing fears, concerns about rejection, alterations in lifestyle; identifies means to cope with feelings; client demonstrates ease in interacting with others; client has increased contact with staff and other clients; client derives comfort from supportiveness of others
Self-care deficit: related to bathing, hygiene, applying medication	Achieve independence	Teach method of care to client and family	Client demonstrates self-care by performing treatment and applying medication

Care of Skin With a Dermatosis

A major concern for any nurse will be to formulate an actual therapeutic plan for the skin disorder, whether it involves a single lesion or major portions of the body surface. Special baths (balneotherapy) may be prescribed by the physician. Table 78–5 identifies the various types and purposes for which these baths may be utilized.

Topical treatment usually involves the use of wet dressings or soaks or application of medications in an appropriate base. The type of skin disorder and whether the condition is acute, subacute, or chronic determine the

Table 78−5   Therapeutic Baths

Type	Action	Purpose	Nursing Implications
Colloidal oatmeal (Aveeno)	Demulcent-emollient	To soothe and protect skin against irritation; to decrease itching	Avoid eye contact or slipping in tub
Oil	Emollient	To provide lubrication of skin and prevent excess evaporation	Avoid slipping in tub
Starch	Demulcent	To provide analgesia, soothe irritation, and absorb excessive moisture	Avoid slipping in tub; observe for yeast infection in intertriginous areas (yeasts thrive on starch)
Tar	Keratolytic	To soften skin keratin and facilitate removal of epidermal scaling	Dry thoroughly; may stain skin or clothing

basis of therapy, rather than the causative factors. Several guidelines are used by physicians to determine treatment, and nurses should also be aware of them. Moist, inflamed, and infected lesions are usually kept wet. Dry, scaling, lichenified lesions are covered with a medication, such as an ointment, to retard further drying. The skin must be closely observed during therapy because subsequent responses may require prompt changes in therapeutic modalities.

Open wet dressings are commonly used with inflammations that involve oozing, ulcers, erosions, or vesicular skin conditions that do not cover a large surface area. The purpose of the dressing is to cause local vasoconstriction during the cooling and drying process and thereby reduce inflammation. Wound drainage, exudate, and crusts are removed when the dressing is changed.

Several solutions may be used to wet the dressing other than sterile water or saline solution. Aluminum acetate (Burow's) solution, which is commonly used, acts as an astringent and mild antiseptic. Acetic acid soaks reduce microbial counts in wound infections, particularly those containing *Pseudomonas* organisms. Silver nitrate solutions have been used effectively in the treatment of burns and are discussed in Chapter 15.

When a continuous wet dressing is required, sterile dressings (gauze, Kerlix) or clean cloths (soft toweling, linen, diapers) may be used to cover the lesion. Because dressings must not be allowed to dry, additional cover layers and frequent moistening may be needed. Nonporous wet or dry dressings should be avoided unless specifically ordered for the purpose of promoting hydration of the skin or penetration of a medication. Coverage with a nonporous wrap may cause heat retention, prevent evaporation, macerate the skin, and promote the overgrowth of bacteria.

Topical medications are suspended in a base that facilitates the penetration and absorption of the drug. Der-

matologists customarily write specific orders fully detailing the composition of a preparation.

The major types of bases or vehicles for therapeutic drugs are creams, lotions, ointments, and powders. Pastes, gels, and aerosols may also be used. Table 78−6 identifies the purpose, clinical indications for, and nursing implications associated with each modality. Medications incorporated into the base substance may act as anti-inflammatory agents, antipruritics, keratolytics, anti-infectives, antiseptics, antiparasitics, emollients, or protectants.

Each type of topical medication requires proper application. The nurse (or client giving self-care) should know the correct amount to use, whether to wear gloves while applying it, how and when to apply it, and how to recognize

Nursing Research Note

Becker L, Goodemote C: Treating pressure sores with or without antacids. *Am J Nurs* 1984; 84:351−352.

Research was conducted to determine whether povidone-iodine or antacids were more effective in treating pressure sores. Two methods were compared. Method 1 consisted of cleansing the wound with povidone-iodine and applying heat with a 60-watt heat lamp 12 to 16 in from the sore for 20 minutes. Method 2 involved cleansing the sore with povidone-iodine and then applying liquid antacids, followed by heat as in method 1.

No significant difference was found in healing of pressure sores regardless of the method used. Both methods were effective in reducing sore width but had no appreciable effect on sore depth.

Nursing preventive actions reduced the number of new pressure sores. Actions instrumental in preventing pressure sore development included nursing assessment for high-risk clients, skin assessment, nutritional assessment, frequent position changes, and frequent cleansing of incontinent clients.

untoward effects. Information is readily available on package inserts, through pharmacists, and in drug textbooks.

A certain number of conditions require systemic or intralesional administration of medication. These drugs may include antibiotics, hormones, corticosteroids, chemotherapy for malignancies, antihistamines, and antipruritics.

Care of Pruritic Skin

Clients may experience numerous sensations and actual pain. Itching is the most common problem, and therapeutic intervention may be required. Therapy is primarily directed at resolving the problem responsible for the pruritus. Unfortunately, situations also exist in which there are no identifiable etiological factors or in which the primary disorder will never be resolved, and pruritus becomes chronic or intractable.

Care should involve hydration of the skin by a cooling bath or use of compresses. The addition of antipruritic colloids such as oatmeal (Aveeno) or starches and use of bath oils are helpful when large body surfaces are involved.

Keeping the skin relatively dry and cool is essential and usually requires climate and humidity controls. The application of local soothing emollients containing camphor, menthol, phenol, salicylic acid, or tars, alone or in combinations, may be prescribed (including some over-the-counter drugs). Topical anesthetics and antihistamines have not proven of value, although systemic antihistamines have some limited utility with histamine-mediated itching. (These drugs may also cause allergic responses that produce itching.) Topical corticosteroids are effective, but long-term use may result in cutaneous side effects and adrenal suppression. Tranquilizers and sedatives may be prescribed when emotional disruptions accompany pruritus or when sleep patterns are disturbed. Itching becomes more intense at night with most cases of pruritus.

Itching seems to demand scratching. Unfortunately, "one scratch is too many, and a thousand is not enough." An itch–scratch cycle can develop that damages the skin further and may lead to infection. A major focus of care in treating severe pruritus is the avoidance of unnecessary stimulation from chemical agents that act as irritants or

Table 78–6	Types of Topical Agents		
Type	**Purpose**	**Clinical Indications**	**Nursing Implications**
Creams	To provide cooling and increase moisture	Moist or dry lesions	Low penetration capacity and may be removed by perspiration or drainage; good for daytime usage
Lotions (suspensions, solutions*)	To provide protective covering after facilitating a drying and cooling process	Acutely inflamed lesions; wet and oozing	Suspensions need shaking; preparations with alcohol may cause excessive drying
Ointments (water-in-oil, oil-in-water)	To lubricate and protect	Dry and scaly lesions	Ointments provide for greatest penetration and absorption because of their occlusiveness; water-in-oil is difficult to remove; may cause skin maceration if occluded; oil-in-water is relatively greaseless and easily absorbed; removable with soap and water
Powders	To promote dryness by absorption of moisture and protect by reducing friction	Intertrigo	Completely dry skin before application; easy removal may necessitate reapplication
Pastes	To protect and lubricate	Intertrigo, chronic skin ulcers	Useful in areas difficult to treat with wet compresses; difficult to remove with soap and water but responsive to mineral oil or vegetable oil
Gels	To provide a dry, greaseless, nonocclusive, nonstaining film	Before blistering, hairy areas	May be painful upon application; cosmetically more favorable
Aerosols	To dry and protect skin	Peristomal hirsute areas and scalp	A substitute for lotions when direct application may be painful

*Suspensions contain insoluble powder in water. Solutions contain active ingredients in a fluid base.

vasodilators (alcohol, coffee, spices); mechanical objects (rough clothing, long fingernails); heat; and psychic stress. The nurse should become aware of all factors that increase or stimulate discomfort and those that lessen or alleviate it. Diversion (reading, watching TV) should be actively explored.

PROVIDING EMOTIONAL SUPPORT

Because skin disorders affect personal appearance and may affect self-image, the nurse must be alert to the emotional implications for the client. Age, sex, social class, occupation, and support systems all may influence the client's adjustment.

Feeling states have to be identified, explored, and dealt with therapeutically. Clients may fear disfigurement, rejection, unemployment, and malignancy. Some clients with chronic skin disorders become depressed, angry, or impotent. The monetary costs of long-term treatment, the time and energy required, and days lost from work for chronic disorders or for long-term treatment of injuries such as severe frostbite or injuries requiring skin grafts can be emotionally distressing. Whenever and wherever possible, the nurse should promote open communication and provide a supportive and accepting atmosphere.

The major nursing activity in providing emotional support should be a genuine willingness to listen and respond. The busy nurse may fail to perceive the client's need to talk about fears or about the effects the condition may have on the client's lifestyle, interpersonal relationships, or employment. Not only does listening often reduce tensions that may have stimulated the itch–scratch cycle, but listening also encourages the client to explore and plan for the adjustments that may be needed.

A second nursing activity important to emotional support is providing information and knowledge that will allow the client to make a more realistic adjustment. For example, a client may have unrealistic expectations about what will happen when a long-standing disfigurement is removed or cleared up, particularly when the condition has been blamed for the client's social deficits. Similarly, a client may be reluctant to tell a physician about unrealistic hopes for cure, mistaken notions about what caused the condition, or problems arising from the desire of family members to try folk remedies.

Nurses should be alert to the need for professional assistance if coping mechanisms are inadequate or there is evidence of psychopathology. Additional assistance may also be needed, for example, when a client leaves the protected environment of the hospital and goes home or when a client faces the end of a remission.

PROTECTING THE SKIN

An important component of nursing care for all clients, but particularly those with integumentary system dysfunction

or those at high risk for developing neoplastic lesions, is protecting the skin from infection and from penetration by ultraviolet rays.

Preventing Infection

Any break in the continuity of skin disrupts the protective mechanism of this organ system and predisposes the client to infection. The plan of care should provide defenses against infection and against external trauma. Nails should be shortened and cleaned if the client is scratching. Wound coverage must be maintained and handled aseptically. Nutritional support will assist the healing and provide for caloric expenditure when cold wet dressings result in extensive heat losses. Room temperature must be low enough to avoid encouraging bacterial growth and fluid loss yet warm enough for comfort. Where changes in sensory nerve endings interfere with the perception of potential hazards, precautions must be taken to prevent injury. Clients may have to be taught to watch themselves carefully instead of depending on perceptions of touch, pain, pressure, and temperature. Remember that any client requires protective measures such as lamb's wool, heel protectors, bed cradles, and the like when appropriate.

Photoprotection

Protecting the skin from ultraviolet radiation is general good practice to avoid injury from sunburn, premature aging, and the development of neoplastic lesions. In recent years, classifications of sun-reactive skin types have been formulated. Table 78–7 lists these types and identifies high-risk individuals who need protective measures to minimize penetration of ultraviolet rays.

Several means may be considered when establishing a protective plan, particularly for those whose skin typing is between I and III. Closer proximity to the equator and high altitude increase the exposure to ultraviolet radiation. It is critical to avoid peak hours of sunshine, even during cloudy days, unless protective clothing and wide brimmed hats are worn. Ultraviolet rays may also be reflected from snow, sand, and concrete. Sunscreens are of great assistance in absorbing or reflecting ultraviolet rays. Unfortunately, many people are more interested in tanning than protecting their skin, even though they may be aware of the aging and carcinogenic effects of sunlight.

Selection of an appropriate sunscreen should be based on a number of factors, which include:

- Type of wave band involved (UV-A, UV-B, or UV-C; see Table 78–8)
- Skin typing and degree of photosensitivity
- Sun protection factor (SPF) offered
- Individual tendency toward drug sensitivity
- Cost

The three broad categories of sunscreens presently available are PABA or para-aminobenzoic acid (Presun, Pabanol);

Table 78–7 Classification of Sun-Reactive Skin Types

Skin Type	Risk	Response to MED*	Characteristics	SPF
I	Greatest	Always burns, never tans	Very light to light skin color (possible freckling); blue eyes; blonde or red hair	10 or more
II	Great	Always burns, sometimes tans	Blue eyes (some may have blue–gray eyes); red or blonde hair (some may have dark brown hair)	10 or more
III	Moderate	Sometimes burns, always tans	White skin; brown hair and eye color	8–10
IV	Low	Rarely burns, always tans	White or light brown skin (Mediterraneans, Orientals, Hispanics); dark hair and eye color	6–8
V	Very low	Rarely burns, tans easily	Heavily pigmented skin (Mediterraneans, Mongolians, American and East Indians, Hispanics)	4
VI	Negligible	Never burns	Black skin	0

*MED (minimal erythema dose) = 15–30 min initial exposure to the summer sun at peak hours, 11 AM–2 PM

Table 78–8 Ultraviolet Light Therapy in Dermatology

Wave Length	Uses	Artificial Sources	Administration	Photobiologic Reaction
UV-A (320–400 nm)* Long-wave radiation	Therapeutic effects obtained when used in conjunction with a circulatory chemical (photosensitizer); called photochemistry	Fluorescent blacklight lamp; high-intensity UV-A fluorescent bulbs	Time of skin exposure (sec or min) and proximity of light source is important to obtain photobiologic effect and to avoid unnecessary hazards. Treatment boxes or booths containing UV-A or UV-B lights are used in clinics and in dermatologists' offices; sunlamps may be used in home settings	Erythema may be absent or minimal at 12–24 h after exposure; may peak 48–72 h or later. Tanning peaks in 5–7 days after exposure and has a longer duration than a naturally obtained tan
UV-B (290–320 nm)* Middle-wave radiation	Responsible for many beneficial effects in phototherapy; comprises the sunburn spectrum of UVL	Fluorescent sunlamp bulbs, sunlamp bulbs, hot quartz lamps	See above	Much more rapid development of erythema necessitates graduated time exposure to obtain minimal erythema dose. Tanning and accommodation to UVL also requires increase in time exposure. Severe burns possible
UV-C (200–290 nm)* Short-wave radiation	Limited use in dermatology; has bactericidal effects	Operating room germicidal lamps, cold quartz lamps		Insignificant tanning follows erythema; mainly causes desquamation of skin

*nm (nanometer) signifies units of wave lengths.

PABA esters and derivatives (Block Out, Pabafilm, Coppertone, Super Shade); the non-PABA chemical agents such as benzophenones, cinnamates, and phenylbenzamidozole (UVAL, Piz Buin); and physical sunscreens or sunblockers containing such substances as titanium dioxide or zinc oxide (A-fil, Shadow, Covermark). The purchaser may determine the length of time protection is being offered by multiplying the SPF shown on the bottle by the time required to obtain the minimal erythema dose (MED). Hypothetically, when a sunscreen with an SPF of 8 is used by a person who displays an MED in 30 minutes, a protection of 240 minutes or 4 hours is provided (8 SPF × 30 min = 240 min).

These products must be applied one hour prior to sun exposure. All exposed areas should be covered. Reapplication is necessary when the sunscreen is removed by perspiration or water.

PHOTOTHERAPY

Several dermatoses are treated with the application of ultraviolet light (UVL) because it temporarily suppresses mitosis in the basal cells of the epidermis. Sunlight not only provides the optimal source of UVL but is inexpensive and most effective. Unfortunately, it is difficult to control and monitor the intensity of natural UVL to ensure safe and efficient therapeutic usage. Artificial sources can be provided and regulated to obtain desired dermatological effects. Both middle-wave length (UV-B) and long-wave length (UV-A) radiation have the most therapeutic benefits for select dermatoses. Table 78–8 provides detailed information on ultraviolet light therapy. Chapter 79 discusses the specific disorders that benefit from phototherapy.

UVL therapy is generally provided in a health care setting where treatments are administered by qualified personnel. In addition to careful monitoring of exposure time and distance, protection should be provided for the eyes (sun goggles, glasses) and for uninvolved skin surfaces (sunscreen). Clients should be instructed to use eye protection with home usage of sun lamps and should be advised to follow time schedules for exposure and avoid falling asleep during self-treatment. Dangers of using UVL for tanning are discussed in Chapter 79.

PROMOTING SELF-CARE

The promotion of self-care for clients with dermatological problems is a major goal, as with any illness. To prepare the client and family for self-care, the nurse will need to explain treatments and health requirements, demonstrate topical care (with client redemonstration), and discuss expected outcomes. A considerable amount of instructing should address measures required to prevent undue stress on the skin. As a health educator, the nurse should also highlight factors that can exacerbate the disorder or convert a relatively benign lesion into a major problem.

Section IV: Evaluation

The goals to be attained by both nurse and client should be specific, realistic, and measurable. The plan of care for the dermatology client may generally focus on impaired skin integrity, discomfort, fluid volume deficits, impaired home maintenance management, potential for injury, knowledge deficits, disturbances in self-concept, and sleep-pattern disturbances. Therefore, client outcomes should demonstrate resolution of the skin disorder; a state of comfort and restfulness; fluid balance; a comprehension of the problem, necessary therapy, and protective measures; administration of self-care; and manifestation of satisfactory emotional coping mechanisms.

Table 78–4 illustrated a sample nursing care plan with nursing diagnoses, the plan of care, and the anticipated outcomes. Chapter 79 will provide information about specific integument disorders, the characteristic skin signs and symptoms, treatment plan, and nursing care. This knowledge is essential so the process of planning care is guided by fact, scientific principles, and proven therapies for each skin disorder.

Chapter Highlights

Complex cause-and-effect relationships related to cutaneous manifestations require skillful use of the nursing process.

Assessment of the integumentary system may reveal possible problems with oxygenation, nutrition, metabolism, elimination, immunity, or hormone imbalances.

Nurses must learn to recognize the natural blend of pigmentation in various types of healthy skin and to examine the buccal mucosa, tongue, lips, nail beds, and sclera to supplement skin information.

Skin should be assessed for color, temperature, texture, turgor, and the presence of edema. The nurse then notes the type, shape, arrangement, and distribution of lesions.

(continued)

Chapter Highlights (continued)

Hair should be examined for color, sheen, texture, pliability, distribution, and amount.

Nails are examined for shape, transparency, bulk, surface texture, and flexibility.

A hand-held magnifying lens and a Wood's light are useful in direct examination of the skin. Patch tests, intradermal skin tests, and skin biopsy with histological study are also used.

Laboratory and diagnostic tests primarily involve direct examination of the lesion, culturing the exudate, skin testing, and histological studies.

Nursing care of clients with a cutaneous disorder focuses on the provision of care (general hygiene, skin and wound care, comfort and emotional support); protection (from further injury, secondary infection, heat losses, fluid and electrolyte imbalances); and teaching self-care and health maintenance.

Skin disorders affect personal appearance and may affect self-image. Clients fear disfigurement, rejection, unemployment, and malignancy.

Client outcomes should demonstrate resolution of the skin disorder; a state of comfort and restfulness; fluid balance; a comprehension of the problem, necessary therapy, and protective measures; administration of self-care; and manifestation of satisfactory emotional coping mechanisms.

Bibliography

Andberg MM, Rudolph A, Anderson TP: Improving skin care through patient and family training. *Top Clin Nurs* (July) 1983; 5:45–54.

Arndt KA: *Manual of Dermatologic Therapeutics With Essentials of Diagnosis*, 3rd ed. Boston: Little, Brown, 1983.

Delancy VL: Skin assessment. *Top Clin Nurs* (July) 1983; 5:5–10.

Fitzpatrick TB, et al: *Dermatology in General Medicine,* 2nd ed. New York: McGraw-Hill, 1979.

Fitzpatrick TB, Polano MK, Suurmonch D: *Color Atlas and Synopsis of Clinical Dermatology.* New York: McGraw-Hill, 1983.

Grimes J, Iannopollo E: *Health Assessment in Nursing Practice.* Monterey, CA: Wadsworth, 1982.

McKay M: Topical dermatologic therapy. *Primary Care* 1983; 10:513–524.

Sauer GC: *Manual of Skin Diseases,* 4th ed. Philadelphia: Lippincott, 1980.

Turner ML: Skin changes after forty. *Am Fam Physician* (June) 1984; 29:173–181.

Malkiewicz J: The integumentary system. *RN* (Dec) 1984; 44:55–60. The author provides a comprehensive guide to the assessment of the integumentary system. Precise terminology aids in identification of lesions, and methods of examining and palpating the skin are presented.

Neilley LK, DarEllis RA: Nailing down a diagnosis. *Nurse Pract* (May) 1984; 9:26–34. In this excellent article, the authors discuss how the nails can act as a barometer of health, offer clues to nutritional problems, and serve as windows through which capillary changes associated with systemic disease can be viewed. They emphasize the importance of assessing the nails when evaluating any client.

Rubin BA: Black skin: Here's how to adjust your assessment and care. *RN* (March) 1979; 42:31–35. This article identifies pertinent observations to make in assessing black skin and points of care. Pictures help to illustrate dermatological conditions.

Suggested Readings

Anders JE: Topicals. *RN* (Sept) 1982; 45:32–42. Informative article with practical application. Pictures illustrate methods of drug administration. Vehicles are described; examples given; and effects, advantages, special considerations, and disadvantages are highlighted.

Anders JE, Leacin EE: Sun versus skin. *Am J Nurs* 1983; 83:1015–1020. The authors effectively present the hazards of sunlight on skin and suggest protective measures.

Black skin problems. *Am J Nurs* 1979; 79:1092–1094. This article discusses skin conditions seen more often in black clients. Assessment, prevention, and treatment are covered. Color photographs of each condition are presented.

Resources

SELF-HELP GROUPS AND OTHER ORGANIZATIONS

Acne Research Institute
1587 Monrovia Ave.
Newport Beach, CA 92663
  Educational services to professionals and to persons with acne are provided through this organization.

Bald Headed Men of America
P.O. Box "BALD"
211 N. King St.
Dunn, NC 28334
Phone: (919) 726-1004
  Building self-pride and discouraging discrimination against persons who have lost their hair are the goals of this organization founded in 1973.

National Alopecia Areata Foundation
P.O. Box 5027
Mill Valley, CA 94941

This association provides a support network for persons with alopecia areata and also keeps them medically informed. It also provides for public awareness of the disease and raises funds for research.

National Psoriasis Foundation
6415 S.W. Canyon Dr., Suite 200
Portland, OR 97221

This organization provides services to both lay and professional persons through education, research, publications, and facilitating communication between persons with psoriasis.

Society for the Rehabilitation of the
Facially Disfigured
550 First Ave.
New York, NY 10016
Phone: (212) 679-1534

Clients with facial disfigurement from severe burns, congenital malformation, or cancer will find this organization useful in promoting self-esteem, providing sur-gical help and rehabilitation services for those unable to afford private care, and providing public education.

NURSING ORGANIZATIONS

American Society of Plastic and Reconstructive
Surgical Nurses
23341 Milwaukee Ave.
Half Day, IL 60069
Phone: (312) 634-1405

The membership of this nursing organization is composed of nurses (RNs and LVNs) working with plastic surgeons or interested in plastic and surgical reconstructive nursing. Their official journal is *Plastic Surgical Nursing*. Dues, $30.

Dermatology Nurses' Association
Box 56
Pitman, NJ 08071

An organization for nurses with a special interest in dermatological nursing. Membership is RNs and other interested health care workers. Dues, $40.

Chapter 79

Specific Disorders of the Integumentary System

Carolyn Gorczyca

Objectives

When you have finished studying this chapter, you should be able to:

Give examples of common dermatoses that occur in adults because of congenital/genetic defects, multifactorial causes, immune hypersensitivity, infections/infestations, neoplasia, and trauma.

Compare and contrast common dermatoses that may be prevented, cured, or become chronic.

Assess the client for characteristic subjective and objective data common to selected dermatoses.

Describe therapeutic measures used to prevent and treat selected skin disorders.

Assume an active role in case finding for common dermatological disorders.

Explain the therapeutic, comforting, teaching, and protecting roles of the nurse in the prevention and management of common dermatological disorders.

Identify appropriate nursing interventions to assist the client in adjusting to psychosocial problems resulting from disorders of the integument.

There are over 2000 skin disorders, and it is essential for the nurse to become familiar with those conditions that commonly occur in adults. The nurse needs to know the characteristic features of dermatoses to provide services aimed at health preservation and early detection of lesions. Much of the monitoring will take place in community settings where the nurse may function in a variety of roles—professional health care provider, friend, or neighbor. Less frequently, the nurse will encounter clients with primary dermatological problems in an acute care setting.

Understanding the pathogenesis of skin disorders allows nurses to teach clients to use measures that can avoid the onset of a disease state or prevent subsequent complications. A major nursing concern involves the client's comprehension of the prognosis of each disorder. Many skin diseases result in lifelong problems requiring frequent or intermittent medical supervision, periodic adjustments in treatment, and constant supportive care. Nurses who understand how and when to intervene effectively can assist a client with a dermatosis to attain problem resolution and restore skin integrity, or to control manifestations and prevent complications when a cure is not possible. In addition, the effective nurse goes beyond the skin disease and recognizes the client as a person who is affected both physiologically and psychosocially by the pathological state.

Classification of a dermatological condition under a single etiologic category is difficult and may be debated. For this text, placement has been determined by the most outstanding influential causative factor.

Section I: Congenital/Genetic Disorders

Disorders discussed here are those dermatoses that are present at birth, become evident relatively soon afterward, or indicate a familial tendency. Skin texture, hair distribution, and glandular activity are greatly influenced by genetic programming. Excess dryness or oiliness, hair loss or gains, and hyperactivity of the sebaceous glands are frequent problems associated with skin disorders such as acne, alopecia, hypertrichosis, and ichthyosis.

Besides the examination of the presenting lesions and review of the subjective data, some clients may require hormonal studies as part of the diagnostic process. Because some of these problems are inevitable, become chronic conditions, or occur during significant periods of growth and development, emotional support is a crucial nursing role.

ACNE VULGARIS

Acne vulgaris (common acne) is a frequent, chronic, inflammatory disorder affecting the pilosebaceous units of the integument. This disorder occurs predominantly in adolescence when the sebaceous glands are activated. Acne can extend into young adulthood, particularly in women. Males tend to be more severely affected than females, and Caucasians have a higher incidence than Orientals and blacks (Fitzpatrick, 1979).

Many factors contribute to the cause or exacerbation of acne. Familial tendencies have been demonstrated, indicating a genetic linkage. Irritation has been attributed to a combination of increased sebum production and bacterial activity associated with the *Propionibacterium (Corynebacterium)* acnes, a normal organism of the hair follicle. Other contributing factors include endocrine imbalances; use of oral contraceptives; hormonal therapy (corticosteroids, androgens); other drugs (Dilantin, lithium); emotional stress; lack of cleanliness; exposure to comedogenic (lesion-producing) substances such as cosmetics, heavy oils, greases, and tars; and mechanical trauma of the lesions. Although some dermatologists cite dietary implications, no conclusive scientific evidence exists about the cause of acne. Flare-ups are seasonal and seen mostly in the fall and winter, although hot humid weather coupled with inadequate hygiene may also exacerbate the lesions.

Clinical Manifestations

Acne vulgaris is characterized by both noninflammatory and inflammatory skin lesions, primarily on the face and, to a lesser extent, on the neck, upper arms, and trunk (Figure 79–1). **Comedones** (blackheads and whiteheads), the classic noninflammatory lesions of acne, result from blockage of the follicle by lipid and keratin debris. An open comedo (blackhead) develops when the lipid oxidizes; its coloring comes from the presence of melanin. A whitehead is a closed comedo. Typical inflammatory lesions associated with acne vulgaris include papules and pustules. In severe cases, nodules and cysts may occur along with pitting and hypertrophic scarring. **Seborrhea,** an increase in the amount of sebum excreted (and possibly a change in the sebum itself), is commonly seen with acne, usually on the scalp and face.

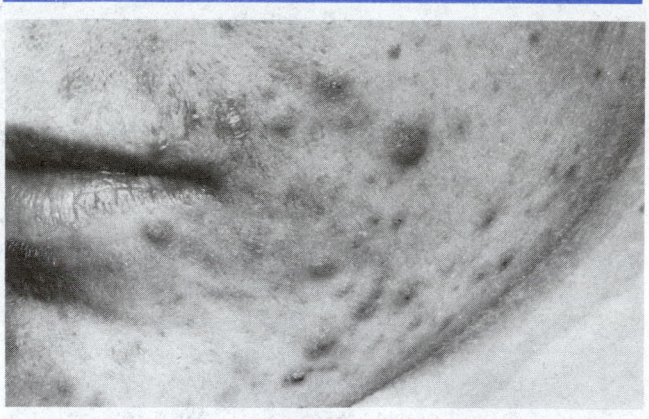

Figure 79–1

Acne vulgaris. Erythematous papules and pustules.
SOURCE: Binnick SA: *Skin Diseases: Diagnosis and Management in Clinical Practice.* Baltimore, MD: Williams & Wilkins, 1982.

Therapeutic Measures

Therapy is determined primarily by the presence or absence of inflammation and by the individual responses during the course of treatment. The treatment of acne has been revolutionized by retinoid therapy. Retinoids, analogues of vitamin A, have shown favorable results in treating acne and several other dermatological conditions. If retinoid treatment is begun early, disfigurement from scarring can be largely prevented even in clients with severe cystic acne. Because more effective treatments have been found, UVL and vitamin A are no longer common in the treatment of acne.

The treatment plan may combine several measures to resolve the problem. Among them are the following:

- Comedo extraction
- Abrasive cleansers
- Comedolytics
- Retinoids
- Antibiotics
- Estrogens
- Corticosteroids
- Antiseborrheic shampoos
- Dermabrasion

Treatment of noninflammatory lesions is directed toward removal of the obstructions and prevention of new comedo formation. These goals may be attained in part by regular atraumatic expression of comedones (removal of the plug) to prevent lesions from becoming irritated and progressing to an inflammatory stage. A comedo extractor in the hands of a skilled care provider allows gentle removal without risk of trauma (and scarring) or further irritation. Abrasive cleansers may be used to remove surface debris.

Comedolytic (comedo dissolving) and peeling agents assist in the removal of the comedo plugs. Topical preparations containing a single drug or combination of sulfur, resorcinol, or salicylic acid have been used, although these substances are giving way to the use of retinoic acid (tretinoin). Tretinoin is not only effective on existing lesions but ultimately prevents the formation of new comedones and the development of inflammation. Use of retinoic acid also facilitates the resolution of pustules by unroofing (removing the upper surface of) the lesions to allow spontaneous drainage. Favorable results usually become evident at about 12 weeks; clients may receive maintenance therapy for several years to prevent relapses. Topical application will cause some feeling of warmth, redness, slight tingling, and scaling at the site. The client must be informed that the medication may have to be discontinued temporarily or the dosage readjusted if the reaction becomes severe. Other instructions must also be given. Use of strong or medicated cosmetics, soap, or skin cleansers should be avoided. The area must be thoroughly dry before retinoic acid is applied, avoiding contact with the eyes, mouth, and mucous membranes. Exposure to sunlight or ultraviolet rays must be minimized; treatment may have to be delayed if the skin receives a burn. Benzoyl peroxide may be included in the treatment plan—either alone or in combination with retinoic acid. In addition to its comedolytic effect, benzoyl peroxide provides a bacteriostatic action.

Systemic retinoids have been incorporated into the therapeutic regimen for severe inflammatory disease. Isotretinoin (Accutane), the newest synthetic drug, decreases the size and activity of sebaceous glands, reducing sebum production. Side effects require serious consideration because the drug not only produces significant skin problems such as cheilitis (inflammation of the lip) and dry hair, but can cause conjunctivitis, hypertriglyceridemia, and musculoskeletal pain. Blood and hepatic laboratory studies are necessary to monitor cell counts, enzymes, and lipids. Because toxic effects are increased by vitamin A, the client should avoid excessive intake of vitamin A. Isotretinoin causes embryonic deformities in animals, and sexually active women of childbearing age must use contraceptive measures during treatment and for a month after drug discontinuance.

Presence of an inflammatory process warrants the use of antibiotics; the degree of involvement determines whether they will be used topically or systemically. Clindamycin, erythromycin, and tetracycline are the drugs of choice. The first two are most effective topically and may be used prophylactically to decrease the likelihood of inflammatory lesions. Tetracycline is the drug of choice for systemic use because it is relatively inexpensive, has minimal side effects, and may safely be given (in low doses of 250 mg daily) for the long-term therapy required in treating acne.

Dilute triamcinolone acetonide (Aristocort, Kenalog) may be injected into lesions to manage severe acne in which cysts and nodules develop. Such therapy produces rapid involution of lesions and reduces the occurrence of scarring. The medication is injected into the lesion with a 30-gauge needle to minimize discomfort. Atrophy of the skin in the involved area may be an untoward effect, and the client should be made aware of this potential outcome. Systemic corticosteroids such as prednisone or dexamethasone are reserved for cases refractory to all other modalities of treatment. Side effects and adverse reactions require discriminating use of these anti-inflammatory agents.

Estrogen therapy and the use of anovulatory drugs may be selected for women, primarily postadolescents, who fail to show significant improvement from aggressive conventional acne treatment. The estrogens suppress the androgenic hormones that have activated the sebaceous glands. Appropriate doses of mestranol or ethinyl estradiol are found to be most effective (Enovid-E, Ovulen). Favorable results from these drugs may be anticipated within 2 months and marked improvement in 4 months. Estrogen treatment, which entails the hazard of thrombosis, may be contraindicated in women who smoke and those with a history of thrombophlebitis, thromboembolitic disorders, cerebral apoplexy, liver disorders, and abnormal vaginal bleeding.

Dermabrasion is a surgical procedure used to lessen the disfiguring effects that may have resulted from the inflammatory process. Dermabrasion is discussed in Chapter 80.

Specific Nursing Measures

The greatest concern of the nurse is to encourage the client to make a major commitment to following the prescribed therapeutic plan. The client should understand the basic pathophysiology and the course of remissions and exacerbations involved in acne. Instructions for treatment must be explicit and understandable. Clients must learn of potential problems and how to protect the skin from further injury.

Sunlight, for example, may be used therapeutically but only if the skin is kept dry and exposure is not contraindicated by any of the drugs used. Irritation and subsequent inflammation may result from undue pressure, friction, rubbing, or squeezing of the affected areas. Clothing made from wool or roughly textured fabrics should be avoided. Athletes in contact sports or who perspire excessively under heavy clothing may need to stop playing temporarily. Undue pressure on the involved areas of the face, possibly caused by resting it against a hand while studying or listening to a classroom lecture, forceful expression (squeezing) of acne lesions, or a variety of other manipulations may activate the inflammatory process and lead to scarring. Anger or embarrassment over having blemishes may provoke squeezing that traumatizes the skin.

Hygiene is important to prevent external irritants from exacerbating the inflammatory process. Mild soaps and thorough drying of the skin should be encouraged when comedolytics are being used. Treatment may also require shampooing with a soap that controls the seborrhea. Clients whose work exposes them to oils, grease, and tars should be instructed to cleanse their skin frequently and particularly to wash off heavy perspiration.

Consideration must be given to avoiding substances that encourage comedones. Cosmetics containing heavy oil bases should be replaced with a thinner, water-based preparation. Cleansers, astringents, toners, and moisturizers should be selected that avoid excess oil but do not cause more dryness than desired. Major cosmetic companies perform comedogenic studies, and results are available upon request. Topical medications can be tinted so they do not have to be covered by cosmetics.

Body image is a critical component of the self-concept, and any disturbance in appearance may greatly impede a normal emotional passage through adolescence or young adulthood. For many individuals, much time is spent grooming, dressing, and improving sexual attractiveness. The appearance of even one "pimple" could prove to be a crisis, let alone the development of severe acne vulgaris or cystic acne. A person may also become the victim of others who openly display their own fears, pity, repulsion, or curiosity about the condition. Emotionally, fear of rejection, failure to belong to peer groups, to secure a job, or to be dating may result in depression, anger, worthlessness, aggressiveness, and a complexity of behavioral responses. Teenagers who develop acne should be observed for increasing social isolation and potential suicidal tendencies. A teenage client may believe that acne skin lesions are a punishment for a lack of control over sexual impulses or for sexual activities such as masturbation that are contrary to the mores and teachings of some families, religions, or cultural groups.

Any person with acne needs to be able to express feelings freely to someone who is able to see beyond "you'll grow out of it" and recognize the underlying dynamics the stress of acne may have triggered. Showing acceptance and sincere concern may encourage open communication and client trust that can enhance the relationship between nurse and client. Provide time in the nursing care plan to facilitate interactions with the client and family or friends. (See the case study of a client with acne at the end of this chapter.)

ACNE ROSACEA

Acne rosacea is a chronic dermatosis involving the pilosebaceous glands of the face. It is characterized by intermittent erythema that can progress to persistent flushing and telangiectasis, and by the presence of acneiform lesions. The condition is most common in light-skinned, fair-complexioned persons between the ages of 30 and 50. Although women are affected three times more frequently, men may develop a more severe form of the disorder (Arndt, 1983).

Although no basic cause has been determined, most people affected by this disorder have oily, pale skin and tan with difficulty. Ingestion of hot liquids and hot food and the consumption of alcohol contribute to the problem by increasing the vasodilation.

Clinical Manifestations

Papules, pustules, and nodules are the primary lesions that may appear amid the telangiectases, usually in a symmetrical distribution on the cheeks, chin, midforehead, and nose. Rhinophyma, a hyperplastic process of the soft tissue of the nose, develops more frequently in men. The skin, usually commencing in the lower portion of the nose, becomes bright red to purplish red, and irregularly thickened. Serious cases of acne rosacea may involve the eye and cause blepharitis, conjunctivitis, and keratitis.

Therapeutic Measures

Treatment involves the administration of systemic antibiotics and topical preparations containing benzoyl peroxide. Oral tetracycline has been found the most effective drug and is given long term. Recurrences are common, but the disorder may have a spontaneous resolution after several years. Argon laser surgery may be used to destroy large telangiectatic blood vessels and surgical shaving, dermabrasion, or electrosurgery to reduce rhinophyma.

Specific Nursing Measures

Because of the need to prevent unnecessary vasodilation, it is important to instruct the client to avoid any stimuli that would increase the likelihood of flushing. Foods and liquids should be eaten at no more than a warm temperature. Alcohol and use of excessive seasoning should be avoided, along with exposure to emotional stress, excessive activities, sunlight, and extremes of environmental heat and cold.

ICHTHYOSIS VULGARIS

Dry skin is a common dermatological problem. However, in the pathological conditions known as *ichthyosiform dermatoses,* scales characteristically accumulate on the cutaneous surface. In extreme cases, the integument may be patterned somewhat like a fish or snake skin. Ichthyosis vulgaris, the most common type of dry skin disorder, is the least severe. Although the keratinocytes grow at a normal rate, the cells in the stratum corneum fail to slough off individually.

All forms of ichthyosis are genetically linked. In ichthyosis vulgaris, the mode of inheritance is as a dominant autosomal trait. A family history of atopy usually exists, marked by disorders such as hay fever, eczema, asthma, or urticaria (hives).

Clinical Manifestations

Ichthyosis vulgaris appears in early childhood and remains lifelong. Small, white scales appear primarily on the exten-

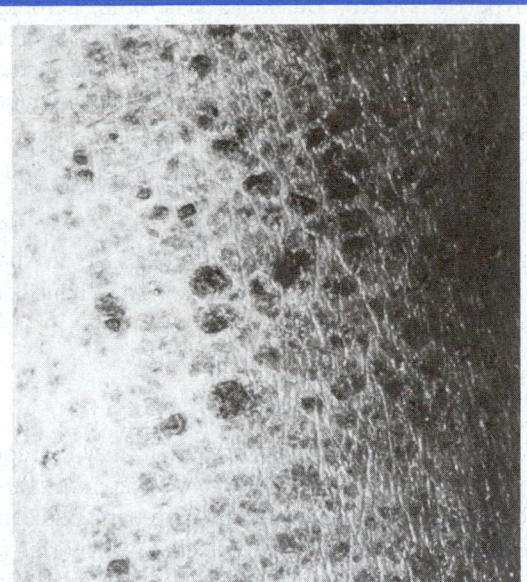

Figure 79–2

Ichthyosis vulgaris.

SOURCE: Binnick SA: *Skin Diseases: Diagnosis and Management in Clinical Practice.* Baltimore, MD: Williams & Wilkins, 1982.

sor surface of the extremities and on the trunk, forehead, cheeks, and scalp. The texture of the skin becomes rough. Hyperkeratosis and exaggerated skin markings are seen on the palms and soles (Figure 79–2). Exacerbations occur during cold, dry temperatures, and the client develops a winter pruritus. Problems are usually not evident during the summer.

Therapeutic Measures

Treatment of ichthyosis vulgaris (and dry skin in general) requires the maintenance of a hydrated, soft, cutaneous surface. This goal is best accomplished by providing moisture and preventing its subsequent evaporation. Hydration may be facilitated by soaking the affected area or bathing for 5 to 10 minutes in water between 43°C and 46°C (110°F and 115°F), followed immediately by the application of water-in-oil or fatty hydrophobic medications (Aquaphor, Eucerin, lanolin, petrolatum). Urea-containing lotions (Aquacare, Calmurid, Carmol) are also recommended because of the water-binding capacity of urea.

Specific Nursing Measures

Clients should be counseled to provide an environment that protects the moisture content of the skin. Living in a humid, tropical climate is ideal but not feasible for all those concerned. Therefore, room temperature should be kept comfortably low (to keep down evaporation), and moisture content should be maintained through use of light clothing and humidification when dryness is extreme. Excessive bathing

and exposure to drying soaps, solvents, or compounds should be avoided. Bath oils (Keri, Domol, Lubath) should be added to bath water, applied in a dilute preparation after bathing, or used as a substitute for a bath.

In more severe cases of ichthyosis, more intense or prolonged emotional support may be required because of gross disfigurement. These clients may be objects of curiosity to others. Some have even been exhibited in carnivals as freaks ("alligator man" or "snake-skinned lady"). Genetic counseling may be recommended because of the inherited characteristics of this disorder.

ALOPECIA

Alopecia is the loss of body hair (primarily on the scalp) with the presence of bald spots or total baldness. Alopecia may be patchy or diffuse, scarring or nonscarring. In cases where scar tissue forms, regrowth of hair becomes impossible because the follicles have been permanently destroyed.

Causes for hair loss are multiple. The most common type of alopecia, male pattern baldness, is hereditary. Female pattern baldness occurs in a small percentage of women, usually around the age of 50.

Alopecia areata is a common disorder of asymptomatic, noninflammatory, nonscarring hair loss. The etiological basis is unknown, although a family history has been implicated, as has autoimmune disease. Emotional stress, particularly a life crisis, has also been known to precipitate the loss. Alopecia areata affects both sexes equally, and the initial attack is frequently seen in clients under the age of 25. A significant incidence occurs in persons with Down's syndrome (Fitzpatrick, 1979).

Loss of hair may also occur from repeated friction; cutaneous infection; drugs and chemicals; trauma (frostbite, burns); skin disease and neoplasms; nutritional deficiencies (loss of large amounts of amino acids and trace elements); x-ray; endocrine imbalances; and acute and chronic systemic illness.

Clinical Manifestations

Male pattern baldness most often begins with receding of the hairline in front, followed by lessening of hair on the crown of the head and in the temporal areas.

The losses associated with alopecia areata appear gradually over several weeks and may be localized (areas on the scalp, eyelids, or cheeks) or extensive (Figure 79–3). Baldness over the entire head is called alopecia totalis, and if the entire body becomes hairless, it is alopecia universalis. Regrowth is often spontaneous, but a less favorable prognosis exists when the onset occurs before puberty or if the losses are extensive. Recurrence is quite common.

Therapeutic and Specific Nursing Measures

Treatment for alopecia is relatively limited and is contingent on the etiological factors, whether scarring has result-

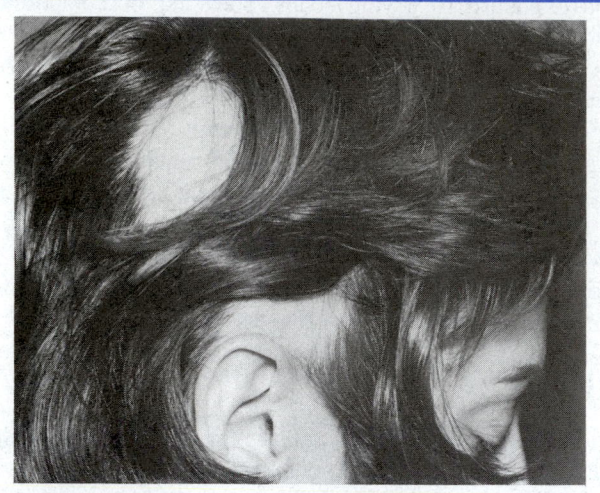

Figure 79–3

Alopecia areata.
SOURCE: Binnick SA: *Skin Diseases: Diagnosis and Management in Clinical Practice.* Baltimore, MD: Williams & Wilkins, 1982.

ed, and whether regrowth is genetically possible. Topical, intralesional, or systemic corticosteroids, repeated applications of topical photosensitizers (DNCB), and prolonged photochemotherapy have been used to treat alopecia areata. The major therapy may be directed toward assisting the individual in coping with any emotional disturbances caused by the alopecia, particularly if the condition becomes chronic with no possibility of inducing regrowth. Use of wigs or hair transplantation or replacement may be encouraged if at all possible (refer to Chapter 80). Artificial implants have not been successful to date, may cause infection and scarring, and should be discouraged. Research into the potential use of minoxidil, a vasodilator used as an antihypertensive, is ongoing.

HYPERTRICHOSIS/HIRSUTISM

Hypertrichosis and hirsutism involve the abnormal growth of hair. Hypertrichosis is a generalized or localized excess of hair on any body part or intradermal nevus (male). Hirsutism, which develops in women and children, is androgen-dependent and is confined to adult male patterns of hair distribution.

There may be familial tendencies to develop excess hair, but no strong indications exist. Increased hair growth is associated with hormonal changes, especially during pregnancy and menopause, and also in hypothyroid-

ism, hyperthyroidism, Cushing's syndrome, acromegaly, Stein–Leventhal syndrome, and adrenogenital syndrome. Trauma, chronic inflammation, anorexia nervosa and other wasting diseases, and some drugs can result in hypertrichosis or hirsutism.

Clinical Manifestations

Coarse or fine hair may appear in excess on any part of the body. The most prominent areas of growth include the face, chest, breast, and back.

Therapeutic Measures

If no curable disease is found, treatment may be required to suppress androgen production with appropriate hormones. Otherwise, use of bleaching preparations containing a 6% solution of hydrogen peroxide; depilatories (Nair, Neet, Nudit, Magic Shaving Powder, Royal Crown Shaving Powder); depilating waxes; plucking; and shaving are the methods most often used. None of these will destroy the blood supply to the hair follicles, so regrowth is inevitable within 8 to 13 weeks. Although it is costly and time-consuming, electrolysis offers a means of permanent hair removal. The process entails destruction of the hair-nourishing blood vessels by use of a high frequency current and/or chemical cauterization. To ensure proper and effective treatment without scarring, the procedure must be performed by a skilled electrologist.

Specific Nursing Measures

Disfigurement from the appearance of abnormal amounts and distribution of hair is likely to be psychosocially disruptive for either men or women and should be recognized as a source of emotional stress. It is important for the nurse to direct the client to appropriate medical attention to identify any hormone imbalances that could be treated to reduce the excess of hair. The nurse should also be able to instruct the client in the use of either permanent or temporary methods to remove hair. Women need to be aware that although the use of plucking, waxing, and depilatories removes hair for longer periods of time than shaving, hairs could become darker and coarser. If permanent removal is preferred, the client should be informed that the speed of results is contingent on the degree of damage done to the follicles by previous methods of removal and the amount and type of hair involved. Electrolysis may be costly, but the permanent elimination of unwanted hair usually makes it emotionally rewarding.

Section II: Disorders of Multifactorial Origin

Many dermatological problems are categorized as acquired or idiopathic dermatoses, and usually represent a group of pathological conditions in which no definite or singular

etiological factor can be identified. A dermatosis may also be labeled as acquired if there is no congenital or genetic basis. The disorders to be discussed here include seborrheic dermatitis, psoriasis, pityriasis rosea, chloasma, and vitiligo. These dermatoses cause a diversity of pathophysiological problems and could involve an increased rate of keratinocyte production, alterations in pigmentation, the development of an inflammatory process, or all of these. Long-term treatment, a significant stressor in itself, may be required.

SEBORRHEIC DERMATITIS

Seborrheic dermatitis is a chronic inflammatory condition characterized by red, scaling eruptions in areas where sebaceous glands are highly concentrated, such as the scalp, face, and trunk. The cause is basically unknown, although a familial tendency is suggested. Emotional and physical stress are also responsible for recurrence of the problem. Increased production of sebum has not been found to have any significant pathophysiological influence. Some individuals develop dandruff, a minor condition that involves excessive desquamation (shedding of dead cells), without any evidence of inflammation.

Clinical Manifestations

The onset of seborrheic dermatitis is gradual. The condition has a tendency to worsen in colder weather because of decreased indoor humidity and lack of summer sunlight. Pruritus is a common complaint. Varying sized white or yellowish-red macules and papules may appear on the scalp, eyelids, eyebrows, paranasal area, ears, moustache, beard, presternal area, and in body folds (Figure 79–4). The lesions may be dry or greasy and may develop crusts or fissures.

Therapeutic Measures

Therapy will be aimed at reducing any inflammatory process and/or decreasing epidermal proliferation. Shampoos that contain 2% selenium sulfide (Exsel, Iosel, Selsun Blue) are effective antiseborrheics. Similar responses may be obtained from preparations that contain 1% to 2% zinc pyrithione (Danex, Head & Shoulders, Zincon). Shampoos containing salicylic acid with sulfur (Ionil, Sebulex) or tar (Sebutone, Zetar) are less effective. Keratolytic gels may be applied overnight to remove thick crusts. Topical medications may include corticosteroids and sulfur-containing substances.

Specific Nursing Measures

Because seborrheic dermatitis is chronic, nursing care should help prepare the client to plan for long-term management and control. Shampooing schedules and techniques and the administration of topical medications in the prescribed vehicle should be explained and demonstrated. Because stress plays a major role in the exacerbation of this condition, the client needs to recognize the need to develop effective coping mechanisms whenever possible and to practice the stress management techniques discussed in Chapter 2.

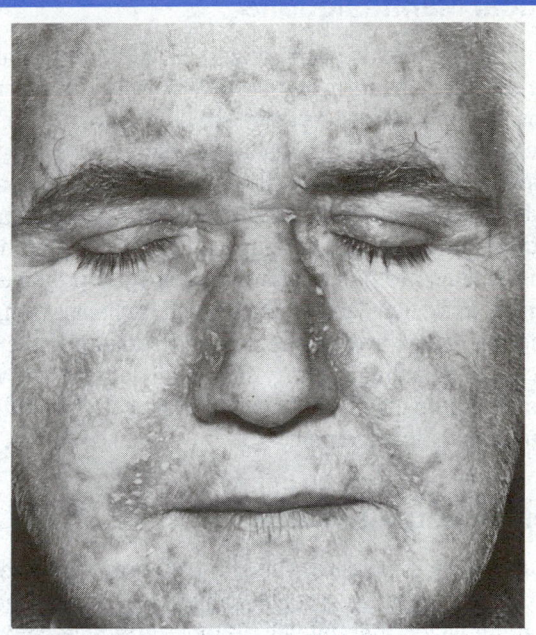

Figure 79–4

Seborrheic dermatitis.
SOURCE: Binnick SA: *Skin Diseases: Diagnosis and Management in Clinical Practice.* Baltimore, MD: Williams & Wilkins, 1982.

PSORIASIS

Psoriasis is a common recurring disorder indicative of an overly rapid proliferation of epidermal cells in which characteristic scaling, papules, and plaques appear, most frequently on the elbows, knees, and scalp. No cure exists. Much time, human resources, and money are spent in controlling the manifestations.

Between 2 and 8 million Americans are afflicted with psoriasis (Arndt, 1983). Onset occurs generally during adulthood, although a significant number of cases are known to appear before the age of 20, with equal frequency in both sexes. Additionally, a significant number of people with psoriasis (5% to 10%) also have an associated arthritic condition to manage.

The reason why keratinocytes mature in 3 or 4 days in psoriasis instead of the normal 28 days remains unknown. Familial tendencies have been associated with approximately 30% of clients. Significant immunologic abnormalities have also been demonstrated. A form of acute psoriasis has also been known to follow several days after streptococcal pharyngitis. Exacerbations have been correlated with alcohol ingestion, excessive exposure to sunlight, stress, obesity, and use of certain drugs such as systemic corticosteroids, lithium, and chloroquine. Cutaneous trauma related to scratching, surgical wounds, and other superficial injuries may result in the formation of a new patchy lesion in clients with psoriasis.

Clinical Manifestations

The initial appearance of psoriasis usually is gradual and generally takes the form of elevated, sharply circumscribed lesions covered by white-silvery scales (Figure 79-5). The shape and arrangements of psoriatic lesions vary: they may be limited to one or a localized group of lesions, may be distributed over a region, or distribution may be general, including not only the skin but also the nails. Cutaneous manifestations are most common over bony prominences and in intertriginous areas. Excoriation, lichenification, and oozing may occur with some cases. Psoriasis of the nails may cause crumbling, pitting, and distal detachment of the plates. Pruritus may be anticipated, particularly with scalp and anogenital involvement.

Therapeutic Measures

Because there is no cure, the aim of therapy is to reduce the proliferation rate to a controllable state. Several factors determine which therapy will be most effective, and individualization of care is important. Most therapies include a combination of drugs, the use of natural or artificial UVL, or both. Psoriatic lesions affecting the nails have no specific therapy and often disappear spontaneously or when treatment of the skin is effective.

The use of corticosteroids for management of psoriasis aims at inhibiting mitosis (formation of new cells), thereby reducing scaling and thickening of the skin. These drugs may be administered topically, systemically, or intralesionally. Fluorinated corticosteroids (Kenalog, Cordran, Synalar, Valisone) may be prescribed for topical usage on localized lesions. The mode of administration may include several daily applications of a cream-based drug followed by an overnight plastic occlusive dressing. A continual 24-hour occlusive coverage may also be used. Prolonged use of these drugs may result in atrophy of the skin, striae, and telangiectasis. If systemic corticosteroids are used, clients should be informed that initial improvement is maintained only by increasing the dosage, and that rebound reactions are likely when treatment ends. Intralesional injections of triamcinolone acetonide (Aristocort, Kenalog) may be prescribed for solitary resistant plaques and possibly for psoriatic lesions of the nails.

Coal tar preparations have long had a significant role in the treatment of psoriasis. In addition to removing scales and plaque, these drugs inhibit DNA synthesis in both normal and hyperplastic skin. The preparation is usually used in conjunction with corticosteroids, other keratolytic agents such as salicylic acid and sulfur, or with phototherapy. Coal tar preparations, in the form of ointments, bath oils, emulsions, shampoos and lotions, may be specifically compounded from a physician's prescription or bought over the counter. The medication is usually applied to the lesions or to bath water if involvement is extensive.

Phototherapy or actinotherapy provides a regulated exposure to natural UVL (sunlight), or artificial sources of middle-wave length UVL (UV-B), to reduce basal cell production in mild to moderate cases of psoriasis. Therapeutic regimens require three treatments a week for an average of twenty-three exposures. More aggressive phototherapy includes exposures ranging from five to seven times per week (Arndt, 1983).

Goeckerman's regimen, usually performed on hospitalized clients, combines coal tar and UV-B. A tar bath (Zetar, Balnetar) or overnight application of a gel (Estar) is the first step in the procedure. Complete removal of any remaining drug is essential before the client is exposed to the light. The exposure time, which is regulated to produce minimal erythema in 12 hours, begins with a few seconds or minutes for artificial UVL, which is equal to 20 to 30 minutes of natural sunlight. Exposure time is increased gradually, but mild phototoxicity should be anticipated. Following a bath to remove any scales, coal tar or steroids may be applied to the involved areas. Prolonged remission usually requires a 2 to 3 week course of therapy.

Photochemotherapy currently offers the most promising treatment for widespread, severe psoriasis. The mechanism involves administration of a chemical sensitizer followed by exposure to long-wave length UVL (UV-A) approximately 2 hours later. A group of drugs known as psoralens act as the photosensitizers and, in conjunction with UV-A, reduce the accelerated rate of cell production seen in psoriasis. This combination of a psoralen with UV-A is known by the acronym PUVA. A course of treatment usually involves 10 to 20 exposures over 4 to 8 weeks. Remission is maintained by using PUVA twice monthly (Arndt, 1983).

Methoxsalen (Oxsoralen), the most commonly used psoralen derivative, is available for oral administration as well as topical application. The client is exposed to UV-A when peak photosensitivity is most likely. Erythematous

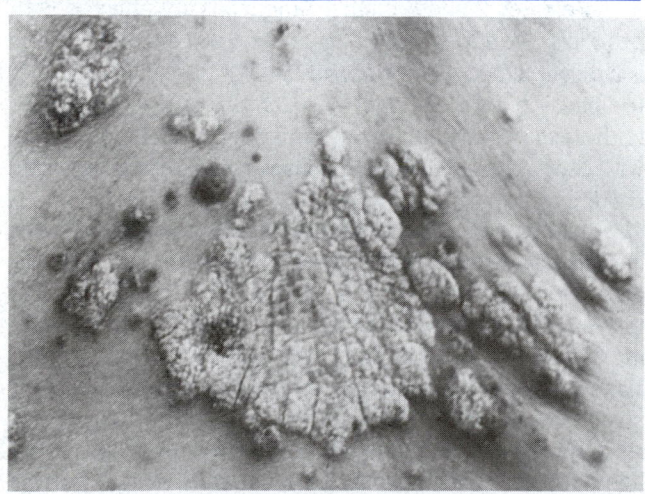

Figure 79-5

Generalized psoriasis. (Courtesy of Millard Fillmore Hospital, Buffalo, NY)

responses are delayed much longer with long-wave ultraviolet light than with UV-B and may not be totally visible until peak effects are reached in 48 to 72 hours. Overexposure may result in swelling, blistering, itching, pain, and scaling of the skin. Therefore, it is essential that medication dosages and time exposure be carefully calculated by the dermatologist and that the client be closely monitored for untoward reactions. Degree of skin pigmentation, photosensitivity, hepatic insufficiency, and systemic lupus erythematosus require caution in the use of this method of therapy or the therapy may be contraindicated.

Effective treatment for widespread psoriatic lesions may be obtained from the use of anthralin (dithranol, Cignolin, Lassar's paste), a drug with cytotoxic and cytostatic actions. Several modalities of treatment may be used in which cool tar baths, application of corticosteroid creams, UVL, or PUVA are combined with the anthralin paste method. Applying the paste over a petrolatum base is recommended because the medication may be more precisely applied to the psoriatic plaques. The unaffected skin must be observed for blistering and erythema because of the irritating property of anthralin. Clothing, skin, and blonde hair are also stained by this drug.

Methotrexate (Amethopterin) or hydroxyurea (Hydrea) may be selected in the treatment of clients who have severe psoriasis that has become resistant to other forms of therapy. The purpose of using antimetabolites is to inhibit DNA synthesis and obtain remission of cell proliferation. Clients are carefully screened for hepatic, renal, and hematologic abnormalities because of the potential risks of this type of chemotherapy. Treatment is closely supervised and discontinued if a toxic reaction becomes evident, such as diarrhea or ulcerative stomatitis. Clients seek such treatment to gain control over a disease that has proved costly physically, emotionally, and financially.

A new retinoid, etretinate (Tregrison) has been found to be useful in the treatment of psoriasis. Studies are continuing to measure its effectiveness alone and in combination with adjunctive therapy such as ultraviolet radiation and PUVA.

Specific Nursing Measures

Psoriasis is one of the few dermatoses that may require hospitalization, most likely because of a need for more intense or assisted therapy. Day care centers have also been established to provide closer supervision and aid with therapeutic measures without requiring 24-hour confinement.

Nursing care is directed at restoring skin integrity through the administration of the prescribed treatment. Be aware of and understand the responsibilities involved in drug therapy, particularly effective application and removal of topical drugs. Proper coverage of lesions is essential and usually requires airtight dressings or use of plastic wrap (Saran Wrap) so that penetration of lesions is effective. As each component of therapy is implemented, incorporate a teaching plan that will promote client self-care.

Potential for injury is ever present. Clients with psoriasis should be cautioned to avoid rubbing or scratching the skin because trauma may initiate the development of new lesions. Excoriated areas may also be a port of entry for bacteria, and secondary infections may ensue. Various methods of alleviating the itch–scratch cycle may have to be initiated, as discussed in Chapter 78.

Protection of the eyes and uninvolved skin is essential when artificial UVL is used. Teach the client to avoid overexposure to sunlight and additional cutaneous injury. Clients should always follow safety precautions in self-treatment and be certain that anyone administering UVL therapy, if not a physician, nurse, or recognized therapist, is experienced and technically competent. Commercial establishments offering UVL for tanning do not follow medically precise techniques and may be a source of injury. (See Chapter 78 for sources of artificial UV-B and nursing implications.)

Psoriasis is a classic example of a skin disorder that can be emotionally upsetting to the client. Whether generalized or local, lesions are usually visible and may cause feelings of humiliation and embarrassment. The chronicity and recurrent flare-ups; the tedious skin care; the staining of skin, nails, clothing, and bedding; and the financial drain may weaken coping mechanisms so that additional counseling may be required. As discouraged as someone may become with psoriasis, it is essential that treatments be continued and exacerbating factors avoided. The support that can be given by an individual, whether a lay person or professional, and by a mutual support group may prove highly valuable in motivating the client to persevere.

PITYRIASIS ROSEA

Pityriasis rosea is a moderately common maculopapular disorder seen primarily in adolescents and young adults. It occurs most commonly during the spring and fall. Although the cause of this condition is said to be a virus, proof has not been established.

Clinical Manifestations

The onset of pityriasis is characterized by a "herald" patch, a red scaly plaque 2 to 5 cm across, which may appear on any part of the body. In a week or two, oval erythematous discrete lesions become visible, primarily over the chest, trunk, upper arms, and thighs.

Therapeutic Measures

Pityriasis rosea is self-limiting, and spontaneous remission often occurs within 4 to 6 weeks. Most persons do not require treatment. Sunlight and UVL will provide relief from pruritus and may facilitate involution of the lesions. Topical or systemic corticosteroids may be required in more severe inflammatory reactions. Itching may be alleviated by antipruritics, lotions, emollients, or antihistamines.

CHLOASMA

Chloasma or melasma is a disorder in which increased melanin production produces brownish patchy discolorations on the skin. It is a common dermatosis with a higher incidence in dark-skinned Caucasians, predominantly women.

The etiology of this type of hyperpigmentation is unknown. Hormonal influences are suspected because alterations have occurred during pregnancy (mask of pregnancy) and menopause, with the use of oral contraceptives, and in the presence of ovarian disorders or tumors. Discolorations have also been associated with chronic illness and may follow a cutaneous inflammatory process. Chloasma is distinct from freckles, which represent a genetically determined hyperpigmentation in which enlarged melanocytes form excess melanin.

Clinical Manifestations

Subjective complaints identified with chloasma, or any increase in pigmentation, are limited to concerns about alterations in appearance. No symptoms are present, unless the hyperpigmentation is secondary to a systemic illness or other dermatosis.

Large macular lesions usually appear on the face, generally on the forehead, cheeks, upper lip, and the sides of the neck. The color may range from yellowish-brown to a very dark brown. (Freckles are much smaller in diameter and are scattered over the body, most prominently in sun-exposed areas.)

Therapeutic Measures

Some types of hyperpigmentation of the skin need no therapeutic intervention because the discoloration fades. Chloasma does not fade by itself, and bleaching of the skin becomes the recommended mode of treatment. Preparations containing hydroquinone (Artra, Eldoquin, Esotérica) are used to inhibit tyrosine conversion in melanin synthesis. Subsequently, this altered process results in a more rapid fading of hyperpigmented areas. Topical application several times a day should produce improvement within 8 weeks. Clients must be cautioned to discontinue therapy if the skin becomes irritated or a rash develops.

Specific Nursing Measures

Avoiding exposure to ultraviolet rays is essential to prevent further darkening. Clients should be instructed to cover the affected skin, either with clothing or with sunscreening or sunblocking preparations. (See specific information on sunscreens and sunblockers presented in Chapter 78.)

VITILIGO

Vitiligo is a disorder in which temporary or permanent depigmentation develops. It may involve the hair as well as the skin because of gradual melanocytic destruction. The condition affects children and adults equally. Although vitiligo occurs in all racial groups, an increased incidence has been recorded in India, Pakistan, and the Far East. Vitiligo has many psychosocial ramifications. In India, for instance, a woman with this condition is considered unmarriageable. Other psychosocial implications are discussed later in this section.

The pathogenesis is unknown, and vitiligo is classified as an acquired idiopathic disorder. Approximately 30% of persons with vitiligo have a family history of this skin disorder (Arndt, 1983). Cases have been noted with monozygomatic twins in which both or only one twin has been affected. An associated depigmentation also occurs with systemic illnesses such as pernicious anemia, diabetes mellitus, and thyroid disease. Screening procedures for any of these conditions may be involved in the diagnostic process for vitiligo.

Clinical Manifestations

Lesions are macular, pure white, often symmetrical, and frequently develop over bony prominences (elbow, knee, ankle, wrist) and about body openings (Figure 79–6). Alterations are usually progressive and may be limited to

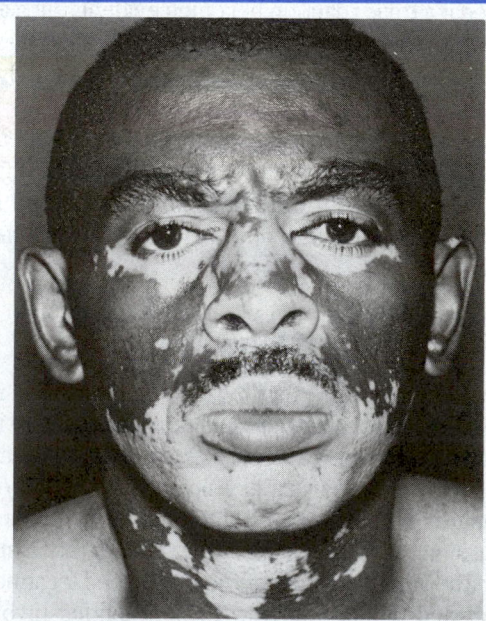

Figure 79–6

Vitiligo.

SOURCE: Binnick SA: *Skin Diseases: Diagnosis and Management in Clinical Practice.* Baltimore, MD: Williams & Wilkins, 1982.

an isolated lesion or become localized, generalized, or universal. Illumination from a Wood's light is useful in determining the presence of melanin within the area.

Therapeutic Measures

Several methods are available to treat vitiligo, although none alters the pathophysiological process. The prime objective, therefore, is to improve cosmetic appearance.

The use of PUVA is the most effective therapy at this time. Depending on the degree of skin involvement, either a systemic or a topical psoralen preparation is administered. Exposure to UV-A light is highly individualized and contingent on the complexion and tanning abilities of the client. Those with light complexions may not require treatment because depigmentation is not as obvious a problem as with dark-brown or black-skinned people. If PUVA is used, the unaffected skin should be covered with sunscreens to prevent excessive tanning. Reestablishing desired pigmentation may take as long as 2 years.

Depigmentation through chemical bleaching is recommended for clients over 40 years of age with more than 40% of their skin area showing vitiligo that has proved recalcitrant to PUVA. Female clients must not be pregnant or lactating. Because of the social implications of skin color in many cultures and societies throughout the world, people with highly pigmented skin should not receive this treatment, unless they are emotionally prepared to accept the color change. Remedy of the physiological problem must also consider the psychosocial adjustment that might be required. Topical application of monobenzone or hydroquinone ointment (Benoquin) results in depigmentation.

Because treatment results are slow, cosmetics may be employed as a temporary camouflage. A solution of potassium permanganate has been used to paint vitiliginous areas in brown-skinned clients. Cosmetic coverups (Vita-Dye, Dy-O-Derm) and makeup (Covermark, Reflecta) are also available.

Specific Nursing Measures

Because no pathophysiological disturbance becomes manifest during the depigmentation process unless an associated systemic illness is present, the major focus of nursing concern is likely to be the psychosocial aspects. Many clients may not know about or understand vitiligo and may have developed myths or unscientific rationales about the cause. Information that the pathogenesis is unknown must be made clear along with the chronic nature of the depigmentation. Options for treatment may need to be identified when clients have not received medical assistance, to prevent the search for a nonexistent cure. Clients should be cautioned to apply sunscreen to normal skin when exposed to the sun so that contrast between the two areas is not increased.

Psychosocial disturbances may be covert, and the nurse must plan to explore the emotional implications with the person, particularly those with highly pigmented skin. Serious disfigurement may already have deterred employment opportunities, interpersonal relationships, and personal growth. Support systems must be developed and strengthened so that the individual may adjust emotionally to the stresses imposed by vitiligo.

Section III: Immune Hypersensitivity Disorders

Eczematous dermatitis or eczema is a general term covering various forms of eruptive inflammatory disease of the integument that result from an immediate or delayed hypersensitivity reaction after exposure to an exogenous, endogenous, or unknown substance. The body attempts to destroy the antigen but cannot make effective use of humoral or cellular immune mechanisms. The resulting cutaneous cytological and vascular alterations give evidence that a pathophysiological state exists. Contact and atopic dermatitis, urticaria, drug reactions, and pemphigus vulgaris are disorders that involve an immune hypersensitivity reaction.

One-third of the clients who seek the help of a dermatologist are troubled with eczematous dermatitis (Fitzpatrick, 1979). These disorders occur readily within occupational, household, and recreational settings. Within the hospital, drug reactions are a leading cause for seeking a dermatological consultation. The various forms of eczematous disease have proven costly, not only in the loss of time and productivity, lost wages, and medical expenses, but in the human suffering incurred.

General Nursing Implications

Nurses play an integral role in teaching preventive measures to those who develop an immune hypersensitivity, whether the dermatosis is acute, subacute, or chronic. Care of clients with allergic reactions may not be limited to the cutaneous manifestations; the nurse may be involved with life-saving measures when an anaphylactic reaction occurs.

Another important aspect of nursing deals with the administration of drugs that may be responsible for a hypersensitivity reaction. Knowledge about the medications most likely to create difficulties and a recognition of manifestations of problems or side effects is required of every nurse. Specific cutaneous responses associated with drug therapy are discussed later in this chapter (see Drug Eruptions).

CONTACT DERMATITIS

Contact dermatitis, a common inflammatory dermatosis seen in acute, subacute, and chronic forms, involves the epidermal and dermal layers of the skin. Causative agents responsible for the reaction act either as a primary irritant or an allergic sensitizer. Primary irritants are external or exogenous agents that cause an immediate inflammatory reaction when direct contact is made with the integument. Substances that act as antagonists include chemicals, clothing, shoes, rubber, metals (nickel), dyes, preservatives, plants, solvents, topical medications, soaps, insect sprays, industrial oils, perfumes, cosmetics, and toiletries.

Allergic sensitizers involve a cell-mediated reaction that results in a delayed hypersensitivity response. Lymphocytes, specifically the T-cells, become sensitized when contact is made with allergens such as poison ivy or poison oak. An initial response may develop within 5 to 21 days, or a latent period may occur. Upon subsequent exposure, skin eruptions appear within 12 to 48 hours, depending on the potency of the allergen, duration of exposure, permeability of the skin, and the development of immunity.

Certain topical and systemic medications are known to be sensitizing agents and therefore, should be prescribed and used with caution. Unfortunately, some of the products may be sold over the counter, and the user may not be aware of the precautions. One such drug is benzocaine, a substance found in hundreds of compounds and used to produce local anesthesia. Neomycin and ethylenediamine are also common sensitizers. Ethylenediamine is a component of frequently used medications such as aminophylline and hydroxyzine hydrochloride (Vistaril, Atarax). Some antihistamines must be monitored for their own cutaneous side effects even though they may be ordered for allergic responses that involve skin manifestations. A client who is receiving diphenhydramine (Benadryl) and tripelennamine hydrochloride (Pyribenzamine) may develop urticaria, whereas use of promethazine (Phenergan) may evoke photosensitivity. A pharmacology textbook will give an extensive list of drugs that may cause sensitization. In the diagnostic process, it may be difficult for the dermatologist to distinguish between a primary irritation and an allergic reaction.

Clinical Manifestations

The inflammation with contact dermatitis may range from mild to severe, and the resultant lesions indicate the acuteness or chronicity of the response. Generally, the client will complain of pruritus (which varies in intensity), pain, and burning. Mild reactions will display erythema, microvesicles, and oozing. In an acute contact dermatitis, the degree of redness increases, and lesions may progress to the size of bullae, become eroded, or develop into ulcerations. The extent of the cutaneous lesion may be localized to the exact area of contact or generalized if an allergen was internalized. Edema in various parts of the body may become evident, as well as signs of systemic involvement (fever, general malaise, weakness).

Chronic exposure to irritants and allergens causes areas of skin to redden, dry, scale, lichenify, fissure, and at times

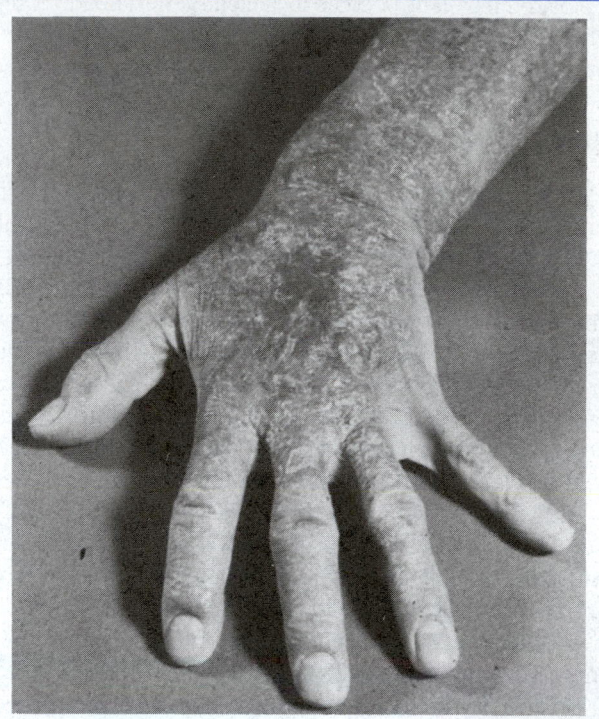

Figure 79–7

Contact dermatitis. (Courtesy of Millard Fillmore Hospital, Buffalo, NY)

to become hypopigmented and hyperpigmented (Figure 79–7).

Therapeutic Measures

Treatment is based on the severity of the response. The primary objective in all cases is to identify and remove the irritant or allergen. Acute contact dermatitis may take several weeks to resolve and may require rest along with the prescribed therapeutic measures. (Pruritus can cause sleep disturbances, and antihistamines may have a sedative effect.) Wet dressings soaked with aluminum acetate (Burow's) solution may be applied several times a day until vesiculation and oozing cease. Corticosteroids may be given systemically using prednisone, triamcinolone, or betamethasone if the allergic response or inflammation is severe; otherwise, topical application of fluocinonide, triamcinolone, or fluocinolone is started when vesicles have disappeared. Balneotherapy using Aveeno baths to soothe and protect the skin may be ordered if the problem is generalized and severe (see Chapter 78). Antibiotics may be necessary to combat any superimposed infection.

In chronic conditions, the application of a nonwater-soluble emollient (petrolatum) is used to prevent dryness and soften the skin, possibly in conjunction with topical corticosteroid ointments. Medical supervision may be required for a lengthy period of time to control the manifestations.

Specific Nursing Measures

Care of the client with contact dermatitis, beyond the prescribed medicinal treatment of the lesions and subjective complaints, should center on teaching of preventive measures. The goal will be to increase the knowledge base so that the client can directly control his or her skin integrity. Specific points to be included in the instructions to the client are listed in Box 79–1.

A concern that may have to be addressed involves contagion. Clients should be made aware that contact dermatitis is not transmissible, not even with poison ivy or poison oak, unless the oils of the plant are still on the skin or clothing.

ATOPIC DERMATITIS

Atopic dermatitis is a common pruritic inflammatory dermatosis seen most often as a chronic, recurring problem in persons with a hereditary predisposition toward allergy. Although this disorder usually appears first during infancy or childhood, it often extends into adolescence and adulthood.

Atopic dermatitis has been attributed to an immunologic defect because a significant percentage of clients have a personal or family history of allergic disease. Presence of conditions such as hay fever, asthma, and allergic rhinitis have been closely linked with the development of atopic dermatitis.

Attacks of atopic dermatitis may be set off or made worse by several factors. An episode of pruritus may develop from irritating or occlusive topical medications, items of clothing such as wool or silk, rapid changes or extremes in temperature, or too much bathing. Approximately 10% of the clients with atopic dermatitis respond allergically to foods, inhalation of allergens, and direct contact with irri-

| Box 79–1 | Self-Care Instructions for the Client With Contact Dermatitis |

Limit exposure to household or occupational irritants if possible

Wear protective clothing or gloves when contact cannot be avoided

Wash new clothing and bed linens before use

Avoid clothing made from synthetics known to cause irritation and wear as many natural fabrics as possible

Avoid any natural fabrics such as wool or silk if they are allergens

Use hypoallergenic cosmetics, jewelry, etc.

Avoid abrasive soaps

Lubricate skin to prevent cracking

Wear protective creams

Become aware of drugs known to cause sensitization, and monitor contents of any medication being used

Wash skin and clothing thoroughly after exposure to allergens

tants. Emotional stress, which triggers anxiety, frustration, aggression, and hostility, is a key factor known to precipitate symptom recurrence.

Clinical Manifestations

No distinct primary lesions may be apparent in adulthood. The skin is usually markedly dry and contains papular lichenified plaques, excoriations, erosions, and crusts (Figure 79–8). Areas of involvement include cubital and popliteal fossae, anterior and lateral aspects of the neck, forehead, face, wrists, and dorsa of the hands and feet. Hand dermatitis is common.

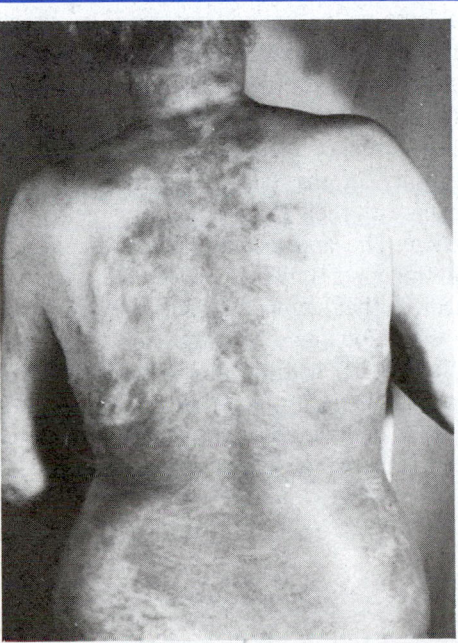
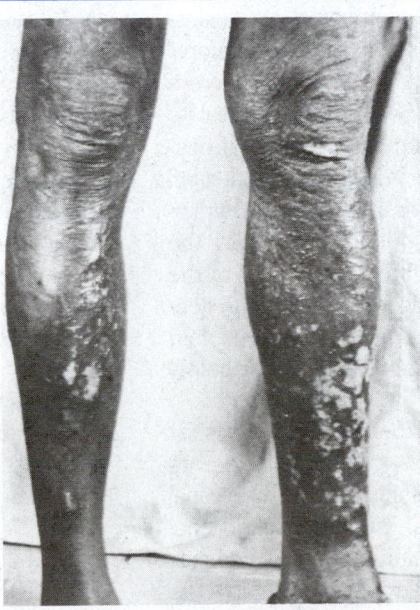

Figure 79–8

Atopic dermatitis. **Left.** Acute atopic dermatitis with erythema. **Right.** Chronic atopic dermatitis with lichenification. (Courtesy of Millard Fillmore Hospital, Buffalo, NY)

The most outstanding feature in atopic dermatitis is the presence of intense pruritus. A vicious cycle develops in which the client feels an itch, scratches it, a rash develops, and the rash itches. Lichenification, which involves the thickening of skin from repeated rubbing and scratching over an extended period, further reduces the skin's threshold to withstand irritation, and the cycle becomes more permanent.

Lesions are vulnerable to invasion by microorganisms. Bacterial infections from staphylococci and streptococci are likely, as is contamination by the herpes simplex virus.

Therapeutic Measures

Treatment of adult-type atopic dermatitis aims at eliminating precipitating factors and pruritus, suppressing the inflammatory process, lubricating the skin, and providing essential emotional support. Management of this condition is highly individualized and takes into account the usual necessity for long-term therapy.

The mainstay of treatment for atopic dermatitis is the use of topical corticosteroids. Specific drugs and strengths must be individually determined and altered according to the regression or resolution of the symptoms. Fluorinated corticosteroids may be used short term to initiate healing, but replacement by other anti-inflammatory agents is important to avoid untoward skin changes. Ointments and occlusive therapy are preferred because penetration is faster. Because of keratolytic actions, coal tar preparations may be used as adjuvant therapy along with the corticosteroids.

Antibiotic therapy is used whenever the presence of bacteria is confirmed. Wet dressings are prescribed when a draining lesion appears. Ultraviolet light has beneficial effects, and sunlight or an artificial UVL source may be used judiciously.

Dealing with the pruritus that accompanies atopic dermatitis may be difficult and require a multidimensional approach to both physiological and psychological factors (see Chapter 78). Covering the affected areas has no value, and lesions often appear beyond the borders of the dressing. Emollients (petrolatum, Eucerin, Nivea) can lessen the dryness. Antihistamines such as hydroxyzine hydrochloride (Atarax, Vistaril) may be incorporated into the regimen, although the benefits are limited. Because of the effects of prostaglandin, a pathogenic factor in itching, acetylsalicylic acid (aspirin) may be administered on a full dosage scale (300–600 mg daily with increases to just below the level causing tinnitus).

Tranquilizers and sedatives may be prescribed to assist in the alleviation of psychic stress or emotional factors influencing the dermatosis. If drugs and normal emotional supports do not resolve problems, further professional counseling may be required to decondition the learned pattern of response to the pathologic cycle or to assist the client in recognizing and coping with emotional stressors. As identified by Griesemer and Nadelson, pruritus is often

---

Box 79–2   Self-Care Instructions for the Client With Atopic Dermatitis

Provide a climate and humidity-controlled environment to avoid overwarming, chilling, sweating, and excessive dryness

Wear clothing that is absorbent and nonirritating

Launder clothing with bland soaps

Rest and relax

Avoid excessive bathing and use of irritating soaps

Avoid known allergens or sensitizers, especially topical anesthetics or antihistamines

Protect skin from secondary infection

Avoid vaccinations or contact with persons who have been vaccinated (Kaposi's varicelliform eruptions, a viral disease, may develop.)

Avoid contact with persons who have herpetic lesions (Disseminated eruptions may occur from self-inoculation.)

Practice stress management techniques

---

used to release tension, particularly resulting from anger or guilt (Fitzpatrick, 1979). The perception of itching becomes more obvious when an individual is experiencing fear, stress, boredom, and depression.

Specific Nursing Measures

The instructions in Box 79–2 will facilitate the client's understanding and ability to prevent recurrence and complications when treated in other health care settings. Clients with atopic dermatitis may need hospitalization when a therapeutic environment is required to disrupt the ravages of pruritus or when self-care is not feasible.

The supportive care given to these clients is important because problems with atopic dermatitis may extend through a lifetime. If the disease has had its beginnings in infancy or early childhood, the adult may have long-standing behavior patterns that need recognition. There may be an inability to respond pleasurably to touch or to accept the appearance of the body. Sometimes people become preoccupied with their skin disorder or the potential for exacerbation. The appearance of skin manifestations may provide the opportunity to receive the attention of others or to receive other secondary gains. For example, an eczematous condition may excuse an adolescent who feels inept from participating in sports. Job-related dermatitis may provide an adult with an excuse to seek out a less strenuous position. Identifying the needs and feelings of each client is important before adaptability can be fostered.

URTICARIA

Urticaria, or hives, is a common vascular dermatosis characterized by the appearance of transient wheals; it may be acute or chronic. Deeper involvement of the dermis and subcutaneous tissue is referred to as angioedema.

Urticaria is most frequently caused by drugs (penicillin, salicylates, sulfonamides); foods (strawberries, chocolate, tomatoes, shellfish, pork, cheese, and spices); insect bites; and inhalants. Special types of urticaria have been associated with exposure to physical agents (cold, natural, and artificial sunlight); increased body temperature (cholinergic urticaria); and with systemic illnesses such as autoimmune disease, internal malignancy, and infection. Brisk stroking of the skin or a constant pressure is known to cause the appearance of wheals and is referred to as *dermagraphism*. Although emotional stress has also been closely linked with the occurrence of chronic urticaria, a vast number of recurring cases are labeled idiopathic.

Clinical Manifestations

Lesions form because the histamine released during the immune response causes localized or generalized vasodilation, increased capillary permeability, and subsequent extravasation of proteins and fluids into the tissues. Inspection reveals local, regional, or generalized papules and edematous plaques, which vary in size and number. Larger lesions have a blanched center with a reddened halo. The trunk, hands, feet, lips, and ears are the sites most commonly affected.

The client with urticaria will have pruritus, often intense, along with stinging, prickling, numbness, and a feeling of flushing. True urticaria usually disappears within 24 hours. Persistence of the lesions indicates more extensive problems. In addition to cutaneous manifestations, other signs and symptoms may indicate the presence of anaphylaxis or serum sickness. (Refer to Chapter 13 for a discussion of anaphylaxis.)

Therapeutic and Specific Nursing Measures

The prime objective in treatment is the removal (or the future avoidance) of the precipitating factor. This may require that the nurse help the client to plan a method of identifying the contributing cause or causes, such as keeping a personal record. Administration of antihistamines is the other important component of therapy, whether given for a short duration or prophylactically for recurring problems. In addition to hydroxyzine hydrochloride (Atarax, Vistaril), chlorpheniramine maleate (Chlor-Trimeton), cyproheptadine hydrochloride (Periactin), or diphenhydramine hydrochloride (Benadryl) may be prescribed. Side effects such as drowsiness and dry mouth may become a problem when dosages are increased to the limit of tolerance. Colloidal or tepid baths, cool or ice water compresses, and antipruritic lotions or emulsions (calamine) may be used to treat subjective complaints.

The nurse is primarily involved in the prevention of future episodes by providing appropriate client instruc-

tions; however, the nurse must be alert for urticarial manifestations provoked by drugs the client is receiving. Additional support may be necessary when emotions play a role in the pathogenesis.

DRUG ERUPTIONS

The skin is frequently affected by adverse drug reactions. As many as 40% of hospitalized clients will develop adverse reactions as a result of therapeutic usage of multiple drugs (Fitzpatrick, 1979). A cause for the cutaneous eruptions is basically unknown, but mechanisms of drug reactions have been attributed in some degree to allergy, pharmacologic factors (overdosage, drug interactions), and unexplained client idiosyncracies.

Clinical Manifestations

Lesions may occur immediately after taking the drug or be delayed for several days. Initially, the reaction may begin in a localized area and progress to a generalized state, in which the total surface of the body is involved.

In addition to anaphylaxis, serious and life-threatening situations can develop in which multiple bullous lesions appear, although this is rare. Toxic epidermal necrolysis, in which the full thickness of the epidermis is detached—a syndrome that mimics systemic lupus erythematosus—and exfoliative dermatitis, a generalized scaling eruption (Figure 79–9), are also major untoward effects.

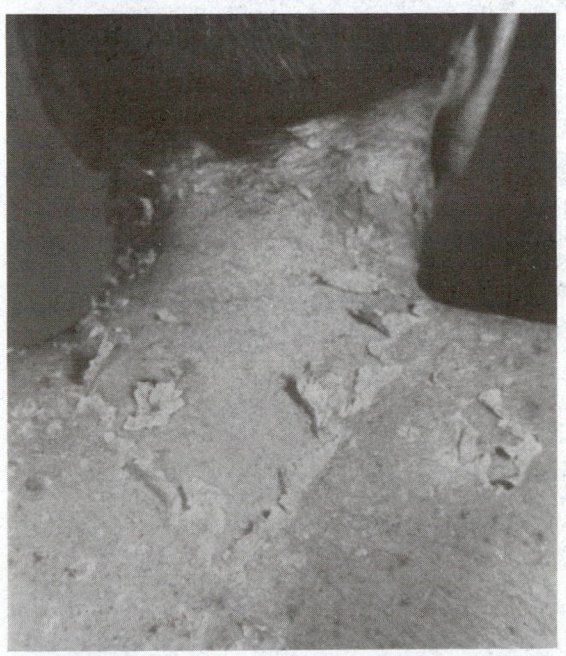

Figure 79–9

Exfolliative dermatitis from reaction to penicillin. (Courtesy of Millard Fillmore Hospital, Buffalo, NY)

Table 79–1 lists selected cutaneous manifestations and the drugs known to produce these adverse reactions. A pharmacology or dermatology text will provide more detailed information.

Therapeutic and Specific Nursing Measures

The drug or drugs responsible for the eruptions must be discontinued. Treatment is similar to that of urticaria. A careful history of drug allergies and idiosyncrasies elicited upon admission and clearly noted on the client's chart is an important preventive tool. The following questions should be answered: Have you ever developed any allergic reactions when using prescribed or over-the-counter drugs? Were they taken orally; used topically; or administered by injection, inhalation, instillation, or suppository? What kind of reaction did you have? Can you describe the skin changes? If the allergic response occurred during the client's hospitalization, a list of drugs received on a routine, stat, or p.r.n. basis must be identified in addition to any anesthetic and diagnostic agents. Management of allergies includes discontinuing the offending drugs followed by treatment of symptoms. If serious damage and losses of the integument occur, the focus of concern becomes preventing fluid and electrolyte loss, infection, and major metabolic alteration.

PEMPHIGUS VULGARIS

A number of dermatological disorders involve the appearance of bullous eruptions that are of limited consequence. Pemphigus vulgaris, however, is a serious chronic condition of the skin and mucous membranes that could prove fatal if not properly treated or if very severe.

The disorder results from an autoimmune response that disrupts the basement membrane of the skin and may be seen in persons who already have an autoimmune disease. It occurs with notable frequency among those of Jewish and Mediterranean ancestry, usually after the age of 40.

Table 79–1	Adverse Cutaneous Manifestations Associated With Drug Therapy
Cutaneous Manifestations	**Drugs**
Urticaria (most common)	Acetylsalicylic acid Blood and blood products Codeine Diazepam Morphine Penicillins and related antibiotics Radiopaque media Serum Sulfonamides
Exanthema (rash resembling measles or scarlet fever)	Allopurinol Para-aminosalicylic acid Penicillins and related antibiotics
Photosensitivity	Chlorothiazides Demeclocycline Phenothiazines Psoralens Sulfonamides Sulfonylureas
Fixed drug reactions (circumscribed hyperpigmented or purplish-red lesions, macular to bullous, which recur at the same site with each readministration)	Barbiturates Phenolphthalein Phenylbutazone Sulfonamides
Bullae	Barbiturates Bromides Iodides Phenylbutazone Sulfonamides
Purpura	Indomethacin Phenylbutazone Quinidine
Acneiform	ACTH Androgenic hormones Diphenylhydantoin Glucocorticoids Lithium
Alopecia	Coumarin derivatives Cytotoxics

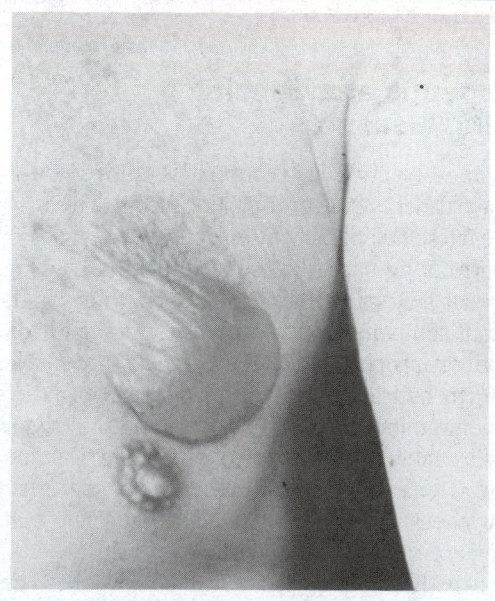

Figure 79–10

Bulla in pemphigus vulgaris. (Courtesy of Millard Fillmore Hospital, Buffalo, NY)

Clinical Manifestations

Cutaneous eruptions may develop on any part of the body although a predilection for the scalp, face, chest, axillae, groin, and umbilicus has been recognized. Bullous lesions appear as tense, fluid-filled sacs that erupt easily, ooze, and bleed (Figure 79–10). Erosions also develop on the mucous membranes of the mouth, nose, pharynx, larynx, vagina, and gastrointestinal tract. Pemphigus vulgaris may begin with a localized area, progressing to a generalized state.

Therapeutic Measures

Prognosis is directly related to the institution of therapy and the scope of surface involvement. Clients are given immunosuppressants such as azathioprine (Imuran) in combination with systemic corticosteroids or cytotoxic drugs such as cyclophosphamide (Cytoxan) until remission has occurred. Maintenance on steroids is then necessary.

Specific Nursing Measures

Major nursing concerns focus on the prevention and treatment of life-threatening problems. Localized infections may progress to septicemia, and extensive losses of skin may subject the client to fluid imbalances sufficient to produce a hypovolemic crisis. Hospitalization is often required so that a protective environment can be provided, fluid replaced, and nutrition supplemented. Intensive nursing care may become necessary along with the definitive therapeutic regimen to treat the lesions. Several of the principles related to burn care apply to the client with severe pemphigus vulgaris.

Section IV: Infections and Infestations

An infection generally results from direct bacterial, viral, or fungal invasion of the integument. Cutaneous manifestations and the systemic communicable diseases they represent are not addressed here because they occur primarily in childhood or no longer exist as common adult problems. The exception is herpes zoster. Skin lesions associated with sexually transmitted disease are discussed with disorders of the reproductive system in Chapters 64 and 67.

Secondary infections of the skin may develop in an area weakened by a primary dermatosis; by degeneration of the circulatory system (causing stasis dermatitis, leg ulcers); by trauma; by insect bites; or by the presence of neurologic deficits (causing decubitus ulcers following spinal cord injuries). In the integument, infestations involve the habitation or invasion of skin and hair by arthropods classified as mites and insects, protozoans, and helminths.

Because the surface area of the body is constantly exposed to a multitude of pathogenic organisms, the skin is a potential target area for infection. If the body's defenses fail, a superficial infection may begin and possibly lead to serious systemic involvement. The keratinized cells of the epidermis prove highly resistive to infectious disease until the host defenses are disturbed, permeability of the skin increases, or the virulence of the microorganism increases. Some factors that increase vulnerability to a skin infection are: poor health; poor hygiene; malnutrition; a warm humid climate; obesity; use of systemic steroids, antibiotics and chemotherapy; immunodeficiencies; the presence of dysglobulinemia, leukemia, or diabetes; and a break in the continuity of the skin (accidental, intentional, or pathogenic).

The skin supports normal flora of various kinds. Those that flourish on the exposed areas such as the face, neck, and hands differ from those on the moist cutaneous surface of the axilla, groin, perineum and between the toes or those on the upper arm, trunk, and legs. *Staphylococcus aureus*, for example, is found more abundantly on the exposed areas of the skin, whereas gram-negative bacilli are usually located in moist areas. Organisms may become pathogenic when they are picked up on the hands and moved to a surface not prepared to resist them. Antibiotics, topical medications, soaps, and deodorants may alter the skin's innate protective mechanisms and allow pathogenesis. Organisms may spread to deeper levels of the integument when an increased temperature dilates pores.

General Nursing Implications

Prevention of infections and infestations should be a foremost nursing goal. Skin that is allowed to become moist, warm, and permeable to pathogens becomes a fertile area for infection. The risk of infection also increases significantly when the skin has multiple folds and crevices that are not accessible to light and to good aeration to facilitate drying.

Good hygiene is an important therapeutic goal because it will discourage most skin infections as well as some types of infestations. Cleanliness, adequate aeration, optimal moisturization, and provision of protective measures for high-risk persons must be included in a nursing plan of care, whether the client is in a hospital, an outpatient clinic, an ambulatory care setting, a place of work, or wherever the nurse has occasion to promote health and prevent illness.

SPECIFIC NURSING MEASURES FOR BACTERIAL SKIN INFECTIONS

The normal skin is inhabited by gram-positive cocci, primarily staphylococci (S epidermidis, S albus) and gram-positive diphtheroids or bacilli (Corynebacterium acnes,

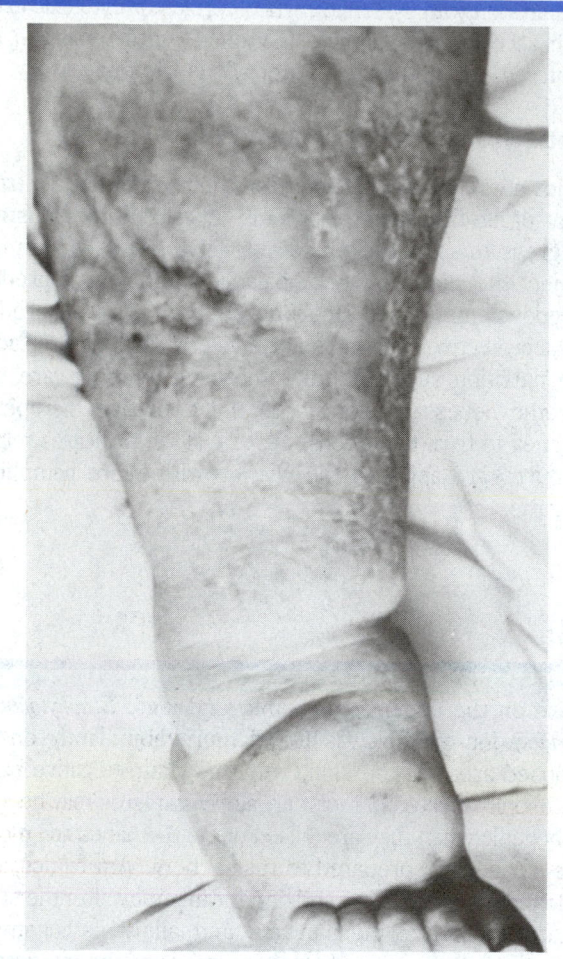

Figure 79–11

Cellulitis. (Courtesy of Millard Fillmore Hospital, Buffalo, NY)

Propionibacterium acnes). Gram-negative bacteria *(E coli, Proteus, Enterobacter, Pseudomonas)* are not commonly found on the skin surface except in the warm, moist intertrigenous areas. Most pyodermas are caused by staphylococci and a few by streptococci. These bacteria may penetrate as deep as the subcutaneous tissue. Skin infections caused by bacterial organisms include impetigo, folliculitis, furuncles, carbuncles, erysipelas, and cellulitis (Figure 79–11). These specific skin infections and their incidence, causative agent, manifestations, duration, and treatment measures are described in Table 79–2.

A plan of care involves preventive measures as well as therapy to prevent recurrence and to protect others. Contagion is associated with impetigo, and contamination of other family members is not uncommon. Staphylococci colonize more readily in moist cutaneous lesions; therefore, maintenance of dry skin is an important nursing consideration. Removing crusts associated with impetigo is

critical because beta hemolytic organisms thrive under semiaerobic conditions.

Bacteria may arrive on the skin from sites that normally harbor potential pathogens, such as the upper airways. Antibiotic creams or ointments may be instilled into the anterior nares daily until the problem is resolved. Hygiene is important so bathing and shampooing with bactericidal (providone-iodine) or bacteriostatic (hexachlorophene) soaps are necessary, especially for family members who may have direct contact with the infected person or may be at high risk because of immunosuppression or breaks in the continuity of the skin.

Use of separate towels, washcloths, and bed linens and daily laundering are recommended. Handkerchiefs should be replaced by disposable paper tissues. Because those who work with oils and greases show an increased incidence of follicular infections, they should be informed that drying of the skin and avoidance of irritating and occlusive clothing may help avoid problems.

SPECIFIC NURSING MEASURES FOR VIRAL SKIN INFECTIONS

Cutaneous viral infection develops below the stratum corneum and depends on the ability of the virus to adapt within the host cell. If the parasitic virus interferes with normal cellular structure and function, a local inflammatory process along with the formation of lesions and cell destruction may develop. The disorder need not become manifest and could remain latent because the organism is not sufficiently virulent to produce pathologic alterations in the host cells.

Herpesvirus hominis type I causes cutaneous facial manifestations known as "cold sores" or "fever blisters" and herpetic whitlow, an infection involving the nail margins (paronychia), fingers, and hands. Herpes zoster, another form of viral-induced dermatosis, results from reactivation of latent varicella-zoster virus. This virus is called varicella-zoster because it is indistinguishable from the virus that causes varicella (chicken pox). Warts, or veruccae, although considered to be intraepidermal tumors, are caused by infection with the human papilloma virus. The viral skin infections, their incidence, causative agent, clinical manifestations, duration, and treatment measures are discussed in Table 79–3 and illustrated in Figure 79–12.

Contagion is a prime nursing concern with viral skin infections. Protective efforts become critical when a client has a medical disorder or is receiving drugs that interfere seriously with the immune response. Prevention of contact is essential because exposure to infected individuals may prove life threatening, particularly to immunocompromised persons.

Inoculation herpes (herpetic whitlow) should be a concern for dental, medical, and nursing personnel because herpetic lesions may develop through direct hand or finger contact with the vesicular fluid of the area of involvement

Table 79-2 Bacterial Skin Infections

Condition and Causative Agent	Incidence/Comments	Clinical Manifestations	Duration	Treatment Measures
Impetigo (group A *Streptococcus, Staphylococcus,* or mixed)	Very common and contagious; seen primarily in children and young adults; approximately 5% of cases may be complicated by post-streptococcal glomerulonephritis	Erythematous macules, oozing vesicles; usually seen on face, arms, and legs; varying degrees of pruritus	Days	Penicillin (long acting or divided doses); oxacillin for staphylococcal infection; erythromycin soak 3–4 times a day with warm water, saline, or soap solution to remove crusts
Folliculitis (*Staphylococcus*)	Common infection of hair follicles; serious implications with scalp, nasal, and eye involvement	Superficial or deep pustules may be scattered or discrete; frequently seen on the face; also appears on trunk and extremities; pain	Self-limited	Topical hygiene and antibiotics; remove predisposing factors (oils, tar)
Furuncle (*Staphylococcus*)	Deep follicular abscess; may have progressed from folliculitis; commonly found on hair-bearing skin where friction and sweating occur; seen in children, adolescents, and young adults	Firm, red, hard nodule that ruptures and discharges a purulent core; may ulcerate; usually seen on face, scalp, neck, buttocks, and axilla; highly tender and may cause throbbing pain	Days	Moist heat; topical or systemic antibiotics sensitive to *Staphylococcus* (penicillin, erythromycin); recurrence may require long-term therapy and consideration for bacterial interference therapy
Carbuncle (*Staphylococcus*)	Collection of furuncles; commonly seen in thick inelastic skin	Similar to furuncles but with multiple points of drainage; usually appear on neck, back, and thighs; very painful; systemic signs such as fever, malaise	Heal slowly and produce scarring	Similar to furuncles; surgical incision only if absolutely necessary
Erysipelas (beta hemolytic *Streptococcus*)	Acute highly inflammatory infection involving subcutaneous tissue; uncommon; occurs in very young and elderly	Bright red, tender, hot, sharply defined bordered plaque, which may develop superficial vesicles and bullae; usually seen on face and around the ears; pain at the site of infection	2–3 wks; recurrence common	Bed rest; oral or parenteral antibiotics (penicillin, erythromycin); local cool, wet dressing for comfort
Cellulitis (gram-positive bacillus: *Streptococcus, Staphylococcus*); (gram-negative bacillus: *Escherichia coli, Proteus, Klebsiella*)	Deep subcutaneous tissue involvement; usually a complication of ulcerations, decubiti, wounds, dermatitis	Dependent on causative organism; extensive erythema and tenderness with gram-positive; warmth and slight redness, brawny edema (increasing as infection progresses) with gram-negative; malaise, fever, chills, enlarged lymph nodes		Bed rest; systemic antibiotic specific for causative organism; surgical drainage; treatment of primary disease

Table 79-3 Viral Skin Infections

Condition and Causative Agent	Incidence/Comments	Clinical Manifestations	Duration	Treatment Measures
Herpes simplex type 1 (cold sores, fever blisters, canker sores caused by *Herpesvirus hominis*)	Common disorder; primary infection occurs in young children; recurrence usually associated with adults; frequently seen in women; herpesencephalitis is a possible complication	Clusters of vesicles or vesicopustules on an erythematous base; may ulcerate or crust; appears on lips near mucocutaneous junction, cheek; burning, itching, tingling may develop	5-8 days; recurrent	Symptomatic treatment because of self-limiting nature; keep lesions dry (70% alcohol, Blistex); topical antibiotic; topical anesthetic
Herpetic whitlow or inoculation herpes (caused by *Herpesvirus hominis*)	Primary or recurrent; occurs on damaged or broken skin (burns, needle punctures; often seen in health personnel who come in contact with oral secretions or lesions of infected clients	Lesions of fingers, paronychia, and hands; erythema and edema develop with multiple discrete vesicles at the margins of the lesion; tingling sensation followed by intense, throbbing pain; lymphadenopathy and lymphangitis; possibility of fever, chills, and malaise	3-4 wks; recurrence possible	Analgesics for pain; topical acyclovir (Zovirax)
Herpes zoster (shingles) caused by activation of latent varicella-zoster virus	Majority over age 40; initially infected with varicella virus (chickenpox); organism resides in dorsal root of cranial and spinal nerve ganglia; 50% of clients develop ophthalmic involvement	Erythematous papules that progress into vesicles, pustules, and crusts; seen unilaterally, primarily on dermatomes of the thorax and less frequently in cervical, trigeminal, and lumbosacral areas; pain along the course of a peripheral sensory nerve can precede the eruptions; postherpetic neuralgia	Approximately 3 wks	Symptomatic treatment with analgesics; for vesicular stage use cool compresses with Burow's solution, drying lotion, splinting of area with dressing to relieve pain; systemic corticosteroids in selected acute cases; ophthalmic corticosteroids with keratoconjunctivitis involvement; immunosuppressed clients may receive cytosine arabinoside, interferon, acyclovir, zoster immune globulin (ZIG)
Verrucae (warts) caused by human papilloma virus	Benign epidermal tumors; any age but most commonly seen at 12-16 yr; spread by contact or autoinoculation	All warts manifest a local epidermal proliferation and keratinization	Many warts are self-limiting to within a few weeks, months or years because of spontaneous involution	Common keratolytic therapy; painting of lesions with salicylic acid and lactic acid mixtures (SAL, Duofilm, Keralyt); cryosurgery; light electrosurgery; avoid treatment that scars; immunotherapy less common

Condition and Causative Agent	Incidence/Comments	Clinical Manifestations	Duration	Treatment Measures
				but used with resistive lesions (DNCB application); topical or oral vitamin A; topical 5-fluorouracil; intralesional bleomycin
a. V. vulgaris (common wart)		Firm papules; hyperkeratotic surface with vegetation; isolated or clustered on hands, fingers, knees		
b. V. plantaris (plantar or palmar wart)	Often follows trauma	Small papules and plaques with a rough, hyperkeratotic surface; isolated; many (mosaic pattern) at pressure points, particularly on feet; may become painful		
c. V. planae (flat wart)		Flat-surfaced papules, usually numerous, closely set on face, dorsa of hand, shins, or knees		
d. Condylomata acuminata (moist or anogenital wart) (see also Chapters 64 and 67)	Young adults with increasing frequency	Minute papules appearing in cauliflowerlike masses or clusters; may enlarge significantly; isolated or multiple lesions within anorectal area, urethral meatus, and on the cervical and vaginal mucosa	Weeks to yrs; spontaneous remissions; recurrence possible	Topical podophyllum resin, 5-fluorouracil, DNCB therapy; cryosurgery; electrocautery; surgical excision with large lesions

or by contamination from oral–pharyngeal–tracheal secretions. Use of gloves is recommended when caring for or treating clients with suspected lesions or those who have a potential to develop herpetic lesions.

Prevention of recurring herpes simplex should be incorporated into a treatment plan. Emotional stress, exposure to sunlight, illness, menstruation, and fatigue have been identified as precipitating factors. Proper use of sunscreens and maintenance of healthful living are basic to avoidance of recurrence.

With increased frequency, herpes zoster is being complicated by postherpetic neuralgia in the elderly. Pain becomes chronic and difficult to alleviate. Use of antipsychotic drugs and transcutaneous electrical stimulators may be necessary in severe cases.

Plantar warts are known to occur more readily on surface areas that are moist and sustain friction. The importance of drying the feet and cushioning these areas should be stressed. Many people apply keratolytic agents to warts with or without the direction of a health care provider. Drugs that destroy cutaneous lesions may also be injurious to healthy skin, and users need to know this. Instruct clients to protect the surrounding skin with petroleum jelly and to make sure that a small amount of the keratolytic has been applied to the lesion only. Nursing measures for genital warts are discussed in Chapters 64 and 67.

SPECIFIC NURSING MEASURES FOR FUNGAL SKIN INFECTIONS

Superficial mycoses or fungal infections of the skin are among the most common types of dermatoses. Mycoses are caused by vegetative cellular organisms known as *der-*

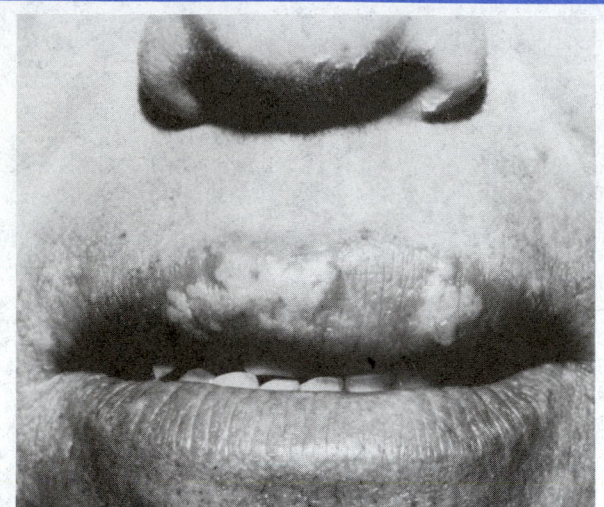

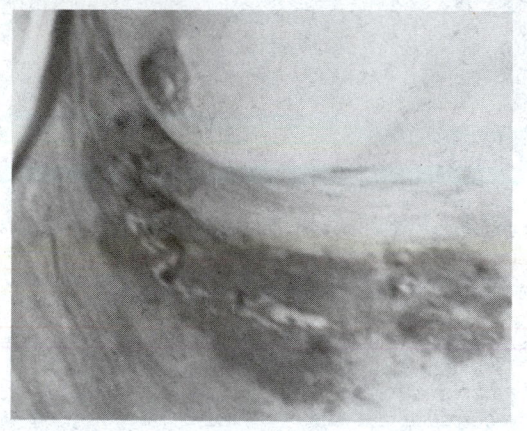

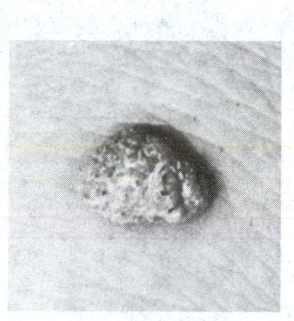

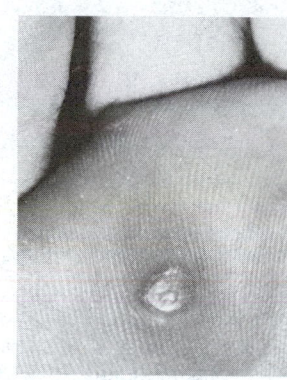

Figure 79–12

Viral skin infections. **A.** Herpes labialis ("cold sore," "fever blister"). **B.** Herpes zoster showing distribution along nerve. **C.** Verruca vulgaris, the common wart. **D.** Verruca plantaris, plantar wart on the sole of the foot.

SOURCE: **A, C, D:** Binnick SA: *Skin Diseases: Diagnosis and Management in Clinical Practice*. Baltimore, MD: Williams & Wilkins, 1982; **B:** Courtesy of Millard Fillmore Hospital, Buffalo, NY.

matophytes, which can survive on the dead horny layers of the skin and some of the appendages such as the nails (Figure 79–13). Because of strong host resistance in a healthy integument, the overall incidence of fungal infection is kept relatively low.

Dermatophytosis, commonly referred to as tinea or ringworm, results from superficial fungal invasion usually limited to a depth of 1 or 2 mm. The hair and nails may also be affected. Tinea versicolor is another type of superficial infection that primarily involves the trunk of the body. Candidiasis or moniliasis is a deeper fungal dermatosis that involves a localized or generalized infection of mucocutaneous tissue. Common sites affected include the margin of the nails, intertriginous areas, oral and vaginal mucosa, and the corners of the mouth.

Blastomycosis, coccidioidomycosis, and histoplasmosis are all deep fungal infections that produce cutaneous lesions in addition to systemic involvement. The major port of entry is the lung, and additional information is available in Chapter 20.

Sources of infecting agents include soil, animals, and

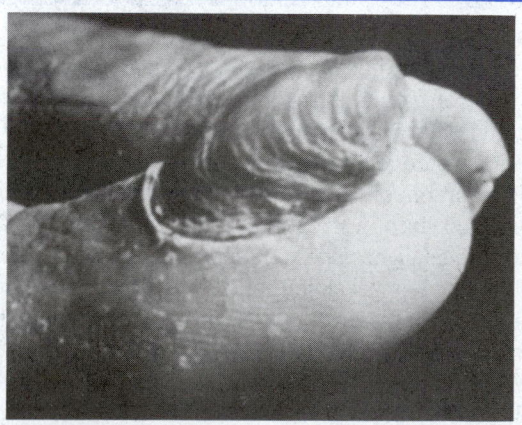

Figure 79–13

Fungal infection of the toenail (onychomycosis). The nail is thick, ridged, and brown. (Courtesy of Millard Fillmore Hospital, Buffalo, NY)

other humans. Besides direct contact with other infected persons, the coexistence of poor nutrition and poor hygiene, hot and humid climates, the presence of debilitating and certain neoplastic diseases, the use of immunosuppressants and long-term use of topical corticosteroids predispose the skin to the development of fungal lesions.

In the case of tinea pedis, or athletes' foot, the addition of minor trauma to the skin is thought to be necessary for infection to occur.

Candida albicans, a yeastlike fungus, is normally found on mucous membranes, skin, and within the gastrointestinal tract and the vagina. However, given the right set of circumstances, the organisms have a potential for causing candidiasis. Predisposing factors include a hot and humid environment that allows unaerated skin surfaces to become excessively moist; macerated skin from occlusive dressings or clothing; systemic use of antibiotics, corticosteroids, or contraceptives; pregnancy; diabetes, Cushing's disease; and poor general health. Fungal skin infections, their incidence, causative agent, clinical manifestations, duration, and treatment measures are discussed in Table 79–4.

Prophylactic measures are the first line of defense against fungal infections and become more important when the predisposing factors are numerous. Intertriginous and interdigital areas must be kept clean and dry. Bathing and application of a simple talc or antifungal powder at least once a day may prevent initial irritation. Shoes and clothing should allow for proper aeration and not build up moisture as plastic footwear, sneakers, wool, and synthetic fibers do. Advise clients to wear nonocclusive shoes and absorbent socks, preferably made of cotton. Wool socks worn by hikers and skiers tend to trap moisture. Frequent changes of apparel along with proper laundering in hot water are also important.

Use of griseofulvin (Fulvicin-U/F, Grifulven V), a fungistatic and fungicidal antibiotic, has been effective in the treatment of dermatophytes, especially when topical antifungals fail to resolve the condition. Clients with liver failure or penicillin sensitivity should not receive this drug. Anyone using griseofulvin must be cautioned to avoid direct sunlight to prevent photosensitivity and to watch for possible allergic manifestations, gastrointestinal intolerance, and headache.

Although griseofulvin is used to treat tineal infections, onychomycosis is rarely cured by this drug or other therapy. The length of treatment, the unsightliness of the hands, and the catching of nails on clothing may become discouraging to clients, who often need emotional support.

Several cutaneous fungal infections have a tendency to recur. Clients should understand their role in prevention and continuance of prescribed care.

SPECIFIC NURSING MEASURES FOR PARASITIC INFESTATIONS

Dermatologic parasites are an extensive problem around the world because of bites and skin invasion by protozoans, helminths, and arthropods. The focus in this discussion will be on scabies, pediculosis, and tick bites because they are a common cause of dermatologic problems.

At one time, scabies and pediculosis were associated with the poor and with unclean living conditions. A freer sexual climate has changed this picture significantly. Sexual transmission has joined low socioeconomic status as an influencing factor in the transmission of scabies.

Ticks can become attached to anyone because they inhabit wooded areas, brush, and grass. Ticks may also attach to other mammals, birds, and reptiles, making them carriers of ticks. The parasitic skin infestations, their incidence, causative agents, clinical manifestations, duration, and treatment measures are discussed in Table 79–5.

As much as possible, transmission of pediculoses and scabies must be halted once the problem has been identified. Pesticides must be used to destroy the parasites. In addition, clothing, bed linens, and toweling require washing in boiling water, dry cleaning, ironing, or dusting with appropriate pesticides to prevent reinfestation from parasites and their ova. Those who have come in intimate contact with an infested client or who share clothing, hair brushes, combs, or bed linens may need treatment as well.

Protection against ticks may be obtained by applying insect repellents containing diethyltoluamide (Mosquitone lotion, Off liquid, Cutter Insect Repellent Cream) to skin and clothing. Wearing protective clothing in wooded areas is also a preventive measure. Proper removal of ticks is discussed in Table 79–5.

Section V: Neoplasia

The abnormal proliferation of cells within the various layers of skin is a common dermatological problem. Many integumentary lesions are benign, with a few classified as precancerous. The three major types of malignancies originate either in the epidermal layer of skin or the melanocyte.

Neoplasms of the skin provoke great concern about disfigurement when lesions occur on the head and neck. Of added importance is the fact that a significant per-

centage of people will develop primary carcinomas of the integument.

Skin cancer is the most frequent malignancy estimated at more than 400,000 new cases per year (American Cancer Society, 1985). Malignant melanoma is expected to account for 22,000 of these cases. Although the mortality is minimal compared to the death rate from primary tumors of other organs, and the systemic involvement is

Table 79–4 Fungal Skin Infections

Condition and Causative Agent	Incidence/Comments	Clinical Manifestations	Duration	Treatment Measures
Tinea (ringworm) caused by *Microsporum, Trichophyton, Epidermophyton*		All tinea infections involve an inflammatory process; pain and itching may be present	All, except those involving the nails, are of short duration when adequate treatment is given	Hygienic measures; topical antifungal solutions or creams treat most superficial fungal infections of the skin: clotrimazole (Lotrimin); miconazole (Monistat-Derm); haloprogin (Halotex); tolnaftate (Tinactin); may be combined with a keratolytic agent to soften and exfoliate skin; systemic griseofulvin for widespread or rapidly progressing infection, recalcitrant (hair, nails), or recurrent lesions
a. T. capitis (scalp)	Rare after puberty; highly contagious	Scaling patches with hair loss or breaking of the shafts		
b. T. barbae (beard)	Rare; seen in adult men, such as farmers in contact with contaminated cattle	Sharp scaling, loss of hair; kerion formation (inflamed purulent lesion) in a deeper infection		
c. T. corporis (non-hairy smooth skin)	Most common in children	Inflamed circinate patches or plaques common on exposed areas, face, arms		
d. T. cruris (groin)	Very common, mainly in men; may occur concomitantly with T. pedis	Scaly patches or plaques, usually symmetrical; may extend into gluteal folds and buttocks		
e. T. manuum (hands)	Usually seen with T. pedis and onychomycosis	Unilateral mild erythema with hyperkeratosis and scaling on palmar surface		
f. T. pedis (athlete's foot)	Most common fungal infection; generally seen in adults	Scaling, maceration, and fissures of toe webs; occasional vesicles and bullae; secondary bacterial infection	Recurrent	
g. T. onychomycosis (nails)	40% of cases have fungal infection elsewhere	Whitish discoloration and thickening of nail plate with possible separation from nail bed	Difficult to cure	
h. T. versicolor; caused by *Pityrosporon furfur*	Represents 5% of all fungal infection; common to young adults, usually in summer months	Lesions varying in color (white, pinkish-brown); macular scaling patches usually found on trunk and upper arms; light and	Recurrent; untreated conditions last for years	Wide range of treatment; topical application to affected areas with selenium sulfide (Selsun), 25% sodium hyposulfite, keratolytic

Condition and Causative Agent	Incidence/Comments	Clinical Manifestations	Duration	Treatment Measures
		dark pigmentary changes		creams (Keralyt Gel), imidazole creams and lotions (Lotrimin, Monistat-Derm, Halotex, Tinactin); hygienic measures
Candidiasis caused by *Candida albicans*				
a. Monilial paronychia (skin surrounding nails)	Occurs often in house-wives from frequent water immersion of hands	Painful swelling around nail plate		Gloves and cotton liner to protect hands; wet Burow's solution soaks for inflammation
b. Monilial intertrigo	Common	Pruritus, burning; red eroded patches with axillary, inframammary, umbilical, anogenital, or interdigital involvement		Topical antifungal agents; amphotericin B (Fungizone); nystatin (Mycostatin)
c. Perlèche (may also be caused by streptococci or staphylococci)	A form of cheilosis	Cracks or erythematous fissures at corners of mouth		Carbol-fuchsin solution (Castellani's paint)

Table 79–5 Skin Infestations

Condition and Causative Agent	Incidence/Comments	Clinical Manifestations	Duration	Treatment Measures
Scabies (mites) caused by *Sarcoptes scabiei*	Children, young adults; epidemics in a 30-yr cycle, the latest occurring in the 1970s; associated with skin-to-skin contact and with crowded and poor living conditions, sexual intimacy, or a nosocomial outbreak	Ridges, small linear threadlike lines; characteristic burrows; possible vesicles, nodules, or secondary infections; lesions appear on hands (interdigital webs), wrists, axillary folds, penis, scrotum, buttocks, nipples, abdomen; intense pruritus, especially when skin increases in warmth (eg, while sleeping)	Life cycle: Female mite excavates into skin for 1–2 months laying 10–25 eggs; incubation 3 wks	Bathe or shower and apply the pesticide gamma benzene hexachloride cream or lotion (Kwell, Gamene) to entire skin from neck down for 8–12 h, then bathe; repeat application in another week; apply crotamiton (Eurax), scabicide and antipruritic agent; apply 5%–10% precipitated sulfur; antipruritics
Pediculosis (lice infestation)	Incidence has increased	Extreme pruritus	Life cycle: Adult female lives approximately 1 month, laying up to 10 eggs daily; incubation 7–9 days; grows to adult louse in 1 wk	Shampoos or topical application of pesticide (Kwell, Gamene), pyrethrins (RID Liquid)

(continued)

Table 79-5 Skin Infestations (continued)				
Condition and Causative Agent	**Incidence/Comments**	**Clinical Manifestations**	**Duration**	**Treatment Measures**
a. Pediculosis corporis (body) caused by *Pediculus humanus corporis*		Scratch marks; eczematous changes; reddened papules		
b. Pediculosis capitis (head) caused by *Pediculus humanis capitis*		Ova (nits) visible on hairs, above ears		After treatment, use fine-tooth comb to remove nits and dead lice
c. Pediculosis pubis (genital) caused by *Phthirus pubis*	Frequently coexists with other sexually transmitted diseases	Ova visible on pubic and thigh hairs; difficult to locate insect on skin; may be in seams of clothing		
Tick bite from Argasidae (soft-bodied ticks) and Ixodidae (hard-bodied ticks)	Large mites attach to human skin and engorge on blood; transmit several rickettsial and viral diseases	Pruritus after several days of attachment; presence of tick may resemble wart or vascular tumor; bite appears as a small nodule surrounded by a necrotic ring; fever, headache, abdominal pain, malaise occur from secreted toxins from female tick; granulomas may form	Tick may drop off spontaneously; lesions persist 1-2 wks	Ensure removal of entire tick; remove by touching with a hot nail, extinguished match head or applying a few drops of chloroform, gasoline, or turpentine

proportionately limited, the lesions cause their own set of physiological and psychosocial stressors. Malignancies of the skin increase with age and are the most common dermatosis that bring the elderly to the dermatologist.

General Nursing Implications

The nurse plays an important role in the prevention of cutaneous lesions that develop predominantly from extrinsic factors known to cause damage to the normal integument. Many neoplasms are preventable or controllable when individuals, particularly those in high-risk groups, practice basic health principles that protect the skin and are alert to significant changes that require medical attention. A nurse should assume an active role in case finding. Because the integument is highly apparent and many of the lesions occur in unclothed areas, the nurse may have opportunities to make critical observations in industrial settings, hospitals, other health agencies, or simply as a friend or neighbor. Knowing that the majority of clients with skin cancer have a good prognosis should encourage early problem identification and treatment.

An important component of nursing care focuses on the protection of skin, particularly for those with a high

risk of developing neoplastic lesions (see Chapter 78 and Table 78-7). Teaching people who have precancerous lesions to monitor for significant change in the lesion is also important. Media warnings to seek medical attention for sores that do not heal or a change in a wart or mole may encourage many to act. The nurse, however, should know the specific danger signals that indicate malignant changes in pigmented nevi, the most serious of all cutaneous carcinomas. These lesions should be observed for the alterations noted later in this chapter.

A teaching plan should include preventing chronic irritation of any lesion. Constant rubbing may occur from clothing, straps, belts, or eye glasses, for example. A physician may decide to remove the lesion prophylactically if cellular changes suggest a potential change to malignancy.

SEBORRHEIC KERATOSIS

Seborrheic keratosis is a common benign epidermal growth of keratinocytes and melanocytes and is most frequent in persons over 40. Aging skin characteristically contains an isolated lesion or several scattered lesions.

Seborrheic keratoses are genetically transmitted as an autosomal dominant trait. Individuals with oily acne or seborrheic-type skin may also be more likely to develop these lesions. Heavily pigmented people have a low incidence of occurrence.

Clinical Manifestations

The growth initially appears as a small, slightly elevated papule or plaque, possibly containing some pigmentation. Enlargement takes place slowly with the surface becoming rough or warty. Color varies from yellow to brown or may even be black. Keratotic lesions generally appear on the face, scalp, trunk, and upper extremities. The most common complaint involves cosmetic disfigurement.

Therapeutic Measures

Simple curettage provides the easiest removal and causes the least cosmetic defect. Electrodesiccation also allows for easy removal but may result in minor scarring. Ethyl chloride, carbon dioxide, or liquid nitrogen may be used to freeze the lesions and facilitate easier scraping or allow sloughing.

KELOIDS/HYPERTROPHIC SCARRING

A **keloid** is a benign proliferative growth of fibrous tissue at the site of an injury or incision that extends beyond the confines of the wound. Hypertrophic scarring, which is the more common scarring problem, results in a much smaller dermal lesion. Both lesions represent a disequilibrium between the anabolic and catabolic phases of wound healing. A normal balance is usually reached at about 3 to 4 weeks after the injury. With abnormal scar formation, collagen is produced faster than it can be assimilated into the wound.

Although the basic etiology is unknown, the increased production of connective tissue has shown a correlation with trauma, a higher degree of inflammation, and infection. Wounds with excessive or poorly aligned tension because of location or suturing, burns, and the introduction of foreign substances into the skin are also considered to be some of the provocative factors. Young adults, particularly blacks and others with highly pigmented skin, show a predisposition for keloids and hypertrophic scarring.

Clinical Manifestations

Hypertrophic scars appear to correspond in size and shape to the underlying wound but become more raised, wider and thicker than anticipated, and remain reddened. Keloids may take several months to extend beyond the hypertrophic stage and develop into larger, smooth, hard, irregularly shaped, hyperpigmented lesions (Figure 79–14). The presternum, shoulders, upper back, lower legs, head, and neck are the most frequent areas of involvement. Problems may also develop in ear lobes following piercing for cosmetic purposes. Both types of lesions usually cause

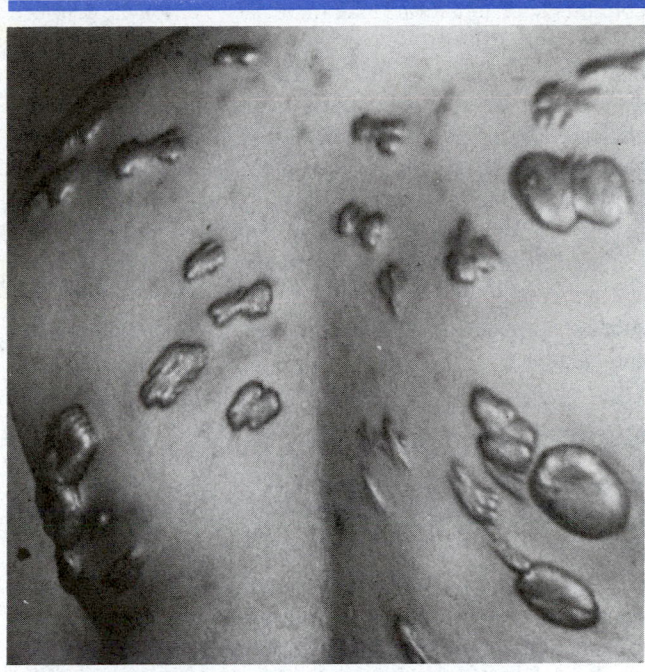

Figure 79–14
Keloids on the upper back. (Courtesy of Millard Fillmore Hospital, Buffalo, NY)

minimal sensory effects, although pruritus and pain may be noted on occasion with keloid formation.

Therapeutic Measures

Treatment of lesions may result in additional problems with cellular proliferation, especially when simple surgical excision is used. The most important therapeutic step for persons at high risk is to avoid injury or incisions that would stimulate unchecked cell growth. When surgery must be performed, problems are less apt to develop in early childhood or in late adulthood. When surgery is necessary in a high-risk period, the direction of a scar may be changed by use of a Z- or Y-shaped incision line to reduce tension.

Hypertrophic scars may resolve spontaneously within 1 year of formation. Intralesional injections with corticosteroids (such as triamcinolone acetate or diacetate), coupled with cryosurgery, have been recommended. Precautions must be taken to deter atrophy, telangiectasia, and depigmentation of healthy tissue when intralesional steroids are used. A combination of x-ray therapy and surgical excision may be elected for large keloids. Pressure dressings and garments have been helpful; the continuous force can prevent collagen fibers from abnormal development.

EPITHELIAL CYST

Several types of cystic lesions may develop within the various layers of the skin; they consist of a sac or capsule that contains lipid and keratinous materials. Although the more common growths may be termed *sebaceous cysts,* the actual histologic classification further identifies the lesions as epidermoid or pilar cysts (wens). They have an unknown etiology. *Milia* are firm, pinhead-sized, asymptomatic, white globular lesions that develop spontaneously after trauma to the skin (burns, incisions, dermabrasion) or following dermatosis. They are normal in newborns. *Dermoid cysts* occur in the subcutaneous tissue and are congenital, originating from embryonic tissue. Besides epithelial cells and cutaneous appendages, dermoid cysts may also contain bone and cartilage.

Clinical Manifestations

Sebaceous cysts appear to be globular, elevated, and firm. Lesions may range from 0.2 to 5 cm, and any enlargement may be attributed to an increase in soft, yellow-white material that fills the sac. These cysts commonly appear on the scalp, face, neck, and back. Milia, in addition to forming in traumatized areas, also appear around the eyes and on the forehead. Dermoid cysts have more diversified locations and may develop at the lateral ends of the eyebrows; sublingually; on the neck; and in the sternal, perineal, scrotal, and sacral areas. These cysts grow as large as 10 cm.

Therapeutic Measures

Complete surgical excision is the treatment of choice. Regrowth may be possible in some cases if the cystic capsule is not entirely removed. Milia and small cysts may be treated by simple incision and expression of the contents. Any sac may be removed with a hemostat.

LIPOMA

Lipomas, common benign tumors generally encapsulated in the subcutaneous layer of skin, are composed of adipose tissue. An individual may have one or several lesions on the body that vary in size and often feel rubbery or compressible. Lipomas are seen most frequently on the buttocks, thighs, back, forearms, and neck of adults. Surgical excision is limited to cases in which functional interference or obvious disfigurement develops.

NEUROFIBROMATOSIS

The appearance of multiple cutaneous tumors stemming from nervous tissue occurs with von Recklinghausen's disease, a condition that is transmitted genetically (see Chapter 37). In addition to cellular proliferation along the course of peripheral nerves, alteration in pigmentation occurs. Irregular tan to brown macules known as café-au-lait spots, may be seen as regional freckling, diffuse bronzing, or graying of the skin. Surgical removal of neurofibromatoses is limited to isolated, problematic lesions (see Chapter 39).

HEMANGIOMA

Referred to as a vascular nevus or birthmark, a hemangioma is a congenital lesion appearing at birth or within the neonatal period. Lesions differ in the extent to which they involve the vasculature within the cutis and subcutis. The depth of the hemangioma is indicated by the presenting color. The three major types of lesions are the nevus flammeus (port-wine stain), angiomatous nevus (strawberry nevus), and the cavernous hemangioma.

Clinical Manifestations

Port-wine stains are irregularly shaped macules that may range from red to reddish purple. Lesions are present at birth, and the capillary dilatation or ectasia will remain through a lifetime. Although the most common sites are the face and the occiput area of the scalp, these lesions may appear elsewhere on the body. Concomitant occurrence of convulsions, mental retardation, and glaucoma indicates a more extensive involvement of the vasculature with serious neurological and/or ocular involvement. The port-wine stain alters in color and appearance with age, progressing to a deeper purple and possibly developing a cobblestone texture.

A strawberry nevus is a soft or moderately firm lesion with a red to bluish-red color that appears at birth or shortly thereafter. It may occur on any portion of skin surface but is more common on the face, trunk, or legs, or on the oral and vaginal mucosa. Enlargement can be anticipated during the first year. Most strawberry nevi involute spontaneously by the fifth year, leaving virtually no residual effects. Deeper lesions may be the exception.

Cavernous hemangiomas (Figure 79–15) usually involve

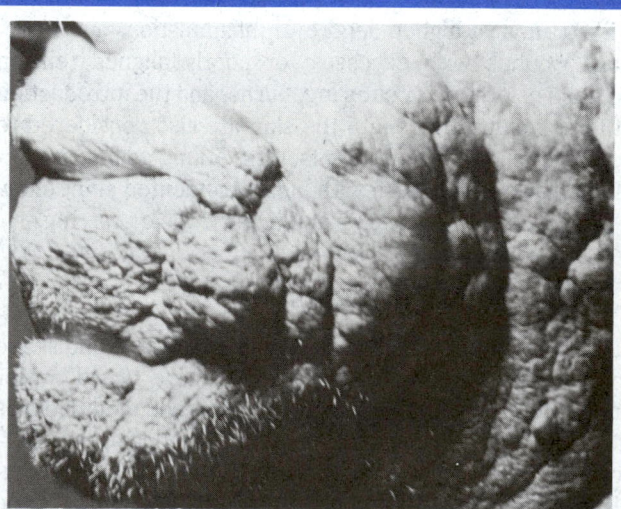

Figure 79–15

Cavernous hemangioma. (Courtesy of Millard Fillmore Hospital, Buffalo, NY)

the subcutaneous layer of the skin and appear to be soft, rounded masses. Lesions may be skin colored or may range from red to blue or purple in hue. As with the strawberry nevus, the cavernous hemangioma is expected to involute without treatment during early childhood.

Therapeutic Measures

Because of the anticipated resolution of both the strawberry nevus and the cavernous hemangioma, treatment is not usually a prime consideration. Parents must be given adequate explanations to prevent undue worrying and the necessary supports to accept the lesions until they eventually disappear.

Port-wine stains, however, require some type of therapy. Until recently, little could be done to alter the appearance of the lesion. Electrodesiccation, cryosurgery, dermabrasion, excision, grafting, and camouflage by tattooing with flesh-colored pigments have provided cosmetic benefits. Skin-colored waterproof cosmetics (Covermark) are used to cover lesions. Individuals can become adept at disguising unsightly stains.

Argon laser surgery offers new hope for clients with port-wine stains. Further discussion of laser surgery and the nursing implications can be found in Chapter 80.

Specific Nursing Measures

Care of these clients should include emotional support, which helps facilitate self-acceptance despite the presence of a distorted appearance. If love and acceptance have been provided through the client's lifetime, the client may not be hindered by major emotional obstacles. Pre- and postoperative nursing care are discussed in Chapter 80.

PIGMENTED NEVUS CELL TUMOR

Pigmented nevus cell tumors involve cellular proliferation of the pigment-producing melanocytes. Melanocytic nevi, also referred to as moles, are classified histologically as a junctional, compound, or dermal nevus, depending on the layer of skin in which the aggregation of cells has occurred. A cytologic exam is needed to make this determination. A junctional nevus, the most superficial lesion, arises from melanocytes above the basement membrane at the dermal–epidermal border. Because of the high activity level of these cells, this type of nevus is considered to be potentially malignant. Danger signals that indicate malignant changes in pigmented nevi are listed in Box 79–3.

Compound nevi contain cells from both the deep dermis and the lining of the epidermal junction (Figure 79–16). Intradermal or resting nevi arise solely in the dermal layer of skin and are unlikely to become cancerous. Specific examples of these lesions include the giant hairy nevus, blue nevus, halo nevus, and juvenile nevus.

Studies have indicated that pigmented growths show a hereditary tendency (Fitzpatrick, 1983). Nevi arise from

---

Box 79–3 Danger Signals That Indicate Malignant Changes in Pigmented Nevi

Color and uniformity (red, white, or blue areas)

Pigmentation (mottled shades of black or brown)

Diameter (sudden enlargement)

Border (development of irregular border or extension of lesion)

Surface characteristic (presence of erosion, bleeding, ulceration, inflammation, blistering, and serous drainage)

Sensation (onset of pain, itching, tingling)

Consistency (softening or friable consistency)

Shape (uneven elevation)

---

cells present since embryonic life, with only a small percentage being apparent at birth. These lesions may appear across the life span of an individual but usually become evident in early childhood with an increasing occurrence during puberty and pregnancy. Melanocytic nevi are common among Caucasians and are seen less frequently in highly pigmented people.

Clinical Manifestations

Nevi that appear in childhood tend to be flat and only slightly elevated compared to the more distinct conformations that develop in adulthood. Lesions vary considerably in size, color, surface appearance, and form. Dimensions may range from 1 or 2 mm to a growth that covers a large portion of the body surface. Color may vary from a normal skin tone through a spectrum of browns to black and depends in some degree on the exact depth of origin. Surface appearance may be smooth or rough, slightly to markedly elevated, hairy, or hairless. The shape may be round, domelike, polypoid, or papillomatous. Increased or decreased pigmentation around the periphery of the lesion presents a halo effect. Nevi can appear anywhere on the body. Those located on the palms, soles, and genitalia are most likely to be junctional and should be closely observed for significant changes.

Therapeutic Measures

Biopsy is critical before any major decisions are made. Dermatologists recommend that histologic samples be obtained by excision, when possible, to allow for complete examination of the lesion. Once the diagnosis is confirmed, subsequent therapy may involve total surgical excision with possible skin grafting or the use of electrosurgery.

Removal of all pigmented nevi to prevent the development of malignant melanoma is not practical because the skin may contain many lesions. Prophylactic surgery may be elected when a nevus develops in an area where malignant melanoma has an increased likelihood of occurrence,

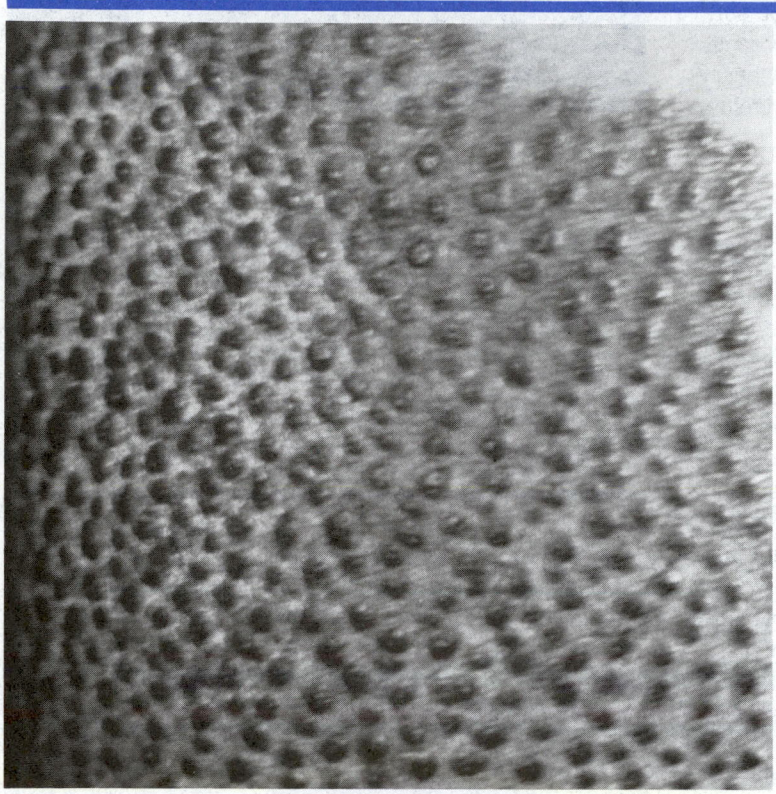

Figure 79—16

Compound nevus.

SOURCE: Binnick SA: *Skin Diseases: Diagnosis and Management in Clinical Practice.* Baltimore, MD: Williams & Wilkins, 1982.

if the lesion is biologically active, or if chronic irritation is a problem.

ACTINIC KERATOSIS

Considered a precancerous growth, actinic, senile, or solar keratosis is a common disorder involving the development of single or multiple cutaneous lesions from chronic exposure to sunlight. Susceptible persons include those with skin types I to III (refer to Table 78–7 in Chapter 78). Rarely is the neoplastic disorder seen in people who tan easily. Farmers, ranchers, sailors, and those who participate in outdoor sports have an increased likelihood of actinic lesions—more so if they are genetically predisposed. Actinic keratosis occurs predominantly in middle and later years, but solar lesions may develop earlier when risk factors and exposure are high.

Clinical Manifestations

Actinic keratoses usually appear as flat, hard, dry, scaly, firmly attached lesions. The color may range from skin tone to yellow, brown, or black and are contingent on the amount of horny materials that adhere. Sites of predilection include the face, ears, neck, forearms, and dorsa of the hands.

Therapeutic Measures

Use of 5-fluorouracil cream or solution (Efudex, Fluoroplex) in prescribed strengths has proven to be an effective treatment. An experimental antimitotic drug, cycloheximide (Acti-dione), may become an alternative. Cryosurgery, electrosurgery and curettage, dermabrasion, and/or chemical peeling have also been used to treat actinic keratoses. Nodules should be excised surgically. Prevention of actinic keratosis is the most important component of care whether by sunscreens, protective clothing, change in occupation, or an alteration in lifestyle and climate. The ultimate goal would be to markedly decrease sun exposure.

Specific Nursing Measures

When fluorouracil has been prescribed, instruct the individual about appropriate and safe application of the drug. If gloves are not worn, hands must be washed immediately after fluorouracil has been handled to avoid effects on uninvolved skin and mucous membranes. The involved area must never be occluded, and the medication must be applied cautiously near the eyes, nose, and mouth. In addition, inform clients that the treatment may make the area unsightly because of erythema, scaling, hyperpigmentation, dermatitis, suppuration, and swelling. Complete healing may not occur for 1 or 2 months after chemotherapy has ended. Leukopenia, thrombocytopenia, bleeding stomatitis, and gastrointestinal ulcerations may occur with systemic absorption.

ARSENICAL KERATOSIS

Chronic exposure to the chemical element arsenic, whether industrially, environmentally, or medicinally, may cause precancerous changes in normal skin. Individuals who work with herbicides, insecticides and pesticides, metal smelting and castings, certain ceramics, dyes, decorative pigments, and wood preservatives may have long-term contact with this carcinogen. Contamination of drinking water obtained from underground wells is a potential problem in certain areas of the world where arsenic is found in abundance. Although not in prominent use today, certain medications (known as Fowler's solution and Asiatic pills) used to treat instances of resistant psoriasis contain sufficient arsenic to become problematic.

Clinical Manifestations

Hyperpigmentation occurs, especially on the trunk, with some degree of hypopigmentation and alopecia. Keratotic lesions initially appear on the palms and soles; however, if chronic exposure continues, lesions become more widespread, and basal cell or squamous cell carcinoma may develop.

Systemically and in more acute forms, the client will manifest malaise, anorexia, weight loss, nausea, vomiting, and diarrhea. Arsenic intoxication may be detected by the examination of urine, hair, and nails.

Therapeutic Measures

Drug therapy with dimercaprol (BAL) is reserved for systemic involvement and has no effect on already existing keratoses or malignant lesions. Prevention and early case finding are important considerations in the treatment plan. Change in occupation may be a necessary consideration.

Local destruction is the treatment of choice, but complete removal may not be feasible because of the number of lesions. Electrodesiccation and curettage, topical application of 5-fluorouracil, and cryosurgery have been used to alleviate the disorder.

BASAL CELL CARCINOMA

Basal cell epithelioma, the most common form of skin cancer, arises from the germinative layer of the epidermis or the appendages. This lesion carries the most favorable prognosis because cellular proliferation is slow, detection and treatment frequently occur in the early stage, and metastasis is extremely rare. Basal cell carcinoma is seen in adults, usually after age 40, and with a slightly higher prevalence in males (Fitzpatrick, 1979).

Basal cell carcinoma is closely linked with chronic exposure to strong solar ultraviolet radiation, particularly in those with skin types I and II (refer to Table 78–4 in Chapter 78). Incidence is highest in regions where sunlight is most abundant and intense, such as the southern United States and Australia. X-ray irradiation, scars, and chemical carcinogens can also be implicated as causative agents.

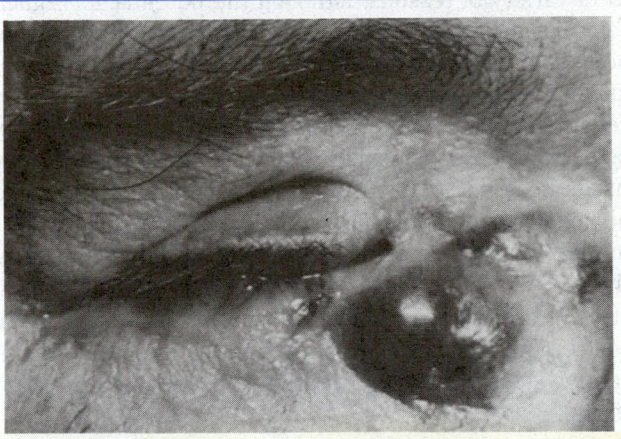

Figure 79–17
Basal cell carcinoma. (Courtesy of Millard Fillmore Hospital, Buffalo, NY)

Clinical Manifestations

Nodular-ulcerative basal cell carcinoma is the most common type. The lesion begins as a papule, progresses to the nodular stage, and can develop a depressed ulcerated center. The borders of the tumor are raised, appear waxy or pearly, and may contain fine telangiectatic vessels (Figure 79–17). Basal cell carcinomas may also be referred to as rodent ulcers because they characteristically invade the subcutis, bone, and other underlying tissue. Areas of predilection include the nose, eyelids, and cheek (that is, exposed parts of the head). Superficial basal cell carcinoma appears frequently on the trunk, often involving multiple tumors. These lesions appear to be barely elevated plaques whose centers are crusted and erythematous.

Therapeutic Measures

Several methods have been employed to treat basal cell carcinoma. The ultimate determination is based on the location, size, depth of the tumor, and age of the client. Surgical excision, curettage and electrodesiccation, radiation therapy, cryotherapy, and microscopically controlled excision (Mohs' procedure, MCE) are all used. The primary aim is to eliminate the tumor and prevent irregular local extension of the lesion into the deeper tissues, but without destroying healthy cells and causing major cosmetic defects. High cure rates for basal cell malignancies allow more options in the selection of a method. However, the initial treatment must be sufficiently aggressive to be curative because recurrent lesions do not respond favorably to subsequent therapy.

Curettage and electrodesiccation, although convenient, expeditious, less costly, and less destructive of tumor-free tissue are limited to uncomplicated lesions no greater than 1 cm in diameter. Surgical excision may be elected for a variety of reasons, although the potential for significant disfigurement becomes a disadvantage. Skin flaps can be used to cover tissue losses only after pathologic examinations confirm that the skin margins are free of tumor cells. Radiation therapy has shown high cure rates and may be selected for tumors where minimal destruction of healthy tissue is essential. Cryosurgery, through the use of liquid nitrogen, allows for a quick, effective, inexpensive, cosmetically positive mode of treatment and is considered as the approach of choice in a limited number of cases. Mohs' surgery has achieved the highest cure rate in treating basal cell tumors, and use of this method has increased significantly. Details of the procedure are presented in Chapter 80.

Specific Nursing Measures

The nurse plays a major role in the prevention and case finding of basal cell lesions. Many clients are treated on an outpatient basis, and the role of the nurse is often limited to preoperative teaching and immediate postoperative care. Health teaching should stress the need for regular health care follow-ups. The care of clients who require surgery is discussed in Chapter 80.

SQUAMOUS CELL CARCINOMA

The second most common malignancy of the skin involves the prickle or squamous cell, cells which evolve in the maturation process of the keratinocytes. Tumors may also be referred to as prickle cell, epithelioma, or epidermoid carcinoma. This neoplasm grows more rapidly than a basal cell carcinoma, is much more invasive, and carries a higher mortality rate because of its metastatic nature. Squamous cell epitheliomas are seen predominantly in males over 55.

Like basal cell carcinoma, squamous cell malignancies develop in proportion to excesses in sunlight exposure and inherent genetic tendencies (skin type and color). This type of neoplasm has frequently developed from other lesions. In addition to actinic keratosis, unstable thermal burn scars, ulcerations, chronic sinus tracts (draining a suppurative cavity to the skin surface or between cystic or abscess cavities), therapeutically irradiated skin, and discoid lupus erythematosus can develop squamous cell carcinoma. Chronic exposure to coal tar derivatives, arsenicals, and some other chemicals may also be contributory.

Clinical Manifestations

The lesion may appear as a papule, plaque, or nodule. Crusts, erosions, or ulcerations are characteristic, as is an irregular border (Figure 79–18). Lesions appear mostly on the exposed area of the head (cheek, lip, ears) but may frequent the neck, forearms, and backs of the hands, or appear on the legs of women. Regional lymph nodes may enlarge because of the metastatic process.

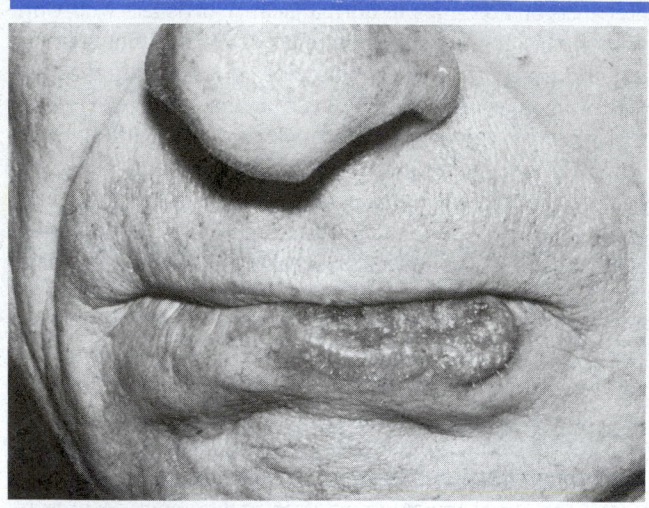

Figure 79–18

Squamous cell carcinoma.
SOURCE: Binnick SA: *Skin Diseases: Diagnosis and Management in Clinical Practice.* Baltimore, MD: Williams & Wilkins, 1982.

Therapeutic and Specific Nursing Measures

Treatment of squamous cell carcinoma is basically similar to the method used for basal cell epitheliomas. Staging of the lesion will help the physician to determine the exact approach to use. Occurrence of squamous cell carcinoma in the elderly necessitates an assessment of their general health status because any major illness or chronic illness will influence the modality and extensiveness or treatment. Prevention of recurrence requires the elimination or minimization of exposure to carcinogens. The nursing measures are similar to those for basal cell carcinoma.

MALIGNANT MELANOMA

Melanoma, a malignancy arising from melanocytes, is the least frequent of primary skin cancers but the most serious. Because of a high degree of metastasis generally involving major organs, the 5-year survival rate for Caucasians (82%) is lower than the survival rate (95%) for clients with other types of skin cancer (American Cancer Society, 1985). Rates for blacks could not be calculated because of an insufficient number of cases. Malignant melanomas are responsible for 5500 of the 7400 deaths from skin cancer annually (American Cancer Society, 1985).

Incidence of melanoma increases with age. Rare in children, notable occurrence begins in young adults with the peak frequency in the fourth and fifth decades of life. Since after World War II, the appearance of malignant melanoma, specifically the superficial spreading type, has markedly increased in younger persons (Fitzpatrick, 1983).

Exposure to intense sunlight, even intermittently, plays

a key role in pathogenesis, especially with skin types I to III (refer to Table 78–7 in Chapter 78). Although it is rare, melanoma may develop in those with more highly pigmented skin—Asians, American Indians, blacks, and persons who tan readily.

Congenital or acquired nevi may be labeled as precursors to malignant melanomas, but because of inconclusive evidence, this remains controversial. Familial tendencies have been found in 2% to 5% of cases (Fitzpatrick, 1979).

The occurrence of certain clinical phenomena has given credibility to the fact that the defenses of the immune system are reduced in the development of malignant melanomas. Spontaneous remissions, the prolonged period of time that occurs between recurrence or invasiveness of lesions, and the effects of immunotherapy tend to confirm that host immunity has a significant endogenous impact on the control of melanomatous cells.

Clinical Manifestations

Characteristics of a malignant melanoma relate closely to the histologic type of lesion. The four classifications of melanoma, in order of frequency, include the (1) superficial spreading melanoma (SSM), (2) nodular melanoma (NM), (3) lentigo maligna melanoma (LMM), and (4) acral lentiguous melanoma (ALM).

The lesional changes identified in Box 79–3 are indicative of malignant melanomas. Color changes may include a variety of browns, black, blue-black, white, pink (amelanotic), red, purple, or gray. The lesion may be slightly raised, as with SSM, or may have a marked elevation as with NM (Figure 79–19).

Melanoma can occur on any part of the body (head, trunk, extremities, and anogenital area). Lentigo maligna melanoma, generally associated with the elderly, may develop from Hutchinson's melanotic freckles, a multifocal atypical collection of melanocytes that appear on the face, neck, forearms, and backs of the hands. Acral lentiguous melanoma represents the small percentage of lesions that appear on the palms, soles, or subungually (nail bed). This last type of malignancy shows increased incidence in blacks and Orientals.

The most serious prognosis involves the nodular type because it rapidly invades the dermis and subcutaneous tissue. Superficial spreading and lentigo maligna melanomas are less serious. Any melanomatous tumor has the potential to metastasize through the lymphatic and vascular channels or to develop satellite extensions. The lungs, liver, bone, heart, stomach, small intestines, brain, and kidney may be invaded and result in the appropriate symptomatology for the organ. Added concern for metastasis exists when a melanoma develops on the hands, feet, and anogenital area.

During the diagnostic process, tumors are ranked by their level of penetration. Level I indicates an intradermal, noninvasive melanoma, whereas Level V signifies extension into the subcutaneous adipose tissue.

Therapeutic Measures

A total excisional biopsy, whenever possible, and staging of the melanoma are essential before a treatment plan is determined. Factors in the decision-making process include the level of tumor invasiveness, type of melanoma, host response, and the degree of metastasis. Surgical removal offers the best chance of cure. A wide and deep excision is usually performed to remove all cancerous cells. A regional lymph node dissection is included when findings are positive for lymphatic metastasis but is still considered controversial as an elective component of treatment. More extensive surgery such as amputation of a digit or a limb, abdominal perineal resection, or vulvectomy may be performed because of the extent and location of the malignant melanoma.

Radiation therapy may be used with other modalities to treat the primary tumor, but melanomatous cells have not proven radiosensitive to any great degree. Radiation may be instituted for management of metastatic lesions.

Chemotherapy is useful in adjuvant treatment and when dissemination of melanoma has occurred. Dacarbazine (DTIC) has proven to be the most beneficial chemotherapeutic agent, although the nitrosoureas (BCNU, CCNU, MeCCNU) may also be used. Isolated regional limb hyperthermic perfusion (RLHP), considered investigational, has a 5-year survival rate of 75% to 80% compared to a 21% to 33% rate associated with the use of amputation to treat in-transit metastatic disease (Loescher & Leigh, 1984). Malignant melanomas are considered in-transit when tumor cells arise between the primary site and regional lymph nodes. Although several chemotherapeutic agents have been used, phenylalanine mustard (L-PAM, or Melphalan) has proven effective in RLHP.

Research has also demonstrated that melanoma cells are destroyed by high temperatures and that a synergistic effect is obtained when L-PAM and hyperthermia are used in combination with RLHP. The procedure requires 1 to 2 hours and is performed under general anesthesia. Vascular cannulation provides for arterial inflow and venous outflow. A tourniquet is applied to the involved limb to prevent systemic leakage, allowing higher doses of the drug to be

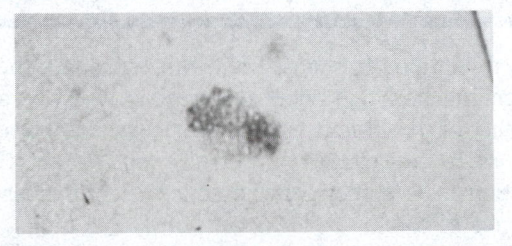

Figure 79–19

Malignant melanoma. (Courtesy of Millard Fillmore Hospital, Buffalo, NY)

administered. The perfusate is oxygenated by pump oxygenator and heated to 41°C (105.8°F) while the temperature of the extremity is raised to 39°C (102.2°F) by use of heat lamps or Aquamatic K-pad. When the desired temperatures are reached, the drug is introduced into the venous outflow line. The residual cytotoxic drug is washed out from the system and the appropriate amount of blood replaced before the procedure is completed.

Immunotherapy has also been used in adjuvant therapy for advanced disease. It has not proven to be significantly effective, however. The immunotherapeutic approach has made use of the bacillus Calmette-Guerin (BCG) antigen to encourage the client's immune system to destroy the cancerous melanoma cells. BCG may be administered intralesionally, intradermally, or both. Other methods of activating the host defense mechanisms include injecting the client with melanomatous cells that have been mixed with other antigens or transfusing with lymphocytes procured from another melanoma client.

At present, no one treatment is the answer to eradicating a melanomatous lesion, and the trend is toward a combined approach.

Specific Nursing Measures

The increased number of therapeutic interventions and the lethal implications of malignant melanoma make the role of the nurse more important. Although the diagnosis may be already confirmed, the client could be faced with more extensive testing before a decision can be made as to the scope and depth of surgery or subsequent therapy.

Emotional support is a critical part of nursing care. A client with malignant melanoma may be fully aware of the overall prognosis associated with the disorder but may need opportunities for expression of feelings and more information to facilitate a realistic adjustment. Coping mechanisms need to be assessed and assistance given to both client and family during the initial adjustment period and when further admissions are necessitated. Anxiety and fears may become evident as the client considers the following possibilities: loss of body parts, mutilation, recurrence of disease, and psychosocioeconomic constraints.

Because surgical excision is usually involved in the initial treatment and may be used for metastatic lesions, nursing care will revolve around the operative procedure. Some clients may need minimal assistance, whereas others may become totally dependent on the nurse for maintenance of physiological needs and emotional support, particularly when the melanoma has metastasized to another organ.

If chemotherapy is instituted, the nurse must become aware of the potential hazards. Dacarbazine (DTIC) is likely to cause leukopenia, thrombocytopenia, severe nausea and vomiting, anorexia, and a flulike syndrome. Using L-PAM with RLHP may cause mild edema, erythema, reversible limb hyperpigmentation, alopecia, and a rare occurrence of blistering or ulceration. Clients may also develop myelosuppression and nausea or vomiting if systemic leakage occurs. High doses of L-PAM may prolong wound healing.

Clients who have received RLHP must be closely monitored for disruption in arterial and venous circulation to the involved extremity. Heparin is administered both during the perfusion procedure and postoperatively to prevent clotting problems. The involved limb should be kept elevated and the client should wear antiembolic elastic stockings. Blood and Doppler studies monitor the potential problems. Transient neuropathy may develop in the perfused limb from tourniquet pressure, causing the client to experience numbness and tingling. Instruct the client to protect the extremity from potential trauma such as burns and lacerations that result from sensory loss.

Clients who receive immunotherapy must be assessed for any untoward effects. Although the majority of clients tolerate BCG vaccinations well, a common febrile response (up to 40°C or 104°F) may occur, accompanied by malaise, vomiting, arthralgia, myalgia, and headache. Three types of serious toxic complications may occur in the form of disseminated BCG infection, reactivation of an old, dormant, acid-fast infection, or anaphylactic hypersensitivity reactions (Dorr & Fritz, 1980).

Clients should be reminded of the need for regular checkups to monitor remission and recurrence of melanoma.

Section VI: Trauma

A traumatic injury involves disruptive or destructive damage to the various cutaneous layers and appendages of healthy skin because of direct physical force, external penetration by objects, extreme heat, or extreme cold.

Trauma to the skin and underlying tissue is a common disorder that frequently brings a person to the hospital for emergency treatment. Minor problems may be cared for at the site of injury, but extensive wounds may require hospitalization for more involved therapy and rehabilitation.

Prevention of trauma to the skin should be the most outstanding nursing concern because of the overall vulnerability of this organ system to external stressors. Accidents are leading causes of morbidity and mortality; health education and common sense practice can often lessen the incidence of injury.

A nursing assessment and subsequent first-aid treatment may be provided at the scene of the accident. A knowledgeable nurse recognizes the need for further professional medical assistance and directs the injured person or family member to the appropriate facilities. Chapter 13 includes a discussion of trauma care and identifies the nursing role in management of the problem. Chapter 15 discusses burns; skin grafting is discussed in Chapter 80.

COLD INJURY

Several types of dermatological problems may result from exposure to freezing and near-freezing temperatures. Humidity, wind, and high altitudes also become influential. Damage from cold injury may be minor or extensive enough to cause loss of a body part. The hands, feet, nose, and ears are the most commonly involved structures.

Individuals with a history of peripheral vascular disease (from arteriosclerosis, diabetes mellitus, or Raynaud's syndrome) have a higher susceptibility to cold injury. Persons who smoke or drink excessive amounts of alcohol are also at high risk. Alcohol causes heat loss from vasodilation, and the warmth generated may prevent adequate body coverage during inclement weather. Nicotine, on the other hand, causes vasoconstriction, thus diminishing peripheral circulation.

Chilblain (erythrocyanosis) is a mild chronic disorder that involves a localized paradoxical vascular response to cold or cooling temperatures 0° to 15.5°C (32° to 60°F) in which initial vasoconstriction is followed by brief intense vasodilation. It is more common in women, particularly in individuals with a familial tendency.

Immersion or trench foot develops from continued exposure to wetness and non-freezing coldness under conditions in which the feet are usually immobile and in a dependent position for long periods. Although seen primarily in soldiers during wartime, the problem may occur in anyone in a situation of prolonged exposure (eg, construction workers whose shoes and socks are wet, skiers who do not keep their feet dry, and outdoorsmen).

Frostbite is an injury in which tissue is damaged by freezing, either superficially or sufficiently deep to cause death to the skin and underlying muscle, bone, nerves, and blood vessels. Frostbite may be accompanied by hypothermia, a generalized cooling of the body below the core temperature of 37°C (98.6°F).

Degrees of tissue trauma caused by cold may be used to describe the severity of the effects. A first-degree injury results in erythema after rewarming, whereas patchy blistering characterizes a second-degree involvement. Third-degree penetration causes necrosis of the skin and may progress to fourth-degree injury where soft tissue loss and gangrene of digits or an extremity may result.

Clinical Manifestations

Chilblain involves the appearance of red edematous areas on the dorsal surface of the hands, feet, lower legs, nose and ears, generally with the onset of cold, damp weather.

Color varies with ambient temperature and the degree of elevation of the extremity. The client may complain of pruritus and burning, usually with increased warming of the part. Blistering and ulceration may develop. The lesions may remain for several days or weeks with complete remission during warm weather.

Immersion or trench foot may be recognized by the appearance of pale, cold, swollen feet. The individual has pain upon weight bearing, tingling, and paresthesia. Clinical manifestations become more apparent as warming begins. Tinea infection may also accompany the primary problem.

The symptoms in frostbite depend on the depth of involvement. Initially, a frostbitten part may appear blanched or actually frozen, and the person may experience a sharp aching pain or have no sensation except at the edge of the affected area. During thawing from ice crystallization, the affected area may become erythematous, deep purple, or black. Within 48 hours after warming of the superficial injury, plasma and intracellular fluid extravasate into the interstitial spaces causing blistering, bullae formation, or edema. A resultant hemoconcentration and decreased lumen of the blood vessels cause vascular sludging, increasing the likelihood of thrombosis in the smaller capillaries. Larger blood vessels may remain in a state of spasm and further decrease distal circulation. Another fluid shift occurs within 5 to 10 days when reabsorption takes place and the formation of eschar becomes evident. Viable tissue will appear as the eschar begins to separate during the subsequent weeks of the healing process (Figure 79–20).

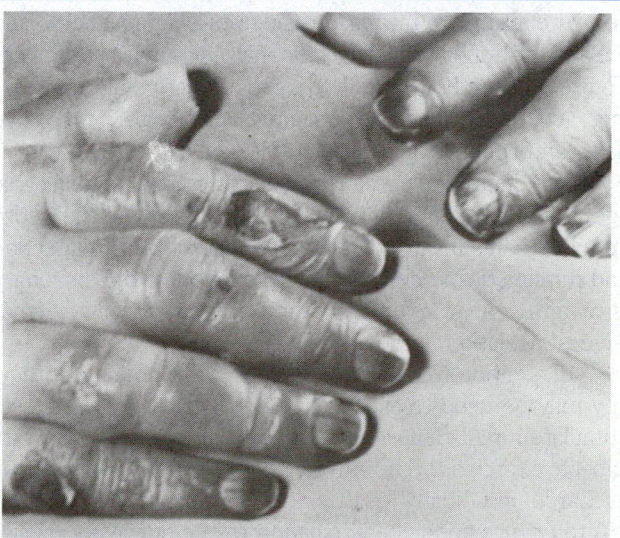

Figure 79–20

Frostbite to the hands. Scarring, eschar formation, and sloughing of tissue are occurring simultaneously. (Courtesy of Millard Fillmore Hospital, Buffalo, NY)

It is difficult to assess the degree of injury until the remaining blood supply has been fully established. If an area remains unchanged, with persistent blanching, anesthesia, lack of edema, and cyanosis, the nurse may then see necrosis develop. In the presence of a dry gangrene that has resulted from a very deep frostbite, autoamputation is possible.

Therapeutic Measures

Chilblain responds poorly to any therapy and is treated by general measures such as the wearing of warm clothing and maintenance of a warm environment. Ultraviolet light, vasodilators, and sympathectomies have been used in some cases.

Immersion or trench foot must be treated by immediate removal of wet clothing and careful rewarming of involved extremities. If possible, bed rest with moderate elevation of the legs is recommended. Otherwise, provision of adequate foot rest is the other alternative. Keeping the feet dry and cleansing between the toes are essential to prevent the development of secondary infection.

The most immediate treatment for frostbite is to rewarm the affected area gradually. Shelter the person and avoid refreezing once first aid measures are begun. Treatment for hypothermia takes precedence over localized involvement, and warm clothing and beverages may prove helpful.

The involved area should be immersed in a water bath with a temperature ranging between 100° and 108°F (17.7° and 42°C) until the part is entirely flushed (DeLapp, 1980). Nonsubmergible structures such as ears and areas on the face should be treated with a warm moist cover. Rewarming causes a great deal of pain. The involved area should be protected from hitting the sides of warming tubs, and the administration of sedatives or analgesics may be required. To prevent further injury by tissue destruction or refreezing, avoid the application of snow, cold water, excessive heat, and rubbing or vigorous massages.

The injured part is carefully dried, an antibacterial agent applied, digits individually separated, and the entire area dressed similarly to a burn to protect it from infection and further tissue destruction. Elevation of the extremity is maintained. If an open method of treatment is elected, reverse isolation is required.

In addition to daily wound care, whirlpool hydrotherapy may be used to aid the natural debridement process, stimulate circulation, and provide buoyancy so that joints can be exercised. The physician may need to incise the eschar longitudinally (escharotomy is described in Chapter 15) to ensure adequate circulation to the surviving tissue. Surgery may be required to assist with debridement when the natural process is retarded and infection threatens. Other surgical interventions are used only when amputation or grafting is required.

Arteriograms, Doppler studies, and plethysmographic determinations may be needed to measure the vascular response to the injury (they are discussed in Chapter 26). A vasodilator such as reserpine (Serpasil) may be injected into a vasoplastic artery to cause a local medical sympathectomy. Anticoagulent therapy has some value but is not ordered routinely.

Specific Nursing Measures

Prevention is a foremost nursing concern with cold injuries. Industrial and school nurses may have the greatest occasion to provide information about how to avoid overexposure. Nurses who care for the elderly or for clients with peripheral vascular diseases or alcohol dependency should incorporate a list of precautions in a teaching program. The instructions for all susceptible persons include:

- Minimizing exposure to excess cold, wet, and high altitudes
- Dressing warmly with several layers of clothing
- Changing to dry clothing at once whenever necessary
- Wearing mittens, caps, and boot liners
- Avoiding alcohol and tobacco
- Inspecting the skin for color changes
- Being aware of altered sensations

Treatment of hospitalized clients with severe frostbite can be a challenge to the nurse because of the length of time needed for injured tissue to become revitalized and for the amount of permanent damage to be determined.

Protecting the wound from infection is important because of the altered circulation and ultimate loss of nonviable tissue. Medical and surgical asepsis should be maintained, not only during dressing changes, but when bathing, turning, or touching the client. Comfort is of prime importance during the warming phase and may cause concern during tissue repair. Usually, clients who have sustained frostbite develop a high sensitivity to colder temperatures because of a resultant ischemic neuritis and tend to experience pain in the hands and feet.

When the limbs are involved, active and passive motion of the joints is essential, and the care plan should include a daily exercise program. When injuries are extensive and body function is adversely affected or parts have been lost, a physical and occupational therapist may join the health team to provide rehabilitation services.

During the days when the extent of damage is uncertain, clients may require a great deal of emotional support. Initially, the client may be relieved to have survived. However, when the ultimate outcome is more obvious and loss of a body part becomes inevitable, the grieving process may begin. It is important to encourage expression of feelings and to provide an atmosphere in which acceptance and independence are fostered. Planning for the future may also require vocational counseling when loss of body function or loss of a body part prevents the client returning to his or her job.

Chapter Highlights

Many skin disorders are the result of several factors that may combine an unknown etiology, an intrinsic predisposition, or extrinsic elements.

Long-term exposure to the sun is responsible for alterations in the skin that may precede or result in serious disorders or cause the exacerbation of some dermatoses.

Drugs may be responsible for adverse cutaneous reactions.

Each dermatosis has a characteristic set of cutaneous clinical manifestations that include various changes in vasculature, pigmentation, configuration, density, texture, turgor, sensation, and temperature, with gains or losses of skin or hair and the appearance of fluid excesses and drainage.

Treatment of dermatologic disorders is highly individualized.

Clients with skin disorders are frequently seen in schools, occupational health settings, clinics, summer camps, and other ambulatory care facilities where the nurse may be closely involved with diagnosis and treatment.

Pharmacologic agents are major components in the treatment of dermatoses and require proper administration or application to be effective.

Anti-infectives, anti-inflammatory agents, antihistamines, comedolytics, keratolytics, retinoids, pesticides, antipruritics, photosensitizers, immunosuppressants, and cytotoxics represent major classifications of drugs used to treat skin disorders.

Natural sunlight or artificial sources of ultraviolet light may be of therapeutic use in selected dermatoses.

Clients with skin disorders that involve an immune hypersensitivity should be made aware of factors causing allergic sensitization or cutaneous irritation as a part of the treatment plan.

Chronic skin conditions require heavy expenditures of time, human resources, and costly supplies.

Health teaching is an important concern in dermatological nursing because many dermatoses may be prevented or managed through communication of pertinent information.

Skin disorders that cause disfigurement and affect the emotional well-being of an individual may require psychosocial intervention.

Personal hygiene, climate and humidity control, appropriate clothing, cleaning agents, toiletries, cosmetics, and sunscreens should be considered in the prevention or treatment of skin disorders.

Diseased skin should be protected from further injury and secondary dermatoses.

Bibliography

American Cancer Society. *Cancer Facts and Figures 1985.* New York: American Cancer Society, 1985.

Arndt KA: *Manual of Dermatologic Therapeutics With Essentials of Diagnosis,* 3rd ed. Boston: Little, Brown, 1983.

Binnick SA: *Skin Diseases: Diagnosis and Management in Clinical Practice.* Baltimore, MD: Williams & Wilkins, 1982.

DeLapp TD: Taking the bite out of frostbite and other cold weather injuries. *Am J Nurs* 1980; 80:56–60.

Domonkos AN, Arnold HL, Odom RB: *Andrew's Diseases of the Skin; Clinical Dermatology,* 7th ed. Philadelphia: Saunders, 1982.

Dorr RT, Fritz WL: *Cancer Chemotherapy Handbook.* New York: Elsevier North Holland, 1980.

Emmett AJ, O'Rourke MG: *Malignant Skin Tumors.* Edinburgh: Livingstone, 1982.

Fitzpatrick TB et al: *Dermatology in General Medicine,* 2nd ed. New York: McGraw-Hill, 1979.

Fitzpatrick TB et al: *Update: Dermatology in General Medicine.* New York: McGraw-Hill, 1983.

Fitzpatrick TB, Polano MK, Suurmond D: *Color Atlas and Synopsis of Clinical Dermatology.* New York: McGraw-Hill, 1983.

Grant HD, Murray RH Jr, Bergeron JD: *Emergency Care,* 3rd ed. Bowie, MD: Brady, 1982.

Gumport SL: The diagnosis and management of common skin cancers. *CA* 1981; 31:79–90.

Larrow L, Noe JM: Port wine stain hemangiomas. *Am J Nurs* 1982; 82:786–790.

Lawlis GF, Achterberg J: Acne: The disease and stress. *Top Clin Nurs* (July) 1983; 5:23–31.

Loescher LJ, Leigh S: Isolated regional limb hyperthermic perfusion as treatment for melanoma. *Cancer Nurs* 1984; 7:461–467.

Lucey J, Baroni M: Herpetic whitlow. *Am J Nurs* 1984; 84:60–61.

Maddin S (editor): *Current Dermatologic Therapy.* Philadelphia: Saunders, 1982.

Miaskowski C: Potential and actual impairments in skin integrity related to cancer and cancer treatment. *Top Clin Nurs* (July) 1983; 5:64–71.

Sauer GC: *Manual of Skin Diseases,* 4th ed. Philadelphia: Lippincott, 1980.

Tyler G: Treatment of special burns. In: *Clinical Burn Therapy:*

A Management and Prevention Guide. Hummel RC (editor). Boston: John Wright PSG, 1982.

Suggested Readings

DeLapp TD: Taking the bite out of frostbite and other cold weather injuries. *Am J Nurs* 1980; 80:56–60. A comprehensive article, this reading offers a practical application for prevention and treatment of cold weather injuries.

Koren ME, Hermmann CS: Cancer immuno-therapy: What, why, when, how. *Nurs 81* (Jan) 1981; 11:34–41. Immune mechanisms and the purpose of immunotherapy in the treatment of select cancers are described. The role of the nurse in the use of this therapeutic method is highlighted, with a case presentation of a client with malignant melanoma.

Loescher LJ, Leigh S: Isolated regional limb hyperthermic perfusion as treatment for melanoma. *Cancer Nurs* 1984; 7:461–467. This article reports on the research being conducted in the treatment of melanoma with isolated regional limb hyperthermic perfusion and includes a detailed account of the procedure itself as well as the nursing implications.

The Client With Acne

I. Descriptive Data	This is Mary Dixon's first visit to the University Adolescent Outpatient Clinic. She was initially referred by a school nurse and is accompanied by her mother. Mrs Dixon was present during the first part of the health history and then left the room. Additional information was sought from Mary alone, as is Adolescent Clinic policy. Mrs Dixon was not present during the physical examination.

II. Personal Data

Date and Time:	Jan 5, 1986
Full Name:	Mary Therese Dixon
Social Security Number:	000-00-0000
Address:	920 Kings St., Apt. #110, Los Angeles, CA 90715
Sex:	Female
Age:	15 years, 6 months
Birthdate:	6-3-70
Marital Status:	Single
Race/Culture:	Caucasian
Occupation:	Student
Usual Health Care Provider:	Martha Donovan, RN, nurse practitioner, Adolescent Clinic

III. Health History

Source of Information:	Client and mother
Reliability of Informants:	Reliable
Chief Concern:	"I want to get rid of these pimples."
History of Present Illness:	This is a 15½-year-old, white adolescent female with a 1-year history of acne that has gradually worsened. Client has sought no previous medical care, initially believing the pimples would go away with a proper diet and face washing. Six months ago began reducing intake of chocolate and fried foods without any noted improvement in complexion. In addition to a daily shower, began to wash face twice a day with Dial soap followed by "lots" of rubbing alcohol applied to all pimples. Around that same time, she noted that the whiteheads and blackheads on her face were becoming larger, more reddened in appearance, and were spreading to her neck and shoulders. Four weeks ago, Mary started "picking" at the pimples on her forehead, resulting in some hard pus-filled whiteheads.
	No past problems with skin rashes. Uses no lotions (prescription or over the counter), creams, or cosmetics (except lipstick and eye shadow) on her face. Denies any relationship between acne and menstrual periods. Has a "best" boyfriend but is not sexually active. Mother had a "bad case" of acne as a teenager resulting in some facial scarring. Mary relates that she is now becoming embarrassed by her acne and is self-conscious about her "ugly face."
Past Health History:	
Pregnancy/Labor/Delivery:	Product of a normal, spontaneous vaginal delivery at term; birth weight, 7 lb, 8 oz; no neonatal complications
Childhood Illnesses:	Mumps, age 4 yr
Immunizations:	Booster Td, age 14 yr; primary DTP and TOPV series completed; measles and rubella vaccine, age 2.
Hospitalizations:	Four-day stay for dehydration due to gastroenteritis, age 4 mo
Surgeries:	T&A, age 5

(continued)

Case Study written by Margaret Brady.

The Client With Acne

Allergies: Mold and cats (skin-testing positive) manifested by allergic rhinitis

Medications: Multivitamin 1 q.d.; chlorpheniramine (Chlor-Trimeton) sustained-release tabs, 8 mg q. 8–12 h p.r.n. for allergy symptoms; ASA for dysmenorrhea

Family History: Father, age 36, living; alcoholic (divorced from mother, 1983)
Mother, age 35, A&W; acne as a teenager, bronchial asthma
Sister, age 14, A&W
Brother, age 11, A&W; bronchial asthma, heart murmur
MGM, maternal aunt, both with history of asthma
No other significant family health problems

Personal/Social History: Lives with mother, sister, and brother in a two-bedroom apartment. Close-knit family. Generally gets along well with her sister and brother, although they do fight on occasion. Feels that she needs to help her mother more as she is the oldest child. No extended family members live close by. Mother employed as a clerk in a grocery store and is gradually working off debts incurred by ex-husband. Parents divorced 3 years ago. Mary says she loves her dad but fears his drinking. He has moved out of state, sends no support money, and has not been in touch with them for the last 2 years.

Mary is a sophomore in high school; maintains a C+ average in required math, English, and biology courses. Does B work in social sciences and history. Mary asked the school nurse for help with her acne, and a referral was made to the clinic because Mrs Dixon's health insurance does not cover outpatient physician visits. Mrs Dixon had wanted to seek medical help for Mary earlier but felt she could not afford care and did not know that Mary could be seen on a sliding-scale payment basis.

Habits: Sleeps average 8 hours a night; runs at least 2 to 4 miles per day for girl's track team training; bites nails; drinks no alcohol; denies cigarette smoking and marijuana use (has tried smoking cigarettes twice); denies nonprescription and "street" drug use; uses car seat belts regularly.

Sexual Education: Feels fairly comfortable talking about sex with her mother. Shares information with "best" girlfriend. Knowledgeable about sexual intercourse, conception, and some contraception practices. Has no plans to become sexually active in the near future.

Nutrition: Eats from basic four food groups with a three-meal pattern plus frequent snacking on cookies and diet soft drinks. Favorite meal—hamburger, coke, and fries. Averages 16 to 24 oz of milk per day.

Review of Systems: States her overall health is excellent; has high energy level; only health concern is acne

Skin: See history of present illness

Eyes: Vision just tested at school, 20/20 OU; no history of infections, eye pain, or decreased vision

Ears: External otitis media 6 months ago, no further problems; passed school audiometric testing this year

Nose/Throat: Allergic rhinitis three to four episodes per year; responds well to chlorpheniramine; dental visit 2 months ago

Respiratory: Occasional cold; denies dyspnea/wheezing on exercising

Gynecological: Menarche: 14 yr, 3 mo; cycle regular 28 days; mild cramping first 24—36 h, responds to ASA, 650 mg q. 4—6 h p.r.n.; never had pelvic examination

Musculoskeletal: Denies leg and joint pains; screened annually in school for scoliosis, no curvature noted

Psychological: No recent major changes in mood or behavior; generally feels positive about self except for "acne"; normal adolescent concerns noted

Physical Assessment:

Height: 5 ft, 5 in (45th percentile for age)

Weight: 114 lb (6th percentile for age)

Vital Signs: Temperature 98^8F (oral); pulse 72; respirations 20; B/P 100/60 right arm, sitting

General Appearance: Well-developed, well-nourished, smiling adolescent female with obvious facial acne

Skin: Numerous open and closed comedones over face, neck, and shoulders; occasional nodules and inflammatory papules on shoulders; several small pustules on forehead; no cysts; no scarring noted; no excessive oiliness noted

HEENT: Conjunctiva clear, no redness, no exudate; left tympanic membrane slightly retracted but movable on pneumatic otoscopy, landmarks visible; light reflex normal; nasal turbinates with slightly bluish and boggy appearance, nostrils patent bilaterally; pharynx without exudate or redness; teeth, good hygiene and in good repair

Respiratory: Lungs clear to auscultation, no rales, no rhonchi

Breasts: Tanner Stage 5; no masses palpable, equal size bilaterally

Cardiovascular: PMI at 5 LICS, slightly medial to MCL; S1, S2 normal, no murmurs; femoral pulses strong and equal bilaterally

Genitourinary: Tanner Stage 5 pubic hair; normal external female genitalia

Musculoskeletal: Spine straight; no thoracic hump, no sacral tilt, scapulae level, flank angles equal on scoliosis screening examination

III. Diagnostic Data Routine initial examination/laboratory screening showed a normal CBC, urinalysis, and negative tine test.

IV. Summary Mary was placed on tetracycline, 500 mg PO, once daily plus the following topical keratolytic agents: Tretinoin (Retin-A) 0.05% cream in the morning and benzoyl peroxide gel 5% at bedtime. The purpose, action, and side effects of each drug were outlined, and a drug information sheet was given to Mary. Additional information was presented on proper skin hygiene and avoidance of squeezing the lesions. Common myths surrounding acne were also addressed. Issues of increasing sexual identity/awareness and body image concerns were discussed at this first visit. Mary was scheduled to return to the Adolescent Clinic to see her primary health care provider who would be in charge of Mary's long-term acne management and adolescent health care needs.

V. Nursing Care Plan

Nursing Diagnoses	Client Care Goals	Plan/Nursing Implementation	Expected Outcomes
Skin integrity, impairment of: related to acne	Involve self actively in skin care regimen; ask questions freely	Instruct regarding skin hygiene and practices that worsen the skin problem (eg, squeezing pimples,	Assumes responsibility for skin hygiene measures and taking medications as pre-

(continued)

V. Nursing Care Plan (continued)

Nursing Diagnoses	Client Care Goals	Plan/Nursing Implementation	Expected Outcomes
		oil-based cosmetics, rubbing alcohol); assess knowledge of the prescribed pharmacologic management plan: tetracycline, 500 mg, once daily, application of tretinoin 0.05% cream in AM and benzoyl peroxide gel 5% at bedtime; give personal medication profile sheet covering purpose, side effects (including teratogenic), and contraindications; discuss plan for long-term follow-up care necessary for acne control	scribed; reduces practices that are irritating to the skin (eg, squeezing pimples, using creams, rubbing alcohol); continues to use cosmetics sparingly; reduction in numbers of pustules and inflammatory papules within 1 to 2 months; describes correctly the rationale behind pharmacologic and hygiene treatment plan
Self-concept, disturbance in: body image and self-esteem	Express feelings of frustration over physical appearance due to acne	Assign primary health care provider to coordinate medical and psychosocial care; encourage attendance at clinic-sponsored adolescent group meetings where adolescents come to discuss various developmental concerns; encourage to share feelings with peers	Reduction in number of negative comments about complexion; continues to maintain friendships with peers and normal activities (no drastic change in behavior pattern)
Coping, potential for ineffective individual: related to emerging sexuality issues	Understand the physical and psychosocial changes occurring during adolescence; readily discuss these issues	Facilitate discussion of sexuality issues and sex education; encourage reading of clinic pamphlets and booklets on sexual issues relevant to adolescence	Seeks out information and readily brings up concerns regarding sex education and sexual identity
Coping, ineffective family: compromised	Learn to express anger over father's alcoholism; participate with mother in setting up realistic schedule of activities and household duties for all members of family	Encourage family to discuss their mutual concerns and worries (eg, finances, household duties, father's absence); refer mother to clinic social worker	Reduction in amount of tension at home (reports of family squabbles to decrease); family to increase network of social supports (eg, church groups, community organizations)

Chapter 80

Surgical Approaches to Integumentary System Dysfunction

Carolyn Gorczyca

Objectives

When you have finished studying this chapter, you should be able to:

Describe surgical approaches used to treat dermatological problems.

Describe plastic and reconstructive surgery for skin disorders.

Identify indications for each surgical approach as well as any contraindications.

Explain the role of the nurse in the perioperative management of clients who are having dermatological or plastic and reconstructive surgery.

Teach clients their responsibilities for the care of the integument following a surgical procedure on the skin.

Anticipate the physiological alterations in the skin and complications that may occur as a result of surgery.

Anticipate the psychosocial and lifestyle implications that result from surgery on the integumentary system.

Surgery is a major therapeutic component in management of some skin problems, whether the pathogenesis is related to a congenital, genetic, or acquired disorder; infection; neoplasia; trauma; or the normal aging process. Surgery may range from a minor operation to a complex set of surgical procedures and may be performed by a dermatologist, a general surgeon, or a plastic surgeon. Procedures may be performed as an ambulatory care service in a physician's office or a clinic, or may require hospitalization for several days. For clients admitted to the hospital for traumatic injuries, such as burns, surgery is only a part of the treatment regimen.

Recent technological advances have expanded the number of surgical approaches to dermatological problems. For example, surgeons are able to transplant skin and tissue flaps using an operating microscope to reattach the finer blood vessels and increase success. All of the fine instruments used in this delicate surgery are small enough to fit into a teacup. Laser surgery has also made an impact in the treatment of a number of skin disorders. Surgical intervention to remedy skin disorders or defects requires not only a vast range of technical skills but also artistic ability. Plastic surgery can reach beyond the cutaneous layers to include reconstruction of underlying musculoskeletal structures in repairing deformities and defects of the integument. It includes the field of cosmetic or aesthetic surgery, which has grown as techniques have developed to remedy visible defects that often impose both an emotional and economical burden.

This chapter discusses both dermatological surgery for the treatment of cutaneous lesions, as well as plastic and reconstructive surgery.

Section I: General Considerations in Surgery of the Integument

Whether elective or required, surgery is chosen when an alternative treatment would not be as effective and when the risks do not outweigh the benefits. Before consenting to the procedure, the client must be informed of the possible alterations in skin color, texture, configuration, sensory perception, or all of these. Selection of the surgeon is important, and clients should be encouraged to investigate available options. Clients should also be aware of the surgeon's expertise and whether the surgeon is as concerned with aesthetics as with the functional restoration of the part. (Refer to the resources list at the end of Chapter 78.) Clients should also understand what their health insurance covers because some plans do not cover surgery that is considered cosmetic.

Extensive surgery or any procedure that may produce significant changes in appearance must be carefully planned beforehand and discussed in detail with the client. The surgeon may use photographs and drawings to illustrate the proposed outcomes and to identify the various stages of repair, if more than one is required. Clients should be clearly informed when surgery does not offer a permanent resolution of the problem. During these initial sessions, the physician also attempts to establish a trusting relationship with the client to identify motivational factors, personality traits, and the effects of social and cultural influences on the person's feelings about body image. Care providers must establish effective communication and correctly assess the psychological state of each client so any unrealistic expectations about aesthetic gains or losses can be clarified before the surgeon proceeds. This relationship is especially critical when dissatisfaction with cosmetic surgery can lead to legal action. Surgery may be avoided in situations where a perceptive care provider recognizes that elective correction of a physical defect may not have the desired psychological effect and may even compound the emotional distress of the client.

The nurse should be fully informed about both the surgical procedure and the expected outcome to be able to care for the client knowledgeably, to be supportive, and to assist the client in attaining the desired goal. Preoperatively, clients have many fears about disfigurement and recovery that can be alleviated through effective communication. Clients with malignant lesions may feel that surgery has been imposed on them and may need to express their concerns about the quality as well as the quantity of life that will remain.

To promote healing, minimize disfigurement, and prevent complications, the surgeon who operates on the skin considers numerous factors. Scarring and the formation of hematomas and seromas are avoided by careful planning of incisional lines; by avoiding the use of aspirin or aspirin-containing compounds for two weeks before and after surgery; by limiting destruction of healthy tissue and remov-

ing devitalized tissue; by using appropriate suturing or closure materials and inserting drains; and finally, by applying an appropriate dressing. In addition, healing occurs faster in areas with a good blood supply. Preventing nausea and vomiting also reduces stress on facial incisions.

Because of the circulation, facial incisions normally require only 3 to 5 days to heal, whereas legs and feet may take 2 to 4 weeks. Prompt suture removal is useful in preventing irritation but timing will differ with the procedure. Infection, always a potential problem, is limited by preoperative cleansing with a bactericidal soap, effective asepsis, promotion of wound healing, and appropriate use of antibiotics. Infections or inflammatory conditions of the skin must be treated before performing elective surgery. Scarring is minimized by judicious wound care and by avoiding unnecessary dermatological surgery on young persons and on areas such as the presternum, shoulders, upper back, lower legs, head and neck that are vulnerable to hypertrophic reactions and the development of keloids (see Chapter 79).

Postoperatively, the potential for life-threatening problems becomes a serious concern with extensive reconstructive surgery, skin transplantation, and any surgery requiring general anesthesia. The age of the client, premorbid health status, and precipitating factors necessitating surgery should be considered in planning for monitoring and maintenance of vital functions. Early mobility is critical in preventing systemic problems; however, strict regulation and proper positioning of the affected part may be required to ensure good healing.

Although the hospitalized client may depend on the nurse for wound management, self-care should be taught as soon as possible in preparation for discharge, which often occurs in a few days. A plan of care must deal with the anticipated effects from the operative procedure, such as ecchymosis, edema, discomfort, and sensory deficits. Each client must be made aware of the time needed for various stages of healing, not only to avoid discouragement, but to prevent the client from putting undue stress on the wound. Nutrition is an integral part of healing, and supplements must be provided when protein and vitamin deficits exist. A client who does not require hospitalization and who must assume responsibility for preoperative and postoperative care needs clear explanations and written instructions on preoperative preparation, how to facilitate wound closure, and how to prevent any injury to the skin. It may be necessary to instruct a family member or friend who will assist the client at home.

Even the client who has been carefully prepared for the aesthetic effects of surgery must be closely monitored by the nurse and physician to assess behaviors indicating emotional adjustment during recovery. A nurse should be present when an extensive or highly disfiguring wound is viewed for the first time and should have developed a plan to elicit the client's feelings then and throughout hospitalization. Anxiety and depression are common reactions and may be evidenced by eating and sleeping disturbances, crying, and withdrawal from routine activities (see Chapter 6). The true surgical outcome may not become obvious during the early postoperative period.

Whenever dermatological surgery affects the general appearance, the client needs to integrate the altered body image. The client's behaviors may indicate either acceptance or rejection of the change. Fears may become evident as the client prepares for discharge and socialization beyond the protective hospital environment. The family may need instruction in how to observe for major emotional difficulties and to notify the health care provider when coping becomes too stressful. Although external wounds heal, the psyche may need more time and possibly assistance for the repair process to be fully integrated.

Section II: Dermatological Surgery

Most dermatological surgery for the treatment of cutaneous lesions can be carried out in an ambulatory care facility in a relatively brief period of time. Although often classified as "minor" surgery because of these factors, they may be anxiety provoking and not always perceived as minor by the client.

The surgical procedures discussed here are dermabrasion, cryosurgery, electrosurgery, surgical excision, microscopically controlled excision, and laser surgery. Chemical peeling is also included for discussion in this section. Although not technically a surgical procedure, it shares many of the physiological and psychosocial/lifestyle implications for the client that dermatological surgical procedures do and therefore is included in this chapter.

CHEMICAL PEELING

Chemical peeling (chemical planing, chemabrasion, or chemexfoliation) involves the use of caustics to destroy the epidermis and upper portion of the dermis by chemical coagulation.

The ultimate outcome of chemical peeling is a smoother skin and permanent lightening of pigmentation. Therefore, one of the major purposes of this procedure is to rejuvenate aging skin by removing fine facial wrinkles, lentigines (flat brown pigmented spots), and actinic lesions. Superficial scars from acne can be eradicated, and the discoloration from freckling or chloasma can also be effectively reduced with chemical peeling. Chemabrasion is often used in conjunction with dermabrasion to obtain a more effective cosmetic improvement.

The ideal client who is less likely to scar or develop hyperpigmentation during healing has dry skin, blue eyes, and a fair complexion. The procedure is used cautiously or is even contraindicated in those who are darkly pigmented, have pigment disturbances, are taking birth control pills, or tend to scar.

Surgical Procedure

Several cauterants may be used for chemical peeling. Liquid phenol, or Bakers' formula (a 50% phenol solution),

though effective in treating aging skin, is known to cause renal, hepatic, and even cardiac toxicity when absorbed. Trichloroacetic acid (TCA) is also effective but less hazardous. Combes' formula, a combination of resorcinol, salicylic acid, lactic acid, and ethanol, has been recently introduced as a cauterant.

After the skin is cleansed to remove surface oils and debris, the selected chemical is meticulously applied with cotton applicators, either to the entire face or to segmented areas such as the forehead and perioral areas, the cheeks, eyelids, or the upper and lower lips, avoiding contact with the eyes. Because of an increased tendency for scarring and hyperpigmentation on the neck, treatment of this location is contraindicated. Following application of the caustic agent, the treated area is taped with waterproof adhesive tape, which is left in place for 24 to 48 hours to improve the penetration process.

Implications for the Client

Physiological Implications

Cauterants cause an uncomfortable burning sensation for 30 to 45 minutes after application followed by edema that begins within about 8 hours and gradually subsides in 3 to 4 weeks. The eyelids are particularly susceptible to edema. During the first 2 days and during separation of the crust, the client may be uncomfortable and sleep may be disturbed. The denuded area is susceptible to infection. The most serious problem may result from a herpes simplex infection, which can travel readily over the denuded tissue. Mild untoward effects include sensitivity to sunlight, prolonged redness, talangectasia, and the development of milia even after healing. Complications may result from phenol toxicity.

Psychosocial/Lifestyle Implications

When chemical peeling removes or reduces superficial scars, actinic lesions, and areas of discoloration or rejuvenates aging skin, clients' self-concept and body image improve. Initially, however, clients must contend with edema, disfiguring crusts, and erythema. The erythema may take as long as 6 to 12 weeks to disappear. Clients may be reluctant

Table 80–1 Chemical Peeling: Implications for the Client	
Physiological Implications	**Psychosocial/Lifestyle Implications**
Burning for 30–45 min after application of cauterant	Improvement in self-concept and body image with successful treatment
Postoperative edema beginning within about 8 h and lasting for 3–4 wk	Edema and crusting may cause initial anxiety
Postoperative discomfort and interference with sleep possible for the first 2 days posttreatment and during separation of the crust	Limitations on general activity as well as chewing, drinking, talking, and facial expressions until the crust resolves
Possibility of infection in denuded area (herpes simplex is the most serious)	Prolonged erythema (6–12 wk) may affect usual social activities
Possibility of mild untoward effects such as sensitivity to sunlight, prolonged redness, telangiectasia, and milia	
Possibility of phenol toxicity	

to engage in their usual social activities until they feel more comfortable with their appearance.

The crusts that form over the denuded area may interfere with chewing, drinking, talking, and facial expression. The client is required to restrict activities and alter the diet to avoid injuring the healing area. Complications such as unwanted pigmentary changes and scarring may cause disfigurement. Table 80–1 summarizes client implications for chemical peeling.

Nursing Implications

Preoperative Care
Preoperative care should include thorough explanations of the procedure and healing process. Clients will be asked to cleanse the facial area thoroughly with a hexachlorophene-based liquid soap for a few days prior to surgery to help prevent infection and to avoid any soap that produces an oily skin residue.

A total peel, or one-stage peel, may require hospitalization, or the surgery may be performed on an ambulatory basis. The amount of preoperative sedation is individualized and gauged by the degree of burning sensation the client is likely to experience 30 to 45 minutes following topical application of the cauterant.

Postoperative Care
The potential toxic effects from phenol warrant close monitoring of cardiac function and blood pressure in the immediate postoperative period.

Elevating the head of the bed will decrease edema and is helpful in lessening discomfort during the first 2 postoperative days. Narcotic analgesics and hypnotics may be necessary to provide comfort and rest. When the adhesive tape is removed, sedation is usually given to minimize pain. Thymol iodine powder is then applied several times over the denuded area to protect against infection and to aid in the formation of a crust.

To promote a smoother epithelialization, the client must be instructed to avoid splitting the crust formed over the wound. A liquid diet minimizes chewing, and written communication or hand signals limits talking. General activity is minimized to lessen movement.

Approximately 3 to 5 days after the crust has formed, it may be softened by gently washing the area with mild soap and water and applying an ointment containing 5% boric acid or vitamins A and D. Some surgeons prefer liberal coverage with petrolatum jelly or cold cream to facilitate crust removal and do not permit washing the face until 12 to 14 days after surgery. Encourage the client to allow spontaneous sloughing of the crust with whatever procedure is prescribed. Cool tap water compresses, steroid creams, analgesics, and tranquilizers may relieve the itching or burning sensation that occurs when the crust separates.

Clients should be instructed to use sunscreen and avoid direct exposure to sunlight for 3 to 6 months. Water-based makeup may be used to cover the erythema when the wound area has healed. The client should expect the redness to fade gradually over 6 to 12 weeks.

DERMABRASION

Dermabrasion (or surgical planing) involves the removal of the epidermis and the upper dermis by an abrasive instrument to eliminate superficial irregularities and discolorations. Dermabrasion is used mainly for aesthetic rather than therapeutic purposes. The face and scalp are most often treated because they contain more of the glands and follicles needed for reepithelialization.

The prime candidates for skin planing have been persons with shallow or moderate scarring, generally from acne vulgaris or a pox virus. The procedure may be used to remove fine facial wrinkles from aging skin. Traumatic or surgical scars may be flattened and made less conspicuous, and tattoos may be removed by dermabrasion. Clients who demand perfection are not usually considered good candidates for dermabrasion. Also not considered good candidates are clients with a history of hypertrophic scarring or keloid formation, clients with an active pyoderm, warts, or a prior severe or recurrent herpes simplex infection, and clients with highly pigmented skin where dermabrasion may alter pigmentation.

Surgical Procedure

Dermabrasion may be performed in the physician's office or other outpatient health care facility, but extensive planing usually requires hospitalization. General or local anesthesia may be used.

Dermabrasion is accomplished through use of a motor-driven rotary instrument consisting of fine stainless steel wires or coarse diamond burrs. The superficial layer of skin is sanded until irregular surfaces are minimized. The area is irrigated during and following abrasion with copious amounts of saline solution to provide an observable field and to remove any debris that would interfere with healing.

An experienced surgeon may perform the procedure in less than one half hour. The abraded area may be coated with an antibiotic ointment, left exposed, or covered with Owen's gauze (saponified cellulose acetate), petrolatum gauze, or a nonadhering dressing (Telfa). Additional coverage may include dry fluffed gauze and a pressure dressing. Use of a thrombin paste is an alternate method; besides controlling bleeding, the paste forms a protective coat over the abraded area once it dries. The outer dressing is usually removed after 24 to 48 hours. Because the wound exudes not only blood and serum but clotting substances such as fibrin and thromboplastin, excessive bleeding is not usually a major problem.

Implications for the Client

Physiological Implications

Clients usually develop marked edema immediately after surgery, which may last for 3 to 6 weeks. Pain occurs while exudate oozes from the abraded area for approximately the first 48 hours forming a thick crust. As the crust forms and the exudate tightens, the client may experience discomfort increased by chewing and talking. The crust loosens in 7 to 10 days and sloughs spontaneously in about 2 weeks. Erythema may last for 6 to 12 weeks. Pruritus is common during this period.

Excess pigmentation and depigmentation are potential untoward effects. More commonly, a brownish discoloration that varies in intensity may appear in the abraded area. Infection, the development of milia, spreading of existing warts or herpes simplex, and hypertrophic scarring are potential complications. The skin may be sensitive to sunlight.

One dermabrasion treatment may be insufficient to accomplish the goal. Some conditions may require up to three sessions to attain the desired effects. Although this procedure offers cosmetic improvement, it may never totally eliminate defects.

Psychosocial/Lifestyle Implications

Clients who understand that dermabrasion may not completely eliminate a defect are usually pleased with the cosmetic improvement that results. Self-esteem is increased, and body image is enhanced.

The crusting requires restrictions on talking, chewing, and other facial movements as well as dietary alterations for foods requiring less chewing.

The initial disfigurement and discoloration may be upsetting and cause the client to limit socialization for the 6 to 12 weeks while the erythematous skin returns to its normal color and texture. Most clients return to work in approximately 2 weeks or when the crust has sloughed.

Complications such as pigmentary changes and scarring may cause emotional distress and adversely affect the client's self-esteem and body image. Table 80–2 summarizes client implications related to dermabrasion.

Nursing Implications

Preoperative Care

The preoperative preparation should focus on reinforcement of teaching and client discussion regarding the aesthetic outcomes, description of the actual procedure, and self-care instruction. Thorough cleansing of the skin with liquid hexachlorophene (pHisoHex) is begun several days before dermabrasion. Male clients must shave on the day of surgery. Preoperative medication is based on the needs of the client.

Postoperative Care

Encourage the client to keep the head elevated to help reduce the marked edema that follows surgery. The measures identified for chemical peeling should be instituted to prevent premature cracking and separation of the crust. The last layer of dressing covering the wound is removed by the third day; removal may be facilitated by showering. Applying cocoa butter, mineral oil, lanolin, or cold creams will assist in removing the crust, lessen the discomfort associated with tightening of the exudate, and lubricate the skin.

Pain, which usually dissipates as the crust forms, may be alleviated by analgesics or sedatives. Keeping the area dry and free from injury will assist in preventing infection until healing is complete. Itching may become a problem, and clients may need to be instructed in how to avoid scratching and prevent infection from fingernail damage (see Chapter 78). Instruct clients to avoid direct exposure to sunlight without protective coverage.

Table 80-2   Dermabrasion: Implications for the Client

Physiological Implications	Psychosocial/Lifestyle Implications
Marked edema immediately after surgery; edema may last for 3–6 wk	Cosmetic improvement
Pain for approximately 48 h postoperatively; discomfort from tightening of the exudate	Increased self-esteem and enhanced body image
Crust takes 7–10 days to loosen, sloughing spontaneously in about 2 wk	Limitations on talking, chewing, facial movements, and alteration of diet because of crusting
Pruritus common	Edema and erythema may be distressing and cause the client to limit social activities for 6–12 wk postoperatively
Excess pigmentation, depigmentation, or brownish discoloration may occur	Return to work in approximately 2 wk or after crust sloughs
Potential complications are infection, development of milia, spread of existing warts or herpes simplex, hypertrophic scarring	Complications may cause emotional distress and adversely affect self-esteem and body image
Abraded skin is sensitive to sunlight	
Repeat treatments may be necessary	

CRYOSURGERY

Cryosurgery freezes tissue, either superficially or at a deeper level, to produce necrosis. It is a simple, safe, and fast procedure that has been effective in the treatment of superficial basal cell carcinoma, seborrheic and actinic keratoses, leukoplakia, and warts.

Surgical Procedure

The lesion is frozen using solid carbon dioxide (dry ice), liquid nitrogen, or Freon 114. Depending on the agent, administration involves direct application by a large loosely wound cotton swab, a spray, or a closed cryoprobe system.

Cryonecrosis begins when tissue temperature reaches −20° to −30°C. The duration of freezing is usually a matter of seconds.

Implications for the Client

Physiological Implications

The client may experience moderate to marked pain during the freezing and thawing process and for the first 24 hours after treatment. A blister forms as the area thaws. It subsequently dries, crusts, and sloughs off in 10 to 14 days. Some localized edema may also develop. Complications such as hemorrhage and infections are rare, and little wound care is required. Major complications such as hypertrophic scarring or pigmentary changes are unlikely if cryosurgery has been superficial. The client may be required to return for evaluation in 2 weeks, when the procedure may be repeated if necessary (eg, when the lesion is deep) to eradicate the dermatological problem.

Psychosocial/Lifestyle Implications

Clients generally have a favorable attitude toward cryosurgery because it can be performed on an ambulatory basis, is a brief procedure, and has few postoperative restrictions and complications. The client may feel uncomfortable about the blister or crust, especially if it is located in a visible area such as the face or hand. There may be anxiety, apprehension, or frustration if the client is concerned that all the dysfunctional tissue may not have been destroyed and the procedure may have to be repeated or that an incompletely removed malignant lesion continues to grow. Table 80-3 summarizes client implications for cryosurgery.

Nursing Implications

Preoperative Care

Because most cryosurgery on skin is performed in a physician's office, many nurses may have limited opportunity for direct client contact. The client should be prepared for the surgery and know what to expect during and after the surgery.

Postoperative Care

Because hemorrhage and infections are rare, wound coverage is not necessary, but the area must be kept clean and dry. The client may be required to return in 2 weeks for an evaluation to determine whether further cryosurgery is necessary.

ELECTROSURGERY

Electrosurgery involves the use of electrical currents to destroy tissue selectively by thermocauterization. Electrosurgical instruments containing a wire loop, blade, needle,

Table 80–3 Cryosurgery: Implications for the Client	
Physiological Implications	**Psychosocial/Lifestyle Implications**
Marked to moderate pain during the freezing-thawing process and first 24 h postoperatively	Improvement in body image
Minimal edema possible	Reduction of anxiety associated with presence of lesion
Blister formation during thawing; dries, crusts, and sloughs off in 10 to 14 days	Minimal wound care and little or no restrictions on usual activity
Complications are rare	Embarrassment in regard to blister or crust if highly visible
May need to be repeated if lesion not completely eradicated	Anxiety or frustration if repeat procedure is necessary or malignant lesion not completely removed

or ball can be used for cutting, cauterizing, and coagulating. A local anesthetic is administered unless the procedure can be done quickly.

Small basal cell and squamous cell epitheliomas, actinic and seborrheic keratoses, leukoplakia, skin tags, cutaneous horns, warts, and hypertrichosis are a number of dermatological conditions that can be treated by some form of electrosurgery.

Surgical Procedure

Electrodesiccation involves the dehydration of tissues through use of a single (monoterminal) needle electrode. The current is transmitted through a spark directly into the area or by a lightning effect when the needle is held a short distance away. This method is usually followed by curettage to remove the destroyed tissue. Electrocoagulation and electrosurgical excision require a more intense heat than the desiccation process to be effective. Therefore, caution must be taken to avoid burning of normal tissue. Because alternating (biterminal) currents are used, the client must be in firm contact with a ground, usually along the broad expanse of the back, before the procedure can begin.

Implications for the Client

Physiological Implications
Edema and erythema may occur at the operative site and will probably subside in 2 to 3 days. The rate of healing depends on the depth and extent of the electrosurgery as well as on the site involved. Facial wounds heal the fastest, taking from 1 to 6 weeks. Wounds in other areas may take longer to heal. Repeated treatment may be required.

No suturing is necessary. In addition, there is a high cure rate and little or no bleeding. Infection is uncommon because the electrical currents sterilize the wound. Because bleeding is minimal, dressings are not usually required.

Scarring may be a postoperative complication and is more likely to occur when there is full-thickness skin loss.

A realistic assessment can be made 2 to 3 months after the surgery. Depending on the depth and extent of the electrosurgery, full-thickness skin loss is a potential complication.

Electrosurgery is contraindicated in clients who have demand pacemakers because it could deactivate the pacemaker cycle.

Psychosocial/Lifestyle Implications
Electrosurgery is a simple, convenient procedure that requires little or no alteration in a client's lifestyle. Clients may be concerned about their appearance until healing is completed if the operative site is highly visible. The potential for substantial scarring may cause apprehension and alter the client's body image. Table 80–4 summarizes client implications related to electrosurgery.

Nursing Implications

Preoperative Care
Electrosurgery is readily performed in outpatient health care facilities, and a preoperative medication is not required. The skin is cleansed and allowed to dry. The nurse's role is supportive and educative.

Postoperative Care
Dressings may not be required because bleeding and infection are not common problems. If dressings are used, they should be nonadherent. Clients should be informed about edema, erythema, and healing requirements. Instruct clients to return to their health care provider in 2 to 3 months to have healing evaluated.

SURGICAL EXCISION

Surgical excision involves the sharp dissection of an abnormal cutaneous growth with immediate closure of the wound so primary healing can occur. Aesthetics are considered, but removing enough tissue to prevent regrowth is the most important goal.

Table 80–4 Electrosurgery: Implications for the Client	
Physiological Implications	**Psychosocial/Lifestyle Implications**
Edema and erythema at operative site usually subsides in 2–3 days	Requires little or no alteration in lifestyle
Rate of healing depends on depth and extent of procedure and on site involved	Concern about appearance if operative site is highly visible
No suturing	Apprehension about possibility of scarring
High cure rate	Severe scarring may adversely affect body image
Little or no bleeding	
Infection uncommon	
Potential for severe scarring when the lesion is deep	
Contraindicated for clients with demand pacemakers	

Although microscopically controlled surgical excision also involves cutting primarily with scalpel and scissors, there are several major differences. Therefore, microscopically controlled surgical excision is discussed separately.

Many types of benign and malignant skin lesions are removed by excision, including basal cell and squamous cell carcinomas, melanomas, sarcomas, nevi, lipomas, fibromas, and cysts. In select cases, scars and keloids are also treated by this approach. Tissue is also excised from the integument for biopsy.

Some minor lesions may be resected on an ambulatory basis. Hospitalization is warranted for more complex procedures, clients at risk because of age or health status, and when there is need for postoperative supervision. The extent of preplanning depends on the area involved. Further reconstructive surgery may also be required.

Surgical Procedure

Under a local or general anesthesia, the lesion is dissected. Besides the conventional approach, a variety of excisions such as elliptical, wedge, or circular may be employed. (Z-plasty and other forms of skin transplantation may be required to place healthy tissue over a defective area or to provide wound coverage.) Wide resections are performed when the primary site allows for more extensive removal. More radical surgery is done when malignancies extend beyond the integument and involve critical structures within the head and neck region. A detailed discussion of this type of surgery is in Section III of this chapter and in Chapter 21.

Implications for the Client

Physiological Implications
The extensiveness of the excision determines the phys-

iological implications for the client. The major goal is to remove sufficient diseased tissue to achieve a cure. Likewise, the potential for infection and bleeding and the rate of tissue healing depend on the anatomical site involved and the extent of surgery. Extensive excision may require several surgical procedures for reconstruction.

Psychosocial/Lifestyle Implications
Aesthetic considerations are secondary to the primary goal of removing enough tissue to effect a cure in the case of malignancy. This means that disfigurement and the need for reconstructive surgery vary with each client's individual situation. Table 80–5 summarizes client implications related to surgical excision.

Nursing Implications

Preoperative Care
Although the preoperative care is often routine, the client should be prepared for the experiences that may be foreign and frightening. Additional psychological support may be required no matter how minor the procedure appears to be.

Postoperative Care
Excised areas will probably be covered and should be observed for bleeding. Compression dressings, tissue drains, or wound suction will be employed to prevent the accumulation of blood, serum, or other drainage from interfering with the healing process. The wound may be closed with sutures, skin tape, or clips. How long the sutures remain depends on the rate of healing and the intent to prevent undue scarring in visible areas.

Table 80–5 Surgical Excision and Microscopically Controlled Excision: Implications for the Client

Physiological Implications	Psychosocial/Lifestyle Implications
Surgical excision:	
Potential for bleeding and infection, other complications, and rate of healing contingent on anatomical site involved and extent of surgery	Because aesthetic considerations are secondary, disfigurement may result
	Potential alteration of body image
Further surgical procedures for reconstructive purposes may be required	Anxiety over reconstructive surgery if needed
	Apprehension while awaiting biopsy results
Microscopically controlled excision (MCE):	
Pain from application of zinc chloride paste in Mohs' classic technique	Surgery takes 2 days with Mohs' classic technique, 1 day with fresh tissue technique
Precision preserves healthy tissue	May need to be repeated if the lesion is not completely removed
Wounds that heal by secondary intention may take longer	Fear of disfigurement, especially if lesion is located in a highly visible area although disfigurement is less than with surgical excision in certain instances
High cure rate	
Complications such as infection and bleeding are rare	

MICROSCOPICALLY CONTROLLED EXCISION

Microscopically controlled excision (MCE) involves the removal of a precisely mapped epithelioma in serial fashion and the careful examination of the entire undersurface of each segment for malignant cells. The classic method, Mohs' technique, used a chemical fixative as part of the procedure. A more recent approach to MCE that eliminates the fixative is called the *fresh tissue technique* and has replaced the classic Mohs' technique. It is, however, often referred to as "Mohs' surgery, fresh tissue technique."

The types of tumors for which MCE is recommended include resistive or recurrent squamous cell or basal cell carcinomas, tumors greater than 2 cm in diameter (Robinson, 1982), and epitheliomas around the nose, ear, and eye. According to Tromovitch (Maddin, 1982), microscopically controlled excision offers the highest cure rate of any technique for these tumors.

Surgical Procedure

MCE can be performed under either general or local anesthesia, in the hospital or on an ambulatory basis. The classic Mohs' technique involved the application of dichloroacetic or trichloroacetic acid to the visible skin lesion. A layer of zinc chloride paste was subsequently applied to fixate and preserve the cellular detail of the lesion and an occlusive dressing to cover the area was applied. The second step, scalpel surgery, was usually performed within 24 hours after the fixative was applied. The actual excision involved undercutting and flattening the central portion of the lesion to eliminate loss of normal tissue. A finely detailed anatomic map of the removed tissue, with number and color codes allowed careful microscopic determination of the exact location of any remaining malignant cells. If malignant cells were found on the undersurface of any segment, the entire procedure was repeated as often as necessary to remove the entire tumor. (A fixated area provides for a bloodless field of operation.)

The fresh tissue technique provides several advantages over the classic method. Because a chemical fixative is not required, the surgery can be completed in 1 day, tissue contact with a caustic agent is avoided, and the client does not experience the pain associated with zinc chloride application. (The other steps remain the same as in the classic technique.) Immediate reconstruction of the excised area may be performed because the wound has little edema and is usually free from suppuration or tissue necrosis.

Implications for the Client

Physiological Implications
The caustic effect of zinc chloride causes pain upon application when Mohs' classic technique is used. This technique also requires a 24-hour wait before the surgical procedure can be completed. The fresh tissue technique can be performed in 1 day.

The precision of the anatomic mapping preserves healthy tissue, keeping the area of excision smaller. Wounds that heal by secondary intention may take longer. Complications such as infection and bleeding are rare.

Psychosocial/Lifestyle Implications

Surgery can be accomplished in 1 day with the fresh tissue technique or 2 days with Mohs' technique with minimal disruption of usual activities. Clients may fear disfigurement, especially if the operative site is visible. Disfiguration with this procedure is less in certain instances than with surgical excision (Robinson, 1982). Mohs' technique may require more than one surgery until the lesion is removed. Table 80–5 summarizes the client implications related to MCE.

Nursing Implications

Preoperative Care

The uniqueness of this surgery should have been explained by the surgeon, but the nurse may need to clarify aspects of the procedure the client hasn't understood. The client is likely to be under stress, which may become more evident during preoperative interactions. The presence of a malignancy, particularly on the face, provokes fears of disfigurement. Fears of a negative prognosis must also be addressed prior to treatment.

Postoperative Care

Wounds may be surgically closed or allowed to heal by secondary intention depending on size. A bandage or nonadherent dressing may provide sufficient coverage. Clients who have been treated on an ambulatory basis should be given oral and written instructions for dressing change and cleansing of the wound. Dressings are usually changed twice daily and the wound cleansed with half-strength hydrogen peroxide. Although secondary infection is rare, topical antibiotic ointments may be prescribed for prophylaxis. Soft tissue slough generally occurs in 7 days and should show a healthy granulating base. Clients return for checkups several times during the first 12 months and then yearly for 5 years.

LASER SURGERY

Selected skin lesions have been treated primarily by argon and carbon dioxide lasers. (Laser surgery is described in Chapter 14.) Argon lasers cause thermocoagulation in the dermal layer of the skin without removing or destroying overlying tissue and have proven useful for vascular lesions and removal of tattoos. Port-wine stains have responded by lightening in color, flattening, appearing smoother, and decreasing in size because of skin contraction. A halt in the evolution of port-wine stains also becomes evident as the lesion ceases to darken. Other vascular lesions treated with the argon laser include spider ectasia, ectatic vessels associated with rosacea, telangiectasia, and selected vascular tumors. The carbon dioxide laser affects the superficial layer of the skin and has been used in the treatment of warts, malignant skin tumors, leukoplakia, and actinic keratosis. Burns and decubitus ulcers have also been debrided by this surgical approach.

Surgical Procedure

Laser surgery for dermatological conditions may be performed on an ambulatory basis and with the use of local anesthesia. Both the carbon dioxide and argon lasers can be focused on the skin lesion with millimeter accuracy, and the depth can be controlled to minimize damage to surrounding tissue and the skin's glandular appendages.

Implications for the Client

Physiological Implications

Skin effects from laser surgery can range from a mild reddening to blistering or even charring. The extent of the thermal damage to the skin depends on a number of factors—wavelength of the laser, absorption and scattering rates, beam size, duration of time exposure, size of the area treated, and cooling abilities of the involved tissues. Edema lasting for several hours or days should be anticipated. Marked swelling of the eyelids occurs when surgery is performed in the periorbital area.

Healing occurs fastest with the carbon dioxide laser because of the diminished blood loss and the sealing effect of the beam on the wounds. A port-wine stain treated with the argon laser tends to weep for 1 to 3 weeks and may or may not subsequently form a crust or scab. The skin may take from 2 to 9 months, and in some cases up to 2 years, to lighten.

The most significant pain that occurs during skin laser surgery is from the injection of relatively large amounts of lidocaine 2% (Xylocaine) as a local anesthetic during treatment of a port-wine stain. Its purpose is to decrease the pain produced by thermocoagulation over a large skin area.

Studies have reported marked lightening without scarring in 70% to 85% of the clients treated by argon laser for port wine stains, and significant scarring in 4% to 6% (Dixon, 1983). Pigmentation changes do occur because melanin also absorbs light; changes may range from a whitening to a brownish discoloration. The most favorable results have been obtained in adults in whom the blood vessels in the lesion have become dilated or ectatic and when the color of the port-wine stain has progressed from pink to purple. Clients with olive-colored or highly pigmented skin and clients with increased potential for scarring (children or individuals with a history of hypertrophic scarring) are not considered good candidates for argon laser treatment. In addition, scarring is more likely to occur when lesions have been located in the area of the upper lip, chin, or the angle of the mandible.

Psychosocial/Lifestyle Implications

Some lifestyle changes are involved with laser surgery for port-wine stains. Clients need to provide wound care until healing occurs. The use of cosmetics, as well as shaving, should be delayed until healing is complete. Direct exposure to sunlight should be avoided for at least 10 weeks

Table 80–6 Laser Surgery: Implications for the Client

Physiological Implications	Psychosocial/Lifestyle Implications
Laser surgery in general:	
Skin effects ranging from mild erythema to blistering or charring	Must care for wound until it heals
Edema for several hours or days postoperatively	Use of cosmetics and shaving delayed until site is healed
Faster healing with carbon dioxide laser	
Eye damage is a hazard to both client and operating room personnel; protective safety gear should be worn	
Port-wine stain:	
Port-wine stain wounds weep for 1–3 wk and may or may not form a scab	Direct exposure to sunlight without sunscreen protection should be avoided for at least 10 wk
Atrophic and hypertrophic scarring and pigmentation changes are potential complications	Altered body image image and emotional distress if scarring and discoloration occur
Treatment usually requires several surgeries; depends on size of lesion	Direct exposure of the port-wine stain to sunlight should be avoided for 3 wk preoperatively
Pain associated with injection of local anesthetic	Lightening, flattening, and smoothing of skin, especially in visible areas, reduces emotional distress and improves self-esteem and body image
Skin usually takes 2 to 9 mo to lighten; may take as long as 2 yr	

after surgery unless sunscreen protection is used. Sunscreen should not be applied until healing has taken place. Scarring and discoloration may alter the body image and cause emotional distress. Removal or improvement of appearance of the lesion reduces anxiety and increases the client's self-esteem and improves body image. Table 80–6 summarizes client implications of laser surgery.

Nursing Implications

Preoperative Care

Alleviation of preoperative fear associated with laser therapy and health teaching regarding postoperative care are prime responsibilities of the nurse. Clients who are having laser surgery for port-wine stains are requested to avoid direct exposure to the sun for 3 weeks preoperatively because the erythema could inhibit the treatment effects. Drugs containing aspirin or other anticoagulating agents are contraindicated for a week prior to surgery to lessen postoperative bleeding.

In the case of port-wine stains, a 2 cm patch test may be performed before actual treatment so the physician and the client can realistically assess the healing time needed,

the positive and negative aesthetic outcomes, and the physiological and psychosocial effects that accompany treatment. The client should also be made aware of the anticipated duration of the treatment because a number of sessions will be required for complete removal of the lesion or to attain the desired outcomes.

Postoperative Care

Application of ice packs to the eyelids, elevation of the head, and forced winking to activate ocular muscles may all assist in decreasing postoperative edema.

The wound with port-wine stains, which may weep for 1 to 3 weeks, must be kept clean and dry. During this phase, the area should be washed at least three times a day, rinsed well, gently patted dry, and covered with nonadherent dressings or Band-Aids to prevent trauma to the site or premature separation of the crust. Although infection is uncommon, precautions may be taken by topical application of antibiotics until the wound is healed.

The client should return to the surgeon for evaluation of healing. A reasonable evaluation of the effectiveness of treatment of a port-wine stain can be made in approximately 4 months.

Section III: Plastic and Reconstructive Surgery

Contrary to the tendency to think of plastic and reconstructive surgery as purely cosmetic, most plastic surgical procedures are done to improve body function. The defects being treated often involve more structures than the skin

alone. This section includes procedures to improve body function as well as procedures to improve body appearance.

Taking skin or other tissues from other areas of the body or even exogenous sources to cover wounds or other

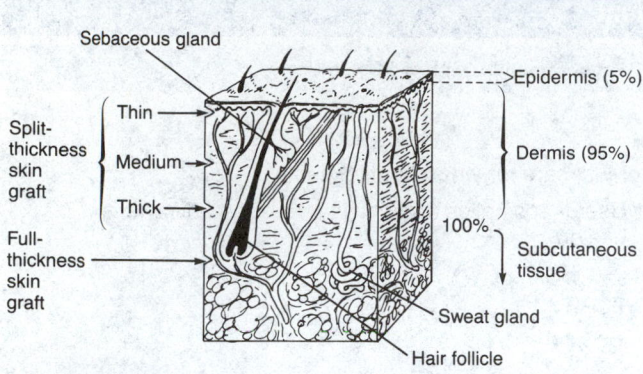

Figure 80-1

Skin graft thickness. A split-thickness graft includes the epidermis and a portion of the dermis. A full-thickness graft includes the entire epidermis and dermis.

integumentary defects is accomplished by several methods of transplantation and reconstruction that involve grafting, formation of a flap, or microsurgical free-flap transfer. These procedures have different applications and perioperative concerns and are discussed in this section.

Cosmetic surgery specifically related to the integument and discussed here includes rhytidoplasty (face-lift), blepharoplasty (eyelid surgery), body contouring by liposuctioning, and hair transplantation. Dermabrasion and chemical peeling, two other cosmetic procedures, were discussed earlier in this chapter. Rhinoplasty (nose reshaping) is discussed in Chapter 21; and breast augmentation (enlargement), breast reduction, and breast and nipple reconstruction are discussed in Chapter 65.

Nursing Research Note

Kravitz M, Green J, Langston L, Epstein B, Worden G: Improperly sterilized fine-mesh gauze associated with donor site infections in skin-grafted burn patients. *Am J Infect Control* 1985; 13(3):178–182.

An increased number of donor site infections during a 4-month period motivated a team of investigators to examine the cause. Ironically, neither the skin grafts themselves nor the ungrafted burn sites became infected. Many factors were examined. Ultimately, it was found that the strips in the inner half of the fine mesh gauze roll were not affected by sterilization procedures. When cultured, the strips were found to be contaminated by *Staphylococcus*.

In some cases, only exhaustive, repeated review of basic procedures can uncover reasons for some hospital infections. Nurses must follow basic infection control practices in all routine aspects of nursing care as well as isolation procedures when appropriate. Policy manuals for infection control in individual hospitals should be read and followed by all personnel.

SKIN GRAFTING

Skin grafting entails the surgical removal of varying depths of cutaneous tissue from its vascular, nervous, and lymphatic connections and its transfer to a designated area without direct attachment to the underlying surface. The graft may be either a split-thickness or full-thickness graft (Figure 80-1). A split-thickness graft includes the entire epidermis and a thin (0.008 to 0.012 in), intermediate (0.012 to 0.014 in), or thick (0.015 to 0.024 in) portion of the dermis. A full-thickness graft includes the epidermis and the entire dermal layer. Grafts are also classified by source:

- *Autograft,* from the same person
- *Isograft,* from a genetically identical person (identical twin)
- *Allograft* or *homograft,* from the same species but genetically dissimilar, as from a cadaver
- *Xenograft* or *heterograft* from a different species, as from a pig (porcine graft)

New techniques of cloning the client's skin in vitro are under development, as are techniques of making artificial skin and culturing allograft skin cells in ways that reduce the likelihood of rejection. Except for autografts and isografts, skin from other sources provides only temporary wound coverage and in time will be rejected by the client's immune system.

Many clients who receive skin grafts have sustained trauma producing an acute or chronic skin loss—generally, thermal and chemical burns. (Refer to Chapter 15.) Grafts are also performed when insufficient skin is available during excision of cutaneous tumors or to repair wound dehiscence. Skin ulcerations caused by infection, inadequate arterial or venous circulation, and pressure may also require skin grafts. Because a vascular bed and healthy underlying tissue are essential, skin grafts are not indicated over denuded bone, tendon or cartilage; on heavily irradiated tissue; or for chronically ulcerated lesions. In these instances, other techniques such as skin flaps or free flap transfers may be indicated (these are discussed later in this chapter).

Most skin grafts are split thickness because vascularization occurs much more successfully. Full-thickness grafts, which allow closer matching of skin color, texture, and hair growth, are used when full-thickness loss has occurred and may be selected when cosmetic appearance is the prime consideration. Donor sites from which full dermal layers have been harvested usually require split-thickness grafts because the denuded areas lack the regrowth powers normally generated from the epithelial cells found in the lining of the sebaceous glands, sweat glands, and hair follicles extending into the dermis.

Surgical Procedure

Before any skin can be transplanted, the recipient bed must reflect the appropriate type of granulation tissue and the necessary vascularity. Mechanical debridement (refer to the earlier discussion in Chapter 15) will probably begin at the bedside several days prior to surgery. The purpose is to remove devitalized tissue, encourage epithelialization, and prevent bacterial colonization. Methods include wet-to-dry dressings, hydrotherapy, enzymatic preparations, and cutting with instruments. At the time of surgery, the wound must demonstrate less than 100,000 bacteria per gram of tissue and the absence of streptococcal infection.

Once the client is anesthetized, a more aggressive debridement process is begun that usually entails tangential excision or the removal of devitalized tissue until pinpoint bleeding starts. Blood losses during debridement may be prohibitive if extensive areas are being grafted and blood must be immediately replaced. The recipient bed must show hemostasis adequate for the graft to succeed, or surgery must be delayed. Electrocautery, temporary clamping, use of fine absorbable sutures, direct pressure, and topical application of thrombin inhibit excessive bleeding.

When selecting the donor site, the surgeon considers the color, vascularity, texture, visibility, and the potential for and effects of scarring. The exception is wound coverage for burn clients when maintenance of life takes precedence over cosmetic concerns. Common donor sites include the thighs, abdomen, buttocks, arms, and chest (Figure 80–2), but the selection is always contingent on the availability of viable skin.

Grafts are harvested by several methods and are usually acquired after the client has received local or general anesthesia.

- *Pinch grafts,* no longer common, are "islands of skin" approximately 1 cm in diameter that have been trans-

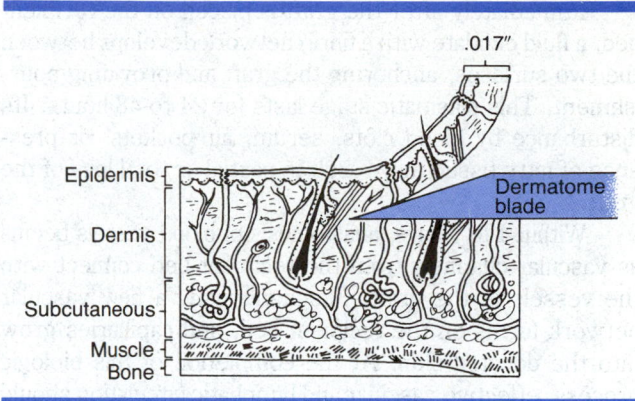

Figure 80–3

Removing a medium split-thickness graft with a dermatome blade.

planted to the denuded area. The surgeon obtains the graft by cutting the portion of skin picked up with fine tissue forceps or a sharp straight needle.

- *Sheet grafts* are solid pieces of skin used when the amount of donor tissue can exactly cover the recipient area. These grafts may be obtained freehand using a surgical knife or razor blade. The Humby knife and a variety of hand or electric dermatomes provide calibration that allows for precise regulation of thickness. The dermatomes are widely used, particularly the electric models, because the faster procurement of skin allows a reduction in anesthesia time (Figure 80–3).

- *Meshed* or *expanded grafts* may be used to: (1) allow hematomas, seromas, and air to escape without need for disturbing the transplant; (2) cover large areas when donor sites are limited; (3) conform to irregular surfaces; and (4) decrease skin contractures (Figure 80–4). A major disadvantage is the initial cosmetic effects of the lack of uniformity in the appearance of the skin.

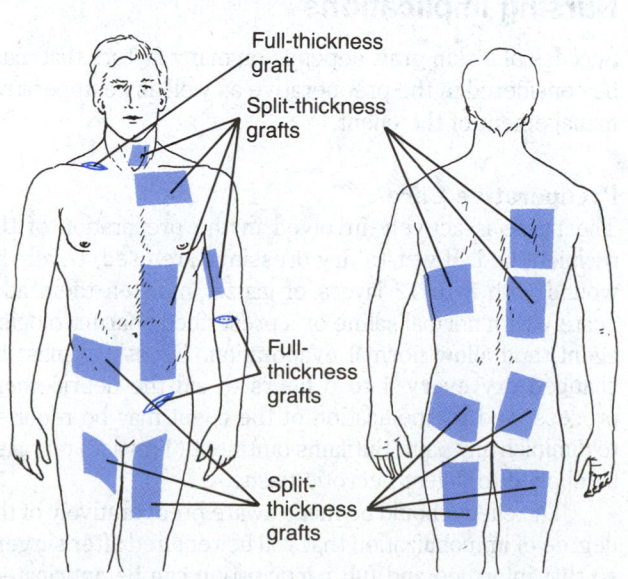

Figure 80–2

Donor sites for skin grafts.

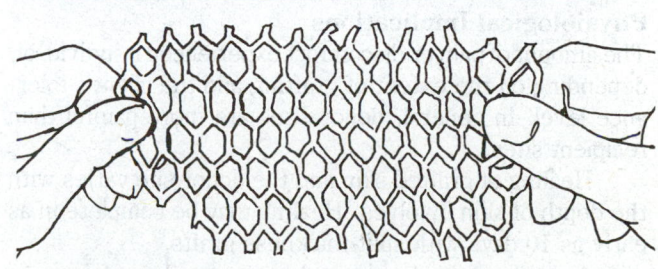

Figure 80–4

Meshed or expanded graft.

Immediately after the graft is placed on the recipient bed, a fluid exudate with a fibrin network develops between the two surfaces, anchoring the graft and providing nourishment. This plasmatic stage lasts for 24 to 48 hours. Its disturbance by blood clots, serum, air pockets, or presence of fatty tissue may result in partial or total loss of the graft.

Within 4 to 7 days, anastomosis of blood vessels begins as vascular channels from the recipient bed connect with the vessels in the graft. Simultaneously, a new vascular network forms on the recipient bed, and capillaries grow into the donated skin. At the completion of this biologic process, effective vascular and lymphatic circulation should be established. This process of successful vascularization is called a "take."

To promote successful transplantation, the graft must be immobilized to prevent any dislodgment that would disrupt the take. Fixation may be accomplished by suturing (running, interrupted, multiple quilting) and use of metal staples, self-adherent tape (Steri-strips), tie-over dressings (stinting), and numerous other means. If the client is not being treated by the open method, the graft site may be covered with petrolatum gauze (Xeroform), antibiotic gauze (Furacin), or a single layer of fine- or coarse-mesh gauze followed by additional wet (warm saline) or dry dressings and roller bandage to protect the area. Ace bandages or Elastoplast may be used for the outer layer. Regional immobilization may be required by splinting, casting, wiring of joints, or use of skeletal traction. Restriction of movement is especially important when the hands, axillae, neck, ankles, and extremities have been grafted.

The donor site may be similarly covered with a fine-mesh gauze or parachute silk and then dressed with multiple layers of moist or dry gauze to absorb blood and serum that ooze from the wound. A transparent polymer membrane (OpSite) that may also be used for coverage allows the wound to be seen.

Any unused portions of skin, if properly moistened and protected, can be stored at 4°C, a normal refrigeration temperature, and held for 14 to 21 days.

Implications for the Client

Physiological Implications

The amount of pain or discomfort experienced is individual, depending on the extent of grafting and the client's tolerance level. In general, donor sites are more painful than recipient sites.

Healing of grafted skin and the donor site varies with the depth of skin involved. Healing may be complete in as early as 10 days with split-thickness grafts.

A successful take depends on a number of factors: The recipient bed must be prepared properly; the wound should be free from streptococcal infection and have a low bacteria count; bleeding must be controlled; the graft must be successfully immobilized; hematomas and seromas must be prevented or eliminated; adequate venous circulation must exist; and infection must be prevented. More successful vascularization occurs with split-thickness grafts.

A number of long-term problems are associated with skin grafting. Skin contractures, hypertrophic scarring, and keloid formation are possible. The grafted skin may be dry and itchy; the pigmentation may be altered; hair loss or decrease may occur; sweating ability and sebaceous glands may be lost; and sensations of pain, touch, and temperature may be altered.

Psychosocial/Lifestyle Implications

How favorable the cosmetic effects are depend also on a number of factors such as the client's skin color and texture, the potential for scarring, and whether the graft is highly visible. Whenever possible, aesthetics are considered in decisions made about grafting; this may not be possible when extensive burns are involved. Body image disturbances may result from disfigurement because of contractures or scarring, pigmentary or skin texture changes, or the need to wear unsightly garments or appliances postoperatively.

Lifestyle disruptions in school, work, or friend relationships may occur when treatment and hospitalization are extensive and lengthy. Family relationships and roles are also affected when the client is absent from the home for long periods of time. In addition, much of the severely burned client's psychic energy is directed toward survival and the need to cope with the physiological changes involved. Clients may have little energy left to invest in others. Table 80–7 summarizes the client implications of skin grafting.

Nursing Implications

Success of a skin graft depends on many factors that must be considered in the preoperative as well as postoperative management of the client.

Preoperative Care

The nurse is actively involved in the preparation of the recipient bed. If wet-to-dry dressings are used, cover the wound with 8 to 12 layers of gauze, moisten them adequately with normal saline or a prescribed pharmacological agent, and allow normal evaporation. Dressings must be changed dry every 4 to 6 hours to aid the debridement process, and premedication of the client may be required to diminish any pain. Sutilains ointment (Travase) may also be applied to digest necrotic tissue.

The client should be made aware preoperatively of the degree of immobilization that will be required after surgery so that informed and full participation can be anticipated. The emotional implications can be dealt with early in treatment, and discussion of cosmetic and physiological effects should be considered critical.

Table 80–7   Skin Grafting, Skin Flap or Pedicles, and Free Skin Grafts: Implications for the Client

Physiological Implications	Psychosocial/Lifestyle Implications
Skin grafting:	
Pain, especially in donor site	Aesthetic considerations may not always be possible, (eg, when extensive burns are involved)
Length of healing varies; split-thickness grafts heal faster	Body image disturbances from disfigurement or need to wear unsightly garments or appliances
Successful takes depend on a variety of factors such as proper preparation of recipient bed, absence of high bacterial count or streptococcal infection in wound, control of bleeding, immobilization of graft, prevention or elimination of hematomas and seromas, adequate venous circulation, prevention of infection	Disruptions in education, career, or interpersonal relationships with family and friends when extensive or multiple grafting is required
Vascularization more successful with split-thickness grafts	Absence from the home for treatment may result in role change
Long-term problems may exist: skin contractures; hypertrophic scarring; keloid formation; dryness and itching; altered pigmentation; hair loss or decrease; loss of sweating ability; loss of sebaceous glands; alteration in sensations of pain, touch, and temperature	Emotional energy directed toward survival and coping; little is left over for others
Skin flaps:	
Vascularization takes 4–6 wk	Aesthetic effects considered whenever possible
Original skin color and texture usually maintained if flap is local	A number of operations may be necessary
Hair growth and sebaceous gland secretion continue	Lifestyle disruptions, body image disturbances, and coping patterns similar to those discussed above
Loss of sensation and sweating ability may be temporary	
Flap growth occurs in proportion to body growth	
Flap necrosis is a possible complication for as long as 3 yr	
Older adults requiring head and neck reconstruction may face serious postoperative problems	
Free flap transfer:	
Surgery is lengthy, requiring 3–8 h; increased potential for postoperative complications	Smoking and substances containing caffeine must be restricted for 1 wk preoperatively and several months postoperatively
Success depends on immediate vascularization	Fewer restrictions on activity and positioning; shorter period of immobilization
Potential vascular complications are arterial and venous thromboses and leaking at the site of an anastomosis; require immediate surgical correction	Performed in one stage
Graft survival threatened by hematoma formation and external compression	Reduction in hospitalization time, cost, and morbidity
Postoperative pain in donor site; no pain in recipient site	Lifestyle disruptions tend to be less serious
Sensory deficits in skin flap for several months	Initial bulkiness and loss of contouring at recipient site can be disruptive to body image
	Debulking and shaping the flap may be necessary 3–4 mo after tissue transplant
	Donor site can usually be hidden by clothing
	Body image ultimately improved

Postoperative Care

The most immediate postoperative nursing concerns are the restoration and maintenance of vital body functions. The age of the client, area of involvement, and presurgical health status contribute to the intensity of care involved. The nurse will also be concerned with two wounds (donor and recipient) when the client returns from surgery. The ultimate aim for the recipient site is revascularization. A successful take is accomplished when the graft turns from pale white-yellow to pink. This goal may be aided by preventing any movement of or pressure on the graft, therapeutic management of any hematomas or seromas that may form, and by inhibiting infection.

If an open method of treatment or meshed grafts are not employed, the recipient bed should be inspected within 24 to 72 hours for the presence of hematomas or seromas that would interfere with vascularization if any salvaging of a disturbed skin transplant is likely. The dressing must be removed carefully by a qualified physician or nurse. Hematomas or seromas are removed by gently rolling a cotton-tipped applicator over the area, or creating a fish-mouth opening with fine scissors and either flushing with saline or aspirating the fluid.

In addition to avoiding any movement of the graft, the client must avoid continuous pressure on the graft site. Elevation of the involved part will facilitate venous circulation, and elastic bandages may also be prescribed. Whenever the arms and legs are bandaged, it is essential to assess the digits for color, temperature, and swelling to determine the circulatory status. If bed rest is prolonged when the legs have received grafts, problems related to immobilization must be actively deterred. Elastic stockings are not generally used because they may disrupt the graft. Ambulation should be performed slowly and carefully to prevent venous engorgement of grafted dependent areas.

Infection is prevented by maintaining good asepsis during wound management. An increase in temperature and an odor emanating from the graft around the fourth postoperative day may indicate infection. With sepsis, the blood pressure may drop and blood cultures will be positive. Early treatment with soaks and debridement may be necessary to preserve portions of the graft and decrease scarring. The treatment of sepsis is described in Chapter 15.

Proper care of the donor site is also imperative; the site should be treated as a partial or full-thickness burn. The nursing goals are to promote healing and to prevent infection. The outer dressing may be removed within 24 to 72 hours after surgery. The fine-mesh gauze or innermost covering is allowed to fall off spontaneously, usually within 2 weeks.

Donor sites may be more painful than recipient areas because the donor sites have exposed nerve endings. Until the crust forms, wound coverage lessens the discomfort by preventing contact with air currents, clothing, and bedding. Bed cradles will help, and analgesics should be administered accordingly.

If donor sites become infected, treatment may incorporate topical antimicrobials such as those used in burn care. These include mafenide (Sulfamylon), silver sulfadiazine (Silvadene), silver nitrate, gentamicin (Garamycin), nitrofurazone (Furacin), povidone-iodine (Betadine), or polymyxin B-bacitracin (Polysporin).

Healing of the graft and donor sites, which varies with the depth of the transplanted skin, may be complete in as few as 10 days if a thin split-thickness graft has been used. The client's nutritional status, premorbid condition, and present homeostatic balance have a great influence on the repair process. Maintenance of a positive nitrogen balance is critical for fast and effective healing.

Long-term problems associated with skin grafting should be addressed, and the client should be taught how to treat the alterations. Skin lotions, lanolin-containing ointments, vaseline, or any lubricating product should be applied to the cutaneous surface regularly to avoid or reduce dryness and itching when sebaceous glands are lost.

Contraction of grafts and the development of hypertrophic scars or keloids are potential problems. An active program of prevention is usually undertaken when the likelihood of scarring is increased because the client is younger or has highly pigmented skin, joints or high-risk areas on the body are involved, infection has occurred, or split-thickness grafts have been used. Braces, splints, pressure dressings or garments, or orthotic devices may have to be worn to prevent contracture for a number of years until the scars have matured.

Pigmentation may be altered by reduction or increase in color, although the grafted skin usually maintains its original characteristics. Hair growth depends on the thickness of the graft. Loss of hair follicles with split-thickness grafts may result in an absence of hair or a decrease in amount. The ability to sweat is lost in most skin grafts, although some return is possible. Sensations of pain, touch, heat, and cold return in proportion to the nerve potential of the recipient bed. The replaced skin should be actively protected until the client is aware of what new or restored sensations can be perceived. Active protection consists of avoiding temperature extremes and physical injury. If physical injury does occur, the skin surface must be closely monitored for untoward changes indicating interruption of vascularization or healing.

Emotional responses to skin grafts vary. A person highly influenced by physical attributes is likely to find the alterations in color and texture of the grafted skin upsetting. Clients who have been traumatized and close to death may respond positively despite the cosmetic alterations. Whatever the response, major disfigurement that requires reconstructive surgery may leave the client in need of intense psychological support.

Behavioral maladjustments may become more apparent when the client has been discharged since most hospital environments support unusual behavior. After discharge, the stressors may be related to inabilities to adjust socially and an inability to cope with the long-term treatment of skin contracture and scarring. Whenever any emotional problems can be alleviated through verbal communication, the creation of a therapeutic milieu, and family support, the nurse should become a major facilitator. However, the nurse must also recognize the need for professional counseling and refer the client when appropriate.

SKIN FLAPS

Skin flaps involve the transplantation of both cutaneous and subcutaneous tissue and may include fascia and muscle in a manner that preserves the blood supply of the donor site until vascularization is established at the recipient site and detachment is completed. Skin flaps are indicated to achieve the following goals:

- Providing bulk or padding when tissue has been lost over bony prominences through trauma or disease, such as a fingertip injury or a decubitus ulcer
- Closing defects that cannot be effectively sutured or when vascularization is poor, such as tissue losses with head and neck cancer, radiated tissue, or avulsion wounds
- Covering wounds that will require later surgery, such as bone, cartilage, tendon, or nerve repair
- Reconstructing normal body contour after surgical excision, as for the breast, eyelid, nose, or face
- Protecting underlying structures such as carotid arteries that may have become surgically exposed during head and neck surgery or because of tumor erosion
- Restoring the lumen of the food and air passages

Myocutaneous flaps have an additional muscle attachment and are used in areas that have a poor blood supply.

Surgical Procedure

Because skin flaps involve more than one surgical procedure, a critical component is preplanning. The tissue being utilized for transplantation will require a blood supply adequate to ensure viability and to accomplish the goal and is carefully assessed preoperatively.

Preplanning includes the selection of the donor site and whether to design a local or distant flap. A local flap is considered when tissue adjacent to the defect has a good blood supply, is sufficiently elastic, and can be feasibly transferred. The local flap also provides better aesthetic effect because skin color and texture are more closely matched. When distant flaps are necessary, they may be chosen from an area that can be concealed by clothing.

A delayed graft may have to be considered when vascular efficiency is questionable in a client who has a history of arteriosclerosis, diabetes, radiation damage, or who is elderly. Rather than immediate transfer and attachment, a "training" period of approximately 1 to 1½ weeks is allotted for the involved blood vessels to increase their effectiveness.

An incision is made in the form of the flap except at the base or stem area. The graft tissue is undermined and the incision sutured. Circulation to the potential flap becomes totally dependent on the competence of the blood vessels remaining in the attached base.

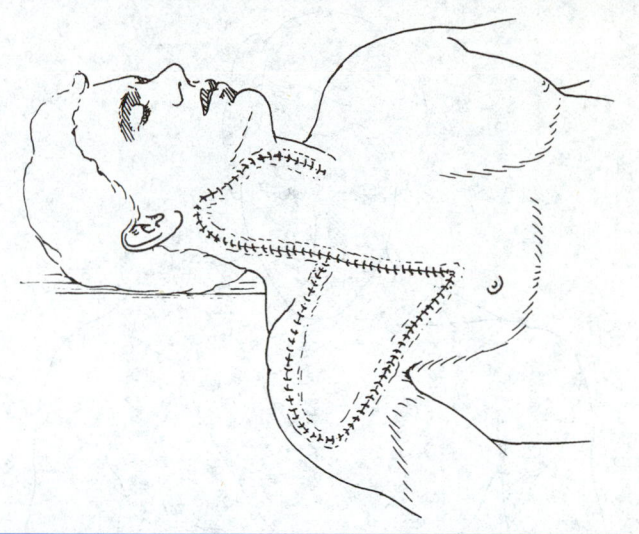

Figure 80–5

Direct transfer of a skin flap.

Flaps may be moved by straight advancement or at a pivot point. They may be attached directly to the wound (Figure 80–5) and the entire flap used to cover the defect, or they may be attached through an indirect method that uses a carrier, or migration, process in which a tube pedicle is formed when the raw surfaces are closed (Figure 80–6). The carrier method uses a temporary attachment, such as the wrist, in the eventual movement of the pedicle to the defect. The pedicle migrates or travels its own length in the necessary number of steps to reach the final destination. Once vascularization has been established within the recipient bed, the unused portion of the tube can be returned to the donor site or used for further reconstructive surgery. Denuded donor sites may require skin grafts to provide necessary coverage.

Skin flaps are procured from a number of areas on the body. Reconstructive surgery involving the face may utilize a temporal forehead flap or the sternomastoid myocutaneous flap. One of the most commonly used sources is the deltopectoral flap. The deltopectoral, acromiothoracic, groin, and hypogastric flaps are taken from the trunk. Pedicle grafts taken from the extremities are usually used to repair defects on the contralateral leg or arm.

Throughout the operative procedure, the surgeon is careful to prevent any factors that might cause eventual flap necrosis. To avoid undue internal pressure from capillary bleeding or the accumulation of fluid or air (dead space), drainage tubes or suction catheters are placed in the wound. External pressure is reduced by keeping the flaps free of dressings and tape or removing them within 24 hours.

After vascularization has been established, the flap or tube can be separated at the base or along the tube. (Additional reconstruction may still be needed.)

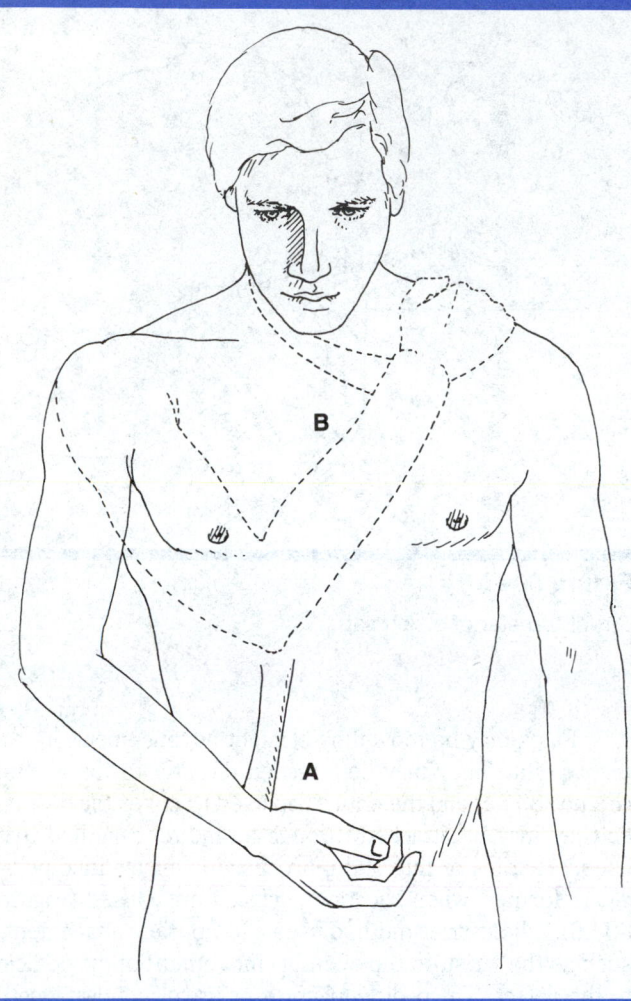

Figure 80–6

Indirect transfer of a tube pedicule by migration. The abdominal tube pedicle is migrated to the wrist **(A).** At a later operation, the upper end of the tube pedicle is detached and migrated to the side of the neck **(B).** Eventually the lower end will be detached and transplanted to the opposite side of the neck, and then opened throughout its length to replace scar contractures on the neck after they have been excised.

Implications for the Client

Physiological Implications

Successful grafting of skin flaps depends on establishing and maintaining a blood supply to the graft. Vascularization takes 4 to 6 weeks. The client can anticipate that skin color and texture will be maintained if the skin flap is a local one. Hair growth and sebaceous gland secretion will continue in the graft. Although loss of sensation and sweating occur immediately after surgery, return is possible in several weeks or perhaps as long as 3 years after. Flap growth will be proportional to body growth.

Flap necrosis occurring as long as 3 years after grafting is a postoperative complication. The potential for life-threatening postoperative problems exists in older adults who require head and neck reconstruction.

Psychosocial/Lifestyle Implications

Cosmetic effects are considered in preplanning whenever possible. Treatment usually involves a number of operations to attain the desired goal. Being aware of the stages is crucial to the client's ability to cope with the stresses, discomfort, and strict immobilization required. Lifestyle disruptions and body image disturbances are similar to those discussed in relation to skin grafting. Table 80–7 summarizes the client implications of skin flaps.

Nursing Implications

Preoperative Care

Survival of the skin flaps begins with the preoperative teaching program. Clients need a clear explanation of the nursing care involved in the perioperative period and the eventual self-care to be attained. After the surgeon has explained the surgical procedures and the expected outcomes, the nurse should discuss with the client any puzzling points, and any questions about the immediate and long-term physiological effects. Provide a supportive environment that will help bring to the surface any psychosocial difficulties. Client anxieties will be intensified when gross disfigurement is involved.

Postoperative Care

The most immediate focus of care will be on avoiding or dealing with life-threatening problems related to pulmonary and cardiovascular sequelae. Frequently, pedicle grafts involve head and neck surgery on an elderly client with major health problems involving the lungs, heart, blood vessels, or metabolism.

Two key nursing objectives with this type of surgery involve (1) maintenance of circulation to and from the graft and (2) prevention of infection. Because a baseline reference point is critical, the nurse must begin an immediate assessment of flap color, temperature, skin appearance, and capillary filling. Observations are required every 2 hours for the first 72 hours and then every 4 hours. The normal findings include a pink and warm flap that immediately recovers from a blanching test and shows no lines of demarcation, shininess, or engorgement. Any significant alteration should be promptly brought to the attention of the physician.

Care must be taken to prevent any tension, overstretching, twisting, kinking, or pressure on the flap. Avoid placing tape, tracheostomy collars, ties, or tubes on any portion of the flap. Sometimes, tracheostomy tubes are sutured in place instead. For correct positioning, body parts, particularly the head and neck, should be supported by towel rolls or sand bags.

The promotion of venous circulation is an important nursing concern. Because edema will be a normal postoperative occurrence, gravity drainage should be instituted. Although a semi-Fowler's position will assist upper body involvement, prolonged periods of elevation without attention may also cause the flap to pull on the suture line or against a rigid bony surface. Drainage catheters should be monitored frequently to be sure they are functioning properly and the tubings gently milked (or Hemovacs emptied) as needed so internal pressures are reduced.

In addition to sluggish circulation, any inflammatory process in the area of the flap may potentiate a wound infection and possible flap necrosis. A program of incisional care is usually instituted to remove crusts and dried exudate. Half-strength hydrogen peroxide is applied with cotton applicators to the incision and completely swabbed off with normal saline or sterile water to prevent any chemical irritation. Antimicrobial ointment may also be applied. If areas of necrosis develop, treatment with acetic or boric acid soaks and wet-to-dry dressings promotes debridement. Sutures may be removed in 10 days if healing progresses smoothly.

Maintenance of an optimum nutritional intake for the client is important, and a high protein and high calorie diet may be helpful. An alteration in the consistency of the food or the route of delivery (such as tube or intravenous feedings) may also be necessary if the client is undergoing surgery of the head or neck.

Clients should be informed about the characteristics the skin flap will possess (refer to physiological implications). Instruct the client to take precautions to protect the grafted area until the sensory nerve endings are reestablished.

Emotional responses to flap surgery are individual, especially when gross disfigurement is involved. Surgery on the head and neck can result in extensive losses of tissue with the need for major reconstruction and use of prosthetic devices. Some clients will undergo an emotional crisis because of the disfigurement or because of a long period of immobilization. Nurses need to be keenly perceptive of the psychosocial adaptive mechanisms each client employs. Elderly clients may need additional support and time to reestablish independence or to return to their premorbid level of activity.

Incorporate the appropriate nursing care into the preoperative regimen if a split-thickness graft or full-thickness graft was required at the donor site (see earlier discussion).

FREE FLAP TRANSFER

In free flap transfer or transplant, a completely detached portion of cutaneous and subcutaneous tissue that may include fascia and muscle is moved to a distant recipient site with immediate establishment of vascularization by microsurgical anastomosis of blood vessels.

The advent of the operating microscope and microsurgery has given a new dimension to skin and tissue transplantation. A transfer of this type may be considered when

the other two methods (skin grafts or skin flaps) do not provide for a satisfactory replacement. Specifically, a free flap transfer may be used to:

- Replace skin and tissue losses associated with tumors, radiation, and ulceration
- Reconstruct areas damaged by trauma
- Reconstruct scar tissue secondary to burns
- Restore surface contours

This method of skin and tissue replacement is advantageous because the surgery can be performed in a one-stage operation, will result in minimal flap fibrosis, allows clients to assume a more comfortable position postoperatively, and requires a shorter period of immobilization. The total result is a decrease in hospitalization time, cost, and morbidity. Disadvantages include the length of time the surgery takes and the need for immediate reoperation if vascular complications develop.

Surgical Procedure

Presurgical planning is integral to transplanting a free flap. A complete assessment of the vascular supply (including arteriogram or venogram if necessary) within the donor and recipient areas is made before this approach is selected. On the day before surgery, critical vessels are identified by ultrasound Doppler and mapped on the surface of the skin.

The surgery requires approximately 3 to 8 hours and may use two operative teams: one to focus on preparation of the recipient site and the other to raise the flap from the donor area. The initial step is to verify the suitability of the vasculature in the recipient bed. Next, the recipient bed may need debridement, resection, or release of skin contractures. Donor tissue is isolated from one of numerous sites, the iliofemoral (groin) flap being the most common. The flap is placed carefully in the recipient bed so microsurgical vascular attachments can be made. Gentle handling of the tissue during the entire surgery is essential to the success of the transplant.

The wound is closed when revascularization is complete and no complications are apparent. Suturing is done meticulously to minimize tension. Drainage catheters must be inserted without disturbing the anastomosed vasculature. A dressing or Xeroform gauze may be applied over the suture line only to prevent wound contamination and to absorb drainage. Excessive coverage would interfere with effective monitoring of vascular integrity and may cause flap compression when drainage hardens. Donor sites may have a primary closure and contain drainage catheters, or they may be covered with skin grafts.

Implications for the Client

Physiological Implications

Since the surgery is long, there is increased potential for respiratory and circulatory complications, wound infection, and pressure sores. The success of the surgery depends on whether vascularization is established immediately by microsurgical anastomoses. Potential vascular complications include arterial and venous thromboses and leaking at the site of an anastomosis. These complications hamper graft survival and require immediate surgery to restore circulation. Hematoma formation and external compression will also hamper graft survival.

Postoperative pain in the flap is not anticipated because the flap is denervated during transfer. Donor sites, however, are painful. Sensory deficits in the grafted area are expected for several months after surgery. If the donor site requires a split-thickness graft, then the appropriate physiological implications in Table 80–7 apply as well.

Psychosocial/Lifestyle Implications

One lifestyle modification is necessary both before and after surgery. Smoking and substances containing caffeine must be restricted for 1 week preoperatively and for several months postoperatively to facilitate optimal postoperative vascularization.

The free flap transfer allows the client to assume a more comfortable position after surgery. In addition, it is performed in a single stage and requires a shorter period of immobilization. There is ultimate reduction in hospitalization time, cost, and morbidity. Lifestyle restrictions are apt to be less serious.

Body image is ultimately improved by the repair of the physical defect. Initially, however, the flap appears bulky and lacks contour, and its appearance may be disturbing to the client. Although some shrinkage does occur, a minor operative procedure may be necessary in 3 to 4 months (once vascularization has been established) to debulk and shape the flap. Body image changes in relation to donor sites are likely to be less disturbing. Because many of the donor sites can be easily hidden by clothing, there is less visible disfigurement. Table 80–7 summarizes the client implications of free flap transfers.

Nursing Implications

Preoperative Care

Instruct clients to avoid substances containing caffeine and to avoid smoking for 1 week preoperatively. These restrictions help to ensure flap survival by decreasing the risk of vascular spasms and clotting problems in the blood vessels of the flap and should be continued for several months postoperatively.

The long surgical procedure makes the client more vulnerable to pneumonia, pulmonary emboli, wound infection, and pressure sores. Therefore, the preoperative preparation of the client includes a thorough assessment to detect any covert health problems that could increase the hazards as well as a thorough assessment of the vascular supply. Clients should be taught the necessary ventilatory measures and exercises and should be prepared

to expect the necessary postoperative neurovascular assessments.

Postoperative Care

Postoperative prophylaxis includes use of antibiotics, coughing and deep breathing, tracheal suctioning if necessary, air mattresses or water beds, antiembolic stockings, and mobilization as soon as possible.

Close observation of the flap is crucial, and assessment is performed every 15 minutes for 48 hours, and then every 4 hours for 5 days. The major portion of the transplanted tissue is usually visible, facilitating assessment. Initially, the surgeon and recovery room nurse simultaneously evaluate color, capillary refill, and tissue turgor to establish a mutual baseline and to ensure minimal variance in the subjectivity of subsequent assessments. Temperature readings, a source of objective data, are provided by a digital telethermometer. A surface probe on the flap and a second probe on a surface area distal to the flap provides a control measure. Simultaneous assessments should also be made whenever the responsibility for monitoring the flap is transferred from one nurse to another.

Distinctions can be made between arterial and venous problems by alterations in parameters being measured. Arterial complications will be indicated by a pale or white color and a decrease in tissue turgor (shallow depression or concavity), temperature (a 2° deviation from baseline is abnormal), and capillary refill (normal is 1 to 3 seconds). Venous difficulties cause cyanosis, flap distention or fullness (slight edema may be normal), minimal temperature change, and a rapid capillary refill. Because alterations may be subtle, any uncertainties should be brought to the surgeon's attention immediately, along with overt manifestations. Nurses have a crucial role in the early detection of these postoperative complications. Bonavita (1985) has reported that these vital nursing observations were crucial in salvaging 4% of the free flap transfers at her facility.

Vascular complications include arterial and venous thromboses and leaking at the site of an anastomosis. These problems require immediate surgery for restoration of circulation. Use of anticoagulant therapy or vasodilators is not a routine procedure and is determined by the individual needs of the client. Grafts must also be monitored for hematoma formation and effective function of drainage equipment. External compression on the transplant must be prevented by properly positioning the client off the flap and allowing the transplant to be unencumbered by equipment, bed linens, or unauthorized wound coverage.

Clients are usually immobilized for 7 to 10 days and the recipient site elevated to facilitate venous circulation. If a lower extremity has received a free flap transplant, elastic bandages are applied before the client ambulates. The client should dangle the affected leg first before ambulating to allow the leg to become accustomed to the change in circulation. Keep the leg elevated when the client is out of bed. Clients should be instructed to take precautions with the flap because a sensory deficit will exist for several months after surgery.

Care of the donor site will be geared toward measures that promote repair by primary intention or reepithelialization if a split-thickness graft was required. Administer analgesics as necessary.

RHYTIDOPLASTY

Rhytidoplasty is the use of plastic surgery to remove wrinkles from the face. The procedure is often referred to as a "face lift" (Figure 80–7). This type of surgery is performed primarily because of the degenerative effects of the aging process on the skin, particularly the face and neck. Wrinkles frequently appear on the forehead, cheeks, around the eyes (crow's-feet), and around the mouth. The loss of subcutaneous tissue, muscle mass, and strength as well as diminished skin elasticity result in the formation of jowls, double chins, neck folds, and redundancy of periorbital fat and skin.

Surgical Procedure

The client may receive either local or general anesthesia. Several approaches may be used, but a C-shaped incision extending from the temporal area of the scalp downward and posterior to the earlobe is most common. The skin is undermined and dissected, creating a facial flap that is raised upward and backward. Excess tissue is removed so the desired tautness can be achieved. The surgeon may also need to excise fatty tissue to restore facial contour, especially in the area of the chin (mentoplasty). Blepharoplasty or chemical peeling may be performed concurrently.

Implications for the Client

Physiological Implications
Facial edema is expected after rhytidoplasty and will be increased if additional cosmetic procedures are performed concurrently. Ecchymosis of the conjunctiva and the operative site is also normal and may take a few weeks to resolve. Potential complications include hematoma formation and damage to the facial nerve (CN VII). Some hair loss may occur if hair follicles have been destroyed.

Psychosocial/Lifestyle Implications
Once edema and bruising subside and healing is completed, clients experience enhanced self-esteem and improved body image. The results lack permanency lasting for 5 to 10 years because degenerative integumentary changes continue with aging. Scarring is uncommon in later adulthood and is also related to the skill of the surgeon. Hair loss, if it occurs, may cause some body image problems.

Activities in general, and facial movement in particular, should be limited for at least 2 days after surgery.

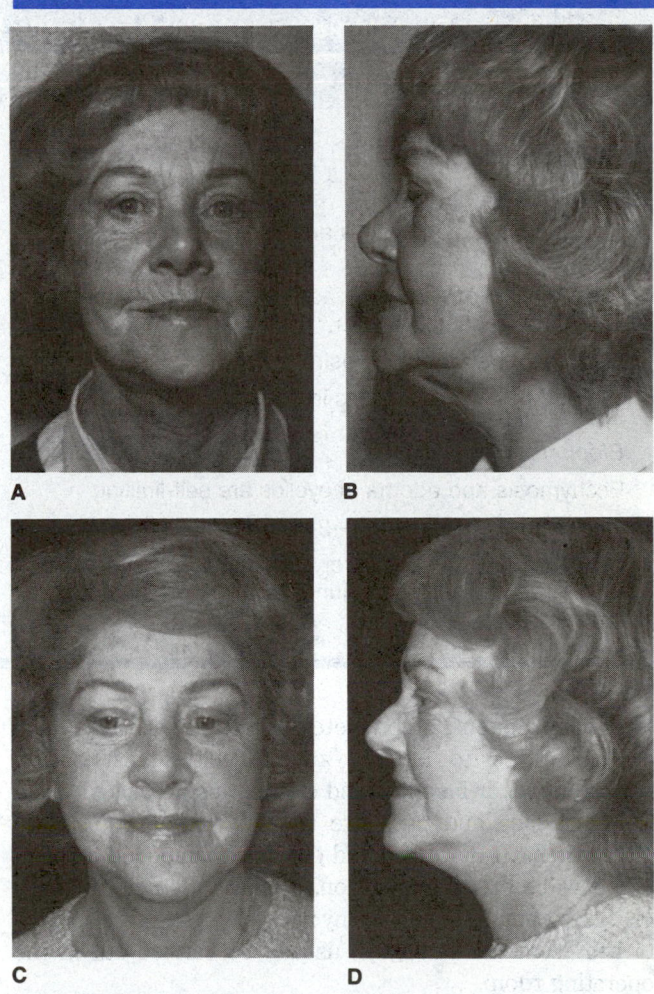

Figure 80–7
Client who has had rhytidoplasty and blepharoplasty.
A, B. Before views. **C, D.** After views.

Other activities that can stress or injure the suture line (combing and brushing the hair or excess jaw movements) should be limited until wound healing has taken place. The usual diet is usually altered to a liquid diet. Excessive weight loss after surgery could affect the appearance of the operative area. Dressings are in place only briefly, and sutures are removed from 3 days to 2 weeks after surgery, depending on their location. Table 80–8 summarizes the client implications of rhytidoplasty.

Nursing Implications

Preoperative Care
Each client will be individually evaluated and the desired outcome carefully plotted by the plastic surgeon before hospitalization. The client must be made aware that the effects are not permanent—skin sagging continues. A preoperative weight reduction program may be essential so that later weight losses do not markedly alter the repair. Because clients are in an age range where medical prob-

Table 80–8 Rhytidoplasty and Blepharoplasty: Implications for the Client	
Physiological Implications	**Psychosocial/Lifestyle Implications**
Rhytidoplasty:	
Facial edema	Enhanced self-esteem and improved body image
Ecchymosis of conjunctiva and operative site lasting for weeks	Improvement not permanent because of aging
Hematoma formation and facial nerve (CN VII) damage are potential complications	Body image difficulties if scarring or hair loss occur
	Activity limitations and diet alteration temporary and minimal
Hair loss if hair follicles destroyed	Excessive weight loss after surgery can have untoward effects
Temporary sensory deficits in operative site	
Blepharoplasty:	
Ecchymosis and edema of eyelids are self-limiting	Increased anxiety because of occlusive dressing
Occlusive dressing for 12–24 h	Enhanced self-esteem and improved body image
Corneal injury, temporary or permanent ptosis, ectropion, asymmetry, and conjunctival injury are potential complications	Alteration in body image and increased emotional discomfort if complications occur

lems are frequent, a complete physical examination must be performed to identify any difficulties, particularly hypertension or bleeding and clotting disturbances.

The face and neck are usually washed with hexachlorophene (pHisoHex) and the hair shampooed for several days before the operation. Men are required to shave on the morning of surgery. Any necessary cutting or removal of hair from the scalp will usually be carried out in the operating room.

Postoperative Care

Clients return from the operating room with a firm dressing in place. They may have cotton padding around the ears to minimize discomfort and to protect the auricular cartilage from trauma.

Use of tissue drains and slight pressure exerted by roller gauze or Ace bandage help to prevent hematomas and limit edema. Edema can be decreased by keeping the upper body elevated in a semi-Fowler's position. Any abnormal increase in the anticipated swelling around the eye or mouth, specifically asymmetrical swelling, should be reported to the surgeon immediately, as should any client complaints about heightening discomfort from tightening of the skin. They may indicate hematoma formation. Ecchymosis in the conjunctiva and in the operative area is normal and will not resolve for a number of weeks.

Partial damage to a branch of facial nerve (CN VII) is a serious complication, but one that rarely occurs. The nurse may test for nerve integrity by having the client smile, whistle, wrinkle the nose, wrinkle the forehead, or close the eyelids. Use of drops and ointment may be necessary to protect the eyes from corneal abrasions or conjunctival irritation (see also Figure 76–5).

Limitation of activity for at least 2 days will reduce stress on the surgical site. To reduce facial movement, the client should receive a liquid diet and limit talking. The client should also avoid tipping the head forward.

The bulky dressing is removed after approximately 48 hours. Preauricular sutures may be removed in 3 to 5 days; incisions in hair-bearing areas require 2 weeks for healing.

Discharge from the hospital may be allowed after the pressure dressings are removed. Showering may be allowed to help cleanse the area of drainage and the operative antiseptic. Instruct the client to exercise care in combing and brushing hair in the area of the incision and to avoid excess jaw movements until wound healing is complete. Shampooing, hair coloring, and makeup may also be restricted. Hair dryers and earrings should be used with caution until sensation returns.

BLEPHAROPLASTY

Blepharoplasty is the excision of redundant eyelid tissue. Anyone who develops an excess of skin in the eyelids or protrusion of periorbital fat may become a candidate for blepharoplasty. Normal aging produces a loss of elasticity and a relaxation of the eyelid skin. (Tissue excess seen in young and middle-aged persons can be the result of a hereditary tendency.) Because periocular manifestations occur with allergies and are associated with cardiovascular and thyroid disease, a complete medical evaluation is essential before surgery is decided on.

Besides aesthetic reasons, surgery may be indicated because a drooping eyelid obstructs the client's vision. The client's visual field should be examined preoperatively to provide baseline information for postoperative comparison should any problems arise.

Surgical Procedure

Careful planning precedes surgery, and appropriate markings are made before the actual surgical preparations begin. This step is particularly important when local anesthesia is being used because infiltration of the area may significantly distort the contour of the tissue. Corrective blepharoplasty may include resection of the upper and lower eyelids, removal of protruding orbital fat, or minor trimming of the lid skin (Figure 80–7).

Implications for the Client

Physiological Implications

Ecchymosis and edema of the eyelids are expected and are self-limiting. The client will have an occlusive dressing for 12 to 24 hours. Complications may include injury to the cornea during surgery or postoperatively because swelling of the eyelids prevents closure. Other possible complications include temporary or permanent ptosis, ectropion (particularly of the lower eyelid), asymmetry in appearance, and conjunctival injury.

Psychosocial/Lifestyle Implications

The client may experience heightened anxiety while the occlusive dressing is in place. Once the edema and ecchymosis have subsided (in approximately 10 days), the appearance may be evaluated for improvement. Anxiety is relieved and body image is enhanced when appearance or vision are improved because excess tissue has been removed or drooping has been corrected. The complications outlined above will adversely affect the client's body image and increase emotional discomfort. Table 80–8 summarizes the client implications related to blepharoplasty.

Nursing Implications

Preoperative Care

The face is cleansed preoperatively as prescribed. The client may require additional emotional support because of a fear of injury to the eyes.

Postoperative Care

An occlusive dressing may be maintained for 12 to 24 hours to minimize swelling, bleeding, or hematoma formation, and to rest the eyes. Subsequently, the area may be left exposed or covered with small dressings. The application of cold or iced saline dressings may also help to control the extent of swelling and bleeding. Precautions should be taken to prevent drying, irritation, and injury to the cornea because the edema will hinder complete closure of the lids. Skin sutures may be removed as early as the third or fourth postoperative day, depending on the area of involvement.

BODY CONTOURING BY LIPOSUCTIONING

Body contouring or sculpturing using liposuctioning involves the surgical removal of excessive adipose tissue by regional fat aspiration through a minimal number of small incisions. The standard dermolipectomy utilizes excision and plication to remove redundant fatty tissue and skin, but this approach results in longer scars, greater morbidity, and requires longer hospitalization.

Liposuctioning is relatively recent and is gaining in popularity. It is recommended for treatment of localized excesses of fat in particular anatomical regions (ankles, calves, medial and lateral aspects of the knees, thorax, abdomen, thighs, gluteals, upper arms, and face) that have not been responsive to dieting or exercise. It is not a method appropriate to generalized weight loss. Clients must have good skin tone so skin will more readily contract to the newly contoured frame. Therefore, the young adult is most commonly treated with this method.

Surgical Procedure

The original surgery, referred to as lipoexeresis (removal of fat), was developed by Schruddle, a German physician who pioneered body contouring in the early 1960s (Grazer, 1983). His method employs curetting and suction irrigation of the fat particles, whereas more recent techniques employ curettage instruments with suctioning attached. Suction-assisted lipectomy may also be performed as a wet procedure. Known as *body contouring by lipolysis aspiration*, this approach involves local infiltration of a hypotonic solution into the fatty deposits followed by the suctioning process. A combination of normal saline and distilled water, with the addition of hyaluronidase (Wydase) to assist in the diffusion of the solution, emulsifies the adipose tissue.

Surgery is most frequently performed under general anesthesia, but epidural blocks or local infiltration may be used. Each technique involves 1 to 2 cm incisions strategically placed in the area being treated (Figure 80–8). Insertion and manipulation of the instrument varies and may involve tunneling or fan-shaped honeycombing in back-and-forth movements along the desired plane. Care must be taken to avoid injury to blood vessels and lymphatics, which could lead to tissue necrosis.

The amount of adipose tissue removed may vary from a few ounces or grams to as much as 2 to 4 lb (1 to 2 kg). An increase in platelet aggregation may occur when free fatty acids are increased in the bloodstream. Because this can lead to thrombosis, some surgeons who perform liposuctioning infuse the client with dextrose in 5% alcohol during the operation to reduce the free fatty acids and prevent complications (Grazer, 1983).

Placement of wound catheters (Hemovac) and tissue drains is essential to facilitate healing. Use of a compres-

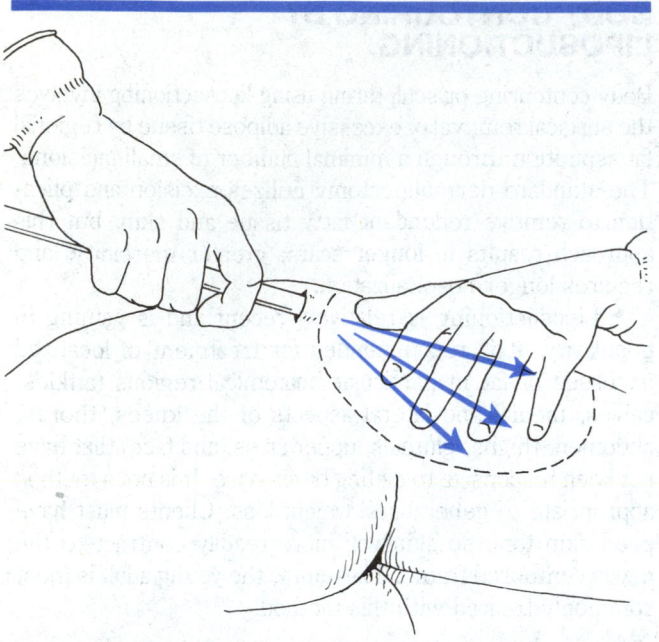

Figure 80–8
Trochanteric suction-assisted lipectomy.

sion bandage (Elastoplast, Sparelast) also plays an integral role in molding the desired shape of the surgical area.

Implications for the Client

Physiological Implications

Compression dressings and wound drainage systems are required for at least 48 hours and possibly as long as 2 weeks to curtail the formation of hematomas or seromas and the accumulation of lymphatic drainage. Compression dressings also assist in molding the body part to its desired shape and may involve wearing Ace bandages, elastic stockings, support hose, or a girdle for 6 to 8 weeks.

Edema and ecchymosis are expected in the operative area; they gradually resolve over a 2- to 3-week period. Edema in the abdomen and inner thighs is usually present for 3 to 6 weeks and may last as long as 6 months. Infection is rare.

Thrombosis is a potential complication when free fatty acids are released into the bloodstream. Vascular stress may occur when large amounts of fat and fluid (1000 cc) are removed, requiring the preoperative administration of IV crystalloid solutions or intraoperative or postoperative administration of an autogenous blood transfusion or plasma. Postoperative adhesions, an irregular contour, sagging skin, and regional dysesthesia (impairment of sensation) or anesthesia are other potential complications.

Psychosocial/Lifestyle Implications

The client must actively participate in self-care to help achieve healing and the desired contour. The client may need to wear special compression bandages or garments, possibly limiting the client's choice of clothing and social activities. Massaging the area may also be required. Exposure to the sun and temperature extremes may need to be avoided for 3 to 6 months.

Clients may be concerned about the postoperative edema and ecchymosis. The edema, in particular, may be discouraging to clients who see minimal difference between the original problem and the apparent results of the treatment. Clients may impose limitations on their social contacts if they are uncomfortable with visible bruising or swelling.

Body image and self-esteem are enhanced when the surgical results are positive. Adverse effects on body image and self-esteem may result from the complications described earlier.

Clients may be incapacitated for 1 to 2 weeks, and full recovery requires approximately 6 weeks. Table 80–9 summarizes the implications of liposuctioning for the client.

Nursing Implications

Preoperative Care

In discussing the procedure with the client preoperatively, the surgeon should clearly identify the ultimate goal of the surgery and explain the immediate and long-range effects of contour surgery. The nurse may need to reemphasize that liposuctioning is not a means to general weight reduction. An intravenous crystalloid solution may be administered if appropriate. Antibiotics may be prescribed prophylactically. Remind clients to bring any special compression garments (girdle, support hose, etc.) when they are to be discharged the same day.

Postoperative Care

The postoperative care depends on the area involved surgically and the amount of adipose tissue removed. Closer monitoring for pulmonary and cardiovascular complications is required when the procedure has been extensive and lengthy. The average length of hospitalization in this case is 2 to 4 days, and clients are discharged before wound healing is complete. Liposuctioning is now performed as an outpatient procedure whenever possible.

Bed rest may be advised for the first 12 to 24 hours, but early ambulation is important to prevent complications. The initial compression dressing and the drainage system may be left intact for 48 hours or for as long as 2 weeks. Ace bandages, full-length elastic stockings, support panty hose, or a girdle may also be worn for 6 to 8 weeks following surgery on the abdomen, buttocks, or legs.

Most clients experience discomfort. The abdominal area appears to be the most sensitive after liposuctioning. Analgesics, emotional support, and relaxation techniques will help. Although formation of hematomas or seromas and the accumulation of lymphatic fluid will be curtailed by

Table 80–9 Liposuctioning: Implications for the Client

Physiological Implications	Psychosocial/Lifestyle Implications
Ecchymoses and edema in the operative area for 2–3 wk; edema of the abdomen and inner thighs may last for 3–6 wk or up to 6 mo	Compression bandages or garments may be required for as long as 6–8 wk
Thrombosis, adhesions, irregular contour, and regional dysesthesia or anesthesia are potential complications	Self-imposed limitation on social activities if client is uncomfortable with appearance
Vascular stress may result from the removal of large amounts of fat	Temporary limitation on exposure to sun and temperature extremes for 3–6 mo
	Enhanced self-esteem and body image
	Discouragement and lowered self-esteem with unsatisfactory results
	Incapacitation for 1–2 wk; full recovery in approximately 6 wk

the dressing-drainage measure, these potential problems remain a major concern.

Postoperatively, again explain the healing process and the role of the client in self-care. Clients should be taught to expect ecchymoses in the operative area that gradually resolve over 2 to 3 weeks. Remind clients that postoperative adhesions and an irregular contour can be reduced by gentle massage of the area beginning approximately 10 to 15 days after surgery. Physical therapy may also be prescribed. Because regional dysesthesia or anesthesia is common following body sculpturing, clients should be instructed to protect the involved area from temperature extremes and sun exposure for at least 3 to 6 months. Discharge instructions should specify wound care, hygiene, activity allowances, and the importance of a scheduled follow-up.

HAIR TRANSPLANTATION

Hair transplantation is the placement of autografts into areas of baldness. Although hair may be transplanted by the use of hair plugs, strip grafts, or scalp flaps from unaffected areas, this discussion will be limited to the first method. At present, hair transplantation is the most common surgical approach used for hair restoration.

Male pattern baldness is the most common condition for which transplant therapy is recommended. Androgenetic alopecia in women and hair losses from traumatic injuries such as burns or avulsions may also be considered for transplantation. Selection of candidates also depends on the availability of scalp donor sites and quality of hair, on the potential for future losses, and on the extent of degenerative changes in the scalp and head. Because the client may require 3 to 4 transplants several weeks apart and must await regrowth of functional hair for several months postoperatively, emotional stability is a major concern. Any bleeding tendencies, healing difficulties, general infection, or scalp disorders may also contraindicate surgery.

Surgical Procedure

Under local anesthesia, the donor tissue is obtained by a punch excision. The surgeon must be careful not to destroy the follicles or the capillaries in the papillae that provide the blood supply to the hair. These plugs, which contain 10 to 15 hair follicles each, are carefully cleansed of any debris, trimmed of excess fat, and placed into recipient holes created by the same or a smaller punch. Preplanning will have determined the number of sessions required to provide for sequential placement of hair plugs so that there is a gradual filling of the defect.

Implications for the Client

Physiological Implications
The client can expect to experience mild discomfort, numbness or paresthesia, edema of the scalp, swelling of the eyelids when the frontal scalp is involved, and bleeding immediately after surgery. Edema generally subsides in about 3 days. Crusts will form and slough spontaneously. The crusts may cause pruritus. Vascularization of the autografts takes about 10 days. Occasionally, a plug may fall out and need to be replaced.

Complications are rare and may include infection and hypertrophic scarring or keloid formation. A cobblestoning or raising effect is common in the graft site but usually flattens in several months. The grafted hair will fall out in a month and regenerate in approximately 3 months.

Psychosocial/Lifestyle Implications
Immediately after surgery strenuous activity is restricted for the first week and alcoholic beverages are restricted for the first 24 hours to promote vascularization and avoid disturbing the graft. Minimal wound care is required.

Clients may be uncomfortable with postoperative restrictions on not combing or brushing over the transplanted area for 10 days and may limit their social activities

Table 80–10 Hair Transplantation: Implications for the Client	
Physiological Implications	**Psychosocial/Lifestyle Implications**
Mild discomfort, numbness or paresthesia, swelling of scalp and eyelids for 3 days, bleeding immediately after surgery	Alcoholic beverages restricted for 24 h
Vascularization takes 10 days	Strenuous activities restricted for 1 wk
Plugs may dislodge and require replacement	Combing and brushing over the transplanted area restricted for 10 days; shampooing restricted for 5 days
Complications such as infection and hypertrophic scarring or keloid formation are rare	Three to four transplantations may be required several weeks apart; the length of time may be discouraging
Cobblestoning or raising of graft site common; flattens in several months	Increased self-esteem and body image
Grafted hair falls out in 1 mo and regenerates in 3 mo	

accordingly. Hair may not be shampooed for 5 days, and then carefully without massage.

The process is a long one when several transplants are required. The client may need 3 to 4 transplantations performed several weeks apart and regrowth may take from 3 to 4 months for each transplantation. Clients may find the length of time discouraging or frustrating. After the process is completed, increased self-esteem and a more positive body image usually result. Table 80–10 summarizes the client implications of hair transplantation.

Nursing Implications

Preoperative Care
This method of hair transplantation is almost always performed on an ambulatory basis, and the client is responsible for perioperative care. Instructions for both preoperative and postoperative care must be explicit, both in writing and with oral explanations. Aspirin or aspirin-containing products should be avoided preoperatively to

prevent excessive bleeding. Instruct the client to shampoo his hair the morning of surgery.

Postoperative Care
A nonadherent dressing is left in place overnight to provide hemostasis. If bleeding continues or resumes and does not respond to direct pressure or a pressure dressing, the client should notify the physician immediately. Wound care will include the application of an antibiotic ointment to the graft sites with light dressing coverage until healing is complete.

If a plug falls out, the client may be instructed by some surgeons to thoroughly rinse the graft in normal saline, replace it in the correct direction of hair growth, and return to the surgeon for evaluation. Another alternative is to wrap the graft in saline-soaked gauze and return to the surgeon for reimplantation. Still other surgeons instruct the client to discard the plug. The client continues to provide wound care to both grafted and donor sites and to adhere to the postoperative restrictions discussed earlier (see physiological implications).

Chapter Highlights

A variety of surgical approaches including plastic and reconstructive surgery may be used to treat dermatoses and disfigurement from alterations of the integument and to transplant skin and hair.

Several procedures require a preplanning phase to allow careful plotting of the desired outcome.

With selected procedures, the emotional well-being of a client is evaluated to determine problems that could influence postoperative recovery.

Select surgical approaches may be contraindicated

in clients who are young, highly pigmented, readily scar, have an active dermatosis, or have unrealistic expectations regarding the results of the surgery.

The rate of wound healing involving the skin primarily varies with the type of surgical approach and the blood supply to the anatomical area being treated.

Appropriate wound closure, drainage equipment, and dressings have a significant influence on the prevention of postoperative complications such as hematomas, seromas, infections, and scarring.

Alterations in the color, texture, configuration, and sensory perception of the skin may result from surgery involving the integument.

The nurse plays an important role in the viability of skin and tissue transplants by monitoring and maintaining circulation and preventing infection.

Many surgical procedures can be performed on an ambulatory basis or require minimal hospitalization. Clients therefore often assume responsibility for wound care.

A teaching program for clients includes the identification of postoperative manifestations such as ecchymosis, erythema, drainage, edema, discomfort, sensory deficits, the anticipated duration of any physiological or psychosocial alterations, self-care requirements, and measures to prevent injury to the skin.

Alterations in the appearance and/or function of the skin from surgery or complications may have a significant impact on the client's emotional adjustment.

Bibliography

Acres C, Kraft ER: Skin transplantation. *Am J Nurs* 1981; 81:1466–1467.

Barrett BM (editor): *Manual of Patient Care in Plastic Surgery.* Boston: Little Brown, 1982.

Bonavita L: Free tissue transfer. *Am J Nurs* 1985; 85:384–387.

Converse JM (editor): *Reconstructive Plastic Surgery: Principles and Procedures in Correction, Reconstruction, and Transplantation,* 2nd ed. Philadelphia: Saunders, 1977.

Dixon JA: *Surgical Application of Lasers.* Chicago: Yearbook Medical Publishers, 1983.

Fidler JP: Debridement and grafting of full-thickness burns. In: *Clinical Burn Therapy: A Management and Prevention Guide.* Hummel RP (editor). Boston: John Wright PSG, 1982.

Fourmer PF, Otteni FM: Lipodissection in body sculpturing: The dry procedure. *Plast Reconstr Surg* 1983; 72:598–609.

Grabb WC, Smith JW: *Plastic Surgery.* 3rd ed. Boston: Little, Brown, 1979.

Grazer FM: Suction-assisted lipectomy, suction lipectomy, lipolysis and lipexeresis. *Plast Reconstr Surg* 1983; 72:620–623.

Illouz YG: Body contouring by lipolysis: A 5-year experience with over 3000 cases. *Plast Reconstr Surg* 1983; 72:591–597.

Kesselring UK: Regional fat aspiration for body contouring. *Plast Reconstr Surg* 1983; 72:610–619.

Lyons RJ: Promoting healing of skin flaps and grafts. *AORN J* 1982; 35:1174–1183.

Maddin S (editor): *Current Dermatologic Therapy.* Philadelphia: Saunders, 1982.

McIntire SN, Cioppa AL: *Cancer Nursing: A Developmental Approach.* New York: Wiley, 1984.

Noe JM, Barsky SH, Geer DE, Rosen S: Port-wine stains and the response to argon laser therapy: Successful treatment and the predictive role of color, age, and biopsy. *Plast Reconstr Surg* 1980; 65:130–136.

Robinson JK: Mohs' surgery for skin cancer. *Am J Nurs* 1982; 82:282–283.

Suggested Readings

Bonavita L: Free tissue transfer. *Am J Nurs* 1985; 85:387. The nursing implications in perioperative care of the client undergoing a free tissue transfer are discussed and highlighted with photos and illustrations.

Conlee D: Cosmetic surgery patients. *Nurs 81* (Nov) 1981; 11:90–95. The author uses a decade of experience to highlight problems associated with cosmetic surgery and important nursing measures.

Larrow L, Noe JM: Port wine stain hemangiomas. *Am J Nurs* 1982; 82:786–790. Treatment of port-wine stains through the use of the argon laser is presented in detail. The reading includes implications for the nurse and the care involved.

Lyons RJ: Promoting healing of skin flaps and grafts. *AORN J* 1982; 35:1174–1183. The author effectively presents the differences between skin flaps and grafts and the nursing care that is necessary to assist in the healing process.

Markland A: Nursing care of the suction lipectomy patient. *Plast Surg Nurs* (Summer) 1984; 2:44–46. Nursing care for the suction lipectomy client is described, from the initial consultation through the perioperative period and postoperative office visits.

Robinson JK: Mohs' surgery for skin cancer. *Am J Nurs* 1982; 82:282–283. The procedure is described with illustrations to demonstrate the surgical approach and the outcomes.

Severo R: *Lisa H.* New York: Harper & Row, 1985. This is the story of a young woman with neurofibromatosis primarily involving the face and the eyes. It details both physiological and psychosocial effects of the disfigurement as well as the radical reconstructive facial surgery she undergoes.

Common Abbreviations and Acronyms

Acronym or Abbreviation	Definition
AAL	anterior axillary line
AC	air conduction
ADL	activities of daily living
AIDS	acquired immune deficiency syndrome
AP	anteroposterior; anterior and posterior
ARDS	adult respiratory distress syndrome
ASA	acetylsalicylic acid (aspirin)
ASHD	arteriosclerotic heart disease
ATN	acute tubular necrosis
A:V ratio	artery to vein ratio
AVM	arteriovenous malformation
A&W	alive and well
BC	bone conduction
BCG	Bacillus Calmette-Guerin (TBC vaccine)
BDR	background diabetic retinopathy
BGM	blood glucose monitoring
BM	bowel movement
BP	blood pressure
BPH	benign prostatic hyperplasia
BS	bowel sounds or breath sounds
BSE	breast self-examination
c̄	with
Ca	cancer
CAD	coronary artery disease
CAPD	continuous ambulatory peritoneal dialysis
CAT	computed axial tomography
CC	chief concern
CHF	congestive heart failure
CM	costal margin
CN	cranial nerve
CNS	central nervous system
COPD	chronic obstructive pulmonary disease
CSF	cerebrospinal fluid
CT	computed tomography
CTT	computed transverse tomography
CV	cardiovascular
CVA	costovertebral angle; cerebrovascular accident
CVP	central venous pressure
D/C	discontinued
DES	diethylstilbestrol
DIC	disseminated intravascular coagulation

Acronym or Abbreviation	Definition
DIP	distal interphalangeal
DJD	degenerative joint disease
DKA	diabetic ketoacidosis
DM	diabetes mellitus
DOE	dyspnea on exertion
DRGs	diagnosis-related groups
DTRs	deep tendon reflexes
Dx	diagnosis
ECG	electrocardiogram
EENT	eye, ear, nose, and throat
EOMs	extraocular movements
ESRD	end-stage renal disease
ETOH	alcohol
EUA	exam under anesthesia
FB	foreign body
FH	family history
Fx	fracture
G	gravida
GI	gastrointestinal
GU	genitourinary
gyn	gynecology
HDL	high density lipoproteins
HEENT	head, eye, ear, nose, and throat
HHNK	hyperglycemic hyperosmolar nonketotic
HJR	hepatojugular reflux
HMO	health maintenance organization
H or E	hemorrhages or exudates
HPI	history of the present illness
HTN	hypertension
Hx	History
I & D	incision and drainage
I & O	intake and output
ICP	intracranial pressure
ICS	intercostal space
IDDM	insulin-dependent diabetes mellitus
IOP	intraocular pressure
IPPB	intermittent positive pressure breathing
IU	international unit
IUD	intrauterine device
IVP	intravenous pyelogram

JVD	jugular venous distention		**PPDR**	preproliferative diabetic retinopathy
JVP	jugular venous pressure		**PPO**	preferred provider organization
			PTA	prior to admission
KUB	kidney, ureter, bladder			
			RICS	right intercostal space
LBCD	left border of cardiac dullness		**RLL**	right lower lobe
LDL	low density lipoproteins		**RLQ**	right lower quadrant
LICS	left intercostal space		**RML**	right middle lobe
LLQ	left lower quadrant		**R/O**	rule out
LMP	last menstrual period		**ROM**	range of motion
LOC	level of consciousness		**ROS**	review of systems
LP	lumbar puncture		**RSB**	right sternal border
LSB	left sternal border		**RSR**	regular sinus rhythm
LUQ	left upper quadrant		**RUL**	right upper lobe
			RUQ	right upper quadrant
MAL	midaxillary line		**Rx**	treatment
MCL	midclavicular line			
MGF	maternal grandfather		**s̄**	without
MGM	maternal grandmother		**S₁**	first heart sound
MI	myocardial infarction		**S₂**	second heart sound
MSL	midsternal line		**S₃**	third heart sound
			S₄	fourth heart sound
NAD	no acute distress		**SI**	systems international
NIDDM	noninsulin-dependent diabetes mellitus		**SLE**	systemic lupus erythematosus
nl	normal limits		**SOAP**	subjective, objective, assessment, plan
NPO	nothing by mouth		**SOB**	shortness of breath
NSR	normal sinus rhythm		**S/P**	status post
N&V	nausea and vomiting		**SQ**	subcutaneous
			S&S	symptoms and signs
ō	none			
OB	occult blood		**T&A**	tonsillectomy and adenoidectomy
OC	oral contraceptives		**TBC**	tuberculosis
OD	right eye		**Td**	tetanus diptheria
OR	operating room		**TIA**	transient ischemic attack
OS	left eye		**TM**	tympanic membrane
OTC	over-the-counter		**TMJ**	temporomandibular joint
OU	both eyes		**TPN**	total parenteral nutrition
			TSE	testicular self-exam
PA	posteroanterior		**TSS**	toxic shock syndrome
PAL	posterior axillary line			
Pap smear	Papanicolaou smear		**URI**	upper respiratory infection
PDR	proliferative diabetic retinopathy		**UTI**	urinary tract infection
PE	physical exam; pulmonary embolism			
PERRLA	pupils equal, round, reactive to light and accommodation		**VD**	venereal disease
			VFs	visual fields
PGF	paternal grandfather		**VLDL**	very low density lipoproteins
PGM	paternal grandmother		**VS**	vital signs
PH	past history			
PI	present illness			
PID	pelvic inflammatory disease		**WD**	well developed
PIP	proximal interphalangeal		**WN**	well nourished
PMD	private medical doctor		**wnl**	within normal limits
PMI	point of maximal impulse		**w/fe**	white female
PMP	previous menstrual period		**w/m**	white male
PND	paroxysmal nocturnal dyspnea; postnasal drip			
POR	problem oriented record		**⊕**	positive
PPD	packs per day (cigarettes); purified protein derivative (tuberculin)		**⊖**	negative
			ō	none
			ⓜ	murmur

Glossary

abiotrophic diseases   diseases which are not present at birth, but manifest themselves later in life

accommodation   the process by which the eye adjusts for distance, maintaining a clear visual image with a shift in gaze

acholic (clay-colored) stools   stools absent of brown coloration; indicative of biliary dysfunction

acini   the terminal respiratory units of the lungs formed by the respiratory bronchioles, alveolar ducts, and alveoli

action potential   the process of cardiac depolarization and repolarization

active immunity   occurs when the host produces antibodies in response to antigenic stimulation

active transport   the movement of small particles across cell membranes from an area of greater to lesser concentration

adenohypophysis   the anterior lobe of the pituitary gland

afterload   the tension the ventricles must develop in systole to pump against pressure in the aortic valve and aorta

agnosia   the inability to recognize familiar objects in the environment through the senses of touch and vision

allergens   substances capable of inducing hypersensitivity

allergy   an altered bodily state in which an exaggerated response occurs with exposure to an antigen

alopecia   the loss of body hair (primarily on the scalp) with the presence of bald spots or total baldness

amaurosis fugax   a transient loss of vision in one eye

amenorrhea   the absence of menstruation

anabolism   building up of the system by changing simple compounds into complex substances; constructive phase of metabolism

angina   chest pain that results from myocardial ischemia

anhidrosis   the absence of sweat

anosmia   loss of smell

antigen   a foreign protein or protein complex capable of stimulating a specific immune response when present in the body

anxiety   state of uneasiness, discomfort; feeling of apprehension

aphagia   inability to swallow

aphakia   the absence of the lens of the eye

apheresis   the process of separating whole blood into its four major components and removing one for use

apraxia   the inability to carry out a learned, voluntary act when motor function is intact

arcus senilis   a peripheral corneal opacity common in clients over age 60

arteriovenous (AV) fistula   the internal anastomosis of an artery to a vein

arteriovenous (AV) shunt   the external connection of an artery to a vein using two pieces of synthetic tubing and a connector

arthroscopy   the examination of a joint through a special fiberoptic endoscope (an arthroscope)

ascites   the accumulation of protein-rich serous fluid in the peritoneal cavity

asterixis   a flapping tremor of the hand characteristic of ammonia toxicity

asthenopia   ocular discomfort related to an uncorrected refractive error

astigmatism   irregularities in the surface of the lens or cornea

ataxia   lack of muscle coordination

athetosis   slow, twisting, snakelike movements in the upper extremities

atrophy   a wasting away

auscultatory gap   a silent interval between the systolic and diastolic pressure in some hypertensive clients

autodigestion   digestion of tissues (especially in the stomach and pancreas) by their own secretions

azotemia   the accumulation of urea and other nitrogenous substances (uric acid and creatinine) in the blood

B-lymphocytes (B cells)   cells which mature in the bone marrow and, when triggered by an antigen, differentiate into antibody-producing cells

ballottement   a palpatory technique used when the presence of fluid is suspected

band keratopathy   calcium deposits in the cornea

bitemporal hemianopia   the loss of the peripheral visual fields

body image   a person's concept of the size, shape, and functioning of the body and its parts

borborygmi   hyperactive bowel sounds

bradycardia   a pulse rate below 60 beats per minute

brawny induration   edema which acquires a "woody" feeling because of increased connective tissue in the subcutaneous tissue

bruit   an audible murmur in a blood vessel secondary to turbulent blood flow

bulbar paralysis   paralysis of the lips, tongue, mouth, pharynx, and larynx

bunion   inflammation and thickening of the bursa on the medial side of the first metatarsal head of the great toe

cachexia   the "wasting away" associated with chronic disease and cancer characterized by anorexia, weakness, and emaciation

café au lait spots   spots of light brown patchy skin pigmentation

calculi   stones

carcinoma in situ   noninfiltrating carcinoma

cardiac output   the amount of blood the heart pumps per minute

cardiac reserve   the difference between cardiac output at rest and cardiac output when the physiological limit is reached

cardiac tamponade   an accumulation of fluid in the pericardial sac which prevents the heart from filling and reduces cardiac output

cardinal directions of gaze   the six directions in which the globe of the eye can move depending on which muscle is acting predominantly

cardiopulmonary bypass   the use of a heart-lung machine during surgery, which allows the heart to be stopped and maintains a bloodless surgical field

cardiopulmonary resuscitation (CPR)   artificial respiration combined with external cardiac compression to provide for oxygenation of vital tissues until cardiac function is restored

carpopedal spasm   a spasm of the hands and feet associated with tetany

catabolism   breaking down of the system by changing complex substances into simple compounds; destructive phase of metabolism

cavitary seeding   the inadvertent transfer of tumor cells to a new site during surgery

cell-mediated immunity   immunity depending on the local action of the T-lymphocyte after becoming sensitized by contact with a specific antigen

cerumen   a yellowish-brown wax formed by secretions from the sebaceous and apocrine glands

cheilosis   fissures and dry scaling of lips and at corners of the mouth

chemosis   edema of the conjunctiva around the cornea

cholecystectomy   a resection of the gallbladder

cholecystitis   inflammation of the gallbladder

cholecystostomy   the surgical formation of an opening in the gallbladder

choledochostomy   incision of the common bile duct for removal of biliary calculi and insertion of a T-tube

choledocolithiasis   obstruction of the common bile duct by gallstones

cholelithiasis   gallstones

chondrocalcinosis   calcification of the articular cartilage

chorea   involuntary twitching of the limbs or facial muscles

Chvostek's sign   twitching of the facial muscles when the facial nerve is percussed; seen in tetany

chylomicrons   particles of lipids

chyme   the food bolus after being mixed with gastric juices and churned by the stomach's musculature

circadian rhythms   diurnal variation; a pattern based on a cycle consisting of 24 hours

climacteric   the period of premenopausal changes

clinical death determination of death according to medical standards usually linked to irreversible cessation of circulatory and respiratory function or neurologic function

clonus a series of involuntary muscle contractions precipitated by a sudden passive stretch of muscle

cogwheel rigidity rhythmic jerking fluctuations in the intensity of muscle tone on passive range of motion

colic intermittent fluctuating pain caused by smooth muscle spasm

comedones blackheads and whiteheads

compromised host a client whose host defenses against infection are impaired

confabulate to fill memory gaps with imagined experiences

contracture the shortening and fixing of muscle fibers which limits a joint's range of motion

convergence the medial movement of the two eyeballs so they are both directed toward the object being viewed

crepitation a coarse, crackling sensation with palpation of the subcutaneous tissue caused by escape of air from the lungs into the tissue; also the grating sound and sometimes a palpable vibration when a joint is moved, produced by the roughened synovium in arthritic disease

cretinism a condition of severe congenital hypothyroidism marked by retardation of both growth and mental development

cross-tolerance the tolerance to one pharmacologic agent which then requires larger doses of similar drugs to achieve the desired effect

cyanosis a blue tinge to the skin that appears when hemoglobin oxygen saturation is reduced

cycloplegia paralysis of the ciliary muscle causing paralysis of ocular accommodation

debridement the removal of tissue or eschar prior to healing or any skin-grafting procedure

decerebrate posturing the hyperextension of both the upper and lower extremities

decorticate posturing hyperflexion of the upper extremities and hyperextension of the lower extremities

dehiscence disruption of the superficial layers of a wound

depolarization the flow of electrical impulses that leads to contraction of the heart muscle

dialysate a solution composed of water, glucose, sodium, chloride, potassium, calcium, and acetate or bicarbonate that passes through the semipermeable membrane in dialysis

dialysis removal of elements from the blood through a semipermeable membrane

diapedesis the passage of leukocytes through the unruptured wall of a capillary

diastasis recti a separation of the two rectus abdominis muscles

diffusion the mixing of molecules caused by their tendency to move continuously and randomly in a solution or gas

diplopia double vision

diverticuli a pouch or sac created by herniation of lining mucous membrane through the muscular coat of a tubular structure such as the large intestine

drug dependence a condition in which a person requires the effects of a specific drug to function

drusen yellow deposits visualized as mounds on Bruch's membrane

dysarthria poorly articulated speech

dyskinesias defects in voluntary movement resulting in fragmentary or incomplete movement

dysmenorrhea painful menstruation

dysmetria the inability to measure distance properly in muscular acts

dyspareunia pain associated with intercourse

dyspepsia indigestion

dysphagia difficulty swallowing

dyspnea difficult breathing

dysrhythmias disturbances in the heart's rhythm

dystonia intense, irregular torsion muscle spasms

ecchymoses irregular hemorrhagic areas larger than petichiae that can be dark purplish, brown, yellow, or greenish in color; bruises

echolalia the parrotlike repetition of words spoken by others

ectopic beats cardiac impulses originating outside the SA node

ectropion turning outward of the eyelid margin; usually of the lower eyelid

edema a local or general accumulation of excess fluid in the body tissues

effector T cells killer cells, helpers, and suppressors; essential in regulating the body's fight against invasive organisms

effusion swelling of a joint caused by an increase in synovial fluid or the presence of blood in the joint capsule

egophony a change from an "ee" to a long "a" sound heard when auscultating over an area of lung consolidation

ejection fraction the percentage of left ventricular end-diastolic volume that is pumped

electromyogram (EMG) a test to measure the electric currents produced by muscles, both at rest and during contraction

endotoxins part of the outer cell wall, usually of gram-negative bacteria, and released only upon its destruction

enophthalmos recession of the eye within the orbit; characterized by a drooping upper eyelid

enterotoxins exotoxins that impair intestinal absorption and provoke secretion of electrolytes and water

entropion inversion of the eyelid margin

epicritic (discriminating) pain sharp, localized, pricking pain produced by A-delta fibers

epiphora excessive watering of the eye

eructation belching; usually associated with the swallowing of air

erythropoietin a protein produced in the kidneys that stimulates red blood cell production

eschar necrotic burned skin

euthanasia mercy killing

euthyroidism a normal state of thyroid functioning

evisceration complete disruption of the surgical wound, with protrusion of the viscera

exophthalmos bilateral protrusion of the eyeball; often indicates a thyroid disorder

exotoxins particularly lethal toxins, usually produced by gram-positive bacteria, released by the bacteria itself

extra-anatomic bypass (EAB) the extension of a Dacron graft from one femoral artery to another

extravasation the leakage of a fluid (IV solutions, drugs) into surrounding tissues

fasciculations fine, rapid, twitching movements originating in small groups of muscle fibers

fecalith a hard mass of dry stool

feedback mechanisms a closed-loop mechanism driven by plasma concentrations of a specific hormone which, in turn, regulates its secretion

festination a shuffling and propulsive gait

fetor hepaticus a sweet breath odor resembling acetone or old wine

first-degree burn a burn which damages only the epidermal layer of skin

flaccidity decreased or absent muscle tone

flank the part of the body between the ribs and the ilium of the pelvis

floaters deposits of protein or cells suspended in the vitreous humor that float across the visual field

fortification a visual aura which includes colored patterns with a dark center and jagged edges

fracture a break in the continuity of a bone

full-thickness burn the equivalent of third-degree burns

fundus (of the eye) the retinal area

gallop rhythm an S_3 or S_4 heard along with S_1 and S_2, causing triplets of heart sounds resembling a horse's gallop

genogram a diagram of the family tree

glycemic index the blood glucose levels produced by various foods

glycogen stored carbohydrate

glycogenesis the synthesis of glycogen from glucose

glycogenolysis the conversion of glycogen to glucose

glycosuria glucose in the urine

goiter the enlargement of the thyroid gland

graft-versus-host disease (GVHD) a tissue incompatibility syndrome in which competent T-lymphocytes from the donor circulate and attack host tissue

gynecomastia enlarged, feminine-appearing breasts in males

habitus physical appearance

health risk appraisal (HRA) quantitative measure estimating an individual's probability of dying from a particular cause within a specified time

heart rate the number of strokes per minute

hematemesis bloody vomitus

hematochezia passage of stools containing bright red blood that originates high in the GI tract

hemodialysis dialysis in which an artificial kidney contains the semipermeable membrane

hemoptysis purulent, bloody, or blood-tinged sputum

hepatomegaly enlargement of the liver

heterozygous denotes two different alleles at the same locus

hirsutism excessive hair growth, especially of male hair patterns in women

HLA antigens a complex of antigens related to susceptibility to certain diseases and rejection of transplanted tissues

homonymous hemianopia the loss of half of the visual field

homozygous denotes two identical alleles at the same locus

hormone a chemical substance synthesized by an endocrine gland, secreted directly into the bloodstream, and carried to other sites where its physiological actions are exerted

hormone-receptor binding the process by which certain hormones bind to specific target cell receptors

hormone-target cell specificity the capability of certain cells to respond to a specific hormone

hospice a facility that specializes in caring for the terminally ill and their families

humoral immunity immunity mediated by antibodies that circulate in the blood and are present in the body fluids

hypercapnia above-normal levels of carbon dioxide in the blood

hyperopia farsightedness

hyperorality an insatiable need for oral stimulation by chewing or tasting objects

hyperplasia an increase in the number of cells

hypersensitivity an altered bodily state in which an exaggerated response occurs with exposure to an antigen

hypertonic (solution) a solution with a greater osmolality than blood plasma, causing a rapid influx of water from cells into the plasma

hypertrichosis excess growth of hair

hypertrophy an increase in the size of an organ or structure due to an increase in the size of its cells

hyphema blood in the anterior chamber between the cornea and iris resulting from a tear in the ciliary body

hypoacusia a hearing loss

hypotonia flaccidity of muscle

hypotonic (solution) a solution with a lower osmolality than blood plasma, causing water to move from the plasma into the cells

hypoxemia below-normal levels of oxygen in the blood

iatrogenic a condition or disorder induced by medical treatment

icterus jaundice

idiopathic a condition without recognizable cause

immunoglobulin (Ig) a specialized plasma protein (antibody) produced by the B-lymphocytes in response to the presence of an antigen

impotence an impairment of penile erectile function

injection congestion of blood vessels

interferon a protein produced by T-lymphocytes and many other cells in response to the presence of viruses and other parasites that stimulates noninfected cells to produce an antiviral protein that inhibits viral multiplication

intermittent claudication a cramping pain in a muscle brought on by exercise and relieved by rest

intertriginous areas apposed surfaces of the skin, such as the creases of the neck, breasts, groin, or buttocks

ischemia deficiency of blood because of a constricted or obstructed blood vessel

isometric contraction occurs when a muscle becomes tense while remaining the same length

isotonic (solution) a solution with the same osmolality as blood plasma

isotonic contraction occurs when a muscle shortens during contraction

jaundice yellow coloration of skin and sclerae

Kayser-Fleischer ring a rusty-brown corneal accumulation of copper characteristic of hepatolenticular degeneration

keloid a benign proliferative growth of fibrous tissue at the site of an injury or incision extending beyond the wound itself

ketosis accumulation of ketones

kwashiorkor protein malnutrition resulting from a protein-poor diet or protein loss because of physiological stress

kyphosis an increased convex curve of the thoracic spine (hunchback)

lacrimation the production of tears

laser a device that transforms light of various frequencies into a finely focused beam capable of great heat and power

leukoplakia white thickened plaques that form on mucous membranes

LeVeen shunt peritoneal-jugular shunt which provides a route for reinfusion of ascitic fluid into the venous system

lichenification localized thickening of skin resulting from everyday mechanical pressures or chronic irritation

lipolysis the breakdown of fat

living will a document stating a person's desires about care and intervention to prolong life artificially if he or she becomes unable to communicate

lordosis an increased concave curve of the lumbar spine (swayback)

lymphadenitis inflamed lymphatic vessels coupled with inflamed lymph nodes

lymphadenopathy lymph node enlargement

lymphangitis inflamed lymphatic vessels

lymphedema edema resulting from improper function or obstruction of the lymphatics

macrophages cells of the reticuloendothelial system that can engulf foreign particles

malnutrition the reduced intake or utilization of nutrients, particularly protein and calories, in relation to requirements

malocclusion imperfect alignment of teeth that affects how they meet during chewing (the "bite")

marasmus protein and calorie malnutrition resulting from a chronic reduction of protein and calorie intake

mastication (chewing) the initial preparation of food for the digestive process, when it is ground into a pulp and mixed with saliva

melanin a brown-black pigment that gives color to skin and hair

melena (tarry stools) usually associated with bleeding of the upper GI tract; the natural red color is lost during passage through the bowel

memory cells a subgroup of B cells which signal the immune system that previous exposure to an antibody has occurred

menarche the onset of menstruation

menopause the cessation of the menstrual cycle

menorrhagia excessive menstrual flow of greater than usual duration

metastasis spread of disease when malignant cells detach from the parent tissue and migrate to other body tissues

metrorrhagia bleeding between menstrual periods

microaneurysms minute aneurysms

micrographia handwriting which is cramped and small with signs of tremor

micturition urination

miosis the constricting of the pupil

mittelschmerz ovulatory pain

morbidity illness

mortality death

murmurs sounds resulting from vibrations produced by turbulence of blood flow in the heart

muscle tone the tension in the resting muscle or the response of a limb to movement

mydriasis the dilation of the pupil

myelosuppression the suppressive alteration in the function of the bone marrow; a side effect of most antineoplastic agents

myoclonus spasm of a muscle or muscle groups

myopia nearsightedness

myxedema hypofunction of the thyroid

neoplasm tumor

neovascularization the formation of new blood vessels

nephrolithiasis renal calculi

neuralgia an uncomfortable, painful, burning sensation that extends along the course of one or more nerves

neuritis pain and tenderness along the course of the nerve resulting from inflammation, trauma, or infection

neurohypophysis the posterior lobe of the pituitary gland

nociceptive impulses impulses giving rise to sensations of pain

normal sinus rhythm (NSR) the orderly rhythm of the healthy heart, whose rate at rest is between 60 and 100 beats per minute

nutrient deficiency specific vitamin and mineral deficiency states

nystagmus an abnormal involuntary movement of both eyes either horizontally, vertically, diagonally, or circularly

obesity an excess of relative body fat

obtunded lethargic, drowsy

oligomenorrhea markedly diminished menstrual flow

oncogenes genetic material that can spur malignant transformation and is thought to be latent in the chromosomes of some

opportunists normally harmless organisms which, under certain circumstances, can become pathogenic

orthopnea difficulty breathing when not in an upright position

osmol measures the amount of work dissolved particles can do in drawing fluid through a semipermeable membrane

osmolality the number of osmols per liter of solvent

osmolarity the number of osmols per liter of solution

osmosis the movement of water through a semipermeable membrane from an area of lesser to greater particulate concentration

osmotic pressure the force exerted by particles in solution to stop osmosis

ossification the process by which rapidly forming cells in the epiphyseal plates are gradually replaced by bone cells

overweight an excess in body weight

ovulation the rupture of an ovarian follicle and release of the ovum

pacemaker a device that supplies electrical impulses to the heart muscle to stimulate heartbeat

pallalia the involuntary repetition of sentences

palpitation an unpleasant awareness of a rapid or irregular heartbeat

papilledema edema and inflammation of the optic nerve at its point of entrance into the eyeball

paraplegia the paralysis of both legs and possibly other areas of the trunk

paresthesia an abnormal sensation such as numbness, tingling, burning, or prickling

paroxysmal nocturnal dyspnea (PND) a sudden attack of dyspnea that awakens the client from sleep

partial-thickness burn the equivalent of first- and/or second-degree burns

passive immunity acquired when antibody and complement are transferred to a person without the body's active participation

pericardial effusion an accumulation of fluid in the pericardial sac

peritoneal dialysis dialysis in which the client's peritoneal lining serves as the semipermeable membrane

perseveration the repetition of a motor or verbal action

petechiae red to brownish pinpoint hemorrhages in the skin or mucous membranes

phagocytosis the engulfing of foreign particles by macrophages

phlebothrombosis the formation of a blood clot in a vein, usually in the legs

photophobia ocular discomfort induced by bright light

photopsia the appearance of flashing lights

physical dependence occurs when a person experiences physiological symptoms of withdrawal when use of a drug is discontinued

pinguecula yellow raised fatty plaques on the bulbar conjunctiva usually seen nasally

plasma osmolality the concentration of particles (electrolytes and nonelectrolytes) in the plasma

plethoric round and full, with congestion of blood vessels; a red florid complexion

pleural friction rub leathery, grating sound produced when inflamed or roughened pleural surfaces rub together

pleximeter in indirect percussion, the middle finger of the nondominant hand

plexor in indirect percussion, the tip of the middle finger of the dominant hand

pneumoperitoneum air or gas in the peritoneal cavity

point of maximal impulse (PMI) the systolic thrust of the cardiac apex, which is sometimes visible and/or palpable

Poiseuille's law the flow rate of a fluid through a tube is proportional to pressure differences and the diameter of the tube in relation to the length of the tube and the viscosity of the fluid

polyp a pedunculated growth found on the mucosal surface of vascular organs

postural hypotension a drop in blood pressure when moving from a lying or sitting to a standing position

precordium the area of the anterior chest overlying the heart

preload the degree of stretch of myocardial fibers before contraction

premature ejaculation the inability to exert any voluntary control over the timing of the ejaculatory reflex

presbycusis a slowly progressive bilateral hearing loss related to aging

presbyopia a loss of ability to focus clearly on objects close to the eye

primary intention the healing of approximated and closed surgical wounds with minimal formation of granulation or scar tissue

Prinzmetal's angina angina that occurs at rest

prognathism the lengthening, thickening, and protruding of the mandible

proinsulin a precursor to insulin

proptosis a downward displacement, as with the eyeball in exophthalmos

prostaglandins compounds synthesized from unsaturated fatty acids with an apparent role in acute and chronic inflammatory reactions

protopathic (undiscriminating) pain slow, diffuse, burning, aching, poorly localized pain produced by C fibers

pruritus itching

psychological dependence occurs when a person has a compulsion to continue using a drug in order to maintain self-esteem and well-being

ptosis the drooping or dropping of an organ or a part, as in the drooping of the upper eyelid

pulmonary edema engorgement of the pulmonary vasculature with accumulation of fluid in the interstitial spaces and alveoli

pulmonary surfactant a fluid produced by the secretory glands of the alveolar wall which reduces its surface tension

pulse pressure the difference between the systolic and diastolic blood pressures

quadriplegia the paralysis of all four extremities

rales sounds auscultated heard over the smaller bronchi or alveoli and caused by the passage of air through bronchi containing fluid

rebound a palpatory technique often used for assessment of peritoneal inflammation with appendicitis

rebound tenderness pain felt after withdrawal of pressure during palpation; a reliable sign of peritoneal inflammation

recombinant DNA the artificial introduction of DNA into a cell to alter it and the subsequent replication of the new and natural DNA

reflux backward or return flow

reflux nephropathy the directing back of urine from the bladder toward the renal pelvis through the ureters during voiding

refraction the passage of light rays from a transparent medium into a second transparent medium with a different density

renal osteodystrophy a serious bone pathology resulting from chronic disease of the kidneys

repolarization the return to the resting membrane potential resulting from the presence of potassium ions in the cardiac cell membrane

resting membrane potential the electrically negative charge of the inside of the cardiac cell membrane in relation to the outside

retinopathy pathological changes in the retina of the eye

retrograde ejaculation the backflow of ejaculate into the bladder

rhonchi gurgling sounds originating in the larger air passages and heard on auscultation; also called coarse rales

rigidity a pronounced increase in muscle tone

root pain pain caused by disease of the dorsal roots of the spinal nerves and felt in the cutaneous areas supplied by the affected roots

scanning speech speech that is slow and deliberate, punctuated with pauses between syllables

scoliosis a lateral curve of the spine

scotomas blind gaps in the visual fields

sebum a lipid substance produced by the sebaceous gland which provides some lubrication of hair and epidermis

seborrhea excess production of sebum

secondary intention the healing of an infected incision or one purposely left open, with greater formation of granulation or scar tissue

second-degree burn a burn which damages the epidermal layer and part of the dermal layer of skin

self-concept the total set of beliefs and feelings one holds about one's self

self-esteem the personal value placed on oneself

semen the collective product of the male accessory sex glands

sialolithiasis formation of salivary calculi; may cause parotitis if a stone lodges in the parotid gland

singultus hiccups

skin turgor the normal fullness and elasticity of the skin

smegma the cheesy secretion of sebaceous glands found chiefly beneath the prepuce

spasticity increased resistance of muscles to passive stretch with rapid extension or flexion of a joint

spermatogenesis the formation of sperm

splenic sequestration the trapping of sickled erythrocytes by the spleen

station the manner in which one stands

steatorrhea (fatty stools) frequent, frothy, foul, and floating stools; caused by altered digestion and absorption of fat

steatosis fatty infiltration of the liver which often precedes cirrhosis

striae streaks or lines

stroke volume the amount of blood the heart pumps with each stroke

substance abuse the continued use of chemical agents despite the emotional, social, legal, and health problems their use creates

sulcus (of the prostate) a midline groove that separates the two lobes of the prostate

superinfection a secondary infection resulting from overgrowth of normal flora during antibiotic treatment

sympathetic ophthalmia inflammation of the uveal tract of an uninjured eye

syncope a transient loss of consciousness associated with muscle weakness and an inability to stand; fainting

synechiae adhesions of parts, especially the iris to the lens or the cornea

T-lymphocytes (T cells) a heterogeneous group of cells that mature in the thymus gland and differentiate into a variety of effector T cells (killer cells, helper cells, and suppressor cells)

tachycardia a pulse rate greater than 100 beats per minute

tactile fremitus a palpable vibration of air through the airways as a person speaks

target cells cells that are sites for the physiological effect of specific hormones

teichopsia a visual aura which includes flashing lights zigzagging across the visual fields

tertiary intention healing which involves debridement of large infected or contaminated wounds followed by mechanical skin closure

third-degree burn a burn which damages both the epidermal and dermal layers of skin

thrills palpable vibrations over the precordium similar to those felt on the throat of a purring cat

thrombophlebitis inflammation of a vein with thrombus formation

tinnitus a ringing, buzzing, or hissing in the ear or head

tolerance the need for increasingly larger amounts of a drug to produce the same effects; comes with repeated exposure

torticollis twisting of the head to one side in response to muscle contraction; wryneck

torus palatinus a midline bony outgrowth on the hard palate

total parenteral nutrition (TPN) the intravenous infusion of all necessary nutrients

toxins poisonous substances

traction pulling force applied to a fractured limb to overcome muscle spasm and realign the fracture

trigone an area of the posterior wall of the bladder defined by the urethra and the two ureteral slits

Trousseau's sign carpopedal spasm with inability to open the hand when a blood pressure cuff is placed on the arm, elevated over the systolic reading, and left in place for 2 to 3 minutes

twitching localized, spasmodic contraction of a single muscle group

universal donor type O blood, which can be transfused into clients without causing reactions because it lacks antigens

universal recipient type AB blood, which has both A and B antigens and can accept transfusions of any blood type

uremia azotemia with clinical symptoms

uremic fetor a urinelike breath odor

uremic frost the crust of urate crystals that can accumulate on the skin as a result of uremia

ureteral stent a hollow tubelike device made of silicone placed within a ureter to maintain ureteral flow

vertigo a sensation of disturbed motion as if the person was revolving in space

visual field the area within which stimuli produce sight when the eye is looking straight ahead

vitiligo skin patches that lack pigment

wheezes whistling sounds resulting from the narrowing of respiratory passages

whispered pectoriloquy whispered syllables heard clearly when auscultating over an area of lung consolidation

xanthelasmas (xanthomas) flat or slightly raised yellowish lesions on the upper or lower eyelids in the elderly; often associated with elevated cholesterol levels

xerostomia dryness of the mouth

Drug Index

female sexual development and, 1815
gluten-free, 1510
   sprue and, 1509
health history and, 136
hearing loss and, 2091
heart failure and, 803–804
hepatic-biliary dysfunction and, 1564–1565
hyperlipidemia and, 780, 781
integumentary system and, 2158
intestinal hernia and, 1498
lactose-restricted, 1494
mitral valve commissurotomy and, 827
musculoskeletal system and, 1635
myocardial infarction and, 788, 793
nephrolithiasis and, 1057
peripheral vascular disease and, 842–843, 851
polyps and, 1513
stomach cancer and, 1513
urinary system and, 990
urolithiasis and, 1057
weight reduction, 215
Dietary fiber
anorectal fissure and, 1501
cancer and, 46, 324, 325
diabetic diet and, 1329, 1330
hemorrhoids and, 1501
intestinal hernia and, 1499
Dietary history, 192, 1438
cardiovascular, 732
hematologic system and, 884
peripheral vascular disease and, 843
Diet counseling, gastrointestinal disorders and, 1492
Diet therapy, peptic ulcer disease and, 1495–1496
Diethylstilbestrol, 1865–1866
Diffuse toxic goiter, 1350
Diffusion, 77, 1427
capillary membrane and, 712
dialysis and, 1020
impairment of, 521
tubular reabsorption and, 983
Digestion, 1427
changes in, 1430
enzymes of, 1421, 1428
secretions and, 1429
Digital subtraction angiography, cardiovascular system and, 747–748
1,25-Dihydroxycholecalciferol, 1286
Dilatation and curettage, 1902–1903, 1903
Dipeptidases, actions of, 1428
Diphtheria, 593–594
artificial active immunity and, 22
causative agent of, 273
death rate for, 43
epidemiology of, 281
exotoxins in, 288
immunization and, 300
incubation period of, 273
prevention of, 281
Diphtheroids, normal habitat of, 271
Diplococcus pneumoniae, 915
Diplopia, 1129, 1993, 2001, 2005
blow-out fracture and, 2052
botulism and, 291
cataract and, 2041
endocrine dysfunction and, 1290, 1294
head and neck trauma and, 600

hematologic disease and, 883
polycythemia vera and, 940
respiratory tract cancer and, 597
suboccipital craniectomy and, 1242, 1247
Wernicke's encephalopathy and, 243
Disaccharidases, actions of, 1428
Disaccharides, 1492
Disaster, 364
Disease. See also specific type
definitions of, 17–18
hierarchy of, 18
hot-cold, 57, 58
Disease control, epidemiology and, 279–300
Disease-producing agents, 270–272, 273
Disease vectors, 272
Diskectomy
anterior cervical, 1261–1262, 1262
microlumbar, 1258–1261, 1260
Dislocation, 1739
Disorientation
hypomagnesemia and, 87
poisoning and, 390
shock and, 94
Displacement, 116–117
Dissections, aortic, surgical repair of, 836–838, 837
Disseminated intravascular coagulation, 922–923
bleeding time and, 889
burn client and, 441
cancer and, 353
fibrin degradation products and, 718
partial thromboplastin time and, 889
prothrombin time and, 889
Rocky Mountain spotted fever and, 298
septic shock and, 288
shock and, 98
Distributive shock, 94, 97–98
Diurnal variation, hormone regulation and, 1278
Diverticuli, 1496, 1497
esophageal, 1474, 1475
perforated, peritonitis and, 1504
Diverticulitis, 1496–1498
barium studies and, 1448
colon conduit and, 1086
intestinal obstruction and, 1511
Diverticulosis, 1496–1498
gastrointestinal bleeding and, 1503
Divorce, 3–4
DJD. See Degenerative joint disease
DKA. See Ketoacidosis, diabetic
DNA, aging and, 30
DOE. See Dyspnea on exertion
Domestic violence, 1894–1895
Dominance, 26
Dopamine, 1106, 1279
appetite regulation and, 210
Doppler ultrasonography. See Ultrasonography, Doppler
Dorsal position, 420, 420
Dorsalis pedis pulse. See Pulse, dorsalis pedis
Down's syndrome, 28
leukemia and, 323
periodontal disease and, 1475
DPT vaccine. See Vaccines, DPT
DRGs. See Diagnosis-related groups
Drooling, oral cancer and, 1482

Drowning, 34, 364, 385–386
cardiac arrest and, 369
neurologic insult and, 372
Drug abuse, 225
acquired immune deficiency syndrome and, 926
conditions associated with, 60
drowning and, 34
hepatic-biliary dysfunction and, 1564
infective endocarditis and, 806
surgical risk and, 402
young adults and, 61
Drug addiction, 212
Drug dependence, 232. See also Physical dependence, Psychological dependence
Drug overdose, 364
acute respiratory failure and, 645
adult respiratory distress syndrome and, 618
cardiac arrest and, 369
neurogenic shock and, 94
Drug reactions
alcohol and, 240–241
drug abuse and, 60
Drug screening, 257
Drug therapy
anaphylactic shock and, 97
bone marrow and, 723
cutaneous manifestations of, 2194
erythropoiesis and, 720
hematologic system and, 883
hyperthyroidism and, 1353
infection and, 277–278
leukopenia and, 720
malnutrition and, 191–192
nutrient deficiencies and, 185
nutritional status and, 186–188
obesity and, 218
Raynaud's phenomenon and, 857
thrombocytopenia and, 720
Drunk driving, 364
Drusen, 2042
DSA. See Digital subtraction angiography
DST. See Dexamethasone suppression test
DTRs. See Deep tendon reflexes
DUB. See Uterine bleeding, dysfunctional
Dubin-Johnson syndrome, 1562, 1586
Duchenne dystrophy, 1151
Ductus deferens, 1822
Dumping syndrome, 1430
vagotomy and, 1528
Duodenal ulcers. See Ulcers, duodenal
Duodenoscopy, 179, 1448
Duodenostomy, 1460
Duodenum, 1421, 1422
absorption in, 1427
barium studies and, 1447
peptic ulcer disease and, 1493
secretions of, 1426
Dura mater, 1115
DVT. See Thrombophlebitis, deep-vein
Dwarfism, pituitary, 1377–1378, 1378
Dye clearance, hepatic-biliary dysfunction and, 1572–1573
Dying. See also Death
assessment and, 484–490
development levels and, 485–487
ethical issues and, 498–503
evaluation and, 498

family and, 485
fear and, 479–480
intervention and, 495–497
nursing diagnosis and, 490–491
planning and implementation and, 491–495
research and, 503
social and cultural values and, 484–485
views of, 478–479
Western culture and, 487–480
Dying client
physical care of, 491
physiological needs of, 492
psychological care of, 491–495
resuscitation of, 499
spiritual care of, 495
Dynorphin, appetite regulation and, 210
Dysarthria, 1130
Dysentery. See specific type
Dysequilibrium, 2095
Dysgerminoma, 1884
Dyskinesia, 1125
Parkinson's disease and, 1174
Dysmenorrhea, 1838
adenomyosis and, 1870
endocrine dysfunction and, 1294
endometriosis and, 1838, 1866, 1871
primary, 1866–1867
Dysmetria, multiple sclerosis and, 1183
Dyspareunia, 1831, 1838, 1931
endometriosis and, 1871
hysterectomy and, 1906
malnutrition and, 199
Sjogren's syndrome and, 1733
Dyspepsia, 1438
nonsteroidal antiinflammatory agents and, 106
Dysphagia, 1130, 1428–1429
botulism and, 291
conditions associated with, 1431
dermatomyositis and, 1675
epiglottitis and, 595
esophageal achalasia and, 1473
esophageal cancer and, 1483
esophageal diverticula and, 1474
esophagitis and, 1479
goiter and, 1359, 1360
iron deficiency and, 883
laryngotracheal trauma and, 604
oral cancer and, 1480, 1482
radiation therapy and, 347
respiratory dysfunction and, 529
respiratory tract cancer and, 596
suboccipital craniectomy and, 1244
Dysphasia, superior vena cava syndrome and, 354–355
Dysphonia, dermatomyositis and, 1675
Dyspnea, 528
acquired immune deficiency syndrome and, 928
acute respiratory failure and, 645
adult respiratory distress syndrome and, 618, 619
bronchiectasis and, 635
bronchogenic carcinoma and, 647
cardiac tumors and, 810
cardiovascular disease and, 730
chest trauma and, 650
chronic bronchitis and, 640
congestive heart failure and, 797

potassium imbalance and, 84
preoperative, 401
subarachnoid hemorrhage and,
1157
thoracic aneurysms and, 861
Electrocoagulation, gastrointestinal
bleeding and, 1502
Electrodessication
basal cell carcinoma and, 2209
hemangioma and, 2207
seborrheic keratosis and, 2205
Electroencephalography, 178,
1132–1133
Huntington's chorea and, 1153
seizure disorders and, 1160
Electrolyte imbalances, 82–87
apheresis and, 907
burns and, 442
kidneys and, 985–986
near-drowning and, 386
nephrectomy and, 1070
premature ventricular complexes
and, 776
protein-sparing modified fast and,
214
pyelolithotomy and, 1072
Electrolytes, 76–77
absorption of, 1422, 1427
burns and, 452
cardiovascular system and,
740–741
gastrointestinal, 1452
kidney transplantation and, 1077
measurement and distribution of,
77
movement of, 77–78
pancreas and, 1424
preoperative, 401
trauma client and, 379
urinary, 1003
Electromagnetic receptors, 1098
Electromyography, 178, 1006, 1136
muscular dystrophy and, 1151
musculoskeletal assessment and,
1648
suboccipital craniectomy and, 1242
Electroneurography, 178
Electronystagmography, 178, 2101
vestibular function and, 2098
Electroretinography, 178
Electrosurgery, 2226–2227, 2228
condylomata acuminata and, 1950
Elimination
alterations in, 1427, 1430–1431,
1451, 1935
burn client and, 452, 453, 456,
458–459
endocrine dysfunction and, 1316
malnutrition and, 199
postoperative, 431, 433–434
spinal cord injury and, 1431–1432
Embolectomy, 950–951, 950
Embolism, 722
air, 722
hemodialysis and, 1023
lung biopsy and, 547
total parenteral nutrition and,
203
aortic resection and, 837
arterial bypass and, 954, 955
cardiac trauma and, 810
cerebral, 1168
cerebrovascular accident and, 1168
cholesterol, 722
coronary artery disease and, 780

embolectomy and, 950
fat, 722
fractures and, 1714
pulmonary, 722
atrial flutter and, 773
breast reconstruction and, 1924
burn client and, 442
chest pain and, 731
fractures and, 1714
free flap transfer and, 2240
hip fracture and, 1755
infective endocarditis and, 806
intracaval filter and, 960
pericarditis and, 807
postoperative, 431
pulmonary blood flow and, 721
thrombophlebitis and, 870
wasted ventilation and, 521
ventricular aneurysmectomy and,
829
Embolization
arterial occlusion and, 868
arteriovenous fistula and, 857
cardiac tumors and, 810
gastrointestinal bleeding and, 1502,
1503
infective endocarditis and, 806
peripheral arterial aneurysms and,
861
Embryonic carcinoma, 1955
Emergency care. See also Trauma
ABCs of, 369–371
assessment and, 377–380
documentation of, 367
evaluation and, 384
implementation and, 380–384
legal considerations in, 366–367
nurse and, 367–369
nursing diagnosis and, 380,
381–383
pharmacologic intervention in, 374
trends in, 364–365
Emergency client
clinical appraisal of, 378–379
nursing care plan and, 380
nursing diagnosis and, 381–383
Emergency Department Nurses'
Association, 367, 368, 380
Emergency medical services systems, 365
Emergency medical technicians, prehospital trauma care and, 366
Emergency nursing, 364
prehospital trauma care and, 366
standards and guidelines for, 368
EMG. See Electromyography
Emigrants, morbidity/mortality and,
41–43
Emmetropia, 2006
Emotion, limbic system and, 100
Emphysema, 154, 155, 641–645, 643
acute respiratory failure and, 645
airflow obstruction and, 536
blow-out fracture and, 2052
centrilobular, 642, 642
chest trauma and, 650
client characteristics and, 640
esophageal trauma and, 1484
hypoxia and, 548
laryngotracheal trauma and, 604
lobectomy and, 692
panlobular, 642–643, 642
pneumothorax and, 652
pulsus paradoxus and, 735
respiratory acidosis and, 89

segmental resection and, 692–693
smoking and, 60, 251
thoracic surgery and, 693
tracheobronchial injury and, 653
wasted ventilation and, 521
Empyema, 631–632
pneumonia and, 622, 623, 624
staphylococcal infection and, 290
thoracic surgery and, 693
EMSSs. See Emergency medical services systems
EMTs. See Emergency medical
technicians
Enabling, substance abuse and,
253–254
Encephalitis, 1186–1187
epidemiology of, 282
prevention of, 282
respiratory alkalosis and, 91
Encephalopathy
uremic, 988
ureterosigmoidostomy and, 1088
Wernicke's, 243
Endarterectomy, 950, 952, 952
kidney revascularization and, 1073
Endemic disease, 274, 275
Endocardial pacing, transvenous,
834, 834
Endocarditis, 806–807
aortic insufficiency and, 796
aortic regurgitation and, 737
bacterial, 734
cardiac pacing and, 835
infective, 806
hypertrophic cardiomyopathy
and, 809
petechiae and, 734
pulmonic insufficiency and, 794
prosthetic, aortic resection and,
836
staphylococcal, 290, 623
subacute bacterial, dental extraction and, 1477
valve replacement and, 828
Endocardium, tumors of, 809–810
Endocrine function, intracranial surgery and, 1239
Endocrine glands, 1272
structure of, 1272–1273
Endocrine system
burns and, 442
cardiovascular system and, 724
diagnostic testing and, 1297–1315,
1297–1302
disorders of
assessment of, 1293–1315
evaluation and, 1320
nursing care plan and,
1317–1319
nursing diagnosis and,
1315–1316
planning and implementation and,
1316–1320
duodenal ulcer and, 1493
eyes and, 1995
female reproductive system and,
1812
functions of, 1273–1278
gastrointestinal system and, 1433
integumentary system and,
2156–2157
interrelationships of, 1271–1286
obesity and, 213–214
pathophysiology of, 1286–1289
preanesthesia history and, 400

psychosocial factors and,
1290–1291
regulatory functions of, 1278–1286
related systems and, 1289–1290
Endolymph, 2087
Endolymphatic hydrops, 2115–2117
Endometrial cancer, 1882
dilatation and curettage and, 1902
risk factors in, 333
signs and symptoms of, 333
staging of, 1882
Endometriosis, 1870–1871, 1870
dysmenorrhea and, 1838, 1866,
1871
hysterectomy and, 1906
oophorectomy and, 1910
Endophthalmitis, blow-out fracture
and, 2052
Endoplasmic reticulum, 714
Endorphins, 100, 1107
acupuncture and, 104
appetite regulation and, 210, 210
Endoscope, 178
Endoscopy, 178
common procedures, 179
esophageal cancer and, 1483
esophageal perforation and, 1485
gastrointestinal, 1448–1449
gastrointestinal bleeding and,
1502, 1503
hiatal hernia and, 1473
inflammatory bowel disease and,
1509
laryngeal injury and, 604
pancreatic cancer and, 1514
polyps and, 1513
Endotoxins, 288
Endotracheal intubation
acute respiratory failure and, 646
epiglottitis and, 595–596
laryngeal injury and, 604
nosocomial infection and, 278
postoperative, 425–426
respiratory acidosis and, 91
superinfection and, 309
tracheobronchial injury and, 653
Endotracheal tube, 415, 556–558,
557
inhalation anesthesia and, 414–415
suctioning and, 558, 563
Enema, 1453
Energy balance, weight gain/loss and,
210
ENG. See Electronystagmography
Enkephalins, 100, 1107
appetite regulation and, 210, 210
Enmeshment, eating disorders and,
224
Enophthalmos, 2006
blow-out fracture and, 2052
Entamoeba histolytica, 299
pericarditis and, 808
Enteritis, regional. See Crohn's
disease
Enterobacter cloacae, aspiration pneu-
monia and, 624
Enterobacter spp.
normal habitat of, 271
skin and, 2196
Enterobiasis, 299
Enterobius vermicularis, 299
Enterocele, posterior colporrhaphy
and, 1915
Enterococci, habitat of, 271
Enterotoxins, 291

Fluid volume excess
  burn client and, 459–460
  urinary system/kidney dysfunction
    and, 1009, 1014, 1017–1018
Flukes, 299
Fluorescein angiography, visual system and, 2010
Fluorescein staining, corneal,
  2009–2010
Fluorescent treponemal antibody
  absorption test, 1850, 1932,
  2099
Fluoroscopy, 177
  cardiac, 745
    percutaneous transluminal angio-
      plasty and, 824
  gastrointestinal system and,
    1447–1448
  hiatal hernia and, 1473
Fogarty catheter, 950
Folate deficiency, erythrocyte indices
  and, 887
Foley catheter, 421–422, 422, 579,
  1059, 1061, 1063, 1503, 1915,
  1953
Folic acid deficiency, 194
  erythropoiesis and, 720
  reticulocytosis and, 888
  tongue and, 1442
Follicle cysts, 1888–1889
Follicle-stimulating hormone, 1276,
  1279
  female sexual development and,
    1806
Folliculitis, 143
Food additives, cancer and, 46
Food handling, infectious disease and,
  302–303
Food intolerance, peptic ulcer disease
  and, 1496
Food poisoning, 391
  bacterial, 291
    epidemiology of, 282
  gastritis and, 1505
  infectious gastroenteritis and, 1510
  prevention of, 282
  seasonality of, 39
  staphylococcal, 290
Food record form, 219
Food spoilage, temperature and, 302
Foot drop, 419, 1221
Forced expiratory volume, preoperative, 401
Forced vital capacity, 537
Forebrain, 1099
Foreign bodies, ocular, 2051–2052
Formication, cocaine abuse and, 249
Fovea centralis, 1989
Fractures, 1694–1715. See also Casts
  blow-out, 2052
  endocrine dysfunction and, 1290,
    1294
  external fixation of, 1751–1754,
    1753
  facial, 600–601
  healing of, 1626–1627, 1629
  hyperparathyroidism and, 1363
  internal fixation of, 1749–1751,
    1750, 1751
  orbital, 2052
  pathological, hypercalcemia and, 86
  rib, 650
  skull, 1197
  sternal, 650
  types of, 1695, 1696–1698

Frank-Starling law, 706
FRC. See Functional residual capacity
Freckles, 2155
Free fatty acids
  appetite regulation and, 210
  fat digestion and, 208
Free flap transfer, 2239–2241
Fremitus, 155
Fresh tissue technique, 2229
Frontal lobe, 1099
Frontal sinuses, 513
  assessment and, 147–148, 147
  sinusitis and, 588
  surgical procedures and, 677
Frontal trephination, 677
Frontoethmoidectomy, 588
Frostbite, 34, 388, 2126, 2213–2214,
  2213
Frost suture, 2075, 2075
Frozen section technique, 330
FSH. See Follicle-stimulating hormone
FTA-ABS. See Fluorescent trepone-
  mal antibody absorption test
Functional residual capacity, 537
  asthma and, 637
Fundoscopy, cardiovascular disease
  and, 734
Fundus, of eye, 144, 145
Fungi, 270
  conjunctivitis and, 2046
  keratitis and, 2047
  lung abscess and, 631
  pericarditis and, 807
  skin infection and, 2199–2201,
    2202–2203
Funnel breast, 1662, 1662
Furstenberg diet, Meniere's syn-
  drome and, 2116
Furuncles, 143, 290
Furunculosis, 2119–2121, 2119
Fusiform bacilli, Vincent's angina and,
  593
Fusobacterium spp.
  aspiration pneumonia and, 624
  habitat of, 271
FVC. See Forced vital capacity

Gag reflex, 1429
  regional anesthesia and, 419
  suboccipital craniectomy and, 1244
Gait, neurologic assessment and,
  1128
Gallbladder
  cancer of, 1594
  functions of, 1559
  structure of, 1558, 1558
  surgical procedures and,
    1613–1616
  trauma and, 1596
  ultrasonography and, 1573
Gallop rhythm, 160
Gallstones. See Cholelithiasis
Gamma globulin, hepatitis A and,
  1590
Gamma-glutamyl transpeptidase,
  hepatic-biliary dysfunction and,
  1571
Gamma radiation, 345–346
Ganglia, 1098
Ganglioglioma, 1192
Gangrene, 2157. See also Gas
  gangrene
  arterial insufficiency and, 843
  arterial occlusion and, 868
  arterial trauma and, 874

arteriovenous fistula and, 857
bowel, peritonitis and, 1504
Buerger's disease and, 858
peripheral arterial aneurysms and,
  861
polyarteritis nodosa and, 864
Raynaud's disease and, 858
Gardner's syndrome, 1513, 1514
Gardner-Wells tongs, 1201
Gardnerella vaginalis, vaginal infection and, 166, 1876
GAS. See General adaptation
  syndrome
Gas dilution method, 537
Gas exchange, 572
  burn client and, 452, 455, 459, 460
  hematologic disease and, 892,
    896–897, 899
  hepatic-biliary dysfunction and,
    1561–1561, 1577, 1580–1581,
    1582
  impaired, 548
  kidneys and, 986
  mechanical ventilation and,
    567–571
  urinary system/kidney dysfunction
    and, 1009–1010, 1015–1016,
    1018
Gas gangrene, 292
  causative agent of, 273
  exotoxins and, 288
  incubation period of, 273
Gastrectomy
  pernicious anemia and, 921
  subtotal, 1528
  total, 1528
Gastric acid, caffeine and, 249
Gastric air bubble, 157, 163
Gastric analysis, 1450
  hematologic disease and, 890
  pernicious anemia and, 921
Gastric cancer
  gastritis and, 1505
  pernicious anemia and, 921
Gastric disorders, surgical procedures
  and, 1527–1531
Gastric-inhibitory peptide, 1286
  actions of, 1427
Gastric motility. See Motility
Gastric mucosa
  absorption in, 1427
  cells of, 1421
Gastric reflux, 1421, 1429
  hiatal hernia and, 1473
Gastric resection, 1527–1530, 1529
Gastric ulcers. See Ulcers, gastric
Gastrin, 1286, 1426
  actions of, 1427
  irritable bowel syndrome and, 1498
  Zollinger-Ellison syndrome and,
    1495
Gastrinoma, duodenal ulcer and, 1495
Gastritis, 23, 1505–1506
  alcohol abuse and, 244, 1434
  barium studies and, 1447
  gastric ulcer and, 1493
  gastrointestinal bleeding and, 1501
  nonsteroidal antiinflammatory
    agents and, 106
  stomach cancer and, 1513
  subtotal gastrectomy and, 1528
  uremia and, 989
Gastroduodenostomy, 1528
Gastroenteritis
  contaminated water and, 1435

death rate for, 43
infectious, 270, 291, 1510
Gastrointestinal bleeding
  alcoholic coma and, 260
  amyloidosis and, 1676
  anemia and, 1432
  aplastic anemia and, 920
  bone marrow transplantation and,
    967
  coronary artery bypass surgery
    and, 822
  esophageal cancer and, 1483
  graft-versus-host disease and, 968
  hypovolemic shock and, 94
  lower, 1503
  peptic ulcer disease and, 1495
  polyarteritis nodosa and, 865
  suboccipital craniectomy and, 1244
  thrombocytopenia and, 882
  trauma and, 1516
  upper, 1501–1503
    causes of, 1501
  uremia and, 987
Gastrointestinal bypass, 1531, 1531
Gastrointestinal fluid, electrolytes in,
  1452
Gastrointestinal hormones. See also
  specific type
  actions of, 1427
Gastrointestinal secretions,
  1425–1426
  changes in, 1429
Gastrointestinal surgery
  infective endocarditis and, 806
  nutrient absorption and, 185
Gastrointestinal system, 1420
  alcohol abuse and, 244
  amyloidosis and, 1676
  burns and, 442–443
  disorders of
    assessment and, 1438–1450
    evaluation and, 1464
    infectious, 1504–1511
    inflammatory, 1504–1511
    neoplastic, 1511–1516
    nursing diagnosis and,
      1450–1453
    obstructive, 1511–1516
    planning and implementation and,
      1453–1462
    psychosocial factors and,
      1433–1435
    traumatic, 1516–1517
  endocrine system and, 1290
  female reproductive system and,
    1812
  hypokalemia and, 84
  integumentary system and, 2157
  interrelationships of, 1419–1427
  laboratory tests and, 1446–1447
  nursing care plan and, 1454–1456
  pathophysiology of, 1428–1431
  preoperative period and, 405
  regulatory functions of, 1286,
    1425–1427
  related systems and, 1431–1433
  respiratory system and, 522
  sensory nerves of, 997
  urinary system and, 988–989
Gastrojejunostomy, 1528
Gastroplasty, 1531, 1532
  obesity and, 218
Gastroscopy, 179, 1448
  polyps and, 1513
Gastrostomy, 1460, 1530–1531, 1530

Immune system, 21–24
  aging and, 30
  cancer and, 323–324
  infection and, 276
  nosocomial infection and, 278
Immunity, 22, 275
  cellular, corneal allograft reaction
    and, 2044
  influenza and, 297
  tetanus and, 292
Immunization, 22, 275, 300–301
  burn client and, 386
  diphtheria and, 593
  DPT, 292, 593
  health history and, 134
  influenza and, 297
  middle-age and, 62
  mortality rates and, 43
  rabies and, 297
  tetanus, 292
    oral/esophageal trauma and, 1485
Immunoglobulin, 22. See also
    Antibodies
  assays, multiple myeloma and,
    938–939
  asthma and, 637
  characteristics of, 23
  classes of, 22
  hematologic disease and, 889
  immediate hypersensitivity and, 23
  plasma levels of, 25
  respiratory function testing and, 543
Immunoglobulin E, anaphylactic shock
    and, 97
Immunoglobulin G
  agammaglobulinemia and, 929
  hyperthyroidism and, 1350
Immunologic agents, 293–296
Immunosuppression
  septic shock and, 97
  stomatitis and, 1478
Immunotherapy
  cancer and, 351–352
  lung cancer and, 648
  malignant melanoma and, 2212
Impedance audiometry, 2100
Impedance plethysmography. See
    Plethysmography, impedance
Impetigo, 291
Implant surgery, 7
  artificial heart, 832–833
  cardiac pacemakers and, 834–836
  cochlear, 2139–2140, 2140
  ventricular assist devices and, 834
Implied consent, emergency care and,
    367
Impotence, 1830–1831, 1937
  alcohol abuse and, 244
  arterial bypass and, 955
  arteriosclerosis obliterans and, 870
  diabetes mellitus and, 1341
  endocrine dysfunction and, 1290
  hypertension and, 726
  hypopituitarism and, 1286
  multiple sclerosis and, 1183
  penile implant and, 1969
  peripheral vascular disease and,
    842, 849
IMV. See Intermittent mandatory
    ventilation
Incarceration, intestinal, 1498
Incisional biopsy. See Biopsy,
    incisional
Incisional hernia. See Hernia,
    incisional

Incontinence
  fecal, 1431
  ileostomy and, 1540
  nervous system dysfunction and,
    1139, 1144
  spinal cord compression and, 354
  spinal cord injury and, 1431–1432
  stress, anterior colporrhaphy and,
    1915
  urinary, 989, 1041, 1938
    cystitis and, 1051
    cystocele and, 1873, 1874
    prostatectomy and, 1960, 1962
Incus, 2084–2085
Independence, eating disorders and,
    225
Independent practice, 14
Indigestion. See also Dyspepsia
  endocrine dysfunction and, 1290,
    1294
Infant botulism, 291
Infant mortality, ethnic differences
    in, 4
Infarction. See specific type
Infection, 24–25, 269–314
  abdominal aortic aneurysms and,
    860
  acquired immune deficiency syn-
    drome and, 928
  adult respiratory distress syndrome
    and, 618
  agammaglobulinemia and, 929
  aneurysms and, 859
  aplastic anemia and, 920
  auditory system and, 2094,
    2118–2123
  bone, 1691–1693
  bone marrow transplantation and,
    965–966, 967
  burn client and, 453, 457, 460
  cancer and, 328
  casts and, 1709–1710
  central nervous system and,
    1185–1190
  chain of, 271
  chemical peeling and, 2223
  chronic obstructive pulmonary dis-
    ease and, 644
  coronary artery bypass surgery
    and, 822
  cranioplasty and, 1252
  disseminated intravascular coagula-
    tion and, 923
  focal, 275
  fractures and, 1712
  granulocytopenia and, 925
  hearing loss and, 2090
  heart transplantation and, 830
  hematologic disease and, 893, 897,
    899
  hemodialysis and, 1023
  hepatic-biliary system and, 1562,
    1589–1593
  Hodgkin's disease and, 937
  hysterectomy and, 1907
  integumentary system and, 2155,
    2173, 2195–2201
  intracranial surgery and, 1239
  joints and, 1734–1736
  kidneys and, 986, 1049–1054
  leukemia and, 893, 933
  leukocytosis and, 888
  local, 275
  male reproductive system and,
    1937–1938, 1945–1952

malnutrition and, 189, 199
mastectomy and, 1921
microlumbar diskectomy and, 1259
multiple myeloma and, 938
musculoskeletal system and, 1633
myocarditis and, 807
nervous system and, 1118–1119
pelvic exenteration and, 1912
peripheral arterial aneurysms and,
    861
peripheral nervous system and,
    1217–1218
pernicious anemia and, 893
posterior laminectomy and, 1266
primary, 274
pyelolithotomy and, 1072
salpingoplasty and, 1910
secondary, 274
sickle cell anemia and, 915
skin grafting and, 2236
stress ulcer and, 1495
subclinical, 274
surgical risk and, 402
susceptibility to, 275–278
systemic, 275
thoracic surgery and, 693
total hip replacement and, 1767
total parenteral nutrition and, 203
transurethral prostatectomy and,
    1962
upper respiratory tract and,
    586–596, 620–634
urinary system and, 1049–1054,
    1050
urinary system/kidney dysfunction
    and, 1008–1009, 1011–1014, 1017
visual system and, 2044–2048
vulvectomy and, 1911
Infection control, 278
Infectious arthritis. See Arthritis,
    infectious
Infectious disease
  antimicrobial therapy and, 309–310
  assessment and, 303–305, 303
  bacterial, 288–292
  classification of, 274–275
  diagnostic studies and, 304–305
  food handling and, 302–303
  helminthic, 299–300
  hygiene and sanitation and,
    301–302
  immunization and, 300–301
  isolation precautions and, 310–313
  physiologic support and, 309
  protozoal, 298–299
  viral, 292–297
Infectious hepatitis. See Hepatitis,
    infectious
Infectious mononucleosis. See Mono-
    ucleosis, infectious
Inferior vena cava, plication of,
    960–962, 961
Infertility, 1829–1830
  female, 1867–1868
    dilatation and curettage and,
      1902
    endometrial cancer and, 1882
    endometriosis and, 1871
    ovarian cancer and, 1884
  hypothyroidism and, 1356
  male, 1938
  situational, 1830
Infertility studies, 1844–1847
Infestation, integumentary system
    and, 2155, 2195–2201

Infiltration anesthesia, 418
Inflammation, 25–26
  chemical mediators of, 25–26, 26
  coronary artery disease and, 780
  musculoskeletal system and,
    1632–1633, 1641
  nervous system and, 1118–1119
  neutrophils and, 718
Inflammatory bowel disease,
    1508–1509
  carcinoembryonic antigen and, 330
  colorectal cancer and, 1514
Influenza, 269, 275, 292, 296–297
  age and, 40
  causative agent of, 273
  epidemiology of, 284
  incubation period of, 273
  myocarditis and, 807
  pericarditis and, 807
  prevention of, 284
  staphylococcal infection and, 290
Influenza virus
  acute rhinitis and, 580
  pneumonia and, 623
Informed consent
  client checklist for, 404
  diagnostic testing and, 177
  emergency care and, 367
  surgery and, 403
Inguinal hernia. See Hernia, inguinal
Inhalation anesthesia, 414–415
Inhalation injury, 441, 452
Inhalation therapy, nosocomial infec-
    tion and, 278
Inheritance patterns, 27, 27
Inhibiting factors, 1279
Injury, malnutrition and, 199
Insect bites
  angioneurotic edema and, 585
  auditory system injury and, 2126
Insect stings
  anaphylactic shock and, 97
  symptoms and nursing prescrip-
    tions for, 386–387
  tetanus and, 292
Insomnia
  barbiturates and, 245
  caffeine and, 249
  marijuana withdrawal and, 253
  nonsteroidal antiinflammatory
    agents and, 106
Inspection, 139
  auditory system and, 2096
  breasts and, 152
  ears and, 146
  male reproductive system and, 164,
    1930–1931
  posterior chest and, 154–155
  respiratory system and, 530–532
  urinary system and, 996–997
Inspiration, deviated nasal septum
    and, 583
Inspiratory capacity, 537
Inspiratory reserve volume, 537
Institute of Medicine, 14–15
Insula, function of, 1107
Insulin, 1273, 1284–1285, 1289,
    1327–1328, 1333, 1341–1342
  administration of, 1328, 1333
    sites for, 1333
  alcohol metabolism and, 240
  appetite regulation and, 210, 210
  classification of, 1327
  hyperglycemia and, 1446
  kidney failure and, 984

Some SI Units Applicable to Health

Quantity	SI Unit	Symbol	Customary Unit	Typical Application
Length	kilometer	km	mile,	Distance,
	meter	m	yard, foot,	distance in
	centimeter	cm	inch	visual acuity,
	millimeter	mm (10^{-3} m)		body linear
	micrometer	μm (10^{-6} m)		measurement, size of bacteria
Surface area	square			Surface area
	centimeter	cm^2	square inch	Body surface
	square meter	m^2	square foot	area
Mass	kilogram	kg	lb, oz	Body mass,
	gram	g		pharmaceuti-
	milligram	mg		cal and
	microgram	μg		chemical products
Temperature	degree Celsius*	°C	°F or degree Fahrenheit	Body temper- ature, clinical thermometer
Time	day	d		Expression of
	hour	h		point in time in
	minute	min		a health record,
	second	s		24 h clock, time of medication
Volume and capacity	liter	L	qt	Fluid or gas,
	milliliter	mL	cc or fluid oz, teaspoon	measuring vessel, baby formula, oral dosage
Power	watt	W	horsepower	Mechanical power, bicycle ergometer tests

* **The degree Celsius:** Note that the unit of temperature is the degree Celsius (not degree centigrade). This has been accepted because the kelvin has limited application in medicine. The symbol for degree Celsius is °C. Although the scale origins of kelvin and Celsius differ, the degree Celsius equals the kelvin in magnitude, thus, a rise in body temperature of 1.0 k is equivalent to a rise of 1.0 °C. 0 °C is defined as 273.15 K, 98.6 °F-37 °C-310.15 K.

† Not yet an approved SI unit